Blaustein's Pathology of the Female Genital Tract

Fourth Edition

Wonderful is he who can teach . . . and
wise is he who can be taught.

KATHA-UPANISHAD

Robert J. Kurman

Editor

Blaustein's Pathology of the Female Genital Tract

Fourth Edition

With 1339 Illustrations in 1501 Parts, 10 in Full Color

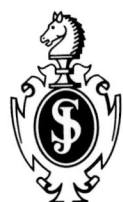

Springer-Verlag

New York Berlin Heidelberg London Paris
Tokyo Hong Kong Barcelona Budapest

ROBERT J. KURMAN, M.D.
Departments of Gynecology and Obstetrics and Pathology
The Johns Hopkins Hospital and The Johns Hopkins University
  School of Medicine
Baltimore, MD 21287, USA

Library of Congress Cataloging-in-Publication Data
Blaustein's pathology of the female genital tract.—4th ed. / Robert
  J. Kurman, editor.
      p.   cm.
    Includes bibliographical references and index.
    ISBN 0-387-96452-5. — ISBN 0-387-94166-5. — ISBN 3-540-94166-5
    1. Pathology, Gynecological.   I. Kurman, Robert J.
  II. Blaustein, Ancel, 1919–1984.   III. Title: Pathology of the female
  genital tract.
    [DNLM: 1. Genitalia, Female—pathology.   WP 100 B645 1994]
  RG77.P37   1994
  618.1′07—dc20   93-23252

Printed on acid-free paper.

Production managed by Bill Imbornoni; manufacturing supervised by Rhea Talbert.
Typeset by ATLIS Graphics & Design, Inc., Mechanicsburg, PA.
Color insert prepared by Arcata Graphics/Kingsport Press, Kingsport, TN.
Printed and bound by Arcata Graphics/Kingsport Press, Kingsport, TN.
Printed in the United States of America.

9 8 7 6 5 4 3 2 1

ISBN 0-387-94166-5 Springer-Verlag   New York   Berlin   Heidelberg
ISBN 3-540-94166-5 Springer-Verlag   Berlin   Heidelberg   New York

*In memory of my mother
and to Carole*

Preface

The conceptual framework and methodologies that direct the practice of a particular discipline and form the basis for scientific inquiry in that area have been referred to by Kuhn as "paradigms."[1] Research conducted within the context of the paradigm inevitably leads to observations that are inconsistent with the paradigm or that cannot be explained by it. This requires formulation of a new paradigm. Scientific progress can be viewed as the continuing replacement of one paradigm by another, each one more closely approximating "reality." Although scientific progress is generally regarded as an evolutionary process, Kuhn views it as a revolutionary one. According to Kuhn, science advances through periods of straightforward research, during which time a field is relatively stable, punctuated by quantum leaps in "understanding" that lead to the introduction of a new paradigm. The ideas that lead to the development of a new paradigm are based on an entirely new way of perceiving reality and as such are revolutionary. Kuhn goes on to note that scientific textbooks expound a particular set of paradigms that represent what the scientific community is committed to at a given point of time. Accordingly, as paradigms are replaced, textbooks must be rewritten.

There are several examples of paradigm shifts that have occurred in gynecologic pathology over the last few years. For example, in earlier editions of this text, endometrial hyperplasia was regarded as a precursor of endometrial carcinoma and the relationship of unopposed estrogenic stimulation to the development of endometrial carcinoma was not clear. In the present edition simple hyperplasia is interpreted as a response to unopposed estrogenic stimulation and atypical hyperplasia as a precursor of endometrial carcinoma. Furthermore, although it is now widely acknowledged that many endometrial carcinomas are related to estrogenic stimulation it is also appreciated that others are not.

Introduction of new paradigms is generally met with skepticism by most scientists working in the field who are loathe to give up a set of ideas with which they are familiar and comfortable. For example, the recent proposal to classify squamous intraepithelial lesions (SIL) of the cervix using a two-tier system as opposed to a three- or four-tier system has been highly controversial. The two-tier system is based on the view that intraepithelial lesions subsume both banal human papillomavirus (HPV) infections (low-grade SIL) and precursors of invasive squamous

carcinoma (high-grade SIL). This is a major departure from the preceding paradigm, as espoused in the previous edition of this text, in which all intraepithelial
lesions (i.e., cervical intraepithelial neoplasia [CIN] 1, 2, 3) were regarded as
constituting a histologic spectrum that shared a common etiology, biology, and
natural history. The paradigm shift was based on the introduction of the Bethesda
System, which divides SILs into low and high grade, and morphologic, molecular
biologic, and epidemiologic studies showing that certain HPV infections are a
major causal factor in the development of cervical cancer. Specifically, a prospective study has shown that 28% of women with normal cervical smears but with
HPV 16 detected in cervical swabs develop high-grade SIL (CIN 2/3) within 2
years without ever manifesting low-grade SIL (CIN 1).[2] These findings strongly
suggest that high-grade lesions develop de novo, rather than evolving from low-
grade lesions. The results of this study, in conjunction with others showing that the
vast majority of low-grade lesions spontaneously regress,[3] support the two-tier
division of SILs into viral infections and cancer precursors. Curiously, the new
paradigm more closely reflects the 1960s paradigm of a two-disease system, dysplasia and carcinoma-in situ, rather than the paradigm of the 1970s and 1980s, in
which intraepithelial lesions were regarded as a single disease. This underscores
Kuhn's view that scientific advances do not necessarily progress in a straightforward incremental fashion.

Since the previous edition of this textbook, the International Federation of
Gynecology and Obstetrics (FIGO) has revised the tumor staging systems, the
Bethesda System for cervical cytology has been introduced, and the World Health
Organization (WHO) and International Society of Gynecological Pathologists
(ISGYP) have revised the histologic classifications of tumors involving the entire
female genital tract. The new classifications have been utilized by all the authors of
the various chapters, many of whom served on the committees responsible for
their development. Clinicians often accuse pathologists of continually changing
the names of lesions without necessarily shedding new insight into their diagnosis
and management. Classifications reflect our attempt to place various morphologically recognized entities into some type of order based on our current understanding of the disease process. As our understanding of a disease changes, so do our
classifications. Is there an end in sight to the continually changing classifications
and evolving paradigms? If we draw the analogy of classification of disease to the
cosmologists' paradigms of our universe, Harrison provides a thought-provoking
response:

I hold the view that we alone create and organize the universe in which we live, and no other
universe is or ever can be the Universe. Yesterday a universe, today another, and tomorrow
yet another. Each universe presents a conceptual scheme that organizes human thoughts
and shapes human understanding. Generally, within each universe the end to the search for
all knowledge at last looms in sight. Each universe in its day flourishes as an awe-inspiring,
self-consistent scheme of thought, yet each is doomed to be superseded by another and
perhaps grander scheme.[4]

Methodology is an integral part of a paradigm but it is important to remember
that the observations disclosed by the methods we employ are representations of
reality and should not be confused with reality itself. As noted by Heisenberg,
"what we observe is not nature itself, but nature exposed to our method of
questioning."[5] For example, the mitotic level of a uterine smooth muscle tumor
weighs heavily in the pathologic diagnosis. A tumor with 5 mitotic figures/10
high-power fields and minimal cytologic atypia is classified as a *smooth muscle
tumor of uncertain malignant potential*, whereas one with 6 mitotic figures/10
high-power fields is classified as a *leiomyosarcoma*.[6,7] It is obvious that this count is
subject to many variables including such factors as promptness of fixation, thickness of the section, and the subjective interpretation by the observer who

performs the mitotic count. It is not likely that the behavior of these two tumors, based on the microscopic assessment, is as different as the diagnostic labels would imply.

New methods and the insights gleaned from their application play an important role in changing our paradigms. For example, molecular biologic studies have led to the development of a new model of carcinogenesis. In this model, carcinogenesis is viewed as a multistep process characterized by a series of defined genetic events. These genetic events include activation of oncogenes coupled with inactivation of suppressor genes, which are involved in cell adhesion, signal transduction, transcription, translation, and cell cycle regulation.[8] Despite the important advances in research at the molecular level, a complete understanding of disease and its impact on society requires an integration of molecular biology with morphology and epidemiology. Thus, Potter poses the question, "What gets cancer — the genes, the cell, the organ, the organism, or even perhaps the population?"[9]

In this edition of the textbook, the overall format has been changed to reflect the importance of methodology on the science and practice of gynecologic pathology. Accordingly, the various techniques used in gynecologic pathology are included in a separate section entitled "Adjunctive Methods." Subjects included in this section are immunohistochemistry, molecular biology, flow cytometry, and epidemiology. The first part of each of these chapters is devoted to a general discussion of the subject focusing on specific aspects of the methodology, including limitations and factors that must be considered in interpretation. The remainder of the chapter then describes the application of the technique to specific gynecologic diseases. Cytopathology and gross examination are not adjunctive techniques but are included in this section because they are involved with all aspects of gynecologic pathology and therefore relate to all of the individual chapters.

The format of the main body of the text has remained essentially unchanged. A minor revision is the inclusion of the chapter on embryology with that on abnormal sexual development; the subjects covered in both chapters are closely related and combining them into one chapter permits a more concise, less redundant presentation. The previous single chapter devoted to vulvar diseases has been separated into two chapters, one dealing with benign and the other with malignant diseases, because of our increased understanding of diseases that affect this organ. Considerable effort has gone into maintaining a uniform format for all of the individual chapters in order to facilitate reading and retrieval of specific information. Specific entities begin with general features that include a discussion of etiology and epidemiology followed by the clinical features, pathologic findings, differential diagnosis, clinical behavior, and treatment. As in the past, ultrastructure and immunohistochemistry are considered in the context of conventional light microscopy and are included where they are useful in differential diagnosis or in elucidating pathogenesis. Whereas the overall format has undergone only minor changes, the content of the various chapters—from the standpoint of photographs, text, and references—has undergone considerable change. Approximately two-thirds of the book has been extensively revised from the previous edition.

As in previous editions, the text is intended to provide an authoritative reference for the practicing pathologist and obstetrician/gynecologist and to present a readable account of gynecologic pathology for medical students and residents in training. The emphasis is on pathophysiology and clinical–pathologic correlation. This has been the approach to research, teaching, and clinical practice in the Department of Gynecology and Obstetrics at The Johns Hopkins Hospital and Medical School since the turn of the century and was exemplified in *Novak's Gynecologic and Obstetric Pathology*. *Blaustein's Pathology of the Female Genital Tract* continues in that tradition.

I am indebted to Mrs. Sue Skierkowski and Shirley Myers for secretarial assistance and to Mr. Raymond Lund and Norman Barker for the photomicrography of several of the chapters that I have written. As with the previous edition, the assistance of the staff at Springer-Verlag has been greatly appreciated. The task of editing was facilitated by the superb group of contributors, many of whom were involved with previous editions. Close cooperation with them has been one of the most gratifying aspects of working on this project. I am also grateful to my mentors, the late Dr. William Ober and Drs. Henry Norris and Robert Scully, as well as to my colleagues in the Departments of Pathology and Gynecology and Obstetrics at The Johns Hopkins Hospital who have contributed directly and indirectly to my ability to undertake and execute this project. I have been fortunate to work with an outstanding staff, Drs. Kathleen Cho and Lora Hedrick, both junior faculty members in the Division of Gynecologic Pathology, the fellows in the Division, and the residents who rotate on the Gynecologic Pathology Service. My association with all of these individuals has been a continuing intellectual challenge and an ongoing educational experience. Finally, I am grateful to my wife, Carole, without whose support, patience, and encouragement this endeavor would not have been possible.

Baltimore, Maryland   ROBERT J. KURMAN
1993

References

1. Kuhn TS (1970) The structure of scientific revolutions, 2nd ed. Chicago, The University of Chicago Press
2. Koutsky LA, Holmes KK, Critchlow CW, et al. (1992) A cohort study of the risk of cervical intraepithelial neoplasia grade 2 or 3 in relation to papillomavirus infection. N Engl J Med 327: 1272–1278
3. Nasiell K, Roger V, Nasiell M (1986) Behavior of mild cervical dysplasia during long term follow-up. Obstet Gynecol 67: 665–669
4. Harrison E (1985) Masks of the universe. New York, Macmillan Publishing Co
5. Heisenberg W (1959) Physics and philosophy. New York, Harper and Row
6. Kempson RL, Hendrickson MR (1987) Pure mesenchymal neoplasms of the uterine corpus. In: Fox H (ed) Haines and Taylor, Obstetrical and gynaecological pathology, 3rd ed. Edinburgh, Churchill Livingstone, pp 411–456
7. Silverberg SG, Kurman RJ (1992) Tumors of the uterine corpus and gestational trophoblastic disease. Atlas of Tumor Pathology, Third Series Fascicle 3, Washington, D.C., Armed Forces Institute of Pathology, pp 130–140
8. Vogelstein B, Fearon ER, Hamilton SR, et al. (1988) Genetic alterations during colorectal tumor development. N Engl J Med 319: 525–532
9. Potter JD (1992) Reconciling the epidemiology, physiology, and molecular biology of colon cancer. JAMA 268: 1573–1577

Preface to the First Edition

This text is written for the obstetrician, gynecologist, pathologist, and for residents training in these disciplines. It is a multiauthored book and the editor is aware of the problems this can create, but the expansion of information in the field of gynecologic pathology renders single authorship obsolete.

The format is largely traditional but the contents include topics that have not appeared in past texts. Clear cell adenocarcinoma of the vagina and vaginal and cervical adenoses are discussed in detail in a separate chapter. A chapter on embryology and congenital anomalies is written by an embryologist and the advantage of its inclusion is self evident. Ovarian neoplasms in childhood and adolescence are fortunately rare occurrences, but information concerning them is generally not readily available in existing texts. It is of sufficient importance to deserve a separate chapter. Amniotic fluid analysis for fetal viability is now commonly used and for this reason a detailed discussion of this subject is presented.

A chapter is included on gross description and preparation of gynecologic specimens. It contains the input and review of several directors of gynecologic-pathology laboratories.

The text contains many electron micrographs taken by transmission and scanning electron microscopy. Their inclusion is not an absolute necessity in gynecologic pathology, but is informative because they offer another perspective and are now a commonly used modality for studying tissue. The present day literature is replete with descriptions of specimens by electron microscopy, and it is hoped that the text will enable the readers to familarize themselves with electron microscopy as used in this specialty.

Experimentation in the field of obstetrics and gynecology has become more sophisticated over the years and for this reason the chapter on animal models of tumors of the ovaries and uterus is included. The contributions that comparative pathology can make to understanding disease mechanisms justify the addition of the chapter on comparative uterine and ovarian tumors in the animal kingdom.

The authors include a mixture of clinicians, pathologists, and basic scientists, and it is hoped that this gives the book the balance between the experience of the clinician and the pathologist.

ANCEL BLAUSTEIN, M.D.

Contents

Contributors

NORIO AZUMI, M.D., Ph.D.
Associate Professor of Pathology
Medical Director, Molecular Diagnostic Laboratory
Georgetown University School of Medicine
Washington, D.C., USA

DEBRA A. BELL, M.D.
Associate Professor of Pathology
Harvard Medical School
Associate Pathologist
Massachusetts General Hospital
Boston, Massachusetts, USA

REX BENTLEY, M.D.
Assistant Professor of Pathology
Duke University Medical Center
Durham, North Carolina, USA

PETER F. BERNHARDT, M.D.
Pathologist
Department of Pathology
Alexian Brothers Medical Center
Elk Grove Village, Illinois, USA

LOUISE A. BRINTON, Ph.D.
Chief, Environmental Studies Section
Environmental Epidemiology Branch
Epidemiology and Biostatistics Program
National Cancer Institute
Rockville, Maryland, USA

KATHLEEN R. CHO, M.D.
Assistant Professor of Pathology, Gynecology
    and Obstetrics, and Oncology
The Johns Hopkins University School of Medicine
Baltimore, Maryland, USA

PHILIP B. CLEMENT, M.D.
Clinical Professor of Pathology
University of British Columbia
Vancouver Hospital and Health Sciences Center
Vancouver, British Columbia, Canada

BERNARD CZERNOBILSKY, M.D.
Professor of Pathology
Medical School of the Hebrew University and Hadassah
Jerusalem, Israel
Chief, Department of Pathology
Kaplan Hospital
Rehovot, Israel

ALEX FERENCZY, M.D.
Professor of Pathology, Obstetrics and Gynecology
McGill University and The Sir Mortimer B.
    Davis-Jewish General Hospital
Montreal, Quebec, Canada

DEBORAH J. GERSELL, M.D.
Professor of Pathology
Washington University School of Medicine
Division of Surgical Pathology
Barnes Hospital
St. Louis, Missouri, USA

LORA HEDRICK, M.D.
Assistant Professor of Pathology, Gynecology
   and Obstetrics, and Oncology
The Johns Hopkins University School of Medicine
Baltimore, Maryland, USA

FREDERICK T. KRAUS, M.D.
Professor (Visiting Staff) of Pathology
Washington University School of Medicine and
Director of Placental and Perinatal Pathology
St. John's Mercy Medical Center
St. Louis, Missouri, USA

ROBERT J. KURMAN, M.D.
Richard W. TeLinde Professor
Gynecology, Obstetrics and Pathology
The Johns Hopkins University School of Medicine
Director of Gynecologic Pathology
The Johns Hopkins Hospital
Baltimore, Maryland, USA

MICHAEL T. MAZUR, M.D.
Clinical Professor of Pathology
SUNY Health Science Center at Syracuse
Associate Pathologist
Crouse Irving Memorial Hospital
Syracuse, New York, USA

HENRY J. NORRIS, M.D.
Pathologist
Arnold Palmer Hospital for Women and Children and
   Orlando Regional Health Center
Orlando, Florida, USA

TIM PARMLEY, M.D.
Professor of Obstetrics and Gynecology and Pathology
University of Arkansas
School of Medical Sciences
Little Rock, Arkansas, USA

STANLEY J. ROBBOY, M.D.
Professor of Pathology, Obstetrics and Gynecology
Director, Gynecologic Pathology
Duke University Medical Center
Durham, North Carolina, USA

PETER RUSSELL, M.D., B.Sc. (Med.), F.R.C.P.A.
Clinical Professor of Pathology
Sydney University and Royal Prince Alfred Hospital
Sydney, Australia

MARK H. SCHIFFMAN, M.D.
Clinical Investigator, Environmental Studies Section
Environmental Epidemiology Branch
Epidemiology and Biostatistics Program
National Cancer Institute
Rockville, Maryland, USA

ROBERT E. SCULLY, M.D.
Emeritus Professor of Pathology
Harvard Medical School
Pathologist
Massachusetts General Hospital
Boston, Massachusetts, USA

MARK E. SHERMAN, M.D.
Assistant Professor of Pathology
The Johns Hopkins University School of Medicine
Division of Cytopathology
The Johns Hopkins Hospital
Baltimore, Maryland, USA

ALEKSANDER TALERMAN, M.D., Ph.D., F.R.C. Path.
Peter A. Herbut Professor of Pathology and Cell Biology
Thomas Jefferson University School of Medicine
Philadelphia, Pennsylvania, USA

JAMES E. WHEELER, M.D.
Professor of Pathology and Laboratory Medicine
Hospital of the University of Pennsylvania
Philadelphia, Pennsylvania, USA

EDWARD J. WILKINSON, M.D.
Professor of Pathology and Laboratory Medicine
University of Florida College of Medicine
Gainesville, Florida, USA

THOMAS C. WRIGHT, M.D.
Assistant Professor of Pathology
Associate Director, Division of Ob/Gyn Pathology and
   Department of Pathology
College of Physicians and Surgeons of Columbia
   University
New York, New York, USA

ROBERT H. YOUNG, M.D., F.R.C. Path.
Associate Professor of Pathology
Harvard Medical School
Director of Surgical Pathology
Massachusetts General Hospital
Boston, Massachusetts, USA

RICHARD J. ZAINO, M.D.
Professor of Pathology
M.S. Hershey Medical Center
Penn State University
Hershey, Pennsylvania, USA

CHARLES ZALOUDEK, M.D.
Professor of Clinical Pathology
University of California, San Francisco, School of
  Medicine
San Francisco, California, USA

I

Pathology of the Female Genital Tract

1

Embryology of the Female Genital Tract and Disorders of Abnormal Sexual Development

Stanley J. Robboy, M.D., Peter F. Bernhardt, M.D., and Tim Parmley, M.D.

An appreciation of the embryologic development of the genital tract provides the background for understanding many pathologic conditions encountered in the female. Among these are disorders of abnormal sexual development, which are closely linked with abnormalities occurring in early embryological development.

Embryology

Most of the female genital tract is of mesodermal origin. The germ cells are of endodermal origin and the vulva and the epithelial lining of the vagina are of ectodermal origin. The chronology and sequence of events that underlie the development of the female genital tract are summarized in Table 1.1.

Gonadal Development

In humans and other mammals, the karyotype "XY" genetically defines the sex as male, whereas "XX" defines the female sex. Sex is determined by the presence or absence of a signal from a substance called the *testis determining factor* (TDF), which is found on the Y chromosome. Testes are formed if this gene is expressed by the embryo before the differentiation of the urogenital ridge. Further male development occurs under the influence of hormones secreted later by the testes (Fig. 1.1). Without TDF, the gonads differentiate as ovaries and the embryo develops as a female. The timely expression of TDF is critical to the development of male sex; in its absence, the embryo develops a female phenotype by "default," regardless of genetic sex.[34]

Extensive efforts have been expended during the past two decades to identify TDF and its products. Several candidates, such as H-Y antigen, have been proposed and

Table 1.1. Synopsis of stages of normal embryologic development

Crown–rump length (mm)	Week after ovulation	CR length/day	Description of event
3	3.3	2.5/24	Pronephric tubules form; pronephric (mesonephric) duct arises and grows caudad as solid cord
7	4	3–5/27	Pronephros degenerated, but mesonephric duct reaches cloaca
12	5	7–9/33	Cloaca divides into rectum and UGS
18	6	8–11/37	Müllerian ducts appear as funnel-shaped opening of coelomic epithelium; indifferent gonad bulges into coelom
23	7	17/48	Müllerian ducts about 1/2 distance to UGS
		20–30 mm	Testis anatomically distinct with seminiferous tubules
29	8	51 d+	Müllerian ducts elongate and near UGS
			51 d Ducts approach each other
		23–28 mm	54 d Ducts in apposition; sinusal tubercle appears
		27–31 mm	56+ d Ducts fuse and in contact with UGS
43	9	30? mm 56? d	So-called ambisexual stage ends; experimental data for dating müllerian duct regression unclear; experimentally, müllerian duct is sensitive to MIS through 25+ mm CR size; ducts in older embryos not sensitive. Clinically, embryos 31–35 mm before effect observed; regression completed by 43–55 mm
			Leydig cells appear
		50? mm	Testes and ovaries acquire capacity to secrete characteristic hormones at same stage of development; testosterone coincides with histologic development of Leydig cells and immediately precedes virilization of genital tract; ovary not yet differentiated; rate-limiting step is appearance of 3-beta-OH-steroid-dehydrogenase, which is 50-fold more abundant in testis than ovary; ovary converts T to estradiol, which testis cannot do; later regulation shifted to pituitary placenta gonadotropins where T→estradiol controlled by conversion of cholesterol to pregnenolone
60	10	56 mm	Müllerian ducts completely fused (entire septum gone); caudal aspect proliferates; epithelium lining canal stratifies (2–3 cells layers thick)
		70 d	Anogenital distance lengthens
71	11	71 d	T synthesis sufficient to induce development of mesonephric duct into definitive structures (epididymis, vas deferens, and seminal vesicle); subsequently, T converted peripherally into 5-DHT, which causes: UGS→prostate Genital tubercle→glans penis Genital folds→penis (only 3.5 mm long) Genital swelling→scrotum
		72–4 d	Fusion of labioscrotal folds Closure of median raphe Closure of urethral groove
			Phallus in both sexes 3 mm long; thereafter grows in males 0.72 mm/wk and females 0.20 mm/wk
		75 d	Mesonephric ducts regress if not stimulated by T
		60+ mm	Vaginal plate first seen distinctly (complete at 140 mm; wk 17); initially, upper uterovaginal canal is large and oval in cross-section, mostly lined by pseudostratified columnar epithelium; extensive growth begins caudally; cells stratify
		68 mm	Uterovaginal canal occluded caudally, progresses cranially
93	12	77 mm	Extensive uterovaginal growth continues caudally
105	13	100–120 mm	Cervical glands appear; wavy, but undifferentiated
		105 mm	Vaginal rudiment approaches vestibule
			True ovarian organogenesis begins with onset of meiotic prophase
116	14		
130	15	126 mm	Primary folds of mucosa give uterine lumen "W"-shaped appearance on cross-section
		130 mm	Vaginal rudiment reaches level of vestibular glands; uterovaginal canal (15 mm total length) divisible into vagina (3/6ths), cervix (2/6ths), and corpus (1/6th); boundaries ill-defined
			Isthmus readily distinguishable
			Stromal layers of uterus begin definition
			Solid epithelial anlage of anterior and posterior fornices appear
			Vagina begins to show slight estrogen effect
142	16	139 mm	Fallopian tube begins active growth phase, begin to coil
		140 mm	Vaginal plate completed; lower end reaches vestibule; upper end extends into endocervical canal
			Female urogenital sinus becomes shallow vestibule
153	17	151 mm	Vaginal plate longest and begins to canalize; corpus glands appear as slight outpouchings
164	18	160 mm	Palmate folds of cervix appear (forerunner adult cervix)
		162 mm	Mucoid development of cervix begins
			Smooth muscle of uterus appears
			Estrogen effect apparent throughout vagina
		162 mm	Cavitation of vaginal canal completed
177	19	170 mm	Fornices hollow

Table 1.1. *Continued*

Crown–rump length (mm)	Week after ovulation	CR length/day	Description of event
186	20	185 mm	Dramatic increase in growth and coiling of fallopian tube (about 3 mm/wk to week 34)
197	21		
208	22		
230	24	210 mm	Differentiation of muscular layer of uterus complete
		227 mm	Fundus well marked; uterus assumes adult form
250	26		
270	28		
290	30		
328	34		
362	38	266 d	Birth

UGS, urogenital sinus; MIS, müllerian-inhibiting substance; T, testosterone; d, day; 5-DHT, 5-alpha-dihydrotestosterone; wk, week; CR, crown–rump.

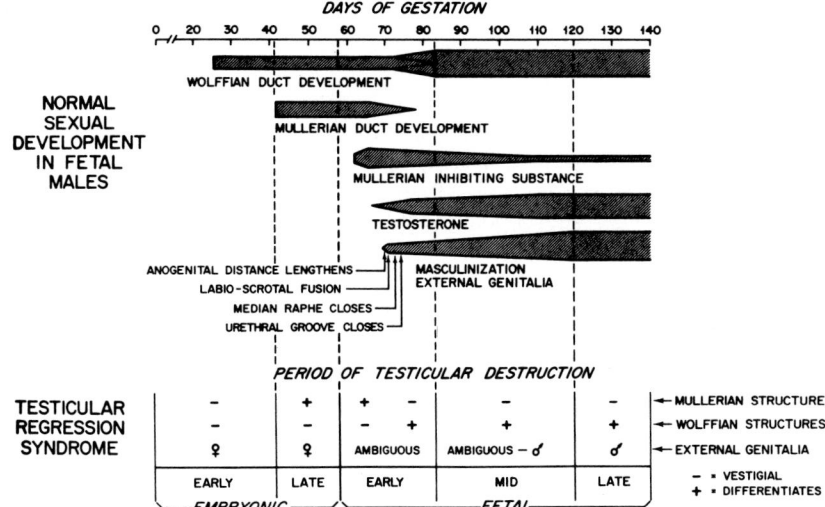

FIG. 1.1. Normal sexual development. Embryological development is determined by several factors, all of which are time specific during embryogenesis. The abnormalities that accompany the testicular regression syndrome are related to the normal sequence of events. (From Welch and Robboy, ref. 67, with permission of Pediatric Andrology.)

later discarded. The current candidate is a gene called SRY (*sex determining region Y*), located in region 1A1 adjacent to the pseudoautosomal pairing region at the distal end of the short arm of the Y chromosome.[54] It encodes for a DNA binding protein, the binding activity product of which is believed to regulate sexual differentiation.[20] Evidence supporting this thesis includes: the SRY gene is absent from the normal X chromosome, the SRY gene is present on the X chromosome of "sex-reversed" XX human males,[54] the homologous gene in the mouse is initially expressed just before sexual differentiation normally occurs,[16] and genetic splicing of the SRY gene into the chromosomally female embryo causes it to develop as a male.[24]

During the development of both male and female human embryos, the primordial germ cells, characterized by large clear cells with vesicular nuclei, migrate from the yolk sac to the urogenital ridges via the hindgut approximately 3 weeks after fertilization (Figs. 1.2, 1.3). The mesodermal epithelium on the medial surface of the urogenital ridge begins to proliferate, resulting in the epithelium of the eventual gonad, while the gonads themselves begin

to differentiate. In males, the testis is anatomically distinct with early tubular formation and immature Sertoli cells by day 44. In females, ovarian differentiation, characterized by the development of primordial follicles, begins some five weeks later. The initial stages of both testicular and ovarian development appear independent of whether the primordial germ cells are present or absent in the gonad or have proliferated normally.[33]

In the presence of TDF the proliferating surface cells differentiate into so-called sex cords, which are cords of epithelial cells that extend from the surface of the gonad into the medulla (Fig. 1.4). Subsequently, a capsule (tunica albuginea) develops and separates these epithelial cords from the surface. The cords become the testicular tubules as the epithelial cells differentiate into the tall, clear, flask-shaped Sertoli cells of the testis and the gonadal stromal cells become the interstitial or Leydig cells (Fig. 1.5). In normal development, the germ cells are incorporated completely within the tubules.

If TDF is absent (i.e., normal 46 XX females), the dividing germ cells are incorporated into a proliferating mass of

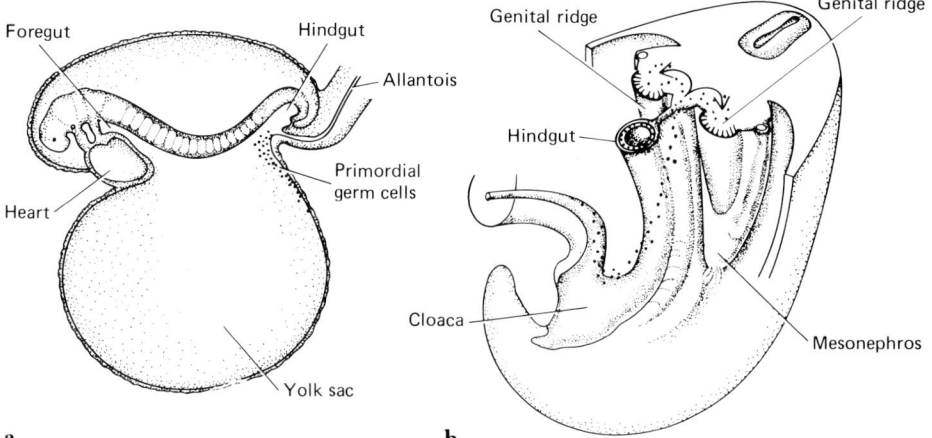

a   **b**

Fig. 1.2. Three-week embryo. Drawings showing: **a**: Curved embryo with primordial germ cells in the wall of the yolk sac, close to the allantoic attachment. **b**: Migration path of primordial germ cells along the wall of the hindgut and dorsal mesentery into the genital ridge. (From Sadler, ref. 47, with permission of Williams & Wilkins Co.)

surface epithelial cells, which results in a thickened cortex that presages the organization of the adult ovary (Fig. 1.6). From the second to the early third trimester, this thickened cortical mass of proliferating epithelial and germ cells divides into small groups demarcated by strands of stromal tissue extending from the medulla to the cortex. The small groups of germ cells and epithelial cells are further subdivided into primordial follicles composed of single germ cells surrounded by a layer of epithelial cells, the primitive granulosa cells. In normal development, each germ cell is characteristically encapsulated in its own follicle. This is associated with entry into meiosis and cessation of further proliferation.

If the normal male genetic constitution (46 XY) is present, some of the early epithelial proliferation contributes to the connection between the sex cord and the mesonephric tubules. Where gonads are destined to become

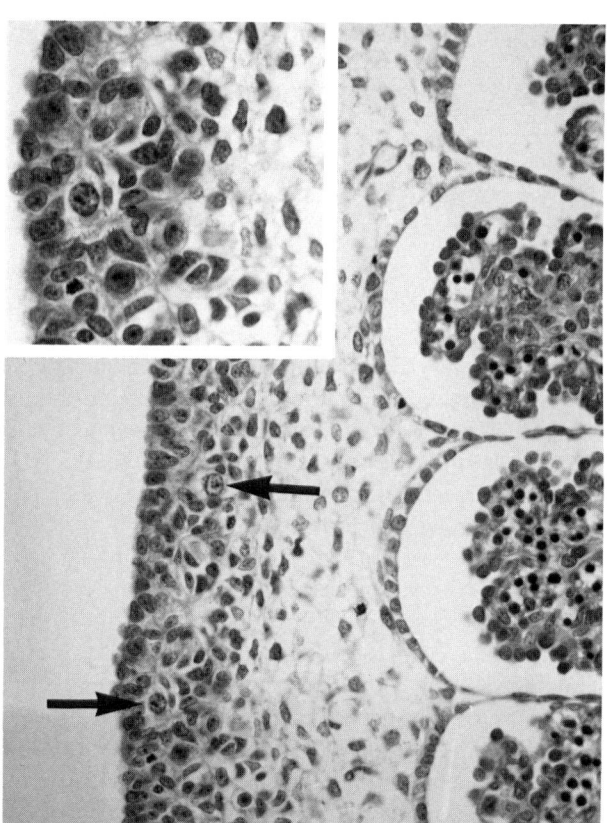

Fig. 1.3. Urogenital ridge. A thickened layer of cells that invests two germ cells (*arrows*) lies beneath the surface epithelium. The mesonephric glomeruli are below. *Inset*: A compact layer of cells closely resembling the surface layer surrounds the germ cells.

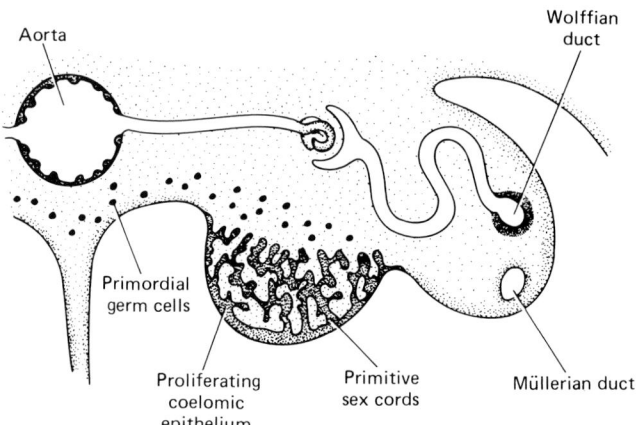

Fig. 1.4. Transverse section through the lumbar region of a six-week embryo. The indifferent gonad in which the primitive sex cords appear derive from the proliferating coelomic epithelium is shown. Cells of the primitive sex cords surround some of the primordial germ cells. (From Sadler, ref. 47, with permission of Williams & Wilkins Co.)

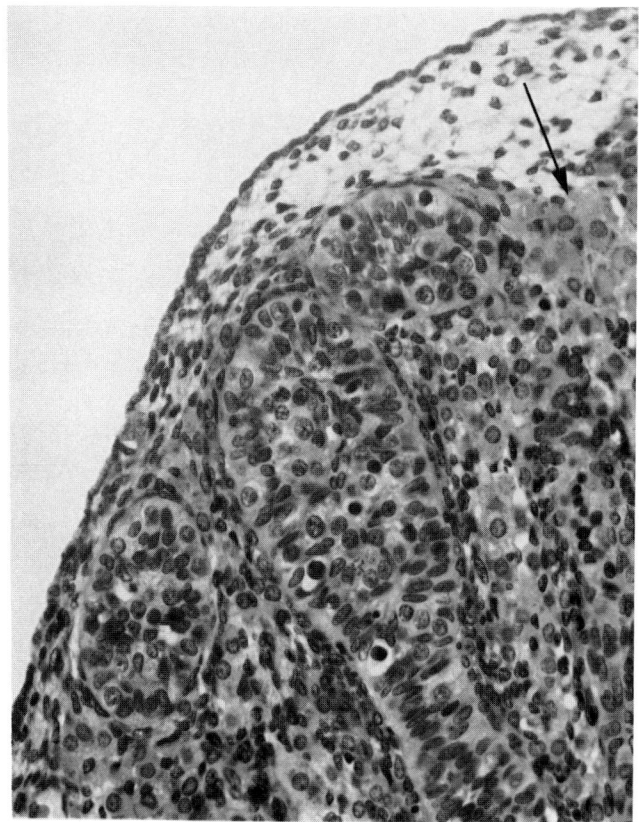

FIG. 1.5. **Fetal testis.** Epithelial cords are destined to become the testicular tubules and contain Sertoli cells. Interstitial cells, some of which contain abundant eosinophilic cytoplasm characteristic of Leydig cells (*arrow*), lie between the cords. The surface is differentiating into a capsule.

ovary, early proliferation degenerates in the ovarian hilum, leaving a few tubules, the rete ovarii. Interstitial (Leydig) cells develop extensively in the stromal tissue of the second-trimester female gonad, but degenerate in most cases by term. The few found in the hilum of the adult ovary are called hilus cells. Thus, the gonad develops primarily from mesodermal tissues, with the exception of the germ cells, which are endodermal in origin.

Müllerian and Wolffian Duct Development

Once the male pathway of development has begun, two hormones produced by the fetal testis then control the differentiation of the male phenotype. The first is müllerian inhibiting substance (MIS), a large glycoprotein that the Sertoli cells produce early during fetal life.[9,26] The gene responsible for this substance is on chromosome 19. The primary function of MIS is to cause regression of the müllerian (paramesonephric) ducts in the male fetus. In the female, MIS is produced in insignificant amounts during fetal life (as there are no testes); in the absence of this substance, the müllerian ducts develop passively to form the fallopian tubes, uterus, and vaginal wall. MIS is first secreted in effective amounts 56 to 62 days after fertilization, and the process of müllerian regression is normally completed by about day 77, after which the müllerian tissue is no longer sensitive to MIS. The MIS receptor in müllerian tissue appears to reside in stromal cells[60]; the mechanism by which müllerian tissue loses its sensitivity to MIS is not understood. MIS has a local action and inhibits development of the ipsilateral fallopian tube. To prevent

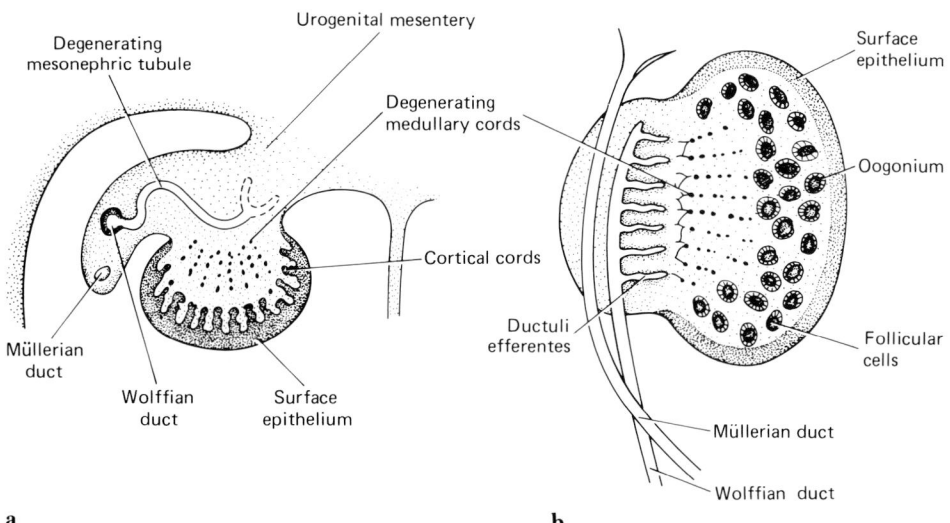

a

b

FIG. 1.6. **a: Transverse section through the ovary at seven weeks gestation.** The primitive (medullary) sex cords are undergoing degeneration and cortical cords are forming. **b: Five-month fetus.** The ovary and genital ducts have degenerative medullary cords. The excretory mesonephric tubules (ductuli efferentes) lack communication with the rete. Groups of oogonia surrounded by follicular cells lie in the cortical zone of the ovary. (From Sadler, ref. 47, with permission of Williams & Wilkins Co.)

development of both the uterus and vagina, both testes must secrete adequate amounts of MIS. Thus, a patient with a testis and a contralateral streak, ovary, or ovotestis generally has a uterus and vagina and a single fallopian tube on the side with the streak or ovary.

Additional functions of MIS have recently been discovered. In the female, ovarian granulosa cells begin producing MIS only after the müllerian-derived tissues (fallopian tubes, uterus, and vagina) are well developed and no longer susceptible to the regressive effects of MIS. Serum MIS levels in girls rise slowly after birth from nearly undetectable levels until they reach a plateau after 10 years of life equivalent to the adult male serum MIS concentration. In contrast, the male serum MIS concentration is relatively high at birth, peaks at 4–12 months of age, and then falls progressively to a baseline low adult level by about 10 years of age.[21] A major action of MIS in the young female may be to inhibit oocyte meiosis in the developing follicle.[64] Dramatically high levels of MIS have been found in women with ovarian sex cord tumors.[18] Secondary actions of MIS in males may be to initiate testicular descent[69] and regulate germ cell maturation.[57]

The second hormone that the fetal testis secretes is testosterone. This androgenic steroid, which is critical for male development, is required for the wolffian (mesonephric) duct to differentiate into the epididymis, vas deferens, and seminal vesicle. Leydig cells appear in the testis around day 54 to 64 and shortly thereafter begin to produce testosterone. Leydig cell activity is probably stimulated by increased production of chorionic gonadotropin by the placenta at that time. Testosterone acts locally on the ipsilateral wolffian duct by binding to a specific high affinity intracellular receptor protein. This receptor hormone complex binds DNA to regulate transcription of specific genes that govern further development. In the absence of a testis or inability of a testis to produce testosterone in adequate amounts by 10–12 weeks, or insensitivity of the wolffian duct anlage to testosterone, the epididymis, vas deferens, and seminal vesicle do not differentiate. Only rarely are abnormally elevated testosterone levels reached sufficiently early during embryogenesis in a female fetus to cause the wolffian duct to differentiate into definitive male organs (androgen administration to the mother during pregnancy, or congenital adrenogenital syndrome).

By the sixth week of embryonic life, the coelomic epithelium invaginates at several points on the lateral surface of the paired urogenital ridges and coalesces to form the paired tubes termed the *müllerian* or *paramesonephric duct* (Fig. 1.7). Each duct extends caudally in the urogenital ridge immediately lateral to and using the wolffian duct as a guidewire. For proper müllerian duct migration to occur, it is essential that the wolffian duct be present. Spatially lateral to the cranial aspect of the wolffian ducts, the müllerian ducts cross over caudally to lie medial to

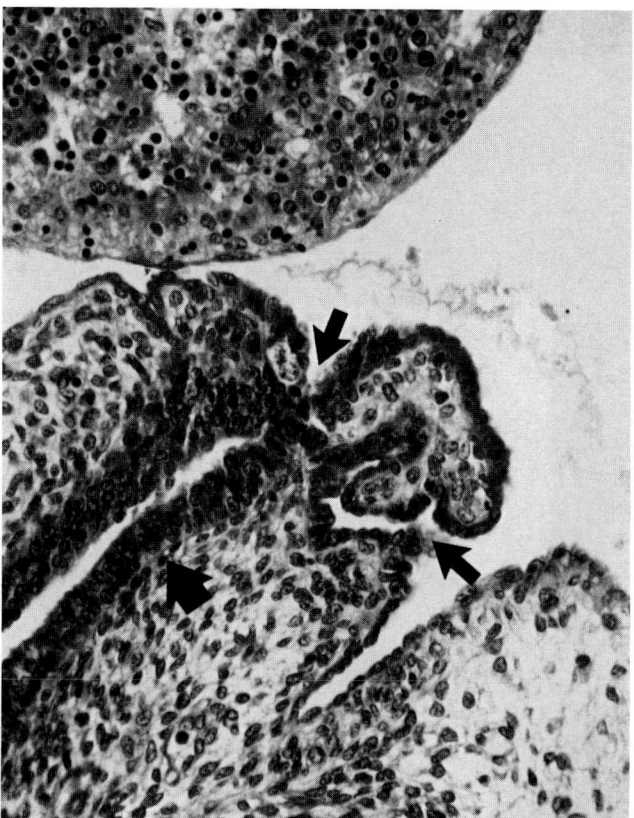

FIG. 1.7. Lateral surface of the urogenital ridge. The coelomic epithelium on the surface is proliferating and forming several invaginations (*narrow arrows*), that coalesce to form the müllerian duct (*wide arrow*).

them as they enter the pelvis (Figs. 1.8, 1.9). By about the end of the eighth week of embryonic life, the müllerian ducts between the two wolffian ducts fuse to form a single structure, which is the anlage of the common uterovaginal canal (Figs. 1.10, 1.11). The tip of the müllerian duct abuts on the posterior wall of the urogenital sinus immediately between the two orifices of the wolffian ducts (Fig. 1.12). The point where the tip of the müllerian duct abuts on the posterior wall of the urogenital sinus is within the patch of mesoderm inserted into the wall of the sinus by the wolffian ducts. This point defines the site of the future vaginal orifice, the hymenal membrane (Fig. 1.13).

The patch of mesodermal urogenital sinus epithelium lying between the orifices of the two wolffian ducts, in response to the apposition of the müllerian duct tip, begins to proliferate. A column of squamous epithelial cells is formed, termed the *vaginal plate*, which displaces the tip of the müllerian duct from the wall of the urogenital sinus. Recent studies suggest that the vaginal plate and müllerian duct are patent early in the second trimester. The vaginal plate gives rise to the epithelium that ultimately lines the vagina.

The development of the stromal component of the genital canal is little studied, but is clearly of major impor-

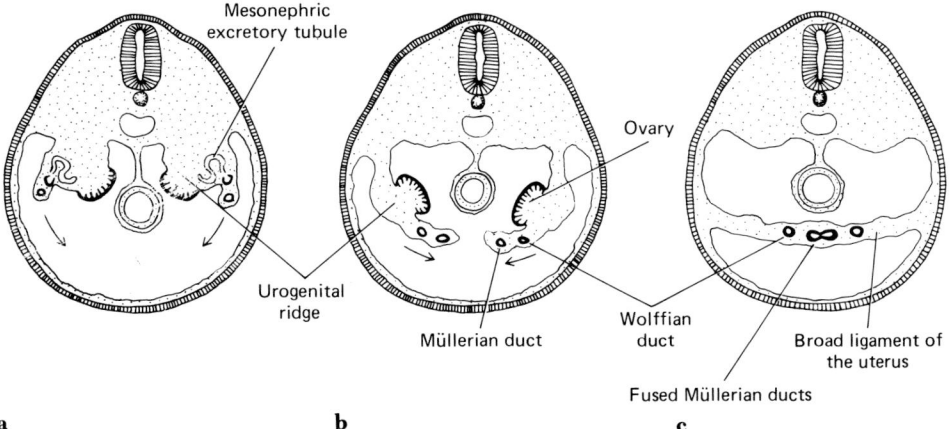

a　　　　　　　　b　　　　　　　　c

FIG. 1.8. Transverse section through urogenital ridge at progressively lower levels (a,b,c). The müllerian ducts approach each other in the midline and fuse. As a result, a transverse fold, the broad ligament of the uterus, forms in the pelvis. The gonads come to lie at the posterior aspect of the transverse fold. (From Sadler, ref. 47, with permission of Williams & Wilkins Co.)

tance.[5,6] In addition to its role in the development of the walls of the tubular muscular organs, there is extensive experimental evidence to indicate that the stroma directs epithelial development as well. Thus, the entire structure of the vagina, cervix, uterus, and tubes is determined by stromal–epithelial interaction.

Smooth muscle appears in the walls of the genital canal between 18 and 20 weeks, and by approximately 24 weeks, the muscular position of the uterine wall is well developed. Vaginal, uterine, and tubal muscular walls develop around the müllerian duct alone, so that the wolffian duct remnants are external to the true wall of

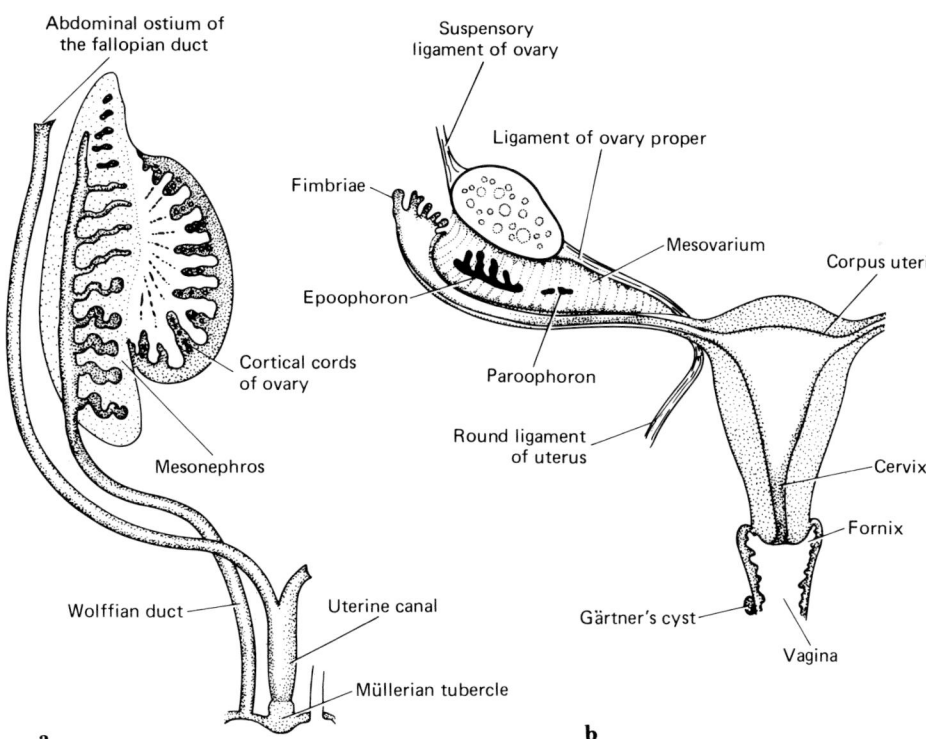

a　　　　　　　　　　　　　　b

FIG. 1.9. Eight-week female fetus. a: Genital ducts showing the müllerian tubercle and formation of the uterine canal. **b:** Genital ducts after descent of ovary. The only parts remaining of the mesonephric system are the epoophoron, the paroophoron, and Garner cyst. Also present are the suspensory ligament, the ligament of the ovary proper, and the round ligament of the uterus. (From Sadler, ref. 47, with permission of Williams & Wilkins Co.)

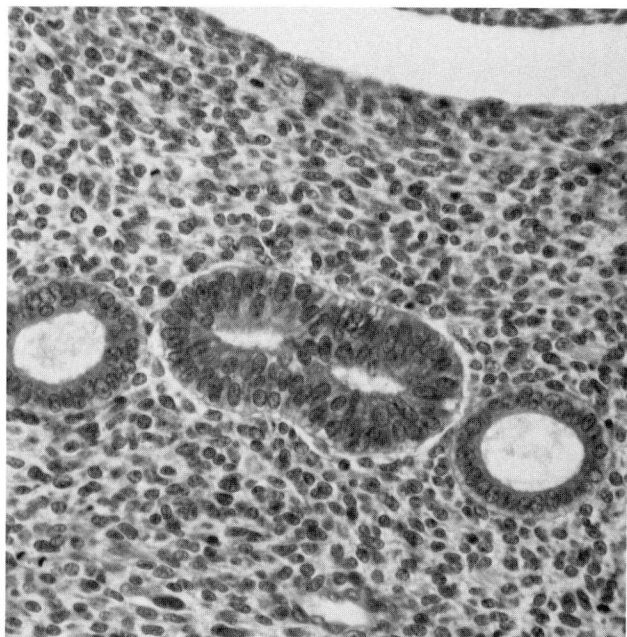

Fig. 1.10. Müllerian and wolffian ducts in a six-week fetus. Two müllerian ducts lie between the two wolffian ducts and are fusing.

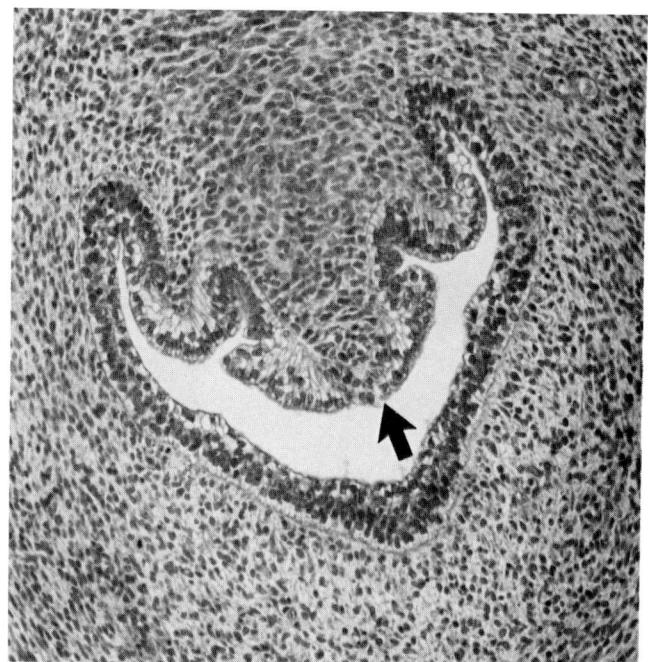

Fig. 1.12. Urogenital sinus at level of the müllerian tubercle. The müllerian ducts contact the urogenital sinus at this site (*arrow*). The epithelium of the anterior and posterior walls of the sinuses is dissimilar.

the canal. Cervical glands appear at about 15 weeks and rudimentary endometrial glands by 19 weeks, but the endometrium is not well developed even at term in most infants.

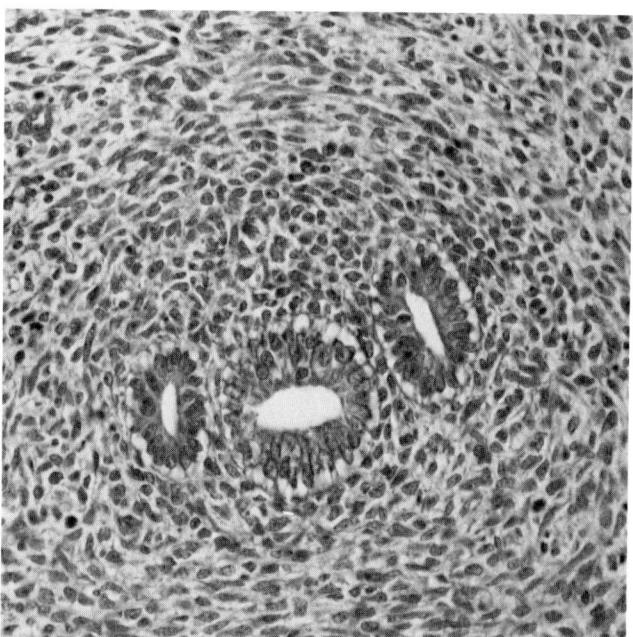

Fig. 1.11. The müllerian and wolffian ducts in a seven-week fetus. The müllerian ducts have fused into a single structure, which lies between the two wolffian ducts.

External Genitalia Development

Testosterone also acts as a prohormone for dihydrotestosterone (DHT), the substance ultimately responsible for initiating masculinization of the external genitalia and differentiation of the prostate. The enzyme 5-alpha-reductase, found in the tissues of the external genitalia and urogenital sinus, mediates the conversion of testosterone to DHT. DHT causes (1) the genital tubercle to enlarge and form the glans penis, (2) the genital folds to enlarge and fuse to form the penile shaft with migration of the urethral orifice along the lower border of the shaft to the tip of the glans, (3) the genital swellings to fuse and form a scrotum, and (4) the urogenital sinus tissues to differentiate into prostate. Failure of the external genitalia to develop in males in the presence of testes may be due to a lack of adequate testosterone secretion into the systemic circulation, deficient enzyme (5-alpha-reductase) at the end-organ level to convert testosterone to DHT, or complete end-organ insensitivity (testicular feminization). Lesser degrees of deficiency or end-organ insensitivity may result in partial male development characterized by a small penis, hypospadias, deficient formation of the scrotum, or a persistent urogenital sinus (vaginal opening into urethra). The effects of DHT begin about day 70, with fusion of the labioscrotal folds and closure of the median raphe, and continue at day 74 with closure of the urethral groove. External genital development is complete by day 120–140 (18th-20th week).

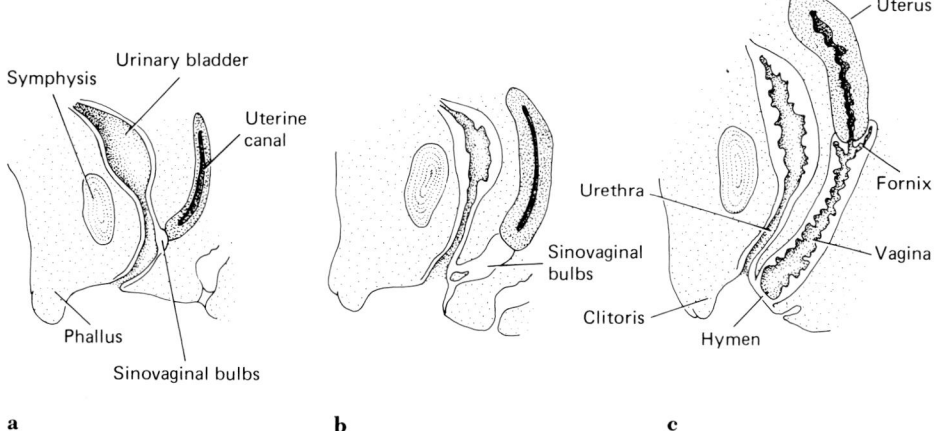

FIG. 1.13. Sagittal sections during different times in the formation of the uterus and vagina. The fused müllerian duct gives rise to the upper third of the vagina, the cervix, and the fundus of the uterus. (From Sadler, ref. 47, with permission of Williams & Wilkins Co.)

The urogenital sinus into which the vagina opens enlarges as the embryo grows, so that it becomes the vestibule of the adult external genitalia. Consequently, the vestibule is lined, except for a variable portion anterior to the urethral orifice, by the endodermal epithelium of the urogenital sinus. This is clinically important as the endodermal-derived epithelium differs not only morphologically from the mesodermal and ectodermal-derived epithelium, but responds differently to a variety of stimuli, notably sex steroids.

The form of the external genitalia results from events that begin during the fourth embryonic week in the mesodermal stroma immediately lateral and ventral to the cloacal plate. Just ventral to the plate, the stroma produces paired elevations of the ectoderm, which fuse to form the genital tubercle (Fig. 1.14). Immediately lateral to the cloacal plate on each side, two parallel folds develop by the same mechanism. The more medial, the urogenital fold, is destined to become the labium minus. The more lateral is the labioscrotal fold, which becomes the labium majus.

The labioscrotal fold extends cranially around the genital tubercle and fuses with its partner on the other side, becoming the mons pubis. At the end of the sixth week, the urorectal septum fuses with the cloacal plate, thus dividing this structure into the anal membrane posteriorly and the urogenital membrane ventrally. The lateral folds are distributed primarily in relation to the urogenital membrane. In both the male and female, the lateral folds fuse across the midline in front of the anus. In the male, the fusion moves ventrally in zipper-like fashion. The urogenital folds fuse to form a portion of the wall of the penile urethra, and the labioscrotal folds fuse to form the scrotum (Fig. 1.15). As female differentiation reflects the absence of this fusion, it may be difficult to detect, although by the end of the first trimester, significant fusion should have occurred in a male fetus.

Summary of Genital Development

In summary, female internal organs and external genitalia develop in the absence of hormones secreted by the fetal ovary, and differentiate even when gonads are absent. Unless interrupted by the regressive influence of MIS, differentiation of the müllerian ducts proceeds cephalocaudally to form fallopian tubes, a uterus, and a vagina. In the absence of the masculinizing effect of DHT, the undifferentiated external genital anlage develops into the vulva. The genital tubercle develops into the clitoris, the genital folds into the labia minora, and the genital swellings into the labia majora. Thus, the infant with ovaries or streak gonads has female internal and external genitalia at birth. Only if the female fetus has systemically elevated levels of

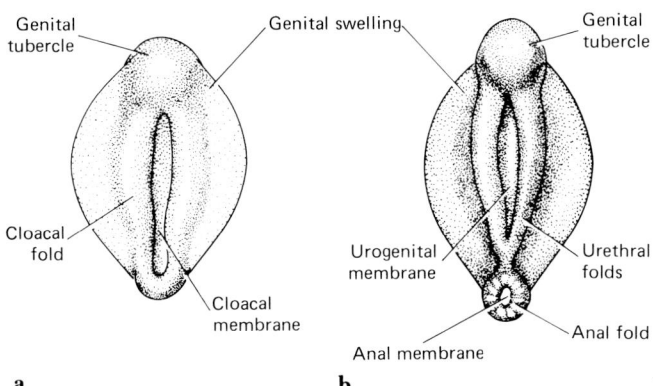

FIG. 1.14. Development of the external genitalis. a: The indifferent stage of the external genitalia at approximately four weeks. **b**: At approximately six weeks. (From Sadler, ref. 47, with permission of Williams & Wilkins Co.)

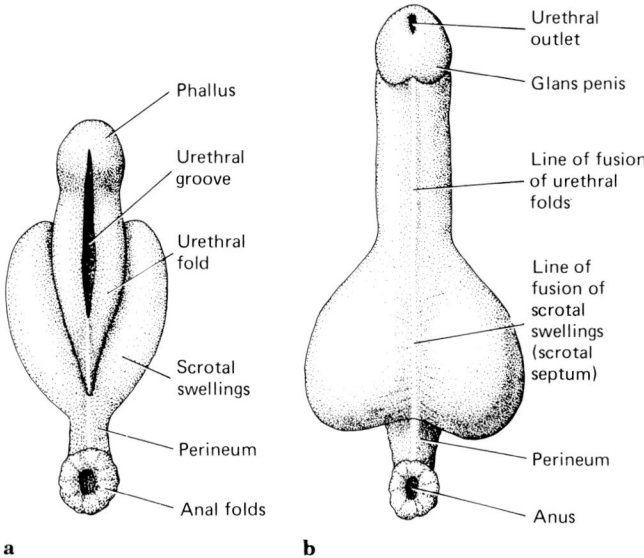

Phallus
Urethral groove
Urethral fold
Scrotal swellings
Perineum
Anal folds

Urethral outlet
Glans penis
Line of fusion of urethral folds
Line of fusion of scrotal swellings (scrotal septum)
Perineum
Anus

a   b

FIG. 1.15. **Male external genitalia. a**: At ten weeks gestation a deep urethral groove is present which is flanked by urethral folds. **b**: In the newborn. (From Sadler, ref. 47, with permission of Williams & Wilkins Co.)

androgens before the 10th–12th week of gestation does any degree of internal male development occur. In such cases the external genitalia may appear ambiguous or may resemble that of a normal phenotypic male; the vagina in these instances opens into the membranous portion of the urethra. If the androgens are not elevated until after the 20th week, by which time the external genitalia have fully formed, the only virilizing effect is an enlarged clitoris.

Intersexual Disorders

New insights into the biology of sexual development and advances in chromosome analysis have led to early identification and prompt treatment of the intersexual patient, which facilitates a more normal life for affected individuals. Based on these advances, a classification of abnormal sexual development has been developed that correlates the gonadal and genital anatomy with the chromosomal findings and specific genetic or metabolic defects[51,67] (Table 1.2). This permits an integrated approach to this complex group of disorders according to the manner by which patients present as well as on the pathophysiologic basis of the defect. The classification also groups patients who are at high risk for development of gonadal neoplasia.

Gender Identification Disorders with a Normal Chromosome Constitution

FEMALE PSEUDOHERMAPHRODITISM

Female pseudohermaphroditism occurs as a result of relative androgen excess in utero in an individual with two

Table 1.2. Classification of intersexual disorders

Disorders associated with a normal chromosome constitution
  Female pseudohermaphroditism
    Adrenogenital syndrome (testosterone overproduction due to adrenocorticoid insufficiency)
      21 alpha-hydroxylase deficiency
      11 beta-hydroxylase deficiency
    Maternal ingestion of progestins or androgens
    Maternal virilizing tumor
  Male pseudohermaphroditism
    Gonadal defects
      Testicular regression syndrome (gonadal destruction)
      Leydig cell agenesis
        Defective hCG-LH receptor
      Defects in testosterone synthesis
        Testosterone and adrenocorticoid insufficiency
          20, 22-demolase deficiency
          3 beta-hydroxylase dehydrogenase deficiency
          17 alpha-hydroxylase deficiency
        Testosterone insufficiency only
          17-20-desmolase deficiency
          17 beta-hydroxysteroid (17-ketosteroid reductase) dehydrogenase deficiency
      Defect in müllerian-inhibiting substance (persistent müllerian duct syndrome)
    End-organ defects
      Disordered androgen receptor binding
        Androgen insensitivity syndrome (testicular feminization)
        Incomplete androgen insensitivity syndrome (Reifenstein syndrome)
      Disordered testosterone metabolism
        5 alpha-reductase deficiency
Disorders associated with an abnormal sex chromosome constitution
  Sexual ambiguity infrequent
    Klinefelter syndrome
    Turner syndrome
    XX male syndrome
    Pure gonadal dysgenesis (some forms)
  Sexual ambiguity frequent
    Mixed gonadal dysgenesis, including:
      Pure gonadal dysgenesis (some forms)
      Dysgenetic male pseudohermaphroditism
    True hermaphroditism

"Idiopathic" or "unclassified" conditions exist within each major category. We assume that each category of male pseudohermaphroditism with defects in specific protein products or receptors has forms in which the abnormality is total or partial, or where the defect results from a qualitatively abnormal structure. hCG-LH, human chorionic gonadotropin–luteinizing hormone.

ovaries and two X chromosomes (46 XX). The elevated level of androgen present during embryogenesis usually results in genital ambiguity and may result in the appearance of a phenotypic male. Tumors, if they appear, are virtually always benign.[42a]

Adrenogenital Syndrome

Congenital adrenal hyperplasia, unlike all other conditions responsible for the appearance of ambiguous genitalia in

FIG. 1.16. Biosynthesis of mineralocorticoids, glucocorticoids, and sex steroids. (From Saenger et al., ref. 48, with permission of Pediatric Andrology.)

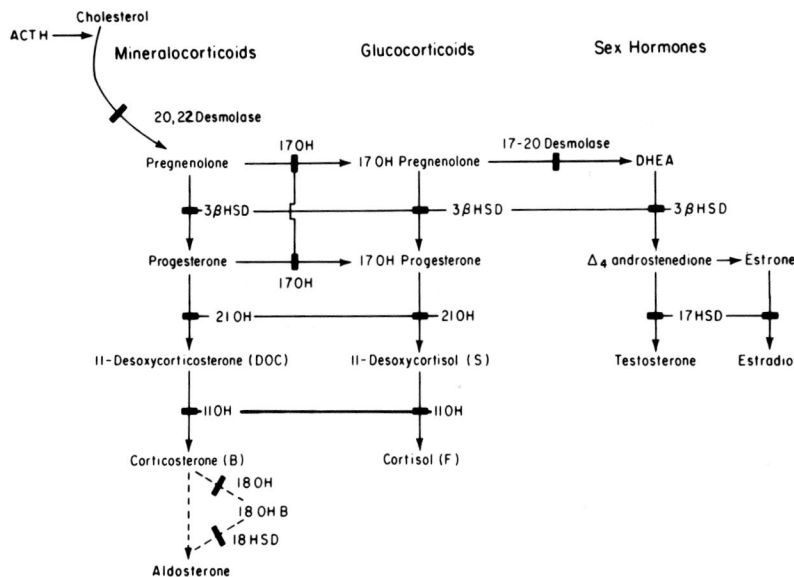

the newborn, may be life-threatening because of a lack of synthesis of specific adrenal steroids. Prompt diagnosis and institution of appropriate therapy are therefore essential. With early treatment normal external genitalia and fertility can be achieved. The manifestations of the adrenogenital syndrome in the XX individual are summarized most easily through an understanding of the biosynthetic pathways of mineralocorticoid, glucocorticoid, and sex steroids (Fig. 1.16). Two enzymes, 21-hydroxylase and 11-beta-hydroxylase, participate in the formation of the glucocorticoids, desoxycorticosterone and cortisol, and the mineralocorticoid, aldosterone, but not of testosterone or the estrogens, estrone or estradiol. Deficiency of either enzyme in the 46 XX female leads to elevated adrenocorticotropic hormone (ACTH) products and hence elevated levels of testosterone and other strongly androgenic intermediates, which may result in sexual ambiguity or marked virilization of the newborn's external genitalia.[39] 3-Beta-hydroxysteroid dehydrogenase is required for testosterone formation. In its absence, the principal androgen to form is the weak androgen, dehydroepiandrosterone (DHEA), which has 1/20th the potency of testosterone. Patients with deficiency of this enzyme, therefore, show signs of only mild virilization, usually on clitoral hypertrophy but not with labial fusion or anterior displacement of the urethral orifice.

21-Hydroxylase deficiency is inherited as an autosomal recessive trait caused by a lesion of the gene coding for cytochrome $P_{450}c21$. It accounts for more than 95% of cases of congenital adrenal hyperplasia, occurring once in 50,000 births. Heterozygote carriers can be identified through use of ACTH stimulation. Present data suggest that a series of allelic genes on the short arm of chromosome 6, between the HLA-B and -DR loci, code for the 21-hydroxylase enzyme and that these allelic variants, in-

cluding rearrangements, deletions, or point mutations explain the occurrence of the wide variation in symptomatology observed in these patients.[35,56] The extent to which signs of virilization evolve depends on which time during fetal life the disease began. If the onset begins after the 16th week of gestation, the clitoris may be enlarged; if androgen excess occurs earlier, the vagina and urethra may open into a common urogenital sinus. More marked clitoral enlargement and an opening of the urogenital sinus at the clitoral base may mimic penile hypospadias and suggest an even earlier temporal effect. On occasion, the changes have been of such severity that the female infants have been misdiagnosed as cryptorchid males with or without hypospadias.

Males have no evidence of genital ambiguity but may have an enlarged phallus and a hyperpigmented rugated scrotum. Bilateral testicular nodules, composed of interstitial cells resembling Leydig cells or cells of adrenal rest origin, occasionally develop (Fig. 1.17).

Maternal Ingestion of Progestins or Androgens

Maternal ingestion of synthetic progestins was implicated as a cause of female pseudohermaphroditism in the late 1950s when such treatment was employed for threatened or habitual abortion; subsequently, progestins have also been implicated in the development of hypospadias in male offspring.[53] Most cases of female pseudohermaphroditism in this category developed after maternal ingestion of Ethisterone (17-alpha-ethinyl-testosterone) or Norlutin (17-alpha-ethinyl-19-nortestosterone), but occasionally after the ingestion of Enovid, diethylstilbestrol, androgens, or the intramuscular administration of progesterone. Masculinization usually consists of phallic enlargement and variable degrees of labioscrotal fusion, depending on the

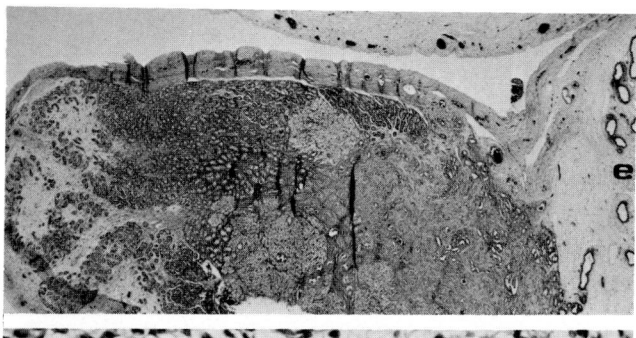

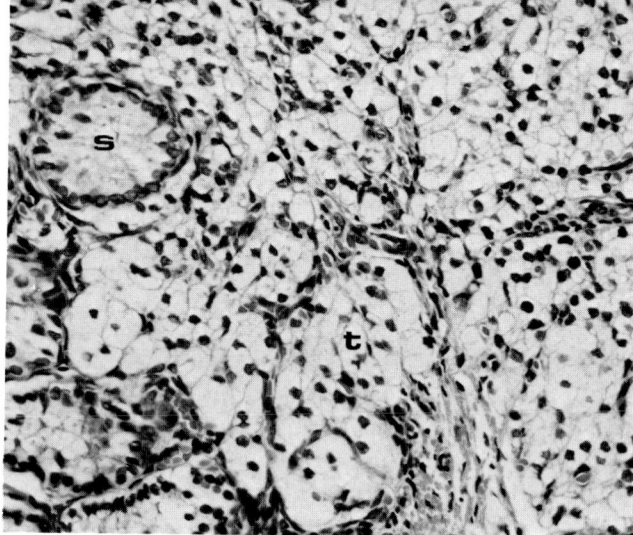

FIG. 1.17. **Interstitial cell tumor of the testis in a 4-year-old child with adrenogenital syndrome.** The tumor cells (*T*), which are illustrated at high magnification adjacent to immature seminiferous tubules (*S*) in the inset, resemble adrenocortical cells more closely than Leydig cells. The epididymis (*E*) is adjacent to the testis. (From Welch and Robboy, ref. 67, with permission of Pediatric Andrology.)

time during gestation when the therapy was administered. Although the degree of masculinization usually is less than that associated with the adrenogenital syndrome, the sexual ambiguity in female infants has been of such severity in some instances as to result in male sex assignment. The degree of virilization does not progress with age. The gonads and internal genital organs are unaffected, and ovulation, menstruation, and normal secondary female characteristics appear at puberty.

Maternal Virilizing Tumors

A variety of benign and malignant tumors, primary as well as metastatic to, the ovary have been associated on rare occasions with virilization of the mother and her female offspring[44a,50a] (see Chapters 16, 19, 22). The luteoma of pregnancy, by far the most common lesion that causes maternal virilization during pregnancy, is discussed as the prototype of this category. Rarer conditions include

Krukenberg tumors arising from primary adenocarcinomas of the stomach and mucinous tumors primary in the ovary. The common thread among all such lesions is the development of hormonally active cells, usually as theca cells, which secrete androgenic hormones.

The pregnancy luteoma is a benign hyperplastic lesion of the ovary that is encountered most often as an incidental finding at the time of cesarean section or postpartum sterilization, usually in women who are multiparous. Elevated levels of human chorionic gonadotropin (hCG) are thought to induce hyperplasia of theca-lutein or stroma-lutein cells. A small percentage of the female infants have become masculinized, with mild enlargement of the clitoris and occasionally minimal degrees of labioscrotal fusion or rugate, hyperpigmented ("scrotal") labia. The nature of these changes indicates that the ovarian nodules do not function until the second half of gestation, which is in accord with the occasional onset of masculinization in the mother during the third trimester.

At operation, one and often both maternal ovaries are enlarged by one or more soft, yellow-brown nodules that are well circumscribed but not encapsulated. Although most are less than 2 cm in diameter, they may be as large as 20 cm in greatest dimension. On microscopic examination, the nodules consist of large, polygonal cells with granular, eosinophilic cytoplasm, which are smaller and more eosinophilic than the luteinized granulosa cells of the corpus luteum but larger than the theca-lutein cells. Intracellular lipid is sparse, if at all present. Mitoses may be observed, but only rarely are they numerous.

Elevated plasma and tissue levels of testosterone, DHT, androstenedione, and DHEA have been detected in virilized patients; the plasma levels return to normal once the tumor is extirpated. Even without treatment, the nodules regress and disappear soon after delivery. Rarely, a functional luteoma may reoccur during a subsequent pregnancy.[63] Other primary functioning tumors of the ovary that may lead to virilization of the female offspring as well as metastatic tumors to the ovary that induce the stroma to function during pregnancy are discussed elsewhere in this book.

MALE PSEUDOHERMAPHRODITISM

The term *male pseudohermaphroditism* is applied to a heterogeneous group of intersex conditions that are characterized by an intrauterine state of relative functional androgen deficiency, an apparently normal 46 XY karyotype, and either identifiable testes or evidence that testes were present during fetal development. The external genitalia are usually female or ambiguous, although in certain categories (e.g., testicular regression syndrome) they may appear as phenotypically male. The defect may be in the gonad, leading to deficiency in androgens, MIS, or both. Alternatively, end-organ defects in which developing tissues are unresponsive to androgens or MIS may lead to the abnormal phenotype. Tumors, if they occur, are sometimes malignant.[42a]

Primary Gonadal Defects

A primary defect of the gonad in an XY karyotype individual may lead to male pseudohermaphroditism by any one of the following mechanisms: regression (destruction) of the gonads or their anlage during intrauterine life, agenesis of the Leydig cells, a specific enzymatic defect in testosterone synthesis, or a defect in elaboration or action of MIS.

Testicular Regression Syndrome. Testicular regression follows the irreparable destruction of the testes at a critical stage of fetal development in an XY individual.[4] The phenotype of the affected individual reflects the specific stage of fetal development during which the testes were damaged. In general, gonadal regression that occurs during embryonic life, before the elaboration of MIS and/or androgenic steroids by the testes, leads to a female phenotype. Regression of the testes during late embryonic through mid–fetal life permits a masculine phenotype to develop (Fig. 1.1). The testicular regression syndrome has a variety of etiologies, some possibly as diverse as inherited genetic defect, intrauterine infection, or infarction. The heterogeneity of presentation of this syndrome and its relative rarity have led to numerous and sometimes confusing terms for this disorder, including *true agonadism, testicular dysgenesis, rudimentary testis, vanishing testis,* and *complete bilateral anorchia.* The terms *pure gonadal dysgenesis* and *Swyer syndrome* have been used for the testicular regression syndrome by some authors. We avoid these latter terms so as not to confuse them with other conditions similarly named and discussed below.

At one end of the spectrum of the testicular regression syndrome, the internal genitalia and gonads are absent and the external genitalia are female. Presumably, the urogenital ridge was destroyed in its entirety during early embryonic life, even before the müllerian ducts began to differentiate (before day 42).

At the other end of the spectrum, which approximates the end point of normal genital development, the patients are phenotypic males with infantile to nearly normal male external genitalia, normally differentiated wolffian duct structures, and completely inhibited müllerian duct development. Often in these cases no genital tissue is identified, but an area of fibrosis, hemorrhage, or hemosiderin deposition is found at the expected site of the gonad near residual vas deferens or epididymis. Occasionally, atrophic seminiferous tubules may be found amid a fibrous stroma. Testicular regression presumably occurred during the late fetal period (after 120 days), when müllerian structures had already atrophied under the influences of MIS and testosterone and DHT had exerted a major influence on the normal development of internal and external genitalia.

Torsion and infarction of improperly descended testes has been suggested.[55]

Intermediate in the spectrum of the testicular regression syndrome are patients with ambiguous genitalia and various combinations of wolffian and/or müllerian duct development. Testes that regressed during the late embryonic period (day 43–59) will have secreted insufficient testosterone to affect the wolffian duct. The production of MIS will have been variable, resulting in poorly differentiated or rudimentary müllerian structures (incomplete inhibition). In the absence of systemic androgens, the external genitalia appear female.

Regression of the testes during the early fetal period (day 59–84) after Sertoli cell (MIS) and Leydig cell (testosterone) function have begun or about to begin results in an individual with ambiguous external genitalia and various combinations of wolffian and müllerian development depending on the duration of androgen secretion and müllerian inhibition.

Regression of the testes during the mid–fetal period (day 84–120) results in more advanced masculinization of the external genitalia, although degrees of ambiguity are usually present. Since müllerian duct inhibition is normally completed by day 80, the müllerian structures will have been suppressed and wolffian structures develop.

Leydig Cell Agenesis. Leydig cell agenesis is a very rare cause of male pseudohermaphroditism.[31] Affected individuals have a 46 XY karyotype and testes with interstitial fibrosis, but no mature Leydig cells. Tubules with Sertoli cells and, sometimes, immature spermatogonia are found. The müllerian structures are absent, indicating appropriate testicular production of MIS during fetal life. The wolffian duct system is developed either partially or fully such that identifiable vasa deferentia and epididymides are present. The phenotype varies and is usually female with unremarkable or ambiguous external genitalia, although unambiguous males with evidence of primary hypogonadism have been reported. The presence of wolffian duct development and the variable degrees of masculinization of the external genitalia indicate that some Leydig cells must have differentiated and functioned during early fetal life. Luteinizing hormone levels are elevated in affected individuals. The underlying defect in this disorder is believed to be an absence or defect of the luteinizing hormone (LH)-hCG receptor on the Leydig cell or with some other, unknown, factor arresting Leydig cell development.

Defects in Testosterone Synthesis. Congenital deficiency of any enzyme involved in the production of testosterone in the testis or adrenal gland results in a state of androgen deficiency (relative estrogen excess)[32] (Fig. 1.16). The histologic appearance of the testicular tissue is variable. It has been described occasionally to be "normal," but the photomicrographs in some reports have disclosed large clusters of Leydig cells surrounding tubules lined only by Sertoli cells. In general, the number of gonads studied for any of the conditions and the range of ages studied (infancy, childhood, adulthood) have been limited. Mullerian structures are absent, but wolffian duct structures may be present. The degree to which the external genitalia develop depends on the type and severity of the defect.

Three inherited enzymatic defects involve both the synthesis of adrenal mineralocorticoid and glucocorticoid hormones as well as adrenal and testicular sex hormones. The most severe defect, which involves the conversion of cholesterol intermediates to pregnenolone (20,22-desmolase), almost always ends lethally from a salt-wasting crisis if untreated during infancy.[48] Although the external genitalia in the male are ambiguous or female, sufficient testosterone must be secreted during embryogenesis since the internal genitalia are male. The testes in the infant disclose immature seminiferous tubules with spermatogonia. The germ cells disappear by several years of age.

The deficiency of 3-beta-hydroxylase dehydrogenase, like the 20,22-desmolase deficiency, results in decreased synthesis of mineralocorticoid and glucocorticoid hormones as well as adrenal and testicular sex hormones, and may lead to life-threatening salt wasting in infancy. DHEA, which is a weak androgen secreted in high amounts, results in slight clitoral enlargement in the female, but rarely completely masculinizes the external genitalia in males. Hence, the male may be born with ambiguous genitalia and may resemble a virilized female. Males in whom the defect is partial may be born with hypospadias, but at puberty develop gynecomastia. The testes in older boys generally are immature, exhibiting seminiferous tubules with spermatogenic arrest and diminished numbers of Leydig cells.

In contrast to the early age of diagnosis in the above two syndromes, the diagnosis in most patients with 17-alpha-hydroxylase deficiency is not suspected until the anticipated time of puberty or later. Recently, however, the de- tailed steroid analysis of the urine of a newborn male presenting with ambiguous genitalia has shown that the correct diagnosis can be made in the young.[7]

Deficiencies of two enzymes, 17,20-desmolase and 17-hydroxysteroid dehydrogenase (17-ketosteroid reductase), result in deficient testosterone synthesis but do not affect the production of either mineralocorticoids or glucocorticoids. The former defect (conversion of 17-hydroxypregnenolone to DHEA) is extremely rare. The patients reported presented with ambiguous external genitalia and inguinal or intraabdominal testes. Spermatogonia were present in the testis of infants but were absent in the biopsies of their older teenage relatives. All had third degree hypospadias, but normal male internal ductal differentiation.

Genetic males with 17-hydroxysteroid dehydrogenase (17-ketosteroid reductase) deficiency have almost all been raised as females because of incomplete masculinization.

Most are diagnosed at or after puberty when signs of virilization such as clitoromegaly and hirsutism become apparent. Müllerian duct derivatives are absent, consistent with normal antimüllerian hormone action. Wolffian duct differentiation, indicative of testosterone secretion during embryogenesis, is normal. The testes present in the inguinal canal or labia majora contain rare to no spermatogonia, and may exhibit numerous Leydig cells.

Defect in Müllerian-inhibiting Substance (Persistent Müllerian Duct Syndrome). The persistent müllerian duct syndrome, also known as *hernia uteri inguinalis*, is a rare form of male pseudohermaphroditism characterized by the presence of müllerian duct structures in 46 XY phenotypic males. These patients usually present when young with unilateral or bilateral cryptorchid testes, normal or almost normal male external genitalia, and an inguinal hernia into which prolapses an infantile uterus and fallopian tubes. The testes are histologically normal, wolffian duct structures are developed, the pubertal development is normal, and a rare patient has been fertile. Treatment is surgical, consisting of orchiopexy and herniorrhaphy with hysterectomy and bilateral salpingectomy. If at operation any patient has a streak gonad or a tumor rather than bilateral testes, the diagnosis of mixed gonadal dysgenesis should be considered.[43] In most cases of persistent müllerian duct syndrome, the vas deferens is tightly adherent to the residual uterus or upper vagina, and in some cases the müllerian structures must be left intact to preserve the vas deferens.[11] Malignant testicular tumors have been reported in the very rare cases of adult patients with persistent müllerian duct syndrome and uncorrected cryptorchid testes.[61] The persistent müllerian duct syndrome seems to be a heterogeneous group of disorders, caused by different defects in the müllerian-inhibiting system. Familial cases have been reported. Some patients produce no MIS, whereas others produce normal amounts of biologically active MIS, suggesting either end organ insensitivity to MIS or an abnormality of the timing of MIS secretion.[17] Some patients might produce a biologically inactive form of MIS.

End-organ Defects

The normal development of the wolffian duct derivatives and the external genitalia requires that these structures be responsive to androgen and that the enzyme, 5-alpha-reductase, be present in the anlage of the prostate and external genitalia to convert testosterone to DHT. A molecular defect of the androgen receptor system (e.g., unstable androgen receptor or lack of androgen receptor) leads to impaired development of both wolffian duct structures and external genitalia in 46 XY individuals. If only 5-alpha-reductase is absent or defective, the abnormalities in the reproductive tract are confined to the external genitalia and prostate.

Androgen Receptor Disorders (Androgen Insensitivity Syndromes). Disorders of androgen receptor function result in a variety of phenotypes ranging from phenotypic women with intraabdominal testes to individuals with ambiguous genitalia to phenotypic men with minimal clinical abnormalities. Because androgen receptor defects lead to such a variety of different clinical disorders, much nosological confusion exists in the literature regarding subclassification of the androgen resistance syndromes. In Griffin's classification scheme,[15] the five categories in order of increasing virilization (decreasing feminization) are: complete and incomplete testicular feminization, Reifenstein syndrome, infertile male syndrome, and undervirilized male syndrome. All share an X-linked recessive inheritance, the result of a defect in the androgen receptor gene, which has been localized to the long arm of the X chromosome, position Xq11.2-q12.[29] A variety of different mutations of this gene have been characterized, most of which are limited to individual families. These mutations may lead to absence of the androgen receptor because of deletion of the gene. Alternatively, only the hormone-binding region of the receptor may be deleted or altered such that testosterone binding is absent or impaired. Finally, some mutations alter the DNA binding region of the receptor, leaving testosterone binding intact while rendering the receptor unable to carry out its function as a regulatory protein.[15]

Complete Testicular Feminization. Complete testicular feminization is the most common form of male pseudohermaphroditism. The external genitalia are phenotypically female and, for this reason, the condition is rarely diagnosed before puberty unless an inguinal hernia or labial mass is encountered or unless the disease is known to be familial. Primary amenorrhea is the most common complaint leading to evaluation and subsequent diagnosis. The medical history usually reveals that breast development occurred as expected at puberty. Pubic and axillary hair are scant, the vagina is shortened, and the epididymides, vasa differentia, seminal vesicles, and prostate are absent. As a rule, both the cervix and the body of the uterine corpus are absent. A fragment of fallopian tube may be found in up to one-third of cases.[46] The testes are cryptorchid and may be located in the inguinal canal, the pelvis, or rarely the labia. In the complete or almost complete form of the syndrome, the individual exhibits a truly female consciousness gender identity, with normal extragenital erotogenic sensitivity and normal maternal attitude.

The gonads in infants and young children are relatively normal but by age 5 years, they show abnormalities.[36] By young adulthood, the gonad often is involved with benign or malignant tumors as described below. If tumors are not present by this age, the gonad is usually small and on section is tan to brown and traversed by thin white bands. A 1- to 2-cm firm, white nodule of hyalinized smooth muscle is usually present at one pole of the testes. Theories regarding what this nodule might represent include an abnormally hypertrophied gubernaculum or rudimentary uterine structure. Microscopic examination of the testicular parenchyma discloses immature seminiferous tubules usually sparsely distributed or clustered in small aggregates. Spermatogonia may be present, but spermatogenesis is absent. The number of spermatogonia that are found is age-dependent, diminishing as the patient ages.[36] The interstitium is usually abundant and often resembles ovarian stroma (Fig 1.18). Fetal-type Leydig cells may be abundant. The findings indicate that Leydig cells are active hormone producers. The Leydig cells in individuals with testicular feminization have an ultrastructure typical of cells involved in active hormone synthesis[42]; the systemic androgen levels in these individuals are characteristically elevated. These findings indicate that the pathologic defect in the testicular feminization syndrome is an end-organ defect and not a lack of hormone production by the testes.

Most testes of affected individuals contain multiple benign nodules that are discrete, firm, yellow to brown, and bulge above the sectioned surface (Fig. 1.18). Hamartomatous nodules may be present, usually bilaterally, in virtually every case the authors have examined. The typical size varies from 1 mm to 1 cm, and to 4 cm in the series of Rutgers and Scully.[46] The bulk of the nodule usually comprises seminiferous tubules lacking lumina; spermatogonia may be present. Sertoli cell adenomas are hamartomas composed predominantly or exclusively of closely packed immature seminiferous tubules lacking lumina and lined by immature, uniform Sertoli cells. The adenomas average 3 cm in diameter, ranging up to 25 cm. The interstitium in the testes of affected patients often resembles ovarian stroma, and frequently contains Leydig cells. On rare occasions, Leydig cell nodules form, and have been considered benign tumors. In summary, the name applied to each type of nodule is somewhat arbitrary and depends largely on the types of components present as well as their number and size. Most nodules are classified as hamartomas, Sertoli cell adenomas, or rarely as Leydig cell tumors.

Malignant gonadal tumors develop with increasing frequency with age in patients with testicular feminization. Seminoma is the most commonly encountered gonadal malignancy in this syndrome. Intratubular germ cell neoplasia is sometimes seen, either independently or in association with seminoma. Other malignant germ cell tumors and malignant sex cord tumors are also rarely encountered. Unlike mixed gonadal dysgenesis in which tumors develop in young individuals, the risk of malignancy in patients with testicular feminization is only 4% by the age of 25 years,[30] but reaches 33% by 50 years. Since malignant tumors rarely develop before completion of puberty, castration can usually be delayed until after adolescence, thus permitting the patient to undergo a normal pubertal spurt and develop female secondary sex characteristics.

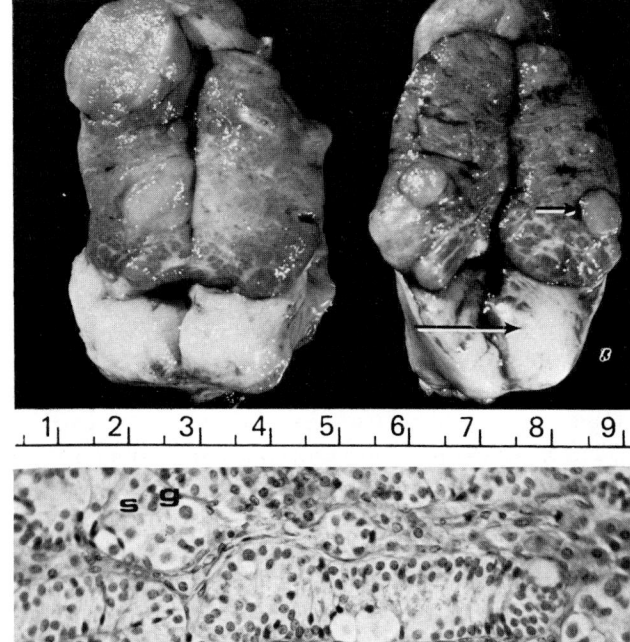

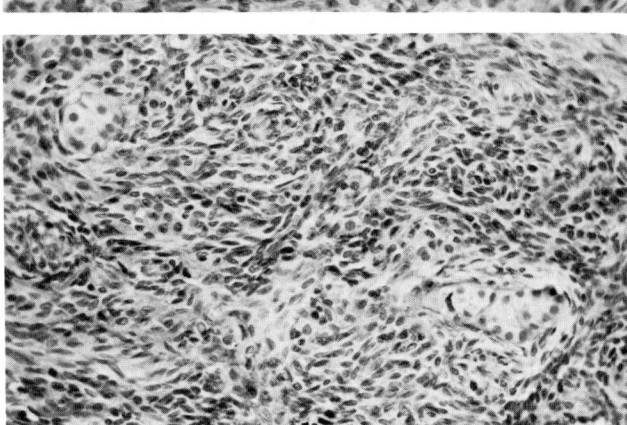

FIG. 1.18. Testis in the complete form of androgen insensitivity (testicular feminization) syndrome. *Top*: Testis in a 17-year-old with the complete form of androgen insensitivity (testicular feminization) syndrome. Numerous Sertoli cell adenomas (*short arrows*) are present in the parenchyma. The mass near one pole (*long arrow*) may represent an abnormally hypertrophied gubernaculum. *Middle*: Hamartoma with immature seminiferous tubules (*S*), numerous germ cells (*G*), and numerous Leydig cells (*L*) in the interstitium. *Bottom*: Contralateral testis with scattered immature seminiferous tubules embedded in a dense ovarian-type cortical stroma. Occasional interstitial cells (*arrows*) are present. (From Welch and Robboy, ref. 67, with permission of Pediatric Andrology.)

Incomplete Testicular Feminization. About 10% of patients with androgen insensitivity syndrome have incomplete testicular feminization. It resembles complete testicular feminization except that there is partial fusion of the labioscrotal folds and usually some clitoromegaly at birth. Also, underdeveloped wolffian duct derivatives are often present. If the diagnosis is established during childhood, gonadectomy should be performed before puberty, since virilization may accompany breast development at puberty. Estrogen therapy should be given at the appropriate time to initiate feminization. The pathologic findings are similar to those described for the complete form of testicular feminization.[36]

Other Forms. Reifenstein syndrome, infertile male syndrome, and undervirilized male syndrome are other forms of incomplete androgen insensitivity in which the phenotype is male. There are few reports describing the microscopic findings of the gonads.

Men with Reifenstein syndrome usually present with gynecomastia and severe hypospadias, and children or teenagers with perineoscrotal hypospadias. However, the phenotypic spectrum is wide, even within the same affected family with a single androgen receptor abnormality in all affected family members. The usual abnormalities include hypospadias, breast development at puberty, female habitus, azoospermia, cryptorchidism, and hypoplasia or absence of wolffian duct structures. The "infertile male syndrome" is a rare androgen receptor defect characterized by a phenotypically normal man with infertility caused by azoospermia. Finally, in the "undervirilized male syndrome" the individual is a male with gynecomastia, a small penis, decreased beard and body hair, a normal male urethra, a normal sperm density, and an identifiable androgen receptor defect. Most affected individuals are infertile.

DISORDERED TESTOSTERONE METABOLISM

5 Alpha-reductase Deficiency. Deficiency of the enzyme 5-alpha-reductase impairs the conversion of testosterone to DHT, the hormone that masculinizes the indifferent urogenital sinus and induces development of the prostate.[15,22,59] The disorder has an autosomal recessive inheritance and is rare. Most reported cases come from family clusters found in three relatively isolated geographic locations in the Dominican Republic, southern Turkey, and Papua New Guinea.

Affected males typically are phenotypically female with female to ambiguous external genitalia at birth (pseudovaginal perineoscrotal hypospadias). The small clitoris-like phallus lacks a urethral orifice. In most affected individuals the urogenital sinus opens on the perineum and within the sinus an anterior orifice leads to the urethra and a posterior orifice to a blind vaginal pouch. The testes are in the inguinal canals or labia. The müllerian derived structures are absent whereas wolffian-derived structures (vas deferens, epididymis, and seminal vesicle), the anlage of which respond to testosterone, are normal.

At puberty, virilization occurs and the breasts fail to develop. The penis lengthens, the bifid scrotum grows and becomes rugated and hyperpigmented, and the testes enlarge and descend. Testicular biopsy specimens reveal spermatogenesis and tubular atrophy in some individuals, complete spermatogenic arrest and Leydig cell hyperplasia in others. The prostate fails to develop and remains impalpable. Erection, ejaculation, and orgasm are possible in some affected individuals; these individuals are not fertile, however.

Neonates with this disorder frequently go unrecognized and are raised as females. After the virilization that accompanies puberty, individuals raised as girls sometimes reverse their sex roles and function as men, often with a stormy period of adjustment. Individuals with a male gender identity benefit from surgical correction of hypospadias and cryptorchidism. High doses of testosterone enhance virilization. Persons raised as females who elect to continue to function as females into adulthood benefit from orchiectomy before the onset of puberty to avoid the accompanying virilization. Estrogen therapy is useful to promote feminization.

Gender Identification Disorders with an Abnormal Sex Chromosome Constitution

Additions, deletions, or mosaicism of the sex chromosomes characterize individuals in this category. The appearance of the gonads is variable and ranges from the presence of a streak gonad to a nearly normal female or male gonad on both gross and microscopic examination. These disorders are subdivided into two broad categories depending on the frequency with which sexual ambiguity occurs.

Sexual Ambiguity Infrequent

Klinefelter Syndrome

Klinefelter syndrome occurs in about 1 of every 1000 live newborn males.[49] The karyotype is usually 47 XXY which, in most cases, results from nondysjunction occurring during meiosis of either paternal or maternal gametes. Less frequently, a 47 XXY/46 XY mosaic karyotype is found, caused by nondysjunction during mitosis of the developing zygote. The diagnosis is usually first suspected at adolescence when the patient presents with gynecomastia, obesity, or signs of eunuchism. The testes are small. The beard and body hair frequently are sparse. Most patients are tall with long legs resulting in a diminished upper lower body segment ratio. Laboratory tests reveal low testosterone levels, elevated gonadotropic levels (postpuberty), and azoospermia. Frequently associated clinical findings include learning disabilities, behavioral disorders, reduced economic striving, and limited sexual drive. The diagnosis also may be established at other stages of life because of evaluation of age-related clinical concerns. Genetic screening programs identify the fetus with Klinefelter syndrome. Although infants with Klinefelter syndrome usually have normal external male genitalia at birth, the syndrome is sometimes discovered during evaluations of newborns with hypospadias, micropenis, and small soft testes or cryptorchidism. In adults, Klinefelter syndrome may be discovered during an evaluation for infertility or malignancy.

The Klinefelter testis is morphologically normal at birth in most cases. Primary spermatogonia are already greatly reduced in number by late childhood. Shortly before the expected time of puberty, the seminiferous tubules begin to degenerate. The absence of elastic fibers in the tubular wall indicates that the process of atrophy began prepubertally. The testes in adult 47 XXY individuals are small and rarely exceed 2 cm in maximal dimension (Fig. 1.19). On microscopic examination, they are largely atrophic, have hyalinized seminiferous tubules, and a relative increase in the number of Leydig cells. Some tubules may be preserved, but lined only by Sertoli cells. Rarely, an occasional seminiferous tubule of the adult testis contains germ cells in varying stages of maturation. If sperm are detected, mosaicism, most likely of the 46 XY/47 XXY pattern, should be suspected. Patients with this mosaic karyotype are sometimes fertile.

The Leydig cells become pronounced in number sometime after puberty. Although they appear hyperplastic relative to the atrophic appearance of the other elements, it is uncertain whether the absolute volume is greater than in normal testes. Functionally, the Leydig cells are abnormal as evidenced by low levels of serum testosterone in the setting of elevated levels of serum LH and follicle-stimulating hormone (FSH) and subnormal increase in response to administration of hCG.

A variety of neoplasms have been associated with Klinefelter syndrome. Both gonadal and extragonadal germ cell tumors develop with increased frequency. Most extragonadal tumors occur in the mediastinum as teratoma and embryonal cell carcinoma (teratocarcinoma) or choriocarcinoma.[27] In the testis, seminoma, teratoma, and embryonal cell carcinoma have been encountered. The risk of breast carcinoma in men with Klinefelter syndrome may be 20% higher than in normal men. Hematologic malignancies have also been reported, including acute leukemia, Hodgkin's disease, malignant lymphoma, and chronic myelogenous leukemia.

Turner Syndrome

In the classic form, Turner syndrome is a disorder in which sexually immature phenotypic females of short stature have various congenital anomalies and streak gonads. The

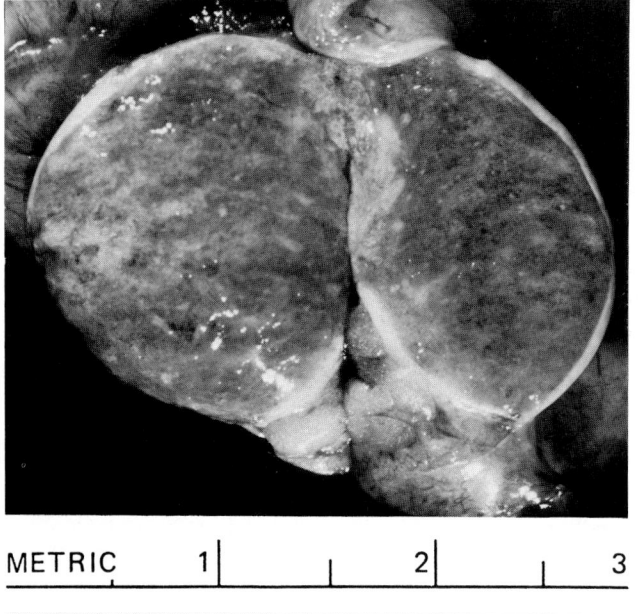

METRIC   1   2   3

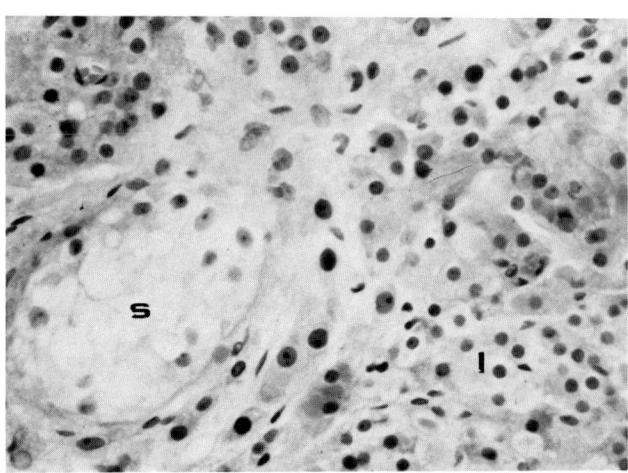

FIG. 1.19. The testis in Klinefelter syndrome. *Top*: The parenchyma of the 2-cm testis is golden yellow to slightly brown. *Bottom*: Clusters of Leydig cells (*L*) surround a seminiferous tubule (*S*). (From Welch and Robboy, ref. 67, with permission of Pediatric Andrology.)

cytogenetic hallmark is the 45 X karyotype with a sporadic, nonfamilial pattern of inheritance. Other karyotypes identified less frequently in this syndrome include mosaic 45 X/46 XX and 46 XX with isochrome X (duplication of one arm of the X chromosomes with the loss of the other arm). Patients with a 45 X/46 XY mosaic karyotype (considered in mixed gonadal dysgenesis) usually present with obvious sexual ambiguity, but sometimes present as phenotypic females with the clinical stigmata of Turner syndrome. A significant difference between patients with 45 X/46 XY mosaic karyotype and those with classic 45 X Turner syndrome is that gonadoblastoma and malignant germ cell tumors are common in patients with the former and rare in the latter. Thus, all patients who are evaluated for Turner

syndrome and who have a negative buccal smear should have karyotypic analysis to rule out the presence of a Y chromosome.

About 98% of fetuses with a 45 X karyotype abort; the frequency of Turner syndrome is about 1:3000 liveborn females. In the newborn, the overt findings are related to lymph stasis, which manifests itself as edema of the dorsum of the hands or feet or, less frequently, as swellings of the nape of the neck (cystic hygroma). Later in childhood and in adult life, webbing of the neck or elevation of the distal portion of the nails are residua of more marked swellings present during fetal life and may still provide a clue to the correct diagnosis. A rare, but important, major presentation is hydronephrosis due to ureteropelvic stenosis; all female neonates with a ureteropelvic obstruction should have a buccal smear. Congenital anomalies of other organ systems are associated with Turner syndrome and include a short fourth metacarpal, hypoplastic nails, multiple pigmented nevi, and coarctation of the aorta. The full range of somatic anomalies (more than 40) associated with this condition is presented elsewhere.[19,28]

Patients who reach adolescence undiagnosed often present with primary amenorrhea. Examination reveals underdeveloped secondary sex characteristics and a small uterus. Urinary gonadotropins are always elevated and the vaginal smear lacks cornified cells. The buccal smear in a 45 X individual reveals few if any Barr bodies; in those 20% of patients with mosaic karyotype (usually 45 X/46 XX or 45 X/47 XXX, the smear discloses a subnormal number of chromatin positive cells (about 5–15% for a female). Only rare patients with Turner syndrome have become pregnant and most of these have a 46 XX cell line.

At laparotomy, the internal genitalia are female and, although small, are in normal relation to one another. The adult gonads appear as white fibrous streaks, 2–3 cm long and 0.5 cm in diameter, and are located in the position normally occupied by the ovary (Fig. 1.20). On microscopic examination a streak consists of an attenuated cor-

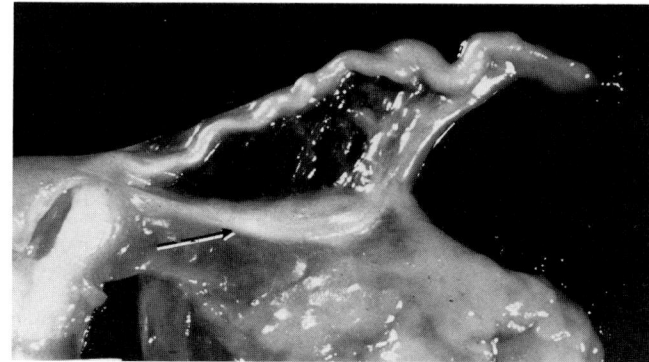

FIG. 1.20. Streak ovary (*arrow*) in Turner syndrome. The streak gonad is thin, fibrous, and lacks germ cells. (From Welch and Robboy, ref. 67, with permission of Pediatric Andrology.)

tex, a medulla, and a hilus. The cortex is composed of characteristic ovarian stroma in which the cells are elongated, wavy, and comprise conspicuous nuclei and scant cytoplasm. Rete tubules (rete ovarii) and hilar cells are typically present in the hilus region. Oocytes are almost always absent in adults with Turner syndrome. Oocytes are present in normal numbers in 45 X embryos before the 12th week of gestation. In older fetuses and young children, the number of oocytes falls progressively relative to the normal number for the age until the number reaches zero, usually before the time of normal menarche, thus leading to primary amenorrhea. These findings suggest that the second X chromosome is necessary for granulosa cell development and primary follicular formation; in the absence of this X chromosome, granulosa cells fail to differentiate and, as a result, the oocytes degenerate.

Gonadal tumors are exceedingly rare. Tumors of germ cell origin are undoubtedly rare because of the paucity of germ cells. Development of neoplasms of the so-called common epithelial type suggest that the coelomic epithelium encapsulating the gonad can undergo malignant change even if the gonad is a streak.[37] Endometrial carcinoma may develop occasionally in those patients who have had long-term exogenous estrogen therapy to foster the appearance of the female secondary sex characteristics. Both natural estrogens and synthetic nonsteroidal estrogens have been implicated. The duration of usage usually exceeds 3 years. Extragonadal tumors, most often of neurogenic origin, have been reported in children and young adults.[68]

XX Male Syndrome

The XX male syndrome is a disorder characterized by a nearly normal but infertile phenotypic male with a 46 XX karyotype that frequently contains a fragment of Y chromosome on which the testis determining factor (TDF) is located.[3] This syndrome, one of the rarest of all sex chromosome anomalies, occurs in about 1 of 24,000 newborn males.[70] XX males share many characteristics of men with Klinefelter syndrome. Both have a generally masculine appearance, normal or near normal external genitalia, male psychosexual orientation, normal to weak secondary sexual characteristics, normal to low androgen levels, and azoospermia. The testes are small, with prominent Leydig cells and tubules lined only by Sertoli cells. The most common reasons for referral are similar to those with Klinefelter syndrome, namely infertility or abnormal secondary sexual characteristics. XX males also tend to differ clinically from men with Klinefelter syndrome: the former are generally shorter in height, and the frequency of hypospadias and gynecomastia is higher. The frequency of impaired intelligence is not increased in XX males relative to the general population.

The XX male syndrome potentially results from at least three distinctly different mechanisms.[1,3,13,14,70] About 70% of these patients have a small portion of paternally derived Y chromosome, which contains the SRY gene, the TDF present abnormally on the X chromosome. These patients are called Y(+) by some. The SRY gene normally is found on the short arm of the Y chromosome adjacent to the pseudoautosomal pairing region. During meiosis in the father, an abnormal exchange sometimes leads to the transfer onto the X chromosome of the entire pseudoautosomal region plus the adjacent portion of the Y chromosome with the SRY gene. Inheritance of such an X chromosome from the father leads to the Y(+) XX male syndrome. The inheritance pattern of this form of the syndrome is sporadic. These patients have normal male external genitalia. Hypospadias and ambiguous genitalia are virtually never found. Apparently, the presence of the SRY gene is adequate to lead to normal male phenotype. Azoospermia in these patients results from the lack of other genes normally found on the Y chromosome necessary for sperm development.

Some patients with the XX male syndrome lack Y-derived DNA. Such Y(−) XX males might result by two different mechanisms. The first accounts for the familial transmission of an autosomal dominant or X-linked inheritance of XX maleness. These patients usually have ambiguous genitalia. This indicates that genes exist, probably downstream from TDF, that can trigger testis determination when mutated. Nothing specific is known about these putative genes, but their phenotypic effect seems slightly different from that of TDF. A second potential mechanism that might lead to the Y(−) condition is chromosomal mosaicism with a prevalent XX lineage. In such patients, the Y-containing cell line might simply be technically too difficult to identify because of the small number of such cells. Alternatively, a 47 XXY zygote might lose its Y chromosome by nondysjunction early in ontogeny, thus allowing a 46 XX cell line to persist; the 47 XXY cell line may have persisted long enough to induce male gonadal development. Such patients, just as patients with familial Y(−) XX maleness, often present with sexual ambiguity suggesting that patients with Y(−) XX male syndrome are closely related both phenotypically and etiologically to XX true hermaphrodites, who present with both testicular and ovarian tissue.

Pure Gonadal Dysgenesis

Pure gonadal dysgenesis is a term that historically has been encompassed in a number of diverse conditions, including testicular regression syndrome. In the context defined herein, pure gonadal dysgenesis refers to a phenotypic female without genetic ambiguity in whom the internal genitalia include müllerian structures (uterus and fallopian tubes) and generally streak gonads, the constellation of which probably still encompasses a multitude of diverse conditions. The patients may appear phenotypically normal or have hypoplastic external genitalia. The pure gonadal dysgenesis syndrome occurs with both 46 XX and 46 XY karyotypes and has both familial and sporadic patterns of inheritance.

The 46 XX-type pure gonadal dysgenesis is either an autosomal recessive disorder or, less frequently, an abnormality of the X chromosome. Such patients have greater ovarian development than those with 46 XY pure gonadal dysgenesis or Turner syndrome and present more often with signs of ovarian dysfunction (secondary amenorrhea or infertility) rather than primary gonadal failure (primary amenorrhea). Deletions of either the short or long arm of an X chromosome have been identified in 46 XX pure gonadal dysgenesis.[25,51]

The 46 XY-type pure gonadal dysgenesis is more common than the 46 XX form of the disorder. The 46 XY type may be caused by deletion of the TDF gene,[8] an inactive TDF, or a defect in some TDF co-factor.[12] The syndrome may be sporadic or familial, with either X-linked recessive or autosomal recessive patterns of inheritance.[45] Some patients have a mosaic 45 X/46 XY karyotype.

Patients with 46 XX pure gonadal dysgenesis, as those with Turner syndrome, only rarely develop gonadal tumors. Hilus cell hyperplasia and hilus cell tumors with the usual associated virilizing effects have been reported.[51] Patients with 46 XY pure gonadal dysgenesis are at high risk for gonadoblastoma and other germ cell tumors, as is true of all patients with streak gonads and a Y chromosome.

SEXUAL AMBIGUITY FREQUENT

Patients in this category exhibit a wide range of phenotypic appearances and internal genitalia. A Y chromosome is often present, usually as part of a mosaic complement. Sexual ambiguity is a common finding.

Mixed Gonadal Dysgenesis

Mixed gonadal dysgenesis (MGD) is a heterogeneous syndrome characterized usually by a 45 X/46 XY or 46 XY karyotype, persistent müllerian duct structures, an abnormal testis, and a contralateral streak gonad. The functional deficit imposed by the abnormal testis is expressed as incomplete inhibition of müllerian development, incomplete differentiation of wolffian duct structures, and incomplete male development of the external genitalia. Often, incomplete mediation of the testicular descent occurs, resulting in both internal and external asymmetry of the genitalia and a mixture of male and female features in an individual in whom neither gonad is normal. About two thirds of the affected individuals are raised as females and the remainder as males. Some patients with MGD exhibit phenotypic features of Turner syndrome. Elsewhere, we have suggested that the syndrome of MGD should be enlarged to incorporate some patients with bilateral streak gonads (described above as 46 XY type pure gonadal dysgenesis) or bilateral abnormal testes with mosaic 45 X/46 XY karyotype (dysgenetic male pseudohermaphroditism), because the clinical, pathological, and chromosomal features of these syndromes closely resemble each other.[43]

The underlying genetic and karyotype abnormalities leading to the syndrome of mixed gonadal dysgenesis are currently under investigation. A variety of different genetic abnormalities appear to result in MGD, thus leading to the phenotypic heterogeneity of MGD. Partial deletions of both the short and long arms of chromosome Y have been detected in these individuals.[2,52] Cases of dicentric Y and no detectable Y chromosomal anomaly have also been observed.[52,66]

Clinically, MGD is usually detected in the neonate because of ambiguity of the external genitalia. Frequently, a palpable testis bulges through an indirect inguinal hernia or descends completely into the labioscrotal fold, resulting in asymmetry of the genital swellings. This clinical appearance has prompted some investigators to name the syndrome *asymmetric gonadal dysgenesis*. If the gonads are intraabdominal, the labioscrotal folds may appear as normal labia or as empty scrotal sacs. The condition is likely to go unrecognized unless the clitoris is sufficiently enlarged to mandate investigation, which is common. The gonad that descends is almost always a testis, and the streak gonads are always intraabdominal unless dragged into a "hernia uteri inguinale."

Organs derived from the müllerian duct persist in 95% of cases (Fig. 1.21). The uterus is usually infantile or rudimentary. The fallopian tubes are frequently bilateral. If a testis is grossly near normal size and well differentiated, the fimbriated end of the ipsilateral tube may be absent, but in only one-third of cases is the ipsilateral tube entirely absent. Organs of wolffian duct derivation also may be present, but the frequency is variable. The epididymis is identified in two-thirds of cases and is usually present on the side where there is a testis. The vas deferens is encountered less frequently. The seminal vesicle is identified only rarely probably because tissue near the bladder/prostate region is not usually removed.

The gonad may be a testis or a streak. Streak gonads may be partially differentiated toward ovary or testis. Bilateral gross testes, frequently of an asynchronous degree of maturity, are found in about 15% of cases whereas a unilateral gross testis is found in 60%. The testis is consistently abnormal architecturally, its organization being divided into three zones, each of which reflects the quantity and type of cellular components present. The three zones, which are described below in detail, include (1) the region of the tunica albuginea or cortex, which exhibits widely spaced seminiferous tubules or differentiation toward ovary, (2) the medulla, which is composed of normal or near-normal seminiferous tubules and interstitium, and (3) a hilar region with poorly differentiated seminiferous tubules that are only partly differentiated toward testis.

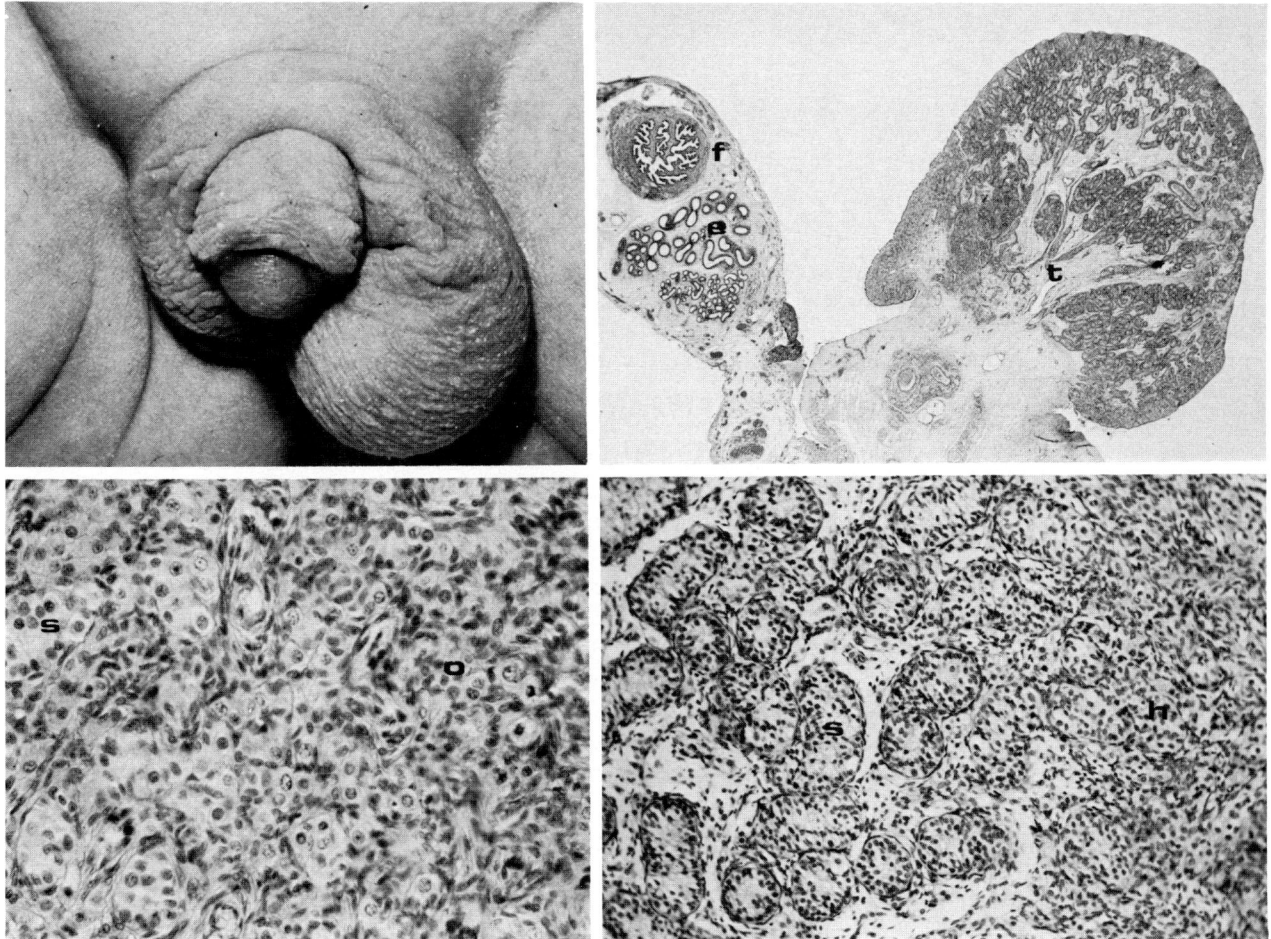

Fig. 1.21. Mixed gonadal dysgenesis. *Top left*: External genitalia in MGD. The left testis had descended into the scrotum; the right streak was in the abdominal cavity. Because of this characteristic appearance, some investigators prefer the name "asymmetric gonadal dysgenesis" rather than mixed gonadal dysgenesis. *Top right*: Testis (*T*) and adjacent fallopian tube (*F*) and epididymis (*E*). The medulla contains immature seminiferous tubules with germ cells and interstitial cells whereas the region nearer the cortex resembles fetal ovary with immature sex cords and rare primordial follicles. *Bottom left*: Cortex of gonad in which testicular seminiferous tubules (*S*) merge into fetal type ovary (*Q*). *Bottom right*: The medullary parenchyma of the testis is composed of normal immature seminiferous tubules (*S*) with germ cells and occasional interstitial cells, whereas the parenchyma in the region of the hilus (*H*) near the rete testis appears less committed as testis and is characterized by abnormal, pleomorphic seminiferous tubules. The photograph is taken at the junction of the two zones. (From Robboy et al., ref. 43, with permission of Human Pathology.)

The superficial cortex may contain seminiferous tubules that are often widely separated by edematous, undifferentiated stroma. Sometimes the tubules penetrate the incompletely formed tunica albuginea and open onto the serosa. Occasionally, broad zones of cortex differentiate slightly toward the ovary, even displaying rare primordial follicles. Mice that spontaneously develop chromosomal mosaicism as a result of nondysjunction often show gonads with ovarian tissue at the periphery and seminiferous cords centrally.[10]

The central zone (medulla) of the macroscopic infant testis is architecturally and cytologically normal. Narrow closed seminiferous tubules are lined by Sertoli cells with abundant cytoplasm. The number of spermatogonia vary; advanced forms of spermatogenic maturation are not observed. Leydig cells are present in small clusters of varying size. The nuclei of the Leydig cells contain finely dispersed chromatin, and the cytoplasm varies from minimal and amphophilic or slightly basophilic to abundant and eosinophilic. In older patients, the medulla is atrophic and the tubules are lined only by Sertoli cells (Fig. 1.22). The basement membranes are often thickened. Prominent clusters of Leydig cells fill the interstitium.

The architecturally disorganized hilar region discloses seminiferous tubules that are swollen by increased numbers of Sertoli cells and are lined by indistinct basement

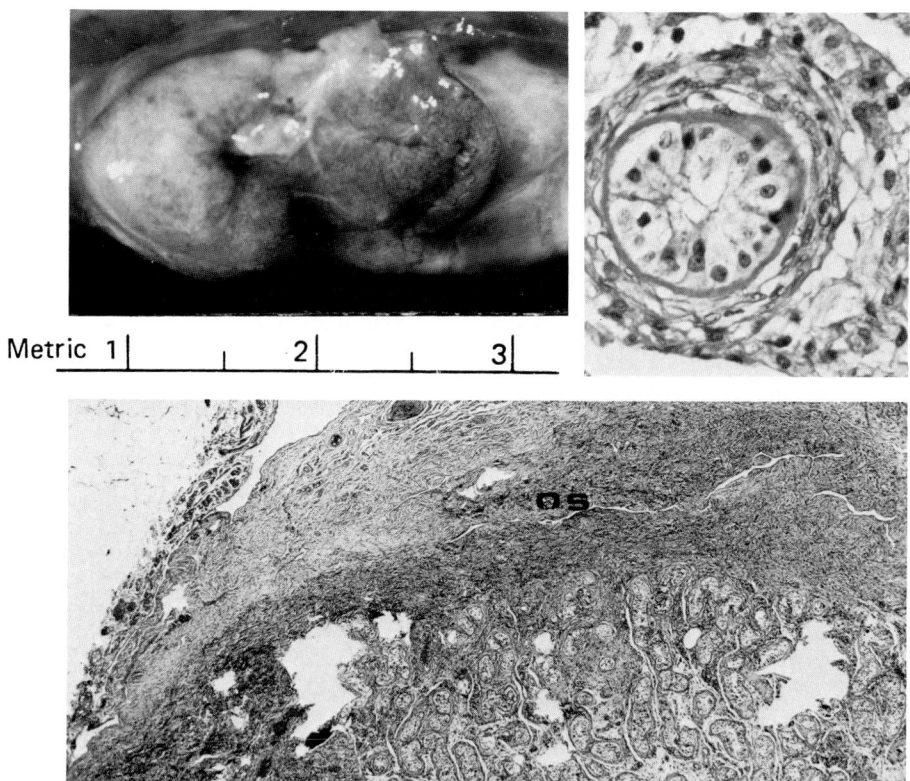

FIG. 1.22. Testis in mixed gonadal dysgenesis. *Upper left*: The tunica albuginea from the testis of a 35-year-old phenotypic man is tan and maximally 1 mm thick; the parenchyma is golden yellow. *Lower*: Cross-section of tunica albuginea, which is composed of stroma resembling the stroma of ovarian cortex (*OS*) and medulla with seminiferous tubules. *Upper right*: Detail of seminiferous tubules lined only by Sertoli cells. The interstitium is filled with Leydig cells. (From Robboy et al. ref. 43, with permission of Human Pathology.)

membranes. These tubules also merge with the surrounding stroma, imparting the appearance of a homogeneous blend of Leydig cells, germ cells, Sertoli cells, and an indeterminate type of interstitial stroma. The region resembles neither fetal ovary nor testis.

The streak gonads appear similar to those found in Turner syndrome. We have not observed a gonad that has been identifiable grossly as an ovary or has been shown microscopically to contain graafian follicles, corpora lutea, or corpora albicantia. The presence of rare primordial follicles or, as in the fetal ovary, aggregates of germ cells partially surrounded by immature granulosa cells are evidence that a streak gonad can differentiate toward the ovary. Morphologic changes may occur over time in the streak gonads. Myriads of germ cells present in a streak of an infant may degenerate and disappear by puberty, resulting in a gonad composed exclusively of fibrous tissue and a few rete tubules (Fig. 1.23); similar changes occur in the streak gonads of Turner syndrome (45 X karyotype).

Approximately one-third of patients with MGD develop gonadoblastoma, a tumor found almost exclusively in patients with an intersex syndrome and a Y chromosome.[40,50,51] Gonadoblastoma accounts for three-fourths of the gonadal tumors arising in dysgenetic gonads and is usually discovered during the first to fourth decades of life. Many of the isolated reports of gonadoblastoma associated with other forms of hermaphroditism described clinically and pathologically actually may be examples of MGD.

About 20% of gonadoblastomas arise in a streak gonad and another 20% arise in a dysgenetic testis; in the remaining cases, the nature of the underlying gonad cannot be determined with certainty because it is replaced by tumor. The gross appearance of the gonad with gonadoblastoma varies according to the size of the neoplasm, the presence of calcification, and whether the gonadoblastoma has been overgrown by a malignant form of germ cell tumor (usually germinoma) (Fig. 1.24). Approximately one-fifth of gonadoblastomas are discovered solely because a streak gonad was examined microscopically (Fig. 1.25). The contralateral gonad also contains a gonadoblastoma in more than one-third of patients.[45,51]

On microscopic examination, the gonadoblastoma appears as circumscribed nests of neoplastic germ cells having the cytologic properties of germinoma (dysgerminoma and seminoma) and that are encompassed individually or in groups by sex cord derivatives with inconspicuous cyto-

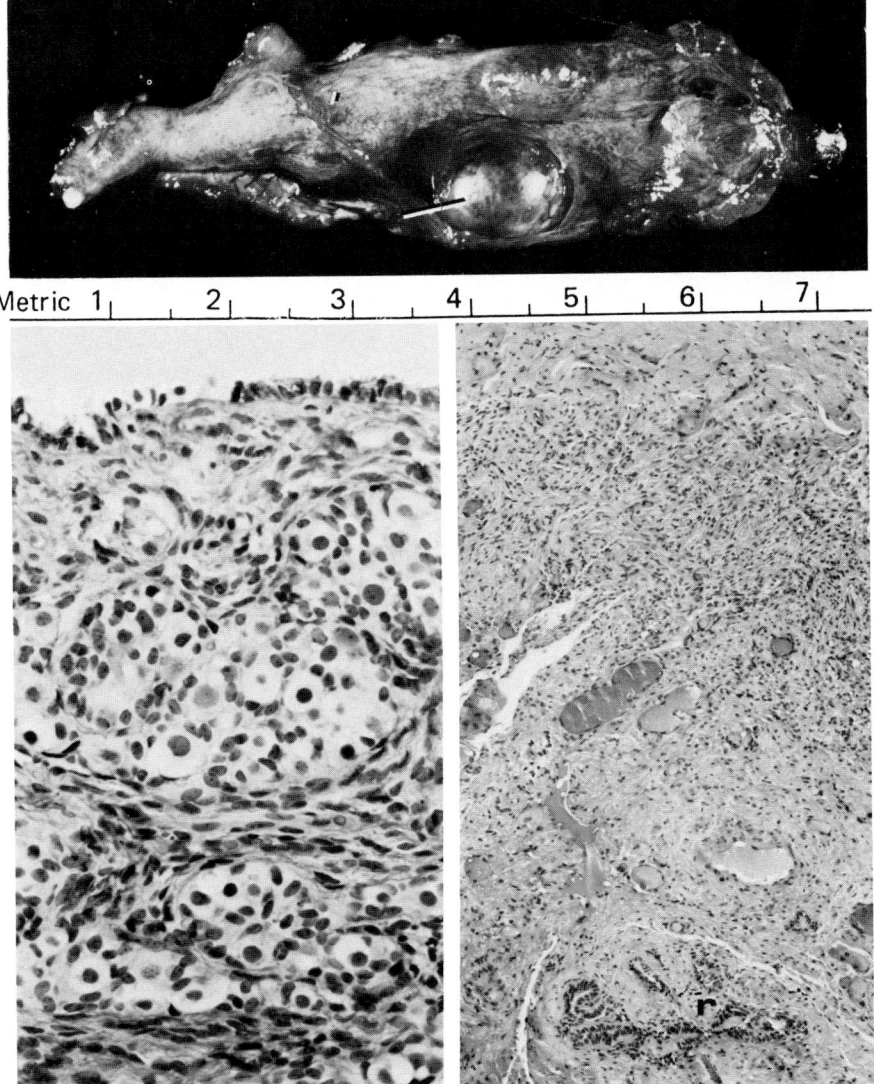

Metric 1 2 3 4 5 6 7

FIG. 1.23. Mixed gonadal dysgenesis. When the patient was an infant, the streak gonad resembled a fetal ovary with germ cells and immature sex cords (*lower left*). When the streak gonad was removed in its entirety 13 years later (*top; arrows*), it existed only as several microscopic areas of whispy ovarian-type cortical stroma and rete ovarii (*R*) (*lower right*). (From Robboy et al. ref. 43, with permission of Human Pathology.)

plasm and small round to oval nuclei resembling immature Sertoli cells.[44] Hyaline, composed of basement membrane material, is found along the margin or as nodules within the nests of tumors. In four-fifths of cases the hyaline material is calcified, initially appearing as small, laminated spheres, which eventually fuse and coalesce into large mulberry-like masses. Not infrequently, the only evidence that a dysgerminoma originated in a gonadoblastoma is the presence focally of mulberry-like calcifications. Hormonally active cells that resemble lutein and Leydig cells are found interspersed among the nests of tumor in about two-thirds of cases. These hormonally active cells are found least frequently in nonvirilized phenotypic females, more often in virilized females, and most frequently in phenotypic males. To some degree, their appearance may be related to the postpubertal age of the patient when the gonad is examined.

Approximately 30% of gonadoblastomas are overgrown by a malignant germ cell tumor, usually the germinoma; 8% are overgrown by endodermal sinus tumor, immature teratoma, embryonal carcinoma, or choriocarcinoma. Although the gonadoblastoma itself does not metastasize and therefore can be considered as an in situ malignancy, the typically malignant behavior of the other tumors makes early prophylactic removal of the gonads in all patients advisable. Also, to avoid the consequences of onset of virilization if the patient is to be raised as a female, it is important that gonadectomy be performed before the patient reaches puberty. Patients who have been treated with long-

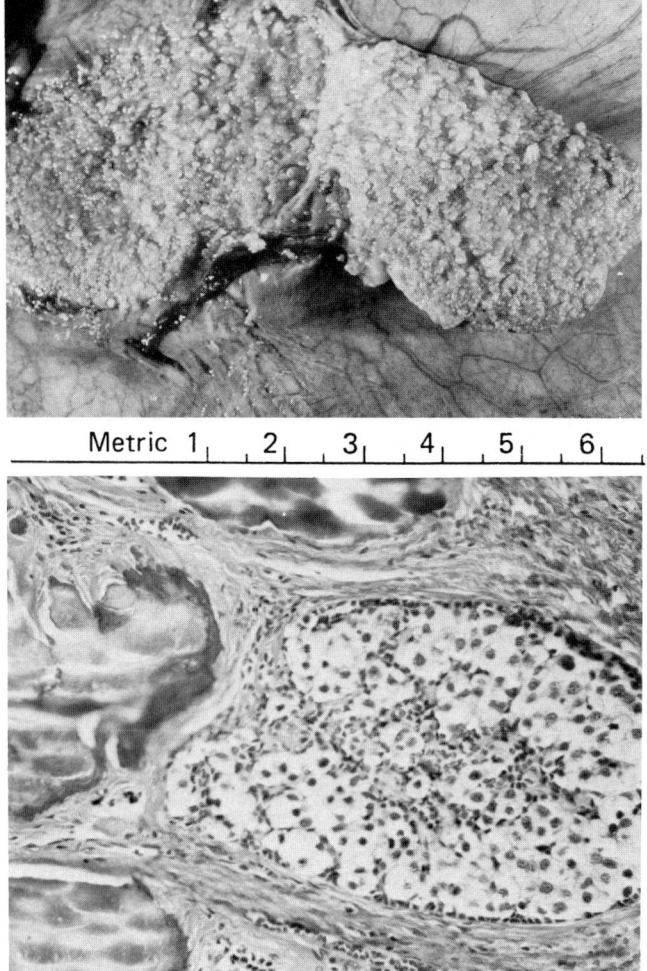

Metric 1   2   3   4   5   6

FIG. 1.24. Gonadoblastoma in mixed gonadal dysgenesis.
Top: 15-cm gonadal tumor composed largely of dysgerminoma.
At one pole is a 5 × 2 × 0.5 cm calcified gonadoblastoma. *Bottom*: Gonadoblastoma. Multiple mulberry-like calcific masses
partially replace the tumor nests composed of germ cells surrounded by sex cord derivatives. (From Welch and Robboy, ref.
67, with permission of Pediatric Andrology.)

term administration of estrogen may on occasion develop
endometrial carcinoma. Congenital cardiovascular anomalies
have also been reported in patients with MGD.[65]

True Hermaphroditism

True hermaphroditism is defined as the presence of both
testicular and ovarian tissue in a patient. Affected individuals may have either a female or male phenotype with a
variable degree of sexual ambiguity. Because the wavy,
cortical-type stroma typically seen in the female gonad can
be found in both female and male gonads and therefore is
nonspecific, follicular structures must be identified to classify gonadal tissue as ovarian and seminiferous tubules to

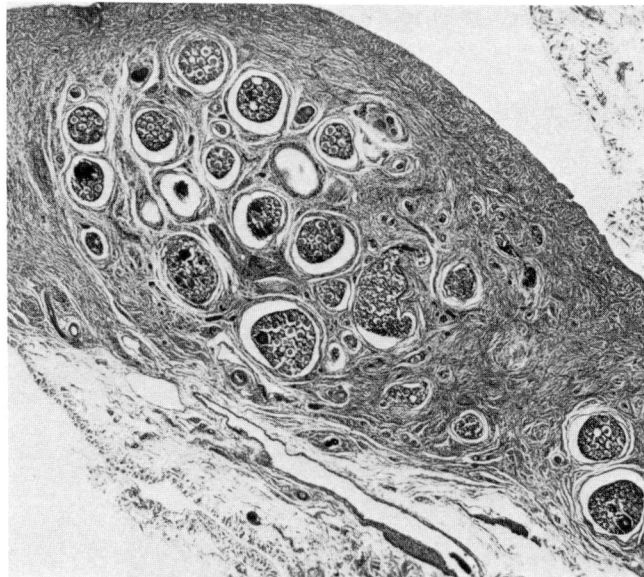

FIG. 1.25. Gonadoblastoma occupying a gonadal streak.
(From Scully, ref. 50, with permission of Cancer.)

classify the tissue as testicular. In true hermaphrodites, the
gonads may be ovary and testis separately or combined in
an ovotestis.

The ovotestis is the most frequently encountered gonad
in true hermaphroditism. In four-fifths of cases the ovarian
and testicular tissues are arranged in an end-to-end fashion. The ovarian portion of an ovotestis has a convoluted
surface whereas the testicular portion is smooth and glistening. Frequently, a distinct line demarcates the two tissues. The firm nature of the palpable ovarian tissue and the
soft texture of the testis are valuable clinical signs when
evaluating the nature of a gonad in an infant with ambisexual external genitalia.[62]

An ovary, which preferentially develops on the left side,
is the second most common gonad in true hermaphrodites.
Every patient over 15 years of age in the series of van
Niekerk[62] had either a corpus luteum or a corpus albicans.
The testis, which is the gonad least often encountered,
develops preferentially on the right.

The location of the gonad is influenced by the type
and quantity of gonadal tissue present. Increasing amounts
of ovarian tissue increase the probability that the gonad
will be in an ovarian position. When a gonad with the
macroscopic features of an ovary is situated in the inguinal
canal or in the labioscrotal fold, the possibility of it
being an ovotestis should be seriously considered. The
position of the testis is less constant. Most (63%) reside
in the scrotum, 14% in the inguinal region, 1% in the
internal inguinal ring, and 22% in a normal ovarian position.

The nature of the genital organ adjacent to a gonad in
true hermaphroditism depends on the nature of the gonad,

which is in contrast to MGD, in which a fallopian tube is often adjacent to the gonad, regardless of whether it is a testis or streak. In true hermaphroditism a fallopian tube is adjacent to an ovary and an epididymis or vas deferens is adjacent to a testis. Either a müllerian or wolffian structure, but not both, is adjacent to an ovotestis. MIS appears to be functional. Ninety-five percent of fallopian tubes adjacent to ovotestes have closed ostia. Only 10% of uteri are normal; the other patients have absent uteri (13%), unicornuate uteri (10%), absent cervix (14%), or uterine hypoplasia (46%).

The most common karyotypes in true hermaphroditism are 46 XX (60%), 46 XY (12%), and mosaic (28%), usually 46 XX/46 XY, 46 XY/47 XXY, or least frequently 45 X/46 XY. Patients with a "Y" chromosome have a two- to threefold increased frequency of having a testis as opposed to an ovotestis. Nearly 75% of true hermaphrodites with an ovary and ovotestis have a 46 XX karyotype.

As in other subclasses of intersex, the causes of true hermaphroditism at the genetic level are under investigation. Chromosome Y specific genes (e.g., SRY) have been detected in some but not all 46 XX true hermaphrodites, suggesting several potential mechanisms for the development of XX true hermaphroditism, similar to individuals with XX male syndrome.[23,38,41]

The clinical presentations of true hermaphrodites vary to some extent depending on the patient's age at the time of diagnosis. Until recently, the condition often went undetected until adolescence, when phenotypic male patients were evaluated for gynecomastia and phenotypic female patients were evaluated for amenorrhea or failure to develop secondary sex changes. Thus, in the series of van Niekerk and Retief,[62] three-fourths of patients were raised as males and one-fourth as females. Many patients, however, menstruated and a few became pregnant. Phenotypic males may experience monthly hematuria because of menstruation into a persistent urogenital sinus. With an increased awareness of intersex states, the condition is recognized more often in infants because of ambiguous genitalia, usually in the form of a small phallus (enlarged clitoris). Like MGD, the scrotum may be asymmetric, with the larger, more normal-appearing hemiscrotum containing a testis. Among 160 patients the external genitalia were asymmetric in three-fourths (labioscrotal folds in 63% and hemiscrotums in 13%).

On microscopic examination, the gonadal tissue often appears normal if the patient is young. In infants the ovarian tissue contains numerous follicles, whereas the testicular parenchyma discloses normal-appearing seminiferous tubules with spermatogonia. Patients in the reproductive years may have ovarian tissue with structures indicative of ovulation, for example, follicles, corpora lutea, and corpora albicantia, but spermatogenesis is rare in the testicular portion. The testicular portion of an ovotestis is usually abnormal with incomplete development, loss of germ cells, and tubular

sclerosis. Scrotal testes in these patients show less severe changes, sometimes showing faulty spermatogenesis.[51]

At times, distinction between true hermaphroditism and MGD can be difficult. In the newborn, asymmetric ambiguous genitalia may be observed in both conditions. If a streak gonad from a patient with MGD is serially sectioned, a rare primordial follicle may be encountered in what otherwise appears to be a fetal-type ovary admixed with testis with well developed seminiferous tubules.[43] If the term *true hermaphroditism* is restricted to those patients in whom the ovarian and testicular tissue are both apparent grossly, it should be possible to segregate more clearly those individuals in whom the ovarian tissue may be functional.

Gonadal tumors occur in less than 3% of affected individuals. Germinoma is the most common type of tumor, but gonadoblastomas and a variety of other tumors have been reported.[45,58]

References

1. Abbas NE, Toublanc JE, Boucekkine C, Toublanc M, Affara NA, Job JC, Fellous M (1990) A possible common origin of "Y-negative" human XX males and XX true hermaphrodites. Hum Geneti 84: 356–360

2. Cantrell MA, Bicknell JN, Pagon RA, Page DC, Walker DC, Saal HM, Zinn AB, Disteche CM (1989) Molecular analysis of 46,XY females and regional assignment of a new Y chromosome specific probe. Human Genetics. 83: 88–92

3. de la Chapelle A, Hastbacka J, Korhonen T, Maenpaa J (1990) The etiology of XX sex reversal. Reprod Nutr Devel Suppl 1: 39s–49s

4. Coulam CB (1979) Testicular regression syndrome. Obstet Gynecol 53: 44–49

5. Cunha GR, Alarid ET, Turner T, Donjacour AA, Boutin EL, Foster BA (1992) Normal and abnormal development of the male genital tract. Role of androgens, mesenchymal-epithelial, and growth factors. J Androl 13: 465–475

6. Cunha GR, Young P (1992) Role of stroma in oestrogen-induced epithelial proliferation. Epithel Cell Biol 1: 18–31

7. Dean HJ, Shackleton CHL, Winter JSD (1984) Diagnosis and natural history of 17-hydroxylase deficiency in a newborn male. J Clin Endocrinol Metabol 59: 513–520

8. Disteche CM, Casanova M, Saal H, Friedman C, Sybert V, Graham J, Thuline H, Page DC, Fellous M (1986) Small deletions of the short arm of the Y chromosome in 46,XY females. Proc Natl Acad Sci 83: 7841–7844

9. Donahoe PK (1992) Mullerian inhibiting substance in reproduction and cancer. Mol Reprod Dev 32: 168–172

10. Eicher EM, Beamer WG, Washburn LL, Whitten WK (1980) A cytogenetic investigation of inherited true hermaphroditism in BALB/cWt mice. Cytogenet Cell Genet 28: 104–115

11. Fernandes ET, Hollabaugh RS, Young JA, Wilroy SR, Schriock EA (1990) Persistent müllerian duct syndrome. Urology 36: 516–518

12. Fil C, Scully RE (1990) Case records of the Massachusetts General Hospital, case 13-1990. Eng J Med 322: 917–925

13. Furguson-Smith MA, Cooke A, Affara NA, Boyd E, Tomlie

JL (1990) Genotype-phenotype correlations in XX males and their bearing on current theories of sex determination. Hum Genet 84: 198–202

14. Fuse H, Satomi S, Kazama T, Katayama T, Nagabuchi S, Tamura T, Nakahori Y, Nakagome Y (1991) DNA hybridization study using Y-specific probes in an XX-male. Andrologia 23: 237–239

15. Griffin JE (1992) Androgen resistance—the clinical and molecular spectrum. N Engl J Med 326: 61–68

16. Gubbay J, Collignon J, Koopman P, Capel B, Economan A, Musterberg A, Vivian N, Goodfellow PN, Lovell-Badge R (1990) A gene mapping to the sex determining region of the mouse Y chromosome is a member of a novel family of embryonically expressed genes. Nature 346: 245–250

17. Guerrier D, Tran D, Vanderwinden JM, Hideux S, van Outrive L, Legeai L, Bouchard M, van Vliet G, de Haet MH, Picard JY, Kahn A, Josso N (1989) The persistent müllerian duct syndrome: A molecular approach. J Clin Endocrinol Metab 68: 46–52

18. Gustafson ML, Lee MM, Scully RE, Moncure AC, Hirakawa T, Goodman A, Muntz HG, Donahoe PK, MacLaughlin DT, Fuller AF (1992) Mullerian inhibiting substance as a marker for ovarian sex cord tumor. N Engl J Med 326: 466–471

19. Hall JC, Gilchrist DM (1990) Turner syndrome and its variants. Pediat Clin North Am 37: 1421–1440

20. Harley VR, Jackson DI, Hextall PJ, Hawkins JR, Berkovitz GD, Sockanathan S, Lovell-Badge R, Goodfellow PN (1992) DNA binding activity of recombinant SRY from normal males and XY females. Science 255: 453–456

21. Hudson PL, Dougas I, Donahoe PK, Cate RL, Epstein J, Pepinsky RB, MacLaughlin DT (1990) An immunoassay to detect human müllerian inhibiting substance in males and females during normal development. J Clin Endocrinol Metab 70: 16–22

22. Imperato-McGinley J, Miller M, Wilson JD, Peterson RE, Schackleton C, and Gajdusek DC (1991) A cluster of male pseudohermaphrodites with 5 alpha-reductase deficiency in Papua New Guinea. Clin Endocrinol 34: 293–298

23. Jager RJ, Epensperger C, Fraccaro M, Scherer G (1990) A ZFY negative 46,XX true hermaphrodite is positive for the Y pseudoautosomal boundary. Hum Genet 85: 666–668

24. Koopman P, Gubbay J, Vivian N, Goodfellow P, Lovell-Badge R (1991) Male development of chromosomally female mice transgenic for Sry. Nature 351: 117–21

25. Krauss CM, Turksoy RN, Atkins L, McLaughlin C, Brown LG, Page DC (1987) Familial premature ovarian failure due to an interstitial deletion of the long arm of the X chromosome. N Engl J Med 317: 125–131

26. Kuroda T, Lee MM, Ragin RC, Hirobe S, Donahoe PK (1991) Mullerian inhibiting substance production and cleavage is modulated by gonadotropins and steroids. Endocrinology 129: 2985–2992

27. Lee MW, Stephens RL (1987) Klinefelter's syndrome and extragonadal germ cell tumors. Cancer 60: 1053–1055

28. Lippe B (1990) Turner syndrome. Endocrinol Metab Clin North Am 20: 121–152

29. Mandel JL, Monaco AP, Nelson DL, Schlessinger D, Willard HF (1992) Genome maps III (X Chromosome). Science 258: 87–102

30. Manuel M, Katayama KP, Jones HW Jr (1976) The age of occurrence of gonadal tumors in intersex patients with a Y chromosome. Am J Obstet Gynecol 124: 293–300

31. Martinez-Mora J, Saey JM, Toran N, Isnard R, Perez-Libarme MM, Egozcue J, Audi L (1991) Male pseudohermaphroditism due to Leydig cell agnesia and absence of testicular LH receptors. Clin Endocrinol 34: 485–491

32. Mastroyannis C, Wallach EE (1987) Male pseudohermaphroditism: Inborn errors in testosterone biosynthesis. Semin Reprod Endocrinol : 26–276

33. McCoshen JA (1982) In vivo sex differentiation of congeneic germinal cell aplastic gonads. Am J Obstet Gynecol 142: 83–88

34. McLaren A (1991) Development of the mammalian gonad: The fate of the supporting cell lineage. Bioessays 13: 151–156

35. Morel Y (1991) Gene heterogeneity in adrenal 21-hydroxylase. Presse Med 20: 945–949

36. Muller J (1984) Morphometry and histology of gonads from 12 children and adolescents with the androgen insensitivity (testicular feminization) syndrome. J Clin Endocrinol Metab 59: 785–789

37. Murphy GF, Welch WR, Urcuyo R (1979) Brenner tumor and mucinous cystaderoma of borderline malignancy in a patient with Turner's syndrome. Obstet Gynecol 54: 660–663

38. Nakagome Y, Seki S, Fukutani K, Nagafuchi S, Nakahori Y, Tamura T (1991) PCR detection of distal Yp sequences in an XX true hermaphrodite. Am J Med Genet 41: 112–114

39. New MI (1992) Genetic disorders of adrenal hormone synthesis. Horm Res 37 (suppl 3): 22–33

40. Page DC (1987) Hypothesis: A Y-chromosomeal gene causes gonadoblastoma in dysgenetic gonads. Development 101 (suppl): 151–155

41. Pereira ET, Cabal de Almeida JC, Gunha ACYRG, Patton M, Taylor R, Jeffery S (1991) Use of probes for ZFY, SRY, and the Y pseudoautosomal boundary in XX males, XX true hermaphrodites and an XX female. J Med Genet 28: 591–595

42. Pierre-Louis ML, Kovi J, Sampson CC, Worrell RG, Rosser SB (1983) Ultrastructure of the gonads in the testicular feminization syndrome. J Natl Med Assoc 75: 1177–1184

42a. Porter S, Gilles CB (1993) Genomic imprinting. A proposed explanation for the different behaviours of testicular and ovarian germ cell tumors. Med Hypoth 41: 37–41.

43. Robboy SJ, Miller T, Donahoe PK, Jahre C, Welch WR, Haseltine FP, Miller WA, Atkins L, Crawford JD (1982) Dysgenesis of testicular and streak gonads in the syndrome of mixed gonadal dysgenesis: Perspective derived from a clinicopathologic analysis of twenty-one cases. Hum Pathol 13: 700–716

44. Roth LM, Eglen DE: Gonadoblastoma (1989) Immunohistochemical and ultrastructural observations. Int J Gynecol Pathol 8: 72–81

44a. Russell P, Bannatyne P. (1989) Surgical pathology of the ovaries. New York, Churchill Livingstone, p 492

45. Rutgers JL (1991) Advances in the pathology of intersex conditions. Hum Pathol 22: 884–891

46. Rutgers JL, Scully RE (1991) The androgen insensitivity syndrome (testicular feminization). A clinicopathologic study of 43 cases. Int J Gynecol Pathol 10: 126–144

47. Sadler TW (1985): Langman's Medical Embryology, 5th ed. Baltimore: Williams & Wilkins

48. Saenger P, Levine LS, New MI (1981) Male pseudohermaphroditism due to abnormal testosterone biosynthesis and metabolism. Clin Androl 7: 87–97

49. Schwartz ID, Root AW (1991) The Klinefelter syndrome of testicular dysgenesis. Endocrinol Metab Clin North Am 20: 153–163

50. Scully RE (1970) Gonadoblastoma. A review of 74 cases. Cancer 25: 1340–1356

50a. Scully RE (1987) Ovarian tumours with functioning stroma. In Fox H, Obstetrical and gynaecological pathology, 2nd ed Churchill Livingstone, New York, 1987; 724–736

51. Scully RE (1991) Gonadal pathology of genetically determined diseases. In Kraus FT, Damjanov (eds), The pathology of reproductive failure (International Academy of Pathology Monograph No. 33). Baltimore, Williams and Wilkins. pp 257–285

52. Shinobara M, Minowada S, Aso Y, Yamada K, Nakahori Y, Tamura T, Nakagome Y (1991) A t(Y;15) translocation with a deletion of the proximal Yq in a boy with mixed gonadal dysgenesis. Hum Genet 86: 422–423

53. Simpson JL, Golbus MS (1992) Genetics in obstetrics and gynecology, 2nd ed, Philadelphia, WB Saunders, 350

54. Sinclair AH, Berta P, Palmer MS, Hawkins JR, Griffiths BL, Smith MJ, Foster JW, Frischauf AM, Lovell-Badge R, Goodfellow PN (1990) A gene for the human sex determining region encodes a protein with homology to a conserved DNA binding motif. Nature 346: 240–244

55. Smith NM, Byard RW, Bourne AJ (1991) Testicular regression syndrome—a pathological study of 77 cases. Histopathology 19: 269–272

56. Strachan T, White PC (1991) Molecular pathology of steroid 21-hydroxylase deficiency. J Steroid Biochem Mol Biol 40: 537–543

57. Taketo T, Saeed J, Nishioka Y, Donahoe PK (1991) Delay of testicular maturation in the B6.Y (Dom) ovotestis demonstrated by immunohistochemical staining for müllerian inhibiting substance. Devel Biol 146: 386–395

58. Talerman A, Verp MS, Senekjian E, Gilewski T, Vogelzang N (1990) True hermaphrodite with bilateral ovotestes, bilateral gonadoblastomas and dysgerminomas, 46 XX/46 XY karyotype, and a successful pregnancy. Cancer 66: 2668–2672

59. Thigpen AE, Davis DL, Gautier T, Imperato-McGinley J, Russell DW (1992) The molecular basis of steroid 5 alpha-reductase deficiency in a large Dominican kindred. N Engl J Med 327: 1216–1219

60. Tsuji M, Shima H, Yonemura CY, Brody J, Donahoe PK, Cunha GR (1992) Effect of human recombinant müllerian inhibiting substance on isolated epithelial and mesenchymal cells during müllerian duct regression in the rat. Endocrinology 131: 1481–1488

61. van Haarhoven CJHM, Juttmaran JR, Pypers PM, Roukema JA (1991) A testicular tumor in the left adnexa. The persistent müllerian duct syndrome with testicular malignancy. Eur J Surg Oncol 17: 97–98

62. van Niekerk WA, Retief AE (1981) The gonads of human true hermaphrodites. Human Genet 58:117–122

63. Van Slooten AJ, Rechner SF, Dodds WG (1992) Recurrent maternal virilization during pregnancy caused by benign androgen-producing ovarian lesions. Am J Obstet Gynecol 167: 1342–1344

64. Voutilainen R, Miller WL (1989) Potential relevance of müllerian inhibiting substance to ovarian physiology. Semin Reprod Endocrinol 7: 88–93

65. Wallace TM, Levin HS (1990) Mixed gonadal dysgenesis. Arch Pathol Lab Med 114: 679–688

66. Weckworth PF, Johnson HW, Pantzar JT, Coleman GU, Masterson JST, McGillivray B, Tze WJ (1988) Dicentric Y chromosome and mixed disgenesis. J Urol 139: 91–94

67. Welch WR, Robboy SJ (1981) Abnormal sexual development: A classification with emphasis on pathology and neoplastic conditions. Pediatr Androl 7:71–85

68. Wertelecki W, Fraumeni JF, Mulvihill JJ (1970) Nongonadal neoplasia in Turner's syndrome. Cancer 26: 485–488

69. Yamanaka J, Baker M, Metcalfe S, Hutson JM (1991) Serum levels of müllerian inhibiting substance in boys with cryptorchidism. J Pediatr Surg 26: 621–623

70. Zakharia G, Krauss DJ (1990) Sex reversal syndrome (XX male). Urology 36: 322–324

2

Benign Diseases of the Vulva

Edward J. Wilkinson, M.D.

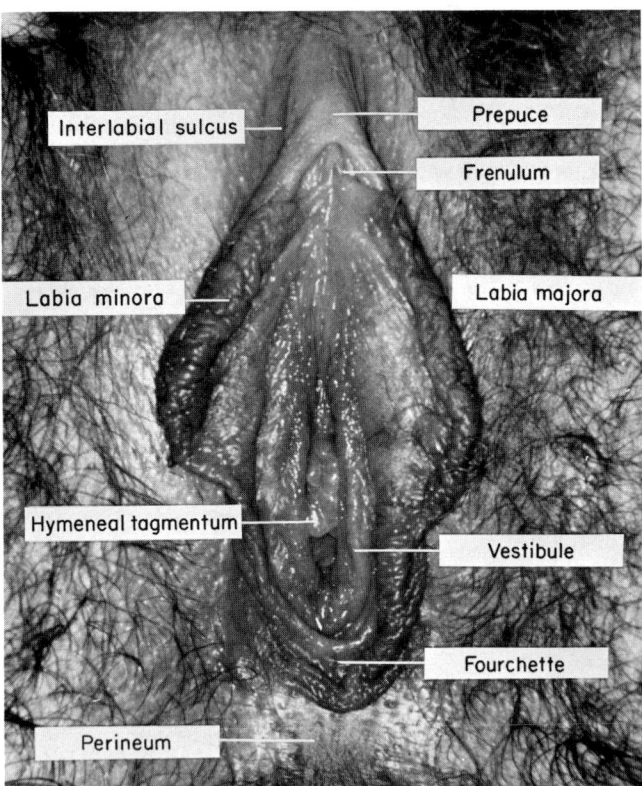

Fig. 2.1. **Topography of the vulva, normal adult.**

Anatomy

The external female genitalia include the mons pubis, labia majora and minora, prepuce, frenulum, clitoris, and vestibule. The orifices of the Skene and Bartholin glands, as well as those of the minor vestibular glands and the urethral meatus, open into the vestibule (Fig. 2.1). After adrenarche, the mons pubis and lateral aspects of the labia majora acquire increased amounts of subcutaneous fat and develop the coarse, curly surface hair characteristic of the adult. During adolescence, the labia acquire a characteristic hyperpigmentation and the clitoris undergoes some enlargement. The entire vulva, with the exception of the vulvar vestibule, is covered by keratinized, stratified squamous epithelium.[95] The labia majora contain both smooth muscle and fat, whereas the labia minora are devoid of adipose tissue but are rich in elastic fibers and blood vessels.[171] Within the lateral aspects of the labia

majora, sebaceous glands associated with hair follicles are evident. Toward the medial aspects of the labia majora the hair follicles are absent and sebaceous glands open directly to the surface epithelium. Similar sebaceous gland elements are seen on the perineum posterior to the vestibule. The labia minora typically do not contain glandular elements, although sebaceous glands without hair follicles may be found within the interlabial sulcus and at the lateral base of the labia minora.

The apocrine glands of the labia majora, prepuce, posterior vestibule, and perineal body, like the apocrine glands of the axilla, develop their secretory function at adrenarche, whereas the eccrine sweat glands, primarily involved in heat regulation, function before puberty.[105] The apocrine glands are homologous to the scent glands of lower animals and secrete via a process of decapitation.

The vestibule is bounded medially by the external portion of the hymenal ring, posteriorly and laterally by the line of Hart, and anteriorly by the frenulum of the clitoris. The line of Hart is the junction between the nonkeratinized mucous membrane epithelium of the vestibule, the thinly keratinized epithelium of the medial aspects of the labia minora, the posterior aspects of the labia majora, and the perineal body. The mucosa of the vestibule is glycogenated in women of reproductive age, or those on estrogen, and resembles vaginal mucosa (Fig. 2.2). The

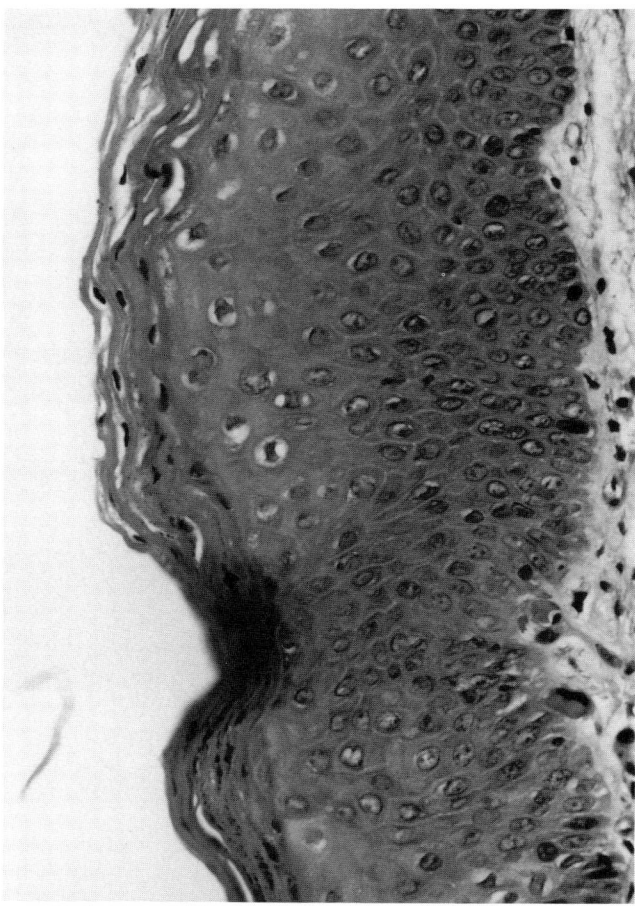

FIG. 2.2. Vulvar vestibule. At the junction of the vestibule nonkeratinized squamous epithelium merges with the keratinized squamous epithelium of the fourchette.

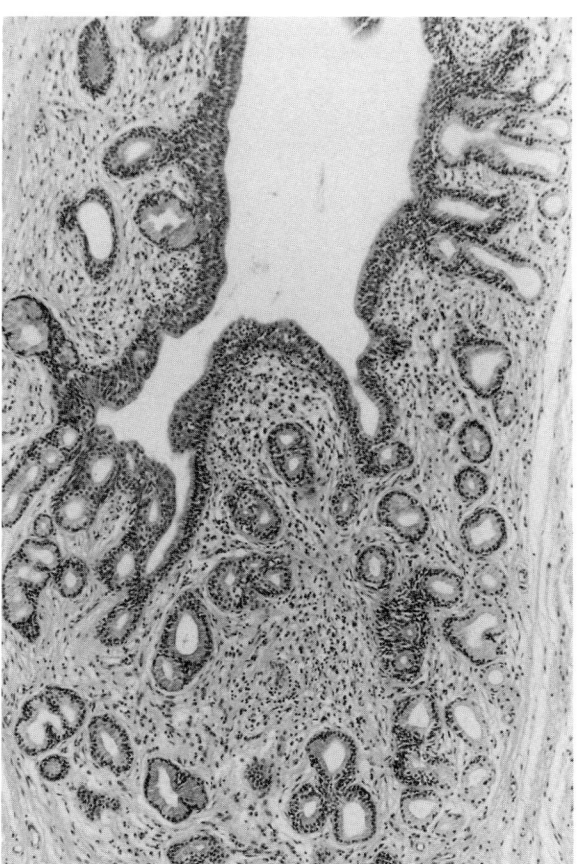

FIG. 2.3. Bartholin duct and gland. The terminal bartholin duct has a transitional epithelial-type lining that merges with the simple columnar mucous-secreting epithelium of the Bartholin's gland acini. The glands are tubuloalveolar and racemose. The surrounding fibrous stroma is somewhat more cellular than the peripheral stroma.

linea vestibularis is located in the posterior portion of the vestibule, and is a white streak or spot in the midline of the posterior vestibule extending nearly to the posterior commissure.[118] It is seen in approximately one-quarter of newborn female infants. The squamous epithelium of the vestibule merges with the transitional epithelium at the urethral meatus, and the duct openings of the paraurethral glands, the major vestibular (Bartholin) glands, and the minor vestibular glands.

The paired external openings of the paraurethral (Skene) glands are found on either side of the urethral meatus and along the posterior and lateral aspects of the urethra itself.[104] The ducts are lined by transitional epithelium, whereas the glands are composed of pseudostratified mucous-secreting columnar epithelium.

The major vestibular glands of Bartholin are bilateral racemose, tubuloalveolar glands, with acini composed of simple, columnar, mucous-secreting epithelium (Fig. 2.3). Each gland is drained by a duct measuring approximately

2.5 cm in length, and lined proximally by mucous-secreting epithelium and distally by transitional epithelium. The duct exits just external to the hymenal ring on the posterolateral aspect of the vestibule where it is lined by squamous epithelium. Thus, depending on the location within the Bartholin duct, there are three types of epithelial linings.

The minor vestibular glands are composed of acini lined by simple columnar mucous-secreting epithelium. They lie within 1–2.5 mm of the superficial epithelium and communicate with the vestibular surface. Squamous metaplasia often occurs within these glands and may obliterate them completely, resulting in the formation of a vestibular cleft (Figs. 2.4, 2.5). These minor glands ring the vestibule and extend from the frenulum on both sides of the meatus, around the external base of the hymenal ring, to the fourchette.[82,202]

Specialized glands referred to as *anogenital sweat glands* have been described within the vulvar interlabial sulcus and in the medial aspects of the labia majora. They also are

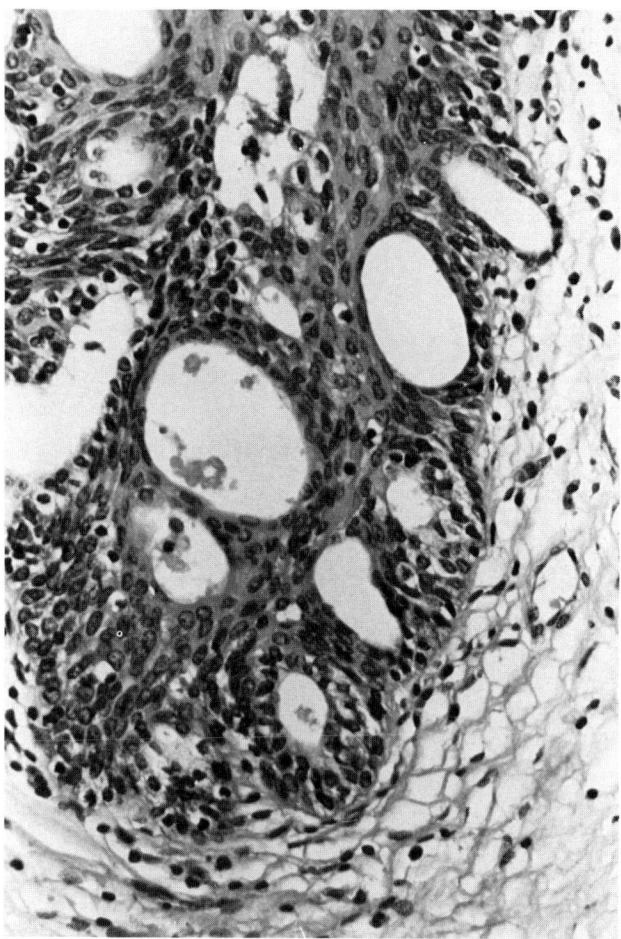

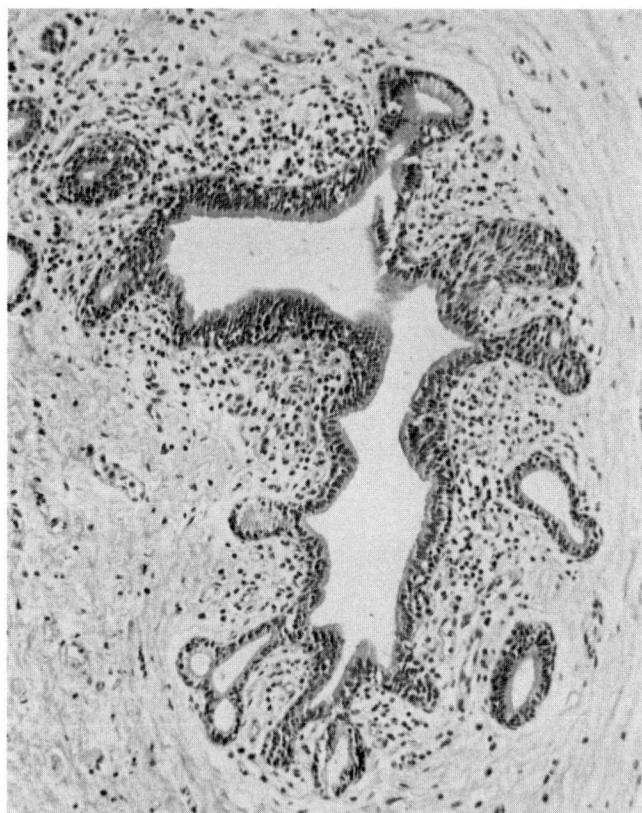

FIG. 2.5. Vulvar vestibular gland with associated vulvar vestibulitis. A complex minor vestibular gland is seen in the superficial submucosa of the vestibule. Low cuboidal epithelium lines the gland. Note the chronic inflammatory cells within the adjacent submucosa. The inflammatory infiltrate consists predominately of lymphocytes and plasma cells, with some mast cells.

FIG. 2.4. Minor vestibular gland with squamous metaplasia. Some low columnar, mucous-secreting cells line gland lumens and are associated with metaplastic squamous epithelium.

found in lesser numbers within the perineum and about the anus. The glands have long and wide coiled ducts that open to the surface, and have a simple columnar epithelium with apical snouts and myoepithelium beneath the glandular epithelium.[236,237]

The clitoris is covered by thinly keratinized stratified squamous epithelium. No sebaceous, apocrine, or eccrine sweat glands are present. Within the stroma of the clitoris are two conjoined corpora cavernosa, which branch near the base of the clitoris and lie along the pubic rami as divided crura. They are invested in a loose fibrous tissue sheath with an incomplete center septum.

The dermis and stroma of the vulva are rich in collagen, blood vessels, and myofibroblastic-type cells that are typically immunoreactive for desmin.[245] Within the superficial subepithelial stroma myxoid-like changes may be seen that have been reported extending from the ectocervix to the vulva. Atypical-appearing multinucleated cells may be observed in this subepithelial myxoid area.[1]

The femoral and inguinal lymph nods receive all the lymphatic drainage from the vulva with the exception of the clitoris, which may have a minor secondary lymphatic pathway.[178,186] A meshwork of delicate intercommunicating lymphatic vessels extends from the labia minora, clitoral prepuce, and vestibule, anteriorly and superiorly bypassing the clitoris. The lymphatic bed of the labia majora drains in an anterior, superior direction toward the mons. These anastomose with the lymphatic vessels from the labia minora and prepuce and drain into the ipsilateral inguinal and femoral nodes. Some contralateral flow also may occur into the superior medial nodes of the femoral group.[216] The superficial inguinal lymph nodes are the major nodes that drain the vulva and therefore are included in a radical vulvectomy specimen.[108,161] They consist of 8–10 nodes on each side, which are divided into a superior oblique and inferior ventral group. The superior oblique group is found about Poupart ligament, and the inferior ventral group lies above the junction of the saphenous vein and fascia lata.

Lymphatic drainage from the clitoris and midline perineum proceeds bilaterally.[108] Lymphatic flow from other sites on the vulva usually proceeds to the ipsilateral groin and pelvic lymph nodes. Injection studies using Tc-colloid have demonstrated that both ipsilateral and contralateral pelvic lymph nodes receive lymphatic drainage from unilateral labial injection in more than 67% of cases.[108]

A second minor lymphatic pathway from the glans clitoris joins the lymphatics of the urethra, traverses the urogenital diaphragm, and merges with the lymphatic plexus on the anterior surface of the bladder. From here the drainage is to the interiliac, obturator nodes and external iliac nodes. No direct pathway of lymphatic flow from the clitoris to the pelvic nodes could be demonstrated by in vivo colloid injection.[108] This finding correlates with the observation that in cases of clitoral carcinoma, in which the inguinofemoral lymph nodes are free of tumor, it is highly unlikely that the pelvic nodes are involved.

The superficial and deep external pudendal arteries branch from the femoral artery. The internal pudendal arteries branch from the internal iliac arteries. These branches from the femoral and internal iliac arteries provide the major blood supply to the vulva via the anterior and posterior labial branches. The clitoris, including the crura and corpora cavernosa, is supplied separately by the deep arteries of the clitoris, whereas the anterior vaginal artery supplies blood flow to the vestibule and the Bartholin glands. The venous return parallels the arterial supply.

The nerve supply to the vulva includes sensory nerves, special receptors, and autonomic nerves to the vessels and various glands. The major nerves of the vulva derive from the anterior (ilio-inguinal) and posterior (pudendal) labial nerves. The clitoris is innervated by the dorsal nerve of the clitoris and the cavernous nerves of the clitoris, which also supply the vestibule.[128]

Developmental Abnormalities

The normal range of clinical measurements for the clitoris in adult women measures 16.0 ± 4.3 mm in length, with a transverse diameter of 3.4 ± 1.0 mm and longitudinal diameter of 5.1 ± 1.4 mm. Parous women have slightly larger measurements than nulliparous women, but height and weight do not influence clitoral size.[240] Clitoral enlargement may occur independently or in association with generalized vulvar enlargement. Clitoral enlargement in the newborn suggests adrenogenital syndrome, exogenous maternal androgen therapy, or some form of hermaphroditism. A clitoral mass from an infant has been identified with chromosomal mosaicism where the clitoral skin had a hyperdiploid chromosomal abnormality with normal chromosomes being found in the ovary. This is an example of ambiguous genitalia resulting from a somatic cell mutation with maldevelopment of the clitoris.[215] Clitoral enlarge-

ment also has been reported associated with Lawrence–Seip syndrome.[110] Besides developmental abnormalities, a variety of tumors including granular cell tumors, hemangiomas, and vascular, neural, and smooth muscle tumors may cause clitoral enlargement.[52,117,225]

Hypertrophy and asymmetry of the labia minora may occur without demonstrable etiology and, in some cases, may be associated with chronic irritation, as may be seen in women wearing indwelling urethral catheters. True hypoplasia occurs infrequently and may be a sign of defective steroidogenesis.

Imperforate hymen is remarkably rare, with a reported frequency of 0.014%, and usually is discovered between the onset of menarche and 10–18 years of age. Surgical excision of the hymen is the usual treatment.

Slight fusion of the labia minora may be seen in infants without apparent cause and typically responds to topical estrogen cream. Labial fusion, like clitoral hypertrophy, also may be present with intersex disorders. In these situations, the defect is developmental, but such fusion also may be acquired secondary to lichen sclerosus, lichen planus, or inflammatory conditions, with subsequent adhesion formation.[33,55,71] A low transverse vaginal septum may occlude the vaginal lumen and result in hematocolpos with the onset of menstruation. Excision of the septum is the usual therapy of choice.

Duplication of the vulva is extremely rare and usually is associated with duplication of the internal müllerian system and rectum as well. In müllerian agenesis, the hymen and vagina usually are represented by only a depression in the vestibular area. Congenital absence of the clitoris[67] and external genitalia also have been described.[60] The urethra may open into the vagina rather than into the vestibule. Ectopic urethral orifices are seen occasionally adjacent to the hymen.[54]

Infectious Diseases

The most prevalent infectious diseases of the vulva in North America include human papillomavirus (HPV), typically manifested as condylomata acuminata, herpes genitalis, syphilis, and molluscum contagiosum (Table 2.1). Clinical diagnosis does not necessarily require specific organism characterization in all these conditions.

Human Papillomavirus Infection

GENERAL FEATURES

HPV is responsible for benign tumors, that is, condylomata acuminata and precursor lesions of certain types of vulvar carcinoma (i.e., vulvar intraepithelial neoplasia, VIN).[173,190] The latter are described in Chapter 3, Premalignant and Malignant Tumors of the Vulva.

Table 2.1. Infectious diseases of the vulva

Disease	Causative microorganism	Salient histopathological features	Diagnostic methods
Condyloma acuminatum	Papillomavirus	Acanthosis, hyperkeratosis parakeratosis, papillomatosis perinuclear halo (koilocyte)	Histopathology Immunohistochemistry Molecular hybridization
Herpes genitalis	Herpes simplex hominis Type II	Intranuclear inclusions	Cytopathology, culture, serology
Syphilitic chancre	*Treponema pallidum*	Ulceration, chronic inflammation, vasculitis	Darkfield, fluorescence, silver stain, serology
Condyloma lata	*Treponema pallidum*	Like chancre, with epithelial hyperplasia	Same as syphilitic chancre
Molluscum contagiosum	DNA poxvirus group	Intracytoplasmic inclusions	Cytopathology, histopathology
Granuloma inguinale	*Calymmatobacterium granulomatis*	Donovan bodies, granulomatous reaction without caseation, pseudoepitheliomatous hyperplasia	Giemsa stain, silver stain
Lymphogranuloma venereum	*Chlamydia* (TRIC agent)	Granulomatous reaction without caseation	Serology
Tuberculosis	*Mycobacterium tuberculosis*	Acid-fast bacilli (AFB), granulomatous reaction with caseation	AFB stain, AFB culture
Chancroid	*Hemophilus ducreyi*	Granulomatous reaction without caseation	Culture, gram stain

Condylomata acuminata (genital warts) are sexually transmitted benign neoplasms that may involve the vulva, vagina, cervix, urethra, anal canal, and perianal skin.[16,139,177] From 1966 to 1981, the estimated number of consultations for genital warts reported by office-based private physicians in the United States increased from 169,000 to 946,000, whereas in 1981, the number of consultations for genital herpes was 295,000.[30] In England the estimated incidence of genital warts was 23.42 per 100,000 in 1972 rising to 52.90 per 100,000 in 1982.[201] The prevalence of HPV infection varies greatly, depending on the population studies. In most studies, clinically evident vulvar involvement is less common than cervical HPV infection.[29,243]

Molecular biologic methods employing hybridization have identified HPV-6 as the most common HPV type in typical genital condylomata acuminata.[16,92,93] HPV-11 has been found in approximately one-fourth of genital warts.[93]

CLINICAL FEATURES

Clinically, condylomas present as papillary, verrucous, or papular lesions of the skin and mucous membrane that are nearly always multiple and frequently confluent (Fig. 2.6). Most lesions are asymptomatic unless secondarily infected.

Condylomata acuminata are commonly associated with vaginitis, pregnancy, diabetes mellitus, oral contraceptive use, poor perineal hygiene, immunosuppression, and sexual activity with multiple partners.[137,241] Approximately

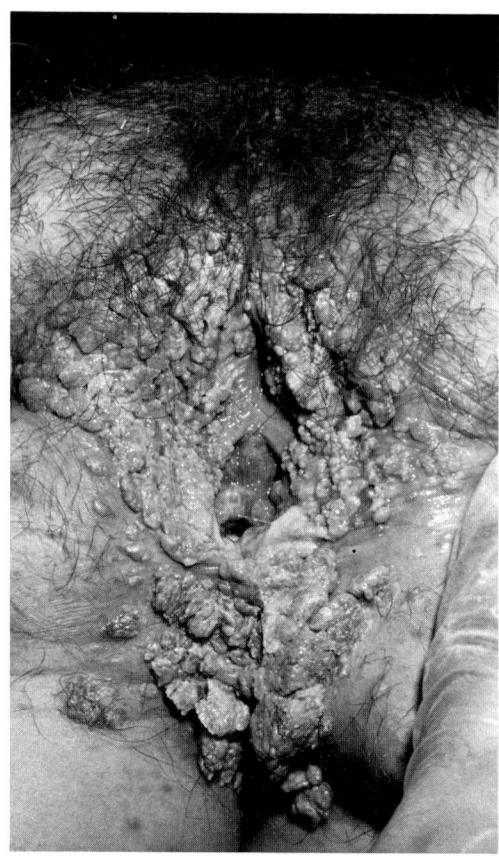

FIG. 2.6. **Condylomata acuminata.** Widespread involvement of vulva and perianal region.

30–50% of women with vulvar condyloma acuminatum have associated cervical HPV infection.[243] The presence of vulvar condyloma acuminatum in children may be related to sexual abuse.[53]

Gross Findings

On gross inspection, condylomata acuminata usually present as discrete papillary growths, arising from a central stalk or as large sessile lesions. Condylomata acuminata may be slightly raised, roughened, irregular bordered areas on the cervix, vagina, or vulva. Small lesions are best appreciated with application of 3–5% acetic acid for 3–5 minutes and colposcopic examination. Lesions that are detectable by colposcopic magnification only, or by performing HPV testing on the tissue in question, are considered subclinical.[44]

Microscopic Findings

Histologically, there is acanthosis, dyskeratosis, parakeratosis, hyperkeratosis, and a prominent granular layer. A superficial chronic inflammatory infiltrate often is present in the dermis. Typical perinuclear cytoplasmic "halos," with "raisinoid" pyknotic nuclei or slightly enlarged nuclei (koilocytosis), are commonly present in the superficial epithelial cells, and binucleated and multinucleated squamous cells often are found (Fig. 2.7). Parabasalar hyperplasia with accentuated intracellular bridges may be seen. Enlarged parabasal cells with "foamy" or "ground glass"–appearing nuclear chromatin may be present. Electron microscopic studies have demonstrated the presence of the intranuclear viral particles in condylomata; the number of identifiable particles is related to the age of the wart, reaching a peak after 6–12 months of growth, and decreasing after 2–3 years.[176,177]

Differential Diagnosis

Condylomata acuminata at times may be difficult to distinguish from VIN. Condylomata are typically verrucous or papillary, and have normal or no mitosis, koilocytosis, parabasal hyperplasia, accentuated intracellular bridges, dyskeratosis, accentuation of the granular layer, and hyperkeratosis.[47] In contrast, the presence of flat macular growth, abnormal mitoses, cytologically atypical nuclei, marked variation in nuclear size and shape, and hyperchromasia are characteristics of VIN lesions. Unlike VIN, condylomas usually are diploid; however, atypia may be seen related to tetraploidy or octoploidy. Unlike VIN, this atypia is characterized by large polyploid cells with moderate nuclear pleomorphism and some degree of hyperchromasia, but without abnormal mitosis. Tetraploidy and octoploidy

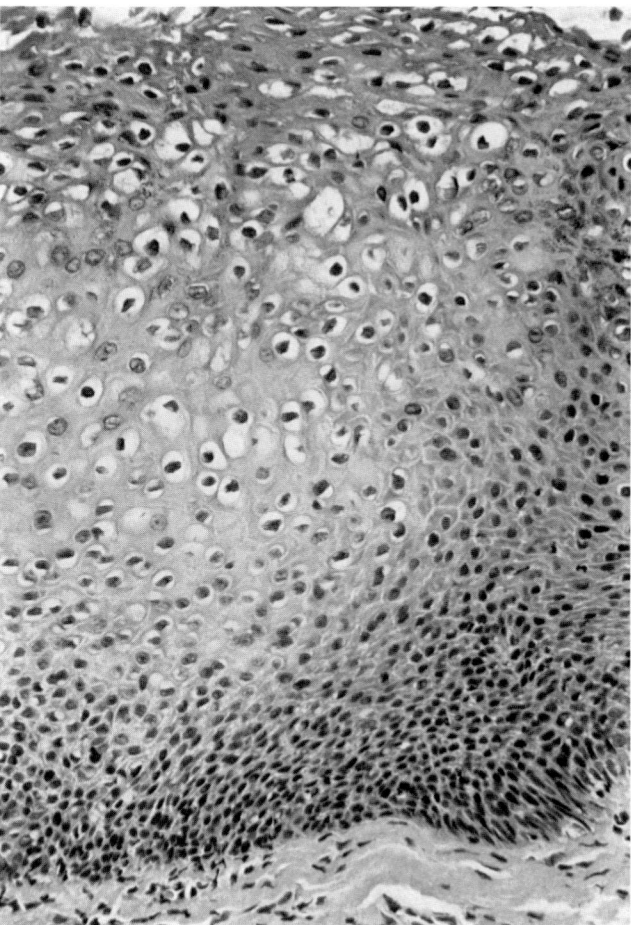

Fig. 2.7. **Condyloma acuminatum.** Parabasalar hyperplasia is seen with prominent intracellular bridges between some cells. Above the basilar layer koilocytotic cells with prominent perinuclear halos are found in the more superficial epithelium.

(variates of normal polyploidy) results in the cells having 26 × 4 or 26 × 8 chromosomes but this is not aneuploidy and does not reflect a premalignant process.[167,218] Typical condylomas will be HPV antigen positive by immunoperoxidase techniques in approximately 50% of cases whereas VIN will be immunoreactive in less than 10% of cases; however, such testing is not of value in distinguishing these two entities.[132]

In a given case of VIN, a spectrum may be found from typical VIN 3 to adjacent changes that may have the morphologic changes of condyloma acuminatum. As a matter of practice, the first diagnosis given on the pathology report is that of the most serious lesion identified, with subsequent diagnosis following. In our present state of understanding, it is acceptable to classify flat condylomata acuminata (condyloma plana) of the vulva as VIN 1 (see Vulvar Intraepithelial Neoplasia in Chapter 3).

Regressing or early flat condylomata acuminata also may resemble lichen simplex chronicus or squamous cell hyperplasia; however, the prominent granular layer, accenuated intracellular bridges, parabasalar hyperplasia, and koilocytosis are typically lacking. If this cannot be resolved by histopathological examination, molecular biologic methods such as polymerase chain reaction (PCR) or in situ hybridization, to detect HPV, may be applicable and are of value in establishing the diagnosis of HPV-associated changes when virus is identified.

Vulvar vestibular papilloma are differentiated from condylomata in that the epithelium lacks hyperkeratosis and other typical microscopic features of condyloma and are confined to the vulva vestibule.[15] Fibroepithelial polyps may have the shape of large condylomas; however, the epithelium also lacks the microscopic features of condyloma. Condylomata lata may resemble condylomata acuminata clinically; however, on biopsy, the deep inflammatory infiltrates with plasma cells and the presence of spirochetes on a Warthin–Starry silver stain distinguishes these lesions.

CLINICAL BEHAVIOR AND TREATMENT

The natural history of HPV infections of the vulva usually is one of a long protracted course and may be influenced by immunologic factors.[276] Regression has been noted after pregnancy. Presentation following radiation therapy has been observed.[137] Progression of condyloma acuminatum of the vulva to VIN has been documented.[37,47] Malignant transformation to squamous cell carcinoma also has been observed.[127]

Oncogenesis secondary to papillomavirus is well recognized in experimental animals. The earliest evidence of the transformation of genital condylomata into carcinoma is the observation, using DNA microspectrophotometry, of transition areas in condylomata wherein aneuploid neoplastic cell populations are found adjacent to the more normal polyploid cells of the condyloma.[109a]

The association of vulvar and vaginal condylomata acuminata with invasive squamous cell carcinoma has been documented in women with Fanconi anemia, and has been observed in women with Hodgkin disease as well as with other causes of immunosuppression[246] (see Chapter 3, Premalignant and Malignant Tumors of the Vulva).

The topical application of dilute podophyllin,[242] or the judicious application of concentrated halogenated acetic acid (trichloroacetic acid), are common approaches to the treatment of small vulvar condylomata. Electrodesiccation, surgical excision, cryosurgery, and hot wire loop excision, or laser ablation, have been used for large lesions.[139,197] Interferon, usually injected intralesionally, has been used for intractable condylomata; however, the long-term success of this form of therapy is uncertain. Podophyllin and interferon are contraindicated in pregnancy.[17]

HPV has been identified by Southern blot hybridization in morphologically normal skin adjacent to condyloma acuminatum, and its presence in normal adjacent skin is associated with a significantly higher recurrence rate as compared with patients without HPV present in the adjacent normal skin.[68]

Approximately 40–60% of children with laryngeal papillomatosis are born from mothers with a history of genital HPV infection.[139,144,191] However, the true incidence of infection of the larynx of the newborn infant, from a mother with genital papillomavirus infection, is unknown, but probably low. No correlation has been shown between the volume of maternal wart tissue and occurrence of infantile laryngeal papillomata. Employing DNA hybridization techniques, it has been observed that approximately one-half of laryngeal papillomas contain HPV-11.[93] This finding supports the view that laryngeal papillomas of infancy and childhood are acquired at the time of vaginal delivery.

Herpes Virus Infection

GENERAL FEATURES

The causative agent is the herpes simplex virus (HSV) (var. hominis Type 2), although in some instances the Type I virus may be involved. The incidence of herpes virus infection in the United States has been reported as 126 per 100,000. Approximately 600,000 new cases of genital herpes occur each year in the United States. Although approximately 20% of the U.S. population has been infected by HSV 2, the frequency of vulvar involvement is unknown.[140]

CLINICAL FEATURES

The initial clinical presentation frequently includes dysuria and/or urinary retention with vulvar pain that may be incapacitating. Systemic symptoms, including generalized malaise and fever, are frequently seen along with a mild inguinal lymphadenopathy. The sequential appearance of vesicles, pustules, and painful shallow ulcers that often are infected secondarily with bacteria characterize the clinical findings. The vesicles (Fig. 2.8; see color insert) usually are asymptomatic, whereas the ulcers are extremely painful. The lesions can involve the anus, urethra, bladder, cervix, and vagina, as well as the vulva. The acute ulcers heal in approximately 16 days.[46,140] Of the women who are culture positive for HSV, diagnostic genital vesicles and ulcers are present in approximately two-thirds; the remainder of the women have nondetectable or atypical lesions, or are asymptomatic.[115,126]

MICROSCOPIC FINDINGS

An early intact herpes simplex vesicle extends deeply into the epidermis. The histological transformation of the HSV-infected epithelial cell begins with a homogenization of the nuclear chromatin resulting in a "ground glass" appear-

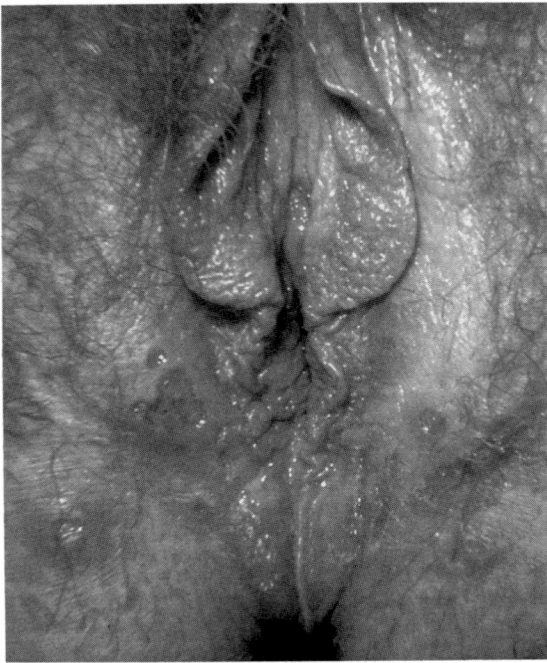

FIG. 2.8. **Herpes simplex ulcer.** HSV infection, untreated, 7 days after the onset of symptoms. Multifocal ulceration is present. (See color insert.)

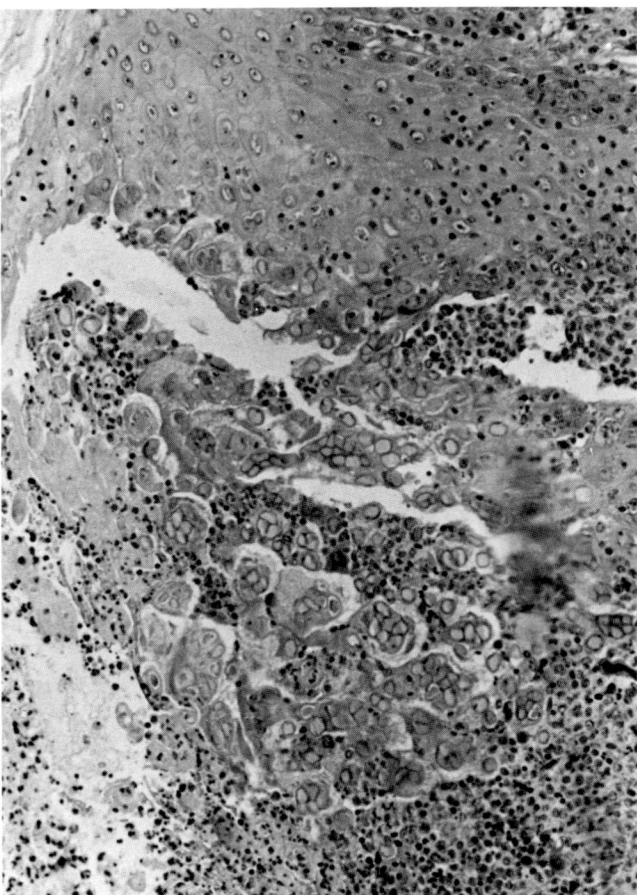

FIG. 2.9. **Herpes simplex ulcer.** Crater margin shows multinucleated clusters with distinctive intranuclear homogenization and inclusion bodies.

ance, which then progresses to the more typical eosinophilic intranuclear inclusion body.[89] The characteristic intranuclear inclusions are seen at the periphery of the lesion (Fig. 2.9). Subsequently, the cells undergo karyorrhexis and lysis. A biopsy taken in the late ulcerative phase, therefore, does not always show the intranuclear inclusions. Cytological evaluation of the scraping of the base and edges of a fresh ulcer, or freshly opened vesicle, usually will show the multinucleated cells with viral cytopathic effects, characteristic of HSV infection. Cytological examination of vesicular aspirate is an effective method of identifying the cytopathological changes of HSV, and is almost as sensitive as virus isolation. Moistening the ulcer with a saline-soaked sponge and then scraping the ulcer with a wooden spatula may improve the diagnostic yield from ulcerative lesions. Whether the sample is from an ulcer or a freshly opened vesicle, the specimen should be smeared on a clean slide, rapidly fixed in 95% ethanol, or with spray fixative, and stained with Papanicolaou stain. Morphologic changes seen with HSV infection are not reliable in separating primary from secondary infection, or in distinguishing HSV Type I from Type II infection. Furthermore, herpes zoster can involve the vulva and may have similar cytological findings.

ADJUNCTIVE METHODS

HSV-specific fluorescein conjugated antiserum may be placed on smears of ulcers or vesicles to identify HSV antigens. Immunoperoxidase techniques, employing HSV-specific antibodies, may be of value if the histopathological findings are nonspecific and can be employed on paraffin-embedded tissue.

Isolation of HSV, Types I or II, can be achieved by the inoculation of tissue culture monolayers, such as WI-38 human embryonic lung fibroblasts or monkey kidney cells. Both types of HSV produce characteristic cytopathic changes on these cell lines, which are confirmed by direct immunofluorescence employing monoclonal antibodies to HSV.[126] Virus isolation can be achieved within 4 days.[46] Rapid viral culture over 24 hours, followed by a search for HSV antigen using immunoperoxidase technique, can give results in less than 2 days. PCR technique, employing HSV-specific primers, is another approach to the positive identification of HSV infections.[32,206]

Serologic studies on acute and convalescent serum samples are of value in distinguishing primary from recurrent infection. In primary infection, significant rises (more than fourfold dilution) are found. In recurrent infection the patient is seropositive at presentation and antibody titers will not rise consistently. Serologic methods are not reliable in separating HSV Type I from Type II.[46] Asymptomatic viral shedding of HSV has been documented in 1.5–3% of women who are seropositive for HSV Type II.[3,126] HSV infection may have some oncogenic potential; however, this relationship remains to be defined.[188,259,260]

CLINICAL BEHAVIOR AND TREATMENT

Recurrent episodes of hepatic vulvitis are common after primary infection; recurrences decrease in frequency over time, whether or not acyclovir is given prophylactically. Acyclovir may reduce the severity of infection if given early in the course of illness.[115a,140]

Varicella (Herpes Zoster) (Vulvar Shingles)

Varicella infection of the vulva is rare. The prodromal pain within the vulva, without apparent physical findings, may simulate vestibulitis. The subsequent development of vesicles and ulcers assists in making the distinction because vestibulitis is not associated with vesicles and ulcers. The patients usually are postmenopausal, and the vesicles are characteristically unilateral.[10,249] The cytological findings from scrapings of opened vesicles, as well as the histological findings, are those of a herpes virus infection. Therapy with acyclovir is reported to reduce pain significantly if begun within 48 hours of the presentation of the rash.[180] The protracted neuralgia and recurrent bouts of vesicles are as described for shingles.

Cytomegalovirus Infection

Cytomegalovirus (CVM) vulvitis, like Herpes type II vulvitis, presents with an ulcerated vulvovaginitis. The histopathological findings are similar, although the viral inclusions are both intranuclear and intracytoplasmic. Viral inclusions also may be seen involving vascular endothelial cells, as well as the epithelial cells. CMV infection has been associated with vulvar ulcers in a woman with acquired immunodeficiency syndrome (AIDS). Culture or immunoperoxidase studies using specific antibodies to CMV, or PCR employing CMV-specific primers, are necessary to establish the diagnosis.[75]

Epstein–Barr Virus Infection

Epstein–Barr virus (EBV) has been cultured from painful ulcers on the labium minus of a woman during a primary infection of infectious mononucleosis. The ulcers slowly healed over 32 days.[187] EBV infection may be a sexually transmitted disease.[187]

Molluscum Contagiosum

Molluscum contagiosum is a moderately contagious viral disease that, in adults, is often related to intimate and/or

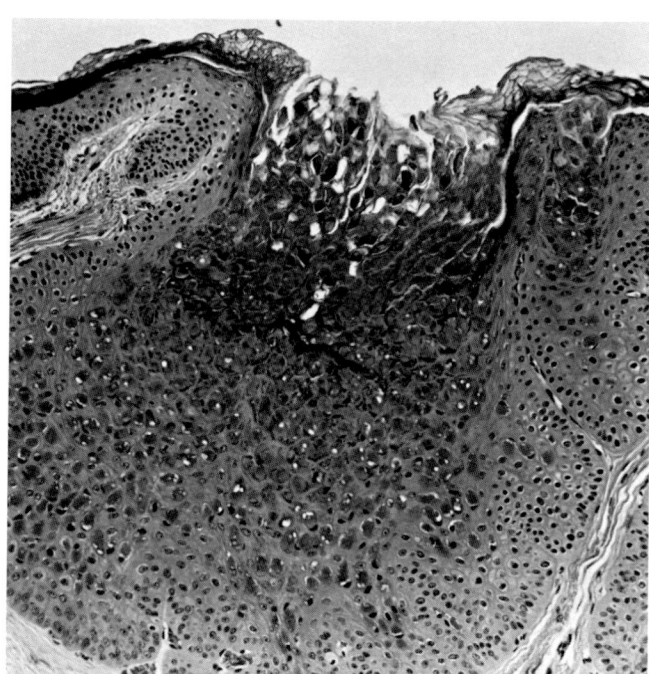

FIG. 2.10. Molluscum contagiosum. Cells within the acanthotic nest show increasing density of intracytoplasmic inclusions as the surface umbilication is approached.

sexual contact.[194] Molluscum contagiosum usually is asymptomatic; however, perianal lesions frequently become pruritic or secondarily infected. The lesions are small, smooth papules (3–6 mm in diameter) with a central punctum or umbilication. They generally are multiple and separate, although they may be single. Rare plaque formations, made up of 50–100 individual clustered lesions, also have been described. The incubation period varies between 14 and 50 days. Clinical diagnosis usually does not require biopsy. Cytological identification of the typical intracytoplasmic inclusion bodies (molluscum bodies) within scrapings from the interior of the molluscum papule are adequate to confirm the diagnosis.

Histological examination demonstrates marked acanthosis and the characteristic intracytoplasmic viral inclusions (Fig. 2.10). Recently infected cells contain an eosinophilic cytoplasmic inclusion (molluscum body). With aging, the cytoplasmic bodies take on a more basophilic appearance preceding lysis of the cell.[194] The central dimple of the lesion is seen histologically if the lesion is carefully bisected. Within the dermis there often is a marked vascular response with endothelial proliferation and perivascular inflammation. Electron microscopy has demonstrated that the virus is brick-shaped and contains a DNA core with a two-layered protein coat measuring 300 nm × 210 nm.[20] Most lesions regress spontaneously; untreated lesions may persist for years, during which time they may be spread by close contact.

Syphilis

CLINICAL FEATURES

Syphilis is a venereal disease caused by the spirochete *Treponema pallidum*. The primary lesion is the chancre, a painless, indurated, shallow, clean-appearing ulcer with raised edges. The chancre usually presents within 3 weeks after initial contact; the range, however, is 7–90 days. If secondarily infected, the chancre may become soft and painful and show an ulcerated surface. Although chancres are generally single, they may be multiple. Chancres may occur on inconspicuous surfaces, such as the cervix, anal mucosa, or oral pharynx. In approximately 50% of women and 30% of men the primary lesion is never seen. Lymphadenopathy presents 3 to 4 days after the chancre. The nodes are nontender, freely moveable, and rubbery.[59]

Left untreated in the primary phase, the chancre will heal within 2–6 weeks and typically does not leave a scar.[163] The secondary stage of the disease will become evident within 6 weeks to 6 months. At this point, the patient may present with a skin rash that often involves mucous membranes as well as the palms of the hands and soles of the feet.[248] On occasion, the secondary lesions are papular, especially about the vulva, presenting as elevated plaques up to 3 cm in diameter. These are known as condylomata lata, and clinically may mimic condylomata acuminata (Fig. 2.11; see color insert). Such lesions also may occur on other mucocutaneous borders. The tertiary gumma of syphilis is rarely seen on the vulva.

MICROSCOPIC FINDINGS

If syphilis were not considered in the clinical differential, the diagnosis may be quite difficult from histological material alone. Microscopically, the diagnosis of syphilis may be difficult. The primary chancre is characterized by ulceration of the epidermis with acute and chronic inflammation within the dermis. There is a marked perivascular inflammatory response, characterized by the presence of large numbers of plasma cells (Fig. 2.12). Histological examination of condylomata lata reveals marked acanthosis and hyperkeratosis (Fig. 2.13). The inflammatory response within the dermis is similar to that in the primary chancre with a marked, predominantly plasmacytic inflammatory infiltrate. The arteritis in both lesions may be sufficiently severe to result in obliteration of the smaller vessels. Dieterle or Warthin–Starry silver stains for spirochetes are always of value if there is any suspicion of syphilis, but may be negative with active infection. Serologic studies for syphilics should be performed if

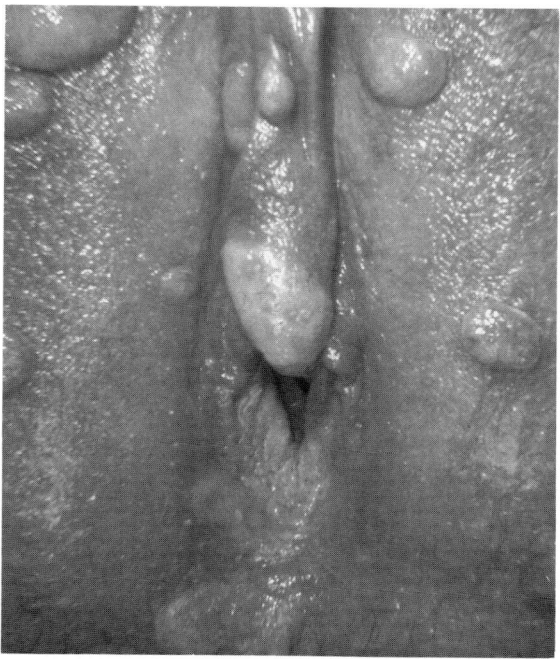

FIG. 2.11. Condyloma lata. Multiple papules are present. (See color insert.)

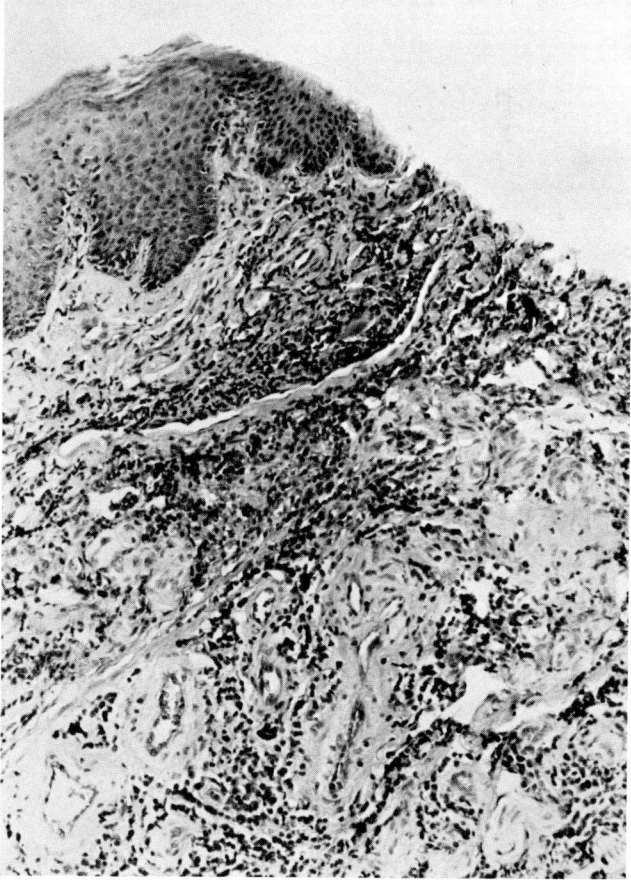

FIG. 2.12. Lymphogranuloma venereum. The slightly ulcerated epithelium is associated with a marked superficial and deep chronic inflammation that is most intense about the dermal vessels and lymphatics. The inflammatory infiltrates consist predominantly of plasma cells and lymphocytes.

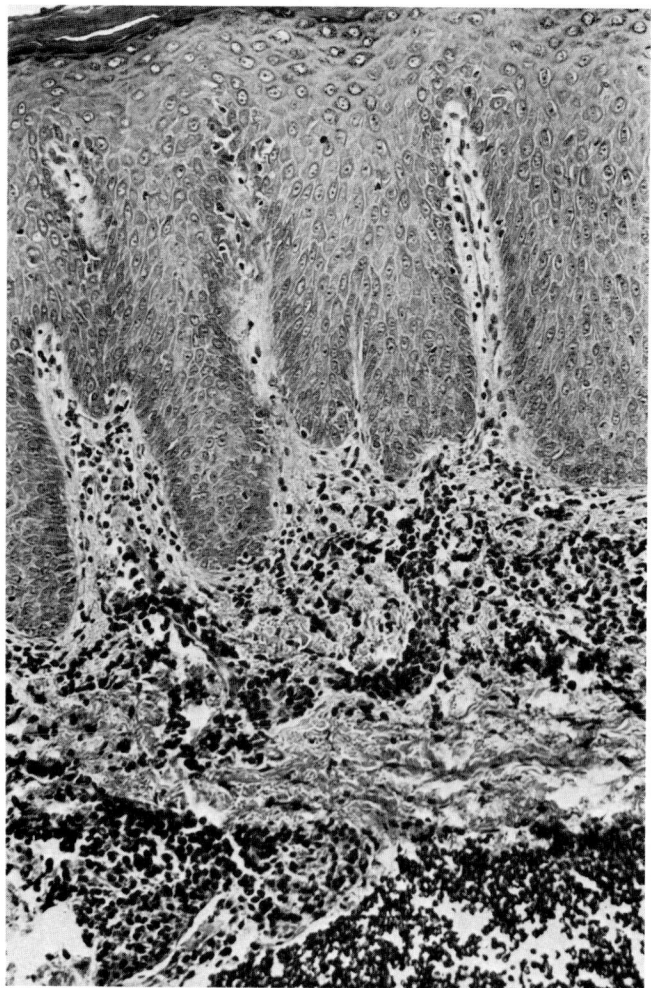

FIG. 2.13. **Condyloma latum.** Prominent acanthosis is present with a marked dermal perivascular inflammatory cell infiltrate that consists primarily of plasma cells and lymphocytes, with some neutrophils. Vascular endothelial proliferation is present with associated arteritis.

syphilis is considered clinically or from the pathological findings.

ADJUNCTIVE METHODS

The primary chancre, as well as the condyloma latum and other secondary lesions, are rich in spirochetes. Therefore, when a chancre or secondary lesion of syphilis is suspected, an attempt to identify spirochetes within the lesion should be made. This is accomplished through either dark-field examination of serum expressed from the base of the ulcer or by the fluorescent conjugated antibody technique, which employs a dried smear preparation. The organism measures up to 15 μm in length and 0.20 μm in thickness.

It is spiral in shape, with 6–14 coils. Motility, characterized by flexion, rotation about the long axis, and random movement is noted on dark-field examination of fresh sera from an active lesion. These methods for identification of spirochetes are far more sensitive and specific than is silver stain on paraffin-embedded tissue. The chancre may be present for weeks before serologic tests become reactive. More than 70% of patients with dark-field–positive lesions have a reactive serology at the time of initial diagnosis. The most common serologic testing methods are based on the identification of reagin. These tests become positive approximately 1 month after the disease is contracted. Common reagin testing methods employ microflocculation testing and include the Venereal Disease Research Laboratory (VDRL) and Rapid Plasma Reagin (RPR).[174] These two tests have similar specificity and can be quantitated to evaluate the course of the disease and response to therapy. The fluorescent Treponema antibody, absorbed (FTA-ABS) test is highly sensitive and is ordered if the resin tests are nonreactive, weakly reactive, or if there is a possibility of a false-positive result. Biologic false positive can occur in lupus erythematosus, virus infection, cirrhosis of the liver, pregnancy, malaria, and other inflammatory or autoimmune diseases. Once the FTA-ABS becomes positive, it can remain so for the life of the patient. If the FTA-ABS is positive, spinal fluid serologic evaluation will be necessary to rule out neurosyphilis. A false-positive FTA-ABS is rare and, if detected, requires *T. pallidum* mobilization testing and careful follow-up.[59,163]

CLINICAL BEHAVIOR AND TREATMENT

Approximately 30% of patients with primary syphilis will undergo spontaneous remission of the disease. Those who are not treated or who do not achieve spontaneous remission may progress to tertiary syphilis with its well-recognized cardiovascular and central nervous system effects. Untreated syphilis may prove fatal in 10% of those afflicted. Penicillin or another appropriate systemic antibiotic is the treatment of choice.

Granuloma Inguinale

Granuloma inguinale (Donovanosis, Granuloma venereum) is caused by *Calymmatobacterium granulomatous,* a gram-negative heavily encapsulated rod considered to be in the bacterial family Enterobacteriaceae. Granuloma inguinale occurs with approximately equal frequency in men and women. Primary lesions may occur on the vulva, vagina, or cervix and may present as painless papules or necrotizing ulcers with rolled borders and a friable base. Inguinal adenopathy usually is absent.[57,209] The lesions usually appear within 1 week to a month of exposure; anal coitus or fecal contamination of the vulva or vagina have been incriminated as modes of transmission.[163] Granuloma inguinale extends primarily by local infiltration, although lymphatic permeation may occur during later stages of the disease. Chronic lymphatic infiltration and fibrosis frequently result in a massive brawny edema of the external genitalia. There is controversy as to the true origin of the edema, because dye injection studies suggest that the lymphatic drainage is intact. With involvement of the cervix, the disease may advance via the cervical lymphatics to involve parametrial tissues.[130]

The clinical diagnosis of granuloma inguinale depends on the identification of the Donovan bodies within the tissue. This is best accomplished by preparing smears or a biopsy from the edge of the ulcer and pressing this biopsy tissue between two slides. The tissue imprints are air dried, fixed in methanol, and stained with Giemsa stain.[216] Any antibiotic treatment may obscure the diagnosis, necessitating biopsy at a later date to identify organisms.

Histologically, the main portion of the lesion consists of granulation tissue associated with an extensive chronic inflammatory cell infiltrate and endarteritis. An ulcer usually is covered with a fibrinous exudate and necrosis may be present. The surface epithelium, adjacent to the ulcer, may show prominent pseudoepitheliomatous hyperplasia. Necrosis and microabscesses may be seen within the epidermis.[57,216] Within the granulation tissue there is a dense mixed inflammatory cell infiltrate, consisting predominantly of plasma cells and mononuclear cells with few lymphocytes, which extends into the dermis. Large vacuolated histiocytes that contain the characteristic encapsulated bacilli, Donovan bodies, within their cytoplasm frequently are present (Fig. 2.14). They can be demonstrated with a Warthin–Starry stain or Giemsa stain. The Donovan bodies may be found extracellularly, as well as intracellularly, and may appear coccoid, coccobacillary, or bacillary.[216] Ultrathin plastic-embedded sections, as well as electron microscopy, may be of value in diagnosis.[130,216]

Calymmatobacterium granulomatous may be cultured by special techniques. The diagnosis depends on the clinical findings and documenting the organism within a tissue specimen or by culture. Syphilis, chancroid, and herpes virus infection usually are included in the differential diagnosis.[58]

Lymphogranuloma Venereum

Lymphogranuloma venereum (LGV) is caused by *Chlamydia,* and occurs approximately three times more frequently in men than in women. The disease has three phases: (1) erosion of the skin, (2) adenitis, and (3) fibrosis and destruction.[58] Lymphogranuloma venereum is spread primarily via the lymphatics. The initial ulcers, which generally are not tender or painful, often are ignored. Adenitis

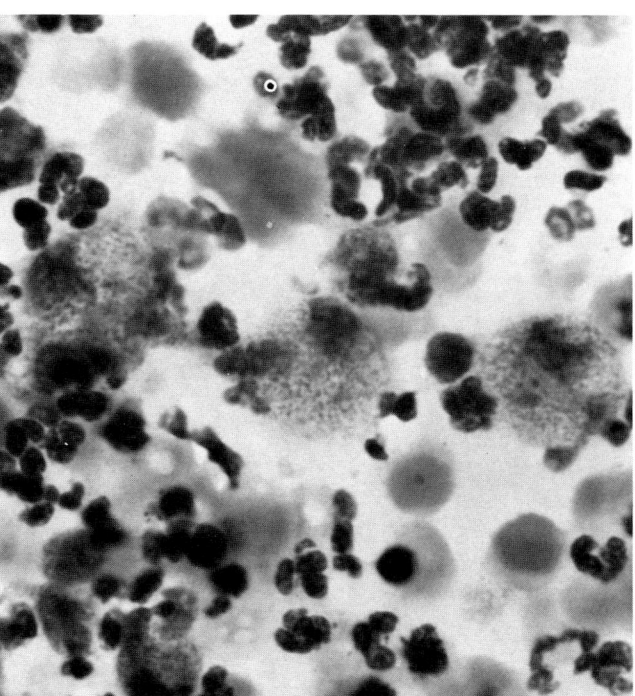

FIG. 2.14. **Granuloma inguinale.** Large histiocytes obtained by smear show numerous intracytoplasmic Donovan bodies.

may evolve into painful superficial groin nodes, or buboes, that frequently rupture through the skin with exudation of a purulent discharge. The third phase of the disease often results in stricture and fibrosis of the vagina and rectum.[248] During this phase, chronic lymphatic obstruction is responsible for the characteristic nonpitting edema of the external genitalia.

The histology of LGV is not diagnostic and reveals no characteristic viral inclusions or identifiable organisms by the usual modes of investigation. Smears and biopsy specimens should be evaluated for organisms (spirochetes, Donovan bodies, etc.) to rule out other diseases with a similar presentation. Histologically, giant cells may be seen along with lymphocytes and plasma cells (Fig. 2.15). Older lesions may exhibit extensive fibrosis of the dermis and sinus tracts. The diagnosis is based on the typical clinical presentation, along with positive complement fixation tests. Culture, as well as other specific immunohistochemical tests, can assist in the diagnosis of LGV. Treatment is systemic tetracycline or doxycycline.[163]

Chancroid

Chancroid is relatively rare and presents with a genital ulcer that usually is tender, nonindurated, and has a friable

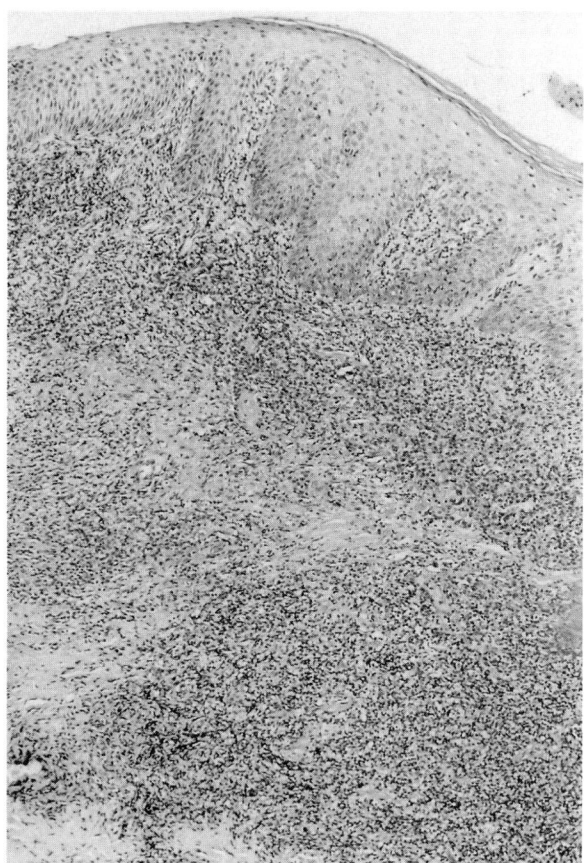

Fig. 2.15. Lymphogranuloma venereum. An intense superficial and deep chronic inflammatory infiltrate is present, composed predominantly of lymphocytes and plasma cells. A few multinucleated giant cells are present.

purulent erythematous base. Primary lesions may be single or multiple and tend to be small, mesauring approximately 1–2 mm in diameter. Coalescence of the lesions leads to ulcers approaching up to 3 cm in diameter. Tender inguinal adenopathy with flocculent nodes may be present. The incubation period may be as short as 10 days.[211] The clinical differential diagnosis includes herpes virus infection and primary syphilis.[211]

Chancroid is caused by the organism *Haemophilus ducreyi,* a gram-negative, nonmotile bacillus, which in culture grows in pairs and parallel chains. Skin tests and biopsies may not be diagnostic. Identification of the organism by culture is necessary for accurate diagnosis.[168] Selective Agar medium has been developed for the organism, which has improved culture isolation. Histological examination of the tissue demonstrated a granulomatous-type reaction with chronic inflammatory cells consisting primarily of lymphocytes and plasma cells, and the presence of the gram-negative organisms, which may be present in large numbers and in parallel chains.[134]

Tuberculosis

Tuberculosis of the vulva is rare. It usually is associated with tuberculosis of other genital sites, primarily fallopian tube, and endometrium. Genital involvement usually is associated with pulmonary tuberculosis. Autoinoculation by hematogenous or direct spread therefore is the most common method of transmission to the vulva. Primary inoculation or sexual transmission of tuberculosis is most uncommon. Immunosuppression may play a role in susceptibility. Vulvar tuberculosis has been described in a renal transplant patient.[231]

The usual organism is *Mycobacterium tuberculosis;* however, atypical mycobacteria also have been incriminated. Diagnosis usually can be made by biopsy of the involved tissues. Caseating granulomas with Langhan giant cells are found and acid-fast stains usually reveal the mycobacterium (Fig. 2.16). Confirmation of the diagnosis can be made by culture techniques. Appropriate long-term systemic antibiotics are the recommended therapy.

Giant cells of the foreign body type are encountered frequently in vulvar tissues in which a previous biopsy has been performed (Fig. 2.17). These giant cells, associated with noncaseating granulomas, often result from embedded suture occasionally seen in prior biopsied areas, and should not be confused with tuberculosis. Vulvar ulceration, secondary to sarcoidosis, has been reported and should be included in the differential diagnosis of granulomatous ulcerations of the vulva.[166]

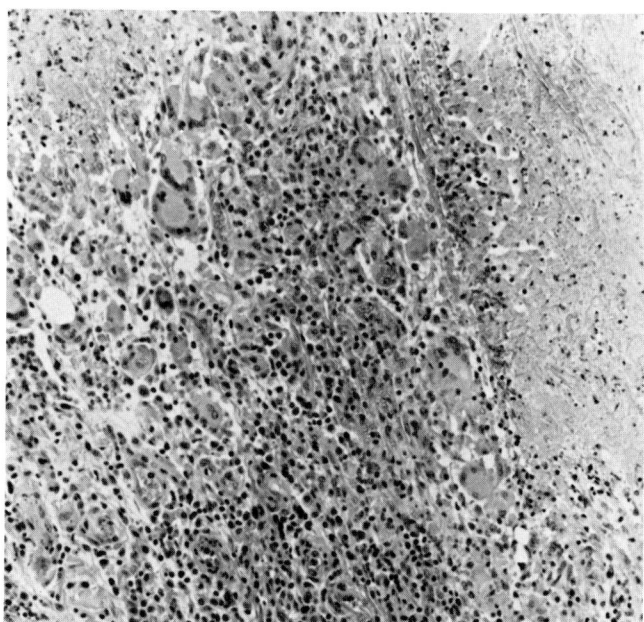

Fig. 2.16. Vulvar tuberculosis. Caseating granulomas with Langhan giant cells.

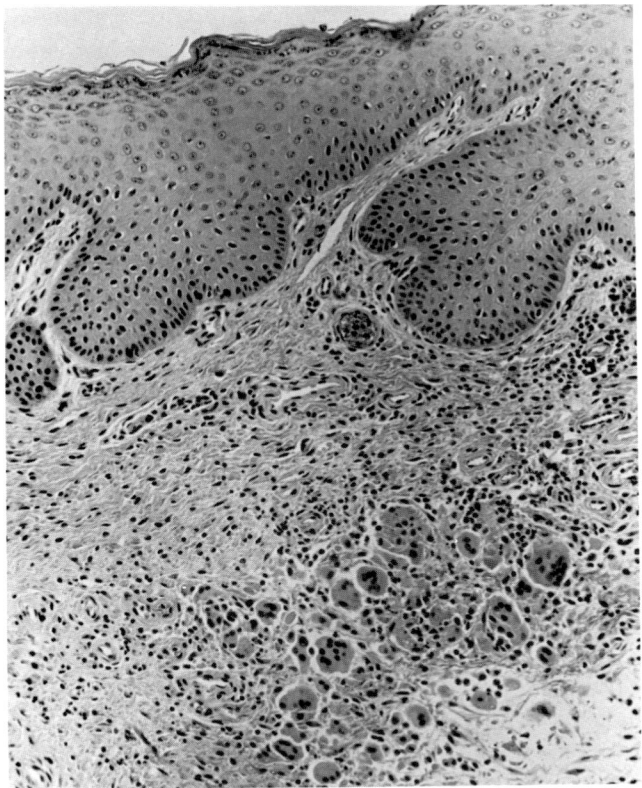

FIG. 2.17. Foreign body giant cell. Multinucleated giant cells are present, but caseation is lacking.

Miscellaneous Infectious Diseases

Chronic inflammatory conditions of the vulvar and perianal skin without concomitant ulceration often are caused by fungal infections, although a variety of irritants, unrelated to infection, may be responsible.[24] *Candida* and dermatophytes are frequent pathogens. Such conditions rarely require biopsy, and accurate diagnosis generally can be accomplished by microscopic examination of skin scrapings placed in 10% potassium hydroxide, or by appropriate culture methods. Topical antifungal creams are the usual therapy.

Chronic and acute vaginitis related to trichomonas, *Chlamydia, Candida* species, or other infectious agents may be associated with inflammation of the vulva, especially the vulvar vestibule. The histological findings usually are not diagnostic. Vulvar candidiasis usually can be diagnosed by employing silver stains for fungus, with recognition of the fungal organisms within the keratin, or superficial epithelium.

Bacterial infections may produce clinical findings similar to those seen with fungus infections. Erythrasma is a chronic bacterial infection of the genitocrural area that shows a coral-red fluorescence under Wood's light. The disease is most common in obese diabetes. Scrapings of these lesions, when stained with Gram stain, demonstrate the causative gram-positive bacteria, *Corynebacterium minutissimum,* in rods, filaments, and coccoid forms.[134]

Parasitic Infections

Enterobius vermicularis (pinworm, seatworm) is a relatively common intestinal parasite. The female worm measures 8–13 mm in length and 0.5 mm in diameter. The male is approximately one-fourth as long as the female, and has the same diameter. Infected children frequently present with complaints of severe vulvovaginal pruritus, which may awaken them at night. Other complaints include lower abdominal pain, diarrhea, restlessness, and nocturia. Studies for fungus and bacteria are not diagnostic, and examination of the vulvar vestibule and vagina reveal marked inflammation. Occasionally, an adult female helminth found on the vestibule or perineal areas is brought to the laboratory. More commonly, the pathologist is presented with a cellulose-tape-slide preparation for identification of the typical embryonated eggs of *E. vermicularis.*[80] A granuloma secondary to *Enterobius* eggs has been reported involving the vulva.[228]

Vulvar schistosomiasis, usually *Schistosoma mansoni,* is well documented and primary skin lesions on the vulva from penetration of the infective *Cercariae* may be seen. When biopsied, the parasite may be found within the epidermis.[157]

Cutaneous myiasis of the vulva, secondary to infestation of the larval form of the muscoid fly and sarcophaga, has been reported. Recognition of the larva extracted from the vulvar tissues is diagnostic.[41,125]

Nonneoplastic Epithelial Disorders

To establish a standardized system of nomenclature based on histopathological findings, the International Society for the Study of Vulvar Disease (ISSVD) and International Society of Gynecological Pathologists (ISGP) recommended in 1986 that all such lesions be classified as nonneoplastic epithelial disorders and classified as lichen sclerosus, squamous cell hyperplasia, and other dermatoses (Table 2.2).[106a]

The vast majority of lesions of the vulva have no premalignant potential. Both the clinician and the pathologist have been confused by such diagnoses as kraurosis vulvae, leukoplakia, and atrophic vulvitis.[115a] Such vague terminology reflects the prior use of terms based on gross rather than microscopic features. Historically, the term *dystrophy* was first proposed to describe a clinically related group of disorders of epithelial growth that usually present as white lesions of the vulva, and that microscopically are characterized by alterations of the epithelial and dermal

Table 2.2. Classification of vulvar
nonneoplastic disorders

1975–1986[a]	1987[b]
Lichen sclerosus	Lichen sclerosus
Hyperplastic dystrophy	Squamous cell hyperplasia
Mixed dystrophy	Other dermatoses

[a] Developed by the International Society for the Study of
Vulvar Disease (ISSVD).
[b] Developed by the ISSVD and the International Society
of Gynecological Pathologists.

architecture. Two basic clinical varieties of dystrophy were
recognized by the ISSVD in 1976: lichen sclerosus and
hyperplastic dystrophy.[115a] When both co-existed on different areas of the same vulva, it was recommended that
the lesion be classified as a mixed dystrophy. The term
mixed dystrophy has been discontinued because it is now
recognized that lichen sclerosus is commonly associated
with variable degrees of squamous cell hyperplasia (formerly called *hyperplastic dystrophy*) and this reflects the
spectrum of changes seen in lichen sclerosus, rather than
the presentation of two distinctive epithelial disorders.

It is not always possible to distinguish clinically the various forms of nonneoplastic epithelial disorders on the basis
of their gross appearance alone. All may be white, scaly,
and fissured (Fig. 2.18). Although biopsy may not be nec-

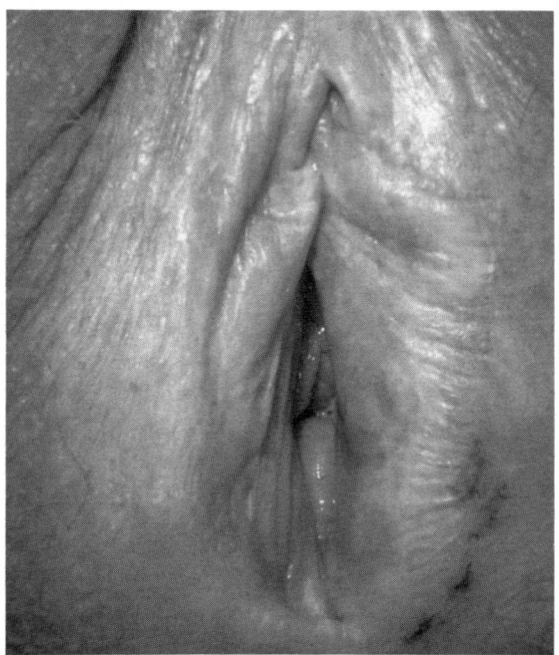

FIG. 2.18. Lichen sclerosus. White epithelium with focal subcutaneous ecchymosis is seen. The labia minora are somewhat
atrophic. (See color insert.)

essary in all cases, especially in children with typical findings of lichen sclerosus, multiple representative biopsies to
sample the entire lesion usually are very informative. On
the basis of the histological findings, the pathologist can
separate white lesions of a neoplastic type from nonneoplastic epithelial disorders.

Lichen Sclerosus (Lichen Sclerosus et Atrophicus)

GENERAL FEATURES

Lichen sclerosus is a dermatosis of unknown etiology characterized by progressive thinning of the epithelium, subepithelial edema with fibrin deposition, and an underlying
zone of chronic inflammation within the dermis. It is a
common cause of white epithelial changes on the
vulva.[99,136] As a cutaneous disease, it may affect the trunk
or extremities, but is found most frequently on the genitalia. The exact prevalence is unknown and awaits a definitive large-scale study. The disease is not racially confined,
and although it is noted most commonly in postmenopausal Caucasian women, cases may first present in children as young as 18 months of age.[18,77,136]

In a study of 30 untreated women with lichen sclerosus,
serum levels of dihydrotestosterone were observed to be
below normal values for their age.[81] This was true for the
reproductive age group as well as those in their postmenopausal years. At the same time, free testosterone levels
were found to be elevated, suggesting a block in the enzymatic conversion of testosterone to dihydrotestosterone.
The pathophysiology of this disorder thus remains obscure.

A genetic aspect is present; 15 families have now been
recorded in which successive generations have manifested
lichen sclerosus. For the most part, these have been
mother/daughter pairs, but in one instance both mother
and father were affected, as was their young daughter.
Within such families, there is a tendency toward a similar
age of onset for affected individuals. Human leukocyte
antigen (HLA) types were found to be prevalent in one
study, supporting the genetic aspect.[79]

CLINICAL FEATURES

In children, symptoms include dysuria, painful defecation,
and rectal bleeding.[18] Lichen sclerosus can lead to anal
fissures and genital and perianal ulcers, which may be
confused with child sexual abuse. In adult women, the
clinical findings typically are thinned and whitened epithelium, which usually is symmetrical and involves the labia
minora, clitoris, prepuce, frenulum, and perineal body.
Perirectal involvement is common. In advanced cases, loss
and agglutination of the labia minora, frenulum, prepuce,
and adhesions of the clitoris are found. Stenosis of the
introitus is common. In men, the glands of the penis and

prepuce frequently are involved and distal urethral stricture and phimosis may occur. Under these circumstances, the condition is clinically known as *balanitis xerotica obliterans*.

GROSS FINDINGS

The vulvar lesions of lichen sclerosus typically are pale white, flat, plaque-like areas that in advanced cases may be associated with thinned parchment-like epithelium and focal areas of ecchymosis and superficial ulceration (Fig. 2.18; see color insert). The vaginal mucosa is not involved.

MICROSCOPIC FINDINGS

The microscopic findings of lichen sclerosus can vary considerably, related to age of the lesion, excoriation, and treatment.[99] The principal histological changes include blunting or loss of the rete ridges and the concomitant development of homogeneous subepithelial edema of variable thickness within the dermis (Fig. 2.19). The homogeneous zone has been described as collagenized or edematous and usually shows a reduction or absence of elastic fibers. Beneath this zone, a band of scattered lymphocytes usually is seen. The epithelium is thinned, but hyperkeratosis may be present in some cases. The basal cell layer often is disorganized and spongiosis may be evident. There is both an absence of melanosomes in the keratinocytes

and a disappearance of the melanocytes. This lack of pigment, as well as edema contribute to the white clinical appearance. Mitotic figures are rare or absent. In some cases, the mechanical trauma of rubbing and scratching will have produced bullous areas of lymphedema and subepithelial lacunae filled with erythrocytes (Fig. 2.20). Areas of ulceration and acute inflammation also may be seen.

DIFFERENTIAL DIAGNOSIS (SEE DIFFERENTIAL UNDER LICHEN PLANUS)

ULTRASTRUCTURAL FINDINGS

Ultrastructural studies have shown that collagen metabolism is abnormally active and the number of capillaries is reduced. The basal lamina is thickened and discontinuous. Degenerate dermal and collagenous material can be found between the cells of the epidermis, and melanocytes are rare.[148]

IMMUNOHISTOCHEMICAL AND RELATED STUDIES

The presence of an elastase-type protease in vulvar fibroblasts from lichen sclerotic tissue has been reported that may be responsible for the loss of elastic tissue so frequently seen.[94] An increased concentration of collagenase inhibitor also has been reported. Tissue studies of glucose metabolism as well as alkaline phosphatase and adenosine

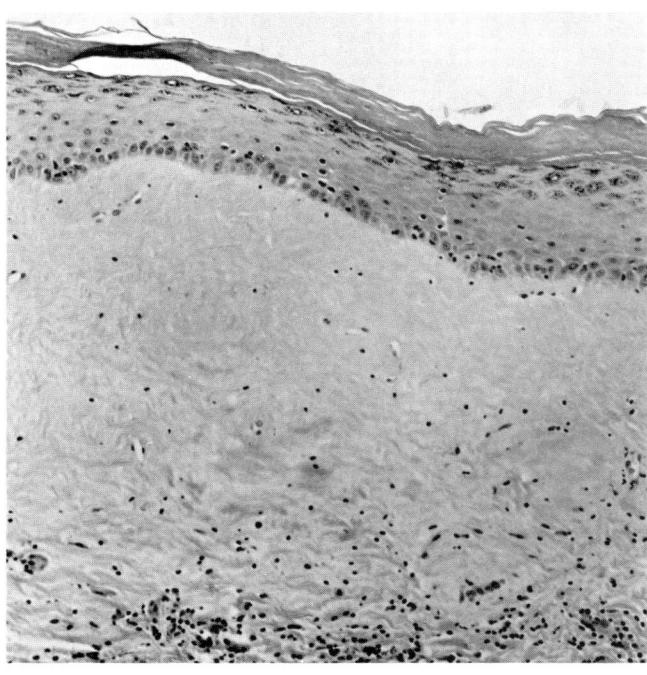

FIG. 2.19. **Lichen sclerosus.** Hyperkeratosis is present along with loss of rete pegs and homogenization of the dermis.

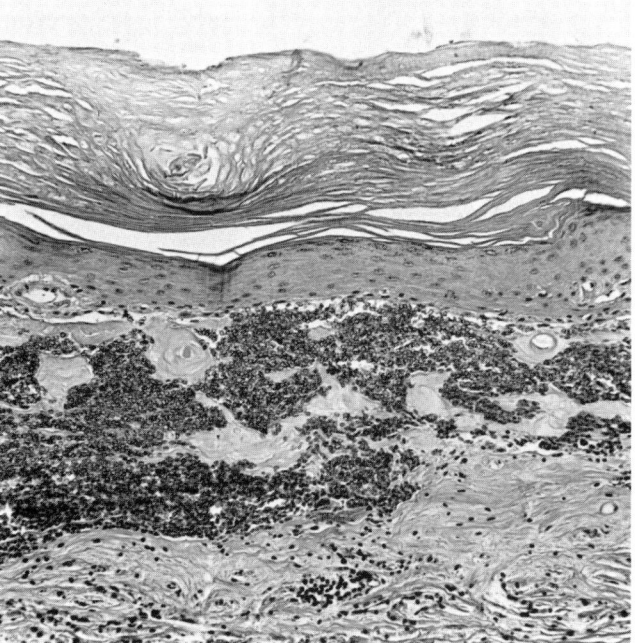

FIG. 2.20. **Lichen sclerosus.** Marked hyperkeratosis with extravasation of blood in the dermis.

triphosphatase have shown a surprisingly high rate of activity, equal to that seen in hyperplastic specimens and greater than that found in normal menopausal skin. The cell cycle protein Ki-67 is present in the basal and many parabasal epithelial cells involved by lichen sclerosus.[98a] These findings are consistent with other in vitro work that has demonstrated that the uptake of tritiated thymidine by such epithelium is greater than normal, despite the lack of mitoses.[115a] An apparent premature maturation of all cells above the basal layer has been reported based on their high concentration of involucrin.[51]

There is a growing body of evidence that an autoimmune mechanism may be involved. Patients with lichen sclerosus have been noted to have an increased number of organ-specific antibodies and more autoimmune disease than the normal population.[34,55,94,98] On a histological level, direct immunofluorescence studies have shown a deposit of fibrin along the dermoepidermal junction in 75% of the specimens studied.[28] With an indirect fluorescent technique, IgM and C3 were heavily concentrated along the basal lamina of the epithelium.[55] Studies on activated T cells within lichen sclerosus have identified activated (HLA-Dr+) T cells and increased epidermal CD1a+ Langerhan cells, evidence of persistent activation of lymphoid cells and epidermal antigen presenting cells, respectively.[34]

Clinical Behavior and Treatment

Traditional management has relied on the long-term topical application of testosterone or progesterone. Recent studies have reported good results with topical, high-potency corticosteroids.[49] In children, clearing or improvement of the anogenital lesions has been reported at puberty.[71,136] Topical testosterone has been reported to arrest the symptoms and progress of the disease; however, it cannot be used in children because it is systemically absorbed. Topical corticosteroids are used frequently in the early course of therapy to relieve symptoms. In a controlled prospective study of 67 women with vulvar lichen sclerosus, without associated squamous cell hyperplasia, who were treated with topical 2% testosterone propionate or 0.35% progesterone for up to 8 weeks, more than half the study group had complete relief of symptoms and regression of physical findings. Approximately one-fifth of the patients had no significant response in either symptoms or findings. No differences were found between progesterone or testosterone therapy; however, some control patients responded to the lubricant base alone.[36] Current therapy includes the initial use of topical high-potency corticosteroids to relieve symptoms. Opinion varies as to long-term therapy. Topical corticosteroid alone or long-term typical testosterone or progesterone have been advocated.

Lichen sclerosus sometimes is associated with vulvar squamous carcinoma, however, it is not considered to be a premalignant intraepithelial neoplasm (see Chapter 3, Premalignant and Malignant Tumors of the Vulva). In a recent report of vulvar squamous cell carcinoma, 61% had lichen sclerosus. Forty-three of the 47 cases with lichen sclerosus were not recognized to have vulvar lichen sclerosus until the time of the tumor diagnosis.[133a] In a prospective study of 350 women with lichen sclerosus, Ridley et al. observed the subsequent occurrence of vulvar squamous cell carcinoma in 3.5% of the patients.[154,201] Aneuploidy by flow cytometry has been reported in 4 of 17 cases of lichen sclerosus.[167] In cases where lichen sclerosus is associated with vulvar squamous cell carcinoma, squamous cell hyperplasia usually is observed adjacent to the carcinoma.[205]

Women with lichen sclerosus required continued therapy and follow-up because, although it is not a disease that requires vulvectomy or is cured by local excision or ablative treatment, such as laser therapy or cryotherapy, over time it is associated with a small but significant risk of vulvar carcinoma in postmenopausal women. In these cases, tumor development occurs in the field of lichen sclerosus, and typically is associated with visible tumor or hyperplastic changes that indicate biopsy to establish the diagnosis of tumor. With improved therapy, it is expected that the frequency of tumor may be decreased.

Squamous Cell Hyperplasia (Formerly Hyperplastic Dystrophy)

General Features

Squamous cell hyperplasia is an epithelial disorder characterized by acanthosis and variable hyperkeratosis without atypia, significant associated inflammation, or evidence of a specific dermatosis. Squamous cell hyperplasia is a descriptive term applicable both clinically and histologically to an epithelial thickening of the vulva that cannot be otherwise specifically classified. It is considered to be a nonspecific response of the genital skin to a wide variety of irritants. Squamous cell hyperplasia is typically found in adult women, most commonly occurring in women between 30 and 60 years of age. There is no racial predilection. Clinically, the most common presenting complaint is pruritus confined to a focal area on the vulva that usually can be pointed to by the patient.

Gross Findings

The involved vulvar area usually is not symmetrical, as is often seen with lichen sclerosus, and may be confined to a focal area, usually involving the labia majora. The involved area appears gray-white, or reddened with adjacent gray-white epithelium. The skin markings often are accentuated, a sign of intradermal edema; excoriations and fissures frequently bear witness to the intensity of the itching. There is no shrinkage, stenosis, or agglutination of the labia, as occurs in lichen sclerosus. The condition is clinically indistinguishable from what has previously been called *neurodermatitis* or *eczema*.

Microscopic Findings

The histopathological features of squamous cell hyperplasia are epithelial thickening with acanthosis. Hyperkeratosis and parakeratosis may be present. There typically is no significant inflammatory infiltrate, although some lymphocytes may be seen in the superficial dermis. There is no significant dermal fibrosis or thickening. The changes are otherwise nonspecific and the diagnosis is arrived at by exclusion of other dermatoses (Fig. 2.21). The individual squamous cells are regular with distinct intercellular bridges. The nuclei are round to oval and contain finely

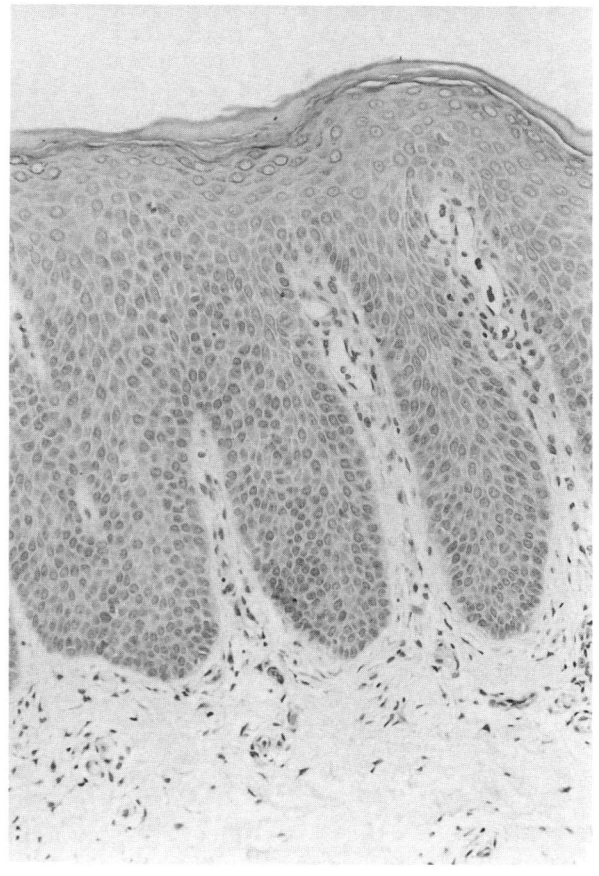

Fig. 2.21. Squamous cell hyperplasia. Epithelial thickening with acanthosis and mild hyperkeratosis is evident. No nuclear atypia is present and no dermal fibrosis or thickening is identified within the superficial dermis. There is no significant inflammation.

distributed chromatin. Nucleoli may be prominent; however, there is progressive maturation of the cells as they approach the superficial layers. Mitotic figures, if present, are normal and confined to the basal layer. Hyperkeratosis may be seen associated with accentuation of the granular layer. Although parakeratosis may be present in otherwise typical areas of hyperplasia, its presence should prompt a careful search for cellular atypia, and VIN of the differentiated type (see Vulvar Intraepithelial Neoplasia in Chapter 3). In the absence of atypia or lichen sclerosus, there is no evidence of risk of carcinoma from this process. The diagnosis of squamous hyperplasia is one of exclusion. The differential diagnosis includes lichen simplex chronicus, fungal infection, human papillomavirus infection, and VIN (see differential under Lichen Simplex Chronicus).

Clinical Behavior and Treatment

Treatment is based on limiting or preventing exposure of the vulva to potential irritants in conjunction with the use of topical corticosteroids and antipruritics. Symptoms usually abate within 2–3 weeks.[36] Occasionally, local excision or laser ablation of the hyperplastic area may be effective in unresponsive cases.

The significance of squamous cell hyperplasia found adjacent to squamous cell carcinoma, as seen in approximately 50% of women with vulvar carcinoma, is not well understood. In some cases, there is associated lichen sclerosus or VIN.[205]

Lichen Simplex Chronicus

Lichen simplex chronicus (LSC) has been considered to be equivalent to squamous cell hyperplasia by some dermatopathologists.[184] The microscopic diagnosis of lichen simplex chronicus, however, includes the finding of a superficial dermal chronic inflammatory infiltrate with collagenization of the superficial dermis immediately beneath the epidermis (Fig. 2.22). The treatment is essentially the same as for squamous cell hyperplasia.

Differential Diagnosis

The differential diagnosis of squamous cell hyperplasia and LSC includes chronic candidiasis or dermatophyte infection of the vulva that usually can be differentiated by a silver stain for fungus or periodic acid-Schiff (PAS) stain for the organisms. The fungal organisms usually are present in the keratin layer. The finding of inflammatory exocytosis, with acute inflammatory cells within the epithelium, is a clue that fungal infection may be a factor. Regressing or early flat condylomata acuminata also may resemble LSC or squamous cell hyperplasia; however, the prominent granular layer, accentuated intracellular

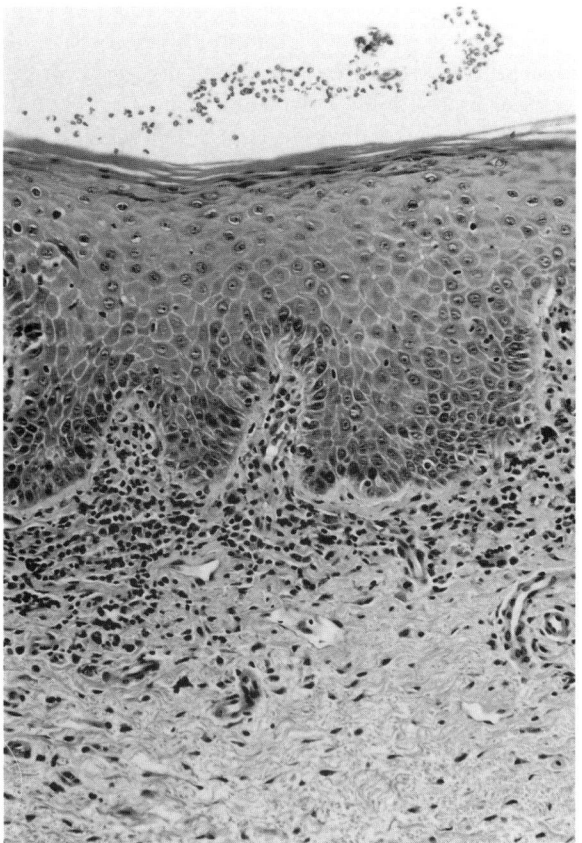

FIG. 2.22. Lichen simplex chronicus. The epithelium is slightly thickened; however, no hyperkeratosis is present. Within the superficial dermis there is a prominent chronic inflammatory cell infiltrate. In this example, there is minimal fibrosis within the superficial dermis.

bridges, parabasalar hyperplasia, and koilocytosis typically are lacking. If this cannot be resolved by histopathological examination, molecular biologic methods, such as PCR or in situ hybridization (to detect HPV) may be helpful in establishing the diagnosis of HPV-associated changes when virus is identified. Psoriasis or lichen planus may be included in the differential diagnosis; however, they represent distinct entities that are clinically and histologically identifiable.

Other Dermatoses

Lichen Planus

GENERAL FEATURES

Lichen planus (LP) has a wide age distribution; however, it presents most commonly in women over 40 years of age.[62,146,180] Vulvar pruritis and burning are common symptoms; however, the patient may be asymptomatic. White, lace-like plaques involving the oral and vaginal mucosa also may be present. Involvement of all three sites is referred to as the *vulvo-vaginal-gingival syndrome* reported by Pelisse. The syndrome is recognized as an erosive form of LP.[180] Patients with this condition experience vulvar pain, dyspareunia, and burning. Postcoital bleeding also has been reported.[180] LP can result in severe introital and vaginal adhesions, scarring, and stenosis.

GROSS FINDINGS

The clinical appearance may be highly variable on the vulva, ranging from delicate reticulated papules to an erosive desquamative process involving the vagina and vulva. Within the vulva, the erosive process is typically confined to the vulvar vestibule and commonly involves the vagina. With advancing disease, there is loss and agglutination of the labia minora and prepuce, associated with thinned epithelium, postinflammatory hypopigmentation, and shrinkage with stenosis of the vaginal introitus. In advanced stages, it may be difficult to distinguish LP from advanced lichen sclerosus (LS). Vaginal involvement with adhesions and synechiae clinically characterizes LP, as does the finding of mucous membrane lesions outside the vulva.

MICROSCOPIC FINDINGS

The histopathological features may be highly variable depending on the age of the lesion as well as its location. Mucous membrane lesions may differ considerably from those occurring on vulvar skin.[134] In the skin there are two important microscopic features: a band-like chronic inflammatory infiltrate that is predominantly lymphocytic, with no or rare plasma cells. The inflammation is lichenoid, involving the upper dermis and immediate overlying epidermis (Fig. 2.23). Liquification necrosis of the basal epithelial cells is seen and these cells typically are admixed with chronic inflammatory cells. Degenerated keratinocytes result in colloid body formation. Within the vulvar skin, the involved epithelium may show acanthosis and hyperkeratosis. Immunofluorescent studies usually are not contributory. The epithelial changes are variable within mucous membranes and include thinning of the epithelium, with ulceration and bullous formation. In contrast to the findings within the skin, plasma cells may be evident with mucosal involvement.

DIFFERENTIAL DIAGNOSIS

LS can be distinguished from LP by the absence of the lichenoid inflammatory infiltrate at the dermal–epidermal junction in LS. Colloid bodies also are common in LP. LP typically involves mucosal as well as nonmucosal sites, whereas LS does not involve the vagina or oral mucosa. In advanced cases, mucosal involvement may be the most important distinguishing feature.

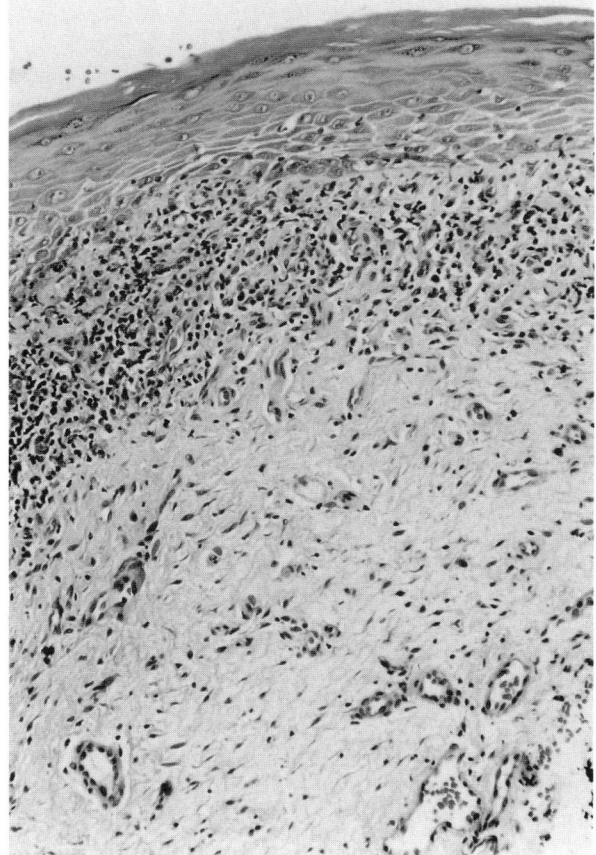

Fig. 2.23. Lichen planus. The epithelium is somewhat thinned with loss of rete ridges. A prominent granular layer is evident without significant hyperkeratosis in this example. There is a prominent band-like chronic inflammatory infiltrate consisting almost entirely of lymphocytes, which is lichenoid and involves the basal layer. Liquification necrosis of the basal cells with colloid body formation is evident. (Courtesy of J. L. Thomasen, M.D., Milwaukee, WI.)

Cicatricial pemphigoid and LP may both cause scarring and stenosis of the vulvar vestibule and vagina. Lichen planus has the characteristic lichenoid inflammatory pattern with colloid bodies within the epithelium. Cicatricial pemphighoid forms subepithelial blisters and a positive Nikotsky sign is present clinically. Immunofluorescence demonstrates linear IgA deposits, which are absent in LP.

Morphea (scleroderma) may be included in the differential diagnosis in that a band-like chronic inflammatory infiltrate may be seen with epithelial thinning; however, the subepithelial edema with interdermal inflammation, as seen in LS, typically is not seen in morphea. Morphea usually involves other sites, especially the back. Unlike LP, the inflammation in morphea typically is perivascular and deep within the dermis. Lymphocytic infiltrates are seen about the skin adnexa. Sclerosus of the dermis results in dermal thickening and loss of fat about skin appendages, as well as loss of skin appendages.

CLINICAL BEHAVIOR AND TREATMENT

Adhesion formation can lead to scarring and agglutination of the labia minora.[62] Topical cortical steroids are the usual form of treatment; fluorinated corticosteroids may be needed initially to provide relief. Additional therapy may include topical and/or oral cyclosporine, oral dapsone, and oral griseofulvin.[63]

Psoriasis

Psoriasis is inherited as a simple autosomal dominant trait with incomplete penetrance. Psoriasis affects approximately 2% of the population of the United States. On the vulva, the disease typically involves the lateral aspects of the labia majora and genitocrural areas.[201] The lesions present as silvery-topped erythematous papules. When this loose silvery scale is removed, several punctate bleeding points can be seen (Auspitz sign). Coalescence of papules results in plaque formation. The lesions frequently are symmetric and may persist for years. At times, new psoriatic lesions develop at sites of trauma within 7–30 days after the trauma. This is referred to as *Koebner phenomenon*.

Histological findings include hyperkeratosis, parakeratosis, uniform acanthosis (elongation of the rete ridges to an even length), diminution of the granular layer, and collections of polymorphonuclear leukocytes within the epidermis (Munro abscesses) (Fig. 2.24). Mitotic activity increases within the epidermis, reflecting the significantly increased rate of epithelial turnover. The dermal papillae are clubbed and edematous. Prominent vessels are seen within the papillae, and there is a minimal chronic inflammatory cell infiltrate with the dermis.[134,185]

Contact Dermatitis

Vulvar contact dermatitis may be of an allergic type, which is a cell-mediated response to sensitizing agents such as nickel or rubber, or an irritant related to exposure to chemical or physical agents that damage the skin. Urinary incontinence is a common cause of irritation. Irritant dermatitis is the more common of the two. The lesions typically are confined to the area of exposure and usually persist for some time after the exposure.[183]

The pathological findings may be quite variable, depending on the severity and duration of the process and whether or not there is an associated allergic response. The most constant histopathological findings are epidermal intracellular edema with microvesiculation. The superficial perivascular inflammatory response consists predominantly of lymphocytes and histiocytes; eosinophils may be present. Superficial erosion or ulceration may be present and in long-standing contact dermatitis, epithelial thickening with parakeratosis and hyperkeratosis also occurs.

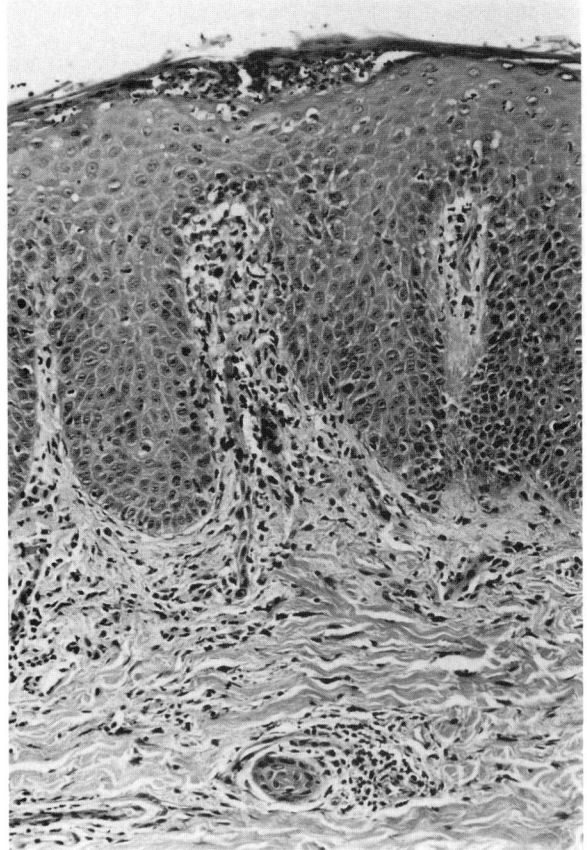

Fig. 2.24. Psoriasis. Prominent uniform acanthosis is present. A superficial intraepidermal abscess (Munro abscess) is evident. The dermal papillae are clubbed and infiltrated by chronic inflammatory cells.

Fixed Drug Eruption (Dermatitis Medicamentosa)

Fixed drug eruptions constitute a complex group of cutaneous manifestations of drug allergic reactions that are subclassified as Types I through IV. Type I is mediated through IgE antibodies and usually presents as urticaria. Type II is mediated through IgG and IgM antibodies and may be manifested as drug purpura or a bullous drug eruption. Type III is related to immune complexes and may be expressed as a maculopapular eruption, exanthem, urticaria, and/or vasculitis. Type IV is cell mediated and may manifest as contact dermatitis, an exanthem, and/or a maculopapular eruption. The histopathological findings may be suggestive or supportive of a fixed drug eruption. Skin or patch testing, indirect and direct Coombs tests, and other specific laboratory testing, as well as a detailed clinical history, are necessary to diagnose precisely, such cases.[162]

Atopic Dermatitis

Women with atopic dermatitis may have involvement of the vulva, with associated pruritis and burning.[183] The physical findings may be limited to dryness and scaling, but thickening of the skin with localized excoriations may be evident if the vulva has been irritated by scratching.

Vulvar biopsies are rarely performed on these patients and the pathological findings often are that of squamous cell hyperplasia, or are nonspecific. Histopathological features include epidermal edema with spongiosis. Within the dermis, lymphocytes and macrophages are present and the density of the infiltrate tends to correlate with the severity and chronicity of the process. Eosinophils and basophils also may be identified. Immunofluorescent studies have demonstrated IgE on epidermal Langerhan cells.[26]

Plasma Cell Vulvitis (Vulvitis of Zoon)

This type of vulvitis usually presents with symptoms of pruritus and burning. It is characterized by erythematous macules that usually have focal hemorrhagic areas. The lesions may be multiple.[183] On microscopic examination the epithelium is thinned, with flattening of rete ridges and lack of a granular layer or keratinized surface. Parabasal keratinocytes have a horizontal orientation with marked spongiosis. The inflammatory infiltrate is lichenoid in type, consisting predominantly of plasma cells. Prominent dermal blood vessels are evident with associated intradermal hemorrhage and hemosiderin.[223] The differential diagnosis includes syphilis, because of the perivascular plasma cell infiltrate, as well as lichen planus and other chronic dermatosis. The etiology is unknown; however, local irritation and poor hygiene may be contributing factors. Perineal hygiene, supportive care, and topical corticosteroids are the usual treatment.

Fox–Fordyce Disease

Fox–Fordyce disease is a disorder of the apocrine glands; 90% of cases occur in women. The disease generally begins at puberty and presents as a pruritic papular eruption usually involving the axillae, vulva, and perianal regions.

On microscopic examination, the center of the papule often contains a hair follicle and apocrine sweat gland duct plugged by keratin. There may be an associated rupture of the interepithelial portion of the duct with subsequent vesicle formation within the epidermis. These vesicles cannot be seen unless serial sections are performed.[105] Chronic inflammatory changes are present in the dermis and there is dilatation of the apocrine gland acini (Fig. 2.25). In addition, there is epidermal acanthosis and spongiosis. Deposition of mucin may be found in the ducts, glands, and tissues surrounding the skin appendages.

Fox–Fordyce disease is a chronic condition that may progress somewhat during pregnancy or after menopause; however, no definite therapy is known. In women of reproductive age, oral contraceptives may relieve symptoms and reduce somewhat the severity of the process. Systemic antibiotics and topical, as well as locally injected corticos-

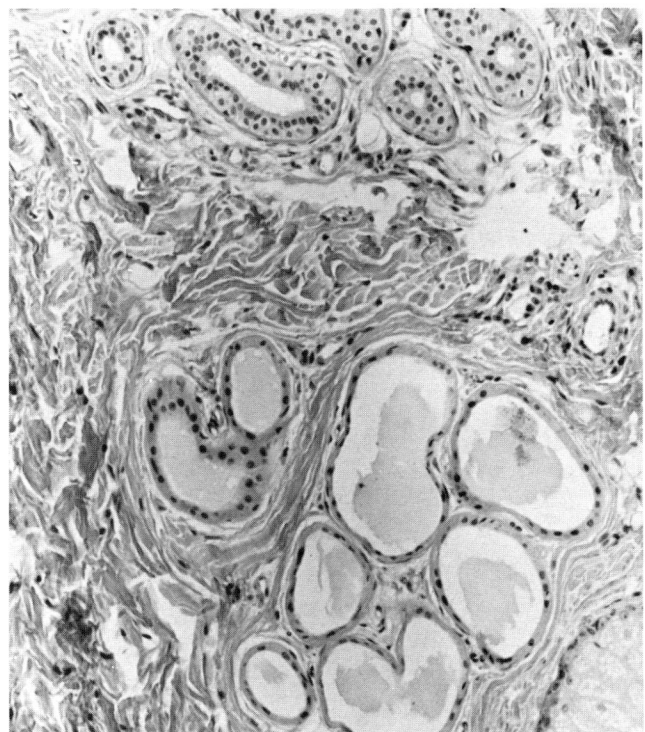

FIG. 2.25. **Fox–Fordyce disease.** Dilated apocrine glands show inspissated secretion.

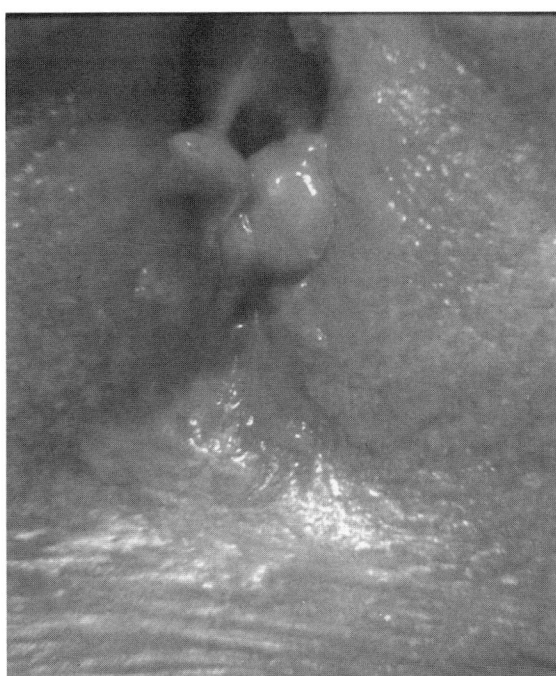

FIG. 2.26. **Vulvar vestibulitis.** Marked inflammation is present adjacent and external to the hymenal ring. Point tenderness was present over these areas. (See color insert.)

teroids and antipruritics, relieve symptoms. Hidradenitis suppurativa as well as folliculitis may complicate the clinical course.

Vulvar Vestibulitis (Vulvar Vestibular Syndrome)

GENERAL FEATURES

Vulvar vestibulitis is a clinical disorder of unknown etiology associated with inflammation of the vulvar vestibule, severe vestibular tenderness to pressure, and entry dyspareunia. This condition is characterized clinically by slight edema of the hymen and redness around the gland openings in the vestibule, with marked "pin point" tenderness to pressure[252,253] (Fig. 2.26; see color insert). Bacterial, chlamydial, and viral studies from affected areas have not supported an infectious etiology.[78,155]

Vulvar vestibulitis is a clinical complex that represents part of a spectrum of vulvar pain–related disorders. Chronic candidiasis, as well as vulvar papillomatosis, may be associated with dyspareunia and vulvar pain. A number of vulvar dermatoses may cause vulvar pain. In addition, there is a condition described as essential vulvodynia that is of unknown etiology and is a diagnosis of exclusion.[155]

MICROSCOPIC FINDINGS

Histopathological features include areas of mild to moderate inflammatory response, characterized by a superficial chronic inflammatory infiltrate that is composed predominantly of lymphocytes (Fig. 2.27). Approximately two-thirds of the cases also have plasma cells within the infiltrate. Polymorphonuclear leukocytes and eosinophils are rare. The stromal tissue beneath the vestibular epithelium is involved most prominently and the minor vestibular glands may be surrounded by the inflammatory process (Fig. 2.5). Inflammatory cells occasionally are found within the glandular epithelium or within the acini or ductal lumina. These patients rarely have clinically or morphologically evident condyloma acuminatum or VIN.[189,247]

ADJUNCTIVE METHODS

Studies for HPV employing PCR have demonstrated that HPV is rarely detected in the vestibular epithelium in these cases; HPV types 6, 11, 16, and 18 are infrequently identified, with HPV type 11 being found in two, and HPV 16 in 1 of 32 patients in one study.[247] The finding of these HPV types is similar to what has been identified in control groups.[247] Although there have been studies suggesting some association, normal flora, background contamination, and lack of control groups limit interpretation.[147,235] Currently, there is no evidence linking HPV with vestibulitis.

CLINICAL BEHAVIOR AND THERAPY

The natural history of vulvar vestibulitis is poorly understood and no long-term controlled prospective studies have

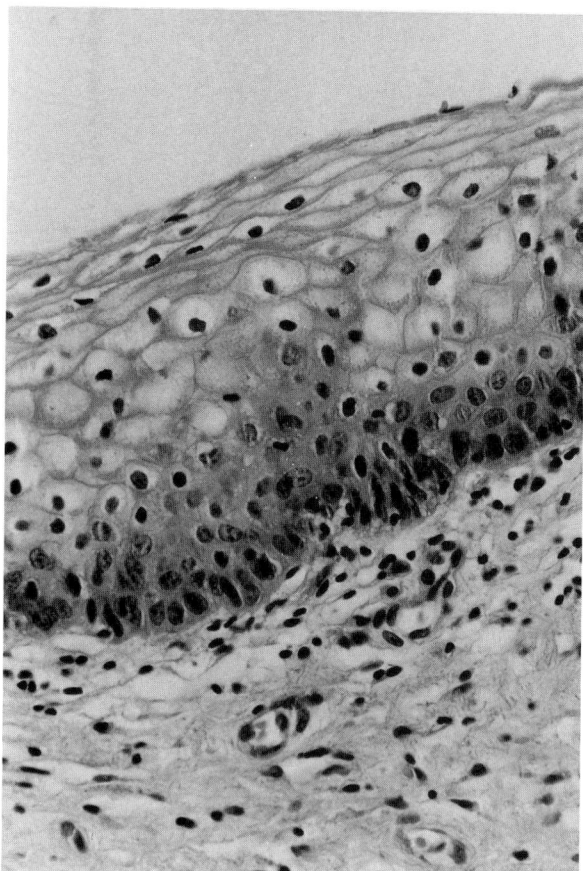

FIG. 2.27. **Vulvar vestibulitis.** The epithelium is nonkeratinized and glycogen rich in this case. The perinuclear clearing is typical and not representative of HPV effect (PCR for HPV was negative in this case). There is a mild superficial chronic inflammatory cell infiltrate that consists predominantly of lymphocytes (see Fig. 2.5).

been reported to date. Many of these patients move from physician to physician seeking relief. Local excision of the vestibule has been advocated; however, the recurrence rate, with follow-up up to 5 years, reveals that recurrent symptoms after surgery is relatively common, occurring in more than one-half the cases in some series. Antibiotics produce no response, nor can the symptoms be alleviated by corticosteroids. Nonvaporization laser ablation of the superficial submucosal ectatic blood vessels has been proposed, especially in cases having recurrent symptoms after surgery.[149] Interferon has been advocated with some response; however, long-term follow-up data after such therapy currently is not available.[149] A number of additional topical treatments have been suggested, including topical testosterone. More than one-half of these patients initially will obtain some relief from topical therapy. Management is long term and supportive; clinical studies are ongoing.

Vulvitis Granulomatosa

This cutaneous granulomatous process, resembling cheilitis granulomatosa Miescher–Melkersson–Rosenthal syn-

drome, is of unknown etiology and rarely involves the vulva.[97] Clinically, the labia majora are indurated, swollen, and erythematous without tenderness. The labia minora, as well as the perineum and perianal areas, also may be involved. Mild regional lymphadenopathy typically is present. The process remains localized but is slowly progressive.

Histopathological findings include a chronic granulomatous inflammatory infiltrate composed of histiocytes and giant cells, as well as lymphocytes and plasma cells. The infiltrate involves the dermis and extends to the epithelium. The differential diagnosis includes other granulomatous inflammatory processes.[97]

Factitial Vulvitis

Factitial vulvitis is uncommon but may present as a chronic inflammatory process, often with associated superficial ulceration. In such cases the pathological findings often are nonspecific. The ulcers typically are superficial with minimal inflammation.[183] The correct diagnosis may become apparent after a detailed clinical history, usually after numerous studies and repeat visits to the clinician have been made.

Behçet Syndrome

Behçet syndrome refers to the triad of oral ulcers, genital ulcers, and ophthalmologic inflammation.[101] Ocular changes may be absent in mild cases. Other findings include acne, cutaneous nodules, thrombophlebitis, encephalopathy, and colitis.[169] Behçet syndrome causes deep ulcerations on the vulva that may result in fenestration of the labia and lead to gangrene of the labia. The ulcerations characteristically heal and relapse, and are associated with simultaneous oral ulcers.

Histologically, necrotizing arteritis frequently is seen and can be considered a cardinal pathological finding. A chronic inflammatory infiltrate may be perivascular or involve the vessel wall with homogenization of the arterial media. Endothelial cell swelling also occurs and may result in arteriolar occlusion, as well as venous thrombosis.

Crohn Disease

Crohn disease is a chronic noncaseating granulomatous disease of unknown etiology that can involve, besides the gastrointestinal tract, the vulva and perineum in adults and children.[233] Cutaneous ulcerations occur in areas where there is close apposition of skin, such as the vulva and submammary areas. When Crohn disease involves the vulva, the resulting ulcers often are slit-like, multiple, deep, and secondarily infected. Vulvar and perianal erythema, induration, and/or ulceration may be the presenting signs of Crohn disease.[129,179] Involvement of the colon, rectum, or small bowel is not always present when the vulva is involved. Perianal fistulas, as well as fistulas to other sites in the female genital tract, are complications of Crohn disease. When perianal draining sinuses and abscesses occur, they often drain a fluid resembling small bowel contents.

Microscopically, the disease is characterized by a noncaseating granulomatous inflammation within the dermis, which usually is deep and associated with fissures and sinus tracts. Studies for acid-fast bacteria and fungi are negative. A marked granulation tissue response frequently is seen surrounding the ulcers but significant lymphadenitis is rare.

Pyoderma Gangrenosum

Pyoderma gangrenosum is a progressive necrotic and ulcerative condition of the skin, of uncertain etiology. Most case reports of pyoderma gangrenosum occur on the legs and are associated with chronic ulcerative colitis. Pyoderma gangrenosum of the vulva may present some time after treatment for colitis, ileostomy, or abdominal perineal resection of the colon and rectum. The microscopic findings reveal epithelial ulceration with severe acute and chronic inflammation. If the biopsy is from the ulcer edge, the sharply demarcated ulcer is adjacent to hyperplastic squamous epithelium. Organisms are not identified within the inflammatory process. Systemic corticosteroid therapy usually is effective. Wide local excision, with skin grafting, may be necessary.[256]

Necrotizing Fasciitis (Includes Synergistic Bacterial Infection)

Postoperative, post-traumatic, or necrotizing fasciitis is a life-threatening infection that usually is secondary to a polymicrobial infection that may develop after episiotomy or other types of vaginal, vulvar, or abdominal surgery.[4,226,229] Diabetes mellitus predisposes to necrotizing fasciitis.[4] The clinical presentation is that of a rapidly progressing inflammatory process that may initially appear as mild cellulitis or edema with inflammation. Delay in diagnosis without therapy carries a nearly 50% mortality. Prompt radical excision of the infected tissue and broad spectrum systemic antibiotic therapy offers the only chance of cure.[226]

Hidradenitis Suppurativa

Hidradenitis suppurativa is a chronic inflammatory disorder of the apocrine glands.[232] Deep-seated, painful, subcutaneous nodules are found in areas containing apocrine glands, especially the axilla and vulva. The lesions commonly progress subcutaneously, producing confluent masses that subsequently ulcerate the epidermis and result in draining sinuses and extensive scarring. The condition may co-exist with Fox–Fordyce disease. Total excision of involved areas may be necessary in advanced cases, although laser ablation and unroofing the sinuses has been reported as effective.[217,232] Histologically, in the early stages hidradenitis suppurativa demonstrates a perifolliculis with an acute and chronic infiltrate within the dermis. The later stages of the disease result in destruction of the epithelial appendages with sinus tract formation[134] (Fig. 2.28).

Acute Idiopathic Vulvar Ulcer

An acute, single, painful ulcer of the medial portion of the labia minora has been described in women within 24 hours of coitus.[23] Evaluation of these ulcerations shows no causative agent to date, and they most probably are traumatic.

Mites and Lice

A variety of mites are capable of producing local and limited chronic skin infections of the perineal area, including scabies.[100] Mites must be specifically considered, because they are not demonstrable by the usual skin-scraping or culture techniques.[100,165] Mites are small arachnids and

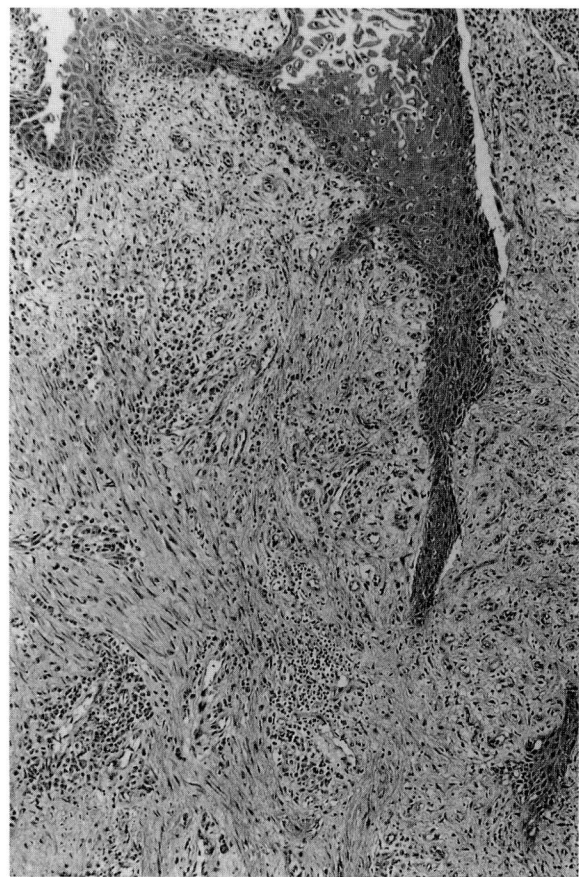

Fig. 2.28. Hidradenitis supprativa. There is a severe acute and chronic inflammatory cell infiltrate within the dermis with involvement and destruction of the skin appendages. (Courtesy of N. Sisson Hardt, M.D., Gainesville, FL.)

belong to the order Acarina. They differ from lice, which are insects. Mites have a fused head and thorax, devoid of primary segmentation, and four pairs of legs. Mites burrow within the epidermis, inducing severe pruritus. The overt skin lesions are papular and, when examined under a magnifying lens, reveal an adjacent burrow. Scrapings from the burrow or specimens obtained from the patient's clothing can be fixed in an alcohol-ether-acetic acid-formalin mixture and analyzed microscopically for mites.

Lice are associated with irritation of the skin due to secondary infection of feeding sites. The pubic louse, *Phthirius pubis* of the class Insecta, is the usual offender and can be diagnosed by identifying the louse and nits on the hair shaft (Fig. 2.29).

Spider Bite

A brown recluse (*Loxosceles reclusa*) spider bite on the vulva has been reported, associated with a protracted ulceration and infection of the vulva. Although secondary infection may occur with such ulcers, slow and progressive healing over several months is the usual clinical course.[141]

Bullous Diseases

Although virtually any dermatologic disease can involve the vulva, the following bullous diseases bear discussion, as they may first be observed and biopsied by the gynecolo-

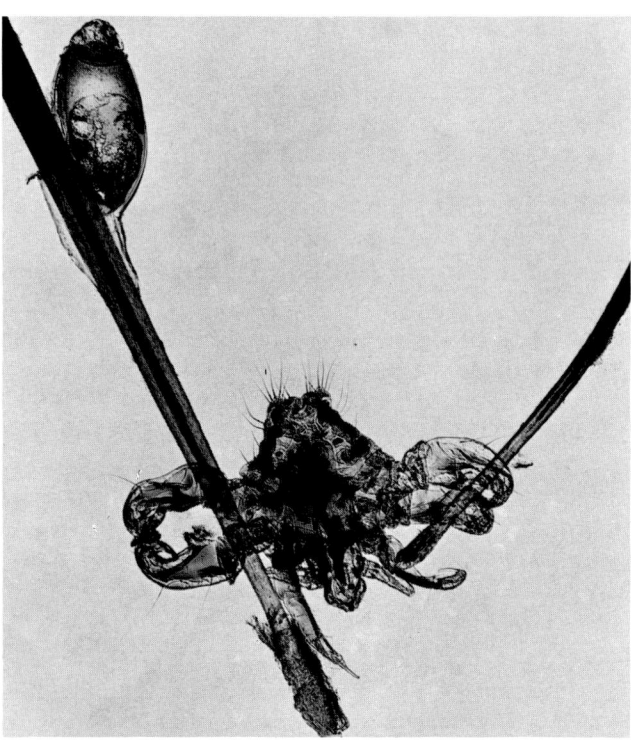

FIG. 2.29. Pubic louse with nit. Phthirius pubis clings, head down, to a hair shaft with attached egg.

gist. Definitive diagnosis of most bullous diseases requires clinical and pathological correlation, and in some cases the clinical findings are essential in distinguishing these cutaneous diseases that otherwise have very similar or identical histopathological findings. The key histopathological features and differential diagnosis of bullous and bullous-like diseases are summarized in Table 2.3.

Pemphigus (Pemphigus Vulgaris)

Pemphigus vulgaris initially may present on the vulva as recurrent superficial ulcers and erosions. Associated oral lesions usually are present in these patients, and rectal lesions also may occur.[183] The disease is life-threatening and biopsy of a fresh vulvar vesicle of ulceration usually is diagnostic. Microscopic findings include acantholysis with intraepithelial, suprabasal vesicle formation (Fig. 2.30) (Table 2.3). Direct immunofluorescent studies demonstrate IgG deposited on the epithelial intercellular substance. Circulating antibodies to epithelial intracellular components can be detected and are valuable in diagnosis. Therapy includes high doses of corticosteroids and supportive measures.

Pemphigus Vegitans

This variant of pemphigus may present as a localized, indurated, inflamed area with vesicles. The pathological as well as immunofluorescent and immunologic findings are similar to pemphigus vulgaris, although eosinophils are a prominent component of the inflammatory infiltrate.[183] The presence of eosinophils, as well as the localized and self-limited character of the disease, distinguish it from pemphigus.

Pemphigoid (Bullous Pemphigoid)

Pemphigoid can involve the vulva and is characterized by moist, tender ulcers that involve the labia minora, majora, and perianal areas. At times, fluid-filled bullae also are present. Biopsies of fresh ulcers, including normal adjacent skin, typically show the characteristic subepidermal bullae (Fig. 2.31) (Table 2.3). In advanced stages, biopsy of ulcerated areas may show only granulation tissue.

Cicatricial pemphigoid that, unlike pemphigoid, results in scarring and stenosis has been reported involving the vulva secondary to drug hypersensitivity.[238] The disease prevents as erosions, erythema, and small blisters of the vulva, perianal, and anal mucosa, associated with chronic burning pain and painful ulcers. The origin of the recurrent scarring of the vulva may not be apparent until the presentation of ocular involvement secondary to cicatricial pemphigoid.[84] Severe cicatrization with shrinkage, suggesting advanced vulvar lichen sclerosus, or lichen planus, characterizes the process. In contrast to lichen sclerosus or lichen planus, cicatricial pemphigoid is associated with

Table 2.3. Differential diagnosis of vesicular bullous and bullous-like diseases of the vulva

Disease	*Location of vesicle* Subepidermal	*Location of vesicle* Intraepidermal suprabasal	Acantholysis of suprabasal cells	Significant systemic manifestations	Immunofluorescent localization
Pemphigus vulgaris	No	Yes	Yes	Yes	IgG Intercellular
Pemphigus vegitans	No	Yes	Yes	No	IgG Intercellular
Pemphigoid (bullous) (cicatricial pemphigoid)	Yes	No	No	Yes, localized scarring (sometimes debilitating)	IgG linear along basement membrane IgA, IgM, C_3, C_5 may be in basement membrane
Herpes gestationis	Yes	No	No	Yes	C_3 Linear along basement membrane. IgG may also be present. IgM, IgA is rare
Polymorphic eruption of pregnancy, pruritic urticarial plaques and papules in pregnancy (PUPPP)	Yes	No	No	Yes	Negative
Darier disease	No	Yes	Yes, 3+ dyskeratosis	Yes	Negative
Warty dyskeratoma	No	Yes	Yes	No	Negative
Erythema multiforme (Stevens–Johnson syndrome)	No	Yes, necrotic keratinocytes, Hydropic degeneration of basal keratinocytes	No	Yes	IgM Complement in and about superficial dermal vessels in some cases
Hailey–Hailey	No	Yes	Yes, 4+ No dyskeratosis	No	Negative
Localized acantholytic disease of the vulva	No	Yes	Yes	No	Negative
Benign chronic bullous disease of childhood (linear IgA disease)	Yes	No	Microabscesses in dermal papillae	No, flu-like symptoms may precede presentation	IgA linear along basement membrane (C_3, IgA, IgG, IgM also may be present)
Dermatitis herpetiformis	Yes	No	No	No, Severe pruritus in some cases	IgA deposits in the tips of dermal papillae and/or along the basement membrane

small blisters and a positive Nikolsky phenomenon (slippage and detachment of the superficial epidermis from the underlying dermis when the examining finger is slid over the skin surface).

Microscopically, there is subepithelial blister formation with a mixed inflammatory cell infiltrate within the dermis (Fig. 2.31). Direct immunofluorescence demonstrates linear IgG, and occasionally complement C3 and C5, along the basement membrane. Immunoglobulins IgA and IgM may or may not be present[224,238] (Table 2.3). Systemic or topical corticosteroids may be of value. If the condition is drug related, the offending medication should be discontinued.

Herpes Gestationis

This vesiculobullous disease is unique to pregnant women, with an estimated incidence of approximately 0.6 per 100,000 pregnancies. Presenting signs and symptoms often are severe pruritus and a macular erythematous rash that leads to blistering and superficial ulcerations. The lesions may involve the vulva and pubic area in addition to the anterior abdomen and chest. Involvement of the extremities is less common. The process usually presents in the second trimester and spontaneous regression follows soon after delivery, although regression may occur in the late third trimester.

Histopathological findings include a subepidermal blister that may contain eosinophils, lymphocytes, and histiocytes. There is a perivascular superficial dermal inflammatory infiltrate that also is rich in lymphocytes and eosinophils. Immunofluorescent studies demonstrate C3 as a linear basement membrane deposit (Table 2.3). Approximately one-quarter of the cases also have immunoglobulin deposition within the basement membrane. Serologic studies demonstrate circulating complement-fixing IgG antibodies in most cases.

The main differential diagnosis is polymorphic eruption

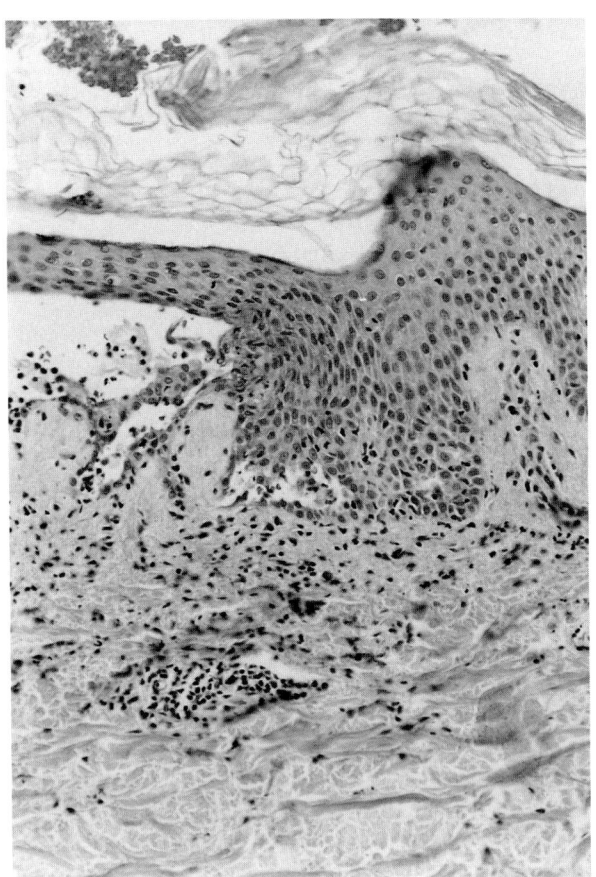

2.30

Fig. 2.30. Pemphigus (pemphigus vulgaris). Suprabasal vesicle formation is evident with prominent acantholysis. A small suprabasal acantholytic area is present in the rete, adjacent to the larger vesicle.

Fig. 2.31. Bullous pemphigoid. A subepidermal bullae is evident, with intact epithelium separated from the underlying dermis. An intense inflammatory infiltrate of lymphocytes, neutrophils, and eosinophils is seen within the dermis with some inflammatory cells within the bullae.

of pregnancy, which typically presents in the late third trimester and may have essentially the same histopathological findings.[113] In contrast to herpes gestationis, the immunofluorescent studies are uniformly negative in polymorphic eruption of pregnancy (Table 2.3). Prurigo of pregnancy and pruritic folliculitis of pregnancy may be included in the differential of dermatosis associated with pregnancy but are not bullous diseases.[102,156]

Darier Disease (Keratosis Follicularis)

Darier disease is inherited as an autosomal dominant trait, although spontaneous cases also may occur. Patients present anytime after late childhood. The disease frequently involves the vulva. Although it usually is not con-

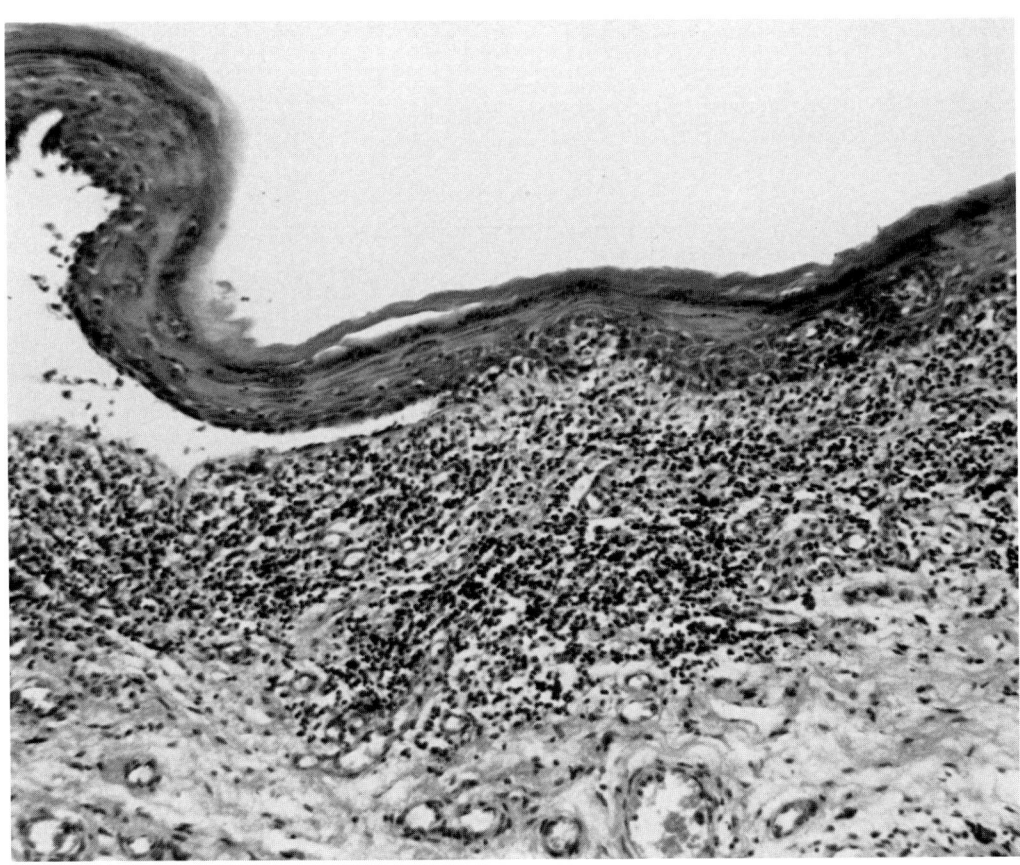

2.31

sidered a bullous disease, it is listed herein because a bullous microscopic appearance is a relatively common observation. On clinical examination, the lesions are crusted, hyperkeratotic papules that often appear darker than the surrounding skin. The papules may be secondarily infected.[134,201]

Histologically, acantholysis of the suprabasal epithelial cells results in clefts that extend from the basal layer through the granular layer. Acantholytic cells are seen within the clefts. Corps ronds and nuclear grains can be found in the graular layer and individual cell keratinization may be present, reflecting dyskeratosis (Table 2.3). Hyperkeratosis, acanthosis, and papillomatosis are seen along with keratotic plugs. Rarely, epithelial basal cell budding into the adjacent dermis may be seen. The inflammatory cell infiltration within the dermis usually is minimal, unless the lesions are secondarily infected.[134] The main differential diagnosis is warty dyskeratoma, Hailey–Hailey disease, and localized acantholytic disease of the vulva (Table 2.3).

Warty Dyskeratoma

Warty dyskeratoma of the vulva typically presents with a histological picture essentially identical to Darier disease (Fig. 2.32). Distinguishing clinical features are that Darier disease usually is congenital, and carried as an autosomal dominant, whereas dyskeratoma is not (Table 2.3). Darier disease is multifocal and may involve the trunk and extremities as well as the face. Warty dyskeratoma, however, usually involves the head, neck, or vulva as a single lesion.[61]

Erythema Multiforme (Stevens–Johnson Syndrome)

Vulvar involvement has been reported in association with Stevens–Johnson syndrome, which is the severe form of erythema multiforme. Involvement of the mouth, eyes, and skin, with associated high fever and other systemic symptoms, characterizes the syndrome. This disease may be associated with herpes virus or mycoplasma infection, drug therapy, malignancy, or radiotherapy.

The histopathological features are complex, depending on the age of the lesion. Major features include necrotic keratinocytes with cellular edema and intraepithelial vesicle formation. Separation of the epithelium from the dermis is associated with hydropic degeneration of the basal keratinocytes (Table 2.3). Within the dermis there is a prominent chronic inflammatory infiltrate consisting of lymphocytes and histiocytes. Extravasated red blood cells may be present within the dermal inflammatory process, as well as within the epidermis. Intravascular complement and IgM deposition may be seen within the superficial dermal vessels by immunofluorescent staining.[156]

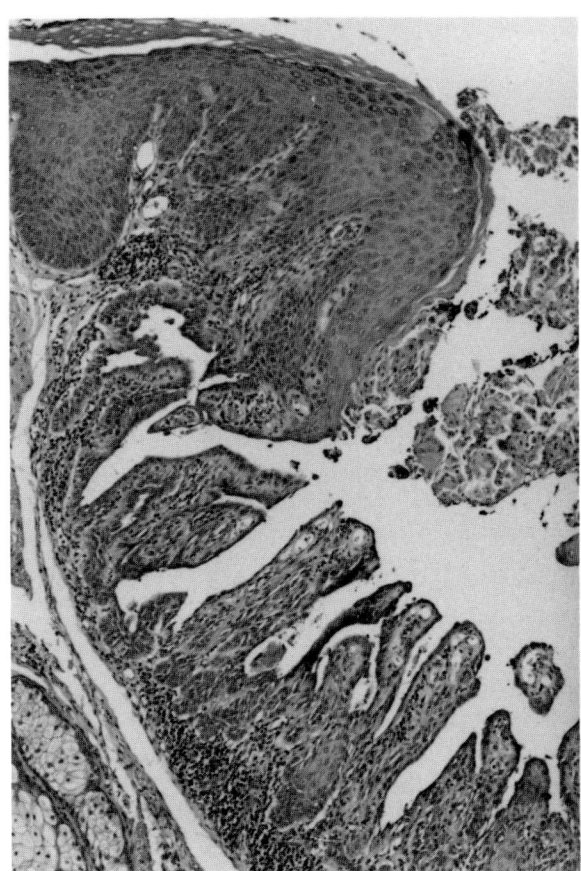

Fig. 2.32. **Warty dyskeratoma.** Acantholysis of the suprabasal epithelial cells, with intraepithelial clefts extending from the basal layer through the granular layer. Acantholytic cells are within the clefts and there is evidence of dyskeratosis. (Courtesy of David Dolson, M.D., Philadelphia, PA.)

There are case reports of "introital adenosis" occurring 1 to 3 years after the diagnosis of Stevens–Johnson syndrome, characterized clinically by erosions within the vulvar vestibule and medial aspects of the labia minora. On histopathological examination, glandular epithelium has been identified within these areas associated with submucosal inflammation.[22,150] The epithelium was described in one case as columnar epithelium of tubal-endometrial type, having secretory, ciliated, and intercalary type cells.[150] The term *mucinous metaplasia* of the vulva has been described for these changes, which are consistent with columnar cell metaplasia.[43]

Hailey–Hailey Disease (Familial Benign Pemphigus)

Hailey–Hailey disease is inherited as an autosomal dominant trait; approximately one-third of patients, however, have no family history of the disease. Onset of the disease often occurs during adolescence. Intertriginous areas usually are involved, but several cases in which the lesions are confined exclusively to the vulva have been reported.[231] The usual clinical presentation is of recurrent clusters of vesicles that develop, rupture, and result in crusted, moist papules that later coalesce to form plaques. Presentation as an isolated white plaque on the labia majora may occur.[65]

Histologically, there is acantholysis with resultant suprabasalar lacunae. Unlike Darier disease, vesicles and bullae also are found (Fig. 2.33) (Table 2.3). Acantholytic cells, which maintain their nuclear detail, can be seen within the vesicles and the acantholysis is more marked than in Darier disease. Basal cells maintain their orientation to the basement membrane. Rarely, corps ronds are seen in the granular layer. There is minimal, if any, dyskeratosis in Hailey–Hailey disease, in contrast to Darier disease. Strands of epidermal cells may proliferate into the dermis, but little dermal inflammatory infiltrate exists unless secondary infection is present.

Darier disease and Hailey–Hailey disease (familial benign pemphigus) must be distinguished not only from one another, but they also must be distinguished from pemphigus vulgaris, pemphigus vegetans, and warty dyskeratoma.[61,134] Table 2.3 summarizes the major distinguishing features.

Localized Acantholytic Disease of the Vulva

This disease of unknown etiology can involve the labia majora as well as the adjacent upper medial thighs. The lesions usually are papular and multiple, although solitary lesions may occur. The microscopic findings are characterized by acantholytic dyskeratosis or acantholysis alone (Table 2.3). Hyperkeratosis and papillomatosis may be present, as well as a mild perivascular lymphocytic infiltrate in the superficial dermis. The differential diagnosis includes Darier disease, Hailey–Hailey disease, and warty dyskeratoma. Excision is therapeutic and diagnostic in most cases.[45]

Benign Chronic Bullous Disease of Childhood (Linear IgA Disease)

This disease commonly involves the lower abdominal, pelvic, inguinal, and genital areas, presenting as clusters of annular lesions that usually are pruritic and typically evolve over the course of 24 hours. The annular lesions evolve to tense bullae that, if ruptured, ulcerate and become crusted. Patients may have fever and anorexia. In up to one-half the cases a bacterial or viral infection precedes the eruption.[250] Because of the location and striking and abrupt appearance of the lesions, they may be mistaken for evidence of child abuse.

Biopsy of an early bullous lesion reveals subepithelial vesicles that may contain granulocytes and eosinophils within the vesicular fluid. Microabscesses may occur within the epidermis. The diagnostic finding is the identification of a linear deposition of IgA in the basement membrane (Table 2.3). Other immunoglobulins and complement C3 also may be found.[250] The differential diagnosis includes dermatitis herpetiformis and bullous pemphigoid. Dermatitis herpetiformis is distinguished by having granular rather than linear IgA deposits, whereas bullous pemphigoid has linear IgG basement membrane deposits.[151] Therapy includes systemic corticosteroids, dapsone, and sulfapyridine.[250]

Depigmentation Disorders

Hypopigmented Conditions

The vulvar skin, especially that of the perineal body and lateral labia majora, in adult women usually is more pigmented than is the general body surface. Biopsies of the normal vulva show dendritic melanocytes scattered along

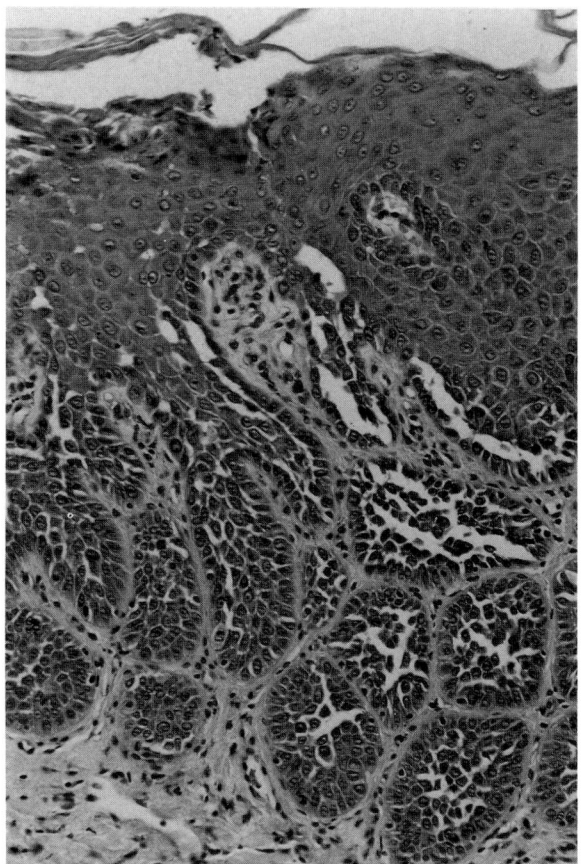

FIG. 2.33. Hailey-Hailey disease (benign familial pemphigus). Acantholysis is present in the suprabasal area and lower dermis. The mid- and upper epidermis remain intact, although some acantholysis is present.

the basal layer of the epithelium as well as squamous keratinocytes containing variable concentrations of melanin granules. Areas of the vulvar skin that appear hypopigmented therefore are clinically remarkable. There are three basic conditions that result in vulvar hypopigmentation: vitiligo, albinism, and postinflammatory depigmentation (leukoderma).

Vitiligo

Vitiligo is an inherited disorder in which the melanocytes are lost from areas of skin that were previously normally pigmented. This condition frequently affects the vulva, and biopsies from vitiliginous areas show a remarkable absence of both basilar melanocytes and melanin granules.

Albinism

Albinism, an inherited genetic disorder, is characterized by an inability of the melanocytes to produce pigment. There is an absence of melanin granules in the keratinocytes. Large pale cells may be present within the basal layer, representing incompetent melanocytes.

Postinflammatory Depigmentation (Leukoderma)

In areas of previous ulceration, recently healed skin will temporarily lack a normal population of melanocytes. Such postinflammatory depigmentation, or leukoderma, is common after herpes infection, syphilitic ulceration, burns, and deep laser or cryotherapy. Histologically, the skin appears thinned, metabolically active, and lacks the usual amount of pigment. On careful microscopic inspection, some melanin usually will be evident.

Pigment Disorders of Melanocytic Origin and Nevi

In a prospective study of 301 women, 37 (12%) were found to have a pigmented lesion of the vulva. Of these women, all were white and only 26% of the patients were aware that they had a pigmented lesion. More than 50% of the pigmented lesions were lengito simplex (lengitines), seven patients had nevi of which one had the histological features of a dysplastic nevus, five patients had postinflammatory hyperpigmentation, two cases represented hemangiomas, and one patient had a pigmented lesion that proved to be VIN with ulceration.[204]

Lentigo Simplex

The most common hyperpigmented lesion occurring on the vulva is lentigo simplex (lentigines), which may occur on the mucous membranes as well as the skin. The lesion is typically small, 4 mm or less in diameter, flat, and uniformly pigmented. Histologically, lentigo simplex is a localized circumscribed area of slightly hyperplastic epidermis that contains a population of functioning melanocytes associated with hyperpigmentation. Extreme degrees of epidermal pigmentation may be present, with numerous squamous cells exhibiting cytoplasmic melanin granules, usually in highest concentration near the epithelial–stromal junction (Fig. 2.34). There may be mild acanthosis and slight clubbing of the rete ridges, and heavily pigmented melanophages may be present in the upper dermis. At times, a minimal superficial dermal inflammatory cell infiltrate is noted, but this is by no means constant. Clinically, lentigines closely resemble junctional nevi and, therefore, are frequently biopsied. Except for the rare leopard syndrome, in which thousands of lentigines are present all over the body, lentigo simplex is essentially devoid of clinical significance. In contrast to lentigo simplex, actinic lentigines usually are seen on sun-exposed areas only.[12,138]

Vulvar Melanosis

Vulvar melanosis is characterized by prominent brown to black pigmented macular areas with irregular borders that may be solitary or multiple and located on the labia minora or labia majora as well as on the vaginal introitus and perineum. The pigmented areas vary in size up to 45 cm in diameter. Vulvar melanosis typically occurs in women of reproductive age and is asymptomatic.[143,210]

The microscopic findings are essentially similar to lentigo simplex, although epithelial hyperplasia usually is not seen and the lesions typically are larger than lentigo, which

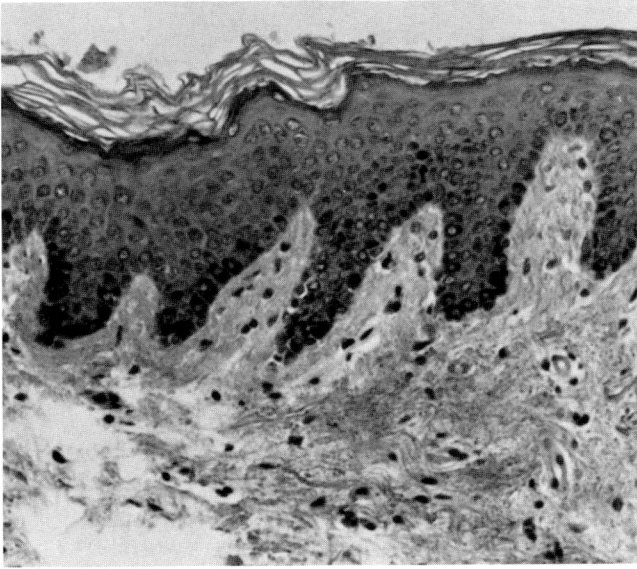

FIG. 2.34. **Lentigo simplex.** Note the heavy concentration of deeply pigmented melanocytes at the tips of the accentuated rete ridges.

characteristically are not more than 4 mm in diameter. Unlike typical nevi or melanoma, there is no junctional nesting of nevus cells and no atypia within the melanocytes. The pigmentation may be intense within the basal layer and, although melanocytes may be slightly increased in number, they are arranged in a single cell layer within the dermal–epidermal junction.[210,219]

Congenital and Giant Nevomelanocytic Nevi

Congenital nevi are found in approximately 10% of newborns and usually are less than 4 mm in diameter. Giant nevomelanocytic nevi (>20 cm in diameter) (garment type), although rare, carry an increased risk of developing malignant melanoma in prepubertal individuals.

Junctional, Compound, and Intradermal Nevi

Vulvar melanocytic nevi may be junctional, compound, or intradermal. These nevomelanocytic types occur on the vulva with nearly equal distribution.[74] Clinically they usually are well defined, papular, uniformly pigmented and typically under 10 mm in diameter.[204] As described by Pinkus and Mehregan, the typical nevus cell is characterized mainly by its negative attributes.[185] The cells are somewhat larger than melanocytes and have round or ovoid nuclei. Dendrites are not present, and intercellular connections are not visible. The cells may lie singly within the dermis, but more commonly they tend to form nests. Unless they contain melanin, their cytoplasm is clear without granulations or fibrils.

In pure junctional nevi, which are identified relatively infrequently on the vulva, the nevus cells are located within the epidermis and at the dermal–epidermal junction. Individual cells, or cell nests, bulge downward from the tips of the rete ridges. There is no connective tissue noted between the nevus cells and the adjacent squamous keratinocytes. Such nevi are young and somewhat undifferentiated. With age, the basement membrane of the epidermis surrounding the nests disappears, and reticulum, collagen, and elastic fibers envelop the nests, pushing the epidermis upward. During this process, the lesion is clinically noted to be elevated above the level of the surrounding skin.

Histologically, nevus cells are within both the epidermis and the dermis. Such lesions are called *compound nevi* (Fig. 2.35). Further differentiation results in complete enclosure of the nevus cells and nests by connective tissue elements such that the lie wholly intradermal; no activity is seen at the dermoepidermal junction. These nevi are referred to as *intradermal*. Most nevi biopsied on the vulva are either compound or intradermal in type. With time, nevi may regress completely or may result in a fibrous papule or acrochordon.[182]

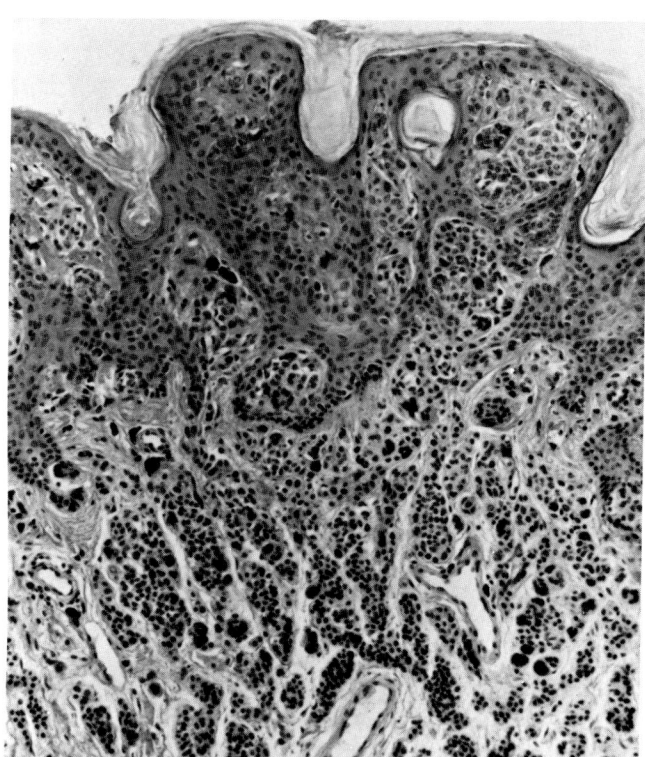

Fig. 2.35. Compound nevus. Nests of nevus cells are evident within the epithelium as well as within the dermis.

Atypical Vulvar Nevi

The so-called atypical vulvar nevus has many clinical and histopathological features in common with acquired dysplastic nevi. The atypical vulvar nevus occurs in young women ranging from 20 to 30 years of age. Although not considered specifically as dysplastic by some authors, or associated with dysplastic nevi in other sites, the atypical vulvar nevus demonstrates prominent variable-sized junctional melanocytic nests. Although some features may suggest a diagnosis of melanoma, the lesion is small, well circumscribed, and lacks pagetoid spread, necrosis, or mitotic activity in the dermis[40,74] (Fig. 2.36).

Dysplastic Nevi

Dysplastic melanocytic nevi are seen most often in young women of reproductive age. Rare on the vulva, they present as pigmented, elevated lesions greater than 0.5 cm in diameter with irregular borders. Microscopic examination reveals large epithelioid or spindle-shaped nevus cells with nuclear pleomorphism and prominent nucleoli. The nevus cells are clustered in intraepithelial nests and are present in skin appendages, including hair shafts and the ducts of sweat glands.[2,40,74,182] They often have a low-power microscopic appearance of a large junctional nevus, with a dermal component that has spindle- or epithelioid-

Acanthosis Nigricans and Pseudoacanthosis Nigricans

Acanthosis nigricans has been reported involving the vulva, although other sites where skin folds are found, including the axilla and submammary area, are more commonly involved. The clinical presentation is a diffuse, velvet-like, brown to gray-black skin change that is characteristically symmetrical and may involve all the keratinized epithelium of the vulva, including the inguinal gluteal folds as well as the medial aspects of the upper thighs. Within the vulva, the pigmentation usually involves the labia majora and lateral labia minor as well as the pubis.[156] In adults, acanthosis nigricans may be associated with adenocarcinoma of the stomach or other visceral malignancies. Its presentation should prompt the search for gastric and other tumors, especially if it occurs with sudden onset and is associated with pruritis and the appearance of multiple seborheic keratosis.[109]

A second variant of this type of skin change recognized in adults is pseudoacanthosis nigricans. This lesion has been reported in obese individuals as well as those with autoimmune or endocrine disorders or lipodystrophy. A third variant of acanthosis nigricans occurs in children. It is not associated with any of the disorders described in adult variants.[48]

The microscopic features are characterized by prominent papillomatosis with acanthosis and hyperkeratosis. Keratinous horn cysts may be seen within the epidermis. Increased melanin typically is seen within the basal layer. No significant inflammation or distinctive dermal changes are found.

Cysts

Bartholin Cyst and Abscess

The Bartholin ducts are prone to obstruction at their vestibular orifice. Such obstruction results in subsequent accumulation of secretion with associated cystic dilatation of the duct.[207,212,255] The content of an uninfected Bartholin cyst is a mucoid, clear, translucent liquid that, when cultured, fails to grow bacteria. The secretion stains with mucicarmine, PAS before and after diastase digestion, and Alcian blue at pH 2.5, consistent with sialomucin. The epithelium lining the cyst may be squamous, transitional, or low cuboidal mucinous epithelium. In some cases it is flattened and otherwise not classifiable (Fig. 2.37). Generally, there is minimal, if any, inflammatory response within the adjacent tissue. The epithelium of the cyst is immunoreactive for carcinoembryonic antigen (CEA).

Bartholin cysts may be recurrent, and occasionally are associated with primary infection of the Bartholin gland, in which case they require marsupialization. In postmeno-

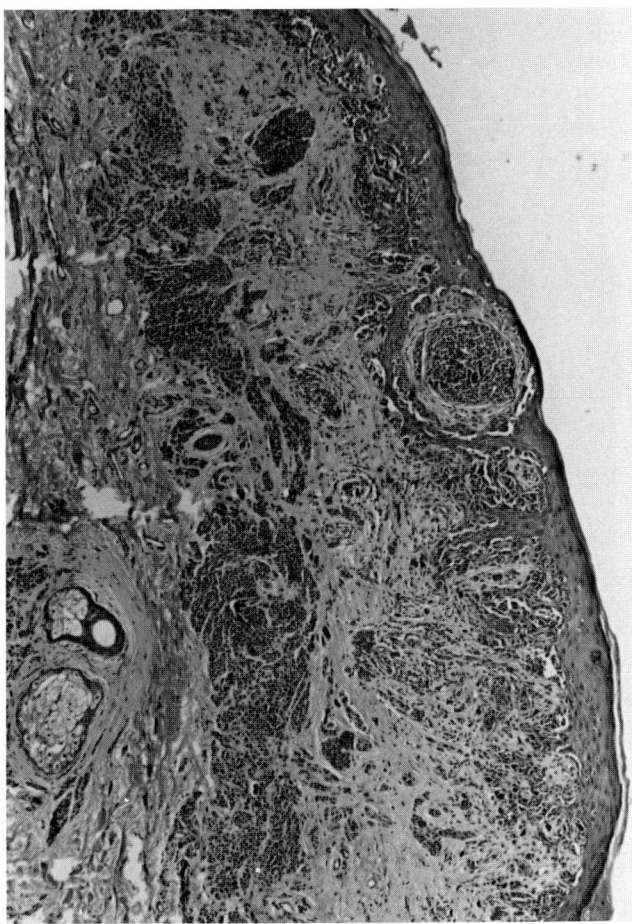

FIG. 2.36. Atypical vulvar nevus. This acquired atypical nevus has marked cytoatypia in the superficial and junctional areas with small, benign-appearing nevus cells within the dermis. (Courtesy of KK. Pierson, M.D., Gainesville, FL.)

type nevus cells in nests or isolated within the papillary and reticular dermis. Three features distinguish a dysplastic nevus from melanoma: (1) symmetrical growth, which is evident on microscopic examination of a full cross-section of the nevus. This can be determined by visualizing a line drawn perpendicular to the surface of the center of the nevus. The halves should be mirror images of each other; (2) the presence of the most atypical cells in the superficial levels of the nevus, with smaller and more uniform cells in the deeper areas; (3) pagetoid spread of single melanocytes with little or no involvement of the upper one-third of the epithelium.[2,25,74,82,182,199] Besides malignant melanoma, a lesion of the dysplastic nevus syndrome should be included in the differential diagnosis. Individuals with dysplastic nevus syndrome have multiple large nevi, usually greater than 0.5 cm in diameter, which may be found on the vulva and on the trunk and extremities. Individuals with dysplastic nevus syndrome have a high risk of subsequent malignant melanoma, whereas women with isolated atypical nevi of the vulva do not.

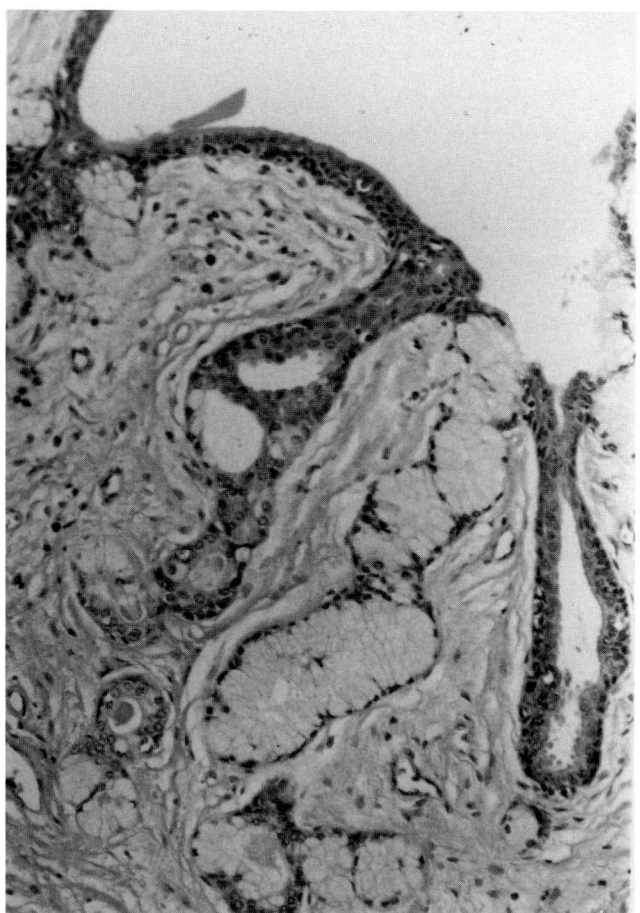

FIG. 2.37. **Bartholin cyst.** The dilated duct has a flattened transitional epithelial lining. The adjacent tissue has a few scattered inflammatory cells. Bartholin glandular elements are adjacent to the cyst (also see Fig. 2.3).

pausal women, recurrent cysts or a palpable mass after cyst drainage should be excised surgically because of the possibility of associated carcinoma of the Bartholin gland. (see Chapter 3, Premalignant and Malignant Tumors of the Vulva). Bartholin adenocarcinomas, when present, tend to be in the tissues adjacent to the cyst wall.

Bartholin abscess is an acute process often associated with *Neisseria* gonorrheal infection, although it may be related to *Staphylococcus* or to other anaerobic organisms. Microscopically, the Bartholin duct abscess demonstrates a striking acute inflammatory reaction within the stroma surrounding the duct. A purulent exudate is present within the lumen of the abscess wall. Excision, drainage, and antibiotics are the treatments of choice. Occasionally, the infection subsides without abscess formation or becomes chronic. Bartholin duct cysts, resulting from distal obstruction of the duct secondary to chronic inflammation and scarring, may be a late sequelae of chronic infection.

Mucocele-like changes have been reported in the Bartholin glands. The patient presents with tenderness and swelling in the Bartholin gland area with nodularity or a deep palpable cystic mass. On gross examination the tissue is nodular and may be partially cystic. Microscopically, dilated ducts and distended gland elements contain mucinous-like material. This material, along with foamy histiocytes, may be seen within the stroma.[73]

Keratinous Cyst (Epithelial Inclusion Cyst)

Keratinous cysts frequently are seen on the vulva and generally are located on the labia majora. They typically are superficial and range in size from 2 to 5 mm, but may be larger. They may occur at any age, including newborns.[160] Keratinous cysts usually contain a white to pale yellow grumous or cheesy material without hair. Foreign body–type giant cells may be seen in the tissue adjacent to the cyst wall, secondary to keratinous material leaking into the adjacent dermis. The lining of the cyst is characterized by a relatively flattened, stratified squamous epithelium that is immunoreactive for high molecular weight keratin (Fig. 2.38). Whether or not these cysts represent primary keratinous cysts, unrelated to sebaceous glands, or are actually occluded sebaceous glands that have undergone squamous metaplasia, is debatable. Step sections through the cysts may show communication with the surface epithelium and underlying or adjacent sebaceous glands, in some cases. An unusually high frequency of vulvar kerati-

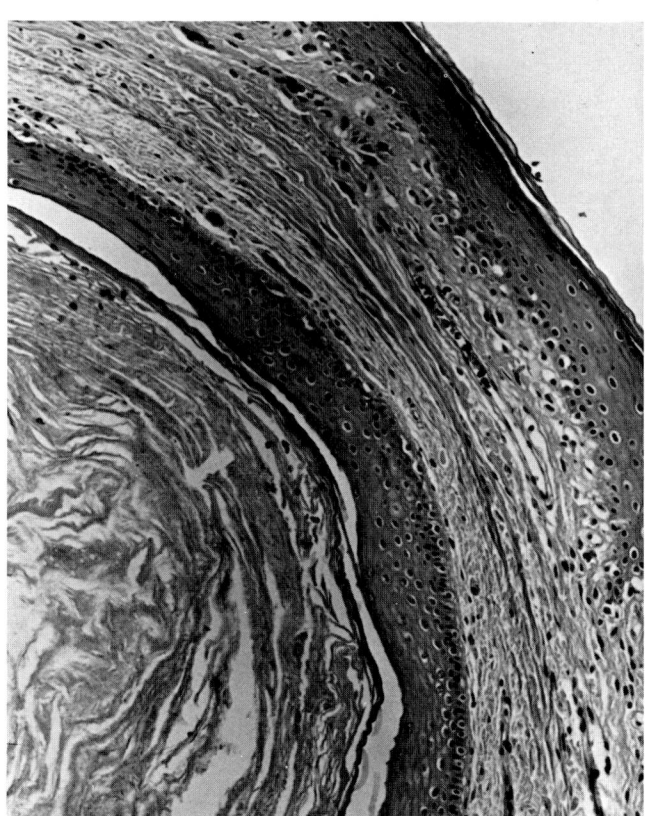

FIG. 2.38. **Keratinous cyst.** Stratified squamous epithelial lining is evident.

nous cysts has been reported in Nigerian children, related to female circumcision.[112] Such cysts are not considered premalignant, although carcinoma arising in keratinous cysts may occur. Treatment usually is not necessary; however, surgical excision may be necessary for diagnosis or if the cysts are enlarging, symptomatic, or secondarily infected.

Mucous Cyst

Mucous cysts usually are seen within the vestibule and are lined by mucous-secreting, cuboidal to columnar epithelium without peripheral muscle fibers or evidence of myoepithelial cells (Fig. 2.39). Squamous metaplasia may be present. Histochemical studies demonstrate that the epithelial cells lining the cyst stain with both alcian blue and Mayer mucicarmine, whereas the epithelial lining of cysts of mesonephric origin do not exhibit these reactions.[82] The cysts probably develop from occlusion of minor vestibular glands (Fig. 2.40).[82,172,202] Electron microscopic studies of mucinous cysts of the vestibule have demonstrated that these cysts have an epithelium consistent with an origin from urogenital sinus endoderm.[172,202] Since the vulvar vestibule arises embryologically primarily from the urogenital sinus, the origin of these cysts from minor vestibular glands is not inconsistent with a urogenital sinus origin.

Mucinous metaplasia of the vulva has been described, presenting as a solitary depressed red area of the labia minora.[43] In one reported case this responded to topical estrogen cream. The finding of columnar cell metaplasia of the nonkeratinized squamous epithelium of the vulva vestibule or vagina, to columnar epithelium of mucinous or tubal-epithelial type, also has been described after Stevens–Johnson syndrome as well as after laser and 5-flu-orouracil (5-FU) therapy[150] (see below).

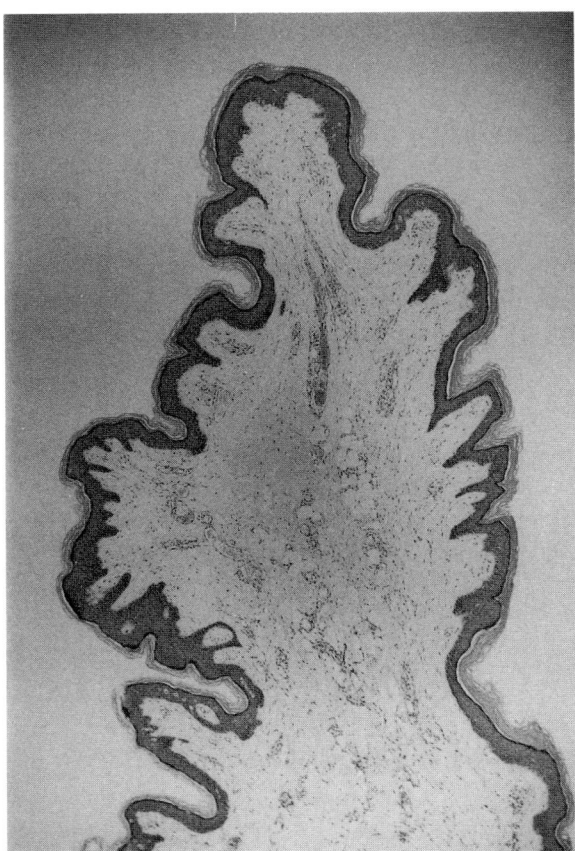

FIG. 2.40. **Fibroepithelial polyp.** This polyp is primarily stromal, with prominent vessels within the central stalk. The epithelial surface is keratinized, stratified squamous epithelium. No inflammation or glandular elements are evident.

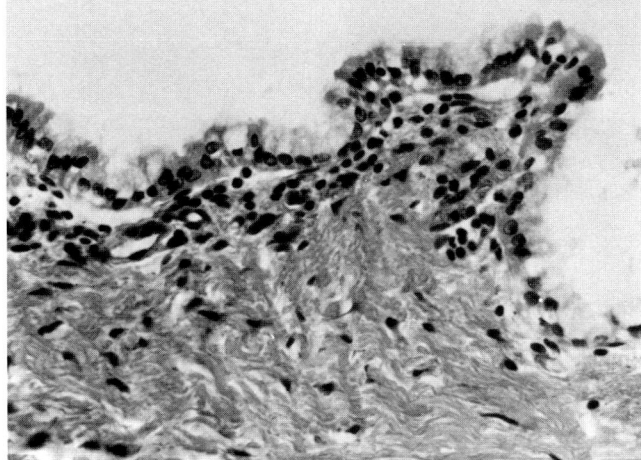

FIG. 2.39. **Mucous cyst of the vestibule.** Simple columnar mucous-secreting cells rest on the basement membrane. Note absence of underlying smooth muscle layer.

Ciliated Cysts of the Vulvar Vestibule: Vestibular Adenosis

Ciliated cysts, lined with columnar epithelium resembling müllerian epithelium (tubal-endometrial epithelium), consisting of ciliated, secretory, and undifferentiated type cells, have been reported occurring within the vulvar vestibule in women with chronic inflammation of the vestibule associated with Stevens–Johnson syndrome, as well as in women who have had extensive laser or 5-FU therapy of the vagina and vestibule secondary to columnar cell metaplasia.[150,214] The cysts within the vestibule are believed to be acquired, since the müllerian system does not contribute to the development of the vestibule. The cysts are distinguished from endometriosis by the absence of associated endometrial stroma or hemosiderin-laden macrophages. In the vagina such changes, when associated with 5-FU, slowly regress over time by a process of squamous metaplasia. In the vestibule, such cysts may be followed by observation over time; if persistent and/or symptomatic, they can be excised.

Mesonephric-like Cyst (Wolfian-like Duct Cyst)

Mesonephric-like cysts are encountered occasionally on the lateral aspects of the vulva and vagina. They are thin-walled, translucent, and contain a clear fluid. The lining epithelium usually is cuboidal to columnar, and is not ciliated. Immunohistochemical techniques show smooth muscle in the submucosal areas.[112]

Cyst of the Canal of Nuck (Mesothelial Cyst)

Cysts of the canal of Nuck are generally found in the superior aspect of the labia majora or inguinal canal and are believed to arise from inclusions of the peritoneum at the inferior insertion of the round ligament into the labia majora. As such, they are analogous to the hydrocele of the spermatic cord. These cysts can achieve substantial size and must be distinguished from inguinal herniae, with which they are associated in approximately one-third of cases.[131]

Benign Solid Tumors and Tumor-like Lesions

The benign solid tumors of the vulva, although rare, comprise a complex group. For convenience, the lesions may be divided into those that are of epithelial origin, of which there are squamous lesions and glandular lesions, and those that originate from vulvar soft tissue (mesenchymal origin).

Squamous Epithelial Tumors

Fibroepithelial Polyp (Acrochordon)

A fibroepithelial polyp, or "skin tag," is a relatively uncommon benign polypoid tumor of the vulva. In contrast to the vestibular papilloma, the fibroepithelial polyp occurs on the hair-bearing skin of the vulva. These tumors vary in their clinical appearance from small, flesh-colored or hyperpigmented, papillomatous growths resembling condylomata to large pedunculated tumors that often are hypopigmented. On cut section, fibroepithelial polyps are soft and fleshy. Small tumors may resemble nevi; large lesions may present cosmetic problems, but generally they are clinically insignificant. They usually arise in hair-bearing skin but may be found on the labia minora.[35] Their origin is most probably from a regressing nevus.

Histologically, their epithelial surface varies from a thickened layer with papillomatosis, hyperkeratosis, and acanthosis to an attenuated flattened layer exhibiting multiple primary folds (Fig. 2.40). Fibroepithelial polyps may be of two distinct morphologic types, one that is predominantly epithelial and another that is primarily stromal. The

connective tissue stalk is composed of loose bundles of collagen with moderate numbers of blood vessels. The stroma may be edematous and hypocellular. The stromal cells usually have relatively uniform nuclei; however, marked atypia may be seen in some cases.[35]

Vulvar Vestibular Papilloma (Micropapilloma Labialis)

The vestibular papilloma is a benign papillary lesion that is composed of a delicate fibrovascular connective tissue core covered by squamous epithelium. In contrast to fibroepithelial polyps, vestibular papilloma typically occur on the vestibule. They are relatively common lesions. In a study of women presenting for colposcopy, 25% were found to have vestibular papillae.[31] When multiple, they also may involve the medial aspects of the labia minora and posterior medial labia majora. They occur almost exclusively in women of reproductive age. Vestibular papillae are small, usually less than 5 mm in length, with a diameter of 1–2 mm. Solitary lesions usually are seen adjacent to the hymen, whereas multiple, papillomas typically occur in clusters, usually on the lateral–posterior aspects of the vestibule. They may be asymptomatic and associated with pruritis.[96] In some cases they may be seen in women with vulvar vestibulitis. Vulvar vestibular papilloma, associated with vestibular pruritus, burning, and/or dyspareunia, has been identified as a clinical complex. Initial reports described an association with HPV; however, newer studies fail to show a significant association.[15,164,244] The etiology of vestibular papillomatosis is unknown in most cases.[15] In those cases with solitary papillae, it appears that papillae may be an anatomic variant.[31]

On microscopic examination, vestibular papillae typically have a stratified squamous nonkeratinized epithelial surface, which is glycogen rich in women of reproductive age. They may have a thin keratin layer. The papillae have a fibrovascular core, often with a prominent central vessel (Fig. 2.41). Usually inflammation is not present. The glycogen-rich squamous epithelium may be confused with HPV changes, but can be distinguished from koilocytosis of HPV infection by the normal-sized nuclei and lack of other features of HPV infection including dyskeratosis, parabasalar hyperplasia, accentuation of intracellular bridges, and multinucleation.

Seborrheic Keratosis

Seborrheic keratosis is a benign epithelial growth characterized by acanthotic epidermis associated with papillomatosis, hyperkeratosis, and epithelial invaginations forming horn cysts. The lesions are raised with irregular borders occurring on hair-bearing skin of the vulva. They vary from pale brown to brownish black, and appear to be stuck onto the skin surface. Although clinically insignificant, their gross appearance often mimics that of a nevus or mela-

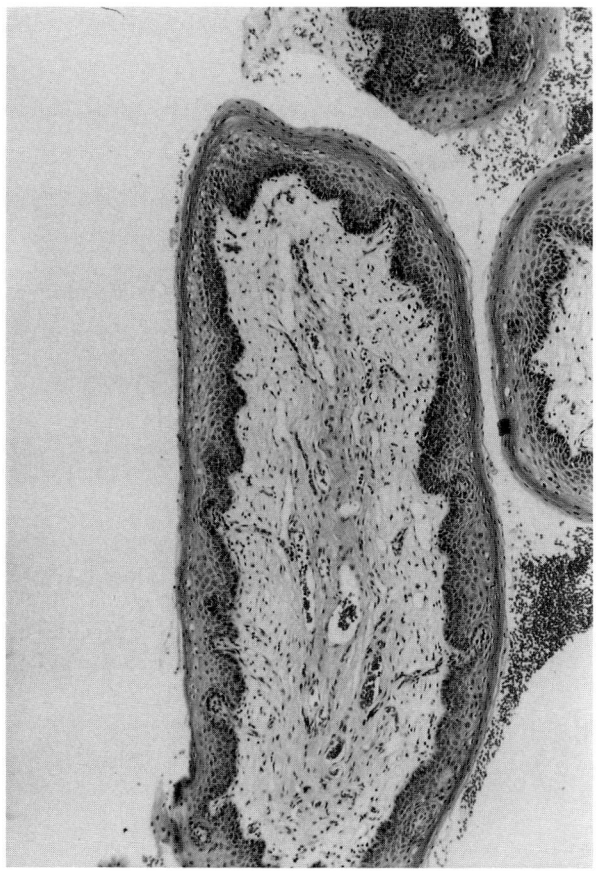

FIG. 2.41. Vestibular papilloma. This papilloma is small and has prominent central nonmuscular vessels oriented to the long axis of the papilloma. The epithelium is nonkeratinized, stratified squamous epithelium. A few lymphocytes are present immediately beneath the epithelium.

noma. Multiple seborrheic keratosis presenting over a short period of time may be associated with internal malignancy (Leser–Trelat syndrome).[193] This association is especially strong when associated with acanthosis nigricans.

Histologically, hyperkeratosis, acanthosis, and papillomatosis are seen. On low-power examination the entire keratosis appears to be above a straight line drawn from the normal epidermis at one side of the lesion to the normal epidermis at the other side. Both mature squamous cells and basal type cells are noted in strands and cords surrounding numerous horny keratin cysts (Fig. 2.42). Varying degrees of hyperpigmentation may be present.

Keratoacanthoma

Keratoacanthomas are rapidly growing, self-limited proliferations of the squamous epithelium in which horny masses of keratin are pushed upward while tongues of squamous epithelium invade the dermis, resembling

squamous cell carcinoma. These tumors may occur on hair-bearing skin of the vulva.[134,198]

Glandular Tumors

Papillary Hidradenoma (Hidradenoma Papilliferum)

CLINICAL FEATURES

Papillary hidradenoma is a benign tumor of apocrine sweat gland origin, composed of epithelial and myoepithelial cells lining complex delicate fibrovascular branching stalks. Papillary hidradenoma usually presents as a small, dome-shaped tumor less than 2 cm in size. The lesion generally arises from the labia majora, interlabial sulci, or lateral surface of the labia minora. The tumors usually are asymptomatic; however, ulceration of the overlying surface may produce bleeding. Papillary hidradenomas have not been described before puberty and almost all cases have occurred in Caucasian women.[13]

Most authorities maintain that the tumor is of sweat gland origin; however, the hidradenoma does not contain carcinoembryonic antigen as do sweat gland tumors. There is evidence that they arise from anogenital "sweat" glands.[235,236]

MICROSCOPIC FINDINGS

Histologically, under low-power examination, an adenomatous pattern simulates a well-differentiated adenocarcinoma (Fig. 2.43). Stromal compression often results in the formation of a well-circumscribed pseudocapsule. At times, epithelial cells become entrapped within the compressed connective tissue, creating a pseudoinfiltrative appearance. The tumor is composed of numerous tubules and acini lined by a single or double layer of cuboidal cells, the outer layer representing myoepithelial cells (Fig. 2.44). At times, the cells lining the lumen of the adenomatous structures are large and pale, exhibiting the morphologic and staining characteristics of apocrine sweat gland secretory cells.[254] An inflammatory reaction is unusual unless secondary infection is present. These benign tumors cannot be distinguished histologically from intraductal papillomas arising from ectopic breast tissue unless the adjacent breast tissue is identified.[237] Mitotic figures are rare and only mild degrees of cellular and nuclear pleomorphism are present.

CLINICAL BEHAVIOR AND TREATMENT

Clinically, the hidradenoma is benign; however, an intraductal carcinoma resembling mammary-type apocrine epithelium has been described arising in a hidradenoma.[181] Local excision, including the base of the mass, is sufficient therapy.

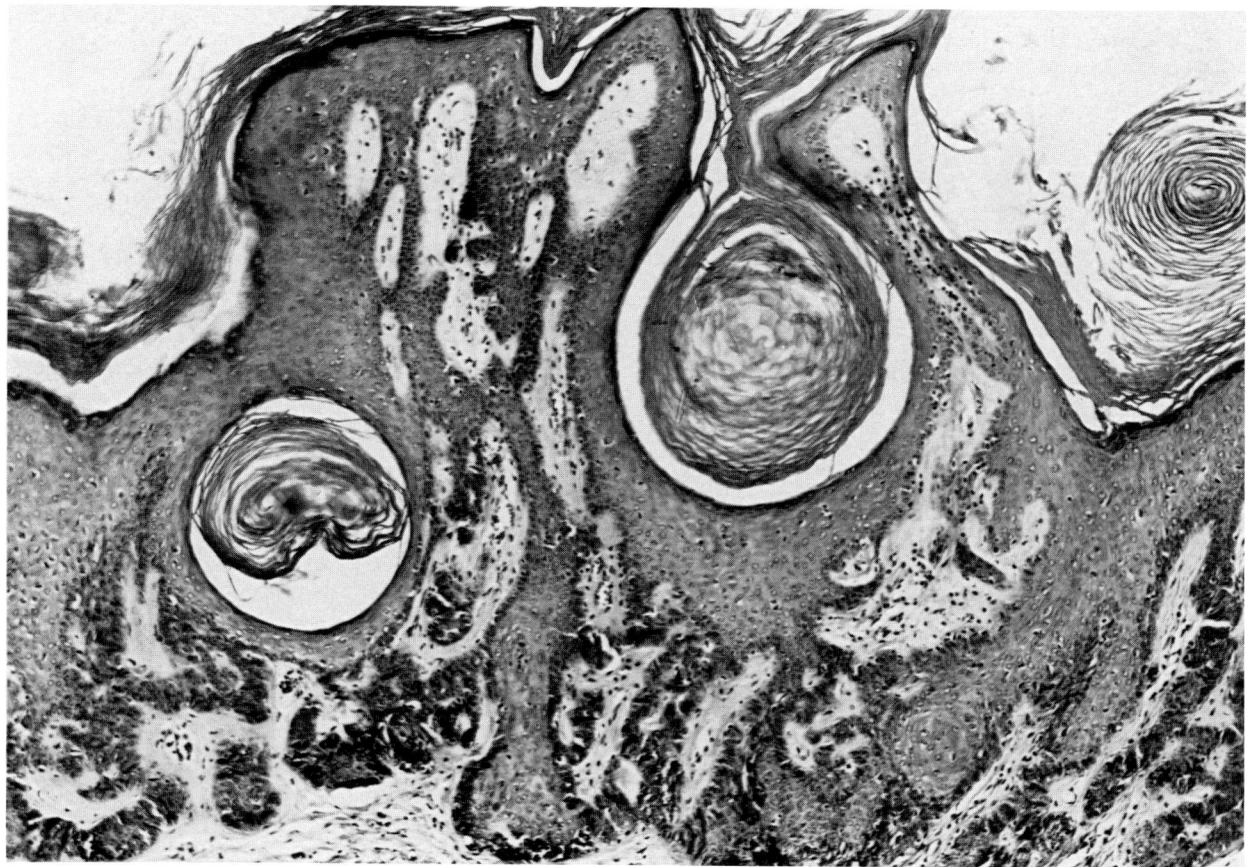

FIG. 2.42. Seborrheic keratosis, pigmented. When pigmented, these lesions may mimic VIN or melanoma on the vulva. Note that the diameter of the lesion is substantially greater than its thickness. The melanocytic hyperplasia and hyperpigmentation is present primarily in the basal layers. Keratin pearls are present.

Nodular Hidradenoma (Clear Cell Hidradenoma, Clear Cell Myoblastoma, Solid Cystic Hidradenoma, Eccrine Acrospiroma, Eccrine Sweat Gland, Adenoma of Clear Cell Type)

The nodular hidradenoma is a benign tumor of eccrine sweat gland origin composed of distinctive small cells with clear cytoplasm. It is not a variant of the papillary hidradenoma, but rather represents a distinctive and unusual tumor of the epidermal adnexa. Isolated examples of this tumor have been found occasionally on the vulva. This tumor is believed to be derived from the epithelial matrices in eccrine sweat gland primordia.

Histologically, the nodular hidradenoma is largely solid and does not resemble the papillary hidradenoma. Lobules or segments of large clear cells are divided by strands of reticular connective tissue. The characteristic cell is large and polygonal, and the cytoplasm appears clear. The relatively small nucleus is round to oval and may exhibit an irregular outline. The chromatin frequently is clumped, and a single nucleolus often is seen. Mitotic figures are unusual (Fig. 2.45). Wide local excision is considered adequate therapy.[254]

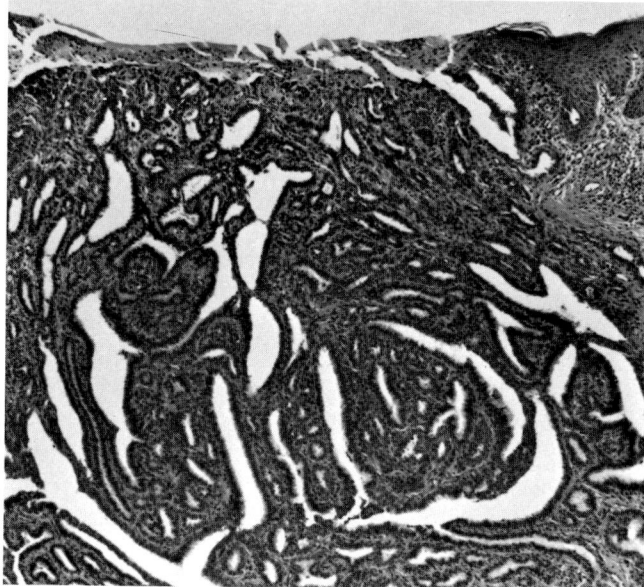

FIG. 2.43. Papillary hidradenoma. Low-power pattern of this adenomatous tumor ulcerating through skin surface. At low magnification this benign tumor can be misinterpreted as adenocarcinoma.

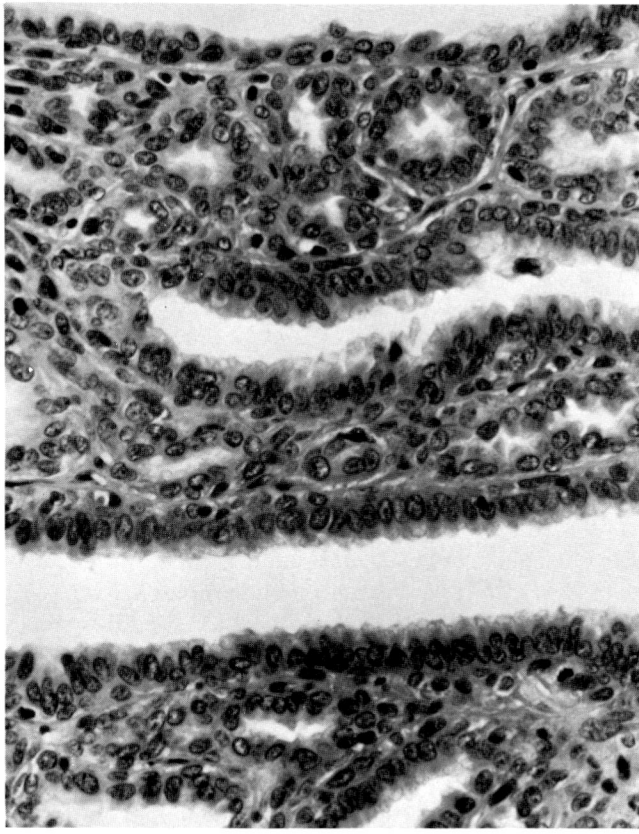

FIG. 2.44. **Papillary hidradenoma.** High-power examination shows tubules and acini lined with a single or double layer of bland cuboidal to columnar cells.

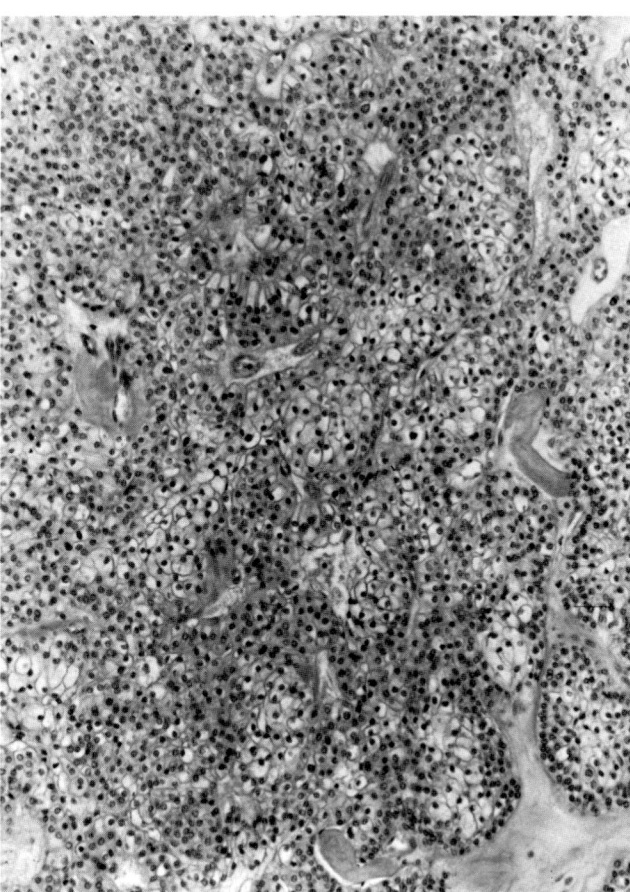

FIG. 2.45. **Nodular hidradenoma (clear cell hidradenoma).** The sheets of large clear cells are separated by occasional collagen bands and blood vessels.

Syringoma

The syringoma is a benign tumor of eccrine ductal origin characterized by multiple small and relatively uniform epithelial-lined tubules and cysts within a fibrous stroma. It is assumed to be an adenoma of the eccrine ducts. These lesions occur on the vulva as well as the eyelids, cheeks, axillae, and abdomen. Clinically, multiple clustered flesh-colored papules are noted within the deeper skin layers of the labia majora bilaterally. They often are asymptomatic, although pruritis may occur.[107,257] Histologically, the tumor lacks a clearly defined border. Within the dermis, numerous small, dilated duct spaces are seen. These spaces usually are lined by two rows of epithelial cells that appear flat, secondary to pressure atrophy. The comma-like formation of these glandular spaces is characteristic (Fig. 2.46).

Mixed Tumor of the Vulva (Pleomorphic Adenoma)

Mixed tumor of the vulva is a rare neoplasm that usually presents as a solid, subcutaneous tumor involving the labia majora and/or the Bartholin gland area. The histopathological findings are similar to those of mixed tumors of the

parotid and other salivary glands. The tumor consists of epithelial cells arranged in tubules or nests, mixed with a fibrous stroma with chondromatous, osseous, and myxoid elements. These stromal-like elements are believed to arise from pluripotential myoepithelial cells that, in the vulva, are found in the Bartholin glands, sweat glands, and from accessory breast tissue.[208]

Although these tumors are considered benign, local recurrence, as well as malignant mixed tumors, have been reported.[175] When metastasis occurs from a malignant mixed tumor, usually it is composed of only epithelial elements. There are insufficient cases of vulvar mixed tumors to determine the natural history of this tumor in this site. Wide local excision, with free margins, is the recommended therapy of choice for both primary tumor and local recurrences.

Trichoepithelioma

Trichoepithelioma is a benign tumor of hair follicle origin that is rare within the vulva.[39] The tumor presents as single or multiple cutaneous nodules with normal-appearing overlying epithelium. On microscopic examination, the tu-

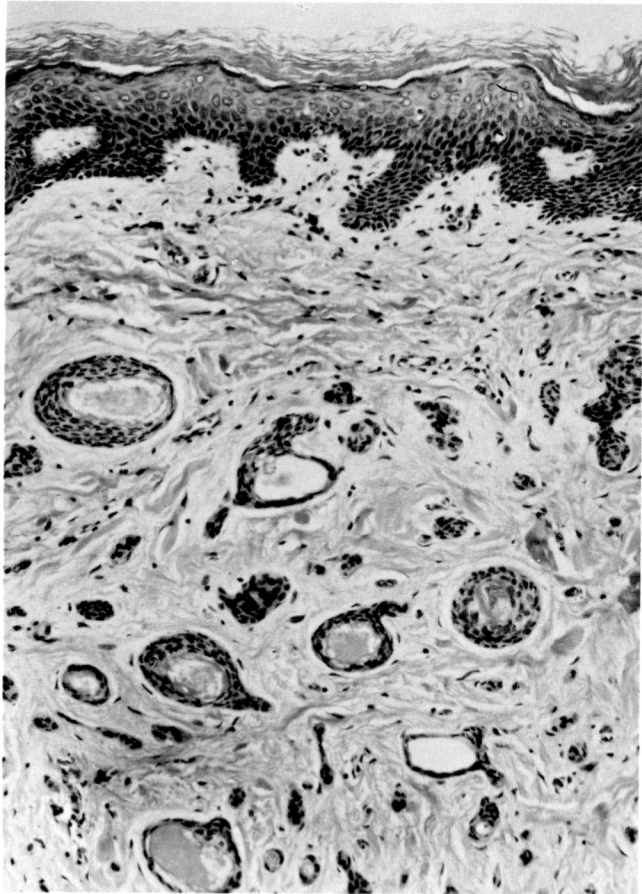

FIG. 2.46. Syringoma. The comma pattern of the eccrine structures is easily appreciated.

mor is composed of complex interconnected nests of basaloid cells, which form small cysts containing keratin "horn cysts." Hair or hair-forming elements are rare. Excision is therapeutic. Trichoepithelioma is distinguished from basaloid carcinoma or basal cell carcinoma, in that it is not infiltrative, contains "horn cysts," may exhibit hair-forming elements, and is not associated with an intraepithelial neoplastic component.

Trichilemmoma

Trichilemmoma is rare on the vulva, occurring in the dermis of the labium majus, where it presents as a slowly growing solid mass.[8] Microscopic examination reveals a lobulated tumor with a pushing border that may show no connection with the overlying epithelium. The tumor cells are palisaded peripherally and have increased cytoplasm as they stratify toward the centers of the nests, which contain amorphous keratin. No granular layer is formed. Nuclear pleomorphism may be present and calcification may occur. Trichilemmal cysts (pilar tumors) also have been described

on the vulva,[27,192] as has trichoblastic fibroma.[91] Local excision is therapeutic.

Adenoma of Minor Vestibular Glands

Adenoma of minor vestibular glands is a rare benign tumor, arising within the vestibule. These lesions are small, ranging from 1 to 2 mm. The tumor is composed of multiple small glands lined by mucin-secreting columnar epithelium.[9,72] Most cases have been found incidentally in vestibulectomy specimens excised for vulvar vestibulitis,[78] and some may represent a nodular hyperplasia.

Endometriosis

Vulvar endometriomas develop from ectopic endometrial epithelium (see Chapter 17, Diseases of the Peritoneum). Decidua implanted in an episiotomy incision at the time of delivery, as well as menstrual endometrium implanting in a small area of trauma, have been implicated in the etiology of this condition. The clinical appearance is variable, ranging from bluish, red, cystic masses to amorphous deep-seated nodules. Endometriomas of the vulva usually are located near the posterior fourchette. Cyclic enlargement and regression often are noted. Fine-needle aspiration may be of value in the diagnosis, demonstrating benign glandular and stromal cellular elements.[142] Histologically, both endometrial glands and stroma are present with a fibrotic response. A foreign body–giant cell reaction and hemosiderin-laden macrophages may be noted, especially in cases in which the onset was preceded by recent surgery.

Mesenchymal Tumors

Vascular Tumors

Capillary Hemangioma (Strawberry Hemangioma, Juvenile Hemangioma, Nevus Vasculosis)

Capillary hemangioma is typically encountered in infants or young children. It is a well-demarcated, superficial, slightly elevated, usually irregularly surfaced, red to violet lesion that is rarely ulcerated or associated with bleeding. Biopsy is not indicated because of the very typical appearance, which usually is diagnostic. Observation over time demonstrates regression of the lesion; therapy generally is unnecessary. The pathological findings consist of numerous clustered endothelial-lined small capillaries within a fibrous tissue matrix.

Cavernous Hemangioma

Cavernous hemangioma is rare on the vulva, although its occurrence in young children has been documented.[117] This benign vascular lesion may be relatively large, complex, and deep in comparison to capillary hemangiomas. It also may be associated with deep pelvic hemangioma. Distortion of the vulva may be present and clitoral involvement may resemble clitoral hypertrophy.[117] Cavernous hemangioma of the vulva in children, as a rule, does not require therapy because it regresses over time. Like capillary hemangioma, cavernous hemangiomas may ulcerate and bleed, and on rare occasion may require therapy.[117]

Acquired Hemangioma of Adults (Senile Hemangioma)

Acquired hemangioma is far more common than other hemangiomata on the vulva. They typically are multiple, small (1–3 mm), red to purple papules with no known clinical significance. Histologically, acquired hemangiomas have numerous dilated capillaries in the intradermal tissue. These vascular spaces are lined with a single layer of endothelial cells and are separated by connective tissue that may show collagenization.[135] Hemangiomatous-like changes may be found on the vulva after radiotherapy.[258]

DIFFERENTIAL DIAGNOSIS OF HEMANGIOMAS

The differential diagnosis of hemangiomas includes angiokeratoma, pyogenic granuloma, bacterial angiomatosis, hemangiopericytoma, angiosarcoma, and Kaposi sarcoma. All these lesions are highly vascular and must be differentiated from hemangioma.[42,135] Angiokeratomas typically are dark red to black, raised, warty-appearing lesions that have an acanthotic overlying epithelium that is immediately adjacent to the prominent vascular channels of the angiokeratoma. Pyogenic granuloma usually is an elevated red lesion that histologically resembles granulation tissue and may have a collarette of elevated epithelium surrounding it. Hemangiopericytoma is a solid vascular neoplasm that is composed of staghorn-shaped vessels. In addition, there is a distinctive perivascular pericyte proliferation that can be identified with a reticulin stain. Bacterial angiomatosis resembles Kaposi sarcoma but contains the bacteria *Rochalimaea henselae*, which can be identified using Warthin–Starry stain[42,195] Kaposi sarcoma is a malignant vascular tumor composed of malignant spindle cells, some of which form distinct slit-like vascular spaces containing red blood cells.

Angiokeratoma

The angiokeratoma is a variant of hemangioma and occurs almost exclusively on the scrotum and vulva; however, it has been described presenting as an ulcerated tumor of the clitoris.[158] Fabray disease is associated with angiokeratomas; however, vulvar involvement is apparently rare, although it has been observed.[227] Somewhat larger than senile angiomata, these lesions often are purple to brown-black in color and occur primarily in women of childbearing age. Their peculiar appearance often prompts exci-

sional diagnostic biopsy, although they have no clinical significance.[19,106]

Histologically, the dilated epithelial-lined channels are separated by strands and cords of squamous epithelial cells representing downgrowth from the overlying epithelium, which is often hyperkeratotic (Fig. 2.47). Varying degrees of acanthosis and papillomatosis are present, along with a mild inflammatory reaction in the deep dermis. Angiosarcomas and Kaposi sarcoma are included in the differential diagnosis of vascular tumors.[135] These malignant tumors typically are more cellular, have cellular atypia, have less well-formed vascular spaces that are usually slit-like, and are infiltrative, with poorly defined margins.

Pyogenic Granuloma (Granuloma Pyogenicum)

The pyogenic granuloma is a variant of hemangioma that may occur anywhere on the skin. It is analogous to the epulis tumor of pregnancy. Most of the pyogenic granulomas that occur on the vulva do so during gestation. Although previously thought to be secondary to a superficial wound infection, this tumor is recognized as a form of hemangioma characterized by rapid growth. Because the surface is easily traumatized, the lesion often is secondarily infected.

Histologically, a thin ulcerated epidermis is noted covering a mass of granulation tissue. Capillaries are numerous, and secondary inflammatory changes frequently are found within the stroma (Fig. 2.48). Around the periphery of the

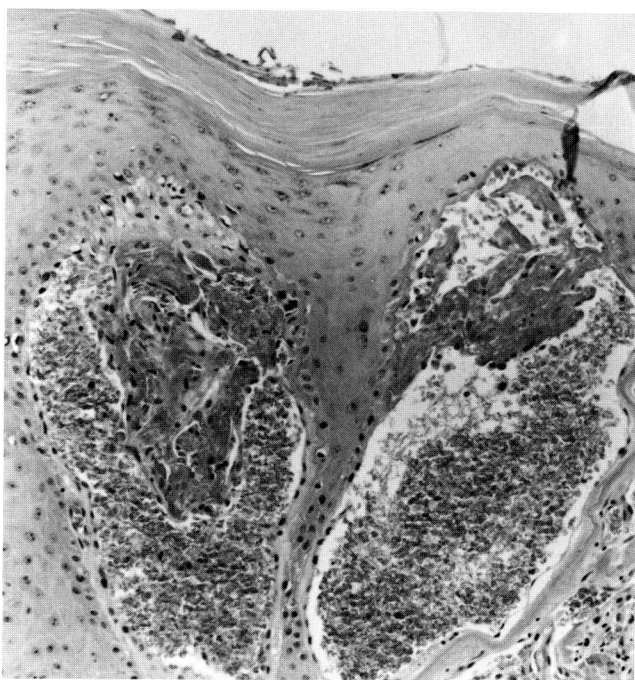

FIG. 2.47. Angiokeratoma. Strands of squamous epithelium surround endothelial lined vascular spaces.

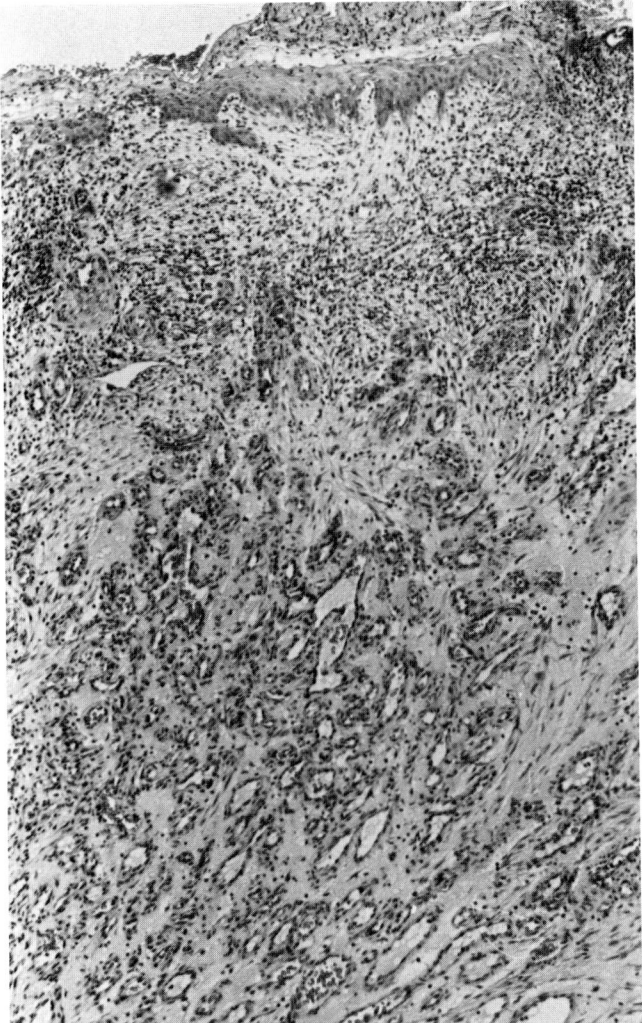

FIG. 2.48. Pyogenic granuloma. Superficial ulceration of the mucosa is present, with a chronic inflammatory infiltrate. Within the submucosa multiple endothelial lined vascular spaces are seen surrounded by a delicate fibrous stroma, resembling granulation tissue.

lesion, there may be a downward growth of the epidermis producing a "collarette."

Lymphangioma

Vulvar lymphangiomas may be congenital or acquired. Congenital lymphangiomas have been reported associated with lower extremity lymphangiomas and may be large, cavernous in type, and associated with deep lymphatics.[111,258] Vulvar lymphangiomas have been reported after radiation therapy to the pelvis.[258]

Histologically, lymphangiomas consists of variable-sized lymphatics, lined with endothelial cells within a fibrous connective tissue without associated smooth muscle. Unlike hemangiomas, which are included in the differential diagnosis, lymphangiomas characteristically do not contain red blood cells. The treatment of vulvar lymphangiomas is highly variable depending on the individual case. No therapy is usually necessary; however, surgical excision is applicable in some cases. Secondary infection is recognized as a potentially severe complication. Recurrence after therapy does not imply malignant transformation.

Lymphangioma Circumscriptum

Lymphangioma circumscriptum is a relatively rare condition that is benign and thought to be secondary to a localized developmental defect of the dermal lymphatics. Initial presentation may be in childhood; however, vulvar cases have been described initially presenting in women in their 30s. The process is characterized by multiple clustered blebs and vesicles that are white to purple in color and may be small, or exceed 2 cm in diameter.[222] The blebs of lymphangioma circumscriptum may become secondarily infected, ulcerated, and macerated, resulting in pain and cellulitis. The diagnosis usually is made by the clinical appearance and biopsy.

The microscopic findings reveal distinctive subepidermal cystic spaces containing lymph that is eosinophilic and acellular. These endothelial-lined cysts, which may be multiloculated, are immediately beneath the basal epithelial layer in the papillary dermis (Fig. 2.49). Dilated lymphatic spaces can be found in the reticular dermis. Some of these deeper lymphatics may be surrounded by a prominent peripheral smooth muscle layer. The overlying epithelium usually is unremarkable but may be eroded or hyperkeratotic. Treatment includes surgical excision or laser therapy.[111]

Angiomyofibroblastoma

Angiomyofibroblastoma is a benign vulvar tumor that may present as a Bartholin cyst or mass, measuring from 0.5 to 12 cm in diameter.[69] The tumor is well circumscribed and composed of spindled to oval stromal cells with bland nuclei and eosinophilic cytoplasm. Mitotic figures are absent to rare. In addition, the tumor contains numerous capillary-like vessels. Some areas, predominantly about vessels, may be cellular, with adjacent hypocellular areas. Plump stromal cells, especially about vessels, are seen with little stromal mucin (Fig. 2.50). Collagen may be prominent and mast cells are present in most cases. The stromal cells may be reactive for vimentin and desmin, but lack actin, S-100 protein, and cytokeratin.

In contrast to aggressive angiomyxoma, angiomyofibroblastoma is more cellular, has more numerous vessels, and the vessels lack vascular wall thickening and hyalinization. Local excision is the treatment of choice.[69]

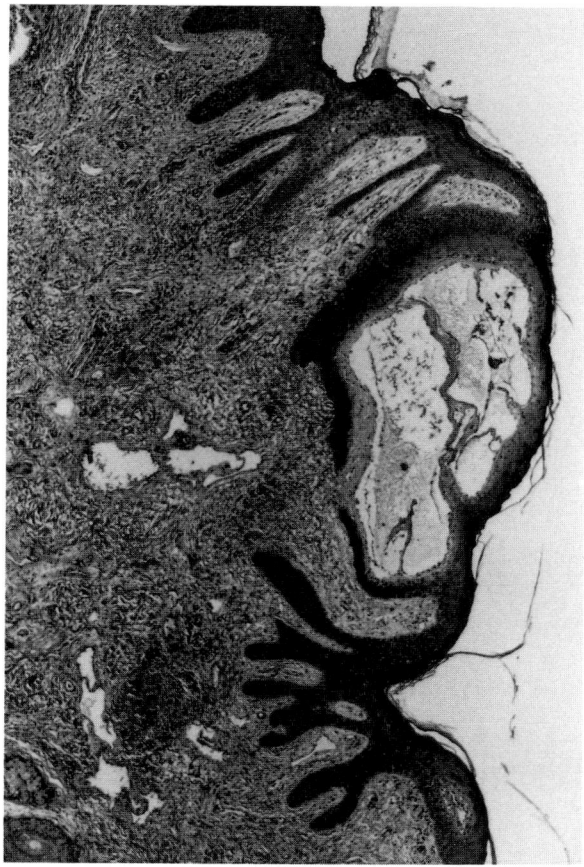

FIG. 2.49. **Lymphangioma circumscriptum.** Subepidermal multiloculated cystic spaces are seen that are filled with acellular eosinophilic lymph. Some slightly dilated deeper lymphatic channels are evident in the deeper dermis. (Courtesy of G. Segal, M.D., Gainesville, FL.)

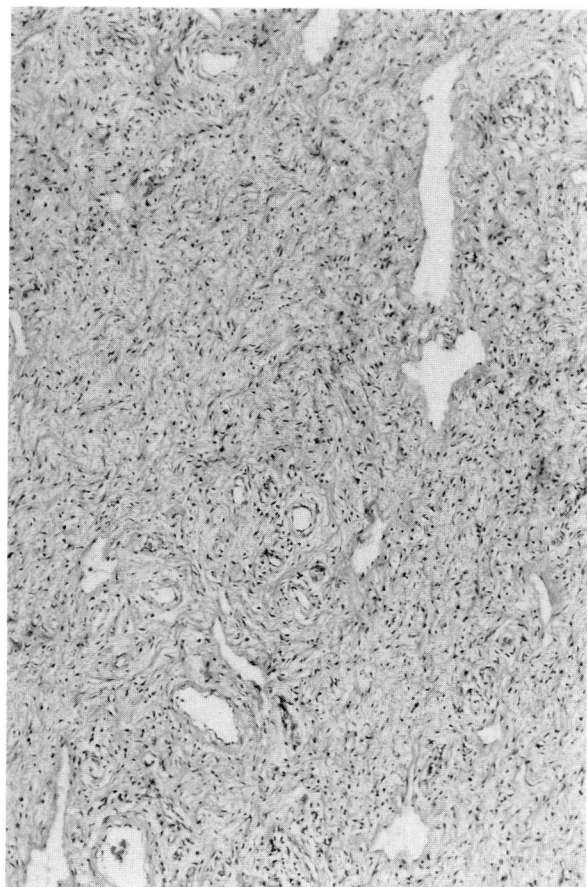

FIG. 2.50. **Angiomyofibroblastoma.** This benign tumor is composed of spindled and oval stroma cells with relatively uniform, bland-appearing nuclei with eosinophilic cytoplasm and infrequent or no mitosis. Numerous capillary-like vessels are present, with variable shapes. (Courtesy of R. Kurman, M.D., Baltimore, MD.)

Muscle Tumors

Leiomyoma

Benign leiomyomas are the most common soft tissue tumors of the vulva. They arise from smooth muscle and may arise from the smooth muscle elements surrounding the crura of the clitoris. Vulvar leiomyomatosis in children associated with esophagogastric leiomyomatosis has been reported.[66]

The tumor is composed of smooth muscle cells having round to oval nuclei with eosinophilic cytoplasm with poorly defined cell boarders (Fig. 2.51). Myxoid change may occur, and has been reported associated with pregnancy.[230] Epithelioid leiomyoma also has been reported in pregnancy.[7]

Leiomyoma can be distinguished from leiomyosarcoma by the lower or absent mitotic activity and lack of evidence of infiltration in leiomyoma. Both will be immunoreactive for desmin, myosin, and actin and do not contain myoglobin as do rhabdomyosarcomas and rhabdomyomas.[135]

Therapy is local excision. Gonadotropin suppression may be useful in rare cases.[66]

Rhabdomyoma

Rhabdomyoma is a benign tumor of striated muscle origin that, although rare in the vulva, has been reported in women of reproductive age.[56] Rhabdomyoma presents as a polypoid mass. On microscopic examination, the tumor contains mature striated muscle cells intermixed with fibrovascular stroma. Rhabdomyomas of the fetal myxoid type must be differentiated from embryonal rhabdomyosarcomas, which have nuclear pleomorphism, mitotic activity, and are infiltrative.

Neural Tumors

Granular Cell Tumor

Granular cell tumor is of peripheral nerve sheath origin and may occur in the vulva in children or adults. This

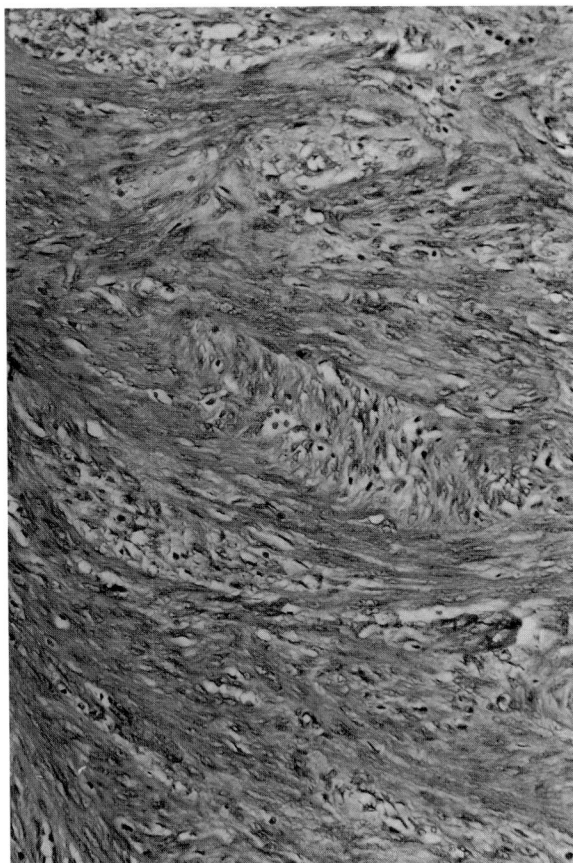

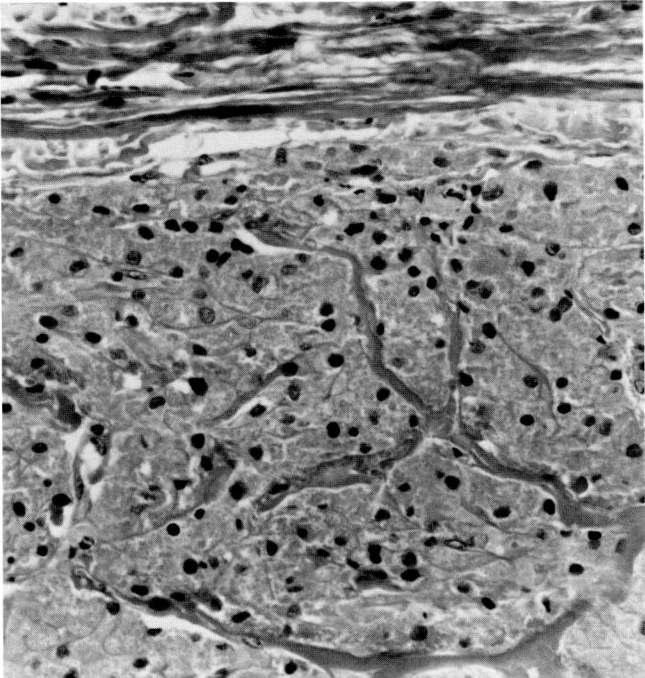

Fig. 2.52. Granular cell tumor. Note nests of polyhedral cells with granular cytoplasm separated by collagenous cords.

Fig. 2.51. Leiomyoma. The tumor is composed of smooth muscle cells with relatively small uniform nuclei without evident mitoses.

tumor presents typically as a painless, slow-growing, subcutaneous mass, usually involving the labia majora, clitoris, or mons pubis.[121,145] The tumor may present as a solitary enlargement of the clitoris, mimicking clitoral hypertrophy.[52,251] Pripism of the crus of the clitoris has been reported related to a locally aggressive granular cell tumor.[220] Approximately 7% of granular cell tumors in women occur on the vulva.[145] They are multiple in approximately 10–15% of the cases.[135]

Histologically, granular cell tumors are not encapsulated and are composed of irregular groups of large polyhedral cells with indistinct cell borders and nuclei that are relatively small and uniform with hyperchromatic chromatin. The cell groups usually are separated by strands of hyalinized stroma. The cytoplasm of these cells is packed with numerous eosinophilic granules (Fig. 2.52). Granular cell tumor contains S-100 protein and myelin basic protein, which can be demonstrated by immunoperoxidase techniques.[165a] Carcinoembryonic antigen and myelin basic protein PO and P2 also have been identified.[135,153] In approximately 50% of granular cell tumors, the overlying squamous epithelium exhibits remarkable pseudoepithe-

liomatous hyperplasia.[251] Extreme degrees of acanthosis are noted, and the nests and cords of hyperplastic squamous cells may mimic an invasive squamous carcinoma.[251] Rapid enlargement of benign granular cell tumors may occur in pregnancy. Malignant vulvar granular cell tumors are rare and usually are not recognized as malignant unless regional aggressive behavior or metastasis are identified.[145] Careful microscopic examination of the margins of the surgical specimen therefore is important. Local recurrences are common. Malignant granular cell tumor, with pulmonary and regional metastasis, with a subsequent fatal outcome has been reported.[145] Wide local excision is the usual treatment for both primary and locally recurrent granular cell tumors.[251]

Neurofibroma

Neurofibroma is a benign tumor of nerve sheath origin that involves the vulva in approximately 18% of women with von Recklinghausen's disease. Approximately one-half of the observed vulvar neurofibromas are found in women with neurofibromatosis.[80,83,213] Neurofibromas are generally under 3 cm in diameter; however, tumors as large as 25 cm have been described.[239] A giant solitary variant of neurofibroma of the labia has been reported.[239] Neurofibromas are rare before puberty. When they present, they may grow rapidly; malignant degeneration to neurofibrosarcoma or malignant Schwannoma may occur.

The tumor is composed of whorls and wavy bundles of slender spindle cells that often exhibit a palisade arrangement of the nuclei. The tumor is not encapsulated and may involve the dermis as well as the underlying fat. The cell borders are indistinct and strands of collagen-rich stroma, with mast cells, are commonly seen. The nuclei typically are small and have pointed poles; some may have a wavy appearance. Large, bizarre nuclei with hyperchromatic nuclear chromatin may be seen, which is a benign finding and is referred to as *ancient change*.[135] Mitosis should not be present in benign neurofibromas, and the presence of only 1 mitotic figure per 10 high-power fields is sufficient evidence for a diagnosis of neurofibrosarcoma.[135]

Nerve stains show long, thin nerve fibers scattered throughout the tumors, and occasionally the intervening collagen may undergo a peculiar mucoid degeneration. Neurofibromas contain S-100 antigen.[165a] Steroid receptors have been reported in some neural tumors in the pelvis and vulva.[38] In patients with neurofibromatosis the tumors are multicellular (polyclonal) in origin, unlike neurofibromas in normal individuals, where they are monoclonal in origin.[123]

When associated with neurofibromatosis there generally is no reason to excise vulvar neurofibromas unless they are rapidly enlarging, ulcerated, or symptomatic. In individuals without neurofibromatosis these tumors present as a subcutaneous mass and excision is both diagnostic and therapeutic. Individuals with hereditary neurofibromatosis also have an increased risk for other tumors, including glioma, ganglioneuroma, pheochromocytoma, meningioma, leukemia, Wilm tumor, and rhabdomyosarcoma.[123]

Schwannoma (Neurilemmoma)

Schwannomas rarely involve the vulva; however, the few cases reported have involved the clitoris and may mimic clitoral hypertrophy.[103] These benign tumors arise from the neuroectodermal nerve sheath and usually are solitary. Histologically, they contain both Antoni Type A and Type B tissue patterns (Fig. 2.53). The cellular (Antoni type A) areas consist of spindle cells with oval or elongated nuclei that have a palisaded and wavy appearance. Verocay bodies often are seen in these areas and are formed by alignment of the nuclei in regular rows that are separated by intervening acellular areas. Hypocellular (Antoni type B) areas contain spindled and small cells with hyperchromatic nuclear chromatin and lipid-laden histiocytes. Collagen fibers and mast cells usually are present. A myxomatous matrix is typically present within which small vessels with prominent thickening of the vessel wall are seen.

These tumors are immunoreactive for S-100 protein and are distinguished from leiomyomas in that they lack desmin (see Malignant Mesenchymal Tumors, Malignant Schwannoma in Chapter 3). Local excision is the treatment of choice.[103]

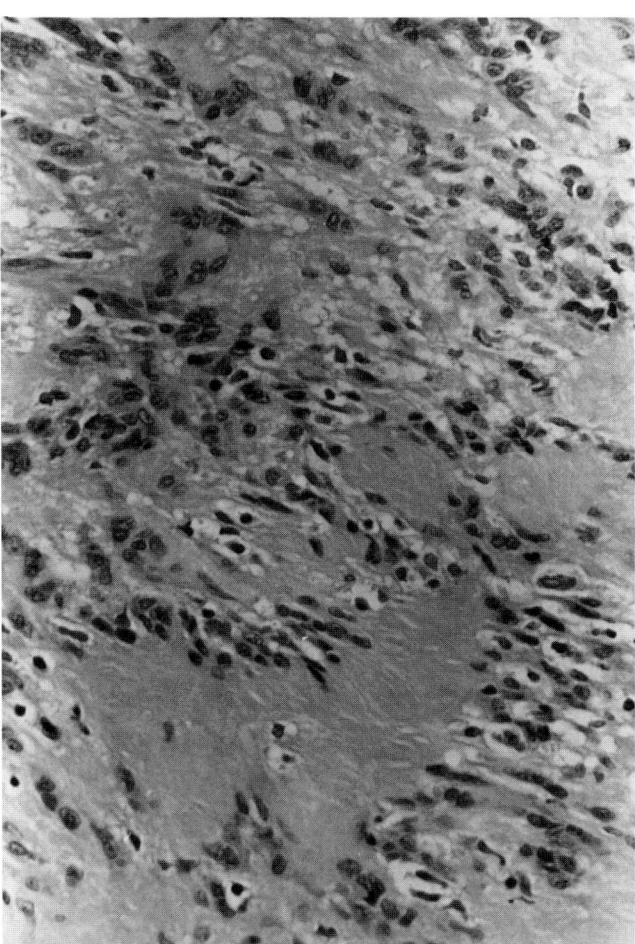

Fig. 2.53. **Schwannoma.** Densely packed spindle cells from Antoni type A areas are admixed with hypocellular Antoni type B areas.

Glomus Tumor

Glomus tumor of the vulva is a rare tumor. However, it has been reported associated with severe introital dyspareunia. The tumor is typically less than 4 cm in diameter, solitary, and the pain is localized to the tumor mass.[114,124] Microscopically, the tumor is composed of epithelioid-like cells forming lobules with surrounding vessels. The stroma about the tumor typically is hyalinized and usually contains identifiable nerves. Mast cells also may be present within this stroma.

Tumors of Fibroblastic or Fibrohistiocytic Origin

Fibroma

Benign fibromas may appear as vulvar masses arising from the deeper connective tissues surrounding the vaginal introitus or adjacent to the perineal body. Rarely do such tumors undergo malignant degeneration; left untreated, however, they can grow to substantial size. On cut section, fibromas are firm and smooth with a white or grayish color. Yellow striae and a somewhat softer consistency signify the admixture of a lipomatous element, which is not uncommon. They do not involve this overlying epidermis. Histologically, parallel bundles of fibrocytes are seen. With large tumors, hyaline, cystic, and hemorrhagic degeneration have been described.[135]

Desmoid Tumor

Desmoid tumors (aggressive fibromatous) are characterized by increased fibroblasts with thickening and fibrosis of the involved tissue. There typically is no associated inflammatory response.[120] Wide local excision is the treatment of choice.

Benign Fibrous Histiocytoma (Dermatofibroma)

Fibrous histiocytomas also have been referred to as *subepidermal nodular fibrosis, histiocytoma,* and *sclerosing hemangioma.* The term *dermatofibroma* is reserved for those tumors 1.5 cm or less in diameter. Masses larger than this, or that are polypoid in appearance, are referred to as *benign fibrous histiocytoma.*[193]

This benign tumor is rare on the vulva; however, the clinical presentation may be as a slightly raised, pale brown to red solitary subcutaneous mass. On microscopic examination, the tumor is composed of fibroblastic-type cells with a fascicular growth pattern that focally may have a storiform appearance. Typically, collagen is evident and may be prominent in some areas. Lymphocytes, foamy histiocytes, and Touton-type giant cells may be found. Typically few if any mitotic figures are present (Fig. 2.54). This benign histiocytic tumor may have associated epithelial hyperplasia; however, it lacks stromal infiltration. In contrast, dermatofibrosarcoma protuberans usually has epithelial thinning and is characterized by infiltrative growth (see Malignant Mesenchymal Tumors, Dermatofibrosarcoma Protuberans in Chapter 3). The tumor cells are immunoreactive for α-1-antichymotrypsin, α-1-antitrypsin, and vimentin. Wide extended local excision is the treatment of choice.

Miscellaneous Tumors and Tumor-like Lesions

Lipoma

Lipomas arising from the vulvar fat pads present as soft, lobulated growths generally attached to the labia majora by broad-base pedicles. Lipomas of the vulva presenting at birth have been reported.[86] Histologically, mature fat cells are seen, often interspersed with strands of fibrous connective tissue. When the fibrotic element is prominent, the tumor should be called a *fibrolipoma.* Lipomas are immunoreactive for S-100 antigen.

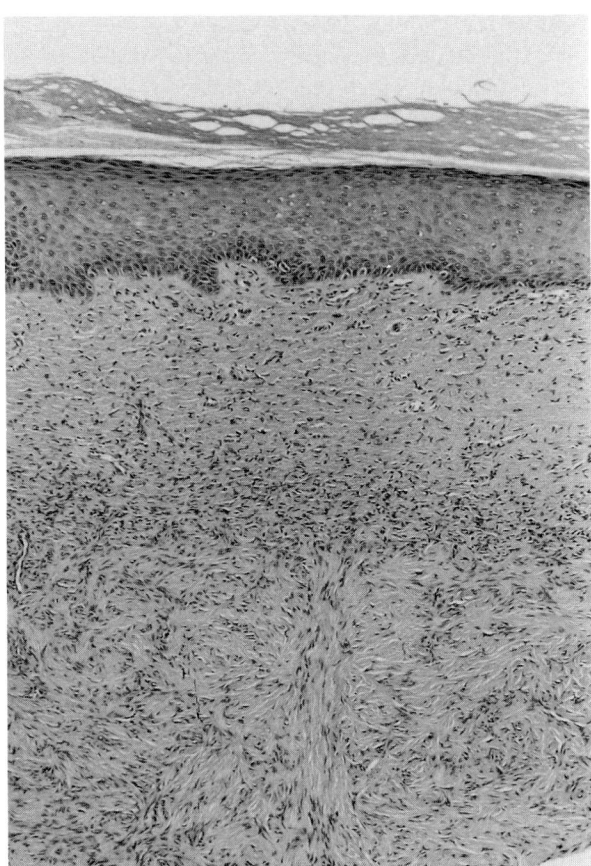

FIG. 2.54. Dermatofibroma. The tumor is beneath the most superficial dermis and is composed of spindled fibroblast type cells with a fascicular storiform pattern. The cell groups are separated in some areas by collagen.

Nevis Lipomatous Superficialis

This distinctive benign tumor of adipose tissue presents as a nodule within the dermis with normal-appearing overlying epithelium. Microscopic examination reveals adipose tissue within the dermis, distinct from the underlying adipose tissue.

Lymphoid Hamartoma

A benign lymphoid hamartoma has been described occurring in the subcutaneous tissue of the labia majora presenting as a symptomatic subcutaneous cystic mass.[119] The histological features include lymphoid tissue within an apparent fibrous capsule in the subcutaneous tissue. Unlike a lymph node, no adjacent lymphoid sinusoides are seen. A "whorled" appearance to the epithelioid-like lymphoid element within the mass resembles Hassel capsules. A chronic anemia with associated hypergammaglobulinemia has been reported with benign lymphoid hamartoma occurring in other sites, but not within the female genital tract. Removal of the mass results in resolution of the laboratory findings and a benign clinical course.

Nodular Fasciitis (Pseudosarcomatous Fasciitis, Proliferative Fasciitis)

Nodular fasciitis is not a neoplasm in the strict sense, but it may present as a mass that clinically, as well as pathologically, mimics a sarcoma. Nodular fasciitis may grow locally as a solid subcutaneous mass that may be attached to underlying tissues. The mass usually is solitary, sometimes tender, and may have been present for several years before medical assistance is sought.

The histopathological features of nodular fasciitis show spindle cell–like growth without encapsulation (Fig. 2.55). The mass may have a collagenous or myxoid matrix. Prominent capillaries and chronic inflammatory cells usually are present. Although mitotic figures may be common in the fibroblasts, abnormal mitoses are not seen. Some cytolysis usually is present. Heterologous elements such as bone

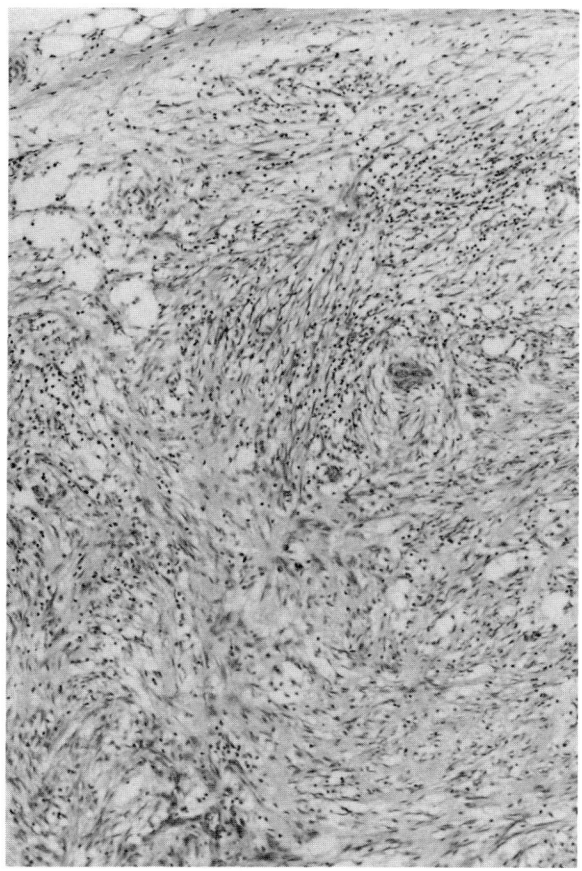

FIG. 2.55. Nodular fasciitis. This nonencapsulated mass is composed of spindle-shaped cells within a somewhat myxoid stroma. Prominent capillaries are within the mass and some lymphocytes are present. (Courtesy of David Dolson, M.D., Philadelphia, PA.)

and cartilage, as well as giant cells, have been reported.[88,203] The mass may be infiltrative and involve muscle. Immunoperoxidase studies contribute only in that the spindle cells have no distinctive immunoreactive antigen and are negative for desmin and myoglobin, to distinguish them from muscle tumors that are immunoreactive for these antigens.[159,165a]

Ectopic Breast Tissue

The occurrence of breast tissue in the vulva is not well understood, but is currently considered to be ectopic.[236,237] The amount and character of breast tissue reported within the labia majora varies from small, isolated nodules of mammary duct epithelium to large, bilateral structures that have been observed to lactate during the puerperium. Clinically, ectopic breast tissue in the vulva presents usually as an amorphous enlargement of the labia, usually first noted in association with pregnancy.[90,196] Benign cystic disease (fibrocystic disease) within the breast tissue, as well as fibroadenomas, lactating adenomas, and intraductal papillomas, have been described.[70,170,200] Fibroadenomas may arise in vulvar ectopic breast tissue and are distinguished from hidradenomas of sweat gland origin by the findings of adjacent ectopic breast tissue and the characteristic features of a fibroadenoma.[70] Intraductal papillomas may mimic hidradenoma to the degree that the two cannot be distinguished.[200] Lactating adenomas also have been described.[170] Histologically, the ectopic breast tissue is identical to ectopic breast tissue occurring elsewhere.

Adenocarcinoma of the ectopic breast tissue of the vulva has been reported. The complete removal of symptomatic ectopic breast tissue is advocated except when such tissue is discovered during pregnancy, in which case excision should be deferred until after puerperal regression is complete, or regression is to the point of the process no longer being symptomatic or associated with a palpable mass.

Ectopic Salivary Gland

Ectopic salivary gland tissue has been observed in the vulva.[152]

Idiopathic Vulvar Calcinosis

Although not a cystic condition, vulvar carcinosis may resemble keratinous cysts on clinical presentation, presenting as small (usually 2 mm or less), firm, subcutaneous nodules involving the majora and fourchette. The vulvar cases reported have occurred predominantly in adolescent women. Histological examination demonstrates normal-appearing overlying epithelium with basophilic acellular superficial subcutaneous nodules measuring from less than 0.1 mm to approximately 2 mm, associated with a chronic inflammatory infiltrate, mast cells, and foreign body giant cells. The acellular material stains with Von Kossa stain and contains acid mucopolysaccharides.[11] The process in rare, benign, and of uncertain etiology but appears similar to idiopathic scrotal calcinosis.[87]

Vulvar Amyloidosis

Nodules within the vulva have been described related to involvement of the vulva in a woman with systemic amyloidosis.[230a]

Urethra

Prolapse

Prolapse of the urethral mucosa may occur at any age, but it is most common in premenarchal children and in postmenopausal women.[14] Redundancy of the mucosa and laxity of the supporting periurethral fascia contribute to the formation of prolapse, which is aggravated by increased abdominal pressure; it may be related to relative lack of estrogen. The prolapsing urethra may present as a large red polypoid mass covered with urethral mucosa with edematous vascular submucosa, protruding from the urethra mimicking a urethral neoplasm. Histologically, the urethral mucosa may exhibit ulceration, and the underlying connective tissue is generally filled with an inflammatory infiltrate. Vascular engorgement usually is present. Cryosurgery is an effective method of treatment.[76,115a]

Urethral Caruncles

Caruncles are sessile or polypoid masses that arise at the urethral meatus in postmenopausal women. They may represent localized areas of prolapse, and are by far the most common lesions of the urethra. Caruncles often are asymptomatic but may cause bleeding or dysuria. Clinical differentiation from urethral carcinoma may be impossible; therefore, excision is indicated for diagnosis. Recurrences may be observed.[21] Histologically, the submucosa of the urethral caruncle may contain large venous channels that often are dilated and engorged. A myxomatous or granulomatous pattern may be present in the supporting tissue, which often is infiltrated densely with chronic inflammatory cells. Excision, with hemostatic destruction of the base of the lesion, is the treatment of choice.

Malacoplakia of the Urethra

Malacoplakia is a chronic granulomatous inflammatory porcess that usually involves the bladder if the urethra is involved. The lesion presents as a polypoid mass at the urethral meatus and on microscopic examination foamy histiocytes with associated lymphocytes, granulocytes, and plasma cells. The diagnostic Michaelis–Gutmann bodies are seen within the cytoplasm of the histiocytes as inclusions having a blue-gray color (Fig. 2.56). The inclusions may appear laminated or targetoid. With PSA stain the Michaelis–Gutmann bodies usually stain pink to red. Many of the adjacent histiocytes also contain PAS-positive cytoplasmic material.[221] Excision may be diagnostic and curative for small lesions within the urethra, although recurrences are not uncommon. Antibiotics also may be of value.

Periurethral Cysts

Periurethral cysts can be subclassified related to their epithelial lining, and are similar to cysts of the vulvar vestibule. The cysts can be classified into four distinctive types: *epithelial inclusion (keratinous) cysts* have a squamous ep-

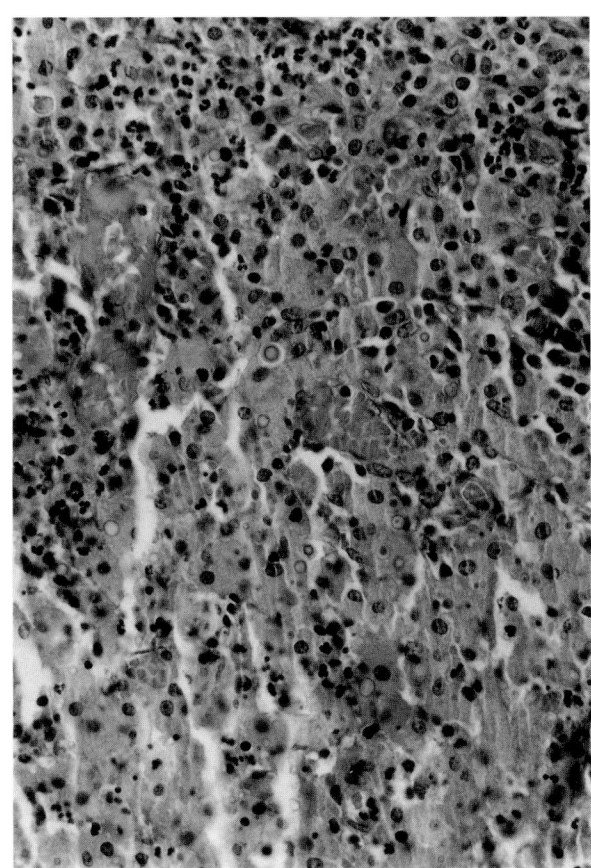

Fig. 2.56. **Malacoplakia of the urethra.** This section, from a polypoid mass within the urethra, demonstrates many foamy histiocytes admixed with lymphocytes, plasma cells, and granulocytes. Round inclusions are present in some of the histiocytes (Michaelis–Gutmann bodies), which are approximately the size of the nuclei of the histiocytes and have a dark periphery and pale center. (Courtesy of J. Emery, M.D., Gainesville, FL.)

ithelial lining, and may arise secondary to trauma or surgical procedures trapping epithelium; *mucous cysts* have a columnar, endocervical-type epithelial lining and may have associated squamous epithelium, secondary to squamous metaplasia. The cytoplasm of the columnar epithelium contains mucin. These cysts appear essentially identical to the mucous cysts of the vulvar vestibule although they have been referred to as müllerian cysts in the urologic literature[50]; *mesonephric-like cysts* have a low cuboidal epithelium that does not stain with mucin; *urothelial cysts* usually are seen in infants and are rare in adults. They are believed to arise from Skene ducts or from proximal urothelial ducts. These cysts have a urothelial epithelial lining, although those near the urethra meatus may have a squamous epithelial lining.[50]

Suburethral Diverticulum

Suburethral diverticula originate from the upper two-thirds of the posterior urethral wall and may extend cephalad to involve the region beneath the vesicle neck. Although a congenital etiology has been proposed for some cases, most are thought to begin as an infection in one of the tubular periurethral glands[104] followed by abscess formation with eventual breakthrough into the urethral lumen.

Urethral Condyloma Acuminatum

Urethral condyloma acuminatum may present like a caruncle or urethral carcinoma, and usually is seen in women of reproductive age and not in older individuals.[5,6] In children urethral and periurethral condylomata may be polypoid and clinically suggest sarcoma botryoides. In adult women they usually are associated with other lower genital infection, especially vulvar vestibular condyloma acuminatum. Some patients may have symptoms of urethritis associated with urethral condyloma acuminatum. In these patients the condyloma may be in the mid- or upper urethra. On biopsy they have a stratified squamous epithelium within which typical features of mucosal HPV infection are seen, including koilocytosis, multinucleation, and parabasalar hyperplasia (Fig. 2.57). HPV types 6 and 16 have been observed in these urethral condyloma.[6]

Leiomyoma of the Urethra

Urethral leiomyoma is a relatively rare, benign, smooth muscle tumor that may be associated with dysuria, hematuria, or infection; approximately one-half of the reported cases observed a external urethral mass. These tumors may enlarge in pregnancy, suggesting hormonal receptors. Microscopically the tumor is composed of smooth muscle cells arranged in a whorled pattern. Malignant change has

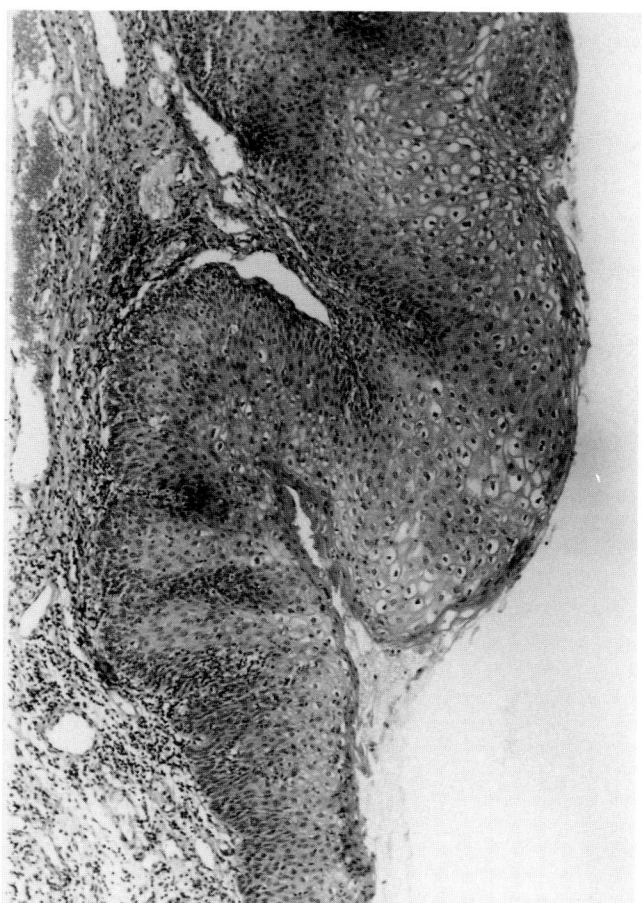

FIG. 2.57. **Urethral condyloma acuminatum.** The stratified squamous epithelium of the urethra has koilocytes within the upper epithelium and there is parabasalar hyperplasia. Mild superficial chronic inflammation is present (this lesion contained HPV 6 by PCR). (Courtesy of Paul Allen, M.D., Pascagula, MS).

not been reported. Local excision is the treatment of choice and usually is curative.[85]

Acknowledgment. The author acknowledges Ms. Sandra Fortier for her secretarial assistance in the preparation of this chapter, and Dr. K Kendall Pierson for his review of some of the dermatopathology-related issues in this chapter.

Dedication. These two chapters on vulvar disease are dedicated in memory of Eduard G. Friedrich, Jr., M.D., friend, colleague, and my collaborator to previous editions of this work.

References

1. Abdul-Karim FW, Cohen RE (1990) Atyipcal stromal cells of lower female genital tract. Histopathology 17: 249–253
2. Ackerman AB, Mihara I (1985) Dysplasia, dysplastic melanocytes, dysplastic nevi, the dysplastic nevus syndrome,

and the relation between dysplastic nevi and malignant melanomas. Hum Pathol 16: 87–91

3. Adam E, Kaufman RH, Mirkovic RR, Melnick JL (1979) Persistence of virus shedding in asymptomatic women after recovery from herpes genitalis. Obstet Gynecol 54: 171

4. Addison WA, Livengood CH, Hill GB, Sutton GP, Fortier KJ (1984) Necrotizing fasciitis of vulvar origin in diabetic patients. Obstet Gynecol 63: 473

5. Allen PM, Davis GD (1992) A new instrument for the visualization of and laser treatment of the female urethra and trigone. Int Urogynecol J 3: 133–136

6. Allen PM, Davis GD, Bowen LW, Sand PK, Habert DB, Wilkinson EJ (1993) Polymerase chain reaction and morphologic studies on inflammatory lesions of the proximal urethra in patients with genital papillomavirus lesions and urethral syndrome: data from a multicenter study group (In preparation)

7. Aneiros J, Belträn E, Gacia del Moral R, Nagoles FF Jr (1982) Epithelioid leiomyoma of the vulva. Diagn Gynecol Obstet 4: 351–356

8. Avinoach I, Zirfkin HJ, Glezerman M (1989) Proliferating trichilemmal tumor of the vulva. Case report and review of the literature. Int J Gynecol Pathol 8: 163/N168

9. Axe S, Parmley T, Woodruff JD, Hlopak B (1986) Adenomas in minor vestibular glands. Obstet Gynecol 68: 16–18

10. Balfour HJ Jr (1988) Varicella zoster virus infections in immunocompromised hosts. Am J Med 85(2A): 68–73

11. Balfour FJT, Vincenti AC (1991) Idiopathic vulvar calcinosis. Histopathology 18: 183–184

12. Barnhill RL, Albert LS, Shama SK, Goldenhersh MA, Rhodes AR, Sober AJ (1990) Genital lentiginosis; A clinical and histopathologic study. J Am Acad Dermatol 22: 453–460

13. Basta A, Madej Jr JG (1990) Hydradenoma of the vulva. Incidence and clinical observations. Eur J Gynecol Oncol 11: 185–189

14. Bayonet-Rivera NP, Magoss I (1970) Vulvar tumor in children due to prolapse of urethral mucosa. Am J Obstet Gynecol 108: 572

15. Bergeron C, Ferenczy A, Richart RM, Guralnick M (1990) Micropapillomatosis labialis appears unrelated to human papillomavirus. Obstet Gynecol 76: 281–286

16. Bergeron C, Nayhashfar Z, Canaan C, et al (1987) Human papillomavirus type 16 in intraepithelial neoplasia and co-existent invasive carcinoma of the vulva. Int J Gynecol Pathol 6: 1–11

17. Bergman A, Bhatia NM, Broen EM (1984) Cryotherapy for treatment of genital condyloma during pregnancy. J Reprod Med 29: 432

18. Berth-Jones J, Graham-Brown RA, Burns DA (1991) Lichen sclerosus et atrophicus—a review of 15 cases in young girls. Clin Exp Dermatol 16: 14–17

19. Blair C (1970) Angiokeratoma of the vulva. Br J Dermatol 83: 409

20. Blank H, Davis C, Collins C (1970) Electron microscopy for the diagnosis of cutaneous viral infections. Br J Dermatol 83: 69

21. Bolduan JP, Farah RN (1981) Primary urethral neoplasms. Review of 30 cases. J Urol 125: 198

22. Bonafe JL, Thibaut I, Hoff J (1990) Introital adenosis associated with the Stevens-Johnson syndrome. Clin Exp Dermatol 15: 356–357

23. Boyce DC, Valpey JM (1971) Acute ulcerative vulvitis of obscure etiology. Obstet Gynecol 38: 440

24. Britz MB, Maibach HI (1979) Human cutaneous vulvar reactivity to irritants. Contact Dermatitis 5: 375

25. Brodell RT, Santa Curz D (1985) Borderline and atypical melanocytic lesions. Semin Diagn Pathol 2: 63–86

26. Bruynzeel-Koomen C, Van Wichen DF, Toonstra J, Berrens L, Bruynzeel PL (1986) The presence of IgE Molecules on epidermal Langerhan's cells in patients with atopic dermatis. Arch Dermatol Rec 278: 199–205

27. Buchler DA, Sun F, Chaprevich T (1978) A pilar tumor of the vulva. Gynecol Oncol 6: 479–486

28. Bushkell LL, Friedrich EG, Jordon RE (1981) An appraisal of routine direct immunofluorescence in vulvar disorders. Acta Derm Venereol 61: 157

29. Butler EB, Stanbridge CM (1984) Condylomatous lesions of the lower female genital tract. Clin Obstet Gynecol 11: 171

30. CDC (1983) Condyloma acuminatum, United States, 1966–1981. MMWR 23: 306

31. Campion MJ, DiPaola FM, Crozier MA, Rathrock R, Vellios F, Franklin EW (1994) Labial micropapillomatosis human papillomavirus infection or anatomic variant. Obstet Gynecol (In press)

32. Cao M, Xiao X, Egbert B, Darragh TM, Benedict TS (1989) Rapid detefction of cutaneous herpes simplex virus infection with the polymerase chain reaction. J Invest Dermatol 82: 391–392

33. Capraro VJ (1971) Congenital anomalies. Clin Obstet Gynecol 14; 988

34. Carli P, Cattaneo A, Pimpinelli N, Cozza A, Bracco G, Giannotti B (1991) Immunohistochemical evidence of skin immune system involvement in vulvar lichen sclerosus et atrophicus. Dermatologica 182: 18–22

35. Carter J, Elliott P, Russell P (1992) Bilateral fibroepithelial polypi of labium minus with atypical stromal cells. Pathology 24: 37–39

36. Cattaneo A, Bracco GL, Maestrini G, et al (1991) Lichen sclerosus and squamous hyperplasia of the vulva. A clinical study of medical treatment. J Reprod Med 36: 301–305

37. Chaung T, Perry HO, Kurland LT, Ilstrup DM (1984) Condyloma acuminatum in Rochester, Minn, 1950–1978. II Anaplasias and unfavorable outcomes. Arch Dermatol 120: 476

38. Chetkowski R, Sakamoto H, MacLusky N, Merino M, Schwartz PE (1985) Solitary pelvic neural tumors with high steroid receptor content. Gynecol Oncol 20: 43

39. Cho D, Woodruff JD (1988) Trichoepithelioma of the vulva. A report of two cases. J Reprod Med 33: 317–319

40. Christensen WN, Friedman KJ, Woodruff JD, Hood AF (1987) Histologic characteristics of vulvar nevocellular nevi. J Cutan Pathol 14: 87–91

41. Cilla G, Pico F, Peris A, Idigoras P, Urbieta M, Perez-Trallero E (1992) Human genital myiasis due to Sarcophaga. Rev Clin Esp 190: 189–190

42. Cockerell CJ, LeBoit EP (1990) Bacillary angiomatosis: a newly characterized, pseudoneoplastic, infectious, cutaneous vascular disorder. J Am Acad Dermatol 22: 501–512

43. Coghill SB, Tyler X, Shaxted EJ (1990) Benign mucinous metaplasia of the vulva. Histopathology 17: 373–375

44. Cone R, Beckmann A, Aho M, Wahlstrom T, Ek M, Corey L, Paavonen J (1991) Subclinical manifestations of vulvar human papillomavirus infection. Int J Gynecol Pathol 10: 26–35

45. Cooper PH (1989) Acantholytic dermatosis localized to the vulvocrural area. J Cutan Pathol 16: 81–84

46. Corey L, Adams HG, Brown ZA, Holmes KK (1983) Genital herpes simplex virus infections: Clinical manifestations, course, and complications. Ann Intern Med 98: 958

47. Crum CP, Fu YS, Levine RU, Richart RM, Towensend DE, Fenoglio CM (1982) Intraepithelial squamous lesions of the vulva: Biologic and histologic criteria for the distinction of condylomas from vulvar intraepithelial neoplasia. Am J Obstet Gynecol 144: 77

48. Curth HO, Aschner BM (1959) Genetic studies on acanthosis nigricans. Arch Dermatol 79: 55

49. Dalziel KL, Mallard R, Wojnarowska F (1991) The treatment of vulvar lichen sclerosus with very potent topical steroid (clobetasol propionate 0.05% cream). Br J Dermatol 124: 461

50. Das SP (1981) Paraurethral cysts in women. J Urol 126: 41–43

51. de Oliveira M, Saleiro V (1986) Involucrin expression in vulvar lesions. J Reprod Med 31: 828

52. Degefu S, Dhurandhar N, O'Quinn AG, Fuller PN (1984) Granular cell tumor of the clitoris in pregnancy. Gynecol Oncol 19: 246

53. Derksen DJ (1992) Children with condylomata acuminata. J Fam Pract 34: 419–423

54. Dewhurst CJ (1968) Congenital malformations of the genital tract in childhood. J Obstet Gynecol Br Common 75: 377

55. Dickie RJ, Horne CH, Sutherland HW, Bewsher PD, Stankler L (1982) Direct evidence of localized immunological damage in vulvar lichen sclerosus et atrophicus. J Clin Pathol 35: 1395

56. diSant'Agnese PA, Knowles DM (1980) Extracardiac rhabdomyom: A clinicopathologic study and review of the literature. Cancer 46: 780

57. Dodson RF, Fritz GS, Hubler WR, Rudolph AH, Knox JM, Chu LW (1974) Donovanosis: A morphologic study. J Invest Dermatol 62: 611

58. Douglas CP (1962) Lymphogranuloma venereum and granuloma inguinale of the vulva. J Obstet Gynecol Br Commun 69: 871

59. Drusin LM (1972) The diagnosis and treatment of infectious and latent syphilis. Med Clin North Am 56: 1161

59a. Dungar CF, Wilkinson EJ (1994) Vaginal columnar cell metaplasia associated with topical 5-Fluorouracil therapy. J Reprod Med (Submitted)

60. Dunn JM (1970) Congenital absence of the external genitalia. J Reprod Med 4: 66

61. Duray PH, Merino MJ, Axiotis C (1983) Warty dyskeratoma of the vulva. Int J Gynecol Pathol 2: 286

62. Edwards L (1989) Vulvar lichen planus. Arch Dermatol 125: 1677–1680

63. Edwards L (1992) Desquamative vulvitis. Dermatol Clin 10: 325–337

64. Ekwo E, Wong YW, Myers M (1979) Asymptomatic cervicovaginal shedding of herpes simplex virus. Am J Obstet Gynecol 134: 102

65. Evron S, Leviatan A, Okon E (1984) Familial benign chronic pemphigus appearing as leukoplakia of the vulva. Int J Dermatol 23: 556

66. Faber K, Jones MA, Spratt D, Tarraza Jr HM (1991) Vulvar leiomyomatosis in a patient with esophagogastric leiomyomatosis: review of the syndrome. Gynecol Oncol 41: 92–94

67. Falk HC, Hyman AB (1971) Congenital absence of clitoris. Obstet Gyencol 38: 269

68. Ferenczy A, Mitao M, Nagai N, Silverstein SJ, Crum CP (1985) Latent papillomavirus and recurring genital warts. N Engl J Med 313: 784

69. Fletcher CD, Tsang WY, Fisher C, Lee KC, Chan JK (1992) Angiomyofibroblastoma of the vulva: A benign neoplasm distinct from aggressive angiomyxoma. Am J Surg Pathol 16: 373–382

70. Floushee JH, Pruitt AB Jr (1967) Vulvar fibroadenoma from aberrant breast tissue. Report of 2 cases. Obstet Gynecol 29: 819–823

71. Flynt J, Gallup DG (1979) Childhood lichen sclerosus. Obstet Gynecol 53: 79S

72. Fowler WC Jr, Lawrence H, Edelman DA (1981) Paravestibular tumor of the female genital tract. Am J Obstet Gynecol 139: 109

73. Freedman SR, Goldman RL (1978) Mucocele-like changes in Bartholin's glands. Hum Pathol 9: 111

74. Friedman RJ, Ackerman B (1981) Difficulties in the histologic diagnosis of melanocytic nevi on the vulvae of premenopausal women. In: Ackerman AB (ed) Pathology of malignant melanoma. New York, Mason, pp 119–127

75. Friedmann W, Schafer A, Kretschmer R (1990) CMV virus infection of the vulva and vagina. Geburtshilfe-Frauenheilkd 50: 729–730

76. Friedrich EG Jr (1977) Cryosurgery for urethral prolapse. Obstet Gynecol 50: 359

77. Friedrich EG Jr (1976) Lichen sclerosus. J Reprod Med 17: 147

78. Friedrich EG Jr (1987) Vulvar vestibulitis syndrome. J Reprod Med 32: 110–114

79. Friedrich EG Jr, MacLaren NK (1984) Genetic aspects of vulvar lichen sclerosus. Am J Obstet Gynecol 150: 161

80. Friedrich EG Jr, Burch K, Bahr JP (1979) The vulvar clinic: An eight year appraisal, Am J Obstet Gynecol 135: 1036

81. Friedrich EG Jr, Kalra PS (1984) Serum levels of sex hormones in vulvar lichen sclerosus, and the effect of topical testosterone. N Engl J Med 310: 488

82. Friedrich EG Jr, Wilkinson EJ (1973) Mucous-cysts of the vulvar vestibule. Obstet Gynecol 42: 407

83. Friedrich EG Jr, Wilkinson EJ (1985) Vulvar surgery for neurofibromatosis. Obstet Gynecol 65: 135

84. Frith P, Charnock M, Wojnarowska F (1991) Cicatricial pemphigoid diagnosed from ocular features in recurrent severe vulvae scarring. Two case reports. Br J Obstet Gynecol 98: 482–484

85. Fry M, Wheeler Jr JS, Mata JA, Culkin DJ, St Martin E, Venable DD (1988) Leiomyoma of the female urethra. J Urol 140:613–614

86. Fukamizu H, Matsumoto K, Inouek K, Moriguchi T (1982) Large vulvar lipoma. Arch Dermatol 118: 447

87. Fukaya Y, Ueda H (1991) A case of idiopathic vulvar calcinosis. The first in Japan. J Dermatol 18: 680–683

88. Gaffney EF, Majmuder B, Bryan JA (1982) Nodular fasciitis (pseudosarcomatous fasciitis) of the vulva. Int J Gynecol Pathol 1: 307

89. Galloway DA, McDougall JK (1990) Alterations in the cellular phenotype induced by herpes simplex viruses. J Med Virol 31: 36–42

90. Garcia JJ, Verkauf BS, Hochberg CJ, Ingram JM (1978) Aberrant breast tissue of the vulva: A case report and review of the literature. Obstet Gynecol 52: 225–228

91. Gilks CB, Clement PB, Wood WS (1989) Trichoblastic fibroma. A clinicopathologic study of three cases. Am J Dermatopathol 11: 397–402

92. Gissmann L, deVillers EM, Zur Hausen H (1982) Analysis of human warts (condylomata acuminata) and other genital tumors for human papilloma virus type 6 DNA. Int J Cancer 29: 143

93. Gissmann L, Wolnik L, Ikenberg H, Koldovsky V, Schnurch HG, Zur Hausen H (1983) Human Papillomavirus types 6 and 11 DNA sequences in genital and laryngeal papillomas and in some cervical cancers. Proc Natl Acad Sci 80: 560

94. Godeau G, Frances C, Hornebeck W, Brechemier D, Robert L (1982) Isolation and partial characterization of an elastase-type protease in human vulva fibroblasts: Its possible involvement in vulvar elastic tissue destruction of patients with lichen sclerosus et atrophicus. J Invest Dermatol 78: 270

95. Williams PL (ed) (1989) Gray's textbook of anatomy, 37th ed. New York, Churchill Livingstone

96. Growdon WA, Fu Y, Lebherz TB, Rapkin A, Mason GD, Parks G (1985) Pruritic vulvar squamous papillomatosis: Evidence for human papillomavirus etiology. Obstet Gynecol 66: 564

97. Hackel H, Hartmann AA, Burg G (1991) Vulvitis granulomatosa and anoperineitis granulomatosa. Dermatologica 182: 128–131

98. Harrington CI, Dunsmore IR (1981) An investigation into the incidence of autoimmune disorders in patients with lichen sclerosus et atrophicus. Br J Dermatol 104: 563

98a. Hendricks J, Wilkinson EJ (1994) KI-67 expression in lichen sclerosus of the vulva. (In manuscript)

99. Hewitt J (1986) Lichen sclerosus. J Reprod Med 31: 781

100. Hewitt M, Barrow GI, Miller DC, Turk F, Turk S (1973) Mites in the personal environment and their role in skin disorders. Br J Dermatol 89: 401

101. Hewitt AB (1971) Behcet's disease. Br J Vener Dis 47: 52

102. Holmes RC, Black MM (1983) The specific dermatoses of pregnancy. J Am Acad Dermatol 8: 805–812

103. Huang HJ, Yamabe T, Tagawa H (1983) A solitary neurilemmoma of the clitoris. Gynecol Oncol 15: 103–110

104. Huffman JW (1948) The detailed anatomy of the paraurethral ducts in the adult human female. Am J Obstet Gynecol 55: 86

105. Hurley HJ, Shelley WB (1960) The human apocrine sweat gland in health and disease. Charles C Thomas

106. Imperial R, Helwig EB (1967) Angiokeratoma of the vulva. Obstet Gynecol 29: 307

106a. International Society for the Study of Vulvar Disease (1976) New nomenclature for vulvar disease I. Obstet Gynecol 47: 122

107. Isaacson D, Turner ML (1979) Localized vulvar syringomas. J Am Acad Dermatol 1: 352

108. Iversen T, Aas M (1983) Lymph drainage from the vulva. Gynecol Oncol 16: 179

109. Jacobs MI, Rigel DS (1981) Acanthosis nigricans and the sign of Leser–Trélat associated with adenocarcinoma of the gall bladder. Cancer 48: 328

110. Janakiv JK, Dremalatha S, Rughuveera N, Thambiah AS (1980) Lawrence-Seip syndrome. Br J Dermatol 103: 693

111. Johnson TL, Kennedy AW, Segal GH (1991) Lymphangioma circumscriptum of the vulva. A report of two cases. J Reprod Med 36: 808–812

112. Junard TA, Thomas SM (1981) Cysts of the vulva and vagina: A comparative study. Int J Gynecol Obstet 19: 239

113. Jurecka W, Holmes RC, Black MM, McKee PH, Das AK, Bhogal B (1983) An immunoelectron microscopic study of the relationship between herpes gestationis and polymorphic eruption of the pregnancy. Br J Dermatol 108: 147–151

114. Katz VL, Askin FB, Bosch BD (1986) Glomus tumor of the vulva: A case report. Obstet Gynecol 67: 43–45S

115. Kaufman RH, Faro S (1985) Herpes genitalis: Clinical features and treatment. Clin Obstet Gynecol 28: 152

115a. Kaufman RH, Friedrich EG Jr, Gardner HL (1990) Benign diseases of the vulva and vagina. Chicago, Yearbook Med Publishers

116. Kaufman RH, Friedrich EG Jr (1985) The carbon dioxide laser in the treatment of vulvar disease. Clin Obstet Gynecol 28: 220

117. Kaufman RH, Friedman K (1981) Hemangioma of the clitoris confused with adrenogenital syndrome: Case report. Plast Reconstruct Surg 62: 452–454

118. Kellogg ND, Parra JM (1991) Linea vestibularis. Pediatrics 87: 926–929

119. Kernen JA, Morgan ML (1970) Benign lymphoid hamartoma of the vulva. Obstet Gynecol 35: 290

120. Kfuri A, Rosenshein N, Dorfman H, Goldstein P (1981) Desmoid tumor of the vulva. J Reprod Med 26: 272

121. King DF, Bustillo M, Broen EN, Hiros FM (1979) Granular cell tumors of the vulva. A report of 3 cases. J Dermatol Surg Oncol 5: 794

122. King LS, Sullivan M (1947) Effects of podophyllin and of colchicine on normal skin, on condyloma acuminatum, and on verruca vulgaris. Arch Pathol 43: 374

123. Knudson AG (1985) Hereditary cancer oncogenes, and antioncogenes. Cancer Res 45: 1437

124. Kohorn EI, Merino MJ, Goldenhersh M (1986) Vulvar pain and dyspareunia due to glamus tumor. Obstet Gynecol 67: 41–42S

125. Koranantakul O, Lekhakula A, Wansit R, Koranantakul Y (1991) Cutaneous myiasis of vulva caused by the muscoid fly (Chrysomyia genus). Southeast Asian J Trop Med Public Health 22: 458–460

126. Koutsky LA, Stevens CE, Holmes KK, et al (1992) Underdiagnosis of genital herpes by current clinical and viral-isolation procedures. N Engl J Med 326: 1533–1539

127. Kovi J, Tillman RL, Lee SM (1974) Malignant transforma-

tion of condyloma acuminatum: A light microscopic and ultrastructural study. Am J Clin Pathol 61: 702

128. Krantz KE (1958) Innervation of the human vulva and vagina. Obstet Gynecol 12: 382

129. Kremer M, Nussenson E, Steinfeld M, Zuckerman P (1984) Crohn's disease of the vulva. Am J Gastroenterol 79: 376

130. Kuberski T (1980) Granuloma inguinale (Donovanosis). Sex Trans Dis 7: 29

131. Kucera PR, Glazer J (1985) Hydrocele of the canal of nuck: A report of four cases. J Reprod Med 30: 439

132. Kurman RJ, Shah KH, Lancaster WD, Jenson AB (1981) Immunoperoxidase localization of papillomavirus antigens in cervical dysplasia and vulvar condylomas. Am J Obstet Gynecol 140: 9321

133. Kurman RJ, Potkul RK, Lancaster WD, Lewandowski G, Weck PR, Delgato G (1990) Vulvar condylomas and squamous vestibular micropapilloma: Differences in appearance and response to treatment. J Reprod Med 35: 1019–1022

133a. Leibowitch M, Neill S, Pelisse M, Moyal-Baracco M (1990) The epithelial changes associated with squamous cell carcinoma of the vulva: a review of the clinical, histological and viral findings of 78 women. Br J Obstet Gynaecol 97: 1135–1139

134. Lever WF, Schaumburg-Lever G (1990) Histopathology of the skin, 6th ed. Philadelphia, JB Lippincott

135. LiVolsi VA, Brooks JJ (1987) Soft tissue tumors of the vulva. In: Wilkinson EJ (ed) Contemporary issues in surgical pathology. Pathology of the vulva and vagina, vol 9. New York, Churchill Livginstone, pp 209–238

136. Loening-Baucke V (1991) Lichen sclerosus et atrophicus in children. Am J Dis Child 145: 1058–1061

137. Lowell DM, LiVolsi VA, Ludwig ME (1983) Genital condyloma virus infection following pelvic radiation therapy: Report of seven cases. Int J Gynecol Pathol 2: 294

138. Lucky AW (1988) Pigmentary abnormalities in genetic disorders. Dermatol Clin 6: 193–197

139. Lynch PJ (1985) Condylomata acuminata (anogenital warts). Obstet Gynecol 28: 142

140. Maccato ML, Kaufman RH (1992) Herpes genitalis. Dermatol Clin 10: 415–422

141. Magrine JR, Masterson BJ (1981) Loxosceles reclusa spider bite: A consideration in the differential diagnosis of chronic, nonmalignant ulcers of the vulva. Am J Obstet Gynecol 140: 343

142. Mahmud N, Kusuda N, Ichenose S, et al (1992) Needle aspiration biopsy of vulvar endometriois. A case report. Acta Cytol 36: 514–516

143. Maize JC (1988) Mucosal melanosis. Dermatol Clin 6: 283–293

144. Majmudar B, Hallden C (1986) The relationship between juvenile laryngeal papillomatosis and maternal condylomata acuminata. J Reprod Med 31: 804

145. Majmudar B, Castellano PZ, Wilson RW, Siegel RJ (1990) Granular cell tumors of the vulva. J Reprod Med 35: 1008–1014

146. Mann MS, Kaufman RH (1991) Erosive lichen planus of the vulva. Clin Obstet Gynecol 34: 605–613

147. Mann MS, Kaufman RH, Brown D, Adam E (1992) Vulvar

vestibulitis: Significant clinical variables and treatment outcome. Obstet Gynecol 79: 122–125

148. Mann PR, Cowan MA (1973) Ultrastructural changes in four cases of lichen sclerosus et atrophicus. Br J Dermatol 89: 223

149. Marinoff SC, Turner MLC (1991) Vulvar vestibulitis syndrome: An overview. Am J Obstet Gynecol 165: 1228–1233

150. Marquette GP, Su B, Woodruff JD (1985) Introital adenosis associated with Stevens–Johnson Syndrome. Obstet and Gynecol 66: 143–145

151. Marsden RA, McKee PH, Bhogal B, Black MM, Kennedy LA (1980) A study of benign chronic bullous dermatosis of childhood and comparison with dermatitis herpetiforms and bullous pemphigoid occurring in childhood. Clin Exp Dermatol 5: 159–172

152. Marwah S, Bergman ML (1980) Ectopic salivary gland in the vulva (choristoma): Report of a case and review of the literature. Obstet Gynecol 56: 398

153. Matthews J, Mason G (1983) Granular cell myoblastoma: An immunoperoxidase study using a variety of antisera to human carcinoembryonic antigen. Histopathology 7: 77

154. McKendrick MW, McGill JI, White JE, Wood MJ (1986) Oral acyclovir in acute herpes zoster. Br Med J Clin Res 293: 1529–1532

155. McKay M, Frankman O, Horowitz B, et al (1991) Vulvar vestibulitis and vestibular papillomatosis. Report of the ISSVD Committee on vulvodynia. J Reprod Med 36: 413–415

156. McKee PH (1989) Pathology of the skin with clinical correlations. Jowett M, Smillie (ed) Philadelphia, JB Lippincott

157. McKee PH, Wright E, Hutt MSR (1983) Vulvar schistosomiasis. Clin Exp Dermatol 8: 189

158. McNeely TB (1992) Angiokeratoma of the clitoris. Arch Pathol Lab Med 116: 880–881

159. Meister P, Buckmann FW, Konrad E (1978) Nodular fasciitis. Analysis of 100 cases and review of the literature. Pathol Res Pract 162: 133

160. Merlob P, Bahari C, Liban E, Reisner SH (1978) Cysts of the female external genitalia in the newborn infant. Am J Obstet Gynecol 132: 607

161. Milbrath JR, Wilkinson EJ, Friedrich EG Jr (1975) Xerographic evaluation of radical vulvectomy specimens. Am J Roentgenol Radiat Ther Nucl Med 125: 486

162. Millikan LE (1985) Drug eruptions (dermatitis medicamentosa). In: Moschella SL, Hurley HJ (eds) Dermatology, 2nd ed. Philadelphia, WB Saunders, pp 425–463

163. Morse SA (1990) Atlas of Sexually Transmitted Diseases. Philadelphia, JB Lippincott

164. Moyal-Barracco M, Leibowitch M, Orth G (1990) Vestibular papillae of the vulva. Lack of evidence for human papillomavirus etiology. Arch Dermatol 126: 1594–1598

165. Muller G, Jacobs PH, Moore NE (1973) Scraping for human scabies. Arch Deramtol 107: 70

165a. Nadji M, Ganjei P, Penneys NS, Morales AR (1984) Immunohistochemistry of vulvar neoplasms: A brief review. Int J Gynecol Pathol 3: 41

166. Neill SM, Smith NP, Eady RA (1984) Ulcerative sarcoido-

sis: A rare manifestation of a common disease. Clin Exp Dermatol 9: 277

167. Newton JA, Camplejohn RS, McGibbon DH (1987) A flow cytometric study of the significance of DNA aneuploidy in cutaneous lesions. Br J Dermatol 117: 169–174

168. Oberhofer TR, Back AE (1982) Isolation and cultivation of *Haemophilus Ducreyi.* J Clin Microbiol 15: 625

169. O'Duffy JD, Carney JA, Deodhar S (1971) Behcet's disease. Ann Intern Med 75: 561

170. O'Hara MF, Page DL (1985) Adenomas of the breast and ectopic breast under lactational influences. Hum Pathol 16: 707–712

171. O'Rahilly R, Muller F (1992) Human embryology and teratology. New York, J Wiley & Sons

172. Oi RH, Munn R (1982) Mucous cysts of the vulvar vestibule. Hum Pathol 13: 584

173. Okagaki T, Clark BA, Zachow KR, et al (1984) Presence of human papillomavirus in verucous carcinoma (Ackerman) of the vagina. Arch Pathol Lab Med 108: 567

174. Olansky S (1972) Serodiagnosis of syphilis. Med Clin North Am 56: 1145

175. Ordonez NG, Manning JT, Luna MA (1981) Mixed tumor of the vulva: A report of two cases probably arising in Bartholin's gland. Cancer 48: 181

176. Oriel JD, Almeida JD (1970) Demonstration of virus particles in human genital warts. Br J Vener Dis 46: 37–42

177. Oriel JD (1971) Natural history of genital warts. Br J Vener Dis 47: 1

178. Parry-Jones E (1963) Lymphatics of the vulva. J Obstet Gynecol Br Commun 70: 751

179. Patton LW, Elgart ML, Williams CM (1990) Vulvar erythema and induration. Extraintestinal Crohn's disease of the vulva. Arch Dermatol 126: 1351–1354

180. Pelisse M (1989) The vulva-vaginal-gingival syndrome. A new form of erosive lichen planus. Int J Dermatol 28: 381–384

181. Pelosi G, Martignoni G, Bonetti F (1991) Intraductal carcinoma of mammary-type apocrine epithelium arising within a papillary hidradenoma of the vulva. Report of a case and review of the literature. Arch Pathol Lab Med 115: 1249–1254

182. Pierson KK (1987) Malignant melanomas and pigmented lesions of the vulva. In: Wilkinson EJ (ed) Contemporary issues in surgical pathology. Pathology of the Vulva and Vagina, vol 9. New York, Churchill Livingstone, pp 155–179

183. Pincus SH (1992) Vulvar dermatoses and pruritus vulva. Dermatol Clin 10: 297–308

184. Pincus SH, Stadecker MJ (1987) Vulvar dystrophies and noninfectious inflammatory conditions. In: Wilkinson EJ (ed) Contemporary issues in surgical pathology. Pathology of the Vulva and Vagina, vol 9. New York, Churchill Livingstone, pp. 11–24

185. Pinkus H, Mehregan AH (1981) A guide to dermatohistopathology. New York, Appleton-Century-Crofts

186. Plentl AA, Friedman EA (1971) Lymphatic system of the female genitalia. Philadelphia, WB Saunders

187. Portnoy J, Ahronheim GA, Ghibu F, Clecner B, Joncas JH (1984) Recovery of Epstein–Barr virus from genital ulcers. N Engl J Med 311:966

188. Prakash SS, Reeves WC, Sisson GR, et al (1985) Herpes simplex virus type 2 and human papillomavirus type 16 in cervicitis, dysplasia and invasive cervical carcinoma. Int J Cancer 35: 51

189. Pyka RE, Wilkinson EJ, Friedrich EG Jr, Croker BP (1988) The histopathology of vulvar vestibulitis syndrome. Int J Gynecol Pathol 7: 249–257

190. Quan MB, Moy RL (1991) The role of human papillomavirus in carcinoma. J Am Acad Dermatol 25: 698–705

191. Quirk CA, Krzyzek RA, Watts SL, Faras AJ (1980) Relationship between condylomata and laryngeal papillomata. Clinical and molecular virological evidence. Ann Otol 89: 467

192. Ramesh V, Iyengar B (1990) Proliferating trichilemmal cysts over the vulva. Cutis 45: 187–189

193. Reed RJ (1990) Neoplasms of the skin. In: Silverberg SG (ed) Principles and practice of surgical pathology, 2nd ed. New York, Churchill Livingstone, p 193–254

194. Reed RJ, Parkinson RP (1977) The histogenesis of molluscum contagiosum. Am J Surg Pathol 1: 161

195. Reed JA, Brigati DJ, Flynn SD, McNutt NS, Min K, Welch DF, Slater LN (1992) Immunocytochemical identification of Rochalimaea henselae in bacillary (epithelioid) angiomatosis, parenchymal bacillary peliosis, and persistent fever with bacteremia. Am J Surg Pathol 16: 650–657

196. Reeves KO, Kaufman RH (1980) Vulvar extopic breat tissue mimicking periclitoral abscess. Am J Obstet Gynecol 137: 509

197. Reid R (1985) Superficial laser vulvectomy: The efficacy of extended superficial ablation for refractory and very extensive condylomas. Am J Obstet Gynecol 151: 1047

198. Rhatigan RM, Nuss RC (1985) Keratoacanthoma of the vulva. Gynecol Oncol 21: 118

199. Rhodes AR, Mihm MC Jr, Weinstock MA (1989) Dysplastic melanocytic nevi. A reproducible histologic definition emphasizing cellular morphology. Mod Pathol 2: 306–319

200. Rickert RR (1980) Intraductal papilloma arising in supernumerary vulvar breast tissue. Obstet Gynecol 55: 84–87S

201. Ridley CM (1975) The vulva. Philadelphia, WB Saunders

202. Robboy SJ, Ross JS, Prat J, Keh PC, Welch WR (1978) Urogenital sinus origin of mucinous and ciliated cysts of the vulva. Obstet Gynecol 51: 347

203. Roberts W, Daly JW (1981) Pseudosarcomatyous fasciitis of the vulva. Gynecol Oncol 11: 383

204. Rock B, Hood AF, Rock JA (1990) Prospective study of vulvar nevi. J Am Acad Dermatol 22: 104–106

205. Rodke G, Friedrich EG Jr, Wilkinson EJ (1988) Malignant potential of mixed vulvar dystrophy (lichen sclerosis associated with squamous cell hyperplasia). J Reprod Med 33: 545–550

206. Rogers BB, Josephson SL, Mak SK, Sweeney PJ (1992) Polymeras chain reaction amplification of herpes simplex virus DNA from clinical samples. Obstet Gynecol 79: 464–469

207. Rorat E, Ferenczy A, Richart RM (1975) Human Bartholin gland, duct and duct cyst. Arch Pathol 99: 367

208. Rorat E, Wallach RC (1984) Mixed tumors of the vulva: Clinical outcome and pathology. Int J Gynecol Pathol 3: 323

209. Rosen T, Tschen JA, Ramsdell W, Moore J, Markham B (1984) Granuloma inguinale. J Am Acad Dermatol 11: 433

210. Rudolph RE (1990) Vulvar melanosis. J Am Acad Dermatol 23: 982–984

211. Salzman RS, Kraus SJ, Miller RG, Scottnek FO, Kleris GS (1984) Chancroidal ulcers that are not chancroid. Arch Dermatol 120: 636

212. Sarrel PM, Steege JF, Maltzer M, Bolinsky D (1983) Pain during sex response due to occlusion of the Bartholin gland duct. Obstet Gynecol 62: 261

213. Schreiber MN (1963) Vulvar von Recklinghausen's disease. Arch Dermatol 88: 136

214. Sedlacek TV, Riva JM, Magen AB, Mangan CE, Cunnane MF (1990) Vaginal and vulvar adenosis. An unsuspected side effect of CO_2 laser vaporization. J Reprod Med 35: 995–1001

215. Seely JR, Bley Jr R, Altmiller CJ (1984) Localized chromosomal mosaicism as a cause of dysmorphic development. Am J Hum Genet 36: 899

216. Sehgal VN, Shyamprasad AL, Beohar PC (1984) The histopathological diagnosis of donovanosis. Br J Vener Dis 60: 45

217. Sherman AL, Reid R (1991) CO_2 laser for supperative hidradenitis of the vulva. J Reprod Med 36: 113–117

218. Shevchuk MM, Richart RM (1982) DNA content of condyloma acuminatum. Cancer 49: 489

219. Sison-Torre EQ, Ackerman AB (1985) Melanosis of the vulva. Am J Dermatopathol 7S: 51–60

220. Slavin RE, Christie JD, Swedo J, Powell LC Jr (1986) Locally aggressive granular cell tumor causing priapism of the crus of the clitoris. A light and ultrastructural study, with observations concerning the pathogenesis of fibrosis of the corpus cavernosum in priapism. Am J Surg Pathol 10: 497–507

221. Sloane BB, Figueroa TE, Ferguson D, Moon TD (1988) Malacoplakis of the urethra. Urology 139: 1300–1301

222. Sood M, Mandal AK, Ganesh K (1991) Lymphangioma circumscriptum of the vulva. J Indian Med Assoc 89: 262–263

223. Souteyrand P, Wong E, MacDonald DM (1981) Zoon's balinitis (balanitis circumscripta plasmacellularis). Br J Dermatol 105: 195–199

224. Stage AH, Humeniuk JM, Easley WK (1984) Bullous pemphigoid of the vulva: A case report. Am J Obstet Gynecol 150: 169

225. Stenchever MA, McDivitt RW, Fisher JA (1973) Leiomyoma of the clitoris. J Reprod Med 10: 75

226. Stephenson H, Dotters DJ, Katz V, Droegemueller W (1992) Necrotizing fasciitis of the vulva. Am J Obstet Gynecol 166: 1324–1327

227. Stone K (1994) Angiokeratomas of the vulva associated with Fabray's disease. (In manuscript)

228. Sun T, Schwartz NS, Sewell C, Lieberman P, Gross S (1991) Enterobius egg granuloma of the vulva and peritoneum: Review of the literature. Am J Trop Med Hyg 45: 249–253

229. Sutton GP, Smirz LR, Clark DH, Bennett JE (1985) Group B streptococcal necrotizing fasciitis arising from an episiotomy. Obstet Gynecol 66: 733

230. Tavassoli FA, Norris HJ (1979) Smooth muscle tumors of the vulva. Obstet Gynecol 53: 213–217

230a. Taylor SC, Baker E, Grossman ME (1991) Nodular vulvar amyloid as a presentation of systematic amyloidosis. J Am Acad Dermatol 24: 139

231. Tham SN, Choong HL (1992) Primary tuberculous chancre in a renal transplant patient. J Am Acad Dermatol 26; 342–344

232. Thomas R, Barnhill D, Bibro M, Hoskins W (1985) Hidradenitis suppurativa: A case presentation and review of the literature. Obstet Gynecol 66: 592

233. Tuffnell D, Buchan PD (1991) Crohn's disease of the vulva in childhood. Br J Clin Pract 45: 159–160

234. Turner ML, Marinoff SC (1991) Pudendal neuralgia. Am J Obstet Gynecol 165: 1233–1236

235. Umpierre SA, Kaufman RH, Adam E, Wood KV, Adler-Storth ZK (1992) Human papillomavirus DNA in tissue biopsy specimens of vulvar vestibulitis patients treated with interferon. Obstet Gynecol 78: 693–695

236. Vander Putte SCJ (1991) Anogenital "sweat" glands. Histology and pathology of a gland that may mimic mammary glands. Am J Dermatopathol 13: 557–567

237. Van der Putte SCJ (1994) Mammary-like glands of the vulva and their disorders. Int J Gynecol (In press)

238. Van Joost TH, Faber WR, Manuel HR (1980) Drug-induced anogenital cicatricial pemphigoid. Br J Dermatol 102: 715

239. Venter PF, Röhm GF, Slabber CF (1981) Giant neurofibromas of the labia. Obstet Gynecol 57: 128–130

240. Verkauf BS, Von Thron J, O'Brien WF (1992) Clitoral size in normal women. Obstet Gynecol 80: 41–44

241. Von Krogh G (1979) Varts: Immunological factors of prognostic significance. Int J Dermatol 18: 195

242. Wade TR, Ackerman AB (1985) The effects or resin podophyllin on condyloma acuminatum. Am J Dermatopathol 6: 1009

243. Walker PG, Colley NV, Grubb C, Tejerina A, Oriel JD (1983) Abnormalities of the uterine cervix in women with vulvar warts. A preliminary communication. Br J Vener Dis 59: 120

244. Wang AC, Hsu JJ, Hseuh S, Sun CF, Tsao KC (1991) Evidence of human papillomavirus deoxyribonucleic acid in vulvar squamous papillomatosis. Int J Gynecol Pathol 10: 44–50

245. Wilkinson EJ (1991) Pathology of the vagina. Curr Opin Obstetr Gynecol 3: 553

246. Wilkinson EJ (1992) Normal histology and nomenclature of the vulva, and malignant neoplasms, including VIN. Dermatol Clin 10: 283–296

247. Wilkinson EJ, Guerrero E, Daniel R, et al (1993) Vulvar vestibulitis is rarely associated with human papillomavirus infection types 6, 11, 16 or 18. Int J Gynecol Pathol 12: 344–349

248. Wisdom A (1973) Color atlas of venereology. Chicago, Year Book Medical Publishers

249. Kent HL, Wisniewski PM (1990) Interferon for vulvar vestibulitis. J Reprod Med 35: 1138–1140

250. Wojnarowska F (1988) Chronic bullous disease of childhood. Semin Dermatol 7: 58–65

251. Wolber RA, Talerman A, Wilkinson EJ, Clement PB (1991) Vulvar granular cell tumors with pseudocartinomatous hyperplasia: A comparative analysis with well-differentiated squamous carcinoma. Int J Gynecol Pathol 10: 59–66

252. Woodruff JD, Friedrich EG (1985) The vestibule. Clin Obstet Gynecol 28: 134

253. Woodruff JD, Parmley TH (1983) Infection of the minor vestibular gland. Obstet Gynecol 62: 609

254. Woodworth H, Dockerty MB, Wilson BB, Pratt JH (1971) Papillary hidradenoma of the vulva: A clinicopathologic study of 69 cases. Am J Obstet Gynecol 110: 501

255. Word B (1968) Office treatment of cyst and abscess of Bartholin's gland duct. South Med J 61: 514

256. Work BA (1980) Pyoderma gangrenosum of the perineum. Obstet Gynecol 55: 126

257. Young AW, Herman EW, Tovell HMM (1980) Syringoma of the vulva: Incidence, diagnosis, and cause of pruritus. Obstet Gynecol 55: 515

258. Young AW, Wind RM, Tovell HMM (1980) Lymphangioma of the vulva. NY State J Med 80: 987

259. Zur Hausen H, Gissman L, Schlehofer JR (1984) Viruses in the etiology of human genital cancer. Prog Med Virol 30: 170

260. Zur Hausen H (1982) Human genital cancer: Synergism between two virus infections or synergism between a virus infection and initiating events? Lancet 2: 1370

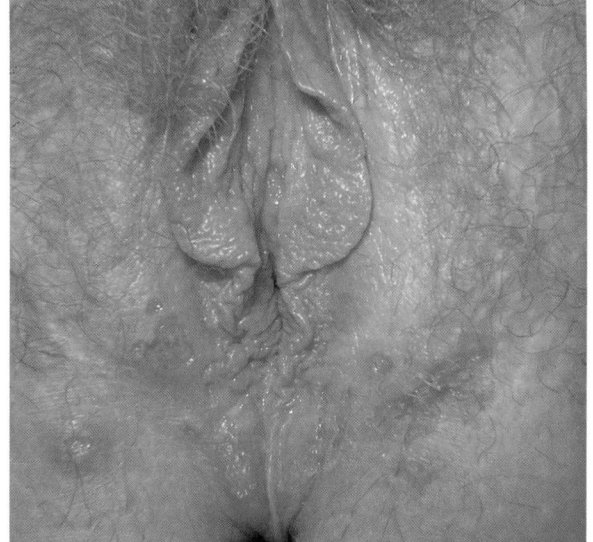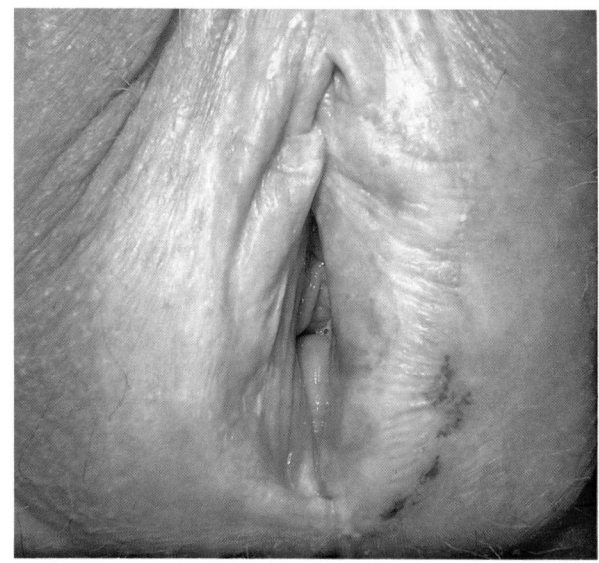

Plate 1

FIG. 2.8

FIG. 2.18

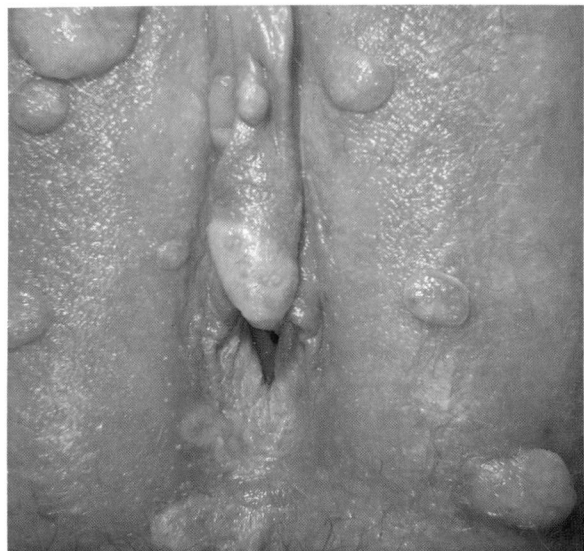

FIG. 2.11

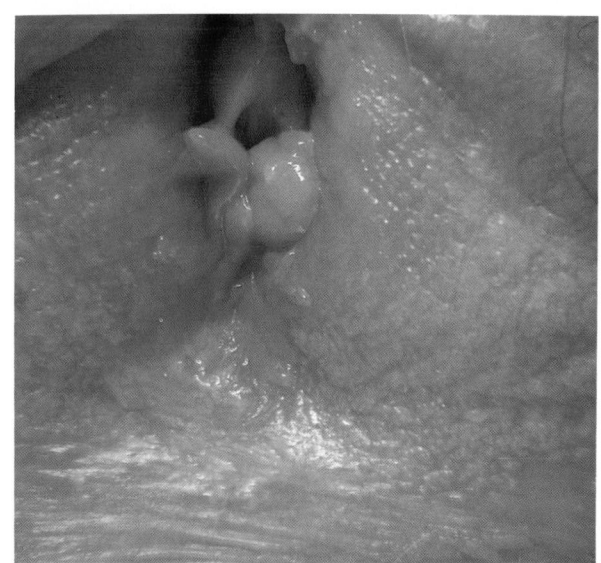

FIG. 2.26

FIG. 2.8. Herpes simplex ulcer. HSV infection, untreated, 7 days after the onset of symptoms. Multifocal ulceration is present.

FIG. 2.11. Condyloma lata. Multiple papules are present.

FIG. 2.18. Lichen sclerosus. White epithelium with focal subcutaneous ecchymosis is seen. The labia minora are somewhat atrophic.

FIG. 2.26. Vulvar vestibulitis. Marked inflammation is present adjacent and external to the hymenal ring. Point tenderness was present over these areas.

FIG. 3.1. VIN. Multiple macular and plaque-like white areas are seen about the labia majora.

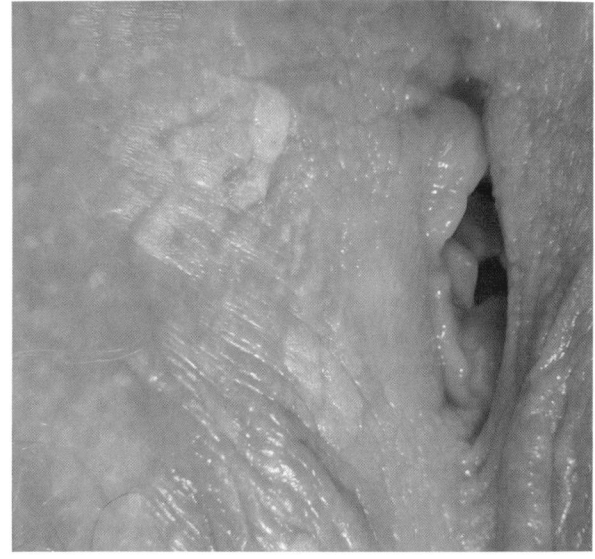

FIG. 3.1

Plate 2

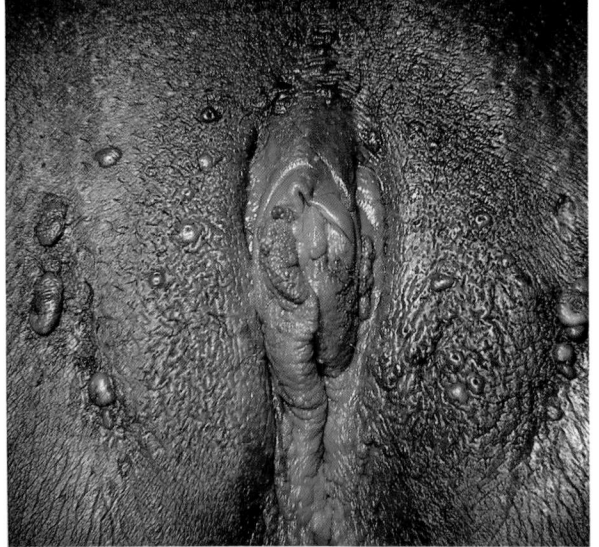

FIG. 3.2

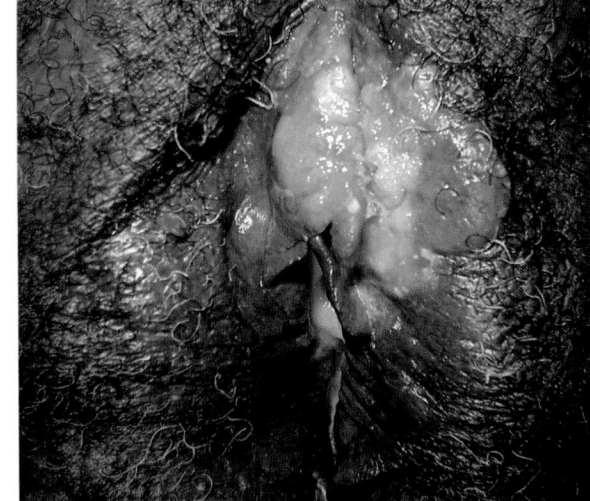

FIG. 3.15

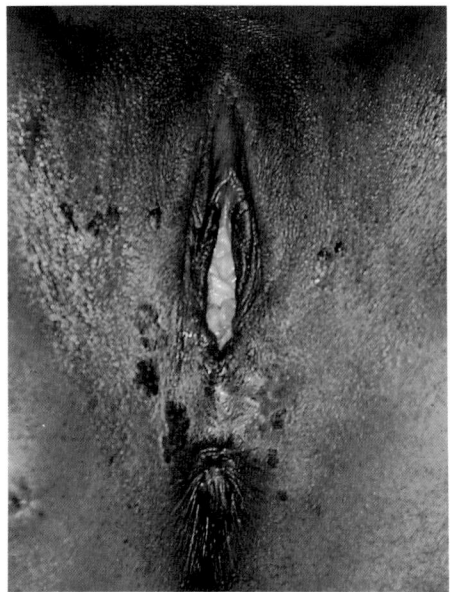

FIG. 3.3

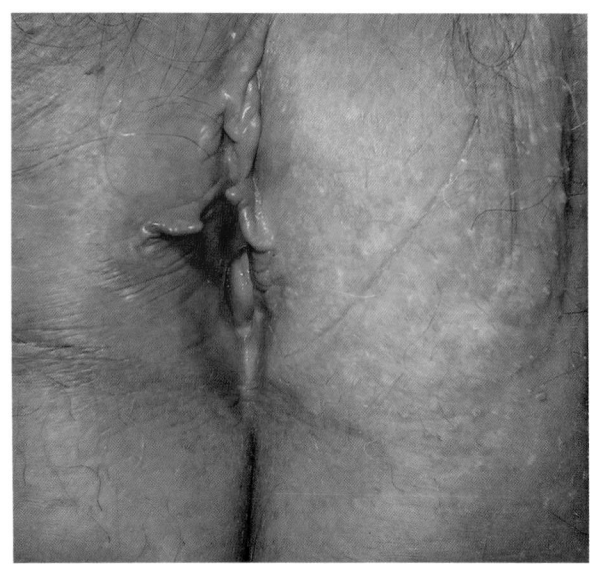

FIG. 3.33

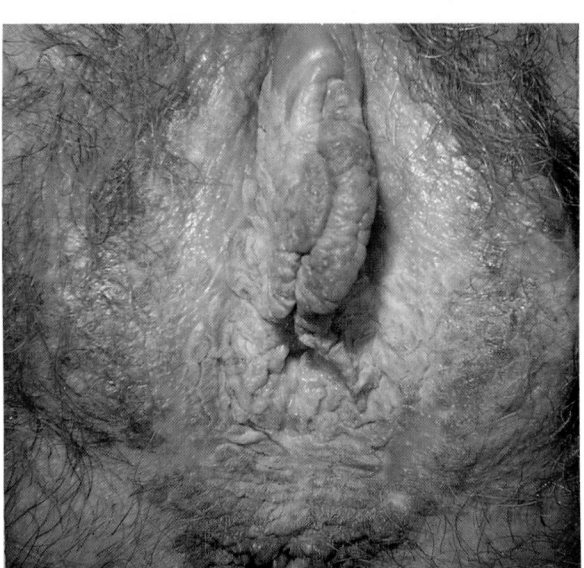

FIG. 3.4

FIG. 3.2. VIN. Multiple pigmented papules are noted about the labia majora in this young pregnant woman. Clinically, this lesion has been termed *bowenoid papulosis*.

FIG. 3.3. VIN. Multiple pigmented macular areas are present about the vulva and perianal area.

FIG. 3.4. VIN. Confluent distribution of pigmented, slightly raised, rough-surfaced areas are seen involving the labia majora and minora.

FIG. 3.15. Squamous cell carcinoma. The tumor involves the medial aspect of the left anterior labium majus and clitoris.

FIG. 3.33. Paget disease. An eczematoid, slightly raised area is noted on the medial anterior surface of the left labium majus.

3

Premalignant and Malignant Tumors of the Vulva

Edward J. Wilkinson, M.D.

Vulvar Intraepithelial Neoplasia (Dysplasia, Carcinoma In Situ)

GENERAL FEATURES

The incidence of vulvar intraepithelial neoplasia (VIN) (dysplasia, in situ carcinoma) has nearly doubled when comparing recorded cases between 1973 and 1976, and 1985 and 1986.[242] Several investigators suggest that it is becoming more frequent in young women 20–35 years of age.[9,21,39,58,133,208] The true incidence of VIN probably is higher than reported, because generally only a subset, carcinoma in situ (VIN 3) cases, is reported. Approximately 50% of these women will have other neoplasia involving the genital tract, most often cervical intraepithelial neoplasia (CIN).[34,136,283] Approximately one-half will exhibit a history of a preexisting or concomitant sexually transmitted disease, of which condylomata acuminata is the most frequent.[115] Some patients are asymptomatic, although many complain of pruritus.

Current terminology for VIN, as proposed by the International Society for the Study of Vulvar Disease (ISSVD), the World Health Organization (WHO), and the International Society of Gynecological Pathologists (ISGYP), is shown in Table 3.1.[214] Lesions of the vulva that are distinctly papular or verrucoid have been clinically termed *bowenoid papulosis* by some authors, but they are histologically indistinguishable from other forms of intraepithelial neoplasia and behave in a similar fashion.[263] The separate term *bowenoid papulosis* therefore is not included in the ISSVD, WHO, and ISGYP classification.

CLINICAL FEATURES

The lesions of VIN typically present clinically with a raised surface. Approximately one-quarter of the lesions are pigmented. VIN 3 is, in fact, the second most common cause of pigmented vulvar lesions.[89] Approximately one-half of the patients with VIN have white lesions, or lesions that are distinctly acetowhite, after the application of topical 3–5% acetic acid. The remainder of VIN lesions may be pink, gray, or red. Lesions involving the nonkeratinized mucous membrane of the vestibule appear red. Such red lesions have been called *erythroplasia of Queyrat*, but like bowenoid papulosis are not designated separately and are included within the VIN category. The lesions may be macular (Fig. 3.1) or papular (Fig. 3.2) and they may be single or multiple (Fig. 3.3). Confluent growth may be seen with plaques (Figs. 3.1, 3.4) forming a diffuse pattern (Fig. 3.4).[89,92,208,278] (See insert for color photos of Figs. 3.1–3.4.) The anal skin and squamous mucosa of the anal canal are the most frequently involved secondary sites.[64]

Table 3.1. International Society for the Study of Vulvar Disease classification of intraepithelial neoplasia

Prior terminology 1976–1983	Present terminology 1985
Mild atypia	VIN 1 Mild dysplasia
Moderate atypia	VIN 2 Moderate dysplasia
Severe atypia	VIN 3 Severe dysplasia
Carcinoma in situ	VIN 3 Carcinoma in situ
Paget disease	Paget disease

VIN, vulvar intraepithelial neoplasia.

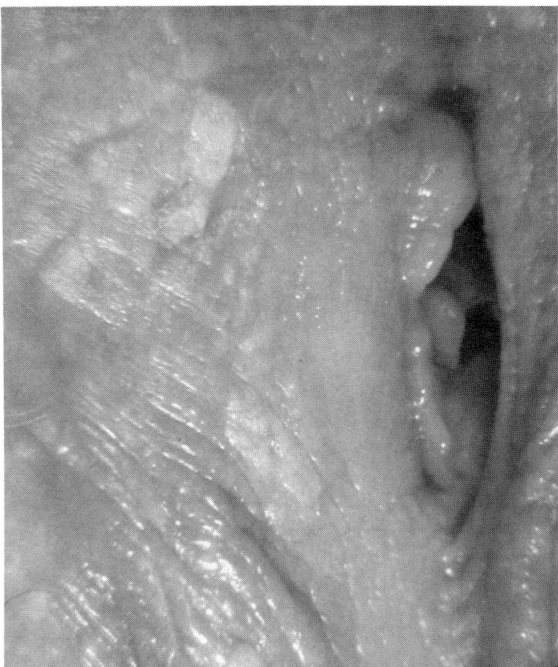

FIG. 3.1. VIN. Multiple macular and plaque-like white areas are seen about the labia majora. (See color insert.)

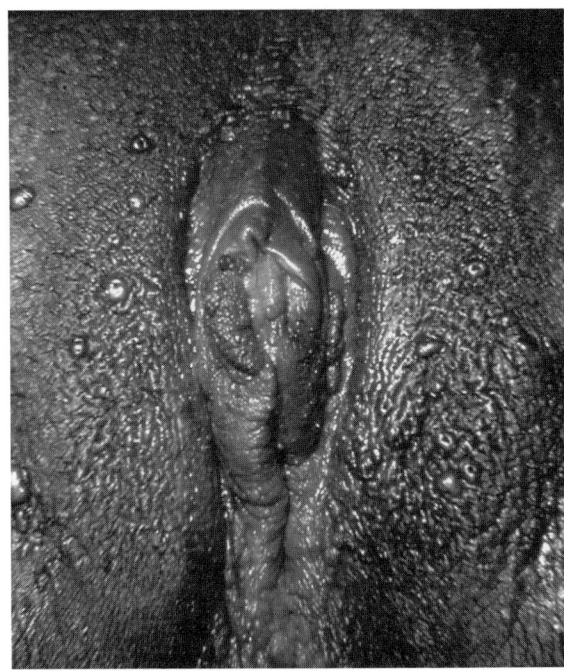

FIG. 3.2. VIN. Multiple pigmented papules are noted about the labia majora in this young pregnant woman. Clinically, this lesion has been termed *bowenoid papulosis*. (See color insert.)

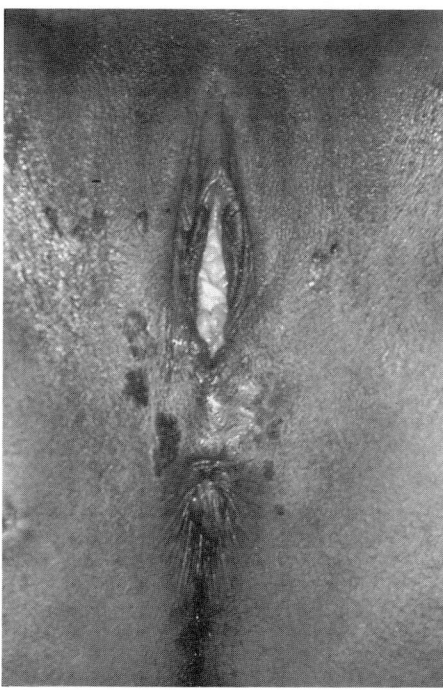

FIG. 3.3. VIN. Multiple pigmented macular areas are present about the vulva and perianal area. (See color insert.)

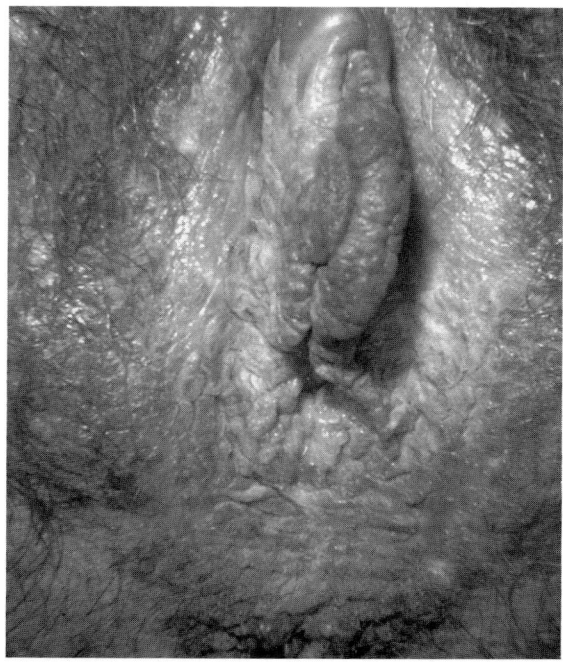

FIG. 3.4. VIN. Confluent distribution of pigmented, slightly raised, rough-surfaced areas are seen involving the labia majora and minora. (See color insert.)

MICROSCOPIC FINDINGS

The epithelial cells of VIN typically lack keratinocyte maturation and exhibit high mitotic activity, high nuclear/cytoplasmic ratio, and lack cytoplasmic differentiation in the upper layers of the epithelium (Fig. 3.5). The cells may show evidence of altered maturation with multinucleation and dyskeratosis, including the formation of intraepithelial squamous pearls within acanthotic rete ridges (Fig. 3.6). Nuclear pleomorphism and hyperchromasia are present; however, nucleoli are uncommon. Radial dispersion of nuclear chromatin and coarse clumping of the chromatin are further suggestions of DNA abnormalities. The coarse nuclear chromatin seen in the epithelial cells of VIN corresponds to an increased number of interchromatinic and perichromatinic granules that are sometimes clustered in globular structures.[143] The so-called individual cell keratinization seen within the epithelium is attributed to the

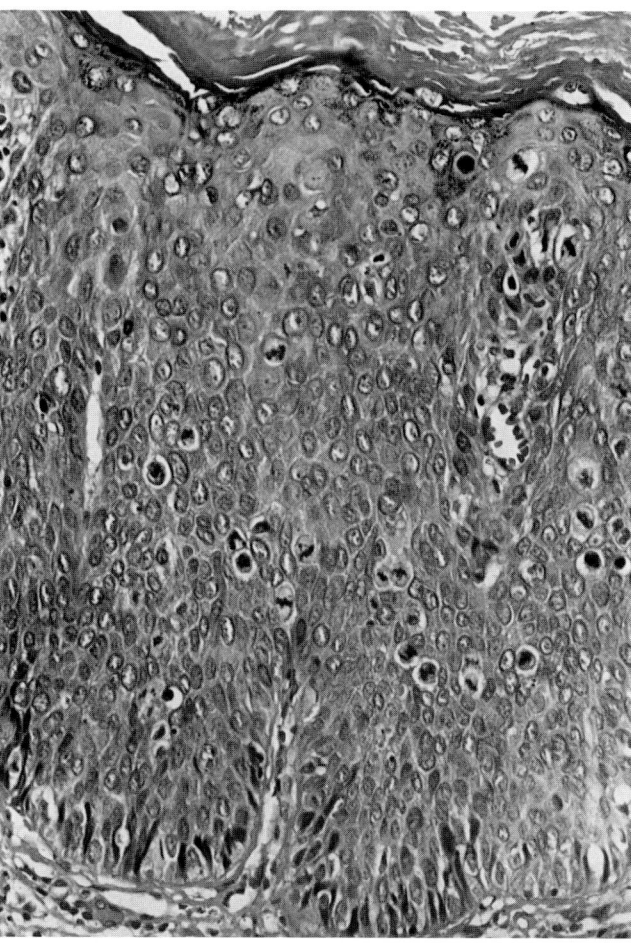

FIG. 3.5. VIN 2. Hyperchromatic, pleomorphic cells are present in the lower two-thirds of the epithelium, which are crowded, vertically oriented, and show lack of maturation except near the surface. Many mitotic figures are present, some of which are abnormal.

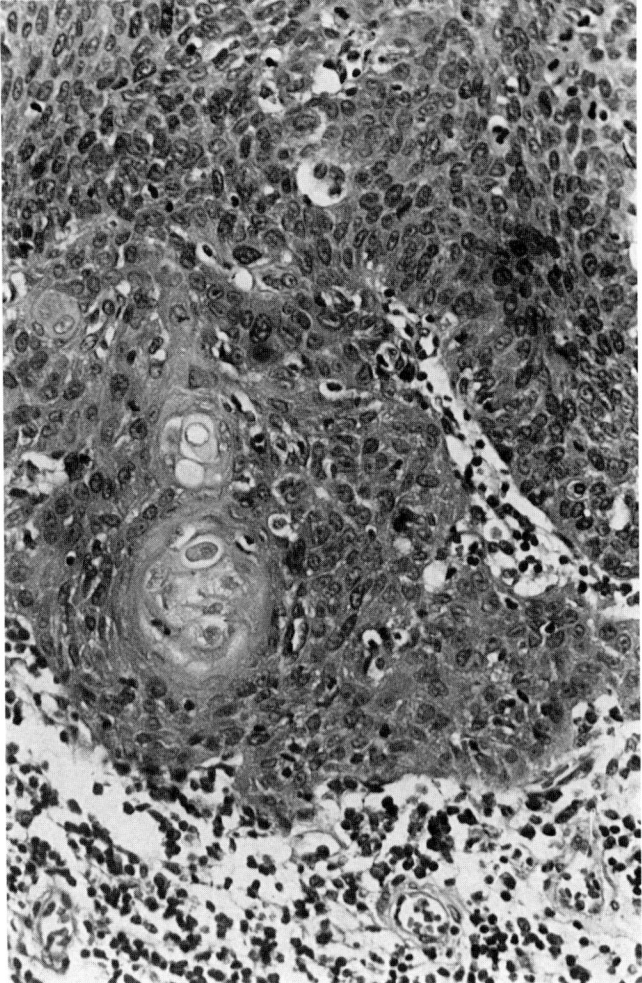

Fig. 3.6. **VIN 3 with superficial invasion.** The prominent cells have eosinophilic cytoplasm and nuclear chromatin with clearing near the basal layer.

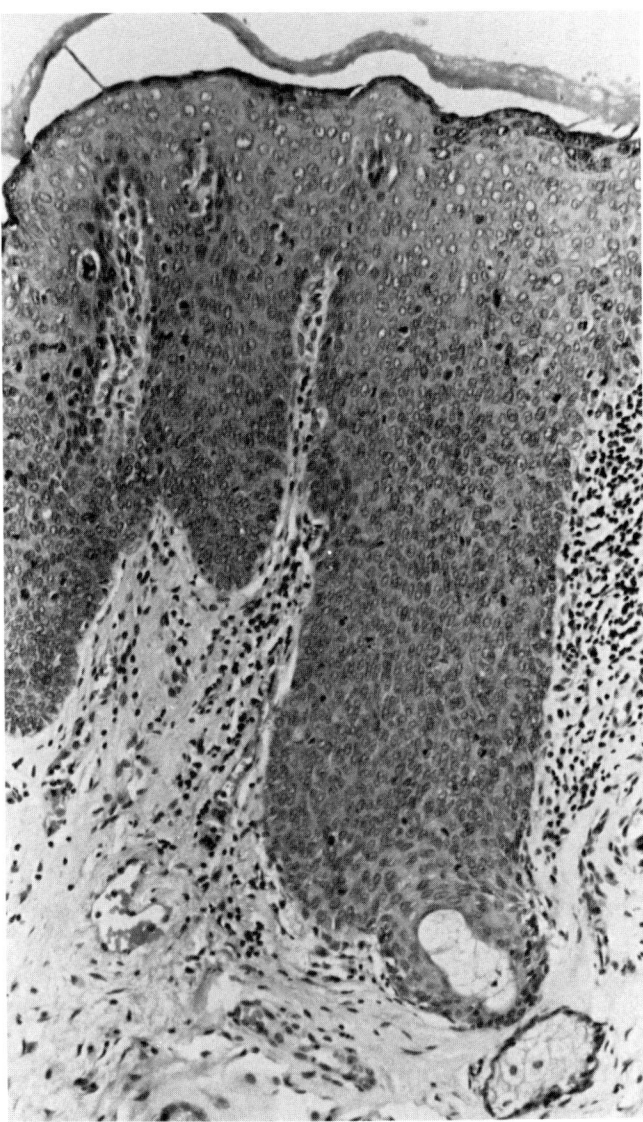

Fig. 3.7. **VIN 3, involving a skin appendage.** Cellular disarray with lack of maturation is seen within the epithelium. Part of a sebaceous gland is seen at the base of the lesion.

presence of aggregated tonofiliments that may be produced in the process of abnormal cell division.[227] Parakeratosis is seen when keratinocytes fail to form granules of prekeratin and retain nuclear material at the epithelial surface.

Both intracellular and extracellular pigment granules may be distributed throughout the epidermis. Dermal melanophages often are prominent beneath the basal layer and within the dermal papillae.

VIN involves the skin appendages in more than 50% of the cases studied.[173] Skin appendage involvement by VIN should not be confused with early invasion (Fig. 3.7). It may be found within skin appendages as deep as 2.7 mm in hair-bearing areas.[230] In non–hair-bearing areas the skin appendages and minor vestibular glands are more superficial. The thickness of the epithelium involved by VIN may range from 0.10 to 1.90 mm, with a mean of 0.52 ± 0.23 mm.[19]

Microscopic Grading

When grading VIN, one should consider the quality and quantity of the individual cellular atypicalities, the relative density and percentage of the abnormal cell population, as well as the overall architecture of the epithelium. When such changes are few in number and confined to the lower third of the epithelium, VIN 1 (mild dysplasia) is reported (Fig. 3.8). Flat condyloma acuminatum of the vulva may be included in the VIN 1 category because the biologic difference between VIN 1 and flat condyloma is unknown and the morphologic distinction is unreliable. VIN may be associated with typical condyloma acuminatum.[191] A lesion is classified as VIN 2 (moderate dysplasia) if the changes described above extend through approximately one-half to

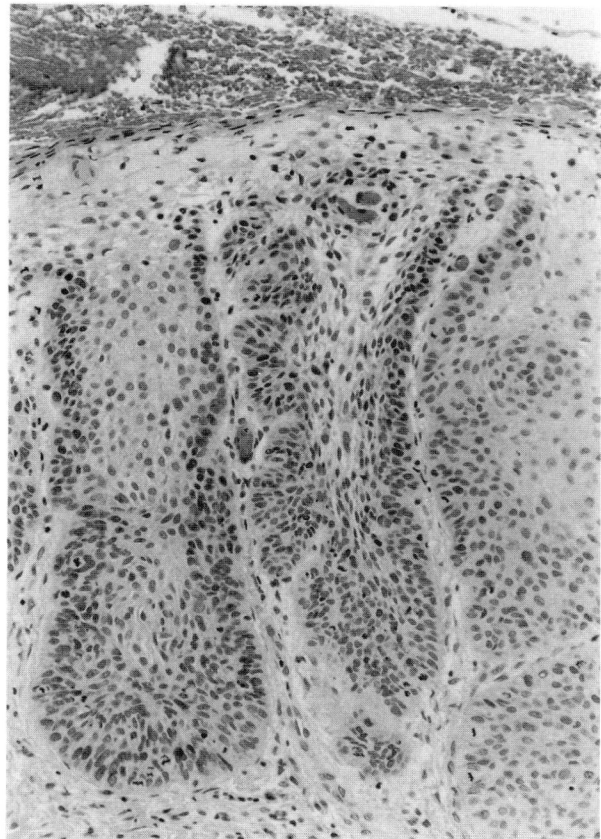

FIG. 3.8. VIN 1, mild dysplasia. There is crowding of the basal and parabasal cells with some cellular disarray and loss of maturation within the lower one-third of the epithelium. Some nuclear pleomorphism is present.

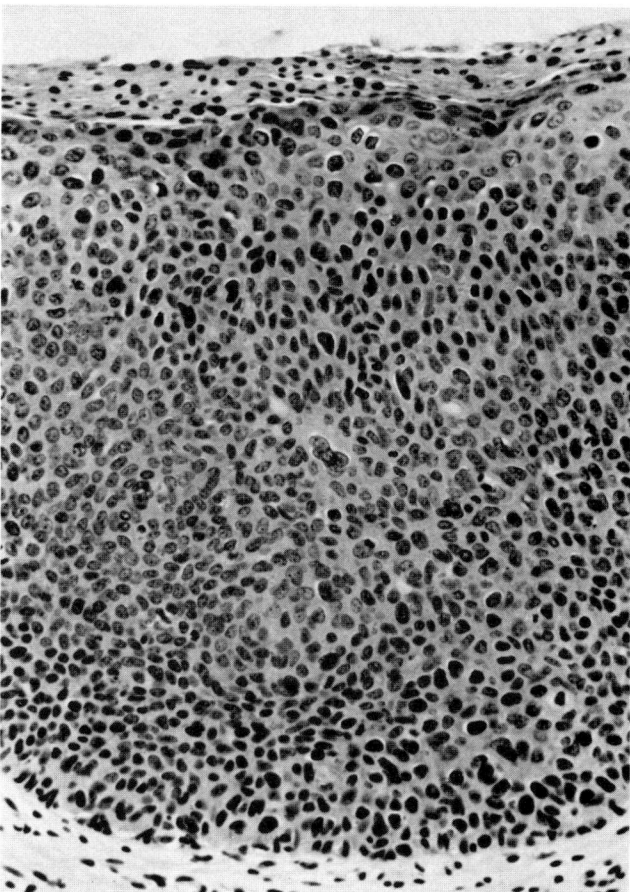

FIG. 3.9. VIN 3 (carcinoma in situ), basaloid type. Complete replacement of the epithelium with overlying parakeratosis resembling carcinoma in situ of the cervix.

two-thirds of the epithelium, and individually keratinized cells and mitoses within this lower two-thirds of the epithelium may be seen (Fig. 3.5). When cellular atypia involves more than two-thirds of the full thickness of the epithelium, disregarding the keratin layer, the diagnosis is VIN 3 (severe dysplasia) or VIN 3 (carcinoma in situ) if the change is essentially full thickness but does not necessarily include the surface layers above the granular zone (Figs. 3.9, 3.10). On rare occasions, cells show prominent eosinophilic cytoplasm with nuclear chromatin clearing and prominent nucleoli.[3] This cellular type is classified as the *well-differentiated type* of VIN, and should be classified as a VIN 3 lesion. This cellular change also is commonly seen adjacent to invasive vulvar carcinoma (Fig. 3.6). (See below, Histologic Subtypes of VIN.)

Abnormal mitoses are nearly always present in VIN 2 and 3 lesions and may be seen in all but the most superficial layers of the epithelium. Lack of abnormal mitoses should raise the question as to whether or not a lesion belongs in the VIN 2 or 3 category. A spectrum of epithelial changes may be seen extending from VIN 1 to VIN 3, with variable degrees of cellular differentiation.

HISTOLOGIC SUBTYPES OF VIN

Nuclear size within VIN may be large and pleomorphic (Figs. 3.5, 3.10) or relatively small and more uniform (Fig. 3.9). Accordingly, VIN has been subclassified into three types, *basaloid*, *warty*, and *well differentiated*, based largely on these nuclear features. The *basaloid type* of VIN has relatively small, uniform cells with hyperchromatic and coarse nuclear chromatin. Nucleoli are rare and abnormal mitoses usually are found. There is little or no maturation of the keratinocytes similar to carcinoma in situ of the cervix; however, some keratinization or parakeratosis may be seen at the surface (Fig. 3.9). The *warty type* of VIN has larger cells with greater nuclear pleomorphism. The nuclear chromatin is coarse and clumped and nucleoli are seen infrequently, although abnormal mitosis usually can be identified. Toward the surface the keratinocytes have features of condyloma acuminatum with koilocytosis, and binucleation or multinucleation. A prominent granular layer, with associated dyskeratosis, parakeratosis, and/or hyperkeratosis usually is present[192] (Fig. 3.10). The *well-*

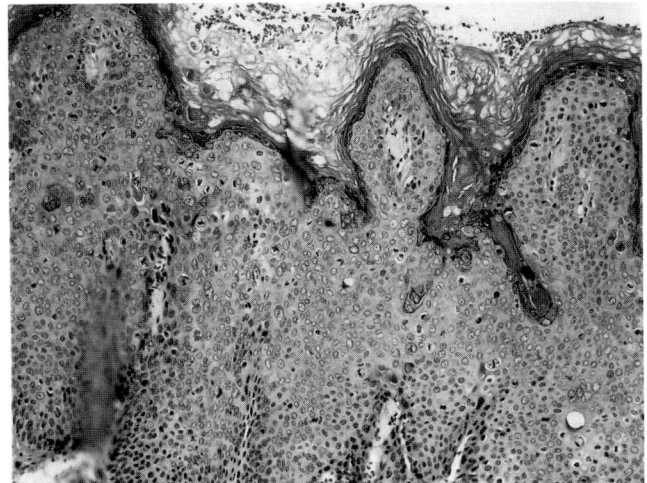

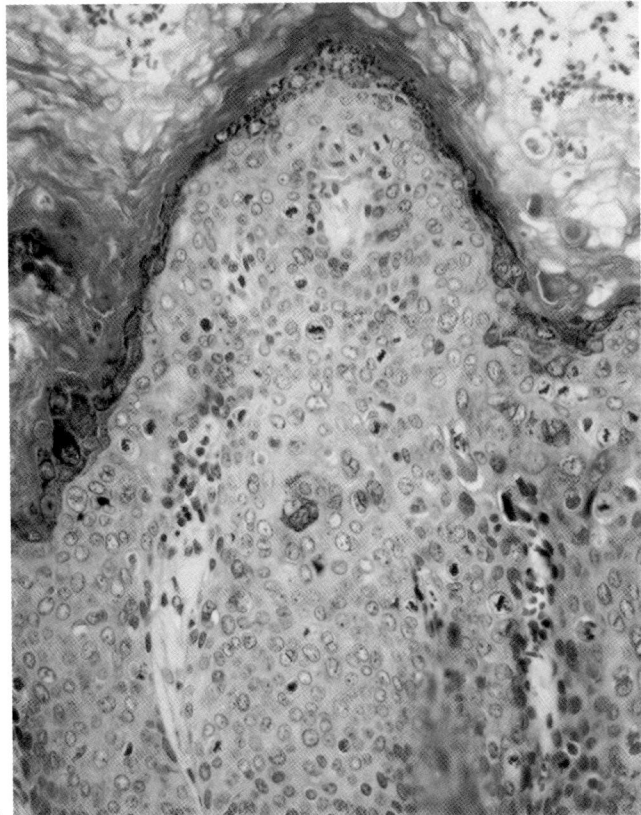

FIG. 3.10. a: VIN 3, warty (condylomatous) type. The surface of the lesion is spiked with marked hyperkeratosis. A prominent granular layer is evident. **b: VIN 3, warty (condylomatous) type.** There is marked cellular disarray with prominent nuclear pleomorphism. Several multinucleated keratinocytes are present.

differentiated type of VIN has a large and pleomorphic keratinocytic cell population with minimal nuclear hyperchromasia or coarse nuclear chromatin (Fig. 3.11). This lesion has been previously referred to as *carcinoma in situ,*

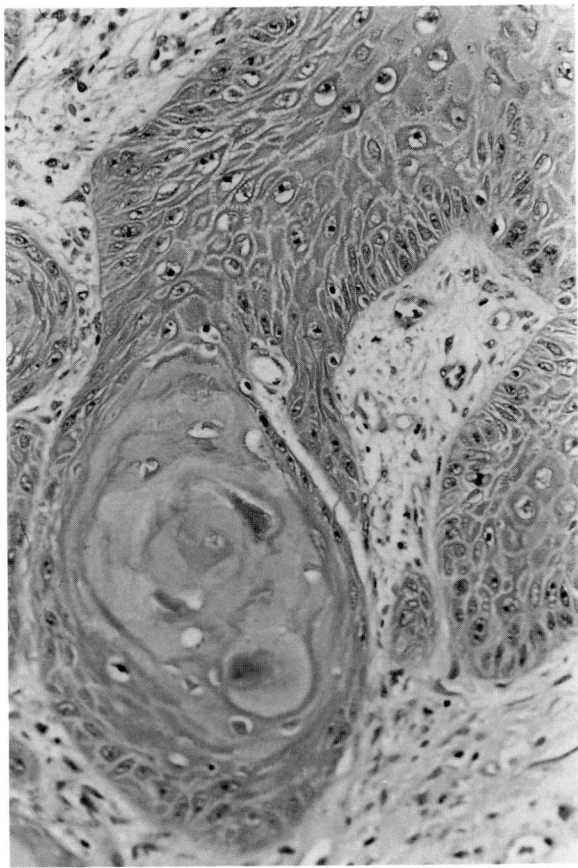

FIG. 3.11. VIN 3, well-differentiated type. The epithelium has slight cellular disarray and the keratinocytes have prominent cytoplasm. The nuclei are somewhat enlarged. Within the parabasal area of the rete ridge, the cells have increased eosinophilic cytoplasm with dyskeratosis in this example.

simplex type[3] (Fig. 3.11). The cells of well-differentiated VIN typically have a relatively large amount of eosinophilic cytoplasm, as compared to the other two types of VIN, and typically contain nucleoli. The distinctive feature is the prominent increased eosinophilic cytoplasm within the keratinocytes at the base of some of the rete ridges, with the cells in these areas also having larger nuclei than the overlying epithelium, with prominent large nucleoli.[3,275] A similar lesion, but lacking the distinctive increased eosinophilic cytoplasm of the base of the rete ridges, has been designated by some as atypical squamous hyperplasia because this lesion histologically resembles squamous hyperplasia (see Chapter 2, Benign Diseases of the Vulva) more closely than it does the other types of VIN.[152] However, despite the association with keratinizing squamous carcinoma, there are no longitudinal studies demonstrating that either of these findings is a precursor of squamous carcinoma. It is not infrequent for an individual case to show more than one pattern of VIN. Mixtures of basaloid and warty patterns are particularly frequent. These "mixed" cases can be classified according to the predominant component or simply as VIN, not otherwise specified.

Differential Diagnosis

The differential diagnosis of VIN includes basal cell carcinoma, superficial spreading malignant melanoma, and Paget disease. Immunoperoxidase methods to assist in distinguishing these are summarized in Table 3.2.

The possibility that podophyllin effect on condylomata of the vulva could result in their being misinterpreted as VIN is highly improbable because the changes from short-term podophyllin use are quite different from VIN. Mitotic arrest with cells in metaphase seen after podophyllin contrasts with the abnormal mitotic figures seen in VIN. Nuclear karyorrhexis is rarely present with VIN, whereas it can be found in at least 90% of condyloma cases.[264] In VIN the nuclear size is variable and nuclear chromatin usually is coarse, with little cellular swelling. These changes are uncommon in podophyllin effect. The cellular changes from a single application of podophyllin will regress within 1–2 weeks, whereas VIN will persist (see Chapter 2, Benign Diseases of the Vulva).

Adjunctive Studies

Most VIN lesions contain aneuploid populations of cells, that is, they contain a DNA content other than (23 × 2) or multiples of 23 (i.e., 46, 69, 92, etc.).[58,93,278] Aneuploidy is common in high-grade genital intraepithelial neoplasia, although not all malignant epithelial neoplasms of the genital tract are aneuploid. The larger cells found in VIN lesions usually have a higher cellular DNA content and often are aneuploid in the near triploid or tetraploid range, whereas VIN lesions with smaller cells tend to be aneuploid in the near diploid range.[278] Keratin expression provides evidence for the lack of cellular maturation.[79]

In most cases VIN lesions are multifocal. DNA analysis by microspectrophotometry suggests that separate lesions have arisen from separate stem cells, forming distinguishable clones. Large spreading lesions may result from centrifugal growth from a single cell line or by confluence of

Table 3.2. Immunohistochemical localization of HPV, CEA, and S-100 protein in the differential diagnosis of some vulvar diseases

	Condyloma	VIN	Paget disease	Melanoma
Human papilloma (HPV) antigen	+[a]	−/+[b]	−	−
Carcino-embryonic antigen (CEA)	−	−	+	−
S-100 protein	−	−	−	+

[a] Detected in approximately 50% of cases.
[b] Detected in up to 10% of cases.

separate and distinct clones.[278] In single VIN lesions approximately half have different stem cells by DNA microspectrophotometry, suggesting that such lesions may undergo clonal evolution.[278] Evidence for HPV in VIN based on molecular biologic studies, including DNA in situ hybridization, has been demonstrated in most cases.[200] HPV-16 is the predominant type found and is identified more commonly in the warty and basaloid types of VIN than in the well-differentiated type.[59,60,100,124,158,192,221] Viral structural proteins are found in a small proportion of VIN, mainly in the low-grade lesion. Viral particles usually are not identifiable by electron microscopy in VIN.

Clinical Behavior and Treatment

VIN associated with vulvar invasive squamous carcinoma is reported in 2–18% of larger series that have specifically examined for this association.[42,141] In evaluation of epithelial changes adjacent to vulvar squamous cell carcinoma, 60–80% of superficially invasive carcinomas and 25% of deeply invasive carcinomas have adjacent VIN.[158,292] Invasion, if present, occurs most commonly in postmenopausal women, although it may occur in women of reproductive age.[9,35,38,58,208] Spontaneous regression of VIN may occur; however, no long-term prospective studies have evaluated this. Regression appears to be most common in young women and those who are pregnant, whereas women of advanced age, those who are severely immunosuppressed, and women with Fanconi anemia are at a greater risk for invasion.[41,281] Significantly lowered lymphocyte transformation responses have been reported in unselected women with carcinoma in situ of the vulva as compared to control subjects.[225]

Conservative therapy is now recommended for VIN and most cases are managed with local excision; laser ablation also may be appropriate for selected patients.[88,118,137,275]

Squamous Cell Carcinoma

Vulvar squamous cell carcinomas are divided into two categories: superficially invasive carcinoma and frankly invasive carcinoma. Superficially invasive squamous cell carcinomas invade to a depth of 1 mm or less and a diameter of 2 cm or less. Tumors that exceed these dimensions are classified as *invasive squamous carcinoma*.

Vulvar squamous carcinoma has an overall incidence of approximately 1.5/100,000 women in the United States, which increases with advancing age to as high as 20/100,000 women.[113,292] Unlike VIN, the incidence of vulvar squamous cell carcinoma has not increased significantly when comparing 1973 to 1976 and 1985 to 1987.[242] Overall, it has been shown that approximately 40% of all vulvar squamous carcinomas are associated with HPV.[192,201,254,267,294] Current evidence, however, supports the view that vulvar carcinoma can be separated in two broad groups. One group consists of younger women (mean age, 55 years) who have VIN associated with squamous cell carcinoma. These women also have a high rate of cervical and vaginal neoplasia. HPV is detected in approximately 75% of these tumors. HPV 16 is the most common type found in these tumors. These women also tend to be heavy cigarette smokers, and their vulvar squamous tumor types are predominantly of the warty or basaloid types. The second population of women with vulvar carcinoma are older (mean age, 77 years) and do not have associated VIN or a history of heavy cigarette smoking. Their tumors rarely contain HPV and typically they are well-differentiated squamous cell carcinomas.[152,254] These women often have associated vulvar dermatoses, especially lichen sclerosus or squamous hyperplasia.[59,106,152] Other epidemiologic factors associated with vulvar squamous cell carcinoma include chronic granulomatous disease, most notably granuloma inguinale.[107] Cigarette smoking is associated with an increased odds ratio of having vulvar carcinoma, the risk increasing with the number of cigarettes smoked.[62] In addition to cigarettes, other carcinogen exposure also increases risk.[164,187,265] Suppressed immunocompetence also is recognized as a risk factor.[41,281] Diabetes mellitus[187] and achlorhydria[266] have been associated with a slight increased risk of vulvar carcinoma. Poor perineal hygiene also has been implicated. Vulvar carcinoma may occur during pregnancy, although parity does not appear to be a significant risk factor.[233]

Superficially Invasive Squamous Cell Carcinoma (ISSVD Stage IA)

GENERAL FEATURES

In 1983, the ISSVD accepted the concept of superficially invasive squamous cell carcinoma of the vulva, and suggested that: "Stage 1A carcinoma of the vulva be defined as a single lesion measuring 2 cm or less in diameter and with a depth of invasion of 1 mm or less." Patients with more than one site of invasion are not to be included.[146,214] This definition includes cases that have capillary-like space involvement, provided that the tumor does not invade deeper than 1 mm. Tumor diameter alone is not an adequate indicator of prognosis.

The identification of a subset of invasive vulvar squamous cell carcinoma, that would not be at risk for metastasis to inguinal or regional lymph nodes, has progressed through a series of definitions of microinvasion that have been proposed by numerous investigators. Until more definitive criteria are established for microinvasive cancer, it is suggested that the term *microinvasive carcinoma* not be used in reporting vulvar carcinoma, but rather that the diameter of the tumor, the depth of invasion, the thickness of the tumor, the presence or absence

of vascular space involvement, and the status of surgical margins be reported. These findings will influence treatment options.

CLINICAL FEATURES

Superficially invasive squamous cell carcinoma may present as an ulcer, red macule or papule, or white hyperkeratotic plaque. It may be associated with VIN and present as a VIN lesion, including as a pigmented brown or black macule or papule. Although the presence of invasion associated with VIN may be heralded by the finding of an associated ulcer, irregularly contoured elevated mass, abnormal vascularity, or marked hyperkertosis, no specific clinical findings definitively separate VIN from VIN with superficial invasion.[42]

MICROSCOPIC FINDINGS

Accurate measurements require a calibrated ocular or comparable measuring device. For clarity, the measurement from the surface of the tumor, or from the base of the granular layer if a keratin layer is present, to the deepest point of invasion is defined as the "thickness of the tumor." The measurement from the epithelial stromal junction of

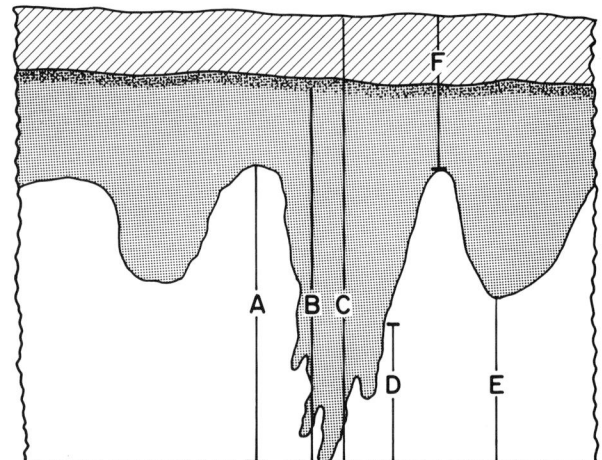

FIG. 3.12. **Methods of measuring depth of invasion of squamous cell carcinoma of the vulva.** The tumor thickness is defined as the measurement from the granular layer (*B*) or surface if nonkeratinized (*C*) to the deepest point of invasion. The depth of invasion is defined as the measurement from the epithelial stromal junction of the adjacent most superficial dermal papillae to the deepest point of invasion (*A*). Measurement of the depth of invasion also can be accomplished by measuring from the surface to the deepest point of invasion and subtracting the measurement from the surface to the epithelial stromal junction of the most superficial dermal papillae (*F*) (*A* = *C* − *F*). Other measurements have included measurements from the rete ridge (*D*) and from the deepest tip of the adjacent rete ridge (*E*). (Reprinted by permission of Wilkinson EJ.)

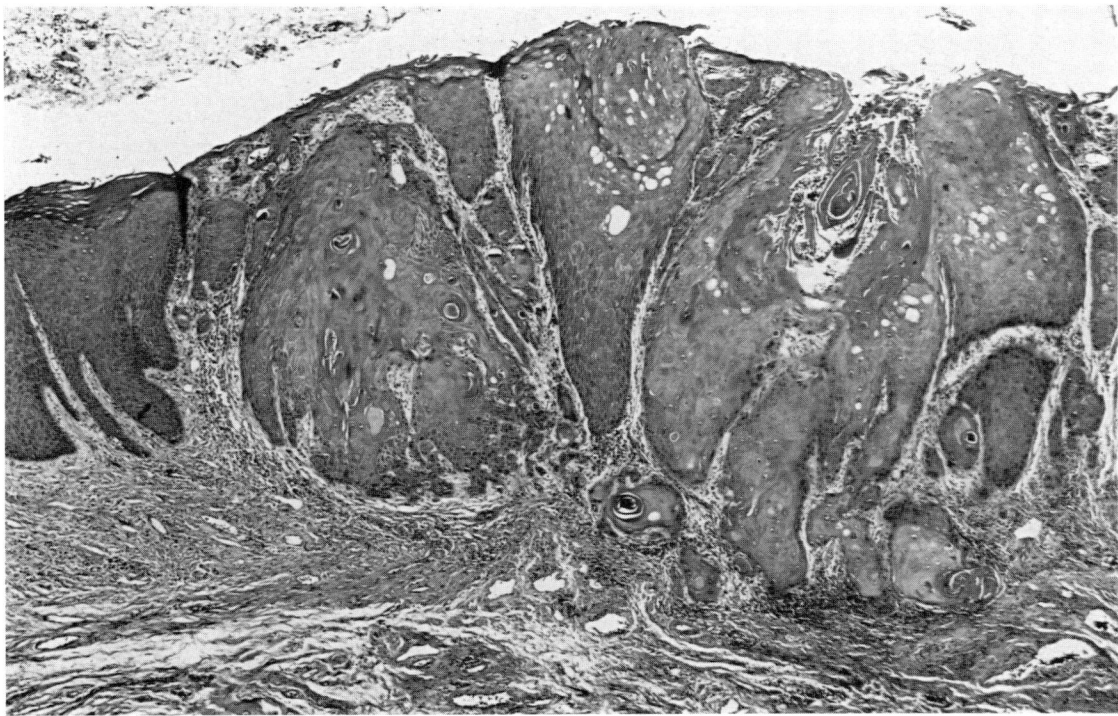

Fig. 3.13. Squamous cell carcinoma. The depth of invasion is 2.7 mm from the most superficial adjacent dermal papillae to the deepest point of invasion.

the adjacent dermal papillae to the deepest point of invasion is defined as the "depth of invasion" (Fig. 3.12). Methods of measurement require a description along with the measurement within the pathology report.[274] The depth of invasion also can be measured by measuring the thickness of the tumor and subtracting the epithelial measurement from the surface to the epithelial stromal junction of the immediately adjacent dermal papillae.[103,104] In general, both measurements can be made when the tumor is superficial or 3 mm or less in depth (Figs. 3.6, 3.13). In larger tumors, the diameter and dimensions of the tumor may be too great to include an adjacent dermal papillae; however, this often can be overcome by appropriate sectioning. Both measurements are valuable because in cases where there is marked acanthosis, the thickness of the epithelium may give an overestimate of the tumor's size. If the tumor is ulcerated the thickness measurement may underestimate the true tumor size.

The ISGYP recommends that the following information should always be included in the surgical pathology report because it is crucial to therapeutic decisions: depth of invasion in millimeters, thickness of the tumor in millimeters, method of measurement of the depth of invasion and thickness, presence or absence of vascular space involvement by tumor, diameter of the tumor (as measured from the specimen), and clinical measurement of the tumor diameter, when available. When there is a question as to whether or not invasion is present, and additional sectioning does not resolve the question, it is recommended that invasion not be diagnosed.

CLINICAL BEHAVIOR AND TREATMENT

In patients meeting the ISSVD criteria of Stage 1A carcinoma of the vulva, recommended therapy is wide local excision of the lesion, without vulvectomy. Sampling of the ipsilateral groin nodes, or bilateral groin nodes if the tumor is midline, has been suggested. However, with 1 mm or less of invasion, the probability of node metastasis is extremely small, and node sampling or resection is not contributory in most cases.

In a recent study, 36 (18%) of 190 patients with 2 cm or smaller tumor had lymph node metastasis. Of those with node metastasis, the relative 5-year survival was 78.6% compared with 97.9% for those with negative nodes.[119] Initial studies, following work that had been done on the cervix, used 5-mm depth of invasion as the basis of separation.[85,271] Using the 5-mm depth of invasion, it has subsequently been found that on average approximately 15% of these women will have inguinal lymph node metastasis (Fig. 3.14).° The microscopic evaluation of lymph nodes for detection of metastatic squamous carcinoma may be

---

°Refs. 10,15,27,37,64,69,70,72,76,104,116,128,142,146,151,167, 193,224,271,274,276,282.

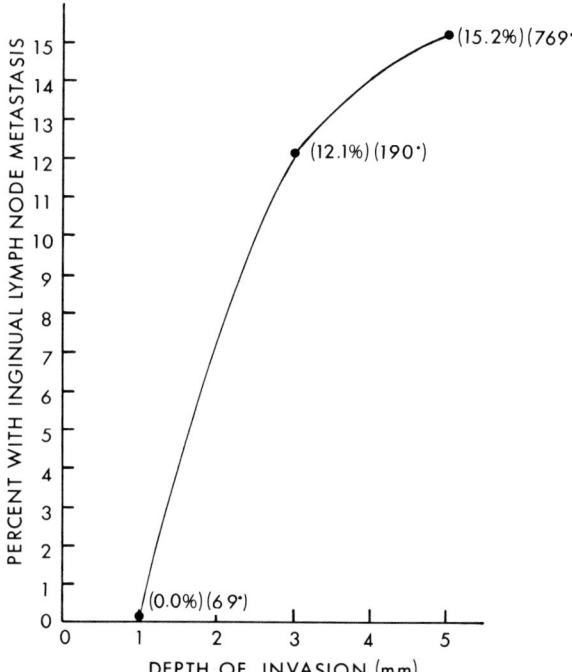

FIG. 3.14. Percent of women who underwent lymphadenectomy with inguinal lymph node metastasis plotted against the depth of invasion of their tumor. The frequency of lymph node metastasis rises rapidly with depth of invasion beyond 1 mm. (Reprinted by permission of Wilkinson, EJ, ref. 282.)

augmented by use of a polyclonal keratin antibody.[13] In a study evaluating both depth of invasion and tumor thickness, more than 40% of the cases had groin metastasis when the thickness of the tumor exceeded 4 mm[23] and therefore a 3-mm depth of invasion has been suggested. However, this depth of invasion was found to be associated with inguinal lymph node metastasis in approximately 10% of cases.* Selected patients with tumors of this depth may be treated by wide local excision with ipsilateral regional node dissection.[98] There are insufficient studies specifically evaluating tumors with a depth of invasion of 2 mm or less; however, the risk of lymph node metastasis in these cases appears very low. In two small studies specifically examining tumors with invasion of 1 mm to 2 mm, without vascular space involvement, none had node metastasis.[23,209] Until more data are available on tumors that invade between 1 and 2 mm, definitive therapeutic recommendations cannot be made. For now it is safe to say there is little risk, if any, of inguinal lymph node metastasis, with invasion less than 1 mm in depth.†

---

*Refs. 10,23,27,37,47,76,103,116,128,132,146,184,276,282, 288,289.
†Refs. 10,23,37,47,76,98,103,108,128,142,144,209,218,224, 240,271,274,282

Invasive Squamous Cell Carcinoma

CLINICAL FEATURES

Invasive squamous carcinoma may present as an exophytic papillomatous mass or as an endophytic ulcer. The tumor usually is located on the labia minora or majora; however, the clitoris is primarily involved in approximately 5–15% of cases.[86,103,150] The tumor is typically solitary (Fig. 3.15; see color insert), with less than 10% of cases presenting with multifocal tumors (Figs. 3.16, 3.17).[292]

Aberrant hormonal activity has been reported in vulvar carcinoma.[229,241] Gynecological tumors were responsible for 20.5% of malignancy-associated hypercalcemia in one series.[241] After the ovary, the vulva is the second most common gynecological tumor associated with hypercalcemia. Vulvar squamous carcinomas, with associated hypercalcemia, usually are large, well differentiated, and without bony metastasis.[188] Surgical excision of the tumor results in the serum calcium levels returning to normal. The hypercalcemia results from secretion of parathyroid hormone (PTH) or PTH-like substance by the tumor; however, serum levels of PTH usually are within normal limits, as are levels of 1,25 dehydroxyvitamin D and 29 hydroxyvitamin D.[241] Nevertheless, the hypercalcemia associated with a vulvar carcinoma that is neither metastatic nor involves bone may still be secondary to tumor production of PTH. PTH has been demonstrated by immunoperoxidase techniques within carcinomas associated with hypercalcemia in lung, bladder, and parotid tu-

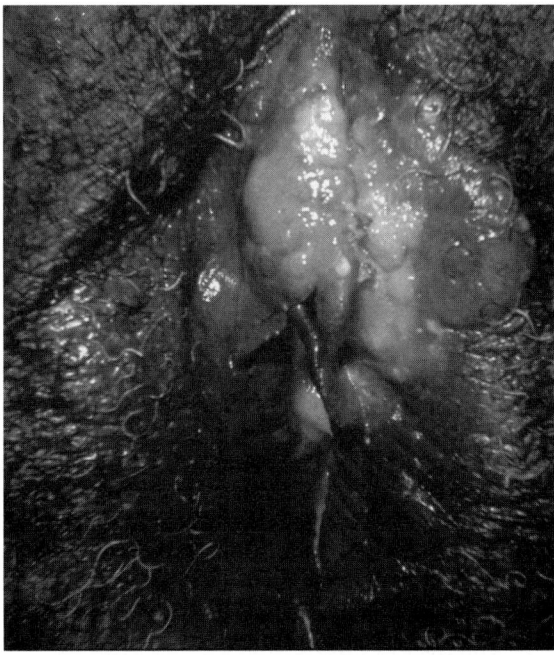

FIG. 3.15. Squamous cell carcinoma. The tumor involves the medial aspect of the left anterior labium majus and clitoris. (See color insert.)

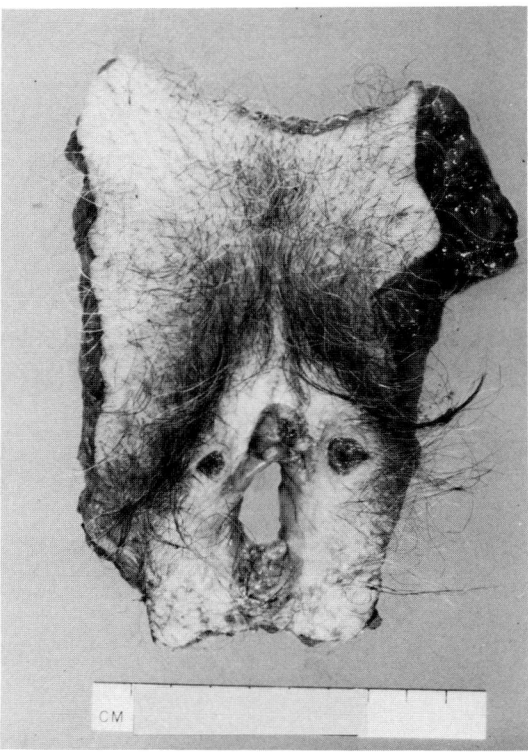

FIG. 3.16. "Mirror image" squamous cell carcinomas. The tumor involves the medial aspects of the labia majora bilaterally.

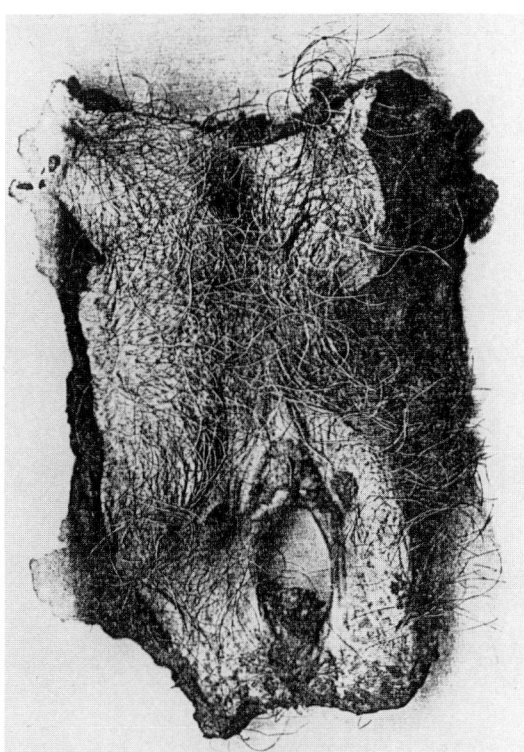

FIG. 3.17. Total vulvectomy with "mirror image" squamous carcinoma. A photocopy of the specimen in Fig. 3.16 was made by placing the specimen, skin surface down, on a photocopy machine. Skin detail, with the bilateral tumors, are evident. This may be used in specimen preparation and may become part of the permanent record to document from where sections were taken.

mors even though the serum levels of PTH were normal in these patients.[125]

MICROSCOPIC FINDINGS

The Gynecologic Oncology Group (GOG) has advised grading of squamous cell carcinomas according to the percentage of undifferentiated cells. The latter are small cells with scant cytoplasm showing little or no differentiation and infiltrating the stroma either in elongated cords or small clusters[223] (Fig. 3.18). This grading system can be reduced to three grades. Grade 1 tumors have no undifferentiated cells, grade 2 tumors have undifferentiated cells comprising less than half the tumor, and grade 3 tumors contain half or more of the poorly differentiated component. Grade 1 tumors have little risk of regional lymph node metastasis; the risk is higher with increasing grade.[123,223] Currently, tumor grading is not routinely performed. Additional factors that may be of significance in prognosis and in the probability of lymph node metastasis include the diameter of the lesion, the presence of vascular space invasion,[37,128,129,153] and tumor ulceration.[153] Confluent growth, defined as anastomosing cords or tumor, or tumor in the dermis exceeding 1 mm³ (Figs. 3.19, 3.20) does not correlate with the occurrence of node metastasis,[72,193] but is not found in tumors having 1 mm or less of invasion.[274] Clinical pathological studies support the same recommendations of the ISGYP in reporting frankly inva-

sive squamous cell carcinoma as for superficial invasive squamous cell carcinoma: (1) depth of invasion in millimeters, (2) thickness of the tumor in millimeters, (3) presence or absence of vascular space involvement by the tumor, (4) diameter of the tumor measured from the specimen in the fresh or fixed state, and (5) clinical measurement of the tumor diameter, when available.

CHROMOSOMAL STUDIES

Cytogenetic studies on short-term cultures and early established cell lines of vulvar carcinomas have demonstrated that these tumors are genetically complex with multiple chromosome rearrangements that remain karyotypically stable in culture. The tumors typically are heterogeneous with multiple, but closely related, clonal populations. Both development and progression are apparent sequelae of altered gene expression.[287] A recent study on vulvar carcinomas employing flow cytometry and image analysis demonstrated a high frequency of aneuploidy with a predominance of tumors within the hypertetraploid range.[75] Immunohistochemical studies employing monoclonal antibodies to Ki 67, a proliferation-associated marker, has

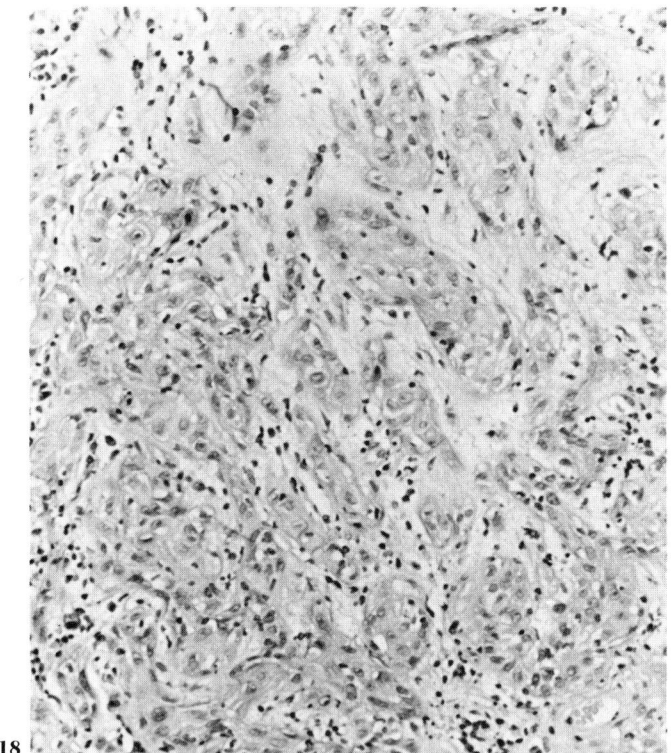

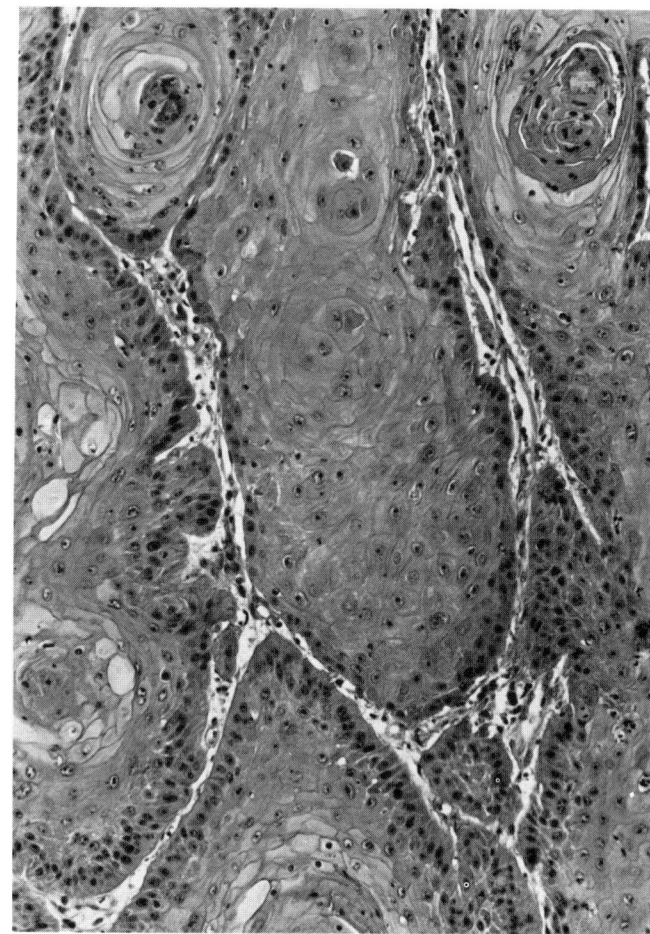

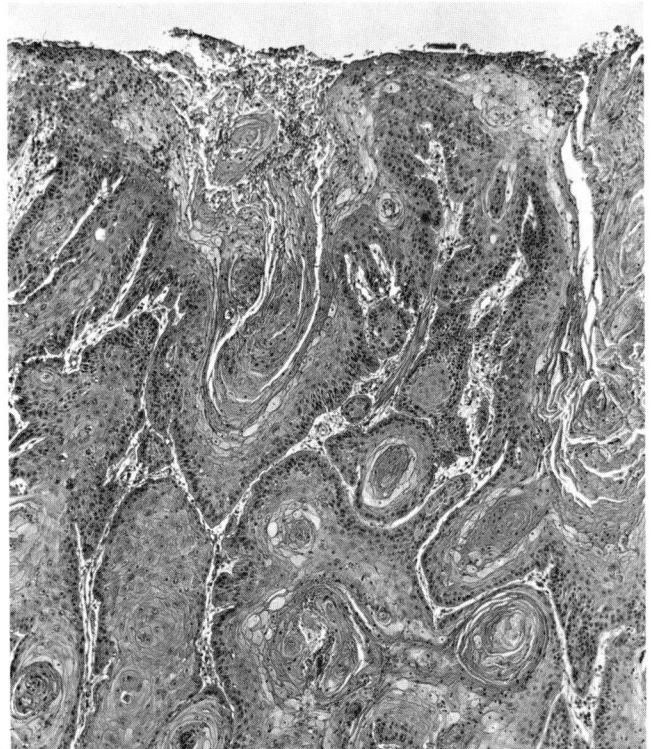

demonstrated two distinct tumor labeling patterns, diffuse and localized, that appear to be associated with prognosis; the diffuse pattern is associated with poor prognosis.[109]

CLINICAL BEHAVIOR AND TREATMENT

The clinical staging of vulvar carcinoma is summarized in Table 3.3.[87,149,150] Inguinal–femoral lymph node status[117,223] and the diameter of the tumor are independent prognostic factors. The overall 5-year relative survival, related to stage, is reported in a series of 588 patients with vulvar carcinoma as follows: stage I, 98%; stage II, 87%; stage III, 75%; stage IV, 29%.[119] The distance between the

---

FIG. 3.18. **Invasive squamous carcinoma, poorly differentiated.** Small nests of invasive cells not clearly squamous in origin are seen.

FIG. 3.19. **Invasive squamous cell carcinoma, well differentiated.** The tumor is keratinized and has a confluent growth pattern.

FIG. 3.20. **Invasive squamous cell carcinoma, well differentiated.** Tongues of well-differentiated squamous epithelium with keratinization are evident.

Table 3.3. Staging of vulvar carcinoma (F.I.G.O., 1989)

Stage 0	
Tis	Carcinoma in situ, intraepithelial carcinoma
Stage I[a]	
T1 N0 M0	Tumor confined to the vulva and/or perineum, 2 cm or less in greatest dimension, nodes are not palpable
Stage II	
T2 N0 M0	Tumor confined to the vulva and/or perineum, more than 2 cm in greatest dimension, nodes are not palpable
Stage III	
T3 N0 M0	Tumor of any size with 1) Adjacent spread to
T3 N1 M0	the lower urethra and/or the vagina, and/or
T1 N1 M0	the anus, and/or 2) unilateral regional
T2 N1 M0	lymph node metastasis
Stage IVA	
T1 N2 M0	Tumor invades any of the following: upper
T2 N2 M0	urethra, bladder mucosa, rectal mucosa,
T3 N2 M0	pelvic bone, and/or bilateral regional node
T4 any N M0	metastasis
Stage IVB	
Any T	Any distant metastasis including pelvic lymph
Any N M1	nodes

F.I.G.O., International Federation of Gynecology and Obstetrics.
[a] International Society for the Study of Vulvar Disease stage I is defined as a solitary tumor ≤2 cm in greatest diameter, with a depth of invasion of ≤1 mm.[146,214]

tumor and the surgical margin is a significant predictor of local recurrence. A surgical margin of 8 mm or less is associated with a 50% chance of local recurrence.[108] In a GOG study of 121 eligible patients with stage I vulvar carcinoma with a tumor thickness of 5 mm or less without vascular space invasion by tumor and negative lymph nodes, 19 patients (15.7%) experienced recurrence of tumor and there were seven deaths (5.8%) from tumor, of which five were related to recurrence in the groin nodes.[240] In cases beyond 1-mm invasion, more extensive surgery can be planned, including groin node dissection.[36,87,98,103,144,265,266]

Terminology for surgical procedures and characterization of depth of invasion of vulvar tumors has been developed by the ISSVD and is shown in Table 3.4.[130]

The reliability of clinical evaluation in the determination of whether tumor is present in inguinal nodes is reviewed in Table 3.5. It is recognized that pathological evaluation of lymph nodes for metastasis also may be falsely negative, and all lymph node tissue should be submitted for microscopic analysis.[279,280] In assessing groin nodes, fine-needle aspiration may be the first step if suspicious nodes are present because the technique is rapid, safe, cost effective, and will detect gross metastasis. Bone metastasis may be present.[1] Current oncologic thought has become conservative, attempting to define high- and low-risk groups requiring individualization of therapy.[36,70,104,128,129] Many patients are now offered immediate reconstructive surgery as

Table 3.4. Surgical procedures and characterization of depth of invasion of vulvar tumors[a]

Vulvectomy
Partial vulvectomy: removal of a part of the vulvar/perineal integument independent of depth.
Total vulvectomy: removal of the whole vulva and appropriate integument of the perineum independent of depth.
Depth of excision
Superficial: Removal of the most superficial layer with a variable amount of dermis and subcutaneous tissue.
Deep: Removal of the vulva to the superficial aponeurosis of the urogenital diaphragm and/or pubic periosteum

[a] Developed by the International Society for the Study of Vulvar Disease.

part of the initial procedure.[98] Radiation techniques are now available that allow skin-sparing treatment of the groin nodes and have been used successfully in both primary and adjunctive treatment.[33,82,168]

Histologic Subtypes of Vulvar Squamous Cell Carcinoma

Squamous cell carcinoma of the vulva can be subdivided into several morphologically distinct subtypes, which are summarized in Table 3.6. Histologically, invasive squamous cell carcinomas that are not otherwise specified (NOS) usually are well-differentiated tumors, but moderately and poorly differentiated varieties are found in 5–10% of the cases (Figs. 3.13, 3.18–3.20).[128,167,205,265]

Table 3.5. False-positive and false-negative clinical assessment of inguinal nodes

	False positive (%)	False negative (%)
Way (1948)	44	61
Franklin and Rutledge (1971)	8	21
Boyce et al. (1985)	6	21

Table 3.6. Histologic subtypes of squamous vulvar carcinoma

Squamous cell carcinoma (NOS)
Basaloid carcinoma
Warty (condylomatous) carcinoma
Verrucous carcinoma
Giant cell carcinoma
Spindle-cell carcinoma
Acantholytic squamous cell carcinoma (adenoid squamous carcinoma)
Lymphoepithelioma-like carcinoma
Basal cell carcinoma
    Metatypical basal cell carcinoma (Basosquamous carcinoma)
    Adenoid basal cell carcinoma
    Sebaceous cell carcinoma

NOS, not otherwise specified.

Basaloid Carcinoma

Recent studies have shown an elevated prevalence of human papillomavirus (HPV), mainly type 16, with certain types of invasive squamous carcinomas of the vulva. Among these are basaloid carcinomas, which occur in young women (mean age, 54 years), compared with typical keratinizing squamous cell carcinomas (mean age, 77 years). Basaloid carcinomas frequently are associated with adjacent VIN, usually of the basaloid type. In contrast to typical squamous cell carcinomas, basaloid carcinomas are associated with synchronous or metachronous squamous neoplasms of the cervix and vagina.[152]

On gross examination, basaloid carcinomas are similar to typical squamous cell carcinomas. Microscopically, they are characterized by variable-sized nests of immature squamous cells showing little, if any, squamous maturation. Some tumors are composed of small, irregularly shaped clusters and cords of cells surrounded by a densely hyalinized stroma. The basal-type cells within the nests and cords resemble those in the classic type of carcinoma in situ of the cervix (Figs. 3.21, 3.22). Characteristically, they are ovoid and relatively uniform in size, with scant cyto-

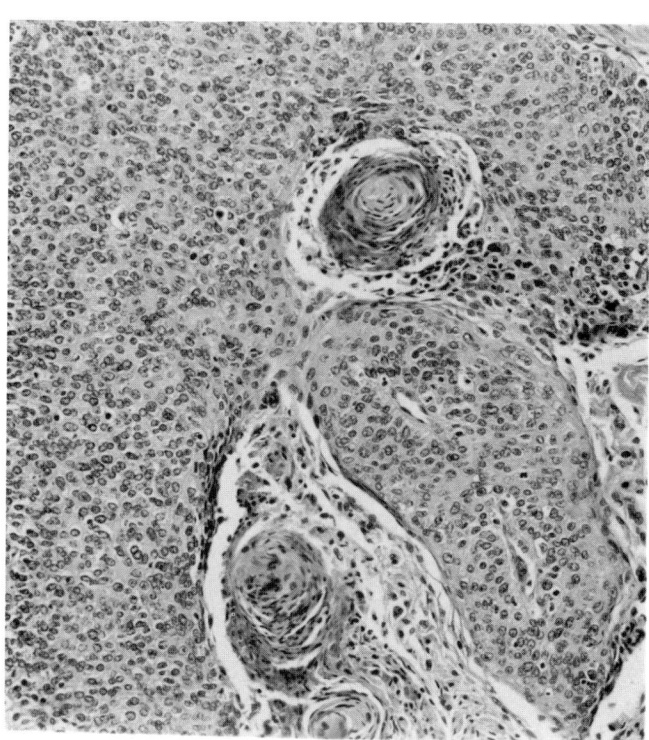

FIG. 3.22. Basaloid carcinoma. The tumor is composed of relatively small cells with hyperchromatic, slightly pleomorphic nuclei. There is cellular disarray throughout the neoplasm; however, some keratinization is evident. (Courtesy of R.J. Kurman, M.D., Baltimore, MD.)

plasm and a high nuclear cytoplasmic ratio and, therefore, they appear undifferentiated. Nuclei contain evenly distributed coarsely granular chromatin, creating a stippled appearance. A moderate degree of mitotic activity usually is evident. Occasionally, the cells in the center of a nest show evidence of maturation and contain more abundant cytoplasm. Keratinization may be evident in the center of the nests and keratin pearls occasionally are present. Desmosomes usually are not evident. The behavior of basaloid carcinoma appears to be similar to typical keratinizing squamous carcinomas but there is insufficient experience at this point to draw firm conclusions.[152] Basaloid carcinoma at times may be difficult to distinguish from basal cell carcinoma. In contrast to basaloid carcinoma, basal cell carcinomas tend to be more circumscribed and have a lobular appearance. The characteristic palisading of the outermost layer of cells in the nests of basal cell carcinoma is lacking in basaloid carcinoma. The differential diagnosis of basaloid carcinoma also includes metastatic small cell carcinoma and Merkel cell tumor. These tumors have a more diffusely infiltrative pattern characterized by ill-defined nests, trabeculae, and individual cells invading the stroma rather than the broad anastomosing bands and well-defined nests typical of basaloid carcinoma. Small cell tumors usually are immunoreactive for neuroendocrine

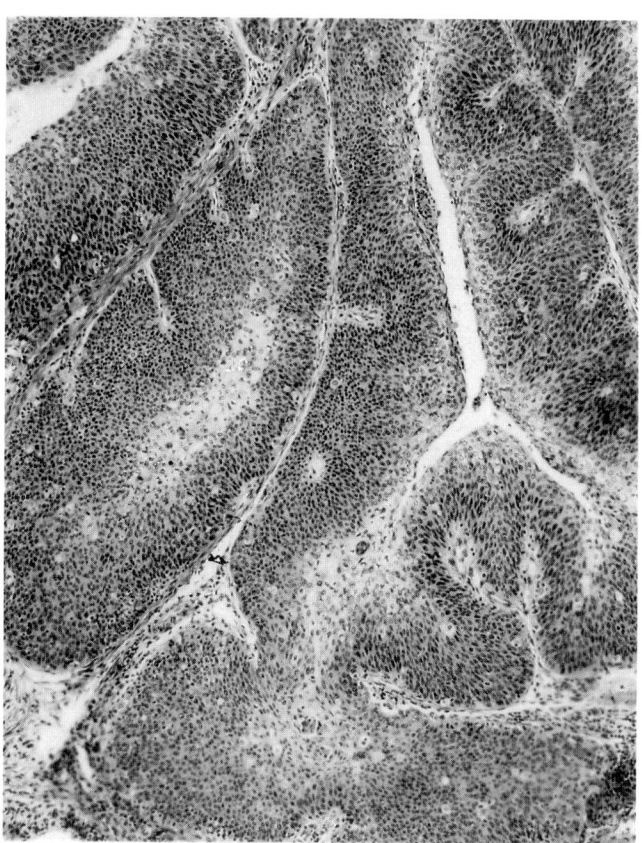

FIG. 3.21. Basaloid carcinoma. The tumor is composed of immature-appearing keratinocytes without significant maturation or keratinization. The surrounding stroma appears fibrous. (Courtesy of R.J. Kurman, M.D., Baltimore, MD.)

markers; Merkel cell tumors have a characteristic perinuclear cytoplasmic "dot" that is immunoreactive for cytokeratins.

Warty Carcinoma (Condylomatous Carcinoma)

Warty carcinoma is found predominantly in younger women (mean age, 55 years) and presents clinically as a papillary tumor that may resemble condyloma acuminatum. Vulvar squamous cell carcinoma may arise associated with condyloma acuminatum, and these tumors usually are warty or verrucous carcinomas.[68,74,228] On microscopic examination the tumor has multiple papillary projections with a keratinized epithelial surface and fibrovascular cores (Figs. 3.23, 3.24). Cytological atypia is seen, especially within the basal and parabasal cells, where there is nuclear pleomorphism and nuclear hyperchromasia. Multinucleation may be present. Mitotic figures usually can be found, but may not be atypical. Cytoplasmic perinuclear clearing and varying degrees of nuclear atypia resembling koilocytosis is present in a substantial number of cells. It is the most characteristic feature. At the junction

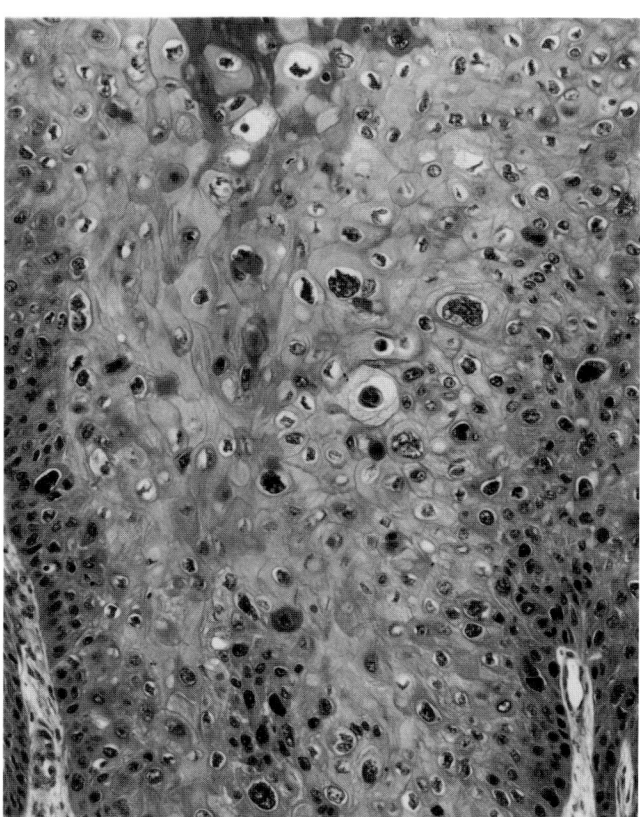

FIG. 3.24. Warty (condylomatous) carcinoma. Cells with pleomorphic nuclei and vacuolated cytoplasm resembling koilocytes are present within the neoplastic epithelium. There is nuclear pleomorphism. The cells have prominent eosinophilic cytoplasm. (Courtesy of R.J. Kurman, M.D., Baltimore, MD.)

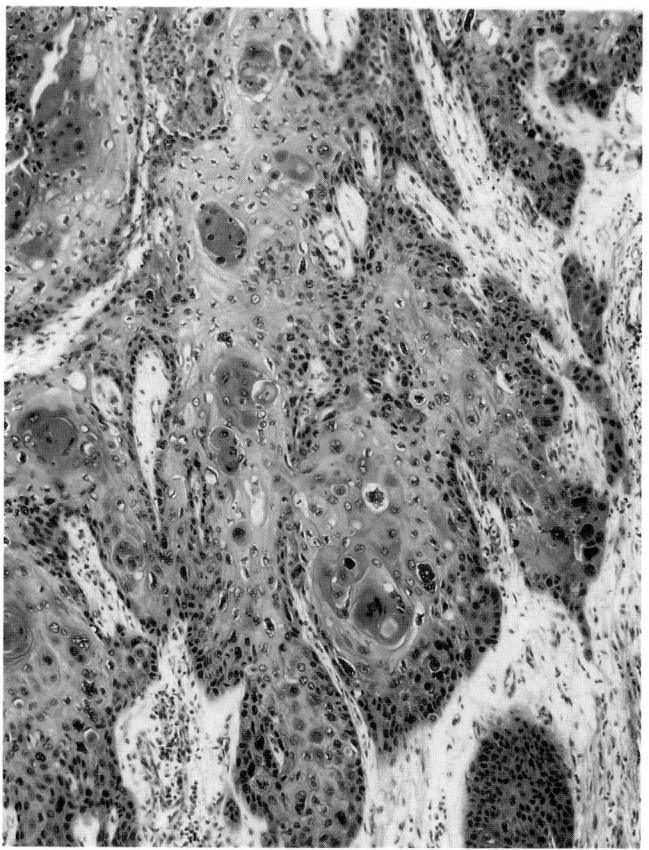

FIG. 3.23. Warty (condylomatous) carcinoma. The cords of neoplastic cells are separated by a fibrovascular stroma. Keratinization is present. (Courtesy of R.J. Kurman, M.D., Baltimore, MD.)

between the exophytic portion of the tumor and the underlying stoma, irregular-shaped nests of epithelium are present that may be associated with keratin pearls and dyskeratotic cells. In this area the tumor resembles a keratinized squamous cell carcinoma. In some cases these areas are small and focal. This tumor frequently is associated with HPV type 16.[74,190,152,254] The clinical course of warty carcinoma appears generally good; however, lymph node metastasis may occur. The prognosis appears intermediate between verrucous carcinoma and squamous cell carcinoma of the usual type.[254] Approximately 80% of warty and basaloid carcinomas have adjacent warty or basaloid VIN. About one-quarter of the warty and basaloid carcinomas are associated with other genital tract squamous neoplasias.[152]

Verrucous Carcinoma

Verrucous carcinoma is highly differentiated squamous carcinoma that has a verrucous pattern and invades with a pushing border in the form of bulbous pegs of neoplastic cells.[31,134] The term *giant condyloma of Buschke-Lowen-*

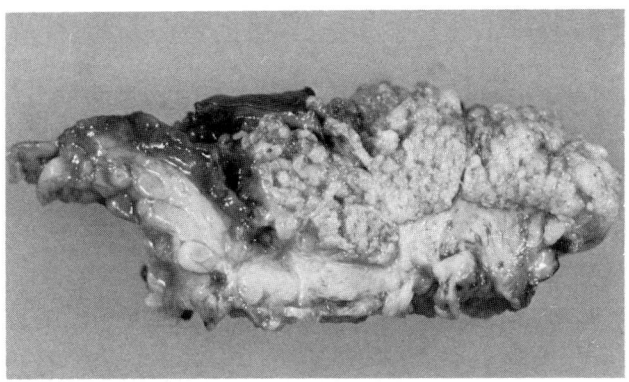

FIG. 3.25. **Verrucous carcinoma in cross-section.** This tumor was 5 cm in diameter. It has a broad, well-defined margin of infiltration involving the underlying fibrofatty tissue.

stein is considered to be a synonym for verrucous carcinoma, but it is confusing and therefore is not recommended. Squamous cell carcinomas at times may have some of the architectural features of verrucous carcinoma but, if they lack a high degree of differentiation, they should not be designated verrucous carcinoma.[4,145]

Verrucous carcinoma is a papillary exophytic growth that may have the appearance of an exophytic, broad-based condyloma acuminatum, and distort or completely obscure the vulva[11] (Fig. 3.25). Secondary infection may be associated with a malodorous discharge. Regional lymph nodes usually are not enlarged. Condyloma acuminatum and squamous cell carcinoma may be adjacent to verrucous carcinomas.[68,74] Verrucous carcinoma has been reported to be associated with HPV, typically type 6, or variants of type 6.[211,212,258]

The microscopic features of verrucous carcinoma include prominent acanthosis with a pushing tumor–dermal interface and bland cytological features[147,202] (Fig. 3.26). The deep advancing margin is characterized by large bulbous nests of squamous epithelium. There is minimal nuclear pleomorphism, with the greatest degree of nuclear atypia nearest the dermal interface. The nuclei may have coarse chromatin and variable-sized nucleoli, distinguishing them from normal adjacent keratinocytes. Mitotic figures are rare and when present are normal. The abundant cytoplasm of the tumor cells is eosinophilic, without dyskeratosis. Koilocytosis is not a feature of this tumor. Parakeratosis and/or hyperkeratosis usually are present, and

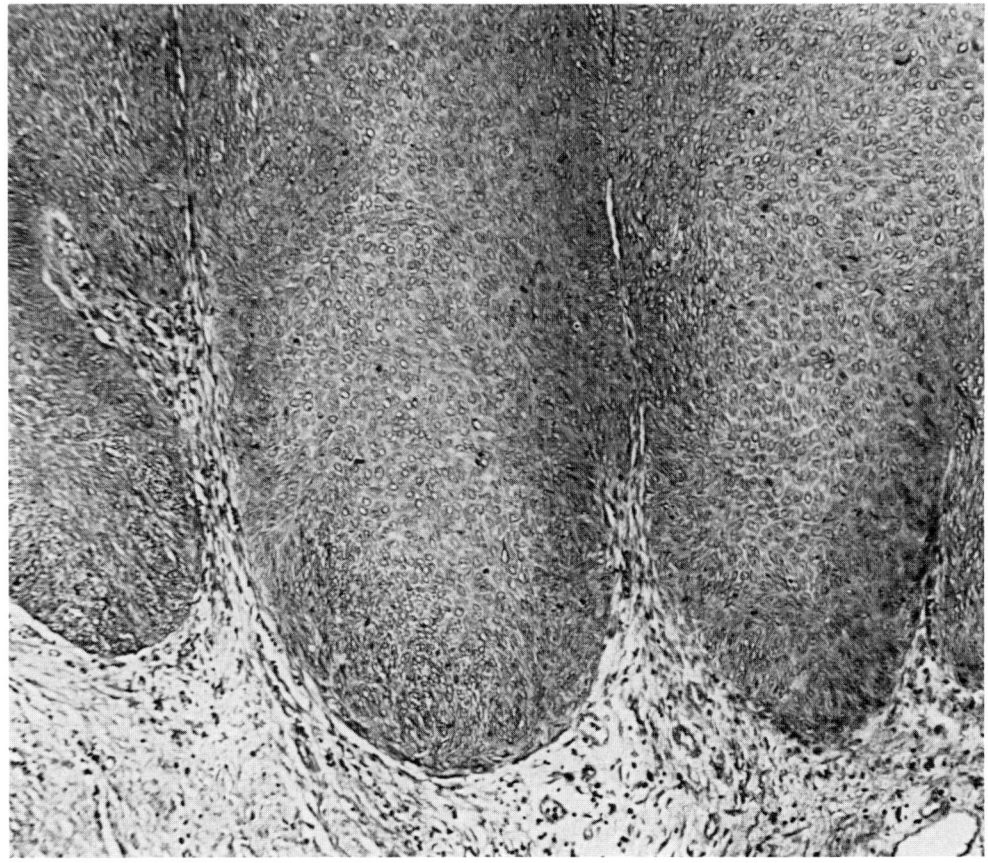

FIG. 3.26. **Verrucous carcinoma.** A section from the specimen in Fig. 3.25. There is a well-defined tumor–stromal interface. The cells are well differentiated and a prominent chronic inflammatory infiltrate is present within the stroma.

may be prominent. There is an absence of fibrovascular cores separating the bulbous epithelial downgrowths. An inflammatory infiltrate within the dermis usually is present. These tumors typically are diploid.

The differential diagnosis includes the typical variety of squamous cell carcinoma, warty carcinoma, and condyloma acuminatum. Squamous cell carcinoma of the usual type (keratinizing squamous carcinoma) has greater nuclear pleomorphism and a more irregular type of infiltration of the stroma compared with the bulbous rete pegs of verrucous carcinoma. Warty carcinoma, despite its verruciform appearance, has fibrovascular cores within the papillary fronds, unlike verrucous carcinoma. In addition, these tumors display greater nuclear atypia, koilocytosis, and, at their deep margin, invade like typical squamous cell carcinomas. Condyloma acuminatum is characterized by a complex branching papillary architecture with vascular papillae, lacks bulbous downgrowths, and typically shows koilocytosis.

Verrucous carcinomas may recur locally after excision. Lymph node metastasis is extremely rare, and its presence should prompt re-evaluation of the lesion for areas of the usual type of squamous cell carcinoma. Wide local excision and total vulvectomy without lymph node dissection are the most common methods of therapy. If the tumor is excised completely, the prognosis is excellent. The role of radiotherapy in these tumors is not well studied, but may be applicable in very advanced cases.

Giant Cell Carcinoma

Squamous cell carcinoma with tumor giant cells is a variant of squamous cell carcinoma characterized by multinucleated tumor giant cells, large nuclei with prominent nucleoli, and prominent eosinophilic cytoplasm (Fig. 3.27). This tumor variant is relatively rare and is associated with a poor prognosis.[265,266] The most important differential diagnosis is malignant melanoma, which may not be melanin producing and commonly forms multinucleated tumor giant cells.[265,277] Melanomas typically have intranuclear inclusions and prominent nucleoli. Unlike giant cell carcinoma, melanomas are typically S-100 and melanoma antigen (HMB45) immunoreactive.[277]

Spindle-cell Squamous Cell Carcinoma

Spindle-cell carcinoma of the vulva may mimic a sarcoma or be associated with sarcoma-like stroma[50,238] (Fig. 3.28). However, the neoplastic spindle cells are immunoreactive for keratin.[182,222] Spindle-cell carcinoma may be associated with tumor giant cells, which are also immunoreactive for keratin.[222] Spindle-cell carcinoma must be distinguished from mesenchymal spindle cell tumors including leiomyosarcoma, malignant fibrous histiocytoma and fibrosarcoma, as well as spindle-cell malignant melanoma and transitional cell carcinoma with spindle-cell features.

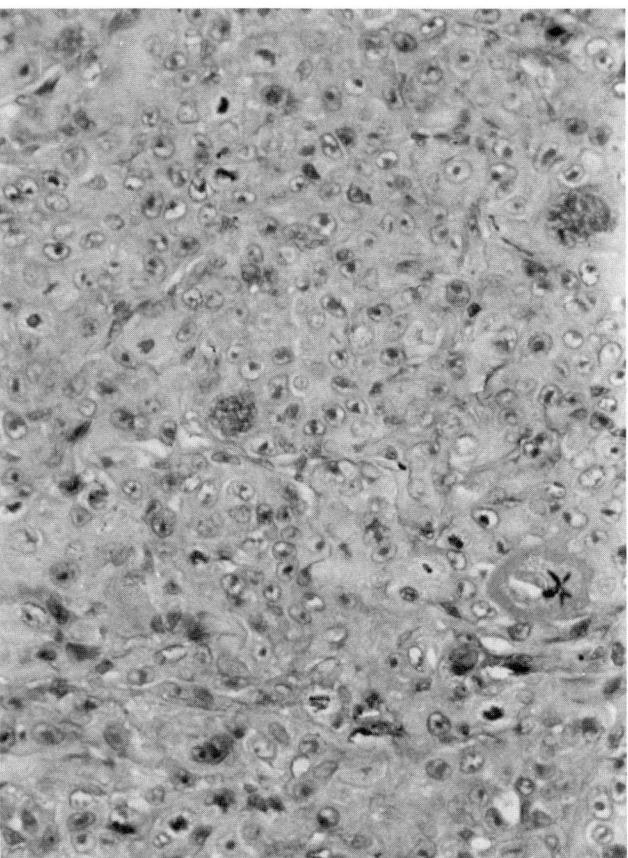

Fig. 3.27. **Giant cell carcinoma of the vulva.** Multinucleated tumor giant cells are evident. The cells contain nuclei with prominent nucleoli and abundant eosinophilic cytoplasm.

Acantholytic Squamous Cell Carcinoma (Adenoid Squamous Carcinoma)

The acantholytic squamous tumor forms rounded spaces, or pseudoacini, lined with a single layer of squamous cells.[156,260] Dyskeratotic and acantholytic cells are sometimes present in the central lumen (Fig. 3.29). These changes are focal in most cases, and may occur within otherwise well-differentiated squamous tumors.[140] The adenoid architecture does not correlate with lymph node involvement or the clinical course of the tumor.

Lymphoepithelioma-like Carcinoma

These tumors are recognized within the skin and may occur rarely on the vulva in older individuals.[40] The tumor consists of nests or syncytial groups of epithelioid-appearing cells mixed with, and surrounded by, a dense lymphocytic infiltrate (see Ch. 8, Carcinoma and Other Tumors of the Cervix). The epithelial cells are immunoreactive for high molecular weight cytokeratins, which distinguishes them from inflammatory processes and malignant large cell lymphomas. Lymphomas, including Ki-1 lymphomas,

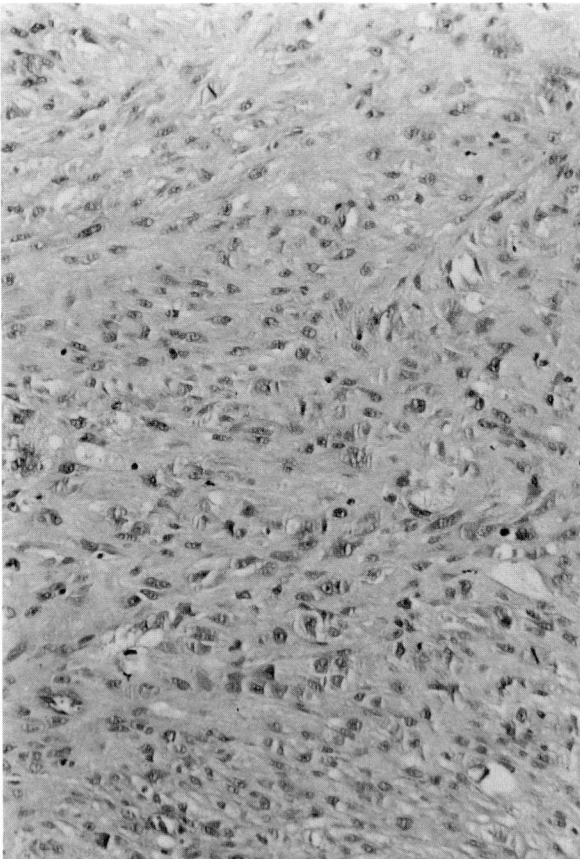

FIG. 3.28. Spindle-cell squamous carcinoma. The tumor cells are dispersed within the dermis and have a spindle shape. Some nuclear pleomorphism is evident within the tumor cells.

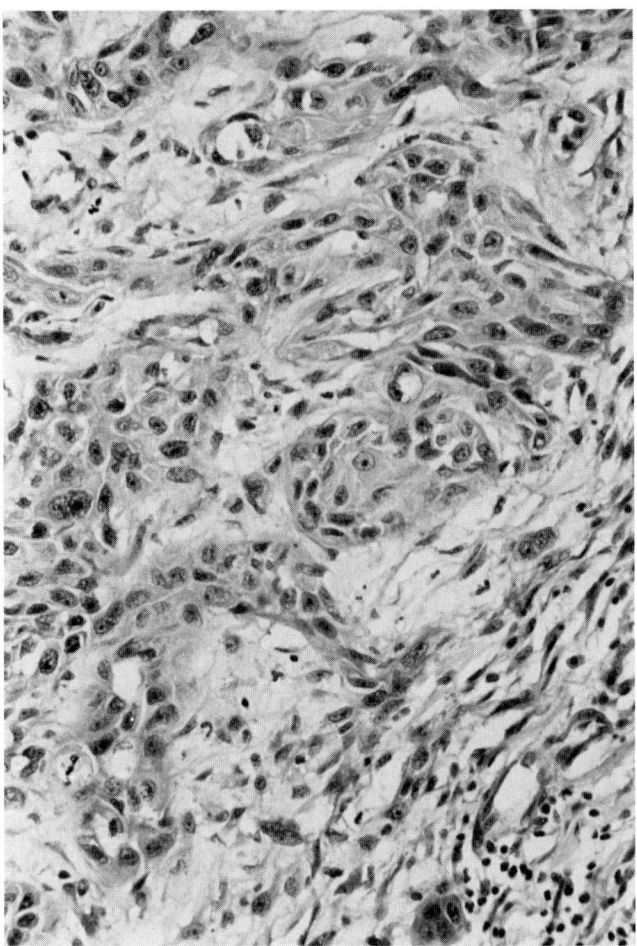

FIG. 3.29. Acantholytic squamous carcinoma. Nests of poorly differentiated squamous cell carcinoma are arranged in a crude acinar manner. Some of the central acini are vacuolated.

which are immunoreactive for lymphocytic markers, contain an immunophenotypic monoclonal population of neoplastic lymphocytic cells. The therapy is wide local excision with or without local radiation therapy.[40]

Basal Cell Carcinoma

Although basal cell carcinomas of the skin are extremely common, they rarely occur on the vulva, a site not often exposed to actinic radiation. Breen et al. have shown that when such vulvar tumors do arise, they are found primarily in elderly white women, whose symptomatology consists of itching or the presence of a mass.[25] Most lesions are confined to the labia majora.

The histological pattern resembles that of basal cell carcinomas occurring elsewhere on the skin (Fig. 3.30). Small, elongated cells with deeply basophilic nuclei are present; a large variety of architectural patterns can be recognized ranging from slight palisading of the basal layer of the epidermis to the formation of large club-shaped masses of pleomorphic basal cells. The connective tissue response frequently consists of a chronic inflammatory cell infiltrate and occasionally shows a mucoid or myxomatous change.

A local recurrence rate of 20% is noted after wide local excision. Metastasis to regional lymph nodes occurs on rare occasion.[61] The overall prognosis for these tumors, however, is excellent, and no patients have been found to expire as a result of the disease.

Metatypical Basal Cell Carcinoma (Basosquamous Carcinoma)

Metatypical basal cell carcinoma, or basosquamous carcinoma, represents a mixture of both squamous and basal cell neoplastic elements. In these cases the squamous cells have nuclear atypia (Fig. 3.31). The clinical significance of such change is unclear.[226] Basosquamous carcinoma are locally aggressive and may metastasize.

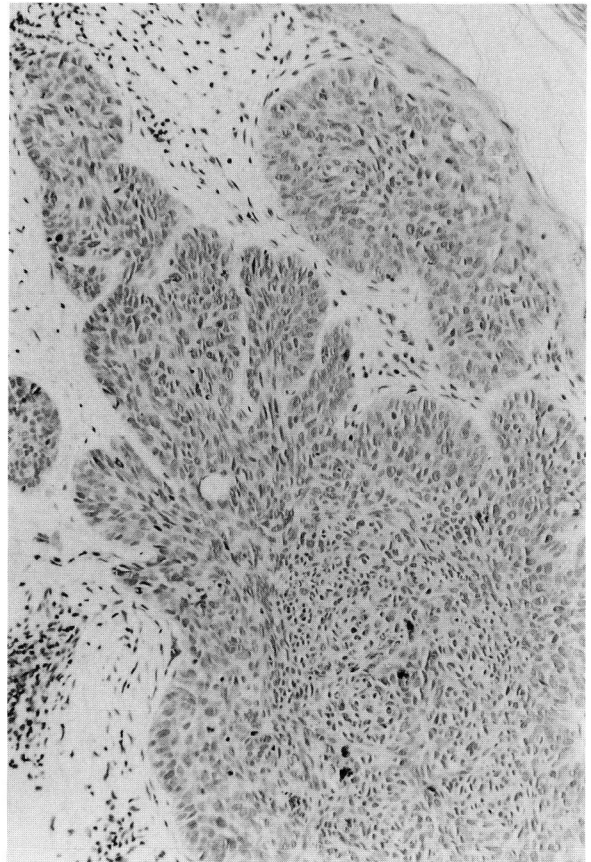

FIG. 3.30. **Basal cell carcinoma.** The tumor cells are small, uniform, lack maturation, and show characteristic palisading at the periphery of the involved rete ridges. The rete ridges are branched and extend in a pushing manner into the adjacent dermis.

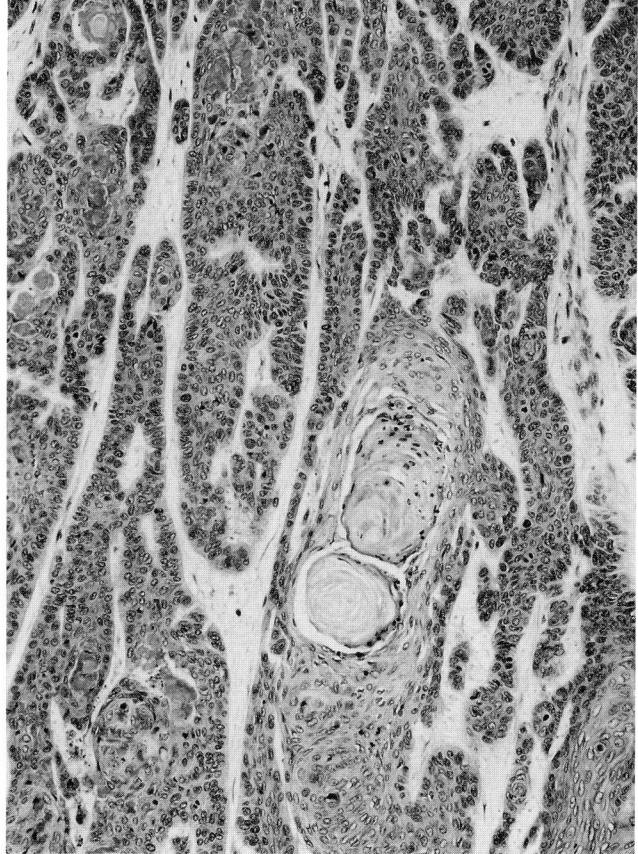

FIG. 3.31. **Basosquamous carcinoma (metatypical basal cell carcinoma).** The cells show increased cytoplasm in the areas of squamous carcinoma. (Courtesy of R.J. Kurman, M.D., Baltimore, MD.)

Adenoid Basal Cell Carcinoma

Adenoid basal cell carcinoma is a variant of basal cell carcinoma in which tubular and gland-like differentiation is seen within a tumor that otherwise is a characteristic basal cell carcinoma.

Sebaceous Cell Carcinoma

Sebaceous cell carcinoma is a tumor with features of basosquamous cell carcinoma that also has sebaceous differentiation (Fig. 3.32). This tumor type has been associated with vulvar intraepithelial neoplasia.[131]

Adenocarcinoma

Adenocarcinomas of the vulva are rare vulvar malignancies. Many previous reports of this entity have been shown retrospectively to represent benign hidradenomas or foci of adnexal Paget disease. Most adenocarcinomas of the vulva arise as primary malignant tumors of the Bartholin gland; however, they also may arise from sweat glands or other skin appendage origin, the urethra, Skene gland, and from Paget disease.[249,273] Primary adenocarcinoma of the vulva arising in cloacal tissue has been reported.[253]

Paget Disease

GENERAL FEATURES

Paget disease is characterized by a primary intraepithelial proliferation of atypical glandular-type cells that may invade the dermis, or by an intraepithelial proliferation of similar cells secondary to an underlying adenocarcinoma.

Friedrich et al. have found that 14% of all reported cases of vulvar Paget disease were associated with a carcinoma of the breast.[91] Urinary tract malignancy has been found with genital Paget disease.[207] Cases with associated adenocarcinoma of the Bartholin gland and squamous cell carcinoma

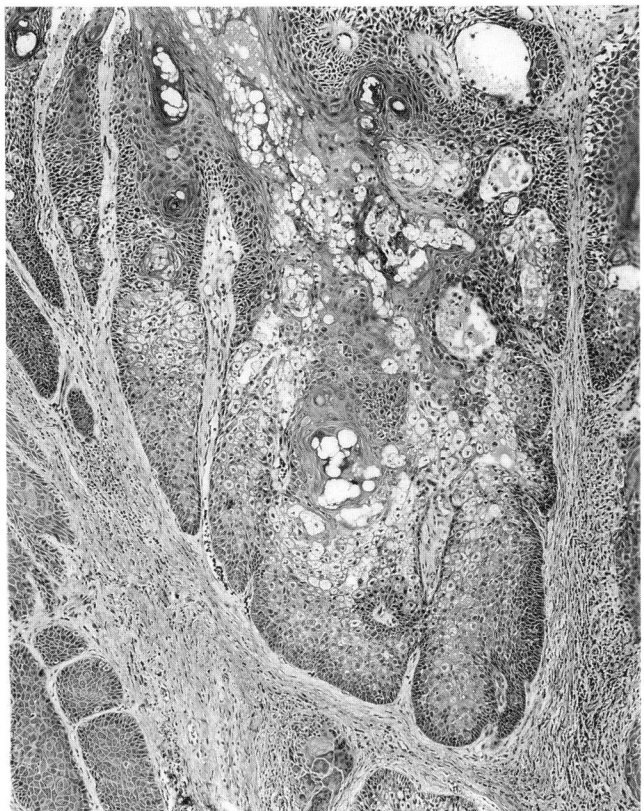

FIG. 3.32. **Sebaceous carcinoma.** The tumor is composed of cords and nests of basaloid-appearing cells, which, in the larger tumor areas, are associated with sebaceous cells that are present in pagetoid nests in the parabasal areas and in larger clusters near the epithelial surface. (Courtesy of R.J. Kurman, M.D., Baltimore, MD.)

of the vulva also have been reported.[283] Perianal involvement by Paget disease is associated with a high frequency of adenocarcinoma of the rectum.[111]

Extensive work on the ultrastructure of the Paget cell has generally revealed features consistent with adenocarcinoma.[84,174] Some Paget cells contain the organelles associated with apocrine cells,[186] whereas others resemble eccrine cells[83] and still others resemble squamous keratinocytes.[84,239] In some instances more than one type of cell has been identified in the same case. These findings are all consistent with the concept that the Paget cell represents an aberrant differentiation from a multipotent cell derived from the embryonic stratum germinativum of the epidermis. Primitive stem cells destined to form basal keratinocytes may differentiate into Paget cells with some of the ultrastructural characteristics of keratinocytes; stem cells that differentiate into apocrine anlage may form Paget cells with apocrine organelles, and so forth. Such an interpretation accounts for the observation that Paget cells are often first noted just above the basal layer of the epithe-

lium and that they may be located within any of the skin adnexae.

The finding of Paget-like cells in foci of metastatic tumors of either squamous or glandular origin suggests that the malignant tumor cell is still capable of aberrant differentiation into a Paget cell. Dermal invasion by previous intraepithelial Paget cells has been documented.[194] Vulvar Paget disease is therefore properly classified as a form of intraepithelial neoplasia that may become invasive. Of importance is the frequency with which the epidermal changes are associated with separate invasive carcinomas. Early investigators noted underlying adnexal adenocarcinoma beneath the skin in the vicinity of Paget disease in many extramammary cases.[111] This led some to conclude that Paget cells in the epidermis represented an intradermal migration of neoplastic cells from an underlying tumor, as occurs in the breast. However, it now seems clear that Paget cells in extramammary sites arise de novo in the epidermis or epidermally derived adnexal structures, where their presence may or may not be associated with a separate and often subjacent independent carcinoma (Fig. 3.33; see color insert).

Clinically, vulvar Paget disease appears as a red to pink eczematoid area with white islands of hyperkeratosis (Fig. 3.34). Pruritus is present in more than half the patients. Almost all are postmenopausal Caucasian women,[16,29] although a case of vulvar Paget disease has been reported in a 24-year-old black woman.[236]

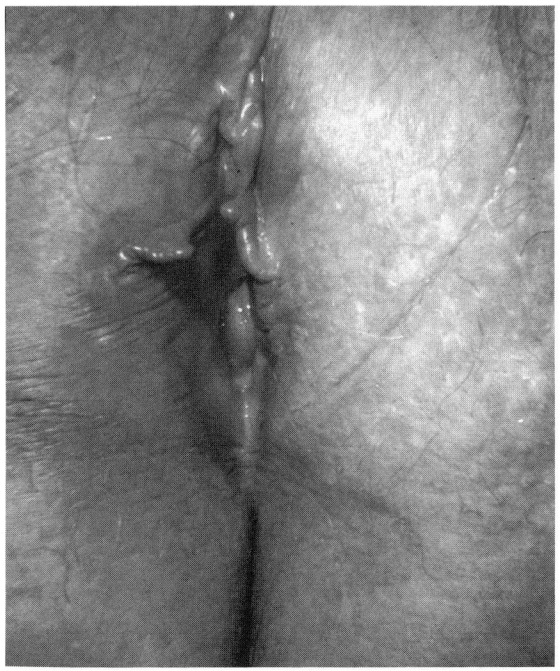

FIG. 3.33. **Paget disease.** An eczematoid, slightly raised area is noted on the medial anterior surface of the left labium majus. (See color insert.)

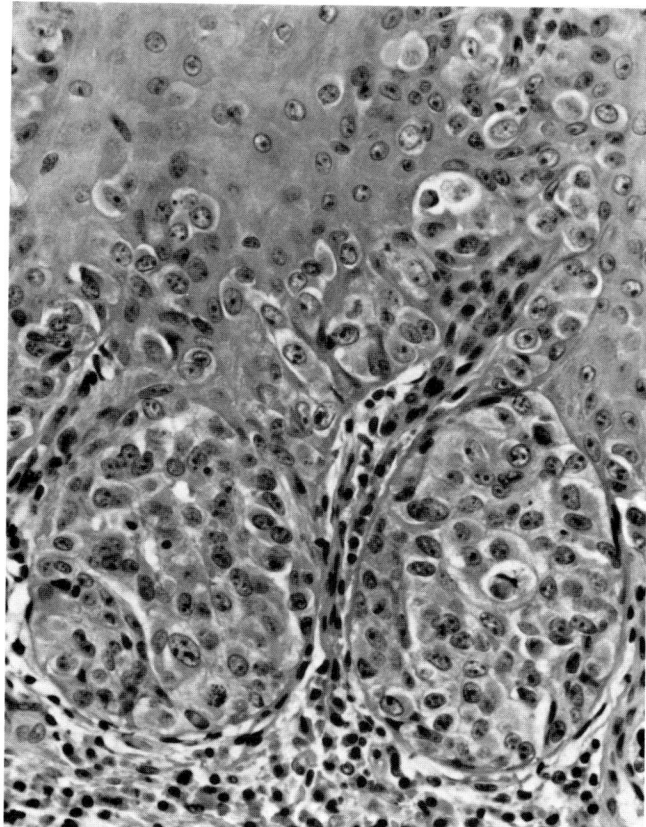

FIG. 3.34. Paget disease. Paget cells are present singly and in nests. Their pale cytoplasm easily differentiates them from surrounding keratinocytes.

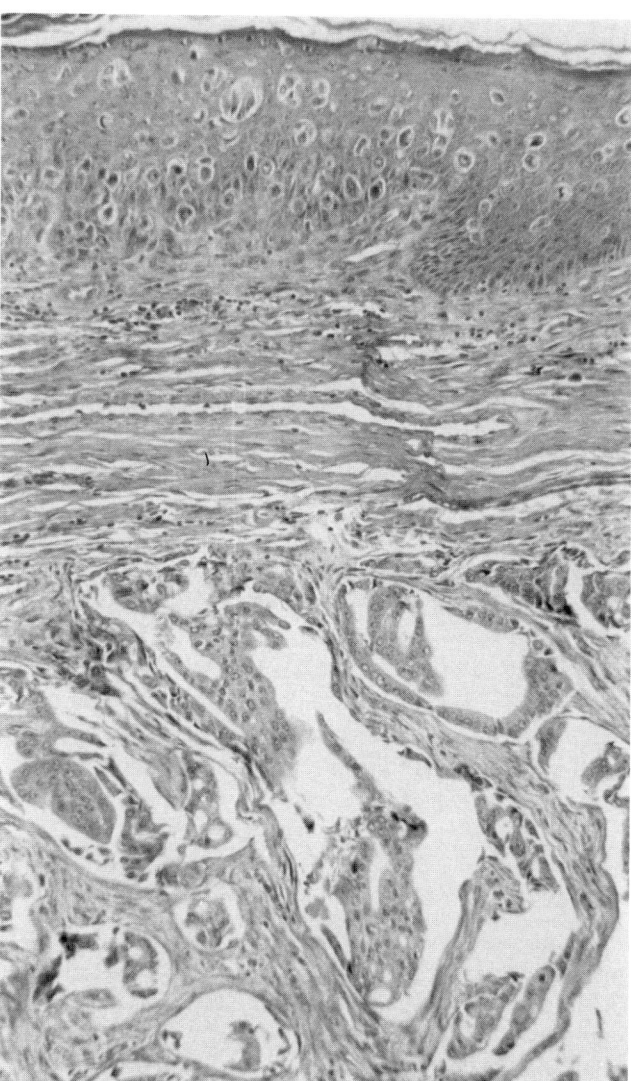

FIG. 3.35. Paget disease with underlying adenocarcinoma. Paget cells are present in the overlying epithelium. The adenocarcinoma consists of neoplastic glands within the dermis.

GROSS FINDINGS

Not all involved areas are visibly altered on physical examination. In a careful topographic study, Gunn and Gallager[102] demonstrated that the outline of the histologically involved area was highly irregular and of much greater extent than the visible lesion. In addition, multicentric foci, some occurring in grossly normal-appearing skin, were noted. This accounts for the frequent "recurrences" of disease despite seemingly adequate excision. Fluorescein has been used clinically to assit in visualization of the extent of Paget disease before excision.[176]

MICROSCOPIC FINDINGS

The early histopathological findings consist of intraepithelial, Paget cells occurring singly and in groups (Fig. 3.35). The cells may involve skin appendages and the surface epithelium. Typically, they are grouped predominantly within the basal and parabasal zones, with fewer cells present superficially. The cells are generally larger and have paler cytoplasm than the adjacent keratinocytes. Their cytoplasm is finely granular and amphophilic to ba-

sophilic, and may be vacuolated, forming signet-ring cells. Occasionally, gland spaces are formed within cell groups. The nuclei of the Paget cells are round to oval and may be the same size or larger than those of the adjacent keratinocyte nuclei. The nuclear chromatin may vary from vesicular and finely granular to coarsely hyperchromatic. Generally, one or more enlarged nucleoli are present. Mitotic figures may be found but are not frequent. Paget cells can be identified on cytological examination of scrapings from saline-moistened areas.[66,185] Adenocarcinoma may be found beneath the Paget disease and occurs in approximately 10–20% of the cases reported (Fig. 3.33). Its origin may be from underlying skin appendages, Bartholin gland, or as a consequence of invasive Paget disease.

DIFFERENTIAL DIAGNOSIS AND ADJUNCTIVE STUDIES

Paget cells are PAS positive (diastase resistant), mucicarmine positive, aldehydefuchsin positive, and alcian blue positive.[111] The cells stain pink against a background of greenish blue with Movat stain. In addition, Paget cells, as well as the cells and secretions of normal eccrine and apocrine glands, are rich in carcinoembryonic antigen (CEA) demonstrable by immunoperoxidase techniques.[178,183] Paget cells are immunoreactive for low molecular weight keratin 35 beta.[14] These reactions distinguish Paget cells from the large pale cells sometimes seen in VIN or in superficial spreading malignant melanoma, and may be useful in defining Paget-free surgical margins of resection (Table 3.2).[14,94] The dopa reaction on fresh tissue has been studied and found to be negative in Paget disease. This indicates an inability of the cell to produce melanin and again distinguishes it from a melanoma cell. Melanoma is distinguished further by being immunoreactive for HMB-45, which is absent in Paget cells.[14] Paget cells, however, may contain granules of melanin, demonstrable with Fontana–Masson stain, but these probably are produced by neighboring melanocytes and are engulfed only secondarily by the Paget cell. Paget cells have not been demonstrated to be associated with common genital human papillomaviruses.[234]

CLINICAL BEHAVIOR AND TREATMENT

Paget disease usually is a slowly progressive, indolent, superficial process. The treatment and prognosis of Paget disease of the vulva depends on whether an associated underlying invasive adenocarcinoma is present, and patients may be divided into two groups on this basis.[57,250,285] Consequently, it is incumbent on the pathologist to make a diligent search through all submitted tissue to identify, or rule out, an underlying invasive adenocarcinoma. Current therapy is wide local excision of the visible Paget disease, with excision to the fascia to exclude underlying adenocarcinoma. Microscopic Paget disease peripheral to the primary lesion with normal-appearing epithelium does not appear to harbor the same risks of underlying adenocarcinoma and can be treated by a more conservative approach, such as superficial laser ablation.[81]

Bartholin Gland Tumors

GENERAL FEATURES

A wide variety of tumors may arise from the Bartholin gland. The criteria for the diagnosis of a tumor of Bartholin gland origin are that the neoplasm must (1) arise at the site of Bartholin gland, (2) be consistent histologically with a primary neoplasm of Bartholin gland, and (3) not be metastatic.[43,292] Adenocarcinomas account for approximately 40% of Bartholin gland carcinomas, but others include squamous cell carcinoma (40%), adenoid cystic carcinoma (15%), transitional cell carcinoma (less than 5%), adenosquamous carcinoma (less than 5%), and poorly differentiated adenocarcinomas.[43,292]

CLINICAL FEATURES

Carcinoma of the Bartholin gland usually presents as an enlargement in the gland area and may be mistaken for a cyst. The average age of women with this tumor is 50 years, with most of them between 40 and 70 years of age.

GROSS FINDINGS

Bartholin gland tumors are typically solid, deeply infiltrative, and occupy the site of the gland, occasionally obscuring its presence. They range in size from 1 to 7 cm in diameter.

MICROSCOPIC FINDINGS

Adenocarcinomas of the Bartholin gland usually are nonspecific in type, but mucinous and papillary types have been described.[43] The tumors usually contain intracytoplasmic mucin and are immunoreactive for CEA.[181,182] Fine-needle aspiration cytology may be of value in initial diagnosis.[126] The differential diagnosis of Bartholin gland adenocarcinoma includes adenocarcinoma of skin appendage origin and metastatic adenocarcinoma. These tumors typically do not involve the Bartholin gland and the tumor type may not be consistent with a primary tumor of Bartholin gland.

Squamous cell carcinomas arising in the Bartholin gland have the same microscopic appearance as those arising elsewhere in the vulva. These tumors are typically immunoreactive for CEA.[182]

Adenoid cystic carcinomas arising in the Bartholin gland are similar to those occurring in salivary glands, the upper respiratory tract, and skin. They are composed of uniform, small cells arranged in cords and nests with a cribriform pattern. Variable-sized cysts filled with an amphophilic or eosinophilic acellular basement membrane–like material also may be encountered (Fig. 3.36).[2,5,22] Keratin and S-100 antigen are detectable by immunohistochemical techniques.[181] The S-100 reactivity may demonstrate a myoepithelial cell element. Ultrastructural features include basement membrane–like material within the cysts.[154]

The differential diagnosis of adenoid cystic carcinoma includes adenocarcinoma, basal cell carcinoma, metastatic atypical carcinoid, and small cell carcinoma. Adenocarcinomas lack the uniform acinar arrangement and intraluminal basement membrane material of adenoid cystic carcinoma. Basal cell carcinomas are more solid and lack the

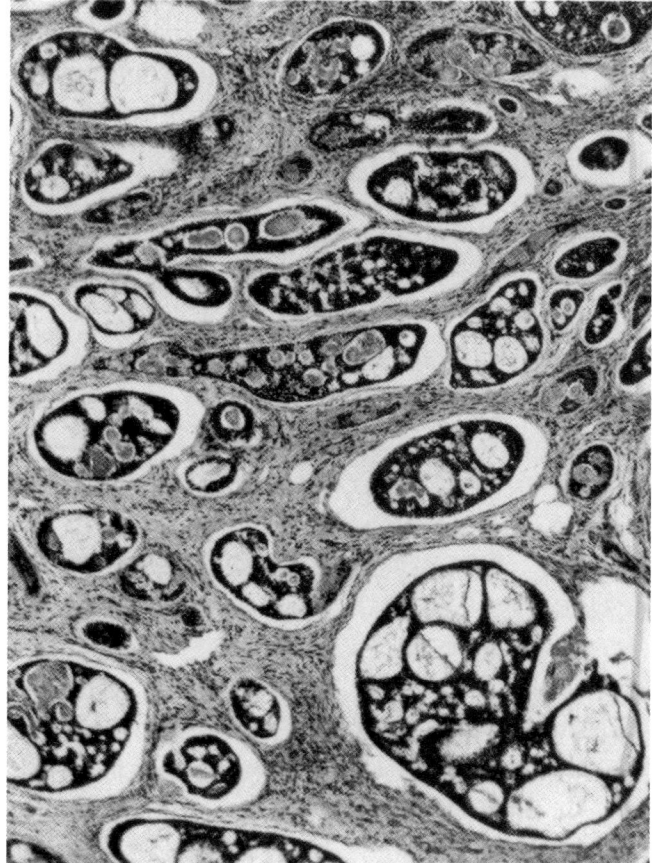

FIG. 3.36. Adenoid cystic carcinoma. The tumor is composed of relatively small hyperchromatic cells arranged in well-circumscribed masses within the stroma. Well-defined cystic spaces are evident in this tumor. (Courtesy of R.J. Kurman, M.D., Baltimore, MD.)

cystic spaces and the intracystic basement membrane–like material. Metastatic carcinoids and small cell carcinomas are more solid, have fewer lumens, contain argyrophil cells, and stain for neuron-specific enolase in most cases. Carcinoids almost always react with antibodies against chromogranin and other neuroendocrine markers.

Adenosquamous carcinoma of the Bartholin gland contain a mixture of squamous cells identified by keratin formation and intracellular bridges and glandular cells that typically contain mucin.[140,260]

Transitional cell carcinoma arising in the Bartholin gland is composed of uniform polyhedral or rounded epithelial cells often lining broad papillary fronds. Rare areas of glandular or squamous differentiation may be found. The differential diagnosis includes poorly differentiated squamous cell carcinoma and adenocarcinoma. If more than rare foci contain glands or show keratinization, the tumor is of mixed cell type and should be so designated with a listing of the different tumor types.

CLINICAL BEHAVIOR AND TREATMENT

The primary treatment for a Bartholin gland carcinoma is wide excision to the fascia, radical hemivulvectomy, or total vulvectomy. Ipsilateral or bilateral inguinal–femoral lymph node dissection is necessary, regardless of the type of primary excision.[53,159,272] Adjunctive radiation therapy to the vulva and regional lymph nodes also has been advocated.[53]

Approximately 20% of carcinomas of the Bartholin gland are associated with metastases to the inguinal–femoral lymph nodes. The overall 5-year survival of patients with Bartholin gland carcinomas is approximately 50% when the groin nodes are free of tumor, but decreases to 18% when two or more nodes are involved.[43,159,272] If the groin nodes are involved there is a 20% probability that pelvic lymph node metastasis also will be present, but if the groin nodes are free of metastasis, there is essentially no risk of pelvic node metastasis.[43]

Therapy for adenoid cystic carcinoma of the Bartholin gland is wide local excision with ipsilateral inguinal–femoral lymphadenectomy.[54] There is sufficient evidence to state that survival is better with adenoid carcinoma than with other forms of carcinoma of the Bartholin gland.

The treatment of vulvar adenosquamous carcinoma is similar to that of squamous cell carcinoma.[260] Adenosquamous carcinomas have a poorer prognosis than squamous cell carcinomas. The poorer prognosis is related in part to the higher frequency of lymph node metastasis.

Breast Carcinoma and Other Tumors Arising in Ectopic Mammary-like Tissue

Both benign and malignant tumors, as well as fibrocystic disease, have been described within the ectopic breast tissue.[46] Only a few cases of adenocarcinoma of ectopic vulvar breast tissue have been reported.[46,101,232] These tumors have histopathological features identical to those of breast adenocarcinomas and have been associated with breast adenocarcinoma.[101] Most of them are infiltrating ductal carcinomas. In some cases an intraductal carcinoma component has been identified. In one case, an intraductal carcinoma of mammary type was found arising in a papillary hidradenoma of the vulva.[196] It now appears that hidradenomas may arise from mammary-like anogenital glands.[262] Metastasis to inguinal lymph nodes from adenocarcinoma arising in vulvar ectopic breast tissue has been observed.[46] These adenocarcinomas contain secretory material similar to that of breast adenocarcinomas, including α-lactalbumin and milk fat globulin protein, and also may contain estrogen and progesterone receptors as well.[46,232] Cystosarcoma phyllodes arising in ectopic vulvar breast tissue also has been described.[174]

Metastatic carcinoma may be difficult to exclude, but if breast tissue or ductal in situ carcinoma is also evident, the lesion is a primary carcinoma of ectopic breast tissue. Unlike carcinomas arising in ectopic breast tissue, metastatic carcinomas to the vulva are not associated with adjacent breast tissue and usually are larger.[7,166]

The development of a malignant tumor within ectopic breast tissue requires a radical surgical operation: either total vulvectomy or radical wide local excision and inguinal–femoral lymphadenectomy.

Carcinomas of Sweat Gland Origin

Carcinomas of vulvar sweat gland origin are rare, comprising less than 1% of all vulvar carcinomas.[273] Presenting symptoms usually are delayed until the formation of a painless vulvar mass.[174] In addition to undifferentiated sweat gland adenocarcinomas, ductal eccrine carcinoma, eccrine porocarcinoma, and eccrine hidradenocarcinoma have been reported.[273] Apocrine adenocarcinoma has been described with vulvar Paget disease.[174] Adenocarcinoma resembling breast adenocarcinoma has been described that may have arisen from skin adnexa. In addition, ductal eccrine adenocarcinoma, eccrine porocarcinoma, and clear cell hidradenocarcinoma of the vulva have been reported.[67,273] A number of vulvar apocrine carcinomas have been associated with vulvar Paget disease.[174] Apocrine carcinoma is composed of tumor cells with the distinctive eosinophilic granular cytoplasm of the cells of origin, and may be associated with apocrine decapitation-type secretion. The tumor may have solid, glandular, or papillary areas. Nuclear pleomorphism and hyperchromasia are present.

Other Adenocarcinomas

Rare adenocarcinomas of the vulva may arise from Skene glands[249] or ectopic cloacal tissue.[253]

Malignant Mesenchymal Tumors

Malignant mesenchymal tumors are relatively rare neoplasms within the vulva and are generally encountered more commonly in other sites.[70] Most sarcomas arise from the labia majora, and a wide age range (6–64 years) is noted.[63,71,162] The clinical course is unpredictable and is only somewhat dependent on the histological type. The following discussion of these tumors is applicable to the vulva; however, the reader is referred to the referenced articles or comprehensive texts on soft tissue tumors for a more detailed discussion of these neoplasms. Table 3.7 summarizes some of the differential diagnostic features of myxoid soft tissue tumors that may occur in the vulva.

Leiomyosarcoma

Leiomyosarcoma is the most common sarcoma involving the vulva.[63] In one series of 32 patients with vulvar leiomyosarcoma the mean age of presentation was 35 years, with a range from 18 to 66 years of age. All patients presented with a mass in the vulva.[246] The tumor may arise in the labium majus, Bartholin gland area, the clitoris, and the labium minus in decreasing order of frequency. The tumors often are 5 cm in diameter or larger when first detected. Local pain and an enlarging mass are the most common presenting symptoms.[189,246]

Leiomyosarcoma is composed of interlacing smooth muscle cells that, when sectioned on long axis, have a perinuclear clear area, or halo, that may be of diagnostic value (Fig. 3.37). Epithelioid leiomyosarcomas also have been described in this site.[246] Leiomyosarcomas generally are larger, have infiltrative margins, cellular atypia, and higher mitotic activity than leiomyomas; however, aggres-

Table 3.7. Differential histopathological features distinguishing tumors with myxoid change in the vulva

	In children	Cambium layer	Sheets of immature cells	Gland elements	Prominent vascularity	Atypical fibroblasts	Nuclear pleomorphism	Mitotic figures	Cross-striations straplike muscle cells
Fetal myxoid rhabdomyoma	−	−	−	−	−	−	−	−	+
Aggressive angiomyxoma	−	−	−	+	+	−	−	±	−
Embryonal rhabdomyosarcoma (sarcoma botyroides)	+	+	+	−	+	−	+	+	+
Benign pseudosarcomatous polyps	−	−	−	−	+	+	±	−	−
Vulvar polyps with myxoid stroma	−	−	−	−	−	+	±	−	−
Leiomyoma with myxoid change (in pregnancy)	−	−	−	−	−	−	±	±	−
Nodular (pseudosarcomatous) fasciitis	±	−	−	−	−	±	−	+	−

+, present, −, absent, ±, occasionally seen.

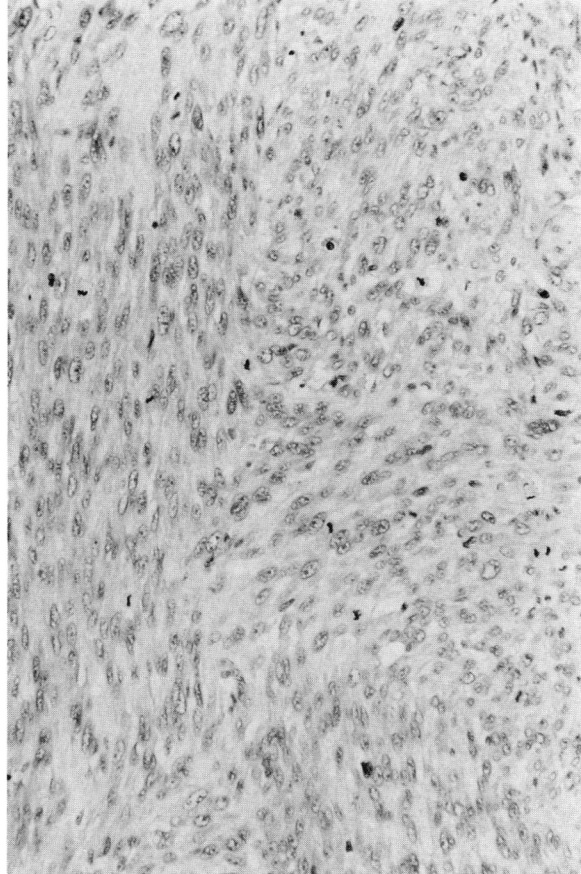

FIG. 3.37. **Leiomyosarcoma.** The tumor is composed of spindle-shaped cells arranged in an interwoven pattern. Minimal nuclear pleomorphism is present; however, many mitotic figures are evident.

sive behavior, with recurrence and metastasis, may prove the main distinguishing feature in a given case. Generally, leiomyosarcomas will have a mitotic count exceeding 10 mitoses per 10 high-power fields.[63] However, smooth muscle tumors with infiltrative margins and a mitotic rate greater than 5 per 10 high-power fields have a higher recurrence rate than tumors with well-circumscribed margins. In addition, tumors 5 cm or larger in diameter have a higher recurrence rate than those under 5 cm.[63] The diagnosis of leiomyosarcoma is straightforward when there is nuclear atypia, cellular pleomorphism, and there are 5 or more mitosis per 10 high-power fields.[246] When nuclear atypia is absent or slight, the diameter is more than 5 cm, the margin is infiltrative, and the mitotic count is 5 per 10 high-power fields or higher, the risk or recurrence is uncertain.

Leiomyosarcoma may recur locally, or metastasize, with pulmonary and hepatic metastasis being more common sites.[12,63,71] Wide extended local excision or partial or total excision is the usual initial approach provided.

Embryonal Rhabdomyosarcoma (Sarcoma Botyroides)

Embryonal rhabdomyosarcoma is a malignant tumor of striated muscle origin that grows in a distinctive polypoid manner. Within the vulva the tumor typically occurs in infants and is rare beyond 10 years of age, although it has been reported in young women.[55,71] Embryonal rhabdomyosarcoma has been described arising from the labia majora and hymenal area in infants. The tumor usually presents with bleeding, secondary to tumor ulceration.[52,243] In cases where the tumor involves the vagina as well as the labia minora, the tumor should be considered of vaginal origin.

These tumors grow in a polypoid manner, usually presenting as a solid mass if within the vulva, but may present as a fleshy, violet to skin colored, grape-like mass. On microscopic examination the tumor has a thin squamous epithelial surface overlying the edematous or myxomatous tumor (see Chapter 4, Diseases of the Vagina). Within the subepithelial area a denser cellular area forming the "cambium zone" is found that is composed of spindle or round cells. These tumor cells may be found within the overlying epithelium. Embryonal rhabdomyoblasts, which are round to spindle-shaped with prominent eosinophilic cytoplasm, and hyperchromatic, pleomorphic nuclei are frequently observed. Rhabdomyoblasts with cellular cross striation may be found being in approximately 15% of the cases.[177] Electron microscopy can be of value in identifying cross-striations within the cytoplasm of rhabdomyoblasts.[162] In one series actin filaments were found in all cases studied, although only 41% of the tumors contained both actin and myosin filaments.[177] In addition, spindle-shaped cells with small nuclei and dense nuclear chromatin are seen intermingled within the tumor cell population. The cytoplasm of the tumor cells usually are immunoreactive for myoglobin, desmin, actin, and vimentin. Although myoglobin is skeletal muscle specific, it is not always immunoreactive in this tumor.[56]

Local growth with late metastasis to regional nodes and distant sites is the usual pattern of spread. The tumors typically grow rapidly and metastasize early. In early tumors combination systemic chemotherapy, including vincristine, actinomycin, and cyclophosphamide (VAC), followed by local excision or radiation therapy, has provided a relatively high cure rate and preserves fertility.[114] Overall 5-year survival is reported from 25% to 50%, although significantly better survival is expected with early tumors and improved therapy.[52,55,114]

Dermatofibrosarcoma Protuberans

Dermatofibrosarcoma protuberans is an aggressive tumor of histiocytic origin that usually presents as a solitary, firm, brownish subcutaneous nodular or multinodular mass. It occurs most often in postmenopausal women.[25] Clinically this tumor may be confused with a large nevus.

Histologically, the tumor is characterized by intradermal growth, with a broad junction between the tumor and the adjacent epithelium, resulting in an elevated epithelial surface (Fig. 3.38). The tumor is densely cellular, with the cells arranged in a characteristic storiform pattern. The cells, unlike malignant fibrous histiocytoma, show little cytological atypia, rare mitosis, and no tumor giant cells.[162] In the base of the tumor an infiltrative growth pattern may be seen. Wide local excision, with a deep margin, is necessary because recurrence is not unusual, although metastasis is rare. Apparent transformation to malignant fibrous histiocytoma has been reported.[162]

Malignant Fibrous Histiocytoma

Malignant fibrous histiocytoma (MFH) arises from histiocytes that have undergone fibroblastic differentiation. It is rare on the vulva, but nonetheless is the second most common sarcoma in this site.[63] It usually presents as a large solitary mass in middle-aged women.[112,248]

Malignant fibrous histiocytoma is typically a solid tumor that is white to yellow on section. Areas of necrosis and focal hemorrhage may be seen. The tumor is typically deep and not immediately beneath the skin, as seen with dermatofibrosarcoma protuberans.

MFH is characterized by infiltrative growth and marked nuclear pleomorphism with giant cells and multinucleated cells. Cells with large nuclei containing multiple prominent nucleoli and abundant eosinophilic cytoplasm are admixed with smaller round to spindle-shaped cells with moderate nuclear pleomorphism. Mitotic figures usually are present and commonly atypical. The spindle cells may be arranged in a storiform pattern or in interlacing bundles (Fig. 3.39). The cells of MFH usually contain α-1-antichymotrypsin and/or α-1-antitrypsin, one or both of which can be identified in approximately 80% of cases.[172]

A number of subtypes of MFH have been described. These include an inflammatory type, which contains many

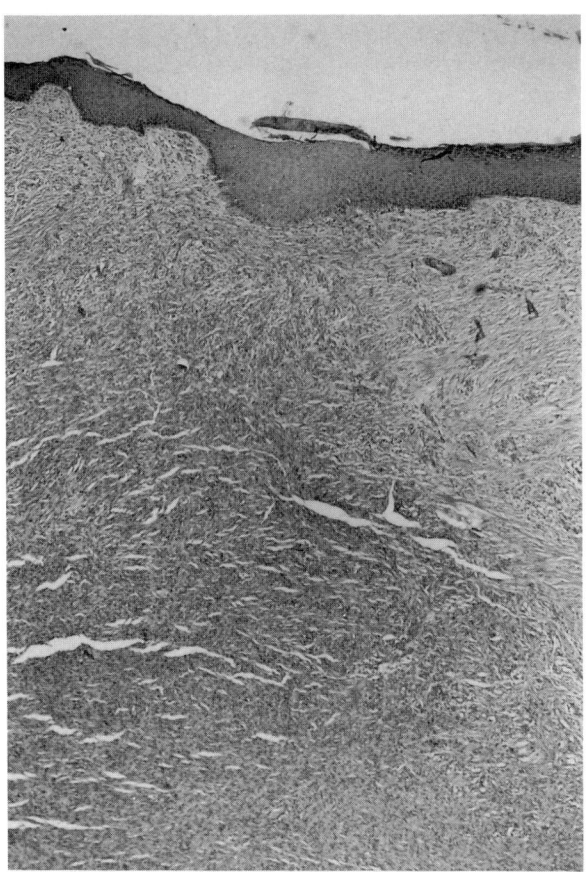

FIG. 3.38. **Dermatofibrosarcoma protuberans.** The tumor lies beneath the epithelium and is separated by a margin of normal-appearing dermis (Grentz zone) in the case. The tumor cells are arranged in a storiform pattern without prominent nuclear pleomorphism, hyperchromasia, or associated vascularity. The tumor characteristically extends deeper than the adjacent dermis. (Courtesy of David Dolson, MD, Philadelphia, PA.)

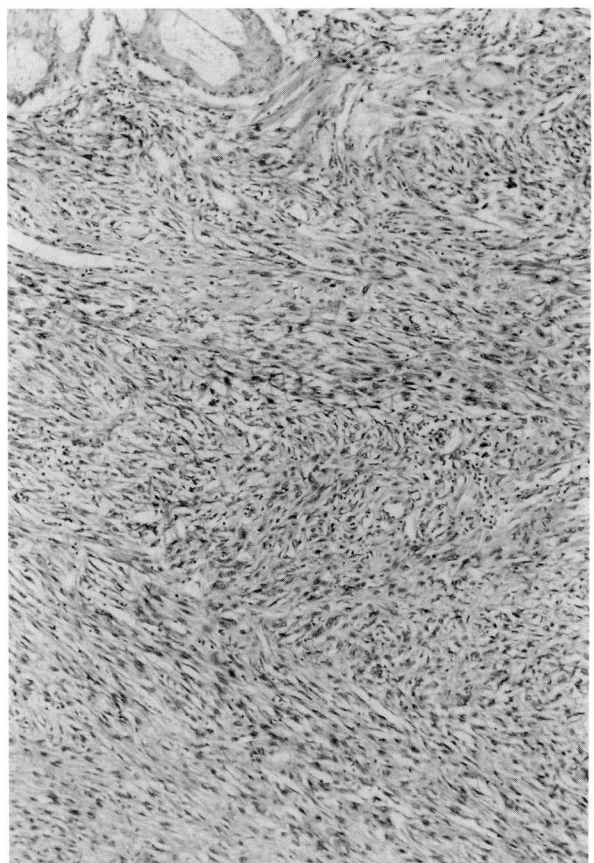

FIG. 3.39. **Malignant fibrous histiocytoma.** The tumor is deep to the sebaceous glands and is composed of markedly pleomorphic spindled cells arranged in an interdigitated "storiform" pattern.

acute inflammatory cells; a giant cell variant (giant cell tumor of soft parts), which contains giant cells with osteoclast-like features but no osteoid or bone; a myxoid variant containing a prominent hypocellular myxoid component; and an angiomatoid variant containing prominent blood vessels and blood-filled spaces.[155,269,270]

Characteristically, MFH is locally invasive. Involvement of the underlying fascia increases the risk of local or distant metastasis.[63,269] The treatment is wide local excision or radical vulvectomy. Lymphadenectomy is reserved for those cases with clinical evidence of regional node involvement. Postoperative radiotherapy is believed of value in reducing local recurrence. An insufficient number of cases have been described in the vulva to permit a definitive statement about the prognosis, but approximately half the patients reported have had recurrences or died of metastatic disease.

Epithelioid Sarcoma

The histogenesis of epithelioid sarcomas is obscure. The tumor is believed to arise primarily from the reticular dermis, although it may occur in deeper soft tissue.[105,259] These tumors typically occur in young individuals and have been observed presenting in the labia majora and in the subclitoral area.

Microscopically, the epithelioid sarcoma has a granuloma-like appearance with areas of necrosis. The tumor is composed of polygonal cells arranged in sheets and nests. The cells have abundant eosinophilic cytoplasm, giving some cells an epithelial appearance (Fig. 3.40). Cartilage and bone also may be found, which is thought to reflect metaplasia. There is moderate nuclear pleomorphism and frequent mitotic figures are generally noted. Epithelioid sarcomas contain keratin by immunoperoxidase study and have immunohistochemical findings essentially the same as found in malignant rhabdoid tumor.[44,197]

These tumors usually are indolent, although local recurrence with associated distant metastasis has been seen with unusual frequency compared with other sites, suggesting that vulvar epithelioid sarcoma acts more aggressively.[259] Vascular space invasion is associated with recurrence. Therapy is wide local extended excision with inguinal–femoral lymphadenectomy and local radiation therapy.[105]

Malignant Rhabdoid Tumor

Malignant rhabdoid tumor is of uncertain origin and is rare within the vulva. It has been reported presenting as a Bartholin mass in a young adult woman.[197] The tumor presents as a deep subcutaneous mass that may involve the deep dermis.

On microscopic examination the tumor has a multinodular, lobulated appearance with poorly defined margins. Areas of hemorrhage and vascularity may be present. The

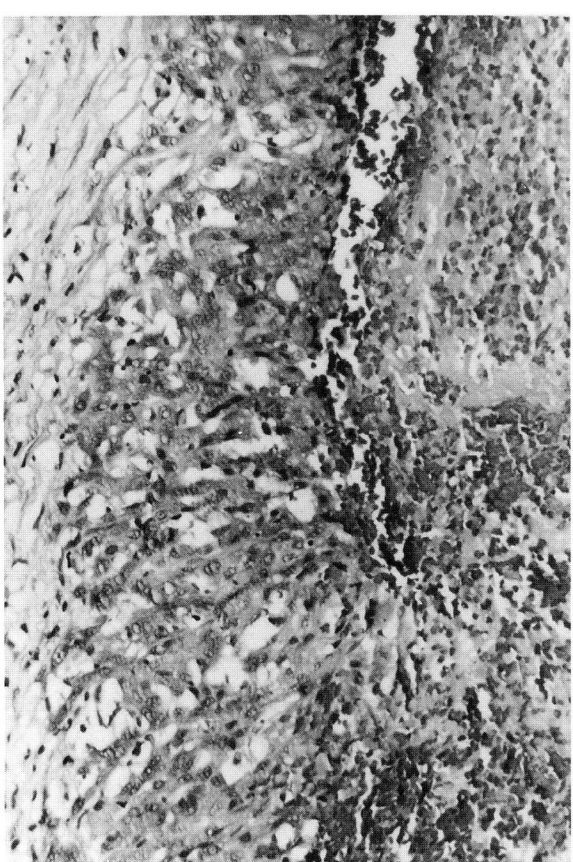

FIG. 3.40. **Epithelioid sarcoma.** The tumor is composed of relatively large epithelial-like cells with eosinophilic cytoplasm and pleomorphic nuclei. The cells are loosely cohesive and arranged in a nodular manner, resembling a granuloma. (Courtesy of Teresa Perrone, M.D., St. Louis, MO.)

tumor cells are large with pleomorphic nuclei that have vesicular chromatin and prominent nucleoli; mitosis is common (Fig. 3.41). The cytoplasm is eosinophilic, and because of their polygonal shape the cells may resemble squamous cells or rhabdomyoblasts. The cells have a distinctive eosinophilic cytoplasmic inclusion that has been demonstrated by electron microscopy to be composed of intermediate filaments. Because of the inclusion, and indenting of the nucleus by the inclusion, the cells may have a signet-ring appearance. Immunohistochemical studies demonstrate immunoreactivity to antibodies directed to cytokeratins and epithelial membrane antigen. The cells also may be immunoreactive to actin, CEA, and human milk fat globulin-2. The tumor cells typically are not immunoreactive to desmin or S-100 antigen. The primary differential diagnosis is epithelioid sarcoma, which essentially has the same immunoreactivity but lacks the lobulated growth pattern and the large cells with nuclear pleomorphism and distinctive cytoplasmic inclusions. In addition, malignant rhabdoid tumor lacks necrosis or the granulomatous appearance of epithelioid sarcoma.

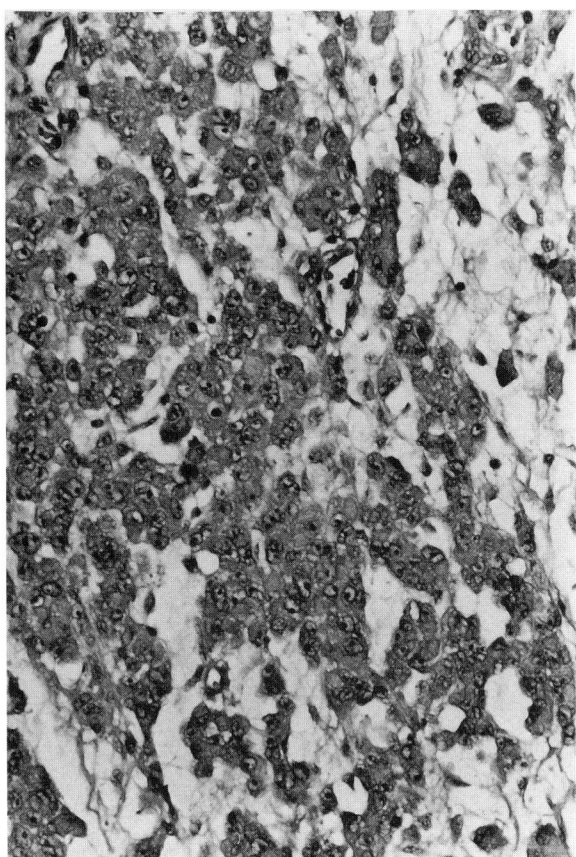

FIG. 3.41. Malignant rhabdoid tumor. The cells are arranged in nests and cords. The tumor cells are large with prominent eosinophilic cytoplasm and large nuclei with vesicular chromatin and prominent nuclei. The nuclei are eccentric within the cells, and in many cells are displaced by an eosinophilic cytoplasmic inclusion, which may indent the nucleus. (Courtesy of Teresa Perrone, M.D., St. Louis, MO.)

Malignant rhabdoid tumor is locally aggressive and may metastasize. Total vulvectomy, or wide local excision, with bilateral inguinal–femoral lymphadenectomy has been recommended, although there are few cases available for study.[197]

Aggressive Angiomyxoma

Although aggressive angiomyxoma is included in the category of malignant mesenchymal tumors, it is locally aggressive only and therefore is not a sarcoma. Aggressive angiomyxoma presents as a subcutaneous mass, and may present within the vulva as a mass within the Bartholin gland area. The tumor usually presents in adult women under 40 years of age. It may involve contiguous sites including the vagina and buttocks.[45]

On gross examination, the aggressive angiomyxoma has a soft myxoid appearance, and on cut section, small vessels may be visible. The tumor may appear to have well-defined

margins that may prove to be involved on microscopic examination (Fig. 3.42).

On microscopic examination aggressive angiomyxoma has a distinctive myxoid appearance with numerous muscular medium-sized vessels that are typically clustered. The tumor cells are spindle-shaped fibroblasts and myofibroblasts that lack significant nuclear pleomorphism or mitotic figures (Fig. 3.43). The tumor may contain epithelial elements that form glands and contain mucin. The neoplasm may invade fat and entrap neural elements. The spindle cells are immunoreactive to muscle actin, but are negative for S-100 antigen. The endothelial elements of the vessels are immunoreactive for Factor VIII; however, the spindle cell elements do not express this antigen. The primary differential diagnosis is myxoid MFH and angiomyofibroblastoma. MFH has a storiform pattern and is immunoreactive for α-1-antitrypsin and α-1-antichymotrypsin. Angiomyofibroblastoma is cellular and has well-defined tumor margins without prominent clustered muscular arterioles.

Aggressive angiomyxoma usually has a benign course; however, locally aggressive infiltrative growth and local recurrence are not uncommon. Metastasis has not been reported.

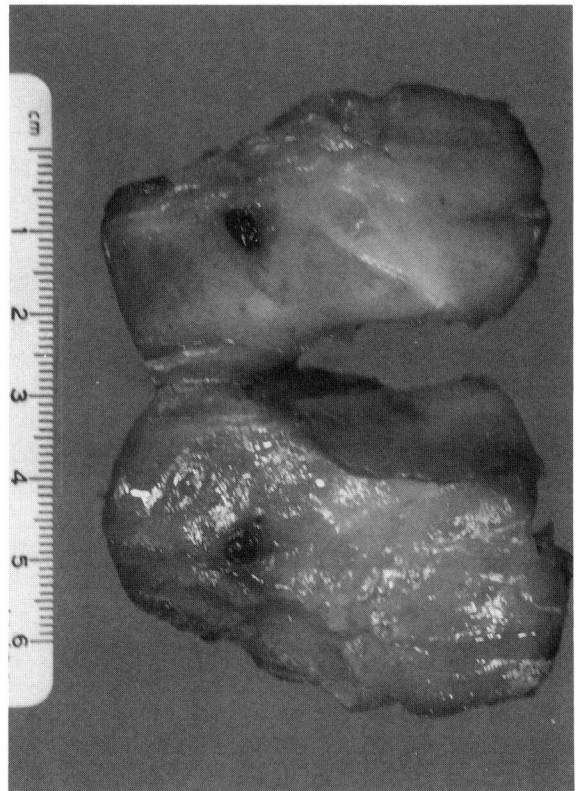

FIG. 3.42. Aggressive angiomyxoma. The tumor has a uniform gelatinous appearance with poorly defined margins. Within the translucent gelatinous-like mass, vessels of various sizes can be seen clustered within the tumor. (Courtesy of R.J. Kurman, M.D., Baltimore, MD.)

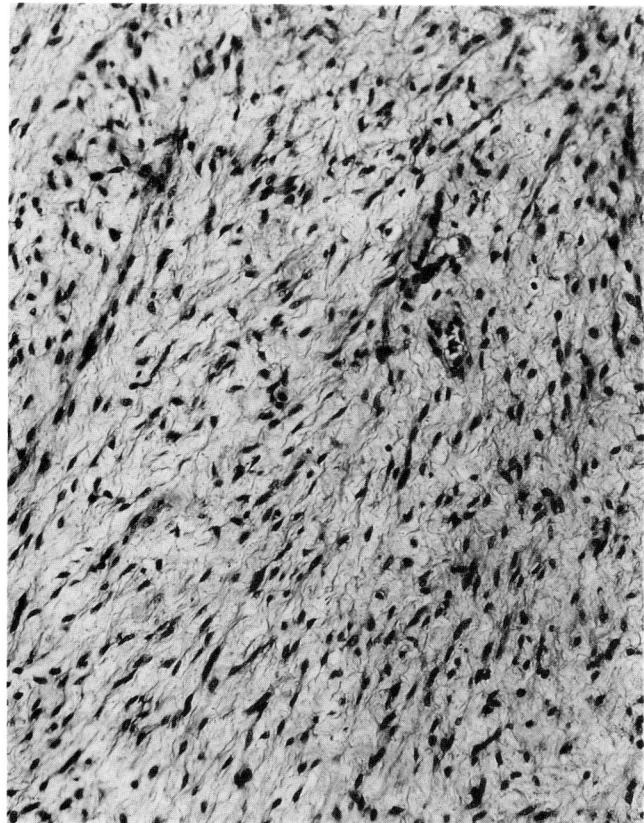

FIG. 3.43. Aggressive angiomyxoma. The stroma of the tumor is myxoid with vessels of various sizes, many of which are clustered. The cells within the stroma have nondiscernable cell borders and small spindle-shaped nuclei.

Recurrences as early as 1 year and as late as 14 years after surgery have been reported. Wide local excision without lymphadenectomy is the therapy of choice.[20,162,237]

Angiosarcoma and Lymphangiosarcoma

Primary angiosarcoma involving the vulva has been reported as a primary perianal tumor after radiation therapy to the pelvis.[63,165] Lymphangiosarcoma has been reported in the thigh after radiation therapy for vulvar carcinoma.[120]

On gross examination these tumors typically are solid and have poorly defined margins. Angiosarcomas usually are deep red. On microscopic examination the angiosarcoma is composed of complex slit-like vessels of irregular size lined by cells with large pleomorphic nuclei; mitotic activity usually is evident. In poorly differentiated areas, the tumor may be relatively solid. The tumor cells are typically immunoreactive for Factor VIII and *Ulex Europeaus* lectin antigen (UEA).

Hemangiopericytoma

Hemangiopericytoma has been reported occasionally as a primary tumor of the vulva. Metastasis to bone 14 years after therapy for vulvar hemangiopericytoma has been observed.[63,291] The tumor presents as a subcutaneous, partially cystic mass within the labia majus and fourchette.

Microscopically, the tumor is composed of small spindle-shaped pericytes with slightly eosinophilic cytoplasm and relatively large nuclei with minimal pleomorphism. Nucleoli may be evident. The mitotic count usually is low, with fewer than 4 mitotic figures per 10 high power fields. There is an associated complex capillary component, with the tumor cells each surrounded by a reticulin network peripheral to the vascular spaces. Necrosis or hemorrhage generally is not present within the tumor.[162] Although nuclear pleomorphism with numerous mitoses, high cellularity, and necrosis may characterize some aggressive lesions, benign hemangiopericytomas tend to be small, have a mitotic count of fewer than 4 per 10 high-power fields, and lack areas of necrosis or hemorrhage.[162]

The primary differential diagnosis includes monophasic synovial sarcoma, angiosarcoma, and metastatic endometrial stromal sarcoma. The pericytes of hemangiopericytoma are not immunoreactive for cytokeratins or S-100, as seen in synovial sarcoma, or Factor VIII, as seen in angiosarcoma.[162] Electron microscopy is of value to identify the subendothelial pericytes and distinguish this tumor from endometrial sarcoma. Differentiation from other malignant angiomatous tumors can be facilitated by the use of reticulum stains, which show the pericytes to be external to the reticulin network surrounding the individual blood vessels.[63,160,162] A malignant vulvar hemangiopericytoma has been reported to have metastasized to the femur. Treatment usually is wide local excision.[291]

Kaposi Sarcoma

Among the tumors of endothelial origin that may involve the vulva, Kaposi sarcoma is important because of its association with acquired immunodeficiency syndrome (AIDS). Although this tumor has been described within the vulva, it is rarely reported in this site.[6,162] Over time, the clinical presentation of the tumor evolves from a skin patch to a plaque to a nodular stage. Usually more than one skin lesion is present. There is debate as to whether this is a primary malignant neoplastic process or a reactive process to some infectious agent. HPV has been described associated with Kaposi sarcoma, the reproducibility and significance of which remains to be determined.[78]

When presenting as a patch, microscopic examination reveals the tumor within the dermis to have increased vascularity with irregular-shaped vascular spaces. Mononuclear cells are seen about the vascular spaces. In later stage lesions, more numerous vessels, which often are shaped irregularly, are associated with atypical spindle cells within the dermis (Fig. 3.44). In the advanced, or nodular stage, the tumor is a highly vascular spindle-cell neoplasm.

The differential diagnosis includes bacillary (epithelioid) angiomatosis, tumors of fibrohistiocytic origin, benign vascular tumors, scar, and a variety of other skin changes.[24] Bacillary angiomatosis contains the bacteria *Rochalimaea henselae*. The organism can be identified as bacterial rods using the Warthin–Starry stain or other immunohistochemical techniques in fresh or formalin-fixed tissue, employing bacteria-specific antibodies. The organism also may be cultured.[213] Tumors of fibrohistiocytic origin typi-cally are immunoreactive for α-1-antitrypsin or α-1-anti-chymotrypsin, have a storiform appearance, and lack irregular vascular spaces. Benign vascular tumors are well circumscribed and have well-defined vascular spaces. Scars are characterized by lack of skin appendages and a more fibrous and less vascular dermis. The gross appearance is also usually distinctive as compared with Kaposi sarcoma.

Alveolar Soft Part Sarcoma

Alveolar soft part sarcoma may arise within the vulva and has been reported as a primary tumor within the right labium minus in a 62-year-old woman.[231] These tumors usually occur in the deep tissue of the extremities of young adults.

The histopathology of the tumor is characterized by loosely arrayed polygonal cells with granular cytoplasm on delicate to thick fibrovascular and fibrocollagenous stalks. In some areas the tumor cells form alveolar-like structures. No true glands or secretory products are seen, although the tumor cells do protrude into the tumor luminal spaces. Mitoses are rare and the tumor tends to have a pushing border. Metastatic renal cell or clear cell tumors may mimic this tumor.[162]

These tumors have an indolent course, although metastasis to lymph nodes and distant sites may occur. Local recurrence is reported in 30–42% of cases and the reported survival ranges from 30% to 50% in nonvulvar sites.[231]

Recommended therapy is wide local excision with resection of the regional lymph nodes. Radical surgery does not appear to improve survival, but chemotherapy and/or immunotherapy may be of value.[231]

Malignant Schwannoma

Malignant schwannoma may arise within the labia minora or labia majora, as well as other sites within the vulva. The tumor characteristically occurs in women of reproductive age. Although this tumor occurs with higher frequency in individuals with von Recklinghausen neurofibromatosis, approximately half the reported cases within the vulva are unrelated to neurofibromatosis.[63,71,157,251]

The tumor presents as a subcutaneous mass and on gross examination is a relatively solid fibrous mass. A nerve trunk typically is associated with the tumor.

On microscopic examination the tumor is typically cellular with nuclear palisading. Mitotic figures are easily identified. Heterologous elements may be present including cartilage, striated muscle, and epithelial glandular elements. Approximately one-half of the cases are immunoreactive for S-100 antigen. Electron microscopy may be of value in establishing the diagnosis if branching, nontapered, cytoplasmic processes and microtubules can be identified.[162,247]

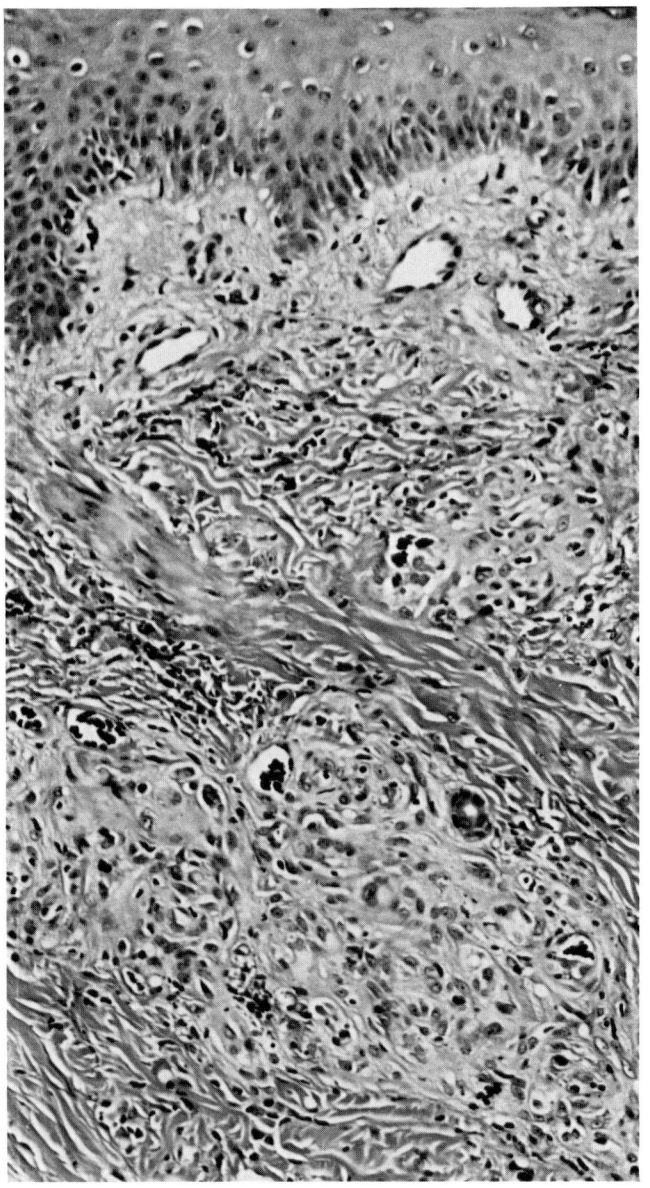

FIG. 3.44. Kaposi sarcoma. Many vessels, some of which are irregularly shaped, are seen within the dermis. Atypical spindle cells surround the vessels.

There are insufficient cases reported to determine the prognosis of this tumor within the vulva; however, local recurrence, as well as pulmonary metastasis, have been reported. Wide extended excision of the primary tumor without regional lymphadenectomy or radiation therapy has been advocated for tumors confined to the vulva.[251]

Granular Cell Tumor

A malignant granular cell tumor of the vulva has been described. This case was recognized primarily by local recurrence and infiltrative growth (see Chapter 2, Benign Diseases of the Vulva).[217]

Liposarcoma

Liposarcoma is a rare tumor within the vulva.[32,95] These tumors typically present as soft tissue tumors, without involvement of the overlying epithelium.

On microscopic examination the tumor may be well differentiated and composed of neoplastic adipocytes in a lobular pattern. The nuclei of the tumor usually are pleomorphic and atypical. The vessels within liposarcoma are arranged in a "chicken wire" pattern.[32]

Two subtypes of liposarcoma may present significant variations in gross and/or microscopic appearance. Myxoid liposarcoma grossly has a gelatinous appearance and on microscopic examination is composed of lipoblasts with relatively uniform nuclei within an extensively myxoid stroma. In contrast, the round cell liposarcoma is cellular and composed of relatively uniform neoplastic adipocytes with prominent eosinophilic cytoplasm. Liposarcoma may be immunoreactive for S-100 antigen, but this is not a uniform finding.

Langerhans Granulomatosis (Histiocytosis X), Including Eosinophilic Granuloma

Langerhans granulomatosis (histiocytosis X) is recognized to have three clinical types: Letterer–Siwe disease, Hand–Schuller–Christian disease (a chronic progressive form), and eosinophilic granuloma (a benign localized form).[96] Of these, eosinophilic granuloma has been well documented involving the vulva.[127,162,252,293] Eosinophilic granuloma may be localized entirely to the vulva, although most cases reported have involved other sites as well, including the pituitary gland, resulting in diabetes insipidis.[127]

The clinical presentation typically is a cutaneous pigmented papule or subcutaneous nodule. The surface of the mass may be ulcerated. The skin lesions typically present between 5 and 13 years of age, although the initial presentation may be in early adulthood.[96,293] Regional lymphadenopathy, secondary to nodal involvement, may occur; however, systemic symptoms are uncommon.

Microscopic examination reveals a cell population consisting predominantly of Langerhans-type cells intermixed with inflammatory cells. Eosinophils, granulocytes, lymphocytes, and plasma cells may all be present and an acute inflammatory cell infiltrate may be seen about the mass. Necrosis may be present within the tumor, but usually is localized. The Langerhans-type cells within the mass are immunoreactive for S-100 antigen.[182]

Localized Langerhans cell histiocytosis usually can be treated by radiation therapy. More advanced disease may require chemotherapy.

Malignant Melanoma

GENERAL FEATURES

Melanomas account for approximately 9% of all malignant tumors of the vulva, occurring predominantly in white women, with the highest frequency in the sixth and seventh decades; approximately one-third occur in women under 50 years of age. A vulvar mass is the most common presentation, although pruritus and bleeding also are frequent. In some cases, the melanoma has arisen from a pre-existing benign or atypical pigmented lesion.[48,135,179,180,286] Melanomas occur on the clitoris, labia minora, and labia majora with approximately equal frequency.[121] The mass usually is elevated slightly or nodular and may be pigmented or nonpigmented (Fig. 3.45). Pigmented epithelium may be seen adjacent to the mass and satellite nodules may be present. Clinically, malignant melanoma may resemble melanosis vulva, nevi, pigmented VIN or, if nonpigmented, squamous cell carcinoma.

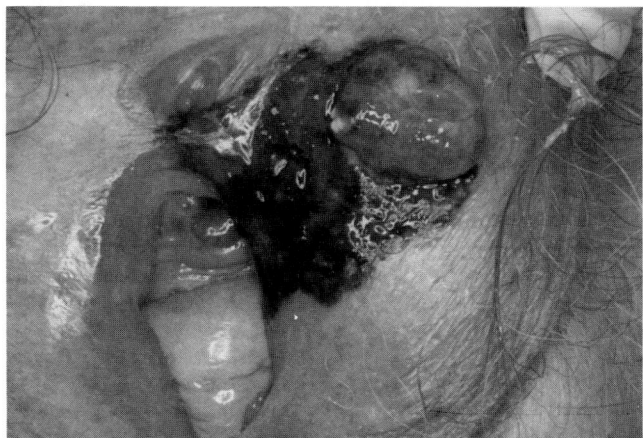

FIG. 3.45. Malignant melanoma. This represented a superficial spreading malignant melanoma with vertical growth within the field of a superficial tumor. (Courtesy of Linda S. Morgan, M.D., Gainesville, FL.)

MICROSCOPIC FINDINGS

Vulvar melanomas are of three distinct histopathologic types: superficial spreading melanoma (Fig. 3.46), nodular melanoma (Fig. 3.47), and acral lentiginous melanoma (Fig. 3.48).[18,175,204,245] The relative frequency of these types differs in various reports. Acral lentiginous melanoma was the most common type identified in one series, accounting for 10 of the 16 cases (63%); nodular melanoma accounted for 3 of 16 (18.6%).[18] In another series of 14 patients who died of vulvar melanoma, 65% had nodular melanoma, 21% had superficial spreading melanoma, and 14% had acral lentiginous melanoma.[139] Some of this variation may relate to differences in the criteria used to distinguish superficial spreading melanoma from nodular melanoma. Superficial spreading melanoma usually can be differentiated from nodular melanoma by evaluating the adjacent epithelium. If the radial growth of a melanoma or atypical melanocytes involves four or more adjacent rete ridges, the tumor should be classified as superficial spreading melanoma (Fig. 3.46).[199] Acral lentiginous melanomas have both vertical growth, as is seen in nodular melanoma, and radial growth, as is seen in superficial spreading melanoma. Atypical melanocytes usually can be identified within the epithelium adjacent to acral lentiginous and superficial spreading melanomas.

Malignant melanomas may consist predominantly of epithelioid, dendritic (nevoid), or spindle-cell types, either pure or mixed, within a given tumor. The cells may contain no melanin or variable amounts, ranging from minimal to very large quantities. The histopathological features vary considerably and certain features can be correlated with the subtype of the melanoma. Within the invasive area of a superficial spreading melanoma, the malignant melanocytic cells usually are large and have relatively uniform nuclei with prominent nucleoli. Similar melanocytic cells can be found within the adjacent epithelium, representing the radial growth phase of the tumor. Junctional melanocytes are numerous and distributed within the epithelium in a pagetoid distribution. In nodular melanomas an intraepithelial component may be present in addition to an invasive component, but without an adjacent radial growth phase. The cells of nodular melanomas may be polygonal (epithelioid) or spindle shaped. The polygonal cells contain abundant eosinophilic cytoplasm, large nuclei, and prominent nucleoli. The dendritic cells have tapering cytoplasmic extensions resembling nerve cells and show moderate nuclear pleomorphism. Spindle cells have smaller, oval nuclei and may be arranged in sheets or bundles.

Acral lentiginous melanomas of the vulva arise most commonly within the vestibule. They may show little or no pagetoid spread and are characterized by spindle cells within the junctional zone with extension into the adjacent dermis in a diffuse pattern (Fig. 3.48). The spindle cells are uniform with little nuclear pleomorphism. Within the subepithelial tissue, the tumor cells usually evoke a desmoplastic response.

Both the level of invasion of a malignant melanoma and its thickness have prognostic significance.[30] The Clark classification of cutaneous melanomas into five levels of inva-

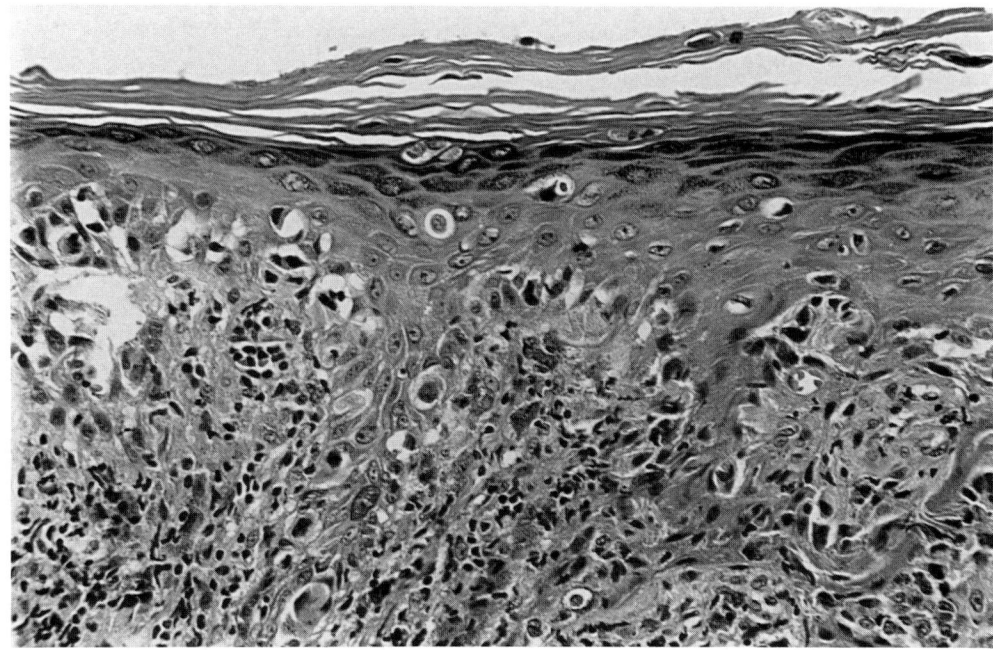

FIG. 3.46. Superficial spreading malignant melanoma. Pagetoid spread of the melanoma cells into the upper third of the epidermis is seen. Markedly atypical melanocytic cells are seen within the epithelial–stromal junctional area. No invasion is present. (Courtesy of K.K. Pierson, M.D., Gainesville, FL.)

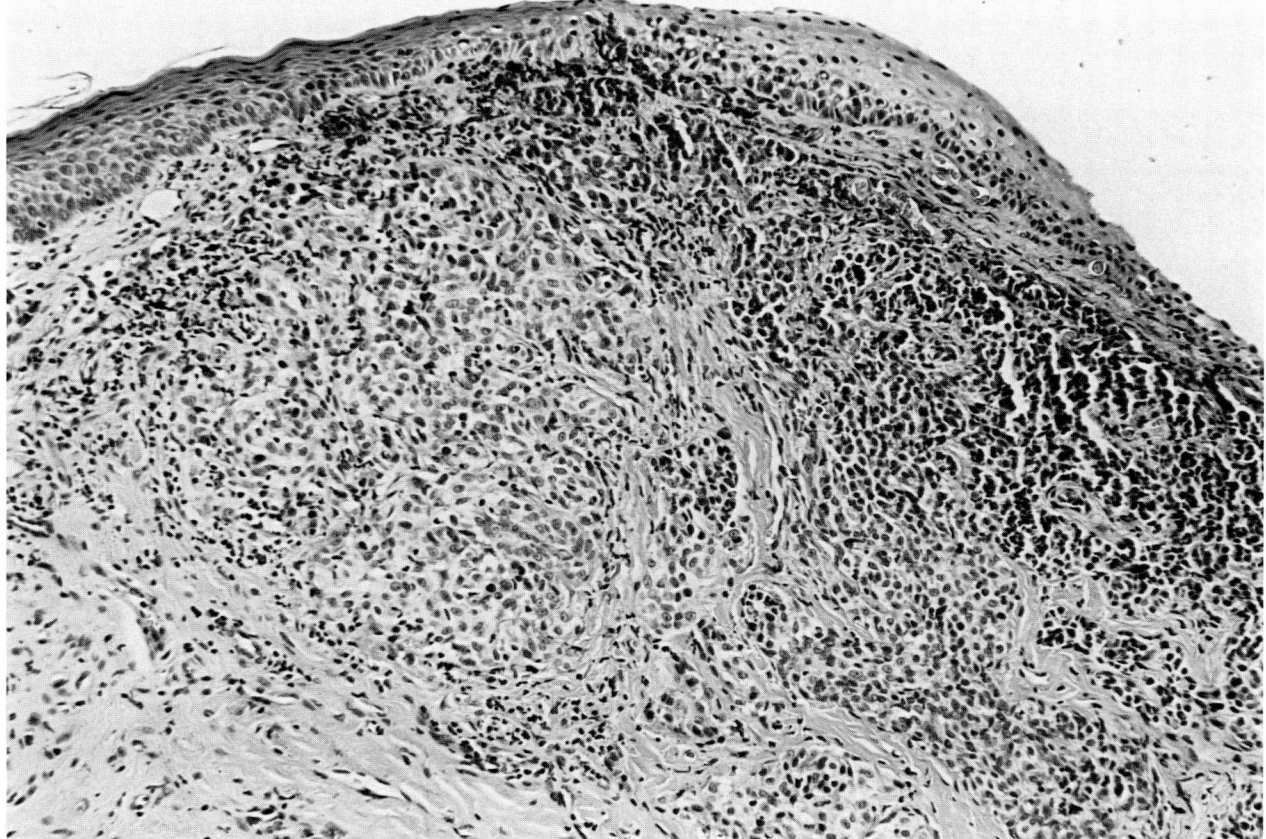

FIG. 3.47. **Nodular melanoma.** The nodular melanoma is entirely within the dermis, with an elevated, intact epithelium overlying the tumor. The melanoma cells are large and polygonal; arranged in nests, sheets, and cords within the dermis. (Courtesy of KK. Pierson, M.D., Gainesville, FL.)

sion is well accepted and can be applied to most melanomas of the vulva, with the exception of those arising within mucocutaneous areas. This system has been modified somewhat to accommodate vulvar melanomas (Fig. 3.49).[48] A level I melanoma is a melanoma in situ; level II melanoma extends into the superficial papillary dermis; level III melanoma fills and expands the papillary dermis; level IV melanoma invades the reticular dermis; level V melanoma invades beyond the reticular dermis into fat or other deeper tissues. Thickness measurements for cutaneous malignant melanomas as proposed by Breslow[30] require measurement from the deep border of the granular layer of the overlying epithelium to the deepest point of tumor invasion. If a lesion is less than 0.76 mm in thickness, it has little or no metastatic potential. Correlations between the thickness and the level of a vulvar melanoma can be made.[48] Level I melanomas have no measurable thickness. In one study, it was observed that level II melanomas had a thickness of 1 mm or less, level III melanomas had a thickness exceeding 1 mm up to 2 mm, and level IV melanomas had a thickness exceeding 2 mm but did not involve subcutaneous fat or adjacent deeper structures.[48]

DIFFERENTIAL DIAGNOSIS

Superficial spreading malignant melanoma must be distinguished from Paget disease, VIN, and dysplastic nevi.[215] The cells of Paget disease usually are larger than superficial spreading melanoma, have more cytoplasm, and are clustered with occasional gland formation. Some of the cells almost always contain mucin. Immunohistochemical studies to distinguish these include studies for CEA, S-100 protein, HMB-45, and cytokeratins. Paget disease is immunoreactive for CEA whereas melanomas are not (Table 3.2).[181,182] Melanomas usually are immunoreactive for S-100 protein and HMB-45, whereas the nonmelanocytic tumors are negative.[97] Melanin stains are not of value because Paget cells may contain melanin pigment, and amelanotic melanomas do not contain detectable melanin. Melanomas do not contain cytokeratins 54-dK, which are identified in Paget cells. Electron microscopy is of value in this differential diagnosis because melanoma cells contain melanosomes and other cytoplasmic ultrastructural features that are not present in Paget cells.

Squamous cell carcinomas with tumor giant cells, or those predominantly composed of spindle cells, may re-

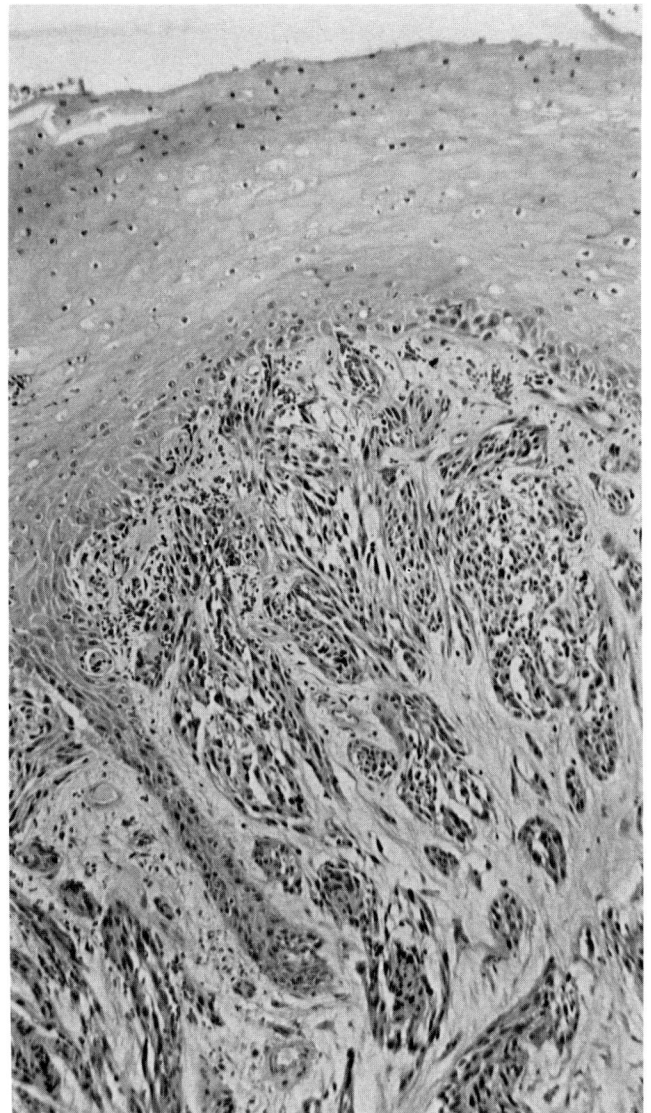

FIG. 3.48. Mucosal acral lentiginous melanoma. This histological variant of malignant melanoma is characterized by a radial component with a lentiginous pattern at the mucosal–stromal interface. In this case, spindle cells are seen within the submucosa near the junctional zone and within the deeper dermis with an associated desmoplastic response. The cytological uniformity is characteristic. No pagetoid spread is evident. This type of malignant melanoma usually is found within the vulvar vestibule. (Courtesy of KK. Pierson, M.D., Gainesville, FL.)

semble malignant melanoma. Typical squamous cell carcinoma may be identifiable adjacent to the giant-cell or spindle-cell component. Immunohistochemical studies are of value in the differential diagnosis.[277] Spindle-cell tumors of soft tissue origin, large cell lymphomas, and metastatic tumors including choriocarcinoma, may be included in the differential diagnosis. In these cases, review of the clinical history and physical and radiologic findings, as well as thorough sectioning of the submitted tissue and a panel of immu-

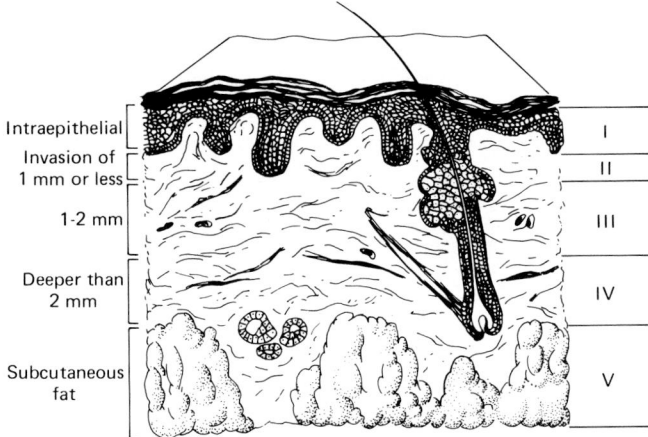

FIG. 3.49. Levels of vulvar melanoma invasion. (Reprinted by permission of The American College of Obstetricians and Gynecologists. Obstetrics and Gynecology 45: 638, 1975.)

noperoxidase tests, usually will provide sufficient evidence to permit an accurate diagnosis. The immunoperoxidase panel should include a spectrum of antibodies, including epithelial markers (e.g., AE1/3, 54-kD, EMA), hematopoietic markers (e.g., leukocyte common antigen [LCA]), muscle markers (e.g., desmin, actin), fibrohistiocytic markers (e.g., α-1-antitrypsin, α-1-antichymotrypsin), neural and neuroendocrine tumor markers (e.g., S-100, chromogranin, synaptophsin), common adenocarcinoma markers (e.g., CEA), and melanoma markers (e.g., HMB-45, S-100).

It should be emphasized that when faced with a poorly differentiated vulvar tumor that defies classification on initial microscopic examination, melanoma should be placed first on the list of the differential diagnosis.

CLINICAL BEHAVIOR AND TREATMENT

Factors that adversely influence survival include a tumor thickness exceeding 2 mm, Clark level V, a mitotic count exceeding $10/mm^2$, surface ulceration, and a minimal or absent inflammatory reaction.[139,255,286] Vascular space invasion and tumor necrosis also are associated with a poorer prognosis and are seen more commonly with large melanomas.[199] No recurrences of vulvar melanoma have been observed when the thickness was 0.75 mm or less.[198,286] An excellent prognosis has been associated with melanomas at Clark level II or less and those with a thickness of 1.49 mm or less. A tumor volume of less than $100 \ mm^3$ also correlates with an excellent prognosis.[17]

Vulvar melanomas may recur locally, or in the cervix, urethra, vagina, or rectum.[204] Distant metastasis may be the first sign of recurrence. Metastases to the lungs, brain, urinary bladder, bone marrow, and abdominal wall have all been observed.[139] The prognosis after recurrence is guarded, with a 5-year survival of only 5%.[204]

The usual treatment for vulvar melanomas with a thickness of 0.75 mm or less is wide local excision with a 2-cm circumferential and deep margin. Melanomas of greater thickness are treated by wide excision to the fascia or partial or total vulvectomy.[255] Depending on the size of the tumor, the surgical procedure may include bilateral inguinal lymphadenectomy.[286] Radical vulvectomy does not appear to improve survival when compared to radical local excision with bilateral groin lymphadenectomy.[235]

Other Malignant Tumors of the Vulva

Yolk Sac Tumor (Endodermal Sinus Tumor)

Endodermal sinus tumor (EST) is primarily a germ cell tumor occurring in ovary and testis (see Chapter 20, Germ Cell Tumors of the Ovary). Its occurrence in extragonadal sites is rare. In women, the vagina, pelvis, and vulva have been reported as primary sites.[148,219,261]

The histopathological features are well described and EST may present with one of several recognized patterns of growth. Characteristic Schiller–Duval bodies and eosinophilic hyaline droplets may be seen within the undifferentiated tumor (see Chapter 20). Confusion with adenocarcinoma may occur if these characteristic features are not seen. Immunoperoxidase studies to demonstrate the presence of alpha-fetoprotein (AFP) and an elevated serum level of AFP confirm the diagnosis.

Recommended therapy for vulvar EST is wide local excision and chemotherapy. Regional lymphadenectomy may be applicable in selected cases. Chemotherapy has markedly improved survival in patients with this tumor.

Primary Malignant Lymphoma

Malignant lymphoma may present as a destructive neoplasm, or as a mass that may mimic a Bartholin gland neoplasm, clitoral enlargement, or other tumor types.[203,256] Kappa-positive lymphoplasmacytic lymphoma, angiocentric small and large mixed-cell lymphoma, as well as plasmocytoma have been reported in the vulva.[73,256] The diagnosis of lymphoma is confirmed by immunoperoxidase studies for specific lymphocyte markers to identify the neoplastic cell population.

The differential diagnosis includes inflammatory conditions and dermatoses as well as lymphoepithelioma-like carcinoma. Dermatoses and benign inflammatory processes, unlike lymphomas, contain mixed populations of lymphocytes and other inflammatory cells. Lymphoepithelioma-like carcinomas contain epithelial cells that express high molecular weight cytokeratins and lack evidence of a monoclonal lymphocytic population.[40] Large cell lymphomas, including Ki-1 lymphomas, may mimic poorly differentiated carcinoma and immunoperoxidase studies, including LCA; specific lymphocyte markers as well as epithelial markers are of value to distinguish these.

Appropriate aggressive chemotherapy is the treatment of choice for most lymphomas.[256]

Merkel Cell Tumor

Merkel cell tumor of the vulva is rare, and few cases have been reported.[49,51,122] These tumors typically present as an intradermal nodule or nodules with erythema of the overlying skin.[26,51,122] These tumors may be associated with VIN or squamous cell carcinoma.[26,244]

Three distinctive histopathological types of Merkel cell tumor are recognized, namely the trabecular or carcinoid-like type, the intermediate cell type, and the small cell or oat cell–like type. The histopathological features are that of a poorly differentiated neoplasm composed of diffuse, unorganized population of relatively small, uniform, hyperchromatic cells usually without prominent nucleoli. Immunocytochemistry demonstrates a distinctive perinuclear cytoplasmic dot employing cytokeratin-specific antibodies. Neuronspecific enolase (NSE) usually is immunoreactive, although chromogranin may be negative. Electron microscopy is of value in identifying neurosecretory granules.

Merkel cell tumors are clinically very aggressive with regional node metastasis and subsequent widespread metastasis often occurring within a year of diagnosis. Therapy includes wide local excision with regional lymphadenectomy, local radiation therapy, and chemotherapy.[49]

Metastatic Tumors

Metastatic tumors comprise approximately 8% of all tumors of the vulva. The metastases were identified concurrent with the diagnosis of the primary tumor in 27% of cases in one series.[65] Tumors of the genital tract are common sites of the primary tumor with squamous carcinoma of the cervix being the most frequent tumor metastatic to the vulva followed by carcinomas of the endometrium and ovary.[65] Other common primary tumor sites include the bladder and urethra.[65,170] Other primary tumors that have metastasized to the vulva include carcinoma of the vagina, breast, kidney, melanoma, stomach, gestational choriocarcinoma, lung, and neuroblastoma.[65,170,199,206,210] Malignant lymphomas also may metastasize to the vulva[77] and Bartholin gland.[203,292] The vulva may be involved by direct extension of tumors arising in the vagina, urethra, bladder, or rectum.

Metastatic tumors typically involve the dermis and overlying epithelium and consequently are often associated with ulceration.[65]

Patients with metastatic carcinoma to the vulva generally have a poor prognosis. Treatment is primarily palliative and radical surgical approaches are not indicated.

Tumors of the Urethra

Urethral Carcinoma

Urethral carcinoma constitutes less than 1% of malignancies affecting the female genitalia and occurs almost exclusively in the elderly age group.[99,138] Urethral bleeding, frequency, and dysuria are the most frequent presenting complaints.[161,257,268] Tumors in the distal urethra usually give rise to symptoms early in their course.[8]

The vast majority of these tumors arise in the distal urethra and are squamous cell carcinomas.[99,161,169] Squamous cell carcinomas and transitional cell carcinomas may be papillary, forming papillomas or papillary carcinomas, or nonpapillary, presenting as carcinoma in situ of urothelial or squamous type, or as solid high-grade urothelial carcinomas or squamous cell carcinomas. Transitional cell carcinomas may be seen in the distal as well as proximal urethra and have been described arising within a urethral diverticulum. Adenocarcinomas of the urethra are relatively rare, accounting for approximately 10% of all primary urethral carcinomas.[171] They occur in the proximal urethra as well as within urethral diverticuli.[80,195,216] Primary adenocarcinoma arising in Skene glands also have been reported.[249] Histopathological types of adenocarcinoma include columnar/mucinous, clear cell carcinoma, and colloid types.[163,171,290] The growth pattern may be papillary or glandular. Pagetoid carcinomatous involvement of the distal urethral epithelium may be associated with urothelial carcinoma of the bladder. Both urethral squamous carcinomas and adenocarcinomas are immunoreactive for CEA.[182] Periurethral glands are immunoreactive for prostate-specific antigen (PSA), which is expected in that they are homologous to the male prostate. It would be anticipated that tumors arising from these glands would be PSA immunoreactive. Although a staging system for tumors of the urethra has been proposed, no uniformly accepted staging system currently exists.[99,292]

The prognosis related to urethral carcinoma is relatively poor, with a 5-year overall survival with anterior urethral tumors being 51%, and with posterior tumors or entire urethral involvement being only 6%. The overall survival has been reported from 22% to 27%, with a 5-year disease-free survival of only 27%.[99,292] Survival in urethral carcinoma is influenced by the fact that 20–50% of women with urethral carcinoma will have metastasis to superficial and/or deep pelvic nodes when first seen.[99,161] Improved and individualized surgical and radiotherapy techniques may substantially increase survival.[268]

Other Malignant Tumors of the Urethra

Lymphoma, melanoma, and sarcoma have all been reported arising within the urethra.[216,292]

References

1. Abdul-Karim FW, Kida M, Wentz WB, et al (1990) Bone metastasis from gynecologic carcinomas: A clinicopathologic study. Gynecol Oncol 39: 108–114
2. Abell MR (1963) Adenocystic (pseudoadenomatous) basal cell carcinoma of vestibular glands of vulva. Am J Obstet Gynecol 86: 470–482
3. Abell MR (1965) Intraepithelial carcinoma of epidermis and mucosa of vulvar and perineum. Surg Clin North Am 45: 1170
4. Ackerman LV (1948) Verrucous carcinoma of the oral cavity. Surgery 23: 670–678
5. Addison A, Parker RT (1977) Adenoid cystic carcinoma of Bartholin's gland. Gynecol Oncol 5: 196
6. Agarossi A, Vago L, Lazzarin A, et al (1991) Vulvar Kaposi's sarcoma. A case report (letter) Ann Oncol 2: 609–610
7. Ahmed W, Beasley WH (1979) Carcinoma of stomach with a metastasis in the clitoris. J Pak Med Assoc 29: 62–63
8. Ampil FL (1985) Primary malignant neoplasm of the female urethra. Obstet Gynecol 66: 799
9. Andreasson B, Bock JE (1985) Intraepithelial neoplasia in the vulvar region. Gynecol Oncol 21: 300
10. Andreasson B, Nyboe J (1985) Predictive factors with reference to low risk of metastases in squamous carcinoma of the vulvar region. Gynecol Oncol 21: 196
11. Andreasson B, Bock JE, Strom KV, Visfeldt J (1983) Verrucous carcinoma of the vulvar region. Acta Obstet Gynecol 62: 183
12. Audet-LaPointe P, Paquin F, Geurard MJ, Charbonneau A, Methot F, Morand G (1980) Leiomyosarcoma of the vulva. Gynecol Oncol 10: 350–355
13. Auger M, Colgan TJ (1990) Detection of metastatic vulvar and cervical squamous carcinoma in regional lymph nodes by use of a polyclonal keratin antibody. Int J Gynecol Pathol 9: 337–342
14. Bacchi CE, Goldfogel GA, Greer BE, Gown AM (1992) Paget's disease and melanoma of the vulva. Use of a panel of monoclonal antibodies to identify cell type and to microscopically define adequacy of surgical margins. Gynecol Oncol 46: 216–221
15. Barnes AE, Crissman JD, Schellhas HF, Azoury RS (1980) Microinvasive carcinoma of the vulva: A clinicopathologic evaluation. Obstet Gynecol 56:234
16. Beecham CT (1976) Paget's disease of the vulva. Obstet Gynecol 47: 61
17. Beller U, Demopoulos RI, Beckman EM (1986) Vulvovaginal melanoma. A clinicopathologic study. J Reprod Med 31: 315–319
18. Benda JA, Platz CE, Anderson B (1986) Malignant melanoma of the vulva: a clinical-pathologic review of 16 cases. Int J Gynecol Pathol 5: 202–216
19. Benedet JL, Wilson PS, Matisic J (1991) Epidermal thickness and skin appendage involvement in vulvar intraepithelial neoplasia. J Reprod Med 36: 608–612

20. Bëgin LR, Clement PB, Kirk ME, Jothy S, McCaughey WT, Ferenczy A (1985) Aggressive angiomyxoma of pelvic soft parts: a clinicopathologic study of nine cases. Hum Pathol 16:621–628

21. Bernstein SG, Kovacs BR, Townsend DE, Morrow CP (1983) Vulvar carcinoma in situ. Obstet Gynecol 61: 304

22. Bernstein SG, Voet RL, Lifshitz S, Buchsbaum HJ (1983) Adenoid cystic carcinoma of Bartholin's gland. Case report and review of the literature. Am J Obstet Gynecol 147: 385

23. Binder SW, Huang I, Fu YS, Hacker NF, Berek JS (1990) Risk factors for the development of lymph node metastasis in vulvar squamous cell carcinoma. Gynecol Oncol 37: 9–16

24. Blumenfeld W, Egbert BM, Sagebiel RW (1985) Differential diagnosis of Kaposi's sarcoma. Arch Pathol Lab Med 109: 123

25. Bock JE, Andreason B, Thorn A, Holck S (1985) Dermatofibrosarcoma protuberans of the vulva. Gynecol Oncol 20: 129

26. Bottles K, Lacey CG, Goldberg J, Lanner-Cusin K, Horn J, Miller TR (1984) Merkel cell carcinoma of the vulva. Obstet Gynecol 63: 61–65S

27. Boyce J, Fruchter RG, Kasambilides E, Nicastri AD, Sedlis A, Remy JC (1985) Prognostic Factors in carcinoma of the vulva. Gynecol Oncol 20: 364

28. Breen JL, Neubecker RD, Greenwald E, Gregori CA (1975) Basal cell carcinoma of the vulva. Obstet Gynecol 46: 122

29. Breen JL, Smith CI, Gregori CA (1978) Extramammary Paget's disease. Clin Obstet Gynecol 21: 1107

30. Breslow A (1975) Tumor thickness, level of invasion and node dissection in stage I cutaneous melanoma. Ann Surg 182:572–575

31. Brisigotti M, Moreno A, Murcia C, Matias-Guiu X, Prat J (1989) Verrucous carcinoma of the vulva. A clinicopathologic and immunohistochemical study of five cases. Int J Gynecol Pathol 8: 1–7

32. Brooks JJ, LiVolsi VA (1987) Liposarcoma presenting on the vulva. Am J Obstet Gynecol 156: 73–75

33. Bryson SCP, Colgan TJ, Vernon CP (1986) Invasive squamous cell carcinoma of the vulva: Delineation of high-risk group requiring adjuvant radiotherapy. J Reprod Med 31: 976

34. Buchler DA (1975) Multiple primaries and gynecologic malignancies. Am J Obstet Gynecol 123: 376

35. Buckley CH, Butler EG, Fox H (1984) Vulvar intraepithelial neoplasia and microinvasive carcinoma of the vulva. J Clin Pathol 37: 1201

36. Burke TW, Stringer CA, Gershenson DM, Edwards CL, Morris M, Wharton JT (1990) Radical wide excision and selective inguinal node dissection for squamous cell carcinoma of the vulva. Gynecol Oncol 38: 328–332

37. Buscema J, Stern JL, Woodruff JD (1981) Early invasive carcinoma of the vulva. Am J Obstet Gynecol 140: 563

38. Buscema J, Woodruff JD, Parmley TH, Genadry R (1980) Carcinoma in situ of the vulva. Obstet Gynecol 55:225

39. Caglar H, Tamer S, Hreshchyshyn MM (1982) Vulvar intraepithelial neoplasia. Obstet Gynecol 60: 346

40. Carr KA, Bulengo S, Weiss LM, Nickoloff BJ (1992) Lymphoepitheliomalike carcinoma of the skin. Am J Surg Pathol 16: 909–913

41. Caterson RJ, Furber J, Murray J, McCarthy W, Mahony JF, Shell AGR (1984) Carcinoma of the vulva in two young renal allograft recipients. Transplant Proc 16: 559

42. Chafe W, Richards A, Morgan LS, Wilkinson EJ (1988) Unrecognized invasive carcinoma in vulvar intraepithelial neoplasia (VIN). Gynecol Oncol 31:154–165

43. Chamlian DL, Taylor HB (1972) Primary carcinoma of Bartholin's gland. A report of 24 patients. J Obstet Gynecol 39: 489–494

44. Chase D, Enzinger F, Weiss SW (1984) Keratin in epithelioid sarcoma. An immunohistochemical study. Am J Surg Pathol 8: 435

45. Cheung TH, Chan MK, Chang A (1991) Aggressive angiomyxoma of the female perineum: case reports. Aust N Z J Obstet Gynaecol 31: 285–287

46. Cho D, Buscema J, Rosenshein NB, Woodruff JD (1985) Primary breast cancer of the vulva. Obstet Gynecol 66s: 79–81

47. Chu J, Tamimi HK, El M, Figge DC (1982) Stage I vulvar cancer: Criteria for microinvasion. Obstet Gynecol 59: 716

48. Chung AF, Woodruff JM, Lewis JL (1975) Malignant melanoma of the vulva: A report of 44 cases. Obstet Gynecol 45: 638–646

49. Cliby W, Soisson AP, Berchuck A, Clarke-Pearson DL (1991) Stage I small cell carcinoma of the vulva treated with vulvectomy, lymphadenectomy, and adjuvant chemotherapy. Cancer 67: 2415–2417

50. Copas P, Dyer M, Comas FV, Hall DJ (1982) Spindle cell carcinoma of the vulva. Diag Gynecol Obstet 4:235

51. Copeland LJ, Cleary K, Sneige N, Edwards CL (1985) Neuroendocrine (Merkel cell) carcinoma of the vulva: A case report and review of the literature. Gynecol Oncol 22:367–378

52. Copeland LJ, Gershenson DM, Saul PB, Sneige N, Stringer CA, Edwards CL (1985) Sarcoma botryoides of the female genital tract. Obstet Gynecol 66: 262

53. Copeland LJ, Sneige N, Gershenson DM, McGuffe VB, Abdul-Karim F, Rutledge FN (1986) Bartholin gland carcinoma. Obstet Gynecol 67: 794–801

54. Copeland LJ, Sneige N, Gershenson DM, Saul PB, Stringer CA, Sesk JC (1986) Adenoid cystic carcinoma of Bartholin's gland. Obstet Gynecol 67: 115–120

55. Copeland LJ, Sneige N, Stringer CA, Gershenson DM, Saul PB, Kavanagh JJ (1985) Alveolar rhabdomyosarcoma of the female genitalia. Cancer 56: 849

56. Corson JM, Pinkus GS (1981) Intracellular myoglobin: A specific marker for skeletal muscle differentiation in soft tissue sarcomas. An immunoperoxidase study. Am J Pathol 103: 384–389

57. Creasman WT, Gallager HS, Rutledge F (1975) Paget's disease of the vulva. Gynecol Oncol 3: 133

58. Crum CP, Braun LA, Shah KV, et al (1982) Vulvar intraepithelial neoplasia: Correlation of nuclear DNA content and the presence of a human papillomavirus (HPV) structural antigen. Cancer 49: 468

59. Crum CP (1992) Carcinoma of the vulva: Epidemiology and pathogenesis. Obstet Gynecol 79: 448–454

60. Crum CP, Liskow A, Petras P, Keng WC, Frick HC (1984) Vulvar intraepithelial neoplasia (severe atypia and carcinoma in situ). Cancer 54: 1429

61. Cruz-Jimenez PR, Abell MR (1975) Cutaneous basal cell carcinoma of the vulva. Obstet Gynecol 36: 1860–1868

62. Daling JR, Sherman KJ, Hislop TG, et al (1992) Cigarette smoking and the risk of anogenital cancer. Am J Epidemiol 135: 180–189

63. Davos I, Abell M (1976) Soft tissue sarcoma of the vulva. Gynecol Oncol 4: 70–86

64. Dean RE, Taylor ES, Weisbrod DM, Martin JW (1974) The treatment of premalignant and malignant lesions of the vulva. Am J Obstet Gynecol 119: 59

65. Dehner LP (1973) Metastatic and secondary tumors of the vulva. Obstet Gynecol 42: 47

66. Dennerstein GJ (1968) The cytology of the vulva. J Obstet Gynecol Br Commonwlth 75: 603–609

67. Di Bonito L, Patriarca S, Falconieri G (1992) Aggressive "breast-like" adenocarcinoma of vulva. Pathol Res Pract 188: 211–214

68. Dinh TV, Powell LC, Hanninan EV, Yang HL, Wirt DP, Yandall RB (1988) Simultaneously occurring condylomata acuminata, carcinoma in situ and verrucous carcinoma of the vulva and carcinoma in situ of the cervix in a young woman. J Reprod Med 33: 510–513

69. DiSaia P (1985) Management of superficially invasive vulvar carcinoma. Clin Obstet Gynecol 28: 196–203

70. DiSaia PJ, Creasman WT, Rich WM (1979) An alternate approach to early cancer of the vulva. Am J Obstet Gynecol 133: 825–832

71. Di Saia PJ, Rutledge F, Smith JP (1971) Sarcoma of the vulva. Obstet Gynecol 38:180

72. Donaldson ES, Powell DE, Hanson MB, Van Nagell JR (1981) Prognostic parameters in invasive vulvar cancer. Gynecol Oncol 11:184

73. Doss LL (1978) Simultaneous extramedullary plasmacytomas of the vagina and vulva. Cancer 41:2468

74. Downey GO, Okagaki T, Ostrow RS, Clark BA, Twiggs LB, Faras AF (1988) Condylomatous carcinoma of the vulva with special reference to human papillomavirus DNA. Obstet Gynecol 72: 68–73

75. Drew PA, Orlando CA, Wilkinson EJ, Hendricks JB (1994) Prognostic factors in carcinoma of the vulva by flow cytometric DNA analysis. (In manuscript)

76. Dvoretsky PM, Bonfiglio TA, Helmkamp BF, Ramsey G, Chuang C, Beecham JB (1989) The pathology of superficially invasive, thin vulvar squamous cell carcinoma. Int J Gynecol Pathol 3: 331

77. Egwuatu VE, Ejeckam GC, Okaro JM (1980) Burkitt's lymphoma of the vulva. Case report. Br J Obstet Gynecol 87: 827

78. Ensoli B, Nakamura S, Salahuddin SZ et al (1989) AIDS-Kaposi's sarcoma-derived cells express cytokines with autocrine and paracrine growth effects. Science 243: 223

79. Esquius J, Brisigotti M, Matas-Guiu X, Prat J (1991) Keratin expression in normal vulva non-neoplastic epithelial disorders, vulvar intraepithelial neoplasia, and invasive squamous cell carcinoma. Int J Gynecol Pathol 10: 341–355

80. Evans KJ, McCarthy MP, Sands JP (1981) Adenocarcinoma of a female urethral diverticulum: A case report and review of the literature. Urology 126: 124–126

81. Ewing TL (1991) Paget's disease of the vulva treated by combined surgery and laser. Gynecol Oncol 43: 137–140

81a. F.I.G.O. News (1989) Annual report on the results of treatment in gynecological cancer. Int J Gynaecol Obstet 28: 189

82. Fairey RN, MacKay PA, Benedet JL, Boyes DA, Turko M (1985) Radiation treatment of carcinoma of the vulva. Am J Obstet Gynecol 151: 591

83. Ferenczy A, Richart RM (1972) Ultrastructure of perianal Paget's disease. Cancer 29: 1141

84. Fetherston WC, Friedrich EG (1972) The origin and significance of vulvar Paget's disease. Obstet Gynecol 39: 735

85. Franklin EW (1972) Clinical staging of carcinoma of the vulva. Obstet Gynecol 40: 277

86. Franklin EW, Rutledge FD (1972) Epidemiology of epidermoid carcinoma of the vulva. Obstet Gynecol 39:165

87. Franklin EW, Rutledge FD (1971) Prognostic factors in epidermoid carcinoma of the vulva. Obstet Gynecol 37: 892

88. Friedrich EG Jr (1972) Reversible vulvar atypia. Obstet Gynecol 39: 173

89. Friedrich EG Jr, Burch K, Bahr JP (1979) The vulvar clinic: An eight year appraisal. Am J Obstet Gynecol 135: 1036

90. Friedrich EG Jr, Julian CC, Woodruff JD (1964) Acridine orange fluorescence in vulvar dysplasia. Am J Obstet Gynecol 90: 1281

91. Friedrich EG Jr, Wilkinson EJ, Steingraeber PH, Lewis DJ (1975) Paget's disease of the vulva and carcinoma of the breast. Obstet Gynecol 46: 130

92. Friedrich EG Jr, Wilkinson EJ, Fu YS (1980) Carcinoma in situ of the vulva: A continuing challenge. Am J Obstet Gynecol 136: 830

93. Fu YS, Reagan JW, Townsend DE, Kaufman RH, Richard RM, Wentz WB (1981) Nuclear DNA study of vulvar intraepithelial and invasive squamous neoplasms. Obstet Gynecol 57: 643

94. Ganjei P, Giraldo KA, Lampe B, Nadji M (1990) Vulvar Paget's disease. Is immunocytochemistry helpful in assessing the surgical margins? J Reprod Med 35: 1002–1004

95. Genton CY, Maroni ES (1987) Vulval liposarcoma. Arch Gynecol 240: 63–66

96. Gianotti F, Caputo R (1985) Histiocytic syndromes: A review. J Am Acad Dermatol 13: 383–404

97. Glasgow BJ, Wen DR, Al-Jitawi S, Cochran AJ (1987) Antibody to S-100 protein aids the separation of pagetoid melanoma from mammary and extramammary Paget's disease. J Cutan Pathol 14: 223–226

98. Gordon AN (1991) Current concepts in the treatment of invasive vulvar carcinoma. Clin Obstet Gynecol 34: 587–598

99. Grabstald H (1973) Proceedings: Tumors of the urethra in men and women. Cancer 32: 1236–1255

100. Gross G, Hagedorn M, Ikenberg H, et al (1985) Bowenoid papulosis. Arch Dermatol 121: 858

101. Guerry RL, Pratt-Thomas HR (1976) Carcinoma of supernumerary breast of vulva with bilateral mammary cancer. Cancer 38: 2570–2574

102. Gunn RA, Gallager HS (1980) Vulvar Paget's disease: A topographic study. Cancer 46: 590–594

103. Hacker NF, Berek JS, Lagasse LD, Nieberg RK, Leuchter

RS (1984) Individualization of treatment for stage I squamous cell vulvar carcinoma. Obstet Gynecol 63: 155

104. Hacker NF, Nieberg RK, Berek JS, et al (1983) Superficially invasive vulvar cancer with nodal metastases. Gynecol Oncol 15:65

105. Hall DJ, Grimes MM, Goplerud DR (1980) Epithelioid sarcoma of the vulva. Gynecol Oncol 9: 237–246

105a. Hart WR, Millman JB (1977) Progression of intraepithelial Paget's disease of the vulva to invasive carcinoma. Cancer 40: 2333

106. Hart WR, Norris HJ, Helwig EB (1975) Relation of lichen sclerosus et atrophicus of the vulva to development of carcinoma. Obstet Gynecol 45: 369

107. Hay DM, Cole FM (1970) Postgranulomatous epidermoid carcinoma of the vulva. Am J Obstet Gynecol 108: 479

108. Heaps JM, Fu YS, Montz FJ, Hacker NF, Berek JS (1990) Surgical-pathologic variables predictive of local recurrence in squamous cell carcinoma of the vulva. Gynecol Oncol 38: 309–314

109. Hendricks JB, Wilkinson EJ, Drew PA, Blaydes SM, Kubilis P, Munakata S (1994) Ki-67 expression in vulvar carcinoma. Int J Gynecol Pathol (in press)

110. Hendricks JB, Wilkinson EJ, Pharis PG, Sapi Z, Braylan RC (1993) Quantitative morphologic assessment of nuclei extracted from paraffin for DNA flow cytometry. Mod Pathol 6: 565

111. Helwig EB, Graham JH (1963) Anogenital (extra-mammary) Paget's disease. Cancer 16:387–403

112. Hensley GT, Friedrich EG (1973) Malignant fibroxanthoma: A sarcoma of the vulva. Am J Obstet Gynecol 116: 289–291

113. Henson D, Tarone R (1977) An epidemiologic study of cancer of the cervix, vagina, and vulva based on the Third National Cancer Survey in the United States. Am J Obstet Gynecol 129: 525

114. Hicks ML, Piver MS (1992) Conservative surgery plus adjuvant therapy for vulvovaginal rhabdomyosarcoma, diethylstilbestrol clear cell adenocarcinoma of the vagina, and unilateral germ cell tumors of the ovary. Obstet Gynecol Clin North Am 19: 219–233

115. Hilliard GD, Massey FM, O'Toole RV (1979) Vulvar neoplasia in the young. Am J Obstet Gynecol 135: 185

116. Hoffman JS, Kumar NB, Morley GW (1983) Microinvasive squamous carcinoma of the vulva: Search for a definition. Obstet Gynecol 61: 615

117. Hoffman JS, Kumar NB, Morley GW (1985) Prognostic significance of groin lymph node metastases in squamous carcinoma of the vulva. Obstet Gynecol 66: 402

118. Hoffman MS, Pinelli DM, Finan M, Roberts WS, Fiorica JV, Cavanagh D (1992) Laser vaporization for vulvar intraepithelial neoplasia III. J Reprod Med 37: 135–137

119. Homesley HD, Bundy BN, Sedlis A, et al (1991) Assessment of current International Federation of Gynecology and Obstetrics staging of vulvar carcinoma relative to prognostic factors for survival (a Gynecologic Oncology Group study). Am J Obstet Gynecol 164: 997–1003

120. Huey GR, Stehman FB, Roth LM, Ehrlich CE (1985) Lymphangiosarcoma of the edematous thigh after radiation therapy for carcinoma of the vulva. Gynecol Oncol 20: 394

121. Hulagu C, Erez S (1973) Juvenile melanoma of clitoris. J Obstet Gynaecol Br Commw 80: 89–91

122. Husseinzadeh N, Whesseler T, Newman N, Shbaro I, Ho P (1988) Neuroendocrine (Merkel Cell) carcinoma of the vulva. Gynecol Oncol 29: 105–112

123. Husseinzadeh N, Zaino R, Nahhas WA, Mortel R (1983) The significance of histologic findings in predicting nodal metastasis in invasive squamous cell carcinoma of the vulva. Gynecol Oncol 16: 105

124. Ikenberg H, Gissmann L, Gross G, Grussenford-Conen EI, Zur Hausen H (1983) Human papillomavirus type 16 related DNA in genital Bowen's disease and in Bowenoid papulosis. Int J Cancer 32: 563

125. Ilardi CF, Faro JC (1985) Localization of parathyroid hormone-like substance in squamous cell carcinomas. An immunoperoxidase study with ultrastructural localization. Arch Pathol Lab Med 109: 752

126. Imachi M, Tsukamoto N, Shigematsu T, Nakano H (1992) Cytologic diagnosis of primary adenocarcinoma of Bartholin's gland. A case report. Acta Cytol 36: 167–170

127. Issa PY, Salem PA, Brihi E, Azoury RS (1980) Eosinophilic granuloma with involvement of the female genitalia. Am J Obstet Gynecol 137: 608

128. Iversen T (1985) New approaches to treatment of squamous cell carcinoma of the vulva. Clin Obstet Gynecol 28: 204

129. Iversen T, Abeler V, Aalders J (1981) Individualized treatment of stage I carcinoma of the vulva. Obstet Gynecol 57: 85

130. Iversen T, Andreasson B, Bryson SCP, et al (1990) Surgical-procedure terminology for the vulva and vagina. A report of an International Society for the Study of Vulvar Disease Task Force. J Reprod Med 35: 1033–1034

131. Jacobs DM, Sandles LG, Leboit PE (1986) Sebaceous carcinoma arising from Bowen's disease of the vulva. Arch Dermatol 122: 1191–1193

132. Jafari K, Cartnick EN (1976) Microinvasive squamous cell carcinoma of the vulva. Gynecol Oncol 4: 158

133. Japaze H, Garcia-Bunuel R, Woodruff JD (1977) Primary vulvar neoplasia: A review of in situ and invasive carcinoma. Obstet Gynecol 49: 404

134. Japaze H, vanDinh T, Woodruff JD (1982) Verrucous carcinoma of the vulva: Study of 24 cases. Obstet Gynecol 60: 462

135. Jaramillo BA, Ganjei P, Averette HE, Sevin BU, Lovecchio JL (1985) Malignant melanoma of the vulva. Obstet Gynecol 66: 398

136. Jimerson GK, Merrill JA (1970) Multicentric squamous malignancy involving both cervix and vulva. Cancer 26: 150

137. Jobson VW, Homesley HD (1983) Treatment of vaginal intraepithelial neoplasia with the carbon dioxide laser. Obstet Gynecol 62: 90

138. Johnson DE, O'Connell JR (1983) Primary carcinoma of female urethra. Urology 21: 42

139. Johnson TL, Kumar NB, White CD, Morley GW (1986) Prognostic features of vulvar melanoma: A clinicopathologic analysis. Int J Gynecol Pathol 5: 110–118

140. Johnson WC, Helwig EB (1981) Adenoid squamous cell carcinoma. Cancer 19:1639

141. Jones RW, McLean MR (1986) Carcinoma in situ of the vulva: A review of 31 treated and 5 untreated cases. Obstet Gynecol 68: 499–503

142. Kabulski Z, Frankman O (1978) Histologic malignancy

grading in invasive squamous cell carcinoma of the vulva. Int J Obstet Gynecol 16: 233

143. Karasek J, Smetana K, Oehlert W, Konrad B (1970) The ultrastructure of Bowen's disease: Nuclear and nucleolar lesions. Cancer Res 30: 2791

144. Kelley JL III, Burke TW, Tornos C, et al (1992) Minimally invasive vulvar carcinoma: An indication for conservative surgical therapy. Gynecol Oncol 44: 240–244

145. Kluzak TR, Krause FT (1987) Condylomata, papillomas and verrucous carcinomas of the vulva and vagina. In: Wilkinson EJ, (ed.) Pathology of the vulva and vagina. New York: Churchill Livingstone, pp 49–77

146. Kneale BL (1984) Microinvasive cancer of the vulva: Report of the International Society for the Study of Vulvar Disease Task Force, VIIth Congress. J Reprod Med 29: 454

147. Kraus FT, Perez-Mesa C (1966) Verrucous carcinoma. Cancer 19: 26

148. Krishnamurthy SC, Sampat MB (1981) Endodermal sinus (yolk sac) tumor of the vulva in a pregnant female. Gynecol Oncol 11: 379

149. Krupp PJ, Lee FY, Batson HW, Allen PM, Collins JH (1973) Carcinoma of the vulva. Gynecol Oncol 1: 345

150. Krupp PJ, Lee FY, Bohm JW, Batson HW, Diem JE, Lemire JE (1975) Prognostic parameters and clinical staging criteria in epidermoid carcinoma of the vulva. Obstet Gynecol 46: 84

151. Kunscher A, Kanbour AI, David B (1978) Early vulvar carcinoma. Am J Obstet Gynecol 132: 599

152. Kurman RJ, Toki T, Schiffman MH (1993) Basaloid and warty carcinomas of the vulva. Distinctive types of squamous cell carcinoma frequently associated with HPV. Am J Surg Pathol 17: 133–145

153. Kurzl RG, Messerer D, Baltzer J, Lohe KJ, Zander J (1986) Vulvar Carcinoma: A clinical, histologic and morphometric study of 197 patients with squamous cell carcinoma of the vulva. J Reprod Med 31: 980

154. Kuzuya K, Matsuyama M, Nishi Y, Chihara T, Suchi T (1981) Ultrastructure of adenocarcinoma of Bartholin's gland. Cancer 48: 1392–1398

155. Kyriakos M, Kempson RL (1976) Inflammatory fibrous histiocytoma, an aggressive and lethal lesion. Cancer 37: 1584–1606

156. Lasser A, Cornorg JL, Morris JM (1974) Adenoid squamous cell carcinoma of the vulva. Cancer 33: 224

157. Lawrence WD, Shingleton HM (1978) Malignant schwannoma of the vulva: A light and electron microscopic study. Gynecol Oncol 6: 527–537

158. Leibowitch M, Neill S, Pelisse M, Moyal-Baracco M (1990) The epithelial changes associated with squamous cell carcinoma of the vulva. Br J Obstet Gynaecol 97: 1135–1139

159. Leuchter RS, Hacker NF, Voet RL, Berek JS, Townsend DE, Lagasse LD (1982) Primary carcinoma of the Bartholin gland: A report of 14 cases and review of the literature. Obstet Gynecol 60: 361–368

160. Lever WF, Schaumburg-Lever G (1990) Histopathology of the skin, 7th ed, Philadelphia, JB Lippincott

161. Levine RL (1980) Urethral cancer. Cancer 45: 1965

162. LiVolsi VA, Brooks JJ (1987) Soft tissue tumors of the vulva. In: Wilkinson EJ (ed) Contemporary issues in surgical pathology. Pathology of the Vulva and Vagina, vol 9. New York, Churchill Livingstone, p 209–238

163. Loo KT, Chan JKC (1992) Colloid adenocarcinoma of the urethra associated with mucosal in situ carcinoma. Arch Pathol Lab Med 116: 976–977

164. Mabuchi K, Bross DS, Kessler II (1985) Epidemiology of cancer of the vulva. A case control study. Cancer 55: 1843

165. Maddox JC, Evans HL (1981) Angiosarcoma of the skin and soft tissue. Cancer 48: 1907–1921

166. Mader MH, Friedrich EG Jr (1982) Vulvar metastasis of breast carcinoma. A case report. J Reprod Med 27: 169–171

167. Magrina JF, Webb MJ, Gaffey TA, Symmonds RE (1979) Stage I squamous cell cancer of the vulva. Am J Obstet Gynecol 134: 453

168. Malmstrom H, Janson H, Simonsen E, Stenson S, Stendahl U (1990) Prognostic factors in invasive squamous cell carcinoma of the vulva treated with surgery and irradiation. Acta Oncol 29: 915–919

169. Mayer R, Fowler Jr, Clayton M (1987) Localized urethral cancer in women. Cancer 60: 1548–1551

170. Mazur MT, Hsueh S, Gersell DJ (1984) Metastases to the female genital tract: Analysis of 325 cases. Cancer 53: 1978

171. Meis JM, Ayala AG, Johnson DE (1987) Adenocarcinoma of the urethra in women. A clinicopathologic study. Cancer 60: 1038–1052

172. Meister P, Natharth W (1981) Immunohistochemical characterization of histiocytic tumors. Diagn Histopathol 4: 79–87

173. Mene A, Buckley CH (1985) Involvement of the vulval skin appendages by intraepithelial neoplasia. Br J Obstet Gynecol 92: 634

174. Michael H, Roth LM (1987) Paget's disease, skin appendage tumors, and congenital and acquired cysts of the vulva. In: Wilkinson EJ (ed) Pathology of the vulva and vagina, vol 9. New York, Churchill Livingstone, pp 25–48

175. Mihm MC, Clark WH, From L (1971) The clinical diagnosis, classification and histogenetic concepts of the early stages of cutaneous malignant melanomas. N Eng J Med 284: 1078

176. Misas JE, Cold CJ, Hall FW (1991) Vulvar Paget disease: Fluorescein-aided visualization of margins. Obstet Gynecol 77: 156–159

177. Morales AR, Fine G, Horn RC Jr (1972) Rhabdomyosarcoma: An ultrastructural appraisal. Pathol Annu 7: 81–106

178. Morales AR, Gould EW, Nadji M (1985) Immunocytochemistry in tumor diagnosis. Boston, Martinus Nijhoff

179. Morgan L, Joslyn P, Chafe W, Ferguson K (1988) A report on 18 cases of primary malignant melanoma of the vulva. Colposcopy Gynecol Laser Surg 4: 161–170

180. Morrow CP, Rutledge FN (1972) Melanoma of the vulva. Obstet Gynecol 39: 745–752

181. Nadji M, Ganjei P (1987) The application of immunoperoxidase techniques in the evaluation of vulvar and vaginal disease. In: Wilkinson EJ (ed) Contemporary issues in surgical pathology. Pathology of the Vulva and Vagina, vol 9. New York, Churchill Livingstone, pp 239–248

182. Nadji M; Ganjei P, Penneys NS, Morales AR (1984) Im-

munohistochemistry of vulvar neoplasms: A brief review. Int J Gynecol Pathol 3: 41

183. Nadji M, Morales AR, Girtanner RE, Ziegels-Weissman J, Penneys NS (1982) Paget's disease of the skin: A unifying concept of histogenesis. Cancer 50: 2203–2206

184. Nakao CY, Nolan JF, diSaia PJ, Futoran R (1974) Microinvasive epidermoid carcinoma of the vulva with an unexpected natural history. Am J Obstet Gynecol 120: 1122

185. Nauth HF, Schilke E (1982) Cytology of the exfoliative layer in normal and diseased vulvar skin: Correlation with histology. Acta Cytol 26: 269–283

186. Neilson D, Woodruff JD (1972) Electron microscopy in in-situ and invasive vulvar Paget's disease. Am J Obstet Gynecol 113: 719

187. Newcomb PA, Weiss NS, Daling JR (1981) Incidence of vulvar carcinoma in relation to menstrual, reproductive and medical factors. J Natl Cancer Inst 73: 391

188. Niebyl JR, Genadry R, Friedrich EG, Wilkinson EJ, Woodruff JD (1974) Vulvar carcinoma with hypercalcemia. Obstet Gynecol 45: 343

189. Nirenberg A, Slavin J, Ostor AG (1993) Primary vulvar sarcomas. Int J Gynecol Pathol (Submitted)

190. Okagaki T (1981) Warty carcinoma of the vulva: A probable implication of human papillomavirus at the causative agent. Lab Invest 44: 49A

191. Oriel JD, Whimster IW (1971) Carcinoma in situ associated with virus-containing anal warts. Br J Dermatol 84: 71

192. Park JS, Jones RW, McLean MR, et al (1991) Possible etiologic heterogeneity of vulvar intraepithelial neoplasia. A correlation of pathologic characteristics with human papillomavirus detection by in situ hybridization and polymerase chain reaction. Cancer 67: 1599–1607

193. Parker RT, Duncan I, Rampone J, Creasman W (1975) Operative management of early invasive epidermoid carcinoma of the vulva. Am J Obstet Gynecol 123: 349

194. Parmley TH, Woodruff JD, Julian CG (1975) Invasive vulvar Paget's disease. Obstet Gynecol 46: 341

195. Patanaphan V, Prempree T, Sewchand W, Hafiz MA, Jaiwatana J (1983) Adenocarcinoma arising in female urethral diverticulum. Urology 22: 259

196. Pelosi G, Martignoni G, Bonetti F (1991) Intraductal carcinoma of mammary-type apocrine epithelium arising within a papillary hydradenoma of the vulva. Report of a case and review of the literature. Arch Pathol Lab Med 115: 1249–1254

197. Perrone T, Swanson PE, Twiggs L, Ulbright TM, Dehner LP (1989) Malignant rhabdoid tumor of the vulva: is distinction from epithelioid sarcoma possible? A pathologic and immunohistochemical study. Am J Surg Pathol 13: 848–858

198. Phillips GL, Twiggs LB, Okagaki T (1992) Vulvar melanoma: A microstaging study. Gynecol Oncol 14: 80–88

199. Pierson KK (1987) Malignant melanomas and pigmented lesions of the vulva. In: Wilkinson EJ (ed) Contemporary issues in surgical pathology. Pathology of the vulva and vagina, vol 9. New York, Churchill Livingstone, pp 155–179

200. Pilotti S, Rilke F, Shah K, Torre GD, DePalo G (1984) Immunohistochemical and ultrastructural evidence of papillomavirus infection associated with in situ and microinvasive squamous cell carcinoma of the vulva. Am J Surg Pathol 8:751

201. Pilotti S, Rotola A, D'Amato L, Di-Luca D, Shah KV, Cassai E, Rilke F (1990) Vulvar carcinomas: Search for sequences homologous to human papillomavirus and herpes simplex virus DNA. Mod Pathol 3:442–448

202. Pinkus H, Mehregan AH (1981) A Guide to Dermatohistopathology. New York, Appleton-Century-Crofts

203. Plouffe L, Tulandi T, Rosenberg A, Ferenczy A (1984) Non-Hodgkin's lymphoma in Bartholin's gland: Case report and review of literature. Am J Obstet Gynecol 148: 608

204. Podratz KC, Gaffey TA, Symmonds RE, Johansen KL, O'Brien PC (1983) Melanoma of the vulva: An update. Gynecol Oncol 16: 153–168

205. Poulsen HE, Taylor CW, Sobin LH (1979) Histologic typing of female genital tract tumors. In: International Histologic Classification of Tumors, No. 13: WHO, Geneva, Switzerland

206. Powell CS, Jones PA (1983) Carcinoma of the bladder with a metastasis in the clitoris. Br J Obstet Gynecol 90: 380

207. Powell FC, Bjornsson J, Doyle JA, Cooper AF (1985) Genital Paget's disease and urinary tract malignancy. J Am Acad Dermatol 13: 84

208. Powell LC, Dinh TV, Rajaraman S, et al (1986) Carcinoma in situ of the vulva: A clinicopathologic study of 50 cases. J Reprod Med 31: 808

209. Preti M, Micheletti L, Barbero M, et al (1993) Histologic parameters of vulvar invasive carcinoma and lymph node metastases. J Reprod Med 38: 28–32

210. Radman HM (1981) Metastatic melanoma of the vulva. Md State Med J 30:60

211. Rando RF, Sedlacek TV, Hunt J, Jenson AB, Kurman RJ, Lancaster WD (1986) Verrucous carcinoma of the vulva associated with an unusual type 6 human papilloma virus. Obstet Gynecol 67: 70–75S

212. Rastkar G, Okagaki T, Twiggs LB, Clark BA (1982) Early invasive and in situ warty carcinoma of the vulva: Clinical, histologic, and electron microscopic study with particular reference to viral association. Am J Obstet Gynecol 143: 814–820

213. Reed JA, Brigati DJ, Flynn SD (1992) Immunocytochemical identification of Rochalimaea henselae in bacillary (epithelioid) angiomatosis, parenchymal bacillary peliosis, and persistent fever and bacteremia. Am J Surg Pathol 16: 650–657

214. Report of the ISSVD Terminology Committee (1986) Proc VIII World Congress, Stockholm, Sweden. J Reprod Med 31: 973

215. Rhodes AR, Mihm MC Jr, Weinstock MA (1989) Dysplastic melanocytic nevi. A reproducible histologic definition emphasizing cellular morphology. Mod Pathol 2: 306–319

216. Roberts TW, Melicow MM (1977) Pathology and natural history of urethral tumors in females. Review of 65 cases. Urology 10: 583

217. Robertson AJ, McIntosh W, Lamont P, Guthrie W (1981) Malignant granular cell tumor (myoblastoma) of the vulva: Report of a case and review of the literature. Histopathology 5: 69

218. Ross MJ, Ehrmann RL (1987) Histologic prognosticators

in stage I squamous cell carcinoma of the vulva. Obstet Gynecol 70: 774–784

219. Roth LM, Panganiban WG (1978) Gonadal and extragonadal yolk sac carcinomas. A clinicopathologic study of 14 cases. Cancer 37: 812

220. Roth LM, Lee SC, Ehrlich CE (1977) Paget's disease of the vulva. A histogenetic study of five cases including ultrastructural observations and review of the literature. Am J Surg Pathol 1: 193

221. Rusk D, Sutton GP, Look KY, Roman A (1991) Analysis of invasive squamous cell carcinoma of the vulva and vulvar intraepithelial neoplasia for the presence of human papillomavirus DNA. Obstet Gynecol 77: 918–922

222. Santeusanio G, Schiaroli S, Anemona L, et al (1991) Carcinoma of the vulva with sarcomatoid features: A case report with immunohistochemical study: Case report. Gynecol Oncol 40: 160–163

223. Sedlis A, Homesley H, Bundy BN, et al (1987) Positive groin lymph nodes in superficial squamous cell vulvar cancer. A gynecologic oncology group study. Am J Obstet Gynecol 156: 1159–164

224. Sedlis A, Marshall R, Homesley H, Bundy B (1984) Positive groin lymph nodes in vulvar cancer with superficial tumor penetration. Society of Gynecologic Oncology, Miami, Florida, February 7

225. Seski JC, Reinholter ER, Silva J (1978) Abnormalities of lymphocyte transformations in women with intraepithelial carcinoma of the vulva. Obstet Gynecol 52: 332

226. Schueller EF (1965) Basal cell cancer of the vulva. Am J Obstet Gynecol 93: 199

227. Seiji M, Mizuno F (1969) Electron microscopic study of Bowen's disease. Arch Dermatol 99: 3

228. Shafeek MA, Osman ME, Hussein MA (1979) Carcinoma of the vulva arising in condylomata acuminata. Obstet Gynecol 54: 120

229. Shane JM, Naftolin F (1975) Aberrant hormone activity by tumors of gynecologic importance. Am J Obstet Gynecol 121: 133

230. Shatz P, Bergeron C, Wilkinson EJ, Arseneau J, Ferenczy A (1989) Vulvar intraepithelial neoplasia and skin appendage involvement. Obstet Gynecol 74: 769–774

231. Shen JT, D'Ablaing G, Morrow CP (1982) Alveolar soft part sarcoma of the vulva: Report of first case and review of literature. Gynecol Oncol 13: 120

232. Simon KE, Dutcher JP, Runowicz CD, Wiernik PH (1988) Adenocarcinoma arising in vulvar breast tissue. Cancer 62: 2234–2238

233. Sivanesaratnam V, Pathmanathan R (1990) Carcinoma of the vulva in pregnancy: A rare occurrence. Asia Oceania J Obstet Gynaecol 16: 207–210

234. Snow SN, DeSouky S, Lo JS, Kurtycz D (1992) Failure to detect human papillomavirus DNA in extramammary Paget's disease. Cancer 69: 249–251

235. Sondergaard K, Schou G (1985) Survival with primary cutaneous malignant melanoma evaluated from 2012 cases. A multivariate regression analysis. Virchows Arch [A] 406: 179–195

236. Stapleton JJ (1984) Extramammary Paget's disease of the vulva in a young black woman. J Reprod Med 29: 444

237. Steeper T, Rosai J (1983) Aggressive angiomyxoma of the female pelvis and perineum. Report of nine cases. Am J Surg Pathol 7: 463

238. Steeper TA, Piscioli F, and Rosai J (1983) Squamous cell carcinoma with sarcoma-like stroma of the female genital tract. Clinicopathologic study of four cases. Cancer 52: 890

239. Stegner HE (1986) Ultrastructure of preneoplastic lesions of the vulva. J Reprod Med 31: 815

240. Stehman FB, Bundy BN, Dvoretsky PM, Creasman WT (1992) Early stage I carcinoma of the vulva treated with ipsilateral superficial inguinal lymphadenectomy and modified radical hemivulvectomy: A prospective study of the gynecologic oncology group. Obstet and Gynecol 79: 490–497

241. Stewart AF, Romero R, Schwartz PE, Kohorn EI, Broadus AE (1982) Hypercalcemia associated with gynecologic malignancies: Biochemical characterization. Cancer 49: 2389

242. Sturgeon SR, Brinton LA, Devesa SS, Kurman RJ (1992) In situ and invasive vulvar cancer incidence trends (1973 to 1987). Am J Obstet Gynecol 166: 1482–1485

243. Talerman A (1973) Sarcoma botryoides presenting as a polyp on the labium majorus. Cancer 32: 994

244. Tang CK, Toker C, Nedwich A, Zaman AN (1982) Unusual cutaneous carcinoma with features of small cell (oat cell) and squamous cell carcinomas. A variant of Merkel cell neoplasm. Am J Dermatopathol 4: 537–548

245. Tasseron EW, van der Esch EP, Hart AA, Brutel de la Riviere G, Aartsen EJ (1992) A clinicopathological study of 30 melanomas of the vulva. Gynecol Oncol 46: 170–175

246. Tavassoli FA, Norris HJ (1979) Smooth muscle tumors of the vulva. Obstet Gynecol 53: 213

247. Taxy JB, Battifora H, Trujillo Y, et al (1981) Electron microscopy in the diagnosis of malignant schwannoma. Cancer 48: 1381–1391

248. Taylor RN, Bottles K, Miller TR, Braga CA (1985) Malignant fibrous histiocytoma of the vulva. Obstet Gynecol 66: 145–148

249. Taylor RN, Lacey CG, Shuman MA (1985) Adenocarcinoma of Skene's duct associated with a systemic coagulopathy. Gynecol Oncol 22: 250–256

250. Taylor PR, Stenwig JT, Klausen H (1975) Paget's disease of the vulva. Gynecol Oncol 3: 46

251. Terada KY, Schmidt TW, Roberts JA (1988) Malignant schwannoma of the vulva. A case report. J Reprod Med 33: 969–972

252. Thomas R, Barnhill D, Bibro M, Hoskins W, Hambidge W (1986) Histiocytosis X in gynecology. A case presentation and review of the literature. Obstet Gynecol 67: 46–49S

253. Tiltman AJ, Knutzen VK (1978) Primary adenocarcinoma of the vulva originating in misplaced cloacal tissue. Obstet Gynecol 51: 30–33S

254. Toki T, Kurman RJ, Park JS, Kessis T, Daniel RW, Shah KV (1991) Probable nonpapillomavirus etiology of squamous cell carcinoma of the vulva in older women: A clinicopathologic study using in situ hybridization and polymerase chain reaction. Int J Gynecol Pathol 10: 107–125

255. Trimble EL, Lewis JL Jr, Williams LL, et al (1992) Management of vulvar melanoma. Gynecol Oncol 45: 254–258

256. Tuder RM (1992) Vulvar destruction of malignant lymphoma. Gynecol Oncol 45: 52–57

257. Turner AG, Hendry WF (1980) Primary carcinoma of the female urethra. Br J Urol 52: 549

258. Ubben K, Krzyzek R, Ostrow R, et al (1979) Human papilloma virus DNA detected in two verrucous carcinomas. J Invest Dermatol 72: 195

259. Ulbright TM, Brokow SA, Stehman FB, Roth LM (1983) Epithelioid sarcoma of the vulva. Evidence suggesting a more aggressive behavior than extragenital epithelioid sarcoma. Cancer 52: 1462

260. Underwood JW, Adcock LL, Okagaki T (1978) Adenosquamous carcinoma of skin appendages (adenoid squamous cell carcinoma, pseudoglandular squamous cell carcinoma, adenoacanthoma of sweat glands of Lever) of the vulva. A clinical and ultrastructural study. Cancer 42: 1851–1858

261. Ungerleider RS, Donaldson SS, Warnke RA, Wilbur JR (1978) Endodermal sinus tumor. The Stanford experience and the first reported case arising in the vulva. Cancer 41: 1627

262. Van der Putte SCJ (1993) Mammary-like glands of the vulva and their disorders. Int J Gynecol Pathol (In press)

263. Wade TR, Kopf AW, Ackerman AB (1978) Bowenoid papulosis of the penis. Cancer 42: 1890

264. Wade TR, Kopf AW, Ackerman AB (1979) Bowenoid papulosis of the genitalia. Arch Dermatol 115: 306

265. Way S (1960) Carcinoma of the vulva. Am J Obstet Gynecol 79: 692

266. Way S (1982) Malignant disease of the vulva. Edinburgh, Scotland, Churchill Livingstone

267. Weed JC, Lozier C, Daniel SJ (1983) Human Papillomavirus in multifocal, invasive female genital tract malignancy. Obstet Gynecol 62: 835

268. Weghaupt K, Gerstner GJ, Kucera H (1984) Radiation therapy for primary carcinoma of the female urethra: A survey over 25 years. Gynecol Oncol 17: 58

269. Weiss SW, Enzinger FM (1978) Malignant fibrous histiocytoma, an analysis of 200 cases. Cancer 41: 2250–2266

270. Weiss SW, Enzinger FM (1977) Myxoid variant of malignant fibrous histiocytoma. Cancer 39: 1672–1685

271. Wharton JT, Gallager S, Rutledge FN (1974) Microinvasive carcinoma of the vulva, Am J Obstet Gynecol 118: 159

272. Wheelock JB, Goplerud DR, Dunn LJ, Oates JF (1984) Primary carcinoma of the Bartholin gland: A report of ten cases. Obstet Gynecol 63: 820

273. Wick MR, Goellner JR, Wolfe JT III, Su WPD (1985) Vulvar sweat gland carcinoma. Arch Pathol Lab Med 109: 43–47

274. Wilkinson EJ (1991) Superficially invasive carcinoma of the vulva. Clin Obstet Gynecol 34: 651–661

275. Wilkinson EJ (1992) Normal histology and nomenclature of the vulva and malignant neoplasms, including VIN. Dermatol Clin 10: 283–296

276. Wilkinson EJ (1987) Superficially invasive carcinoma of the vulva. In: Wilkinson EJ (ed) Contemporary issues in surgical pathology. Pathology of the vulva and vagina, vol 9. New York, Churchill Livingstone, pp 103–117

277. Wilkinson EJ, Croker BP, Friedrich EG Jr, Franzini DA (1988) Two distinct pathologic types of giant cell tumor of the vulva. A report of two cases. J Reprod Med 33: 519–522

278. Wilkinson EJ, Friedrich EG, Fu YS (1981) Multicentric nature of vulvar carcinoma in situ. Obstet Gynecol 58: 69

279. Wilkinson EJ, Hause L (1974) Probability in lymph node sectioning. Cancer 33: 1269

280. Wilkinson EJ, Hause LL, Hoffman RG, et al (1982) Occult axillary lymph node metastases in invasive breast carcinoma: Characteristics of the primary tumor and significance of the metastases. Pathol Annu 17: 67

281. Wilkinson EJ, Morgan LS, Friedrich EG (1984) Association of Franconi's anemia and squamous-cell carcinoma of the lower female genital tract with condyloma acuminatum. J Reprod Med 29: 447

282. Wilkinson EJ, Rico MJ, Pierson KK (1982) Microinvasive carcinoma of the vulva. Int J Gynecol Pathol 1: 29

283. Woodruff JD (1985) Carcinoma in situ of the vulva. Clin Obstet Gynecol 28: 230

284. Woodruff JD, Borkowf HI, Holzman GB, Arnold EA, Knaack J (1965) Metabolic activity in normal and abnormal vulvar epithelia. Am J Obstet Gynecol 91: 809

285. Woodruff JD, Richardson EH (1957) Malignant vulvar Paget's disease. Obstet Gynecol 10: 10

286. Woolcott RJ, Henry RJ, Houghton CR (1988) Malignant melanoma of the vulva. Australian experience. J Reprod Med 33: 699–702

287. Worsham MJ, VanDyke DL, Grenman SE, et al (1991) Consistent chromosome abnormalities in squamous cell carcinoma of the vulva. Genes Chromosome Cancer 3: 420–432

288. Yazigi R, Piver MS, Tsukada Y (1978) Microinvasive carcinoma of the vulva. Obstet Gynecol 51: 368

289. Yoonessi M, Goodell T, Satchidanand S, Fett W, Solis F (1983) Microinvasive squamous carcinoma of the vulva. J Surg Oncol 24: 315

290. Young RH, Scully RE (1985) Clear cell adenocarcinoma of the bladder and urethra. Am J Surg Pathol 9: 816

291. ZaKut H, Lotan M, Lipnilsky M (1985) Vulvar hemangiopericytoma. A case report and review of previous cases. Acta Obstet Gynecol Scand 64: 619–621

292. Zaino RJ (1987) Carcinoma of the vulva, urethra and Bartholin's gland. In: Wilkinson EJ (ed) Contemporary issues in surgical pathology. Pathology of the vulva and vagina, vol 9. New York, Churchill Livingstone, pp 119–153

293. Zinkham WH (1976) Multifocal eosinophilic granuloma. Natural history, etiology and management. Am J Med 60: 457–463

294. Zur Hausen H, Gissman L, Schlehofer JR (1984) Viruses in the etiology of human genital cancer. Prog Med Virol 30: 170

4

Diseases of the Vagina

Richard J. Zaino, M.D., Stanley J. Robboy, M.D.,
Rex Bentley, M.D., and Robert J. Kurman, M.D.

The vagina, like other orifices that interface between external environment and the interior milieu, acts as a barrier to many potentially invasive microorganisms. It is thus not surprising that the vagina is the site of a variety of infections, both sexually and nonsexually transmitted, and this, in fact, represents the predominant type of pathology of this organ. In contrast, neoplasms are relatively unusual in this site, which is somewhat unexpected in view of the relationship between infection (e.g., human papilloma virus infection) and the development of carcinoma of the vulva and cervix.

Because of its profound effects on the development of the vagina, the pathology of in utero diethylstilbestrol (DES) exposure has been integrated into the Developmental Disorders and Malignant Neoplasms sections of this chapter. In few other areas of medicine have the interrelationships of embryology, anatomy, physiology, and neoplasia been so well defined. The astute reader will note, however, that the failure to identify many aspects relating to the pathogenesis of many other diseases of the vagina reflects our current state of ignorance.

Development

Debate over the embryologic origins of the vagina has persisted for more than 50 years. These differences reflect the complex and dynamic interrelationship of tissues derived from different germ cell layers and the lack of an animal model that parallels human vaginal development. Nonetheless, the discovery of specific epithelial and stromal abnormalities in the lower genital tract of women exposed to DES in utero emphasizes that pathologic changes in the adult may be a consequence of disordered embryogenesis. A brief review of vaginal development therefore follows (for a more detailed discussion see Chapter 1, Embryology and Disorders of Abnormal Sexual Development).

It is generally agreed that both the müllerian ducts and the urogenital sinus contribute to the formation of the vagina.[57,249] The müllerian ducts first appear as funnel-shaped openings of the coelomic epithelium in the meso-

nephric ridge about postconception day 37.[57,84,291] They grow caudally as paired tubes, extending to meet the posterior wall of the urogenital sinus. At about day 54, the caudal portions of the müllerian ducts fuse, forming a straight uterovaginal canal that is lined by simple columnar epithelium. The uterovaginal canal continues to elongate caudally until about day 66. Shortly thereafter, the epithelium from the caudal tip of the canal to the external cervical os changes to a stratified squamous type. This results from a migration of squamous cells from the urogenital sinus, rather than from squamous metaplasia of the native müllerian columnar epithelium.[291] Continued stratification of the squamous epithelial lining progressively occludes the more caudal portion of the canal leading to the development of a solid vaginal plate. In the 16th week, the squamous epithelium of the vagina and ectocervix begins to mature, becoming glycogenated and thickened. Desquamation subsequently results in canalization of the vaginal plate. Vaginal development is essentially complete by the 18th–20th week. A band of subepithelial stroma extending from the endocervix to the vulva has been described, but the role of the vaginal stroma in induction of mucosal changes remains unclear.[57,74,297]

In the past, our knowledge of vaginal embryology was derived from classic dissections of the fetus. Several experiments of nature in humans (in utero exposure to DES, transverse vaginal septation, and partial vaginal agenesis) and in mice (testicular feminization syndrome and agenesis of the lower vagina)[57] as well as recent studies using human fetal grafts transplanted into the nude mouse[58,291] have provided the opportunity for elegant studies of altered development. They reaffirm that the vagina is of dual origin, with a native lining of müllerian columnar cells that are retained unless there is a contribution of squamous cells from the urogenital sinus.

Anatomy

The vagina is a partially collapsed, midline, tubular structure that extends from the vestibule of the vulva to the uterine cervix. The vagina is posterior to the urinary bladder and anterior to the rectum, with an angle of more than 90° between the axis of the vagina and that of the uterus (Fig. 4.1). In the adult, the vagina is about 9 cm in length. The anterior and posterior walls are in contact with each other, with the exception of the cranial (proximal) end where the vagina surrounds the ectocervix. Here, there are vault-like recesses between the vaginal walls and the cervix termed *fornices*, which are deepest posteriorly. In contrast to the slack anterior and posterior walls, the lateral walls are relatively rigid, resulting in a somewhat compressed lumen with an H shape in transverse sections.[288,298]

The vagina is in contact anteriorly with the uterine cervix, the base of the bladder, and the urethra. The proximal

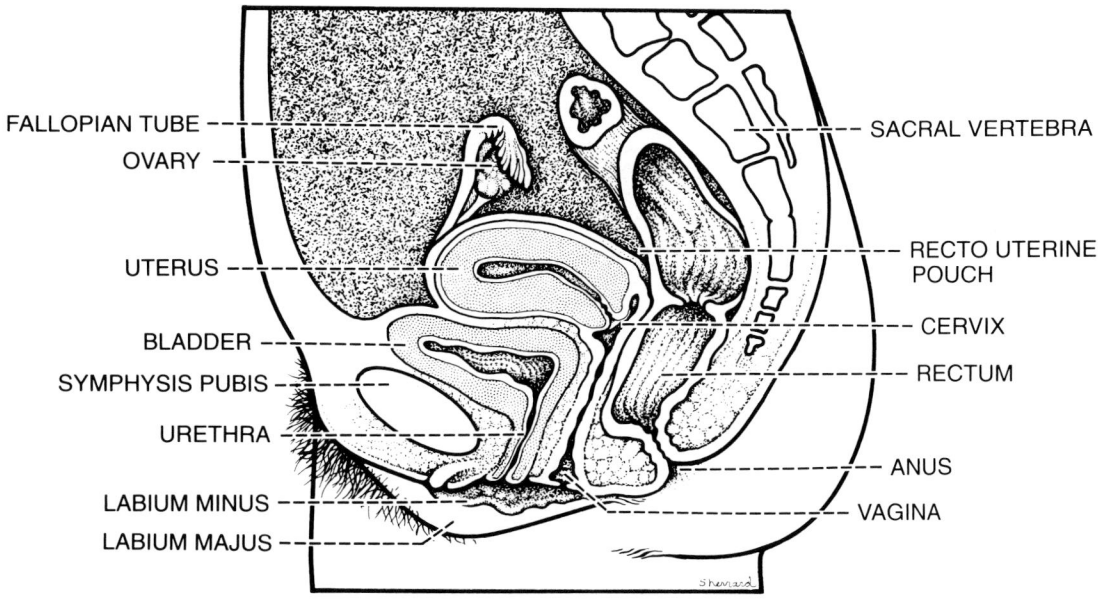

FALLOPIAN TUBE

OVARY

UTERUS

BLADDER

SYMPHYSIS PUBIS

URETHRA

LABIUM MINUS

LABIUM MAJUS

SACRAL VERTEBRA

RECTO UTERINE POUCH

CERVIX

RECTUM

ANUS

VAGINA

FIG. 4.1. **Median sagittal section of the female pelvis.**

third of the urethra is separated from the vagina by loose connective tissue; it enters into the vaginal wall distally where their fasciae fuse into a single dense layer. Posteriorly, the upper fourth of the vaginal wall is bounded by peritoneum, and forms the anterior part of the cul-de-sac or pouch of Douglas. The rectovaginal septum connects the adventitia of the middle half of the vagina with the rectum, whereas the perineal body and anal and rectal sphincters separate the remaining more caudal portion from the anal canal. Laterally, each ureter, crossed by the uterine artery and vein, runs just above the lateral fornix. Caudally (distally), the levator ani and bulbocavernosus muscles partially surround the vagina, which ultimately opens into the vestibule (Fig. 4.2).

Blood is supplied to the vagina primarily by branches of the internal iliac artery, including the uterine, vaginal, middle rectal, and internal pudendal arteries.[262,298] Extensive anastomoses provide alternate routes of flow, which minimize the possibility of ischemic damage. A complex network of veins surrounds the vagina, forming a plexus with the uterine, pudendal, and rectal veins, which drain into the interior iliac vein.

The lymphatic drainage of the vagina is complex and variable.[8] The lymphatics of the proximal anterior vagina and vaginal vault join those of the cervix, and drain primarily into the external iliac lymph nodes. The posterior portion of the vagina drains into the inferior gluteal, sacral, and anorectal lymph nodes, whereas the distal part of the vagina, like the vulva, drains into the femoral lymph nodes. It is important to note that, as a consequence of extensive anastomotic channels, any pelvic, anorectal, or femoral node may be involved in the lymphatic drainge of any part of the vagina.

The innervation of the vagina is principally from the superior hypogastric plexus of the autonomic nervous system. This plexus bifurcates and is joined by branches of the second through fifth sacral nerves, forming the pelvic plexuses.[49,229]

Histology and Physiology

The vaginal wall consists of three layers: mucosa, muscularis, and adventitia (Fig. 4.3). The vaginal mucosa is thrown into ill-defined laterally oriented folds or rugae of about 2–5 mm in thickness (Fig. 4.4). The thickness of the folds varies according to location and hormonal stimulation. The mucosal lining is a stratified squamous epithelium that is normally glycogenated and nonkeratinizing.[288] Subdivision of the epithelium into layers is somewhat arbitrary but useful, since it provides a basis for understanding the variable appearance of squamous cells in vaginal cytologic smears (Fig. 4.5). The basal layer consists of a single layer of columnar cells, with the principal axis of the cells perpendicular to the basement membrane. The nuclei are oval and uniformly hyperchromatic, and are surrounded by relatively scant cytoplasm, resulting in a high nuclear/cytoplasmic ratio. The parabasal layer usually consists of two to five layers of cells of cuboidal shape, with a centrally located, round, uniformly hyperchromatic nucleus. Mitoses usually are confined to the basal and parabasal layers. The intermediate layer is of variable thickness. The cells in this layer contain moderate quantities of slightly flattened cytoplasm and oval nuclei with finely dispersed chromatin. The long axis of both nucleus and cytoplasm is parallel to the basement membrane. The superficial layer also varies

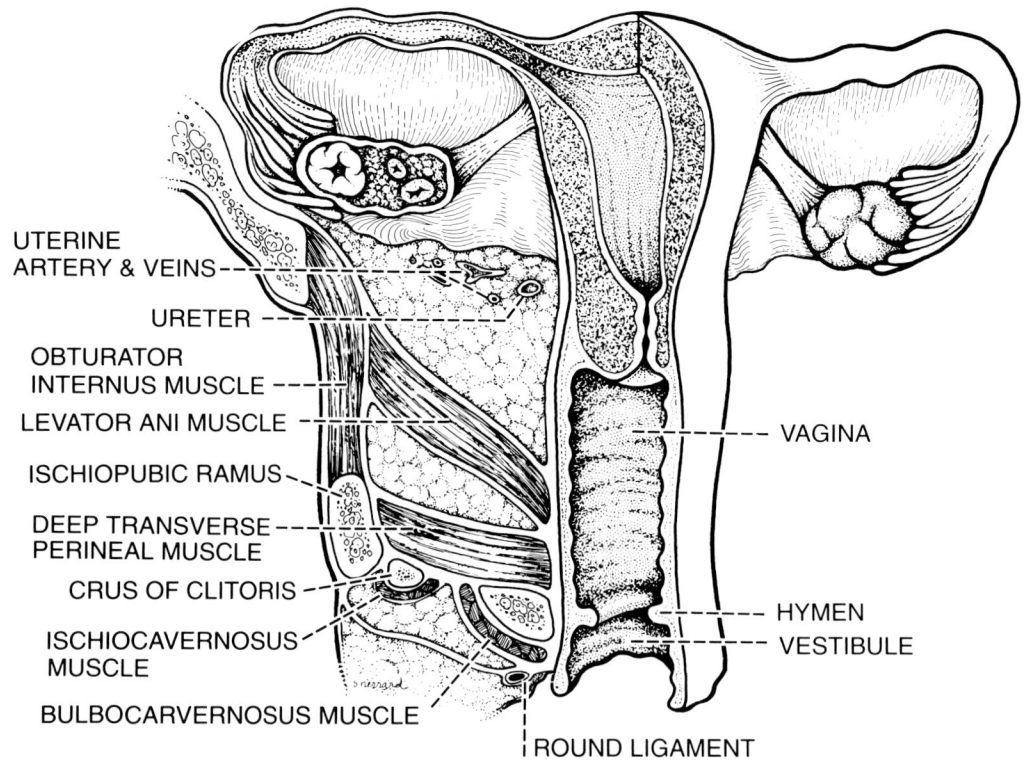

UTERINE
ARTERY & VEINS

URETER

OBTURATOR
INTERNUS MUSCLE

LEVATOR ANI MUSCLE

ISCHIOPUBIC RAMUS

DEEP TRANSVERSE
PERINEAL MUSCLE

CRUS OF CLITORIS

ISCHIOCAVERNOSUS
MUSCLE

BULBOCARVERNOSUS MUSCLE

VAGINA

HYMEN

VESTIBULE

ROUND LIGAMENT

FIG. 4.2. Vagina, uterus, and supporting structures of the pelvis.

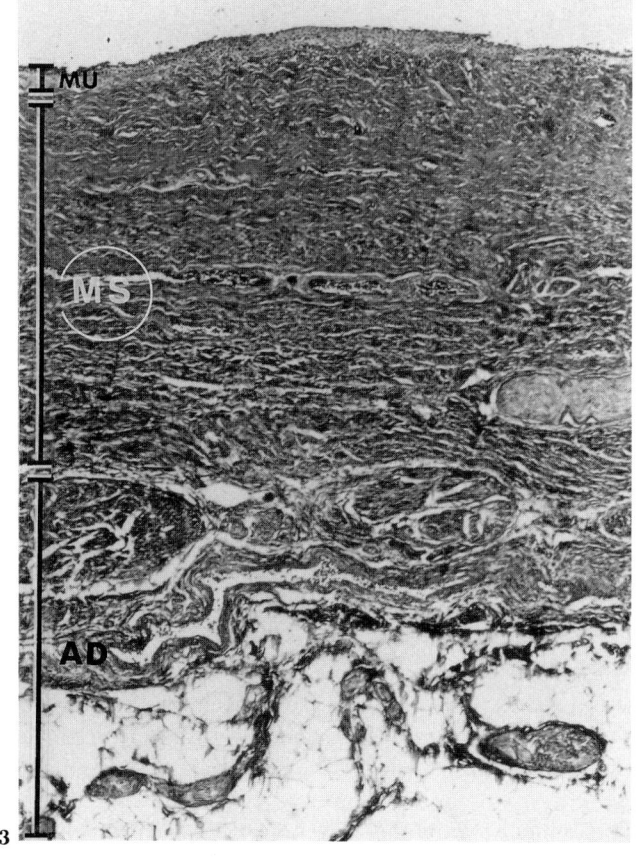

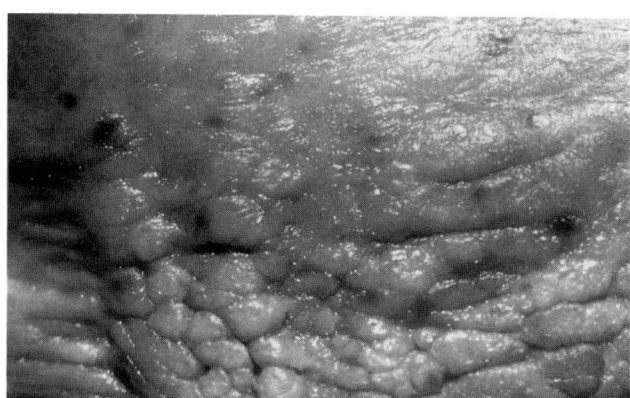

FIG. 4.3. **Vaginal wall.** Mucosa, (*MU*), muscularis (*MS*), and adventitia (*AD*). The smooth muscle bundles are of variable thickness and ill-defined. The adventitia contains numerous blood vessels and nerves within adipose tissue.

FIG. 4.4. **Vaginal mucosa.** The mucosa is composed of ill-defined, laterally oriented folds or rugae.

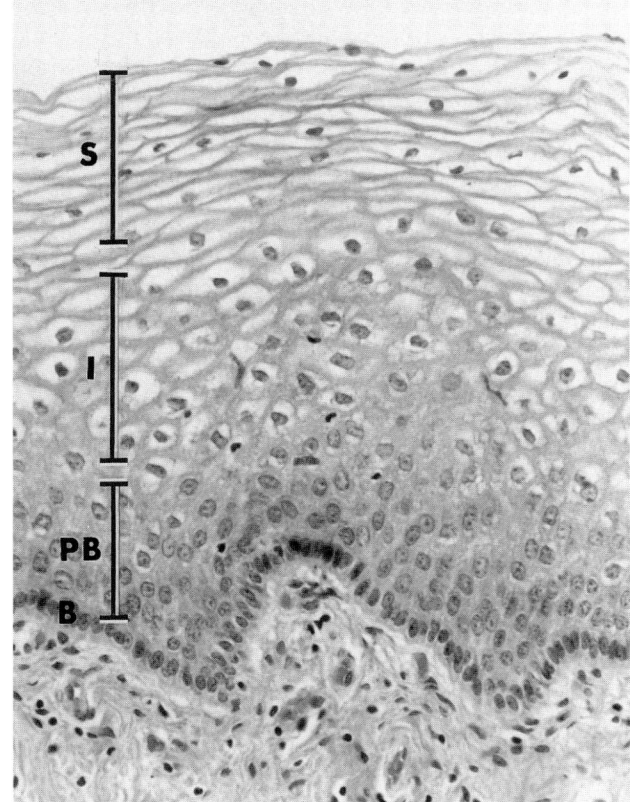

FIG. 4.5. Mature vaginal squamous epithelium. The epithelium is composed of a basal layer (*B*), several layers of parabasal cells (*PB*), and multiple layers of intermediate (*I*) and superficial (*S*) cells that progressively accumulate glycogen.

in thickness. The cells contain pyknotic nuclei, which are small, round, and hyperchromatic. The cytoplasm is abundant, with an orientation similar to intermediate cells. The three-dimensional configuration of these cells is that of a highly attenuated disc, resulting in a flattened appearance when viewed in cross-section.

Variable quantities of glycogen may be present in the intermediate and superficial cell layers. The glycogen accumulates initially in a perinuclear location within intermediate cells, resulting in a clear zone around the nucleus. This appearance may cause confusion with the perinuclear clearing of koilocytes. However, the presence of nuclear membrane irregularity in koilocytes, and the characteristic location of these normal cells in the middle rather than superficial third of the epithelium, are helpful distinguishing features. Melanocytes have been identified as a normal constituent of the basal layer in about 3% of women.[234]

The lamina propria, which lies beneath the squamous epithelium, consists of a loose fibrovascular stroma containing elastic fibers and nerves. A band of stroma extends from the endocervix to the vulva, which contains atypical polygonal to stellate stromal cells with scant cytoplasm. Some of these cells are multinucleated or have multilobu-

lated nuclei (Fig. 4.6).[74] The muscularis consists of poorly delineated, inner circular, and outer longitudinal bundles of smooth muscle. Some of the outer longitudinal layers of muscle pass into the lateral pelvic wall to contribute to the inferior portion of the cardinal ligaments,[288] whereas fibers of the bulbocavernosus form a sphincter around the distal vagina. The adventitia is a thin coat of dense connective tissue that merges with the loose connective tissue of the surrounding pelvis, which contains the lymphatic and venous plexuses and nerve bundles.[80]

The squamous cells of the vagina contain intranuclear steroid receptors and represent a target tissue for sex steroids. The thickness and maturation of the epithelium varies throughout the menstrual cycle. Since the vagina is rarely biopsied but frequently sampled cytologically, the latter procedure has contributed greatly to our knowledge of normal and aberrant maturation.[179] During the proliferative phase the epithelium progressively proliferates and matures fully in response to estrogens. The addition of progesterone during the secretory phase is associated with an arrest of maturation at the intermediate cell level and a decrease in epithelial thickness. Although glycogen is

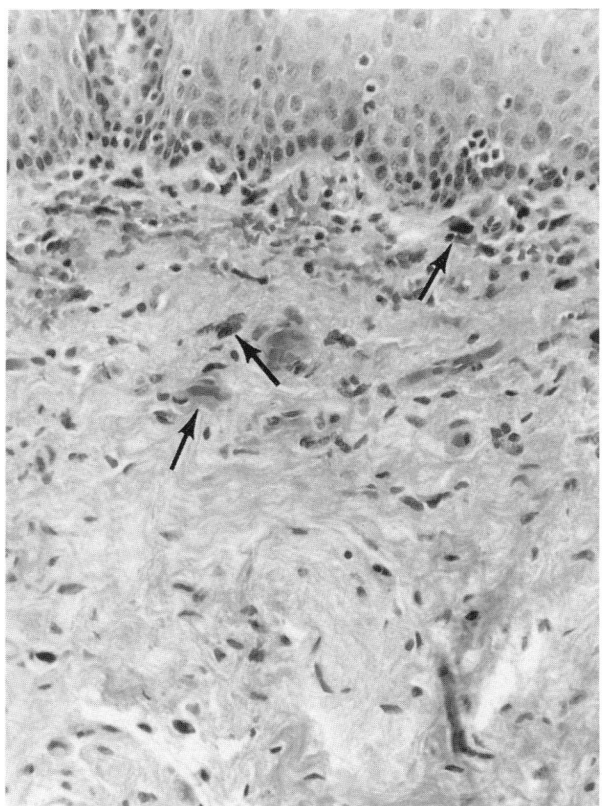

FIG. 4.6. Lamina propria of the vagina. Beneath the squamous epithelium of the vagina is an ill-defined zone of large, stellate, or spindle stromal cells (*arrows*), which extends from the cervix to the vulva. These stromal cells may be the source of the bizarre cells identified in some vaginal fibroepithelial polyps.

found in the intermediate and superficial cells throughout the menstrual cycle,[122] it is particularly abundant during pregnancy. Transient vaginal atrophy is found in some women postpartum, particularly those who are lactating.[369] After menopause, a gradual reduction in the thickness of the epithelium occurs, first with a loss of superficial cells, followed by intermediate cells, such that the mucosa of late menopausal women may be reduced to only six to eight layers of parabasal cells (Fig. 4.7). As a consequence, a normal postmenopausal atrophic pattern may be confused with a high-grade intraepithelial lesion unless care is taken to identify other nuclear abnormalities. Newborn infants, having been exposed to maternal steroids in utero, have a fully mature-appearing epithelium that rapidly regresses to atrophy within about 4 weeks.[179,245] A gradual maturation of the epithelium follows the onset of menarche.[123] Exposure of the postmenopausal vagina to estrogen leads to squamous maturation comparable to that observed in the proliferative phase of reproductive age women. It is interesting to note that in one study, the time required for a vaginal squamous cell to make the transition from progenitor cell through desquamation was about 5 days for both cycling and postmenopausal women.[9]

There are scant data concerning vaginal function during coitus or parturition.[212] Distension and lengthening of the proximal two-thirds of the vagina occurs during the early phases of sexual response, followed by constriction of the distal third. The anterior portion of the levator ani, the pubococcygeus muscle, appears to be involved in orgasmic function, but the mechanism is speculative.[115,212] Even the source of vaginal fluids that are present during arousal has been disputed. Glands are not normally present in the

vagina, and candidate sources include secretions from sebaceous, sweat, Bartholin and Skene glands, or the endocervix. Fine droplets appear scattered throughout the rugal folds of the vaginal wall during arousal, followed by a rapid coalescence.[212] The fluid is believed to represent a transudate resulting from associated vasoconstriction within the venous plexus.[80,126,212,288] The fluid usually is acidic, with a pH around 4.6, but rises during the sexual response.[126,162] This fluid contains a variety of enzymes, enzyme inhibitors, and immunoglobulins, which may play a role in liquefaction of coagulated semen and capacitation of spermatocytes, or have antimicrobial activity.[126] The immunoglobulin A levels are highest during the late proliferative phase,[117] but the significance of this observation is unclear. During pregnancy and immediately postpartum, edema, vascular congestion, and loss of collagen have been noted in the lamina propria, which may serve to increase elasticity of vaginal tissues during delivery.[206]

Developmental Disorders

Lesions Related to In Utero Exposure to DES

Diethylstilbestrol and the chemically related drugs, hexestrol and dienestrol, are synthetic, nonsteroidal estrogens that were administered frequently to gravid women who were thought to be at high risk for early pregnancy loss during the 1940s through the 1960s. In 1971, the rare development of clear cell adenocarcinoma of the vagina in young women was linked to their exposure in utero to these drugs.[144] Subsequently, a number of nonneoplastic changes were identified in the genital tract of DES-exposed daughters, such as adenosis (glandular epithelium or its secretory products in the vagina), cervical ectropion, various types of cervicovaginal ridges, and structural abnormalities of the uterine corpus and fallopian tube. Recommendations for the identification and management of exposed daughters,[285,286] possible sequelae in mothers,[120] daughters, and sons,[16,108,190,308,312,324] and animal models for the study of DES exposure are presented elsewhere.*

Gross Structural Changes of the Vagina and Cervix

Approximately one-fifth of DES-exposed women demonstrate gross structural changes in the cervix or vagina.[143] Descriptive designations have included coxcomb (hood), collar (rim), pseudopolyp, and ridge. The pseudopolyp is caused by a peripheral concentric cervical band that gives the portio vaginalis central to it the appearance of a protruding cervical polyp; however, the presence of the exter-

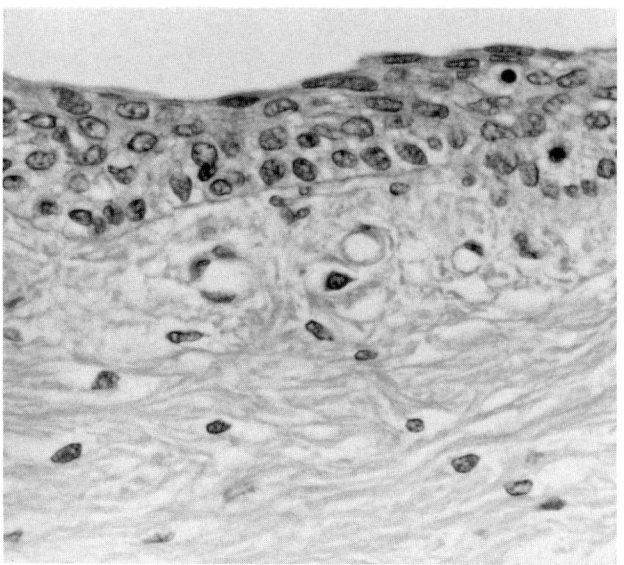

FIG. 4.7. Vaginal atrophy. The epithelium is reduced to only a few layers of parabasal and basal cells.

*Refs. 27,30,33,58,59,65,130,202,217,218,230,231,260,261,266, 291,297,331,332,360.

nal os at its center differentiates it from a true polyp. The cervix may be hypoplastic, the vaginal fornices may be obliterated, or the vagina may be traversed by a ridge (septum) consisting of fibrous connective tissue covered by squamous epithelium (Fig. 4.8). The natural history of the structural abnormalities is not well understood, although some ridges have been observed to disappear as the cervix and vagina undergo remodeling with age.

Vaginal Epithelial Changes: Adenosis and Squamous Metaplasia

Vaginal adenosis and metaplastic squamous epithelium—vaginal epithelial changes (VECs)—are common in DES-exposed females. During the pre-DES era, vaginal adenosis was a clinical rarity, detected only occasionally in women, usually in their 30s or 40s, who often complained of an excessive mucous discharge from the vagina.[164,185]

The adenosis found in non–DES women is identical microscopically to that of young women who were so exposed in utero.[283] Clinically, adenosis should be suspected when the vaginal mucosa contains red granular spots or patches (Fig. 4.8) and does not stain with an iodine solution (Fig. 4.9). On colposcopy, adenosis appears as glandular or metaplastic epithelium replacing the native squamous epithelium of the vaginal mucosa.

Adenosis, with or without squamous metaplasia, involves the upper third of the vagina in 34% of DES-exposed women. The anterior wall is involved most frequently and the posterior wall least frequently. These changes extend into the middle third of the vagina in 9% and the lower third in 2% of exposed women. In unexposed women, adenosis is rare,[357] although during late prenatal life and childhood, glandular epithelium extends well onto the exocervix in up to a third of persons, and rarely even onto the vagina.

Mucinous columnar cells, which by light and electron microscopy resemble those of the normal endocervical mucosa, comprise the glandular epithelium most frequently encountered as adenosis (62% of biopsy specimens with vaginal adenosis).[284] This epithelium, which most frequently lines the surface of the vagina, is the type of glandular epithelium most commonly seen by colposcopy (Fig.

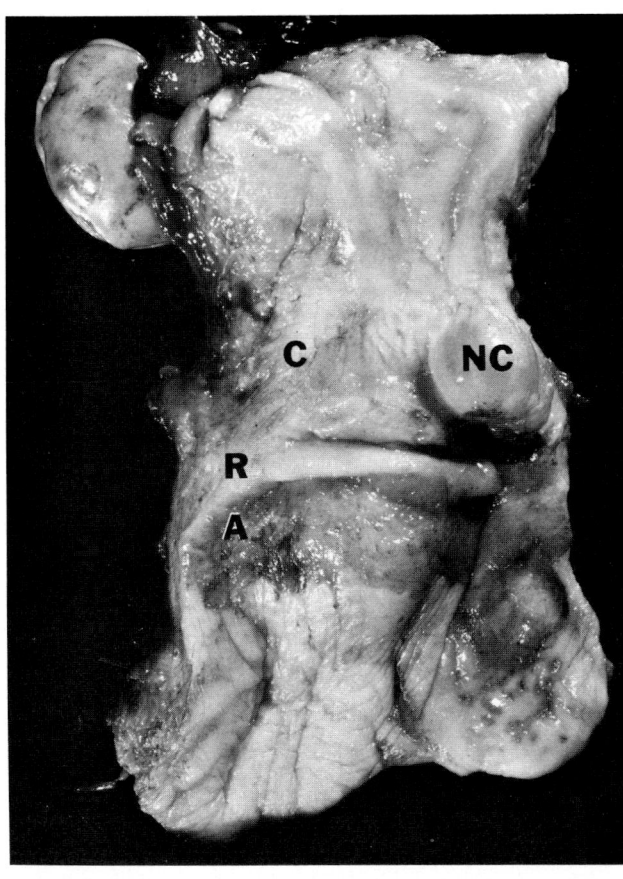

METRIC 1 | 2 | 3 | 4 | 5 | 6 | 7 | 8 |

Fig. 4.8. Opened uterus and vagina from a woman exposed to DES in utero. Transverse vaginal ridge (*R*), cervix (*C*), and zone of adenosis (*A*) that macroscopically appears as a red granular patch. Nabothian cyst (*NC*) of cervix is also visible along right margin of specimen. (Reprinted by permission of Herbst et al., N Engl J Med 287:1259–1264, 1972.)

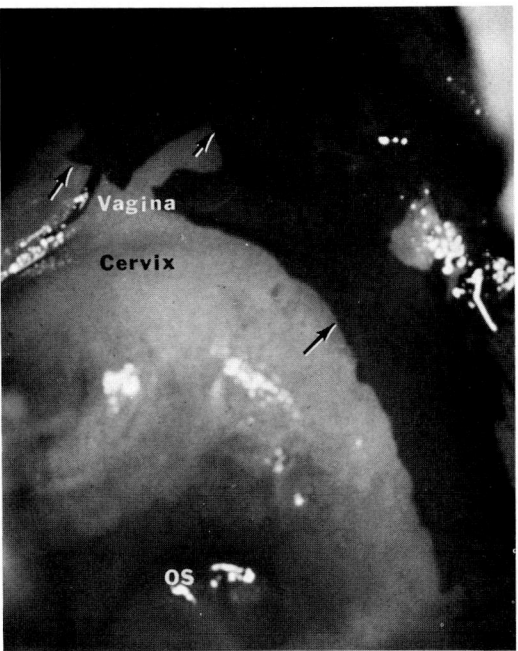

Fig. 4.9. Abnormal iodine (Schiller) stain in which aglycogenated (nonstaining) areas in both vagina and cervix appear white in photograph and represent the transformation zone. Glycogenated vaginal epithelium stains black. *Arrows* demarcate staining from nonstaining areas. (Reprinted by permission of Robboy et al., J Reprod Med 15: 13–18, 1975.)

4.10). Commonly, the mucinous columnar cells also line glands in the lamina propria (Fig. 4.11).

Dark cells and light cells, often ciliated and resembling the lining cells of the fallopian tube and endometrium, are found in 21% of specimens with adenosis (Fig. 4.12).

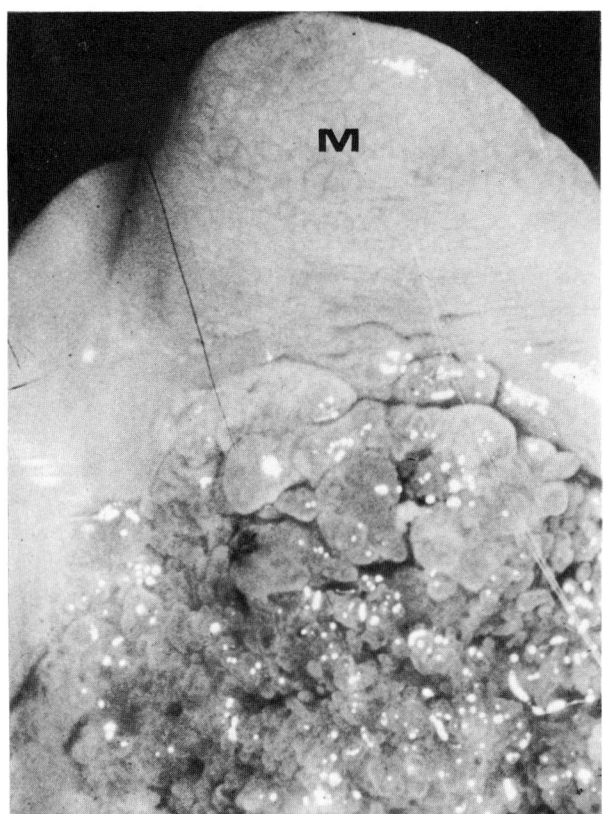

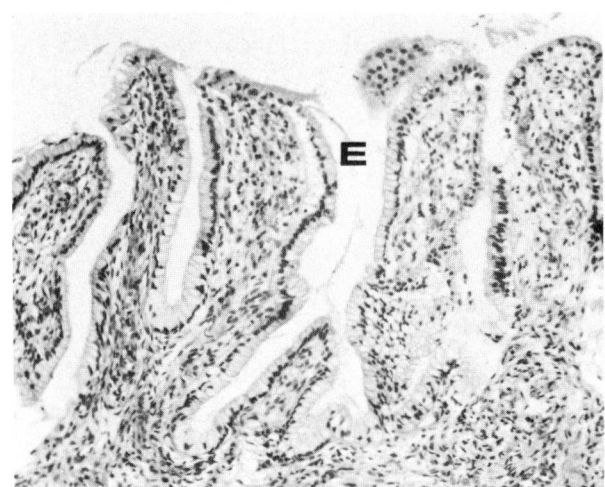

FIG. 4.10. Cervical ectropion. *Top:* Colpophotograph of anterior cervical cockscomb covered with metaplastic squamous epithelium in mosaic pattern (*M*). Grape-like structures along inner half of cervix are composed of fibrovascular cores covered by mucinous columnar epithelium (ectropion). *Bottom:* Photomicrograph of mucinous columnar cells (*E*) lining fibrovascular papillae. Same microscopical pattern in vagina is called *adenosis*.

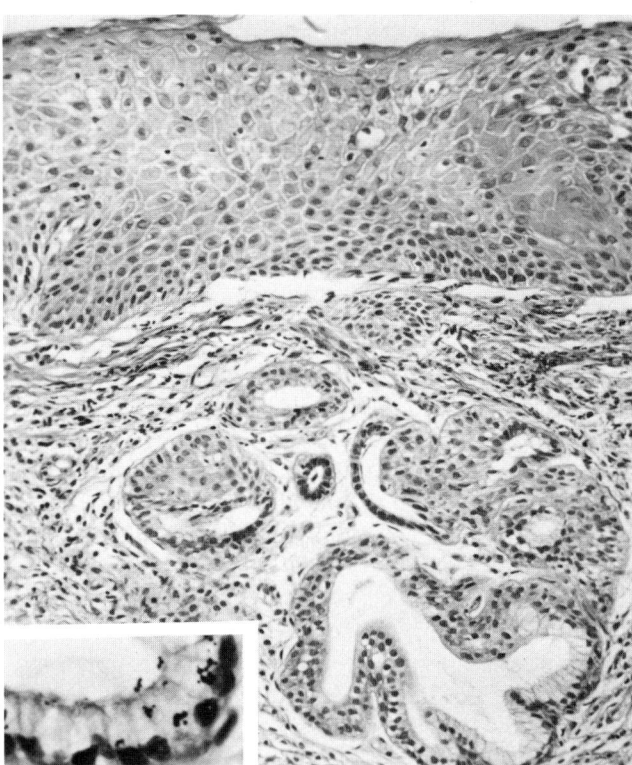

FIG. 4.11. Vaginal adenosis. Mucinous gland with focal squamous metaplasia in lamina propria. *Inset:* Detail of individual mucinous columnar cells.

These cells usually are found in glands in the lamina propria and not on the surface of the vagina. Although adenosis in the lower vagina is rare, the percentage of biopsy specimens with adenosis that exhibit tuboendometrial cells in comparison with mucinous cells increases markedly in frequency. Mucinous glands and mucinous pools or droplets are encountered frequently in the same biopsy specimen; mucinous and tuboendometrial cells are found together only occasionally in biopsy material.

In most biopsy specimens, metaplastic squamous cells replace adenosis to some degree (Fig. 4.11), indicating the manner by which adenosis regresses. Squamous metaplasia, a reactive and physiologic process, begins as reserve cell proliferation, then progresses through immature and mature stages. The glandular epithelium gradually disappears, and intercellular pools of mucin and droplets remain as the final vestiges of adenosis. When completely replaced by squamous epithelium, obliterated glands appear in the lamina propria as squamous pegs, which are continuous with the metaplastic squamous epithelium covering the surface (Fig. 4.13). Eventual maturation of the metaplastic squamous epithelium with acquisition of glycogen makes it indistinguishable from the normal (native) squamous epithelium.

Follow-up studies in which the same subjects have been examined repeatedly over a period of several years have

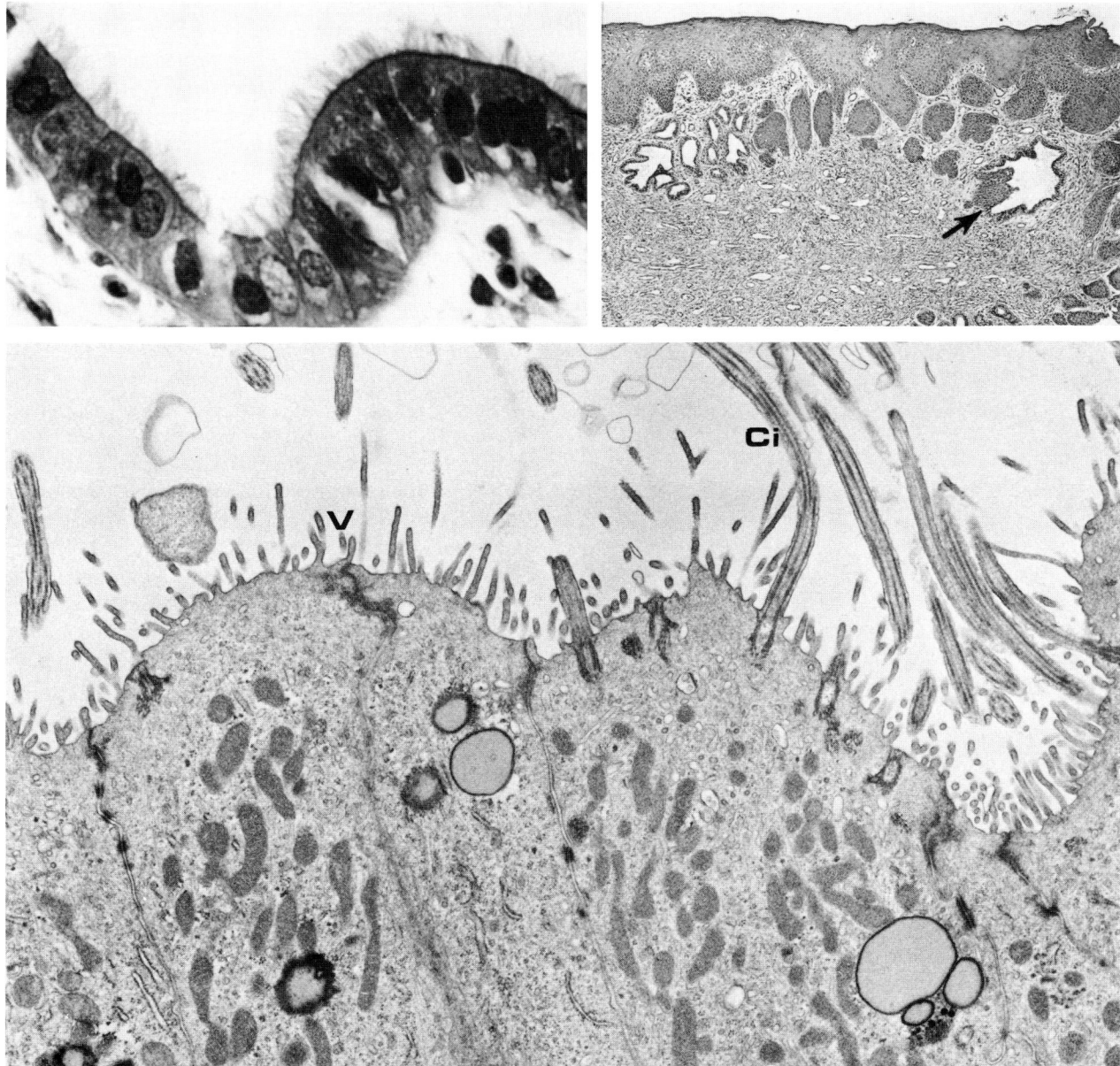

Fig. 4.12. Vaginal adenosis. *Upper right:* Glands lined by ciliated dark cells similar to tubal or endometrial epithelium are present in inflamed lamina propria and merge with squamous pegs (*arrow*). Surface epithelium is composed of glycogen-free squamous cells, accounting for abnormal iodine staining. *Upper left:* Detail of ciliated dark (tuboendometrial) cells. *Bottom:* Tu-boendometrial cells are tall columnar and have orderly arrangement and distribution of organelles, some, e.g., mitochondria, in a supranuclear location. Many cilia (*Ci*) are in apex. Microvilli (*V*) are numerous and regularly distributed along luminal surface. (Reprinted by permission of Dickersin et al., ref. 68.)

indicated that adenosis, structural changes, and VECs may regress spontaneously.[7,238,290] After 3 years of follow-up, the hoods had disappeared in more than half the participants (Fig. 4.14). The extent of VEC did not increase with time. Because VECs disappear spontaneously, they should not be treated.

THE EMBRYOLOGIC BASIS OF VAGINAL ADENOSIS AND CERVICAL ECTROPION

The DES experience and the experimental studies it has fostered have provided new insights into the development of the normal lower genital tract and the effects caused by

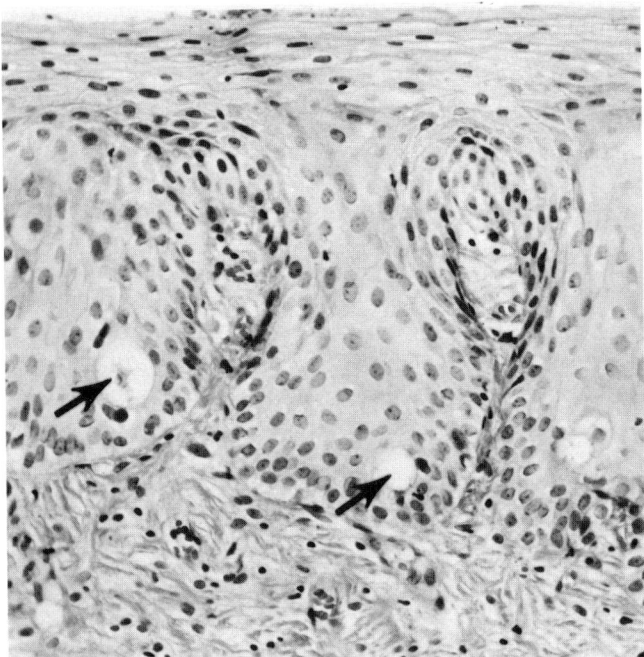

FIG. 4.13. Squamous pegs. Nests of metaplastic squamous cells are present in lamina propria and are continuous with surface epithelium. Intracellular droplets of mucin (*arrows*) represent final vestiges of healing process of adenosis. (Reprinted by permission of Robboy et al., ref. 284.)

prenatal DES exposure.[281] In brief, the embryonic transitional squamous epithelium of the urogenital sinus is now believed to extend up the vagina and exocervix, replacing the original columnar (müllerian) epithelium lining these organs. Estrogen appears to affect the stroma, which then inhibits the upgrowth, and hence leads to the development of adenosis from persistent residual embryonic glandular epithelium. The stroma of the vaginal wall (like the uterine corpus and fallopian tube) induces the growth of a tuboendometrial-type epithelium. The stroma of the superficial endocervix favors mucinous columnar epithelium. In the DES-exposed woman, the embryonic müllerian epithelium that has not been replaced by sinus epithelium differentiates into predominantly mucinous epithelium in the upper vagina and predominantly tuboendometrial epithelium in the lower vagina. In DES-exposed fetal organs, the stromal components of the uterine wall fail to segregate normally into an outer layer of smooth muscle and an inner layer of endometrial stroma.[291,332]

Imperforate Hymen

Imperforate hymen probably represents the most common significant congenital anomaly of the vagina. Its frequency is reported to be about 1 in 2000 female patients. The presence of a thick mucoid secretion that distends the vagina may provide a clue to diagnosis in the neonate, but often an imperforate hymen is not recognized until puberty, when there is retention of menstrual detritus. If not corrected promptly, infertility may result from endometriosis and pelvic adhesions associated with retrograde menstruation.[351]

Vaginal Agenesis

Complete vaginal agenesis is relatively rare, occurring in about 1 in 5000 female births.[71] As an isolated defect it results from incomplete caudal development and fusion of the lower part of the müllerian ducts (müllerian dysgenesis). The external genitalia usually appear normal, except for the introitus, where a short blind pouch may be present.[351]

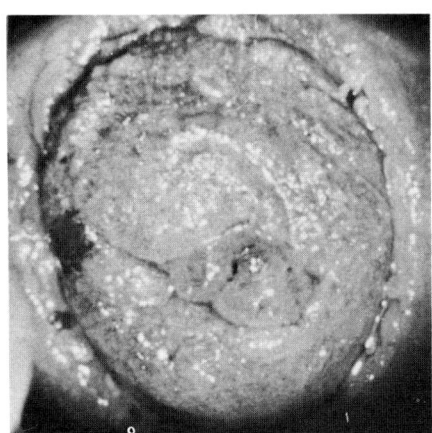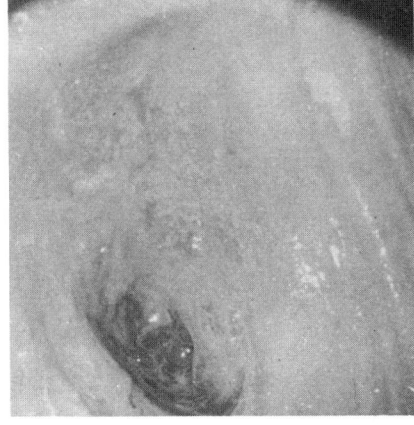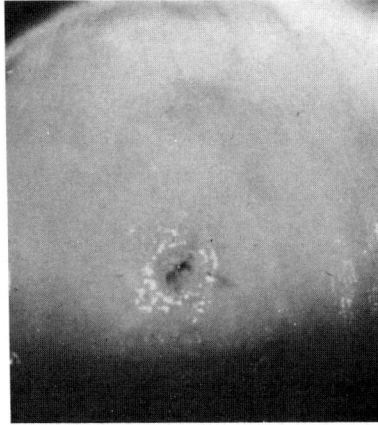

FIG. 4.14. Serial colpophotographs of cervix. *Left:* Portio of cervix displaying extensive ectropion. Cervical rim is circumferential and covered with columnar epithelium. Note prominent groove demarcating it from portio vaginalis. *Middle:* After 24 months, much of rim has disappeared and 70% of the ectropion has been replaced by metaplastic epithelium. Groove is obliterated between 9 and 4 o'clock. *Right:* Forty-two months after initial observation, entire portio vaginalis covered by metaplastic epithelium, with rim completely obliterated. (Reprinted by permission of Antonioli et al., ref. 7.)

Therapy usually involves construction of an artifical vagina. Although this rarely results in a specimen for pathologic examination, the defect often is associated with the absence of the uterus and fallopian tubes (müllerian agenesis or Mayer–Rokitansky–Kuster–Hauser syndrome),[83] and with anomalies of the urinary tract.[242] The latter syndrome provides insight into embryologic development and demonstrates that an intact mesonephric duct is required for the growth and caudal lengthening of the müllerian duct during fetal life. Since the gonads are not of müllerian origin, they usually are normal. About 25% of women with vaginal agenesis have a uterus and they may have complications from retrograde menstruation.

Transverse Vaginal Septum

A transverse vaginal septum is uncommon, occurring anywhere within the vagina, but most frequently at the junction of the cranial and middle thirds.[251,351] It presumably results from incomplete migration or excavation of the vaginal plate. A complete vaginal septum results in obstructive symptoms similar to an imperforate hymen, whereas a partial septum may allow passage of menstrual flow, but cause dyspareunia or laceration during childbirth. The microscopic appearance of the septum is typically that of a fibrovascular stroma covered on two surfaces by epithelium. Although the caudal surface is covered by a stratified nonkeratinizing squamous epithelium, the cranial aspect is covered typically by glandular epithelium, as might be predicted from the embryologic development.

Miscellaneous Congenital Disorders

Complete duplication of the vagina with a septum including muscularis extending to the introitus is rare, and typically is accompanied by cervical and uterine duplication. Longitudinal septa that lack a muscular layer are more common. They often are clinically asymptomatic. Congenital rectovaginal fistulas often are associated with an imperforate anus. Typically, the anus opens into the posterior caudal portion of the vagina, near the forchette.[251,351]

Infectious Inflammatory Disorders

The normal vaginal flora is varied and changes from birth through menarche to menopause. Although it has long been evident that Lactobacilli split glycogen to form lactic acid, thus reducing the pH of the vagina, this does not provide a complete explanation for the regulation of the vaginal flora. The ecosystem reflects a delicate balance that includes the interplay of steroid hormones, vascularity, vaginal acidity, and glycogen.[98] It can be upset easily by commonly occurring mechanical, chemical, or hormonal manipulation. Approximately 10^9 obligate anaerobic and 10^8 facultative bacteria are present in a gram of vaginal secretion, of which Lactobacilli probably are the most common.[209] Three hundred and forty five organisms were represented in 52 specimens collected from healthy adults, including the following anaerobes: *Peptococcus, Bacteroides, Peptostreptococcus, Lactobacillus, Eubacterium* spp., and aerobes: *Stapylococcus epidermidis, Corynebacterium* spp., and *Lactobacillus* sp.[15,98] The proportion of aerobic organisms decreases about 100-fold during the week before menses. During pregnancy, more Lactobacilli and yeast, but fewer anaerobic bacteria, are present.[200] On the third day after parturition, there is a dramatic increase in the number of anaerobic bacteria. Postmenopausal women also have a relatively larger proportion of anaerobes, with more Lactobacilli recovered from those treated with estrogen.[188] Organisms that at times are associated with vaginitis may colonize the vagina of healthy, asymptomatic women.[128]

Vaginitis

Vaginitis is the most common reason for a patient to visit her gynecologist, accounting for more than 10 million office visits each year.[174] Abnormal colonization or invasive infection has been reported for practically all major types of organisms, including viruses, bacteria, fungi, and parasites. It is difficult to determine the most common organism responsible for vaginitis, since frequency lists vary according to age, sexual activity, and method of microbial identification.[82,89,104,307,317] Currently, more than 20 bacterial, viral, and protozoan agents are considered to be responsible for sexually transmitted diseases (STDs) (Table 4.1). Since notification that one has an STD frequently evokes a strong emotional response, it is important to remember that the distinction between sexually and nonsexually transmitted disease is at times arbitrary. Whereas many infectious agents make use of the opportunity afforded by close apposition of mucous membranes or secretions in order to spread, there is variability in the stringency of their demands.

The clinical diagnosis of vaginitis frequently is based on the presence of a vaginal discharge. Reliance on this finding alone may lead to overdiagnosis, since the production of vaginal fluid is a physiologic event caused by transudation of fluid through the vaginal wall, with additional contributions by cervical and uterine secretions, exfoliated epithelial cells, bacteria, and bacterial products. This is particularly noticeable at midcycle when cervical mucus becomes watery and profuse, and often is interpreted erroneously as a "discharge." Other relatively nonspecific criteria of vaginitis include subjective assessment of the color, odor, quantity, or quality of the discharge.[82] In contrast to discharge caused by vaginitis, normal vaginal secretions are floccular rather than homogeneous, and neither malodorous nor associated with pruritis. Although accurate diagno-

Table 4.1. Sexually
transmitted pathogens

Bacterial agents
  N. gonorrhoeae
  C. trachomatis
  M. hominis
  U. urealyticum
  T. pallidum
  G. vaginalis
  H. ducreyi
  Shigella
  Campylobacter
  Group B Streptococcus
Fungal agents
  C. albicans
Viral agents
  Herpes simplex virus
  Hepatitis B virus
  Cytomegalovirus
  Human papilloma virus
  Molluscum contagiosum virus
Protozoan agents
  T. vaginalis
  E. histolytica
  G. lamblia
Ectoparasites
  P. pubis
  S. scabiei

Saline or potassium hydroxide suspensions of a discharge containing blastospores and pseudohyphae permit a presumptive microscopic diagnosis to be made immediately. Unfortunately, the sensitivity of wet prep exam is only about 65%,[221] and the morphologic appearance is not entirely specific. In one study, Papanicolaou-stained smears demonstrated the organism in 46% of infected patients, compared with 85% for the wet prep and 94% for culture.[220] In daily practice, it is the experience of the examiner that seems to be the most critical determinant for accurate recognition of the organism. Definitive identification of the fungus is made by culture.

Biopsies, which are rarely obtained, contain relatively dense infiltrates of primarily mononuclear inflammatory cells and congested blood vessels in the stroma, with exocytosis of neutrophils into the overlying epithelium (Figs. 4.15, 4.16).[170] Candida generally are not identifiable unless the discharge remains adherent, where the organisms are visualized as yeast and pseudohyphae intertwined among the desquamated squamous cells.[21] First-line therapy of topical imidazole derivatives, sometimes coupled with initial topical application of gentian violet, has been used for the past 20 years.[89] The recent introduction of triazols

sis of vaginitis does not require a biopsy, some infectious agents cause highly specific tissue reactions, with which the pathologist should be familiar.

Candida

Candida albicans probably is the most common potential or active pathogen in the female genital tract.[159] Between 1980 and 1990 the frequency has nearly doubled. *C. albicans* is found frequently in the colon of healthy individuals, and spread from the contaminated perineum probably is the usual method of introduction of the organism into the vagina.[149,160] Interestingly, fomites from bathtubs or toilet seats do not appear to be a common mechanism for transmission.[6] Sexual transmission plays a role in some patients, resulting from either penile–genital or oral–genital transmission.[89] About 4% of healthy, asymptomatic women harbor candida in the vagina. Factors associated with an increased risk of developing symptomatic infection include pregnancy, oral contraceptive use, antibiotic therapy, diabetes mellitus, and tight-fitting clothes. A deficient cellular immune response has been identified in some women with chronic candidal vaginitis.[330] Changes in the vaginal flora likely play a role in the development of candidiasis.

Vulvar pruritis is the typical presenting symptom, often accompanied by a white, granular, vaginal discharge. The vagina appears reddened, and superficial erosion of the mucosa may be evident after removal of a pseudomembrane of adherent granular debris.

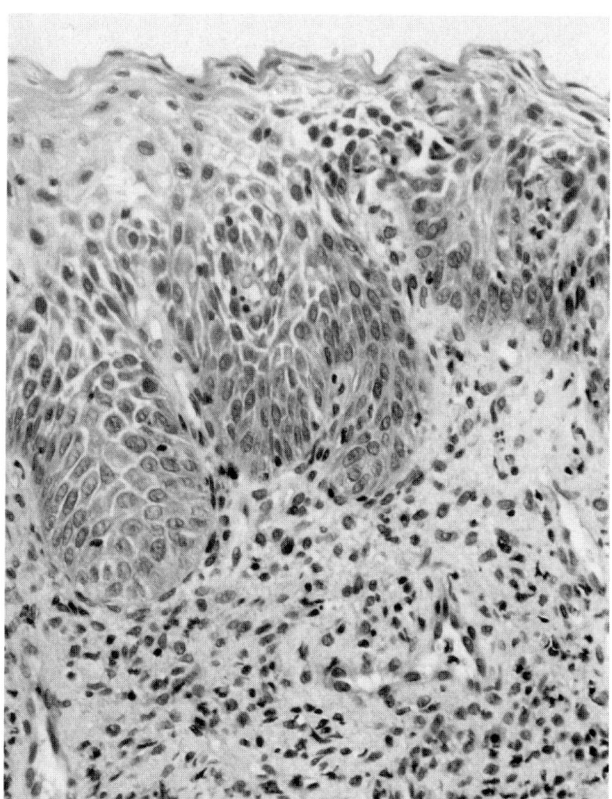

FIG. 4.15. Vaginitis due to *Candida* or *Trichomonas.* The histologic changes, including variably dense infiltrates of mononuclear inflammatory cells in the stroma and neutrophils in the epithelium, are similar for both organisms.

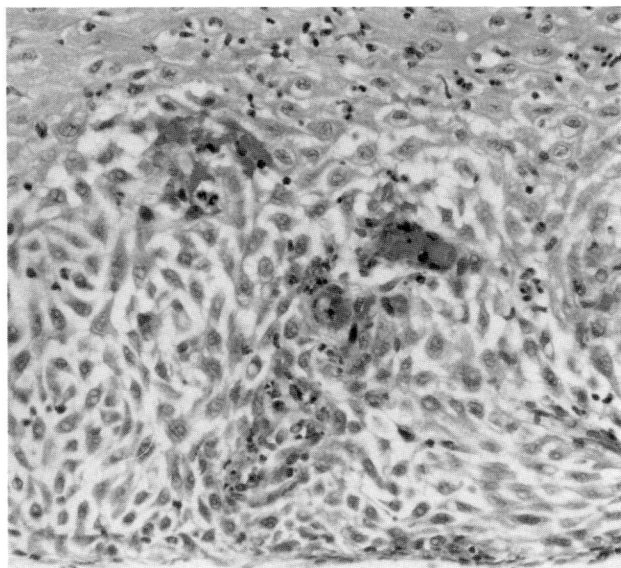

Fig. 4.16. Vaginitis due to *Candida* or *Trichononas*. Pronounced intercellular edema (spongiosis) of the vaginal and cervical squamous epithelium with exocytosis of acute inflammatory cells may occur with infection by either *Candida* or *Trichomonas*.

permits equally effective therapy of shorter duration. However, recurrence remains common and is not confined to those with predisposing conditions.

Candidal species other than *C. albicans* are responsible for at least one-third of cases of fungal vaginitis,[156,173,340] and infection with *C. tropicalis* is associated with a high rate of recurrence.[156] *C. glabrata* typically produces milder symptoms than *C. albicans*,[23] but *C. glabrata* has been reported to cause a severe ulcerative vaginitis simulating malignancy.[46] The microscopic appearances of most candida species are similar, but *C. glabrata* produces only yeasts (blastospores), which are slightly smaller than those of *C. albicans*.[23,340]

Bacterial Vaginosis

Organisms such as trichomonas and candida have long been known to produce vaginitis; however, until recently there have been a substantial number of women who have a copious vaginal discharge or pruritis in the absence of a readily identifiable pathogen. The diagnosis of bacterial vaginosis is made if three of the following four criteria are present: (1) homogeneous, thin, malodorous discharge, (2) vaginal pH >4.5, (3) vaginal epithelial cells with numerous attached bacteria ("clue" cells), and (4) fishy odor upon alkalinization of vaginal secretions.[4] In the past, this condition was designated nonspecific vaginitis, but the term *bacterial vaginosis* currently is preferred, since evidence of inflammation is typically absent.[209] *Gardnerella*, a gram-

negative bacillus, has been isolated from women with vaginosis at a higher rate than asymptomatic women, and thus was considered to be responsible for nonspecific vaginitis.[103,104,197] However, more recent studies cast doubt on this concept, since this organism and "clue" cells have been identified at times with similar frequency in healthy women without vaginal discharge.[195,215,320] Currently, it is believed that bacterial vaginosis is not an infection by a single organism, but rather an overgrowth of multiple colonizing bacteria including *Gardnerella* and a variety of anaerobes.[258,339,358] The flora typically found in affected women includes not only disproportionately large numbers of *Gardnerella vaginalis*, but also abundant *Bacteroides bivius*, *Mycoplasma hominis*, *Mobiluncus mulieris*, and *Mobiluncus curtisii*.[148,209,335] In an animal model, the inoculation of *Gardnerella* and *Mobiluncus* together caused the clinical disease, although neither alone was capable of doing so.[210] The diagnosis usually is confirmed by elimination of other pathogens, combined with identification of gram-negative to gram-variable bacilli and "clue" cells on wet mount or smears, or by culture.[110,170,337,365] No specific histopathologic features have been described.

Efforts to restore the local environment by topical administration of acetic acid, estrogen, or fermented milk products have been ineffective. In contrast, antimicrobial therapy with metronidazole or intravaginal clindamycin produces clinical cure in most women, further supporting the concept that anaerobes acting with *Gardnerella* produce bacterial vaginosis.[320] The initiating cause remains unknown, but sexual transmission occurs in some instances.[170,189,320] Although the disease usually carries no appreciable morbidity, bacterial vaginosis during pregnancy has been significantly associated with premature rupture of membranes and chorioamnionitis.[189]

Trichomonas Vaginalis

Trichomoniasis is responsible for more than 2.5 million infections per year in the United States, and about 180 million infections worldwide.[338] It is found in about 10% of asymptomatic women, and almost 50% of those attending STD clinics.[327] The organism is almost always sexually transmitted,[227] although trichomonads reportedly may survive in tap water, soap water, and chlorinated swimming pools.[89] The mechanism by which *Trichomonas* causes disease is unknown, but the organisms are found both in the vaginal lumen and adherent to squamous, but not columnar, epithelial cells.[277] Invasion of the squamous mucosa does not occur. *Trichomonas* is a strict anaerobe and there frequently is an alteration in the associated vaginal flora, with increased anaerobic bacteria.[353] Although the role of sex steroids is unclear, infection is generally lower in women taking oral contraceptives.[28]

Symptoms of infection include vaginal discharge, intense pruritis, and dyspareunia, with exacerbations often temporarlly related to menses. However, in one study, only 17% of culture-positive women noted pruritis, and more than one-third did not even complain of a vaginal discharge.[219] When present, the vaginal discharge usually is copious, homogeneous, yellow green to gray, and malodorous. Typically, the vaginal mucosa is erythematous and punctate hemorrhages may be present, particularly on the cervical mucosa, leading to what is unfortunately described as a "strawberry cervix."

The diagnosis usually is made by the microscopic identification of motile organisms accompanied by many neutrophils in a saline preparation. The protozoan is ovoid, about 10–20 μm in diameter, with polar flagella. Active motility, in the form of a jerky swaying motion, is provided by the flagella and undulating membrane. If the wet prep diagnosis is based on the presence of motile organisms, the specificity approaches 100%. Trichomonads also may be found in Papanicolaou-stained vaginal smears in about 70% of cases, a sensitivity similar to that of the wet prep.[204,318] Culture methods are available,[233] expensive, and generally unnecessary. The organism is not detectable in biopsy specimens from culture-positive women, although an inflammatory response of variable intensity may be seen, including dilated vessels in the stroma, accompanied by dense infiltrates of plasma cells and lymphocytes (Fig. 4.15). The ectocervical as well as vagina mucosa is commonly spongiotic (Fig. 4.16).[177] Neutrophils frequently are present in large numbers among the squamous cells, sometimes forming intraepithelial abscesses. There may be irregular acanthosis of the epithelium, with pseuodepitheliomatous hyperplasia. A fibrinopurulent exudate composed of necrotic debris, neutrophils, and lymphocytes is found in foci of ulceration. Metronidazole provides effective therapy, although recurrence is common if the typically asymptomatic male partner is not also treated.

Acquired Immunodeficiency Syndrome

Currently, acquired immunodeficiency syndrome (AIDS) is one of the leading causes of death among women of reproductive age in the United States (Fig. 4.17). Between 1981 and 1991, there were 168,000 cases of AIDS reported in the United States, about 10% of which occurred in females.[44] Although there are no gross or histopathologic changes of AIDS specific to the vagina, the pathologist should be aware that about one-third of adult women with AIDS have acquired the disease through heterosexual contact. The proportion due to heterosexual transmission is increasing, and worldwide probably accounts for the great majority of human immunodeficiency virus (HIV) infections.[198] Most HIV infections resulting from heterosexual contact have occurred in women who reported only vaginal intercourse.[253] The virus has been identified in both semen and cell-free seminal fluid.[198] Certain sexually transmitted diseases are considered to be risk factors for sexual transmission of HIV, particularly those that cause ulceration of the vaginal mucosa, permitting access of the virus to the blood.[44] By use of polymerase chain reaction (PCR)–amplified in situ hybridization, HIV has been identified in macrophages of the submucosal and deep stroma near the transformation zone of the cervix (J. Nuovo, personal communication). Recently, localization of simian immunodeficiency virus (SIV) in dendritic cells of the monkey vagina has been demonstrated in an experimental model, suggesting that heterosexual transmission of HIV may occur across an intact mucosa.[223]

Group B Streptococcus

Group B streptococci (*Streptococcus agalactiae*) can be found in 5–35% of normal females[11,73,154,374] and thus are

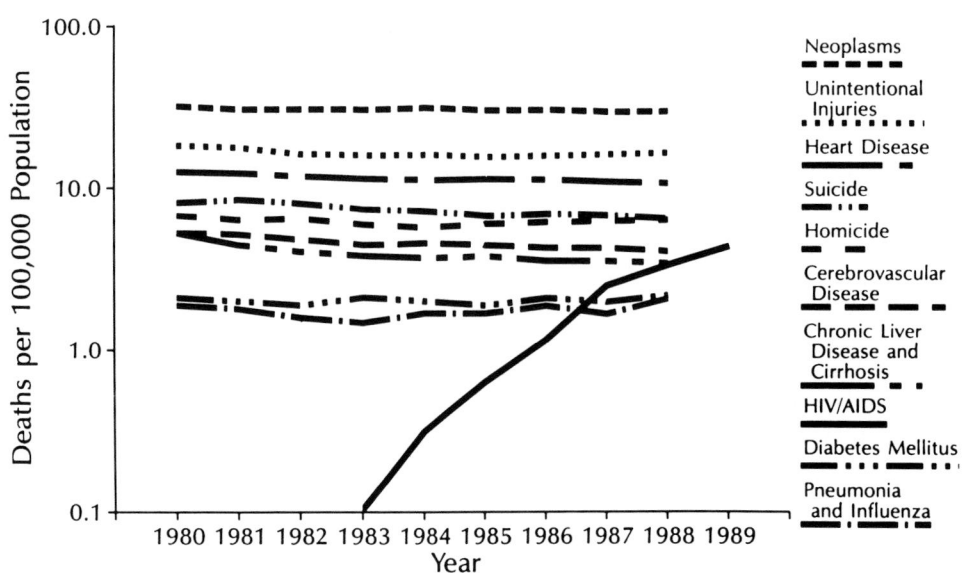

FIG. 4.17. **Leading causes of death among women 25–44 years of age in the United States, 1981–1989.** Data source: National Vital Statistics, NCHS, CDC. (From Epidemiology of HIV in the United States, in *AIDS: Etiology, Diagnosis, Treatment, and Prevention,* Philadelphia, JB Lippincott, 1992.)

considered to be part of the normal vaginal flora. These bacteria frequently are sexually transmitted,[147] although they also can ascend from the lower intestinal tract, which may serve as a reservoir.[69] Although Group B streptococcal colonization of the vagina or urethra usually causes little morbidity to the adult female, a vaginitis at times may occur.[147] Histopathologic changes resulting from vaginal infection by Group B streptococci have not been well described. More significantly, this organisms is a frequent cause of abortion, chorioamnionitis, premature rupture of membranes, perinatal death, and intrapartum and postpartum bacteremia.[153,328] For reasons that currently are unknown, only a small proportion of colonized mothers or infants develop symptomatic infection.[328]

Actinomycetes

Actinomycetes have been implicated in upper genital tract infections in women wearing intrauterine contraceptive devices, but also are found in the vagina of about one-quarter of women without such devices. These organisms represent part of the normal oral and colonic flora, from which it may be introduced into the vagina. Vaginitis subsequently occurs when overgrowth is favored by the presence of a foreign body.[60,125] Actinomycetes are recognized in Papanicolaou-stained smears and tissue sections as a dense mass of fine, blue, filamentous bacteria, using radiating from a central core.

Malacoplakia and Xanthogranulomatous Pseudotumor

Malacoplakia and xanthogranulomatous pseudotumor of the vagina are closely related entities resulting from infection by gram-negative bacilli, usually *Escherichia coli*.[176,199,322,354] Typically, yellow polypoid nodules arise from the vaginal mucosa, at times accompanied by a discharge. The microscopic findings are identical to those described in other body sites, and include the presence of large collections of histiocytes with abundant granular to pale foamy cytoplasm (von Hansemann cells), with interspersed plasma cells and lymphocytes. Both intracellular and extracellular, concentrically laminated basophilic masses (Michaelis–Gutmann bodies) are present in variable numbers. The clinical suspicion of tumor may lead the pathologist to the misdiagnosis of a rare neoplasm such as a granular cell tumor, unless care is taken to consider this lesion. The correct diagnosis may be confirmed by the finding of numerous gram-negative rod-like bacteria on tissue gram stain, silver stain, or by electron microscopy.

Tuberculosis

Genital tract tuberculosis is no longer frequent in the United States, but remains a significant problem in Third World nations. The vagina is involved in about only 1% of these women, and patients present with localized ulceration.[235] Characteristic microscopic features include necrotizing granulomata containing Langhans giant cells underlying an ulcerated epithelium.[50]

Emphysematous Vaginitis

Emphysematous vaginitis is a rare entity (about 200 reported cases), characterized by multiple, discrete, gas-filled cystic cavities in the vaginal mucosa. Most patients present with symptoms of vaginal discharge, although some are aware of popping sounds associated with the rupture of the cysts during intercourse. The dramatic presentation and physical findings have prompted an interest disproportionate to the frequency or significance of the disease. There is evidence that it is an unusual manifestation of a common infection in an immunocompromised host.[166,341] No single organism has been identified as the causative agent, although both *Trichomonas vaginalis* and *G. vaginalis* have been implicated.[105] Chemical analyses of the lesions have disclosed a wide variety of gases, including ammonia, hydrogen sulfide, nitrogen, oxygen, carbonic acid, and trimethylamine. The microscopic findings are variable, with cysts in the stroma lined by either multinucleated giant cells, squamous cells, or both. A scattering of chronic inflammatory cells accompanies the cysts.[105,152,179] Bacterial or protozoan production of gas with transmucosal passage into the stroma has been suggested, but the pathogenesis remains obscure.[105,311]

Unusual Types of Bacterial Vaginitis

Occasionally, vaginitis may be caused by bacteria that are commonly pathogenic in other sites. Shigella vulvogaginitis has been identified primarily as a cause of a chronic, sanguinous, purulent vaginal discharge in children, unassociated with intestinal infection.[62,274,305] *Haemophilus influenzae*, *Corynebacterium diphtheria*, and *Neisseria meningitidis* also rarely cause vaginitis in children,[39,77,78,326] but the histologic changes have not been documented. Staphylococcal infection of the vagina after systemic antibiotic therapy was reported more than 30 years ago, and thought to result from a disturbed indigenous flora[187] (see the section on Toxic Shock Syndrome).

Parasitic Vaginitis

Parasitic infection of the vagina, although currently rare in the United States, almost certainly will be encountered more frequently because of greater global travel.

Vaginal amebiasis due to *Entamoeba histolytica* has been reported in Mexico, South Africa, and India, where the infection is endemic.[137,151,226,352] Most patients present with a bloody vaginal discharge. The gross appearance mimics carcinoma, with one or more ulcerated, necrotic growths typically involving the vagina and cervix. Microscopically, the lesions are characterized by ulceration of the epithelium with replacement by a fibrinopurulent exudate containing trophozoites of 15–60 μm in diameter. In cytologic preparations they appear somewhat larger than histiocytes, and approximate the size of parabasal cells. Positive staining with periodic acid-Schiff (PAS) stain or acid phosphatase provides further support for the diagnosis.

Eggs of *Enterobius vermicularis* or *Trichuris trichiura* usually are found after incidental contamination of the vagina associated with intestinal infestation by these worms.[225,345] Eggs and worms of *Schistosoma mansoni* and hematobium have been identified in pelvic tissues including the vagina, presumably reflecting anastomoses between hemorrhoidal and hypogastric veins.[40,107] They elicit a striking host inflammatory response, ultimately resulting in dense fibrosis.

Toxic Shock Syndrome

GENERAL FEATURES

In 1978 Todd et al. described an acute, potentially life-threatening disease characterized by fever, hypotension, headache, confusion, rash, vomiting, diarrhea, and oliguria. The disease was termed *toxic shock syndrome* (TSS) because it was associated with infection with strains of *Staphylococcus* that produced a unique epidermal toxin.[343] By 1980, more than 98% of cases had been related to the use of tampons during menses.[86] The incidence is about 6 cases per 100,000 menstruating women per year. Although *S. aureus* rarely inhabits the vagina normally, it has been isolated from about 75% of women with TSS.[61,216] More recently it has become evident that children or adults with any focal staphylococcal infection are also at risk for TSS, and about 11% of all reported cases are nonmenstrual.[278]

PATHOGENESIS

There is a strong relationship between localized infection with *S. aureus* and the development of TSS. Studies of patients with TSS as well as experimental systems have revealed that some staphylococci elaborate a protein of about 22 kDa termed *toxic shock syndrome toxin 1* (or staphylococcal enterotoxin F), which produces essentially all of the systemic biologic effects.[22] However, TSS can occur in the the absence of this toxin, and other staphylococcal entertotoxins, streptococcal exotoxins, and endotoxins from gram-negative bacteria have been implicated in some cases of TSS.[278,336] The mechanism by which tampon use during menses predisposes to TSS remains some-

what unclear, but it is believed that microulcerations of the vaginal mucosa caused by tampons (see below, Tampon Ulcer) permit the growth of toxin-producing staphylococci. A diminished host immune response to the toxin, access of toxin through a denuded endometrial mucosa, and the normal menstrual phase decrease in lactobacilli that are inhibitory to the growth of staphylococci may facilitate the process.[86,96,134,304] A multifactorial sequence is supported by the observation that some women harbor toxin-producing strains in the vagina without symptoms, whereas other women have recurrent episodes of the illness. A dramatic reduction in the incidence of TTS occurred when Rely superabsorbant tampons were withdrawn from the market in 1980.[182]

CLINICAL FEATURES

The diagnosis of TSS is based on a constellation of clinical features, as follows: fever, hypotension, palmar or diffuse erythroderma followed by desquamation, hyperemia of conjunctivae or mucous membranes of vagina or pharynx, and multisystem dysfunction: vomiting, diarrhea, impaired renal, cerebral, or hepatic function, cardiopulmonary dysfunction, thrombocytopenia, elevated creatine phosphokinase, and decreased serum calcium and phosphate.[61] Vaginal erythema, erosions, or vaginitis, sometimes accompanied by a purulent exudate, typically are present.[275,359] Abdominal or bilateral adnexal tenderness is present in about half of cases.[138]

GROSS AND MICROSCOPIC FINDINGS

The disease is systemic, with pathologic abnormalities described in lung, liver, and kidney, as well as genital tract.[1,246] Ulceration and discoloration of the vaginal and cervical mucosa are present focally. Microscopically, there is extensive desquamation of the epithelium, with underlying subacute vasculitis, perivascular inflammatory cell infiltrates, and platelet thrombi.[1,246] Rare gram-positive cocci have been found in the fibrinopurulent exudate associated with ulcers. Deep tissue invasion by the organisms has not been described.[246]

CLINICAL BEHAVIOR AND TREATMENT

The spectrum of severity of TSS varies from a relatively mild to a rapidly fatal illness, with a mortality rate of about 4%.[329] The treatment includes beta-lactamase–resistant antistaphylococcal antibiotics, and aggressive, supportive measures for systemic manifestations related to shock.[278,359] Intravenous immunoglobulin therapy also has been effective, supporting the concept that the symptoms of TSS result from a toxin that may be neutralized by infused antibodies.[14]

Noninfectious Inflammatory Diseases

The vagina occasionally is the site of involvement by a systemic disease, a generalized disease of squamous mucosa, or by extension from a disease elsewhere in the pelvis.

Desquamative Inflammatory Vaginitis

Desquamative inflammatory vaginitis is the term that has been applied to an unusual process in which bright red, well-delineated areas replace portions of the normal mucosa of the cranial half of the vagina. A pseudomembrane at times replaces the ulcerated mucosa.[102,171,214] A copious, purulent to hemorrhagic vaginal discharge is present, smears of which display numerous neutrophils and a high proportion of parabasal cells. The women usually are premenopausal, and have normal serum estrogen levels. The etiology is unknown, and no single bacterial or viral agent has been identified. A history of tampon use was not provided in the cases described. There typically is little response to antibiotic or estrogen therapy.

Ligneous Vaginitis

Ligneous conjunctivitis is a rare, chronic inflammatory condition of unknown pathogenesis that usually involves the conjunctivae beginning in childhood. In the acute phase there frequently is an associated nasopharyngitis or vulvovaginitis. The chronic phase is characterized by asymptomatic sessile or pedunculated yellow-white to red firm masses on the conjunctiva. Histologically, these represent subepithelial accumulations of eosinophilic material, which may be accompanied by granulation tissue or chronic inflammatory cell infiltrates. Electron microscopic examination reveals electron-dense homogeneous and fibrillary material. Histologically identical lesions have been reported to coexist in the vagina and cervix.[145,319]

Allergic Reactions to Seminal Fluid

A few women display allergic reactions after exposure to seminal fluid.[37,127,194] The severity of the response varies from localized vulvovaginal urticarial reactions to generalized urticaria and bronchospasm. The onset of symptoms immediately follows contact with seminal fluid, and the duration of the reaction is between 2 and 72 hours.

Crohn Disease

Rectovaginal fistulas occur in some patients with Crohn disease,[79] and in situ squamous carcinoma has been reported in the vaginal and perineal mucosa of a 36-year-old woman with Crohn disease involving the vagina.[270] Vagi-

nal fistulae with the sigmoid colon or cecum after perforation of a diverticulum have been identified in about 1% of women with diverticulosis.[10]

Bullous Dermatoses

Vaginal stenosis may develop as a sequela of severe bullous erythema multiforme (Stevens–Johnson syndrome) in which extensive vulvar and vaginal ulceration occurred.[116] Acantholytic intraepithelial bullae may be found when there is vaginal involvement by familial benign chronic pemphigus (Hailey–Hailey disease).[350]

Giant Cell Arteritis

Giant cell arteritis is not always limited to the temporal arteries, and may be associated with either generalized or limited visceral involvement. A panarteritis, with fragmentation and destruction of the internal elastic lamella, and phagocytosis of elastic material by multinucleated giant cells may be seen in the vagina as part of limited female genital tract involvement.[18,306]

Thrombotic Thrombocytopenic Purpura

Massive, acute hemorrhagic necrosis of the vagina has been reported as one of the initial manifestations of thrombotic thrombocytopenic purpura.[100] The disease usually is characterized by the pentad of fever, microangiopathic hemolytic anemia, thrombocytopenia, neurologic symptoms, and renal dysfunction. Numerous thrombi are found microscopically in the vaginal stroma, accompanied by superficial hemorrhage and necrosis and sloughing of the epithelium.

Lesions That Follow Trauma, Surgery, and Radiation

Atrophic Vaginitis

Atrophy of the squamous epithelium of the vagina, accompanied by loss of glycogen and an increase in the pH, are physiologic events in postmenopausal women that reflect estrogen deprivation. The response also includes a change in the vaginal flora, with a reduction in the lactobacilli that ordinarily inhibit other potential pathogens. The thin epithelium seems to offer little resistance to an altered flora which may include streptococci, staphylococci, *E. coli*, and diphtheroids.[17] As a result, minor trauma may facilitate a transition from simple atrophy to atrophic vaginitis. Many patients are asymptomatic, but there may be minor vaginal bleeding, pruritis, dysuria, or dyspareunia, accompanied at times by a watery discharge. Atrophy of the vagina produces a pale-appearing mucosa, with petechiae and loss of rugal folds. Microscopically, there is a variable reduction or loss of the superficial and intermediate cell layers. Small ulcers with acute inflammation and granulation tissue may be interspersed among regions of intact epithelium. Elsewhere, the submucosa is infiltrated by lymphocytes and plasma cells (Fig. 4.18).[171] Although the histologic changes are relatively straightforward, occasionally there is confusion of atrophy with a high grade squamous intraepithelial lesion (see below, Vaginal Intraepithelial Neoplasia). There usually is a good response to estrogen replacement, with epithelial cell maturation and a return to premenopausal flora and pH. Antibiotic therapy rarely is necessary.

Tampon Ulcer

Although tampons have been in use for 60 years, there had been little interest in their effects on the vagina until about 1980, when mucosal ulceration and TSS were related to their use. In several series of cases, the women presented with abnormal vaginal discharge or intermenstrual bleeding. Typically, a single ulcer with an irregular border of granulation tissue was identified in one of the vaginal fornices. After neoplasms and infectious etiologies were excluded, a more detailed history revealed the frequent use of tampons. Microscopically, some of the ulcers contained fibrillar foreign bodies within the exudate.[163] The lesions healed spontaneously within 2–3 months after discontinuation of tampon usage.[131,163] Subsequently, Friedrich

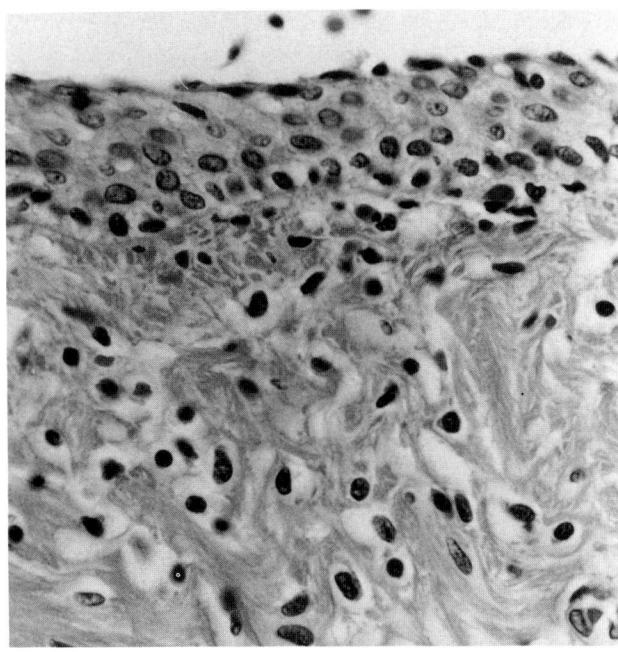

Fig. 4.18. Atrophic vaginitis. In addition to profound atrophy of the epithelium, there is dense infiltration of the stroma by chronic inflammatory cells.

studied the vagina during tampon use, and characterized a sequence of clinically asymptomatic, colposcopic, and microscopic changes as follows: (1) mucosal dehydration, (2) layering or intraepithelial cleavage, and (3) microulceration.[88,90] Ultrastructural findings include a widening of the intercellular spaces separating squamous cells and a marked reduction in the number of desmosomes. He suggested that these changes resulted from a fluid shift across the vaginal epithelium due to the absorbant qualities of the tampon. This hypothesis explains the higher frequency of mucosal alteration with the use of superabsorbant tampons. The great frequency with which tampons induce clinically inapparent vaginal microulcerations helps to explain their relationship to superficial staphylococcal infections and the development of TSS.

Postoperative Spindle Cell Nodule

In 1984, Proppe et al. described a lesion of the lower genitourinary tract that closely simulated a sarcoma histologically, but was benign.[271] The term *postoperative spindle cell nodule* was applied to the lesion because typically it arose within 1–3 months of surgery in the region, and usually presented as polypoid, poorly defined nodules. The microscopic appearance is characterized by intersecting fascicles of plump spindle cells with a delicate network of small blood vessels, sometimes accompanied by extravasated blood or hemosiderin (Fig. 4.19). Superficial ulceration may be present, and chronic inflammatory cells are scattered in the deeper portions of the lesions. The spindle cells have oval, elongated nuclei with evenly dispersed chromatin and abundant eosinophilic cytoplasm. Since mitotic figures are numerous and the lesions are poorly circumscribed, they may easily be confused with sarcoma (Fig. 4.20). Helpful distinguishing features include the lack of nuclear pleomorphism or nuclear hyperchromasia, absence of abnormal mitotic figures, and the clinical history of a recent surgical procedure in the region of the lesion.[271] Local recurrence has not been reported, even after incomplete resection.[124,271] Lesions of similar histologic appearance have been reported in the urinary tract in the absence of a clinical history of surgery or instrumentation.[372]

Vaginal Vault Granulation Tissue

Vaginal vault granulation tissue is a common finding after hysterectomy.[121] One or more small, red, granular to polypoid lesions may be seen grossly, which microscopically are composed of ulcerated, edematous, granulation tissue containing numerous neutrophils superficially and lymphocytes and plasma cells in the deeper stroma. Occasionally, scattered bizarre stromal cells may cause confusion with a malignant neoplasm (Fig. 4.21), particularly if the hysterectomy has been performed for a cervical or corpus tumor.

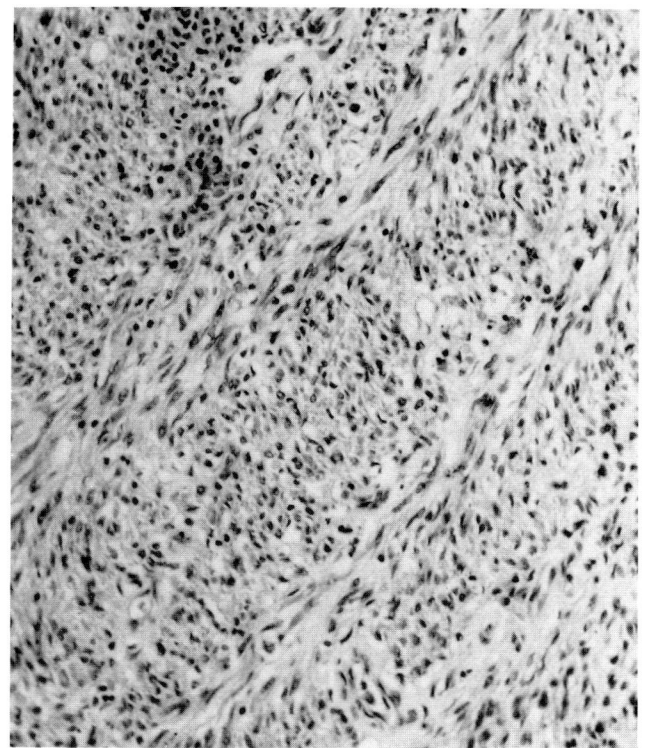

FIG. 4.19. **Postoperative spindle cell nodule.** The lesion is characterized by intersecting fascicles of plump spindle cells. (Courtesy of Robert E. Scully, M.D., Boston, MA)

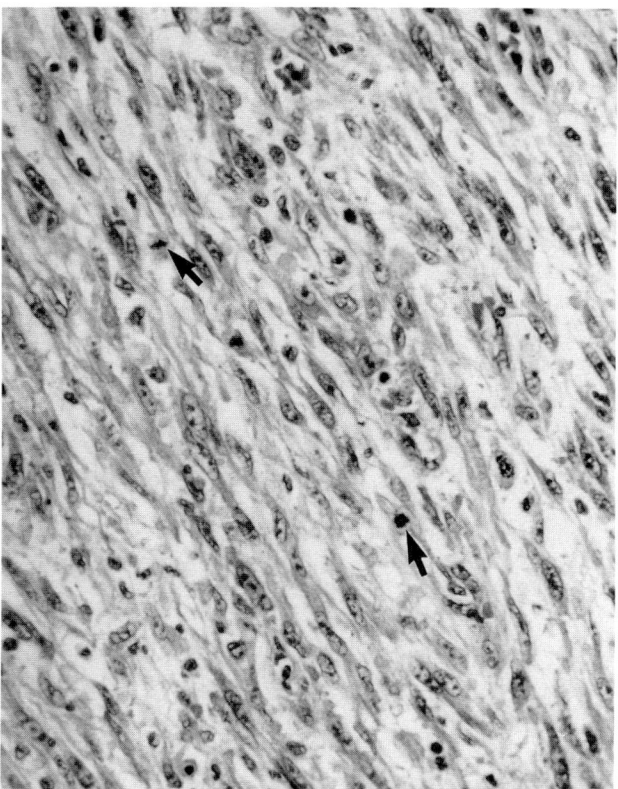

FIG. 4.20. **Postoperative spindle cell nodule.** The cells contain oval nuclei with delicate chromatin and distinct nucleoli. There are numerous mitotic figures (*arrows*). (Courtesy of Robert E. Scully, M.D., Boston, MA.)

Fistula

Vesicovaginal and ureterovaginal fistulas may occur as a complication of hysterectomy, resulting from ischemic necrosis secondary to interruption of the vascular supply.[211,333] The surgical correction usually yields small fragments of tissue with variable amounts of granulation tissue, fibrosis, chronic inflammation, and little or no epithelium. Rarely calculi are present. These are composed of urinary salts that develop in the vagina because of continuous leakage of urine from a vesicovaginal fistula.[273] Vesicovaginal fistula and vaginal laceration also may be a consequence of coitus.[81,240]

Radionecrosis

Radiation therapy to the vulva, vagina, or uterine cervix may cause necrosis, ulceration, or stenosis of the vagina.[131,296] The mechanism by which this injury develops reflects the sensitivity of endothelial cells to radiation, with thrombosis, and subsequent stenosis or obliteration of small blood vessels, stromal fibrosis, and epithelial ulceration. The formation of granular to polypoid masses, particularly in the vaginal vault, may clinically simulate recurrent cervical carcinoma. In addition to the vascular changes, dense infiltrates of plasma cells, granulation tis-

sue, and bizarre stromal cells with pleomorphic, hyperchromatic nuclei may be sprinkled through the stroma. Even in the absence of a gross lesion, one may anticipate extreme atrophy of the vaginal squamous mucosa as a consequence of radiation therapy combined with cessation of ovarian function (Fig. 4.22).[171] Careful examination of nuclear detail helps to distinguish radiation atrophy from intraepithelial carcinoma. Atrophic cells have high nuclear/cytoplasmic ratios such as those of intraepithelial carcinoma, but have a regular, round to oval nuclear shape with a uniform distribution of chromatin that may appear smudged, in contrast to the irregular nuclear contours and clumped chromatin of vaginal intraepithelial neoplasia. Occasionally, radiation may result in partially obliterated vascular channels lined by plump endothelial cells containing large nuclei with vesicular chromatin, which simulate cords of invasive carcinoma. The distinction may be assisted by immunohistochemistry. Although a positive immunostaining reaction is not always present, the localization of Factor VIII antigen in the atypical cells coupled with the absence of staining for keratins provides evidence for reactive endothelial rather than epithelial cells.

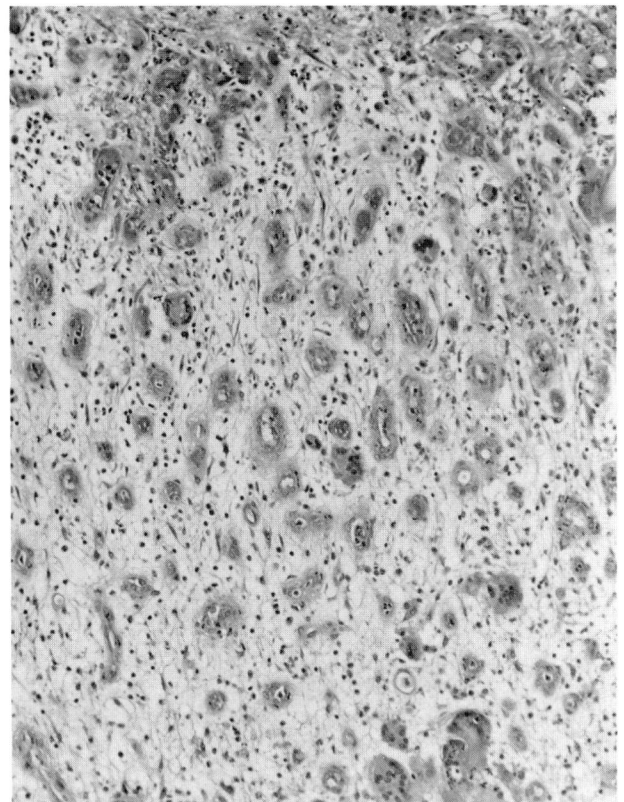

FIG. 4.21. **Granulation tissue.** Scattered bizarre stromal cells and prominent endothelial cells may simulate adenocarcinoma.

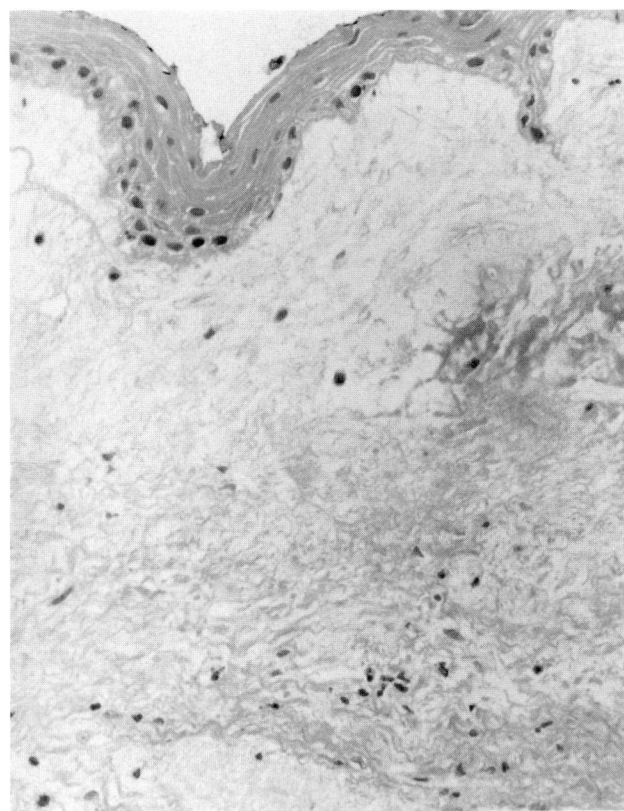

FIG. 4.22. **Radiation change.** Long-term consequences of irradiation to the vagina include atrophy of the squamous epithelium, edema, fibrosis within the stroma, and obliteration of vascular channels.

Vaginal Prolapse

Cystocele, rectocele, and vaginal prolapse may occur after multiple vaginal deliveries.[17] The surgical correction may include removal of elliptical fragments of vaginal mucosa in which variable degrees of acanthosis, hyperkeratosis, or parakeratosis are present (Fig. 4.23).

Fallopian Tube Prolapse

Prolapse of the fallopian tube into the vagina is a relatively uncommon complication of either vaginal or abdominal hysterectomy.[315,366] Patients often present with abdominal pain, vaginal discharge, or vaginal bleeding. A red, granular mass usually is present at the vaginal apex, which grossly may be confused with granulation tissue or carcinoma. Manipulation of the prolapsed tube typically causes extreme pain. Microscopically, a complex pattern of tubular, glandular, and papillary structures may be present (Fig. 4.24). Nuclear crowding and stratification are common, and ciliated or secretory columnar cells of typical tubal-type may be difficult to locate (Fig. 4.25).[315] There often is associated inflammation and granulation tissue. Fimbriae

rarely are identifiable, and both diligence and an awareness of the condition are required to avoid the misdiagnosis of adenocarcinoma.

Cysts

Cysts of the vagina are relatively uncommon. Several classifications for cystic lesions have been proposed, reflecting a combination of good microscopic descriptions, an incomplete knowledge of embryology, and an assumption that histologic differentiation mirrors histogenesis.[67,76,172,265] A functional classification scheme follows: squamous inclusion cysts, mesonephric cysts, müllerian cysts, and Bartholin gland cysts.

Squamous Inclusion Cyst

Squamous inclusion cysts probably are the most common of the vaginal cysts, resulting from entrapment of fragments of mucosa during repair of a vaginal laceration or episiotomy.[67,172] These cysts often are asymptomatic and vary from a few millimeters to several centimeters in diam-

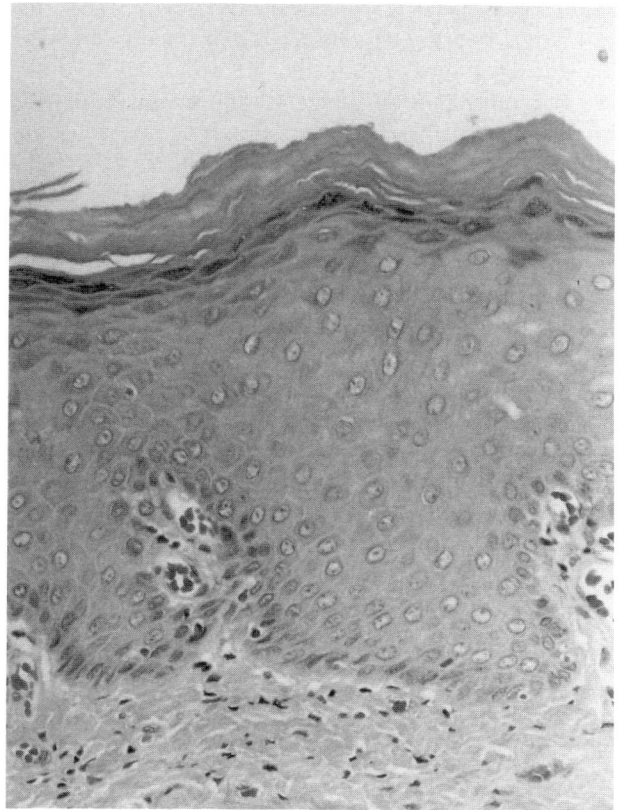

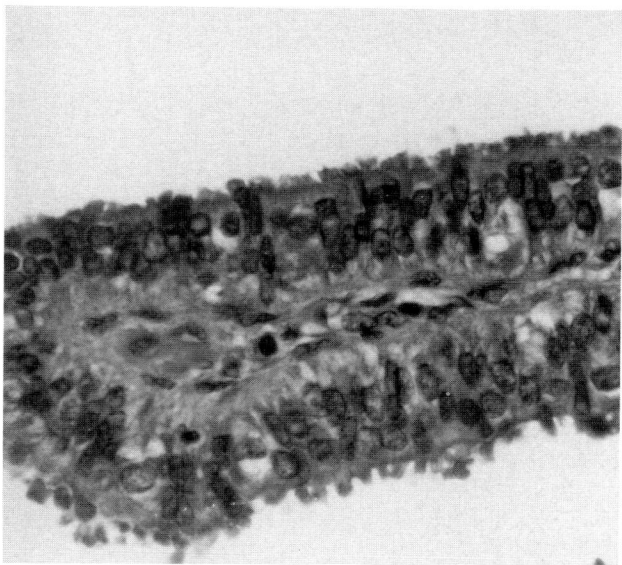

FIG. 4.25. Fallopian tube prolapse. At high magnification, nuclear enlargement and stratification may suggest the possibility of adenocarcinoma. However, many of the cells are ciliated, confirming that the structure is fallopian tube.

FIG. 4.23. Vaginal prolapse. Acanthosis and hyperkeratosis of the squamous epithelium is present.

eter. The microscopic appearance is that of a cyst wall formed by a stratified squamous epithelium, lacking rete ridges, with a central mass of keratin from desquamated cells.

Mesonephric Cyst

Mesonephric cysts, also termed Gartner's duct cysts, most often are located along the anterolateral wall of the vagina, following the route of the mesonephric duct. It is assumed that mesonephric cysts result from secretion by small isolated epithelial remnants after incomplete regression of the mesonephric duct. Mesonephric cysts are lined by low cuboidal, non–mucin-secreting cells, which are devoid of cytoplasmic mucicarmine or PAS-positive material (Fig. 4.26).

Müllerian Cyst

The genesis of the müllerian cysts is poorly understood; perhaps some are derived from islands of adenosis.[172] They are located anywhere within the vagina. Grossly, they are indistinguishable from mesonephric duct cysts, usually less than 2 cm in diameter. The distinction is made on microscopic examination. Müllerian cysts may be lined by any of the epithelia of the müllerian duct, including mucinous endocervical, endometrial, and ciliated tubal types (Fig. 4.27). Tall columnar mucin-secreting cells of endocervical type are most common, and squamous metaplasia may be observed.

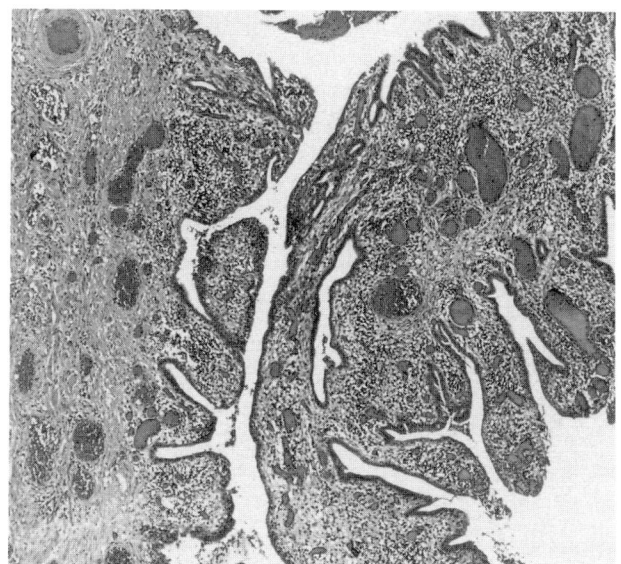

FIG. 4.24. Fallopian tube prolapse. When the plicae are blunt, there may be confuson with adenocarcinoma. Note the preserved muscularis visible on the left.

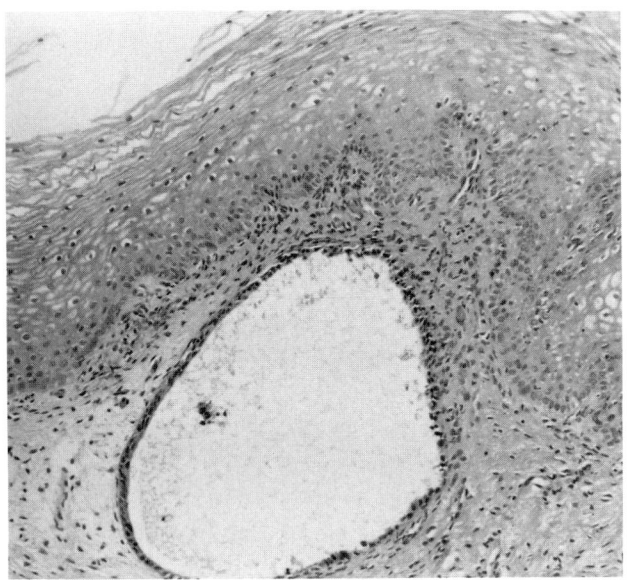

FIG. 4.26. Mesonephric cyst. The cyst is typically small and lined by a simple cuboidal epithelium, lacking cilia or intracellular mucin.

Bartholin Gland Cyst

Bartholin gland cysts occur in the region of the ducts of Bartholin glands, near the opening of the primary duct into the vestibule. The pathogenesis is incompletely understood, but usually involves occlusion of the duct, associated with either a highly viscous thick mucoid secretion or in-

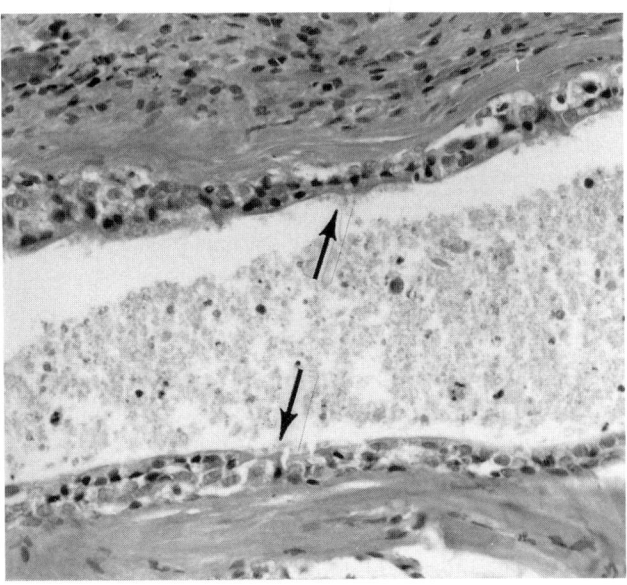

FIG. 4.27. Müllerian cyst. The cyst is lined by cuboidal or columnar cells, which may be of endocervical, tubal, or endometrial type. Note the cilia (*arrows*) along the apical border of scattered cells.

fection of the gland.[172] The cyst may enlarge rapidly and cause dyspareunia. The cyst lining varies from mucin-secreting to squamous or "transitional," reflecting the different types of epithelium lining the duct and gland. Histochemical and ultrastructural studies of the mucinous cells of normal Bartholin glands, as well as these cysts, reveal no differences from the cells of the endocervix.[300] The Bartholin gland is of urogenital sinus origin whereas the cervix is of müllerian derivation; therefore, the weakness of a histogenetic classification of vaginal cysts based on histologic features is reinforced further by this observation. Cysts of identical histologic appearance may occur elsewhere in the vestibule, reflecting the presence of numerous minor vestibular glands of urogenital sinus origin.[35,91,295] The treatment of vaginal cysts usually is excision, although marsupialization may be indicated for some Bartholin gland cysts.[172]

Benign Neoplasms

Squamous Papilloma

Squamous papillomas may be single but frequently are multiple. These lesions usually are only a few millimeters in diameter, and most commonly occur in clusters near the hymenal ring, resulting in a condition referred to as *squamous papillomatosis*.[183] The lesions usually are asymptomatic, but may be associated with vulvar burning or dyspareunia. Squamous papillomas may be difficult to distinguish from condylomas by gross inspection. Colposcopic and microscopic examination reveal the squamous papilloma to be composed of a single papillary frond with a central fibrovascular core (Fig. 4.28). It lacks the complex arborizing architecture and koilocytes of the condyloma. In contrast to the condyloma, the squamous papilloma probably is not sexually transmitted or related to infection by human papilloma virus (HPV). However, it is important to note that there may be a time during the evolution of condylomas when koilocytes are not easily identifiable.

Condyloma Acuminatum

An extensive discussion of the features of condylomas is provided in Chapter 2, Benign Diseases of the Vulva, and Chapter 6, Benign Diseases of the Cervix. Since the biologic and pathologic characteristics of vaginal condylomas are similar to those in the cervix and vulva, they are not described here.

Müllerian Papilloma

Ulbright et al. have described a papillary tumor arising in the wall of the upper vagina in a 5-year-old girl. Microscopically, it was composed of a complex arborizing fibrovascu-

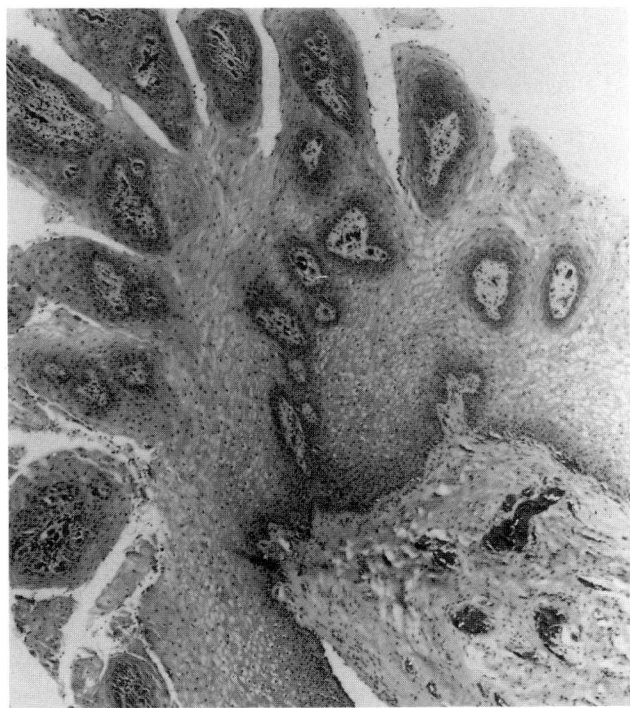

Fig. 4.28. Squamous papilloma. In contrast to a condyloma, this lesion lacks koilocytes and complex branching papillae.

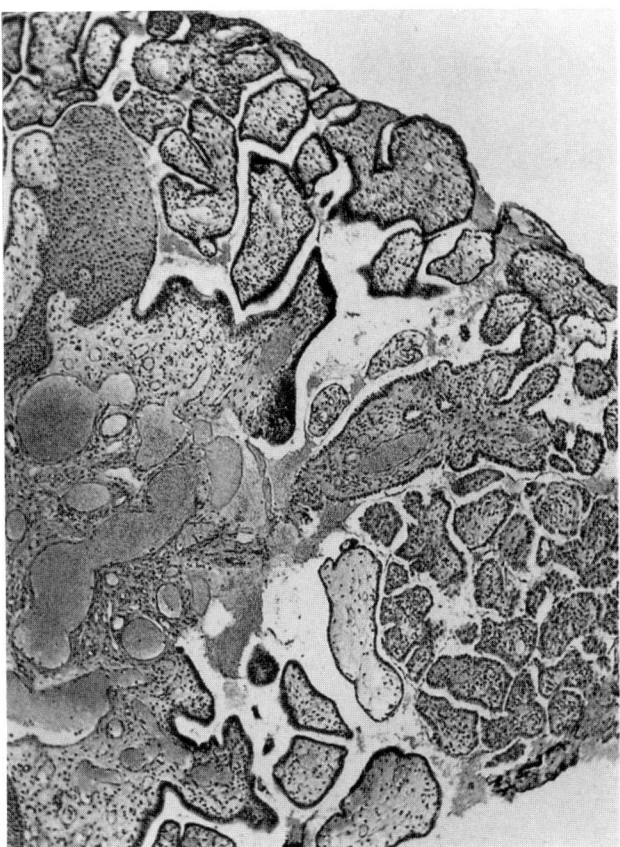

Fig. 4.29. Müllerian papilloma. Complex, branching, thick fibrovascular cores are covered by a bland low columnar epithelium.

lar core that supported bland-appearing epithelial cells that in some areas formed both solid masses and glandular lumina (Fig. 4.29).[232] The ultrastructural features, including microvilli, perinuclear arrays of microfilaments, tonofilaments, and complex cytoplasmic interdigitations, were interpreted as evidence of müllerian origin. Similar tumors, displaying an exophytic growth pattern and covered by mucin-secreting, hobnail, or eosinophilic cells have been described in both the vagina and cervix of young girls, and have been classified as mesonephric papillomas. Although their behavior clearly is benign, their embryologic origin remains uncertain.

Fibroepithelial Polyp (Mesodermal Stromal Polyp)

The fibroepithelial polyp or mesodermal stromal polyp is an uncommon hamartomatous or benign neoplastic polypoid mass of the vagina that evokes a level of interest in pathologists disproportionate to its frequency or significance. Because of the presence of bizarre stromal cells, the lesion also has been referred to as *pseudosarcoma botryoides*, reflecting the potential for confusion with sarcoma botryoides. The mean age at diagnosis is about 40 years, with an age range extending from the newborn to 77 years.[43,222,224,239,243,272] About 25% of the patients are pregnant at the time of diagnosis. The lesions usually are asymptomatic, and discovered incidentally during pelvic examination, on the lateral wall of the lower third of the vagina. The size varies from 0.5–4 cm, and the gross configuration may be that of a single edematous soft polyp resembling an acrochordon, a papillary lesion with finger-like projections or a cerebriform mass (Fig. 4.30). Microscopically, an edematous fibrovascular stroma is covered by stratified squamous epithelium. Within the stroma are variable numbers of fibroblasts. About half the polyps contain large cytologically atypical stromal cells with hyperchromatic, pleomorphic nuclei, and abundant cytoplasm with sharply tapered cytoplasmic processes (Fig. 4.31). Multinucleated bizarre cells are not uncommon, and mitotic activity is variable, but generally low. Ultrastructural and immunohistochemical studies have shown evidence of fibroblastic or smooth muscle differentiation and localization of desmin but not smooth muscle actin.[132,133,222,224] Cells with a similar histologic appearance have been described in a band-like subepithelial stromal zone extending from the endocervix to the vulva of normal females, and may represent the origin of these atypical cells.[74] The immunolocalization of steroid receptors in these bizarre cells and frequent relationship to pregnancy raises the possibility that fibroepithelial polyps are hormonally induced.

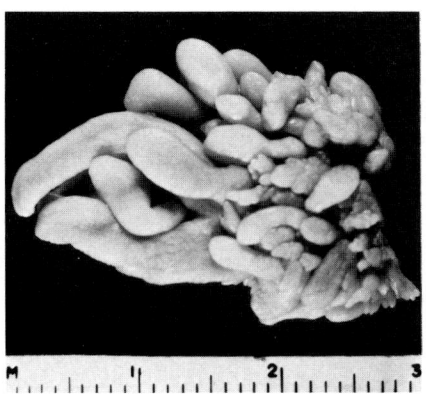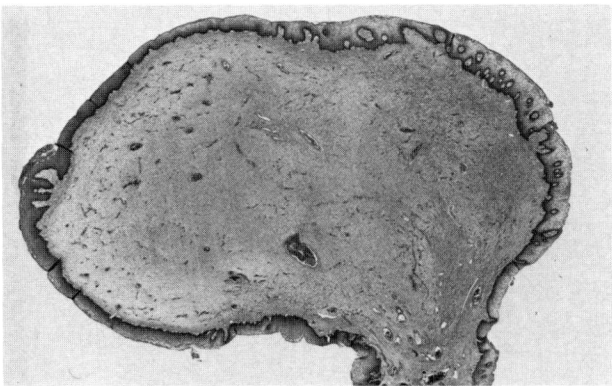

FIG. 4.30. **Fibroepithelial polyp.** *Left:* Gross; note finger-like projections. *Right:* Microscopic view; note squamous epithelial lining. (Courtesy of Henry J. Norris, M.D., Washington, D.C.)

The bizarre cells may create concern about a malignant mesenchymal neoplasm, particularly sarcoma botryoides; however, the fibroepithelial polyp lacks a "cambium layer," small undifferentiated stromal cells, rhabdomyoblasts, or invasion of the overlying squamous epithelium, which are typical features of sarcoma botryoides. The vast majority of fibroepithelial polyps occur in women over the age of 20, whereas sarcoma botryoides is confined almost always to children less than 5 years of age.

Leiomyoma

The most common mesenchymal neoplasm in the vagina of adult women is the leiomyoma.[21,94] The mean age at detection is about 40 years, with a reported range of 19–72 years.[94,334] The tumor may occur anywhere within the vagina, usually in a submucosal location. Vaginal leiomyomas vary from 0.5 to 15 cm in diameter, averaging about 3

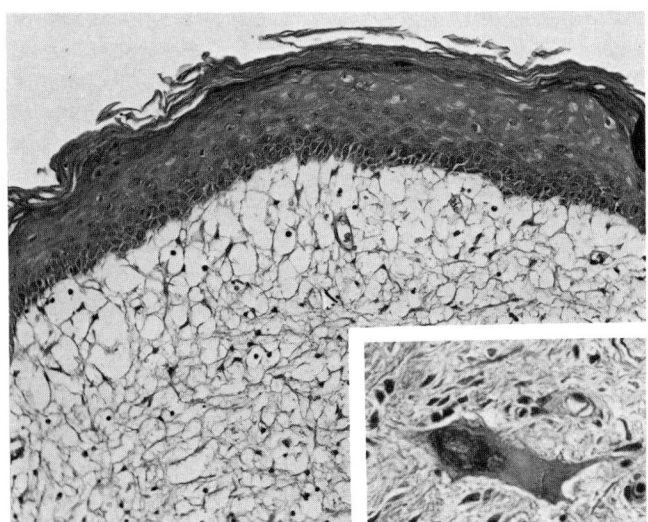

FIG. 4.31. **Fibroepithelial polyp.** High-power view of an atypical stromal cell. (Courtesy of Henry J. Norris, M.D., Washington, D.C.)

cm.[334] Since most are relatively small, they often are asymptomatic. Larger tumors may produce pain, hemorrhage, dystocia, or dyspareunia.

The gross and microscopic appearances of vaginal leiomyomas resemble those of their uterine counterparts. They are well circumscribed, firm masses that occasionally may contain foci of necrosis, edema, or hyalinization. Microscopically, they are composed of interlacing fascicles of spindle-shaped cells, with elongated, oval nuclei and little or no mitotic activity or nuclear pleomorphism. Of 60 cases of smooth muscle tumors of the vagina reviewed by Tavassoli and Norris, only 7 contained more than 5 mitoses per 10 high power fields (HPF). Five patients developed recurrence after local excision. All of the recurrent tumors were in the subset with high mitotic activity and generally moderate to marked nuclear atypia.[334] Accordingly, it is recommended that the diagnosis of vaginal leiomyoma be reserved for those tumors with fewer than five mitoses per 10 HPF. However, it also should be noted that increased mitotic activity in the absence of aggressive behavior may be present in vaginal leiomyomas during pregnancy.

Rhabdomyoma

Rhabdomyoma is a rare benign tumor displaying skeletal muscle differentiation, about 20 cases of which have been reported arising within the vagina.[35,97,112,192] The average age at diagnosis is about 45 years, with a range extending from 34 to 57 years. Patients typically present with a solitary, polypoid to nodular mass that varies from 1 to 11 cm in diameter. The overlying mucosa usually is intact.

Microscopically, rhabdomyomas are composed of benign-appearing fetal- or adult-type skeletal muscle cells surrounded by variable quantities of fibrous stroma (Fig. 4.32). The cells are of spindle to oval shape, with plump oval nuclei and abundant granular, eosinophilic cytoplasm. Mitotic activity and nuclear pleomorphism are absent. The diagnosis is confirmed by identification of intracytoplasmic fibers with cross-striations (Fig. 4.33), staining for which

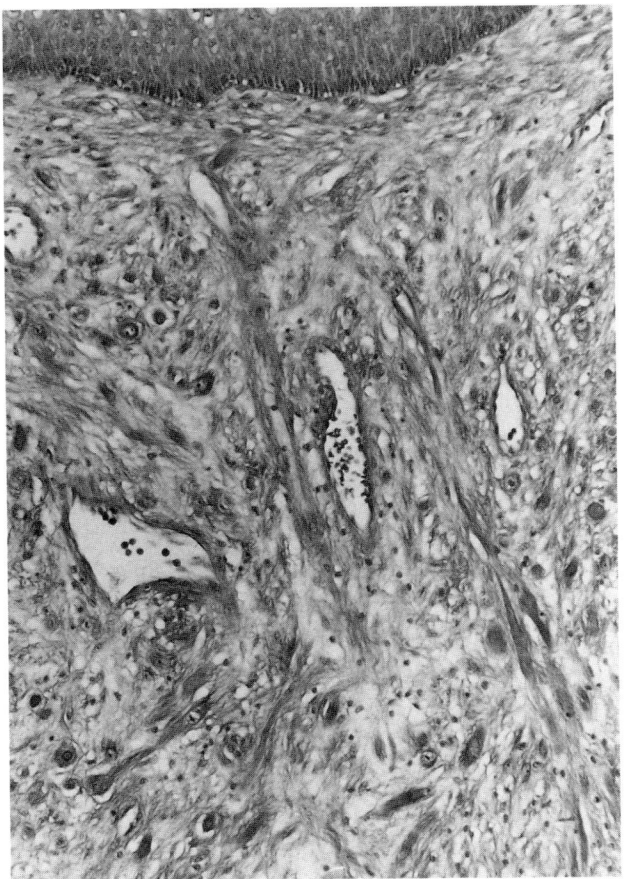

FIG. **4.32. Vaginal rhabdomyoma.** At low magnification, a nonencapsulated mass of plump, elongated cells is visible.

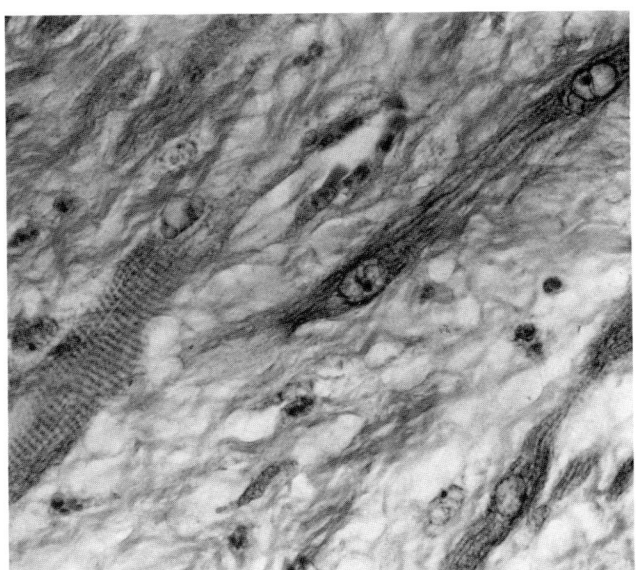

FIG. **4.33. Vaginal rhabdomyoma.** At higher magnification, cross-striations are enhanced by staining with PTAH.

may be enhanced by PTAH or trichrome preparations. Immunohistochemistry and electron microscopy usually are not needed to confirm the presence of skeletal muscle differentiation.[112,192] It is important not to confuse vaginal rhabdomyoma with embryonal rhabdomyosarcoma, but this is generally not difficult because there are differences in the age at presentation and at gross and microscopic appearances (see below, Embryonal Rhabdomyosarcoma). The behavior of rhabdomyoma is benign, and local excision provides adequate therapy.

Benign Mixed Tumor

Tumors that histologically bear some resemblance to salivary gland neoplasms are classified as benign mixed tumors. These neoplasms are rare, and usually present as a slowly growing painless mass that may occur anywhere in the vagina, but most frequently near the hymenal ring.[28a,34,41,316,367] The mean age at diagnosis is 30 years. Since the tumors are well circumscribed but nonencapsulated within the submucosa, they often are diagnosed preoperatively as a polyp or cyst (Fig. 4.34). They range in size from 1.5 to 5 cm.

Microscopically, the neoplasm is characterized by a biphasic proliferation of stromal and epithelial cells (Fig. 4.35). The spindle cells are arranged in intersecting fascicles and contain small, oval nuclei with finely granular chromatin and usually only rare mitotic figures. The epithelial component includes nests of bland-appearing glycogenated, stratified squamous cells and occasional glands lined by a mucin-secreting epithelium.[28a,316] The behavior is benign, and recurrences have not been reported after local excision.

Endometriosis

It is not uncommon for endometriosis to involve the vagina, either superficially implanted in the squamous mucosa or involving the deep stroma, particularly of the rectovaginal septum.[101,175,207,355,368] A complete discussion of endometriosis is provided in Chapter 17, Diseases of the Peritoneum.

Adenosis

A lesion similar in appearance to adenosis associated with in utero DES has been reported following laser vaporization or 5-fluorouracil treatment of vaginal condylomas.[308a] It probably develops as a healing response to the denudation of the squamous epithelium by the ablative treatment.

Miscellaneous Benign Tumors and Tumor-like Lesions

In addition to those tumors that are highly characteristic for the vagina, sporadic cases of benign neoplasms and

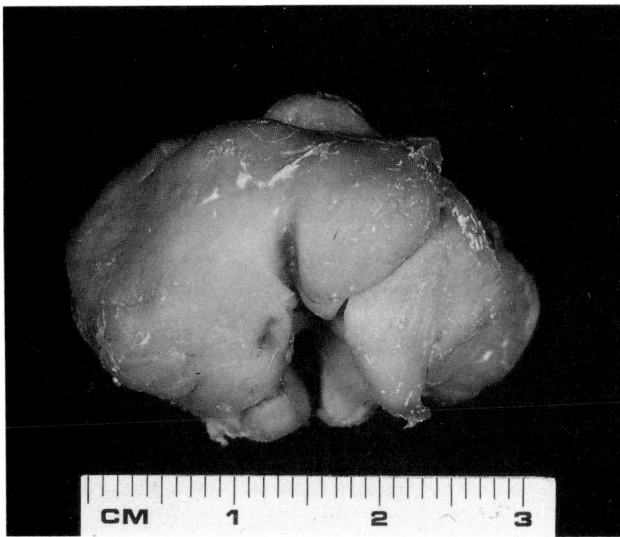

Fig. 4.34. Benign mixed tumor of the vagina. The tumor typically is well circumscribed, but nonencapsulated. (Courtesy of Henry J. Norris, M.D., Washington, D.C.)

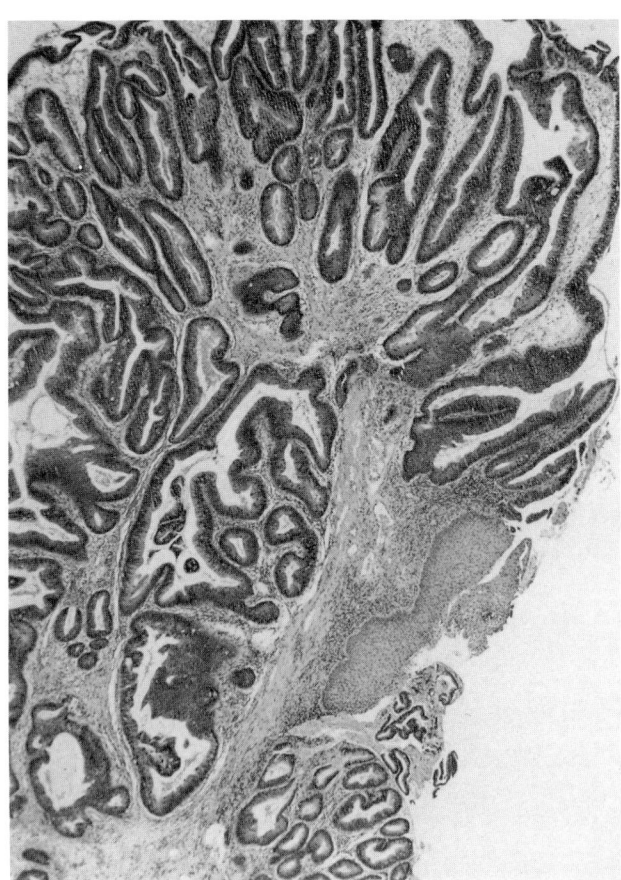

Fig. 4.36. Villous adenoma of the vagina. The lesion presented as a polypoid mass. It is histologically identical to villous adenoma in the colon.

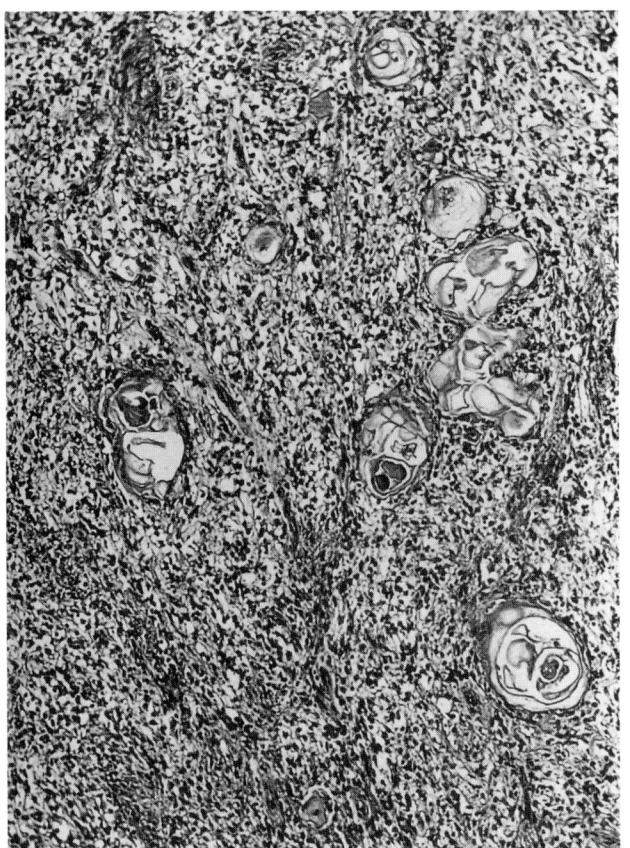

Fig. 4.35. Benign mixed tumor of the vagina. Nests of stratified squamous cells are surrounded by irregular fascicles of spindle stromal cells.

tumor-like processes have been reported, including adenomatoid tumor,[203] villous adenoma (Fig. 4.36),[85] mature cystic teratoma,[184] Brenner tumor,[42] hemangioma,[113] granular cell tumor,[109,177] neurofibroma,[66,111] paraganglioma,[257] glomus tumor,[321] blue nevus,[342] and eosinophilic granuloma.[375] Thyroid and parathyroid glands have been described in the vaginal wall of a 3-year-old girl, but probably these represented monodermal differentiation within a benign vaginal teratoma.[184]

Malignant Neoplasms

Vaginal Intraepithelial Neoplasia

In contrast to the high prevalence of intraepithelial lesions of the cervix and vulva, vaginal intraepithelial neoplasia (VAIN) is relatively rare. The reason for this discrepancy is unknown, but may prove pivotal to understanding carcinogenesis involving the squamous epithelium of the lower female genital tract. The terminology for intraepithelial neoplasia of the vagina continues to evolve, reflecting conceptual refinements, and parallels that for the cervix and vulva. According to the recommendations of the Bethesda System, lesions previously recognized as VAIN 1 or mild dysplasia are designated low-grade squamous intrepithelial lesion (LSIL), whereas VAIN 2 or 3, or moderate or severe dysplasia or carcinoma in situ, should be designated as high-grade squamous intraepithelial lesion (HSIL).

General Features

The incidence of in situ carcinoma of the vagina is reported to be about 0.20 cases per 100,000 in Caucasian females, and 0.31 cases per 100,000 in black females. This is less than 1% of the incidence for the same disease in the cervix.[55,139] The highest incidence rates are observed in women over the age of 60, with the mean age at diagnosis of VAIN 3 about 53 years. These figures are 10 or more years greater than the age of detection of cervical intraepithelial neoplasia (CIN) 3.[157] Risk factors for the development of VAIN include immunosuppression, HPV infection or squamous neoplasia elsewhere in the lower genital tract, irradiation, and in utero exposure to DES. Almost 75% of women with VAIN have preceding or coexisting squamous carcinomas of the cervix or vulva.[20,168,191,301,314] These observations have generated the concept of a field effect, in which the squamous epithelium of the entire lower female genital tract is at risk for neoplastic transformation. This hypothesis is appealing, since the squamous epithelia of these sites do share a common embryonic derivation from the urogenital sinus, and all are susceptible to infection by various HPVs.

Radiation therapy for cervical carcinoma results in exposure of the vagina to ionizing radiation, and women who have had pelvic radiation for benign as well as malignant diseases are at increased risk for development of VAIN.[8,20,106,168,191,301]

During the mid 1970s it was first suggested that DES-exposed offspring might be at risk for increased rates of dysplasia because of the extent of metaplastic tissue present in both the cervix and vagina. Multiple studies subsequently conducted of prevalence rates indicated that the frequency of dysplasia in both the exposed and unexposed populations was approximately the same. In 1984 the DESAD Project amplified its findings on the frequency of dysplasia. The incidence rates were slightly higher in exposed women. The new occurrence of squamous cell dysplasia in women under observation developed twice as frequently in DES-exposed women in contrast to those that were never exposed in utero.[25,287] Some believe that the DESAD findings may not be valid and that the increased rates of dysplasia, especially of mild form, may be caused by over- or misinterpretation of the HPV-infected tissue for dysplasia,[280] especially as the DESAD study was conducted before many of the histologic intricacies of HPV infection were fully appreciated.

Regardless of interpretation, DES itself is not felt to be the etiologic cause of dysplasia. Possibly, the metaplastic squamous epithelium, which is more extensive in the vagina in DES-exposed women, may be more susceptible to agents that give rise to dysplasia, but even this is speculative.

Recent reports have suggested that in utero exposure to DES may impair the immune system, and that this may influence development of squamous cell lesions.[26] Treatment of mice with DES introduces a significant long-term inhibitory effect of all components of the immune system, especially on the natural killer (NK) cell system. Clinical studies have reported that exposed women also have biochemical alterations.[236,362] It has been suggested that a selective suppression of the immune system might allow for the development of squamous cell neoplasia in the cervix and vagina by permitting higher susceptibility to infection with HPV and herpes simplex virus. Without further evidence, such consideration must be viewed as speculative.

Gross Findings

Women with VAIN usually are asymptomatic, and in most instances there is no grossly identifiable lesion in the vagina. Occasionally, the epithelium appears raised, roughened, and white or pink.[99,119] More often, the diagnosis is made by a colposcopically directed biopsy (Fig. 4.37) subsequent to an abnormal cytologic diagnosis in which sampling of the vagina as well as the cervix has been per-

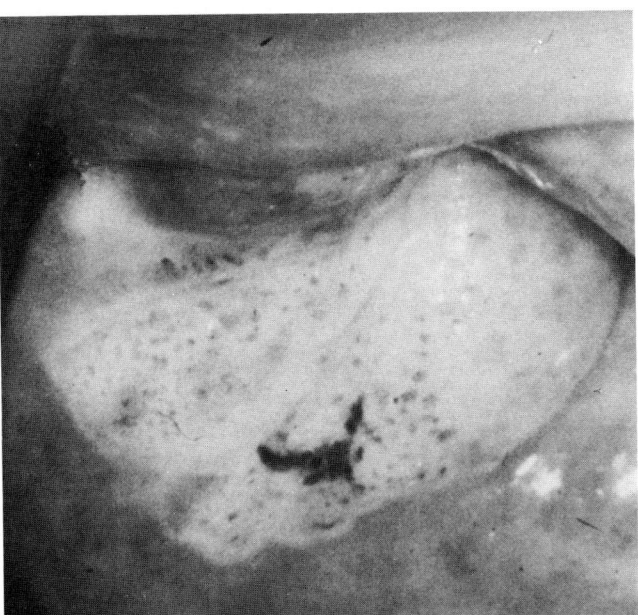

Fig. 4.37. VAIN 3 of the vaginal vault, colposcopic appearance. The lesion was detected after a hysterectomy for cervical intraepithelial neuroplasia. It appears as a raised white plaque with a punctate pattern resulting from engorged subepithelial capillaries. (Reprinted by permission of Frederick Sillman, M.D., New York, NY.)

formed, or in vaginal samples after hysterectomy. The process is multifocal or diffuse in almost half of the cases, and usually is located in the proximal third of the vagina.[20,191,301]

MICROSCOPIC FINDINGS

The microscopic features of VAIN are analogous to those of CIN (see Chapter 7, Precancerous Lesions of the Cervix). VAIN is characterized histologically by the presence of nuclear abnormalities including enlargement with irregular shape, hyperchromasia, and irregular condensation of chromatin. Lesions are graded from VAIN 1 to 3 (corresponding to mild, moderate, and severe dysplasia, carcinoma in situ) or as LSIL and HSIL. The grade is inversely related to the retention of the ability of the cells to differentiate as they progress through the epithelium, as manifested by acquisition of cytoplasmic organelles, appropriate cell polarity, and loss of mitotic activity (Figs. 4.38–4.41). SIL (VAIN) lesions nearly always display some loss of squamous maturation as well as disordered maturation, frequently including increased mitotic activity, abnormal mitotic figures, acanthosis, and dyskeratosis.

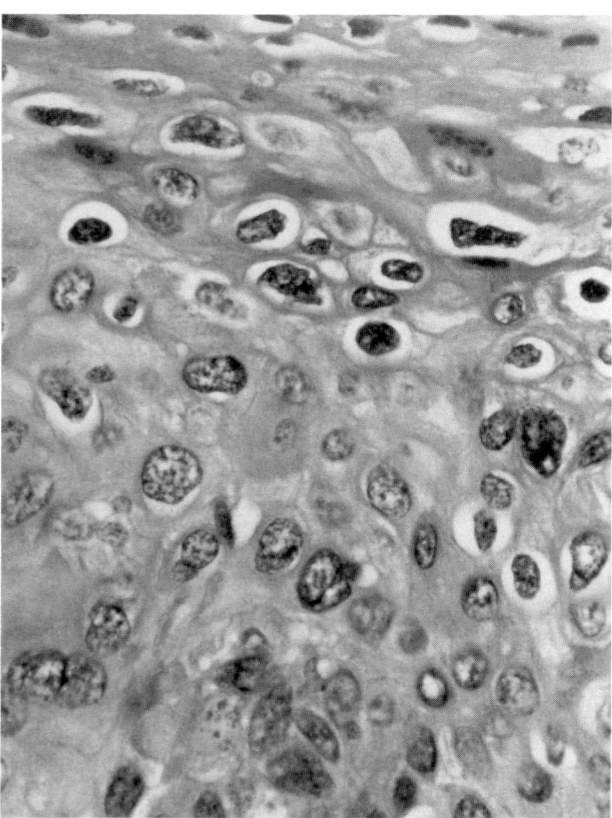

FIG. 4.39. **Low-grade SIL (VAIN 1).** At high magnification, the nuclear features of intraepithelial neoplasia are evident. This includes nuclear enlargement, pleomorphism, coarse chromatin, and irregular nuclear contours. Koilocytosis is also evident.

The differential diagnosis of SIL (VAIN) includes atrophy, radiation change, and immature squamous metaplasia in women with adenosis, all of which may display loss of glycogen and a relative increase in cellularity. The distinction rests primarily on the characteristic nuclear features of SIL (VAIN), which are absent in the other conditions. Radiation changes include nuclear enlargement, smudged chromatin, multinucleation, and vacuolization of cytoplasm, with lack of mitotic activity.[93] Occasionally, there may be significant nuclear atypia associated with inflammatory and reactive processes, but usually this is expressed as regular nuclear enlargement with vesicular chromatin and moderate-sized nucleoli. Such changes are referred to as *reactive squamous atypia* (Fig. 4.42).

CLINICAL BEHAVIOR AND TREATMENT

The natural history of SIL (VAIN) is uncertain. In one study, about 5% of SIL (VAIN) progressed to invasive carcinoma, with sequential changes documented by serial biopsies.[301] Therapy generally is local excision, although

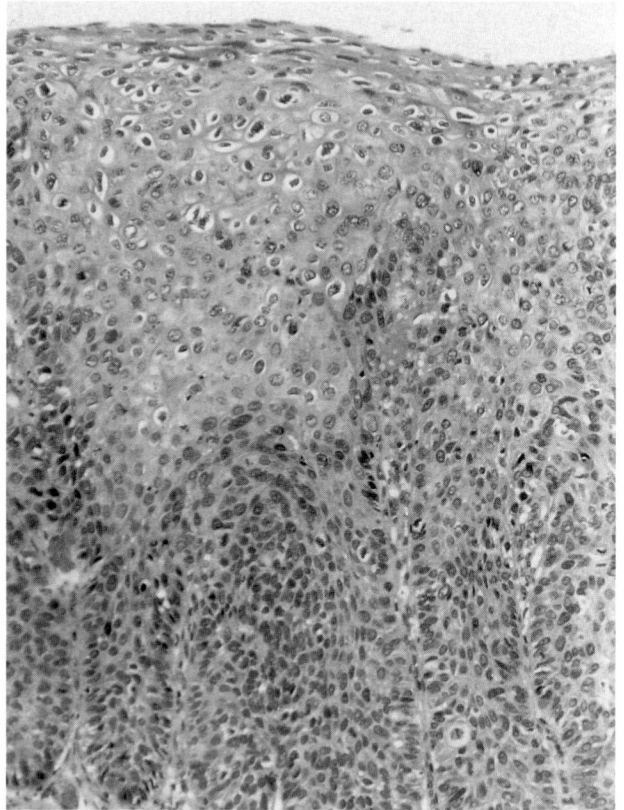

FIG. 4.38. **Low-grade SIL (VAIN 1).** There is irregular acanthosis of this epithelium in addition to koilocytosis and nuclear features of intraepithelial neoplasia. The extensive cytoplasmic differentiation is diagnostic of VAIN 1 (low-grade SIL).

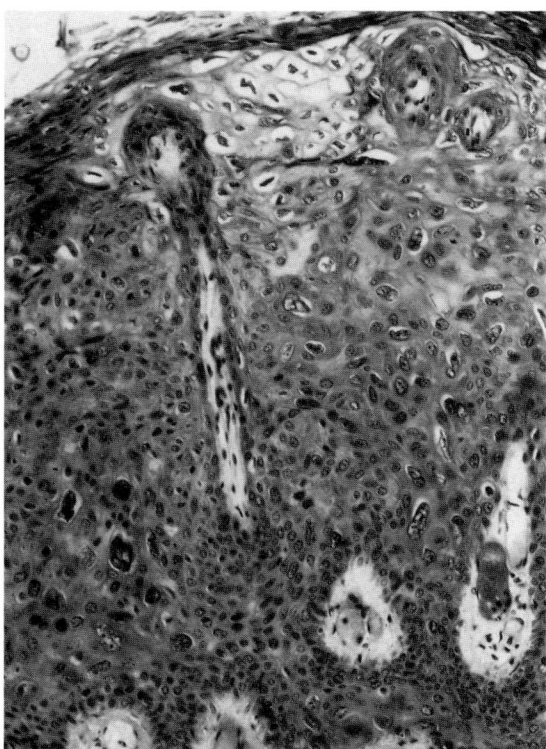

Fig. 4.40. **High-grade SIL (VAIN 2).** This intraepithelial process is characterized by enlargement and pleomorphism of nuclei, but preservation of some features of cytoplasmic differentiation is noted in cells of the intermediate and superficial layers. (Reprinted by permission of Kurman et al., ref. 183.)

topical 5-fluorouracil, laser vaporization, vaginectomy, and irradiation also have been successfully used.[32,99,323,370]

Squamous Cell Carcinoma

GENERAL FEATURES

Squamous cell carcinoma represents about 90% of malignant neoplasms primary to the vagina. The incidence is 0.42 cases per 100,000 in Caucasian women and 0.93 per 100,000 in black women,[55] which is about one-fiftieth the incidence of cervical squamous cell carcinoma.[227] Only 1% of malignant neoplasms of the female genital tract are classified as squamous cell carcinoma originating in the vagina.[64,142,209] The incidence reflects both the relative rarity of squamous cell carcinoma at this site and the extremely rigid criteria for diagnosis of vaginal as compared with cervical carcinoma, which results in underestimation of its true frequency. The International Federation of Gy-

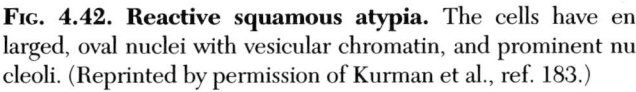

Fig. 4.42. **Reactive squamous atypia.** The cells have enlarged, oval nuclei with vesicular chromatin, and prominent nucleoli. (Reprinted by permission of Kurman et al., ref. 183.)

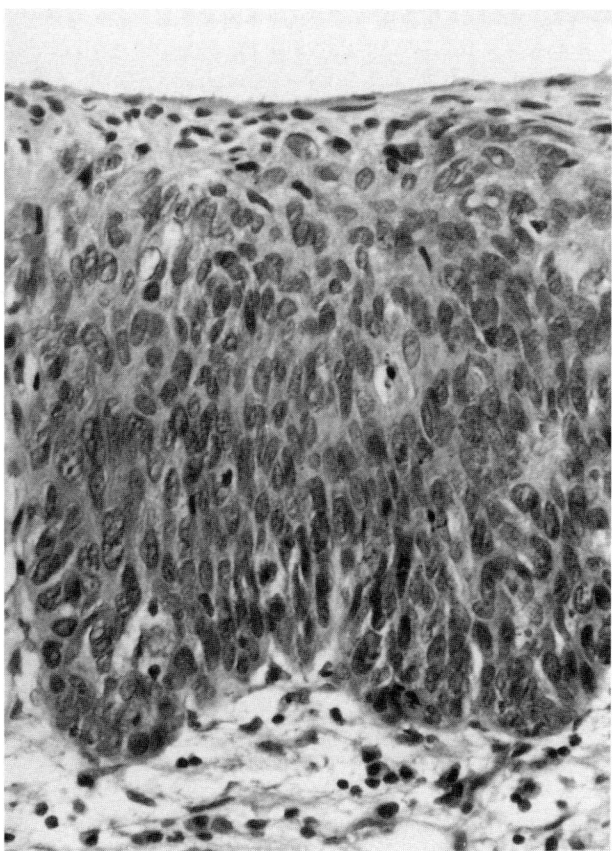

Fig. 4.41. **High-grade SIL (VAIN 3).** Cytoplasmic differentiation is limited to the uppermost layers of the squamous epithelium. The remaining cells have a high nuclear/cytoplasmic ratio, with a longitudinal nuclear axis perpendicular to the basement membrane.

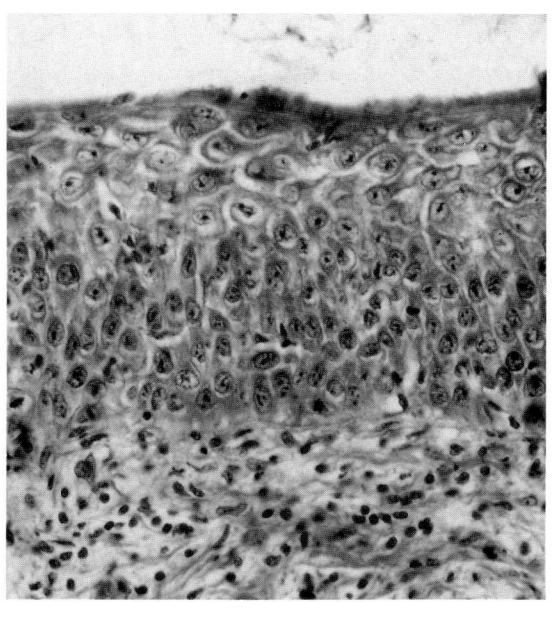

necology and Obstetrics (FIGO) staging of vaginal cancer is analogous to that of cervical cancer and is based on clinical rather than pathologic examination (Table 4.2). In order to be considered a primary tumor of the vagina the neoplasm must be located in the vagina, without clinical or histologic evidence of involvement of the cervix or vulva. Thus, bulky tumors located in the upper vagina that have extended onto the portio vaginalis of the cervix are classified as primary cervical carcinoma. Similarly, squamous cell carcinoma occurring in the vagina within 5 years of therapy for cervical carcinoma is considered to be recurrent cervical carcinoma rather than a new primary carcinoma of the vagina.[255] It is thus not surprising that only 10–20% of vaginal malignancies are classified as primary neoplasms of the vagina.[93] The risk factors for invasive squamous carcinoma of the vagina are the same as those for SIL (VAIN).[29,361] Occasionally, squamous cell carcinomas also have been reported in young women with congenital absence of the vagina 8 to 25 years after the creation of a neovagina.[155,299]

CLINICAL FEATURES

The mean age at diagnosis of invasive vaginal squamous carcinoma is 64 years.[183] The presenting symptoms usually are painless vaginal bleeding or discharge, dysuria, or frequency.[3,361] There is a relationship between duration of symptoms and the size and spread of tumor. Unfortunately, about 20% of patients with vaginal cancer delay more than 7 months from onset of symptoms to initiation of therapy.[264]

Most of the tumors arise in the proximal third of the vagina,[264] with 57% involving the posterior wall and 27% located on the anterior wall.[263]

GROSS FINDINGS

Vaginal squamous carcinomas vary in size from clinically occult to larger than 10 cm. The gross configuration is similarly variable and includes polypoid, fungating, indurated, and ulcerated lesions.

Table 4.2. FIGO staging of vaginal carcinoma (1978)

Stage	Clinical status
0	Intraepithelial
I	Limited to vaginal wall
II	Extends to subvaginal tissue but not to pelvic side wall
III	Extends to pelvic side wall
IV	Extends beyond the true pelvis or involves mucosa of the bladder or rectum (bullous edema does not consign the patient to stage IV)
IVa	Adjacent organs involved
IVb	Distant organs involved

MICROSCOPIC FINDINGS

Squamous cell carcinomas of the vagina resemble those arising in the cervix (Fig. 4.43). Histologic grade using either the method of Broders or Reagen and Wentz has not been related to prognosis.[70,244,247] Microinvasive carcinoma is not currently a defined entity in the vagina; however, superficially invasive tumors, with less than 3 mm of stromal invasion and no vascular space invasion, appear to have a low likelihood of nodal metastasis.[256] The distinction of early invasive carcinoma from intraepithelial carcinoma is based on a constellation of findings, including the presence of angulated narrow cords of squamous cells at the stromal interface, frequently with acquisition of more abundant eosinophilic cytoplasm, and a desmoplastic or inflammatory host response. Unfortunately, these features are not present in every case of early invasive squamous carcinoma.

CLINICAL BEHAVIOR AND TREATMENT

The clinical stage is the single most important indicator of prognosis.[70,248] Direct spread into the soft tissues of the pelvis or to the mucosa of the bladder or rectum occurs

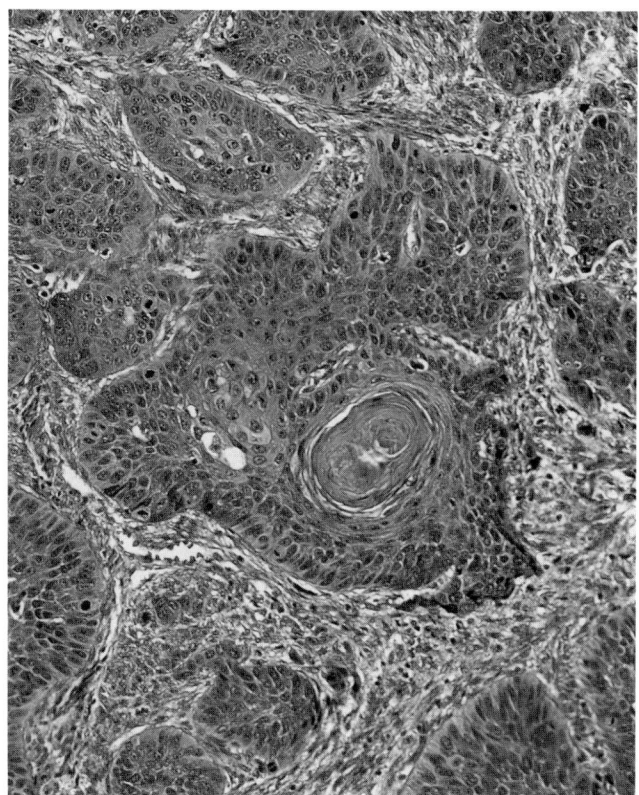

FIG. 4.43. Squamous cell carcinoma of the vagina. Keratin pearl formation is evident.

early because the wall of the vagina is thin and is separated from these organs by only a few millimeters of connective tissue. As discussed in the section on anatomy, the lymphatic drainage of the vagina is complex and variable, and any of the inguinal or pelvic lymph nodes may be the site of metastasis, although there is some relationship to the location of the tumor within the vagina.[208]

Radiation therapy is the modality used primarily to treat vaginal squamous carcinoma, although radical vaginectomy may be indicated in selected instances.[250] A review by Benedot et al. indicated that the survival rate at 5 years is as follows: stage I—71%, stage II—47%, stage III—25%, and stage IV—8%.[19] Recently, several studies have indicated a considerably better survival rate, comparable to that for cervical squamous carcinoma.[70,249,250,268] Although metastases may be discovered ultimately in the lungs or supraclavicular lymph nodes, recurrent disease typically is local and occurs within 2 years of diagnosis.[183]

Verrucous Carcinoma

The use of the term *verrucous carcinoma* should be reserved for those rare vaginal tumors that display the characteristic features described by Ackerman.[2,56] Grossly, they are exophytic, fungating masses with a coarsely granular or undulating surface. Microscopically, the characteristic feature of verrucous carcinoma is the presence of squamous cells with bland cytological features. At the deep margin of the tumor, the squamous cells invade in a pushing fashion as broad bulbous masses, creating a so-called baggy pants appearance (Fig. 4.44). On the surface of the tumor, hyperkeratosis and acanthosis are common. The distinction of verrucous carcinoma from condyloma or pseudoepitheliomatous hyperplasia may be difficult and may not be possible in a superficial biopsy specimen. Some authors have indicated that verrucous carcinoma does not display the koilocytosis or surface papillae formed of fibrovascular cores covered by squamous cells, which are typical of condylomata or warty carcinomas,[161,180,181,183] but other investigators disagree.[72,205] This issue, however, is not of primary importance because the diagnosis rests on the presence of bland cytological features in the broad bulbous masses of squamous cells at the stromal interface. Verrucous carcinomas display a relatively indolent growth potential, with frequent local recurrence after incomplete excision. Lymph node metastasis occurs rarely, if ever. Since verrucous carcinomas not only are resistant to therapeutic irradiation but actually may transform to conventional squamous carcinoma after radiation therapy, the treatment usually is wide local or radical surgery.[2,93,181] Tumors with a mixed pattern of both verrucous and conventional squamous carcinomas behave with the aggressiveness of typical squamous cancer, and should be classified as such.

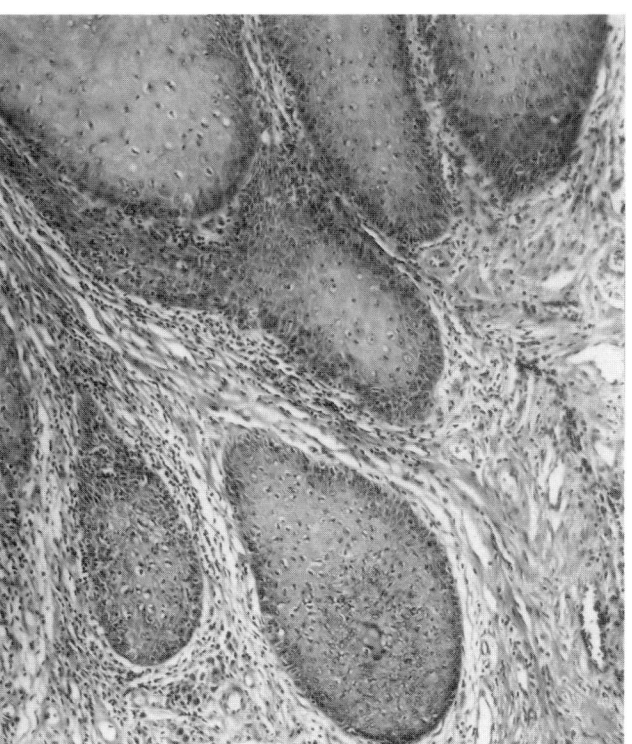

FIG. 4.44. **Verrucous carcinoma.** The tumor is characterized by a proliferation of cytologically bland squamous cells arranged in broad bulbous masses, which have a smooth interface with the stroma.

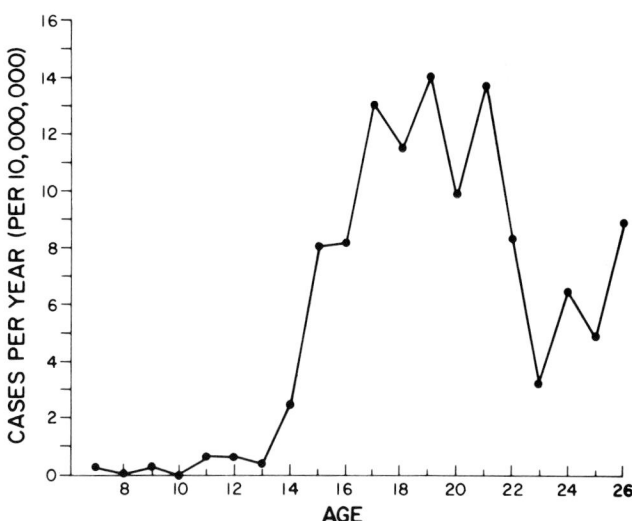

FIG. 4.45. **Incidence of clear cell adenocarcinoma by age at diagnosis among native-born white women.** (Reprinted by permission of Herbst AL, Cole P, Norusis MJ, et al. (1980) Epidermologic aspects and factors related to survival in 384 registry cases of clear cell adenocarcinoma of the vagina and cervix. Am J Obstet Gynecol 135:876.)

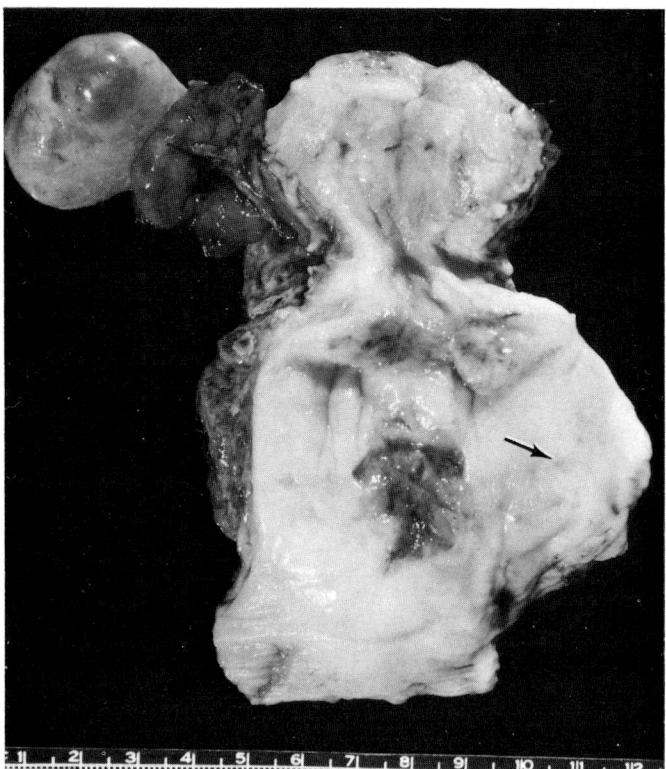

Fig. 4.46. Flat clear cell carcinoma of vagina. *Left:* In addition to tumor, several patches of adenosis (*arrow*) are present in the vagina. Vaginal adenosis and extensive ectropion of the cervix appear red in the fresh state. *Right:* Cross-section of the vagina with deeply invasive tumor and vascular invasion (*arrow*).

Warty Carcinoma

Squamous cell carcinomas in which many of the cells contain nuclear abnormalities and perinuclear cytoplasmic cavitation similar to the koilocytes in intraepithelial neoplasms have been designated *warty carcinoma*. These

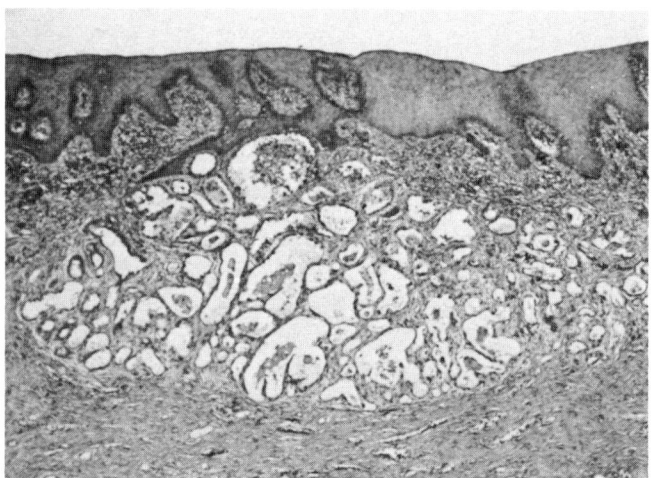

Fig. 4.47. Clear cell carcinoma confined to lamina propria. The tumor is palpable, but cannot be seen with the colposcope.

changes are not typically present in verrucous carcinoma. In addition, warty carcinomas have greater nuclear pleomorphism than verrucous carcinomas, as well as multinucleation, and an infiltrative pattern at the stromal interface. A detailed clinicopathologic analysis of warty carcinomas in the vagina has not been reported. Preliminary data from similar tumors in the vulva indicate that they behave in a low-grade malignant fashion, although metastases to regional lymph nodes occur occasionally (see Chapter 3, Premalignant and Malignant Tumors of the Vulva).[186]

Clear Cell Adenocarcinoma

GENERAL FEATURES

More than 580 cases of clear cell adenocarcinoma of the vagina or cervix in young girls and women had been accessioned by the beginning of 1992 by the Registry for Research on Hormonal Transplacental Carcinogenesis.[140] Approximately 60% of the patients have had documented exposure in utero to DES, hexestrol, or dienestrol; another 12% were exposed to an unknown form of medication, usually for a high-risk pregnancy. The records in several cases indicate only exposure to steroidal estrogens or progesterone, but there is no evidence of an association of clear

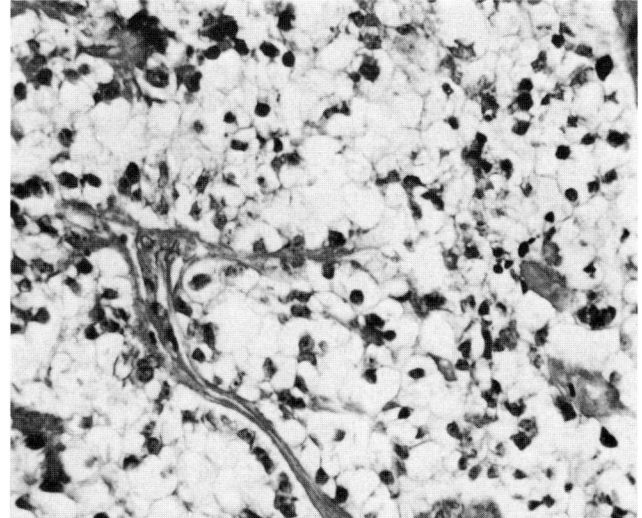

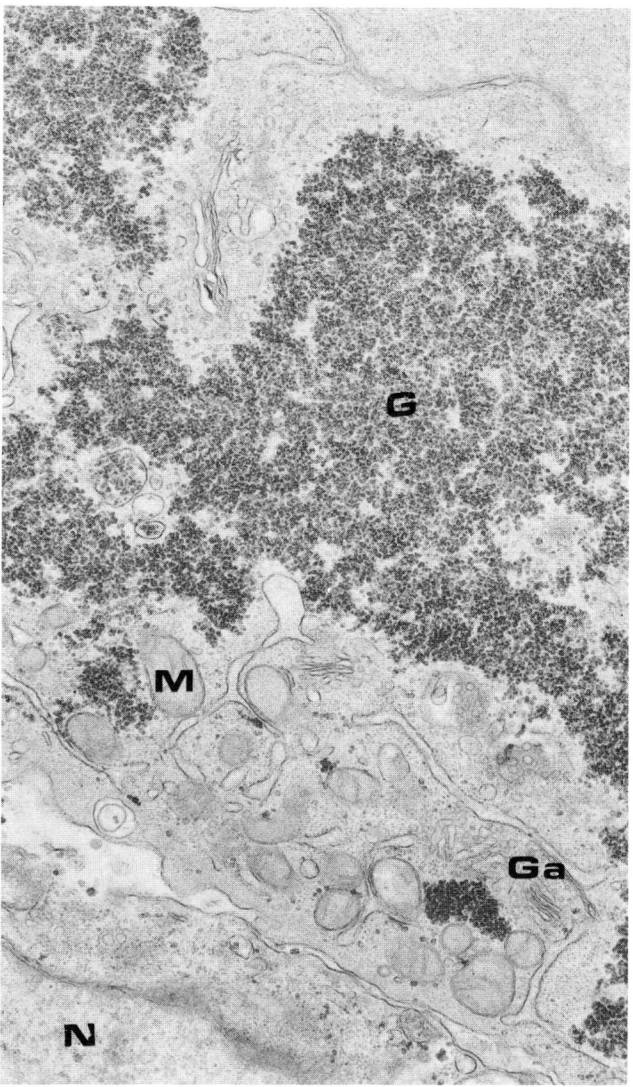

FIG. 4.48. **Clear cell carcinoma.** *Top:* Solid pattern of tumor, resembling clear cell carcinoma of ovary and endometrium. *Bottom:* Special processing of specimen for electron microscopy demonstrates glycogen particles (*G*) in large collections in cytoplasm. Nuclei (*N*) and cytoplasmic organelles, such as mitochondria (*M*) and Golgi apparatus (*Ga*), are less electron dense by this technique. Osmium tetroxide. ×12,000. (Reprinted by permission of (*top*) Scully et al. Ann Clin Lab Sci 4:222–233, 1974; (*bottom*) Dickersin et al., ref. 122.)

◁————————————————————

cell adenocarcinoma with prenatal exposure to these hormones.[169] The proportion of negative to positive histories of DES exposure is greater for cervical tumors than for vaginal tumors, a finding consistent with the observation that clear cell adenocarcinoma of the cervix in young women was a recognized but rare entity before the DES era, whereas clear cell adenocarcinoma of the vagina was exceedingly rare, limited only to a few case reports.

The median age at the time of diagnosis is 19 years (Fig. 4.45). Although a rare patient has been as young as 7 years of age, only after the age of 14 years does the age-incidence curve rise sharply. It plateaus between ages 17 and 21 years and then declines rapidly. Clear cell adenocarcinoma develops in about 0.014–0.14% of exposed girls and women up to the age of 24 years. The rarity of the neoplasm has been confirmed in multiple studies in which no tumors were encountered among large groups of women specifically examined because of their history of prenatal DES exposure.[237,259,356] The greatest number of DES-exposed patients with these tumors were born in 1951–1953, the years when the drug was prescribed most frequently for pregnancy support. It is anticipated that the final estimate of incidence may rise somewhat because many cases have been misclassified and therefore not reported,[158] and because new tumors have been discovered in several of many thousands of DES-exposed women while they were under medical observation.[303] The risk of tumor development is higher when the drug was started early in pregnancy.[141] In a rare case, the tumor has developed in only one of two monozygotic twins,[302] suggesting that factors other than DES exposure play a role in carcinogenesis.

CLINICAL FEATURES

The tumor may involve any portion of the vagina and/or cervix. Approximately 60% of lesions have been confined to the vagina (Fig. 4.46). The remainder have been limited to the cervix or involved both the cervix and vagina. Most vaginal tumors arise on the anterior wall, usually in the upper third, corresponding to the most frequent site of adenosis.

Tumors also have been found on the wall opposite the

main tumor, presumably a result of implantation ("kissing lesions"). Unlike the larger tumors, which almost always cause symptoms such as vaginal bleeding or discharge, many small tumors are asymptomatic and have been detected only as more young women have sought examination because of their known exposure to DES.

On occasion, multicentric tumors have been demonstrated on microscopic examination. Whereas a multicentric origin has been suspected grossly in some larger tumors, submucosal continuity often has been found on microscopic examination in these cases.

GROSS FINDINGS

Tumors have varied in size from microscopic to large. Most of the larger cancers are polypoid and nodular, but some are flat or ulcerated, having a granular or indurated surface. Small tumors, currently being seen more frequently, usually are palpable. They may be invisible on colposcopic examination if confined to the lamina propria and if covered by intact, normal, or metaplastic squamous epithelium. Although most cancers are superficial and invade only a few millimeters into the vaginal or cervical wall (Fig. 4.47), some penetrate far more deeply or extend more centrifugally than might be anticipated on gross examination.

MICROSCOPIC FINDINGS

By light and electron microscopy, the DES-associated clear cell adenocarcinoma is identical to the clear cell adenocarcinoma of the ovary and endometrium, which occur sporadically in older women. Several histologic patterns may be observed, either alone or in combination. A characteristic pattern, for which the tumor is named, consists of solid sheets of clear cells (Fig. 4.48), the clear appearance of the cytoplasm being caused by the dissolution of glycogen when the specimen is processed for microscopic examination. A second (and the most frequent) pattern, the tubulocystic pattern, is characterized by tubules and cysts lined by hobnail cells (Fig. 4.49), by flat cells (Fig. 4.50), or by cells that resemble to varying degrees müllerian type epithelium. The hobnail cell is characterized by a bulbous nucleus that protrudes into the lumen beyond the apparent cytoplasmic limits of the cell. Flat cells often appear innocuous. When only this type of epithelium is present in a small biopsy, it may be difficult to differentiate tumor from adenosis. Less common patterns include a papillary pattern (Fig. 4.51), a tubular pattern resembling endometrial carcinoma (Fig. 4.52), and a pattern composed of cords of cells with eosinophilic cytoplasm (Fig. 4.53). Mitoses usually are rare. In any of these patterns, the lumen may contain mucin. The cytoplasm, however, is mucin free.

Atypical adenosis, characterized by glands with cellular stratification, nuclear pleomorphism, hyperchromasia, and prominent nucleoli (Fig. 4.54), has been identified near the periphery of most clear cell carcinomas in which the excised vagina has been serially blocked for microscopic examination. Atypical cells with nuclei that are larger and more irregular in outline than those seen in normal endocervical cells or the cells lining the glands of the adenosis have been identified in approximately 0.5% of cervical and vaginal smears from DES-exposed women.[282,290] The frequent finding of the tuboendometrial type of glandular cell and the rarity of the mucinous type of cell adjacent to the tumors suggest that the clear cell adenocarinoma arises

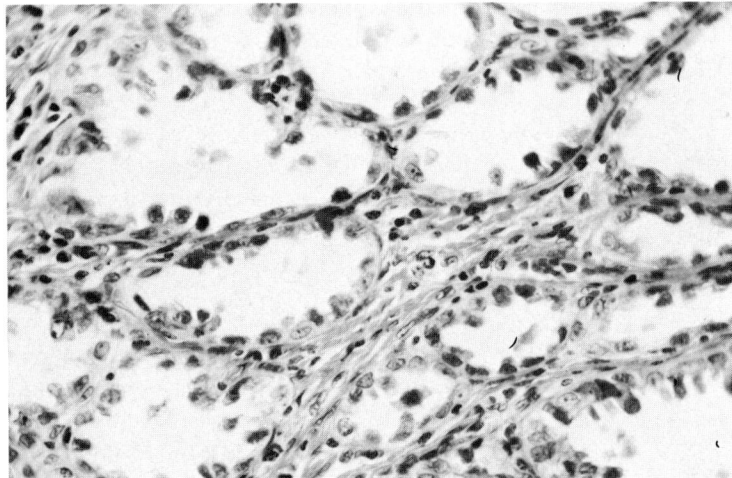
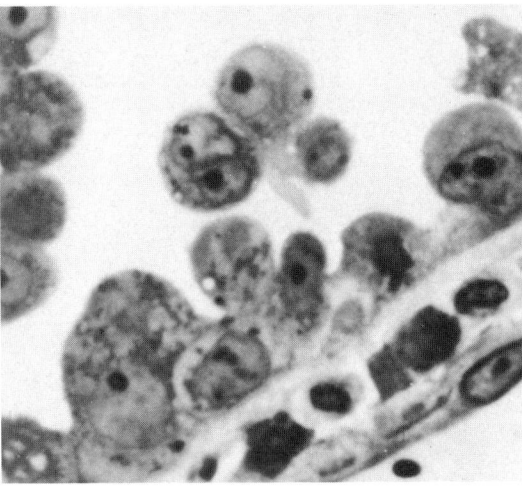

FIG. 4.49. Clear cell carcinoma. *Left:* Tubulocystic pattern of tumor in which small tubules are lined by neoplastic hobnail, columnar, or cuboidal cells. *Right:* Detail of hobnail cells showing luminal protrusion of nucleus and scant apical cytoplasm. (Reprinted by permission of Dickersin et al., ref. 68.)

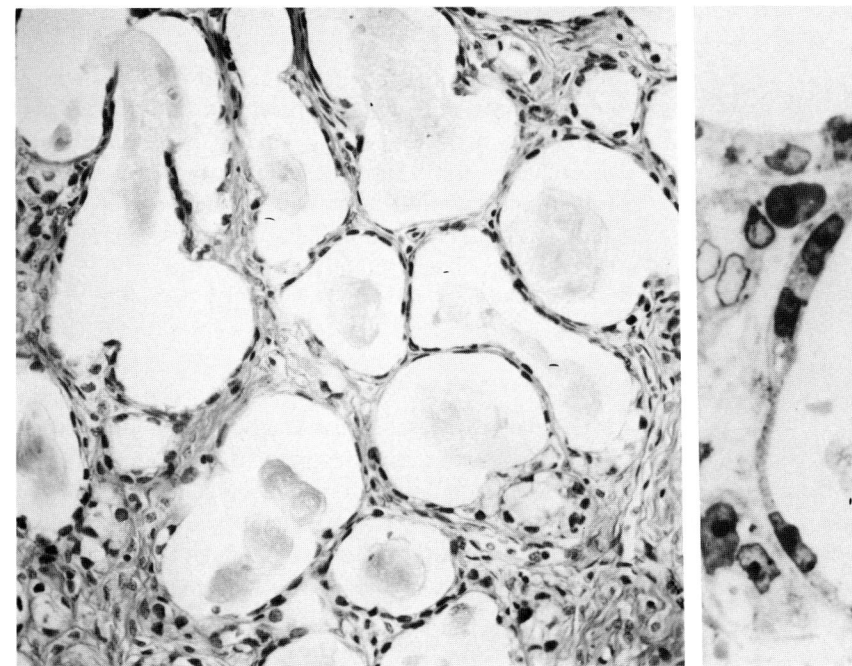

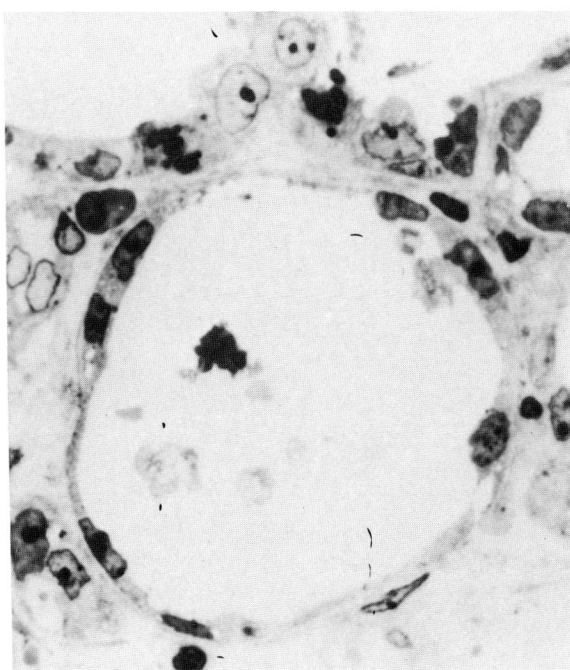

FIG. 4.50. Clear cell carcinoma. *Left:* Tubulocystic pattern characterized by dilated cysts lined by flat cells. *Right:* Detail of flat cells, one of which has an atypical mitosis. Small clear spaces in cytoplasm are vestiges of glycogen. (Reprinted by permission of Dickersin et al., ref. 68.)

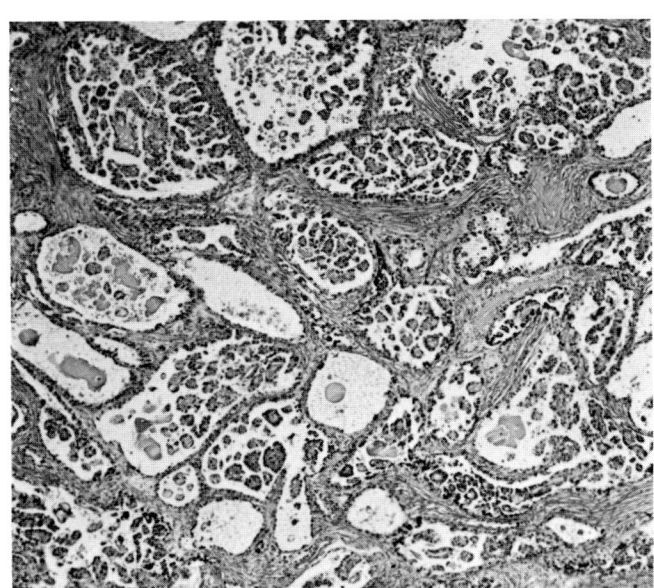

FIG. 4.51. Clear cell carcinoma. Papillary pattern of tumor.

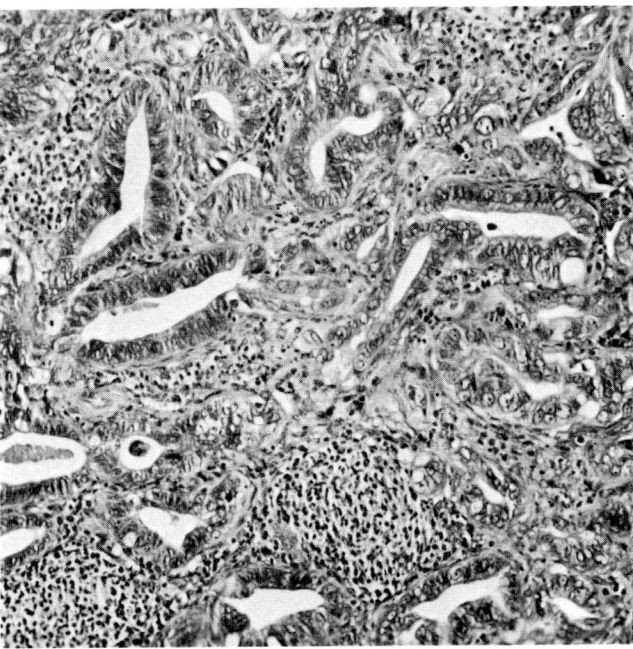

FIG. 4.52. Clear cell carcinoma. The tumor is composed of tubules lined by stratified columnar cells resembling endometrial carcinoma. This is a very rare pattern.

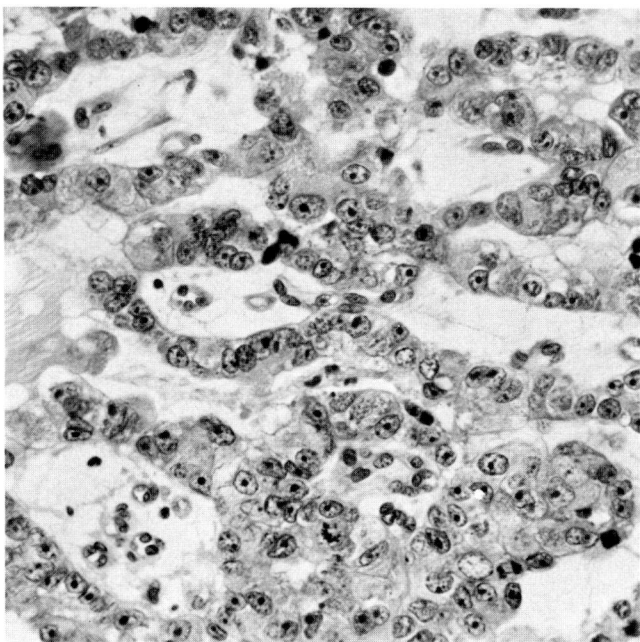

FIG. 4.53. Clear cell carcinoma. Cords and solid masses of cell with deeply eosinophilic cytoplasm and nuclei with prominent nucleoli. This is a rare pattern.

from the tuboendometrial cells.[293,294] Similarly, there are no mucinous cells adjacent to clear cell carcinoma arising from the endometrium in elderly women. The studies of nuclear DNA content show that (1) atypical forms of tu-

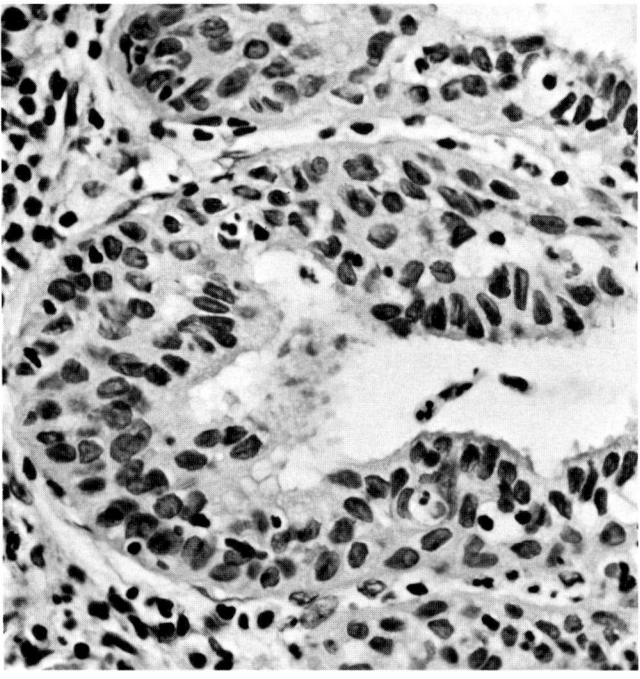

FIG. 4.54. Atypical adenosis. Nuclei vary both in size and shape; cells are stratified.

boendometrial-type cells may have an aneuploid pattern, (2) tuboendometrial cells demonstrate greater proliferative activity (more often in a tetraploid state) than do endocervical-type cells, and (3) polyploid patterns are associated with active-appearing vaginal adenosis. However, there has been no case yet where, over time, microscopically proven atypical adenosis has progressed to carcinoma and, consequently, proof that atypical adenosis is a precursor of clear cell carcinoma is lacking.

DIFFERENTIAL DIAGNOSIS

Microglandular hyperplasia is a benign condition that can resemble adenocarcinoma on gross and microscopic examination. Usually associated with the use of oral contraceptives or occasionally with pregnancy, it is rarely observed in their absence. Although microglandular hyperplasia almost always develops in the cervix, cases also have been described arising in foci of vaginal adenosis. Most of the young women had histories of exposure prenatally to DES.[292] Initially, the lesions were misinterpreted as a clear cell adenocarcinoma. Grossly, the lesion is soft, granular, tan-yellow, and usually flat. Occasionally, it may be cauliflower-like and multicentric (Fig. 4.55). Microscopic examination demonstrates many small, closely packed glands devoid of intervening stroma (see Chapter 6, Benign Diseases of the Cervix). The presence of extensive nests of metaplastic squamous cells with pale eosinophilic cytoplasm may make the lesion difficult to distinguish from the solid pattern of clear cell carcinoma. A clue to the diagnosis is the presence of clefts lined by mucinous epithelium that course through the metaplastic squamous epithelium. The fact that the glands have been observed in continuity with the clefts suggests that the glands result from budding and arborization of the mucinous epithelium that constitutes one type of vaginal adenosis as well as the lining of the normal endocervix. Microglandular hyperplasia has not been shown to arise from the tuboendometrial type of adenosis. The lesion generally is reversed when oral contraceptives are discontinued.

The Arias–Stella reaction (see Chapter 9, Anatomy and Histology of the Uterine Corpus) usually occurs in pregnant women and must be distinguished from clear cell adenocarcinoma. Although usually seen in the endometrium, the Arias–Stella reaction has been observed in the endocervix and occasionally in vaginal adenosis of the tuboendometrial type. Characteristically, hypersecretory glands are lined by cells with markedly enlarged nuclei resembling hobnail cells. However, in clear cell adenocarcinoma, the presence of sheets of clear cells or prominent papillae should enable the two lesions to be distinguished. In addition, the hobnail-like nuclei in the Arias–Stella reaction commonly are smudged, lack mitotic activity, and appear to be degenerative.

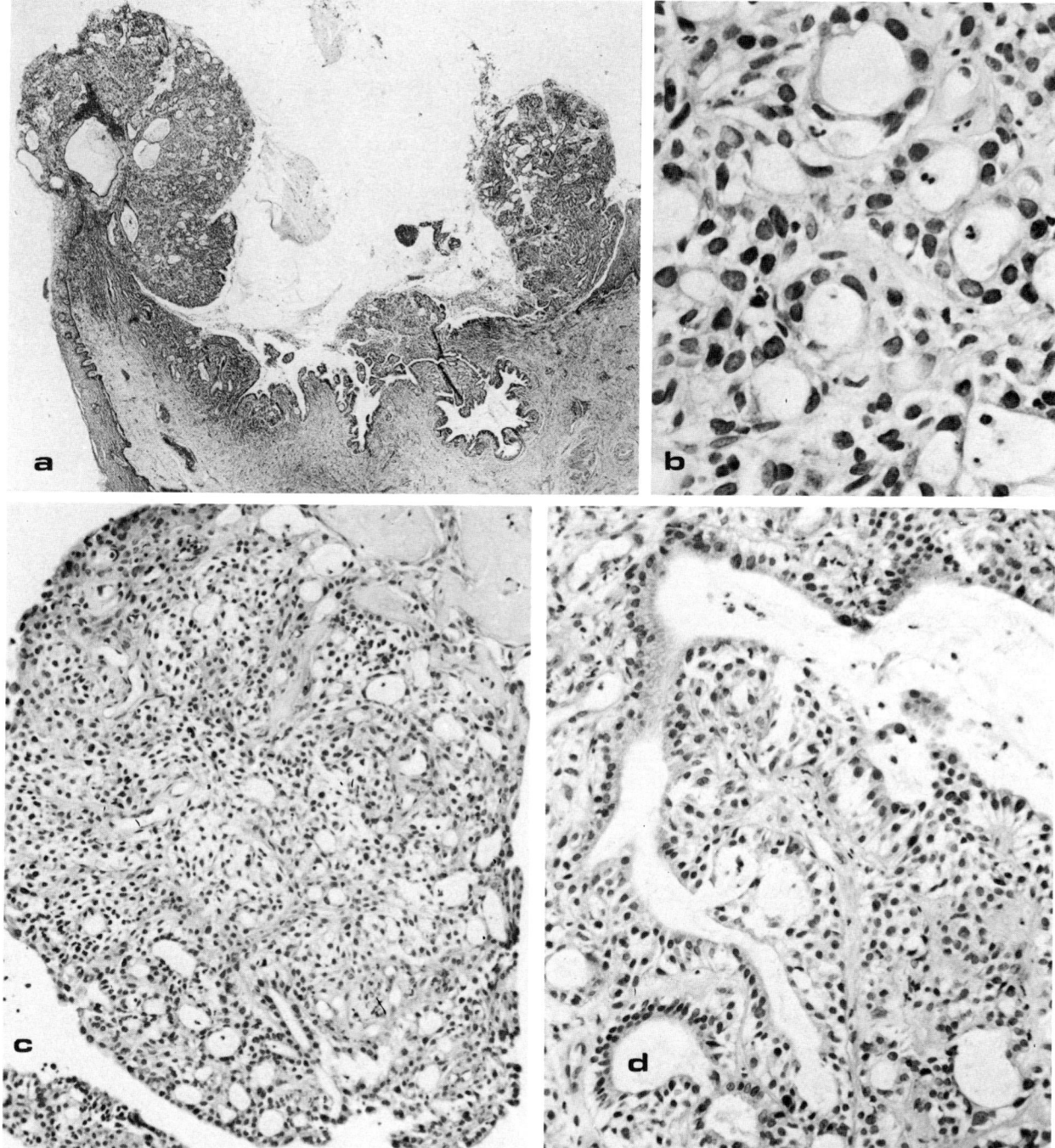

FIG. 4.55. Microglandular hyperplasia. a: Polypoid mass with irregular clefts lined by mucinous columnar cells merges into mucinous glandular epithelium of adenosis in lamina propria of vagina. **b:** Detail of glands closely packed and separated by little or no stroma. Nuclei are uniform and have relatively fine, evenly dispersed chromatin. **c:** Nests composed largely of metaplastic squamous cells. **d:** Cleft and small glandular spaces lined by mucinous cells. (Reprinted by permission of Robboy et al., ref. 292.)

ULTRASTRUCTURE

By electron microscopy, the neoplastic cells from each of the patients are of the same basic type, with glycogen and microvilli being prominent features (Fig. 4.48).[68] Intracellular glycogen is abundant in clear cells in the solid areas and is present in varying but lesser amounts in the other cell types, including areas in which it is not apparent at the light microscopic level.

CLINICAL BEHAVIOR AND TREATMENT

The tumor spreads locally and also metastasizes via lymphatics and blood vessels. Approximately one-sixth of tumors confined clinically to the vagina or cervix (stage I) are discovered on exploration to have metastasized to the pelvic lymph nodes. The frequency of nodal involvement reaches approximately 50% when stage II tumors are considered. Clear cell carcinoma extends outside the abdominal cavity more frequently than does squamous cell carcinoma of the vagina or cervix. Thirty-six percent of the initial recurrences of clear cell carcinomas are in the lung or a supraclavicular lymph node, in contrast to less than 10% for squamous cell carcinomas.

The 5-year actuarial survival rates for all patients with clear cell adenocarcinoma is high. It is about 93% at 5 years and 87% at 10 years when the tumor is stage I.[140] When tumors cause no symptoms or are discovered during the course of an examination because of a history of DES exposure, survival with appropriate therapy approaches 100%. Other factors associated with a better prognosis are an older age (19 years or older) at the time of diagnosis and a tubulocystic microscopic pattern. Large size and/or deep invasion into the wall are associated with a poorer prognosis, but small or superficial tumors also may recur or metastasize. The presence of aneuploidy appears to have no effect on prognosis,[364] but nuclear atypia may be associated with a worse prognosis.[129] Pregnancy at the time of diagnosis does not appear to affect outcome adversely.[309] Recurrences develop most often within 3 years after primary therapy; however, recurrences as late as 19 years after treatment have been observed.[34a,144a] After treatment of the recurrence, approximately one-fifth of the patients survive an additional 3 years or more.

Embryonal Rhabdomyosarcoma (Sarcoma Botryoides)

GENERAL FEATURES

The most common malignant neoplasm of the vagina in infants and children is embryonal rhabdomyosarcoma, most of which are of the subtype designated sarcoma botryoides.[12,53,232] Nearly 90% of cases are diagnosed before 5 years of age.[87,146] This is a rare tumor of unknown etiology and pathogenesis. Certainly the distribution of embryonal rhabdomyosarcomas does not correlate with the mass of skeletal muscle, since most of these neoplasms arise in or near the mucosa of either the head and orbit or the lower urogenital system.

CLINICAL FEATURES

The mean age at diagnosis is 2 years, with a range extending from birth to 41 years.[87,146,193] Most children present with symptoms of a vaginal mass or bleeding. The tumors usually are located along the anterior wall of the vagina, and appear as papillae, small nodules, or pedunculated or sessile soft, polypoid masses with an intact overlying mucosa. Larger tumors may protrude through the introitus (Fig. 4.56). The tumors usually are staged according to the Intergroup Rhabdomyosarcoma Study (IRS) classification, which is based on combined features of extent of disease, resectibility, and microscopic evaluation of margins of excision (Table 4.3).[213]

GROSS FINDINGS

Soft gray or tan, edematous, and nodular tumors are typical. The polypoid gross configuration is thought to result

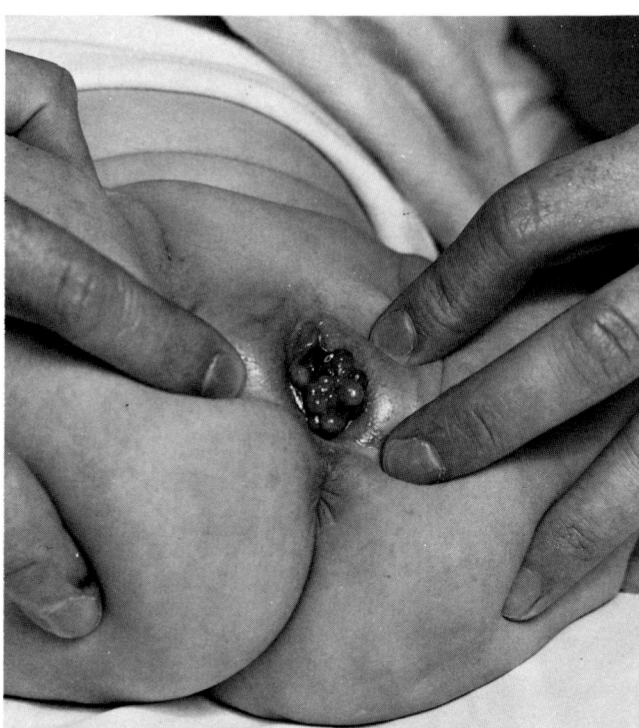

FIG. 4.56. Sarcoma botryoides of the vagina. The gross appearance is that of a polypoid mass protruding through the vaginal introitus and resembling a bunch of grapes. (Reprinted by permission of Hilgers R, Malkasian GD Jr, Soule EH (1970) Embryonal rhabdomyosarcoma (botyroid type) of the vagina: A clinicopathologic review. Am J Obstet Gynecol 107:484.)

Table 4.3. Intergroup rhabdomyosarcoma study (IRS) clinical grouping system

Group I	Localized disease, completely resected
	Regional nodes not involved
	Confined to muscle or organ of origin
	Contiguous involvement—infiltration outside the muscle or organ of origin, as through fascial planes
Group II	Regional disease
	Grossly resected tumor with microscopic residual disease. No evidence of gross residual tumor. No clinical or microscopic evidence of regional node involvement
	Regional disease, completely resected (regional nodes involved completely resected with no microscopic residual)
	Regional disease with involved nodes, grossly resected, but with evidence of microscopic residual
Group III	Incomplete resection or biopsy with gross residual disease
Group IV	Metastatic disease present at onset

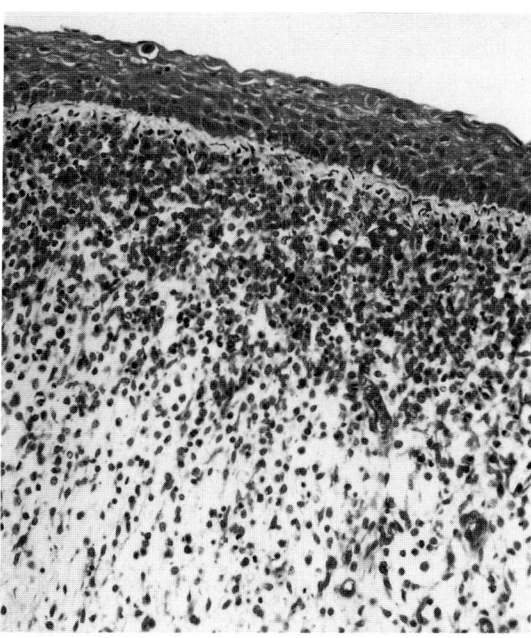

FIG. 4.58. Embryonal rhabdomyosarcoma, botryoide type. A densely cellular, submucosal, cambium layer is typically present. (Reprinted by permission of Kurman et al., ref. 183.)

from relatively unrestricted growth into the lumen of a hollow organ (Fig. 4.57).

MICROSCOPIC FINDINGS

Sarcoma botryoides is characterized by a polypoid growth pattern with a dense cambium layer of tumor cells immediately subjacent to the surface epithelium (Fig. 4.58). The term *cambium* was chosen as an analogy to the peripheral actively growing layer in tree trunks and branches. Beneath the cambium layer, small neoplastic cells are scattered in a loose myxoid or dense collagenous stroma. The tumor cells are of round to spindle shape, with oval nuclei, an open chromatin pattern, and inconspicuous nucleoli.[346]

Focal evidence of rhabdomyogenesis may be evident in any of the patterns, with eosinophilic cytoplasm containing fibers in which cross-striations are present (Fig. 4.59). However, in cases that lack such features, ultrastructural examination is useful for identification of both thick and thin fibrils, and occasionally Z bands.[94] Immunohistochemical staining with antibodies directed against muscle-specific actin, desmin, or myoglobin also may be helpful in establishing the diagnosis.[12,31,54,75,167,183] Although the first two antibodies are more sensitive than myoglobin, they are not specific for skeletal muscle differentiation.

The differential diagnosis includes fibroepithelial polyps, müllerian papillomas, and rhabdomyomas. The correct diagnosis can be made by considering the age at presentation and the microscopic features as described above. After radiation or chemotherapy, occasionally there is difficulty in determining whether scattered mature-appearing skeletal muscle fibers represent residual tumor cells, which are refractory to therapy, or radiated benign muscle fibers of the pelvis.

CLINICAL BEHAVIOR AND TREATMENT

The tumor initially grows into the vaginal wall and soft tissue of the pelvis, bladder, or rectum and subsequently metastasizes to lymph nodes, lungs, liver, and bone. Prognosis is

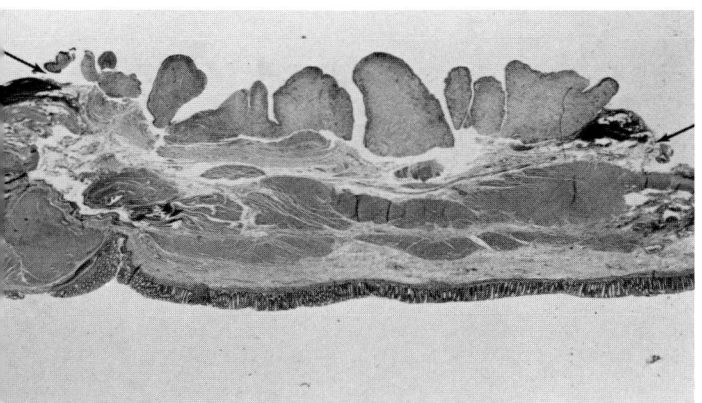

FIG. 4.57. Sarcoma botryoides of the rectovaginal septum. Note the polypoid appearance of the tumor outlined by *arrows*.

related to histologic type and clinical stage. Metastatic tumor is detected in between 24% and 41% of patients with genitourinary and pelvic tumors.[51,252] Historically, the prognosis after radical surgery was poor, with survival rates of less than 20%.[51,94] The introduction of combined multiagent chemotherapy with vincristine, actinomycin, and cyclophosphamide in addition to surgery has dramatically improved the probability of survival.[51,232] The overall 3-year survival for all anatomic sites reported by the IRS I and II was 66% for embryonal rhabdomyosarcoma and 85% for sarcoma botryoides.[232] A recent study suggests that the outcome is even more favorable for vaginal rhabdomyosarcoma, with only 1 death due to tumor reported in 24 evaluable cases.[136]

Melanoma

GENERAL FEATURES

About 120 cases of vaginal melanoma have been reported, representing less than 5% of the malignant neoplasms of the vagina and less than 1% of all melanomas.[45] The mean age at diagnosis is 57 years, with a range from 22 to 83

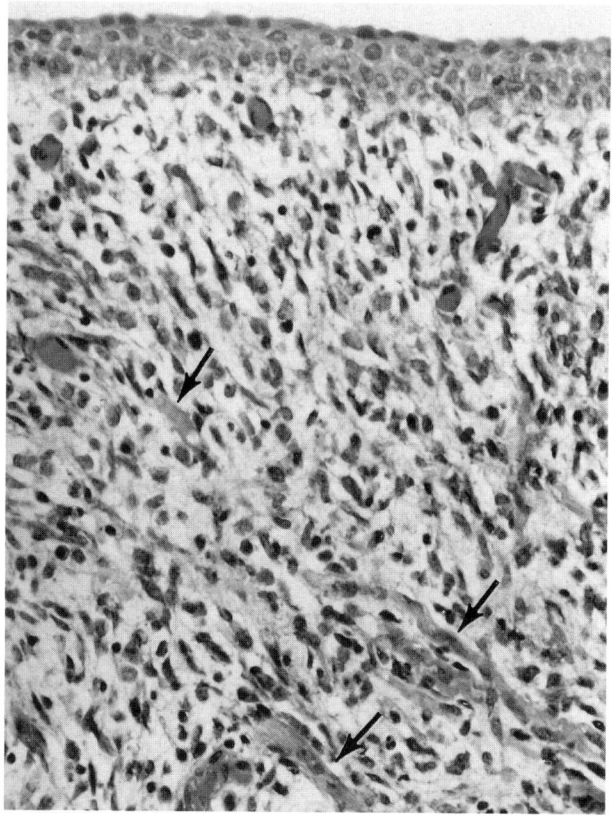

FIG. 4.59. **Embryonal rhabdomyosarcoma, botryoide type.** In contrast to the vaginal rhabdomyoma, the embryonal rhabdomyosarcoma contains densely cellular regions composed of small primitive cells. Interspersed strap cells (*arrows*) confirm the skeletal muscle differentiation.

years.[196] Presenting symptoms include vaginal bleeding, discharge, and a mass. Although the tumors may arise anywhere within the vagina, there is a predilection for the distal third.[45] The etiology and pathogenesis are unknown, but a disproportionately large number of vaginal melanomas have occurred in Japanese women, followed in frequency by Caucasian and then black women.[45,135,196] In one autopsy study, melanocytes were identified in the basal layer of the vagina of 3 of 100 women.[234] It has been suggested that such a condition, referred to as *benign melanosis,* is the setting from which melanoma occasionally may arise,[135,347] and we have seen localized regions of melanosis in the vagina remote from melanomas. Unfortunately, the term *melanosis* also has been used to designate melanophages in the stroma and lentigo malignum-like lesions in mucosal tissues, further obscuring interpretation of the scant available literature.

GROSS FINDINGS

Melanomas may appear as nodular, polypoid, or fungating gray or black soft masses that vary from 0.5 to 8 cm in diameter.[45,201] Frequently, there is ulceration of the overlying epithelium.

MICROSCOPIC FINDINGS

Vaginal melanomas have no microscopic characteristics that are distinctive for this site. The diagnosis usually rests on a constellation of features. In addition to junctional activity, the presence of highly atypical melanocytes, either singly or in clusters, extending through the squamous epithelium is common (Fig. 4.60). The infiltrating neoplastic cells may be epithelioid, spindled, or mixed. Melanin is common within both neoplastic melanocytes and benign melanophages. The lateral spread is typically of the lentiginous type, with single, spindled cells containing pleomorphic nuclei at the epithelial–stromal interface.[45] Rarely, a pagetoid junctional component consisting of epithelioid melanocytes in nests is present.[45]

Since Clark's levels are not appropriate for mucosal sites of melanoma, a system based entirely on tumor thickness has been proposed by Chung et al., as follows: level I—tumor confined to the surface epithelium, level II—invasion of 1 mm or less, level III—invasion of 1–2 mm, and level IV—invasion greater than 2mm.[45] Unfortunately, most of the tumors are deeply invasive. In a group of 19 patients, only 1 was at level III; the remainder were at level IV.[45]

DIFFERENTIAL DIAGNOSIS

The diagnosis usually is straightforward, since most vaginal melanomas are large, with gross and microscopic pigmentation. The differential diagnosis may include melanoma metastatic from other sites, poorly differentiated

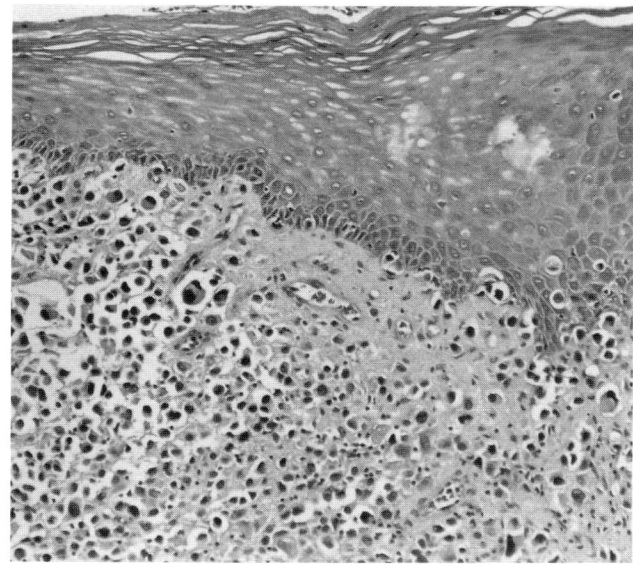

FIG. 4.60. Melanoma. Junctional involvement (right side of field) is frequently identified peripheral to ulcerated or intact central region of deep stromal invasion in primary vaginal melanomas.

squamous carcinoma, sarcoma, and blue nevus. Since primary vaginal melanoma is rare, it is important to rule out metastasis from other sites. The presence of an extensive lateral junctional component is typical in melanomas arising in the vagina, but relatively uncommon in metastases. A complete history is essential, and some cases can be confirmed only by post mortem examination. When large ulcerated lesions are devoid of pigment, immunohistochemistry and ultrastructural examination may permit discrimination of melanoma from other poorly differentiated neoplasms. Positive staining of malignant cells with antibodies directed against S-100 protein is a sensitive, but not specific, marker of melanocytic or neural differentiation. HMB-45 is a less sensitive but more specific indicator of melanoma, and staining for keratan or desmin should be absent. Ultrastructural findings include premelanosomes and melanosomes, as well as abundant rough and smooth endoplasmic reticulum.[135] A high degree of nuclear atypia and numerous mitotic figures usually permit discrimination of melanoma from the rare benign vaginal nevus.

CLINICAL BEHAVIOR AND TREATMENT

The prognosis for vaginal melanoma is poor, with 5-year survival rates of less than 10–20%.[45,196] Undoubtedly, this reflects the inherent aggressiveness of melanoma coupled with the typically deep invasion found at the time of diagnosis.[45,276] In one study, survival was inversely related to the mitotic activity.[24] Both lymphatic and hematogenous metastases are common, with the vagina and groin being the most common initial sites of spread. Primary therapy usually includes wide local or radical excision. The value of groin node dissection, radiation, and chemotherapy remains unknown.[196,250]

Yolk Sac Tumor

Although the yolk sac (endodermal sinus tumor [EST]) usually arises in the gonads, about 56 cases have been reported in the vagina.[48] It is appealing to consider that these tumors originate from germ cells that have failed to complete migration normally in the embryo from the hindgut to the gonad. However, this hypothesis does not provide an obvious explanation for the absence of other malignant germ cell tumors in the vagina, or the predilection of EST for the vagina.

All vaginal ESTs have been diagnosed in children of less than 4 years of age. The presenting symptom usually is a bloody vaginal discharge. The gross and microscopic features of vaginal EST closely resemble those of ovarian origin. Polypoid or sessile, soft, tan or white vaginal masses of 1–5 cm in diameter are typical.[183] A variety of histologic patterns may be present including the microcystic, reticular, papillary, and solid types of EST. Schiller–Duval bodies, composed of papillary arrangements of columnar cells separated from central vascular channels by an acellular zone of connective tissue, are characteristic findings (Fig. 4.61). Extracellular hyaline droplets also are common. Although the histologic findings usually are typical, the diagnosis may not be considered initially because of the rarity of EST in the vagina. The differential diagnosis includes clear cell adenocarinoma, from which EST may be distinguished by the younger age and positive immunohistochemical reactions for alpha-fetoprotein and alpha-1-antitrypsin.[371]

EST is an extremely aggressive tumor. In the past, the median survival was 11 months, and the survival rate at 5 years was less than 25%.[52,250] Most patients developed recurrence and died within 2 years, even after radical surgery.[52,183] The addition of multiagent chemotherapy usually consisting of vincristine, actinomycin, and cyclophosphamide since 1970 has resulted in a 95% disease-free survival at 2 years.[5,52,371] Preliminary data suggest that combination chemotherapy and conservative surgery may permit preservation of future sexual function and fertility as well as an excellent cure rate.[250]

Leiomyosarcoma

About 40 leiomyosarcomas of the vagina have been reported.[254] The frequency and behavior have been difficult to establish because the pathologic criteria separating benign from malignant smooth muscle tumors have varied. Currently, it is recommended that smooth muscle tumors of greater than 3 cm diameter, with five or more mitotic figures per 10 HPFs, moderate or marked cytologic atypia,

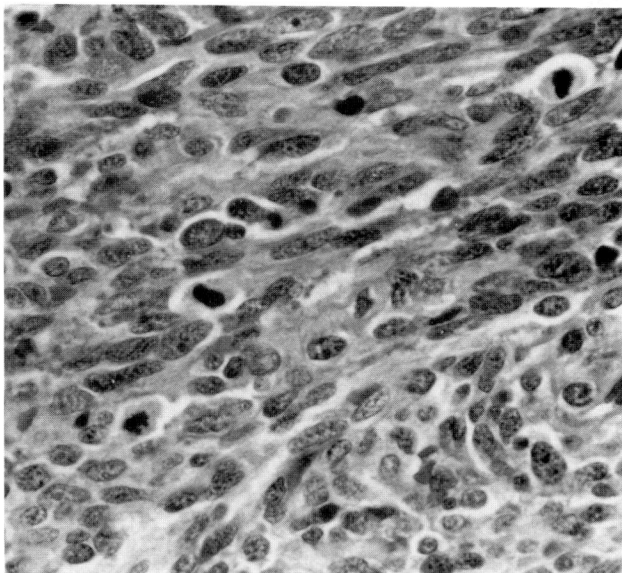

Fig. 4.62. Vaginal leiomyosarcoma. The tumor resembles that of uterine origin, with fascicles of spindle cells having moderate or marked nuclear pleomorphism with increased mitotic activity.

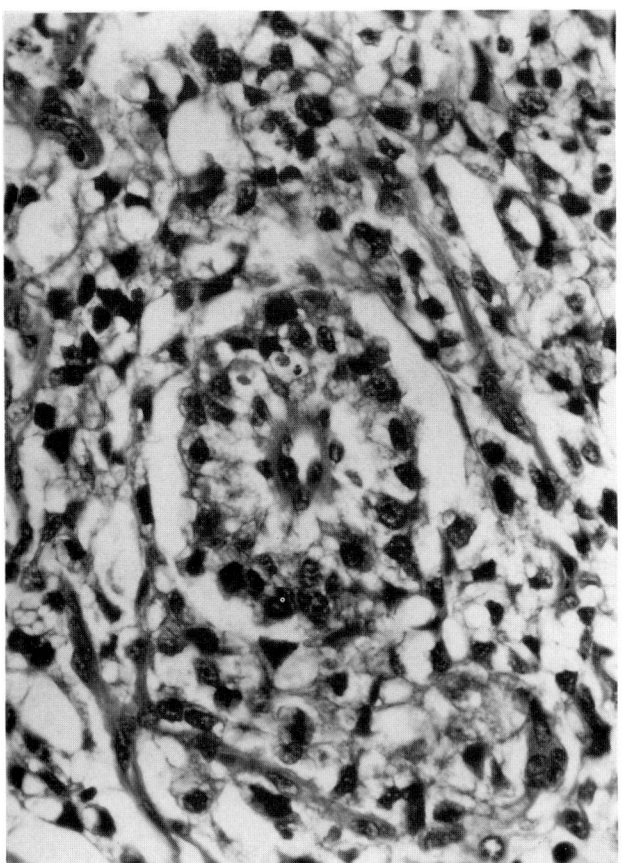

Fig. 4.61. Yolk sac tumor. The centrally located Schiller–Duval body is characterized by a papillary arrangement of columnar cells separated from a central vascular core by a zone of acellular connective tissue. (Courtesy of Henry J. Norris, M.D., Washington, D.C.)

and infiltrating margins be classified as leiomyosarcoma (Fig. 4.62).[334] The age range extends from 25 to 86 years. Vaginal bleeding is the most common presenting symptom. The gross and microscopic features resemble those of uterine leiomyosarcoma, but the spread of tumor is by local invasion and hematogenous metastasis. The 5-year survival rate is about 35%.[254] The primary therapy is surgical, and exenteration may be required to provide an adequate margin around larger tumors.

Malignant Mixed Tumor

Probably unrelated to the benign vaginal mixed tumor is the reportedly malignant mixed tumor, which resembles either synovial sarcoma or a malignant tumor arising from mesonephric rests.[241,313] Two of these rare tumors occurred in women 24 and 33 years old, who presented with a polypoid nodule in the lateral vaginal fornix. The microscopic appearance is of an intact vaginal squamous mucosa with a subjacent mixture of solid nests of polyhedral-

shaped cells and flattened epithelial cells in acinar or tubular arrays, bordered peripherally by smaller bundles of spindle cells resembling fibroblasts (Fig. 4.63). Ultrastructural features resembling synovial sarcoma were noted in one case.[241,313] The presence of mitotic activity as great as eight mitoses per 10 HPFs coupled with nuclear pleomorphism and moderate-sized nucleoli suggested that the process was malignant. However, the biologic potential remains uncertain in the absence of long-term follow-up.

Secondary Neoplasms

Although primary neoplasms of the vagina are quite rare, secondary spread of malignant neoplasms to the vagina by direct extension or lymphatic or hematogenous metastasis is quite common. Fu and Reagan found that only 58 (16%) of 355 invasive carcinomas involving the vagina represented primary neoplasms.[94] Spread from primary carcinoma of the cervix was most common (32%), followed by endometrium (18%), colon and rectum (9%), ovary (6%), vulva (6%), and urinary tract (4%). Even among the squamous carcinomas found in the vagina, only a minority prove to be primary to this site. About 75% are secondary, arising in either the cervix (79%) or vulva (14%).[94]

Miscellaneous Malignant Neoplasms

Endometrioid adenocarinomas, stromal sarcomas, and malignant mixed müllerian tumors occasionally originate in the vagina, at times arising from a background of endo-

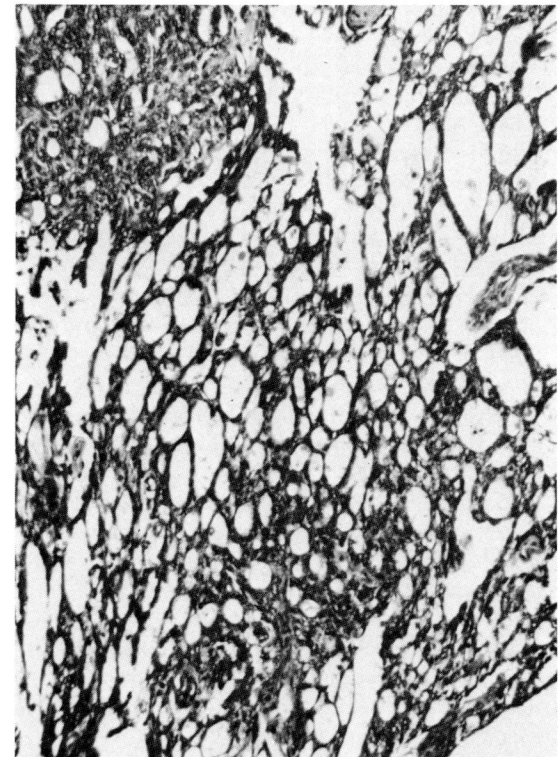

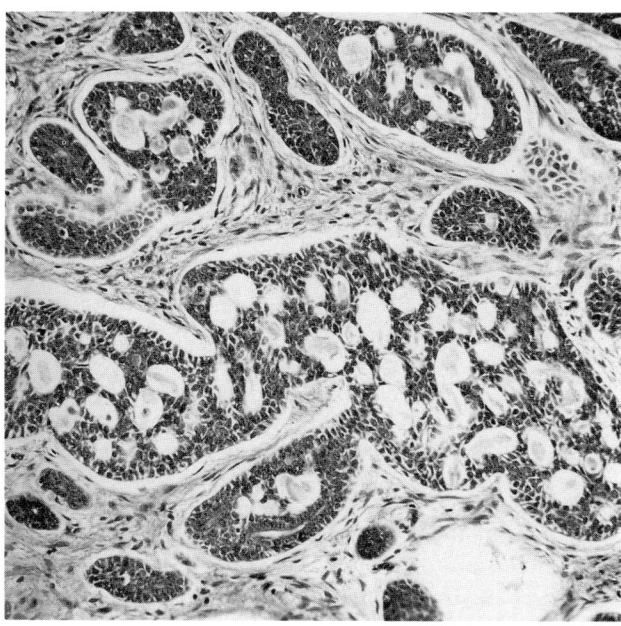

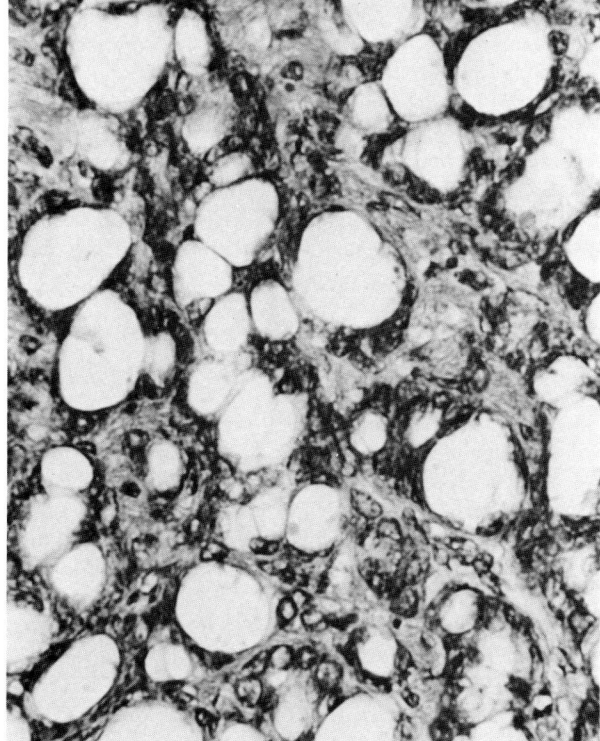

FIG. 4.64. Adenoid cystic carcinoma of the vagina. The tumor resembles that found in the uterine cervix, with solid and cribriform arrangements of well-delineated cell masses. (Courtesy of Henry J. Norris, M.D., Washington, D.C.)

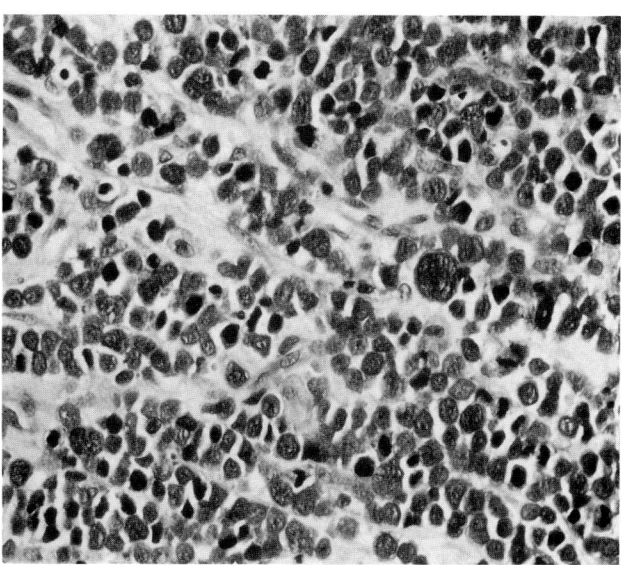

FIG. 4.63. Malignant tumor of the vagina resembling synovial sarcoma. *Top:* In this area, the tumor is predominantly acinar. Mucin stains showed positive reactions in inspissated material in lumina and in some of the cells. *Bottom:* High-power view of the acini. The nuclei of cells are prominent, whereas cytoplasmic borders are indistinct. (Reprinted by permission of Okagaki et al., ref. 241.)

FIG. 4.65. Small cell carcinoma of the vagina. The tumor shares histologic features with small cell carcinomas arising elsewhere. The cell of origin remains unknown. (Reprinted by permission of Kurman et al., ref. 183.)

metriosis.[114,254] In addition, there are occasional reported cases of primary vaginal adenocarcinoma in situ,[47] intestinal-type adenocarcinoma,[92] adenosquamous carcinoma,[279,310,325] adenocarcinoma arising in mesonephric duct remnants,[150,373] adenoid basal cell carcinoma,[228] adenoid cystic carcinoma (Fig. 4.64),[183] carcinoid tumor,[95] small cell carcinoma (Fig. 4.65),[165,267] malignant schwannoma,[63] fibrosarcoma,[244] malignant fibrous histiocytoma,[363] angiosarcoma,[269,344] and alveolar soft part sarcoma.[38]

References

1. Abdul-Karim FW, Lederman MM, Carter JR, et al. (1981) Toxic shock syndrome: Clinicopathologic findings in a fatal case. Hum Pathol 12: 16–22

2. Ackerman LV (1948) Verrucous carcinoma of the oral cavity. Surgery 23: 670–678

3. Al-Durdi M, Monaghan JM (1977) Thirty-two years experience in management of primary tumors of the vagina. Br J Obstet Gynecol 127: 513

4. Amsel R, Totten PA, Spiegel CA, et al. (1983) Nonspecific vaginitis: Diagnostic criteria and microbial and epidemiologic associations. Am J Med 74: 14–22

5. Anderson WA, Sabio H, Durso N, et al. (1985) Endodermal sinus tumor of the vagina. The role of primary chemotherapy. Cancer 56: 1025–1027

6. Andrew DE, Bumstead E, Kempton AG. (1975) The role of fomites in the transmission of vaginitis. Can Med Assoc J 112: 1181–1183

7. Antonioli DA, Burke L, Friedman EA (1980) Natural history of diethylstilbestrol-associated genital lesions: Cervical ectopy and cervicovaginal hood. Am J Obstet Gynecol 137: 847

8. Arbitol MM, Davenport JH (1974) The irradiated vagina. Obstet Gynecol 44: 249

9. Averette HE, Weinstein GD, Frost P (19709) Autoradiographic analysis of cell proliferation kinetics in human genital tissues. I. Normal cervix and vagina. Am J Obstet Gynecol 108: 8–17

10. Bacon HE, Ross ST, Malvar P (1972) Sigmoidovaginal and cecovaginal fistula as a complication of peridiverticulitis: Report of eight cases. Dis Colon Rectum 15: 41–48

11. Baker CJ (1977) Summary of the workshop on perinatal infections due to group B streptococcus. J Infect Dis 136: 137

12. Bale PM, Parsons RE, Stevens MM (1983) Diagnosis and behavior of juvenile rhabdomyosarcoma. Hum Pathol 14: 596–611

13. Barrett KF, Bledsoe S, Greer BE, Droegemueller W (1977) Tampon-induced vaginal or cervical ulceration. Am J Obstet Gynecol 127: 332–333

14. Barry W, Hudgins L, Donta ST, Pesanti EL (1992) Intravenous immunoglobulin therapy for toxic shock syndrome. JAMA 267: 3315–3316

15. Bartlett JG, Onderdonk AB, Drude E, et al. (1977) Quantitative bacteriology of the vaginal flora. J Infect Dis 136: 271–277

16. Beard CM, Melton LJ III, O'Fallon WM, et al. (1984) Cryptorchism and maternal estrogen exposure. Am J Epidemiol 120: 707

17. Beecham CT (1980) Classification of vaginal relaxation. Am J Obstet Gynecol 136: 957–958

18. Bell DA, Mondschein M, Scully RE (1986) Giant cell arteritis of the female genital tract. A report of three cases. Am J Surg Pathol 10: 696–701

19. Benedet JL, Murphy KJ, Fairey RN, et al. (1983) Primary invasive carcinoma of the vagina. Obstet Gynecol 62: 715

20. Benedet JL, Sanders BH (1984) Carcinoma in situ of the vagina. Am Obstet Gynecol 148: 695–700

21. Bennett HG, Ehrlich HM (1941) Myoma of the vagina. Am J Obstet Gynecol 42: 314

22. Bergdoll MS, Reiser RF, Crass BA, et al. (1981) A new staphylococcal enterotoxin, enterotoxin F, associated with toxic-shock-syndrome staphylococcus aureus isolates. Lancet 1: 1017–1021

23. Boquet-Jiménez E, Alvarez San Cristóbal A (1978) Cytologic and microbiologic aspects of vaginal torulopsis. Acta Cytol 22: 331–334

24. Borazjani G, Prem KA, Okagaki T, et al. (1990) Primary malignant melanoma of the vagina: A clinicopathological analysis of 10 cases. Gynecol Oncol 37: 264–267

25. Borgno G, Bersani R, Micheletti L, et al. (1988) Colposcopic findings before sexual activity. Cervix Low Female Genital Tract 6: 69–73

26. Bornstein J, Adam E, Adler-Storthz K, Kaufman RH (1988) Development of cervical and vaginal squamous cell neoplasia as a late consequence of in utero exposure to diethylstilbestrol. Obstet Gynecol Surv 43: 15–21

27. Boutin EL, Battle E, Cunha GR. The germ layer origin of mouse vaginal epithelium restricts its competence: Prostatic induction. Submitted

28. Bramley M, Kinghorn G (1979) Do oral contraceptives inhibit *Trichomonoas vaginalis?* Sex Transm Dis 6: 261–263

28a. Branton PA, Tavassoli FA (1993) Spindle cell epithelioma, the so-called mixed tumor of the vagina. Am J Surg Path 17: 509–515

29. Brinton LA, Nasca PC, Mallin K, et al. (1990) Case-control study of in situ and invasive carcinoma of the vagina. Gynecol Oncol 38: 49

30. Brody JR, Cunha GR (1989) Histologic, morphometric and immunocytochemical analysis of myometrial development in rats and mice: II. Effects of DES on development. Am J Anat 1986: 21–42

31. Brooks JJ (1982) Immunohistochemistry of soft tissue tumors. Myoglobin as a tumor marker for rhabdomyosarcoma. Cancer 50: 1757

32. Brown GR, Fletcher GH, Rutledge FN (1971) Irradiation of in situ and invasive carcinoma of the vagina. Cancer 28: 1278

33. Bullock BC, Newbold RR, McLachlan JA (1988) Lesions of testis and epididymis associated with prenatal diethylstilbestrol exposure. Environment Health Perspect 77: 29–31

34. Buntine DW, Henderson PR, Biggs JSG (1979) Benign mullerian mixed tumor of the vagina. Gynecol Oncol ε 21–26

34a. Burks RT, Schwarz AM, Wheeler JE, Antoniolli D (1990) Late recurrence of clear cell adenocarcinoma of the cervix: Case report. Obstet Gynecol 76:525–527

35. Carinelli SG, Carinelli I, Merlo D-N (1984) Mucinous cysts of the vulva. Cervix & l.f.g.t. 2: 143–148

36. Ceremshak RJ (1969) Benign rhabdomyoma of the vagina. Am J Clin Pathol 52: 604–606

37. Chang T-W (1976) Familial allergic seminal vulvovaginitis. Am J Obstet Gynecol 126: 442–444

38. Chapman GW, Benda JO, Williams T (1984) Alveolar soft part sarcoma of the vagina. Gynecol Oncol 18: 125–129

39. Charles V, Charles SX (1978) A case of vulvo-vaginal diphtheria in a girl of seven years. Indian J Pediatr 15: 257–258

40. Chaves E, Palitot P (1964) Pelvic schistosomiasis. Am J Obstet Gynecol 89: 1000–1002

41. Chen KTK (1981) Benign mixed tumor of the vagina. Obstet Gynecol 57: 89S–90S

42. Chen KTK (1981) Brenner tumor of the vagina. Diag Gynecol Obstet 3: 255

43. Chirayil SJ, Tobon H (1981) Polyps of the vagina: A clinicopathologic study of 18 cases. Cancer 47: 2904–2907

44. Chu SY, Berkelman RL, Curran JW (1992) Epidemiology of HIV in the United States. In: DeVita VT, Hellman S, Rosenberg SA (eds) AIDS: Etiology, diagnosis, treatment, and prevention, Chapter 7. Philadelphia, JB Lippincott, pp 99–109

45. Chung AF, Casey MJ, Flannery JT, et al. (1980) Malignant melanoma of the vagina—Report of 19 cases. Obstet Gynecol 55:720–727

46. Clark JFJ, Faggett T, Peters B, Sampson CC (1978) Ulcerative vaginitis due to torulopsis glabrata: A case report. J Natl Med Assoc 70: 913–914

47. Clement PB, Benedet JL (1979) Adenocarcinoma in situ of the vagina. A case report. Cancer 43: 2479–2485

48. Clement PB, Young RH, Scully RE (1988) Extraovarian pelvic yolk sac tumors. Cancer 62: 620–626

49. Clemente CD (ed) (1985) Gray's anatomy of the human body, 30th ed. Philadelphia, Lea & Febiger

50. Coetzee LF (1972) Tuberculous vaginitis. South Afr Med J 46: 1225–1226

51. Coffin CM, Dehner LP (1992) The soft tissue. In: Stocker JT, Dehner LP (eds) Pediatric pathology, Vol 2, Chapter 29. Philadelphia, JB Lippincott, pp 1091–1132

52. Copeland LJ, Sneige N, Ordonez NG (1985) Endodermal sinus tumor of the vagina and cervix. Cancer 55: 2558–2565

53. Copeland LJ, Sneige N, Stringer CA, et al. (1985) Alveolar rhabdomyosarcoma of the female genitalia. Cancer 56: 849–855

54. Corson JM, Pinkus GS (1981) Intracellular myoglobin—a specific marker for skeletal muscle differentiation in soft tissue sarcomas: An immunoperoxidase study. Am J Pathol 103: 384

55. Cramer DW, Cutler SJ (1974) Incidence and histopathology of malignancies of the female genital organs in the United States. Am J Obstet Gynecol 118: 443–460

56. Crowther ME, Lowe DG, Shepherd JH (1988) Verrucous carcinoma of the female genital tract: A review. Obstet Gynecol Surv 43: 263–280

57. Cunha GR (1975) The dual origin of vaginal epithelium. Am J Anat 143: 387–392

58. Cunha GR, Taguchi O, Namikawa R, et al. (1987) Teratogenic effects of clomiphene, tamoxifen, and diethylstilbestrol on the developing human female and genital tract. Hum Pathol 18: 1132–1143

59. Cunha GR, Taguchi O, Sugimura Y, et al. (1988) Absence of teratogenic effects of progesterone on the developing genital tract of the human female fetus. Hum Pathol 19: 777–783

60. Curtis EM, Pine L (1981) Actinomyces in the vaginas of women with and without intrauterine contraceptive devices. Am J Obstet Gynecol 140: 880–884

61. Davis JP, Chesney PJ, Wand PJ, LaVenture M (1980) Toxic-shock syndrome. Epidemiologic features, recurrence, risk factors, and prevention. N Engl J Med 303: 1429–1435

62. Davis TC (1975) Chronic vulvovaginitis in children due to Shigella flexneri. Pediatrics 56: 41–44

63. Davos I, Abell MR (1976) Sarcomas of the vagina. Obstet Gynecol 47(3): 342–350

64. Daw E (1971) Primary carcinoma of the vagina. J Obstet Gynecol Br Commonwealth 78: 853

65. DeCherney AH, Cholst I, Naftolin F (1981) Structure and function of the fallopian tubes following exposure to diethylstilbestrol (DES) during gestation. Fertil Steril 36: 741

66. Dekel A, Avidan D, Bar-ziv J, et al. (1988) Neurofibroma of the vagina presenting with urinary retention. Review of the literature and report of a case. Obstet Gynecol Surv 43: 325–327

67. Deppisch LM (1975) Cysts of the vagina: Classification and clinical correlations. Obstet Gynecol 45: 632–637

68. Dickersin GR, Welch WR, Erlandson R, Robboy SJ (1980) Ultrastructure of 16 cases of clear cell adenocarcinoma of the vagina and cervix in DES-exposed young women. Cancer 45: 1615

69. Dillon HC Jr, Gray E, Pass MA, Gray BM (1982) Anorectal and vaginal carriage of group B streptococci during pregnancy. J Infect Dis 145: 794–799

70. Dixit S, Singhal S, Baboo HA (1993) Squamous cell carcinoma of the vagina: A review of 70 cases. Gynecol Oncol 48: 80–87

71. Droegemueller W, Herbst AL, Mishell DR, Jr, Stenchever MA (1987) Comprehensive Gynecology. St. Louis, CV Mosby, p 974

72. Dvoretsky PM, Bonfiglio TA (1986) The pathology of vulvar squamous cell carcinoma and verrucous carcinoma. In: Sommers SC, Rosen PP, Fechner RE (eds) Pathology annual, Part 2, Vol 21. Connecticut, Appleton-Century-Crofts, pp 23–45

73. Eickhoff TC, Klein JO, Daly AL, et al. (1964) Neonatal sepsis and other infections due to group B beta-hemolytic streptococci. N Engl J Med 271: 1221–1228

74. Elliott GB, Elliott JDA (1973) Superficial stromal reactions of lower genital tract. Arch Pathol 95: 100–101

75. Eusebi V, Ceccarelli C, Gorza L, et al. (1986) Immunocytochemistry of rhabdomyosarcoma. The use of four different markers. Am J Surg Pathol 10: 293

76. Evans DMD, Hughes H (1961) Cysts of the vaginal wall. J Obstet Gynaecol Br Comm 68: 247–253

77. Fallon RJ, Robinson ET (1974) Meningococcal vulvovaginitis. Scand J Infect Dis 6: 295–296

78. Farrand RJ (1971) Haemophilus influenzae infections of the genital tract. J Med Microbiol 4: 357–358

79. Faulconer HT, Muldoon JP (1975) Rectovaginal fistula in patients with colitis: Review and report of a case. Dis Colon Rectum 18: 413–415

80. Fawcett DW (ed) (1986) Bloom and Fawcett's textbook of histology, 11th ed. Philadelphia, WB Saunders

81. Fish SA (1956) Vaginal injury due to coitus. Am J Obstet Gynecol 72: 544–548

82. Fleury FJ (1979) The diagnosis of vaginitis. Am J Diagn Gynecol Obstet 1: 209–216

83. Fliegner JR (1987) Congenital atresia of the vagina. Surg Gynecol Obstet 165: 387–391

84. Forsberg J-G (1973) Cervicovaginal epithelium: Its origin and development. Am J Obstet Gynecol 7: 1025–1043

85. Fox H, Wells M, Harris M, et al. (1988) Enteric tumors of the lower female genital tract: a report of three cases. Histopathology 12: 167–176

86. Friedell S, Mercer LJ (1986) Nonmenstrual toxic shock syndrome. Obstet Gynecol Surv 41: 336–341

87. Friedman M, Peretz BA, Nissenbaum M, Paldi E (1986) Modern treatment of vaginal embryonal rhabdomyosarcoma. Obstet Gynecol Surv 41: 614–618

88. Friedrich EG (1981) Tampon effects on vaginal health. Clin Obstet Gynecol 24: 395–406

89. Friedrich EG (1985) Vaginitis. Am J Obstet Gynecol 152: 247–251

90. Friedrich EG, Siegesmund KA (1980) Tampon-associated vaginal ulcerations. Obstet Gynecol 55: 149–156

91. Friedrich EG, Wilkinson EJ (1973) Mucous cysts of the vulvar vestibule. Obstet Gynecol 42: 407–414

92. Frick HC, Jacox HW, Taylor HC (1968) Primary carcinoma of the vagina. Am J Obstet Gynecol 101: 695–703

93. Fu YS, Reagan JW (1989) Pathology of the uterine cervix, vagina, and vulva, Chapter 7. Philadelphia, WB Saunders, pp 193–224

94. Fu YS, Reagan JW (1989) Pathology of the uterine cervix, vagina, and vulva, Chapter 9. Philadelphia, WB Saunders, pp 336–379

95. Fukushima M, Twiggs LB, Okagaki T (1986) Mixed intestinal adenocarcinoma-argentaffin carcinoma of the vagina. Gynecol Oncol 23: 387–394

96. Fuller AF, Swartz MN, Wolfson JS, Salzman R (1980) Toxic-shock syndrome. N Engl J Med 303: 881

97. Gad A, Eusebi V (1975) Rhabdomyoma of the vagina. J Pathol 115: 179–181

98. Galask RP, Larsen B, Ohm MJ (1976) Vaginal flora and its role in disease entities. Clin Obstet Gynecol 19: 61–81

99. Gallup DG, Morley GW (1975) Carcinoma in situ of the vagina: A study and review. Obstet Gynecol 46: 334

100. Gallup DC, Nolan TE, Martin D, et al. (1991) Thrombotic thrombocytopenic purpura first seen as massive vaginal necrosis. Am J Obstet Gynecol 165: 413–415

101. Gardner HL (1966) Cervical and vaginal endometriosis. Clin Obstet Gynecol 9: 358–372

102. Gardner HL (1968) Desquamative inflammatory vaginitis: A newly defined entity. Am J Obstet Gynecol 102: 1102–1105

103. Gardner HL (1980) Haemophilus vaginalis vaginitis after twenty-five years. Am J Obstet Gynecol 137: 385–391

104. Gardner HL, Dampeer TK, Dukes CD (1957) The prevalence of vaginitis: A study in incidence. Am J Obstet Gynecol 73: 1080–1087

105. Gardner HL, Fernet P (1964) Etiology of vaginitis emphysematosa. Report of ten cases and review of literature. Am J Obstet Gynecol 88:680–694

106. Geelhoed GW, Henson DE, Taylor PT, et al. (1976) Carcinoma in situ of the vagina following treatment for carcinoma of the cervix. A distinctive clinical entity. Am J Obstet Gynecol 124: 510

107. Gelfand M, Ross MD, Blair DM, Weber MC (1972) Distribution and extent of schistosomiasis in female pelvic organs, with special reference to the genital tract, as determined at autopsy. Am J Trop Med Hyg 20: 846–849

108. Gershman ST, Stolley PD (1988) A case-control study of testicular cancer using Connecticut tumor registry data. Int J Epidemiol 17: 738–742

109. Geschicter CF (1934) Tumors of muscle. Am J Cancer 22: 378–410

110. Goei SH, Wells JI (1981) Corynebacterium vaginale in non-purulent vaginitis. Med J Aust 1: 470–472

111. Gold BM (1971) Neurofibromatosis of the bladder and vagina. Am J Obstet Gynecol 113: 1055–1056

112. Gold JH, Bossen EH (1976) Benign vaginal rhabdomyoma. A light and electron microscopic study. Cancer 37: 2283–2294

113. Gompel C, Silverberg SG (1977) Pathology in gynecology and obstetrics. Philadelphia, JB Lippincott

114. Goyert G, Budev H, Wright C, et al (1987) Vaginal Müllerian stromal sarcoma. A case report. J Reprod Med 32: 129–130

115. Graber B, Kline-Graber G (1979) Female orgasm: Role of pubococcygeus muscle. J Clin Psychiatry 40: 348–351

116. Graham-Brown RAC, Cochrane GW, Swinhoe JR, et al. (1981) Vaginal stenosis due to bullous erythema multiforme (Stevens-Johnson syndrome). Br J Obstet Gynaecol 88: 1156–1157

117. Grant TD, Mace KD (1977) Quantitation of secretory immunoglobulin A in vaginal secretions. J Am Coll Health 26: 81–84

118. Gravett MG, Nelson HP, DeRouen T, et al. (1986) Independent associations of bacterial vaginosis and Chlamydia trachomatis infection with adverse pregnancy outcome. JAMA 256: 1899

119. Gray LA, Christopherson MM (1969) In-situ and early invasive carcinoma of the vagina. Obstet Gynecol 34: 226

120. Greenberg ER, Barnes AB, Resseguie L, et al. (1984) Breast cancer in mothers given diethylstilbestrol in pregnancy. N Engl J Med 311: 1393

121. Greenhalf JO (1972) Vaginal vault granulation tissue following total abdominal hysterectomy. Br J Clin Pract 26: 247–249

122. Gregoire AT, Kandil O, Ledger WJ (1971) The glycogen content of human vaginal epithelial tissue. Fertil Steril 22: 64–68

123. Gompel C, Silverberg SG (1985) Pathology in gynecology and obstetrics, 3rd ed. Philadelphia, JB Lippincott

124. Guillou L, Gloor E, De Grandi P, Costa J (1989) Postoperative pseudosarcoma of the vagina. A case report. Pathol Res Pract 185: 245–248

125. Gupta PK, Hollander DH, Frost JK (1976) Actinomycetes in cervicovaginal smears: An association with IUD usage. Acta Cytol 20: 295–297

126. Hafez ESE (1977) The vagina and human reproduction. Am J Obstet Gynecol 129: 573–584

127. Halpern BM, Ky T, Robert R (1967) Clinical and immuno-

logical study of an exceptional case of reaginic type sensitization to human seminal fluid. Immunology 12: 247

128. Hammerschlag MR, Alpert S, Onderdonk AB, et al. (1978) Anaerobic microflora of the vagina in children. Am J Obstet Gynecol 131: 853

129. Hanselaar AG, Van Leusen ND, DeWilde PCM, Vooijs GP (1991) Clear cell adenocarcinoma of the vagina and cervix. A report of the Central Netherlands Registry with emphasis on early detection and prognosis. Cancer 67: 1971–1978

130. Haney AF, Newbold RR, Fetter BF, McLachlan JA (1986) Paraovarian cysts associated with prenatal diethylstilbestrol exposure. Am J Pathol 124: 405–411

131. Hartman P, Diddle AW (1972) Vaginal stenosis following irradiation therapy for carcinoma of the cervix uteri. Cancer 30: 426–429

132. Hartmann C-A, Sperling M, Stein H (1990) So-called fibroepithelial polyps of the vagina exhibiting an unusual but uniform antigen profile characterized by expression of desmin and steroid hormone receptors but no muscle-specific actin or macrophage markers. Am J Clin Pathol 93: 604–608

133. Hartmann CA, Sperling M, Stein H (1990) So-called fibroepithelial polyps of the vagina exhibiting an unusual but uniform antigen profile characterized by expression of desmin and steroid hormone receptors but no muscle-specific actin or macrophage markers. Am J Clin Pathol 93: 604–608

134. Harvey M (1981) Absorption of staphylococcal toxin in toxic-shock syndrome (Letter to the Editor). N Engl J Med 305: 1652–1653

135. Hasumi K, Sakamoto G, Sugano H, et al (1978) Primary malignant melanoma of the vagina. Study of four autopsy cases with ultrastructural findings. Cancer 42: 2675–2686

136. Hays DM, Shimada H, et al. (1985) Sarcomas of the vagina and the uterus: The Intergroup Rhabdomyosarcoma Study. J Pediatr Surg 20: 718

137. Heinz KPW (1973) Amoebic infection of the female genital tract. A report of three cases. South Afr Med J 47: 1795–1798

138. Helms CM, Lengeling RW, Pinsky RL, et al. (1981) Toxic shock syndrome: A retrospective study of 25 cases from Iowa. Am J Med Sci 282: 50–60

139. Henson D, Tarone R (1977) An epidemiologic study of cancer of the cervix, vagina, and vulva based on the Third National Cancer Survey in the United States. Am J Obstet Gynecol 129: 525–532

140. Herbst AL (1992) Vaginal clear cell cancer: Incidence, survival and screening. In: Long-term effects of exposure to diethylstilbestrol (DES) (NIH Workshop), April 22–24, Falls Church, VA, pp 19–20

141. Herbst AL, Anderson S, Hubby MM, et al. (1986) Risk factors for the development of diethylstilbestrol-associated clear cell adenocarcinoma: A case-control study. Am J Obstet Gynecol 154: 814–822

142. Herbst AL, Green TH Jr, Ulfelder H (1970) Primary carcinoma of the vagina. Am J Obstet Gynecol 106: 210

143. Herbst AL, Poskanzer DC, Robboy SJ, et al. (1975) Prenatal exposure to stilbestrol: A prospective comparison of exposed female offspring with unexposed control. N Engl J Med 292: 334

144. Herbst AL, Ulfelder H, Poskanzer DC (1971) Adenocarcinoma of the vagina: Association of maternal stilbestrol therapy with tumor appearance in young women. N Engl J Med 284: 878

144a. Herbst AL (personal communcation)

145. Hidayat AA, Riddle PJ (1987) Ligneous conjunctivitis: A clinicopathologic study of 17 cases. Ophthalmology 94: 949–959

146. Hilgers RD, Malkasian GD Jr, Soule EH (1970) Embryonal rhabdomyosarcoma (botryoid type) of the vagina: A clinicopathologic review. Am J Obstet Gynecol 107: 484

147. Hill HR (1984) Group B streptococcal infections. In: Holmes KK, Mårdh P-A, Sparling PF, Wiesner PJ (eds) Sexually transmitted diseases. New York, McGraw-Hill, p 397–407

148. Hillier SL, Critchlow CW, Stevens CE, et al. (1991) Microbiological, epidemiological and clinical correlates of vaginal colonisation by Mobiluncus species. Genitourin Med 67: 26–31

149. Hilton AL, Warnock DW (1975) Vaginal candidiasis and the role of the digestive tract as a source of infection. Br J Obstet Gynaecol 82: 922–926

150. Hinchey WM, Silva EG, Guarda LA, et al. (1983) Paravaginal wolffian duct (mesonephros) adenocarcinoma: A light and electron microscopic study. Am J Clin Pathol 80: 539–544

151. Hingorani V, Mahapatra LN (1964) Amebiasis of vagina and cervix. J Int Coll Surgeons 42: 662–667

152. Hoffman DB, Grundfest P (1959) Vaginitis emphysematosa. Am J Obstet Gynecol 78: 428–430

153. Hood M, Janney A, Dameron G (1961) Beta hemolytic streptococcus group B associated with problems of the perinatal period. Am J Obstet Gynecol 82: 809

154. Hoogkamp-Korstanje JAA, Gerrards LJ, Cats BP (1982) Maternal carriage and neonatal acquisition of group B streptococci. J Infect Dis 145: 800–803

155. Hopkins MP, Morley GW (1987) Squamous cell carcinoma of the neovagina. Obstet Gynecol 69: 525–527

156. Horowitz BJ, Edelstein SW, Lippman L (1985) Candida tropicalis vulvovaginitis. Obstet Gynecol 66: 229–232

157. Hummer WK, Mussey E, Decker DG, Dockerty MB (1970) Carcinoma in situ of the vagina. Am J Obstet Gynecol 108: 1109–1116

158. Horwitz RI, Viscoli CM, Merino M, et al. (1988) Clear cell adenocarcinoma of the vagina and cervix. Incidence, misclassified disease, and diethylstilbestrol. J Clin Epidemiol 41: 593–597

159. Hurley R, Leask B, Faktor JA, de Fonseka CJ (1973) Incidence and distribution of yeast species and of trichomonas vaginalis in the vagina of pregnant women. J Obstet Gynaecol Br Commonw 80: 252

160. Hurley R, de Louvois J (1979) Candida vaginitis. Postgrad Med J 55: 645–647

161. Japaze H, Dinh TV, Woodruff JD (1982) Verrucous carcinoma of the vulva: Study of 24 cases. Obstet Gynecol 60: 462–466

162. Jaszczak S, Hafez ESE (1978) The vagina and infertility. In: Hafez ESE, Evans TN (eds) The human vagina, Chapter 15. Amsterdam, Elsevier/North-Holland Publishing Company, p 223

163. Jimerson SD, Becker JD (1980) Vaginal ulcers associated with tampon usage. Obstet Gynecol 56: 97–99

164. Johnson LD, Driscoll SG, Hertig AT, et al. (1979) Vaginal adenosis in stillborns and neonates exposed to diethylstilbestrol and steroidal estrogens and progestins. Obstet Gynecol 53: 671

165. Joseph RE, Enghardt MH, Doering DL, et al. (1992) Small cell neuroendocrine carcinoma of the vagina. Cancer 70: 784–789

166. Josey WE, Campbell WG (1990) Vaginitis emphysematosa. J Reprod Med 35: 974–977

167. Kahn HJ, Yeger H, et al. (1983) Immunohistochemical and electron microscopic assessment of childhood rhabdomyosarcoma: Increased frequency of diagnosis over routine laboratory methods. Cancer 51: 1897

168. Kanbour AI, Klionski B, Murphy AI (1974) Carcinoma of the vagina following cervical cancer. Cancer 34: 1838–1841

169. Katz Z, Lancet M, Skornik J, et al. (1985) Teratogenicity of progestogens given during the first trimester of pregnancy. Obstet Gynecol 65: 775

170. Kaufman RH (1980) The origin and diagnosis of "nonspecific vaginitis." N Engl J Med 303: 637–638

171. Kaufman RH, Friedrich EG, Gardner HL (1989) Atrophic, Desquamative, and Postradiation Vulvovaginitis. In: Benign diseases of the vulva and vagina, 3rd ed, Chapter 16. Chicago, Year Book Medical Publishers, pp 419–434

172. Kaufman RH, Friedrich EG, Gardner HL (1989) Cystic tumors. In: Benign diseases of the vulva and vagina, 3rd ed, Chapter 9. Chicago, Year Book Medical Publishers, pp 237–285

173. Kearns PR, Gray JE (1963) Mycotic vulvovaginitis. Incidence and persistence of specific yeast species during infection. Obstet Gynecol 22: 621–625

174. Kent HL (1991) Epidemiology of vaginitis. Am J Obstet Gynecol 165: 1168

175. Keyzer C, Lilford R, Gordon W, Bloch B (1982) Pyoderma gangrenosum, vesicovaginal fistula and endometriosis. A case report. South Afr Med J 61: 843–845

176. Khan AR (1979) Malakoplakia of vagina. J Ind Med Assoc 72: 254–255

177. Kiviat NB, Paavonen JA, Wølner-Hanssen P, et al. (1990) Histopathology of endocervical infection caused by Chlamydia trachomatis, herpes simplex virus, Trichomonas vaginalis, and Neisseria gonorrhoeae. Hum Pathol 21: 831–837

178. Koskela O (1964) Granular cell myoblastoma of the vagina. Ann Chir Gynaec Fenn 53: 270–273

179. Koss LG (1992) Diagnostic cytology and Its histopathologic bases, Vol 1, 4th ed. Philadelphia, JB Lippincott

179. Kramer K, Tobin H (1987) Vaginitis emphysematosa. Arch Pathol Lab Med 111: 746–749

180. Kraus FT (personal communication)

181. Kraus FT, Perez-Mesa C (1966) Verrucous carcinoma. Clinical and pathologic study of 105 cases involving oral cavity, larynx and genitalia. Cancer 19: 26–38

182. Krause RM (1992) The origin of plagues: Old and new. Science 257: 1073–1078

183. Kurman RJ, Norris HJ, Wilkinson E (1992) Tumors of the vagina. In: Atlas of Tumor Pathology, 3rd Series, Fascicle 4. Tumors of the cervix, vagina, and vulva. Washington, DC, Armed Forces Institute of Pathology, pp 141–178

184. Kurman RJ, Prabha AC (1973) Thyroid and parathyroid glands in the vaginal wall: Report of a case. Am J Clin Pathol 59: 503–507

185. Kurman RJ, Scully RE (1974) The incidence and histogenesis of vaginal adenosis: An autopsy study. Hum Pathol 5: 265

186. Kurman RJ, Toki T, Schiffman MH (1993) Basaloid and warty carcinomas of the vulva. Distinctive types of squamous cell carcinoma frequently associated with human papillomaviruses. Am J Surg Pathol 17(2): 133–145

187. Lang WR, Israel SL, Fritz MA (1958) Staphylococcal vulvovaginitis. A report of two cases following antibiotic therapy. Obstet Gynecol 11: 352–354

188. Larsen B, Galask RP (1980) Vaginal microbial flora: Practical and theoretic relevance. Obstet Gynecol 55: 100S–113S

189. Larsson P-G, Platz-Christensen J-J, Sundström E (1991) Is bacterial vaginosis a sexually transmitted disease? Int J STD AIDS 2: 362–364

190. Leary FJ, Resseguie LJ, Kurland LT, et al. (1984) Males exposed in utero to diethylstilbestrol. JAMA 252: 2984

191. Lenehan PM, Meffe F, Lickrish GM (1986) Vaginal intraepithelial neoplasia: biologic aspects and management. Obstet Gynecol 68: 333–337

192. Leone PG, Taylor HB (1973) Ultrastructure of a benign polypoid rhabdomyoma of the vagina. Cancer 31: 1414–1417

193. Levene M (1960) Congenital retinoblastoma and sarcoma botryoides of the vagina. Cancer 13: 532

194. Levine BB, Sriaganian RP, Schenkein I (1973) Allergy to human seminal plasma. N Engl J Med 288: 894

195. Levison ME, Trestman I, Quach R, et al. (1979) Quantitative bacteriology of the vaginal flora in vaginitis. Am J Obstet Gynecol 133: 139–144

196. Levitan Z, Gordon AN, Kaplan AL, Kaufman RH (1989) Primary malignant melanoma of the vagina: Report of four cases and review of the literature. Gynecol Oncol 33: 85–90

197. Lewis JF, O'Brien SM, Ural UM, Burke T (1971) Corynebacterium vaginale vaginitis in pregnant women. Am J Clin Pathol 56: 580–583

198. Lifson AR (1992) Transmission of the Human Immunodeficiency Virus. In: DeVita VT, Hellman S, Rosenberg SA (eds) AIDS: Etiology, diagnosis, treatment, and prevention, Chapter 8. Philadelphia, JB Lippincott, pp 111–117

199. Lin JI, Caracta PF, Chang CH, et al. (1979) Malakoplakia of the vagina. South Med J 72: 326–328

200. Lindner JGEM, Plantema FHF, Hoogkamp-Korstanje JAA (1978) Quantitative studies of the vaginal flora of healthy women and of obstetric and gynaecologic patients. J Med Microbiol 11: 233

201. Liu L-Y, Hou Y-J, Li J-Z (1987) Primary malignant melanoma of the vagina: A report of seven cases. Obstet Gynecol 70: 569–572

202. Long-Term Effects of Exposure to Diethylstilbestrol (DES) (NIH Workshop), April 22–24, 1992, Falls Church, VA, pp 1–94

203. Lorenz G (1978) Adenomatoid tumor of the ovary and vagina. Zent Gynakkol 100: 1412–1416

204. Lossick JG, Kent HL (1991) Trichomoniasis: Trends in diagnosis and management. Am J Obstet Gynecol 165: 1217–1222

205. Lucas WE, Benirschke K, Lebherz TB (1974) Verrucous carcinoma of the female genital tract. Am J Obstet Gynecol 119: 435–440

206. Manabe Y, Yoshida Y (1986) Collagenolysis in human vaginal tissue during pregnancy and delivery: A light and electron microscopic study. Am J Obstet Gynecol 155: 1060–1066

207. March CM, Israel R (1976) Rectovaginal endometriosis: An isolated enigma. Am J Obstet Gynecol 125: 274–275

208. Marcus SL (1960) Primary carcinoma of the vagina. Obstet Gynecol 15: 673

209. Mårdh P-A (1991) The vaginal ecosystem. Am J Obstet Gynecol 165: 1163–1168

210. Mårdh P-A, Holst E, Moller BR (1984) The Grivet monkey as a model for study of vaginitis. In: Mårdh P-A, Taylor-Robinson D (eds) Bacterial vaginosis. Stockholm, Almquist and Wiksell International, p 201

211. Mascasaet MA, Lu T, Nelson JH (1976) Ureterovaginal fistula as a complication of radical pelvic surgery. Am J Obstet Gynecol 124: 757–760

212. Masters WH (1960) The sexual response cycle of the human female. I. Gross anatomic considerations. West J Surg, Obstet Gynecol (Jan-Feb), pp 57–72

213. Maurer HM, Moon TE, Donaldson M, et al. (1977) The Intergroup Rhabdomyosarcoma Study: A preliminary report. Cancer 40: 2015–2026

214. McCormack WM (1990) Unusual vulvovaginal conditions: Interstitial cystitis, focal vulvitis and desquamative inflammatory vaginitis. In: Sobel JD (ed) Vulvovaginal infections: Current concepts in diagnosis and therapy. New York, Academy Professional Information Services, Inc., pp 149–160

215. McCormack WM, Hayes CH, Rosner B, et al. (1977) Vaginal colonization with *Corynebacterium vaginale (Haemophilus vaginalis)*. J Infect Dis 136: 740–745

216. McKenna UG, Meadows JA, Brewer NS, et al. (1980) Toxic shock syndrome, a newly recognized disease entity. Report of 11 cases. Mayo Clin Proc 55: 663–672

217. McLachlan JA, Newbold RR (1987) Estrogens and development. Environment Health Perspect 75: 25–27

218. McLachlan JA, Newbold RR, Shah HC, et al. (1982) Reduced fertility in female mice exposed transplacentally to diethylstilbestrol. Fertil Steril 38: 364

219. McLellan R, Spence MR, Brockman M, et al. (1982) The clinical diagnosis of trichomoniasis. Obstet Gynecol 60: 30

220. McLennan MT, Smith JM, McLennan CE (1972) Diagnosis of vaginal mycosis and trichomoniasis: Reliability of cytologic smear, wet smear and culture. Obstet Gynecol 40: 231–234

221. Merkus JMWM, Bisschop MPJM, Stolte LAM (1985) The proper nature of vaginal candidosis and the problem of recurrence. Obstet Gynecol Surv 40: 493–504

222. Miettinen M, Wahlström T, Vesterinen E, Saksela E (1983) Vaginal polyps with pseudosarcomatous features. A clinicopathologic study of seven cases. Cancer 51: 1148–1151

223. Miller CJ, Vogel P, Alexander NJ (1992) Localization of SIV in the genital tract of chronically infected female rhesus macaques. Am J Pathol 141: 655–660

224. Mucitelli DR, Charles EZ, Kraus FT (1990) Vulvovaginal polyps. Histologic appearance, ultrastructure, immunocytochemical characteristics and clinicopathologic correlations. Int J Gynecol Pathol 9: 20–40

225. de Mundi Zamorano A, del Alamo CM, de Blas LL, San Cristobal AA (1978) Egg of *Trichuris trichiura* in a vaginal smear. Acta Cytol 22: 119–120

226. Munguia H, Franco E, Valenzuela P (1966) Diagnosis of genital amebiasis in women by the standard Papanicolaou technique. Am J Obstet Gynecol 94: 181–188

227. Murad TM, Durant JR, Maddox WA, Dowling EA (1975) The pathologic behavior of primary vaginal carcinoma and its relationship to cervical cancer. Cancer 35: 787–794

228. Naves AE, Monti JA, Chichoni E (1980) Basal cell-like carcinoma of the upper third of the vagina. Am J Obstet Gynecol 137: 136–137

229. Netter FH (1965) Innervation of internal genitalia. In: Oppenheimer E (ed) The CIBA collection of medical illustrations. A compilation of paintings on the normal and pathologic anatomy of the reproductive system, Vol 2. New Jersey, CIBA Pharmaceutical Company of CIBA-GEIGY Corporation, p 103

230. Newbold RR, Bullock BC, McLachlan JA (1983) Exposure to diethylstilbestrol during pregnancy permanently alters the ovary and oviduct. Biol Reprod 28: 736

231. Newbold RR, Tyrer S, Haney AF, McLachlan JA (1983) Developmentally arrested oviduct—A structural and functional defect in mice following prenatal exposure to diethylstilbestrol. Teratology 27: 417

232. Newton WA, Soule EH, Hamoudi AB, et al (1988) Histopathology of childhood sarcomas, intergroup rhabdomyosarcoma studies I and II: Clinicopathologic correlation. J Clin Oncol 6: 67–75

233. Nielsen R (1973) *Trichomonas vaginalis*. II. Laboratory investigations in trichomoniasis. Br J Vener Dis 49: 531–535

234. Nigogosyan G, de la Pava S, Pickren JW (1964) Melanoblasts in vaginal mucosa: Origin for primary malignant melanoma. Cancer 17: 912–913

235. Nogales-Ortiz F, Tarancón I, Nogales F (1979) The pathology of female genital tuberculosis. Obstet Gynecol 53: 422–428

236. Noller KL, Blair PB, O'Brien PC, et al. (1988) Increased occurrence of autoimmune disease among women exposed in utero to DES. Fertil Steril 49: 1080–1082

237. Noller KL (1990) DES update. Clin Pract Gynecol V2, p 149

238. Noller KL, Townsend DE, Kaufman RH, et al. (1983) Maturation of vaginal and cervical epithelium in women exposed in utero to diethylstilbestrol (DESAD Project). Am J Obstet Gynecol 146: 279

239. Norris HJ, Taylor HB (1966) Polyps of the vagina. A benign lesion resembling sarcoma botryoides. Cancer 19:227–232

240. O'Collins JP, Butler B (1973) Vesico-vaginal fistula after sexual intercourse. Med J Aust 1: 299

241. Okagaki T, Ishida T, Hilgers RD (1976) A malignant tumor of the vagina resembling synovial sarcoma. A light and electron microscopic study. Cancer 37: 2306–2320

242. Opitz JM (1987) Editorial comment: Vaginal atresia (von

Mayer-Rokitansky-Küster or MRK anomaly) in hereditary renal adysplasia (HRA). Am J Med Genet 26: 873–876

243. Östör AG, Fortune DW, Riley CB (1988) Fibroepithelial polyps with atypical stromal cells Pseudosarcoma botryoides) of vulva and vagina. A report of 13 cases. Int J Gynecol Pathol 7: 351–360

244. Palmer JP, Biback SM (1954) Primary cancer of the vagina. Am J Obstet Gynecol 67: 377–397

245. Parker CE, Johnson FC (1963) The effect of maternal estrogens on the vaginal epithelium of the newborn. Clin Pediatr 2: 374–377

246. Paris AL, Herwaldt LA, Blum D, et al. (1982) Pathologic findings in twelve fatal cases of toxic shock syndrome. Ann Intern Med 96: 852–857

247. Perez CA, Arneson AN, Dehner LP, et al. (1974) Radiation therapy in carcinoma of vagina. Obstet Gynecol 44: 862

248. Perez CA, Bedwinek JM, Breaux SR (1983) Patterns of failure after treatment of gynecologic tumors. Cancer Treat Symp 2: 217

249. Perez CA, Camel HM, Galakatos AE, et al. (1988) Definitive irradiation in carcinoma of the vagina: Long-term evaluation of results. Int J Radiat Oncol Biol Phys 15: 1283

250. Perez CA, Gersell DJ, Hoskins WJ, McGuire WP III (1992) Vagina. In: Hoskins WJ, Perez CA, Young RC (eds) Principles and practice of gynecologic oncology, Chapter 26. Philadelphia, JB Lippincott, pp 567–590

251. Perrin EVD (1978) Pathobiology of vaginal malformations. In: Hafez ESE, Evans TN (eds) The human vagina, Chapter 16. Amsterdam, Elsevier/North-Holland Publishing Company, p 245

252. Perrone TL, Manivel JC, Dehner LP (1992) The female reproductive system. In: Stocker JT, Dehner LP (eds) Pediatric pathology, Vol 2, Chapter 22. Philadelphia, JB Lippincott, pp 873–904

253. Peterman TA, Stoneburner RL, Allen JR, et al. (1988) Risk of human immunodeficiency virus transmission from heterosexual adults with transfusion-associated infections. JAMA 259: 55

254. Peters WA, Kumar NB, Anderson WA, Morley GW (1985) Primary sarcoma of the adult vagina: A clinicopathologic study. Obstet Gynecol 65: 699–704

255. Peters WA, Kumar NB, Morley GW (1985) Carcinoma of the vagina: Factors influencing treatment outcome. Cancer 55: 892

256. Peters WA, Kumar NB, Morley GW (1985) Microinvasive carcinoma of the vagina: A distinct clinical entity? Am J Obstet Gynecol 153: 505–507

257. Pezeshkpour G (1981) Solitary paraganglioma of the vagina. Report of a case. Am J Obstet Gynecol 139: 219–221

258. Pheifer TA, Forsyth PS, Durfee MA, et al. (1978) Nonspecific vaginitis. Role of Haemophilus vaginalis and treatment with metronidazole. N Engl J Med 298: 1429–1434

259. Piver MS, Lele SB, Baker TR, Sandecki A (1988) Cervical and vaginal cancer detection at a regional diethylstilbestrol (DES) screening clinic. Cancer Detect Prevent 11: 197–202

260. Plapinger L (1981) Morphological effects of diethylstilbestrol on neonatal mouse uterus and vagina. Cancer Res 41: 4667

261. Plapinger L, Bern HA (1979) Adenosis-like lesions and other cervico-vaginal abnormalities in mice treated perinatally with estrogen. J Natl Cancer Inst 63: 507

262. Platzer W, Poisel S, Hafez ESE (1978) Functional anatomy of the human vagina. In: Hafez ESE, Evans TN (eds) The human vagina, Chapter 3. Amsterdam, Elsevier/North-Holland Publishing Company

263. Plentl AA, Friedman EA (1971) Lymphatic system of the female genitalia: The morphologic basis of oncologic diagnosis and therapy. Philadelphia, WB Saunders, pp 51–74

264. Podczaski E, Herbst AL (1986) Cancer of the vagina and fallopian tube. In: Knapp RC, Berkowitz RS (eds) Gynecologic oncology, Chapter 13. New York, Macmillan, pp 399–424

265. Pradhan S, Tobon H (1986) Vaginal cysts: A clinicopathological study of 41 cases. Int J Gynecol Pathol 5:35–46

266. Prahalada S, Castrancane VD, Hendricks AG, Goldzieher JW (1988) Diethylstilbestrol-induced cervical and vaginal adenosis using the neonatal mouse model. J Biol Reprod 38: 935–943

267. Prasad CJ, Ray JA, Kessler S (1992) Primary small cell carcinoma of the vagina arising in a background of atypical adenosis. Cancer 70: 2484–2487

268. Prempree T, Amornmarn R (1985) Radiation treatment of primary carcinoma of the vagina: Patterns of failure after definitive therapy. Acta Radiol Oncol 24: 51

269. Premptee T, Tang C-K, Hatef A, et al. (1983) Angiosarcoma of the vagina: A clinicopathologic report. Cancer 51: 618–622

270. Prezyna AP, Kalyanaraman U (1977) Bowen's carcinoma in vulvovaginal Crohn's disease (regional enterocolitis). Report of first case. Am J Obstet Gynecol 128: 914–916

271. Proppe KH, Scully RE, Rosai J (1984) Postoperative spindle cell nodules of genitourinary tract resembling sarcomas. A report of eight cases. Am J Surg Pathol 8: 101–108

272. Pul M, Yilmaz N, Gürses N, Ozoran Y (1990) Vaginal polyp in a newborn—A case report and review of the literature. Clin Pediatr 29: 346

273. Raghavaiah NV, Devi AI (1980) Primary vaginal stones. J Urol 123: 771–772

274. Rajkumar S, Narayanaswamy G, Laude TA (1979) Shigella vulvovaginitis in childhood: A case report. J Natl Med Assoc 71: 1005–1006

275. Raum ME, Friedrich EG, Slaff JI (1980) Toxic shock syndrome with vaginal ulceration. J Florida Med Assoc 67: 935–936

276. Reid GC, Schmidt RW, Roberts JA, et al. (1989) Primary melanoma of the vagina: A clinicopathologic analysis. Obstet Gynecol 74: 190–199

277. Rein MF, Müller M (1990) Trichomonas vaginalis. In: Holmes KK, Mårdh P-A, Sparling PF, Wiesner PJ (eds) Sexually transmitted diseases, 2nd ed. New York, McGraw-Hill

278. Resnick SD (1990) Toxic shock syndrome: Recent developments in pathogenesis. J Pediatr 116: 321–328

279. Rhatigan RM, Mojadidi Q (1973) Adenosquamous carcinomas of the vulva and vagina. Am J Clin Pathol 59: 208–217

280. Richart RM (1986) The incidence of cervical and vaginal dysplasia after exposure to DES. JAMA 255: 36–37

281. Robboy SJ (1983) A hypothetic mechanism of diethyl-

stilbestrol (DES)-induced anomalies in prenatally exposed women. Hum Pathol 14: 831

282. Robboy SJ, Friedlander LM, Welch WR, et al. (1976) Cytology of 575 young females exposed prenatally to diethylstilbestrol (DES). Obstet Gynecol 48: 511

283. Robboy SJ, Hill EC, Sandberg EC, Czernobilsky B (1986) Vaginal adenosis in women born prior to the diethylstilbestrol (DES) era. Hum Pathol 17: 488

284. Robboy SJ, Kaufman RH, Prat J, et al. (1979) Pathologic findings in young women enrolled in national cooperative diethylstilbestrol adenosis (DESAD) project. Obstet Gynecol 53: 309

285. Robboy SJ, Noller KL, Kaufman RH, et al. (1980) Prenatal diethylstilbestrol (DES-exposure): Recommendations of the Diethylstilbestrol Adenosis (DESAD) project for the identification and management of exposed individuals. DHEW publication No. 80-2049

286. Robboy SJ, Noller KL, Kaufman RH, et al. (1982) An atlas of findings in the human female after intrauterine exposure to diethylstilbestrol. DHEW publication No. 82-2344

287. Robboy SJ, Noller KL, O'Brien P, et al. (1984) Increased incidence of cervical and vaginal dysplasia in 3,980 diethylstilbestrol (DES)-exposed young women: Experience of the National Collaborative DES-Adenosis (DESAD) Project. JAMA 252: 2979

288. Robboy SJ, Prade M, Cunha G (1992) Vagina. In: Sternberg SS (ed) Histology for pathologists, Chapter 45. New York, Raven Press Ltd, pp 881–892

289. Robboy SJ, Scully RE, Herbst AL (1975) Pathology of vaginal and cervical abnormalities associated with prenatal exposure to diethylstilbestrol. J Reprod Med 15: 13

290. Robboy SJ, Szyfelbein WM, Goellner JR, et al. (1981) Dysplasia and cytologic findings in 4,589 young women enrolled in diethylstilbestrol-adenosis (DESAD) project. Am J Obstet Gynecol 140: 579

291. Robboy SJ, Taguchi O, Cunha GR (1982) Normal development of the human female reproductive tract and alterations resulting from experimental exposure to diethylstilbestrol. Human Pathol 13: 190–198

292. Robboy SJ, Welch WR (1977) Microglandular hyperplasia in vaginal adenosis associated with oral contraceptives and prenatal diethylstilbestrol (DES) exposure. Obstet Gynecol 49: 430

293. Robboy SJ, Welch WR, Young RH, et al. (1982) Topographic relation of adenosis, clear cell adenocarcinoma and other related lesions of the vagina and cervix in DES-exposed progeny. Obstet Gynecol 60: 546

294. Robboy SJ, Young RH, Welch WR, et al. (1984) Atypical (dysplastic) adenosis: Forerunner and transitional state to clear cell adenocarcinoma in young women exposed in utero to diethylstilbestrol. Cancer 54: 869

295. Robboy SJ, Ross JS, Prat J, et al. (1978) Urogenital sinus origin of mucinous and ciliated cysts of the vulva. Obstet Gynecol 51: 347–351

296. Roberts WS, Hoffman MS, LaPolla JP, et al. (1991) Management of radionecrosis of the vulva and distal vagina. Am J Obstet Gynecol 164: 1235–1238

297. Roberts DK, Walker NJ, Parmley TH, Horbelt DV (1988) Interaction of epithelial and stromal cells in vaginal adenosis. Hum Pathol 19: 855–861

298. Romanes GJ (1981) Cunningham's textbook of anatomy, 12th ed. London, Oxford University Press

299. Rotmensch J, Rosenshein N, Dillon M, et al. (1983) Carcinoma arising in the neovagina: Case report and review of the literature. Obstet Gynecol 61: 534

300. Rorat E, Ferenczy A, Richart RM (1975) Human Bartholin gland, duct, and duct cyst. Histochemical and ultrastructural study. Arch Pathol 99: 367–374

301. Rutledge F (1967) Cancer of the vagina. Am J Obstet Gynecol 97: 635–655

302. Sandberg EC, Christian JC (1980) Diethylstilbestrol-exposed monozygotic twins discordant for cervicovaginal clear cell carcinoma. Am J Obstet Gynecol 137: 220

303. Sander R, Nuss RC, Rhatigan R (1986) Diethylstilbestrol-associated vaginal adenosis followed by clear cell adenocarcinoma. Int J Gynecol Pathol 5: 362–370

304. Sanders CC, Sanders WE, Fagnant JE (1982) Toxic shock syndrome: An ecologic imbalance within the genital microflora of women? Am J Obstet Gynecol 142: 977–982

305. Sanders DY, Wasilauskas BL (1973) Shigella vaginitis. Clinical notes on two childhood cases. Clin Pediatr 12: 54–55

306. Schneider V (1981) Visceral giant cell arteritis limited to the female genital tract. A case report. J Reprod Med 26: 328–331

307. Schneider GT, Geary WL (1971) Vaginitis in adolescent girls. Clin Obstet Gynecol 14: 1057–1076

308a. Sedlacek TV, Riva JM, Magen A, Morgen CE, Cunnane MG (1990) Vaginal and vulvar adenosis. An unsuspected side effect of CO_2 laser vaporization. J Reprod Med 35: 995–1001

308. Schumacher GFB, Gill WB, Hubby MM, et al. (1981) Semen analysis in male exposed in utero to diethylstilbestrol (DES) or placebo. IRSC Med Sci 9: 100

309. Senekjian EK, Hubby M, Bell DA, et al. (1986) Clear cell adenocarcinoma (CCA) of the vagina and cervix in association with pregnancy. Gynecol Oncol 24: 207–219

310. Sheets JL, Dockerty MD, Decker DG, Welch JS (1964) Primary epithelial malignancy in the vagina. Am J Obstet Gynecol 89: 121–128

311. Shenker L, Blaustein A (1963) Emphysematous vaginitis. A theory of its pathogenesis and report of a case. Obstet Gynecol 22: 295–300

312. Sherry ME (1992) The effects of diethylstilbestrol on human prostate development. Thesis, Univ Calif San Francisco

313. Shevchuk MM, Fenoglio CM, Lattes R (1978) Malignant mixed tumor of the vagina probably arising in mesonephric rests. Cancer 42: 214–223

314. Sillman FH, Sedlis A, Boyce JG (1985) A review of lower genital intraepithelial neoplasia and the use of topical 5-fluorouracil. Obstet Gynecol Surv 40: 190–220

315. Silverberg SG, Frabler WJ (1974) Prolapse of fallopian tube into vaginal vault after hysterectomy. Histopathology, cytopathology, and differential diagnosis. Arch Pathol 97: 100–103

316. Sirota RL, Dickerson GR, Scully RE (1981) Mixed tumors of the vagina: A clinicopathologic analysis of eight cases. Am J Surg Pathol 5: 413–422

317. Sobel JD (1990) Vaginal infections in adult women. Med Clin North Am 74: 1573–1602

318. Spence MR, et al. (1980) The clinical and laboratory diagnosis of *Trichomonas vaginalis* infection. Sex Transm Dis 7: 168

319. Spencer LM, Straatsma BR, Foos RY (1968) Ligneous conjunctivitis. Arch Ophthal 80: 365–367

320. Spiegel CA, Amsel R, Eschenbach D, et al. (1980) Anaerobic bacteria in nonspecific vaginitis. N Engl J Med 303: 601–607

321. Spitzer M, Molho L, Seltzer VL, et al. (1985) Vaginal glomus tumor: Case presentation and ultrastructural findings. Obstet Gynecol 66: 86S–88S

322. Strate SM, Taylor WE, Forney JP, Silva FG (1983) Xanthogranulomatous pseudotumor of the vagina: Evidence of a local response to an unusual bacterium (mucoid *Escherichia coli*). Am J Clin Pathol 79: 637–643

323. Stuart GCE, Flagler EA, Nation JG, et al. (1988) Laser vaporization of vaginal intraepithelial neoplasia. Am J Obstet Gynecol 158: 240–243

324. Sugimura Y, Cunha GR, Yonemura CU, Kawamura J (1988) Temporal and spatial factors in diethylstilbestrol-induced squamous metaplasia of the developing human prostate. Hum Pathol 19: 133–139

325. Sulak P, Barnhill D, Heller P, et al. (1988) Nonsquamous cancer of the vagina. Gynecol Oncol 29: 309–320

326. Sunderland WA, Harris HH, Spence DA, Lawson HW (1972) Meningococcemia in a newborn infant whose mother had meningococcal vaginitis (Letter to the Editor). J Pediatr 81: 856

327. Sweet RL, Gibbs RS (1985) Infectious Vulvovaginitis. In: Infectious Diseases of the female genital tract, Chapter 6. Balitmore, Williams & Wilkins, pp 89–96

328. Sweet RL, Gibbs RS (1985) Perinatal infections. In: Infectious diseases of the female genital tract, Chapter 13. Baltimore, Williams & Wilkins, pp 206–214

329. Sweet RL, Gibbs RS (1985) Toxic Shock Syndrome. In: Infectious diseases of the female genital tract, Chapter 5. Baltimore, Williams & Wilkins, pp 78–88

330. Syverson RE, Buckley H, Gibian J, Ryan GM (1979) Cellular and humoral immune status in women with chronic *Candida* vaginitis. Am J Obstet Gynecol 134: 624–627

331. Taguchi O, Cunha GR, Lawrence WD, Robboy SJ (1984) Timing and irreversibility of müllerian duct inhibition of the embryonic reproductive tract of the human male. Dev Biol 106: 394

332. Taguchi O, Cunha GR, Robboy SJ (1983) Experimental study of the effect of diethylstilbestrol (DES) on the development of the human female reproductive tract. Biol Res Prac 4: 56

333. Tancer ML (1980) The post-total hysterectomy (vault) vesicovaginal fistula. J Urol 123: 839–840

334. Tazvassoli FA, Norris HJ (1979) Smooth muscle tumors of the vagina. Obstet Gynecol 53: 689–693

335. Teo C, Kwong L, Benn R (1987) Incidence of motile, curved anaerobic rods (*Mobiluncus* species) in vaginal secretions. Pathology 19: 193–196

336. The Working Group on Severe Streptococcal Infections (1993) Defining the Group A streptococcal toxic shock syndrome. Rationale and consensus definition. JAMA 269: 390–391

337. Thomason JL, Anderson RJ, Gelbart SM, et al. (1992) Simplified Gram stain interpretive method for diagnosis of bacterial vaginosis. Am J Obstet Gynecol 167: 16–19

338. Thomason JL, Gelbart SM (1989) Trichomonas vaginalis. Obstet Gynecol 74: 536–541

339. Thomason JL, Gelbart SM, Anderson RJ, et al. (1990) Statistical evaluation of diagnostic criteria for bacterial vaginosis. Am J Obstet Gynecol 162: 155–160

340. Timonen S, Salo OP, Meyer B, Haapoja H (1966) Vaginal mycosis. Acta Obstet Gynecol Scand 45: 232–247

341. Tjugum J, Jonassen F, Olsson JH (1986) Vaginitis emphysematosa in a renal transplant patient. Acta Obstet Gynecol Scand 65: 377, 378

342. Tobon H, Murphy AI (1977) Benign blue nevus of the vagina. Cancer 40: 3174

343. Todd J, Fishaut M, Kapral F, Welch T (1978) Toxic-shock syndrome associated with phage-group-I staphylococci. Lancet 2: 1116–1118

344. Tohya T, Katabuchi H, Fukuma K, et al (1991) Angiosarcoma of the vagina. A light and electronmicroscopy study. Acta Obstet Gynecol Scand 70: 169–172

345. de Torres EF, Benitez-Bribiesca L (1973) Cytologic detection of vaginal parasitosis. Acta Cytol 17: 252–257

346. Tsokos M, Webber BL, Parham DM, et al. (1992) Rhabdomyosarcoma. A new classification scheme related to prognosis. Arch Pathol Lab Med 116: 847–855

347. Tsukada Y (1976) Benign melanosis of the vagina and cervix. Am J Obstet Gynecol 124: 211–212

348. Ulbright TM, Alexander RW, Kraus FT (1981) Intramural papilloma of the vagina: Evidence of Müllerian histogenesis. Cancer 48: 2260–2266

349. Ulfelder H, Robboy SJ (1976) The embryologic development of the human vagina. Am J Obstet Gynecol 126: 769–776

350. Václavínková V, Neumann E (1981) Vaginal involvement in familial benign chronic pemphigus (Morbus Hailey-Hailey). Acta Dermatovener (Stockholm) 62: 80–81

351. Valdes CT, Malinak LR, Franklin RR (1989) Developmental anomalies of the vulva and vagina. In: Kaufman RH, Friedrich EG, Gardner HL (eds) Benign diseases of the vulva and vagina, 3rd ed, Chapter 3. Chicago, Year Book Medical Publishers, Inc, pp 26–54

352. van Coeverden de Groot HA (1963) Amoebic vaginitis. South Afr Med J 37: 246–247

353. van der Meijden WI, Duivenvoorden HJ, Both-Patoir HC, et al. (1988) Clinical and laboratory findings in women with bacterial vaginosis and trichomoniasis versus controls. Eur J Obstet Gynecol Reprod Biol 28: 39–52

354. van der Walt JJ, Marcus PB, de Wet JJ, Burger AJJ (1973) Malacoplakia of the vagina. First case report. South Afr Med J 47: 1342–1344

355. Venter PF, Anderson JD, Van Velden DJJ (1979) Postmenopausal endometriosis. A case report. South Afr Med J 56: 1136–1138

356. Vessey MP, Fairweather DVI, Norma-Smith B, Buckley JA (1983) A randomized double-blind controlled trial of the value of stilbestrol therapy in pregnancy: Long-term follow-up of mothers and their offspring. Br J Obstet Gynecol 90: 1007–1017

357. de Virgiliis G, Sideri M, Rossi A, et al. (1985) "DES-Like" anomalies. I. Biological and clinical problems. A study on 12,285 cases. Cervix Low Female Genital Tract 3: 297–312

358. Vontver LA, Eschenbach DA (1981) The role of gardnerella vaginalis in nonspecific vaginitis. Clin Obstet Gynecol 24: 439–460

359. Wager GP (1983) Toxic shock syndrome: A review. Am J Obstet Gynecol 146: 93–102

360. Walker BE (1989) Animal models of prenatal exposure to diethylstilbestrol. IARC Sci Pub (Lyon) 96: 349–364

361. Way S (1948) Primary carcinoma of the vagina. J Obstet Gynaecol Br Emp 55: 739

362. Ways SC, Mortola JF, Zvaifler NJ, et al. (1987) Alterations in immune responsiveness in woman exposed to diethylstilbestrol in utero. Fertil Steril 48: 193–197

363. Webb MJ, Symmonds RE, Weiland LH (1974) Malignant fibrous histiocytoma of vagina. Am J Obstet Gynecol 119: 190–192

364. Welch WR, Fu YS, Robboy SJ, Herbst AL (1983) Nuclear DNA content of clear cell adenocarcinoma of the vagina and cervix and its relations to prognosis. Gynecol Oncol 15: 230

365. Wells JI, Goei SH (1981) Rapid identification of *Corynebacterium vaginale* in non-purulent vaginitis. J Clin Pathol 34: 917–920

366. Wheelock JB, Schneider V, Goplerud DR (1985) Prolapsed fallopian tube masquerading as adenocarcinoma of the vagina in a postmenopausal woman. Gynecol Oncol 21: 369–375

367. Whelton JA (1962) Mixed tumor arising in the vagina. Obstet Gynecol 19: 803–805

368. Williams GA (1965) Postsurgical and post-traumatic tumors. Clin Obstet Gynecol 8: 1020–1034

369. Wisniewski PM, Wilkinson EJ (1991) Postpartum vaginal atrophy. Am J Obstet Gynecol 165: 1249–1254

370. Woodruff JD, Parmley TH, Julian CG (1975) Topical 5-fluorouracil in the treatment of vaginal carcinoma in situ. Gynecol Oncol 3: 124–125

371. Young RH, Scully RE (1984) Endodermal sinus tumor of the vagina: A report of nine cases and review of the literature. Gynecol Oncol 18: 380–392

372. Young RH, Scully RE (1987) Pseudosarcomatous lesions of the urinary bladder, prostate gland, and urethra. A report of three cases and review of the literature. Arch Pathol Lab Med 111: 354–358

373. Yousem HL (1961) Adenocarcinoma of Gartner's duct cyst presenting as a vaginal lesion. A case report. Sinai Hosp J, pp 112–114

374. Yow MD, Leeds LJ, Thompson PK, et al. (1980) The natural history of group B streptococcal colonization in the pregnant woman and her offspring. I. Colonization studies. Am J Obstet Gynecol 137: 34–38

375. Zinkham WH (1976) Multifocal eosinophilic granuloma. Natural history, etiology and management. Am J Med 60: 457

5

Anatomy and Histology of the Cervix

Alex Ferenczy, M.D., and Thomas C. Wright, M.D.

Gross Anatomy

The uterus is best divided into corpus, isthmus, and cervix. The cervix (term taken from the Latin, meaning *neck*) is the most inferior portion of the uterus, protruding into the upper vagina. The transition between the endocervix and the lower portion of the uterine corpus is termed the *isthmus* or *lower uterine segment*. The latter is used for descriptive purposes during gestation and labor and is an important landmark for the pathologist when describing cancers of the uterine corpus. The muscular layer in the region of the isthmus is less well developed than in the corpus, a feature that facilitates effacement and dilation during labor. The vagina is fused circumferentially and obliquely to the distal part of the cervix and is divided into an upper, supervaginal, and lower vaginal portion.[28] The cervix measures 2.5–3.0 cm in length in the adult nulligravida, and when normally positioned it is angled slightly downward and backward. The vaginal portion (portio vaginalis) of the cervix, also referred to as the *exocervix*, is delimited by the anterior and posterior vagina fornices and has a convex elliptical surface. The portio may be divided into anterior and posterior lips, of which the anterior is shorter and projects lower than the posterior lip. In the center of the exocervix is the external os. This external os is circular in the nulligravida and slit-like in the parous woman (Fig. 5.1). The external os is connected with the isthmus of the uterus by the cervical canal (endocervix). The canal is an elliptical cavity, measuring 8 mm in its greatest diameter and contains longitudinal mucosal ridges, the plicae palmatae (Fig. 5.2).

The blood supply of the cervix is provided by the descending branches of the uterine arteries, reaching the lateral walls along the upper margin of the paracervical ligaments (cardinal ligaments of Mackenrodt). These ligaments and the uterosacral ligaments, which attach the supervaginal portion of the cervix to the second through fourth sacral vertebrae, are the main sources of fixation, support, and suspension of the organ. The venous drainage parallels the arterial system, with communication between the cervical plexus and neck of the urinary bladder. The lymphatics of the cervix have a dual origin: coursing beneath the mucosa and deep in the fibrous stroma.[44] Both systems collect into two lateral plexuses in the region of the isthmus and give origin to four efferent channels running toward the external iliac and obturator nodes, the hypogastric and common iliac nodes, the sacral nodes, and the nodes of the posterior wall of the urinary bladder. The innervation of the cervix is chiefly limited to the endocervix and peripheral deep portion of the exocervix.[28] This distribution is responsible for the relative insensitivity to pain of the inner two-thirds of the portio vaginalis. The cervical nerves are derived from the pelvic autonomic system and the superior, middle, and inferior hypogastric plexuses.

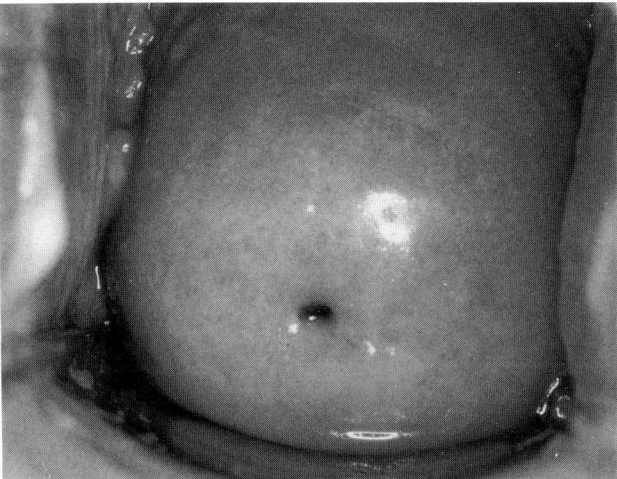 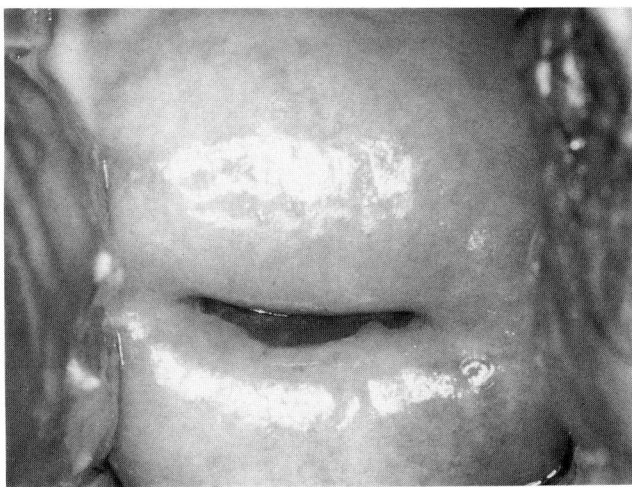

FIG. 5.1. **Normal cervix uteri.** *Left:* Nulliparous cervix with a circular external os. *Right:* Parous cervix with a slit-like external os.

Histology and Physiology

The cervix is composed of an admixture of fibrous, muscular, and elastic tissue and is lined by columnar and squamous epithelium. Fibrous connective tissue is the predominant component. Smooth muscle comprises 15% of the substance and is located mainly in the endocervix, the portio vaginalis being nearly devoid of smooth muscle fibers.[18] In contrast, at the isthmus 50–60% of the supportive tissue consists of concentrically arranged smooth muscle, which acts as a sphincter.

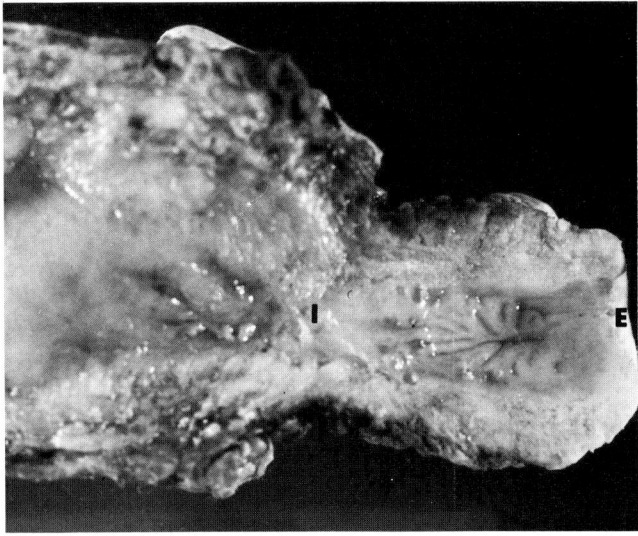

FIG. 5.2. **Normal cervix uteri.** Transected multiparous uterus. The endocervical canal is delimited by the isthmus *(I)* and external os *(E)*. Note prominent mucosal folds of endocervical canal.

Squamous Epithelium

Histologically, the mature nonkeratinized squamous epithelium of the exocervix is similar to the vaginal epithelium but under normal circumstances lacks the rete pegs seen in the vagina. It is divided into three zones: the basal or germinal cell layer, which is responsible for continuous epithelial renewal; the midzone or stratum spinosum, the dominant portion of the epithelium; and the superficial zone, containing the most mature cell population (Fig. 5.3).

The basal or germinal layer contains two types of cells. One type is the true *basal cell* which is about 10 μm in diameter, with scant cytoplasm and oval nuclei oriented perpendicularly to the underlying basal lamina (Fig. 5.3). The other type of cell is termed the *parabasal cell* because of its geographic placement. Parabasal cells are larger than basal cells and have more cytoplasm.

Ultrastructurally, the parabasal cells are attached by numerous tonofilament–desmosomal complexes and contain some intracytoplasmic glycogen. Phosphorylase and amylo-1-6-glucosidase, enzymes essential for glycogen synthesis, are localized in the parabasal region.[14] Epithelial regeneration appears to be the major function of the basal layer. Accordingly, epidermal growth factor receptors and HER-2/neu, which is a growth factor receptor structurally related to the epidermal growth factor receptor, are found predominantly in the basal and parabasal cells.[33,36] The amount of growth factor receptors becomes reduced as the squamous epithelial cells differentiate and move into the intermediate cell layer.[2] Basal cells appear to act as stem or reserve cells whereas parabasal cells comprise the actively replicating compartment. This is supported by the following: (1) mitotic figures usually are found in parabasal but not basal cells, (2) radioautography studies demonstrate a

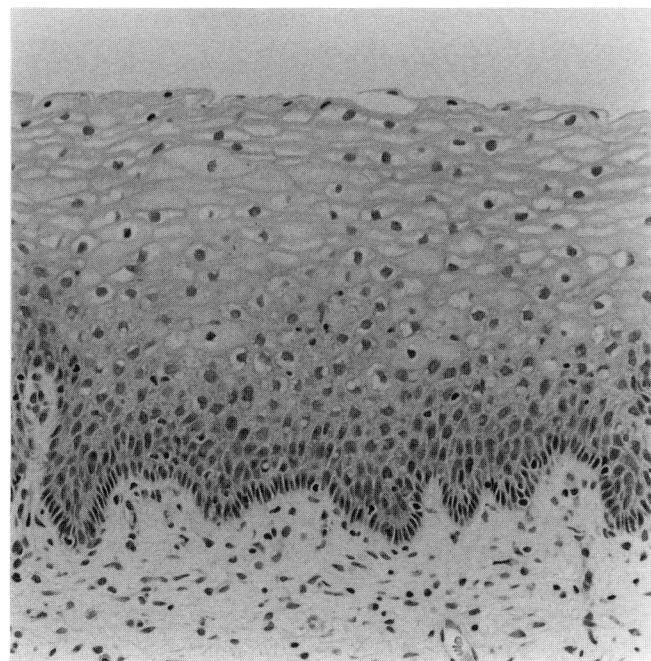

FIG. 5.3. Normal squamous epithelium. The mature squamous epithelium of the portio of the cervix shows a gradual ascending maturation, vacuolization of midzone cells, and a single layer of basal cells in which the nuclei are perpendicularly oriented to the basal lamina. The stromal–epithelial junction contains a finger-like, fibrovascular stromal papilla penetrating the lower portion of the epithelium.

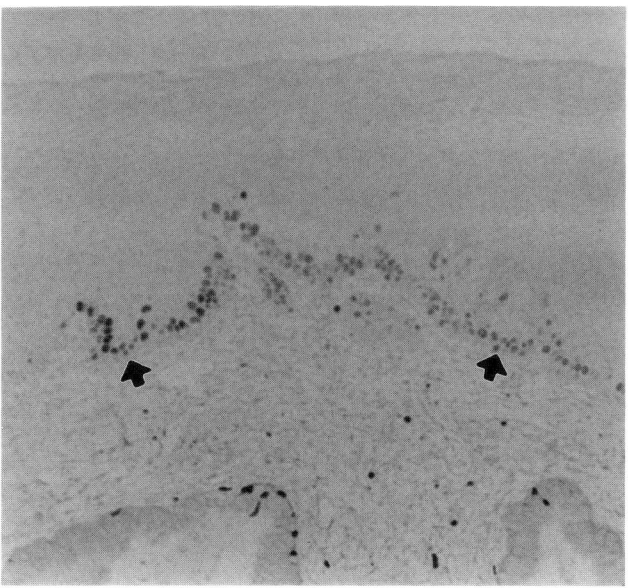

FIG. 5.4. Normal squamous epithelium. Markers for proliferating cells are restricted to the parabasal cell layers (arrows) of the exocervical stratified squamous epithelium. Immunohistochemical staining using antibodies against PCN.

high uptake of tritiated thymidine, one of the best markers for DNA proliferation in the parabasal, but not the basal cell layer,[1] and (3) other markers for actively proliferating cells such as Ki-67 antigen and proliferating cell nuclear antigen (PCN) are localized to parabasal cells (Fig. 5.4).[26] Ki-67 antigen is a nuclear antigen expressed in all phases of the cycle except G_o and PCN is a cellular protein that is present only in the nucleus of cycling cells, not in resting cells. These antigens are excellent markers for cells that are actively replicating.

The midzone is occupied by cells that are undergoing maturation, characterized by a gradual increase in the volume of the cytoplasm. Nuclear size, however, remains stable up to the most superficial cell level. These cells are referred to as *intermediate cells* when they exfoliate. They do not divide. Intermediate cells have abundant periodic acid-Schiff reagent (PAS)-positive, diatase-labile intracellular glycogen, which is responsible for the clear, vacuolated appearance of their cytoplasm.

The superficial zone forms the most differentiated compartment of the squamous epithelium. These cells are flattened and have a larger area of cytoplasm (50 μm in diameter) and smaller pyknotic nuclei than the underlying intermediate cells (Fig. 5.5). The pink, eosinophilic cytoplasm has abundant intermediate filaments, which provide

rigidity (Fig. 5.5, *inset*). Superficial cells also contain occasional membrane-bound keratinosomes. The abundant intermediate filaments form a complex network of microridges seen on the surface of the most superficial and mature cells.[11] The function of the cornified surface is to protect the underlying epithelial cells and subepithelial vasculature from trauma and infection. The microridges are believed to enhance surface adhesion (Fig. 5.6). The paucity of desmosomes between the upper superficial cells explains their loose attachment and easy desquamation.

Biochemical and immunohistochemical analysis of the squamous epithelium of the cervical portio has demonstrated the presence of cytoplasmic proteins specific for terminally differentiated squamous cells corresponding to the orderly vertical maturation process seen histologically and ultrastructurally.[15] Although large bundles of intermediate filaments are identified ultrastructurally in only superficial cells, all cell layers of the stratified squamous epithelium of the cervix express intermediate-sized filaments of the cytokeratin type.[8,17,37,38,40,51] The cytokeratin family of intermediate filaments consists of at least 19 cytokeratin polypeptides with molecular weights between 40 and 70 kDa and isoelectric points between pH 7.8 and 4.9.[37] These 19 cytokeratin polypeptides can be divided into two distinct multigene classes.[19] Type 1 cytokeratins tend to be relatively small and acidic whereas Type 2 cytokeratins tend to be larger and more basic. The expression of different cytokeratin polypeptides can serve as a marker for the state of epithelial differentiation. In the exocervix, the expression of cytokeratin polypeptides is positionally

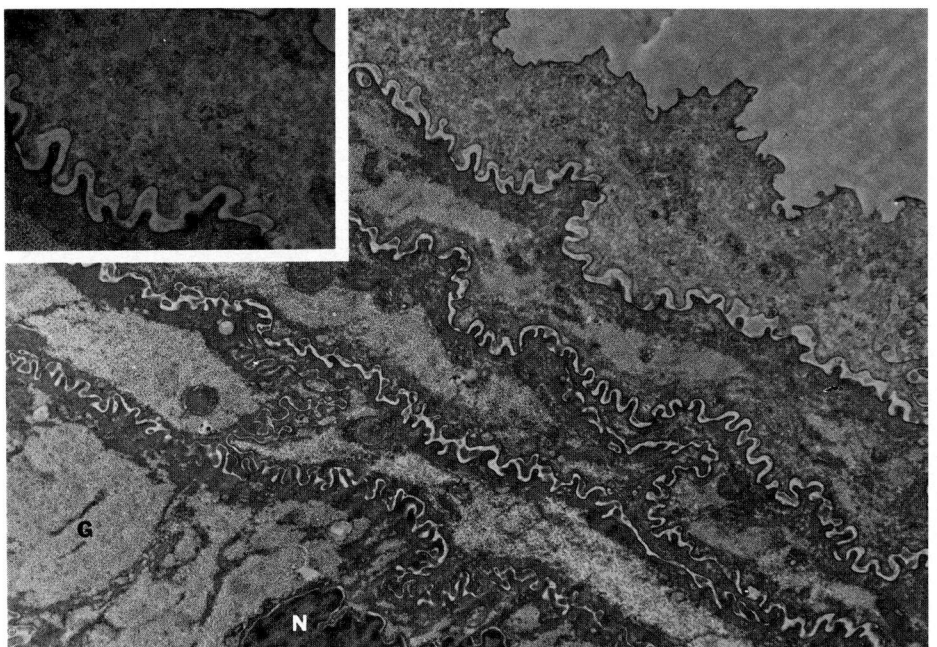

Fig. 5.5. Normal squamous epithelium. Electron microscopy of the superficial cells. They have pyknotic nuclei (N) and flattened cytoplasm packed with glycogen (G). The most superficial cells are rich in microfilaments and contain irregular-surfaced membrane projections. Note the lack of desmosomal attachments between the most superficial cells, a feature facilitating desquamation. ×4795. Inset: Higher magnification of intracytoplasmic microfilaments in the most superficial cells. ×11,370.

regulated. Immunohistochemical studies using monoclonal antibodies directed against specific cytokeratin polypeptides have shown that basal cells express cytokeratins characteristic of simple (nonstratified) types of epithelium.[8,17,51] These are specifically cytokeratins 18 and 19. Cells in the parabasal, intermediate, and superficial cell layers do not stain with monoclonal antibodies directed against cytokeratins 18 and 19, but do react with monoclonal antibodies directed against cytokeratins 4 and 13, which are characteristic of certain types of stratified epithelium.[8,17,38,51] A number of other cytokeratin polypeptides also are expressed in the stratified epithelium of the cervix, but in varying amounts depending on the location. Thus, near the squamocolumnar junction, large amounts of cytokeratins 4, 5, 6, 13, 14, and 15 are expressed together with minor amounts of cytokeratins 16, 17, and 19. In contrast, closer to the vagina additional cytokeratins, including 1, 2, 10, 11, also are expressed.[17] Involucrin, a precursor of envelope protein necessary for cross-linkage of intermediate and superficial squamous cells, also is present diffusely in the suprabasal layers of the squamous portio epithelium[49,53] (Fig. 5.7). Involucrin serves as a marker of suprabasal differentiation unrelated to keratinization.

The epithelium of the exocervix is remodeled by proliferation, maturation, and desquamation during the reproductive period. The epithelium is completely replaced by a new population of cells every 4–5 days; the process of squamous epithelial maturation can be accelerated to 3 days by the administration of estrogenic compounds.[27,28] Studies using either radiolabeled estrogen or antibodies against estrogen receptor have localized estrogen receptors to nuclei in the basal, parabasal, and intermediate cell layers.[26,29,30,41,43] Compared with the endometrium where marked variations in estrogen receptor content occur during the menstrual cycle, much less cyclical variation of estrogen receptor expression occurs in the cervix.[26,30,41,43] Only a small increase in levels of estrogen receptor occurs during the follicular as compared with the luteal phase. In atrophic and highly inflamed exocervical epithelium, the amount of estrogen receptor is reduced.[29,30] No progesterone receptors are detected immunohistochemically in the exocervical epithelium during the follicular phase of the menstrual cycle, whereas during the luteal phase and during pregnancy, progesterone receptors appear in the parabasal cell layer.[26] Both estrogen and progesterone receptors can be detected in stromal fibroblast-like cells of the exocervix throughout the menstrual cycle.

In general, estradiol-17β stimulates epithelial proliferation, maturation, and desquamation, whereas progesterone inhibits maturation at the upper midzone level of the epithelium. Accordingly, the portio epithelium during the postnatal period is fully mature and contains large amounts of glycogen as a result of maternal estrogen stimulation. Maturation ceases and glycogen disappears rapidly as the serum hormone levels fall. The epithelium remains atrophic during childhood until menarche when, under the stimulatory effect of ovarian hormones, maturation occurs again and glycogen reappears. During pregnancy, when progesterone levels are elevated, superficial cell maturation is absent.

In addition to estrogen and progesterone, the human cervical epithelium also responds to retinoids. Retinoids are a class of steroid molecules that includes naturally occurring compounds with vitamin A activity as well as synthetic analogues of retinol that may or may not have biologic activity. Retinoids play important roles in regulating the growth and differentiation of a variety of epithelia.[54,55] Their role in regulating cellular differentiation may

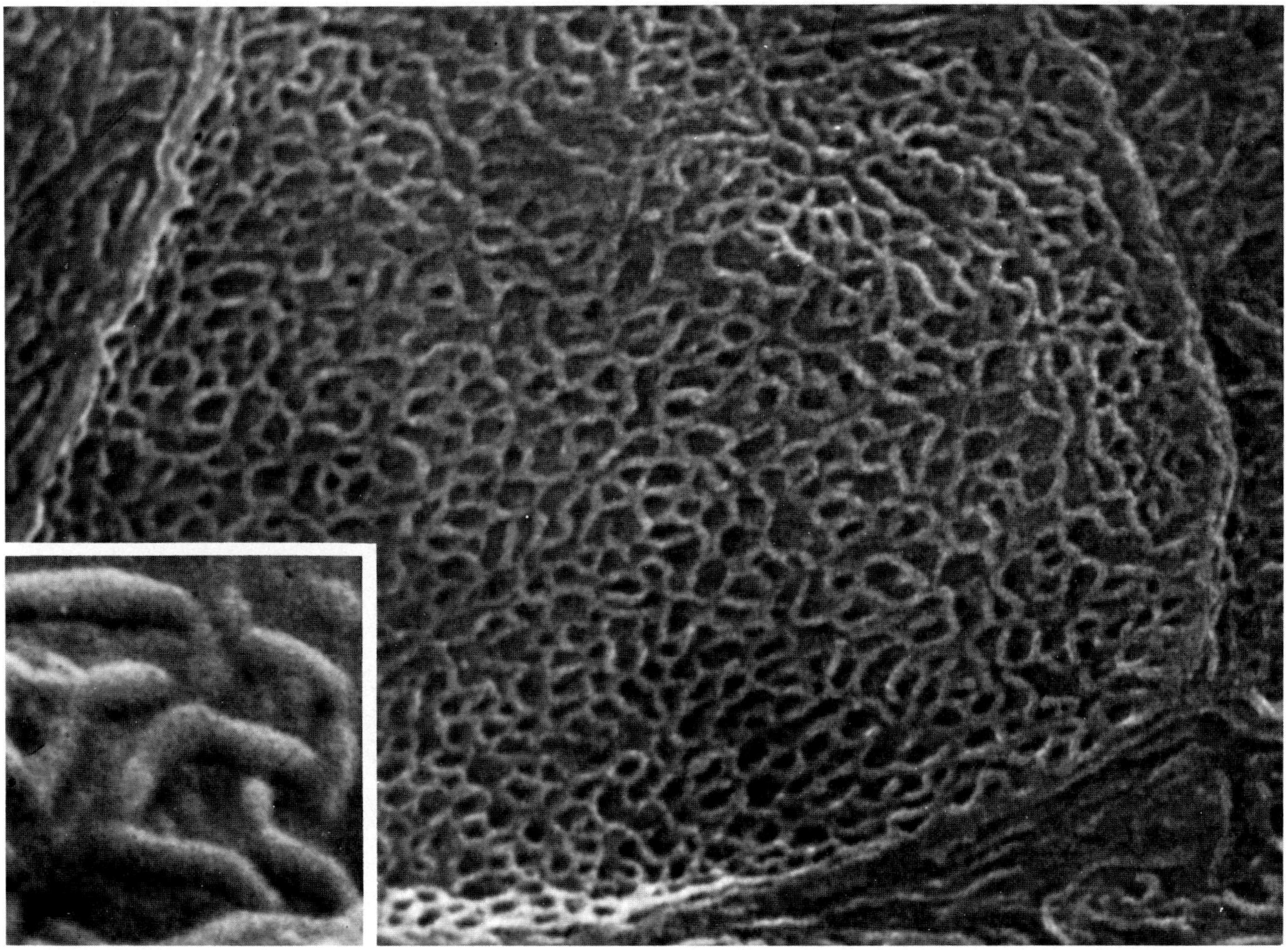

FIG. 5.6. Normal squamous epithelium. Scanning electron micrograph of the most superficial cells of the native squamous portio epithelium. The surface contains an intricate system of microridges. ×8240. *Inset:* Higher magnification of microridges representing nodular evaginations of the surface plasma membrane. ×22,660.

be especially important in the cervix because retinoids modulate squamous and mucinous differentiation. In a variety of target epithelia, vitamin A deficiency results in squamous metaplasia and excessive keratinization,[55] whereas vitamin A excess promotes the formation of mucinous epithelium. Epidemiologic studies have found that women with high dietary intakes of vitamin A and closely related compounds have a reduced risk of developing cervical cancer. Other studies have demonstrated that the topical administration of certain forms of retinoic acid or retinyl acetate can cause regression of squamous intraepithelial lesion (SIL) (CIN).[21,47,52] Retinoid action in target epithelium is mediated by both cellular binding proteins and nuclear receptors.[3,5,32] Immunohistochemical studies have localized a binding protein for retinoic acid called *cellular retinoic acid-binding protein* (CRABP) and a binding protein for retinol called *cellular retinol-binding protein* (CRBP) in the stratified squamous epithelium of the cervix.[22] CRABP is localized predominantly to the basal layer of the epithelium, whereas CRBP is present throughout all layers of the cervical epithelium (Fig. 5.8).

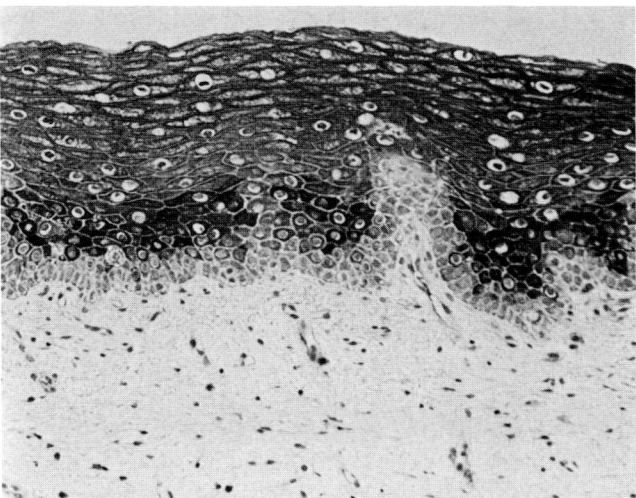

FIG. 5.7. Normal squamous epithelium. Involucrin can be identified in exocervical stratified squamous epithelium using immunohistochemistry. Note intense staining in suprabasal stratum spinosum and absence of staining in the basal cells. (Courtesy of M.J. Warhol, M.D., Philadelphia, PA.)

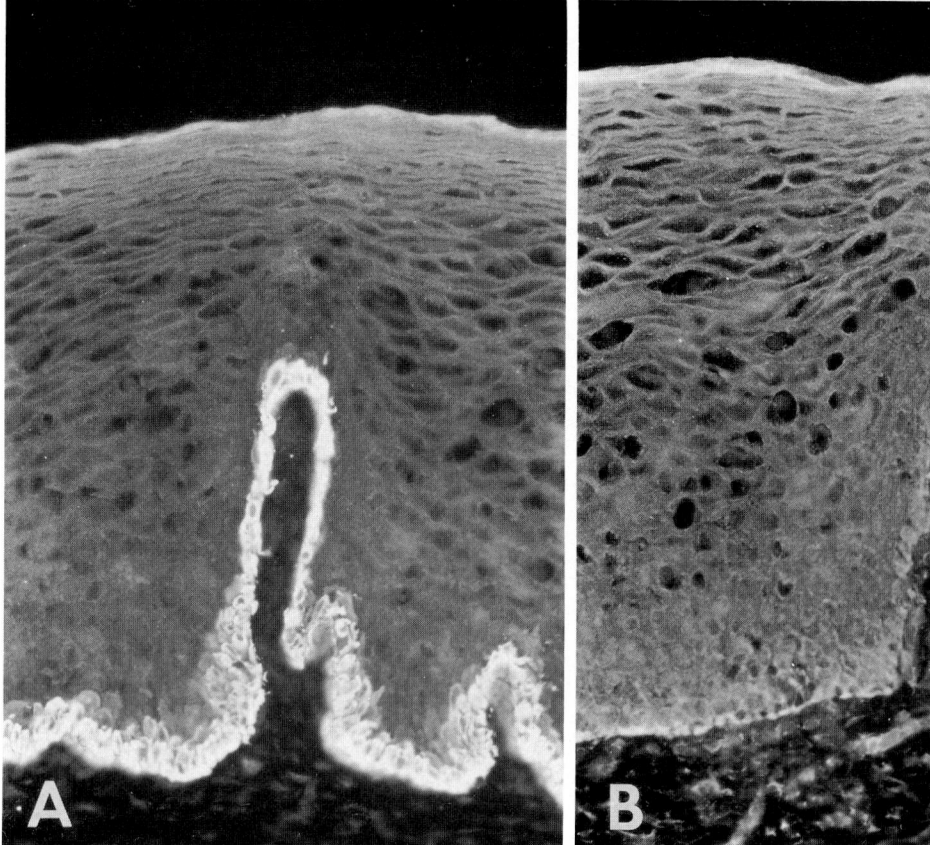

Fig. 5.8. Normal squamous epithelium. Cellular retinoic acid–binding protein and cellular retinal–binding protein can be identified in exocervical stratified squamous epithelium using indirect immunofluorescence. **A:** Cellular retinoic acid–binding protein (CRABP) is present in the basal cells. **B:** Cellular retinol–binding protein (CRBP) is present throughout the entire epithelial thickness. (Reproduced with permission by Hillemanns et al., ref. 22.)

In postmenopausal women, who no longer produce ovarian hormones, the squamous epithelium is atrophic with little or no intracytoplasmic glycogen (Fig. 5.9). Surface epithelial maturation and stromal papillae are absent. These cellular alterations should not be confused with cervical intraepithelial neoplasia (see Chapter 7, Precancerous Lesions of the Cervix). The atrophic epithelial covering does not adequately protect the subepithelial vasculature against trauma, a situation that frequently leads to bleeding and inflammation.

The squamous epithelium of the portio is supported by fibrous connective tissue, devoid of endocervical glands. There is a well-developed capillary network at the stromal–epithelial junction, with occasional finger-like extensions into the epithelium, the stromal papillae (Fig. 5.3).[25] The penetrating vessels within the papillae supply the epithelial cells with nutrients and oxygen. In addition to connective tissue fibers and capillaries, occasional free nerve endings are seen entering the stromal papilla.[28]

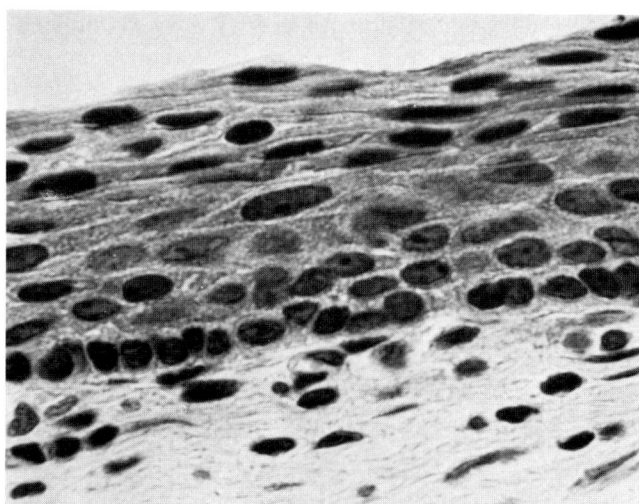

Fig. 5.9. Atrophic squamous epithelium. The epithelium is thin and devoid of glycogen-rich vacuolated cells. The cells in the lower half of the epithelium have prominent nuclei and nucleoli, but cellular cohesion is normal and cytological atypia is absent.

Columnar Epithelium

The mucosa of the cervical canal (endocervix) is composed of a single layer of mucin-secreting, columnar epithelium that lines both the surface and the underlying glandular structures. The latter are traditionally called *compound, tubular,* or *racemose, endocervical glands.* Fluhman,[13] however, using three-dimensional plastic reconstructions from serial histological sections, demonstrated that the endocervical glands actually represent deep, cleft-like infoldings of the surface epithelium with numerous blind, tunnel-like collaterals (Fig. 5.10). Because of the complex architecture of these clefts, or grooves, including oblique, transverse, and longitudinal arrangements, they appear as isolated glands in histological sections (Fig. 5.10). The epithelium lining the clefts is identical with that lining the surface, and consequently the endocervical mucin-producing apparatus is not considered glandular but a complex infolding mucinous membrane. True glands in contrast, have different epithelial lining in their secretory apparatus compared with their ductal and surface epithelial portions.

Especially in multiparous and older women, endocervical glands can appear in histological sections as distinct clusters of up to 50 small glands (Fig. 5.11). Connections between these glands and the endocervical surface may not be apparent. The glands in these clusters are frequently distended by inssispated mucus. Because of distention of the glands by mucus, the lining columnar epithelium fre-

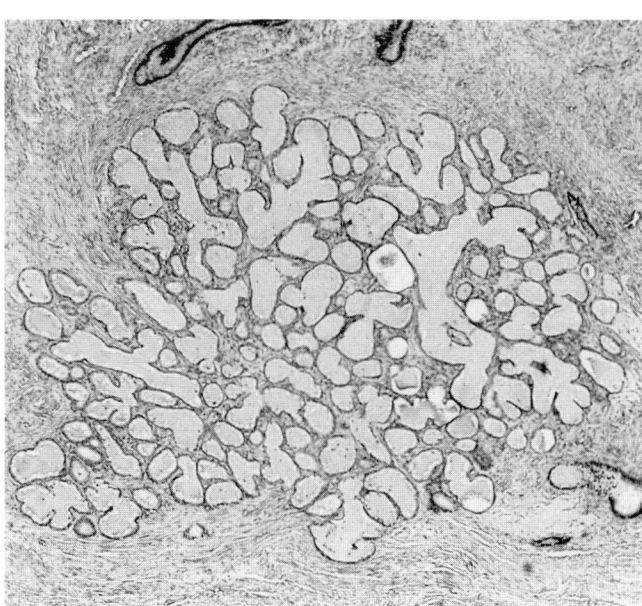

FIG. 5.11. Endocervical tunnel clusters. Small clusters of endocervical glands can develop in the stroma of the older patient and are called *endocervical tunnel clusters.*

quently is quite flattened. Fluhman used the term *tunnel clusters* to refer to these benign clusters of endocervical glands.[13] It is important not to confuse them with well-differentiated, invasive endocervical adenocarcinoma (see Chapter 8, Carcinoma and Other Tumors of the Cervix).

The columnar epithelial cells characteristically have basally placed nuclei and tall, uniform, finely granular cytoplasm filled with mucinous droplets (Fig. 5.12). The droplets have great affinity for alcian blue stains, reflecting their sulfated, sialic acid, mucopolysacchride content.[9] Cells lining the luminal surface have been termed *picket cells* because of their resemblance to a picket fence (Fig. 5.12). Occasionally, nonsecretory cells with cilia are observed[20] (Fig. 5.12, *inset*), the main function of which appears to relate to the distribution and mobilization of endocervical mucus. Isolated neuroendocrine epithelial cells of argyrophil and argentaffin type also may be identified within the endocervical epithelium by histochemical stains.[12,16] The argentaffin-positive cells often contain serotonin, as demonstrated by immunoperoxidase techniques. The physiologic purpose of these rare endocrine endocervical cells is obscure. Biochemically and immunohistochemically, the columnar cells of the endocervix have features of simple epithelia characterized by the presence of only low molecular weight cytokeratins, including cytokeratins 7, 8, 18, 19.[17] However, endocervical cells are not completely homogeneous with regard to cytokeratin expression and occasional endocervical cells express cytokeratin 4, which usually is associated with stratified epithelium. Involucrin is not expressed in the columnar epithelium of the endocervix.[53]

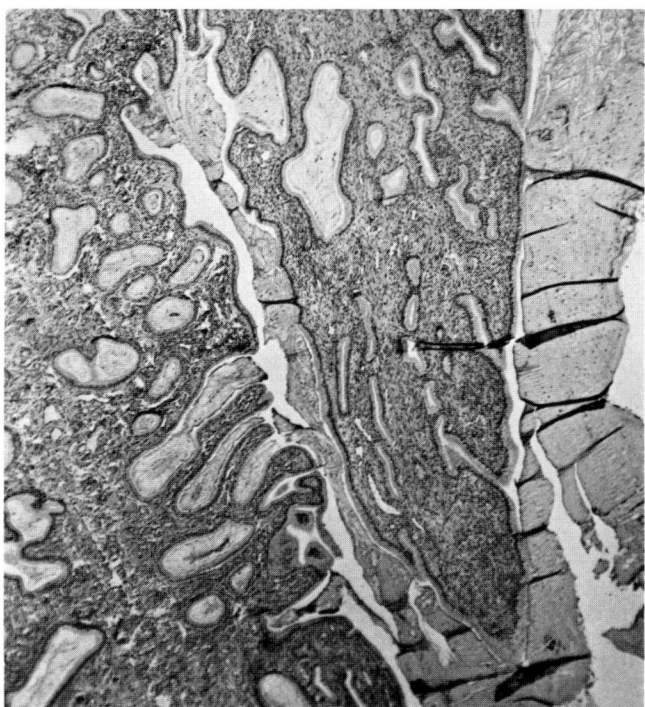

FIG. 5.10. Endocervical mucosa. There are cleft-like infoldings and tunnel-like collaterals. The neighboring gland-like structures represent tangentially sectioned cleft-tunnel complexes.

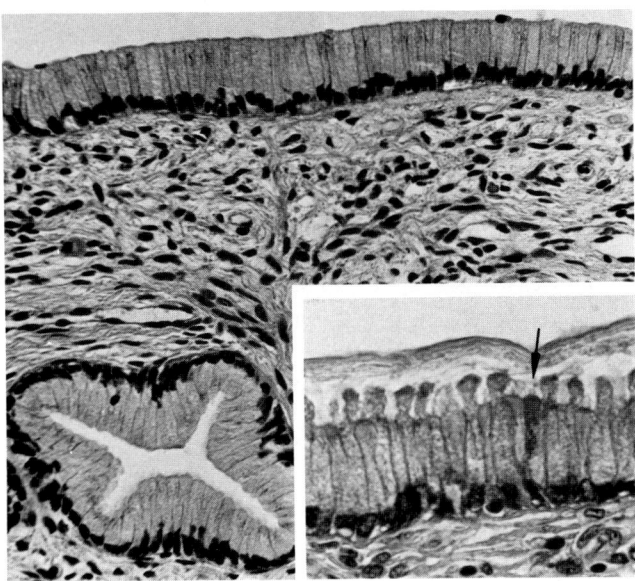

Fig. 5.12. Endocervical mucosa. Tall columnar mucin-filled endocervical cells with basal nuclei. *Inset:* Endocervical cells engaged in apocrine secretion whereby portions of apical cytoplasm are expelled. Ciliated cells are present *(arrow).*

Mitosis in the columnar epithelium is rarely, if ever, observed. It is not known whether regeneration occurs from the underlying subcolumnar reserve cells,[20] which under normal circumstances are seldom seen even at the ultrastructural level, or from the persisting mature endocervical cells. Unlike the attenuated vascular stromal papillae of the original squamous portio epithelium, the subepithelial capillary network in the endocervical mucosa is well developed. Unlike the endocervical epithelium from which it is derived, cervical mucus is subject to profound cyclic changes. Under estrogenic stimulation, the endocervical secretions are profuse, watery, and alkaline, facilitating sperm penetration. During the postovulatory phase, secretions are scant, thick, and acid, containing numerous leukocytes, and act as a barrier to sperm penetration. Biochemical[42] and ultrastructural analyses[4] have shown that cervical mucus is composed of a heterogeneous micellar network of glycoproteins. The intermicellar space occupied by cervical plasma is rich in sodium chloride and potassium, the ions of which are responsible for the crystallization of mucus or ferning (arborization) reaction. Under estrogenic influence, the glycoprotein micelles are arranged parallel to each other at a distance of 5–15 μm, creating a channel system that is favorable to sperm penetration. During progestagenic stimulation, the micellar channel system is replaced by a dense network composed of interlacing micellar fiber bridges that preclude sperm penetration. Ultrastructurally,[11,18] endocervical secretory activity operates by both the apocrine and the merocrine type of expulsion of secretory products. In the former, a portion of apical cytoplasm packed with secretory granules

is detached (Fig. 5.13) whereas, in the latter, secretory products are released from apical granules through pore-like openings of the surface cytoplasmic membrane. Syntheses of mucoproteins is initiated in the Golgi cisternae and perigolgian vesicles.[11,18] The coalescence of perigolgian vesicles leads to the formation of larger secretory units that, by a similar process, form prominent granules with a granulofilamentous content. The Golgi is associated with free ribosomes, granular endoplasmic reticulum, and mitochondria, providing the essential protein matrix and energy for mucoprotein synthesis.

The stroma of the endocervix is comparatively better innervated than that of the exocervix. Fibers run parallel to muscle bundles, but sensory-free endings have not been clearly demonstrated.[28] True lymphoid follicles, with or without germinal centers, are encountered in the subepithelial stroma of both the exocervix and the endocervix.

Lymphoid-derived Cells

Mucosal immunity is an important component of the host's defense mechanism against viral and bacterial pathogens. Components of both the secretory (IgA antibody-mediated) as well as the cellular immune systems are present in the cervix. Cellular local immune responses may be particularly important in determining the outcome of human

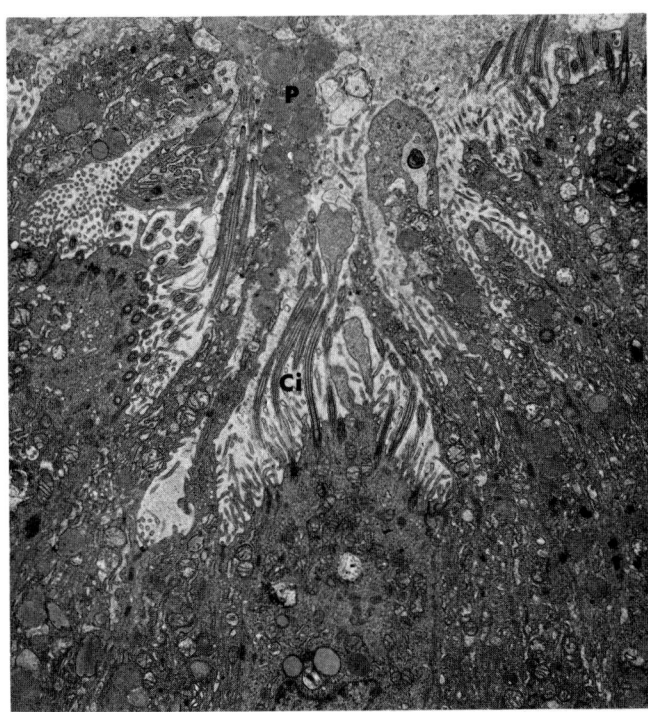

Fig. 5.13. Endocervical mucosa. Electron micrograph of mucin-containing endocervical cells alternating with ciliated cells *(Ci).* Secretion is of the apocrine type, as indicated by intraluminal protrusions *(P)* of apical cytoplasmic substance packed with mucinous droplets and various organelles. ×4030.

papillomavirus (HPV) infections in the cervix. A variety of lymphocyte and dendritic macrophage subsets are present in both the epithelium of the exo- and endocervix as well as the subepithelial stroma.[35] Dendritic macrophages can be identified by their long cytoplasmic processes (Fig. 5.14) and are the predominant antigen-presenting cells in epithelial tissues. They are critical for cellular immunity at mucosal surfaces because they present foreign antigens in conjunction with major histocompatibility (MHC) Class II antigens to T lymphocytes. In the cervix these cells display both topographic and phenotypic heterogeneity.[23,48] Bone marrow–derived dendritic macrophages that react with anti-Leu 6 monoclonal antibodies and contain Birbeck's granules in their cytoplasm by electron microscopy are called *Langerhans' cells*. Langerhans' cells express the CD4 receptor on their surface. They are phagocytic cells that internalize antigens and migrate out of the epithelium to lymph nodes where they present antigens to T and B lymphocytes. Only a small subset of all cervical dendritic macrophages are Langerhans' cells, and the Langerhans' cells are located primarily in the stratified squamous epithelium in the suprabasal cell layers.[23,48] Most dendritic macrophages in the cervix do not react with anti-Leu 6 monoclonal antibodies.[23,48] Leu 6–negative dendritic macrophages are HLA DR–positive and are distributed throughout both the ectocervical epithelium and stroma.

Large numbers of T lymphocytes also are present in the cervix under normal conditions.[35,48] Cytotoxic-suppressor T cells (Leu 2a positive) are the major T-cell subtype present in the cervix. Leu 2a–positive cells can be found in both the epithelium and stroma of either the exocervix and endocervix, but are present predominantly in the subepithelial stroma. Variable numbers of helper T cells (Leu 3a positive) also are present in the exocervical stroma, as are B lymphocytes and plasma cells.[48] These cells participate in the cervical secretory (IgA-mediated) immune system. It should also be pointed out that cervical epithelial cells may play an, as yet, undefined role in mucosal immunity. Not only are MHC Class II antigens expressed on dendritic macrophages, but keratinocytes in areas of squamous metaplasia as well as columnar epithelial cells of the endocervix can express HLA DR on their surfaces.[48]

Because the presence of lymphocytes in the cervix is a normal finding, the diagnosis of chronic cervicitis should be reserved for specimens showing a marked infiltration of lymphocytes.

The Transformation Zone

The squamocolumnar junction of the cervix is defined as the border between the stratified squamous epithelium and the mucin-secreting columnar epithelium of the endocervix. Morphogenetically, there are two different squamocolumnar junctions (Fig. 5.15). One is termed the *original* squamocolumnar junction and is the site at which the native squamous covering of the exocervix abuts the endocervical columnar epithelium at the time of birth. At birth, most females have some mucin-secreting columnar endocervical epithelium present on the portio surface of the cervix that forms an *ectropion* or cervical *ectopy*. The exact location of the original squamocolumnar junction and, therefore, the amount of endocervical ectopy present at birth depends on the extent of inward migration of squamous epithelium from the lower third of the vagina. In women exposed to diethylstilbestrol (DES) in utero, the normal migration of the squamous epithelium is halted prematurely and the original squamocolumnar junction often is located in the vagina rather than on the exocervix.[46] In these DES-exposed women, the entire cervical portio can be covered with endocervical columnar epithelium.

At about the age of 1 year, the cervix begins to elongate. This results in migration of the squamocolumnar junction towards the external os. This migration is frequently incomplete and one colposcopic study of prepubertal girls between the ages of 1 and 13 years found the presence of endocervical ectopy in 43% of these girls.[31] Hormonal and other physical factors influence the size and distribution of the cervical ectopy by altering the shape and volume of the cervical lips. At the time of menarche or during pregnancy both the uterus and the cervix enlarge. Enlargement of the cervix is accompanied by alterations in its shape, which result in more of an "eversion" or rolling outward of endocervical columnar epithelium onto the portio (Fig. 5.15). As a result, in most women during the reproductive period, cervical ectopy is present, and the size of the ectopy is most

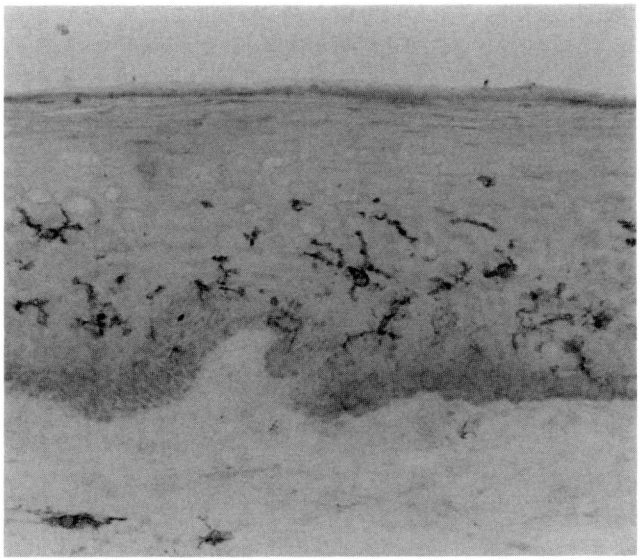

FIG. 5.14. Normal squamous epithelium. Leu 6–positive dendritic macrophages (Langerhans' cells) can be localized using immunohistochemistry and are present predominantly in the intermediate cell layers of the epithelium.

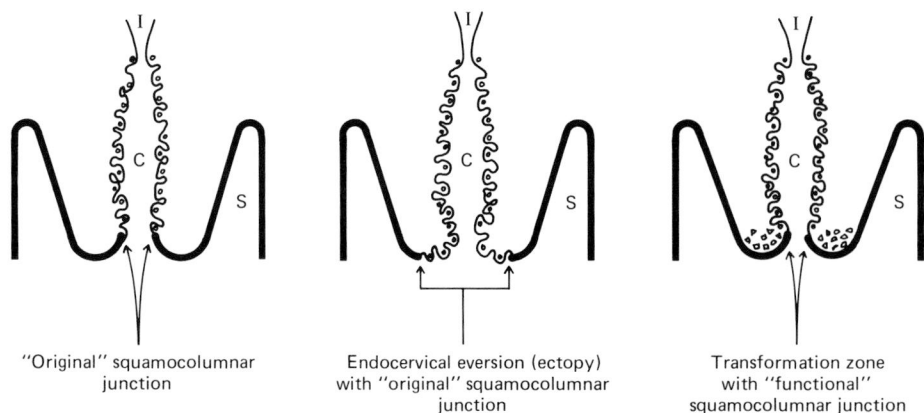

"Original" squamocolumnar
junction

Endocervical eversion (ectopy)
with "original" squamocolumnar
junction

Transformation zone
with "functional"
squamocolumnar junction

FIG. 5.15. The transformation zone. Schematic representation of original and functional squamocolumnar junctions and three basic types of portios. *Left:* Diagram of a portico completely covered with native squamous epithelium. The squamocolumnar junction is at the external os. *Middle:* Denotes cervical ectopy, with the squamocolumnar junction being located on the exocervix below the external os. *Right:* Indicates areas of cervical ectopy that have become covered with squamous epithelium. This area is the cervical transformation zone. The new, or functional, squamocolumnar junction of the transformation zone is at the external os. S, squamous epithelium; C, endocervical columnar epithelium; I, uterine isthmus.

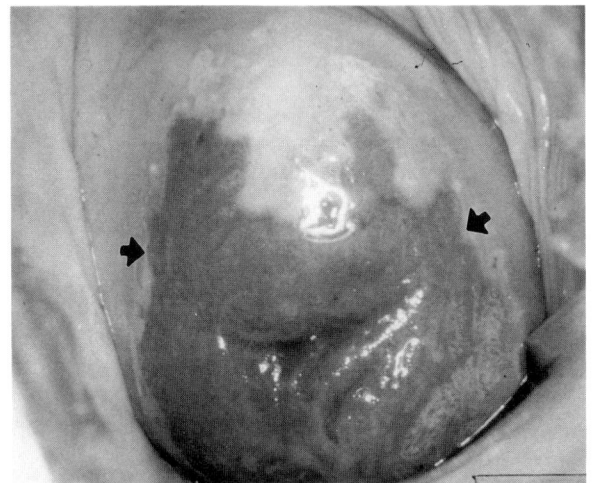

A

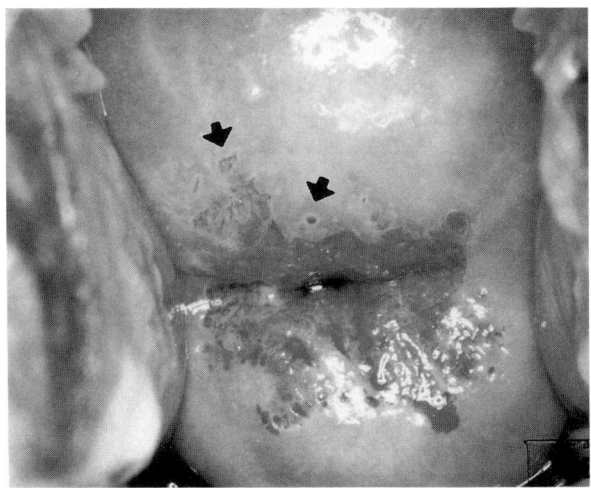

B

FIG. 5.16. The transformation zone. Colpophotographs of endocervical eversion of the transformation zone. **A:** Endocervical mucosa is everted on both the anterior and the posterior lip and surrounds the anatomic external os. The original squamocolumnar junction (SCJ) is on the portio of the cervix *(arrows)*. **B:** Squamous metaplasia is occurring and the new SCJ is now internal to the original SCJ. The area between the original and new SCJ is the transformation zone. Residual endocervical gland mouths are represented by the circular openings *(arrows)*. **C:** The transformation zone is completely mature and the SCJ is inside the endocervical canal. No endocervical gland mouths are present.

C

extensive in younger women (under 20 years of age), after the first pregnancy. Cervical ectopy occurs twice as commonly on the anterior as on the posterior lip, but both lips maybe involved simultaneously.[7] Cervical ectopy may be particularly exaggerated with progestin therapy, typically oral contraceptive users.

When viewed with the naked eye, the endocervical mucosa appears as a red, velvety zone, sharply contrasting with the neighboring pink, translucent squamous portio epithelium (Fig. 5.16A). Because of its gross appearance, the term *cervical erosion* often is used by clinicians to refer to this columnar epithelium. This term is incorrect, however, because there is no epithelial denudation (true erosion).[34] Instead, the red appearance is due to papillary excrescences of varying size, resembling a bunch of grapes when viewed with the colposcope. Histologically these are blunt-ended papillae, lined by endocervical columnar epithelium and supported by a fibrovascular stroma containing numerous chronic inflammatory cells. The cervical ectopy is a normal physiologic finding and should not be construed as a pathological abnormality.

Over time, the columnar epithelium that composes the cervical ectopy is remodeled and replaced by metaplastic squamous epithelium. As this occurs, the histological squamocolumnar junction moves toward the exocervical os. This newly formed squamocolumnar junction is called the *physiologic, functional,* or *new* squamocolumnar junction. Whereas the original squamocolumnar junction usually is quite abrupt (Fig. 5.17), the junction between the columnar and squamous epithelium at the physiologic or functional squamocolumnar junction can be either abrupt or gradual. The region between the neonatal original squamocolumnar junction and the postpubertal functional squamocolumnar junction is termed the *transformation zone*. The transformation zone is characterized histologically by the presence of metaplastic epithelium. The concept of the transformation zone is extremely important for understanding the pathogenesis of squamous cell carcinomas of the cervix and its precursors, because virtually all cervical squamous neoplasia begins at the new squamocolumnar junction and because the extension and limits of cervical cancer precursors coincide with the distribution of the transformation zone.[45] It also is important to remember that during the childbearing years and during pregnancy the transformation zone is located, in almost all instances, on the exposed portion of the cervix. Consequently, the vast majority of cervical neoplasias can be removed for histological diagnosis by punch biopsy.

The transformation zone may be difficult to visualize with the naked eye. Its localization, however, is greatly enhanced with the application of 5% acetic acid and the use of the colposcope (see Chapter 7, Precancerous Lesions of the Cervix). Colposcopically, the transformation zone is characterized by smooth, translucent, slightly white tissue that corresponds to metaplastic squamous epithe-

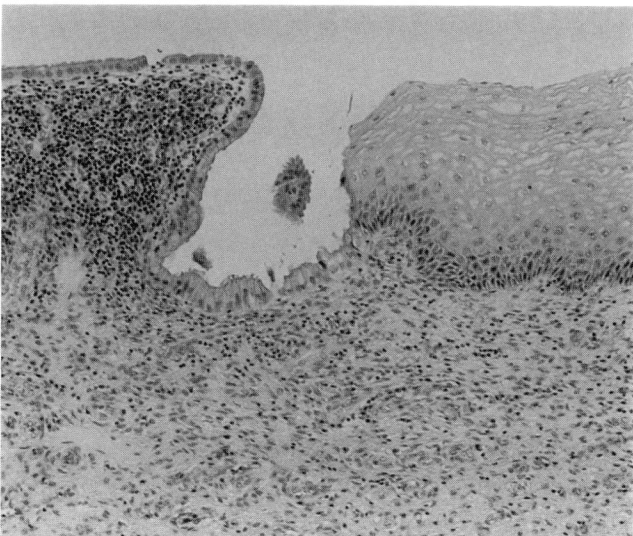

FIG. 5.17. Squamocolumnar junction. Endocervical columnar epithelium meets the native squamous portion epithelium. Note the abrupt transition between the mature squamous epithelium of the portio and the endocervical mucosa. A similar sharp demarcation may be seen at the squamocolumnar junction of the mature transformation zone. The lamina propria of the columnar epithelium is frequently obscured by a chronic inflammatory exudate.

lium with circular openings and spherical bumps of 2–4 mm, which correspond to the underlying endocervical glands and nabothian cysts, respectively (Fig. 5.16B). Nabothian cysts are formed when the mouths of endocervical clefts become obliterated by the proliferating surface metaplastic squamous epithelium. As the flow of mucus is blocked, the secretory products accumulate, leading to cystic glandular dilations, or nabothian cysts. Microscopically, the cystic spaces are lined by low columnar endocervical cells, supported by a distended basal lamina (Fig. 5.18).

Movement of the functional squamocolumnar junction continues throughout the reproductive years (Fig. 5.16C). Therefore, in older and postmenopausal women, the functional squamocolumnar junction is located nearly always above the external os.

Squamous Metaplasia

Metaplasia is defined as the replacement of one type of mature tissue by another equally mature type of tissue. In the cervix, squamous metaplasia is the replacement of the mucin-producing columnar epithelium by stratified squamous epithelium and appears to occur by two different mechanisms (Fig. 5.19). One mechanism consists of direct ingrowth from the native portio epithelium bordering the columnar epithelium, a process frequently referred to as *squamous epithelialization*. The second mechanism

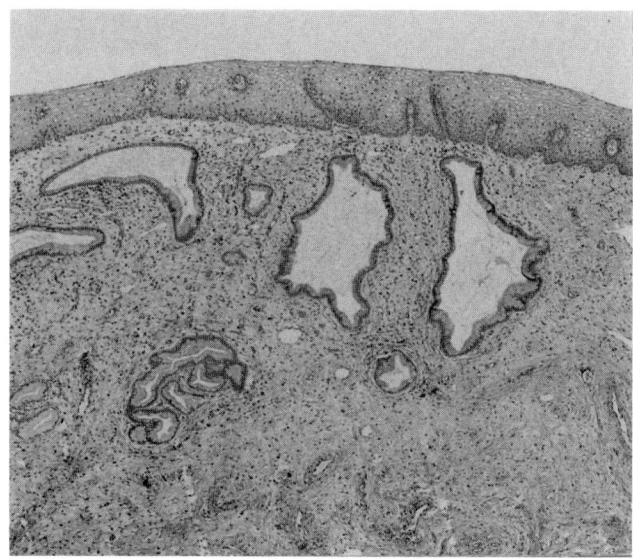

FIG. 5.18. Transformation zone. Microscopic appearance of the outer portio limit of the transformation zone. Mature squamous epithelium covers underlying endocervical glands that are distended with mucin.

involves a proliferation of undifferentiated subcolumnar reserve cells of the endocervical epithelium that differentiate into squamous epithelium. This process has been termed *squamous metaplasia,* but such names as *epidermidization* and *squamous prosoplasia* also are used.[13] The latter term, derived from the Greek meaning *forward* and *to form,* was proposed by Fluhman[13] and probably is the most accurate one, although used rarely today.

The process of squamous epithelialization has been documented by histological, colposcopic, colpomicroscopic, and electron microscopic observations[7,10] that have shown that tongues of native squamous epithelium of the portio grow beneath the adjacent columnar epithelium and expand between the mucinous epithelium and its basement membrane (Fig. 5.20). As the squamous cells expand and mature, the endocervical cells gradually are displaced upward, degenerate, and eventually are sloughed (Fig. 5.21, top). A similar process is observed in the re-epithelialization of true pathological erosion of the endocervix, the so-called ascending healing of Meyer.[34] The progression of squamous transformation of the endocervical ectropion is primarily depending on local (vaginal) environmental fac-

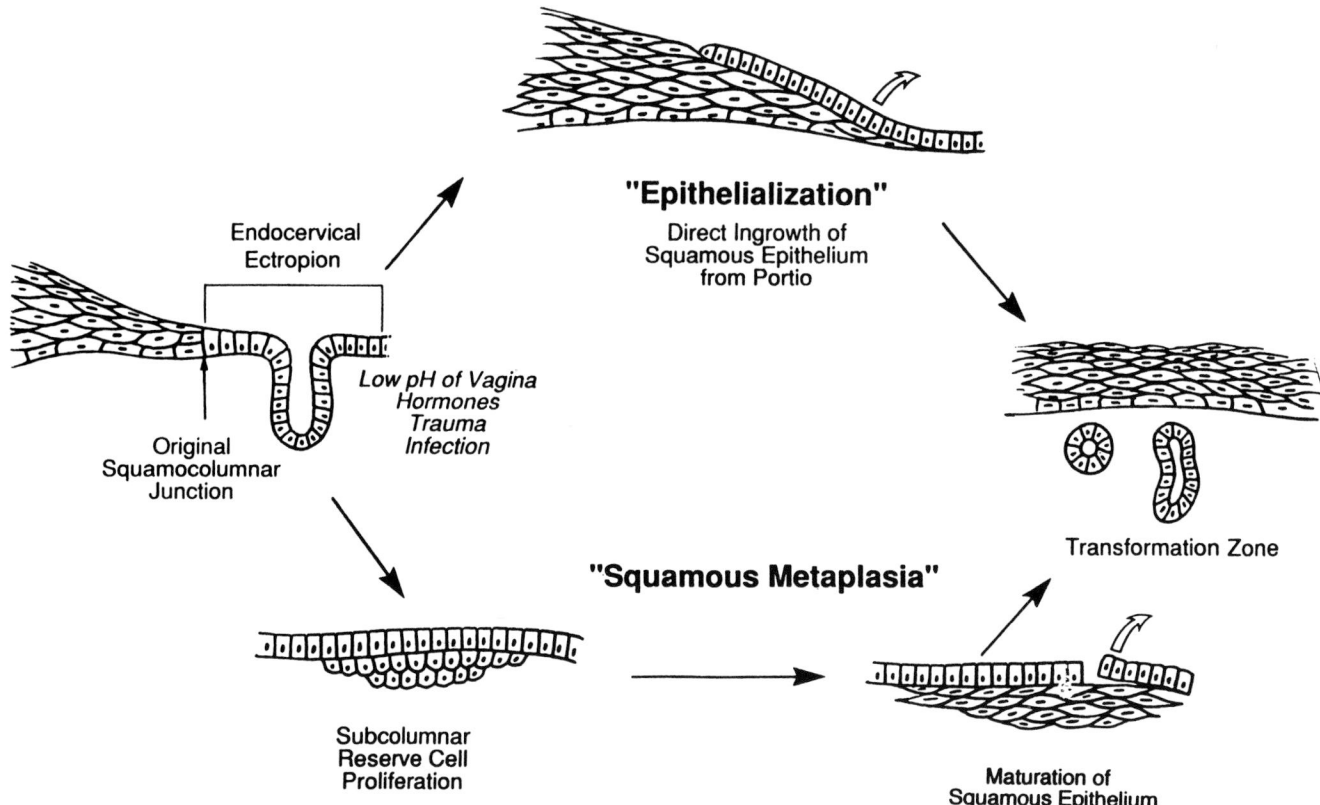

FIG. 5.19. Squamous metaplasia. There are two histogenic mechanisms by which the endocervical mucosa is replaced by squamous epithelium. The first is the direct ingrowth of squamous epithelium from the portio, which is referred to as squamous epithelialization *(top).* The other is through prolifera-tion of subcolumnar reserve cells and their subsequent maturation into a squamous epithelium, which is called squamous metaplasia *(bottom).* Both result in a mature squamous epithelium overlying endocervical mucus-producing glands *(right).*

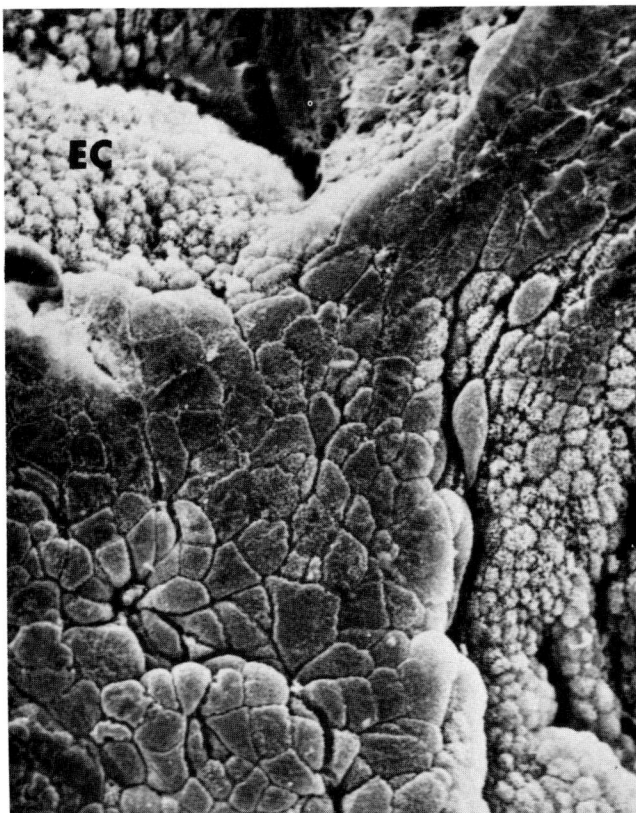

FIG. 5.20. Squamous metaplasia. Scanning electron microscopic appearance of the outer edge of the early transformation zone. Narrow tongues of squamous epithelium with a pavement-like surface pattern extend onto the everted endocervical mucosa (EC). ×4280.

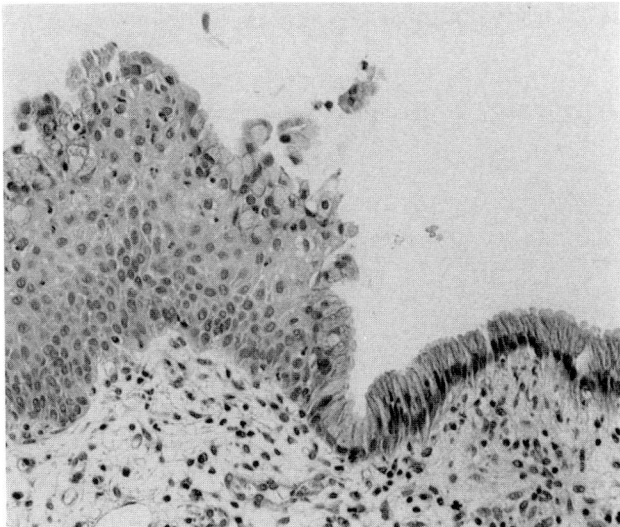

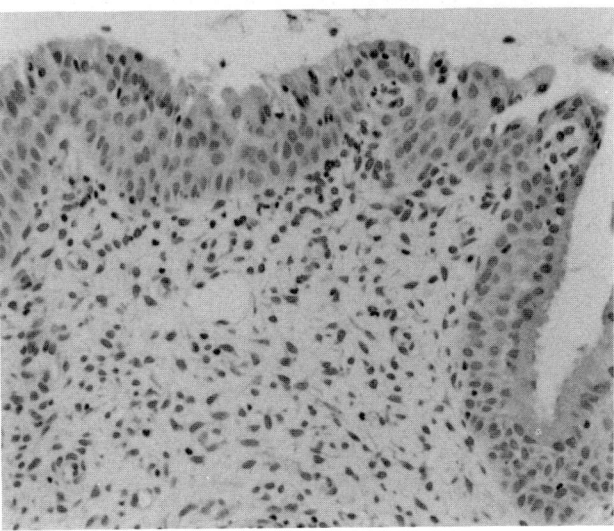

FIG. 5.21. Squamous metaplasia. *Top:* During squamous epitheliation a narrow tongue of squamous epithelium from the portio grows under the everted endocervical mucosa and lifts it off the basement membrane. The endocervical cells then degenerate and are sloughed. *Bottom:* During squamous metaplasia, a layer of cuboidal reserve cells develops between the columnar endocervical cells and the basal lamina.

tors, with the initial stimulus being the low (acid) pH of the vagina after puberty.[6] Trauma, chronic irritation, or cervical infection also play a role in development and maturation of the transformation zone by stimulating repair and remodeling; eventually the ectocervix is covered by a protective surface of mature squamous epithelium (Fig. 5.18). The process of squamous epithelialization is thought to be responsible for the obliteration of the outer two-thirds of endocervical ectopy. Rapid squamous re-epithelialization of the columnar epithelium of the transformation zone also may be produced iatrogenically by electrocautery, cryosurgery, or laser surgery.

The second mechanism involved in replacement of columnar epithelium by a squamous epithelium and the function of the transformation zone is squamous metaplasia (i.e., squamous prosoplasia). This process has been thoroughly documented by Fluhman[13] and others.[7] The first stage of squamous metaplasia is the appearance of small cuboidal cells beneath the columnar mucinous epithelium, the so-called subcolumnar reserve cells (Fig. 5.21, bottom). *Reserve cells* have large, uniformly shaped, round nuclei with faintly granular chromatin and occasional ag-

gregates of chromatin (i.e., chromocenters of reserve cells). The cell borders are poorly defined and the cells have only scant amounts of cytoplasm. There is an increased rate of nucleic acid synthesis in reserve cells when examined by autoradiography[20] and their fine ultrastructural characteristics[10,20] are similar to those of the basal cells of the mature squamous portio epithelium. The origin of subcolumnar reserve cells is controversial. Some investigators suggest a direct derivation from columnar mucinous secretory cells,[13] whereas others favor an origin from the basal cells of the squamous portio epithelium, embryonal rests of urogenital origin, or stromal cells as possible

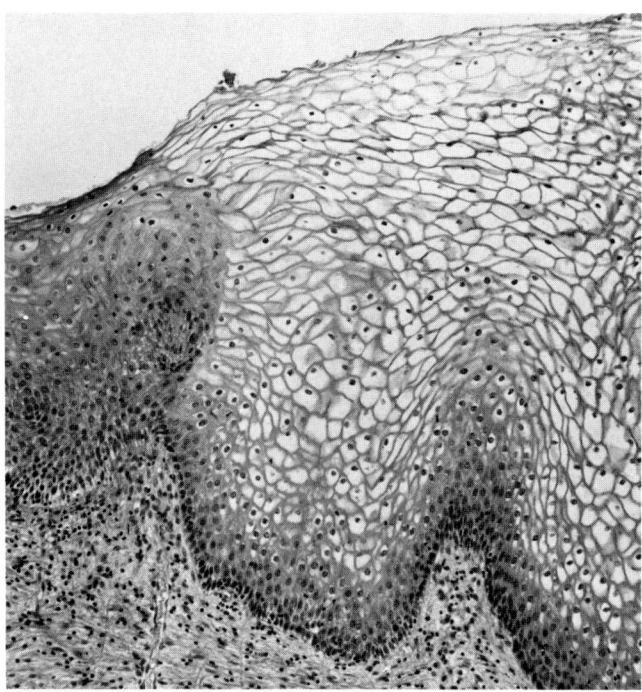

Fɪɢ. 5.22. **Transformation zone epithelium.** On the right, the epithelium has achieved full maturation and is identical to normal native portio epithelium, whereas on the left, squamous differentiation, including glycogenation, is incomplete.

sources.[6] Recent cell culture and implantation experiments in vitro and in vivo combined with immunohistochemical studies show that human endocervical cells can differentiate reversibly and give rise to CK7 and CK8 in positive endocervical mucin-secreting cells or CK13 positive reserve cells. In these experiments, reserve cells were identified to be the origin of squamous metaplastic cells.[51a] Progressive growth and stratification of reserve cells (subcolumnar reserve cell hyperplasia), followed by differentiation into immature squamous, result in the formation of a fully mature squamous epithelium indistinguishable from the native portio epithelium (Fig. 5.18).

Immature squamous metaplastic epithelium is distinguished from its mature counterpart by a lack of surface maturation and inconspicuous intracytoplasmic glycogen. It is, characteristically, sharply demarcated from the native portio epithelium by a perpendicular or oblique line to the surface (Fig. 5.22). As a result, the uninitiated observer may mistake immature squamous metaplasia for a SIL, particularly when the process also involves the underlying glands (Fig. 5.23). In contrast to neoplastic epithelium the immature squamous metaplastic epithelium maintains cell organization and cohesion; nuclear atypia is absent and, usually, a single row of endocervical cells overlies the squamous cells. Ultrastructurally, the immature, squamous metaplastic cells resemble the parabasal cells of the portio epithelium. The superficial cells of the immature transfor-

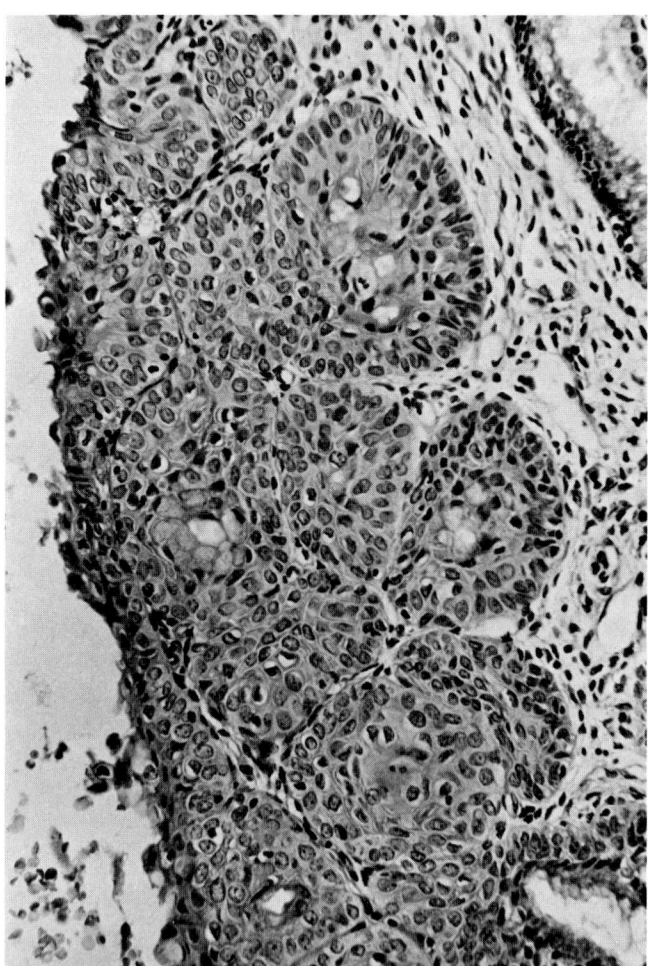

Fɪɢ. 5.23. **Immature squamous metaplasia.** Immature squamous metaplasia can involve both the surface and the deep endocervical glands. Note trapped mucinous endocervical cells in the center of the metaplastic foci. Unlike squamous intraepithelial lesions (SIL) with gland involvement, in squamous metaplasia nuclear atypia is minimal and there is normal cellular cohesion.

mation zone epithelium are covered by numerous microvillous projections rather than surface microridges (Fig. 5.24).[11] Unlike squamous epithelialization, which involves the peripheral regions of the endocervical tissue, squamous metaplasia has a random distribution within the ectropion, reflecting its asynchronous development. The patchy, uneven distribution of squamous metaplasia within the ectropion may be due to the presence of circumscribed, focal stimuli or to differing rates of cell transition and maturation.[10]

Biochemically and immunohistochemically, immature squamous metaplasia shares features of both the mature squamous epithelium and the columnar mucinous epithelium. The keratin intermediate filaments of metaplastic squamous cells are similar to those of terminally differentiated squamous cells but are less complex and fewer in

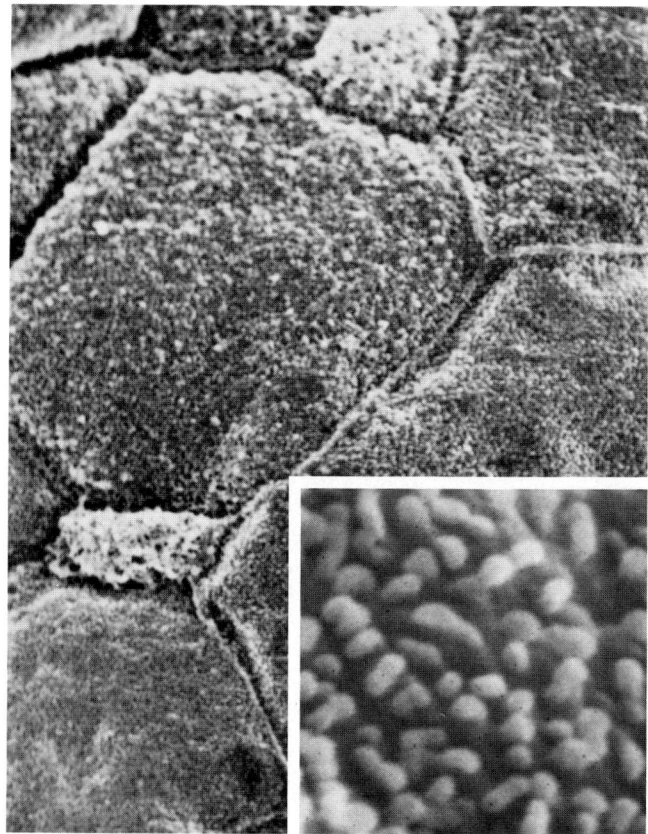

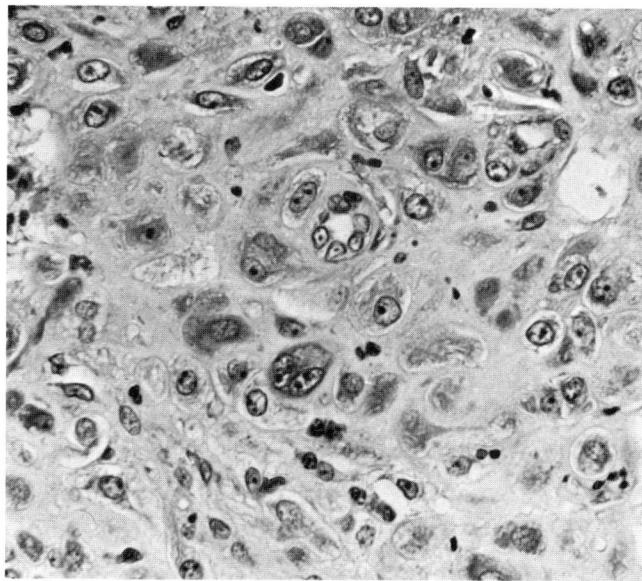

FIG. 5.25. Decidual reaction. A decidual reaction of cervical stromal cells can occur during pregnancy. The cells are identical to gestational decidual cells of the endometrium. Decidual change in the cervix should be distinguished from poorly differentiated invasive squamous cell carcinoma or undifferentiated carcinoma.

FIG. 5.24. Immature squamous metaplasia. Scanning electron microscopy of immature squamous metaplastic cells with well-developed terminal bars. In contrast to the superficial cells of the mature squamous epithelium, which are covered by microridges, the superficial cells of the immature transformation zone are covered by microvilli. Among the squamous cells is an entrapped endocervical cell *(lower left)*. ×2400. *Inset:* Higher magnification of surface microvilli. ×15,000.

number.[8,38,51] Involucrin expression is highly variable and is related to the amount of intermediate and superficial cell maturation present within an area of metaplasia.[49,53] Focal mucin production may be demonstrated by cytoplasmic mucicarmine positivity. The bipotential nature of immature metaplasia is further corroborated ultrastructurally by the finding of individual cells, within islands of metaplasia, that contain both squamous and columnar mucinous cytoplasmic organelles, including varying ratios of tonofibrils, glycogen with secretory granules, and glycocalyces. Cilia occasionally may persist in otherwise mature squamous cells.[10]

With the aid of the colposcope, islands of squamous metaplastic epithelium are seen on the tips of endocervical papillae, expanding centripetally and developing delicate epithelial bridges that fuse with neighboring epithelial proliferations (Fig. 5.16B). Further growth, expansion, and interanastomosis between squamous epithelial islands

eventually lead to complete obliteration of the underlying columnar epithelium (Fig. 5.16C).

Pregnancy and Puerperium

The morphologic alterations that occur in the antepartum or postpartum cervix are not pathognomonic of pregnancy or parturition but are seen more commonly at these times than in the nonpregnant postpartum state. They are related to the stimulatory effects of elevated steroid hormones. The spongy enlargement of the pregnant cervix is caused by increased vascularity and edema of the stroma accompanied by acute inflammation.[39] The massive destruction of collagen fibers and accumulation of extracellular glycoprotein ground substance before labor result in cervical softening and affacement, facilitating dilation of the cervix to about 10 cm during labor. Decidualization of the stroma, either patchy or diffuse, occurs in about one-third of the cervices examined histologically (Fig. 5.25) and disappears by 2 months' postpartum.[24] It is mediated presumably by the high levels of progesterone during pregnancy.

Gestational cervical mucus is thick, tenacious, rich in leukocytes, and forms a mucous plug that obliterates the cervical canal, sealing the endometrial cavity from the vagina and thus preventing bacterial invasion. Squamous metaplasia and lobules of tightly packed, small endocervical glandular units forming polypoid protrusions into the canal often are seen. The term *microglandular endocervical hyperplasia* is used for the latter type of lesion. An identical endocervical proliferation is seen in patients using oral contraceptives (See Chapter 6, Benign Diseases of the Cervix). The intense proliferation of endocervical mucinous cells is associated with enlargement and softening of the portio during the course of gestation and leads to a more exaggerated protrusion of the endocervical ectropion onto the exocervix. This is rapidly replaced by immature squamous epithelium of both native portio and subcolumnar reserve cell origin.[6,13,24,50] As a result, in most primigravidas an immature cervical transformation zone is seen, which often persists for long periods. The squamocolumnar junction of the transformation zone is located nearly always distal to the external os. Subsequent active remodeling of the transformation zone occurs to a comparatively lesser extent in subsequent pregnancies.[13] True pathological erosion during pregnancy is observed to involve the everted endocervix next to the native portio epithelium in about 10% of biopsies.[24] Postpartum injuries, such as lacerations produced during labor, are seen in most primiparous and half of multiparous patients,[24] with a distribution of 2:1 in favor of the anterior lip.[50] The denuded areas are subsequently re-epithelialized by ingrowing native squamous epithelium on the exocervix.

References

1. Averette HE, Weinstein GD, Frost P (1970) Autoradiographic analysis of cell proliferation kinetics in human genital tissues. I. Normal cervix and vagina. Am J Obstet Gynecol 108: 8–17
2. Berchuck A, Rodriguez G, Kamel A, Soper JT, Clarke-Pearson DL, Bast RC JR (1990) Expression of epidermal growth factor receptor and HER-2/Neu in normal and neoplastic cervix, vulva, and vagina. Obstet Gynecol 76: 381–387
3. Blomhoff R, Green MH, Berg T, Norum KR (1990) Transport and storage of vitamin A. Science 250: 399–404
4. Chretien FC, Gernigon C, David G, Psychoyos A (1973) The ultrastructure of human cervical mucus under scanning electron microscopy. Fertil Steril 24: 746–757
5. Chytil F, Ong DE (1987) Intracellular vitamin A-binding proteins Annu Rev Nutr 7: 321–335
6. Coppleson M, Reid BL (1967) Preclinical carcinoma of the cervix uteri. Oxford, Pergamon Press
7. Coppleson M, Pixley E, Reid BL (1971) Colposcopy. A scientific and practical approach to the cervix in health and disease. Springfield, Ill, Charles C Thomas
8. Czernobilsky B, Moll R, Franke WW, et al (1984) Intermediate filaments of normal and neoplastic tissues of the female genital tract with emphasis on problems of differential tumor diagnosis. Pathol Res Pract 179: 31–37
9. Fand SB (1973) The histochemistry of human cervical epithelium. In: Blandau RJ, Moghissi KS (eds) The biology of the cervix. Chicago, University of Chicago Press, pp 103–24
10. Feldman D, Romney SL, Edgcomb J, Valentine T (1984) Ultrastructure of normal, metaplastic and abnormal human uterine cervix: use of montages to study the topographical relationship of epithelial cells. Am J Obstet Gynecol 150: 573–688
11. Ferenczy A, Richart RM (1974) Female reproductive system. Dynamics of scan and transmission electron microscopy. New York, John Wiley & Sons
12. Fetissof F, Berger G, Dubois MP, et al (1985) Endocrine cells in the female genital tract. Histopathology 9: 133–145
13. Fluhman CF (1961) The cervix uteri and its diseases. Philadelphia, WB Saunders
14. Foraker AG, Marino GA (1961) Glycogen-synthesizing enzymes in the uterine cervix. Obstet Gynecol 17: 311–315.
15. Foraker AG, Wingo WJ (1956) Protein-bound sulfhydryl and disulfide group in squamous carcinoma of the uterine cervix. Am J Obstet Gynecol 71: 1182
16. Fox H, Kazzaz B, Langley FA (1964) Argyrophil and argentaffin cells in the female genital tract and in ovarian mucinous cysts. J Pathol Bacteriol 88:479–488
17. Franke WW, Moll R, Achtstaetter T, Kuhn C (1986) Cell typing of epithelial and carcinomas of the female genital tract using cytoskeletal proteins as markers. In Peto R (ed) Banbury Reports 21, cervical cancer. pp 121–144
18. Friedrich ER (1973) The normal morphology and ultrastructure of the cervix. In: Blandau RJ, Moghissi KS (eds) The biology of the cervix. Chicago, University of Chicago Press, pp 79–102
19. Fuchs EV, Coppock SM, Green H, Cleveland DW (1981) Two distinct classes of keratin genes and their evolutionary significance. Cell 27: 75–84
20. Gould PR, Barter RA, Papadimitriou JM (1979) An ultrastructural, cytochemical and autoradiographic study of the mucous membrane of the human cervical canal with reference to subcolumnar cells. Am J Pathol 95: 1–16
21. Graham S (1984) Epidemiology of retinoids and cancer. J Natl Cancer Inst 73: 1423–1428
22. Hillemanns P, Tannous-Khuri L, Koulos JP, Talmadge DA, Wright TC (1992) Localization of cellular retinoid-binding proteins in human cervical intraepithelial neoplasia and invasive carcinoma. Am J Pathol 141: 973–979
23. Hughes RG, Norval M, Howie SEM (1988) Expression of major histocompatibility class II antigens by Langerhans cells in cervical intraepithelial neoplasia. J Clin Pathol 41: 253
24. Johnson LD (1973) Dysplasia and carcinoma in-situ in pregnancy. In: Norris HJ, Hertig AT, Abell MR (eds) The uterus. International Academy of Pathology Monographs. Baltimore, Williams & Wilkins, pp 382–412
25. Kolstad P, Stafl A (1977) Atlas of colposcopy, 2nd ed. Baltimore, University Park Press
26. Konishi I, Fujii S, Nonogaki H, Nanbu Y, Iwai T, Mori T (1991) Immunohistochemical analysis of estrogen receptors, progesterone receptors, Ki-67 antigen, and human papillomavirus DNA in normal and neoplastic epithelium of the uterine cervix. Cancer 68: 1340–1350
27. Koss LG (1979) Diagnostic cytology and its histopathologic bases, 3rd ed. Philadelphia, J B Lippincott
28. Krantz KE (1973) The anatomy of the human cervix, gross and microscopic. In: Blandau RJ, Moghissi K (eds) The biology of the cervix. Chicago, University of Chicago Press
29. Kupryjánczyk J (1990) Epidermal growth factor receptor ex-

pression in the normal and inflamed cervix uteri: a comparison with estrogen receptor expression. Int J Gynecol Pathol 9: 263–271

30. Kupryjánczyk J, Möller P (1988) Estrogen receptor distribution in the normal and pathologically changed human cervix uteri: an immunohistochemical study with use of monoclonal anti-ER antibody. Int J Gynecol Pathol 7: 75–85

31. Linhartova A (1978) Extent of columnar epithelium on the ectocervix between the ages of 1 and 13 years. Obstet Gynecol 52: 451–456

32. Mangelsdorf DJ, Ong ES, Dyck JA, Evans RM (1990) Nuclear receptor that identifies a novel retinoic acid response pathway. Nature 345: 224–229

33. Maruo T, Yamasaki M, Ladines-Llave CA, Mochizuki M (1992) Immunohistochemical demonstration of elevated expression of epidermal growth factor receptor in the neoplastic changes of cervical squamous epithelium. Cancer 69: 1182–1187

34. Meyer R (1941) The basis of the histological diagnosis of carcinoma with special reference to carcinoma of the cervix and similar lesions. Surg Gynecol Obstet 73: 14

35. Miller CJ, McChesney M, Moore PF (1992) Langerhans cells, microphages and lymphocyte subsets in the cervi and vagina of rhesus macaques. Lab Invest 67:628–634.

36. Mittal K, Pearson J, Demopoulos R (1990) Patterns of mRNA for epidermal growth factor receptor and keratin B-2 in normal cervical epithelium and in cervical intraepithelial neoplasia. Gynecol Oncol 38: 224–229

37. Moll R, Franke WW, Schiller DL, Geiger B, Krepler R (1982) The catalog of human cytokeratins: patterns of expression in normal epithelia, tumors and cultured cells. Cell 31:11–24

38. Moll R, Levy R, Czernobilsky B, Hohlweg-Majert P, et al. (1983) Cytokeratins of normal epithelia and some neoplasms of the female genital tract. Lab Invest 49: P599–610

39. Naftolin F, Stubblefield PG (eds) (1980) Dilatation of the uterine cervix. Connective tissue biology and clinical management. New York, Raven Press

40. Nielsen LN, Hørding U, Daugaard S, Rasmussen LP, Norrild B (1991) Cytokeratin intermediate filament pattern and human papillomavirus type in uterine cervical biopsies with different histological diagnosis. Gynecol Obstet Invest 32: 232–238

41. Nogogaki H, Fujii S, Konishi I, Nanbu Y, Ozaki S, Ishikawa Y, Mori T (1990) Estrogen receptor localization in cervical neoplasia. Cancer 66: 26620

42. Odeblad E (1968) The functional structure of human cervical mucus. Acta Obstet Gynecol Scand 47 (Suppl 1): 57–79

43. Press MF, Nousek-Goebl NA, Bur M, Greene GL (1986) Estrogen receptor localization in the female genital tract. Am J Pathol 123: 280–92

44. Reiffenstuhl G (1964) The lymphatics of the female genital organs. Philadelphia, JB Lippincott

45. Richart RM (1973) Cervical intraepithelial neoplasia. In: Sommers SC (ed) Pathology annual. New York, Appleton-Century-Crofts, pp 301–328

46. Robboy SJ, Taguchi O, Cunha GR (1982) Normal development of the human female reproductive tract and alterations resulting from experimental exposure to diethylstilbesterol. Hum Pathol 13: 190–198

47. Romney SL, Dwyer A, Slagle S, et al (1985) Chemoprevention of cervix cancer; Phase I-II: a feasibility study involving the topical vaginal administration of retinyl acetate gel. Gynecol Oncol 20: 109–119

48. Roncalli M, Sideri M, Giè P, Servida E (1988) Immunophenotypic analysis of the transformation zone of human cervix. Lab Invest 58: 141–149

49. Serra V, Ramirez AA, Lara C, Marzo C, Castells A, Bonilla-Musoles F (1990) Distribution of involucrin in normal and pathological human uterine cervix. Gynecol Oncol 36: 34–42

50. Singer A (1976) The cervical epithelium during pregnancy and the puerperium. In: Jordan JA, Singer A (eds) The Cervix London, WB Sanders, p 105

51. Smedts F, Ramaekers F, Troyanovsky S, et al (1992) Basalcell keratins in cervical reserve cells and a comparison to their expression in cervical intraepithelial neoplasia. Am J Pathol 140: 601–612

51a. Tutsumi K, Sun Q, Yasumoto S (1993) In vitro and in vivo analysis of cellular origin of cervical squamous metaplasia. Am J Pathol 143(4): 1150–1158

52. Vecchia C, Franceschi S, Decarli A, et al (1984) Dietary vitamin A and the risk of invasive cervical cancer. Int J Cancer 34: 319

53. Warhol MJ, Anatonioli DA, Pinkus GS, et al (1992) Immunoperoxidase staining for involucrin: a potential diagnostic aid in cervicovaginal pathology. Hum Pathol 13: 1095

54. Wolbach SB, Howe PR (1932) Epithelial repair in recovery of vitamin A deficiency. An experimental study. J Exp Med 57: 511

55. Wolbach SB, Howe PR (1925) Tissue changes following deprivation of fat-soluble A vitamin. J Exp Med 42: 753–777.

6

Benign Diseases of the Cervix

Thomas C. Wright, M.D., and Alex Ferenczy, M.D.

Inflammatory Diseases

Cervicitis can be divided into two categories, based on whether the etiology of the disorder is noninfectious or infectious. Whatever the etiology, the tissue response of the cervix to injury is limited and reflects the basic mechanisms of inflammation and repair. Two types of morphologic changes, however, that are encountered often in association with a variety of inflammatory diseases deserve specific attention. These are *atypia of repair* and *hyperkeratosis and parakeratosis.*

Atypia of Repair

In cases of severe, acute, long-standing chronic inflammation or infection and with epithelial injury of any kind—true erosion, biopsy, or conization—the squamous and endocervical epithelia undergo reactive changes characterized by epithelial disorganization and nuclear atypia (Fig. 6.1). These changes often are confused, histologically[95] and cytologically,[72] with intraepithelial neoplasia. In reactive atypia, the cytoplasmic membrane is better defined, the nuclei are uniform in shape and size, and the chromatin is aggregated in prominent aggregates or clumps. The epithelium often is infiltrated with migrating inflammatory cells. Mitotic figures are normal and are confined to the proliferating basal and parabasal cell populations. Characteristically, the cells in the upper half of the epithelium are not abnormal, and maturation occurs in an orderly fashion. In the endocervical columnar cells, the reparative morphologic alterations include nuclear en-

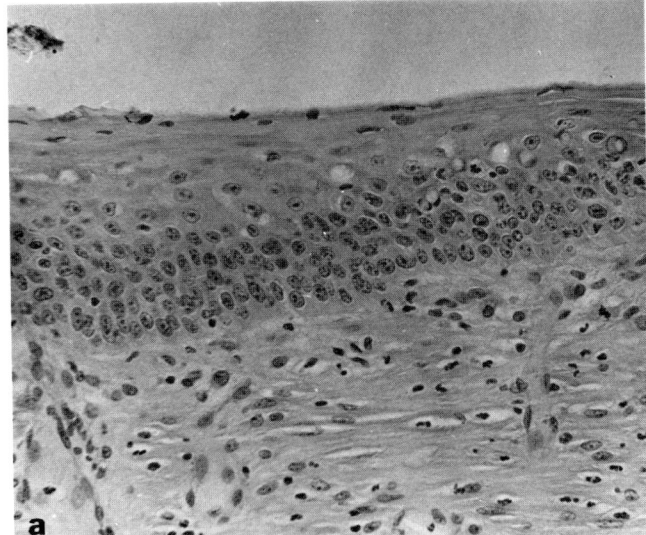

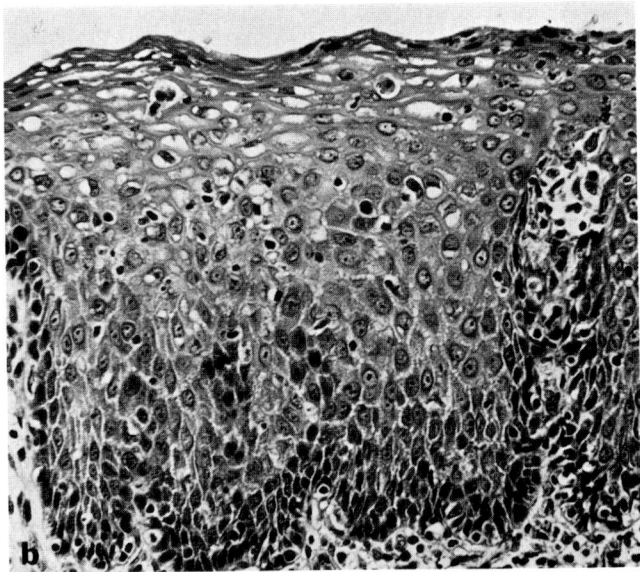

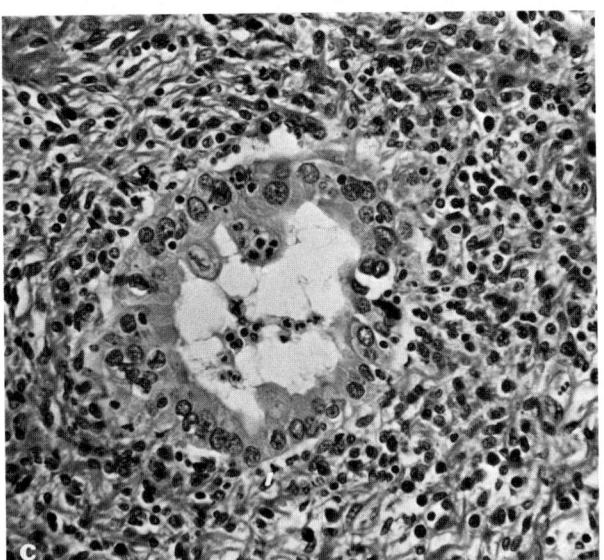

Fig. 6.1. Reparative Atypia. a: Basal cell hyperplasia involving the lower one-third of the squamous epithelium of the cervix. The nuclei contain prominent chromocenters but lack nuclear abnormalities associated with neoplasia. The epithelial cells above the enlarged basal zone display normal maturation. These alterations often are associated with mucosal denudation caused by either trauma or severe inflammation. **b:** Trichomonal cervicitis. The epithelium exhibits intercellular edema, elongation of rete pegs, and poor glycogenization. The lower half is occupied by parabasal-type cells with prominent nucleoli and intercellular bridges. Both the epithelium and the stromal papillae are infiltrated by acute inflammatory cells. **c:** Trichomonal cervicitis. Endocervical epithelium with nuclear enlargement, mitosis, microabscesses, and inconspicuous intracellular mucus. Note the diffuse distribution of nuclear chromatin, the cytoplasmic eosinophilia, and the absence of mitoses, features distinguishing endocervical atypia of inflammation from in situ adenocarcinoma of the cervix.

largement and hyperchromasia with irregularity of nuclear size and shape and smudgy chromatin. There also is cytoplasmic eosinophilia and loss of mucinous droplets (Fig. 6.1). Although this type of glandular epithelium appears highly atypical, the changes are focal, alternating with normal mucinous columnar cells, and are confined to areas with inflammation or mucosal injury. In addition, the deep cytoplasmic eosinophilia (which is presumably caused by an increase in ribosomes and mitochondria) and the absence of abnormal mitoses are features that distinguish the inflammatory lesions from an in situ adenocarcinoma of the endocervix. The atypical cellular changes accompany the increased DNA and RNA synthesis that occurs during the repair of the damaged or inflamed epithelium.

Hyperkeratosis and Parakeratosis

Hyperkeratosis and parakeratosis can be detected cytologically in up to 8% of all women undergoing routine Pap smear screening.[65] Both hyperkeratosis and parakeratosis have the gross appearance of a thickened, white epithelium and can be either focal or diffuse. When diffuse, the entire portio is covered by a thickened, white, and wrinkled epithelial membrane. When focal, a slightly raised white plaque is present. The etiologic and histogenic mechanisms of cervical hyperkeratosis are poorly understood. Most patients with diffuse hyperkeratosis have prolapsed uteri. Focal areas of hyperkeratosis sometimes can be associated with a local chronic irritation.

Microscopically, the whitish plaque corresponds to the presence of a thick keratin layer (hyperkeratosis) that may or may not contain pyknotic nuclei (parakeratosis) (Figs. 6.2, 6.3). The epithelium often is acanthotic and has a well-developed granular layer, prominent intercellular bridges, and elongated rete pegs. Characteristically, the epithelial cells contain sparse glycogen, but cytological atypicality is absent. The reactive nature of hyperkeratosis and parakeratosis is evidenced by a consistent association with epithelial hyperplasia and chronic inflammation.

Although there is neither morphologic nor clinical evidence that hyperkeratosis or parakeratosis represent precursor lesions to cervical neoplasia, both hyperkeratosis and parakeratosis can occur in association with squamous intraepithelial lesion (SIL) (CIN) and invasive cervical cancer. Therefore, there is controversy surrounding the need for further evaluation of women in whom hyperkeratosis or parakeratosis is detected on an otherwise negative Pap smear (see Chapter 25, Cytopathology). Because of the association of hyperkeratosis and parakeratosis with SIL (CIN) and cervical cancer, some experts suggest that all women with Pap smears demonstrating these findings need colposcopy.[25,47] Recently, however, three studies have reported that less than 4% of women with hyperkeratosis or parakeratosis without nuclear atypia on an otherwise negative Pap smear had SIL (CIN) and that in all instances the SIL was low-grade. This suggests that routine

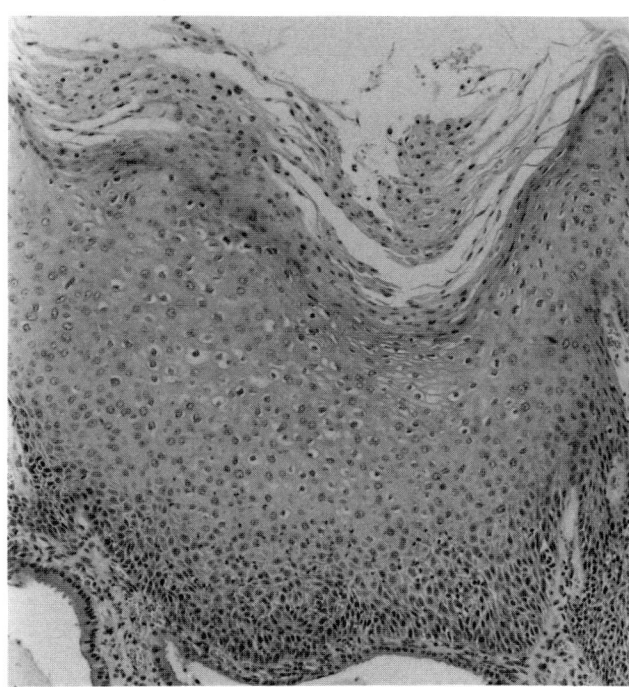

FIG. 6.3. Parakeratosis of the cervix. Parakeratosis is the retention of pyknotic nuclei in the superficial cell layer. Parakeratosis is frequently accompanied by hyperkeratosis and both are present in this patient with low-grade SIL (CIN 1).

colposcopic evaluation is unnecessary in such women.[7,17,65] It should be emphasized, however, that since hyperkeratosis occasionally may overlie invasive carcinomas, all grossly visible white plaques on the portio vaginalis or vaginal epithelium should be biopsied.

Noninfectious Cervicitis

Noninfectious cervicitis is, for the most part, chemical or mechanical in nature, and the inflammatory response is nonspecific. Common causes include chemical irritation secondary to douching or local trauma produced by foreign bodies, including tampons, diaphragms, pessaries, and intrauterine contraceptive devices. Surgical instrumentation and therapeutic intervention are common iatrogenic causes of cervical tissue injury and inflammation. Acute cervicitis is characterized by stromal edema, vascular congestion, and neutrophilic infiltration of the stroma and epithelium. Clinically, the cervix appears swollen, erythematous, and friable, and there may be an associated purulent endocervical discharge. Prolonged or severe acute inflammation eventually leads to degenerative changes in the epithelial surface, loss of endocervical secretory activity, and ulceration.

In chronic cervicitis, round cells, including lymphocytes, plasma cells, and histiocytes, predominate in the inflammatory infiltrate and are associated with varying amounts

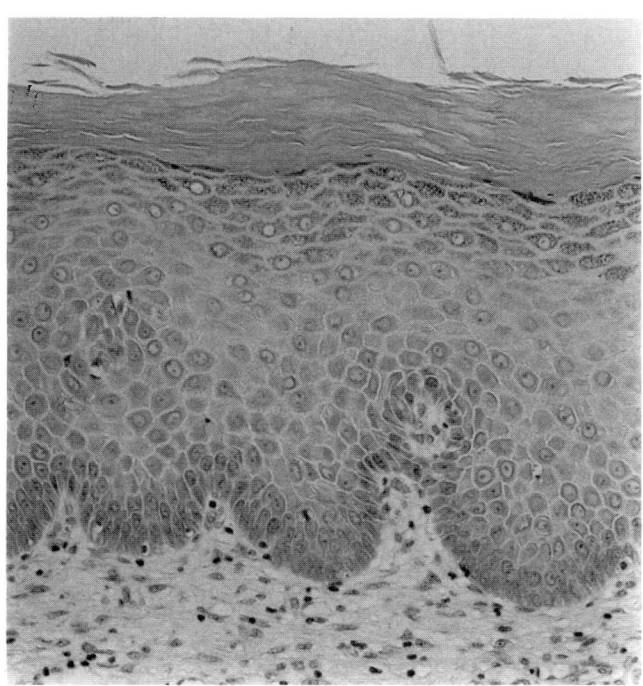

FIG. 6.2. Hyperkeratosis of the cervix. Hyperkeratosis is manifested by a superficial layer of anucleated, keratinized squamous cells, which frequently is accompanied by a thickened granular layer.

of granulation tissue and stromal fibrosis. On gross and colposcopic examination, the cervical mucosa is hyperemic because of an increased number of terminal vessels and may contain true epithelial erosions (ulcerations) or lacerations. The cervical stroma contains a normal, physiologic population of inflammatory cells, and the diagnosis of chronic cervicitis should be reserved for cases in which there is definite clinical and histological evidence of a significant chronic inflammatory process. Otherwise, a histological diagnosis based on the presence of scattered lymphocytes has no clinical significance and is meaningless. Occasionally, lymphoid follicles with germinal centers are found beneath the epithelium in patients with noninfectious cervicitis (Fig. 6.4). The presence of lymphoid follicles beneath the cervical epithelium is frequently referred to as *follicular cervicitis*. In some instances, the lymphoid inflammatory reactions may produce lymphoma-like lesions, raising the question of lymphoma (see below).[131]

Infectious Cervicitis

Table 6.1 summarizes some of the important or pathologically significant etiologic organisms of infectious cervicitis.

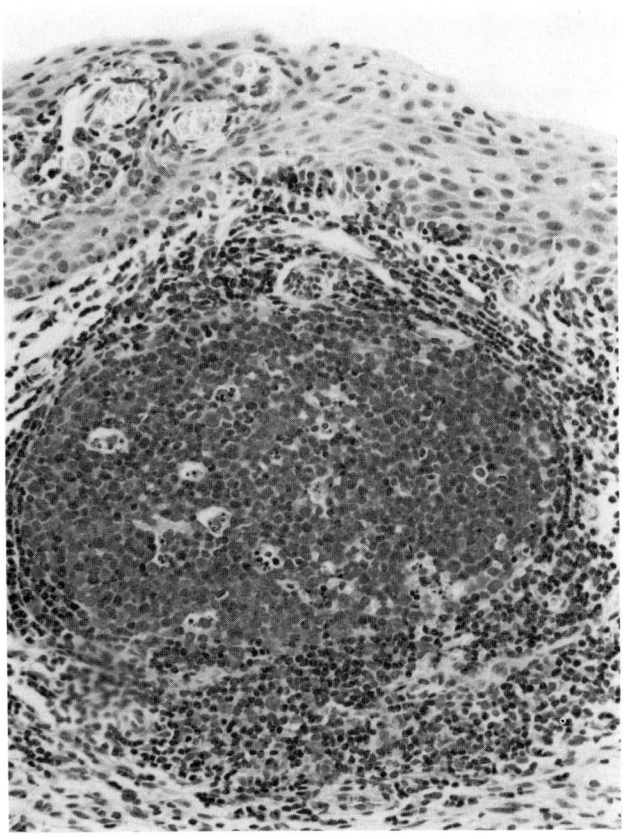

FIG. 6.4. Chronic cervicitis. A subepithelial lymphoid follicle with a prominent germinal center is present. When lymphoid follicles are numerous, the condition is referred to as *follicular cervicitis*.

Table 6.1. Microorganisms causing infectious cervicitis

Bacteria, chlamydia, mycobacteria, polymicrobial, endogenous vaginal aerobes and anerobes
Chlamydia trachomatis
Neisseria gonorrhoeae
Mycoplasma hominis
Group B *Streptococcus*
Ureaplasma ureolyticum
Gardnerella vaginalis
Actinomyces israelii
Mycobacterium tuberculosis
Treponema pallidum
Viruses
Herpes simplex virus
Human papillomavirus
Fungi
Candida
Aspergillus
Protozoa and parasites
Trichomonas vaginalis
Ameba
Schistosomes

It is apparent from this listing that infectious cervicitis is of major epidemiologic importance because of its epidemic proportion and because of its central role in the pathogenesis of sexually transmitted diseases.[61,128] In our current understanding of the pathogenesis of pelvic inflammatory disease, infectious cervicitis is the initial event; it also is the primary infectious focus in related syndromes, such as postpartum and postabortal endometritis. Spontaneous abortion, premature delivery, chorioamnionitis, stillbirth, and neonatal pneumonia and septicemia have been directly related to concurrent bacterial infection of the cervix. Even when asymptomatic, infectious cervicitis can be clinically important since it can act as a source for sexual transmission to male partners as well as ascending infection in the woman and vertical transmission during pregnancy.[109]

Infectious cervicitis can affect either the endocervical-type columnar epithelium producing *endocervicitis* (mucopurulent cervicitis) or affect the stratified squamous epithelium of the exocervix producing *exocervicitis*.[61] The infectious agents that cause endo- and exocervicitis tend to differ, although some agents can cause both. When discussing infectious cervicitis, it is important that clear criteria be used to define the disease and to distinguish clinically apparent disease from asymptomatic disease. Clinically apparent endocervicitis (mucopurulent cervicitis) is defined principally by the presence of a yellow endocervical discharge containing many polymorpholeukocytes, erythema, and friability of the cervical ectropion.[61] Exocervicitis is manifested by either ulcerations and necrosis or the diffuse punctated erythema (colpitis macularis) associated with *Trichomonas vaginalis* infections.

Bacterial and Chlamydial Cervicitis

Bacterial and chlamydial infections of the cervix are the most common cause of infectious cervicitis and are associated with a nonspecific inflammatory response. The columnar epithelium of the endocervix is much more susceptible to bacterial and chlamydial infections than is the surrounding squamous epithelium, and endocervicitis is characteristic. Consequently, patients with a large columnar ectropion, as seen in young women or during pregnancy, are at higher risk for bacterial and chlamydial infections and for developing acute endocervicitis.[60,61,128] Although some degree of cervical involvement commonly occurs in women with bacterial vaginosis, the cervical involvement is rarely important clinically. The infectious agents that most commonly cause clinically significant mucopurulent cervicitis are *Chlamydia trachomatis* and *Neisseria gonorrhoeae*. Infection with either of these two agents requires no predisposing factors and is primarily dependent on exposure and size of the inoculum.[61,128] Although chlamydial and bacterial infections of the cervix are infrequent in older postmenopausal women and are unusual before menarche, both *N. gonorrhoea* and *C. trachomatis* are reported occasionally in children and may affect the atrophic vaginal epithelium as well as the cervix, producing cervicovaginitis.[59] Recent epidemiologic data indicate that *C. trachomatis* infection is the most common sexually transmitted disease in the Western world, with a prevalence far exceeding that of gonorrhea.[26,101,113,124] The prevalence of *C. trachomatis* cervical infection ranges from 3% to 5% of asymptomatic women and up to 40% of women tending sexually transmitted disease (STD) clinics.

In pregnant women and women under 20 years of age, isolation rates for *C. trachomatis* from cervices of asymptomatic patients are as high as 10–22%.[85,103,113] Slightly more than one-third of women with cervical chlamydial infections are symptomatic.[59] Symptomatic women with acute mucopurulent cervicitis, defined by the presence of a visible, yellow-green, endocervical exudate or by the presence of ≥10 neutrophils per (1000×) field in a smear of endocervical mucus have culture-positive *C. trachomatis* infection in 58% of cases.[13] Generalized lower genital tract infection is common, often involving the urethra (so-called urethral syndrome) and the rectum.[61] The high risk of exposure of these patients to multiple STDs is highlighted by the frequent finding of other concurrent bacterial infections, principally gonorrhea, as well as cervicitis of viral etiology.[61,70,113]

Inflammatory and reactive colposcopic patterns in women with *C. trachomatis* cervicitis include hypertrophic cervical ectropion and an atypical transformation zone epithelium that may be confused colposcopically with a low-grade SIL.[58,85,87] Histologically, follicular cervicitis is frequently found in patients with *C. trachomatis* infection and *C. trachomatis* is now presumed to be a major cause of this condition (Fig. 6.4).[33,58,85,87] *C. trachomatis* cervicitis also has been associated with a dense, diffuse inflammatory exudate as well as reactive squamous and endocervical atypia.[33,70,109] Intracytoplasmic inclusions in endocervical columnar or metaplastic cells may be identified in some cases. Immunohistochemical studies have demonstrated that these inclusions are composed of aggregated chamydial organisms at different stages of development (Fig. 6.5).[33,70] However, it should be stressed that the identifica-

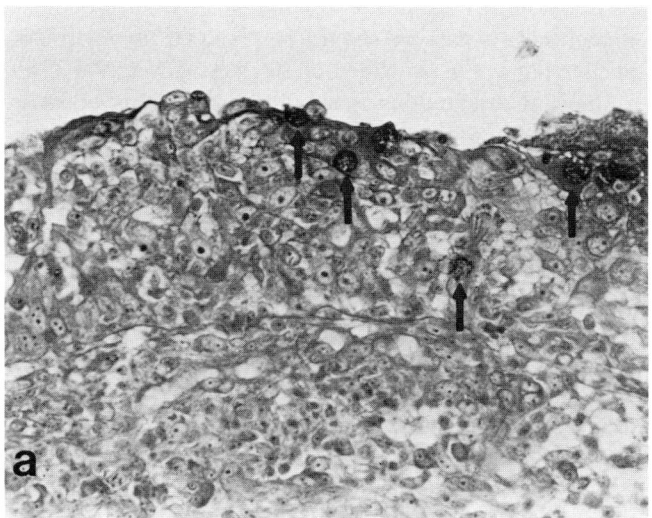 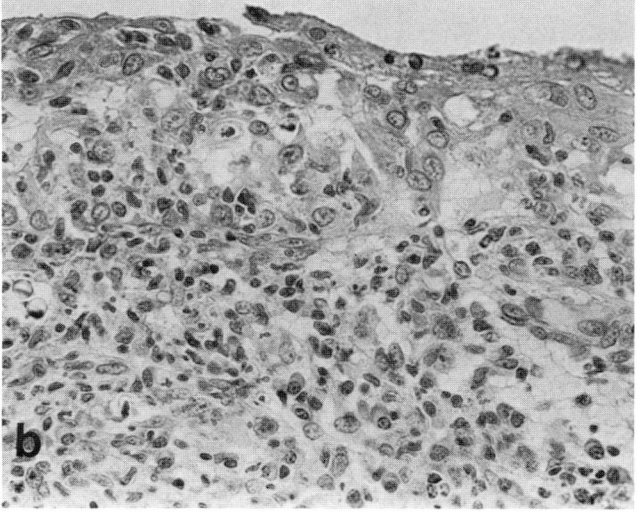

Fig. 6.5. Chlamydial cervicitis. a: Immunoperoxidase staining for chlamydial antigens. Several rounded cytoplasmic inclusions are seen. **b:** The epithelium and stroma are infiltrated by acute and chronic inflammatory cells, partially obscuring the epithelial–stromal junction. The metaplastic epithelium displays reactive atypia. Scattered cytoplasmic vacuoles are present, but the finding is not specific for the definitive diagnosis of chlamydia infection. (Courtesy of C. P. Crum, M. D., Boston, MA.)

tion of these cytoplasmic epithelial inclusions in cervical Papanicolaou smears and biopsies is too insensitive and nonspecific to be of use diagnostically.[50,70,71,92,109,129]

C. trachomatis cervicitis is diagnosed most accurately by culture,[102] by direct immunofluorescence staining of smears using monoclonal antibodies, or by enzyme-linked immunosorbent assay (ELISA) on cervical swabs. Since endometritis and salpingitis (see Chapter 10, Benign Diseases of the Endometrium, and Chapter 14, Diseases of the Fallopian Tube) complicate C. trachomatis cervicitis in approximately 40% and 11% of cases, respectively, and often are subclinical, the patient with C. trachomatis cervicitis and her sexual partner(s) should be treated.[52,86,113] Postinfectious sequelae include pelvic inflammatory disease, tubal infertility, and neonatal pneumonia. Symptomatic infection in the male is manifested more commonly as acute urethritis, but the infection may be asymptomatic.

Actinomycosis

Actinomycosis infection of the female genital organs, including the cervix, is caused by *Actinomyces israelii*.[12,43,96] It results from surgical instrumentation, clinical abortion, intrauterine contraceptive devices (see Chapter 10, Benign Diseases of the Endometrium, and Chapter 14, Diseases of the Fallopian Tube), or direct extension from parametrial and appendiceal lesions or from the anus. More than 300 cases of genital actinomycosis are reported in the literature.[12,43,96] The diagnosis is made by demonstrating the organism (classified between true bacteria and complete fungi) in the center of large abscesses, occasionally with granuloma formation. The lesions appear yellow and granular to the naked eye, hence the term *sulfur granules*. They are composed of branching, gram-positive filaments with peripheral palisading clubs. Chronic infection of the cervix by *Actinomyces* may produce significant fibrosis and scarring.[12,128]

Tuberculosis

Tuberculosis of the cervix is almost invariably secondary to tuberculous salpingitis and endometritis and is typically associated with pulmonary tuberculosis (see Chapter 10, Benign Diseases of the Endometrium and Chapter 14, Diseases of the Fallopian Tube).[36,104] The prevalence of cervical tuberculosis in a population with genital tuberculosis varies between 2% and 60% with a prevalence of 5% in the United States.[104] Macroscopically, the cervix may appear normal, inflamed, or simulates invasive carcinoma. Histologically, tuberculous infection of the cervix is recognized by the presence of multiple granulomas or tubercles characterized by central caseous necrosis, epithelioid histiocytes, and multinucleated Langerhans giant cells. The periphery of the tubercle contains a heavy lymphoplasmocytic infiltrate (Fig. 6.6). Tuberculous cervicitis may often

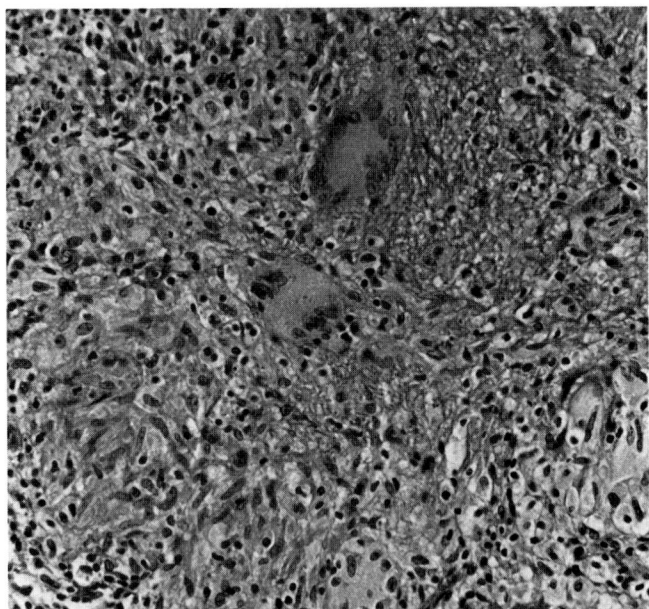

FIG. 6.6. Tuberculous cervicitis. Typical granuloma with palisading epithelial cells, multinucleated Langerhans giant cells, and central caseous necrosis. Acid-fast stain for *Mycobacterium tuberculosis* was positive.

appear as a noncaseating, granulomatous lesion. Since caseating, nontuberculous granulomas due to lymphogranuloma venereum or sarcoidosis may be encountered in the cervix, the unequivocal diagnosis of tuberculous cervicitis requires demonstration of acid-fast *Myobacterium tuberculosis,* a straight, rod-shaped bacillus, by Ziehl-Neelsen–stained sections, by culture, or by animal inoculation of cervical tissue.[40] Because culture or animal inoculation yields far better results than staining of tissue sections, unfixed biopsy material should be obtained for microbiologic testing whenever tuberculosis is suspected. The most common granulomatous lesions to be distinguished from tuberculous cervicitis include foreign body giant cell granulomas secondary to sutures, crystals, or cotton, lymphogranuloma venereum, schistosomiasis, and sarcoidosis. Cervical granuloma occasionally may develop postoperatively as a reaction to local tissue necrosis.[36]

Other Granulomatous Infections

Certain venereally transmitted diseases commonly encountered in the vulva also may involve the cervix (see Chapter 2, Benign Diseases of the Vulva). These include syphilis, either as the primary chancre, secondary mucous patches, or tertiary gumma,[30,36,120] lymphogranuloma venereum,[36] granuloma inguinale,[6,36] and chancroid.[43] All these conditions may resemble carcinoma clinically. This is particularly a problem with granuloma inguinale, which is endemic in areas of Africa that have high prevalences of invasive cervical cancer. Up to 50% of women with granuloma inguinale may be misdiagnosed initially as having carcinoma of the cervix; many of these women are thought to have high-stage tumors because of spread of the infection to the parametrial tissue.[62] In addition to characteristic morphologic features, specific bacteriologic and immunologic techniques are available for identifying each of these diseases.

Viral Diseases

In contrast to bacterial infections of the cervix, the prevalent agents of viral cervicitis—human papillomavirus (HPV) and herpes simplex virus (HSV)—have a predilection for the squamous epithelium and produce characteristic morphologic changes. Cytomegalovirus, although often isolated from cervical secretions, is not typically associated with cervicitis, and its role in cervical infection is poorly understood.[61,90]

Herpes Virus

Although the precise prevalence of cervical HSV infection (herpes genitalis) is not known, it is far greater than generally recognized.[4,5] HSV can be isolated from the genital tract in 0.25–5% of women attending STD clinics.[29,73] However, up to 70% of HSV-2 infections appear to be asymptomatic.[56] This results in wide discrepancies between the prevalence of serologic evidence of infection and clinically recognized infections. HSV-2 antibodies are detected in approximately 80–90% of female prostitutes, 50% of women attending STD clinics, and about 30% of obstetric patients in the United States.[29,56,57] In the United States, serologic evidence of HSV-2 infection is much greater in blacks than in whites, but symptomatic infections are more common in whites. The prevalence of serum antibodies to HSV-2 is strongly associated with socioeconomic status and increases with age. The prevalence of genital HSV infections increased markedly between the 1960s and 1980s in the United States, Europe, Australia, and parts of Africa.[56,57] The Centers for Disease Control estimated that there were 295,000 patient visits for consultation for genital herpes infections in the United States during 1981.[27] Genital herpesvirus infections are caused chiefly by HSV-2. Only 5–15% of primary genital HSV outbreaks are caused by HSV-1.[8]

Herpes simplex viruses types 1 and 2 have several common features, including architecture, size, envelope, mode of multiplication, and double-stranded DNA genetic content. However, HSV-1 is chiefly found in the oropharyngeal region (herpes buccalis) and has different biologic properties and a different distribution than does HSV-2 virus.[80] HSV-2 is a DNA-containing virus that measures 150 nm in diameter.[123] The virions are surrounded by a hexagonal protein capsid and the capsid, in turn, is enveloped by an inner glycoprotein-rich and outer lipid-rich membrane. Viral particles are thought to replicate within the host cell nuclei, where they synthesize viral proteins necessary for replication of viral DNA.[123] HSV-2 is acquired through sexual contact, and most female patients are teenagers or are unmarried. Primary herpetic infections produce symptoms within 3–7 days after exposure. When the vulva is involved, symptoms include severe vulvar pain, tenderness, painful urination, and profuse watery vaginal discharge. The symptoms of recurrent herpes genitalis are comparatively less severe than those experienced during the primary infection. The disease is characterized by the development of multiple, painful vesicles involving the vulva, perineum, vagina, and cervix that rapidly evolve into shallow, painful ulcerations.[29,56,57] Cervical involvement can be detected in 90% of women with primary genital HSV-2 infections. In contrast, only 12–20% of women with recurrent genital herpetic lesions involving the external genitalia have cervical involvement.[29,56,57] In most women with cervical involvement, the cervical lesions are readily observable on the cervix and, occasionally, the ulceronecrotic process is so extensive that a fungating, necrotic mass appears on the cervical portio, which can be mistaken for carcinoma.[115] Shedding of herpesvirus from asymptomatic, clinically unapparent cervical lesions occurs in 4–10% of infected women and serves as a hidden reservoir for propagation of infection.[5]

Herpesvirus infection may be diagnosed by cervical cultures, neutralizing antibodies serology, and Papanicolaou smears. In the Papanicolaou smear, large multinucleated cells with the characteristic intranuclear ground-glass viral inclusions are observed. Occasionally, during the vesicular phase, a biopsy may reveal the presence of suprabasal intraepidermal vesicles filled with serum, degenerated epidermal cells, and multinucleated giant cells, some containing eosinophilic, intranuclear inclusions surrounded by a clear halo (Fig. 6.7). Diagnostic yield by isolation and cytology is most efficient within 2–3 days after the onset of symptoms.[29,56,57]

Herpes genitalis has two important clinical implications. First, it may result in spontaneous abortion, fetal morbidity, and fetal mortality.[28] Second, some studies have suggested that there are associations between HSV infections of the female genital tract and the genesis of cervical carcinoma (see Chapter 7, Precancerous Lesions of the Cervix).

Herpes-like Lesions

Vesicular and bullous lesions of the cervical squamous mucous membrane, other than herpetic cervicitis, have been reported.[11] Pemphigus vulgaris of the cervix is a rather common finding in women with generalized disease.[67] Microscopically there are multiple intraepithelial bullae in a suprabasal location containing the characteristic acantholytic Tzanck cells.

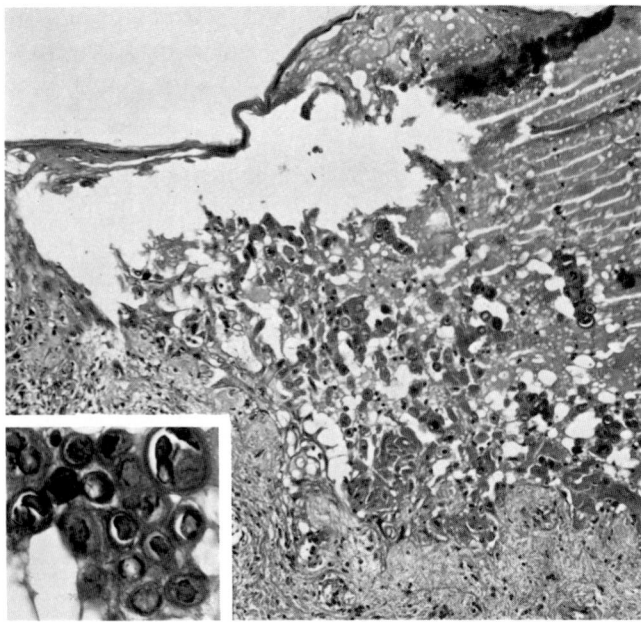

FIG. 6.7. Herpetic cervicitis. Suprabasal herpetic vesicle in squamous epithelium of the portio. *Inset:* High-power view of acantholytic intravesicular epithelial cells with ground-glass intranuclear viral inclusions.

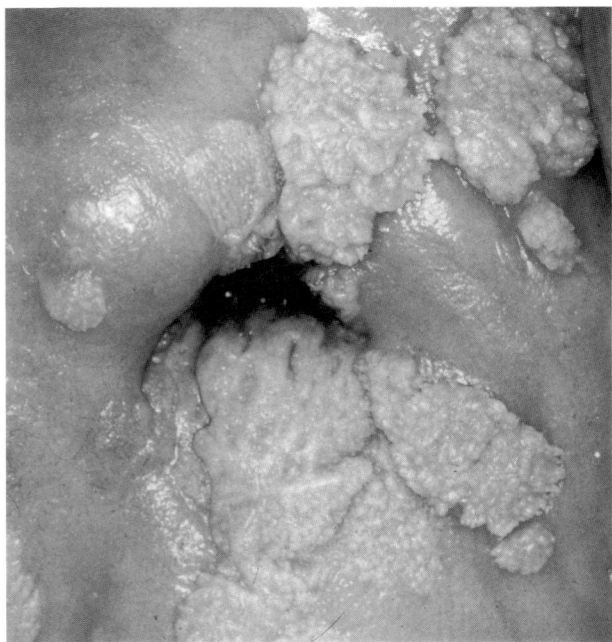

FIG. 6.8. Exophytic condylomata acuminata. The lesions are multifocal and form raised white papillary projections.

Isolated arteritis of the cervix, histologically identical but clinically unrelated to polyarteritis nodosa, rarely may be encountered.[31] The etiology of this condition is unknown. It may be asymptomatic or may be associated with bleeding and may clinically resemble cancer.[75]

Human Papillomavirus

Human papillomavirus (HPV) is a double-stranded DNA tumor virus that is a member of the family Papovaviridae. More than 22 types of HPV can infect the lower anogenital tract and the resulting infections can produce a variety of gross and histological lesions (see Chapter 7, Precancerous Lesions of the Cervix). Exophytic condyloma acuminata are one of the common manifestations of HPV infection of the lower anogential tract and usually are caused by HPV types 6 and 11.[19,32,45] When florid condylomas of the vulva are identified, multicentric disease can occur and internal vaginal or cervical exophytic condylomas occasionally can be identified.[15,53,108] Exophytic condylomas of the cervix are commonly multifocal and may involve the mature squamous epithelium of the native cervical portio as well as the immature squamous epithelium of the transformation zone, including metaplastic squamous epithelium replacing endocervical glands. Extension into the endocervical canal may occur. Grossly and colposcopically, condyloma acuminata appear white, and the degree of whiteness depends largely on the thickness of associated surface hyperkeratosis (Fig 6.8). Other configurations of cervical ex-

ophytic condylomas include myriads of minute, maculopapular, only slightly raised condylomas involving the vagina and the cervix.

Microscopically, the histological features of exophytic cervical condyloma acuminata include architectural alterations such as papillomatosis, acanthosis, parakeratosis, and hyperkeratosis as well as cytological alterations including koilocytosis (manifested by perinuclear cytoplasmic cavitation), nuclear enlargement and atypia. Multinucleation also is frequently observed (Fig 6.9) (see Chapter 2, Benign Diseases of the Vulva, and Chapter 7, Precancerous Lesions of the Cervix).

The natural history of exophytic cervical condyloma acuminata is one of spontaneous regression, good response to conservative therapy, unpredictable recurrence, and sometimes persistence. Lesion regression or apparent cure after biopsy occurs in 20–65% of patients.[46,77–79] The natural history of genital condylomas in general may be modified by host factors, notably immunosuppression and steroid hormone levels.[93] Recurrence of condylomas during early and mid-trimester pregnancy is reported commonly, with the lesions increasing in size and multifocality until term. After delivery, spontaneous regression of the condylomas is the rule. There is increasing concern about genital HPV infection during pregnancy because of the possibility of vertical transmission of infection to the fetus and neonate. There are anecdotal reports of infants born with genital condylomas or developing them in the immediate postnatal period.[79] Of even greater concern is the risk of

taining white flakes, often accompanied by vulvar pruritus. Aspergillus infection of the cervix is reported uncommonly and is prevalent only in the immunosuppressed host.[129]

Protozoal and Parasitic Diseases

Cervical infestation by *T. vaginalis* is frequent and associated most often with concurrent trichomonal vaginitis. A foamy, yellow-green vaginal discharge typically is described. Acute trichomonal cervicitis may provoke an intense inflammatory response with prominent reparative atypia in exfoliated squamous and endocervical cells, with corresponding gross and colposcopic abnormalities.[72] Diagnosis usually is made by a wet mount or by identification of the organism on Papanicolaou smear (see Chapter 4, Diseases of the Vagina).

Rare instances of parasitic infestations, such as echinococcosis or hydatid cysts and ulceronecrotic amebiasis, have been encountered in the cervix (Fig 6.10).[24,74] In contrast, schistosomiasis (bilharziasis) of the cervix, gener-

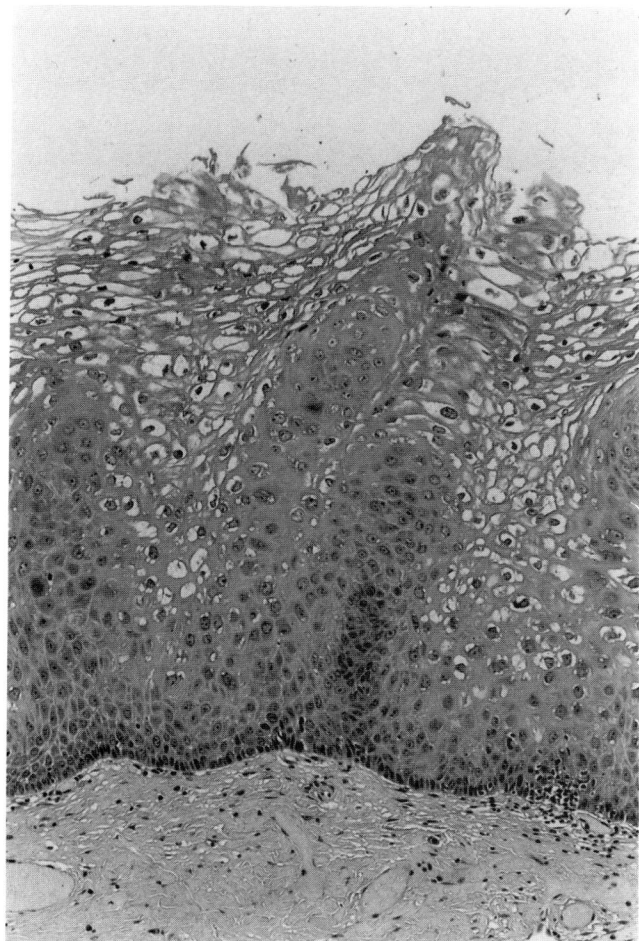

Fig. 6.9. Exophytic condyloma acuminatum. The classic histological features of condyloma acuminatum are papillomatosis with acanthosis, parakeratosis, hyperkeratosis, as well as cytological alterations including multinucleation, koilocytosis, and nuclear atypia.

development of laryngeal papillomatosis because of the morbidity and mortality associated with this disease.[94,116] Although correlated with similar genital HPV types and linked causally to infection in the mother, the factors requisite for the development of laryngeal papillomatosis are not fully understood, and clinically apparent disease occurs in only a relatively small number of children at risk for exposure. Intrauterine infection of the fetus also is possible and there is no clear-cut evidence that delivery via cesarean section reduces the risk of developing laryngeal papillomatosis.[89]

Fungal Diseases

Cervical fungal infection by *Candida albicans* usually occurs as part of a generalized lower genital tract infection involving the vagina and vulva. Alkalinization of vaginal pH, antibiotic therapy, and poorly controlled diabetes mellitus all favor fungal overgrowth.[129] Typically, a *Candida* infection is associated with a viscous vaginal discharge con-

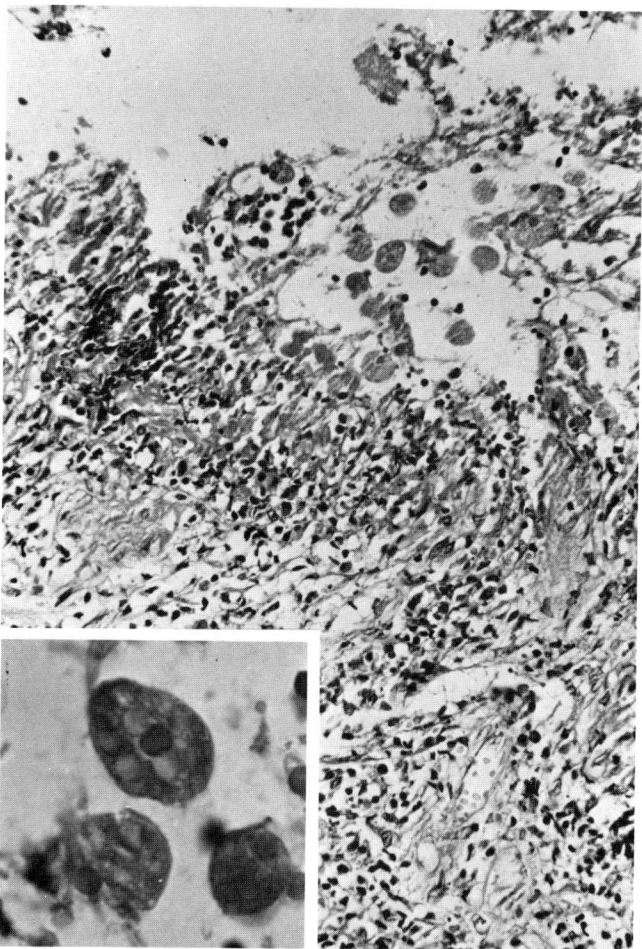

Fig. 6.10. Ulceronecrotic amebiasis of cervix. Numerous amebae are present in the superficial exudate. *Inset:* Detail of *Entamoeba histolytica* with vacuolated cytoplasm.

ally caused by *Schistosoma mansoni,* is very common in Africa (Egypt), South America, Puerto Rico, and several Asian countries.[9,37,105] Many cases of cervical schistosomiasis are associated with urinary schistosomiasis and sterility. The latter condition is presumably related to increased Schistosoma-stimulated antispermatozoal antibodies.[37] Microscopically, noncaseating granulomas (pseudotubercles) with ova surrounded by multinucleated giant cells are seen and the ova often are calcified (Fig. 6.11). *S. mansoni* has a long lateral spine, whereas *S. haematobium* has a short spine extending from one of its poles. Cervical schistosomiasis may be associated with extensive pseudoepitheliomatous hyperplasia of the cervical squamous epithelium, masquerading both clinically and histologically as carcinoma. Chronic, untreated infection has been implicated in the genesis of cervical carcinoma in populations in which schistosomiasis is prevalent.[105]

Cervicovaginitis Emphysematosa

This unusual disease is characterized by multiple, bluegray, subepithelial cysts of the portio vaginalis and vagina (see Chapter 4, Diseases of the Vagina).[49,125] The cause of this condition is unknown, but it often is associated with trichomoniasis.[49,125] Gas-forming bacteria have never been identified. The cysts are dilated connective tissue spaces without lining epithelium that contain air and carbon dioxide. Some of the cysts are surrounded by multinucleated foreign body giant cells, and often the subepithelial veins and lymphatics are dilated. The disappearance of the disease after eradication of trichomoniasis and the experimental production of gas by *T. vaginalis* in subcutaneous tissue of guinea pigs suggest an etiologic relationship.[81]

Benign Tumors

Endocervical Polyps

Endocervical polyps constitute the most common new growths of the uterine cervix.[1,36] Cervical polyps are focal, hyperplastic protrusions of endocervical folds, including the epithelium and substantia propria. Cervical polyps are found most often during the fourth to sixth decades and in multigravidas.[1] They may present with profuse leukorrhea caused by hypersecretion of mucus from inflamed endocervical epithelium or abnormal bleeding from ulceration of the surface epithelium.[1] Clinically, cervical polyps are rounded or elongated, with a smooth or lobulated surface that often is reddened because of increased vascularity. Most polyps are single and measure from a few millimeters to 2–3 cm. In rare instances they may reach gigantic dimensions, protruding beyond the introitus and resembling carcinoma.[76] Many different cervical lesions can have a polypoid gross appearance (Table 6.2). The correct diagnosis is based on microscopic examination and therefore all polypoid cervical lesions should be microscopically evaluated. Microscopically, cervical polyps display a variety of patterns that vary according to the preponderance of one or another of the tissue components (Table 6.3). The most

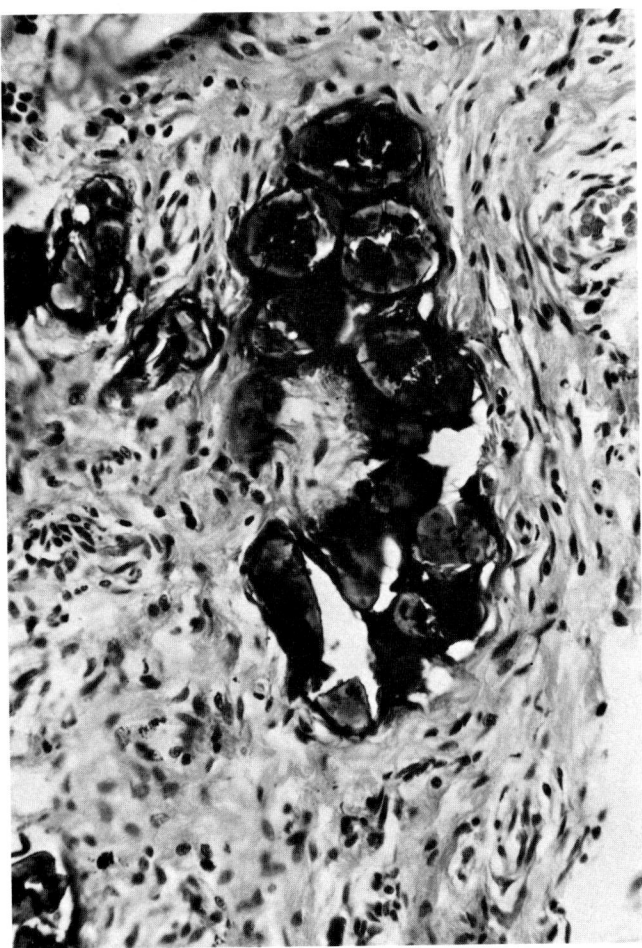

Fig. **6.11. Cervical schistosomiasis.** Note calcified *Schistosoma haematobiium* ova.

Table **6.2.** Differential clinical diagnosis of polypoid lesions of the cervix

Polyp
Microglandular endocervical hyperplasia
Decidua
Granulation tissue
Leiomyoma
Adenomyoma
Fibroadenoma
Squamous papilloma
Condyloma acuminatum
Papillary adenofibroma
Squamous cell carcinoma
Adenocarcinoma
Sarcoma, primary or secondary

Table 6.3. Types of cervical polyps

Endocervical mucosal
Fibrous
Vascular
Mixed endocervical–endometrial
Mesodermal stromal

common type is the endocervical mucosal polyp. It is composed of mucinous epithelium that lines crypts, with or without cystic changes (Fig. 6.12). Occasionally, they may be mainly fibrous, representing an overgrowth of the connective tissue stroma of the portio. In other cases blood vessels predominate and the lesion is called a *vascular polyp.* Squamous metaplasia involving the surface or glandular epithelium of polyps frequently is observed. The supporting connective tissue of polyps is generally loose, with centrally placed feeding vessels, and is almost always infiltrated by a chronic inflammatory infiltrate. Occasion-

ally, such infiltration may be so extensive as to be the principal tissue constituent of the polyp. In these cases, polypoid granulation tissue devoid of surface epithelium is observed. Polyps originating in the isthmus often have an admixutre of endocervical-and endometrial-type epithelial components and are referred to as *mixed polyps* (Fig. 6.13).

Carcinoma, either in situ or invasive (adeno- or squamous), arising in cervical polyps is extremely rare, with a prevalence of 0.2–0.4%.[1] Endocervical polyps with adenocarcinomatous changes must be differentiated from polypoid adenocarcinoma of the endocervix and from endocervical polyps that are involved secondarily by adjacent adenocarcinoma (Fig. 6.14). The most useful criterion for differentiating between the two is to determine whether or not the base of the pedicle of the polyp is involved by carcinoma. The base of a polyp that harbors a primary tumor is free of disease, and the carcinoma usually has a focal distribution within an otherwise benign polyp. In a polypoid carcinoma, the entire mass is malignant, including its base and neigh-

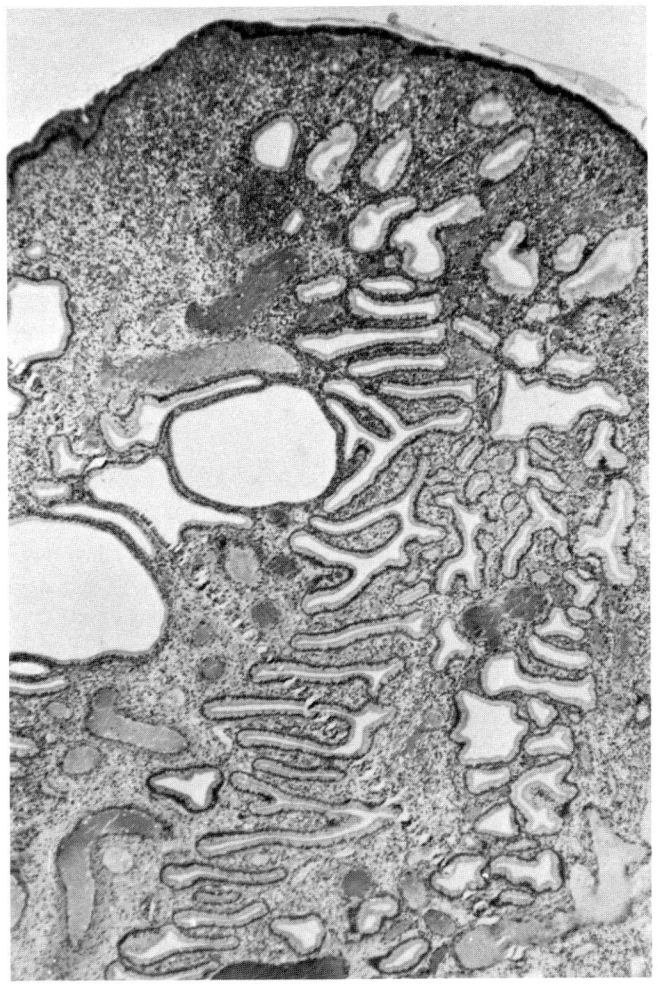

FIG. 6.12. Endocervical polyp. This is the most common histological type of endocervical polyp. Endocervical-type, tall columnar, mucinous epithelium covers the surface and crypts.

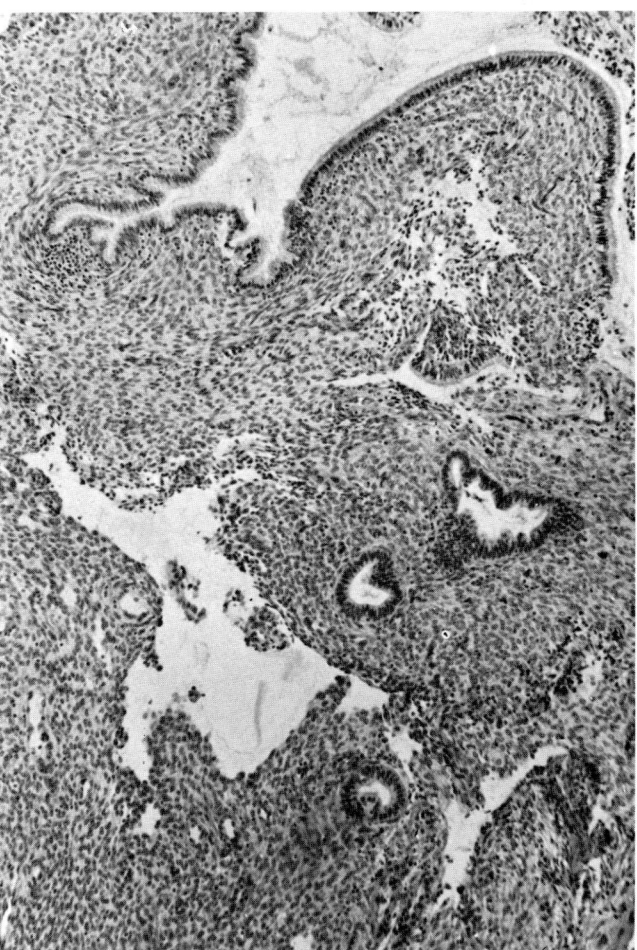

FIG. 6.13. Mixed endocervical–endometrial polyp. This polyp developed from the uterine isthmus. There is endometrial stroma with endometrial glands admixed with mucinous endocervical epithelium (*top*).

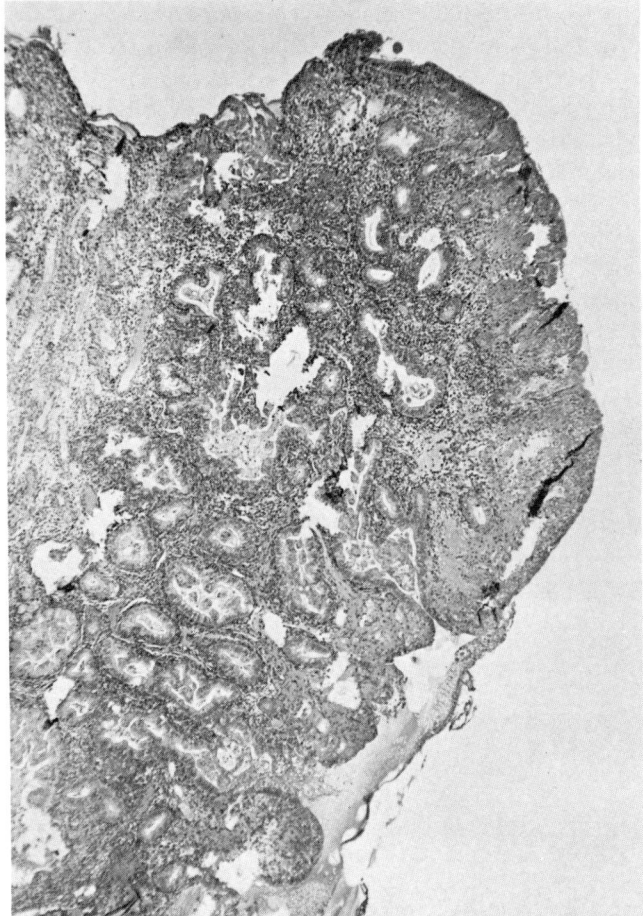

Fig. 6.14. Adenocarcinoma in situ within endocervical polyp. The adenocarcinoma in situ is confined to the superficial area of the polyp.

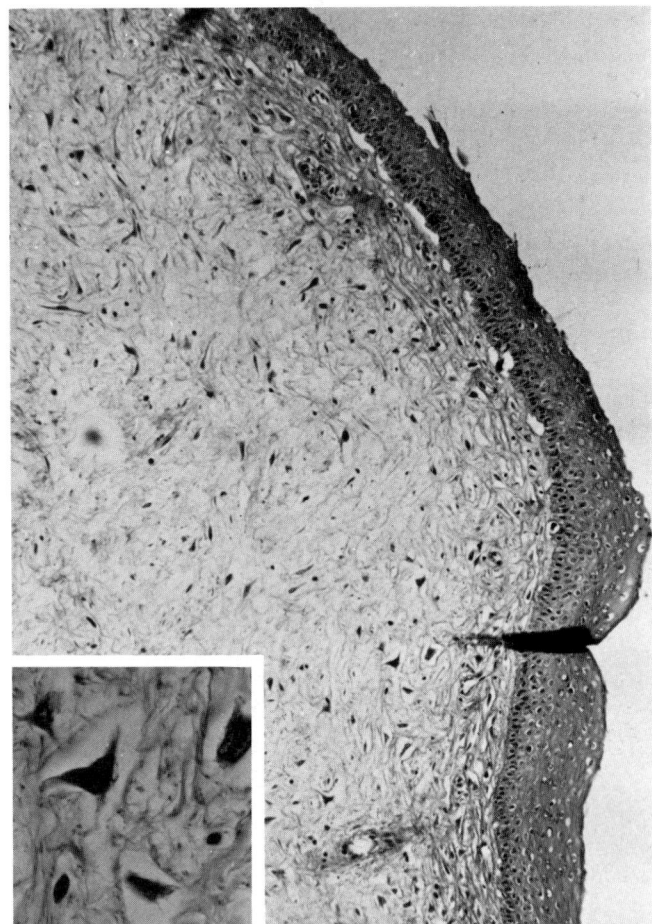

Fig. 6.15. Mesodermal stromal polyp of cervix. Spindle-shaped and stellate fibroblasts are embedded in a loose myxoid stroma simulating sarcoma botryoides. Note absence of subepithelial cambium layer. *Inset:* High magnification of stellate atypical fibroblasts.

boring areas. A focus of carcinoma in a cervical polyp without involvement of its base but associated with similar carcinoma in the adjacent regions should be regarded as a secondary rather than a primary focus. Adenocarcinoma confined to a polyp has an excellent prognosis.[3]

Mesodermal Stromal Polyp (Pseudosarcoma botryoides)

Mesodermal stromal polyps are benign, exophytic proliferations of stroma and epithelium that can occur in the vagina and cervix of women of reproductive age. These lesions are seen most frequently in pregnant patients and arise more commonly from the vagina (see Chapter 4, Diseases of the Vagina) than from the cervix.[39,83] Histologically, these polyps are composed of an edematous stroma that is covered by a benign-appearing stratified squamous epitheliium (Fig 6.15). The stromal component usually is comprised of bland-appearing plump stromal fibroblasts. However, in some cases there can be focal areas of bizarre fibroblasts with irregular, occasionally multinucleated hyperchromatic nuclei that resemble the fibroblasts in radiation reactions.[21] These areas can be quite alarming on causal inspection because they may simulate the appearance of sarcoma botryoides (Fig. 6.15).[38,39] These lesions differ from sarcoma botryoides by the absence of mitotic figures, lack of rhabdomyoblasts, and lack of a cambium layer.

Decidual Pseudopolyp

During gestation, the stroma of the cervix can undergo focal decidual changes. This decidual change is identical to that which occurs in the lamina propria of the fallopian tube or on the serosal surface of the uterus during pregnancy. Histologially, the decidualized cells are present just underneath the surface epithelium and have oval, bland nuclei with large amounts of pale eosinophilic granular cytoplasm and prominent cytoplasmic membranes (Fig. 6.16). The gross appearance of the decidual change depends on the site. If the change occurs on the exocervix, it frequently presents as a raised plaque or pseudopolyp, which can be mistaken for invasive carcinoma both colposcopically and microscopically. During gestation, cervical polyps also may contain focal stromal decidual changes and rarely massive decidualization of endocervical stroma occurs, producing a polypoid protrusion from the endocervix. Clinically, decidualized polyps need to be differentiated from extruded fragments of decidua, which may indicate an impeding miscarriage. Distinction is made by identifying a stalk for the decidualized polyp whereas expulsed fragments of decidua lack a stalk. Areas of decidualization are microscopically differentiated from invasive nonkeratinizing squamous cell carcinoma by the lack of significant nuclear atypia, as well as lack of mitotic figures, a co-

existing SIL, and continuity with the surface epithelium. In difficult cases, immunohistochemistry using antibodies against cytokeratin proteins can be used to differentiate cytokeratin-negative decidul reactions from cytokeratin-positive nonkeratinizing squamous cell carcinoma.

Placental Site Trophoblastic Nodule

Placental site trophoblastic nodules can be found in the endocervix, immediately beneath the epithelium. These lesions are histologically identical to early implantation sites that can be detected in the endometrium of women of reproductive ages.[132] Microscopically, placental site trophoblastic nodules are well-defined lesions that have a hyalinized appearance and contain intermediate trophoblasts and inflammatory cells (see Chapter 24, Gestational Trophoblastic Disease and Related Lesions). The intermediate trophoblast cells frequently are degenerated and have extensive cytoplasmic vacuolization but lack significant nuclear atypia and mitotic activity. Intermediate trophoblast stains positively with antibodies against cytokeratins and human placental lactogen. The lack of significant nuclear atypia and mitotic activity as well as the presence of staining with antibodies against human placental lactogen allow these lesions to be differentiated microscopically from invasive nonkeratinizing squamous cell carcinomas.

Leiomyoma

Cervical leiomyomas represent about 8% of all uterine myomas.[42] They usually occur singly and produce unilateral enlargement of the cervical portio. At times the lesion may protrude from the canal, resembling an endocervical polyp, and in pregnancy may produce dystocia. Cervical leiomyomas are similar grossly, microscopically, and ultrastructurally to those observed in the myometrium; a variety of histological patterns may be encountered, including atypical (symplastic) leiomyoma, which contains cells with bizarre nuclei (Fig. 6.17) (see Chapter 13, Mesenchymal Tumors of the Uterus). Another variant designated *vascular leiomyoma* is characterized by an abundance of varying-sized, thick-walled, hyalinized blood vessels. Histological continuity between the smooth muscle fibers and the muscular wall of blood vessels often is demonstrated, suggesting that the latter represents the source of the neoplastic growth.

Papillary Adenofibroma

In 1971, Abell described three polypoid lesions of endocervical origin that contained branching clefts and papillary excrescences lined by mucinous epithelium with foci of squamous metaplasia (Fig. 6.18).[2] The epithelium was supported by a compact, cellular, fibrous tissue composed of spindle-shaped and stellate fibroblasts, with an occa-

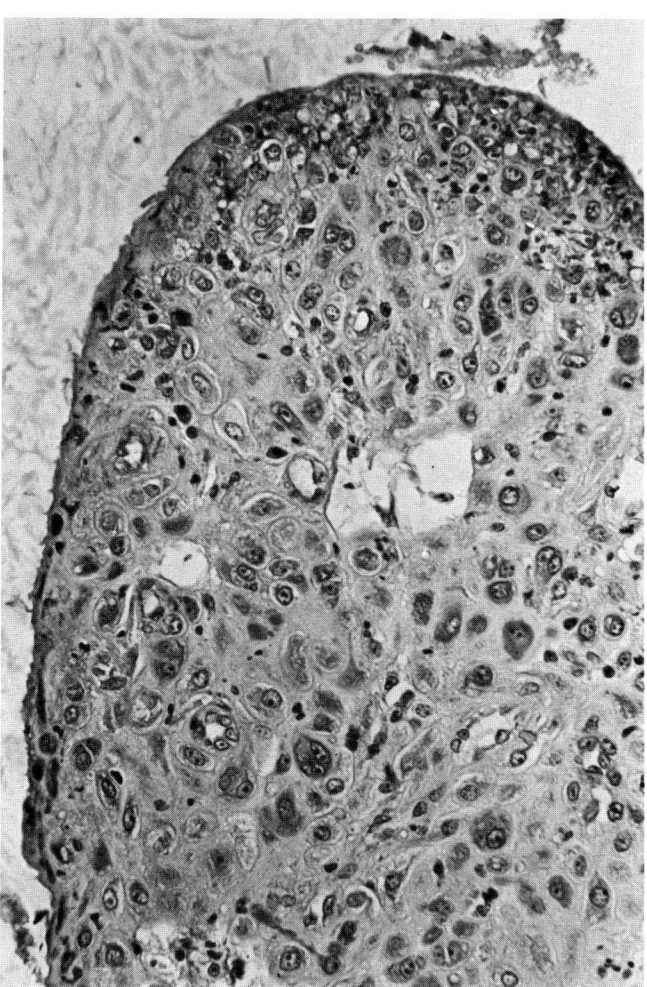

FIG. 6.16. **Decidual pseudopolyp.** These pseudopolyps develop during pregnancy and are composed of typical decidual cells.

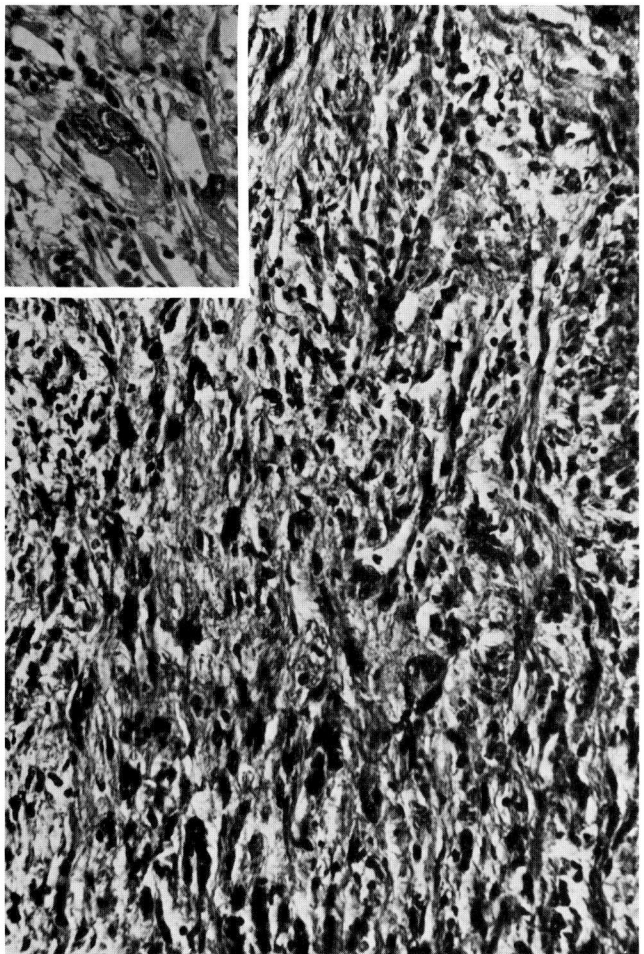

Fig. 6.17. Atypical (symplastic) leiomyoma of the cervix. This atypical leiomyoma developed in a pregnant patient and has atypical giant cells and pleomorphism but no mitotic figures. Such neoplasms should not be interpreted as sarcoma. *Inset:* Detail of atypical neoplastic smooth muscle cells. (Courtesy of Dr. B. Bigelow, New York, NY.)

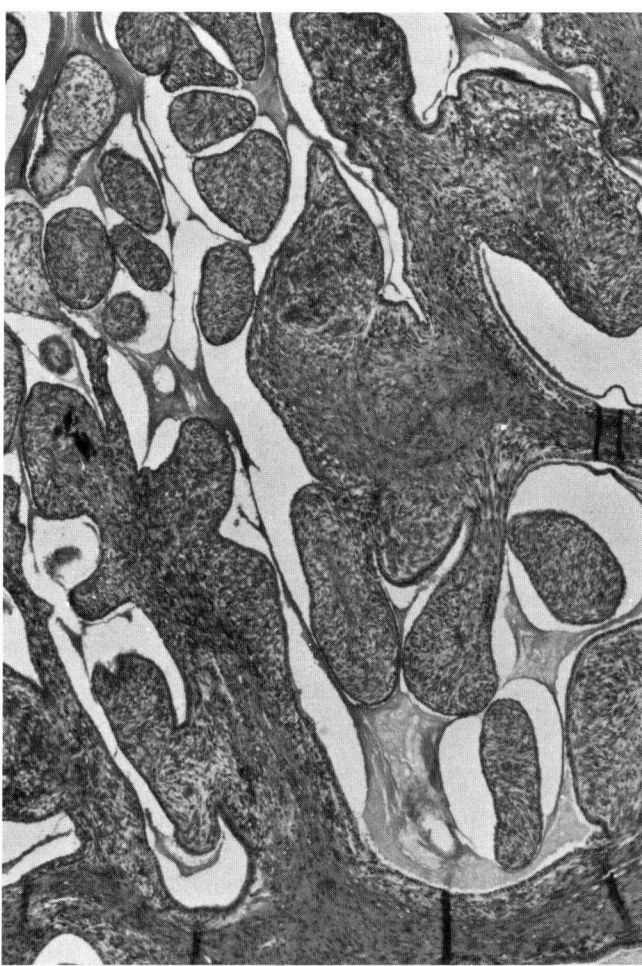

Fig. 6.18. Papillary adenofibroma. Fibroepithelial papillae project into cystic spaces. The endocervical lining epithelium produces abundant mucin.

sional storiform pattern. The stroma was devoid of smooth muscle fibers and mitoses were rare. Because of their resemblance to adenofibroma of the ovary, the term *papillary adenofibroma of the cervix* was suggested.[2] Similar papillary growths have since been reported in the endometrium and fallopian tube.[54,122] Although a focus of adenocarcinoma has been found in one case of papillary adenofibroma of the endometrium, to date all the patients are alive and well. Papillary adenofibroma of the female reproductive tract, including the cervix, occurs exclusively in perimenopausal and postmenopausal women.

The hypercellular stromal component of papillary adenofibroma may resemble cervical adenosarcoma. The latter also is papillary but the stroma is hypercellular. The stromal cells in adenosarcoma may display only mild atypia but there is increased mitotic activity (see Chapter 13, Mesenchymal Tumors of the Uterus).[22]

Adenomyoma and Fibroadenoma

These neoplasms are rare and are composed of an admixture of fibroconnective tissue and smooth muscle elements intermingling with mucinous endocervical epithelium.[54] Depending on the predominance of the fibrous or muscular tissue component, they are classified as adenomyoma or fibroadenoma.

Miscellaneous Tumors

Hemangiomas are rarely found in the cervix. They may be of capillary or cavernous type.[55] A single instance of cervical lymphangioma was reported by Stout and several cases of lipoma of the cervix are on record.[98,117] Neoplasma of neurogenic derivation arising in the cervix are extremely rare and include neurofibroma and ganglioneuroma.[14,42] Benign blue nevi of the endocervix, indistinguishable from those arising in the dermis, occasionally are seen.[35,88] They are composed of melanin-containing fusiform cells with dendritic cytoplasmic processes, located in the stroma of the endocervix.

Cysts

Nabothian Cyst

Nabothian cysts are the most common type of cyst of the cervix and develop within the transformation zone secondary to squamous metaplasia covering over and obstructing endocervical glands. Grossly, these lesions appear as yellow or white cysts that are frequently multiple and can measure up to 1.5 cm in diameter. Microscopically, they are lined by a somewhat flattened, single layer of mucin-producing endocervical epithelium (Fig 6.19). In some cases squamous metaplasia of the lining epithelium occurs. The lining epithelium is almost always at least focally positive with mucicarmine stains, allowing these lesions to be distinguished from traumatic inclusion cysts and mesonephric duct cysts. Although nabothian cysts usually are confined to the superficial portion of the cervix, they have been reported to extend through the wall of the cervix.[23]

Tunnel Clusters

Endocervical tunnel clusters are benign collections of endocervical glands that usually are located close to the surface epithelium of the cervix. Tunnel clusters are quite common and become more prevalent with increasing age. In Fluhmann's original description they were detected in 8% of all adult women and 13% of the postmenopausal women.[43,44] They appear to be more common in pregnant women. These lesions are asymptomatic and are detected as incidental findings in either hysterectomy specimens or cone biopsies obtained for unrelated reasons.[106]

Two types of tunnel clusters originally were described.[43,44] One type represents a cluster of closely packed glands that are noncystic and are lined by tall columnar epithelium. The other type is grossly cystic and lined by a cuboidal or flattened epithelium (Fig 6.20). These collections of glands have a clustered appearance with a rounded margin and do not invade into the deep cervical stroma. The importance of tunnel clusters is that occasionally they are misinterpreted as minimal deviation adenocarcinomas of the cervix.[23,106] However, tunnel clusters do not have nuclear atypia, mitotic activity, and most importantly do not invade into the deep cervical stroma.

Inclusion Cyst

Traumatic inclusion cysts are a form of epidermal inclusion cysts that commonly occur in the vagina at sites of surgical repair of episiotomies or vaginal intrapartum lacerations

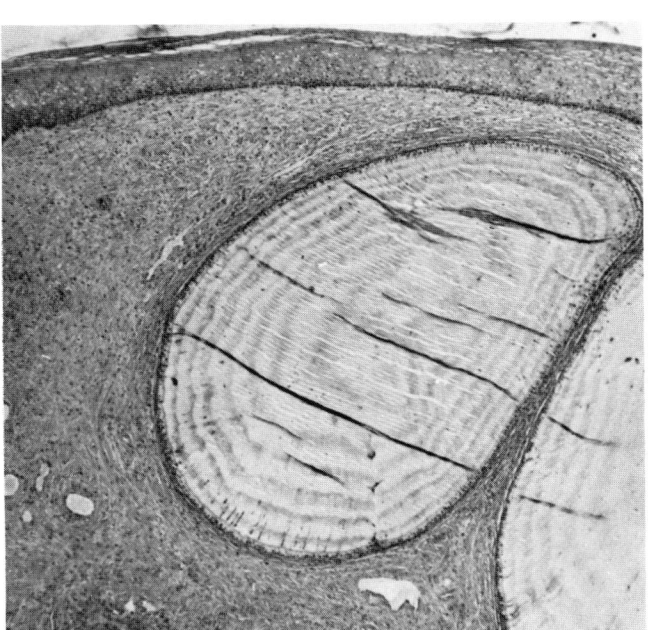

FIG. 6.19. **Nabothian cyst.** Nabothian cysts are lined by a flattened layer of mucin-producing epithelium.

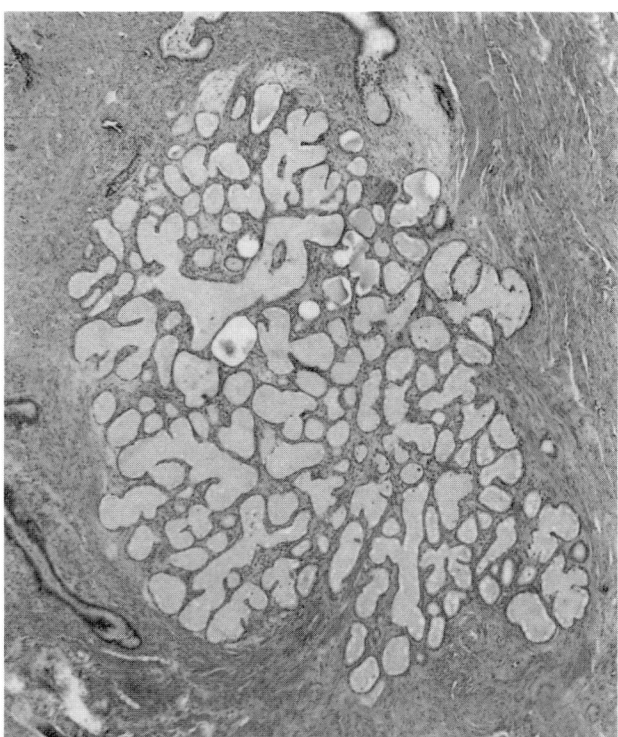

FIG. 6.20. **Endocervical tunnel cluster.** This lesion consists of closely packed cystically dilated glands lined by a flattened epithelium. The lesion is well demarcated and does not extend beyond the depth of the normal endocervical glands.

(see Chapter 4, Diseases of the Vagina). They are thought to develop from viable fragments of epithelium that become entrapped within the stroma at the time of obstetrical trauma or subsequent surgical repair. Inclusion cysts are uncommonly found on the cervix. Grossly, they present as unilocular cystic structures measuring 1–2 cm in diameter beneath the native portio epithelium.[43] Microscopically, traumatic inclusion cysts are lined by a stratified squamous epithelium similar to that of the vaginal mucosa but usually somewhat thinner. The epithelium shows normal maturation with the basal cells oriented away from the cyst cavity, which is filled with desquamated epithelial cells. The cyst contents are identical to those of epidermal inclusion cysts at other sites and are thick, white, and cheesy.

Tumor-like Lesions

Microglandular Hyperplasia

Microglandular hyperplasia is a benign proliferation of endocervical glands. Microglandular hyperplasia is detected frequently as an incidental finding on a cervical biopsy, cone biopsy, or hysterectomy specimen. If clinically apparent, it most often resembles a cervical polyp measuring 1–2 cm in size. These patients may complain of postcoital bleeding or spotting. Microglandular hyperplasia is most common in women of the reproductive ages and has been detected in up to 27% of cone biopsies or hysterectomy specimens.[10,82] In most instances it occurs in patients with a history of oral contraceptive use or in pregnant or postpartum patients.[16,20,82,126] Most, therefore, consider microglandular hyperplasia to be a reflection of progestagenic stimulation, although in occasional cases it is found in women with no known exposure to progestational agents.[20,82] Other authors have described the sporadic occurrence of microglandular hyperplasia in patients with hyperestrogenism or exogenous estrogen therapy.[121,126] Several cases also have been reported in which there was no associated hormonal history. Persistence of the lesion for long periods of time after discontinuation of pills or termination of pregnancy suggests that increased hormone levels are needed for inducing, but not for maintaining, the lesions.[82]

Histologically, microglandular hyperplasia may be single or distributed in multiple foci. It may involve the surface and/or deeper portions of endocervical clefts. Two histological types of microglandular hyperplasia originally were recognized. The most common form, initially termed *microglandular hyperplasia*, consists of tightly packed, varying-sized glandular or tubular units lined by flattened to cuboidal cells with eosinophilic granular cytoplasm containing small quantities of mucin (Fig. 6.21). The glands

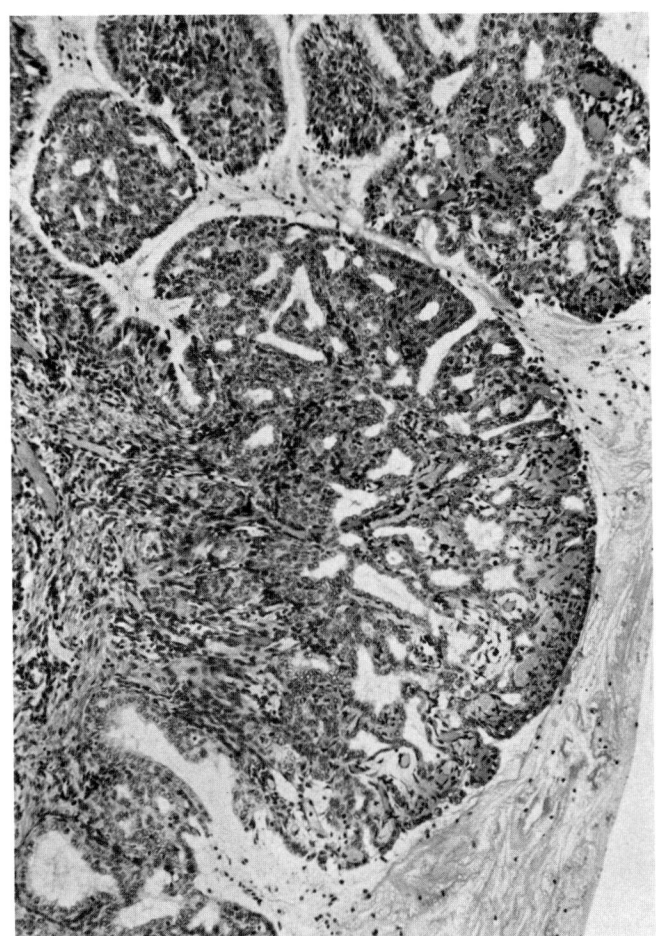

FIG. 6.21. Microglandular hyperplasia. This lesion was associated with oral contraceptive use. There is an adenomatous pattern with cuboidal lining cells and focal squamous metaplasia.

vary in size and shape, from round and small to large irregularly dilated, cystic structures. The stroma separating the glands usually is infiltrated with acute and chronic inflammatory cells. The nuclei of the endocervical cells are uniform, with occasional pleomorphism and hyperchromasia, but mitotic activity is quite low, with only 1 mitotic figure per 10 high-power fields.[133] Associated squamous metaplasia and subcolumnar reserve cell hyperplasia are seen in many cases. Foci with a solid proliferation of cells, including signet-ring cells, also can be present. A second form of microglandular hyperplasia originally was described by Taylor et al. and designated *endocervical hyperplasia*.[119] This is a florid form of microglandular proliferation that is classified simply as part of the histological spectrum of microglandular hyperplasia by most contemporary authors.[133] In florid forms of microglandular hyperplasia the glandular elements are arranged in a reticulated or solid pattern with areas of nuclear hyperchromasia and pleomorphism (Fig. 6.22). These lesions clearly appear to

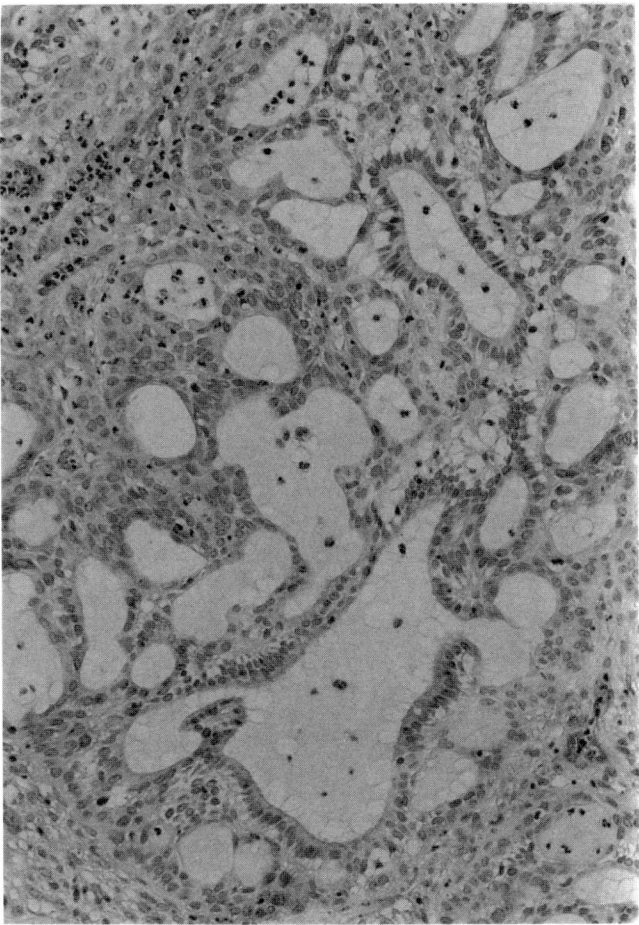

FIG. 6.22. Microglandular hyperplasia. The hyperplastic cells form a reticular pattern of florid microglandular hyperplasia. Note extensive vacuolization, which is caused by cystic dilation of intercellular spaces. There is a paucity of intracellular mucin. Squamous metaplasia surrounds several glands.

be benign because no patients are yet reported to have developed malignant tumors with long-term follow-up.[130] The significance of the florid forms of microglandular hyperplasia is that the irregularly arranged glands can impart an infiltrative appearance and they can be mistaken for adenocarcinoma; in particular, clear cell adenocarcinoma.[99,130,133] Microglandular hyperplasia with solid areas, especially when the solid component predominates or when signet-ring cells are present, also can be difficult to distinguish from adenocarcinomas.[119,133] The benign nature of these florid lesions usually is demonstrable by a lack of clear-cut stromal invasion and the low mitotic activity of microglandular hyperplasia as compared with endocervical adenocarcinoma. More importantly, unlike clear cell carcinoma, microglandular hyperplasia lacks intracellular glycogen and usually contains intracellular mucin. In addition, florid forms of microglandular hyperplasia almost always contain areas with the more typical histological features of

microglandular hyperplasia.[130,133] Immunohistochemistry does not appear to be particularly useful for distinguishing microglandular hyperplasia from adenocarcinoma. Although most cases of microglandular hyperplasia do not react with antibodies against carcinoembryonic antigen (CEA), occasional cases of invasive adenocarcinomas of the cervix also can be CEA negative and in others the positivity may be focal and quite weak (see Chapter 8, Carcinoma and Other Tumors of the Cervix).[34,51,112,114]

Endometriosis and Tubal Metaplasia

Endometriosis refers to lesions that are composed of ectopic endometrial glands and stroma (see Chapter 17, Diseases of the Peritoneum), whereas *tubal metaplasia* refers to endocervical glands that are lined by a müllerian-type epithelium that closely resembles that of the fallopian tube. Endometriosis of the cervix may occur on the portio or in the endocervical canal.[48,97] Most areas of endometriosis of the exocervix appear as one or more small, blue or red nodules, measuring a few millimeters in diameter. Occasionally, however, the lesion may be larger or cystic and may produce abnormal vaginal bleeding. Histologically, the glands and stroma resemble proliferative endometrium. Rarely the glands are secretory and decidua may be seen in pregnancy or with progestin therapy (Fig. 6.23). A case of adenocarcinoma arising within cervical endometriosis has been reported.[18]

The mechanism responsible for the development of endometriosis is unknown but it is clear that cervical endometriosis frequently develops after cervical trauma. Gardner reported that cervical endometriosis developed in 5–15% of patients undergoing cervical cautery or cone biopsy and a more recent analysis of 42 cervices after cone biopsy detected endometriosis in 43%.[48,63] This association has been interpreted by some investigators as evidence supporting Sampson's implantation theory.[97] According to this theory, endometrial tissue is implanted into the cervical mucosa or submucosa after postmenstrual cauterization or during delivery. However, other investigators interpret the frequent occurrence of posttraumatic endometriosis as supporting the view that cervical endometriosis represents a reparative/metaplastic process.[63] Support for the concept that cervical endometriosis develops as a metaplastic process as opposed to direct implantation also comes from the frequent demonstration of glands with either tuboendometrioid or pure tubal metaplasia in posttraumatic cervices.[63]

Ciliated, nonsecretory endocervical epithelial cells are a normal component of the endocervix and are present most frequently high in the endocervical canal. Tuboendometrioid metaplasia of the cervix is a type of metaplasia that is histologically similar to the tubal metaplasia that can develop in the endometrium in patients with unopposed estrogenic stimulation. Endocervical glands demonstrating

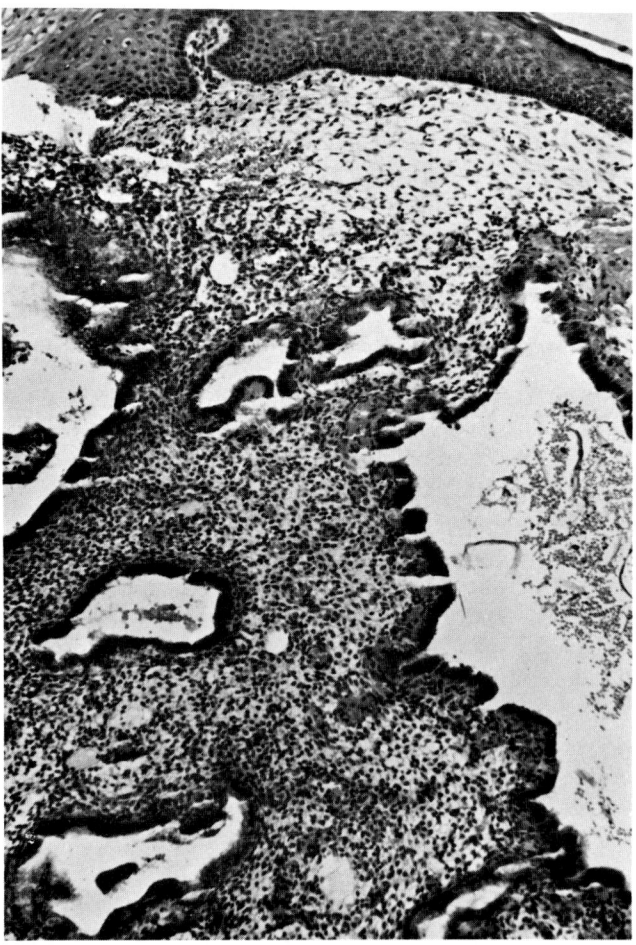

FIG. 6.23. **Endometriosis of the cervix.** Both typical endometrial glands and stroma are present beneath the squamous portio epithelium.

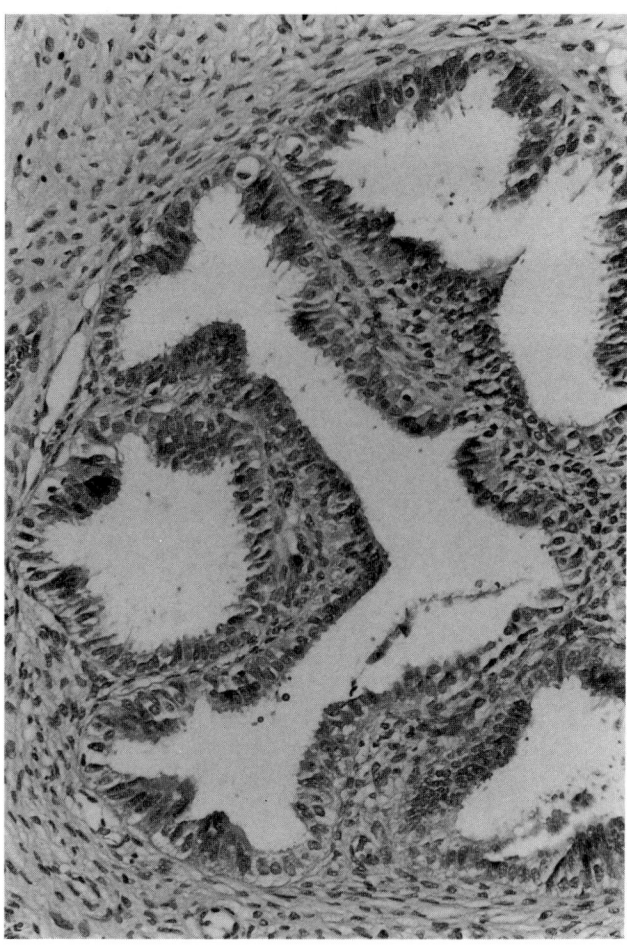

FIG. 6.24. **Tuboendometrioid metaplasia.** The columnar, mucus-producing epithelium has been replaced by a pseudostratified epithelium with a high nuclear-cytoplasmic ratio and cilia.

tuboendometrioid metaplasia are lined by a pseudostratified epithelium composed of columnar cells with a high nuclear-cytoplasmic ratio (Fig. 6.24). Many of these cells are ciliated or have secretory features with apical snouts but the glands lack an associated endometrial stroma. Because of the pseudostratification and high nuclear-cytoplasmic ratio, these glands can be misinterpreted as representing adenocarcinoma in situ. In pure tubal metaplasia, the endocervical glands are lined by an epithelium that resembles more closely that of the fallopian tube and contains many more ciliated cells than are normally present in the endocervical epithelium as well as tubal-type secretory cells and reserve or intercalary cells (Fig 6.25).[66,84,118] Tubal metaplasia can be found in up to 31% of patients and does not appear to be related to the phase of menstrual cycle, the presence of inflammatory changes, or low-grade SIL (CIN 1).[66,84,118] As with tuboendometrioid metaplasia, tubal metaplasia can be quite extensive and can be mistaken for endocervical glandular neoplasia.

Arias Stella Reaction

During pregnancy, the gestational Arias–Stella reaction can develop in both endocervical glands and in ectopic endometrial glands within the cervix. In one study of 191 gravid hysterectomy specimens, the Arias–Stella reaction of endocervical glands, was detected, at least focally, in 9% of the cases. The Arias–Stella reaction of the endocervix usually is focal and is present more commonly in the proximal portion of the endocervix involving superficial as opposed to deeply situated glands. Microscopically, the Arias–Stella reaction that occurs in the endocervical glands during pregnancy is identical to that which occurs in the endometrium. The cells within the affected glands are markedly enlarged with irregular, frequently hyperchromatic nuclei that can project into the glandular lumen in a hobnail pattern. The cells are pseudostratified and have hypersecretory cytoplasmic features with abundant vacuolated cytoplasm (Fig 6.26). Papillary processes with fi-

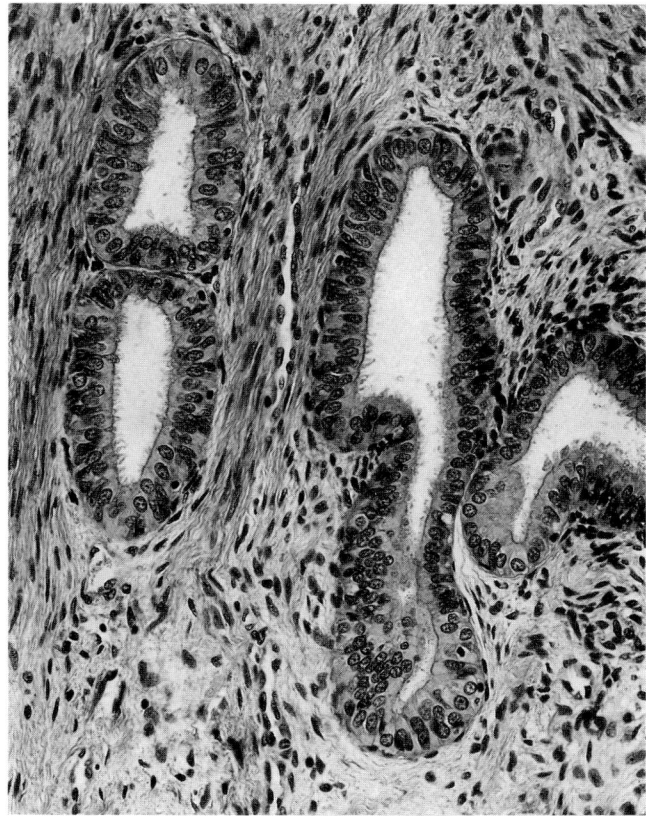

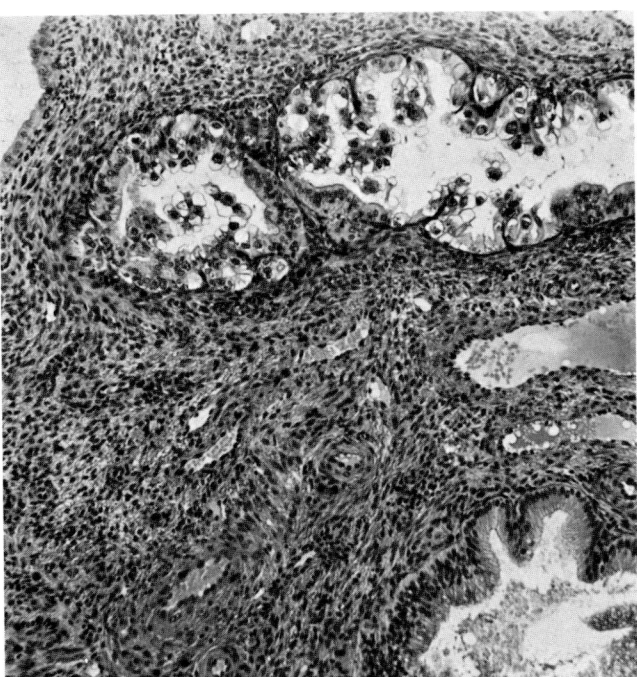

FIG. 6.26. **Arias–Stella reaction.** The Arias–Stella reaction should not be confused with clear cell adenocarcinoma of the cervix.

FIG. 6.25. **Tubal metaplasia.** The columnar, mucus-producing epithelium has been replaced by a tubal type epithelium with ciliated, secretory, and intercalated cells.

brovascular cores lined by enlarged epithelial cells can project into the endocervical gland lumen. The Arias–Stella reaction occasionally can be mistaken for clear cell carcinoma or adenocarcinoma in situ of the cervix. Differentiation from clear cell carcinoma is made by the lack of a mass lesion and clear-cut stromal invasion as well as by the absence of the classic tubular and papillary areas typical of clear cell carcinoma. The cells in adenocarcinoma in situ have more uniform nuclei and less cytoplasmic vacuolization. The Arias–Stella reaction lacks mitotic activity whereas both clear cell carcinoma and adenocarcinoma in situ are mitotically active. Because of the possiblity of confusing Arias–Stella reaction with clear cell carcinoma or adenocarcinoma in situ, the diagnosis of the latter two entities should be made with caution in the pregnant patient.

Mesonephric Remnants and Mesonephric Hyperplasia

The vestigial elements of the distal ends of the mesonephric ducts are found in 1–22% of cervices. The wide variation in the reported prevalence of these remnants appears to be a function of how extensively the cervix is sampled and the site of sampling.[41] Mesonephric remnants are present most commonly in the lateral aspects of the cervix, a region that usually is not sampled on routine hysterectomy specimens. They consist of small tubules or cysts that usually are located deep in the lateral cervical wall.[110] Characteristically, the tubules are arranged in small clusters or have an orderly distribution reminiscent of the ampullary portion of the fetal mesonephric duct. The tubules are lined by nonciliated, low columnar, or cuboidal epithelium.[110] The lining cells contain no glycogen or mucin, features that distinguish mesonephric from endocervical epithelium. The tubular lumen, however, often is filled with pink, homogeneous, periodic acid–Schiff (PAS)-positive secretions (Fig. 6.27). Mesonephric remnants may become hyperplastic, resulting in a florid, tubuloglandular proliferation with transmural involvement of the cervix (Fig. 6.28) and masquerading as a minimal deviation adenocarcinoma of the endocervix (see Chapter 8, Carcinoma and Other Tumors of the Cervix). Florid mesonephric hyperplasia is almost always asymptomatic and is detected on either cervical biopsy, cone biopsy, or hysterectomy specimens.[41] Histological differentiation between mesonephric hyperplasia and mesonephric remnants is quite arbitrary and of little clinical importance. Similarly, the histological subdivision of mesonephric hyperplasia into lobular, diffuse, and ductal forms lacks any known clinical significance.[41] Florid mesonephric hyperplasia is a benign condition and is distinguished from mesonephric

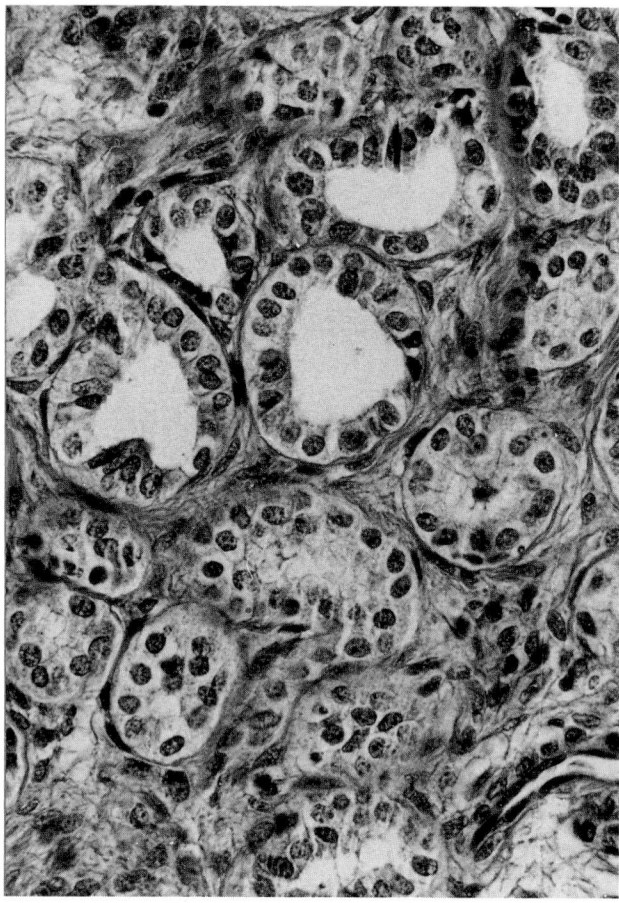

FIG. 6.27. Mesonephric remnants. The mesonephric tubules are lined by cuboidal erythelium with bland nuclei. The lumens contain pink, homogeneous, intraluminal secretions. (Courtesy of R. J. Kurman, M. D., Baltimore, MD.)

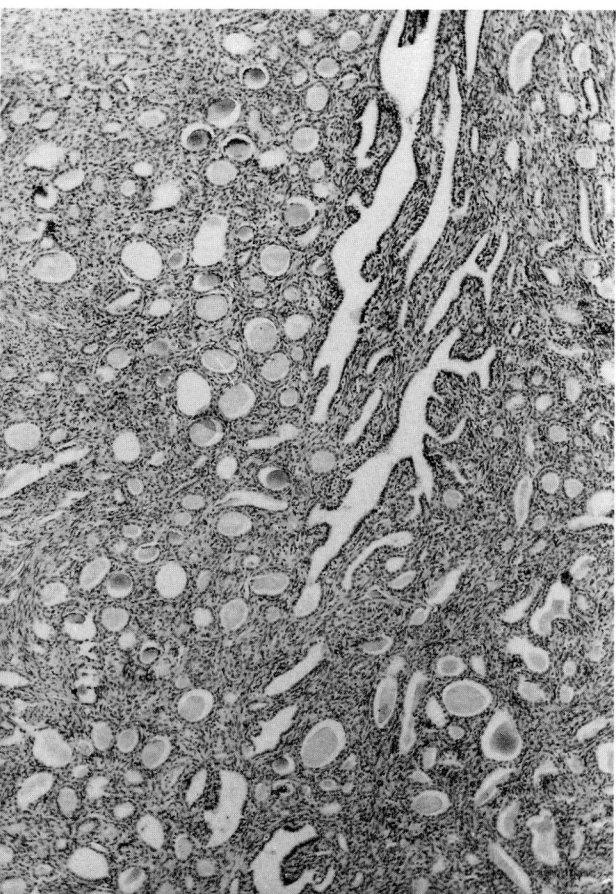

FIG. 6.28. Florid mesonephric hyperplasia. Extensive mesonephric tubular–ductal proliferation deep in the cervix, resembling an invasive adenocarcinoma. Unlike the latter, The lobular architecture is maintained in hyperplasia. Note mesonephric duct in center surrounded by a proliferation of small tubules. (Courtesy of R. J. Kurman, M. D., Baltimore, MD.)

carcinoma by lack of a haphazard glandular pattern and retention of a lobular pattern in which small tubules are clustered around a larger duct. Mitotic activity is very low in florid hyperplasia. In contrast to most cervical adenocarcinomas, CEA is absent in florid mesonephric hyperplasia. In addition, normal mesonephric remnants usually are admixed with the hyperplastic tubules.

Müllerian Papilloma

Rare instances of benign, papillary growth of the cervix in children have been described.[64,69,107] They are composed of complex papillary projections lined by flat cuboidal epithelium with cores of loose fibrovascular tissue. Cytological atypia and mitoses are absent. In the past the lesions were thought to be of mesonephric duct origin, although they have not been encountered in association with meso-

nephric remnants. Although the histogenesis of these lesions remains uncertain, recent studies favor a müllerian origin.

Postoperative Spindle Cell Nodule

Postoperative spindle cell nodules of the cervix are clinically and histologically identical to their more common counterparts of the vulva and vagina.[91] These lesions may develop after either a cervical biopsy or some other form of trauma.[68] They are composed of actively proliferating spindle cells with oval nuclei arranged in interlacing bundles (see Chapter 4, Diseases of the Vagina). The cells may vary slightly in size and mitotic figures often are present. A characteristic feature is the presence of neutrophils and erythrocytes in the lesion, giving it the appearance of granulation tissue.

Lymphoma-like Lesions

Lymphoma-like lesions (pseudolymphomas) are marked inflammatory lesions of the cervix, extensive enough to cause confusion with a lymphoproliferative lesion.[131] Lymphoma-like lesions are composed of a superficial band of large lymphoid cells admixed with mature lymphocytes and plasma cells (Fig. 6.29). The lymphoid infiltrates commonly include macrophages and germinal centers, which help to distinguish them from lymphomas. Another feature that helps to distinguish lymphoma-like lesions from lymphomas is the superficial localization of the infiltrate. Lymphoma-like lesions rarely infiltrate deeper than 3 mm from the surface epithelium, whereas lymphomas of the cervix usually extend beyond the depth of the endocervical glands (see Chapter 8, Carcinoma and Other Tumors of the Cervix).

Heterologous Tissue

Glia

There are 15 recorded cases of neuroglial tissue in the cervix or the endometrium (see Chapter 10, Benign Diseases of the Endometrium).[111] Although the term *glioma* is used for this condition, the high degree of differentiation of the glial tissue, the absence of mitoses, and the absence of recurrence are against its being neoplastic (Fig. 6.30). The lesion should not be confused with a pure heterologous sarcoma or a teratoma. The neural tissue is believed to represent either implantation of fetal cerebral glia at the time of instrumentation of the gravid uterus or heterotopic maldevelopment during embryogenesis.[111] When the cervix is involved, the lesion usually appears as a polyp that bleeds readily.

Skin

Among the pathological curiosities of the cervix are cases of true epidermidization of the cervical mucosa. In these instances sebaceous glands, hair, and sweat glands are found.[127] The presence of these ectodermal structures,

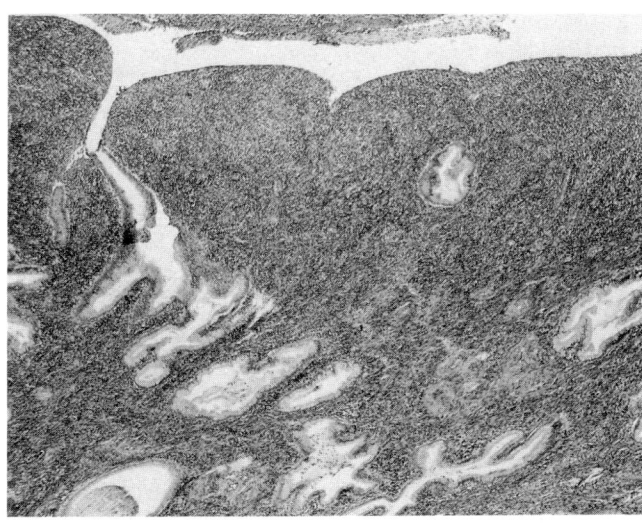

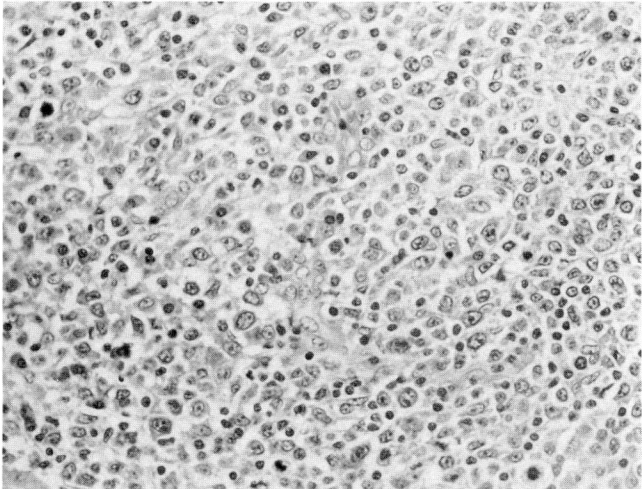

FIG. 6.29. **Lymphoma-like lesion. a:** These lesions are distinguished from lymphoma by their superficial location and the presence of macrophages and germinal centers. **b:** Higher magnification view of the infiltrate. (Courtesy of Dr. R. Young, Boston, MA.)

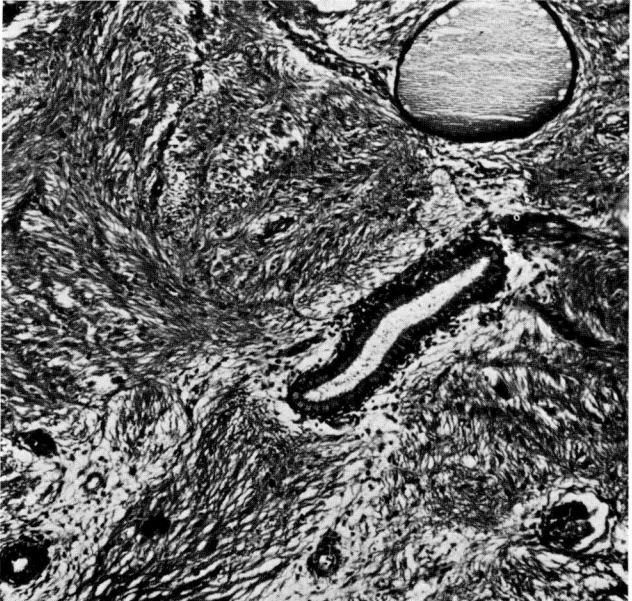

FIG. 6.30. **Glioma of the endocervix.** Bundles of well-differentiated neuroglial tissue intermingle with normal endocervical epithelium. (Courtesy of Dr. Y. Boivin, Montreal, Quebec, Canada.)

which normally are appendages of the epidermis, on a mucous membrane of mesodermal derivation is difficult to explain. It is conceivable, however, that stratified squamous epithelium under certain circumstances, such as long-standing chronic inflammation, can form the appendages of its epidermal analogue.

Cartilage

Four cases of heterotopic mature cartilage in the cervix are on record.[100] The finding of these structures alone has no clinical significance. They should not be confused with a malignant mixed mesodermal tumor.

References

1. Aaro LA, Jacobson LJ, Soule EH (1963) Endocervical polyps. Obstet Gynecol 21: 659
2. Abell MR (1971) Papillary adenofibroma of the uterine cervix. Am J Obstet Gynecol 110: 990–993
3. Abell MR, Gosling JRG (1962) Gland cell carcinoma (adenocarcinoma) of the uterine cervix. Am J Obstet Gynecol 83: 729
4. Adam E, Kaufman RH, Melnick JL, et al (1973) Seroepidemiologic studies of herpesvirus type 2 and carcinoma of the cervix. IV. Dysplasia and carcinoma in situ. Am J Epidemiol 98: 77–87
5. Adam E, Kaufman RH, Mirkovic RR, et al (1979) Persistence of virus shedding in asymptomatic women after recovery from herpes genitalis. Obstet Gynecol 54: 171–173
6. Adams JQ, Packer H (1955) Granuloma inguinale of the cervix. South Med J 48: 27
7. Andrews S, Miyazawa K (1989) The significance of a negative Papanicolaou smear with hyperkeratosis or parakeratosis. 73: 751–753
8. Barton IG, Kinghorn GR, Walker MJ, et al (1981) Association of HSV-1 with cervical infection. Lancet ii: 1108
9. Berry A (1966) A cytopathological and histopathological study of bilharziasis of the female genital tract. J Pathol Bacteriol 9: 325
10. Brown LJR, Wells M (1986) Cervical glandular atypia associated with squamous intraepithelial neoplasia: A premalignant lesion? J Clin Pathol 39: 22–28
11. Burd LI, Esterly JR (1971) Vesicular lesions of the uterine cervix. Am J Obstet Gynecol 110: 887–888
12. Burkman RT, Damewood MT (1985) Actinomyces and the intrauterine contraceptive device. In: Zatuchni GI, Goldsmith A, Sciarra J (eds) Intrauterine contraception. Advances and future prospects. New York, Harper & Row, pp. 427–437
13. Burnham RC, Paavonen J, Stevens CE, et al (1984) Mucopurulent cervicitis: The ignored counterpart in women of urethritis in men. N Engl J Med 311: 1–6
14. Busby JG (1952) Neurofibromatosis of the cervix. Am J Obstet Gynecol 63: 674
15. Byrne MA, Taylor-Robinson D, Anderson MC, et al (1989) Value of colposcopy in STD clinic based on first year's experience. Genitourin Med 64: 316–320
16. Candy J, Abell MR (1968) Progestogen-induced adenomatous hyperplasia of the uterine cervix. JAMA 203: 323
17. Cecchine S, Iossa A, Ciatto S, et al (1990) Colposcopic survey of Papanicolaou test-negative cases with hyperkeratosis or parakeratosis. Obstet Gynecol 76: 857–859
18. Chang SH, Maddox WA (1971) Adenocarcinoma arising within cervical endometriosis and invading the adjacent vagina. Am J Obstet Gynecol 110: 1015–1017
19. Chow LT, Hirochika H, Nasseri M, et al (1987) Human papilloma virus gene expression. In: Steinberg BM, Taichman LB (eds) Papillomaviruses, Cancer Cells. Cold Spring Harbor, Cold Spring Harbor Press, pp 55–73
20. Chumas JC, Nelson B, Mann WJ, et al (1985) Microglandular hyperplasia of the uterine cervix. Obstet Gynecol 66: 406–409
21. Clement PB (1985) Multinucleated stromal giant cells of the uterine cervix. Arch Pathol Lab Med 109: 200–202
22. Clement PB, Scully RE (1974) Mullerian adenosarcoma of the uterus. A clinicopathologic analysis of 10 cases of a distinctive type of mullerian mixed tumor. Cancer 34: 1138–1149
23. Clement PB, Young RH (1989) Deep nabothian cysts of the uterine cervix. A possible source of confusion with minimal-deviation adenocarcinoma (adenoma malignum). Int J Gynecol Pathol 8: 340–348
24. Cohen C (1973) Three cases of amoebiasis of the cervix uteri. J Obstet Gynecol Br Commonw 80: 476
25. Coleman DV, Evans DMD (1988) Biopsy, Pathology and Cytology of the Cervix. London, Chapman and Hall
26. Control CfD (1982) Sexually transmitted diseases treatment guidelines. MMWR 31: 355
27. Control CfD (1983) Condyloma acuminatum—United States, 1966–1981. MMWR 32: 306–308
28. Corey L (1984) Genital herpes. In: Holmes KK, Mardh PA, Sparling PF, Weisner PJ (eds) Sexually Transmitted Diseases. New York, McGraw-Hill Book Company, pp 449–474
29. Corey L, Holmes KK (1983) Genital herpes simplex virus infection: current concepts in diagnosis, therapy and prevention. Ann Intern Med 98: 973–983
30. Crossen RJ (1930) A case of gumma of cervix. Am J Obstet Gynecol 19: 708
31. Crow J, McWhinney H (1979) Isolated arteritis of the cervix uteri. Br J Obstet Gynecol 86: 393–398
32. Crum CP, Egawa K, Levine RU, et al (1985) Human papillomavirus infection (condyloma) of the cervix and cervical intraepithelial neoplasia: A histological and statistical analysis. Gynecol Oncol 15: 88–94
33. Crum CP, Mitao M, Winkler B, et al (1984) Localizing chlamydial infection in cervical biopsies with the immunoperoxidase technique. Int J Gynecol Pathol 3: 191–197
34. Dabbs DJ, Geisinger KR, Norris HT (1986) Intermediate filaments in endometrial and endocervical carcinomas. The diagnostic utility of vimentin patterns. Am J Surg Pathol 10: 568–576
35. De Molnar AMD, Guralnick M, Ferenczy A (1978) Blue nevus of the endocervix. Report of two cases and ultrastructure. Gynecol Oncol 6: 373–382
36. Dougherty CM, Moore WR, Cotten N (1962) Histologic diagnosis and clinical significance of benign lesions of the nonpregnant cervix. Ann NY Acad Sci 97: 683

37. El-Mahgoub S (1972) Antispermatozoal antibodies in infertile women with cervicovaginal schistosomiasis. Am J Obstet Gynecol 112: 781–784

38. Elliott GB, Elliott JDA (1973) Superficial stromal reactions of lower genital tract. Arch Pathol 95: 100–101

39. Elliott GB, Reynolds HA, Fidler HK (1967) Pseudosarcoma botryoides of cervix and vagina in pregnancy. J Obstet Gynecol Br Commonw 74: 728

40. Evans CS, Goldman RL, Klein HZ, et al (1984) Necrobiotic granulomas of the uterine cervix. A probable postoperative reaction. Am J Surg Pathol 8: 841–844

41. Ferry JA, Scully RE (1990) Mesonephric remnants, hyperplasia, and neoplasia in the uterine cervix. Am J Surg Pathol 14: 1100–1111

42. Fingerland A, Sikl H (1938) Ganglioneuroma of cervix uteri. J Pathol Bactrol 47: 631

43. Fluhmann CF (1961) The cervix uteri and its diseases. Philadelphia, W. B. Saunders

44. Fluhmann CF (1961) Focal hyperplasia (tunnel clusters) of the cervix uteri. Obstet Gynecol 17: 206–214

45. Fu YS, Braun L, Shah KV, et al (1983) Histologic, nuclear DNA, and human papillomavirus studies of cervical condylomas. Cancer 52: 1705–1711

46. Fu YS, Reagan J, Richart RM (1981) Definition of precursors. Gynecol Oncol 12: s220

47. Fu YS, Reagan JW (1989) Pathology of the uterine cervix, vagina, and vulva. Philadelphia, W. B. Saunders

48. Gardner HL (1966) Cervical and vaginal endometriosis. Clin Obstet Gynecol 9: 358

49. Gardner HL, Fernet P (1964) Etiology of vaginitis emphysematosa. Am J Obstet Gynecol 88: 680

50. Giampaola C, Murphy J, Benes S, et al (1983) How sensitive is the Papanicolaou smear in the diagnosis of infections with *Chlamydia trachomatis?* Am J Clin Pathol 80: 844–849

51. Gilks CB, Young RH, Aguirre P, et al. (1989) Adenoma malignum (minimal deviation adenocarcinoma) of the uterine cervix. A clinicopathological and immunohistochemical analysis of 26 cases. Am J Surg Pathol 13: 717–729

52. Gjonnaess JH, Dalaker K, Anestad G, et al (1982) Pelvic inflammatory disease: Etiologic studies with emphasis on chlamydial infection. Obstet Gynecol 59: 550–555

53. Griffiths M, Sanderson D, Penna LK (1992) Cervical epithelial abnormalities among women with vulval warts—no more common than among controls. Int J Gynecol Cancer 2: 49–51

54. Grimalt M, Arguelles M, Ferenczy A (1975) Papillary cystadenofibroma of endometrium. A histochemical and ultrastructural study. Cancer 36: 137–144

55. Gudson JT (1965) Hemangioma of the cervix. Am J Obstet Gynecol 91: 204

56. Guinan ME, Wolinsky SM, Reichman RC (1985) Epidemiology of genital herpex simplex virus infection. Epidemiol Rev 7: 127–46

57. Guinan ME, MacCalman J, Kern ER, et al (1981) The course of untreated recurrent genital herpes simplex infection in 27 women. N Engl J Med 304: 759–763

58. Hare MJ, Toone E, Taylor-Robinson D, et al (1981) Follicular cervicitis—colposcopic appearances and association with *Chlamydia trachomatis.* Br J Obstet Gynecol 88: 174–180

59. Harrison HR, Costin M, Meder JB, et al (1985) Cervical chlamydia trachomatis infection in university women. Relationship to history, contraception, ectopy and cervicitis. Am J Obstet Gynecol 153: 244–251

60. Hobson D, Karayiannis P, Byng RE, et al (1980) Quantitative aspects of chlamydial infection of the cervix. Br J Vener Dis 56: 56

61. Holmes KK (1990) Lower genital tract infections in women: Cystitis/urethritis, vulvovaginitis and cervicitis. In: Holmes KK, Mardh PA, Sparling PF, Weisner PJ (eds) Sexually transmitted diseases. New York, McGraw-Hill Book Company, pp 557–589

62. Hoosen AA, Draper G, Cooper K (1990) Granuloma inguinale of the cervix: A carcinoma look-alike. Genito Med 66: 380–382

63. Ismail SM (1991) Cone biopsy causes cervical endometriosis and tubo-endometrioid metaplasia. Histopathology 18: 107–114

64. Janovski MS, Kadson EJ (1963) Benign mesonephric papillary and polypoid tumors of the cervix in childhood. J Pediatrics 63: 211

65. Johnson CA, Lorenzette LA, Liese BS, et al (1991) Clinical significance of hyperkeratosis on otherwise normal Papanicolaou smears. J Family Pract 33: 354–358

66. Jonasson JG, Wang HH, Antonioli DA, et al (1992) Tubal metaplasia of the uterine cervix: A prevalence study in patients with gynecologic pathologic findings. Int J Gynecol Pathol 11: 89–95

67. Kaufman RH, Watts JM, Gardner HL (1969) Pemphigus vulgaris genital involvement. Obstet Gynecol 33: 264

68. Kay S, Schneider V (1985) Reactive spindle cell nodule of the endocervix simulating uterine sarcoma. Int J Gynecol Pathol 4: 255–257

69. Kistner RW, Hertig AT (1955) Papillomas of the uterine cervix—the malignant potentiality. Obstet Gynecol 6: 147

70. Kiviat NB, Paavonen JA, Brockway J, et al (1985) Cytologic manifestations of cervical and vaginal infections. I. Epithelial and inflammatory cellular changes. JAMA 253: 989–996

71. Kiviat NB, Peterson M, Kinney-Thomas E, et al (1985) Cytologic manifestations of cervical and vaginal infections. II. Confirmation of *Chlamydia trachomatis* infection by direct immunofluorescence using monoclonal antibodies. JAMA 253: 997–1000

72. Koss LG, Wolinska WH (1959) *Trichomonas vaginalis* cervicitis and its relationship to cervical cancer: A histocytological study. Cancer 12: 1171

73. Koutsky LA, Holmes KK, Critchlow CW, et al (1992) A cohort study of the risk of cervical intraepithelial neoplasia grade 2 or 3 in relation to papillomavirus infection. N Engl J Med 327: 1272–1278

74. Langley FG (1943) Primary echinococcal cyst of the uterus. Br J Surg 30: 278

75. Lauritzen AF, Meinecke G (1987) Isolated arteritis of the uterine cervix. Acta Obstet Gynecol Scand 66: 659–660

76. Lippert LJ, Richart RM, Ferenczy A (1974) Giant benign endocervical polyp: Report of a case. Am J Obstet Gynecol 118: 1140–1142

77. Meisels A, Fortin R (1976) Condylomatus lesions of the cervix and vagina. I. Cytological patterns. Acta Cytol 20: 505–509

78. Meisels A, Fortin R, Roy M (1977) Condylomatous lesions of the cervix: II. Cytologic, colposcopic and histopathologic study. Acta Cytol 21: 379–390

79. Meisels A, Roy M, Fortier M (1981) Human papillomavirus (HPV) infection of the cervix: The atypical condyloma. Acta Cytol 25: 7–16

80. Nahimias AJ, Roizman B (1973) Infection with herpes simplex viruses 1 and 2. N Engl J Med 289: 667–674

81. Newton WL, Reardon LV, DeLeva AM (1960) A comparative study of the subcutaneous inoculation of germ-free and conventional guinea pigs with two strains of *Trichomonas vaginalis*. Am J Trop Med Hyg 9: 56

82. Nicolas RM, Fidler HK (1971) Microglandular hyperplasia in cervical cone biopsies taken for suspicious and positive cytology. Am J Clin Pathol 56: 424–429

83. Norris HJ, Taylor HB (1966) Polyps of the vagina: A benign lesion resembling sarcoma botryoides Cancer 19: 226

84. Novotny DB, Maygarden SJ, Johnson DE, et al (1991) Tubal metaplasia. A frequent potential pitfall in the cytologic diagnosis of endocervical glandular dysplasia on cervical smears. Acta Cytol 36: 1–10

85. Paavonen JA, Brunham R, Kiviatt N, et al (1982) Cervicitis—etiologic, clinical and histopathologic findings. In: Mardhl PA, Holmes KK, Oriel JD, et al (eds) Chlamydial infections. New York, Elsevier, pp 141–146

86. Paavonen JA, Kiviat N, Brunham RC, et al (1985) Prevalence and manifestations of endometritis among women wtih cervicitis. Am J Obstet Gynecol 152: 280–286

87. Paavonen JA, Vesterinen E, Meyer B, et al (1982) Colposcopic and histological findings in cervical chlamydial infection. Obst Gynecol 59: 712–715

88. Patel DS, Bhagavan BS (1985) Blue nevus of the uterine cervix: Hum Pathol 16: 79–86

89. Patsner B, Baker DA, Orr JW (1990) Human papillomavirus genital tract infections during pregnancy. Clin Obstet Gynecol 33: 258–267

90. Pereira LH, Embil JA, Haase DA, et al (1990) Cytomegalovirus infection among women attending a sexually transmitted disease clinic: Association with clinical symptoms and other sexually transmitted diseases. Am J Epidemiol 131: 683–692

91. Proppe KH, Scully RE, Rosai J (1984) Postoperative spindle cell nodules of genitourinary tract resembling sarcomas. A report of eight cases. Am J Surg Pathol 8: 101–108

92. Purola E, Paavonen JA (1982) Routine cytology as a diagnostic acid in chlamydial cervicitis. Scand J Infect Dis B345: 55

93. Purtilo DT (1974) Defective immune surveillance in viral carcinogenesis. Lab Invest 51: 373–385

94. Quick CA, Watts SL, Krzyzek RA, et al (1980) Relationship between condylomata and laryngeal papillomata. Ann Otol 89: 467–471

95. Richart RM (1973) Cervical intraepithelial neoplasia. In: Sommers SC (ed) Pathology annual. New York, Appleton-Century-Crofts, pp 301–328

96. Richter GA, Pratt JH, Nicolas DR, et al (1972) Actinomycosis of the female genital organs. Minn Med 55: 1003

97. Ridley JH (1968) The histogenesis of endometriosis. A review of facts and fancies. Obstet Gynecol Surv 23: 1

98. Rilke F, Cantaboni A (1964) Lipomas of the uterus. Presentation of 2 cases and review of the recent literature. Ann Obstet Gynecol 86: 646

99. Robboy SJ, Welch WR (1977) Microglandular hyperplasia in vaginal adenosis associated with oral contraceptives and prenatal diethylstilbestrol exposure. Obstet Gynecol 49: 430–434

100. Roth E, Taylor HB (1966) Heterotopic cartilage in the uterus. Obstet Gynecol 27: 838

101. Schacter J (1978) Chlamydial infections. N Engl J Med 298: 490–495

102. Schacter J (1984) Biology of *Chlamydia trachomatis*. In: Holmes KK, Mandh PA, Sparling PF, Weisner PJ (eds) Sexually transmitted diseases. New York: McGraw-Hill Book Co, pp 243–257

103. Schacter J, Stoner E, Moncada J (1983) Screening for chlamydial infections in women attending family planning clinics. West J Med 138: 375

104. Schaefer G (1970) Tuberculosis of female genital tract. Clin Obstet Gynecol 13: 965–998

105. Schwartz DA (1984) Carcinoma of the uterine cervix and schistosomiasis in West Africa. Gynecol Oncol 19: 365–370

106. Segal GH, Hart WR (1990) Cystic endocervical tunnel clusters. A clinicopathologic study of 29 cases of so-called adenomatous hyperplasia. Am J Surg Pathol 14:895–903

107. Selzer F, Nelson HM (1982) Benign papilloma (polypoid tumor) of the cervix uteri in children: Report of two cases. Am J Obstet Gynecol 84: 165

108. Sfameni SF, Ostor AG, Chanen W, et al (1986) The association between vulvar condylomata acuminata, cervical wart virus infection and cervical intraepithelial neoplasia. Aust NZ J Obstet Gynecol 26: 149–151

109. Shafer MA, Chen WKL, Kromhout LK, et al (1985) Chlamydial endocervical infections and cytologic findings in sexually active female adolescents. Am J Obstet Gynecol 151: 765–771

110. Sherrick JC, Vega JG (1962) Congenital intramural cysts of the uterus. Obstet Gynecol 19: 486

111. Slavutin L (1979) Uterine gliosis and ossification. Am J Diag Gynecol Obstet 1: 351

112. Speers WC, Picaso LG, Silverberg SG (1983) Immunohistochemical localization of carcinoembryonic antigen in microglandular hyperplasia and adenocarcinoma of the endocervix. Am J Clin Pathol 79: 105–107

113. Stamm WE, Holmes KK (1984) *Chlamydia trachomatis* infections of the adult. In: Holmes KK, Mardh PA, Sparling PF, Weisner PJ (eds) Sexually transmitted diseases. New York, McGraw-Hill Book Co, pp 258–269

114. Steeper TA, Wick MR (1986) Minimal deviation adenocarcinoma of the uterine cervix ("adenoma malignum"). An immunohistochemical comparison with microglandular endocervical hyperplasia and conventional adenocarcinoma. Cancer 58: 1131–1138

115. Stein BJ, Siciliano A (1966) Necrotizing herpes simplex viral infection of the cervix during pregnancy: Mimic of squamous cell carcinoma. Am J Obstet Gynecol 94: 249

116. Steinberg BM, Topp WC, Schneider PS, et al (1983) Laryngeal papillomavirus infection during clinical remission. N Engl J Med 308: 1261–1264

117. Stout AP (1943) Hemangioendothelioma: A tumor of blood

vessels featuring vascular endothelial cells. Ann Surg 118: 445

118. Suh K-S, Silverberg SG (1990) Tubal metaplasia of the uterine cervix. Int J Gynecol Pathol 9: 122–128

119. Taylor HB, Irey NS, Norris HJ (1967) Atypical endocervical hyperplasia in women taking oral contraceptives. JAMA 202: 637

120. Tchertkoff V, Ober WB (1066) Primary chancre of the cervix uteri. N Y State J Med 66: 1921

121. Tsukada Y, Piver MS, Barlow JT (1977) Microglandular hyperplasia of the endocervix following long-term estrogen treatment. Am J Obstet Gynecol 127: 888–889

122. Vellios F, Ng ABP, Reagan JW (1973) Papillary adenofibroma of the uterus. A benign mesodermal mixed tumor of mullerian origin. Am J Clin Pathol 60: 543–551

123. Wagner EK (1974) The replication of herpesviruses. Am Sci 62: 584–593

124. Westrom L, Mardh PA (1972) Genital chlamydial infections in the female. In: Mardh PA, Holmes KK, Oriel JD (eds) Chlamydial infections. New York, Elsevier, pp 121–141

125. Wilbanks GD, Carter B (1963) Vaginitis emphysematosa. Obstet Gynecol 22: 301

126. Wilkinson E, Dufour DR (1976) Pathogenesis of microglandular hyperplasia of the cervix uteri. Obstet Gynecol 47: 189–195

127. Willis RA (1962) The borderland of embryology and pathology, 2nd ed. Washington, D.C., Butterworths

128. Winkler B, Crum CP (1986) *Chlamydia trachomatis* infection of the female genital tract: Pathogenetic and clinicopathologic considerations. In: Sommers SC, Fechner RE, Rosen PP (eds) Pathology annual. Norwalk, CT, Appleton-Century-Crofts

129. Winkler B, Richart RM (1985) Cervical/uterine pathologic considerations in pelvic infection. In: Zatuchni GI, Goldsmith A, Sciarra JJ (eds) Intrauterine contraception: Advances and future prospects. New York, Harper & Row, pp 438–449

130. Young RH, Clement PB (1991) Pseudoneoplastic glandular lesions of the uterine cervix. 8: 234–249

131. Young RH, Harris NL, Scully RE (1985) Lymphoma-like lesions of the lower female genital tract: A report of 16 cases. Int J Gynecol Pathol 4: 289–299

132. Young RH, Kurman RJ, Scully RE (1988) Proliferations and tumors of intermediate trophoblast of the placental site. Semin Diagn Pathol 5: 223–237

133. Young RH, Scully RE (1989) Atypical forms of microglandular hyperplasia of the cervix simulating carcinoma. Am J Surg Pathol 13: 50–56

7

Precancerous Lesions of the Cervix

Thomas C. Wright, M.D., Robert J. Kurman, M.D., and Alex Ferenczy, M.D.

Precursors of Squamous Cell Carcinoma

Terminology and Historical Perspective

The histopathological classification of a disease should reflect both current concepts of its pathogenesis as well as its clinical behavior. Over the last 50 years our understanding of the pathobiology and behavior of cervical cancer precursors has evolved considerably. As a result, the terminology used to classify preinvasive lesions of the cervix has frequently changed.[40] Although these changes in nomenclature and the resulting lack of a uniform terminology have been an ongoing source of confusion to both gynecologists and pathologists, each change has actually reduced the number of specific pathological categories and has made clinical decision-making more straightforward.

The existence of precursor lesions for invasive cervical cancer has been recognized for more than 50 years. As early as 1886, Sir John Williams commented on the presence of noninvasive epithelial abnormalities adjacent to invasive squamous cell carcinomas of the cervix.[387] The spatial relationships and histological appearance of these noninvasive epithelial lesions were better described by Cullen in 1900, who recognized that these intraepithelial lesions histologically resembled the adjacent invasive cancers.[73,313] In the 1930s, Broders reintroduced the term *carcinoma in situ* that was first used by Schottlander and Kermauner to refer to these intraepithelial cervical lesions.[36,192] A temporal relationship between carcinoma in situ and invasive cancer was subsequently reported by Smith and Pemberton, who diagnosed carcinoma in situ in several patients months to years before the development of invasive cervical cancer.[268,343] The recognition that there was both a spatial and temporal relationship between carcinoma in situ and invasive squamous cell carcinoma led to the hypothesis that invasive squamous cell carcinoma develops from a histologically well-defined precursor lesion.[36,323] This hypothesis was subsequently substantiated by long-term follow-up studies, which clearly demonstrated that a significant proportion of untreated patients with carcinoma in situ will subsequently develop invasive squamous cell carcinoma.[188,193]

Once it was accepted that carcinoma in situ was a precursor to invasive squamous cell carcinoma, population-based cytological screening programs were begun to detect and treat precursor lesions before the actual development of cancer. As large numbers of women began to be screened for cervical disease, it became apparent that many women had cervical epithelial abnormalities that were cytologically/histologically less severe than carcinoma in situ. These lesions formed a histological spectrum that ranged from lesions in which the majority of the cells had the cytological features of carcinoma in situ to those in which the degree of atypicality was much less. In 1956 Reagan and co-workers introduced the term *dysplasia* to refer to this spectrum of cervical abnormalities with features intermediate between those of carcinoma in situ and normal cervical epithelium.[283] Dysplasia actually means "abnormality of development," and was used by Reagan to refer to a proliferation of abnormal squamous epithelial cells that superficially resemble those of the basal layer but that have nuclear atypia, nuclear enlargement with resulting changes in the nuclear-cytoplasmic ratio, and a disorganized arrangement or loss of normal polarity. Depending on the extent to which the thickness of the epithelium displayed these changes, dysplasia was subclassified as mild, moderate, or severe. This classification was thought to reflect the biological potential of the lesions for progressing to carcinoma in situ and, eventually, invasive squamous cell carcinoma of the cervix.

In 1961, at the First International Congress on Exfoliative Cytology, the Committee on Histological Terminology for Lesions of the Uterus Cervix defined carcinoma in situ as follows: "Only those cases should be classified as carcinoma in situ which, in the absence of invasion, show a surface lining epithelium in which, throughout its whole thickness, no differentiation takes place. The process may involve the lining of the cervical glands." It is recognized that the cells of uppermost layers may show some slight flattening. The very rare case of an otherwise characteristic carcinoma in situ that shows a greater degree of differentiation belongs to the exceptions for which no classification can provide. Dysplasia of the cervix was defined as ". . . all other (than carcinoma in situ) disturbances of differentiation of the squamous epithelial lining of surface and glands . . . They may be characterized as of high or low degree, terms which are preferable to suspicious and nonsuspicious, as the proposed terms describe the histological appearance and do not express an opinion."[379] Therefore, the key distinguishing feature of dysplasia was that the atypical cells did not extend through the full thickness of the epithelium or invade the basement membrane. Although most clinicians used the term dysplasia, occasionally, lesions with this histology were termed *basal cell hyperplasia* or *atypical hyperplasia*. In the cytological nomenclature, dysplasia was considered to be a benign to possibly malignant squamous epithelial atypia, whereas carcinoma in situ was designated as positive for malignant cells.

The separation of noninvasive cervical lesions into two groups, dysplasia and carcinoma in situ, implied that there was a biologic distinction between these two entities and that the two could be reproducibly distinguished from each other. In most centers dysplasia was considered to be a potentially reversible process and therefore was either ignored, followed, or treated depending on a variety of clinical factors whereas carcinoma in situ was considered to be

a highly significant lesion and patients with this diagnosis usually were treated with hysterectomy. This classification of noninvasive precursor lesions into dysplastic and carcinoma in situ lesions was based solely on arbitrary histological differences that often were quite subtle.[41,191] For example, the diagnosis of severe dysplasia as opposed to carcinoma in situ was based on the presence of a single layer of flattened epithelial cells on the surface of the lesion and, based on the appearance of this single layer of cells, a patient might be treated either conservatively or by hysterectomy. In the 1960s several studies of inter-and intraobserver variability of histological diagnosis demonstrated that pathologists could not reproducibly distinguish between severe dysplasia and carcinoma in situ.[63,180,339] This called into question the justification of basing marked differences in clinical management solely on subjective histological criteria.[296]

Subsequently, a number of studies in the late 1960s suggested that the cellular changes of dysplasia and carcinoma in situ were qualitatively similar and remained constant throughout the histological spectrum.[296] Both dysplasia and carcinoma in situ were found to be monoclonal proliferations of abnormal squamous epithelial cells with an aneuploid nuclear DNA content.[115,116,295] Quantitative differences in the extent of maturation and variable rates of cell cycle turnover were considered to be evidence of differing degrees of differentiation, but to be of limited value in clinical management.[301] On the basis of these descriptive biologic studies, Richart introduced the concept that all types of precursor lesions to squamous cell carcinoma of cervix represented a single disease process, which he termed *cervical intraepithelial neoplasia* (CIN).[296,294]

The CIN terminology divided cervical cancer precursors into three groups. CIN 1 corresponded to lesions previously diagnosed as mild dysplasia, CIN 2 corresponded to moderate dysplasia, and CIN 3 to both severe dysplasia and carcinoma in situ, since pathologists could not reproducibly distinguish between the two. At the time of its introduction, CIN was thought to define a spectrum of histological changes that shared a common etiology, biology, and natural history. Furthermore, the diagnostic term CIN implied that such lesions, if untreated, had a significant, albeit individually unknown, risk of developing into invasive carcinoma in the future. As a corollary, it was presumed that when the histological changes of CIN were diagnosed and the lesion adequately treated, the development of invasive cancer could be prevented. Although the CIN terminology allowed lesions to be subdivided into three separate categories, it was anticipated that the use of a unified concept of a single disease process would deemphasize lesion grade as a determinate of clinical management.[40,296]

The CIN terminology provided information that allowed the clinician to manage patients in an appropriate manner, and it became the most widely used histological terminology for cervical cancer precursors. However, over the last decade there has been an explosion of information about the etiology of cervical cancer and its precursor lesions. It is now widely accepted that both invasive squamous cell carcinomas and adenocarcinomas of the cervix as well as their respective precursor lesions are caused, at least in part, by specific types of human papillomavirus (HPV) that infect the anogenital tract.[195,393,402] Unfortunately, the identification of HPV in cervical condyloma, cervical cancer precursor lesions, and invasive carcinomas led to the introduction of a plethora of terms such as *flat condyloma, atypical condyloma, condyloma planum, subclinical papillomavirus infection, koilocytotic atypia, condylomatous atypia*, and *warty atypia*, which caused considerable confusion in the classification of intraepithelial lesions.[23,68,104] More importantly, as our understanding of the pathogenesis of cervical cancer precursors grew, it became clear that the basic premise underlying the CIN terminology is incorrect; the spectrum of histological changes that are referred to as CIN do not represent a single disease process at different stages in its development but instead two distinct biological entities, one a productive viral infection and the other a true neoplastic process confined to the epithelium.

The productive HPV infection of the cervical squamous epithelium is self-limited in most patients and commonly results in a flat lesion and less frequently in an exophytic one (condyloma acuminatum). The flat lesion can be caused by any of the more than 22 different types of HPV that infect the human anogenital tract.° Typically these lesions are diploid or polyploid. Flat lesions in which there is productive viral infection display cytoplasmic cavitation and nuclear abnormalities. These lesions have been designated in the past *koilocytotic atypia, koilocytosis, flat condyloma, mild dysplasia* or *CIN 1*.[104]

The other entity subsumed within the morphologic CIN spectrum is histologically "high grade."[116,113,385] These high-grade lesions frequently are aneuploid and true intraepithelial neoplasia with a potential to progress to invasive squamous cell carcinoma if left untreated. High-grade lesions are composed of proliferating basal-type atypical cells with a high nuclear-cytoplasmic ratio and have been designated *moderate, dysplasia , severe dysplasia, carcinoma in situ*, or *CIN 2* or *CIN 3*. In contrast to low-grade intraepithelial lesions, which are very heterogeneous with regard to associated HPV types, high-grade intraepithelial lesions are associated with only a limited number of high "oncogenic risk" HPV types including HPV 16, 18, and 31.[17,69,109,170,212,216,386] There is a common misconception that low-grade lesions are "viral" whereas high-grade lesions are not. The prevalence of HPV in both low- and high-grade lesions is similar, approximately 90%. In low-grade lesions viral particles are produced and consequently the virus is infectious, that is, there is productive infection. In high-grade lesions the viral DNA is present but infectious viral particles are rarely produced or are produced in low amounts.

Recently it has been suggested that the terminology used to refer to cervical cancer precursors be changed to reflect better the biologic processes that underlie the histological patterns. One modification has been proposed by Richart, who suggests that the original CIN 1, 2, 3 terminology be abolished and replaced with the terms *low-grade cervical intraepithelial neoplasia (Lo-CIN)* (including lesions previously classified as flat condyloma and CIN 1) and *high-grade cervical intraepithelial neoplasia (Hi-CIN)* (including CIN 2 and 3 lesions).[298,395] Another modification of the terminology has been incorporated into the Bethesda System of cytological diagnosis and uses the terms *low-grade squamous intraepithelial lesion (L-SIL)* for lesions previously classified as koilocytotic atypia and CIN 1 and *high-grade squamous intraepithelial lesion (H-SIL)* for lesions previously called CIN 2 and CIN 3.[1,215] The two terminologies are essentially the same except for the use of "lesion" rather than "neoplasia" in the Bethesda System. There are pros and cons to both and neither is perfect. Specifically, the use of the term *neoplasia* when referring to low-grade lesions is misleading since, for the most part, these are self-limited HPV infections that only rarely progress to invasive squamous cell carcinoma if untreated. *Intraepithelial lesion* better describes these low-grade viral infections than does the term *intraepithelial neoplasia*. Unfortunately, use of the term *lesion* is imprecise when referring to high-grade neoplasia, which is frequently aneuploid and has the potential for progressing to invasive cancer. Use of the term *intraepithelial lesions* to describe the low-grade abnormalities and *intraepithelial neoplasia* when referring to the high-grade precursors would be more precise, but would lead to even further confusion during this transition from a multitier to a two-tier system. Among the several advantages of the two-tier system are that it accurately reflects the biology of the lesions as we currently view it, it can be used for both cytological and histological diagnosis, and it reflects current clinical management, since many clinicians now follow selected patients with low-grade SIL (CIN 1) but treat patients with high-grade SIL (CIN 2, 3). The use of a uniform terminology for both cytological and histological diagnoses should minimize the misunderstanding that inevitably occurs when different terminologies are used for cytological and histological diagnosis. In this chapter the same terms used for histological diagnosis are the same as those used in the Bethesda System for cytological diagnosis, that is, *low-grade squamous intraepithelial lesion* and *high-grade squamous intraepithelial lesion*. Correlations

---

°Refs. 17,69,113,116,170,212,216,385,386.

between this system and the previous terminologies are shown in Table 7.1.

GENERAL FEATURES

Prevalence

SIL (CIN) is predominantly a disease of women in their reproductive years, with a large population impact and risk factors characteristic of a sexually transmitted disease (STD). An accurate estimate of the prevalence of SIL (CIN) in the United States is not available. This is caused by many factors, which include (1) SIL (CIN) is not a reportable disease, (2) different data sets use incompatible classifications of cancer precursors and therefore are not comparable, (3) apparent prevalence rates are dependent on the extent to which a population is screened, and (4) the prevalence rate in a specific population will be dependent on the prevalence of other causative factors for cervical neoplasia. Nonetheless, it is clear from a variety of sources that cytological evidence of SIL (CIN) is much more common than overt genital condyloma acuminata. Cytological screening of attendees at Planned Parenthood Clinics Nationwide between 1981 and 1983 detected cytological evidence of SIL (CIN) in 2.3% of all patients.[316] CIN 1 and 2 were detected in 2.2% of all smears, whereas CIN 3 was detected in only 0.2% of the smears. The prevalence of CIN in this particular population decreased with increasing age. The prevalence of CIN 1 and 2 peaked at 2.6% in women 25–29 years of age and decreased to 0.9% in women over the age of 50 years. The peak prevalence of CIN 3 was 0.5% and occurred in smears from women 35–39 years old. A similar age dependency but a higher prevalence of low-grade SIL (CIN 1) has been reported in a recent Canadian study.[230] In the Canadian study, cytological changes suggestive of HPV infection (equivalent to low-grade SIL) were detected in 6% of smears from women 20–24 years old and in 2.6% from women over 34 years old. Better estimates of the prevalence of cervical disease can be obtained from large, population-based surveys. Unfortunately, only a few such studies are available. One recent, population-based survey of women in a socioeconomically deprived region of Kentucky reported an average, annual, age-adjusted incidence rate of 195 per

100,000 women for all grades of "dysplasia" and 38 per 100,000 women for carcinoma in situ.[112] Estimates of the prevalence of CIN 3 in the United States as a whole can be obtained from the Surveillance, Epidemiology, and End Results (SEER) Program which is a population-based tumor registry that accrues data from several locations in the United States. Although the SEER data set probably underestimates the true prevalence of CIN 3 since not all centers report both severe "dysplasia" and carcinoma in situ, this is the best data available at the national level. According to the SEER data set, the average annual age-adjusted incidence rate per 100,000 females for CIN 3 in 1986–1987 was 31.5 for white females and 31.2 for black females.[112]

The clinical scope and epidemiology of SIL (CIN) has undergone dramatic changes over the past few decades. SIL (CIN) appears to be becoming increasingly common. A review of cervical smears over a 10-year period at one medical center from southern Australia found that the prevalence of cytological evidence of low-grade SIL (CIN 1) increased from 0.6% in 1978 to 5.6% in 1988.[93] The mean age at diagnosis of high-grade SIL (CIN 2, 3) is decreasing, as both the incidence and prevalence of high-grade SIL (CIN 2, 3) increase in teenagers and women under 30.[3,10,19,304,315] In studies from the 1950s, dysplasia was rarely documented in women younger than 25 years and the mean age of patients with CIN 3 ranged between 35 and 40.[62,267] Cytological evidence of high-grade SIL (CIN 2, 3) can now be found in women under the age of 15 years and the age-specific incidence for CIN 3 currently peaks in the 25–29-year-old group and decreases with advancing age thereafter.[321] The prevalence of low-grade SIL (CIN 1) and high-grade SIL (CIN 2, 3) combined in teenagers and young adults aged 15–19 years is 18.8 per 1000.[315] Similarly, studies of Jewish Israeli women have indicated a substantial increase in the incidence of CIN and invasive cervical cancer in that population,[11,355] historically at low risk for the development of cervical malignancy.[362] The incidence of cervical cancer in all ages of Israeli-born Jewish women rose from 2.7/100,000 in 1960–1966 to 4.6/100,000 in 1972–1976.[11,355] These epidemiologic changes have been attributed to changes in sexual behavior patterns and corroborate previous epidemiologic data suggesting a direct causal relationship between sexual activity and the pathogenesis of cervical neoplasia. They also underscore the importance of performing cytological screening in sexually active teenagers.

Etiology

Epidemiologic studies have identified a number of possible risk factors for the development of both cervical cancer and its precursor lesions, which include early age at first intercourse, age at first pregnancy, number of sexual partners, a history of cigarette smoking, oral contraceptive use,

Table 7.1. Terminologies for cervical cancer precursor lesions

WHO/ISGYP[a] classification	Bethesda System terminology
Mild dysplasia (CIN 1)	Low-grade squamous intraepithelial lesion
Moderate dysplasia (CIN 2)	High-grade squamous intraepithelial lesion
Severe dysplasia/carcinoma in situ (CIN 3)	

[a] World Health Organization and International Society of Gynecological Pathologists.

Table 7.2. Risk factors associated with SIL (CIN) in various epidemiologic studies

Sexual activity
    Number of sexual partners
    Early sexual activity (especially less than 16 years of age)
Sexually transmitted diseases
    Human papillomavirus
    Herpes simplex virus
Early age of first pregnancy
Parity
Low socioeconomic class
Cigarette smoking
Human immunodeficiency virus
Immunosuppression from any cause
Vitamin deficiencies
Interval since last Pap smear
Oral contraceptive use

SIL, squamous intraepithelial lesion; CIN, cervical intraepithelial neoplasia.

socioeconomic class, interval since the last Pap smear, a history of abnormal Pap smears, parity, nutritional variables, immunosuppression, and infection with either herpes simplex virus Type 2 or specific types of human papillomavirus (i.e., types 16 and 18) (Table 7.2).[*] Although the risk factors for cervical cancer and its precursors are similar, the strength of association between these risk factors and cervical cancer is generally stronger than the strength of association between the risk factors and SIL (CIN). The two major independent risk factors in recent case control studies of cervical cancer precursors have been lifetime number of sexual partners and a history of cigarette smoking.[166,266] Some studies, but not others, have identified early sexual activity during the period of active development of the cervical transformation zone to be an important risk factor.[141,166,266] There also are many co-variables that are believed to be secondarily related to the incidence of cervical carcinoma because they are a common feature of the population that has early, multiple sexual contacts.

The concept that cervical cancer (and presumably its precursors) is a sexually transmitted disease is further substantiated by the epidemiologic characterization of the high-risk male. These studies document the relevance of the male partner's sexual history in determining a woman's risk for the development of cervical carcinoma and support the concept that a transmissible agent is responsible, in part, for the pathogenesis of cervical cancer.[†] Historically, a variety of sexually transmitted pathogens including *Chlamydia trachomatis, Neisseria gonorrhoeae, Gardnerella vaginalis, Mycoplasma hominis, Trichomonas vagina-*

[*]Refs. 7,32,34,35,82,107,131,132,147,149,166,176, 178,203,264,326,332,372,374.
[†]Refs. 33,47,49,130,177,178,185,218,341,344,362.

lis, and cytomegalovirus have been proposed as being the etiologic agent for cervical cancer. However other studies, including a large case-control study, of the prevalence of these pathogens in women with cervical cancer precursors have found that none are present more frequently in patients than in controls when analyzed independently of sexual activity. Therefore, the associations of infections by these particular pathogens with cervical cancer and its precursors seem to characterize the sexual history of the population at risk rather than playing an etiologic role themselves.[51,137,195,374] Over the past 15 years attention has focused on HPV as the primary etiologic agent in the multifactorial pathogenesis of cervical cancer.

HUMAN PAPILLOMAVIRUSES

In the late 1970s, zur Hausen suggested that there might be an association between HPV and cervical cancer.[400] Many epidemiologic, clinicopathologic, and molecular studies have subsequently linked the presence of specific types of HPV to the development of anogenital cancers and their precursors and there is little doubt that HPVs play a central, if not critical, role in the pathogenesis of most cervical cancers and their precursor lesions.[321,393,402] Koss and Durfee coined the term *koilocytotic atypia* in 1956 to describe abnormal squamous epithelial cells that were characterized by prominent perinuclear vacuolizaton (koilocytes) and were detected in Pap smears of patients with dysplasia and invasive carcinoma.[190] In 1976 both Meisels and co-workers as well as Purola and Savia published papers suggesting that the cells in condyloma acuminata that contained viral particles compatible with HPV by electron microscopy were cytologically identical to the "koilocytes" that had been described by Koss and Durfee.[231,280] Soon after this, several groups detected viral particles using electron microscopy or HPV capsid proteins using immunohistochemistry in low-grade SIL (CIN 1) (Fig. 7.1).[202,199,208] With the application of molecular techniques to the study of cervical disease, rapid progress was made in understanding the relationships between HPV and cervical cancer in the mid-1980s. Several groups of investigators demonstrated that specific types of HPV DNA could be identified by Southern blot hybridization in most invasive squamous cell carcinomas of the cervix and a substantial number of cervical cancer precursors.[90,125,126,127] Shortly thereafter, HPV DNA was isolated in tissues from metastatic cervical carcinoma[207] and in tumor cell lines established from cervical carcinoma, indicating that the HPV was an integral component of the tumors.[28] Since these initial studies, similar findings have been reported from numerous laboratories throughout the world and more than 22 types of HPV capable of infecting the anogenital tract have been isolated and characterized.[78]

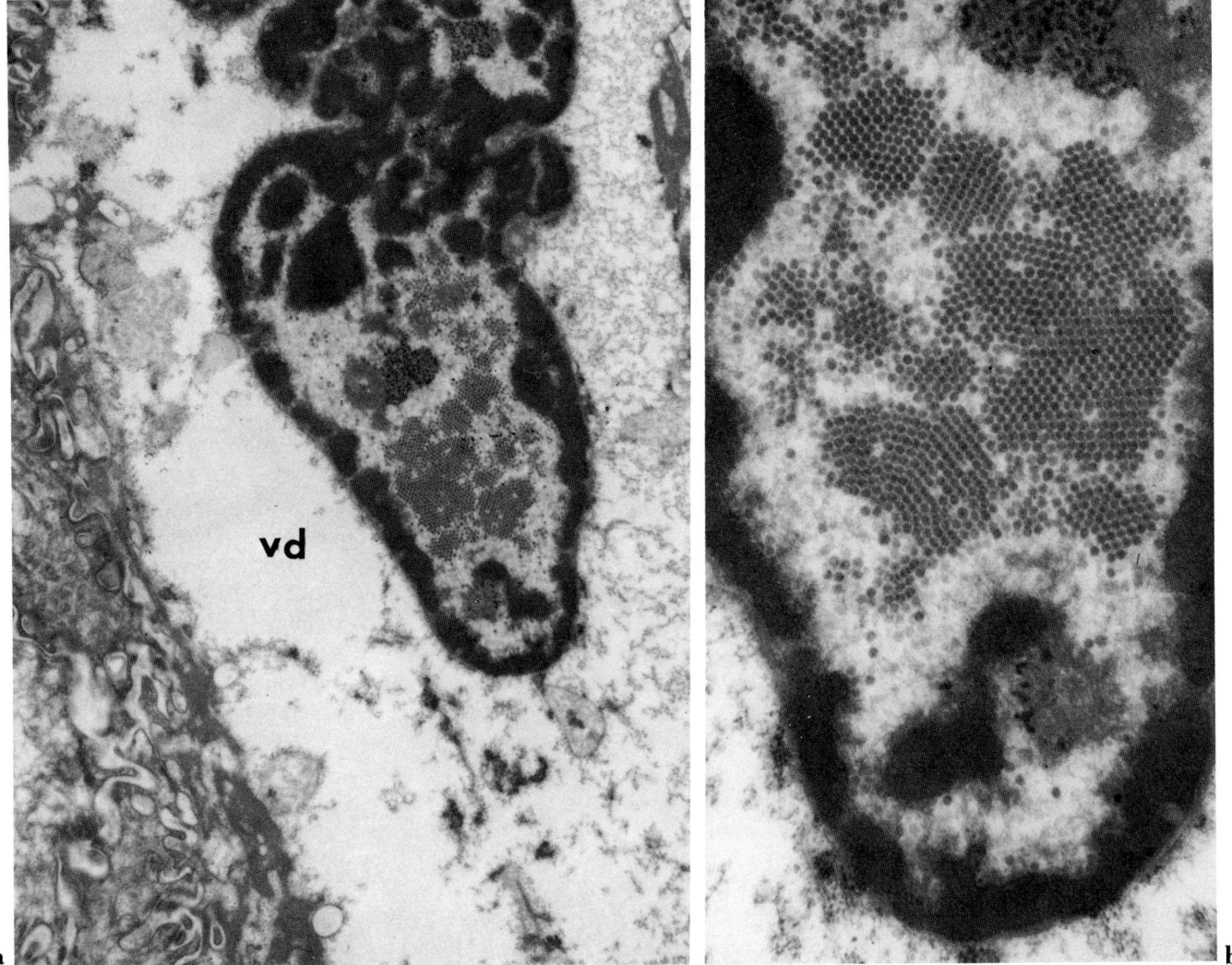

FIG. 7.1. HPV-infected cells. Electron microscopy of cells productively infected with HPV. **a:** There are intranuclear aggregates of HPV in a koilocytotic, superficial cell of a low-grade SIL (CIN 1). The marginated nuclear chromatin is agglutinated, and the cytoplasmic substance displays vacuolar degeneration (*vd*). The latter corresponds to koilocytotic ballooning on light microscopy. **b:** Higher magnification of HPV particles in the nucleus.

Classification of HPV and Association with Specific Types of Anogenital Lesions

Papillomaviruses are classified as members of the family Papovaviridae, which includes Simian virus 40 (SV40) and polyoma virus as well as the papillomaviruses. All members of Papovaviridae are DNA tumor viruses that are dissimilar at the DNA level and lack shared antigens but have similar biologic effects on their hosts.[124,152,271,272,401] Papillomaviruses are characterized by a double-stranded DNA genome of approximately 8000 base pairs in length, a nonenveloped virion that measures 45–55 nm in diameter, and an icosahedral capsid. Papillomaviruses are widely distributed throughout nature. There are bovine, canine, avian, rabbit, deer, and human papillomaviruses. They are all highly species specific: viruses that infect one species do not infect other species. Papillomaviruses are classified on the basis of the species that they infect and the relatedness of their genomes as determined by DNA hybridization.[56,153]

Papillomaviruses are epitheliotrophic viruses that predominantly infect skin and mucous membranes and produce characteristic epithelial proliferations at the sites of infection.[37,38,271,272,273] These benign epithelial proliferations or papillomas have the capacity to undergo malignant transformation under certain circumstances. Examples of this in animals include the papillomas induced in domestic rabbits by the cottontail rabbit papillomavirus (CRPV), which can progress to invasive squamous cell carcinomas when treated with topical applications of methylcholantrene and alimentary tract papillomas induced in cattle by bovine papillomavirus (BPV), which undergo malignant transformation when the animals eat radiomimetic bracken ferns.[159,197,256,338] In humans, HPV infections occur on the skin and mucous membranes, in the conjunctiva, oral cavity, larynx, tracheobronchial tree, esophagus, bladder, anus, and genital tract of both sexes. HPVs appear to be fastidious in their growth requirements and replicate only in the nucleus of infected cells. Because of their fastidiousness, only limited success has been achieved in obtaining viral replication in model systems.[198]

In addition to being species specific, papillomaviruses are also relatively tissue and site specific.[64,78,135,136,271,272] For example, HPV 1 preferentially infects the stratified squamous epithelium of the sole of the foot and produces plantar warts (verruca plantaris), whereas HPV 2 and 4 preferentially infect the stratified epithelium of the fingers to produce common warts termed verruca vulgaris. Other types such as 6 and 11 almost exclusively infect the stratified epithelium of mucosal surfaces of the oral and anogenital tract and produce condyloma acuminata and laryngeal papillomatosis.[125,126] Unlike many other viruses in which specific viral isolates have capsid proteins with different antigenic structures, the capsid proteins of papillomavirus are highly conserved and antibodies directed against BPV capsid proteins cross-react with human papillomaviruses.[163,200] Therefore, specific types of HPV cannot be identified serologically (serotypes) and DNA sequence is used to identify different viral types (genotypes). A papillomavirus isolate is considered to be a new type and given a sequential number if its DNA is less than 50% homologous with the DNA of other known isolates from the same species as determined by DNA hybridization.[56]

To date, more than 60 types of HPV have been isolated.[78] These viruses can be divided into three general groups (Table 7.3). A mucocutaneous group contains types that infect the skin and the oral epithelium. Another group includes viruses isolated from patients with epidermodysplasia verruciformis, a rare, genetic disorder of cellular immunity in which patients frequently develop HPV associated skin lesions that can progress to invasive squamous cell carcinomas when exposed to the sun.[257-259,261] The third group of more than 22 types of HPV infects the anogenital tract. These target cell associations are not absolute, however, and some cutaneous HPVs such as type 2 also can infect mucosal epithelium and HPV 16, which is considered to be a genital-type HPV, has been found in association with squamous cell carcinomas of the conjunctiva and subungual region.[150,224,225,243] The specific associations of 17 of the anogenital HPV types are shown in Table 7.3.

Table 7.3. Classification of human papillomaviruses (HPV)

HPV Type	Lesion
Mucocutaneous Group	
1	Verruca plantaris
2	Verruca vulgaris
	Verruca plantaris
3	Verruca plana
4	Verruca vulgaris
	Verruca plantaris
7	Butcher's warts
10	Verruca plana
13	Focal epithelial hyperplasia
28	Verruca plana
29	Verruca vulgaris
32	Focal epithelial hyperplasia
38	Verruca vulgaris
41	Squamous carcinoma
Epidermodysplasia Verruciformis Group	
5, 8, 9, 12, 15, 17, 19–21, 23–25, 36, 46, 47	Macular warts
Genital (Cervical) Group	
6, 11	Condyloma acuminatum; Low-grade SIL (CIN 1)
16	All grades of SIL; Squamous cell carcinoma;
18	All grades of SIL; Adeno- and squamous cell carcinoma
30	All grades of SIL
31, 33, 35, 39	All grades of SIL; Squamous cell carcinoma
40	All grades of SIL
42, 43, 44	Low-grade SIL (CIN 1)
45	All grades of SIL; Squamous cell carcinoma
51, 52, 56	All grades of SIL; Squamous cell carcinoma

Modified from ref. 78.
SIL, squamous intraepithelial lesion; CIN, cervical intraepithelial neoplasia.

Based on their associations with specific types of lesions, the most prevalent anogenital HPVs have been divided into three "oncogenic risk" groups (Table 7.4).[212,213,288] The low oncogenic risk group includes HPVs 6 and 11. These viruses are considered to be of low oncogenic risk since they usually are associated with condyloma acuminata of the anogenital tract and occasionally associated with low-grade SIL (CIN 1) but only rarely associated with high-grade SIL (CIN 2, 3) and almost never associated with invasive squamous cell carcinomas of the cervix. HPVs 42, 43, and 44 are included in the low oncogenic risk viruses because they have the same distribution as HPVs 6 and 11. The intermediate oncogenic risk HPVs frequently are associated with all grades of SIL (CIN), but only infrequently with invasive cancers. This group includes types 31, 33, 35, 51, and 52. The high oncogenic risk HPVs are

Table 7.4. Oncogenic-risk grouping of anogenital human papillomavirus.

Low oncogenic risk: 6, 11, 42, 43, 44
Intermediate oncogenic risk: 31, 33, 35, 51, 52
High oncogenic risk: 16, 18, 45, 56

types 16, 18, 45, and 56. These are considered high oncogenic risk viruses because they are the type most frequently associated with invasive squamous cell carcinomas of the anogenital tract.

The clinical significance of grouping HPV types into three oncogenic risk groups has not yet been realized. When this grouping originally was proposed, it was anticipated that histology would predict HPV type and that low-grade SIL (CIN 1) lesions of the cervix usually would be associated with low oncogenic-risk HPVs.[70,213] However, it is now known that low-grade SIL (CIN 1) lesions are extremely heterogeneous with regard to their associated HPV types. A study by Lungu et al. that used polymerase chain reaction (PCR) to detect and type HPV DNA in 278 cervical biopsies from SIL (CIN) lesions of all grades found that 22% of low-grade SIL (CIN 1) were associated with multiple HPV types (Table 7.5).[216] Only 15% of low-grade SIL (CIN 1) were associated with low oncogenic risk HPVs (6, 11, 42, 43, and 44), 19% were associated with unknown or "novel" HPV types, and 29% with HPV 16, 18

and 33. Similar results have been reported by Willet et al. and by Bergeron et al., who used high stringency Southern blots with a large number of type-specific probes to type 188 cervical biopsies (Table 7.5).[17,386] In Bergeron's study, low oncogenic risk HPV types were very infrequently associated with low-grade SIL (CIN 1). HPV 16 and 18 were detected in 25% of the low-grade SIL (CIN 1), novel HPV types in 25%, and multiple types in 9%. These studies clearly indicate that histology does not correlate with HPV type for low-grade SIL (CIN 1).

In contrast, there is a much closer correlation between histology and associated HPV type in high-grade SIL (CIN 2, 3) (Table 7.6). In the PCR study of Lungu et al., only 7% of high-grade SIL (CIN 2, 3) contained more than one HPV type and 88% were associated with HPV types 16, 18, or 33.[216] Similar results were reported by Willet et al. and by Franquemont et al., who used in situ hybridization to type HPV and detected HPV 16 in more than 70% of high-grade SIL (CIN 2, 3).[109,386] Bergeron et al. detected HPV 16 and 18 in 61% of high-grade SIL (CIN 2, 3) using high stringency Southern blot hybridization.[17]

Genomic Organization of HPV

The genomic organization of the different types of HPV appears to be similar (Fig. 7.2)[37,38] (see Chapter 28, Molecular Biology). The viral genome can be divided into three regions: the upstream regulatory region (URR), the early region, and the late region.[333] The URR is a noncod-

Table 7.5. Human papillomavirus (HPV) types associated with low-grade SIL (CIN 1)

	Number (%) HPV DNA (+) lesions associated with HPV type						
	6/11	16	18	30s	Others	Novel[a]	Multiple HPV types
Bergeron et al.	0	11 (21)	2 (4)	10 (19)	15 (28)	13 (25)	5 (9)
Lungu et al.	15 (15)	16 (16)	3 (3)	18 (18)	7 (7)	19 (19)	22 (22)
Willet et al.	7 (27)	8 (31)	1 (4)	3 (12)	—	7 (25)	—

[a] "Novel" represents viral types other than those listed in Table 7.3.
Multiple HPV types represent lesions containing more than a single type of HPV.
Modified with permission from refs. 17, 216, 386.
SIL, squamous intraepithelial lesion; CIN, cervical intraepithelial neoplasia.

Table 7.6. Human papillomavirus (HPV) types associated with high-grade SIL (CIN 2, 3)

	Number (%) HPV DNA (+) lesions associated with HPV type						
	6/11	16	18	30s	Others	Novel[a]	Multiple HPV types
Bergeron et al.	0	30 (57)	2 (4)	4 (8)	4 (8)	11 (21)	2 (4)
Franquemont et al.	0	20 (77)	0	0	0	0	0
Lungu et al.	1 (1)	127 (72)	6 (3)	19 (11)	2 (1)	7 (4)	13 (7)
Willet et al.	3 (27)	20 (71)	0	0	—	1 (4)	—

[a] "Novel" represents viral types other than those listed in Table 7.3.
Multiple HPV types represent lesions containing more than a single type of HPV.
Modified from refs. 17, 109, 216, 386.
SIL, squamous intraepithelial lesion; CIN, cervical intraepithelial neoplasia.

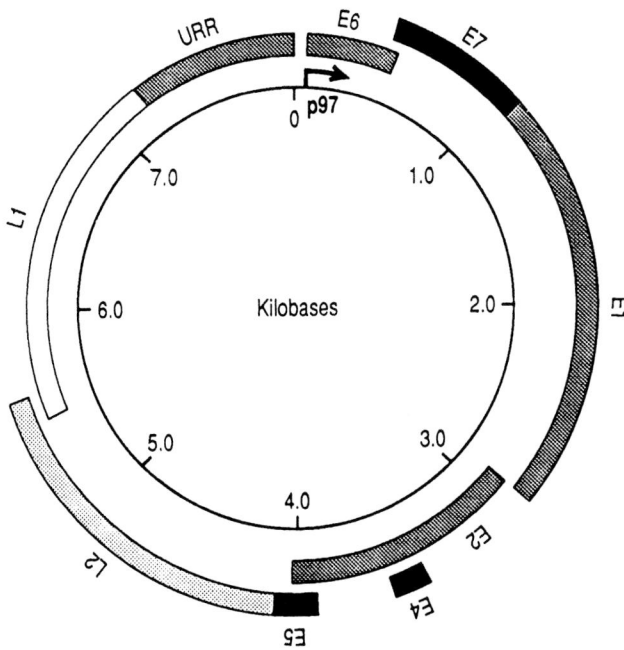

FIG. 7.2. **HPV genome.** HPV is a double-stranded, circular, DNA tumor virus whose genome can be divided into three regions; the upstream regulatory region (*URR*), the early region, and the late region.

ing region of the viral genome that is important in regulating viral replication and transcription of downstream sequences in the early region. Both the early region and the late region contain a series of open reading frames (ORFs), which are regions of the genome lacking stop codons and, therefore, are potentially translatable into proteins. The early region is transcribed early in the viral life cycle (hence its name) and encodes predominantly for proteins that are important in viral replication, whereas the late region encodes for viral structural proteins that are produced late in the viral life cycle.[37,53,71,103,205,217]

The URR is a highly complex regulatory region whose exact functions and role in the life cycle of the virus are still not completely known. This region contains binding sites for various transcription factors including activator protein 1 (AP 1) and a keratinocytic-specific transcription factor 1 (KRF 1) as well as for virally derived transcriptional factors.[219,255] Binding of these and other transcription factors regulates transcription of the early region ORFs.

The early region ORFs encode for proteins required for viral replication and maintenance of a high viral copy number in infected cells.[205,217] The early region also includes the transforming regions of the HPV genome. Six different ORFs, which are designated E1, E2, E4, E5, E6, and E7, have been identified in the early region of HPV.[37] The E2 ORF encodes for two proteins that are DNA binding pro-

teins that regulate transcription.[376] These proteins are important for regulating the expression of the early region ORFs.[20] They act by binding to specific DNA sequences in the URR.[122,123,206,347] One of these transcription regulators is encoded by the entire E2 ORF and transactivates (i.e., stimulates transcription of) the early region, whereas the other E2-encoded transcriptional regulator is smaller, and encodes a protein that transrepresses (i.e., inhibits transcription of) the early region. The E6 and E7 ORFs encode for the major transforming genes of HPV (see below, Transforming Properties). The E5 ORF of HPV encodes a protein with weak transforming activity. The E4 ORF encodes for a series of proteins that appear to be important for maturation of the virus and viral replication.[85–87,263] E4-derived proteins are extremely abundant in lesions such as planter warts, which produce large amounts of virus and may be important in altering the normal cytokeratin matrix of infected cells so as to allow viral particles to be released from the cells.

The late region of HPV contains two ORFs designated L1 and L2, which encode capsid proteins. The L1-encoded protein is the major capsid protein and is highly conserved among papillomaviruses from all species.[276] The L2-encoded protein is a minor capsid protein that is much more variable among viral types.[189] Transcription from the L1 and L2 ORFs occurs as a late event in the viral life cycle at a time when infectious virus is being produced.[103] Transcription from the late region appears to be regulated by cell-derived, transcriptional regulators that are produced only by the differentiated cells of the intermediate and superficial layers of the squamous epithelium. Therefore, large amounts of L1- and L2-encoded capsid proteins can be detected in condyloma acuminata and in low-grade SIL (CIN 1), but these proteins are present in only low amounts in high-grade SIL (CIN 2, 3) or cervical cancers.[103,200]

Life Cycle of HPV

Although the HPV life cycle is not completely characterized, the rough outlines of the process are known (Fig. 7.3).[401,402] The initial site of infection is thought to be either basal cells or primitive "basal-like" cells of the immature squamous epithelium. Following the introduction of the virus into the epithelium, two types of infections can occur. Under one set of conditions, the virus establishes a *latent infection,* which is defined as maintenance of a viral infection without the production of infectious virus.[325] In latent infections viral DNA remains in the nucleus in a free circular form called an *episome.* Replication of the episomal DNA in latent infections is tightly coupled to the replication of the epithelial cells and occurs only in concert with replication of the host cell's chromosomal DNA. Since complete viral particles are presumably not produced in latent infections, the characteristic cytopathic

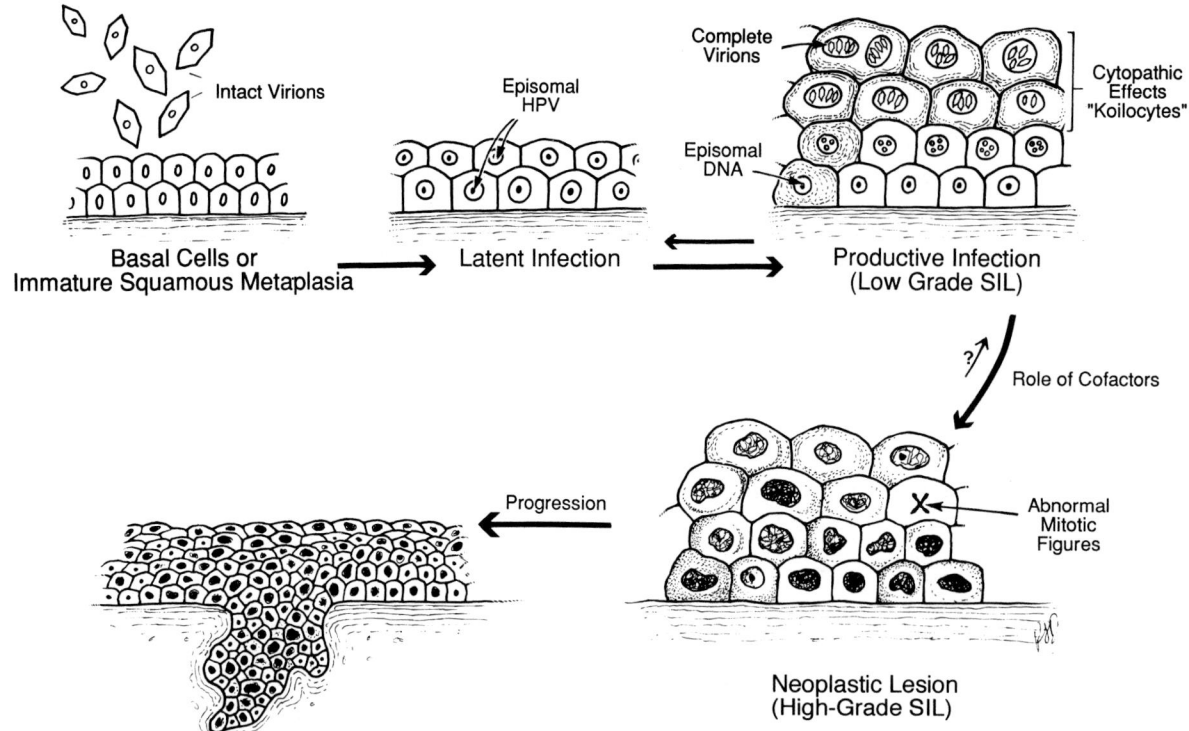

FIG. 7.3. Life cycle of HPV. The first step in an HPV infection is contact of intact virions with basal cells or immature squamous metaplastic cells. This can produce either a latent infection or a productive infection. In a latent infection HPV DNA remains as an episomal form in the nucleus of the infected basal cell. In productive infections, viral replication becomes uncoupled from cellular DNA synthesis and large amounts of viral DNA and proteins are made in the intermediate and superficial cell layers of the epithelium, producing the characteristic cytopathic effects of HPV. During the development of high-grade SIL and invasive squamous cancers, additional cellular and viral events take place resulting in the formation of a "true" cancer precursor. These can include the generation of aneuploid stemlines and integration of HPV DNA into the chromosomal DNA.

effects of a HPV infection are not present and HPV can be identified only by using molecular methods. Latently infected squamous epithelium displays no morphologic abnormality. The other type of infection is a *productive viral infection*. In productive viral infectiions, viral DNA replication occurs independently of host chromosomal DNA synthesis. This independent viral DNA replication produces large amounts of viral DNA and results in infectious virions. Viral DNA replication takes place predominantly in the intermediate and superficial cell layers of the stratified squamous epithelium. As the virally infected epithelial cells mature and move toward the epithelial surface, cell-derived, differentiation-specific transcriptional factors produced by the epithelium stimulate the production of viral capsid proteins. This allows large amounts of intact virions to be formed (Fig. 7.1) and produces the characteristic cytopathic effects of HPV that can be detected cytologically and histologically (Fig. 7.4) in cells from the superficial layers of positively infected epithlium. These cytopathic effects include acanthosis, cytoplasmic vacuolization, nuclear atypia, and multinucleation.

Epidemiologic studies suggest that many women come in contact with anogenital HPVs, presumably through sexual contact (see Table 7.7).[162,164] In many of these women, latent infections develop that can be detected using molecular hybridization techniques, but no clinical or cytological manifestations develop.[14,182,184,240,310] Shedding of sufficient quantities of HPV DNA to be detected with hybridization methods such as dot blots or Southern blot hybridization occurs only transiently in these latently infected women and therefore there is considerable variation in detection of HPV DNA when multiple tests are performed over time.[241] Eventually most of these women spontaneously resolve their infections, as evidenced by the low prevalence of latent HPV infections in women over the age of 35 years.[239] In a small subset of latently infected women, productive infection develops and the patients develop cytological and histological evidence of low-grade SIL (CIN 1). Although the exact factors that regulate the transition from a latent to a productive infection are unknown, immunological factors and viral type probably are important.[110]

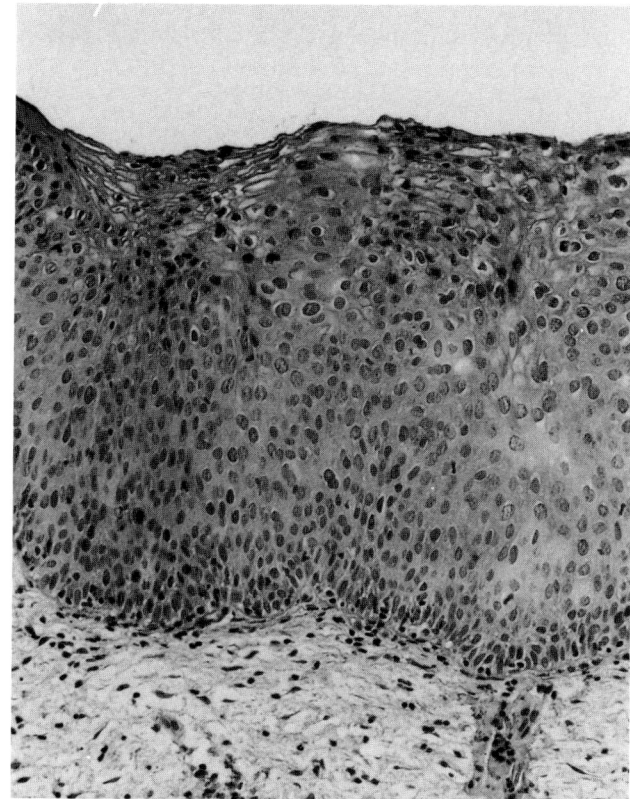 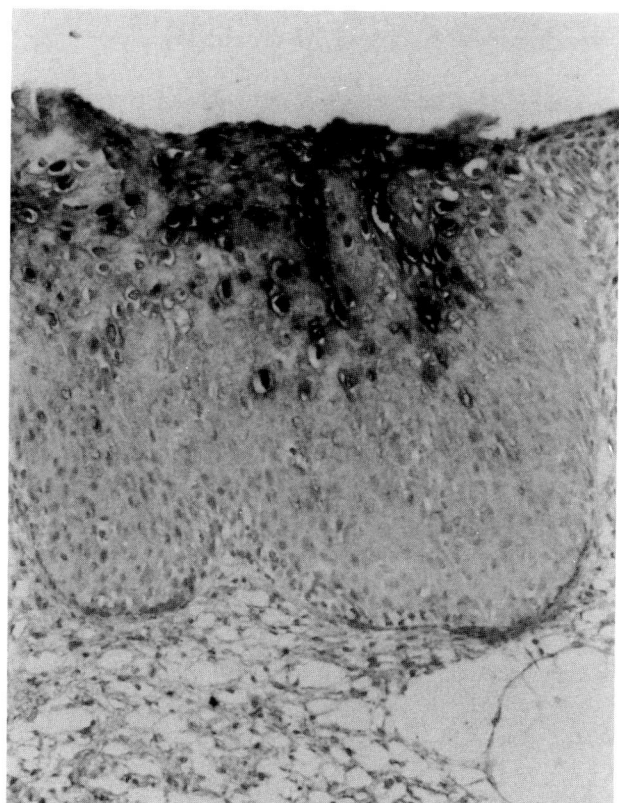

a

b

FIG. 7.4. **Productive HPV infection.** In productive HPV infections large amounts of viral DNA and capsid proteins are produced in the intermediate and superficial cell layers resulting in the characteristic cytopathic effects. **a:** Histological and cytological features of productive HPV infections include acanthosis, cytoplasmic vacuolization, nuclear atypia (koilocytosis), and multinucleation. **b:** In situ hybridization using a probe directed against HPV DNA detects large amounts of viral DNA in the superficial epithelial cells that demonstrate cytopathic effects.

Mechanism of Malignant Transformation

In vitro studies using tissue culture cells have provided insight into the mechanism by which HPV transforms (i.e., induces the properties of malignancy in) the cervical epithelium. The E6 and E7 ORFs represent the principal transforming genes of HPV.[15,16,171,277,345] Expression of the E6 and E7 ORFs from high oncogenic risk HPVs such as 16 and 18 but not of low "oncogenic risk" HPVs such as 6 and 11 in established tissue culture cell lines causes the cells to become completely transformed.[16,171,274] A high efficiency of transformation of these already immortalized (i.e., have already have acquired an infinite lifespan in culture) tissue culture cell lines requires that both E6 and E7 be present. The two viral genes complement each other and are only weakly active when introduced alone. In addi-

Table 7.7. Prevalence of cervical HPVs in the general population

Author, year	Country	Method	HPV types probed for	% HPV (+)
Bauer et al., 1991	United States	PCR	All anogenital	33
		Dot blot	6, 11, 16, 18, 33, 35	7
de Villiers et al., 1987	Germany	FISH	6, 11, 16, 18	10
Kjaer et al., 1988	Denmark	FISH	6, 11, 16, 18	13
	Greenland	FISH	6, 11, 16, 18	9
Kiviat et al., 1989	United States	Dot blot	6, 11, 16, 18, 31	11
van de Brule, 1989	Netherlands	PCR	6, 11, 16, 18, 33	22
		FISH	6, 11, 18, 31, 33	3

Data from refs. 14, 80, 182, 184, 367.
FISH, filter in situ hybridization; PCR, polymerase chain reaction; HPV, human papillomavirus.

tion to having in vitro transforming activity, both E6 and E7 are almost always actively transcribed in cervical cancers, suggesting that the over- or unregulated expression of these genes is required for the maintenance of the transformed malignant phenotype.[328,330,331,397] This has been confirmed by studies demonstrating that inhibition of E6 and E7 expression by antisense mRNA leads to reversion to a nontransformed phenotype.[65] One way overexpression of the E6 and E7 ORFs might occur is through loss of E2 expression. The E2-encoded proteins regulate transcription of the early region, generally repressing E6 and E7 transcription.[376] In low-grade SIL (CIN 1) and in most high-grade SIL (CIN 2, 3), HPV is episomal and the E2 ORF is intact.[72,223] However, in most cancers, the HPV DNA is integrated into the cellular DNA.[72,118,223] Integration occurs in the E1/E2 region, leading to disruption and inactivation of the ORFs. The control of E6 and E7 is therefore lost, resulting in overexpression of E6 and E7, which is important for malignant transformation.

Many insights into how E6 and E7 act to cause transformation are being gathered and are described in detail in Chapter 28, Molecular Biology. In brief, these transforming genes appear to act by disrupting the normal control processes that regulate cellular growth. The E6 protein of HPV 16 binds to and causes the rapid degradation of the p53 protein, which is an important regulator of cellular growth and differentiation[92,102,319,382] and the E7 protein appears to deregulate cell growth by binding to cyclin A, p107, and p105RB (retinoblastoma gene product), which regulate the progression of cells from the G_1 phase of the cell cycle into the S phase.[91,244] This causes the loss of important cellular constraints to cell proliferation, thereby resulting in a loss of growth control.[402]

The above model of cervical cancer pathogenesis based on E2 inactivation secondary to integration with resultant E6 and E7 overexpression is too simplistic and cannot fully explain the development of cervical cancer. For example, even though the vast majority of cervical cancers have HPV DNA integrated into the cellular DNA, in some invasive cancers only episomal HPV DNA is detected.[72,118,223] Likewise, fusion of HPV-associated transformed cervical epithelial cells with nontransformed cells results in the formation of nonmalignant hybrids despite the fact that there is continued overexpression of the E6 and E7 ORFs.[27] In vivo, there is, on average, a 10-year delay between an initial HPV infection and the development of cancer and only a small fraction of the patients exposed to high oncogenic risk HPVs will subsequently develop cancer. In vitro, cultured human epithelial cells expressing the E6 and E7 ORFs are nonmalignant at early passages but become fully malignant at later passages.[143,244,378] This suggests that additional events/factors probably are important for the development of cervical cancer, which may include induction of chromosomal instability with the de-

velopment of aneuploidy, the site specific at which HPV integrates into the genome, and loss of cellular signals that regulate the expression of the E6 and E7 ORFs (see Chapter 28, Molecular Biology).[175,187,390,402]

Epidemiologic Evidence Linking Human Papillomavirus to the Development of Cervical Cancer and Its Precursors

The molecular data linking HPV to the development of SIL (CIN) and cervical cancer have, until recently, been more compelling than the epidemiologic data.[247,321] To implicate HPV clearly as the causative agent of SIL (CIN) and cervical cancer, epidemiologic studies must demonstrate that there is consistently a strong relationship between HPV infection and cervical neoplasia, that the temporal sequence of events is correct (i.e., infection is followed by neoplasia), that the association between HPV and neoplasia is relatively specific, and that the epidemiologic evidence is consistent with what is known about the biology and natural history of cervical neoplasia (see Chapter 29, Epidemiology).[108]

Although many epidemiologic studies have implicated a venereally transmitted agent as the causative factor for cervical neoplasia and HPV DNA has consistently been identified more frequently in women with cervical neoplasia than in controls, the association between HPV and cervical neoplasia has been too weak in most older studies to allow HPV to be identified as the causative factor.[79,80,229,285] Moreover, some epidemiologic studies have found that women with multiple sexual partners remain at risk for the development of SIL (CIN) and cervical cancer even after controlling for the presence of HPV infections, suggesting that additional venereally transmitted factors may be important etiologic agents.[84,286] Other studies have failed to find an association between measures of sexual activity and risk of infection with HPV.[186,286,371]

It is important to be aware that results of epidemiologic studies may be flawed unless various factors are taken into account and controlled for (see Chapter 29, Epidemiology). Among the most important factors in studies of HPV and cervical neoplasia is the method by which HPV status is determined.[108] The early studies describing associations between HPV and cervical disease used either Southern blot hybridization (SBH) or filter in situ hybridization (FISH) to detect and type HPV DNA. SBH is relatively sensitive and highly specific and is considered by many to be the "gold standard" for detecting HPV DNA.[210,211] Although well suited for small-scale studies, SBH is too time consuming and labor intensive to be used for large epidemiologic studies and, therefore, many studies have used the more rapid and economical dot blot methodologies, such as FISH or commercial dot blot kits, for detecting

HPV DNA. FISH is relatively insensitive and detects only 4 of the more than 22 types of HPV that infect the anogenital tract and frequently has high, nonspecific binding. Studies that have used FISH therefore should be viewed with considerable caution.[81,210,211] Commercial dot blot kits based on RNA-DNA hybridization with probes against the seven most common anogenital HPV types (ViraPap, ViraType) were introduced several years ago and have replaced FISH for large-scale studies. Although these newer dot blot methods for detecting HPV DNA are more specific and sensitive than FISH, it appears that in the near future they will be replaced by even more sensitive and specific methods. One method that is currently being introduced is based on solution hybridization and uses fluorescence instead of radioactivity to detect the hybridization product (Hybrid Capture).[311] Another detection method is the PCR. This is an enzymatic technique that amplifies the target DNA sequences a millionfold.[317] The amplified product can then be detected in a variety of ways including nucleic acid hybridization. Because of its exquisite sensitivity, PCR is capable of detecting very small amounts of a target DNA and has the advantage of being quick and easy to perform.[221,336,367] The disadvantage of PCR is that it is highly susceptible to cross-contamination and occasionally produces false-positive results.

The more recent epidemiologic studies have used better controlled HPV DNA detection methods and, in contrast to the earlier studies, have consistently reported that: (1) the vast majority of SIL (CIN) and cervical cancer are strongly associated with HPV and (2) that many of the traditional risk factors for the development of SIL (CIN) and cervical cancer such as number of lifetime sexual partners, age at first intercourse, and lower socioeconomic status act as surrogates of HPV infection.[209,240,245,246,310,322] For example, a recent study of 467 women attending a university health service found that HPV DNA positivity as detected using PCR was strongly and independently associated with traditional risk factors for SIL including increasing number of sexual partners, young age, black race, and use of oral contraceptives.[209] The prevalence of HPV infection in women with 10 or more lifetime sexual partners was 69% compared with 21% among women with only a single sexual contact (odds ratio of 11.2). Similarly, another study of young women that used the modified dot blot to detect HPV DNA reported that number of sexual partners was strongly associated with HPV DNA positivity.[240]

In several recent case-control studies HPV DNA positivity has been associated with a significantly increased risk for the concomitant presence of SIL (CIN) and cervical cancer. One case control study of HPV and SIL (CIN) from the United States reported that at least 76% of the cases of SIL (CIN) could be attributed to infection with HPV and in this study the traditional risk factors for the development of SIL (CIN) all disappeared when HPV infection was controlled for, suggesting that sexual behavior risk factors act predominantly as surrogates of HPV infection.[322] Similarly, two large case-control studies of HPV and cervical cancer that used PCR also have reported strong associations between HPV and invasive cervical cancer. One study investigated 436 women with cervical cancer and 387 control women from Colombia and Spain and found the presence of HPV to be the strongest risk factor for invasive cervical cancer (OR = 23.8).[26] In this study the number of lifetime sexual partners, but not age at first intercourse, was eliminated as a risk factor when HPV was controlled for. In another PCR study from China, not only was a strong association between HPV and invasive cervical cancer documented, but the risk factors considered showed an independent effect after allowing for the strong HPV effect.[269] Finally, in a prospective study of cytologically/colposcopically negative women enrolled from a sexually transmitted diseases clinic, it has been reported that approximately 30% of women who are HPV 16 DNA positive developed high-grade SIL (CIN 2, 3) over a 2-year period.[196] Taken together, these more recent epidemiologic studies clearly document a strong and consistent association between HPV DNA and both SIL (CIN) and invasive cervical cancer as well as temporal relationships between HPV infection and the development of cervical neoplasia consistent with HPV being a causative agent. These data, together with the large amount of molecular evidence linking HPV to the development of SIL (CIN) and cervical cancer, clearly indicate that HPV infection acquired through sexual exposure is causal in the development of both SIL (CIN) and invasive cervical cancer.[321,322] However, the long latency between the initial exposure to HPV and the development of cervical cancer as well as the fact that only a small fraction of women exposed to HPV develop cervical disease suggest that other co-factors are necessary in the pathogenesis of cervical neoplasia.

HERPES SIMPLEX VIRUS, TYPE 2

Herpes simplex virus type 2 (HSV-2) previously received considerable attention in relation to the etiology of SIL (CIN), with both biological and epidemiological studies linking HSV-2 to SIL (CIN) and cervical carcinoma.[177,249] Herpes virus antigens have been detected by immunofluorescence in exfoliated cervical squamous carcinoma cells,[312] and the virus has been identified sporadically at the ultrastructural level in cervical carcinoma cells grown in tissue culture. However, whole viral particles consistent with HSV-2 virions have not been visualized in genital tract carcinoma. Herpes simplex virus has been demonstrated to transform cultured cell lines and produce malignant tumors when injected into newborn hamsters and nude mice.[120,158,227] Aurelian[8] demonstrated the presence of a tumor-specific antigen, AG-4, in cervical cancers and showed that AG-4 is an HSV-related structural polypeptide located on the cell surface. In situ hybridization studies have shown that cervical biopsies containing SIL (CIN), when probed with fragments of radiolabeled DNA from HSV-2, hybridized with the corresponding viral RNA within the cells in the absence of active infection.[226] HSV-2 genomic sequences are neither consistently retained nor expressed in experimental models, with the result that no particular transcriptional product could be assigned to maintenance of the transformed state.[120]

Well-controlled, retrospective seroepidemiologic studies have shown that patients with invasive and noninvasive cancers of the cervix have a higher frequency of neutralizing antibodies against HSV-2 than do controls matched for race, age, and socioeconomic status.[75,149,237,249,342] A recent case control study of 766 women with invasive cervical and 1532 controls of women from Latin America found a possible interaction between HPV 16/18 and HSV-2 in the development of invasive cervical carcinoma. The presence of HSV-2 antibodies by themselves was associated with a relative risk of 1.6 for the development of invasive cervical cancer.[149] Although this relative risk was much less than that associated with the presence of HPV 16 or 18 DNA, it persisted independent of other risk factors. Most importantly, patients who had antibodies against HSV-2 and also were HPV 16/18 DNA positive had a twofold greater risk for developing cervical cancer than patients who were only HPV 16/18 DNA positive, suggesting a possible interaction between the two viruses.

Several hypotheses have been proposed for possible mechanisms by which HSV could act as a co-factor with HPV in the pathogenesis of cervical cancer. A hit-and-run mechanism for HSV has been hypothesized by Galloway and McDougall,[120] postulating that HSV may cause transformation without continued viral presence or expression by activating cellular oncogenes, mediating gene amplification, or acting as a mutagen. zur Hausen has suggested that HSV may act synergistically as an initiator or promoter in HPV-stimulated epithelium, providing for more efficient cellular transformation.[400] HPV DNA integration into host cell DNA is facilitated in cells that have been infected previously with HSV, and in vitro transformation studies have found HPV 16 to be fully transforming in human genital keratinocytes that have been previously immortalized by HSV-2.[83,156] Despite evidence to suggest associations between HSV-2 and the development of invasive cervical cancer, many epidemiologists are not convinced that these associations are important. In contrast to the retrospective studies, a prospective serologic study of Czechoslovakian women, with a follow-up of at least 4 years, found no difference in the prevalence of HSV-2

antibody between patients with CIN and invasive carcinoma and matched controls.[373] No differences were observed in the prevalence of HSV-2 antibody titers between patients having disease at entry and those developing disease during the study.[372] However, proponents of HSV-2 as a factor have criticized this study for overmatching and small numbers of cases,[149] and further studies are needed to define better the role of HSV-2 infection in the pathogenesis of cervical cancer.

IMMUNOSUPPRESSION AND HUMAN IMMUNODEFICIENCY VIRUS

Our understanding of carcinogenesis is now based on the interaction of initiators and promoters, with neoplastic transformation developing as the result of a series of multiple, synergistic events. The host's immune system plays an important role in this multifactorial process. Immune suppression provides a background for the development of neoplasia by predisposing to infection by oncogenic viruses and by allowing neoplastic proliferations to escape immune surveillance and other host regulatory mechanisms.[281] With respect to cervical carcinogenesis, there is evidence for an interaction with the immune system. HPV infection is increased in frequency in immunosuppressed individuals, and the condylomas in immunosuppressed patients tend to be larger in size, multicentric, and refractory to treatment.[340] Vulvovaginal neoplasia, SIL (CIN), and cervical carcinoma are also more common in patients on immunosuppressive therapy.[139,327,340] It has been proposed that the cytostatic and cytotoxic effects of therapeutic agents, such as azathioprine, corticosteroids, and alkylating agents, potentiate the effects of the already compromised immune system.[389] In renal transplant patients, the relative risk (RR) of cervical cancer is increased by 5.4. This increased relative risk for cervical cancer should be compared with a 1.5- to 2.5-fold increased relative risk for the development of epithelial cancers on other mucosal surfaces that are unassociated with a viral etiology.[270]

A number of studies have clearly documented that there is a high prevalence of cytological abnormalities in women infected with the human immunodeficiency virus (HIV) and cervical cancer has recently been classified as an acquired immunodeficiency syndrome (AIDS) case-defining illness by the U.S. Centers for Disease Control, U.S.* One of the early studies of HIV infection and cervical disease in women enrolled in a methadone maintanence program in the Bronx, New York, reported that 6 of 45 HIV-seronegative women (13%) had cytological evidence of SIL (CIN) compared with 3 of 18 (17%) of HIV-infected women without AIDS and 14 of 33 (42%) of HIV-infected women

---

*Refs. 31,59,95,204,220,222,318,361,369,391.

with AIDS.[369] Similarly, in a study of prostitutes from Zaire, the prevalence of cytological evidence of SIL (CIN) was 27% in HIV-infected women compared with 3% in HIV-uninfected women.[204] Although many of the early studies had small sample sizes and failed to confirm cytological abnormalities by colposcopy and cervical biopsy,[58] the finding of a high prevalence of SIL (CIN) in HIV-infected women has been confirmed by other studies that have addressed these issues. In one recent study of 398 HIV-infected women and 357 demographically similar HIV-seronegative women enrolled from New York City, the prevalence of biopsy-proven SIL (CIN) was 5 times higher in the seropositive women and increased as the CD4+ T-lymphocyte count decreased.[391] In this study most SIL (CIN), both in HIV-infected and uninfected women, were found to be attributable to HPV infection even after controlling for sexual factors with either agent.

Rapidly progressive invasive cervical cancers also have been reported in HIV-infected women and two studies have suggested that there is a high prevalence of invasive cervical cancer in HIV-infected women.[289,318,329] However, other large cross-sectional studies, one of 270 cervical cancer patients and 359 control women from Tanzania and one of 398 HIV-infected women from New York City have failed to detect an association between HIV-infection and invasive cervical cancer.[361,391]

OTHER ETIOLOGIC FACTORS

Besides infectious agents, other etiologic co-factors, including iatrogenic and environmental carcinogens and nutritional influences, have been studied. Barrier methods of contraception, particularly condoms and diaphragms, appear to decrease the risk of cervical neoplasia.[290] Oral contraceptive (OCP) users have been reported in several studies to have an increased incidence of SIL (CIN) and cervical carcinoma.[57,132,236,370] Other studies have suggested that OCP use, although not directly implicated in the development of SIL (CIN), may influence its natural history by accelerating lesion progression.[236,370] However, these findings are controversial because other investigators have been unable to substantiate any causal relationship between OCPs and SIL (CIN).[55,265,356] A recent review of this subject concluded that there appears to be a weak association between OCP use and SIL, but that this association is so weak that it may be due to bias and confounding.[32]

Correlations between prenatal diethylstilbestrol (DES) exposure and cervicovaginal intraepithelial neoplasia have been similarly conflicting. Despite early observations to the contrary,[305] a study by the Diethylstilbestrol Adenosis (DESAD) Project of 3980 DES-exposed women in the United States described a two- to fourfold increased incidence rate of SIL (CIN) in DES progeny compared with matched controls.[304] However, the DESAD project data must be interpreted with caution because immature squamous metaplasia in the DES offspring often is confused with SIL (CIN), even by expert pathologists. Such diagnostic pitfalls might have contributed to the relatively high incidence of SIL (CIN) in the DES offspring.

Cigarette smoking[35,55,166,266,365] may be associated, independently of sexual activity, with an increased risk of SIL (CIN) and the risk may be duration and dose dependent in women who smoke more than a half pack of cigarettes per day. It is possible, although not proved, that carcinogens in cigarette smoke may act in concert with certain HPVs, leading to the development of SIL (CIN). Smoke-derived products, including nicotine and cotenoids, have been isolated from cervical mucus of smokers and passive smokers, and there is a reduction in the number of Langerhan's cells in smokers, suggesting that there may be a localized defect in cell-mediated immunity.[145,320]

Nutritional and dietary factors also have been investigated as co-variables in the development of cervical carcinoma. Deficiencies of vitamins A and C in women with SIL (CIN) have been documented in some studies and are hypothesized to interact with the metaplastic epithelium of the transformation zone.[262,309,377] However, other studies have failed to find a relationship between SIL (CIN) and the dietary intake of retinol and beta-carotene.[77] Folate deficiency also has been implicted as a possible co-variable for the development of SIL (CIN). Although previous studies on the role of folate deficiency were viewed with skepticism since folate deficiency can cause a benign cytomegaly of the squamous and columnar epithelia that can sometimes resemble SIL (CIN),[368,379,383] a recent case-control study found that folate deficiency enhances the effect of other risk factors such as parity, HPV 16 infection and cigarette smoking on the development of SIL (CIN).[45] This study also suggested that oral contraceptives can cause low blood folate levels, thereby linking these two risk factors for the development of SIL (CIN).[44,354,383]

CLINICAL FEATURES

SIL (CIN) occurs on the anterior lip of the cervix twice as commonly as on the posterior lip and is rarely seen at the lateral cervical angles. This distribution is similar to the distribution of both the everted endocervical epithelium and the transformation zone during the postpartum period.[291,384] SIL (CIN) may expand horizontally and involve the entire transformation zone, but it stops abruptly at the junction with the native portio epithelium.[291,295] The area of the transformation zone, therefore, predetermines the distribution and extent of SIL (CIN) on the exposed portion of the cervix.[293] The endocervical extension of SIL (CIN) is not restricted and extension along the entire endocervical canal and into the uterus can rarely occur.[76,99] The size and endocervical distribution of SIL (CIN) tend to vary directly with increasing severity of grade. High-grade SIL (CIN 2, 3) lesions usually have the largest surface area and more frequently involve the endocervical canal.

The mechanism by which SIL (CIN) grows and extends into normal squamous epithelium and into the columnar epithelium of the endocervix is a matter of contention. In the 1960s and early 1970s many investigators studied this process and two separate theories were developed. One view was that SIL (CIN) is multicellular in origin and spreads by transformation of cells from normal to neoplastic in a vertical direction.[60,61,284] This multicellular theory predicts that SIL (CIN) will arise in predetermined areas containing an abnormal cell population. The primary lesion grows and expands by transforming the adjacent normal epithelium into neoplastic epithelium or by the coalescence of multiple predetermined neoplastic fields, producing a larger lesion.[42,60,61,165,284] The contrasting theory was that SIL (CIN) is unicellular in origin and begins in a single cell or at most in an extremely circumscribed group of cells. According to the unicellular theory, SIL (CIN) spreads horizontally along the basement membrane by mechanically lifting the adjacent normal squamous and endocervical columnar cells.[98,291] These theories were both developed before the recognition that the biology/virology of low-grade SIL (CIN 1) and high-grade SIL (CIN 2, 3) are quite different. In light of our current understanding of the pathogenesis of SIL (CIN), it would be expected that low-grade SIL (CIN) is most likely multicellular in origin, since it develops within a field of latently infected cervical epithelium and frequently is associated with multiple types of HPV. In contrast, high-grade SIL (CIN 2, 3) usually is associated with only a single type of HPV, is frequently aneuploid, and may contain integrated HPV DNA. Therefore, high-grade SIL would be expected to be of unicellular origin.

There is no unanimous opinion on the cellular origin of SIL (CIN). Three cellular sites of origin have been proposed: basal cells of the squamous epithelium of the portio, basal cells of the transformation zone epithelium, and reserve cells of the endocervix.[165] Most SIL (CIN) begins at the squamocolumnar junction of the transformation zone, with one edge of the lesion bordering the endocervical columnar epithelium.[292] Only about 10% of SIL (CIN) will involve the endocervical canal without involving the squamocolumnar junction.[2,105,279] In general, the portion of SIL (CIN) on the exocervical portio surface is low-grade whereas the portion of SIL (CIN) that extends into the endocervical canal is high-grade (Fig. 7.5). From these observations it is now proposed that most SILs (CIN) arise in the basal cells of the transformation zone epithelium, which is formed by the coalescence of squamous metaplastic epithelium with native squamous epithelium.

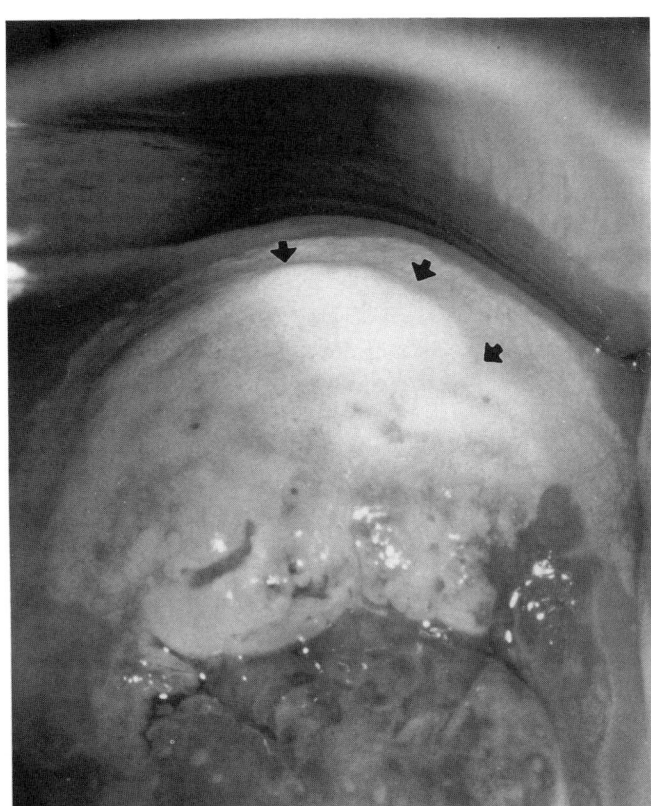

Fig. 7.5. High-grade SIL (CIN 2, 3). Colposcopic appearance of high-grade SIL (CIN 2, 3) arising within a low-grade SIL (CIN 1). High-grade SIL (CIN 2, 3) usually develops internally to the low-grade SIL (CIN 1), presents with an internal margin (*arrows*), and extends into the endocervical canal.

PATHOLOGICAL FINDINGS

SIL (CIN) is characterized by abnormal cellular proliferation, maturation, and cytological atypia. The cytological abnormalities include hyperchromatic nuclei, abnormal chromatin distribution, nuclear pleomorphism, and increased nuclear-cytoplasmic ratio. Nuclear atypia is the hallmark of SIL (CIN). The nuclear borders are irregular, and the chromatin is coarse, granular (salt and pepper), or filamentous throughout the nuclear mass. The nuclear alterations are found in all levels of the epithelium regardless of the degree of cytoplasmic maturation. Increased mitotic activity at all epithelial levels and the presence of morphologically abnormal mitotic figures also are typical of SIL (CIN).[115,116,242,275,388]

Ultrastructurally, both the nuclear and cytoplasmic alterations of SIL (CIN) are consistent with a progressive lack of normal differentiation.[337] There is a decrease in glycogen, tonofilaments, desmosomes, and specialized junctional units with increasing histological dedifferentiation (Fig. 7.6). These alterations are correlated with a progressive decrease in cellular adhesions, basal pseudopodia,

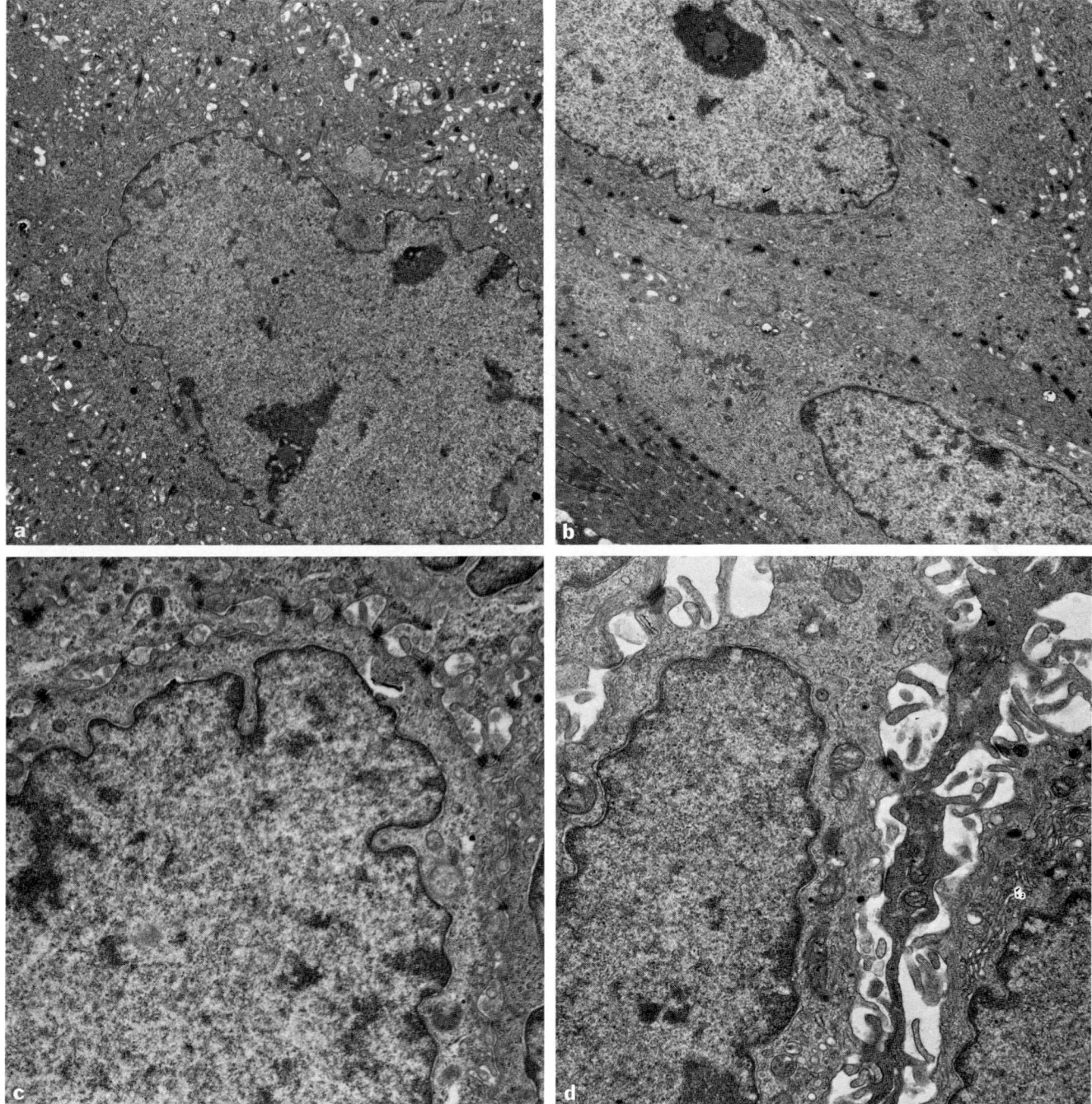

Fig. 7.6. SIL (CIN 2, 3). Electron micrographs of neoplastic cells from the middle third of the epithelium in (**a**) low-grade SIL (CIN 1) and (**b,c,d**) high-grade SIL (CIN 2, 3). The common features include increased nucleus-cytoplasm ratio, irregular nuclear contour, prominent nucleoli, and abundant free and bound ribosomes. Note the gradual decrease in the number of desmosomes, tonofilaments, and glycogen particles from **a–d**. **a**. ×5000. **b**. ×5000. **c**. ×10,200. **d**. ×10,200.

and cell contact inhibition demonstrated by time-lapse cinematography in cells grown in vitro.[300,301] The surface ultrastructure of cervical cancer precursors also differs from the normal architecture. The most outstanding feature is the absence of surface microridges and the presence of abundant microvilli (Fig. 7.7).

The traditional grading of intraepithelial neoplasia was based on the proportion of the epithelium occupied by basaloid, undifferentiated cells, reflecting a progressive loss of epithelial maturation and decreasing glycogenization with increasing lesion severity.[296] The spectrum of epithelial alterations that comprises SIL (CIN) therefore

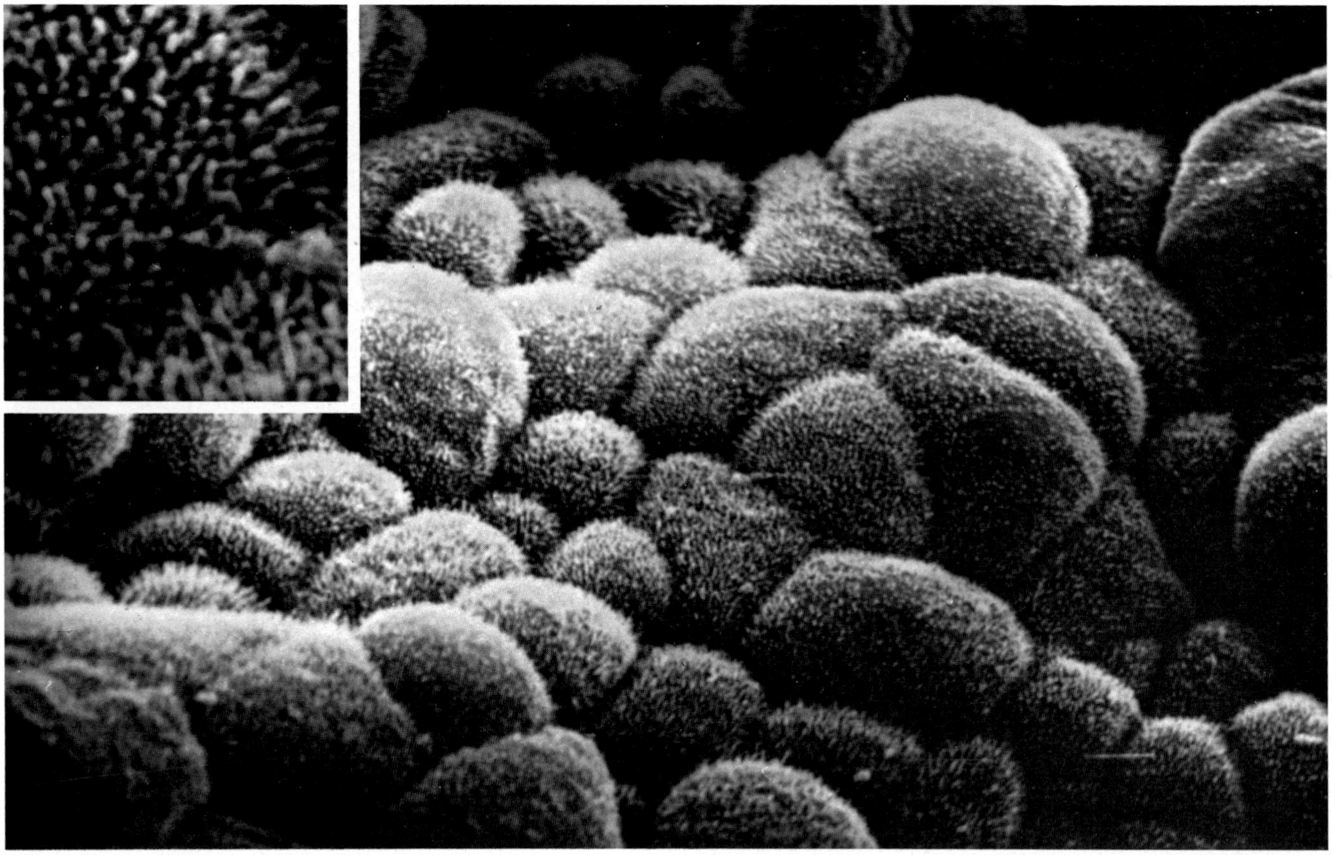

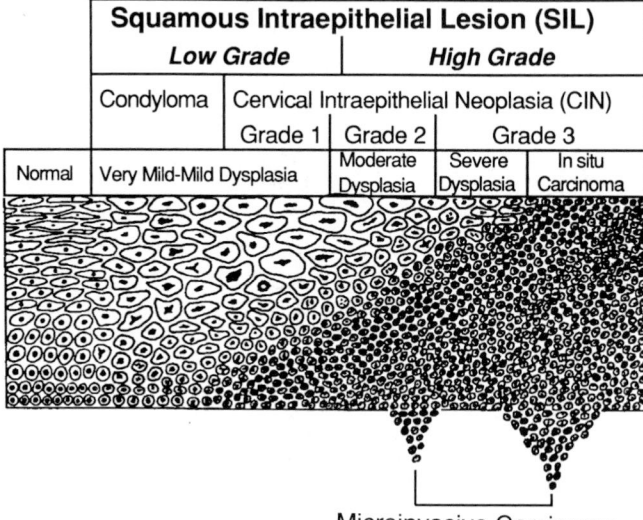

Fig. 7.7. High-grade SIL (CIN 2, 3). Scanning electron microscopy of the surface of high-grade SIL (CIN 2, 3). Note cellular disorganization, pleomorphism, and bulging microvillous surface membranes and lack of intercellular terminal bars. ×2280. *Inset:* Higher magnification of tightly packed surface microvilli. ×9120.

were classified semiquantitatively into three categories: CIN grade 1—neoplastic, basaloid cells occupying the lower third of the epithelium; CIN grade 2—basaloid cells occupying the lower third to two-thirds of the epithelium; CIN grade 3—basaloid cells occupying two-thirds to full thickness of the epithelium (Fig. 7.8). Adoption of The Bethesda System nomenclature to histological classification results in a two-tier rather than a three-tier grading system.

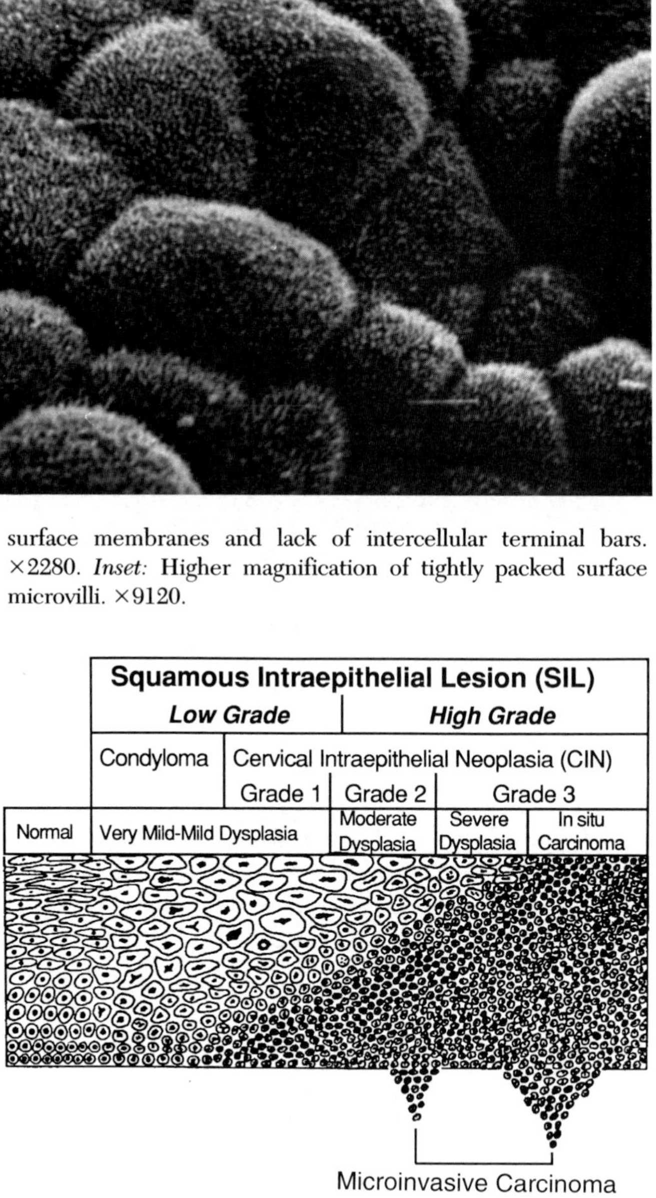

Low-grade Squamous Intraepithelial Lesion (CIN 1)

In 1977 Meisels et al. introduced the term *flat condyloma* to describe a flat HPV-induced cervical lesion that closely resembled the typical exophytic appearance of a cervical condyloma acuminatum.[232] Implicit in the use of this term was the belief that flat cervical condylomata could be distinguished from CIN 1 on a histological basis and that there was a different distribution of HPV types in the two lesions. Flat condylomas, like exophytic condylomas, would contain HPV 6 and 11. CIN 1 would contain HPV 16, like carcinoma. Flat condylomata were defined as le-

Squamous Intraepithelial Lesion (SIL)				
Low Grade		**High Grade**		
Condyloma	Cervical Intraepithelial Neoplasia (CIN)			
	Grade 1	Grade 2	Grade 3	
Normal	Very Mild-Mild Dysplasia	Moderate Dysplasia	Severe Dysplasia	In situ Carcinoma

Microinvasive Carcinoma

Fig. 7.8. Cervical squamous carcinoma precursors. Schematic representation of cervical cancer precursors and the the different terminologies that have been used to refer to them. The risk of developing microinvasion from different states of SIL (CIN) is arbitrarily represented and is not necessarily proportional to that illustrated in this scheme.

sions with a marked HPV cytopathic effect and an orderly basal cell layer whereas CIN 1 lesions had a marked HPV cytopathic effect accompanied by a loss of polarity, crowding, overlapping, and disorganization of the basal cell layer.[233,235] The introduction of the flat condyloma terminology caused considerable confusion among clinicians and pathologists. This was due, in part, to the fact that the histological features of CIN 1 and flat condylomata overlapped to such a degree that it was frequently impossible for the pathologist to distinguish between them using conventional criteria.

To clarify possible differences between cervical flat condyloma and CIN 1 lesions, several studies analyzed these lesions for nuclear DNA content and associated HPV type.[18,114,117,335] Using computerized imaging cytometry, Fu and co-workers compared ploidy levels in cervical lesions diagnosed as either cervical condyloma or CIN 1 and found similar ploidy levels in both.[113,117] All lesions histologically classified as flat condyloma and 67% of lesions histologically classified as CIN 1 had diploid, and occasionally polyploid, DNA patterns.[113] Similarly, Jacobsen et al. using flow cytometry reported diploid DNA patterns in almost all lesions classified as mild and moderate dysplasia.[157] Although early studies suggested differences in HPV distribution in these lesions, several subsequent studies have reported that there were no differences in the HPV types associated with "flat condylomas" and CIN 1 (see above, Classification of HPV and Association with Specific Types of Anogenital Lesions), indicating that lesions with the histological appearances of flat condyloma or CIN 1 should be grouped into a single entity, that is, low-grade SIL (CIN 1).[169,386]

The architectural abnormalities associated with low-grade SIL (CIN 1) are due to a proliferation of basal and parabasal cells in the infected epithelium. The resultant hyperplasia can be highly variable and takes many forms but is characterized most commonly by papillomatosis and acanthosis. One of the more common patterns of the acanthosis is that of moderate epithelial thickening and an undulating, slightly raised surface (Fig. 7.9). In the older literature, cervical lesions with HPV-associated cytopathic effects and only a moderate degree of epithelial thickening were referred to as *condyloma planum*. Using the newer, Bethesda terminology, such lesions, when they occur on the cervix, are designated low-grade SIL (CIN 1). Other types of epithelial hyperplasia that can occur in productive HPV infection are multiple papillary fronds containing fibrovascular cores and pointed epithelial spikes arising from the epithelium (Fig 7.10). Colposcopically the latter have prominent, fine surface spikes and are frequently referred to in the colposcopic literature as *spiked condyloma*. The surface of low-grade SIL (CIN 1) frequently has a layer of parakeratosis and somewhat less commonly hyperkeratosis with an associated granular layer (Fig. 7.10). When gland involvement by the HPV-infected epithelium and acanthosis predominate, the histological pattern ap-

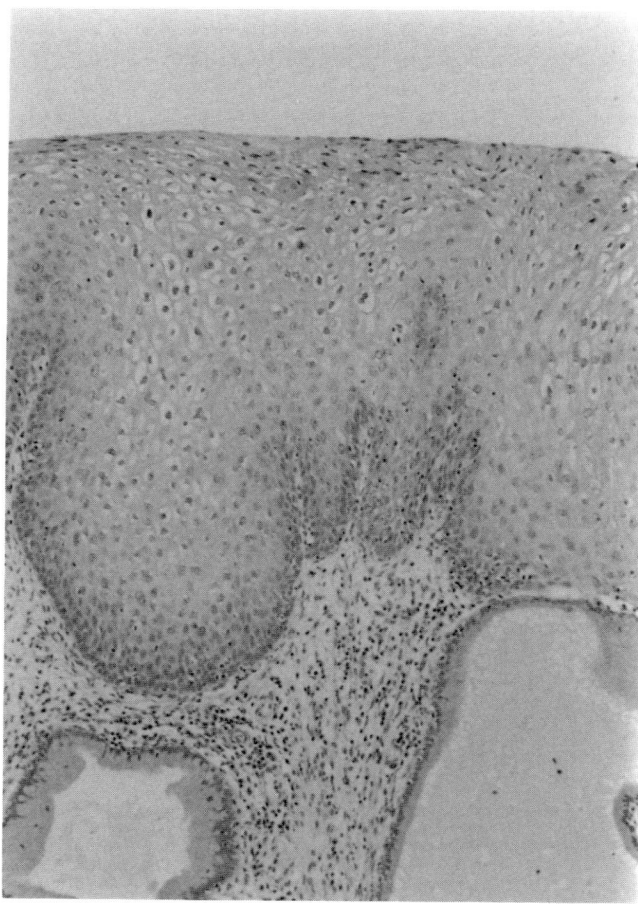

Fig. 7.9. Low-grade SIL (CIN 1). Papillomatosis and acanthosis frequently are found in low-grade SIL (CIN 1). Most commonly papillomatosis and acanthosis are manifested as a slightly thickened epithelium with an undulating surface.

pears endophytic and superficially resembles that of an inverted nasal papilloma (Fig. 7.11).

It is now recognized that low-grade SIL (CIN 1) is the morpologic manifestation of productive HPV infections of the cervical squamous epithelium, which can be caused by any of the anogenital types of HPV. In productive HPV infection, many viral particles are produced and the infected squamous cells demonstrate the cytopathic effects of HPV.[50,208] These cytopathic effects are considered the most characteristic cytological/histological features of low-grade SIL (CIN 1) and include perinuclear cytoplasmic cavitation with thickening of the cytoplasmic membrane, nuclear atypia, and anisocytosis (Fig 7.12). Nuclear atypia is characterized by enlargement, hyperchromasia, and irregularity and wrinkling of the nuclear membrane. Cells near the surface may have nuclei that are somewhat smaller and pyknotic. The combination of nuclear atypia and cytoplasmic cavitation has been termed *koilocytosis* or

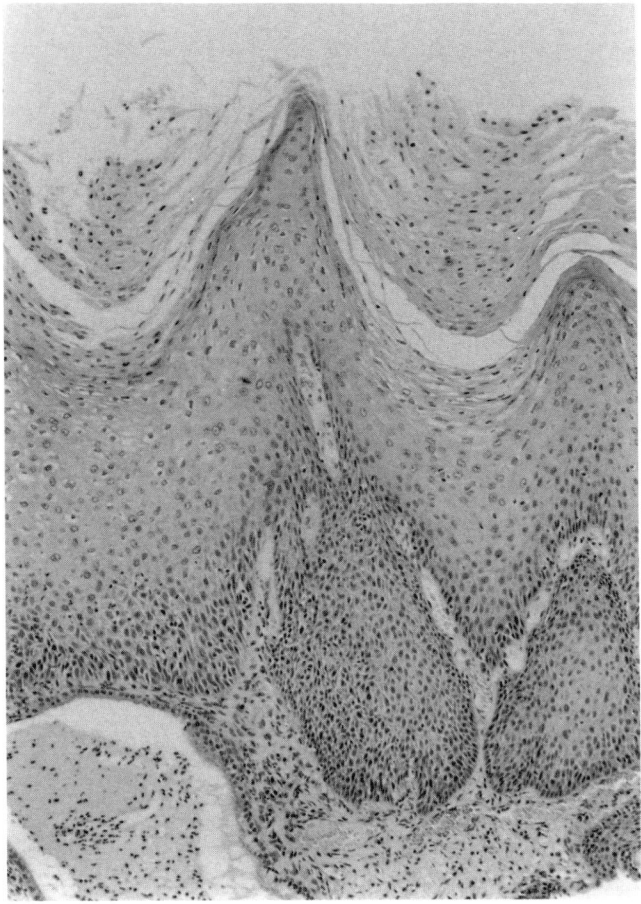

FIG. 7.10. Low-grade SIL (CIN 1). Acanthosis, parakeratosis, and hyperkeratosis frequently occur in SIL (CIN). Acanthosis and papillomatosis also can produce pointed spikes with fibrovascular cores, the so-called spiked condyloma.

koilocytotic atypia. The cells productively infected with HPV typically are polyploid and many also are binucleated or multinucleated.[113] Polyploid cells are cytologically atypical and are readily recognized as being "abnormal" on either cytology or histology. This atypia is characterized predominantly by anisonucleosis; to a lesser extent there is nuclear enlargement and an increase in nuclear-cytoplasmic ratio. Taken together, the histological and cytological features of koilocytosis, nuclear atypia, architectural abnormalities, and multinucleation are pathognomonic of an HPV-infected epithelium at any site in the lower genital tract and are especially prominent in low-grade SIL (CIN 1) lesions. It must be emphasized that nuclear abnormalities must be present. Cytoplasmic vacuolization in the absence of nuclear atypia is a nonspecific change that may occur as a reflection of atrophy-related vacuolar degeneration, in non–HPV-related infections, such as trichomoniasis, *G. vaginalis,* and candidiasis, and at times in normal squamous epithelium containing abundant amounts of glycogen.

The microscopic features of low-grade SIL (CIN 1) are a direct result of productive HPV infection, which induces cytoskeletal abnormalities and mitotic spindle abnormalities. Recent studies have shown that the E4 protein of HPV interacts with filaggrin, a cytokeratin binding protein, and expression of the E4 protein in keratinocytes causes specific cytokeratin proteins to be lost from the cells and a collapse of the cytokeratin matrix.[85,88] This may lead to cytoplasmic cavitation, which is one of the features of koilocytosis. Mitotic spindle abnormalities that occur in productive HPV infections appear to interfere with mitosis and cytokinesis. This leads to the polyploidy and bi- or multinucleated cells that usually are present in productive HPV infections. Although the mechanism responsible for the interference by HPV of mitosis and cytokinesis is unknown, recently it has been found that the capsid proteins of a closely related DNA tumor virus, polyoma, directly bind to the mitotic spindle of infected cells and may interfere with mitosis through this mechanism.[358]

DIFFERENTIAL DIAGNOSIS

The most common problem in the differential diagnosis of low-grade SIL (CIN 1) is the overinterpretation of koilocytosis and flat condyloma. This is due largely to the indiscriminate use of this term for squamous epithelium showing the slightest hint of "cytoplasmic vacuolization" in the absence of nuclear atypia. Normal metaplastic squamous epithelium with prominent glycogen vacuolization often is confused with low-grade SIL (CIN 1). In contrast to the focal distribution of koilocytes in low-grade SIL, cells of normal squamous epithelium that have perinuclear clearing are not sharply demarcated, the nuclei are not enlarged or atypical, and multinucleated cells are infrequent. Cytoplasmic vacuolization in the absence of nuclear atypic is a nonspecific change that may occur as a reflection of atrophy-related vacuolar degeneration, in non–HPV-related infections, such as trichomoniasis, *G. vaginalis,* and candidiasis. In addition to the absence of nuclear atypia, normal stratification and maturation are maintained in such conditions, whereas in HPV-associated lesions, there is some degree of cellular disorganization, particularly near the surface, and there is disturbance in the normal pattern of maturation.

Studies measuring interobserver variability of histological diagnosis of cervical lesions demonstrate that although agreement between pathologists is excellent for invasive lesions, and moderately good for high-grade SIL (CIN 2, 3), it is poor for low-grade SIL (CIN 1).[155,306,334] The most significant discrepancies are in the ability of the pathologists to distinguish low-grade SIL (CIN 1) from reactive squamous proliferations. This suggests that the morphologic criteria routinely used to distinguish these two lesions have serious shortcomings. The importance of nuclear aty-

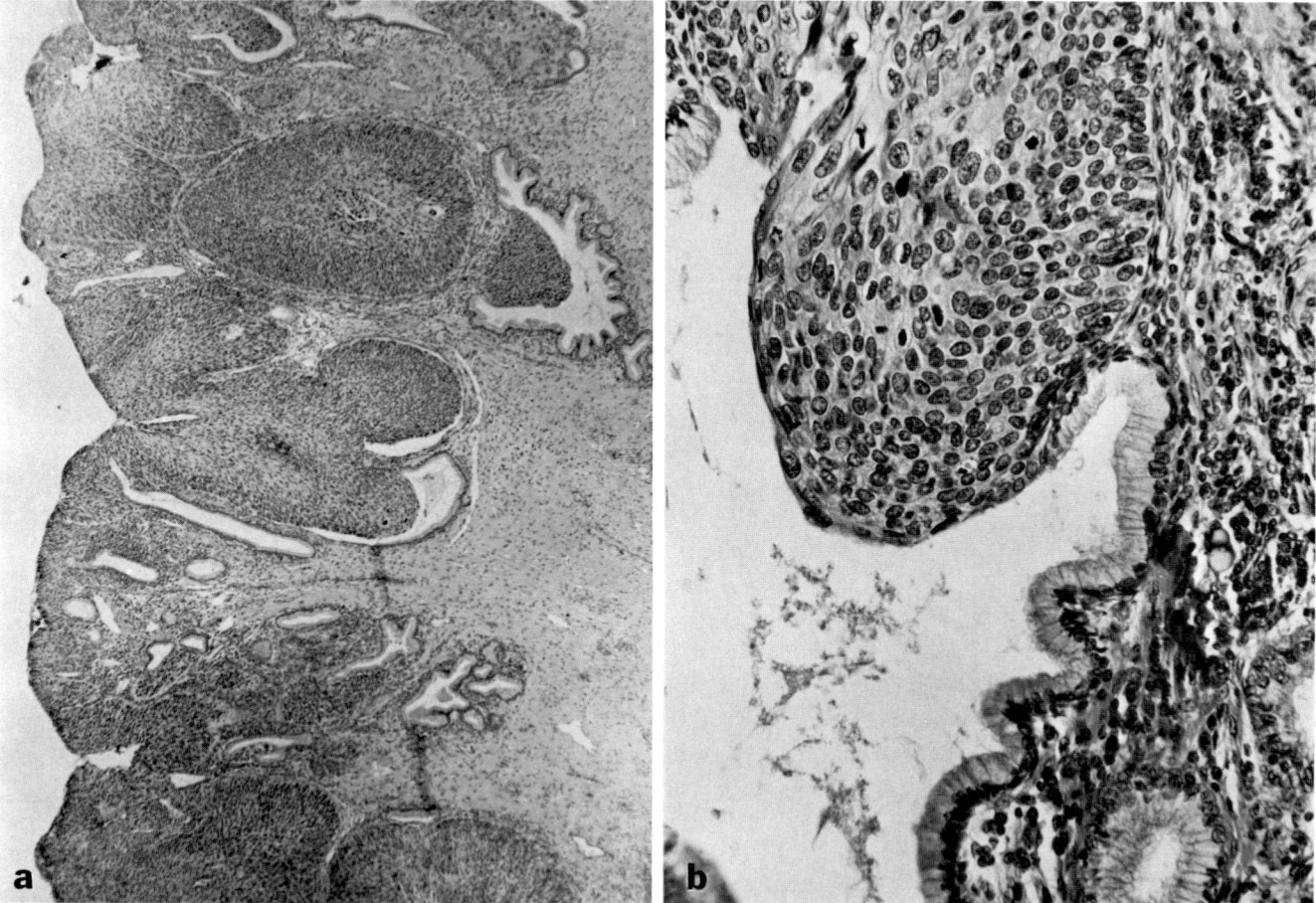

Fig. 7.11. **Low-grade SIL (CIN 1). a:** SIL can grow into and distend endocervical clefts. Note the smooth margins of ingrowing SIL retaining the normal configuration of endocervical mucosa. **b:** SIL grows between the endocervical epithelium and its basal lamina.

pia in the distinction of low-grade SIL (CIN 1) from reactive lesions is confirmed by a number of studies. Correlation of HPV DNA with specific cytological/histological findings have uniformly found that perinuclear halos in the absence of significant nuclear atypia are nonspecific features.[109,238,375] Therefore, the diagnosis of low-grade SIL (CIN 1) should be made only when significant nuclear atypia accompanies perinuclear halos.

Since low-grade SIL (CIN 1) is a manifestation of productive HPV infection and reactive atypias are not, one approach the pathologist can use to assist in the diagnosis of low-grade SIL (CIN 1) is to perform in situ hybridization for HPV DNA.[302] Commercially available in situ hybridization kits have a sensitivity of approximately 50 copies of HPV DNA per cell and are sensitive enough to detect HPV DNA in approximately 80–90% of cervical lesions with the histological features of low-grade SIL (CIN 1).[52,66,210] Although HPV DNA can be detected in cervical swabs of cytologically normal women by PCR or Southern blot hybridization, HPV is not detected in normal or reactive epithelium by in situ hybridization.[302]

Therefore, these kits can be used to distinguish low-grade SIL from reactive processes that histologically mimic low-grade SIL. Since the in situ hybridization kits require a certain degree of technical expertise, pathologists should send specimens to be tested to reference laboratories if these tests are not performed routinely at their own institution. When in situ hybridization is used it is important that the specimens be fixed in neutral buffered formalin or alcohol formalin and not be fixed in acidic fixatives such as Bouin's solution or Zenker's solution, which degrade the DNA and reduce sensitivity.[254]

High-grade Squamous Intraepithelial Lesion (CIN 2, 3)

In high-grade SIL (CIN 2, 3) , immature basal-type cells should occupy more than the lower third of the epithelium. In addition, there is nuclear crowding, pleomorphism, and loss of the normal cell polarity (Fig. 7.13). The nuclei of the

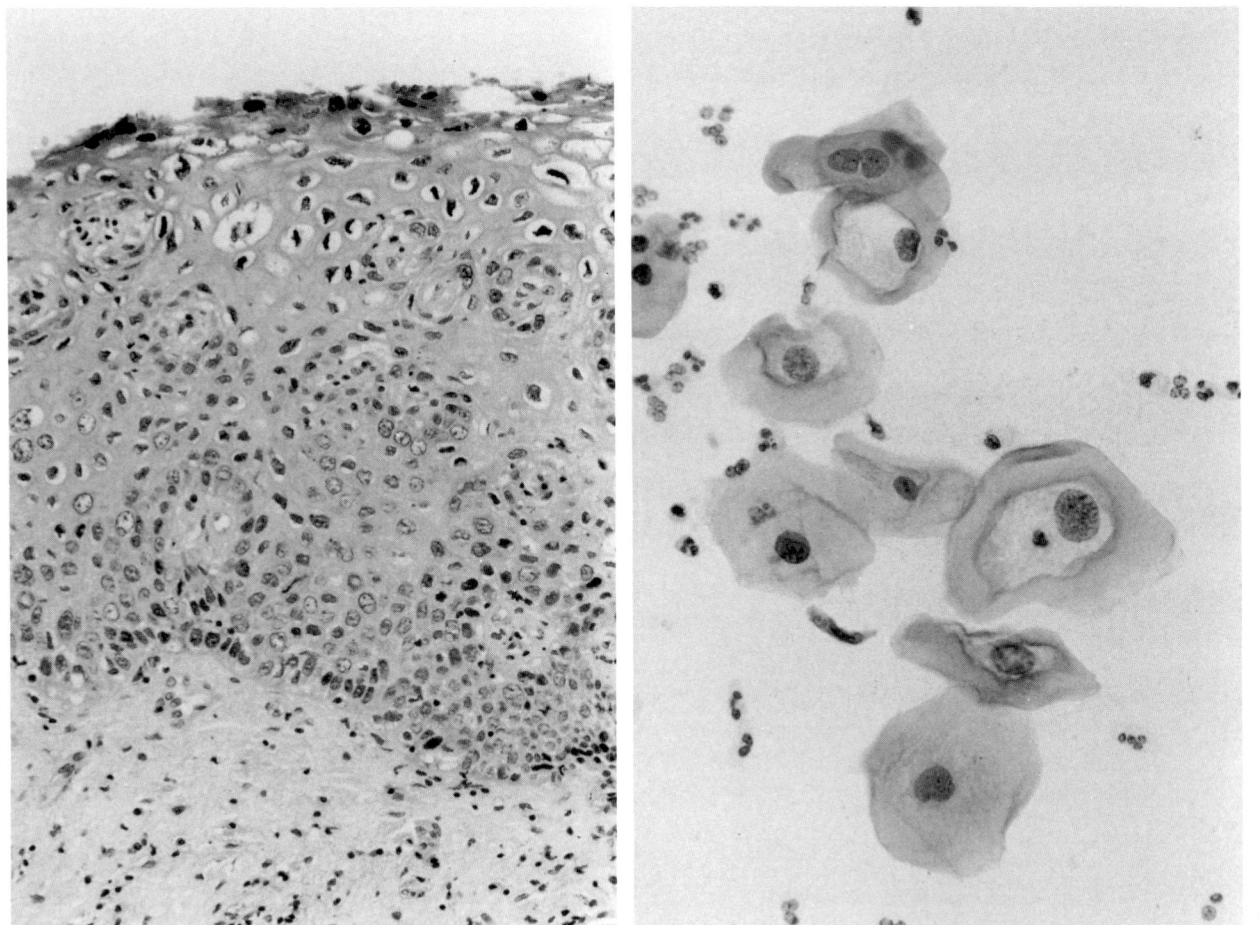

FIG. 7.12. Cytopathic effects of HPV. The cytopathic effects of HPV include nuclear enlargement, nuclear pyknosis or hyperchromaticity, anisocytosis, multinucleation, and perinuclear cyto- plasmic vacuolization. **a:** Histological features on cervical biopsy. **b:** Cytological features on Pap smear.

immature basal-type cells are enlarged when compared with the nuclei of cells at comparable levels of the normal epithelium. This nuclear enlargement frequently is most pronounced in the lower half of the epithelium, although in all cases the superficial cells demonstrate some degree of nuclear enlargement. In contrast to low-grade SIL (CIN 1), the nuclear chromatin is more coarsely granular. Prominent nuclei or chromocenters are uncommon. Normal and abnormal mitotic figures are present. Cytoplasm usually is scant, resulting in an increase in the nuclear-cytoplasmic ratio. Cell borders between the primitive cells usually are indistinct. The cells overlying the basal-type cells also have atypical nuclei but have more cytoplasm and therefore lower nuclear-cytoplasmic ratios, more distinct cell boundaries, and can have prominent HPV cytopathic effects including perinuclear halos and bi- or multinucleation. In the superficial layers of the epithelium, individual dyskeratotic cells may be seen. These cells are small with pyknotic hyperchromatic nuclei and dense acidophilic cytoplasm. Another characteristic feature of high-grade SIL (CIN 2, 3) is the variability in nuclear size (anisonucleolis). It should be stressed, however, that this is a variable histological feature. In some high-grade SIL (CIN 2, 3) lesions, particularly those that were previously termed carcinoma in situ, the nuclei at first glance appear relatively uniform in size, although careful scrutiny will reveal some variation in nuclear size and shape.

A subset of high-grade SIL (CIN 2, 3) has been further subdivided by some investigators into three cytological subtypes: small cell anaplastic, large cell keratinizing, and large cell nonkeratinizing CIN 3.[267,283] The small cell variety usually is found within the external os or endocervical canal and is composed of small, undifferentiated, malignant cells of the basal cell type (Fig. 7.14). The large cell keratinizing lesion originates on the exposed portion of the cervix and displays prominent intercellular bridges, macronucleoli, and extensive surface keratinization (Fig. 7.15). Large cell nonkeratinizing lesions are composed of undif-

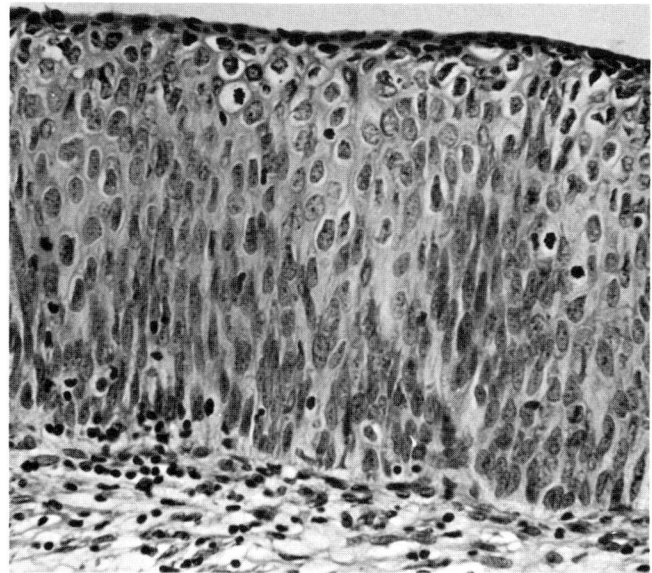

FIG. 7.13. High-grade SIL (CIN 2, 3). Undifferentiated neoplastic cells replace 50% or more of the epithelium. The nuclear-cytoplasmic ratio is increased and the cytoplasmic membranes and the basal layer are indistinct. A few koilocytes are present in the superficial layers.

ferentiated cells the size of normal parabasal cells (Fig. 7.16). Individual cell keratinization may be encountered. Because accurate studies concerning the invasive potential of each of these subtypes are lacking, prediction of the likelihood of progression to invasive carcinoma should not be based on the above subclassification.

In most tissues aneuploidy is a marker of malignant potential. Chromosomal karyotyping studies as well as studies directly measuring the DNA content of lesional tissue support the concept that aneuploid SIL (CIN) lesions are true cervical cancer precursors.[116,181,385] By either Feulgen microspectroscopy or flow cytometry, most low-grade SILs (CIN 1) are diploid or polyploid whereas most high-grade SILs (CIN 2, 3) are aneuploid.[114,115,157,287] In both prospective and retrospective studies, ploidy has been a good predictor of clinical behavior—most SILs (CIN) that progress or persist have been aneuploid whereas most of those that regress are diploid or polyploid.[22,116,251] A number of studies have compared histological features with ploidy levels and found that cervical lesions with diploid or polyploid DNA contents generally retain polarity of the basal cell layer and lack abnormal mitotic figures, whereas aneuploid lesions have more marked nuclear atypia and more cellular disorganization.

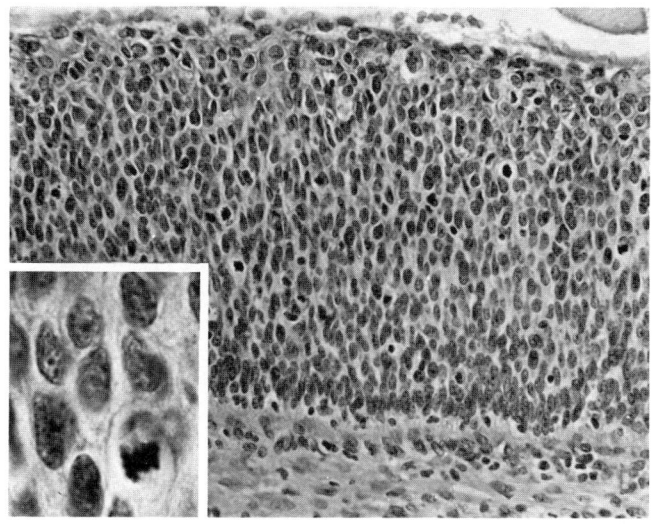

FIG. 7.14. High-grade SIL (CIN 2, 3). The full thickness of the epithelium is composed of small, undifferentiated neoplastic cells. This is the classic *small cell carcinoma in situ*. Note numerous mitotic figures, loss of cellular maturation and organization, and lack of koilocytes. *Inset:* Aggregated nuclear chromatin and mitosis. Characteristically, cell membranes are ill-defined.

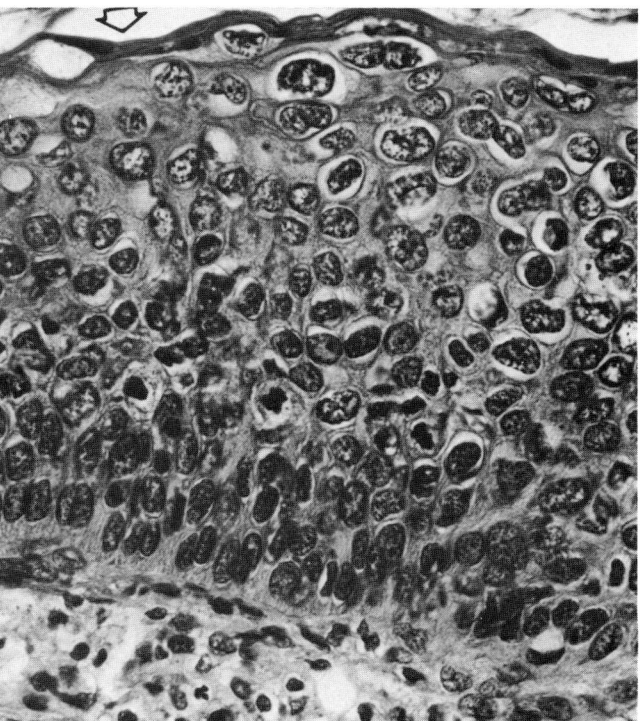

FIG. 7.15. High-grade SIL (CIN 2, 3). This type of high-grade SIL has been referred to as *large cell keratinizing carcinoma in situ*. Note cellular prominence, well-defined cytoplasmic membranes, occasional koilocytes, and fine surface keratinization (*arrow*).

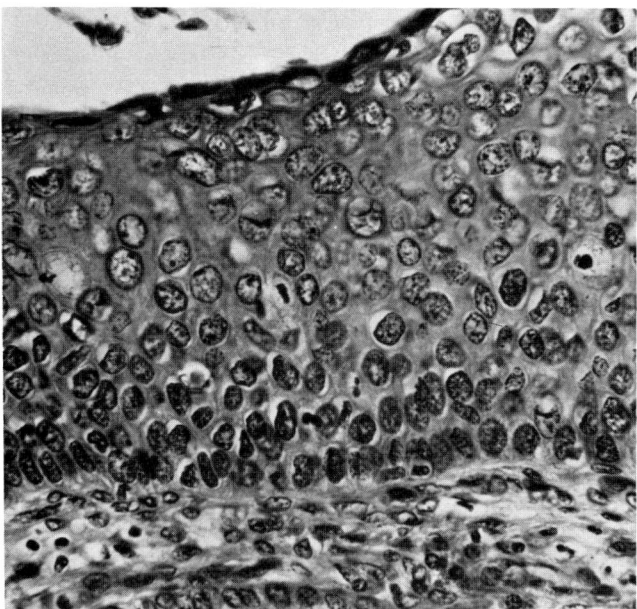

FIG. 7.16. High-grade SIL (CIN 2, 3) This type of high grade SIL has been referred to as *large cell nonkeratinizing carcinoma in situ*. The neoplastic cells have hyperchromatic nuclei with clumping of chromatin. There is a high degree of cellular disorder and cytoplasmic membranes are indistinct.

The best histological correlate of aneuploidy is *abnormal mitotic figures* (AMF) (Fig. 7.17).[18,114,388]

Therefore some authors have suggested that AMFs other than multipolar and dispersed metaphases are an accurate histological surrogate of aneuploidy and can be used as a histological determinate for discriminating between low-grade SIL (CIN 1) and high-grade SIL (CIN 2, 3).[298,388] However, AMFs should not be used as the sole criteria for discriminating between low-grade SIL (CIN 1) and high-grade SIL (CIN 2, 3) for several reasons: (1) AMFs can be difficult to distinguish from karyorrhexis, (2) detection of AMFs is influenced by variables that are independent of ploidy level, including size of biopsy, quality of fixation, quality of the microscopic section, and number of levels examined, and (3) some high-grade SIL (CIN 2, 3) lesions, and even some invasive cancers, lack AMFs and are not aneuploid.[22,140,242] Therefore, although a lesion showing the above features with unequivocal AMFs should be classified as high-grade SIL (CIN 2, 3), the converse is not true. Lesions with the other histological features of a high-grade SIL (CIN 2, 3) should be classified as such even in the absence of AMFs. It is also important to point out that using these criteria, some high-grade lesions will have cells with prominent HPV cytopathic effects similar to those seen in low-grade SIL (CIN 1) (Fig. 7.18). The

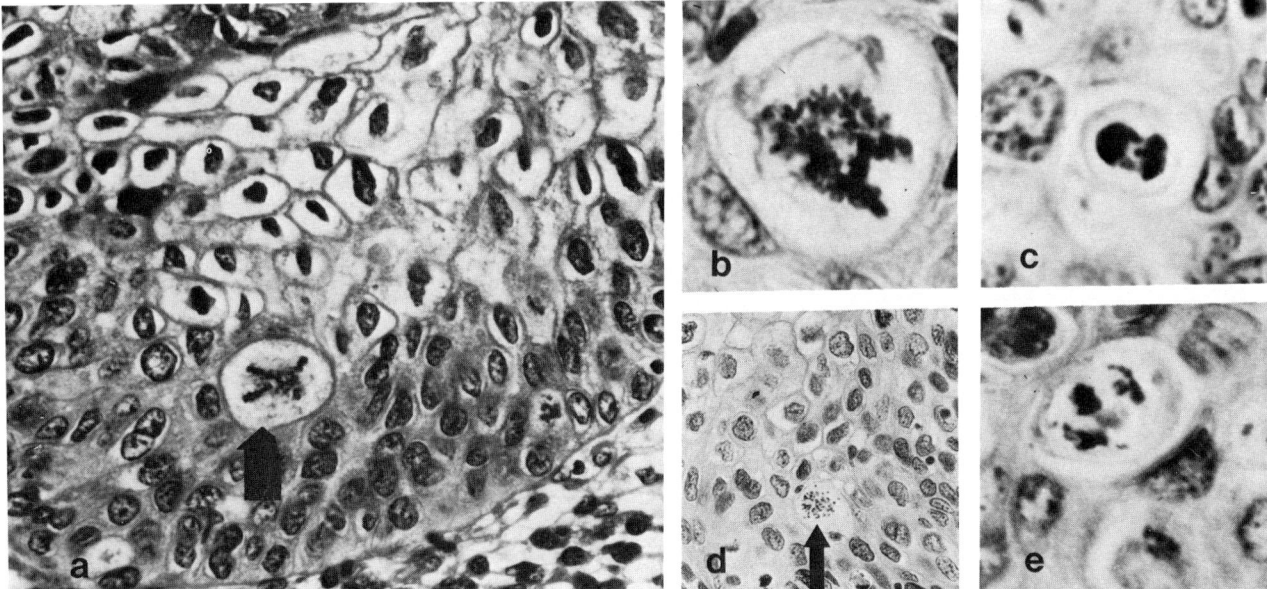

FIG. 7.17. Abnormal mitotic figures. Morphologic variability of abnormal mitotic figures in aneuploid SIL (CIN) lesions. **a:** Quadripolar mitotic figure in a lesion with extensive koilocytosis. **b:** Bizarre mitotic figure with Y shape and numerous poorly organized chromosomes. **c:** Two-group metaphase. **d:** Dispersed mitotic figure (*arrow*) with finely distributed chromosomes. **e:** Three-group metaphase.

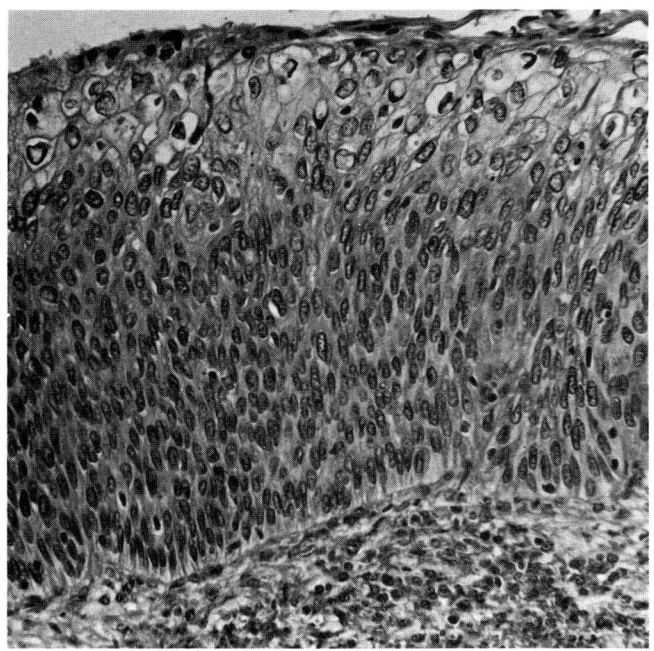

Fig. 7.18. High-grade SIL (CIN 2, 3). Even though the upper third of the epithelium is occupied by single and multinucleated koilocytes, this is a high-grade SIL (CIN 2,3) with undifferentiated basal-type cells replacing approximately two-thirds of the epithelium.

presence of such cells should not be taken as evidence that the lesion is low grade if other features of a high-grade lesion are present. Therefore, the criteria used for distinguishing low-grade SIL (CIN 1) from high-grade SIL (CIN 2, 3) include other parameters such as the distribution of immature, basal-type cells and mitotic figures in the epithelium, the extent of abnormalities of differentiation and polarity, and the degree of nuclear atypia (Table 7.8).

DIFFERENTIAL DIAGNOSIS

Immature metaplasia and atrophy are the most common lesions mistaken for high-grade SIL (CIN 2, 3). In immature metaplasia, the full thickness of the epithelium is composed of immature parabasal cells with a high nuclear-cytoplasmic ratio (Fig 7.19). The cells usually are vertical, and the nuclei are only slightly hyperchromatic. The most helpful feature in distinguishing high-grade SIL (CIN 2, 3) from immature metaplasia is the absence of nuclear pleomorphism in the latter. Immature metaplasia may have mitotic activity, but abnormal mitotic figures are not present. The chromatin in metaplastic squamous epithelium is finer and more evenly distributed than in high-grade SIL (CIN). In addition, cellular polarity is retained, cell membranes are clearly defined, and cellular crowding is not marked. Finally, mucinous epithelium often is present on the surface of immature metaplastic squamous epithelium but rarely overlies SIL (CIN) (Fig 7.19). Sometimes there may be nuclear atypia within immature metaplasia (Fig 7.20). Such lesions are designated by some as *atypical immature metaplasia.*[67] The use of this term is not generally recommended unless clarified with a note because it is not widely accepted and may be confusing to clinicians.

Reparative processes also may be misinterpreted as high-grade SIL (CIN 2, 3) (Fig 7.21). In reparative processes, atypical basal cells occupy the lower half of the epithelium but the cells have a regular nuclear outline, prominent nucleoli, and usually have distinct cell membranes. In addition, dense acute and chronic inflammatory infiltrates usually are present. Atrophic epithelium occasionally is difficult to distinguish from high-grade SIL (CIN 2, 3) because it is composed of basal and parabasal cells showing no differentiation. Although there is a high nuclear-cytoplasmic ratio, atrophic epithelium is thin and shows no nuclear pleomorphism, mitotic activity, atypia, or lack of polarity. In older women, in whom it is difficult to distinguish atrophy from a high-grade SIL (CIN 2, 3), a repeat biopsy after a course of topical, daily estrogen should resolve the problem by inducing maturation in the atrophic epithelium. In contrast, estrogen administration does not alter the appearance of SIL (CIN). Finally, high-grade SIL (CIN 2, 3), particularly with extensive gland involvement, may be confused with microinvasive carcinoma (see Chapter 8, Carcinoma and Other Tumors of the Cervix).

Table 7.8. Distinguishing features of low-grade SIL (CIN 1) and high-grade SIL (CIN 2, 3)

Feature	Low-grade SIL (CIN 1)	High-grade SIL (CIN 2, 3)
HPV types	Any anogenital HPV	Predominantly 16, 18, 31, 33
Koilocytosis	Frequently present	Occasionally present
Ploidy	Mostly diploid or polyploid	Usually aneuploid
Abnormal mitotic figures	Absent	Frequent
Location of undifferentiated cells and mitotic figures	Lower third	Upper two-thirds

HPV, human papillomavirus; SIL, squamous intraepithelial lesion; CIN, cervical intraepithelial neoplasia.

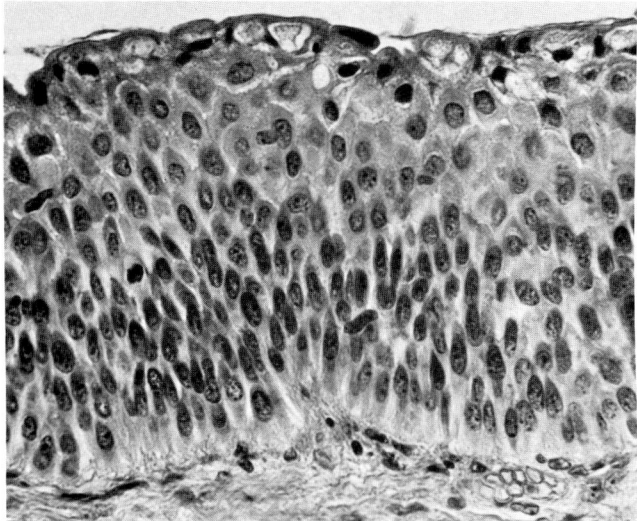

Fig. 7.19. Immature squamous metaplastic epithelium. Metaplastic squamous cells proliferate beneath the mucinous endocervical cells. These may be confused with koilocytes; however, their vacuolar features are due to mucinous-vacuolar degeneration secondary to their separation from the basal lamina rather than papillomavirus infection. Note the hyperplasia of the basal cells with occasional mitotic figures and attempt at cytoplasmic maturation in the upper half of the epithelium. The cells in the upper strata of the epithelium are regularly orientated, with uniformly dispersed nuclear chromatin and cellular borders. Intercellular bridges are well defined.

BEHAVIOR

The behavior of SIL (CIN) has been studied extensively.[165,180] Large-scale studies with follow-up using cytology and colposcopy alone, without biopsy altering the natural course of the disease, are particularly useful.[106,154,192,293] In one of the earliest, large-scale studies, Richart and colleges studied women with SIL (CIN) ascertained initially by two or three consecutive abnormal smears. These women were followed using only cytology and colpomicroscopy for 9 years and about 50% of women with CIN 1 progressed to CIN 3.[12,13,299] In the remaining cases, the lesions either progressed to CIN 2 or remained persistent at the same grade (28%). Although spontaneous regressions did occur, they were confined to patients with "very mild dysplasia," and their number was negligible (6%) when compared with the progression rates. Follow-up examinations showed that the rate of progression increased and the transit time became shorter with increasing severity of CIN. Therefore, the probability that an untreated lesion will progress to CIN 3 is directly dependent on the grade of the lesion. These observations suggested that lesions develop progressively from a better to a lesser differentiated state. The media transit time to CIN 3 was approximately 58 months for CIN 1, 2 years for CIN 2, and 4 years for all the CIN 1–2 lesions taken

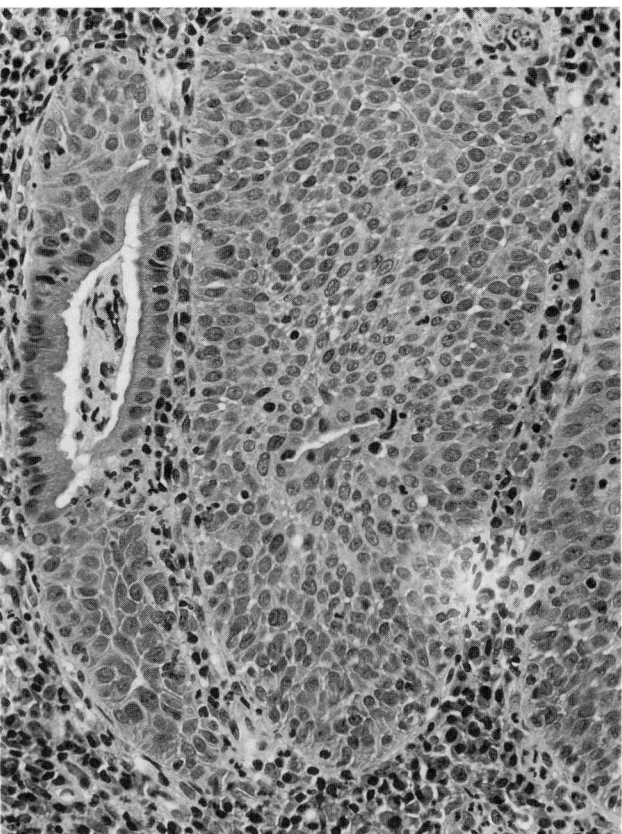

Fig. 7.20. Atypical squamous metaplasia. This lesion is composed of proliferating metaplastic squamous cells that have nuclear atypia but to a lesser degree than usually associated with SIL.

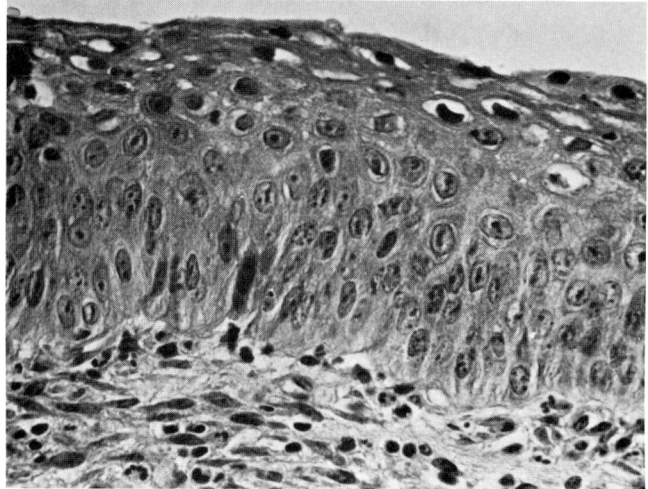

Fig. 7.21. Atypia of repair. Note disorganization of normal maturation. Atypical basal cells occupy the lower half of the epithelium, simulating a high-grade SIL (CIN 2, 3) lesion with koilocytosis. Unlike SIL (CIN), however, the basal cells in atypia of repair have a regular nuclear outline, prominent nucleoli, and distinct cell membranes. Additionally, cells in the upper half of the epithelium are not koilocytotic but contain degernerative perinuclear elliptoid-shaped halos.

Table 7.9. Natural history of low-grade SIL (CIN 1)

Study	No. of patients	Regressed (%)	Persisted (%)	Progressed (%)
Campion et al.	100	7	67	26
Greenberg et al.	176	46	46	9
Hall and Walton	100	62	24	13
Heinzl et al.[a]	2417	46	44	10
Kataja et al.[a]	532	43	39	16
Meisels et al.	110	91	0	9
Nasiell et al.	555	62	22	16
Richart and Barron	557	6	44	50
Robertson et al.	1347	57	27	15
Total	5894	47	37	16

[a] Includes both CIN 1 and CIN 2.
Modified from refs. 46, 133, 138, 144, 173, 234, 252, 299, 307.
SIL, squamous intraepithelial lesion; CIN, cervical intraepithelial neoplasia.

together. However, it is important to point out that there are a number of aspects of this study that may reduce the applicability of its conclusions to patients today. First, the patients enrolled in this study were unusual by today's standards in that all had two to three persistently abnormal Pap smears before entry into the study. Second, an unusual grading system was used to classify the Pap smears in that smears were classified as CIN 1 even when up to 10% of the atypical cells were of the basal type. By today's standards such smears would be classified as high grade. Finally, the actual number of patients in each category was rather small, and therefore complex mathematical models had to be used to project transit times.

Significantly lower rates of persistence and progression and higher rates of regression have been reported in other large-scale studies of the "natural history" or behavior of mild and moderate dysplasia (Table 7.9).* This is not surprising since various studies have used different entry criteria, different diagnostic criteria for categorizing lesions as SIL (CIN), and different study designs. For example, some studies have used punch biopsy and endocervical curettage to establish the diagnosis. These diagnostic methods may remove (treat) lesions and therefore may interfere with long-term analysis by increasing the frequency of spontaneous regression and decreasing the frequency of progression.[250,293]

One of the largest long-term follow-up studies of women with SIL (CIN) was carried out in Sweden by Nasiell and co-workers. In this study, 555 women with mild dysplasia and 894 women with moderate dysplasia were followed on average for 39 and 78 months, respectively.[250,252] In 62% of the women with mild dysplasia, regression to normal occurred; in 22%, there was persistence of mild or moderate dysplasia; and in 16% there was progression of mild dysplasia to severe dysplasia or carcinoma in situ. In women with moderate dysplasia followed without biopsy

for an average of 51 months, spontaneous regression occurred in 28% and progression to severe dysplasia or carcinoma in situ occurred in 50%. Many other prospective follow-up studies of low-grade SIL (CIN 1) have found rates of regression, progression, and persistence similar to those reported by Nasiell et al. (Table 7.9). Taken together, these studies clearly demonstrate that although approximately 16% of low-grade SIL (CIN 1) lesions have the potential for progressing to high-grade SIL (CIN 2, 3) and about 37% persist, many of these lesions (approximately 47%) regress spontaneously if left untreated.

High-grade SIL (CIN 2, 3) has a much greater potential for progressing (Table 7.10).* In a prospective analysis reported by McIndoe et al., carcinoma in situ progressed to invasive carcinoma in 29% of patients followed from 1 to 20 years, and the rate of progression increased directly with the length of follow-up, peaking at 34.6% in patients followed for 14 years.[228] In another study Kohmeir reported, 71% of women with carcinoma in situ developed invasive carcinoma during a minimum follow-up period of 12 years.[194] Other long-term retrospective studies have demonstrated progression of carcinoma in situ to invasive cancer in 22–60% of cases.[30,119,193,346,348]

The prospective follow-up data are in agreement with epidemiologic investigations. The prevalence of low-grade SIL (CIN) proportionally decreases with age.[41,352] New lesions arise in the form of low-grade SIL (CIN 1) instead of high-grade SIL (CIN 2, 3), as determined by calculations of the incidence rate, and there is a 1000–2000 times higher annual incidence of high-grade SIL (CIN 2, 3) in women with previously documented low-grade SIL (CIN) than in those with normal cytological findings.[41,352] In animals, cervical lesions also develop through progressive stages of SIL (CIN) to frankly invasive carcinoma.[314] Richart and co-workers contend that high grade SIL (CIN) usually begins as a small focus within a low-grade SIL (CIN

*Refs. 46,121,133,138,144,168,173,179,234,250,252,307,357.

*Refs. 100,101,165,180,191,193,194,228.

Table 7.10. Natural history of carcinoma in situ

Study	No. of patients	Follow-up	Regressed (%)	Persisted (%)	Progressed (%)
Gad	16	0.5–17 yrs		31	41
Kottmeier	30	>12 yrs			72
Koss et al.	67	6 yrs	25	61	6
McIndoe et al.	131	1–28 yrs	8	69	22
Sorensen et al.	127	>5 yrs		35	
Spriggs et al.	37	>2 yrs		41	60

Modified from refs. 119, 193, 194, 228, 346, 348.

1).[291,292] This small focus then gradually expands and replaces the low-grade SIL (CIN 1). According to this theory, the transition from a low-grade SIL (CIN 1) to a high-grade SIL (CIN 2, 3) represents a monoclonal event within HPV-infected epithelium. That such transitions can occur has been shown by a chromosomal study of SIL (CIN) and microinvasive carcinoma in a single patient, in whom both lesions had a similar abnormal modal number and marker chromosomes.[349]

It should be pointed out, however, that several lines of evidence suggest that high-grade SIL (CIN 2, 3) may develop as an independent event without progressing from low-grade SIL (CIN1). Based primarily on mapping studies, Burghart and co-workers, as well as Koss, have argued that high-grade SIL does not develop by a direct transformation from low-grade SIL.[41,192] Instead, they have suggested that high-grade SIL develops de novo from the epithelium adjacent to low-grade SIL. A recent long-term follow-up study of women visiting an STD clinic also supports the view that high-grade SIL (CIN 2, 3) develops independently from low-grade SIL (CIN 1). This study found that most cases of high-grade SIL (CIN 2, 3) arose de novo in this population in the absence of a cytologically detectable, low-grade SIL (CIN 1) precursor.[196] On the basis of this and other data, some authors have challenged the entire concept that low-grade SIL (CIN 1) is a precursor to high-grade SIL (CIN 2, 3).[183]

MANAGEMENT

Current management of SIL (CIN) depends on a combination of cytology, colposcopy, and directed biopsy as outlined in Figure 7.22.[297,394,395] This management protocol provides a logical approach to therapy based on lesion size, distribution, and grade. The primary objectives both for the clinician treating the patient and the pathologist examining the specimens are: (1) to rule out invasive cancer, and (2) to determine the extent and distribution of noninvasive lesions. Once these objectives have been met, the clinician treating the patient may select from a variety of options for managing women with SIL (CIN). Although an extensive discussion of the work-up and management of women with cervical disease is beyond the purview of this chapter, the pathologist should have a basic understanding of this work-up if he/she is to provide information that will facilitate patient management.

Colposcopy and Cervical Biopsy

If the clinician feels that a woman with an abnormal Pap smear has a significant chance of having SIL (CIN), a glandular lesion, or cancer, colposcopy generally will be performed. The colposcope is a stereoscopic binocular magnifying instrument that provides a three-dimensional image of the tissue surfaces examined. Morphologic changes of the epithelium and vascular pattern that accompany SIL (CIN) and invasive cancer can be visualized and magnified from 4 to 40 times. Before colposcopic examination, a 3–5% solution of acetic acid is applied to the cervix, which removes mucus and dehydrates cells. In areas that microscopically display abnormal surface keratinization, epithelial hyperplasia, or nuclear crowding, the mucosa appears white.

Colposcopic examination of the cervix is limited to the portio and outer third of the endocervical canal. It is inadequate for the evaluation of endocervical neoplasms. The entire transformation zone and lesion, if present, must be visualized for the colposcopic examination to be considered satisfactory. Colposcopic diagnosis is based on the evaluation of the surface contour, color tone (degree of opacity), and border of the lesions.[5,43] Besides the epithelial abnormalities, the subepithelial vascular network undergoes profound alterations in association with SIL (CIN).[350] The flat capillary network, which is found beneath the normal cervical epithelium, becomes tortuous and compressed vertically by the actively growing epithelium, with extension close to the surface (Fig 7.23) producing a colposcopic pattern of punctation (Fig. 7.24). Further proliferation and interconnection of proliferating masses of epithelium result in compression of the vascular network into basket-like structures around the abnormal epithelium, producing a colposcopic mosaic (Fig 7.24). Because of severe compression, some of the capillaries eventually disappear, resulting in an increase in the intercapillary distance. In early invasive carcinoma, a system of new capillaries is generated running parallel to the surface of the abnormal epithelium; this is the so-called horizontal

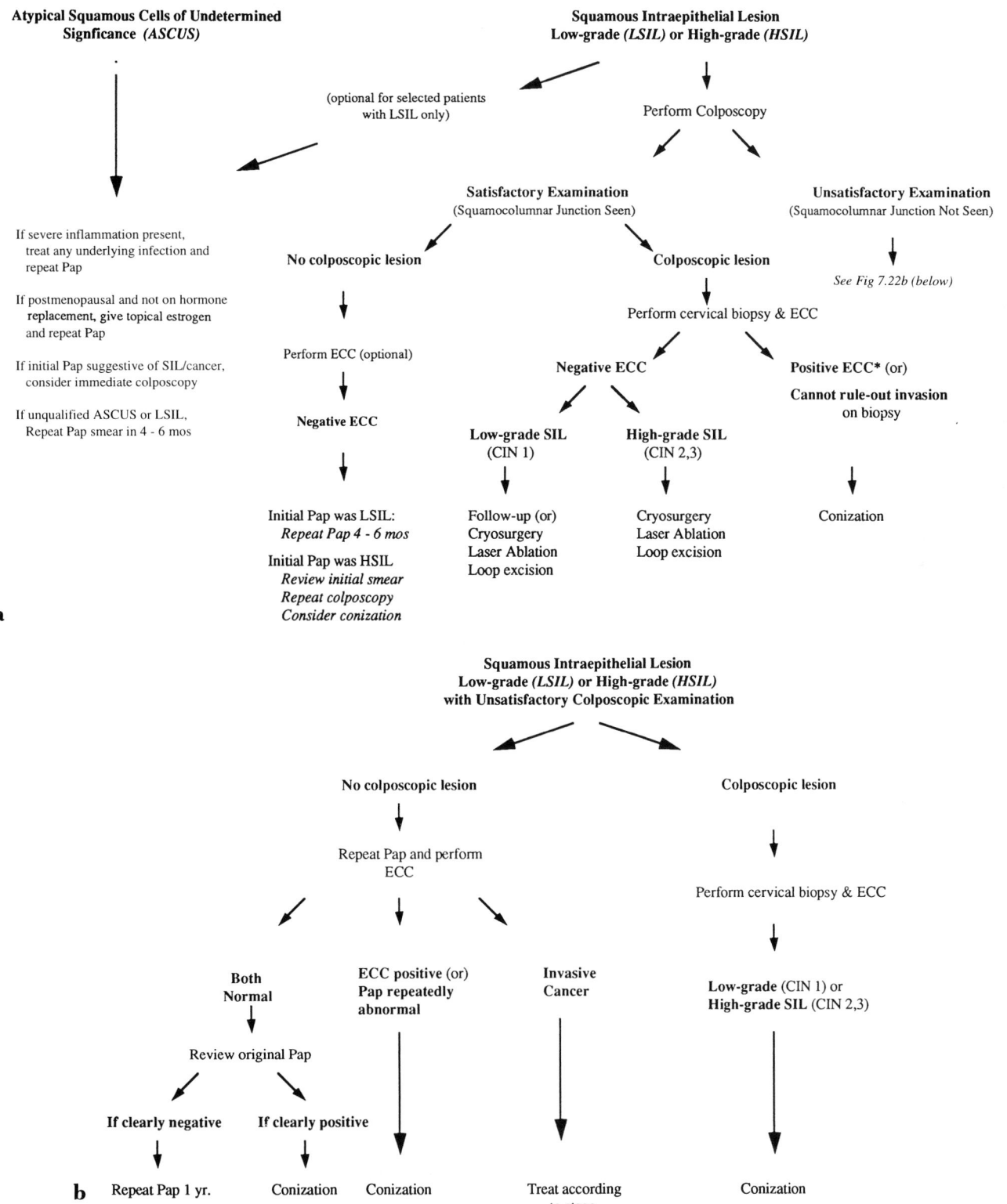

Fig. 7.22. Triage for abnormal Papanicolaou smear. a: Evaluation and management of women with ASCUS or SIL Papanicolaou smear who have a satisfactory colposcopic examination. (If only one or two fragments of SIL are present, this may be a contaminant from the exocervix. A repeat colposcopic evaluation is suggested.) **b:** Evaluation of woman with a SIL Papanicolaou smear who has an unsatisfactory colposcopic examination.

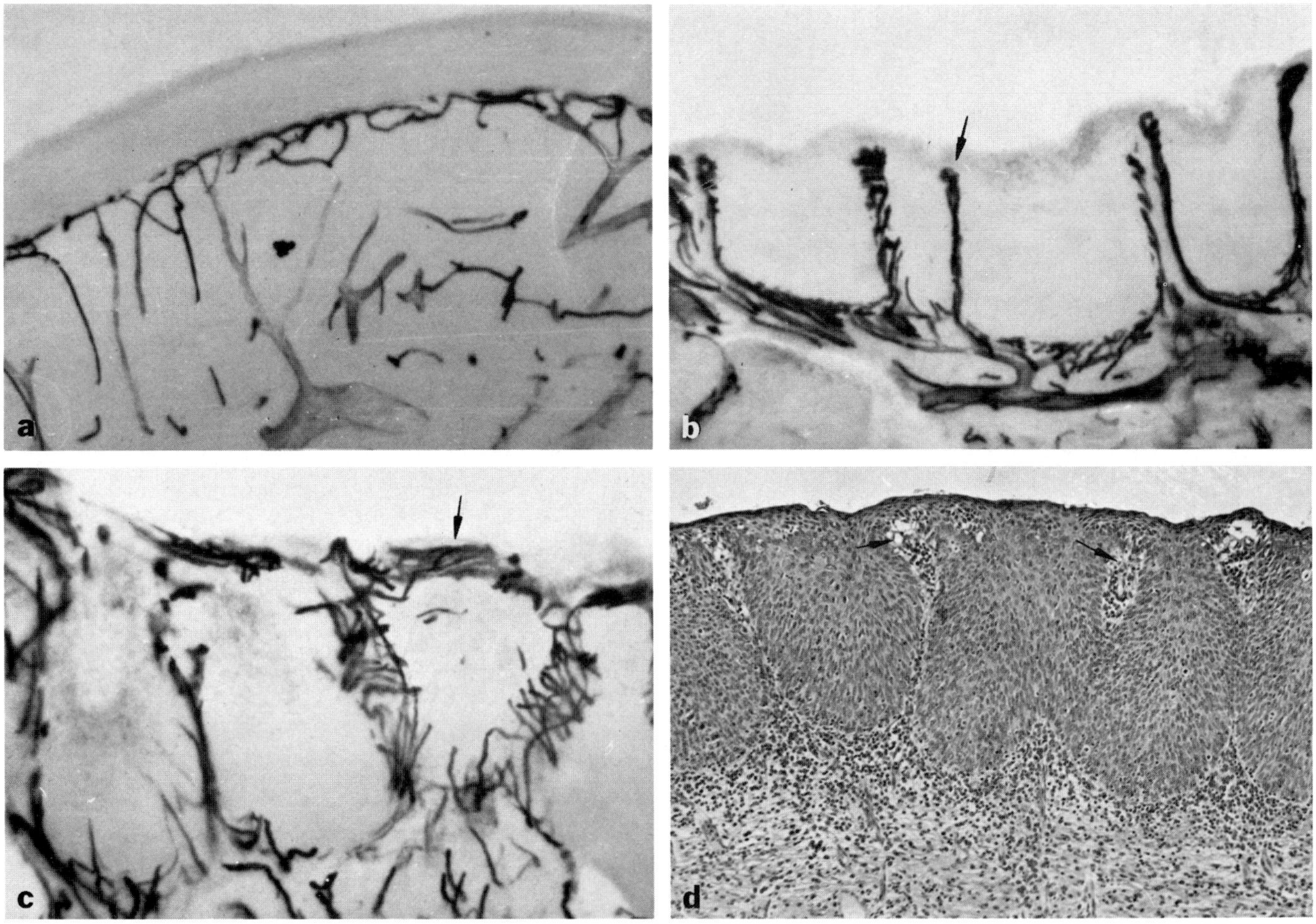

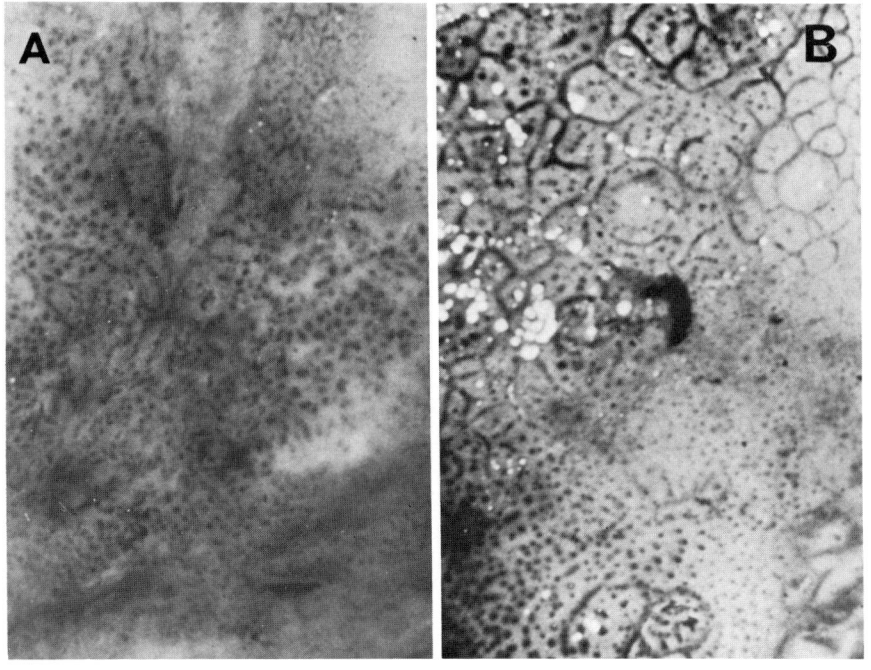

7.23

7.24

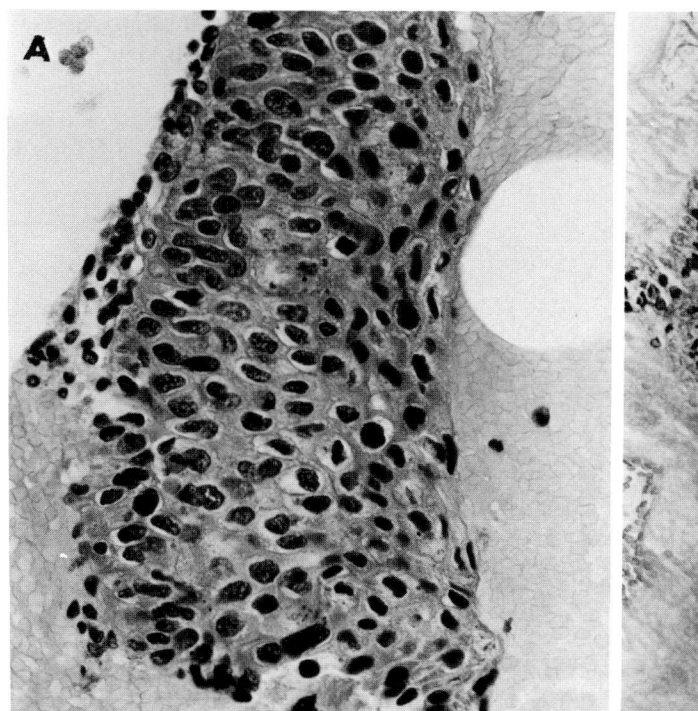

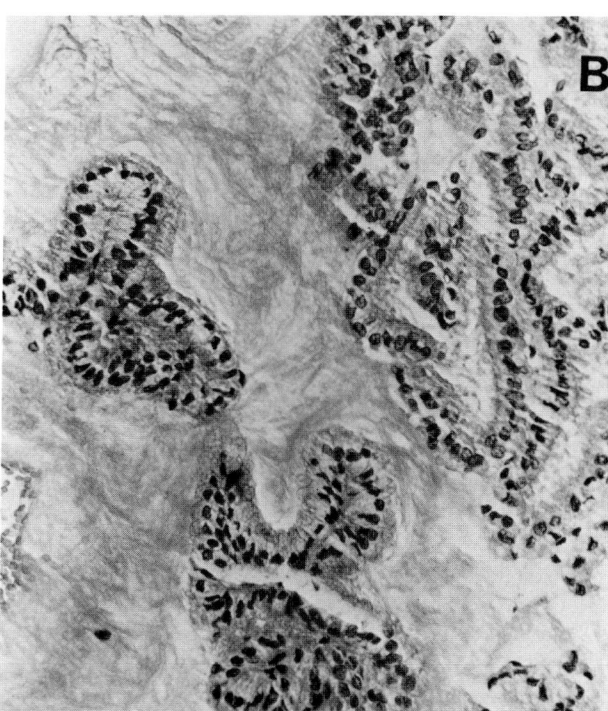

FIG. 7.25. **Endocervical curettings. A: Positive endocervical curettings with a strip of atypical epithelium.** The latter lacks orientation and underlying stroma. As a result, grading cannot be performed, and invasion cannot be ruled out. **B: Negative endocervical curettings with fragments of endocervical epithelium.**

capillary network. These vascular changes and variation in the intercapillary distance are the most important diagnostic colposcopic criteria that serve to distinguish noninvasive from invasive cervical squamous carcinoma.[5,43] Areas with the most pronounced colposcopic abnormality are sampled using a small punch biopsy instrument, such as the square-jawed Kevorkian biopsy punch.

FIG. 7.23. **Histochemical preparations of the terminal vascular network of the cervix. a:** Flat capillary network beneath normal squamous epithelium. **b:** Abnormal vascular growth (*arrow*) in advanced SIL (CIN), producing colposcopic mosaic pattern. **c:** Abnormal horizontal vascular pattern (*arrow*) in early invasive carcinoma of cervix. **d:** Histology of high-grade SIL (CIN 2, 3) in which the vascular stroma papillae are compressed vertically by masses of neoplastic cells, with extension near the surface (*arrows*) producing a colposcopic pattern of punctation (Courtesty of Dr. A. Stafl, Milwaukee, WI.)

FIG. 7.24. **Colposcopic appearances of SIL (CIN). A:** Colposcopic pattern of punctation. Note variation in size of punctate vessels and intercapillary distance. **B:** Colposcopic pattern of mosaic. The epithelium is compartmentalized into irregular baskets and is associated with a coarse punctation pattern.

Endocervical Curettage

Many clinicians perform an endocervical curettage during colposcopic evaluation of the cervix. Endocervical curettage (ECC) is performed to evaluate lesion distribution and morphology within the endocervical canal and to exclude the presence of invasive carcinoma, unsuspected cervical adenocarcinoma in situ, and invasive adenocarcinoma. Endocervical curettage contributes to the diagnostic accuracy of the colposcopic evaluation, particularly in patients in whom no exocervical lesion can be visualized or in whom the squamocolumnar junction is within the endocervical canal.[89,142] With the introduction of endocervical brushes, some clinicians are now using this method instead of the endocervical curettage to evaluate the endocervical canal. The endocervical curettage specimen consists of endocervical tissue fragments, blood, mucus, and when positive, strips of atypical epithelium (Fig. 7.25). To avoid the loss of tiny tissue fragments during processing, the clinician should collect and concentrate the sample, including mucus and blood, on a small square of lens paper and immediately place it in the fixative. By this method, even the smallest tissue fragments can be recovered easily in the laboratory, embedded, and sectioned entirely.

In most instances, when atypical epithelium is detected in the endocervical curettage it lacks underlying stroma and orientation is not possible. As a result, the pathologist can neither rule out underlying invasion nor grade an intraepithelial lesion. In other cases, where the atypical epithelium is well oriented, the pathologist is able to grade the lesion if desired. However, it should be reemphasized that a basic principle of colposcopy is that unless a SIL (CIN) lesion is visualized in its entirety during the examination, cancer has not been ruled out and a cone biopsy is required regardless of grade of the SIL (CIN). It also is helpful if the pathologist conveys an estimate of the amount of atypical epithelium that is present in the endocervical currettings. If only a few small fragments of atypical epithelium are present in the endocervical currettings these may represent "pick-ups" from a lesion that actually is confined to the portio and does not extend into the endocervical canal. In such cases it is preferable to reexamine the patient with the colposcope rather than proceed directly with conization. If the lesion is fully visualized, the endocervical curettage should be repeated under colposcopic visualization to avoid sampling lesional tissue on the portio in the endocervical curettage. Frequently the second, carefully performed curettage yields no atypical epithelium and the patient may be managed on a conservative, outpatient basis. Conversely, the pathologist should be careful not to discount or overlook a few or even a single fragment of atypical epithelium in an endocervical curettage. In a recent review of 21 women who developed invasive cancer after cryotherapy, 7 out of 18 endocervical curettages taken before cryotherapy were found on review to contain SIL (CIN) that had been missed at the time of original diagnosis.[324]

Cervical Conization

Cervical conization is performed as a diagnostic procedure under a number of different circumstances (Table 7.11). A cervical conization specimen represents a conically shaped section of cervix performed for both diagnostic and therapeutic purposes. The cone size varies according to lesion distribution and corresponding operative plan: shallow conization for a predominantly exocervical lesion or a deep cone for a predominantly endocervical lesion. The apex and base of the sample represent the endocervical and exocervical margins, respectively. The technique for processing the specimen is discussed in Chapter 30, Gross Description, Processing, and Reporting of Gynecological and Obstetric Specimens.

TREATMENT

It should be stressed that the observations on the behavior of SIL (CIN) described previously apply only to a population and provide no objective means to predict the potential of regression, persistence, or progression of SIL (CIN) in the individual patient. Since it is impossible to predict which patients will progress to invasion with a given SIL (CIN) at a given time, many clinicians feel that these lesions, once detected, regardless of degree or morphologic severity, should be treated to prevent the development of invasive carcinoma. However, as increasing numbers of patients are diagnosed with low-grade SIL (CIN 1), other clinicians are now taking a more conservative approach and are following patients with low-grade SIL (CIN 1).[167,179,395] In contrast, in almost all instances a diagnosis of high-grade SIL (CIN 2, 3) will result in the patient being treated with ablative (cryosurgical or laser surgical) or excisional (electrosurgical loop excision or cone biopsy) therapy.

Cryosurgery as a method for ablating CIN was introduced in the 1970s and is one of the techniques used most frequently for treating lesions limited to the portio. The failure or residual rate (5–10%) and the long-term recurrence rate (1 of 1000 women per year develops a new CIN after successful cryotherapy) in experienced hands do not exceed that of therapeutic conization.[174,364] Cure rates are not affected by the grade of lesion treated, with only lesion size and quality of freeze proving to be prognostic variables of statistical significance.[6,97] Furthermore, complications and costs of cryosurgery are negligible compared with those of conization.[303] Cryodestruction of cervical tissue is caused by freezing tissue below $-22C°$ with a cryoprobe applied to the cervix. Intracellular and extracellular crystallization leads to dehydration of cells. This results in high electrolyte concentrations that produce biochemical injury associated with lysosomal enzyme release and cell destruction. The only significant end point for successful cryosurgical management of CIN is that the margins of the iceball extend 5 mm and preferably 10 mm beyond the limits of the lesion. Postcryotherapy cervical epithelium quickly sloughs, and healing is generally completed within 12 weeks.

The carbon dioxide (CO_2) laser is another treatment modality for noninvasive neoplasms of the cervix, vagina, and vulva. Unlike conventional light, which is emitted in all directions and has a low energy, laser light is composed of parallel beams of uniform wave lengths (10.6 μm). As a

Table 7.11. Indications for cone biopsy

Normal colposcopy,[a] persistent abnormal cytology, or positive endocervical curettage
Abnormal cytology, squamocolumnar junction not visualized
Limits of lesion not visualized
Microinvasive carcinoma on biopsy or colposcopy suspicious of invasive carcinoma
Adenocarcinoma in situ on biopsy or endocervical curettage
Lack of correlation among cytological, colposcopic, and histological findings[b]

[a] Including the vagina, vulva, and urethra.
[b] i.e., low-grade squamous intraepithelial lesion (SIL) on biopsy and colposcopy with high-grade SIL or invasive cancer on cytology.

result, the laser beam can be directed onto a small spot, where it produces a very high energy density. In the CO_2 laser a mixture of CO_2, nitrogen, and helium is excited by an electrical discharge, and the excited CO_2 molecules give off photons of light energy in the infrared (invisible) part of the spectrum. The light energy is amplified, focused, and directed by a luminous spot of the target beam. Energy output ranges from 1 to 100 W. The laser beam energy is absorbed by the intracellular and extracellular water in tissues, and tissue temperatures rise instantaneously above 100°C. The tissue fluids boil and expand, and the exploded cells are evaporated. As a result, CO_2 laser treatment produces considerably less necrosis than cryosurgery. Evaporation of tissues permits more rapid healing with less vaginal discharge than is associated with cryosurgery.[351] The failure and recurrence rates of laser treatment of cervical lesions are similar to those of cryosurgery.[9,351,364] The expensive equipment cost is its major disadvantage when compared with cryotherapy. Extensive cervical lesions and associated vaginal or vulvar lesions can be treated more easily and appropriately by laser surgery than by cryotherapy.[96]

Recently the loop electrosurgical excision procedure has been used increasingly to treat patients with SIL CIN.[48,278,392] With this technique a tissue specimen is obtained using thin wire loop electrodes that simultaneously cut and cauterize tissue. The technique is both diagnostic as well as therapeutic. As with cervical biopsies, the role of pathological examination of this specimen is to rule out invasive cancer and rule in the presence of SIL (CIN). Because this technique is performed under colposcopic guidance, the colposcopist can determine whether or not the "true" surgical margin of excision is free of disease at the time the procedure is performed and the pathologist need not report margins (see Chapter 30, Gross Description, Processing, and Reporting of Gynecological and Obstetric Specimens).

Precursors of Cervical Adenocarcinoma

Over the last two decades endocervical glandular lesions have received increasing attention, attributable to a variety of factors. One factor is a perception that the prevalence of adenocarcinomas of the cervix and its precursor lesions is increasing. There has been a documented absolute increase in the prevalence of invasive adenocarcinomas in specific groups of women in both the United States and Europe. This may be due in part to the increased routine use of cytobrushes in screening and the widespread adoption of excisional methods for treating SIL (CIN) lesions such as shallow laser conization and the loop electrosurgical excision procedure (LEEP) which permit pathological

examination of the entire transformation zone. In addition, there is an increased recognition of these lesions by pathologists, and an awareness by colposcopists that certain types of glandular lesions cannot be recognized colposcopically.

TERMINOLOGY AND HISTORICAL PERSPECTIVE

In 1957 Stewart stated that "every infiltrative cervical cancer must come from in situ cancer, there being no other thing it could come from".[353] Although this statement is universally accepted, more than three decades after it was made little is known about the natural history of precursors of invasive endocervical adenocarcinoma.

The first indication that precursor lesions exist came in 1952 when Helper described highly atypical neoplastic cells lining architecturally normal endocervical glands adjacent to frankly invasive endocervical adenocarcinomas.[146] Shortly thereafter, Friedell and McKay described two patients with atypical glandular lesions of the cervix and designated these lesions *adenocarcinoma in situ* (AIS) because of their histological resemblance to invasive endocervical adenocarcinoma.[111] One of these patients had a co-existent invasive adenocarcinoma of the cervix and one, squamous carcinoma in situ. Although endocervical glandular lesions with this morphology had been alluded to by Hauser in 1894 and Meyer in 1930, before the descriptions by Helper, Friedell, and McKay, these lesions were not considered to be precursors of endocervical adenocarcinomas.

By analogy to squamous cell cervical cancer precursors, which demonstrate a wide spectrum of histological changes, some authors have proposed parallel classification schemas for endocervical adenocarcinoma precursors that include lesions with a lesser degree of abnormality than AIS.[29,39,128,214] Such low-grade putative glandular precursor lesions originally were termed *endocervical dysplasia* by Bousfield et al.,[29] but other terms such as *atypical hyperplasia* also are used to refer to lesions that resemble AIS but have a somewhat lesser degree of nuclear atypia and mitotic activity.[151,201] Recently Gloor and associates have suggested that the term *cervical intraepithelial glandular neoplasia* (CIGN) be used to refer to both endocervical glandular dysplasia and AIS and that endocervical glandular dysplasia be classified as either CIGN grade 1 or 2 and AIS be classified as CIGN grade 3.[128] Because of the relative rarity of endocervical glandular dysplasia, the subjective nature of the morphologic criteria used to distinguish it from AIS, and the infrequent co-existence of endocervical glandular dysplasia with AIS, the significance of endocervical glandular dysplasia is not known.[151,160,381] Because glandular dysplasia implies a relationship to AIS and invasive carcinoma that has not been documented, we prefer the more noncommittal term *atypical endocervical hyperplasia.* for these atypical proliferations that fall short of AIS.

EPIDEMIOLOGY AND ETIOLOGY

The prevalence of AIS is not known but it is considerably less common than SIL (CIN). In most series, the ratio between AIS and CIN 3 high-grade SIL (CIN 2/3) has ranged from 1:26 to 1:237. One of the best estimates for the prevalence of AIS comes from the Kentucky Cervical Cancer Tumor Registry, a population-based tumor registry encompassing 4,877,301 patient-years at risk, which includes 4350 cervical cancers (including 2391 cases of squamous carcinoma in situ).[112] In this registry, only 16 cases of AIS were documented. Nine occurred in association with squamous carcinoma in situ and seven occurred as pure AIS. For comparison, there were 121 invasive adenocarcinomas of the cervix. Although no population-based data are available on the prevalence of atypical endocervical hyperplasia, in the first large histological study of this lesion it was detected in 15% of 105 cone biopsies or hysterectomies performed for CIN 3 (high-grade SIL).[39] In that study, atypical endocervical hyperplasia was 16 times more common than AIS. This prevalence is considerably higher than that reported in most other series in which most patients with endocervical atypical hyperplasia also have AIS.[128,214]

The mean age at diagnosis for endocervical atypical hyperplasia is 37 years.[39,214] The mean age at diagnosis of women with AIS ranges from 39 to 46 years and is about 10 years lower than the mean age at which invasive adenocarcinoma of cervix is diagnosed.[21,25,29,214] The age relationship between AIS and invasive adenocarcinoma is similar to that of high-grade SIL (CIN 3) and invasive squamous cell carcinoma, suggesting that AIS is a precursor lesion.[359] However, unlike squamous lesions of the cervix in which high-grade precursors occur more frequently than invasive cancer, exactly the opposite relationship exists for AIS and invasive adenocarcinoma of the cervix. Invasive glandular lesions are more common than noninvasive glandular lesions. A number of reasons have been proposed for this apparent discrepancy, including the fact that AIS is more difficult to detect both cytologically and colposcopically than is SIL (CIN) and, therefore, might not be detected before the development of invasive adenocarcinoma.

Additional support implicating AIS as a precursor of invasive adenocarcinoma comes from several anecdotal case reports and two small series of patients who had cytological or histological evidence of AIS several years before the detection of invasive adenocarcinoma.[24,25,172] In a cytological study, Boddington et al. found that 6 of 13 women with invasive adenocarcinoma had previous Pap smears containing atypical endocervical cells 2–8 years before the diagnosis of cancer.[24] Similarly, Boon et al. found that 5 of 18 women with invasive adenocarcinomas had unrecognized AIS on cervical biopsies 3–7 years before detection of the invasive lesion.[25] Although these studies have been interpreted as indicating that AIS is a precursor lesion, it is conceivable that an unrecognized invasive cancer was present at the time of the original Pap smear or cervical biopsy.

The proportion of AIS that occurs in association with SIL (CIN) ranges from 24% to 75%.[4,54,74,214,363,380] This suggests that the two types of lesions may share a common etiology. Using in situ hybridization, Tase and co-workers examined eight cases of AIS for the presence of HPV DNA and found that five of the cases contained HPV but that, unlike SIL (CIN) lesions analyzed with the same method, most AIS was associated with HPV 18 as opposed to HPV 16 in SIL (CIN).[359] Since this initial report, two other groups have analyzed AIS for the presence of HPV DNA and it appears clear that most AIS is associated with HPV DNA. Farnsworth et al. detected HPV DNA in 89% of AIS and the ratio of HPV 18 to HPV 16 in positive cases was 2:1.[94] In a series of eight cases Griffin et al., using PCR, detected HPV in 63% of AIS but HPV 18 was not detected.[134] Associations between atypical endocervical hyperplasia and HPV are more controversial. In the original study by Tase et al., only 2 of 36 cases of atypical endocervical hyperplasia contained HPV DNA.[360] However, in a more recent study, Higgins et al. reported that 94% of atypical endocervical hyperplasias were associated with HPV DNA and 75% were associated with HPV 18.[148]

CLINICAL FEATURES

Up to 83% of women with AIS or atypical hyperplasia are asymptomatic and the lesions are detected either during cytological screening or fortuitously on an endocervical currettage, cervical punch biopsy, or cone or loop excisional biopsy performed during the work-up for SIL (CIN).[4,253,282,363] In women who are symptomatic, the most common complaint is abnormal vaginal bleeding, either postcoital, postmenopausal, or out of phase. Rarely do symptomatic patients present with an abnormal discharge.

AIS and atypical hyperplasia are difficult to detect both cytologically and colposcopically. In a recent histological study of 51 women with atypical hyperplasia or AIS, only 53% of the women had atypical glandular cells detected cytologically on the prediagnosis Pap smears.[74] The other cases were detected fortuitously on biopsies taken to evaluate SIL (CIN). Similarly, in another study of 36 women with AIS, glandular abnormalities were detected on the prediagnosis Pap smear in only one-half the women.[4] The detection of AIS on endocervical currettage also can be difficult.[4]

The distribution of AIS in the cervix is important for determining the most appropriate clinical management of these patients. AIS involves both the surface and glands in almost all cases. In 65% of cases, AIS involves the transformation zone[4,21,363] and in the vast majority of cases it is unifocal. AIS can extend for a distance of up to 3 cm into the endocervical canal.[21,74,260]

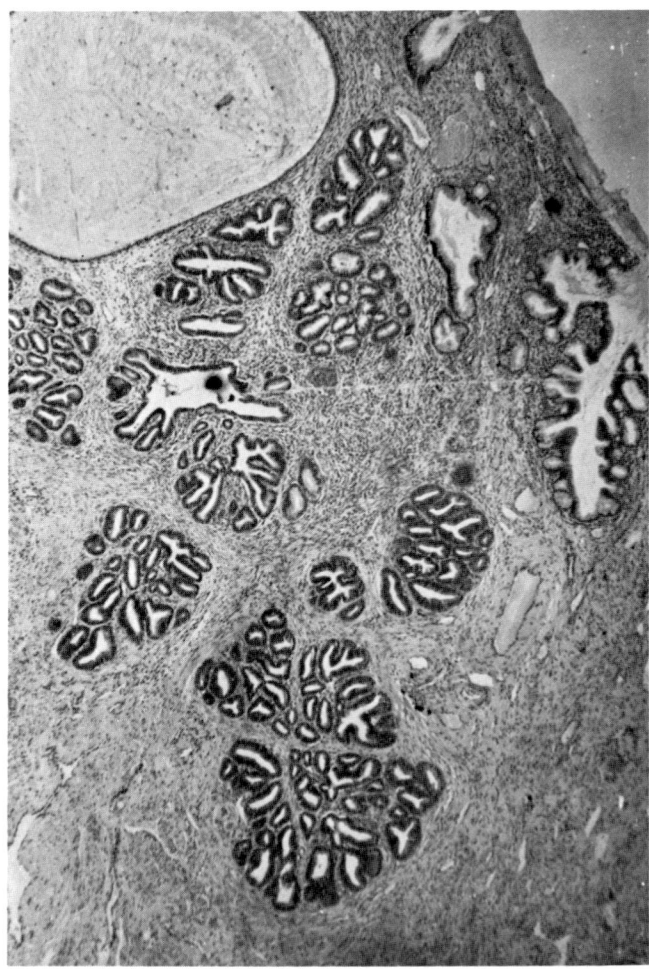

FIG. 7.26. **Adenocarcinoma in situ.** AIS is characterized at low magnification by the presence of endocervical glands that have numerous outpouchings and complex papillary infoldings.

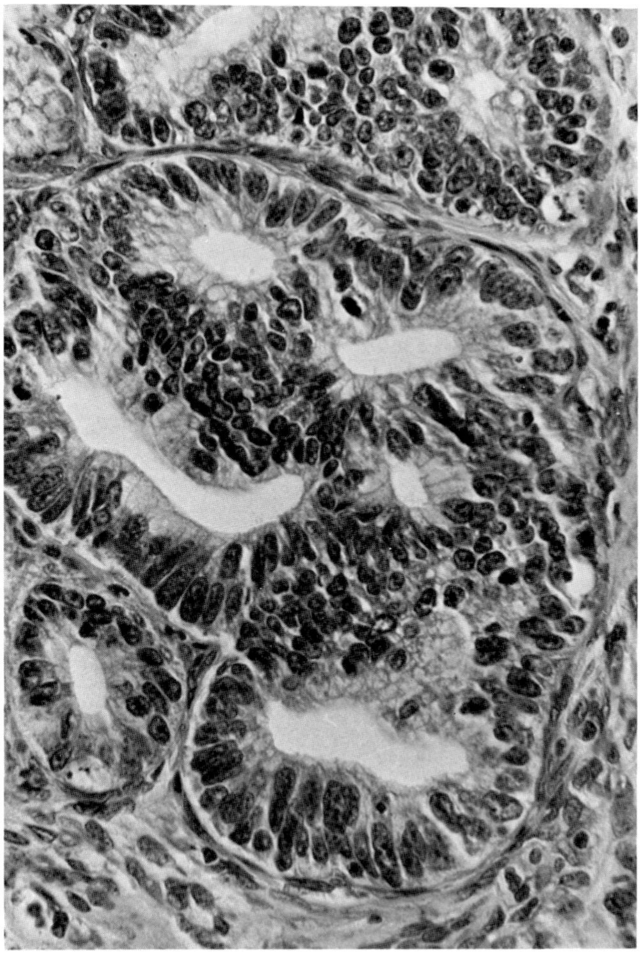

FIG. 7.27. **Adenocarcinoma in situ.** The endocervical glands are lined by atypical columnar cells that are pseudostratified and have elongated, hyperchromatic nuclei with coarsely granular chromatin and frequent mitotic figures. A cribriform appearance can be focally present.

PATHOLOGICAL FINDINGS

AIS is characterized by the presence of endocervical glands lined by atypical columnar epithelial cells that cytologically resemble the cells of invasive adenocarcinoma but that occur in the absence of invasion (Fig. 7.26). These cells have elongated, cigar-shaped, hyperchromatic nuclei with granular chromatin (Fig. 7.27). The amount of cytoplasm is greatly reduced and there is only minimal intracellular mucin. The cells are crowded and pseudostratified, forming two or more rows. AIS may involve glands either focally, multifocally, or diffusely. Typically some glands show an abrupt transition between normal epithelium and AIS (Fig. 7.28). Mitotic figures, including AMFs, are common. Architecturally, the glands of AIS can have numerous outpouchings and complex papillary infoldings and may display a cribriform pattern focally (Fig. 7.29).

Ostor et al. have described two histological types of AIS.[260] One is the typical endocervical-type of AIS described above. The other has features of a colonic, as opposed to endocervical, mucosa with prominent goblet cells (Fig. 7.30). The colonic type is uncommon and usually occurs in association with typical endocervical AIS. The goblet cells in colonic AIS contain o-acetylated sialomucin, which is a marker of intestinal differentiation. Some intestinal types of AIS also contain argentaffin and Paneth cells.[160,366] Endometrioid types of AIS also occur. Rare examples of adenosquamous and clear cell AIS have been described.[129,161]

Invasion should be suspected if the involved glands extend beyond the glandular field or beyond the deepest uninvolved endocervical crypt. In addition, in AIS there should be no desmoplasia or stromal reaction around the involved glands. Other worrisome features that can be

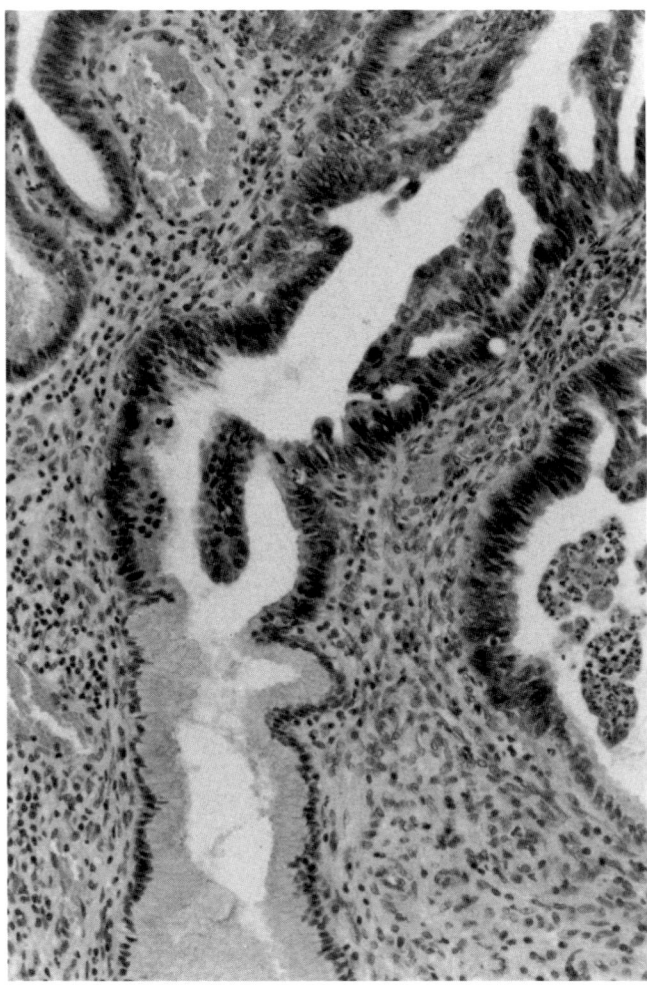

FIG. 7.28. Adenocarcinoma in situ. AIS frequently demonstrates an abrupt change within single glands between neoplastic (*right side*) and normal-appearing glandular epithelium (*left side*).

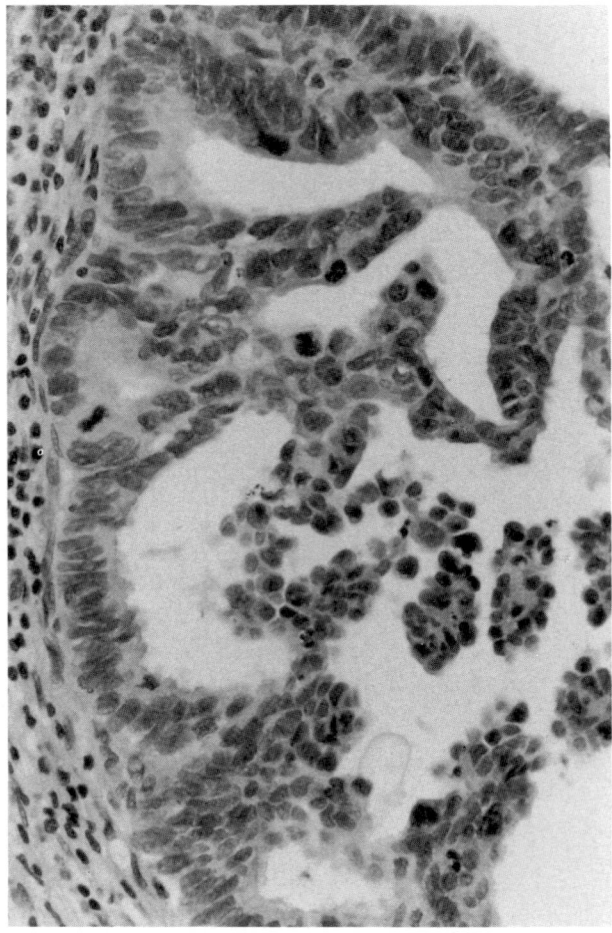

FIG. 7.29. Adenocarcinoma in situ. The glands of AIS may have complex papillary infoldings and a cribriform appearance focally.

associated with invasion are exuberant glandular budding, an extensive cribriform pattern, foci in which the glands become confluent or back-to-back, and the formation of papillary projections from the endocervical surface.[308]

The histological criteria used for diagnosing atypical hyperplasia include hyperchromatic nuclei with only occasional mitotic figures and minimal pseudostratification (Fig. 7.31). Atypical endocervical hyperplasia usually lacks cribriform areas and papillary projections. Some authors have suggested that the number of glands involved in the process is a distinguishing feature between AIS and atypical hyperplasia.[201] If only a single gland is involved, even if there is marked nuclear atypia, a diagnosis of atypical hyperplasia rather than AIS is made. The use of this criterion may decrease the possibility of overdiagnosing reactive, reparative endocervical processes as AIS.

DIFFERENTIAL DIAGNOSIS

The differential diagnosis of AIS and atypical hyperplasia includes reparative/reactive glandular atypias secondary to inflammation, radiation or viral infections, Arias–Stella reaction, microglandular hyperplasia, endometriosis, tubal metaplasia, mesonephric remnants, and invasive adenocarcinoma. Endocervical glands may display a wide range of cytological and architectural changes in response to inflammation and radiation. In reactive/reparative atypia, the nuclei become enlarged and have prominent nucleoli, but have nuclear clearing and lack hyperchromasia (Fig. 7.32). Nuclei may be pleomorphic but the chromatin usually is smudged and degenerative in appearance. Mitotic activity usually is absent or minimal, as is pseudostratification. Care must be taken to distinguish between true pseudo-

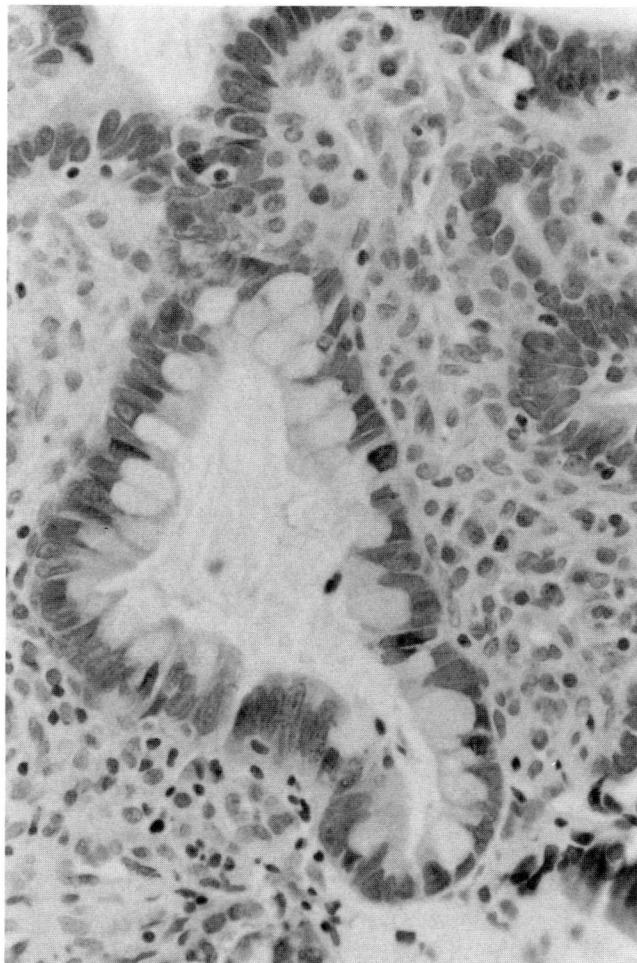

FIG. 7.30. Adenocarcinoma in situ. Colonic-type AIS contains prominent goblet cells and usually occurs in association with typical endocervical AIS.

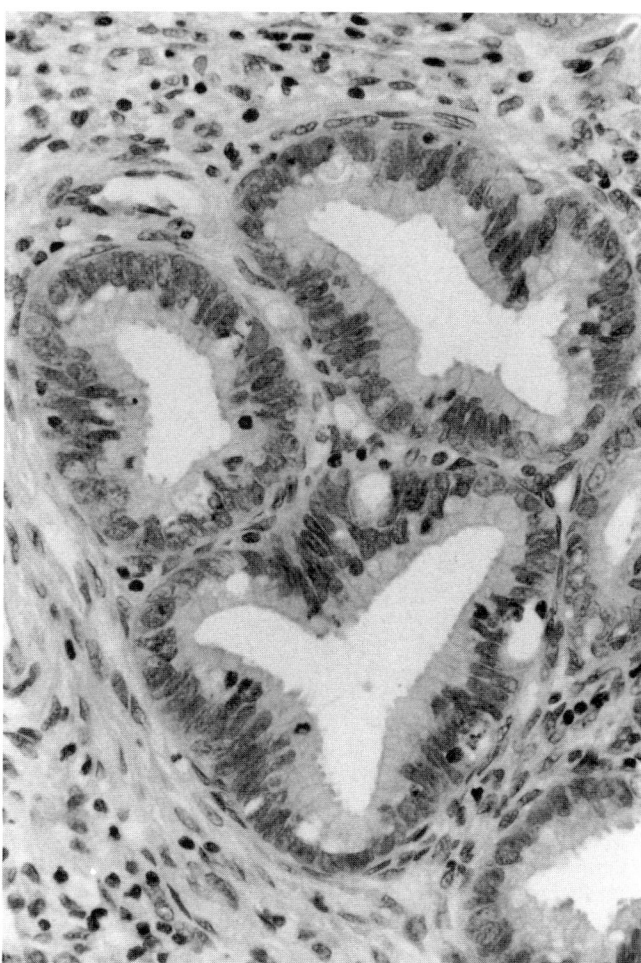

FIG. 7.31. Atypical hyperplasia. Compared with AIS, atypical hyperplasia has less pseudostratification (usually only two rows of cells) and fewer mitotic figures. Endocervical glandular dysplasia also lacks cribriform areas and papillary projections.

stratification and tangential sectioning through glands that can appear as pseudostratification. Although intraglandular papillary projections should not occur in reactive/reparative processes, exaggerated endocervical papillary projections that project into the endocervical canal can occur. These stromal projections contain infiltrates of chronic inflammatory cells and are lined by a single layer of endocervical cells. This entity has been termed *papillary endocervicitis*[398] Endocervical atypias secondary to repair characteristically have a dense acute and chronic inflammatory infiltrate surrounding the glands and polymorpholeukocytes may infiltrate into the epithelium.

Reactive glandular atypia secondary to irradiation is characterized by nuclear enlargement and pleomorphism, but the cytoplasm frequently is vacuolated or granular. Pseudostratification and mitotic figures are absent. Atypia due to irradiation has much more cell to cell variation in size and shape than is typical of AIS or atypical hyperplasia (Fig 7.33).

Glands with the Arias–Stella reaction have a single layer of hyperchromatic, enlarged nuclei that frequently protrude into the gland lumen (i.e. hobnail cells). Typically, Arias–Stella reactions involve only a portion of a gland and mitotic activity is absent. Although microglandular hyperplasia occasionally can be confused with AIS, microglandular hyperplasia lacks significant nuclear atypia and pseudostratification, and has few mitotic figures. Moreover, microglandular hyperplasia has a characteristic pattern of many small, closely packed, uniform glands. Atypical forms of microglandular hyperplasia have been described that form solid masses of epithelium and have significant degrees of cytological atypia.[399] These lesions almost always contain areas of typical microglandular hyperplasia, which allow them to be identified as atypical forms of microglandular hyperplasia (see Chapter 6, Benign Diseases of the Cervix). Similarly, endometriosis of the cervix usually is readily recognizable and easily distinguished from AIS.

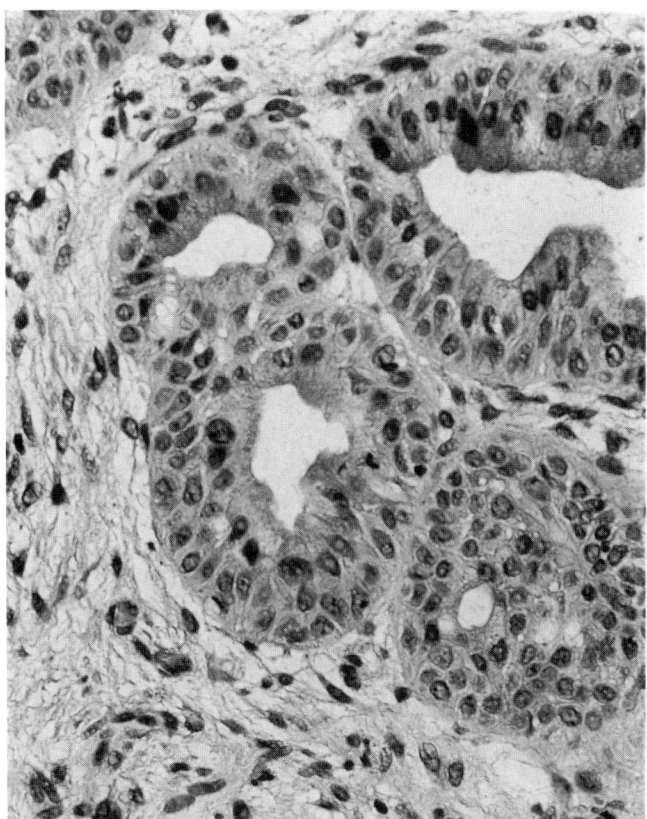

FIG. 7.32. Reactive endocervical atypia. The nuclei are enlarged but the chromatin is smudged. Mitotic activity is either absent or minimal.

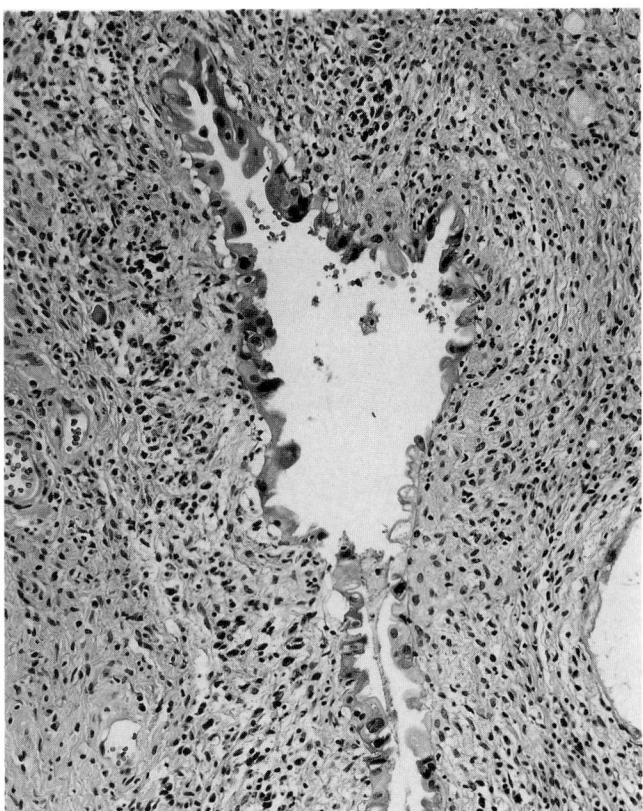

FIG. 7.33. Radiation-induced endocervical atypia. Endocervical atypia induced by irradiation lacks pseudostratification and mitotic figures and is accompanied by degenerative cytoplasmic changes and more cell to cell variation than glandular neoplasia.

Typical endometriosis consists of glands and a prominent stroma. The cells lining the glands are basally located endometrial-type cells that can be pseudostratified and mitotically inactive. Both tubal metaplasia and mesonephric remnants should not be mistaken for AIS since they have bland nuclei that lack mitoses and other histological features that allow them to be recognized (see Chapter 6, Benign Diseases of the Cervix).

CLINICAL BEHAVIOR AND TREATMENT

Because of the relative rarity of AIS, no natural history studies have been published and therefore the evidence that these lesions are precursors for invasive endocervical adenocarcinoma remains circumstantial. Despite this, until recently the treatment of choice was simple hysterectomy. Recently, however, there have been several series of patients with AIS who have been followed after cone biosies.[74,214,248] In one of the largest of these series, Cullimore et al. followed for at least 12 months 42 patients with AIS who were treated by cervical conization only and de-

tected no recurrences in patients in whom the margins of resection were clear. Based on this and other studies, conservative management now appears to be an option in women desirous of maintaining their fertility.

References

1. National Cancer Institute Workshop (1989) The 1988 Bethesda system for reporting cervical/vaginal cytologic diagnoses. JAMA 262: 931–934
2. Abdul-Karim FW, Fu YS, Reagan JW, et al (1982) Morphometric study of intraepithelial neoplasia of the uterine cervix. Obstet Gynecol 60: 210–214
3. Alawattegama AB (1984) Screening for cervical intraepithelial neoplasia and cancer in the Sheffield STD clinic. Br J Vener Dis 60: 117–120
4. Andersen ES, Arffmann E (1989) Adenocarcinoma in situ of the uterine cervix: A clinico-pathologic study of 36 cases. Gynecol Oncol 35: 1–7
5. Anderson M, Jordan J, Morse A, et al (1991) A text and atlas of integrated colposcopy. St. Louis, Mosby Year Book
6. Arof HM, Gerbie MV, Smeltzer J (1984) Cryosurgical treat-

ment of cervical intraepithelial neoplasia: Four-year experience Am J Obstet Gynecol 150: 865

7. Audet-Lapointe P (1971) Detection of cervical cancer in a women's prison. Can Med Assoc 104: 509–511

8. Aurelian L (1976) Sexually transmitted cancers? The case for genital herpes. J Am Vener Dis Assoc 2: 10

9. Baggish JS (1980) High-power density carbon dioxide laser therapy for early cervical neoplasia. Am J Obstet Gynecol 139: 117

10. Bamford PN, Barber M, Beilby JOW (1982) Changing patterns of cervical intraepithelial neoplasia seen in a family planning clinic. (Letter) Lancet i: 747–827

11. Baram A, Schacter A (1982) Cervical carcinoma: Disease of the future for Jewish women. Lancet i: 747

12. Barron BA, Richart RM (1968) A statistical model of the natural history of cervical carcinoma based on a prospective study of 557 cases. J Natl Cancer Inst 41: 1343

13. Barron BA, Richart RM (1970) A statistical model of the natural of cervical carcinoma. II. Estimates of the transition time from dysplasia to carcinoma in situ. J Natl Cancer Inst 45: 1025

14. Bauer HM, Ting Y, Greer CE, et al (1991) Genital human papillomavirus infection in female university students as determined by a PCR-based method. JAMA 265: 472–477

15. Bedell MA, Jones KH, Grossman SR, et al (1989) Identification of human papillomavirus type 18 transforming genes in immortalized and primary cells. J Virol 63: 1247–1255

16. Bedell MA, Jones KH, Laimins LA (1987) The E6-E7 region of human papillomavirus type 18 is sufficient for transformation of NIH 3T3 and rat −1 cells J Virol 61: 3635–3640

17. Bergeron C, Barrasso R, Beaudenon S, et al (1992) Human papillomaviruses associated with cervical intraepithelial neoplasia. Great diversity and distinct distribution in low- and high-grade lesions. Am J Surg Pathol 16: 641–649

18. Bergeron C, Ferenczy A, Shah K, et al (1987) Multicentric human papillomavirus infections of the female genital tract. Correlation of viral types with abnormal mitotic figures, colposcopic presentation, and location. Obstet Gynecol 69: 736–742

19. Berkowitz RS, Ehrmann RL, Lavizzo-Mourey R, et al (1979) Invasive cervical carcinoma in young women. Gynecol Oncol 8: 311–316

20. Bernard BA, Bailly C, Lenoir MC, et al (1989) The human papillomavirus type 18 (HP18) E2 gene product is a repressor of the HPV18 regulatory region in human keratinocytes. J Virol 63: 4317–4324

21. Bertrand M, Lickrish GM, Colgan TJ (1987) The anatomic distribution of cervical adenocarcinoma in situ: implications for treatment. Am J Obstet Gynecol 157: 21–25

22. Bibbo M, Dytch HE, Alenghat E, et al (1989) DNA ploidy profiles as prognostic indicators in CIN lesions. Am J Clin Pathol 92: 261–265

23. Binder MA, Cates GW, Emson HE, et al (1985) The changing concepts of condyloma. A retrospective study of colposcopically directed cervical biopsies. Am J Obstet Gynecol 151: 213–219

24. Boddington MM, Spriggs AI, Cowdell RH (1976) Adenocarcinoma of the uterine cervix: Cytological evidence of a long preclinical evolution. Br J Obstet Gynecol 83: 900–903

25. Boon ME, Baak JPA, Kurver PJH, et al (1981) Adenocarcinoma in situ of the cervix: An underdiagnosed lesion. Cancer 48: 768–773

26. Bosch FX, Munoz N, de SanJose S, et al (1992) Risk factors for cervical cancer in Columbia and Spain. Int J Cancer 52: 750–758

27. Bosch FX, Schwarz E, Boukamp P, et al (1990) suppression in vivo of human papillomavirus type 18 E6-E7 gene expression in non-tumorigenic HeLa fibroblast hybrid cells. J Virol 64: 4743–4754

28. Boshart M, Gissman L, Ikenberg H, et al (1984) A new type of papillomavirus DNA, its presence in genital cancer biopsies and in cell lines derived from cervical cancer. EMBO J 3: 1151–1157

29. Bousfield L, Pacey F, Young Q, et al (1980) Expanded cytologic criteria for the diagnosis of adenocarcinoma in situ of the cervix and related lesions. Acta Cytol 24: 283–296

30. Boyes DA, Fidler HK, Lock DR (1963) The significance of in situ carcinoma of the uterine cervix. In Proceedings of First International Congress on Exfoliative Cytology. JB Lippincott, Philadelphia, PA

31. Bradbeer C (1987) Is infection with HIV a risk factor for cervical intraepithelial neoplasia? Lancet ii: 1277–1278

32. Brinton LA (1991) Oral contraceptives and cervical neoplasia. Contraception 43: 581–595

33. Brinton LA (1992) Epidemiology of cervical cancer-an overview. In: Munoz N, Bosch FX, Shah K, Meheus A (eds). The epidemiology of cervical cancer and human papillomavirus. Lyon, IARC Scientif Publication, pp 3–22

34. Brinton LA, Fraumeni JF (1986) Epidemiology of uterine cervical cancer. J Chron Dis 39: 1051–1065

35. Brinton LA, Schairer C, Haenszel W, et al (1986) Cigarette smoking and invasive cervical cancer. JAMA 255: 3265–3269

36. Broders AC (1932) Carcinoma in situ contrasted with benign penetrating epithelium JAMA 99: 1670–1674

37. Broker TR (1987) Structure and genetic expression of papillomaviruses. Obstet Gynecol North Am 14: 329–348

38. Broker TR, Botchan M (1986) Papillomaviruses: Retrospectives and prospectives. In: Botchan TG, Sharp PA (eds) Cancer cells/DNA tumor viruses. Cold Spring Harbor, Cold Spring Harbor Laboratory, pp 17–36

39. Brown LJR, Wells M (1986) Cervical glandular atypia associated with squamous intraepithelial neoplasia: a premalignant lesion? J Clin Pathol 39: 22–28

40. Buckley CH, Butler EB, Fox H (1982) Cervical intraepithelial neoplasia. J Clin Pathol 35: 1–13

41. Burghardt E (1973) Early histological diagnosis of cervical cancer. Stuttgart, Georg Thieme Verlag

42. Burghardt E, Ostor AG (1983) Site and origin of squamous cervical cancer: A histomorphologic study. Obstet Gynecol 62: 117–127

43. Burke L, Antonioli DA, Ducatman BS (1991) Colposcopy: Text and Atlas, Norwalk, Conn, Appleton & Lange

44. Butterworth CE, Hatch KD, Gore H, et al (1982) Improvement in cervical dysplasia associated with folic acid therapy in users of oral contraceptives. Am J Clin Nutr 35: 73–82

45. Butterworth CEJ, Hatch KD, Macaluso M, et al (1992) Folate deficiency and cervical dysplasia. JAMA 267: 528–533

46. Campion MJ, Cuzick J, McCance DJ, et al (1986) Progres-

sive potential of mild cervical atypia: Prospective, cytological, colposcopic, and virologic study. Lancet ii: 237–240

47. Campion MJ, Singer A, Clarkson PK, et al (1985) Increased risk of cervical neoplasia in consorts of men with penile condylomata acuminata. Lancet i: 97

48. Cartier R (1984) Practical Colposcopy, 2nd ed. Paris, Laboratore Cartier

49. Cartwright RA, Sinson JD (1981) Carcinoma of penis and cervix. Lancet i: 97

50. Casas-Cordero M, Morin C, Roy M, et al (1981) Origin of the koilocyte in condylomata of the human cervix. Ultrastructural study. Acta Cytol 25: 383–392

51. Cevenini R, Costa S, Rumpianes F, et al (1981) Cytological and histopathological abnormlaities of the cervix in genital *Chlamydia trachomatis* infections. Br J Vener Dis 57: 334–337

52. Chapman WB, Lorincz AT, Willett GD, et al (1993) Evaluation of two commercially available in situ hybridization kits for detection of human papillomavirus DNA in cervical biopsies: Comparison to Southern blot hybridization. Mod Pathol 6: 73–79

53. Chow LT, Hirochika H, Nasseri M, et al (1987) Human papilloma virus gene expression. In: Steinberg JLB, Taichman LB (eds) Papillomaviruses, Cancer Cells. Cold Spring Harbor, Cold Spring Harbor Press

54. Christopherson WM, Nealon N, Gray LA (1979) Noninvasive precursor lesions of adenocarcinoma and mixed adenosquamous carcinoma of the cervix uteri. Cancer 44: 975–983

55. Clarke EA, Hatcher J, McKeown-Eyssen GE, et al (1985) Cervical dysplasia: Association with sexual behavior, smoking and oral contraceptive use? Am J Obstet Gynecol 151: 612–616

56. Coggin JR, zur Hausen H (1979) Workshop on papillomaviruses and cancer. Cancer Res 39: 545–546

57. Collaborative Study of Neoplasia and Steroid Contraception - WHO (1985) Invasive cervical cancer and combined oral contraceptives. Br Med J 290: 961–965

58. CDC (1990) Risk for cervical disease in HIV-infected women—New York City. MMWR 39: 846–849

59. CDC (1993) 1993 Revised classification system for HIV infection and expanded surveillance case definition for AIDS among adolescents and adults. MMWR 41: 1–20

60. Coppleson M (1970) The origin and nature of premalignant lesions of the cervix uteri. Int J Gynecol Obstet 8: 539

61. Coppleson M, Reid B (1967) Preclinical carcinoma of the cervix uteri. Oxford, Pergamon Press

62. Cramer DW, Cutler SJ (1974) Incidence and histopathology of malignancies of the female genital organs in the United States. Am J Obstet Gynecol 118: 443

63. Crocker J, Fox H, Langley FA (1968) Consistency in the histological diagnosis of epithelial abnormalities of the cervix uteri. J Clin Pathol 21: 67

64. Croissant OF, Breitburd F, Orth G (1985) Specificity of cytopathic effect of cutaneous human papillomaviruses. Clin Dermatol 3: 43

65. Crook T, Morgenstern JP, Crawford L, et al (1989) Continued expression of HPV 16 E7 protein is required for maintenance of the transformed phenotype of cells co-transformed by HPV 16 plus EJ-ras. EMBO J 8: 513–519

66. Crum C, Nuovo G, Friedman D, et al (1988) A comparison of biotin and isotope labeled ribonucleic acid probes for in situ detection of HPV 16 ribonucleic acid in genital precancers. Lab Invest 58: 354–359

67. Crum CP, Egawa K, Fu YS, et al (1983) Atypical immature metaplasia (AIM): A subset of human papillomavirus infection of the cervix. Cancer 51: 2214–2219

68. Crum CP, Levine RU (1984) Human papillomavirus infection and cervical neoplasia: New perspectives. Int J Gynecol Pathol 3: 376–386

69. Crum CP, Mitao M, Levine RU, et al (1985) Cervical papillomaviruses segregate within morphologically distinct precancerous lesions. J Virol 54: 675–681

70. Crum CP, Nagai N, Mitao M, et al (1985) Histological and molecular analysis of early cervical neoplasia. In: Howley P, Broker T (eds) Papillomaviruses: Molecular and Clinical Aspects. New York, New York, pp 19–29

71. Crum CP, Nuovo G, Freidman D, et al (1988) Accumulation of RNA homologous to human papillomavirus type 16 open reading frames in genital precancers. J Virol 62: 84–90

72. Cullen AP, Reid R, Campion M, et al (1991) A analysis of the physical state of different human papillomavirus DNAs in intraepithelial and invasive cervical neoplasia. J Virol 65: 606–612

73. Cullen TS (1900) Cancer of the Uterus, New York, Appleton and Company

74. Cullimore JE, Luesley DM, Rollason TP, et al (1992) A prospective study of conization of the cervix in the management of cervical intraepithelial glandular neoplasia (CIGN)—a preliminary report. Br J Obstet Gynecol 99: 314–318

75. Dale GE, Coleman RM, Best JM, et al (1988) Class-specific herpes simplex virus antibodies in sera and cervical secretions from patients with cervical neoplasia: A multi-group comparison. Epidemiol Int 100: 455–465

76. Daniele E, Perino A, Catinella E (1985) Superficial endometrial involvement by cervical intraepithelial neoplasia detected by intrauterine cytology. Acta Cytol 29: 411–413

77. de Vet HC, Knipschild PG, Grol ME, et al (1991) The role of beta-carotene and other dietary factors in the aetiology of cervical dysplasia: results of a case control study. Int J Epidemiol 20: 603–610

78. de Villiers EM (1989) Heterogeneity of the human papillomavirus group. J Virol 63: 4898–4903

79. de Villiers EM, Schneider A, Gross G, et al (1986) Analysis of benign and malignant urogenital tumors for human papillomavirus infection by labelling cellular DNA. Med Microbiol Immunol 174: 281–286

80. de Villiers EM, Wagner D, Schneider A, et al (1987) Human papillomavirus infections in women with and without abnormal cervical cytology. Lancet i: 703–706

81. de Villiers EM, Wagner D, Schneider A, et al (1992) Human papillomavirus DNA in women without and with cytological abnormalities: Results of a 5-year follow-up study. Gynecol Oncol 44: 33–39

82. Devesa SS (1984) Descriptive epidemiology of cancer of the uterine cervix. Obstet Gynecol 63: 605

83. DiPaolo JA, Woodworth CD, Popescu NC, et al (1990) HSV–2 induced tumorigenicity in HPV 16 immortalized human genital keratinocytes. Virology 177: 777–779

84. Donnan SP, Wong FW, Ho SC, et al (1989) Reproductive and sexual risk factors and human papilloma virus infection in cervical cancer among Hong Kong Chinese. Int J Epidemiol 18: 32–36

85. Doorbar J (1991) An emerging function for E4. Papillomavirus Reports 2: 145–147

86. Doorbar J, Campbell D, Grand RJA, et al (1986) Identification of the human papilloma virus–1a E4 gene products. EMBO J 5: 355–362

87. Doorbar J, Coneron I, Gallimore PH (1989) Sequence divergence yet conserved physical characteristics among the E4 proteins of cutaneous human papillomaviruses. Virology 172: 51–62

88. Doorbar J, Ely S, Sterling J, et al (1991) Specific interaction between HPV 16 E1-E4 and cytokeratins results in collapse of the epithelial cell intermediate filament network. Nature 352: 824–827

89. Drescher CW, Peters WA, Roberts JA (1983) Contribution of endocervical curettage in evaluating abnormal cervical cytology. Obstet Gynecol 62: 343–347

90. Durst M, Kleinheinz A, Hotz M, et al (1985) The physical state of human papillomavirus type 16 DNA in benign and malignant genital tumors. J Gen Virol 66: 1515–1522

91. Dyson N, Howley PM, Munger K, et al (1989) The human papillomavirus 16 E7 oncoprotein is able to bind to the retinoblastoma gene product. Science 243: 934–937

92. Eliyahu D, Michalovitz D, Eliyahu S, et al (1989) Wild type p53 can inhibit oncogene mediated focus formation. Proc Natl Acad Sci 86: 8763–8767

93. Evans S, Dowling K (1990) The changing prevalence of cervical human papillomavirus infection. Aust NZ J Obstet Gynaecol 30: 375–377

94. Farnsworth A, Laverty C, Stoler MH (1989) Human papillomavirus messenger RNA expression in adenocarcinoma in situ of the uterine cervix. Int J Gynecol Pathol 8: 321–330

95. Feingold AR, Vermund SH, Burk RD, et al (1990) Cervical cytologic abnormalities and papillomavirus in women infected with human immunodeficiency virus. J AIDS 3: 896–903

96. Ferenczy A (1985) Comparison of cryo- and carbon dioxide laser therapy for cervical intraepithelial neoplasia Obstet Gynecol 66: 793–798

97. Ferenczy A (1985) Comparison of cryo- and carbon dioxide laser therapy for cervical intraepithelial neoplasia. Obstet Gynecol 66: 793

98. Ferenczy A, Richard RM (1974) Female reproductive system. Dynamics of scan and transmission electron microscopy. New York, John Wiley & Sons

99. Ferenczy A, Richart RM, Okagaki T (1971) Endometrial involvement by cervical carcinoma in situ. Am J Obstet Gynecol 110: 590–592

100. Fidler HK, Boyes DA, Nichols TM, et al (1970) Cervical cytology in the control of cancer of the cervix. Mod Med Can 25: 9

101. Fidler HK, Boyes DA, Worth AJ (1968) Cervical cancer detection in British Columbia. J Obstet Gynecol Br Commonw 75: 392

102. Finlay CA, Hinds PW, Levine AJ (1989) The p53 proto-oncogene can act as a suppressor of transformation. Cell 57: 1083–1093

103. Firzlaff JM, Kiviat NB, Beckmann AM, et al (1988) Detection of human papillomavirus capsid antigens in various squamous epithelial lesions using antibodies directed against the L1 and L2 open reading frames 164: 467–477

104. Fletcher S (1983) Histopathology of papillomavirus infection of the cervix uteri: The history, toxonomy, nomenclature and reporting of koilocytic dysplasias. J Clin Pathol 36: 616–624

105. Foote FW, Stewart FW (1948) The anatomical distribution of intraepithelial epidermoid carcinomas of cervix. Cancer 1: 431–440

106. Fox CH (1967) Biologic behavior of dysplasia and carcinoma in situ. Am J Obstet Gynecol 99: 960

107. Franceschi S, LaVecchia C, Decarli A (1986) Relation of cervical neoplasia with sexual factors, including specific venereal diseases. Cold Spring Harbor, NY, Cold Spring Harbor Laboratory pp 65–78

108. Franco EL (1991) The sexually transmitted disease model for cervical cancer; Incoherent epidemiologic findings and the role of misclassification of human papillomavirus infection. Epidemiology 2: 98–106

109. Franquemont DW, Ward BE, Anderson WA, et al (1989) Prediction of "high-risk" cervical papillomavirus infection by biopsy morphology Am J Clin Pathol 92: 577–582

110. Frazer IH, Tindle RW (1992) Cell-mediated immunity to papillomaviruses. Papillomavirus Reports 3: 53–55

111. Friedell GH, McKay DG (1953) Adenocarcinoma in situ of endocervix. Cancer 6: 887–897

112. Friedell GH, Tucker TC, McManmon E, et al (1992) Incidence of dysplasia and carcinoma of the uterine cervix in an Appalachian population. J Natl Cancer Inst 84: 1030–1032

113. Fu YS, Braun L, Shah KV, et al (1983) Histologic, nuclear DNA, and human papillomavirus studies of cervical condylomas Cancer 52: 1705–1711

114. Fu YS, Huang I, Beaudenon S, et al (1988) Correlative study of Human papillomavirus, DNA, histopathology and morphometry in cervical condyloma and intraepithelial neoplasia. Int J Gynecol Pathol 7: 297–307

115. Fu YS, Reagan J, Richart RM (1981) Definition of precursors. Gynecol Oncol 12: s220

116. Fu YS, Reagan JW, Richart RM (1983) Precursors of cervical cancer Cancer Surv 2: 359–382

117. Fujii T, Crum CP, Winkler B, et al (1984) Human papillomavirus infection and cervical intraepithelial neoplasia. Histopathology and DNA content. Obstet Gynecol 63: 99–104

118. Fukushima M, Yamakawa Y, Shimano S, et al (1990) The physical state of human papillomavirus 16 DNA in cervical carcinoma and cervical intraepithelial neoplasia. Cancer 66: 2155–2161

119. Gad C (1976) The management and natural history of severe dysplasia and carcinoma in situ of the uterine cervix. Br J Obstet Gynecol 83: 554–559

120. Galloway DA, McDougall JK (1983) The oncogenic potential of herpes simplex viruses: Evidence for a "hit and run" mechanism. Nature 302: 21–23

121. Garutti P, Segala V, Folegatti MR, et al (1991) Evolution of cervical intraepithelial neoplasia grades I and II: A two year follow-up of untreated and treated cases. Cervix 9: 21–24

122. Giri I, Yaniv M (1988) Structural and mutational analysis of E2 transactivating proteins of papillomaviruses reveals three distinct functional domains. EMBO J 7: 2823–2829

123. Giri I, Yaniv M (1988) Study of the E2 gene product of the cottontail rabbit papillomavirus reveals a common mechanism of transactivation among papillomaviruses. J Virol 62: 665–672

124. Gissmann L (1984) Papillomaviruses and their association with cancer in animals and in man. Cancer Surv 3: 161–181

125. Gissmann L, de Villiers EM, zur Hausen H (1982) Analysis of human genital warts (condylomata acuminata) and other genital tumors for human papillomavirus type 6 DNA. Int J Cancer 29: 143–146

126. Gissmann L, Wolnik L, Ikenberg H, et al (1983) Human papillomavirus types 6 and 11 DNA sequences in genital and laryngeal papillomas and in some cervical cancers. Proc Natl Acad Sci USA 80: 560–563

127. Gissmann L, zur Hausen H (1980) Partial characterization of viral DNA from human genital warts (condylomata acuminata). Int J Cancer 25: 605–609

128. Gloor E, Hurlimann J (1986) Cervical intraepithelial glandular neoplasia (adenocarcinoma in situ and glandular dysplasia). A correlative study of 23 cases with histologic grading, histochemical analysis of mucins and immunohistochemical determination of the affinity for four lectins. Cancer 58: 1272–1280

129. Gloor E, Ruzicka J (1982) Morphology of adenocarcinoma in situ of the uterine cervix: A study of 14 cases. Cancer 49: 294–302

130. Graham S, Priore R, Graham M, et al (1979) Genital cancer in wives of penile cancer patients. Cancer 44: 1870–1874

131. Gram IT, Austin H, Stalsberg H (1992) Cigarette smoking and the incidence of cervical intraepithelial neoplasia, grade III, and cancer of the cervix. Am J Epidemiol 135: 341–346

132. Gram IT, Macaluso M, Stalsberg H (1992) Oral contraceptive use and the incidence of cervical intraepithelial neoplasia. Am J Obstet Gynecol 167: 40–44

133. Greenberg M, Reid R, Husain M, et al (1992) A prospective natural history study of minor grade cervical lesions: a preliminary report. In: Abstracts, Fifth Human Papillomavirus Meeting, Chicago, IL

134. Griffin NR, Dockey D, Lewis FA, et al (1991) Demonstration of low frequency of human papillomavirus DNA in cervical adenocarcinoma and adenocarcinoma in situ by the polymerase chain reaction and in situ hybridization. Int J Gynecol Pathol 10: 36–43

135. Gross G, Ikenberg H, Gissmann L, et al (1985) Papillomavirus infection of the anogenital region: Correlation between histology, clincal picture and virus type. Proposal of a new nomanclature. J Invest Dermatol 85: 147

136. Gross G, Pfister H, Hagedorn M, et al (1982) Correlation between human papillomavirus (HPV) type and histology of warts. J Invest Dermatol 78: 160–164

137. Guijon FB, Paraskevas M, Brunham R (1985) The association of sexually transmitted diseases with cervical intraepithelial neoplasia: A case-control study. Am J Obstet Gynecol 151: 185–190

138. Hall JE, Walton L (1968) Dysplasia of the cervix: A prospective study of 206 cases Am J Obstet Gynecol 100: 662–671

139. Halpert R, Fruchter RG, Sedlis A, et al (1986) Human papillomavirus and lower genital neoplasia in renal transplant patients. Obstet Gynecol 150: 251–258

140. Hanselaar AG, Vooijs GP, Oud PS, et al (1988) DNA ploidy patterns in cervical intraepithelial neoplasia grade III, with and without synchronous invasive squamous cell carcinoma: Measurements in nuclei isolated from paraffin-embedded tissue. Cancer 62: 2537–2545

141. Harris RWC, Brinton LA, Cowdell RH, et al (1980) Characteristics of women with dysplasia or carcinoma in situ of the cervix uteri. Br J Cancer 42: 359–369

142. Hatch KD, Shingleton HM, Orr JW, et al (1985) Role of endocervical curettage in colposcopy. Obstet Gynecol 65: 403–408

143. Hawley-Nelson P, Vousden KH, Hubbert NL, et al (1989) HPV16 E6 and E7 proteins cooperate to immortalize human foreskin keratinocytes. EMBO J 8: 3905–3910

144. Heinzl S, Szalmay G, Jochum L, et al (1982) Observations on the development of dysplasia. Acta Cytol 26: 453–456

145. Hellberg D, Nilsson S, Haley NJ, et al (1988) Smoking and cervical intraepithelial neoplasia: Nicotine and cotinine in serum and cervical mucus in smokers and non-smokers. Am J Obstet Gynecol 158: 910–913

146. Helper TK, Dockerty MB, Randall LM (1952) Primary adenocarcinoma of the cervix. Am J Obstet Gynecol 63: 800–808

147. Herrero R, Grinoton LA, Reeves WC, et al (1990) Sexual behavior, venereal diseases, hygiene practices, and invasive cervical cancer in a high risk population. Cancer 65: 380–386

148. Higgins GD, Phillips GE, Smith LA, et al (1992) High prevalence of human papillomavirus transcripts in all grades of cervical intraepithelial glandular neoplasia. Cancer 70: 136–146

149. Hildesheim A, Mann V, Brinton LA, et al (1991) Herpes simplex virus type 2: a possible interaction with human papillomavirus types 16/18 in the development of invasive cervical cancer. Int J Cancer 49: 335–340

150. Hirsch-Behnam A, Delius H, de Villiers E-M (1990) A comparative sequence analysis of two human papillomavirus (HPV) types 2a and 57. Virus Res 18: 81–97

151. Hopkins MP, Roberts JA, Schmidt RW (1988) Cervical adenocarcinoma in situ. Obstet Gynecol 842–844

152. Howley PM (1982) The human papillomaviruses. Arch Pathol Lab Med 106: 429–432

153. Howley PM (1986) On human papillomaviruses. N Engl J Med 315: 1089–1090

154. Hulka BS (1968) Cytologic and histologic outcome following an atypical cervical smear. Am J Obstet Gynecol 101: 190–199

155. Ismail SM, Colelough AB, Dinnen JS, et al (1989) Observer variation in histopathological diagnosis and grading of cervical intraepithelial neoplasia. Br Med J 298: 707–710

156. Iwasaka T, Yokoyama M, Hayashi Y, et al (1988) Combined herpes simplex virus type 2 and human papillomavirus type 16 or 18 deoxyribonucleic acid leads to oncogenic transformation. Am J Obstet Gynecol 159: 1251–1255

157. Jakobsen A, Kristensen PB, Poulsen HK (1983) Flow cytometric classification of biopsy specimens from cervical intraepithelial neoplasia. Cytometry 4: 166–169

158. Jariwalla RJ, Aurelian L, Ts'O POP (1979) Neoplastic transformation of cultured Syrian hamster embryo cells by DNA of herpes simplex virus type 2. J Virol 30: 404–409

159. Jarrett WFH, Murphy J, O'Neil BW, et al (1978) Virus-

induced papillomas of the alimentary tract of cattle. Int J Cancer 22: 323–328

160. Jaworski RC (1990) Endocervical glandular dysplasia, adenocarcinoma in situ, and early invasive (microinvasive) adenocarcinoma of the uterine cervix. Semin Diagn Pathol 7: 190–204

161. Jaworski RC, Pacey NR, Greenberg ML, et al (1988) The histologic diagnosis of adenocarcinoma in situ and related lesions of the cervix uteri. Adenocarcinoma in situ. Cancer 61: 1171–1181

162. Jenison SA, Yu X-P, Valentine JM, et al (1990) Evidence of prevalent genital type human papillomavirus infections in adults and children. J Infect Dis 162: 60–69

163. Jenson AB, Rosenthal JD, Olson C, et al (1980) Immunologic relatedness of papillomavirus from different species J Natl Cancer Inst 64: 495–500

164. Jochmus-Kudielka I, Schneider A, Braun R, et al (1989) Antibodies against the human papillomavirus type 16 early proteins in human sera: Correlation of anti-E7 reactivity with cervical cancer. J Natl Cancer Inst 81: 1698–1704

165. Johnson LD (1969) The histopathological approach to early cervical neoplasia. Obstet Gynecol Surv 24: 735–767

166. Jones CJ, Brinton LA, Hamman RF, et al (1990) Risk factors for in situ cervical cancer: results from a case-control study. Cancer Res 50: 3657–3662

167. Jones MH, Jenkins D, Cuzick J, et al (1992) Mild cervical dyskaryosis; safety of cytological surveillance. Lancet 339: 1440–1443

168. Jordan SW, Smith NL, Dike LS (1981) The significance of cervical cytologic dysplasia. Acta Cytol 25: 237–244

169. Kadish A, Burk R, Kress Y, et al (1986) Human papillomavirus of different types in precancerous lesions of the uterine cervix: histologic, immunocytochemical and ultrastructural studies. Hum Pathol 17: 384–392

170. Kadish AS, Hagan RJ, Ritter DB, et al (1992) Biologic characteristics of specific human papillomavirus types predicted from morphology of cervical lesions. Hum Pathol 23: 1262–1269

171. Kanda T, Furuno A, Yoshiike K (1988) Human papillomavirus type 16 open reading frame E7 encodes a transforming gene for rat 3Y1 cells J Virol 62: 610–613

172. Kashimura M, Shinohara M, Oikawa K, et al (1990) An adenocarcinoma in situ of the uterine cervix that developed into invasive adenocarcinoma after 5 years. Gynecol Oncol 36: 128–133

173. Kataja V, Syrjanen K, Syrjanen S, et al (1990) Prospective follow-up of genital HPV infections; survival analysis of the HPV typing data. Eur J Epidemiol 6: 9–14

174. Kaufman RH, Irwin JF (1978) The cryosurgical therapy of cervical intraepithelial neoplasia. III. Continuing follow-up. Am J Obstet Gynecol 131: 381

175. Kaur P, Mcdougall JK (1988) Characterization of primary human keratinocytes transformed by human papillomavirus type 18. J Virol 62: 1917–1924

176. Keighley E (1968–69) Carcinoma of the cervix among prostitutes in a women's prison. Br J Vener Dis 44: 254

177. Kessler II (1974) Perspectives on the epidemiology of cervcical cancer with special reference to the herpes virus hypothesis. Cancer 34: 1091

178. Kessler II (1977) Venereal factors in human cervical cancer: Evidence from marital clusters. Cancer 39: 1912–1919

179. Kirby AJ, Spiegelhalter DJ, Day NE, et al (1992) Conservative treatment of mild/moderate cervical dyskaryosis: long-term outcome. Lancet 339: 828–831

180. Kirkland JA (1963) Atypical epithelial changes in the uterine cervix. J Clin Pathol 16: 150–154

181. Kirkland JA, Stanley MA, Cellier KM (1967) Comparative study of histologic and chromosomal abnormalities in cervical neoplasia. Cancer 20: 1934–1952

182. Kiviat N, Koutsky LA, Paavonen J, et al (1989) Prevalence of genital papillomavirus infection among women attending a college student health clinic or a sexually transmitted disease clinic. J Infect Dis 159: 293–302

183. Kiviat NB, Critchlow CW, Kurman RJ (1992) Reassessment of the morphological continuum of cervical intraepithelial lesions; does it reflect different stages in the progression to cervical carcinoma? In: Munoz N, Bosch F, Shah K, Mehens A (eds) The Epidemiology of Cervical Cancer and Human Papillomavirus. Lyons, I.A.R.C., pp 59–66

184. Kjaer SK, de Villiers EM, Haugaard BJ, et al (1988) Human papillomavirus, herpes simplex virus and cervical cancer incidence in Greenland and Denmark. A population-based cross-sectional study. Int J Cancer 41: 518–524

185. Kjaer SK, deVilliers E-M, Dahl C, et al (1991) Case-conrol study of risk factors for cervical neoplasia in Denmark. I: Role of the "male factor" in women with one lifetime sexual partner. Int J Cancer 48: 39–44

186. Kjaer SK, Engholm G, Teisen C, et al (1990) Risk factors for cervical human papillomvavirus and herpes simplex virus infections in Greenland and Denmark: a population-based study. Am J Epidemiol 131: 669–682

187. Koi M, Morita H, Yamada H, et al (1989) Normal human chromosome 11 suppresses tumorigenicity of human cervical tumor cell line SiHa. Mol Carcinog 2: 12–21

188. Kolstad P, Klem V (1979) Long-term follow-up of 1121 cases of carcinoma in situ. Obstet Gynecol 48: 125–133

189. Komly CA, Breitburd F, Croissant O, et al (1986) The L2 open reading frame of human papillomavirus type 1a encodes a minor structural protein carrying type-specific antigens. J Virol 60: 813–816

190. Koss L, Durfee GR (1956) Unusual patterns of squamous epithelium of uterine cervix: Cytologic and pathologic study of koilocytotic atypia. Ann NY Acad Sci 63: 1245–1261

191. Koss LG (1978) Dysplasia. A real concept of a misnomer? Obstet Gynecol 51: 374

192. Koss LG (1992) Diagnostic Cytology and Its Histopathologic Basis. New York, J. B. Lippincott Co

193. Koss LG, Stewart FW, Foote FW, et al (1963) Some histological aspects of behavior of epidermoid carcinoma in situ and related lesions of the uterine cervix Cancer. 16: 1160–1211

194. Kottmeier HL (1961) Evolution et traitement des epitheliomas. Rev Fran Gynecol d'Obstet 56: 821–826

195. Koutsky LA, Galloway DA, Holmes KK (1988) Epidemiology of genital human papillomavirus infection. Epidemiol Rev 10: 122–163

196. Koutsky LA, Holmes KK, Critchlow CW, et al (1992) A cohort study of the risk of cervical intraepithelial neoplasia grade 2 or 3 in relation to papillomavirus infection. N Engl J Med 327: 1272–1278

197. Kreider JW, Bartlett GL (1985) Shope rabbit papilloma-

carcinoma complex: A model system of HPV infections. Clin Derm 3: 20

198. Krieder JW, Howett MK, Leure-Dupree AE, et al (1987) Laboratory production in vivo of infectious human papillomavirus type 11. J Virol 61: 590–593

199. Kurman RJ, Jenson AB, Lancaster WD (1983) Papillomavirus infection of the cervix. II. Relationship to intraepithelial neoplasia based on the presence of specific viral structural proteins. Am J Surg Pathol 7: 39

200. Kurman RJ, Jenson AB, Sinclair CF, et al (1984) Detection of human papillomaviruses by imunocytochemistry. In: DeLellis RA (eds) Advances in Immunohistochemistry. Chicago, Year Book Medical Publishers, pp 201–221

201. Kurman RJ, Norris HJ, Wilkinson E (1992) Atlas of Tumor Pathology, Third Series, Fascicle 4, Tumors of the Cervix, Vagina and Vulva. Washington, D.C., Armed Forces Institute of Pathology

202. Kurman RJ, Sanz LE, Jenson AB, et al (1982) Papillomavirus infection of the cervix. I. Correlation of histology with viral structural antigens and DNA sequences. Int J Gynecol Pathol 1: 17–28

203. La Vecchia C, Franceschi S, DeCarli A, et al (1986) Sexual factors, venereal diseases, and the risk of intraepithelial and invasive cervical neoplasia. Cancer 58: 935–941

204. Laga M, Icenogle JP, Marsella R, et al (1992) Genital papillomavirus infection and cervical dysplasia—opportunistic complications of HIV infection. Int J Cancer 50: 45–48

205. Lambert PF, Howley PM (1988) Bovine papillomavirus type IE1 replication-defective mutants are altered in their transcriptional regulation. J Virol 62: 4009–4015

206. Lambert PF, Spalholz BA, Howley PM (1987) A transcriptional repressor encoded by BPV–1 shares a common carboxy-terminal domain with the E2 transactivator. Cell 50: 69–78

207. Lancaster WD, Castellano C, Santos C, et al (1986) Human papillomavirus deoxyribonucleic acid in cervical carcinoma from primary and metastic sites. Am J Obstet Gynecol 154: 115

208. Laverty CR, Russell P, Hills E, et al (1978) The significance of noncondylomatous wart virus infection of the cervical transformation zone: A review with discussion of two illustrative cases. Acta Cytol 22: 195–201

209. Ley C, Bauer HM, Reingold A, et al (1991) Determinants of genital human papillomavirus infection in young women. J Natl Cancer Inst 83: 997–1003

210. Lorincz AT (1987) Detection of human papillomavirus infection by nucleic acid hybridization Obstet Gynecol Clinics North Am 14: 451–469

211. Lorincz AT (1990) Human papillomavirus detection methods. In: Holmes KK, Mardh P-A, Sparling PF, Wiesner PJ (eds) Sexually Transmitted Diseases, 2nd ed. New York, McGraw-Hill Information Services Company

212. Lorincz AT, Reid R, Jenson AB, et al (1992) Human papillomavirus infection of the cervix: Relative risk associations of 15 common anogenital types. Am J Obstet Gynecol 79: 328–337

213. Lorincz AT, Temple GF, Kurman RJ, et al (1987) Oncogenic association of specific human papillomavirus types with cervical neoplasia. J Natl Cancer Inst 79: 671–677

214. Luesley DM, Jordan JA, Woodman CBJ, et al (1987) A retrospective review of adenocarcinoma-in-situ and glandular atypia of the uterine cervix. Br J Obstet Gynecol 94: 699–703

215. Luff RD (1992) The Bethesda System for reporting cervical/vaginal cytologic diagnoses: Report of the 1991 Bethesda Workshop. Hum Pathol 23: 719–721

216. Lungu O, Sun XW, Felix J, et al (1992) Relationship of human papillomavirus type to grade of cervical intraepithelial neoplasia. JAMA 267: 2493–2496

217. Lusky M, Botchan M (1984) Characterization of the bovine papilloma virus plasmid maintenance sequences. Cell 36: 391–401

218. MacGregor JE, Innes G (1980) Carcinoma of penis and cervix. Lancet i: 1246–1247

219. Mack DH, Laimins LA (1991) A keratinocyte-specific transcription factor, KRF–1 interacts with AP–1 to activate expression of human papillomavirus type 18 in squamous epithelial cells. Proc Natl Acad Sci 88: 9102–9106

220. Maiman M, Fruchter RG, Serur E, et al (1990) Human immunodeficiency virus infection and cervical neoplasia. Gynecol Oncol 38: 377–382

221. Manos MM, Ting Y, Wright DK, et al (1989) Use of polymerase chain reaction amplification for the detection of genital human papillomaviruses Cancer Cells 7: 209–214

222. Marte C, Kelly P, Cohen M, et al (1992) Papanicolaou smear abnormalities in ambulatory care sites for women infected with human immunodeficiency virus. Am J Obstet Gynecol 166: 1232–1237

223. Matsukura T, Koi S, Sugase M (1989) Both episomal and integrated forms of human papillomavirus type 16 are involved in invasive cervical cancers. Virology 172: 63–72

224. McDonnell JM, Mayr AJ, Martin WJ (1989) DNA of human papillomavirus type 16 in dysplastic and malignant lesions of the conjunctiva and cornea. N Engl J Med 320: 1442–1446

225. McDonnell JM, Wagner D, Ng ST, et al (1991) Human papillomavirus type 16 DNA in ocular and cervical swabs of women with genital tract condylomata. Am J Ophthalmol 112: 61–66

226. McDougall JK, Galloway DA, Fenoglio CM (1980) Cervical carcinoma: Detection of herpes simplex virus RNA in cells undergoing neoplastic change. Int J Cancer 25: 1–8

227. McDougall JK, Nelson JA, Myerson D, et al (1984) HSV, CMV, and HPV in human neoplasia. J Invest Dermatol 83: 72S–76S

228. McIndoe WA, McLean MR, Jones RW, et al (1984) The invasive potential of carcinoma in situ of the cervix. Obstet Gynecol 64: 451–458

229. Meanwell C, Cox M, Blackledge G, et al (1987) HPV 16 DNA in normal and malignant cervical epithelium: implications for the aetiology and behaviour of cervical neoplasia. Lancet i: 703–707

230. Meisels A (1992) Cytologic diagnosis of human papillomavirus. Influence of age and pregnancy stage. Acta Cytol 36: 480–482

231. Meisels A, Fortin R (1976) Condylomatous lesions of the cervix and vagina. I. Cytologic patterns. Acta Cytol 20: 505–509

232. Meisels A, Fortin R, Roy M (1977) Condylomatous lesions of the cervix: II. Cytologic, colposcopic and histopathologic study. Acta Cytol 21: 379–390

233. Meisels A, Morin C, Casas-Cordero M (1982) Human papillomavirus infection of the uterine cervix. Int J Gynecol Pathol 1: 75–94

234. Meisels A, Morin C, Casas-Cordero M (1984) Lesions of the uterine cervix associated with papillomaviruses and their clinical consequences. Adv Clin Cytol 2: 1–31

235. Meisels A, Roy M, Fortier M, et al (1979) Condylomatous lesions of the cervix: Morphologic and colposcopic diagnosis Am J Diagn Gynecol Obstet 1: 109

236. Melamed MR, Flehinger BJ (1973) Early incidence rates of precancerous cervical lesions in women using contraceptives. Gynecol Oncol 1: 290–298

237. Melnick JL, Adam E, Rawls WE (1974) The causative role of herpesvirus type 2 in cervical cancer. Cancer 34: 1375–1385

238. Mittal KR, Chan W, Demopoulos RL (1990) Sensitivity and specificity of various morphological features of cervical condylomas. Arch Pathol Lab Med 114: 1038–1041

239. Morrison EA, Ho GYF, Vermund SH, et al (1991) Human papillomavirus infection and other risk factors for cervical neoplasia: a case-control study. Int J Cancer 49: 6–13

240. Moscicki A-B, Palefsky J, Gonzales J, et al (1990) Human papillomavirus infection in sexually active adolescent females: Prevalence and risk factors. Pediatr Res 28: 507–513

241. Moscicki A-B, Palefsky JM, Gonzales J, et al (1992) Colposcopic and histologic findings and human papillomavirus (HPV) DNA test variability in young women positive for HPV DNA. J Infect Dis 166: 951–957

242. Mourits MJE, Pieters WJ, Hollema H, et al (1992) Three-group metaphase as a morphologic criterion of progressive cervical intraepithelial neoplasia. Am J Obstet Gynecol 167: 591–595

243. Moy RL, Eliezri YD, Nuovo GJ, et al (1989) Human papillomavirus type 16 DNA in periungual squamous cell carcinomas. JAMA 261: 2669–2673

244. Munger K, Werness BA, Dyson N, et al (1989) Complex formation of human papillomavirus E7 proteins with the retinoblastoma tumor suppressor gene product. EMBO J 8: 4099–4105

245. Munoz N (1992) Review of case-control and cohort studies. In: Munoz N, Bosch FX (eds) Human Papilloma Virus and Cervical Cancer. Lyons, IARC

246. Munoz N, Bosch FX, de-SanJose S, et al (1992) The causal link between human papillomavirus and invasive cervical cancer: A population-based case-control study in Colombia and Spain. Int J Cancer 52: 743–749

247. Munoz N, Bosch X, Kaldor JM (1988) Does human papillomavirus cause cervical cancer: The state of the epidemiological evidence. Br J Cancer 57: 1–5

248. Muntz HG, Bell DA, Lage JM, et al (1992) Adenocarcinoma in situ of the uterine cervix. Obstet Gynecol 80: 935–939

249. Nahmias AJ, Roizman B (1973) Infection with herpes-simplex viruses 1 and 2. N Engl J Med 289: 667–674, 719–725, 781–789

250. Nasiell K, Nasiell M, Vaclavinkova V (1983) Behavior of moderate cervical dysplasia during long-term follow-up. Obstet Gynecol 61: 609–614

251. Nasiell K, Naslund I, Auer G (1984) Cytomorphologic and cytochemical analysis in the differential diagnosis of cervical epithelial lesions. Anal Quant Cytol 6: 196–200

252. Nasiell K, Roger V, Nasiell M (1986) Behavior of mild cervical dysplasia during long-term follow-up. Obstet Gynecol 67: 665–669

253. Nicklin JL, Wright RG, Bell JR, et al (1991) A clinicopathological study of adenocarcinoma in situ of the cervix. The influence of cervical HPV infection and other factors, and the role of conservative surgery. Aust NZ J Obstet Gynecol 31: 179–183

254. Nuovo GJ, Silverstein SJ (1988) Comparison of formalin, buffered formalin, and Bouin's fixation on the detection of human papillomavirus deoxyribonucleic acid from genital lesions. Lab Invest 59: 720–724

255. Offord EA, Beard P (1990) A member of the activator protein 1 family found in keratinocytes but not in fibroblasts required for transcription from a human papillomavirus type 18 promoter. J Virol 64: 4792–4798

256. Olson C, Gordon DE, Robl MG, et al (1969) Oncogenicity of bovine papillomavirus. Arch Environ Health 19: 827

257. Orth G (1986) Epidermodysplasia verruciformis: a model for understanding the oncogenicity of human papillomaviruses. In: Evered D, Clark S (eds) Papillomaviruses. New York, John Wiley & Sons, pp 157–174

258. Orth G, Favre M, Breitburg F, et al (1980) Epidermodysplasia verruciformis: A model for the role of papillomaviruses in human cancer. In: Essex. M, Todaro G, Hausen. HZ (eds) Viruses in Naturally Occurring Cancer. Cold Spring Harbor, NY. Cold Spring Harbor Laboratory Press, pp 259

259. Orth G, Jablonska S, Jarzabek-Chorzelska M, et al (1979) Characteristics of the lesions and risk of malignant conversion associated with the type of human papillomavirus involved in epidermodysplasia verruciformis. Cancer Res 39: 1074–1082

260. Ostor AG, Pagano R, Davoren RAM, et al (1984) Adenocarcinoma in situ of the cervix. Int J Gynecol Pathol 3: 179–190

261. Ostrow RS, Bender M, Niimura M, et al (1982) Human papillomavirus DNA in cutaneous primary and metastasized squamous cell carcinomas from patients with epidermodysplasia verruciformis. Proc Natl Acad Sci USA 79: 1634–1638

262. Palan PR, Mikhail M, Basu J, et al (1988) Decreased plasma B-carotene levels in women with uterine cervical dysplasias and cancer. J Natl Cancer Inst 80: 454–455

263. Palefsky JM, Winkler B, Rabanus J-P, et al (1991) Characterization of in vivo expression of the human papillomavirus type 16 E4 protein in cervical biopsy tissues. J Clin Invest 87: 2132–2141

264. Parazzini F, La Vecchia C (1990) Epidemiology of adenocarcinoma of the cervix. Gynecol Oncol 39: 40–46

265. Parazzini F, La Vecchia C, Negri E, et al (1990) Oral contraceptive use and invasive cervical cancer. Int J Epidemiol 19: 259–263

266. Parazzini F, LaVecchia C, Negri E, et al (1992) Risk factors for cervical intraepithelial neoplasia. Cancer 69: 2276–2282

267. Patten SF Jr. (1969) Diagnostic Cytology of the Uterine Cervix. Baltimore, Williams & Wilkins

268. Pemberton FA, Smith GV (1929) The early diagnosis and prevention of carcinoma of the cervix: A clinical pathologic study of borderline cases treated at the Free Hospital for women. Am J Obstet Gynecol 17: 165

269. Peng H, Liu S, Mann V, et al (1991) Human papillomavirus

types 16 and 33, herpes simplex virus type 2 and other risk factors for cervical cancer in Sichuan Province, China. Int J Cancer 47: 711–716

270. Penn I (1986) Cancers of the anogenital region in renal transplant recipients. Cancer 58: 611–616

271. Pfister H (1984) Biology and biochemistry of papillomaviruses. Rev Physiol Biochem Pharmacol 99: 112–131

272. Pfister H (1987) Papillomaviruses: General Description, Taxonomy, and Classification. New York, Plenum pp 1–38

273. Pfister H (1990) General introduction to papillomaviruses, properties of the virions and classification. In: Pfister H (eds) Papillomaviruses and Human Cancer. Boca Raton, CRC Press, pp 2–4

274. Phelps WC, Yee CL, Mungei K, et al (1988) The human papillomavirus type 16 E7 gene encodes transactivation and transforming functions similar to those of adenovirus E1A Cell 58: 539–547

275. Pieters WJ, Koudstaal J, Ploem-Zaajer JJ, et al (1992) The three group metaphase as morphologic indicator of high ploidy cells in cervical intraepithelial neoplasia. Anal Quant Cytol Histol 14: 227–232

276. Pilacinski WP, Glassman DL, Kazysek RA (1984) Cloning and expression in E. coli of the bovine papillomavirus type L1 and L2 open reading frames. Biotechnology 2: 356

277. Pirisi L, Yasumoto S, Feller M, et al (1987) Transformation of human fibroblasts and keratinocytes with human papillomavirus type 16 DNA. J Virol 61: 1061–1066

278. Prendiville W, Cullimore J, Norman S (1989) Large loop excision of the transformation zone (LLETZ). A new method of management for women with cervical intraepithelial neoplasia. Br J Obstet Gynecol 96: 1054–1060

279. Przybora LA, Plutowa A (1959) Histological topography of carcinoma in situ of cervix uteri. Cancer 12: 263–277

280. Purola E, Savia E (1977) Cytology of gynecologic condyloma acuminatum. Acta Cytol 21: 26–31

281. Purtilo DT (1974) Defective immune surveillance in viral carcinogenesis. Lab Invest 51: 373

282. Qizilbash A-H (1975) In situ and microinvasive adenocarcinoma of the uterine cervix. J Clin Pathol 64: 155–170

283. Reagan JW, Hamonic MJ (1956) The cellular pathology in carcinoma in situ; a cytohistopathological correlation. Cancer 9: 385

284. Reagan JW, Ng ABP, Wentz WB (1969) Concepts of genesis and development in early cervical neoplasia. Obstet Gynecol Surv 24: 860

285. Reeves WC, Brinton LA, Brenes MM, et al (1985) Case-control study of cervical cancer in Herrera Province, Republic of Panama. Int J Cancer 36: 55

286. Reeves WC, Brinton LA, Garcia M, et al (1989) Human papillomavirus infection and cervical cancer in Latin America. N Engl J Med 320: 1437–1441

287. Reid R, Fu YS, Herschman BR, et al (1984) Genital warts and cervical cancer VI. The relationship between aneuploid and polyploid cervical lesions. Am J Obstet Gynecol 150: 189–199

288. Reid R, Greenberg M, Jenson AB, et al (1987) Sexually transmitted papillomaviral infections I. The anatomic distribution and pathologic grade of neoplastic lesions associated with different viral types. Am J Obstet Gynecol 156: 212–222

289. Rellihan MA, Dooley DP, Burke TW, et al (1990) Rapidly progressing cervical cancer in a patient with human immunodeficiency virus infection. Gynecol Oncol 36: 435–438

290. Richardson AC, Lyon JB (1981) The effect of condom use on squamous cell cervical intraepithelial neoplasia. Am J Obstet Gynecol 140: 909–913

291. Richart RM (1965) Colpomicroscopic studies of the distribution of dysplasia and carcinoma in-situ on the exposed portion of the human uterine cervix. Cancer 18: 950

292. Richart RM (1966) Colpomicroscopic studies of cervical intraepithelial neoplasia. Cancer 19: 395

293. Richart RM (1966) The influence of diagnostic and therapeutic procedures on the distribution of cervical intraepithelial neoplasia. Cancer 19: 1635

294. Richart RM (1968) Natural history of cervical intraepithelial neoplasia. Clin Obstet Gynecol 10: 748–784

295. Richart RM (1969) A theory of cervical carcinogenesis. Obstet Gynecol Surv 24: 874

296. Richart RM (1973) Cervical intraepithelial neoplasia: A review. In: Sommers SC (eds) Pathology Annual. East Norwalk, CT, Appleton-Century-Crofts, pp 301–328

297. Richart RM (1987) Causes and management of cervical intraepithelial neoplasia. Cancer 60: 1951–1959

298. Richart RM (1990) A modified terminology for cervical intraepithelial neoplasia. Obstet Gynecol 75: 131–133

299. Richart RM, Barron BA (1969) A follow-up study of patients with cervical dysplasia. Am J Obstet Gynecol 105: 386–393

300. Richart RM, Lerch V (1966) Time lapse cinematographic observations of normal human cervical epithelium, dysplasia and carcinoma in situ. J Natl Cancer Inst 37: 317

301. Richart RM, Lerch V, Baron B (1967) A time-lapse cinematographic study in vitro of mitosis in normal human cervical epithelium, dysplasia and carcinoma in situ. J Natl Cancer Inst 39: 571

302. Richart RM, Nuovo GJ (1989) HPV DNA in-situ hybridization can be used for the quality control of diagnostic biopsies Obstet Gynecol 75: 223–226

303. Richart RM, Sciarra JJ (1968) Treatment of cervical dysplasia by outpatient electrocauterization Am J Obstet Gynecol 101: 200–205

304. Robboy SJ, Noller KL, O'Brien P, et al (1984) Increased incidence of cervical and vaginal dysplasia in 3,980 diethylstilbestrol (DES) exposed young women: Experience of the National Collaborative DES-Adenosis (DESAD) Project. JAMA 252: 2979–2983

305. Robboy SJ, Szyfelbein WM, Goellner JR, et al (1981) Dysplasia and cytologic findings in 4,489 young women enrolled in diethylstillbesterol-adenosis (DESAD) project. Am J Obstet Gynecol 140: 579

306. Robertson AJ, Anderson JM, Beck JS, et al (1989) Observer variability in histo-pathological reporting of cervical biopsy specimens. J Clin Pathol 42: 231–238

307. Robertson JH, Woodend BE, Crozier EH, et al (1988) Risk of cervical cancer associated with mild dyskaryosis. Br Med J 297: 18–21

308. Rollason TP, Cullimore J, Bradgate MG (1989) A suggested columnar cell morphological equivalent of squamous carcinoma in situ with early stromal invasion. Int J Gynecol Pathol 8: 230–236

309. Romney SL, Palan PR, Dattagupta C, et al (1981) Retinoids

and the prevention of cervical dysplasias. Am J Obstet Gynecol 141: 890–894

310. Rosenfeld W, Vermund SH, Wentz SJ, et al (1989) High prevalence rate of human papillomavirus infection and association with abnormal Papanicolaou smears in sexually active adolescents. Am J Dis Child 143: 1443–1447

311. Rothrock RS (1992) Hybrid capture system: an innovative non-isotopic method for human papillomavirus detection. Eur Clin Lab October: 12

312. Royston I, Aurelian L (1970) Immunofluorescent detection of herpes virus antigens in exfoliated cells from human cervical carcinoma. Proc Natl Acad Sci 67: 204

313. Rubin IC (1910) The pathological diagnosis of incipient carcinoma of the uterus. Am J Obstet Gynecol 62: 668–676

314. Rubio CA, Lagerlof B (1974) Studies on the histogenesis of experimentally induced cervical carcinoma. Acta Pathol Microbiol Scand 82: 153

315. Sadeghi SB, Hsieh EW, Gunn SW (1984) Prevalence of cervical intraepithelial neoplasia in sexually active teenagers and young adults. Am J Obstet Gynecol 148: 726

316. Sadeghi SB, Sadeghi A, Robboy SJ (1988) Prevalence of dysplasia and cancer of the cervix in a nationwide Planned Parenthood population. Cancer 61: 2359–2361

317. Saiki RK, Sharf S, Falcona F, et al (1987) Enzymatic amplification of beta globin genomic sequences and restriction site analysis for diagnosis of sickle cell anemia. Science 230: 1350–1354

318. Schafer A, Friedmann W, Mielke M, et al (1991) The increased frequency of cervical dysplasia-neoplasia in women infected with the human immunodeficiency virus is related to the degree of immunosuppression. Am J Obstet Gynecol 164: 593–599

319. Scheffner M, Werness BA, Huibregtse JM, et al (1990) The E6 oncoprotein encoded by human papillomavirus types 16 and 18 promotes the degradation of p53. Cell 63: 1129–1136

320. Schiffman M, Brinton L, Holly E, et al (1987) Regarding mutagenic mucus in cervix of smokers. J Natl Cancer Inst 78: 590–591

321. Schiffman MH (1992) Recent progress in defining the epidemiology of human papillomavirus infection and cervical neoplasia. J Natl Cancer Inst 84: 394–398

322. Schiffman MH, Bauer HM, Hoover RN, et al (1993) Epidemiologic evidence that human papillomavirus infection causes most cervical intraepithelial neoplasia. J Natl Cancer Inst 85: 958–964

323. Schiller W (1928) Uber fruhstadien des portiocarcinoms und ihre diagnose. Arch Gynakol 133: 211–283

324. Schmidt C, Pretorius RG, Bonin M, et al (1992) Invasive cervical cancer following cryotherapy for cervical intraepithelial neoplasia or human papillomavirus infection. Obstet Gynecol 80: 797–800

325. Schneider A (1990) Latent and subclinical genital HPV infections. Papillomavirus Report 1: 2–5

326. Schneider A, Shah K (1989) The role of vitamins in the etiology of cervical neoplasia: An epidemiological review. Arch Gynecol Obstet 246: 1–13

327. Schneider V, Kay S, Lee HM (1983) Immunosuppression as a high-risk factor in the development of condyloma acuminatum and squamous neoplasia of the cervix. Acta Cytol 27: 220–224

328. Schneider-Gädicke A, Schwarz E (1986) Different human cervical carcinoma cell lines show similar transcription patterns of human papillomavirus type 18 early genes. EMBO J 5: 2285–2292

329. Schwartz LB, Carcangiu ML, Bradham L, et al (1991) Rapidly progressive squamous cell carcinoma of the cervix coexisting with human immunodeficiency virus infection: clinical opinion. Gynecol Oncol 41: 255–258

330. Schwarz E, Freese UK, Gissman L, et al (1985) Structure and transcription of human papillomavirus sequences in cervical carcinoma cells. Nature 314: 111–114

331. Schwarz E, Schneider-Gädicke A, zur Hausen H (1987) Human papillomavirus type–18 transcription in cervical carcinoma cell lines and in human cell hybrids. Cancer Cells 5: 47–53

332. Sebastian JA, Leeb BO, See R (1978) Cancer of the cerivix-a sexually transmitted disease. Cytologic screening in a prostitute population. Am J Obstet Gynecol 131: 620–623

333. Seedorf K, Krammer G, Rowekamp W, et al (1985) Human papillomavirus type 16 DNA sequence. Virology 145: 181–185

334. Sherman ME, Schiffman MH, Erozan YS, et al (1992) The Bethesda system. A proposal for reporting abnormal cervical smears based on the reproducibility of cytopathologic diagnosis. Arch Pathol Lab Med 116: 1155–1158

335. Shevchuk MM, Richart RM (1982) DNA content of condyloma acuminatum. Cancer 49: 489–492

336. Shibata D, Arnheim N, Martin W (1988) Detection of human papilloma virus in paraffin-embedded tissue using the polymerase chain reaction 167: 225–230

337. Shingleton HM, Richart RM, Wiener J, et al (1968) Human cervical intraepithelial neoplasia. Fine structure of dysplasia and carcinoma in situ. Cancer Res 28: 695

338. Shope RE, Hurst EW (1933) Infectious papillomatosis of rabbits; with a note on histopathology. J Exp Med 58: 607

339. Siegler EE (1956) Microdiagnosis of carcinoma in situ of the uterine cervix: A comparative study of pathologist's diagnoses. Cancer 9: 463

340. Sillman F, Stanek A, Sedlis A, et al (1984) The relationship between human papillomavirus and lower genital intraepithelial neoplasia in immunosuppressed women. Am J Obstet Gynecol 150: 300–308

341. Singer A, Reid BL, Coppleson M (1976) A hypothesis: The role of a high risk male in the etiology of cervical carcinoma. a correlation of epidemiology and molecular biology. Am J Obstet Gynecol 126: 110–115

342. Slattery ML, Overall JC, Abbott TM, et al (1989) Sexual activity, contraception, genital infections, and cervical cancer: Support for a sexually transmitted disease hypothesis. Am J Epidemiol 130: 248–258

343. Smith GV, Pemberton FA (1934) The picture of very early carcinoma of the uterine cervix. Surg Gynecol Obstet 59: 1–8

344. Smith PG, Kinlen LJ, White GC, et al (1980) Mortality of wives of men dying with cancer of the penis. Br J Cancer 41: 422–428

345. Smotkin D, Wettstein FO (1986) Transcription of human papillomavirus type 16 early genes in a cervical cancer and a cancer-derived cell line and identification of the E7 protein. Proc Natl Acad Sci USA 83: 4680–4684

346. Sorensen HM, Petersen O, Nielsen J, et al (1964) The spontaneous course of premalignant lesions of the vaginal portion of the uterus. Acta Obstet Gynecol Scand 43: 103–104

347. Spalholz BA, Lambert PF, Yee CL, et al (1987) Bovine papillomavirus transcriptional regulation: Localization of the E2-responsive elements of the long control region. J Virol 61: 2128–2137

348. Spriggs AI, Boddington MM (1980) Progression and regression of cervical lesions: Review of smears from women followed without initial biopsy or treatment. J Clin Pathol 33: 517–525

349. Spriggs AI, Bowey CE, Cowdell RH (1971) Chromosomes of precancerous lesions of the cervix uteri. Cancer 27: 1239

350. Stafl A, Mattingly RF (1975) Angiogenesis of cervical neoplasia. Am J Obstet Gynecol 121: 845–852

351. Stafl A, Wilkinson EJ, Mattingly RF (1977) Laser treatment of cervical and vaginal neoplasia Am J Obstet Gynecol 128: 128

352. Stern E, Neely PM (1963) Carcinoma and dysplasia of the cervix. A comparison of rates for new and returning populations. Acta Cytol 7: 357–361

353. Stewart FW (1957) Factors influencing curability of cancer. In: Conference Proceedings of the Third National Cancer Conference. Philadelphia, J. B. Lippincott, pp 62–73

354. Streiff RR (1970) Folate deficiency and oral contraceptives. JAMA 214: 105–108

355. Suprun HZ, Schwartz J, Spira H (1985) CIN and associated condylomatous lesions. A preliminary report on 4,764 women from northern Israel. Acta Cytol 29: 334–340

356. Swan SH, Brown WL (1981) Oral contraceptive use, sexual activity and cervical carcinoma. Am J Obstet Gynecol 139: 52–57

357. Syrjanen K, Saarikoski S, Vayrynen M, et al (1989) Factors associated with the clinical behaviour of cervical human papillomavirus infections during a long-term prospective follow-up. Cervix 7: 131–143

358. Talmage DA, Freund R, Dubensky T, et al (1992) Heterogeneity in state and expression of viral DNA in polyoma virus-induced tumors of the mouse. Virology 187: 734–747

359. Tase T, Okagaki T, Clark BA, et al (1989) Human papillomavirus DNA in adenocarcinoma in situ, microinvasive adenocarcinoma of the uterine cervix and coexisting cervical squamous intraepithelial neoplasia. Int J Gynecol Pathol 8: 8–17

360. Tase T, Okagaki T, Clark BA, et al (1989) Human papillomavirus DNA in glandular dysplasia and microglandular hyperplasia: Presumed precursors of adenocarcinoma of the uterine cervix. Obstet Gynecol 73: 1005–1008

361. ter Meulen J, Eberhardt HC, Luande J, et al (1992) Human papillomavirus (HPV) infection, HIV infection and cervical cancer in Tanzania, East Africa. Int J Cancer 51: 515–521

362. Terris M, Wilson F, Nelson JH (1973) Relation of circumcision to cancer of the cervix. Am J Obstet Gynecol 117: 1056

363. Tobon H, Dave H (1988) Adenocarcinoma in situ of the cervix. Int J Gynecol Pathol 7: 139–151

364. Townsend DE, Richart RM (1983) Cryotherapy and carbon dioxide laser management of cervical intraepithelial neoplasia: A controlled comparison. Obstet Gynecol 61: 75–78

365. Trevathan E, Layde P, Webster LA, et al (1983) Cigarette smoking and dysplasia and carcinoma in situ of the uterine cervix. JAMA 250: 499

366. Trowell JE (1985) Intestinal metaplasia with argentaffin cells in the uterine cervix. Histopathology 9: 561–569

367. Van den Brule AJC, Class ECJ, du Maine M, et al (1989) Use of anticontamination primers in the polymerase chain reaction for the detection of human papillomavirus genotypes in cervical scrapes and biopsies. J Med Virol 29: 20–29

368. VanNiekerk WA (1962) Cervical cells in megaloblastic anemia of puerperium. Lancet 1: 1277

369. Vermund SH, Kelley KF, Klein RS, et al (1991) High risk of human papillomavirus infection and cervical squamous intraepithelial lesions among women with symptomatic human immunodeficiency virus infection. Am J Obstet Gynecol 165: 392–400

370. Vessey MF (1984) Exogenous hormones in the aetiology of cancer in women. J Roy Soc Med 77: 542

371. Villa LL, Franco EL (1989) Epidemiologic correlates of cervical neoplasia and risk of human papillomavirus infection in asymptomatic women in Brazil. J Natl Cancer Inst 81: 332–340

372. Vonka V, Kanka J, Hirsch I, et al (1984) Prospective study on the relationship between cervical neoplasia and herpes simplex type 2 virus. II. Herpes simplex type 2 antibody presence in sera taken at enrollment. Int J Cancer 33: 61

373. Vonka V, Kanka J, Jelinek I, et al (1984) Prospective study on the relationship between cervical neoplasia and herpes simplex type–2 virus. I. Epidemiological characteristics. Int J Cancer 33: 49

374. Vonka V, Kanka J, Roth Z (1987) Herpes simplex type 2 virus and cervical neoplasia Adv Cancer Res 49: 149–191

375. Ward BE, Burkett BA, Peterson C, et al (1990) Cytological correlates of cervical papillomavirus infection. Int J Gynecol Pathol 9: 297–305

376. Ward P, Coleman DV, Malcolm DB (1989) Regulatory mechanisms of the papillomaviruses Trends Genet 5: 97–98

377. Wassertheil-Smoller S, Romney SL, Wylie-Rosset J, et al (1981) Dietary vitamin c and uterine cervical dysplasia. Am J Epidemiol 114: 714

378. Watanabe S, Kanda T, Yoshiike K (1989) Human papillomavirus type 16 transformation of primary human embryonic fibroblasts requires expression of open reading frames E6 and E7. J Virol 63: 965–969

379. Weid GL (1961) Proceedings of the First International Congress on Exfoliative Cytology., Philadelphia, J.B. Lippincott

380. Weisbrot IM, Stabinsky C, Davis M (1972) Adenocarcinoma in situ of the uterine cervix. Cancer 29: 1179–1187

381. Wells M, Brown LJR (1986) Glandular lesions of the uterine cervix: the present state of our knowledge. Histopathology 10: 777–792

382. Werness BA, Levine AJ, Howley PM (1990) Association of human papillomavirus types 16 and 18 E6 proteins with p53. Science 248: 76–79

383. Whitehead N, Reyner F, Lindenbaum J (1973) Megaloblastic changes in the cervical epithelium. Association of oral contraceptive therapy and reversal with folic acid. JAMA 266: 1421

384. Wilbanks GD, Richart RM (1967) The peurperal cervix, injuries and healing: A colposcopic study. Am J Obstet Gynecol 97: 1105

385. Wilbanks GD, Richart RM, Terner JY (1967) DNA content

of cervical intraepithelial neoplasia studied by two wavelength Feulgen cytophotometry. Am J Obstet Gynecol 98: 792–799

386. Willet GD, Kurman RJ, Reid R (1989) Correlation of the histological appearance of intraepithelial neoplasia of the cervix with human papillomavirus types. Int J Gynecol Pathol 8: 18–25

387. Williams J (1888) Cancer of the uterus: Harveian Lectures for 1886. London, H.K. Lewis

388. Winkler B, Crum CP, Fujii T (1984) Koilocytotic lesions of the cervix: The relationship of mitotic abnormalities to the presence of papillomavirus antigens and nuclear DNA content. Cancer 53: 1081–1087

389. Winkler B, Norris HJ, Fenoglio CM (1982) The female genital tract. In: Ridell RH (eds) Pathology of Drug-induced and Toxic Diseases. New York, Churchill Livingstone

390. Woodworth CD, Waggoner S, Barnes W, et al (1990) Human cervical and foreskin epithelial cells immortalized by human papillomavirus DNAs exhibit dysplastic differentiation in vivo. Cancer Res 50: 3709–3715

391. Wright TC, Ellerbrock TE, Chiasson MA, et al (1993) Comparison of cervical intraepithelial neoplasia in human immunodeficiency virus-infected and uninfected women: Prevalence, Pap smear validity and epidemiological risk factors. Submitted

392. Wright TC, Gagnon MD, Richart RM, et al (1992) Treatment of cervical intraepithelial neoplasia using the loop electrosurgical excision procedure. Obstet Gynecol 79: 173–178

393. Wright TC, Richart RM (1990) Role of human papillomavirus in the pathogenesis of genital tract warts and cancer. Gynecol Oncol 37: 151–164

394. Wright TC, Richart RM (1992) Pathogenesis and diagnosis of preinvasive lesions of the lower genital tract. In: Hoskins WJ, Perez CA, Young RC (eds) Principles and Practice of Gynecologic Oncology. Philadelphia, J. B. Lippincott, pp 509–536

395. Wright TC, Richart RM (1993) Controversies in the management of low grade cervical intraepithelial neoplasia. Cancer 71: 1413–1421

396. Yasumoto S, Burkhardt AL, Doniger J, et al (1986) Human papillomavirus type 16 DNA-induced malignant transformation of NIH 3T3 cells. J Virol 57: 572–577

397. Yee C, Krishnan-Hewlett Z, Baker CC, et al (1985) Presence and expression of human papillomavirus sequences in human cervical carcinoma cell lines. Am J Pathol 119: 361

398. Young RH, Clement PB (1991) Pseudoneoplastic glandular lesions of the uterine cervix. Semin Diag Pathol 8: 234–249

399. Young RH, Scully RE (1989) Atypical forms of microglandular hyperplasia of the cervix simulating carcinoma. Am J Surg Pathol 13: 50–56

400. zur Hausen H (1977) Human papillomaviruses and their possible role in squamous cell carcinomas. Curr Top Microbiol Immunol 78: 1–30

401. zur Hausen H (1987) Papillomaviruses in human cancer. Cancer 59: 1692–1696

402. zur Hausen H (1991) Human papillomaviruses in the pathogenesis of anogenital cancer. Virology 184: 9–13

8

Carcinoma and Other Tumors of the Cervix

Thomas C. Wright, M.D., Alex Ferenczy, M.D., and Robert J. Kurman, M.D.

The World Health Organization (WHO) classification for tumors of the cervix has been revised recently in collaboration with the International Society of Gynecological Pathologists. Three general categories of epithelial tumors of the cervix are now recognized: squamous cell carcinoma, adenocarcinoma, and "other" epithelial tumors (Table 8.1.)[307] The latter category encompasses adenosquamous carcinoma and glassy cell carcinoma, tumors that have been grouped in the past with mucoepidermoid carcinoma and classified as "mixed" carcinomas. The "other" epithelial tumor category also includes adenoid basal cell carcinoma and adenoid cystic carcinomas as well as carcinoid-like carcinoma and small cell carcinoma, which were classified previously as neuroendocrine carcinoma (Table 8.1). The relative proportions of these different types of carcinoma varies from study to study, but ingeneral, approximately 60–80% of invasive carcinomas of the cervix are classified as squamous cell carcinomas.[1,40,43,58,60,314] Mesenchymal tumors including smooth muscle and stromal tumors and mixed epithelial and mesenchymal tumors, such as adenosarcoma and malignant mixed mesodermal tumors, are similar in appearance and behavior to those occurring in the uterine corpus and are discussed in detail in Chapter 13, Mesenchymal Tumors of the Uterus.

The most widely accepted staging system for carcinomas of the cervix is that of the International Federation of Gynecologists and Obstetricians (FIGO) (Table 8.2). This staging system divides invasive carcinoma into four stages. Stage I includes all tumors confined to the cervix and is

Table 8.1. Modified World Health Organization histological classification of epithelial tumors of the uterine cervix

Squamous cell carcinoma
   Microinvasive squamous cell carcinoma
   Invasive squamous cell carcinoma
   Verrucous carcinoma
   Warty (condylomatous) carcinoma
   Papillary squamous cell (transitional) carcinoma
   Lymphoepithelioma-like carcinoma
Adenocarcinoma
   Mucinous adenocarcinoma
      Endocervical type
      Intestinal type
      Signet-ring type
   Endometrioid adenocarcinoma
      Endometrioid adenocarcinoma with squamous metaplasia
   Clear cell adenocarcinoma
   Minimal deviation adenocarcinoma
      Endocervical type (adenoma malignum)
      Endometrioid type
   Serous adenocarcinoma
   Mesonephric carcinoma
   Well-differentiated villoglandular adenocarcinoma
Other epithelial tumors
   Adenosquamous carcinoma
   Glassy cell carcinoma
   Mucoepidermoid carcinoma
   Adenoid cystic carcinoma
   Adenoid basal carcinoma
   Carcinoid-like tumor
   Small cell carcinoma
   Undifferentiated carcinoma

divided into two broad categories, microinvasive and more deeply invasive carcinomas.[270] Stage II tumors extend beyond the cervix but not to the pelvic sidewall and do not involve the lower third of the vagina. Stage III tumors include those that extend to the pelvic sidewall, cause hydronephrosis or a nonfunctioning kidney or involve the lower third of the vagina. Stage IV tumors extend beyond the true pelvis or clinically involve the mucosa of the bladder or rectum.

Squamous Cell Carcinoma

Microinvasive Squamous Cell Carcinoma

The concept of microinvasive carcinoma (MICA) of the cervix was first introduced in 1874 by Mestwerdt.[234] Microinvasive carcinoma is considered a preclinical stage in the progressive spectrum of high grade squamous intraepithelial lesions (SIL), previously referred to as cervical intraepithelial neoplasia (CIN) and frank clinical invasive carcinoma of the cervix uteri. The most appropriate definition of MICA is controversial despite numerous studies.[25,33,54,95,184] The main subjects of contention are the maximum depth of stromal invasion and the significance of vascular invasion, tumor volume, and confluency of neo-

plastic epithelium, as related to the frequency of pelvic lymph node metastasis, vaginal recurrence, and survival. Most patients who die of disseminated squamous cell carcinoma have either lymphatic channel involvement, tumors measuring more than 5 mm in greatest extent, or tumors more than 2.5 cm in volume.[35,46,184,187] Accordingly, FIGO has defined stage IA tumors as tumors that invade to a depth of *not more than 5 mm taken from the base of the epithelium, either surface or glandular, from which it originates and a second dimension, the horizontal spread, must not exceed 7 mm* (Table 8.2).[193,220] Stage IA tumors frequently are referred to as MICA. Tumors that qualify as stage IA are further subdivided into those with a measurable depth of invasion, Stage IA2, and those with minimal microscopic invasion, too shallow to be measured accurately, stage IA1.

Because some patients with stage IA tumors as defined by FIGO have had lymph node metastases, the Society of Gynecological Oncologists (SGO) in the United States has proposed a more restricted definition of MICA. The definition of MICA proposed in 1974 by the Committee on Nomenclature for the SGO states: *A microinvasive lesion should be defined as one in which neoplastic epithelium invades the stroma in one or more places to a depth of 3 mm or less below the basement membrane of the epithelium and in which lymphatic or blood vascular involvement is not demonstrated.*[67] According to this definition, histologically detected lesions with 3.1–5 mm deep stromal invasion or with vascular space invasion but less than 3.1 mm deep stromal invasion represent stage 1B carcinomas. Lesions that fulfill the SGO definition of MICA have virtually no potential for either metastases or recurrence and therefore this definition appears to be the most appropriate one for guiding clinical management. It is important to stress that because the lesion cannot be visualized on gross inspection, the diagnosis of MICA is *always* based on histological examination of a cone biopsy specimen that *includes the entire lesion.*

General Features

Most MICAs are found in patients in their early 40s, between two extremes of age, early 20s and 70s.[100] According to various investigators, the frequency of MICA in patients with SIL (CIN) varies from less than 1% to more than 50%.[205] This wide variation in prevalence reflects differences in the definition of MICA, methods of sampling of cervical specimens, and the criteria used for diagnosing invasion. A 4% prevalence of MICA has been demonstrated in serial step sections of specimens with SIL (CIN).[8,35,181,360] It is important to note, however, that patients included in these series were treated with traditional cold knife cone biopsy and usually had high-grade SIL (CIN 2,3). For example, in Anderson's series of patients treated with cold knife cone biopsies, 91% of the patients were classified as having CIN 3.[8] Estimates of the inci-

Table 8.2. 1988 modification of International Federation of Gynecologists and Obstetricians (FIGO) staging of carcinoma of the cervix uteri

Stage	
0	Carcinoma in situ, intraepithelial carcinoma
I	The carcinoma is strictly confined to the cervix (extension to the corpus should be disregarded)
IA	Preclinical carcinomas of the cervix, that is, those diagnosed only by microscopy
IA1	Minimal microscopically evident stromal invasion
IA2	Lesions detected microscopically that can be measured. The upper limit of the measurement should not show a depth of invasion of more than 5 mm taken from the base of the epithelium, either surface or glandular, from which it originates, and a second dimension, the horizontal spread, must not exceed 7 mm; larger lesions should be classified as stage IB
IB	Lesions of greater dimensions than stage IA2, whether seen clinically or not. Performed space involvement should not alter the staging but should be specifically recorded so as to determine whether it should affect treatment decisions in the future
II	The carcinoma extends beyond the cervix but has not extended to the pelvic wall. The carcinoma involves the vagina but not as far as the lower third
IIA	No obvious parametrial involvement
IIB	Obvious parametrial involvement
III	The carcinoma has extended to the pelvic wall. On rectal examination, there is no cancer-free space between the tumor and pelvic wall; the tumor involves the lower third of the vagina; all cases with hydronephrosis or nonfunctioning kidney are included unless they are known to be due to other causes
IIIA	No extension to the pelvic wall
IIIB	Extension to the pelvic wall and/or hydronephrosis or nonfunctioning kidney
IV	The carcinoma has extended beyond the true pelvis or has clinically involved the mucosa of the bladder or rectum; a bullous edema as such does not permit a case to be allotted to stage IV
IVA	Spread of the growth to adjacent organs
IVB	Spread to distant organs

Notes: Stage IA carcinoma should include minimal microscopically evident stromal invasion as well as small cancerous tumors of measurable size. Stage IA should be divided into those lesions with minute foci of invasion visible only microscopically as stage IA1 and macroscopically measurable microcarcinomas as stage IA2, in order to gain further knowledge of the clinical behavior of these lesions. The term *IB occult* should be omitted.

The diagnosis of both stage IA1 and IA2 cases should be based on microscopic examination of removed tissue, preferably a cone, which must include the entire lesion. The lower limit of stage IA2 should be measurable macroscopically (even if dots need to be placed on the slide before measurement), and the upper limit of stage IA2 is given by measurement of the two largest dimensions in any given section. The depth of invasion should not be more than 5 mm taken from the base of the epithelium, either surface or glandular, from which it originates. The second dimension, the horizontal spread, must not exceed 7 mm. Vascular space involvement, either venous or lymphatic, should not alter the staging but should be specifically recorded, as it may affect treatment decisions in the future.

Lesions of greater size should be classified as stage IB.

As a rule, it is impossible to estimate clinically whether a cancer of the cervix has extended to the corpus or not. Extension to the corpus should therefore be disregarded.

Modified from International Federation of Gynecology and Obstetrics. Annual report on the results of treatment in gynecological cancer. Vol 20. Stockholm: FIGO, 1988.

dence and prevalence of MICA in the general population can be obtained from population-based cervical cancer registries. A population-based registry from British Columbia, Canada, estimates the incidence of MICA to be 4.8 per 100,000 women screened. In this same registry, the incidence of carcinoma in situ was 316 per 100,000 women screened.[23]

With the widespread adoption of shallow laser excisional conization and loop electrosurgical excision procedure (LEEP) as methods for treating SIL (CIN), better estimates of the prevalence of MICA in patients with all grades of SIL (CIN) have been obtained. In an analysis of shallow laser excisional conization specimens from 196 patients with SIL (CIN) that did not extend into the endocervical canal, McIndoe et al. detected colposcopically unsuspected MICA in two (1%) of the patients.[229] Larger studies of specimens obtained by loop electrosurgical excision are currently reporting colposcopically undetected MICA in 0.4–3% of all patients with CIN.[147,216,246,247] In assessing the probability of MICA developing in women

with SIL (CIN), the size as well as grade of the lesion seems to be important. Microinvasive squamous cell carcinoma appears to be associated most commonly with extensive high-grade SIL (CIN 2,3) involving either the surface of the cervix or the endocervical crypts.[345]

CLINICAL FEATURES

Most patients with MICA are asymptomatic and the tumors generally are discovered on a routine cervical smear. The cervix demonstrates a grossly normal appearance or nonspecific findings, such as chronic cervicitis or true erosion. A definitive diagnosis of microinvasion is made on histological evaluation of cervical tissue removed by conization or at hysterectomy. For many years it has been taught that cytopathologists and colposcopists are able to predict early stromal invasion with a high degree of accuracy. Ng et al., on the basis of cellular characteristics in Pap smears, correctly predicted 27 of 31 patients with proved MICA, an accuracy of 87%.[250] However, more recent cytological studies have failed to predict accurately the presence of microinvasion.[190,298] Colposcopically, areas of MICA usually display a marked degree of whiteness consistent with CIN and contain one or more foci of bizarre surface-branching vessels (Fig. 8.1).[23,33,328] Therefore, the recommended approach to establish the diagnosis of microinvasion has been to obtain a colposcopically directed punch biopsy of the area suspicious for microinvasion, followed by a conization to exclude more advanced disease. The cone is sampled completely for microscopic examination, and the pathologist evaluates the surgical margins, depth of stromal invasion, the greatest lateral extent of the lesion, and whether vascular space invasion is present.

More recent studies have shown, however, that microinvasion frequently cannot be detected accurately using colposcopy or cytology. For example, in a study that correlated colposcopic appearances with histological findings of a large number of loop excision specimens, Murdoch et al. demonstrated that the accurate colposcopic detection of

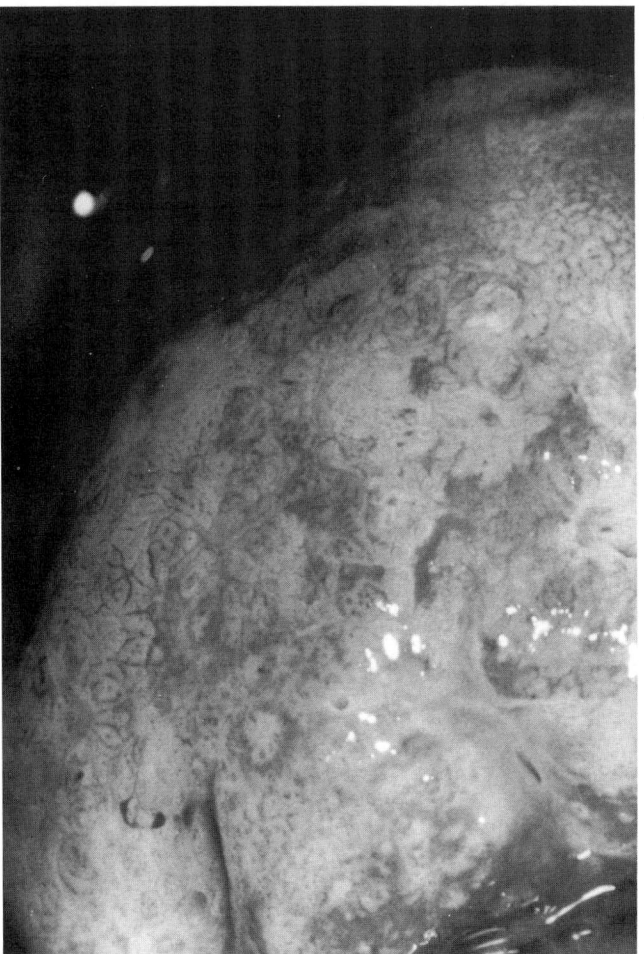

FIG. 8.1. Microinvasive squamous cell carcinoma of the cervix. The colposcopic lesion is densely acetowhite with a prominent mosaic vascular pattern and coarse branching vessels. (Photograph courtesy of Dr. Duane Townsend, Sacramento, CA.)

MICA requires invasion of greater than 1 mm into the cervical stroma.[247]

PATHOLOGICAL FINDINGS

The diagnosis of MICA is based on the presence of one or more tongues of malignant cells penetrating through the basement membrane of the squamous epithelium (Fig. 8.2). The latter invariably demonstrates a SIL (CIN) of varying severity, and in most instances the underlying endocervical glands are replaced extensively by the intraepithelial disease. Typically in the microinvasion foci, the cells are better differentiated with abundant eosinophilic cytoplasm and prominent nucleoli as compared with the associated SIL (CIN). Occasionally, small foci of keratinization are seen within the microinvasive foci. Because of focal disruption of the basement membrane, the margin of the invading nests is ragged, flanked by intact basement membrane on either side (Figs. 8.2 and 8.3). This irregular contour probably is the most reliable criterion for the diagnosis of MICA. It is easily distinguished from the smooth and regular contour or masses of neoplastic cells that represent endocervical gland involvement by high-grade SIL (CIN 2, 3). There often is a conspicuous lymphoplasmacytic infiltrate surrounding the tips of the invasive epithelial prongs, and frequently there is a desmoplastic response in the adjacent stroma. Two additional histological features that are reported to be helpful for diagnosing MICA, particularly when there is a marked inflammatory infiltrate, are apparent duplication or folding of the neoplastic epithelium and scalloping of the margins of the epithelium at the dermal–epidermal interface.[71]

Roche and Norris defined lymphatic space invasion as endothelial-lined (capillary-like) spaces containing tumor cells that are contiguous with the stroma (Fig. 8.4).[296]

—————————————————————————⊳

FIG. 8.2. Microinvasive squamous carcinoma of the cervix. a: Tongues of neoplastic epithelium project into the stroma from an area of high-grade SIL that has replaced a preexisting endocervical gland. Stromal extension is less than 1 mm in depth. **b:** Higher magnification of the microinvasive focus, which characteristically displays an irregular margin and better differentiated neoplastic cells than those above the basal lamina. The stromal epithelial junction of the invasive focus is typically infiltrated by chronic inflammatory cells. (Reprinted with permission from Kurman RJ, et al, ref. 199.)

FIG. 8.3. Microinvasive squamous cell carcinoma of the cervix. Irregularly shaped nests of epithelium invade the stroma. This is an unusual type of squamous carcinoma in which the epithelium overlying the area of invasion is mature and lacks atypia. Note abnormal mitotic figures (*arrows*).

FIG. 8.4. Microinvasive squamous cell carcinoma of the cervix. Neoplastic cells adhere to the endothelial lining of a lymphatic capillary space.

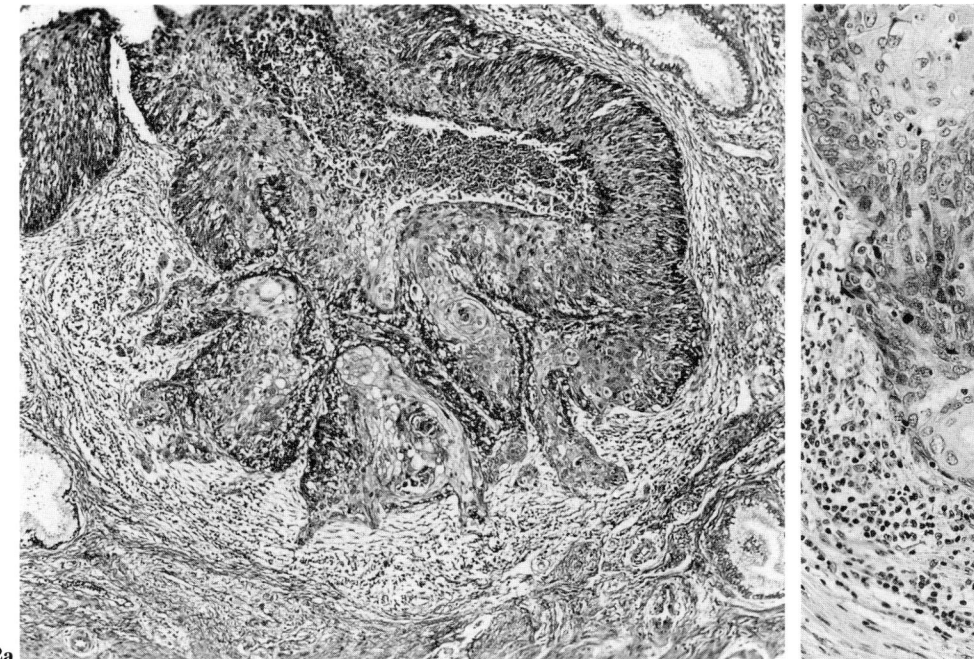

8.2a

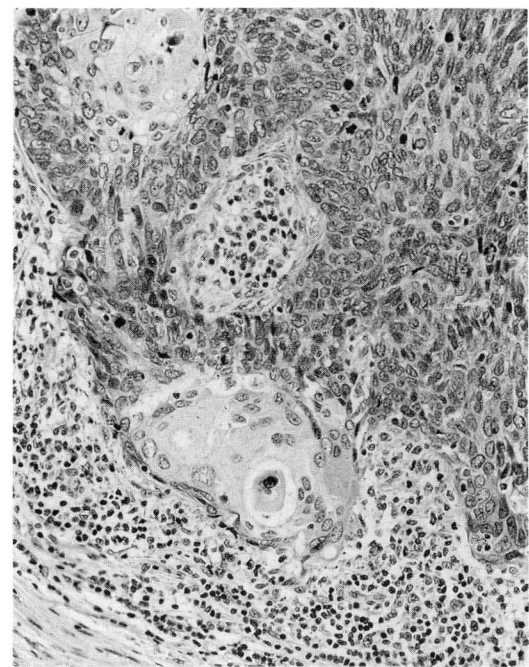

8.2b

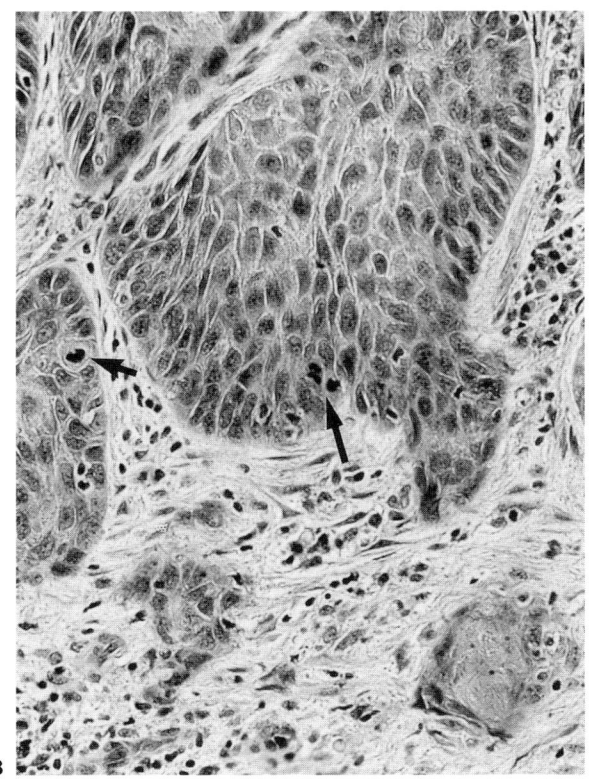

8.3

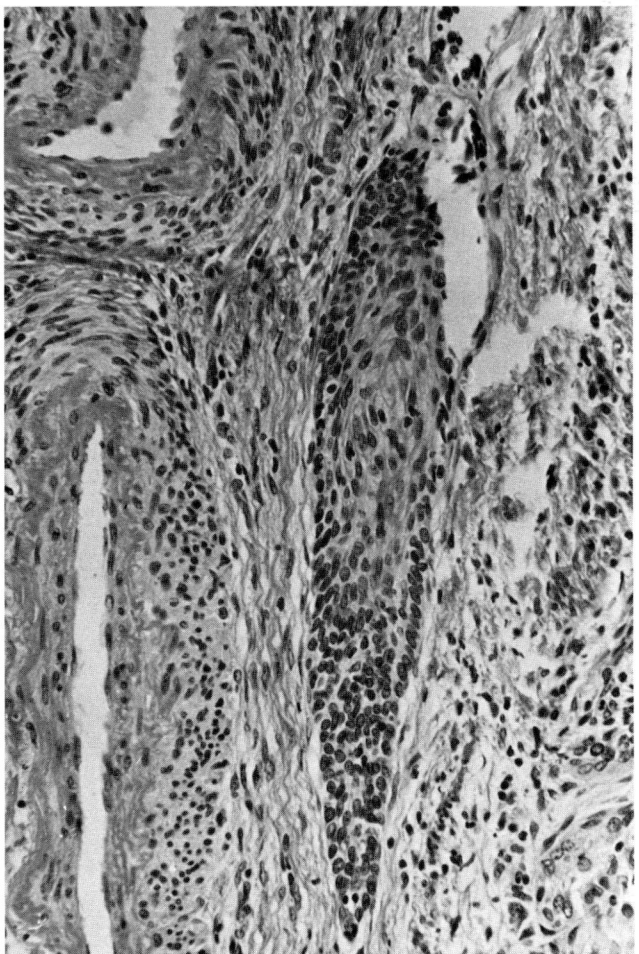

8.4

Identification of early lymphatic and vascular space invasion, particularly in the cervical stroma adjacent to the overlying epithelium, may be difficult and often is hampered by technical processing artifacts (Fig. 8.5). Staining endothelial cells using either antibodies against Factor VIII or with *Ulex agglutinin* sometimes is helpful for distinguishing between true lymphvascular space involvement and processing artifacts. In view of the difficulties in distinguishing small blood vessels and capillaries from small lymphatic channels, the term *lymphvascular space(s)* is used in this chapter.

For consistency in the measurement of the depth of stromal invasion, the following guidelines are recommended. The depth of neoplastic projections should not exceed 3 mm from the initial site of invasion either from the basal lamina of the surface epithelium or from endocervical glands replaced by intraepithelial neoplasia (Fig.

8.6). There are cases, however, in which a direct histological continuity between invasive foci and SIL cannot be demonstrated, even in deeper cuts of the paraffin block. In such instances, it is assumed that invasion originated from the basal cells of the overlying SIL (CIN). As a result, depth of invasion is measured arbitrarily from the basal lamina of the surface SIL (CIN) (Fig. 8.6).

The most accurate method to measure the depth of stromal penetration is with a calibrated slide or ocular microscale.[277,280] A more convenient, but perhaps less accurate, method of establishing the size and depth of penetrating foci consists of using a microscopic field that corresponds to a diameter of 1 mm. This may be determined by direct microscopic visualization with a transparent metric ruler. Although variation in microscopic objective and ocular lenses exists, in general a microscopic field of 160× measures a little more than 1 mm in diameter. The depth of penetration also depends on the angle at which sections are prepared, and efforts should be made to secure vertically sectioned tissue samples. The lateral extent of MICA is measured as described for the depth of stromal penetration. Measurements are made between the two points where the neoplastic epithelium (regardless of whether it is microinvasive or SIL) meets the adjacent normal epithelium.

IMMUNOHISTOCHEMICAL FINDINGS

At the site of initial stromal invasion, disruption of the basement membrane has been identified using electron microscopy. Therefore, a number of studies have attempted to use immunohistochemistry and antibodies directed against basement membrane constituents such as laminin or type IV collagen as a way of enhancing the

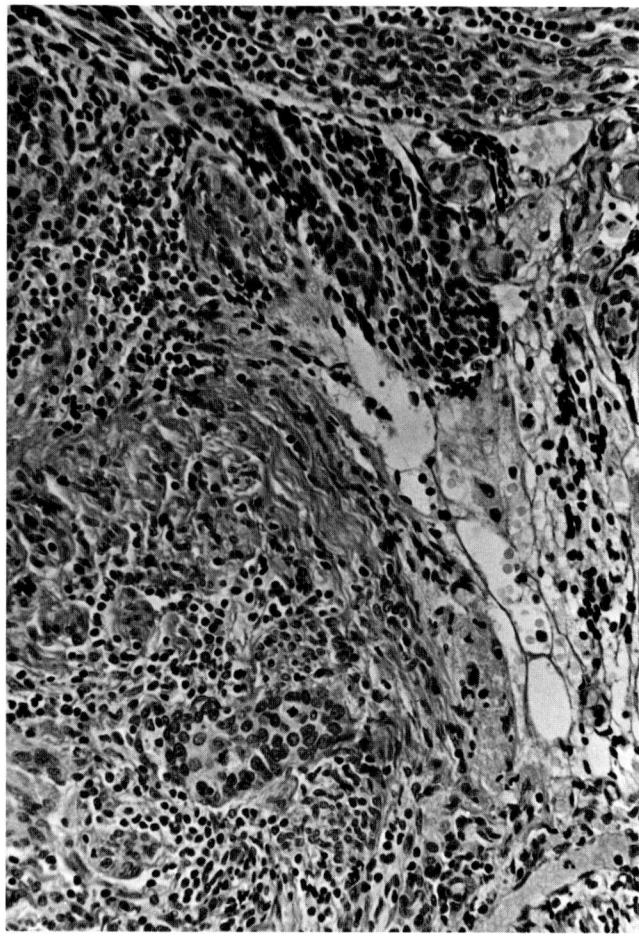

FIG. 8.5. **Squamous intraepithelial lesion (SIL) simulating microinvasive carcinoma.** Implanted nests of neoplastic epithelium are present at the site of previous biopsy site. Note artifact of shrinkage characterized by irregular outline and absence of endothelial lining of the space surounding tumor cells. Edema, extravasated red blood cells, and inflammatory exudate indicate response to injury.

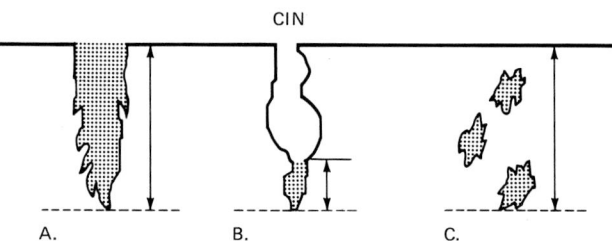

FIG. 8.6. **Methods of measuring depth of invasion of microinvasive squamous carcinoma of the cervix.** The pattern of stromal invasion determines the stromal depth measurement that is most appropriate. **A:** Origin of invasion at surface SIL (CIN)—depth of stromal invasion is measured from point of origin of invasion downward to the last cell of the invasive focus. **B:** Origin of invasion at SIL (CIN) with gland involvement—depth of stromal invasion is measured from site of origin downward to the last cell of the invasive focus. **C:** Origin of invasion not seen—depth of stromal invasion is measured from basal lamina of surface SIL (CIN) downward to the last cell of the invasive focus.

recognition of early stromal invasion in cervical carcinomas. In one of the first studies using this approach, Barsky et al. used antibodies against laminin and type IV collagen and demonstrated that benign and in situ lesions from a number of sites including breast, pancreas, skin, and prostate had a continuous basement membrane whereas microinvasive lesions at these sites had a loss of basement membrane staining.[20] However, other investigators have found that small basement membrane disruptions (as defined by laminin and type IV collagen staining) frequently occur in both the normal cervical epithelium and in squamous intraepithelial lesions that lack microinvasion, especially in areas with severe stromal inflammatory infiltrates.[74,353] In addition, foci of basement membrane staining frequently occur in areas of invasion and the amount of staining tends to increase as the degree of differentiation of the invading tumor increases.[89] In a recent test of the usefulness of type IV collagen immunoreactivity in assessing questionable early stromal invasion, Stewart and McNicol found the technique to be of limited diagnostic value.[333]

Differential Diagnosis

MICA is frequently misdiagnosed. Of 265 purported cases of MICA submitted to a group of reference pathologists of the Gynecologic Oncology Group, 132 cases (approximately 50%) were rejected.[309] Special attention should be paid to the interpretation of recently biopsied conization specimens. These often harbor individual nests of neoplastic epithelium buried within the cervical stroma at the site of a previous punch biopsy (Fig. 8.5). Such nests represent clusters of intraepithelial disease that may be disrupted and incorporated into the stroma by the punch biopsy and masquerade as MICA. Therefore, a diagnosis of microinvasion should be made with caution when such a phenomenon is seen at or near a recent biopsy site. SIL (CIN) or immature squamous metaplasia with extensive gland involvement also should be distinguished from MICA. A prominent stromal desmoplastic response, abundant eosinophilic cytoplasm, and an irregular margin or scalloping of the epithelial nest are features associated with invasive foci.

Risk Factors

Factors that have been reported to increase an individual's risk for nodal metastases, recurrence, and death are: (1) depth and pattern of stromal invasion, (2) presence of lymphvascular space involvement, (3) tumor volume, and (4) status of the resection margin. However, the lack of a uniform definition and methodology for measuring the depth of invasion together with different lengths of follow-up and treatment methods make interpretation of the published data difficult. For example, the maximal depth of stromal invasion in studies of MICA varies from 1 to 5 mm.[33,95,184] Some studies characterize microinvasion by the absence of confluency of invasive foci[33] and/or the absence of vascular permeation,[33,68] whereas in others lymphatic involvement[68,296] and confluency[296] do not exclude the diagnosis of MICA. It is not surprising, therefore, that the frequency of pelvic node metastasis associated with MICA varies from 0 to 7%.[25,31]

Depth and Pattern of Invasion

Depth of stromal invasion is a major factor in determining the outcome of patients with MICA. Early studies reported that no residual carcinoma was detected in the hysterectomy specimen when MICA invaded 1 mm or less in the cone biopsy. In contrast, residual carcinoma was detected in a significant proportion of cases when MICA detected on cone biopsy invaded 3 mm or more into the stroma. Pathological analysis of lymph nodes removed at the time of radical surgery demonstrates a clear relationship between the depth of stromal invasion and the presence of lymph node metastases (Table 8.3).[62,64,67,80,131,151,221,319,351] Only two patients with lymph node metastases have been reported out of 382 patients with 3 mm or less stromal invasion. In contrast, the prevalence of lymph node metastases is 5.3% in women with between 3.1 and 5 mm of invasion, 16% in women with stage 1B invasive cervical squamous cell carcinoma invading to a depth of 6–10 mm, and 24% in women with stage 1B carcinoma invading to a depth of 11–15 mm.

The development of recurrent disease or death from cervical cancer in women with less than 1 mm of stromal invasion who have been managed with either a cone biopsy or a simple hysterectomy is infrequent.[14,47,62,64,187] In three recent, long-term follow-up studies involving 403 women, not a single patient with less than 1 mm of stromal invasion treated with a cone biopsy or simple hysterectomy died of their tumor (Table 8.4).[47,64,187] Similarly, recurrent disease occurs in approximately 1% of patients when tumors invade less than 3 mm (Table 8.5).[67,62,221,309,312,319,222] Recurrence occurs in

Table 8.3. Pelvic node metastasis with early invasive carcinoma according to depth of stromal penetration

Depth of invasion (mm)[a]	No. of patients	% of patients with (+) lymph nodes
≤3	382	0.5
3.1–5	399	5.3
5.1–10	329	15.8
10.1–15	179	23.5
15.1–20	121	38.0

[a] Depth of stromal invasion regardless of presence or absence of vascular invasion and confluency.
Modified from refs. 62, 67, 80, 131, 140, 207, 221, 312, 319, 351.

Table 8.4. Outcome of women with microinvasive squamous cell carcinoma with 1 mm or less invasion managed by cone biopsy or simple hysterectomy

Author	No. of patients	No. of deaths from tumor
Burghardt et al.	259	0
Coppleson et al.	54	0
Koldstad	90	0
Total	403	0

Modified from refs. 47, 64, 187.

Table 8.6. Relationship between depth of invasion and presence of lymphvascular space involvement

Depth of invasion (mm)	No. of patients	Percentage of cases showing lymphvascular space involvement	
		Mean	Range
<1.0	353	3	0–8
1.0–3.0	416	16	9–29
3.1–5.0	312	22	12–43

Adapted from refs. 62, 67, 187, 207, 221, 309.

approximately 5% of patients when there is 3.1–5 mm of invasion (Table 8.5).

Confluency of neoplastic epithelium in MICA is not associated with pelvic node metastases, vaginal recurrence, or cancer death.[131,207,296,319] In summary, clinical outcome is strongly influenced by the depth but not pattern of invasion.

LYMPHVASCULAR SPACE INVOLVEMENT

The relationship between lymphvascular space involvement and clinical outcome in women with early invasive squamous cell carcinoma is less clear-cut than the relationship between depth of invasion and lymph node metastases. Lymphvascular space involvement is reported to occur in 0–8% of early squamous cell carcinomas that invade less than 1 mm into the stroma and in 9–29% of tumors invading 1–3 mm into the stroma (Table 8.6).[47,67,187,207,221,309,312] The large variation between the different reports is due to several factors, including the number of pathological sections evaluated and interobserver variability in determining lymphvascular space involvement. Shrinkage of stroma surrounding invasive nests can result in the formation of artifactual spaces that can be

interpreted erroneously as vascular invasion. One study of early invasive squamous cell carcinoma reported that the frequency of detection of lymphvascular space involvement increased from 30% to 57% when step sections were cut through the site of invasion.[296] Despite the problems with recognizing lymphvascular space involvement, most studies have found a relationship between increasing depth of invasion and an increased frequency of lymphvascular space invasion (Table 8.6).

The clinical significance, however, of lymphvascular space involvement in patients with early invasive cervical cancer is controversial. Although several series of patients with 5 mm or less invasion have reported no direct relationship between the presence of lymphvascular space involvement and the presence of lymph node metastases, other studies have found lymphvascular space involvement to be an adverse prognostic indicator.[47,207,221,309,351] For example, in a recent study by Burghardt et al., three of the four patients with 3 mm or less of invasion who developed recurrent disease after simple hysterectomy or cone biopsy had lymphvascular space involvement.[47] Similarly, in a study by Koldstad of 232 patients with stage 1A1 and 411 patients with stage 1A2 squamous cell carcinoma, three of four patients who died of recurrent cancer after therapy had lymphvascular space involvement.[187] Vascular invasion also appears to be a predictor of the presence of invasive carcinoma in the subsequent hysterectomy specimen.[80] Invasive carcinoma has been found in 80% of subsequent hysterectomy specimens when vascular invasion was present in the cone biopsy. Therefore, it is the prevailing opinion in the United States that lymphvascular space involvement should be assessed in women with early invasive squamous cell carcinoma and that the presence of lymphvascular space involvement excludes a diagnosis of MICA.

Table 8.5. Invasive cancer recurrences after any type of therapy for early invasive squamous cell carcinoma of the cervix in patients with differing depths of invasion

Author	No. of patients with recurrent invasive cancer/ total patients (%)	
	<3.0 mm of invasion[a]	3.1–5.0 mm of invasion[a]
Copeland et al.	8/552 (1.4%)	3/121 (2.5%)
Maiman et al.	0/65	0/30
Sedlis et al.	1/111 (0.9%)	1/21 (4.7%)
Sevin et al.	0/7	44/36 (11%)
Simon et al.	0/43	0/26
van Nagell et al.	2/145 (1.4%)	6/32 (19%)
Total	11/923 (1.2%)	14/266 (5.3%)

[a] Irrespective of presence or absence of lymphvascular space involvement or horizontal extent of tumor.
Modified from refs. 62, 221, 309, 312, 319, 351.

TUMOR VOLUME AND HORIZONTAL EXTENT

In recent years, the morphologic evaluation of the volume of MICA has been emphasized by some authors. Burghardt and Holzer have introduced the concept of tumor volume as applied to MICA and have reported no pelvic node metastases in patients with 420 mm^3 of cancer

Table 8.7. Residual invasive tumor in postconization hysterectomy specimens according to lateral extent of carcinoma with up to 5 mm stromal invasion

Lateral extent of invasion	No. of patients	% with residual disease in postconization hysterectomy specimen
<4	55	2
>4 mm <8 mm	26	27
>8 mm	23	35

Adapted from ref. 309.

or less, with the exception of one case in which vascular invasion was noted.[48] However, their method of measuring volume by serially sectioning cone specimens is both cumbersome and time-consuming and is unlikely to become a routine laboratory method. Other investigators have used lateral extent of spread as a surrogate for measuring tumor volume. The lateral extent of spread of early invasive squamous cell carcinoma has been correlated with the frequency of residual neoplasia in the postcone hysterectomy specimens (Table 8.7).[309] In another series of 134 patients, 3 women with tumor diameters of up to 10 mm died of their disease.[212]

Surgical Margins

Perhaps one of the most important contributions of the pathologist to the appropriate management of early invasive squamous cell carcinoma is evaluating surgical margins of conization specimens.[67,120,207,309,311] In fact, the status of cone margins may well be the most important single parameter in deciding the therapeutic approach to patients with early invasive squamous cell carcinoma. In most studies women with cone margins positive for either SIL (CIN) or invasive disease are much more likely to have residual invasive disease in the hysterectomy specimens than are women with negative margins. Furthermore, the residual invasion may actually be deeper that that found in the cone biopsy specimen (Table 8.8).

Table 8.8. Relationship between status of cone biopsy margin in patients with early invasive squamous cell carcinoma of the cervix and residual disease in the postcone hysterectomy specimen

Author	Negative margins No. of patients (% with residual cancer)		Positive margins No. of patients (% with residual cancer)	
Creasman et al.	45	(4.4)	13	(77)
Greer et al.	17	(24)	33	(82)
Leman et al.	24	(0)	23	(39)
Sedlis et al.	85	(4)	15	(80)
Total	171	(5.3)	84	(69)

Adapted from refs. 67, 120, 207, 309.

Treatment

The therapy for MICA is as controversial as the definition of this lesion. The trend is in the direction of more conservative management, with attempts at individualization of treatment based on (1) the definition of the lesion, (2) lateral extent, and (3) involvement of cone margins. The data on risk factors for nodal metastases, recurrence, and death, although incomplete, suggest that lesions with 3 mm or less stromal penetration, measured from the point of origin in invasion and without lymphvascular space involvement, have virtually no potential for metastasis or recurrences. On the other hand, those invading 3 mm or less but with vascular invasion may potentially metastasize, although the risk is small (about 3.5%). Therefore, most authorities believe that women with less than 3 mm of stromal invasion and lacking lymphvascular space involvement can be managed with procedures less radical than those required for stage IB invasive squamous cell carcinomas.[268,342] Patients who are to be managed with less radical procedures should not have colposcopically overt carcinoma and should have had a diagnostic conization that removed the entire lesional tissue with negative lines of resection together with a negative endocervical curettage obtained at the time of conization.

At most centers the recommended therapy for MICA that fulfills the SGO definition is a simple hysterectomy. Most authorities now agree that women with MICA who are desirous of maintaining fertility can be managed safely with conization provided they are willing to undergo careful, periodic follow-up and provided they clearly understand that there is a measurable (albeit low) risk of developing pelvic lymph node metastases or recurrent disease.

Invasive Squamous Cell Carcinoma

General Features

Incidence

Despite advances in the detection and management, cervical cancer continues to be a significant health problem on a worldwide scale. In 1980 cervical cancer was the second most frequent cancer in women throughout the world, accounting for 15% of all malignancies in women.[347] It has been estimated that 465,000 cases of invasive cervical cancer occurred throughout the world in 1980.[347] Because of widespread differences in the availability of screening programs and the prevalence of risk factors, there continue to be marked differences in the relative frequency of cervical cancer in developed and undeveloped countries.[125] Cervical cancer is the most frequent type of cancer in women in the developing world whereas it is the 10th most frequent type of cancer in much of the developed world.[262] The regions of the world where the incidence is greatest include sub-Saharan Africa, Central and South America, and Southeast Asia. The highest incidence rate has been reported from parts of Brazil, where there is an age-standardized rate of 83.2 and in Colombia where there is an age-standardized rate of 48.2.[262] The lowest reported incidence rates are from parts of the Middle East, with an age-standardized rate of 3.9 in Kuwaitis living in Kuwait and 3.0 in non-Jews living in Israel.[347]

The average age of patients with invasive squamous cell carcinoma is 51.4 years, 15–23 years older than patients with high-grade SIL (CIN 2,3) and 8 years older than patients with microinvasive carcinoma.[65,287] Cervical cancer occurs, however, at almost any age between 17 and 90 years. In recent years there has been increasing recognition that cervical cancer can occur in women under the age of 35 years. Women under the age of 35 years account for up to 24.5% of all patients with invasive cervical cancer at some institutions in the United States. In certain areas of the United Kingdom increases in the incidence of invasive cervical cancer in women in this age group have been noted.[26,61] The increase in the United Kingdom is most likely related to multiple factors including a failure to provide adequate cytological screening programs for sexually active young women and a change in the demographics of the population being screened.[61,316] Recently similar increases in the incidence of invasive squamous cell carcinoma of the cervix in women under age 50[202a] have been detected in the United States.

There is little doubt that cytological screening programs play a major role in reducing both the incidence and mortality of invasive cervical cancer. This has been demonstrated most conclusively by data from the Nordic countries, Canada, and parts of Scotland.[124,217,238] The incidence of cervical cancer in the Nordic countries between 1945 and 1980 is directly correlated with the extent of cytological screening.[124,125] Cytological screening was

introduced into Iceland and Finland in the mid-1960s and was rapidly accepted and widely used. In both of these countries a marked decrease in the incidence of cervical cancer occurred after the introduction of screening programs. In contrast, Denmark and Sweden introduced widespread screening more slowly and less uniformly and experienced less of a decline in the incidence of cervical cancer. In Norway no cytological screening program was introduced and the incidence of invasive cervical cancer actually increased over this time period.

Reductions in the incidence and mortality of invasive cervical cancer also have occurred in the United States and Canada since the widespread introduction of cytological screening. According to the American Cancer Society, only 30% of all U.S. women had ever had a Pap smear in 1961 but this number increased to 87% by 1987 (Fig. 8.7).[276] In 1940 the incidence of invasive cervical cancer in the United States was 32.6 per 100,000 women, which is similar to that currently seen in the developing world whereas by 1984 the incidence was 8.3 per 100,000 women. The reduction in incidence was paralleled by a reduction in mortality.[83] In 1991 there were only 13,500 cases of invasive cervical cancer diagnosed in the United States and 4500 cervical cancer deaths.[322] Despite the low incidence of invasive cervical cancer in the United States, cervical cancer continues to be a problem among selected groups of women. The incidence among black women is almost three times the incidence of white women in the United States and there are significant geographic variations.[16,66,105,362] A significant proportion of the remaining cases of invasive cervical carcinoma could be prevented if all women at risk underwent routine cytological screening and colposcopic evaluation of significant cytological abnormalities. In a review of women diagnosed with invasive cervical cancer in British Columbia from 1985 to 1988, it

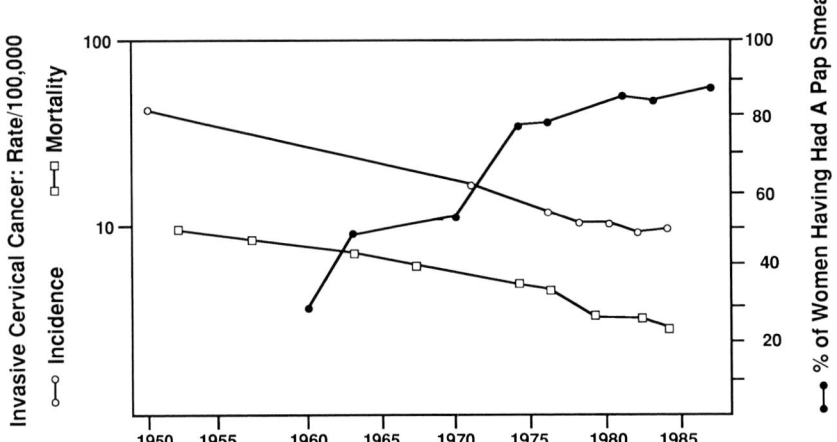

FIG. 8.7. Rate of cytological screening (*curve with black dots*) versus the incidence and mortality of invasive cervical cancer in the United States, 1940–1984. As the rate of screening increased, the incidence and mortality of invasive cancer decreased. (Modified from refs. 83 and 276.)

was found that 39% of the women who developed invasive cervical cancer had never had a Pap smear and that another 11% had had their last Pap smear more than 3 years previously.[7]

HISTOGENESIS AND ETIOLOGY

A considerable body of evidence has been accumulated suggesting that invasive squamous cell carcinoma develops from SIL (CIN). Patients with invasive squamous cell carcinoma have similar epidemiologic characteristics to those with preinvasive precursor lesions (see Chapter 7, Precancerous Lesions of the Cervix). Most women with invasive cancer of the cervix are from lower socioeconomic groups, have begun heterosexual activity early in life, marry early, are multiparous, and have many sexual partners.[38] Most of these are co-variables and are related to sexual intercourse. Moreover, significantly more women (8 times as many as expected) with cervical cancer are observed among spouses of men with cancer of the penis.[119,177]

The molecular evidence linking human papillomavirus (HPV) to invasive squamous cell carcinoma of the cervix is considerable. HPV DNA has been detected in the vast majority of squamous cell carcinoma of the cervix and in most cervical carcinomas cell lines.[°] In patients with metastatic cervical carcinoma, HPV DNA also can be identified in lymph node metastases, with viral DNA hybridization patterns frequently, but not always, matching those of the primary cervical tumor.[150,200] Almost all of the recent studies from well-established laboratories analyzing tissues for multiple types of HPV have detected HPV DNA in more than 80% of invasive squamous cell carcinomas or have found a surprisingly consistent prevalence of HPV 16 in 42–55% of cases.[†] The failure to detect HPV DNA in a small subset of invasive squamous cell carcinomas could be due to a number of factors including failure to sample the lesion adequately, presence of a HPV type other than those assayed for, loss of part of the HPV genome from the malignant cells, or the existence of a type of invasive squamous cell carcinoma that is truly unassociated with HPV DNA. This issue currently remains unresolved.

There is also considerable epidemiologic evidence linking HPV to invasive squamous cell carcinoma of the cervix. Five large case control studies using widely varying methodologies for detecting HPV DNA have found strong associations between specific types of HPV, mainly HPV 16 and 18, and invasive cervical squamous carcinoma.[34,86,244,266,285,304] Two of the most recent of these studies used polymerase chain reaction (PCR) and found that none of the the standard sexual risk factors were independently associated with the development of invasive cervical cancer after controlling for the effect of HPV. This suggests that sexual behavior risk factors are surrogates for HPV infection.[34,266] Taken together, the molecular and epidemiologic evidence now clearly indicates that infection with certain types of HPV is a major causal factor of cervical carcinoma.

It has been estimated that approximately 1–5% of untreated low-grade SIL (CIN 1) will eventually progress to invasive cancer.[63,100,190,257] The percentage of carcinoma in situ that has progressed to invasive squamous cell carcinoma has been between 6% and 74% in the various follow-up series (see Chapter 7, Precancerous Lesions of the Cervix).[190,192,194,230,257] The estimated average duration of preclinical microinvasive disease to to overt clinical carcinoma is about 10 years.[287]

Although some high-grade SIL may develop from low-grade SIL, there are some investigators who believe that generally high-grade lesions do not evolve from low-grade ones but are established at the outset as high-grade lesions.[45,185] These investigators maintain that lesional grade is influenced by location, namely that HPV infection of the ectocervix results in a low-grade lesion whereas infection of the endocervical canal results in a high-grade lesion.

CLINICAL FEATURES

The presenting symptoms of patients with invasive carcinoma of the cervix of all histological types appear to be dependent on the size and stage of the lesion.[276] Early series from the 1950s through the 1970s were composed predominantly of patients with bulky, late-stage disease. Nearly all of these patients had clinically visible cancers and nearly all complained of abnormal vaginal bleeding. The most significant and common feature was bleeding after intercourse or douching. Intermittent spotting, serosanguinous discharge, and frank hemorrhage also were frequently encountered. Ten to 20 percent of the patients complained of bloody malodorous discharge and pain, often radiating to the sacral region. More recent studies include a much higher percentage of patients with stage I disease. Patients with stage I disease frequently are asymptomatic and detected on the basis of an abnormal Pap smear.[276] Weakness, pallor, weight loss, edema of the lower extremities, rectal pain, and hematuria are symptoms and signs of either locally advanced or metastatic disease.

Means for accurate detection and diagnosis of frank invasive carcinoma include cytology, colposcopy, and colposcopically directed punch biopsy.[268] Rectovaginal examination, intravenous pyelography (IVP), cystoscopy, proctosigmoidoscopy, and skeletal survey are used to assess the clinical stage of the disease.

Invasive carcinoma of either the squamous or glandular type develops in the cervical stump that remains after subtotal hysterectomy in 0.1–1.9% of patients.[180,273,365] In a study of 173 women with carcinoma of the cervical

---

°Refs. 79,114,136,160,213,286,291,308,356,369,379.
†Refs. 79,136,158,176,183,213,291,356.

stump, Wolff et al. divided their patients into those in whom the neoplasm was found within 2 years of the subtotal hysterectomy and those in whom the lesion appeared more than 2 years after the operation.[365] The 5-year survival of patients of the first group was worse (30%) than either those of the second group (49%) or those with cancer of the cervix in general. Based on these observations, it has been suggested that cervical stump cancers occurring within the first 2 years after surgery represent residual malignancy, whereas those discovered after 2 years are "new" cancers arising de novo from the cervical stump.[365]

Although 3–10% of cervical cancers occur in pregnant women, invasive carcinoma of the cervix is relatively uncommon during gestation, occurring approximately once in 2200 pregnancies.[32,94,122,256,267] Nevertheless, routine cervical cytology should be part of the initial prenatal examination. The mean age of pregnant women with invasive cervical cancer is 34 years, which is considerably lower than that of women in the general population with invasive cervical cancer and women who are pregnant usually present with early stage tumors.[122] In one series of pregnant patients with invasive cervical disease, 74% were stage I.[141] The treatment of pregnant patients with invasive cervical cancer depends on the clinical stage of the disease and, in general, prognosis is not altered by pregnancy.[122,128,141]

Gross Findings

Invasive squamous cell carcinoma displays a wide range of gross appearances. Early lesions may be focally indurated, ulcerated, or present as a slightly elevated and granular area that bleeds readily on touch. Colposcopic examination usually reveals atypical, tortuous vessels varying widely in size and configuration. Approximately 98% of early carcinomas are localized within the transformation zone, with variable degrees of encroachment onto the neighboring native portio. More advanced tumors have two major types of gross appearance: endophytic and exophytic. Endophytic carcinomas are either ulcerated or nodular (Fig. 8.8). They tend to develop within the endocervical canal and frequently invade deeply into the cervical stroma to produce an enlarged, hard, barrel-shaped cervix. In some patients with endophytic carcinomas the cervix grossly appears normal. The exophytic varieties of cervical carcinomas have a polypoid or papillary appearance (Fig. 8.9).

Microscopic Findings

Microscopically, invasive squamous cell carcinomas have considerable heterogeneity. Many are characterized by anastomosing tongues or cords of neoplastic epithelium infiltrating the fibrous stroma of the cervix (Fig. 8.10). Characteristically, the contour of the infiltrating nests and clusters is irregular and ragged. In other cases the tumor

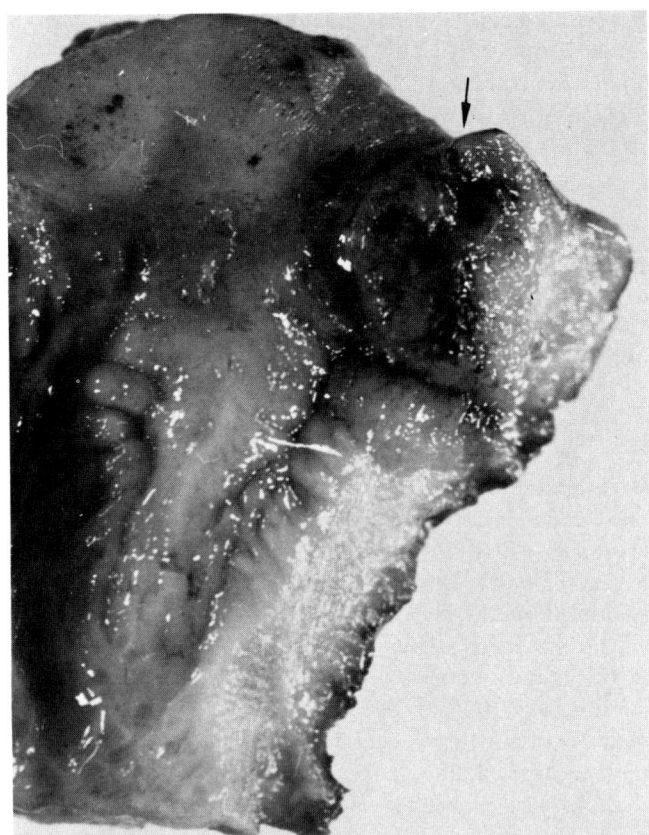

Fig. 8.8. Squamous carcinoma of the cervix. Note the circumscribed margin of this endophytic tumor that elevates the squamous portio epithelium (arrow), which is not ulcerated.

invades either as individual cells or almost completely replaces the stroma with large masses of neoplastic squamous cells. Cells in the center of the invading nests frequently become necrotic or undergo extensive keratinization (Fig. 8.11). Individual cells generally are polygonal or oval with eosinophilic cytoplasm and prominent cellular membranes. Intracellular bridges may or may not be visible. In some cases the nuclei are relatively uniform whereas in others they are quite pleomorphic. In most cases, the chromatin is coarse and clumped and mitotic figures, including abnormal forms, commonly are encountered.

Fig. 8.9. Squamous carcinoma of the cervix. A bulky friable exophytic mass projects from the external os. (Courtesy of Dr. B. K. Chun, Washington, D.C.)

Fig. 8.10. Invasive squamous carcinoma of the cervix. Note the irregular contour of infiltrative nests. There is an inflammatory exudate at the epithelial–stromal junction.

Fig. 8.11. Well-differentiated (grade 1) invasive squamous carcinoma of the cervix. Keratin pearl formation is evident.

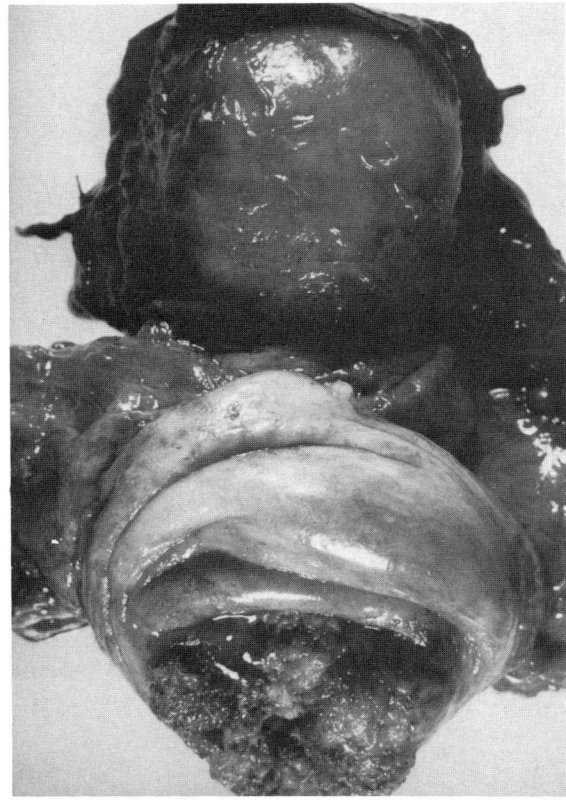

8.9

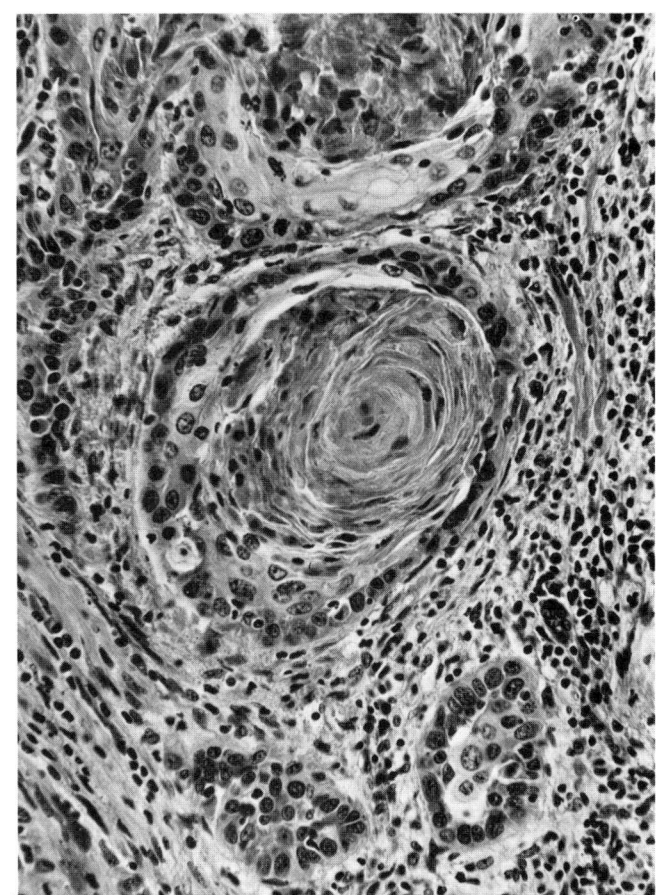

8.11

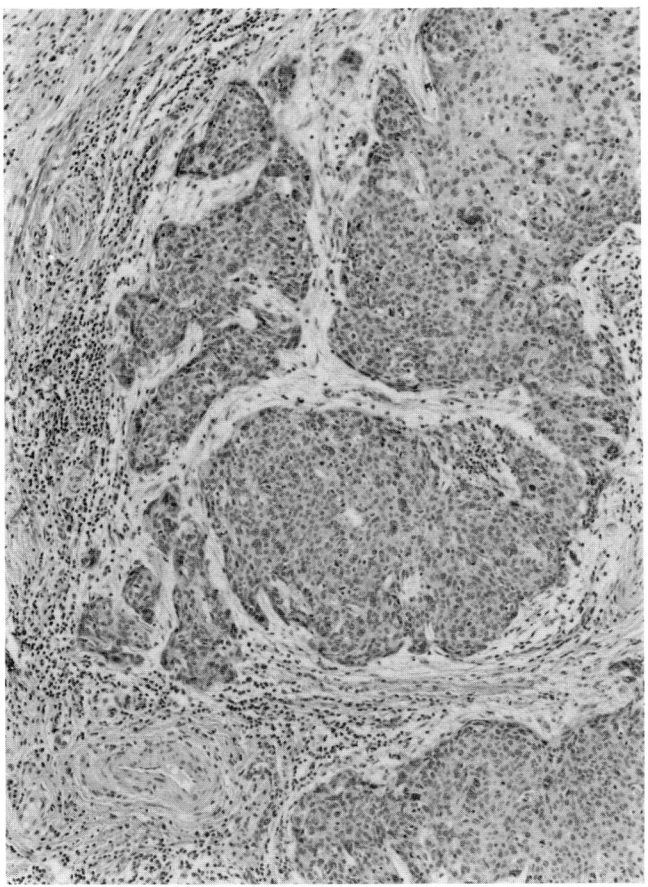

8.10

HISTOLOGICAL TYPING

One of the earliest approaches to classifying cervical squamous cell carcinomas was based on the predominant cell type.[284] This classification separated squamous cell carcinomas into large-cell keratinizing, large cell nonkeratinizing, and small-cell nonkeratinizing. In the experience of Wentz and Reagan, the best 5-year survival rate after radiation therapy was associated with large-cell nonkeratinizing carcinomas (68.3%), followed by the large-cell keratinizing type (41.7%), whereas small-cell carcinomas had a 20% 5-year survival rate.[359] Because there has been frequent confusion between the small-cell nonkeratinizing squamous cell carcinomas described by Wentz and Reagan and small-cell undifferentiated carcinomas with neuroendocrine features similar to those described in the lung, the current WHO classification of invasive cervical cancers places small-cell undifferentiated carcinoma with neuroendocrine features in a separate category and divides invasive squamous cell carcinomas into two groups, keratinizing and nonkeratinizing.

Keratinizing carcinomas are characterized by the presence of well-differentiated squamous cells that are arranged in nests or cords that vary greatly in size and configuration. One of the most characteristic features of keratinizing carcinomas is the presence of keratin "pearls" within the epithelium (Fig. 8.11). These "pearls" are composed of clusters of squamous cells that have undergone keratinization and are arranged in a concentric nest. The presence of a single keratin "pearl" is sufficient to classify a tumor as a keratinizing carcinoma. The neoplastic squamous cells not forming keratin "pearls" frequently have abundant eosinophilic cytoplasm and prominent intracellular bridges. The nuclei often are enlarged but mitotic figures are not numerous.

Nonkeratinizing squamous cell carcinomas are characterized by nests of neoplastic squamous cells that frequently undergo individual cell keratinization but, by definition, do not form keratin "pearls" (Fig. 8.12). These cells have relatively indistinct cell borders. The nuclei tend to be round to oval with coarsely clumped chromatin. Mitotic figures are frequent. Other nonkeratinizing squamous cell carcinomas are composed of masses and nests of small basaloid cells with scant cytoplasm and hyperchromatic uniform nuclei with frequent mitotic activity. These tumors are similar to the basaloid carcinomas of the vulva and vagina.

Although some investigators have reported that this classification has prognostic significance in patients being treated with radiotherapy,[102,282,336] others have found no significant difference in prognosis between patients with large-cell nonkeratinizing and large-cell keratinizing squamous carcinomas when treated with radical surgery.[117,161]

MICROSCOPIC GRADING

Several attempts have been made to classify cervical carcinomas according to the degree of differentiation. The first method used for grading squamous cell carcinomas of the cervix was that originally proposed in the 1920s by Broders for grading squamous cell carcinomas of the lip.[41] This method was based on the proportion of the tumor that was undergoing keratinization with the formation of squamous pearls and the number of mitoses. A modification of the Broder method that is based on the degree of differentiation currently is the most widely used histological grading system. Using this method, squamous cell carcinomas are graded as well differentiated (grade 1), moderately differentiated (grade 2), and poorly differentiated (grade 3). Most squamous cell carcinomas are moderately differentiated (grade 2), followed by poorly differentiated (grade 3) and well differentiated (grade 1).

In well differentiated (grade 1 tumors), the most striking feature is abundant keratin, which is deposited as concentric whorls (keratin pearls) in the centers of neoplastic epithelial nests (Fig. 8.11). The cells appear mature, with abundant eosinophilic cytoplasm. Individual cell keratinization (dyskeratosis) characterized by intense cytoplasmic

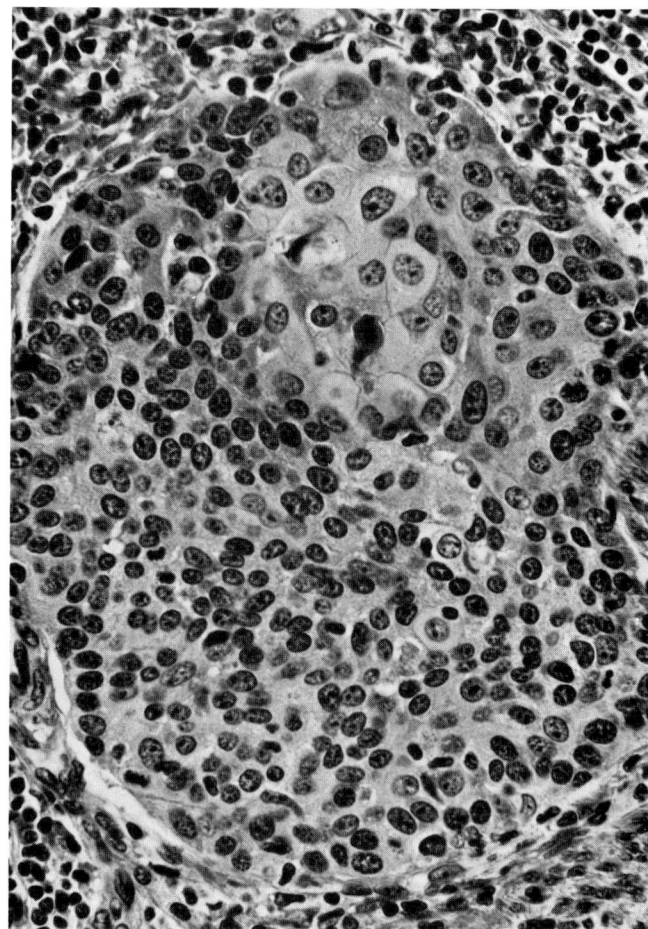

FIG. 8.12. Moderately differentiated (grade 2) squamous carcinoma of the cervix. Abortive keratinization but no pearl formation. Accordingly, this tumor can be classified as a nonkeratinizing squamous carcinoma.

eosinophilia also may be present. The cells are packed tightly and have well-developed intercellular bridges. The nuclei are large, irregular and hyperchromatic, with numerous chromocenters. Mitotic figures are present, with maximum concentration at the periphery of the advancing epithelial nests. The stroma often is infiltrated by chronic inflammatory cells, and occasionally a foreign body giant cell reaction is observed.

In moderately differentiated (grade 2) squamous cell carcinomas, the neoplastic cells are more pleomorphic than in grade 1 tumors, are characterized by large irregular nuclei, and have less abundant cytoplasm. The cellular borders, as well as intercellular bridges, appear indistinct. Keratin pearl formation is virtually nonexistent, but individual cell keratinization is seen in the center of nests of tumor cells. Mitotic figures are more numerous than in grade 1 carcinomas (Fig. 8.12).

Poorly differentiated (grade 3) squamous cell carcinomas generally are composed of cells with hyperchromatic oval nuclei and scant indistinct cytoplasm, resembling the malignant cells of high-grade SIL (CIN 2, 3) (Fig. 8.13). Clear-cut squamous differentiation manifested by keratinization may be difficult to find. Mitoses and areas of necrosis are abundant. Poorly differentiated lesions occasionally are composed of large, pleomorphic cells with giant, bizarre nuclei and abnormal mitotic figures. In rare instances, the neoplastic cells assume a spindle-shaped configuration resembling a sarcoma (Fig. 8.14). Immunohistochemical staining for epithelial membrane antigen (EMA) and cytokeratins demonstrates the epithelial nature of the spindle cell component in these cases.

Studies analyzing the effect of tumor grade on prognosis are difficult to compare because of wide differences in the stage of the patients and the therapies used. A study by Chung et al. of early-stage squamous cell carcinomas found that poorly differentiated tumors were associated with a higher frequency of tumor recurrence and a worse 2-year survival.[56] Although this finding has been confirmed by some,[101,321] most studies have failed to confirm that histopathological grade, as determined by the degree of differentiation, influences clinical outcome and have found a high degree of interobserver variability in the grade assigned to a particular tumor.[49,137,203,249,275,376] Because histopathological grade has failed to predict clinical outcome in these studies, more comprehensive grading systems have been developed that take into account the tumor–host interactions including the degree of tumor keratinization, nuclear differentiation, number of mitosis,

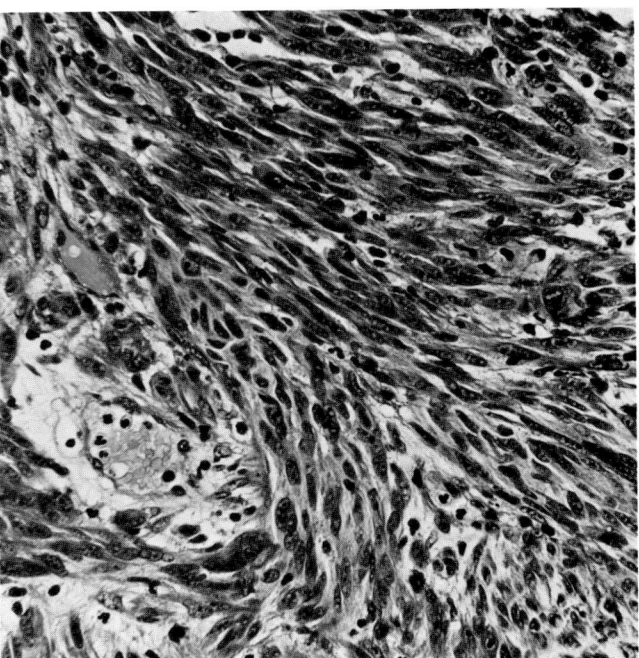

Fig. 8.14. Invasive squamous carcinoma with spindle-shape features. Note fusiform configuration of cells, resembling a sarcoma. This area merged into moderately differentiated squamous carcinoma.

cell size, nuclear-cytoplasmic ratio, inflammatory response to the tumor, stromal response to the tumor, vascular invasion, and the pattern of invasion of the tumor into the underlying stroma. First introduced by Stendall et al., this approach has been termed the *malignancy grade score* (MGS) and was found to be of highly significant prognostic value in early studies.[258,330,331,332] However, even these more comprehensive methods of determining tumor grade have failed to provide significant prognostic information in other large, well-controlled studies.[69,70,323] In summary, there has been no conclusive demonstration that a histological grading or histological typing sysem (see above) reliably predicts prognosis.

IMMUNOHISTOCHEMICAL FINDINGS

Squamous cell carcinomas of the cervix express a complex variety of keratins differing in pattern and number depending on the grade of histological differentiation.[73,240,320] Differentiated, keratinizing cervical carcinomas have the most complex pattern of keratin intermediate filaments and contain polypeptides characteristic of terminally differentiated cervical keratinocytes including 4, 5, 6, 8, 13, 14, 16, 17, 18 and 19.[320] Nonkeratinizing cervical squamous cell carcinomas express keratins 6, 14, 17, and 19 in all cases and keratins 4, 5, 7, 8, 10, 13, 16, and 18 occasionally.[320] The heterogeneous intermediate filament patterns expressed in cervical carcinoma indicate that

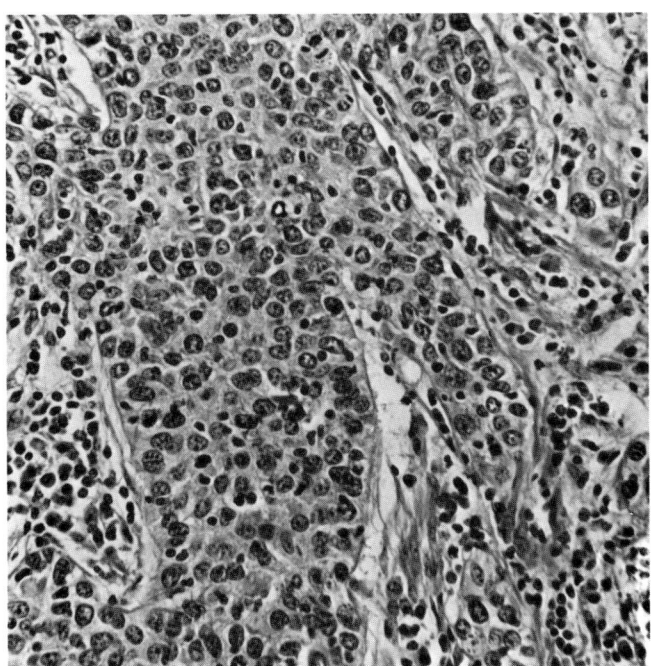

Fig. 8.13. Poorly differentiated (grade 3) squamous carcinoma. There is anisonucleosis, scant cytoplasm, and indistinct cell membranes.

some sets of keratin polypeptides are conserved during malignant transformation whereas the expression of other keratin polypeptides reflects a selection of a minor cell type or clone during carcinogenesis or even de novo expression.[240] Involucrin, a marker for squamous differentiation distinct from keratin, also can be identified in differentiated areas of squamous cell carcinoma in 93% of patients, indicating conservation of this protein during transformation.[303] The distribution of keratin polypeptides and involucrin in invasive squamous cell carcinomas of the cervix has not been shown to assist in histological diagnosis.

Monoclonal antibodies derived from cervical carcinomas include a tumor-associated antigen, referred to as *squamous cell carcinoma antigen* or *TA-4*, which is glycoprotein of 48,000 molecular weight. Elevations of serum TA-4 have been observed in women with cervical carcinoma and can be used to monitor the effects of therapy and detect tumor recurrence.[173,224] In tissue sections, TA-4 is localized in differentiated and keratinized cells in normal cervical squamous epithelium and malignant tumors. Antigen expression in carcinomas is linked to differentiation and cannot be identified in small-cell undifferentiated tumor.[224] For additional discussion of immunohistochemical findings see Chapter 26, Immunohistochemistry.

Ultrastructural Findings

The ultrastructural hallmarks of neoplastic cells of squamous origin include intracytoplasmic bundles of tonofilaments, desmosome–tonofilament complexes, and finger-like intercellular microvilli.[96] These alterations are identified readily in well- and moderately differentiated neoplasms.[96] The tonofilaments may be aggregated and form large globular masses (Fig. 8.15). In the lesser differentiated lesions, tonofilaments and desmosomal plates are reduced and poorly developed. Loss of demosomal attachments and separation of desmosomal–tonofilament complexes lead to loss of cellular cohesion. Another characteristic feature of squamous carcinoma cells is the profound decrease in gap–junction nexuses compared with normal cervical squamous epithelium.[232]

Differential Diagnosis

Histologically, the lesions most commonly confused with invasive squamous cell carcinomas are squamous metaplasia and high-grade SIL (CIN 2, 3) with extensive endocervical gland involvement, gestational decidual reaction with degenerative features, condylomata acuminata, and reparative changes associated with chronic granulomatous diseases such as lymphogranuloma venereum and granuloma inguinale. With the exception of high-grade SIL (CIN 2, 3), these lesions can all be differentiated from invasive

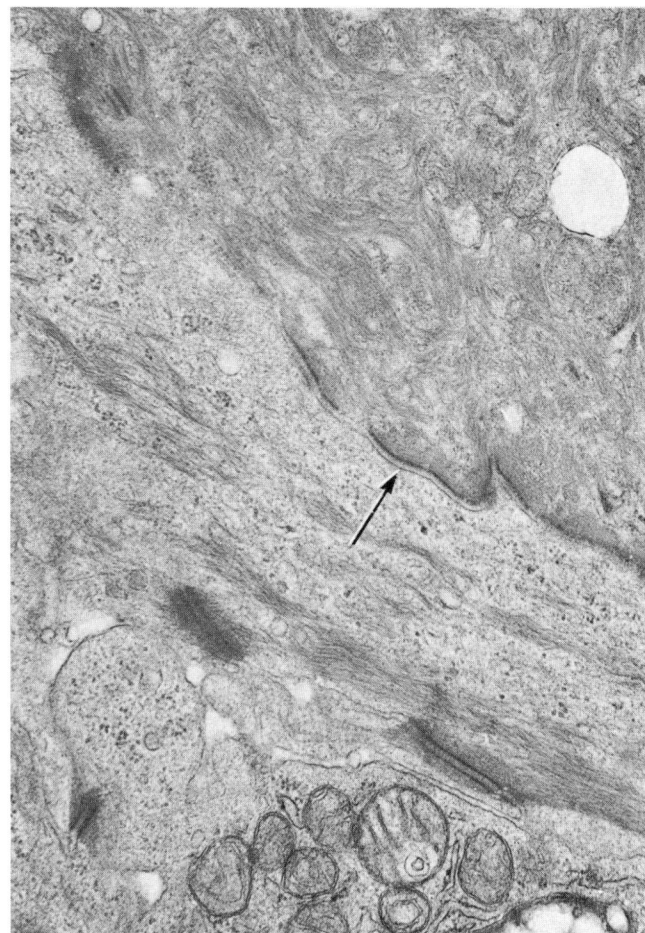

Fig. 8.15. Well-differentiated invasive squamous carcinoma of the cervix. Individual cells undergoing keratinization (dyskeratosis) contain lobular masses of tonofilaments that are responsible for intense eosinophilia on light microscopy. Separation and retraction of desmosomal tonofilament attachments is present (*arrow*). The intercellular space (I) contains interdigitating microvilli. ×7438.

squamous cell carcinoma by the absence of significant nuclear atypia and their low mitotic activity.

Both squamous metaplasia and high-grade SIL (CIN 2, 3) are frequently extensive and extend into endocervical glands. Even though a low level of mitotic activity can be present in squamous metaplasia, careful evaluation of the cytological appearance of the metaplastic cells reveals their benign nature since the cells are relatively uniform in size and shape and lack significant nuclear atypia. Moreover, the borders of endocervical glands involved with either squamous metaplasia or high-grade SIL (CIN 2, 3) are rounded and distinct and lack the irregular margins, scalloping, and the desmoplasia and dense inflammatory infiltrate that occasionally contains foreign body giant cells in the stroma adjacent to the nests (Fig. 8.16).

A decidual reaction with degenerative features lacks mitotic activity and in difficult cases can be differentiated from invasive squamous cell carcinomas by the use of immunohistochemical staining because decidual cells do not contain cytokeratin. Placental-site nodules or plaques represent incompletely resorbed hyalinized implantation sites and appear as well-circumscribed nodules or plaques containing intermediate trophoblastic cells. These cells lack mitotic activity and are arranged in nests surrounded by hyaline material. Again, in difficult cases immunohistochemistry can be used to determine the true nature of these lesions because the intermediate trophoblast within these well-circumscribed nodules usually contain placental lactogen (see Chapter 24, Gestational Trophoblastic Disease and Related Lesions).

Squamous cell carcinomas that contain large amounts of cytoplasmic glycogen sometimes can be confused with clear cell carcinomas (Fig. 8.17). Like clear cell carcinomas, cells in these tumors have clear cytoplasm and distinct cell membranes. However, squamous cell carcinoma with clear cytoplasm lacks the characteristic hobnail cells and the papillary or tubulocystic areas that are typical of clear

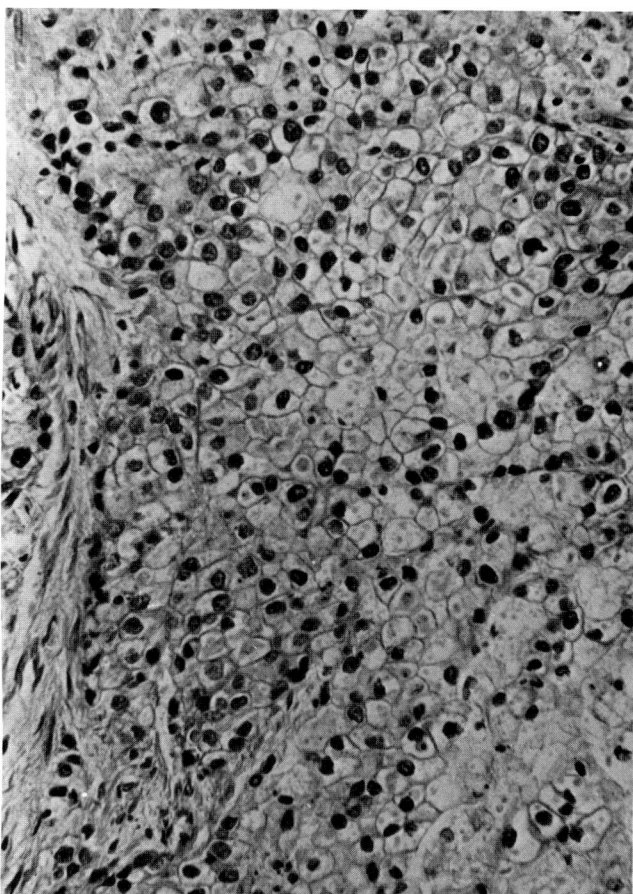

FIG. 8.17. **Invasive squamous carcioma of the cervix with clear cell features.** The cells are rich in glycogen, which results in their clear cytoplasmic appearance. The cellular borders are well defined.

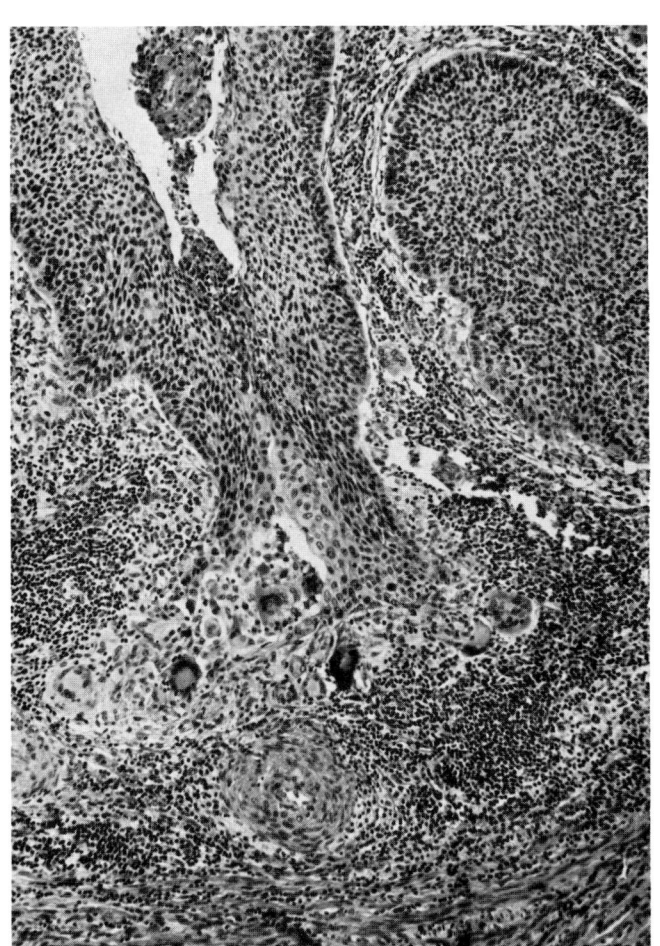

FIG. 8.16. **Moderately differentiated (grade 2) squamous carcinoma of the cervix.** Note foreign body giant cell reaction to infiltrating tumor cells.

cell carcinomas. In squamous cell carcinomas a careful search of multiple sections usually will detect areas with unambiguous squamous differentiation.

It also can be difficult to distinguish between poorly differentiated squamous cell carcinomas composed of small, basaloid cells and small cell (undifferentiated) carcinomas of the neuroendocrine type. Small cell carcinomas of the neuroendocrine type typically invade the stroma diffusely as individual cells or as small discohesive nests and show extensive crush artifact. They frequently form rosettes or trabeculae and the cells characteristically have smudged, intensely hyperchromatic nuclei and lack nucleoli. In contrast, poorly differentiated squamous cell carcinomas invade as cohesive nests and the cells have oval nuclei with granular chromatin. In difficult cases electron microscopy or immunohistochemistry can be used to demonstrate neurosecretory granules in small cell carcinomas of the neuroendocrine type. Unfortunately, there is overlap of this feature between the two types of neoplasms. In the final analysis, conventional microscopic features are the most useful in distinguishing these tumors.[6]

RISK FACTORS

Stage is the most important prognostic factor in cervical carcinoma. Histological typing and grade have little direct influence on survival within any stage (see Microscopic Grading).[56,137,203,249,275,376] Within a particular stage, other prognostic factors include tumor size (volume), vascular invasion, depth of invasion,[151,376] and size or bulk of lymph node metastases.[152,376] Accordingly, in reporting squamous cell carcinomas, the depth of invasion (in millimeters or the proportion of the wall invaded), the presence or absence of vascular invasion, and the size of the tumor (greatest tumor dimension) should be reported. In contrast, histological grading and typing into keratinizing and nonkeratinizing are of less clinical value.

AGE

Another factor that influences prognosis is patient age. In 1952, Lindell demonstrated that survival of women with cervical cancer increases with increasing age.[210] This was later confirmed by Kottmeir and others who also reported poorer survival rates for young women with cervical cancer.[195,275,299] However, there are a number of other large studies, including one of Meanwell et al. from the United Kingdom that analyzed more than 10,000 women with invasive cervical cancer, that have actually reported younger women to have a better prognosis than older women.[166,233] In general it appears that there is little difference in prognosis between younger and older women with stage I or IIA tumors, but that younger women with higher stage disease have a poorer survival.[265,299]

HPV DNA STATUS

Several studies have assessed the role of HPV type on outcome but the results are conflicting. Initial studies found a significant correlation between tumor grade and the presence of HPV 18. In one study of 30 patients, 83% of tumors associated with HPV 18 were poorly differentiated.[18] Weaker associations were noted between the presence of HPV 18 and lymph node involvement and young age. Similarly, Walker et al. analyzed 100 invasive cervical cancers for HPV DNA using Southern blot and found that 45% of the tumors associated with HPV 18 recurred compared with a 16% recurrence rate in HPV 16–associated tumors.[356] Women with HPV 18–associated tumors were 8 years younger than women whose tumors were associated with HPV 16 but HPV status was not significantly associated with tumor size, presence of parametrial involvement, or lymph node status.[356] Subsequent studies have failed to confirm that specific types of HPV are associated with

either adverse prognostic indicators or clinical outcome.[136,158,175,183,291,308] Three recent studies have found that tumors in which HPV DNA is not detectable have a poorer prognosis than those in which it is.[79,136,291]

DNA PLOIDY

The clinical importance of tumor ploidy is currently unclear. Using flow cytometry, 33–80% of invasive cervical carcinomas have an aneuploid DNA distribution.[88,129,157,158,175,335,377] There is little agreement, however, as to whether DNA ploidy level is an independent prognostic factor. Although several studies have demonstrated associations between aneuploidy and poor prognostic indicators such as lymph node metastases, higher stage, or increased age,[88,158] three other flow cytometry studies have all failed to demonstrate any significant effect (independent of stage) of DNA ploidy status on clinical outcome.[77,158,175] When considering DNA ploidy measurements made by flow cytometry it must be pointed out that tumors that are "diploid" by flow usually have chromosomal aberrations and therefore are actually aneuploid (but at a level too low to be detected by flow cytometry). Large cytogenetic studies have found that all invasive cervical cancers contain chromosomal aneuploidy when defined as numerical and/or structural aberrations and that euploid cervical cancers either do not exist or are extremely uncommon.[13,327]

CELLULAR ONCOGENES

Alterations in either the expression or function of cellular genes that control cell growth and differentiation are being actively investigated as prognostic markers in cervical cancer (see Chapter 28, Molecular Biology). Both specific point mutations of the first exon of *ras* genes as well as amplifications of *ras* genes[17] occur in invasive carcinomas of the cervix. Overexpression of *ras* genes is found using immunohistochemical methods in 57% of keratinizing squamous cell carcinomas and 54% of large-cell nonkeratinizing carcinomas.[300] Overexpression of the *ras* gene product, p21, is associated with a poor prognosis[300] and an increased frequency of lymph node involvement.[133,300] Overexpression of p21 appears to be due to amplification of Ha-*ras* genes, which occurs in 66% of cervical squamous cell carcinomas.[290,294] Mutations and loss of heterozygosity of Ha-*ras* genes also occur in invasive cervical carcinomas.[289] Although loss of heterozygosity of the cHa-*ras* gene in squamous cell carcinomas was not associated with advanced stage disease, mutations were associated with a poor prognosis. In contrast, mutations of the Ki-*ras* gene have been detected in only a small percentage of invasive cervical adenocarcinomas and are not significantly associated with stage, grade, or survival.[196]

Alterations in the c-*myc* oncogene also have been associated with a poor prognosis in some studies. The c-*myc* oncogene is amplified from 3 to 30 times in 21% of cervical squamous cell carcinomas[254,293] and is more frequent in high-stage (stage III and IV) tumors than in low-stage tumors.[293] Overexpression of c-*myc* has been associated with a worse clinical outcome.[156,292,293]

BEHAVIOR

Squamous cell carcinoma of the cervix spreads principally by direct local invasion of adjacent tissues and lymphatics and less commonly through blood vessels. Initially, the tumor grows by extending along tissue spaces of least resistance, such as the perineural and perivascular tissues, into the paracervical and parametrial areas and into the cardinal and uterosacral ligaments. Ultimately, lateral spread may reach the bony pelvis, encompassing and obstructing one or both ureters. Direct extension also may involve the uterine cavity and vagina, with extension into the urinary bladder and rectum, resulting in vesicovaginal and rectovaginal fistulas.

The spread of cervical cancer via lymphatics occurs relatively early in the course of the disease, occuring in 25–50% of patients with stage IB and II carcinomas.[52,178] The most common sites of lymph node metastases are the internal iliac, obturator, external iliac, and common iliac lymph nodes.[271] Later in the course of the disease, extension to the lateral sacral, para-aortic, and inguinal nodes can occur. Isolated invasion of the sacral, external iliac, and hypogastric nodes occasionally is observed. Distant lymph node metastases above the diaphragm including the supraclavicular lymph nodes are uncommon and are a feature of widespread disease.[84] In these cases, cancer cells are transported from the para-aortic nodes into the mediastinum and then into the thoracic duct.

Hematogenous dissemination is the least common metastatic pathway of cervical carcinoma, although nearly 50% of surgically removed specimens may contain histological evidence of blood vessel invasion.[110] Blood-borne metastases to the lung, liver, bone, heart, skin, and brain are generally seen in stage IV tumors or when the local growth has previously been irradiated.

Ureteral obstruction caused by tumor invasion of the ureteral wall or by compression due to tumor in periureteral lymphatics leads to hydroureter, hydronephrosis, hydronephrotic renal atrophy, pyelonephritis, and loss of renal function. Obstruction of both ureters results in uremia and is a leading cause of death.[324] Although the frequency of ureteral involvement was unchanged between the 1930s and 1960s and the 1970s, advances in radiation therapy that occurred in the 1970s have reduced the number of patients dying of ureteral obstruction and uremia from 28% to 6.7%.[174] Peritonitis caused by obstruction and perforation of large or small bowel, respiratory failure asso-

ciated with pulmonary metastasis, or massive edema, hemorrhage, cardiac failure, massive venous thrombosis, pulmonary embolism, and complications of radiation therapy represent the major causes of death.

TREATMENT

The three basic therapeutic modalities for squamous cell carcinoma are radiation, surgery, or a combination of radiation and surgery. At present, radical hysterectomy with pelvic lymphadenectomy is considered the most appropriate therapeutic approach for most stage IA2 squamous cell carcinomas of the cervix invading more than 3 mm into the stroma or with lymphvascular space involvement. The operative death rate has declined considerably and now approaches zero.[268] In stage IB and early stage II cases, radical hysterectomy and bilateral pelvic lymphadenectomy is preferred but results of radical surgery and radiation therapy are essentially similar.

The preferred treatment for most stage II and all stage III patients is combined external and intracavitary radiotherapy. Radiation of invasive squamous cell carcinoma of the cervix produces a decrease in tumor size and eventual regression. In one study, 90% of 493 patients of all stages had no gross tumor 12 weeks after termination of combined external radiation (^{60}Co, 5000 R) and intracavitary radium (4000 R) therapy.[223] Tumor regression is generally faster in neoplasms of small size and in those confined to the cervix (stage I) than in larger advanced stage lesions. The rapidity of tumor regression apparently is unrelated to histological patterns and degree of differentiation.

Morphologic changes in cervical squamous carcinoma cells that are considered evidence of response to ionizing radiation are cellular differentiation with keratinization, cell degeneration with cytoplasmic vacuolization, pyknosis, and nucleomegaly.[116] Nuclear polyploidy (i.e., generation of multiple double sets of DNA) is the result of arrest of mitotic activity caused by radiation. Radiation-induced changes in adenocarcinoma of the cervix include nuclear shrinkage and pyknosis, cytoplasmic vacuolization, decrease in mucin synthesis, and a striking abundance of intracytoplasmic cytophagosomes.

Modern techniques of radiotherapy use a variety of intracavitary radium applicators and low-intensity needles. External megavoltage with ^{60}Co is required for adequate radiation of the pelvis. The total cancercidal dose of both radium and x rays to control squamous cell carcinoma of the cervix is on the order of 6000–7000 rads. The most common complications, in decreasing frequency, are proctitis, vault necrosis, hemorrhagic cystitis, peritonitis resulting from obstruction, perforation, necrosis of the bowel, vesicovaginal fistula, and profuse hemorrhage.[268] The frequency of major complications associated with radical surgery is about 3% and includes ureterovaginal and vesicovaginal fistulas, bladder atony and hypotonic bladder dysfunction, ureteral strictures, thrombophlebitis, cuff abscesses, and hematoma.

Chemotherapy using a variety of regimens, most of which use *cis*platin either alone or in combination with other drugs such as bleomycin and methotrexate, has been used for primary chemotherapy followed by local therapy, for postoperative adjuvant therapy in high-risk patients, or combined with pelvic radiotherapy.[342] Forty to 70 percent of patients with metastatic or recurrent cancer previously treated with surgery or patients with locally advanced disease being treated for the first time will respond to *cis*platin-containing regimens, but the proportion of patients with prolonged responses is considerably less.[342]

The 5-year survival for treated stage I patients is 90–95%, 50–70% for stage II, 30% for stage III, and less than 20% for patients with stage IV disease.[187,193,201,299] The survival rates are reduced even in patients with low-stage disease when metastases to lymph nodes are present and survival rate appears to correlate with the number of positive nodes.[153,178] Metastatic node involvement occurs in 8–25% of stage I, 21–38% of stage II, and 32–46% of stage III lesions.[178,251] Typically, most recurrences appear within 2 years after initial therapy.

Verrucous Carcinoma

Verrucous carcinoma is a rare variant of squamous cell carcinoma. In the female genital tract, the most commonly involved region is the vulva, but well-documented cases have been described in the cervix.[81,92,159,172,197,214,264] In the past, this tumor has been reported as *giant condyloma acuminatum of Buschke and Lowenstein* but the implication that this tumor is a type of condyloma is erroneous and confusing and therefore the term no longer is used.[263,264] Clinically, verrucous carcinoma appears as a large, sessile tumor that grossly resembles a condyloma. Verrucous carcinoma is a slow-growing, locally invasive malignant tumor. Because it is frequently diagnosed incorrectly, it may become quite advanced and lead to death. Five of eight patients in one series of the cervix died of verrucous carcinoma or the cervix shortly after the diagnosis was made.[214] Histologically, cervical verrucous carcinomas are identical to the more common vulvar tumors and are predominantly exophytic and characterized by frond-like papillae with or without surface keratinization (see Chapter 3, Premalignant and Malignant Tumors of the Vulva). The epithelium lacks significant cytological atypia and mitotic activity, although in some cases mitoses may be found in the deep layers. The base of the tumor is composed of invasive nests of epithelium that are broad and expansile, with a well-circumscribed pushing margin. There is a conspicuous inflammatory reaction at the epithelial stromal junction. Verrucous carcinoma of the vulva has been associated with HPV 6 infection.[3,206,255]

Verrucous carcinoma should be distinguished from warty carcinoma (see below) and condyloma acuminata.[263,264] Unlike condyloma acuminatum, verrucous carcinoma lacks the central fibroconnective tissue cores in the epithelial papillae that are charactersitic of condylomata.[197] Typically these tumors recur locally but do not metastasize unless they are inadequately radiated, in which case accelerated growth and metastasis may occur.[3,51,172] The most appropriate therapy is wide local excision, if possible. However, these lesions frequently can be deeply invasive, even extending into the endometrium or adjacent pelvic tissues.[24,326,346] Regional lymph nodes are rarely involved, and distant metastases are exceedingly rare.[214]

Warty (Condylomatous) Carcinoma

Warty (condylomatous) carcinoma is a variant of squamous cell carcinoma of the cervix that has marked condylomatous changes.[199] These tumors have been described recently and are histologically identical to the warty carcinoma of the vulva.[283] Unlike verrucous carcinoma, warty carcinomas demonstrate features of a typical squamous cell carcinoma at the deep margin. In addition, many of the malignant cells have cytoplasmic vacuolization and nuclear changes closely resembling koilocytotic atypia (see Chapter 3, Premalignant and Malignant Tumors of the Vulva). Although clinical experience with these tumors is limited, they appear to behave less aggressively than typical well-differentiated squamous cell carcinomas of the cervix.

Papillary Squamous (Transitional) Cell Carcinoma

Papillary squamous cell carcinoma is a rare variant of squamous cell carcinoma of the cervix that has a histological resemblence to transitional cell carcinoma of the urinary bladder.[281] These tumors are composed of papillary projections that are covered by several layers of atypical basaloid cells resembling those of a high-grade SIL (CIN 2, 3) (Fig. 8.18). The cells have hyperchromatic, oval nuclei and minimal amounts of cytoplasm. Mitoses are frequent. Focally there usually are areas of squamous differentiation. Typical invasive squamous cell carcinoma usually can be identified at the base of the tumor, appearing as well-circumscribed nests of epithelium in continuity with papillae that extend deeply into the stroma. Focal invasion of the papillae themselves also is sometimes present. The behavior of papillary squamous (transitional) cell carcinoma is similar to that of invasive squamous cell carcinoma with the exception that late recurrences have been reported.[281]

Papillary squamous cell carcinoma can be mistaken for a papillary squamous cell carcinoma in situ on a superficial

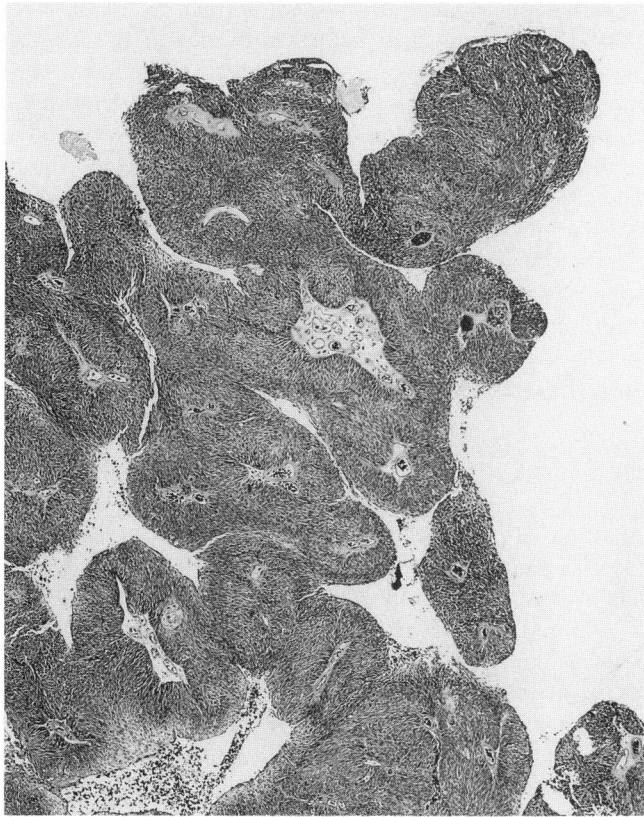

FIG. 8.18. Papillary squamous (transitional) cell carcinoma. The tumor is composed of papillary projections covered by basaloid cells resembling high-grade SIL (CIN 2, 3).

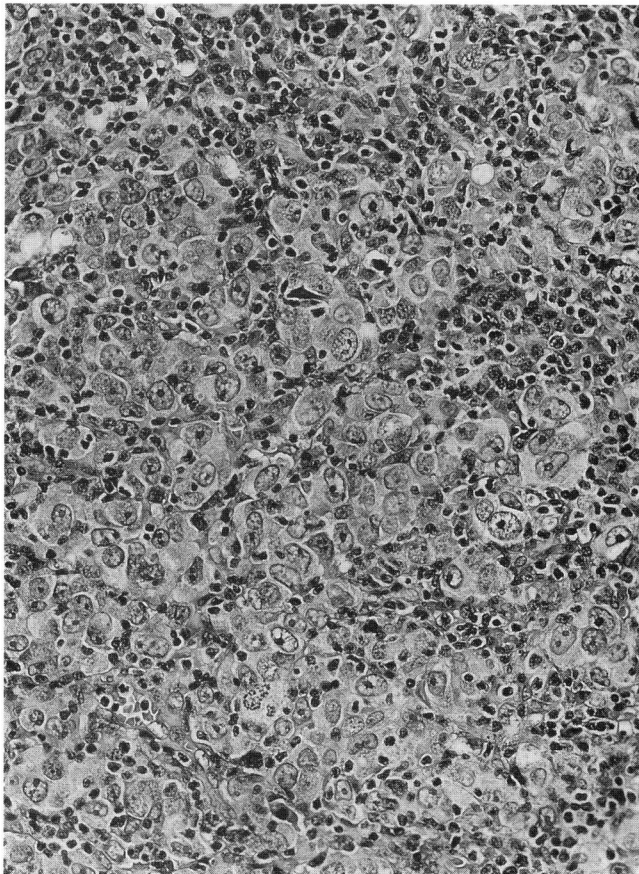

FIG. 8.19. Lymphoepithelioma-like carcinoma. The tumor is composed of sheets of undifferentiated cells surrounded by a stromal inflammatory infiltrate. The individual cells have abundant cytoplasm, indistinct cell borders, and uniform vesicular nuclei.

biopsy.[278] Since papillary squamous cell carcinoma is capable of acting aggressively and metastasizing, it is important that a cone biopsy be performed to rule out invasion whenever a papillary squamous cell carcinoma in situ is diagnosed. These tumors also can be diagnosed mistakenly as verrucous carcinoma or as condyloma acuminatum with atypia. Papillary squamous cell carcinomas lack the condylomatous changes and degree of cytoplasmic differentiation present in the other lesions.

Lymphoepithelioma-like Carcinoma

Lymphoepithelioma-like carcinomas are a distinctive subset of squamous cell carcinomas of the cervix that typically are well circumscribed and composed of undifferentiated cells surrounded by a marked stromal inflammatory infiltrate.[123,127,132] These tumors account for up to 5.5% of cervical cancers in some series and are histologically similar to lymphoepitheliomas arising in the nasopharynx, salivary glands, breast, and thymus.[132] The cells composing this tumor are relatively undifferentiated but have abundant cytoplasm and uniform vesicular nuclei (Fig. 8.19).

The cell borders tend to be indistinct and form what has been described as a syncytium.[239] The nests of undifferentiated cells are surrounded by a marked chronic inflammatory infiltrate composed of lymphocytes, plasma, cells and eosinophils. In the cervix a consistent relationship to Epstein-Barr virus has not been demonstrated, but only a few cases have been studied.

Lymphoepithelioma-like carcinomas can be mistaken for either glassy cell carcinomas or true lymphoproliferative disorders. In contrast to lymphoepitheliomas like carcinoma, glassy cell carcinomas have a poor prognosis and are characterized by prominent cell borders, ground-glass cytoplasm, and prominent nucleoli. Lymphoproliferative disorders can be differentiated easily from lymphoepithelioma-like carcinoma through the use of immunohistochemical staining with antibodies against leukocyte common antigen, cytokeratin, and epithelial membrane antigen.

Adenocarcinoma

Adenocarcinomas of the cervix comprise a heterogeneous group of neoplasms (Table 8.1) that display a variety of histological patterns. Because these cell types and patterns frequently are admixed, the histological classification of these tumors is based on the predominant cell type. If additional histological components comprise at least 10% of the tumor, some authors recommend classifying the tumor according to the predominant pattern and listing the individual components as part of the diagnosis.

The most commonly encountered type of cervical adenocarcinoma is the mucinous type.[149,186,301,343] Although some studies have found endometrioid adenocarcinomas to be more prevalent than endocervical adenocarcinomas, in almost all series these two histological types taken together account for between 66% and 90% of all invasive cervical adenocarcinomas.[27,279] In one recent series of 136 invasive adenocarcinomas, mucinous adenocarcinomas accounted for 57% of the tumors, endometrioid adenocarcinomas for 30%, and clear cell adenocarcinomas for 11%. The other types combined accounted for only 3% of the tumors.[301]

PREVALENCE

The relative proportions and absolute incidences of squamous cell carcinomas and adenocarcinomas of the cervix have been changing in the United States and Western Europe over the last 40 years since the introduction of widespread cytological screening programs. In the 1950s and 1960s, approximately 95% of all invasive cervical carcinomas were classified as squamous cell carcinomas and only 5% as adenocarcinomas.[134,236] However, in series of invasive cervical cancers published since the early 1970s, squamous cell carcinomas have accounted for only 75–80% of the cases[7,11,78,82,108,145] whereas the remainder, 20–25%, included various types of adenocarcinomas, adenosquamous carcinomas, and undifferentiated carcinomas.[78,142] In the clinical series of Shingleton et al. the percentage of adenocarcinomas to total cervical cancers increased from 7% in the period from 1974 to 1978 to 19% in the 1979–1980 period.[313] Similarly, in the clinical series of Hopkins and Morley, the percentage of adenocarcinomas to total cervical cancers increased from 19% in 1970–1973 to 27% in 1982–1985.[139] Cancer registries from the United States, Finland, and Norway have all reported increases in the ratio of adenocarcinomas to squamous cell carcinomas over the same period.[90,208,260,269,305] In the Finnish Cancer Registry, 88% of all cervical cancers were classified as squamous cell carcinoma and 6% as adenocarcinoma in 1953–1957 whereas 81% were classified as squamous cell carcinoma and 17% as adenocarcinoma in 1978–1982.[208] The increase in the ratio of adenocarcinomas to squamous cell carcinomas over this time period

does not appear to be due to an absolute increase in prevalence. Data from four cancer registries in the United States, United Kingdom, and Norway all indicate that there has been no significant change in the overall incidence of adenocarcinoma over the last two decades.[53,90,260,269,305] All four registries do, however, report that the incidence of invasive adenocarcinoma in women 35 years or younger increased in the 1970s, but the total number of women 35 years or younger diagnosed with adenocarcinoma is quite small compared with the number of women over the age of 35 years.[53,90,260,269,305]

HISTOGENESIS AND RISK FACTORS

The cell of origin of invasive cervical adenocarcinoma is thought to be the pluripotential subcolumnar reserve cell of the columnar endocervical epithelium and adenocarcinoma in situ is regarded as the immediate precursor to invasive endocervical adenocarcinoma (see Chapter 7, Precancerous Lesions of the Cervix).

Although it has been reported that invasive adenocarcinoma is more prevalent than invasive squamous cell carcinoma in younger women,[28] most studies have failed to confirm a significant difference in the age distribution of the two types of cancers and the mean age of patients with invasive adenocarcinoma of the cervix is between 47 and 53 years.* Similarly, many of the epidemiologic risk factors for the development of adenocarcinoma of the cervix are similar to those described for invasive squamous cell carcinomas.[40,260] Both are frequently associated with SIL (CIN)[219,277] and both are associated with a more than 5-year interval since the last Pap smear (relative risk of 2.7 and 3.6 for adenocarcinoma and squamous cell carcinomas respectively), multiple sexual partners (more than 10 partners has a relative risk of 10.9 and 2.9, respectively, for adenocarcinoma and squamous cell carcinoma) and a young age at first intercourse (intercourse under the age of 15 has a relative of risk of 2.0 for both adenocarcinoma and squamous cell carcinoma).[40] In addition, HPV, particularly type 18, has been found in association with most invasive adenocarcinomas.[118,340,363,364]

Even though the use of oral contraceptives, particularly those with a large progestational component, for more than 10 years has been shown to be a risk factor for invasive cervical adenocarcinoma in some studies; these findings have not been confirmed by others.[72,163,269] Most recent studies comparing the risk factors for invasive adenocarcinomas with those of squamous cell carcinomas have revealed no significant differences in oral contraceptive use between the two groups of women.[40,139,145,261,317] Controlled prospective studies correlating the type of oral contraceptive or gestagen used, dosage, and duration of use with endocervical glandular changes are required before

---

*Refs. 11, 40, 139, 155, 208, 261, 338, 352.

any relationship between oral contraceptives and progestins and endocervical adenocarcinoma can be substantiated.

A genetic predisposition to invasive cervical adenocarcinoma has been documented in women with Peutz–Jeghers syndrome in whom minimal deviation adenocarcinoma of the cervix occurs more frequently than in the general population.[228,272,375] It also appears that a generalized predisposition to the development of adenocarcinoma of the ovary and cervix can occur since dual primary cervical and ovarian adenocarcinomas develop in some women.[171,371] Mucinous tumors of the ovary appear to be particularly prevalent in women with minimal deviation mucinous adenocarcinomas of the cervix.[171]

CLINICAL FEATURES

The presenting symptom of invasive cervical adenocarcinoma is abnormal vaginal bleeding in about 75% of patients.[149,208,301] Occasional women present with vaginal discharge or with pelvic pain.[149,208,301] Most invasive cervical adenocarcinomas arise in the transformation zone and on gross examination 50% of patients have a fungating, polypoid, or papillary mass.[343] In approximately 15% of patients the cervix is either diffusely enlarged or nodular. In another 15% no gross lesions are visible. Even though most patients with grossly inapparent tumors have early-stage adenocarcinomas, some have deep invasion because the carcinoma arose deep within the endocervical canal.[1,301,343] Adenocarcinoma of the cervix is confined to the cervix (stage I) or the parametrium/vagina (stage II) in 80% of women at the time of diagnosis.[2,78,107,134,149] The diagnostic accuracy of cytopathology in the detection of cervical adenocarcinoma varies according to the expertise of the pathologist and the sampling techniques used. Although in some series only a minority of the tumors have been detected through cytological screening,[10] in most large series the majority of patients with cervical adenocarcinomas have had cytological abnormalities.[208,343,301,343]

Mucinous Adenocarcinoma

PATHOLOGICAL FINDINGS

Mucinous adenocarcinoma is the most common type of invasive cervical adenocarcinoma.[149,186,301,343] There are three histological variants of mucinous adenocarcinomas that can occur either alone or as an admixture. One type is composed of cells that resemble the columnar cells of the normal endocervical mucosa and is referred to as the *endocervical type*. Endocervical-type adenocarcinomas are composed of cells that have basal nuclei and abundant pale granular cytoplasm that stains positively with mucicarmine stains. Most of the endocervical-type mucinous adenocarcinomas are well to moderately differentiated[2] and the

glandular elements are arranged in a complex, racemose, glandular pattern simulating the cleft-tunnel configuration of the normal endocervical mucosa (Figs. 8.20, 8.21). Complex papillary projections may project into the gland lumens and from the surface of the tumor. At times invasive glands may have a cribriform arrangement. They often are surrounded by a reactive, desmoplastic stroma (Fig. 8.22). Cells typically are stratified and there may be considerable nuclear atypia with variation in nuclear size, coarsely clumped chromatin, and prominent nucleoli (Fig. 8.21). Mitoses usually are numerous. Large amounts of mucin may be found in the stroma, forming mucin lakes or pools. In less differentiated tumors, the cells contain less cytoplasm but usually still form recognizable glandular structures.

The second type of mucinous adenocarcinoma of the cervix is termed the *intestinal type* and is composed of cells similar to those present in adenocarcinomas of the large intestine (Fig. 8.23). These tumors frequently contain goblet cells and more rarely argentaffin cells and Paneth cells.[2]

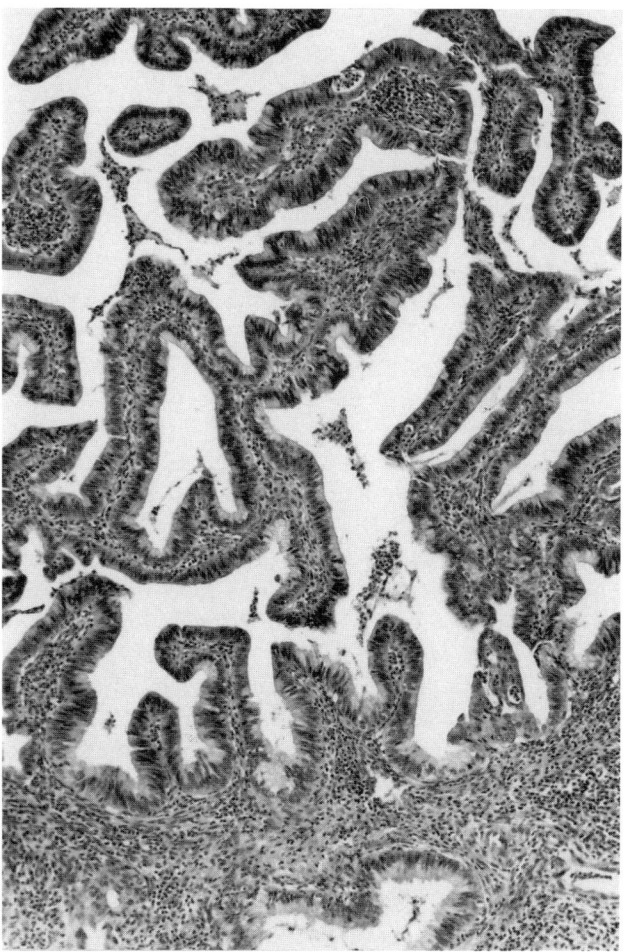

FIG. 8.20. Adenocarcinoma of endocervical type. The tumor is composed of complex glandular structures.

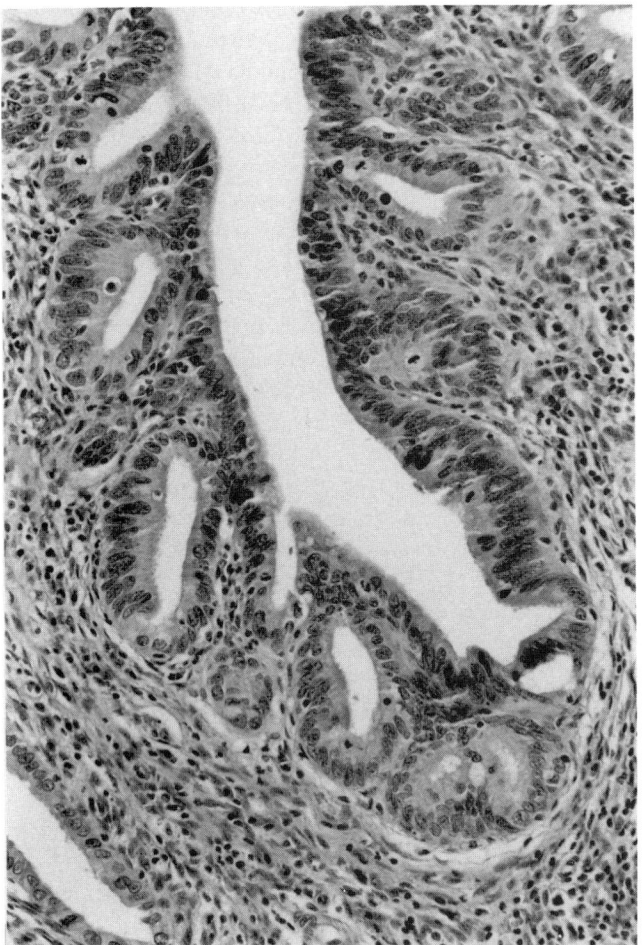

FIG. 8.21. Adenocarcinoma of endocervical type. The cells lining the glands are pseudostratified and have hyperchromatic nuclei with coarse chromatin, mitoses, and reduced intracytoplasmic mucin.

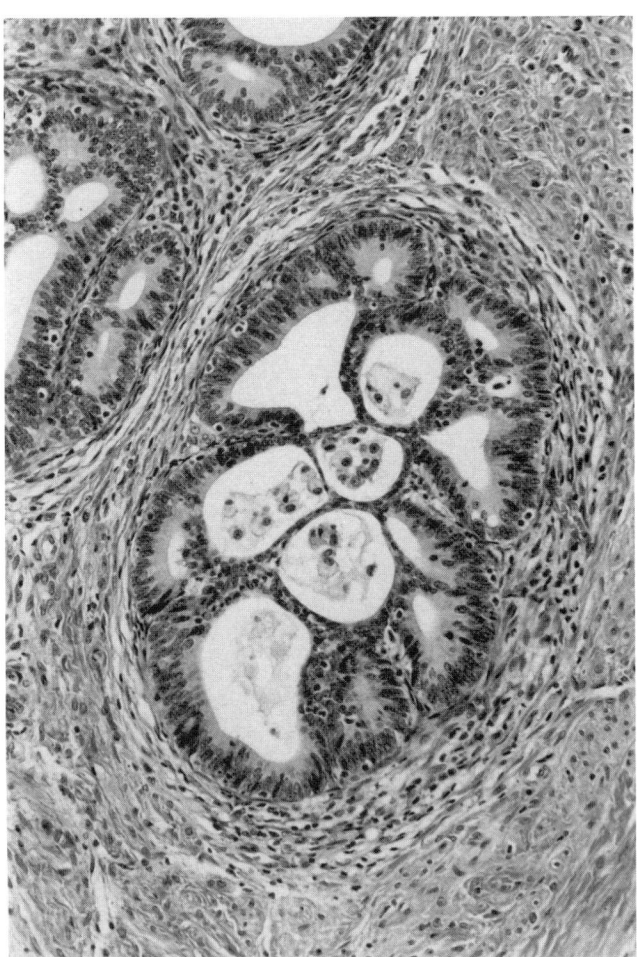

FIG. 8.22. Adenocarcinoma of endocervical type. Invasive glands may have a cribriform arrangement and be surrounded by an altered, desmoplastic stroma.

In the intestinal type, the tumor cells tend to be pseudostratified and contain only small amounts of intracellular mucin. They can either form glands with papillae or infiltrate throughout the stroma in a pattern similar to that of colonic adenocarcinoma. The third form of mucinous adenocarcinoma is composed mainly of signet ring cells and is designated the *signet-ring* form. Signet-ring carcinomas rarely occur in a pure form and usually are admixed with intestinal or endocervical adenocarcinomas.

Mucinous adenocarcinomas of the cervix are graded on the basis of either architectural features in a manner similar to that used for endometrial adenocarcinomas or on the basis of nuclear grade.[27,149,199] Using an architectural grading system, well-differentiated tumors are defined as those in which less than 10% of the tumor volume is composed of solid sheets of cells, the remainder of the tumor being glandular; in moderately differentiated tumors, 11–50% of the tumor is composed of solid sheets of cells; and

in poorly differentiated tumors more than 50% of the tumor is solid.

IMMUNOHISTOCHEMICAL FINDINGS

Because it can be difficult to distinguish between primary endometrial and cervical adenocarcinomas on the basis of histological parameters alone, a number of investigators have studied the utility of special stains for mucin and immunohistochemistry for discriminating between these two types of tumors[78,242] (see Chapter 26, Immunohistochemistry). It is now clear that even though more cervical adenocarcinomas than endometrial adenocarcinomas stain strongly positive with alcian blue, there is sufficient overlap between the staining patterns of the two tumors to render alcian blue staining of little diagnostic value (Table 8.9).[59,73] Immunostaining patterns with carcinoembryonic antigen (CEA) also have been suggested as a way of dis-

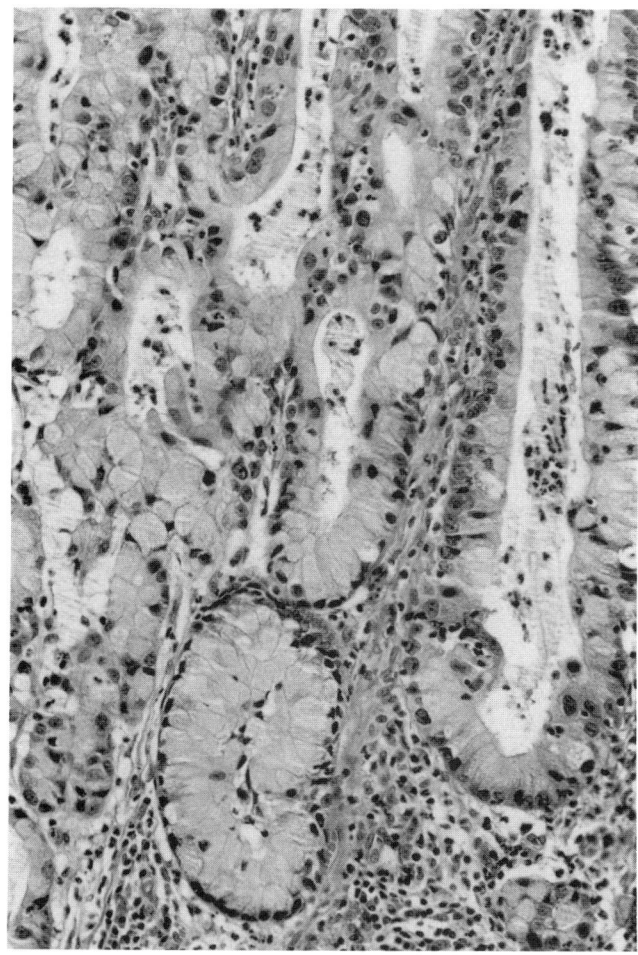

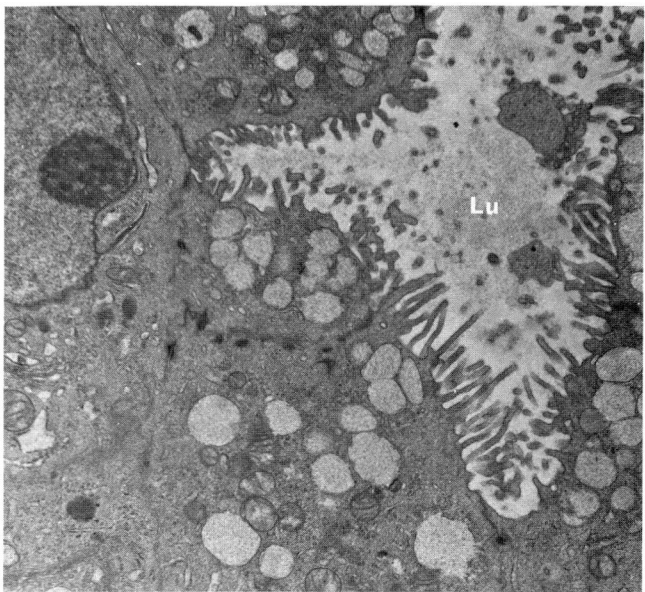

FIG. 8.24. **Adenocarcinoma of endocervical type.** By electron microscopy the neoplastic endocervical cells have apical, mucin-containing secretory granules. Mucinogenesis is reduced in neoplastic as compared with normal endocervical epithelium. *Lu*, lumen. ×6810.

FIG. 8.23. **Adenocarcinoma of intestinal type.** Goblet cells are interspersed among the neoplastic glands.

criminating between endometrial and cervical primaries. In one early study, 80% of endocervical tumors stained positively with CEA compared with 8% of primary endometrial adenocarcinomas.[354] More recent studies, however, have found CEA staining to be limited value in distinguishing an endocervical from an endometrial primary in the individual case (Table 8.9).[198,218] CEA immunocytochemistry also is of limited value for distinguishing invasive adenocarcinomas from atypical, but benign, glandular lesions of the endocervix because CEA positivity can be detected in squamous metaplasia and in normal cervical glandular epithelium and some endocervical adenocarcinomas are negative or only weakly positive.[103,235,325,329]

Several other immunohistochemical stains may be of value in distinguishing primary cervical adenocarcinomas from endometrial carcinomas (Table 8.9). Primary cervical adenocarcinomas stain relatively weakly with antibodies directed against vimentin whereas approximately 60% of primary endometrial adenocarcinomas stain strongly.[75,339] IC5 is a monoclonal antibody developed against a human

cervical adenocarcinoma cell line. The IC5 antibody stains 90% of cervical adenocarcinomas cytoplasmically but does not stain the cytoplasm of endometrial adenocarcinomas.[198] Instead, staining of endometrial adenocarcinomas is restricted to the luminal surface cell membrane and occurs in only 40% of the tumors.[198] Panels of monoclonal antibodies directed against the mucus-specific antigens M1, M2, and M3 also may be helpful in selected cases. One study demonstrated that 56% of cervical adenocarcinomas contain both the M1 and M3 mucus-associated antigens whereas no primary endometrial adenocarcinomas stained for both types of antigen (Table 8.9).[218]

Table 8.9. Differentiating primary endometrial from primary cervical adenocarcinomas

	Percentage of primary tumors that stain	
Stain or antigen	Endocervical	Endometrial
Alcian blue[218]	100	77
CEA[198,218,354]	59–80	8–50
Vimentin[339]	0	66
IC5[198]	90 (cytoplasmic)	40 (luminal)
M1 and M3[218]	56	0

Adapted from refs. 198, 218, 339, 354.
CEA, carcinoembryonic antigen; M1, M3, and IC5, monoclonal antibodies derived against either endocervical adenocarcinoma cells or mucus-associated proteins.

ULTRASTRUCTURAL FINDINGS

Transmission electron microscopy confirms the light microscopic and histochemical observations of a gradual decrease and an eventual loss of mucin production in increasingly dedifferentiated adenocarcinoma of the cervi (Fig. 8.24).[96]

DIFFERENTIAL DIAGNOSIS

The major benign lesions that must be distinguished from invasive mucinous adenocarcinoma of the cervix are microglandular hyperplasia, hyperplastic mesonephric remnants, and the Arias–Stella reaction. Microglandular hyperplasia tends to occur in younger women and frequently is polypoid. Unlike invasive adenocarcinomas, which extend beyond the depth of normal endocervical glands, microglandular hyperplasia is confined to the normal endocervical glands.[372] In addition, microglandular hyperplasia is composed of relatively uniform, small glands lined by a simple layer of bland epithelium with few mitoses. Mesonephric remnants are tubular, retain a clustered arrangement associated with a mesonephric duct, and usually are deep in the cervical stroma. The epithelium lining the tubules usually is cuboidal and not stratified. Cytological atypia is minimal.[98] The Arias–Stella reaction is distinguished from clear cell adenocarcinoma by the distinctive cytonucleomegaly and lack of mitoses. In addition, the clear cytoplasmic appearance of Arias–Stella reaction is not caused by an accumulation of glycogen but by an increased cytoplasmic matrix in which the organelles are dispersed. The presence of other changes of pregnancy, such as decidua, confirms the diagnosis.

The malignant lesions that must be distinguished from invasive adenocarcinoma of the cervix include adenocarcinoma in situ (AIS), primary endometrial adenocarcinoma with extension into the endocervical canal, and metastatic adenocarcinoma. Adenocarcinoma in situ of the cervix is distinguished from invasive cervical adenocarcinoma by the lack of extension beyond the depth to which normal endocervical glands extend, lack of desmoplasia surrounding the glands, and lack of foci of closely packed glands.[277] The normal endocervical glandular architecture is maintained in AIS.

Metastatic adenocarcinoma to the cervix usually occurs in the setting of a patient with a known, widely metastatic primary lesion and is characterized histologically by a lack of surface involvement and widespread lymphvascular involvement. In assessing whether a carcinoma is of primary endocervical origin or is metastatic to the cervix, the pathologist should evaluate the following morphologic features: (1) neoplastic growth pattern, (2) co-existent in situ changes, (3) cell type, and (4) histochemical characteristics. Transition between in situ and invasive carcinoma[277] provides the strongest evidence for a primary origin and is found in up to 43% of primary cervical adenocarcinomas.[2]

RISK FACTORS

Major prognostic indicators for cervical adenocarcinoma include tumor diameter, depth of invasion, involvement of lymphvascular spaces, stage, and presence or absence of lymph node metastases.[10,27,91,189,279] Depth of invasion can be expressed either in millimeters of distance from the endocervical lumen or as percentage of the total thickness of the wall that is involved.

Poor prognostic features include tumor size greater than 3 cm, uterine enlargement, and high grade. Ploidy level (nuclear DNA content) has been correlated with histological grade and may have prognostic significance.[12,107] Low ploidy level, with stem cell modal values less than triploid, are associated with well-differentiated adenocarcinoma, whereas poorly differentiated adenocarcinomas are associated with high ploidy, and greater than triploid stem cell modal values. Moreover, women with hypotriploid tumors have a significantly higher survival rate (45–55%) than women with hypertriploid tumors (10–18%).[107]

CLINICAL BEHAVIOR AND TREATMENT

Adenocarcinoma of the cervix spreads in a fashion similar to squamous cell carcinoma and, in general, both squamous and adenocarcinomas are treated similarly. The two most commonly used therapeutic modalities for stage I and II adenocarcinoma are radiation alone or radiation followed by simple hysterectomy.[167,274] Only a few studies have directly compared the therapeutic results achieved with invasive squamous cell and adenocarcinomas over the same time period and from the same institution and these studies have produced conflicting data. In one report, Hopkins and Morley found that local extension as well as lymph node metastases occurred comparatively earlier in adenocarcinomas than in squamous cell carcinoma.[142] Similar results have been reported by others who have found that the overall 5-year survival rates are lower for adenocarcinoma (48–56%) than for squamous cell carcinoma patients (68%).[27,91,107,142] However, other comparison studies, as well as several population-based studies, have failed to confirm that prognosis and survival are affected by histological type.[11,126,208]

Endometrioid Adenocarcinoma

As in endometrial and ovarian neoplasms, endometrioid adenocarcinomas of the cervix are defined as tumors composed of cells that resemble those of typical adenocarcinomas of the uterine corpus. Endometrioid carcinomas account for up to 30% of endocervical adenocarcinomas. The cells of endometrioid adenocarcinomas tend to be stratified and have oval nuclei that are arranged with their long axis perpendicular to the basement membrane of the gland (Fig. 8.25). The cells contain very little or no mucin and have less cytoplasm than do the cells of mucinous adenocarcinomas. Endometrioid adenocarcinomas frequently contain small foci of squamous epithelium. However, at times it can be difficult to differentiate endometrioid adenocarcinoma from less well-differentiated mucinous adenocarcinomas of the endocervical type and many tumors classified as endometrioid adenocarcinomas actually may represent poorly differentiated mucinous tumors that have lost their capacity to produce mucin.

It can also be difficult to differentiate between an endometrioid carcinoma primary in the cervix and a primary endometrial adenocarcinoma. Primary uterine corpus tumors are usually bulky tumors that invade the myometrium by the time they extend to the cervix and therefore cause uterine enlargement. In contrast, primary cervical adenocarcinomas often cause cervical enlargement in the absence of uterine enlargement. Even with large destructive primary cervical adenocarcinomas, differentiation from primary endometrial adenocarcinoma can be made if normal endometrium is present on either a fractional dilation and curettage or an endometrial biopsy. Contamination, however, of the endometrial sample while passing the curette or biopsy instrument through the involved endocervical canal can occur. In these cases a careful search through multiple sections may reveal atypical endometrial hyperplasia in primary endometrial tumors and either AIS, SIL (CIN), or foci with features of a typical endocervical carcinoma in primary endocervical tumors.

Clear Cell Adenocarcinoma

Clear cell carcinomas account for approximately 4% of adenocarcinomas of the cervix.[252] Although clear cell adenocarcinoma of the cervix has been reported in young women with a history of in utero exposure to diethylstilbestol (DES),[135,295] these tumors also can develop in the absence of exposure to DES.[93,130,169] Tumors that develop in the absence of DES exposure occur most commonly in postmenopausal women whereas those that occur in women exposed to DES tend to be young. The sporadically developing tumors arise in either the exocervix or endocervix whereas the tumors developing in DES-exposed women develop predominantly on the exocervix. The microscopic features of clear cell carcinoma with or without DES exposure are the same as in older women with no known exposure to DES and are described in detail in Chapter 4, Diseases of the Vagina. There are three basic microscopic patterns; solid, tubulocystic, and papillary. The cells comprising the tumor have an abundant clear cytoplasm because of the accumulation of glycogen or a granular eosinophilic cytoplasm. In addition, there are cells with prominent with hyperchromatic and pleomorphic nuclei that project into the lumen of the cysts and tubules to form hobnail cells (Fig. 8.26). Tubules typically are lined by a single layer of relatively bland cells.

The differential diagnosis of clear cell carcinomas includes other types of cervical adenocarcinomas as well as benign processes such as Arias–Stella reaction and microglandular hyperplasia. Distinguishing between these entities can be difficult, especially on small biopsy samples. Microglandular hyperplasia usually lacks the degree of nuclear atypia of clear cell carcinoma and it also usually contains mucin. Arias–Stella reactions can be differentiated on the basis of lack of mitotic activity, lack of the classic patterns of clear cell carcinoma, and the clinical history of pregnancy.

Minimal Deviation Adenocarcinoma

Minimal deviation adenocarcinoma is an extremely well-differentiated variant of cervical adenocarcinoma in which the cells composing the tumor lack the typical cytological features of malignancy. These tumors were originally re-

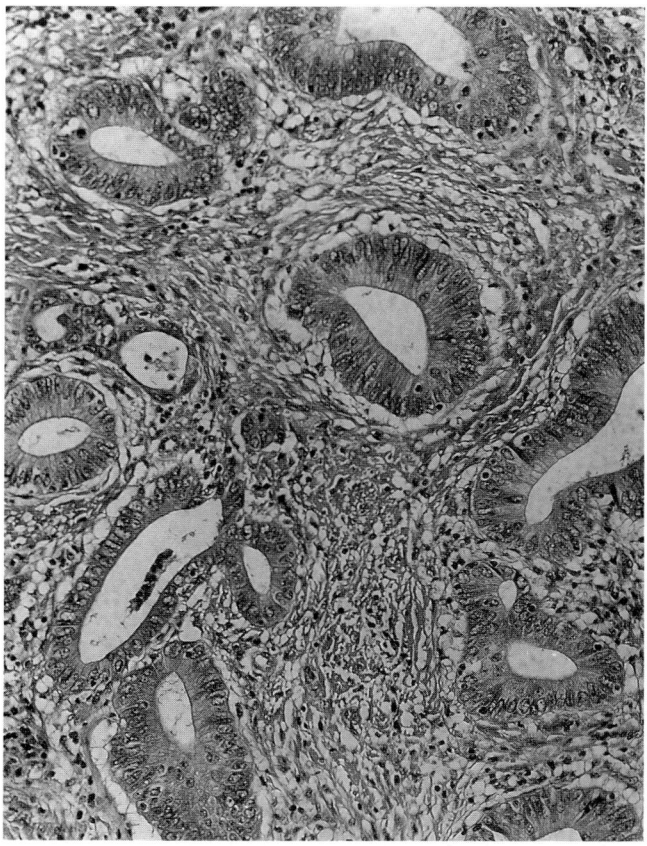

Fig. 8.25. Adenocarcinoma of endometrioid type. These tumors are similar to the typical endometrial adenocarcinoma.

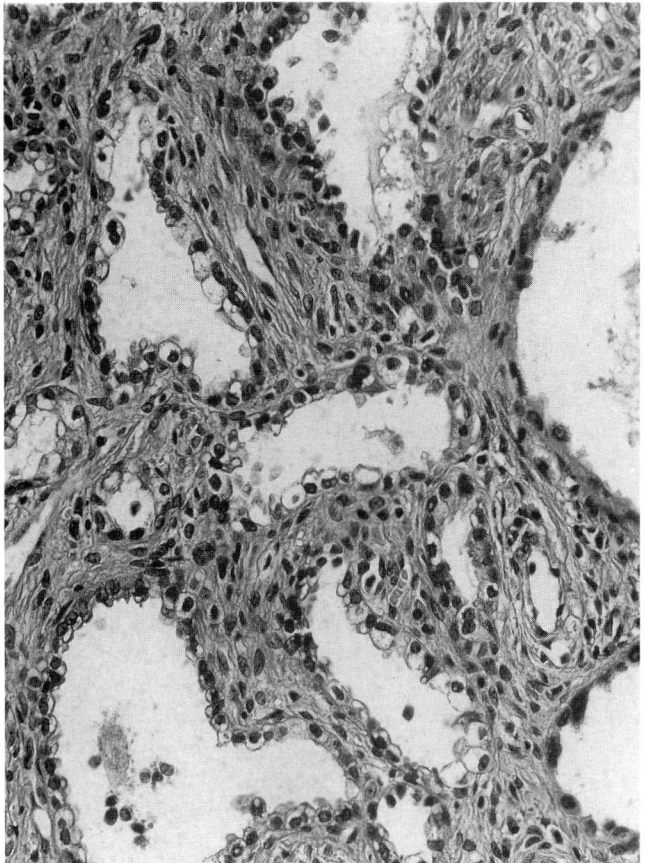

FIG. 8.26. **Clear cell carcinoma.** Clear cells and hobnail cells are lining tubules and cysts.

ferred to as *adenoma malignum*. Because of their close cytological resemblance to normal endocervical glands, in 1975 Silverberg and Hurt introduced the term *minimal deviation adenocarcinoma* (MDA) for these lesions.[231,318] Although all of the tumors in the original description were extremely well-differentiated mucin-producing adenocarcinomas, more recently MDA has been expanded to include endometrioid and clear cell variants.[170,343,374]

Minimal deviation adenocarcinomas are uncommon tumors and account for only 1–3% of all cervical adenocarcinomas.[170] These tumors are more likely than other types of cervical adenocarcinomas either to precede or develop coincidentally with an ovarian carcinoma. The ovarian neoplasms with which MDA is most likely to be associated include mucinous adenocarcinomas and sex cord tumors with annular tubules. Both MDA of the cervix and ovarian sex cord tumors with annular tubules have been strongly associated with Peutz–Jeghers syndrome.[228,375] In one series, 4 of 27 women with Peutz–Jeghers syndrome developed MDA.[375] Therefore, close clinical surveillance of women with Peutz–Jeghers syndrome is recommended, including careful endocervical cytological examination and periodic endocervical curettage.

Minimal deviation adenocarcinomas frequently are associated with either a profuse watery or mucinous vaginal discharge and some cases are associated with abnormal endocervical cells on Pap smear.[337] Grossly and colposcopically, cervices with early forms of MDA can appear normal. In more advanced cases, polypoid lesions or irregularities of the cervix sometimes can be noted. In other cases there are cervical ulcerations or only cervical stenosis without an obvious lesion.

The characteristic microscopic features of MDA are the presence of cytologically low-grade, but architecturally atypical, glands that vary in size, shape, and location (Fig. 8.27). In the mucin-producing forms, the glands are lined by a single layer of tall columnar epithelium that usually has minimal, if any, nuclear atypia (Fig. 8.28). The nuclei are bland, lack prominent nucleoli, and are located at the base of the epithelium. In the endometrioid type, the cells lining the glands resemble either normal proliferative or hyperplastic endometrium. Although some glands may exhibit a similar branching arrangement to that of the normal endocervical glands, characteristically glands with bizarre

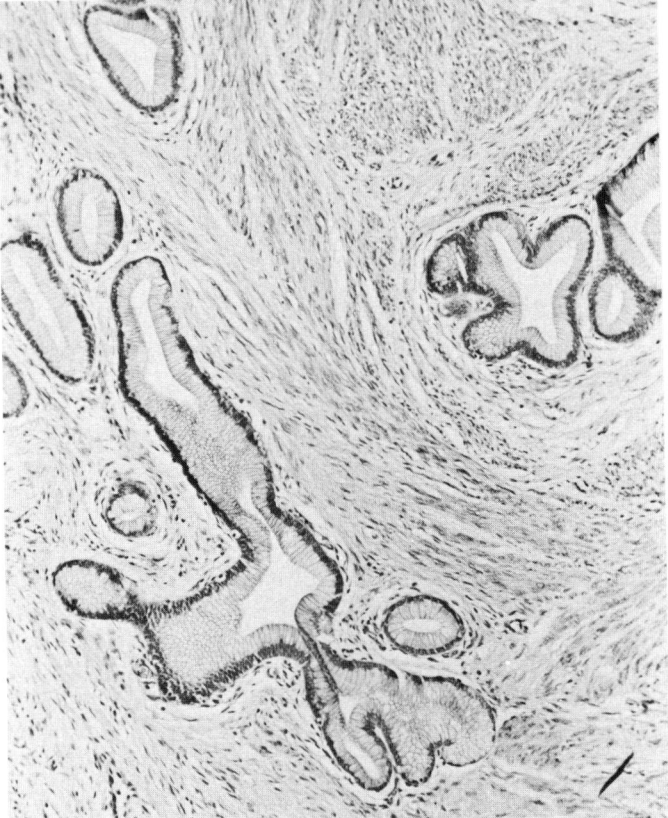

FIG. 8.27. **Minimal deviation adenocarcinoma.** There is an irregular glandular, branching pattern that differs from normal endocervical glands despite close resemblance of lining cells to normal endocervical epithelium. A discrete rim of periglandular stromal edema is present around the glands.

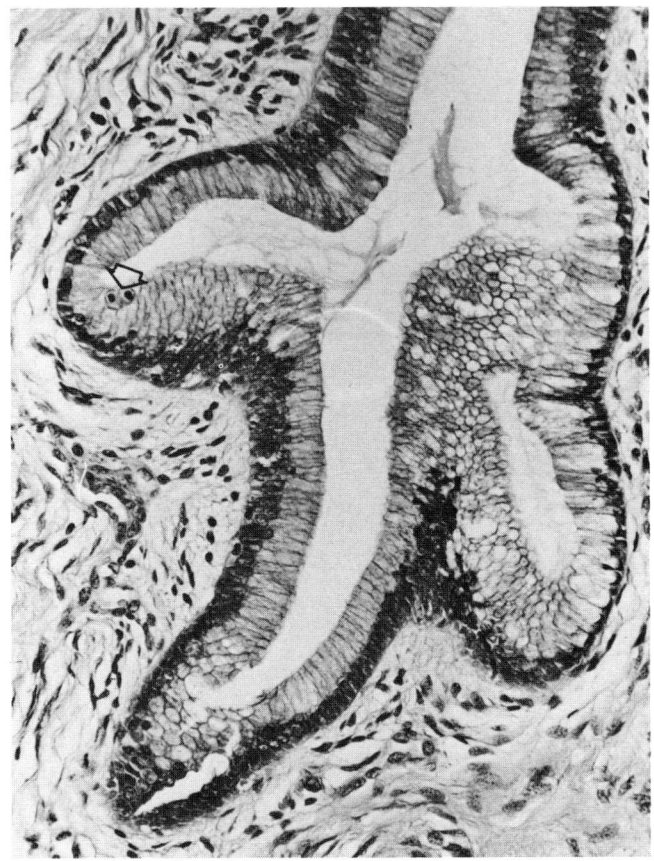

FIG. 8.28. Minimal deviation adenocarcinoma. Slightly enlarged nuclei in a basal position and occasional mitotic figures (*arrow*) are present.

angular outpouchings that vary greatly in size are present.[113,168,235] Desmoplasia frequently is present surrounding the angular outpouchings of MDA. However, the most reliable criteria to assess the malignant nature of MDA is the haphazard arrangement of glands that extend beyond the level of normal endocervical glands and the presence of occasional mitoses in glandular cells.[9] Mitoses are quite uncommon in the normal, nonneoplastic, endocervical epithelium and the presence of mitoses should alert the pathologist to the possible presence of MDA. However, occasional mitotic figures in otherwise normal-appearing glands should not be taken as sufficient for a diagnosis of MDA. Minimal deviation adenocarcinoma often involves more than two-thirds of the thickness of the cervical stroma extending beyond the normal endocervical crypts and tunnels which can range up to 5–7 mm in maximum depth.[113,170] Because the depth of penetration of the glands is a key histological feature of MDA, in most cases the diagnosis cannot be made on a superficial cervical biopsy, but instead requires either a cone biopsy or hysterectomy specimen. Immunohistochemical studies using CEA have found a highly variable staining with only focal areas of positivity within these tumors.[44,113]

The differential diagnosis of MDA includes several conditions in which nonneoplastic glands extend beyond 7 mm from the surface. These conditions include endocervical tunnel clusters, deeply situated nabothian cysts, and mesonephric hyperplasia. The glands of endocervical tunnel clusters, mesonephric hyperplasia and deep nabothian cysts usually are much more uniform in size than are the glands of MDA and lack the bizarre branching and irregular outpouchings characteristic of the glands of MDA. The benign processes also lack a desmoplastic response.

Although earlier reports and several of the more recent series have suggested an extremely poor prognosis for women with MDA,[113,168,231] other series have found survival rates similar to those of women with well-differentiated ordinary adenocarcinoma.[170,318] The discrepancy in observations may be due to a number of factors including undertreatment of MDA because deep invasion by the tumor was not appreciated. In some cases, minimal deviation adenocarcinomas have not been diagnosed correctly even in hysterectomy specimens before the development of recurrent disease.

Serous Adenocarcinoma

Serous adenocarcinoma of the cervix is an extremely rare form of cervical adenocarcinoma that histologically is identical to serous adenocarcinomas arising in the ovary or endometrium. These tumors are composed of papillary tufts and complex papillae lined by cells with pleomorphic, high-grade nuclei (Fig. 8.29). In the only report describing

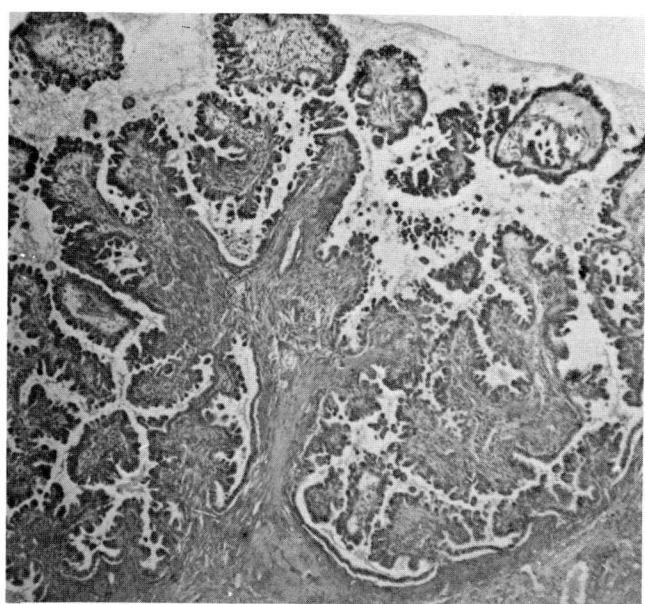

FIG. 8.29. Serous adenocarcinoma. There are branching papillae lined by atypical epithelium and supported by connective tissue stroma resembling papillary serous carcinoma of the ovary.

these tumors, none of the three tumors were deeply invasive, but two of the patients had pelvic node metastasis.[112]

Mesonephric Carcinoma

Mesonephric duct remnants are detected in up to 20% of cervices removed during routine hysterectomy and adenocarcinomas can rarely develop in these remnants.[148] Mesonephric carcinomas are very rare and in the past were confused with clear cell carcinomas of the cervix. In contrast to the superficial location of cervical clear cell adenocarcinomas, true mesonephric adenocarcinomas develop deep in the lateral wall of the cervix, in a site corresponding to the location of mesonephric duct remnants.[21,202,350] The tumor is composed of closely packed tubular-shaped glands that diffusely infiltrate the stroma (Figs. 8.30, 8.31). The cells of mesonephric carcinoma are not clear and have a negligible amount of intracytoplasmic glycogen.[130,169,202,297] They form a single layer and the cytoplasm of mesonephric carcinoma cells is more granular than the cells of clear cell carcinoma. A diagnosis of mesonephric carcinoma should be made only if the tumor is located deep in the wall of the cervix, the endocervical mucosa is uninvolved, and there is no evidence that the patient was exposed to DES. Distinguishing mesonephric

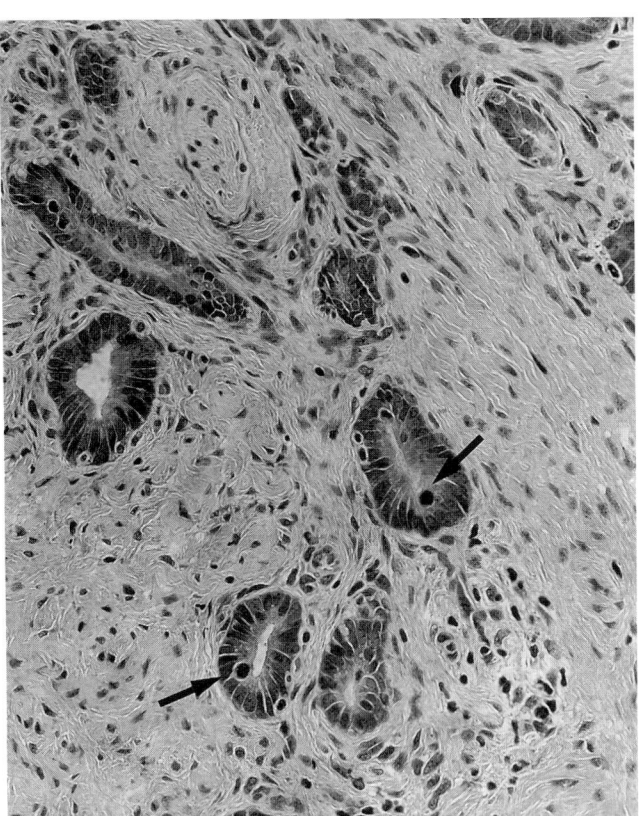

FIG. 8.31. Mesonephric carcinoma. Haphazardly arranged tubular glands with minimal nuclear atypica. Note mitotic activity (*arrows*).

carcinoma from florid mesonephric hyperplasia can be difficult since most carcinomas develop in the setting of a diffuse form of mesonephric hyperplasia (see Chapter 6, Benign Diseases of the Cervix).[98] In contrast to mesonephric hyperplasia, the carcinoma does not have a lobular architecture and the nuclei appear cytologically malignant.

Well-differentiated Villoglandular Adenocarcinoma

Villoglandular adenocarcinoma is a well-differentiated form of cervical adenocarcinoma that occurs predominantly in young women and has an excellent prognosis.[144,164,373] The characteristic features of this tumor are a surface component that is composed of papillae lined by epithelium that has only mild cytological atypia (Figs. 8.32, 8.33). The epithelial cells lining the papillae can have either endocervical, endometrioid, or intestinal features (including goblet cells). Because of the large number of surface papillae, these tumors frequently form an exophytic, friable tumor mass. Most of the papillae have central cores containing spindle-shaped stromal cells resembling those of the normal cervical stroma and a variable number of inflammatory cells. The papillae can be either long and thin or thick and short. Small papillary tufts composed

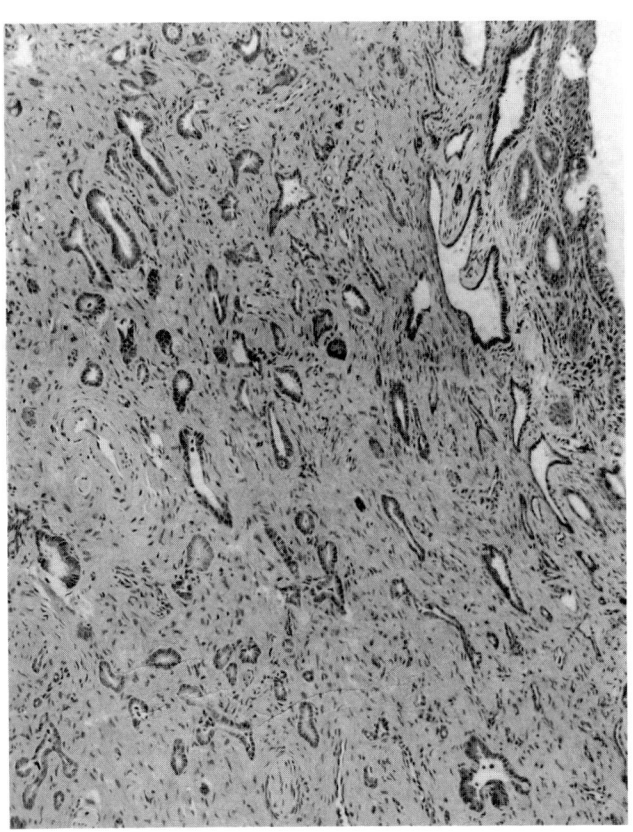

FIG. 8.30. Mesonephric carcinoma. The tumor is composed of tubular glands that diffusely infiltrate the stroma.

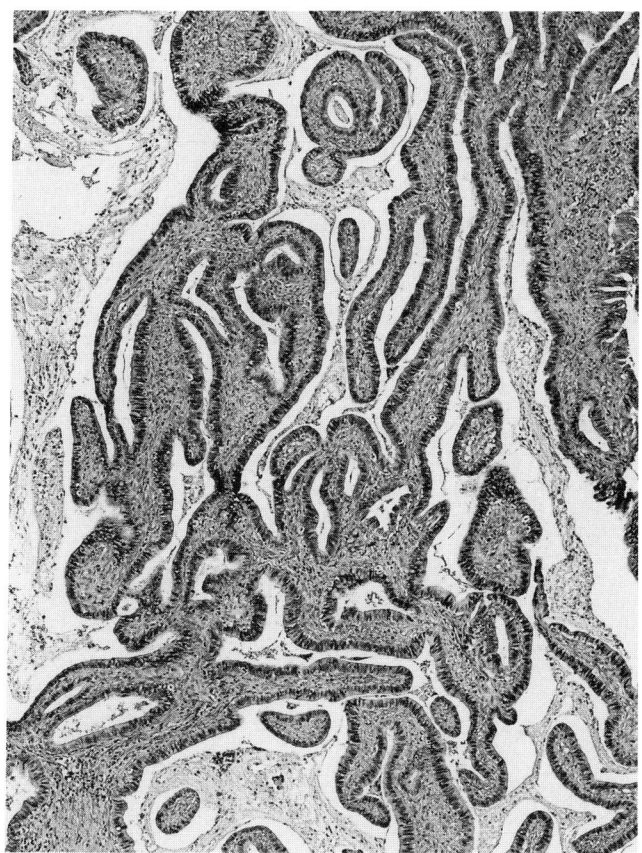

Fig. 8.32. Well-differentiated villoglandular adenocarcinoma. The tumor is composed of long, thin papillae. (Used with permission from Jones MW, et al., ref. 164.)

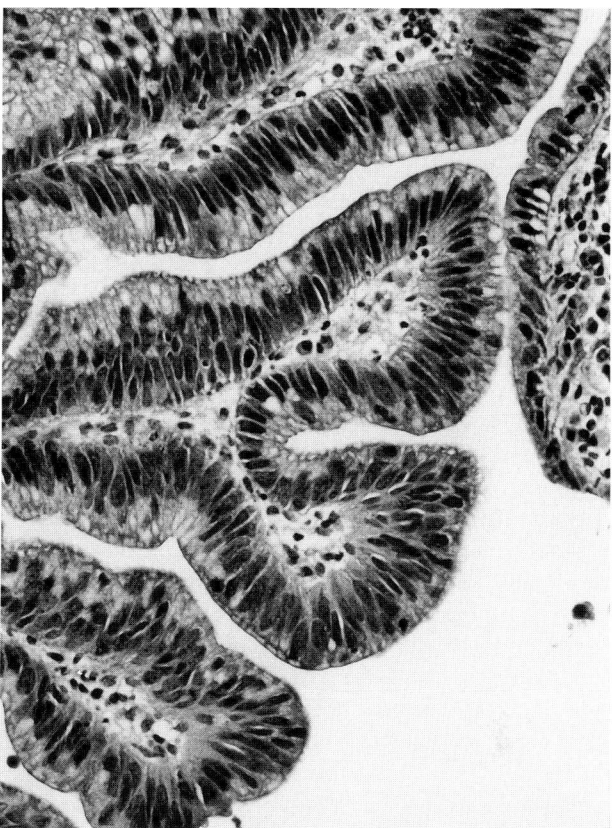

Fig. 8.33. Well-differentiated villoglandular adenocarcinoma. The cells lining the papillae are pseudostratified and have minimal cytological atypia. (Used with permission from Jones MW, et al., ref. 164.)

entirely of epithelial cells of the type characteristic of serous carcinomas of the ovary are absent. Beneath the papillary surface, the infiltrating portion of the tumor is composed of irregular branching glands that are surrounded typically by only a minimal desmoplastic response.

The differential diagnosis of these tumors include papillary endocervicitis, papillary adenofibromas of the cervix, and the müllerian papilloma.[370,373] All three of these lesions lack the degree of cellular atypia that is present in villoglandular adenocarcinomas. The müllerian papilloma is a lesion of children whereas the age of patients with villoglandular adenocarcinomas ranges from 23 to 54 years, with a mean of 37 in one series.

Villoglandular adenocarcinomas have been associated frequently with the use of oral contraceptives before diagnosis.[164] In most cases the tumor is superficially invasive, although deep invasion with extension into the uterine corpus may occur. In the cases published to date, the clinical outcome of patients with villoglandular adenocarcinomas has been excellent.[144,164,373] All patients, including those who were treated by simple excisional biopsy or cone

biopsy, were alive and well with no evidence of recurrent disease after 7–77 months of follow-up.[164,373]

Other Epithelial Tumors

Adenosquamous Carcinoma

Adenosquamous carcinomas are defined as tumors that contain an admixture of histologically malignant squamous and glandular cells.[87,315,361,366] Glucksmann and Cherry, who originally emphasized the importance of adenosquamous carcinomas, used the term *mixed cervical carcinomas* to refer to adenosquamous carcinomas as well as glassy cell carcinomas and signet-ring carcinomas.[115] In the recent WHO classification, the term *mixed carcinomas* has been deleted and adenosquamous carcinomas are now classified under *other epithelial tumors* (Table 8.1).[307]

Adenosquamous carcinomas account for between 5% and 25% of all cervical cancers.[40,126,282,313,338,368] They occur in both young and old women and can be associated with pregnancy. The squamous component generally includes areas that are well differentiated and contain either keratin "pearls" or sheets of cells with individual cell keratinization. To make the diagnosis of adenosquamous carcinoma, there must be sufficient differentiation of the adenocarcinomatous component so that glands are histologically recognizable. Although the well-differentiated forms usually are recognized easily, when the adenocarcinomatous component is less well differentiated and present in relatively small amounts, it can be easily overlooked. The term *adenosquamous carcinoma* is not used for adenocarcinomas that contain bland (nonmalignant)-appearing squamous differentiation. Instead, such tumors are classified as endometrioid adenocarcinomas of the cervix with squamous metaplasia (see above, Endometrioid Carcinoma).

Lesions with mixed patterns of epithelial differentiation are thought to arise from the pluripotential subcolumnar reserve cells of the endocervical mucous membrane and represent biphasic differentiation.[2,42] The epidemiologic risk factors associated with adenosquamous carcinomas of the cervix are more similar to those of squamous cell carcinomas than of adenocarcinomas.[40] The prevalence of adenosquamous carcinomas may be increased in young women[28,37,126,338,352] and these tumors metastasize to pelvic lymph nodes twice as frequently as squamous cell carcinomas or adenocarcinomas.[126,313] Despite the increase in pelvic lymph node metastases, the prognosis in patients with adenosquamous carcinomas has not been significantly worse than that of patients with squamous cell carcinomas in some studies,[126,143,241,368] although other series have reported a poorer prognosis associated with these tumors.[30,109,301]

Glassy Cell Carcinoma

A poorly differentiated form of adenosquamous carcinoma has been referred to as glassy cell carcinoma.[115] Glassy cell carcinoma comprises less than 1% of cervical cancers and has been reported to have an extremely aggressive clinical course, with a poor response to radiation and surgery.[109,211,220,310] Although the existence of poorly differentiated adenosquamous carcinomas with this histology is widely accepted, it has been argued that classifying these tumors as a separate entity is unwarranted since, compared with other types of poorly differentiated carcinomas, these tumors do not have a significantly different clinical course.[220,358]

On gross examination these tumors are commonly large and produce a barrel-shaped cervix (Fig. 8.34). The major microscopic features of glassy cell carcinomas include (1) rather uniform large polygonal cells with finely granular ground glass-type cytoplasm, hence the name *glassy cell*, (2) distinct cell membranes, and (3) prominent nucleoli

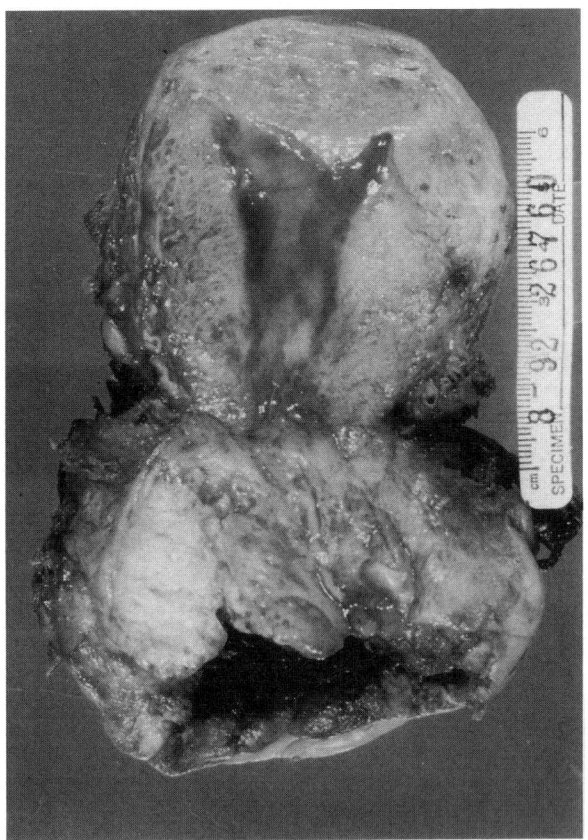

FIG. 8.34. Glassy cell carcinoma. The tumor has diffusely infiltrated the cervix to form a barrel-shaped cervix.

(Fig. 8.35).[253,288,366] In addition, the cells lack intercellular bridges, dyskeratosis, and intracellular glycogen. Mitotic figures are abundant. The stroma is characteristically heavily infiltrated by lymphoplasmacytic and eosinophilic inflammatory cells. Occasionally, areas of keratin pearl and abortive lumen formation are seen together with signet-ring cells and intracellular mucin. The overlying surface squamous epithelium may be normal or may contain SIL (CIN). Ultrastructurally, the adenosquamous nature of glassy cell carcinoma is evidenced by rare abortive glandular lumen formation together with well-developed tonofilament–desmosomal complexes, interdigitating microvilli, and cytoplasmic microfilaments.[288]

Mucoepidermoid Carcinoma

Buckley and Fox have argued that all cervical carcinomas should be stained with a mucin stain such as mucicarmine before classification because a considerable number of cervical squamous cell carcinomas lacking recognizable glands still produce mucin that can be detected with special stains.[42,43] They and others use the term *mucoepidermoid carcinoma* to refer to these mixed squamous cell carcino-

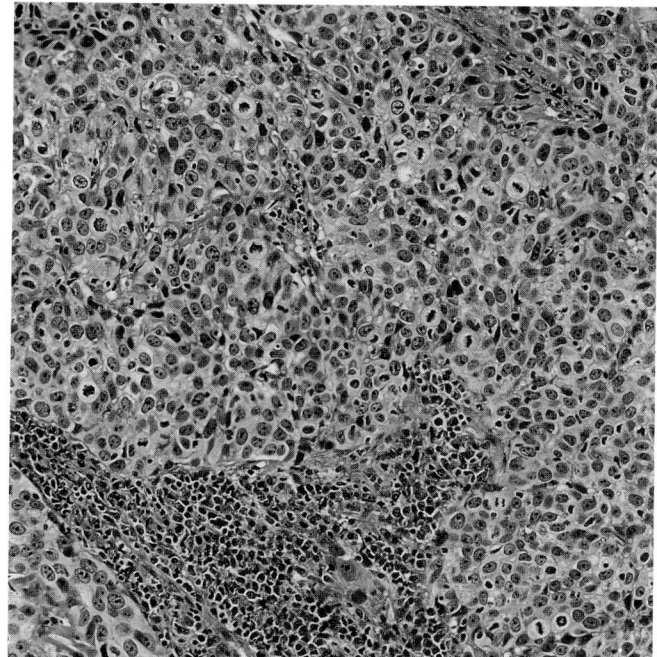

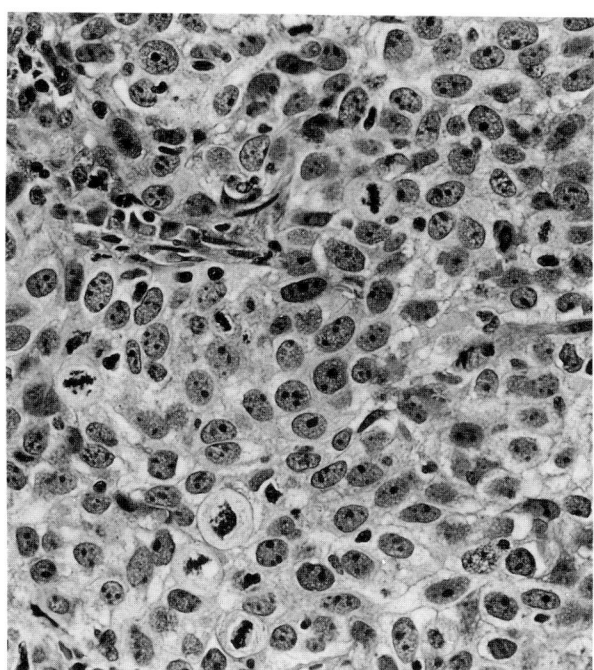

FIG. 8.35. **Glassy cell carcinoma.** **a:** The tumor has neither apparent squamous nor glandular differentiation and is arranged in lobules. The stroma contains an abundant chronic inflammatory exudate. **b:** The neoplastic cells have a granular glassy cytoplasm, well-defined cytoplasmic membranes, and prominent nucleoli.

mas that produce mucin but lack recognizable glands.[42,43,344] Mucoepidermoid carcinomas are a common form of cervical carcinoma, accounting for up to 20% of cervical carcinomas in some series.[22,60,87,259] In mucoepidermoid carcinoma the squamous component usually is large cell nonkeratinizing or focally keratinizing and the mucin-producing cells frequently are localized in the center of nests of squamous cell carcinoma (Fig. 8.36). The mucinous component includes goblet or signet-ring type cells which contain mucinocarminophilic, periodic acid–Schiff (PAS)-positive, diastase-resistant mucopolysaccharides. The mucin from these cells is extruded into the intercellular spaces or fibrous stroma, where it may collect in small or large lakes.

In some studies, mucoepidermoid carcinomas have been more common in younger patients and have been associated with an increased risk of lymph node metastases.[22,42,43,126,154] This has led some authors to propose that these tumors have a distinctive clinical presentation and contribute to a subset of young women with highly aggressive cervical cancers.[42,43] However, most studies have failed to detect a significant clinical difference between patients with mixed carcinomas and those with pure squamous cell carcinomas of the cervix.[22,39,50,60,126,338,352] Therefore, these tumors are not included as a separate entity

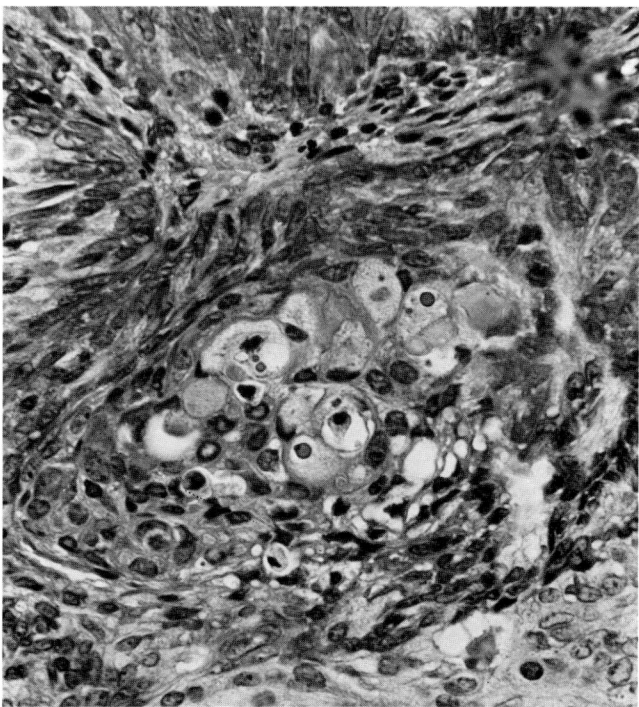

FIG. 8.36. **Mucoepidermoid carcinoma.** There are pale, mucin-containing cells within masses of neoplastic squamous cells.

in the most recent WHO classification, but are included within the category of adenosquamous carcinoma.[307]

Adenoid Cystic Carcinoma

Adenoid cystic carcinoma of the cervix is a relatively uncommon tumor, accounting for less than 1% of all cervical adenocarcinomas. It is characterized by cylindrical hyaline bodies and/or small acini or cysts lying within solid nests or between anastomosing cords of uniform basaloid tumor cells.[104,146,183,226,237,248] The nuclei of these cells are small and relatively uniform and there are frequent mitotic figures. Focal squamous differentiation and necrosis may be present. In cross-section, the hyaline cylinders appear round or ovoid, giving the neoplasm a sieve-like appearance (Fig. 8.37). At the electron microscopic level, the hyaline material is partly composed of coalesced masses of basal lamina produced by the epithelial tumor cells and partly of fine precollagen and collagen fibers of fibroblastic origin.[191,226] However, unlike adenoid cystic carcinomas of other sites, cervical adenoid cystic carcinomas contain few myoepithelial cells as detected by electron microscopy or S-100 and actin immunohistochemical stains.

Adenoid cystic carcinoma may be associated with squamous adenocarcinoma of the cervix.[2,97] The tumor is seen most often in patients between the sixth and seventh decades and is more common in blacks than whites. It is relatively commonly associated with mucinous ovarian neoplasms. Adenoid cystic carcinoma often forms hard palpable masses in the cervix that can be ulcerated or friable. Lymphatic involvement is common and the tumor behaves aggressively with frequent local recurrences or metastatic spread.[85,97,104,182,237] Adenoid cystic carcinoma of the cervix should be differentiated from adenoid basal carcinoma of the cervix (see below).

Adenoid Basal Carcinoma

Adenoid basal carcinoma is frequently confused with adenoid cystic carcinoma because both have common histological features. Adenoid basal carcinomas are composed of small, uniform cells that resemble basal cell carcinomas of the skin and lack significant nuclear atypia.[15,76] These cells are arranged in small nests and cords (Fig. 8.38). At the periphery of the nests, there is palisading of the nuclei and some of the nests have central cystic spaces that can be filled with necrotic debris. In the center of the nests there also can be either squamous or glandular differentiation. Adenoid basal carcinoma usually can be distinguished from adenoid cystic carcinoma by the lack of the characteristic intraluminal hyaline material frequently present in adenoid cystic carcinomas, the presence of smaller, less pleo-

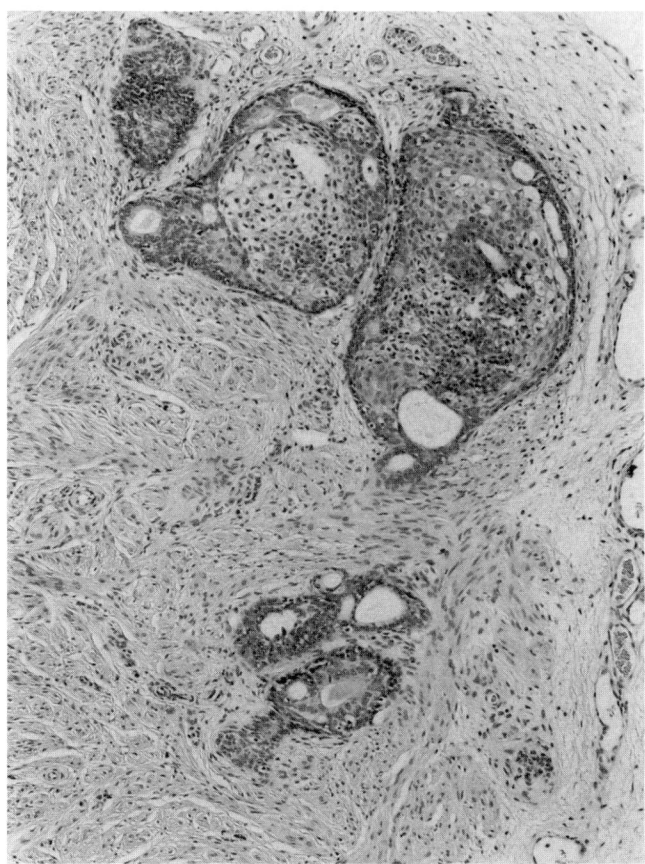

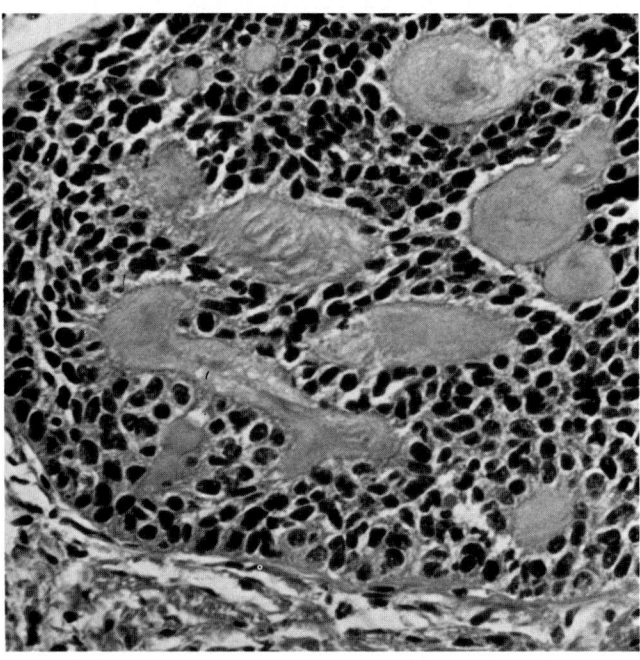

FIG. 8.37. Adenoid cystic carcinoma. Cylindrical hyaline bodies are present within solid nests of basaloid tumor cells.

FIG. 8.38. Adenoid basal carcinoma. Small uniform cells display palisading of the nuclei at the periphery of the nests. The appearance simulates basal cell carcinoma.

morphic nuclei, and less mitotic activity than is characteristic of adenoid cystic carcinomas.[15,85,97] Both adenoid basal and adenoid cystic carcinomas are associated frequently with SIL (CIN) and can have squamous differentiation in the center of the invading nests of cells. Therefore, these features should not be used to distinguish between the two types of tumors. Electron microscopy can be used to distinguish between adenoid basal and adenoic cystic carcinomas. Adenoid basal carcinomas usually lack the redundant basal lamina and true lumens with microvilli that are characteristic of adenoid cystic carcinomas.[226]

Adenoid basal carcinomas are uncommon neoplasms that account for less than 1% of cervical adenocarcinomas and usually are found in postmenopausal, especially black, women.[85,97] The mean age of patients with adenoid basal carcinoma is approximately 60 years. Adenoid basal carcinoma behaves much less aggressively than adenoid cystic carcinoma. Patients with adenoid basal carcinoma almost always have low-stage disease and are asymptomatic without grossly detectable masses. Adenoid basal carcinomas usually are detected as unexpected findings in patients undergoing hysterectomy or cone biopsy for a co-existent SIL.

Carcinoid-like Tumors and Small Cell Carcinomas (Neuroendocrine Carcinoma)

Three histological types of neuroendocrine carcinomas of the cervix have been described. One type usually is classified as a cervical adenocarcinoma that contains neuroendocrine granules and is histologically similar to intestinal carcinoid tumors. The two other histological types resemble either pulmonary atypical carcinoid tumors (intermediate cell neuroendocrine carcinomas) or pulmonary small undifferentiated (oat cell) carcinoma. These latter two types usually are classified together as small cell (undifferentiated) carcinomas of the cervix.

The exact cellular origin of neuroendocrine tumors of the cervix is unknown. Small numbers of argyrophil cells are present in the exocervical epithelium of approximately 40% of women[99] and in the endocervical epithelium in about 20% of women.[341] Argyrophil cells also are detected in about 60% of minimal deviation adenocarcinomas of the cervix and in 14% of other types of cervical adenocarcinomas or adenosquamous carcinomas.[306]

Carcinoid-like Tumor

Tumors that have been categorized as well-differentiated carcinoid tumors of the cervix originally were described by Albores-Saavedra et al. and were classified as carcinoid tumors because they contained neuroendocrine granules and were histologically similar to intestinal carcinoid tumors.[4,5,19,367] Microscopically, these well-differentiated tumors grow in solid sheets and trabeculae and glandular

lumina are found scattered throughout the tumor (Figs. 8.39, and 8.40). The neoplastic cells have round to oval spindle-shaped nuclei and finely granular cytoplasm. Tumors with foci of squamous differentiation and crystal violet and Congo red–positive amyloid stroma are commonly seen. Mitoses may be numerous, and vascular invasion is common. Using immunohistochemistry, somatostatin, calcitonin, vasoactive intestinal polypeptide, antidiuretic hormone (ADH), adrenocorticotropin hormone (ACTH), glucagon, gastrin, serotonin, histamine, amylase, and beta-melanocyte-stimulating hormone (β-MSH) all have been shown to be produced by these tumors.[111,225,306,367] Although early reports suggested that these tumors had a relatively good prognosis, more recent reports clearly demonstrate that these tumors can act in a malignant fashion with local and distant metastasis. To date, none of the cases has been associated with the carcinoid syndrome.

Tumors that have been described previously in the literature as well-differentiated cervical carcinoid tumors actually appear to be adenocarcinomas of the cervix, which in areas resemble carcinoid tumors of the intestinal tract and have neuroendocrine differentiation. Neurosecretory granules can be identified in many carcinomas of the cervix if diligently searched for, at present it is unclear whether

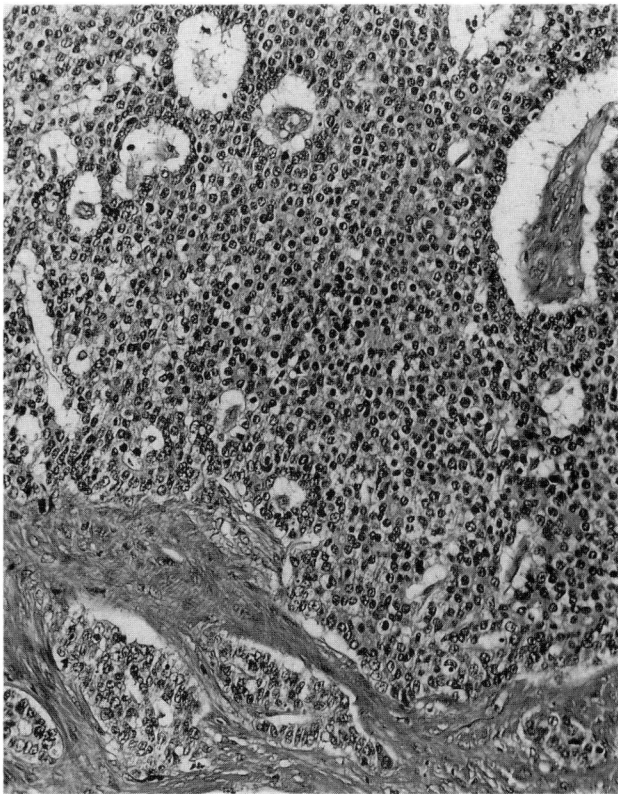

FIG. 8.39. Carcinoid-like tumor. Solid masses and acini composed of small uniform cells.

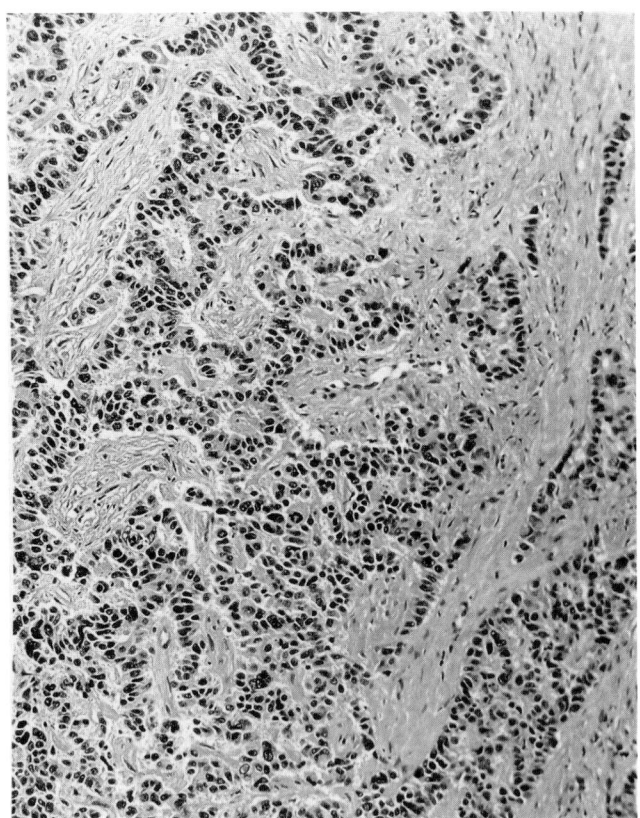

FIG. 8.40. **Carcinoid-like tumor.** Small uniform cells in a trabecular pattern.

pure carcinoid tumors of the cervix exist or whether all these tumors actually represent adenocarcinomas.[199]

Small Cell Carcinoma

Small cell carcinomas of the cervix are histologically identical to their counterparts at other sites such as the lung.[121] These tumors are characterized by small anaplastic cells that have scant amounts of cytoplasm, finely stippled chromatin, and inconspicuous nucleoli. They should be distinguished from adenocarcinomas with carcinoid features and poorly differentiated nonkeratinizing squamous cell carcinomas composed of small cells. Small cell carcinomas account for between 2% and 5% of all cervical tumors. In one of the larger series, patients ranged in age from 25 to 87 years with a median age of 42 years.[111] In another study comparing small cell carcinoma with nonkeratinizing squamous carcinoma composed of small cells, the mean age of women with small cell carcinoma was 36 years compared with 50 years for the squamous carcinomas.[6] Grossly, these tumors range in size from small, clinically inapparent lesions to large ulcerated tumors measuring more than 6 cm in diameter.[111] Small cell carcinomas are deeply infiltrative more frequently than are squamous or adenocarcinomas and frequently presented as a barrel-shaped cervix.[199]

Microscopically, small cell carcinomas are composed of sheets and cords of closely packed, small cells that diffusely infiltrate the stroma (Fig. 8.41). The cells have inconspicuous cytoplasm and closely resemble the cells of oat cell carcinoma of the lung. The cells have hyperchromatic nuclei, high nuclear-cytoloplasmic ratios, and a high mitotic rate with 3 or more mitoses present in most high power fields. The nuclear shape varies from round to spindled and nuclear molding is a characteristic feature. Nuclear detail and nucleoli frequently are obscured by smudging of the nucleus and, as with their pulmonary counterparts, histological sections frequently demonstrate extensive crush artifact (Fig. 8.41). Small areas of either squamous or glandular differentiation can be present, but should account for less than 5% of the total tumor volume.[111]

Neuroendocrine dense-core granules can be detected using Grimelius staining or electron microscopy in most cases. Although these tumors have been associated with ectopic ACTH,[29,162] insulin,[179] and gastrin production,[306,367] this appears to be an uncommon event.[111] By immunohistochemistry, neuroendocrine markers such as neuron-specific enolase, chromogranin, or synaptophysin

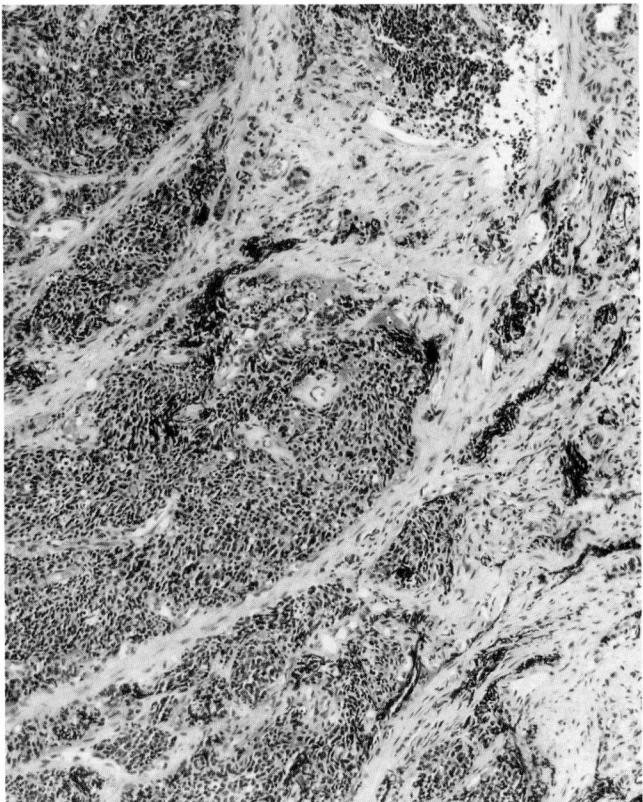

FIG. 8.41. **Small cell carcinoma.** Small cells with hyperchromatic nuclei and scant, indistinct cytoplasm diffusely infiltrate the stroma. A characteristic type of crush artifact is present in the center and right.

are present in most cases; however, calcitonin, insulin, somatostatin, and serotonin are only uncommonly detected.

Small cell carcinoma of the cervix is a highly aggressive tumor. The prognosis for this tumor is worse than that of its well-differentiated carcinoid counterpart[4,5] and also is worse than that of stage-comparable, poorly differentiated small cell squamous carcinoma.[6,35,111,121] In the series of Walker et al., 9 of 12 patients died as a direct result of their tumor and the median duration of those dying of disease was only 12.5 months.[355] Similarly, in the series of Gersell et al. 10 of 15 patients died as a direct result of their tumor.[111] Recently these tumors have been analyzed for the presence of HPV DNA using in situ hybridization. In one study 14 of 18 neuroendocrine-positive cases contained HPV 18.[334] Comparison of the distribution of HPV 16 to HPV 18 in small cell carcinoma and nonkeratinizing squamous cell carcinomas composed of small cells revealed that HPV 16 was found more frequently in the squamous carcinomas (56% vs 20%), whereas small cell carcinoma had a higher frequency of HPV 18 (60% vs 36%).[6]

Differentiation between small cell carcinoma and nonkeratinizing squamous carcinoma with small cells can be difficult. The diagnosis of small cell carcinoma should be reserved to tumors composed of small cells in which squamous or glandular differentiation is absent or very minor. Women with small cell carcinoma tend to be younger than women with nonkeratinizing squamous carcinoma with small cells. Histologically, cells of nonkeratinizing squamous carcinoma with small cells resemble those of high-grade SIL (CIN 2, 3) and lack the nuclear molding and extensive crush artifact present in most small cell carcinomas. Small cell carcinomas invade the stroma diffusely in trabeculae and poorly defined nests. In contrast, nonkeratinizing squamous carcinoma with small cells invade the stroma in discrete nests. In an individual case immunocytochemistry for neuroendocrine markers may not be helpful because 40% of nonkeratinizing squamous carcinoma with small cells are positive for neuroendocrine markers and 40% of small cell carcinomas are positive for cytokeratins.[6] Immunohistochemical staining with antibodies against leukocyte common antigen and neuroendocrine markers can be useful for differentiating between small cell carcinoma from lymphoproliferative disorders.

Mesenchymal and Mixed Epithelial and Mesenchymal Tumors

Malignant mesenchymal tumors that can arise in the cervix include leiomyosarcoma, endocervical stromal sarcoma, embryonal rhabdomyosarcoma (botryoid type), alveolar soft-part sarcoma, and osteosarcomas (see Chapter 13, Mesenchymal Tumors of the Uterus). Primary cervical sar-

comas are very rare; the most common form is the leiomyosarcoma, of which 20 cases have been reported. Primary cervical mixed epithelial and mesenchymal tumors include two reported cases of cervical adenosarcoma, rare cases of malignant mixed mesodermal tumor (MMMT), and a single reported case of Wilm's tumor.

Miscellaneous Tumors

Examples of synchronous adenocarcinoma and squamous cell carcinoma occurring independently in the cervix have been reported.[96,365] They may be either invasive or in situ. In the invasive form, one carcinoma often invades the other, resulting in a collision tumor. Although such tumors closely resemble adenosquamous carcinomas, the different neoplastic components remain histologically distinct, separated from each other by narrow stroma or their respective basal lamina. Because direct transition from one cell type into another, as occurs in adenosquamous carcinoma, is not seen, these tumors are best considered separate primary carcinomas.

Primary malignant melanoma is among the least common of the malignant tumors that arise in the cervix. Twenty four patients have been reported.[55,138,243,302] The prognosis of primary malignant melanoma is quite poor, with only a 40% 5-year survival for patients with stage I disease and a 14% 5-year survival for patients with higher stage disease.[165] Approximately 50% of cases involve the vagina at the time of diagnosis and are stage II or above. Common presenting signs include vaginal bleeding, frequently of short duration. In most instances the lesion is pigmented and dark brown. The diagnosis of primary melanoma of the cervix is based on the histological demonstration of junctional changes in the squamous epithelium and the absence of similar lesions elsewhere in the body. Morphologically it is identical to melanoma arising in the skin and extragenital mucous membranes; it frequently contains intracytoplasmic melanin pigment granules. The pathogenesis of malignant melanoma of the cervix is unclear, although its origin may be ascribed to the melanin-containing cells from the schwannian sheath in the normal cervix.[57]

Primary choriocarcinoma in the cervix is rare and presumably results from a preexisting cervical pregnancy or displaced intrauterine molar tissue. Nearly 50 such cases are recorded in the literature.[348] The gross and microscopic appearance, as well as the clinical course, are identical with those found in the uterine corpus.

Lymphomas and leukemias both can involve the cervix. More often these disorders are secondary, a manifestation of systemic disease. Leukemic infiltration of the cervix, especially of the granulocytic type, is a rather common occurrence at autopsy in women with leukemia.[215] Granulocytic sarcomas, which are well demarcated extramedullary tumors composed of malignant granulocytic precursor cells, also have been reported in the cervix.[106] Granulocytic sarcomas should be differentiated from granulocytic leukemic infiltrates and can either accompany or precede the development of acute myelogenous leukemia. Secondary lymphomatous involvement of the cervix is reported in 6% of women dying with generalized disease.[204] Primary lymphomas occasionally can arise in the cervix and usually present in premenopausal women as abnormal vaginal bleeding. Seventy percent of these tumors are of the diffuse large cell type and 20% are lower grade follicular lymphomas.[245]

Primary cervical germ cell tumors have been described. These include both the mature teratomas and yolk sac tumors.

Secondary Tumors

Direct extension from local pelvic tumor is the most common source of cervical involvement by secondary carcinoma, often originating in the endometrium, rectum, or bladder. Intrapelvic and intragenital, lymphatic, or vascular metastases to the cervix occur less often but are associated with ovarian carcinoma, endometrial adenocarcinoma, and uncommonly with transitional cell carcinoma of the bladder.[36,188,209] Another lesion that has a relatively high rate of cervical metastasis is choriocarcinoma. Sarcomas of the uterine corpus also may involve the cervix. Metastases to the cervix from distant primary foci are rare;[36] the most common sites are the gastrointestinal tract (colon and stomach),[209,378] the ovary,[209] and the breast.[188,357] Instances of metastatic carcinoma of the kidney, gall bladder, pancreas, lung, thyroid,[209,349] and malignant melanoma also have been described.[36,188,227,378] On occasion, metastases may occur primarily as cervical involvement and pose a differential diagnostic problem. Unusual gross appearance or histologic patterns (e.g., signet-ring cell carcinoma or clear cell carcinoma) may provide a clue to the possibility of origin in a distant primary site.

References

1. Abell MR (1973) Invasive carcinoma of the uterine cervix. In: Norris HJ, Hertig AT, Abell MR (eds) The Uterus. Baltimore, Williams and Wilkins, pp 413–456
2. Abell MR, Gosling JRG (1962) Gland cell carcinoma (adenocarcinoma) of the uterine cervix. Am J Obstet Gynecol 83: 729
3. Abramson AL, Brandsman JBS, et al (1985) Verrucous carcinoma of the larynx, possible human papillomavirus etiology. Arch Otolaryngol 111: 709–715
4. Albores-Saavedra J, Larraza O, Poucell S, et al (1976) Carcinoid tumors of the uterine cervix. Cancer 38: 2328–2342
5. Albores-Saavedra J, Rodriguez-Martinez HA, Larraza-Hernandez O (1979) Carcinoid tumors of the cervix. Pathol Annu 14: 273
6. Ambros RA, Park J-S, Shah KV, et al (1991) Evaluation of histologic, morphometric, and immunohistochemical criteria in the differential diagnosis of small cell carcinoms of the cervix with particular reference to human papillomavirus types 16 and 18. Mod Pathol 4: 586–593
7. Anderson GH, Benedet JL, LeRiche JC, et al (1992) Invasive cancer of the cervix in British Columbia: A review of the demography and screening histories of 437 cases seen from 1985–1988. Obstet Gynecol 80: 1–4
8. Anderson MC (1987) Are we vapourising microinvasive lesions? Colpo Gynecol Laser Surg 3: 33–36
9. Anderson MC, Hartley RB (1980) Cervical crypt involvement by intraepithelial neoplasia Obstet Gynecol 55: 546–550
10. Angel C, DuBeshter B, Lin JY (1992) Clinical presentation and management of stage I cervical adenocarcinoma: A 25 year experience. Gynecol Oncol 44: 71–78
11. Anton-Culver H, Bloss JD, Bringman D, et al (1992) Comparison of adenocarcinoma and squamous cell carcinoma of the uterine cervix: A population based epidemiologic study. Am J Obstet Gynecol 186: 1507–1514
12. Atkin NB (1976) Prognostic significance of ploidy level in human tumors. I. Carcinomas of the uterus. J Natl Cancer Inst 56: 909
13. Atkin NB, Baker MC, Fox MF (1990) Chromosome changes in 43 carcinomas of the cervix uteri. Cancer Genet Cytogenet 44: 229–241
14. Averette HE, Nelson JH, Ng AP, et al (1976) Diagnosis and management of microinvasive (stage IA) carcinoma of the uterine cervix. Cancer 38: 414–425
15. Baggish M, Woodruff JD (1971) Adenoid basal lesions of the cervix. Obstet Gynecol 37: 807
16. Baquet CR, Horm JW, Gibbs T, et al (1991) Socioeconomic factors and cancer incidence among Blacks and Whites. J Natl Cancer Inst 83: 551–557
17. Barbacid M (1987) ras Genes Annu Rev Biochem 56: 779–827
18. Barnes WE, Delgado G, Kurman RJ, et al (1988) Possible prognostic significance of human papillomavirus type in cervical cancer. Gynecol Oncol 29: 267–273
19. Barrett RJ, Davos I, Leuchter RS, et al (1987) neuroendocrine features in poorly differentiated and undifferentiated carcinomas of the cervix. Cancer 60: 2325–2330
20. Barsky SH, Siegel GP, Jannotta F, et al (1983) Loss of basement membrane components by invasive tumors but not by their benign counterparts. Lab Invest 49: 140–147
21. Barter RA (1961) Carcinoma of the cervix arising from remnants of Gartner's duct. Aust NZ J Obstet Gynecol 1: 64–72
22. Benda JA, Platz CE, Bushsbaum H, et al (1985) Mucin production in defining mixed carcinoma of the uterine cervix: A clinicopathologic study. Int J Gynecol Pathol 4: 314–327
23. Benedet JL, Anderson GH, Boyes DA (1985) Colposcopic accuracy in the diagnosis of microinvasive and occult invasive carcinoma of the cervix. Obstet Gynecol 65: 5557
24. Benedet JL, Clement PB (1987) Verrucous carcinoma of the cervix and endometrium. Diagn Gynecol Obstet 2: 197

25. Benson WL, Norris HJ (1977) A critical review of the frequency of lymph node metastasis and death from microinvasive carcioma of the cervix. Obstet Gynecol 49: 632

26. Beral V, Booth M (1986) Predictions of cervical cancer incidence and mortality in England and Wales. Lancet 1: 495

27. Berek JS, Hacker NF, Fu YS, et al (1985) Adenocarcinoma of the uterine cervix: Histologic variables associated with lumph node metastases and survival. Obstet Gynecol 65: 46

28. Berkowitz RS, Ehrmann RL, Lavizzo-Mourey R, et al (1979) Invasive cervical carcinoma in young women. Gynecol Oncol 8: 311–316

29. Berthelot P, Benhamon JP, Fauvert R (1961) Hypercorticisme et cancer de l'uterus. Nouv Presse Med 69: 1899

30. Bethwaite P, Yeong ML, Holloway L, et al (1992) The prognosis of adenosquamous carcinomas of the uterine cervix. Br J Obstet Gynecol 99: 745–750

31. Bohm JW, Krupp PJ, Lee FYL, et al (1976) Lymph node metastasis in microinvasive epidermoid cancer of the cervix. Obstet Gynecol 48: 65

32. Bokhman JV, Urmancheyeva AF (1989) Cervix uteri cancer and pregnancy. Eur J Gyncol Oncol 10: 406–411

33. Boronow RC, Averette HE, Nelson JHJ, et al (1975) Defining cervical microinvasive carcinoma. Contemp OB/Gyn 5: 121

34. Bosch FX, Munoz N, de SanJose S, et al (1992) Risk factors for cervical cancer in Columbia and Spain. Int J Cancer 52: 750–758

35. Boyes DA, Worth AJ, Fidler HK (1970) The results of treatment of 4389 cases of preclinical squamous carcinoma. J Obstet Gynecol Br Commonw 77: 769

36. Brady LW, O'Neill EA, S.H. F (1977) Unusual sites of metastasis. Semin Oncol 4: 59

37. Brand E, Berek JS, Hacker NF (1982) Controversies in the management of cervical adenocarcinoma. Obstet Gynecol 71: 261–269

38. Brinton LA (1992) Epidemiology of cervical cancer-an overview. In: Munoz N, Bosch FX, Shah K, Meheus A (eds) The Epidemiology of Cervical Cancer and Human Papillomavirus. Lyon, IARC Scientif Publication, pp 3–23

39. Brinton LA, Fraumeni JF (1986) Epidemiology of uterine cervical cancer. J Chron Dis 39: 1051–1065

40. Brinton LA, Tashima K, Lehman HF, et al (1987) Epidemiology of cervical cancer by cell type. Cancer Res 47: 1706–1711

41. Broders AC (1920) Squamous-cell epithelioma of the lip: A study of five hundred and thirty-seven cases. JAMA 74: 656–664

42. Buckley CF, Fox H (1992) Pathology of clinical invasive carcinomas of the cervix. In: Coppleson M (eds) Gynecologic Oncology. Churchill Livingston, Edinburgh, pp 649–662

43. Buckley CH, Beards CS, Fox H (1988) Pathological prognostic indicators in cervical cancer with particular reference to patients under the age of 40 years. Br J Obstet Gynaecol 95: 47–56

44. Bulmer JN, Griffin NR, Bates C, et al (1990) Minimal deviation adenocarcinoma (adenoma malignum) of the endocervix: A histochemical and immunohistochemical study of two cases. Gynecol Oncol 36: 139–146

45. Burghardt E (1991) Colposcopy–Cervical Pathology, 2nd ed. New York, Thieme Medical Publishers 46. Burghardt E, Baltzer J, Tulusan H, et al (1992) Results of surgical treatment of 1028 cervical cancers studied with volumetry. Cancer 70: 648–655

47. Burghardt E, Girardi F, Lahousen M, et al (1991) Microinvasive carcinoma of the uterine cervix (International Federation of Gynecology and Obstetrics stage IA). Cancer 67: 1037–1045

48. Burghardt E, Holzer E (1977) Diagnosis and treatment of microinvasive carcinoma of the uterine cervix. Obstet Gynecol 4: 59

49. Burke TW, Hoskins WJ, Heller PG, et al (1987) Prognostic factors associated with radical hysterectomy failure. Gynecol Oncol 26: 153–159

50. Carmichael JA, Clarke DH, Moher D, et al (1986) Cervical carcinoma of women aged 34 and younger. Am J Obstet Gynecol 154: 264–269

51. Cherry CP, Glucksmann A (1955) Lymphatic embolism and lumph node metastasis in cancers of vulva and of uterine cervix. Cancer 8: 564

52. Cherry CP, Glucksmann A (1955) Lymphatic embolism and lumph node metastasis in cancers of vulva and of uterine cervix. Cancer 8: 564

53. Chilvers C, Mant D, Pike MC (1987) Cervical adenocarcinoma and oral contraceptives. Br Med J 295: 1446–1447

54. Christophersen WM, Parker JE (1964) Microinvasive carcinoma of the uterine cervix: A clinical-pathological study. Cancer 17: 1123

55. Chua S, Viegas OA, Wee A, et al (1989) Malignant melanoma of the cervix. Gynecol Obstet Invest 27: 107–109

56. Chung CK, Stryker JA, Ward SP, et al (1981) Histologic grade and prognosis of carcinoma of the cervix. Obstet Gynecol 57: 636–642

57. Cid JM (1959) La pigmentation melanique de l'endocervcix Ann Anat Pathol 4: 617

58. Clement PB, Scully RE (1982) Carcinoma of the cervix: histologic types. Semin Oncol 9: 251–264

59. Cohen C, Shulman G, Budgeon LR (1982) Endocervical and endometrial adenocarcinoma. Am J Surg Pathol 6: 151–157

60. Colgan TJ, Auger M, McLaughlin JR (1993) Histopathologic classification of cervical carcinomas and recognition of mucin-secreting squamous carcinomas. Int J Gynecol Pathol 12: 64–69

61. Cook GA, Draper GL (1984) Cancer and carcinoma in situ in Great Britain. Br J Cancer 50: 367–375

62. Copeland LJ, Silva EG, Gershenson DM, et al (1992) Superficially invasive squamous cell carcinoma of the cervix. Gynecol Oncol 45: 307–312

63. Coppleson M (1970) The origin and nature of premalignant lesions of the cervix uteri. Int J Gynecol Obstet 8: 539

64. Coppleson M (1992) Early invasive squamous and adenocarcinoma of the cervix (F160 stage 1a): clinical features and management. In Coppleson M (eds) Gynecologic Oncology. Churchill Livingston, Edinburgh, pp 631–648

65. Cramer DW (1974) The role of cervical cytology in the declining morbidity and mortality of cervical cancer. Cancer 34: 2018–2027

66. Cramer DW, Cutler SJ (1974) Incidence and histopathol-

ogy of malignancies of the female genital organs in the United States. Am J Obstet Gynecol 118: 443

67. Creasman WF, Fetter BF, Clarke-Pearson DL, et al (1985) Management of stage IA carcinoma of the cervix. Am J Obstet Gynecol 153: 164–172

68. Creasman WT, Rutledge F (1972) Carcinoma in-situ of the cervix. Obstet Gynecol 39: 373–380

69. Crissman JD, Budhraja M, Aron BS, et al (1987) Histopathologic prognostic factors in stage II and III squamous cell carcinoma of the uterine cervix: An evaluation of 91 patients treated primarily with radiation therapy. Int J Gynecol Pathol 6: 97–103

70. Crissman JD, Makuch R, Budhraja M (1985) Histopathologic grading of squamous cell carcinoma of the uterine cervix: An evaluation of 70 stage IB patients. Cancer 55: 1590–1596

71. Crum CP (1993) Papillomavirus-related changes and premalignant and malignant squamous lesions of the uterine cervix. In: Clement PB, Young RH (eds) Tumors and Tumorlike Lesions of the Uterine Corpus and Cervix. New York, Churchill Livingstone, pp 51–83

72. Czernobilsky B, Kessler I, Lancet M (1974) Cervical adenocarcinoma in a woman on long-term contraceptives. Obstet Gynecol 1974: 517–521

73. Czernobilsky B, Moll R, Franke WW, et al (1984) Intermediate filaments of normal and neoplastic tissues of the female genital tract with emphasis on problems of differential dianosis. Pathol Res Pract 179: 31

74. D'Ardenne AJ (1989) Use of basement membrane markers in tumour diagnosis. J Clin Pathol 42: 449–457

75. Dabbs DJ, Geisinger KR, Norris HT (1986) Intermediate filaments in endometrial and endocervical carcinomas. Am J Surg Pathol 10: 568–576

76. Daroca PJ, Dhurandhar HN (1980) Basaloid carcinoma of the uterine cervix. Am J Surg Pathol 4: 235–239

77. Davis JR, Aristizabal S, Way DL, et al (1989) DNA ploidy, grade and stage in prognosis of uterine cervical cancer. Gynecol Oncol 32: 4–7

78. Davis JR, Moon LB (1975) Increased incidence of adenocarcinoma of uterine cervix. Obstet Gynecol 45: 79

79. DeBritton RC, Hildesheim A, DeLao SL, et al (1993) Human papillomaviruses and other influences on survival from cervical cancer in Panama. Obstet Gynecol 81: 19–24

80. Delgado G, Bundy BN, Fowler WC, et al (1989) A prospective surgical pathological study of stage I squamous carcinoma of the cervix: A Gynecologic Oncology Group study. Gynecol Oncol 35: 314–320

81. Demian SDE, Bushkin FL, Echevarria RA (1973) Perineural invasion and anaplastic transformation of verrucous carcinoma. Cancer 32: 395–401

82. Devesa SS (1984) Descriptive epidemiology of cancer of the uterine cervix. Obstet Gynecol 63: 605

83. Devesa SS, Young JL, Brinton LA, et al (1989) Recent trends in cervix uteri cancer. Cancer 64: 2184–2190

84. Diddle AW (1972) Carcinoma of the cervix uteri with metastases to the neck. Cancer 29: 452

85. Dinh TV, Woodruff JD (1985) Adenoid cystic and adenoid basal carcinomas of the cervix. Obstet Gynecol 65: 705–709

86. Donnan SP, Wong FW, Ho SC, et al (1989) Reproductive and sexual risk factors and human papilloma virus infection in cervical cancer among Hong Kong Chinese. Int J Epidemiol 18: 32–36

87. Doughtery CM, Cotten N (1964) Mixed squamous-cell and adenocarcinoma of the cervix: Combined, adenosquamous and mucoepidermoid types. Cancer 17: 1132

88. Dyson JED, Joslin CAF, Rothwell RI, et al (1987) Flow cytofluorometric evidence for the differential radioresponsiveness of aneuploid and diploid cervix tumors. Radiother Oncol 8: 263–272

89. Ehrmann RL, Dwyer IM, Yavner D, et al (1988) An immunoperoxidase study of laminin and type IV collagen distribution in carcinoma of the cervix and vulva. Obstet Gynecol 72: 257–262

90. Eide TJ (1987) Cancer of the uterine cervix in Norway by histologic type, 1970–1984. J Natl Cancer Inst 79: 199–205

91. Eifel PJ, Morris M, Oswald J, et al (1990) Adenocarcinoma of the uterine cervix. Cancer 65: 2507–2514

92. Faaborg LL, Smith ML, Newland JR (1979) Case report: Uterine cervical and vaginal verrucous squamous cell carcinoma. Gynecol Oncol 8: 104

93. Fawcett KJ, Dockerty MB, Hunt AB (1966) Mesonephric carcinomas and adenocarcinomas of the cervix in children. J Pediatr 69: 104

94. Fay RA, Crandon AJ, Hudson CN, et al (1982) Cervical carcinoma associated with pregnancy. Lancet 2: 1213

95. Fennell RHJ (1978) Microinvasive carcinoma of the uterine cervix. Obstet Gynecol Surv 33: 406

96. Ferenczy A, Richard RM (1974) Female reproductive system. Dynamics of scan and transmission electron microscopy. New York, John Wiley & Sons

97. Ferry JA, Scully RE (1988) "Adenoid cystic" carcinoma and adenoid basal carcinoma of the uterine cervix. A study of 28 cases. Am J Surg Pathol 12: 134–144

98. Ferry JA, Scully RE (1990) Mesonephric remnants, hyperplasia, and neoplasia in the uterine cervix. A study of 49 cases. Am J Surg Pathol 14: 1100–1111

99. Fetissof F, Serres G, Arbeille B, et al (1991) Argyrophilic cells and ectocervical epithelium. Int J Gynecol Pathol 10: 177–190

100. Fidler HK, Boyes DA, Worth AJ (1968) Cervical cancer detection in British Columbia. J Obstet Gynecol Br Commonw 75: 392

101. Figge DC, Tamimi HK (1981) Patterns of recurrence of carcinoma following radical hysterectomy. Am J Obstet Gynecol 140: 213–220

102. Finck FM, Denk M (1970) Cervical carcinoma: relationship between histology and survival following radiation therapy. Obstet Gynecol 116: 339–343

103. Flint A, McCoy JP, Schade W, et al (1988) Cervical carcinoma antigen: distribution in neoplastic lesions of the uterine cervix and comparison to other tumor markers. Gynecol Oncol 30: 63–70

104. Fowler JWC, Miles PA, Surwit EA, et al (1978) Adenoid cystic carcinoma of the cervix—report of nine cases and a reappraisal. Obstet Gynecol 52: 337–342

105. Friedell GH, Tucker TC, McManmon E, et al (1992) Incidence of dysplasia and carcinoma of the uterine cervix in an Appalachian population. J Natl Cancer Inst 84: 1030–1032

106. Friedman HD, Adelson MD, Elder RC, et al (1992) Granulocytic sarcoma of the uterine cervix—literature review of

granulocytic sarcoma of the female genital tract. Gynecol Oncol 46: 128–137

107. Fu YS, Regan JW, Fu AS, et al (1982) Adenocarcinoma and mixed carcinoma of the uterine cervix. II. Prognostic value of nuclear DNA analysis. Cancer 49: 2571–2577

108. Gallup DG, Abell MR (1977) Invasive adenocarcinoma of the uterine cervix. Obstet Gynecol 49: 596–603

109. Gallup DG, Harper RH, Stock RJ (1985) Poor prognosis in patients with adenosquamous cell carcinoma of the cervix. Obstet Gynecol 65: 416–422

110. Gardner HL, Parsons L (1962) Blood vessel invasion in cancer of the cervix. Cancer 15: 1269

111. Gersell DJ, Mazoujian G, Mutch DG, et al (1988) Small-cell undifferentiated carcinoma of the cervix. A clinicopathologic, ultrastructural, and immunocytochemical study of 15 cases. Am J Surg Pathol 12: 684–698

112. Gilks CB, Clement PB (1992) Papillary serous adenocarcinoma of the uterine cervix: A report of three cases. Mod Pathol 5: 426–431

113. Gilks CB, Young RH, Aguirre P, et al (1989) Adenoma malignum (minimal deviation adenocarcinoma) of the uterine cervix. A clinicopathological and immunohistochemical analysis of 26 cases. Am J Surg Pathol 13: 717–729

114. Girardi F, Fuchs P, Haas J (1992) Prognostic importance of human papillomavirus type 16 DNA in cervical cancer. Cancer 69: 2502–2504

115. Glucksmann A, Cherry CP (1956) Incidence, histology and response to radiation of mixed carcinomas (adenocanthomas) of the uterine cervix. Cancer 9: 971

116. Glucksmann A, Spear FG (1945) The qualitative and quantative histological wxamination of biopsy material from patients treated by radiation for carcinoma of the cervix uteri. Br J Radiol 18: 313

117. Goellner JR (1976) Carcinoma of the cervix. Clinicopathologic correlation of 196 cases. Am J Clin Pathol 66: 775–785

118. Gordon AN, Bornstein J, Kaufman RH, et al (1989) Human papillomavirus associated with adenocarcinoma and adenosquamous carcinoma of the cervix: Analysis by in situ hybridization. Gynecol Oncol 35: 345–348

119. Graham S, Priore R, Graham M, et al (1979) Genital cancer in wives of penile cancer patients. Cancer 44: 1870–1874

120. Greer BE, Figge DC, Tamimi HK, et al (1990) Stage IA2 squamous carcinoma of the cervix: Difficult diagnosis and therapeutic dilemma. Am J Obstet Gynecol 162: 1406–1411

121. Groben P, Reddick R, Askin F (1985) The pathologic spectrum of small cell carcinoma of the cervix. Int J Gynecol Pathol 4: 42–57

122. Hacker NF, Berek JS, Lagasse LD, et al (1982) Carcinoma of the cervix associated with pregnancy. Obstet Gynecol 59: 735–746

123. Hafiz MA, Kragel PJ, C. T (1985) Carcinoma of the uterine cervix resembling lymphoepithelioma. Obstet Gynecol 66: 829–831

124. Hakama (1982) Trends in the incidence of cervical cancer in the Nordic countries. In: Magnus K (eds) Trends in Cancer Incidence. Causes and Practical Implications. New York, Hemisphere, pp 279–292

125. Hakama M, Miller AB, Day NE (eds) (1986) Screening for Cancer of the Uterine Cervix. Vol 76, Lyons. IRAC Scientific Publications.

126. Hale RJ, Wilcox FL, Buckley CH, et al (1991) Prognostic factors in uterine cervical carcinoma: a clinicopathological analysis. Int J Gynecol Cancer 1: 19–23

127. Halpin TF, Hunter RE, Cohen MB (1989) Lymphoepithelioma of the uterine cervix. Gynecol Oncol 34: 101–105

128. Hannigan EV (1990) Cervical cancer in pregnancy. Clin Obstet Gynecol 33: 837–845

129. Hanselaar AG, Vooijs GP, Oud PS, et al (1988) DNA ploidy patterns in cervical intraepithelial neoplasia grade III, with and without synchronous invasive squamous cell carcinoma: Measurements in nuclei isolated from paraffin-embedded tissue. Cancer 62: 2537–2545

130. Hart WR, Norris HJ (1972) Mesonephric adenoarcinomas of the cervix. Cancer 29: 106–113

131. Hasumi K, Sakamoto A, Sugano H (1980) Microinvasive carcinoma of the uterine carvix. Cancer 45: 928

132. Hasumi K, Sugano H, Sakamoto G, et al (1977) Circumscribed carcinoma of the uterine cervix with marked lymphocytic infiltration. Cancer 39: 2503–2507

133. Hayashi Y, Hachisuga T, Iwasaka T, et al (1991) Expression of ras oncogene product and EGF receptor in cervical squamous cell carcinomas and its relationship to lymph node involvement Gynecol Oncol 40: 147–151

134. Helper TK, Dockerty MB, Randall LM (1952) Primary adenocarcinoma of the cervix. Am J Obstet Gynecol 63: 800–808

135. Herbst AL, Cole P, Norusis MJ, et al (1979) Epidemiologic aspects and factors related to survival in 384 registry cases of clear cell adenocarcinoma of the vagina and cervix. Am J Obstet Gynecol 135: 876–886

136. Higgins GD, Davy M, Roder D, et al (1991) Increased age and mortality associated with cervical carcinomas negative for human papillomvavirus RNA. Lancet 338: 910–913

137. Himmelmann A, Willen R, Iosif S, et al (1992) Prospective histopathologic malignancy grading to indicate the degree of postoperative treatment in early cervical carcinomas. Gynecol Oncol 46: 37–41

138. Holmquist ND, Torres J (1988) Malignant melanoma of the cervix. Report of a case. Acta Cytol 32: 252–256

139. Hopkins MP, Morley GW (1991) A comparison of adenocarcinoma and squamous cell carcinoma of the cervix. Obstet Gynecol 77: 912–917

140. Hopkins MP, Morley GW (1991) Stage 1B squamous cell cancer of the cervix: clinicopathologic features related to survival. Am J Obstet Gynecol 164: 1520–1529

141. Hopkins MP, Morley GW (1992) The prognosis and management of cervical cancer associated with pregnancy. Obstet Gynecol 80: 9–13

142. Hopkins MP, Schmidt RW, Roberts JA, et al (1988) Gland cell carcinoma (adenocarcinoma) of the cervix. Obstet Gynecol 72: 789–795

143. Hopkins MP, Schmidt RW, Roberts JA, et al (1988) The prognosis and treatment of stage I adenocarcinoma of the cervix. Obstet Gynecol 72: 915–921

144. Hopson L, Jones MA, Boyce CR, et al (1990) Papillary villoglandular carcinoma of the cervix. Gynecol Oncol 39: 221–224

145. Horowitz IR, Jacobson LP, Zucker PK, et al (1988) Epidemiology of adenocarcinoma of the cervix. Gynecol Oncol 31: 25–31

146. Hoskins WJ, Averette HE, Ng AB, et al (1979) Adenoid cystic carcinoma of the cervix uteri: Report of six cases and review of the literature. Gynecol Oncol 7: 371–384

147. Howe DT, Vincenti AC (1991) Is large loop excision of the transformation zone (LLETZ) more accurate than colposcopically directed punch biopsy in the diagnosis of cervical intraepithelial neoplasia? Br J Obstet Gynaecol 98: 588–591

148. Huffman JW (1948) Mesonephric remnants in the cervix. Am J Obstet Gynecol 56: 23–40

149. Hurt WG, Silverberg SG, Frable WJ, et al (1977) Adenocarcinoma of the cervix: Histopathologic and clinical features. Am J Obstet Gynecol 129: 304–315

150. Ikenberg H, Teufel G, Schmitt B, et al (1993) Human papillomavirus DNA in distant metastases of cervical cancer. Gynecol Oncol 48: 56–60

151. Inoue R (1984) Prognostic significance of the depth of invasion relating to nodal metastases, parametrial extension and cell types. Cancer 54: 1714

152. Inoue T, Chihara R, Morita K (1984) The prognostic significance of the size of the largest nodes in metastic carcinoma from the uterine cervix. Gynecol Oncol 19: 187

153. Inoue T, Morita K (1990) The prognostic significance of number of positive nodes in cervical carcinoma stages IB, IIA, and IIB. Cancer 65: 1923–1927

154. Ireland D, Cole S, Kelly P, et al (1987) Mucin production in cervical intraepithelial neoplasia and stage 1B carcinoma of cervix with pelvic lymph node metastases. Br J Obstet Gynaecol 94: 467–472

155. Ireland D, Hardiman P, Monaghan JM (1985) Adenocarcinoma of the uterine cervix: A study of 73 cases. Obstet Gynecol 65: 82–85

156. Iwasaka T, Yokoyama M, Oh-Uchida M, et al (1992) Detection of human papillomavirus genome and analysis of expression of c-myc and Ha-ras oncogenes in invasive cervical cancers. Gynecol Oncol 46: 298–303

157. Jacobsen A (1983) Ploidy level and short time prognosis of early cervix cancer. Radiother Oncol 1: 271–275

158. Jarrell MA, Heintz N, Howard P, et al (1992) Squamous cell carcinoma of the cervix: HPV 16 and DNA ploidy as predictors of survival. Gynecol Oncol 46: 361–366

159. Jennings RH, Barclay DL (1972) Verrucous carcinoma of the cervix. Cancer 30: 430–434

160. Ji HX, Syrijanen S, Klemi P, et al (1991) Prognostic significance of human papillomavirus (HPV) type and nuclear DNA content in invasive cervical cancer. Int J Gynecol Cancer 1: 59–67

161. Johansson O, Johansson JE, Lindberg LG, et al (1976) Prognosis recurrences and metastases correlated to histologic cell type in carcinoma of the uterine cervix. Acta Obstet Gynecol Scand 55: 255–259

162. Jones HW, Plymate S, F.B. G, et al (1976) Small cell nonkeratinizing carcinoma of the cervix associated with ACTH production. Cancer 38: 1629–1635

163. Jones MW, Silverberg SG (1989) Cervical adenocarcinoma in young women: Possible relationship to microglandular hyperplasia and use of oral contraceptives. Obstet Gynecol 73: 984–989

164. Jones MW, Silverberg SG, Kurman RJ (1992) Well-differentiated villoglandular adenocarcinoma of the uterine cervix: A clinicopathological study of 24 cases. Int J Gynecol Pathol 12: 1–7

165. Jones WH, Droegemueller W, Makowski ELA (1971) A primary melanocarcinoma of the cervix. Obstet Bynecol 111: 959

166. Junor EJ, Symonds RP, Watson ER, et al (1989) Survival of younger cervical carcinoma patients treated by radical radiotherapy in the West of Scotland 1964–1984. Br J Obstet Gynecol 96: 522–528

167. Kagan AR, Nussbaum H, Chan PY, Ziel HK (1973) Adenocarcinoma of the uterine cervix. Am J Obstet Gynecol 117: 464–468

168. Kaku T, Enjoji M (1983) Extremely well-differentiated adenocarcinoma ("adenoma malignum") of the cervix. Int J Gynecol Pathol 2: 28–41

169. Kaminski PF, Maier RC (1983) Clear cell adenocarcinoma of the cervix unrelated to diethylstilbestrol exposure. Obstet Gynecol 62: 720–727

170. Kaminski PF, Norris HJ (1983) Minimal deviation carcinoma (adenoma malignum) of the cervix. Int J Gynecol Pathol 2: 141–152

171. Kaminski PF, Norris HJ (1984) Coexistence of ovarian neoplasms and endocervical adenocarcinoma. Obstet Gynecol 64: 553–556

172. Kashimura M, Tsukamoto N, Matsukuma K, et al (1984) Verrucous carcinoma of the uterine cervix: Report of a case with follow-up of 6 1/2 years. Gynecol Oncol 19: 204–215

173. Kato H, Morioka H, Aramaki S, et al (1983) Prognostic significance of tumor antigen TA–4 in squamous cell carcinoma of the uterine cervix. Am J Obstet Gynecol 145: 350–354

174. Katz HJ, Davies JNP (1980) Death from cervix uteri carcinoma: The changing pattern. Gynecol Oncol 9: 86–89

175. Kenter GG, Cornelisse CJ, Aartsen EJ, et al (1990) DNA poidy level as a prognostic factor in low stage carcinoma of the uterine cervix. Gynecol Oncol 39: 181–185

176. Kenter GG, Cornelisse CJ, Jiwa NM, et al (1993) Human papillomavirus type 16 in tumor tissue of low-stage squamous carcinoma of the uterine cervix in relation to ploidy grade and prognosis. Cancer 71: 397–401

177. Kessler II (1977) Venereal factors in human cervical cancer: Evidence from marital clusters. Cancer 39: 1912–1919

178. Ketcham AS, Hoye RC, Taylor PT, et al (1971) Radical hysterectomy and pelvic lymphadenectomy for carcinoma of the uterine cervix. Cancer 28: 1272–1277

179. Kiang DT, Bauer GE, Kennedy BJ (1973) Immunoassayable insulin in carcinoma of the cervix associated with hypoglycemia. Cancer 31: 801–805

180. Kilkku P, Gronroos M (1982) Perioperative electrocoagulation of endocervical mucosa and later carcinomas of the cervical stump. Acta Obstet Gynecol Scand 61: 265–267

181. Killackey MA, Jones WB, Lewis JL (1986) Diagnostic conization of the cervix; Review of 460 consecutive cases. Obstet Gynecol 67: 766–770

182. King LA, Talledo OE, Gallup DG, et al (1989) Adenoid cystic carcinoma of the cervix in women under age 40. Gynecol Oncol 32: 26–30

183. King LA, Tase T, Twiggs LB, et al (1989) Prognostic significance of the presence of human papillomavirus DNA in patients with invasive carcinoma of the cervix. Cancer 63: 897–900

184. Kirk ME (1974) Carcinoma of the cervix, stage Ia. Hum Pathol 5: 253

185. Kiviat NB, Critchlow CW, Kurman RJ (1992) Reassessment of the morphological continuum of cervical intraepithelial lesions; does it reflect different stages in the progression to cervical carcinoma? In: Munoz N, Bosch F, Shah K, Mehens A (eds) The Epidemiology of Cervical Cancer and Human Papillomavirus. Lyons, I.A.R.C. pp 59–66

186. Kleine W, Rau K, Schwoeorer D, et al (1989) Prognosis of the adenocarcinoma of the cervix uteri: A comparative study. Gynecol Oncol 35: 145–149

187. Koldstad P (1989) Follow-up study of 232 patients with stage IA1 and 411 patients with stage IA2 squamous cell carcinoma of the cervix (microinvasive carcinoma). Gynecol Oncol 33: 265–272

188. Korhonen M, Stenback F (1984) Adenocarcinoma metastatic to the uterine cervix. Gynecol Obstet Invest 17: 57–65

189. Korhonen MO (1984) Adenocarcinoma of the uterine cervix. Prognosis and prognostic significance of histology. Cancer 53: 1760

190. Koss LG (1992) Diagnostic Cytology and Its Histopathologic Basis. New York, J. B. Lippincott Co

191. Koss LG, Brannan CD, Ashikari R (1970) Histologic and ultrastructural features of adenoid cystic carcinoma of the breast. Cancer 26: 1271

192. Koss LG, Stewart FW, Foote FW, et al (1963) Some histological aspects of behavior of epidermoid carcinoma in situ and related lesions of the uterine cervix Cancer 16: 1160–1211

193. Kottmeier, H-L (1976) Annual report on the results of treatment in carcinoma of the uterus, vagina and ovary. Vol 16, F160, Stockholm

194. Kottmeier HL (1961) Evolution et traitment des epitheliomas. Rev Fran Gynecol d'Obstet 56: 821–826

195. Kottmeier HL (1964) Surgical and radiation treatment of carcinoma of the uterine cervix. Acta Obstet Gynecol Scand 43 (suppl 2): 1–49

196. Koulos J, Wright TC, Follen MM, et al (1993) Relationships between cKi-ras mutations, HPV types and prognostic indicators in invasive endocervical adenocarcinomas. Gynecol Oncol 48:364–369

197. Kraus FT, Perez-Mesa C (1966) Verrucous carcinoma. Cancer 19: 26

198. Kudo R, Sasano H, Koizumi M, et al (1990) Immunohistochemical comparison of new monoclonal antibody IC5 and carcinoembryonic antigen in the differential diagnosis of adenocarcinoma of the uterine cervix. Int J Gynecol Pathol 9: 325–336

199. Kurman RJ, Norris HJ, Wilkinson E (1992) Atlas of Tumor Pathology, Third series, Fascicle 4, Tumors of the Cervix, Vagina and Vulva, Washington, D.C., Armed Forces Institute of Pathology 200. Lancaster WD, Castellano C, Santos C, et al (1986) Human papillomavirus deoxyribonucleic acid in cervical carcinoma from primary and metastic sites. Am J Obstet Gynecol 154: 115–119

201. Lanciano RM, Won M, Hanks GE (1992) A reappraisal of the International Federation of Gynecology and Obstetrics staging system for cervical cancer. A study of patterns of care. Cancer 69: 482–487

202. Lang G, Dallenbach-Hellweg G (1990) The histogenetic origin of cervical mesonephric hyperplasia and mesonephric adenocarcinoma of the uterine cervix studied with immunohistochemical methods. Int J Gynecol Pathol 9: 145–157

202a. Larsen NS (1994) Invasive cervical cancer rising in young white females. J Natl Cancer Inst 86: 6–7

203. Larsson G, Alm P, Gullberg B, et al (1983) Prognostic factors in early invasive carcinoma of the uterine cervix: A clinical, histopathologic, and statistical analysis of 343 cases. Am J Obstet Gynecol 146: 145–153

204. Lathrop JC (1967) Views and reviews: Malignant pelvic lymphomas. Obstet Gynecol 30: 137

205. Latour JPA (1961) Results in the management of preclinical carcinoma of the cervix. Am J Obstet Gynecol 81: 511

206. Lehn H, Ernst TM, Sauer G (1984) Transcription of episomal papillomavirus DNA in human condylomata acuminata and Buschke-Lowenstein tumors. J Gen Virol 65: 2003–2010

207. Leman MH, Benson WL, Kurman RJ, et al (1976) Microinvasive carcinoma of the cervix. Obstet Gynecol 48: 571

208. Leminen A, Paavonen J, Forss M, et al (1990) Adenocarcinoma of the uterine cervix. Cancer 65: 53–59

209. Lemoine NR, Hall PA (1986) Epithelial tumors metastatic to the uterine cervix. A study of 33 cases and review of the literature. Cancer 57: 2002–2005

210. Lindell A (1952) Carcinoma of the uterine cervix: Incidence and influence of age. A statistical study. Acta Radiother 92 (suppl): 1–102

211. Littman P, Clement PB, Henriksen B, et al (1976) Glassy cell carcinoma of the cervix. Cancer 37: 2238–2246

212. Lohe KJ (1978) Early squamous cell carcinoma of the uterine cervix. I. Definition and histology. Gynecol Oncol 6: 10

213. Lorincz AT, Reid R, Jenson AB, et al (1992) Human papillomavirus infection of the cervix: Relative risk associations of 15 common anogenital types. Am J Obstet Gynecol 79: 328–337

214. Lucas WE, Benirschke K, Lebherz RB (1974) Verrucous carcinoma of the female genital tract. Am J Obstet Gynecol 119: 435

215. Lucia SP, Mills H, Lowenhaupt E, et al (1952) Visceral involvement in primary neoplastic diseases of the reticuloendotelial system. Cancer 5: 1193

216. Luesley DM, Cullimore J, Redman CWE, et al (1990) Loop diathermy excision of the cevical transformation zone in patients with abnormal cervical smears Br Med J 300: 1690–1693

217. MacGregor JE, Moss SM, Parkin DM, et al (1985) A case-control study of cervical cancer screening in northeast Scotland. Br Med J 290: 1543–1546

218. Maes G, Fleuren GJ, Bara J, et al (1988) The distribution of mucins, carcinoembryonic antigen, and mucus-associated antigens in endocervical and endometrial adenocarcinomas. Int J Gynecol Pathol 7: 112–122

219. Maier RC, Norris HJ (1980) Coexistence of cervical intraepithelial neoplasia with primary adenocarcinoma of the endocervix. Obstet Gynecol 56: 361–364

220. Maier RC, Norris HJ (1982) Glassy cell carcinoma of the cervix. Obstet Gynecol 60: 219–224

221. Maiman M, Fruchter RG, DiMaio TM, et al (1988) Superficially invasive squamous cell carcinoma of the cervix. Obstet Gynecol 72: 399–403

222. Maiman M, Fructer RG, Segur E, et al (1988) Prevalence of

human immunodeficiency virus in a colposcopy clinic. JAMA 260: 2214–2215

223. Marcial WA, Bosch A (1970) Radiation-induced tumor regression in carcinoma of the uterine cervix. Prognostic significance. Am J Roentgenol 108: 113

224. Maruo T, Shibata K, Kimura A, et al (1985) Tumor-associated antigen, TA–4, in the monitoring of the effects of therapy for squamous cell carcinoma of the uterine cervix. Serial determinations and tissue localization. Cancer 56: 302–308

225. Matsuyama M, Inoue T, Ariyoshi Y, et al (1979) Argyrophil cell carcinoma of the uterine cervix with ectopic production of ACTH, B-MSH, Serotonin, histamine and amylase. Cancer 44: 1813–1823

226. Mazur MT, Battifora HA (1982) Adenoid cystic carcinoma of the uterine cervix: Ultrastructure, immunofluorescence and criteria for diagnosis. Am J Clin Pathol 77: 494–500

227. Mazur MT, Hsueh S, Gersell DJ (1984) Metastases to the female genital tract, analysis of 325 cases. Cancer 53: 1978–1984

228. McGowan L, Young RH, Scully RE (1980) Peutz-Jeghers syndrome with "adenoma malignum" of the cervix. A report of two cases. Gynecol Oncol 10: 125–133

229. McIndoe G-A, Robson MS, Tidy JA, et al (1989) Laser excision rather than vaporization: the treatment of choice for cervical intraepithelial neoplasia. Obstet Gynecol 74: 165–168

230. McIndoe WA, McLean MR, Jones RW, et al (1984) The invasive potential of carcinoma in situ of the cervix. Obstet Gynecol 64: 451–458

231. McKelvey JL, Goodlin RR (1963) Adenoma malignum of the cervix; a cancer of deceptively innocent histologic pattern. Cancer 16: 549

232. McNutt NS, Weinstein RS (1969) Carcinoma of the cervix. Deficiency of nexus intercellular junctions. Science 165: 597

233. Meanwell CA, Kelly KA, Wilson S, et al (1988) Young age as a prognostic factor in cervical cancer: Analysis of population based data from 10,022 cases. Br Med J 296: 386–391

234. Mestwerdt G (1947) Probeexzision und kolpposkopie in des fruhdiagnose des portiokarzinoms. Zentr Gynak 4: 326

235. Michael H, Grawe L, Kraus FT (1984) Minimal deviation endocervical adenocarcinoma: clinical and histologic features, immunohistochemical staining for carcinoembryonic antigen, and differentiation from confusing benign lesions. Int J Gynecol Pathol 3: 261–276

236. Mikuta JJ, Celebre JA (1969) Adenocarcinoma of the cervix. Obstet Gynecol 33: 753

237. Miles PA, Norris HJ (1971) Adenoid cystic carcinoma of the cervix: An analysis of 12 cases. Obstet Gynecol 38: 103

238. Miller AB, Lindsay J, Hill GB (1976) Mortality from cancer of the uterus in Canada and relationship to screening for cancer of the cervix. Int J Cancer 17: 602–612

239. Mills SE, Austin MB, Randall ME (1985) Lymphoepithelioma-like carcinoma of the uterine cervix. A distinctive, undifferentiated carcinoma with inflammatory stroma. Am J Surg Pathol 9: 883–889

240. Moll R, Levy R, Czernobilsky B, et al (1983) Cytokeratins of normal epithelial and some neoplasms of the female genital tract. Lab Invest 49: 599–610

241. Monaghan JM, Ireland D, Mor-Yosef S, et al (1990) Role of centralization of surgery in stage IB carcinoma of the cervix: a review of 498 cases. Gynecol Oncol 37: 206–209

242. Moore RB, Reagan JW, Schoenberg MD (1959) The mucins of the normal and cancerous uterine mucosa. Cancer 12: 215–221

243. Mordel N, Mor-Yosef S, Ben-Baruch N, et al (1989) Malignant melanoma of the uterine cervix: case report and review of the literature. Gynecol Oncol 32: 375–380

244. Munoz N, Bosch FX, de-SanJose S, et al (1992) The causal link between human papillomavirus and invasive cervical cancer: A population-based case-control study in Colombia and Spain. Int J Cancer 52: 743–749

245. Muntz HG, Ferry JA, Flynn D, et al (1991) Stage IE primary malignant lymphomas of the uterine cervix. Cancer 68: 2023–2032

246. Murdoch JB, Grimshaw RN, Monaghan JM (1991) Loop diathermy excision of the abnormal cervical transformation zone. Int J Gynecol Cancer 1: 105–111

247. Murdoch JB, Grimshaw RN, Morgan PR, et al (1992) The impact of loop diathermy on management of early invasive cervical cancer. Int J Gynecol Cancer 2: 129–133

248. Musa AG, Hughes RR, Coleman SA (1985) Adenoid cystic carcinoma of the cervix: A report of 17 cases. Gynecol Oncol 22: 167–173

249. Ng ABP, Atkin NB (1973) Histological cell type and DNA value in the prognosis of squamous cell cancer of uterine cervix. Br J Cancer 28: 322–331

250. Ng ABP, Reagan JW, Lindner EA (1972) The cellular manifestations of microinvasive squamous cell carcinoma of the uterine cervix. Acta Cytol 16: 5–13

251. Nogales F, Bottela-Llusia J (1965) The frequency of invasion of the lumph nodes in cancer of the uteri cervis: A study of the degree of extension in relation to the histological type of tumor. Am J Obstet Gynecol 93: 91

252. Noller KL, Decker GG, Dockerty MB, et al (1974) Mesonephric (clear cell) carcinoma of the vagina and cervix. a retrospective analysis. Obstet Gynecol 640–644

253. Nunez C, Abdul-Karim FW, Somrak TM (1985) Glassy cell carcinoma of the uterine cervix. Acta Cytol 29: 303

254. Ocadiz R, Sauceda R, Cruz M, et al (1987) High correlations between molecular alterations of the c-myc oncogene and carcinoma of the uterine cervix. Cancer Res 47: 4173–4177

255. Okagaki R, Clark BA, Zachow KR, et al (1984) Presence of human papillomavirus in verroucous carcinoma (Ackerman) of the vagina. Arch Pathol Lab Med 108: 567

256. Orr JW, Shingleton HM (1983) Cancer in pregnancy. In: Cancer VIII. Chicago, Year Book Medical Publishers

257. Ostor AG (1993) Natural history of cervical intraepithelial neoplasia: A critical review. Int J Gynecol Pathol 12: 186–192

258. Pagnini CA, Palma PD, DeLaurentiis G (1980) Malignancy grading in squamous carcinoma of the cervix treated by surgery. Br J Cancer 41: 467–480

259. Papadia S (1962) Mucinous patterns in epidermoid carcinomas. Gynecologia 153: 337

260. Parazzini F, La Vecchia C (1990) Epidemiology of adenocarcinoma of the cervix. Gynecol Oncol 39: 40–46

261. Parazzini F, La Vecchia C, Negri E, et al (1988) Risk factors for adenocarcinoma of the cervix: a case-control study. Br J Cancer 57: 201–204

262. Parkin MD (1988) Estimates of the worldwide frequency of sixteen major cancers in 1980. Int J Cancer 41: 184–197

263. Patridge EE, Murad R, Shingletonn HM, et al (1980) Verrucous lesions of the female genitalia. I. Giant condylomata. Am J Obstet Gynecol 137: 412–418

264. Patridge EE, Murad T, Shingleton HM, et al (1980) Verrucous lesions of the female genitalia. II. Verrucous carcinoma. Am J Obstet Gynecol 137: 419–424

265. Peel KR, Khoury GG, Joslin CAF, et al (1991) Cancer of the cervix in women under 40 years of age, a regional survey, 1975–1984. Br J Obstet Gynecol 98: 993–1000

266. Peng HQ, Liu SL, Mann V, et al (1991) Human papillomavirus types 16 and 33, herpes simplex virus type 2 and other risk factors for cervical cancer in Sichuan Province, China. Int J Cancer 47: 711–716

267. Pepe F, Pepe G, Guarnuto V, et al (1989) Cancer and pregnancy. Retrospective study on the frequency in 57,393 deliveries. G Ital Oncol 9: 77–79

268. Perez CA, Kurman RJ, Stehman FB, et al (1992) Uterine cervix. In: Hoskins W, Perez C, Young R (eds) Principles and Practice of Gynecologic Oncology. Philadelphia, J. B. Lippincott

269. Peters RK, Chao A, Mack TM, et al (1986) Increased frequency of adenocarcinoma of the uterine cervix in young women in Los Angeles County. J Natl Cancer Inst 76: 423–428

270. Peterson F (ed) (1989) Annual report on results of treatment in gynecologic cancer. F160 Vol 20, Stockholm

271. Plentyl AA, Friedman E (1971) Lymphatic system of the female genitalia. In: Cohen, MR. The Morphologic Basis of Oncologic Diagnosis and Therapy. Philadelphia, W. B. Saunders

272. Podczaski E, Kaminski PF, Pees RC, et al (1991) Peutz-Jeghers syndrome with ovarian sex cord tumor with annular tubules and cervical adenoma malignum. Gynecol Oncol 42: 74–78

273. Pratt JH, Jefferies JA (1976) The retained cervical stump. A 25 year experience. Obstet Gynecol 48: 711

274. Prempree T, Amornmarn R, Wizenberg MJ (1985) A therapeutic approach to primary adenocarcinoma of the cervix. Cancer 56: 1264–1268

275. Prempree T, Patanaphan V, Sewchand W, et al (1983) The influence of patients' age and tumor grade on the prognosis of carcinoma of the cervix. Cancer 51: 1764–1771

276. Pretorius R, Semrad N, Watring W, et al (1991) Presentation of cervical cancer. Gynecol Oncol 42: 48–53

277. Qizilbash A-H (1975) In situ and microinvasive adenocarcinoma of the uterine cervix. J Clin Pathol 64: 155–170

278. Qizilbash AH (1974) Papillary squamous tumors of the uterine cervix. A clincial and pathologic study of 21 cases. Am J Clin Pathol 61: 508–520

279. Raju KS, Kjorstad KE, Abeler V (1991) Prognostic factors in the treatment of stage 1B adenocarcinoma of the cervix. Int J Gynecol Cancer 1: 69–74

280. Rampone JF, Klem W, Kolstad P (1973) Combined treatment of stage 1b carcinoma of the cervix. Obstet Gynecol 41: 163

281. Randall ME, Andersen WA, Mills SE, et al (1986) Papillary squamous cell carcinoma of the uterine cervix: a clinicopathologic study of nine cases. Int J Gynecol Pathol 5: 1–10

282. Randall ME, Constable WC, Hahn SS, et al (1988) Results of the radiotherapeutic management of carcinoma of the cervix with emphasis on the influence of histologic classification. Cancer 62: 48–53

283. Rastkar G, Okagaki T, Twiggs LB, et al (1982) Early invasive and in situ warty carcinoma of the vulva: Clinical, histologic, and electron microscopic study with particular reference to viral association. Am J Obstet Gynecol 143: 814–820

284. Reagan JW, Ng ABP (1973) The cellular manifestations of uterine carcinogenesis. In: Norris NJ, Hertig AT, Abell MR (eds) The Uterus. Baltimore, Williams & Wilkins Co., pp 320–347

285. Reeves WC, Brinton LA, Garcia M, et al (1989) Human papillomavirus infection and cervical cancer in Latin America. N Engl J Med 320: 1437–1441

286. Reid R, Greenberg M, Jenson AB, et al (1987) Sexually transmitted papillomaviral infections I. The anatomic distribution and pathologic grade of neoplastic lesions associated with different viral types. Am J Obstet Gynecol 156: 212–222

287. Report TW (1982) Report of the Task Force of the Department of Health and Welfare of Canada. Cervical Cancer Screening Programs. The Walton Report. Can Med Assoc J 127: 581

288. Richard L, Guralnick M, Ferenczy A (1981) Ultrastructure of glassy cell carcinoma of cervix. Diagn Gynecol Obstet 3: 31

289. Riou G, Barrois M, Sheng ZM, et al (1988) Somatic deletions and mutations of c-Ha-ras gene in human cervical cancers. Oncogene 3: 329–333

290. Riou G, Barrois M, Tordjman I, et al (1984) Presence of papillomavirus genomes and amplification of the c-myr and s-Ha-ras oncogenes in invasive cancers of the uterine cervix. Can Roy Acad Sci (III) 299: 575–580

291. Riou G, Favre M, Jeannel D, et al (1990) Association between poor prognosis in early-stage invasive cervical carcinomas and non-detection of HPV DNA. Lancet 335: 1171–1174

292. Riou G, Le MG, Le Doussal V, et al (1987) c-myc proto-oncogene expression and prognosis in early carcinoma of the uterine cervix. Lancet ii: 761–763

293. Riou GF (1988) Protooncogenes and prognosis in early carcinoma of the uterine cervix. Cancer Surv 7: 441–456

294. Riou GF, Barrois M, Dutronquay V, et al (1985) Presence of papillomavirus DNA sequences, amplification of c-myc and c-Ha-ras ocogenes and enhanced expression of c-myc in carcinomas of the uterine cervix. In: Howley P, Broker T (eds) Papillomaviruses: Molecular and Clinical Aspects. New York, Alan R Liss, pp 47–56

295. Robboy SJ, Herbst AL, Scully RE (1974) Clear-cell adenocarcinoma of the vagina and cervix in young females: Analysis of 37 tumors that persisted or recurred after primary therapy. Cancer 34: 606

296. Roche WD, Norris HJ (1975) Microinvasive carcinoma of the cervix. The significance of lymphatic invasion and confluent patterns of stromal growth. Cancer 36: 180–186

297. Rosen Y, Dolan TE (1975) Carcinoma of the cervix with cylindromatous features believed to arise in mesonephric duct. Cancer 36: 1739–1747

298. Rubio CA (1974) Cytologic studies in cases with carcinoma in situ and microinvasive carcinoma of the uterine cervix. Acta Pathol Microbiol Scand A82: 161–168

299. Rutledge FN, Mitchell MF, Munsell m, et al (1992) Youth as a prognostic factor in carcinoma of the cervix: A matched analysis. Gynecol Oncol 44: 123–130

300. Sagae S, Kuzumaki N, Hisada T, et al (1989) ras Oncogene expression and prognosis of invasive squamous cell carcinomas of the uterine cervix. Cancer 63: 1577–1582

301. Saigo PE, Cain JM, Kim WS, et al (1986) Prognostic factors in adenocarcinoma of the uterine cervix. Cancer 57: 1584–1593

302. Santosa JT, Kucera PR, Ray J (1990) Primary malignant melanoma of the uterine cervix; two case reports and a century's review. Obstet Gynecol Surv 45: 733–740

303. Sassoon AF, Said JW, Nash G, et al (1985) Involucrin in intraepithelial and invasive squamous cell carcinomas of the cervix: An immunohistochemical study. Human Pathol 16: 467

304. Schmauz R, Okong P, deVilliers EM, et al (1989) Multiple infections in cases of cervical cancer from a high-incidence area in tropical Africa. Int J Can 43: 805–809

305. Schwartz SM, Weiss NS (1986) Increased incidence of adenocarcinoma of the cervix in young women in the United States. Am J Epidemiol 124: 1045–1047

306. Scully RE, Aguirre P, DeLellis RA (1984) Argyrophilia, serotonin, and peptide hormones in the female genital tract and its tumors. Int J Gynecol Pathol 3: 51–70

307. Scully RE, Poulson H, Sobin LH (1994) International histological classification and histologic typing of female genital tract tumors. Springer-Verlag, Berlin, in press

308. Sebbelov AM, Kjorstad KE, Abeler VM, et al (1991) The prevalence of human papillomavirus type 16 and 18 DNa in cervical cancer in different age groups: a study on the incidental cases of cervical cancer in Norway in 1983. Gynecol Oncol 41: 141–148

309. Sedlis A, Sall S, Tsukada Y, et al (1979) Microinvasive carcinoma of the uterine cervix: A clinical-pathologic study. Am J Obstet Gynecol 133: 64–74

310. Seltzer V, Sall S, Castadot MJ, et al (1979) Glassy cell cervical carcinoma. Gynecol Oncol 8: 141–151

311. Seski JC, Abell MR, Morley GW (1977) Microinvasive squamous carcinoma of the cervix. Definition, histologic analysis, late results of treatment. Obstet Gynecol 50: 410–414

312. Sevin BU, Nadji M, Averette HE, et al (1992) Microinvasive carcinoma of the cervix. Cancer 70: 2121–2128

313. Shingleton HM, Gore H, Bradley DH, et al (1981) Adenocarcinoma of the cervix. I. Clinical evaluation and pathologic features. Am J Obstet Gynecol 139: 799–814

314. Shorrock K, Johnson J, Johnson IR (1990) Epidemiological changes in cervical carcinoma with particular reference to mucin-secreting subtypes. Histopathology 17: 53–57

315. Sidhu GS, Koss LG, Barber HRK (1970) Relation of histologic factors to the response of stage I epidermoid carcinoma of the cervix to surgical treatment: Analysis of 115 patients. Obstet Gynecol 35: 329–338

316. Silcocks PBS, Moss SM (1988) Rapidly progressive cervical cancer: Is it a real problem? Br J Obstet Gynaecol 95: 1111–1116

317. Silcocks PBS, Thornton-Jones H, Murphy M (1987) Squamous and adenocarcinoma of the uterine cervix: a comparison using routine data. Br J Cancer 55: 321–325

318. Silverberg SG, Hurt WG (1975) Minimal deviation adenocarcinoma ("adenoma malignum") of the cervix: A reappraisal. Am J Obstet Gynecol 121: 971–975

319. Simon NL, Gore H, Shingleton HM, et al (1986) Study of superficially invasive carcinoma of the cervix. Obstet Gynecol 68: 19–24

320. Smedts F, Ramaekers F, Troyanovsky S, et al (1992) Keratin expression in cervical cancer. Am J Pathol 141: 497–511

321. Smiley LM, Burke TW, Silva EG, et al (1991) Prognostic factors in stage IB squamous cervical cancer patients with low risk for recurrence. Obstet Gynecol 77: 271–275

322. Society AC (1991) Cancer Facts and Figures—1991, Atlanta, American Cancer Society 323. Sorensen FB, Bichel P, Jakobsen A (1992) DNA level and stereologic estimates of nuclear volume in squamous cell carcinomas of the uterine cervix. A comparative study with analysis of prognostic impact. Cancer 69: 187–199

324. Sotto LSJ, Graham JB, Pickren JW (1960) Post-mortem findings in cancer of the cervix. Am J Obstet Gynecol 80: 106–168

325. Speers WC, Picaso LG, Silverberg SG (1983) Immunohistochemical localization of carcinoembryonic antigen in microglandular hyperplasia and adenocarcinoma of the endocervix. Am J Clin Pathol 79: 105–107

326. Spratt DW, Lee SC (1977) Verrucous carcinoma of the cervix. Am J Obstet Gynecol 129: 699–700

327. Sreekantaiah C, De Braekeleer M, Haas O (1991) Cytogenetic findings in cervical carcinoma. A statistical approach. Cancer Genet Cytogenet 53: 75–81

328. Stafl A, Mattingly RF (1975) Angiogenesis of cervical neoplasia. Am J Obstet Gynecol 121: 845–852

329. Steeper TA, Wick MR (1986) Minimal deviation adenocarcinoma of the uterine cervix. An immunohistochemical comparison with microglandular endocervical hyperplasia and conventional adenocarcinoma. Cancer 58: 1131–1138

330. Stendahl U, Willen H, Willen R (1979) Classification and grading of invasive squamous cell carcinoma of the uterine cervix. Acta Radiol Oncol 18: 481–496

331. Stendahl U, Willen H, Willen R (1980) Invasive squamous cell carcinoma of the uterine cervix. I. Definition of parameters in a histolopathologic malignancy grading system. Acta Radiol Oncol 19: 467–480

332. Stendahl U, Willen H, Willen R (1981) Invasive squamous cell carcinoma of the uterine cervix: II. Reproducibility of a histopathologic malignancy grading system. Acta Radiol 20: 65–70

333. Stewart CJR, McNicol AM (1992) Distribution of type IV collagen immunoreactivity to assess questionable early stromal invasion. Clin Pathol 45: 9–15

334. Stoler MH, Mills SE, Gersell DJ, et al (1991) Small-cell neuroendocrine carcinoma of the cervix. Am J Surg Path 15: 28–32

335. Strang P, Stendahl U, Frankendal B, et al (1986) Flow cytometric DNA patterns in cervical carcinoma. Acta Radiol Oncol 25: 249–254

336. Swan DS, Roddick JW (1973) a clinical-pathologic correla-

tion of cell type classification for cervical cancer. Am J Obstet Gynecol 116: 666–670

337. Szyfelbein WM, Young RH, Scully RE (1984) Adenoma malignum of the cervix. Cytologic findings. Acta Cytol 28: 691–698

338. Tamimi HK, Frigge DC (1982) Adenocarcinoma of the uterine cervix. Gynecol Oncol 13: 335–344

339. Tamimi HK, Gown AM, Kim-Deobald J, et al (1992) The utility of immunocytochemistry in invasive adenocarcinoma of the cervix. Am J Obstet Gynecol 166: 1655–1662

340. Tase T, Okagaki T, Clark BA, et al (1988) Human papillomavirus types and localization in adenocarcinoma and adenosquamous carcinoma of the uterine cervix: a study by in situ hybridization. Cancer Res 48: 993–998

341. Tateishi R, Wada A, Hayakawa K, et al (1975) Argyrophil cell carcinomas (Apudomas) of the uterine cervix. Light and electron microscopic observations of 5 cases. Virch Arch [A] 366: 257–274

342. Tattersall MHN, Coppleson M, Elliott PM (1992) Clinical invasive carcinoma of cervix: integration of chemotherapy with local treatment. In: Coppleson M (eds) Gynecologic Oncology. Edinburgh, Churchill Livingston

343. Teshima S, Shimosata Y, Kishi K, et al (1985) Early stage adenocarcinoma of the uterine cervix. Histopathologic analysis with consideration of histogenesis. Cancer 56: 167–172

344. Thelmo WL, Nicastri AD, Fruchter R, et al (1990) Mucoepidermoid carcinoma of the uterine cervix stage IB. Long-term follow-up, histochemical and immunohistochemical study. Int J Gynecol Pathol 9: 316–324

345. Tidbury P, Singer A, Jenkins D (1992) CIN 3: The role of lesion size in invasion. Br J Obstet Gynecol 99: 583–586

346. Tiltman AJ, Atad J (1982) Verrucous carcinoma of the cervix with endometrial involvement. Int J Gynecol Pathol 1: 221–226

347. Tomatis L (1990) Cancer: Causes, Occurrence and Control, Lyon, World Health Organization International Agency for Research on Cancer

348. Tsukamoto N, Nakamura M, Kashimura M, et al (1980) Primary cervical choriocarcinoma. Gynecol Oncol 9: 99–107

349. Twombley GH, Di Palma S (1951) Growth and spread of cancer of cervix uteri. Am J Roentgenol 65: 691–697

350. Valente PT, Susin M (1987) Cervical adenocarcinoma arising in florid mesonephric hyperplasia; report of a case with immunocytochemical studies. Gynecol Oncol 27: 58–68

351. van Nagell JR, Greenwell N, Powell DF, et al (1983) Microinvasive carcinoma of the cervix. Am J Obstet Gynecol 145: 981–991

352. Vesterinen E, Forss M, Nieminen U (1989) Increase of cervical adenocarcinoma: A report of 520 cases of cervical carcinoma including 112 tumors with glandular elements. Gynecol Oncol 33: 49–53

353. Vogel HP, Mendelsohn G (1987) Laminin immunostaining in hyperplastic, dysplastic, and neoplastic lesions of the endometrium and uterine cervix. Obstet Gynecol 69: 794–799

354. Wahlstrom T, Lindgren J, Korhonen M, et al (1979) Distinction between endocervical and endometrial adenocarcinoma with immunoperoxidase staining of carcinoembryonic antigen in routine histological tissue specimens. Lancet 2: 1159

355. Walker AN, Mills SE, Taylor PT (1988) Cervical neuroendocrine carcinoma; a clinical and light microscopic study of 14 cases. Int J Gynecol Pathol 7: 64–74

356. Walker J, Bloss JD, Liao S-Y, et al (1989) Human papillomavirus genotype as a prognostic indicator in carcinoma of the uterine cervix. Obstet Gynecol 74: 781–785

357. Way S (1980) Carcinoma metastatic to the cervix. Gynecol Oncol 9: 298

358. Wells M, Brown LJR (1986) Glandular lesions of the uterine cervix: The present state of our knowledge. Histopathology 10: 777–792

359. Wentz WB, Reagan JW (1959) Survival in cervical cancer with respect to cell type. Cancer 12: 384–388

360. Wheeler JD, Hertig AT (1955) The pathologic anatomy of carcinoma of the uterus. I. Squamous carcinoma of the cervix. Am J Clin Pathol 25: 345–375

361. Wheeless CR, Graham R, Graham JB (1970) Prognosis and treatment of adenoepidermoid carcinoma of the cervix. Obstet Gynecol 35: 928–932

362. White JE, Enterline JP, Alam A, et al (1980) Cancer among blacks in the United States—recognizing the problem. In: Mettlin C, Murphy G (eds) Cancer Among Black Populations. New York, Alan R Liss, pp 35–53

363. Wilczynski SP, Bergen S, Walker J, et al (1988) Human papillomavirus and cervical cancer: Analysis of histopathological features associated with different viral types. Hum Pathol 19: 697–704

364. Wilczynski SP, Walker J, Liao SY, et al (1988) Adenocarcinoma of the cervix associated with human papillomavirus. Cancer 62: 1331–1336

365. Wolff JP, Lacour J, Chassagne D, et al (1972) Cancer of the cervical stump. A study of 173 patients. Obstet Gynecol 39: 10–16

366. Yajima A, Fukuda M, Noda K (1984) Histopathological findings concerning the morphogenesis of mixed carcinoma of the uterine cervix. Gynecol Oncol 18: 157–164

367. Yamaski M, Tateishi R, Hongo J, et al (1984) Argyrophil small cell carcinomas of the uterine cervix. Int J Gynecol Pathol 3: 146–152

368. Yazigi R, Sandstad J, Munoz AK, et al (1990) Adenosquamous carcinoma of the cervix: Prognosis in stage IB. Obstet Gynecol 75: 1012–1015

369. Yee C, Krishnan-Hewlett Z, Baker CC, et al (1985) Presence and expression of human papillomavirus sequences in human cervical carcinoma cell lines. Am J Pathol 119: 361

370. Young RH, Clement PB (1991) Pseudoneoplastic glandular lesions of the uterine cervix. Semin Diagn Pathol 8: 234–249

371. Young RH, Scully RE (1988) Mucinous ovarian tumors associated with mucinous adenocarcinomas of the cervix. A clinicopathological analysis of 16 cases. Int J Gynecol Pathol 7: 99–111

372. Young RH, Scully RE (1989) Atypical forms of microglandular hyperplasia of the cervix simulating carcinoma. Am J Surg Pathol 13: 50–56

373. Young RH, Scully RE (1989) Villoglandular papillary adenocarcinoma of the uterine cervix. A clinicopathologic analysis of 13 cases. Cancer 63: 1773–1779

374. Young RH, Scully RE (1993) Minimal deviation endo-

metrioid adenocarcinoma of the uterine cervix: A report of five cases of a distinctive neoplasm that may be misinterpreted as benign. Am J Surg Pathol 17:660–665

375. Young RH, William R, Welch WR, et al (1982) Ovarian sex cord tumor with annular tubules. Review of 74 cases including 27 with Peutz-Jeghers syndrome and four with adenoma malignum of the cervix. Cancer 50: 1384–1402

376. Zaino RJ, Ward S, Delgado G, et al (1992) Histopathologic predictors of the behavior of surgically treated stage IB squamous cell carcinoma of the cervix. Cancer 69: 1750–1758

377. Zanetta G, Katzmann JA, Keeney GL, et al (1992) Flow-cytometric DNA analysis of stages IB and IIA cervical carcinomas. Gynecol Oncol 46: 13–19

378. Zhang YC, Zhang PF, Wei YH (1983) Metastatic carcinoma of the cervix uteri from the gastrointestinal tract. Gynecol Oncol 15: 287–290

379. zur Hausen H (1991) Human papillomaviruses in the pathogenesis of anogenital cancer. Virology 184: 9–13

9

Anatomy and Histology of the Uterine Corpus

Alex Ferenczy, M.D.

The first comprehensive description of the external anatomy of the human uterus was made by the Greek physician Soranus of Ephesus in the second century A.D.[77] Until the Renaissance in Europe, several misconceptions prevailed about the function and internal anatomy of the uterus. For example, it was believed that the cervix had a spongy consistency similar to that of the lungs and served the function of respiration. The theory of a multicompartmentalized uterus with seven chambers was held for centuries, until the anatomy of the uterus became better known when dissection of cadavers became a part of medical practice. Leonardo da Vinci in the 15th century and Vesalius in the 16th century demonstrated that the human uterus had a

single cavity lined by decidua and supported by muscular layers. In the 18th century, William Hunter described the gestational uterus including the placenta and the uteroplacental vascular system. Development of histology and microscopy led to an explosive growth of knowledge of the uterus, with detailed descriptions of the embryology by Müller in the 19th century and hormone-mediated cyclic endometrial changes by Hitschmann and Adler and later by Robert Schroeder in the early 20th century.

Embryology and Anatomy

The endometrium and myometrium are of mesodermal origin, and both structures are formed secondary to fusion of the müllerian ducts between the eighth and ninth postovulatory weeks.[68] Until the 20th week of gestation, the endometrium is composed of a single layer of columnar epithelium supported by a thick layer of fibroblastic stroma. By the 20th gestational week, the surface epithelium invaginates into the underlying stroma, forming glandular structures that extend toward the underlying myometrium. At birth the uterus measures about 4 cm in length, much of which is made up of the cervix (Fig. 9.1A). The endometrial surface and glands are lined by a low columnar to cuboidal epithelium, which in general is devoid of either proliferative or secretory changes; it resembles the inactive endometrium in menopausal or in castrated premenopausal women (Fig. 9.1B). The endometrial mucosa measures less than 0.5 mm in thickness.

During the prepubertal period, the endometrial mucosa

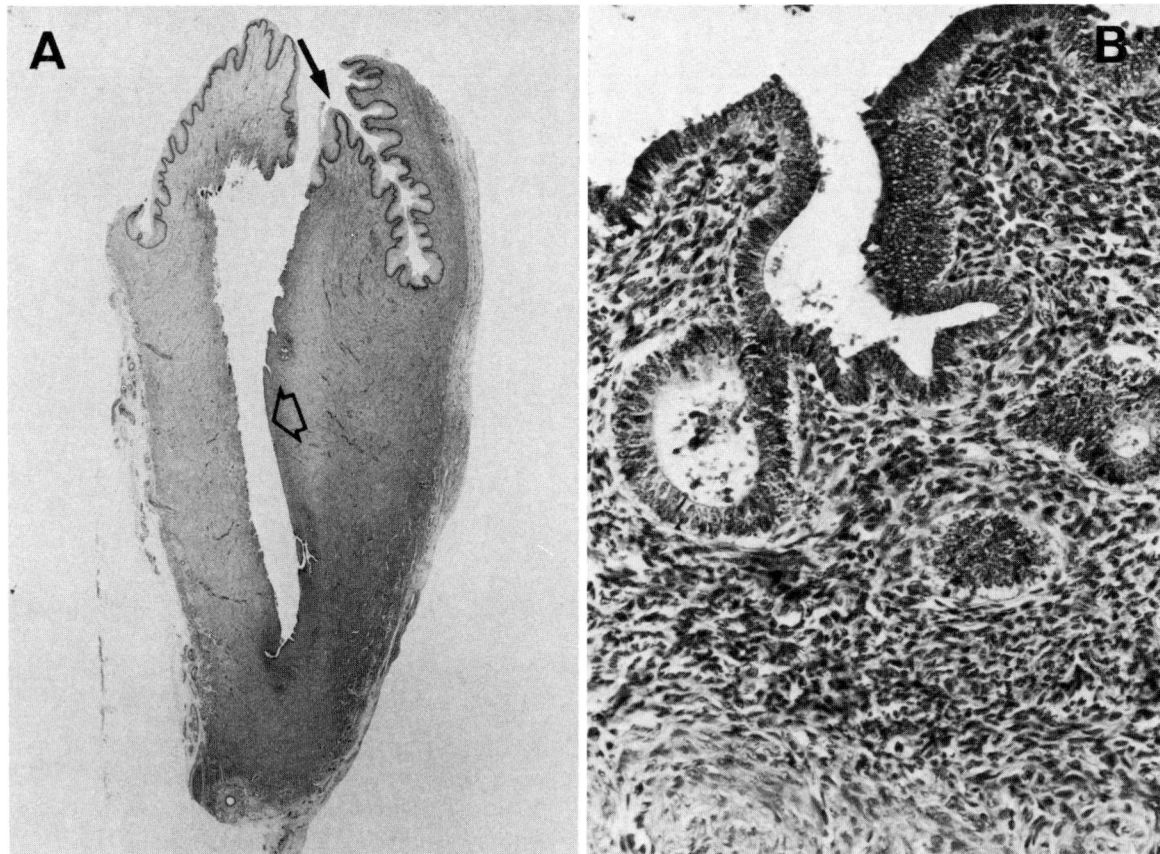

Fig. 9.1. Neonatal uterus. A: Whole mount section of a 4-day-old baby's uterus. The cervix (*narrow and open arrows*) is the dominant part of the uterus. **B:** The endometrium is thin and has few glands. The endometrial lining epithelium is of the inactive type. The stroma is dense and compact, resembling the basalis layer of the endometrium during the postpubertal period.

remains inactive, and the cervix comprises the predominant portion of the uterus. In the reproductive years, the size and weight of a normal uterus vary according to parity. In nulliparous women, it measures 8 cm in length, 5 cm in width at the fundus level, and 2.5 cm in thickness and weighs between 40 and 100 g. Multigravid uteri (four deliveries or more) measure about 10–12 cm × 5–7 cm × 2.5–3.5 cm and weight up to 250 g.[58] The corpus uterus is divided into fundus, corpus, and isthmus regions. The uterus is located between the rectum (posteriorly) and urinary bladder (anteriorly); it is supported by the round and utero-ovarian ligaments and is covered by the pelvic peritoneum. The endometrium during the reproductive period undergoes cyclic morphologic changes. These are particularly evident in the upper two-thirds of the mucosa, the so-called functionalis layer. Morphologic alterations are minimal in the lower one-third of the basalis layer. In postmenopausal life, the endometrium recapitulates the neonatal-fetal period, being thin with relatively few glands and lined by cuboidal epithelium that is devoid of proliferative or secretory activity (see section on inactive and atrophic endometrium).

Vascular Anatomy

The endometrial mucosa has an abundant vascular supply originating from the radial arteries of the underlying myometrium (Fig. 9.2). These penetrate the endometrium at regular intervals and give rise to the basal arteries. These in turn divide into horizontal and vertical branches, the former providing the blood supply to the basal layer of the endometrium and the latter to the overlying functionalis layer. The endometrial vessels in the functionalis layer are referred to as *spiral arterioles* (Fig. 9.2). Their development and arborization near the surface and their connections with the subsurface epithelial precapillary system, as well as extreme coiling during the menstrual cycle (Figs. 9.2, 9.3), are influenced by the ovarian steroid hormones and, presumably, prostaglandins.[7]

Histologically, the feature differentiating the endometrial and myometrial arteries is the absence of subendothelial elastica in the endometrial arteries except for the basal portion and its presence in the myometrial arteries (Fig. 9.4). Veins and lymphatics are closely associated with the endometrial arteries and glands, respectively. Uterine lym-

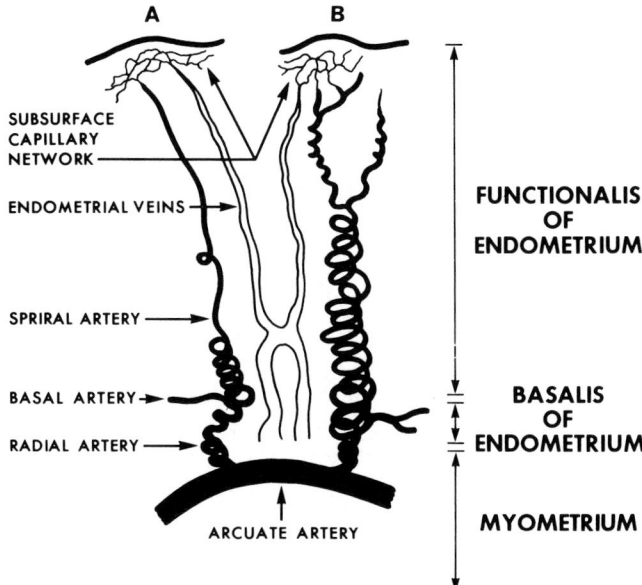

FIG. 9.2. Endometrial vessels. The coiled endometrial spiral arteries originate from the myometrial arcuate arteries and have connections with the subsurface capillary network, which in turn is drained by dilated veins. Arborization and coiling of spiral arteries are amplified in the postovulatory period (**B**) compared with the preovulatory phase (**A**) of the menstrual cycle.

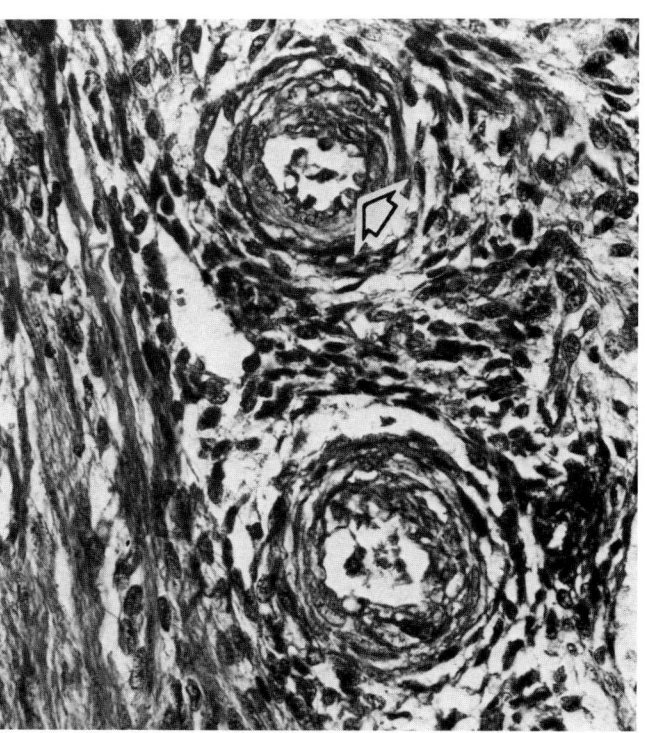

FIG. 9.4. Basal endometrial and myometrial arcuate arteries. Both arterial systems contain fine Weigert stain-positive elastic membranes (*arrow*) that presumably contribute to vascular constriction and ischemic necrosis during periods of menstruation. Elastica is absent in arteries of the endometrial functionalis.

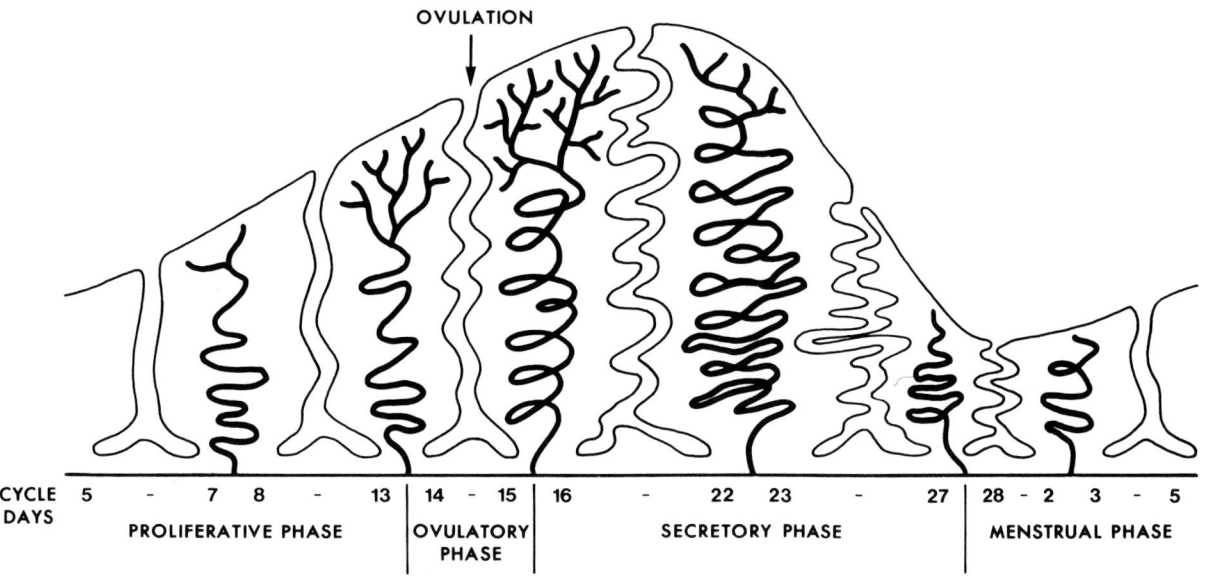

FIG. 9.3. Diagrammatic representation of endometrial vascular alterations during the menstrual cycle. There is a gradual increase in the arborization and coiling of spiral arteries during the preovulatory–ovulatory and postovulatory periods up to cycle days 23–25. The spiral arterial growth parallels the gradual increase in length and coiling of endometrial glands (*hollow tu-* *bules*). During the late secretory phase and menstrual period, collapse of the vascular and glandular systems predominates, whereas both the vessels and glands remain essentially unchanged in the lower one-third of the basal layer throughout the menstrual cycle.

phatics drain from subserosal uterine plexuses to the pelvic and periaortic lymph nodes.

Steroid Hormone, Receptor, and Immunopeptide Interactions in the Endometrial Cycle

The endometrial cycle in women follows a series of morphologic and physiologic events characterized by proliferation, secretory differentiation, degeneration, and regeneration of the uterine lining (Fig. 9.5). These alterations are controlled by cyclically released ovarian estradiol (E_2) and progesterone (P). The endometrium thus is a highly sensitive indicator of the hypothalamopituitary–ovarian axis and serves to determine whether the infertile patient has ovulatory cycles.[57] Steroid hormone control of endometrial, epithelial, stromal, and presumably endothelial cells is mediated by estrogen receptors (E_2R) and progesterone receptors (PgR). These steroid receptors are proteins concentrated in the nuclei of endometrial cells that have high affinity to bind E_2 and P, respectively.[52] Because they are sex steroid hormone (ligand)–specific, a particular receptor may display high affinity for a closely related class of hormones, and the same class may compete for available binding sites. For example, E_2R effectively binds not only E_2 but also estrone (E_1), as well as synthetic estrogens, such as diethylstilbestrol (DES).

Although E_2 has a crucial role in the proliferation of endometrial cells in vivo, E_2 alone is not able to induce

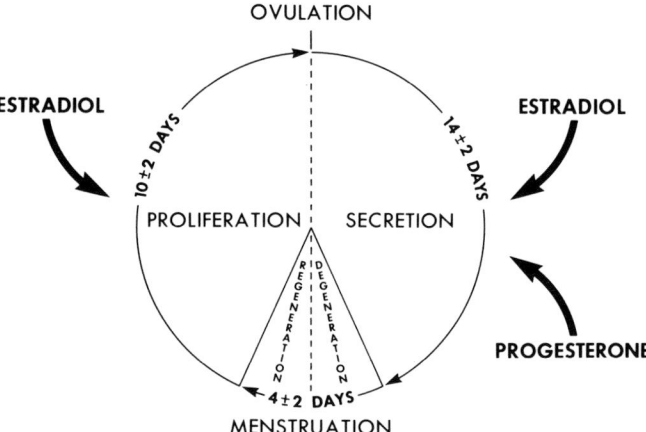

FIG. 9.5. Schematic representation of steroid hormone–morphologic interactions during the endometrial cycle. Estradiol promotes endometrial proliferation, whereas after ovulation, progesterone converts estradiol-primed endometrium into secretory tissue. Postovulatory estradiol amplifies the progesterone effect, and after withdrawal of both estradiol and progesterone, the endometrial mucosa degenerates and regenerates within the period of menstruation. (Reprinted by permission of Ferenczy A and Guralnick M (1983) Endometrial microstructure: Structure function relationships throughout the menstrual cycle. Semin Reprod Endocrinol 1:205.)

proliferation of endometrial cells in primary culture. Recent studies suggest that the mitogenic action of E_2 is mediated indirectly (paracrine) by a polypeptide growth factor, epidermal growth factor (EGF).[92] EGF promotes the transition of cells from G0 to G1 phase of the cell cycle.[37,82] Human endometrial cells have EGF receptors and m-RNA for EGF. EGF-like immunoreactivity is seen in both the endometrial glands and stromal cells, with higher concentrations in the glands than stroma, and parallels the fluctuation of cyclic sex steroids during the menstrual cycle. It appears that the regulation of EGF receptor content is regulated by ovarian estradiol and progesterone secretion (autocrine control). Indeed, EGF alone fails to influence cell proliferation but in combination with E_2 increases mean gland but not stromal cell counts more than 50% in vitro. The immunolocalization of EGF in normal human endometrium (Table 9.1) and the stimulation of gland cell proliferation in cultures by EGF and E_2 provide support for a role of EGF in uterine growth.[41,92]

Another proliferation-related protein is MAb 1BE12 antigen. This high molecular weight (>900 kDa) glycoprotein detects a breast cancer–associated protein and is detected also in the apical cytoplasm of normal proliferative but not secretory endometrial gland cells both in frozen and paraffin-embedded endometrium (Table 9.1). As a result, MAb 1BE12 activity is considered to be a cell proliferation marker.[13] MAb 1BE12 activity also shows some similarities with MSN-1MAb, an antibody raised against human endometrial carcinoma cells.[66] In one study, immunoreactivity with MAb 1BE12 was greater in carcinoma and atypical hyperplasia than in hyperplasia without significant cytologic atypia and normal proliferative endometrium.[13]

The concentrations of E_2R and PgR in the normal endometrium vary during the normal menstrual cycle according to fluctuating plasma levels of E_2 and P. The highest values of E_2R (400 fmol/mg protein) and PgR (1000 fmol/mg protein) concentrations occur during the midproliferative phase (8th–10th day of the cycle)[40,97] and correspond to rising plasma levels of E_2 during the preovulatory and early postovulatory secretory phases of the cycle. E_2 promotes the synthesis of both E_2R and PgR,[52] whereas P inhibits the synthesis of E_2R. Monoclonal antibodies to E_2R (estrophilin) derived from MCF-7 human breast cancer cell lines permit[39] the precise intracellular localization of E_2R by means of immunohistochemistry in frozen tissue sections.[10] Most of E_2R is localized in the nuclei rather than the cytoplasm of endometrial epithelial and stromal cells (Fig. 9.6). Endothelial cells fail to stain with antiestrophilin antibody. The concept of the mechanisms of sex steroid hormone–receptor action in target cells is illustrated in Fig. 9.7 and includes the following major steps: (1) circulating and unbound (from sex hormone–binding globulin) steroid hormone molecules are taken up from the cytoplasmic membrane presumably by cytoplasmic receptors, (2) the hormone molecules enter the nucleus, which contains most (90–95%) of the cellular receptors, (3) the

Table 9.1. Immunoreactivity of human endometrium during the menstrual cycle[a]

Antigen	Proliferative phase		Secretory phase		Presumed function
	Glands	Stroma	Glands	Stroma	
E$_2$R	+	+	+	+	Proliferation
PgR	+	+	+	+	Secretory differentiation
				(decidua +++)	
EGF	+	+	±	+	Proliferation
IGF-1	+	+	±	+	Proliferation
Ki67	+	±	+	+	Proliferation
			(POD 3)	(decidua +++)	
1BE12	+	−	−	−	Proliferation
pHER-2/neu	+	−	±	−	Proliferation
Cathespin	+	−	±	−	Proliferation
p.myc/RAS	−	−	−	−	—
HLA-DR	+	−	−	−	Proliferation
VLA-1	−	−	+	+	Proliferation
				(decidua +++)	
B72.3 (TAG-72)	−	−	+	−	Secretory differentiation
Placental protein 14	−	−	+		
Carbohydrate—type 3 chains (ABO)					Secretory differentiation (glycolysation)
A	+	−	−	−	
H	+	−	+	−	Secretory differentiation (glycolysation)
Sialyl T	+	−	+	−	Secretory differentiation (glycolysation)
Sialyl TN	−	−	+	−	Secretory differentiation (glycolysation)
Relaxin	+	−	+	+	Collagenolysis
				(decidua +++)	
CD13, CD10	−	+	−	+	Immunomodulators
				(decidua +++)	
Keratins (AE 1/3, CAM 5.2)	+	−	+	−	Cytoplasmic support
EMA	+	−	+	−	Epithelial differentiation
Vimentin	+	+	+	+	Cytoplasmic support
Desmin	−	+	−	+	
MSA	−	+	−	+	Mesenchymal cell migration and integrity?
α-SMA	−	+	−	+	Mesenchymal cell migration and integrity?
S-100	−	−	−	−	Mesenchymal cell migration and integrity?

[a] Heterogeneous distribution.
MSA, muscle-specific actin; α-SMA, smooth muscle actin; IGF-1, insulin-like growth factor 1 (evaluated in rats).
E$_2$R, estrogen receptor; PgR, progesterone receptor; EGF, epidermal growth factor; EMA, epithelial membrane antigen.

intranuclear hormone molecules induce conversion of the inactive (nonfunctional) 4S form of receptor to active (functional) 5S form of receptor, (4) the hormonally activated 5S receptor binds to acceptor genes in the nucleus and influences gene expression by stimulating RNA polymerase and thus messager RNA (mRNA) transcription, and (5) the newly formed mRNA is transported to the cytoplasm, where it is translated into proteins, including anabolic and catabolic enzymes as well as new receptors (receptor replenishment). According to this concept, the most significant effect of sex hormones is intranuclear activation of receptors that in turn initiate a sequence of events that lead to alterations in physiologic functions of target cells.

Morphology and Physiology of the Normal Endometrium

An awareness of the morphologic variation of the endometrium throughout the cycle is essential for documenting whether ovulation has occurred and to diagnose specific causes of infertility such as luteal phase defect. Endometrial dating, even in expert hands, is not highly reproducible. A discrepancy of 1–2 days in endometrial dating in relation to the calendar day on which subsequent menses occurs is generally acceptable. Unfortunately, in less experienced hands, diagnostic inconsistencies between evaluators of the same biopsies may be as high as 65%; the same pathologist even may be inconsistent in reading the same biopsy at different times in up to 27% of cases.[38] To avoid bias, the pathologist should read the clinical information, including the date of the last menstrual period, after evaluating the histologic section. The first day of bleeding is considered day 1 of the cycle (Fig. 9.8).[65]

The major morphologic features that occur in the endometrium throughout the cycle are shown in Fig. 9.8. During the proliferative phase, daily morphologic alterations are not sufficiently obvious to permit accurate dating. On the other hand, the daily changes in the endometrium during the postovulatory period are sufficiently distinct to permit accurate evaluation of the endometrial cycle.[42,65]

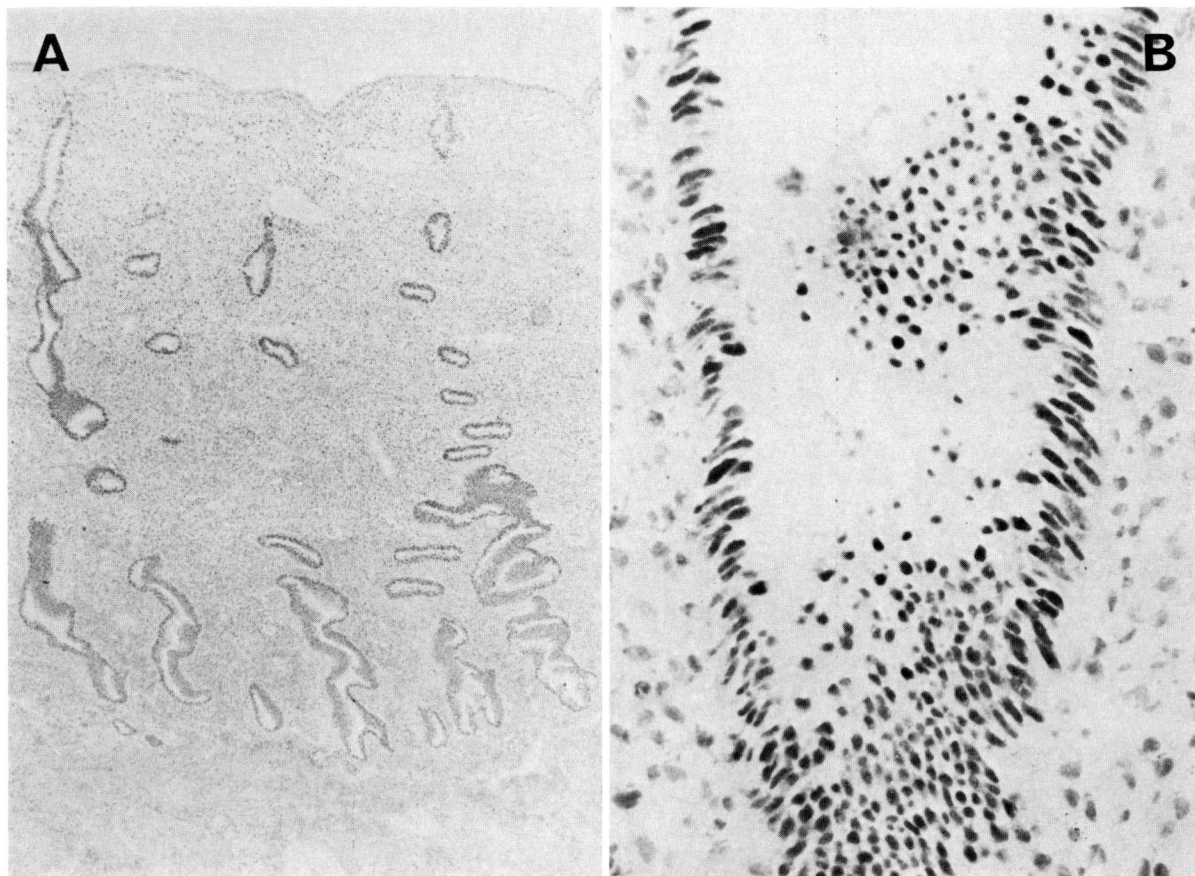

FIG. 9.6. Immunohistochemical localization of estrogen receptor (estrophilin). A: Estrogen receptors are present in midproliferative phase endometrium, as indicated by the dark (*gray to black*) diaminobenzidine reaction product within cell nuclei.

B: Receptors are localized to epithelial and stromal cell nuclei, although the intensity of specific staining is stronger in most epithelial cell nuclei than in most stromal cell nuclei. (Reprinted by permission of Press et al., ref. 75.)

Proliferative Phase

The preovulatory endometrium is characterized by proliferation of gland cells, stromal cells, and vascular endothelial cells, leading to an increase in the volume of the uterine mucosa. Synthesis of nuclear DNA is increased[22] (Fig. 9.9A), and mitoses are numerous (Fig. 9.9B). As a result, the straight glands in the early proliferative phase (Fig. 9.9C) become progressively more voluminous and tortuous (Fig. 9.10) during the mid- and late phases of proliferation. Increased nuclear DNA synthesis and mitotic activity in gland cells correlates with high levels of nucleolar organizer regions (NORs). These can be demonstrated by silver stains and are found on chromosomes 13–15, 21, and 22 as loops of DNA.[103] They are transcribed to ribosomal RNA and serve as an index of gland cell growth. The changes are under the influence of E_2, which stimulates the DNA-promoter enzyme, thymidilate synthetase.[27] The endometrium demonstrates zonal variations in its response to hormonal stimuli. For example, DNA synthesis is greater in the upper two-thirds of the functionalis of the fundus and corpus than in the lower third, the isthmic and cornual regions, and the basalis layer.[27] Both Ki67 and

HLA-DR as detected by immunostaining parallel the mitotic activity in gland cells during the preovulatory cycle and until the third postovulatory day. Expression of Ki67 is

---→

FIG. 9.7. Schematic representation of sex steroid hormone–receptor interaction in target cells. Circulating, free hormone molecule(s) following their passage through cell membranes are bound to cytoplasmic 4S receptors; the hormone–receptor complex is transported (*A*) to and in the nucleus, where the biologically active 5S steroid receptor complex is formed (*B*) from either the inactive 4S cytoplasmic steroid–receptor complex or by interaction of the 4S nuclear receptor with the steroid dissociated from 4S cytoplasmic receptor. The 5S receptor stimulates RNA polymerase and transcription (*C*) of messenger RNA; mRNA is transported (*D*) to cytoplasm, where it is translated (*E*) into new proteins related to physiologic cell functions. Most cellular receptors are intranuclear and are in equilibrium with small amounts of cytoplasmic receptors.

FIG. 9.8. Endometrial morphologic alterations during the menstrual cycle. (Adapted by permission of Noyes et al., ref. 65.)

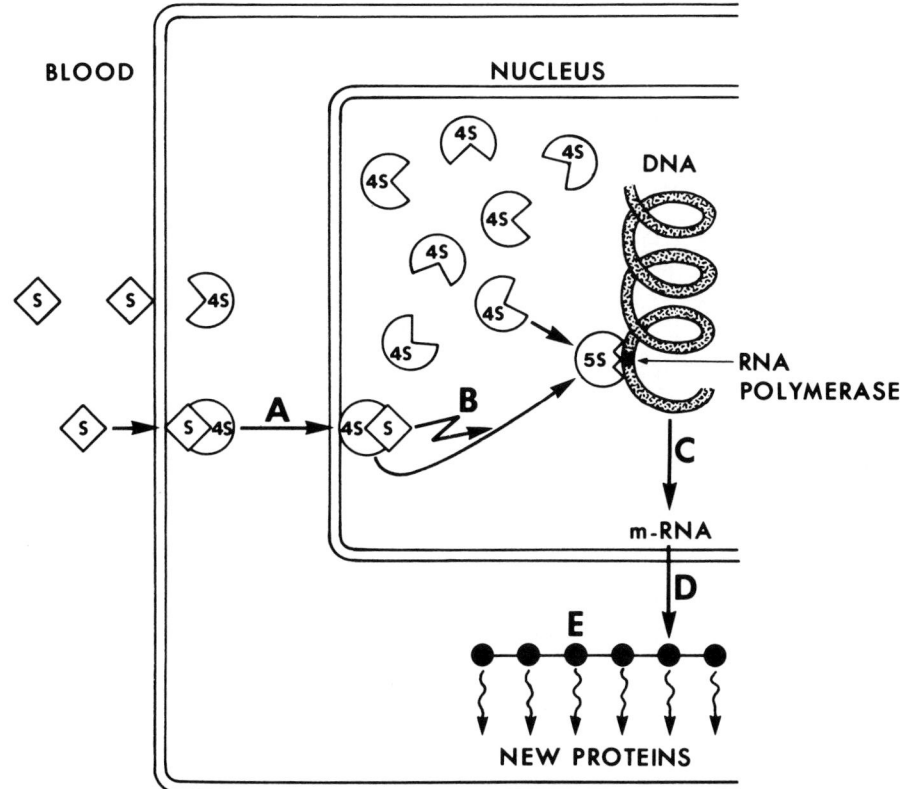

9.7

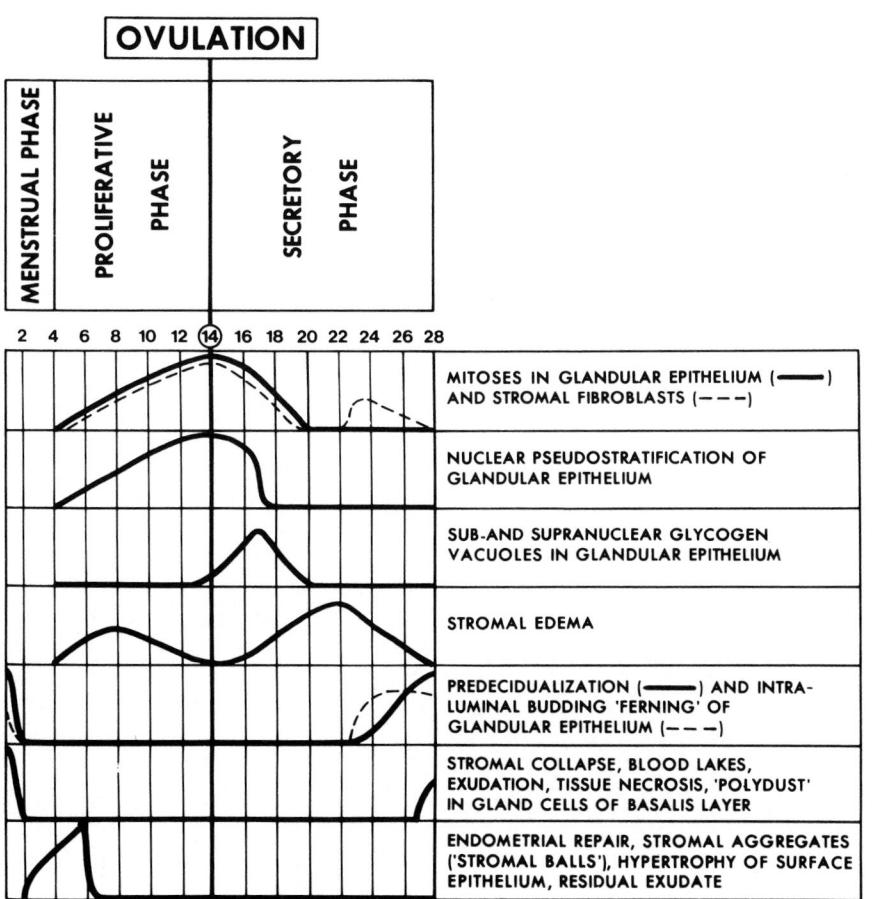

9.8

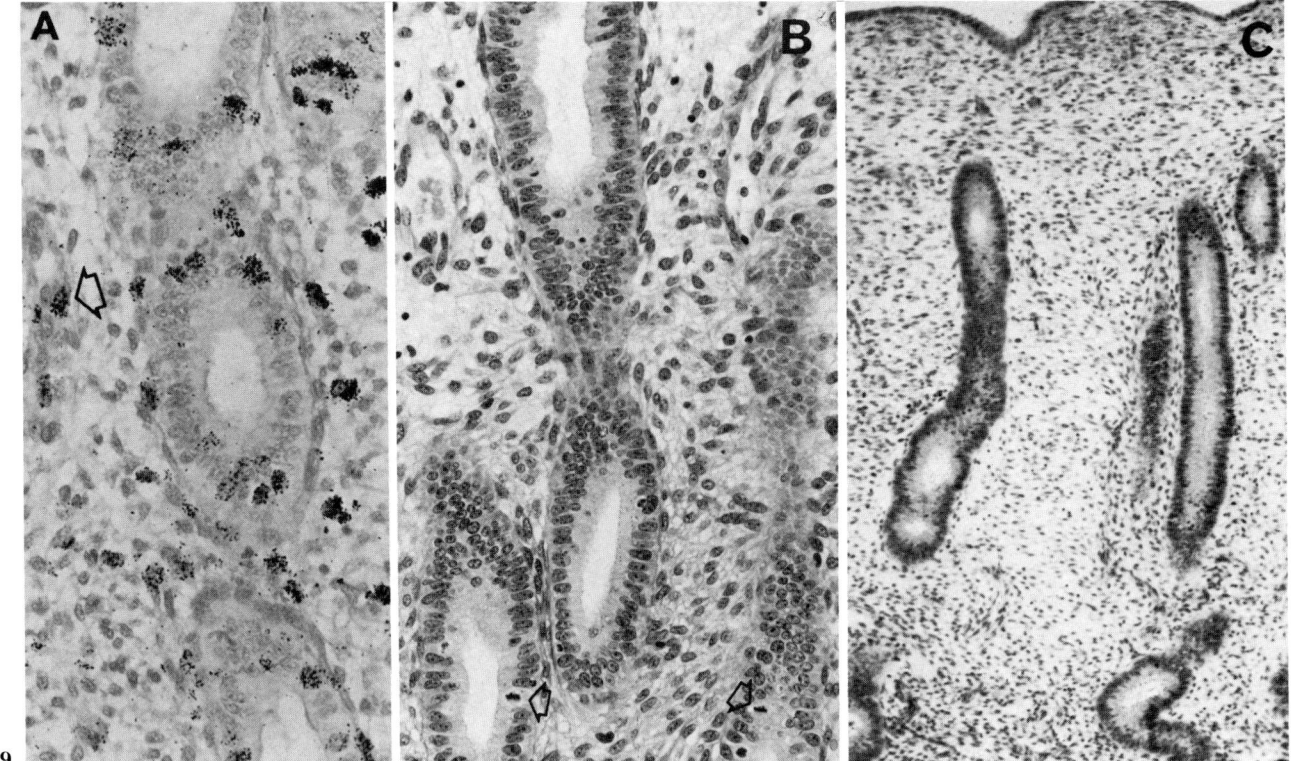

9.9

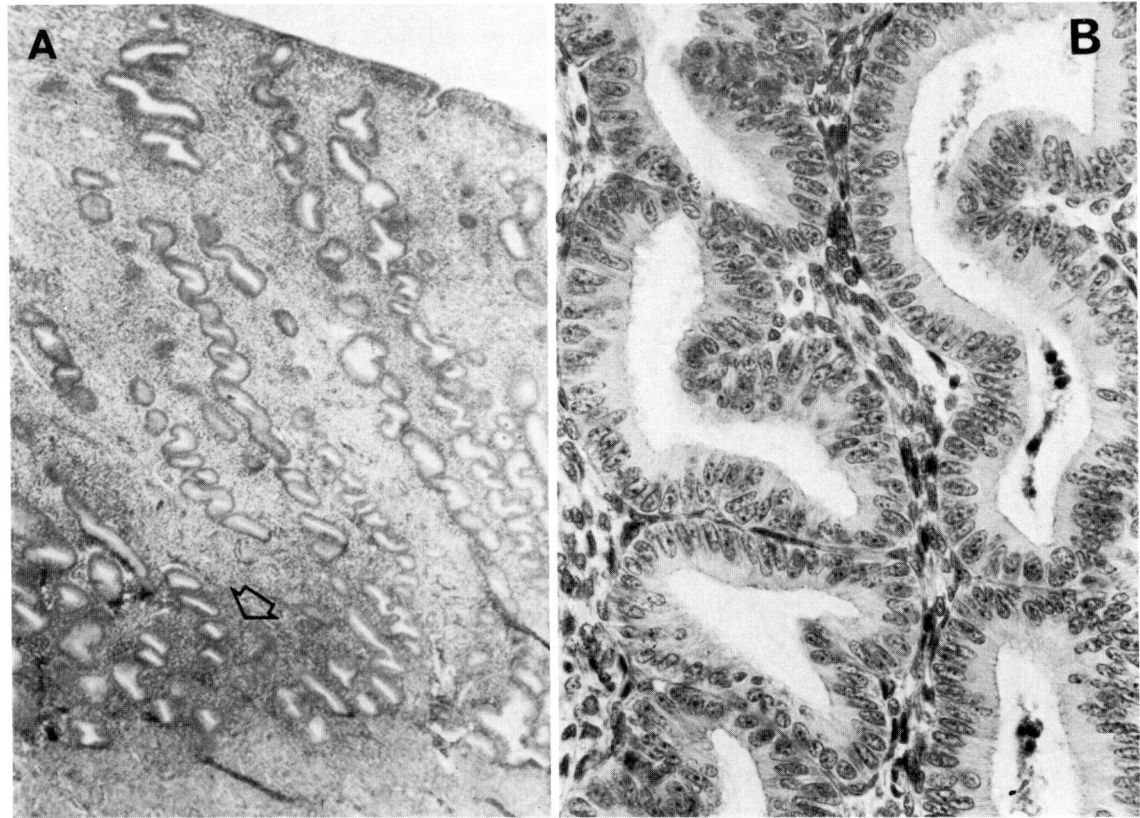

9.10

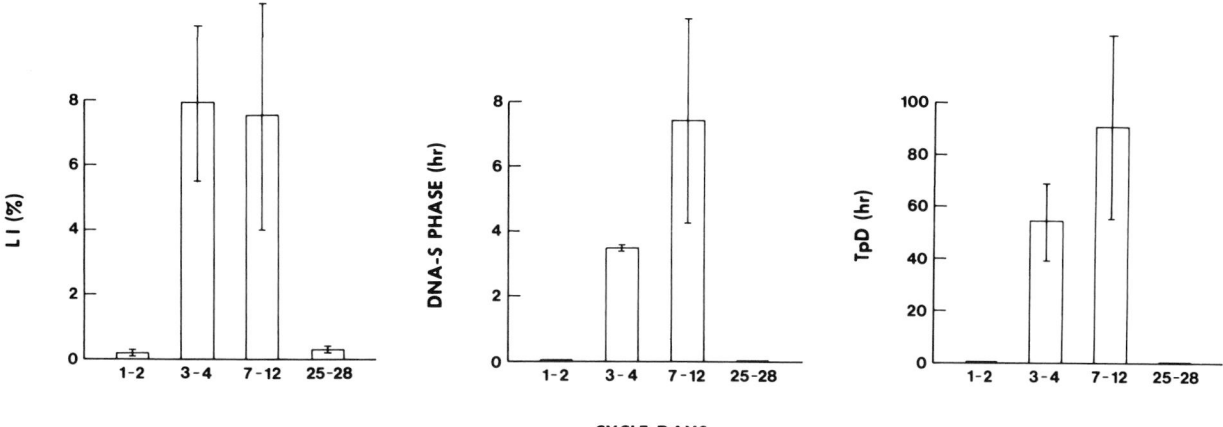

CYCLE DAYS

FIG. 9.11. Kinetic characteristics of the endometrium during the menstrual cycle according to in vitro historadioautography using the double-labeling technique with ³H-thymidine. Labeling index (*LI*), DNA synthesis phase (*DNA-S phase*), and potential doubling time (*TpD*) are negligible during the premenstrual and early menstrual periods. Note the sudden increase in LI and shortening of the DNA-S phase and tissue turnover time during the regenerative period on cycle days 3–4. The postregenerative period (cycle day 5 on) is characterized by prolongation of both the DNA-S phase and tissue turnover time. (Reprinted by permission of Ferenczy, ref. 26.)

comparatively greater in the functionalis than the basalis endometrium, whereas HLA-DR, one of the major class II histocompatibility antigens, is more evident in the basalis.[91] The geographic variation in the sensitivity of the endometrium to hormonal stimulation correlates with different biologic functions. The upper functional layer serves as the implantation site, providing an appropriate metabolic and physical environment for the implanted blastocyst. The lower functionalis provides the integrity of the endometrial mucosa. The maximum number of endometrial cells engaged in DNA synthesis is seen between cycle days 8 and 10 (Fig. 9.11) and corresponds to maximal mitotic activity, peak plasma E_2 levels, and maximum concentration of E_2R. The decline in the E_2-promoted DNA activity by days 11–14 (Fig. 9.11) when P levels are low is possibly related to endometrial refractoriness to relative hyperstimulation of the preovulatory endometrium by E_2. In addition to E_2, insulin-like growth factor (IGF-1) as well as agents that increase intracellular cyclic adenosine monophosphate (cAMP) stimulate PgR synthesis.[4]

In addition to growth promotion, E_2 stimulates the formation of ultrastructural organelles in gland cells and stromal cells as well as the vascular endothelium.[27] These include free and bound ribosomes, adenosine triphosphate (ATP)–rich mitochondria, and Golgi and primary lysosomes (Fig. 9.12A). These structures provide a protein matrix, energy, and synthesis and storage of enzymes, respectively. Endometrial enzymes, such as the Golgi-related lactate dehydrogenase, hexokinase, pyruvate kinase, and glucose-6-phosphatase (the last is especially abundant in the granular endoplasmic reticulum),[106] are all involved in carbohydrate metabolism during the postovulatory phase of the menstrual cycle. Acid phosphatase and presumably B-glucuronidase confined within membrane-bound primary lysosomes derived from the golgi complex contribute to endometrial destruction during the menstrual period.[43] Experimental studies[90] in animals reveal that sex steroid molecules may be transported from the cytoplasm into the nucleus by endometrial lysosomes that migrate into the nucleus. Some aspects of the glycosylation pattern in normal cyclic endometrium have been investigated by the use of monoclonal antibodies against mucin type 3 chain ABO-related antigens and their precursors.[79] Expression of these antigens is influenced not only by the erythrocyte ABO blood type, but also by the secretory genes (SE, se) and, in the endometrium, they may be hormonally regulated. Glands in the functionalis of proliferative endometrium express type 3 chain A, H, and

<hr />

FIG. 9.9. Proliferative endometrium. A: Historadioautography of proliferative endometrium, cycle day 12. Radiothymidine granules are heavily incorporated into the nuclei of endometrial gland cells, stromal fibroblasts, and capillary endothelium (*arrow*). **B:** Routine histologic staining of proliferative glands lined by columnar cells with pseudostratified, pencil-shaped nuclei. Mitoses (*arrows*) are seen. (Reprinted by permission of Ferenczy and Guralnick, ref. 24.) **C:** Cycle day 8. Straight glands with narrow lumens oriented perpendicular to the surface. The stroma is edematous and well vascularized.

FIG. 9.10. Proliferative endometrium, cycle day 12. A: Rows of voluminous, tortuous glands arranged at regular intervals characterize the preovulatory endometrium. The somewhat edematous stroma of the functionalis layer contrasts with the dense, compact stroma of the lower basalis layer (*arrow*). **B:** The glands have an S-shaped configuration, are closely apposed, and the lining cells have pseudostratified nuclei.

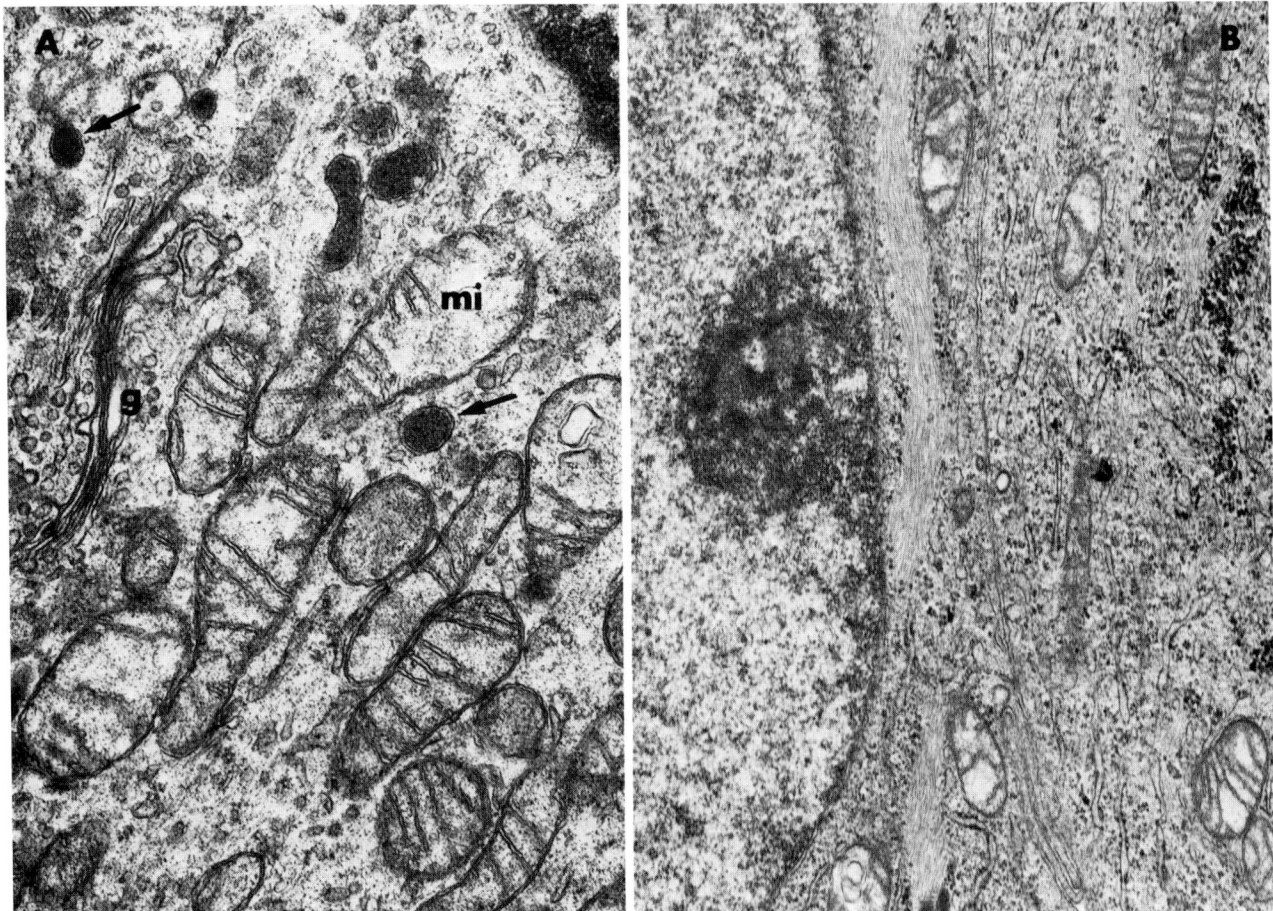

Fig. 9.12. Proliferative endometrium, cycle day 10. A: Gland cells have well-developed intracytoplasmic mitochondria (*mi*). The Golgi complex (*g*) has periogolgian vesicles from which originate membrane-bound, hydrolytic enzyme-containing electron-dense primary lysosomes (*arrows*) Free and bound ribosomes provide for basic proteins. ×32,000. **B:** Bundles of inter-mediate filaments serve as a cytoskeleton to tall, late proliferative endometrial gland cells. ×9000. (Reprinted by permission of Ferenczy A and Guralnick M (1983) Endometrial microstructure: Structure function relationships throughout the menstrual cycle. Semin Reprod Endocrinol 1:205.)

sialated T antigens, whereas in secretory glands, sialyl-T and sialyl TN antigens are observed (Table 9.1). Antigen expression is focal and is consistent with the increased synthesis of galactose, mannose, sialic acid, fucose, etc., and the apocrine and merocrine secretion of carbohydrates in glands in the secretory phase of the cycle.[79]

Characteristically, both the proliferative- and secretoary-type epithelial cells stain positively for cytokeratin and vimentin (AE 1-3 and CAM 5.2),[19] although vimentin is absent in glands of the late secretory phase endometrium (Table 9.1; Figs. 9.12B and 9.13).

Also, the surface and gland cells acquire numerous cilia and microvilli (Fig. 9.14A). Ciliary shafts have a strong forward and slow recovery ciliary beat pattern, and cilia are particularly numerous around gland openings (Fig. 9.14B).[23,24,26] These findings are consistent with their role in facilitating mobilization and distribution of endometrial secretions during the progestational phase of the menstrual cycle.[28] Surface microvilli are extensions of the cyto-plasmic substance and serve to increase the overall cell surface. This situation enhances excretory, secretory, and adsorptive functions of gland cells. Unlike endometrial ep-

Fig. 9.13. Immunohistochemistry of cyclic endometrium. A: Proliferative endometrium, intense transepithelial staining is observed only in gland cells. **B:** Secretory endometrium, cycle day 25 (POD 11), staining remains intense in the glnds, whereas none is found in the adjacent predecidual cells. Cytokeratin AE 1/3. **C:** In the proliferative endometrium, all elements including stromal fibroblasts, vessels, and to a lesser extent, the base of gland cells, demonstrate immunostaining. **D:** Secretory endometrium, cycle day 26 (POD 12). Staining is confined to predecidual and endothelial cells. Vimentin. **E:** Early secretory endometrium, 17th day (POD 3), staining is prominent in the apical portion of some gland cells (×500). **F:** Secretory endometrium, cycle day 26 (POD 12). Immunostaining is confined to the luminal surface membranes of gland cells B72.3.

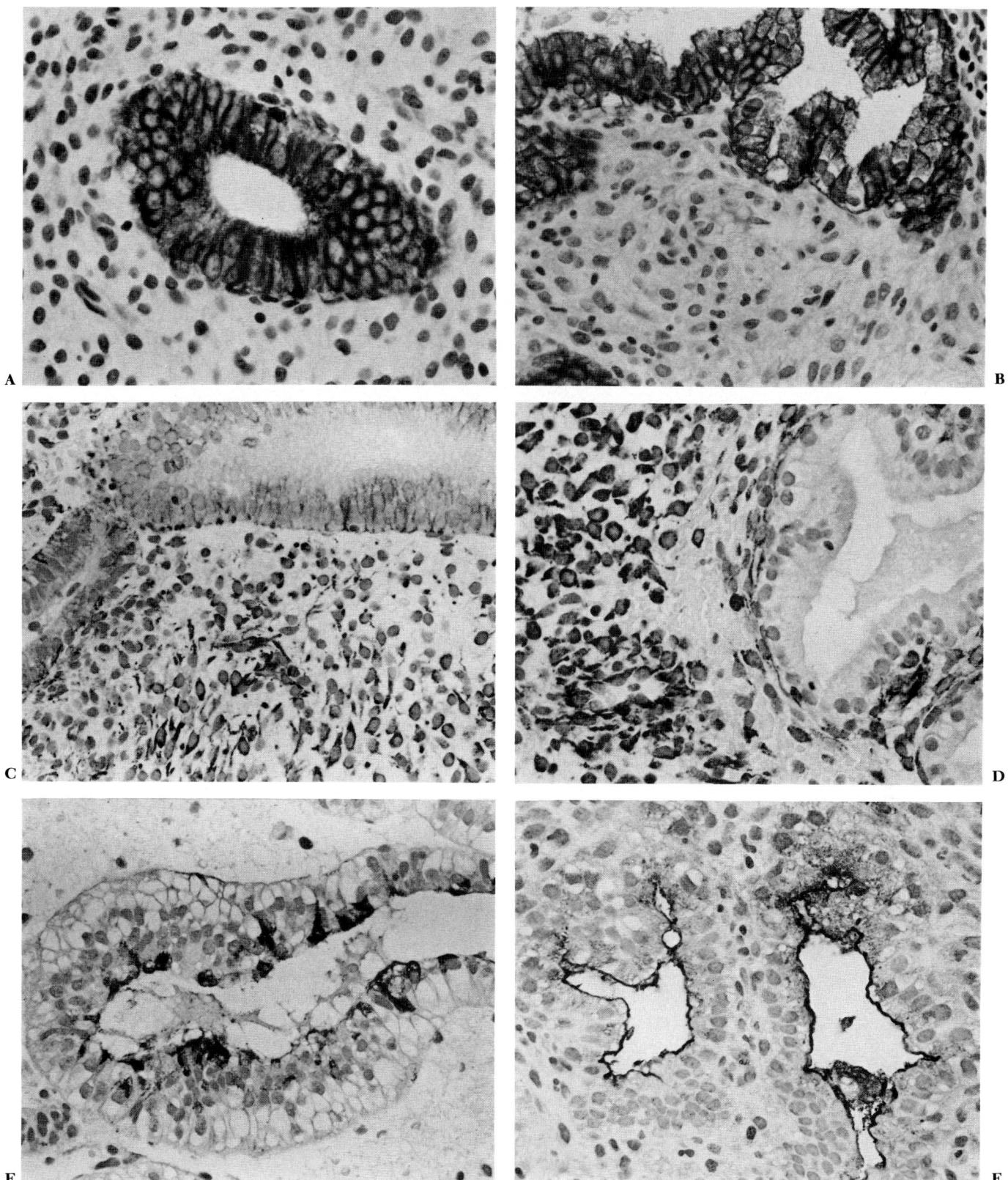

9.13

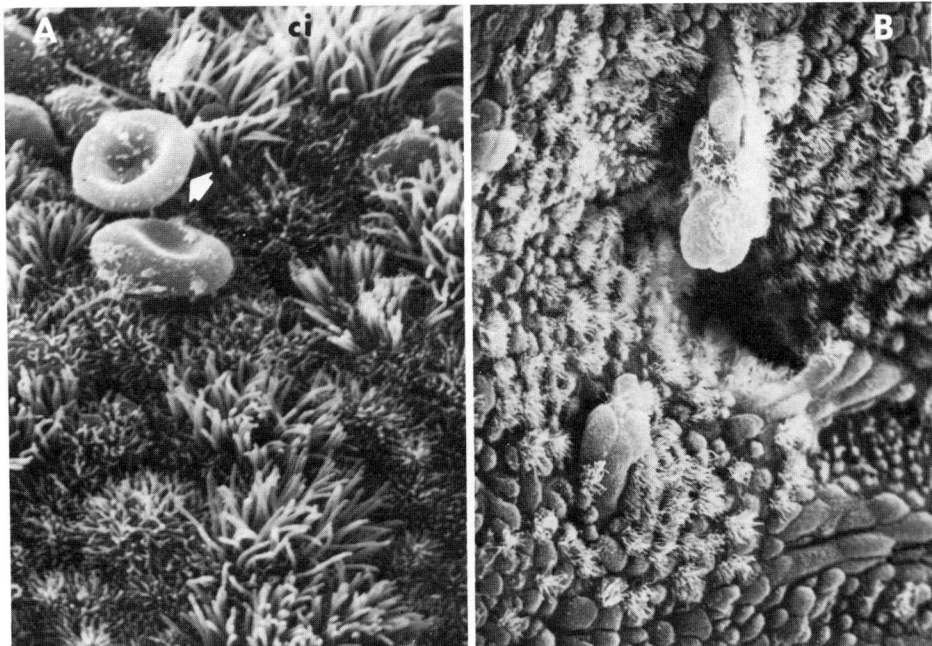

FIG. 9.14. Proliferative endometrium, cycle day 12. A: Scanning electron microscopy of surface epithelium with ciliated cells (*ci*) and microvillous cells. Red blood cells 7 μm in size (*arrow*) are seen. ×3000. B: On cycle days 5–6 the surface is completely repaired, and the gland openings are surrounded by ciliated cells. ×1000. (Reprinted by permission of Ferenczy A and Guralnick M (1983) Endometrial microstructure: Structure function relationships throughout the menstrual cycle. Semin Reprod Endocrino 1:205.)

ithelial cells, stromal cells do not react with cytokeratin but only with vimentin (Fig. 9.13) and smooth muscle–related antigens (Table 9.1).

Lymphoid aggregates resembling follicles (Fig. 9.15A) may be seen in the endometrial stroma, particularly during the proliferative phase of the cycle. Although they stain for IgA, IgM, or IgG, they are unlikely to play a significant role, if any, in the local secretory immune system. Indeed, endometrial epithelial cells synthesize negligible amounts of immunoproteins,[80] have few Langerhans' cells, and IgG-containing plasma cells are absent in normal endometria. The observations are consistent with the sterile nature of normal endometrium.

Secretory Phase

POSTOVULATION DAYS 1–3

After ovulation, under the influence of P, the E_2-primed endometrium undergoes rapid secretory differentiation.[27,65] The morphologic alterations that are used to date the endometrium are shown in Table 9.2. During cycle days 14 and 15 (postovulation day, POD 1), the morphology of the endometrium is not significantly different from that seen in the late proliferative phase of the menstrual cycle. On the 16th day (POD 2) of the cycle, small cylindrical vacuoles appear in the base of the gland cells in the functional layer. Otherwise, the epithelium is indistinguishable from that of the late proliferative phase; the

gland cells remain tall and the nuclei pseudostratified (Fig. 9.15B). Similar changes may be produced by estrogens alone in the absence of ovulation. As a result, incomplete or abortive subnuclear vacuolization is not considered specific to ovulation. Coinciding with the appearance of subnuclear vacuoles, the secretory gland endometrium acquires B72.3 and the very late antigen-1 (Table 9.1). The latter are heterodimers and belong to the integrin receptor super family and are related to maintaining cell shape, function, and integrity. Very late antigen-1 also is demonstrated in the predecidual cells during the secretory phase of the cell cycle. The first reliable histologic alterations that are considered specific to ovulation are seen on the 17th day (POD 3) of the cycle.[65] These include well-developed subnuclear glycogen vacuoles in gland-lining cells and palisading of gland-cell nuclei. Both phenomena involve every cell in a given gland (Fig. 9.16A, B).

Ultrastructurally[27,103] and histochemically,[79] the vacuoles correspond to pools of glycogen granules (Fig. 9.17A). Accumulation of glycogen and its synthesis are unique phenomena of the endometrium in that this occurs in the absence of excessive glycogen intake or exercise. Mitochondrial gigantism, with increased numbers of cristae (Fig. 9.17B), occurs in response to the increased demand for energy for glycogen metabolism.[103] The intracellular glycogen is broken down by enzymes of oxidative phosphorylation into glycoproteins and synthesized via the Golgi complex in the supranuclear region.

At the ultrastructural level, ovulation is manifested by

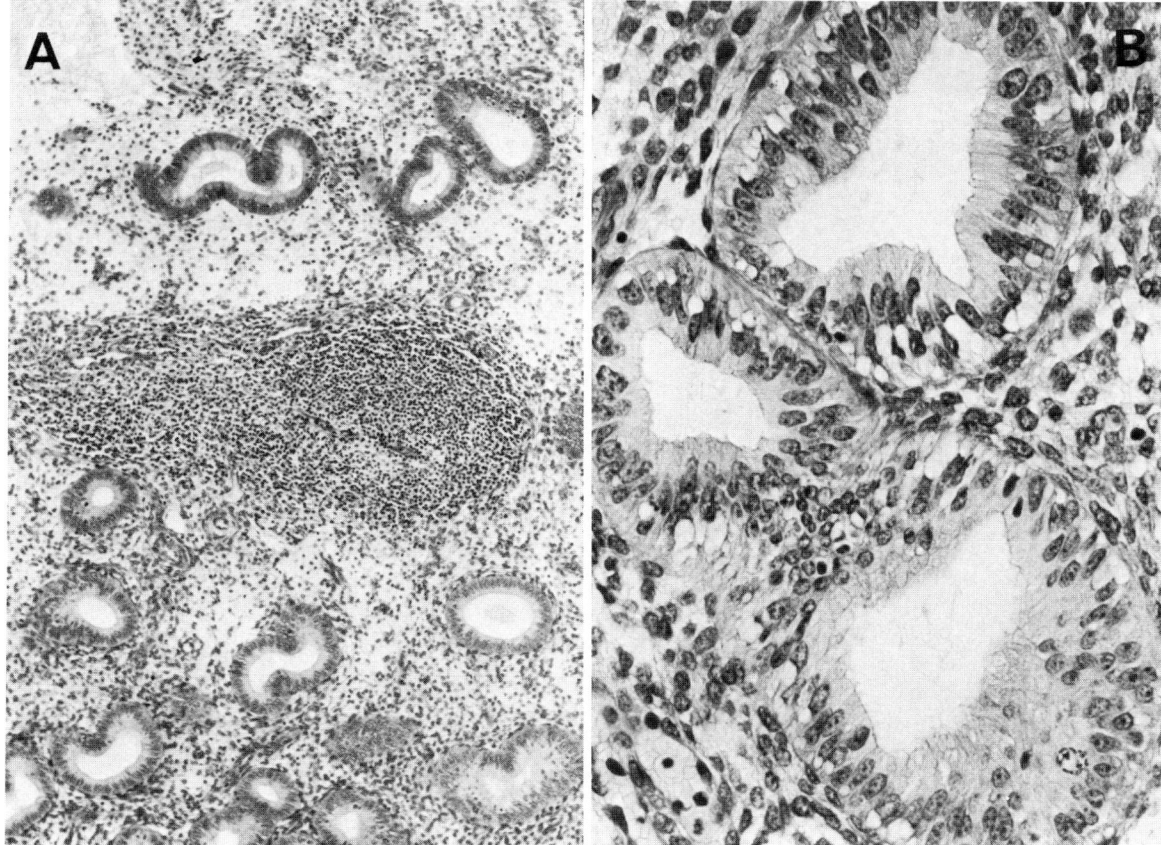

Fig. 9.15. Proliferative endometrium. A: Aggregates of mature lymphocytes forming lymphoid follicle-like structures in the basalis layer of the endometrium. **B:** Day 16 endometrium. Gland cells with small, abortive, subnuclear glycogen vacuoles. Many gland cells are devoid of vacuoles, and nuclear pseudostratification is maintained. The overall histology is that of glands of the late proliferative rather than the postovulatory phase. Similar changes may be seen in anovulatory endometrium.

the appearance of giant mitochondria and the so-called nucleolar channel system (NCS) formed by the helical infolding of the nuclear membranes into the nuclear or nucleolar substance[64] in glands cells (Table 9.1, Fig. 9.18A, B). NCS is seen as early as the 15th day of the cycle, but its significance is not known. These structures are unique to women and are seen only during the postovulatory phase.[103] However, NCS may be produced both in vivo and in vitro by progesterone or its synthetic variants,[76] and has been described in two cases of pelvic endometriosis.[47]

MAb B72.3 recognizes an epitope associated with a high molecular weight, mucin-like glycoprotein TAG-72;[96] intense B72.3 immunoreactivity is observed in the fundal endometrium only during the postovulatory phase of the cycle (Fig. 9.13), whereas staining is sporadic in the lower uterine segment (Table 9.1). In the latter, immunoreactivity is unrelated to cycle days. TAG72/B72.3 is thus a marker of ovulation in cyclic endometrium.[70] Another protein marker of secretory endometrium is placental protein 14 (PP14), which is synthesized in the endometrial glandular cells.[101]

Table 9.2. Morphologic evidence of ovulation

Morphology	Cycle days
Nucleolar channel system[a] in gland cells	15–25
Subnuclear vacuolization with nuclear palisading of gland cells	17–18
Stromal edema with ferning of glandular epithelium	22–23
Perivascular and stromal predecidualization	23–28
Diffuse predecidual and glandular necrosis, inflammation, and vascular thrombosis	1–2
Inflammatory exudate, aggregates of stromal cells (stromal balls) with or without hypertrophic surface epithelial cells, diffuse	2–4

[a] At transmission electron microscopic level.

POSTOVULATION DAYS 4–6

On cycle day 18 (POD 4) supranuclear vacuolization is established (Fig. 9.19A), and between days 19 and 20 (POD 5 and 6), the glycoprotein-rich and mucopolysaccharide-rich supranuclear cytoplasmic products are expelled into the glandular lumen by apocrine-type secretion.[103] This is characterized by protrusion and eventual detach-

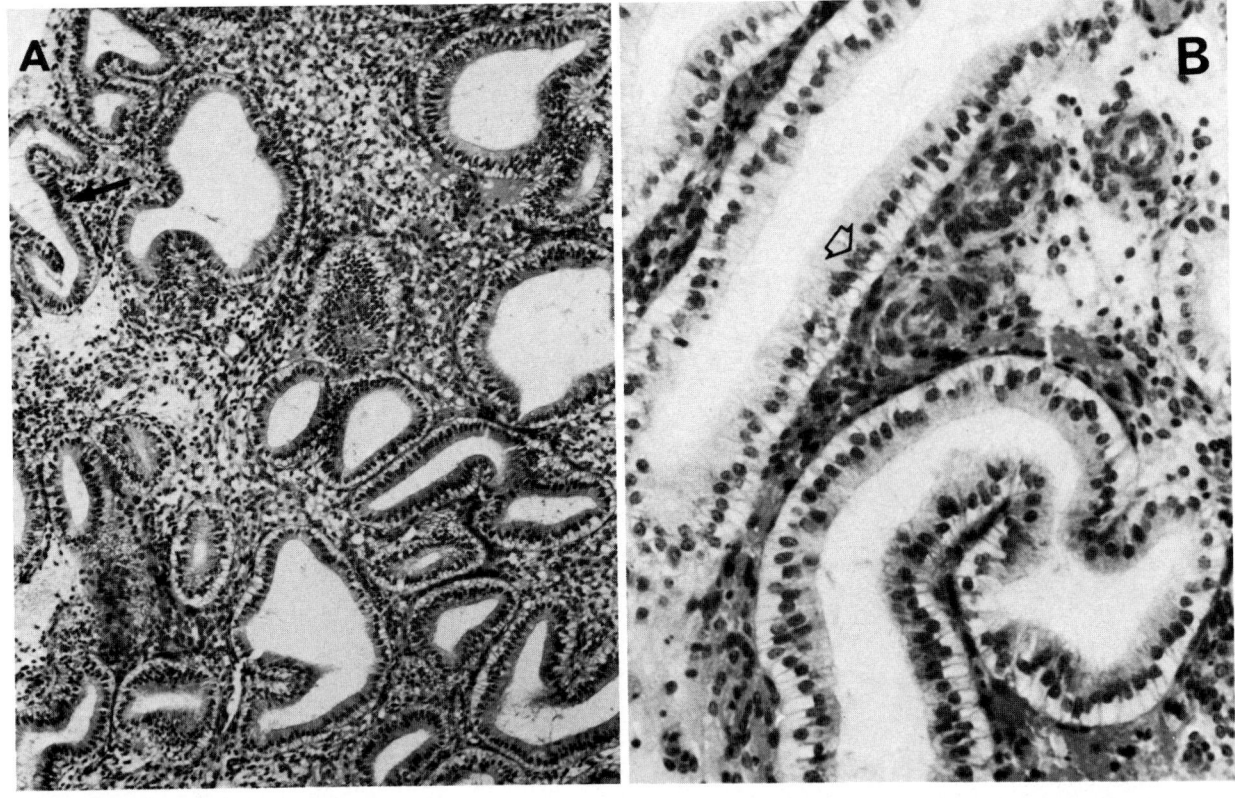

9.16

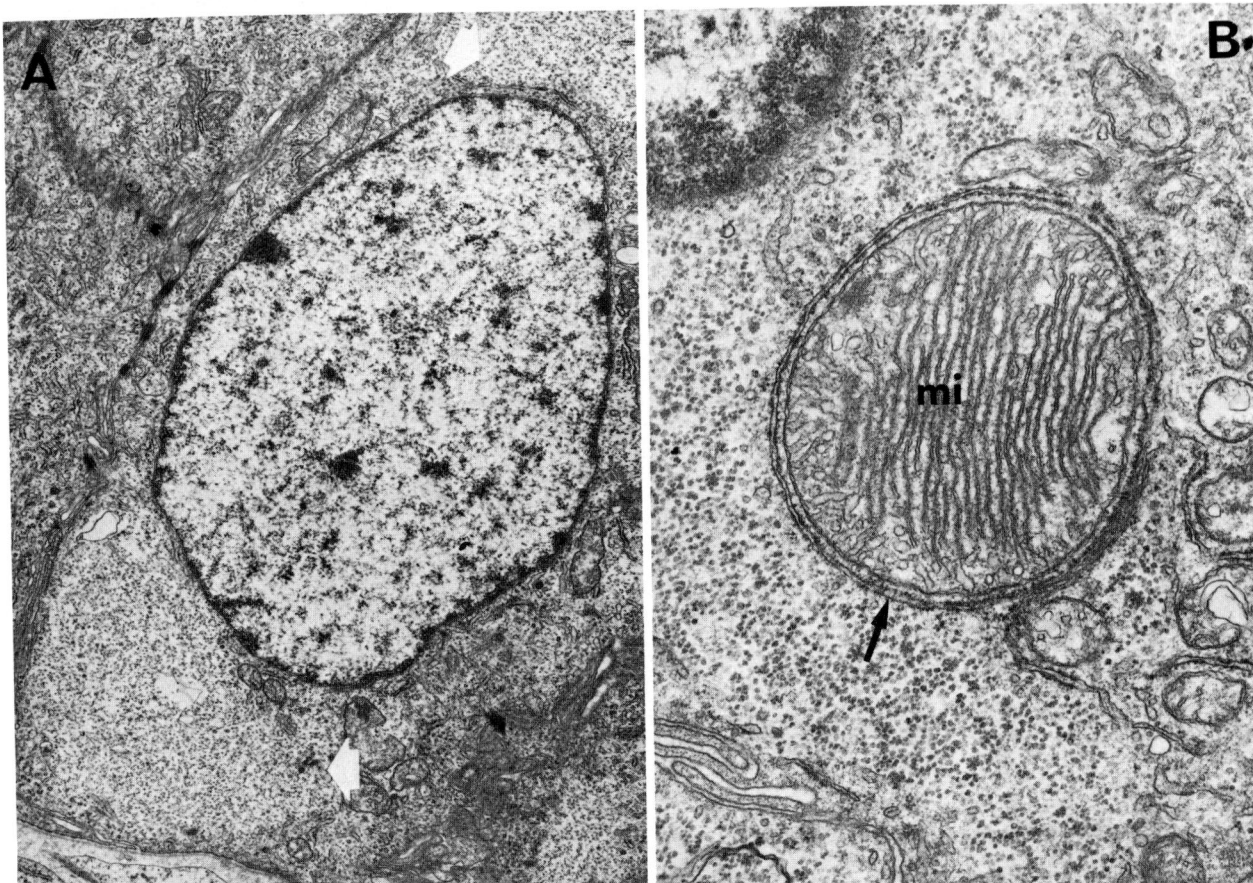

9.17

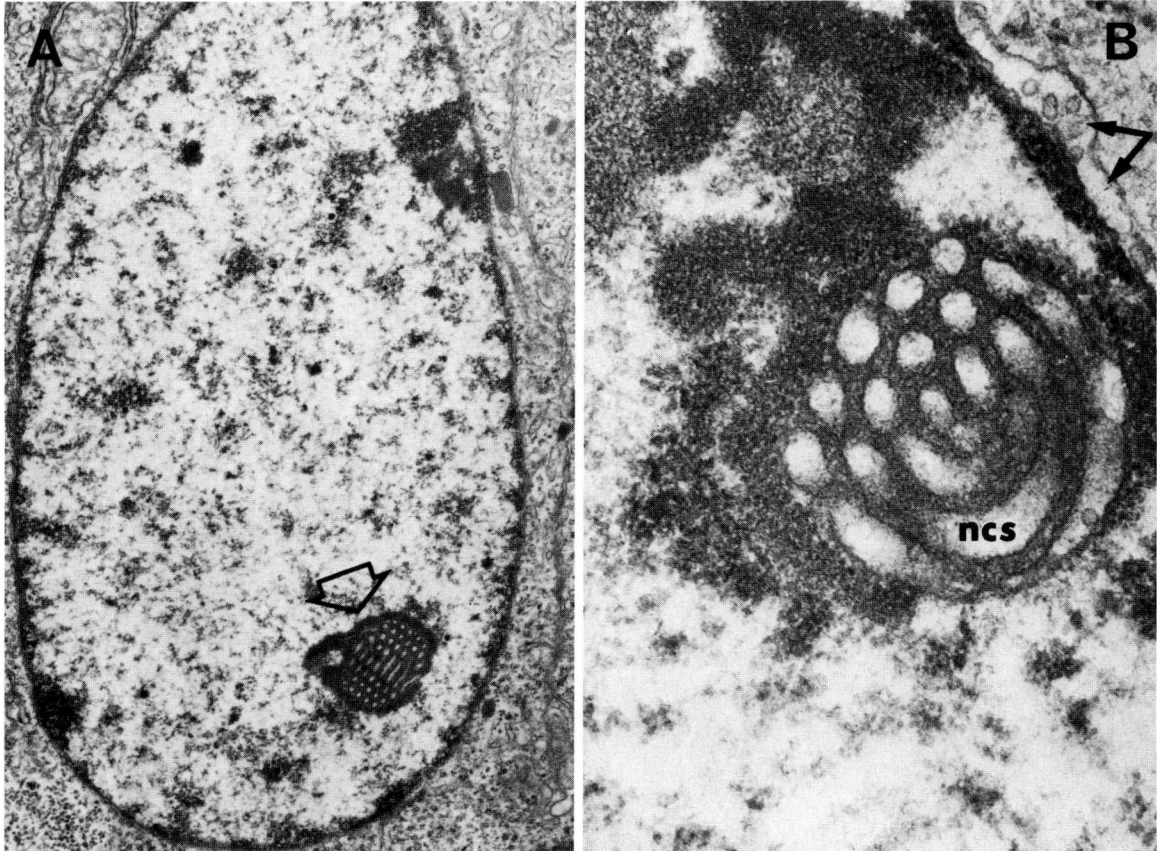

FIG. 9.18. Postovulatory secretory endometrium, cycle day 17 (POD 3). A: Gland cell with a nucleolar channel system (*arrow*), subnuclear glycogen, and giant mitochondria enveloped by parallel membranes of glandular endoplasmic reticulum. These ultrastructural features are typical of postovulatory endo-metrium. ×8000. B: Detailed view of nucleolar channel system (*ncs*) made of hollow, membrane-bound tubules embedded in dark granular nucleolonema. Vesicular structures seen in ncs are also seen between the inner and outer nuclear membrane (*arrows*). ×60,000.

FIG. 9.16. Postovulatory, secretory endometrium. A: Many glands on cycle day 17 (POD 3) have S-shaped configurations (*arrow*), conspicuous subnuclear vacuolization, and nuclear pali-sading. The stroma is relatively edematous. B: Detailed view of the 17th day secretory endometrium. Each gland cell has a well-developed subnuclear vacuole. As a result, the nuclei are pushed up to the center of the cells producing nuclear palisading (*arrow*). These are the first morphologic features in the menstrual cycle that are indicative of ovulation.

FIG. 9.17. Postovulatory, secretory endometrium, cycle day 18. A: Ultrastructure of gland cells with abundant sub- and supranuclear glycogen granules (*arrows*). ×11,000. B: Detailed view of glycogen–giant mitochondria (*mi*)–granular endoplasmic reticulum (*arrow*) complex. Their close ultrastructural relation-ship is geared for glycoprotein synthesis. ×23,000. (Reprinted by permission of Ferenczy and Guralnick, ref. 24.)

ment of the apical portion of cells (Fig. 9.19B). Uterine secretory fluids also contain plasma transudates derived from circulating blood in the endometrial mucosa. The peak of intraglandular secretions coincides with the time of implantation of the free blastocyst, on cycle day 21 (POD 7) if fertilization takes place.

DNA synthesis and cell divisions in gland cells cease (Figs. 9.11, 9.19B) concomitantly with the initiation of apocrine secretory activity by day 19.[27] Mitosis is inhibited further by the rising levels of postovulatory P. Progester-one antagonizes the action of E_2 by interfering with either the recycling or replenishment or both of cytoplasmic E_2R[52] and through the action of the P-specific enzyme 17β-hydroxydehydrogenase (E_2DH).[40] E_2DH converts the potent uterotropic E_2 into relatively weak E_1, which rapidly leaves the cell without significantly stimulating the nuclei of target cells. As a result, an increase in E_2DH lowers the intracellular concentration of E_2 and its recep-tors. Progesterone prevents the epithelial cells from enter-ing the premitotic (G_1 and S) phases of the cell cycle.[108]

POSTOVULATION DAYS 7–10

From cycle day 20 on, the changes in the stroma rather than the glands are evaluated in dating the endometrium

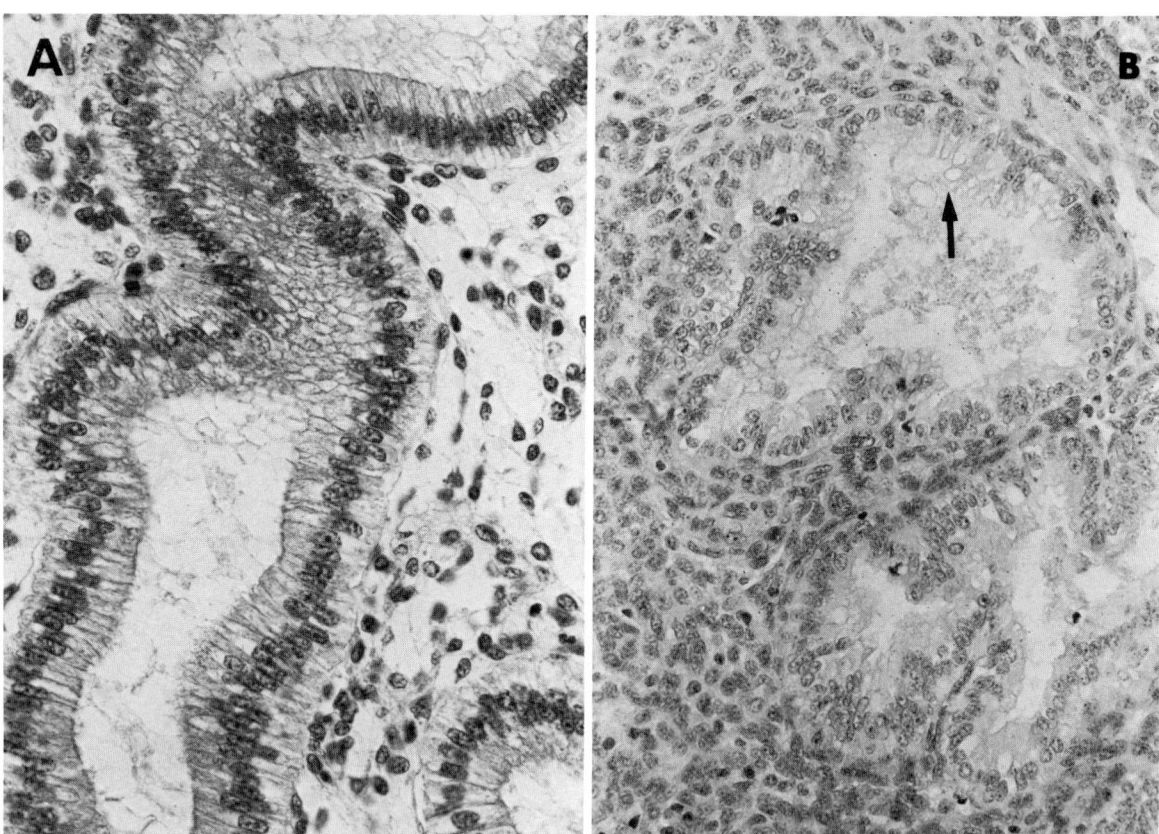

FIG. 9.19. Postovulatory secretory endometrium, cycle day 18 (POD 4). A: Endometrial gland cells have well developed sub- and supranuclear vacuoles, and nuclear palisading is evident. Many cells contain finely granular cytoplasmic substance, and intraluminal vacuolated secretory products are abundant. **B:** His-toradioautograph of secretory endometrium. Lack of uptake of radiothymidine by gland cells coincides with conspicuous apocrine secretory activity (*arrow*) and accumulation of intraluminal secretory products.

(see Table 9.1). The changes are edema (days 20–23), coiling of spiral arterioles (days 22–25), and predecidualization of the stroma (days 23–28). These alterations are mediated by prostaglandin F_2 (PGF_2) and PGE_2.[89] The elevated concentrations of midluteal phase E_2 on cycle day 22 (POD 8) increase the synthesis of the enzyme, cyclooxygenase, responsible for PG production.[1] PGE_2 in turn promotes capillary permeability,[26] leading to maximal stromal edema on day 22 (POD 10) (Fig. 9.20A). Experimental studies have shown that PGE_2 and leukotrienes are potent vasoactive agents that promote vascular permeability as well as stromal decidualization in progesterone-primed endometrium. PGE_2, LTC_4, or both elicit a marked decidual/vascular response in hypophysectomized progesterone-primed pseudopregnant rats; conversely, inhibitors of PGs and LTs such as indomethacin and FPL 55712, respectively, reduce decidualization.[93] E_2 triggers production of PGE_2 and leukotrienes.[94] The increasing concentration of E_2 in the early to mid-postovulatory period may play a role in preparing the endometrium for implantation of the blastocyst through these arachidonate

metabolites.[89] Endometrial vascular arborization is best visualized by Factor VIII immunostaining. PGE_2 presumably also promotes vascular endothelial mitotic activity, perivascular concentrations of filaments (Fig. 9.20B), and mitoses that are first seen in the postovulatory endometrium on day 22 of the cycle (Fig. 9.20C). Endothelial proliferation leads to coiling of the arterial system of the endometrium (Fig. 9.21A), a phenomenon that produces vascular clusters in the upper functionalis layer, seen in histologic sections (Fig. 9.21B). The PGE-mediated vascular growth concept is substantiated further by the fact that immunohistochemically the vascular endothelium is devoid of receptors of estradiol and progesterone.[72]

Vascular permeability and edema of the stroma are the essential prerequisites for the predecidual transformation (Fig. 9.21B) of uncommitted stromal cells.[84] The role of endometrial histamine,[17] bradykinin, and serotonin[98] in these biologic events is not completely understood.

In rare instances, endocrine type cells with positive immunostaining for serotonin and somatostatin are encountered in proliferative and secretory phase endometrial

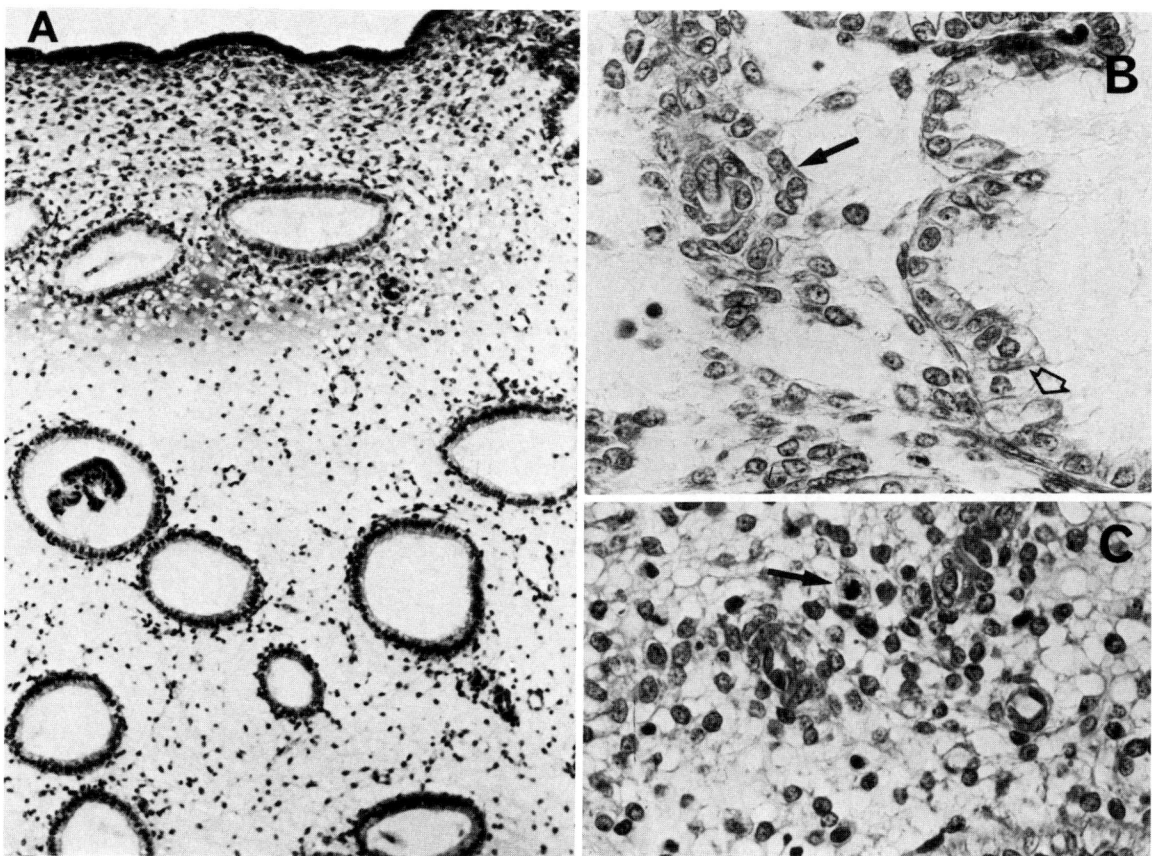

FIG. 9.20. Postovulatory, secretory endometrium, cycle day 22 (POD 8). A: There is marked stromal edema producing a naked gland–stromal cell pattern. The glands have somewhat dilated lumens with secretions, and the lining epithelium is low, columnar, and devoid of intraluminal projections. B: Detailed view of perivascular thickening due to hypertrophy of perivascular stromal cells (arrow). The gland cells are low columnar to cuboidal and have apical apocrine secretory protuberances (open arrow). C: Mitoses (arrow) in perivascular stromal cells reappear on late 22nd–early 23rd day of the menstrual cycle.

glands.[85] In experimental animal systems, release of histamine from mast cells and the subsequent edematous response occur within a few hours of E_2 stimulation.[50] Endometrial cell membranes and blastocyst membranes in the rabbit and rat, respectively, have receptors for histamine.[50] It is also possible that histamine is synthesized by the implanted blastocyst itself as well as the endometrium, and it may facilitate the implantation process. In the human endometrium, the role of mast cells is yet to be determined. In other tissue systems they may modulate immunologic and inflammatory responses. The human endometrium contains few mast cells even when the endometrium is fixed in basic lead citrate and stained with Toluidine blue for 4–5 days.[18] They are located chiefly in the basal layer; their number is unchanged through the cycle but drops with age, with a marked decrease in the menopause. Although they contain heparin-rich granules and mast cells are increased in endometria with an intrauterine contraceptive device (IUCD) in place, they have no relationship with abnormal uterine bleeding. In addition, antihistamines do not prevent stromal edema, whereas indomethacin does.[17] These observations suggest that histamine may act on the endometrium indirectly by the production of PG.[50] Endometrial vascular proliferation at the implantation site is related to the blastocyst rather than to histamine or PGE_2. The blastocyst has a unique biologic property that is shared only with tumor cells producing the so-called angiogenesis factor, a substance capable of inducing growth of new capillaries.[32]

An important immunosuppressive mechanism that operates at the chorio–decidual interface is provided by trophoblast-derived E_2 and P. The concentrations of both sex steroids are increased at this area, and P has been shown to effectively suppress interleukin-2–activated lymphocyte cytotoxicity.[74] This paracrine immunosuppressive effect of P is dose-dependent and confers resistance to lysis to trophoblast by cytotoxic mononuclear cells.[22] Because cytotoxic cells are stimulated by IL-1 and because P suppresses in vitro IL-1 production by monocytes, P-related immunosuppression may operate by decreasing macrophage IL-1 production and the subsequent activation of cytotoxic lymphocytes.[22]

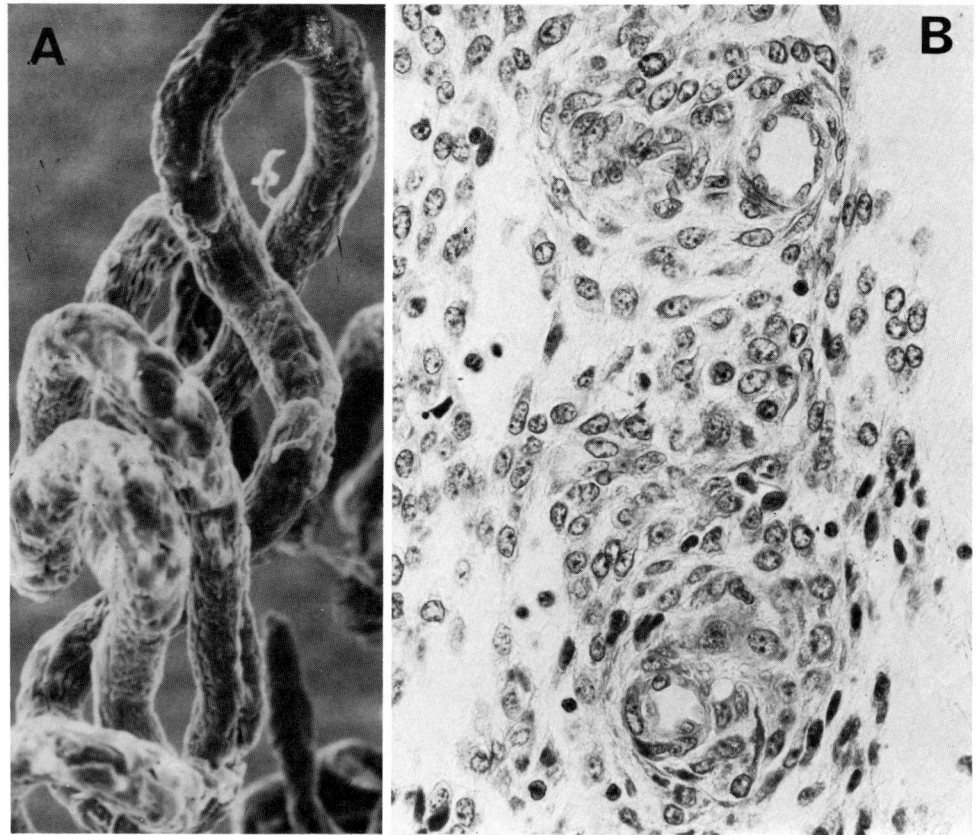

FIG. 9.21. Postovulatory, secretory endometrium, cycle day 23 (POD 9). A: Vascular preparation of spiral arteries seen with scanning electron microscopy. B: Predecidual thickening around spiral arteries can better be appreciated on cycle day 23. This is due to enlargement and rounding of the cytoplasm and nuclei of perivascular stromal cells. (Reprinted by permission of Ferenczy A and Guralnick M (1983) Endometrial microstructure: Structure function relationships throughout the menstrual cycle. Semin Reprod Endocrinol 1:205.)

EGF and its receptor EGF/R) are immunolocalized predominantly in the cytoplasm of syncytiotrophoblast but also in intermediate trophoblast during human implantation.[46] EGF has a differentiating effect on trophoblast, stimulating synthesis and secretion of human chorionic gonadotropin (hCG), human placental lactogen (hPL), and P. EGF/R is similar to ERB/β oncogene,[82,87,8] and it is possible that it also contributes to the controlled trophoblastic invasion of the decidua.

Stromal predecidualization (not pseudodecidualization; the prefix "pre" refers to decidual transformation of stromal cells before their further decidual development during pregnancy) begins by day 22–23 (POD 8–9) (see Table 9.1) around spiral arterioles and capillaries of the functional layer (Fig. 9.21B). Coinciding with the beginning of the predecidual reaction on cycle day 23, the glands form intraluminal epithelial projections, so-called ferning (see Table 9.1; Fig. 9.22A). Perivascular predecidualization is more obvious on day 24 (POD 10) and is characterized by the conversion of uncommitted spindle-shaped stromal cells into plump epithelial-like cells with enlarged nuclei and increased cytoplasm.

Predecidual cells increase in size not only by cellular hypertrophy but also by mitosis and endoreduplication. The latter may be recognized by enlarged nuclei or double nucleation (tetraploidy). Proliferation of predecidual cells is mediated by growth-related peptides, as well as prostaglandins[9] and presumably Ki67. Predecidual cells are devoid of E_2 receptors by immunohistochemistry,[10] their growth thus seems not to be stimulated by circulatory E_2. Progesterone receptors, on the other hand, are present,[10] which together with the high midsecretory phase serum progesterone levels may play a role in cytoplasmic differentiation of predecidual cells. Ki67 is expressed only in the nucleus of cycling proliferative but not in resting cells,[36] and its expression is up-regulated by progesterone.[91] In endometrial stromal cells, PgR is expressed both in the proliferative and secretory phases of the cycle; however, Ki67 immunoreactivity in endometrial stromal cells is weak during the proliferative phase but is increased in

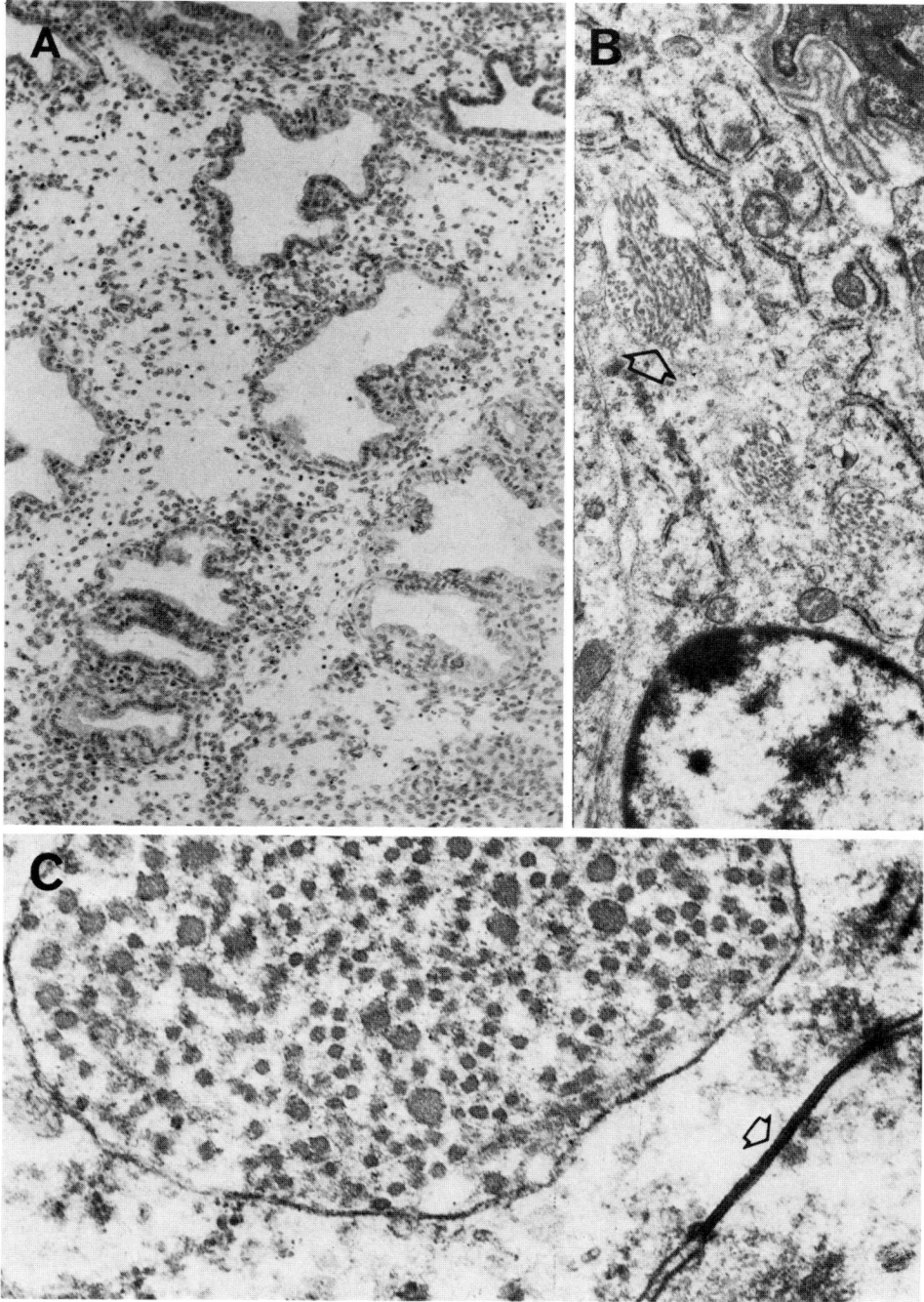

Fig. 9.22. Postovulatory, secretory endometrium, cycle day 23 (POD 9). A: In addition to predecidual vascular cuffing, intraluminal epithelial projections (glandular ferning) and stromal edema are typical features of cycle day 23. **B:** Predecidual stroma cells with membrane-bound heterocytophagolysosomes (*arrow*) containing extracellular collagen fibers. ×7000. **C:** Higher magnification of heterocytophagolysosome with cross-sectioned, partially digested, extracellular collagen fibers. A tight junctional nexus (*arrow*) is seen in between predecidual cells. ×10,000. (Reprinted by permission of Ferenczy A and Guralnick M (1983) Endometrial microstructure: Structure function relationships throughout the menstrual cycle. Semin Reprod Endocrinol 1:205.)

secretory phase endometrium (Table 9.1). Decidualized cells show strong reactivity for both PR and often for Ki67 (Fig. 9.23). Decidual transformation also may occur in extrauterine locations chiefly during periods of pregnancy in the subcoelomic mesenchyme of the pelvic peritoneum, ovary, and omentum.[44] Decidualization also can be triggered by electrical, mechanical, or chemical stimulation in progesterone-primed rodent uteri and fallopian tubes.[56,107] Ultrastructurally, predecidual cells lack the typical features of epithelial cells, such as bundles of intermediate tonofilaments, glandular lumens, or desmosomal connections. On the other hand, they have intercellular gap-junction nexuses (Fig. 9.22C). The latter are composed of hexagonal microtubules forming an open-channel system between adjacent cells that facilitates passage of electrolytes and molecules and plays a role in cell contact inhibition.[59,103] Histochemically, the predecidual cells contain glycogen and PAS-positive mucosubstances. Despite their epithelial-like appearance, predecidual cells often stain with vimentin (Fig. 9.13) and desmin but not with cytokeratins or epithelial membrane antigen (Table 9.1). The immunoreactivity of predecidual cells is consistent with their stromal cell derivation. Predecidual cells represent precursor forms of gestational decidual cells (decidus vera). The cells have several metabolic functions related either to pregnancy or, if conception has not occurred, to menstrual breakdown of the endometrium. For example, the decidual cells have phagocytotic properties (Fig. 9.22B, C) and digest extracellular collagen matrix.[59] Decidual phagocytosis may facilitate the development of the decidual reaction by removing collagen from the endometrial stroma. The latter may represent a mechanical obstacle to proliferating and expanding predecidual cells. If conception does not occur, predecidual cells, by removing collagen, may contribute to menstrual breakdown of the endometrial stroma (Fig. 9.22B, C).

POSTOVULATION DAYS 11–13

Predecidual transformation of stromal cells under the surface epithelium is achieved by day 25 (POD 11), producing the compacta layer (Fig. 9.24). On days 26 and 27 (POD 12 and 13), the upper two-thirds of the functionalis becomes predecidualized, and the glands demonstrate coiling and ferning (Fig. 9.25A). The endometrial stroma during days 26 and 27 is infiltrated by extravasated polymorphonuclear leukocytes and the so-called metrial cells or granulocytes (Fig. 9.25B) Metrial granulocytes resemble eosinophils, except that they have a single, kidney-shaped nucleus (Fig. 9.25B, C). Endometrial stromal granulocytes (EGs), also named Körnchenzellen or "K" cells, are abundant in the late secretory phase of the menstrual cycle, more so in early pregnancy, after which they decline in number and are virtually absent at term.[12] Histologically, it was suggested by immunofluorescence technique that EGs derived from undifferentiated endometrial cells and their secretory granules contained relaxin.[20] However, later studies failed to support the view that EGs are a source of relaxin, and more recently immunohistochemical evidence has been presented that EGs are in fact members of the large granular lymphocyte series.[12] In both formalin-fixed and acetone-fixed decidual tissues, EGs stain positive with LCA, CD-2, MT1, UCHL1, and Leu-19 but fail to stain with CD 16, Leu-7, CD 3, CD 5, CD 7, and HLADR. In view of the gradual increase in the number of EGs during the postovulatory secretory phase of the menstrual cycle and their maximum concentration during the first trimester of pregnancy, they are believed to be under hormonal control and their immunocompetent phenotypic characteristics suggest that they may play an important role in implantation and placentation.

Relaxin (disulfide homologue of insulin) is considered to be an autocrine/paracrine hormone that is believed to be involved in collagenolysis. Monoclonal antibodies to human relaxin and polyclonal antiserum to porcin relaxin identified this hormone predominantly in the glands of both proliferative and secretory phase endometria. The

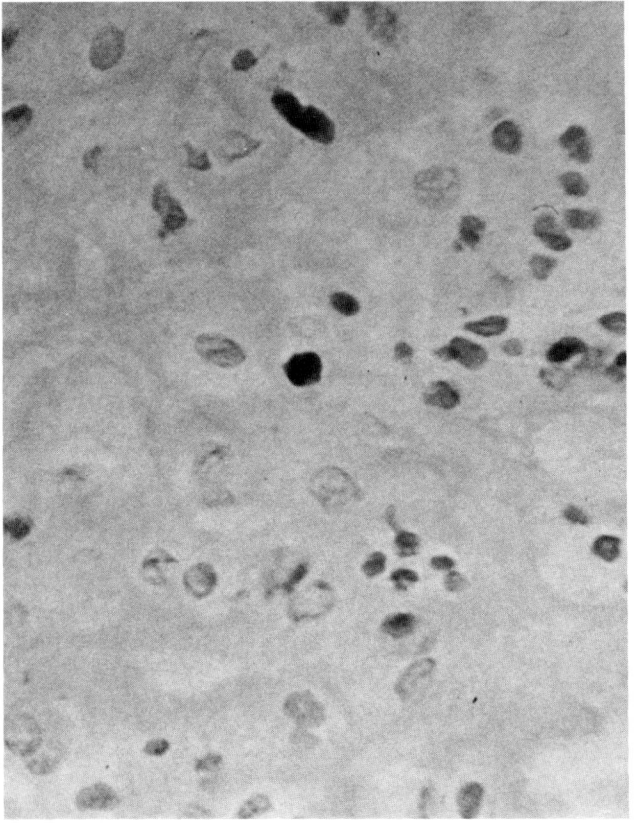

FIG. 9.23. **Occasional gestational decidual cells have intense nuclear staining with Ki67.** (Courtesy of Shingo Fujii, M.D., Matsumoto, Japan.)

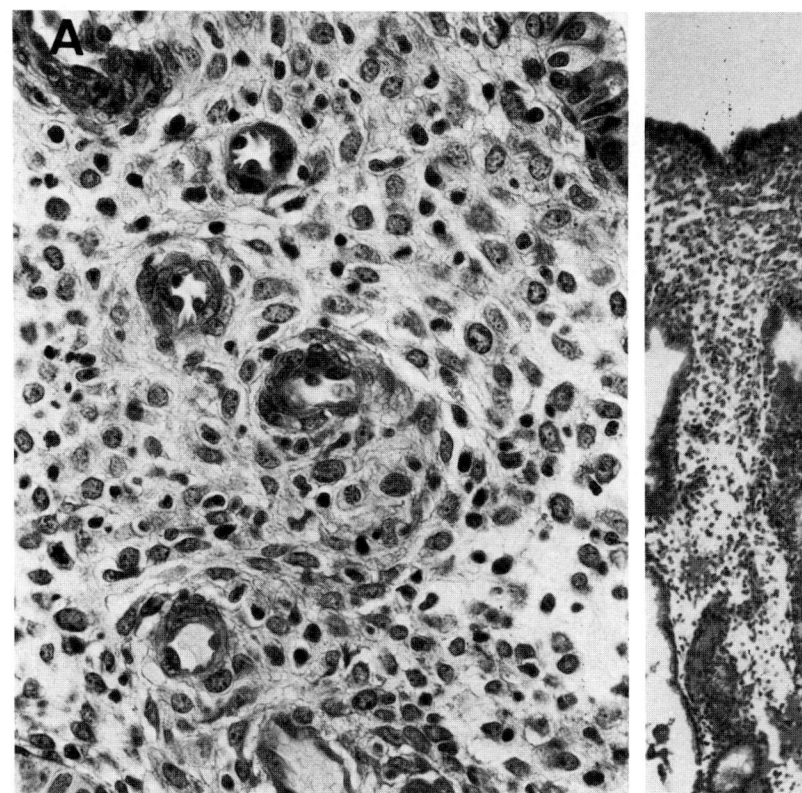

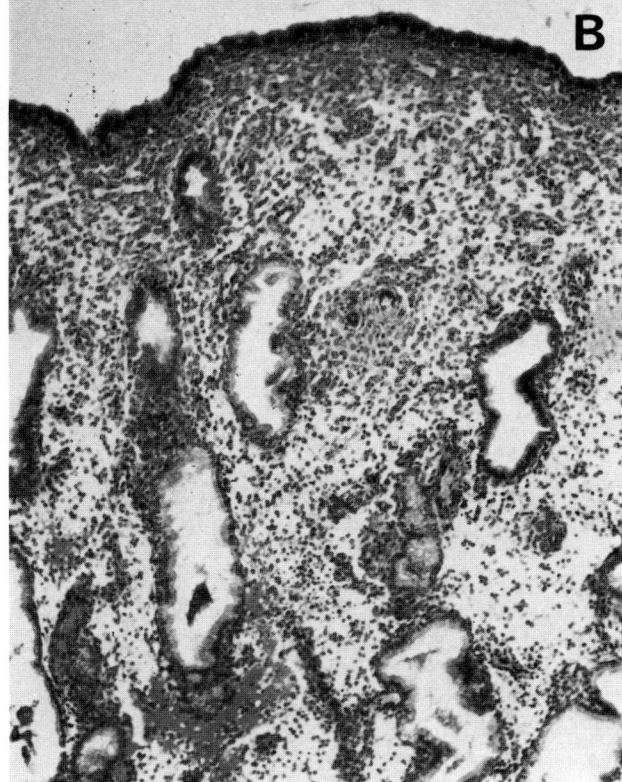

FIG. 9.24. Postovulatory, secretory endometrium, cycle days 24 and 25. **A:** On cycle day 24 (POD 10), predecidual transformation of perivascular stromal cells is evident. Note the well-defined cytoplasmic membranes and round nuclei of prede-

cidual cells resembling epithelial cells. **B:** On cycle day 25 (POD 11), predecidualization of fibroblasts beneath the surface epithelium produces a band-like cellular plate, the so-called compacta layer.

predecidual cells in the late secretory phase, and particularly early gestational decidua parietalis stain heavily, and relaxin genes appear to be transcribed in both the endometrial glands and stroma.[11] Whether they are translated as well has to be determined, but if so, they may be involved in the preparation and maintenance of early pregnancy by increasing collagenase and tissue plasminogen activators to break down collagen. Relaxin also is produced by syncytiotrophoblast, and trophoblast-derived relaxin also may facilitate penetration of decidua. This may cause weakening, rupture, and eventual detachment of fetal membranes, as well as contribute to cervical dilation.[30] If conception does not occur, relaxin may affect the endometrial stroma, facilitating breakdown of menstrual tissue. Degenerated nuclear debris of acute and chronic inflammatory cell origin often is seen to be phagocytosed by intact gland cells of the lower spongiosa and basalis layers on cycle days 28, 1, and 2 (Fig. 9.26B).

Menstrual Phase

A normal menstrual period lasts 4 days ± 1 day. During this time, the endometrial mucosa rapidly degenerates, and 50% of the menstrual detritus is expelled in the first 24

hours of menses. Tissue shedding is followed by regeneration. The upper two-thirds of the endometrium on cycle days 28–2 contains fissures and degenerative predecidual cells admixed with epithelial glandular cells as well as acute and chronic (lymphoid) inflammatory cells (Figs. 9.27, 9.28).

Ultrastructural enzyme tracing studies[43,103] of the upper two-thirds of late secretory endometrium show that it gradually involutes, degenerates, and undergoes necrosis (Fig. 9.28C). The mechanisms by which degeneration occurs are shown in Fig. 9.29. During endometrial proliferation, E_2 stimulates the development of Golgi-derived, primary lysosomes in the epithelial, stromal, and endothelial cells of the functional layer of the endometrium.[26,43] These contain highly potent proteolytic enzymes. During the first half of the postovulatory period, lytic enzymes, including acid phosphatase, are confined to membrane-bound lysosomes by the action of P that stabilizes lysosomal membranes.[102] Coinciding with the fall of E_2 and P by day 25, the integrity of lysosomal membrane is no longer maintained. As a result, lysosomal enzymes are released intracellularly as well as into the intercellular space. Acid hydrolases digest the cytoplasmic elements, intercellular desmosomes, and ultimately the entire cellular system.[43]

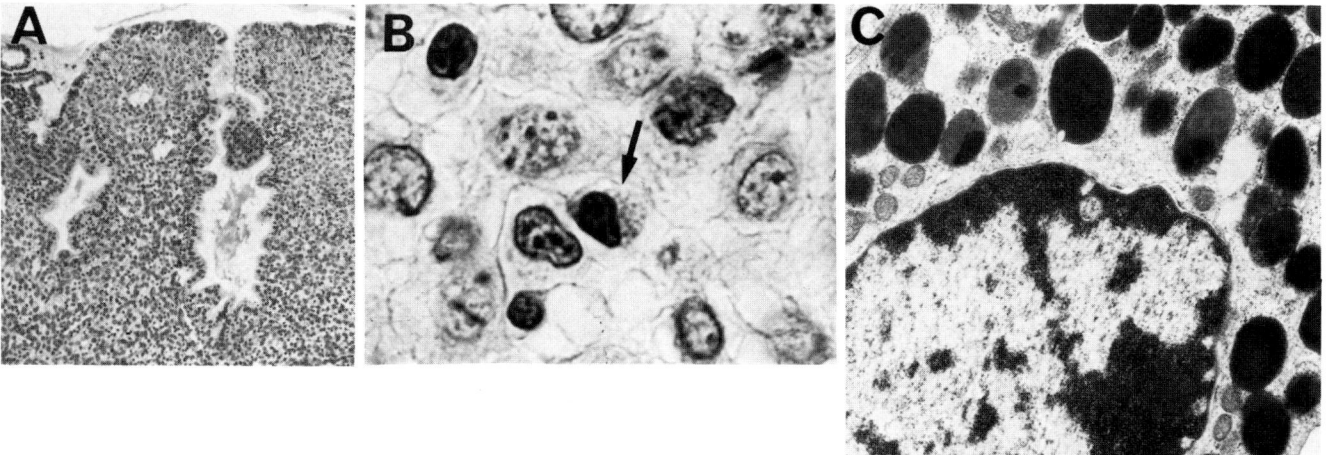

FIG. 9.25. Postovulatory, secretory endometrium, cycle day 26 (POD 12). A: The entire functionalis layer is occupied by predecidual cells secondary to expansion and confluency between the surface epithelial predecidual compacta and perivascular predecidua. The glands demonstrate secretory exhaustion, with inspissated intraglandular secretions. **B:** granular lymphocyte (*arrow*) with a unilobed nucleus and eosinophilic granular cytoplasm. **C:** Ultrastructure of a granular with membrane-bound, presumably relaxin-containing, electron-dense granules. ×12,000. (Reprinted by permission of Ferenczy A and Guralnick M (1983) Endometrial microstructure: Structure function relationships throughout the menstrual cycle. Semin Reprod Endocrinol 1:205.)

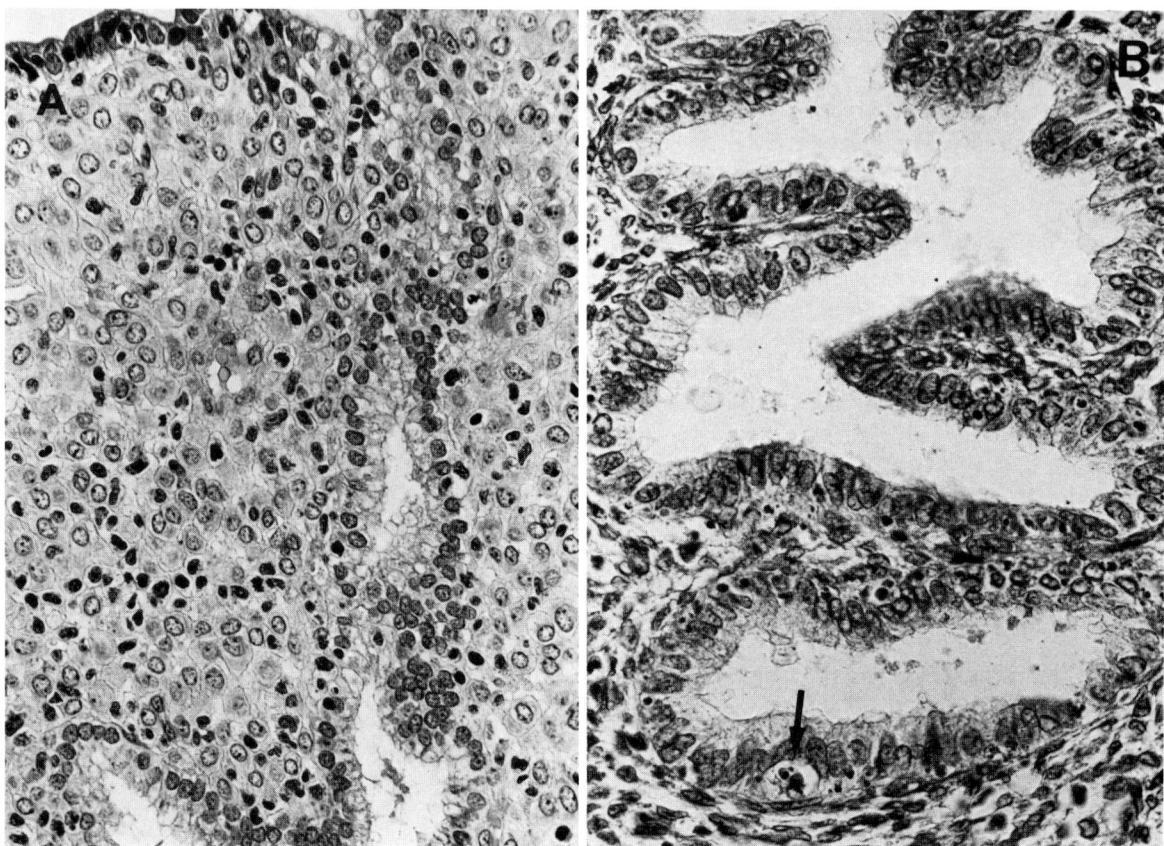

FIG. 9.26. Postovulatory secretory endometrium, cycle day 27 (POD 13). A: The predecidua is scattered with inflammatory cells; they are more conspicuous on cycle day 27 than day 26. **B:** Polydust (*arrow*) in gland cells and the stroma is a typical feature of impending (cycle day 28) or ongoing (cycle days 1 and 2) menstrual degeneration. Polydust has been phagocytosed by gland cells of the lower functionalis and basal layers.

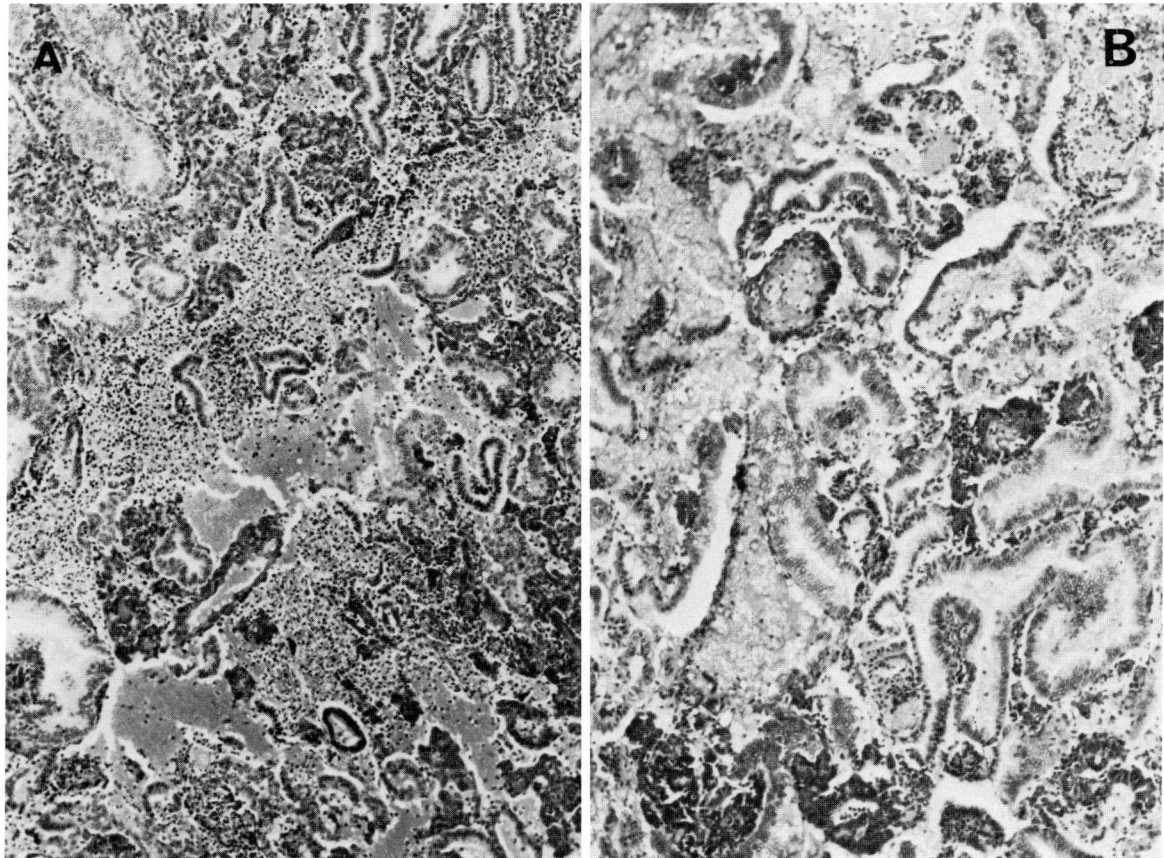

FIG. 9.27. **Menstrual endometrium, degenerative phase.** **A:** On cycle days 1–2, the endometrium contains collapsed stroma, ruptured glands with secretory exhaustion, degenerated predecidua, and inflammatory cells. **B:** Menstrual endometrium in a 42-year-old woman. The glands are larger and less exhausted than in **A:** however, degeneration is diffuse, a feature typical of estrogen–progestogen withdrawal type of bleeding endometrium.

Lysosomal autodigestion destroys the glandular and stromal cells and also the vascular endothelium. Vascular luminal surface membrane injury promotes platelet deposits.[16] These alterations presumably are mediated by prostaglandin–thromboxane, and the final results are manifest by multiple minute foci of ischemic tissue necrosis.[16] In addition, acute swelling of the endothelial cells of endometrial arterioles contributes to obliteration of the vascular lumen.[43] Paralleling these events, PGE_2 and particularly PGF_2 significantly increase in the late secretory endometrium and reach maximum concentrations during the menstrual period.[30] It has been speculated that the high levels of PGF_2 also may release acid hydrolases from lysosomes and, during menstruation, stimulate the onset of ischemic necrosis via vasoconstriction of myometrial and basal arteries. Expulsion of degenerated endometrium is enhanced by PGF_2-mediated myometrial contractions.[30] The menstrual fluid is composed of autolyzed tissue admixed with a heavy polymorphonuclear exudate, red blood cells, and proteolytic enzymes.[8] One of the latter is blood protease plasmin, a potent fibrinolytic agent that prevents

clotting of menstrual blood and facilitates expulsion of the degenerated functionalis. The fibrinolytic activity of the endometrium, which characteristically disappears during the implantation period (cycle day 21), may play a role in preventing this process from occurring during the menstrual period. Plasminogen activators, which convert plasminogen into plasmin, are found in and released from degenerated endometrial vascular endothelium.[55]

Menstrual bleeding is controlled by vasoconstriction of the ruptured basal arteries in the denuded basal layer and radial and arcuate arteries in the myometrium. Rapid denudation of the basal layer reduces menstrual blood loss considerably. The arteries of the functionalis layer lack elastin and consequently cannot contract. In addition, they are shed with the functionalis and fail, therefore, to contribute to uterine hemostasis.[16]

On days 2–4, the functionalis becomes gradually detached from the underlying basalis.[23–26,65] Detachment starts from the fundus and slowly extends toward the isthmus, as observed by hysteroscopy.[61] The cleaved mucosa rolls on itself until it is detached from the basalis and is

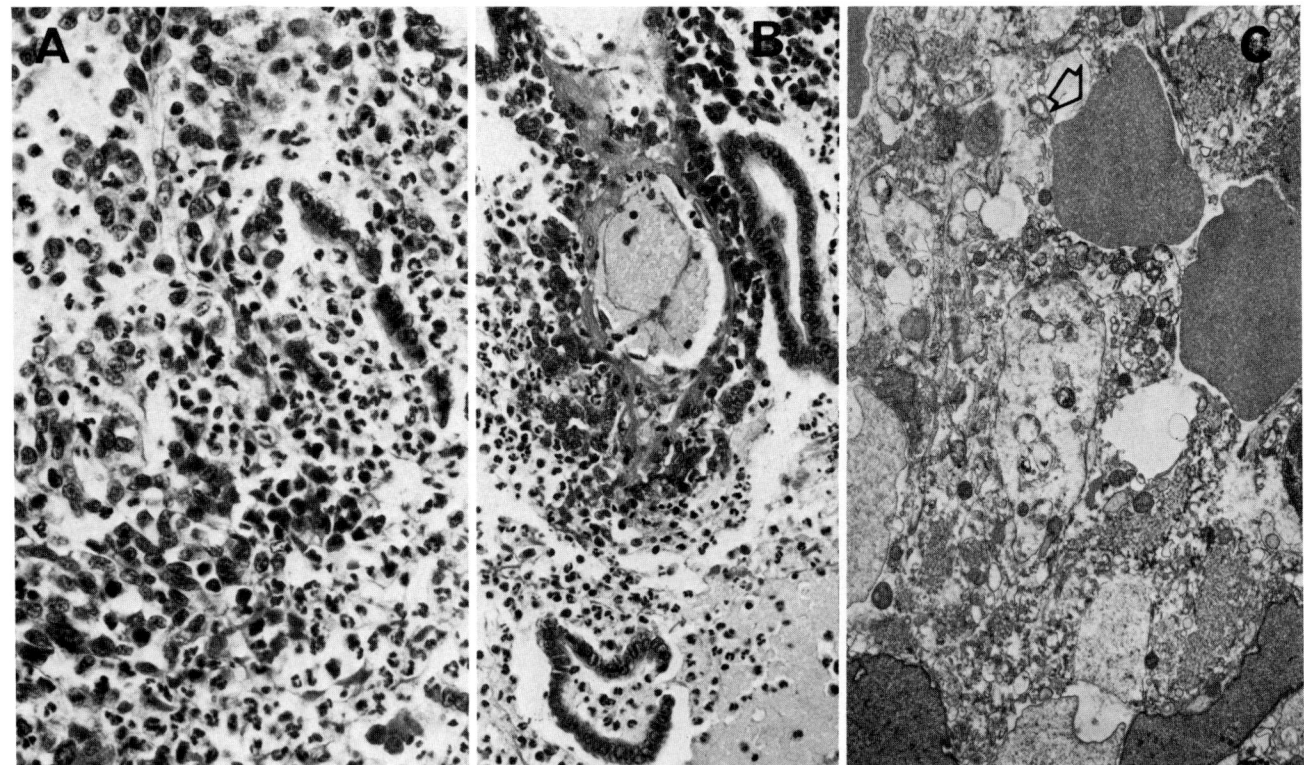

FIG. 9.28. Menstrual endometrium, degenerative phase.
A: Ruptured, collapsed, exhausted glands and degenerative stromal cells intermingling with acute inflammatory cells, edema, and red blood cells. **B:** Ruptured endometrial vessel with fibrinoid deposit surrounded by degenerated predecidua and polymorphs. **C:** Ultrastructurally, there is severe cytologic, organellar, and nuclear degeneration, consistent with irreversible cell injury. Red blood cells (*arrow*) are seen. (Reprinted by permission of Ferenczy A and Guralnick M (1983) Endometrial microstructure: Structure function relationships throughout the menstrual cycle. Semin Reprod Endocrinol 1:205.)

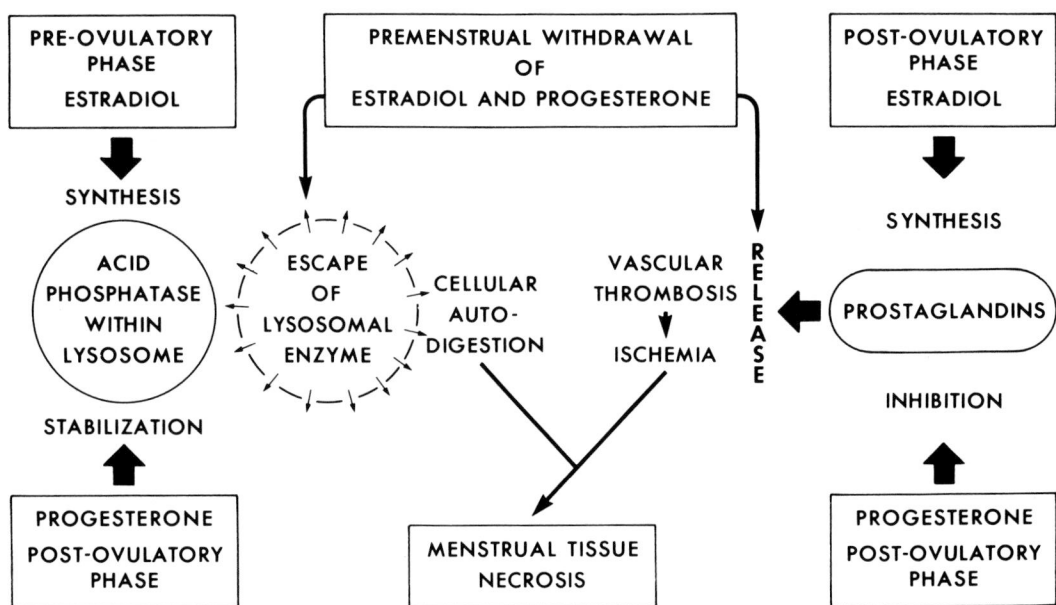

FIG. 9.29. Schematic representation of the morphobiochemical events that lead to the menstrual breakdown of the endometrium. The *large arrows* indicate the stimulatory effects of ovarian hormones. (Reprinted by permission of Ferenczy (1981) Contemp Obstet Gynecol 18: 115.)

shed from the endometrial cavity. Shedding is most prominent during the first 2 days of the menstrual period, and endometrial biopsy or curettage yields abundant tissue. On the other hand, the next 2 days are dominanted by proliferation of the residual basal gland epithlium in areas of complete denudation,[23–26] and the material obtained for histology during these days is generally scant. Reepithelialization occurs by extension of the residual glandular epithelium over the denuded surface (Fig. 9.30A). Essentially similar phenomena are observed in the spontaneously menstruating monkey and in the rabbit[25] in which the endometrium has been artificially denuded. The peripheral regions of the endometrial cavity, such as the isthmus and peritubal ostium, both of which remain intact during the menstrual period,[23,24] also contribute to resurfacing the epithelium. These converging epithelial proliferations interanastomose, leading to a new surface epithelium by cycle day 5 (Fig. 9.30B). Bleeding ceases when the surface has been completely reepithelialized (see Fig. 9.14B).

Epithelial cell migration followed by replication characterizes the biodynamics of endometrial surface repair.[26] Normal proliferative and secretory phase stromal cells are immunopositive for vimentin, muscle-specific actin (MSA), alpha–smooth muscle actin (α-SMA), and rarely desmin (Table 9.1). None of the epithelial-type antibodies (i.e., cytokeratin, epithelial membrane antigen) react with stromal cells.[34] The immunohistochemical findings indicate the potential for smooth muscle differentiation of endometrial stromal cells. The light microscopic, immunohistochemical, and ultrastructural features of endometrial stromal cells are consistent with their similarity to myofibroblasts. Both stromal cells and myofibroblasts participate in normal wound healing. Endometrial stromal cells of the basal layer proliferate to replace shed endometrium and later in the cycle play a supportive role in maintaining endometrial integrity. The first-generation, resurfacing epithelial cells are flattened (Fig. 9.31) and have abundant surface microvilli, intracellular intermediate filaments, microtubules, and pseudopodial projections. These alterations reflect ameboid motility promoted by cyclic adenosine monophosphate and by the interaction of actin-containing filaments with myosin-containing plasma membranes. Nuclear and nucleolar enlargement (Fig. 9.32C) in regenerative cells also promotes cellular motility by providing increased DNA and RNA, respectively. After the initial epithelial spread, mitosis and migration operate simultaneously until a confluent surface layer has been regenerated on cycle day 5. The sudden increase in DNA synthesis and the shortened DNA synthesis phase of regenerative cells provide for accelerated tissue turnover (see Fig. 9.11). The cellular migration and the rapid wound healing capability observed in the human endometrium together with the kinetic and ultrastructural data do not support the view that new endometrial surface and glandular epithelium are regenerated directly from persistent, secretory spongiosa[31] or stromal cells.[6] The latter are be-

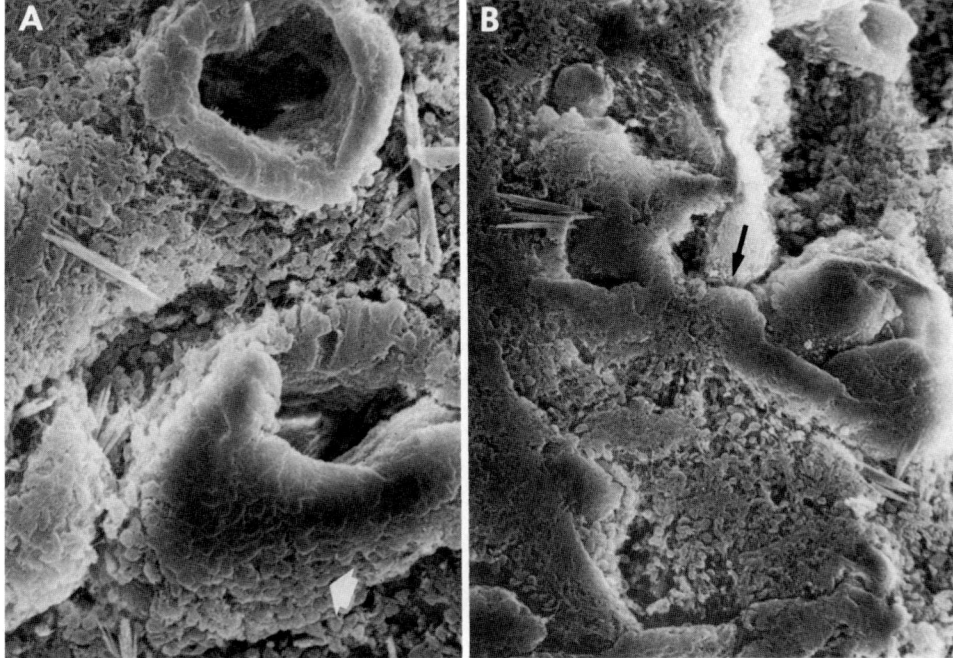

FIG. 9.30. Menstrual endometrium, reparative phase. A: Scanning electron microscopy of regenerative endometrium. On cycle day 3, gland stumps of residual basal glands have epithelial extensions (*arrow*) onto denuded stroma. B: Cycle day 4 is dom-inated by anastomoses of epithelial membranes (*arrow*) from adjacent basal gland opening. (Reprinted by permission of Ferenczy A (1981) The endometrial cycle. In: Sciarra JJ (ed) Gynecology and obstetrics. New York, Harper & Row, vol. 5, pp 1–14.)

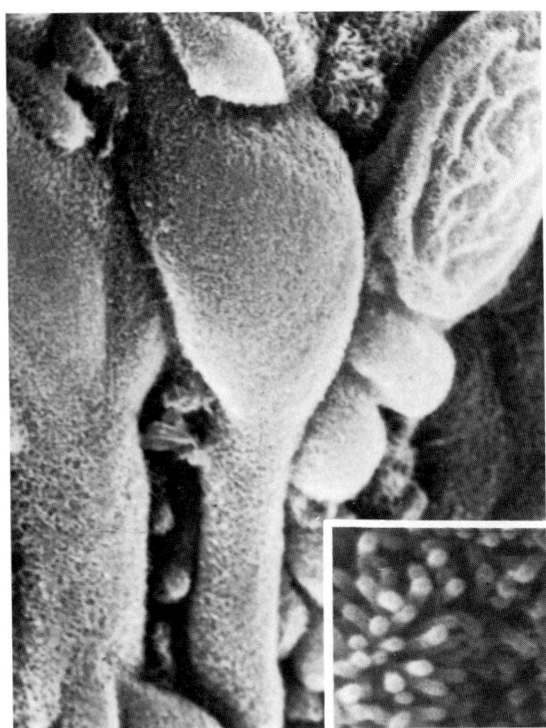

FIG. 9.31. Menstrual endometrium, regenerative phase. On cycle days 3 and 4, the newly formed epithelial cells have flattened cytoplasm and prominent pseudopodial projections. ×24,000. *Inset:* Higher magnification of hair-like surface microvilli. ×50,000. (Reprinted by permission of Ferenczy, ref. 26.)

lieved to contribute to endometrial epithelial repair[25] indirectly, presumably by their positive influence on growth factors[92] and by providing cellular support to the newly resurfacing surface epithelial cells. The latter event is recognized by aggregates of stromal cells beneath resurfacing epithelial cells. These so-called stromal "blue" balls (Fig. 9.32B, C) are typical features of endometrial stromal breakdown after uterine bleeding associated with tissue regeneration (see Fig. 9.8). The deep blue staining characteristic of aggregated stromal cells with H&E stain is due to their prominent nuclei and scant cytoplasm. Tenascin, an extracellular matrix protein, has been immunolocalized around proliferative gland cells and vessels but not secretory-type glands.[99] Tenascin is thought to enhance epithelial migration and proliferation during periods of postmenstrual repair by inhibiting cell attachment to fibronectin.[14] Experimental studies demonstrated that epithelial growth is stimulated and maintained by the adjacent or subjacent supportive fibroblasts.[14] The stromal aggregates are not pathognomonic of postovulatory menstrual regeneration, since they are also seen in endometrium after anovulation, estrogen or progestogen breakthrough bleeding, or withdrawal of exogenous estrogen and progestogens.

Postmenstrual endometrium repair is not induced by E_2. During cycle days 3 and 4, despite increased DNA

synthesis, circulating estrogens and receptors for E_2 and P are low, unchanged from the premenstrual values.[26] In experimental endometrial regeneration in the rabbit, similar proliferative and morphologic patterns are observed, regardless of whether the animals are ovariectomized or have intact ovaries.[25] On cycle days 7–12, however, there is a marked increase in DNA synthesis (see (Fig. 9.11) and mitotic activity in all cell components of the regenerated human endometrium. This coincides with an increase in plasma estrogens and E_2R–PgR concentrations and a slight decrease in serum pituitary hormones. These alterations reflect target cell sensitivity and response to preovulatory E_2.

Morphology of Gestational Endometrium

Glandular Epithelium

If pregnancy occurs, the secretory phase endometrium undergoes further morphophysiologic development and achieves its raison d'être, that is, to provide an appropriate environment for the conceptus. Between days 22 and 28, the endometrium displays hypertrophic and hypersecretory features that many refer to as "gestational hyperplasia."[45] The endometrium is characterized by (1) glandular ferning with epithelial and intraluminal secretions, (2) stromal edema and vascular congestion, and (3) transmucosal predecidual reaction devoid of inflammatory exudate (Fig. 9.33A). The changes are similar to but quantitatively exaggerated from nongestational 22–26-day secretory endometrium. In the latter, each of the above alterations is prominent on a given day of the secretory phase, whereas during early pregnancy, they occur simultaneously. However, gestational hyperplasia is not diagnostic of early pregnancy unless a 9–13-POD ovum is seen implanted in the endometrium or an elevated serum hCG is detected.[5,42] The presence of fibrinoid with syncytial giant cells representing the placental site is diagnostic. Indeed, morphologic modification similar to gestational hyperplasia also may be found in association with double (twin) corpora lutea[45] and persistent corpus luteum cyst.[42] The only pathognomonic feature of intrauterine pregnancy is chorionic tissue, embryonic tissue, or a fibrinoid layer with trophoblastic cells (Fig. 9.33B).

The gestational endometrium becomes distinctive by the fourth week of gestation. Many gestational glands display intraluminal epithelial projections (ferning), and often they are lined with large cells with clear or eosinophilic cytoplasm and varying-sized nuclei (Fig. 9.34). Exaggeration of these cytonuclear alterations produces the so-called Arias–Stella reaction (ASR),[3] characterized by voluminous cells with large hyperchromatic nuclei and irregular nu-

FIG. 9.32. **Menstrual endometrium, regenerative phase. A:** After expulsion of the functionalis layer, the basalis appears denuded (*arrow*) and is cleaved from the upper residual degenerated endometrial mucosa. The latter is made of stromal aggregates, ruptured glands, and inflammatory cells. **B:** Aggregates of residual stromal fibroblasts (stromal balls) are typical of late degenerative–early regenerative phase endometrium. **C:** Endometrial stromal fibroblasts forming the stromal balls are surrounded by resurfacing regenerative epithelial cells, which typically have flattened cytoplasm, enlarged nuclei and nucleoli consistent with repair, and nuclear polyploidy.

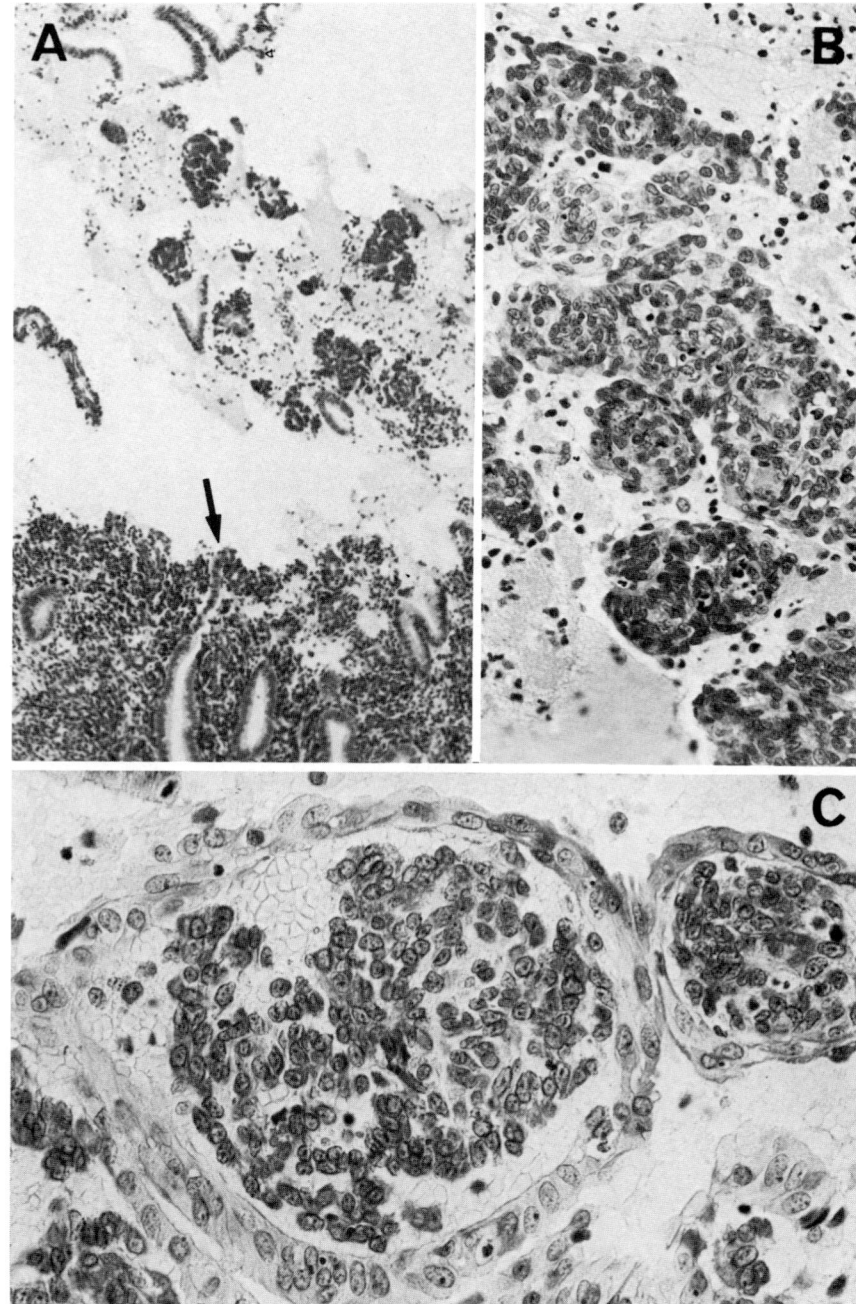

clear membranes. The cytoplasm often is clear and vacuolated. ASR, when extensive, may be confused with clear cell carcinoma. Unlike clear cell carcinoma, ASR is typically focal, and the adjacent endometrium shows normal gestational changes, that is, a prominent decidual reaction. In addition, in the malignant clear cells, there is a high nucleocytoplasmic (N/C) ratio, whereas ASR cells have normal N/C ratios, both the cytoplasm and nucleus being enlarged (cytonucleomegaly) (Fig. 9.35). Nuclear enlargement in ASR is a consequence of nuclear polyploidy, which presumably occurs by endomitosis and subsequent fusion of divided nuclei.[100] This is in contrast with the near diploid or aneuploid nuclear DNA content of endometrial carcinoma. ASR is a hormonally related gland cell hypertrophy associated with intra- or extrauterine pregnancy or trophoblastic disease.[86] The hormones involved are presumably chorionic gonadotropin, estrogen, and progesterone. ASR also may be seen in the glandular epithelium of the cervix, the fallopian tube, endometriosis, or vaginal adenosis.[86] In spontaneous abortion or later gestation, ASR demonstrates nuclear aberrations consistent with degenerative features, including agglutinated nuclear DNA, cytoplasmic vacuolization, and apical nuclear position (hobnail cells) (Fig. 9.35). These observations suggest that ASR in

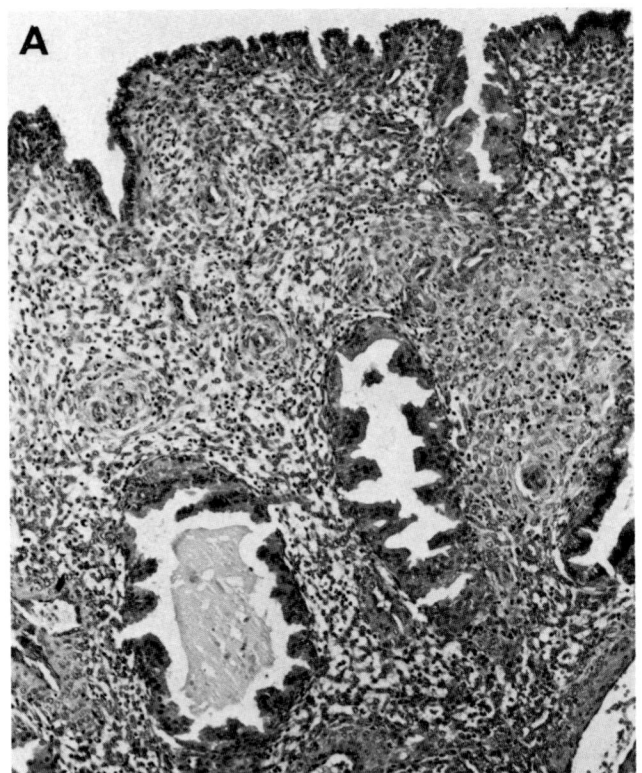

9.33A

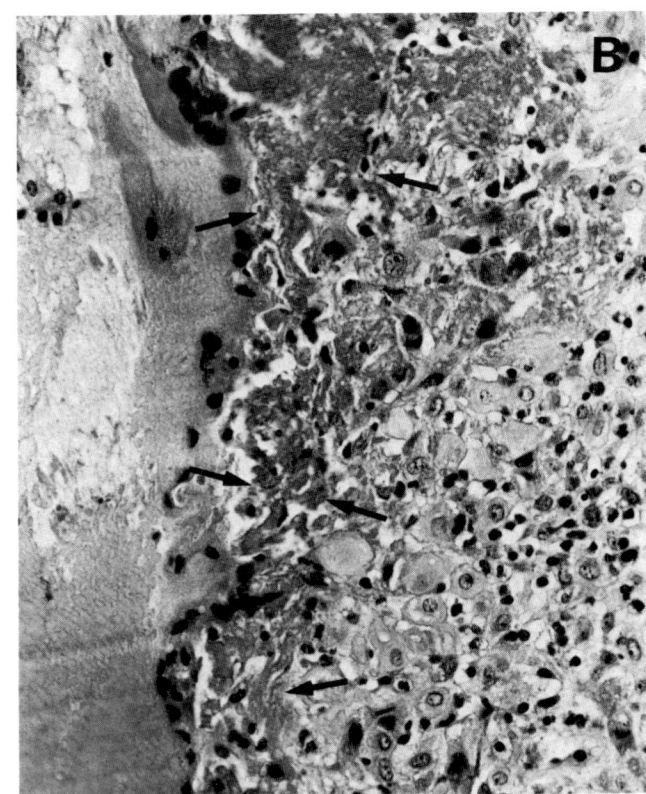

9.33B

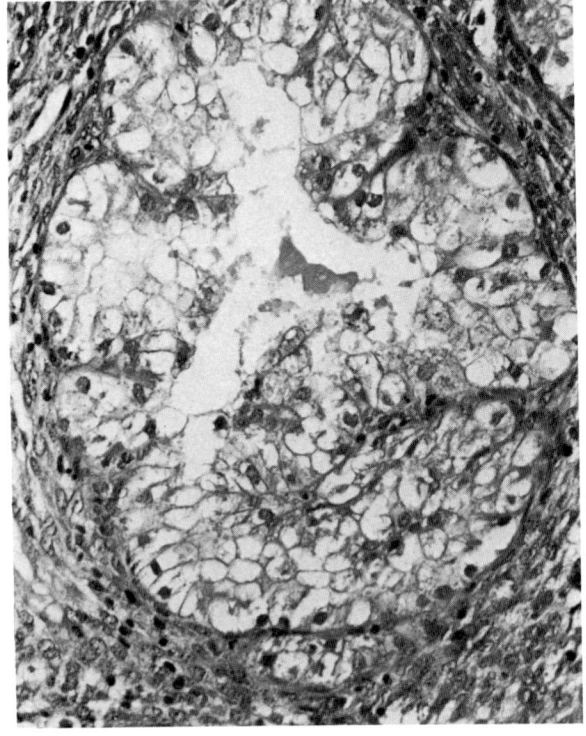

9.34

Fig. 9.33. Gestational endometrium. A: Voluminous secretory glands with numerous, prominent intraluminal epithelial projections and secretions are associated with dense predecidua (*right*), stromal edema (*left*), and a well developed arterial system. When these changes are seen in the upper one-third of the spongiosa layer, they are suggestive but not diagnostic of early gestation. **B:** Fibrinoid (Nitabuch's) layer (*arrows*), with placental site multinucleated syncytial cells on one side (*left*) and gestational decidua vera cells on the other side (*right*), is pathognomonic of intrauterine pregnancy.

Fig. 9.34. Hypersecretory gland with thickened, hypertrophic, pseudostratified cells with clear cytoplasm and blunt-ended epithelial projections into the lumen. The nuclei are round, and unlike those in the Arias–Stella reaction, are small. Both the glandular and cellular alterations are suggestive but not pathognomonic of early pregnancy.

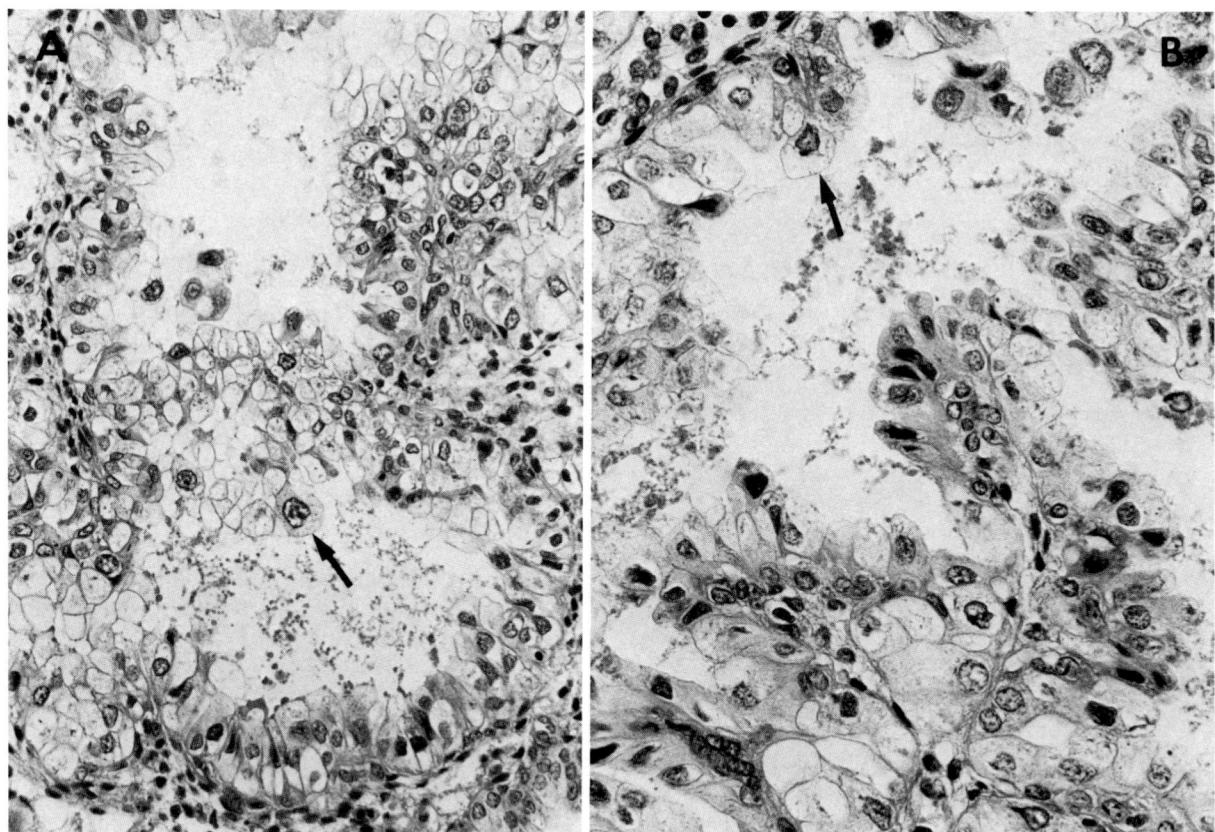

FIG. 9.35. **Gestational endometrium with Arias–Stella reaction (ASR). A:** Voluminous gland in which some of the lining cells demonstrate ASR (*arrow*), characterized by cytonucleomegaly, hyperchromatic nuclei, and enlarged nucleoli. Note the well preserved, finely granular cytoplasmic substance and nuclear chromatin of ASR cells. These are seen in the early developmental phase of ASR. **B:** ASR cells with shrunken, degenerated nuclei and vacuolated cytoplasm (*arrow*). This is the degenerative phase of ASR and is seen in missed abortions.

endometrial gland cells results from hyperstimulation induced by high levels of gestational hormones. These changes regress and disappear after withdrawal of hormonal stimulation.

Another distinctive feature in endometrial gland cells associated with intrauterine pregnancy and trophoblastic disease is nuclear vacuolization, so-called optically clear nuclei (Fig. 9.36), resembling the ground-glass appearance of herpes virus inclusions.[62] Ultrastructurally, however, nuclear clearing corresponds to strands of 70–80-AZ thick filaments. This in turn may correspond to a filamentous presentation of nuclear chromatin, secondary to gestational hormonal hyperstimulation.

Stroma

As discussed earlier, the predecidual cells are transformed into larger epithelioid decidual cells termed *decidua vera*. They are particularly prominent in the upper one-third of the endometrium and produce the compacta layer. Ultra-

structurally, gestational decidual cells contain comparatively more organelles, including intermediate filaments, cigar-shaped mitochondria, and granular endoplasmic reticulum, than their predecidual nongestational counterparts.[59,103] Whereas predecidual cells are interconnected by tight junctional nexuses, the gestational variant has nexuses between cytoplasmic filipodial projections (Fig. 9.37). The gestational decidual reaction is not pathognomonic of intrauterine pregnancy in general, since similar changes may be seen in ectopic pregnancy or as a result of exogenous progestational therapy.

Near the implantation site, cells resembling decidual cells often contain significant nuclear atypia. However, immunohistochemistry localizes human placental lactogen in these cells, incidating that they are intermediate-type trophoblast rather than decidual cells (see Chapter 23, Diseases of Placenta and Chapter 24, Gestational Trophoblastic Disease and Related Lesions).[57] This is also true for the so-called placental site reaction, which is produced by trophoblastic cells infiltrating the decidua near the implan-

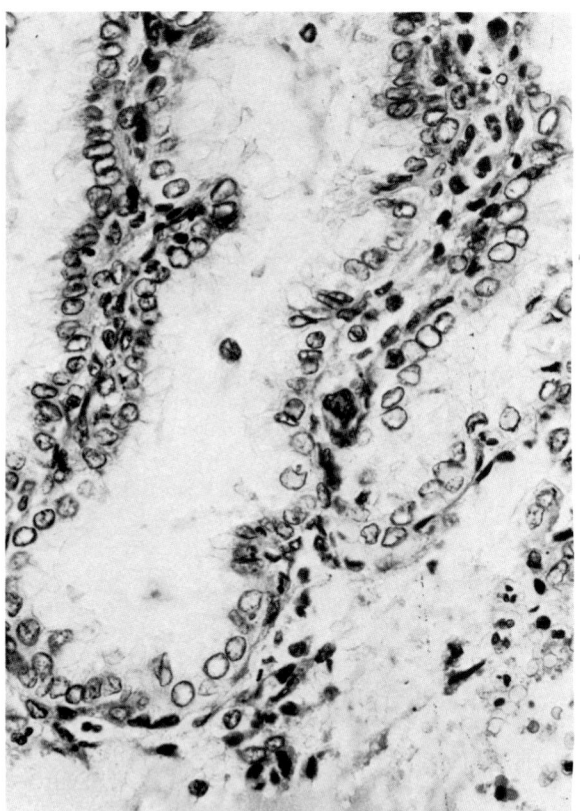

FIG. 9.36. Gestational endometrium. Intranuclear clearing resembling the ground-glass appearance of nuclei with herpes simplex virus inclusions. In gestational endometrial gland cells, however, the nuclei contain thread-like filaments rather than viral particles.

tation site. In both instances, the atypical cytologic features often are those of degeneration with agglutinated nuclear DNA and are focal. The neighboring endometrium contains gestational decidual cells and displays glandular secretory features. Occasionally, however, cytologic atypia seems to be a reflection of active trophoblastic cells that extend into the decidua. The decidual cells have phagocytic properties (see Fig. 22B, C) and digest the extracellular collagen matrix.[59] Decidual phagocytosis may facilitate the development of the decidual reaction by removing collagen from the endometrial stroma, which may represent a mechanical obstacle to proliferating and expanding decidual cells and also infiltrating trophoblastic cells.

Another important function of decidual cells is related to the maintenance of the fetal allograft (fetus).[71] Indeed, it is likely that decidual cells control the invasive nature of the normal trophoblast. Lack of a decidual reaction in the endometrium as occurs in the isthmus or in the fallopian tubal mucosa is accompanied by deep myometrial implantation of the placenta (placenta accreta) and invasion of the myosalpinx, respectively. An abdominal pregnancy may be viable because the subcoelomic mesenchymal cells of the

pelvic and abdominal peritoneum are capable of decidual transformation.[67] The factors that control decidual transformation in different sites are unknown; however, immunologic mechanisms may be involved.[11] Soon after implantation, decidual cells develop direct contact with semiallogenic fetal antigens and are considered to play an important role(s) in maintaining successful implantation and pregnancy. Both endometrial stromal cells and decidual cells have been shown immunohistochemically to express hemopoietic cell-associated CD13 and CD10 antigens in all respects similar to granulocytes, monocytes, and lymphoid cells (Table 9.1).[49] CD13 and CD10 antigens are peptidases; CD13 is an ectoenzyme identical to aminopeptidase, which also is found in intestinal and kidney brush border membrane. It hydrolyzes peptides such as bradykinin and enkephalin. CD10 antigen is similar to endopeptidase and is expressed in lymphoid and kidney cells and also is an ectopeptidase. It has been speculated that endometrial met-enkephalin and interleukin-1 (IL-1),[74] an immunomodulator and an inhibitor of decidualization, respectively,[73] may be degraded by CD13 or CD10, thereby contributing to a favorable environment for successful pregnancy.[49] The immunologic role of decidua is suggested by its suppression of the antibody response of spleen cultures to DNP–polylysine, as well as its suppression of the mixed lymphocyte reaction and proliferative response of lymphocytes to allogeneic graft cells and to T-cell mitogens.[53]

Earlier studies using hemopoietic cell-associated antigens suggested the bone marrow derivation of decidual cells.[53] However, most recent studies provide evidence that this may not be the case.[33,49] Both endometrial stromal cells and decidual cells express CD13 and CD10 surface antigens in all respects similar to granulocytes, monocytes, and lymphoid cells (Table 9.1); however, they are clearly distinguished from the latter by immunohistochemical tracing studies.[49] Also, decidual cells fail to express specific surface antigens of hematopoietic cells such as CD2, CD20, CD11b, and CD14.[51] The human nongestational and, particularly, gestational decidua also has been reported to have endocrinologic functions,[11] which apparently synthesize and release prolactin (PRL) that is immunologically identical to pituitary PRL. Although decidual cells lack ultrastructural similarity to pituitary cells and are devoid of secretory granules, prolactin was localized both in the predecidua and decidua in vitro by immunoblotting and its production is stimulated by progesterone and relaxin.[48] Furthermore, prolactin production was demonstrated exclusively in nongestational stromal cell cultures but not in gland cell cultures, and is induced and maintained by P and E_2.[78] Earlier observations identified gestational decidua synthesizing de novo prolactin and was the source of amniotic fluid prolactin.[81] The basement membrane of decidual cells resembles other basement membranes in the body and may contribute to the formation of

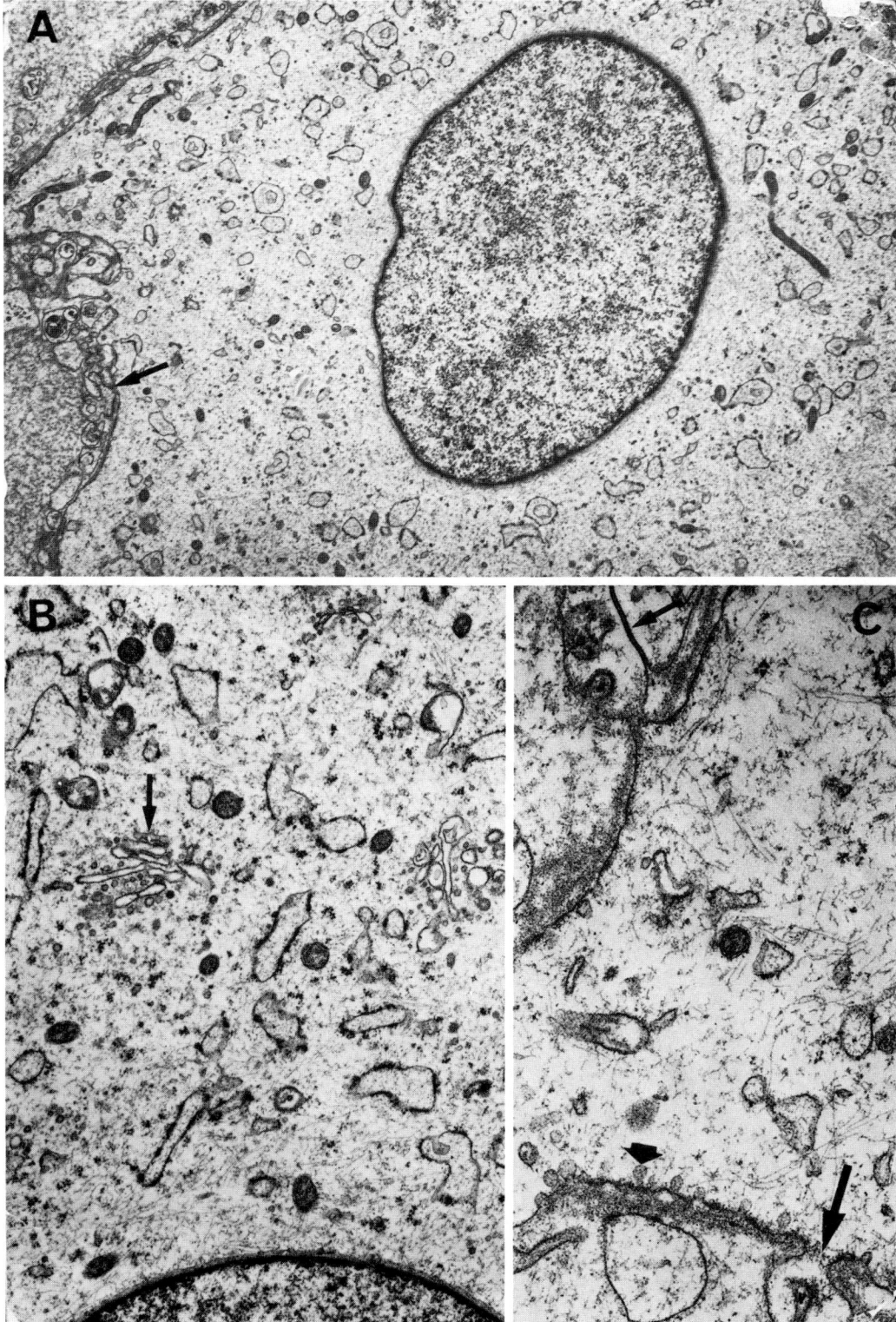

FIG. 9.37. Ultrastructure of 10-week-old gestational decidual cells. A: The prominent cytoplasm is centered by a round nucleus and contains scattered organelles. The cytoplasmic membrane contains club-shaped filopodial processes (*arrow*) projecting into the extracellular space. ×6000. **B:** Detail of organelles including the Golgi complex (*arrow*), intermingling with intermediate filaments. ×12,000. **C:** The cytoplasmic membrane contains micropinocytic vesicles (*short arrow*) and club-shaped cytoplasmic processes (*long arrow*). A tight junctional nexus (*fine arrow*) connects to cytoplasmic projections. ×22,000.

the laminin-rich Nitabuch's layer, in the placental implantation site. Both predecidual cells and cytotrophoblast produce laminin-containing basement membrane[53,54] and intermediate intracytoplasmic fibroblasts,[105] providing for their rigidity and supportive role to endometrial glands. Decidual cells also are suspected of synthesizing PGF_2 from archidonic acid released from intracellular stores of phospholipids.[30] Phospholipase A_2 that releases arachidonic acid is found in intracytoplasmic lysosomes. Release of PGF_2 from gestational decidual cells may play a role in the initiation of labor.

Spiral arteries are larger and their walls are thicker than those found in nongestational secretory endometrium. Some of them display acute atherosis, with concentric intimal proliferation of myofibroblasts and foamy cells (Fig. 9.38). These alterations apparently occur in response to trophoblastic invasion of endometrial vessels; they are focal and are more frequent in primigravidas.[95] They are not associated with preeclampsia, eclampsia, diabetes, or hypertension.[60] After delivery, the endometrial vessels near the implantation site undergo thrombosis and later hyalinization, as does the surrounding decidua. These alterations produce fibrohyaline nodules, so-called placental site nodules, typical of recent to remote (several years) intrauterine pregnancy (Fig. 9.39). When the pla-

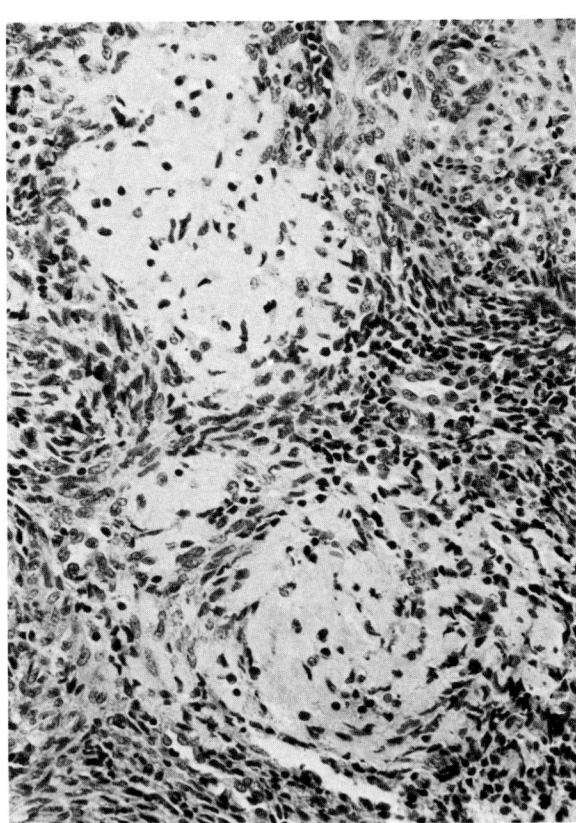

FIG. 9.39. Fibrohyaline nodules scattered with fibroblasts. These structures represent obliterated endometrial arteries at a previous placental site. This patient delivered 8 weeks before a curettage for postpartum bleeding.

cental site becomes acutely or chronically inflamed, the partially hyalinized and thrombosed vessels cannot contract, which leads to postpartum bleeding of the subinvoluting uterus.

Morphology of Inactive and Atrophic Endometrium

An endometrium that is as thick as early to midproliferative phase endometrium but is devoid of morphologic features of either active proliferation or secretion may be considered inactive as far as its response to hormonal stimuli is concerned. The glands and stroma resemble proliferative endometrium, but the glands usually are oriented parallel rather than perpendicular to the surface epithelium. The surface epithelium as well as that lining the glands is columnar to cuboidal and contains pseudostratified nuclei without mitoses, and occasional ciliated cells are seen. The stroma generally is dense throughout, without a clear-cut separation between the basalis and functionalis layer (Fig. 9.40). Such endometrial changes are found in most menopausal and postmenopausal women,[2] in whom ovarian hor-

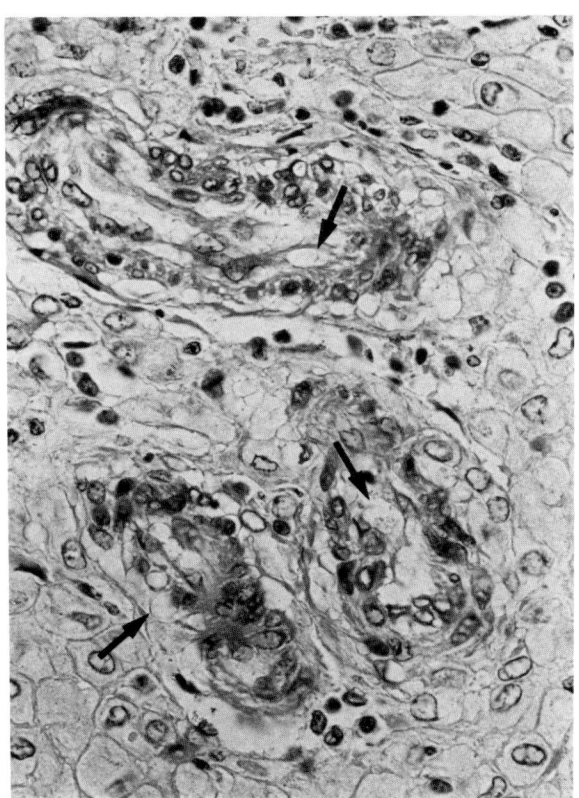

FIG. 9.38. Gestational endometrium. Atherosis of endometrial vessels with foamy vacuolization (*arrows*) of endothelial cells.

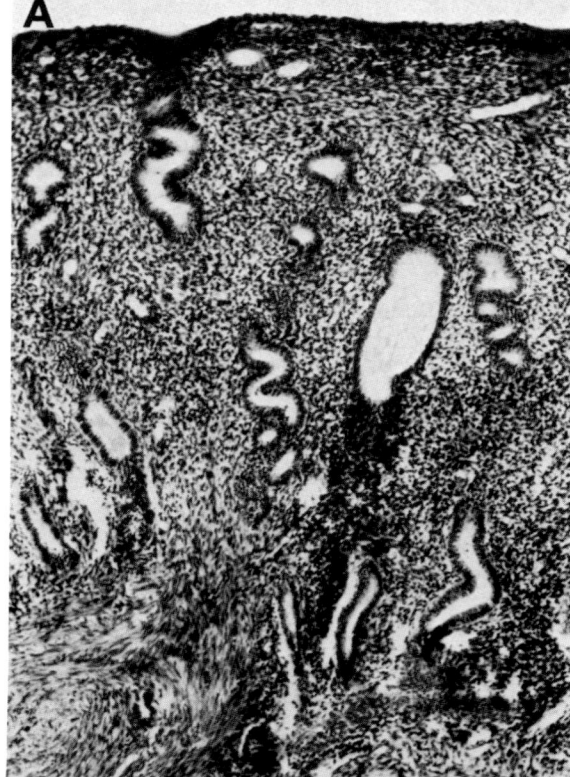

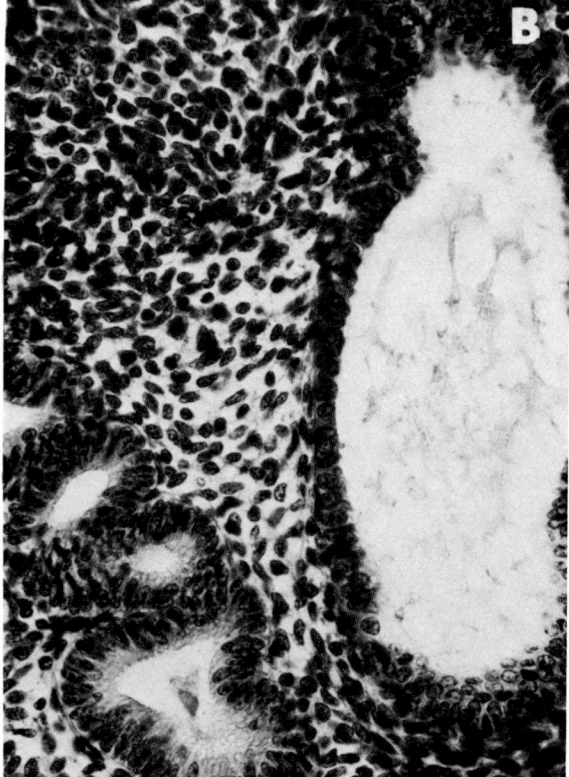

9.40

monal stimuli have decreased to levels not sufficient to induce endometrial proliferation. Nuclear DNA synthesis and E_2R are maintained in the senescent, inactive but not in the severely atrophic endometrium.[75] This phenomenon explains why exogenous estrogens can "revitalize" the inactive endometrium, and both glandular and stromal cells acquire receptors for P. As a result, unopposed estrogens in the menopause may lead to hyperplasia,[35] whereas P therapy either may convert hyperplasia to secretory endometrium or presents the development of hyperplasia.[29]

There are several morphologic manifestations of atrophic endometrium, but all have in common a thin mucosa that measures about half or less the thickness of a basal layer of cyclic endometrium (less than 0.5 mm). Typically, in the curettings, the entire atrophic endometrial mucosa, including its basalis layer, can be seen within a microscopic field of ×250. There is a further decrease in the number and volume, respectively, of glands and stroma and most commonly the glands are oriented parallel to the surface (Fig. 9.41). The lining epithelium of both the surface and glands is low and cuboidal and devoid of cilia, although cilia may be quite frequent in surface epithelial cells. The stroma often is collagenized and resembles the stroma of the isthmus or lower uterine segment in premenopausal women. Endometrial vascular alterations are seldom seen in women with atrophic endometrium, including those with abnormal uterine bleeding. In fact, in more than 50% of patients, no pathology is found in the uterus.[15,63] The most frequent morphologic changes that can be related to clinical bleeding are (1) arteriosclerosis of the myometrial arteries, including the arcuate and radial arteries, with medial hypertrophy and calcification and narrowing of the lumen, and (2) rupture of dilated and engorged endometrial veins secondary to uterine prolapse or compression by dilated atrophic endometrial cysts.[10,63] The former condition when associated with cardiovascular collapse may lead to hemorrhagic necrosis of the endometrial mucosa, producing apoplexia uteri.[21] At other times, coexistent chronic endometritis, submucous leiomyomata, or endometrial polyps may be the organic causes of uterine bleeding.

Often, atrophic endometrium has cystically dilated glands. Whether these represent the atrophic variants of

◁—————————————————

FIG. 9.40. Inactive endometrium. A: The endometrial stroma is uniformly dense without clear-cut separation between the upper functionalis and the lower basalis layers. The glandular architecture is similar to that of midproliferative phase endometrium; however, there are fewer glands, and some of them are oriented parallel to the surface. **B:** Inactive glandular epithelium has pseudostratified nuclei devoid of mitoses, and the surrounding stroma is dense and cellular, resembling the stroma of the basalis layer of cyclic endometrium.

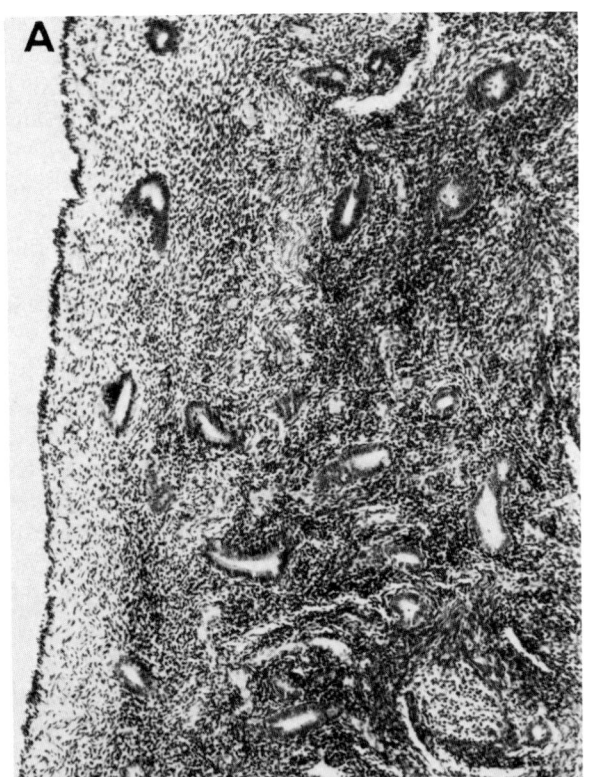

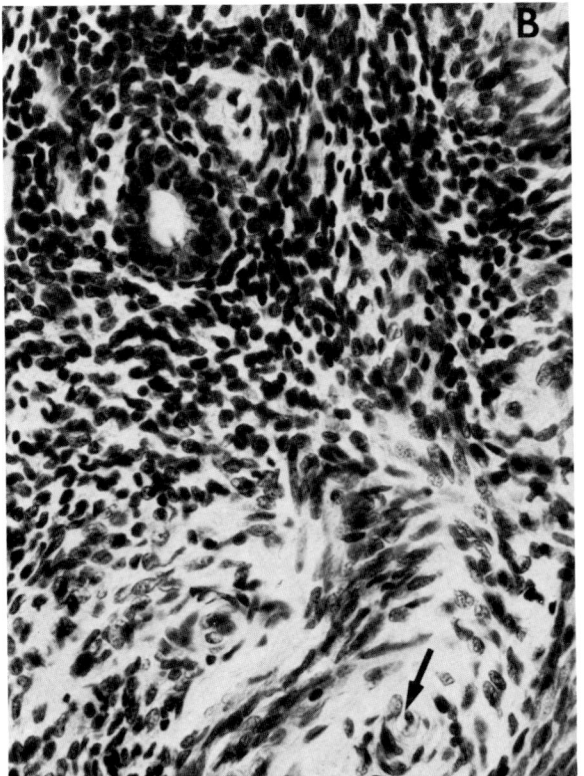

9.41

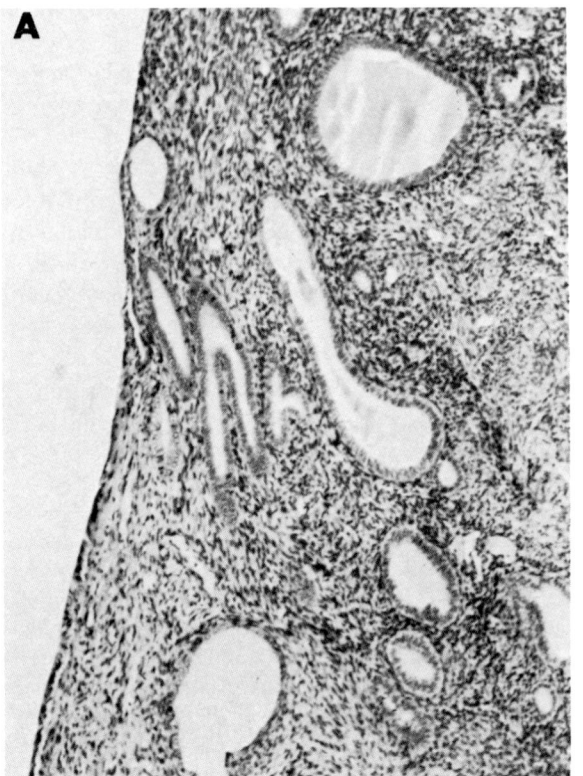

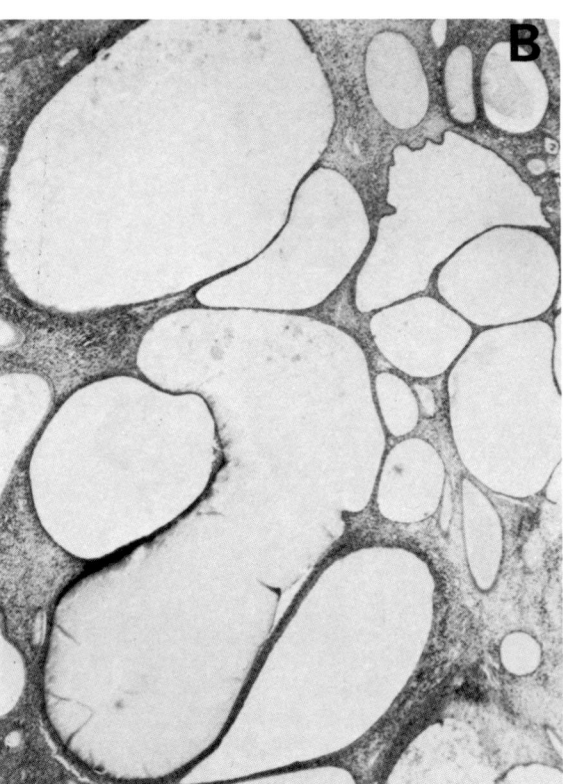

9.42

cystically dilated glands that are seen in the lower functionalis in virtually all women aged 35 years and over[52] is not clear. However, the condition is often referred to as *cystic atrophy* (Fig. 9.42A). Cystically dilated glands also are seen in cystic glandular hyperplasia with retrogressive atrophy. In this case the endometrial mucosa retains the thickness of an otherwise active hyperplasia, but the glandular epithelium is atrophic and the stroma is collagenized (Fig. 9.40B). On occasion, both the surface and glandular epithelium is composed of tall columnar to cuboidal cells, including ciliated cells resembling those seen in hyperplasia. Unlike true hyperplasia, this form of atrophy lacks mitotic figures, the mucosa is thin, and the stroma is relatively rich in collagen fibers (Fig. 9.43A). It is possible that the changes reflect the estrogenic response of otherwise atrophic endometrial epithelium that has been under either endogenous or exogenous estrogenic stimulation. The morphologic changes, furthermore, appear to be confined to the epithelial cells without stromal cell participation. In extreme atrophy, there is endometrial stromal fibrosis, and only the surface epithelium and rare glands remain lined by low cuboidal cells (Fig. 9.43B). In such cases, the isthmic ostium (internal os), as well as the external cervical os, may be completely stenotic, resulting in pyometra. In response to long-standing irritation by the chronic inflammatory exudate, the surface epithelium may undergo squamous metaplasia, which in extreme cases lines the entire endometrial cavity, resulting in the condition referred to as *ichthyosis or psoriasis uteri*.

Technical Consideration and Pitfalls in Interpretation of Biopsies

Accurate morphologic interpretation is achieved when either the biopsy sample or the curetting is taken from the body or fundus region and fixed immediately in either Bouin's solution or 10% buffered formalin. Bouin's solution is preferred because it preserves cytologic characteristics, whereas formalin is a tissue fixative that yields comparatively poor cytologic details.° If Bouin's solution is used, the jaw of the curette should not be immersed in the fixative, because Bouin's solution contains highly corrosive glacial acetic acid, which quickly blunts the cutting edge of the curette. Instead, the specimen should be removed from the curette with forceps, placed on a lens paper, and immersed in the fixative. The specimen adheres to the lens paper, thereby minimizing the possibility that the tissue may be lost during processing (see Chapter 27, Gross Description and Processing).

Morphologic interpretation, including dating of the endometrium, is based on the assessment of the functionalis of the endometrium, which is identified by its covering surface epithelium (see Figs. 9.24B, 9.25A). An endometrial specimen devoid of surface epithelium may lead to an inaccurate diagnosis because, in many instances, such endometrium represents the basalis layer, which does not respond to cyclic hormonal stimuli, and the specimen cannot be dated. In addition, since it often contains voluminous glands and compact stroma, with clusters of basal arteries (Fig. 9.44A), it may be confused with an endometrial polyp or hyperplasia. The endometrium in hysterectomy specimens often contains autolytic artifacts, which are due to the high proteolytic enzyme content of the endometrium.[8,55] This high enzyme content quickly produces autolytic changes if the specimen is not fixed immediately after removal of the uterus. The major morphologic autolytic artifacts include gland and stromal cell retractions (Fig. 9.44B). The best time to confirm ovulation is on cycle day 22 (POD 8) or later. Some investigators, including myself, advocate endometrial sampling at the onset of uterine bleeding.[5] By obtaining samples at the time of early uterine bleeding, the pathologist is able to determine whether the bleeding is caused by breakdown of postovulatory, secretory endometrium, focal necrosis of the endometrium associated with anovulation or other pathologic states, or exogenous sex steroid hormone administration. In addition, since with a few exceptions (inadequate luteal phase) the secretory phase of the cycle is constant in length (14 days ± 2 days), the time of ovulation can be estimated if the endometrium is of the normal menstrual type. During the period of bleeding, both the external os and the lower uterine segment are dilated, facilitating introduction of an endometrial aspirator into the endometrial cavity, thereby minimizing the discomfort associated with the endometrial biopsy. When the pathologist is confronted often with the morphology of menstrual endometrium, his diagnostic expertise of this condition is considerably improved. This, in turn, prevents the confusion of menstrual endo-

---

FIG. 9.41. **Atrophic endometrium. A:** The endometrial mucosa is thin and made of dense fibrocellular stroma and a few small glands with narrow lumens. **B:** Detailed view of endometrial arteries in basalis layer. There is severe obliterative endarteritis with minute lumens (*arrow*). The gland in the upper left is the size of a capillary, has a narrow lumen, and is lined by low cuboidal cells.

FIG. 9.42. **Atrophic endometrium. A:** Several cystically dilated glands, particularly at the endomyometrial junction, are often seen in otherwise atrophic endometrium. Their significance, if any, is unknown, but they are not considered to reflect previous hyperplasia. **B:** Cystic glandular dilation characterized by a relatively tall endometrial mucosa in which there are multiple cystic spaces lined by atrophic epithelium and surrounded by dense fibrous stroma.

°Formalin solution is superior to Bouin's solution if one plans DNA or immunohistochemical studies.

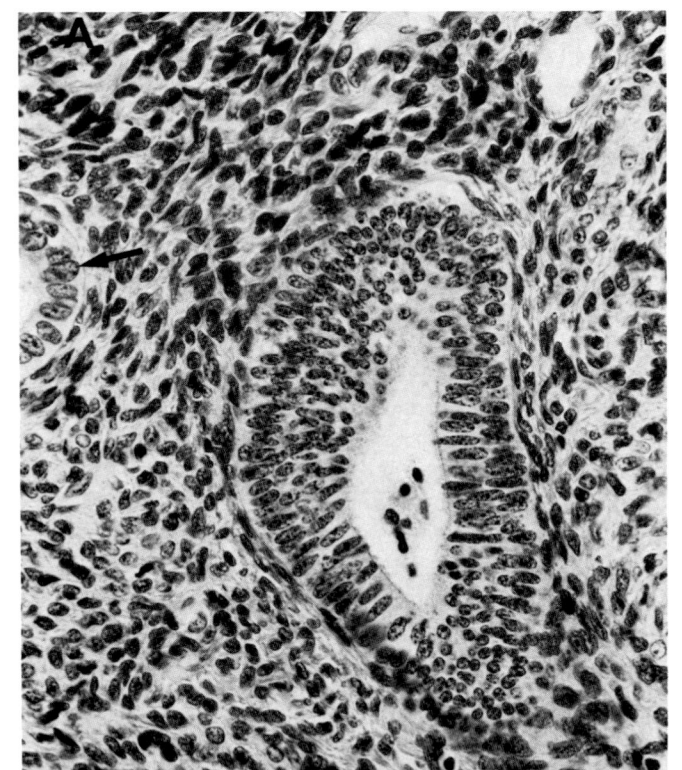
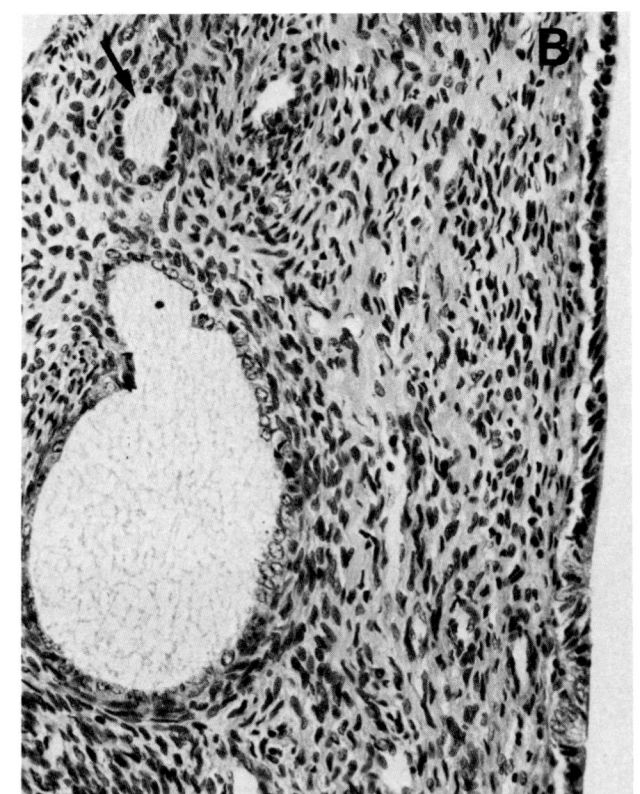

9.43

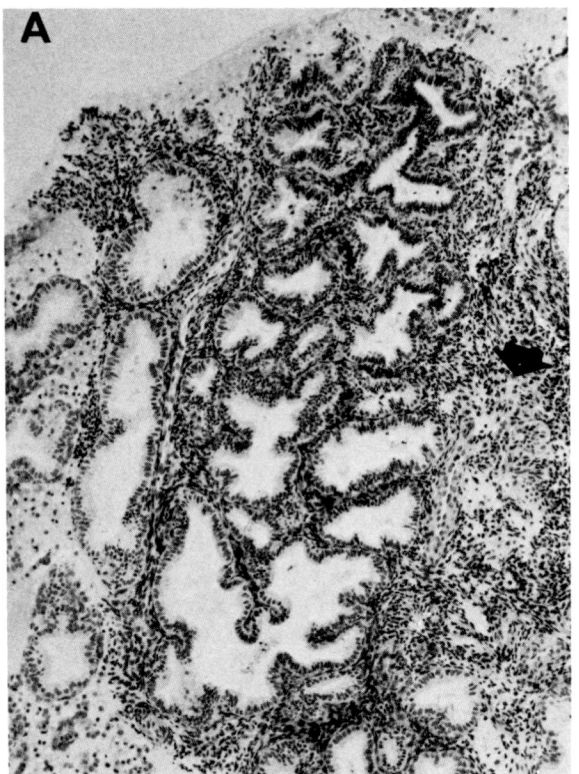
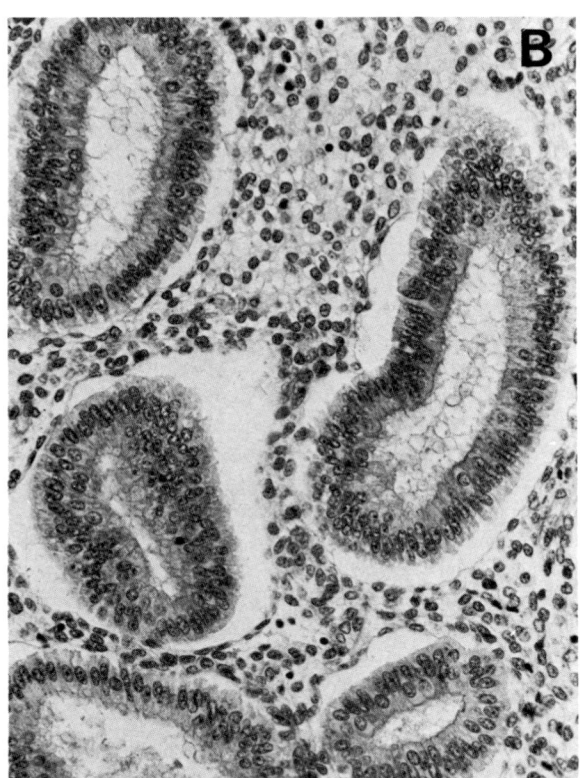

9.44

Fig. 9.43. Atrophic endometrium. A: The gland-lining cells are tall, columnar, with pencil-shaped pseudostratified nuclei and cilia resembling those found in endometrial hyperplasia. However, the endometrium is thin, and the stroma is dense, with many glands lined by atrophic epithelium (*arrow*). **B:** On the other end of the spectrum, in severe glandulostromal atrophy, both the surface- and gland-lining epithelium is low cuboidal, and the stroma is collagenous. Some of the glands resemble capillaries (*arrow*).

Fig. 9.44. Basalis endometrium. A: Clusters of tortuous glands in a back-to-back position masquerading as hyperplasia. The glandular aggregate is focal and flanked by clusters of basal arteries (*right*) (*arrow*) and degenerative spongiosa (*left*). Note the absence of surface epithelium. **B:** Delayed fixation artifact of endometrial specimens results in separation of glands from the supportive stroma, producing periglandular spaces. Such endometrium is difficult to date accurately.

---

metrium with endometrial carcinoma. Such a mistake is seen somewhat frequently in routine pathology practice.[104] Secretory endometrium may be relatively more difficult to date precisely than menstrual endometrium. Indeed, secretory endometrium often demonstrates subtle changes and combinations of morphologic patterns that may result in errors of ±4–5 days. This can be improved to ±2 days, however, by basing the date on the endometrial alterations that represent the most advanced phase of the menstrual cycle. For example, an endometrial biopsy may show changes consistent with the 16th, 17th, and 18th days of the cycle; the diagnosis should be based on the most advanced date and, therefore, reported as 18th-day secretory endometrium instead of averaging cycle days and reporting 17th-day secretory endometrium.

References

1. Abel MH, Baird DT (1980) The effect of 17β-estradiol and progesterone on prostaglandin production by human endometrium maintained in organ culture. Endocrinology 106: 1599

2. Archer DF, McIntyre-Seltman K, Wilborn WW, et al (1991) Endometrial morphology in asymptomatic postmenopausal women. Am J Obstet Gynecol 165: 317–322

3. Arias-Stella J (1972) Atypical endometrial changes produced by chorionic tissue. Hum Pathol 3: 450

4. Aronica SM, Katzenellenbogen BS (1991) Progesterone receptor regulation in uterine cells: stimulation by estrogen, cyclic adenosine 3″, 5″-monophosphate, and insulin-like growth factor I and suppression by antiestrogens and protein kinase. Endocrinology 128: 2045–2052

5. Arronet GH, Berquist GA, Parekh MC, et al (1973) Evaluation of endometrial biopsy in the cycle of conception. Int J Fertil 18: 220

6. Baggish MS, Pauerstein CJ, Woodruff JD (1967) Role of stroma in regeneration of endometrial epithelium. Am J Obstet Gynecol 99: 453

7. Bartelemez GW (1957) The form and the functions of the uterine blood vessels in the rhesus monkey. Contrib Embryol Carnegie Inst Wash 36: 153

8. Beller FK, Schweppe KW (1979) Review on the biology of menstrual blood. In: Beller FK, Schaumacher GFB (eds), The biology of the fluids of the female genital tract. Amsterdam, New York, Elsevier-North Holland Press, pp 231–245

9. Berchuck A, Soisson AP, Olt GJ, et al (1989) Reactivity of epidermal growth factor receptor monoclonal antibodies with human uterine tissues. Arch Pathol Lab Med 113: 1155–1158

10. Bergeron C, Ferenczy A, Toft DO, Schneider W, Shyamala G (1988) Immunocytochemical study of progesterone receptors in the human endometrium during the menstrual cycle. Lab Invest 59: 862–869

11. Bryant-Greenwood GD (1991) The human relaxins: consensus and dissent. Molec Cell endocrinol 79: C125–C132

12. Bulmer JN, Hollings D, Ritson A (1987) Immunocytochemical evidence that endometrial stromal granulocytes are granulated lymphocytes. J Pathol 153: 281–288

13. Charpin C, Pancino G, Blanc B, et al (1991) Monoclonal antibody 1BE12 immunoreactivity with human endometrium. Int J Gynecol Pathol 10: 380–393

14. Chiquet-Ehrismann R, Kalla P, Pearson CA (1989) Participation of tenascin and TGF-beta in reciprocal epithelial-mesenchymal interactions of MCF 7 cells and fibroblasts. Cancer Res 49: 4322–4325

15. Choo YC, Mak KC, Hsu C, Wong TS, Ma HK (1985) Postmenopausal uterine bleeding of nononcogenic cause. Obstet Gynecol 66: 225

16. Christiaens GCML, Sixma JJ, Haspels AA (1980) Morphology of haemostasis in menstrual endometrium. Br J Obstet Gynecol 87: 425

17. Clark KE, Farley DB, Van Orden DE, Brody MJ (1977) Estrogen-induced uterine hyperemia and edema persist during histamine receptor blockade. Proc Soc Exp Biol Med 156: 411

18. Crow J, Wilkins M, Howe S, More L, Helliwell P (1991) Mast cells in the female genital tract. Int J Gynecol Pathol 10: 230–237

19. Dabbs DJ, Geisinger KR, Norris HT (1986) Intermediate filaments in endometrial and endocervical carcinomas: the diagnostic utility of vimentin patterns. Am J Surg Pathol 10: 568–576

20. Dallenbach FD, Dallenbach G (1964) Immunohistologische untersuchungen zur lokalisation des relaxins in menschlichen placenta und decidua. Virchows Arch [Pathol Anat] 337: 301

21. Daly JJ, Balogh K Jr (1968) Hemorrhagic reaction of the senile endometrium ("apoplexia uteri"). Relation to superficial hemorrhagic necrosis of the bowel. N Engl J Med 278: 709

22. Feinberg BB, Tan NS, Gonik B, Brath PC, Walsh SW (1991) INcreased progesterone concentrations are necessary to suppress interleukin-2-activated human mononuclear cell cytotoxicity. Am J Obstet Gynecol 165: 1872–1876

23. Ferenczy A (1976) Studies on the cytodynamics of human endometrial regeneration: I. Scanning electron microscopy. Am J Obstet Gynecol 124: 64–74

24. Ferenczy A (1976) Studies on the cytodynamics of human

endometrial regeneration: II. Transmission electron microscopy and histochemistry. Am J Obstet Gynecol 124: 582–595

25. Ferenczy A (1977) Studies on the cytodynamics of experimental endometrial regeneration in the rabbit. Historadioautography and ultrastructure. Am J Obstet Gynecol 128: 536–545

26. Ferenczy A (1980) Regeneration of the human endometrium. In: Fenoglio CM, Wolff M (eds) Progress in surgical pathology. New York, Masson Publishing USA Inc., Vol 1, pp 157–173

27. Ferenczy A, Bertrand G, Gelfand MM (1979) Proliferation kinetics of human endometrium during the normal menstrual cycle. Am J Obstet Gynecol 133: 859–867

28. Ferenczy A, Richart RM, Agate FJ Jr, Purkerson ML, Dempsey EW (1972) Scanning electron microscopy of the endometrial surface. Fertil Steril 23: 515–521

29. Ferenczy A, Gelfand M (1989) The biologic significance of cytologic atypia in progestogentreated endometrial hyperplasia. Am J Obstet Gynecol 160: 126–131

30. Fitzpatrick RL, Liggins GC (1980) Effects of prostaglandins on the cervix of pregnant women and sheep. In: Naftolin F, Stubblefield PF (eds) Dilatation of the uterine cervix. New York, Raven Press, pp 287–300

31. Flowers CE Jr, Wilborn WH (1978) New observations on the physiology of menstruation. Obstet Gynecol 51: 14–16

32. Folkman J (1976) The vascularization of tumors. Sci Am 234: 58

33. Fowlis DJ, Ansell JD (1985) Evidence that decidual cells are not derived from bone marrow. Transplantation 39: 445–446

34. Franquemont DW, Frierson HF, Mills SE (1991) An immunohistochemical study of normal endometrial stroma and endometrial stromal neoplasms. Am J Surg Pathol 15: 861–870

35. Gelfand MM, Ferenczy A (1989) A prospective 1-year study of estrogen and progestin in postmenopausal women. Effects on the endometrium. Obstet Gynecol 74: 398–401

36. Gerdes GL, Lemke H, Baisch H, et al (1984) Cell cycle analysis of a cell proliferation associated human nuclear antigen defined by the monoclonal antibody Ki67. J Immunol 133: 1710–1715

37. Gerdes J, Pickartz H, Brotherton J, et al (1987) Growth fractions and estrogen receptors in human breast cancers as determined in-situ with monoclonal antibodies. Am J Pathol 129: 486–492

38. Gibson M, Badger GJ, Byrn F, et al (1991) Error in histologic dating of secretory endometrium: variance component analysis. Fertil Steril 56: 242–247

39. Greene GL, Nolan C, Engner JP, Jensen EW (1980) Monoclonal antibodies to human estrogen receptors. Proc Natl Acad Sci USA 77: 5115

40. Gurpide E, Tseng L, Gusberg SB (1977) Estrogen metabolism in normal and neoplastic endometrium. Am J Obstet Gynecol 129: 809

41. Haining REB, Cameron IT, van Papendorp C, et al (1991) Epidermal growth factor in human endometrium: proliferative effects in culture and immunocytochemical localization in normal and endometriotic tissues. Human Reprod 6: 1200–1205

42. Hendrickson MR, Kempson RL (1980) Surgical pathology of the uterine corpus. In: Bennington JL (ed) Major problems in pathology. Philadelphia W.B. Saunders, Vol 12, pp 36–98

43. Henzl MR, Smith RE, Boost G, Tyler ET (1972) Lysosomal concept of menstrual bleeding in humans. J Clin Endocrinol Metab 34: 860

44. Herr J (1978) Decidual cells in the human ovary at term. Am J Anat 152: 7–28

45. Hertig AT (1964) Gestational hyperplasia of endometrium. A morphologic correlation of ova, endometrium and corpora lutea during pregnancy. Lab Invest 13: 1153

46. Hofmann GE, Drews MR, Scott RT (1992) Epidermal growth factor and its receptor in human implantation trophoblast: immunohistochemical evidence for autocrine/paracrine function. J Clin Endocrinol Metab 74: 981–988

47. Horbelt DV, Roberts DK, Walker N, Delmore JE (1986) Nucleolar canalicular structure in extrauterine endometriosis. Human Pathol 17: 924–925

48. Huang JR, Tseng L, Bischof P, Janne OA (1987) Regulation of prolactin production by progestin, estrogen and relaxin in human endometrial stromal cells. Endocrinology 121: 2011–2017

49. Imai K, Maeda M, Fujiwara H, et al (1992) Human endometrial stromal cells and decidual cells express cluster of differentiation (CD) 13 antigen/aminopeptidase N and CD10 antigen/neutral endopeptidase. Biol Reprod 46: 328–334

50. Johnson DC, Dey SK (1980) Role of histamine in implantation: Dexamethasone inhibits estradiol-induced implantation in the rat. Biol Reprod 22: 1136

51. Kamat BR, Isaacson PG (1987) The immunocytochemical distribution of leukocytic subpopulations in human endometrium. Am J Pathol 127: 66–73

52. Katzenellenbogen BS (1980) Dynamics of steroid hormone receptor action. Ann Rev Physiol 42: 17

53. Kearns M (1983) Life history of decidual cells: A review. Am J Reprod Immunol 3: 78–82

54. Kliman HJ, Coutifaris C, Feinberg RF, Strauss JF III, Haimowitz JE (1989) In: Blastocyst Implantation, Yoshinaga K (ed) Boston, Adams, pp 19–83

55. Kok P (1979) Separation of plasminogen activators from human plasma and a comparison with activators from human uterine tissue and urine. Thromb Haemost 4: 734

56. Krehbiel RH (1937) Cytochemical studies of the decidual reaction in the rat during early pregnancy and in the production of deciduomata. Physiol Zool 10: 212–235

57. Kurman RJ, Young RH, Norris HJ, et al (1984) Immunocytochemical localization of placental lactogen and chorionic gonadotropin in the normal placenta and trophoblastic tumors, with emphasis on intermediate trophoblast and the placental site trophoblastic tissue. Int J Gynecol Pathol 3: 101

58. Langlois PL (1970) The size of the normal uterus. J Reprod Med 4: 220

59. Lawn AM, Wilson EW, Finn CA (1971) The ultrastructure of human decidual and predecidual cells. J Reprod Fertil 26: 85

60. Lichtig C, Deutch M, Barnes J (1984) Vascular changes of endometrium in early pregnancy. Am J Clin Pathol 81: 702

61. Lindeman HJ (1979) Hysteroscopic data during menstruation. In: Beller FK, Schaumacher GFB (eds) The biology of the fluids of the female genital tract. Amsterdam, New York, Elsevier-North Holland Press, pp 225–229

62. Mazur MT, Hendrickson MR, Kempson RL (1983) Optically clear nuclei. An alteration of endometrial epithelium in the presence of trophoblast. Am J Surg Pathol 7: 415

63. Meyer WC, Malkasian GD, Dockerty MB, Decker DG (1971) Postmenopausal bleeding from atrophic endometrium. Obstet Gynecol 38: 731

64. More IAR, Armstrong EM, McSeveney D, Chatfield WR (1974) The morphogenesis and fate of the nucleolar channel system in the human endometrial glandular cells. J Ultrastruc Res 47: 74

65. Noyes RW, Hertig AT, Rock J (1950) Dating the endometrial biopsy. Fertil Steril 1: 3

66. Nozawa S, Sakayori M, Ohta K (1989) A monoclonal antibody MSN-1 against a newly established uterine endometrial cancer cell line (SNGII) and its application to immunohistochemistry and flow cytometry. Am J Obstet Gynecol 161: 1079–1086

67. Ober WB (1979) Carcinosarcoma of the ovary. Case report, review of literature and comment on the subcoelomic mesenchyme. Am J Diag Gynecol Obstet 1: 73

68. O'Rahilly R (1977) Prenatal human development. In: Wynn RM (ed) Biology of the uterus. New York, Plenum Press, pp 35–57

69. Orcel L, Smadj A, Roland J, Minh HN (1973) Nouvelle hypothèse sur le mecanisme intime de la menstruation. Rev Fr Gynecol 68: 477

70. Osteen KG, Anderson TL, Schwartz K, Hargrove JT, Gorstein F (1992) Distribution of tumor-associated glycoprotein-72 (TAG-72) expression throughout the normal female reproductive tract. Int J Gynecol Pathol 11: 216–220

71. Parhar RS, Kennedy TG, Lala PK (1988) Suppression of lymphocyte alloreactivity by early gestational human decidua. Cell Immunol 116: 392–410

72. Perrot-Applanat M, Groyer-Picard MT, Garcia E, Lorenzo F, Milgrom E (1988) Immunocytochemical demonstration of estrogen and progesterone receptors in muscle cells of uterine arteries in rabbits and humans. Endocrinology 123: 1511–1519

73. Pierart ME, Najdovski T, Appelboom TE, Deschodt-Lanckman MM (1988) Effect of human endopeptidase 24.11 ("enkephalinase") on IL-1 induced thymocyte proliferation activity. J Immunol 140: 3808–3811

74. Polan ML, Loukides J, Nelson P, et al (1989) Progesterone and estradiol modulate interleukin-1 beta messenger ribonucleic acid levels in cultured human peripheral monocytes. J Clin Endocrinol Metab 69: 1200–1206

75. Press MF, Nousek-Goebl N, King WJ, Herbst AL, Greene GL (1984) Immunohistochemical assessment of estrogen receptor distribution in the human endometrium throughout the menstrual cycle. Lab Invest 51: 495–503

76. Pryse Davies J, Ryder TA, Mackenzie ML (1979) In vivo production of the nucleolar channel system in postmenopausal endometrium. Cell Tissue Res 203: 493

77. Ramsey EM History. In: Wynn RM (ed) Biology of the uterus. New York, Plenum Press, pp 1–34

78. Randolph JF Jr, Peegel H, Ansbacher R, Menon KMJ (1990) In vitro induction of prolactin production and aromatase activity by gonadal steroids exclusively in the stroma of separated proliferative human endometrium. Am J Obstet Gynecol 162: 1109–1114

79. Ravn V, Teglbjaerg CS, Visfeldt J (1992) Mucin-type carbohydrates (type 3 chain antigens) in normal cycling human endometrium. Int J Gynecol Pathol 11: 38–46

80. Rebello R, Green FHY, Fox H (1975) A study of the secretory immune system of the female genital tract. Br J Obstet Gynaecol 82:812

81. Riddick DH, Kusmik WF (1977) Decidua: a possible source of amniotic fluid prolactin. Am J Obstet Gynecol 127: 187–190

82. Sainsbury JRC, Farndon JR, Needham GK, Malcolm AJ, Harris AL (1987) Epidermal growth factor receptor status as predictor of early recurrence of and death from cancer. Lancet 1398–1402

83. Sakbun V, Ali SM, Greenwood FC, Bryant-Greenwood GD (1990) Human relaxin in the amnion, chorion, decidua parietalis, basal plate and placental trophoblast by immunocytochemistry and northern analysis. J Clin Endocrinol Metab 70: 508–514

84. Sananes N, Baulieu EE, LeGoascogne C (1976) Prostaglandin(s) as inductive factor of decidualization in the rat uterus. Mol Cell Endocrinol 6: 153

85. Satake T, Matsuyama M (1987) Argyrophil cells in normal endometrial glands. Virchows Arch A 410: 449–454

86. Silverberg SG, Arias-Stella J (1972) Phenomenon in spontaneous and therapeutic abortion. Am J Obstet Gynecol 112: 777

87. Slamon DJ, Clark GM, Wong SG, et al (1987) Human breast cancer: correlation of relapse and survival with amplification of the HER-2/neu proto-oncogene. Science 235: 177–182

88. Slamon DJ, Goldolphin W, Jones LA, et al (1989) Studies of the HER -/neu protooncogene in human breast and ovarian cancer. Sciences 244: 707–712

89. Smith SK, Abel MH, Baird DT (1984) Effect of 17β-estradiol and progesterone on the levels of prostaglandin $F_{2\alpha}$ and E_2 in human endometrium. Prostaglandins 27: 591–597

90. Szego CM (1972) Lysosomal membrane stabilization and antiestrogen action in specific hormonal target cells. Gynecol Invest 3: 63

91. Tabibzadeh S (1990) Immunoreactivity of human endometrium: correlation with endometrial dating. Fertil Steril 54: 624–631

92. Taketani Y, Masahiko M (1991) Evidence for direct regulation of epidermal growth factor receptors by steroid hormones in human endometrial cells. Human Reprod 6: 1365–1369

93. Tawfik OW, Huet YM, Malathy PV, Johnson DC, Dey SK (1987) Release of prostaglandins and leukotrienes from the rat uterus is an early estrogenic response. Prostaglandins 34: 805–814

94. Tawfik OW, Sagrillo C, Johnson DC, Dey SK (1987) Decidualization in the rat: role of leukotrienes and prostaglandins. Prostagland Leukotri Med 29: 221–227

95. Taylor PV, Hancock KW (1975) Antigenicity of trophoblast and possible antigen-marking effects during pregnancy. Immunology 28: 973

96. Thor A, Viglione MJ, Muraro R, et al (1987) Monoclonal antibody B72.3 reactivity with human endometrium: a study of normal and malignant tissues. Int J Gynecol Pathol 6: 235 247

97. Tseng L (1979) Physiologic changes in binding and metabolism of estradiol and progesterone in human endometrium during the menstrual cycle. Obstet Gynecol Annu 8: 1

98. Van Orden DE, Clancey CJ, Farley DB (1981) Uterine serotonin and receptor blockage during estrogen-induced uterine hyperemia. Proc Soc Exp Biol Med 167: 469

99. Vollmer G, Siegal GP, Chiquet-Ehrismann R, et al (1990) Tenascin expression in the human endometrium and in endometrial adenocarcinomas. Lab Invest 62: 725–730

100. Wagner D, Richart RM (1968) Polyploidy in the human endometrium with the Arias-Stella reaction. Arch Pathol 85: 475

101. Waites GT, James RFL, Bell SC (1988) Immunohistological localization of the human endometrial secretory protein pregnancy-associated endometrial α_1-globulin, an insulin like growth factor-binding protein during the menstrual cycle. J Clin Endocrinol Metab 67: 1100–1104

102. Weissman G (1964) Labilization and stabilization of lysosomes. Fed Proc 23: 1038

103. Wilikinson N, Buckley CH, Chawner L, Fox H. Nucleolar organiser regions in normal, hyperplastic and neoplastic endometrium. Int J Gynecol Pathol 9: 55–59, 1990

104. Winkler B, Alvarez S, Richart RM, Crum CP (1984) Pitfalls in the diagnosis of endometrial neoplasia. Obstet Gynecol 64: 185

105. Winter S, Yarrasch ED, Schmid E, Franke WW (1980) Differences in polypeptide composition of cytokeratin filaments, including filaments from different epithelial tissues and cells. Eur J Cell Biol 22: 371

106. Wynn RM (1989) Histology and ultrastructure of the human endometrium. In: Wynn RM, Jollie WP (eds) Biology of the uterus. New York, Plenum Press, pp 289–329

107. Zaytsev P, Taxy JB (1987) Pregnancy-associated ectopic decidua. Am J Surg Pathol 11: 526–530

108. Zhinkin LD, Samoshkina NA (1967) DNA synthesis and cell proliferation during formation of deciduomata in mice. J Embryol Exp Morphol 17: 598

10

Benign Diseases of the Endometrium

Robert J. Kurman, M.D., and Michael T. Mazur, M.D.

A wide variety of benign diseases, from rare infections to commonplace polyps, occur in the endometrium. Furthermore, since the uterus is a target organ for hormonal stimulation, morphologic changes involving the endometrium may reflect disorders in the hypothalamic–pituitary–ovarian axis and the effects of exogenous hormone medications. The histological alterations are typically manifested by abnormal uterine bleeding, and an endometrial biopsy or curettage is commonly performed to determine its cause and to control excessive bleeding. The endometrial biopsy also continues to be an important and integral part of the infertility work-up. Consequently, it is necessary to be aware of the wide variety of benign diseases as well as hyperplasia and carcinoma that may affect the endometrium. This chapter considers various benign, congenital, and acquired conditions involving the uterine corpus. For a more comprehensive discussion of the interpretation of these various diseases in endometrial biopsies and curettings, the reader is directed to a text that specifically addresses these issues.[146]

Congenital Abnormalities

Congenital abnormalities of the uterus are uncommon.[16] Many of these abnormalities are due to the effects of exogenous hormones, such as diethylstilbestrol (DES)[118] in utero or endogenous hormones associated with abnormal gonads and chromosomal defects. The latter group of congenital disorders is described in Chapter 1, Embryology of the Female Genital Tract and Disorders of Abnormal Sexual Development, and the upper and lower genital tract structural abnormalities associated with in utero DES exposure are discussed in Chapter 4, Diseases of the Vagina. Another group of müllerian duct abnormalities occurs in genotypically normal females with normal gonads. These developmental aberrations, such as defects in the fusion of the müllerian ducts, are due to faulty morphogenesis and are similar to those occurring in other organ systems of the embryo. Little is known of their precise etiology. Some may result from abnormal hormonal stimulation, and others may be of genetic origin. These disorders may be quite complex and frequently are associated with malformations in the urinary system and the distal gastrointestinal tract (see Chapter 1). For practical purposes, these müllerian duct abnormalities can be divided into two categories: (1) abnormalities of fusion and (2) abnormalities due to atresia.

Fusion Defects of the Müllerian Ducts

Normally, the upper one-third of the vagina and the uterus are formed by fusion of the paired müllerian ducts. After fusion, the intervening wall degenerates, forming the endometrial cavity and upper vaginal canal. Two types of abnormalities can occur, depending on whether fusion or subsequent degeneration is the pathologic process. Nonfusion of the müllerian ducts gives rise to the *uterus bicornis* (Figs. 10.1c, 10.2). Persistence of the fused ducts with failure of degeneration results in the development of a septum. If the defect is minor or confined to the fundus, the uterus is referred to as *arcuatus* (Fig. 10.1b). If the septum persists throughout the full length of the uterus and upper vagina, a *uterus didelphys* with a partially double vagina results (Fig. 10.1a). These congenital anomalies may cause infertility or spontaneous abortion and therefore require surgical correction.[89,254]

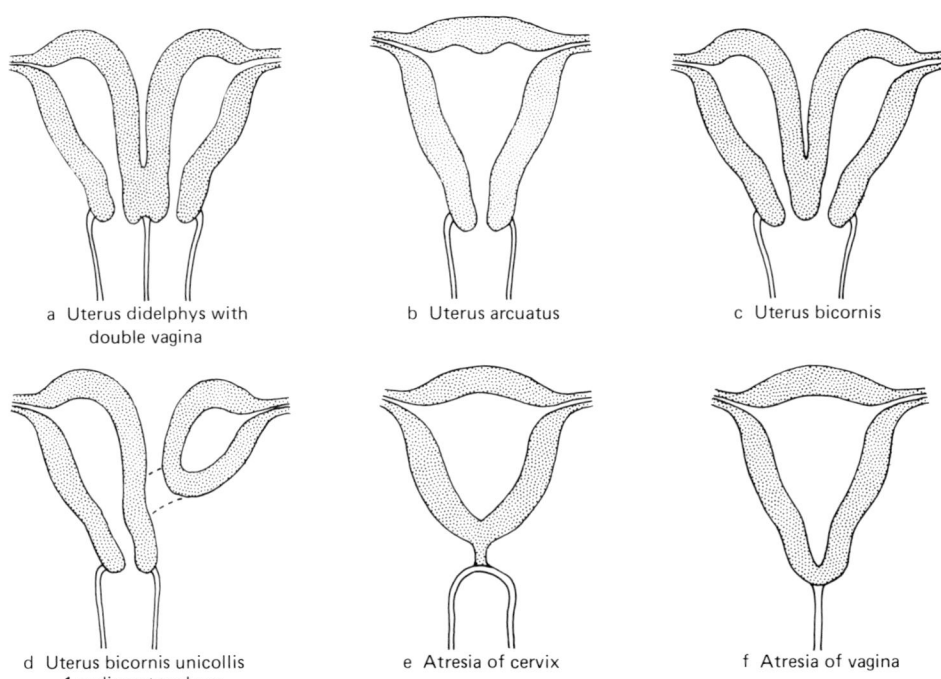

a Uterus didelphys with
   double vagina

b Uterus arcuatus

c Uterus bicornis

d Uterus bicornis unicollis
   1 rudimentary horn

e Atresia of cervix

f Atresia of vagina

FIG. 10.1. **Schematic representation of the main congenital abnormalities of the uterus and vagina.** These abnormalities are caused by persistence of the uterine septum or obliteration of the lumen of the uterine canal. (Reprinted by permission of Sadler, ref. 205a.)

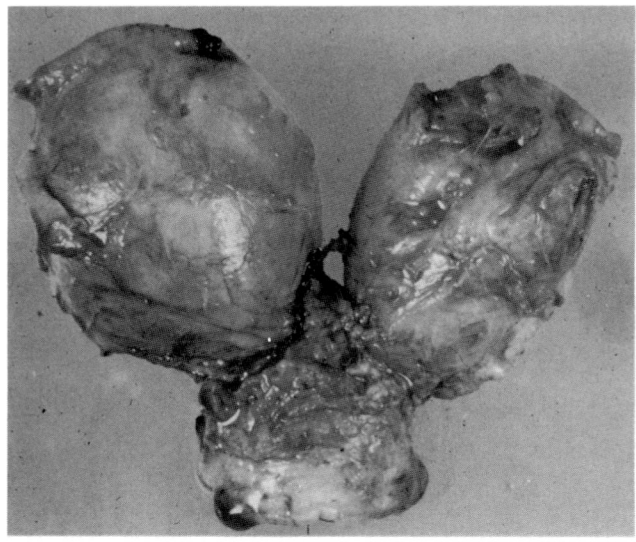

FIG. 10.2. **Bicornuate uterus.** The specimen is unopened.

Atresia of the Müllerian Ducts and Vagina

Atresia can be partial or complete, but a wide range of intermediate degrees of atresia may be encountered. The etiology of this condition is obscure, although a genetic cause sometimes is apparent because siblings may be affected. The pattern of inheritance may be autosomal recessive[116,267] or dominant.[21]

If just one of the müllerian ducts is involved, only the fimbriae and a small muscular mass at the pelvic side wall will form. Occasionally, a rudimetary structure remains as an appendage attached to the unaffected side, giving rise to what is referred to as *uterus bicornis unicollis with a rudimentary horn* (Fig. 10.1d). With bilateral atresia, the upper genital tract may consist of bilateral noncanalized strands of muscular tissue located on the lateral pelvic walls. In severe defects, there is müllerian and vaginal aplasia. This abnormality, referred to as the *Rokitansky–Kuster–Hauser syndrome*, frequently is associated with urinary tract anomalies, such as a pelvic kidney or absence of a kidney. Vertebral and other skeletal abnormalities also may occur, suggesting a severe generalized morphogenetic abnormality involving several organ systems simultaneously.

Patients with these conditions are endocrinologically normal and have complete gonadal development. If the anomaly results in obstruction of the vagina with functional endometrial tissue present, hydrocolpos may be present at birth, or adolescents may present with primary amenorrhea. If only one müllerian duct is affected, giving rise to a rudimentary horn of a uterus bicornis unicollis, a young woman may have regular menstrual cycles associated with a pelvic mass and cyclic pelvic pain. A number of multiple malformation syndromes have been associated with müllerian or vaginal agenesis, such as the Winter syndrome. This syndrome is characterized by vaginal agenesis, renal agenesis, and middle ear anomalies[266] and is inherited in an autosomal recessive manner.

Treatment of patients with complete vaginal atresia requires surgery to create a neovagina. If the anomaly is isolated *vaginal atresia* (Fig. 10.1f), as most commonly occurs, the patient usually will be fertile if a normal uterus and fallopian tubes are present.

Inflammation

Endometritis is divided into acute and chronic forms, depending on the type of inflammatory infiltrate. Chronic endometritis is subdivided into nonspecific and specific types, depending on whether specific morphologic changes or an etiologic agent can be recognized. A diagnosis of endometritis depends on the presence of specific cellular findings because under normal circumstances a wide variety of hematopoietic cells are present in the endometrium. Accordingly, a brief review of their distribution is presented.

Normal Hematopoietic Cells of the Endometrium

Immunohistochemical studies have demonstrated that B lymphocytes occur in lymphoid aggregates in the basalis but are rarely found in the functionalis.[28,184] Occasional lymphoid follicles can be found in otherwise normal endometria. T lymphocytes are relatively uncommon in the proliferative phase but increase during the secretory and menstrual phase.[28] Recently it has been shown that a population of phenotypically unusual lymphocytes (CD2+, CD3−) are found in mid- and late secretory endometrium that localizes to areas with a predecidual reaction. In the past these cells were designated *endometrial stromal granulocytes*, but more recently they have been identified as *granulated lymphocytes*.[27,122] In addition, polymorphonuclear leukocytes (PMNs) are present in small numbers throughout the cycle but do not become evident in large numbers before tissue breakdown and necrosis, that is, menses, occurs.[189] Thus, lymphocytes and PMNs are normally present in different phases of endometrial growth and maturation. In contrast, plasma cells are not normally present in the endometrium.

Mast cells may be found in the endometrium and myometrium. Using toluidine-blue staining[48] it has been shown that mast cells are relatively scant in the endometrium, where they tend to be confined to the basalis. Mast cells are distributed randomly in the myometrium but generally within areas of fibroconnective tissue. They also have been observed within endometrial polyps and leiomyomas. These cells show a trend to decrease in both the endometrium and myometrium with advancing age, suggesting that their presence is hormonally mediated.

Although mast cells contain heparin and have been found in patients with an intrauterine device, their presence has not been associated with menorrhagia.[48]

Acute and Chronic (Nonspecific) Endometritis

The cervix acts as a barrier to the entry of microorganisms into the endometrial cavity. Except for rare forms of endometritis established by hematogenous implantation or descending infection from the fallopian tubes (e.g., tuberculosis), most types of endometritis result from ascending infection through the cervix. The usually impervious cervical barrier is compromised during menses, abortion, parturition, and instrumentation (curettage, insertion of an intrauterine device, cervical conization). In such instances, bacteria, some of which comprise the normal vagina flora, gain access to the endometrial cavity but usually without colonizing or producing infection.

A study analyzing the histological findings in the endometrium of women with documented upper genital tract infection (UGTI) and laparoscopically confirmed acute salpingitis suggests that the traditional classification of "acute" and "chronic" endometritis based on the type of inflammatory infiltrate may not be valid.[124] In this study it was found that the endometria of women with acute salpingitis usually did not contain large numbers of PMNs in the stroma. In fact, PMNs comprising at least 30% of the inflammatory cells occurred in only 27% of the cases. PMNs were found in the superficial endometrium but, in addition, large numbers of lymphocytes and plasma cells were identified in the stroma. Thus, according to convention these women with acute salpingitis would have been classified as having chronic endometritis. Since this study was performed in women suspected of having pelvic inflammatory disease, it is possible that many of these patients with acute salpingitis also had a low-grade, smoldering chronic infection that was clinically silent. Thus, although these women appeared to have an acute infectious process they, in fact, had underlying chronic endometritis.

CLINICAL FEATURES

Clinically significant acute endometritis usually is associated with pregnancy or abortion. The complex clinical aspects of postpartum and postabortal endometritis are beyond the scope of this presentation and are detailed elsewhere.[131,158] Most acute endometritis is caused by hemolytic *Streptococcus*, *Staphylococcus*, *Neisseria gonorrhoeae*, and *Clostridium welchii*.

PATHOLOGIC FINDINGS

Chronic endometritis has been observed in 3–10% of women undergoing an endometrial biopsy for irregular bleeding.[90,202] Patients may have menometrorrhagia, mucopurulent cervical discharge, uterine tenderness, or an elevated erythrocyte sedimentation rate and/or white blood cell count, but some women are asymptomatic. Chronic endometritis has been associated with an abortion in 41%, with salpingitis in 25%, with an intrauterine device in 14%, and with a recent pregnancy in 12%.[30] It also is associated with necrotic tissue, such as an infarcted polyp or carcinoma, or cervical stenosis secondary to radiation or cryosurgery.

Endometritis associated with pregnancy and abortion is characterized by an acute inflammatory infiltrate. Identification of a specific microorganism is based on culture. Since the presence of necrosis, hemorrhage, and a PMN infiltrate is a normal physiologic event occurring in menstrual endometrium, the histological diagnosis of acute endometritis is based on finding moderate to large numbers of PMNs in nonbleeding endometrium[189] or in focal aggregates in the stroma, that is, forming microabscesses or disrupting and filling gland lumens (Fig. 10.3). Occasionally, isolated glands in otherwise normal endometrium contain PMNs and debris in their lumens (Fig. 10.4). The etiology of this is not known; it may represent entrapped menstrual detritus. This finding should not be interpreted as evidence of acute endometritis.

The inflammatory infiltrate in chronic endometritis is composed of variable numbers of plasma cells, lymphocytes, PMNs, and macrophages, but the diagnosis rests on the identification of plasma cells[24,30,66,202] (Fig. 10.5). Plasma cells may be difficult to distinguish from lymphocytes and endometrial stromal cells. In contrast to lympho-

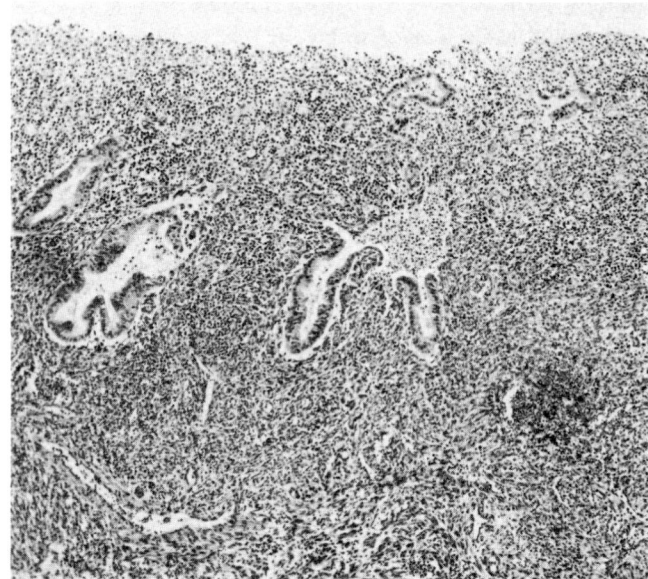

FIG. 10.3. Acute endometritis. A profuse infiltrate of polymorphonuclear leukocytes destroys and fills gland lumens. A microabscess is present on right.

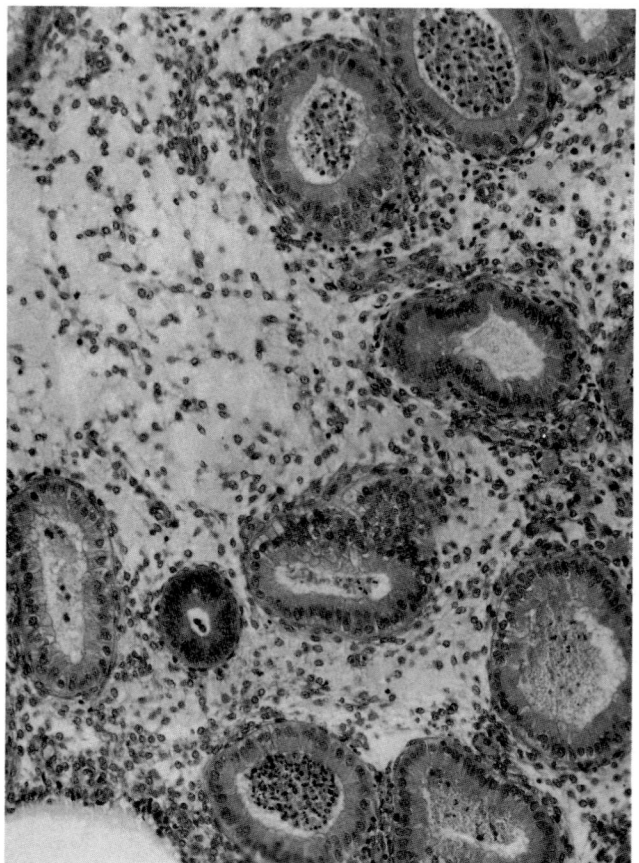

FIG. 10.4. **Endometrial glands with luminal debris.** Tubular glands near the surface contain neutrophils and debris in the lumens. There was no evidence of endometritis in the specimen. This change should not be misinterpreted as acute endometritis.

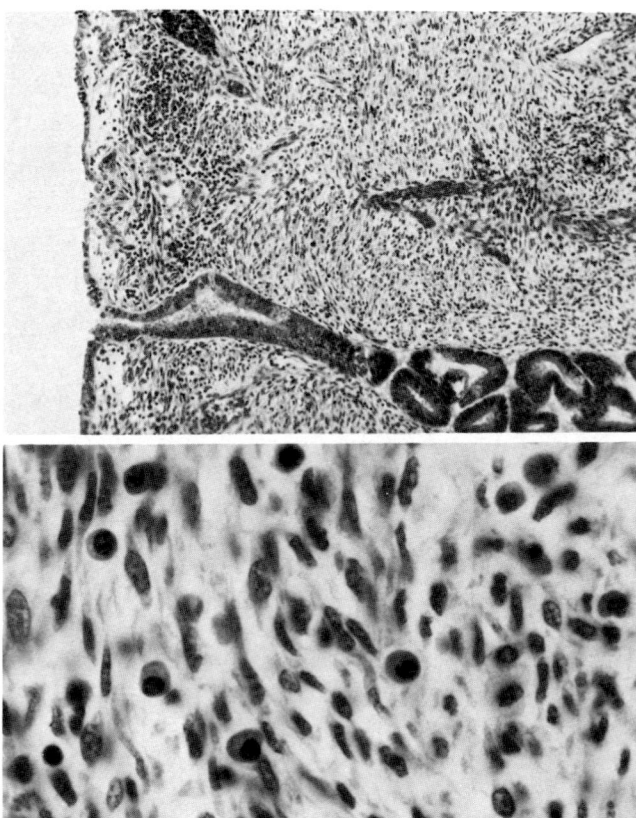

FIG. 10.5. **Chronic endometritis.** *Top:* Chronic endometritis characterized by aggregates of lymphocytes and plasma cells. *Bottom:* Plasma cells with eccentrically placed nuclei and clockface chromatin pattern.

cytes and stromal cells, plasma cells have an eccentrically placed nucleus with a clockface chromatin pattern and pale-staining cytoplasm. Methyl green pyronin or immunohistochemical stains for immunoglobulins may be helpful in their identification, but these are rarely necessary in routine clinical practice.

In chronic endometritis, plasma cells may be scant and every endometrial biopsy cannot be scrutinized for plasma cells under high magnification. Two helpful clues that suggest the presence of chronic endometritis under low power are (1) a characteristic spindle-cell alteration of the stromal cells (Fig. 10.6) and (2) an inability to date secretory endometrium. The problem in dating usually is manifested by a disparity between the appearance of the glands and stroma. Some glands are inactive and it may be difficult to decide whether they are proliferative or secretory. At other times extensive tissue fragmentation associated with chronic inflammation precludes dating. This finding is associated more frequently with *N. gonorrhoeae*.[124] The spindle-cell alteration is characterized by a tendency of the endometrial stromal cells to palisade around glands in a

pinwheel arrangement (Fig. 10.6). The usual oval nuclei of the stromal cells are more spindle-shaped and may be slightly enlarged. Occasionally, regenerative activity is more pronounced, and the glandular cells become stratified, with enlarged rounded nuclei and prominent nucleoli. Squamous metaplasia may be found in association with chronic endometritis, especially along the surface epithelium.

In a study of women with acute salpingitis and upper genital tract infection (UGTI) confirmed laparoscopically, it was found that small numbers of plasma cells had low specificity for predicting UGTI.[124] In this study two findings [one or more plasma cells per ×120 field in the endometrial stroma and five or more PMNs per ×400 in the surface epithelium (Fig. 10.7)] had a sensitivity of 94% and a specificity of 85% for the diagnosis of UGTI. The authors questioned the clinical significance of finding rare plasma cells in asymptomatic women because in an unpublished series of 29 endometrial biopsies from women undergoing an infertility work-up they found rare plasma cells in two women. These women had normal hysterosalpingograms

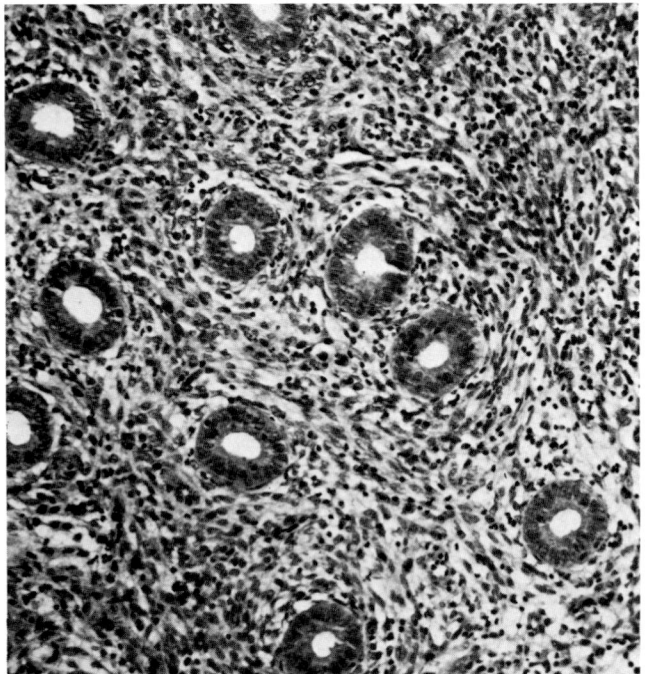

FIG. 10.6. Chronic endometritis. Note the spindle-shaped stromal cells surrounding glands in a pinwheel arrangement.

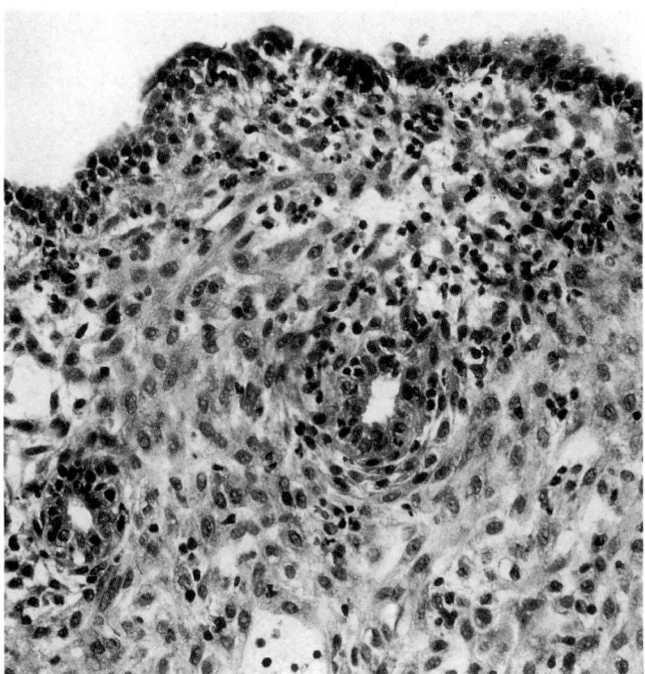

FIG. 10.7. Chronic endometritis. Numerous neutrophils in addition to lymphocytes are present involving the surface of the endometrium, glands, and stroma. Plasma cells were present elsewhere in the specimen.

and did not have antibodies to *C. trachomatis*. Further studies are needed to clarify the significance of small numbers of plasma cells in asymptomatic women.

CLINICAL BEHAVIOR AND TREATMENT

Cultures from the endometrium, tubes, or cul de sac performed at the time of diagnosis of chronic endometritis reveal that *C. trachomatis* and *N. gonorrhoeae* are the most common upper genital tract pathogens found. Other less common isolates are *Escherichia coli*, *Streptococcus agalactiae*, and *Peptostreptococcus magnus*.[124] Accordingly, the histological diagnosis of chronic endometritis in an asymptomatic patient should be followed by an endocervical culture for gonococci and *Chlamydia*.

The diagnosis of endometritis on a biopsy specimen often is an indicator of the presence of pelvic inflammatory disease. In a study comparing endometrial biopsy, clinical examination, and laparoscopy in the diagnosis of acute pelvic inflammatory disease, Paavonen et al.[183] found that the presence of chronic endometritis in the endometrial biopsy correlated with the presence of acute salpingitis at laparoscopy in 89% of patients, compared to only a 67% correlation between bimanual examination and laparoscopy. These findings, in conjunction with the high correlation of mucopurulent cervicitis and endometritis with salpingitis, suggest that chronic endometritis represents an intermediate stage of pelvic inflammatory disease between

cervicitis and salpingitis. The importance of the endometrial biopsy as a predictor of pelvic inflammatory disease is underscored by the observation that significant pelvic adhesions can be found at laparoscopy despite normal hysterosalpingography.[139] Since chronic endometritis is found in the absence of salpingitis,[183] it is conceivable that early endometritis can cause infertility. Thus, the endometrial biopsy can serve as a method for directing specific therapy or as an indicator of the need for laparoscopic examination.

Chronic Endometritis—Specific Types

Chlamydia

CLINICAL FEATURES

C. trachomatis infection as defined by a positive culture or a high serologic antibody titer is associated with 50–60% of cases of salpingitis in several Western European countries and the United States.[96] The risk of infertility after an episode of salpingitis rises from 11% after one episode to 54% after three or more episodes.[261] It has been reported that most patients undergoing tuboplasty for tubal stenosis or adhesions and in whom there is evidence of an infectious origin have never had pain, bleeding, or any clinical sign that would have led to a diagnosis of salpingitis.[96] It therefore appears that *C. trachomatis*, possibly in association with other microorganisms, causes an acute salpingitis or a chronic "silent" salpingitis that is recognized only during the course of an infertility work-up.

PATHOGENESIS

Animal experiments have convincingly demonstrated that *C. trachomatis* by itself can cause salpingitis and tubal obstruction. In one study 100 guinea pigs were inoculated in one tube with *C. trachomatis*. This resulted in the development of a unilateral salpingitis and pyosalpinx in all the animals in the inoculated tube. *C. trachomatis* was found on culture.[210]

PATHOLOGIC FINDINGS

In women with culture proven *C. trachomatis* the findings at surgery include the presence of adhesions and a viscous effusion in the pouch of Douglas. The peritoneal surfaces are reddened and shiny. Mesothelial cysts ranging from a few millimeters to large cysts can be encountered (see Chapter 17, Diseases of the Peritoneum). Cytological examination of the peritoneal fluid reveals a marked inflammatory infiltrate consisting of lymphocytes and plasma cells admixed with clusters of reactive mesothelial cells. The fallopian tubes can show a wide range of findings from acute to chronic salpingitis (see Chapter 14, Diseases of the Fallopian Tube).

Chronic endometritis due to *C. trachomatis* displays a mixed inflammatory infiltrate composed of plasma cells, lymphocytes, and PMNs (see above, Acute and Chronic Endometritis). In a correlated histopathologic and microbiological study it was reported that compared with gonococcal infection, endometritis resulting from *C. trachomatis* displayed a significantly greater number of plasma cells.[124] In addition, lymphoid follicles containing transformed lymphocytes were found only in cases of Chlamydia infection; they were never found in association with gonococcal infection.[124] High concentrations of plasma cells also were found in an immunoperoxidase study performed on paraffin-embedded tissue.[265] In this study Chlamydia was found in only 4% of 90 endometrial biopsies showing chronic endometritis but the percentage rose to 57% in biopsies of patients with severe chronic endometritis and superimposed acute inflammation. Cases positive for Chlamydia also were associated with stromal necrosis and reparative cytological atypia in the glandular and surface epithelium. In this study Chlamydial inclusions were difficult to identify because they were obscured by the inflammatory infiltrate.[265] In another study elementary bodies of *C. trachomatis* were identified by direct immunofluorescence in 75% of cases and typical intracellular Chlamydia inclusions were found in more than 60%.[123]

CLINICAL BEHAVIOR AND TREATMENT

Chlamydia infection usually responds well to tetracycline treatment. Because of the insidious nature of the disease, patients with a histological diagnosis of chronic endometritis should be cultured for Chlamydia and treated appropriately. If the infection is diagnosed and treated at an early stage tubal damage can be minimized and fertility maintained. Patients undergoing tuboplasty also should be cultured and treated before surgery because women with positive cultures have a significantly lower rate of intrauterine pregnancy after microsurgery compared with women with negative cultures.[96]

Mycoplasma

Mycoplasma infection of the endometrium has been associated with infertility and fetal wastage.[24,244,245] Three species of mycoplasma, *Mycoplasma hominis*, *Mycoplasma fermentans*, and *Ureaplasma urealyticum*, have been demonstrated in the lower female genital tract.[34,77,78,181,244] Genital mycoplasias generally are transmitted by sexual contact but the organisms have been cultured from prepubertal girls and women who have denied sexual contact, suggesting that other modes of transmission, such as autoinfection from the anal canal, may occur.[66a]

Although mycoplasma species, especially *U. urealyticum*, appear to have a role in some cases of unexplained infertility, the relationship of this organism to endometrial infection is controversial.[34,35,91] Data regarding both the culture of the organism from the endometrium and the association of positive cultures with an inflammatory endometrial response have been conflicting.[34,35,91,101] The differences in isolation rates in infertile women may be due to cervical contamination because mycoplasmas frequently colonize the lower genital tract.[244] Significant endometrial infection with *U. urealyticum* should cause an identifiable inflammatory response. Horne et al. have identified a lesion termed *subacute focal inflammation* (SFI) associated with *U. urealyticum*.[101] The lesion is characterized by focal collections of lymphocytes; plasma cells and PMLs are rarely seen. The lymphoid aggregates may be small and few in number, making their detection, at times, difficult. They are most easily identified in the secretory phase from the 20th to the 23rd (postovulation day 6–9) days of the cycle, when there is maximal stromal edema. The lesions usually are without germinal centers and tend to be localized just beneath the surface endometrium, adjacent to glands, or around spiral arterioles. In our experience SFI is a relatively rare finding.

The effect of ureaplasmas on infertility may be indirect in women. For example, in a study of 262 patients, it was reported that 87% of women with SFI had pelvic adhesions evident at laparoscopy compared with only 11% who did not have SFI ($p = .0001$).[29] It has been postulated that ureaplasmas, if they cause the lesions, may be responsible for producing adhesions or may place the patient at risk for developing more severe adhesions. Cervicovaginal isolation of *U. urealyticum* was associated with male factor infertility in one study,[35] suggesting that the organism may be a more significant pathogen in males, where it can interfere with spermatogenesis and reduce spermatozoa motility[35] rather than affecting the endometrium.

Tuberculosis

Tuberculosis endometritis caused by *Mycobacterium tuberculosis* is a manifestation of a systemic disease; its frequency parallels that of pulmonary tuberculosis in the population. Rare in the United States, Germany, and Eastern Europe, tuberculous endometritis is more common in Spain and India.[21,107,163,173,237] It is generally found in women during their reproductive years, but it also occurs in postmenopausal women. Clinical manifestations of genital tuberculosis include a pelvic mass or lower abdominal pain. Sometimes, genital tuberculosis is discovered during the course of an investigation for infertility. Often the diagnosis is not made until the time of hysterectomy, when caseating granulomas are found in the fallopian tubes.

The endometrium is affected in one-half to three-quarters of patients with genital tuberculosis.[173] It is the second most commonly infected site in the female genital tract after the fallopian tubes. Endometrial involvement generally occurs from seeding by organisms draining from the fallopian tubes directly. Infection in the fallopian tubes is acquired by hematogenous or, rarely, lymphatic spread from a primary focus in the lungs or gastrointestinal tract.[95]

The extent of the inflammatory involvement in tuberculous endometritis varies from a focal process with very few granulomas to a diffuse process with ulceration of the mucosa and extensive caseous necrosis. Typical granulomatous inflammation with Langhans giant cells (Fig. 10.8) is not always present. The process may be manifested only by a nonspecific endometritis with focal or diffuse infiltrates of plasma cells and lymphocytes.[54] Frequently, destruction of glands occurs, with the inflammatory infiltrate filling gland lumens, as in nonspecific endometritis. The inflammation usually is confined to the superficial and intermediate portion of the endometrium, with transmural involvement occurring only in very severe infections.[173] A reactive proliferative epithelial response with cellular stratification, mild nuclear atypia, and squamous metaplasia may occur. This atypical proliferation should not be confused with a neoplastic process.

Histological diagnosis of tuberculosis is difficult because granulomas often are focal and take up to 2 weeks to develop, and the functionalis, where granulomas usually occur, is shed every 4 weeks.[173] Thus, if tuberculosis is suspected, a curettage, rather than an endometrial biopsy, should be performed during the late secretory or menstrual phase of the cycle. Specific diagnosis requires culture or identification of acid-fast organisms, because other microorganisms may be associated with granulomatous in-

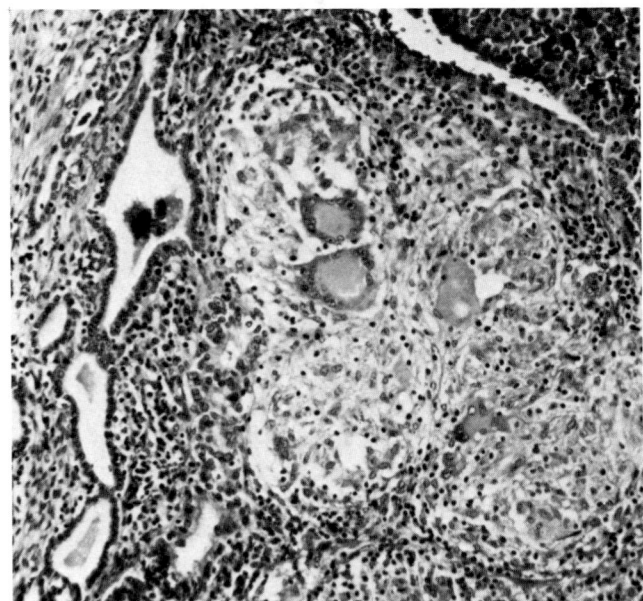

FIG. 10.8. Tuberculous endometritis. Tuberculous endometritis with a nonnecrotizing granuloma containing Langhans giant cells.

flammation. Acid-fast bacilli are rarely demonstrated, even when cultures are positive.[173]

Patients with tuberculous endometritis are nearly always sterile because endometrial involvement develops secondarily from tubal infection. After appropriate antimicrobial therapy, granulomas become hyalinized, but the inflammatory infiltrate may persist for years. In the rare instance of subsequent fertility, implantation is likely to occur in the fallopian tube. Intrauterine pregnancy may terminate in fatal miliary tuberculosis.

Sarcoidosis

A few cases of sarcoid have had endometrial involvement in association with systemic sarcoidosis.[98,242] In contrast to tuberculosis, the granulomas in sarcoidosis are noncaseating, and acid-fast bacilli are not identified. Since these features also may be absent in tuberculous endometritis, every effort should be made to distinguish sarcoidosis from tuberculosis in view of the different prognosis and approach to treatment.

Fungal Infections

Blastomycosis (*Blastomyces dermatitidis*)[70] and coccidioidomycosis (*Coccidioides immitis*)[93,208] may produce granulomatous endometritis as part of a disseminated infection. There have been case reports of mycotic infection consistent with Candida[199] and cryptococcosis (*Cryptococcus glabratus*)[129] in the endometrium. The Gomori silver-methenamine and periodic acid–Schiff (PAS) stains are helpful for identifying the organisms.

Viral Infections

Herpes virus (HSV),[2,67,86,196,213] cytomegalovirus (CMV),[58,147,257] and human papillomavirus (HPV)[251] are the only viruses known to infect the endometrium. Both acute,[2,86,213] and latent[196] HSV infection have been reported. Acute herpes endometritis may occur as an ascending infection or as a result of disseminated viremia.[2,67,213] In acute herpes infection, the glandular cells have ground-glass nuclei that are enlarged and contain round eosinophilic inclusions surrounded by a halo. There is associated patchy necrosis, acute inflammation, and multinucleated giant cells.[67,213] In latent infection there is no histological evidence of herpes infection; virus particles are not identifiable by transmission electron microscopy and cultures are negative.[196] In latent infection, detection of the virus is based on the presence of HSV-specific virion and nonvirion antigens by immunohistochemistry.[196] Care must be used in immunohistochemical analysis to ensure that endogenous biotin is not misinterpreted as specific immunostaining using the avidin-biotin-peroxidase method.[271] The significance of apparent "latent" infection is not known at the present time.

CMV infection when detected by cervical culture has been estimated to occur in 14% of women during pregnancy.[159] In contrast, it is identified only rarely, usually as an incidental finding, in nonpregnant healthy women by microscopic examination.[257] CMV endometritis has been reported in immunocompromised women[22,209] with systemic CMV infection and as a primary infection in nonimmunocompromised patients.[147] It also has been detected in the endometrium in pregnancy, where it has been implicated as a possible cause of spontaneous abortion.[31] Because of its occult presentation, the frequency of CMV infection of the endometrium probably is underestimated. Typically, CMV infection is characterized by an inflammatory infiltrate composed of lymphocytes and plasma cells. The endometrial epithelial cells are markedly enlarged, and contain large, round basophilic nuclear and cytoplasmic inclusions (Fig. 10.9). In a recent report CMV was detected from DNA extracted from a paraffin block using the polymerase chain reaction in an endometrial specimen showing chronic endometritis and ill-defined nonnecrotizing granulomas but without any of the other features of CMV infection.[76] The patient has systemic CMV infection and CMV in the endocervix.

The Arias–Stella reaction (see Chapter 9, Anatomy and Histology of the Uterine Corpus) may be confused with CMV because of the marked nuclear enlargement. In contrast to the Arias–Stella reaction, CMV endometritis has a plasma cell infiltrate and nuclear inclusions and lacks the associated features of gestational endometrium, such as decidua.

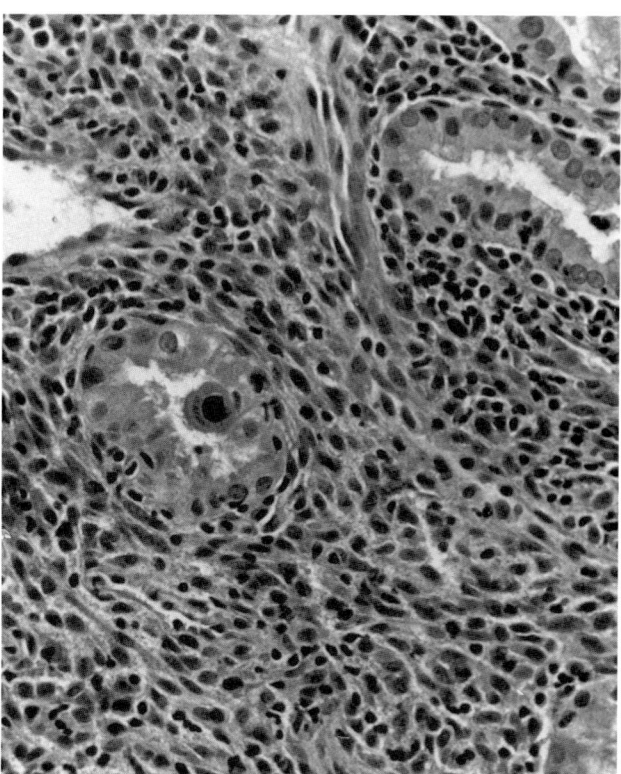

Fig. 10.9. **Cytomegalovirus endometritis.** An enlarged glandular cell contains a large, round, basophilic inclusion.

HPV infection of the endometrium manifested by diffuse condylomatous involvement secondary to cervical infection with HPV has been reported.[251] The histological features are the same as those observed in the cervix (see Chapter 6, Benign Diseases of the Cervix). The differential diagnosis includes rare examples of verrucous carcinoma and well-differentiated squamous cell carcinoma of the endometrium (see Chapter 12, Endometrial Carcinoma).

Parasitic Infections

Schistosoma,[17,162,264] *Enterobius vermicularis*,[211] and *Echinococcus granulosus*[255] are rare causes of endometritis in the United States, but schistosomiasis is endemic in Central America, Africa, the Middle East, and the Far East. Patients usually present with amenorrhea and infertility. The infection may be mild or severe and is characterized by granulomatous inflammation with lymphocytes, plasma cells, eosinophils, and histiocytes closely simulating a tubercle. The endometrial surface may ulcerate and be replaced by granulation tissue. Diagnosis is made by identifying the ova in tissue sections or in smears of vaginal secretions.

Toxoplasmosis (*Toxoplasma gondii*)[193,235] produces a nonspecific inflammation of the endometrium. The microorganism can be identified by immunofluorescence. Fragmentary data implicate this organism in the endometrium as a cause of congenital toxoplasmosis and habitual abortion.

Xanthogranulomatous Inflammation

There have been several reported cases of xanthogranulomatous or histiocytic endometritis.[25,26,129,204,218] The lesion involves the endometrium but may extend into the myometrium and is characterized by an extensive accumulation of foamy histiocytes.

Thus far, all the patients reported have been postmenopausal and many have been radiated previously for endometrial or cervical carcinoma. Patients present with vaginal bleeding or discharge and on pelvic examination have cervical stenosis and pyometria. It has therefore been suggested that the lesion results from obstruction associated with hematometria, inflammation, and perhaps some factors specifically related to radiation-induced tumor necrosis, such as the generation of free radicals and lipid peroxidation.[204]

Microscopically, xanthogranulomatous endometritis is characterized by numerous histiocytes with foamy, granular, or eosinophilic cytoplasm and variable numbers of multinucleated giant cells, lymphocytes, and plasma cells (Fig. 10.10). Although the foam cells are referred to as histiocytes or macrophages, they appear to be endometrial stromal cells in which the cytoplasm has become distended with lipid, hemosiderin, or ceroid after erythrocyte breakdown from nonphysiologic hemorrhage. PAS stains are positive at times. The nuclei of the foam cells are small and bland and exhibit no mitotic activity. In addition to the foam cells, cholesterol crystals, calcification, and necrotic debris typically are present.

Rarely, talc or another foreign substance may elicit a foreign body reaction in the endometrium.[54] Talc may be introduced into the endometrial cavity by instruments contaminated with talcum powder or by gloves during a pelvic examination. Patients may be asymptomatic or may have menorrhagia. Microscopically, the extent of the granulomatous inflammatory reaction depends on the quantity of the talc inoculated. The infiltrate is characterized by histiocytes and foreign body multinucleated giant cells surrounding the talc crystals, along with lymphocytes and plasma cells. The crystals appear as refractile, birefringent, needle-like, or fan-shaped splinters in polarizing light.

Miscellaneous Infections

Two rare forms of endometritis of probable bacterial origin that produce specific morphologic changes are pneumopolycystic endometritis[185] and malakoplakia.[191,248] The former is characterized by the presence of multiple thin-walled cysts and vesicles lined by flattened cells. Multinucleated giant cells occasionally are present. A similar con-

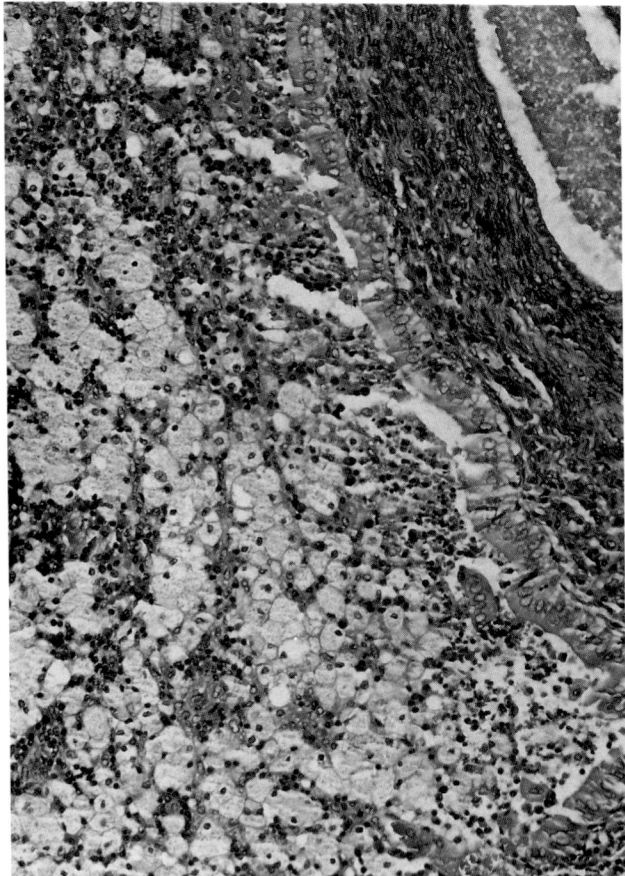

Fig. 10.10. Xanthogranulomatous endometritis. Large numbers of endometrial stromal cells with foamy cytoplasm. Lymphocytes and plasma cells also are present.

dition can be seen in the vagina (see Chapter 4, Diseases of the Vagina). The disease in the vagina is thought to result from infection by *Haemophilus vaginalis* or *Trichomonas*, but the precise origin of this condition in the endometrium is not known.

Malakoplakia most often involves the urinary bladder, only rarely affecting the genital tract. Of the 21 reported cases of genital malakoplakia, 8 have involved the endometrium.[*]

Patients with malakoplakia involving the genital tract range in age from 29 to 84 years (mean 62 years). All those women with disease involving the endometrium have presented with vaginal bleeding. On gross examination, the lesion consists of soft, yellow, gray-brown plaques and nodules. Microscopically, malakoplakia is characterized by a monomorphic population of histiocytes containing eosinophilic or clear cytoplasm (Von Hansemann cells) and may, therefore, simulate xanthogranulomatous endometritis or clear cell carcinoma. The diagnosis of malakoplakia is

---

[*] Refs. 37,39,119,157,191,246,248,252,263.

made by the identification of intracellular and extracellular calcified spherules (Michaelis–Gutman bodies).

In most cases *Escherichia coli* but occasionally *Klebsiella* and *Proteus spp* have been cultured from the lesions. It is thought that a defect in the phagocytic function of monocyte–macrophages leads to persistence of bacteria, which calcify to form Michaelis–Gutman bodies.

Management consists of antibiotic treatment and surgical excision. Recurrences may occur.

Dysfunctional Uterine Bleeding

The endometrium is a sensitive bioassay for estrogen and progesterone. During the reproductive years, the endometrium in response to physiologic changes in estrogen and progesterone levels proliferates, differentiates, and sheds in a cyclical, generally predictable fashion. In ovulatory cycles, the luteal phase is 14 days in length, whereas the follicular phase is variable and may range from 10 to 20 days, yielding a wide range of cycle lengths among normal, ovulating women. After menarche cycle length tends to be long and irregular, shortening over the next 5–7 years to attain a regular pattern through the reproductive age. Cycles begin to lengthen again when a woman is in her 40s before gradually ceasing in the perimenopausal years. Cycle length is based on the rate and quality of follicular growth, which is in turn mediated by follicle-stimulating hormone (FSH) and inhibin.[134]

Abnormalities along the hypothalamic–pituitary–ovarian axis may result in a derangement of follicular maturation, ovulation, or corpus luteum development, with subsequent abnormal hormone secretion. These alterations in the normal hormonal patterns are manifested by abnormal uterine bleeding, infertility, or both.

Dysfunctional uterine bleeding (DUB) is a clinical term used to describe bleeding not attributable to an underlying organic pathologic condition.° DUB, therefore, generally is synonymous with abnormal uterine bleeding resulting from derangement in the magnitude or duration of estrogen and progesterone effects on the endometrium.[230] The term, however, is applied loosely and some regard heavy, prolonged bleeding at the time of menses, that is, menorrhagia, as DUB also. Many uterine lesions can produce bleeding, and these should be excluded before making the diagnosis of DUB.[146] Conditions that can cause abnormal bleeding include endometrial polyps, adenomyosis, leiomyomas, endometritis, atrophy, intrauterine devices, oral contraceptive use, abortion, ectopic pregnancy, hyperplasia, malignant tumors, gestational trophoblastic disease, blood dyscrasias, certain drugs (particularly anticoagulants), and severe renal or liver disease. In addition, hypothyroidism or hyperthyroidism may be first manifested by abnormal menstrual cycles.

Bleeding as a result of anovulatory cycles probably is the most common cause of DUB in women in the reproductive age group. In addition, early decline of the corpus luteum and failure of the corpus luteum to regress at the appropriate time are less common causes of DUB. Bleeding associated with these latter conditions results from abnormal progesterone stimulation of the endometrium. Although not truly regarded as DUB, bleeding from an atrophic endometrium without an organic lesion is the most common cause of postmenopausal uterine bleeding. Finally, when menorrhagia is regarded as a manifestation of DUB the underlying pathophysiology does not appear to be related to sex steroid hormones. The abnormal bleeding in this disorder is due to local abnormalities in the clotting mechanism associated with enhanced fibrinolysis and alterations in prostaglandin synthesis, which inhibits platelet aggregation.

Glandular and Stromal Breakdown Associated with Anovulation

Anovulatory cycles occur when there is development of one or more follicles in the ovary with estradiol synthesis by granulosa and theca cells. The estradiol promotes endometrial proliferation; however, there is no ovulation and subsequent progesterone production by a corpus luteum. Consequently, the endometrium fails to undergo stromal and glandular differentiation, which normally occurs in the secretory phase. The follicles may persist and continue to produce estradiol, or they may regress, ending the estrogen production. When estrogen levels decline, the endometrium can no longer be maintained, and bleeding ensues. A rough correlation exists between the amount of estrogenic stimulation of the endometrium and the pattern of bleeding. Relatively minimal estrogenic stimulation results in intermittent spotting that may be prolonged. Sustained stimulation by high levels of estrogen leads to prolonged amenorrhea followed by precipitous, heavy bleeding. Both of these patterns have been referred to as *estrogen breakthrough bleeding*.[230]

CLINICAL FEATURES

DUB as a result of anovulatory cycles can occur at any time during the reproductive years, but characteristically occurs at menarche and at menopause.[174] Nearly 60% of all cycles in the first year after menarche are anovulatory. For the vast majority of these women, ovulatory cycles ensue, but some women never establish normal cycles.[228] Women in this latter group have infrequent, irregular periods, occasionally marked by extremely heavy bleeding, which may require hospitalization. Typically, these women also are obese, infertile, and hirsute and are considered to have polycystic ovarian

---

°Refs. 4,5,14,106,116,174,190,214,225.

disease (Stein–Leventhal syndrome) (see Chapter 16, Non-neoplastic Lesions of the Ovary). Many women in the reproductive age group with anovulatory cycles, however, do not manifest these classic clinical features. Most of the cycles in a patient with polycystic ovarian disease are anovulatory, but as many as 25% of the cycles may be ovulatory, as documented by the presence of a corpus luteum.

Pathologic Findings

Histological examination of endometrial tissue removed at the time of bleeding may be scanty or abundant, depending on the duration and amount of bleeding that preceded the curettage. The glands are proliferative, but the degree of proliferation depends mainly on the duration of unopposed estrogenic stimulation. Over a period of months to years a variety of metaplasias, hyperplasia, and carcinoma can be produced (see Chapter 11, Endometrial Hyperplasia and Related Cellular Changes and Chapter 12, Endometrial Carcinoma).

When there has been relatively limited estrogenic stimulation the endometrium may appear extensively fragmented (Fig. 10.11). Intact glands and stroma appear as typical proliferative endometrium but frequently most of the glands are fragmented and the stroma is not intact (Fig. 10.12). As the ground substance undergoes dissolution,

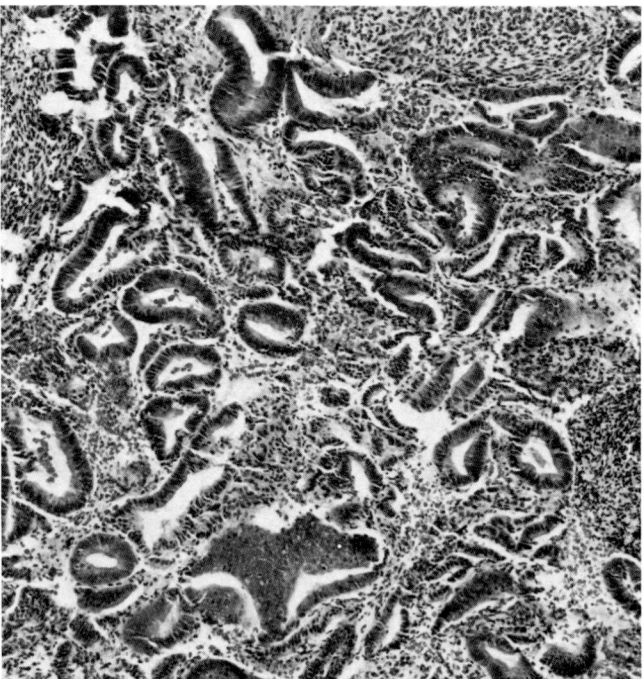

Fig. 10.12. Endometrial glandular and stromal breakdown. There is extensive fragmentation of proliferative glands, stromal necrosis, and hemorrhage.

stromal cells condense and form compact nests of cells with hyperchromatic nuclei and little or no cytoplasm. The normal architecture collapses. Isolated, fragmented glands lie in haphazard disarray without surrounding stroma (Figs. 10.12, 10.13). Nuclear debris from necrotic cells is frequently present as dark granules within the cytoplasm of glandular cells (Fig. 10.13). These features constitute *glandular and stromal breakdown*. When glandular and stromal breakdown is present in a background of proliferative phase endometrium, a comment can be added that the changes are compatible with anovulatory bleeding.

Where there is a greater degree or duration of unopposed estrogenic stimulation the endometrium appears less fragmented, although focal areas similar to those just described may be present. In these cases most of the tissue has a proliferative appearance and such lesions should be classified as *proliferative phase with focal glandular and stromal breakdown* (Fig. 10.14). If in addition to the proliferative endometrium there are focal areas in which the glands are slightly dilatated and are irregularly shaped with

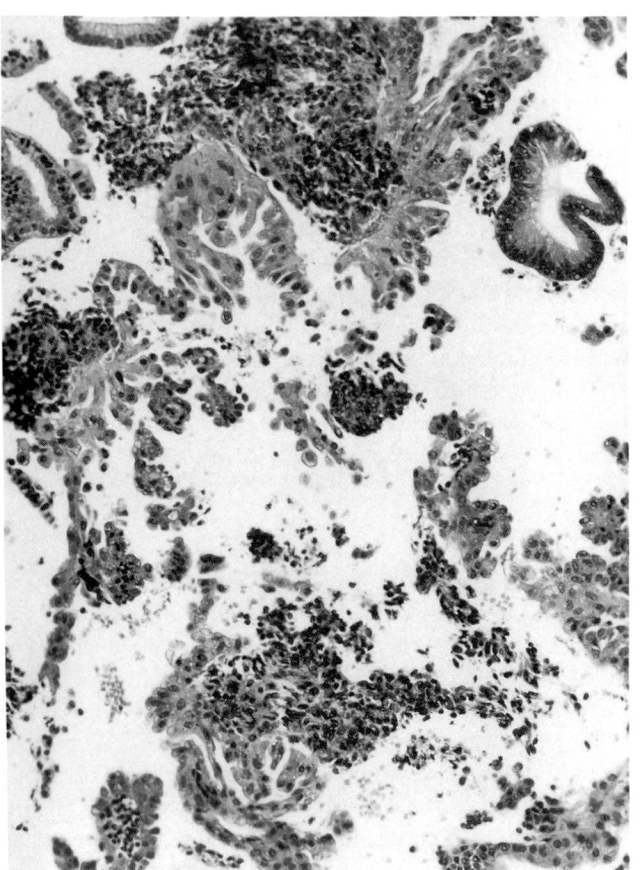

◁

Fig. 10.11. Endometrial glandular and stromal breakdown. There is extensive fragmentation of endometrial glands. Strips of surface epithelium showing eosinophilic syncytial change are present in the upper part of the field. The stromal cells are condensed into tight clusters. These findings are typically found in association with anovulatory cycles.

10.11

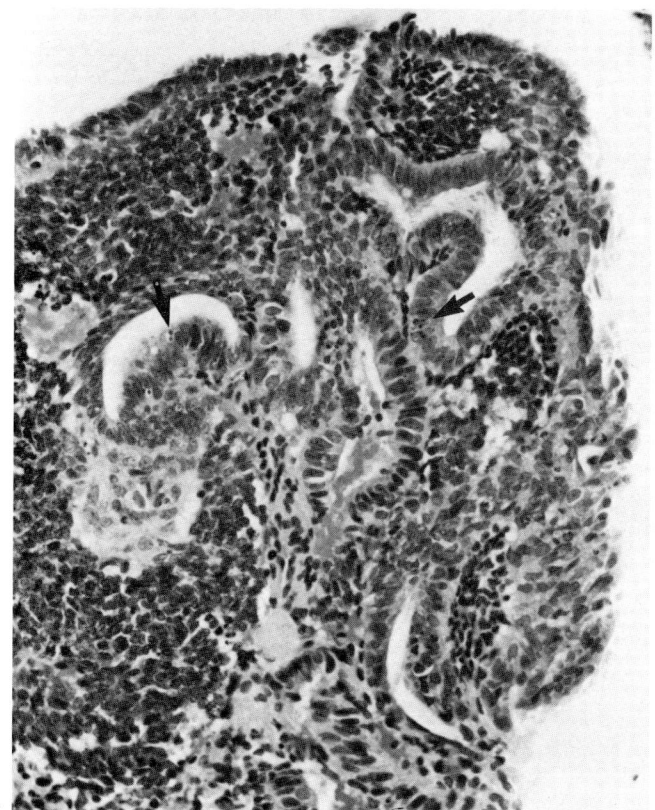

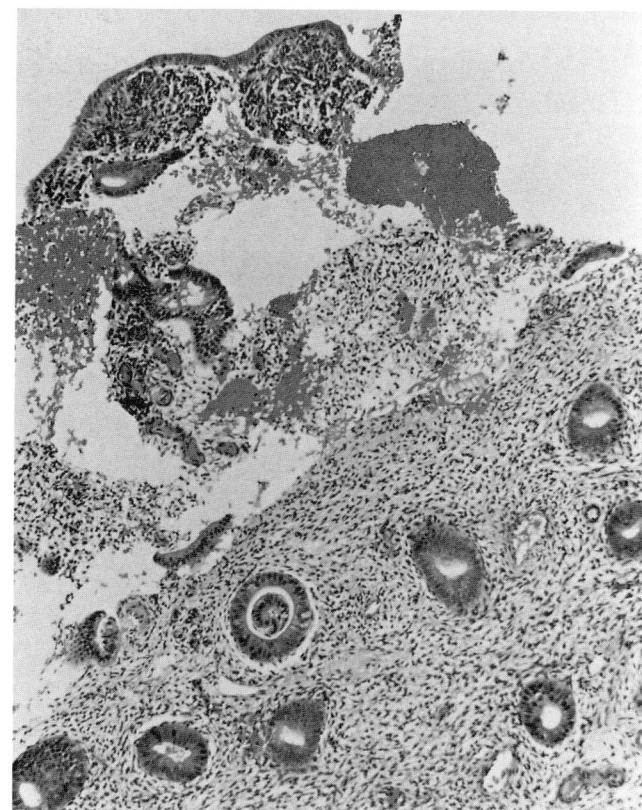

10.13

10.14

focal outpouchings and branching, the lesion may be classified as *disordered proliferative phase*[95] (Figs. 10.15, 10.16). Qualitatively the changes of disordered proliferative phase resemble those of simple hyperplasia but the process is focal. We recommend that the term *disordered proliferative phase* be applied to specimens in which the abnormal glands are focally present in a background of proliferative endometrium (Fig. 10.16). More extensive changes qualify for the diagnosis of *simple hyperplasia* (see Chapter 11, Endometrial Hyperplasia and Related Cellular Changes). Focally, crowded glands with complex invaginations (Fig. 10.17) in an otherwise normal endo

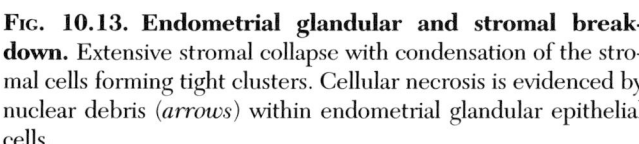

FIG. 10.13. Endometrial glandular and stromal breakdown. Extensive stromal collapse with condensation of the stromal cells forming tight clusters. Cellular necrosis is evidenced by nuclear debris (*arrows*) within endometrial glandular epithelial cells.

FIG. 10.14. Proliferative endometrium with focal breakdown. Most of the endometrium is in the proliferative phase. A focal area of breakdown is present on the surface in the upper part of the field.

FIG. 10.15. Disordered proliferative phase. A few glands are enlarged and irregularly shaped.

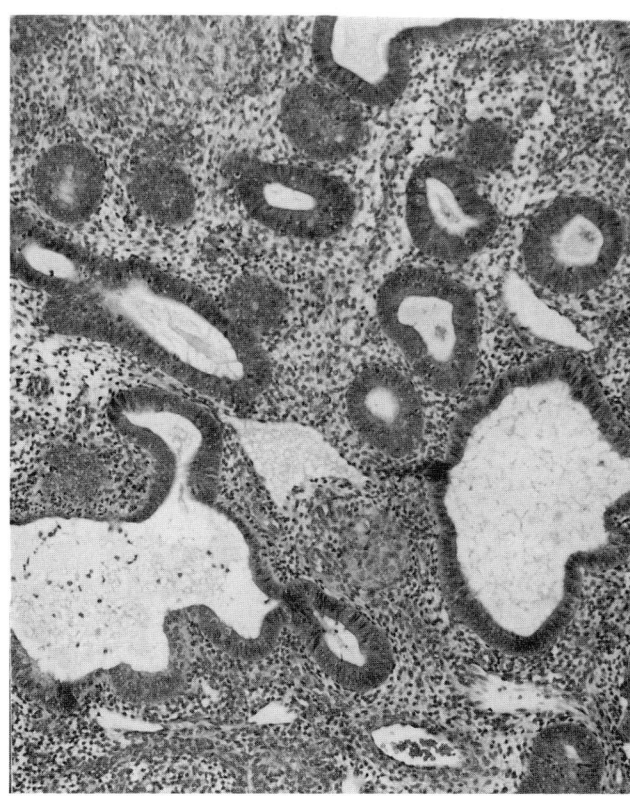

10.15

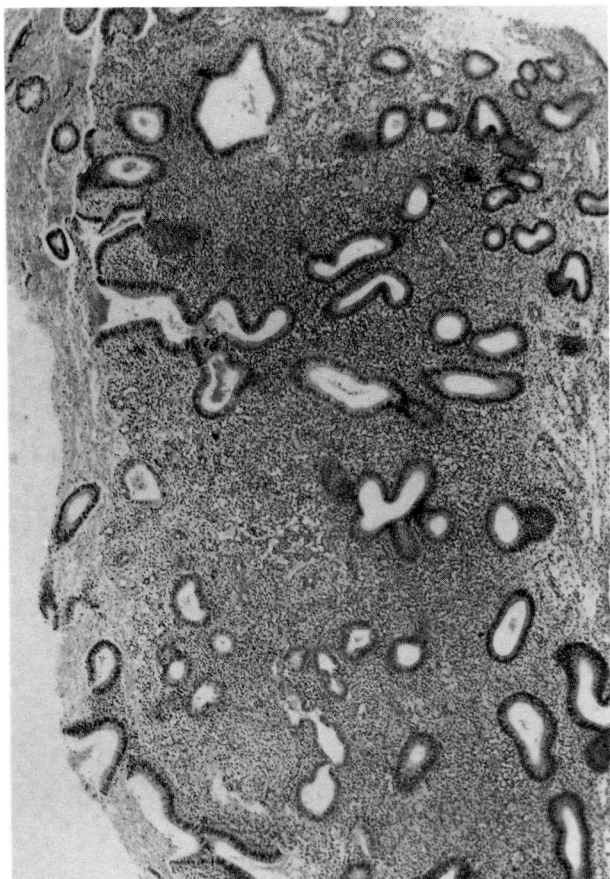

FIG. 10.16. **Disordered proliferative phase.** Most of the endometrium is in the proliferative phase but a few scattered glands that are enlarged and irregularly shaped are present.

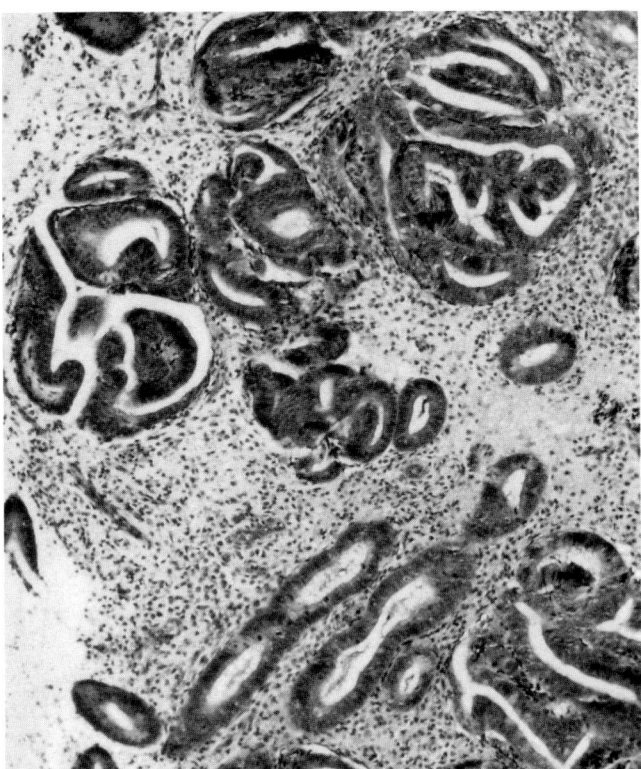

FIG. 10.17. **Focal glandular crowding.** The endometrium is in the proliferative phase. The crowding and the convoluted appearance of the glands are artifactual changes.

metrium is an artifact that should not be confused with disordered proliferative phase or "focal" hyperplasia.

An epithelial change that appears to be related to active breakdown and chronic bleeding has been designated *eosinophilic syncytial change, papillary syncytial change, surface syncytial change,* or *papillary syncytial metaplasia.* Because of its consistent association with breakdown and bleeding, eosinophilic syncytial change appears to be a degenerative/ regenerative rather than a metaplastic process[275] (see Chapter 11, Endometrial Hyperplasia and Related Cellular Changes). Eosinophilic syncytial change typically involves the surface but can also involve glands. The cells often are piled up into papillary projections and overlie clusters of condensed stromal cells (Figs. 10.11, 10.18). Microcystic spaces containing PMNs and nuclear debris frequently are present within the syncytial masses (Fig. 10.18). The cells have prominent eosinophilic cytoplasm, which is frequently vacuolated. The nuclei tend to be round and slightly enlarged but larger, more irregularly shaped nuclei can be observed. Some nuclei contain small nucleoli (Fig. 10.19). This should not be interpreted as "atypia." The chromatin usually is delicate but can be hyperchromatic and smudged, giving a degenerative ap-

pearance. Mitotic activity generally is not evident. Eosinophilic syncytial change may be admixed with other cytoplasmic alterations (metaplasias) including squamous, mucinous, and ciliated change (see Chapter 11, Endometrial Hyperplasia and Related Cellular Changes).

In addition to the stromal and glandular changes, there are profound vascular alterations characterized by the presence of thin-walled ectatic venules. Typically, these blood vessels contain prominent fibrin thrombi (Fig. 10.20), a feature seldom encountered in normal menstrual endometrium. Bleeding during a normal menstrual cycle is a consequence of rhythmic vasospasm and relaxation of the spiral arterioles, resulting in a complete, yet self-limited sloughing of the functionalis (see Chapter 9, Anatomy and Histology of the Uterine Corpus).[198] In anovulatory cycles, spiral arterioles fail to develop adequately, and the dilated, thin-walled venules undergo thrombosis. Stromal necrosis involving random portions of the endometrium results in incomplete shedding. Consequently, the bleeding pattern is asynchronous and highly variable in duration.

DIFFERENTIAL DIAGNOSIS

Because of the profound degree of stromal necrosis and collapse that characterizes endometrial glandular and stro-

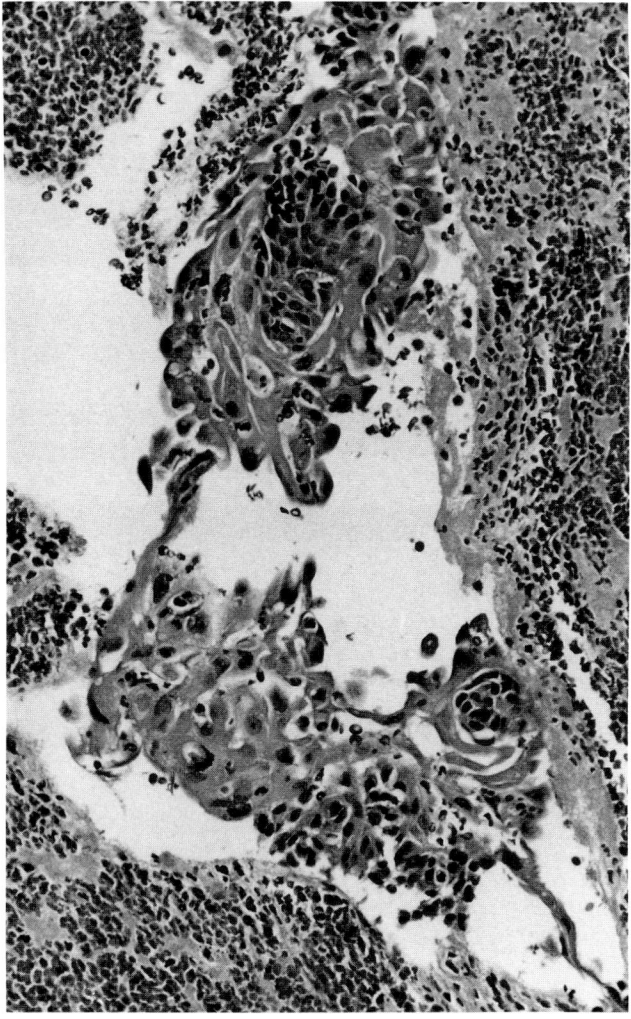

10.18

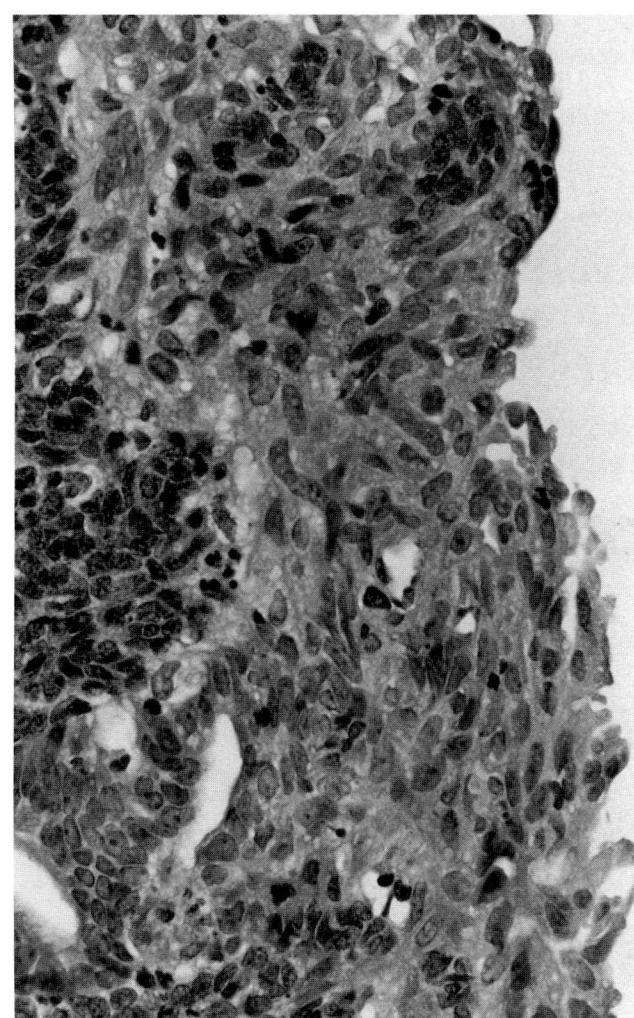

10.19

FIG. 10.18. Eosinophilic syncytial change. Cells with eosinophilic cytoplasm form a syncytium that envelopes clusters of stromal cells. Focal microcystic spaces containing debris are present within the syncytium.

FIG. 10.19. Eosinophilic syncytial change. The lesion is on the surface (*right side* of field) of the endometrium. Cells have slightly enlarged, irregularly shaped nuclei, some of which contain small nucleoli. This change should not be interpreted as "atypia."

FIG. 10.20. Fibrin thrombi in association with glandular and stromal breakdown. Dysfunctional bleeding due to anovulatory cycles may result in mild irregularities in proliferative glands and in the development of thin-walled blood vessels. Bleeding is caused, in part, by disruption of the capillaries that contain fibrin thrombi.

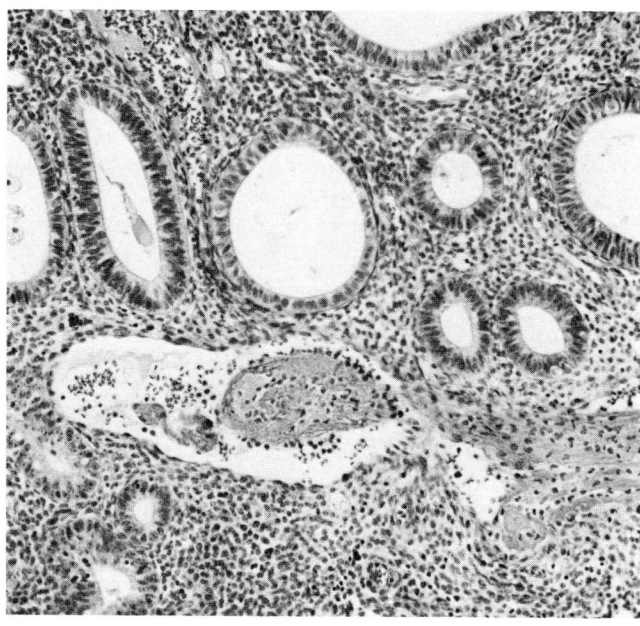

10.20

mal breakdown, the endometrial glands become artificially crowded and there is extensive hemorrhage (Fig. 10.21). It is important not to confuse this appearance with the true glandular crowding of hyperplasia and carcinoma. In contrast to hyperplasia and carcinoma, the glands are fragmented and artifactually are crowded because the surrounding stroma has collapsed. Also in glandular and stromal breakdown the epithelium lacks stratification, atypia, and significant mitotic activity. Glandular and stromal breakdown also occurs in menstrual endometrium, but it is a more diffuse process and the glands show evidence of secretion. In addition, in menstrual endometrium a predecidual reaction is present (Fig. 10.22). Scant focal subnuclear vacuolization may be seen in glandular and stromal breakdown but, with more diffuse vacuolization characteristic of the early secretory phase, does not occur.

The histological pattern in the endometrium reflects the net effect of estrogenic stimulation but is not specific for any particular condition. The histological findings associated with bleeding from anovulatory cycles or replacement hormone therapy are not distinctive.

TREATMENT

Treatment depends on the age of the patient. An acute bleeding episode in a woman under the age of 35 years is best treated the first time with any of the low-dose combi-

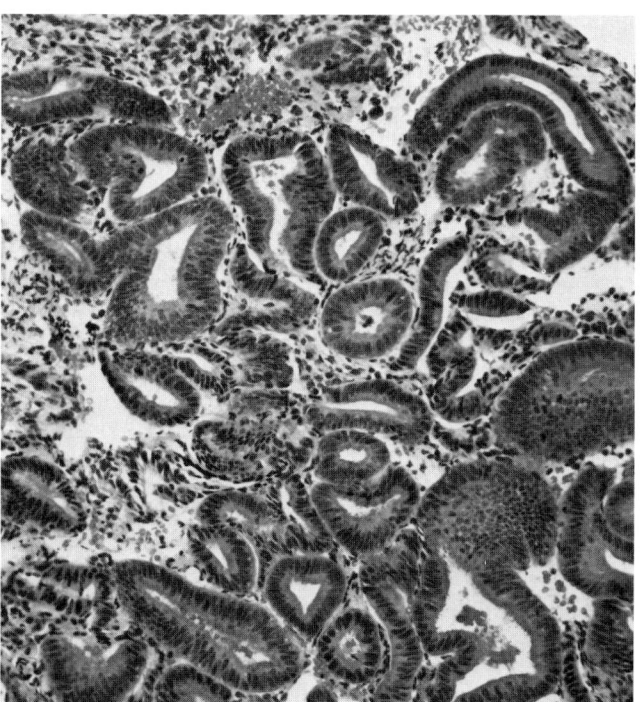

FIG. 10.21. Pseudoglandular crowding in glandular and stromal breakdown. The glandular crowding results from breakdown and dissolution of the intervening stroma. This should not be confused with crowding as a result of hyperplasia.

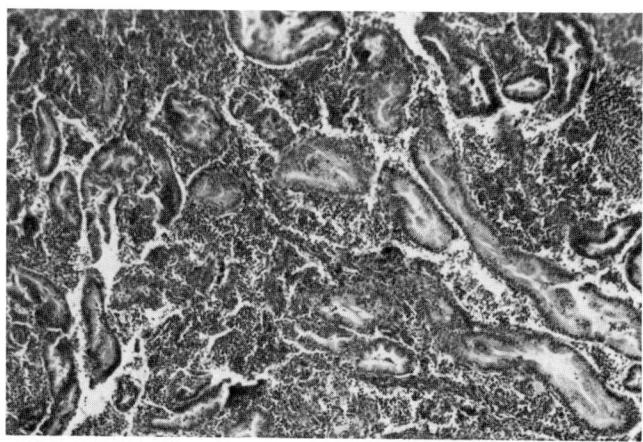

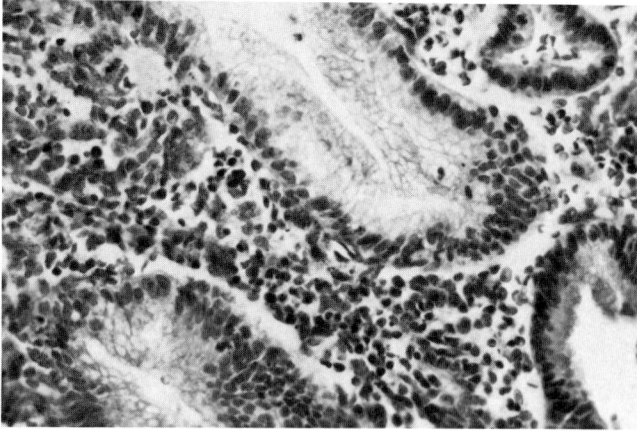

FIG. 10.22. Menstrual endometrium. *Top:* Diffuse hemorhage, necrosis, and stromal breakdown. *Bottom:* Numerous glands containing vacuolated cytoplasm.

nation monophasic birth control pills.[230] One pill two times a day for 5–7 days usually suffices. The progestin stabilizes the uterine vasculature, differentiates the glands and stroma, and results in a complete shedding of the endometrium when therapy is discontinued. Bleeding may be heavy but is self-limited. In women over the age of 35 years and in young women whose bleeding is not controlled with hormones, an endometrial biopsy is necessary to rule out organic pathology. In young women with recurrent anovulatory cycles who are not immediately desirous of childbearing, a week's course of oral medroxyprogesterone acetate (Provera) every 2 months will prevent excessive endometrial buildup and should give controlled withdrawal bleeding. If bleeding occurs in an anovulatory patient who is infertile, induction of ovulation with clomiphene will result in ovulatory cycles and a normal menstrual pattern of bleeding. Bleeding that cannot be controlled by medical treatment requires surgical intervention. Hysterectomy is appropriate for some patients. For those patients who are poor surgical candidates, endometrial ablation using a laser or a resectoscope with a loop or rolling ball electrode is another option.[140]

Atrophy

Bleeding associated with atrophy is manifested by vaginal spotting resulting from no or minimal estrogenic stimulation of the endometrium. This can occur in women on oral contraceptives whose endometria are stimulated inadequately by estrogen, or in postmenopausal women whose endometria are normally atrophic. Atrophic endometria also can occur in reproductive-aged women with premature ovarian failure, or women who have been treated with radiation therapy for advanced cervical carcinoma. Atrophic endometrium is the most common cause of postmenopausal bleeding, accounting for up to 82% of postmenopausal women biopsied for vaginal spotting or bleeding.[40,80,136,152,203,212]

The microscopic appearance of atrophic endometrium is different in hysterectomy and biopsy specimens.[146] In hysterectomy specimens the endometrium is thin and composed of variably sized glands, some of which can show marked cystic dilatation surrounded by compact but diminished stroma compared with endometria from reproductive-aged women. The glands are lined by bland, flattened, or cuboidal nonstratified epithelium. There is no mitotic activity. Under low magnification the cystically dilated glands may be confused with simple hyperplasia. In contrast to atrophy the glandular epithelium in simple hyperplasia is columnar, stratified, and usually mitotic figures are present. In a biopsy or curettage specimen atrophic endometrium is typically scant, consisting of a small amount of mucoid material with a few fragments and strips of glands. Intact glands usually are not found and stroma frequently is absent (Fig. 10.23). Occasionally scattered small clusters of dark stromal cells resembling those seen in anovulatory bleeding are observed. At times the epithelial component is extremely scant, consisting of a few scattered cells. Those specimens should not be diagnosed as being insufficient for diagnosis because this amount of tissue generally is all that is present even after a thorough curettage. Such specimens should be given a descriptive diagnosis, for example, "scant fragments of atrophic endometrial tissue."

Inadequate Luteal Phase

Inadequate luteal phase, also referred to as *luteal phase defect* (LPD), is generally thought to result from inadequate progesterone secretion by the corpus luteum. This disorder is primarily of concern in the evaluation of infertility. It also may be a factor in abnormal uterine bleeding. The pathogenesis of this abnormality is complex and not completely understood. In many cases, LPD develops when the corpus luteum either fails to develop adequately or regresses prematurely. It is postulated that a poorly formed corpus luteum may be due to decreased FSH levels during the follicular phase or to lowered FSH and

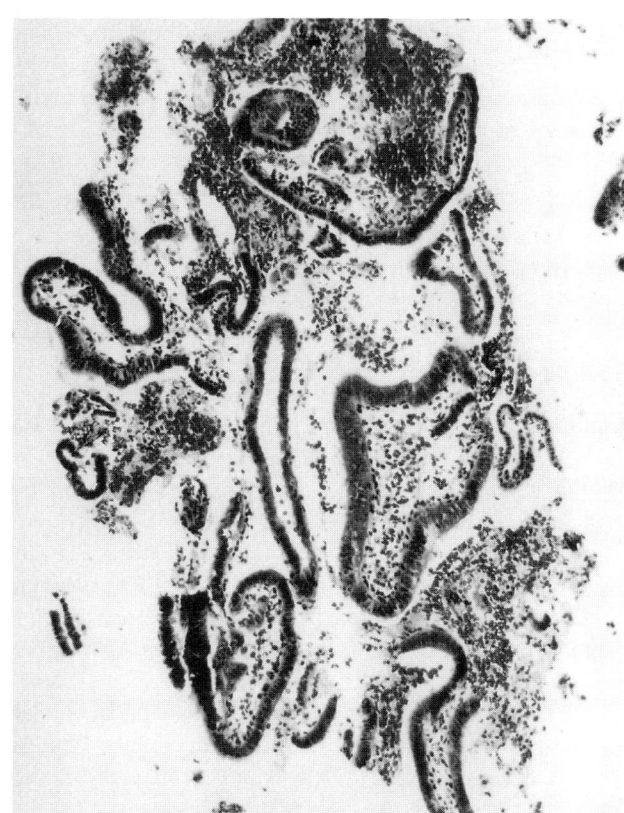

Fig. 10.23. Atrophy. Atrophic endometrium in curettings is characterized by strips of surface endometrium, fragmented glands, and minimal stroma.

luteinizing hormone (LH) peaks at midcycle, resulting in deficient luteinization of the granulosa cells.[230,231] Elevated prolactin levels also may lead to LPD by suppressing progesterone release by the granulosa cells. Any of these processes could result in a reduction of the total amount of progesterone secreted by the corpus luteum. Studies suggest that LPD also may be the result of an end-organ receptor defect, in view of the finding of a reduced number of endometrial progesterone receptor binding sites in some patients with LPD.[127,232] As a result, menses occurs 6–9 days after the LH surge.[112,113,161]

CLINICAL FEATURES

LPD is an uncommon cause of infertility, being found in only 3–5% of infertile women in most studies.[259] The significance of the condition remains controversial because there is a lack of controlled studies evaluating its role in infertility. LPD also has been suggested as a factor in early habitual spontaneous abortions and in abnormal uterine bleeding.[102]

To be significant, LPD must be demonstrated in at least two consecutive cycles because sporadic LPD occurs in normal women.[114] The endometrial biopsy is believed to be one of the best methods of establishing the diagnosis,[7,56,258] but basal body temperature graphs showing a temperature rise that is sustained for less than 10 days and low serum progesterone levels are valuable adjuncts.[51,56,200,230]

PATHOLOGIC FINDINGS

The pathologic features of LPD are not defined completely, mainly because there is no consensus on the exact criteria for the diagnosis. Characteristically, the endometrium in LPD has a normal secretory appearance but shows a lag of more than 2 days from the expected day of the cycle, according to the basal body temperature graph and the onset of menses after biopsy (e.g., a day-22 pattern on day 26).[161,227] In normally cycling women, endometrial dating is, at best, an approximation, with variation from one microscopic field to another and between observers. Reproducibility of endometrial dating is within 2 days of the expected date in about 80% of cases.[175] Consequently, LPD diagnosed by an apparent lag in secretory phase development requires clinical correlation and at least two biopsies showing the lag in development.

The secretory patterns associated with LPD vary, depending on the relative amounts of hormones being secreted. Precise dating is not possible in many instances. In general, the glands and stroma are discordant in their development.[55] Glands may show secretory changes but lack the complex tortuosity expected. The stroma may remain nonreactive, without edema or predecidual development.

The pathologic changes in secretory endometrium attributable to abnormal hormone relationships have not been well studied by careful clinicopathologic correlation of hormone levels, receptor status, and endometrial history. Consequently, although abnormally developed secretory phase endometrium may reflect LPD, the pathologic changes are not diagnostic.

TREATMENT

Various forms of treatment have been used. If LPD is thought to be due to low FSH and LH levels, clomiphene citrate or human menopausal gonadotropin is used to cause an elevation of FSH.[65,230] Progesterone replacement, in the form of daily progesterone vaginal suppositories after the midcycle temperature rise, is another type of treatment, since there is a deficiency of progesterone in LPD.[113,227,260] Alternatively, human chorionic gonadotropin (hCG) is administered to stimulate the corpus luteum to produce progesterone.[230] Bromocriptine, which inhibits prolactin secretion, is used in patients with LPD due to hyperprolactinemia.[60]

Irregular Shedding

Irregular shedding is diagnosed on curettings obtained at least 5 days after the onset of bleeding and is characterized by a mixture of secretory and proliferative patterns (Fig. 10.24). It is a rare cause of abnormal bleeding that develops during the reproductive years, especially between the ages of 24 and 50 years.[148,247] It is characterized by prolonged, heavy bleeding at the time of menses, sometimes lasting longer than 2 weeks.[149,224] Irregular shedding may occur at every menstrual period or only once, such as with a persistent corpus luteum cyst. The continued bleeding appears to be caused by persistent corpus luteum function and continued secretion of progesterone, as irregular shedding can be produced by injecting small doses of progesterone during the menstrual phase of the cycle.[100]

On microscopic examination there is a diverse array of endometrial fragments containing irregular star-shaped secretory glands admixed with early proliferative glands.[54] The stroma around proliferative glands is dense and compact. In areas containing secretory-type glands, the stroma is edematous and the stromal cells may be converted into predecidual cells (Fig. 10.25). Fibrin thrombi may be present. In addition, there is frequent evidence of glandular and stromal breakdown. In contrast to LPD, which

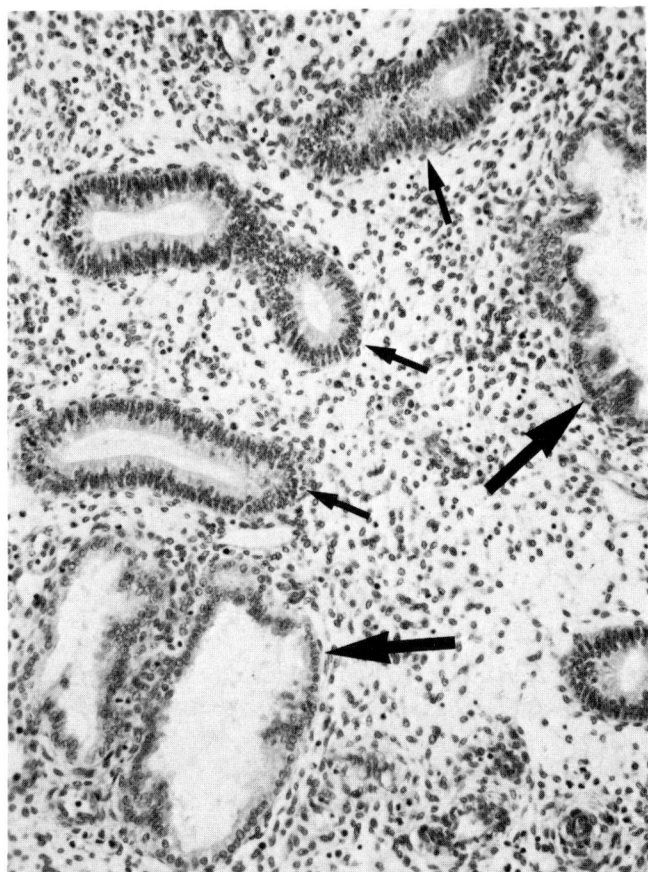

FIG. 10.24. Irregular shedding. Glands showing secretory exhaustion (*large arrows*) are immediately adjacent to proliferative glands (*small arrows*) in an edematous, secretory-type, stroma.

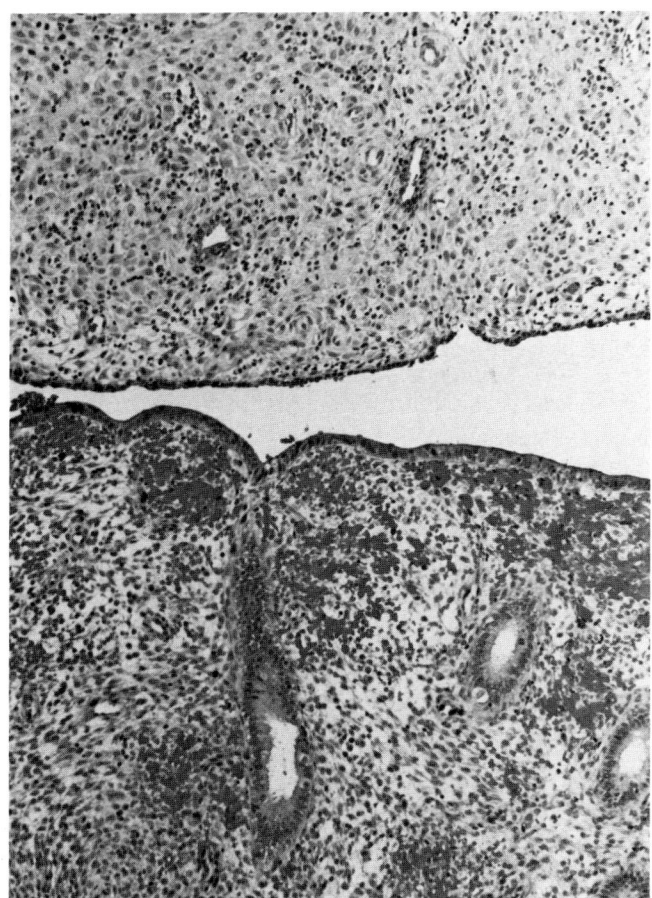

FIG. 10.25. Irregular shedding. *Top:* A secretory pattern with a predecidual reaction. *Bottom:* A proliferative pattern.

shows only secretory changes, irregular shedding demonstrates secretory and proliferative changes.

Other endometrial disorders, including abortions, polyps, and chronic endometritis, may produce bleeding patterns that mimic irregular shedding. In addition, there are abnormal secretory patterns with superimposed bleeding for which there are no specific clinical correlations. Accordingly, these abnormal secretory patterns are best given a descriptive diagnosis.

Unexplained Menorrhagia

In contrast to the above causes of DUB, which are hormonally related, women with unexplained menorrhagia have regular ovulatory cycles. The cause of bleeding appears to be due to local hemostatic factors.[103,250] Normally, at the site of vascular injury platelets adhere to the subendothelium, aggregate, and then degranulate. Fibrin fibers then form between the platelet remnants, forming an occlusive clot. Electron microscopic studies comparing uteri of normally menstruating women with those with menorrhagia disclose the presence of abnormal clots in the latter.

It has been suggested that the unexplained menorrhagia may be due to abnormalities in platelet aggregation related to a shift in prostaglandin synthesis.[3,32] Another mechanism that has been proposed is enhanced fibrinolysis.[205]

Treatment with prostaglandin synthetase inhibitors is highly effective in reducing bleeding in women with menorrhagia. Treatment should begin with the onset of bleeding and be continued for 3–4 days. Intrauterine devices that release progesterone or levonorgestrel also are effective in the treatment of these patients.

Effects of Drugs

Estrogens

Estrogens can stimulate the endometrium even in low concentrations. The duration of exposure rather than the dose of estrogen appears to be more important in the pathologic effect on the endometrium. It has been shown in rabbits that estrogen given over a prolonged period induces endometrial carcinoma,[151] whereas high doses given to monkeys result in atrophy.[94] In humans, prolonged administration of estrogens may result in varying degrees of hyperplasia[178] and, in a small percentage of patients, low-grade carcinoma (see Chapter 11, Endometrial Hyperplasia and Related Cellular Changes and Chapter 12, Endometrial Carcinoma). Estrogen administration also may result in proliferative phase patterns and glandular and stromal breakdown. In these cases the changes are similar to the findings in DUB due to anovulatory cycles. In addition to their proliferative effects, estrogens have other specific morphologic effects on the endometrium, such as various types of epithelial differentiation, including formation of cilia (tubal metaplasia) and cytoplasmic eosinophilia[95] (see Chapter 11, Endometrial Hyperplasia and Related Cellular Changes).

Tamoxifen

Tamoxifen acts as a partial estrogen receptor agonist and has been used as an antiestrogen in the treatment of women with breast cancer. If ongoing clinical trials show that tamoxifen can prevent breast cancer it will undoubtedly be used in millions of healthy women. Despite having been used in the treatment of breast cancer for 20 years, relatively little is known of its effect on the endometrium. Although some epidemiologic studies have shown an increased risk (relative risk of 6.4 at 3–4 years) of developing endometrial carcinoma,[74] other studies have not confirmed this (see Chapter 12, Endometrial Carcinoma). The paradoxical effect of inhibition of breast carcinoma and stimulation of endometrial growth suggest a tissue-specific response to tamoxifen. This differential effect of tamoxifen has been observed in nude mice implanted with breast and endometrial carcinoma cells.[88]

Besides endometrial carcinoma, other uterine abnormalities that have been reported in association with tamoxifen administration include endometrial polyps, hyperplasia, sarcomas, adenomyosis, endometriosis, and leiomyomas.[61,79,168] Endometrial polyps in tamoxifen-treated patients have been reported as having glandular cystic dilatation, hyperplasia, a decidual reaction, and metastatic breast carcinoma.[45] Although recent case-control studies demonstrate increased endometrial thickness and uterine volume and a threefold increase in endometrial polyps in tamoxifen-treated patients compared with controls,[44,130] potentially important confounding factors such as baseline endometrial status and body fat distribution were not taken into account.[168]

Estrogen and Progesterone Therapy in Postmenopausal Women

Many menopausal women are now being treated with hormone replacement therapy because exogenous estrogen administered to these women alleviates the symptoms of menopause and reduces the risk of osteoporotic fractures as well as decreasing the rate of death from coronary artery disease.[57,69] When estrogen is administered alone, the rate of endometrial hyperplasia at 2 years is 40%.[43] The risk of endometrial carcinoma is greater in women on unopposed estrogen as compared with untreated women.[253] For women treated for more than 1 year with estrogen, the risk of endometrial carcinoma may remain increased for more than 10 years after discontinuation of therapy. For all these reasons the current hormonal replacement therapies include the use of a progestational agent, which is given either continuously with estrogen or sequentially for 10–14 days in the latter half of the cycle. By adding a synthetic progestational agent or natural progesterone the rate of hyperplasia is reduced to 2–4% when the dose and duration of treatment are optimized.[43,236,262] Sequential regimens originally were used in doses that were high enough to induce secretory transformation and result in cyclical withdrawal bleeding. Many postmenopausal women, however, find regular bleeding objectionable and consequently compliance is poor with this regimen. Recently, a continuous regimen with a reduced dose of the estrogen and progesterone that results in an atrophic endometrium and amenorrhea has been used. The efficacy of this approach has been evaluated recently in a study of 236 women treated for more than 5 years; there were no cases of hyperplasia or carcinoma.[167] In this study it was found that endometrial growth, assessed by the level of mitotic activity, was controlled by low doses of progesterone. The recovery of adequate amounts of tissue on an endometrial biopsy during the study period correlated with the dose of estrogen and progesterone and the bleeding pattern.

There was 100% recovery of endometrial tissue with high doses but only 18% recovery with low doses. Similarly, no tissue was obtained in 83% of amenorrheic patients but in 93% of women with regular withdrawal bleeding. Hysteroscopic examination of the patients in whom no tissue was obtained revealed that their endometria were atrophic. Furthermore, it was shown that inhibition of endometrial proliferation could be accomplished with low doses of progesterone that failed to induce full secretory maturation. The use of low doses of estrogen and progesterone induced an atrophic endometrium with resulting amenorrhea. This regimen provided equivalent protection from hyperplasia as the higher dose regimens, which resulted in regular bleeding[164,167]

Although it might be presumed that the sequential and combined hormone replacement regimens have similar effects as oral contraceptives, the doses used in the hormone replacement regimens are much lower. Not surprisingly, the histological effects on the endometrium are different. Basically, a wide variety of changes in varying combination can be encountered depending on the dosage, duration of use, whether a combined or sequential administration is used, and the time in the cycle when the biopsy is obtained. Histological changes in the endometria of women on replacement therapy include normal-appearing proliferative or secretory endometrium, mixed proliferative and secretory endometrium, abnormal secretory patterns, and atrophy. Secretory endometria can show variable secretory activity and may or may not display a predecidual change (Figs. 10.26, 10.27). In addition, disordered proliferative phase, hyperplasia, and various types of cytoplasmic changes (metaplasias) can be observed.[59] With the low-dose preparations the endometrium is atrophic or shows weakly secretory patterns that are not developed as fully as those seen in the normal luteal phase.[146]

Although the finding of a decidual reaction in a postmenopausal woman usually indicates the use of a relatively high-dose hormone replacement regimen, rare examples of idiopathic decidual reactions in postmenopausal women have been reported.[41] The pathogenesis of this phenomenon in these patients is unknown.

Contraceptive Steroids (Progestin-Estrogen Agents)

Contraceptive steroids differ chemically from and are metabolized differently than natural hormones and should, consequently, be regarded as inducing a pharmacologic and not a physiologic state. The naturally occurring estrogens are inactivated when administered orally, but by the addition of an ethinyl group at the 17 position, the resulting agent 17-alpha-ethinylestradiol is orally active. This compound and the 3-methyl ether of ethinylestradiol, mestranol, are used as the estrogenic components of oral contraceptives. Mestranol is less potent. These agents have profound progestational activity; some progestins may be

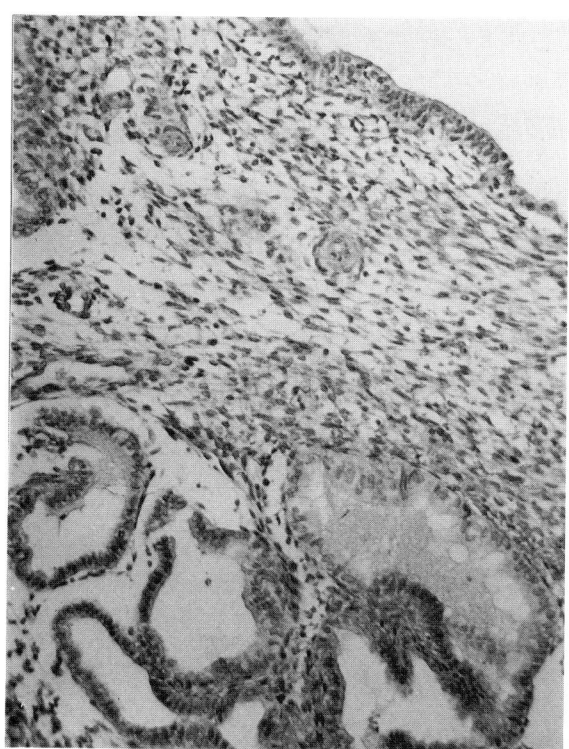

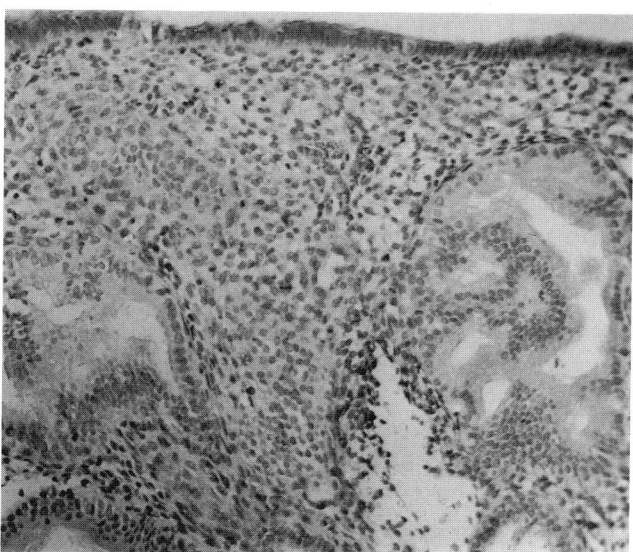

Fig. 10.27. **Estrogen and progesterone hormone replacement therapy.** The endometrium shows full secretory maturation. Glands show secretory exhaustion and the stroma has undergone a predecidual change. (Courtesy of Dr. Dean Moyer, Los Angeles, CA.)

Fig. 10.26. **Estrogen and progesterone hormone replacement therapy.** The glands are variable in appearance. One gland contains secretory material in the lumen and the others are lined by nondescript epithelium. This represents a weak secretory response. The stroma is composed of spindle-shaped cells. There is no evidence of a predecidual reaction. (Courtesy of Dr. Dean Moyer, Los Angeles, CA.)

50 times more potent than natural progesterone. Also, progestational agents are metabolized to estrogenic compounds in the body.[230] The potency of the various progestins varies considerably, and their biologic effect depends mainly on the potency rather than on the dose of drug administered.

The progestational agent in the combination pill prevents ovulation by inhibiting LH secretion through a negative feedback effect on the hypothalamus. Although the estrogenic agent exerts a similar effect on FSH, its primary function is to stimulate the endometrium, thereby preventing breakthrough bleeding, as well as to potentiate the negative feedback action of the progestational agent, thereby permitting reduction in dose of the progestin. This latter effect is attributed to estrogen increasing the intracellular concentration of progesterone receptors.[230,231]

Clinical Features

In the past, contraceptive steroids were administered either as a sequential regimen in which estrogen alone was taken for 14–16 days, followed by 5–6 days during which the estrogen and progestin were given in a single tablet, or as a combined regimen in which a synthetic estrogen is combined with a synthetic progestin in a single tablet taken on day 5 of the cycle and continued for 21 days. The sequential regimen was introduced with the expectation that it would be tolerated better because it more closely simulated a woman's natural endocrine milieu. The sequential pills proved to be less reliable contraceptive agents, as breakthrough ovulations were reported in about 8% of women who used them.[150] They were withdrawn from the market in the United States and Canada in 1976 after reports linking them to endometrial cancer.[120,138,221,222] Evaluation of the women in whom endometrial carcinoma developed while they were using sequential contraceptives demonstrated that 83% used Oracon.[138,221] Weiss and Sayvetz[256] found that women taking Oracon had a risk of endometrial carcinoma substantially higher than did a control group of women who did not use oral contraceptives. The study also provided evidence that the risk of endometrial carcinoma is reduced in women taking combined oral contraceptives, as would be expected from the suppressive effect of progestin-dominated combined regimens. The carcinogenic effect of Oracon does not appear to be attributable to the unopposed estrogen regimen alone because the other sequential pills were not associated with the development of endometrial carcinoma. Oracon, however, used a high dose (100 μg) of the potent estrogen, ethinylestradiol combined with a weak progestin insufficient to mitigate the effect of the estrogen.

Continued use of oral contraceptives, particularly the low-dose preparations (20–35 μg ethinylestradiol), may result in breakthrough bleeding or amenorrhea.[155] Secondary amenorrhea may occur because the low estrogen content of the pill frequently is inadequate to stimulate endometrial growth. Consequently, there is insufficient tissue to produce withdrawal bleeding at the end of a pill cycle. A pill with a slightly higher estrogen content helps in this situation. Prolonged use of oral contraceptives results in the development of thin-walled vascular sinusoids located beneath the endometrial surface, which become ectatic and undergo thrombosis. The endometrial vessels become disrupted and bleed; the surrounding tissue shrinks but is not shed completely; this is manifested clinically as breakthrough bleeding. A 7-day course of conjugated estrogens or ethinylestradiol daily will build up the endometrium and result in uniform withdrawal bleeding.[230]

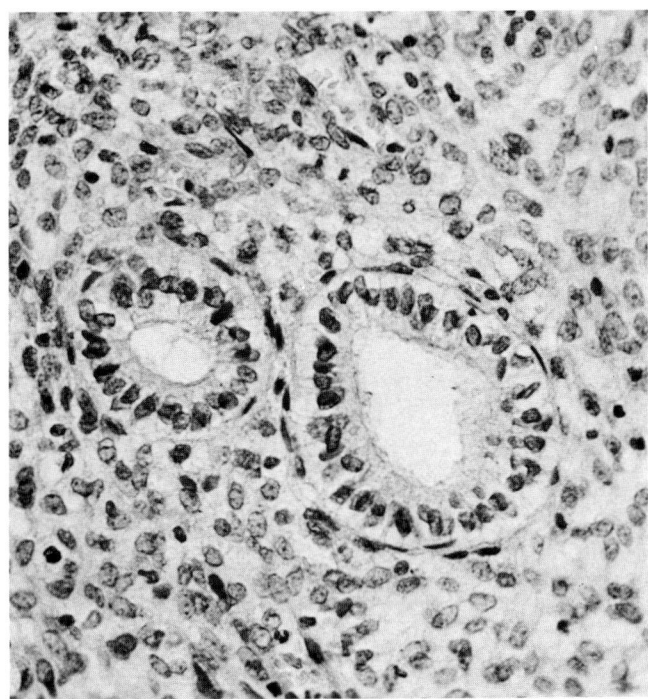

FIG. 10.28. Oral contraceptive therapy. Secretory vacuoles appear prematurely in endometrial glands early during the course of combined oral contraceptive administration.

PATHOLOGIC FINDINGS

The histological alterations produced by exogenous estrogen-progestin oral contraceptives on the endometrium are a function of (1) whether the drugs are administered in the combined or sequential regimen, (2) the dose and duration of drug used, (3) the morphologic appearance of the endometrium before the start of therapy, and (4) the time of the cycle when the tissue is obtained for study.[97,146,176,177]

During the first cycle of the combined regimen in women who had previously been ovulating normally, the proliferative phase is markedly shortened, with an arrest in both the growth and differentiation of the glandular epithelium. The glands remain straight and are lined by a single layer of low, inactive columnar epithelium. Glycogen vacuoles appear prematurely and tend to be randomly distributed (Fig. 10.28). Glandular growth is inhibited, and secretory changes develop slowly, if at all. Stromal edema, which can be striking early in therapy, gives way to a distinct decidual change, and numerous granular lymphocytes appear (Fig. 10.29).

After long-term contraceptive use, there is no evidence of secretory activity. The endometrium undergoes atrophy and is composed of sparse, narrow glands.[38] Most glands disappear, and those remaining are composed of flattened epithelial cells, making the glands difficult to distinguish from capillaries. Changes in the endometrial vasculature also occur, specifically the development of thin-walled vascular sinusoids. The stroma consists primarily of collagenous fibers, and a decidual reaction may not be evident (Fig. 10.30). This is the usual appearance of the endometrium of women using the low-dose formulations.

The ultrastructural features of endometria stimulated by oral contraceptives have been summarized by Cavazos and Lucas.[36] Under the influence of a combined regimen, the estrogen-dependent cell functions are depressed, and an

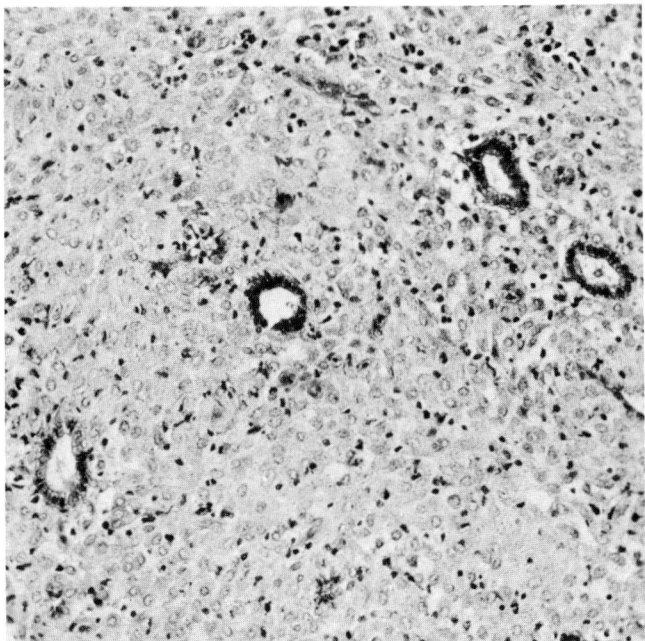

FIG. 10.29. Oral contraceptive therapy. After several cycles of oral contraceptives, the endometrium shows a marked decidual reaction. Glands are small and lined by inactive epithelium.

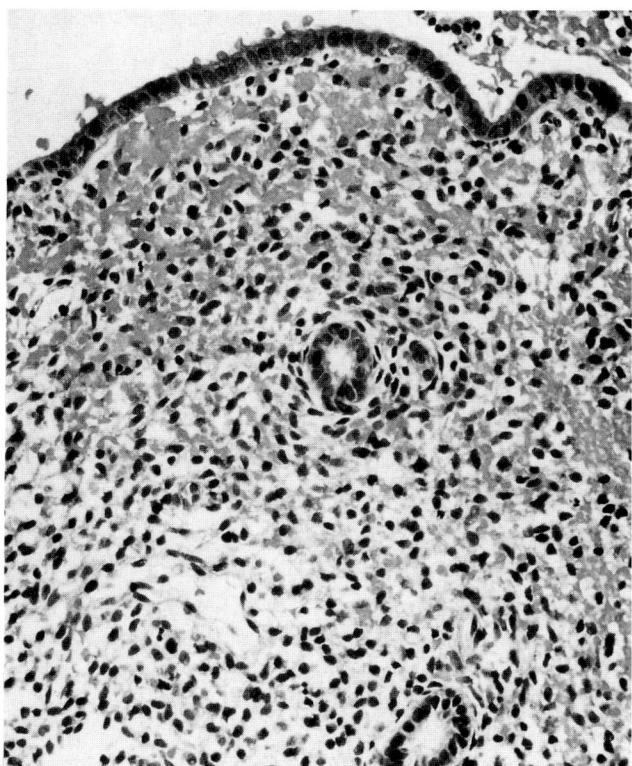

FIG. 10.30. Oral contraceptive effect. Atrophic-appearing endometrium characterized by small glands lined by a single layer of inactive epithelium. The stromal cells are spindle-shaped with no evidence of a decidual change.

intracellular progesterone-type milieu appears. An increase in ribosomal activity and development of the Golgi apparatus is evident during the early phase of the cycle, but the same activities are depressed during the second half of the cycle. Large mitochondria, intranuclear canaliculi, increased glycogen, and rough endoplasmic reticulum characteristic of the secretory phase appear but are suppressed during the latter half of the cycle and do not achieve the development found during the normal postovulatory phase of the cycle.

Progestins, Including Norplant

The effects of these drugs alone on the endometrium are similar to those described for the combined oral contraceptives, but atrophy develops earlier. A marked decidual reaction and glandular suppression of the endometrium may be induced with intramuscular injection of medroxyprogesterone acetate (Depo-Provera). A similar effect is observed with intrauterine devices (IUDs) impregnated with progesterone, but the effect is confined to the superficial portions of the endometrium.

High-dose progestin therapy is used in the medical treatment of endometrial hyperplasia, particularly in

young women who wish to retain their fertility or in older women who are poor surgical candidates. Hyperplastic glands may retain some of their architectural abnormalities but the glandular cells show secretory changes, including the presence of secretory vacuoles. Mitotic activity is decreased and the stroma becomes decidualized. Typically the endometrial response is not uniform, with some foci showing an inhibited appearance whereas other portions of the endometrium may be unaffected. Accordingly, patients treated in this manner must undergo repeated endometrial samples before it can be safely assumed that the hyperplastic process has been completely reverted.

An unusual type of stromal atypia, referred to as *pseudomalignant*[64] or *pseudosarcoma*,[50] has been reported in women receiving high-dose progestational oral contraceptives (Fig. 10.31). Although this lesion is rarely seen now because of the use of low-dose oral contraceptives, the change may be seen in women being treated with proges-

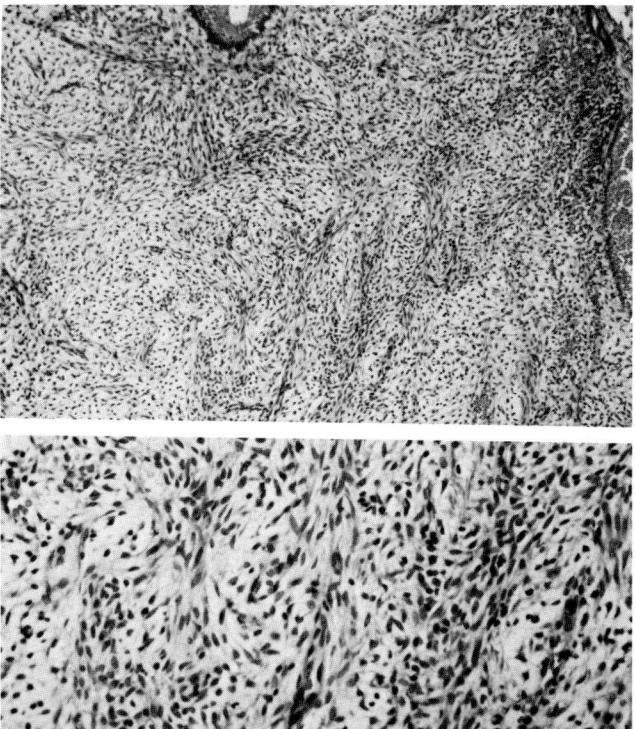

FIG. 10.31. High-dose progesterone effect showing a "pseudosarcomatous" change. *Top:* Low magnification shows a hypercellular spindle-cell stroma. *Bottom:* High magnification shows minimal atypia and an absence of mitotic activity. The lesion mimics low-grade endometrial stromal sarcoma but the stromal cells lack the intimate relationship to small blood vessels characteristic of low-grade stromal sarcoma.

tational agents for endometrial hyperplasia because of the high doses that are used.

Norplant is a long-acting, reversible contraceptive method that is introduced under the skin and releases small amounts of levonorgesterol at a relatively constant rate for up to 5 years. The pregnancy rate during the first 3 years of use is comparable to tubal sterilization.[219] As with other progestins the mechanism of action may be multifactorial: suppression of ovulation, increase in the viscosity of cervical mucus, and suppression of endometrial growth. The main endometrial change is glandular atrophy and stromal decidualization.[49] As with other progestin-only contraceptives, if pregnancy occurs the risk of an ectopic pregnancy is high (20–30%) because of the progestin-induced inhibition of tubal motility.

Danazol

Although structurally related to testosterone, the main metabolite of Danazol is ethisterone, a weak progestin. Danazol mimics the effects of progesterone physiologically and in its effect on the endometrium. It is therefore used in the treatment in endometrosis and endometrial hyperplasia.[226,230]

Early in the course of treatment endometrial glands show weak secretory changes characterized by slight tortuosity, basal nuclei, and cytoplasmic vacuolization; the stroma is hypercellular. After prolonged treatment secretory activity disappears and the endometrium becomes atrophic.[109,141]

Clomiphene Citrate

Clomiphene citrate is an orally active nonsteroidal compound structurally similar to diethylstilbestrol (DES) that binds to extrogen receptors. Clomiphene reduces estrogen receptors in the hypothalamus by inhibiting the process of receptor replacement. Endogenous estrogen levels, therefore, appear to be low, and gonadotropin-releasing hormone is secreted, stimulating pituitary secretion of FSH and LH. When clomiphene is used to induce ovulation, the endometrium displays histological changes that reflect a hypoestrogenic state because of the competitive binding of clomiphene to estrogen receptor. In a review of 710 biopsies it was found that clomiphene induced specific alterations in secretory endometrium.[15] Decreased gland/stroma ratio was the most consistent finding. Gland lumens were reduced in size and glandular tortuosity was diminished. Secretory activity was decreased and there was diminished stromal decidualization. The overall amount of stroma that normally becomes decidualized was reduced and the size of the predecidual cells was decreased. Another investigator reported a discrepancy in the maturation of glands and stroma. Specifically, the glands appeared to lag stromal development by about 7 days. For example, a specimen in which the glands had the appearance of day 16 or 17 contained stroma with an appearance that was consistent with day 23 or 24.[59] Not all studies, however, have shown consistent effects on secretory development.

Gonadotropin-releasing Hormone Agonists

Gonadotropin-releasing hormone agonists (GnRH) are used mainly to suppress the endometrium before resectoscopic ablation or to decrease the size of leiomyomas before myomectomy. After GnRH treatment the endometrium becomes markedly atrophic.[23] At times GnRH is combined with a progestin. In this situation the endometrium shows secretory effects.[133]

Human Menopausal Gonadotropin/Human Chorionic Gonadotropin

Human menopausal gonadotropin (hMG)(Pergonal) and chorionic gonadotropin (hCG) are used often in the treatment of infertility in anovulatory women with polycystic ovarian disease. The two hormones are used together to enhance the LH surge after initial treatment with clomiphene.

The histological effects on the endometrium are unclear. Some studies have reported retarded secretory maturation,[31,194] whereas others have described more highly developed secretory changes than expected for the chronological date of the cycle.[82,215] There are no specific morphologic changes that can be correlated with the effects of these hormones.

RU 486

RU 486 is a synthetic steroid with a high affinity for progesterone receptors. As such, it blocks the action of progesterone on the endometrium. It has been used mainly for voluntary interruption of early pregnancy but is also being evaluated as a possible contraceptive. As a result of its antiprogesterone effect, the endometrium demonstrates inhibition of glandular secretory activity; mitotic activity in the stroma is increased.[238] In postmenopausal women on estrogen therapy it appears to act as a protesterone agonist causing endometrial effects simulating the action of progesterone.[135,233,238]

Prostaglandins

Prostaglandin production by the endometrium increases through the secretory phase. Primary dysmenorrhea is thought to be caused by myometrial contractions induced by prostaglandins. This correlates with the association of dysmenorrhea with ovulatory cycles and may explain the beneficial effect of oral contraceptives on primary dysmenorrhea because the resulting atrophic endometrium has lower prostaglandin levels. Little is known of the morphologic effects of prostaglandins on the endometrium in humans. In rats prostaglandins appear to induce decidualization.[239,240]

Effects of Intrauterine Devices

The IUD is a method of contraception that is best suited for older parous women who are in a stable monogamous relationship and who have no history of pelvic inflammatory disease or ectopic pregnancy.

PATHOLOGIC FINDINGS

The histological effects on the endometrium depend on the composition of the IUD. The plastic devices induce a focal acute and chronic inflammatory response (Fig. 10.32) composed of leukocytes, lymphocytes, plasma cells, macrophages, and rarely, foreign body giant cells.[165,166,179] A significant degree of chronic inflammation is observed in 25–40% of IUD users and may be related to the duration of use.[179] Squamous metaplasia occasionally is present, and a premature predecidual reaction, thought to be related to local trauma from the device, also occurs.[179,268,269] The endometrium immediately beneath the device may show focal fibrosis and pressure atrophy, whereas surrounding regions may be completely unaffected. With copper-bearing devices, inflammatory reactions occur slightly less frequently. Leukocytes are commonly confined to the gland lumens, with exudation on the endometrial surface

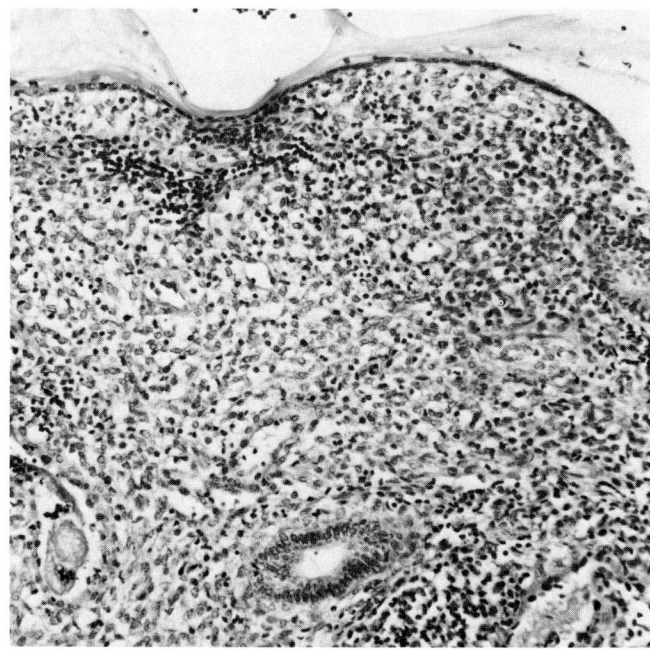

FIG. 10.32. Intrauterine device effect. Endometrium in the vicinity of an intrauterine device shows chronic inflammation.

and sparing of the endometrial stroma. Devices impregnated with progesterone released in a slow, continuous fashion produce a marked, but sharply demarcated, decidual reaction in the endometrium immediately adjacent to the device.[144]

Electron microscopic studies of the effects of the plastic devices reveal giant mitochondria in the glandular epithelial cells during the proliferative phase and premature predecidual changes during the secretory phase.[269,270] An ultrastructural study[87] of endometria in which the copper devices were used shows an increase in the number of mitochondria and lysosomes. The mitochondria show vacuolization of the matrix. Myelin figure formation occurs in 70–80% of the epithelial cells. Specific vascular effects include endothelial degeneration, necrosis, and formation of defects between endothelial cells and adjacent basement membranes.[99] This effect, together with the increase in vessel density,[216] may account for the increased bleeding associated with IUD use.

MECHANISM OF ACTION

The mechanism by which the IUD prevents pregnancy is not entirely clear. Three possible mechanisms that have been suggested are: (1) inhibition of sperm transport from the cervix to the tube, (2) inhibition of sperm capacitation, and (3) interference with implantation.[6] Of these, probably only the latter is affected by IUD-induced changes in the endometrium. For the plastic devices, the inflammatory reaction, in conjunction with an asynchronous premature decidual reaction, results in an unfavorable local environment of implantation of the blastocyst. In addition to these effects, copper ions released by the copper-bearing devices may have direct metabolic effects on endometrial cells, inhibiting several enzyme systems.[182] The mechanism of action for the progesterone-releasing devices is the induced decidual reaction that probably hinders implantation and the local progesterone effect on cervical mucus that may render the cervix impermeable to sperm.

COMPLICATIONS

The IUD, unlike barrier methods, does not protect against sexually transmitted diseases. Shortly after insertion of an IUD there is an increased risk of pelvic infection probably because of the introduction of bacteria at that time, but these are cleared within 24 hours; endometrial cultures 30 days after insertion are sterile.[57] After this period of time any increased risk of upper genital tract infection probably is related to sexually transmitted diseases and not the IUD per se[121,132] as there is no increased risk of infertility among IUD users who are in a monogamous relationship.[47] After elective removal of an IUD for women desiring to become pregnant the pregnancy rates are similar to those in women discontinuing use of other contraceptive devices.[195,207]

A rare infection associated with IUD use is caused by *Actinomyces*, an anerobic, gram-positive organism classified between true bacteria and complete fungi. The presence of any type of IUD, regardless of its duration of use, predisposes a patient to colonization or infection with *Actinomyces*.[92] The typical sulfur granules, composed of a dense central basophilic mass of tangled hyphae surrounded by peripheral radiating filaments, is characteristic (Figs. 10.33, 10.34). The organism can be demonstrated in Papanicolaou-stained cervical vaginal smears.[18]

Actinomyces is not normally found in the cervix and vagina but is part of the normal flora of the oral cavity and gastrointestinal tract. It is likely that the organism is introduced into the lower genital tract during coitus. Because this organism does not ordinarily invade mucosal surfaces, the presence of a foreign body, that is, the IUD, associated tissue injury, and decreased oxygenation may promote colonization by *Actinomyces* and other anaerobic organisms. When tuboovarian abscesses occur in association with the IUD, they tend to be unilateral, especially when associated with *Actinomyces*.[170]

A serious but rare complication of the IUD is perforation through the uterus, with involvement of the omentum and possible bowel obstruction. Bowel obstruction is more likely to occur with copper devices because they are more reactive in the peritoneal cavity than are plastic IUDs. In one study, all seven copper devices that perforated into the abdominal cavity required laparotomy to be removed because of the intense peritoneal reaction, in contrast to

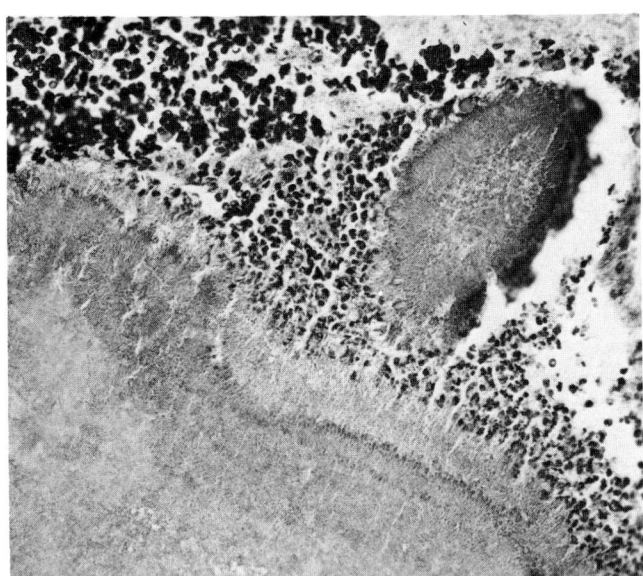

FIG. 10.34. *Actinomyces* **in a patient with an intrauterine device.** Sulfur granules are composed of a dense central basophilic mass of tangled hyphae surrounded by peripheral radiating filaments.

noncopper devices, which could be removed during laparoscopy.[180]

Finally, among women who become pregnant while using an IUD there is a 2–3% risk that the pregnancy is ectopic.[239]

Effects of Curettage

Curettage of the nonpregnant uterus does not appear to have an adverse effect on the endometrium. A slight but significant increase in neutrophils is observed during the first 7 days after a curettage, which then disappears. This is thought to reflect a regenerative process rather than an infectious one.[111] For the first 2 days after a curettage the endometrium is dormant but, beginning with the third day, the endometrial surface is covered by flattened attenuated cells. The basalis contains a serosanguinous exudate with PMNs that is cleared completely in 7–9 days. In one large study, it was found that after curettage more than 83% of women had their menstrual period on schedule, whereas in 10% it was delayed and in 7% it was early.[113,115]

A lesion characterized by extensive eosinophilic infiltration of the endometrium and myometrium, so-called eosinophilic endomyometritis, thought to be secondary to curettage has been reported.[20,63,153] Generally, there is no association with an allergic reaction or parasitic diseases and there is no peripheral eosinophilia. In one study of unselected specimens from the female genital tract a striking eosinophilic infiltrate was found in approximately 1% of cases.[63] The eosinophilic infiltrate usually is associated

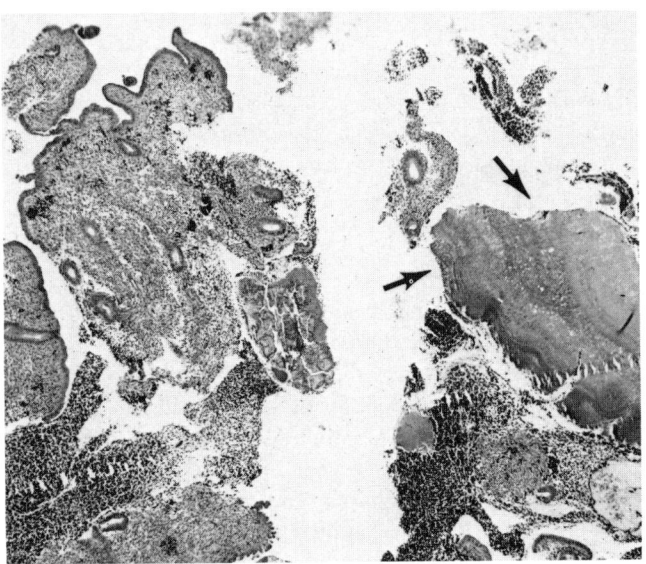

FIG. 10.33. *Actinomyces* **in a patient with an intrauterine device.** Sulfur granules (*arrows*) can be identified under low magnification in endometrial curettings infected with *Actinomyces*.

with other inflammatory cells, especially lymphocytes. The infiltrate typically forms dense aggregates in the endometrium. In the myometrium the infiltrate tends to be in the connective tissue between muscle bundles and in a perivascular location. It has been suggested that the eosinophilic infiltrate results from the release of chemotactic agents from mast cells in the myometrium after tissue injury, specifically a curettage.[153]

Hypomenorrhea or amenorrhea and infertility may follow injury to the endometrium, so-called Asherman syndrome.[10,33,105,110] This condition may develop after a curettage performed during the postpartum or postabortal period, particularly if uterine infection is present. Rarely, tuberculous endometritis or myomectomy is the predisposing factor.

Curettings obtained from women with Asherman syndrome usually contain scant tissue. The uterine synechiae seen at the time of hysteroscopy consist of fibrous tissue or smooth muscle (Fig. 10.35), with no significant inflammation.

The diagnosis of Asherman syndrome is made by hysterography or hysteroscopy, which demonstrates bands of tissue traversing, but rarely obliterating, the endometrial cavity.[73] Many cases of Asherman syndrome show poor correlation between the diminution of menstrual bleeding and the surface area of the endometrium involved by the adhesions. The lack of correlation appears even more exaggerated when the cervicoisthmic area is involved. In the latter cases, after penetration of the obliterated endocervical canal at the time of cervical dilatation and hysteroscopy, a normal endometrial cavity without abnormal accumulation of blood is encountered.[249] It also has been postulated that the intrauterine adhesions are a manifestation of a more widespread process in which the endomyometrium is replaced by fibrous tissue.[270]

Treatment of Asherman syndrome consists of curettage to break the synechiae and placement of an IUD to keep apart the endometrial surfaces.[33] Cyclic estrogen-medroxyprogesterone treatment is administered to induce endometrial proliferation. This form of treatment is curative in most patients, but occasionally intrauterine adhesions reform.[249]

Effects of Laser Surgery

Endometrial ablation using the Nd:YAG laser has been used to treat women with dysfunctional uterine bleeding not controlled by hormonal treatment. Histological examination of uteri that have been subsequently removed is relatively limited and interpretation may be biased as these uteri may have been removed because of intractable bleeding.[85,192] Reepithelization of the sloughed endometrium appears to be complete somewhere between 3–5 months. There is little acute or chronic inflammation present but foreign body giant cells surrounding carbon particles may be observed. Parts of the endometrium show glandular regeneration and in other areas the uterine cavity is lined by a simple cuboidal epithelium overlying a fibrous stroma or directly applied to the myometrium. The appearance is similar to that of Asherman's syndrome (see above).

Effects of Radiation

The morphologic changes induced by radiation are described in Chapter 12, Endometrial Carcinoma. Briefly, the nuclear changes include enlargement, pleomorphism, and hyperchromasia (Fig. 10.36). The cytoplasm of irradiated cells is often granular and vacuolated. A more detailed

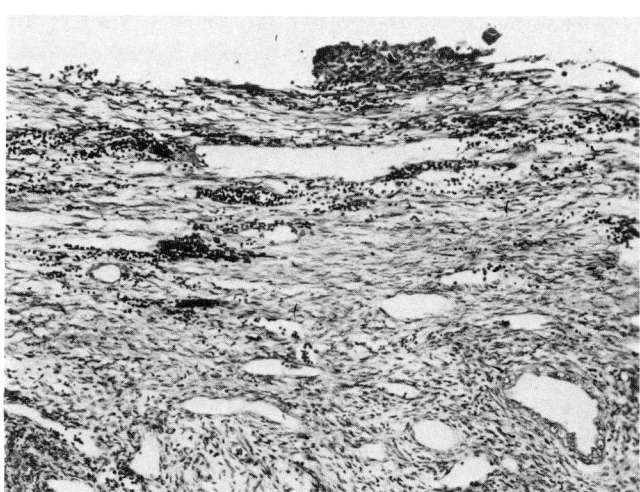

FIG. 10.35. **Asherman syndrome.** The endometrium is characterized by atrophy and fibrosis.

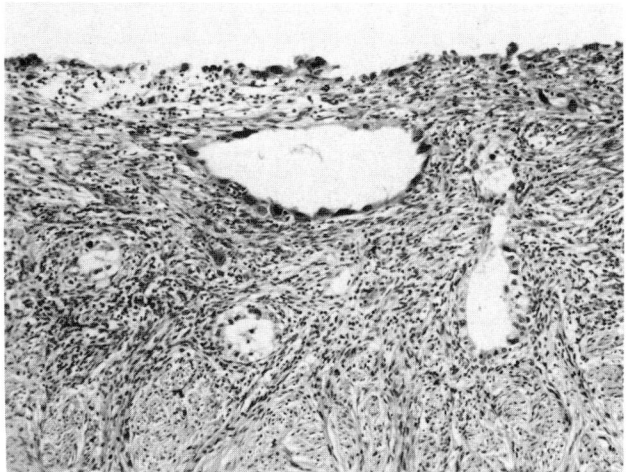

FIG. 10.36. **Radiation effect.** The glands and the surface endometrium are lined by cells showing nuclear atypia.

discussion of radiation-induced endometrial changes is presented by Kraus.[125]

Benign Tumors

Endometrial Polyps

Endometrial polyps are common. They originate as focal hyperplasias of the basalis and develop into benign, localized overgrowths of endometrial tissue covered by epithelium and containing a variable amount of glands, stroma, and blood vessels.

CLINICAL FEATURES

Polyps are encountered most commonly in women between 40 and 50 years of age. Rare before menarche, polyps occur relatively frequently after the menopause. The prevalence of polyps in the general population is about 24%. The most common clinical presentation is abnormal bleeding. During the reproductive years, intermenstrual bleeding or menometrorrhagia is the usual presenting symptom. For some patients, polyps may be the cause of infertility.[75,254] A polyp should always be considered if abnormal bleeding persists after curettage because polyps on a delicate, pliable stalk may be easily missed by the curette.

PATHOLOGIC FINDINGS

Polyps may be broad-based and sessile, pedunculated, or attached to the endometrium by a slender stalk. Furthermore, they vary in size from 1.0 mm to a mass that fills and expands the entire endometrial cavity (Fig. 10.37). Large polyps may extend down the endocervical canal and through the cervix, being visible on physical examination. The surface is tan and glistening, but occasionally the tip or the entire polyp is hemorrhagic due to irritation or infarction. Polyps are generally solitary, but about 20% are multiple. They may originate anywhere in the uterine cavity, but most occur in the fundus, usually the cornual region. Polyps sometimes arise in the lower uterine segment. Upper endocervical polyps and mixed endometrial–endocervical polyps contain glandular epithelium from both components.

Characteristically, a varying proportion of the glands of a polyp are out of phase with the endometrium.[146] The glands usually show some degree of irregularity in outline. In addition, fibrous tissue and sometimes smooth muscle are observed. A polyp with significant amounts of smooth muscle is referred to as an *adenomyomatous polyp*. Hyperplasia (Fig. 10.38) and, occasionally, even carcinoma can occur. Several of the carcinomas that have been reported

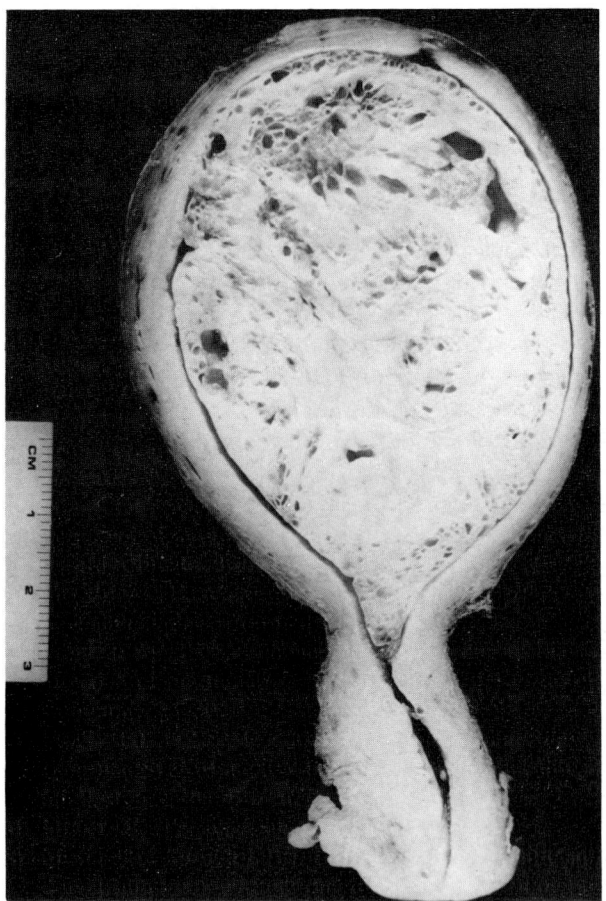

FIG. 10.37. Large endometrial polyp. The polyp entirely fills and distends the endometrial cavity.

are serous and clear cell carcinomas[126,217,220] (Fig. 10.38). Examples of carcinosarcomas[13,62,117,223] confined to an otherwise benign polyp also have been reported. Secretory changes in the glandular epithelium of a polyp are seldom encountered. Rarely, these are seen focally in women with secretory endometrium. Various types of metaplasia, most often squamous metaplasia, of the epithelium also may occur. The endometrial stroma surrounding the glands usually is more fibrotic than the stroma of proliferative endometrium more closely resembling the stroma in the lower uterine segment. A decidual reaction in the stroma, rarely described in polyps when patients have received progestins, is even less common in women with normal cycles.[95] The blood vessels lying at the base of a polyp usually are thick-walled but sometimes are abundant and dilated, simulating a hemangioma.

Because of their morphologic diversity, polyps have defied subclassification to any great extent. Most polyps can be placed into one of three broad groups: hyperplastic, atrophic, or functional.

In hyperplastic polyps, the glands resemble those encountered in diffuse hyperplasia of the endometrium,

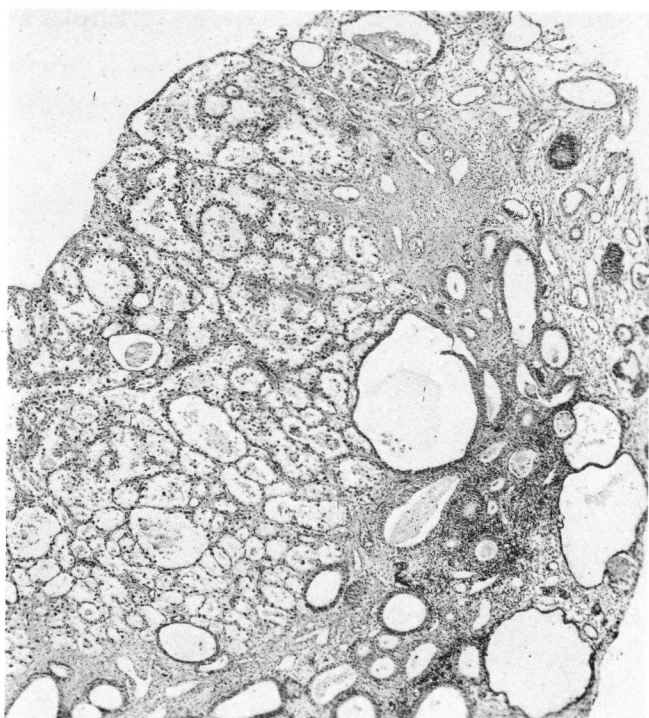

FIG. 10.38. Clear cell carcinoma in the tip of an endometrial polyp. The tumor shows a tubulocystic pattern and is confined to an endometrial polyp. (Reprinted by permission of Kurman and Scully, ref. 126.)

showing active growth and irregular shapes and sizes (Figs. 10.39, 10.40). This is a frequent form of polyp because these tumors are derived from the basalis, which is sensitive to estrogens but much less so to progesterone. Consequently, the varying degrees of proliferative and hyperplastic changes occurring in these polyps result from estrogen stimulation during successive menstrual cycles.

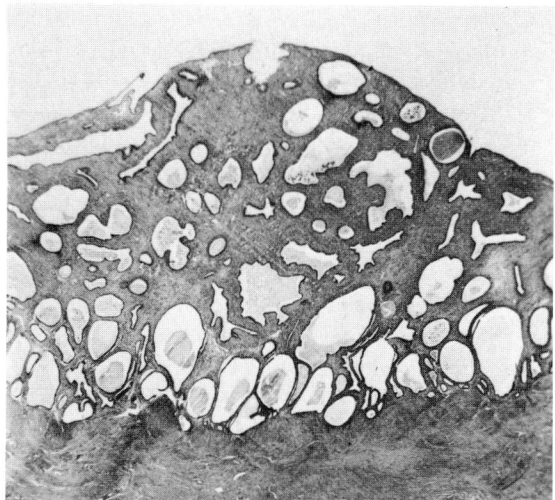

FIG. 10.39. Hyperplastic polyp. The polyp is broad-based and is comprised of irregularly shaped, crowded, hyperplastic glands.

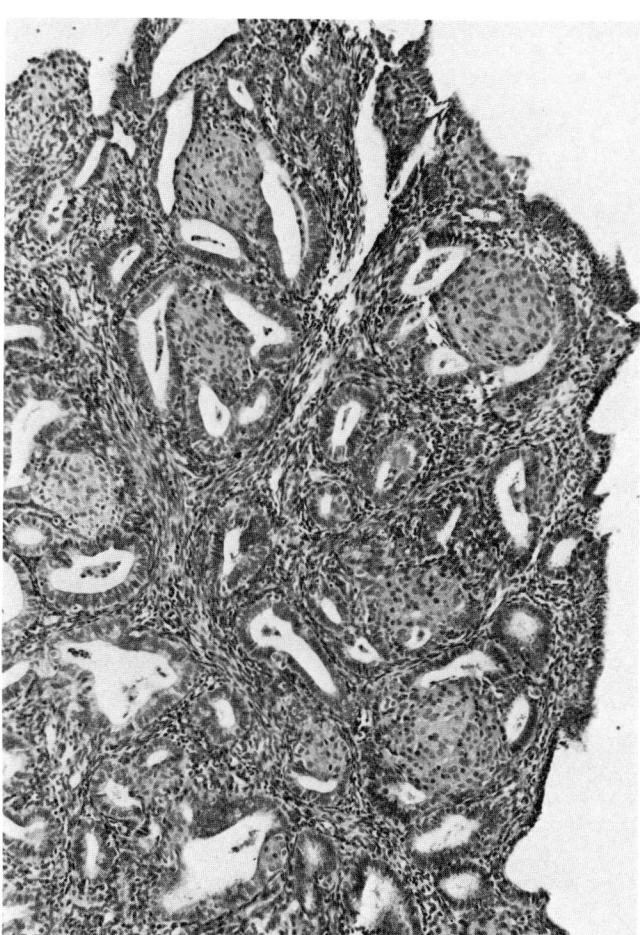

FIG. 10.40. Hyperplastic polyp. This polyp contains crowded irregular glands, some of which show squamous change.

Atrophic polyps show atrophic glandular epithelium that is low columnar to cuboidal. The glands tend to be enlarged and cystically dilated. This form of polyp typically is found in the postmenopausal patient and probably represents regressive changes in a hyperplastic or functional polyp.

Functional polyps are the least frequent. These polyps show glandular changes resembling those of the surrounding endometrium because they respond to hormones of the menstrual cycle (Fig. 10.41).

Polyps may be difficult to recognize in curettage specimens.[146] Ideally, they appear as polypoid-shaped fragments of tissue, with epithelium on three sides. This criterion is difficult to fulfill in many cases, however, because of fragmentation of the specimen or sampling of only a portion of the lesion. In addition, normal endometrium has an irregular surface that may appear polypoid with surface epithelium on three sides when sectioned tangentially; therefore, a polypoid configuration in itself is rarely a suitable diagnostic feature. Other clues to the recognition of a polyp include irregular glands that do not resemble those

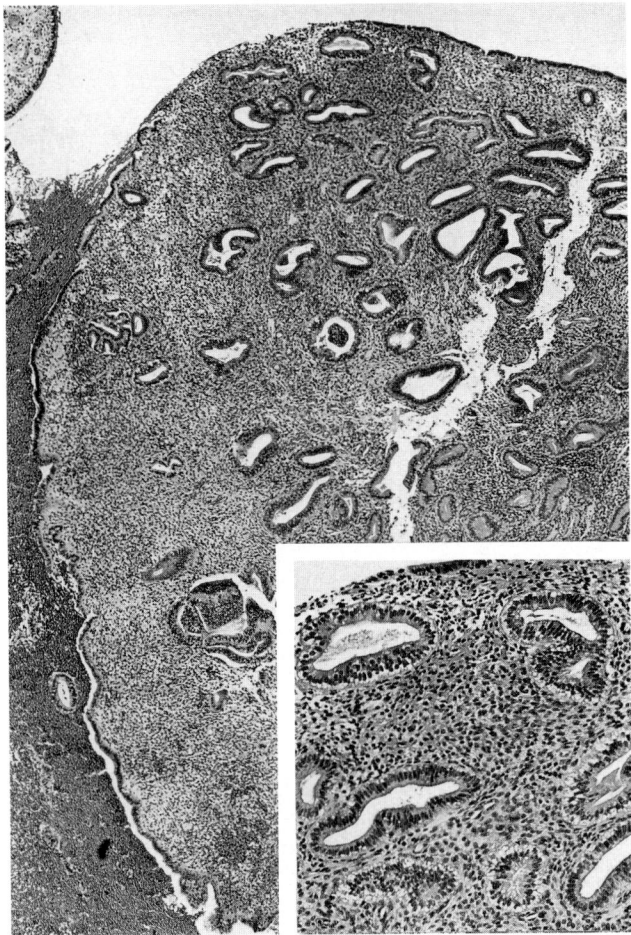

FIG. 10.41. Functional polyp. This polyp contains secretory glands surrounded by dense stroma. *Inset:* Secretory glands with subnuclear vacuoles.

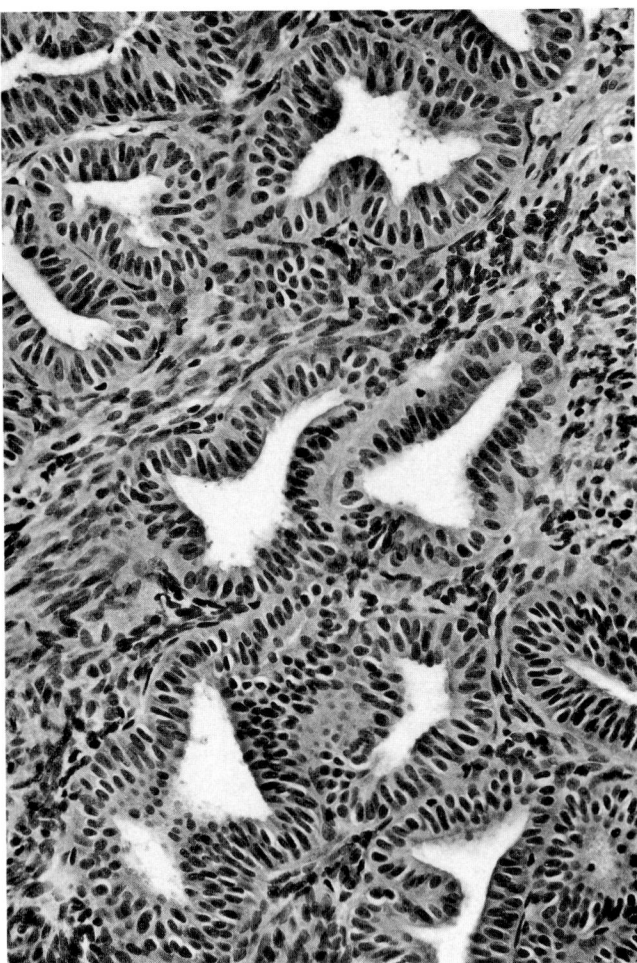

FIG. 10.42. Endometrial polyp. Typically the stroma of a polyp is fibrotic.

of the surrounding endometrium, dense or fibrous stroma (Fig. 10.42), and thick-walled vessels. These features should be seen in fragments of tissue with surface epithelium attached because glands, stroma, and vessels of the basalis can resemble those seein in polyps.

CYTOGENETIC FINDINGS

Three recent cytogenetic studies have shown an inverted chromosome 6 at bands p21 and q22 in endometrial polyps.[52,53,229] This finding suggests that the chromosomal abnormality may play a role in the development of endometrial polyps and targets this region of the chromosome for further molecular analysis.

DIFFERENTIAL DIAGNOSIS

The differential diagnosis of polyps includes hyperplasias, polypoid adenocarcinomas, adenofibromas, and adenosarcomas. Hyperplasias are most likely to cause difficulty in

the differential diagnosis because these abnormalities may have polypoid growth when they are florid. In contrast to benign polyps, however, hyperplasias are diffuse abnormalities; when encountered in curettings, all, or most of, the tissue should show hyperplastic changes—in contrast to the focal change found in polyps. Adenocarcinomas with polypoid growth will retain diagnostic features of malignancy. Adenosarcoma is distinguished from a benign polyp by the distinctive characteristics of the stroma. The stromal cells demonstrate increased mitotic activity and cytological atypia and tend to be closely applied to the glands. In addition, adenosarcomas display a leaf-like pattern unlike polyps that is evident on low magnification (see Chapter 13, Mesenchymal Tumors of the Uterus).

CLINICAL BEHAVIOR AND TREATMENT

The occurrence of carcinoma in benign polyps has been reported to be no more than 0.5%; however, polyps have been found in 12–34% of uteri with endometrial carcinoma.[186,206] A long-term prospective study[9] of patients with endometrial polyps reported that endometrial carcinoma ultimately developed in 3.5% of the patients, but nearly one-half the women in whom carcinoma developed had been treated earlier with intracavitary radium. From these data it appears that women with polyps may be at greater risk for carcinoma than is anticipated for women of the same age. The increased risk stems from the general proliferative trend of endometria harboring polyps. There is no evidence to suggest that polyps have a greater propensity for developing carcinoma than has the adjacent endometrium.

For perimenopausal or postmenopausal women in whom atypical hyperplasia or carcinoma is present in a polyp, hysterectomy is indicated. For lesser degrees of hyperplasia in a polyp, the only treatment needed is polypectomy and curettage. In young women, if the atypical hyperplasia or carcinoma is confined to the polyp, that is, the adjacent endometrium is uninvolved, and the gynecologist is confident that the entire endometrial cavity has been curetted (if hysteroscopy was performed after the curettage), polypectomy probably is curative.

Atypical Polypoid Adenomyoma

The atypical polypoid adenomyoma (APA) occurs in the reproductive years and the perimenopausal period, although rare cases have been seen in postmenopausal women. The lesion has been reported in patients with Turner's syndrome who have been on estrogen replacement therapy.[42] The lesion, like other polyps, usually presents with abnormal uterine bleeding.

The APA grossly resembles an endometrial polyp (Fig. 10.43) and often involves the lower uterine segment. Microscopically, the APA is composed of irregularly shaped hyperplastic glands that are arranged haphazardly within smooth muscle[145,247] (Fig. 10.44). Squamous change is common within the glands, complicating the gland patterns. Central necrosis may be present in the nests of squamous epithelium. The glandular cells display nuclear atypia, loss of polarity, and cytoplasmic eosinophilia (Fig. 10.45). The smooth muscle is composed of short interlacing fascicles, in contrast with the elongated muscle bundles of normal myometrium.

The lesion may be difficult to identify in curettings and must be distinguished from hyperplasia, infiltrating carcinoma, or a malignant mixed mesodermal tumor. The focal nature of the APA and the presence of smooth muscle around the glands distinguish this lesion from atypical hyperplasia (see Chapter 11, Endometrial Hyperplasia and Related Cellular Changes). Infiltrating adenocarcinoma is associated with a reactive fibrous stroma, in contrast to the smooth muscle that surrounds glands in APA (see Chapter 12, Endometrial Carcinoma). Carcinomas usually show more marked atypia and frequently cribriform bridging that contrasts with the milder degree of atypia of APA. Furthermore, in curettings carcinomas rarely show evi-

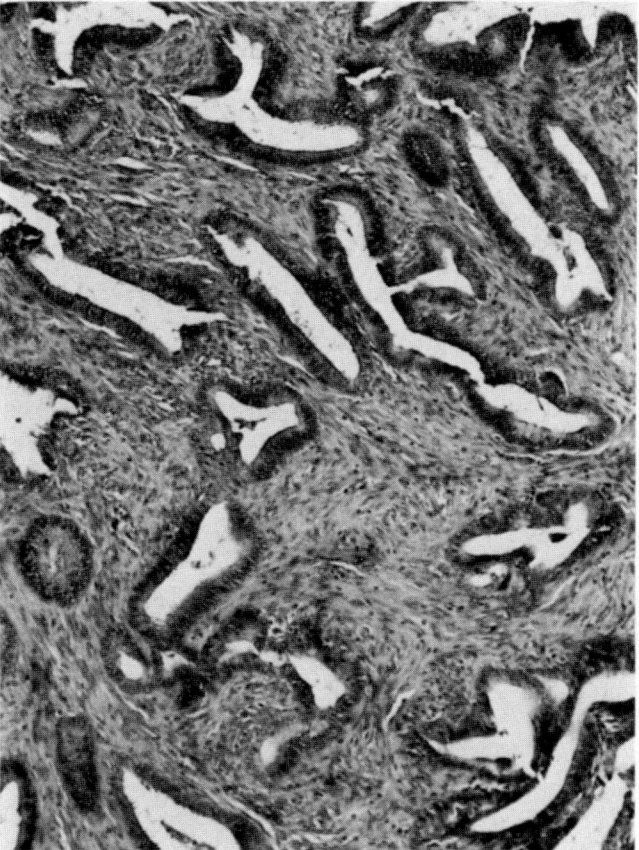

FIG. 10.44. **Atypical polypoid adenomyoma.** Large and atypical glands are surrounded by smooth muscle. (Reprinted by permission of Mazur, ref. 145.)

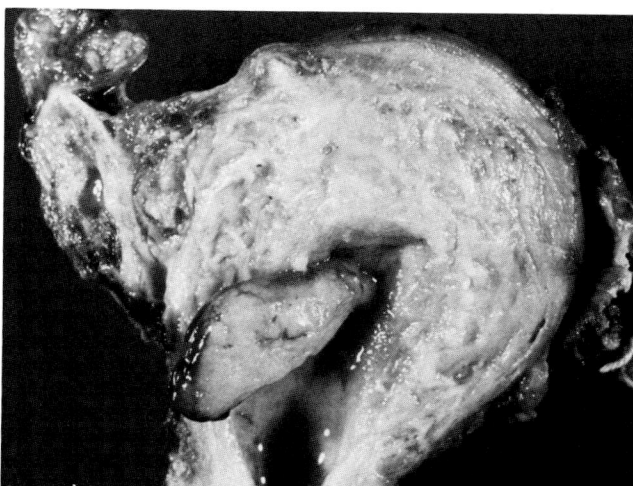

FIG. 10.43. **Atypical polypoid adenomyoma.** The lesion is a discrete pedunculated polypoid mass within the uterine cavity.

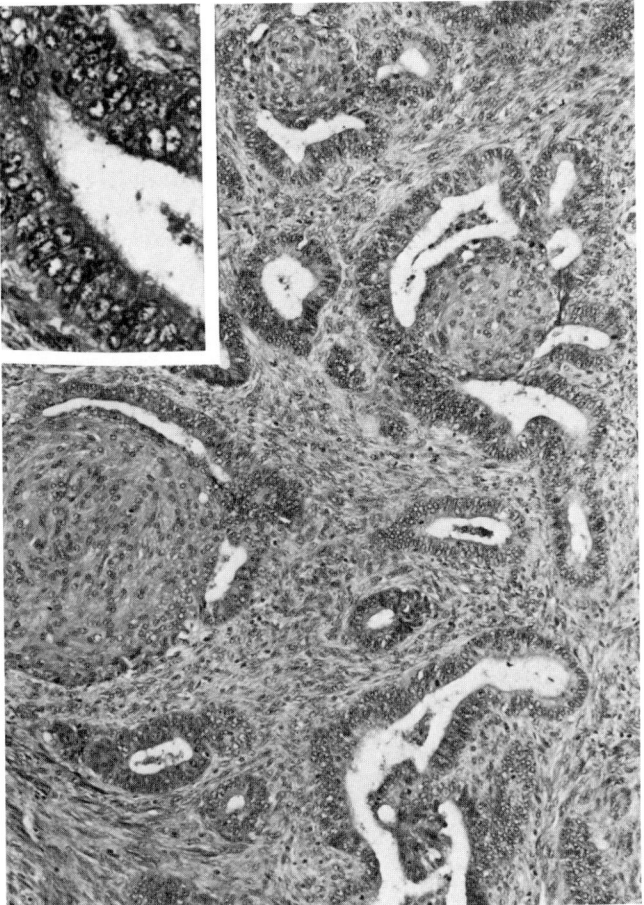

FIG. 10.45. **Atypical polypoid adenomyoma.** The lesion contains irregular glands with foci of squamous differentiation. Smooth muscle surrounds the glands. *Inset:* Cytological atypia is characterized by enlarged nuclei with prominent nucleoli.

dence of myometrial invasion. Accordingly, the presence of atypical glands surrounded by smooth muscle indicates the presence of an APA. Both adenocarcinomas and APA (Fig. 10.45) can show bland squamous differentiation in glands, and this feature is not helpful in separating these entities. In rare instances, it may not be possible to distinguish an APA from a well-differentiated carcinoma, and a hysterectomy will be necessary. The smooth muscle of APA may show focal mitotic activity, but this is generally less than 2 mitoses per 10 high power fields, in contrast to higher rates in sarcomatous patterns. The uniformity of the smooth muscle cells and the lack of high mitotic activity are important features that separate APA from mixed mesodermal tumors (see Chapter 13, Mesenchymal Tumors of the Uterus).

Despite the atypical cytological features of APA, this lesion does not display aggressive behavior. Follow-up has shown that a curettage may be curative in premenopausal women who wish to preserve their fertility, and pregnancy

has followed a curettage.[145,274] There has been one report of an endometrial adenocarcinoma in association with an APA[234]; we have seen similar cases.

Teratoma

Primary benign teratomas of the uterus are extremely rare[128,143,243] and immature teratomas are even more unusual.[95] These must not be confused with the more common types of metaplasia, inherent in the uterus, and implantation of fetal tissues. Nearly 20 teratomas have been reported, but most of those in the older literature are of dubious authenticity. Nicholson[171] concluded in 1956 that only four cases were acceptable, and since then three additional cases have been reported. Microscopically, the appearance of the uterine tumor is similar to that of its ovarian counterpart. The neoplasm is lined by squamous epithelium and contains respiratory epithelium, adipose tissue, and sebaceous glands[143] (Fig. 10.46). A remnant of an embryo should be excluded, and placental and decidual tissue in the surrounding endometrium should be absent.

Brenner Tumor

One tumor with the histological features of a Brenner tumor located in the myometrium immediately beneath the uterine serosa has been reported.[8] The lesion was described as arising from a metaplasia of peritoneal epithelium within the uterus, and not as an endometrial growth. Other examples of ectopic Brenner tumor have been paracervical.

Papillary Serous Tumor

Small papillary tumors lined by tubal type epithelium resembling ovarian serous surface tumors may occur in the endometrium (Fig. 10.47). The few cases we have seen behaved in a benign fashion.

Miscellaneous Lesions

Inflammatory Pseudotumor

Inflammatory pseudotumor, also referred to as *plasma cell granuloma* or *inflammatory myofibroblastic tumor*, is a rare lesion that is believed to be reactive in nature. It most commonly involves the lungs but has been reported in a wide variety of other sites including the liver, stomach, pancreas, spleen, kidney, bladder, spinal cord, and brain. Two cases have been described in the uterus.[84] In this location the lesions presented as leiomyoma-like masses. On microscopic examination these lesions are well circum-

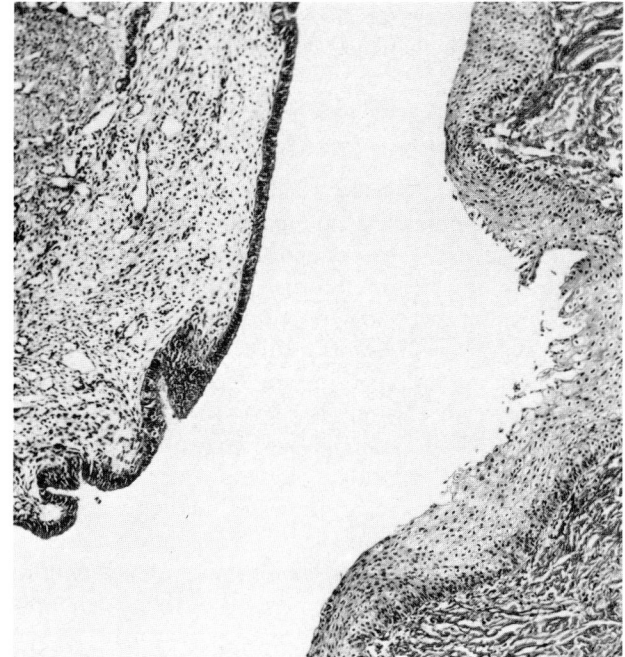

a

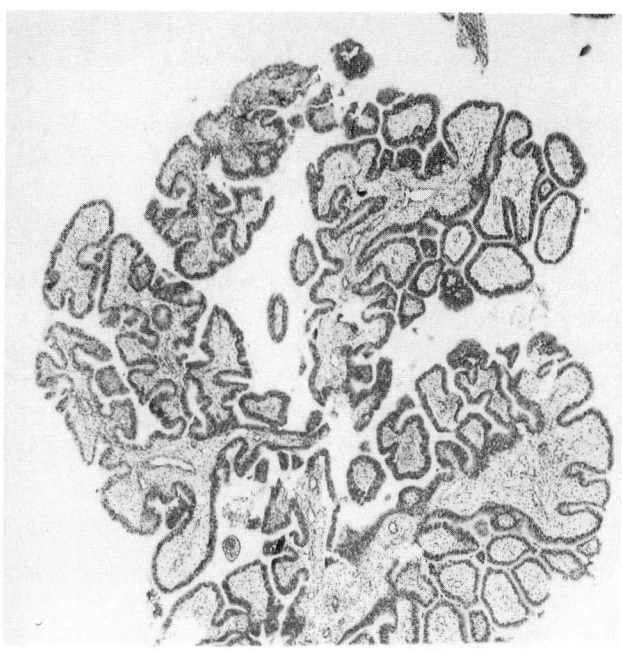

FIG. 10.47. **Benign serous tumor.** The lesion is composed of papillary fronds lined by bland-appearing tubal-type epithelium. The lesion resembles a serous surface tumor of the ovary.

scribed and composed of bland spindle cells that have the appearance of fibroblasts or myofibroblasts. Immunohistochemical stains for actin and vimentin have been positive and ultrastructural studies have confirmed the myofibroblastic nature of the spindle cells. Mitotic figures are rare. There is a marked accompanying inflammatory infiltrate composed mainly of plasma cells but in addition large numbers of PMNs and small and large lymphocytes are present. Rare eosinophils and mast cells also are present. Both patients with uterine lesions are alive and well after 4 years of follow-up.[84]

Postoperative Spindle-cell Nodule

The postoperative spindle-cell nodule is composed of a dense cellular population of spindle cells, small blood vessels, and inflammatory cells. It is a benign lesion that develops as a reparative response to a site of injury. Because of the high level of mitotic activity, it can be confused with a sarcoma but unlike a sarcoma there is no cytological atypia. The lesion occurs more often in the vagina (see Chapter 4, Diseases of the Vagina) but has been described in the endometrium[42] (see Chapter 13, Mesenchymal Tumors of the Uterus).

Lymphoma-like Lesion

A lymphoma-like lesion characterized by aggregates of large lymphoid cells with only rare plasma cells and PMNs has been described in the cervix (see Chapter 6, Benign

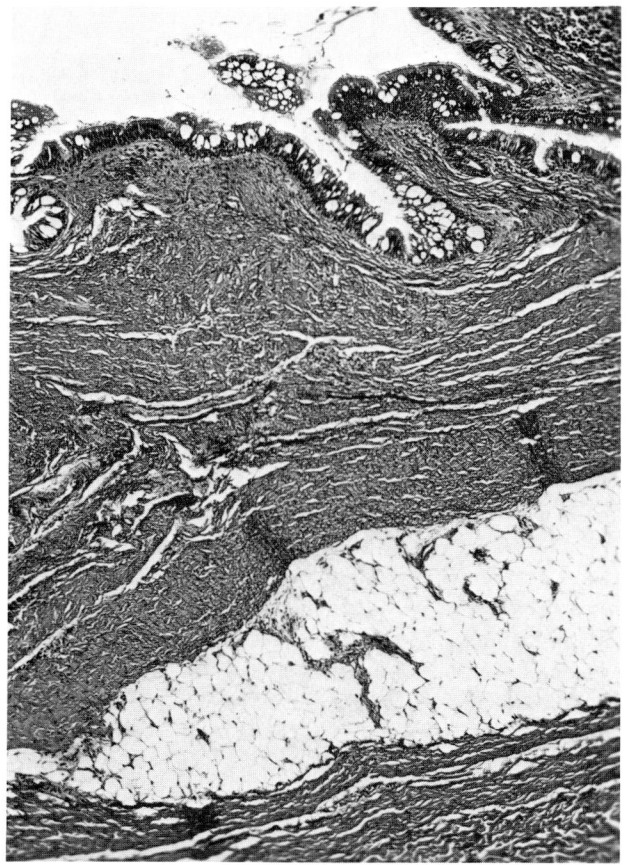

b

FIG. 10.46. **Mature teratoma. a.** Squamous and glandular epithelium are present. **b.** Respiratory epithelium and adipose tissue present elsewhere in the tumor.

Diseases of the Cervix) and endometrium.[273] The aggregates of lymphoid cells resemble reactive germinal centers but lack a peripheral layer of mature lymphocytes. The large lymphoid cells include cleaved and noncleaved follicular center cells and immunoblasts; most of these cells do not stain for anti–light chain antibodies. A mixed inflammatory infiltrate is present at the periphery of the aggregates. Typically the lesions arise on a background of chronic endometritis. The polymorphic infiltrate and associated chronic endometritis as well as the absence of a gross mass and the presence of germinal centers within the lymphoid aggregates assist in the distinction from a lymphoma involving the uterus (see Chapter 13, Mesenchymal Tumors of the Uterus).

Massive Lymphocytic Infiltration in Leiomyomas

Massive lymphocytic infiltration in leiomyomas has been reported.[71] In addition to a moderate to dense infiltration of small lymphocytes, plasma cells, rare eosinophils, and occasional germinal centers are present. The endometrium and adjacent myometrium are devoid of the infiltrate. The underlying cause of this condition is unknown and all the patients with this condition are alive and well with follow-up to 12 years. This lesion is distinguished from a lymphoma involving the uterus on the basis of characteristic gross and microscopic findings. In contrast to a lymphoma which is soft, fleshy, and poorly circumscribed, a leiomyoma with a dense lymphocytic infiltrate has the gross appearance of a typical leiomyoma being firm and well circumscribed. On microscopic examination the leiomyoma contains a population of small lymphocytes as well as plasma cells and occasionally eosinophils. Lymphomas involving the uterus usually are of the diffuse, large-cell type and have a monomorphic rather than a heterogeneous cell population.

Langerhans Cell Histiocytosis

Langerhans cell histiocytosis can either involve the female genital tract as part of a systemic disease or be limited to the genital tract. The endometrium is rarely involved; the vulva is the most common site of genital tract involvement.[11] The lesion is characterized by clusters and sheets of Langerhans cells with grooved and folded vesicular nuclei. There is no correlation between the clinical presentation, extent of involvement, histological appearance, and outcome of the genital lesions, which may undergo complete regression, persistence, or recurrence.

Intravascular Menstrual Endometrium

Occasionally menstrual detritus consisting of clusters of epithelial and or spindle cells can be identified in uterine and parametrial blood vessels. The cytologically bland appearance of the cells serves to distinguish this lesion from an intravascular malignancy.[12]

Giant Cell Arteritis

Giant cell arteritis typically is a localized process with clinical sequelae dependent on the organ that is involved. There have been 17 cases reported involving the female genital tract, of which the uterus was involved in 12.[142] Of these 17 patients, 11 had generalized disease and 6 had no systemic symptoms. Lesions involving the uterus most often occur in asymptomatic postmenopausal women. Microscopically, large numbers of vessels show narrowing and complete obliteration of the lumens by a marked inflammatory infiltrate. The inflammatory infiltrate is sharply localized to the blood vessels and consists of epithelioid histiocytes, lymphocytes, eosinophils, occasional neutrophils, and giant cells. There is no evidence of fibrinoid necrosis. Asymptomatic patients with no laboratory abnormalities probably do not require treatment. Steroids are helpful for symptomatic patients. Acute necrotizing arteritis also may involve the female genital tract.[137] In contrast to giant cell arteritis, necrotizing arteritis is characterized by fibrinoid necrosis, a more acute inflammatory infiltrate, and an absence of giant cells.

Arteriovenous Malformations

Uterine arteriovenous malformations are vascular fistulas composed of an admixture of arterial, venous, and capillary-like channels involving the myometrium and at times the endometrium. These lesions are relatively rare; approximately 35 cases have been reported.[72] Arteriovenous malformations may be congenital or acquired. Although most are thought to be hamartomatous in origin, a frequent history of prior curettage suggests that this procedure may predispose to acquired lesions.

Patients range in age from 23 to 61 years and present with heavy vaginal bleeding. Curettage does not successfully control the hemorrhage and may in fact result in exacerbation of the bleeding. Clinical examination is generally unrevealing but pelvic angiography or ultrasonography can facilitate the diagnosis.

On pathologic examination the lesion may be circumscribed or diffuse in the myometrium with or without endometrial involvement. Microscopically, arteriovenous malformations are composed of a varying proportion of thick- and thin-walled vessels. The thick-walled muscular vessels often show fibrous intimal thickening and represent both arteries and veins.

When the lesion erodes into the endometrium the cause of the bleeding is obvious but in some cases with minor bleeding the malformation is entirely intramural. Hysterectomy usually is necessary to control bleeding, but re-

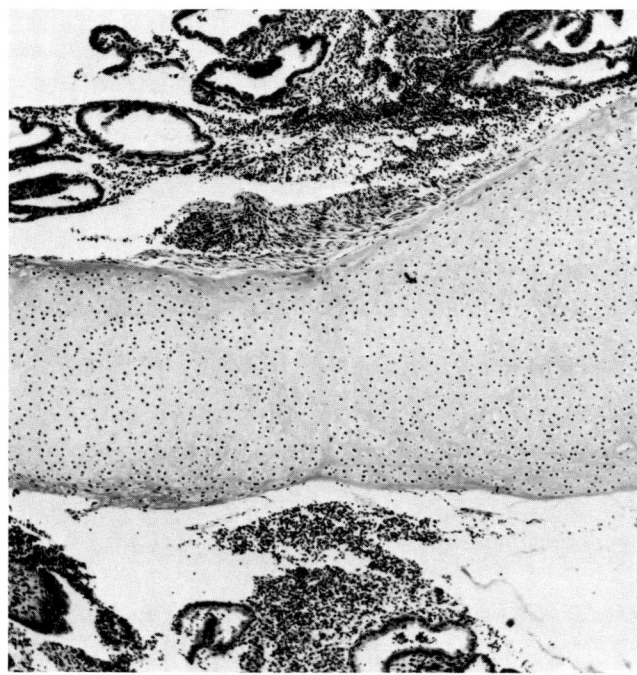

FIG. 10.48. **Heterotopic cartilage.** A well-circumscribed fragment of cartilage is surrounded by otherwise normal-appearing endometrium.

cently some cases have been managed successfully by intraarterial embolization.[188]

Heterologous Tissues

Heterologous tissues are defined as those not native to the endometrium. There have been reports of benign heterologous bone,[46,81,83,104,169] cartilage,[1,83,169,201] smooth muscle,[19] and glial tissue.[169,172,197,276] The two theories advanced to account for their presence are metaplastic transformation of the endometrial stromal cell and implantation of fetal tissue after abortion and instrumentation, with the fetal tissue persisting and growing as a homograft. Before making the diagnosis of benign heterologous tissue, the pathologist should determine if the element is benign or malignant, the latter being a component of a malignant mixed mesodermal tumor.

Heterotopic bone in the endometrium is characteristically found in women with a history of repeated abortions and endometritis.[46,81,104,169] In rare instances, the bone represents a metaplastic phenomenon of the endometrial stroma, triggered by the inflammatory reaction. In most cases the strong association with prior pregnancy, the immaturity of the heterologous element, and the rarity of osseous metaplasia in other types of endometritis indicate that it represents implantation from fetal parts.

Heterotopic cartilage in the endometrium (Fig. 10.48) frequently is associated with a history of prior abortion and

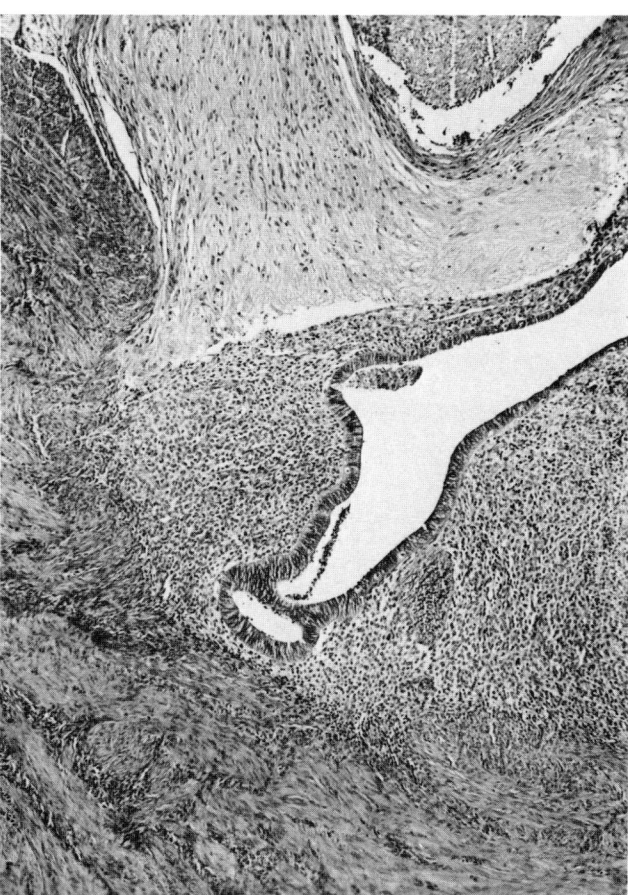

FIG. 10.49. **Mature glia.** A well-circumscribed glial implant is present in the top of the field just above an endometrial gland.

is, therefore, caused by implantation of fetal tissue.[169] In a few patients there is no history of pregnancy and, furthermore, in the series reported by Roth and Taylor,[201] the age of the patients ranged to 52 years. Microscopically, the cartilage was mature, and a transition from endometrial stromal cells to chondrocytes was found in some, suggesting that a metaplastic phenomenon also occurs.

Smooth muscle is heterologous only in relation to the endometrium, as it is obviously a normal component in the myometrium. Occasionally, fascicles and even nodules of benign smooth muscle occur within the endometrium. Some develop without continuity to the underlying myometrium. It is likely that they develop as a metaplastic process from endometrial stromal cells, as the two have a common analage.[19]

Forty-three examples of mature glial tissue in the endometrium have been reported.[42,172,197,276] Microscopically, these occur as multiple foci of mature glial tissue, with an absence of mitotic activity (Fig. 10.49). These foci often are surrounded by a lymphocytic and plasma cell infiltrate, as in a graft rejection. Most cases have a history of instrumented termination of pregnancy. This history,

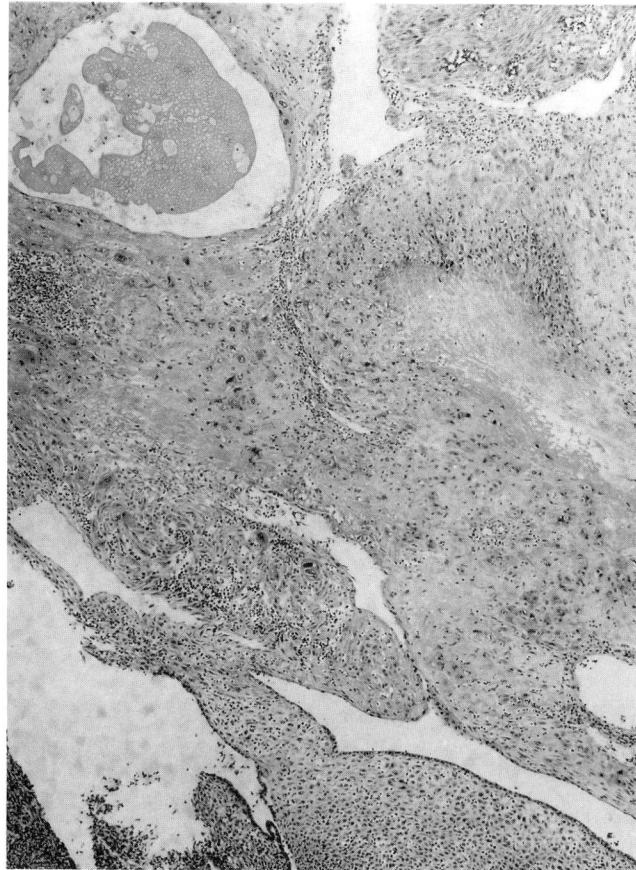

FIG. 10.50. **Subinvolution of the uterus.** A partially involuted placental site composed of enlarged vessels with intermediate trophoblastic cells and fibrinoid replacing the vascular walls. The underlying endometrium has enlarged, dilated glands and a decidualized stroma.

together with the unlikely occurrence of endometrial tissue undergoing metaplasia exclusively into glial tissue or monophytic differentiation of germ cells, supports the theory that the presence of glial tissue in the endometrium is a result of fetal implantation. Rarely, the glial tissue may be a true neoplasm, which is then referred to as a *glioma* of the uterus. In the one case reported, the follow-up was uneventful.[272]

Other rare heterologous tissues that have been found in the endometrium include skin, retina, skeletal muscle, liver, and kidney.[42,243] Like the previously described heterotopic tissues, they probably are of fetal origin after an abortion.

Subinvolution of the Uterus

Normally after delivery of the placenta the uterus decreases in size dramatically over a period of 6–8 weeks. Failure of the uterus to return to its normal size is referred to as *subinvolution*. On clinical examination the uterus, which normally should be firm and close to its size before

pregnancy, is enlarged, soft, and boggy. Although at times the uterus is considerably enlarged, usually it is 6–8 weeks in size. On gross examination the serosal surface has a slightly bluish cast. The cut surface reveals a thickened wall with enlarged blood vessels projecting from the surface. On microscopic examination remnants of the placental site, containing intermediate trophoblastic cells and enlarged vessels enmeshed in eosinophilic fibrinoid along with necrotic decidua, are present (Fig. 10.50). Inflammatory cells also may be present. A retained placental site may serve as a nidus for infection and the subsequent development of postpartum endometritis.

References

1. Aabye R (1955) Cartilage in the endometrium. Acta Obstet Gynecol Scand 34: 105
2. Abraham AA (1978) Herpesvirus hominis endometritis in a young woman wearing an intrauterine contraceptive device. Am J Obstet Gynecol 3: 340
3. Adelanto JM, Rees MRP, Lopez Bernal A, Turnbull AC (1988) Increased uterine prostaglandin E receptors in menorrhagic women. Br J Obstet Gynaecol 99: 162
4. Aksel S, Jones GS (1974) Etiology and treatment of dysfunctional uterine bleeding. Obstet Gynecol 44: 1
5. Altchek A (1977) Dysfunctional uterine bleeding in adolescence. Clin Obstet Gynecol 20: 633
6. Alvarez F, Brache V, Fernandez E, et al (1988) New insights on the mode of action of intrauterine contraceptive devices in women. Fertil Steril 49: 768–773
7. Annos T, Thompson IE, Taymor ML (1980) Luteal phase deficiency and infertility: Difficulties encountered in diagnosis and treatment. Obstet Gynecol 55: 705
8. Arhelger RB, Bocian JJ (1976) Brenner tumor of the uterus. Cancer 38: 1741
9. Armenia CC (1967) Sequential relationship between endometrial polyps and carcinoma of the endometrium. Obstet Gynecol 30: 524
10. Asherman JG (1948) Amenorrhoea traumatica (atretica). J Obstet Gynaecol Br Emp 55: 23
11. Axiotis CA, Merino MJ, Duray PH (1991) Langerhans cell histiocytosis of the female genital tract. Cancer 67: 1650–1660
12. Banks ER, Mills SE, Frierson HF Jr (1991) Uterine intravascular menstrual endometrium simulating malignancy. Am J Surg Pathol 15(4): 407–412
13. Barwick KW, LiVolsi VA (1979) Heterologous mixed mullerian tumor confined to an endometrial polyp. Obstet Gynecol 53: 512–514
14. Beer AE (1970) Differential diagnosis and clinical analysis of dysfunctional uterine bleeding. Clin Obstet Gynecol 13: 434
15. Benda JA (1992) Clomiphene's effect on endometrium in infertility. Int J Gynecol Pathol 11: 273–282
16. Benirschke K (1973) Congenital anomalies of the uterus with emphasis on genetic causes. In: Norris HT, Hertig AT, Abel MR (eds) International Academy of Pathology Monograph No. 14, The uterus. Baltimore, Williams and Wilkins, pp 68–79

17. Berry A (1966) A cytopathological and histopathological study of biharziasis of the female genital tract. J Pathol Bacteriol 91: 325

18. Bhagavan BS, Gupta PK (1978) Genital actinomycosis and intrauterine contraceptive devices. Hum Pathol 9: 567

19. Bird CC, Willia RA (1965) The production of smooth muscle by the endometrial stroma of the adult human uterus. J Pathol Bacteriol 90: 75

20. Bjersing L, Borglin NE (1962) Eosinophilia in the myometrium of the human uterus. Acta Pathol Microbiol Scand 54: 353–364

21. Botella-Llusia J (1967) Tuberculosis of the endometrium. In: Bertelli A, Houck JC (eds) Proceedings of the 5th World Congress on Fertility and Sterility, Stockholm 1966. Amsterdam, Excerpta Medica, International Congress Series 188, p 514

22. Brodman M, Deligdisch L (1986) Cytomegalovirus endometritis in a patient with AIDS. Mt Sinai J Med (NY) 53: 673–675

23. Brooks PG, Serden SP, Davos I (1991) Hormonal inhibition of the endometrium for resectoscopic endometrial ablation. Am J Obstet Gynecol 164: 1601–1608

24. Brudenell JM (1955) Chronic endometritis and plasma cell infiltration of the endometrium. J Obstet Gynaecol Br Emp 62: 269

25. Buckley CH, Fox H (1980) Histiocytic endometritis. Histopathology 4: 105

26. Budny NN (1972) Pyometra with massive foam cell reaction: A case report. Am J Obstet Gynecol 112: 126

27. Bulmer JN, Hollings D, Ritson A (1987) Immunocytochemical evidence that endometrial stromal granulocytes are granulated lymphocytes. J Pathol 153: 281–288

28. Bulmer JN, Lunny DP, Hagin SV (1988) Immunohistochemical characterization of stromal leucocytes in nonpregnant human endometrium. Am J Reprod Immunol Microbiol 17: 83–90

29. Burke RK, Hertig AT, Miele CA (1985) Prognostic value of subacute focal inflammation of the endometrium, with special reference to pelvic adhesions as observed on laparoscopic examination. An eight-year review. J Reprod Med 30: 646

30. Cadena D, Cavanzo FJ, Leone CL, Taylor HB (1973) Chronic endometritis. A comparative clinicopathologic study. Obstet Gynecol 41: 733

31. Campbell BF, Phipps WR, Nagel TC (1988) Endomerial biopsies during treatment with subcutaneous pulsatile gonadotrophin releasing hormone and luteal phase human chorionic gondotropins. Int J Fertil 33: 329

32. Cameron IT, Kelly RW, Baird DT (1985) Prostaglandins in the human uterus: An interaction between endometrium and myometrium. Prostaglandins Leukotrienes Med 17: 329

33. Carmichael DE (1970) Asherman's syndrome. Obstet Gynecol 36: 922

34. Cassell GH, Cole BC (1981) Mycoplasms as agents of human disease. N Engl J Med 304: 80

35. Cassell GH, Younger JB, Brown MB, et al (1983) Microbiologic study of infertile women at the time of diagnostic laparoscopy. N Engl J Med 308: 502

36. Cavazos F, Lucas FV (1973) Ultrastructure of the endometrium. In: Norris HJ, Hertig AT, Abel MR (ed) International Academy of Pathology Monograph No. 14, The uterus. Baltimore, Williams and Wilkins, pp 136–174

37. Chadha S, Vuzevski VD, ten Kate FJW (1985) Malakoplakia of the endometrium: A rare cause of postmenopausal bleeding. Eur J Obstet Gynecol Reprod Biol 20: 181

38. Charles D (1964) Iatrogenic endometrial patterns. J Clin Pathol 17: 205

39. Chen KTK, Hendricks EJ (1985) Malakoplakia of the female genital tract. Obstet Gynecol 65: 84s

40. Choo YC, Mak KC, Hsu C, Wong TS, Ma HK (1985) Postmenopausal uterine bleeding of nonorganic cause. Obstet Gynecol 66: 225–228

41. Clement PB, Scully RE (1988) Idiopathic postmenopausal decidual reaction of the endometrium. Int J Gynecol Pathol 7: 152–161

42. Clement PB (1993) Tumor-like lesions of the uterine corpus. In: Clement PB, Young RH (eds) Tumors and tumor-like lesions of the uterine corpus and cervix. New York, Churchill Livingstone, pp 139–179

43. Clisham PR, Cedars MI, Greendale G, Fu YS, Gambone J, Judd HL (1992) Long-term transdermal estradiol therapy: Effects on endometrial histology and bleeding patterns. Obstet Gynecol 79: 196–201

44. Cohen I, Rosen DJ, Shapria J, et al (1993) Endometrial changes in postmenopausal women treated with tamoxifen for breast cancer. Br J Obstet Gynaecol 100: 567–570

45. Corley D, Rowe J, Curtis MT, Hogan WM, Noumoff JS, LiVolsi VA (1992) Postmenopausal bleeding from unusual endometrial polyps in women on chronic tamoxifen therapy. Obstet Gynecol 79: 111–116

46. Courpas AS, Morris JD, Woodruff JD (1964) Osteoid tissue in utero. Report of 3 cases. Obstet Gynecol 24: 636

47. Cramer DW, Schiff I, Schoenbaum SC, et al (1985) Tubal infertility and the intrauterine device. N Engl J Med 312: 941–947

48. Crow J, Wilkins M, Howe S, More L, Helliwell P (1991) Mast cells in the female genital tract. Int J Gynecol Pathol 10: 230–237

49. Croxatto HD, Diaz S, Pavez M, Croxatto HB (1984) The endometrium during continuous use of levonorgestrel. In: Zatuchni GI, Goldsmith A, Shelton JD, Sciarra JJ (eds). Long-acting contraceptive delivery systems. Philadelphia, Harper & Row, p 290

50. Cruz-Aquino M, Shenker L, Blaustein A (1967) Pseudosarcoma of the endometrium. Obstet Gynecol 29: 93

51. Cumming DC, Honore LH, Scott JZ, Williams KP (1985) The late luteal phase in infertile women: Comparison of simultaneous endometrial biopsy and progesterone levels. Fertil Steril 43: 715

52. Dal Cin P, Brosens I, Van Den Berghe H (1991) Involvement of 6p in an endometrial polyp. Cancer Genet Cytogenet 51: 279–280

53. Dal Cin P, De Wolf F, Klerckx P, van den Berghe H (1992) The 6p21 chromosome region is nonrandomly involved in endometrial polyps. Gynecol Oncol 46: 393–396

54. Dallenbach-Hellweg G (1981) Histopathology of the endometrium, 3rd ed. New York, Heidelberg, Berlin, Springer-Verlag

55. Dallenbach-Hellweg G (1984) The endometrium in infertility. Pathol Res Pract 178: 527

56. Daly DC, Walters CA, Soto-Albors CE, Riddick DH (1983) Endometrial biopsy during treatment of luteal phase defects is predictive of therapeutic outcome. Fertil Steril 40: 305

57. Dawson-Hughes B (1991) Calcium supplementation and bone loss. A review of controlled clinical trials. Am J Clin Nutrition 54(1):274S-280S

58. Dehner LP, Askin FB (1975) Cytomegalovirus endometritis. Report of a case associated with spontaneous abortion. Obstet Gynecol 45: 211–214

59. Deligdisch L (1993) Effects of hormone therapy on the endometrium. Mod Pathol 6: 94

60. Del Pozo E, Wyss H, Tolis G, Aleaniz J, Campana A, Naftolin F (1979) Prolactin and deficiency luteal function. Obstet Gynecol 53: 282

61. De Muylder X, Neven P, De Somer M, Van Belle Y, Vanderick G, De Muylder E (1991) Endometrial lesions in patients undergoing tamoxifen therapy. Int J Gynecol Obstet 36: 127–130

62. Dinh TV, Slavin RE, Bhagavan BS, Hannigan EV, et al (1989) Mixed mullerian tumors of the uterus: A clinicopathologic study. Obstet Gynecol 74: 388–392

63. Divack DM, Janovski NA (1962) Eosinophilia encountered in female genital organs. Am J Obstet Gynecol 84: 761–763

64. Dockerty MB, Smith RA, Symmonds RE (1950) Pseudomalignant endometrial changes induced by administration of new synthetic progestins. Proc Mayo Clin 34: 321

65. Downs KA, Gibson M (1983) Basal body temperature graph and the luteal phase defect. Fertil Steril 40: 466

66. Dumoulin JG, Hughesdon PE (1951) Chronic endometritis. J Obstet Gynaecol Br Emp 58: 222

67. Duncan DA, Varner RE, Mazur MT (1989) Uterine herpes virus infection with multifocal necrotizing endometritis. Hum Pathol 20: 1021–1024

68. Edwards JA, Gale RF (1972) Camptobrachydactyl: A new autosomal dominant trait with two probably homozygotes. Am J Hum Genet 24: 464

69. Evans RA, Somers NM, Dunstan CR, Royle H, Kos S (1993) The effect of low-dose cyclical etidronate and calcium on bone mass in early postmenopausal women. Osteoporosis Int 3: 71–75

70. Farber ER, Leahy MS, Meadows TR (1968) Endometrial blastomycosis acquired by sexual contact. Obstet Gynecol 32: 195

71. Ferry JA, Harris NL, Scully RE (1989) Uterine leiomyomas with lymphoid infiltration simulating lymphoma. Int J Gynecol Pathol 8: 263–270

72. Fleming H, Ostor AG, Pickel H, Fortune DW (1989) Arteriovenous malformations of the uterus. Obstet Gynecol 73: 209

73. Foxi A, Bruno RO, Davison T, Lema B (1966) The pathology of post-curettage intrauterine adhesions. Am J Obstet Gynecol 96: 1027

74. Fornander T, Rutqvist LE, Cedermark B, et al (1989) Adjuvant tamoxifen in early breast cancer. Occurrence of new primary cancers. Lancet i: 117–120

75. Foss BA, Horne HW, Hertig AT (1958) The endometrium and sterility. Fertil Steril 9: 193

76. Frank TS, Himebaugh KS, Wilson MD (1992) Granulomatous endometritis associated with histologically occult cytomegalovirus in a healthy patient. Am J Surg Pathol 16(7): 716–710

77. Friberg J (1978) Genital mycoplasma infections. Am J Obstet Gynecol 132: 573

78. Friberg J (1980) Mycoplasmas and ureaplasmas in infertility and abortion. Fertil Steril 33: 351

79. Gal D, Kopel S, Bashevkin M, Lebowicz J, Lev R, Tancer M (1991) Oncogenic potential of tamoxifen on endometria of postmenopausal women with breast cancer—preliminary report. Gynecol Oncol 42: 120–123

80. Gambrell RD (1974) Postmenopausal bleeding. J Am Geriatr Soc 22: 337–343

81. Ganem KJ, Parsons L, Friedell GH (1982) Endometrial ossification. Am J Obstet Gynecol 83: 1592

82. Garcia JE, Acosta AA, Hsiu J-G, Jones HW Jr (1984) Advanced endometrial maturation after ovulation induction with human menopausal gonadotropin/human chorionic gonadotropin for in vitro fertilization. Fertil Steril 41: 31–35

83. Gerbie AB, Greene RR, Reis RA (1958) Heteroplastic bone and cartilage in the female genital tract. Obstet Gynecol 11: 573

84. Gilks CB, Taylor GP, Clement PB (1987) Inflammatory pseudotumor of the uterus. Int J Gynecol Pathol 6: 275–286

85. Goldfarb HA (1990) A review of 35 endometrial ablations using the Nd:YAG laser for recurrent menometrorrhagia. Obstet Gynecol 76: 833–836

86. Goldman RL (1970) Herpetic inclusions in the endometrium. Obstet Gynecol 36: 603

87. Gonzalez-Angulo A, Aznar-Ramos R (1976) Ultrastructural studies on the endometrium of women wearing TCu-200 intrauterine devices by means of transmission and scanning electron microscopy and X-ray dispersive analysis. Am J Obstet Gynecol 125: 170

88. Gottardis MM, Robinson SP, Satyaswaroop PG, Jordan VC (1988) Contrasting actions of tamoxifen on endometrial and breast tumor growth in the athymic mouse. Cancer Res 48: 812–815

89. Gray SW, Skandalakis JE (1972) Embryology for surgeons: The embryological basis for the treatment of congenital defects. Philadelphia, WB Saunders Co, pp 633–664

90. Greenwood SM, Moran JJ (1981) Chronic endometritis: Morphologic and clinical observations. Obstet Gynecol 58: 176

91. Gump DW, Gibson M, Ashikaga T (1984) Lack of association between genital mycoplasmas and infertility. N Engl J Med 310: 927

92. Hager WD, Douglas B, Majmudar B, Naib ZM, Williams OJ, Ramsey C, Thomas J (1979) Pelvic colonization with Actinomyces in women using intrauterine contraceptive devices. Am J Obstet Gynecol 135: 680

93. Hart WR, Prins RP, Tsai JC (1976) Isolated coccidioidomycosis of the uterus. Hum Pathol 7: 235

94. Hartman CG, Geschickter GF, Speert H (1941) Effects of continuous estrogen administration in very large doses. Anat Rec [Suppl 2] 79: 31

95. Hendrickson MR, Kempson RL (1980) The approach to endometrial diagnosis: A system of nomenclature. In: Bennington JL (ed) Surgical pathology of the uterine corpus. Philadelphia, London, Toronto, WB Saunders Co, pp. 99–157

96. Henry-Suchet J (1988) Chlamydia trachomatis infection and infertility in women. J Reprod Med 33: 912

97. Hilliard GD, Norris JH (1979) The pathologic effects of

oral contraceptives. In: Lingeman C (ed) Recent results in cancer research. Carcinogenic steroids, vol 66. New York, Springer-Verlag, pp 49–71

98. Ho KH (1979) Sarcoidosis of the uterus. Hum Pathol 20: 219

99. Hohnman WR, Shaw ST Jr, Macaulay L, Moyer DL (1977) Vascular defects in human endometrium caused by intrauterine contraceptive devices. Contraception 16: 507

100. Holmstrom EG, McLennan CE (1947) Memorrhagia associated with irregular shedding of the endometrium. Am J Obstet Gynecol 53: 727

101. Horne HW Jr, Hertig AT, Knudsin RB (1973) Sub-clinical endometrial inflammation and T-mycoplasma. Int J Fertil 18: 226

102. Horta JLH, Fernandez JG, Soto de Leon B, Cortes Gallegos V (1977) Direct evidence of luteal insufficiency in women with habitual abortion. Obstet Gynecol 49: 705

103. Hourihan HM, Sheppard BL, Bonnar J (1989) The morphologic characteristics of menstrual hemostasis in patients with unexplained menorrhagia. Int J Gynecol Pathol 8: 221–229

104. Hsu C (1975) Endometrial ossification. Br J Obstet Gynaecol 82: 836

105. Hunt JE, Wallach EE (1974) Uterine factors in infertility: An overview. Clin Obstet Gynecol 17: 44

106. Israel R, Mishell DR Jr, Labudovich M (1970) Mechanisms of normal and dysfunctional uterine bleeding. Clin Obstet Gynecol 13: 386

107. Israel SL, Roitman HB, Clancy C (1963) Infrequency of unsuspected endometrial tuberculosis. JAMA 183: 63

108. Iwasaka T, Wada T, Kidera Y, Sugimori H (1986) Hormonal status and mycoplasma colonization in the female genital tract. Obstet Gynecol 68: 263

109. Jeppsson S, Mellquist P, Rannevik G (1984) Short-term effects of danazol on endometrial histology. Acta Obstet Gynecol Scand Suppl 123: 41–44

110. Jewelewicz R, Khalaf S, Neuwirth RS, Vande Wiele RL (1976) Obstetric complications after treatment of intrauterine synechiae (Asherman's syndrome). Obstet Gynecol 47: 701

111. Johannisson E, Fournier K, Riotton G (1981) Regeneration of the human endometrium and presence of inflammatory cells following diagnostic curettage. Acta Obstet Gynecol Scand 60: 451–457

112. Jones GS (1972) Luteal phase insufficiency. Clin Obstet Gynecol 16: 255

113. Jones GS (1975) Luteal phase defects. In: Behrman SJ, Kistner RW (eds) Progress in infertility, 2nd ed. Boston, Little, Brown, pp 299–324

114. Jones GS, Aksel S, Wentz AC (1974) Serum progesterone values in the luteal phase defects. Effects of chorionic gonadotropin. Obstet Gynecol 44: 26

115. Jorgensen V, Enevoldsen B (1964) The occurrence of the first menstruation after curettage. Acta Obstet Gynecol Scand 42 [Suppl 6]: 159

116. Judd HL (1978) Endocrinology of polycystic ovarian disease. Clin Obstet Gynecol 21: 99

117. Kahner S, Ferenczy A, Richart RM (1975) Homologous mixed müllerian tumors (carcinosarcoma) confined to endometrial polyps. Am J Obstet Gynecol 121: 278

118. Kaufman RH, Binder GL, Gray PN, et al (1977) Upper genital tract changes associated with exposure in utero to diethylstilbestrol. Am J Obstet Gynecol 128: 51

119. Kawai K, Fukuda K, Tsuchiyama H (1988) Malacoplakia of the endometrium: An unusual case studied by electron microscopy and a review of the literature. Acta Pathol Jpn 38: 531

120. Kelly HW, Miles PA, Buster JE, Scragg WH (1976) Adenocarcinoma of the endometrium in women taking sequential oral contraceptives. Obstet Gynecol 47: 200

121. Kessel E (1989) Pelvic inflammatory disease with intrauterine device use: A reassessment. Fertil Steril 51: 1–11

122. King A, Wellings V, Gardner L, Loke YW (1989) Immunocytochemical characterization of the unusual large granular lymphocytes in human endometrium throughout the menstrual cycle. Hum Immunol 24: 195–205

123. Kiviat NB, Wolner-Hanssen P, Peterson M, et al (1986) Localization of *Chlamydia trachomatis* infection by direct immunofluorescence and culture in pelvic inflammatory disease. Am J Obstet Gynecol 154: 865–873

124. Kiviat NB, Eschenbach DA, Paavonen JA, Critchlow CW, Moore DE (1990) Endometrial histopathology in patients with culture-proved upper genital trace infection and laparoscopically diagnosed acute salpingitis. Am J Surg Pathol 14(2): 167–175

125. Kraus FT (1973) Irradiation changes in the uterus. In: Hertig AT, Norris HJ, Abell MR (eds) International Academy of Pathology Monograph No. 14, The uterus. Baltimore, Williams and Wilkins, pp 457–488

126. Kurman RJ, Scully RE (1976) Clear cell carcinoma of the endometrium. An analysis of 21 cases. Cancer 37: 872–882

127. Laatikainen T, Anderson B, Karkkainen J, et al (1983) Progestin receptor levels in endometria with delayed or incomplete secretory changes. Obstet Gynecol 62: 592

128. Lackner JE, Krohn L (1932) Report of a case of teratoma of the uterus. Am J Obstet Gynecol 25: 735

129. Ladefoged C, Lorentzen M (1988) Xanthogranulomatous inflammation of the female genital tract. Histopathology 13: 541

130. Lahti E, Blanco G, Kauppila A, Apaja-Sarkkinen M, Taskinen PJ, Laatikainen T (1993) Endometrial changes in postmenopausal breast cancer patients receiving tamoxifen. Obstet Gynecol 81: 660–664

131. Ledger WJ (1977) Infection in the female. Philadelphia, Lea and Febiger

132. Lee NC, Rubin GL, Borucki R (1988) The intrauterine device and pelvic inflammatory disease revisited: New results from the Women's Health Study. Obstet Gynecol 72: 1–6

133. Lemay A, Jean C, Faure N (1987) Endometrial histology during intermittent intranasal luteinizing hormone-releasing hormone (LH-RH) agonist sequentially combined with an oral progestogen as an antiovulatory contraceptive approach. Fertil Steril 48(5): 775–782

134. Lenton EA, Landgren B, Sexton L, Harper R (1984) Normal variation in the length of the follicular phase of the menstrual cycle. Effect of chronological age. Br J Obstet Gynecol 91: 681

135. Li T-C, Dockery P, Thomas P, et al (1988) The effects of progesterone receptor blockade in the luteal phase of normal fertile women. Fertil Steril 50: 732–742

136. Lidor A, Ismajovich B, Confino E, David MP (1983) Histopathological findings in 226 women with postmenopausal uterine bleeding. Acta Obstet Gynecol Scand 65: 41–43

137. Lombard CM, Moore MH, Seifer DB (1986) Diagnosis of systemic polyarteritis nodosa following total abdominal hysterectomy and bilateral salpingo-oophorectomy: A case report. Int J Gynecol Pathol 5: 63–68

138. Lyon FA, Frisch MJ (1976) Endometrial abnormalities occurring in young women on long-term sequential oral contraception. Obstet Gynecol 47: 639

139. Maathius JB, Horbach JGM, Hall EV (1972) A comparison of the result of hysterosalpingography and laparoscopy in the diagnosis of fallopian tube dysfunction. Fertil Steril 23: 428

140. Magos AL, Baumann R, Lockwood GM, Turnbull AC (1991) Experience with the first 250 endometrial resections for menorrhagia. Lancet 337: 1074–1078.

141. Marchini M, Fedele L, Bianchi S, et al (1992) Endometrial patterns during therapy with danazol or gestrinone for endometriosis—structural and ultrastructural study. Hum Pathol 23: 51–56

142. Marrogi AJ, Gersell DJ, Kraus FT (1991) Localized asymptomatic giant cell arteritis of the female genital tract. Int J Gynecol Pathol 10: 51–58

143. Martin E, Scholes J, Richart RM, Fenoglio CM (1979) Benign cystic teratoma of the uterus. Am J Obstet Gynecol 135: 429

144. Martinex-Manautou J, Maqueo M, Aznar R, Phariss BB, Zaffaroni A (1975) Endometrial morphology in women exposed to intrauterine systems releasing progesterone. Am J Obstet Gynecol 121: 175

145. Mazur MT (1981) Atypical polypoid adenomyoma of the endometrium. Am J Surg Pathol 5: 473

146. Mazur MT, Kurman RJ. (1994) Diagnosis of endometrial biopsies and curettings: A practical approach. Springer-Verlag, New York

147. McCracken AW, D'Agostino AN, Brucks AB, Kingsly WB (1974) Acquired cytomegalovirus infection presenting as viral endometritis. Am J Clin Pathol 61: 556–560

148. McKelvey JL (1942) Irregular shedding of the endometrium. Lancet 2: 434

149. McLennan CE (1952) Current concepts of prolonged or irregular endometrial shedding. Am J Obstet Gynecol 64: 988

150. Mears E (1965) Handbook on oral contraception. London, Churchill Livingstone

151. Meissner WA, Sommers SC, Sherman G (1957) Endometrial hyperplasia, endometrial carcinoma, and endometriosis produced experimentally by estrogen. Cancer 10: 500

152. Meyer WC, Malkasian KGD, Dockerty MB, Decker DG (1971) Postmenopausal bleeding from atrophic endometrium. Obstet Gynecol 38: 731–738

153. Miko TL, Lampe LG, Thomazy VA, Molnar TP, Endes P (1988) Eosinophilic endomyometritis associated with diagnostic curettage. Int J Gynecol Pathol 7: 162–172

154. Mishell DR Jr, Moyer DL (1969) Association of pelvic inflammatory disease with the intrauterine device. Clin Obstet Gynecol 12: 179

155. Moghissi KS (1975) Endometrium and endosalpinx of women treated with microdose progestogens. J Reprod Med 14: 217

156. Mold JW (1969) Benign solid teratoma of uterus. J Pathol 99: 173

157. Molnar JT, Poliak A (1983) Recurrent endometrial malakoplakia. Am J Clin Pathol 80: 762

158. Monif GRR (1974) Infectious diseases in obstetrics and gynecology. New York, Harper and Row

159. Montgomery R, Youngblood L, Medearis DN (1972) Recovery of cytomegalovirus from the cervix in pregnancy. Pediatrics 49: 524–531

160. Moore DE, Spandoni LR, Foy HH, et al (1982) Increased frequency of serum antibodies to Chlamydia trachomatis in infertility due to distal tubal disease. Lancet 1: 574

161. Moszkowski E, Woodruff JD, Jones GS (1962) The inadequate luteal phase. Am J Obstet Gynecol 83: 363

162. Mouktar M (1966) Functional disorders due to bilharzial infection of the female genital tract. J Obstet Gynecol Br Commonw 73: 307

163. Moyer DL (1975) Endometrial lesions in infertility. In: Behrman SJ, Kistner RW (eds) Progress in infertility, 2nd ed. Boston, Little, Brown, pp 91–115

164. Moyer DL (Personal communication)

165. Moyer DL, Mishell DR Jr (1971) Reactions of human endometrium to the intrauterine foreign body. II. Long-term effects on the endometrial histology and cytology. Am J Obstet Gynecol 111: 66

166. Moyer DL, Mishell DR Jr, Bell J (1970) Reactions of human endometrium to the intrauterine device. I. Correlation of the endometrial histology with the bacterial environment of the uterus following short-term insertion of the IUD. Am J Obstet Gynecol 106: 799

167. Moyer DL, de Lignieres B, Driguez P, Pez JP (1993) Prevention of endometrial hyperplasia by progesterone during long-term estradiol replacement: Influence of bleeding pattern and secretory changes. Fertil Steril 59: 992–997

168. Neven P (1993) Tamoxifen and endometrial lesions. Lancet 342: 452

169. Newton CW III, Abell MR (1973) Iatrogenic fetal implants. Obstet Gynecol 40: 686

170. Niebyl JR, Parmley TH, Spence MR, Woodruff JD (1978) Unilateral ovarian abscess associated with the intrauterine device. Obstet Gynecol 52: 165

171. Nicholson GW (1956) Studies of tumour formation: Polypoid teratoma of the uterus. Guy's Hosp Rep 205: 157

172. Niven PAR, Stansfeld AG (1973) "Glioma" of the uterus: A fetal homograft. Am J Obstet Gynecol 115: 434

173. Nogales-Ortiz F, Taranco I, Nogales FF Jr (1979) The pathology of female genital tuberculosis. A 31-year study of 1436 cases. Obstet Gynecol 53: 422

174. Novak E (1933) Recent advances in the physiology of menstruation. Can menstruation occur without ovulation? JAMA 94: 833

175. Noyes RW, Haman JO (1954) Accuracy of endometrial dating. Fertil Steril 4: 504

176. Ober WB (1966) Synthetic progesten-oestrogen preparations and endometrial morphology. J Clin Pathol 19: 138

177. Ober WB (1977) Effects of oral and intrauterine administration of contraceptives on the uterus. Hum Pathol 8: 513

178. Ober WB, Bronstein SB (1967) Endometrial morphology following oral administration of quinestrol. Int J Fertil 23: 210

179. Ober WB, Sobrero AJ, Kurman R, Gold S (1968) Endometrial morphology and polyethylene intrauterine devices. A study of 200 endometrial biopsies. Obstet Gynecol 32: 782

180. Osborne JL, Bennett MJ (1978) Removal of intraabdominal intrautrine contraceptive devices. Br J Obstet Gynecol 85: 868

181. Osborne NG (1977) The significance of mycoplasma in pelvic infection. J Reprod Med 19: 39

182. Oster G, Salgo MP (1975) The copper intrauterine device and its mode of action. N Engl J Med 293: 432

183. Paavonen J, Aine R, Teisala K, et al (1985) Comparison of endometrial biopsy and peritoneal fluid cytologic testing with laparoscopy in the diagnosis of acute pelfic inflammatory disease. Am J Obstet Gynecol 151: 645

184. Payan H, Daino J, Kish M (1964) Lymphoid follicles in endometrium. Obstet Gynecol 23: 570

185. Perkins MB (1960) Pneumopolycystic endometritis. Am J Obstet Gynecol 80: 332

186. Peterson WF, Novak ER (1956) Endometrial polyps. Obstet Gynecol 8: 40

187. Plaut A (1950) Human infection with *Cryptococcus glabratus*. Report of case involving uterus and fallopian tube. Am J Clin Pathol 20: 377

188. Poppe W, Van Assche FA, Wilms G, Favril A, Baert A (1987) Pregnancy after transcatheter embolization of a uterine arteriovenous malformation. Am J Obstet Gynecol 156: 1179–1180

189. Poropatich C, Rojas M, Silverberg SG (1987) Polymorphonuclear leukocytes in the endometrium during the normal menstrual cycle. Int J Gynecol Pathol 6: 230–234

190. Povey WG (1970) Abnormal uterine bleeding at puberty and climacteric. Clin Obstet Gynecol 13: 474

191. Rao NB (1969) Malacoplakia of broad ligament, inguinal region and endometrium. Arch Pathol 88: 85

192. Reid PC, Thurrell W, Smith JHF, Kennedy A, Sharp F (1992) Nd:YAG laser endometrial ablation: Histological aspects of uterine healing. Int J Gynecol Pathol 11: 174–179

193. Remington JS (1973) Toxoplasmosis. In: Charles D, Finland M (eds) Obstetric and perinatal infections. Philadelphia, Lea and Febiger, pp 27–74

194. Reshef E, Segars JH, Hill GA, et al (1990) Endometrial inadequacy after treatment with human menopausal gonadotropin/human chorionic gonadotropin. Fertil Steril 54: 1012–1016

195. Rioux JE, Cloutier D, Dupont P, Lamonde D (1986) Pregnancy after IUD use. Adv Contracept 2: 185–192

196. Robb JA, Benirschke K, Barmeyer R (1986) Intrauterine latent herpes simplex virus infection: I. Spontaneous abortion. Hum Pathol 17: 1196–1209

197. Roca AN, Guajardo M, Estrada WJ (1980) Glial polyp of the cervix and endometrium. Report of a case and review of the literature. Am J Clin Pathol 73: 718

198. Rock J, Garcia CR, Menkin MF (1959) A theory of menstruation. Ann NY Acad Sci 75: 831

199. Rodriguez M, Okagaki T, Richart RM (1972) Mycotic endometritis due to *Candida*. A case report. Obstet Gynecol 39: 292

200. Rosenfeld DL, Chudow S, Bronson RA (1980) Diagnosis of luteal phase inadequacy. Obstet Gynecol 56: 193

201. Roth E, Taylor HB (1966) Heterotopic cartilage in uterus. Obstet Gynecol 27: 838

202. Rotterdam H (1978) Chronic endometritis: A clinicopathologic study. Pathol Annu 13: 209

203. Rubin SC (1987) Postmenopausal bleeding: Etiology, evaluation, and management. Med Clin North Am 71: 59–69

204. Russack V, Lammers RJ (1990) Xanthogranulomatous endometritis. Arch Pathol Lab Med 114: 929–932

205. Rybo G (1966) Plasminogen activators in the endometrium. Acta Obstet Gynecol Scand 45: 411

205a. Sadler TW (1985) Langman's medical embryology, 5th ed. Baltimore, Williams and Wilkins

206. Salm R (1972) The incidence and significance of early carcinomas in endometrial polyps. J Pathol 108: 47

207. Sandmire HF, Cavanaugh RA (1985) Long-term use of intrauterine contraceptive devices in a private practice. Am J Obstet Gynecol 152: 169–175

208. Saw EC, Smale LE, Einstein H, Huntington RW (1975) Female genital coccidioidomycosis. Obstet Gynecol 45: 199

209. Sayage L, Gunby R, Gonwa T, Husberg B, Goldstein R, Klintmalm G (1990) Cytomegalovirus endometritis after liver transplantation. Transplantation 49: 815–817

210. Schachter J, Banks J, Sung M, et al (1982) Hydrosalpinx as a consequence of chlamydial salpingitis in the guinea pig. In: Mardh PA (ed) Chlamydial infections. Amsterdam, Elsevier, pp 371–374

211. Schenken JR, Tamisica J (1956) *Enterobius vermicularis* (pinworm) infection of the endometrium. Am J Obstet Gynecol 72: 913

212. Schindler AE, Schmidt G (1980) Postmenopausal bleeding: A study of more than 1000 cases. Maturitas 2: 269–274

213. Schneider V, Behm FG, Mumaw VR (1982) Ascending herpetic endometritis. Obstet Gynecol 59: 259

214. Scommegna A, DmowskiWP (1973) Dysfunctional uterine bleeding. Clin Obstet Gynecol 16: 221

215. Sharma V, Whitehead M, Mason B, et al (1990) Influence of superovulation on endometrial and embryonic development. Fertil Steril 53: 822–829

216. Shaw ST, Maucaulay LK, Hohman WR (1979) Vessel density in endometrium of women with and without intrauterine contraceptive devices. A morphometric evaluation. Am J Obstet Gynecol 135: 101

217. Sherman ME, Bitterman P, Rosenshein NB, Delgado G, Kurman RJ (1992) Uterine serous carcinoma. A morphologically diverse neoplasm with unifying clinicopathologic features. Am J Surg Pathol 16: 600–610

218. Shintaku M, Sasaki M, Baba Y (1991) Ceroid-containing histiocytic granuloma of the endometrium. Histopathology 18: 169

219. Shoupe D, Mishell DR Jr, Bopp BL, Fielding M (1991) The significance of bleeding patterns in Norplant implant users. Obstet Gynecol 77: 256

220. Silva EG, Jenkins R (1990) Serous carcinoma in endometrial polyps. Mod Pathol 3: 120–128

221. Silverberg SG, Makowski EL (1975) Endometrial carcinoma in young women taking oral contraceptive agents. Obstet Gynecol 46: 503

222. Silverberg SG, Makowski EL, Roche WD (1977) Endometrial carcinoma in young women under 40 years of age: Comparison of cases in oral contraceptive users and nonusers. Cancer 39: 592

223. Silverberg SG, Major FJ, Blessing JA, et al (1990) Carcino-

sarcoma (malignant mixed mesodermal tumor) of the uterus. A gynecologic oncology group pathologic study of 203 cases. Int J Gynecol Pathol 9: 1–19

224. Sinykin MB, Goodlin RC, Barr MM (1956) Irregular shedding of the endometrium. Am J Obstet Gynecol 71: 990

225. Sobrino LG, Kase N (1970) Endocrinologic aspects of dysfunctional uterine bleeding. Clin Obstet Gynecol 13: 400

226. Soh E, Sato K (1990) Clinical effects of danazol on endometrial hyperplasia in menopausal and postmenopausal women. Cancer 66(5): 983–988

227. Soules MR, Wiebe RH, Aksel S, Hammond CB (1977) The diagnosis and therapy of luteal phase deficiency. Fertil Steril 28: 1033

228. Southam AL, Richart RM (1966) The prognosis for adolescents with menstrual abnormalities. Am J Obstet Gynecol 94: 637

229. Speleman F, Dal Cin P, Van Roy N, et al (1991) Is t(6;20)(p21;q13) a characteristic chromosome change in endometrial polyps? Genes, Chromosomes Cancer 3: 318–319

230. Speroff L, Glass RH, Kase NG (1983) Clinical gynecological endocrinology and infertility, 3rd ed. Baltimore, Williams and Wilkins, pp 467–492

231. Speroff L, Glass RH, Kase NG (1989) Clinical gynecologic endocrinology and infertility, 4th ed. Baltimore, Williams and Wilkins

232. Spirtos NJ, Yurewicz EC, Moghisii KS, et al (1985) Pseudocorpus luteum insufficiency: A study of cytosol progesterone receptors in human endometrium. Obstet Gynecol 65: 535

233. Spitz IM, Bardin CW (1993) Mifepristone (RU 486)—a modulator of progestin and glucocorticoid action. N Engl J Med 329: 404–412

234. Staros EB, Shilkitus WF (1991) Atypical polypoid adenomyoma with carcinomas transformation. A case report. Surg Pathol 4: 157–166

235. Stray-Pedersen B, Lorentzen-Styr A-M (1977) Uterine toxoplasma infections and repeated abortions. Am J Obstet Gynecol 128: 716

236. Sturdee DW, Wade-Evans T, Paterson MEL, Thom M, Studd JW (1978) Relations between bleeding pattern, endometrial histology, and oestrogen treatment in menopausal women. Br Med J 1: 1575–1577

237. Sutherland AM (1958) Tuberculosis of endometrium: A report of 250 cases with results of drug treatment. Obstet Gynecol 11: 527

238. Swahn ML, Bygdeman M, Cekan S, et al (1990) The effect of RU 486 administered during the early luteal phase on bleeding pattern, hormonal parameters and endometrium. Hum Reprod 5: 402–408

239. Tatum JH, Schmidt FH, Jain AK (1976) Management and outcome of pregnancies associated with the Copper T intrauterine contraceptive device. Am J Obstet Gynecol 126: 869–879

240. Tawfik OW, Huet YM, Malathy PV, Johnson DC, Dey SK (1987) Release of prostaglandins and leukotrienes from the rat uterus is an early estrogenic response. Prostaglandins 34: 805–814

241. Tawfik OW, Sagrillo C, Johnson DC, Dey SK (1987) Decidualization in the rat: Role of leukotrienes and prostaglandins. Prostaglandins Leukotrienes Med 29: 221–227

242. Taylor AB (1960) Sarcoidosis of the uterus. J Obstet Gynecol Br Emp 67: 32

243. Taylor RN, Welch KL, Sklar DM, et al (1984) Heterotopic skin in the uterus. A report of an unusual case. J Reprod Med 29: 837

244. Taylor-Robinson D, McCormack WM (1980) The genital mycoplasmas. Part 1. N Engl J Med 302: 1003

245. Taylor-Robinson D, McCormack WM (1980) The genital mycoplasmas. Part 2. N Engl J Med 302: 1063

246. Tesluk H, Munn RJ (1984) Malacoplakia of the uterus (letter). Arch Pathol Lab Med 108: 692

247. Thiery M (1955) Irregular shedding of the endometrium. Gynaecologia (Basel) 139: 1

248. Thomas W Jr, Sadeghieh B, Fresco R, Rubenstone AI, Stepto RC, Carasso B (1978) Malacoplakia of the endometrium, a probable cause of postmenopausal bleeding. Am J Clin Pathol 69: 637

249. Toaff R, Ballas S (1978) Traumatic hypomenorrhea-amenorrhea (Asherman's syndrome). Fertil Steril 30: 379

250. Van Eijkeren MA, Christiaens GCML, Gueze JJ, Haspels AA, Sixma JJ (1991) Morphology of menstrual hemostasis in essential menorrhagia. Lab Invest 64: 284

251. Venkataseshan VS, Woo TH (1985) Diffuse viral papillomatosis (condyloma) of the uterine cavity. Int J Gynecol Pathol 4: 370

252. Villaneuva DL (1992) Malakoplakia of the urogenital tract. The Female Patient, 17: July

253. Voigt LF, Weiss NS, Chu J, Daling JR, McKnight B, VanBelle G (1991) Progestogen supplementation of exogenous oestrogens and risk of endometrial cancer. Lancet 338: 274–277

254. Wallach EE (1972) The uterine factor in infertility. Fertil Steril 23: 138

255. Weicker ML, Kaneb GD, Goodale RH (1940) Primary echinococcal cyst of the uterus. N Engl J Med 223: 574

256. Weiss NS, Sayvetz TA (1980) Incidence of endometrial cancer in relation to the use of oral contraceptives. N Engl J Med 302: 551

257. Wenckelbach GFC, Curry B (1976) Cytomegalovirus infection of the female genital tract. Histologic findings in three cases and review of the literature. Arch Pathol Lab Med 100: 1609–1612

258. Wentz AC (1980) Endometrial biopsy in the evaluation of infertility. Fertil Steril 33: 121

259. Wentz AC (1982) Diagnosing luteal phase inadequacy. Fertil Steril 37: 334

260. Wentz AC, Herbert CM, Maxson WS, Garner CH (1984) Outcome of progesterone treatment of luteal phase inadequacy. Fertil Steril 41: 856

261. Westrom L (1980) Incidence, prevalence and trends of acute pelvic inflammatory disease and its consequences in industrialized countries. Am J Obstet Gynecol 138: 880

262. Whitehead MI, King RJB, McQueen J, Campbell S (1979) Endometrial histology and biochemistry in climacteric women during oestrogen and oestrogen/progestogen therapy. J Roy Soc Med 72: 322–327

263. Willen R, Stendahl U, Willen H, Trope C (1983) Malacoplakia of the cervix and corpus uteri: A light microscopic, electron microscopic, and x-ray microprobe analysis of a case. Int J Gynecol Pathol 2: 201

264. Williams A (1967) Pathology of schistosomiasis of the uterine cervix due to *S. haematobium*. Am J Obstet Gynecol 98: 784

265. Winkler B, Reumann W, Mitao M (1984) Chlamydial endometritis. A histological and immunohistochemical analysis. Am J Surg Pathol 8: 771

266. Winter JD, Faiman C, Reyes FI (1978) Normal and abnormal pubertal development. Clin Obstet Gynecol 21: 67

267. Winter JD, Kohn G, Mellinin WJ, et al (1968) A familial syndrome of renal, genital, and middle ear anomalies. J Pediatr 72: 88

268. Wynn RM (1967) Intrauterine devices: Effects on ultrastructure of human endometrium. Science 156: 1508

269. Wynn RM (1968) Fine structural effects of intrauterine contraceptives on the human endometrium. Fertil Steril 19: 867

270. Yaffe H, Ron M, Polishuk WZ (1978) Amenorrhea, hypomenorrhea, and uterine fibrosis. Am J Obstet Gynecol 130: 599

271. Yokoyama S, Kashima K, Inoue S, Daa T, Nakayama I, Moriuchi A (1993) Biotin-containing intranuclear inclusions in endometrial glands during gestation and puerperium. Am J Clin Pathol 99: 13–17

272. Young RH, Kleinman GM, Scully RE (1981) Glioma of the uterus. Am J Surg Pathol 5: 695

273. Young RH, Harris NL, Scully RE (1985) Lymphoma-like lesions of the lower female genital tract: A report of 16 cases. Int J Gynecol Pathol 4: 289–299

274. Young RH, Treger T, Scully RE (1986) Atypical polypoid adenomyoma of the uterus. A report of 27 cases. Am J Clin Pathol 86: 139

275. Zaman SS, Mazur MT (1993) Endometrial papillary syncytial change. Am J Clin Pathol 99: 741–745

276. Zettergren L (1973) Glial tissue in the uterus. Am J Pathol 171: 419

11

Endometrial Hyperplasia and Related Cellular Changes

Robert J. Kurman, M.D., and Henry J. Norris, M.D.

Endometrial hyperplasia constitutes a heterogeneous group of abnormal proliferations, some of which are precursors of endometrial carcinoma. In the 1970s the role of unopposed estrogenic stimulation in the development of endometrial hyperplasia and carcinoma was firmly established on the basis of case-control studies linking these conditions with exogenous unopposed estrogen replacement therapy.[26,28,54,58,72,81] Subsequently, in the 1980s various types of endometrial metaplasia were described.[33,34] As the pathological features of both of these lesions became further characterized, their behavior and relationship to endometrial carcinoma have become more clearly delineated.

Hyperplasia is a proliferative response to estrogenic stimulation and metaplasia is largely a cytoplasmic alteration. Abnormal proliferation is identified by changes in the glandular architecture as compared with the normal proliferative phase. Nuclear atypia may or may not be superimposed on the abnormal structural patterns. Cytoplasmic alterations (metaplasia) are manifested by eosinophilic, ciliated cell (tubal), squamous, secretory/clear, and mucinous changes. Although these changes may develop in response to various stimuli, estrogenic stimulation is the most common. Thus, the morphologic response of the endometrium to estrogenic stimulation is complex and is reflected by a combination of architectural, nuclear, and cytoplasmic alterations. Although classifications separate hyperplasia and the various metaplasias, both are usually intimately associated and cannot always be separately classified.

Endometrial Hyperplasia

DEFINITIONS AND CLASSIFICATION

Endometrial hyperplasia is defined as a proliferation of glands of irregular size and shape with an increase in the gland/stroma ratio compared with proliferative endometrium. The process is diffuse but does not necessarily involve the entire endometrium.

Endometrial hyperplasia is subdivided into two broad categories, hyperplasia without cytological atypia and hyperplasia with cytological atypia (atypical hyperplasia). These proliferative lesions are classified further into *simple*

Table 11.1. Classification of endometrial hyperplasia

Simple hyperplasia
Complex hyperplasia (adenomatous)
Simple atypical hyperplasia
Complex atypical hyperplasia (adenomatous with atypia)

From World Health Organization.

or *complex* according to the extent of glandular complexity and crowding. Thus, both types of hyperplasia, nonatypical and atypical, are classified further as either simple or complex depending mainly on the degree of glandular crowding.

The rationale for this classification is based on the natural history of the disease as shown in long-term follow-up studies.[5,20,48] Fewer than 2% of hyperplasias without cytological atypia progress to carcinoma, whereas 23% of hyperplasias with cytological atypia (atypical hyperplasia) progress to carcinoma. Increasing degrees of glandular complexity and crowding (architectural abnormalities) appear to increase the likelihood of progression to carcinoma but not to the extent that cytological atypia does. The classification proposed by the International Society of Gynecological Pathologists and the World Health Organization (WHO) (Table 11.1), therefore, takes into account both cytological and architectural abnormalities.[68]

CLINICAL FEATURES

Patients with endometrial hyperplasia typically have abnormal bleeding. Occasionally, the lesion is detected fortuitously by endometrial biopsy performed during the course of an infertility work-up or before the start of hormone replacement therapy in postmenopausal women. Hyperplasia develops as a result of unopposed estrogenic stimulation and consequently most patients with hyperplasia have a history of either persistent anovulation or exogenous unopposed estrogen usage. Although anovulation occurs at menarche and in perimenopausal women, hyperplasia is not usually encountered in young women probably because bleeding in menarchial women is seldom evaluated by an endometrial biopsy. The youngest patient reported with hyperplasia was 16 years old.[50] During the reproductive years, hyperplasia is relatively uncommon, typically occurring in women with polycystic ovarian disease (Stein–Leventhal syndrome). These women are anovulatory, obese, infertile, and exhibit hirsutism. However, not all of these features are present in many women with this disorder. Conversely, women who are obese but who do not have polycystic ovarian disease may have hyperplasia presumably as a result of peripheral conversion of androstenedione to estrogen in adipose tissue. The findings of diabetes mellitus and hypertension described in association with endometrial carcinoma may occur in women with hyperplasia, but often none of these associated disorders is

present. Most hyperplasias that occur in perimenopausal women are associated with anovulation.

Postmenopausal women who develop hyperplasia usually are on unopposed estrogen hormone replacement therapy. In these women, the hyperplasia is almost invariably manifested by abnormal bleeding. Although hyperplasia or carcinoma should always be suspected in a postmenopausal woman with bleeding, atrophy is by far the most common cause of abnormal uterine bleeding in this age group. In one study of postmenopausal women with bleeding, 7% had endometrial cancer, 15% had various types of hyperplasia, and 56% had atrophy.[52] Typically, women with hyperplasia or carcinoma have moderate or heavy vaginal bleeding compared with women with atrophic endometria who present with spotting.

GROSS FINDINGS

Hyperplastic endometrium is not distinctive grossly. In hysterectomy specimens, hyperplasia usually presents a velvety, knobby surface of pale, spongy tissue with vague borders. Diffuse thickening is typical, but focal overgrowth may occur and simulate a polyp. The volume of tissue obtained in curettings is usually increased, but it may be quite variable and less than that obtained during the secretory phase of the normal cycle. A diagnosis of hyperplasia, therefore, depends on the histological pattern and not on the volume of tissue. A small volume of tissue may reflect inadequate sampling.

MICROSCOPIC FINDINGS

Hyperplasia is characterized by an increased gland/stroma ratio and a variety of abnormal architectural patterns. Glands typically vary in size and shape. Dilatation and outpouching of glandular epithelium into the stroma characterize the lesser degrees of architectural abnormalities (Figs. 11.1, 11.2). With increasing degrees of architectural abnormality, glands become complex and branched with irregular outlines and infoldings into the lumens. In addition, with increased proliferation glands become crowded, compressing the intervening stroma, resulting in "back-to-back" glandular crowding (Fig. 11.3).

The most important feature in the evaluation of endometrial hyperplasia is the *presence or absence of nuclear atypia*. Cells of a hyperplasia lacking nuclear atypia contain oval, basally oriented, bland nuclei with smooth, uniform contours resembling those in normal proliferative glands (Fig. 11.4). In contrast, cells with nuclear atypia are stratified and show loss of polarity and an increase in the nuclear/cytoplasmic ratio (Fig. 11.5). The nuclei are enlarged, irregular in size and shape, hyperchromatic with coarse chromatin clumping, a thickened irregular nuclear membrane, and have prominent nucleoli. Nuclei tend to be round as compared with the oval nuclei of proliferative endometrium and hyperplasia without atypia. As a result, the nuclei often have a cleared or vesicular appearance with condensation of the chromatin around the nuclear membrane. Nuclear atypia is variable, both qualitatively and quantitatively. Not all glands contain atypical cells and in an individual gland some cells are atypical and others are not. Rare atypical cells should be ignored but if cellular atypia is evident without a diligent search, the diagnosis of atypical hyperplasia should be made. Grading atypia as mild, moderate, or severe is subjective and not reproducible.

Simple Hyperplasia

In simple hyperplasia the glands are cystically dilated, with occasional outpouchings surrounded by an abundant cellular stroma. In other instances, the glands are only minimally dilated but focally crowded. Admixtures of the various patterns frequently occur (Figs. 11.1, 11.2). The cells lining the glands are pseudostratified and columnar with amphophilic cytoplasm. Mitotic activity is variable.

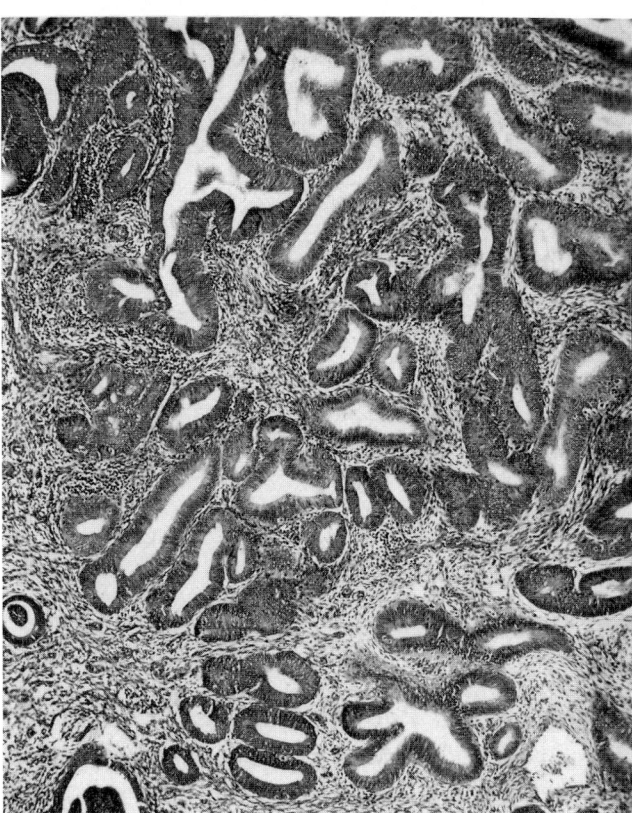

FIG. 11.2. **Simple hyperplasia.** There is slight crowding of glands that are abnormally branched. (Reprinted by permission of Kurman et al., ref. 48.)

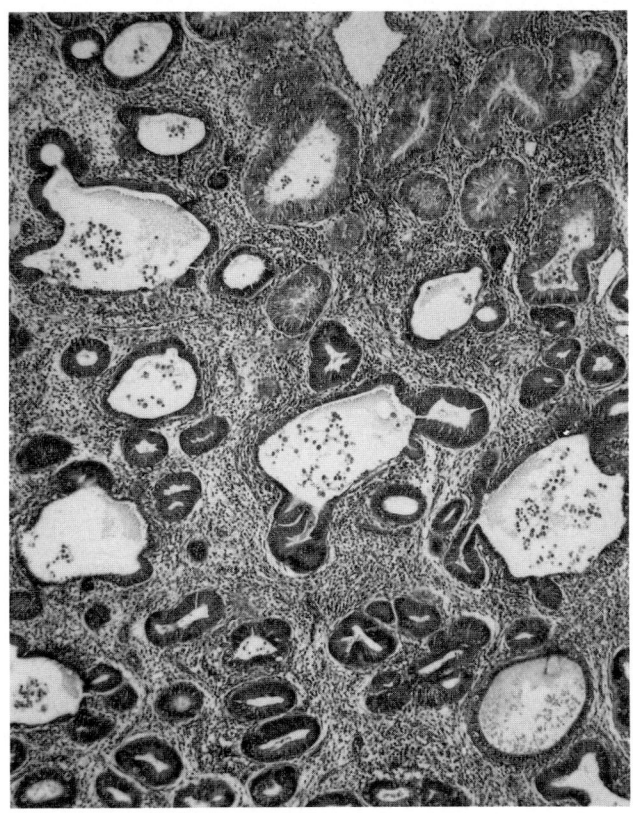

FIG. 11.1. **Simple hyperplasia.** The lesion is characterized by dilated glands with glandular outpouchings. (Reprinted by permission of Kurman et al., ref. 48.)

Complex Hyperplasia

Complex hyperplasia is composed of crowded glands with little intervening stroma[48] (Figs. 11.3, 11.6). Back-to-back glands and papillary intraluminal infoldings are characteristic. Usually the glandular outlines are highly complex but at times are tubular. Epithelial stratification and mitotic activity generally parallel the architectural complexity, but sometimes they are discordant. Epithelial stratification can range from two to four layers, but some glands may exhibit little or no stratification. Mitotic activity is variable and is usually less than 5 mitotic figures per 10 high power fields. Even in highly complex hyperplasia with marked stratification, mitotic figures may be inconspicuous.

Simple Atypical Hyperplasia

The glandular outlines in simple atypical hyperplasia may be relatively simple with minimal complexity or they may be more irregular with intraglandular tufting. They are separated by abundant stroma; back-to-back glands are absent (Fig. 11.7).

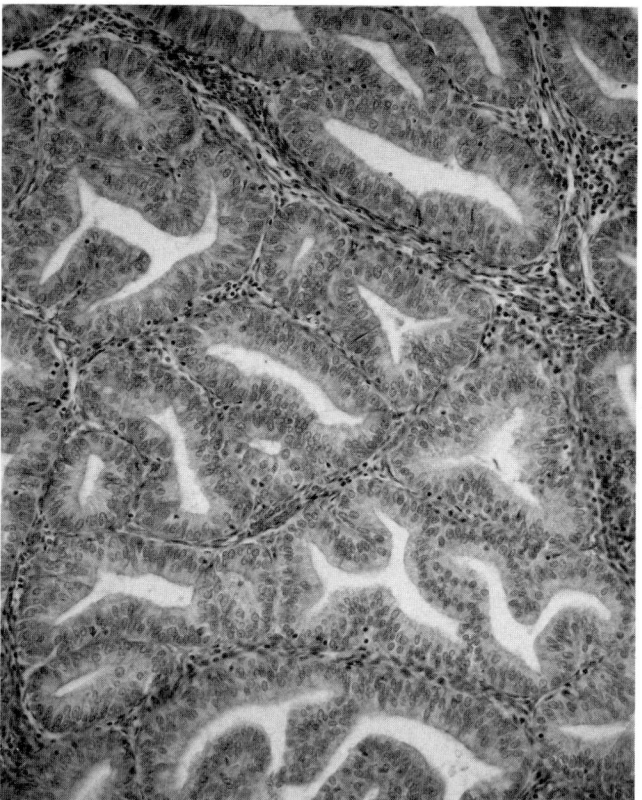

FIG. 11.3. Complex hyperplasia. There is marked glandular crowding resulting in a "back-to-back" appearance.

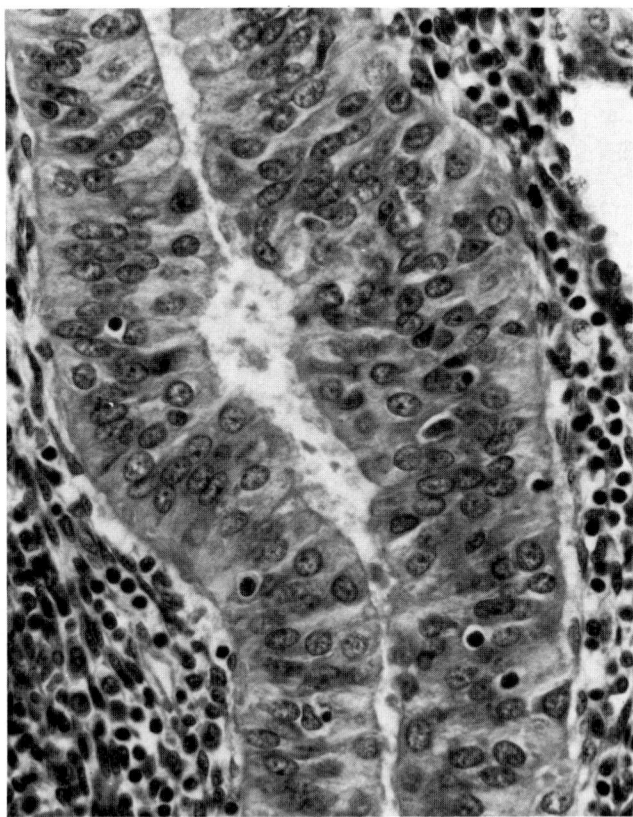

FIG. 11.5. Hyperplasia with atypia. The cells are stratified with loss of polarity. Nuclei are rounded, with granular chromatin and appear vesicular.

Complex Atypical Hyperplasia

In complex atypical hyperplasia the glands almost invariably demonstrate marked structural complexity with irregular outlines and back-to-back crowding (Fig. 11.8). As in hyperplasias without atypia, epithelial stratification and mitotic activity are variable. Papillary infoldings, as in nontypical complex hyperplasia, also are seen. Some atypical hyperplasias may have little stratification and mitotic activity may be inconspicuous.

ENDOMETRIAL STROMA IN HYPERPLASIA

In simple hyperplasia, the stromal cells are more densely packed than in proliferative endometrium. The cells retain their spindle shape but are plump, with enlarged nuclei and indistinct cytoplasm. Mitotic activity in endometrial stromal cells is variable but may be increased. Cytological atypia is rarely observed. In the complex forms of hyperplasia, the stromal cells are spindle-shaped and become compressed by the glandular proliferation. In addition to densely packed stromal cells, clusters of foamy, lipid-laden cells (Fig. 11.9) can occur in the stroma of simple and complex hyperplasia and in approximately one-quarter of

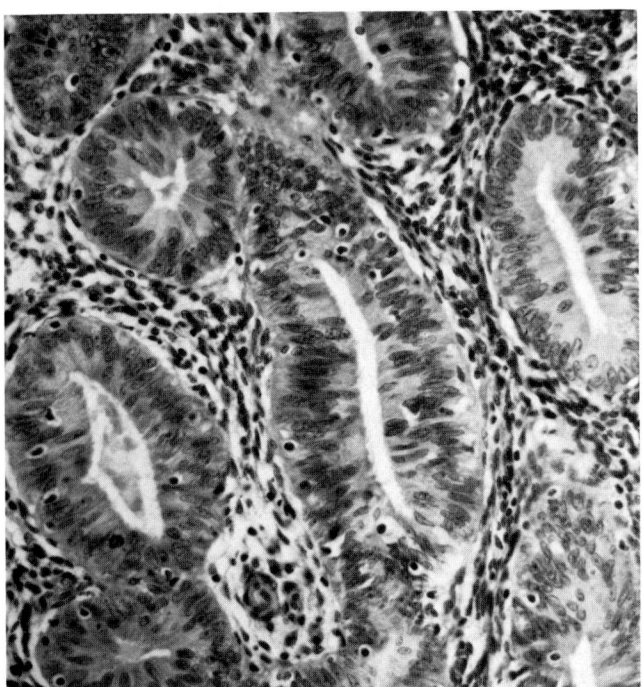

FIG. 11.4. Hyperplasia without atypia. The cells contain nuclei that are cigar-shaped and resemble those in proliferative endometrium.

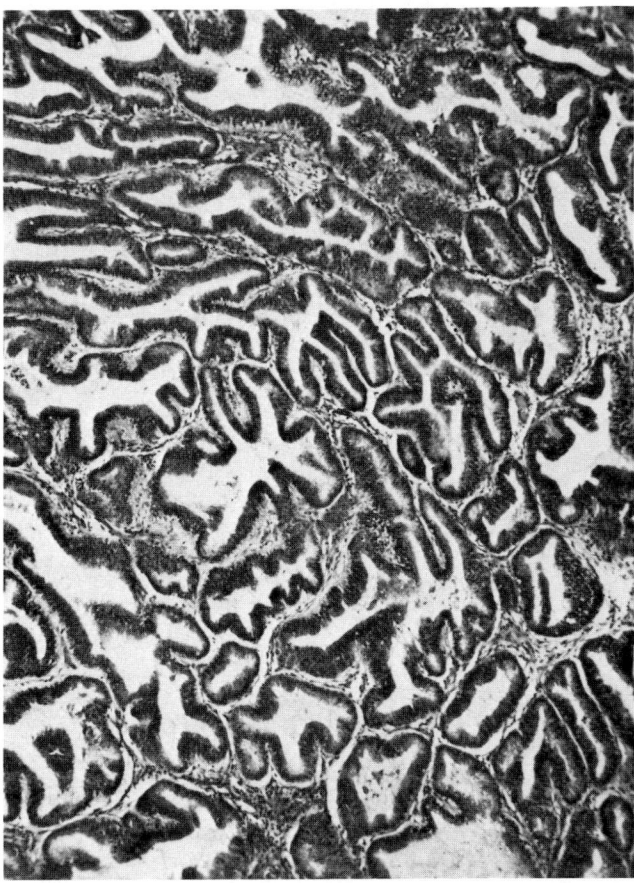

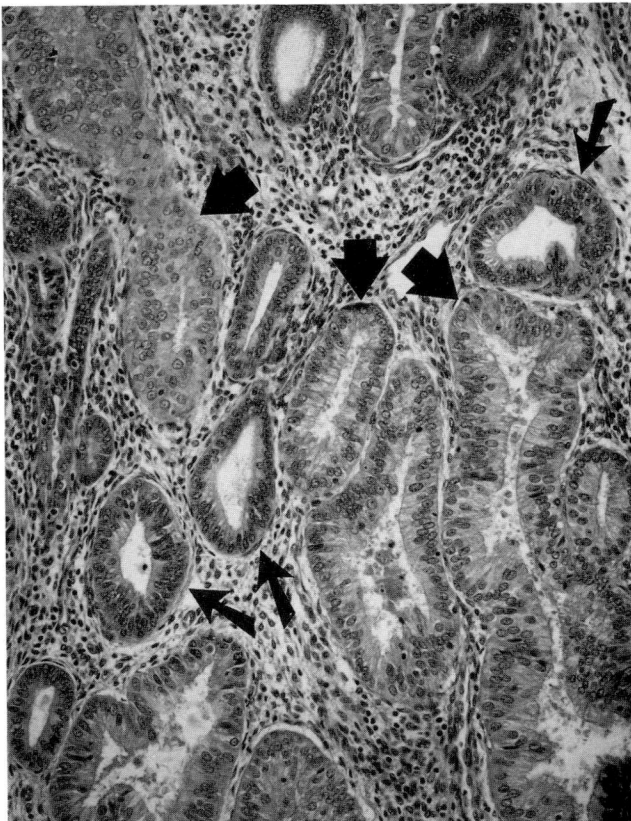

Fig. 11.6. Complex hyperplasia. The lesion is characterized by glands with complex glandular outlines that are markedly crowded. There is no cytologic atypia. (Reprinted by permission of Kurman et al., ref. 48.)

Fig. 11.7. Simple atypical hyperplasia. The glands are lined by atypical cells (*broad arrows*) that are separated by fairly abundant endometrial stroma from glands with no cytologic atypia (narrow arrows). (Reprinted by permission of Kurman et al., ref. 48.)

atypical hyperplasias and well-differentiated adenocarcinomas.[13,14,66] Foam cells have small pyknotic nuclei and cytoplasm that contains lipid droplets but no mucin. The foam cells are altered endometrial stromal cells.[15] Although foam cells may also be observed in atrophic non-neoplastic endometria, their frequent association with hyperplasia or carcinoma serves to warn of these lesions when identified in curettings.

DIFFERENTIAL DIAGNOSIS

Simple and complex hyperplasia must be distinguished from disordered proliferative phase, polyps, ciliated cell change (tubal metaplasia), cystic atrophy, and endometrial glandular and stromal breakdown. *Disordered proliferative phase* is similar qualitatively to simple hyperplasia but is a focal lesion (Fig. 11.10). Disordered proliferative phase is characterized by irregularly shaped and enlarged glands that are focally interspersed among normal proliferative glands. The latter may be focally crowded. The key feature that distinguishes disordered proliferative phase from simple hyperplasia is the focal nature of the glandular abnormality in disordered proliferative phase. The fragments of endometrium containing the disordered glands should not have the appearance of a polyp.

Hyperplastic endometrial polyps often contain areas of simple and complex hyperplasia that are confined to one or just a few fragments of polypoid tissue. The polyp usually stands out as a large rounded tissue fragment in sharp contrast to the remainder of the uninvolved endometrium. Polyps typically have dense fibrous stroma and contain clusters of thick-walled blood vessels near the center of the fragment. The fragments usually are covered on three sides by surface endometrium (see Chapter 10, Benign Diseases of the Endometrium).

Endometrial glands with ciliated cell change are often found in association with simple and complex hyperplasia. When found with hyperplasia the presence of ciliated cell change does not need to be specified. Ciliated glands are usually slightly dilated. When a few isolated glands show ciliated cell change in the absence of hyperplasia, a diagnosis of *ciliated cell change* (tubal metaplasia) is justified (see below).

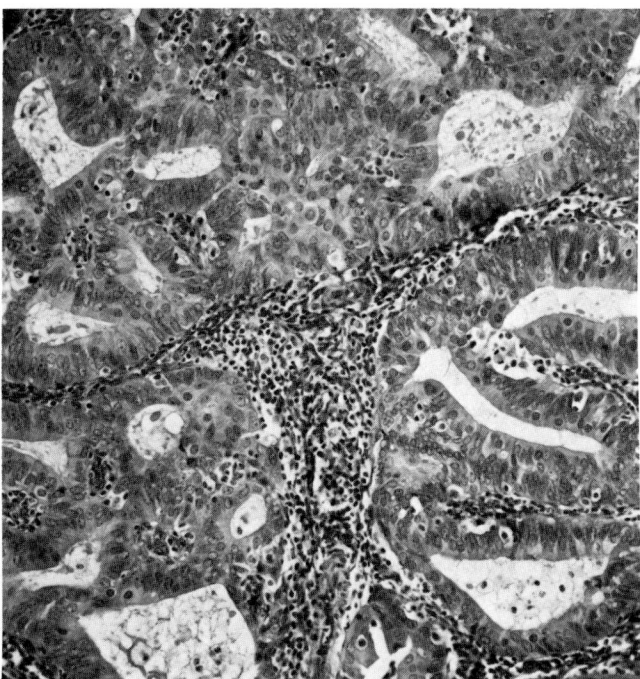

FIG. 11.8. **Complex atypical hyperplasia.** The lesion is characterized by glands with a complex pattern. The cells lining the glands show cytologic atypia.

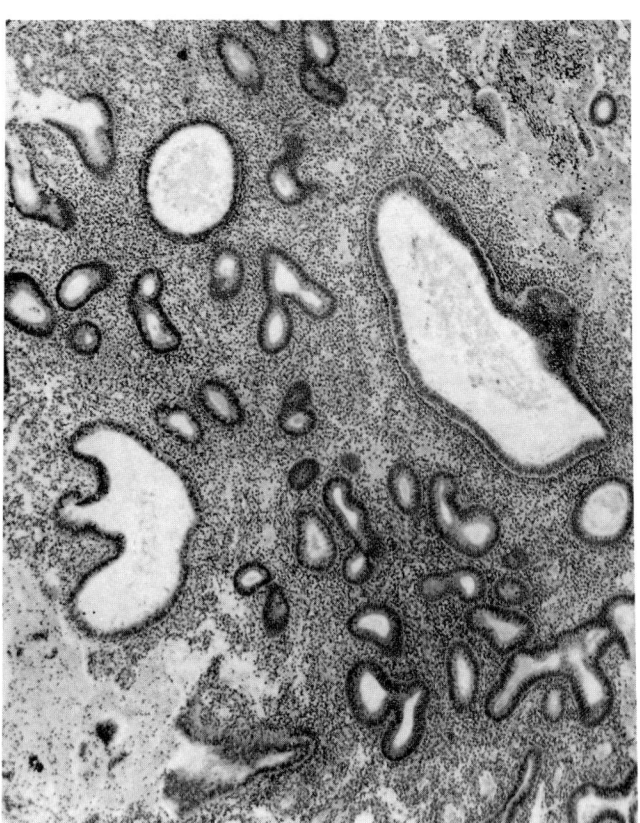

FIG. 11.10. **Disordered proliferative phase.** The lesion is characterized by occasional cystically dilated glands with outpouchings intermixed with normal proliferative endometrial glands.

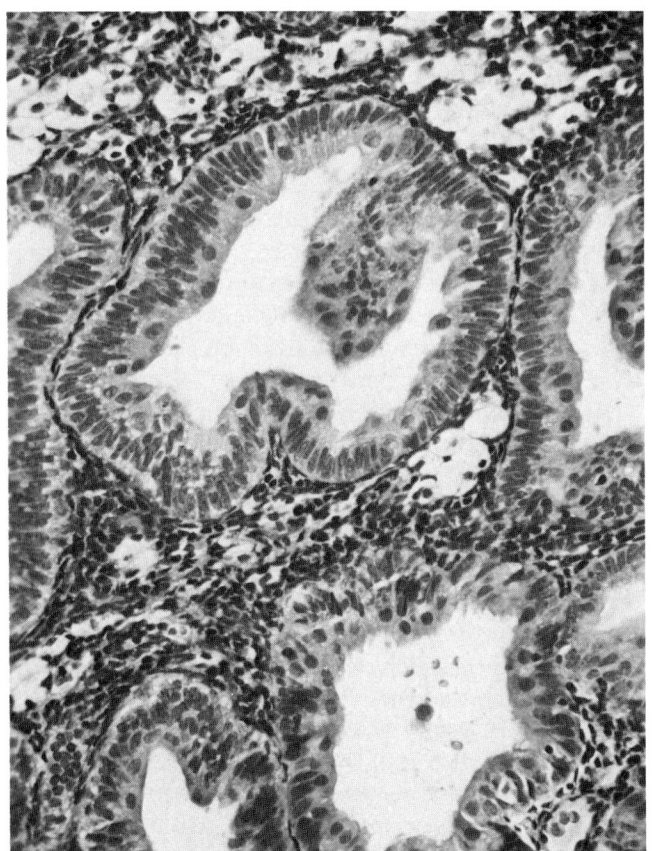

FIG. 11.9. **Complex hyperplasia.** There are clusters of foamy, lipid-laden stromal cells present.

Distinction of cystic atrophy from simple hyperplasia is seldom a problem in curettings because cystically atrophic glands collapse during the procedure because of a paucity of intervening stroma. In hysterectomy specimens, glands are not collapsed but are dilated and lined by a single layer of cells that are often flattened. Mitotic activity is not present. In contrast, in simple hyperplasia there is pseudostratification of columnar epithelial cells. Mitotic activity is variable but present in hyperplasia.

In endometrial glandular and stromal breakdown caused by estrogen withdrawal, proliferative-type glands appear back to back because of loss of intervening endometrial stroma. Glands are often fragmented and nuclear dust typically is present in the cytoplasm. Clusters of stromal cells and fragmented glands surrounded by blood are consistent features (see Chapter 10, Benign Diseases of the Endometrium). In contrast, in complex hyperplasia the glandular outlines are more irregular and complex than the tubular, proliferative-type glands in endometrial glandular and stromal breakdown. Furthermore, glandular fragmentation, nuclear dust, and clusters of stromal cells are usually absent in hyperplasia.

Simple atypical hyperplasia must be distinguished from an atypical polypoid adenomyoma and complex atypical hyperplasia must be distinguished from well-differentiated adenocarcinoma. In contrast to simple atypical hyperplasia, the atypical polypoid adenomyoma is composed of glands that show only a slight degree of architectural complexity. Squamous differentiation in the form of squamous morules is an almost constant feature of the atypical polypoid adenomyoma. Characteristically, the glands in the atypical polypoid adenomyoma are surrounded by smooth muscle in contrast with the dense proliferative stroma found in hyperplasia and the altered or desmoplastic stroma found in association with well-differentiated carcinoma (Fig. 11.11).

Endometrial Stromal Invasion in the Distinction of Atypical Hyperplasia from Well-differentiated Carcinoma

Most endometrial carcinomas are readily identified, but it may be difficult to distinguish some well-differentiated carcinomas from atypical hyperplasia. The two conditions can be separated if specific criteria are used to reduce the subjectivity of the appraisal. The stroma interacts with invasive carcinoma,[39,53] and the morphologic changes it undergoes can serve as a means of identifying carcinoma. The stromal and epithelial alterations associated with invasive carcinoma are referred to collectively as *endometrial*

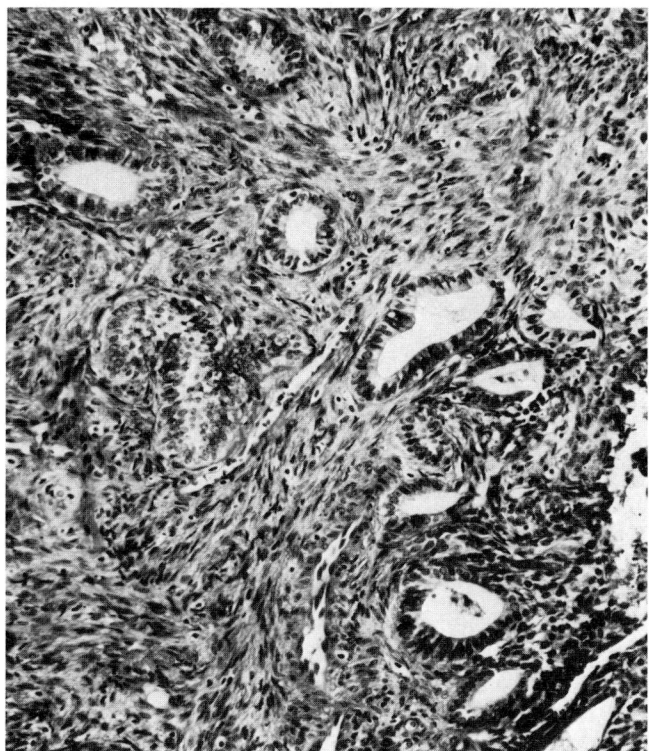

FIG. 11.11. Atypical adenomyomatous polyp. The stroma is composed of smooth muscle and myofibroblasts in bundles and fascicles simulating the desmoplastic response in invasive carcinoma. The glands show minimal atypia and complexity.

stromal invasion. There are three useful criteria, any of which identifies stromal invasion: (1) an irregular infiltration of glands associated with an altered fibroblastic stroma (desmoplastic response), (2) a confluent glandular pattern in which individual glands, uninterrupted by stroma, merge at times creating a cribriform pattern, and (3) an extensive papillary pattern. A process manifesting the features of invasion must be sufficiently extensive to involve half (2.1 mm) of a low-power field 4.2 mm in diameter, to have value in predicting the presence of a biologically significant carcinoma in the uterus.[47,49,59] This criterion, however, should not be applied too rigidly in view of the potential of missing a carcinoma in small samples. If unequivocal evidence of stromal invasion is present in an area measuring somewhat less than one-half a low-power field, a diagnosis of well-differentiated carcinoma should be made. The quantification criterion does not apply to moderately or poorly differentiated carcinomas.

The three criteria for the identification of stromal invasion are described in greater detail below:

1. The altered stroma that reflects invasion contains parallel, densely arranged fibroblasts with more fibrosis than normal endometrial stroma and disrupts the usual glandular pattern (Fig. 11.12). The stromal cells are more spindle-shaped than are the stromal cells of proliferative endometrium, with more elongated nuclei. Collagen compresses the stromal cells so that they have an eosinophilic and wavy appearance (Fig. 11.13), compared with the basophilic naked-nucleus appearance of stromal cells found in proliferative endometrium and hyperplasia (Figs. 11.14, 11.15). In some curettings, fragments of fibrous, relatively glandular polyps or stroma from the lower segment of the uterus may be similar and obscure a diagnosis of carcinoma. Atypical adenomyomatous polyps[56] (see Chapter 10, Benign Diseases of Endometrium) contain smooth muscle and may simulate myometrial invasion (Fig. 11.11). In contrast with the atypical polypoid adenomyoma, smooth muscle is rarely identified in curettings of well-differentiated carcinoma even when there is deep myometrial invasion because only the exophytic portion of the tumor is removed in biopsies and curettings.

2. Confluent glandular aggregates without intervening stroma reflect stromal invasion (Fig. 11.16). Confluent patterns are characterized by glandular configurations in which individual glands are not surrounded by stroma. Instead, glands appear to merge into one another to form a complex labyrinth. Some proliferations are cribriform, resulting from proliferation and bridging of epithelium (Fig. 11.17).

3. Complex papillary patterns represent stromal invasion if multiple, branching, thin fibrous processes lined by epithelium are present (Fig. 11.18). At times these may create a villoglandular pattern. Epithelial papillations lacking a fibrovascular core do not qualify as a feature of invasion.

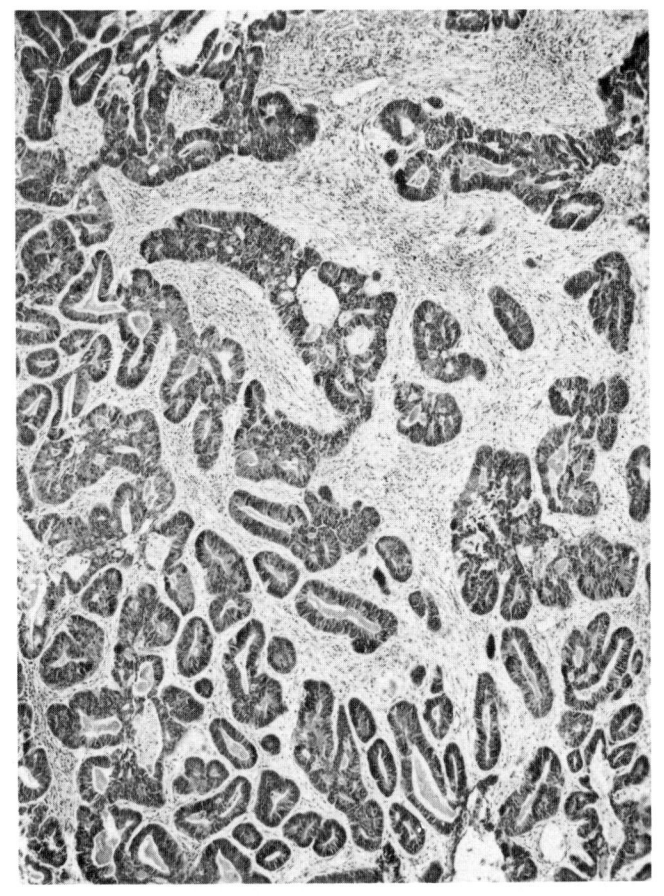

11.12

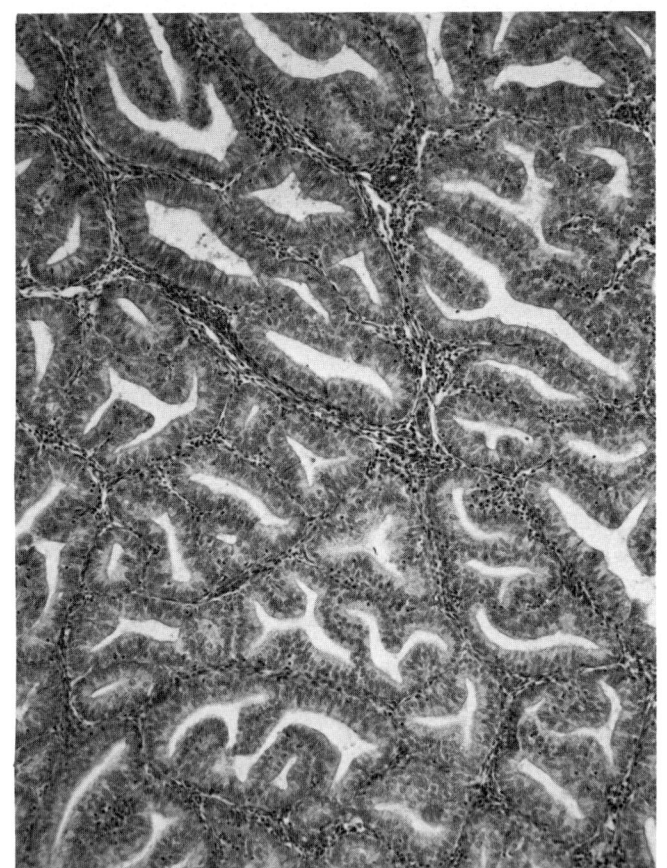

11.14

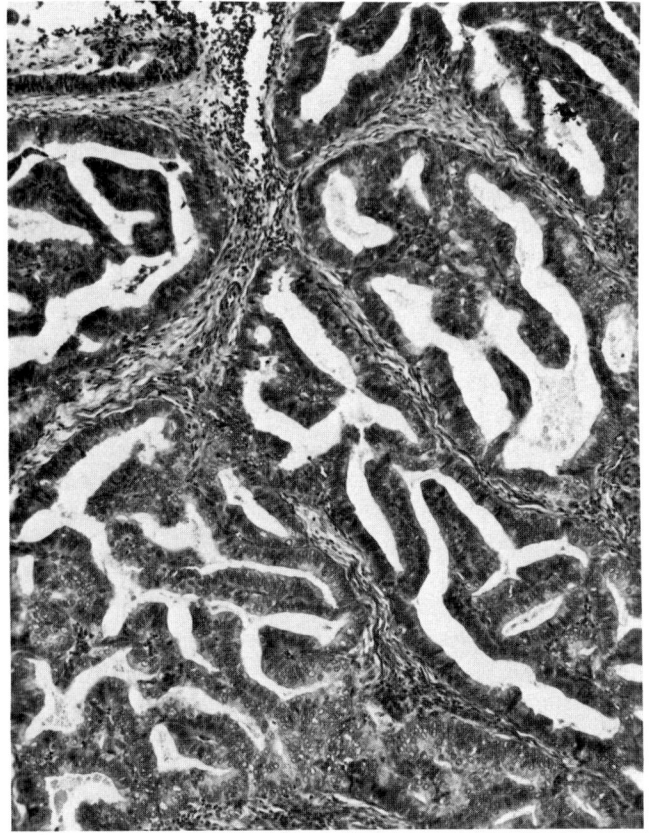

11.13

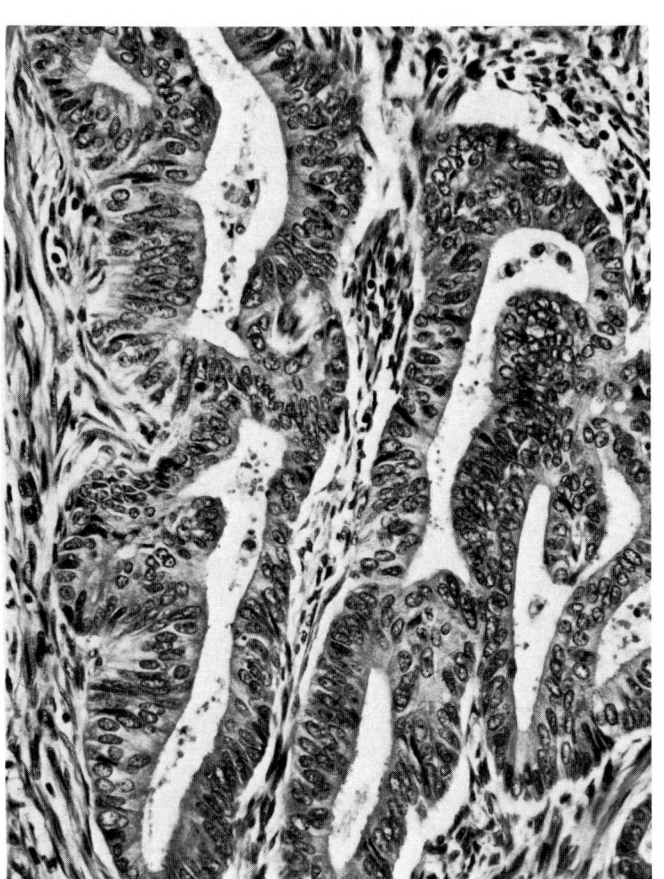

11.15

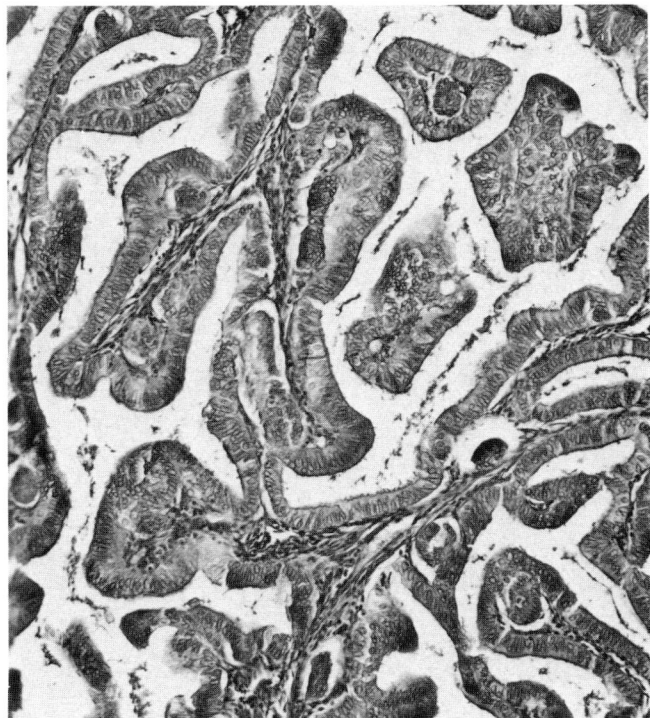

Fig. 11.16. **Well-differentiated carcinoma.** Stromal invasion is manifested by a confluent glandular pattern in which glandular epithelium interconnects one gland with another.

In the past, the presence of masses of squamous epithelium replacing the endometrial stroma was considered a feature of invasion.[47] Masses of squamous epithelium with minimal nuclear atypia that extensively replace the endometrium (over a 2-mm² area) reflect stromal invasion only if they are associated with a desmoplastic response (Fig. 11.19) or a confluent glandular pattern (Fig. 11.20).

Increasing degrees of nuclear atypia, mitotic activity, and stratification of cells in curettings are associated with a higher frequency of carcinoma in the uterus but are of limited value because even a mild degree of these changes is associated with carcinoma in nearly one-third of cases.[47] Even with mild atypia, low mitotic activity, and lesser de-

⬁ ———————————————————

Fig. **11.12. Well-differentiated carcinoma.** An altered stroma (desmoplastic stromal response) results in a haphazard glandular pattern.

Fig. **11.13. Well-differentiated carcinoma.** The altered stroma contains parallel fibroblasts that produce collagen and have an eosinophilic, wavy appearance.

Fig. **11.14. Atypical hyperplasia.** There is marked glandular crowding resulting in compression of the endometrial stroma. The stromal cells are spindle-shaped.

Fig. **11.15. Atypical hyperplasia.** The endometrial stromal cells are spindle-shaped with scant cytoplasm similar to that found in proliferative endometrium.

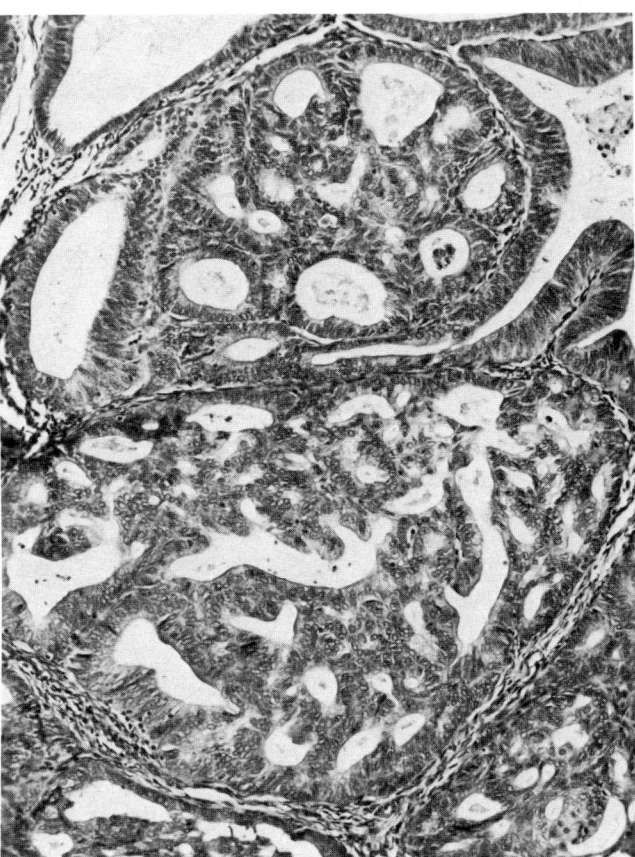

Fig. 11.17. **Well-differentiated carcinoma.** A confluent glandular pattern of stromal invasion creating a cribriform arrangement. (Reprinted by permission of Kurman and Norris, ref. 47.)

grees of stratification in curettings, 20% of residual carcinomas in the resected uterus are moderately or poorly differentiated, and 10% deeply invade the myometrium. These other features in curettings, although useful, therefore are not sufficiently accurate to predict whether a biologically significant lesion is present in the uterus. Unfortunately, assessing varying degrees of nuclear atypia in this borderline group of lesions is subjective and not easily reproduced. In contrast, when stromal invasion is absent in curettings, carcinoma is found in the uterus in only 17% of cases, and all the carcinomas are well differentiated and either confined to the endometrium or only superficially invasive (Table 11.2). If stromal invasion is present in curettings, residual carcinoma is found in the uterus in half; more than one-third of the carcinomas are moderately or poorly differentiated, and a fourth of them invade deeply into the myometrium (Table 11.3). A small proportion (7%) of patients with invasion in curettings will have extrauterine metastases at hysterectomy, and half with metastasis will die of tumor.[47] Thus, the absence of stromal invasion provides the basis for distinguishing atypical hyperplasia from a biologically significant, well-differentiated carcinoma.[43,47,49] The identification of stromal invasion in

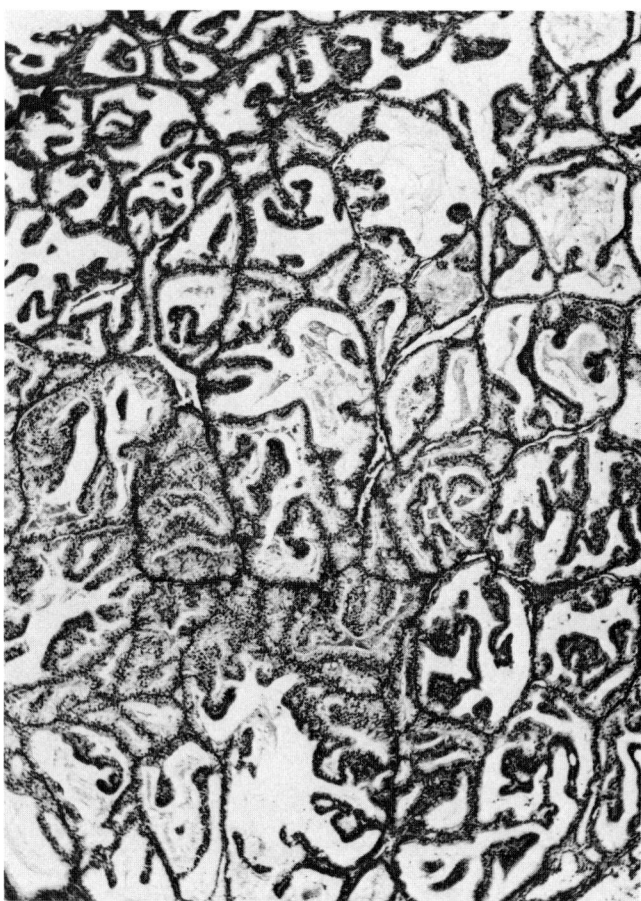

Fig. 11.18. Well-differentiated carcinoma. The complex papillary pattern is extensive enough to indicate stromal invasion.

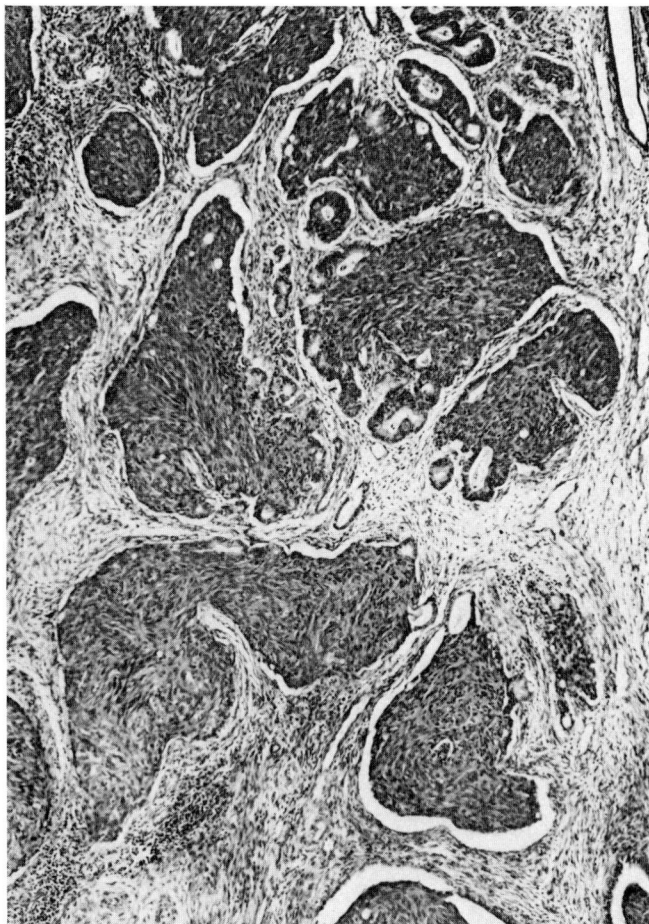

Fig. 11.19. Well-differentiated carcinoma with squamous differentiation (squamous metaplasia). The squamous cells expand out of gland lumens into the surrounding stroma. The diagnosis of stromal invasion is based on the desmoplastic reaction in the stroma.

curettings has two advantages: (1) it is semiquantitative and, therefore, less subjective than other criteria, and (2) it delineates a biologically significant lesion—one having a much greater likelihood of metastasis than one in which invasion is absent.

Experimental studies of neoplasms from the breast, colon, pancreas, and lung lend support to the division of endometrial proliferations into noninvasive and invasive forms based on the histological alterations observed in the endometrial stroma. These studies demonstrate profound molecular and structural alterations in the stroma adjacent to invasive as compared with noninvasive tumors.[39,53,67,69] Invasive tumors can induce a conversion of stromal fibroblasts into myofibroblasts, which elaborate extracellular matrix components, such as type V collagen and proteoglycans, that are increased in desmoplasia and are readily observed by light microscopy using the criteria for stromal invasion as outlined. It has been shown that tumor cells produce growth factors such as platelet-derived growth factor,[65] epidermal-derived growth factor, and insulin-like growth factor,[51] which may play a role in stimulating the growth of stromal cells surrounding tumors.[35]

ELECTRON MICROSCOPY

Scanning and transmission electron microscopic studies[17,18,44,63] reveal that the nonatypical forms of hyperplasia have an increase in the number of estrogen-related organelles in the glandular epithelial cells. These include cilia and microvilli and an increase in free ribosomes, rough endoplasmic reticulum, and complexes of glycogen, Golgi, and mitochondria. Lipid bodies and microfilaments are also increased. These are nonspecific features; ultrastructural analysis does not permit distinction between the cells of nonatypical hyperplasia (Fig. 11.21) and those of normal proliferative endometrium. In hyperplasia with cytological atypia, the changes approach those in carcinoma and estrogen-related features diminish. Cilia and surface microvilli are less frequent, and the mitochondria and rough endoplasmic reticulum are increased and show greater variation. Microfilaments are arranged in a more haphazard fashion than in nonatypical hyperplasia. These

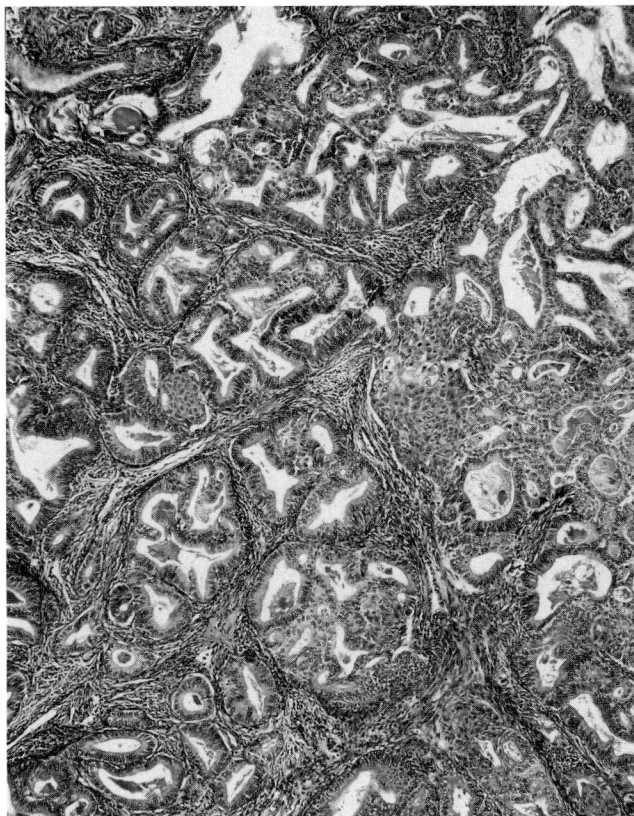

Fig. 11.20. Well-differentiated carcinoma with squamous differentiation. The diagnosis of carcinoma is based on the confluent glandular pattern and altered stroma (desmoplastic response).

bizarre epithelial alterations may closely approach well-differentiated adenocarcinoma but are not so marked (Fig. 11.22). Atypical hyperplasia appears to comprise a heterogeneous population of cells, ranging from those that are indistinguishable from normal proliferative endometrium to those that exist in well-differentiated adenocarcinoma. Estrogen-related characteristics are reduced in carcinoma. Unfortunately electron microscopy, with its limited sample size, does not aid in the distinction between atypical hyperplasia and well-differentiated adenocarcinoma.[16]

QUANTITATIVE MICROSCOPY

Morphometric techniques help distinguish atypical hyperplasia from well-differentiated adenocarcinoma with an accuracy of 95% or better.[1–4,10,22,60] Stereological features in particular are helpful in distinguishing atypical hyperplasia from well-differentiated carcinoma. Glandular size, irregularity of gland lumens, and volume percent of glands and stroma are used to discriminate well-differentiated carcinoma from atypical hyperplasia.[4] Cell count and ploidy, as well as key descriptors of nuclear features such as

Table 11.2. Hysterectomy findings when atypical hyperplasia[a] is present in curettings (89 patients)

Finding	No. (%)
Carcinoma	15 (17)
Grade	
Well differentiated	15 (100)
Moderately differentiated	0
Poorly differentiated	0
Myometrial invasion	
None	8 (53)[b]
Inner one-third	7 (47)[b]
1 mm or less	5
2–4 mm	2

[a] A diagnosis of atypical hyperplasia based on cytological atypia in the absence of endometrial stromal invasion.
[b] The percentages refer to the proportion of carcinomas in the hysterectomy specimen.
Adapted with permission from Kurman and Norris, ref. 47.

Table 11.3. Hysterectomy findings when well-differentiated carcinoma[a] is present in curettings (115 patients)

Finding	No. (%)
Carcinoma	58 (50)
Grade	
Well differentiated	38 (66)[b]
Moderately differentiated	14 (24)[b]
Poorly differentiated	6 (10)[b]
Myometrial invasion	42 (72)[b]
Inner-one-third	28 (48)[b]
Middle and outer third	14 (24)[b]

[a] A diagnosis of well-differentiated carcinoma based on identification of endometrial stromal invasion.
[b] The percentages refer to the proportion of carcinomas in the hysterectomy specimen.
Adapted with permission from Kurman and Norris, ref. 47.

nuclear size, nuclear area, coefficient of nuclear area, and measurements of spherulocity are also helpful.[1,22,60] Morphometric techniques have also been used to assess risk of progression of atypical hyperplasia to carcinoma. At present these have not proved to be more useful as compared with conventional microscopic analysis.[5]

FLOW CYTOMETRY AND IN VITRO HISTOAUTORADIOGRAPHY

Aneuploidy is a feature of malignant cells, with the exception of some carcinomas of endocrine organs.[38,62] Microspectrophotometric studies demonstrate an aneuploid DNA distribution in some atypical hyperplasia,[42,78] although a significant number of well-differentiated endo-

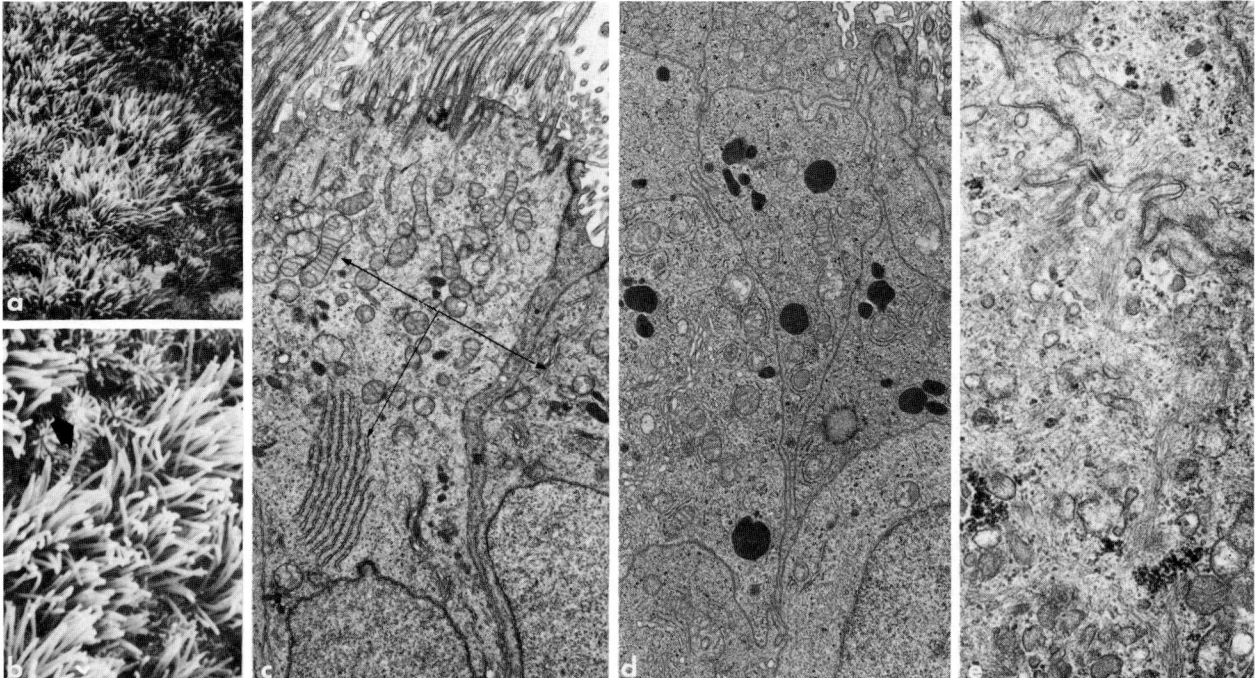

11.21

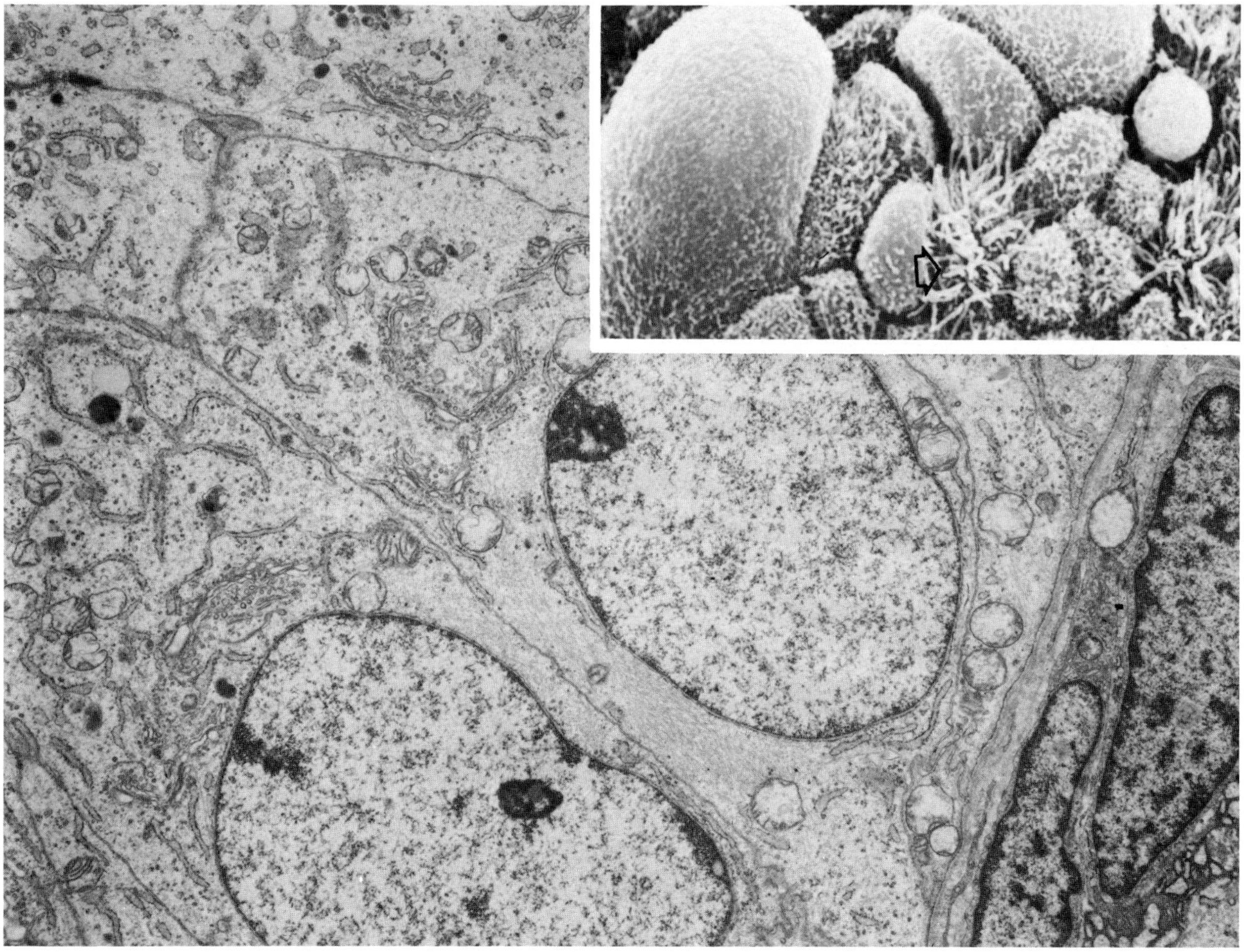

11.22

metrial carcinomas may be diploid or peridiploid.[38,42] Thus, some hyperplasias with a potential to progress cannot be identified or predicted from cell measurements or DNA content.

In vitro DNA labeling with [³H]thymidine or [¹⁴C]thymidine shows atypical hyperplasia to have a prolonged DNA synthesis (S-1 phase) coupled with a shorter cell doubling time, as in carcinoma.[17–19] In this respect, the extreme forms of atypical hyperplasia are similar to those of invasive carcinoma. These techniques may be useful in predicting the likelihood of progression of atypical hyperplasia to carcinoma.

IMMUNOHISTOCHEMISTRY AND MOLECULAR BIOLOGY

Although a variety of antigens have been identified in hyperplastic endometrium, none have been shown to play a significant role in predicting the prognosis of hyperplasia or assisting in the differential diagnosis of atypical hyperplasia versus well differentiated carcinoma (see Chapter 12, Endometrial Carcinoma, and Chapter 26, Immunohistochemistry). Similarly, molecular biologic techniques have not yet proved to be useful in the diagnosis of endometrial hyperplasia or in predicting prognosis (see Chapter 28, Molecular Biology).

BEHAVIOR

It has been noted[79] that most older studies[7–9,30–32,36,37,57,61] including those designed to determine the fate of untreated hyperplasia did not consider cytological and architectural abnormalities separately. This shortcoming was avoided in a retrospective analysis of 170 patients with endometrial hyperplasia in curettings who were followed (mean 13.4 years) without a hysterectomy being performed for at least 1 year.[48] Various histological features were evaluated, and cytological and architectural abnormalities were analyzed independently in an effort to delineate the histological features associated with an increased

risk of progression to carcinoma. A third of the patients with both nonatypical and atypical hyperplasia were asymptomatic after the diagnostic curettage and required no further treatment. Only 2 (2%) of 122 patients with hyperplasia lacking cytological atypia, one with simple and one with complex hyperplasia (Tables 11.4, 11.5), progressed to carcinoma. The two cases of hyperplasia that progressed underwent an alteration to atypical hyperplasia before developing into carcinoma. In contrast, 11 (23%) of the 48 women with atypical hyperplasia progressed to carcinoma ($p = 0.001$) (Table 11.6). Eight percent of patients with simple atypical hyperplasia and 29% of patients with complex atypical hyperplasia progressed to carcinoma (Table 11.7). The presence of glandular complexity and crowding superimposed on atypia, therefore, appears to place the patient at greater risk than does cytological atypia alone. The differences in progression to carcinoma among the four subgroups, however, were not statistically significant. Thus, cytological atypia is the most useful feature in identifying a lesion that might progress to carcinoma. Similar findings have been reported by other investigators.[5,20]

The carcinomas that develop in patients with hyperplasia are relatively innocuous.[31,48] The mean duration of progression of hyperplasia without atypia to carcinoma is nearly 10 years, and it takes a mean of 4 years to progress from atypical hyperplasia to clinically evident carcinoma.[48]

FIG. 11.21. Electron microscopy of hyperplasia without atypia. *a:* Scanning electron microscopy demonstrating abundance of ciliated cells. ×950. *b:* Nonciliated cells are covered by prominent microvillus promontories. ×2850. *c:* A well-developed mitochondria–glandular endoplasmic reticulum–Golgi complex (*arrow*) in gland-lining cells. ×45,600. (Adapted and reprinted by permission of Ferenczy, Ref. 17.)

FIG. 11.22. Electron microscopy of atypical hyperplasia. Note the well-developed Golgi and pleomorphic disposition of microfilaments. Free ribosomes are sparse. ×9300. *Inset:* Scanning electron microscopy showing that ciliated cells (*arrow*) are few and nonciliated cells are pleomorphic with short and sparse microvilli. ×1900. (Reprinted by permission of Ferenczy, ref. 17.)

Table 11.4. Chronological sequence of progression of simple hyperplasia to carcinoma over 11 years in one patient

Age (yr) of patient	Diagnosis, treatment, follow-up
21	Simple hyperplasia; no treatment
26	Term pregnancy
28	Atypical hyperplasia; no treatment
32	Grade 2 adenocarcinoma; TAH
60	Alive and well

TAH, total abdominal hysterectomy.
Adapted with permission from Kurman et al., ref. 48.

Table 11.5. Chronological sequence of progression of complex hyperplasia to carcinoma over 8 years in one patient

Age (yr) of patient	Diagnosis, treatment, follow-up
22	Complex hyperplasia
	Obese, infertile menometrorrhagia
	Clomid, Pergonal, bilateral wedge resection of ovaries
	No pregnancy
26	Atypical hyperplasia; no treatment
30	Grade 1 adenocarcinoma with squamous differentiation; TAH
43	Alive and well

TAH, total abdominal hysterectomy.
Adapted with permission from Kurman et al., ref. 48.

Table 11.6. Follow-up of hyperplasia and atypical hyperplasia in 170 patients

Type of hyperplasia	No. of patients	Regressed		Persisted		Progressed to carcinoma	
		No.	(%)	No.	(%)	No.	(%)
Hyperplasia	122	97	(80)	23	(19)	2	(2)
Atypical hyperplasia	48	29	(60)	8	(17)	11	(23)

Adapted with permission from Kurman et al., ref. 48.

Table 11.7. Follow-up of simple and complex hyperplasia and atypical hyperplasia in 170 patients

Type of hyperplasia	No. of patients	Regressed		Persisted		Progressed to carcinoma	
		No.	(%)	No.	(%)	No.	(%)
Simple	93	74	(80)	18	(19)	1	(1)
Complex	29	23	(80)	5	(17)	1	(3)
Simple atypical	13	9	(69)	3	(23)	1	(8)
Complex atypical	35	20	(57)	5	(14)	10	(29)

Adapted with permission from Kurman et al., ref. 48.

A comparison of the clinicopathological features and behavior of the carcinomas developing after a diagnosis of atypical hyperplasia in women 40 years or younger compared with women over the age of 40 years is shown in Table 11.8. Although all but one of the carcinomas that developed from atypical hyperplasia were well differentiated and minimally invasive, one well-differentiated tumor that extended into the endocervix metastasized to the pelvic peritoneum and a para-aortic lymph node. After abdominal radiation the patient was disease-free 19 years later. These findings and others[5a] suggest that carcinomas associated with hyperplasia are relatively innocuous compared with carcinomas not associated with it.

Table 11.8. Clinical and pathological findings from 11 "untreated" women with progression of atypical hyperplasia to carcinoma

	40 years and younger (8 patients)	Over 40 years (3 patients)
Age range	23–40 years	43–50 years
Polycystic ovarian disease	4 (50%)	0
Obese	4 (50%)	1
Mean time of progression	3.3 years	7.8 years
Grade 1 adenocarcinoma	8 (100%)	2 (66%)
Grade 2 adenocarcinoma	0	1 (33%)
Carcinoma confined to endometrium or superficially invasive	8 (100%)	3 (100%)
Metastatic carcinoma	1[a]	0

[a] Grade 1 adenocarcinoma with squamous differentiation that extended to the endocervix subsequently metastasized to pelvic peritoneum and a para-aortic lymph node. Patient was treated with abdominal radiation and is alive and well 19 years later.
Adapted with permission from Kurman et al., ref. 48.

It has been shown that 17–25% of women with atypical hyperplasia in curettings will have a well-differentiated carcinoma in the uterus if a hysterectomy is performed within 1 month of the curettage.[43,49,76] Increasing degrees of nuclear atypia, mitotic activity, and stratification of cells in curettings are associated with a higher frequency of carcinoma in the uterus. Yet with long-term follow-up, only 11–23% of women with atypical hyperplasia develop carcinoma if a hysterectomy is not done.[31,48] Thus, the lesion designated as well-differentiated carcinoma usually remains stable for a long period of time. Several reasons may account for the relatively low rate of progression to carcinoma in untreated patients with atypical hyperplasia. First, there is a general tendency for the highest grade of atypical hyperplasia to be selected for hysterectomy, leaving the lesser degree of atypia for conservative management. Second, atypical hyperplasia may not be the precursor of all forms of endometrial cancer but only of a type that is slow-growing and slowly progressive. The different forms of endometrial carcinoma and how they relate to hyperplasia are discussed in Chapter 12, Endometrial Carcinoma. Based on these studies it is reasonable to conclude that atypical hyperplasia is a precursor of certain types of endometrial carcinoma. In contrast, hyperplasia without atypia is a benign proliferative response to unopposed estrogenic stimulation, but by itself is not a precursor of endometrial carcinoma.

Management

Management of patients with endometrial hyperplasia is based on a consideration of clinical factors in addition to the microscopic findings.[45] The most important factors are

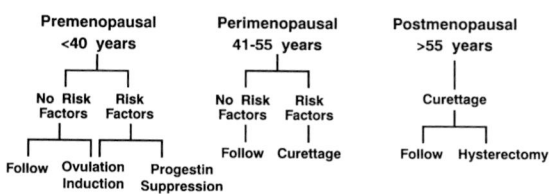

HYPERPLASIA
SIMPLE OR COMPLEX
BASED ON ENDOMETRIAL BIOPSY

FIG. 11.23. Endometrial hyperplasia. Management of simple or complex endometrial hyperplasia.

age and the presence of cytological atypia. Since most women with hyperplasia present with abnormal bleeding, an approach for the evaluation of abnormal bleeding along with the management of hyperplasia is presented (Figs. 11.23, 11.24).

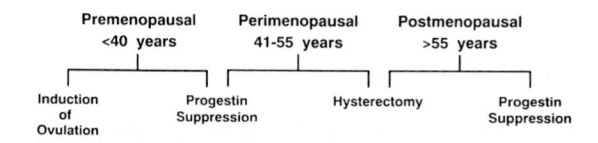

ATYPICAL HYPERPLASIA
SIMPLE OR COMPLEX
BASED ON A CURETTAGE

FIG. 11.24. Atypical hyperplasia. Management of simple or complex aypical hyperplasia.

REPRODUCTIVE-AGE WOMEN (40 YEARS AND YOUNGER)

Most women in the reproductive-age group who present with abnormal bleeding have nonspecific hormonal disorders that are self-limited. These women are at low risk of having carcinoma (Table 11.9). In a study of 460 women 40 years of age and younger, 6 (1.3%) had "mild" hyperplasia (simple hyperplasia) but none had atypical hyperplasia or carcinoma.[41] Therefore, most women in this age group with abnormal bleeding do not require an endometrial biopsy. Women with risk factors for endometrial cancer, such as polycystic ovarian disease or obesity, and women with persistent bleeding should have an endometrial biopsy performed. Traditionally, evaluation of such patients has been by curettage in the operating room but recent reports suggest that office procedures are comparable and are substantially less expensive,[29] with 96% agreement between the biopsy and hysterectomy findings in one study.[75] Even a curettage removes less than half of the endometrium in 60% of cases assessed immediately after the curettage by hysterectomy.[74] Office-based endometrial sampling devices such as the Pipelle device provide adequate specimens, comparable with the Novak biopsy instrument with substantially less patient discomfort.[70,75]

If a diagnosis of simple or complex hyperplasia is made, the patient can be treated conservatively, since these lesions have an extremely low risk (1–2%) of progression to carcinoma. Because the transit time to carcinoma is approximately 10 years and hyperplasia without cytological atypia first progresses through atypical hyperplasia before becoming carcinoma (Tables 11.4, 11.5), follow-up and periodic endometrial biopsies suffice.[48] Conservative management of young women with simple hyperplasia and complex hyperplasia resulted in subsequent pregnancies in 29% and 20% of these women, respectively, in one study[48] (Table 11.10).

Table 11.9. Pertinent findings in endometrium in women with abnormal bleeding according to age

Finding in endometrial specimen[d]	Age					
	Premenopausal[a] <40 years (n = 460)		Perimenopausal[a] 40–55 years (n = 748)		Postmenopausal[b] >55 years (n = 226)	
	No.	(%)	No.	(%)	No.	(%)
Carcinoma	0	(—)	3	(0.4)	15	(7)
Atypical hyperplasia	0	(—)	5	(0.7)	NK[c]	
Hyperplasia	6	(1)	41	(6)	34	(15)
Atrophy	7	(2)	51	(7)	127	(56)
Polyp	6	(1)	13	(2)	19	(8)
Proliferative	139	(29)	273	(36)	31	(14)
Secretory	241	(50)	287	(38)	0	(—)

NK, not known.
[a] Kaminski and Stevens, ref. 41.
[b] Lidor et al., ref. 52.
[c] A category of atypical hyperplasia was not specified in this study.
[d] Not all of the endometrial findings in the study by Kaminski and Stevens are listed and therefore percentages do not total 100%.

Table 11.10. Subsequent pregnancies in "untreated" women with hyperplasia and atypical hyperplasia

Diagnosis	No. of patients <40	No. of patients who became pregnant	No. of full-term pregnancies
Simple hyperplasia	35	10 (29%)	19
Complex hyperplasia	15	3 (20%)	4
Atypical hyperplasia (simple and complex)	24	3 (13%)	4

Adapted from Kurman et al., ref. 48.

Women with atypical hyperplasia on an endometrial biopsy should undergo a curettage in the operating room or a Vabra aspiration in the office to make certain that the endometrial cavity is well sampled. In a review of more than 13,000 curettages and nearly 6000 Vabra aspirations, both methods were 80–90% accurate.[29] The likelihood of carcinoma in the uterus after curettage showing atypical hyperplasia increases with age (Fig. 11.25) and is low in women younger than 40 years of age. Only 2 (12%) of 17 patients under age 40 years with atypical hyperplasia in curettings had carcinoma in the uterus (Table 11.11), and both neoplasms were well differentiated and confined to the endometrium. Therefore, young women with atypical hyperplasia who wish to retain their fertility can have hormonal treatment, either by suppression with progestins or induction of ovulation, but close follow-up and periodic

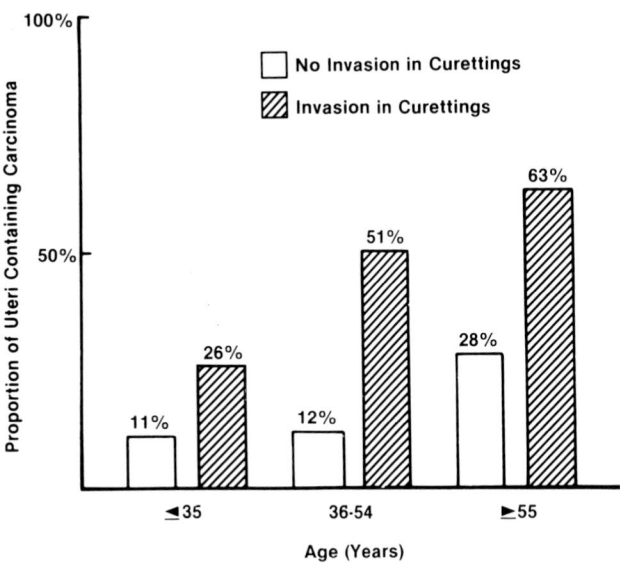

Fig. 11.25. Carcinoma in uterus according to age and presence of stromal invasion in curettings of 204 patients. There is a striking increase in residual carcinoma in the uteri of patients with atypical hyperplasia and well-differentiated adenocarcinoma in curettings with advancing age. (Adapted by permission of Kurman and Norris, ref. 47.)

Table 11.11. Hysterectomy findings according to the presence of atypical hyperplasia or well-differentiated adenocarcinoma in curettings in women under 40 years of age

	Curettings	
Hysterectomy findings	Atypical hyperplasia (n = 17) No.	Well-differentiated carcinoma (n = 35) No.
Carcinoma	2 (12%)	13 (37%)
Grade 1	2	10
Grade 2	0	3
Myometrial invasion		
Endometrium only	2	3
Inner one-third	0	9
Middle one-third	0	1

Adapted from Kurman and Norris, ref. 47.

endometrial biopsies are necessary. A conservative plan of management is justified because the risk of progression to carcinoma in young women is low. Furthermore, the carcinomas that do develop tend to be innocuous, and 13% of those women less than 40 years of age can subsequently become pregnant and have normal deliveries[9,48] (Table 11.10). In contrast, women less than 40 years of age with bona fide well-differentiated carcinoma usually require surgical treatment.

Perimenopausal Women (40 to 55 Years of Age)

Abnormal bleeding in the perimenopausal-age group can be managed in a similar fashion as in younger women because perimenopausal women also are at low risk of having carcinoma (Table 11.9). Most simple and complex hyperplasias in the 40- to 55-year age group are related to anovulation and are self-limited. Women with no risk factors for endometrial carcinoma can be followed, whereas those with risk factors should have a biopsy or Vabra aspiration performed (Figs. 11.23, 11.24). Patients with a diagnosis of atypical hyperplasia can be treated with progestins or a hysterectomy.

Nearly 60% of atypical hyperplasias also regress, but the likelihood of residual carcinoma in the uterus after a curettage increases with age (Fig. 11.25). For patients in the 40- to 55-year age range, treatment should be individualized. Regression occurs frequently, and the risk of residual carcinoma is lower than in older women. Therefore, observation or suppression with progestins monitored by repeat endometrial biopsies every 3 months will suffice. If the lesion persists, a hysterectomy may have to be performed.

Postmenopausal Women (Over the Age of 55 Years)

Women in the postmenopausal-age group with abnormal bleeding have a significant risk of having either carcinoma or atypical hyperplasia (Table 11.9). Accordingly, abnormal bleeding requires immediate evaluation with an endometrial biopsy. A diagnosis of hyperplasia or atypical hyperplasia should be evaluated with a fractional curettage or Vabra aspiration. If the curettings demonstrate hyperplasia without atypia, conservative management is an option because these types of hyperplasia are related to unopposed estrogenic stimulation, either from exogenous hormone treatment or because of peripheral conversion of androgens to estrogen in adipose tissue. Most (80%) hyperplasias treated with cyclic medroxyprogesterone acetate 10 mg a day for 14 days regress; none progressed to carcinoma in a prospective study of 65 postmenopausal women.[20] Conservative management, either observation only or treatment with medroxyprogesterone to produce a medical curettage, therefore, is adequate. Repeated episodes of irregular bleeding that are not responsive to hormone treatment may require a hysterectomy.

Hysterectomy is the treatment of choice for a diagnosis of atypical hyperplasia based on a curettage. In postmenopausal women with surgical risk factors that preclude a hysterectomy, continuous treatment with 20 to 40 mg a day of megestrol acetate can be used effectively to avoid surgery. In a study of 70 women with complex hyperplasia (38 women) and atypical hyperplasia (32 women), surgery was avoided in 93% of patients. With a mean follow-up of more than 5 years the hyperplasias (atypical and nonatypical) completely regressed in 85%. None of the lesions progressed to carcinoma.[23]

For postmenopausal women with hyperplasia or atypical hyperplasia who are receiving exogenous estrogen, termination of the estrogen usually suffices even for atypical hyperplasia, since these proliferations regress after the stimulus for their growth has been removed. Alternatively, cyclic or continuous courses of medroxyprogesterone in women being treated with estrogen substantially reduces the risk of development of endometrial hyperplasia and carcinoma. Using a 7- to 14-day regimen of orally administered 10 mg of medroxyprogesterone to postmenopausal women receiving estrogen, five endometrial carcinomas were detected in 5402 woman-years of continuous estrogen therapy.[27] This incidence is not greater than that of untreated postmenopausal women, in whom the expected incidence of endometrial cancer is 1 to 2 per 1000 woman-years, i.e., 5.4 to 9.8 cases.

Although endometrial biopsy and curettage are the mainstay for the evaluation of women with abnormal bleeding in this age group, preliminary studies suggest that transvaginal ultrasound evaluation may decrease the need for curettage from 50% to 70%.[25,73] These studies have shown that in postmenopausal women who were not on hormone replacement therapy, no carcinomas were found in women whose endometrial thickness was less than 5 mm.[24,25,73] The method is not as accurate, however, for premenopausal women and patients on estrogen replacement treatment.[25,73] The role of transvaginal ultrasound in the evaluation of abnormal bleeding and in screening will require further evaluation.

Table 11.12. Classification of endometrial cellular (cytoplasmic) changes

Eosinophilic (including syncytial change)
Squamous (squamous metaplasia)
Ciliated cell (tubal metaplasia)
Secretory and clear cell
Mucinous

Endometrial Cellular Changes (Metaplasia)

DEFINITIONS AND CLASSIFICATION

Metaplasia is defined as replacement of one type of adult tissue by another type that is not normally found in that location. In the endometrium, most of the changes that are designated as "metaplasia" represent a variety of cytoplasmic alterations that are not encountered in normal proliferative endometrium but do not qualify as true metaplasia. Accordingly, Silverberg has suggested that a more appropriate term is *change*.[71] Use of the term *change* also has the advantage of providing a descriptive designation without employing a specific mechanism of development. In this chapter *change* is used to denote many of the cytoplasmic alterations that have been previously termed *metaplasia*. When these cytoplasmic changes occur in the absence of hyperplasia, they are usually focal. In association with hyperplasia (with or without atypia) they may be diffuse.

The WHO has classified endometrial metaplasia as follows: squamous, mucinous, ciliary, hobnail, clear cell, eosinophilic, surface syncytial, papillary proliferation, and Arias–Stella effect.[68] This classification combines both cytological and architectural alterations, some of which have different etiologies. As previously noted, the endometrial epithelium can undergo a variety of cytoplasmic changes in response to different stimuli that can be observed in both benign and malignant conditions. A simplified classification of these is shown in Table 11.12. It is important to recognize the various cytoplasmic changes because they are benign and can be confused with hyperplasia. When hyperplasia and the cytoplasmic alterations co-exist, as they often do, the hyperplasia should be classified, but it is not necessary to describe the cytoplasmic changes because they do not influence prognosis (see Behavior).

The frequent association of the various endometrial cytoplasmic changes with hyperplasia is probably because both result from a hyperestrogenic state. More than 70% of perimenopausal and postmenopausal women with "metaplasia" had received exogenous estrogen in one study.[33] In addition, the vast majority of young women with "metaplasia" have clinical manifestations of persistent anovulation and primary infertility, features of polycystic ovarian disease.[6,11,33] Besides hyperestrinism, "metaplasia" also may occur in various benign conditions, including polyps, endometritis, trauma, and vitamin A deficiency.[11,21,33,34]

PATHOLOGIC FINDINGS

The various types of endometrial cytoplasmic changes have no distinctive gross features.

Eosinophilic Change

Eosinophilic change is the most common cytoplasmic alteration. Several types of eosinophilic cytoplasmic transformation occur, all of them innocuous. Ciliated cells, squamous cells, oncocytes, and papillary and surface syncytial change all may have eosinophilic cytoplasm. However, eosinophilic cells also occur in association with hyperplasia, particularly atypical hyperplasia (Fig. 11.26).

Glands may be lined partially or completely by eosinophilic cells. Eosinophilic cells that line glands can show considerable variation in shape. They may be columnar when associated with atypical hyperplasia, rounded when associated with ciliated cells, or polygonal forming pavement-like aggregates when they merge with cells that show squamous differentiation (Fig. 11.27). In hyperplastic lesions aggregates of eosinophilic cells often form intraglandular papillary tufts (Fig. 11.27) and bridges (Fig. 11.28) simulating carcinoma. Eosinophilic cells contain variable amounts of cytoplasm that at times can be partially vacuolated (Figs. 11.29, 11.30). The nuclei tend to be round and somewhat stratified. Although at times they appear vesicular, the nuclei are smaller, more uniform, and lack the irregular nuclear membrane, coarse chromatin, and nucleoli that characterize cells with true cytological atypia.

On the endometrial surface, cells with eosinophilic cytoplasm typically merge into a syncytium that either can be flat or more commonly form papillary processes[64] (Fig. 11.27). Typically, the papillary processes lack connective tissue support and contain small cystic spaces filled with polymorphonuclear leukocytes. This lesion has been referred to as *surface syncytial change*, *papillary syncytial change*, or *papillary metaplasia*.[34,71] We prefer the term *eosinophilic syncytial change* because the lesion is characteristically composed of eosinophilic cells forming a syncytium and can involve glands as well as the surface. Eosino-

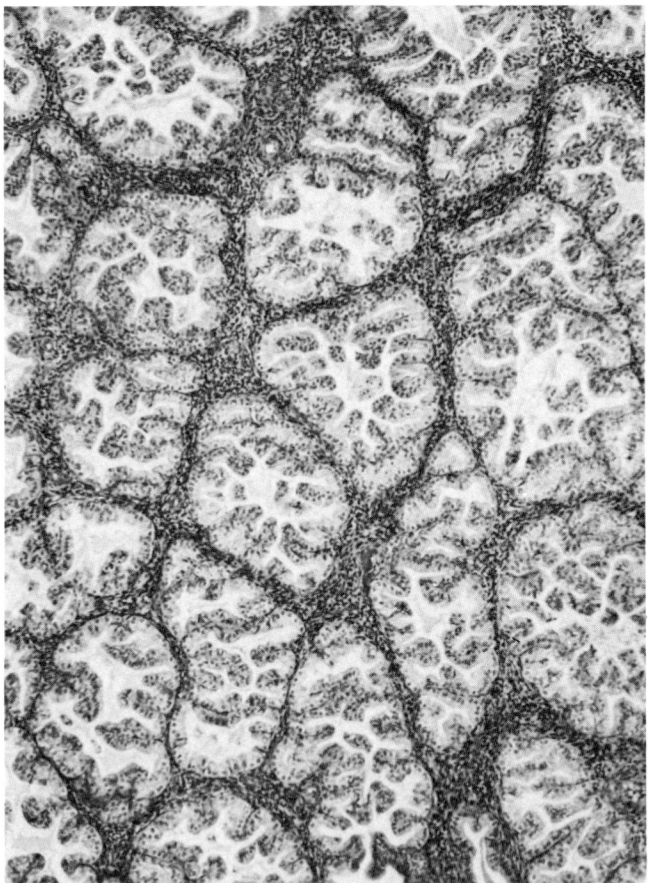

FIG. 11.26. Eosinophilic cell change in an atypical hyperplasia. The cells lining the glands form intraglandular tufts.

philic syncytial change is commonly associated with endometrial stromal breakdown (Fig. 11.29) or inflammation, suggesting that it is a degenerative or a reparative process.[80] The nuclei within the syncytium are arranged haphazardly and piled up. They generally are small and bland but at times may be round and vesicular and display alterations in shape and chromatin texture. Mitotic figures are rare. Hyperchromatic nuclei with smudged chromatin and irregular nuclear membranes appear degenerated whereas enlarged, vesicular nuclei with a prominent nucleolus and smooth nuclear membranes appear reactive (Fig. 11.30). These degenerative and reparative changes should not be interpreted as nuclear atypia.

Squamous Change (Squamous Metaplasia)

Squamous change may occur in all forms of hyperplasia as well as in carcinoma. It is especially common in the more atypical endometrial proliferations (Fig. 11.31) and is rare in normally cycling endometrium or in simple and complex hyperplasias (Fig. 11.32). The squamous cells are usually

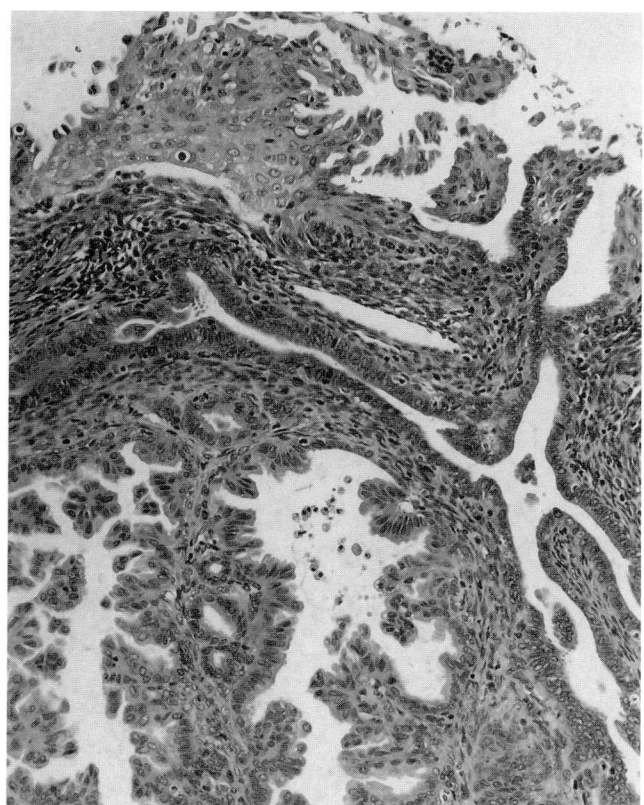

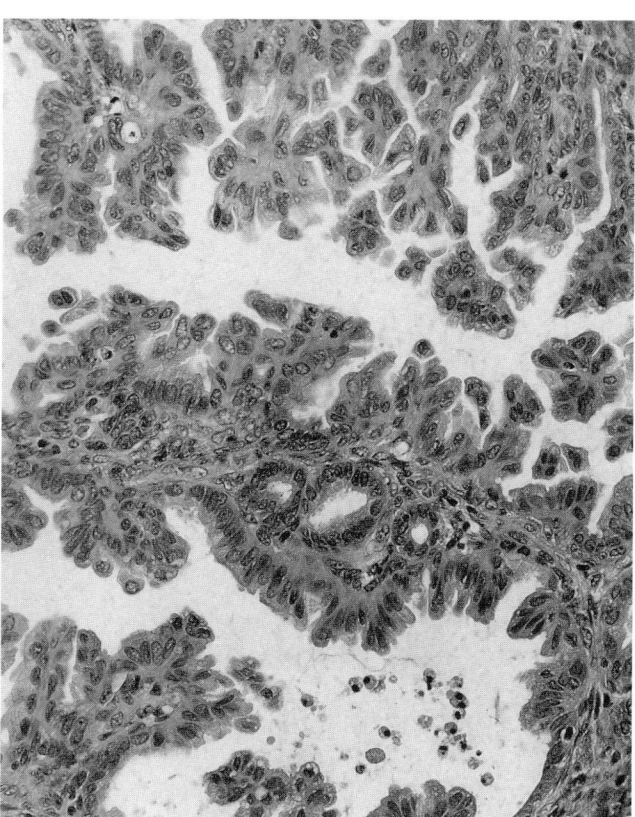

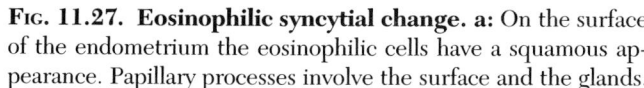

Fig. 11.27. Eosinophilic syncytial change. a: On the surface of the endometrium the eosinophilic cells have a squamous appearance. Papillary processes involve the surface and the glands.

b: The eosinophilic cells form complex intraglandular papillary tufts. There is no cytological atypia.

cytologically bland. The degree of nuclear atypia, when present, generally parallels that of the glandular cells. Typically, the squamous cells have a moderate amount of eosinophilic cytoplasm and are surrounded by a well-defined cell membrane. Often they merge with eosinophilic cells that qualify as eosinophilic change underscoring how these various alterations are intimately related. The squamous cells tend to be rounded or polygonal but may be spindle-shaped, forming a circumscribed nest, the squamous morule, within the gland lumen (Fig. 11.31). Morules reflect immature or incomplete squamous differentiation. The cells are smaller, and the cytoplasm is less prominent than in more completely differentiated squamous cells. Central keratinization and necrosis rarely occur. Eventually, proliferation results in protrusion of the squamous cells into the lumen, leading to replacement of the lumen by nests of squamous cells and coalescence with neighboring glands undergoing the same process. Mitotic activity is rare.

Ciliated Cell Change

Cilia are not usually evident microscopically in proliferative endometrial glandular cells, although they may be observed on the endometrial surface.[55] Ciliated cells occasionally are observed in isolated glands in atrophic or inactive endometria or in polyps in the absence of hyperplasia. The presence of a significant number of ciliated glandular cells is referred to as *ciliated cell change* or *tubal metaplasia* because of the resemblance to epithelium of the fallopian tube. The ciliated cells are often round and slightly enlarged but the nuclear membrane is smooth and uniform and the chromatin is fine and evenly dispersed (Fig. 11.33). There is no nuclear atypia. The ciliated cells may be interspersed singly or in small groups among nonciliated cells, or they may line a larger segment of a gland (Fig. 11.34). Mitotic activity is limited to the adjacent nonciliated cells. Ciliated cell change may occur in glands in the absence of hyperplasia. Dilated venous sinusoids are also frequently present. All of these changes reflect a mild degree of estrogenic stimulation. Ciliated cell change frequently accompanies simple, complex, or atypical hyperplasia (Fig. 11.35).

Secretory and Clear Cell Change

On rare occasions, polygonal cells with clear cytoplasm containing glycogen and bland nuclei are found in glands

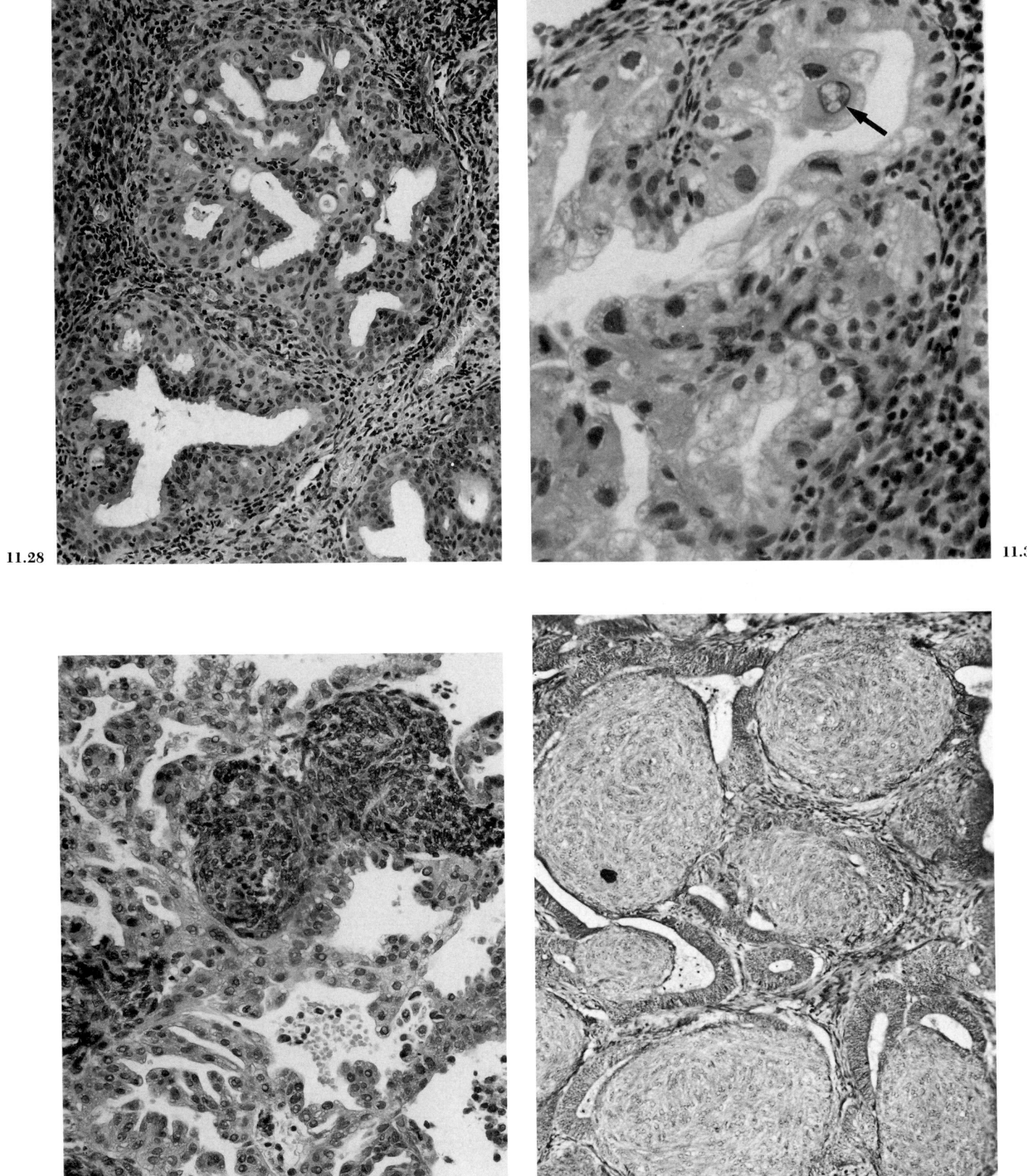

11.28

11.30

11.29

11.3

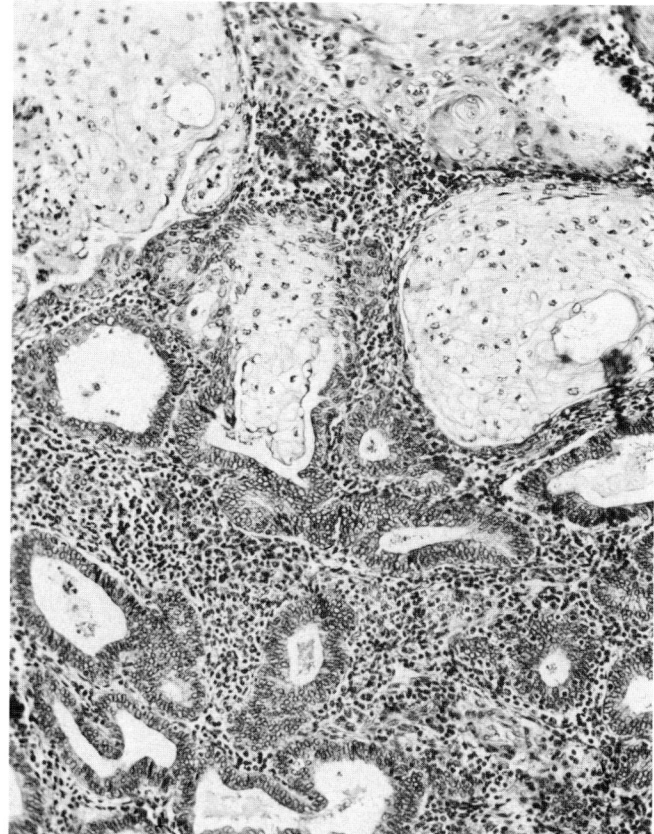

FIG. 11.32. Squamous change (metaplasia) in simple hyperplasia. Both squamous and the glandular cells lack cytological atypia.

or on the surface of the endometrium and have been referred to as *clear cell metaplasia*[33] (Fig. 11.36). In contrast, *secretory effect* is characterized by columnar cells with sub- or supranuclear vacuoles containing clear glycogenated cy-

◁ ———————————————

FIG. 11.28. Eosinophilic change in complex hyperplasia. The cells bridge gland lumens simulating a cribriform pattern (compare with Fig. 11.17).

FIG. 11.29. Eosinophilic syncytial change. The cells with eosinophilic cytoplasm display mild vacuolization, merging to form a syncytium within glands and extending onto the surface. The eosinophilic change envelopes condensed stromal cells (*upper, center*). The latter is a common manifestation of endometrial stromal breakdown.

FIG. 11.30. Eosinophilic change. The cells display varying degrees of cytoplasmic vacuolization and nuclear alterations. Some nuclei are enlarged and hyperchromatic with smudged chromatin and irregular borders. One cell in the upper part of the field has an enlarged, "moth-eaten" nucleus (*arrow*) with chromatin that is indistinct and partially smudged.

FIG. 11.31. Squamous change (metaplasia) in atypical hyperplasia. The squamous cells have almost entirely obliterated gland lumens.

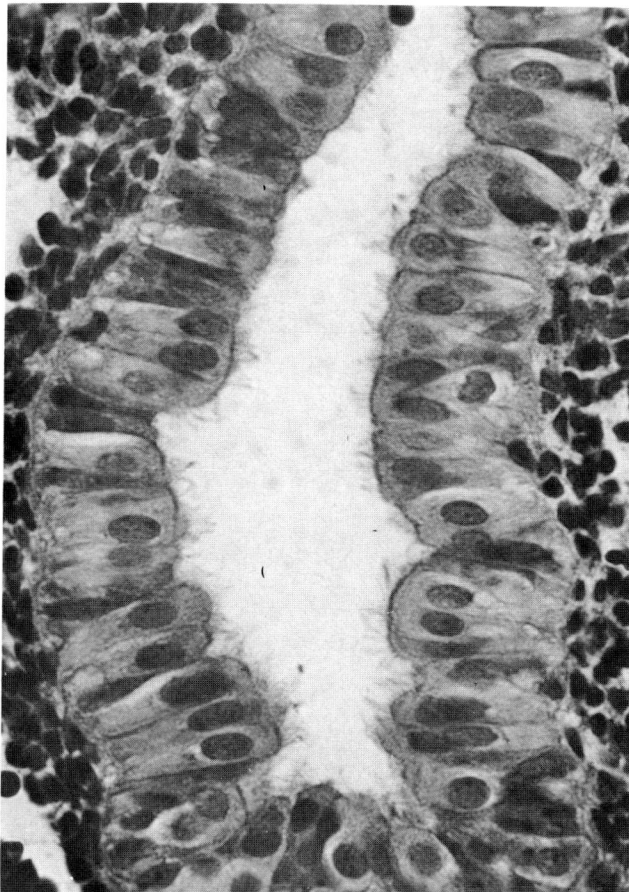

FIG. 11.33. Ciliated cell change. This type of change is characterized by ciliated cells along with intercalated (peg) cells closely resembling the epithelium of the fallopian tube.

toplasm resembling the glandular cells of early secretory endometrium. These also can be observed in nonneoplastic endometria but are seen more often in association with hyperplasia or carcinoma[46,47] (Fig. 11.37). At times secretory change can result from progestational stimulation, but often there is no such association. Columnar cells with secretory change may merge with polygonal-shaped clear cells and with squamous cells containing clear glycogenated cytoplasm. Thus, the accumulation of glycogen can occur in the cytoplasm of a variety of cell types, and is not a true metaplasia but a cytoplasmic alteration.

Mucinous Change

Mucinous change is characterized by mucinous epithelium resembling that of the endocervix cytologically, histochemically, and ultrastructurally.[12] It is one of the least commonly encountered cytoplasmic alterations. the mucinous epithelium tends to be distributed focally and is composed of tall columnar cells with bland, basally oriented nuclei and clear, slightly granular cytoplasm (Figs. 11.38, 11.39).

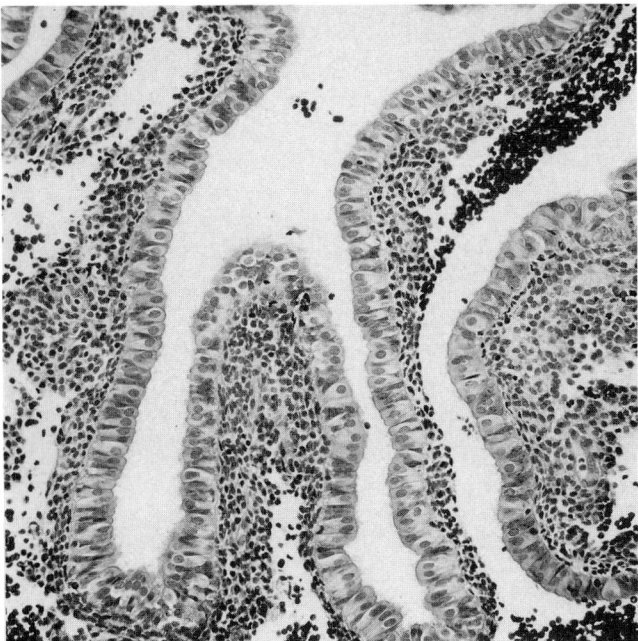

FIG. 11.34. Ciliated cell change. Ciliated cells are present in an enlarged gland with an irregular outline.

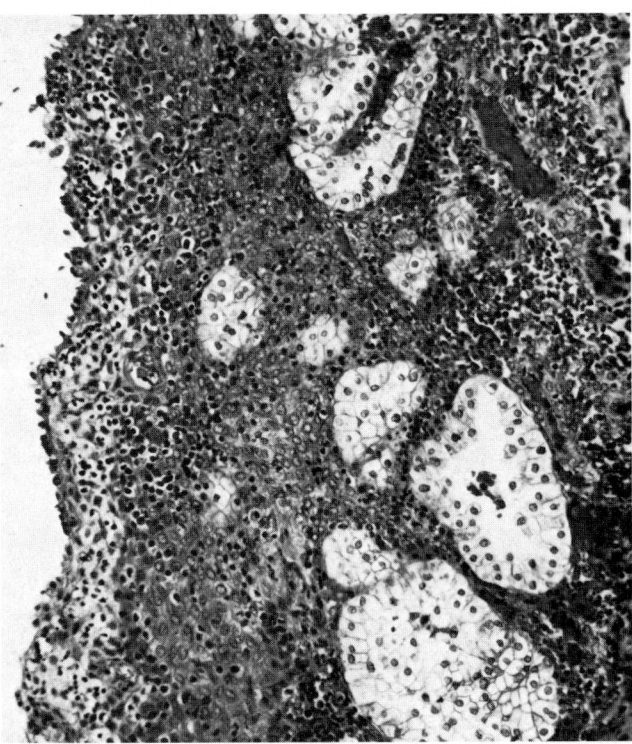

FIG. 11.36. Clear cell change. The clear cells lining endometrial glands contain glycogen.

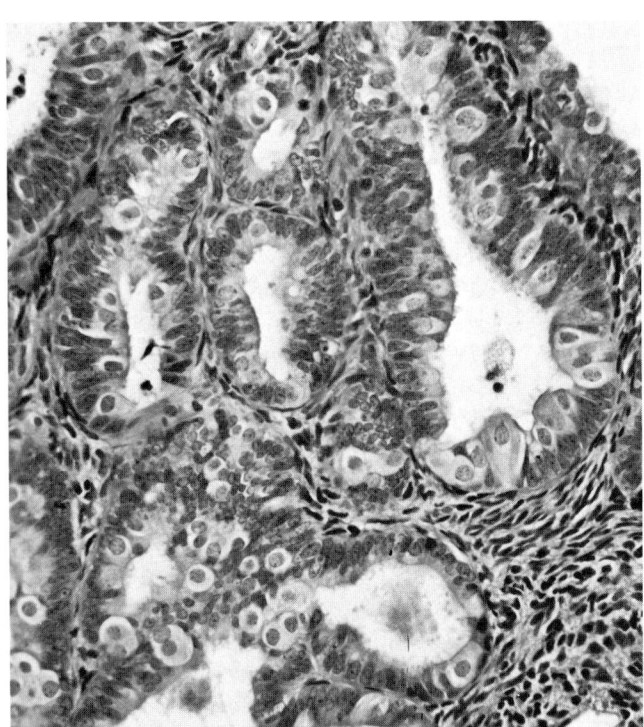

FIG. 11.35. Ciliated change in complex hyperplasia. Numerous ciliated cells with round, bland nuclei and clear cytoplasmic halos are present.

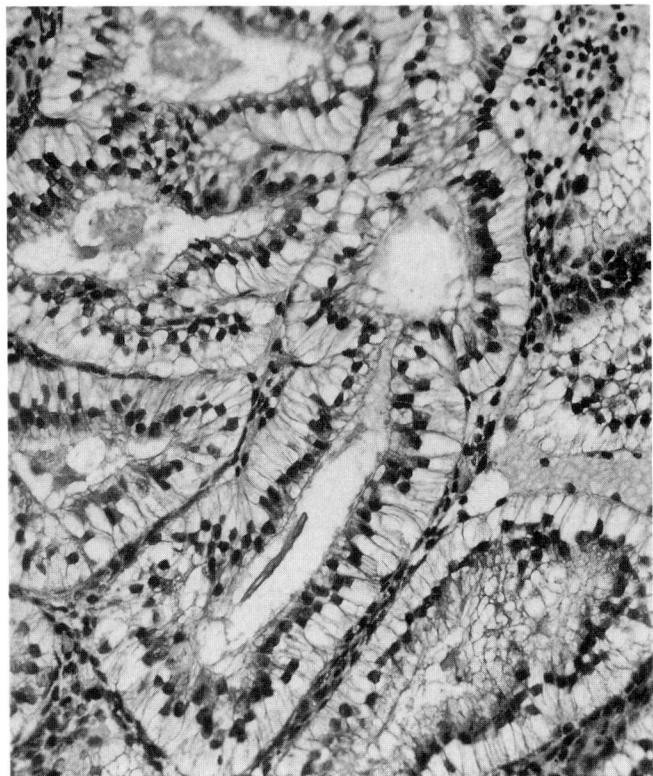

FIG. 11.37. Secretory change in complex hyperplasia. The glands are markedly crowded with little intervening stroma. The cells are columnar with subnuclear vacuoles and the nuclei show no cytological atypia.

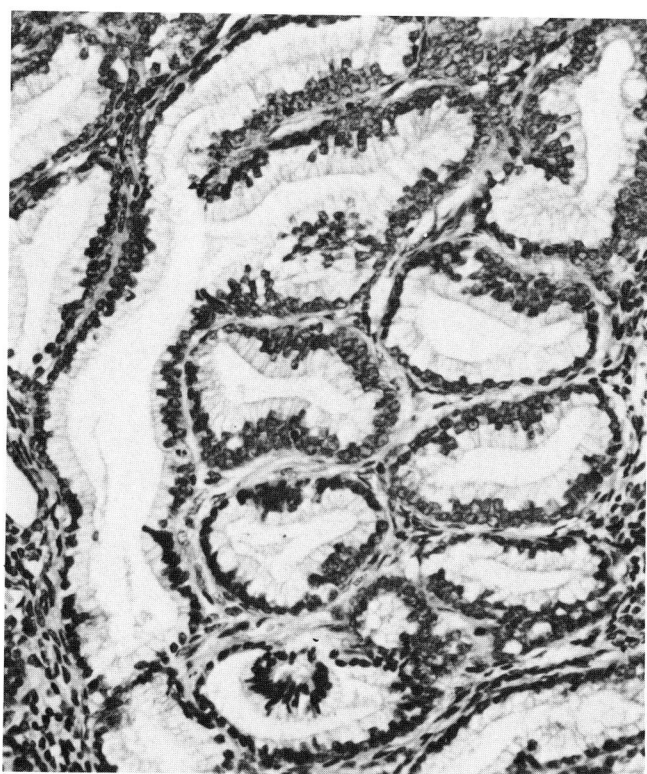

FIG. 11.38. Mucinous changes in complex hyperplasia. The nuclei of the glandular cells are closely applied to the basement membrane. The cytoplasm is clear and intensely positive with mucicarmine stains but contains no stainable glycogen.

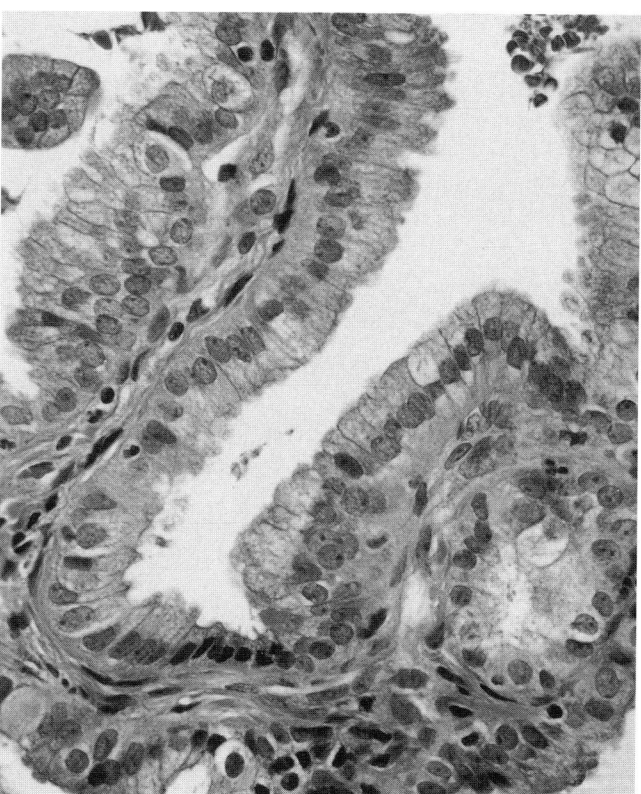

FIG. 11.39. Mucinous change. The mucinous cells form a single layer of columnar epithelium with bland nuclei and granular cytoplasm. The cytoplasm is positive with mucicarmine stains.

At times mucinous change is accompanied by a papillary proliferation. The papillary processes contain normal but compressed stromal cells and are lined by nonstratified columnar epithelium, which is mucinous in areas (Fig. 11.40). Mitotic figures are rare. The cytoplasm is clear in H&E stains because it contains mucin, which is periodic acid-Schiff (PAS) positive and diastase resistant and stains with mucicarmine, toluidine blue, and alcian blue. In contrast to mucinous epithelium, the vacuolated cytoplasm of secretory endometrium contains glycogen. Mucinous change is associated most commonly with atypical hyperplasia. On rare occasion the mucinous epithelium may contain goblet cells and is referred to as *intestinal metaplasia*.

Mixed Cellular Changes

Mixtures of different types of cellular changes are common. Most are closely related and represent different morphologic responses to a variety of stimuli, including estrogenic stimulation.[33] For example, eosinophilic change, especially eosinophilic syncytial change, may resemble squamous epithelium and often is associated with squamous metaplasia. Likewise, eosinophilic and ciliated cell change share many morphologic features and commonly occur together.

DIFFERENTIAL DIAGNOSIS

The most important aspect of the evaluation of the various metaplasias and cellular changes is not to confuse them with hyperplasia or carcinoma. This is best accomplished by evaluating the glandular architecture and cytological features. In hyperplasia, the glandular outlines are irregular and complex and there is stratification of the epithelium reflecting a proliferative process. In contrast, in the various cytoplasmic changes the glandular outlines are regular and have a tubular configuration, although cystic dilatation and slight glandular irregularity occasionally can occur. Although the various cellular changes may be accompanied by slight nuclear enlargement, they lack the abnormal chromatin features of cytological atypia occurring in atypical hyperplasia. At times the various cellular changes may look ominous and suggest carcinoma but evidence of stromal invasion is lacking and therefore a diagnosis of carcinoma is not justified. For example, extensive squamous metaplasia may suggest a diagnosis of carcinoma but without a desmoplastic response or a confluent glandular pat-

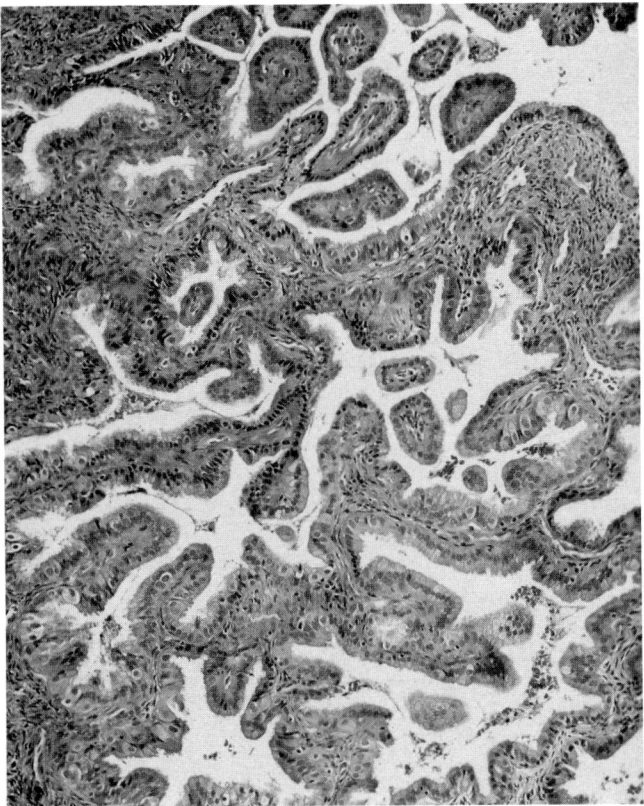

11.40

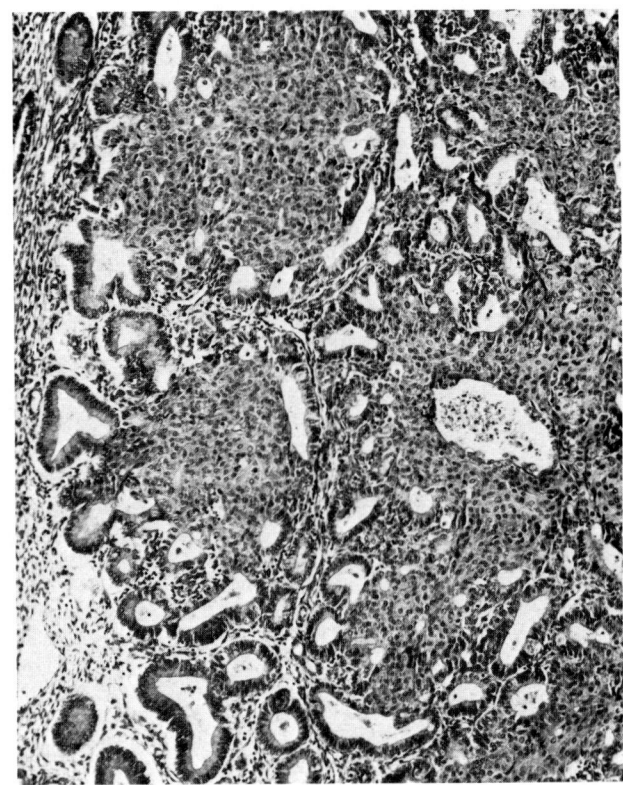

11.41

tern a diagnosis of carcinoma should not be made
(Fig. 11.41). Eosinophilic change associated with hyperplasia can fill and bridge gland lumens but lacks a true
confluent or cribriform pattern (Fig. 11.42). Mucinous
change at times can form complex papillary processes but
the stroma of the papillae are composed of normal endometrial stroma and the epithelium lacks cytological atypia
(Figs. 11.40, 11.43).

Behavior

Cytoplasmic changes, other than eosinophilic syncytial
change, rarely occur in the absence of hyperplasia or carcinoma.[40] In the absence of hyperplasia these changes

**Fig. 11.40. Complex hyperplasia with papillary prolifera-
tion.** The lesion involves the surface of the endometrium (*top of
field*). Most of the glandular epithelium is mucinous.
Fig. 11.41. Complex hyperplasia with squamous change.
There is extensive replacement of the stroma by squamous epithelium. In the absence of an altered (desmoplastic) stroma or a
confluent glandular pattern a diagnosis of carcinoma should not
be made.
Fig. 11.42. Eosinophilic cell change. Cells with eosinophilic
cells fill and bridge the glandular lumen. The microcystic spaces
that result lack the punched-out, hard outlines of a cribriform
pattern (compare with Fig. 11.17).

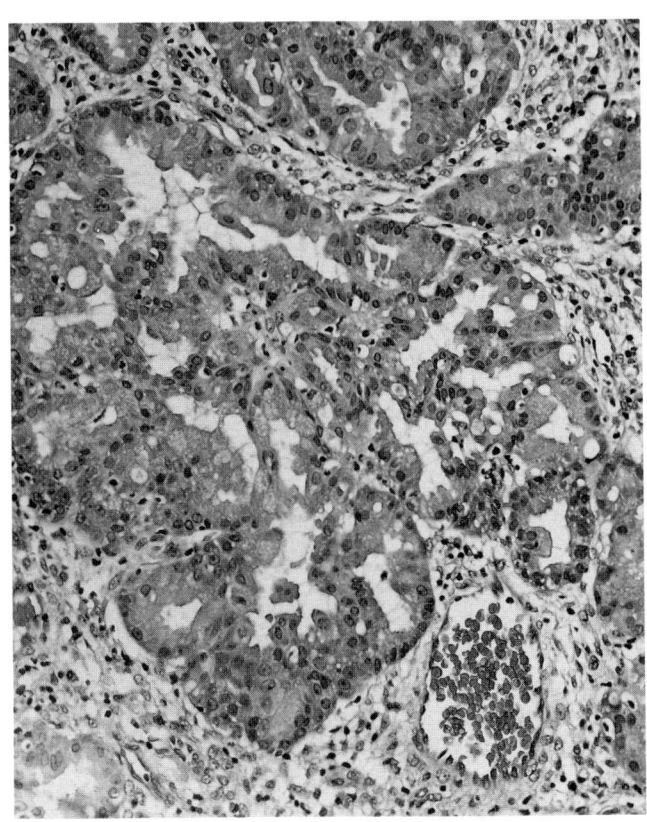

11.4

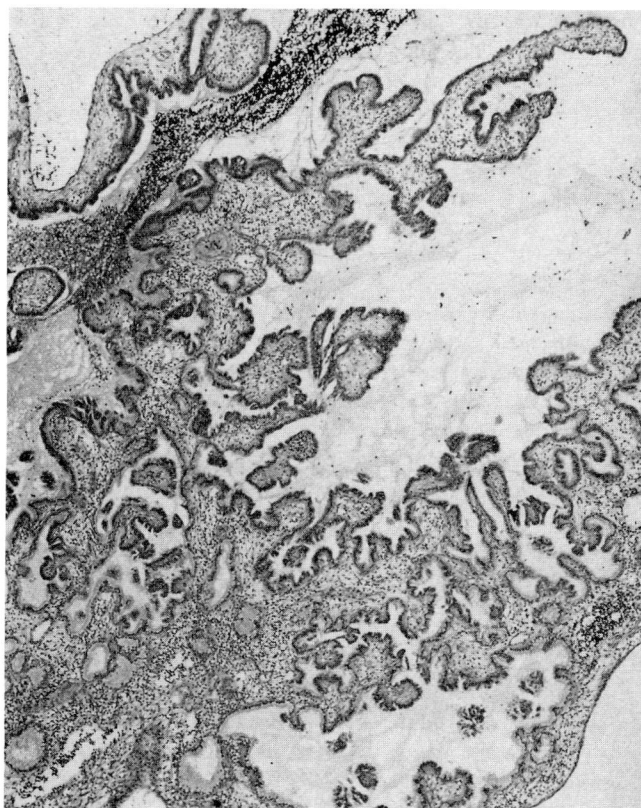

Fig. 11.43. **Papillary mucinous change.** In contrast to the delicate fibrovascular cores of a well-differentiated (endometrioid) carcinoma, the papillae in the papillary mucinous change contain normal endometrial stroma and the epithelial cells are bland.

(metaplasia) had no clinical significance in a study of 89 patients by Hendrickson and Kempson.[33] In a long-term follow-up study of endometrial hyperplasia,[48] 5 of 11 patients with atypical hyperplasia and associated squamous metaplasia eventually developed carcinoma, indicating that atypical hyperplasia with squamous metaplasia has malignant potential.[48] Inasmuch as the cytoplasmic changes by themselves have no prognostic significance, the importance of recognizing them lies in not confusing these benign processes with hyperplasia or carcinoma.

MANAGEMENT

The management of endometrial cytoplasmic changes depends entirely on the nature of the associated proliferative process. If hyperplasia is present it should be managed accordingly. Endometrial cytoplasmic changes without hyperplasia do not require treatment.

References

1. Artacho-Perula E, Roldan-Villalobos R, Roldan-Villalobos A, Vaamonde-Lemos R (1993) Histomorphometry of normal and abnormal endometrial samples. Int J Gynecol Pathol 12: 173–179
2. Ausems WEMA, van der Kamp J-K, Baak JAP (1985) Nuclear morphometry in the determination of the prognosis of marked atypical endometrial hyperplasia. Int J Gynecol Pathol 4: 180–185
3. Baak JPA, Kurver PHJ, Diegenbach PC, Delemarre JFM, Brekelmans ECM, Nieuwlaat JE (1981) Discrimination of hyperplasia and carcinoma of the endometrium by quantitative microscopy—a feasibility study. Histopathology 5: 61–68
4. Baak JPA, Nauta JJF, Wisse-Brekelmans ECM, Bezemer PD (1988) Architectural and nuclear morphometrical features together are more important prognosticators in endometrial hyperplasias than nuclear morphometrical features alone. J Pathol 154: 335–41
5. Baak JPA, Wise-Brekelmans ECM, Fleege JC, van der Putten HWHM, Bezemer PD (1992) Assessment of the risk on endometrial cancer in hyperplasia, by means of morphological and morphometric features. Pathol Res Pract 188: 856–859
5a. Beckner ME, Mori T, Silverberg SG (1985) Endometrial carcinoma: Non-tumor factors in prognosis. Int J Gynecol Pathol 4: 131–145
6. Blaustein A (1982) Morular metaplasia misdiagnosed as adenoacanthoma in young women with polycystic ovarian disease. Am J Surg Pathol 6: 223–228
7. Buehl IA, Vellios F, Carter JE, Huber CP (1964) Carcinoma in situ of the endometrium. Am J Clin Pathol 42: 594–601
8. Campbell PE, Barter RA (1961) The significance of atypical hyperplasia. J Obstet Gynaecol Br Commonw 68: 668–672
9. Chamlian DL, Taylor HB (1970) Endometrial hyperplasia in young women. Obstet Gynecol 36: 659–666
10. Colgan TJ, Norris HJ, Foster W, Kurman RJ, Fox CH (1983) Predicting the outcome of endometrial hyperplasia by quantitative analysis of nuclear features using a linear discriminant function. Int J Gynecol Pathol 1: 347–352
11. Crum CP, Richart RM, Fenoglio CM (1981) Adenoacanthosis of the endometrium. A clinicopathologic study in premenopausal women. Am J Surg Pathol 5: 15–20
12. Demopoulos RI, Greco MA (1983) Mucinous metaplasia of the endometrium: Ultrastructural and histochemical characteristics. Int J Gynecol Pathol 1: 383–390
13. Dewagne MP, Silverberg SG (1982) Foam cells in endometrial carcinoma. A clinicopathologic study. Gynecol Oncol 13: 67–75
14. Fechner RE (1980) Ultrastructure of endometrial stromal foam cells. (Letter) Am J Clin Pathol 73: 731–732
15. Fechner RE, Bossart MI, Spjut HJ (1979) Ultrastructure of endometrial stromal foam cells. Am J Clin Pathol 72: 628–633
16. Fenoglio CM, Crum CP, Ferenczy A (1982) Endometrial hyperplasia and carcinoma. Are ultrastructural, biochemical, and immunocytochemical studies useful in distinguishing between them? Pathol Res Pract 174: 257–284
17. Ferenczy A (1979) Recent advances in endometrial neoplasia. Exp Mol Pathol 31: 226–235
18. Ferenczy A (1982) Cytodynamics of endometrial hyperplasia

and neoplasia. I. Histology and ultrastructure. In: Fenoglio CM, Wolff M (eds) Progress in Surgical Pathology, Vol. 4. New York, Masson Publishing USA, p 95

19. Ferenczy A (1983) Cytodynamics of endometrial hyperplasia and neoplasia. Part II: In vitro DNA histoautoradiography. Hum Pathol 14: 77–82

20. Ferenczy A, Gelfand M (1989) The biologic significance of cytologic atypia in progestogen-treated endometrial hyperplasia. Am J Obstet Gynecol 160: 126–131

21. Fluhman CF (1954) Comparative studies of squamous metaplasia of the cervix uteri and endometrium. Am J Obstet Gynecol 68: 1447–1463

22. Fu YS, Ferenczy A, Huang I, Gelfand MM (1988) Digital imaging analysis of normal, hyperplastic and malignant endometrial cells in endometrial brushing samples. Anal Quant Cytol Histol 10: 139–149

23. Gal D (1986) Hormonal therapy for lesions of the endometrium. Semin Oncol 13: 33–36

24. Goldstein SR, Nachtigal M, Snyder JR, Nachtigal L (1990) Endometrial assessment by vaginal ultrasonography before endometrial sampling in patients with postmenopausal bleeding. Am J Obstet Gynecol 163: 119–123

25. Granberg S, Wikland M, Karlsson B, Norstrom A, Friberg L-G (1991) Endometrial thickness as measured by endovaginal ultrasonography for identifying endometrial abnormality. Am J Obstet Gynecol 164: 47–52

26. Gray LA, Christopherson WM, Hoover RN (1977) Estrogens and endometrial carcinoma. Obstet Gynecol 49: 385–389

27. Greenblatt RB, Gambrell RD Jr, Stoddard LD (1982) The protective role of progesterone in the prevention of endometrial cancer. Pathol Res Pract 174: 297–318

28. Greenwald P, Caputo TA, Wolfgang PE (1977) Endometrial cancer after menopausal use of estrogens. Obstet Gynecol 50: 239–243

29. Grimes DA (1982) Diagnostic dilation and curettage: A reappraisal. Am J Obstet Gynecol 142: 1–6

30. Gusberg SB, Moore DB, Martin F (1954) Precursors of corpus cancer. II. A clinical and pathological study of adenomatous hyperplasia. Am J Obstet Gynecol 68: 1472–1481

31. Gusberg SB, Kaplan AL (1963) Precursors of corpus cancer. IV. Adenomatous hyperplasia as stage 0 carcinoma of the endometrium. Am J Obstet Gynecol 87: 662–678

32. Gusberg SB (1974) Precursors of corpus carcinoma. Estrogens and adenomatous hyperplasia. Am J Obstet Gynecol 54: 905–927

33. Hendrickson MR, Kempson RL (1980) Endometrial epithelial metaplasias—proliferations frequently misdiagnosed as adenocarcinoma: Report of 89 cases and proposed classification. Am J Surg Pathol 4: 525–542

34. Hendrickson MR, Kempson RL (1980) In: Bennington JL (ed) Surgical Pathology of the Uterine Corpus. Major Problems in Pathology. Philadelphia, London, Toronto, W. B. Saunders

35. Herlyn M, Malkowicz SB (1991) Regulatory pathways in tumor growth and invasion. Lab Invest 65: 262–271

36. Hertig AT, Sommers SC (1949) Genesis of endometrial carcinoma. I. Study of prior biopsies. Cancer 2: 946–956

37. Hertig AT, Sommers SC, Bengaloff H (1949) Genesis of endometrial carcinoma. III. Carcinoma in situ. Cancer 2: 964–971

38. Hustin J (1976) Morphology and DNA content of endometrial cancer nuclei under progestogen treatment. Acta Cytol 20: 556–558

39. Iozzo RV (1984) Proteoglycans and neoplastic-mesenchymal cell interactions. Hum Pathol 15: 2–10

40. Kaku T, Tsukamoto N, Tsuruchi N, Sugihara K, Kamura T, Nakano H (1992) Endometrial metaplasia associated with endometrial carcinoma. Obstet Gynecol 80: 812–816

41. Kaminski PF, Stevens CW (1988) The value of endometrial sampling in abnormal uterine bleeding. Am J Gynecol Health II: 33–36

42. Katayma KP, Jones HW (1967) Chromosomes of atypical (adenomatous) hyperplasia and carcinoma of the endometrium. Am J Obstet Gynecol 97: 978–983

43. King A, Seraj IM, Wagner RJ (1984) Stromal invasion in endometrial carcinoma. Am J Obstet Gynecol 149: 10–14

44. Klemi PJ, Gronroos M, Rauramo L, Punnonen R (1980) Ultrastructural features of endometrial atypical adenomatous hyperplasia and adenocarcinomas and the plasma levels of estrogens. Gynecol Oncol 9: 162–169

45. Kraus FT (1985) High-risk and premalignant lesions of the endometrium. Am J Surg Pathol 9(3)(suppl): 31–40

46. Kurman RJ, Scully RE (1976) Clear cell carcinoma of the endometrium. An analysis of 21 cases. Cancer 37: 872–882

47. Kurman RJ, Norris HJ (1982) Evaluation of criteria for distinguishing atypical endometrial hyperplasia from well differentiated carcinoma. Cancer 49: 2547–2559

48. Kurman RJ, Kaminski PF, Norris HJ (1985) The behavior of endometrial hyperplasia. A long-term study of "untreated" hyperplasia in 170 patients. Cancer 56: 403–412

49. Kurman RJ, Norris HJ (1986) Endometrium. In: Henson D, Albores Saavedra J (eds) The Pathology of Incipient Neoplasia. Philadelphia, W. B. Saunders, p 265

50. Lee KR, Scully RE (1989) Complex endometrial hyperplasia and carcinoma in adolescents and young women 15 to 20 years of age. Int J Gynecol Pathol 8: 201–212

51. Leof EB, Wharton W, van Wyk JJ, Pledger WJ (1992) Epidermal growth factor (EGF) and somatomedin C regulate G1 progression in competent BALB/c-3T3 cells. Exp Cell Res 141: 107–115

52. Lidor AB, Ismajovich B, Confino E, David MP (1986) Histopathological findings in 226 women with postmenopausal uterine bleeding. Acta Obstet Gynecol Scand 65: 41–43

53. Liotta LA, Rao CN, Barsky SH (1983) Tumor invasion and the extracellular matrix. Lab Invest 49: 636–649

54. Mack TM, Pike MC, Henderson BE, Pfeffer RI, Gerkins VR, Arthur M, Brown SE (1976) Estrogens and endometrial cancer in a retirement community. N Engl J Med 294: 1262–1267

55. Masterson R, Armstrong EM, Moore IAR (1975) The cyclical variation in the percentage of ciliated cells in the normal human endometrium. J Reprod Fertil 42: 537–540

56. Mazur MT (1981) Atypical polypoid adenomyomas of the endometrium. Am J Surg Pathol 5: 473–482

57. McBride JM (1959) Pre-menopausal cystic hyperplasia and endometrial carcinoma. J Obstet Gynaecol Br Emp 66: 288–296

58. McDonald TW, Anneggers JF, O'Fallon WM, Dockerty MB, Malkasian GD, Kurland LT (1977) Exogenous estrogen and endometrial carcinoma: Case-control and incidence study. Am J Obstet Gynecol 127: 572–580

59. Norris HJ, Tavassoli FA, Kurman RJ (1983) Endometrial hyperplasia and carcinoma. Diagnostic considerations. Am J Surg Pathol 7: 839–846
60. Norris HJ, Becker RL, Mikel UV (1989) A comparative morphometric and cytophotometric study of endometrial hyperplasia, atypical hyperplasia, and endometrial carcinoma. Hum Pathol 20: 219–223
61. Novak E, Rutledge F (1948) Atypical endometrial hyperplasia simulating adenocarcinoma. Am J Obstet Gynecol 55: 46–63
62. Richart RM, Ludwig AS (1969) Alterations in chromosomes and DNA content in gynecologic neoplasms. Am J Obstet Gynecol 104: 463–471
63. Richart RM, Ferenczy A (1974) Endometrial morphologic response to hormonal environment. Gynecol Oncol 2: 180–197
64. Rorat E, Wallach RC (1984) Papillary metaplasia of the endometrium: Clinical and histopathologic considerations. Obstet Gynecol 64: 90S–92S
65. Rozengurt E, Sinnett-Smith J, Taylor-Papadimitriou J (1985) Production of PDGF-like growth factor by breast cancer cell lines. Int J Cancer 36: 247–252
66. Salm R (1962) Macrophages in endometrial lesions. J Pathol Bacteriol 83: 405–409
67. Sawhney N, Garrahan N, Douglas-Jones AG, Williams ED (1992) Epithelial-tromal interactions in tumors. A morphologic study of fibroepithelial tumors of the breast. Cancer 70: 2115–2120
68. Scully RE, Poulson H, Sobin L (in press) World Health Organization—Histologic Typing of Tumors of the Female Genital Tract. Heidelberg, Springer-Verlag
69. Seemayer TA, Schurch W, Lagace R, Tremblay G (1979) Myofibroblasts in the stroma of invasive and metastatic carcinoma. Am J Surg Pathol 3: 525–533
70. Silver MM, Miles P, Rosa C (1991) Comparison of Novak and Pipelle endometrial biopsy instruments. Obstet Gynecol 78: 828–830
71. Silverberg SG, Kurman RJ (1992) Atlas of Tumor Pathology. Tumors of the Uterine Corpus and Gestational Trophoblastic Disease, Third Series, Fascicle 3, Armed Forces Institute of Pathology, Washington, D.C.
72. Smith DC, Prentice R, Thompson DJ, Hermann WL (1975) Association of exogenous estrogen and endometrial carcinoma. N Engl J Med 293: 1164–1167
73. Smith P, Bakos O, Heimer G, Ulmsten U (1991) Transvaginal ultrasound for identifying endometrial abnormality. Acta Obstet Gynecol Scand 70: 591–594
74. Stock RJ, Kanbour A (1975) A prehysterectomy curettage. Obstet Gynecol 45: 537–541
75. Stovall TG, Ling FW, Morgan PL (1991) A prospective, randomized comparison of the Pipelle endometrial sampling device with the Novak curette. Am J Obstet Gynecol 165: 1287–1289
76. Tavassoli FA, Kraus FT (1978) Endometrial lesions in uteri resected for atypical endometrial hyperplasia. Am J Clin Pathol 70: 770–779
77. Tobon H, Watkins GJ (1985) Secretory adenocarcinoma of the endometrium. Int J Gynecol Pathol 4: 328–335
78. Wagner D, Richart RM, Terner JY (1967) Deoxyribonucleic acid content of presumed precursors of endometrial carcinoma. Cancer 20: 2067–2077
79. Welch WR, Scully RE (1977) Precancerous lesions of the endometrium. Hum Pathol 8: 503–512
80. Zaman SS, Mazur MT (1993) Endometrial papillary syncytial change. A nonspecific alteration associated with active breakdown. Am J Clin Pathol 99: 741–745
81. Ziel HK, Finkle WD (1975) Increased risk of endometrial carcinoma among users of conjugated estrogens. N Engl J Med 293: 1167–1170

12

Endometrial Carcinoma

Robert J. Kurman, M.D., Richard J. Zaino, M.D., and Henry J. Norris, M.D.

Epidemiology and Etiology

Endometrial carcinoma is the most common invasive neoplasm of the female genital tract and the fourth most frequently diagnosed cancer in the United States. In 1991 there were an estimated 33,000 new cases and approximately 4000 deaths resulting from this neoplasm.[11,190] World-wide, approximately 150,000 cases are diagnosed each year, making endometrial carcinoma the fifth leading cancer in women.[176] The incidence of endometrial cancer varies widely throughout the world. In developing countries in Asia, Africa, and South America as well as in Japan the incidence is four to five times lower than in industrialized countries in Europe and North America.[67]

Hormonal Stimulation

The strong association between replacement estrogen therapy and the development of endometrial cancer[98,100,153,154,222,267] was demonstrated in a number of case control studies in the late 1970s and was confirmed by the changing incidence rates of endometrial carcinoma in the United States over the past 40 years. The rates parallel the changing drug regimens used for postmenopausal hormone replacement therapy during this period.[103,247] Thus, the average annual age-adjusted incidence rate rose from 23.2 per 100,000 in 1950 to 33.2 in 1975 when unopposed estrogen therapy was used and then declined to 21.3 in 1988 reflecting the addition of progestational agents. It has been shown that women using unopposed estrogen for more than 2 years have a two- to threefold increase in the risk of endometrial cancer, whereas women receiving progestins in conjunction with estrogen have no increased risk.[177] The decline in rates of endometrial cancer since 1975 is confined to women in their 50s, whereas a slight, continuous rise in endometrial cancer rates is observed for women older than 60. The increase in the incidence of endometrial cancer occurring in most countries is thought to be in part due to the aging of the population and probably is not related to estrogen exposure.

The role of unopposed estrogen stimulation in endometrial carcinogenesis is so strong that any factor that mediates this effect, such as obesity or chronic anovulation, increases the risk. For example, although several studies have shown that nulliparity is a risk factor,[179,184,256] a recent study demonstrated that it was not nulliparity per se but rather infertility related to anovulation that is responsible for the increased risk.[79] In contrast, factors that lower the exposure of the endometrium to unopposed estrogen reduce the risk of endometrial cancer, these include the addition of progesterone to hormone replacement regimens, the use of oral contraceptives, or smoking.[85,142] Several case control studies have shown that the use of oral contraceptives for at least 1 year reduces the risk of endometrial carcinoma by 50% and that protection persists at least 15 years after discontinuation.[33] Protection is most profound for women of low parity who are characteristically at higher risk of developing endometrial carcinoma.

Recent studies suggest that tamoxifen may be associated with the development of endometrial carcinoma. Tamoxifen is a nonsteroidal compound that acts by competing with estrogen for estrogen receptors. In reproductive age women it therefore has an antiestrogenic effect but in hypoestrogenic, that is, postmenopausal women, it has weak estrogenic effects. More than 60 cases of endometrial adenocarcinoma in women with breast cancer who have been treated with tamoxifen have been reported.[210] The tumors were International Federation of Gynecology and Obstetrics (FIGO) stage I in 93% of cases, grade 1 in 40%, and grade 2 or 3 in 60%. Carcinoma was reported with dosages as low as 20 mg/day. The duration of treatment was less than 2 years in 57% of patients. In a study of 1800 postmenopausal women with breast cancer who were treated with tamoxifen, there was a statistically significant difference of developing endometrial carcinoma in the treated compared with the control group.[84] The risk of endometrial carcinoma was significantly greater in those women treated for more than 2 years, although most patients developed carcinoma within 2 years. In another study it was shown that, compared with controls, the risk of endometrial carcinoma in the treated group was 1.7–3.3.[12]

Constitutional Factors

Constitutional factors associated with endometrial carcinoma include low parity, obesity, hypertension, and possibly diabetes mellitus.[184,256] Overt diabetes has been reported in less than 2% to more than 40%[96,194] and abnormal glucose tolerance tests from 10% to 65%.[68,194,256] The effect of obesity is related to the enhanced conversion of androstenedione to estrone in fat cells.[15,149,150,204] Again, the overriding effect appears to be unopposed estrogen stimulation, not necessarily obesity. Nonetheless, slender women, ovulating women, and women who are pregnant also may develop endometrial carcinoma.[191] These women represent a subgroup of patients whose endocrine–metabolic profiles are not significantly different from those of control subjects. This suggests that their tumors are not associated with an obvious endocrine or metabolic disorder[150] or that their neoplasms are estrogen-related but arise in progesterone refractory endometrium.[191] These endometrial carcinomas frequently are occult and are not associated with vaginal bleeding.

Diet

The rates of endometrial carcinoma increase in first and second generation Japanese women born in the United States,[104] suggesting that factors such as the high content of animal fat in the Western diet[102] may be an etiologic factor in the development of endometrial carcinoma. Total energy intake and obesity are closely correlated. Although there is some evidence that the intake of animal proteins and fat increase the risk of endometrial cancer and that fresh fruit, vegetables and fibers decrease the risk, the exact role of diet is not clear.[145] Studies analyzing obesity in these patients reveal that after adjusting for age, parity, and smoking status, women with upper body fat have a three-fold higher risk of endometrial cancer than women with lower body fat.[74]

Genetic Aspects

Several studies have shown a high incidence of both endometrial carcinoma and breast cancer among sisters, mothers, and aunts of individuals with endometrial carcinoma,[152,164,251] suggesting a genetic predisposition. More recently it has been proposed that there are two forms of heritable endometrial carcinoma: (1) a cancer family syndrome (Lynch syndrome II) and (2) a predisposition for endometrial carcinoma alone.[26,201] In the Lynch syndrome II, males and females are at an increased risk of developing colon cancer and other adenocarcinomas; females are at an increased risk for ovarian carcinoma and 20–30% of affected women develop endometrial carcinoma.[156]

Two Types of Endometrial Carcinoma

The differences noted in the epidemiology, presentation, and behavior of endometrial carcinoma suggest that there may be two different forms of the disease: an estrogen-related neoplasm that occurs in younger, perimenopausal women and tends to be low grade and a second, more virulent form, unrelated to estrogenic stimulation, that occurs in older postmenopausal women.[25,224] For purposes of this discussion the former is designated type I (estrogen-related) and the latter type II (non–estrogen-related) (Table 12.1).

Several lines of epidemiologic and clinicopathological evidence support the hypothesis that there are two pathogenetic forms of endometrial carcinoma. In one study[192] it was shown that carcinomas in estrogen users are better differentiated than are those in nonestrogen users. Only 4 (12%) of 33 of the estrogen users had poorly differentiated carcinoma compared with 30 (37%) of 81 of the nonusers, suggesting that the development of poorly differentiated adenocarcinoma is unrelated to the use of estrogen. A more recent study showed that compared with nonusers, women on estrogen therapy were younger and had more superficially invasive, lower grade, and lower stage tumors.[172] Further evidence that estrogen plays a role in only the type I tumors also is provided by the finding of significantly higher progesterone receptor levels, which are increased by estrogen, in the type I as compared with the type II group.[65]

There appear to be histological correlates between type I and type II endometrial carcinomas. It has been reported that adenomatous hyperplasia was found more frequently in association with type I as compared with type II tumors.[64] This analysis also showed that endometrioid and mucinous carcinomas segregated into the type I group, whereas "papillary carcinoma" (serous carcinoma), clear cell carcinoma, and anaplastic carcinoma segregated into the type II group. Similar observations were made in a study comparing the histological features of carcinomas in postmenopausal women with and without previous estrogen replacement treatment.[172] In this study the frequency of clear cell and adenosquamous carcinoma was lower in the estrogen users. These findings suggest that the type I tumors are composed of low-grade endometrioid carcinomas including mucinous and secretory carcinomas whereas the type II tumors are composed of serous, clear cell carcinomas, and poorly differentiated carcinomas including adenosquamous carcinoma.

Precursors of Endometrial Carcinoma

Endometrial hyperplasia has long been regarded as a precursor of endometrial carcinoma. Subsequent division of hyperplasia into those with and without cytological atypia provided evidence that hyperplasia without atypia is a manifestation of unopposed estrogenic stimulation but by itself is not a precursor of endometrial carcinoma. This conclusion is based on long-term follow-up studies that reveal that only 2% of hyperplasias without atypia progress to carcinoma. In contrast, nearly one-quarter of atypical hyperplasias progress to well-differentiated endometrial carcinoma, indicating that this lesion is a precursor of endometrioid carcinoma.[138] Furthermore, since no serous carcinomas were found in this study, the findings suggested that atypical hyperplasia is a precursor of type I carcinoma only. A large cytological screening study of 2586 asymptomatic women, however, indicates that a substantial number of endometrioid carcinomas are not preceded by atypical hyperplasia either. Based on the progression rate of atypical hyperplasia to carcinoma, it was expected that there would be eight times as many cases of hyperplasia identified in asymptomatic women compared with carcinoma, but the observed ratio was 1.5:1.[131] The carcinomas detected in this study were endometrioid, not serous carcinomas (Koss LG: personal communication), supporting the view that not all endometrioid carcinomas are preceded by atypical hyperplasia.

In a more recent study, atypical hyperplasia was found adjacent to endometrioid carcinoma in nearly 40% of cases but was not present in association with serous carcinomas. Atypical hyperplasia was distributed equally among all grades of endometrioid carcinoma not concentrated in the low-grade carcinomas. Three-quarters of the serous carcinomas were associated with atrophic endometria compared with only 30% of the endometrioid carcinomas, suggesting that atypical hyperplasia was a precursor of approximately 40% of endometrioid carcinomas but not involved in the genesis of serous carcinoma (Ambros R, et al., unpublished data). Of additional interest was the finding of a lesion designated *endometrial intraepithelial carcinoma* (see below, Serous Carcinoma) in the adjacent endometrium of nearly 90% of serous carcinomas but in only 6% of the endometrioid carcinomas, suggesting that intraepithelial carcinoma may be the precursor of serous carcinoma.

Table 12.1. Endometrial carcinoma: two types

	Type I	Type II
Unopposed estrogen	Present	Absent
Menopausal status	Pre- and perimenopausal	Postmenopausal
Hyperplasia	Present	Absent
Race	White	Black
Grade	Low	High
Myometrial invasion	Minimal	Deep
Specific subtypes	Endometrioid	Serous
		Clear cell
Behavior	Stable	Progressive

Classification

The recent World Health Organization (WHO) and International Society of Gynecological Pathologists (ISGYP) classification of endometrial carcinoma[205] is shown in Table 12.2. The presentation of the various histological types in this chapter adheres closely to this classification. Recent studies, however, indicate that this classification has certain limitations, which are summarized below.

The WHO classification has a category of *serous papillary carcinoma* but does not include *villoglandular* carcinoma as a separate entity. Although uterine serous carcinomas often are designated *papillary*, a papillary growth pattern is not associated with a specific cell type. In addition to serous carcinomas, some endometrioid carcinomas, notably villoglandular carcinoma, as well as mucinous and clear cell carcinomas also may display a papillary pattern. Thus, the designation of "papillary" is ambiguous and misleading. For example, Christopherson et al.[47] included papillary carcinoma containing clear cells in the category of clear cell carcinoma, but papillary tumors displaying endometrioid and serous patterns were included in the category of papillary adenocarcinoma. In contrast, Hendrickson et al.[108] regarded papillary carcinomas with an endometrioid pattern as "villoglandular carcinoma" and those with the serous pattern as "uterine papillary carcinoma," emphasizing that the latter was a highly aggressive subtype. The importance of separating papillary tumors with an endometrioid pattern from those with a serous pattern was confirmed by Chen and associates, who demonstrated a significantly better prognosis for patients with villoglandular as compared with papillary serous carcinoma.[42] Preliminary findings from a Gynecologic Oncology Group (GOG) analysis confirm these findings (RJ Zaino and RJ Kurman, unpublished data). Accordingly, it is important to classify separately serous and villoglandular carcinomas and avoid the term *papillary* entirely.

Serous carcinoma and *clear cell carcinoma* are designated separately in the WHO classification; however, several studies have demonstrated that the two neoplasms frequently co-exist and are associated so intimately that they cannot always be reliably separated.[108,140,211] Endometrial clear cell carcinoma may display tubular, cystic, papillary, and solid patterns.[45,137] Although these patterns often are admixed in ovarian tumors, the tubulocystic pattern predominates in cervical and vaginal clear cell carcinomas whereas the papillary and solid patterns are encountered most frequently in endometrial tumors. Moreover, all of the architectural patterns of clear cell carcinoma can be observed in endometrioid carcinomas. It has been argued that the presence of clear cytoplasm is not a specific finding in endometrial carcinomas[108] and indeed cells with glycogen-rich clear cytoplasm occur in secretory carcinoma, serous carcinoma, and at times in the squamous component of an endometrioid carcinoma. The other type of cell that is commonly found in clear cell carcinoma is the hobnail cell, but this cell is found just as frequently in serous carcinoma.

In addition to the morphologic heterogeneity of clear cell carcinoma, the 5-year survival for all stages as reported in different studies varies from 21%[214] to 75%.[126] Between these extremes, 5-year survivals of 36%,[45] 42%,[3a] 48%,[180] 55%,[137] and 64%[252] have been reported. This wide range in survival and the diverse morphologic findings suggest that tumors currently classified as clear cell carcinoma represent a heterogeneous group of tumors with different clinical and pathological features. In our opinion, clear cell carcinoma of the endometrium as currently defined does not represent a distinct clinicopathological entity. Based on the morphologic features and associations with other endometrial carcinomas, we believe that papillary and solid patterns of clear cell carcinoma with high-grade nuclei should be classified as variants of serous carcinoma. These tumors have a poor prognosis. In contrast, the tubulocystic and the solid pattern of clear cell carcinoma with low-grade nuclei can be regarded as variants of endometrioid carcinoma. These tumors have a relatively good prognosis. Because these concepts have not been evaluated completely, the presentation of clear cell carcinoma in this chapter follows the conventional teaching as delineated in the WHO classification.

Malignant mixed mesodermal tumors (MMMTs) and carcinosarcomas are classified as mixed epithelial and non-epithelial tumors in the WHO classification of uterine tumors but curiously as epithelial tumors in the ovarian tumor classification. This inconsistency reflects the confusion over the histogenesis and classification of carcinosarcomas in different anatomic sites. The debate over whether these biphasic tumors arise from transformation of a single (epithelial) clone with bidirectional differentiation or whether transformation occurs independently from separate epithelial and mesenchymal populations is not resolved fully, but the weight of evidence favors the former view. The literature on this subject is extensive and has

Table 12.2. Classification of endometrial carcinoma[a]

Endometrioid adenocarcinoma
    Villoglandular
    Secretory
    Ciliated cell
    Endometrioid adenocarcinoma with squamous differentiation
Serous carcinoma
Clear cell carcinoma
Mucinous carcinoma
Squamous carcinoma
Mixed types of carcinoma
Undifferentiated carcinoma

[a] Modified World Health Organization and International Society of Gynecological Pathologists Histologic Classification of Endometrial Carcinoma.[205]

been summarized in a symposium devoted to this subject.[254] Briefly, electron microscopic and immunohistochemical studies demonstrate an intimate admixture of cells manifesting both epithelial and mesenchymal properties. Immunohistochemical studies in particular showing cytokeratin and epithelial membrane antigen reactivity in spindle cells within the mesenchymal component that merge with rounded cells showing subtle but clear-cut evidence of glandular differentiation are most persuasive in supporting an epithelial origin of these tumors.[24,63,95,157] Recent cloning studies of MMMT cell lines in which cells with adenocarcinoma and sarcoma features were cloned and propagated independently have confirmed these observations.[76,97] Light microscopic, ultrastructural, and immunohistochemical studies of the tumor derived from the carcinoma clone displayed epithelial and sarcomatous cells as well as transitional-type cells. In contrast, the tumor derived from the sarcoma clone showed no epithelial differentiation. Furthermore, tumors from the adenocarcinoma clone when transplanted into nude mice showed both adenocarcinomatous and sarcomatous components similar to the original neoplasm. Cytogenetic analysis demonstrated common karyotypic abnormalities in both the carcinoma and sarcoma clones, indicating that the two tumor populations were monoclonal in origin. Molecular analysis for c-myc gene amplification revealed that it was present in the original tumor as well as in both the carcinoma and the sarcoma clones.[76]

Finally, the behavior of uterine MMMTs parallels more closely that of highly aggressive endometrial carcinomas than sarcomas, judging from the pattern of spread and the histological appearance of the tumor in vascular channels and in metastatic sites.[24,217] Typically, the tumor in vessels and in metastatic sites is a carcinoma even when most of the primary uterine tumor has a "sarcomatous" appearance. Thus, the data support the view that MMMTs are biphasic tumors demonstrating both epithelial and mesenchymal differentiation but that it is the epithelial component that dictates behavior. Accordingly, these neoplasms are now considered by many investigators as carcinomas and designated sarcomatoid carcinoma. Because this view has not been completely accepted, these neoplasms are presented in Chapter 13, Mesenchymal Tumors of the Uterus, under the designation MMMT.

Clinical and Pathological Features

Endometrioid Carcinoma

This is the most common form of endometrial carcinoma, accounting for more than three-fourths of all cases. These tumors are referred to as *endometrioid* to maintain consistency with the terminology used for describing tumors with the same histological appearance in the cervix, ovary, or fallopian tube. The tumors in this category, by definition, do not contain areas showing more than 10% of squamous, serous, mucinous, or clear cell differentiation. Such foci are common in endometrioid carcinoma and are designated as *mixed* (see Mixed Types of Carcinoma).

CLINICAL FEATURES

Patients with endometrioid carcinoma range in age from the second to the eighth decade, with a mean age of 59 years. Most women are postmenopausal as the disease is relatively uncommon in young women. The prevalence is 3% in women under 40 years and there have been approximately 21 cases reported in women under the age of 30 years, the youngest being 15 years.[82] In young women, the tumor is generally low grade and minimally invasive. However, a poorly differentiated, stage IV carcinoma has been reported in a 25-year-old.[243] Nearly half of women with tumors under the age of 40 years are nulliparous and more than three-quarters are obese. Rarely, endometrioid carcinoma occurs during pregnancy. In half these patients the gestation is at an early stage and is incidental in women known to have carcinoma. In others, the tumor has been detected at the time of a therapeutic or spontaneous abortion.[230] In pregnant women, endometrial carcinomas are nearly always low grade, superficially or noninvasive, and have an excellent prognosis.[112] The tumors generally do not show histological evidence of progesterone-induced changes.

The initial manifestation of endometrial carcinoma usually is abnormal vaginal bleeding, although rarely the patient is asymptomatic and the diagnosis is made fortuitously. In one study 24 asymptomatic women with unsuspected endometrial carcinoma were detected among 8998 women dying of unrelated causes who were autopsied at the Yale–New Haven and Massachusetts General Hospitals. The estimated rates of undetected endometrial carcinoma were 22 and 31 per 10,000, respectively. These rates were four to five times higher than the diagnosis of endometrial carcinoma recorded by the Connecticut State Tumor Registry, indicating that a small number of endometrial carcinomas may be asymptomatic and are undetected during life.[114]

A number of studies have evaluated cytological screening of endometrial cancer. Both direct endometrial sampling as well as examination of cervical cytological smears for the presence of endometrial carcinoma have been performed. In a study of 2586 asymptomatic women the prevalence of occult carcinoma using endometrial cytological sampling was 6.96 per 1000; however, four cases were missed. In addition, the investigators emphasized that endometrial smears were difficult to interpret and that the detection methods were only moderately reliable.[131] About a third of the cases would have been detected using a vaginal pool specimen. In a population-based study from

Australia it was found that when a cervical smear was reported as showing endometrial carcinoma, the lesion was confirmed histologically in only 64% of cases. Conversely, among women with endometrial carcinoma a cervical smear performed in the 2 years preceding the diagnosis predicted the presence of endometrial carcinoma in only 28% of cases.[160] In an attempt to use cytological screening in specific high-risk populations it was reported that among 597 asymptomatic women with diabetes and/or hypertension the diabetic women had a significantly higher rate of atypical or "adenomatous" hyperplasia compared with women with hypertension: 6.3% versus 1.3%, respectively.[101] Since the sensitivity and specificity of cytological examination for the detection of endometrial carcinoma is low, it is not a cost-effective screening tool for endometrial cancer.

Gross Findings

The gross appearance of endometrioid carcinoma is similar to the various other types of endometrial carcinoma with the possible exception of serous carcinoma (see below, Serous Carcinoma). The endometrial surface is shaggy, glistening, and tan and may be focally hemorrhagic. Endometrioid carcinoma is almost uniformly exophytic even when deeply invasive (Fig. 12.1). The neoplasm may be

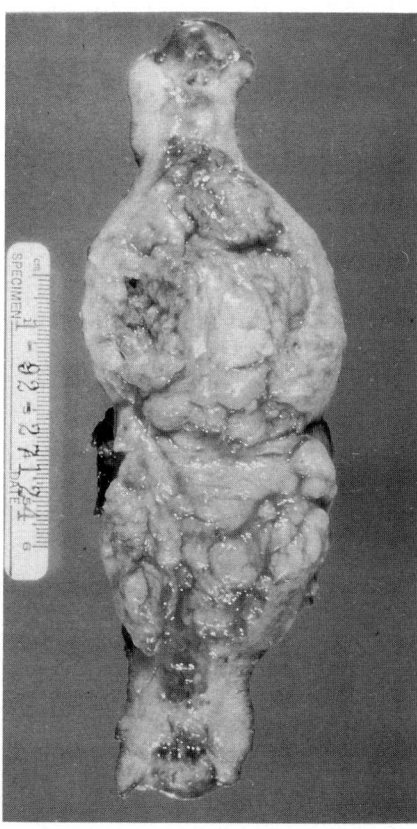

Fig. 12.1. Endometrioid carcinoma. The tumor is exophytic and diffusely involves the endometrium.

focal or diffuse. At times the tumor may appear to be composed of separate polypoid masses. Necrosis usually is not evident macroscopically in well-differentiated carcinomas but may be seen in poorly differentiated tumors, sometimes in association with ulcerated or firm areas. Myometrial invasion by carcinoma may result in enlargement of the uterus, but a small atrophic uterus may harbor carcinoma diffusely invading the myometrium. Myometrial invasion appears as well-demarcated, firm, gray-white tissue with linear extensions beneath an exophytic mass or as multiple, white nodules with yellow areas of necrosis within the uterine wall. Extension to the cervix often occurs.

Microscopic Findings

The microscopic appearance of endometrioid carcinoma is determined by the grade of the tumor. Most endometrioid carcinomas are well differentiated (see Chapter 11, Endometrial Hyperplasia and Related Cellular Changes). The microscopic appearance of higher grade carcinoma reflects the architectural and nuclear alterations associated with increasing grade (see below).

Microscopic Grading

Grading is based on the architectural pattern, nuclear features, or both. The architectural grade is determined by the extent to which the tumor is composed of solid masses of cells as compared with well-defined glands (Table 12.3; Figs. 12.2–12.4). In endometrioid carcinomas with squamous differentiation it is important to exclude masses of squamous epithelium in determining grade, specifically, how much of the tumor is growing in a solid pattern apart from the squamous differentiation. It is not unusual to see low-grade tumors with large masses of bland-appearing squamous epithelium and to include these areas in the evaluation would falsely elevate the grade (see Endometrioid Carcinoma with Squamous Differentiation). The nuclear grade is determined by the variation in nuclear size and shape, chromatin distribution, and size of the nucleoli (Table 12.4; Figs. 12.5–12.7). Mitotic activity is an independent histological variable but it is generally increased with increasing nuclear grade, as are abnormal mitotic figures.

The most recent revision of the FIGO Staging System[58] (Table 12.5) as well as the WHO Histopathologic Classification of uterine carcinoma recommend that tumors be graded using both architectural and nuclear criteria. The grade of tumors that are architecturally grade 1 or 2 should

Table 12.3. Architectural grading of endometrial carcinoma

Grade 1	No more than 5% of the tumor is composed of solid masses
Grade 2	6–50% of the tumor is composed of solid masses
Grade 3	More than 50% of the tumor is composed of solid masses

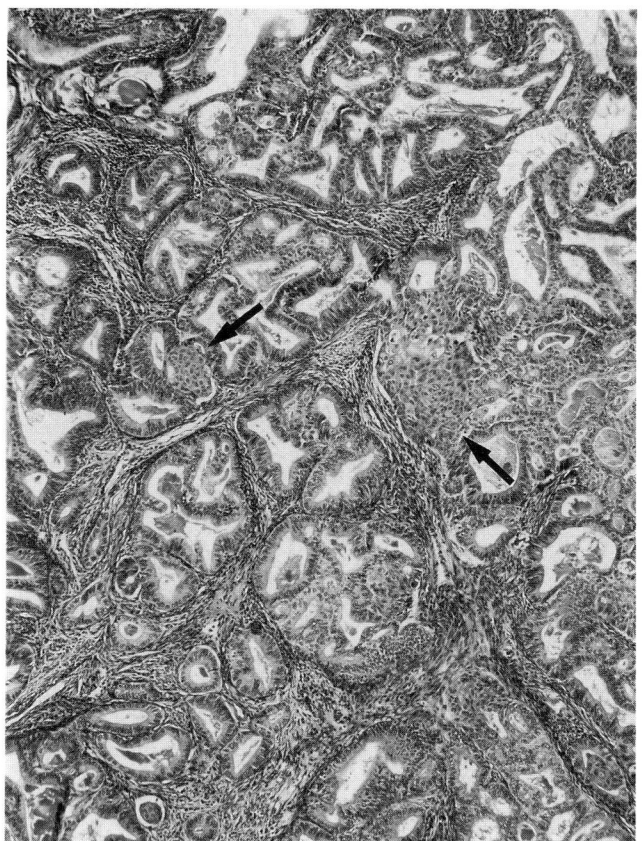

FIG. 12.2. Endometrioid carcinoma, architectural grade 1. The tumor is composed exclusively of well-formed glands. Two small foci of squamous differentiation *(arrows)* are present but because these contribute less than 10% of the tumor, their presence need not be specified.

be increased by one grade in the presence of "notable" nuclear atypia. Notable is not defined but, based on findings from a GOG study, we regard notable as grade 3 atypia.[266] For example, a tumor that is grade 1 by architecture but in which there is marked nuclear atypia (nuclear grade 3) should be upgraded to grade 2. Thus, tumors are graded primarily by their architecture with the overall grade modified by the nuclear grade when there is discordance. Marked differences in architectural grade can be seen within a tumor. It is not unusual to see well-formed glandular elements immediately adjacent to solid masses of cells. When a tumor displays this type of heterogeneity the architectural grade should be based on the overall appear-

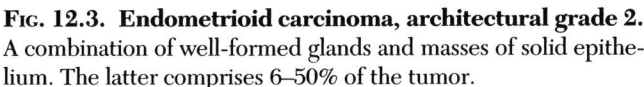

FIG. 12.3. Endometrioid carcinoma, architectural grade 2. A combination of well-formed glands and masses of solid epithelium. The latter comprises 6–50% of the tumor.

FIG. 12.4. Endometrioid carcinoma, architectural grade 3. Only rare gland lumens are present in an otherwise solid proliferation of epithelium.

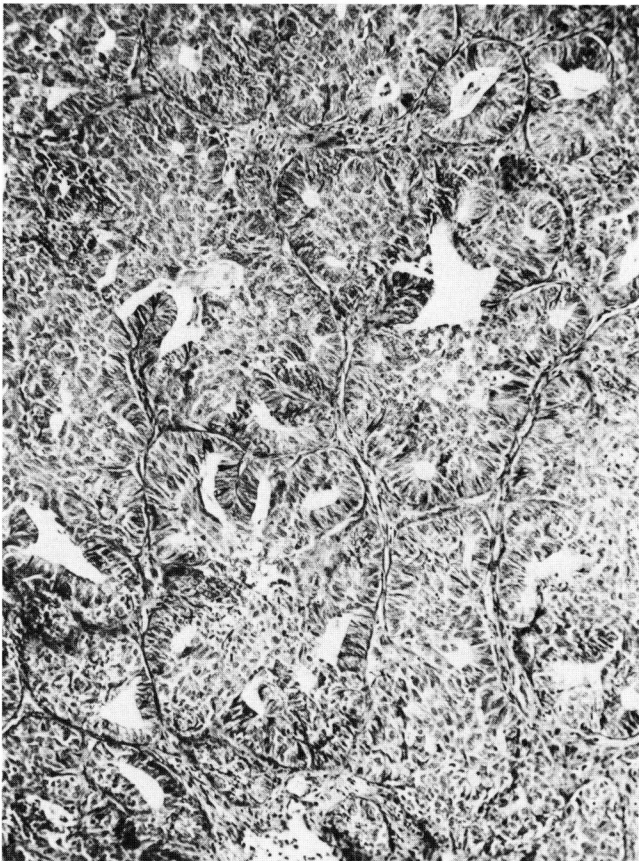

12.3

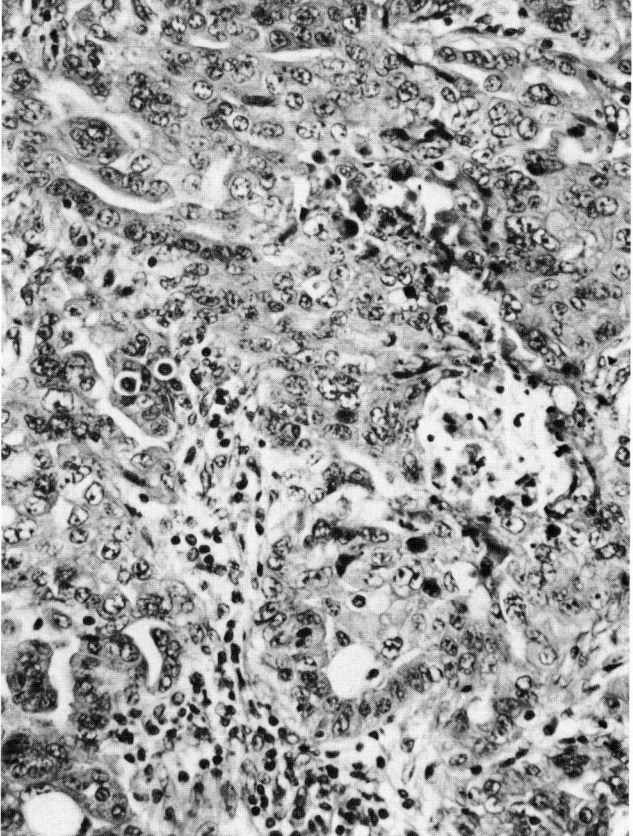

12.4

Table 12.4. Nuclear grading of endometrial carcinoma

Grade 1	Cells with oval nuclei and evenly dispersed chromatin
Grade 2	Cells with nuclei that have features between grades 1 and 3
Grade 3	Cells with markedly enlarged, pleomorphic nuclei displaying irregular coarse chromatin and prominent, eosinophilic nucleoli

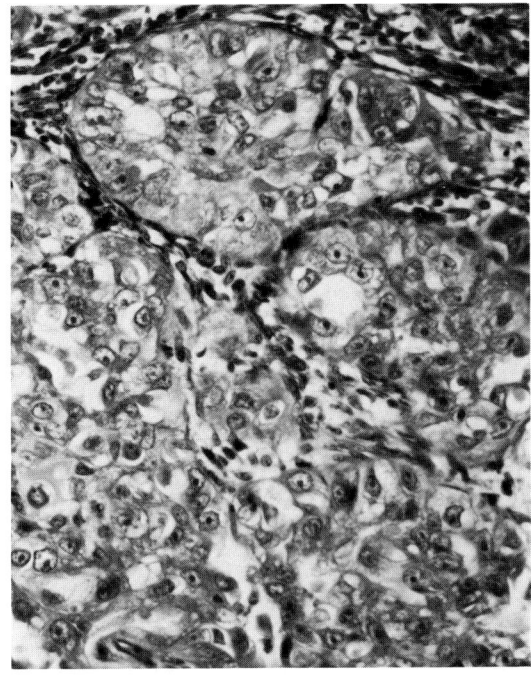

Fɪɢ. 12.5. **Endometrioid carcinoma, nuclear grade 1.** The nuclei are uniform in size, with finely dispersed chromatin.

Fɪɢ. 12.6. **Endometrioid carcinoma, nuclear grade 2.** Nuclei are enlarged relative to nuclear grade 1 and prominent nucleoli are present. The degree of pleomorphism and chromatin clumping is less than nuclear grade 3.

Fɪɢ. 12.7. **Endometrioid carcinoma, nuclear grade 3.** The nuclei are markedly enlarged and pleomorphic with large prominent nucleoli and irregular coarse chromatin.

12.6

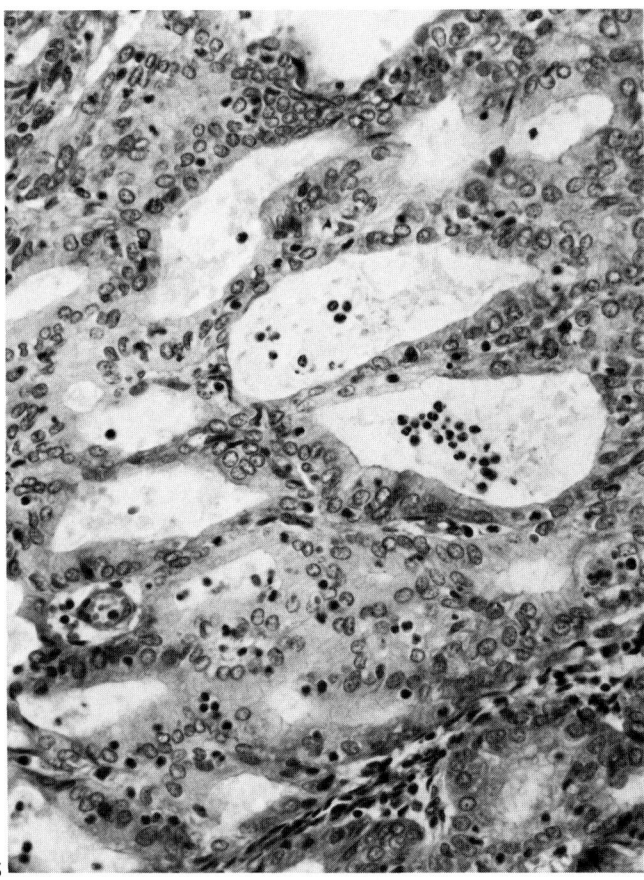

12.5

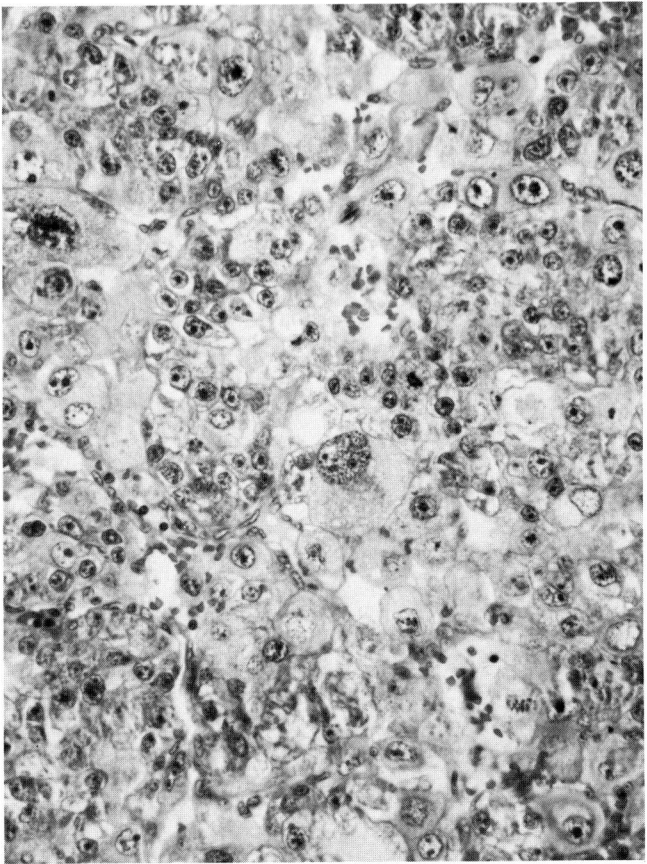

12.7

Table 12.5. International Federation of Gynecology and Obstetrics Staging of Endometrial Cancer, 1988

IA	G1223	Tumor limited to the endometrium
IB	G123	Invasion to <½ myometrium
IC	G123	Invasion to >½ myometrium
IIA	G123	Endocervical glandular involvement only
IIB	G123	Cervical stromal invasion
IIIA	G123	Tumor invades serosa and/or adnexae and/or positive peritoneal cytology
IIIB	G123	Vaginal metastases
IIIC	G123	Metastases to pelvic and/or para-aortic lymph nodes
IVA	G123	Tumor invasion of bladder and/or bowel mucosa
IVB	G123	Distant metastases including intraabdominal and/or inguinal lymph nodes

G1, 5% or less of a nonsquamous or nonmorular solid growth pattern; G2, 6–50% of a nonsquamous or nonmorular solid growth pattern; G3, more than 50% of a nonsquamous or nonmorular solid growth pattern.

Rules on staging:
1. Corpus cancer is now surgically staged. Those patients who do not undergo a surgical procedure should be staged according to the 1971 FIGO clinical staging.
2. Ideally, the thickness of the myometrium should be measured along with the depth of tumor invasion.

Notes on grading:
1. Notable nuclear atypia, inappropriate for the architectural grade, raises a grade 1 or grade 2 tumor by one.
2. In serous adenocarcinomas, clear cell adenocarcinomas, and squamous cell carcinomas, nuclear grading takes precedence.
3. Adenocarcinomas with squamous differentiation are graded according to the nuclear grade of the glandular component.

ance. The heterogeneity in differentiation accounts for the differences in grade that can be observed between the endometrial curettings and the hysterectomy specimen. Discordance between the curettage and hysterectomy specimens ranges between 20% and 30%.[53,62,136,181]

SURGICAL–PATHOLOGICAL STAGING

The stage reflects the extent of disease at the time of diagnosis. It is necessary to determine prognosis and treatment as well as to provide a standardized method of reporting data among different investigators. Effective in 1989, FIGO revised the previous clinical staging to a surgical–pathological system (Table 12.5).[58] The revision in the staging system was based on studies showing that endometrial carcinoma was frequently under- or overstaged clinically[3a] and on new data demonstrating the importance of a variety of histopathological risk factors. The new staging system requires assessment of the pelvic and para-aortic lymph nodes, adnexa, and peritoneal fluid cytology. Pathological analysis includes evaluation of the grade of the tumor, depth of myometrial invasion, and determination of endocervical involvement (see Risk Factors); therefore, it is essential that all of this information is communicated clearly in the surgical pathology report. As a result of

changes in the staging system, procedures such as a fractional curettage that were used in the past are no longer necessary.

RISK FACTORS

The vast majority (75–80%) of women with endometrial carcinoma present with tumor limited to the uterus (stages I and II) and among these women 10–25% eventually will die of disease. One of the most difficult problems in clinical management has been to identify women with stage I disease who have a substantially increased risk of developing recurrence. Based largely on a series of GOG studies,[28,57,163] it has been shown that the risk factors for endometrial carcinoma can be divided into uterine and extrauterine factors. Uterine factors include (1) histological type, (2) grade, (3) depth of myometrial invasion, (4) cervical involvement, (5) vascular invasion, (6) presence of atypical endometrial hyperplasia, (7) progesterone receptor status, and (8) DNA ploidy and S-phase fraction. Extrauterine factors include (1) adnexal involvement, (2) intraperitoneal metastasis, (3) positive peritoneal cytology, and (4) pelvic and para-aortic lymph node metastasis.[163]

Patients with no evidence of extrauterine disease, no cervical involvement, and no evidence of vascular invasion are at a low overall risk of recurrence. For these patients the grade and depth of invasion are important prognostic factors. In contrast to this low-risk group of patients, women with evidence of extrauterine disease, cervical involvement, or vascular invasion constitute a high-risk group. A recent GOG study showed that if one of these three factors was positive, the frequency of recurrence was 20% and increased to 43% for two positive factors and 63% for three factors.[163] In addition to these pathological risk factors, a number of clinical risk factors have been delineated (see below, Other Risk Factors).

GRADE

Grading methods have been discussed above (see Microscopic Grading). Numerous studies have confirmed the value of grading[86,165,168,266] According to a population-based study from the Norwegian Radium Hospital involving nearly 2000 patients, the 5- and 10-year survival rate for patients with grade 1 tumors was 88% and 80%, respectively, with grade 2 tumors 77% and 62%, and with grade 3 tumors 60% and 49%.[3a] The depth of myometrial invasion and the frequency of lymph node metastasis also are related to tumor grade. Only 12% of patients with grade 1 tumors have deep myometrial invasion, whereas 46% of those with grade 3 tumors have deep myometrial invasion.[44] Metastasis to lymph nodes occurs in 5% of patients with well-differentiated tumors but in 26% of those with poorly differentiated carcinoma.[145a]

MYOMETRIAL INVASION

In the past, depth of myometrial invasion has been re-ported as the proportion of the uterine wall invaded by tumor and expressed in thirds. More recently, the revised FIGO staging of endometrial carcinoma limited to the uterus (stage I) incorporates depth of myometrial invasion expressed as inner or outer half. Tumors confined to the endometrium are stage Ia, those involving the inner half of the myometrium are stage Ib, and those involving more than half the uterine wall thickness are stage Ic. In addi-tion, we recommend measuring the maximum depth of invasion in millimeters and expressing this as a percentage of the myometrial thickness. For example, 2 mm of myo-metrial invasion in a uterus measuring 1 cm in thickness would be 20% invasion. Tumor in vascular spaces beyond the deepest point of invasion should not be used for this measurement. An alternate method for assessing depth of invasion is to measure the uninvolved myometrium, in millimeters, from the serosa to the point of maximum tumor invasion.[151] This approach has the advantage of a more accurate measurement because the uterine serosa is readily identified in contrast to the boundary of the endo-myometrium, and a measurement in millimeters may be more easily reproducible.

Endometrial carcinoma may manifest different forms of myometrial invasion.[219] It can invade along a broad push-ing front or it can infiltrate the myometrium diffusely in varying size masses, cords, or in clusters of cells and indi-vidual glands. When it invades along a broad front it may be difficult to determine whether invasion is in fact present unless it can be compared to the adjacent uninvolved en-domyometrium. When the tumor diffusely invades the my-ometrium the neoplastic glands usually elicit a reactive stromal response characterized by loose fibrous tissue ac-companied by a chronic inflammatory infiltrate that sur-rounds the glands. Occasionally, well-differentiated carci-nomas may be deeply invasive with glands directly in contact with surrounding myometrium in the absence of a stromal response (Fig. 12.8). In these cases when myome-trial invasion is superficial the presence of invasion can be identified if a haphazard glandular arrangement is present. Usually this pattern of invasion is found in deeply invasive tumors, however, and therefore recognizing myometrial invasion is not a problem. Finally, carcinoma may be con-fined to the endometrium and invade preexisting endome-trial glands that are beyond the basalis and are in the myometrium. It is important to remember that the endo-myometrial junction is typically irregular and it is not un-usual for endometrial glands to appear to be in the myo-metrium (Fig. 12.9); this can be especially confusing in the cornual area, because of tangential sectioning. Tumors that involve these superficial glands should be reported as be-ing confined to the endometrium.

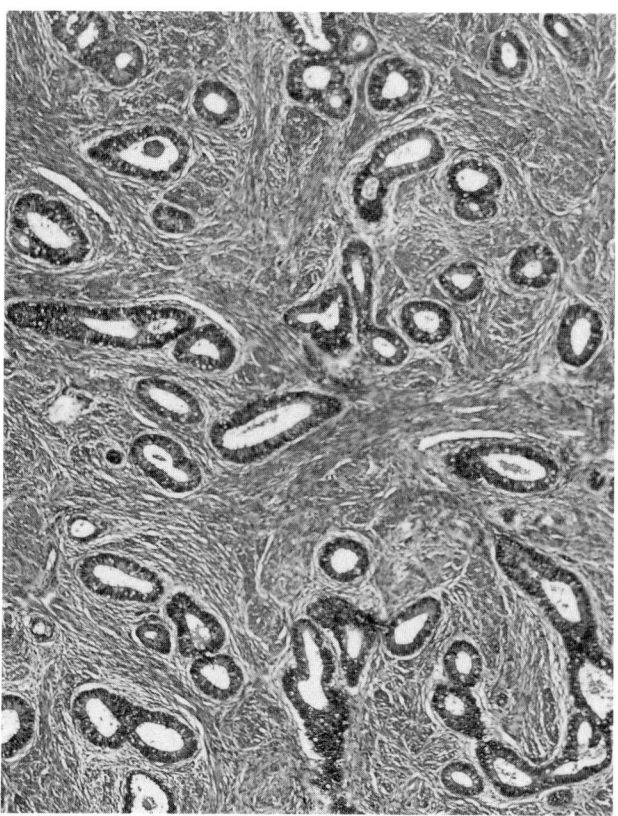

FIG. 12.8. Endometrioid carcinoma, FIGO grade 1. Well-formed glands diffusely invade the myometrium. Surrounding reactive change is minimal.

It may be difficult to distinguish myometrial invasion from extension of the carcinoma into adenomyosis. The distinction, however, is important because the presence of carcinoma in adenomyosis deeper than the maximum depth of true tumor invasion does not worsen the progno-sis.[105,110,120,161] When the carcinoma is surrounded by en-dometrial stroma and residual benign glands are present in these foci, the diagnosis of carcinoma extending into ade-nomyosis is straightforward (Fig. 12.10). At times, how-ever, the distinction from myometrial invasion may be ex-tremely difficult. This is particularly true in older women in whom adenomyosis may have very minimal stroma as a result of fibrosis and atrophy. In these cases it is necessary to evaluate additional features such as the presence of desmoplasia, surrounding edema and inflammation, and the shape of the glands.[120] In contrast to carcinoma involv-ing adenomyosis, true myometrial invasion is characterized by desmoplasia or loosening of the myometrium surround-ing the glands. Often there is accompanying chronic in-flammation and the glandular outline is jagged and irregu-lar as compared to carcinoma involving adenomyosis in which the glands have a smooth, rounded outline and des-moplasia and inflammation are lacking (Fig. 12.11). A re-

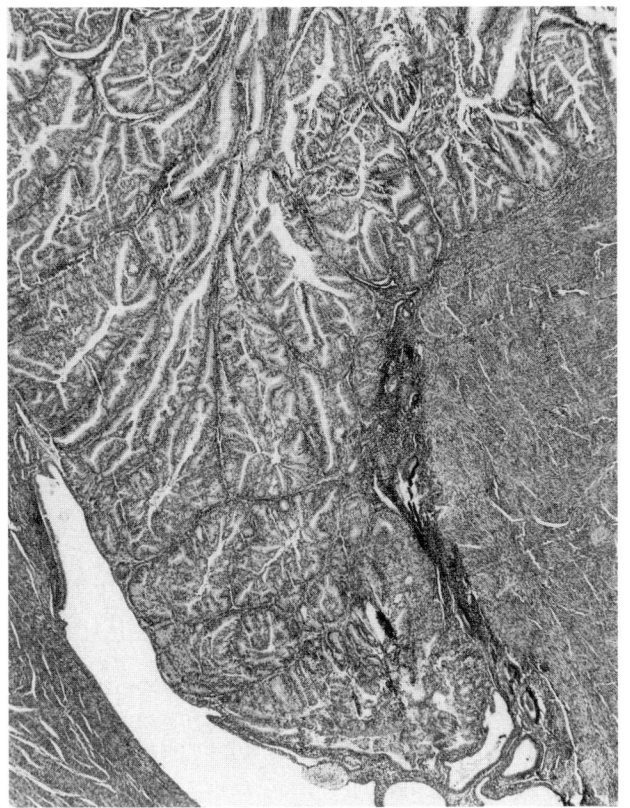

FIG. 12.9. **Endometrioid carcinoma, FIGO grade 1.** The tumor is involving endometrial glands that appear to be in the myometrium. This is because of the irregular endomyometrial junction. The tumor in this case is in the cornual region heightening the appearance of myometrial invasion.

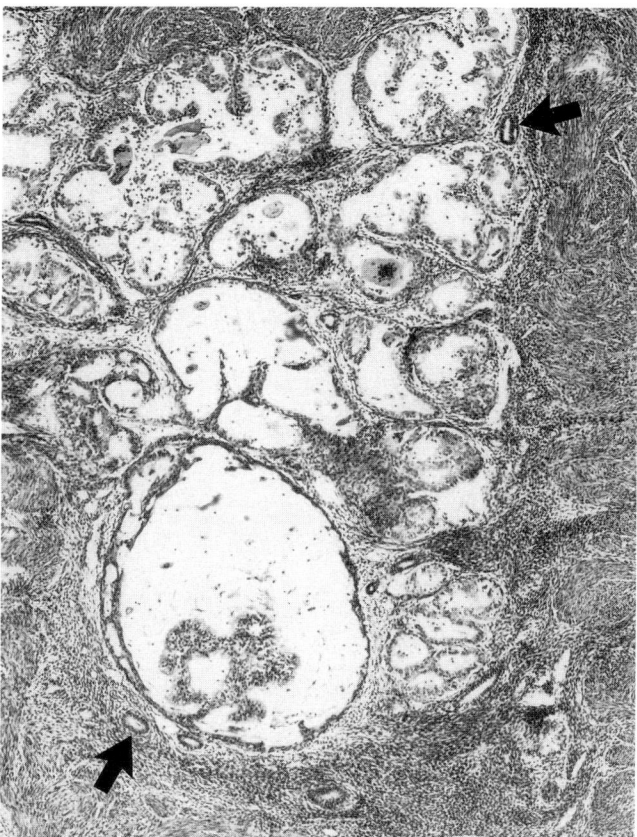

FIG. 12.10. **Endometrioid carcinoma, FIGO grade 1, involving adenomyosis.** The presence of small uninvolved glands (*arrows*) at the periphery of the carcinoma facilitates recognition of the adenomyosis. (Reprinted by permission of Jacques and Lawrence, ref. 120.)

cent study noted that adenocarcinoma involving adenomyosis frequently is associated with preceding estrogen use, low tumor grade, and an excellent prognosis, suggesting that the presence of adenomyosis is linked to type I endometrial carcinomas.[161]

Myometrial invasion, independent of tumor grade, is an important predictor of prognosis. For example, in the GOG experience recurrence developed in only 1 of 99 (1%) patients with no myometrial invasion compared with 15 of 196 (7.7%) with inner third, 8 of 55 (14.5%) with middle third, and 6 of 40 (15%) with outer third invasion when grade was not corrected.[163] In another GOG study it was shown that the 5-year relative survival for endometrioid carcinoma confined to the endometrium was 94%, involving the inner third 91%, inner to middle third 84%, and involving the outer third 59%.[265] The frequency of lymph node metastasis also is related to the depth of myometrial invasion. In clinical stage I endometrial carcinoma, inner third myometrial invasion is associated with lymph node metastasis in 5% of cases, middle third invasion with metastasis in 23%, and outer third invasion with 33%.

When grade and myometrial invasion are analyzed together, grade 1 tumors invading the inner third of the myometrium do not have pelvic node metastasis, but with outer third invasion, pelvic node metastasis occurs in 25%. A similar trend occurs with higher grade tumors. Depth of myometrial invasion probably is the single most important predictor of behavior in stage I and II disease.

CERVICAL INVOLVEMENT

Cervical involvement also has been incorporated into the new FIGO staging system. Tumors confined to the uterus but involving the cervix are stage II. These neoplasms are then staged as IIa if tumor is confined to the surface epithelium or glands and stage IIb if the tumor invades the adjacent stroma. Cervical involvement is associated with a somewhat elevated risk of recurrence, with an overall relapse rate of 16% in the absence of extrauterine disease.[163] Generally, cervical involvement is associated with increasing grade, depth of invasion, and tumor volume so the higher recurrence is not surprising.

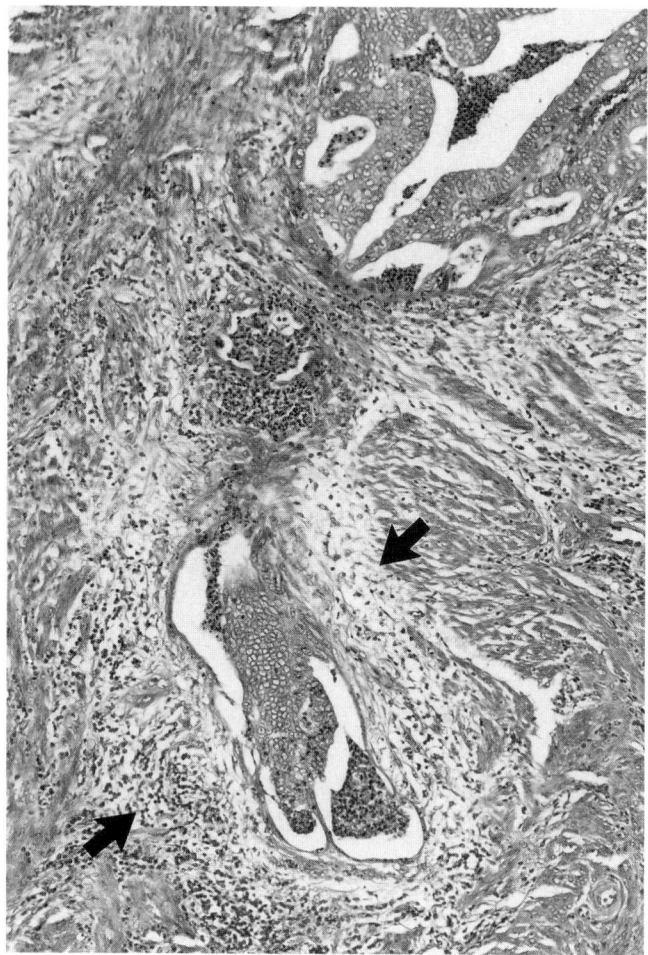

FIG. 12.11. **Endometrioid carcinoma invading the myometrium in association with adenomyosis.** In contrast to carcinoma involving adenomyosis, glands that invade the myometrium are surrounded by a loose stroma with inflammatory cells *(arrows)*. (Reprinted by permission of Jacques and Lawrence, ref. 120.)

VASCULAR INVASION

The presence of vascular invasion should be specified in the surgical pathology report because it is an important predictor of recurrence.[106] In a retrospective study of 379 patients with recurrent endometrial carcinoma,[6] vascular invasion was found in 54%. Usually, vascular invasion is associated with high grade tumors and deep myometrial invasion. A study of stage I endometrial carcinoma, however, revealed a significant correlation between vascular invasion and tumor recurrence independent of differentiation and depth of myometrial invasion.[91,106] In an analysis of stage I grade 1 endometrioid adenocarcinomas with a poor outcome, vascular invasion in addition to myometrial invasion, mitotic index, and absence of progesterone receptor were significant factors that predicted aggressive behavior.[235] In another study aimed at comparing the sig-

nificance of various pathologic risk factors in stage I endometrioid carcinoma, univariate analysis showed that vascular invasion is more important than grade and depth of myometrial invasion in predicting prognosis.[7] Also, the presence of perivascular lymphocytic infiltrates in the myometrium (Fig. 12.12), but not lymphocytic infiltrate at the tumor–myometrial junction, was associated with vascular invasion and is an independent predictor of prognosis. Perivascular lymphocytic infiltrates are thought to be related biologically to vascular invasion and, therefore, either the presence of unequivocal vascular invasion or perivascular lymphocytic infiltrates in the myometrium alone are designated *vascular invasion–associated changes* (VIAC). In view of the close association between VIAC and other variables correlating with recurrence such as deep myometrial invasion and high tumor grade, it is likely that these other factors act by increasing the probability of vascular invasion and subsequent metastasis.

ENDOMETRIAL HYPERPLASIA AND METAPLASIA

Among nontumor risk factors, the presence of atypical endometrial and various metaplasias, especially ciliated cell and eosinophilic change are important in identifying

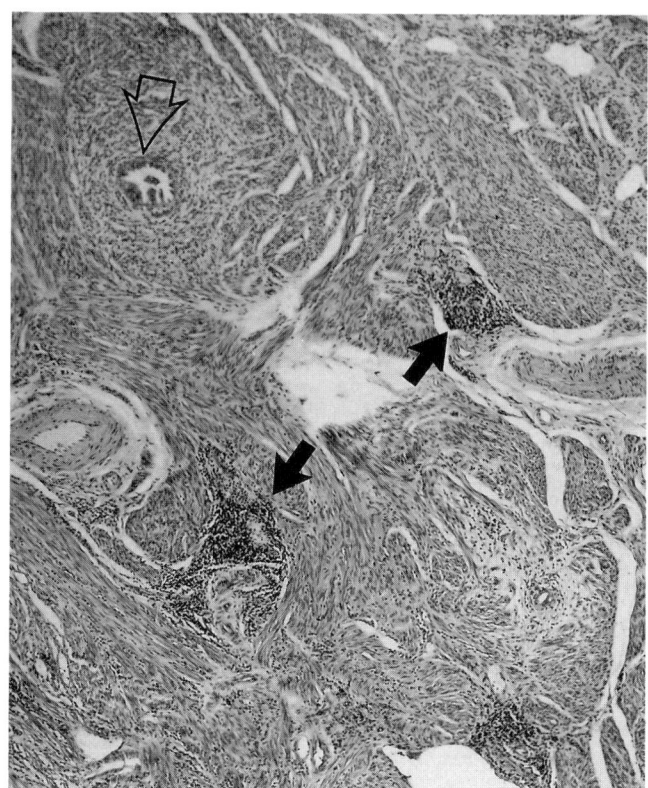

FIG. 12.12. **Vascular invasion–associated changes.** Perivascular lymphocytic infiltration *(dark arrows)* in the myometrium is a useful marker for vascular invasion. An invasive gland is present in the myometrium *(open arrow)*.

patients with a favorable prognosis. The presence of atypical hyperplasia and metaplasia correlates with low tumor grade and lack of myometrial invasion.[18,99,124] In contrast, high-grade tumors are associated more often with an atrophic endometrium.[25]

Peritoneal Cytology

Approximately 11% of patients with stage I disease have positive peritoneal cytology.[155] Positive peritoneal cytology is a risk factor for both abdominal and distant recurrence.[54,258] In the most recent GOG study, among patients with adequate follow-up, 25 (29%) of 86 women developed recurrence compared with 64 (11%) of 611 with negative peritoneal cytology.[163] Even more striking were the results reported from the M. D. Anderson Hospital where among patients with stage I disease only, 7% with negative cytology developed recurrence compared with 32% of the patients with positive peritoneal cytology. The 5-year survival for the two groups also was significantly different (96% vs. 84%).[238] In patients with stage I tumors the frequency of para-aortic lymph node metastasis ranges from 16% to 37%.[57,155,163] It has been suggested that malignant cells may gain access to the peritoneal cavity by either transtubal spread or lymphatic metastasis.[155] The frequent association of positive peritoneal cytology and lymph node metastasis suggests that lymphatic spread is an important route.

Since patients with malignant cells in the peritoneal washings may receive additional treatment, it is important that the pathologist accurately distinguish reactive mesothelial from adenocarcinoma cells. Reactive mesothelial cells may form clusters and have enlarged, atypical nuclei. If there is doubt about the nature of cells in the peritoneal fluid, comparison with the histological appearance of the tumor in the hysterectomy specimen usually resolves the problem.

Estrogen and Progesterone Receptors

Studies of estrogen and progesterone receptors by dextran-coated charcoal analysis have been difficult to interpret. The early studies were compromised by the limited number of cases analyzed and the wide variety of methodologies and experimental conditions used for the assays. In addition, different laboratories use different receptor levels in defining what is a positive result. Evidence now indicates that higher absolute levels than had been used in earlier studies are clinically more meaningful.[175] Immunohistochemical studies using monoclonal antibodies against estrogen and progesterone receptors also have resolved some of the different results by demonstrating that steroid receptors are found not only in benign endometrial epithelium but also in endometrial stromal cells and myometrium of both cycling and postmenopausal women,[22,143,186,208] unlike the breast, where localization of estrogen receptor is found exclusively in epithelial components. This has important implications because the cytosol receptor assays may be falsely elevated because of the contribution of estrogen receptor from associated nonneoplastic endometrial stroma and myometrium.

Measurable amounts of estrogen and progesterone receptor can be detected in varying amounts in most endometrial carcinomas[55,71,72,129,146,175] but in levels lower than in normal cycling endometrium. When the effects of conventional histopathological risk factors are controlled, progesterone receptor status appears to be a more important risk factor than estrogen receptor status.[55,71,72,129,175] In most recent studies positive progesterone receptor correlates with endometrioid carcinoma as compared with serous, clear cell, and adenosquamous carcinomas. In addition, it is associated with low tumor grade, young patient age, low recurrence rate, and greater survival.[55,71,72,129] In contrast, positive estrogen receptor status generally is associated with low recurrence rate but not with survival, grade, or histological type. Neither steroid receptor correlates with stage, myometrial invasion, peritoneal cytology, or retroperitoneal lymph node metastasis.[55,71,72] Most importantly, tumors with positive progesterone receptor have a significantly greater response to progestin treatment than progesterone receptor–negative tumors (60% vs. 19%).[72] Nonetheless, a substantial number of progesterone receptor–positive endometrial carcinomas do not respond to hormone treatment. This may be due to receptor heterogeneity and discordance between the receptor status of the primary and metastatic tumor[27,197] or it may be related to the actual receptor levels. For example, tumors with low positive levels may respond differently from those with high levels.

DNA Ploidy and S-phase Fraction

Approximately two-thirds of endometrial carcinomas are diploid. Aneuploidy occurs in only 16% of stage I tumors. Half of tumors that relapse, however, are aneuploid.[242] Although DNA ploidy correlates with tumor grade, stage, depth of myometrial invasion, and receptor status,[242] by multivariate analysis it is an independent risk factor.[50,117] In one large study it was found that next to clinical stages III and IV, S-phase fraction was the strongest predictor of outcome.[227] Most studies indicate that DNA ploidy and S-phase flow cytometric analysis in endometrial carcinoma are risk factors but the studies are not entirely consistent. The key question is whether these sophisticated and costly techniques provide useful information beyond that obtainable by conventional microscopic analysis. For example, since the frequency of aneuploidy is high in high-grade endometrioid and serous carcinomas and in tumors with a poor prognosis, DNA analysis would not seem to be relevant. On the other hand, it has been shown for low-grade tumors that the 5-year progression–free survival was significantly different between diploid tumors (94%) and aneuploid tumors (64%).[29] A more comprehensive discussion of flow cytometry is presented in Chapter 27, Flow Cytometry.

OTHER RISK FACTORS

Other extrauterine risk factors such as adnexal involvement, intraperitoneal metastasis, and pelvic and para-aortic lymph node metastasis are considered elsewhere (see Clinical Behavior). Age, race, and socioeconomic status are risk factors in endometrial cancer. Some studies have shown that age is the most important risk factor followed by FIGO stage, tumor grade, race, and socioeconomic status.[93,226] Younger women tend to have lower grade and less invasive tumors but age remains an important independent risk factor. The 5-year actuarial survival for white women younger than 55 years with stage I disease was 94% compared with 80% for women 55 years or older in a study from the Surveillance, Epidemiology and End Results (SEER) Program.[226]

Although there is a lower prevalence of corpus cancer in black as compared with white women, white women have a significant survival advantage as compared with black women.[226] Data from the SEER program from 1973–1977 show that the 5-year actuarial survival for white women compared with black women was 84% versus 55%.[226] Black women have a higher proportion of high-grade, high-stage tumors and tend to seek medical attention at a more advanced age compared with white women (median age of 62 years vs. 58). In the Louisville Uterine Cancer Registry, 92% of white women had stage I disease compared with 76% of black women, and 58% of white women had grade I tumors compared with 39% of black women.[48] The survival advantage is reduced but remains statistically significant after adjusting for other risk factors. Removal of stage and income result in the greatest changes in relative risk for race, suggesting that these are the strongest factors that explain the difference in survival. The differences in survival also may be related to the types of cancer found in white and black women. In the United States, a higher frequency of the favorable types of carcinoma (endometrioid as compared with serous, clear cell, and adenosquamous) occur in white women than in black women.[51] In Miyagi Prefecture, Japan, adenosquamous carcinoma represents 41% of all endometrial carcinomas whereas in two different series in the United States, adenosquamous carcinoma represented only 18–23% of endometrial cancers.[215]

MODELS FOR PREDICTING PROGNOSIS

Recent studies reveal that the behavior of a tumor is based on a complex interaction of a number of different factors. Accordingly, models have been developed that assess sev-

Table 12.6. Statistical model of survival predicted by myometrial invasion and vascular invasion–associated changes

		Survival	
Score	No. of cases	No.	%
<1	20	19	95
1–2	45	39	87
2–2.6	17	12	70
>2.6	20	7	35

Score = 0.695 [myometrial invasion (1 if not present, 2 if inner half, 3 if outer half)] + 1.8972 [vascular invasion associated changes (0 if absent, 1 if present)]. Reprinted by permission of Ambros RA and Kurman RJ, ref. 7.

eral factors and permit more accurate prognostication than simply considering one factor alone. For example, by multivariate analysis, the depth of invasion and presence of vascular invasion (VIAC) were found to provide a highly reliable model for predicting outcome (Table 12.6). The model was better able to define patients who were at low and high risk of recurrence as compared with the traditional risk factors using grade and depth of invasion.[7] Inclusion of ploidy into the model permitted even better discrimination of high- and low-risk patients. In a subset of pathological stage I endometrioid carcinoma in whom ploidy analysis was performed, multivariate analysis showed that only the depth of invasion, DNA ploidy, and VIAC were significant risk factors. A statistical model based on these features permitted stratification of patients into four risk groups with 93, 67, 38, and 10% survival, respectively (Table 12.7).[8]

Table 12.7. Statistical model of survival predicted by depth of myometrial invasion, vascular invasion–associated changes, and tumor ploidy

		Survival	
Score	No. of cases	No.	%
<2.2	27	25	93
2.2–2.3	12	8	67
2.4–4.0	8	3	38
>4	10	1	10

Score = 1.91 (vascular invasion associated changes [0 if absent, 1 if present]) + 0.982 [DNA ploidy (0 if peridiploid, 1 if aneuploid)] + 1.13 [depth of myometrical involvement (0 if none, 1 if <50%, 2 if >50%)] Reprinted by permission of Ambros RA and Kurman RJ, ref. 8.

In a preliminary analysis of almost 1000 women with clinical stage I and occult stage II adenocarcinoma of the endometrium entered on a GOG protocol, multivariate analysis has demonstrated that cell type, architectural grade, depth of myometrial invasion, and vascular space involvement are all independent risk factors for recurrence and death from tumor (R.J. Zaino et al., unpublished data). From these data it appears possible to create a model for assignment of the relative risk of death from tumor for individual patients based solely on information gathered by pathological examination of the hysterectomy specimen. For example, if a woman with grade 1 endometrioid carcinoma, with tumor confined to the endometrium and no vascular invasion is arbitrarily assigned a risk of 1, a woman with a grade 2 endometrioid carcinoma, with superficial myometrial invasion and negative vascular space involvement has a relative risk of 2.6, and a woman with a grade 3 endometrioid carcinoma, with middle third myometrial invasion and positive vascular space involvement, has a relative risk of 10. The probability of disease-free survival at 5 years for these three women would be approximately 95%, 90%, and 65%, respectively. Knowledge of the specific risk for each patient would allow better prognostication and, potentially, individually tailored therapy.

DIFFERENTIAL DIAGNOSIS

The main problem in the differential diagnosis of low-grade endometrioid carcinoma is the distinction from atypical hyperplasia, the atypical polypoid adenomyoma, hyperplasia with various types of cytoplasmic alterations (metaplasias), the Arias–Stella reaction, and menstrual endometrium. The distinction from the first three conditions is discussed in Chapter 11, Endometrial Hyperplasia and Related Cellular Changes. At times an extremely atypical Arias–Stella reaction may simulate an adenocarcinoma. In the reproductive age group that Arias–Stella reaction is a much more likely possibility than carcinoma, especially if the clinical history indicates a recent pregnancy. Nonetheless, carcinoma can occur in young women and also in pregnancy. In contrast to a carcinoma, the Arias–Stella reaction tends to be multifocal and is admixed with secretory glands and decidua. The glands in the Arias–Stella may be complex and tortuous but lack confluent or papillary patterns. The stroma does not show a desmoplastic response. The nuclei in the glandular epithelium of the Arias–Stella reaction may be markedly enlarged but the chromatin appears degenerated and smudged and mitotic figures are very unusual.

Menstrual endometrium can be confused with adenocarcinoma because of the extensive tissue breakdown characterized by tissue fragmentation and hemorrhage. The pattern of stromal breakdown results in fragmented glands of varying size and compact clusters of stromal cells haphazardly mixed with blood, which can appear ominous.

The glandular epithelium, however, is bland and shows evidence of secretory activity. Adjacent intact fragments of endometrium with associated predecidual change usually can be identified and assist in the differential diagnosis.

Another problem in differential diagnosis is the distinction of an endometrial from an endocervical primary. Both endometrioid and mucinous carcinomas can arise in either location. The presence of associated endometrial hyperplasia favors a primary site in the endometrium whereas the presence of a squamous intraepithelial lesion suggests cervical origin. The distinction is considered in greater detail in the section on Mucinous Carcinoma. A related problem is the distinction of a primary endometrial carcinoma from a metastasis from an extrauterine site. This is discussed in the section on Tumors Metastatic to the Endometrium.

A high-grade endometrioid carcinoma at times may be difficult to distinguish from a MMMT. MMMTs are highly aggressive neoplasms with a worse prognosis than high-grade endometrioid carcinomas. The diagnosis of a MMMT depends on the identification of a malignant epithelial and mesenchymal component. The latter is characterized by highly atypical spindle cells with increased cellularity and high mitotic activity. The spindle cells may be intimately associated with the carcinomatous component but should in areas be distinct from it. In these cases immunostaining for keratin can be helpful. Although occasional spindle cells may be keratin positive in an MMMT, it is unusual for most of the spindle cells to be positive as they would be in a diffusely infiltrating, poorly differentiated endometrioid adenocarcinoma. The diagnosis of a MMMT usually is not difficult if heterologous elements such as cartilage or rhabdomyoblasts are present. However, rare foci of heterologous tissue, such as cartilage (Fig. 12.13), in what is otherwise a typical endometrioid carcinoma are insufficient for the diagnosis of a MMMT because the latter has a malignant spindle cell component in addition to the heterologous elements. If heterologous elements are not present, the diagnosis of a MMMT depends on clearcut demonstration of biphasic epithelial and mesenchymal components.

ULTRASTRUCTURAL FINDINGS

The neoplastic cells have marked structural variability, paralleling the observations made using light microscopy.[15,36,87,232] Ultrastructurally, endometrioid carcinoma is composed of a heterogeneous population of cells. There are four distinct cell types and two different nuclear forms that differ from normal endometrium. The four cell types are, (1) a large round cell containing a large nucleus and scant cytoplasm with a highly variable content of organelles, (2) an irregularly shaped, elongated cell frequently containing cytoplasmic projections, (3) a clear cell with a paucity of organelles, and (4) a dark cell with dense cytoplasmic contents and pyknotic nucleus. One form of

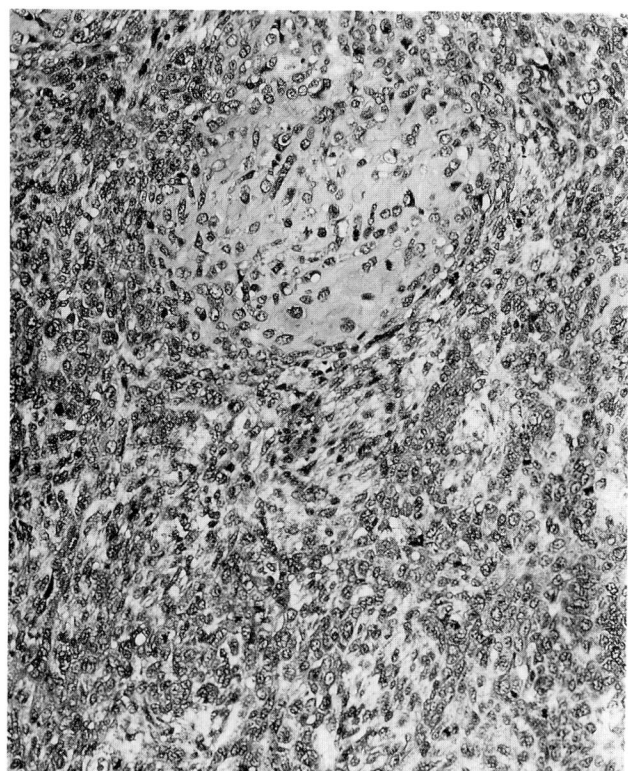

Fig. 12.13. Endometrioid carcinoma, FIGO grade 3. A small focus of cartilage is present in the upper part of the field. In view of its small size and the absence of a "sarcomatous"-appearing mesenchymal component, a diagnosis of malignant mixed mesodermal tumor is not justified.

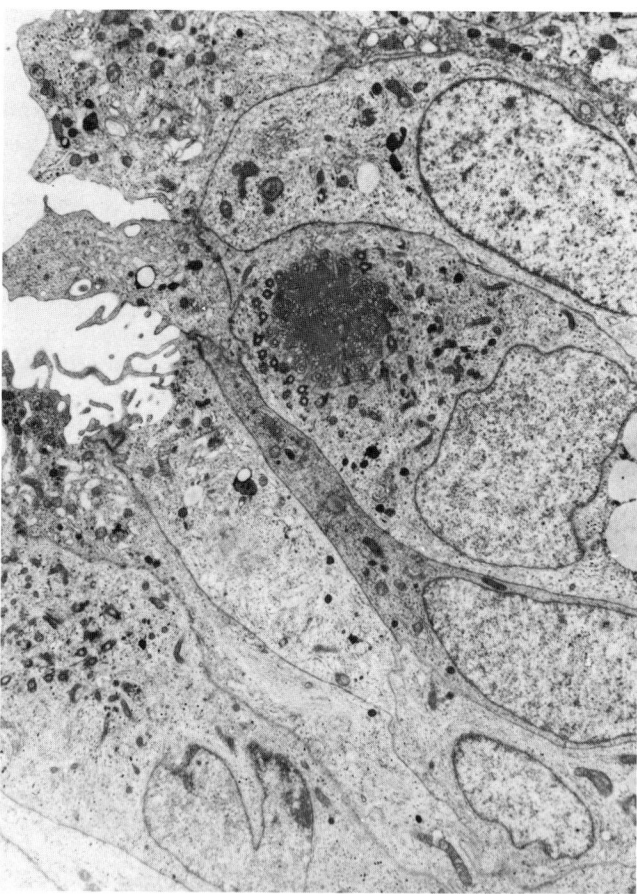

Fig. 12.14. Electron micrograph of endometrioid carcinoma. Ciliated cells with considerable pleomorphism are present. Microvilli are prominent. ×2900. (Reprinted by permission of Cavazos and Lucas, ref. 36.)

nucleus in endometrial carcinoma is a large, rounded nucleus with a relatively smooth margin. The other has an elongated nucleus with numerous deep irregular clefts, producing a lobulated appearance. The nucleolus of these cells is large, but a nucleolar channel system has not been identified.

The cell membrane of adenocarcinoma cells typically has small, sparse microvilli, but occasionally long microvilli are present (Fig. 12.14). The lateral cell membrane is more irregular than in normal cells and tends to undergo dehiscence, leading to the formation of intracellular spaces. The basal cell membrane also is irregular and discontinuous because of the presence of complex cytoplasmic projections irregularly extending into the stroma. There is marked variation in the development of rough endoplasmic reticulum and considerable variation in ribosomal content. Autophagosomes and giant lysosomes are prominent in some cells. Cells may have dense cytoplasm because of the presence of abundant ribosomes, whereas some have clear cytoplasm caused by almost complete absence of ribosomes. The variability in organelle content, size, and

shape exceeds that of endometrial hyperplasia. The Golgi apparatus of endometrial carcinoma cells tends to be poorly developed, and there is scant smooth endoplasmic reticulum as well. Mitochondria show considerable variation in size, shape, and number, and glycogen and lipid are increased. Microtubules and microfibrils are rare, and annulate lamellae are absent.

Immunohistochemical Findings

Most immunohistochemical analyses have been directed at assisting in the distinction of atypical hyperplasia from well-differentiated adenocarcinoma. Other immunohistochemical studies have evaluated different markers in the differential diagnosis of primary endometrial versus endocervical adenocarcinoma (see Mucinous Carcinoma). In addition, studies have used monoclonal antibodies to estrogen and progesterone receptor to determine the distribution of the receptors in the uterus and to compare the utility of the immunohistochemical to the biochemical assays (see above, Estrogen and Progesterone Receptors).

Finally, a few immunohistochemical studies have been performed to evaluate genetic alterations in endometrial cancer. More comprehensive descriptions of the immunohistochemical and molecular biological findings in endometrial carcinoma are presented in Chapter 26, Immunohistochemistry, and Chapter 28, Molecular Biology.

Immunocytochemical investigations of the distribution of cell-cycle–related antigens such as Ki 67 and proliferating cell nuclear antigen,[187] and silver impregnation studies of nucleolar organizer regions,[37,255] have been of no value in distinguishing atypical hyperplasia from well-differentiated adenocarcinoma. Other antibodies that have been studied but have not been particularly useful in the distinction of atypical hyperplasia and well-differentiated adenocarcinoma include those against type IV collagen and laminin that detect defects in basement membrane components.[30,90,244] Antibodies against extracellular matrix proteins such as tenascin,[202] proteolytic enzymes that degrade the extracellular matrix and are associated with tumor invasion such as plasminogen activators and cathepsin D, and tumor-associated antigens, such as TAG-72[225,231] and sialyl-Tn antigen have also been found to be of no value in distinguishing atypical hyperplasia from carcinoma.[118]

Immunohistochemical positivity for estrogen and progesterone receptor has been positively correlated with stage, tumor grade, and survival.[34,38,39,94] Both semiquantitative and quantitative assays using computerized analysis have been performed,[41] but the distribution and intensity of staining varies in different parts of the tumor and even within individual glands, making interpretation difficult and subjective.[23,263] In addition, the immunolocalization of steroid receptors performed on formalin-fixed paraffin-embedded tissue is less sensitive than similar analysis on frozen tissue, which may therefore result in false-negative results. At present there is little value in obtaining immunohistochemical receptor assays on primary endometrial carcinomas. Finally, it should be noted that the presence of steroid receptors by immunohistochemistry in a metastatic tumor does not incriminate the endometrium or breast as the primary site because a wide variety of tumors express these receptors.

Ulex europaeus agglutinin I (Uea-1), a lectin that specifically binds L-fucose, is confined to the luminal surface of benign endometrial glands but is diffusely distributed within the cytoplasm in hyperplastic and neoplastic endometrium, specifically endometrioid carcinoma. High-grade tumors displaying deep myometrial invasion and vascular invasion tend to show more diffuse reactivity than low-grade minimally invasive tumors, but Ulex binding does not appear to be an independent risk factor.[9] There is an increased expression of H and Lewis-b blood group antigens in endometrial carcinoma as compared with benign endometrium regardless of ABO status.[119] The biological significance, if any, of these findings remains to be determined.

A few studies have evaluated cell proliferation markers [Ki-67 and proliferating cell nuclear antigen (PCNA)] in endometrial carcinoma in an effort to correlate the expression of these proteins with various histopathological features. Increased Ki-67 reactivity correlates with architectural and nuclear grade[257] but no correlation was found between PCNA and grade or stage.[169] Lower PCNA reactivity was found in postmenopausal patients on estrogen replacement therapy compared with women who had never received estrogen therapy.[169] The significance of these findings is not clear.

Epidermal growth factor receptor has been identified in endometrial carcinoma with staining generally localized to the cell membrane. There is no correlation between epidermal growth factor receptor expression and grade, stage, or steroid receptor status.[173]

CA-125 and CA-19.9 have both been identified by immunohistochemistry in endometrial carcinomas. Since these proteins also can be identified in serum, they may have value as markers of recurrence.[183]

CYTOGENETIC FINDINGS

Although most endometrial carcinomas are diploid by flow cytometric analysis, this technique has limited sensitivity compared with karyotypic analysis. Using banding techniques after short-term culture, it has been demonstrated that both hypo- and hyper-diploid populations are quite common.[135,221] Trisomy or tetrasomy of the long arm of chromosome 1 is the most common abnormality detected,[52,89] but a variety of other abnormalities including allelic loss of chromosome 17p, translocations, trisomies, and telomere reductions also have been found.[82,113,174,223] The prognostic implications of these genetic changes have not been defined.

ONCOGENES AND SUPPRESSOR GENES

Mutations in codons 12 or 13 of the K-*ras* oncogene have been reported in 10–25% of endometrial carcinomas[77,78,88,148,162] and in 17% of atypical hyperplasias.[78] There is limited correlation between K-*ras* mutations and tumor grade. K-*ras* activation appears to be an early event in endometrial carcinogenesis[77,78] and was found to be an independent unfavorable risk factor in one study.[162]

Both allelic loss, identified by loss of heterozygosity, and point mutations of p53, the most commonly altered suppressor gene in human cancer, have been detected in endometrial carcinoma and atypical hyperplasia. Allelic loss, recognized at the polymorphic site in codon 72 of the p53 gene, was detected in 32% of informative cases of carcinoma and in 25% of atypical hyperplasia.[77,78] Mutations in p53 were significantly more frequent in grade 3 tumors (43%) compared with grade 1 tumors (12%). The frequency of point mutations in atypical hyperplasia is 8%, which does not differ significantly from grade 1 adenocarcinoma. These findings suggest that inactivation of p53 occurs as a later event in endometrial carcinogenesis. Not surprisingly, abnormalities in p53 have been reported particularly frequently in serous carcinomas and those with a poor prognosis.[32,130]

The HER-2/neu oncogene encodes a cell surface glycoprotein similar to the human growth factor receptor. Overexpression of HER-2/neu has been detected in 10–15% of endometrial carcinomas and occurred more frequently in patients with metastatic disease.[21] In another study overexpression of this gene was related to a diminished progression free interval.[111]

Several studies have been unable to detect significant overexpression of C-*myc*, H-*ras*, and N-*ras* oncogenes in endometrial carcinoma.[88,116] High levels of expression of *fms* have been associated with aggressive behavior in one study.[123]

CLINICAL BEHAVIOR

Endometrioid adenocarcinoma spreads by lymphatic and vascular dissemination, direct extension to contiguous organs, and transperitoneal and transtubal seeding.[17] Lymphatic metastasis is three times as common as hematogenous spread,[31] but involvement of the lungs without metastasis to mediastinal lymph nodes suggests that hematogenous spread may occur early in the course of disease. Endometrial carcinoma tends to spread to the pelvic nodes before involving para-aortic lymph nodes. The relative frequency of metastasis to lymph node groups and various organs is shown in Tables 12.8 and 12.9.

In a population-based study from Norway[3a] involving nearly 2000 patients, the 5- and 10-year survival for all stages (surgical–pathological) was 78% and 67%, respectively. Five- and 10-year survival for stage I disease was

Table 12.8. Sites of lymph node metastasis from endometrial carcinoma at autopsy

Lymph nodes	Relative frequency (%)
Para-aortic	64
Hypogastric	61
External iliac	48
Common iliac	40
Obturator	37
Sacral	22
Mediastinal	18
Inguinal	16
Supraclavicular	12

From Hendrickson E (1975) The lymphatic dissemination in endometrial carcinoma. A study of 188 necropsies. Am J Obstet Gynecol 123:570. Reprinted by permission, ref. 107.

Table 12.9. Sites of metastasis from endometrial carcinoma at autopsy

Organ site	Relative frequency (%)
Lung	41
Peritoneum and omentum	39
Ovary	34
Liver	29
Bowel	29
Vagina	25
Bladder	23
Vertebra	20
Spleen	14
Adrenal	14
Ureter	8
Brain or skull	5
Vulva	4
Breast	4
Hand	
Femur	
Tibia	Rare
Pubic bone	
Skin	

From Hendrickson E (1975) The lymphatic dissemination in endometrial carcinoma. A study of 188 necropsies. Am J Obstet Gynecol 123:570. Reprinted by permission, ref. 107.

83% and 71%, for stage II 71% and 60%, for stage III 39% and 34%, and for stage IV 27% and 23%.

Only 3% of women with endometrial carcinoma are diagnosed initially as clinical stage III, and 5% of women thought to have stage I disease clinically have occult involvement of the adnexal areas (pathological stage III) at the time of surgery.[5] These women have a fourfold greater risk of para-aortic lymph node metastases compared with patients without adnexal involvement.[163]

Among the extrauterine risk factors, the presence of positive aortic lymph nodes is most important in predicting prognosis. Only 36% of patients with positive aortic nodes were free of tumor at 5 years compared with 85% with negative aortic nodes.[163] The highest correlation of positive para-aortic lymph nodes is with pelvic lymph nodes. Nearly a third of patients with positive pelvic lymph nodes have positive para-aortic lymph nodes. Other features that correlate with positive aortic nodes are vascular invasion (19%), deep myometrial invasion (17%), positive peritoneal cytology (16%), cervical involvement (12%), and grade 3 tumors (8%).

Despite treatment with surgery and radiotherapy, 50% of stage III tumors recur. Half these patients die with distant metastasis, although local control also is a major problem. About 4% of patients with endometrial carcinoma have stage IV disease. Spread to the lungs occurs in 36% of patients.

The interval for recurrence after initial treatment depends on the histological grade of the tumor and the clinical stage.[199] For grade 1 tumors, the mean time to recurrence is 38 months, for grade 2 tumors it is 21 months, and for grade 3 tumors it is 14 months.[259] Nearly 80% of the failures occur within 3 years, but recurrence can appear as late as 5 years after treatment. One-half of treatment failures occur in the pelvis and one-half at distant sites.[17,71,199]

TREATMENT

The standard treatment for endometrial carcinoma is hysterectomy and bilateral salpingo-oophorectomy. Over the years preoperative or postoperative radiotherapy and chemotherapy have been used in addition to hysterectomy. The current approach is to treat all patients when feasible by hysterectomy supplemented by surgical staging and to administer postoperative radiation to patients with poor prognostic factors that put them at high risk of recurrence. Postoperative estrogen replacement therapy has been advocated for patients with early stage disease and no significant poor prognostic factors.[56] Preliminary reports show that survival is not compromised in patients with low tumor grade (grades 1 and 2), less than 50% myometrial invasion, and no metastases to lymph nodes or other organs.[141]

Because the status of the pelvic and para-aortic lymph nodes are such important prognostic indicators, these nodes should be sampled in patients with no gross evidence of intraperitoneal disease if there is greater than 50% myometrial invasion, grade 3 tumor, cervical involvement, extrauterine spread, serous, clear cell, or undifferentiated carcinoma, or palpably enlarged lymph nodes. Several studies have shown that the depth of myometrial invasion can be assessed by gross inspection and intraoperative frozen section.[66,170,212] In a GOG study only a quarter of patients had these findings but they accounted for the majority of patients with positive aortic lymph nodes.[163]

Postoperatively, patients are classified as low, intermediate, or high risk based on surgical pathological staging. Patients with grade 1 or 2 tumors that are confined to the endometrium or are minimally invasive are defined as low risk and require no further therapy. Patients with pelvic or para-aortic lymph node metastases or involvement of the adnexa or intraperitoneal sites are high risk and receive postoperative radiation (vaginal cuff, pelvis, para-aortic area, or whole abdominal). Radiation appears to be of benefit as the 5-year survival rate for women with positive aortic nodes who were treated with postoperative radiation is nearly 40%.[163] Patients who do not qualify as low or high risk are intermediate in risk. A decision as to whether or not these patients should receive postoperative radiation should be individualized because there are no conclusive data demonstrating a survival benefit for these patients treated with postoperative radiotherapy.

Studies evaluating the use of adjuvant hormonal or cytotoxic chemotherapy have shown no improvement in survival over surgery and radiation and consequently they are currently not recommended as standard treatment. In contrast, radiation, hormone, and cytotoxic chemotherapy are used for management of patients with recurrent tumor. Fifty percent of patients with isolated vaginal vault recurrence treated by irradiation are alive at 3 years.[182]

HISTOLOGICAL EFFECTS OF TREATMENT

RADIATION

The histological changes in neoplastic tissues after intracavitary radiation are nonspecific and variable, showing minor to major alterations from their preirradiated state.[132,250] Similarly, nonneoplastic endometrial or endocervical glands may be affected only minimally or show nuclear and cytoplasmic changes indistinguishable from carcinoma cells.

Because the cytological changes in both neoplastic and nonneoplastic tissue are similar, identification of carcinoma depends largely on the recognition of histological patterns and signs of invasion. Irradiated carcinoma generally retains a haphazard glandular pattern, but nonirradiated, noneoplastic glands tend to maintain their normal architectural arrangement despite radiation effects in the endometrial stroma and myometrium. When radiation effect is evident, nuclei tend to be enlarged, highly pleomorphic, and hyperchromatic, with coarsely clumped chromatin. The cytoplasm often is granular and swollen. Vacuolation can be present in both the nucleus and the cytoplasm (Fig. 12.15). The nuclear changes are due to replication of DNA without cell division. Cytoplasmic vacuolation results from dilatation of various organelles and possible lysis due to damaged lysosomal membranes.[132] In some instances, radiation may enhance cellular differentiation. Occasionally, poorly differentiated carcinomas without squamous differentiation in the curettings may have nests of squamous epithelium in the resected uterus after radiation. Thus, the difference in radiosensitivity of tumor cells and benign cells is due largely to the increased mitotic activity of the neoplastic cells and the better reparative capacity of nonneoplastic cells.[237]

It is in mitosis and the S-phase of the cell cycle that a cell is most susceptible to radiation injury.[237] In view of the variable morphologic response to irradiation, it is often difficult to determine whether irradiated tumor cells are viable or not. It has been shown in animals that some irradiated tumor cells that are morphologically unaltered may, nevertheless, be unable to proliferate when transplanted.[228] This suggests that these cells are no longer viable despite the absence of morphologically recognizable radiation-induced changes. Nonetheless, on a practical basis, if tumor cells are evident after irradiation, it should be assumed that some retain the capacity to persist however abnormal they appear.

Radiation changes in the endometrial stroma and myometrium are greatest in the vicinity of the radiation source.

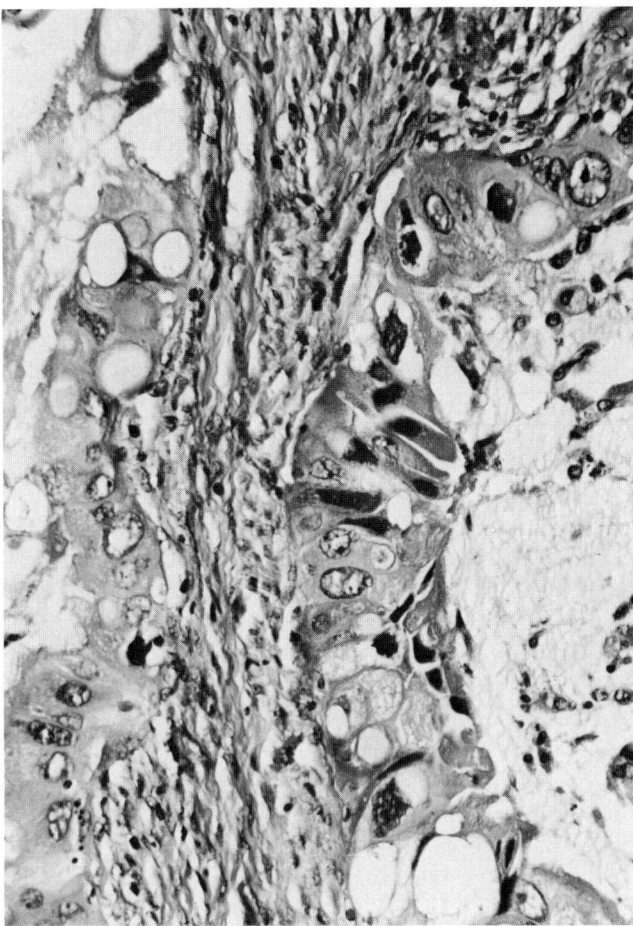

FIG. 12.15. Endometrioid carcinoma with radiation effect. There is marked vacuolation, nuclear hyperchromasia, and pleomorphism within the glandular cells.

The stromal cells are first converted to giant fibroblasts. Early vascular effects include damage to endothelial cells resulting in thrombosis. The stroma undergoes progressive hyalinization, resulting in a collagenous scar. Elastic tissue often is fragmented and frayed, and blood vessels are thickened and sclerotic.[132] Occasionally, changes similar to those found in atherosclerosis may be present in the intima of blood vessels.[128] Foam cells occur in the intima, and myometrial cells may appear granular and swollen, especially in areas close to the radium source. Long-standing radiation effects are characterized by scarring, atrophy, and sclerosis of vessels. The endometrium is thin and easily traumatized, and small blood vessels in the stroma are thin-walled and ectatic. Some blood vessels form plaques of lipid-filled clear cells (lipid cells) in the media, diagnostic of late effects of radiation.

PROGESTINS

Progestin-induced changes include secretory differentiation of glandular cells, mitotic arrest, and decrease in estrogen-related cellular changes, such as ciliogenesis, tissue necrosis, and conversion of spindle-shaped stromal cells to decidual cells[115,189,209] (Fig. 12.16). The earliest evidence of progestin effect is subnuclear vacuolization, observed within 2–3 days of treatment. The vacuoles are a manifestation of glycoprotein synthesis, which is followed by an apocrine-type secretion in which the apical portion of the cytoplasm of the cell is discharged into the gland lumen, with reduction in the size of the cell. Concomitantly, there is a marked decrease in mitotic activity and RNA synthesis, as measured by scintillation radioautographs. Lysosomal autodigestion of cells also is stimulated by progestins.[189]

It has been reported that progestin-induced changes occur only in estrogen and progesterone receptor–positive tumors.[262] These changes included subnuclear and supranuclear PAS-positive vacuoles in well-differentiated tumors and randomly distributed vacuoles in poorly differentiated tumors. Electron microscopic changes included development of Golgi, smooth endoplasmic reticulum, and secretory products resembling both mucin and glycogen in the cytoplasm.

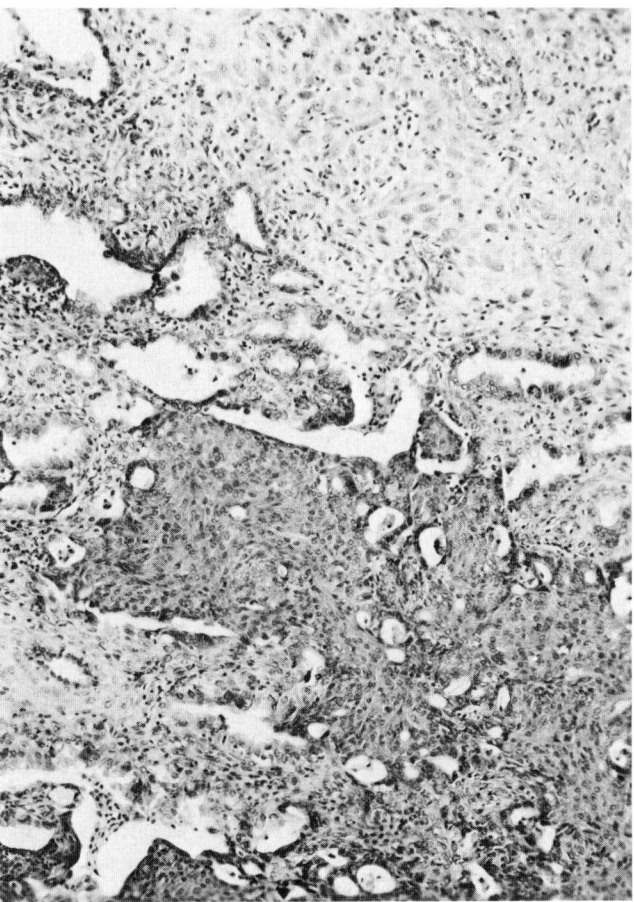

FIG. 12.16. Endometrioid carcinoma with progestin effect. A marked decidual reaction is present in the stroma *(upper portion of field)* after 1 month of high-dose progestin treatment.

Villoglandular Carcinoma

This is a variant of endometrioid carcinoma that displays a papillary architecture in which the papillary fronds are composed of a delicate fibrovascular core covered by columnar cells that generally contain bland nuclei.[42,108]

There is only limited published experience with tumors of this type, and consequently the clinical profile of these patients is sketchy. The mean age is 61 years, similar to that of women with endometrioid carcinoma. All patients reported thus far are white. In all other respects, women with these tumors are similar to patients with low-grade endometrioid carcinoma.

The microscopic appearance of villoglandular is characterized by thin, delicate fronds covered by stratified columnar epithelial cells with oval nuclei that generally display mild to moderate (grade 1 or 2) atypia (Figs. 12.17, 12.18). Occasionally more atypical (grade 3) nuclei may be observed. Mitotic activity is variable, and abnormal mitotic figures are rare.[42,108] Myometrial invasion usually is superficial.

The main consideration in the differential diagnosis is serous carcinoma because both villoglandular and serous carcinomas have a prominent papillary pattern. In contrast to serous carcinomas, villoglandular carcinomas have long delicate papillary fronds and are covered by columnar cells with only mild to moderate nuclear atypia. The cells look distinctly endometrioid with a smooth, luminal border. In fact, minor villoglandular patterns are frequent components of an endometrioid carcinoma. To have significance

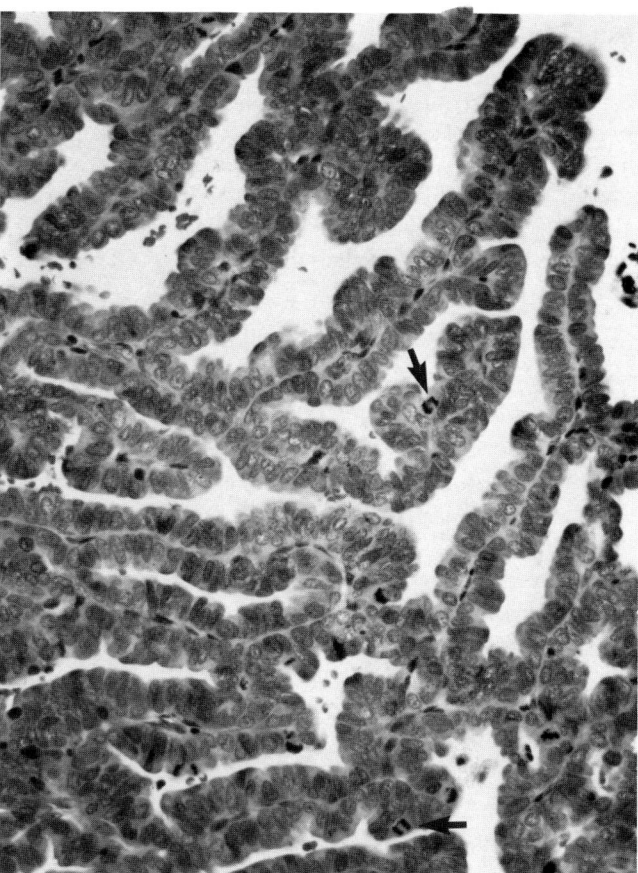

FIG. 12.18. **Villoglandular carcinoma, FIGO grade 1.** The cells covering the fibrovascular cores resemble those in endometrioid carcinoma. There is minimal nuclear atypia. Mitotic activity is present (*arrows*).

as a distinctive entity, the diagnosis is reserved for tumors in which most of the neoplasm has a villoglandular appearance. In contrast to villoglandular carcinomas, serous carcinomas tend to have shorter, thick, densely fibrotic papillary fronds. Probably the most important distinguishing feature is the cytological appearance. The cells of serous carcinoma tend to be rounder, forming small papillary clusters that are detached from the papillary fronds, a finding that is often referred to as *papillary tufts* (see Figs. 12.30, 12.31). As a consequence, the luminal border has a scalloped appearance. The nuclei of serous carcinomas are highly pleomorphic and atypical (grade 3). Macronucleoli typically are present. Many of the cells have a hobnail appearance (see Figs. 12.32, 12.34). It should be noted that considerable nuclear heterogeneity can be observed.

Villoglandular carcinomas generally behave similarly to low-grade endometrioid carcinomas rarely invading deeply or involving the cervix. Consequently, they have an excellent prognosis. Typically, these tumors are at an early stage at the time of diagnosis. Treatment is the same as for

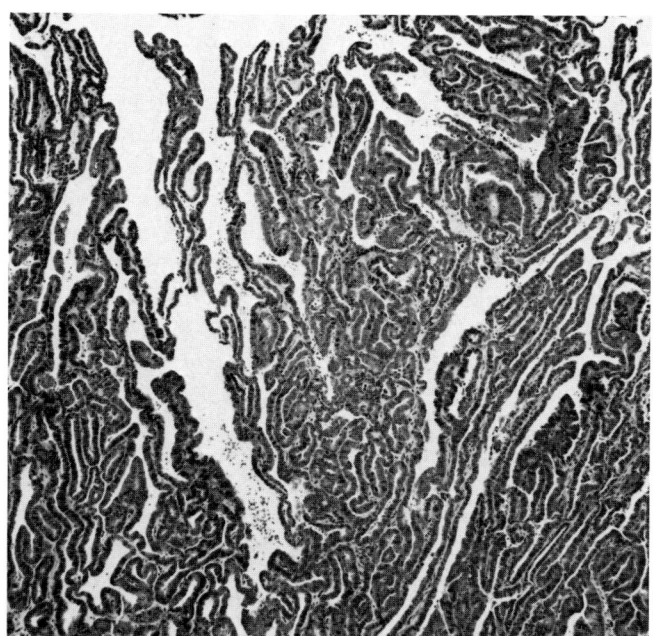

FIG. 12.17. **Villoglandular carcinoma, FIGO grade 1.** The tumor is composed of delicate papillary fronds covered by columnar epithelium that have an endometrioid appearance.

endometrioid carcinoma of comparable stage, grade, and depth of invasion.

At times a typical-appearing villoglandular carcinoma may display marked nuclear atypia. Preliminary data from a GOG analysis reveal that villoglandular carcinomas with grade 3 nuclei are associated with survival that is only slightly worse than those with grade 1 or 2 nuclei (RJ Zaino and RJ Kurman, unpublished data).

Secretory Carcinoma

This is a variant of typical endometrial carcinoma in which the majority of cells exhibit subnuclear or supranuclear cytoplasmic vacuoles resembling early secretory endometrium. A rare pattern, it represents only 1–2% of endometrial carcinomas.[75,137,234]

All patients with secretory carcinoma thus far reported are white. The age range is from 35 to 78 years, with a mean age of 58. Most patients are postmenopausal and experience abnormal bleeding. This histological subtype also may be seen rarely after progestin treatment of an endometrioid carcinoma. In all other respects, including the association of obesity, hypertension, diabetes mellitus, and exogenous estrogen administration, patients with secretory carcinoma are similar to women with endometrioid carcinoma.

Microscopically, secretory carcinoma displays a well-differentiated glandular pattern and is composed of columnar cells, often unstratified, with subnuclear or supranuclear vacuolization closely resembling 16–20-day secretory endometrium (Fig. 12.19). Usually the nuclei are grade 1. The secretory pattern may be focal or diffuse, and it is frequently admixed with endometrioid adenocarcinoma.[75,137]

The endometrium adjacent to secretory carcinoma in young women typically shows a secretory pattern that is more advanced than 17 days, and a corpus luteum is found in most premenopausal patients when a hysterectomy and bilateral salpingo-oophorectomy are performed.[137] Nonetheless, a relationship to progesterone stimulation is not always demonstrable, and most of the women are postmenopausal. The secretory activity in the tumor may be transient because it has been observed in curettings but not in the later hysterectomy specimen.[47] Secretory carcinoma may occur spontaneously in postmenopausal women without exogenous or abnormal levels of progesterone.

It is important to distinguish secretory carcinoma from clear cell carcinoma in view of the excellent prognosis of the former and unfavorable prognosis of the latter. Although both tumors are composed of cells with clear, glycogen-rich cytoplasm, the histological features are distinctive. At times a secretory carcinoma can merge into a clear cell carcinoma (Figs. 12.20, 12.21). The tumors are distinguished by their architectural and cytological appearance. Secretory carcinoma displays a glandular architecture like endometrioid carcinoma and is rarely papillary, cystic, or solid. Clear cell carcinoma, in contrast, frequently has a

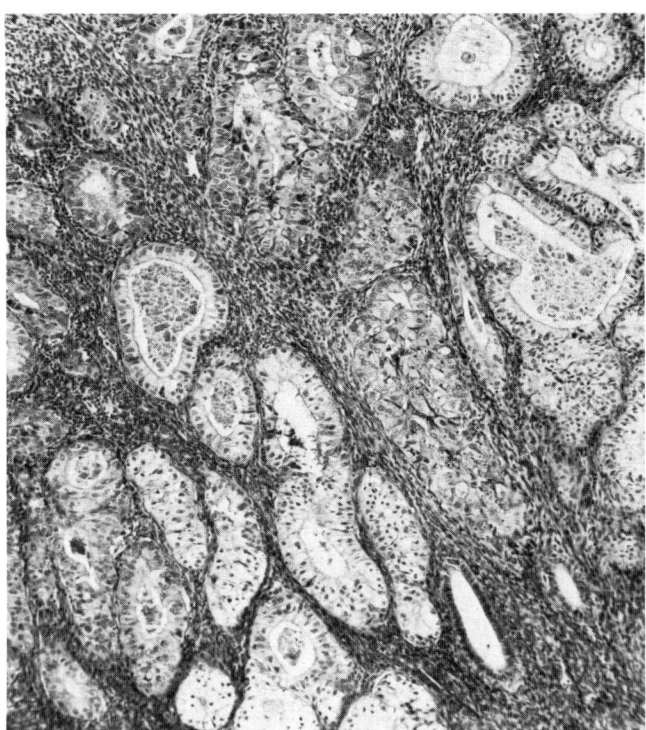

FIG. 12.19. Secretory carcinoma, FIGO grade 1. The tumor is composed of crowded, irregulatory shaped glands lined by cells with relatively bland nuclei. The subnuclear and supranuclear vacuolization is similar to that found in secretory endometrium 2–6 days after ovulation.

papillary or solid pattern and typically is associated with serous differentiation. A well-formed glandular pattern is unusual. The cells of secretory carcinoma are columnar with supranuclear or subnuclear vacuoles. The cells are similar to those in endometrioid carcinoma except for the presence of vacuoles (Fig. 12.21). In contrast, the cells in a clear cell carcinoma are more rounded and the nucleus is generally centrally located; hobnail cells are characteristic. Nuclear atypia is more marked (grade 3) in clear cell carcinoma. A well-formed glandular pattern is unusual.

Cells with clear cytoplasm also may be seen in the squamous component of an endometrioid adenocarcinoma with squamous differentiation. The clear appearance of these cells is also due to the presence of glycogen. Clear squamous cells tend to be polygonal and usually merge with more typical squamous cells with abundant eosinophilic cytoplasm.

The distinction of secretory carcinoma from atypical hyperplasia with secretory effect can be difficult and is based on the presence of stromal invasion in the carcinoma (see Chapter 11, Endometrial Hyperplasia and Related Cellular Changes).

Treatment is the same as that for endometrioid carcinoma of the same stage and grade. Secretory carcinoma usually is low grade, with a 5-year survival of 87%. Death from recurrent disease occurs rarely.[47]

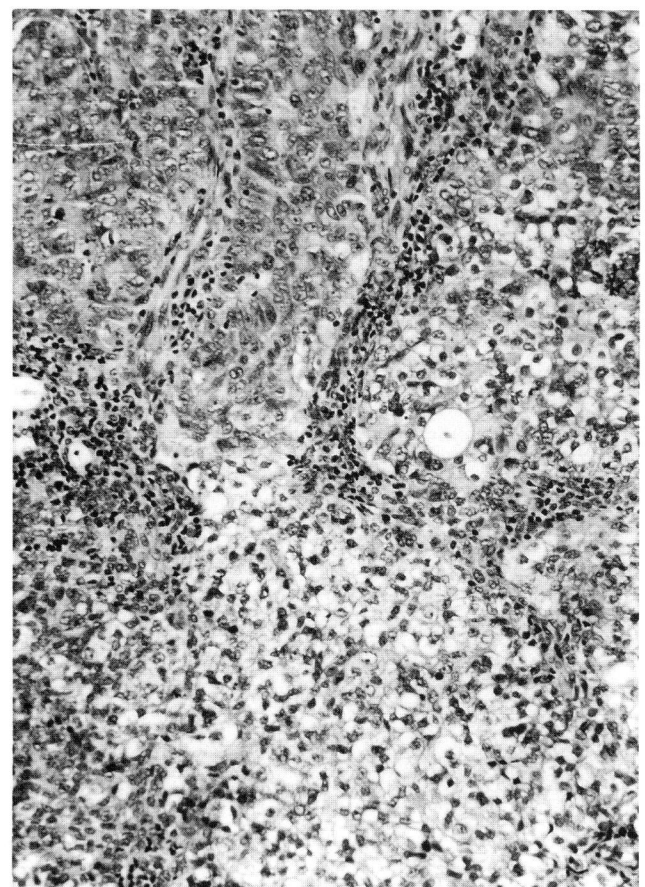

FIG. 12.20. **Mixed clear cell, endometrioid, and secretory carcinoma.** Clear cell carcinoma in the lower part of the field merges with endometrioid carcinoma in the left upper part of field.

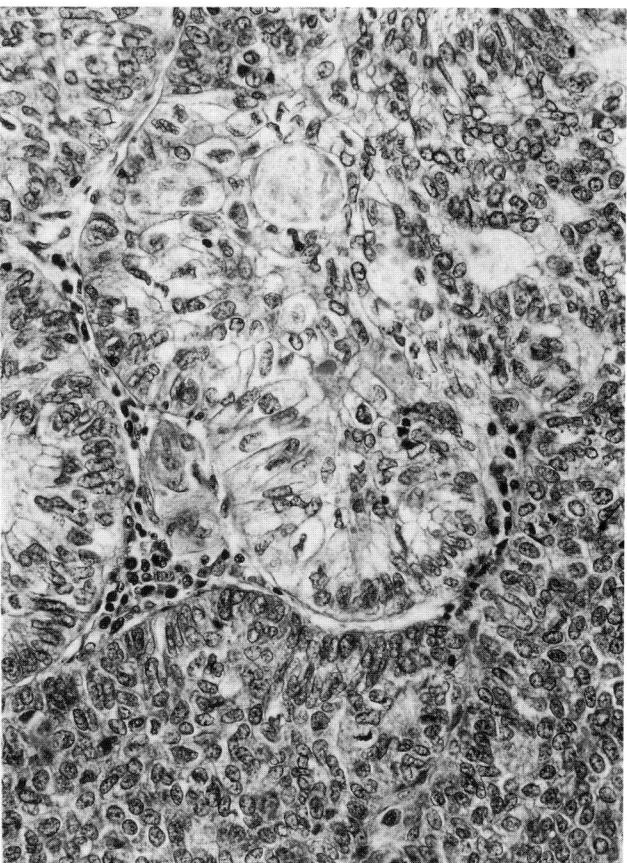

FIG. 12.21. **Mixed clear cell, endometrioid, and secretory carcinoma.** Higher magnification of another field of the same case illustrated in Fig. 12.20. The cells of the secretory carcinoma are columnar with sub- and supranuclear vacuoles. The secretory cells merge with endometrioid carcinoma in the lower part of the field.

Ciliated Carcinoma

This is a rare form of differentiation in low-grade endometrioid carcinoma.[109,193,216] It does not need to be classified separately from endometrioid carcinoma. Its only importance is to remind the pathologist that endometrial proliferations with cilia may still be carcinomas. Estrogen induces cilia formation in the normal endometrium. Despite the prevalence of estrogen use, ciliated carcinoma is an extremely rare carcinoma, and most endometrial proliferations in which cilia are observed represent hyperplasias associated with eosinophilic or ciliated change.

Patients range in age from 42 to 79 years, are postmenopausal, and present with bleeding.[109] Ciliated carcinoma has an association with exogenous estrogen treatment; 4 of 10 patients in one study[109] received estrogen and in another study, ciliated cells were found in 37% of carcinomas in estrogen users compared with 12% of nonusers ($p < .005$).[192]

Microscopically ciliated carcinoma is almost always well differentiated and often displays a cribriform pattern. The gland lumens in the cribriform areas are lined by cells with prominent eosinophilic cytoplasm and cilia (Fig. 12.22).

The nuclei of ciliated cells generally have an irregular nuclear membrane and display coarse nuclear chromatin with prominent nucleoli.[109] In most cases, ciliated carcinoma is admixed with nonciliated endometrioid carcinoma and occasionally areas of mucinous carcinoma.

Although some ciliated carcinomas are moderately differentiated and invade to the middle third of the myometrium, none of the patients has developed recurrence or died of disease. Thus, the presence of cilia in a bona fide carcinoma identifies a low-grade neoplasm.

Endometrioid Carcinoma with Squamous Differentiation

Many endometrioid adenocarcinomas contain squamous epithelium, but the amount of squamous epithelium can vary widely. In a well-sampled neoplasm, the squamous element should constitute at least 10% of a tumor to qualify as an adenocarcinoma with squamous differentiation.

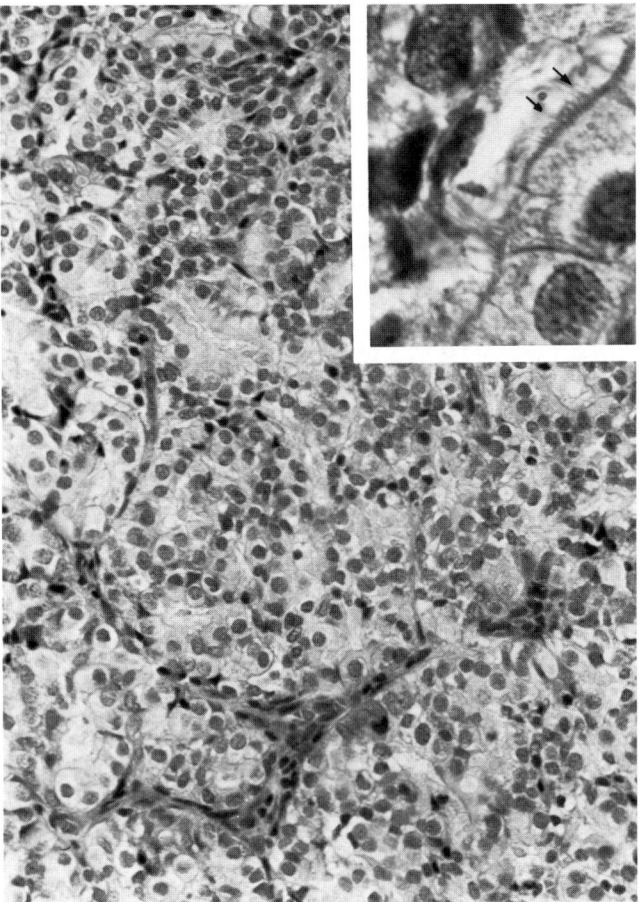

FIG. 12.22. Ciliated carcinoma. The tumor is composed of well-differentiated glands. **Inset:** Cells with minimal nuclear atypia containing cilia *(arrows)* on the luminal surface. The tumor invaded two-thirds into the myometrium. (Courtesy of Michael R. Hendrickson, M.D., Palo Alto, CA.)

Up to the late 1960s an adenocarcinoma containing squamous elements was designated an adenocanthoma. Originally it was thought to be rare and low grade,[171] but when less stringent quantitative criteria were applied, the frequency rose to as high as 44% of endometrial carcinomas.[40] Subsequently, adenocarcinomas with squamous elements were divided into those with benign-appearing squamous differentiation and designated *adenoacanthoma* (AA) whereas those with malignant-appearing squamous epithelium were termed *adenosquamous carcinoma* (AS).[166,167] These neoplasms differ markedly in their behavior; the 5-year survival for AA is 70–87% compared with 19–40% for AS.[4,192,198] This led to the view that AA is a relatively well-differentiated carcinoma with an excellent prognosis whereas AS is a poorly differentiated carcinoma with an unfavorable outlook and that the squamous component was an important factor in determining behavior. Recent studies indicate that the difference in behavior between AA and AS mainly reflects the difference in the grade of these respective neoplasms.[3,264,265] The biological

behavior of adenocarcinomas with squamous elements is similar to endometrioid carcinoma without squamous epithelium. The presence of squamous elements in one study was associated with a slightly increased probability of survival.[265] Categorization of carcinomas with squamous epithelium according to the depth of myometrial invasion and the grade of the glandular component provides more useful prognostic information than the division into AA or AS.[265] The grade of the glandular component generally parallels that of the squamous element. This had led to the view that AA and AS reflect a continuum in the degree of differentiation of the squamous epithelium that parallels the differentiation of the glandular component.[3,264,265] Furthermore, often the squamous component in these neoplasms displays some cytological atypia, and it is difficult to decide whether it is benign-appearing or sufficiently atypical to qualify as malignant. Accordingly, it is recommended that endometrioid carcinomas with squamous epithelium be classified simply as endometrioid carcinoma with squamous differentiation and graded based on the glandular component as well, moderately, or poorly differentiated (grade 1, 2, or 3, respectively).

GENERAL FEATURES

An early report stated that the frequency of adenocarcinomas with squamous epithelium had increased to a point where it represented nearly a third of all endometrial carcinomas in a 5-year period ending in 1971. More recent studies,[3,4,192] however, show that the relative frequency of this tumor has remained relatively constant over the last 30 years.

Population-based studies from different parts of the world show rather striking differences in the prevalence of adenocarcinomas with squamous epithelium. In Iceland the prevalence of AA was 3% and that of AS 1%.[20] In the Miyagi Prefecture the prevalence of AA was 12% and AS 41%,[215] in the Louisville Cancer Registry AA was 22% and AS 7%,[4,51] and in Norway AA was 9% and AS 4%.[3] Although these differences may be due to the criteria used for the histological diagnosis, they also may reflect racial or regional differences.

CLINICAL FEATURES

There are no differences in the clinical features of adenocarcinoma containing squamous epithelium and endometrioid adenocarcinoma. Thus, there are no differences in the frequency of obesity, hypertension, diabetes, and nulliparity among the large series in which this has been analyzed.[4,51,198]

PATHOLOGICAL FINDINGS

These tumors have no distinctive gross findings. Low-grade tumors (grade 1) are composed of glandular and squamous elements but generally the glandular component predominates; the nests of squamous epithelium are confined to gland lumens (Fig. 12.23). The squamous epithelium resembles metaplastic squamous cells of the cervical transformation zone. Frequently, nests of cells with a prominent oval-to-sindle cell appearance, referred to as *morules,* are observed.[46] Intercellular bridges can be identified within the squamous epithelium, and keratin formation is common. The nuclei of the squamous cells are bland, uniform, and lack prominent nucleoli. Mitotic figures are rare.

In higher grade tumors the squamous element is cytologically more atypical and is not confined to gland lumens but often extends out from the glands (Fig. 12.24). At times the squamous cells have a spindle appearance simulating a sarcoma (Fig. 12.25). They may not be in direct continuity with the glandular epithelium, appearing in isolated nests within the myometrium (Fig. 12.26) or in vascular spaces. Keratinization and pearl formation occur to varying degrees. Generally, the glandular component predominates, but masses of undifferentiated cells that may

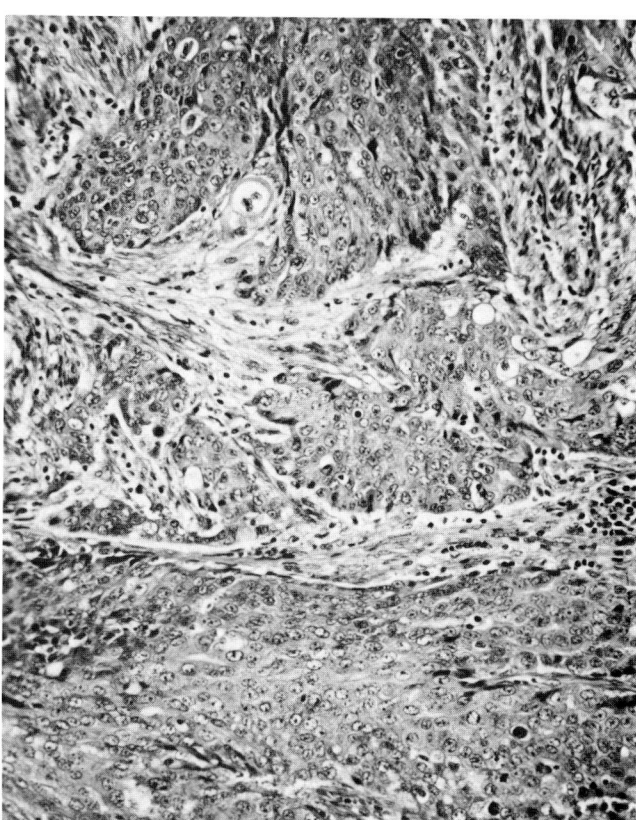

FIG. 12.24. **Endometrioid carcinoma with squamous differentiation, FIGO grade 3.** Sheets of malignant-appearing squamous epithelium diffusely infiltrating the myometrium.

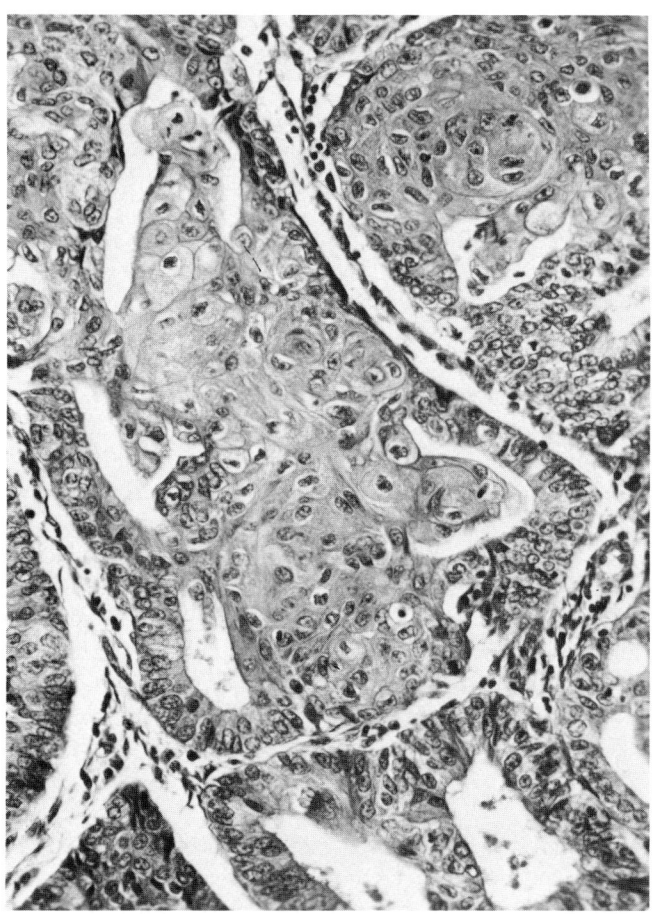

FIG. 12.23. **Endometrioid carcinoma with squamous differentiation, FIGO grade 1.** Both the glandular and squamous elements are grade 1. The squamous nests are confined to the gland lumens.

represent poorly differentiated glandular or squamous cells lie between glands. This undifferentiated epithelium should be considered glandular unless intercellular bridges are demonstrated or the cells have prominent eosinophilic cytoplasm, well-defined cytoplasmic borders, and a sheet-like proliferation without evidence of gland formation. Both the glandular and squamous components display grade 2 or 3 nuclear atypia, an increased nuclear cytoplasmic ratio, and increased mitotic activity. The glandular architecture usually is poorly differentiated. Tumors of intermediate differentiation are common. These neoplasms contain glandular and solid areas in which the squamous cells display a moderate degree of nuclear atypia, defying separation into a "benign" and "malignant" category.

DIFFERENTIAL DIAGNOSIS

The most common problem in the differential diagnosis of the low-grade tumors is with atypical hyperplasia showing squamous metaplasia. To distinguish between the two, the criteria for identifying endometrial stromal invasion should be employed (see Chapter 11, Endometrial Hyperplasia and Related Cellular Changes). At times, a low-grade tumor may be confused with a high-grade carcinoma because

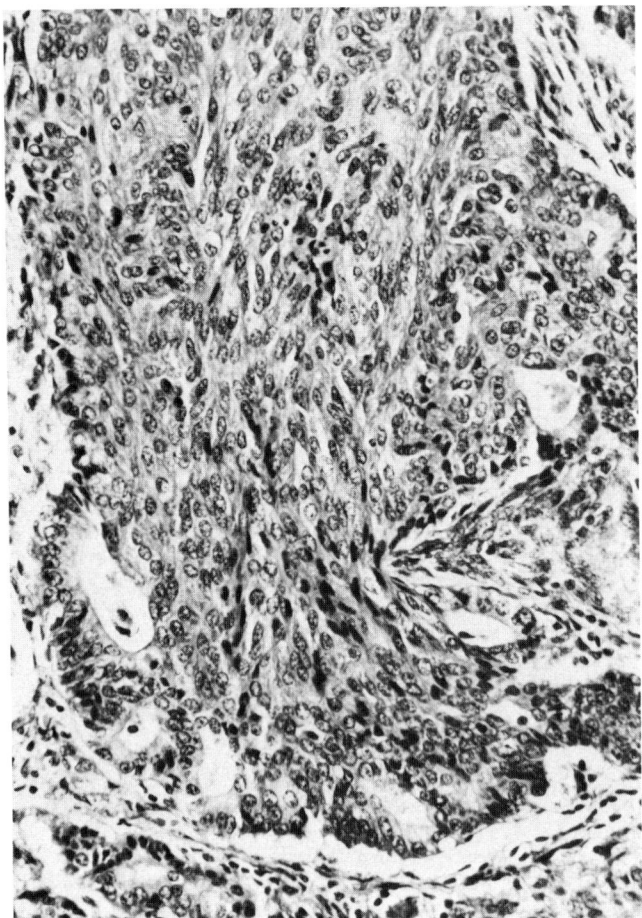

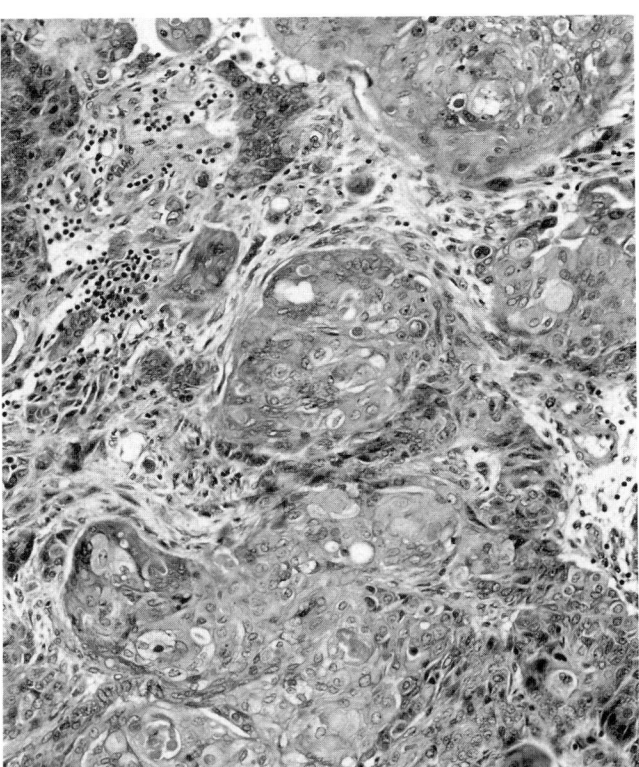

Fig. 12.26. Endometrioid carcinoma with squamous differentiation, FIGO grade 3. Isolated nests of squamous epithelium are diffusely infiltrating the myometrium. (Reprinted by permission of Zaine and Kurman, ref. 264.)

Fig. 12.25. Endometrioid carcinoma with squamous differentiation, FIGO grade 2. The squamous cells have a prominent spindle-cell appearance. This spindle-cell appearance should not be confused with sarcoma.

the masses of squamous epithelium are misconstrued as a solid proliferation of neoplastic cells. The nuclear grade is high in poorly differentiated carcinoma, however. Occasionally, squamous morules may be confused with granulomas, but the presence of foreign body giant cells and an inflammatory infiltrate helps identify the latter. For high-grade adenocarcinomas with squamous epithelium the major problem in differential diagnosis in curettings is distinguishing a primary carcinoma of the endometrium from an adenosquamous carcinoma arising in the endocervix. In the cervix, the squamous component usually predominates, whereas in the endometrium the glandular component predominates. A profusion of cell types, especially mucinous or signet-ring cells, is more characteristic of an endocervical neoplasm.

Immunohistochemical and Ultrastructural Findings

Immunohistochemical studies have reported no qualitative differences in the immunostaining pattern of involucrin and cytokeratin between AA and AS, lending further sup-

port to the view that these tumors reflect different degrees of differentiation in the same neoplasm.[249]

The squamous and glandular elements can be clearly distinguished by electron microscopy. The squamous cells may contain keratohyaline granules, have abundant tonofilaments and tonofibrils, and are joined by numerous desmosomal junctions. Golgi apparatus is scant. In contrast, the glandular cells show luminal formation, have numerous microvilli, and there is a paucity of tonofilaments. Glandular cells also contain abundant Golgi apparatus and vacuoles in the cytoplasm. Cells intermediate between glandular and squamous cells can be seen in clusters extending into gland lumens, suggesting that the two types of cells differentiate from the same stem cell.[87]

Clinical Behavior and Treatment

As described above, when stratified according to stage, grade, and depth of myometrial invasion, there are few differences in the behavior of carcinomas with squamous epithelium compared with endometrioid carcinomas without squamous epithelium.[3,264,265] For example, with stage I, grade 1 disease there are few deaths in patients younger than 50 years.[51] The good prognosis may reflect the younger age of the patients or the biology of the tumor, since the benign-appearing squamous epithelium indicates that the carcinoma has partially differentiated into mature tissue. One of the rare examples of spontaneous regression of endometrial carcinoma was a patient with widespread metastatic grade 1 endometrioid carcinoma with squamous differention.[19] As occurs with endometrioid carcinomas, the low-grade carcinomas with squamous epithelium tend to be only superficially invasive and seldom invade vascular channels as compared with high-grade tumors, which have a high frequency of deep myometrial invasion, vascular space involvement, and pelvic and para-aortic lymph node metastasis.[218] Metastasis of high-grade tumors occurs widely throughout the pelvis and abdomen, involving bowel, mesentery, liver, kidney, spleen, and lymph nodes. Distant metastasis may involve the lungs, heart, skin, and bones.[4] Nearly two-thirds of metastases contain both glandular and squamous elements, but pure adenocarcinoma or squamous carcinoma is encountered in 20% and 8%, respectively.[167] Often it is the squamous component that is identified in vascular channels. Accordingly, the treatment for carcinomas with squamous epithelium is the same as that for endometrioid carcinomas of comparable stage.

A rare finding in patients with adenocarcinoma with squamous differentiation is the presence of keratin granulomas that may involve a wide variety of sites in the peritoneal cavity including the ovaries, tubes, omentum, and serosa of the uterus and bowel.[43,127] Microscopically, these lesions consist of a central mass of keratin and necrotic squamous cells surrounded by a foreign body granulomatous reaction. A proliferation of mesothelial cells also may be present. The granulomas probably result from exfoliation of necrotic cells from the tumor, followed by transtubal spread and implantation on peritoneal surfaces. Thus far, these lesions have not been associated with an unfavorable prognosis.

Mucinous Carcinoma

This uncommon type of endometrial carcinoma has an appearance similar to mucinous carcinoma of the endocervix.[200,233] It occurs as a focal component in up to 42% of endometrioid carcinomas if they are evaluated by mucicarmine stains,[49] but represents the dominant cellular population in only 1–9%.[158,196] To qualify as a mucinous carcinoma, more than one-half the cell population of the tumor must contain PAS-positive, diastase-resistant intracytoplasmic mucin.

CLINICAL FEATURES

Judging from the few published cases, the clinical features of patients with mucinous carcinoma of the endometrium do not differ from those with endometrioid carcinoma. Patients range in age from 47 to 89 years and typically present with vaginal bleeding. In one study more than 40%

had a history of receiving exogenous estrogens.[158] The vast majority of patients present with stage I disease.

PATHOLOGICAL FINDINGS

These tumors do not have distinctive gross features. The most frequent architectural pattern is glandular, often in a villoglandular configuration. The epithelial cells lining the glands and papillary processes tend to be uniform columnar cells with minimal stratification (Fig. 12.27). Cribriform areas are unusual; cystically dilated glands filled with mucin and papillary fronds surrounded by extracellular lakes of mucin, containing neutrophils, are typical (Fig. 12.28). Curiously, mucinous differentiation sometimes is associated with squamous differentiation. Nuclear atypia is mild to moderate and mitotic activity is not prominent. Hyperplasia and mucinous metaplasia sometimes are present in the adjacent endometrium. One study reported that the carcinoma was present in a polyp in 27% of the cases.[158]

The presence of intracytoplasmic mucin can be identified on H&E stains by its distinctive granular, foamy, or

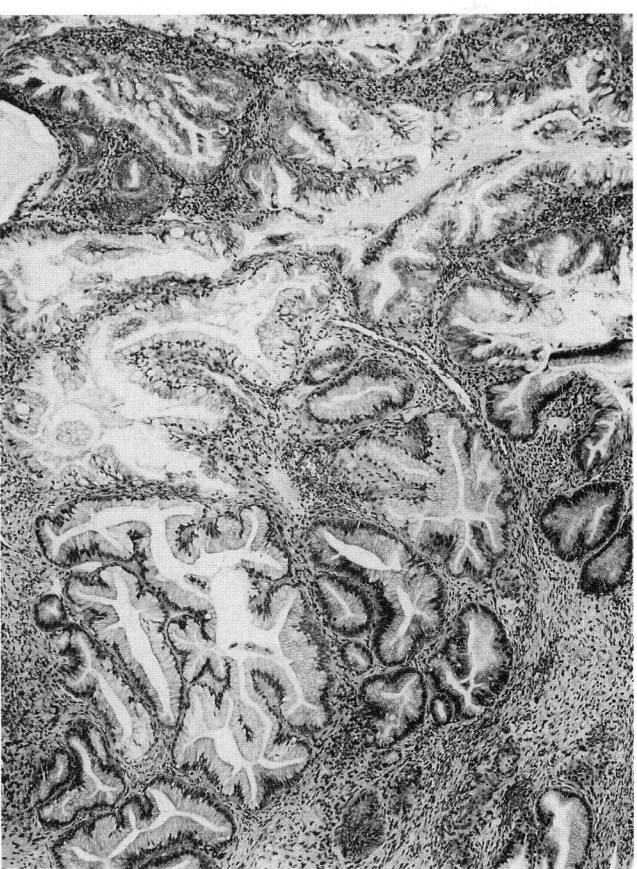

FIG. 12.27. Mucinous carcinoma, FIGO grade 1. The tumor is composed of irregularly shaped glands invading the myometrium. Even under this magnification, uniform columnar cells with basally oriented nuclei can be seen.

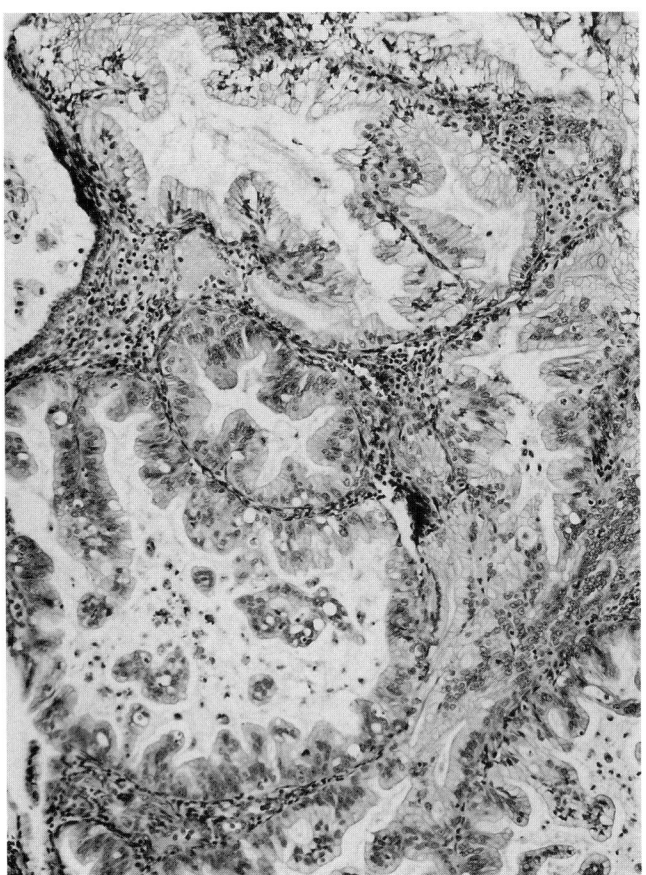

FIG. 12.28. **Mucinous carcinoma, FIGO grade 1.** Higher magnification of same case shown in Fig. 12.27. Papillary projections extend into gland lumens. The latter contain neutrophils. Nuclear atypia is minimal.

bubbly appearance and can be confirmed by PAS, mucicarmine, or alcian blue stains. The intracytoplasmic mucin is variable in both the distribution of mucinous cells in the tumor and in the location of the mucin within individual cells. Mucin may be diffusely present in the cytoplasm, confined to the apical area, or show a combination of both patterns.

DIFFERENTIAL DIAGNOSIS

Endocervical epithelium merges with the endometrium in the lower uterine segment, so it is not surprising that the distinction of primary endocervical from endometrial mucinous carcinoma in currettings can be difficult. There is no histochemical difference in the mucin at either site.[49] Immunohistochemically, carcinoembryonic antigen (CEA) is more common in endocervical than in endometrial carcinomas. Approximately 80% of all endocervical adenocarcinomas show abundant, intracellular CEA whereas only half of typical endometrial carcinomas contain CEA, and this is usually only focal and often confined to the luminal surface.[61,196,245] Mucinous endometrial carcinomas, however, frequently contain immunoreactive CEA. Vimentin is expressed far more commonly in endometrial as compared with endocervical carcinomas. Tumors that are positive for CEA and negative for vimentin are more likely to be endocervical in origin whereas those that are negative for CEA and positive for vimentin are more likely to be primary endometrial carcinomas. Because of the high frequency of CEA in mucinous endometrial carcinomas, immunostaining is not particularly helpful in these instances. Finally, since nearly 80% of endocervical carcinomas contain HPV DNA whereas endometrial carcinomas rarely if ever do, in situ localization of HPV DNA can assist in the differential diagnosis. The presence of an associated endometrial hyperplasia suggests an endometrial primary site. Conversely, the presence of a cervical squamous intraepithelial lesion favors an endocervical primary site.

The distinction of mucinous carcinoma of the endometrium from clear cell or secretory carcinoma is made on the basis of morphology and PAS and mucin stains. The cells in secretory carcinoma are clear (not granular or foamy) because of the presence of glycogen, which is PAS-positive and is removed by diastase treatment. Mucin in these tumors is focal at most. Clear cell carcinoma is almost always papillary or solid in contrast to the glandular pattern of mucinous carcinoma. The cells in clear cell carcinoma tend to be polygonal rather than columnar and hobnail cells are almost invariably present, a cytological feature that is absent in mucinous carcinoma.

Rarely a mucinous carcinoma or a mixed mucinous and endometrioid carcinoma may contain areas that simulate microglandular hyperplasia of the cervix.[261] Such foci are characterized by cells showing mucinous and eosinophilic change with microcystic spaces containing acute inflammatory cells. The patients are in their 50s and 60s, in contrast to women with microglandular hyperplasia, who are young. The complexity of the glandular pattern and the degree of cytological atypia distinguish this carcinoma from microglandular hyperplasia.

CLINICAL BEHAVIOR AND TREATMENT

When stratified by stage, grade, and depth of myometrial invasion, mucinous tumors behave the same as endometrioid carcinomas.[196] Mucinous carcinomas, however, tend to be low grade and minimally invasive and therefore as a group have an excellent prognosis. Treatment is the same as for endometrioid carcinoma. Since most of the tumors are stage I, low grade, and minimally invasive, total abdominal hysterectomy and bilateral salpingo-oophorectomy usually suffices.

Serous Carcinoma

The existence of papillary patterns within endometrial carcinoma has been recognized since the turn of the century.[59] Subsequently, sporadic reports drew attention to the presence of psammoma bodies in primary papillary endometrial carcinomas,[80,139,147] focusing on the similarity with a metastasis from the ovary. Subsequently, Hendrickson et al. reported a series of primary uterine serous carcinomas and identified them as a highly aggressive type of endometrial carcinoma.[108]

As experience with serous carcinoma has increased, it has become apparent that this neoplasm demonstrates considerable diversity in its architectural and cytological features. Although a papillary pattern typically predominates, glandular and solid patterns also occur.[108,140,211] Serous carcinoma originally was described as having thick, short papillae, but subsequent studies have shown that thin papillae may be present in more than half of them.[140,211] The cytological features of these tumors also are quite varied. Polygonal cells with eosinophilic and clear cytoplasm often are seen but hobnail cells are among the most frequently observed cells. A common feature, however, is marked nuclear atypia. Accordingly, serous carcinoma may be defined broadly as a carcinoma in which a papillary or glandular pattern is associated with hobnail cells and high-grade nuclei. Areas containing clear cells do not preclude the diagnosis of serous carcinoma.

CLINICAL FEATURES

The prevalence of serous carcinomas reported from referral centers usually is about 10%; however, in a population-based study from Norway it was only 1%[1] and in Australia 3%.[248] Patients with serous carcinoma range in age from 39 to 93 years but typically are postmenopausal and in contrast to women with endometrioid carcinoma, are older (mean age of 68 years vs. 59 years), are less likely to have received estrogen replacement therapy, and are more likely to have abnormal cervical cytology. There are some data to suggest that women with this neoplasm are less likely to be obese and that a higher proportion of women are black.[69] In other respects, they appear similar.

GROSS FINDINGS

On gross examination, uteri containing these tumors often are small and atrophic. Generally the tumor is exophytic (Fig. 12.29) and has a papillary appearance. Depth of invasion is difficult to assess on macroscopic examination. It is not unusual to find a benign-appearing polyp containing the carcinoma in the hysterectomy specimen after a diagnosis of serous carcinoma has been made on a curetting because these tumors frequently develop within a polyp.

Microscopically, the exophytic component of a serous carcinoma typically has a complex papillary architecture resembling serous carcinoma of the ovary (Fig. 12.30). The papillary fronds may be either short and densely fibrotic (Fig. 12.31) or thin and delicate (Fig. 12.30). The cells covering the papillae and lining the glands form small

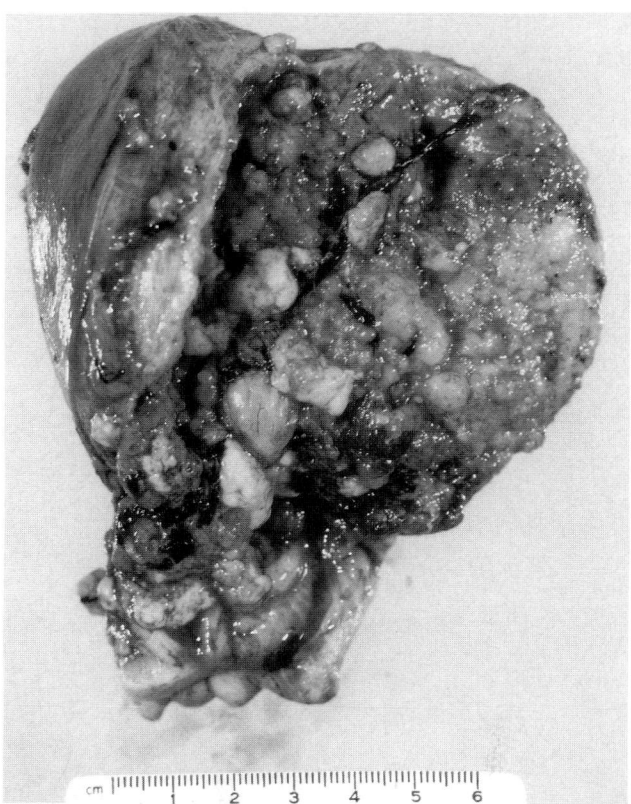

FIG. 12.29. Serous carcinoma. The tumor is exophytic, markedly papillary, and deeply invades the myometrium and cervix.

papillary tufts, many of which are detached and float freely in spaces between the papillae and in gland lumens (Fig. 12.31). The cells are cuboidal or hobnail-shaped (Fig. 12.32) and contain abundant granular eosinophilic or clear cytoplasm. The cells tend to be loosely cohesive. There may be considerable cytological variability throughout the tumor as many cells tend to show marked cytological atypia manifested by nuclear pleomorphism, hyperchromasia, and macronucleoli whereas others are small and not as ominous in appearance. Multinucleated cells, giant nuclei, and bizarre forms occur in half the patients. Lobulated nuclei with smudged chromatin also are frequently encountered (Fig. 12.32). Mitotic activity usually is high and abnormal mitotic figures are easily identified. Psammoma bodies are encountered in a third of cases. The invasive component of the neoplasm can show contiguous downgrowth of papillary processes, or solid masses or glands; the latter often have a gaping appearance. Nests of cells within vascular spaces is a common finding (Fig. 12.33).

The adjacent endometrium is atrophic in almost all cases. Hyperplasia, generally without atypia, is present in 5% of cases.[35,211] In nearly 90% of cases the surface endometrium adjacent to the carcinoma or at other sites away from the neoplasm is replaced by one or several layers of highly atypical cells that overlie atrophic endometrium and

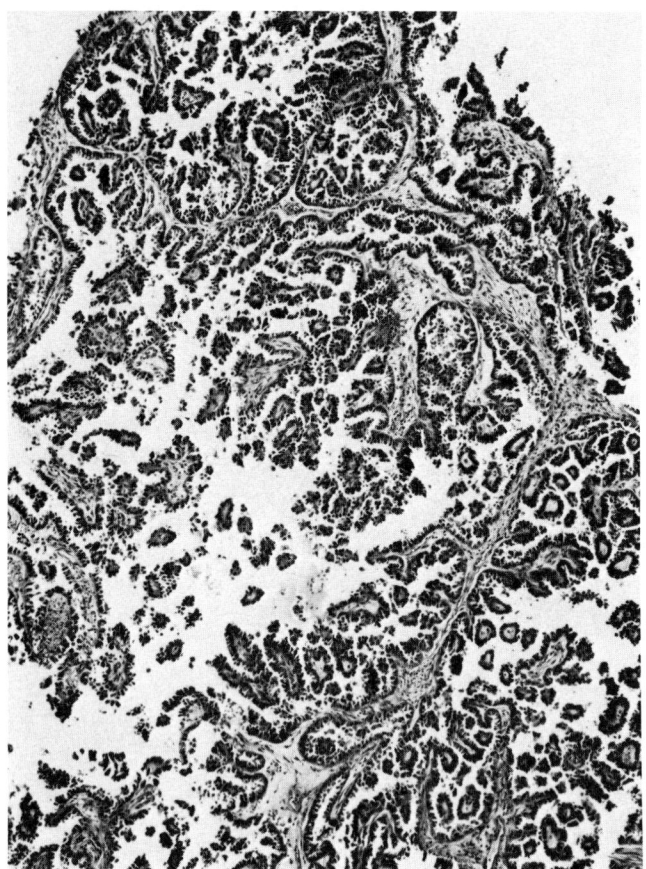

FIG. 12.30. **Serous carcinoma.** The tumor is characterized by a complex papillary architecture resembling serous carcinoma of the ovary.

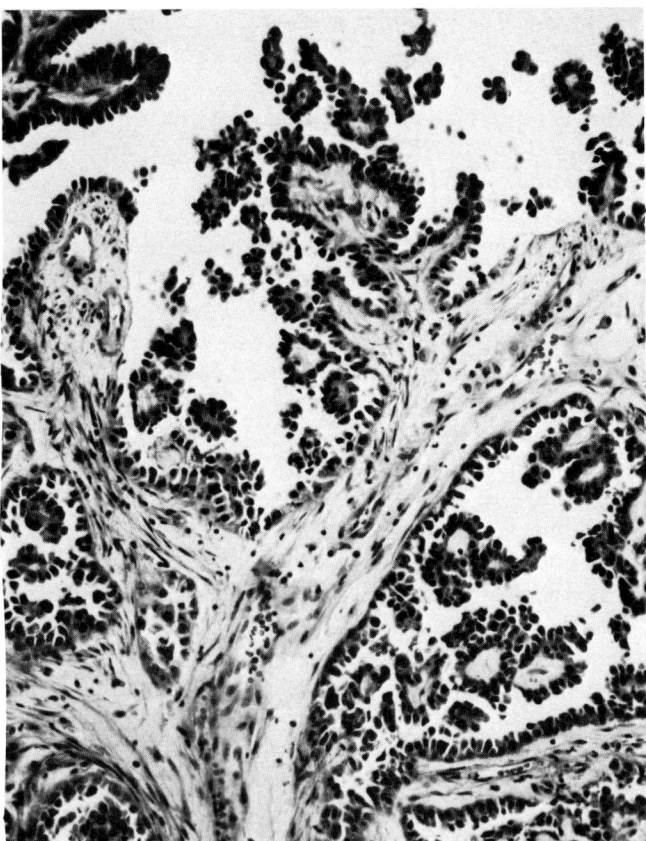

FIG. 12.31. **Serous carcinoma.** Dense fibrotic fibrovascular cores are covered by papillary tufts with many cells having a hobnail appearance. Most of the nuclei in this field are grade 2.

extend into normal glands. These cells are identical to those of the invasive carcinoma and at times form micropapillary processes. This lesion has been designated *endometrial intraepithelial carcinoma*[211] (Figs. 12.34 and 12.35). It is not clear whether this is an in situ precursor or whether it represents surface implantation from the invasive serous carcinoma. It may reflect both processes. The intraepithelial carcinoma can extensively replace the surface endometrium and glands without invasion (Fig. 12.36).

RISK FACTORS

Serous carcinomas tend to invade the myometrium deeply, but the depth of myometrial invasion in pathological stage I tumors does not always correlate with survival. Specifically, in several studies the survival of patients with minimal invasion is similar to that of patients with deep invasion.* Preliminary analysis of a large GOG study indicates a

strong relationship to depth of invasion (RJ Zaino and RJ Kurman, unpublished data). Whereas only 13% of patients with tumor confined to the endometrium died of tumor, the probability increased to 30% with inner-third invasion and to 68% with outer-third invasion. Among 37 cases in

FIG. 12.32. **Serous carcinoma.** Most of the cells covering the papillae are hobnail cells showing marked nuclear atypia (grade 3). Bizarre-shaped nuclei with marked hyperchromasia and smudged chromatin are evident.

FIG. 12.33. **Serous carcinoma.** The tumor extensively involves vascular channels within the myometrium far removed from the tumor mass. The papillary architecture is retained in the intravascular component.

FIG. 12.34. **Endometrial intraepithelial carcinoma.** Highly atypical cells identical to those in serous carcinoma replace the surface epithelium overlying atrophic glands and extend into normal glands (*left side of field*). This lesion was immediately adjacent to an invasive serous carcinoma. (Reprinted by permission of Sherman et al., ref. 211.)

FIG. 12.35. **Endometrial intraepithelial carcinoma.** Another focus of intraepithelial carcinoma on the endometrial surface (*left side of field*) at a remote site from the invasive carcinoma.

*Refs. 1,35,81,140,144,188,211,213.

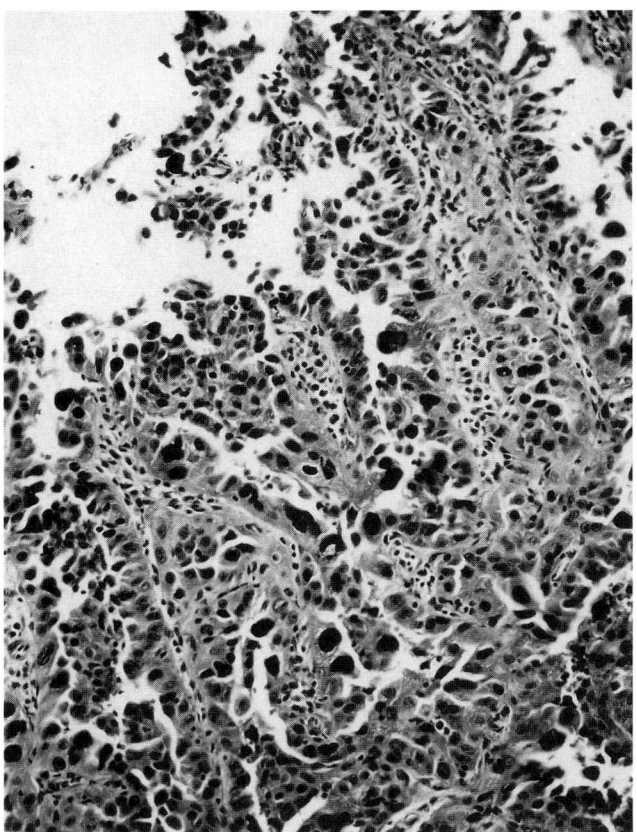

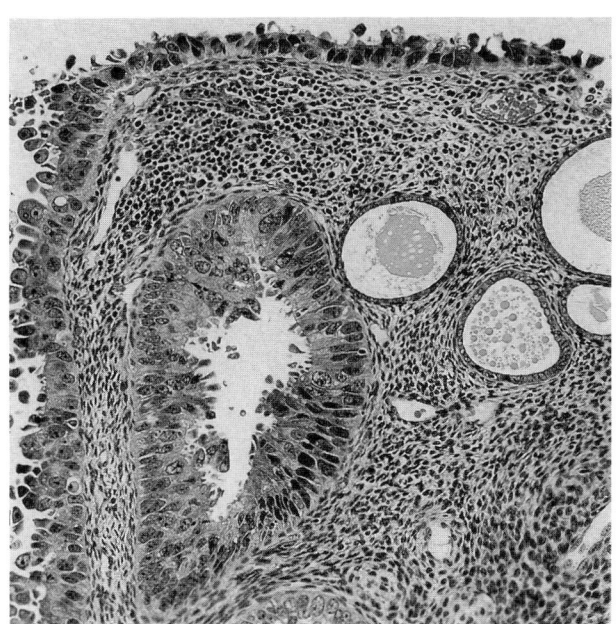

12.34

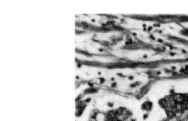

12.32

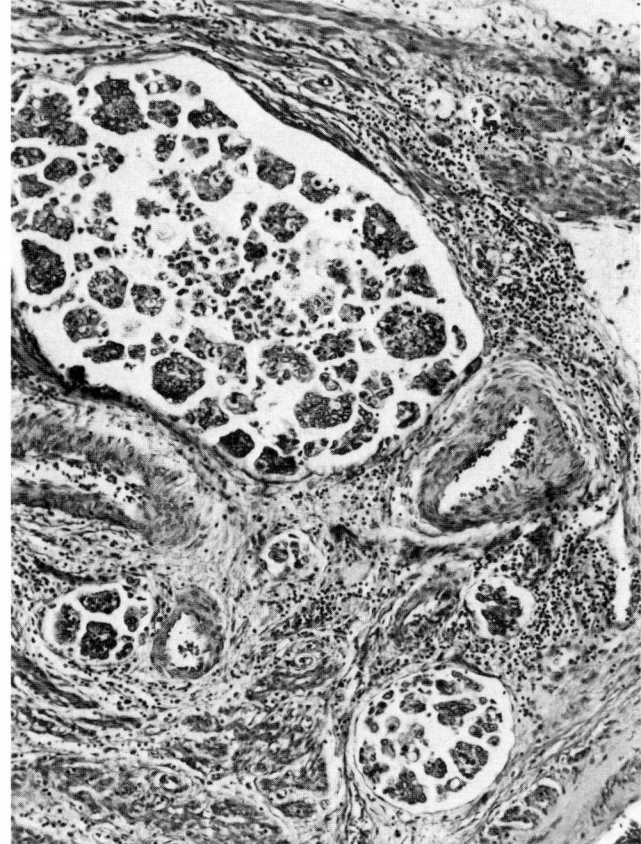

2.33

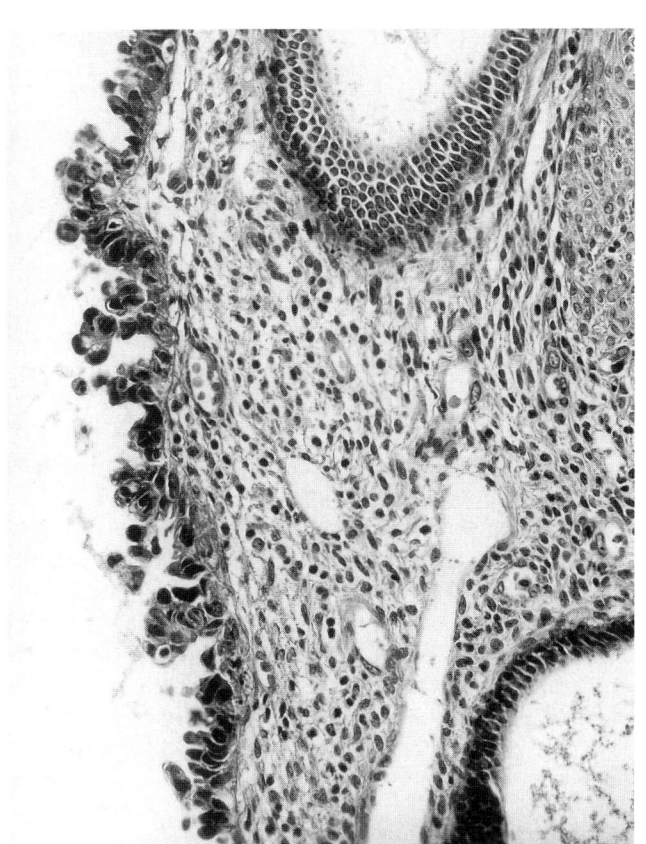

12.35

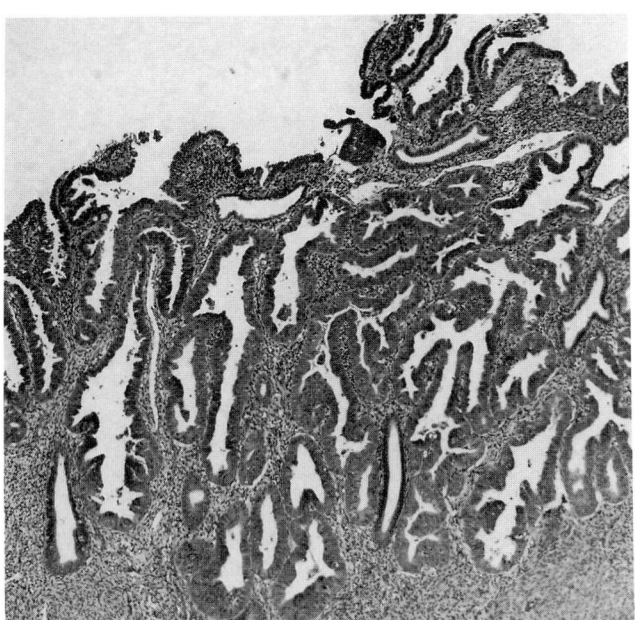

FIG. 12.36. **Endometrial intraepithelial carcinoma.** The neoplasm extensively replaces glands but does not invade the stroma. Elsewhere, an invasive serous carcinoma was present. This appearance can easily be confused with endometrioid carcinoma.

the literature in which serous carcinoma was confined to a polyp or did not invade the myometrium, 22 (59%) recurred.

Nuclear grade does not correlate with survival. This is not surprising because the tumors contain high-grade nuclei by definition. In contrast, an architectural grading system used in the GOG analysis did discriminate prognosis. Thus, based on the extent of solid as compared with papillary patterns, only 30% of patients with grade 1 tumors were dead of disease compared with 44% with grade 2 and 68% with grade 3 neoplasms (RJ Zaino and RJ Kurman, unpublished data). These findings conflict with the FIGO recommendations, which suggest that serous carcinomas be graded according to the nuclear grade. Although the data are preliminary, the GOG findings suggest that architectural grading is of value. Accordingly, we recommend using this method as opposed to nuclear grading for serous carcinoma. Although some investigators have not found a correlation between the presence of vascular invasion and survival[1,35] others have.[92,211] Positive peritoneal cytology was an independent risk factor in one study.[211] Most studies have demonstrated the presence of estrogen and progesterone receptors in serous carcinoma but this has not been useful in either predicting behavior or response to hormone treatment.[92,144,229] Although positive, the receptor levels generally have not been high.

DIFFERENTIAL DIAGNOSIS

Serous carcinoma must be distinguished from villoglandular carcinoma. Unlike serous carcinoma, villoglandular carcinoma is characterized by the predominance of long, delicate papillary fronds that do not display papillary tufting. In addition, the cells are columnar, resembling cells in endometrioid carcinoma and lack high-grade nuclear atypia (see above, Villoglandular Carcinoma).

A serous carcinoma with a prominent glandular pattern that lacks prominent papillary features may be confused with an endometrioid carcinoma. In this case it is the nuclear morphology that aids in the distinction. The glands in an endometrioid carcinoma are lined by columnar cells with nuclei that are grade 1 or 2. Endometrioid carcinomas with grade 3 nuclei are solid, not glandular. In contrast, the glands in a serous carcinoma are lined by cells with high-grade nuclei, some of which are hobnail-shaped (Fig. 12.37). In addition, papillary tufts project or lie detached in the gland lumens.

At times papillary syncytial eosinophilic change, particularly in a small curettage specimen in an older patient, may

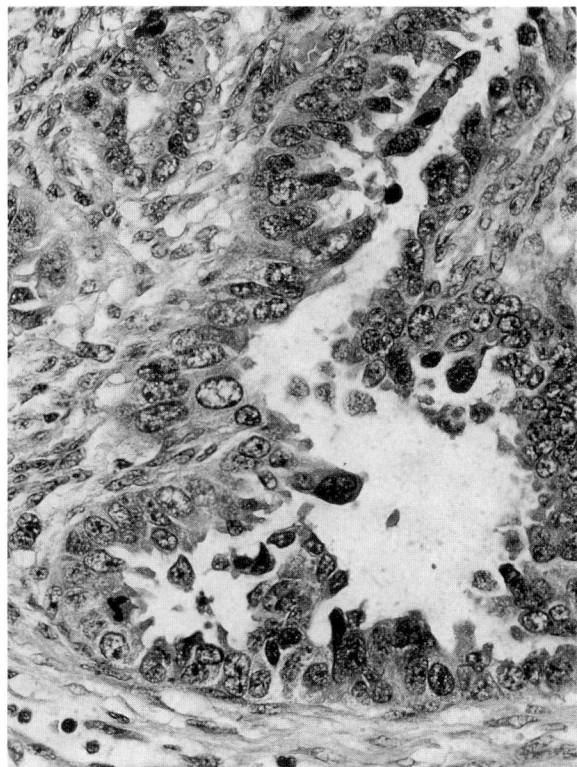

FIG. 12.37. **Serous carcinoma.** Same case as illustrated in Fig. 12.36. A gaping gland lined by cells with high-grade nuclei. Several of the cells are hobnail cells. The high-grade nuclear morphology distinguishes serous carcinoma with a prominent glandular pattern from an endometrioid carcinoma. Endometrioid carcinoma with grade 3 nuclei nearly always displays a solid rather than a glandular architecture.

be difficult to distinguish from serous carcinoma. The papillary processes in eosinophilic change lack fibrovascular support and the cells that form these processes are small and lack significant nuclear atypia or mitotic activity. Typically small microcystic spaces containing neutrophils are present in the syncytial masses.

At times it may not be clear if a serous carcinoma involving the endometrium is primary or metastatic from the ovary. More often than not the uterus is the primary site. A discussion of synchronous tumors involving the endometrium and ovary can be found under Tumors Metastatic to the Endometrium (see below).

Immunohistochemical and Ultrastructural Findings

Strong immunohistochemical staining for p53, which probably reflects genetic mutation of this tumor suppressor gene, has been found in 5 (71%) of 7 serous carcinomas compared with 9 (22%) of 40 endometrioid carcinomas.[32]

In a study comparing the ultrastructural features of serous carcinoma, endometrioid carcinoma, and clear cell carcinoma, Sato et al.[203] found similarities among all three types of neoplasms, particularly between serous carcinoma and clear cell carcinoma. Numerous secretory granules, large nuclei, prominent nucleoli, and a paucity of microfilaments are features that differ from the endometrioid carcinoma and more closely resemble serous carcinoma of the ovary. The ultrastructural findings reflect the poor differentiation of serous carcinoma in contrast to the better differentiated endometrioid carcinoma.

Clinical Behavior and Treatment

Serous carcinoma has a propensity for myometrial and lymphatic invasion (Fig. 12.33). The hysterectomy specimen often discloses tumor in lymphatics extensively within the myometrium, cervix, broad ligament, fallopian tube, and ovarian hilus. In addition, intraepithelial carcinoma similar to that involving the endometrium has been reported on the surfaces of the ovaries, peritoneum, and mucosa of the endocervix and fallopian tube in the absence of gross disease in these sites.[211] Involvement of peritoneal surfaces in the pelvis and abdomen, as in ovarian serous carcinoma, occurs early in the course of disease. Not surprisingly, most studies report that uterine serous carcinoma is clinically understaged in approximately 40% of cases.[35,69] The common finding of widespread disease arising synchronously or asynchronously in the endometrium, ovaries, and peritoneum is interpreted by several investigators as a manifestation of multifocal disease. In patients with high-stage disease, it may be impossible to distinguish a primary serous carcinoma of the ovary from one arising in the uterus. In addition to intraperitoneal spread, serous carcinoma can metastasize to the liver, brain, and skin.

It is not uncommon for serous carcinoma to be confined to an endometrial polyp with no evidence of extrauterine disease at the time of hysterectomy.[35,140,188,211,213] Among 20 cases in which that has been reported, recurrence occurred in 15 (75%). Although vascular invasion or transtubal spread could account for these findings, most investigators regard this as additional evidence supporting multifocal disease. Serous carcinomas secrete CA-125 and serial serum measurements have correlated closely with the course of disease.[144,236]

The 5- and 10-year actuarial survival for all stages was 36% and 18%, respectively, in a study from Norway.[1] Five-year survival for pathological stage I disease is 40%.[35] The median survival for patients who die of disease is 17 months. Patients with mixed endometrial carcinomas containing a component of serous carcinoma that accounted for as little as 25% of the tumor have the same survival as patients with pure serous carcinoma, underscoring the importance of identifying areas of serous carcinoma in uterine carcinomas.[211]

The current approach to treatment is hysterectomy and bilateral salpingo-oophorectomy along with omentectomy, and careful surgical staging including peritoneal cytology and pelvic and para-aortic lymph node sampling. In view of the highly aggressive behavior, adjuvant therapy should be considered for all tumors except those that *minimally* involve the tip of a polyp. Unfortunately, no satisfactory adjuvant therapy is available. In a study evaluating cisplatin, doxorubicin (Adriamycin), and cyclophosphamide (PAC) chemotherapy, which has a 70% response rate in previously untreated ovarian serous carcinoma, the response rate for uterine serous carcinoma was only 20%,[144] suggesting that there are inherent differences in uterine as compared with ovarian serous carcinomas. These tumors also are unresponsive to hormone treatment. Whole abdominal radiation currently is being investigated.

Clear Cell Carcinoma

In the past, clear cell carcinoma was regarded as mesonephric in origin because of its resemblance to renal carcinoma, but the occurrence of clear cell carcinoma in the endometrium, a müllerian derivative, is evidence of its müllerian origin.[137,214]

Clinical Features

The prevalence of clear cell carcinoma ranges from 1% to 5% in most series. Almost all studies report that women with clear cell carcinoma are older than women with endometrioid carcinoma (mean age 67 vs. 59 years). Some studies have reported a higher likelihood of abnormal cytology (58% vs. 5%), a lower frequency of some of the associated constitutional symptoms, such as obesity and diabetes mellitus,[45] and a lack of association of estrogen replacement therapy compared with endometrioid carcinomas, but this has not been confirmed by other studies.[252]

PATHOLOGICAL FINDINGS

These tumors do not have distinctive gross features. Clear cell carcinoma may exhibit solid, papillary, tubular, and cystic patterns (Figs. 12.38–12.42). The solid pattern is composed of masses of clear cells intermixed with eosinophilic cells, whereas papillary, tubular, and cystic patterns are composed predominantly of hobnail-shaped cells with interspersed clear and eosinophilic cells. Cystic spaces frequently are lined by flattened cells. Psammoma bodies can be found in association with papillary areas within the tumor.[137]

The cells typically are large, with clear or lightly stained eosinophilic cytoplasm. The clear cytoplasm is due to the presence of glycogen, demonstrated with a PAS stain and diastase digestion. Cells that have discharged their glycogen and lost most of their cytoplasm are characterized by a

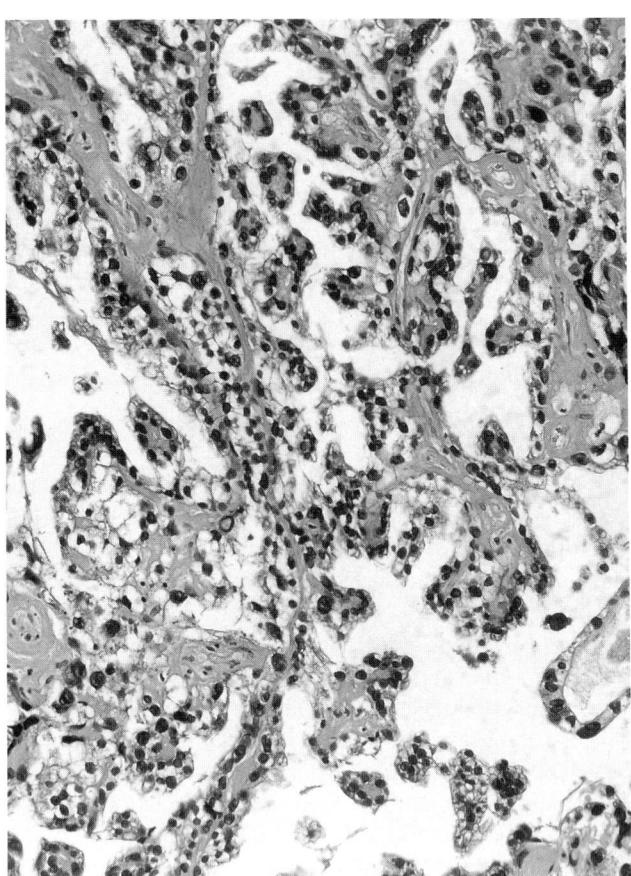

FIG. 12.39. Clear cell carcinoma. The papillae in this neoplasm have hyalinized cores. This feature is seen more frequently in papillary clear cell as compared with serous carcinoma.

naked nucleus, the hobnail cells. Nuclear atypia generally is marked, manifested by pleomorphic, often large, multiple nuclei with prominent nucleoli (Fig. 12.42). Mitotic activity is high, and abnormal mitoses are readily seen. The nuclear grade generally is high.[45,195,214] Because of the diverse histological patterns that are present, clear cell carcinomas are graded based on the nuclear grade only. PAS-positive, diastase-resistant intracellular and extracellular hyaline bodies, similar to those in endodermal sinus tumors, can be found in nearly two-thirds of clear cell carcinomas and serve as a useful identifying feature.[45]

DIFFERENTIAL DIAGNOSIS

The differential diagnosis is between serous carcinoma, secretory carcinoma, and yolk sac tumor. The differential diagnosis of the first two tumors is discussed above (see Secretory and Serous Carcinoma). The distinction from a serous carcinoma is not clinically relevant because their behavior is similar. Yolk sac tumors occur rarely in the endometrium but the patients are young, in contrast to women with clear cell carcinoma who are almost always

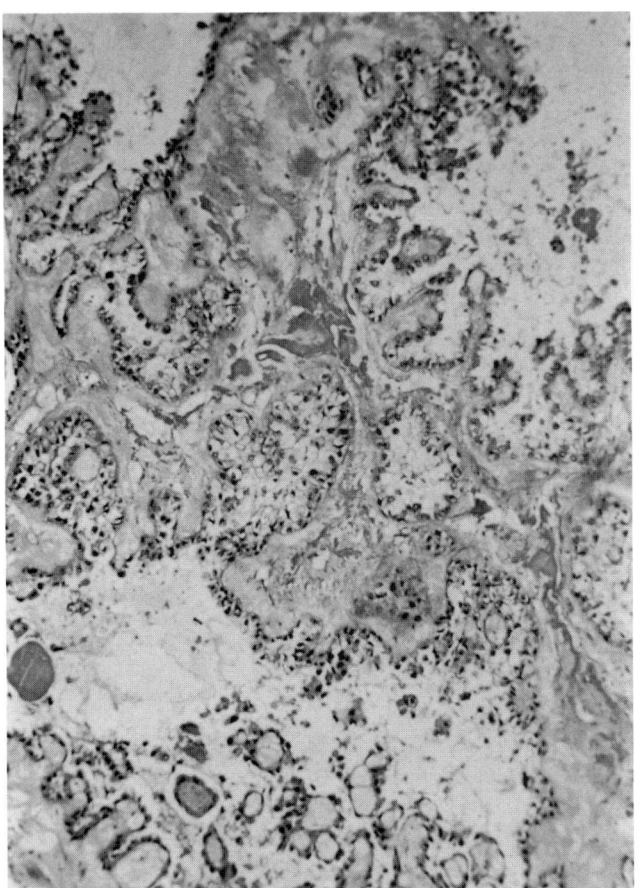

FIG. 12.38. Clear cell carcinoma. The tumor displays a papillary pattern resembling serous carcinoma.

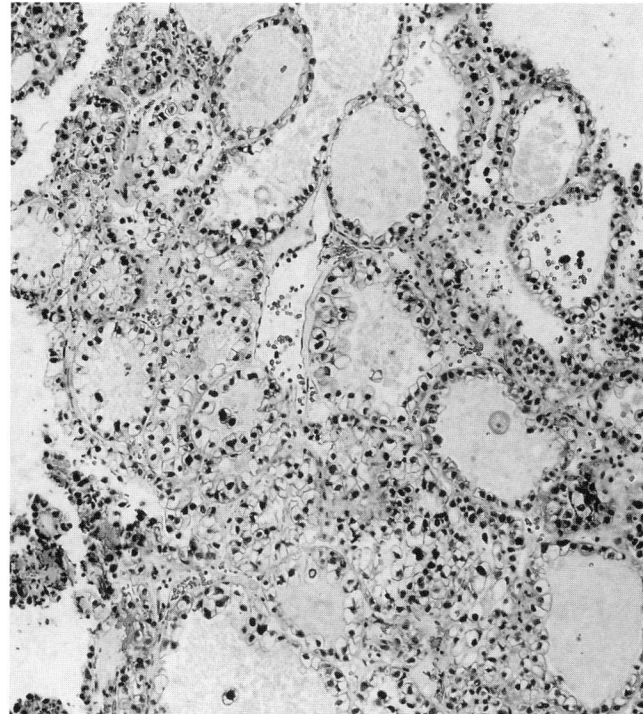

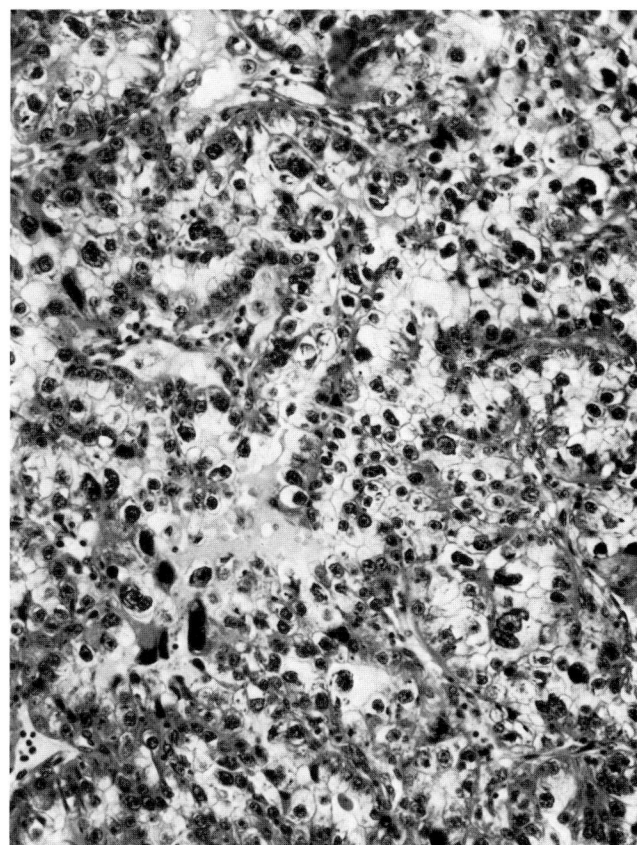

FIG. 12.42. **Clear cell carcinoma.** The tumor is composed of sheets of large clear cells with enlarged, pleomorphic nuclei.

postmenopausal. Microscopically, yolk sac tumors often have a microcystic pattern that can resemble the tubulocystic pattern of clear cell carcinoma. Characteristically, the yolk sac tumor contains Schiller–Duval bodies, which are lacking in clear cell carcinoma. Yolk sac tumors are associated with elevated serum alpha-fetoprotein (AFP) levels and immunohistochemically AFP can be identified in the tumor. We have rarely encountered AFP in clear cell carcinomas (see below).

IMMUNOHISTOCHEMICAL AND ULTRASTRUCTURAL FINDINGS

CA-125 and Leu-M1 have been localized in the cytoplasm of clear cell carcinomas but their presence does not aid in the differential diagnosis.[183,260] We also have observed AFP intracytoplasmically within clear cell carcinoma. This should be considered in the differential diagnosis of clear

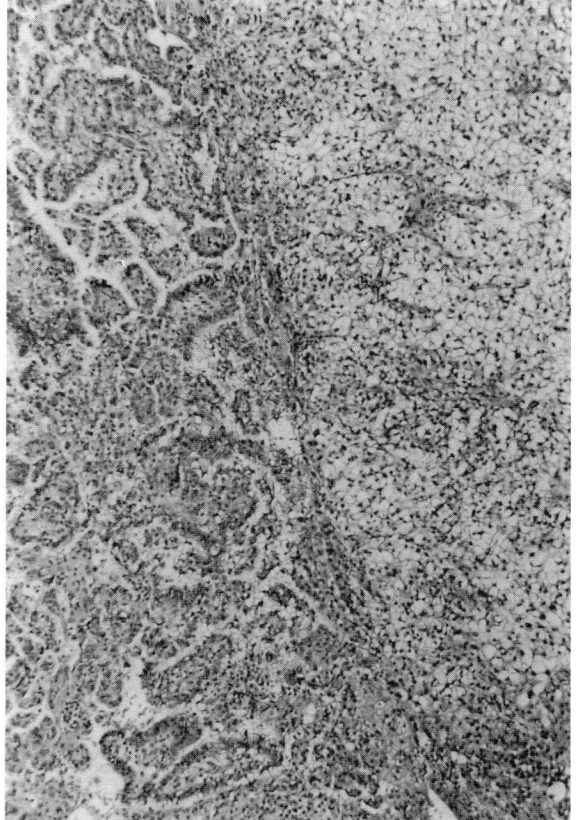

FIG. 12.40. **Clear cell carcinoma.** The tumor displays a tubulocystic pattern resembling endometrioid carcinoma.
FIG. 12.41. **Clear cell carcinoma.** The tumor displays a solid and papillary pattern.

cell carcinoma from yolk sac tumors (see below). An unusual case of a clear cell carcinoma with abundant intracytoplasmic lipid has been reported.[183]

On electron microscopy, the clear cells contain abundant glycogen, parallel stacks of granular endoplasmic reticulum, numerous free ribosomes, and small, uniform rounded mitochondria. Supranuclear Golgi complex and microvesicles are present in some of the cells. Nuclei are irregularly shaped and show shallow indentations. The hobnail-type cells have an abundant supranuclear cytoplasmic matrix and a prominent bulging nucleus.[195,214]

CLINICAL BEHAVIOR AND TREATMENT

Clear cell carcinoma tends to be high grade, deeply invasive, and present in an advanced stage. In one series of 20 patients there were five clear cell carcinomas confined to a polyp. All these women are alive without disease.[126] The reported survival of patients with clear cell carcinoma differs considerably as reported in various series ranging from 21% to 75%.[3a,45,137,180,252] None of the patients with tumor beyond stage I survived for 5 years in the series reported by Christopherson et al.[45] Even in stage I, the 5-year survival was only 44%. In a series of nearly 97 patients the 5-year crude survival was 42% and the 10-year survival 31%.[3a] The mean length of survival for those who fail treatment is 19 months.

Treatment is the same as that for endometrioid carcinoma. The role of adjuvant radiation or chemotherapy is not established at present. In view of the poor prognosis and because these tumors often have high nuclear grade and invade the myometrium deeply, adjuvant radiotherapy often is administered.

Squamous Cell Carcinoma

Squamous carcinoma develops in the endometrium, but it is extremely rare.[159] In a population-based study from Norway the prevalence was 0.1%.[3a] To qualify as primary squamous carcinoma of the endometrium, three criteria must be met: (1) adenocarcinoma is not present in the endometrium, (2) the squamous carcinoma in the endometrium does not have any connection with the squamous epithelium of the cervix, (3) squamous carcinoma is not present in the cervix.[83] By these criteria, only 29 cases of primary squamous carcinoma of the endometrium have been reported.[3a,220] There is a strong association with cervical stenosis, pyometria, and chronic inflammation. The tumor may arise from ichthyosis uteri, a condition in which the endometrium is replaced by keratinized squamous epithelium. In the past, this condition was considered a sequela of the use of steam as treatment for endometritis. With the abandonment of this procedure, ichthyosis uteri has become quite rare.

Microscopically, squamous carcinomas of the endometrium resemble those in the cervix; however, at times they can be extremely well differentiated and therefore difficult to diagnose with certainty in curettings. Sometimes the diagnosis is not established until a hysterectomy is performed (Fig. 12.43).

In addition to typical squamous cell carcinoma, verrucous carcinoma may arise as a primary tumor in the endometrium[114a,197a] (Fig. 12.44). There have been 25 cases of squamous carcinoma in the endometrium reported in association with squamous carcinoma in situ of the cervix[125] (Fig. 12.45). Some of these may have arisen in the endometrium but most probably represent extension from a cervical primary. The prognosis of squamous cell carcinoma is poor with a 5-year survival of 36% for clinical stage I.

Undifferentiated Carcinoma

Tumors that fail to show evidence of either glandular or squamous differentiation are regarded as undifferentiated carcinomas. The prevalence is 1–2%. The mean age of patients with undifferentiated carcinoma is 64 years. The clinical features of women with undifferentiated carcinoma insofar as age, parity, hypertension, and diabetes are concerned are similar to those of endometrioid carcinoma.

In a study of 31 undifferentiated carcinomas these tumors were divided into large cell and small cell/inter-

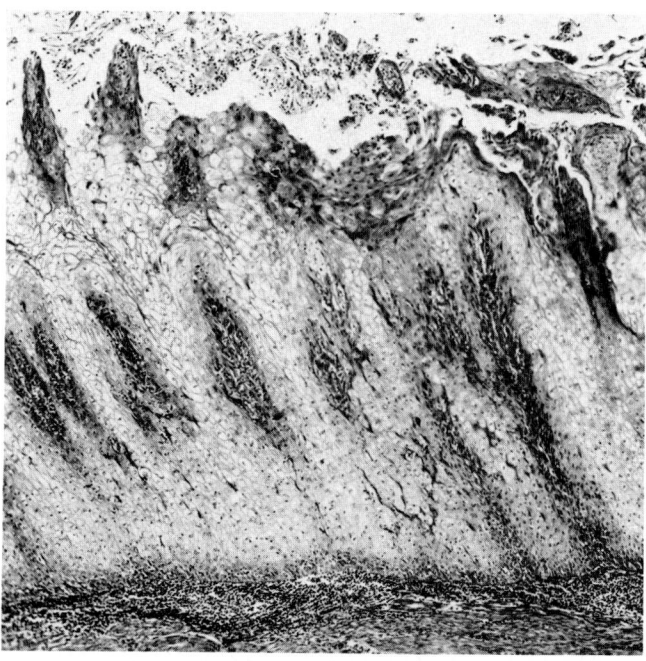

FIG. 12.43. Squamous cell carcinoma. There is complete replacement of the surface endometrium. Elsewhere, the tumor deeply invaded the myometrium.

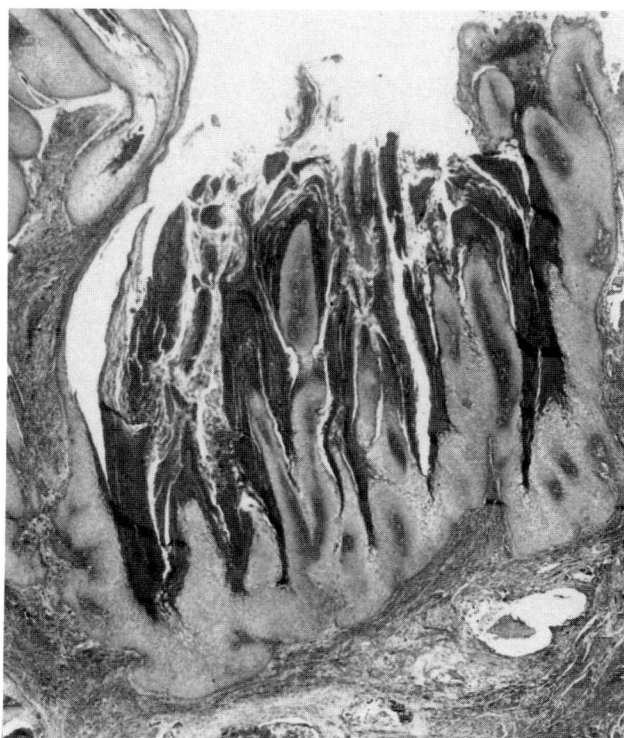

FIG. 12.44. **Verrucous carcinoma.** This tumor arose in endometrial glands and invaded the myometrium superficially. There was no tumor in the cervix, vagina, or vulva.

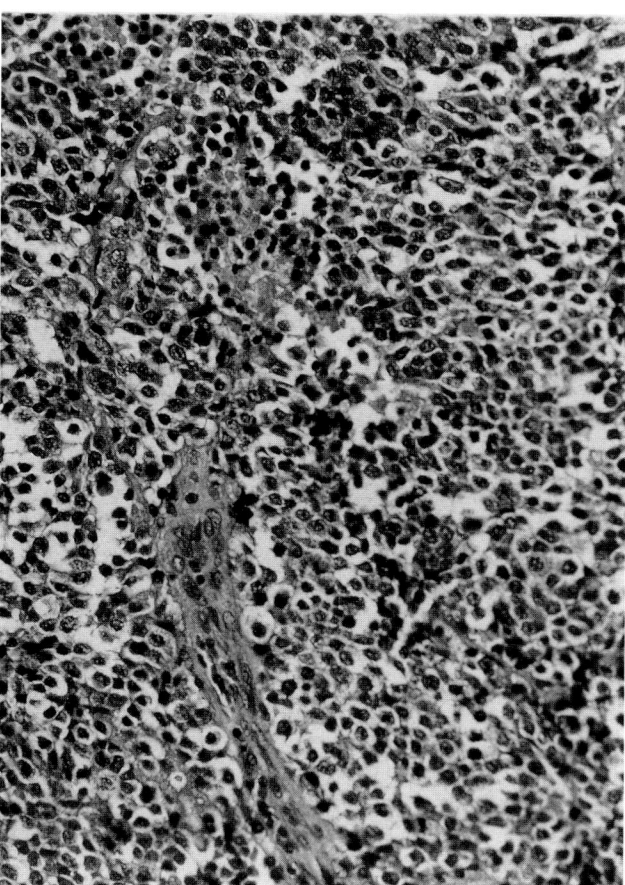

FIG. 12.46. **Small cell carcinoma.** The tumor is composed of undifferentiated small cells resembling neuroendocrine-type small cell carcinoma in other organs.

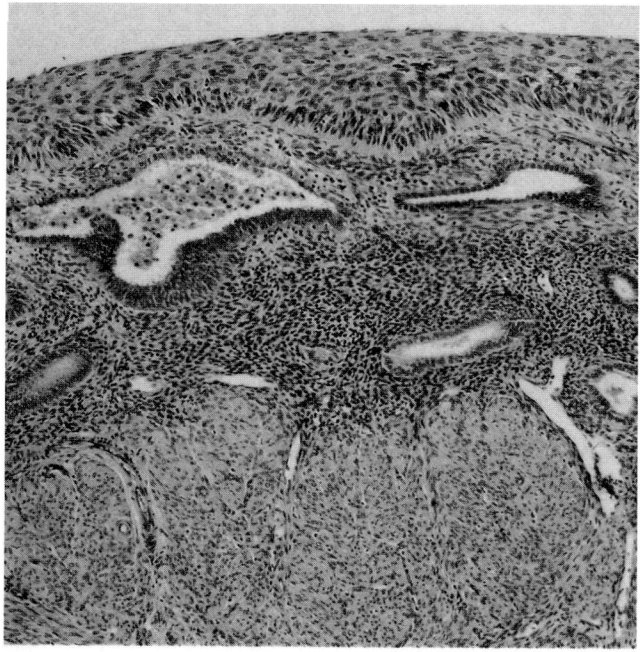

FIG. 12.45. **Cervical high-grade squamous intraepithelial lesion (CIN 3).** The neoplasm grew in a contiguous fashion from the cervix and replaced the endometrium. There was no invasion.

mediate types[2] (Fig. 12.46). Some small cell carcinomas display a trabecular pattern simulating a carcinoid tumor (Fig. 12.47). Typically, these tumors merge into areas with gland formation (Fig. 12.48). Both large and small cell undifferentiated carcinomas in one study reacted uniformly positive with cytokeratin antibodies and 57% co-expressed vimentin.[2] Nearly half the small cell carcinomas were positive for neuron-specific enolase and, of these, synaptophysin and Leu 7 were positive in two-thirds of the cases. In our experience small cell carcinomas have been cytokeratin negative and neuron-specific enolase positive.

In the study of undifferentiated carcinoma by Abelar and associates, the survival difference of the large cell compared with the small-intermediate cell carcinomas was not statistically significant (54% vs. 64%, respectively, at 5 years). As a group the survival of undifferentiated carcinoma at 5 and 10 years was 58% and 48%, respectively, which was similar to grade 3 endometrioid carcinoma.[2]

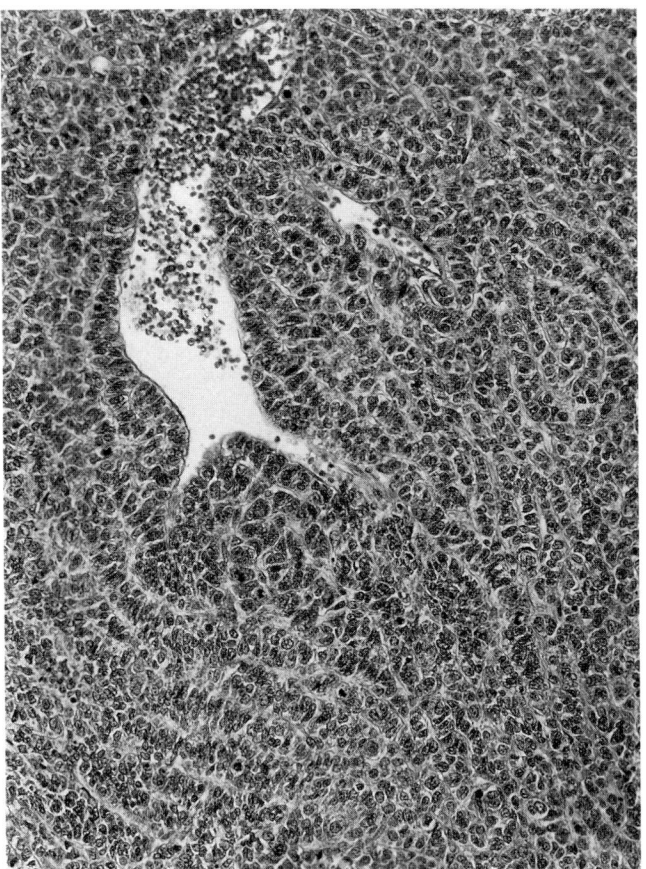

FIG. 12.47. **Small cell carcinoma.** Some case illustrated in Fig. 12.46. The tumor has a trabecular pattern simulating carcinoid.

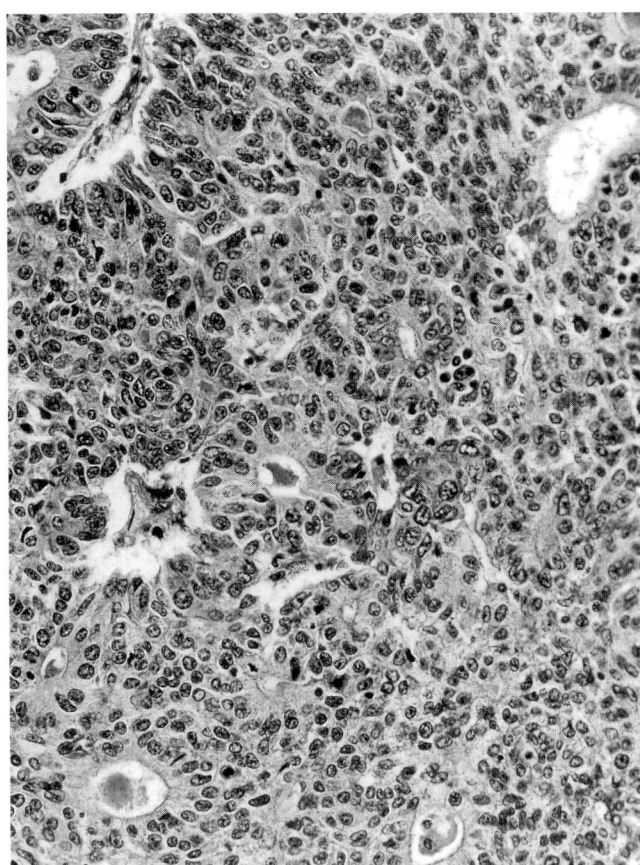

FIG. 12.48. **Small cell carcinoma.** Same case illustrated in Fig. 12.46. The small cell carcinoma forms glandular structures resembling a poorly differentiated endometrioid carcinoma.

Mixed Types of Carcinoma

An endometrial carcinoma may show combinations of two or more of the pure types. By convention, a component comprising 10% or greater has been separately noted. For example, an endometrioid carcinoma containing a clear cell carcinoma that constitutes 10% of the tumor is classified as an endometrioid carcinoma with areas of clear cell carcinoma (Fig. 12.49). Except for a few studies evaluating the significance of foci of serous carcinoma admixed with endometrioid carcinoma, there are no data that can be used as a basis for making valid recommendations concerning what proportion of an additional component that justifies being separately classified. Mixed serous and endometrioid carcinomas containing as little as 25% of a serous component behave as pure serous carcinomas.[211] Except for serous and possibly clear cell components, it is likely that the combination of other tumor types has little if any clinical significance.

Miscellaneous Epithelial Tumors

A number of rare examples of unusual neoplasms arising in the endometrium have been reported, but the data consist largely of case reports precluding a detailed clinicopathological analysis. Some of these are discussed below.

Glassy Cell Carcinoma

Glassy cell carcinoma is regarded as a variant of a mixed adenosquamous carcinoma and occurs in the endometrium.[13,46] First described in the cervix, glassy cell carcinoma is a poorly differentiated neoplasm with little or no glandular or squamous differentiation and is composed of masses and nests of characteristic polygonal cells separated by a fibrous stroma that often contains an abundance of inflammatory cells. The cells have well-defined borders and granular eosinophilic or amphophilic cytoplasm, giving a ground-glass appearance. The nuclei are enlarged and round, with centrally placed, prominent, eosinophilic nucleoli. Mitotic activity, including the presence of abnormal mitotic figures, is high. The behavior, based on a small series of cases, is highly aggressive.

Argyrophilic Cell Carcinoma

Tumors in which the neoplastic cells demonstrate argyrophilia with the Grimelius stain have been termed *argyro-*

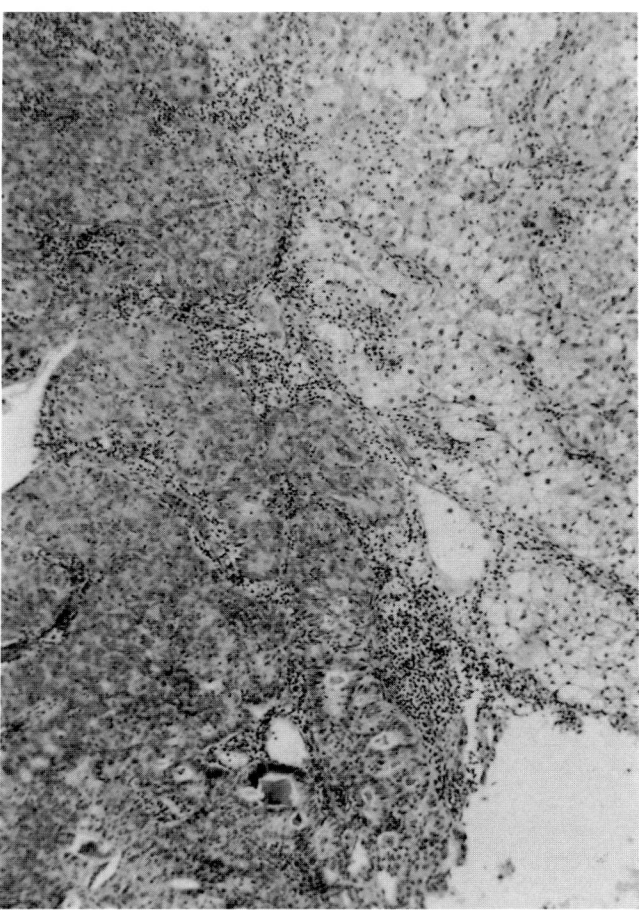

FIG. 12.49. Mixed clear cell and endometrioid carcinoma. The solid clear cell component comprised approximately 25% of the tumor.

philic cell adenocarcinoma.[240] Dense-core granules can be identified by electron microscopy. Immunocytochemical studies reveal peptide hormones and other gastrointestinal hormones in 26–68% of endometrial carcinomas[16,206,240] and argyrophilia can be observed in 8% of normal endometria.[16] Only a small proportion of the argyrophilic cells resemble the hormone-containing cells of the gastrointestinal tract, but it is these cells that stain for serotonin and, less frequently, somatostatin, adrenocorticotropin hormone (ACTH), and calcitonin.[16,206] None of the carcinomas with argyrophilic cells or hormone immunoreactivity have exhibited clinical evidence of hormone activity. These carcinomas do not behave differently from ordinary endometrial carcinoma of the same stage and grade.[239,240]

Yolk Sac Tumor

Four cases of primary yolk sac tumor of the endometrium have been reported.[122] Three of the patients have been in their 20s and one was 42 years of age. Light, immunohis-

tochemical, and ultrastructural studies have shown similar features to yolk sac tumor of the ovary. AFP is elevated in the serum preoperatively and is localized within the cytoplasm of tumor cells. It is thought that these tumors arise in the uterus as a result of aberrant migration of primordial germ cells. All four patients were treated with hysterectomy followed by adjuvant multiagent chemotherapy. Two patients are long-term survivors and two died of disease.

Giant Cell Carcinoma

Rare primary endometrial carcinomas may contain multinucleated giant cells resembling giant cell carcinomas in other sites such as the lung, thyroid, pancreas, and gall bladder.[121] In a report of six cases, the giant cells accounted for a substantial part of the tumor. The remainder of the neoplasm contained undifferentiated carcinoma and areas of more differentiated endometrioid carcinoma. Immunohistochemical studies demonstrated positive immunoreactivity for cytokeratin and epithelial membrane antigen in the giant cell component.[121] Vimentin, desmin, and smooth muscle actin were negative. Four of the six patients in whom the tumor invaded more than superficially developed recurrent tumor and three patients died of disease within 3 years. Tumors with cells resembling osteoclast-like giant cells also have been observed in the endometrium (Fig. 12.50).

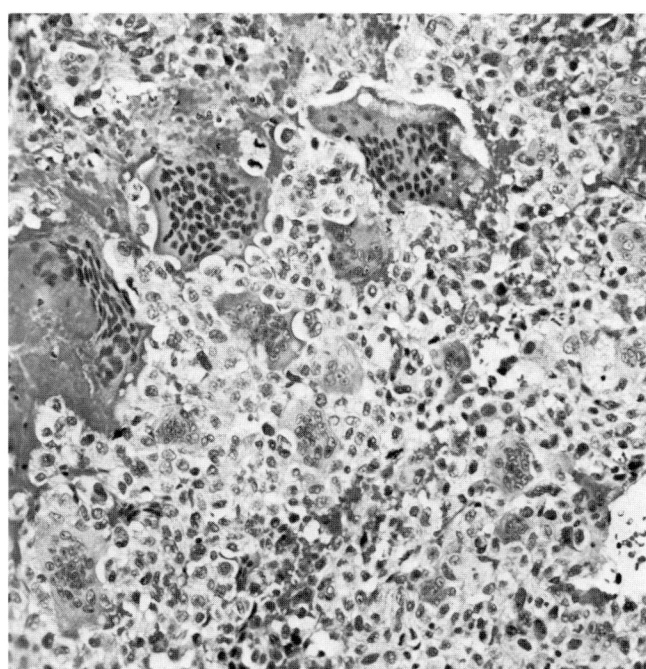

FIG. 12.50. Undifferentiated carcinoma with giant cells. The multinucleated giant cells resemble osteoclastic giant cells.

Choriocarcinoma

Rarely, primary choriocarcinoma of the endometrium may develop in a postmenopausal woman (Figs. 12.51, 12.52), representing a form of differentiation of a carcinoma derived from somatic cells and not a germ cell or trophoblastic neoplasm. Three additional cases in three patients ranging from 48 to 78 years recently have been reported.[178] All three patients had elevated serum human chorionic gonadotropin (hCG) levels and hGC was detected in the syncytiotrophoblastic element in the tumor. All three tumors showed focal glandular differentiation within what was otherwise solid sheets of poorly differentiated cells. All three patients developed recurrent tumor within a year and two died. One patient is alive with disease but follow-up has been brief.[178]

Tumors Metastatic to the Endometrium

OVARIAN CARCINOMA

Simultaneous cancers involving the endometrium and the ovary may represent (1) metastasis from the endometrium to the ovary, (2) metastasis from the ovary to the endometrium, or (3) independent primary tumors (see Chapter 22, Metastatic Tumors of the Ovary). The distinction is

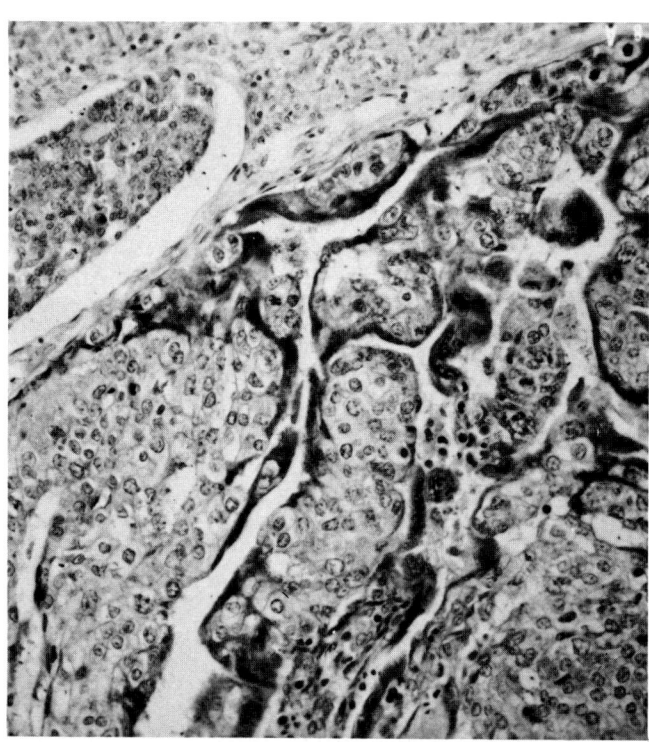

FIG. 12.52. Choriocarcinoma. The same case illustrated in Fig. 12.51. Localization of hCG (*dark black reaction product*) in syncytiotrophoblast.

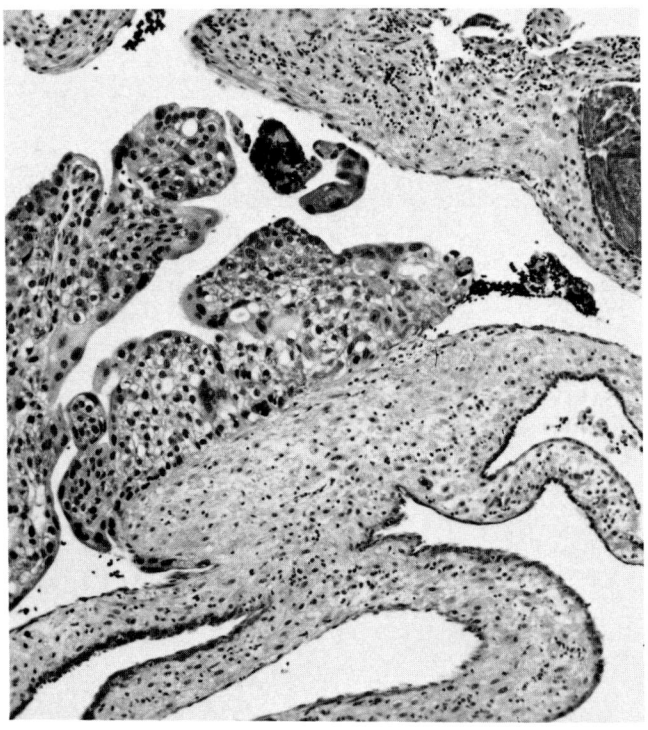

FIG. 12.51. Primary choriocarcinoma. This neoplasm developed in a 64-year-old woman. The tumor appeared to arise from an endometrioid carcinoma with squamous differentiation, FIGO grade 3. The endometrial stroma has undergone a decidual reaction.

important because the prognosis and treatment differ.[207] Scully et al.[207] suggested that when the endometrial carcinoma is small and minimally invasive, the two neoplasms are independent. Eifel et al.[73] found that if the two carcinomas have an endometrioid pattern, the prognosis is good, and therefore the two neoplasms probably are independent. When serous or clear cell carcinoma is found, the prognosis is poor and a primary tumor with metastasis is likely. The primary neoplasm is identified by its larger size or more advanced stage. Ulbright and Roth[241] classified tumors as primary in the endometrium with metastasis to the ovaries when there is multinodular ovarian involvement or at least two of the following criteria are met: (1) small (<5 cm) ovaries, (2) bilateral ovarian involvement, (3) deep myometrial invasion, (4) vascular invasion, or (5) fallopian tube involvement. When these criteria are used, there is a significant difference in the frequency of distant metastasis in the group classified as metastatic versus the group classified as an independent primary. Metastasis from the endometrium to the ovary occurs more often than the reverse. About a third of the cases are independent tumors involving both sites simultaneously. Independent tumors display either well-differentiated endometrioid or nonendometrioid patterns, whereas grade 3 endometrioid carcinoma and MMMTs generally are metastatic when detected.

CARCINOMAS FROM EXTRAGENITAL SITES

When an extragenital tumor metastasizes to the uterus it usually is a manifestation of obvious dissemination.[133] The mean age of patients is 60 years, and they have abnormal bleeding. The diagnosis in curettings may, on rare occasion, be the first clue of an occult primary tumor usually from the breast, stomach, or ovary.[134] Metastatic breast cancer is the most frequent extragenital tumor that metastasizes to the uterus (47%), followed by stomach (29%), melanoma (5%), colon (3%), pancreas (3%), and kidney (3%). In addition, rare examples of metastasis from the gall bladder, appendix, pleura, liver, lung, urinary bladder, and thyroid have been reported.[134]

Metastatic neoplasms to the endometrium frequently infiltrate the endometrium diffusely, sparing the glands (Fig. 12.53). Most neoplasms metastatic to the endometrium are poorly differentiated and lack squamous differentiation, unlike primary endometrial carcinoma. The

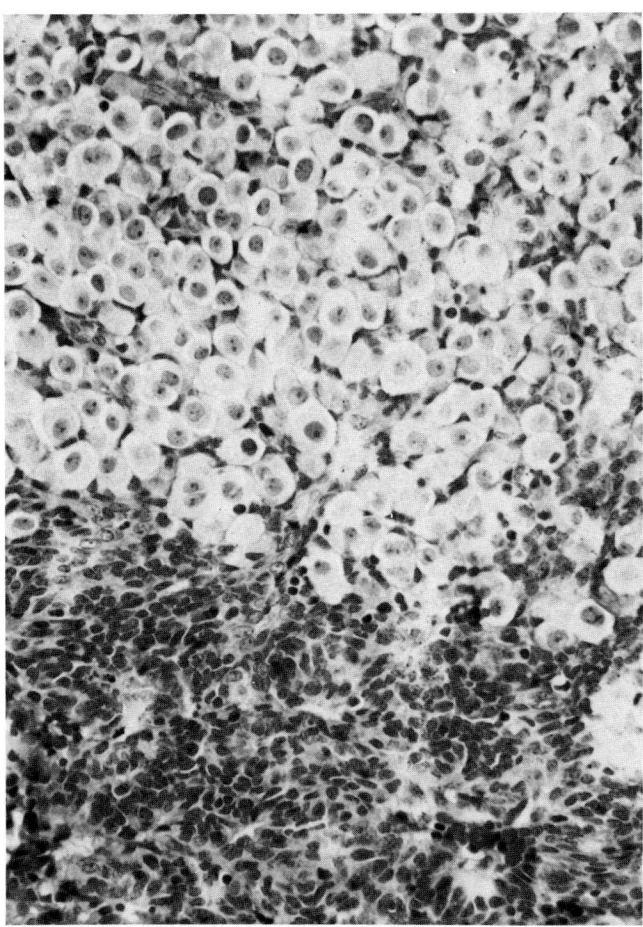

FIG. 12.53. **Metastatic breast carcinoma.** The tumor cells are uniform in size and diffusely infiltrate the endometrium. Metastatic carcinoma should not be mistaken for primary, undifferentiated carcinoma of the endometrium.

myometrium can contain metastatic nodules as well. Mean survival after metastasis to the uterus is 20 months.

References

1. Abeler VM, Kjorstad KE (1990) Serous papillary carcinoma of the endometrium: A histopathological study of 22 cases. Gynecol Oncol 39: 266–271
2. Abeler VM, Kjorstad KE, Nesland JM (1991) Undifferentiated carcinoma of the endometrium. Cancer 68: 98–105
3. Abeler VM, Kjorstad KE (1992) Endometrial adenocarcinoma with squamous cell differentiation. Cancer 69: 488–495
3a. Abeler VM, Kjorstad KE, Berle E (1992) Carcinoma of the endometrium in Norway: A histopathological and prognostic survey of a total population. Int J Gynecol Cancer 2: 9–22
4. Alberhasky RC, Connelly PJ, Christopherson WM (1982) Carcinoma of the endometrium. IV. Mixed adenosquamous carcinoma. A clinicopathological study of 68 cases with long-term follow-up. Am J Clin Pathol 77: 655
5. Alders JG, Abeler V, Kolstad P (1984) Clinical (stage III) as compared to subclinical intrapelvic extrauterine tumor spread in endometrial carcinoma: A clinical and histopathological study of 175 patients. Gynecol Oncol 17: 64
6. Alders JG, Abeler V, Kolstad P (1982) Recurrent carcinoma of the endometrium: A clinical and pathological study of 379 patients. Gynecol Oncol 17: 85
7. Ambros RA, Kurman RJ (1992) Combined assessment of vascular and myometrial invasion as a model to predict prognosis in Stage 1 endometrioid adenocarcinoma of the uterine corpus. Cancer 69: 1424–1431
8. Ambros RA, Kurman RJ (1992) Identification of patients with Stage 1 uterine endometrioid adenocarcinoma at high risk of recurrence by DNA ploidy, myometrial invasion, and vascular invasion. Gynecol Oncol 45: 235–239
9. Ambros RA, Kurman RJ (1993) Association of ulex europaeus agglutinin I binding with invasion in endometrial carcinoma. Int J Gynecol Pathol 12: 301–306
10. Ambros RA, Sherman ME, Zahn CM, Bitterman P, Kurman RJ (unpublished data)
11. American Cancer Society (1991) Cancer statistics. CA 41: 1.
12. Andersson M, Storm HH, Mouridsen HT (1991) Incidence of new primary cancers after adjuvant therapy and radiotherapy for early breast cancer. J Natl Cancer Inst 83: 1013–1017
13. Arends J, Willebrand D, DeKonigs, H, et al (1984) Adenocarcinoma of the endometrium with glassy cell features—immunohistochemical observations. Histopathology 8: 873–879
14. Atkin NB (1976) Prognostic significance of ploidy level in human tumors. I. Carcinoma of the uterus. J Natl Cancer Inst 56: 909
15. Aycock NR, Jollie WP, Dunn LJ (1979) An ultrastructural comparison of human endometrial adenocarcinoma with normal postmenopausal endometrium. Obstet Gynecol 53: 565
16. Bannatyne P, Russell P, Wills EJ (1983) Argyrophilia and endometrial carcinoma. Int J Gynecol Pathol 2: 235

17. Beck RP, Latour JPA (1963) Necropsy reports on 36 cases of endometrial carcinoma. Am J Obstet Gynecol 85: 307

18. Beckner ME, Mori T, Silverberg SG (1985) Endometrial carcinoma: Non-tumor factors in prognosis. Int J Gynecol Pathol 4: 131

19. Beller U, Beckman M, Twombly GH (1984) Spontaneous regression of advanced endometrial carcinoma. Gynecol Oncol 17: 381

20. Benediktsdottir KR, Jonasson JG, Hallgrimsson J (1989) Tumours in Iceland: 12. Malignant tumours of the corpus of the uterus. APMIS 97: 781–786

21. Berchuck A, Rodrigues G, Kinney RB, et al (1991) Overexpression of HER-2/neu in endometrial cancer is associated with advanced stage disease. Am J Obstet Gynecol 164: 15–21

22. Bergeron C, Ferenczy A, Shyamala G (1988) Distribution of estrogen receptors in various cell types of normal, hyperplastic, and neoplastic human endometrial tissues. Lab Invest 58: 338–345

23. Bergeron C, Ferenczy A, Toft DO, Shyamala G (1988) Immunocytochemical study of progesterone receptors in hyperplastic and neoplastic endometrial tissues. Cancer Res 48: 6132–6136

24. Bitterman P, Chun BK, Kurman RJ (1990) The significance of epithelial differentiation in mixed mesodermal tumors of the uterus. A clinicopathologic and immunohistochemical study. Am J Surg Pathol 14: 317–328

25. Bokhman JV (1983) Two pathogenetic types of endometrial carcinoma. Gynecol Oncol 15: 10

26. Boltenberg A, Furgyik S, Kullander S (1990) Familial cancer aggregation in cases of adenocarcinoma corporis uteri. Acta Obstet Gynecol 69: 249–258

27. Borazjani G, Twiggs LB, Leung BS, Prem KA, Adcock LL, Carson LF (1989) Prognostic significance of steroid receptors measured in primary metastatic and recurrent endometrial carcinoma. Am J Obstet Gynecol 161: 1253–1257

28. Boronow RC, Morrow CP, Creasman WT, et al (1984) Surgical staging in endometrial cancer: Clinical-pathologic findings of a prospective study. Obstet Gynecol 63: 825–832

29. Britton LC, Wilson TO, Gaffey TA, Lieber MM, Wieland HS, Podratz KC (1989) Flow cytometric DNA analysis of Stage 1 endometrial carcinoma. Gynecol Oncol 34: 317–322

30. Bulletti C, Galassi A, Jasonni VM, Martinelli G, Tabanelli S, Flamigni C (1988) Basement membrane components in normal, hyperplastic and neoplastic endometrium. Cancer 62: 142–149

31. Bunker M (1959) The terminal findings in endometrial carcinoma. Am J Obstet Gynecol 77: 530

32. Bur ME, Perlman C, Edelmann L, Fey E, Rose PG (1992) p53 expression in neoplasms of the uterine corpus. Am J Clin Pathol 98: 81–87

33. Cancer and Steroid Hormone Study of The Centers for Disease Control and The National Institute of Child Health and Human Development. Combination oral contraceptive use and the risk of endometrial cancer. JAMA (1987) 257: 796–800

34. Carcangiu ML, Chambers JT, Voynick IM, Pirro M, Schwartz PE (1990) Immunohistochemical evaluation of estrogen and progesterone receptor content in 183 patients with endometrial carcinoma. Am J Clin Pathol 94: 247–254

35. Carcangiu ML, Chambers JT (1992) Uterine papillary serous carcinoma: A study on 108 cases with emphasis on the prognostic significance of associated endometrioid carcinoma, absence of invasion, and concomitant ovarian carcinoma. Gynecol Oncol 47: 298–305

36. Cavazos F, Lucas RV (1973) Ultrastructure of the endometrium. In: Norris HJ, Hertig AT, Abel MR (eds) The uterus. Baltimore, Williams and Wilkins Co, p 136

37. Chalas E, Chumas J, Barbieri R, Mann WJ (1991) Nucleolar organizer regions in endometriosis, atypical endometriosis, and clear cell and endometrioid carcinomas. Gynecol Oncol 40: 260–263

38. Chambers JT, MacLusky N, Eisenfield A, Kohorn EI, Lawrence R, Schwartz PE (1988) Estrogen and progestin receptor levels as prognosticators for survival in endometrial cancer. Gynecol Oncol 31: 65–77

39. Chambers JT, Carcangiu ML, Voynick IM, Schwartz PE (1990) Immunohistochemical evaluation of estrogen and progesterone receptor content in 183 patients with endometrial carcinoma. Part II: Correlation between biochemical and immunohistochemical methods and survival. Am J Clin Pathol 94: 255–260

40. Charles D (1967) Endometrial adenoacanthoma. A clinicopathologic study of 55 cases. Cancer 18: 737

41. Charpin C, Andrac L, Habib MC, et al (1989) Immunocytochemical assays in human endometrial carcinomas: A multiparametric computerized analysis and comparison with nonmalignant changes. Gynecol Oncol 33: 9–22

42. Chen J, Trost DC, Wilkinson EG (1985) Endometrial papillary adenocarcinomas: Two clinicopathologic types. Int J Gynecol Pathol 4: 279

43. Chen KTK, Kostich ND, Rosai J (1978) Peritoneal foreign body granulomas to keratin in uterine adenoacanthoma. Arch Pathol Lab Med 108: 359

44. Cheon HK (1969) Prognosis of endometrial carcinoma. Obstet Gynecol 34: 680

45. Christopherson WM, Alberhasky RC, Connelly PJ (1982) Carcinoma of the endometrium: I. A clinicopathologic study of clear-cell carcinoma and secretory carcinoma. Cancer 49: 1511

46. Christopherson WM, Alberhasky RC, Connell PJ (1982) Glassy cell carcinoma of the endometrium. Hum Pathol 13: 421

47. Christopherson WM, Alberhasky RC, Connell PJ (1982) Carcinoma of the endometrium. II. Papillary adenocarcinoma: A clinical pathological study of 46 cases. Am J Clin Pathol 77: 534

48. Christopherson WM, Connelly PJ, Alberhasky RC (1983) Carcinoma of the endometrium. V. An analysis of prognosticators in patients with favorable subtypes and stage I disease. Cancer 51: 1705.

49. Cohen C, Shulman G, Budgeon LR (1982) Endocervical and endometrial adenocarcinoma. An immunoperoxidase and histochemical study. Am J Surg Pathol 6: 151

50. Coleman RL, Schink JC, Miller DS, et al (1993) DNA flow cytometric analysis of clinical stage. I. Endometrial carcinomas with lymph node metastasis. Gynecol Oncol 50: 20–24

51. Connelly PJ, Alberhasky RC, Christopherson WM (1982) Carcinoma of the endometrium. III. Analysis of 865 cases of adenocarcinoma and adeno-acanthoma. Obstet Gynecol 59: 569

52. Coutrier J, Vielh P, Salmon R, et al (1988) Chromosome imbalance in endometrial adenocarcinoma. Cancer Genetic Cytogenet 33: 67–76

53. Cowles TA, Magrina JF, Masterson BJ, et al (1985) Comparison of clinical and surgical staging in patients with endometrial carcinoma. Obstet Gynecol 66: 413

54. Creasman WT, DiSaia PJ, Blessing JA, et al (1981) Prognostic significance of peritoneal cytology in patients with endometrial cancer and preliminary data concerning therapy with intraperitoneal radiopharmaceuticals. Am J Obstet Gynecol 141: 921

55. Creasman WT, Soper JT, McCarty KS Jr, McCarty KS Sr, Hinshaw W, Clarke-Pearson DL (1985) Influence of cytoplasmic steroid receptor content on prognosis of early stage endometrial carcinoma. Am J Obstet Gynecol 151: 922

56. Creasman WT, Henderson D, Hinshaw W, Clarke-Pearson DL (1986) Estrogen replacement therapy in the patient treated for endometrial carcinoma. Obstet Gynecol 67: 326

57. Creasman WT, Morrow CP, Bundy BN, Homesley HD, Graham JE, Heller PB (1987) Surgical pathological spread patterns of endometrial cancer: A Gynecologic Oncology Group study. Cancer 60: 2035–2041

58. Creasman WT (1989) Announcement, FIGO stages: 1988 revisions. Gynecol Oncol 35: 125–127

59. Cullen TS (1900) Cancer of the uterus: Its pathology, symptomatology, diagnosis and treatment. New York, D. Appleton, p 374

60. Czernobilsky B, Katz Z, Lancet M, Galton E (1980) Endocervical-type epithelium in endometrial carcinoma. A report of 10 cases with emphasis on histochemical methods for differential diagnosis. Am J Surg Pathol 4: 481

61. Dabbs DJ, Geisinger KR, Norris HJ (1986) Intermediate filaments in endometrial and endocervical carcinomas. The diagnostic utility of vimentin patterns. Am J Surg Pathol 10: 568–576

62. Daniel AG, Peters WA III (1988) Accuracy of office and operating room curettage in the grading of endometrial carcinoma. Obstet Gynecol 71: 612–614

63. DeBrito PA, Silverberg SG, Orenstein JM (1993) Carcinosarcoma (malignant mixed mullerian [mesodermal] tumor) of the female genital tract: Immunohistochemical and ultrastructural analysis of 28 cases. Hum Pathol 24: 132–142

64. Deligdisch L, Cohen CJ (1985) Histologic correlates and virulence implications of endometrial carcinoma associated with adenomatous hyperplasia. Cancer 56: 1452

65. Deligidish L, Holinka CF (1986) Progesterone receptors in two groups of endometrial carcinoma. Cancer 57: 1385–1388

66. Doering DL, Barnhill DR, Weiser ED, Burke TW, Woodward JE, Park RC (1989) Intraoperative evaluation of depth of myometrial invasion in stage I endometrial adenocarcinoma. Obstet Gynecol 74: 930–933

67. Doll R, Muir C, Waterhouse J (1970) Cancer incidence in five continents. International Union Against Cancer. Berlin, Springer-Verlag, Vol 2, p 44.

68. Dunn LJ, Merchang JA, Bradbury JT, Stone DB (1968) Glucose tolerance and endometrial cancer: A controlled study. Arch Intern Med 121: 246

69. Dunton CJ, Balsara G, McFarland M, Hernandez E (1991) Uterine papillary serous carcinoma: A review. Obstet Gynecol Surv 46: 97–102

70. Dutra F (1959) Intraglandular morules of the endometrium. Am J Clin Pathol 31: 60

71. Ehrlich CE, Young PCM, Cleary RE (1981) Cytoplasmic progesterone receptors in normal, hyperplastic, and carcinomatous endometrium: Therapeutic implications. Am J Obstet Gynecol 141: 539

72. Ehrlich CE, Young PCM, Stehman FB, Sutton GP, Alford WM (1988) Steroid receptors and clinical outcome in patients with adenocarcinoma of the endometrium. Am J Obstet Gynecol 158: 796–807

73. Eifel P, Hendrickson M, Ross J, et al (1982) Simultaneous presentation of carcinoma involving the ovary and uterine corpus. Cancer 50: 163

74. Elliott EA, Matanoski GM, Rosenshein NB, Grumbine FC, Diamond EL (1990) Body fat patterning in women with endometrial cancer. Gynecol Oncol 39: 253–258

75. Elton NW (1942) Morphologic variations in adenocarcinoma of the fundus of the uterus, with reference to secretory activity and clinical interpretations. Am J Clin Pathol 12: 32

76. Emoto M, Iwasaki H, Kikuchi M, Shirakawa K (1993) Characteristics of cloned cells of mixed mullerian tumor of the human uterus. Cancer 71: 3065–3075

77. Enomoto T, Inoue M, Perantoni AO, Teranaka N, Tanizawa O, Rice JM (1990) K-ras activation in neoplasms of the human female reproductive tract. Cancer Res 50: 6139–6145

78. Enomoto T, Fujita M, Inoue M, et al (1991) Alterations of the p53 tumor suppressor gene and its association with activation of the c-K-ras-2 protooncogene in premalignant and malignant lesions of the human uterine endometrium. Cancer Res 51: 5308–5314

79. Escobedo LG, Lee NC, Peterson HB, Wingo PA (1991) Infertility-associated endometrial cancer risk may be limited to specific subgroups of infertile women. Obstet Gynecol 77: 124–128

80. Factor SM (1974) Papillary adenocarcinoma of the endometrium with psammoma bodies. Arch Pathol 98: 201

81. Fanning J, Evans MC, Peters AJ, Samuel M, Harmon ER, Bates JS (1989) Endometrial adenocarcinoma histologic subtypes: Clinical and pathologic profile. Gynecol Oncol 32: 288–291

82. Farhi DC, Nosanchuk J, Silverberg SG (1986) Endometrial adenocarcinoma in women under 25 years of age. Obstet Gynecol 58: 741–745

83. Fluhmann CF (1928) Squamous epithelium in the endometrium in benign and malignant conditions. Surg Gynecol Obstet 47: 309

84. Fornander T, Cedermark B, Mattsson A, et al (1989) Adjuvant tamoxifen in early breast cancer. Occurrence of new primary cancer. Lancet i: 117–119

85. Franks AL, Kendrick JS, Tyler CW Jr (1987) Postmenopausal smoking, estrogen replacement therapy and the risk of endometrial cancer. Am J Obstet Gynecol 156: 20

86. Frick HC, Munnell EW, Richart RM, Berger AP, Lawry MF (1973) Carcinoma of the endometrium. Am J Obstet Gynecol 115: 663

87. Fu YS, Parks PJ, Reagen JW, Wentz WB, Storaasli JP (1979) The ultrastructure and factors relating to survival of endometrial cancers. Am J Diag Gynecol Obstet 1: 55

88. Fujimoto I, Shimizu Y, Hirai Y, et al (1993) Studies on ras oncogene in endometrial carcinoma. Gynecol Oncol 48: 196–202

89. Fujita H, Wake N, Kutsuzawa T, et al (1985) Marker chromosomes of the long arm of chromosome 1 in endometrial carcinoma. Cancer Genet Cytogenet 18: 283–293

90. Furness PN, Lam EW (1987) Patterns of basement membrane deposition in benign, premalignant and malignant endometrium. J Clin Pathol 40: 1320–1323

91. Gal D, Recio FO, Zamubrovic D, Tancer ML (1991) Lymph-vascular space involvement—A prognostic indicator in endometrial adenocarcinoma. Gynecol Oncol 42: 142–145

92. Gallion HH, van Nagell JR, Powell DF, et al (1989) Stage I serous papillary carcinoma of the endometrium. Cancer 63: 2224–2228

93. Gasparini G, Sposetti R, Pozza F, et al (1992) Multivariate analysis of prognostic factors in 232 patients with clinical stage 1 endometrial adenocarcinoma using the new FIGO surgical staging system. Int J Oncol 1: 665–672

94. Geisinger KR, Homesley HD, Morgan TM, Kute TE, Marshall RB (1986) Endometrial adenocarcinoma. A multiparameter clinicopathologic analysis including the DNA profile and the sex steroid hormone receptors. Cancer 58: 1518–1525

95. George E, Manivel JC, Dehner LP, et al (1991) Malignant mixed mullerian tumors. An immunohistochemical study of 47 cases, with histogenetic considerations and clinical correlation. Hum Pathol 22: 215–223

96. Glicksman AS, Rawson RW (1956) Diabetes and altered carbohydrate metabolism in patients with cancer. Cancer 9: 1127

97. Gorai I, Doi C, Minaguchi H (1993) Establishment and characterization of carcinosarcoma cell line of the human uterus. Cancer 71: 775–786

98. Gray LA, Christopherson WM, Hoover RN (1977) Estrogens and endometrial carcinoma. Obstet Gynecol 49: 385

99. Gray LA, Robertson RW, Christopherson WM (1971) Atypical endometrial changes associated with carcinoma. Gynecol Oncol 2: 93

100. Greenwald P, Caputo TA, Wolfgang PE (1977) Endometrial cancer after menopausal use of estrogens. Obstet Gynecol 50: 239

101. Gronroos M, Salmi TA, Vuento MH, et al (1993) Mass screening for endometrial cancer directed in risk groups of patients with diabetes and patients with hypertension. Cancer 71: 1279–1282

102. Gusberg SB (1980) Current concepts in cancer. The changing nature of endometrial cancer. N Engl J Med 302: 729

103. Gusberg SB (1989) Editorial. The rise and fall of endometrial cancer. Gynecol Oncol 35: 124

104. Haenszel W, Kurihara M (1968) Studies of Japanese migrants. I. Mortality from cancer and other diseases among Japanese in the United States. J Natl Cancer Inst 40: 43–66

105. Hall JB, Young RH, Nelson JH (1984) The prognostic significance of adenomyosis in endometrial carcinoma. Gynecol Oncol 17: 32

106. Hanson MB, van Nagell JR Jr, Powell DE, et al (1985) The prognostic significance of lymph-vascular space invasion in stage I endometrial cancer. Cancer 55: 1753

107. Hendrickson E (1975) The lymphatic dissemination in endometrial carcinoma. A study of 188 necropsies. Am J Obstet Gynecol 123: 570

108. Hendrickson M, Ross J, Eifel P, Martinez A, Kempson R (1982) Uterine papillary serous carcinoma. A highly malignant form of endometrial adenocarcinoma. Am J Surg Pathol 6: 93

109. Hendrickson MR, Kempson RL (1983) Ciliated carcinoma—A variant of endometrial adenocarcinoma: A report of 10 cases. Int J Gynecol Pathol 2: 1

110. Hernandez E, Woodruff JD (1980) Endometrial adenocarcinoma arising in adenomyosis. Am J Obstet Gynecol 138: 827

111. Hetzel D, Wilson T, Keeney G, et al (1992) HER-2/neu expression: A major prognostic factor in endometrial cancer. Gynecol Oncol 47: 179–185

112. Hoffman MS, Cavanagh D, Walter TS, Ionata F, Ruffolo EH (1989) Adenocarcinoma of the endometrium and endometrioid carcinoma of the ovary associated with pregnancy. Gynecol Oncol 52: 82–85

113. Horgas G, Grubisic G, Spaventi S (1988) Trisomy and tetrasomy of the long arm of chromosome 1 in a direct preparation of human endometrial adenocarcinoma. Cancer Genet Cytogenet 35: 269–272

114. Horowitz RI, Horowitz SM, Feinstein AR, et al. (1981) Necropsy diagnosis of endometrial cancer and detection-bias in case control studies. Lancet ii: 66

114a. Hussain SF: (1988) Verrucous carcinoma of the endometrium. APMIS 96: 1075–1078

115. Hustin J (1973) Hormonal therapy on endometrial cancer: Effects of large doses given by parenteral or intracavity routes. In: Brush MG, Taylor RW, Williams DC (eds) Symposium on endometrial cancer. London, Cassell Ltd, p 246

116. Ikeda M, Watanabe Y, Nanjob T, Noda K (1993) Evaluation of DNA ploidy in endometrial cancer. Gynecol Oncol 50: 25–29

117. Inoue M, Ogawa H, Tanizawa O, Kobayashi Y, Tsujimoto M, Tsujimura T (1991) Immunodetection of sialyl-Tn antigen in normal, hyperplastic and cancerous tissues of the uterine endometrium. Virchows Arch A Pathol Anat 418: 157–162

118. Ignar-Trowbridge D, Risinger J, Dent G, et al. (1992) Mutations of the Ki-ras oncogene in endometrial carcinoma. Am J Obstet Gynecol 167: 227–232

119. Inoue M, Nakayama M, Tanizawa O (1990) Altered expression of Lewis blood group and related antien in fetal, normal, and malignant tissues of the uterine endometrium. Virchows Arch (A) 416: 221–228

120. Jacques SM, Lawrence WD (1990) Endometrial adenocarcinoma with variable-level myometrial involvement limited to adenomyosis: A clinicopathologic study of 23 cases. Gynecol Oncol 37: 401–407

121. Jones MA, Young RH, Scully RE (1991) Endometrial ade-

nocarcinoma with a component of giant cell carcinoma. Int J Gynecol Pathol 10: 260–270

122. Joseph MG, Fellows FG, Hearn SA (1990) Primary endodermal sinus tumor of the endometrium. Cancer 65: 297–302

123. Kacinski B, Carter D, Mittal K, et al. (1988) High level expression of fms proto-oncogene mRNA is observed in clinically aggressive human endometrial adenocarcinomas. Int J Radiat Oncol Biol Phys 15: 823–829

124. Kaku T, Silverberg SG, Tsukamoto N, et al. (1993) Association of endometrial epithelial metaplasias with endometrial carcinoma and hyperplasia in Japanese and American women. Int J Gynecol Pathol 12: 297–300

125. Kanbour AI, Stock RJ (1978) Squamous cell carcinoma in situ of the endometrium and fallopian tube as superficial extension of invasive cervical carcinoma. Cancer 42: 570

126. Kanbour-Shakir A, Tobon H (1991) Primary clear cell carcinoma of the endometrium: A clinicopathologic study of 20 cases. Int J Gynecol Pathol 10: 67–78

127. Kim K, Scully RE (1990) Peritoneal keratin granulomas with carcinomas of endometrium and ovary and atypical polypoid adenomyoma of endometrium. Am J Surg Pathol 14: 925

128. Kirkpatrick JB (1967) Pathogenesis of foam cell lesions in irradiated arteries. Am J Pathol 50: 291

129. Kleine W, Maier T, Geyer H, Pfleiderer A (1990) Estrogen and progesterone receptors in endometrial cancer and their prognostic relevance. Gynecol Oncol 38: 59–65

130. Kohler MF, Berchuck A, Davidoff AM, et al (1992) Overexpression and mutation of p53 in endometrial carcinoma. Cancer Res 52: 1622–1627

131. Koss LG, Schreiber K, Oberlander SG, Moussouris HF, Lesser M (1984) Detection of endometrial carcinoma and hyperplasia in asymptomatic women. Obstet Gynecol 64: 1–11

132. Kraus FT (1973) Irradiation changes in the uterus. In: Norris HJ, Hertig AT, Abell MR (eds) The uterus. Baltimore, William and Wilkins Co, p 457

133. Kumar A, Schneider V (1983) Metastases to the uterus from extrapelvic primary tumors. Int J Gynecol Pathol 2: 134

134. Kumar NB, Hart WR (1982) Metastases to the uterine corpus from extragenital cancers. A clinicopathologic study of 63 cases. Cancer 50: 2163

135. Kuramoto H, Hamano M (1977) Cytogenetic studies of human endometrial carcinoma by means of tissue culture. Acta Cytol 4: 559–565

136. Kurman RJ, Norris HJ (1982) Evaluation of criteria for distinguishing atypical endometrial hyperplasia from well differentiated carcinoma. Cancer 49: 2547

137. Kurman RJ, Scully RE (1976) Clear cell carcinoma of the endometrium. An analysis of 21 cases. Cancer 37: 872

138. Kurman RJ, Kaminski PF, Norris HJ (1985) The behavior of endometrial hyperplasia. A long-term study of "untreated" hyperplasia in 170 patients. Cancer 56: 403

139. Lauchlan SC (1981) Tubal (serous) carcinoma of the endometrium. Arch Pathol 105: 615

140. Lee KR, Belinson JL (1991) Recurrence in noninvasive endometrial carcinoma. Am J Surg Pathol 15: 965–973

141. Lee RB, Burke TW, Park RC (1990) Estrogen replacement therapy following treatment for stage I endometrial carcinoma. Gynecol Oncol 36: 189–191

142. Lesko SM, Rosenberg L, Kaufman DW, et al (1985) Cigarette smoking and the risk of endometrial cancer. N Engl J Med 313: 593

143. Lessey BA, Killam AP, Metzger DA, Haney AF, Greene GL, McCarty KS Jr (1988) Immunohistochemical analysis of human uterine estrogen and progesterone receptors throughout the menstrual cycle. Endocrinol Metab 67: 334–340

144. Levenback C, Burke TW, Silva E, et al (1992) Uterine papillary serous carcinoma (UPSC) treated with cisplatin, doxorubicin, and cyclophosphamide (PAC). Gynecol Oncol 46: 317–321

145. Levi F, Franceschi S, Negri E, La Vecchia C (1993) Dietary factors and the risk of endometrial cancer. Cancer 71: 3575–3581

145a. Lewis BV, Stallworthy JA, Cowdell R (1970) Adenocarcinoma of the body of the uterus. J Obstet Gynaecol Br Commonw 77: 343

146. Lindahl B, Alm P, Ferno M, Norgren A, Trope C (1984) Plasma steroid hormones, cytosol receptors, and thymidine incorporation rate in endometrial carcinoma. Am J Obstet Gynecol 149: 607

147. LiVolsi VA (1977) Adenocarcinoma of the endometrium with psammoma bodies. Obstet Gynecol 50: 725

148. Long CA, O'Brien TJ, Sanders MM, Bard DS, Quirk JG Jr (1988) A ras oncogene is expressed in adenocarcinoma of the endometrium. Am J Obstet Gynecol 159: 1512–1515

149. Longscope C, Pratt JH, Schneider SH, Fineberg SE (1978) Aromatization of androgens by muscle and adipose tissue in vivo. J Clin Endocrinol Metabl 46: 146

150. Lucas WE, Yen SSC (1979) A study of endocrine and metabolic variables in postmenopausal women with endometrial carcinoma. Am J Obstet Gynecol 134: 180

151. Lutz MH, Underwood PB Jr, Kreutner A Jr, et al (1978) Endometrial carcinoma: A method of classification of therapeutic and prognostic significance. Gynecol Oncol 6: 83

152. Lynch HT, Krush AH, Larsen AL (1967) Heredity and endometrial carcinoma. South Med J 60: 231

153. Mack TM, Pike MC, Henderson BE, et al (1976) Estrogens and endometrial cancer in a retirement community. N Engl J Med 294: 1262

154. McDonald TW, Annegers JF, O'Fallon WM, Dockerty MB, Malkasian GD, Kurland LT (1977) Exogenous estrogen and endometrial carcinoma: Case-control and incidence study. Am J Obstet Gynecol 127: 572

155. McLellan R, Dillon MB, Currie JL, Rosenshein NB (1989) Peritoneal cytology in endometrial cancer: A review. Obstet Gynecol Surv 44: 711–719

156. Mecklin J-P, Jarvinen HJ, Peltopallio P (1986) Cancer family syndrome: Genetic analysis of 22 Finnish kindreds. Gastroenterology 90: 328–333

157. Meis JM, Lawrence WD (1990) The immunohistochemical profile of malignant mixed mullerian tumor. Overlap with endometrial adenocarcinoma. Am J Clin Pathol 94: 1–7

158. Melhem MF, Tobon H (1987) Mucinous adenocarcinoma of the endometrium: A clinicopathological review of 18 cases. Int J Gynecol Pathol 6: 347–355

159. Melin JR, Wanner L, Schulz DM, Cassell EE (1979) Primary squamous cell carcinoma of the endometrium. Obstet Gynecol 53: 115

160. Mitchell H, Giles G, Medley G (1993) Accuracy and survival benefit of cytological prediction of endometrial carcinoma on routine cervical smears. Int J Gynecol Pathol 12: 34–40

161. Mittal KR, Barwick KW (1993) Endometrial adenocarcinoma involving adenomyosis without true myometrial invasion is characterized by frequent preceding estrogen therapy, low histologic grades, and excellent prognosis. Gynecol Oncol 49: 197–201

162. Mizuuchi W, Masims S, Kudo R, et al (1992) Clinical implications of K-Ras mutations in malignant epithelial tumors of the endometrium. Cancer Res 52: 2777–2781

163. Morrow CP, Bundy BN, Kurman RJ, et al (1991) Relationship between surgical-pathological risk factors and outcome in clinical stage I and II carcinoma of the endometrium: A Gynecologic Oncology Group study. Gynecol Oncol 40: 55–65

164. Musubuchi K, Nemoto H (1972) Epidemiologic studies on uterine cancer at Cancer Institute Hospital, Tokyo, Japan. Cancer 30: 268

165. Nahhas WA, Lund CJ, Rudolph JH (1971) Carcinoma of the corpus uteri: A 10-year review of 225 patients. Obstet Gynecol 38: 564

166. Ng ABP (1968) Mixed carcinoma of the endometrium. Am J Obstet Gynecol 102: 506

167. Ng ABP, Reagan JW, Storaasli JP, Wentz WB (1973) Mixed adenosquamous carcinoma of the endometrium. Am J Clin Pathol 59: 765

168. Nielsen AL, Thomsen HK, Nyholm HCJ (1991) Evaluation of the reproducibility of the revised 1988 International Federation of Gynecology and Obstetrics grading system of endometrial cancers with special emphasis on nuclear grading. Cancer 68: 2303–2309

169. Nielsen AN, Nyholm HCJ (1993) Proliferating cell nuclear antigen in endometrial adenocarcinomas of endometrioid type correlated with histologic grade, stage, previous hormonal treatment, and survival. Hum Pathol 24: 1003–1007

170. Noumoff JS, Menzin A, Mikuta J, Lusk EJ, Morgan M, LiVolsi VA (1991) The ability to evaluate prognostic variable on frozen section in hysterectomies performed for endometrial carcinoma. Gynecol Oncol 42: 202–208

171. Novak ER, Nalley WB (1957) Uterine adenoacanthoma. Obstet Gynecol 9: 396

172. Nyholm HCJ, Nielsen AL, Norup P (1993) Endometrial cancer in postmenopausal women with and without previous estrogen replacement treatment: Comparison of clinical and histopathological characteristics. Gynecol Oncol 49: 229–235

173. Nyholm HCJ, Nielsen AL, Ottesen B (1993) Expression of epidermal growth factor receptors in human endometrial carcinoma. Int J Gynecol Pathol 12: 241–245

174. Okamoto A, Sameshima Y, Yamada Y, et al. (1991) Allelic loss of chromosome 17p and p53 mutation in human endometrial carcinoma of the uterus. Cancer Res 51: 5632–5636

175. Palmer DC, Muir IM, Alexander AI, Cauchi M, Bennett RC, Quinn MA (1988) The prognostic importance of steroid receptors in endometrial carcinoma. Obstet Gynecol 72: 388–393

176. Pararzzini F, La Vecchia C, Bocciolone L, Franceschi S (1991) The epidemiology of endometrial cancer. Gynecol Oncol 41: 1–16

177. Persson I, Adami H-O, Bergkvist L, et al. (1989) Risk of endometrial cancer after treatment with oestrogens alone or in conjunction with progestogens: Results of a prospective study. Br Med J 298: 147

178. Pesce C, Merino MJ, Chambers JT, Nogales F (1991) Endometrial carcinoma with trophoblastic differentiation. Cancer 68: 1799–1802

179. Peterson EP (1968) Endometrial carcinoma in young women. A clinical profile. Obstet Gynecol 31: 702

180. Photopulos GJ, Carney CN, Edelman DA, Hughes RR, Fowler WC Jr, Walton LA (1979) Clear cell carcinoma of the endometrium. Cancer 43: 1448–1456

181. Piver MS, Lele S, Barlow J, et al (1982) Parraortic lymph node evaluation in stage I endometrial cancer. Obstet Gynecol 59: 97

182. Podczaski E, Kaminski P, Gursfi K, et al. (1992) Detection and patterns of treatment failure in 300 consecutive cases of early endometrial cancer after primary surgery. Gynecol Oncol 47: 323–327

183. Podczaski E, Kaminski P, Zaino R (1993) CA125 and CA19-9 immunolocalization in normal, hyperplastic and carcinomatous endometrium. Cancer 71: 2551–2556

184. Prem KA, Mensheha NM, McKelvey JL (1965) Operative treatment in adenocarcinoma of the endometrium in obese women. Am J Obstet Gynecol 92: 16

185. Press MF, Nousek-Goebel N, Greene GL (1985) Immunoelectron microscopic localization of estrogen receptor with monoclonal estrophilin antibodies. J Histochem Cytochem 33: 915

186. Press MF, Udove JA, Greene GL (1988) Progesterone receptor distribution in human endometrium. Analysis using monoclonal antibodies to the human progesterone receptor. Am J Pathol 131: 112–124

187. Quinn CM, Wright AA (1990) The clinical assessment of proliferation and growth in human tumors: Evaluation of methods and applications as prognostic variables. J Pathol 160: 93–102

188. Ramirez-Gonzalex CE, Adamsons K, Mangual-Vazquez TY, Wallach RC (1987) Papillary adenocarcinoma in the endometrium. Obstet Gynecol 70: 212–214

189. Richart RM, Ferenczy A (1974) Endometrial morphologic response to hormonal environment. Gynecol Oncol 2: 180

190. Ries LAG, Hankey BF, Miller BA, Hartman AM, Edwards BK (1991) Cancer Statistics Review 1973–1978. National Cancer Institute. NIH Pub. No. 91–2789

191. Risberg B, Grotott O, Westholm B (1983) Origin of carcinoma in secretory endometrium—A study using a whole organ sectioning technique. Gynecol Oncol 15: 32

192. Robboy SJ, Bradley R (1979) Changing trends and prognostic features in endometrial cancer associated with exogenous estrogen therapy. Obstet Gynecol 54: 269

193. Robboy SJ, Miller AW III, Kurman RJ (1982) The pathologic features and behavior of endometrial carcinoma associated with exogenous estrogen administration. Pathol Res Pract 174: 237

194. Roberts DWT (1961) Carcinoma of the body of the uterus at Chelsea Hospital for Women, 1943–1953. J Obstet Gynaecol Br Commonw 68: 132

195. Rorat E, Ferenczy A, Richart RM (1974) The ultrastructure of clear cell adenocarcinoma of endometrium. Cancer 33: 880

196. Ross J, Eifel PH, Cox RS, Kempson RL, Hendrickson MR (1983) Primary mucinous adenocarcinoma of the endometrium. A clinicopathologic and histochemical study. Am J Surg Pathol 7: 715

197. Runowicz CD, Nuchtern LM, Braunstein JD, Jones JG (1990) Heterogeneity in hormone receptor status in primary and metastatic endometrial cancer. Gynecol Oncol 38: 437–441

197a. Ryder DE (1982) Verrucous carcinoma of the endometrium—a unique neoplasm with long survival. Obstet Gynecol 59: 78S–80S

198. Salazar OM, DePapp EW, Bonfiglio TA, Feldstein MK, Rubin P, Rudolph JH (1977) Adenosquamous carcinoma of the endometrium. An entity with an inherently poor prognosis? Cancer 40: 119

199. Salazar OM, Feldstein ML, DePapp EW, et al (1977) Endometrial carcinoma: Analysis of failures with special emphasis on the use of initial preoperative external pelvic radiation. Int J Radiat Oncol Biol Phys 2: 1101

200. Salm R (1962) Mucin production of normal and abnormal endometrium. Arch Pathol 73: 30

201. Sandles LG, Shulman LP, Elias S, et al. (1992) Endometrial adenocarcinoma: Genetic analysis suggesting heritable site-specific uterine cancer. Gynecol Oncol 47: 167–171

202. Sassano H, Nagura H, Watanabe K, et al. (1993) Tenascin expression in normal and abnormal human endometrium. Mod Pathol 6: 323–326

203. Sato N, Mori T, Orenstein JM, Silverberg SG (1984) Ultrastructure of papillary serous carcinoma of the endometrium. Int J Gynecol Pathol 2: 337

204. Schenker JG, Weinstein D, Okon E (1979) Estradiol and testosterone levels in the peripheral and ovarian circulations in patients with endometrial cancer. Cancer 44: 1809

205. Scully RE, Poulson H, Sobin LH (1994) International histological classification and histologic typing of female genital tract tumors. Berlin, Springer-Verlag

206. Scully RE, Aguirre P, DeLellis RA (1984) Argyrophilia, serotonin, and peptide hormones in the female genital tract and its tumors. Int J Gynecol Pathol 3: 51

207. Scully RE, Richardson G, Barlow JF (1966) The development of malignancy in endometriosis. Clin Obstet Gynecol 9: 384

208. Segreti EM, Novotny DB, Soper JT, Mutch DG, Creasman WT, McCarty KS (1989) Endometrial cancer: Histologic correlates of immunohistochemical localization of progesterone receptor and estrogen receptor. Obstet Gynecol 73: 780–784

209. Sekiya S, Takeda B, Kikuchi Y, Sakaguchi S, Takamizawa H (1977) Morphologic and enzyme-cytochemical changes in uterine adenocarcinoma cells of a rat by direct application of progesterone in vitro. Gynecol Oncol 5: 5

210. Seoud M A-F, Johns J, Weed JC Jr (1993) Gynecologic tumors in tamoxifen-treated women with breast cancer. Obstet Gynecol 82: 165–169

211. Sherman ME, Bitterman P, Rosenshein NB, Delgado G, Kurman RJ (1992) Uterine serous carcinoma. A morphologically diverse neoplasm with unifying clinicopathologic features. Am J Surg Pathol 16:600–610

212. Shim JU, Rose PG, Reale FR, Soto H, Tak WK, Hunter RE (1992) Accuracy of frozen-section diagnosis at surgery in clinical stage I and II endometrial carcinoma. Am J Obstet Gynecol 166: 1335–1338

213. Silva EG, Jenkins R (1990) Serous carcinoma in endometrial polyps. Mod Pathol 3: 120–128

214. Silverberg SG, DeGiorgi LS (1973) Clear cell carcinoma of the endometrium: Clinical, pathologic, and ultrastructural findings. Cancer 31: 1127

215. Silverberg SG, Sasano N, Yajima A (1982) Endometrial carcinoma in Miyagi Perfecture, Japan: Histopathologic analysis of a cancer-based series and comparison with cases in American women. Cancer 49: 1504

216. Silverberg SG, Mullen D, Faraci JA, et al. (1980) Endometrial carcinoma: Clinical-pathologic comparison of cases in postmenopausal women receiving and not receiving estrogens. Cancer 45: 3018

217. Silverberg SG, Major FJ, Blessing JA, et al. (1990) Carcinosarcoma (malignant mixed mesodermal tumor) of the uterus. Int J Gynecol Pathol 9: 1–19

218. Silverberg SG (1981) Significance of squamous elements in carcinoma of the endometrium: A review. Prog Surg Pathol 4: 115

219. Silverberg SG, Kurman RJ (1992) Tumors of the uterine corpus and gestational trophoblastic disease. Atlas of tumor pathology. Third Series Fascicle, Armed Forces Institute of Pathology, Washington, DC, p 82

220. Simon A, Kopolovic J, Beyth Y (1988) Primary squamous cell carcinoma of the endometrium. Gynecol Oncol 31: 454–461

221. Slot E (1980) Cytogenetics of carcinoma of the endometrium. I. The study on ploidy. Neoplasia 27: 483–488

222. Smith DC, Prentice R, Thompson DJ, Hermann WL (1975) Association of exogenous estrogen and endometrial carcinoma. N Engl J Med 293: 1164

223. Smith J, Yeh G (1992) Telomere reduction in endometrial adenocarcinoma. Am J Obstet Gynecol 167: 1883–1887

224. Smith M, McCartney AJ (1985) Occult, high-risk endometrial cancer. Gynecol Oncol 22: 154

225. Soisson AP, Berchuck A, Lessey BA, et al. (1989) Immunohistochemical expression of TAG-72 in normal and malignant endometrium: Correlation of antigen expression with estrogen receptor and progesterone receptor levels. Am J Obstet Gynecol 161: 1258–1263

226. Steinhorn SC, Myers MH, Hankey BF, Pelham VF (1986) Factors associated with survival differences between black and white women with cancer of the uterine corpus. Am J Epidemiol 124: 85–93

227. Stendahl U, Strang P, Wagenius G, Bergstrom R, Tribukait B (1991) Prognostic significance of proliferation in endometrial adenocarcinomas: A multivariate analysis of clinical and flow cytometric variables. Int J Gynecol Pathol 10: 271–284

228. Suit HD, Gallagher HS (1964) Intact tumor cells in irradiated tissue. Arch Pathol 78: 648

229. Sutton GP, Brill L, Michael H, Stehman FB, Ehrlich CE (1987) Malignant papillary lesions of the endometrium. Gynecol Oncol 27: 294–304

230. Suzuki A, Konishi I, Okamura H, Makashima N (1984) Adenocarcinoma of the endometrium associated with intrauterine pregnancy. Gynecol Oncol 18: 261–269

231. Thor A, Vigilone MJ, Muraro R, Ohuchi N, Schlom J, Gorstein F (1987) Monoclonal antibody B72.3 reactivity with human endometrium: A study of normal and malignant tissues. Int J Gynecol Pathol 6: 235–247

232. Thrasher TV, Richart RM (1972) An ultrastructural comparison of endometrial adenocarcinoma and normal endometrium. Cancer 29: 1713

233. Tiltman AJ (1980) Mucinous carcinoma of the endometrium. Obstet Gynecol 55: 244

234. Tobon H, Watkins GJ (1985) Secretory adenocarcinoma of the endometrium. Int J Gynecol Pathol 4: 328

235. Tornos C, Silva EG, El-Naggar A, Burke TW (1992) Aggressive stage 1 and grade 1 endometrial carcinoma. Cancer 70: 790–798

236. Tseng PC, Sprance HE, Carcangiu ML, Chambers JT, Schwartz PE (1989) CA 125, NB/70K, and lipid-associated sialic acid in monitoring uterine papillary serous carcinoma. Obstet Gynecol 74: 384–386

237. Tubiana M (1971) The kinetics of tumour cell proliferation and radiotherapy. Br J Radiol 44: 325

238. Turner DA, Gershenson DM, Atkinson N, Sneige N, Wharton AT (1989) The prognostic significance of peritoneal cytology for Stage 1 endometrial cancer. Obstet Gynecol 74: 775–780

239. Ueda G, Yamasaki M, Inoue M, Kurachi K (1979) A clinicopathologic study of endometrial carcinomas with argyrophil cells. Gynecol Oncol 7: 223

240. Ueda G, Sato Y, Yamasaki M, et al (1978) Argyrophil cell adenocarcinoma of the endometrium. Gynecol Oncol 6: 467

241. Ulbright TM, Roth LM (1985) Metastatic and independent cancers of the endometrium and ovary: A clinicopathologic study of 34 cases. Hum Pathol 16: 28

242. Van Dam PA, Watson JV, Lowe DG, Shepherd JH (1992) Flow cytometric DNA analysis in gynecological oncology. Int J Gynecol Cancer 2: 57–65

243. Vardi JR, Tadros GH, Zafaranloo S, Kapadia L, Alderete MN, Shebes ML (1989) Case report. Stage IV endometrial carcinoma in a 25-year-old woman: A case report and review of the literature. Gynecol Oncol 34: 244–248

244. Vogel HP, Mendelsohn G (1987) Laminin immunostaining in hyperplastic, dysplastic and neoplastic lesions of the endometrium and the uterine cervix. Obstet Gynecol 69: 794–799

245. Wahlstrom T, Korhonen M, Lindgren J, Markku S (1979) Distinction between endocervical and endometrial adenocarcinoma with immunoperoxidase staining of carcinoembryonic antigen in routine histologic tissue sections. Lancet 2: 1159

246. Walker AM, Jick H (1979) Cancer of the corpus uteri: Increasing incidence in the United States. Am J Epidemiol 110: 47

247. Walker AM, Jick H (1980) Declining rates of endometrial cancer. Obstet Gynecol 56: 733

248. Ward B, Wright RK (1990) Free papillary carcinoma of the endometrium. Gynecol Oncol 39: 347–351

249. Warhol MJ, Rice RH, Pinkus GS, Robboy SJ (1984) Evaluation of squamous epithelium in adenoacanthoma and adenosquamous carcinoma of the endometrium: Immunoperoxidase analysis of involucrin and keratin localization. Int J Gynecol Pathol 3: 82–91

250. Warren S (1961) The pathology of ionizing radiation. Springfield, Ill, Charles C Thomas

251. Way S (1954) The aetiology of carcinoma of the body of the uterus. J Obstet Gynaecol Br Emp 61: 46

252. Webb GA, Lagios MD (1987) Clear cell carcinoma of the endometrium. Am J Obstet Gynecol 156: 1486–1491

253. Weiner J, Bigelow B, Demopoulis RI (1980) The value of endocervical sampling in the staging of endometrial carcinoma. Diag Gynecol Obstet 2: 265

254. Wick MR, Nappi O (1993) Sarcomatoid carcinomas and carcinosarcomas. Semin Diag Pathol 10: 117–201

255. Wilkinson N, Buckley CH, Chawner L, Fox H (1990) Nucleolar organizer regions in normal, hyperplastic and neoplastic endometria. Int J Gynecol Pathol 9: 55–59

256. Wynder EL, Escher GC, Mantel N (1966) An epidemiological investigation of cancer of the endometrium. Cancer 19: 489

257. Yabushita H, Masuda T, Sawaguchi K, et al (1992) Growth potential of endometrial cancers assessed by a Ki-67 Ag/DNA dual-color flow-cytometric assay. Gynecol Oncol 44: 263–267

258. Yazigi R, Piver MS, Blumenson L (1983) Malignant peritoneal cytology as a prognostic indicator in stage I endometrial cancer. Obstet Gynecol 62: 359

259. Yoonessi M, Anderson DG, Morley GW (1979) Endometrial carcinoma: Causes of death and sites of treatment failure. Cancer 43: 1944

260. Yorishima M, Hiura M, Moriwaki S, et al (1989) Clear cell carcinoma of the endometrium with lipid-producing activity. Int J Gynecol Pathol 8: 286–295

261. Young RH, Scully RE (1992) Uterine carcinomas simulating microglandular hyperplasia. Am J Surg Pathol 16: 1092–1097

262. Zaino RJ, Stayaswaroop PG, Mortel R (1984) Morphology of human uterine cancer in nude mice. Effects of hormone and antihormone treatment. Arch Pathol Lab Med 108: 571–578

263. Zaino RJ, Clarke CL, Mortel R, Satyaswaroop PG (1988) Heterogeneity of progesterone receptor distribution in human endometrial adenocarcinoma. Cancer Res 48: 1889–1895

264. Zaino RJ, Kurman RJ (1988) Squamous differentiation in carcinoma of the endometrium: A critical appraisal of adenoacanthoma and adenosquamous carcinoma. Semin Diagn Pathol 5: 154–171

265. Zaino RJ, Kurman RJ, Herbold D, et al (1991) The significance of squamous differentiation in endometrial carcinoma: Data from a Gynecologic Oncology Group study. Cancer 68: 2293–3202

266. Zaino RJ, Diana KL, Kurman RJ (unpublished data)

267. Ziel HK, Finkle WD (1975) Increased risk of endometrial carcinoma among users of conjugated estrogens. N Engl J Med 293: 1167

13

Mesenchymal Tumors of the Uterus

Charles Zaloudek, M.D., and Henry J. Norris, M.D.

This chapter deals with neoplasms of the uterus in which there is mesenchymal differentiation. Purely mesenchymal tumors, such as those derived from smooth muscle and endometrial stroma, are considered, as are benign and malignant neoplasms in which there are mixtures of epithelium and connective tissue.

The capacity of neoplasms arising in the uterus to form heterologous mesenchymal elements is a reflection of the potentiality of the uterine primordium, which is formed from an anlage of coelomic lining cells and subjacent mesenchymal cells. Within the mesodermal primordium that is to become the uterus, the distinction between duct epithelium and mesenchyme is lost. The müllerian duct epithelial cells seem to form part of the mesenchyme accompanying the duct before the formation of the uterus (see Chapter 1, Embryology of the Female Genital Tract and Disorders of Abnormal Sexual Development). A distinction between the precursors of the endometrium and myometrium is not possible. Neoplasms that subsequently arise in the uterus may express the bipotentiality of their ancestry by forming a mixture of epithelial and mesodermal components as in the biphasic adenofibroma, adenosarcoma, and mixed müllerian tumor.

Mesenchymal tumors of the uterus, other than leiomyomas, are uncommon. Sarcomas, for example, are only 3% of uterine malignancies. A comprehensive classification of nonepithelial neoplasms of the uterus, recently proposed by the World Health Organization (WHO) and the International Society of Gynecological Pathologists (ISGYP), is shown in Table 13.1.[230]

Proper pathologic study of a mesenchymal tumor of the uterus is predicated on careful gross examination and prompt, thorough fixation. If indicated, fresh tissue should be appropriately fixed or frozen for immunohistochemistry, fixed in glutaraldehyde for electron microscopy, or submitted for flow cytometric analysis. Large tumors should be sectioned to ensure adequate penetration of the fixative. After fixation, the tumor should be examined thoroughly, and one block of tissue should be taken for each centimeter of tumor diameter, except from grossly typical leiomyomas. Even the latter may have to be examined extensively if the microscopic appearance is unusual. Three major goals of the pathologic examination of malignant mesenchymal tumors are to determine the type of tumor margin (expansile or infiltrating), to evaluate the depth of myometrial invasion, and to determine whether the tumor involves the serosa or extends beyond the uterus. Tissue samples should be taken with these requirements in mind.

Smooth Muscle Tumors

Leiomyoma

Leiomyomas are the most common uterine neoplasms. They are noted clinically in 20–30% of women older than 30 years of age, and are found in up to three-quarters of hysterectomy specimens when they are systematically searched for.[63] Most leiomyomas are detected in middle-aged women. They are uncommon in women who are younger than 30 years of age; the youngest patient on record was 13 years old. Some leiomyomas apparently regress after the menopause, as they are observed with less frequency in older women. Leiomyomas are more common in black women than in white women.

The growth of leiomyomas is affected by the hormonal milieu. Leiomyomas contain estrogen and progesterone receptors, which can be demonstrated biochemically and immunohistochemically.[234,244] Leiomyomas may increase in size during estrogen therapy and most decrease in size when the patient is treated with a gonadotropin-releasing hormone (GnRH) agonist.[4,237,259] Progestins, progesterone, clomiphene, and pregnancy occasionally are associated with a rapid increase in size and hemorrhagic degeneration of leiomyomas.

Evaluation of a glucose-6-phosphate dehydrogenase marker in leiomyomas of the uterus suggests that they are a proliferation of a single clone of smooth muscle cells. Cytogenetic studies provide further evidence of the clonal nature of the smooth muscle cell proliferation in many leiomyomas.[96,123,139,169,180,196] Some appear to contain several distinct clones of proliferating smooth muscle cells (i.e., they are biclonal or multiclonal).[196]

CLINICAL FEATURES

The clinical presentation depends on the size, location, and number of tumors. Leiomyomas cause many signs and symptoms, the most common of which are pain, a sensation of pressure, and abnormal uterine bleeding. Even small leiomyomas, when submucosal, can cause bleeding, which is caused by compression of the overlying endom-

Table 13.1. Classification of nonepithelial tumors of the uterus and related lesions[a]

Smooth muscle tumors
  Leiomyoma
    Mitotically active leiomyoma
    Cellular leiomyoma
    Hemorrhagic cellular leiomyoma
    Atypical leiomyoma
    Epithelioid leiomyoma
    Myxoid leiomyoma
    Vascular leiomyoma
    Lipoleiomyoma
  Smooth muscle tumor of uncertain malignant potential
  Leiomyosarcoma
    Epithelioid leiomyosarcoma
    Myxoid leiomyosarcoma
  Other smooth muscle tumors
    Metastasizing leiomyoma
    Intravenous leiomyomatosis
    Diffuse peritoneal leiomyomatosis
Endometrial stromal tumors
  Stromal nodule
  Stromal sarcoma (low and high grade)
Mixed endometrial stromal–smooth muscle tumors
Adenomatoid tumor
Other soft tissue tumors (Benign and Malignant)
  Homologous or heterologous
Mixed epithelial–nonepithelial tumors
  Benign
    Adenofibroma
    Adenomyoma
    Atypical polypoid adenomyoma
  Malignant
    Adenosarcoma (homologous or heterologous)
    Mixed müllerian tumor (carcinosarcoma)
      Homologous or heterologous
Miscellaneous tumors
  Sex cord–like tumors
  Lymphomas
  Others

[a] Modified from ref. 227.

etrium and compromise of its vascular supply. In some instances, infertility is attributed to the presence of leiomyomas.

Large tumors can be detected during pelvic examination because they produce uterine enlargement or an irregular uterine contour. Some leiomyomas are pedunculated and protrude through the cervical os. Subserosal pedunculated leiomyomas may undergo torsion, infarction, and separation from the uterus. Secondary infection of leiomyomas can result in fever, leukocytosis, and an elevated sedimentation rate. Among the complications of pregnancy ascribed to leiomyomas are spontaneous abortion, premature rupture of membranes, dystocia, inversion of the uterus, and postpartum hemorrhage.

Gross Findings

Despite the variety of histologic subtypes of leiomyoma, all are grossly similar. Multiple leiomyomas are present in two-thirds of the women with these neoplasms. Leiomyomas are spherical and firm, and they bulge above the surrounding myometrium. The cut surfaces are white to tan in color, with a whorled trabecular pattern. Leiomyomas can be located anywhere in the myometrium. *Submucosal leiomyomas* compress the overlying endometrium. As they enlarge, they may bulge into the endometrial cavity. Rare examples become pedunculated and prolapse through the cervix (Fig. 13.1). *Intramural leiomyomas* are the most common. *Subserosal leiomyomas* can become pedunculated and, upon torsion with necrosis of the pedicle, the leiomyoma can lose its connection with the uterus. Some become attached to another pelvic structure (*parasitic leiomyoma*).

The appearance of a leiomyoma often is altered by degenerative changes. Submucosal leiomyomas frequently are ulcerated and hemorrhagic. Hemorrhage and necrosis are observed in some leiomyomas, particularly in large ones in women who are pregnant or who are undergoing high-dose progestin therapy. Dark red areas represent hemorrhage, and sharply demarcated yellow areas reflect necrosis. The damaged smooth muscle is replaced eventually by firm white or translucent collagenous tissue. Cystic degeneration also occurs (Fig. 13.2), and some leiomyomas become extensively calcified.

Microscopic Findings

Leiomyomas are composed of whorled, anastomosing fascicles of uniform, fusiform, smooth muscle cells. The spindle-shaped cells have indistinct borders and abundant fibrillar, eosinophilic cytoplasm. Nuclei are elongated, with blunt or tapered ends, and have finely dispersed chromatin and small nucleoli. Mitotic figures usually are infrequent. Most leiomyomas are more cellular than the surrounding myometrium. Those that are not are identified by their nodular circumscription and by the disorderly ar-

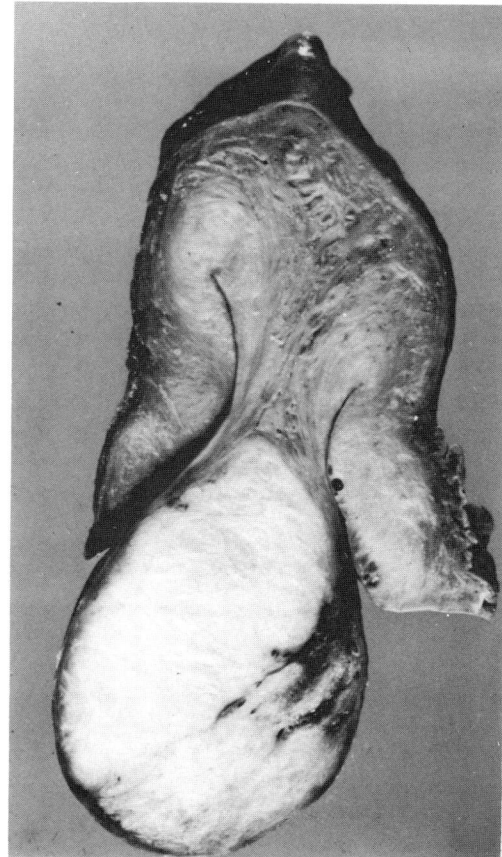

FIG. 13.1. Prolapsed submucosal leiomyoma. Large uterine tumor protrudes through cervix. (Courtesy of Dr. David Taylor, Rotorua, New Zealand.)

rangement of the smooth muscle fascicles within them, out of phase with the surrounding myometrium.

Degenerative changes are common in leiomyomas. Hyaline fibrosis is present in more than 60% of them and edema in about 50%. Marked hydropic change can mimic the appearance of a myxoid smooth muscle tumor, or produce a pattern that can be confused with intravenous leiomyomatosis.[58] There are significant areas of hemorrhage, which tend to be zonal and sharply demarcated, in about 10% of leiomyomas, and cystic degeneration and microcalcification each occur in about 4%. Hemorrhage, edema, myxoid change, hypercellular foci, and cellular hypertrophy occur in leiomyomas in women who are pregnant or taking progestins (see below, Hemorrhagic Cellular Leiomyoma). Progestational agents are associated with a slight increase in mitotic activity, but not to the level observed in a leiomyosarcoma.

Immunohistochemistry

Smooth muscle cells in the myometrium and within smooth muscle tumors react with antibodies to muscle-specific actin, α-smooth muscle actin, and desmin.[87] There

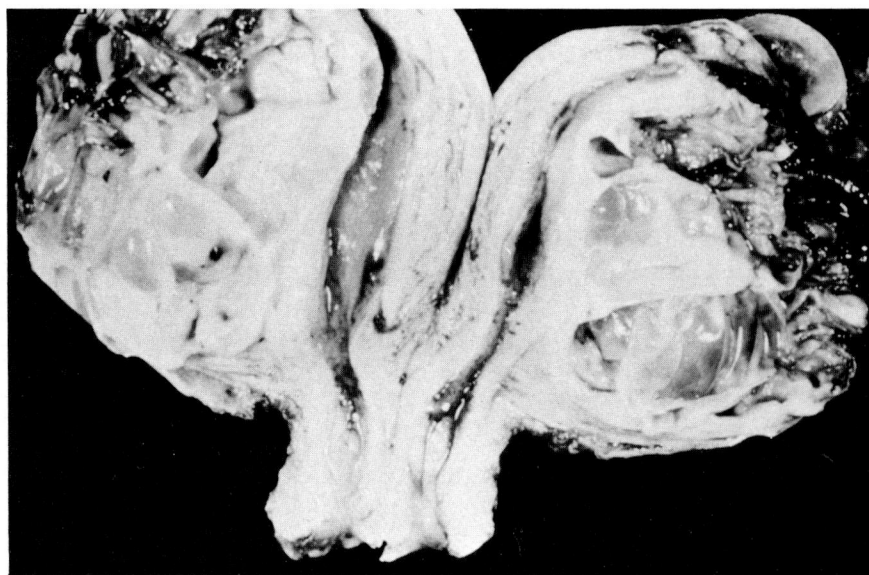

Fig. 13.2. **Cystic change in a subserosal leiomyoma.** The cysts contain serous or hemorrhagic fluid.

is immunoreactivity with vimentin but the intensity of staining and the proportion of cells that stain is less than with the muscle-specific antibodies.[87] Anomalous expression of cytokeratin immunoreactivity is observed frequently in myometrium and in smooth muscle tumors, the extent and intensity of reactivity depending on the antibodies used and the fixation of the specimen.[33,87,112] Epithelial membrane antigen is negative in smooth muscle tumors (see Chapter 26, Immunohistochemistry).

ULTRASTRUCTURE

The smooth muscle cells in leiomyoma have a folded nucleus, an abundance of cytoplasmic myofilaments with dense bodies, dense plaques on the cytoplasmic aspect of the cell membrane, paranuclear aggregates of organelles, pinocytotic vesicles, a well-defined basal lamina, and a prominent extracellular collagenous matrix (Fig. 13.3).[87,92,111,124,167] Intermediate filaments may be distributed around the organelles or they may form prominent paranuclear aggregates that correspond to areas of paranuclear immunostaining with antibodies to desmin, vimentin, or cytokeratin.

CLINICAL BEHAVIOR AND TREATMENT

Many leiomyomas are asymptomatic, and not all require treatment. Leiomyomas need to be treated only if they are symptomatic, interfere with fertility, enlarge rapidly, or pose diagnostic problems. Sometimes they can be excised (myomectomy) but if they are large or multiple, a hysterectomy may be required. Treatment with leuprolide acetate

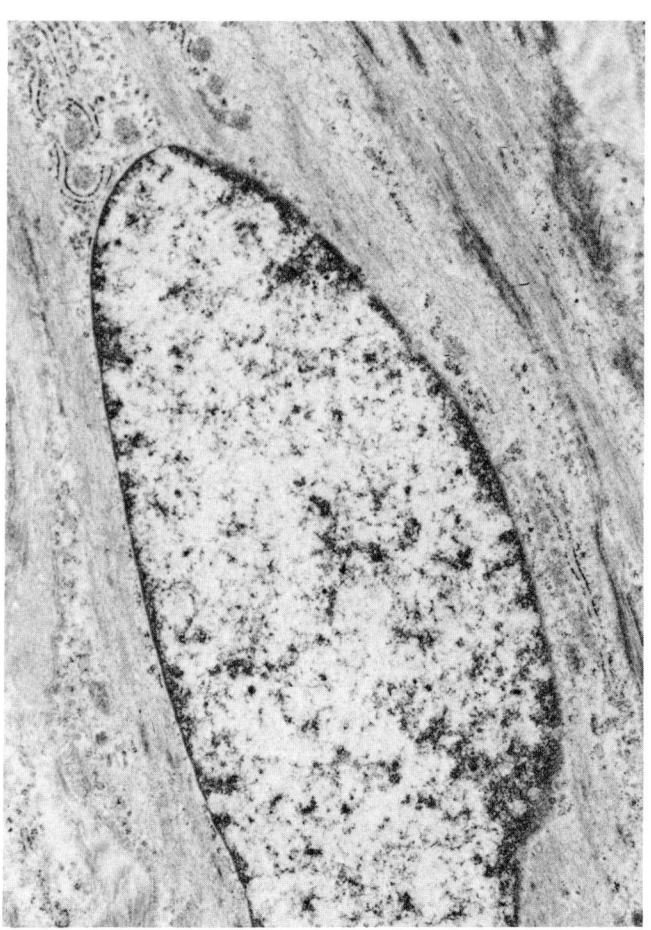

Fig. 13.3. **Ultrastructure of a smooth muscle cell from a typical leiomyoma.** Myofibrils in cytoplasm. ×8000 (Courtesy of George Hilliard, M.D., San Antonio, TX.)

or another gonadotropin-releasing hormone (GnRH) agonist[4,237] results in decrease in size of the leiomyoma, a decrease in uterine volume, and alleviation of the patient's symptoms. The maximum effect is noted after 8–12 weeks. The leiomyomas increase in size again when GnRH agonist therapy is discontinued. Such therapy can be used before surgery to decrease uterine size, facilitating myomectomy or permitting treatment by vaginal rather than abdominal hysterectomy, and to reduce the risk of hemorrhage during surgery.

Specific Subtypes of Leiomyoma

Several specific subtypes of leiomyoma must be distinguished from leiomyosarcoma. These are mitotically active leiomyoma, cellular leiomyoma, hemorrhagic cellular leiomyoma, atypical leiomyoma (leiomyomas with atypical nuclei), and epithelioid leiomyoma.

Mitotically Active Leiomyoma

Occasional leiomyomas that occur in premenopausal women and that have the typical gross and microscopic appearance of a leiomyoma have five or more mitotic figures (MF) per 10 HPF. These are designated as *mitotically active leiomyomas*.[191,199,208] The number of mitotic figures is usually 5–9 MF/10 HPF, but occasional leiomyomas contain 10–15 MF/10 HPF. The clinical evolution is benign, even if the neoplasm is treated by myomectomy.[191,199,208] A diagnosis of mitotically active leiomyoma is inappropriate if the tumor contains atypical cells.

There is a significant increase in mitotic activity in leiomyomas removed during the secretory phase of the menstrual cycle, compared with those removed during menses or during the proliferative phase.[135] Also, leiomyomas removed from women who are taking progestins have a higher mitotic rate than is observed in women who are taking a combination of estrogen and progestin, or who are not taking any exogenous hormones.[254] The patient's hormonal status may play a role in the increased number of mitotic figures seen in mitotically active leiomyomas.[208]

Cellular Leiomyoma

A *cellular leiomyoma* is one that is composed of densely cellular fascicles of smooth muscle with little intervening collagen. The hypercellularity may suggest a leiomyosarcoma, but cellular leiomyoma has fewer mitotic figures (fewer than 5 MF/10 HPF), and usually there is little or no cytologic atypia.[34,45] Palisades of nuclei reminiscent of those seen in the Verocay bodies of a neurilemoma are present in some cellular leiomyomas.[86,107] Electron microscopic evaluation reveals that the cells in these tumors, as in ordinary leiomyomas, contain myofilaments, pinocytotic

vesicles, and other ultrastructural features of smooth muscle cells.[107,166]

A cellular leiomyoma comprising small cells with scanty cytoplasm can be confused with an endometrial stromal tumor. Features that help distinguish a cellular leiomyoma from a stromal tumor are the fusiform shape of the nuclei, the spindled shape of the cells, the reticulin pattern, and the absence of prominent, uniformly distributed blood vessels. Reticulin fibers tend to parallel the fascicles of cells in a leiomyoma, but the reticulin network surrounds individual tumor cells in an endometrial stromal tumor. Immunohistochemistry may not help in this differential diagnosis because smooth muscle cells and stromal cells have a similar immunophenotype.[98] Marked diffuse staining with muscle markers is, however, more suggestive of a smooth muscle tumor than of a stromal neoplasm.

Hemorrhagic Cellular Leiomyoma

A *hemorrhagic cellular leiomyoma*, or "apoplectic" leiomyoma, is a form of cellular leiomyoma that is found in women who are taking oral contraceptives or who are pregnant or postpartum.[179,184] Multifocal stellate hemorrhages are noted grossly. Microscopically, the leiomyoma is cellular and contains patchy areas of hemorrhage and edema. Necrosis generally is not present. Mitotic figures, which may be slightly increased in number, are detected mainly within a narrow zone around the areas of hemorrhage. In contrast with leiomyosarcoma, neither atypical mitotic figures nor significant cytologic atypia is present, and the neoplasm has a circumscribed, noninvasive margin.

Atypical Leiomyoma

A leiomyoma that contains atypical cells is designated as an *atypical leiomyoma*. The atypical cells may be distributed throughout the leiomyoma or they may be clustered. They have enlarged hyperchromatic nuclei with prominent chromatin clumping and, often, smudging (Fig. 13.4). Large intranuclear inclusions of cytoplasm often are present. Multinucleated tumor giant cells can be numerous and prompt the names *bizarre* or *symplastic* leiomyoma.

It may be difficult to distinguish an atypical leiomyoma from a leiomyosarcoma. The main distinguishing feature is that there are fewer than 5 MF/10 HPF in an atypical leiomyoma (Table 13.2).[34,45,86,116] Mitotic figures, when present, are most numerous in cellular areas adjacent to clusters of atypical cells. Atypia, by itself, is not a reliable criterion for malignancy in smooth muscle tumors of the uterus because it occurs in clinically benign smooth muscle tumors, some of which are excised from women taking progestins.[89,207] It is worth noting that leiomyosarcoma can be highly variable in its appearance and may contain areas

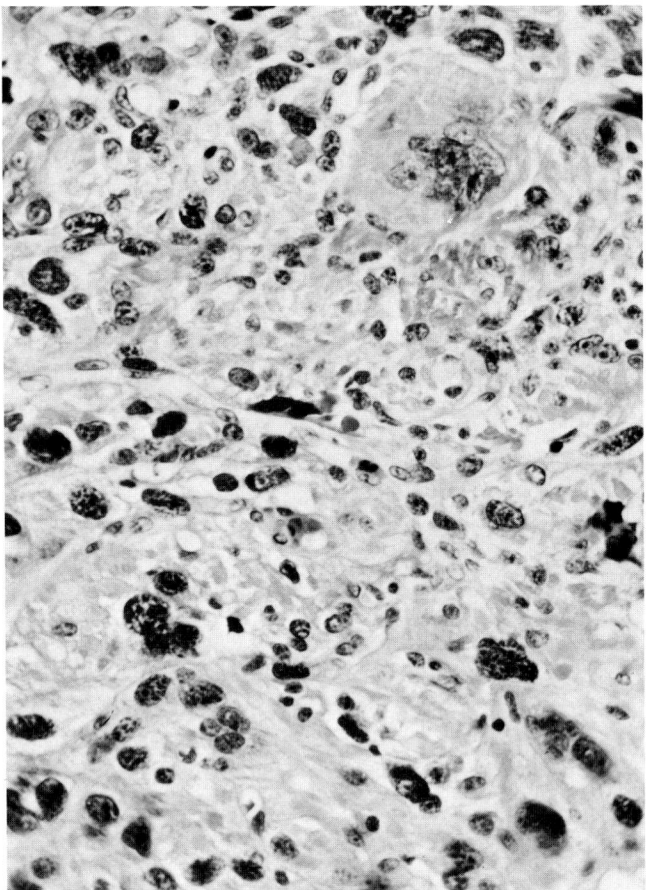

Fig. 13.4. Atypical or symplastic leiomyoma. Single and multinucleated cells have hyperchromatic nuclei with smudged chromafin.

smooth muscle tumor containing atypical cells is detected in an older woman.

Epithelioid Leiomyoma

The category includes leiomyoblastoma, clear cell leiomyoma, and plexiform leiomyoma.[143] Epithelioid smooth muscle tumors have the same histologic appearance in the uterus as in other sites in the body.

The mean age of women with epithelioid leiomyoma is 48 years.[143] Race and parity are similar to that of the normal population. The major symptoms are abnormal bleeding, abdominal or pelvic pain, and abdominal enlargement. The median duration of symptoms is 2 months.

Epithelioid leiomyomas are yellow or gray (Fig. 13.5) and may contain visible areas of hemorrhage and necrosis. They tend to be softer than the usual leiomyoma. Most are solitary, and they can occur in any part of the uterus. The median diameter is 7 cm.

Microscopically, the cells are round or polygonal rather than spinde-shaped, and they are arranged in clusters or cords. The nuclei are round, relatively large, and centrally positioned. There are three basic subtypes of epithelioid leiomyoma: leiomyoblastoma,[32,143,152] clear cell leiomyoma,[38,124,143,167,218] and plexiform leiomyoma.[86,143] Mixtures of the various patterns are common, providing the basis for designating all of them as epithelioid leiomyoma.

Leiomyoblastoma is composed of round cells with eosinophilic cytoplasm (Fig. 13.6) rather than spindle cells. The cells in *clear cell leiomyoma* are polygonal and have abundant clear cytoplasm and well-defined cell mem-

that lack the typical features of hypercellularity, cytologic atypia, and increased mitotic activity. Many sections of an atypical leiomyoma must be studied to be certain that there are no areas in which there is high mitotic activity along with atypia of the cells. The age of the patient also must be considered, as an atypical leiomyoma seldom occurs in a postmenopausal woman. A careful search for other features of leiomyosarcoma is indicated when a

Table 13.2. Histologic criteria for the diagnosis of uterine smooth muscle tumors

MF/10 HPF	Atypia	Cellularity	Diagnosis
0–4	−	Hypercellular	Cellular leiomyoma
0–4	+	Variable	Atypical leiomyoma
5–15	−	Normocellular	Mitotically active leiomyoma
≥5	+	Hypercellular	Leiomyosarcoma
≥5	Minimal	Hypercellular	Uncertain malignant potential

MF, mitotic figures.

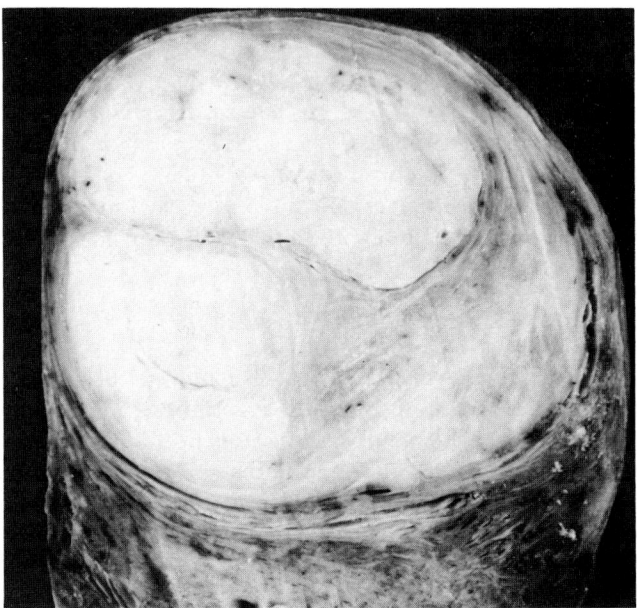

Fig. 13.5. Epithelioid leiomyoma. Cut surface of dense, circumscribed nodule.

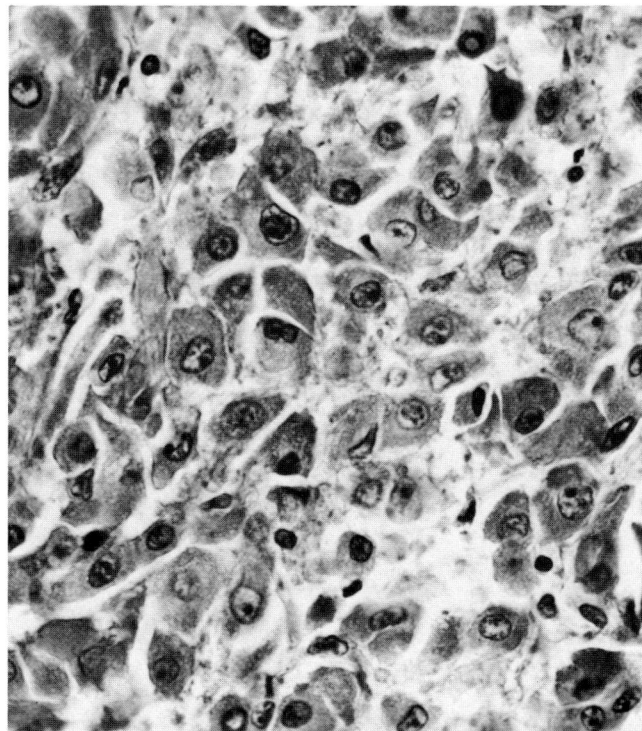

Fig. 13.6. Epithelioid leiomyoma, leiomyoblastoma type. Cellular tumor with little cohesion between cells. (Reprinted by permission from Kurman and Norris, ref. 143)

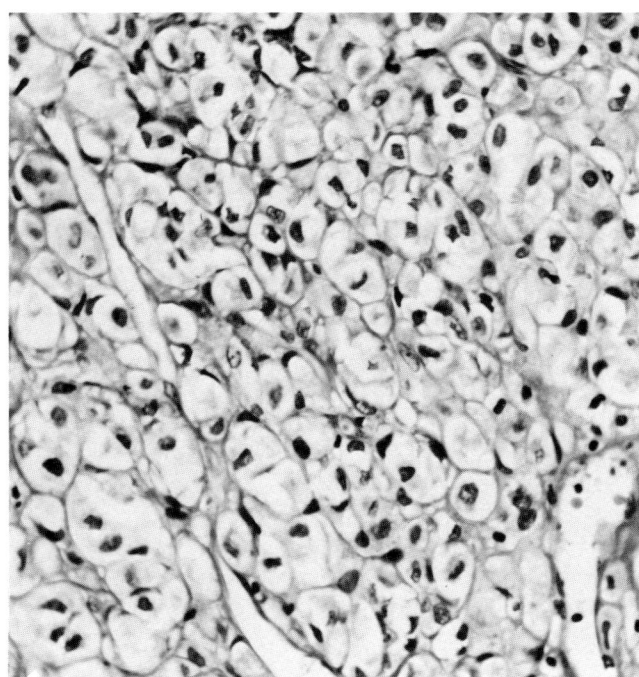

Fig. 13.7. Epithelioid leiomyoma, clear cell type. Nests of cells with abundant clear cytoplasm. (Reprinted by permission from Kurman and Norris, ref. 143)

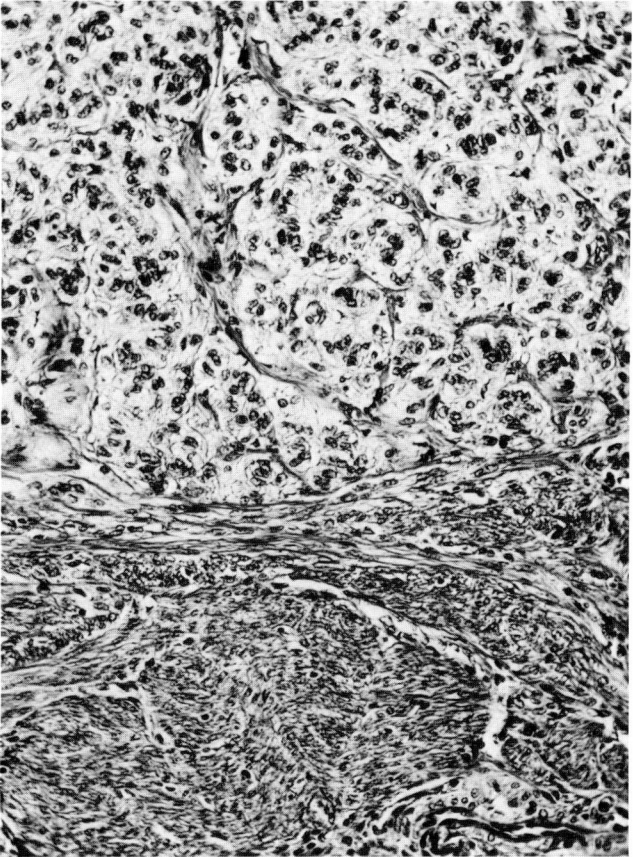

Fig. 13.8. Epithelioid leiomyoma, plexiform type. The tumor is composed of cells in nested and cord-like configurations.

branes (Fig. 13.7). The cells may contain glycogen, but there is minimal lipid and mucin is absent. The nucleus sometimes is displaced to the periphery of the cell, resulting in a signet-ring appearance. *Plexiform leiomyoma* is characterized by cords or nests of round cells with scanty to moderate amounts of cytoplasm (Fig. 13.8). Transition to more typical spindled smooth muscle cells often is identified within an epithelioid leiomyoma. Immunohistochemical study confirms the myogenous phenotype of the tumor cells.[32,74,124] Ultrastructural study reveals features of smooth muscle differentiation such as parallel cytoplasmic filaments, dense bodies, and basal lamina production. The cells in some clear cell leiomyomas contain numerous mitochondria or cytoplasmic vacuoles.[38,124,125,167]

Small plexiform leiomyomas that are detected only on microscopic examination are referred to as *plexiform tumorlets*.[129] These were formerly thought to be angiomas or endometrial stromal tumors, but ultrastructural examination reveals myofilaments and other features of smooth muscle cells (Fig. 13.9),[129,190] and the cells have a myogenous immunophenotype.[74] Plexiform tumorlets usually are solitary and submucosal, but they can occur anywhere in the myometrium and even in the endometrium. Multiple tumorlets are present in some patients.

The behavior of epithelioid leiomyoma of the uterus, like that of similar tumors elsewhere in the body, is diffi-

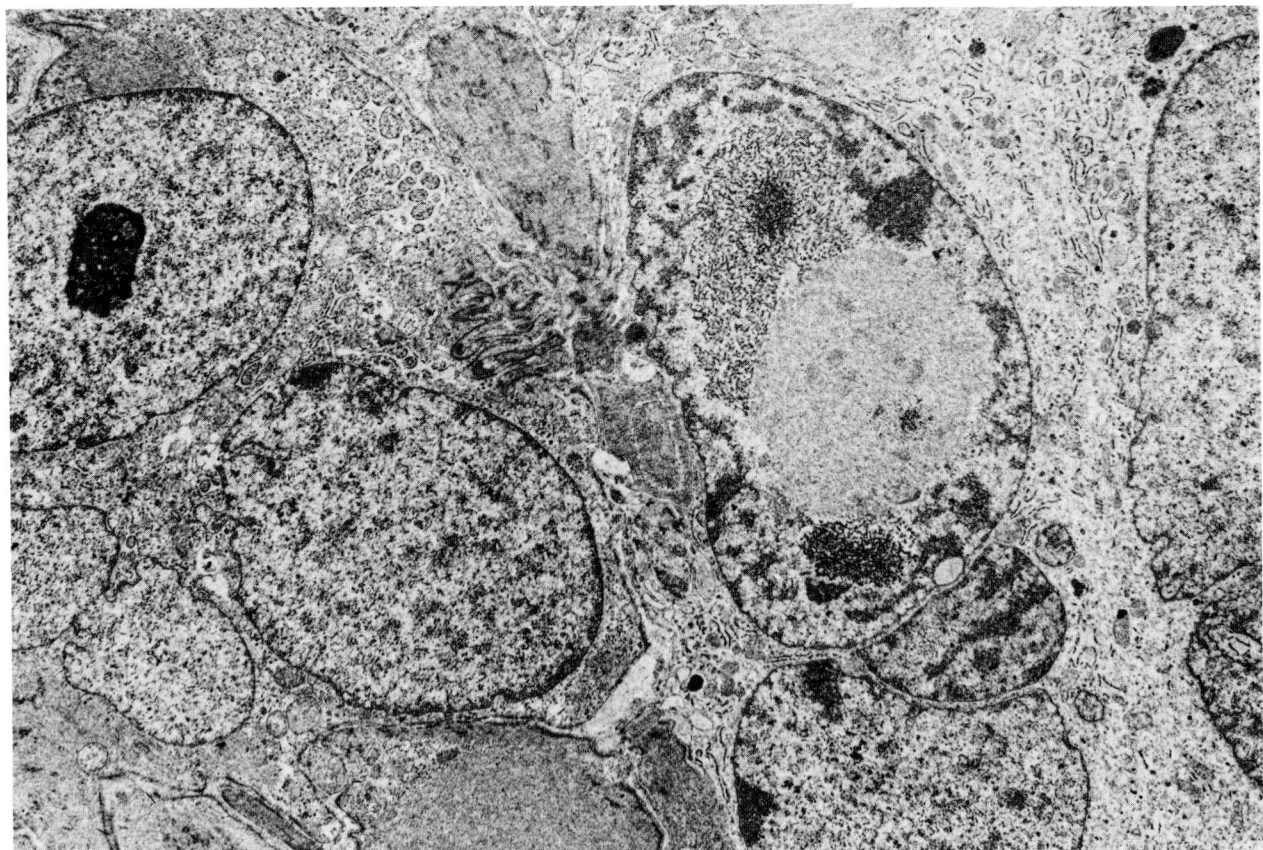

Fig. 13.9. Plexiform leiomyoma. Inclusions of fibrillar cytoplasm within the nucleus. ×5790. (Courtesy of F.A. Tavassoli, M.D., Washington, DC.)

cult to predict. Small tumors in which there is neither cytologic atypia nor significant mitotic activity can be safely regarded as benign.[143] Plexiform tumorlets invariably are benign.[129] Epithelioid leiomyomas with circumscribed margins, extensive hyalinization, and predominance of clear cells generally are benign.[143] The behavior of epithelioid leiomyomas with two or more of the following features is not well established: large size (greater than 6 cm), moderate mitotic activity (2–4 MF/10 HPF), moderate to severe cytologic atypia, and necrosis. Careful follow-up is warranted. Neoplasms with 5 or more MF/10 HPF metastasize with sufficient frequency that all should be regarded as epithelioid leiomyosarcoma.[35,143] Most malignant epithelioid smooth muscle tumors are of the leiomyoblastoma type.

Other Types of Leiomyoma and Related Entities

Myxoid Leiomyoma

Myxoid leiomyomas are soft and translucent. Microscopically, there is abundant amorphous myxoid material between the smooth muscle cells.[166] The margins of a myxoid leiomyoma are circumscribed, and neither cytologic atypia nor mitotic figures are present. Large myxoid smooth muscle tumors and those in which an infiltrating margin, cytologic atypia, or mitotic activity are observed microscopically should be regarded with suspicion. Some myxoid smooth muscle tumors exhibiting these features are clinically malignant even though they do not meet standard criteria for a diagnosis of leiomyosarcoma (see below, Leiomyosarcoma).

Vascular Leiomyoma

A *vascular leiomyoma* contains numerous large-caliber vessels with muscular walls. The distinction between a vascular leiomyoma and a hemangioma or an arteriovenous malformation may be difficult if the vascular component predominates. Vascular leiomyoma is a well-defined, circumscribed neoplasm and contains at least foci of typical spindled smooth muscle cells. Hemangioma is very rare in the uterus, and usually it is of the cavernous type. Hemangioma and arteriovenous malformation tend to be ill-defined grossly and microscopically, lacking the sharp circumscription of a leiomyoma (see Chapter 10, Benign Diseases of the Endometrium).

Lipoleiomyoma

A leiomyoma that contains a significant amount of fat is called a *lipoleiomyoma* (Fig. 13.10) and one that has a vascular component as well is designated as an *angiolipoleiomyoma*. Most occur in middle-aged or elderly women; they may arise in any part of the uterus, including the cervix.[74,122,228] The average diameter is 6 cm and there are soft yellow zones on the cut surface. Fat cells generally are found in circumscribed areas within the leiomyoma, but they may be present diffusely. The smooth muscle component predominates in most instances, and is composed of spindled cells. Other types of leiomyoma, such as epithelioid leiomyoma,[32] also may have a lipomatous component and fatty change is common in intravenous leiomyomatosis. The vascular component of an angiolipoleiomyoma may be venous, arterial, or indeterminate. Pure *lipoma* is extremely rare in the uterus; only a few have been described.[76,206]

Diffuse Leiomyomatosis and Myometrial Hypertrophy

Diffuse leiomyomatosis is an unusual condition in which innumerable small smooth muscle nodules produce symmetrical enlargement of the uterus (Fig. 13.11). The uterus may be greatly enlarged, weighing up to 1000 g. The hyperplastic smooth muscle nodules range from microscopic to 3 cm in size, but most are less than 1 cm in diameter. They are composed of uniform, bland, spindled smooth muscle cells and are less circumscribed than leiomyomas. The clinical course may be complicated by hemorrhage, but the condition is benign.[56,113,145]

Myometrial hypertrophy is a condition in which the myometrium is thickened and the uterus is symmetrically enlarged. No specific gross or microscopic abnormality is noted; the uterus is abnormal only in size. Uterine weight

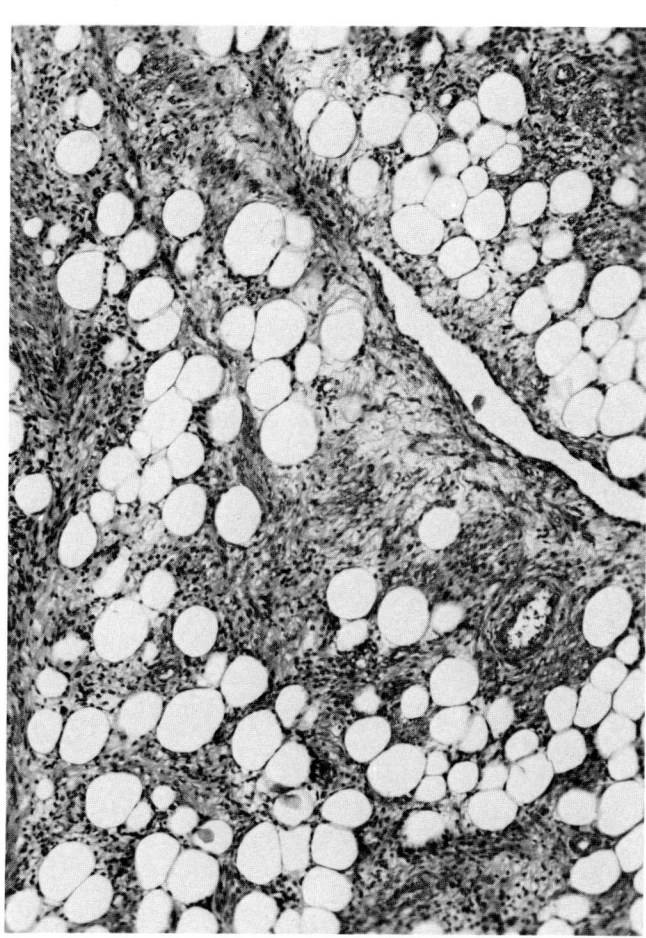

Fig. 13.10. Lipoleiomyoma. The tumor is composed of an intermixture of fat cells, smooth muscle, and collagen.

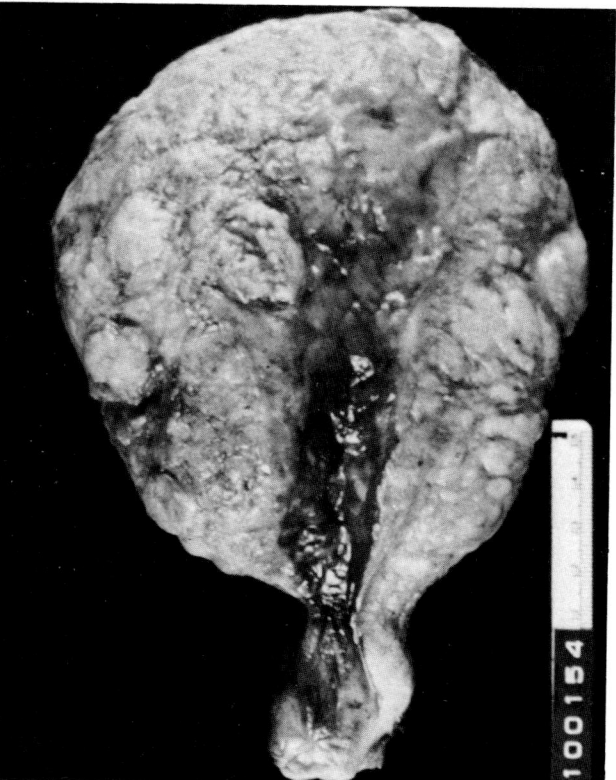

Fig. 13.11. Diffuse leiomyomatosis. The uterus is markedly enlarged, weighing 945 g, and contains innumerable small smooth muscle nodules. (Reprinted by permission from The American College of Obstetricians and Gynecologists, Obstetrics and Gynecology 53[Suppl]:825, 1979.)

increases with age and with increasing parity until the menopause. The average uterine weight decreases after the menopause. The weight beyond which the uterus is abnormally large, indicative of myometrial hypertrophy, is 130 g for the nulliparous uterus, 210 g for parity 1–3, and 250 g for parity of 4 and above.[146]

Intravenous Leiomyomatosis

Intravenous leiomyomatosis is a very rare smooth muscle tumor characterized by nodular masses of histologically benign smooth muscle cells growing within venous channels.[48,183,185]

Women with intravenous leiomyomatosis have a median age of 45 years; few are younger than 40 years. There is no racial predisposition, history of infertility, or decreased parity. The main symptoms are abnormal bleeding and pelvic discomfort. Most patients have a pelvic mass.

Grossly, intravenous leiomyomatosis is a complex coiled or nodular growth within the myometrium with convoluted, worm-like extensions into the uterine veins in the broad ligament or into other pelvic veins (Fig. 13.12). The growth extends into the vena cava in more than 10% of patients, and in some it reaches as far as the heart.[48,59,216,238,255] The worm-like masses vary from soft and spongy to rubbery and firm, and their color is pink-white or gray. The tumor is so uncommon that often it is not recognized on gross examination.

Microscopically, tumor is found within venous channels that are lined by endothelium. Arteries are not involved. The histologic appearance is highly variable, even within the same tumor. The cellular composition of some examples of intravenous leiomyomatosis is similar to a leiomyoma, but most contain prominent zones of fibrosis or hyalinization (Fig. 13.13). Smooth muscle cells may be inconspicuous and difficult to identify. The vascularity of the intravenous growth is so prominent in some cases that it resembles an angiofibroma. Any type of smooth muscle differentiation that occurs in a leiomyoma may be present in intravenous leiomyomatosis.[57] Cellular, atypical, epithelioid, and lipoleiomyomatous growth patterns occur in intravenous leiomyomatosis. These have the same behavior and prognosis as ordinary intravenous leiomyomatosis.[31,57]

Intravenous leiomyomatosis originates in vascular smooth muscle in some cases.[185] The tumor is predominantly or entirely intravascular in this situation (Fig. 13.13), and there are many sites of attachment to the vein walls. Other examples develop by intravascular extension from a leiomyoma.[183,185] The bulk of the tumor is extravascular in these, and sites of origin from a vein wall are not found.

Treatment is by total abdominal hysterectomy and bilateral salpingo-oophorectomy together with excision of any extrauterine extensions. Intravenous leiomyomatosis has a

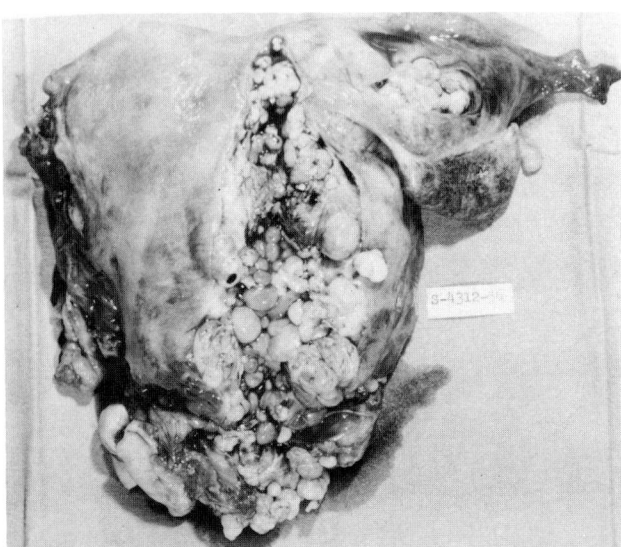

Fig. 13.12. Intravenous leiomyomatosis. Tumor replaces most of the uterus and extends into both broad ligaments and the uterine veins. (Reprinted by permission from Norris and Parmley, ref. 185.)

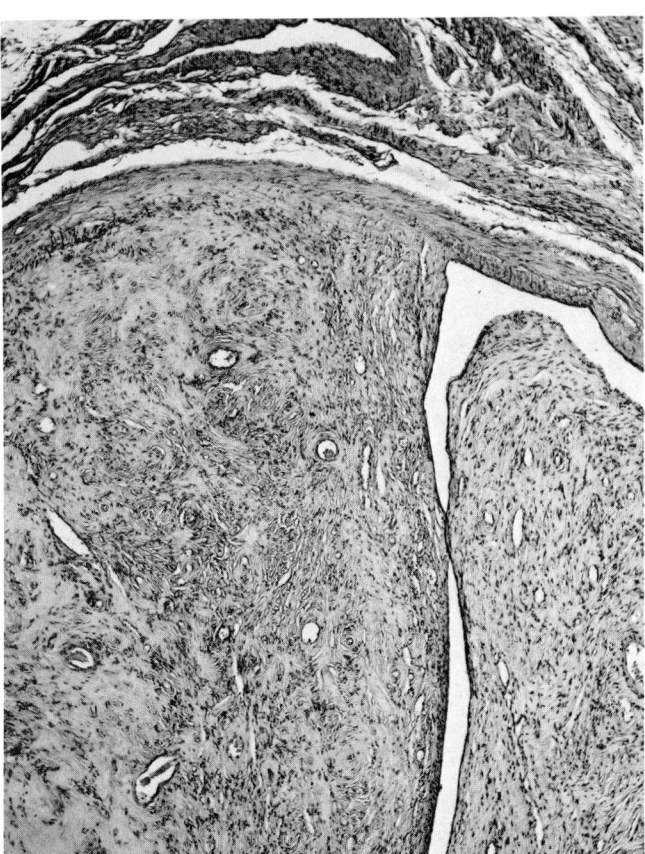

Fig. 13.13. Intravenous leiomyomatosis. Nearly all of the tumor was within the vascular spaces. (Reprinted by permission from Norris and Parmley, ref. 185.)

favorable prognosis even when it is incompletely excised. Pelvic recurrence is infrequent and usually is amenable to surgical excision.[84,185] Residual pelvic tumor may remain stable but progressive growth is possible. Intravenous leiomyomatosis is a hormonally dependent tumor, and progression is more likely in women whose treatment does not include bilateral salpingo-oophorectomy.[48,84,183,185] Long-term survival is possible after removal of plugs of tumor from the vena cava or right atrium, or excision of nodules from the lung.

Benign Metastasizing Leiomyoma

Benign metastasizing leiomyoma is a nebulous condition in which "metastatic" smooth muscle tumor deposits in the lung, lymph nodes, or abdomen appear to be derived from a benign leiomyoma of the uterus. Reports of this condition often are difficult to assess. Almost all cases of benign metastasizing leiomyoma occur in women, most of whom have a history of pelvic surgery. The primary neoplasm, typically removed years before the metastatic deposits are detected, often has been inadequately studied. In some cases, the primary tumor was not examined histologically by the reporting author and in others, the cytologic appearance, including mitotic counts, is not recorded for either the primary tumor or the alleged metastasis. A few examples may represent deportation metastases from intravenous leiomyomatosis that reach the lungs, where they become implanted and grow as multiple intrapulmonary nodules of smooth muscle (Fig. 13.14). Others may represent a multifocal smooth muscle proliferation involving the uterus and extrauterine sites.[42] Most examples of "benign metastasizing leiomyoma," however, appear to be either a primary benign smooth muscle lesion of the lung in a woman with a history of uterine leiomyoma or pulmonary metastases from a previously unrecognized low grade leiomyosarcoma.[101,268]

Disseminated Peritoneal Leiomyomatosis

Disseminated peritoneal leiomyomatosis (DPL) is a rare condition characterized by the presence of multiple smooth muscle, myofibroblastic, and fibroblastic nodules on the peritoneal surfaces of the pelvic and abdominal cavities in women of reproductive age.[12,79,110,173,248] This condition is discussed in connection with leiomyoma of the uterus because it must be distinguished from metastatic leiomyosarcoma.

Most cases are associated with pregnancy, an estrinizing granulosa tumor, or oral contraceptive use.[79,248] The most common presentation is as an unexpected finding at the time of cesarean section. DPL appears as multiple, small, granular white or tan nodules on the pelvic and abdominal peritoneum and on the surfaces of the uterus, adnexa, intestines, and omentum (Fig. 13.15). The nodules are

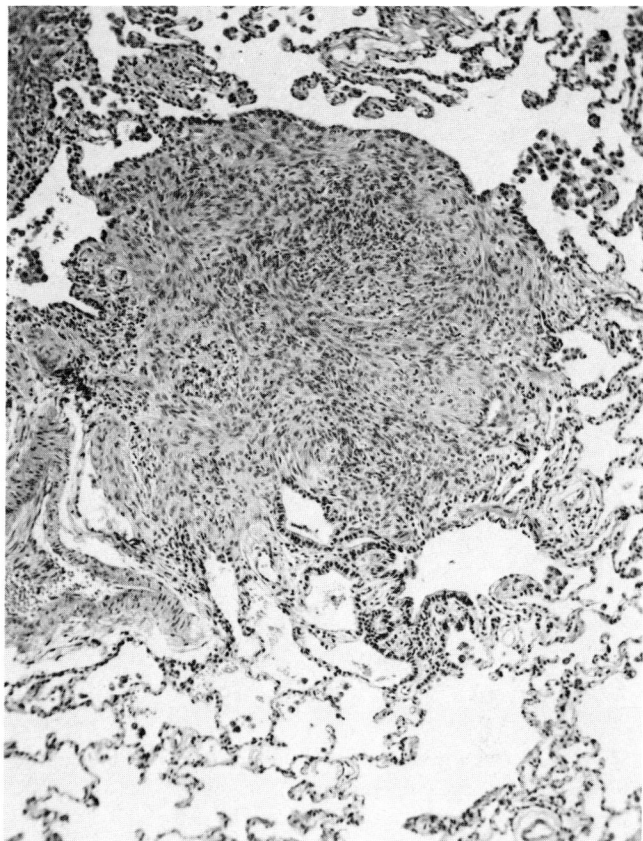

Fig. 13.14. Smooth muscle tumor in lung. The diagnosis was leiomyoma metastatic to lung (benign metastasizing leiomyoma) until the uterus, removed years earlier, was reexamined and found to contain intravenous leiomyomatosis.

distributed randomly and most of them are less than 1 cm in diameter. This contrasts with metastatic leiomyosarcoma, in which the nodules tend to be fewer in number, larger in size, and invasive into adjacent tissues.

Microscopically, the nodules comprise collagen, fibroblasts, myofibroblasts, smooth muscle cells, and, in pregnancy or the postpartum period, decidual cells (Fig. 13.16). Spindled cells usually dominate, raising the possibility that disseminated peritoneal leiomyomatosis may be confused with a metastatic sarcoma. The clinical setting is quite different, however, as is the morphology of the cells. Mitotic figures are infrequent in DPL and nuclear atypia and pleomorphism are minimal or absent. Electron microscopic study shows that most nodules are composed of smooth muscle and decidual cells, although some are mixtures of decidua and fibroblasts or myofibroblasts.[110,182,203,248] DPL illustrates the potential of the connective tissue beneath the peritoneal mesothelium to differentiate into decidua and smooth muscle.

Disseminated peritoneal leiomyomatosis is initiated or promoted by hormonal factors in most cases. Estrogen and progesterone receptors may be demonstrated within DPL

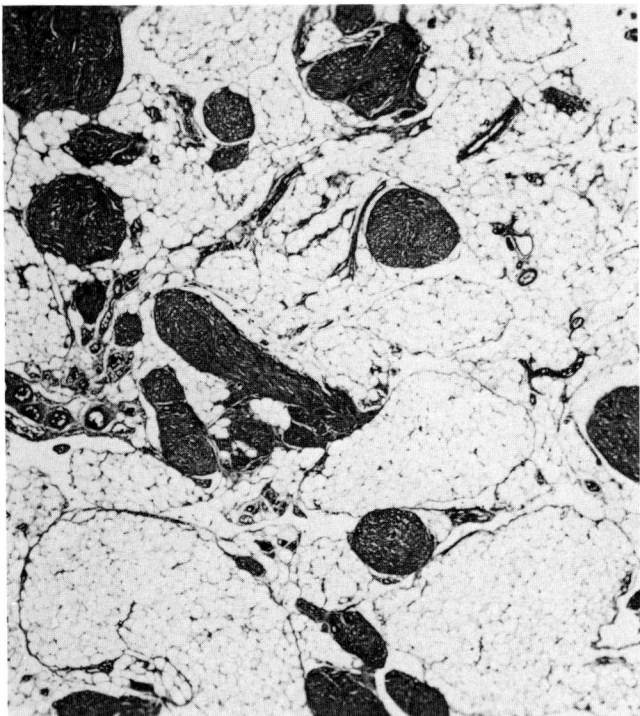

FIG. 13.15. **Disseminated peritoneal leiomyomatosis.** Nodules of smooth muscle in omentum.

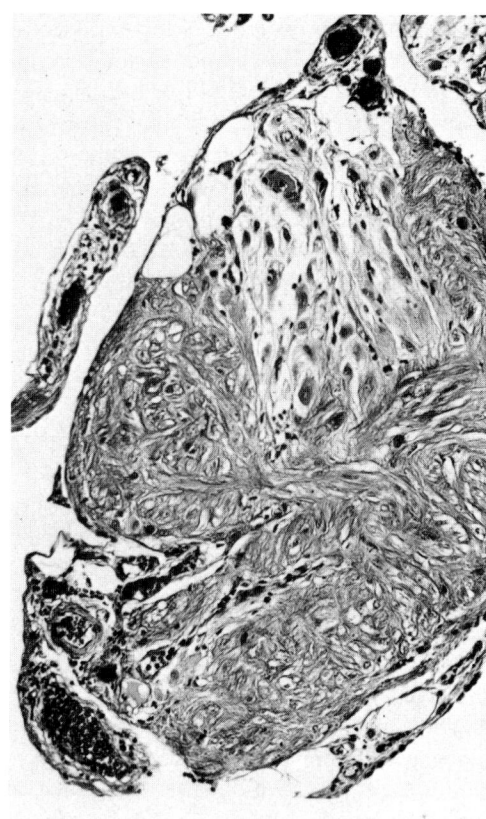

FIG. 13.16. **Disseminated peritoneal leiomyomatosis.** Decidual cells (*top*) are interspersed with collagen and smooth muscle (*bottom*). (Reprinted by permission from Norris and Parmley, ref. 185.)

by biochemical or immunohistochemical methods.[80] DPL generally regresses or remains static after removal of the hormonal stimulus (i.e., after delivery), so radical attempts at excision are unnecessary.[12,248] In keeping with a hormonally dependent process, DPL may regress during therapy with a GnRH agonist.[114] The peritoneal smooth muscle nodules may enlarge again when the GnRH agonist is discontinued or if the patient becomes pregnant.[114,248] Two cases of malignant DPL have been reported. In these, women with no evident uterine leiomyosarcoma and apparently typical DPL subsequently developed malignant smooth muscle tumors of the peritoneum with metastasis.[7,217]

Leiomyosarcoma

Leiomyosarcoma represents about 1.3% of uterine malignancies and about one-third of uterine sarcomas. Approximately 1 of every 800 smooth muscle tumors of the uterus is a leiomyosarcoma, but less than 1% of women thought clinically to have leiomyoma prove to have leiomyosarcoma.[153]

CLINICAL FEATURES

Women with leiomyosarcoma average 52 years of age, nearly a decade older than women with leiomyoma.[18,62,116,266] There is no consistent racial predisposition

nor is there a relationship with gravidity or parity. The clinical presentation is nonspecific. The main symptoms are abnormal vaginal bleeding, lower abdominal pain, or a pelvic or abdominal mass.[62,116,150,220] The average duration of symptoms before diagnosis is 5 months.[150] The rapid growth of a uterine tumor in a postmenopausal woman is suspicious for leiomyosarcoma.[261] Unlike mixed müllerian tumor, leiomyosarcoma is seldom associated with a history of pelvic radiation.[249]

GROSS FINDINGS

Most leiomyosarcomas are intramural and 50–75% are solitary masses in a uterus that does not also contain benign leiomyomas.[34,86,249] A higher proportion involve the cervix than is the case with leiomyoma. Leiomyosarcoma averages 6–9 cm in diameter and is soft or fleshy with poorly defined margins.[18] The cut surface is gray-yellow or pink with areas of necrosis and hemorrhage. Leiomyosarcoma tends to be larger and softer than leiomyoma, it has a more irregular margin, and it is more likely to be hemorrhagic and necrotic (Table 13.3).

Table 13.3. Comparison of the gross pathology of leiomyoma and leiomyosarcoma

Leiomyoma	Leiomyosarcoma
Usually multiple	Often solitary (50–75%)
Variable size, usually 3–5 cm	Large, often >10 cm
Firm, whorled cut surface	Soft, fleshy cut surface
White	Yellow or tan
Hemorrhage and necrosis infrequent	Hemorrhage and necrosis frequent

Microscopic Findings

Leiomyosarcoma is composed of fascicles of spindle cells with abundant eosinophilic cytoplasm (Fig. 13.17). Longitudinal cytoplasmic fibrils, best appreciated with a trichrome stain, frequently are present. The nuclei are fusiform, usually have rounded ends, and are hyperchromatic, with coarse chromatin and prominent nucleoli. Cellular pleomorphism is marked in poorly differentiated neoplasms. Multinucleated tumor cells are found in 50% of leiomyosarcomas and giant cells resembling osteoclasts occasionally are present.[68,86,162] Vascular invasion is identified in 10–22% of leiomyosarcomas.[34] Many leiomyosarco-

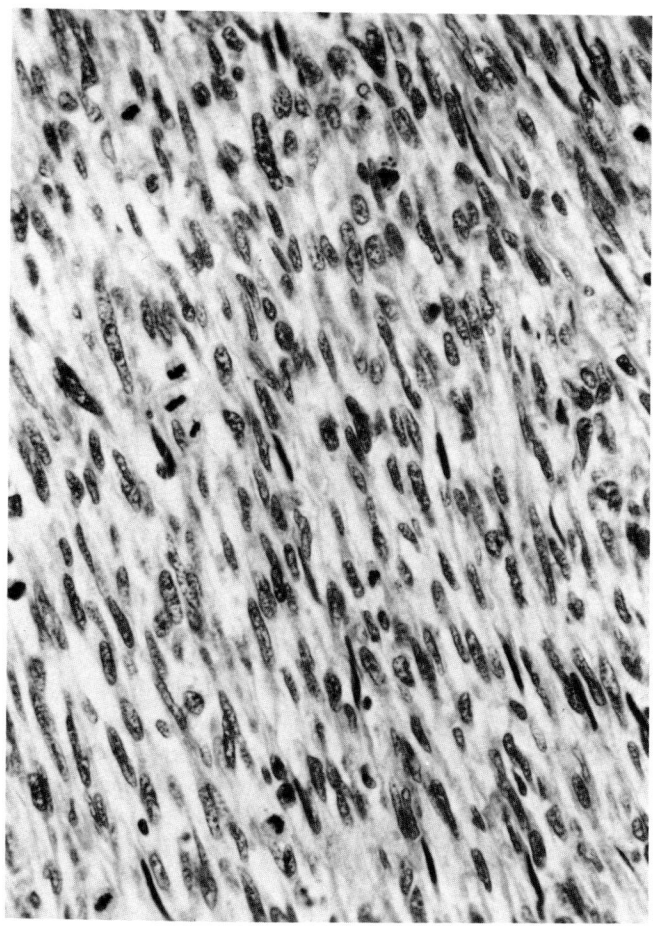

Fig. 13.17. Leiomyosarcoma. The cells are small and uniform but the tumor is hypercellular and there are many mitotic figures.

mas invade the surrounding myometrium, but a leiomyosarcoma with a circumscribed margin can give rise to metastases.

There are three main criteria for the diagnosis of leiomyosarcoma; hypercellularity, significant nuclear atypia, and frequent mitotic figures (Table 13.2).[34] More than 75% of leiomyosarcomas are hypercellular, contain atypical nuclei and have 10 or more MF/10 HPF.[116] Clinicopathologic correlation reveals that a uterine smooth muscle tumor that contains atypical cells and has 5 or more MF/10 HPF is likely to be malignant and should be designated as leiomyosarcoma. Hypercellular and normocellular smooth muscle tumors with no cytologic atypia, but more than 5 MF/10 HPF are designated as mitotically active leiomyomas.

Rare smooth muscle tumors in which there are fewer than 5 MF/10 HPF prove to be a leiomyosarcoma. A smooth muscle tumor that invades beyond the uterus into the adjacent pelvic tissues is designated as a leiomyosarcoma even if it does not exhibit clear-cut microscopic features of malignancy.[137] The presence of abnormal mitotic figures, necrosis (Fig. 13.18),[86] and myometrial or vascular invasion may be helpful in raising the suspicion of leiomyosarcoma when the main criteria do not indicate a clear-cut diagnosis.

Myxoid leiomyosarcoma is a large, gelatinous neoplasm that usually appears to be circumscribed on gross examination.[39,140,197] Microscopically, the smooth muscle cells are widely separated by myxoid material (Fig. 13.19). The low cellularity partly accounts for the presence of only a few MF/10 HPF in most myxoid leiomyosarcomas. In addition to the myxoid appearance, other microscopic features are helpful in identifying the tumor as a leiomyosarcoma. There is microscopic invasion of the surrounding myometrium in most myxoid leiomyosarcomas, and some invade blood vessels. Despite the low mitotic counts, myxoid leiomyosarcoma has the same unfavorable prognosis as typical leiomyosarcoma. Myxoid smooth muscle tumors of the uterus must be regarded with suspicion. Only small, histologically bland, entirely circumscribed examples should be designated as myxoid leiomyoma.

Finally, a rare, otherwise conventional smooth muscle tumor with a low mitotic count proves to be a leiomyosarcoma. Unless the tumor is invasive or contains abnormal mitotic figures or areas of necrosis, there are no grounds for suspecting that it is a leiomyosarcoma until it manifests its true nature by metastasizing. Doubtless, the pulmonary metastases from some "benign metastasizing leiomyomas" originate from neoplasms in this category.

Flow Cytometry

Reports of flow cytometric analysis of malignant uterine smooth muscle tumors are limited and some are difficult to evaluate. One group observed that women with stage I DNA diploid leiomyosarcoma had a significantly more fa-

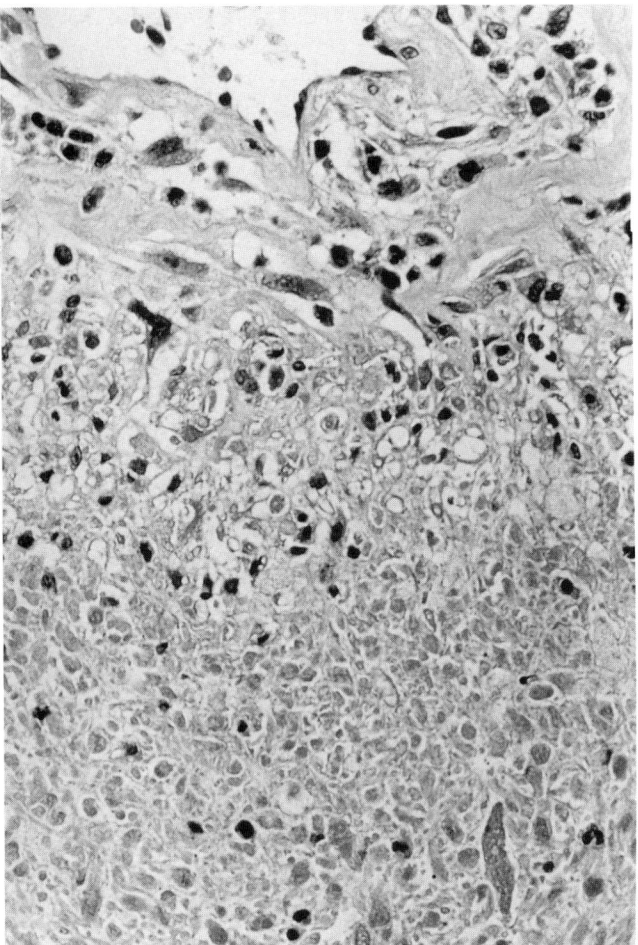

FIG. **13.18. Leiomyosarcoma.** There is extensive necrosis, with viable cells present only around the blood vessel on the top.

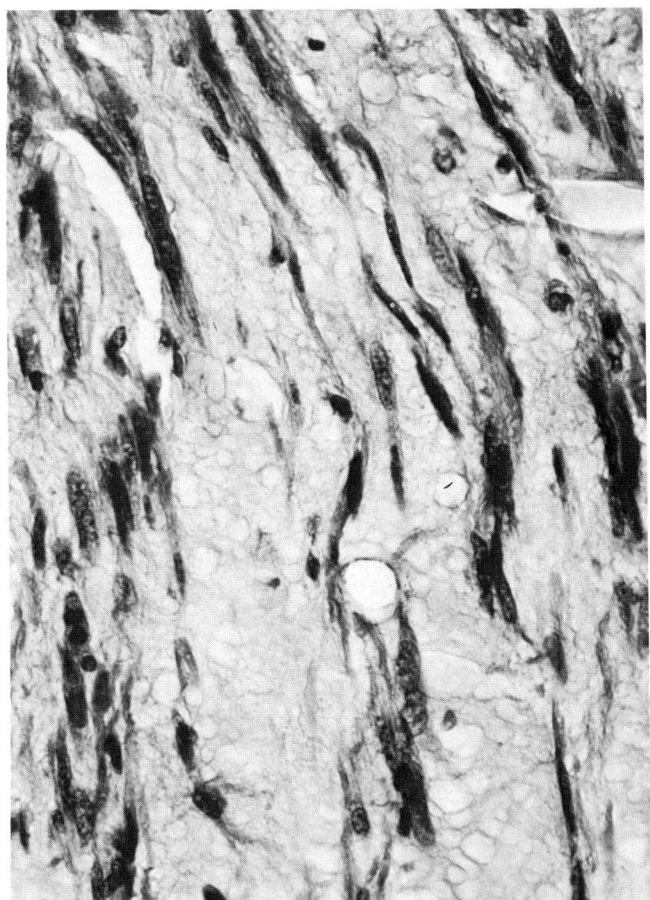

FIG. **13.19. Myxoid leiomyosarcoma.** Some myxoid smooth muscle tumors with this degree of atypia and only a few mitotic figures metastasize.

vorable prognosis than did those whose tumors were DNA nondiploid.[258] Their microscopic diagnostic criteria were unclear, however, and their finding that most leiomyosarcomas were tetraploid or polyploid (vs. diploid or aneuploid) suggests a technical problem. Several other reports indicate that most leiomyosarcomas are DNA aneuploid.[158,201]

ULTRASTRUCTURE

Leiomyosarcoma differs from leiomyoma in that the nuclei are more pleomorphic and the cytoplasmic features are incompletely developed and often disorganized.[30,92] Bundles of thin myofilaments usually are limited to zones along the plasma membranes or parallel to the nuclei. The myofilament bundles contain dense bodies and occasionally they terminate in marginal plaques. Pinocytotic vesicles are present at the plasma membrane. The intermediate filament system of malignant smooth muscle cells is poorly described. A basal lamina surrounds the cells.

CLINICAL BEHAVIOR AND TREATMENT

Leiomyosarcoma is treated by hysterectomy and bilateral salpingo-oophorectomy. Ovarian conservation may be undertaken in premenopausal women because it does not affect the results of therapy.[22,150] Combined therapy (radiation and surgery) does not result in improved survival and is seldom used in the treatment of leiomyosarcoma.[22] The poor results obtained by surgery alone suggest the need for adjuvant chemotherapy, but no active regimen has been identified.[18]

Recurrent or metastatic leiomyosarcoma is difficult to treat. A few patients respond to chemotherapy with doxorubicin,[22] but an effective chemotherapy regimen has yet to be discovered. Localized pelvic or abdominal recurrences and solitary pulmonary metastases occasionally are amenable to surgical resection.

The variation in survival rates reported for leiomyosarcoma is largely a result of the different criteria used for diagnosis. Overall 5-year survival rates in series selected using the criteria described above are

15–25%.[18,22,34,86,150,261,266] When only stage I and II tumors are considered, the 5-year survival rate is 40–70%.[126,150,160] Most recurrences are detected within 2 years.[22,34,116,126] The stage is the most significant prognostic factor.[126,160] Large (>5 cm diameter) leiomyosarcomas tend to have a less favorable prognosis.[86] Some investigators find tumor grade or mitotic activity to be a useful prognostic feature,[150] whereas others find no correlation between tumor grade and clinical behavior.[18,116] Premenopausal women have a more favorable outcome in some series,[126,150,261] but not in others.[18,116]

Endometrial Stromal Tumors

Endometrial stromal tumors occur in two basic forms. The first is the *benign endometrial stromal nodule*, which is a circumscribed, expansile neoplasm that does not infiltrate the myometrium. The second is *endometrial stromal sarcoma*, which infiltrates the myometrium and has metastatic potential. Endometrial stromal sarcoma ranges from a low-grade neoplasm that exhibits an indolent clinical course to a high-grade sarcoma. Low-grade endometrial stromal sarcoma was formerly called *endolymphatic stromal myosis* or *stromatosis*. There are several variants of typical endometrial stromal tumors. These include combined smooth muscle–stromal tumors and uterine tumors that have a histologic appearance reminiscent of an ovarian sex cord–stromal tumor. Most stromal tumors originate within the uterus, but rare examples arise outside the uterus from endometriosis.

Endometrial Stromal Nodule

Endometrial stromal nodules are rare. They represent less than a quarter of endometrial stromal tumors.[37,90,188,251]

CLINICAL FEATURES

Women with endometrial stromal nodules range from 23 to 75 years of age.[247] The median age is 47 years and three-quarters of the neoplasms occur in premenopausal women. There is no unusual racial predisposition. The main symptoms are abnormal bleeding and menorrhagia.[247] The bleeding occasionally is severe enough to cause anemia. Pelvic or abdominal discomfort is a frequent complaint. The duration of symptoms averages 2.2 months. About 10% of patients are asymptomatic, their tumors being found incidentally in hysterectomy specimens.

GROSS FINDINGS

Endometrial stromal nodules are fleshy and yellow or tan. They have a rounded contour (Fig. 13.20) and bulge above the surrounding myometrium. Their size ranges from 0.8 to 15 cm, with a median diameter of 4 cm.[37,90,188,247] Cysts 0.5–5 cm in diameter occasionally are present, but necrosis and hemorrhage are infrequent. Nodules often are polypoid and protrude into the uterine cavity. About 5% of them are multiple. About 50% of endometrial stromal nodules are located entirely within the myometrium in an intramural or subserosal location, with no apparent connection to the endometrium.[37,247] Subserosal stromal nodules rarely become pedunculated, but their external surface may adhere to the round ligament or omentum. Endometrial stromal nodules seldom involve the cervix.

MICROSCOPIC FINDINGS

Endometrial stromal nodules are composed of cells identical to or closely resembling normal proliferative phase endometrial stromal cells (Fig. 13.21).[37,90,188,247,251] Stromal nodules have an expansile, noninfiltrative margin that compresses the adjacent endometrium and myometrium. The neoplastic cells are uniform in size, shape, and staining qualities, and there is minimal cytologic atypia. Decidual change is rare. Mitotic activity ranges from none to 15 MF/10 HPF in the most active areas of the nodule.[247] It usually is very low (fewer than 3 MF/10 HPF), and in about one-half of cases, mitotic figures are not seen in 50 consecutive HPF.[37,90,247] Only 5–10% of stromal nodules have more than 5 MF/10 HPF. The behavior of nodules with high mitotic activity appears similar to that of nodules in which few mitotic figures are identified.

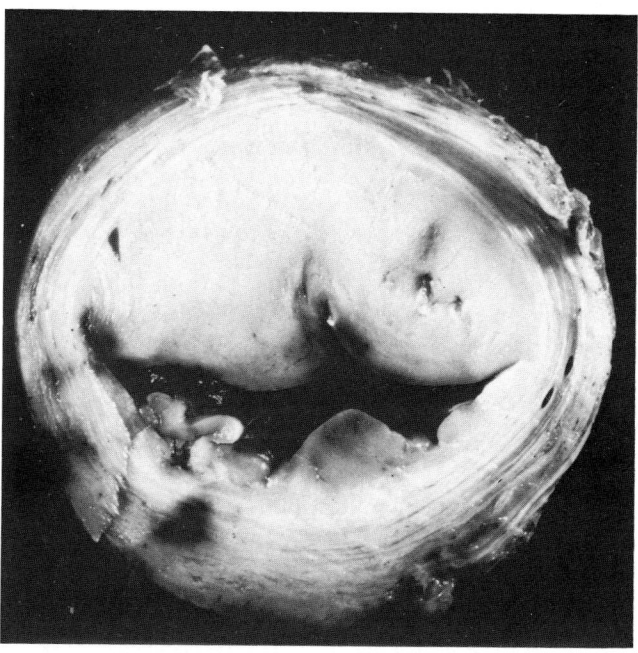

FIG. 13.20. Endometrial stromal nodule. Homogenous cut surface with cystic change. (Reprinted by permission from Zaloudek and Norris, ref. 273a.)

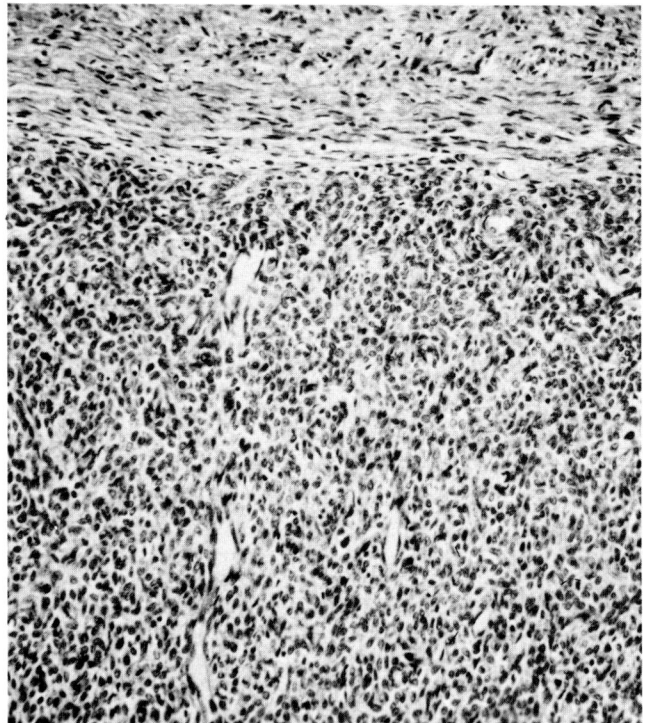

FIG. 13.21. Endometrial stromal nodule. Note the circumscribed, expansile margin that characterizes a stromal nodule. (Reprinted by permission from Tavassoli and Norris, ref. 247.)

A reticulin network encircles individual cells within endometrial stromal nodules. Epithelial-like configurations, such as cords or trabeculae of tumor cells or gland-like structures, occasionally are present (Fig. 13.22). Small areas of necrosis, cysts, foam cells, and occasional calcium deposits also occur. Focal areas of hyalinized collagen having a starburst pattern are present in some neoplasms, and there are minor areas of smooth muscle cell differentiation in about 10% of them.

FLOW CYTOMETRY

Flow cytometric analysis has been performed on a few stromal nodules.[14,83] All are DNA diploid and have a low percentage of cells in S-phase.

CLINICAL BEHAVIOR AND TREATMENT

Hysterectomy is the appropriate therapy for most stromal nodules because the periphery of the nodule must be evaluated to be certain that the tumor is completely circumscribed, with no infiltration of the myometrium. Hysterectomy may not be necessary for small nodules that can be completely excised.[14] Regardless of the extent of surgery, the clinical evolution is benign despite the presence of frequent mitotic figures or minor irregularities of the peripheral margin in a few neoplasms.[14,37,90,188,247,251]

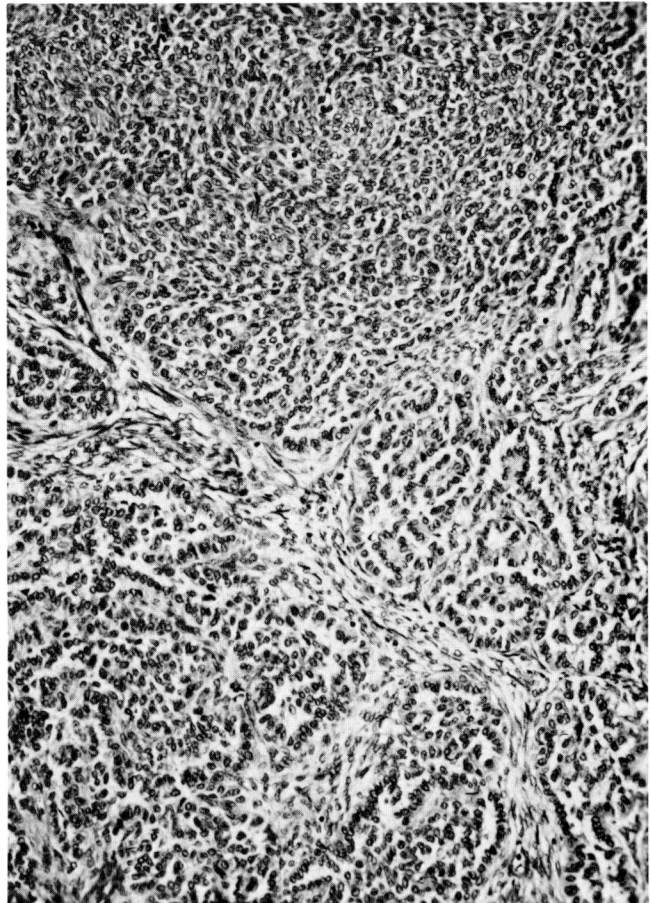

FIG. 13.22. Endometrial stromal nodule. Typical pattern on top, cord-like or tubular pattern on bottom. (Reprinted by permission from Tavassoli and Norris, ref. 247.)

Endometrial Stromal Sarcoma (Low Grade and High Grade)

Endometrial stromal sarcoma (ESS) infiltrates the myometrium. There are two patterns: *low-grade stromal sarcoma* (LGSS) and *high-grade stromal sarcoma* (HGSS).[14,83,90,118,151,188,269] The frequency of endometrial stromal sarcoma is difficult to estimate. Low-grade stromal sarcoma has been excluded from some reports and included in others; some reports include pleomorphic homologous müllerian sarcomas, and benign stromal nodules have even been erroneously included within some reports of endometrial stromal sarcoma. Endometrial stromal sarcoma comprises less than 10% of uterine sarcomas in most large studies; two-thirds are low grade and one-third are high grade. Both forms are included in the following discussion.

CLINICAL FEATURES

Endometrial stromal sarcoma occurs in younger women than does carcinosarcoma, leiomyosarcoma, or endometrial carcinoma. The mean age of women with endometrial stromal sarcoma ranges form 42 to 53 years.° More than 50% of patients are premenopausal, and rare examples of ESS occur in young women and girls.[23,37,90,188] There is no association with endometrial carcinoma risk factors, but a few patients have a history of prior pelvic irradiation.

The main symptoms are abnormal vaginal bleeding, cyclic menorrhagia that gradually becomes more severe, and abdominal pain. The uterus is typically enlarged and has an irregular contour. A few women have bulky polypoid tumors that protrude from the cervical os. The usual clinical impression is that the patient has a uterine leiomyoma that is producing an unusual degree of bleeding. An occasional patient presents with abdominal or pulmonary metastases.[37] Such metastatic deposits may pose a diagnostic problem is they appear before uterine bleeding or enlargement develops and the true nature of the disease is recognized.[3]

Abnormal cells that are diagnostic or suspicious for sarcoma may be detected in the cervicovaginal smear in women with HGSS. Cells shed from a stromal nodule or a LGSS usually are not sufficiently atypical to be distinguished accurately from benign endometrial stromal cells.[163,176]

The diagnosis of HGSS is readily established by the microscopic study of curettings. A low grade stromal tumor can be recognized in curettings but hysterectomy usually is required to distinguish LGSS from a benign stromal nodule. The diagnosis is LGSS if myometrial invasion is identified in the tissue fragments. If the tumor appears circumscribed in the curettings and by magnetic resonance imaging (MRI), and the uterus is small, conservative treatment, based on a presumptive diagnosis of stromal nodule, can be considered if conservation of the uterus is a prime consideration. Curettings are not helpful if the neoplasm is entirely intramural.

At operation, LGSS may resemble intravenous leiomyomatosis or a leiomyoma that has extended into the broad ligament. Frozen section examination permits distinction between these entities.

Gross Findings

The endometrial component of LGSS usually is soft, tan, smooth-surfaced, and polypoid. Intramural growth predominates and exhibits three main patterns. In the first, the myometrium is diffusely thickened but a clearly defined tumor is not evident. In the second, there is a nodular tumor that differs from a leiomyoma in that the cut surfaces are tan or yellow-orange and soft, unlike the white, whorled, firm surface of a leiomyoma. The third, and most familiar, appearance of LGSS is that of a poorly demarcated mass in which pink, tan, or yellow cords and nodules

of tumor permeate the myometrium (Fig. 13.23). LGSS tends to be smaller than HGSS, and its margins are ill-defined and difficult to measure. HGSS is a soft, fleshy, polypoid tumor that bulges into, and often fills, the endometrial cavity. Multiple masses of soft, white-to-tan tumor invade the underlying myometrium on a broad front. Hemorrhage and necrosis frequently are visible.

Both LGSS and HGSS may grow beyond the uterus as infiltrating masses of tan or white tumor than can be palpated as firm, worm-like cords. Pink or tan strands of tumor protrude from the cut surface of the infiltrated tissues and sometimes can be pulled from tissue spaces and vessels.

Microscopic Findings

Low-grade endometrial stromal sarcoma is composed of cells that resemble the stromal cells of proliferative phase endometrium.† There is little variation of the cells in LGSS. They have round or ovoid nuclei with dispersed chromatin and small, inconspicuous nucleoli. The cytoplasm is amphophilic, and the cell border is ill-defined. The uniformity of the cells imparts a monotonous appearance to LGSS. There are typically fewer than 3 MF/10 HPF[37,90,118,188] but there is more mitotic activity in occasional neoplasms that are otherwise typical of LGSS.[14,37,85,243]

Arterioles that resemble the endometrial spiral arterioles are uniformly distributed throughout most LGSS, and capillaries and veins often are conspicuous as well.[37,90] The prominent vascularity is the reason that LGSS can be mistaken for a hemangiopericytoma. Reticulin fibers surround individual cells or small groups of cells, resulting in a basket-weave pattern.[188] Hyalinized zones or plaques are common in LGSS and aggregates of foam cells or foci of necrosis occur in some neoplasms.[37,90] Decidual change is seen occasionally in a stromal tumor as a response to pregnancy or exogenous progesterone.

LGSS invades the myometrium and may extensively permeate it (Fig. 13.24). Invasion of lymphatic and vascular channels is a characteristic of LGSS (Fig. 13.25)[37,90,133,188,241] and is the reason why the neoplasm was formerly called endolymphatic stromal myosis.

Areas of epithelial-like differentiation are present in about one quarter of LGSS.[37,90,154,188] Highly varied in appearance, epithelial-like differentiation can be manifested as trabecular cords of epithelioid cells, mesothelial-like structures, endometrial-type glands, or as glands lined by clear cells (see below, Endometrial Stromal Variants).[51]

High-grade endometrial stromal sarcoma is composed of cells that are more atypical than those in LGSS.[14,188,269] We use the term HGSS for a neoplasm that consists exclu-

---

°Refs. 23,37,85,90,118,133,151,188,204,251,269.

†Refs. 37,83,85,90,118,133,138,188,251.

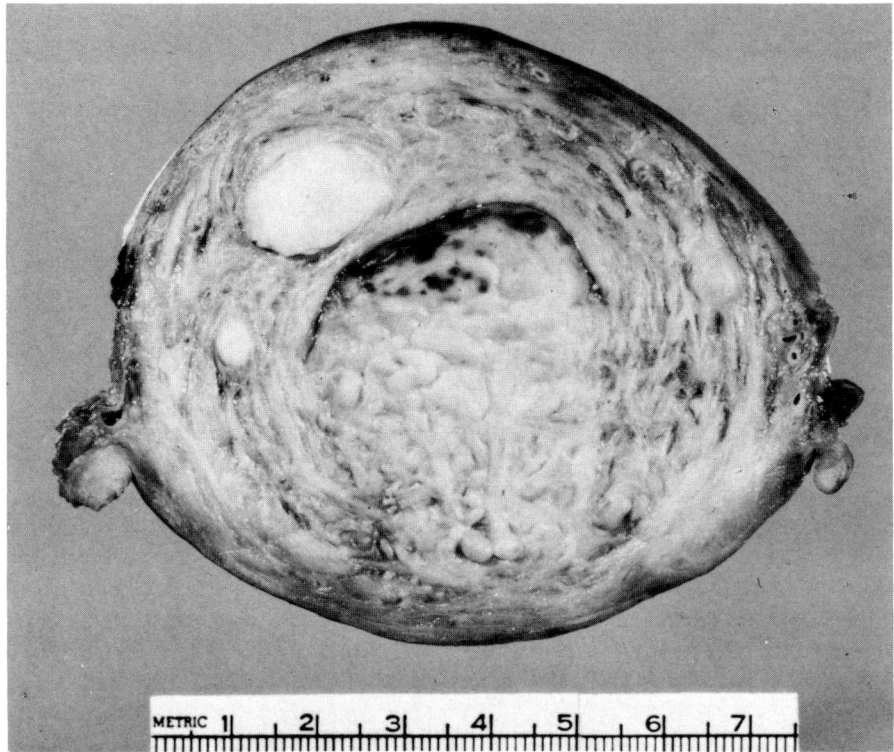

FIG. 13.23. Low-grade endometrial stromal sarcoma. Extensions of tumor (*lower field*) bulge above the cut surface and obliterate the endometrial cavity. Compare with the leiomyomas in the left half of the myometrium. (Reprinted by permission from Norris and Taylor, ref. 188.)

sively of cells that resemble endometrial stromal cells. A variety of sarcomas that do not qualify for this designation arise in the endometrium. Most are pure or mixed sarcomas that resemble the mesenchymal component of a carcinosarcoma.[85] These should be classified separately because grouping them with pure HGSS, as has been done in some studies, obscures the behavior and response to treatment of both types of neoplasms (see below, Homologous and Heterologous Sarcomas).

Compared with the cells in LGSS, those in HGSS have larger, more vesicular nuclei with more prominent chromatin clumps and nucleoli. The cytoplasm is eosinophilic or amphophilic, and the cell borders are indistinct (Fig. 13.26). Mitotic figures are frequent in HGSS. There are almost always 10 or more MF/10 HPF and typically there are 20 or more MF/10 HPF in the most active areas.[90,151,188,269] HGSS infiltrates the myometrium destructively, with areas of hemorrhage and necrosis, in contrast to the myometrial and vascular permeation that typifies LGSS. The vascular pattern and reticulin meshwork are irregular in HGSS.

Some question the need to grade endometrial stromal sarcoma,[37,85] and several recent studies have failed to detect a statistically significant difference in survival between stage I LGSS and HGSS.[23,37,126] We think that there are recognizable pathologic differences between LGSS and HGSS. Pathologists should continue to grade these neo-

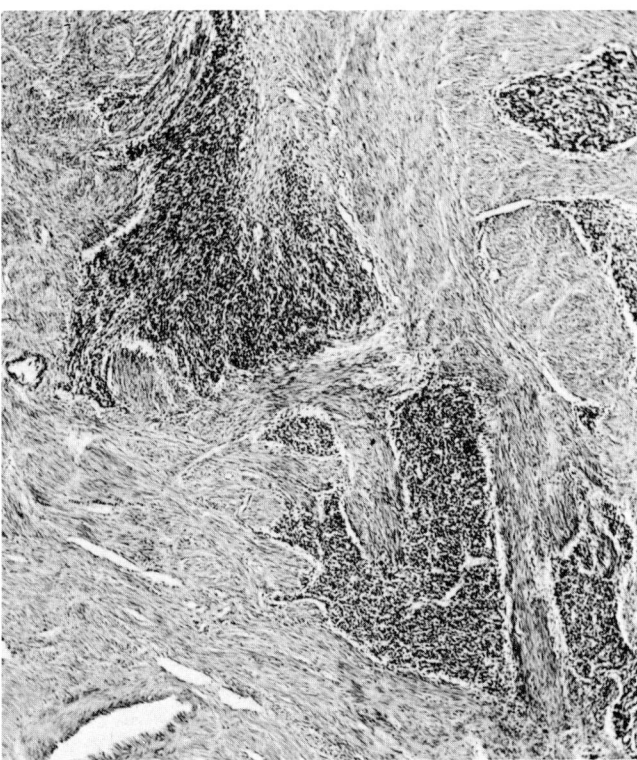

FIG. 13.24. Low-grade endometrial stromal sarcoma. Groups of stromal cells infiltrate the myometrium in a characteristic pattern. (Reprinted by permission from Norris and Taylor, ref. 188.)

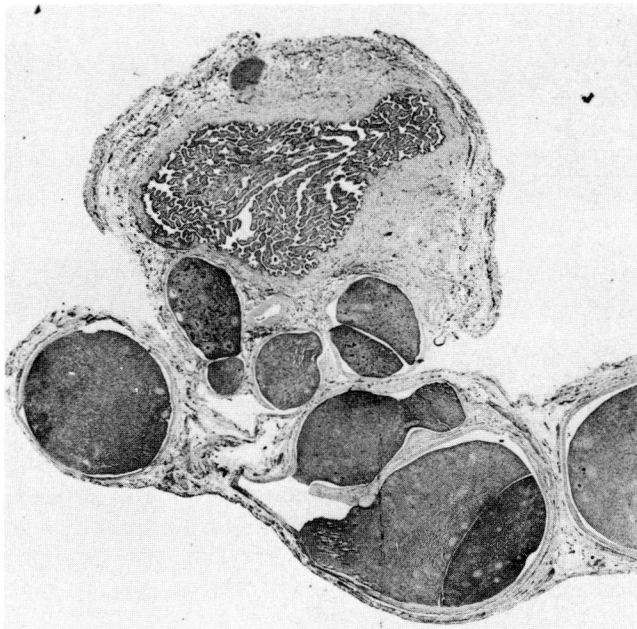

FIG. 13.25. **Low-grade endometrial stromal sarcoma.** Tumor grows in the lymphatics of the mesosalpinx and mesovarium.

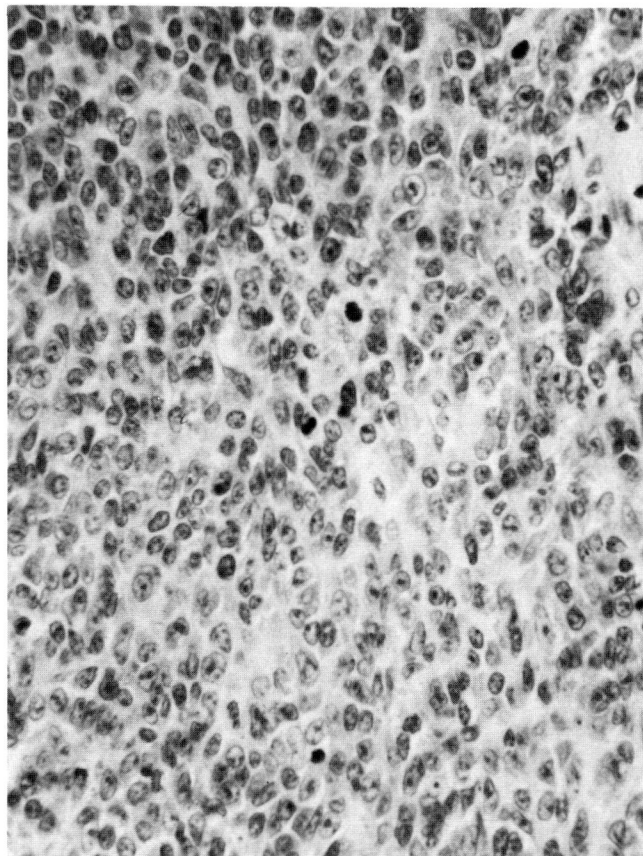

FIG. 13.26. **High-grade endometrial stromal sarcoma.** Note frequent mitotic figures.

plasms pending further study because most reports in the literature suggest that, overall, the behavior of LGSS is different from that of HGSS. It is occasionally difficult to decide whether a stromal sarcoma should be designated as low or high grade. A few neoplasms have frequent mitotic figures but exhibit little atypia and have a growth pattern that is characteristic of LGSS.[14,85,243] Other examples have fewer than 10 MF/10 HPF, but show significant atypia and destructive invasion.[83] A variety of features must be considered when assigning a grade to such stromal sarcomas (Table 13.4). Newer techniques, including flow cytometric analysis, immunohistochemistry, and hormone receptor analysis may be helpful.

FLOW CYTOMETRY

A few endometrial stromal sarcomas have been examined by flow cytometry. LGSS is invariably DNA diploid.[14,81,83,121] Proliferative activity, as measured by the S-phase fraction or a proliferative index that includes both S-phase and G2/M fractions, is generally low in LGSS.[14,81,83] Levels of proliferative activity similar to those obtained in HGSS nevertheless may be observed in some LGSS.[121] In one instance the transition from a LGSS to a HGSS was accompanied by the appearance of a DNA aneuploid cell population.[81] The results of flow cytometric analysis are more varied in HGSS. These may be either DNA diploid or DNA aneuploid.[14,70,83,121] Proliferative activity tends to be greater in HGSS than in LGSS and some have suggested that this may be helpful in grading a stromal sarcoma.[14,83] Flow cytometric data are not absolute criteria for division of stromal sarcoma into low and high grades nor do they always correlate with clinical behavior (see Chapter 27, Flow Cytometry).

IMMUNOHISTOCHEMISTRY

The immunohistochemical staining of endometrial stromal sarcoma varies, depending on the differentiation of the tumor, the fixation of the tissue, the antibodies used, and the technique of staining. Stromal sarcoma cells generally react with antibodies to vimentin.[25,74,88,98,154,219,256] The results of staining with other antibodies are more variable. Stromal sarcoma did not react with antibodies to any other intermediate filaments in one large study.[74] In most reports, however, stromal sarcoma does react with antibodies to intermediate filaments other than vimentin. Some neoplasms contain occasional desmin-positive cells.[88,98,154] In accord with the light microscopic observation of differentiation toward smooth muscle in stromal sarcoma,[37,118] most tumors contain cells that react with muscle-specific actin and α-smooth muscle actin.[88,98,154] Some LGSS contain cells that react with antibodies to cytokeratin,[25,88,98,154] but there is no reaction with antibodies to epithelial membrane antigen. The epithelial-like structures that are present in 25% of LGSS typically stain with cytokeratin but not with

Table 13.4. Typical pathologic findings in endometrial stromal tumors

Diagnosis	MF/10 HPF	Atypia	Vascular pattern	Ploidy	S-phase	ER/PR
Stromal nodule	3<[a]	0–1+	Prominent regular	Diploid	Low %	NA
LGSS	3<[a]	0–1+	Prominent regular	Diploid	Low %	+
HGSS	>10[b]	2+–3+	Inconspicuous irregular	Aneuploid	High %	–

[a] Some have more mitotic figures, including more than 10 MF/10 HPF in occasional tumors.

[b] Rare tumors in this category have fewer than 10 MF/10 HPF.

ER, estrogen receptor; HGSS, high-grade stromal sarcoma; HPF, high-power field; LGSS, low-grade stromal sarcoma; MF, mitotic figures; PR, progesterone receptor; NA, not applicable.

epithelial membrane antigen. They also react strongly with vimentin, muscle-specific actin, and desmin, an immunophenotype that is similar to that of the surrounding stromal cells and to smooth muscle.[154] Endometrial stromal tumors and smooth muscle tumors have a similar immunophenotype,[98] which is not unexpected given their common embryologic derivation (see Chapter 26, Immunohistochemistry).

Steroid hormone receptor assays have been performed on tumor tissue from a few patients with LGSS, and both estrogen and progesterone receptors are present in most neoplasms.[16,81,133,147,219,240,257] Immunohistochemical analysis can be performed if fresh tissue is not available for biochemical testing.[219,256] Progesterone receptors are readily demonstrated by immunohistochemistry (Fig. 13.27), but estrogen receptors may be difficult to identify even when biochemical testing indicates that they are present.[219] Hormone receptors generally are not detected in HGSS.

Ultrastructure

The ultrastructural features of the cells in LGSS are similar to those of stromal cells in early- to midproliferative-phase endometrium and in stromal nodules.[6,28,90,142,165,171] The tumor cells (Fig. 13.28) are irregular or spindle shaped, with round or oval nuclei. The cytoplasm is scanty and usually contains sparsely distributed organelles. Mitochondria, rough endoplasmic reticulum, free ribosomes, microfilaments, and Golgi vesicles are present, but they are less prominent than in smooth muscle cells. Some cells are partly surrounded by a basal lamina, and desmosomes are sparse. The pleomorphism and cytologic atypia seen in HGSS by light microscopy also is observed at the ultrastructural level. The cytoplasmic content is similar to that of LGSS, except that microfilaments are less conspicuous.

Clinical Behavior and Treatment

The type and extent of tumor and the type of operation determine the risk of recurrence. The stage is the most significant prognostic factor.[37,126] Hysterectomy and bilateral salpingo-oophorectomy is the standard treatment for stage I stromal sarcoma. Adnexal spread is not always visi-

ble at operation, and recurrence is more frequent when the adnexal structures are conserved.[23,151] Debulking is recommended when extrauterine tumor is present. Some oncologists recommend long-term postoperative progestin therapy with the hope of reducing the 50% risk of recurrence.[204] Women with stage I LGSS have greater than an 80% long-term survival.[23,37,90,188,204] The best 5-year survival rates reported in stage I HGSS are greater than

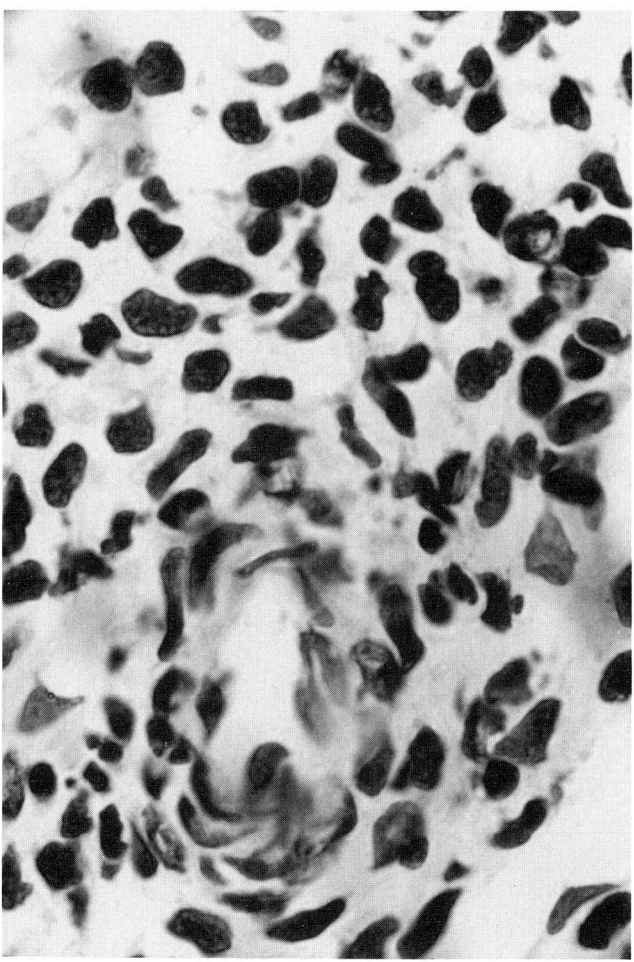

Fig. 13.27. Low-grade endometrial stromal sarcoma. An immunohistochemical stain for progesterone receptors demonstrates a strong positive reaction in the nuclei.

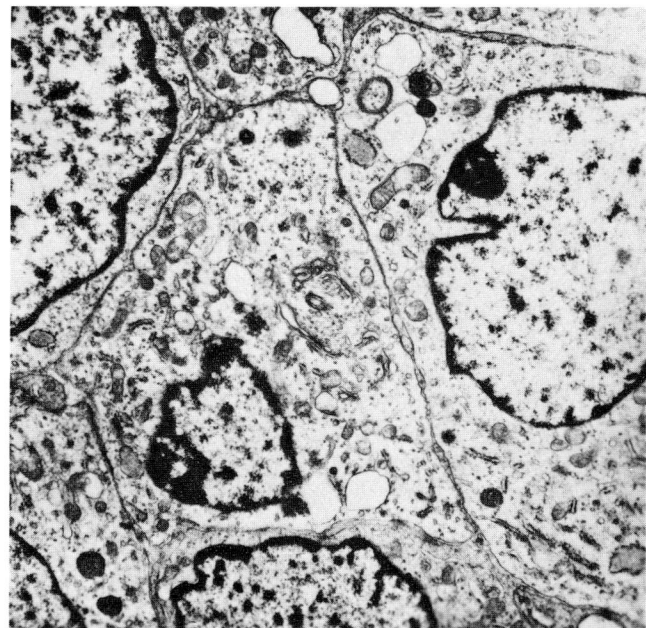

FIG. 13.28. **Low-grade endometrial stromal sarcoma.** The nuclei are rounded, the chromatin is dispersed, and the cytoplasm contains a few organelles and fibrils. ×8000.

50%.[23,151,265] The survival is less favorable (40–50% for LGSS and 0–50% for HGSS) when there is advanced disease at presentation.[23,37,90,151,188,269]

Low-grade stromal sarcoma is slow growing, and recurrence is commonly detected many years after initial treatment.[23,37,85,90,118,151,188] Recurrence usually is in the pelvis and involves the ureter, bladder, vagina, or bowel.[85,204] Metastases beyond the pelvis are distributed over the peritoneal surfaces or omentum. Pulmonary metastases develop in a minority of patients.[37,118,188,204] There is resolution or stabilization of recurrent or metastatic LGSS in more than 50% of patients treated with progestational agents.[136,204,251] Tumors that contain a high level of progesterone receptors are most likely to respond to progesterone therapy, so hormone receptors should be measured in every stromal sarcoma.[16,81,109,133,147,257] Recurrent or metastatic LGSS that does not respond to treatment with progestins sometimes can be treated surgically[23] and radiotherapy also may be used. Chemotherapy is ineffective in LGSS.[23] The median time from diagnosis of LGSS to death is about 11 years.[188] HGSS, in contrast, often exhibits rapid progression. Recurrence usually is evident within 2 years of initial treatment.[90,126,151,188,223,269] Progestational agents generally are ineffective in HGSS. Pelvic recurrences are fewer, and survival is better in patients with low-stage disease treated with combined therapy.[82,202,265] Recurrence outside the radiation field is the most common reason for treatment failure in a patient who has had combined therapy.[62,223] Adjuvant chemotherapy may be a means to control such metastases but an effective adjuvant drug regimen is not available. A few women with metastatic HGSS respond to chemotherapy regimens that contain doxorubicin.[23]

Endometrial Stromal Tumor Variants

There are two neoplasms that contain endometrial stroma that are variants of the usual stromal tumor. One is termed a *uterine neoplasm resembling an ovarian sex cord tumor*,[51] and the other is a *combined smooth muscle–stromal tumor*.

Uterine Neoplasm Resembling an Ovarian Sex Cord Tumor

The *uterine neoplasm resembling an ovarian sex cord tumor* contains a variable quantity of typical endometrial stromal cells. Most neoplasms in this category are endom-

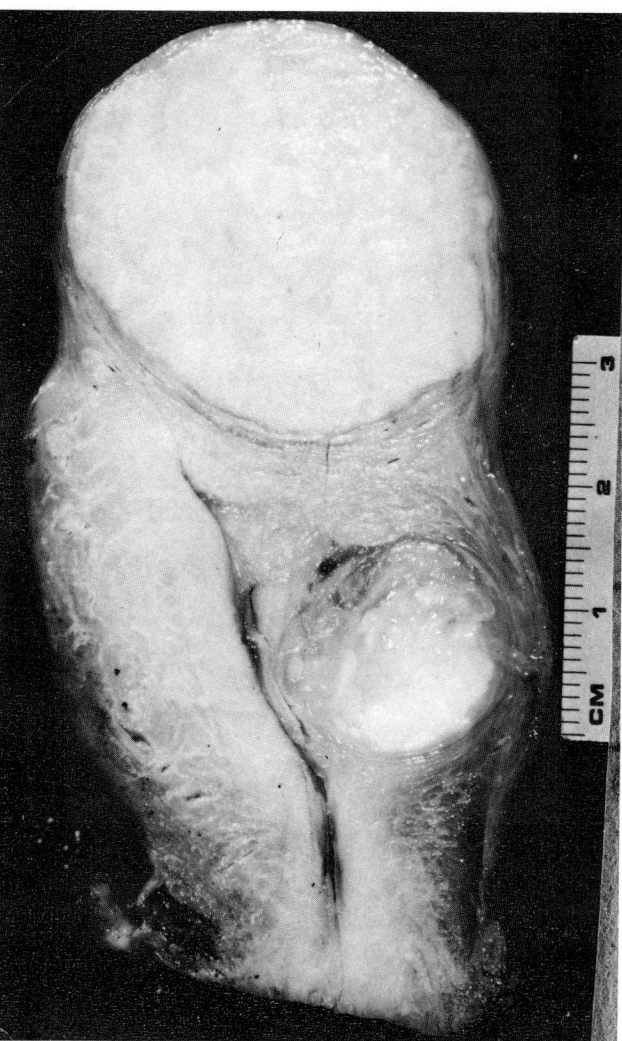

FIG. 13.29. **Endometrial stromal tumor variant resembling a sex cord-stromal tumor (small nodule at lower right).** The large nodule in the fundus is a leiomyoma.

etrial stromal tumors with epithelial-like differentiation in the form of trabeculae, nests, and cords that are reminiscent of growth patterns seen in ovarian sex cord–stromal tumors (Figs. 13.29–13.31). In most examples, the nuclei of the "epithelial" cells are similar to those in the surrounding stromal component. Ultrastructurally, the stromal cells resemble proliferative endometrial stroma and the cells in stromal neoplasms.[91,166] The epithelial-like clusters may[91] or may not[166] contain lumens lined by cells with microvilli. The tumor cells are joined by occasional desmosomes and they contain perinuclear intermediate filaments, raising the question of differentiation toward endometrial glandular structures (Fig. 13.32).[91,166] Features of smooth muscle differentiation such as micropinocytotic vesicles and bundles of filaments with dense bodies are not described.[91] When plexiform and tubular structures dominate the morphologic pattern and endometrial stroma is inconspicuous, the resemblance to other endometrial stromal tumors may be obscure.[51,157] Rarely, "epithelial" differentiation is so prominent that the tumor must be distinguished from endometrial adenocarcinoma or mixed müllerian tumor. Well-formed glands of the type that characterize adenocar-

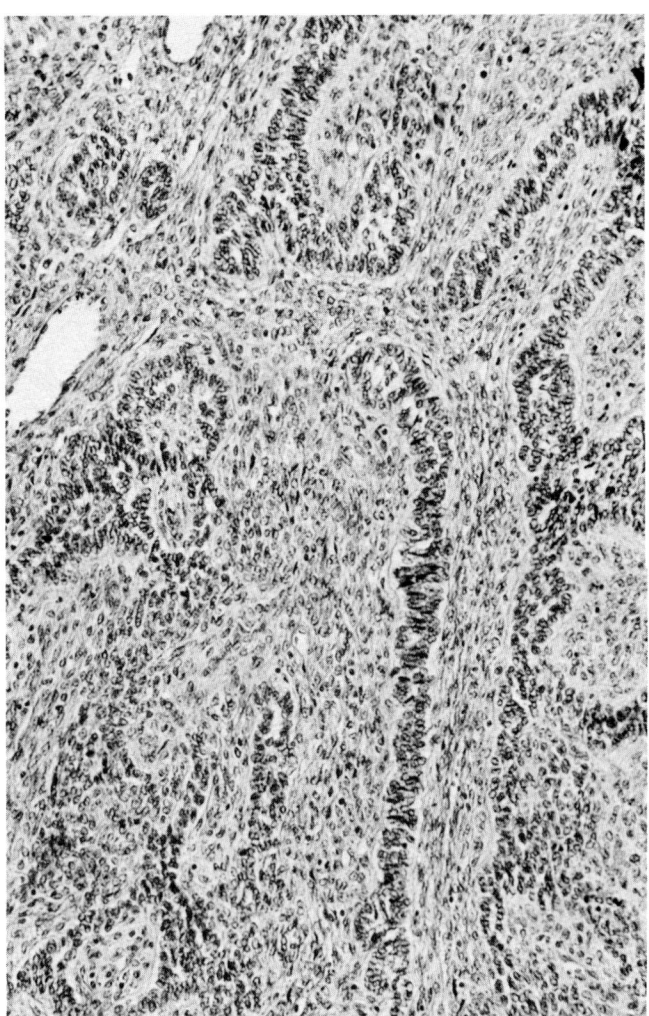

FIG. 13.31. Endometrial stromal tumor variant. The organoid cords look like sex cords to some investigators. (Reprinted by permission from Mazur and Kraus, ref. 166.)

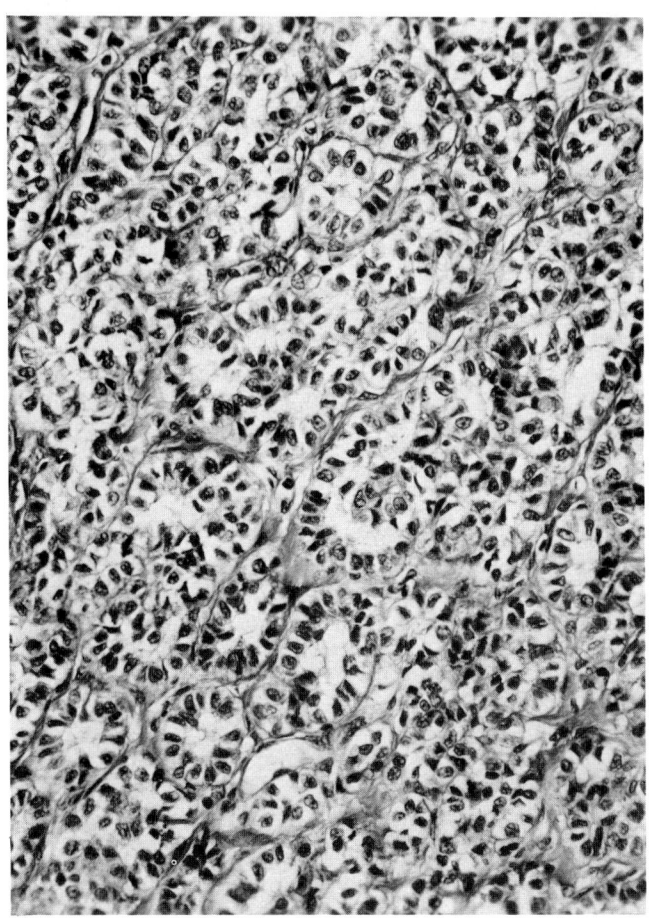

FIG. 13.30. Endometrial stromal tumor variant. The tumor cells grow in a tubular pattern.

cinoma rarely are present, and a recognizable stromal component generally is observed, at least focally. As noted above, the "epithelial" structures in a stromal tumor may express cytokeratin, but usually they also express muscle antigens, and they do not express epithelial membrane antigen. This immunophenotype, together with the absence of heterologous mesenchymal elements and clear-cut carcinoma, helps to distinguish these rare endometrial stromal tumors from a mixed müllerian tumor.

Patients who have uterine stromal tumors with a sex cord pattern are generally of reproductive age, although a few are perimenopausal or postmenopasual.[51] The neoplasms produce abnormal bleeding and uterine enlargement. Although few cases have been reported, the behavior of the tumor, like that of a pure endometrial stromal tumor, probably depends on the cytologic characteristics, the type of margin (i.e., circumscribed versus infiltrating), and the stage.[51,157]

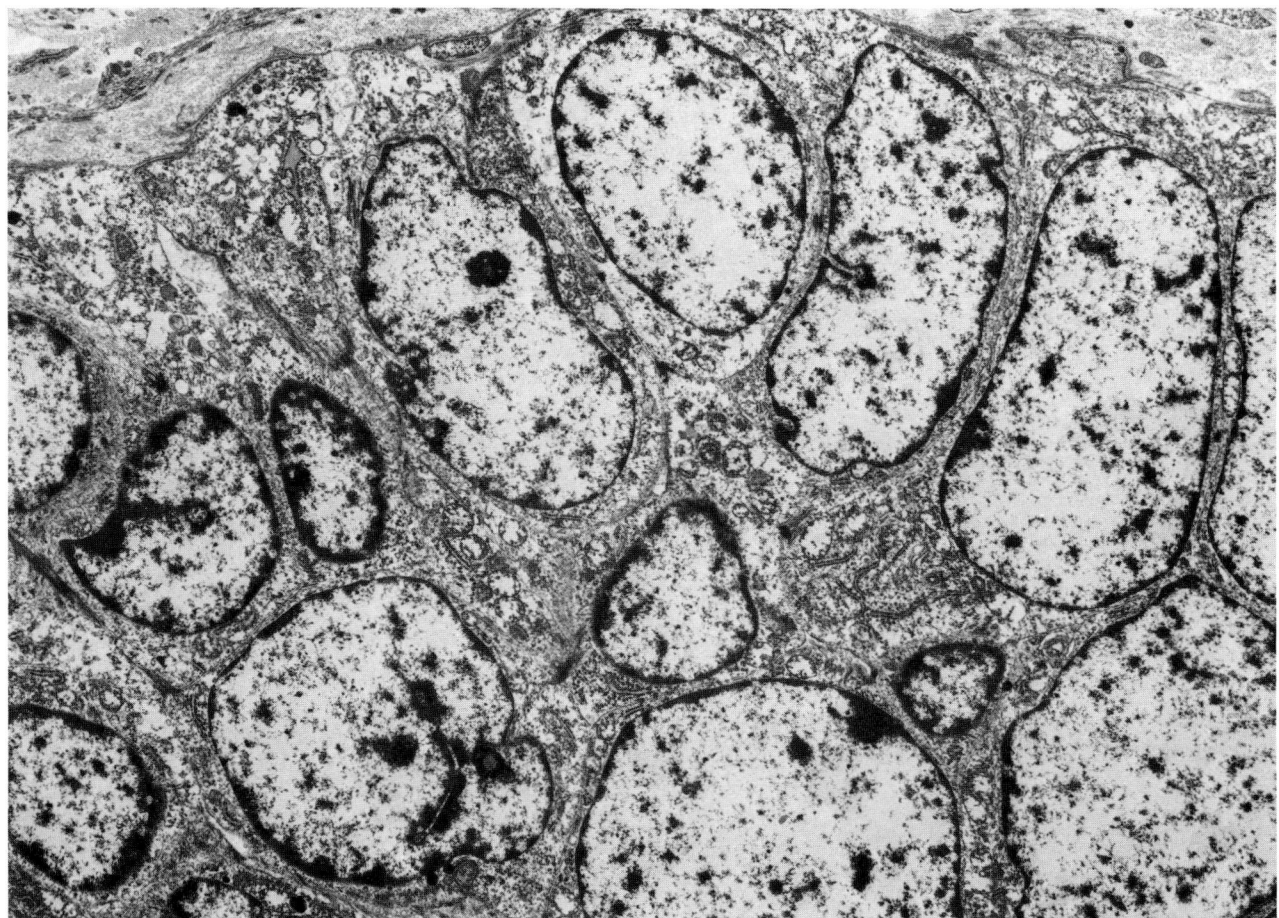

FIG. 13.32. **Endometrial stromal tumor variant (same tumor as shown in Fig. 13.31).** An electron microscopic view of epithelial-like cells within one of the cords. A true lumen is absent. Tonofilaments are present in cell to lower right. (Reprinted by permission from Mazur and Kraus, ref. 166.)

Combined Smooth Muscle–Stromal Tumor

Rare uterine tumors contain significant areas of both smooth muscle and endometrial stromal differentiation. The clinical evolution of such combined smooth muscle-stromal neoplasms is poorly documented, but malignant behavior is possible if the neoplasm is dominated by endometrial stroma and if it has an infiltrating margin. Some neoplasms that were formerly designated as "stromomyomas" are endometrial stromal tumors with trabeculae and cords of cells that exhibit ultrastructural features of smooth muscle differentiation.[166,245] The biphasic features of the "stromomyoma" are not surprising considering that the epithelial-like structures commonly seen in endometrial stromal tumors have a myogenous immunophenotype.[154]

Mixed Epithelial-Mesenchymal Tumors

Mixed epithelial-mesenchymal tumors contain both epithelium and mesenchymal elements as active participants in the neoplastic process. The tumors in this group are morphologically, but perhaps not histogenetically, related. The mixed epithelial-mesenchymal tumor group includes adenofibroma, adenosarcoma, and mixed müllerian tumor (carcinosarcoma) (Tables 13.1, 13.5). There is a gradation of malignant potential ranging from adenofibroma at the benign end of the spectrum, through adenosarcoma, to the highly malignant mixed müllerian tumor. Adenofibroma and adenosarcoma both have a benign glandular component. The stroma is benign in adenofibroma, whereas adenosarcoma has a sarcomatous mesenchymal component. Both stroma and epithelium are malignant in a mixed müllerian tumor. The capacity to form neoplasms with both epithelial and connective tissue differentiation is a result of the embryologic heritage of the epithelium and stroma of the endometrium.

Mixed müllerian tumor is classified as homologous or heterologous, depending on the mesenchymal elements present. Homologous tumors contain mesenchymal cell types that normally are found in the uterus, such as endometrial stromal cells, smooth muscle cells, and fibroblasts. Heterologous tumors exhibit types of mesenchymal differentiation that are not normally observed in the

Table 13.5. Classification of mixed epithelial-mesenchymal tumors

Tumor	Malignant potential	Epithelium	Mesenchymal component
Adenofibroma	None	Benign	Benign, homologous
Adenosarcoma	Low to intermediate	Benign	Low-grade sarcoma, homologous, or heterologous
Mixed müllerian tumor	High	Carcinoma	High-grade sarcoma, homologous, or heterologous

uterus. Heterologous elements include striated muscle, cartilage, osteoid, and fat.

Adenofibroma

CLINICAL FEATURES

This tumor most often arises in the endometrium[50,264] and less often in the cervix[2] or extrauterine locations.[52,131] Women with adenofibroma generally are elderly and most are either peri- or postmenopausal. The median age is 68 years,[273] but patient age varies from 19 years to more than 80 years.[2,8,195,264,273] There is no known racial predilection, nor does adenofibroma have the epidemiologic features of endometrial carcinoma. Abnormal vaginal bleeding is the most frequent complaint. Less common findings include abdominal pain, abdominal enlargement, or a polypoid tumor projecting from the cervix. Some patients give a history of prior removal of polyps.

GROSS FINDINGS

Adenofibroma may arise anywhere in the uterus or in the cervix.[2,5,273] It is a lobulated polypoid neoplasm that varies from soft to firm in consistency. The cut surface is tan or brown with focal hemorrhage. About 50% of adenofibromas contain small cysts that impart a spongy or mucoid appearance. The size ranges from 2 to 20 cm, with a median diameter of 7 cm. A large adenofibroma may fill the endometrial cavity and enlarge the uterus.

MICROSCOPIC FINDINGS

Adenofibroma is composed of histologically bland epithelium and mesenchyme. It originates in the endometrium or cervix and usually does not invade the underlying myometrium (Fig. 13.33) or cervical stroma. Broad papillary fronds covered with epithelium project from the surface and into cystic spaces within the neoplasm. Columnar or cuboidal epithelial cells, most often of endometrioid type, line cysts and cleft-like spaces. Other types of epithelium, such as endocervical, tubal, and squamous epithelium, often occur within the same neoplasm, and the epithelium may be hyperplastic and stratified.

The mesenchymal component usually is fibroblastic (Fig. 13.34), but endometrial stromal cells or mixtures of stromal cells and fibroblasts are present in some neoplasms. The fibrotic stroma is more cellular and uniform than in polyps. The markedly hypercellular periglandular stroma that characterizes adenosarcoma is not seen in adenofibroma. Atypia within the stromal cells generally is absent or mild, and markedly atypical mesenchymal cells are not present. Mitotic figures are rare. There are invariably fewer than 4 MF/10 HPF,[273] and some regard the presence of virtually any countable mitotic activity as indicative of adenosarcoma.[54,128]

CLINICAL BEHAVIOR AND TREATMENT

Hysterectomy is the preferred treatment for an adenofibroma because the neoplasm may recur if it is incompletely curetted or excised.[195,225,273] Hysterectomy ensures complete removal, and it also permits the thorough sampling needed to exclude an adenosarcoma. Conservative therapy, such as repeat curettage, can be considered in young women if imaging studies demonstrate complete removal of the tumor.

Adenofibroma is benign and no tumor-related deaths have been reported. Two unique neoplasms with features of adenofibroma invaded the myometrium, and, in one case, myometrial veins.[55] Both patients were well after

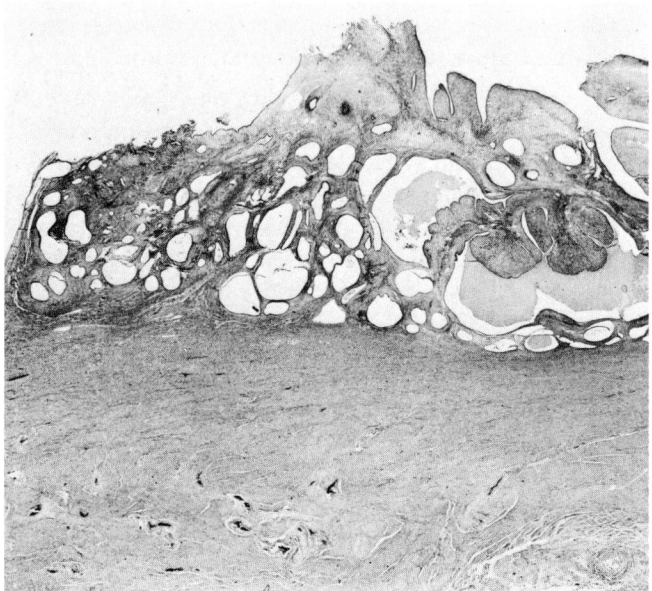

FIG. 13.33. Adenofibroma. A superficial tumor that does not invade the myometrium. (Reprinted by permission from Zaloudek and Norris, ref. 273.)

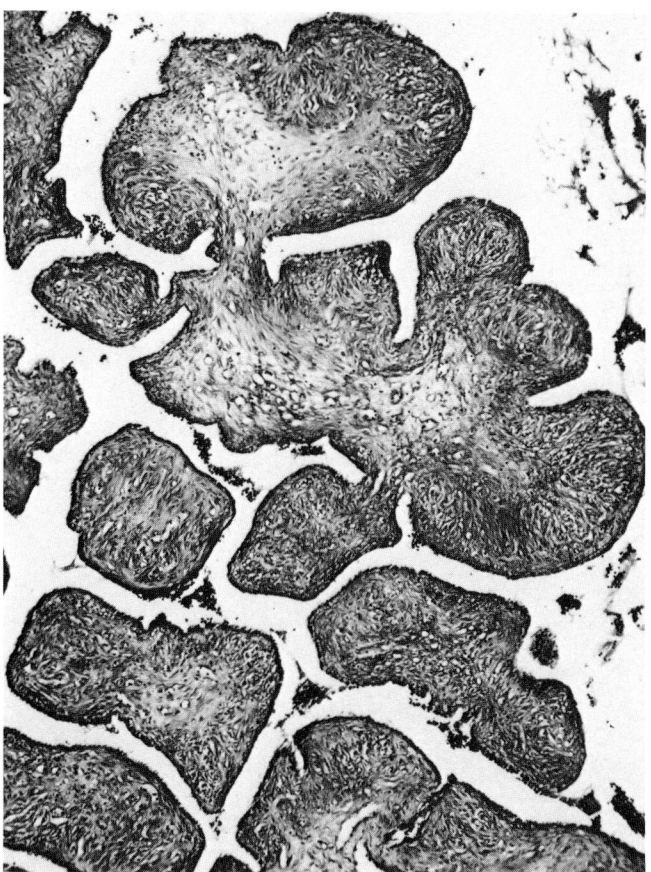

FIG. 13.34. Adenofibroma. Papillae project into cystic spaces and have a hypocellular, collagenous stroma. (Reprinted by permission from Zaloudek and Norris, ref. 273.)

hysterectomy, but a more guarded prognosis is appropriate when an adenofibroma exhibits unusual gross or microscopic features.

Adenosarcoma

This neoplasm most often arises in the endometrium[50,264] but also occurs in cervix[2] or the extrauterine pelvic locations, such as the fallopian tube, ovary, and paraovarian tissues.[52,131] Adenosarcoma occurs in patients of all ages.* The median age is about 57 years, with a range of 14 to 79 years.

Extrauterine adenosarcoma occurs in younger women and is more aggressive than its uterine counterpart. There is no association with obesity or hypertension, nor is there any association with prior pelvic radiation. A minority of patients are diabetic. Some have a history of prior removal of cervical or endometrial polyps.

_____
*Refs. 11,15,54,65,97,108,128,195,263,273.

The most common presenting symptom is abnormal vaginal bleeding. Vaginal discharge, pain, nonspecific urinary symptoms, a palpable pelvic mass, and tumor protruding from the vagina are other common signs and symptoms.

GROSS FINDINGS

Adenosarcoma is a sessile, soft or firm, polypoid neoplasm that fills the endometrial cavity and enlarges the uterus (Fig. 13.35).[54,128,273] A solitary polypoid growth is most characteristic, but some neoplasms grow as multiple papillary or polypoid masses. Adenosarcoma occasionally arises in the cervix.[102,215,246] The cut surface contains small cysts, and it is tan, brown, or gray. Zones of hemorrhage and necrosis are observed in about 25% of adenosarcomas.

MICROSCOPIC FINDINGS

Tubular glands and cleft-like spaces are dispersed throughout the stroma and papillary stromal fronds covered by epithelium project from the surface or into cysts

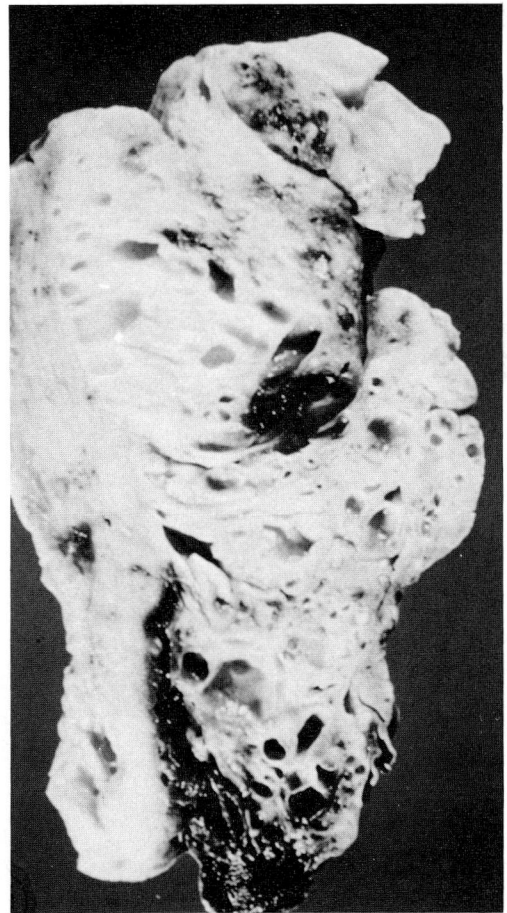

FIG. 13.35. Adenosarcoma in bisected uterus. A polypoid partially infarcted mass containing small cysts fills the endometrial cavity and invades the myometrium.

(Fig. 13.36). The most common type of epithelium resembles inactive or proliferative endometrial epithelium. Secretory, hyperplastic, or atypical hyperplastic endometrioid epithelium is present in some tumors, and adenosarcoma also may contain mucinous, squamous, serous, and clear cell types of epithelium.[54,128,273] Glands and stroma are both present in areas of myometrial invasion, which are observed in 15–20% of adenosarcomas,[54,195,273] suggesting that the epithelium is an actively proliferating part of the neoplasm.

The mesenchymal component of adenosarcoma generally is a homologous sarcoma such as stromal sarcoma or fibrosarcoma; unusual elements such as angiosarcoma[144] are rarely observed in these neoplasms. Periglandular stromal hypercellularity is a characteristic feature of adenosarcoma (Figs. 13.36, 37). The mesenchymal cells show a variable degree of nuclear atypia. Mitotic figures generally are readily identified and number 4 or more MF/10 HPF.[128,273] Rare neoplasms with an atypical stroma characteristic of adenosarcoma, but in which mitotic activity is inconspicuous, recur or metastasize.[54] A neoplasm with an atypical, hypercellular stroma that is condensed around the epithelial elements therefore should be diagnosed as adenosarcoma even if there are only 2–3 MF/10 HPF. Ade-

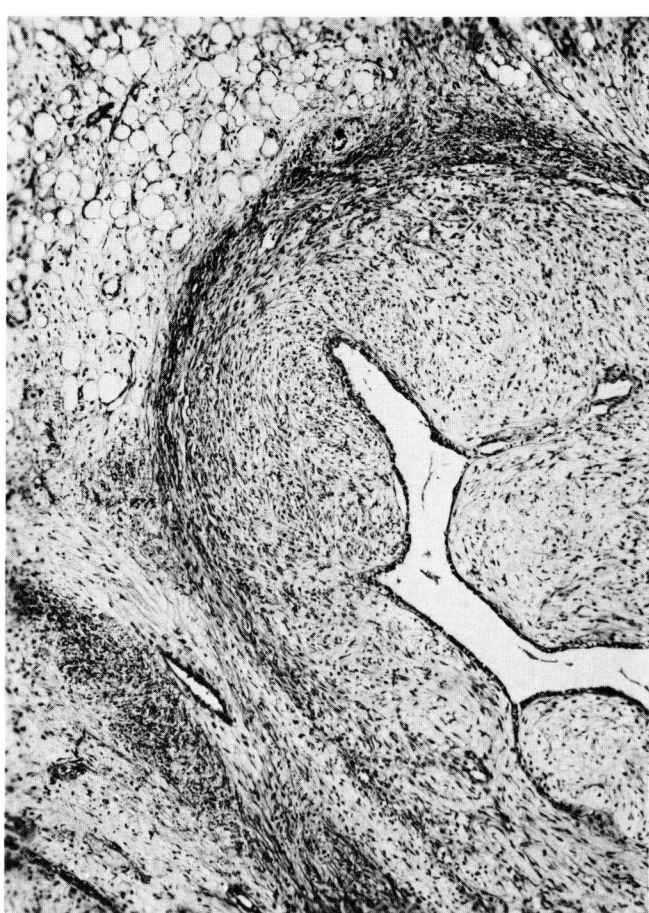

Fig. 13.37. Adenosarcoma. Note periglandular stromal hypercellularity. Fat is present in the upper left. Smooth muscle, cartilage, and striated muscle also occur in adenosarcoma.

nosarcoma often contains bland areas indistinguishable from adenofibroma, so extensive microscopic study may be required to identify a sarcomatous component.[54,273] There are trabecular, insular, or tubular arrangements of plump epithelial-like cells, some of which have abundant foamy cytoplasm, in about 5% of adenosarcomas.[53,120] These structures, which are designated as *sex cord–like elements*,[53] resemble the epithelial-like structures commonly seen in endometrial stromal tumors (see earlier, Endometrial Stromal Tumors).[154]

Heterologous mesenchymal elements are present in 20–25% of adenosarcomas.* Striated muscle (rhabdomyosarcoma) is the most common heterologous element, but cartilage and fat (Fig. 13.37) occasionally are observed. *Sarcomatous overgrowth*, which is observed in 10% of adenosarcomas,[49,128] is characterized by the one-sided proliferation of the sarcomatous component of the tumor. Epithelial elements are absent in the region of sarcoma-

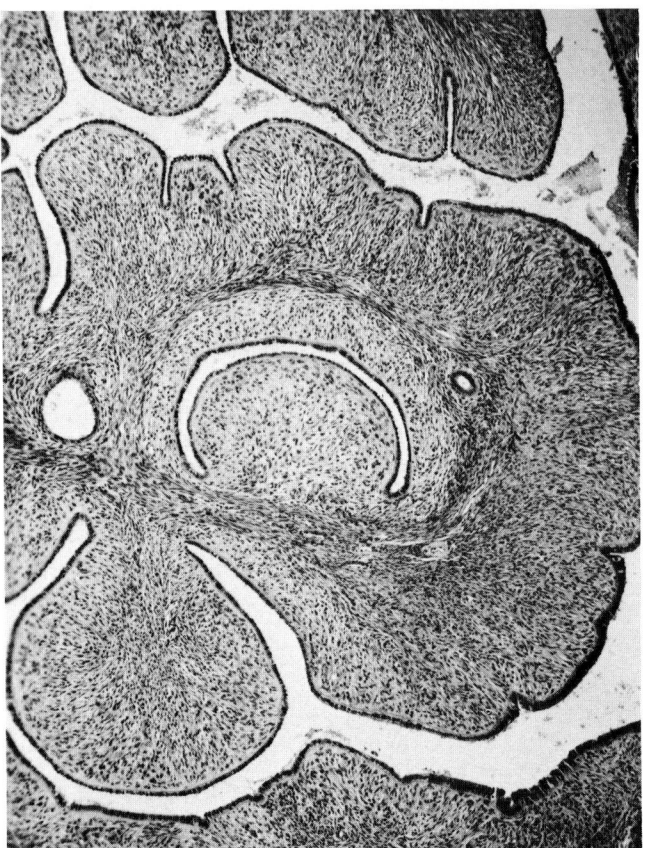

Fig. 13.36. Adenosarcoma. The dense stromal cellularity contrasts with adenofibroma (compare with Fig. 13.34).

---

*Refs. 40,54,97,102,128,144,215,273.

tous overgrowth, which occupies 25% or more of the total tumor volume. The sarcoma typically is of higher grade in the region of sarcomatous overgrowth, with increased cellularity, nuclear atypia, and mitotic activity.[49] Heterologous elements, particularly rhabdomyosarcoma, may be concentrated in the zone of sarcomatous overgrowth.[128]

ULTRASTRUCTURE

Electron microscopic studies[24,67,134,192,194,215] support the impression that two components are present. A distinct basal lamina separates the stromal cells from the epithelium. The epithelium has typical müllerian characteristics, including cilia, microvilli, and basal orientation of the nuclei (Fig. 13.38). The mesenchymal cells often are similar to proliferative phase stromal cells and to the cells in endometrial stromal sarcoma, but in some areas the mesenchymal cells have ultrastructural features of fibroblasts or nonspecific mesenchymal cells.

CLINICAL BEHAVIOR AND TREATMENT

The usual treatment of adenosarcoma is by hysterectomy and bilateral salpingo-oophorectomy. Local excision has been used in a few children and young women. Women with invasive adenosarcoma have a significant risk of pelvic recurrence, but the role of postoperative pelvic radiation is uncertain in this population, as is the effectiveness of chemotherapy.

Adenosarcoma is not as aggressive as mixed müllerian tumor. Recurrence develops in 25–40% of women.[54,128,273] The recurrence is generally in the pelvis or vagina, but distant metastases occur in 5% of patients. Recurrent tumor most often is composed exclusively of the sarcomatous component, but both epithelium and stroma occasionally are present.[54,273] Pathologic features associated with an increased risk of recurrence or metastasis are extrauterine spread at diagnosis, myometrial invasion, especially to the outer half of the myometrium, and sarcomatous overgrowth of the mesenchymal component.[49,54,128,273] Inva-

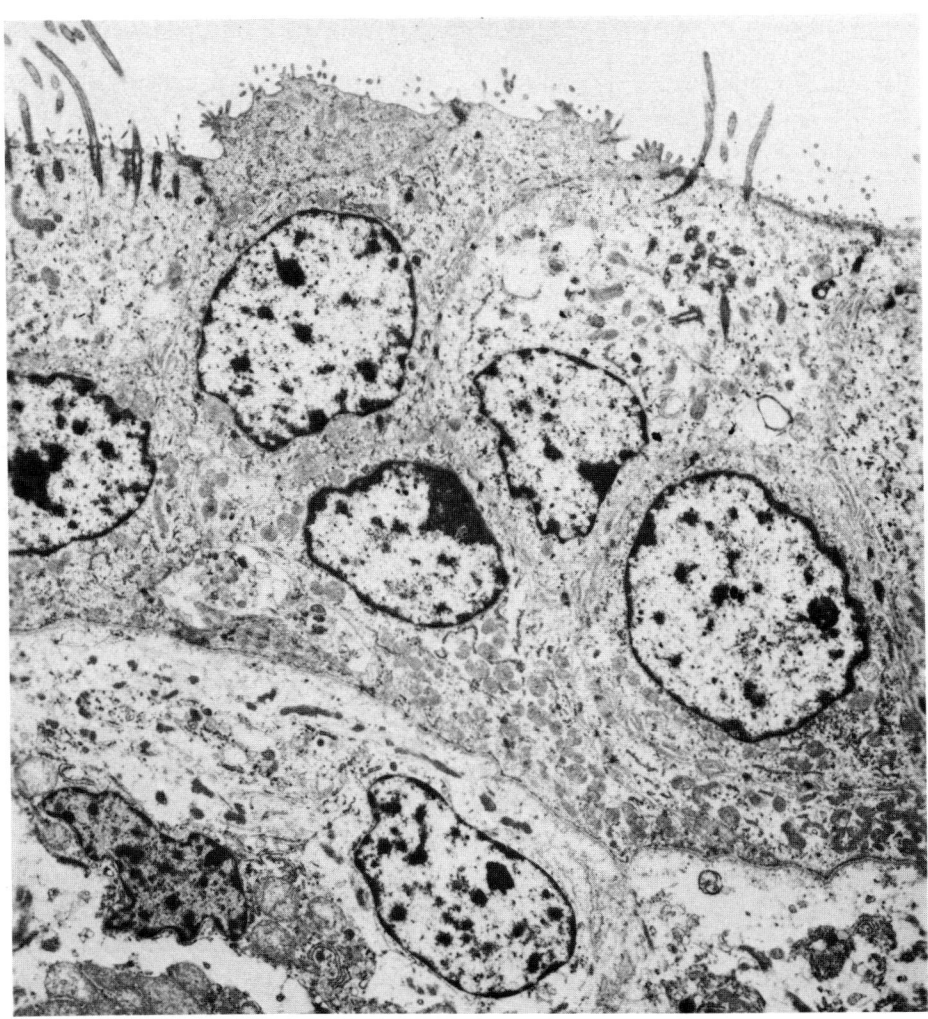

FIG. 13.38. Adenosarcoma. Epithelial cells have microvilli and cilia. Epithelial and stromal cells are separated by a discrete basal lamina. ×4000. (Courtesy of F.A. Tavassoli, M.D., Washington, DC.)

sion of capillary–lymphatic spaces in the myometrium or the presence of rhabdomyosarcoma in zones of sarcomatous overgrowth also portends an unfavorable outcome.[128] Extended clinical observation is necessary because there is typically a long (3.5–5 years) interval between treatment and recurrence.[53,273] About a quarter of patients with adenosarcoma die of tumor, frequently more than 5 years after initial diagnosis.[54,128,273]

Mixed Müllerian Tumor (Carcinosarcoma)

The mixed müllerian tumor (MMT), or carcinosarcoma, is the most common uterine sarcoma.[149,222,266] It is nonetheless rare, constituting less than 1.5% of malignant tumors of the uterus. It is increasing in relative frequency,[78] and it is more common than leiomyosarcoma when stringent criteria are used for the diagnosis of the latter neoplasm.

CLINICAL FEATURES

Most women with MMT are postmenopausal, with a median age of about 65 years.[126,156,186,189,266] The most common symptom is postmenopausal bleeding.[46,202,226] Lower abdominal pain, abdominal distention, and a palpable abdominal mass also are frequent presenting complaints.[160] An enlarged irregular uterus and tumor protruding through the cervical os are common findings.[189,198] Extrauterine spread occurs early, and many patients complain of symptoms caused by gastrointestinal or urinary tract involvement. Few patients are asymptomatic at the time of diagnosis.

Infertility, hypertension, obesity, and diabetes occur in women with MMT, but the association with MMT is not as clear as it is with endometrial carcinoma.[78,156,181] Some women (8–30%) with MMT have a history of prior pelvic irradiation administered as treatment for endometrial bleeding from a benign condition or for invasive cervical cancer.° Norris and Taylor, for example, found 17 postradiation sarcomas in a review of 136 malignant mesenchymal tumors of the uterus, and 13 of the 17 were MMT.[187] The median latent period between pelvic irradiation and the discovery of the sarcoma is about 16 years.[62] Women with postirradiation MMT are younger than those with no radiation history.[187,262] The proportion of patients with a history of radiation is smaller in recent reports on MMT, as radiation is no longer used for benign conditions, and it is used less often to treat cervical cancer.

Curettage can be an effective means of establishing a diagnosis,[226,266] but in some cases the histologic findings are misleading. Curettings may contain only carcinoma or sarcoma, and the biphasic nature of the neoplasm may not become apparent until the entire tumor is studied. The

identification of a heterologous element often requires extensive sampling.

Cytologic studies usually do not play a significant role in the diagnosis of MMT. Most patients have symptoms that mandate curettage, and cytologic evaluation is performed during diagnostic evaluation rather than to detect a tumor in an asymptomatic patient. Malignant cells are identified in most patients,[10,61,126,156,163,250] but usually only malignant epithelial cells are seen,[226] or the malignant cells cannot be classified specifically as epithelial or mesenchymal.[61,78] Rarely, rhabdomyoblasts are identified. Malignant mesenchymal cells in a Pap smear suggest a diagnosis of MMT, as other sarcomas are less common and are rarely evident cytologically.

GROSS FINDINGS

MMT is a sessile or pedunculated polypoid neoplasm that grows into and usually fills the endometrial cavity (Fig. 13.39).[19,224,226] Many are so large that they protrude

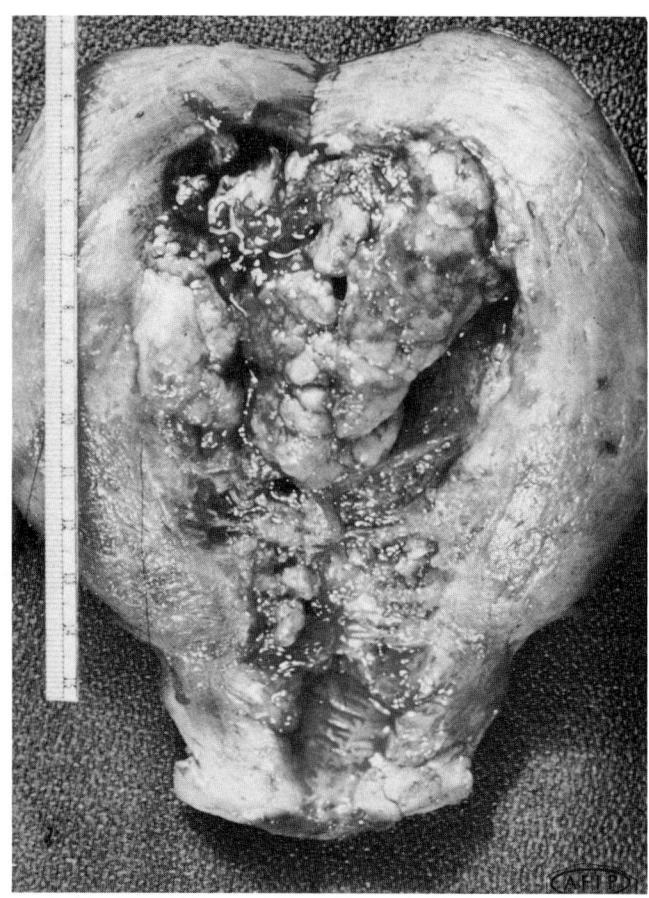

FIG. 13.39. MMT of endometrium. The tumor extends into the myometrium and cervix. (Reprinted by permission from The American College of Obstetricians and Gynecologists. (Obstetrics and Gynecology, 28:57, 1966.))

°Refs. 46,100,170,198,202,226,266.

through the external os. MMT may arise in the cervix, where it grows as a polypoid neoplasm similar to MMT of the endometrium.[1,174,231,270] MMT of the endometrium extends to the endocervix in about a quarter of cases.[231] MMT in the cervix therefore is more likely to represent extension from an endometrial tumor than a primary cervical neoplasm. MMT is soft to firm and has a tan cut surface with areas of hemorrhage and necrosis.[19,186] Gritty or hard areas may reflect the presence of bone or cartilage. Cartilaginous areas often have a translucent appearance. Myometrial invasion usually is apparent on gross examination.

MICROSCOPIC FINDINGS

MMT is composed of an intimate admixture of malignant epithelium and sarcomatous stroma, with the latter usually predominating (Fig. 13.40).[19,46,189] The epithelial component typically is an adenocarcinoma of endometrioid type, but undifferentiated, squamous, clear cell, mucinous, and

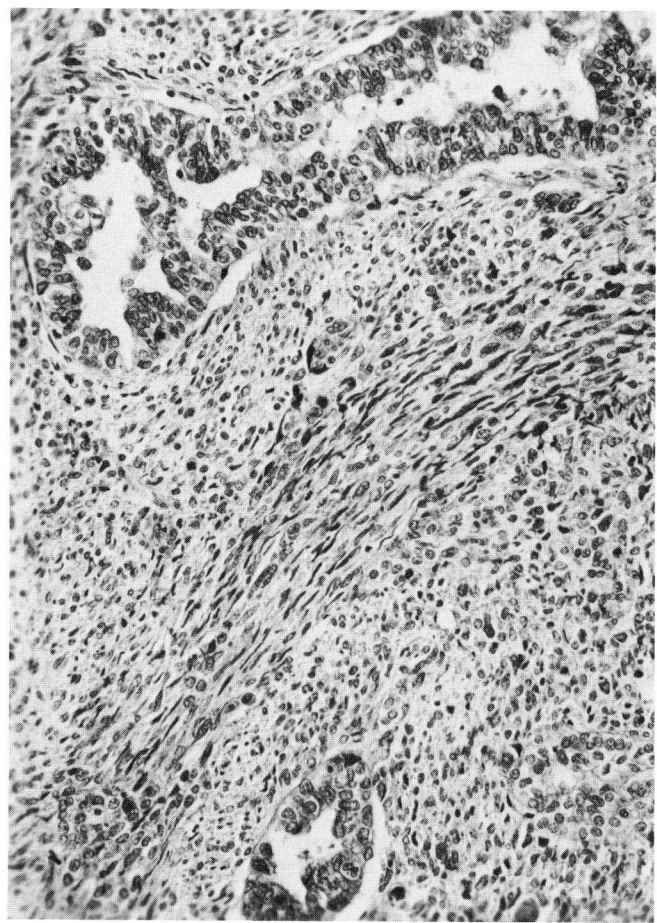

FIG. 13.40. Homologous MMT (carcinosarcoma). Malignant glands are admixed with a sarcomatous stroma.

serous carcinoma are all commonly observed.* Squamous carcinoma is relatively more common in MMT arising in the cervix.

The most common homologous mesenchymal components are endometrial stromal sarcoma and fibrosarcoma (Fig. 13.40).[231] The mesenchymal component of MMT is rarely pure leiomyosarcoma, but some MMTs contain a mixture of leiomyosarcoma, stromal sarcoma, and fibrosarcoma. Heterologous components are found in association with areas of undifferentiated sarcoma or stromal sarcoma. Rhabdomyosarcoma is the most common heterologous element.[19,78,181,231] Rhabdomyoblasts, usually occurring in clusters and associated with undifferentiated sarcoma cells, can be recognized with certainty by routine light microscopy when cytoplasmic cross-striations are identified. Round cells with atypical nuclei and variable amounts of granular or fibrillar acidophilic cytoplasm often are found in association with striated rhabdomyoblasts, and most pathologists regard them as sufficiently characteristic to allow a diagnosis of rhabdomyosarcoma. Immunohistochemical stains for muscle-specific actin, desmin, and myoglobin are useful in the identification of rhabdomyoblasts (see below, Immunohistochemistry). Cartilage is the second most common heterologous element in MMTs (Fig. 13.41).[137,156] Malignant osteoid and fat occasionally are present. Neuroendocrine differentiation, identified by light microscopy,[105,159] or immunohistochemistry,[104] occasionally is noted in MMT.

Rare MMTs are confined to a polyp,[20,127,231] and about a quarter of MMTs are limited to the endometrium. Most invade the myometrium to a variable depth. Capillary–lymphatic spaces within the myometrium commonly are invaded by MMT, usually by the epithelial component of the neoplasm.[27,231]

MMT metastasizes to the pelvic and para-aortic lymph nodes, the pelvic soft tissues, the vagina, the peritoneal surfaces of the upper abdominal cavity, and the lungs.[46,95,186] The histologic appearance of metastatic MMT is variable. Epithelial and mesenchymal components are both present in about a third of metastatic deposits, a third are composed of pure carcinoma, and a third are purely sarcomatous. Metastatic deposits that are evaluated early in the clinical evolution of the disease are likely to be mixed or pure carcinoma,[27,231] whereas combined or sarcomatous metastases are mainly detected late in the course of the disease.[46,95,186]

The histogenesis of MMT has been a source of controversy since it was first described. Many older theories of histogenesis have been discarded in favor of the idea that these tumors develop by neoplastic transformation of the least differentiated cells in the endometrium (primitive stromal cells).[103,104] The müllerian epithelium and mesen-

---

*Refs. 27,78,149,181,186,189,198,231.

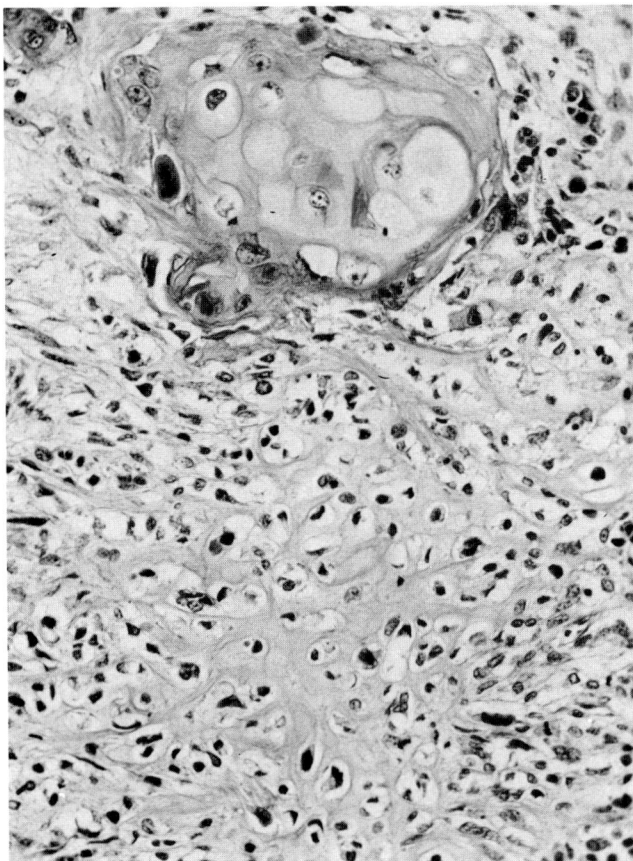

FIG. 13.41. Heterologous MMT. Cartilage (*center*) and squamous epithelium (*top*) are present. (Reprinted by permission from The American College of Obstetricians and Gynecologists. (Obstetrics and Gynecology, 28:57, 1966.))

chyme share a common embryologic background, so neoplastic stromal cells have the potential to differentiate into the rich variety of cell types found in the tumors in this group. The pattern of metastatic spread, the appearance of the metastatic deposits, and the immunophenotype of MMT suggest to others that these neoplasms originate from epithelial cells and that they are a type of metaplastic carcinoma.[27,104,231]

FLOW CYTOMETRY

Only a few MMTs have been analyzed by flow cytometry. Most are DNA aneuploid and have a high S-phase fraction.[158] Too few cases have been studied to determine the prognostic significance of flow cytometric results.

IMMUNOHISTOCHEMISTRY

The malignant epithelial component of MMT is strongly immunoreactive for cytokeratin and epithelial membrane antigen (EMA).[13,27,103,104,168,212] Immunohistochemical staining for cytokeratin and EMA highlights the epithelial component of an MMT (Fig. 13.42), and can be helpful in the diagnosis of MMT when the tumor is composed predominantely of mesenchymal elements. Epithelial cells exhibit variable immunoreactivity with vimentin in at least a third of MMTs.[103,104,168] There is generalized immunoreactivity for vimentin in the mesencymal component of most MMTs,[103,104,168] and occasional mesenchymal cells react with antibodies to muscle-specific actin and α-smooth muscle actin.[104,168] The mesenchymal components of MMT frequently exhibit patchy positive staining of variable intensity with antibodies to cytokeratin and EMA.[27,60,104,168] This staining invariably is less intense and less uniform than is observed in the epithelial component of the tumor. Immunoreactivity with cytokeratin or EMA is not proof of carcinoma unless an epithelial growth pattern also is present.[168] Epithelial antigen expression by the mesenchymal component suggests to some that the sarcomatous stroma develops via metaplasia of the carcinoma.[27,104]

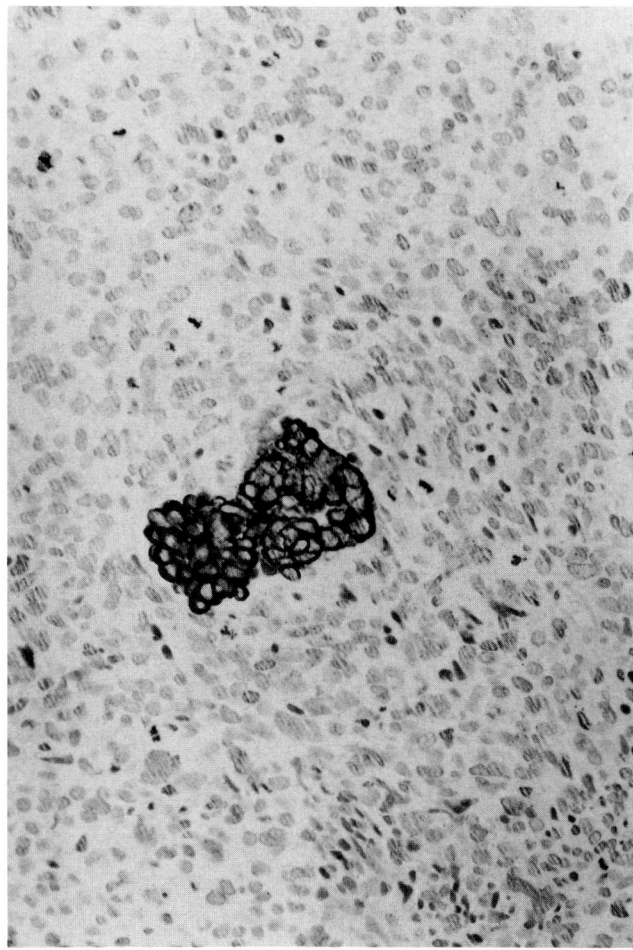

FIG. 13.42. MMT. An immunostain for cytokeratin highlights the epithelial component (*center*) and can be useful in identifying it when the stroma predominates.

Immunohistochemistry may be used to identify heterologous elements in MMT. Myoglobin is the most specific marker of rhabdomyoblastic differentiation,[13,104,177] but it is also the least sensitive.[13,104] In the proper light microscopic context immunoreactivity with desmin or muscle-specific actin also is indicative of rhabdomyosarcoma.[13,104] Areas of chondrosarcoma are reactive with antibodies to S-100 protein, but such areas are identified with equal accuracy by routine light microscopy.[13] Features of neuroendocrine differentiation, which may suggest an unfavorable prognosis, are detected by immunohistochemistry in 15–20% of MMTs (see Chapter 26, Immunohistochemistry).[104]

ULTRASTRUCTURE

The epithelial and mesenchymal compartments of MMT are separated by a basal lamina.[103] The epithelial cells grow in groups and are joined by desmosomes. Zonula occludens junctions are present apically and the surfaces of the cells are covered by short, stubby microvilli.[103,229] The cytoplasm contains glycogen, mitochondria, and an inconspicuous network of intermediate filaments. Prominent tonofilaments, frequently in a perinuclear location, are present in epithelial cells in some MMTs. The mesenchymal cells resemble fibroblasts or stromal cells.[103,229] They contain abundant rough endoplasmic reticulum and a variable number of intermediate filaments. Intercellular junctions are inconspicuous. Rhabdomyoblasts[29,103] and chondroid elements[229] develop from undifferentiated stromal cells. Partially differentiated rhabdomyoblasts contain conspicuous but nonspecific 100-Å filaments in their cytoplasm. Myofilaments are more numerous and better organized in more differentiated rhabdomyoblasts in which well-defined sarcomeric organization and Z bands are present. Cross-striations can be identified at the light microscopic level in only the most differentiated cells.

CLINICAL BEHAVIOR AND TREATMENT

MMTs that are confined to the uterus (stage I and II) are treated by total abdominal hysterectomy and bilateral salpingo-oophorectomy. Dissection of pelvic lymph nodes reveals metastatic tumor in 17% of cases that grossly appear confined to the uterus.[231] Women with stage I–II MMT often are treated with postoperative pelvic radiation, since, in some studies, women treated with combined therapy have less risk of pelvic recurrence.[82,198,223,235,266] The role of postoperative pelvic radiation is unsettled, however, since other studies fail to show a reduced risk of pelvic recurrence in women treated with combined therapy.[78,265] Pelvic irradiation does not affect overall survival because most patients die with distant metastases.[62,82,198,223] Women with early-stage MMT have a 5-year survival of 40–50%.[62,198,224,235,265]

When there is extrauterine tumor spread (stage III–IV) treatment generally is total abdominal hysterectomy, bilateral salpingo-oophorectomy, excision of extrauterine tumor, and postoperative pelvic irradiation. Women with advanced MMT have a 5-year survival rate of only 25–30%, even when treated with combined therapy.[224,235] Pelvic radiation reduces the risk of pelvic recurrence, but death results from metastatic spread beyond the irradiation field to the abdomen, lymph nodes, and lungs. The prognosis is so poor for patients with stage III and IV tumors that, in some instances, they are treated with radiation followed by chemotherapy.[198,235] Occasional patients are cured with this regimen, but survival rates are low.

A variety of pathologic features have been evaluated to learn whether they correlate with prognosis in MMT. The surgical–pathologic stage is the single most significant prognostic factor.[19,78,100,156,181,223,224] When tumor is confined to the uterus (stage I–II) the prognosis is significantly better than when there is extrauterine spread. Positive peritoneal cytology is associated with an unfavorable prognosis, and shows extrauterine spread.[106,130] Small MMTs confined to the tip of a polyp are reported to have a favorable prognosis,[20,78,127] but even when confined to a polyp MMTs can metastasize and cause the patient's death.[231] When tumor is confined to the uterus, some investigators find that large tumor size,[186,189,224] deep myometrial invasion,* extension to the cervix,[231] and capillary–lymphatic space invasion[156,224,231] are associated with increased risk of metastasis and a worse prognosis. Others question the significance of the depth of invasion[27,78,198] or capillary–lymphatic space invasion.[27,181] The presence of high-grade carcinoma or specific types of carcinoma (clear cell, serous) is associated with increased risk of metastasis in some reports,[100,231] whereas in others the appearance of the carcinoma does not correlate with the outcome.[181,224] The pathologic appearance of the sarcomatous mesenchymal component of MMT does not appear to have any bearing on the risk of metastasis or the survival rate.[231] Specifically, the nature of the mesenchymal elements (homologous vs. heterologous),[100,137,156,235,266] the presence or absence of specific heterologous elements (rhabdomyosarcoma or chondrosarcoma), the grade of the sarcomatous component,[149] and the number of mitotic figures in the sarcomatous component[46,149,181] do not correlate with the clinical behavior of the tumor.[231]

The poor survival of patients treated with surgery and radiotherapy, despite control of disease in the pelvis, indicates that occult metastases are present at the time of operation in many patients, even those whose neoplasms are stage I or II. The results obtained in several small studies raise the possibility of improved survival in patients

---

*Refs. 19,137,160,181,202,224,231,265.

with low-stage MMT treated with systemic adjuvant chemotherapy, especially using drug combinations that include cisplatin.[19,200,202] Previous studies using other drug combinations failed to demonstrate improved survival in patients treated with adjuvant chemotherapy.[80,193] Chemotherapy for advanced or recurrent MMT results in a complete or partial response in less than a quarter of patients.[200,239,252] MMT may contain estrogen and progesterone receptors.[148,233,240] Increased receptor levels seem to be associated with improved short-term survival, but women whose tumors are receptor-positive do not have improved long-term survival, nor do they respond to hormonal therapy.[233,240]

Miscellaneous Mesenchymal Tumors and Conditions

Adenomyosis and Adenomyoma

Adenomyosis is a common condition characterized pathologically by the presence of endometrial glands and stroma within the myometrium. Occurring mainly in perimenopausal women, it is detected in 15–20% of uteri. The usual symptoms are abnormal bleeding and dysmenorrhea.

The uterus is enlarged, and as adenomyosis usually is most extensive in the posterior wall, the latter is thickened. The cut surface of the myometrium is trabeculated and contains hemorrhagic foci, but a distinct tumor nodule is not present. Microscopically, there are endometrial glands and stroma within the myometrium (Fig. 13.43).

The lower border of the endometrium is irregular and dips into the superficial myometrium. To avoid misclassifying a normal histologic finding as adenomyosis, some pathologists make the diagnosis only when the distance between the lower border of the endometrium and the adenomyosis exceeds one-half of a low-power field (about 2.5 mm). Adenomyosis exhibits a varied functional response to ovarian hormones. Proliferative glands and stroma generally are observed in the first half of the menstrual cycle. Adenomyosis may not respond to physiologic levels of progesterone, and secretory changes frequently are absent or incomplete during the second half of the cycle.

An adenomyoma is a circumscribed, nodular aggregate of smooth muscle, endometrial glands, and, usually, endometrial stroma. It may be located within the myometrium or it may involve or originate in the endometrium and grow as a polyp. About 2% of endometrial polyps are adenomyomas.

A rare variant of the adenomyoma, the atypical polypoid adenomyoma, appears as an endometrial polyp in premenopausal women (see Chapter 10, Benign Diseases of the Endometrium).[72,77,164,213,271]

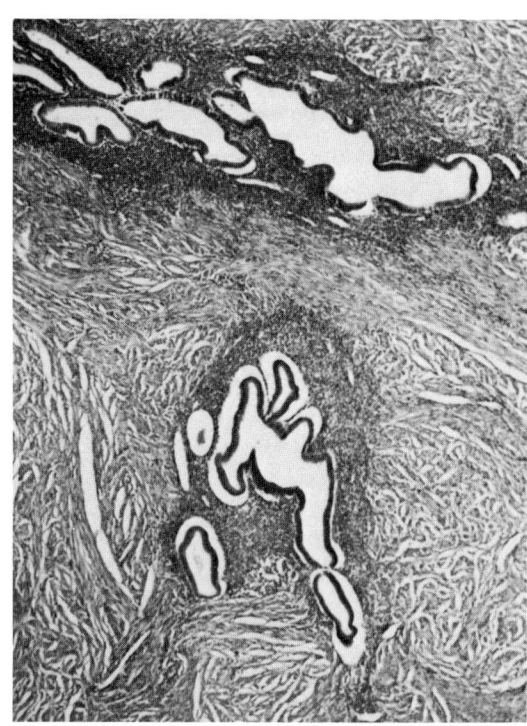

Fig. 13.43. Adenomyosis. Endometrial glands and stroma are present within the myometrium.

Adenomatoid Tumor

This is a distinctive neoplasm of the genital tract. An alternative name, *adenomatoid mesothelioma*, has gained acceptance as histochemical and ultrastructural evidence relating these neoplasms to mesothelium has accumlated.

CLINICAL FEATURES

Adenomatoid tumor usually is an incidental finding in a uterus removed for other causes. About 1% of uteri contain an adenomatoid tumor, but no specific symptoms are attributable to them.[44,161,209,253,272] Less than 10% are multiple. Women with adenomatoid tumor usually are of reproductive age, with a median age of 42 years. There is no known racial predilection or evidence of impairment of fertility. The tumor is benign.

PATHOLOGIC FINDINGS

Adenomatoid tumor typically measures 0.5–1 cm in diameter and is gray or tan, round, and rubbery, with ill-defined margins. Larger adenomatoid tumors occur, but they are rare.[26,71] Usually subserosal and located near the cornu, the adenomatoid tumor resembles a leiomyoma or adenomyoma. Small, uniform cystic spaces may be visible within the tumor.

Microscopically, adenomatoid tumor is composed of spaces lined by flat or cuboidal cells surrounded by a stroma rich in collagen, elastic tissue, and smooth muscle (Fig. 13.44A).[161,209,221,253,272] The smooth muscle fibers may be so prominent that the lesion appears at first glance to be a leiomyoma. Spaces lined by flattened cells resemble lymphatic vessels, reflecting the capacity of mesothelium to resemble endothelium. The cuboidal cells within the lesion often are arranged in cords and tubules. Abundant cytoplasm, round eccentric nuclei, and vacuolation of the cytoplasm may be prominent. The cells may have the appearance of signet cells, resulting in confusion with metastatic signet-ring cell carcinoma. Nuclear atypia, however, is absent or minimal, mitotic figures usually are infrequent, and mucin stains are negative. Adenomatoid tumor may resemble an angioma, but the spaces lack blood.

Histochemically, the cystic spaces in the tumor contain hyaluronic acid. Mucicarmine stains are negative. Immunocytochemical studies reveal that the tumor cells contain cytokeratin (Fig. 13.44B),[236,242] and electron microscopy reveals cells with basal nuclei, dilated intercellular spaces,

microvilli, and bundles of cytoplasmic filaments, all characteristics of mesothelial cells.[221,242]

Homologous and Heterologous Sarcoma

These neoplasms lack the malignant epithelium that is an essential component of MMT. Rare homologous sarcomas arise in the endometrium but differ from endometrial stromal sarcoma by virtue of greater pleomorphism and atypia and lack of clear resemblance to proliferative endometrial stroma.[85] *Rhabdomyosarcoma* is the most common pure heterologous sarcoma of the uterus,[66,117,205,227] but *chondrosarcoma*,[47,141] *osteosarcoma*,[64,75] *liposarcoma*,[17] and tumors containing mixtures of heterologous elements also occur.[260] Neoplasms resembling *malignant fibrous histiocytoma*[43] occur in the uterus, as do *malignant rhabdoid tumors*.[36,41] *Paraganglioma* has been described in the uterus.[21] Histologically benign heterotopic bone, cartilage, and fat occasionally are found in the uterus, and rare be-

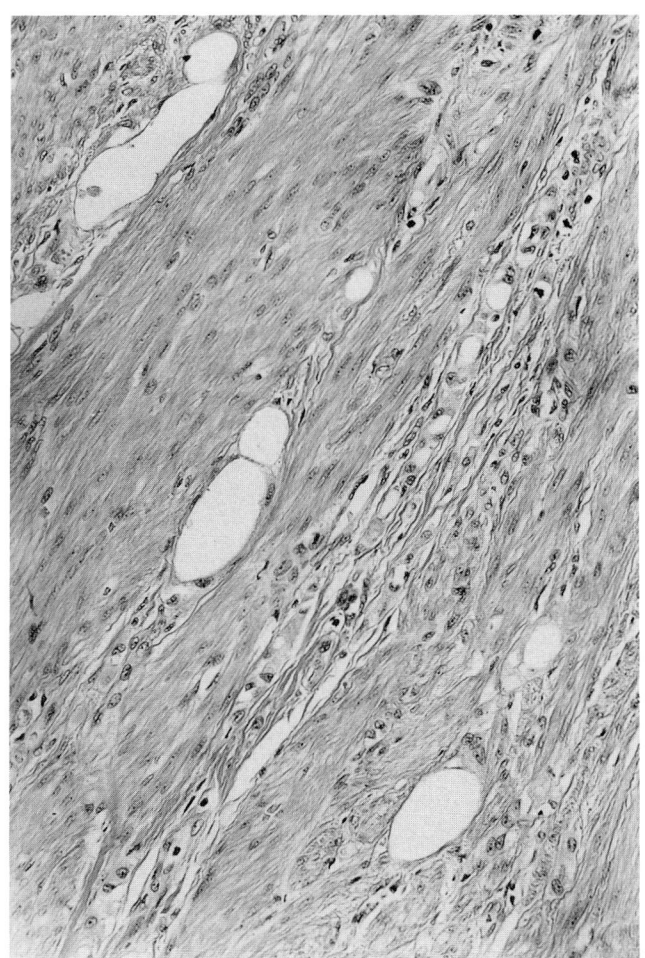

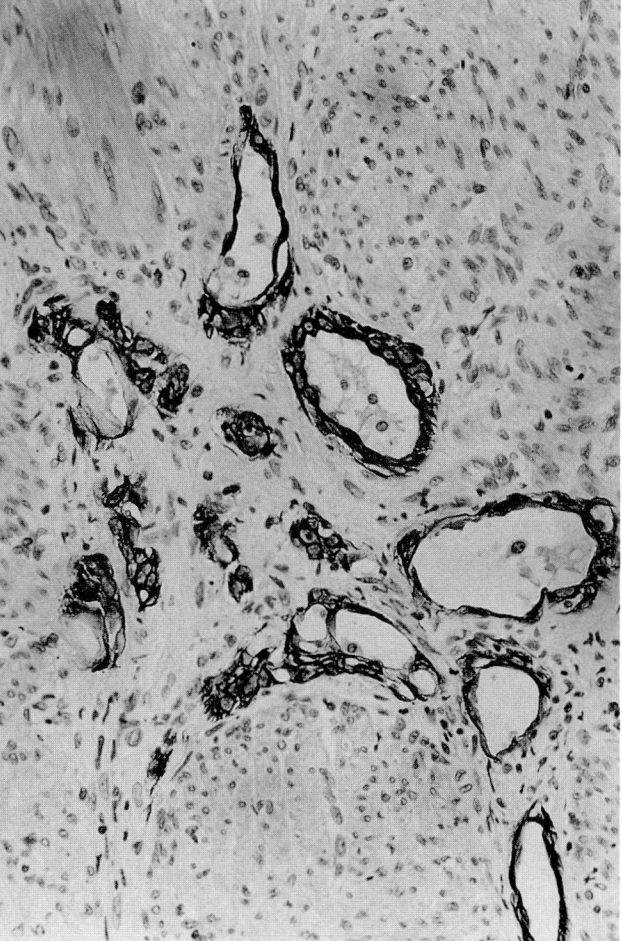

FIG. 13.44. **Adenomatoid tumor. a:** Mesothelial cells arranged in trabeculae, tubules, and microcysts are present among the smooth muscle bundles. **b:** An immunohistochemical stain for cytokeratin highlights the mesothelial component.

nign tumors contain one or more of these elements.[99] They should not be mistaken for a heterologous endometrial sarcoma or a component of a MMT.

Primitive Neuroectodermal Tumor

Rarely, a primitive neuroectodermal tumor (PNET) develops in the uterus.[69,119,175,214] PNET occurs in patients of all ages, but most arise in postmenopausal women. The usual clinical presentation is abnormal vaginal bleeding. The tumor is a soft, fleshy, gray or white polypoid mass that originates in the endometrium and invades the myometrium. Microscopically, PNET of the uterus is composed of small cells with round to oval hyperchromatic nuclei and scanty cytoplasm. Cellular areas merge with fibrillary foci of glial differentiation; ganglion cells may be present. Rosettes, Homer-Wright pseudorosettes, and perivascular ependymal-type rosettes often are noted in PNET. Immunostains for neuron-specific enolase (NSE) generally are positive.[69,175,214] Many PNET also are immunoreactive for other neural or endocrine markers, such as glial fibrillary acidic protein (GFAP), chromogranin, and S-100 protein.[69,214] Electron microscopic study reveals neural processes that contain filaments and microtubules[69,175,214] and, in some examples, neurosecretory granules.[69,119] Too few patients have been studied to define the behavior and most appropriate treatment. The outcome may be favorable in women with stage I neoplasms, but more advanced disease generally leads to death from tumor.[69] MMT may exhibit primitive neuroectodermal differentiation,[105] so a diagnosis of PNET of the uterus is inappropriate if a neoplasm exhibits features of MMT (malignant epithelial and mesenchymal elements).

Vascular Tumors

The most common vascular tumor of the uterus is the *capillary hemangioma* of the cervix. Diffuse ramifying *hemangiomas* of the corpus occur (Fig. 13.45), but are very rare.[9,155] Hemangiomas, which are composed of dilated vascular spaces lined by endothelial cells (Fig. 13.46), may extend through the myometrium and into the broad ligament. In these cases, curettage may lead to bleeding that is difficult to control except by a hysterectomy, which may be associated with marked blood loss. *Arteriovenous malformations* occasionally occur in the uterus, and have a clinical evolution similar to a hemangioma.[94] Rarely, an *angiosarcoma* arises in the uterus.[170,210,267] Composed of anastomosing vascular channels lined by atypical endothelial cells, it infiltrates the myometrium. Poorly differentiated angiosarcoma may contain areas composed of solid sheets of epithelioid cells difficult to recognize as being of vascular origin. Immunohistochemical stains for Factor VIII–related antigen or CD 34 may assist in the diagnosis.

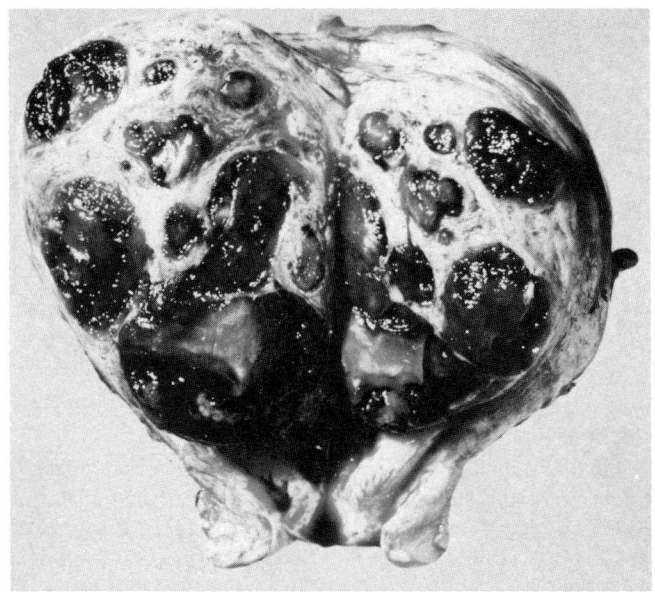

FIG. 13.45. Hemangioma of uterus.

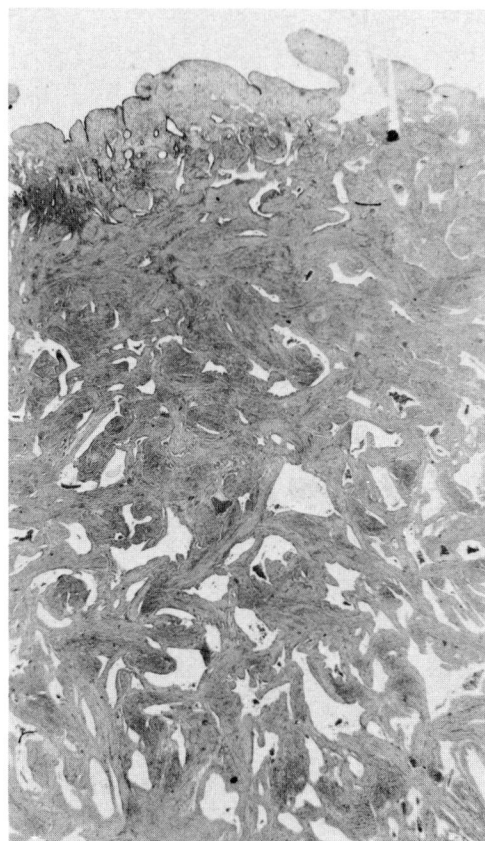

FIG. 13.46. Hemangioma. The tumor is composed of dilated vascular spaces extending throughout the myometrium.

The entity most often reported as *hemangiopericytoma* of the uterus is a misidentified endometrial stromal tumor. Few neoplasms reported as hemangiopericytoma of the uterus closely resemble hemangiopericytoma of the soft tissues. Nonetheless, there is no theoretical reason why a hemangiopericytoma should not occur in the uterus, and a few cases qualify on histologic and ultrastructural grounds.[178,232]

Lymphoma

Lymphoma rarely occurs with uterine involvement as the initial sign or symptom, but when it does, the cervix is the presenting site three times more often than is the endometrium. Lymphoma occurs predominantly in women aged 20 years or older. The major complaints are an abdominal or pelvic mass, abnormal vaginal bleeding, vaginal discharge, and pelvic discomfort. Lymphoma involving the uterus is staged by gynecologic staging criteria and also by a lymphoma-staging classification. The lymphoma usually is a diffuse large cell or a follicular small-cleaved lymphocytic type.[115] Hodgkin's disease rarely involves the uterus.[211] The prognosis of lymphoma presenting in the uterus is more favorable than that of lymphoma presenting in the ovary. An 89% survival rate is reported in patients with localized (Ann Arbor stage IE) lymphoma of the uterus and vagina.[115] The differential diagnosis includes a leiomyoma that contains a heavy lymphocytic infiltrate[93] and lymphoma-like lesions (pseudolymphoma). The latter mainly involve the cervical or endometrial surface, or are just beneath it, whereas lymphoma tends to be larger and more deeply positioned. *Pseudolymphoma* contains a heterogeneous population of lymphoid cells, in contrast to the more monomorphic population seen in most lymphomas, and it does not have the monoclonal immunophenotype that characterizes lymphoma. Uterine involvement as an initial manifestation of leukemia is even rarer than lymphoma at that site.[115,132,274]

References

1. Abdul-Karim FW, Bazi TM, Sorensen K, Nasr MF (1987) Sarcoma of the uterine cervix: clinicopathologic findings in three cases. Gynecol Oncol 26: 103–111
2. Abell MR (1971) Papillary adenofibroma of the uterine cervix. Am J Obstet Gynecol 110: 990–993
3. Abrams J, Talcott J, Corson JM (1989) Pulmonary metastases in patients with low-grade endometrial stromal sarcoma. Clinicopathologic findings with immunohistochemical characterization. Am J Surg Pathol 13: 133–140
4. Adamson GD (1992) Treatment of uterine fibroids: Current findings with gonadotropin-releasing hormone agonists. Am J Obstet Gynecol 166: 746–751
5. Agarwal PK, Husain N, Chandrawati (1991) Adenofibroma of uterus and endocervix. Histopathology 18: 79–80
6. Akhtar M, Kim PY, Young I (1975) Ultrastructure of endometrial stromal sarcoma. Cancer 35: 406–412
7. Akkersdijk GJ, Flu PK, Giard RW, van Lent M, Wallenburg HC (1990) Malignant leiomyomatosis peritonealis disseminata. Am J Obstet Gynecol 163: 591–593
8. Altaras M, Cohen I, Cordoba M, Aderet NB (1984) Papillary adenofibroma of the endometrium: case report and review of the literature. Gynecol Oncol 19: 216–221
9. Alvarez M, Cerezo L (1986) Ovarian cavernous hemangioma. Arch Pathol Lab Med 110: 77–78
10. An-Foraker SH, Kawada CY (1985) Cytodiagnosis of endometrial malignant mixed mesodermal tumor. Acta Cytol 29: 137–141
11. Andrade LALA, Derchain SFM, Vial JS, Alvarenga M (1992) Müllerian adenosarcoma of the uterus in adolescents. Int J Gynecol Obstet 38: 119–123
12. Aterman K, Fraser GM, Lea RH (1977) Disseminated peritoneal leiomyomatosis. Virchows Arch [A] 374: 13–26
13. Auerbach HE, Livolsi VA, Merino MJ (1988) Malignant mixed Müllerian tumors of the uterus. An immunohistochemical study. Int J Gynecol Pathol 7: 123–130
14. August CZ, Bauer KD, Lurain J, Murad T (1989) Neoplasms of endometrial stroma: histopathologic and flow cytometric analysis with clinical correlation. Hum Pathol 20: 232–237
15. Baker TR, Piver MS, Lele SB, Tsukada Y (1988) Stage I uterine adenosarcoma: a report of six cases. J Surg Oncol 37: 128–132
16. Baker VV, Walton LA, Fowler WC, Jr., Currie JL (1984) Steroid receptors in endolymphatic stromal myosis. Obstet Gynecol 63: 72s–74s
17. Bapat K, Brustein S (1989) Uterine sarcoma with liposarcomatous differentiation: report of a case and review of the literature. Int J Gynaecol Obstet 28: 71–75
18. Barter JF, Smith EB, Szpak CA, Hinshaw W, Clarke-Pearson DL, Creasman WT (1985) Leiomyosarcoma of the uterus: clinicopathologic study of 21 cases. Gynecol Oncol 21: 220–227
19. Barwick KW, Livolsi VA (1979) Malignant mixed müllerian tumors of the uterus. A clinicopathologic assessment of 34 cases. Am J Surg Pathol 3: 125–135
20. Barwick KW, Livolsi VA (1979) Heterologous mixed müllerian tumor confined to an endometrial polyp. Obstet Gynecol 53: 512–514
21. Beham A, Schmid C, Fletcher CDM, Auböck L, Pickel H (1992) Malignant paraganglioma of the uterus. Virchows Arch A Pathol Anat Hispathol 420: 453–457
22. Berchuck A, Rubin SC, Hoskins WJ, Saigo PE, Pierce VK, Lewis JL, Jr. (1988) Treatment of uterine leiomyosarcoma. Obstet Gynecol 71: 845–850
23. Berchuck A, Rubin SC, Hoskins WJ, Saigo PE, Pierce VK, Lewis JL, Jr. (1990) Treatment of endometrial stromal tumors. Gynecol Oncol 36: 60–65
24. Bibro MC, Livolsi VA, Schwartz PE (1979) Adenosarcoma of the uterus: ultrastructural observations. Am J Clin Pathol 71: 112–117
25. Binder SW, Nieberg RK, Cheng L, Al-Jitawi S (1991) Histologic and immunohistochemical analysis of nine endometrial stromal tumors: an unexpected high frequency of keratin protein positivity. Int J Gynecol Pathol 10: 191–197

26. Bisset DL, Morris JA, Fox H (1988) Giant cystic adeno-matoid tumour (mesothelioma) of the uterus. Histopathol-ogy 12: 555–558

27. Bitterman P, Chun B, Kurman RJ (1990) The significance of epithelial differentiation in mixed mesodermal tumors of the uterus. A clinicopathological and immunohis-tochemical study. Am J Surg Pathol 14: 317–328

28. Bocker W, Stegner HE (1975) A light and EM study of endometrial sarcomas of the uterus. Virchows Arch A Pathol Anat Hispathol 368: 141–156

29. Bocker W, Stegner HE (1975) Mixed müllerian tumors of the uterus. Ultrastructural studies on the differentiation of rhabdomyoblasts. Virchows Arch A Pathol Anat Hispathol 363: 337–349

30. Bocker W, Strecker H (1975) Electron microscopy of uter-ine leiomyosarcoma. Virchows Arch [A] 367: 59–71

31. Brescia RJ, Tazelaar HD, Hobbs J, Miller AW (1989) Intravascular lipoleiomyomatosis: a report of two cases. Hum Pathol 20: 252–256

32. Brooks JJ, Wells GB, Yeh I-T, Livolsi VA (1992) Bizarre epithelioid lipoleiomyoma of the uterus. Int J Gynecol Pathol 11: 144–149

33. Brown DC, Theaker JM, Banks PM, Gatter KC, Mason DY (1987) Cytokeratin expression in smooth muscle and smooth muscle tumours. Histopathology 11: 477–486

34. Burns B, Curry RH, Bell MEA (1979) Morphologic fea-tures of prognostic significance in uterine smooth muscle tumors: A review of 84 cases. Am J Obstet Gynecol 135: 109–114

35. Buscema J, Carpenter SE, Rosenshein NB, Woodruff JD (1986) Epithelioid leiomyosarcoma of the uterus. Cancer 57: 1192–1196

36. Cattani MG, Viale G, Santini D, Martinelli GN (1992) Malignant rhabdoid tumour of the uterus: An immunohis-tochemical and ultrastructural study. Virchows Arch A Pathol Anat Hispathol 420: 459–462

37. Chang KL, Crabtree GS, Lim-Tan SK, Kempson RL, Hendrickson MR (1990) Primary uterine endometrial stromal neoplasms. A clinicopathologic study of 117 cases. Am J Surg Pathol 14: 415–438

38. Chang V, Aikawa M, Druet R (1977) Uterine leiomyoblas-toma: ultrastructural and cytological studies. Cancer 39: 1563–1569

39. Chen KT (1984) Myxoid leiomyosarcoma of the uterus. Int J Gynecol Pathol 3: 389–392

40. Chen KT (1985) Rhabdomyosarcomatous uterine adeno-sarcoma. Int J Gynecol Pathol 4: 146–152

41. Cho KR, Rosenshein NB, Epstein JI (1989) Malignant rhabdoid tumor of the uterus. Int J Gynecol Pathol 8: 381–387

42. Cho KR, Woodruff JD, Epstein JI (1989) Leiomyoma of the uterus with multiple extrauterine smooth muscle tu-mors: a case report suggesting multifocal origin. Hum Pathol 20: 80–83

43. Chou ST, Fortune D, Beischer NA, McLeish G, Castles LA, McKelvie BA, Planner RS (1985) Primary malignant fibrous histiocytoma of the uterus—ultrastructural and immunocy-tochemical studies of two cases. Pathology 17: 36–40

44. Christensen C (1990) Adenomatoid tumors of the uterus. Eur J Gynaecol Oncol 11: 85–89

45. Christopherson WM, Williamson EO, Gray LA (1972) Leiomyosarcoma of the uterus. Cancer 29: 1512–1517

46. Chuang JT, VanVelden DJ, Graham JB (1970) Carcinosar-coma and mixed mesodermal tumor of the uterine corpus. Review of 49 cases. Obstet Gynecol 35: 769–780

47. Clement PB (1978) Chondrosarcoma of the uterus: report of a case and review of the literature. Hum Pathol 9: 726–732

48. Clement PB (1988) Intravenous leiomyomatosis of the uterus. Pathol Annu 23 Pt 2: 153–183

49. Clement PB (1989) Müllerian adenosarcomas of the uterus with sarcomatous overgrowth. A clinicopathological analysis of 10 cases. Am J Surg Pathol 13: 28–38

50. Clement PB, Scully RE (1974) Müllerian adenosarcoma of the uterus. A clinicopathologic analysis of ten cases of a distinctive type of müllerian mixed tumor. Cancer 34: 1138–1149

51. Clement PB, Scully RE (1976) Uterine tumors resembling ovarian sex-cord tumors. A clinicopathologic analysis of 14 cases. Am J Clin Pathol 66: 512–525

52. Clement PB, Scully RE (1978) Extrauterine mesodermal (Müllerian) adenosarcoma: a clinicopathologic analysis of five cases. Am J Clin Pathol 69: 276–283

53. Clement PB, Scully RE (1989) Müllerian adenosarcomas of the uterus with sex cord-like elements. A clinicopatho-logic analysis of eight cases. Am J Clin Pathol 91: 664–672

54. Clement PB, Scully RE (1990) Müllerian adenosarcoma of the uterus: a clinicopathologic analysis of 100 cases with a review of the literature. Hum Pathol 21: 363–381

55. Clement PB, Scully RE (1990) Müllerian adenofibroma of the uterus with invasion of myometrium and pelvic veins. Int J Gynecol Pathol 9: 363–371

56. Clement PB, Young RH (1987) Diffuse leiomyomatosis of the uterus: a report of four cases. Int J Gynecol Pathol 6: 322–330

57. Clement PB, Young RH, Scully RE (1988) Intravenous leiomyomatosis of the uterus. A clinicopathological analy-sis of 16 cases with unusual histologic features. Am J Surg Pathol 12: 932–945

58. Clement PB, Young RH, Scully RE (1992) Diffuse, peri-nodular, and other patterns of hydropic degeneration within and adjacent to uterine leiomyomas. Problems in differential diagnosis. Am J Surg Pathol 16: 26–32

59. Cooper MM, Guillem J, Dalton J, Marboe CC, Corwin S, Todd GJ, Rose EA (1992) Recurrent intravenous leiomyo-matosis with cardiac extension. Ann Thorac Surg 53: 139–141

60. Costa MJ, Khan R, Judd R (1991) Carcinosarcoma (malig-nant mixed müllerian [mesodermal] tumor) of the uterus and ovary. Correlation of clinical, pathologic, and immu-nohistochemical features in 29 cases. Arch Pathol Lab Med 115: 583–590

61. Costa MJ, Tidd C, Willis D (1992) Cervicovaginal cytology in carcinosarcoma [malignant mixed müllerian (mesoder-mal) tumor] of the uterus. Diagn Cytopathol 8: 33–40

62. Covens AL, Nisker JA, Chapman WB, Allen HH (1987) Uterine sarcoma: an analysis of 74 cases. Am J Obstet Gynecol 156: 370–374

63. Cramer SF, Patel A (1990) The frequency of uterine leio-myomas. Am J Clin Pathol 94: 435–438

64. Crum CP, Rogers BH, Anderson W (1980) Osteosarcoma

of the uterus: case report and review of the literature. Gynecol Oncol 9: 256–268

65. Czernobilsky B, Hohlweg-Majert P, Dallenbach-Hellweg G (1983) Uterine adenosarcoma: a clinicopathologic study of 11 cases with a reevaluation of histologic criteria. Arch Gynecol 233: 281–294

66. Dabbs DJ, Silverman JF, Geisinger KR (1989) Immunohistochemical study of uterine stromal sarcoma and rhabdomyosarcoma. Arch Pathol Lab Med 113: 1151–1154

67. Damjanov I, Casey MJ, Maenza RM, Kennedy AW (1978) Müllerian adenosarcoma of the uterus. Ultrastructure before and after adiation therapy. Am J Clin Pathol 70: 96–103

68. Darby AJ, Papadaki L, Beilby JOW (1975) An unusual leiomyosarcoma of the utrus containing osteoclast-like giant cells. Cancer 36: 495–504

69. Daya D, Lukka H, Clement PB (1992) Primitive neuroectodermal tumors of the uterus: A report of four cases. Hum Pathol 23: 1120–1129

70. De Fusco PA, Gaffey TA, Malkasian GD Jr., Long HJ, Cha SS (1989) Endometrial stromal sarcoma: review of Mayo Clinic experience, 1945–1980. Gynecol Oncol 35: 8–14

71. De Rosa G, Boscaino A, Terracciano LM, Giordano G (1992) Giant adenomatoid tumors of the uterus. Int J Gynecol Pathol 11: 156–160

72. Delprado WJ, Stevens SM, Baird PJ (1985) Atypical polypoid adenomyoma: a case report with ultrastructural examination. Pathology 17: 522–525

73. Demopoulos RI, Denarvaez F, Kaji V (1973) Benign mixed mesodermal tumors of the uterus: a histogenetic study. Am J Clin Pathol 60: 377–383

74. Devaney K, Tavassoli FA (1991) Immunohistochemistry as a diagnostic aid in the interpretation of unusual mesenchymal tumors of the uterus. Mod Pathol 4: 225–231

75. DeYoung B, Bitterman P, Lack EE (1992) Primary osteosarcoma of the uterus: report of a case with immunohistochemical study. Mod Pathol 5: 212–215

76. Dharkar DD, Kraft JR, Gangadharam D (1981) Uterine lipomas. Arch Pathol Lab Med 105: 43–45

77. Di Palma S, Santini D, Martinelli G (1989) Atypical polypoid adenomyoma of the uterus. An immunohistochemical study of a case. Tumori 75: 292–295

78. Dinh TV, Slavin RE, Bhagavan BS, Hannigan EV, Tiamson EM, Yandell RB (1989) Mixed müllerian tumors of the uterus: a clinicopathologic study. Obstet Gynecol 74: 388–392

79. Dryer L, Simson IW, Sevenster CB, Dittrich OC (1985) Leiomyomatosis peritonealis disseminata. A report of two cases and a review of the literature. Br J Obstet Gynaecol 92: 856–861

80. Due W, Pickartz H (1989) Immunohistologic detection of estrogen and progesterone receptors in disseminated peritoneal leiomyomatosis. Int J Gynecol Pathol 8: 46–53

81. Dunton CJ, Kelsten ML, Brooks SE, Viglione MJ, Carlson JA, Mikuta JJ (1990) Low-grade stromal sarcoma: DNA flow cytometric analysis and estrogen progesterone receptor data. Gynecol Oncol 37: 268–275

82. Echt G, Jepson J, Steel J, Langholz B, Luxton G, Hernandez W, Astrahan M, Petrovich Z (1990) Treatment of uterine sarcomas. Cancer 66: 35–39

83. el-Naggar AK, Abdul-Karim FW, Silva EG, McLemore D, Garnsey L (1991) Uterine stromal neoplasms: a clinicopathologic and DNA flow cytometric correlation. Hum Pathol 22: 897–903

84. Evans AT, III., Symmonds RE, Gaffey TA (1981) Recurrent pelvic intravenous leiomyomatosis. Obstet Gynecol 57: 260–264

85. Evans HL (1982) Endometrial stromal sarcoma and poorly differentiated endometrial sarcoma. Cancer 50: 2170–2182

86. Evans HL, Chawla SP, Simpson C, Finn KP (1988) Smooth muscle neoplasms of the uterus other than ordinary leiomyoma. A study of 46 cases, with emphasis on diagnostic criteria and prognostic factors. Cancer 62: 2239–2247

87. Eyden BP, Hale RJ, Richmond I, Buckley CH (1992) Cytoskeletal filaments in the smooth muscle cells of uterine leiomyomata and myometrium: An ultrastructural and immunohistochemical analysis. Virchows Arch A Pathol Anat Hispathol 420: 51–58

88. Farhood AI, Abrams J (1991) Immunohistochemistry of endometrial stromal sarcoma. Hum Pathol 22: 224–230

89. Fechner RE (1968) Atypical leiomyomas and synthetic progestogen therapy. Am J Clin Pathol 49: 697–703

90. Fekete PS, Vellios F (1984) The clinical and histologic spectrum of endometrial stromal neoplasms: a report of 41 cases. Int J Gynecol Pathol 3: 198–212

91. Fekete PS, Vellios F, Patterson BD (1985) Uterine tumor resembling an ovarian sex-cord tumor: report of a case of an endometrial stromal tumor with foam cells and ultrastructural evidence of epithelial differentiation. Int J Gynecol Pathol 4: 378–387

92. Ferenczy A, Richart RM, Okagaki T (1971) A comparative ultrastructural study of leiomyosarcoma, cellular leiomyoma, and leiomyoma of the uterus. Cancer 28: 1004–1018

93. Ferry JA, Harris NL, Scully RE (1989) Uterine leiomyomas with lymphoid infiltrtion simulating lymphoma: a report of seven cases. Int J Gynecol Pathol 8: 263–270

94. Fleming H, Ostor AG, Pickel H, Fortune DW (1989) Arteriovenous malformations of the uterus. Obstet Gynecol 73: 209–214

95. Fleming WP, Peters WA, Kumar NB, Morley GW (1984) Autopsy findings in patients with uterine sarcoma. Gynecol Oncol 19: 168–172

96. Fletcher JA, Morton CC, Pavelka K, Lage JM (1990) Chromosome aberrations in uterine smooth muscle tumors: potential diagnostic relevance of cytogenetic instability. Cancer Res 50: 4092–4097

97. Fox H, Harilal KR, Youell A (1979) Müllerian adenosarcoma of the uterine body: a report of nine cases. Histopathology 3: 167–180

98. Franquemont DW, Frierson HF, Jr., Mills SE (1991) An immunohistochemical study of normal endometrial stroma and endometrial stromal neoplasms. Evidence for smooth muscle differentiation. Am J Surg Pathol 15: 861–870

99. Fukuoka M, Fujii S, Konishi I, Mori T, Parmley TH, Woodruff JD (1987) Fibro-osteochondroma of the uterus. Obstet Gynecol 70: 517–521

100. Gagne E, Tetu B, Blondeau L, Raymond PE, Blais R (1989) Morphologic prognostic factors of malignant mixed

müllerian tumor of the uterus: a clinicopathologic study of 58 cases. Mod Pathol 2: 433–438

101. Gal AA, Brooks JJ, Pietra GG (1989) Leiomyomatous neoplasms of the lung: a clinical, histologic, and immunohistochemical study. Mod Pathol 2: 209–216

102. Gast MJ, Radkins LV, Jacobs AJ, Gersell D (1989) Müllerian adenosarcoma of the cervix with heterologous elements: diagnostic and therapeutic approach. Gynecol Oncol 32: 381–384

103. Geisinger KR, Dabbs DJ, Marshall RB (1987) Malignant mixed müllerian tumors. An ultrastructural and immunohistochemical analysis with histogenetic considerations. Cancer 59: 1781–1790

104. George E, Manivel JC, Dehner LP, Wick MR (1991) Malignant mixed müllerian tumors: an immunohistochemical study of 47 cases, with histogenetic considerations and clinical correlation. Hum Pathol 22: 215–223

105. Gersell DJ, Duncan DA, Fulling KH (1989) Malignant mixed müllerian tumor of the uterus with neuroectodermal differentiation. Int J Gynecol Pathol 8: 169–178

106. Geszler G, Szpak CA, Harris RE, Creasman WT, Barter JF, Johnston WW (1986) Prognostic value of peritoneal washings in patients with malignant mixed müllerian tumors of the uterus. Am J Obstet Gynecol 155: 83–89

107. Gisser SD, Young I (1977) Neurilemoma-like uterine myomas: an ultrastructural reaffirmation of their non-Schwannian nature. Am J Obstet Gynecol 129: 389–392

108. Gloor E (1979) Müllerian adenosarcoma of the uterus. Clinicopathologic report of five cases. Am J Surg Pathol 3: 203–209

109. Gloor E, Schnyder P, Cikes M, Hofstetter J, Cordey R, Burnier F, Knobel P (1982) Endolymphatic stromal myosis. Surgical and hormonal treatment of extensive abdominal recurrence 20 years after hysterectomy. Cancer 50: 1888–1893

110. Goldberg MF, Hurt WG, Frable WJ (1977) Leiomyomatosis peritonealis disseminata: report of a case and review of the literature. Obstet Gynecol 49: 46s–52s

111. Goodhue WM, Susin M, Kramer E (1974) Smooth muscle origin of uterine plexiform tumors: ultrastructural and histochemical evidence. Arch Pathol 97: 263–268

112. Gown AM, Boyd HC, Chang Y, Ferguson M, Reichler B, Tippens D (1988) Smooth muscle cells can express cytokeratins of "simple" epithelium. Immunocytochemical and biochemical studies in vitro and in vivo. Am J Pathol 132: 223–232

113. Grignon DJ, Carey MR, Kirk ME, Robinson ML (1987) Diffuse uterine leiomyomatosis: a case study with pregnancy complicated by intrapartum hemorrhage. Obstet Gynecol 69: 477–480

114. Hales HA, Peterson CM, Jones KP, Quinn JD (1992) Leiomyomatosis peritonealis disseminata treated with a gonadotropin-releasing hormone agonist. Am J Obstet Gynecol 167: 515–516

115. Harris NL, Scully RE (1984) Malignant lymphoma and granulocytic sarcoma of the uterus and vagina. A clinicopathologic analysis of 27 cases. Cancer 53: 2530–2545

116. Hart WR, Billman JK, Jr. (1978) A reassessment of uterine neoplasms originally diagnosed as leiomyosarcomas. Cancer 41: 1902–1910

117. Hart WR, Craig JR (1978) Rhabdomyosarcomas of the uterus. Am J Clin Pathol 70: 217–223

118. Hart WR, Yoonessi M (1977) Endometrial stromatosis of the uterus. Obstet Gynecol 49: 393–403

119. Hendrickson MR, Scheithauer BW (1986) Primitive neuroectodermal tumor of the endometrium: report of two cases, one with electron microscopic observations. Int J Gynecol Pathol 5: 249–259

120. Hirschfield L, Khan LB, Chen S, Winkler B, Rosenberg S (1986) Müllerian adenosarcoma with ovarian sex cord-like differentiation. A light- and electron-microscopic study. Cancer 57: 1197–1200

121. Hitchcock CL, Norris HJ (1992) Flow cytometric analysis of endometrial stromal sarcoma. Am J Clin Pathol 97: 267–271

122. Honore LH (1978) Uterine fibrolipoleiomyoma: report of a case with discussion of histogenesis. Am J Obstet Gynecol 132: 635–636

123. Hu J, Surti U (1991) Subgroups of uterine leiomyomas based on cytogenetic analysis. Hum Pathol 22: 1009–1016

124. Hyde KE, Geisinger KR, Marshall RB, Jones TL (1989) The clear-cell variant of uterine epithelioid leiomyoma. An immunohistologic and ultrastructural study. Arch Pathol Lab Med 113: 551–553

125. Ito H, Sasaki N, Miyagawa K, Tahara E (1986) Bizarre leiomyoblastoma of the cervix uteri. Immunohistochemical and ultrastructural study. Acta Pathol Jpn 36: 1737–1745

126. Kahanpää KV, Wahlström T, Gröhn P, Heinonen E, Nieminen U, Widholm O (1986) Sarcomas of the uterus: a clinicopathologic study of 119 patients. Obstet Gynecol 67: 417–424

127. Kahner S, Ferenczy A, Richart RM (1975) Homologous mixed müllerian tumors (carcinosarcoma) confined to endometrial polyps. Am J Obstet Gynecol 121: 278–279

128. Kaku T, Silverberg SG, Major FJ, Miller A, Fetter B, Brady MF (1992) Adenosarcoma of the uterus: A Gynecologic Oncology Group clinicopathologic study of 31 cases. Int J Gynecol Pathol 11: 75–88

129. Kaminski PF, Tavassoli FA (1984) Plexiform tumorlet: a clinical and pathologic study of 15 cases with ultrastructural observations. Int J Gynecol Pathol 3: 124–134

130. Kanbour AI, Buchsbaum HJ, Hall A (1989) Peritoneal cytology in malignant mixed müllerian tumors of the uterus. Gynecol Oncol 33: 91–95

131. Kao GF, Norris HJ (1978) Benign and low grade variants of mixed mesodermal tumor (adenosarcoma) of the ovary and adnexal region. Cancer 42: 1314–1324

132. Kapadia SB, Krause JR, Kanbour AI, Hartsock RJ (1978) Granulocytic sarcoma of the uterus. Cancer 41: 687–691

133. Katz L, Merino MJ, Sakamoto H, Schwartz PE (1987) Endometrial stromal sarcoma: a clinicopathologic study of 11 cases with determination of estrogen and progestin receptor levels in three tumors. Gynecol Oncol 26: 87–97

134. Katzenstein AL, Askin FB, Feldman PS (1977) Müllerian adenosarcoma of the uterus: an ultrastructural study of four cases. Cancer 40: 2233–2242

135. Kawaguchi K, Fujii S, Konishi I, Nanbu Y, Nonogaki H, Mori T (1989) Mitotic activity in uterine leiomyomas during the menstrual cycle. Am J Obstet Gynecol 160: 637–641

136. Keen CE, Philip G (1989) Progestogen-induced regression in low-grade endometrial stromal sarcoma. Case report and literature review. Br J Obstet Gynaecol 96: 1435–1439

137. Kempson RL, Bari W (1970) Uterine sarcomas. Classification, diagnosis, and prognosis. Hum Pathol 1: 331–349

138. Kempson RL, Hendrickson MR (1988) Pure mesenchymal neoplasms of the uterine corpus: selected problems. Semin Diagn Pathol 5: 172–198

139. Kiechle-Schwarz M, Sreekantaiah C, Berger CS, Pedron S, Medchill MT, Surti U, Sandberg AA (1991) Nonrandom cytogenetic changes in leiomyomas of the female genital tract. A report of 35 cases. Cancer Genet Cytogenet 53: 125–136

140. King ME, Dickersin GR, Scully RE (1982) Myxoid leiomyosarcoma of the uterus: a report of six cases. Am J Surg Pathol 6: 589–598

141. Kofinas AD, Suarez J, Calame RJ, Chipeco Z (1984) Chondrosarcoma of the uterus. Gynecol Oncol 19: 231–237

142. Komorowski RA, Garancis JC, Clowry LJ, Jr. (1970) Fine structure of endometrial stromal sarcoma. Cancer 26: 1042–1047

143. Kurman RJ, Norris HJ (1976) Mesenchymal tumors of the uterus. VI. Epithelioid smooth muscle tumors including leiomyoblastoma and clear cell leiomyoma: a clinical and pathological analysis of 26 cases. Cancer 36: 1853–1865

144. Lack EE, Bitterman P, Sundeen JT (1991) Müllerian adenosarcoma of the uterus with pure angiosarcoma: case report. Hum Pathol 22: 1289–1291

145. Lai FM, Wong FW, Allen PW (1991) Diffuse uterine leiomyomatosis with hemorrhage. Arch Pathol Lab Med 115: 834–837

146. Langlois PL (1970) The size of the normal uterus. J Reprod Med 4: 220–228

147. Lantta M, Kahanpää K, Karkkainen J, Lehtovirta P, Wahlström T, Widholm O (1984) Estradiol and progesterone receptors in two cases of endometrial stromal sarcoma. Gynecol Oncol 18: 233–239

148. Lantta M, Karkkainen J, Wahlström T, Widholm O (1984) Estradiol and progesterone receptors in gynecologic sarcomas. Acta Obstet Gynecol Scand 63: 505–508

149. Larson B, Silfversward C, Nilsson B, Pettersson F (1990) Mixed müllerian tumors of the uterus—prognostic factors: a clinical and histopathologic study of 147 cases. Radiother Oncol 17: 123–132

150. Larson B, Silfversward C, Nilsson B, Pettersson F (1990) Prognostic factors in uterine leiomyosarcoma. A clinical and histopathological study of 143 cases. The Radiumhemmet series 1936–1981. Acta Oncol 29: 185–191

151. Larson B, Silfversward C, Nilsson B, Pettersson F (1990) Endometrial stromal sarcoma of the uterus. A clinical and histopathological study. The Radiumhemmet series 1936–1981. Eur J Obstet Gynecol Reprod Biol 35: 239–249

152. Lavin P, Hajdu SI, Foote FW (1972) Gastric and extragastric leiomyoblastomas. Cancer 29: 305–311

153. Leibsohn S, d'Ablaing G, Mischell DR, Jr., Schlaerth JB (1990) Leiomyosarcoma in a series of hysterectomies performed for presumed uterine leiomyomas. Am J Obstet Gynecol 162: 968–974

154. Lillemoe TJ, Perrone T, Norris HJ, Dehner LP (1991) Myogenous phenotype of epithelial-like areas in endometrial stromal sarcomas. Arch Pathol Lab Med 115: 215–219

155. Lotgering FK, Pijpers L, van Eijck J, Wallenburg HC (1989) Pregnancy in a patient with diffuse cavernous hemangioma of the uterus. Am J Obstet Gynecol 160: 628–630

156. Macasaet MA, Waxman M, Fruchter RG, Boyce J, Hong P, Nicastri AD, Remy JC (1985) Prognostic factors in malignant mesodermal (müllerian) mixed tumors of the uterus. Gynecol Oncol 20: 32–42

157. Malfetano JH, Hussain M (1989) A uterine tumor that resembled ovarian sex-cord tumors: a low-grade sarcoma. Obstet Gynecol 74: 489–491

158. Malmström H, Schmidt H, Persson PG, Carstenen J, Nordenskjöld B, Simonsen E (1992) Flow cytometric analysis of uterine sarcoma: ploidy and S-phase rate as prognostic indicators. Gynecol Oncol 44: 172–177

159. Manivel C, Wick MR, Sibley RK (1986) Neuroendocrine differentiation in müllerian neoplasms. An immunohistochemical study of a "pure" endometrial small-cell carcinoma and a mixed müllerian tumor containing small-cell carcinoma. Am J Clin Pathol 86: 438–443

160. Marchese MJ, Liskow AS, Crum CP, McCaffrey RM, Frick HC (1984) Uterine sarcomas: a clinicopathologic study, 1965–1981. Gynecol Oncol 18: 299–312

161. Marcussen N, Donna A (1988) Adenomatoid tumour of the uterus. Histopathology 13: 582–583

162. Marshall RJ, Braye SG, Jones DB (1986) Leiomyosarcoma of the uterus with giant cells resembling osteoclasts. Int J Gynecol Pathol 5: 260–268

163. Massoni EA, Hajdu SI (1984) Cytology of primary and metastatic uterine sarcomas. Acta Cytol 28: 93–100

164. Mazur MT (1981) Atypical polypoid adenomyomas of the endometrium. Am J Surg Pathol 5: 473–482

165. Mazur MT, Askin FB (1978) Endolymphatic stromal myosis: unique presentation and ultrastructural study. Cancer 42: 2661–2667

166. Mazur MT, Kraus FT (1980) Histogenesis of morphologic variations in tumors of the uterine wall. Am J Surg Pathol 4: 59–74

167. Mazur MT, Priest JB (1986) Clear cell leiomyoma (leiomyoblastoma) of the uterus: ultrastructural observations. Ultrastruct Pathol 10: 249–255

168. Meis JM, Lawrence WD (1990) The immunohistochemical profile of malignant mixed müllerian tumor. Overlap with endometrial adenocarcinoma. Am J Clin Pathol 94: 1–7

169. Meloni AM, Surti U, Contento AM, Davare J, Sandberg AA (1992) Uterine leiomyomas: Cytogenetic and histologic profile. Obstet Gynecol 80: 209–217

170. Meredith RF, Eisert DR, Kaka Z, Hodgson SE, Johnston GA, Boutselis JG (1986) An excess of uterine sarcomas after pelvic irradiation. Cancer 58: 2003–2007

171. Miles PA, Mena H, Ashbaugh PH, Low N (1983) Low grade endometrial stromal sarcoma: report of a case with ultrastructural study. Mil Med 148: 867–868

172. Milne DS, Hinshaw K, Malcolm AJ, Hilton P (1990) Primary angiosarcoma of the uterus: a case report. Histopathology 16: 203–205

173. Minassian SS, Frangipane W, Polin JI, Ellis M (1986) Leiomyomatosis peritonealis disseminata. A case report and literature review. J Reprod Med 31: 997–1000

174. Miyazawa K, Hernandez E (1986) Cervical carcinosarcoma: a case report. Gynecol Oncol 23: 376–380

175. Molyneux AJ, Deen S, Sundaresan V (1992) Primitive neuroectodermal tumour of the uterus. Histopathology 21: 584–585

176. Morimoto N, Ozawa M, Kato Y, Kuramoto H (1982) Diagnostic value of mitotic activity in endometrial stromal sarcoma: report of two cases. Acta Cytol 26: 695–704

177. Mukai K, Varela-Duran J, Nochomovitz LE (1980) The rhabdomyoblast in mixed Müllerian tumors of the uterus and ovary. An immunohistochemical study of myoglobin in 25 cases. Am J Clin Pathol 74: 101–104

178. Munoz AK, Berek JS, Fu YS, Heintz PA (1990) Pelvic hemangiopericytomas: a report of five cases and literature review. Gynecol Oncol 36: 380–382

179. Myles JL, Hart WR (1985) Apoplectic leiomyomas of the uterus. A clinicopathologic study of five distinctive hemorrhagic leiomyomas associated with oral contraceptive usage. Am J Surg Pathol 9: 798–805

180. Nibert M, Heim S (1990) Uterine leiomyoma cytogenetics. Genes Chromosom Cancer 2: 3–13

181. Nielsen SN, Podratz KC, Scheithauer BW, O'Brien PC (1989) Clinicopathologic analysis of uterine malignant mixed müllerian tumors. Gynecol Oncol 34: 372–378

182. Nogales FF, Matilla A, Carrascal E (1978) Leiomyomatosis peritonealis disseminata: an ultrastructural study. Am J Clin Pathol 699: 452–457

183. Nogales FF, Navarro N, Martinez de Victoria JM, Contreras F, Redondo C, Herraiz MA, Seco MA, Velasco A (1987) Uterine intravascular leiomyomatosis: an update and report of seven cases. Int J Gynecol Pathol 6: 331–339

184. Norris HJ, Hilliard GD, Irey NS (1988) Hemorrhagic cellular leiomyomas ("apoplectic leiomyoma") of the uterus associated with pregnancy and oral contraceptives. Int J Gynecol Pathol 7: 212–224

185. Norris HJ, Parmley T (1975) Mesenchymal tumors of the uterus. V. Intravenous leiomyomatosis. A clinical and pathologic study of 14 cases. Cancer 36: 2164–2178

186. Norris HJ, Roth E, Taylor HB (1966) Mesenchymal tumors of the uterus. II. A clinical and pathologic study of 31 mixed mesodermal tumors. Obstet Gynecol 28: 57–63

187. Norris HJ, Taylor HB (1965) Post-irradiation sarcomas of the uterus. Obstet Gynecol 26: 689–694

188. Norris HJ, Taylor HB (1966) Mesenchymal tumors of the uterus. I. A clinical and pathologic study of 53 endometrial stromal tumors. Cancer 19: 755–766

189. Norris HJ, Taylor HB (1966) Mesenchymal tumors of the uterus. III. A clinical and pathologic study of 31 carcinosarcomas. Cancer 19: 1459–1465

190. Nunez-Alonso C, Battifora HA (1979) Plexiform tumors of the uterus: ultrastructural study. Cancer 44: 1707–1714

191. O'Connor DM, Norris HJ (1990) Mitotically active leiomyomas of the uterus. Hum Pathol 21: 223–227

192. Okagaki T, Brooker DC, Adcock LL, Prem KA (1979) Müllerian adenosarcoma of the uterus with rapid progression: an ultrastructural study. Gynecol Oncol 7: 361–370

193. Omura GA, Blessing JA, Major F, Lifshitz S, Ehrlich CE, Mangan C, Beecham J, Park R, Silverberg SG (1985) A randomized clinical trial of adjuvant adriamycin in uterine sarcomas: a Gynecologic Oncology Group study. J Clin Oncol 3: 1240–1245

194. Orenstein HH, Richart RM, Fenoglio CM (1980) Müllerian adenosarcoma of the uterus: literature review, case report, and ultrastructural observations. Ultrasruct Pathol 1: 189–200

195. Ostor AG, Fortune DW (1980) Benign and low grade variants of mixed müllerian tumour of the uterus. Histopathology 4: 369–382

196. Pandis N, Heim S, Bardi G, Floderus U-M, Willen H, Mandahl N, Mitelman F (1991) Chromosome analysis of 96 uterine leiomyomas. Cancer Genet Cytogenet 55: 11–18

197. Peacock G, Archer S (1989) Myxoid leiomyosarcoma of the uterus: case report and review of the literature. Am J Obstet Gynecol 160: 1515–1518

198. Perez CA, Askin F, Baglan RJ, Kao MS, Kraus FT, Perez BM, Williams CF, Weiss D (1979) Effects of irradiation on mixed müllerian tumors of the uterus. Cancer 43: 1274–1284

199. Perrone T, Dehner LP (1988) Prognostically favorable "mitotically active" smooth-muscle tumors of the uterus. A clinicopathologic study of ten cases. Am J Surg Pathol 12: 1–8

200. Peters WA, Rivkin SE, Smith MR, Tesh DE (1989) Cisplatin and adriamycin combination chemotherapy for uterine stromal sarcomas and mixed mesodermal tumors. Gynecol Oncol 34: 323–327

201. Peters WA, III, Howard DR, Andersen WA, Figge DC (1992) Deoxyribonucleic acid analysis by flow cytometry of uterine leiomyosarcomas and smooth muscle tumors of uncertain malignant potential. Am J Obstet Gynecol 166: 1646–1654

202. Peters WA, III, Kumar NB, Fleming WP, Morley GW (1984) Prognostic features of sarcomas and mixed tumors of the endometrium. Obstet Gynecol 63: 550–556

203. Pieslor PC, Orenstein JM, Hogan DL, Breslow A (1979) Ultrastructure of myofibroblasts and decidualized cells in leiomyomatosis peritonealis disseminata. Am J Clin Pathol 72: 875–882

204. Piver MS, Rutledge FN, Copeland L, Webster K, Blumenson L, Suh O (1984) Uterine endolymphatic stromal myosis: a collaborative study. Obstet Gynecol 64: 173–178

205. Podczaski E, Sees J, Kaminski P, Sorosky J, Larson JE, DeGeest K, Zaino RJ, Mortel R (1990) Rhabdomyosarcoma of the uterus in a postmenopausal patient. Gynecol Oncol 37: 439–442

206. Pounder DJ (1982) Fatty tumors of the uterus. J Clin Pathol 35: 1380–1383

207. Prakash S, Scully RE (1964) Sarcoma-like pseudopregnancy changes in uterine leiomyomas. Report of a case resulting from prolonged norethindrone therapy. Obstet Gynecol 24: 106–110

208. Prayson RA, Hart WR (1992) Mitotically active leiomyomas of the uterus. Am J Clin Pathol 97: 14–20

209. Quigley JC, Hart WR (1981) Adenomatoid tumors of the uterus. Am J Clin Pathol 76: 627–635

210. Quinonez GE, Paraskevas MP, Diocee MS, Lorimer SM (1991) Angiosarcoma of the uterus: a case report. Am J Obstet Gynecol 164: 90–92

211. Raggio ML, Bostrom SG, Harden EA (1988) Hodgkin's lymphoma of the uterus presenting as refractory pelvic inflammatory disease. A case report. J Reprod Med 33: 827–830

212. Ramadan M, Goudie RB (1986) Epithelial antigens in malignant mixed müllerian tumours of endometrium. J Pathol 148: 13–18

213. Rollason TP, Redman CW (1988) Atypical polypoid adenomyoma—clinical, histological, and immunocytochemical findings. Eur J Gynaecol Oncol 9: 444–451

214. Rose PG, O'Toole RV, Keyhani-Rofagha S, Qualman S, Boutselis JG (1987) Malignant peripheral primitive neuroectodermal tumor of the uterus. J Surg Oncol 35: 165–169

215. Roth LM, Pride GL, Sharma HM (1976) Müllerian adenosarcoma of the uterine cervix with heterologous elements. A light and electron microscopic study. Cancer 37: 1725–1736

216. Rotter AJ, Lundell CJ (1991) MR of intravenous leiomyomatosis of the uterus extending into the inferior vena cava. J Comput Assist Tomogr 15: 690–693

217. Rubin SC, Wheeler JE, Mikuta JJ (1986) Malignant leiomyomatosis peritonealis disseminata. Obstet Gynecol 68: 126–130

218. Rywlin AM, Recher L, Benson J (1964) Clear-cell leiomyoma of the uterus: report of two cases of a previously undescribed entity. Cancer 17: 100–104

219. Sabini G, Chumas JC, Mann WJ (1992) Steroid hormone receptors in endometrial stromal sarcomas. A biochemical and immunohistochemical study. Am J Clin Pathol 97: 381–386

220. Saksela E, Lampinen V, Precope BJ (1974) Malignant mesenchymal tumors of the uterine corpus. Am J Obstet Gynecol 120: 452–460

221. Salazar H, Kanbour A, Burgess F (1972) Ultrastructure and observations on the histogenesis of mesotheliomas, "adenomatoid tumors", of the female genital tract. Cancer 29: 141–152

222. Salazar OM, Bonfiglio TA, Patten SF, Keller BE, Feldstein M, Dunne ME, Rudolph J (1978) Uterine sarcomas: natural history, treatment and prognosis. Cancer 42: 1152–1160

223. Salazar OM, Bonfiglio TA, Patten SF, Keller BE, Feldstein ML, Dunne ME, Rudolph JH (1978) Uterine sarcomas: analysis of failures with special emphasis on the use of adjuvant radiation therapy. Cancer 42: 1161–1170

224. Schweizer W, Demopoulos R, Beller U, Dubin N (1990) Prognostic factors for malignant mixed müllerian tumors of the uterus. Int J Gynecol Pathol 9: 129–136

225. Seltzer VL, Levine A, Spiegal G, Rosenfeld D, Coffey EL (1990) Adenofibroma of the uterus: multiple recurrences following wide local excision. Gynecol Oncol 37: 427–431

226. Shaw RW, Lynch PF, Wade-Evans T (1983) Müllerian mixed tumour of the uterine corpus: a clinical and histopathological review of 28 patients. Br J Obstet Gynaecol 90: 562–569

227. Siegal GP, Taylor LL, III, Nelson KG, Reddick RL, Frazelle M, Siegfried JM, Walton LA, Kaufman DG (1983) Characterization of a pure heterologous sarcoma of the uterus: rhabdomyosarcoma of the corpus. Int J Gynecol Pathol 2: 303–315

228. Sieinski W (1989) Lipomatous neometaplasia of the uterus. Report of 11 cases with discussion of histogenesis and pathogenesis. Int J Gynecol Pathol 8: 357–363

229. Silverberg SG (1971) Malignant mixed mesodermal tumor of the uterus: an ultrastructural study. Am J Obstet Gynecol 110: 702–712

230. Silverberg SG, Kurman RJ (1992) Tumors of the uterine corpus and gestational trophoblastic disease. Armed Forces Institute of Pathology, Washington, D.C.

231. Silverberg SG, Major FJ, Blessing JA, Fetter B, Askin FB, Liao SY, Miller A (1990) Carcinosarcoma (malignant mixed mesodermal tumor) of the uterus. A Gynecological Oncology Group pathologic study of 203 cases. Int J Gynecol Pathol 9: 1–19

232. Silverberg SG, Willson MA, Board JA (1971) Hemangiopericytoma of the uterus: an ultrastructural study. Am J Obstet Gynecol 110: 397–404

233. Soper JT, McCarty KS, Jr., Hinshaw W, Creasman WT, McCarty KS, Sr., Clarke-Pearson DL (1984) Cytoplasmic estrogen and progesterone receptor content of uterine sarcomas. Am J Obstet Gynecol 150: 342–348

234. Soules MR, McCarty KS, Jr. (1982) Leiomyoma: steroid receptor content. Variation within normal menstrual cycles. Am J Obstet Gynecol 143: 6–11

235. Spanos WJ, Jr., Wharton JT, Gomez L, Fletcher GH, Oswald MJ (1984) Malignant mixed müllerian tumors of the uterus. Cancer 53: 311–316

236. Stephenson TJ, Mills PM (1986) Adenomatoid tumours: an immunohistochemical and ultrastructural appraisal of their histogenesis. J Pathol 148: 327–335

237. Stovall TG, Ling FW, Henry LC, Woodruff MR (1991) A randomized trial evaluating leuprolide acetate before hysterectomy as treatment for leiomyomas. Am J Obstet Gynecol 164: 1420–1423

238. Suginami H, Kaura R, Ochi H, Matsuura S (1990) Intravenous leiomyomatosis with cardiac extension: successful surgical management and histopathologic study. Obstet Gynecol 76: 527–529

239. Sutton G, Blessing JA, Rosenshein N, Photopulos G, DiSaia PJ (1989) Phase II trial of ifosamide and mesna in mixed mesodermal tumors of the uterus (a Gynecologic Oncology Group study). Am J Obstet Gynecol 161: 309–312

240. Sutton GP, Stehman FB, Michael H, Young PC, Ehrlich CE (1986) Estrogen and progesterone receptors in uterine sarcomas. Obstet Gynecol 68: 709–714

241. Suzuki M, Aizawa S, Ushigome S (1989) Endometrial stromal sarcoma of low-grade malignancy. Immunohistochemical and three-dimensional reconstruction study with special emphasis on the inadequate terminology of endolymphatic stromal myosis. Acta Pathol Jpn 39: 260–265

242. Suzuki T, Yoshida Y, Kaku T, Kikuchi K, Mori M (1985) Adenomatoid tumor of the uterus. Ultrastructural, histochemical, and immunohistochemical analysis. Arch Pathol Lab Med 109: 1049–1051

243. Taina E, Maenpää J, Erkkola R, Ikkala J, Söderström O, Viitanen A (1989) Endometrial stromal sarcoma: a report of nine cases. Gynecol Oncol 32: 156–162

244. Tamaya T, Fujimoto J, Okada H (1985) Comparison of cellular levels of steroid receptors in uterine leiomyoma and myometrium. Acta Obstet Gynecol Scand 64: 307–309

245. Tang CK, Toker C, Ances IG (1979) Stromomyoma of the uterus. Cancer 43: 308–316

246. Tang CK, Toker C, Harriman B (1981) Müllerian adenosarcoma of the uterine cervix. Hum Pathol 12: 579–581

247. Tavassoli FA, Norris HJ (1981) Mesenchymal tumors of the uterus. VII. A clinicopathological study of 60 endometrial stromal nodules. Histopathology 5: 1–10

248. Tavassoli FA, Norris HJ (1982) Peritoneal leiomyomatosis (leiomyomatosis peritonealis disseminata): a clinicopathologic study of 20 cases with ultrastructural observations. Int J Gynecol Pathol 1: 59–74

249. Taylor HB, Norris HJ (1966) Mesenchymal tumors of the uterus. IV. Diagnosis and prognosis of leiomyosarcoma. Arch Pathol 82: 40–44

250. Tenti P, Babilonti L, La Fianza A, Zampatti C, Carnevali L, Sonnino P, Franchi M (1989) Cytology of malignant mixed mesodermal tumour of the uterus: experience of 10 cases. Eur J Gynaecol Oncol 10: 125–128

251. Thatcher SS, Woodruff JD (1982) Uterine stromatosis: a report of 33 cases. Obstet Gynecol 59: 428–434

252. Thigpen JT, Blessing JA, Beecham J, Homesley H, Yordan E (1991) Phase II trial of cisplatin as first-line chemotherapy in patients with advanced or recurrent uterine sarcomas: a Gynecologic Oncology Group study. J Clin Oncol 9: 1962–1966

253. Tiltman AJ (1980) Adenomatoid tumours of the uterus. Histopathology 4: 437–443

254. Tiltman AJ (1985) The effect of progestins on the mitotic activity of uterine fibromyomas. Int J Gynecol Pathol 4: 89–96

255. Timmis AD, Smallpeice C, Davies AC, Macarthur AM, Gishen P, Jackson G (1980) Intracardiac spread of intravenous leiomyomatosis with successful surgical excision. N Engl J Med 303: 1043–1044

256. Tosi P, Sforza V, Santopietro R (1989) Estrogen receptor content, immunohistochemically determined by monoclonal antibodies, in endometrial stromal sarcoma. Obstet Gynecol 73: 75–78

257. Tsukamoto N, Kamura T, Matsukuma K, Imachi M, Uchino H, Saito T, Ono M (1985) Endolymphatic stromal myosis: a case with positive estrogen and progesterone receptors and good response to progestins. Gynecol Oncol 20: 120–128

258. Tsushima K, Stanhope CR, Gaffey TA, Lieber MM (1988) Uterine leiomyosarcomas and benign smooth muscle tumors: usefulness of nuclear DNA patterns studied by flow cytometry. Mayo Clin Proc 63: 248–255

259. Upadhyaya NB, Doody MC, Googe PB (1990) Histopathological changes in leiomyomata treated with leuprolide acetate. Fertil Steril 54: 811–814

260. Vakiani M, Mawad J, Talerman A (1982) Heterologous sarcomas of the uterus. Int J Gynecol Pathol 1: 211–219

261. Vardi JR, Tovell HMM (1980) Leiomyosarcoma of the uterus: clinicopathologic study. Obstet Gynecol 56: 428–434

262. Varela-Duran J, Nochomovitz LE, Prem KA, Dehner LP (1980) Postirradiation mixed müllerian tumors of the uterus: a comparative clinicopathologic study. Cancer 45: 1625–1631

263. Vellios F (1980) Papillary adenofibroma-adenosarcoma: the uterine cystosarcoma phyllodes. Prog Surg Pathol 1: 205–219

264. Vellios F, Ng AB, Reagen JW (1973) Papillary adenofibroma of the uterus: a benign mesodermal mixed tumor of müllerian origin. Am J Clin Pathol 60: 543–551

265. Vongtama V, Karlen JR, Piver SM, Tsukada Y, Moore RH (1976) Treatment, results and prognostic factors in stage I and II sarcomas of the corpus uteri. Am J Roentgenol 126: 139–147

266. Wheelock JB, Krebs HB, Schneider V, Goplerud DR (1985) Uterine sarcoma: analysis of prognostic variables in 71 cases. Am J Obstet Gynecol 151: 1016–1022

267. Witkin GB, Askin FB, Geratz JD, Reddick RL (1987) Angiosarcoma of the uterus: a light microscopic, immunohistochemical, and ultrastructural study. Int J Gynecol Pathol 6: 176–184

268. Wolff M, Silva F, Kaye G (1979) Pulmonary metastases (with admixed epithelial elements) from smooth muscle neoplasms: report of nine cases, including three males. Am J Surg Pathol 3: 325–342

269. Yoonessi M, Hart WR (1977) Endometrial stromal sarcomas. Cancer 40: 898–906

270. Young N, Damien M, Schwartz PE, Carter D, Mittal KR (1988) Carcinosarcoma of the uterine cervix initially interpreted as high grade sarcoma. Hum Pathol 19: 605–608

271. Young RH, Treger T, Scully RE (1986) Atypical polypoid adenomyoma of the uterus. A report of 27 cases. Am J Clin Pathol 86: 139–145

272. Youngs LA, Taylor HB (1967) Adenomatoid tumors of the uterus and fallopian tube. Am J Clin Pathol 48: 537–545

273. Zaloudek CJ, Norris HJ (1981) Adenofibroma and adenosarcoma of the uterus: a clinicopathologic study of 35 cases. Cancer 48: 354–366

273a. Zaloudek CJ, Norris HJ (1981) Mesenchymal tumors of the uterus. In: Fenoglio CM, Wolff M (eds), Progress in surgical pathology. Vol III, pp 1–35, New York, Masson Publishing USA, Inc.

274. Zutter MM, Gersell DJ (1990) Acute lymphoblastic leukemia. An unusual case of primary relapse in the uterine cervix. Cancer 66: 1002–1004

14

Diseases of the Fallopian Tube

James E. Wheeler, M.D.

The function of the fallopian tube, transport of sperm and ovum, may be seriously compromised or entirely destroyed by inflammatory processes or tubal pregnancy. Tumors may interfere with normal function or, if malignant, may lead to death. The etiology and pathophysiology of many tubal diseases are imperfectly understood at present.

Anatomy

The normal fallopian tube extends from the area of its corresponding ovary anteriorly and medially to its terminus in the posterosuperior aspect of the uterine fundus. In an adult during the reproductive years, its length is usually between 9 and 11 cm. The tube at the ovarian end opens to the peritoneal cavity and is composed of about 25 irregular finger-like extensions of the tube, the fimbriae. The fimbriae attach to the expanded end of the tube, the infundibulum, which is about 1 cm long and 1 cm in diameter. The infundibulum lies within a few millimeters of the superolateral or tubal end of the ovary. It narrows gradually to about 4 mm in diameter and merges medially with the ampullary portion of the tube, which extends about 6 cm, passing anteriorly as it passes around the ovary. At a point characterized by relative thickening of the muscular wall, the isthmic portion begins and extends some 2 cm to the uterus. Within the myometrium, the tube extends as a 1-cm long intramural segment until it joins the extension of the endometrial cavity at the uterotubal junction.[172]

Throughout its extrauterine course, the tube lies in a peritoneal fold along the superior margin of the broad ligament, the mesosalpinx. The arterial blood supply has a dual origin. A tubal branch of the uterine artery passes in the mesosalpinx laterally from the cornu of the uterus to anastomose with tubal branches of the ovarian artery. Venous drainage parallels the arterial supply via anastomosing tubal branches of uterine and ovarian veins, also located in the mesosalpinx. Tubal lymphatics pass laterally, accompanying the ovarian vessels. Thence, on the right side, lymph drains into nodes in the area of the right renal vein and the inferior vena cava, whereas on the left side, lymph drains into nodes lying between the left ovarian vein and the left renal vein. Lymph also drains into presacral and common ililac nodes. It is apparent that lymphatic spread of tubal malignancy may reach extrapelvic sites in its dissemination.[226]

The nerve supply of the tube is both sympathetic and parasympathetic. Sympathetic fibers from T_{10} through L_2 synapse in the celiac, aortic, renal, inferior mesenteric, cervicovaginal, and possibly presacral plexuses. Postsynaptic fibers pass into the myosalpinx, where they provide adrenergic innervation to the smooth muscle. The fact that isthmic and ampullary tubal muscle is innervated via presacral and ovarian plexuses, respectively, provides a possible neural explanation for differential myosalpingeal activity and formation of a physiologic sphincter. Sensory pain fibers pass along with the sympathetic nerves to the spinal cord at the level of T_{10}–T_{12}. Parasympathetic fibers from the vagus nerve supply the extrauterine tube via postganglionic fibers from the ovarian plexus, whereas the intramural portion is innervated via S_{2-4} parasympathetic fibers synapsing in the pelvic plexuses.[58]

Histology

A mucosal membrane, a wall of smooth muscle, and a serosal coat make up the three histological layers of the tube. The serosa is lined by flattened mesothelial cells. Beneath the mesothelium lies a small amount of connective tissue containing a few collagen fibers and blood vessels. The tubal muscularis generally has two layers: an outer longitudinal layer and an inner circular layer. At the uterine end, beginning in the intramural tube and extending laterally about 2 cm, there is, in addition, an inner longitudinal layer. The outer longitudinal layer is easily overlooked, as it is composed of inconspicuous bundles of smooth muscle interspersed with loose connective tissue containing numerous small blood vessels. The circular layer forms the major muscle mass of the tube. Its thickness varies, being about 0.5 mm in the isthmus and only about 0.1 mm in the ampulla.

The mucosal layer lies directly on the muscularis. It consists of a luminal epithelial lining and a scanty underlying lamina propria containing vessels and spindly or angu-

lar cells. Although these stromal cells seem sparse, they are the cells that lead to focally recognizable decidua in 5–12% of pregnancies (Fig. 14.1)[123,277] and may be seen in 80% of ectopic pregnancies.[111] The mucosa increases significantly in its gross structural complexity as the lumen enlarges from the uterine to the ovarian end. The interstitial and intramural portions each contain about five or six blunt plicae, or folds. In the isthmus, the plicae increase in height to more nearly occupy the larger lumen. A dozen or more plicae, some with secondary folds, are present. In the ampulla, the plicae are frond-like and delicate, and both secondary and tertiary branches may be appreciated. The infundibular plical pattern is similar.

The epithelial layer of the mucosa is composed of at least three histological cell types: ciliated, secretory, and intercalary.[214] About 20–30% of the cells contain prominent cilia,[78] and about 55–65% are secretory (Fig. 14.2).[78] Although some investigators[91] have found the ciliated cells in humans to be apparently randomly and equally distributed throughout the isthmic, ampullary, and fimbriated portions, others[208] have found ciliated cells numerous and preferentially located at the apical portions of the plicae, especially in the fimbriae and ampulla. Ciliated cells in the isthmus are less frequent[76] and occur in short strands. Ciliated cells are even scantier in the intramural tubal segment.

The ciliated cell itself is columnar and approximately 20 to 30 μm long. Electron microscopic study reveals typical ciliary basal bodies and rootlets.[91] The nucleus is oval to round, about 8 to 10 μm in greatest extent, and may lie

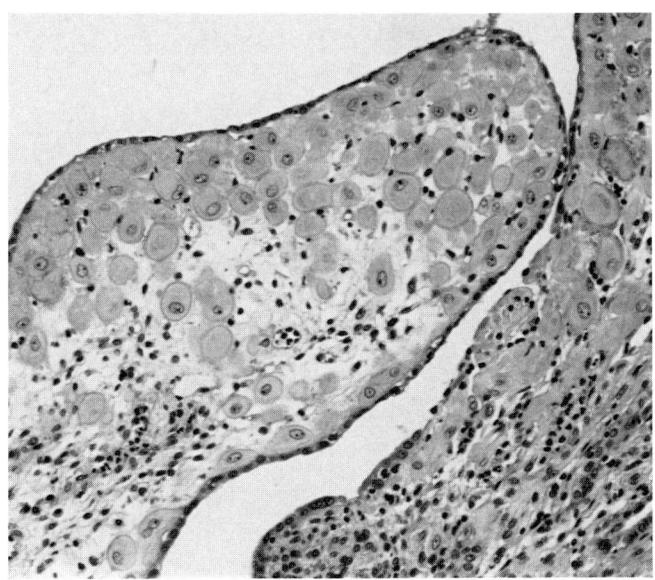

FIG. 14.1. Decidual reaction in tubal mucosa. The endosalpingeal folds are expanded by oval decidualized stromal cells characterized by well-defined cytoplasmic membranes.

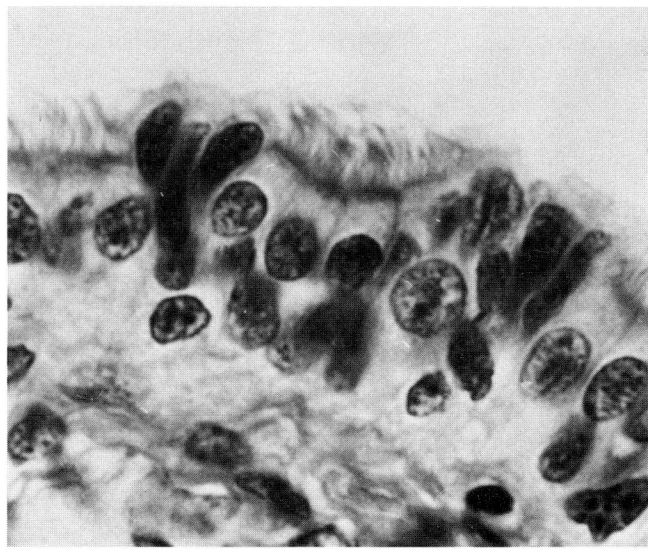

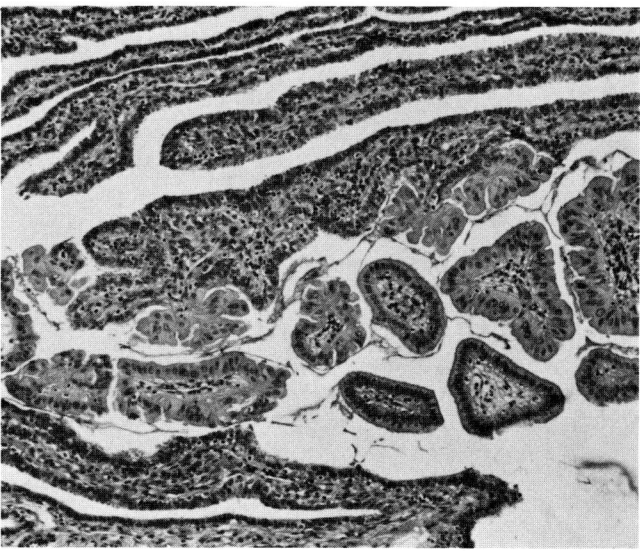

FIG. 14.2. **Tubal epithelium.** Ciliated cells are numerous. Secretory cells with columnar, somewhat compressed nuclei protrude above the level of the ciliated cells. Note vacuolated apical cytoplasm of secretory cells.

FIG. 14.3. **Benign oncocytic (pink cell) metaplasia.** Cells with prominent eosinophilic cytoplasm form papillary projections or line modestly distorted plicae. Scattered lymphocytes are present in plicae.

parallel or perpendicular to the long axis of the cell. The chromatin pattern is moderately granular. A distinct but small nucleolus is present.

The secretory cell also is columnar, approximately the same height as the ciliated cell but often narrower (Fig. 14.2). Its nucleus is ovoid and perpendicular to the long axis of the cell. The chromatin pattern may be somewhat denser than that of the ciliated cell, but its nucleolus is similar.

The intercalary, or peg cell is a columnar cell that appears to be occupied mainly by a thin, dark-staining nucleus. It is likely a morphologic variant of the secretory cell.[202]

In addition to the three epithelial cell types described, scattered lymphocytes may be seen located basally above the basement membrane.[203] Immunohistological analysis of these lymphocytes indicates a preponderance of the T-cytotoxic/suppressor subtype, consistent with formation of mucosal-associated lymphoid tissue (MALT).[192]

The tubal epithelium may undergo metaplastic changes without apparent reason. The metaplastic cells may be squamous or may be columnar and mucin secreting, resembling endocervical epithelium.[212,299] Mucinous metaplasia may be associated with Peutz–Jeghers syndrome.[92] Oncocytic metaplasia with marked cytoplasmic eosinophilia on routine H&E staining may occur. When associated with chronic salpingitis and papillary changes (Fig. 14.3), occasionally it is interpreted as a benign tumor,[237] but there is no convincing evidence that indicates neoplastic behavior. Studies delineating the usual extent of epithelial variability demonstrate that focal nuclear crowding and

tufting are frequent and normal (Fig. 14.4), but mitoses occur infrequently.

Psammoma bodies are an occasional finding in chronic salpingitis but may be seen in otherwise normal-appearing epithelium (Fig. 14.5). Accumulation of lipofuscin in macrophages in the lamina propria has been reported as *pigmentosis tubae*[126] and may be associated with endometriosis.[246]

The wolffian or mesonephric duct develops in close

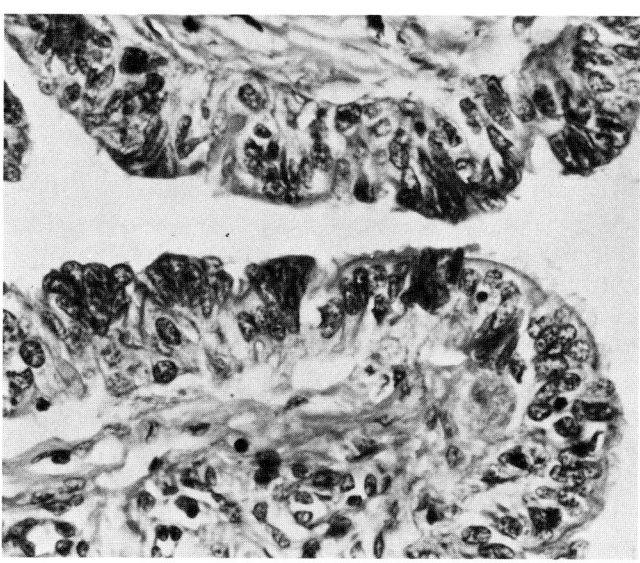

FIG. 14.4. **Tubal epithelium.** Crowding of nuclei and tufting of epithelial cells is a normal variant.

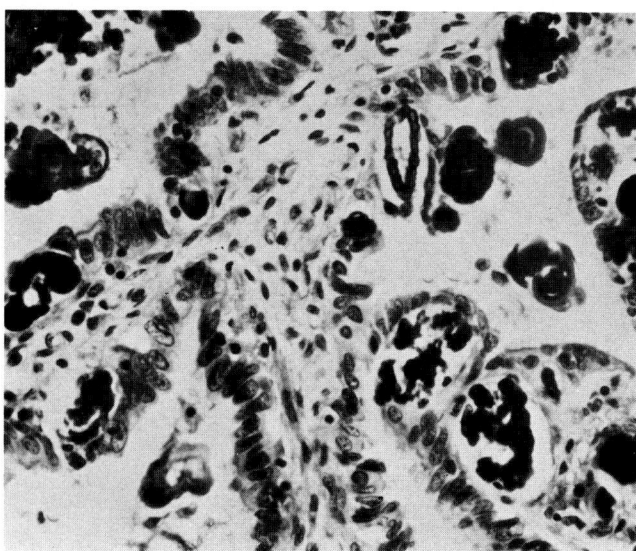

FIG. 14.5. Psammoma bodies in tubal epithelium. These calcific bodies may be found in chronic salpingitis or in relatively normal epithelium containing only rare lymphocytes.

proximity to the fallopian tube, and remnants from it normally persist throughout adult life. These remnants consist of 10 to 15 mesonephric tubules lying in the mesovarium. The tubules are lined by low columnar or cuboidal epithelium containing ciliated and nonciliated cells. There is only a thin, if any, muscular coat.[28] The tubules connect with the mesonephric duct, which runs parallel to the fallopian tube in the mesosalpinx. The duct is lined by nonciliated cuboidal or columnar cells surrounded by a relatively thick layer of first longitudinal and then circular smooth muscle. It is commonly seen on routine histological cross-sections of tube lying outside the circular muscularis (Fig. 14.6).

Physiology with Morphologic Correlation

The morphologic characteristics of the tubal epithelium change during life. Ciliated cells appear during early fetal development[207] and persist until the postmenopausal years. At this time, as circulating estrogen levels drop, the cilia are gradually lost.[102] Estrogen therapy in postmenopausal women, however, restores both the cilia and the ability to transport particulate matter.[102,284] The demonstration of a specific estradiol receptor in the human tube[94] suggests that there is a direct action of estrogen on ciliogenesis.

The characteristics of the tubal epithelium change during the course of the menstrual cycle.[202] Early in the cycle the cells are low, and the secretory cells appear relatively inactive. As ovulation approaches, probably under the influence of an increasing amount of estrogen, the secretory

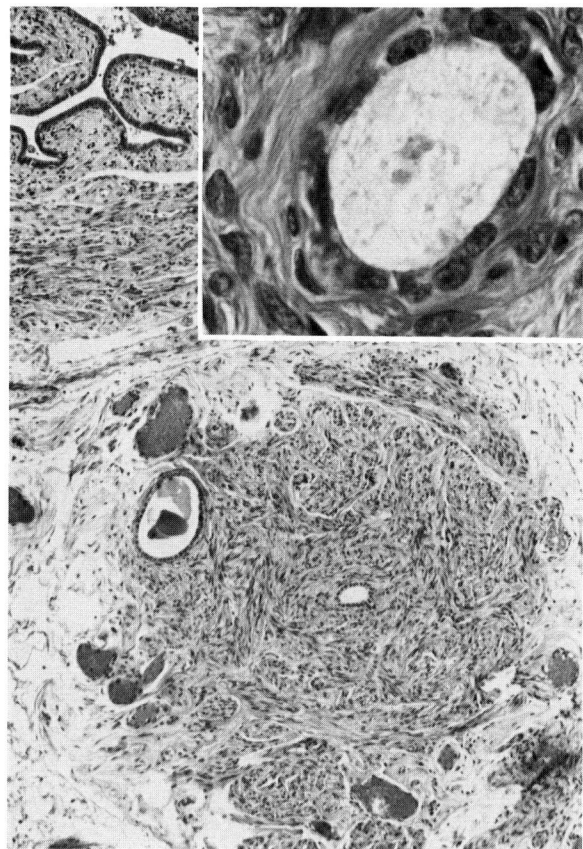

FIG. 14.6. Mesonephric duct remnants. These embryologic rests are commonly found on routine cross-sections. Note tubal lumen and muscularis in *upper left corner.* The nodule of mesonephric remnants *(center)* is composed of simple tubules surrounded by an irregular smooth muscle mass. *Inset:* The tubules are lined by low cuboidal cells.

cells become columnar and actually project beyond the ciliated cells (Fig. 14.2). A discharge of periodic acid-Schiff (PAS)-positive material, probably glycogen, into the tubal lumen has been demonstrated.[98] Changes in cilial maturity and repeated ciliated and deciliation of a minor degree have been documented during the menstrual cycle.[76,283] Other cyclic changes in tubal physiology occur.[139]

The cilia play a dominant role in tubal function at ovulation. The cilia beat in synchronized waves in the direction of the uterus.[101] During the course of ovum pickup, there appears to be a realignment of fimbriae in their relationship to the ovary itself. A distinct fimbria, the fimbria ovarica, runs from the tubal ostium to one pole of the ovary. It is thought that, at the time of ovulation, the muscle of the fimbria ovarica contracts, pulling the tube in the direction of the rupturing follicle. At the same time, some muscular elements in the paraovarian tissue contract, pulling the ovary toward the tubal ostium. This realignment of fimbriae over the rupturing follicle has been observed in several laboratory species, but for technical reasons it has not yet been satisfactorily evaluated in the human. Once the ovum is released from its follicle, surrounded by an entourage of sticky cumulus cells, it is transported along the surface of the fimbriated end of the fallopian tube by the action of the cilia. The ovum is retained within the tube for approximately 3 days,[59] after which it is delivered into the uterus. In Kartagener's syndrome, where cilia are structurally defective and immobile, fertility, although impaired, is preserved. This raises the likelihood that muscular contraction is more important than previously considered. The effect of adrenergic innervation[209] or prostaglandins[55,170] on muscle function and ova transport is not yet well defined.

Spermatozoa are transported upward through the uterus into the fallopian tube. The mechanisms by which they traverse the uterotubal junction and tubal isthmus in the face of a ciliary beat in a downward direction is still not understood. It is known, however, that spermatozoa can reach the tube within minutes after they are placed in the vagina in the human.[249] It is likely that the fertilizing spermatozoa is already present in the fallopian tube at the time the ovum arrives there.

The environment provided within the tubal lumen is of special importance in reproductive function. The fallopian tube does provide a temporary milieu for spermatozoa, the ovum, and finally the fertilized, cleaving zygote during its initial development. The secretory cells certainly must play a role in the provision of suitable conditions for the processes that occur within the tubal lumen. Contents of the tubal fluid have been studied extensively in the rhesus monkey, but only limited observations have been carried out in the human.[63,171] The salient components of oviductal fluid include metabolic substrates, the most important of which are lactate, pyruvate, and bicarbonate, which appears in tubal fluid as a result of carbonic anhydrase in the tubal epithelium, and electrolytes, including calcium.[183] Tubal fluid also contains trypsin inhibitors, which may influence the fertilization process, and a genital tract isoamylase.[251]

The bicarbonate ion is in part responsible for dispersion of cells that surround the ovum. On reaching the level of the zona pellucida (a protein–mucopolysaccharide layer immediately surrounding the egg), the spermatozoan is able to penetrate by virtue of the presence of a trypsin-like enzyme in its head. Trypsin inhibitors appear in high concentration both before and after ovulation, but for a matter of hours after ovulation, they are at their lowest level of concentration.[256] Some investigators have speculated that trypsin inhibitors control the fertilization process so that aged ova that are in the fallopian tube in the presence of a high concentration of inhibitors are not fertilized. Be that as it may, the 3-day residence in the fallopian tube apparently serves a useful function in several experimental mammals. When zygotes are removed prematurely from the tube and placed in the uterus, implantation is less likely.

Most of the work on tubal physiology has focused on its role in reproduction, and only scanty information is available on the tubal immune system and its role in infection. The immunoglobulin IgG is present in tubal fluid. Both subclasses of immunoglobulin A, IgA1 and IgA2, are formed by a scanty population of subepithelial plasma cells[157] with the secretory component contributed by the epithelial cells.[192,225]

Congenital Anomalies

Structural congenital anomalies of the fallopian tube are rare and may be simulated by inflammatory processes or torsion. Tubes associated with uterine abnormalities such as a rudimentary uterine horn or bicornuate uterus may be hypoplastic or partially atretic.[87,152] Bilateral absence of the ampullary muscularis has been reported.[280]

Infertility patients who were exposed in utero to diethylstibestrol (DES) may have shortened, sacculated, and convoluted fallopian tubes despite normal salpingograms. The fimbria are described as constricted and the os as pinpoint.[66] No detailed pathological studies are available. A mouse model of DES exposure produces tubal changes more reminiscent of salpingitis isthmica nodosa.[198]

Apparent congenital absence of a segment of the tube has been reported,[250] as has tubal duplication[64] and accessory tubes.[22] Tubes may be absent in phenotypic females in rare cases.[297]

Torsion, Prolapse, and Intussusception

Among the various anatomic displacements of the tube, torsion is the most common. The usual predisposing factor is cystic enlargement of the ipsilateral ovary. A benign ovarian cyst or tumor is present in 65–80% of patients, and a malignant ovarian tumor is present in 5–15%.[69,165] Paraovarian cysts also are associated with torsion. Tubal enlargement secondary to hydrosalpinx or pyosalpinx[165] or previous gynecological surgery, especially sterilization,[20] are additional causes, but torsion may occur in the absence of apparent adnexal disease.

The typical patient is in the reproductive years, occasionally pregnant,[137] and complains of the sudden onset of lower abdominal pain. At operation, the adnexa on one side is twisted, usually once or twice. Venous outflow is compromised early, and the resulting congestion may lead to arterial compression. The adnexa often is swollen and edematous, with hemorrhagic infarction and gangrene. If surgical intervention is prompt, the tube may be preserved. Undiagnosed torsion in an infant or adult may result in resorption and total disappearance of the infarcted adnexa or in calcification of the necrotic tissue.[21,41]

Tubal prolapse into the vagina may occur rarely as a complication of hysterectomy, usually vaginal[83,240] (see Chapter 4, Diseases of the Vagina). Clinically this is characterized by vaginal discharge, beginning a few days to several years after vaginal hysterectomy. On examination, an excrescence is seen in the vaginal vault, suggestive of granulation tissue or carcinoma. Fimbriae may be apparent grossly. Severe acute and chronic inflammation is present microscopically, and pseudogland formation by the tubal epithelium may mimic adenocarcinoma.[240]

Intussusception of the tube has been reported once.[4] A paraovarian cyst was engulfed by the end of the tube and pulled the fimbriated end into the ampulla. Simple eversion and cystectomy permitted tubal salvage.

Endometriosis and Endosalpingiosis

Endometrial-type tissue may involve the tubal lumen, wall, or serosa. Heterotopic endometrium may entirely replace normal tubal epithelium, with luminal occlusion.[158]

Endosalpingiosis is the ectopic location of tubal-type epithelium involving peritoneal surfaces. Both endometriosis and endosalpingiosis are discussed in detail in Chapter 17, Diseases of the Peritoneum.

Salpingitis

Salpingitis may be divided into three major types: acute, chronic, and granulomatous.

Acute Salpingitis

Acute salpingitis is a purulent inflammatory process usually secondary to the passage of bacteria from the uterine cavity into the tubal lumen.[184b] It is not clear if organisms are carried upward by sperm or trichomonads as vectors or whether some form of passive transport is in effect.[148] Although *Neisseria gonorrhoeae* has been considered the most common causative organism, meticulous bacteriologic studies indicate that the etiology is polymicrobial and that *Chlamydia trachomatis* and anaerobic bacteria, especially *Bacteroides* species and peptostreptococci, frequently are present, as well as such aerobes as *Escherichia coli*.[47,265,268,275,276] The presence in some of these women of serum antibodies against gonococcal pili, however, suggests that gonococci may initiate the process, only to be supplanted by anaerobes.

Elegant in vitro studies by Ward and others[185,288] have clarified the likely initial steps in gonococcal infection, and the molecular mechanisms involved have been reviewed.[33] *N. gonorrhoeae* perfused through the lumen of cultured whole tubes attach only to nonciliated cells. Within 3 hours, microvilli from the cells appear to embrace the gonococci and adhere to them. The bacteria then penetrate both the cells and intercellular junctions, with cell lysis and sloughing. Adjacent ciliated cells are also destroyed but are not invaded directly. After cell lysis, the bacteria penetrate the subepithelial connective tissue. In vivo, this process is considerably modified by the host response. A brisk diapedesis of granulocytes occurs from capillaries into the mucosa and lumen, and there is vascular engorgement and edema of all tubal layers (Fig. 14.7). In severe cases, transudation of plasma proteins results in a fibrinous exudate on the serosal surface, which reddens because of vascular dilatation. As the lumen fills with granulocytes and cellular debris and as the tube distends, pus may be seen dripping from the fimbriated end in patients undergoing laparoscopy. The cell necrosis, distention of the tube, and focal peritonitis lead to abdominal and pelvic pain. The gonococcus gains access to the tube most readily at the time of menstruation. This corresponds to the typical clinical presentation in which the onset of acute pain occurs a few days after menses. The onset of nongonococcal, nonchlamydial acute salpingitis is not, however, clearly related to the recent onset of menses.[266] Over time, repeated invasions result in recurrent symptoms as well as the anatomic changes of chronic salpingitis, discussed below. Acute bacterial salpingitis after tubal ligation is rare.[220]

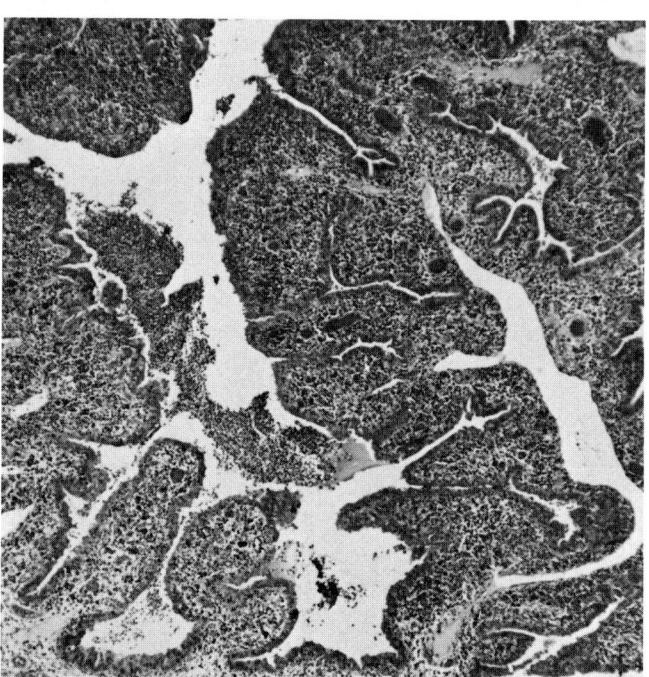

FIG. 14.7. Acute and chronic salpingitis. Plicae are broadened and blunted. Numerous granulocytes, lymphocytes, and plasma cells are present in the mucosa; many granulocytes are present in the lumen.

Although *N. gonorrhoeae* spreads via the epithelial surface and thus causes mucosal changes, other bacteria present in the uterus, such as streptococci, tend to spread into the tube by vascular or lymphatic channels. This results in acute inflammation of the tubal wall, with relative sparing of the mucosa.

Initial reports implicated the intrauterine contraceptive device in the etiology of salpingitis and pelvic inflammatory disease.[150,291] However, newer information eliminating methodologic problems of control groups, ascertainment bias, and confounding factors indicate that any increased risk of infection in a stable monogamous sexual situation may be limited to a few weeks after insertion.[88,164,279,300] Vaginal douching may be a risk factor for acute pelvic inflammatory disease.[244a]

Mycoplasmas have been reported in both acute salpingitis and tuboovarian abscess.[29] Laparoscopically obtained pretreatment cultures from grossly infected tubes occasionally reveal *Mycoplasma hominis*.[180,181] Tubes examined histologically have shown a moderate infiltration with chronic inflammatory cells, some neutrophils, and focal epithelial ulceration.[29] Recent studies suggest that *M. hominis* is not an important cause of salpingitis or infertility.[114,169] *Ureaplasma urealyticum* also may be responsible for acute salpingitis.[267]

C. trachomatis is cultured frequently from the cervix, uterus, and fallopian tubes in women with acute salpingitis.[155,179] The histological appearance of tubes removed during the acute or subacute phase of chlamydial salpingitis is virtually identical to that caused by the gonococcus. There is an initial transmural and mucosal infiltration of polymorphonuclear leukocytes with an intraluminal exudate. Subsequently there is a lymphoplasmacytic response with variable numbers of residual granulocytes.[189,295] Antibodies to chlamydia antigen stain round circumnuclear vacuoles containing granular particles in epithelial cells.[295] On occasion the lymphofollicular response may be so florid as to suggest lymphoma.[287] Long-term tubal damage may be inferred by the finding of distorted tubal folds, areas of mucosa deciliation, and infertility in women with circulating antichlamydia antibody. This occurs whether or not there is a history of overt acute salpingitis.[36,210] Indeed, the frequency of tubal damage appears similar to that caused by the gonococcus.[264] There is a close association with chronic endometritis and, therefore, patients with a diagnosis of chronic endometritis should be evaluated carefully for asymptomatic salpingitis (see Chapter 10, Benign Diseases of the Endometrium). Coxsackie viruses B5 and ECHO 6 have been recovered from tubes with acute salpingitis, but no histological data are available.[181]

An asymptomatic form of acute salpingitis is seen in tubes removed during postpartum ligation. Beginning about 5 hours after delivery and present up to 7 to 10 days later, a small or moderate number of acute or mixed acute

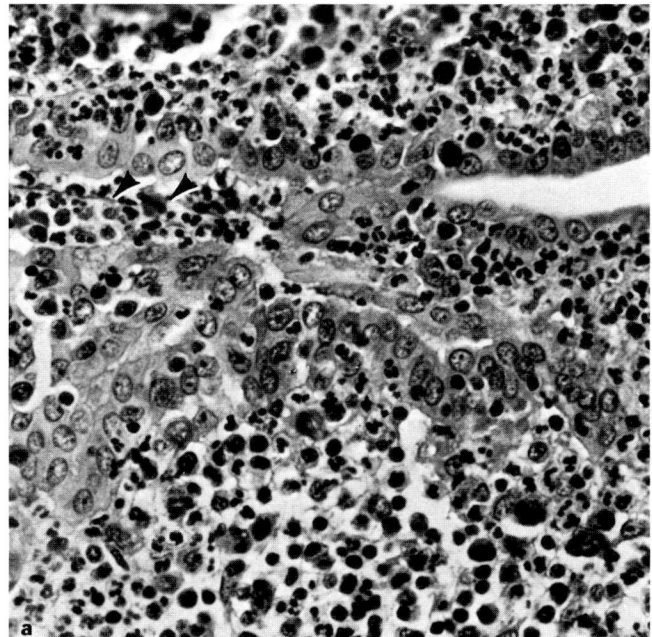

FIG. 14.8a. Acute and chronic salpingitis. Plicae are distended with polymorphonuclear leukocytes, histiocytes, lymphocytes, and plasma cells. Fibrin strands lie in lumen at left *(arrowheads)*. Note approximation of plicae and suggestion of early adhesion at center.

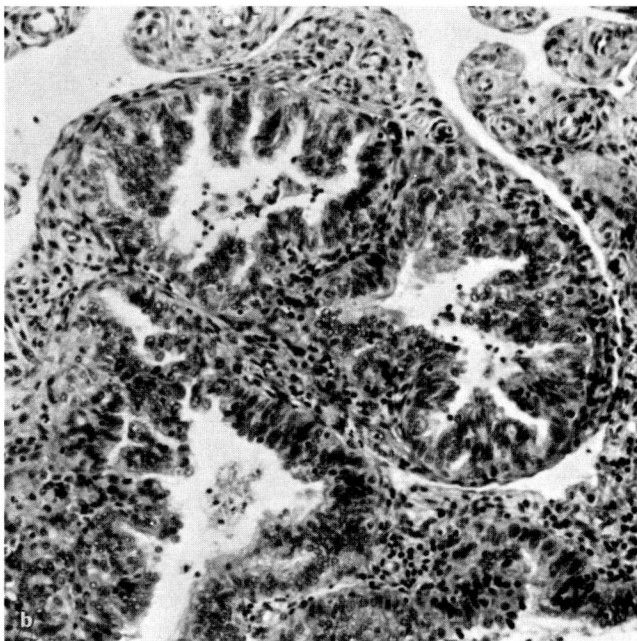

FIG. 14.8b. Chronic salpingitis. Papillary tufts of reactive epithelial cells are prominent, but mitoses are absent. A few lymphocytes may be seen in the stroma. This should not be confused with carcinoma.

and chronic inflammatory cells are found in the mucosa or lumen of 10% or more of specimens.[123,235] Attempts to culture aerobic or anaerobic bacteria[235,255] have been almost uniformly unsuccessful. The process may be regarded as secondary to the trauma of delivery or intrauterine tissue necrosis.

Chronic Salpingitis

When acute salpingitis resolves through agent–host interaction, residual disease may be found in the fallopian tube. With acute inflammation, the mucosal plicae, secondary to surface fibrin deposition, adhere to one another (Fig. 14.8). Healing and organization then lead to permanent bridging between folds. In the classic case, this results in a follicular salpingitis (Fig. 14.9). Plicae may retain much of their size and shape, but present cells, lymphocytes, or both are still present in the mucosa. Often the height of the folds appears lowered, or their intricate pattern, so prominent in the ampulla and infundibulum, is subtly altered. Fibrinous adhesions between the serosa and surrounding peritoneal surfaces may organize into thin fibrous adhesions that, unless routinely sought, are easily overlooked. Peritoneal inflammation may be widespread and thin, violin-string adhesions may form between liver and diaphragm. Agglutination of acutely inflamed fimbriae may be focal or massive. If it is severe enough, the bases of the fimbriae may coalesce in the center, with the fimbriae radiating outward like daisy petals, or the tips of the fimbriae may adhere, blocking the lumen and causing a blunted end, the clubbed tube (Fig. 14.10). The proximity of the ovary to the fimbriae allows multiple tuboovarian

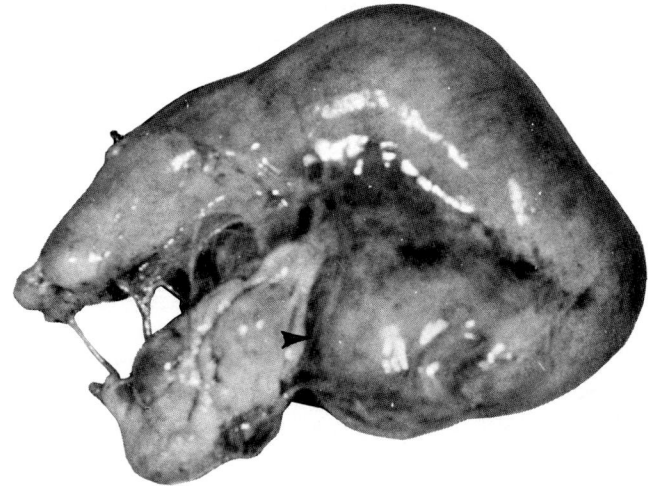

Fig. 14.10. **Chronic salpingitis.** Multiple, thin, fibrous adherences are present between tube and ovary and between ampulla and infundibulum. Distal portion of tube (*arrowhead*) has clubbed appearance because of obliteration of tubal ostium.

adhesions to form, with occlusion of the tubal ostium. The ovary itself may then become more directly involved, and a tuboovarian abscess may result (Fig. 14.11).[273] If the fimbriae close before the ovary is seriously involved, the inflamed, dilated tube forms a pyosalpinx full of acute and chronic inflammatory cells. As the inflammation subsides, the acute and most of the chronic inflammatory cells gradually disappear, and the patient is left with either a severely scarred tube or a hydrosalpinx.

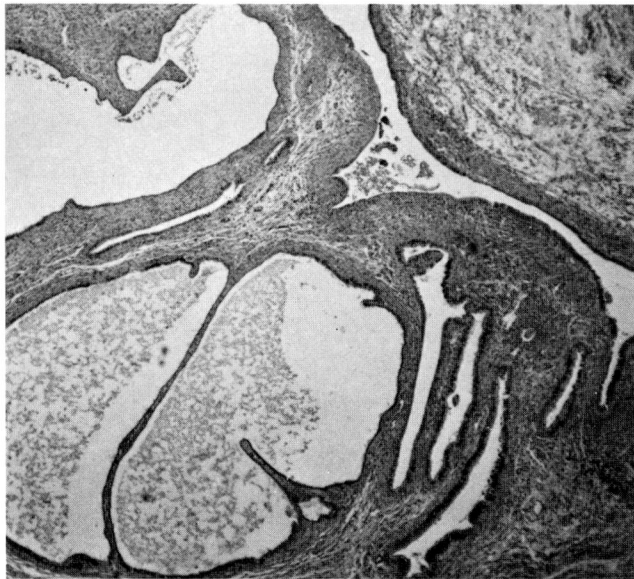

Fig. 14.9. **Salpingitis follicularis.** There is agglutination of plicae with formation of dilated gland-like spaces between them.

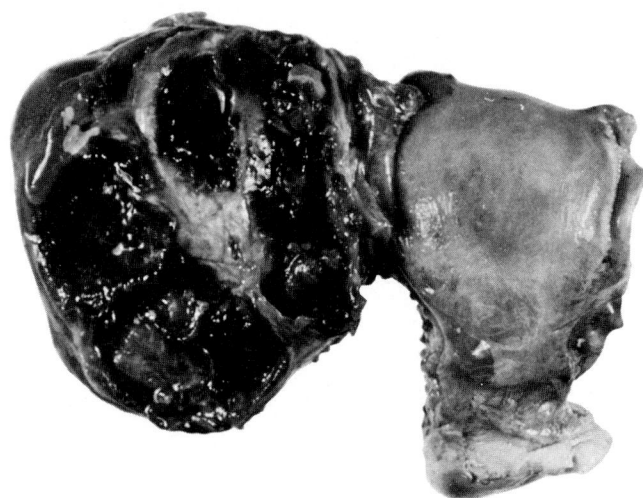

Fig. 14.11. **Tuboovarian abscess.** Posterior view shows bisected tuboovarian abscess involving entire left adnexa. Tube and ovary have been largely destroyed and replaced by a multiloculated mass containing foul-smelling pus.

Both aerobic and anaerobic cultures of any tuboovarian abscess should be obtained in the operating room or laboratory. Prior treatment with antibiotics possibly may eliminate culturable organisms, but with careful technique, anaerobes are isolated in 63–100% of cases.[160] *E. coli, Bacteriodes fragilis, Bacterioides* species, *Peptostreptococcus, Peptococcus,* and aerobic streptococci are the most commonly found organisms; typically, infection is polymicrobial.[159] *Pasturella multocida* also has been isolated recently as a causative agent in a patient with a tuboovarian abscess.[234]

Fungi, including *Blastomyces dermatitidis,* are cultured only rarely from tuboovarian abscesses[195] and may be secondary to hematogenous spread. Tubal coccidioidomycosis also may be found secondary to disseminated disease.[38] Malacoplakia only rarely involves the fallopian tube.[43]

Hydrosalpinx is one of the complications of salpingitis. It is characterized by obliteration of the fimbriated end and dilation of the tube, usually the ampullary and infundibular portions. If the ovary is first involved by tuboovarian adhesions, the ovary may be compressed by the dilated tube. The dilated tube may resemble the chemist's retort, and the wall is generally whitish, thin, and translucent, with occasional fibrous adhesions on its surface (Fig. 14.12). The tube usually contains clear serous fluid with an electrolyte composition similar to serum but with a low protein content.[62,63] Since a luminal communication usually can be demonstrated between dilated and nondilated portions of the tube,[45] the etiology of the dilatation is obscure but it may result in part from a sphincter-like action of the isthmus. The muscle wall is either thin and atrophic or replaced by collagenous connective tissue. Most of the epithelial lining consists of low cuboidal cells, but an occasional plica may persist, with surprisingly intact columnar epithelium with histologically normal ciliated and

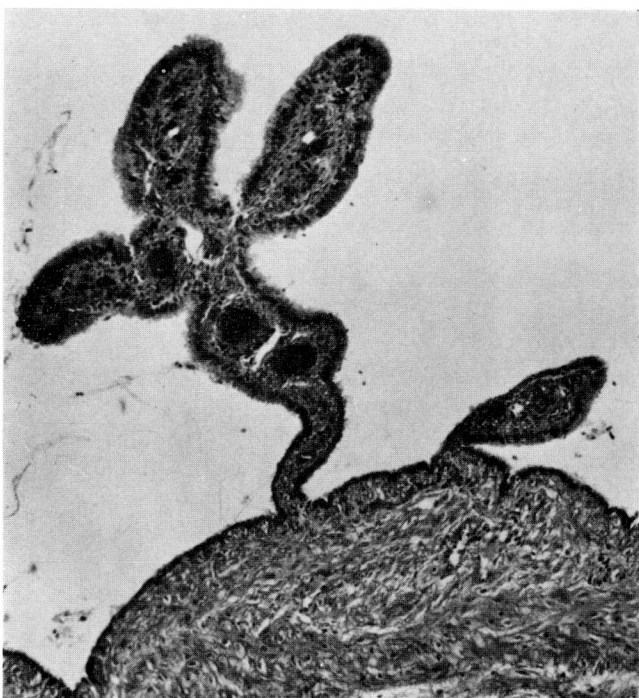

FIG. 14.13. **Hydrosalpinx.** Although most of the luminal epithelium is cuboidal or flattened, occasional plicae may remain with a normal epithelial surface.

secretory cells corresponding morphologically with the menstrual phase (Fig. 14.13). The persistence of healthy-appearing plicae suggests that pressure effects from the luminal fluid may not be responsible for the flattened and absent plicae. Instead, the preceding inflammatory process may have selectively damaged the tubal folds, resulting in uneven scarring and plical disappearance (Fig. 14.14). A few lymphocytes may be found in the wall of the hydrosalpinx but are more commonly absent. Recovery of tubal function, even with expert surgery, is unlikely, and the possibility of tubal torsion with subsequent hemorrhagic infarction remains.[73]

Granulomatous Salpingitis

Granulomatous inflammation of the fallopian tube may result from infection by a number of different organisms, or induced by a variety of noninfectious processes. The histological identification of one or more granulomas calls for immediate communication between pathologist and clinician in order to determine the likely etiology.

Tuberculous Salpingitis

Mycobacterium tuberculosis historically has been the predominant etiologic agent of granulomatous salpingitis. The

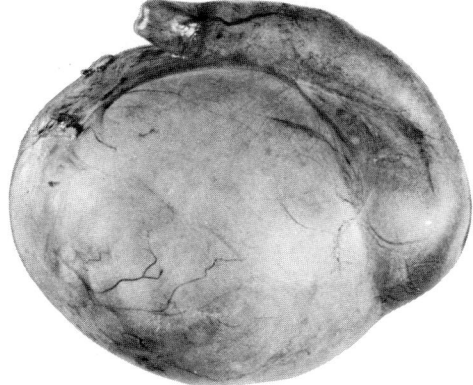

FIG. 14.12. **Hydrosalpinx.** The tube is markedly dilated in the ampullary portion. The fimbriae are obliterated; the wall is thickened but translucent.

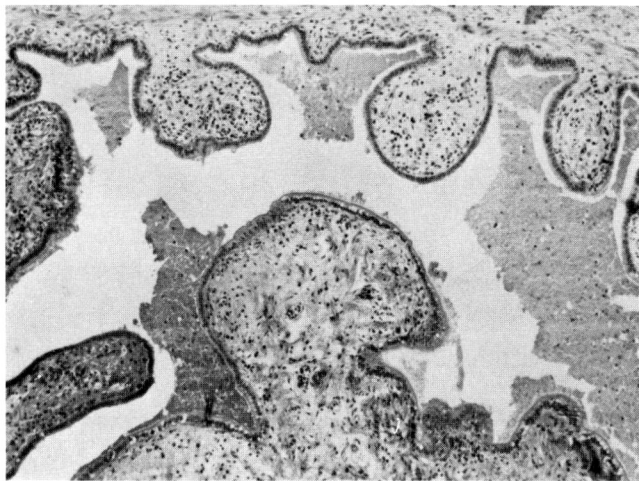

FIG. 14.14. **Chronic salpingitis.** Transitional stage between chronic salpingitis and hydrosalpinx. Marked blunting of plicae; only a scanty residual lymphocytic infiltrate is present.

frequency of tuberculous salpingitis in women studied for infertility ranges from far less than 1% in the United States to more than 10% in India; 10–20% of women who die from tuberculosis have tubal involvement.[241]

Primary infection of the genitalia, as by coitus with a partner with genitourinary tuberculosis, is extremely rare. Secondary spread, usually from a primary pulmonary infection, is the normal route of infection. For reasons still unknown, the blood-borne organism preferentially lodges in the tubes rather than the other parts of the female genital tract. The primary pulmonary lesion may not be radiologically evident, but extrapulmonary involvement of the peritoneum, kidneys, or other site may be present. Lymphatic spread from primary intestinal tuberculosis[110] or direct spread from bladder or gastrointestinal tract may occur.

Although the earliest pathological lesions are microscopic, with advancing disease the tube increases in diameter and may become nodular, mimicking salpingitis isthmica nodosa. In the more common adhesive form of the disease, multiple, dense adhesions may form between the tube and ovary, and the fimbriae and ostium may be obliterated.[115] Frequently, the ostium remains patent and some investigators, in fact, regard the presence of an identifiable ostium and fimbriae in a grossly diseased tube as characteristic of tuberculous salpingitis.[241] With the exudative form of disease, progressive distention mimics bacterial pyosalpinx. Hematosalpinx or hydrosalpinx may be found late in the disease process. In either form, serosal tubercles may be present.

The earliest microscopic lesions are mucosal, with a typical granulomatous reaction of epithelioid cells and lymphocytes arranged in a nodular configuration. Giant cells often are seen, and central caseation, focal or massive, may

be present. Immunosuppressive therapy may modify cellular immunity to a point where granulomas fail to form. With this clinical information, the mere finding of acute and chronic inflammatory cells should lead to consideration of staining for acid-fast organisms. From the mucosa, extension to the muscularis and serosa may occur. As the tubercles enlarge, they may erode through the mucosa and discharge their contents into the tubal lumen (Fig. 14.15). The mucosal inflammatory reaction leads to progressive scarring, with plical distortion and conglutination. Large caseous nodules may form and coalesce, eventually filling the dilated tube. Ectopic calcification may occur in areas of fibrosis. Since tubercles may not be present in a given section, the presence of caseation, fibrosis, or calcification in a tube may be the only histological finding pointing to the necessity for more thorough study. The presence of severe mucosal atypicality in tuberculous salpingitis and confusion with adenocarcinoma have been stressed by numerous authors, but similar atypia may be found in any chronic salpingitis (see Fig. 14.8b). Complications of tuberculous salpingitis are several. Alteration in function is the rule. Sterility is almost universal because of the common bilaterality of the disease. Rarely, successful pregnancies occur, but ectopic tubal nidation is likely in the event that fertilization is successful.[241]

Pelvic pain, sterility, and menstrual irregularities are the most common complaints. Because of repeated seeding of the endometrium from the infected tubes, mycobacterial

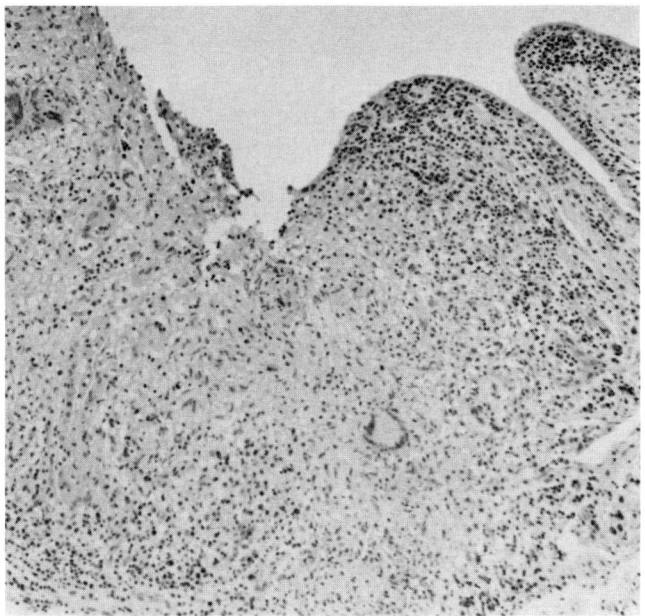

FIG. 14.15. **Tuberculous salpingitis.** Confluent focally necrotizing granulomas occupy most of the endosalpinx except on the far right. There is focal ulceration of the epithelial surface, illustrating a possible mechanism whereby *M. tuberculosis* could reach the tubal lumen and seed the endometrial cavity.

culture and the histological finding on curettage of endometrial tubercles are diagnostically useful (see Chapter 10, Benign Diseases of the Endometrium). Laparoscopy may cause bowel perforation in cases of extensive pelvic and peritoneal tuberculosis.

Actinomycosis

Actinomycotic infections of the tube may occur, many of them associated with intrauterine contraceptive devices (see Chapter 10, Benign Diseases of the Endometrium).[74,263] Recent studies note that actinomycetes probably are part of the indigenous female genital tract flora.[217]

Grossly, a large fibrous mass is present that often includes the ovary. The mass may appear to be a dilated tube or may be more obviously inflammatory, being bound down to pelvic structures with adhesions or fistula formation. Pus is present in the shaggy-walled cavities within the tube. Anaerobic culture is necessary to permit growth of *Actinomyces israelii.* Microscopically, numerous histiocytes, plasma cells, and lymphocytes are present in the abscess wall and gram-positive, filamentous clumps, sulfur granules, may be recognized in the pus. Complications in unrecognized cases may include dissemination to the liver and lung.

Parasitic Salpingitis

Pinworm

The pinworm, *Enterobius vermicularis,* may migrate up the female genital tract, embed in the tube, and cause an inflammatory reaction. The tube may be involved with the ovary in what appears to be a tuboovarian abscess, or a fibrous nodular area may be present. Acute and chronic inflammatory cells may be found together with eosinophils, Charcot–Leyden crystals, and portions of gravid female worm. Ova may be released into the tissue, where they provoke a granulomatous reaction. The ova may be identified by their size (about 20×50 μm) and ovoid asymmetrical shape,[269] but they may be obscured by calcification of granulomas. The ova may be widely disseminated in the peritoneum in the absence of histological tubal involvement, and the fibrous granulomas may simulate metastatic carcinoma.[93]

Schistosomiasis

Although tubal bilharziasis probably is one of the most common causes of granulomatous salpingitis worldwide, it is rare in the United States. In Africa, reported tubal infections occur in as many as 20% of unselected women at autopsy.[99] The ova of *Schistosoma haematobium* are most common, but *Schistosoma mansoni* eggs may be present in some women.[105] If granulomas are present and there is a suspicion of schistosomiasis, sodium hydroxide digestion of the remaining tubal tissue may reveal ova.

Gross findings appear to be related to fibrosis surrounding the ova, producing a nodular or fibrotic tube. Ectopic pregnancy in an infected tube may precipitate its removal, but the granulomas themselves may not always cause sufficient damage to account for abnormal nidation.[24]

Other Parasites

Where the condition is common, hydatid disease secondary to *Echinococcus granulosus* infection may involve the female genital tract, including the adnexae.[107] Cysticercosis also has been described in the tube.[2]

Sarcoid

Sarcoidosis of the tube is rarely reported[115] and appears to accompany disseminated disease. One patient[145] had gross tubal distention, tuboovarian adhesions, an ovarian abscess, and multiple serosal nodules, but bacterial salpingitis was not excluded as a cause. Histologically, noncaseating granulomas may be seen in the mucosa. Culture, special stains, and clinical information are necessary to exclude other granulomatous diseases.

Crohn's Disease

Crohn's disease of the ileum, colon, or appendix may secondarily involve the tube and ovary to produce a granulomatous salpingo-oophoritis.[35,296] Noncaseating granulomas may involve the entire thickness of the tubal muscularis as well as the mucosa. The epithelium may react with severe cellular atypia (Fig. 14.16). Fistulas from bowel to tube also may occur (see Chapter 3, Premalignant and Malignant Tumors of the Vulva).[57]

Xanthogranulomatous Salpingitis

Rare cases of xanthogranulomatous salpingitis are reported[97,126,159,246] in which the tube may be grossly swollen and clubbed or edematous. The mucosal surface may be brown and polypoid because of distention of plicae by lipofusion-laden or foamy macrophages. A mixed chronic inflammatory infiltrate with or without giant cells also may be seen. Although an association with endometriosis is reported,[50,246] this process also might result from salpingitis with bleeding and an atypical host reaction.

Foreign Body

Foreign material may be introduced into the tube in the course of gynecological investigation, especially hysterosalpingography. Lubricant jelly, mineral oil, and starch and talc powder may cause a lipoid or granulomatous salpingi-

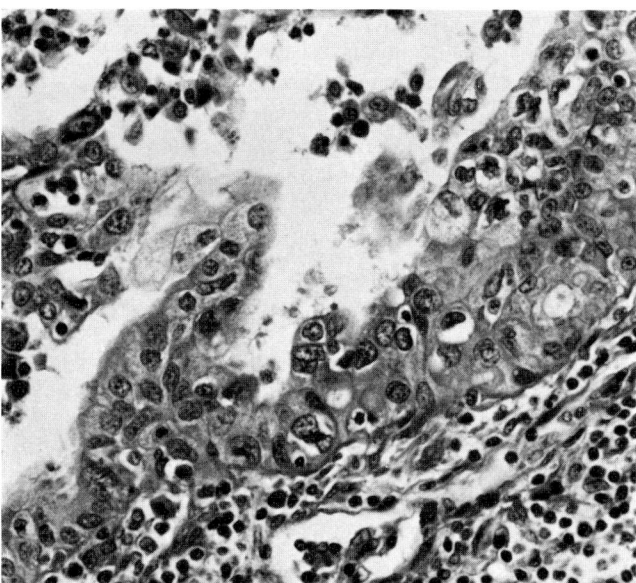

Fig. 14.16. Granulomatous salpingitis secondary to Crohn's disease. Underlying granulomas are not visible here, but severe chronic inflammation is present *(lower right)*. Epithelium is piled up and has marked nuclear atypia. This change should not be confused with carcinoma in situ.

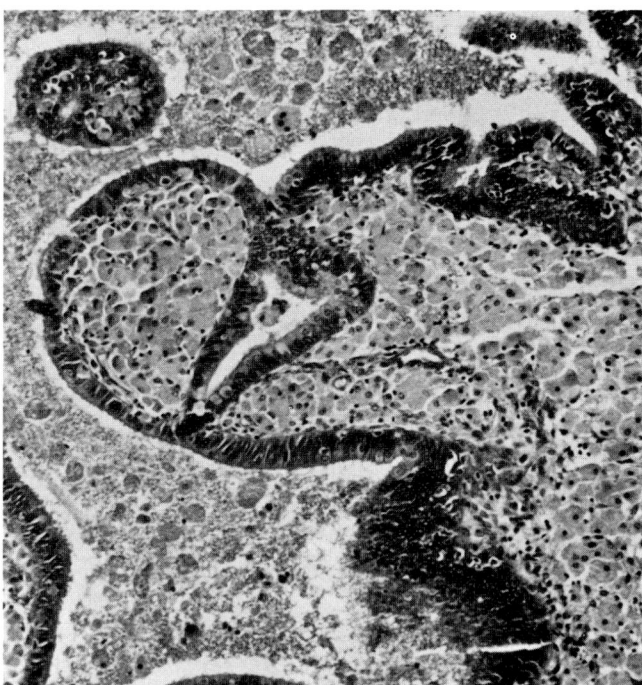

Fig. 14.17. Foreign body reaction in tubal mucosa. Hysterosalpingography or exposure to other foreign material may lead to intense histiocytic reaction, as here, or to formation of foreign body granulomas.

tis.[39,81] An intense phagocytic reaction to introduced lipid material causes accumulation of subepithelial foamy histiocytes (Fig. 14.17). If the patient has received a blood substitute containing polyvinylpyrrolidone (PVP), this foreign material may be ingested by macrophages and deposited in many organs, including the tube.[156] These histiocytes simulate signet-ring cell carcinoma, with mucicarmine-positive vacuolated cytoplasm. An appropriate history and a negative PAS stain should clarify the benign nature of the lesion. Talc may cause mucosal or serosal granulomas. Examination of all granulomas or foreign body reactions under polarized light is useful in the recognition of these processes. Other disease processes in the tube, such as leprosy[299] or amyloidosis,[53] are so infrequent that they are of little clinical or pathological significance. Giant cell arteritis involving the tube has been reported in postmenopausal women, and may be part of a generalized process or an incidental finding.[16]

Salpingitis Isthmica Nodosa

Salpingitis isthmica nodosa consists of one or more outpouchings or diverticula of tubal epithelium in the isthmic region. Involvement is often bilateral, and usually is accompanied by nodular hyperplasia of the surrounding muscularis.

The etiology is unknown. The disease is found in women between the ages of 25 and 60 years (average age at diagnosis is 30 years).[17] Because the lesion is almost unknown before puberty, is not found congenitally, and may be progressive,[184a] attention has focused on other possible causes, including postinflammatory distortion[132,243] and an adenomyosis-like process.[17,301] Against the proposed inflammatory etiology is the usual localization of nodularity in the isthmic portion of the tube or immediately adjacent ampulla.[17] Most of the ampulla is uninvolved, unlike the usual picture in inflammatory salpingitis. When salpingitis isthmica nodosa is associated with inflammatory salpingitis, such as pyosalpinx and hydrosalpinx, the inflammatory process is contralateral nearly as often as it is ipsilateral.[17] Although a few lymphocytes are found in the peridiverticular stroma, scarring usually is absent.

Evidence for a noninflammatory adenomyosis-like origin is more convincing. Moderate or large numbers of endometrial-like stromal cells accompany the diverticula in more than half the patients.[17] As in uterine adenomyosis, the presence of glands appears to stimulate muscular growth, with subsequent mural thickening. Unilateral tubal involvement often is accompanied by uterine adenomyosis on the same side.[301]

The external gross appearance is of one or more nodular swellings in the isthmus up to 1 to 2 cm in diameter. The serosa is smooth. On section, the tissue is firm, and careful inspection may disclose some of the dilated diverticula. Microscopically, the diverticula appear on cross-section as dispersed glands of tubal epithelium surrounded by broad bands of muscularis (Fig. 14.18). Diverticula may closely approach the serosal surface but do not normally connect with it. Endometrial-like stromal cells lying beneath the epithelial outpouchings may be abundant, sparse, or absent. If both glands and stroma are present, a diagnosis of tubal endometriosis may be considered. Because the underlying configuration is diverticular rather than glandular and since the condition is not clearly related to pelvic endometriosis, it seems best to continue using the term *salpingitis isthmica nodosa* until the etiology is better understood.

The most serious clinical and pathological complications of salpingitis isthmica nodosa are infertility and the strong association with ectopic pregnancy.[111,132,216] Inflammatory tubal disease may be associated with it ipsilaterally or contralaterally. A rare complication that we have seen is rupture of a deep diverticulum through the serosa, with subsequent mild intraabdominal bleeding and pelvic pain.

Ectopic Pregnancy

An ectopic pregnancy occurs when the developing blastocyst implants at a site other than in the endometrium of the fundus or lower uterine segment. Since well over 95% of ectopic pregnancies occur in the fallopian tube, the terms

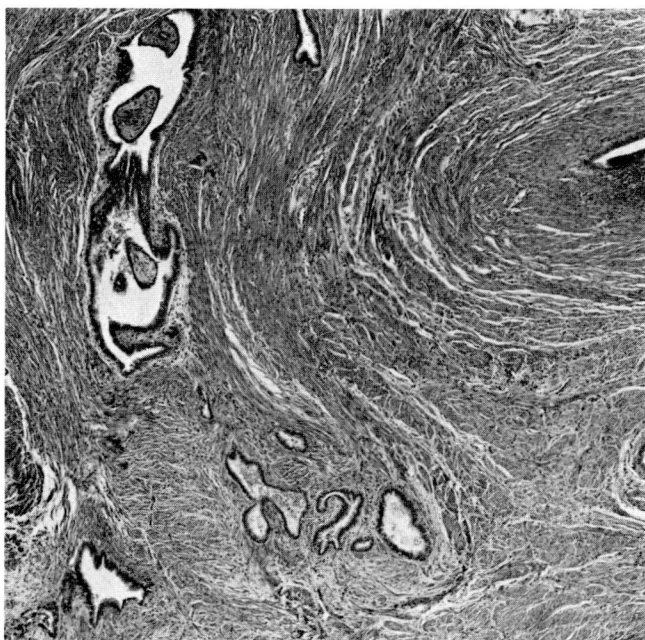

Fig. 14.18. Salpingitis isthmica nodosa. Tubal lumen is partially visible at *upper right*. Cross-sectioned diverticula are widely separated by broad bands of smooth muscle.

ectopic pregnancy and *tubal pregnancy* are nearly synonymous. However, implantation on both tubal fimbriae and ovary, in the abdominal cavity, in the uterine interstitium (intramural pregnancy[186]) or cornu, in the cervix,[30] or in the retroperitoneum[253] also may occur, in descending order of frequency. Hepatic and splenic pregnancy are both extremely rare.[122,282,302] Within the tube, most ectopic pregnancies are found in the ampulla (75–80%), with about 10–15% isthmic and 5% at the fimbriae.[30] Right-sided ectopic pregnancies comprise 52–57% of all tubal pregnancies.[26,30,31,139]

Epidemiologic studies note an increasing incidence of ectopic pregnancy.[10,19,130,236,290,292] Currently 1–2% of all conceptions are ectopic. Histological examination of curettings performed for elective termination of pregnancy reveals an absence of villi in 1 of every 100 women, and each has subsequently been shown to have an unsuspected ectopic pregnancy (personal observations). Ectopic pregnancies may be bilateral; in one series[26] the frequency was 2 of 905. Simultaneous ectopic and intrauterine implantations, so-called combined pregnancy, may occur in 1 in 10,000 to 30,000 pregnancies.[166,294]

ETIOLOGY

The mechanisms responsible for ectopic pregnancy are largely unknown, although any disease process that alters the normal tubal anatomy seems to increase the incidence. Whereas delay in entering the uterine cavity may predispose the blastocyst to tubal nidation, experimentally delayed conceptuses in rabbit, guinea pig, and mouse oviducts degenerate and fail to implant.[34] However, ectopic pregnancy is reported uncommonly in nonhuman primates.[162]

A history of previous pelvic inflammatory disease is the single most common antecedent factor in 35–45% of patients,[31,141,292] and the risk of ectopic pregnancy increases seven times after acute salpingitis.[292] Up to 88% of carefully studied tubes with an ectopic pregnancy also will show chronic salpingitis.[111]

Salpingitis isthmica nodosa,[216] previous pelvic surgery,[31] genital tuberculosis,[116] a history of prenatal DES exposure,[66] and vaginal douching[48] also appear as ectopic risk factors. Although IUDs have been identified in some studies as an independent risk factor for tubal or ovarian ectopic pregnancy,[178,201,224] in general it appears that ectopic rates are lower than in the general population, possibly because the selected population using the device.[118,279,300] The proportion of pregnancies that are ectopic in IUD users is quite high because of the efficacy of prevention of intrauterine pregnancy. Electively induced abortion does not appear to increase the frequency of ectopic pregnancy unless there is postabortal infection.[49] Tubal ectopic pregnancy after tubal sterilization may occur subsequent to tuboperitoneal fistula formation,[258] and repeat ectopic pregnancy on the same or opposite side is common (9%) after one ectopic pregnancy.[119] The increasing use of linear salpingostomy for the removal of an unruptured ectopic pregnancy, especially when only one tube is patent, poses the highest known risk for a repeat ectopic pregnancy (20%) but is tolerated because of the 50–60% chance for intrauterine pregnancy.[67] Ectopic pregnancy after hysterectomy is rare.[306] Abnormalities in the embryo may possibly lead to an increased tendency toward tubal implantation.[37]

CLINICAL FEATURES

Although many women with an ectopic pregnancy still appear as emergency patients with tubal rupture and hemorrhagic shock, because of the increasing frequency, clinicians consider any complaint of pelvic pain with or without menstrual irregularity as possible indication of an ectopic pregnancy. Quantitative, sensitive serum human chorionic gonadotropin (hCG) assays and ultrasonography to identify a gestational sac are subsequently performed.[131,231] Early diagnosis and operation result either in salpingostomy with conceptus removal or salpingectomy for an unruptured ectopic pregnancy. Trophoblastic tissue may persist after salpingostomy and conceptus removal.[174] The remaining tissue may retain its viability and form an ectopic-like tubal mass with a persistent hCG titer, requiring reoperation,[227] or may become implanted on pelvic or uterine serosal surfaces.[42]

PATHOLOGICAL FINDINGS

The unruptured tubal pregnancy is characterized grossly by a somewhat irregular sausage-like dilatation of the tube, with a bluish discoloration due to hematosalpinx (Fig. 14.19). Chorionic villi usually are found in the blood-filled and dilated tubal lumen and, in 75% of cases, appear viable.[199] Nearly two-thirds of cases contain a grossly or microscopically identifiable embryo,[199] and multiple pregnancies may occur.[100]

The extra villous intermediate trophoblast of the conceptus penetrates deep in the tubal wall and into tubal blood vessels. Perhaps because of the limited ability of the endosalpingeal stroma to undergo decidualization, and analogous to a placenta increta, the chorionic villi then invade, first muscularis and then serosa.[213] Another major difference with uterine implantation is the failure of tubal trophoblast to differentiate into chorion frondosum and chorion laeve.[223] Vascular changes in mid-sized tubal arteries adjacent to ectopic pregnancies are similar to those found in the vessels near uterine implantations, with invasion by intermediate trophoblast, proliferation of the vascular intima, and accumulation of foam cells in the intima.[25] Chronic salpingitis is found adjacent to the ectopic pregnancy in nearly half the patients, with a reported range of 29–88%.[111,199] Ultrastructural studies may demonstrate decreased or absent areas of ciliation in the mucosa adja-

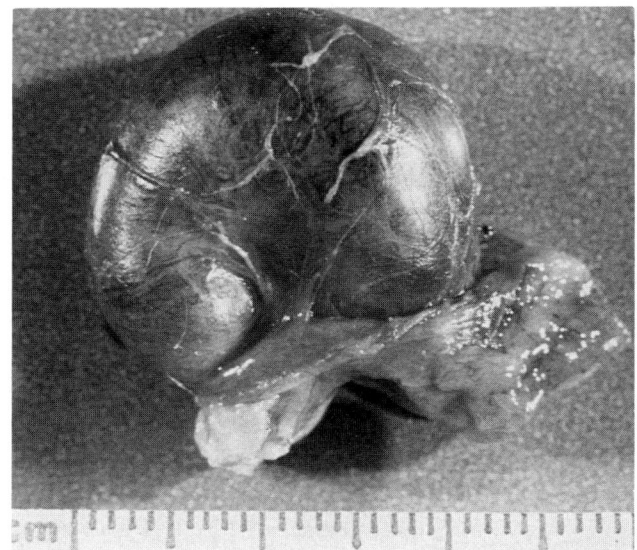

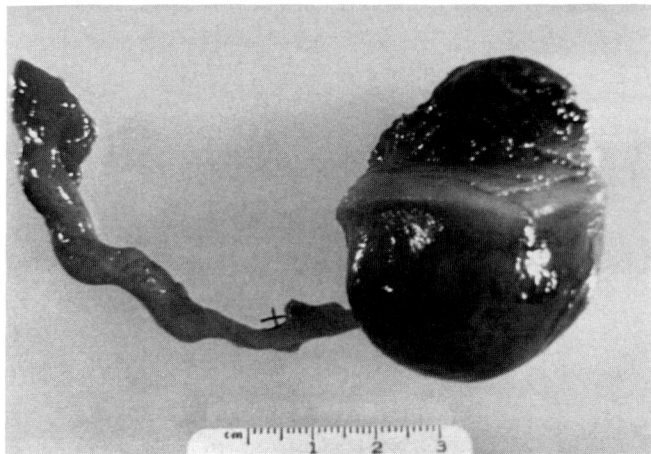

FIG. 14.19. Unruptured ectopic pregnancy. *Top:* Tubal pregnancy. A resected, kinked portion of tube is expanded by the growing pregnancy. Intraluminal blood imparts a bluish discoloration. The thin fibrous peritubal adhesions suggest previous salpingitis. *Bottom:* Cornual pregnancy. The attached tube is normal, but the resected uterine cornu is expanded by the hemorrhagic mass of a nonviable ectopic pregnancy.

cent to the ectopic pregnancy.[281] The tubal wall should be examined microscopically for the diverticula of salpingitis isthmica nodosa.

The pathology of extratubal ectopic pregnancy varies according to the site. Cornual or interstitial pregnancies may expand up to about 12 weeks, when rupture may lacerate one of the uterine arteries as well as the entire side of the uterus. Cervical ectopic pregnancy presents much as an incomplete abortion with bleeding. Because of the fibrous cervical tissue underlying placental implantation, control of bleeding may be difficult.[140]

Ovarian pregnancy is clinically similar to tubal pregnancy, including frequent preoperative rupture.[117] More than half of the patients in one series had a history of previous reproductive tract disease or infertility,[112] and 17–25% had an IUD in place.[85,112]

Macroscopic examination typically reveals a hemorrhagic mass replacing the ovary. The pathological criteria for ovarian pregnancy proposed by Spiegelberg[254] are (1) the tube must be intact and separate from the ovary, (2) the gestational sac must occupy the normal position of the ovary, (3) the gestational sac must be connected to the uterus by the uteroovarian ligament, and (4) ovarian tissue must be demonstrated within the wall of the sac. Pathological documentation of ovarian tissue within the pregnancy may be difficult or impossible if treatment consists of conservative resection or if the pregnancy has extensively replaced the ovarian tissue.

The endometrial glandular changes described by Arias–Stella (see Chapter 9, Anatomy and Histology of the Uterine Corpus) may be found in at least 60% of women with ectopic pregnancy. In addition, very similar changes of nuclear atypia and some cytoplasmic vacuolization occasionally may be found in carefully studied tubes[23,187] (Fig. 14.20).

Sequelae

The natural history of tubal ectopic pregnancy includes spontaneous expulsion from the fimbriated end—tubal abortion—as well as embryonal death and involution of the conceptus. Typically, however, continued growth of the trophoblast leads to increasing dilatation and weakening of the muscularis, with rupture about the eighth week (Fig. 14.21). Because hemorrhage may be massive, it is a major cause of maternal mortality.[77] A few tubal pregnancies have proceeded to term with fetal viability. Peritoneal irritation and formation of dense intestinal adhesions is likely to occur in these patients.[96]

Some tubal pregnancies form a chronic inflammatory mass that, with involution of trophoblast and reestablishment of the menstrual cycle, may present problems in differential diagnosis. The convoluted, blood-filled tube, often with involved ipsilateral ovary, may simulate tumor[135] or an endometriotic mass (Fig. 14.22). Extensive microscopic sampling of a so-called chronic ectopic pregnancy may be required to demonstrate a few ghost villi (Fig. 14.23). In more advanced pregnancy, death of the fetus with retention in the extrauterine location may be followed by calcification of the fetus (lithopedion) or both membranes and fetus (lithokelyphopedion). The mass formed may be discovered only incidentally decades later.[188]

Infertility

Most of the diseases discussed in this chapter may result in sufficient anatomic distortion to cause infertility. In contrast, purely physiological tubal dysfunction is not well defined but may be illustrated by the immotile cilia of Kartagener's syndrome that may lead to reduced fertility;

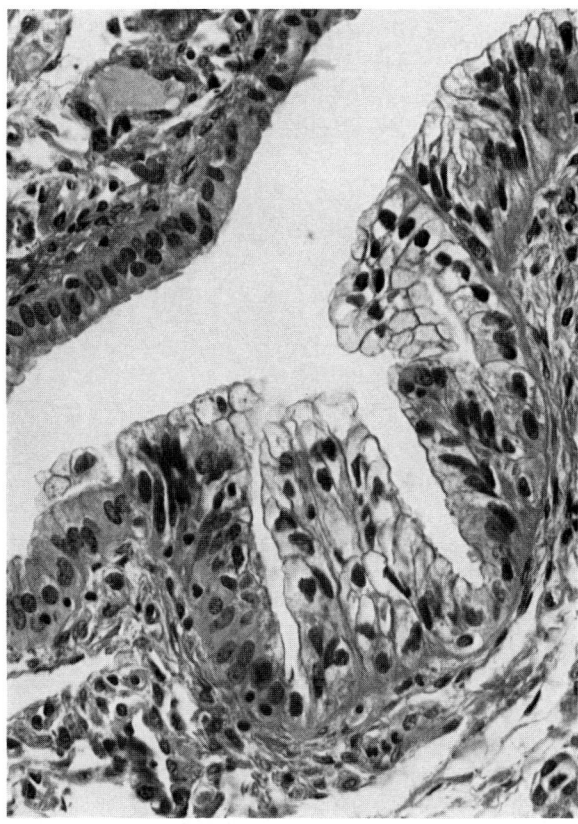

Fig. 14.20. Arias–Stella reaction in tubal epithelium. Note the focally clear epithelial cell cytoplasm, with nuclear enlargement and hyperchromatism.

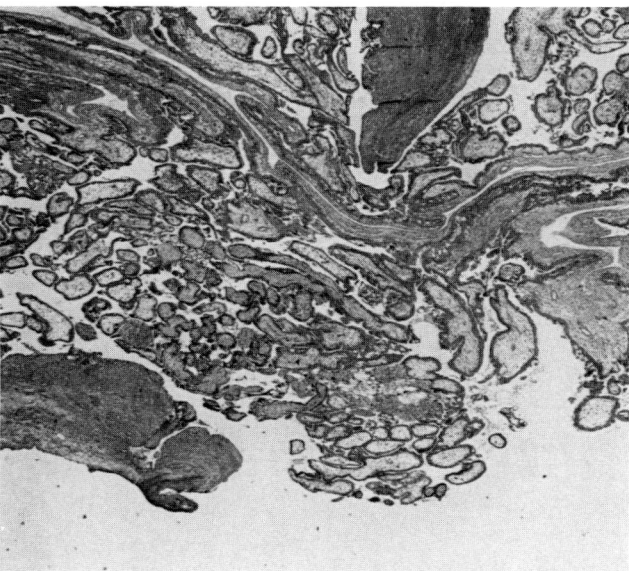

Fig. 14.21. Ruptured tubal pregnancy. After penetration of the tubal musculature by the trophoblastic cells of the ectopic pregnancy, the muscle wall *(top center and bottom left)* weakens and ruptures, with extrusion of chorionic villi.

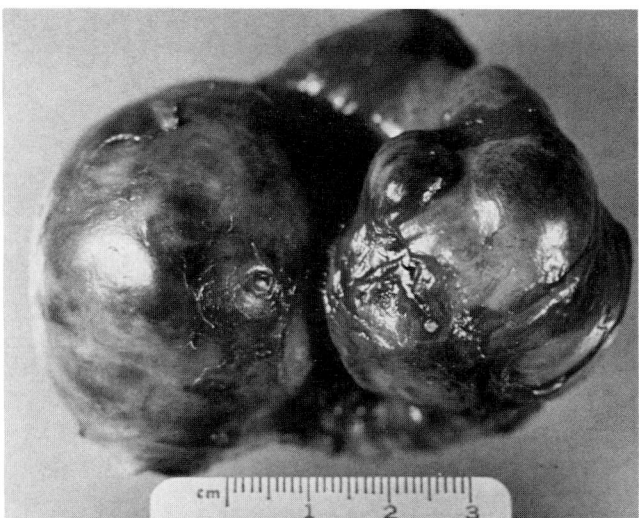

FIG. 14.22. Chronic ectopic pregnancy. This irregularly lobulated mass grossly simulated an ovarian neoplasm.

only 3 of 12 women in one series succeeded in becoming pregnant.[5]

Peritubal adhesions secondary to endometriosis, prior pelvic inflammatory disease, or appendicitis may interfere with normal tubal motility and ovum pickup. Adhesion lysis may be curative. Multiple fimbrial adhesions secondary to gonococcal or other inflammatory tubal disease may be treated by operative lysis and surgical eversion of tubal mucosa. Obliterative fibrosis, possibly secondary to inflammation within the uterus, may lead to obstruction at the uterotubal junction.[95] Resection of the obstruction and microsurgical anastomosis or tubal reimplantation may result in patency rates of about 80–85% and term pregnancy rates of 50%[196] to nearly 80%.[109] Whereas tubal surgery for infertility has been criticized for lack of convincing evidence of effectiveness,[52] untreated complete bilateral tubal obstruction offers no expectation of spontaneous cure, and surgery offers some hope of pregnancy. Typically, tubal patency rates are approximately double the rates for intrauterine pregnancy, and ectopic pregnancy is an ever-present risk.

Tubal patency is commonly checked by hysterosalpingography,[247] using radiopaque dye or intrauterine dye injection with tubal monitoring via laparoscopy (chromopertubation). Cannulation of the tube with a falloposcope of minute diameter and a 0.3-mm lens affords an opportunity to visually assess patency, luminal adhesions, and the state of the epithelial surface.[149] More physiologic methods recently reported[260] may prove useful.

Contraception by interference with tubal function involves procedures designed to damage the tube by caustic chemicals, electrocautery, or surgical removal of a segment of the tube or to obstruct it by placement of a clip.

Intrauterine placement of quinacrine hydrochloride pellets for sterilization leads to necrosis of intramural endosalpingeal mucosa. The associated inflammation and progressive submucosal fibrosis leads to luminal narrowing or obliteration.[82,193] Tubal resection should be confirmed by histological demonstration of a cross-section of tube including the entire tubal lumen. Despite these procedures, spontaneous reanastomosis or fistula formation (Fig. 14.24)

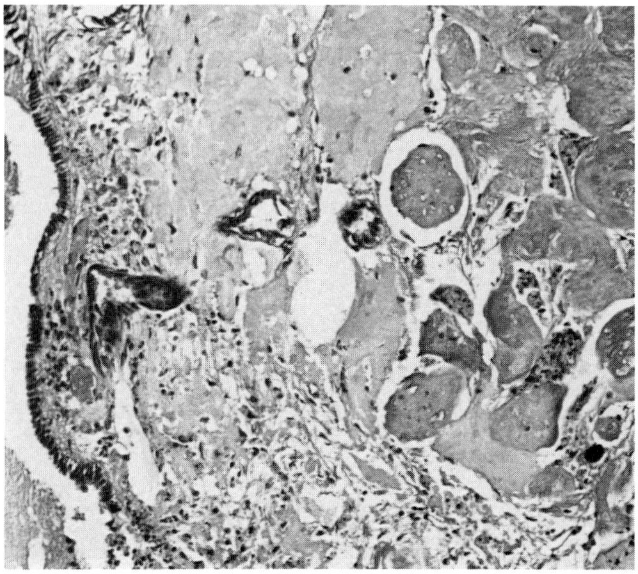

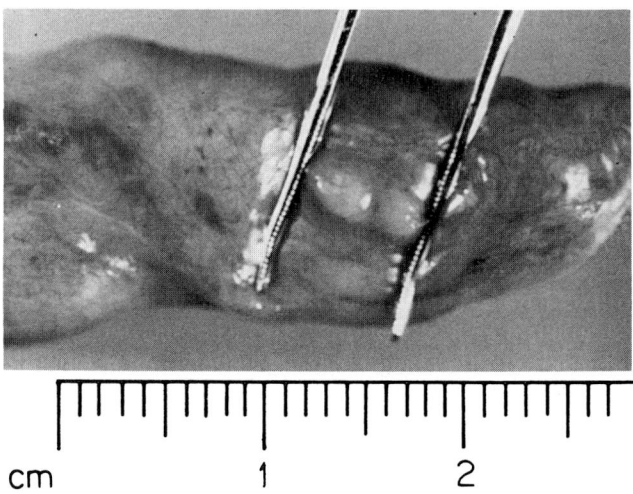

FIG. 14.24. Postligation tubal fistula. This proximal tubal segment was removed simultaneously with an ectopic pregnancy on the opposite side. Slight pressure on the forceps has caused the endosalpingeal mucosa to pout out through a 2- to-3-mm fistulous opening, with the lumen represented by a small dimple in the *center.*

FIG. 14.23. Chronic ectopic pregnancy. Proteinaceous fluid is present in the distorted tubal lumen on the *left.* Fibrotic chorionic villi replacing the normal tubal architecture are present on the *right.*

may occur in approximately 1% of all patients and may lead to fertilization and ectopic or intrauterine pregnancy.[252] Failure rates may be higher in training programs in which clips and rings are more apt to be misapplied.[261] To identify the cause of failure of tubal sterilization procedures, careful gross examination of the specimen, occasionally specimen salpingography, longitudinal orientation of the tubal segment in paraffin, and meticulous sectioning techniques may be necessary.[259] Fistula formation at suture and excision sites appears to be the most common cause of failure after segmental resection. Up to 70% of pregnancies after electrocoagulation are ectopic.[270] Other complications of tubal sterilization have been reviewed recently.[46] The success of surgical reanastomosis in reestablishing a patent lumen varies with the extent of the initial procedure and the skill of the surgeon but is reported to be as high as 80%. Only 25–40% of the patients, however, will subsequently become pregnant. The frequency of ectopic pregnancy after reanastomosis is increased. This may be due to residual fibrosis after the original ligation or to endosalpingeal distortion, which may mimic salpingitis isthmica nodosa.

The American Fertility Society has proposed schemes for the classification of adhesions, tubal occlusions, tubal pregnancies, and müllerian anomalies.[9] The use of standardized nomenclature should make it easier to judge the efficacy of different treatment modalities.

Benign Neoplasms

Both benign and malignant tumors of the fallopian tube are uncommon. They are frequently mistaken for lesions of chronic salpingitis or pyosalpinx, both preoperatively and during the operative procedure itself. Benign tumors are most often of mesodermal origin and usually are small enough to be incidental findings at laparotomy.

Inclusion Cysts and Walthard Nests

The tubal serosa, by invagination, may give rise to a number of benign inclusion cysts. The simplest is a 1- to 2-mm unilocular cyst lying directly beneath the serosal surface lined by mesothelial cells, a mesothelial inclusion cyst. By a process of metaplasia, these cysts may become filled with polygonal epithelial-like cells to form a Walthard nest. On gross examination, a 1- to 2-mm yellowish white nodule lies beneath the serosa. The cells of the Walthard nest often fully occupy it. Their nuclei are irregularly ovoid, and a longitudinal nuclear groove gives them a coffee-bean appearance (Fig. 14.25). Cystic nests may be lined by nonciliated nonmucinous columnar cells. Both mesothelial inclusion cysts and Walthard nests are common incidental findings of no clinical importance.

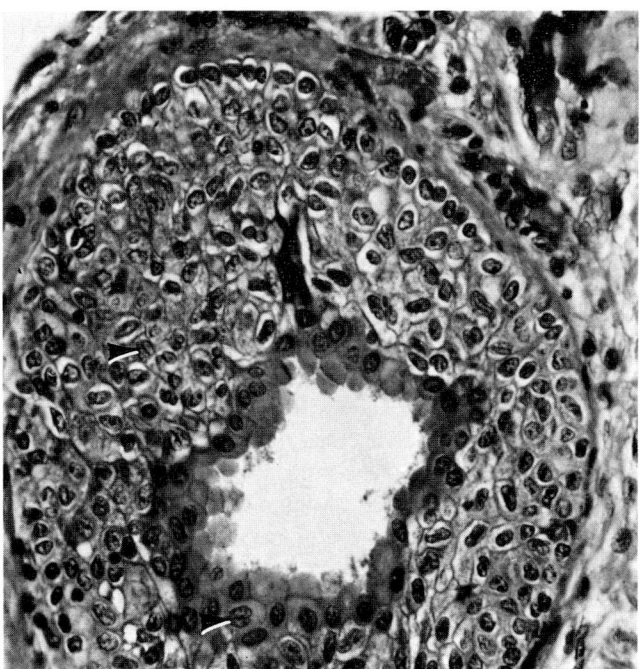

FIG. 14.25. Walthard nest. The most central epithelial cells have undergone columnar metaplasia. Nuclear grooves are visible (*arrowheads*) in other epithelial cells as dark lines in the long axis of ovoid nuclei. Note the serosal surface at *upper left*.

Epithelial Papilloma

Epithelial papillomas or polyps are rare.[108,147] They are composed of a delicate, branching stromal stalk lined by a single layer of nonciliated columnar or oncocytic cells with regular nuclei (Fig. 14.26). Whether or not these lesions have malignant potential is unknown. Because papillary proliferations may accompany salpingitis (see Fig. 14.8b), a

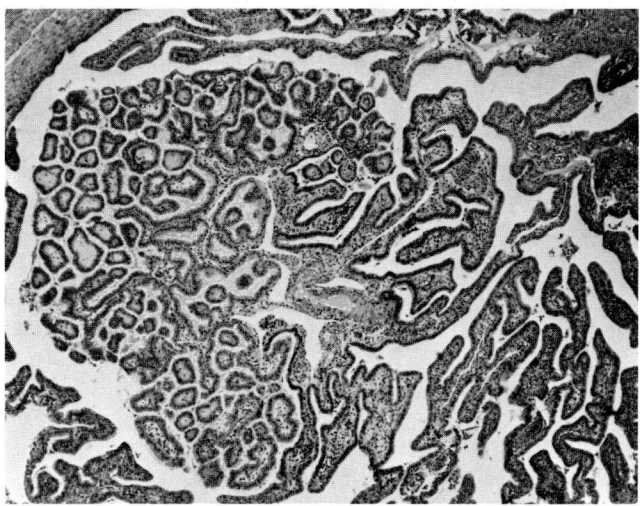

FIG. 14.26. Epithelial papilloma. Single layer of uniform cells lines a delicately branched papillary core.

diagnosis of a papilloma in the presence of inflammation or plical distortion secondary to previous inflammation may not be warranted. The so-called metaplastic papillary tumor of the tube associated with pregnancy[15,237] in most cases appears to represent a papillary oncocytic metaplastic process rather than a true neoplasm.

Leiomyoma and Adenomyoma

Tumors of smooth muscle origin, chiefly leiomyomas, may originate from the tubal muscularis, from smooth muscle of the broad ligament, or from walls of blood vessels in either location. Compared with the frequency of uterine leiomyomas, tubal leiomyomas are quite uncommon.[177,228] Microscopically, they are similar to those found in the uterus, and they can undergo similar degenerative changes. Rarely, benign glands and smooth muscle may be so intimately involved in a tumor that a true adenomyoma is produced (Fig. 14.27).

Adenomatoid Tumor

Adenomatoid tumor (benign mesothelioma) is the most frequent type of benign tubal tumor. Previously reported lymphangiomas[239] probably represent examples of this entity. They are usually only 1 to 2 cm in diameter, appearing as a nodular swelling beneath the tubal serosa, and are yellow or whitish gray on section. They are rarely bilateral.[305] Similar lesions may be found in the uterus,[274] cul-de-sac,[299] or ovary (see Chapter 13, Mesenchymal Tumors of the Uterus, and Chapter 21, Nonspecific Tumors of the Ovary, Including Mesenchymal Tumors and Malignant Lymphoma). Their origin is presumed to be from the cells

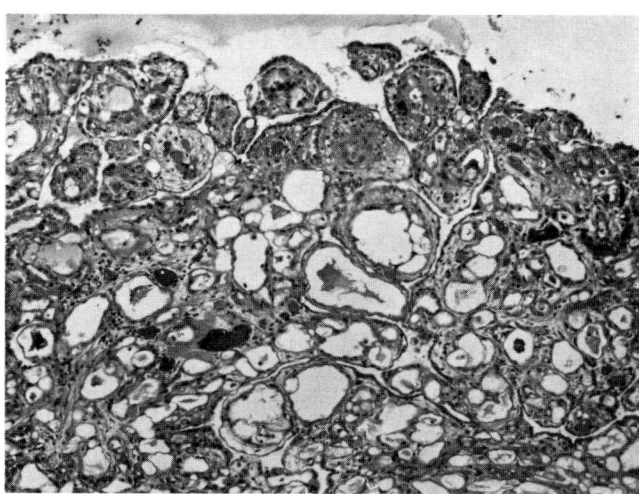

FIG. 14.28. Adenomatoid tumor (benign mesothelioma). Multiple connections with serosal surface are seen at *top*.

of the serosal mesothelium. A fortuitous section may demonstrate a connection between serosa and tumor (Fig. 14.28), but usually the serosa covers the lesion. Microscopically, multiple, small, slit-like or ovoid spaces are lined by a single layer of low cuboidal or flattened epithelial-like cells (Fig. 14.29). The tumor may be large enough to displace the tubal lumen eccentrically and may grow into the supporting stroma of the luminal folds in an infiltrating manner (Fig. 14.30). On frozen section the gynecological pathologist must differentiate the adenomatoid tumor from an infiltrating adenocarcinoma. Histochemical studies[272] have shown hyaluronidase-digestible, alcian blue–positive material in the cells and spaces. No significant

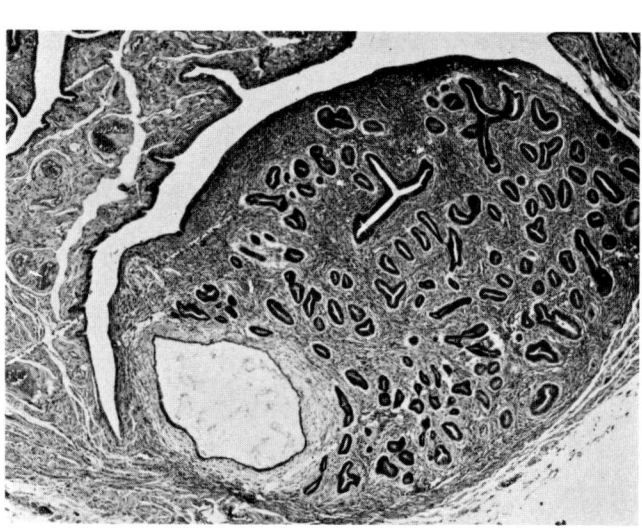

FIG. 14.27. Adenomyoma. A nodule of mixed simple glands and smooth muscle fibers protrudes into the tubal lumen.

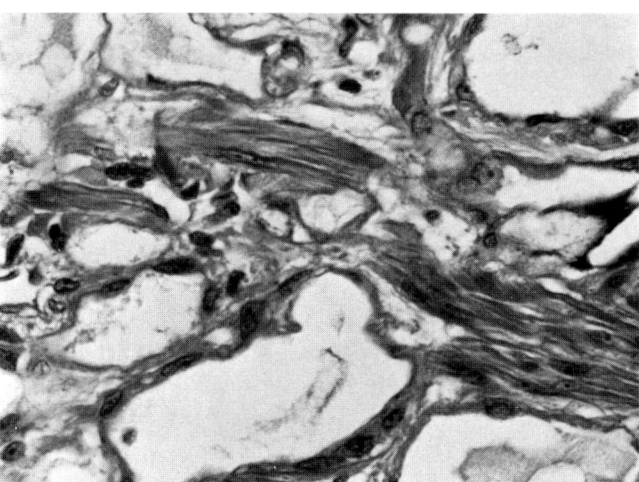

FIG. 14.29. Adenomatoid tumor (benign mesothelioma). Cuboidal or flattened mesothelial cells line dilated slit-like spaces. Infiltration between small bundles of smooth muscle is seen here.

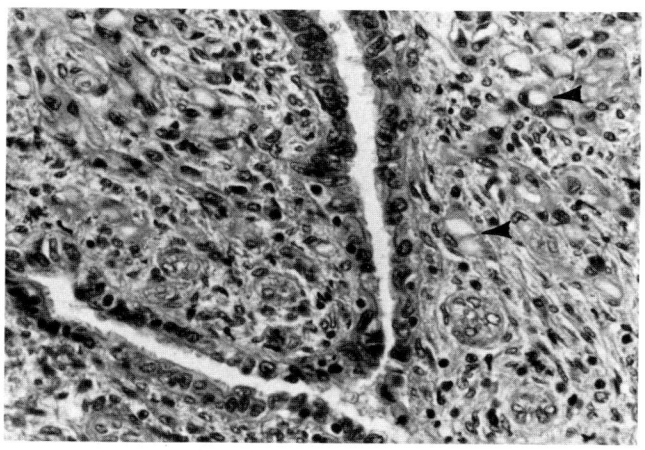

FIG. 14.30. **Adenomatoid tumor (benign mesothelioma).** Tumor infiltrates mucosal folds in a diffuse manner. Vacuolated cells with a signet-ring appearance are evident on the right side of the field *(arrowheads)*. Confusion with carcinoma is possible on frozen section. Note the intact epithelium of the tubal lumen.

glycogen or intracellular mucin is present, as might be found in a tumor of müllerian origin. Electron microscopic[90,272] and immunocytochemical studies support a mesothelial origin for these lesions. Microvilli project from the cell surfaces. Bundles of tonofilaments are present and occasionally are attached to desmosomes. Desmosomes are numerous between cells but are absent along the basal lamina on which the cells lie. These features are not characteristic of endothelial or müllerian epithelium but are seen in benign mesotheliomas[90] as well as in malignant mesotheliomas. Clinically, they are asymptomatic, and rarely, if ever, do they recur after adequate excision.

Other Benign Mesenchymal and Mixed Epithelial–Mesenchymal Tumors

These tumors are rare. Hemangiomas,[79] lipomas,[68] angiomyolipomas,[144] adenofibromas,[44] and neural tumors[204,289] have been reported. Their microscopic appearance is identical to that of similar tumors appearing elsewhere in the body. Occasionally, a benign fibroblastic or fatty tumor will contain a focus of cartilage.[13,205]

Teratoma

Tubal teratomas are rare. Clinically, a patient with a tubal teratoma usually is nulliparous and in the fourth decade.[184] Grossly, the tumors are located most frequently in the lumen, often attached by a pedicle to the inner tubal wall. They may, however, be intramural or attached to the serosa. On section, they are more often cystic than solid and may be small (1–2 cm in diameter) or large (10–20 cm in diameter).[184] As in their ovarian counterparts, ectodermal, mesodermal, and endodermal tissues are represented by

well-differentiated mature elements. One lesion consisting entirely of mature thyroid tissue was described in the tube of a woman without clinical hyperthyroidism.[124] An isolated nodule of pancreatic tissue has been found beneath the tubal mucosa of one patient.[182] Only rare cases of histologically immature tubal teratoma have been described.[14] Although ovarian teratomas appear to originate in abnormally developing ova,[257] only one patient is mentioned in whom ovarian tissue containing ova was found within tubal mucosa.[154]

Malignant Neoplasms

Carcinoma In Situ

Carcinoma in situ (CIS) of the tube is diagnosed accurately only when the epithelial cells of the endosalpingeal lining form papillae with cytologically malignant mitotically active nuclei (Fig. 14.31). CIS may be seen adjacent to invasive tumor in carefully studied cases of tubal carcinoma or in cases of malignant mixed mesodermal tumor, and should not be confused with endosalpingeal seeding from primary ovarian carcinoma (Fig. 14.39).

Previous authors[212,215,299] have illustrated cases in which tubal epithelium showed nuclear crowding and atypia and termed the change *CIS*. It is clear that carefully studied tubes demonstrate similar changes in 18% of routinely accessioned salpingectomy specimens[191] (see Fig. 14.4). Although the lesions are more common in tubes with

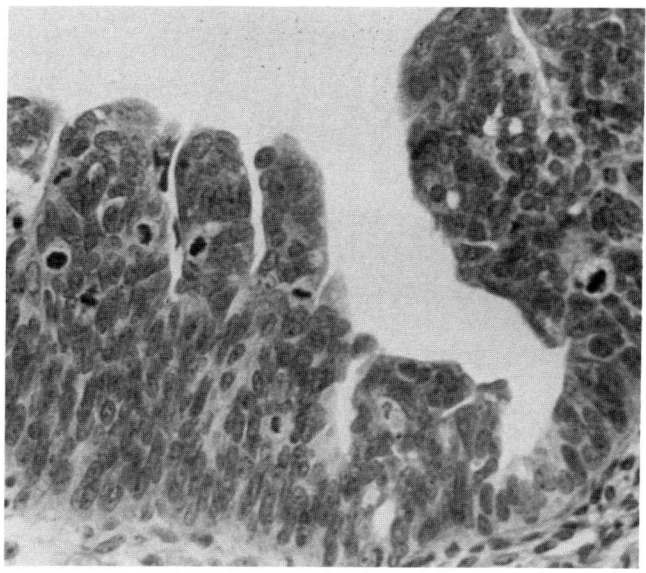

FIG. 14.31. **Carcinoma in situ.** The epithelial cells have lost their polarity and are growing in papillae without stromal cores. Nuclei are hyperchromatic, large, and irregular, and mitoses are numerous. The basement membrane is intact.

salpingitis (see Fig. 14.16), 14% of otherwise normal tubes show changes consisting of nuclear crowding and stratification, loss of polarity, and nuclear atypia. Mitoses are sparse. Frequently, changes are present in only one or two of many sections. Papillary formation with bridging reminiscent of some forms of mammary papillomatosis may occur. Hyperplastic epithelial changes may be more common in patients who have an associated ovarian epithelial tumor.[229] An oncocytic "pink cell" metaplasia with cytoplasmic acidophilia occasionally is present (Figs. 14.3, 14.32). Startling epithelial changes that mimic early papillary adenocarcinoma may be produced by accidental exposure of the specimen to heat.[54]

Invasive Adenocarcinoma

Primary adenocarcinoma of the tube is uncommon. Only 0.2–0.5% of primary female genital malignancies are tubal,[218,303] a prevalence of about 3.6 per million women per year.[233]

Unfortunately, primary tubal carcinoma is rarely found in the in situ stage. The typical patient is usually in her sixth or seventh decade and is rarely younger than 35 years.[233] Nulliparity is present in about 30% of patients.[218,219] The classic signs and symptoms of invasive tubal carcinoma include vaginal bleeding, clear or serosanguinous vaginal discharge (hydrops tubae profluens), pelvic pain, and a pelvic mass.[80,121,218,245,304] The diagnosis is rarely made before operation, but occasionally positive cytology associated with negative endometrial curettage will suggest the correct location of the neoplasm.[18,245]

Grossly, the tube usually is swollen secondary to advanced intraluminal growth. Hydrosalpinx or tuboovarian abscess is ruled out only after the specimen is opened. The lumen usually is filled and dilated by papillary or solid tumor (Fig. 14.33). The fimbriated end is closed in about half the cases.[299]

Bilateral involvement frequently occurs, but the reason for this is unknown. A common carcinogenic stimulus could cause simultaneous development of tumor in both tubes, or a retrograde lymphatic spread after blockage by advanced tubal carcinoma of one side could lead to contralateral metastatic deposits. Subsequent growth might then mimic a second primary tumor. The fact that bilateral tubal carcinoma is present in only 7% of stage 0–II lesions but may be seen in as many as 30% of stage III and IV tumors[244] suggests that metastatic spread in advanced lesions is an important cause of bilaterality.

Microscopically, tubal neoplasms may be classified as epithelial, mixed epithelial–mesenchymal, or mesenchymal (see Table 14.1). The vast majority of tumors are histologically similar to serous adenocarcinomas of the ovary. They are composed of fine branching papillae covered by one or more layers of epithelium with enlarged pleomorphic hyperchromatic nuclei with both increased and abnormal mitoses (Figs. 14.34, 14.35). In poorly differentiated areas the tumor may grow in solid sheets of cells with small or large foci of necrosis.

Abrupt transitions from normal to neoplastic epithelium may be found. Attempts to grade tumor pattern or degree of nuclear atypia have proved to be of limited prognostic value.[71,121,218,219,304] A number of staging schemes have been proposed based on operative or operative combined with pathological findings.[8,84,244] The Oncology Committee of the International Federation of Gynecology and Obstetrics (FIGO) recently has established a staging system for tubal carcinoma based on that for ovarian carcinoma[56] (Table 14.2). Once tumor spreads to the serosa, 5-year survival drops to only one patient in six (Table 14.3),

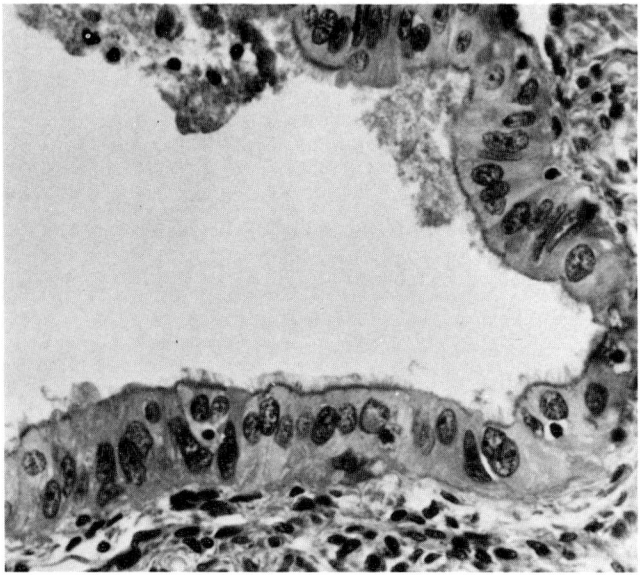

FIG. 14.32. **Benign oncocytic (pink cell) metaplasia.** Nuclear atypia and cell crowding in absence of papillary formations and mitoses should not be confused with early carcinoma.

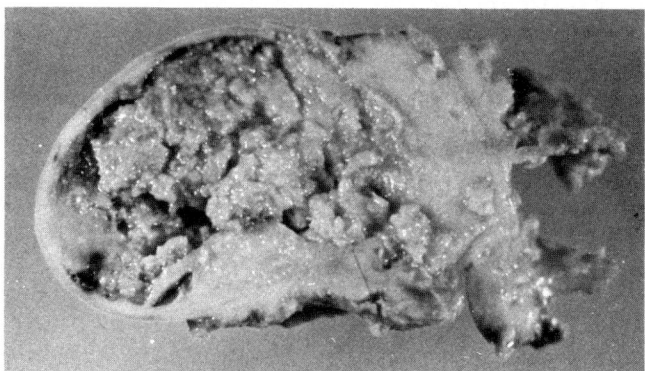

FIG. 14.33. **Primary tubal adenocarcinoma.** Tube is dilated and filled by papillary and solid tumor, which penetrates the muscularis along the lower margin of the specimen.

Table 14.1. Tumors of the fallopian tube (WHO classification)

Epithelial tumors
  Benign
    Adenoma
    Papilloma
    Metaplastic papillary tumor
    Other
  Of borderline malignancy[a]
  Malignant
    Carcinoma in situ
    Serous carcinoma
    Mucinous carcinoma
    Endometrioid carcinoma
    Clear cell carcinoma
    Transitional cell carcinoma
    Squamous cell carcinoma
    Undifferentiated and other
Mixed epithelial–mesenchymal tumors
  Benign
    Adenofibroma
    Adenomyoma
    Adenomatoid
    Other
  Malignant
    Adenosarcoma[a]
    Mesodermal (müllerian) mixed tumor
      Homologous (carcinosarcoma)
      Heterologous
Mesenchymal tumors
  Benign
    Leiomyoma
    Adenomatoid
    Others
  Malignant
    Leiomyosarcoma
    Others

[a] Not reported.

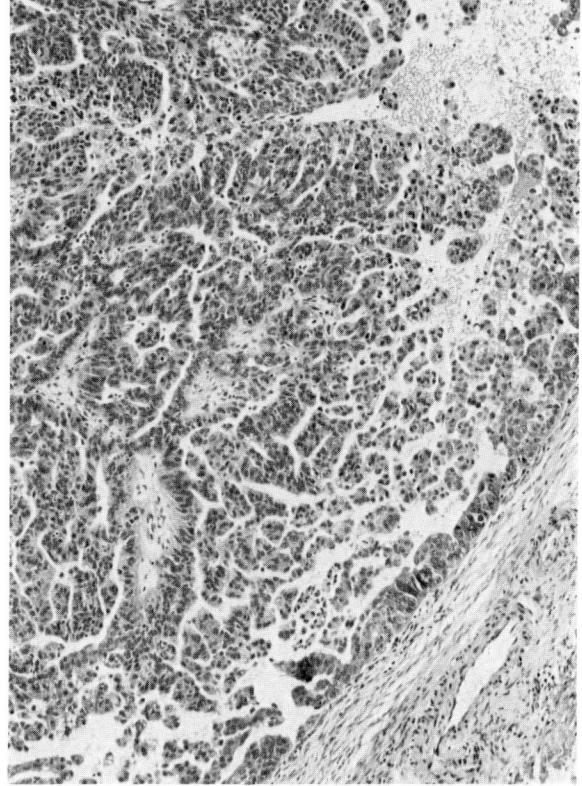

Fig. 14.34. Primary tubal serous carcinoma. The tumor is characterized by a delicate fibrovascular branching core supporting proliferating atypical epithelial cells. Invasion is present in adjacent areas of the wall.

and even 5-year survival is not synonymous with cure.[218,232,244]

Carcinoma subtypes other than serous are uncommon in the tube. Mucinous carcinomas may contain prominent goblet cells on histological examination. Synchronous mucinous primaries have been described in the tube and endocervix.[138] Endometrioid carcinoma may resemble that of the ovary, with or without focal squamous differentiation, or may have an unusual histological appearance suggestive of an adnexal tumor of probable wolffian origin.[65] Primary squamous,[44a,176] adenosquamous,[190] transitional cell,[89] clear cells,[285] and glassy cell[125] carcinomas are rarely seen.

Current treatment by total abdominal hysterectomy and bilateral salpingo-oophorectomy with or without adjuvant radiation or chemotherapy usually fails because of transperitoneal spread.[71] Aggressive cytoreduction and chemotherapy in advanced disease may yield complete responses for more than 3 years.[194] The CA-125 antigenic determinant found in ovarian carcinoma also is characteristic of tubal serous carcinomas[221] and may prove useful in patient follow-up.[200,278] As with other gynecological cancers, tubal carcinoma may cause a variety of paraneoplastic syndromes.[51,128]

Sarcomas and Mixed Epithelial–Mesenchymal Tumors

Sarcomas of the tube may be classified as pure or mixed (Table 14.1). Mixed neoplasms containing cytologically benign epithelial elements are designated adenosarcoma, whereas those containing malignant epithelial areas are designated malignant mixed müllerian tumor. Pure sarcomas may be histologically subtyped if sufficient differentiation is present. Leiomyosarcomas[3] are perhaps the most common type and may arise from the tube or broad ligament. Chondrosarcomas have been described.[3,242] Adenosarcoma arising in the tube has not been reported.

Malignant mixed mesodermal tumors (MMMT) by definition contain both malignant epithelial and malignant mesenchymal elements. The few dozen patients reported

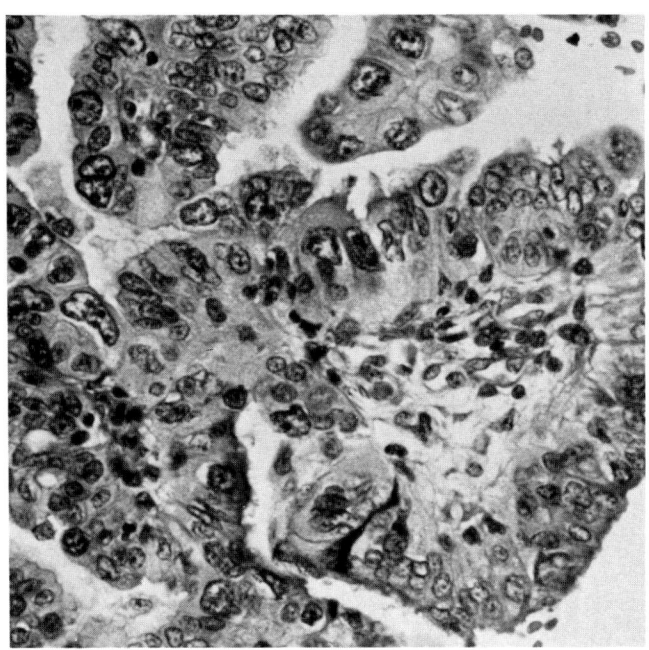

Fig. 14.35. Tubal serous adenocarcinoma. The tumor cells covering the fibrovascular core *(center)* have lost their nuclear polarity. Their nuclei are large, irregular, and hyperchromatic.

Table 14.3. Staging and survival in adenocarcinoma of the fallopian tube

Stage	Definition	No. of patients	Percent 5-year survival without disease
0	Carcinoma in situ	11	82
I	Tumor extends into submucosa or muscularis, not serosa	13	53
II	Tumor extends to serosa	6	16
III	Tumor extends to ovary and/or endometrium	12	8
IV	Tumor extends beyond reproductive organs	34	9

After Schiller and Silverberg, ref. 244.

in the literature are nearly all postmenopausal, with a mean age of 59.[40,151] They may have watery or bloody vaginal discharge and abdominal pain with signs of peritoneal spread. Grossly the tumors distend the tube and usually have spread to adjacent pelvic and abdominal structures. The ovary must be identified clearly to rule out an origin in that organ. The opened tube reveals a shaggy mucosal surface with areas of necrosis and hemorrhage (Fig. 14.36). Microscopically distinct sarcomatous and carcinomatous areas should be identifiable (Figs. 14.37, 14.38). Malignant squamous or glandular foci (or both) lie in an atypical mitotically active spindle-cell background of sarcoma. The sarcoma may consist only of malignant elements homologous to the tube, such as smooth muscle or stroma (for which the term *carcinosarcoma* was formerly used),[120] but commonly malignant cartilaginous areas or foci of osteosarcoma or rhabdomyosarcoma are seen. Areas of mucosal carcinoma in situ may be apparent adjacent to the main tumor mass.[40] The major differential diagnostic pitfall is a poorly differentiated carcinoma with spindle-cell metaplasia. Life expectancy usually is measured in months, but

Table 14.2. International Federation of Gynecologists and Obstetricians (FIGO) fallopian tube tumor staging

Stage 0	Carcinoma in situ (limited to tubal mucosa)
Stage I	Growth limited to fallopian tubes
Stage IA	Growth limited to one tube with extension into submucosa and/or muscularis but not penetrating serosal surface; no ascites
Stage IB	Growth limited to both tubes with extension into submucosa and/or muscularis but not penetrating serosal surface; no ascites
Stage IC	Tumor either Stage 1A or Stage 1B but with extension through or onto tubal serosa or with ascites containing malignant cells or with positive peritoneal washings
Stage II	Growth involving one or more fallopian tubes with pelvic extension
Stage IIA	Extension and/or metastases to uterus and/or ovaries
Stage IIB	Extension to other pelvic tissues
Stage IIC	Tumor either Stage IIA or IIB and with ascites containing malignant cells or with positive peritoneal washings
Stage III	Tumor involving one or both fallopian tubes with peritoneal implants outside pelvis and/or positive retroperitoneal or inguinal nodes. Superficial liver metastasis equals stage III. Tumor appears limited to true pelvis but with histologically proved malignant extension to small bowel or omentum
Stage IIIA	Tumor grossly limited to true pelvis with negative nodes but with histologically confirmed microscopic seeding of abdominal peritoneal surfaces
Stage IIIB	Tumor involving one or both tubes with histologically confirmed implants of abdominal peritoneal surfaces, none exceeding 2 cm in diameter. Lymph nodes are negative
Stage IIIC	Abdominal implants >2 cm in diameter and/or positive retroperitoneal or inguinal nodes
Stage IV	Growth involving one or both fallopian tubes with distant metastases. If pleural effusion is present, cytological fluid must be positive for malignant cells to be Stage IV. Parenchymal liver metastasis equals Stage IV

Note: Staging for fallopian tube carcinoma is by the surgical pathological system. Operative findings designating stage are determined before tumor debulking.

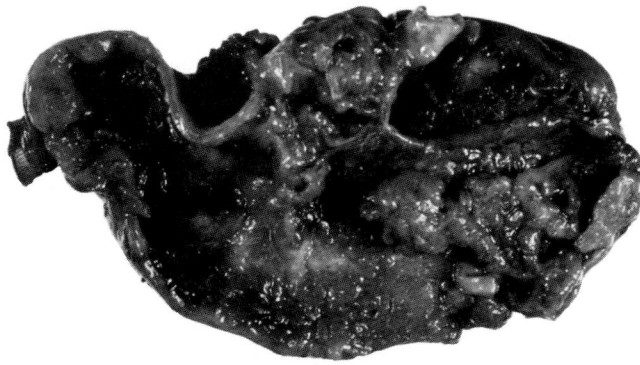

FIG. 14.36. **Primary malignant mixed mesodermal tumor.** Dilated tube has been opened to illustrate the irregular intraluminal projections and a shaggy, irregular mucosal surface.

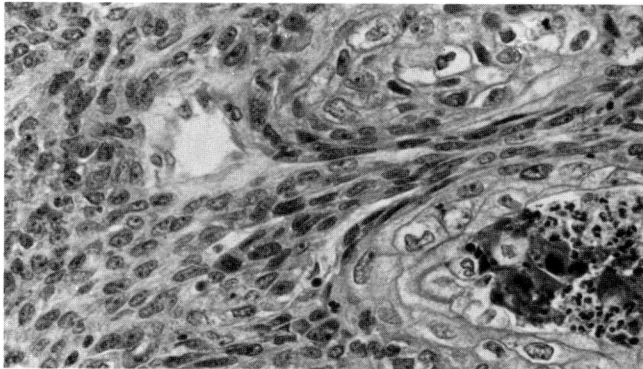

FIG. 14.37. **Primary malignant mixed mesodermal tumor.** Two ovoid islands of malignant squamous epithelium *(right)* lie in the stroma of a leiomyosarcoma.

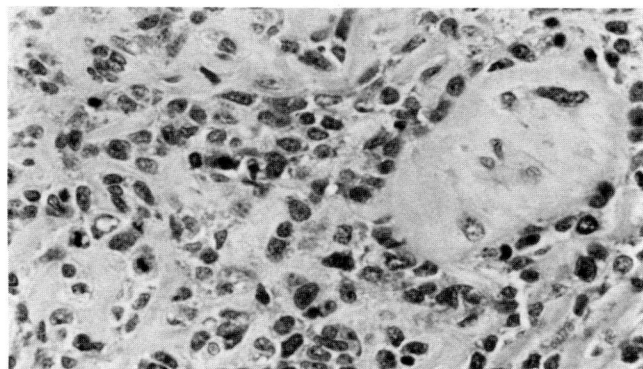

FIG. 14.38. **Primary malignant mixed mesodermal tumor.** At *right*, a relatively acellular nodule of osteoid is seen in a sarcomatous background. Elsewhere, carcinomatous areas are present.

surgery and chemotherapy may lead to longer remission.[40,72,120,151]

Metastatic Tumors

Metastatic tumors involving the tube usually are secondary to spread from carcinomas of the ovary or endometrium.[298] Peritoneal spread involves the serosal surface, whereas lymphatic metastases from adjacent primary sites may involve the mucosa or muscularis as well. Low-grade stromal sarcoma may extend to involve the tubes and ovaries. Spread takes place by the extension of worm-like tongues of tumor along tubal lymphatics. Blood-borne metastases from breast carcinomas or other extrapelvic tumors also may occur. On occasion, squamous carcinoma of the uterine cervix may spread in an in situ manner to involve the endometrial cavity, tubes, and even the ovarian surface.[222] Primary squamous carcinoma is a rarity.[176]

The presence of a large ovarian primary tumor coupled with tumor in the lumen of the fallopian tube and tumor in the endometrial cavity suggests that the tubal lumen may serve as a conduit for tumor spread. Careful study of the tubes removed at surgery for primary ovarian carcinoma reveals that luminal groups of tumor cells may implant onto endosalpingeal surfaces and simulate CIS or early primary tubal carcinoma (Fig. 14.39). Because of frequent secondary involvement of the tubes, Hu et al.[136] suggested that the following criteria be used to determine primary tubal carcinoma: Grossly, the main tumor is in the tube; microscopically, the mucosa is involved and shows a papillary pattern; if the tubal wall is extensively involved, a transition between benign and malignant tubal epithelium should be found. When both tube and ovary are intimately involved by a mass of tumor, the assumption of an ovarian primary tumor may not always be correct.[303] However, since the current surgical and chemotherapeutic treatment for epithelial malignancies of tube and ovary are the same, the distinction is academic.

Lymphoma

Tubal involvement by lymphoma is rare and is associated almost invariably with simultaneous involvement of the ipsilateral ovary.[3] Undifferentiated carcinoma must be ruled out with appropriate immunohistochemical stains.

Trophoblastic Lesions

Trophoblastic tubal lesions are exceedingly uncommon. Patients have risk factors for ectopic pregnancy such as prior salpingitis and tubal occlusion.[197] Hydatidiform moles usually occur as isolated growths but may be associated with intrauterine pregnancy.[262] Clinically, perhaps 1 in 5000 ectopic pregnancies will prove to be a mole.[127] The histological appearance may be that of a complete or a

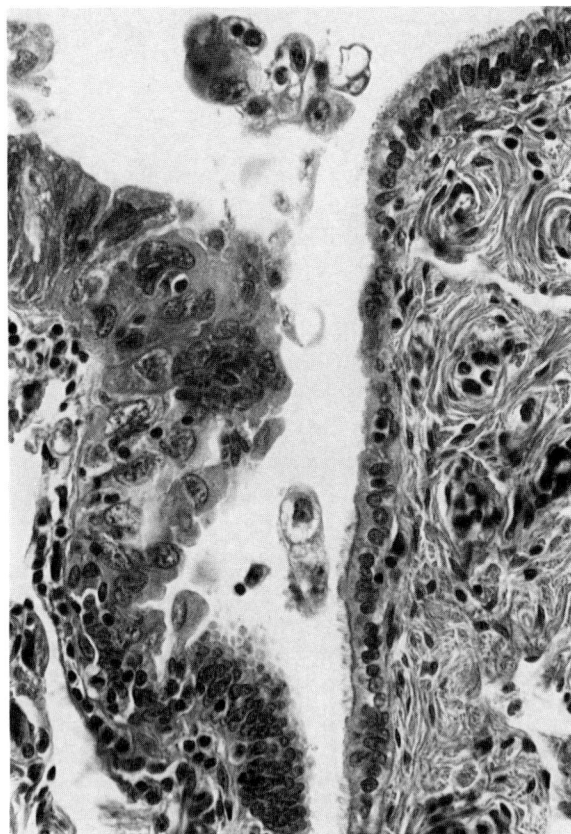

FIG. 14.39. Tubal implantation of ovarian carcinoma. Two clusters of malignant cells from an ipsilateral ovarian carcinoma lie free in the tubal lumen, and on the *left,* carcinoma has implanted and begun to spread over the mucosal surface.

partial mole with clear evidence of trophoblastic proliferation in addition to hydropic swelling of the villi.[197] Choriocarcinoma rarely may arise in the tube.[175] Clinically, the patient is believed to have an ectopic pregnancy. At operation, a large and hemorrhagic, fleshy mass may have largely destroyed the tube. Histologically, the malignant trophoblastic proliferation is similar to that of uterine choriocarcinomas. Response to modern chemotherapy generally has been gratifying[174a,211] (see Chapter 24, Gestational Trophoblastic Disease and Related Lesions).

Paratubal Tumors and Cysts

Adrenal Rests

Adrenal cortical rests, if carefully looked for, may be found in the broad ligament in more than 20% of women. They lie in the ligament "anywhere from its junction with the mesosalpinx to its lateral attachment to the pelvic wall"[86] adjacent to the ovarian vein and just beneath the peritoneum. Grossly, they appear as yellow nodules or disks, but

they may be obscured by fat. Medullary tissue is absent, but microscopically all three cortical layers are recognizable. This accessory tissue may hypertrophy secondary to adrenal destruction[142] or may, rarely, give rise to a functional cortical adenoma.[27,293]

Nests of cells morphologically similar to ovarian hilus cells have been described in the midportion of the tube.[203] In the absence of Reinke crystals, close association with nonmyelinated nerve fibers, or histochemical studies, it is difficult to exclude the possibility of an adrenal rest. Hilus cell nests with Reinke crystals may be seen, however, in fimbrial stroma.[167] These may be the cells responsible for the only case reported of tubal Sertoli–Leydig tumor.[75]

Adnexal Tumor of Probable Wolffian Origin

A small group of distinctive tumors is described as located either within the leaves of the broad ligament or attached to the tube by a pedicle.[143] (These tumors are also described and illustrated in Chapter 21, Nonspecific Tumors of the Ovary, Including Mesenchymal Tumors and Malignant Lymphoma.) Briefly, patients range in age from 29 to 58 years. Either they have abdominal pain and a palpable mass or the tumor is discovered as an incidental finding. The lesions measure from 1.3 to 12 cm in greatest dimension and are lobulated, with gross encapsulation. On section, the consistency may be rubbery or friable, and cysts or calcification may be present.

The microscopic picture varies widely (Fig. 14.40) (see also Figs. 21.19, 21.20). Solid masses of epithelial cells may be present, or tubular areas may be found similar to a well-differentiated Sertoli–Leydig tumor of the ovary (Pick's tubular adenoma). A sieve-like pattern reminiscent of benign tubal mesotheliomas also may be seen. Microscopically, the capsule is often breached by tongues of tumor. Ultrastructural analysis has been interpreted as supporting a mesonephric origin.[70,129,143,271] Although most of these tumors behave in a benign fashion, multiple local recurrences[32] and fatal metastases may occur.[1,271] The differential diagnosis includes the recently described variant of tubal endometrioid carcinoma.[65]

Other Paraovarian Tumors

Other solid paraovarian tumors are most often leiomyomas.[133] Sarcomas and malignant primary epithelial lesions are rare.[60,104] The rare broad ligament adenocarcinomas reported tend to be in women in the reproductive years and are typically low-grade serous lesions.[11,12,230] Overdiagnosis of borderline serous tumors as carcinoma should be avoided.[61] Distinction of a borderline tumor from an invasive serous carcinoma is based on the absence of stromal invasion, using the same criteria that are applied to ovarian serous neoplasms (see Chapter 18, Surface Epithelial–Stromal Tumors of the Ovary). The great majority of

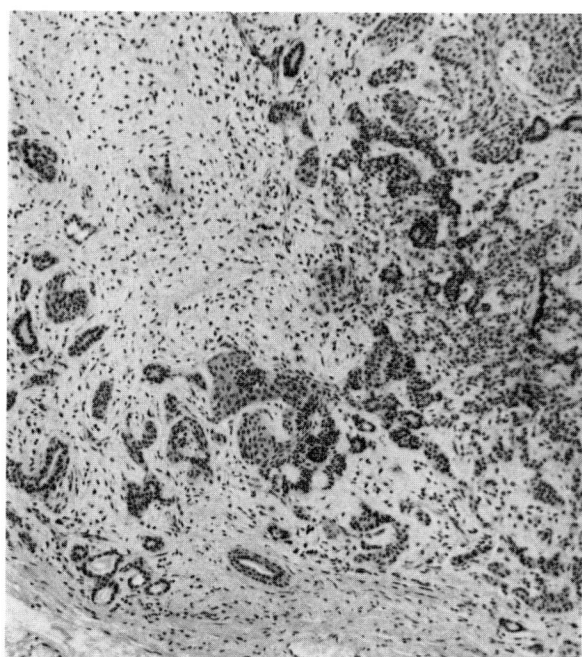 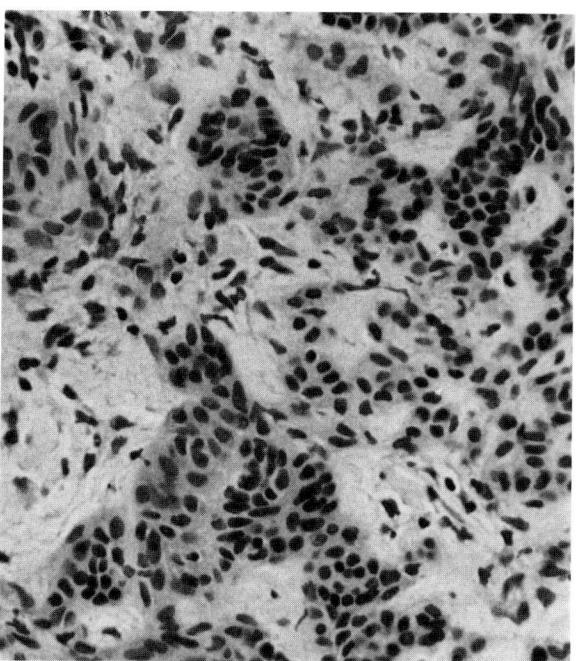

FIG. 14.40. **Paratubal wolffian tumor.** This was an incidentally found, 4-mm mass. *Left:* The tumor has a nonencapsulated pushing border on the *bottom left.* Irregular cords and trabeculae with abortive tubule formation grow haphazardly in a cellular spindle cell stroma. *Right:* The nuclei of the abortive tubules and trabeculae are regular and lack mitotic activity. (Courtesy of Dr. V.A. LiVolsi, Philadelphia, PA.)

broad ligament and paraovarian epithelial tumors are serous neoplasms of low malignant potential.[211,248] The patients range in age from 13 to 76 years (mean, 32–43 years) and present with a pelvic mass with or without ascites or pain.[7,11] At operation there is no involvement of the ovary. Paraovarian cystadenofibromas are occasional, usually incidental findings.[134] Papillary cystadenoma of the broad ligament may be associated with von Hippel–Lindau disease.[153] Extraovarian Brenner tumors,[286] mesosalpingeal choriocarcinoma,[146] broad ligament pheochromocytoma,[6] and extraskeletal Ewing's sarcoma,[173] thecoma[168] and mesovarial ependymoma[113] are among the rare tumors reported adjacent to the tube and ovary.

Paratubal Cysts

Paratubal cysts may arise from mesonephric (wolffian) structures, from paramesonephric (müllerian) structures, or from mesothelial inclusions.[238] Differentiation may be difficult because of compression and atrophy of the lining cells; paramesonephric cysts are lined by epithelium containing numerous ciliated cells. Such cysts also may have papillary infoldings similar to endosalpingeal folds. Mesonephric cysts contain only a few or no ciliated cells and may have a more prominent muscular coat. Ultrastructurally, mesonephric epithelial cells tend to have an inapparent Golgi apparatus, moderate rough endoplasmic reticulum (RER), numerous lysosomes, and minimal glycogen.

Paramesonephric epithelial cells tend to have a prominent Golgi apparatus and RER, prominent glycogen, and only rare lysosomes.[103]

The hydatid of Morgagni is by far the most common paramesonephric cyst. Grossly, it is found dangling from one of the fimbriae. It is ovoid or round, 2 to 10 mm in diameter, and contains clear serous fluid surrounded by a thin translucent wall. Microscopically, it is lined by ciliated and nonciliated cells and may have small epithelial-covered plicae projecting into the lumen. The nonciliated cells undergo cyclic changes.[28] A careful study of paraovarian cysts revealed that 86% of those more than 3 cm in diameter were mesothelial, 14% were paramesonephric, and none was mesonephric.[106]

References

1. Abbot RL, Barlogie B, Schmidt WA (1981) Metastasizing malignant juxtaovarian tumor with terminal hypercalcemia: A case report. Cancer 48: 860–865
2. Abraham JL, Spore WW, Benirschke K (1982) Cysticercosis of the fallopian tube: Histology and microanalysis. Hum Pathol 13: 665–670
3. Abrams J, Kazal HL, Hobbs RE (1958) Primary sarcoma of the fallopian tube. Am J Obstet Gynecol 75: 180–182
4. Adams BE (1969) Intussusception of a fallopian tube. Am J Surg 118: 591–592
5. Afzelius BA, Eliasson R (1983) Male and female infertility

problems in the immotile-cilia syndrome. Eur J Respir Dis 64 (suppl 127):144

6. Al-Jafari MS, Panton HM, Gradwell E (1985) Phaeochromocytoma of the broad ligament. Case report. Br J Obstet Gynaecol 92: 649–651

7. Altaras MM, Jaffe R, Corduba M, et al (1990) Primary paraovarian cystadenocarcinoma: Clinical and management aspects and literature review. Gynecol Oncol 38: 268–272

8. American College of Obstetricians and Gynecologists Committee on Terminology (1972) In: Hughes EC (ed) Obstetric–gynecologic terminology, with section on neonatology and glossary of congenital anomalies. Philadelphia, FA Davis, p 157

9. American Fertility Society (1988) The American Fertility Society classifications of adnexal adhesions, distal tubal occlusion, tubal occlusion secondary to tubal ligation, tubal pregnancies, Mullerian anomalies and intrauterine adhesions. Fertil Steril 49: 944–955

10. Aselton PJ, Stergachis A (1984) Increasing incidence of ectopic pregnancy (Letter). JAMA 251: 469

11. Aslani M, Ahn G-H, Scully RE (1988) Serous papillary cystadenoma of borderline malignancy of broad ligament. Int J Gynecol Pathol 7: 131–138

12. Aslani M, Scully RE (1989) Primary carcinoma of the broad ligament: Report of four cases and review of the literature. Cancer 64: 1540–1545

13. Bachmann FF (1961) Ein chondrolipom des Eileiters. Geburts Frauenheilkd 21: 975

14. Baginski L, Yazigi R, Sandstad J (1989) Immature (malignant) teratoma of the fallopian tube. Am J Obstet Gynecol 160: 671–672

15. Bartnik J, Powell WS, Moriber-Katz S, et al (1989) Metaplastic papillary tumor of the fallopian tube. Case report, immunohistochemical features and review of the literature. Arch Pathol Lab Med 113: 545–547

16. Bell DA, Mondschein M, Scully RE (1986) Giant cell arteritis of the female genital tract. A report of three cases. Am J Surg Pathol 10: 696–701

17. Benjamin CL, Beaver DC (1951) Pathogenesis of salpingitis isthmica nodosa. Am J Clin Pathol 21: 212–222

18. Benson PA (1974) Cytologic diagnosis in primary carcinoma of the fallopian tube. Acta Cytol 18: 429–434

19. Beral V (1975) An epidemiological study of recent trends in ectopic pregnancy. Br J Obstet Gynaecol 82: 775–782

20. Bernardus RE, Van der Slikke JW, Roex AJM, Dijkhuizen GH, Stolk JG (1984) Torsion of the fallopian tube: Some considerations on its etiology. Obstet Gynecol 64: 675

21. Beyth Y, Bar-On E (1984) Turoovarian autoamputation and infertility. Fertil Steril 42: 932–934

22. Beyth Y, Kopolovic J (1982) Accessory tubes: A possible contributing factor in infertility. Fertil Steril 38: 382–383

23. Birch HW, Collins CG (1961) Atypical changes of genital epithelium associated with ectopic pregnancy. Am J Obstet Gynecol 81: 1198–1208

24. Bland KG, Gelfand M (1970) The effects of schistosomiasis on the fallopian tubes in the African female. J Obstet Gynaecol Br Commonw 77: 1024–1027

25. Blaustein A, Shenker L (1967) Vascular lesions of the uterine tube in ectopic pregnancy. Obstet Gynecol 30: 551–555

26. Bobrow ML, Bell HG (1962) Ectopic pregnancy: A 16-year survey of 905 cases. Obstet Gynecol 20: 500–506

27. Boularan, Cahuzac, Salvador, Genesseau (1945) Macrogenitosomie et gynandrie chez un sujet porteu de deux tumeurs cortico-surrenaliennes incluses dans les ligaments larges. Ann Endocrinol (Paris) 6: 57–72

28. Bransilver BR, Ferenczy A, Richart RM (1973) Female genital tract remnants. An ultrastructural comparison of hydatid of Morgagni and mesonephric ducts and tubules. Arch Pathol 96: 255–261

29. Braun P, Besdine R (1971) Tuboovarian abscess with recovery of T. mycoplasm. Am J Obstet Gynecol 117: 861

30. Breen JL (1970) A 21-year survey of 654 ectopic pregnancies. Am J Obstet Gynecol 106: 1004–1019

31. Brenner PF, Roy S, Mishell DR Jr (1980) Ectopic pregnancy. A study of 300 consecutive surgical treated cases. JAMA 243: 673–676

32. Brescia RJ, Cardoso de Almeida PC, Fuller AF Jr, Dickersin GR, Robboy SJ (1985) Female adnexal tumor of probable wolffian origin with multiple recurrences over 16 years. Cancer 56: 1456–1461

33. Britigan BE, Cohen MS, Sparling PF (1985) Gonococcal infection: A model of molecular pathogenesis. N Engl J Med 312: 1683–1694

34. Bronson R, Cunnane M (1975) Transfer of uterine implantation blastocysts to the oviduct in mice. Fertil Steril 26: 455–459

35. Brooks JJ, Wheeler JE (1977) Granulomatous salpingitis secondary to Crohn's disease. Obstet Gynecol 49: 31s–33s

36. Brunham RC, Maclean IW, Binns B, Peeling RW (1985) Chlamydia trachomatis: Its role in tubal infertility. J Infect Dis 152: 1275–1282

37. Busch DH, Benirschke K (1974) Cytogenetic studies of ectopic pregnancies. Virch Arch [Cell Pathol] 16: 319–330

38. Bylund DJ, Nanfro JJ, Marsh WL (1986) Coccidioidomycosis of the female genital tract. Arch Pathol Lab Med 110: 232–235

39. Campbell JS, Nigam S, Hurtig A, Sahasrabudhe MR, Marno I (1964) Mineral oil granulomas of the uterus and parametrium and granulomatous salpingitis with Schaumann bodies and oxalate deposits. Fertil Steril 15: 278–289

40. Carlson JA, Ackerman BL, Wheeler JE (1993) Malignant mixed mullerian tumor of the fallopian tube. Cancer 71: 187–192

41. Case Records of the Massachusetts General Hospital (Case 9–1971) (1971) N Engl J Med 284: 491–496

42. Cataldo NA, Nicholson M, Bihrle D (1990) Uterine serosal trophoblastic implant after linear salpingostomy for ectopic pregnancy at laparotomy. Obstet Gynecol 76: 523–525

43. Chalvardjian A, Picard L, Shaw R, et al (1980) Malacoplakia of the female genital tract. Am J Obstet Gynecol 138: 391–394

44. Chen KTK (1981) Bilateral papillary adenofibroma of the fallopian tube. Am J Clin Pathol 75: 229–231

44a. Cheung ANY, So KF, Ngan HYS, Wong LC (1994) Primary squamous carcinoma of the tube. Int J Gynecol Pathol 13: 92–95

45. Chevallier G, Parent B (1966) L'hydrosalpinx. Etude de 253 cas. Presse Med 74: 2035

46. Chi I-C, Potts M, Wilkens L (1986) Rare events associated with tubal sterilization: An international experience. Obstet Gynecol Surv 41: 7–19

47. Chow AW, Malkasian KL, Marshall JR, Guze LB (1975) The bacteriology of acute pelvic inflammatory disease. Am J Obstet Gynecol 122: 876–879

48. Chow W-H, Daling JR, Weiss NS, Moore DE, Soderstrom R (1985) Vaginal douching as a potential risk factor for tubal ectopic pregnancy. Am J Obstet Gynecol 153: 727–729

49. Chung CS, Smith RG, Steinhoff PG, Mi M-P (1982) Induced abortion and ectopic pregnancy in subsequent pregnancies. Am J Epidemiol 115: 879–887

50. Clement PB, Young RH, Scully RE (1988) Necrotic pseudoxanthomatous nodules of ovary and peritoneum in endometriosis. Am J Surg Pathol 12: 390–397

51. Clement PB, Young RH, Scully RE (1991) Clinical syndromes associated with tumors of the female genital tract. Semin Diag Pathol 8: 204–233

52. Collins JA, Wrixon W, Janes LB, Wilson EH (1983) Treatment-independent pregnancy among infertile couples. N Engl J Med 309: 1201–1206

53. Copeland W Jr, Hawley PC, Teteris NJ (1985) Gynecologic amyloidosis. Am J Obstet Gynecol 153: 555–556

54. Cornog JL, Curie JL, Rubin A (1970) Heat artifact simulating adenocarcinoma of fallopian tube. JAMA 214: 1118–1119

55. Coutinho EM, Maia H Jr, Mattos CER (1975) Contractility of the fallopian tube. Gynecol Invest 6: 146–161

56. Creasman WT (1992) Revision in classification by International Federation of Gynecology and Obstetrics. (Letter) Am J Obstet Gynecol 167: 857–858

57. Crohn BB, Yarnis H (1958) Regional Ileitis, 2nd ed. New York, Grune & Stratton.

58. Crosby EC, Humphrey T, Lauer EW (1962) Correlative Anatomy of the Nervous System. New York, Macmillan

59. Croxatto HB, Diaz S, Feuntealba B, Croxatto HD, Carrillo D, Fabres C (1972) Studies on the duration of egg transport in the human oviduct. I. The time interval between ovulation and egg recovery from the uterus in normal women. Fertil Steril 23: 447–458

60. Czernobilsky B, Lancet M (1972) Broad ligament adenocarcinoma of müllerian origin. Obstet Gynecol 40: 238–242

61. d'Ablaing G, Klatt EC, DiRocco G, Hibbard LT (1983) Broad ligament serous tumor of low malignant potential. Int J Gynecol Pathol 2: 93–99

62. David A, Garcia C-R, Czernobilsky B (1969) Human hydrosalpinx. Histologic study and chemical composition of fluid. Am J Obstet Gynecol 105: 400–411

63. David A, Serr DN, Czernobilsky B (1973) Chemical position of human oviduct fluid. Fertil Steril 24: 435–439

64. Daw E (1973) Duplication of the uterine tube. Obstet Gynecol 42: 137–138

65. Daya D, Young RH, Scully RE (1992) Endometrioid carcinoma of the fallopian tube resembling an adnexal tumor of probable wolffian origin: A report of six cases. Int J Gynecol Pathol 11: 122–130

66. DeCherney AH, Cholst I, Naftolin F (1981) Structure and function of the fallopian tubes following exposure to diethylstilbestrol (DES) during gestation. Fertil Steril 36: 741–745

67. DeCherney AH, Maheaux R, Naftolin F (1982) Salpingostomy for ectopic pregnancy in the sole patient oviduct: Reproductive outcome. Fertil Steril 37: 619–622

68. Dede JA, Janovski NA (1963) Lipoma of the uterine tube. Obstet Gynecol 22: 461–467

69. Demopoulos RI, Bigelow B, Vasa U (1978) Infarcted uterine adnexa: Associated pathology. NY State J Med 78: 2027–2029

70. Demopoulos RI, Sitelman A, Flotte T, Bigelow B (1960) Ultrastructural study of a female adnexal tumor of probable wolffian origin. Cancer 46: 2273–2280

71. Denham JW, Maclennan KA (1984) The management of primary carcinoma of the fallopian tube. Experience of 40 cases. Cancer 53: 166–172

72. Deppe G, Zbella E, Friberg J, Thomas W (1984) Combination chemotherapy for mixed müllerian tumor of the fallopian tube. Cancer 54: 1517–1520

73. Diamant YZ, Aboulafia Y, Raz S (1972) Torsion of hydrosalpinx. Int Surg 57: 303–304

74. Dische FE, Burt JM, Davison NJH, Puntambekar S (1974) Tuboovarian actinomycosis associated with intrauterine contraceptive devices. J Obstet Gynaecol Br Commonw 81: 724–729

75. Dokumov St, Dekov D (1963) A rare case of precocious pseudopuberty due to a Sertoli–Leydig cell tumor originating from the left fallopian tube. J Clin Endocrinol Metab 23: 1262–1266

76. Donnez J, Casanas-Roux F, Caprasse J, Ferin J, Thomas K (1985) Cyclic changes in ciliation, cell height, and mitotic activity in human tubal epithelium during reproductive life. Fertil Steril 43: 554–559

77. Dorfman SF, Grimes DA, Cates W Jr, Binkin NJ, Kafrissen ME, O'Reilly KR (1984) Ectopic pregnancy mortality, United States, 1979 to 1980: Clinical aspects. Obstet Gynecol 64: 386–389

78. Dudkiewicz J (1970) Quantitative and qualitative changes of epithelial cells of fallopian tubes in women according to the phase of menstrual cycle. A cytologic study. Acta Cytol 14: 531–537

79. Ebrahimi T, Okagaki T (1973) Hemangioma of the fallopian tube. Am J Obstet Gynecol 115: 864–865

80. Eddy GL, Copeland LJ, Gershenson DM, et al (1984) Fallopian tube carcinoma. Obstet Gynecol 64: 546–552

81. Elliott GB, Brody H, Elliott KA (1965) Implications of "lipoid" salpingitis. Fertil Steril 16: 541–548

82. El-Kady AA, Mansy MM, Nagib HS et al (1991) Histopathologic changes in the cornual portion of the fallopian tube following a single transcervical insertion of quinacrine hydrochloride pellets. Adv Contracep 7: 1–9

83. Ellsworth HS, Harris JW, McQuarrie HG, Stone RA, Anderson AE (1973) Prolapse of the fallopian tube following vaginal hysterectomy. JAMA 224: 891–892

84. Erez S, Kaplan LA, Wall JA (1967) Clinical staging of carcinoma of the uterine tube. Obstet Gynecol 30: 547–550

85. Evans MI, Angerman NS, Moravec WE, Hajj SN (1979) The intrauterine device and ovarian pregnancy. Fertil Steril 32: 31–35

86. Falls JL (1955) Accessory adrenal cortex in the broad ligament. Cancer 8: 143–150

87. Farber M, Mitchell GW Jr (1979) Bicornuate uterus and partial atresia of the fallopian tube. Am J Obstet Gynecol 134: 881–884

88. Farley TMM, Rosenberg MJ, Rowe PJ, et al (1992) Intrauterine devices and pelvic inflammatory disease: an international perspective. Lancet 339: 785–788

89. Federman Q, Toker C (1973) Primary transitional cell tumor of the uterine adnexa. Am J Obstet Gynecol 115: 863–864

90. Ferenczy A, Fenoglio J, Richart RM (1972) Observations on benign mesotheliomas of the genital tract (adenomatoid tumor). Cancer 30: 244–260

91. Ferenczy A, Richart RM (1974) Female reproductive system: Dynamics of scan and transmission electron microscopy. New York, Wiley, pp 212–253

92. Fetissof F, Berger G, Dubois MP, et al (1985) Female genital tract and Peutz-Jeghers syndrome: An immunohistochemical study. Int J Gynecol Pathol 4: 219–229

93. Fitzgerald TB, Mainwaring AR, Ahmed A (1974) Pelvic peritoneal oxyuriasis simulating metastatic carcinoma. J Obstet Gynaecol Br Commonw 81: 248–250

94. Flickinger GL, Meuchler EK, Mikhail G (1974) Estradiol receptor in the human fallopian tube. Fertil Steril 25: 900–903

95. Fortier KJ, Haney AF (1985) The pathologic spectrum of uterotubal junction obstruction. Obstet Gynecol 65: 93–98

96. Frachtman KG (1953) Unruptured tubal term pregnancy. Am J Surg 86: 161–168

97. Franco V, Florena AM, Guarneri G, et al (1990) Xanthogranulomatous salpingitis. Case report and review of the literature. Acta Eur Fertil 21: 197–199

98. Fredricsson B (1969) Histochemistry of the oviduct. In: Hafex ESE, Blandau RJ (eds) The Mammalian Oviduct. Chicago, University of Chicago Press

99. Frost O (1975) Bilharzia of the fallopian tube. South Afr Med J 49: 1201–1203

100. Fujii S, Ban C, Okamura H, Nishimura T (1981) Unilateral tubal quadruplet pregnancy. Am J Obstet Gynecol 141: 840–842

101. Gaddum-Rosse P, Blandau RJ (1973) In vitro studies on ciliary activity within the oviducts of the rabbit and pig. Am J Anat 136: 91–104

102. Gaddum-Rosse P, Rumery RE, Blandau RT, Thiersch JB (1975) Studies on the mucosa of postmenopausal oviducts: Surface appearance, ciliary activity, and the effect of estrogen treatment. Fertil Steril 26: 951–969

103. Gardner GH, Greene RR, Peckham BM (1948) Normal and cystic structures of broad ligament. Am J Obstet Gynecol 55: 917–939

104. Gardner GH, Greene RR, Peckham B (1957) Tumors of the broad ligament. Am J Obstet Gynecol 73: 536–555

105. Gelfand M, Ross MD, Blair DM, Weber MC (1971) Distribution and extent of schistosomiasis in female pelvic organs with special reference to the genital tract, as determined at autopsy. Am J Trop Med Hyg 20: 846–849

106. Genadry R, Parmley T, Woodruff JD (1977) The origin and clinical behavior of the parovarian tumor. Am J Obstet Gynecol 129: 873–880

107. Georgakopoulos PA, Gogas CG, Sariyannis HG (1980) Hydatid disease of the female genitalia. Obstet Gynecol 55: 555–559

108. Gisser SD (1986) Obstructing fallopian tube papilloma. Int J Gynecol Pathol 5: 179–182

109. Gomel V (1983) An odyssey through the oviduct. Fertil Steril 39: 144–156

110. Gravaller J, Suranyi S, Berensci G (1956) Neue Gesichtpunkte in der Klinik der Genitaltuberkulos. Zentralbl Gynaekol 78: 496

111. Green LK, Kott ML (1989) Histopathologic findings in ectopic tubal pregnancy. Int J Gynecol Pathol 8: 255–262

112. Grimes HG, Nosal RA, Gallagher JC (1983) Ovarian pregnancy: A series of 24 cases. Obstet Gynecol 61: 174–180

113. Grody WW, Nieberg RK, Bhuta S (1985) Ependymoma-like tumor of the mesovarium. Arch Pathol Lab Med 109: 291–293

114. Gump DW, Gibson M, Ashikaga T (1984) Lack of association between genital mycoplasm and infertility. N Engl J Med 310: 937–941

115. Haines M (1958) Tuberculous salpingitis as seen by the pathologist and the surgeon. Am J Obstet Gynecol 75: 472–481

116. Halbrecht I (1951) Cortisone in the treatment of tubal occlusion caused by genital tuberculosis. Fertil Steril 13: 371–379

117. Hallatt JG (1982) Primary ovarian pregnancy: A report of twenty-five cases. Am J Obstet Gynecol 143: 55–60

118. Hallatt JG (1976) Ectopic pregnancy associated with the intrauterine device: A study of seventy cases. Am J Obstet Gynecol 125: 754–758

119. Hallatt JG (1975) Repeat ectopic pregnancy: A study of 123 consecutive cases. Am J Obstet Gynecol 122: 520–524

120. Hanjani P, Petersen RO, Bonnell SA (1980) Malignant mixed müllerian tumor of the fallopian tube. Gynecol Oncol 9: 381–393

121. Hanton EM, Malkasian GD Jr, Dahlin DC, Pratt JH (1966) Primary carcinoma of the fallopian tube. Am J Obstet Gynecol 94: 832–839

122. Harris GJ, Al-Jurf AS, Yuh WTC, et al (1989) Intrahepatic pregnancy. A unique opportunity for evaluation with sonography, computed tomography, and magnetic resonance imaging. JAMA 261: 902–904

123. Hellman LM (1949) Morphology of the human fallopian tube in the early puerperium. Am J Obstet Gynecol 57: 154–165

124. Henriksen E (1955) Struma salpingii. Obstet Gynecol 5: 833–835

125. Herbold DR, Axelrod JH, Bobowski SJ, et al (1988) Glassy cell carcinoma of the fallopian tube. A case report. Int J Gynecol Pathol 7: 384–390

126. Herrera GA, Reimann BEF, Greenberg HL, Miles PA (1983) Pigmentosis tubae, a new entity: Light and electron microscopic study. Obstet Gynecol 61: 80S–83S

127. Hertig AT, Mansell H (1956) Tumors of the female sex organs. Part 1. Hydatiform mole and choriocarcinoma. In: Atlas of tumor pathology, Series 1, Fasc 33, pp 62–63. Washington, DC, Armed Forces Institute of Pathology

128. Hetzel DJ, Stanhope CR, O'Neill BP, et al (1990) Gyneco-

logic cancer in patients with subacute cerebellar degeneration predicted by anti-Purkinje cell antibodies and limited in metastatic volume. Mayo Clin Proc 65: 1558–1563

129. Hinchey WW, Silva EG, Guarda LA, Ordonez NC, Wharton JT (1983) Paravaginal wolffian duct (mesonephros) adenocarcinoma: A light and electron microscopic study. Am J Clin Pathol 80: 539–544

130. Hockin JC, Jessamine AG (1984) Trends in ectopic pregnancy in Canada. Can Med Assc J 131: 737–740

131. Holman JF, Tyrey EL, Hammond CB (1984) A contemporary approach to suspected ectopic pregnancy with use of quantitative and qualitative assays for the beta-subunit of human chorionic gonadotropin and sonography. Am J Obstet Gynecol 150: 151–157

132. Honore LH (1978) Salpingitis isthmica nodosa in female infertility and ectopic tubal pregnancy. Fertil Steril 29: 164–168

133. Honore LH (1981) Parauterine leiomyomas in women: A clinicopathologic study of 22 cases. Eur J Obstet Gynecol Reprod Biol 11: 273–279

134. Honore LH, O'Hara KE (1980) Serous papillary neoplasms arising in paramesonephric parovarian cysts. Acta Obstet Gynecol Scand 59: 525–528

135. Hovadhanakul P, Eachempati U, Cavanagh D (1971) Ureteral obstruction in chronic ectopic pregnancy. Am J Obstet Gynecol 110: 311–313

136. Hu CY, Taymor ML, Hertig AT (1950) Primary carcinoma of the fallopian tube. Am J Obstet Gynecol 59: 58–67

137. Isager-Sally L, Weber T (1985) Torsion of the fallopian tube during pregnancy. Acta Obstet Gynecol Scand 64: 349–351

138. Jackson-York GL, Ramzy I (1992) Synchronous papillary mucinous adenocarcinoma of the endocervix and fallopian tubes. Int J Gynecol Pathol 11: 63–67

139. Jansen RPS (1984) Endocrine response in the fallopian tube. Endocrinol Rev 5: 525

140. Jauchler GW, Baker RL (1970) Cervical pregnancy: Review of the literature and a case report. Obstet Gynecol 35: 870–874

141. Kallenberger DA, Ronk DA, Jimerson GK (1978) Ectopic pregnancy: A 15 year review of 160 cases. South Med J 71: 758

142. Karakascheff KI (1906) Weitere Beitrage zur pathologischen Anatomie der Nebennieren. Beitr Pathol 39: 373

143. Kariminejad MH, Scully RE (1973) Female adnexal tumor of probable wolffian origin. Cancer 31: 671–677

144. Katz DA, Thom D, Bogard P, Dermer MS (1984) Angiomyolipoma of the fallopian tube. Am J Obstet Gynecol 148: 341–343

145. Kay S (1956) Sarcoidosis of the fallopian tubes. J Obsteg Gynaecol Br Emp 63: 871–874

146. Kay S, Schneider V, Litt J (1983) Choriocarcinoma of the mesosalpinx masquerading as congestive heart failure: Ultrastructural observations of the tumor. Int J Gynecol Pathol 2: 72–87

147. Keeney GL, Thrasher TV (1988) Metaplastic papillary tumor of the fallopian tube: A case report with ultrastructure. Int J Gynecol Pathol 7: 86–92

148. Keith LG, Berger GS, Edelman DA, Newton W, Fullan N, Bailey R, Friberg J (1984) On the causation of pelvic inflammatory disease. Am J Obstet Gynecol 149: 215–224

149. Kerin JF, Williams DB, San Roman GA, et al (1992) Falloposcopic classification and treatment of fallopian tube lumen disease. Fertil Steril 57: 731–741

150. Kessel E (1989) Pelvic inflammatory disease with intrauterine device use: A reassessment. Fertil Steril 51: 1–11

151. Kinoshita M, Asano S, Yamashita M, et al (1989) Mesodermal mixed tumor primary in the fallopian tube. Gynecol Oncol 32: 331–335

152. Knab DR, Blanco LJ (1978) Müllerian duct agenesis with a unilateral functioning segment of the rudimentary uterine horn. Am J Obstet Gynecol 132: 222–224

153. Korn WT, Schatzki SC, DiSciullo AJ, et al (1990) Papillary cystadenoma of the broad ligament in Von Hippel–Lindau disease. Am J Obstet Gynecol 163: 596–598

154. Kraus FT (1977) Female genitalia. In: Anderson WAD, Kisane JM (eds) Pathology, 7th ed. St. Louis, CV Mosby, p 1726

155. Kristensen GS, Bollerup AC, Lind K, et al (1985) Infections with Neisseria gonorrhoeae and Chlamydia trachomatis in women with acute salpingitis. Genitourin Med 61: 179

156. Kuo T-t, Hsueh S (1984) Mucicarminophilic histiocytosis. A polyvinyl pyrolidone (PVP) storage disease simulating signet-ring cell carcinoma. Am J Surg Pathol 8: 419–428

157. Kutteh WH, Hatch KD, Blackwell RE, et al (1988) Secretory immune system of the female reproductive tract: I. Immunoglobulin and secretory component-containing cells. Obstet Gynecol 71: 56–60

158. Kuzela DC, Speers WC (1985) Heterotopic endometrium of the fallopian tube. Fertil Steril 44: 552–553

159. Ladefoged C, Lorentzen M (1988) Xanthogranulomatous inflammation of the female genital tract. Histopathology 13: 541–551

160. Landers DV, Sweet RL (1985) Current trends in the diagnosis and treatment of tuboovarian abscess. Am J Obstet Gynecol 151: 1098–1110

161. Landers DV, Sweet RL (1983) Tubo-ovarian abscess: Contemporary approach to management. Rev Infect Dis 5: 876–884

162. Lapin BA, Yakoleva LA (1963) Comparative Physiology in Monkeys. Springfield, Ill, Charles C Thomas, p 215

163. Lauchlan SC (1984) Metaplasias and neoplasias of müllerian epithelium. Histopathology 8: 543

164. Lee NC, Rubin GL, Borucki R (1988) The intrauterine device and pelvic inflammatory disease re-visited: New results from the Women's Health Study. Obstet Gynecol 72: 1–6

165. Lee RA, Welch JS (1967) Torsion of the uterine adnexa. Am J Obstet Gynecol 97: 974–977

166. Levy G, Muller G, Pigaglio O (1987) Grossesses intra-uterine et extra-uterine simultanees. Rev Fr Gynecol Obstet 82: 729–732

167. Lewis JD (1964) Hilus cell hyperplasia of ovaries and tubes. Obstet Gynecol 24: 728–731

168. Lin H-H, Chen Y-P, Lee T-Y (1987) A hormone-producing thecoma of broad ligament. Acta Obstet Gynecol Scand 66: 725–727

169. Lind K, Kristensen GB, Bollerup AC, et al (1985) Impor-

tance of *Mycoplasma hominis* in acute salpingitis assessed by culture and serological tests. Genitourin Med 61: 185

170. Lindblom B, Hamberger L, Wiqvist N (1978) Differentiated contractile effects of prostaglandins E and F on the isolated circular and longitudinal smooth muscle of the human oviduct. Fertil Steril 30: 553–559

171. Lippes J, Ender RG, Pragay OA, Bartholomew WR (1972) The collection and analysis of human fallopian tube fluid. Contraception 5: 85–103

172. Lisa JR, Gioia JD, Rubin IC (1954) Observations on the interstitial portion of the fallopian tube. Surg Gynecol Obstet 99: 159–169

173. Longway SR, Lind HM, Haghighi P (1986) Extraskeletal Ewing's sarcoma arising in the broad ligament. Arch Pathol Lab Med 110: 1058–1061.

174. Lundorff P, Hahlin M, Sjöblom P, et al (1991) Persistent trophoblast after conservative treatment of tubal pregnancy: prediction and detection. Obstet Gynecol 77: 129–133

174a. Lurain JR, Sund PK, Brewer JI (1986) Choriocarcinoma associated with ectopic pregnancy. Obstet Gynecol 68: 286–287

175. Madden S (1950) Chorionepithelioma of the fallopian tube. J Obstet Gynaecol Br Emp 57: 68–70

176. Malinak LJ, Miller GV, Armstrong JT (1966) Primary squamous cell carcinoma of the fallopian tube. Am J Obstet Gynecol 95: 1167–1168

177. Mallory T (1935) Case records of the Massachusetts General Hospital. N Engl J Med 213: 1249–1251

178. Marchbanks PA, Annegers JF, Coulam CB, et al (1988) Risk factors for ectopic pregnancy. A population-based study. JAMA 259: 1823–1827

179. Mårdh P-A, Ripa T, Svensson L, Weström L (1977) *Chlamydia trachomatis* infection in patients with acute salpingitis. N Engl J Med 296: 1377–1379

180. Mårdh P-A, Weström L (1970) Antibodies to *Mycoplasma hominis* in patients with genital infections and in healthy controls. Br J Vener Dis 46: 390–397

181. Mårdh P-A, Weström L (1970) Tubal and cervical cultures in acute salpingitis with special reference to *Mycoplasma hominis* and T-strain mycoplasmas. Br J Vener Dis 46: 179–186

182. Mason TE, Quagliarello JR (1976) Ectopic pancreas in the fallopian tube. Obstet Gynecol 48: 70s–73s

183. Mastroianni L Jr, Komins J (1975) Capacitation, ovum maturation, fertilization and preimplantation development in the oviduct. Gynecol Invest 6: 226–233

184. Mazzarella P, Okagaki T, Richart RM (1972) Teratoma of the uterine tube. Obstet Gynecol 39: 381–388

184a. McComb PF, Rowe TC (1989) Salpingitis isthmica nodosa: Evidence it is a progressive disease. Fertil Steril 51: 542–545

184b. McCormack WM (1994) Pelvic inflammatory disease. N Engl J Med 330: 115–119

185. McGee ZA, Stephens DS, Hoffman LH, Schlech WF III, Horn RG (1983) Mechanisms of mucosal invasion by pathogenic *Neisseria*. Rev Infect Dis 5 (suppl 4): S708.

186. McGowan L (1965) Intramural pregnancy. JAMA 192: 637–639

187. Milchgrub S, Sandstad J (1991) Arias-Stella reaction in fallopian tube epithelium. A light and electron microscopic study with a review of the literature. Am J Clin Pathol 95: 892–895

188. Miller DL, Dillon J (1989) An unusual abdominal mass in an elderly woman. (Letter) N Engl J Med 321: 1613–1614

189. Møller BR, Weström L, Ahrons S, et al (1979) Chlamydia trachomatis infection of the fallopian tubes. Histological findings in two patients. Br J Vener Dis 55: 422–428

190. Moore DH, Woosley JT, Reddick RL, et al (1987) Adenosquamous carcinoma of the fallopian tube. A clinicopathologic case report with verification of the diagnosis by immunohistochemical and ultrastructural studies. Am J Obstet Gynecol 157: 903–905

191. Moore SW, Enterline HT (1975) Significance of proliferative epithelial lesions of the uterine tube. Obstet Gynecol 45: 385–390

192. Morris H, Emms H, Visser T, et al (1986) Lymphoid tissue of the normal fallopian tube—a form of mucosal-associated lymphoid tissue (MALT)? Int J Gynecol Pathol 5: 11–22

193. Mumford SD, Kellel E (1992) Sterilization needs in the 1990s: The case for quinacrine nonsurgical female sterilization. Am J Obstet Gynecol 167: 1203–1207

194. Muntz HG, Tarraza HM, Goff BA, et al (1991) Combination chemotherapy in advanced adenocarcinoma of the fallopian tube. Gynecol Oncol 40: 268–273

195. Murray JJ, Clark CA, Lands RH, et al (1984) Reactivation blastomycosis presenting as a tuboovarian abscess. Obstet Gynecol 64: 828–830

196. Musich JR, Behrman SJ (1983) Surgical management of tubal obstruction at the uterotubal junction. Fertil Steril 40: 423–441

197. Muto MG, Lage JM, Berkowitz RS, et al (1991) Gestational trophoblastic disease of the fallopian tube. J Reprod Med 36: 57–60

198. Newbold RR, Bullock BC, McLachlan JA (1985) Progressive proliferative changes in the oviduct of mice following developmental exposure to diethylstilbestrol. Teratogenesis Carcinogen Mutagen 5: 473–480

199. Niles JH, Clark JFJ (1969) Pathogenesis of tubal pregnancy. Am J Obstet Gynecol 105: 1230–1234

200. Niloff JM, Klug TL, Schaetzl E, Zurawski VR Jr, Knapp BC, Bast RC Jr (1984) Elevation of serum CA125 in carcinomas of the fallopian tube, endometrium and endocervix. Am J Obstet Gynecol 148: 1057–1058

201. Nordenskjöld F, Ahlgren M (1991) Risk factors in ectopic pregnancy. Results of a population-based case-control study. Acta Obstet Gynecol Scand 70: 575–579

202. Novak E, Everett HS (1928) Cyclical and other variations in the tubal epithelium. Am J Gynecol 16: 499–530

203. Odor DL (1974) The question of "basal cell" in oviductal and endocervical epithelium. Fertil Steril 25: 1047–1062

204. Okagaki T, Richart RM (1970) Neurilemmoma of the fallopian tube. Am J Obstet Gynecol 106: 929

205. Outerbridge GW (1914) Polypoid chondrofibroma of the fallopian tube associated with tubal pregnancy. Am J Obstet NY 70: 173

206. Palomaki JF, Blair OM (1971) Hilus cell rest of the fallopian tube. Obstet Gynecol 37: 60–62

207. Patek E, Nilsson L (1973) Scanning electron microscopic

observations on the ciliogenesis of the infundibulum of the human fetal and adult fallopian tube epithelium. Fertil Steril 24: 819–831

208. Patek E, Nilsson L, Johannisson E (1972) Scanning electron microscopic study of the human fallopian tube. Report I. The proliferative and secretory stages. Fertil Steril 23: 459–465

209. Paton DM, Widdicombe JH, Rheaume DE, Johns A (1978) The role of the adrenergic innervation of the oviduct in the regulation of mammalian ovum transport. Pharmacol Rev 29: 67–102

210. Patton DL, Moore DE, Spadoni LR, et al (1989) A comparison of the fallopian tube's response to overt and silent salpingitis. Obstet Gynecol 73: 622–630

211. Patton GW Jr, Goldstein DP (1973) Gestational choriocarcinoma of the tube and ovary. Surg Gynecol Obstet 137: 608–612

212. Pauerstein CJ (1974) The Fallopian Tube: A Reappraisal. Philadelphia, Lea & Febiger

213. Pauerstein CJ, Croxatto HB, Eddy CA, et al (1986) Anatomy and pathology of tubal pregnancy. Obstet Gynecol 67: 301–308

214. Pauerstein CJ, Woodruff JD (1967) The role of the "indifferent" cell of the tubal epithelium. Am J Obstet Gynecol 98: 121–125

215. Pauerstein CJ, Woodruff JD (1966) Cellular patterns in proliferative and anaplastic disease of the fallopian tube. Am J Obstet Gynecol 96: 486–492

216. Persaud V (1970) Etiology of tubal ectopic pregnancy. Radiologic and pathologic studies. Obstet Gynecol 36: 257–263

217. Persson E, Holmberg K (1984) A longitudinal study of *Actinomyces israelii* in the female genital tract. Acta Obstet Gynecol Scand 63: 207–216

218. Peters WA III, Anderson WA, Hopkins MP, et al (1988) Prognostic features of carcinoma of the fallopian tube. Obstet Gynecol 7: 757–762

219. Pfeiffer P, Mogensen H, Amtrup F, et al (1989) Primary carcinoma of the fallopian tube. A retrospective study of patients reported to the Danish Cancer Registry in a five-year period. Acta Oncol 28: 7–11

220. Phillips AJ, D'Ablaing G (1986) Acute salpingitis subsequent to tubal ligation. Obstet Gynecol 67: 55S–58S

221. Puls LE, Davey DD, DePriest PD, et al (1993) Immunohistochemical staining for CA-125 in fallopian tube carcinomas. Gynecol Oncol 48: 360–363

222. Qizilbash AH, DePetrillo AD (1975) Endometrial and tubal involvement by squamous carcinoma of the cervix. Am J Clin Pathol 64:668–671

223. Randall S, Buckley CH, Fox H (1987) Placentation in the fallopian tube. Int J Gynecol Pathol 6: 132–139

224. Raziel A, Golan A, Pansky M, et al (1990) Ovarian pregnancy: A report of twenty cases in one institution. Am J Obstet Gynecol 163: 1182–1185

225. Rebello R, Green FHY, Fox H (1975) A study of the secretory immune system of the female genital tract. Br J Obstet Gynaecol 82: 812–816

226. Reiffenstuhl G (1964) The Lymphatics of the Female Genital Organs. Philadelphia, JB Lippincott

227. Rivlin ME, Meeks GR, Cowan BD, Bates GW (1985) Persistent trophoblastic tissue following salpingostomy for unruptured ectopic pregnancy. Fertil Steril 43: 323–324

228. Roberts CL, Marshall HK (1961) Fibromyoma of the fallopian tube. Am J Obstet Gynecol 82: 364–366

229. Robey SS, Silva EG (1989) Epithelial hyperplasia of the fallopian tube. Its association with serous borderline tumors of ovary. Int J Gynecol Pathol 8: 214–220

230. Rojansky N, Ophir E, Sharony A, Spira H, Suprun H (1985) Broad ligament adenocarcinoma—Its origin and clinical behavior. A literature review and report of a case. Obstet Gynecol Surv 40: 665–671

231. Romero R, Kadar N, Jeanty P, Copel JA, Chervenak FA, DeCherney A, Hobbins JC (1985) Diagnosis of ectopic pregnancy: Value of the discriminatory human chorionic gonadotropin zone. Obstet Gynecol 66: 357–360

232. Rose PG, Piver MS, Tsukada Y (1990) Fallopian tube cancer. The Roswell Park experience. Cancer 66: 2661–2667

233. Rosenblatt KA, Weiss NS, Schwartz SM (1989) Incidence of malignant fallopian tube tumors. Gynecol Oncol 35: 236–239

234. Rowe R, Mikuta J (1992) Cat-scratch salpingitis (letter). New Engl J Med 327: 1395–1396

235. Rubin A, Czernobilsky B (1970) Tubal ligation. A bacteriologic, histologic and clinical study. Obstet Gynecol 36: 199–203

236. Rubin GL, Peterson HB, Dorfman SF, et al (1983) Ectopic pregnancy in the United States, 1970 through 1978. JAMA 249: 1725–1729

237. Saffos RO, Rhatigan RM, Scully RE (1980) Metaplastic papillary tumor of the fallopian tube—A distinctive lesion of pregnancy. Am J Clin Pathol 74: 232–236

238. Samaha M, Woodruff JD (1985) Paratubal cysts: Frequency, histogenesis, and associated clinical features. Obstet Gynecol 65: 691–693

239. Sanes S, Warner R (1939) Primary lymphangioma of the fallopian tube. Am J Obstet Gynecol 37: 316–321

240. Sapan IP, Solberg NS (1973) Prolapse of the uterine tube after abdominal hysterectomy. Obstet Gynecol 42: 26–32

241. Schaefer G (1970) Tuberculosis of the female genital tract. Clin Obstet Gynecol 13: 965–998

242. Scheffey LC, Lang WR, Nugent FB (1941) Clinical and pathologic aspects of primary sarcoma of the uterine tube. Am J Obstet Gynecol 52: 904–916

243. Schenken JR, Burns EL (1943) A study and classification of nodular lesions of the fallopian tube. Am J Obstet Gynecol 45: 624–636

244. Schiller HM, Silverberg SC (1971) Staging and prognosis in primary carcinoma of the fallopian tube. Cancer 28: 389–395

244a. Scholes D, Daling JR, Stergachis A, et al (1993) Vaginal douching as a risk factor for acute pelvic inflammatory disease. Obstet Gynecol 81: 601–606

245. Sedlis A (1961) Primary carcinoma of the fallopian tube. Obstet Gynecol Surv 16: 209–226

246. Seidman JD, Oberer S, Bitterman P, et al (1993) Pathogenesis of pseudoxanthomatous salpingiosis. Mod Pathol 6: 53–55

247. Seigler AM (1983) Hysterosalpingography. Fertil Steril 40: 139–158

248. Seltzer VL, Molho L, Fougner A, et al (1988) Paraovarian cystadenocarcinoma of low-malignant potential. Gynecol Oncol 30: 216–221

249. Settlege DSF, Motoshima M, Tredway DR (1973) Sperm transport from the external cervical os to the fallopian tube in women. A time and quantitation study. Fertil Steril 24: 655–661

250. Silverman AY, Greenberg EI (1983) Absence of segment of the proximal portion of a fallopian tube. Obstet Gynecol 62: 90S–91S

251. Skude G, Mårdh PA, Weström L (1976) Amylases of the genital tract. I. Isoamylases of genital tract tissue homogenates and peritoneal fluid. Am J Obstet Gynecol 126: 652–656

252. Soderstrom RM (1985) Sterilization failures and their causes. Am J Obstet Gynecol 152: 395–403

253. Sotus PC (1977) Retroperitoneal ectopic pregnancy: A case report. (Letter) JAMA 238: 1363–1364

254. Spiegelberg O (1878) Zur Kasuistik der Ovarialschwanagenschaft. Arch Gynakol 13: 73

255. Spore WW, Moskal PA, Nakamura RM, Mishell OR (1970) Bacteriology of postpartum oviducts and endometrium. Am J Obstet Gynecol 107: 572–577

256. Stambaugh R, Seitz HM, Mastroianni L Jr (1974) Acrosomal proteinase inhibitors in rhesus monkey (Macaca mulatta) oviduct fluid. Fertil Steril 25: 352–357

257. Stevens LC, Varnum DS (1974) The development of teratomas from pathogenetically activated ovarian mouse eggs. Dev Biol 37: 369–380

258. Stock RJ, Nelson KJ (1984) Ectopic pregnancy subsequent to sterilization: Histologic evaluation and clinical implications. Fertil Steril 42: 211–215

259. Stock RJ (1983) Histopathologic changes in fallopian tubes subsequent to sterilization procedures. Int J Gynecol Pathol 2: 13–27

260. Stone SC, McCalley M, Braunstein P, Egbert B (1985) Radionuclide evaluation of tubal function. Fertil Steril 43: 757–760

261. Stovall TG, Ling FW, O'Kelley KR, et al (1990) Gross and histologic examination of tubal ligation failures in a residency training program. Obstet Gynecol 76: 461–465

262. Sutherland CG (1953) Tubal mole associated with intrauterine pregnancy. Am J Obstet Gynecol 65: 1146–1148

263. Surur F (1974) Actinomycosis of the female genital tract. NY State J Med 74: 408–411

264. Svensson L, Mårdh P-A, Weström L (1983) Infertility after acute salpingitis with special reference to Chlamydia trachomatis. Fertil Steril 40: 322–329

265. Sweet RL (1975) Anaerobic infections of the female genital tract. Am J Obstet Gynecol 122: 891–901

266. Sweet RL, Blankfort-Doyle M, Robbie MO, Schacter J (1986) The occurrence of chlamydial and gonococcal salpingitis during the menstrual cycle. JAMA 255: 2062–2064

267. Sweet RL, Mills J, Hadley KW, et al. (1979) Use of laparoscopy to determine the microbiologic etiology of acute salpingitis. Am J Obstet Gynecol 134: 68–74

268. Swenson RM, Michaelson TC, Daly MJ, Spaulding EH (1973) Anaerobic bacterial infections of the female genital tract. Obstet Gynecol 42: 538–541

269. Symmers W St C (1950) Pathology of oxyuriasis. Arch Pathol 50: 475–516

270. Tatum HJ, Schmidt FH (1977) Contraceptive and sterilization practices and extrauterine pregnancy: A realistic perspective. Fertil Steril 28: 407–421

271. Taxy JB, Battifora H (1976) Female adnexal tumor of probable wolffian origin. Cancer 37: 2349–2354

272. Taxy JB, Battifora H, Oyasu R (1974) Adenomatoid tumors: A light microscopic, histochemical, and ultrastructural study. Cancer 34: 306–316

273. Taylor ES, McMillian JH, Greeer BE, Droegemueller W, Thompson HE (1975) The intrauterine device and tuboovarian abscess. Am J Obstet Gynecol 123: 338–348

274. Teilum G (1971) Special tumors of the ovary and testis. Copenhagen, Munksgard, p 298–301

275. Thadepalli H, Gorbach SL, Keith L (1973) Anaerobic infections of the female genital tract: Bacteriologic and therapeutic aspects. Am J Obstet Gynecol 117: 1034–1040

276. Thompson C, Allen SD, Stargel MD, Thornsberry C, Benigno BB, Thompson JD, Shulman JA (1980) The microbiology and therapy of acute pelvic inflammatory disease in hospitalized patients. Am J Obstet Gynecol 136: 179–186

277. Tilden IL, Winstedt R (1943) Decidual reactions in fallopian tubes. Am J Pathol 19: 1043–1055

278. Tokunaga T, Miyazaki K, Matsyama S, et al (1990) Serial measurement of CA 125 in patients with primary carcinoma of the fallopian tube. Gynecol Oncol 36: 335–337

279. Treiman K, Liskin L (1988) IUDs–A new look. Population Reports, Series B 16(5):1–31

280. Tulusan AH (1984) Complete absence of the muscular layer of the ampullary part of the fallopian tubes. Arch Gynecol 234: 279

281. Vasquez G, Winston RML, Brosens IA (1983) Tubal mucosa and ectopic pregnancy. Br J Obstet Gynaecol 90: 468–474

282. Veress B, Wallmander T (1987) Primary hepatic pregnancy. Acta Obstet Gynecol Scand 66: 563–564

283. Verhege HG, Bareither ML, Jaffe RC, Akbar M (1979) Cyclic changes in ciliation, secretion and cell height of the oviductal epithelium in women. Am J Anat 156: 505–521

284. Verhege HG, Brenner RM (1975) Estradiol-induced differentiation of the oviductal epithelium in ovariectomized cats. Biol Reprod 13: 104–111

285. Voet RL, Lifshitz S (1982) Primary clear cell adenocarcinoma of the fallopian tube: Light microscopic and ultrastructural findings. Int J Gynecol Pathol 1: 292–298

286. Wagner J, Bettendorf U (1980) Extraovarian Brenner tumor. Case report and review. Arch Gynecol 299: 191–196

287. Wallace TM, Hart WR (1991) Acute chlamydial salpingitis with ascites and adnexal mass simulating a malignant neoplasm. Int J Gynecol Pathol 10: 394–401

288. Ward ME, Watt PJ, Robertson JN (1974) The human fallopian tube: A laboratory model for gonococcal infection. J Infect Dis 129: 650–659

289. Weber DL, Fazzini E (1970) Ganglioneuroma of the fallopian tube. Acta Neuropathol 16: 173–175

290. Weinstein L, Morris MB, Dotters D, Christian CD (1983) Ectopic pregnancy—A new surgical epidemic. Obstet Gynecol 61: 698–701

291. Weström L, Bengtsson LP, Mårdh P-A (1976) The risk of

pelvic inflammatory disease in women using intrauterine contraceptive devices as compared to non-users. Lancet 2: 221–223

292. Westrom L, Bengtsson L PH, Mårdh P-A (1981) Incidence, trends, and risks of ectopic pregnancy in a population of women. Br Med J 282: 15–18

293. Wild RA, Albert RD, Zaino RJ, et al (1988) Virilizing paraovarian tumors: A consequence of Nelson's syndrome? Obstet Gynecol 71: 1053–1056

294. Winer AE, Bergman WD, Fields C (1957) Combined intra- and extrauterine pregnancy. Am J Obstet Gynecol 74: 170–178

295. Winkler B, Reumann W, Mitao M, et al (1985) Immunoperoxidase localization of chlamydial antigens in acute salpingitis. Am J Obstet Gynecol 152: 275–278

296. Wlodarski FM, Trainer TD (1975) Granulomatous oophoritis and salpingitis associated with Crohn's disease of the appendix. Am J Obstet Gynecol 122: 527–528

297. Wong S-LR, Lippe BM, Kaplan SA (1971) The XX.Turner phenotype with unilateral streak gonad and absent uterus. Am J Dis Child 122: 449–451

298. Woodruff JD, Julian CG (1969) Multiple malignancy in the upper genital canal. Am J Obstet Gynecol 103: 810–822

299. Woodruff JD, Pauerstein CJ (1969) The Fallopian Tube. Baltimore, Williams & Wilkins

300. World Health Organization (1987) Mechanism of action, safety, and efficacy of intrauterine devices. WHO Technical Report Series 753, WHO, Geneva

301. Wrork DH, Broders AC (1942) Adenomyosis of the fallopian tube. Am J Obstet Gynecol 44: 412–432

302. Yackel DB, Panton ONM, Martin DJ, et al (1988) Splenic pregnancy-case report. Obstet Gynecol 71: 471–473

303. Yeung HHY, Bannatyne P, Russell P (1983) Adenocarcinoma of the fallopian tubes: A clinicopathological study of eight cases. Pathology 15: 279–286

304. Yoonessi M (1979) Carcinoma of the fallopian tube. Obstet Gynecol Surv 34: 257–270

305. Youngs LA, Taylor HB (1967) Adenomatoid tumors of the uterus and fallopian tube. Am J Clin Pathol 48: 537–545

306. Zolli A, Rocko JM (1982) Ectopic pregnancy months and years after hysterectomy. Arch Surg 117: 962–964

15

Anatomy and Histology of the Ovary

Philip B. Clement, M.D.

This chapter considers the normal macroscopic, microscopic, and ultrastructural morphology of the human ovary and its hormonal function. Since the anatomy and function of the ovary vary considerably at different stages in a woman's life, these aspects are considered during adulthood, childhood, and after the menopause.

The Ovary in Adulthood

GROSS ANATOMY

The ovaries are paired pelvic organs that lie on either side of the uterus close to the lateral pelvic wall, behind the broad ligament and anterior to the rectum. Each ovary is attached along its anterior margin (or hilus) by a double fold of peritoneum, the mesovarium, to the posterior aspect of the broad ligament. Each ovary also is attached at its medial pole to the ipsilateral uterine cornu by the ovarian (or utero-ovarian) ligament, and from the superior aspect of its lateral pole to the lateral pelvic wall by the infundibulopelvic (or suspensory) ligament. The location of the ovary posterior to the broad ligament and a similar relationship of the ovarian ligament to the ipsilateral fallopian tube aid in the determination of the laterality of a salpingo-oophorectomy specimen.

Adult ovaries are ovoid, measure approximately 3.0–5 cm × 1.5–3.0 cm × 0.6–1.5 cm, and weigh 5 to 8 g. Their size and weight, however, vary considerably depending on their content of follicular derivatives. Their pinkish white exterior in early reproductive life usually is smooth (Fig. 15.1), but with time exhibits increasing number of convolutions. Thin-walled, fluid-filled cystic follicles and bright yellow corpora lutea may be partially visible from the external aspect. Three ill-defined zones are discernible on the sectioned surface: an outer cortex, an inner medulla, and the hilus. Follicular structures (cystic follicles, corpora lutea, corpora albicantia) typically are visible in the cortex and medulla (Fig. 15.2).

BLOOD VESSELS

The ovarian artery, a branch of the aorta, courses along the infundibulopelvic ligament and the mesovarial border of the ovary where it anastomoses with the ovarian branch of the uterine artery. Approximately 10 arterial branches arise from this arcade and penetrate the ovarian hilus, becoming markedly coiled and branched as they course through the

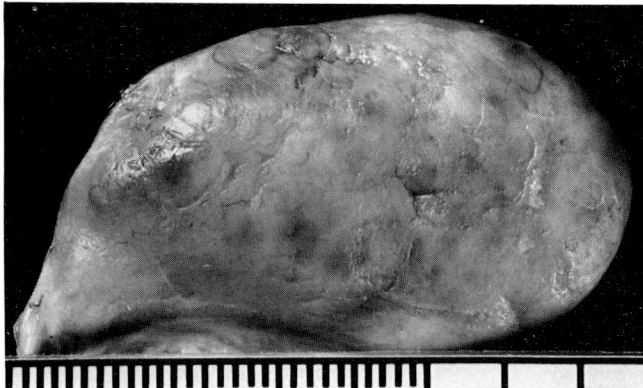

FIG. 15.1. Normal adult ovary from a 25-year-old woman. Except for occasional fibrous adhesions, the external surface is smooth and white.

medulla.[15,117] These helicine arteries have longitudinal ridges of intimal smooth muscle.[15] At the corticomedullary junction, the medullary arteries and arterioles form a plexus from which smaller, straight cortical arterioles arise and penetrate the cortex in a radial fashion, perpendicular to the ovarian surface. These cortical arterioles branch and anastomose several times, forming sets of interconnected vascular arcades.[117] These arcades give rise to capillaries, which form dense networks within the theca layers of the ovarian follicles (Fig. 15.3).

The veins within the ovary accompany the arteries. In the medulla they are large and tortuous. The veins join together in the hilus, forming a plexus that drains into the ovarian veins[15,117]; the latter traverse the mesovarium and course along the infundibulpelvic ligament. The left and right ovarian veins drain into the left renal vein and the inferior vena cava, respectively.

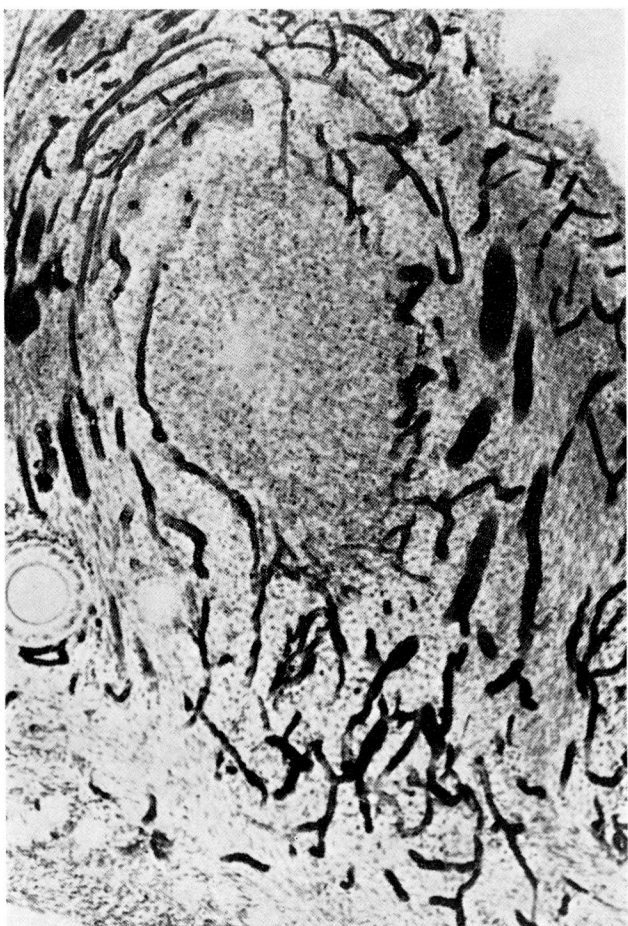

FIG. 15.3. Perifollicular capillary network. Ovarian vessels were injected with colored gelatin before sectioning. (Reprinted by permission of Leeson and Leeson (1970) Histology. Philadelphia, Saunders.)

LYMPHATICS

The lymphatics of the ovary originate predominantly within the theca layers of the follicles. The granulosa layer of a maturing follicle is devoid of lymphatics, in contrast to its counterpart within the corpus luteum, which possesses a rich supply of lymphatics.[110] The lymphatics pass through the ovarian stroma, independent of blood vessels, to drain into larger trunks that form a plexus at the hilus.[110] Within the hilus, the lymphatics and blood vessels converge, with the former coiled around veins in a helicoid fashion.[110] Four to eight efferent channels enter the mesovarium where they converge to form another plexus ("subovarian plexus") that is joined by branches from the fallopian tube and uterine fundus.[110] Leaving the plexus, the drainage trunks diminish in number and size, passing along the free border of the infundibulopelvic ligament in association with the ovarian veins.[110] From there they accompany the ovarian vessels, juxtaposed to the psoas muscle, and drain into the upper para-aortic lymph nodes at the

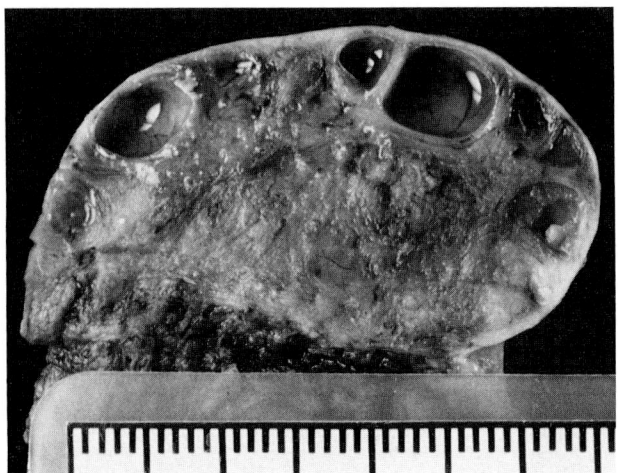

FIG. 15.2. Normal adult ovary (cut surface). Occasional cystic follicles are present in the cortex.

level of the lower pole of the kidney.[38,110,124] The major lymphatic drainage of the ovary is therefore in a cephaloid direction toward the aortic nodes. Accessory channels, however, exist in many women; they bypass the subovarian plexus, passing through the broad ligament to the internal iliac, external iliac, and interaortic lymph nodes, or via the round ligament to the iliac and inguinal lymph nodes.[38,110,124]

NERVES

The nerve supply of the ovary arises from a sympathetic plexus that is enmeshed with the ovarian vessels in the infundibulopelvic ligament.[62] Nerve fibers, which are predominantly nonmyelinated, accompany the ovarian artery, entering the ovary at the hilus. Delicate terminal fibers, many surrounding small arteries and arterioles, penetrate the medulla and cortex to terminate as perifollicular plexuses.[62,103] Adrenergic nerve fibers and terminals have been shown to be in close contact with smooth muscle cells in the cortical stroma and theca externa. The physiological significance of ovarian sympathetic innervation is not clear, although it has been suggested that it may play a role in follicular maturation, follicular rupture, or both.[7,62,94] Substance P, a neuropeptide found within the ovarian thecal and stromal cells, may be supplied by these nerve fibers.[8] In addition, catecholamines can stimulate progesterone production by the ovarian follicles and androgen production by the ovarian stroma in vitro.[37]

Surface Epithelium

HISTOLOGY

The ovary is covered by a single, focally pseudostratified layer of modified peritoneal cells that constitute the surface epithelium. The cells vary from flat to cuboidal to columnar and several types may be seen in different areas of the same ovary (Fig. 15.4). The surface cells are separated from the underlying stroma by a distinct basement membrane. In oophorectomy specimens, the epithelium almost always is denuded as a result of handling by the surgeon and pathologist and a lack of prompt fixation. Preserved epithelium usually is confined to areas protected by surface adhesions or lining sulci.[124] Surface epithelium within these crevices may lose its connection with the surface, giving rise to surface epithelial inclusion glands and cysts (see Chapter 16, Nonneoplastic Lesions of the Ovary).

Histochemical studies have demonstrated glycogen, as well as acid and neutral mucopolysaccharides, within surface epithelial cells.[14,83] Unlike extraovarian mesothelial cells, surface epithelial cells of the ovary have 17β-hydroxysteroid dehydrogenase activity[14] and estrogen,[60] progesterone,[60] and epidermal growth factor[120] receptors. The surface epithelial cells are immunoreactive for cytokeratin, vimentin, and desmoplakin, but not desmin.[11,30,31,92] Several antigens associated with ovarian tumors of surface epithelial origin have been demonstrated with a variable frequency, including CA 125,[68,99,101] anticarbohydrate determinant 19-9 (CA 19-9),[22] and MH99,[24] but not carcinoembryonic antigen.[22,101]

ULTRASTRUCTURE

The ultrastructural appearance of the ovarian surface epithelium is similar to that of the extraovarian peritoneum.[13,41,105] By scanning and transmission electron microscopy the cell surfaces are characterized by dome-shaped apices covered by numerous, often branching, microvilli, an occasional single cilium, and pinocytotic vesicles (Figs. 15.5, 15.6). The cytoplasm contains abundant polysomes, free ribosomes, abundant mitochondria, and bundles of intermediate filaments and tonofilaments. Lipid droplets are sometimes present in the basal cytoplasm. The nuclei have indented nuclear membranes and peripheral nucleoli. Straight or convoluted lateral plasma membranes are reinforced by luminal junctional complexes, scattered desmosomes, and desmosomal–tonofilament complexes. The membranes may be widely separated in areas, creating dilated intercellular spaces.[41] A well-developed basal lamina separates the surface epithelium from the underlying cortical stroma.

Stroma

HISTOLOGY

As the cortical and medullary stroma is continuous and similar in appearance, the boundary between these two zones is ill-defined and arbitrary. Moreover, the amount of stroma in the cortex and medulla varies considerably from one individual to another. Because the stroma of the superficial cortex is typically more fibrotic than elsewhere, it is

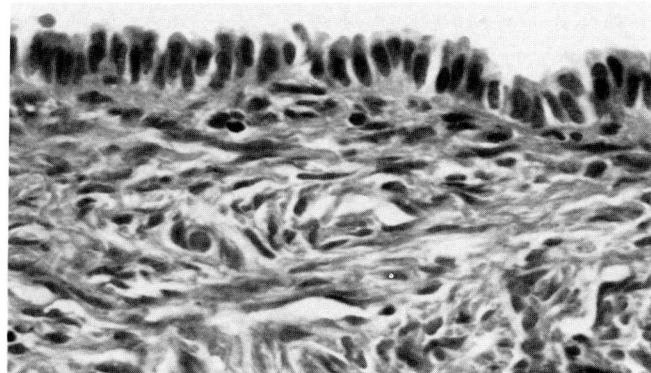

FIG. 15.4. Ovarian surface epithelium. A single layer of columnar cells overlies the ovarian stroma.

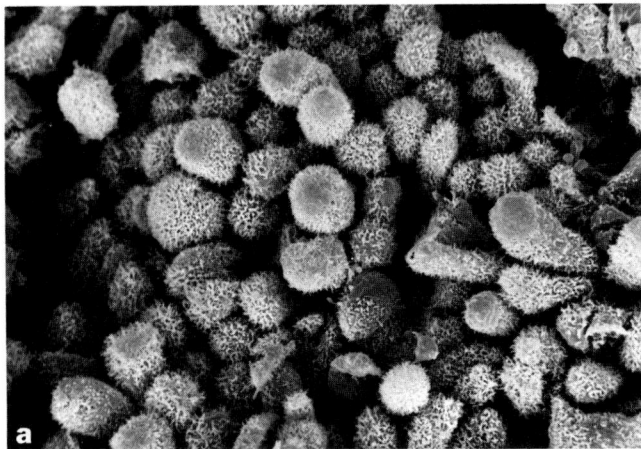

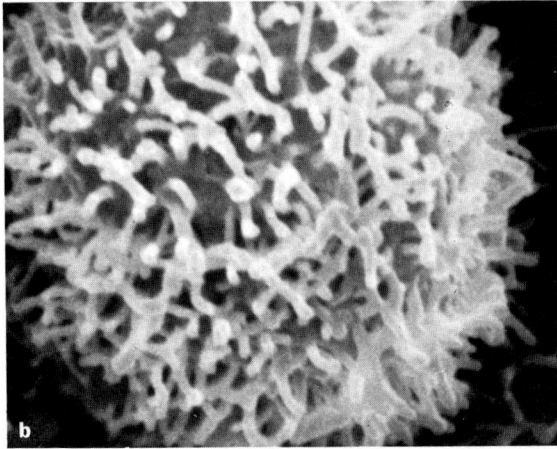

FIG. 15.5. Scanning electron micrograph of ovarian surface epithelium. a: Note dome-shaped apices covered by abundant surface microvilli. ×1140. **b:** Branching surface microvilli. ×12,000. (Reprinted by permission of Ferenczy and Richart, ref. 41. Copyright John Wiley & Sons, Inc., 1974.)

frequently referred to as the *tunica albuginea;* however, it lacks the densely collagenous, almost acellular appearance and sharp delineation of this layer in the testis. The spindle-shaped stromal cells have scant cytoplasm and resemble fibroblasts. They are typically arranged in whorls or a storiform pattern within a dense reticulum network (Fig. 15.7b) and a variable amount of collagen (Fig. 15.7a). Cytoplasmic lipid in the form of fine droplets may be appreciable with special stains, especially in the late reproductive and postmenopausal age groups.[40] The stromal cells are immunoreactive for vimentin, actin, and desmin,[11,31,32,73,92,128] as well as for estrogen, progesterone, and testosterone binding sites.[4] In many women of late reproductive and postmenopausal age, there is a decrease in stromal volume and cellularity, with an increase in collagen (see page 589).

A variety of other cells may be found within the ovarian stroma, most of which probably are derived from the spindle-shaped stromal cells:

1. Luteinized stromal cells are found singly or in small nests at a distance from the follicles, most often in the medulla. They are polygonal with abundant eosinophilic to clear cytoplasm and a central round nucleus with a prominent nucleolus. The cytoplasm contains variable amounts of lipid and may be immunoreactive for testosterone.[95] Luteinized stromal cells increase during pregnancy and after the menopause, probably because of elevated levels of circulating gonadotropins.[17,40] In one autopsy study luteinized stromal cells were demonstrated after diligent searching in 13% of women under the age of 55 years and in one-third of women over that age. More exhaustive sampling might indicate that luteinized stromal cells are a normal finding in the ovary, particularly in later life.[17] In this age group, the presence of luteinized cells usually is not associated with clinical evidence of an endocrine disturbance. In some older women, but more often in younger patients, more striking degrees of stromal luteinization (stromal hyperthecosis) are frequently associated with androgenic or estrogenic manifestations or both (see Chapter 16, Nonneoplastic Lesions of the Ovary).

2. Enzymatically active stromal cells (EASC) are characterized by their oxidative and other enzymatic activity.[40,78,96,124,126] Some EASC correspond to luteinized stromal cells, but most cannot be distinguished from neighboring, nonreactive stromal cells in routine histologic preparations.[124,126] They are typically found in the medulla, and increase in number with age, occurring in more than 80% of postmenopausal women.[126]

3. Decidual cells, representing focal decidual transformation of the ovarian stroma in response to elevated progesterone levels, are found in almost every ovary examined at term. Similar cells also are found occasionally in nonpregnant women (see Chapter 16).[10,12,52,61,132]

4. Endometrial stroma-type cells (ovarian stromatosis) (see Chapter 16).

5. Smooth muscle cells have been demonstrated within the ovarian stroma in otherwise normal ovaries, but also in certain pathological conditions (see Chapter 16).[125] Smooth muscle cells also have been identified on ultrastructural examination within the normal theca externa of the follicles.[102]

6. Fat cells (see Chapter 16).

7. Stromal Leydig cells (see Chapter 16).

Rare cells of neuroendocrine or APUD type, which may be of stromal origin, have been demonstrated within the ovarian stroma in approximately 6% of normal women in one study.[56] The cells occur in small groups in the corticomedullary stromal junction and exhibit argyrophilia and argentaffinity. Their clinical significance and hormonal function, if any, are unknown.

ULTRASTRUCTURE

Typical ovarian stromal cells have slender, spindle-shaped nuclei and complex cytoplasmic processes. Their scant cytoplasm is rich in organelles required for collagen synthe-

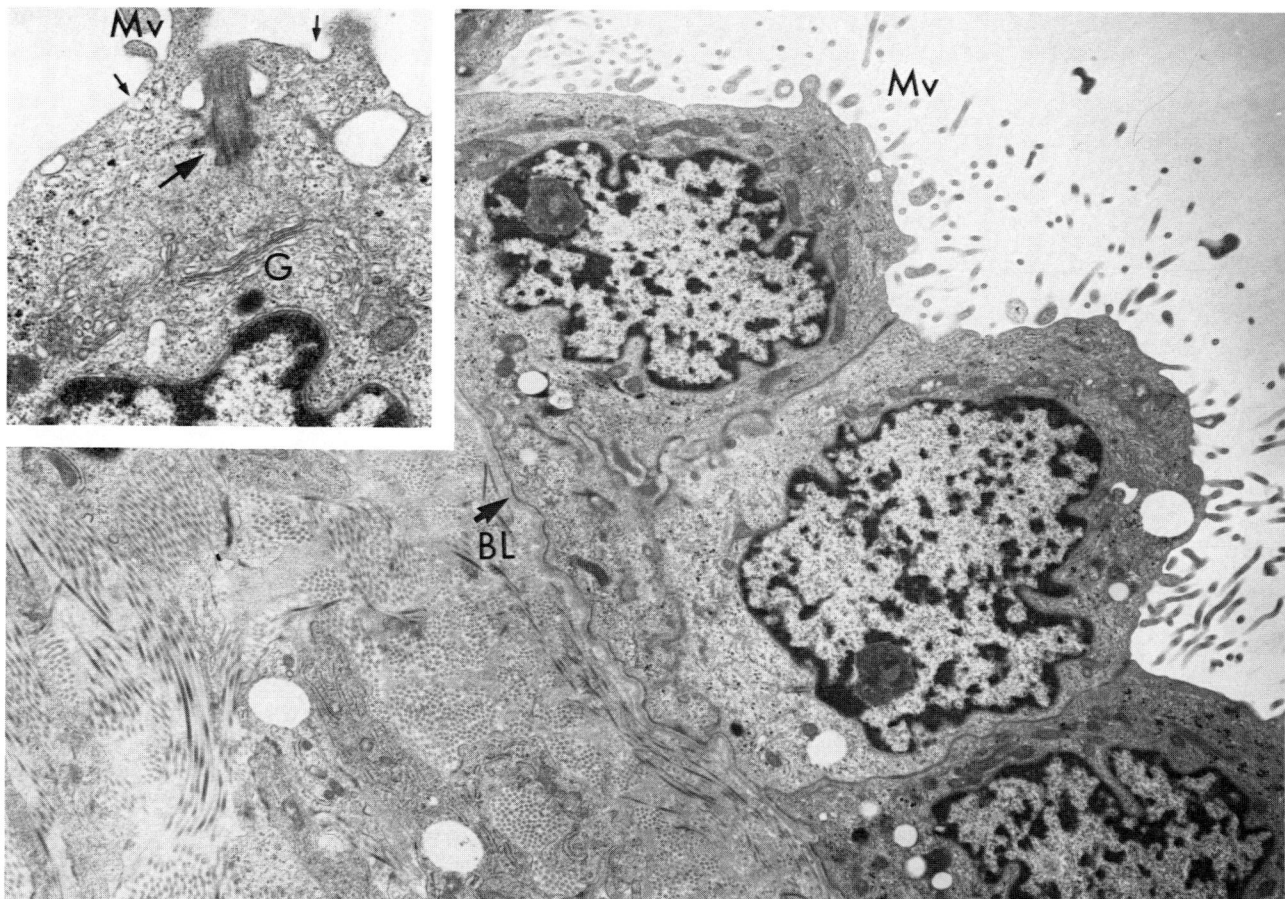

FIG. 15.6. Electron micrograph of ovarian surface epithelium. The cells have numerous microvilli (*Mv*) and well-developed organelles in a perinuclear location. The nuclei have indented membranes and peripheral nucleoli. The lateral plasma membranes are reinforced by luminal junctional complexes and scattered desmosomes but are occasionally widely separated, producing dilated intercellular spaces. A well-defined basal lamina (*BL*) separates the cells from the underlying stroma. *Inset:* The surface microvilli are associated with micropinocytotic vesicles (*short arrows*) and occasional single cilia (*long arrow*). G, Golgi. ×6400. Inset ×22,000. (Reprinted by permission of Ferenczy and Richart, ref. 41.)

sis, including free ribosomes and mitochondria.[41] Tropocollagen, concentrated at the periphery of the cytoplasm, is deposited in the extracellular space and eventually is converted to collagen (Fig. 15.8a).[41] Rows of micropinocytotic vesicles occur along the plasma membrane and desmosome-like attachments may be found between the cells (Fig. 15.8b). Luteinized stromal cells have abundant cytoplasm containing lipid droplets and steroidogenic organelles, including smooth endoplasmic reticulum, mitochondria with tubular cristae, and Golgi complexes.[41,71] Cells with an ultrastructural appearance intermediate in appearance between fibroblastic cells and luteinized cells also are evident.[41] Electron microscopic examination of the argyrophilic stromal cells reveals electron-dense, membrane-bound, cytoplasmic granules measuring from 300 to 750 nm in diameter.[56]

HORMONE SYNTHESIS

Numerous studies have demonstrated the steroidogenic potential and the gonadotropin responsiveness of the ovarian stroma in both pre- and postmenopausal women.[21,35,49,66,67,77,81,86,89,138] In vitro incubation of ovarian stromal tissue indicates that its principal steroid product is androstenedione, in addition to smaller quantities of testosterone and dehydroepiandrosterone.[119] In vitro production of these androgens is enhanced by human chorionic gonadotropin (hCG), pituitary gonadotropins, and insulin, consistent with the presence of receptors for these hormones within the stromal cells.[9,95,96] To what extent the ovarian stroma contributes to the androgen pool in normal premenopausal women is unknown; it is likely the source of small amounts of testosterone.

Primordial Follicles

HISTOLOGY

Approximately 400,000 primordial follicles are present at birth, decreasing progressively through the processes of folliculogenesis and atresia. Their eventual disappearance

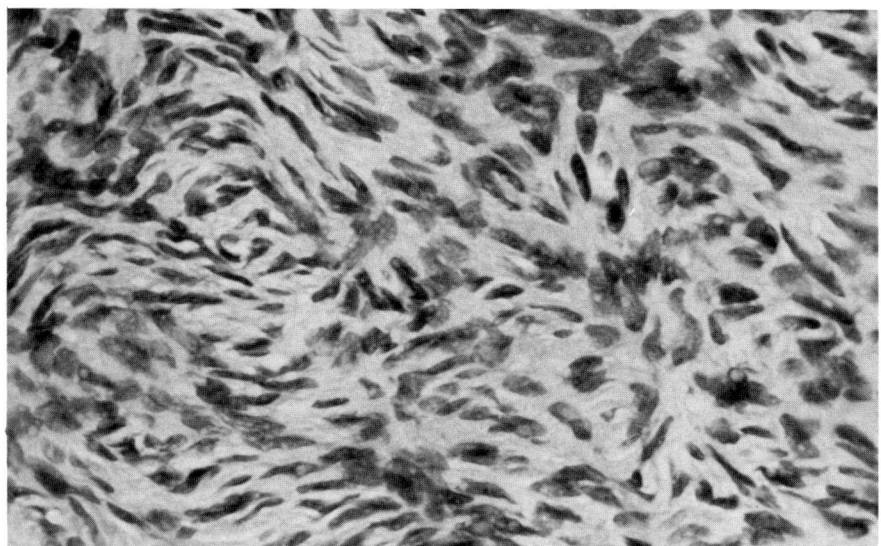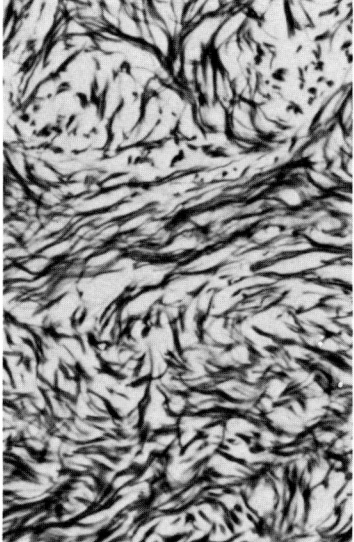

FIG. 15.7. Ovarian stroma. a: Plump, fibroblastic cells are arranged in whorls. **b:** Dense pericellular reticulum pattern is evident (reticulin stain).

corresponds with the end of the menopause. In women of reproductive age, the follicles are irregularly distributed in the superficial cortex. The primordial follicles consist of a primary oocyte, 40–70 μm in diameter, surrounded by a single layer of flattened, mitotically inactive, granulosa cells resting on a thin basal lamina (Fig. 15.9). Rare primordial and maturing follicles contain multiple oocytes.[45] The large spherical nucleus of the oocyte has finely granular, uniformly dispersed chromatin and one or more dense, thread-like nucleoli;[6] rare oocytes have multiple nuclei.[45,79] Within the cytoplasm of the oocyte is a paranuclear, eosinophilic, crescentic zone representing a complex of interrelated organelles ("Balbiani's vitelline body") (Fig. 15.9).[54,55] Within the vitelline body is a dark spot, the centrosome, surrounded by a halo, which in turn is flanked by darker, PAS-positive, granular zones rich in mitochondria.[54,55] The cytoplasm of the oocyte lacks the abundant glycogen and the high alkaline phosphatase activity characteristic of the primordial germ cells and the oogonia of the embryonic gonad.[124]

ULTRASTRUCTURE

The granulosa cells of the primordial follicle have sparse organelles, occasional desmosomal attachments with each other, and microvillous projections that attach to the oocyte through tight apposition (Fig. 15.10).[41] Within the oocyte, the juxtanuclear centrosome of the vitelline body consists of dense granules, closely packed vesicles, and peripheral dense fibers at the periphery of the centrosome (Figs. 15.11, 15.12).[54,55] The centrosome is surrounded by a zone of smooth endoplasmic reticulum (ER) that represents the halo seen by light microscopy. Surrounding the

centrosome and constituting the rest of the vitelline body are a concentration of most of the oocyte's organelles, including multiple Golgi complexes, prominent compound aggregates, numerous mitochondria intimately associated with sparsely granular ER, and annulate lamellae.[54,55] The annulate lamellae are arranged in stacks or concentric arrangements of up to 100 parallel, smooth, paired membranes fused at regular intervals and surround flattened cisternal spaces, 30–50 μm wide (Fig. 15.13).[6,41,54] The annulate lamellae may play a role in nucleocytoplasmic exchange of substances related to metabolic activity or the transfer of genetic information.[41,54]

Maturing Follicles

FOLLICULOGENESIS

Folliculogenesis refers to the continuous process occurring throughout reproductive life whereby cohorts of primordial follicles undergo maturation during each menstrual cycle. Follicular maturation begins during the luteal phase and continues throughout the follicular phase of the next cycle. Each month only one such follicle, the preovulatory or dominant follicle, achieves complete maturation, culminating in the release of the oocyte, that is, ovulation. The other follicles that have begun to mature undergo atresia at earlier stages of their development (see page 582). Folliculogenesis and atresia continue during pregnancy, although the former process does not reach the preovulatory follicle stage.[34,46,80,97]

Follicular maturation begins with enlargement of the oocyte and alteration of the granulosa cells from flat to cuboidal or columnar (*primary follicle*). The granulosa

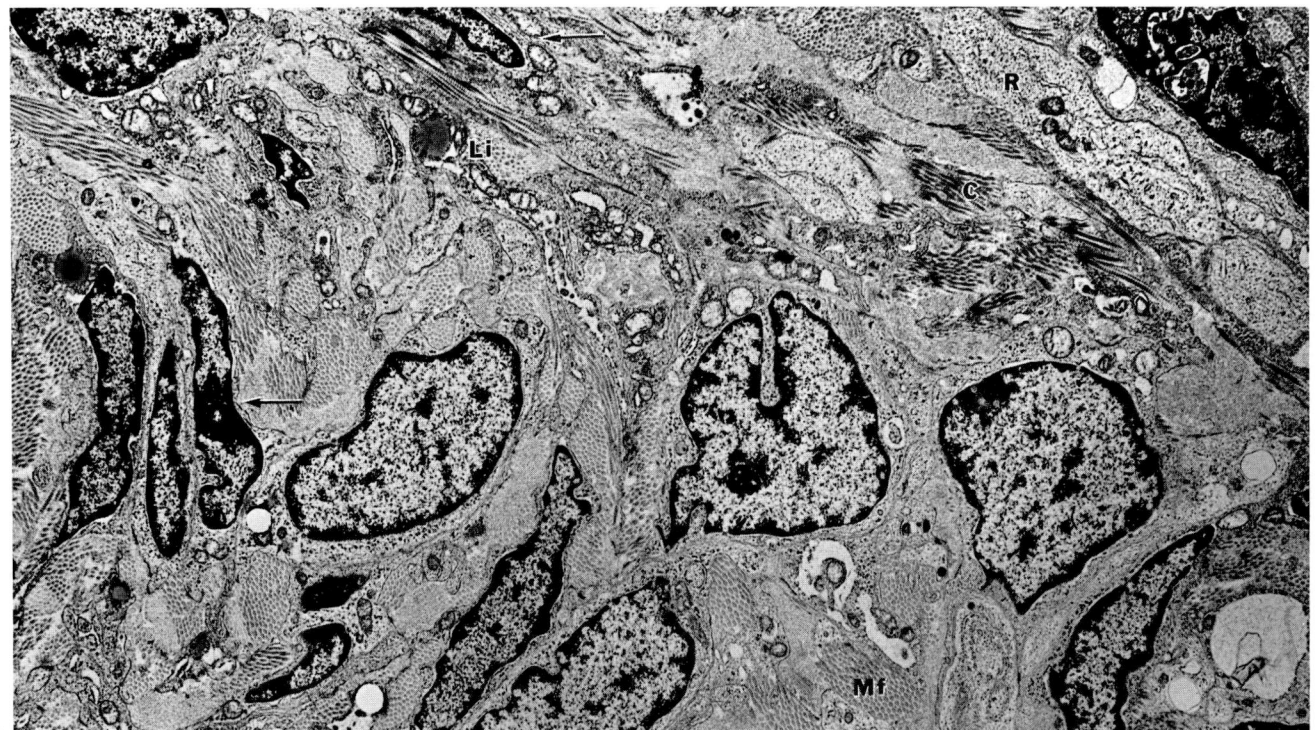

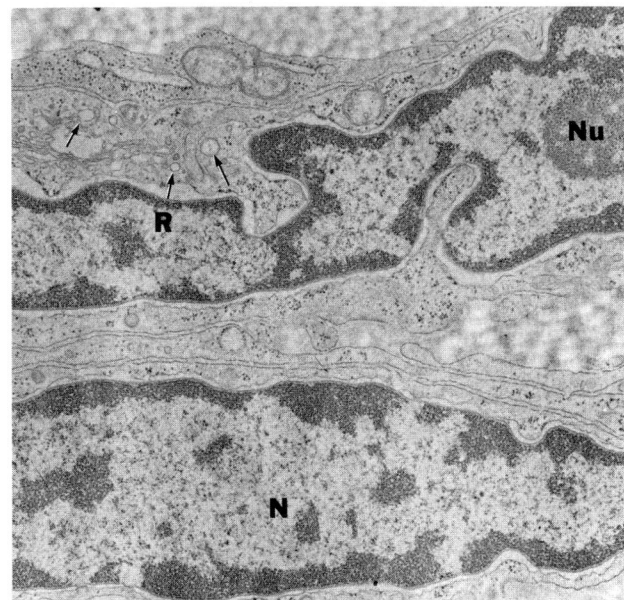

FIG. 15.8. a: Electron micrograph of ovarian stromal cells. The cells are fibroblastic in type. C, collagen fibers. Mf, tropocollagen; R, free ribosomes; Li, lipid inclusions; *upper arrow*, perinuclear clustering of mitochondria. ×3000. **b: Higher power of two stromal cells showing micropinocytotic vesicles (*arrows*).** R, ribosomes; N, nucleus; Nu, nucleolus. ×12,000.

cells proliferate, forming 3–5 concentric layers around the oocyte (*secondary or preantral follicle*) (Fig. 15.14). Preantral follicles measure from 50 to 400 μm in diameter; as they increase in size, they migrate into the more vascularized medulla. Simultaneously, the surrounding ovarian stromal cells become specialized into several layers of theca interna cells and an outer, ill-defined layer of theca externa cells. Secretion of mucopolysaccharide-rich fluid by the granulosa cells results in their separation by fluid-

filled clefts. The latter eventually coalesce to form a single large cavity or antrum lined by several layers of granulosa cells (*tertiary, antral, or vesicular follicle*) (Fig. 15.15). As the follicle enlarges because of continued fluid secretion into the antrum, the oocyte reaches its definitive size and an eccentric position at one pole of the follicle. At this site the granulosa cells proliferate to form the cumulus oophorus that contains the oocyte and protrudes into the antrum (*mature or graafian follicle*) (Fig. 15.16).

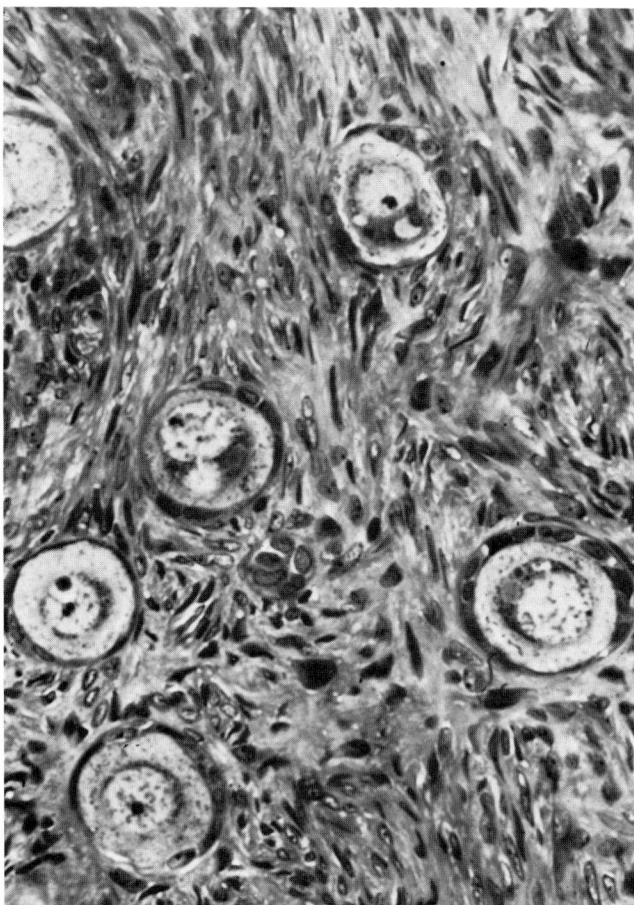

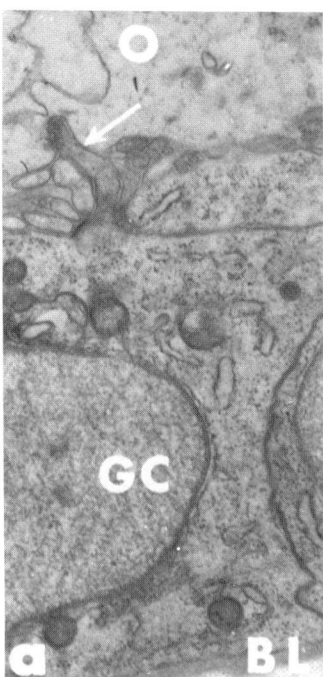

Fig. 15.10. The granulosa cells (*GC*) of the primordial follicle. The granulosa cells have microvillous projections that are attached to the oocyte (*O*) by tight apposition (*arrow*). BL, basal lamina. ×20,000. (Reprinted by permission of Hertig, ref. 54.)

Fig. 15.9. Primordial follicles within ovarian cortex. The primary oocytes are surrounded by a single layer of flattened granulosa cells. Note perinuclear crescentic zones (Balbiani's vitelline body) in the cytoplasm of several of the oocytes. (Reprinted by permission of Baca of Zamboni, ref. 6.)

Ovulation

During each cycle, usually less than four mature follicles in each ovary reach a diameter of 4–5 mm by the middle to late luteal phase; one of them will become the preovulatory follicle of the next cycle.[88] Late in follicular growth, the oocyte, its surrounding zona pellucida, and a single layer of radially disposed, columnar granulosa cells, the corona radiata, detach from the cumulus oophorus and float in the antral fluid. The preovulatory follicle shortly before ovulation reaches a diameter of 15–25 mm.[7,88] It partially protrudes from the ovarian surface at a point that represents the eventual rupture point, or stigma. The surface epithelial and stromal cells in this area become attenuated and degenerate, changes that may be secondary to local ischemia and release of proteolytic enzymes and prostaglandins.[7] The preovulatory follicle then ruptures, possibly aided by contraction of the perifollicular smooth muscle cells, with liberation of the follicular fluid, the oocyte, and its corona radiata into the peritoneal cavity. After ovula-

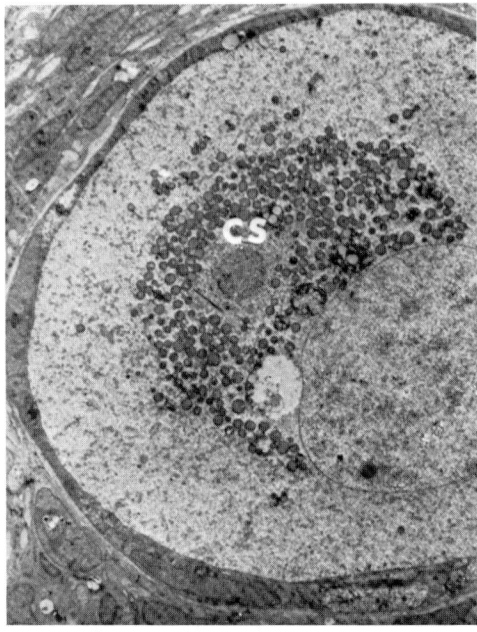

Fig. 15.11. Balbiani's vitelline body. Within a primordial follicle, Balbiani's vitelline body is seen, consisting of a juxtanuclear centrosome (*CS*) surrounded by a condensation of mitochondria, Golgi, endoplasmic reticulum, and lysosomes. ×2400. (Reprinted by permission of Hertig, ref. 54.)

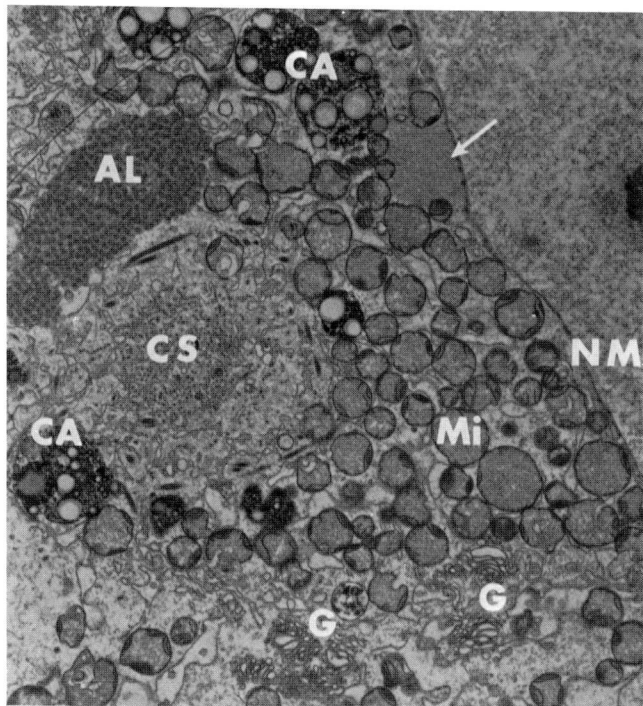

FIG. 15.12. Detailed view of Balbiani's vitelline body. A cluster of closely packed spiral fibrils (*arrow*) is attached to the nuclear envelope (*NM*). The centrosome (*CS*) is composed of dense granules, some arranged periodically on fine fibers, and small vesicles, with a peripheral zone of endoplasmic reticulum and dense fibers. Surrounding the centrosome are masses of mitochondria (*Mi*) and compound aggregates (*CA*). A stack of annulate lamellae (*AL*) is seen tangentially. Note the prominent endoplasmic reticulum in close association with multiple Golgi complexes (*G*) at the periphery of the vitelline body. (Reprinted by permission of Hertig, ref. 54.)

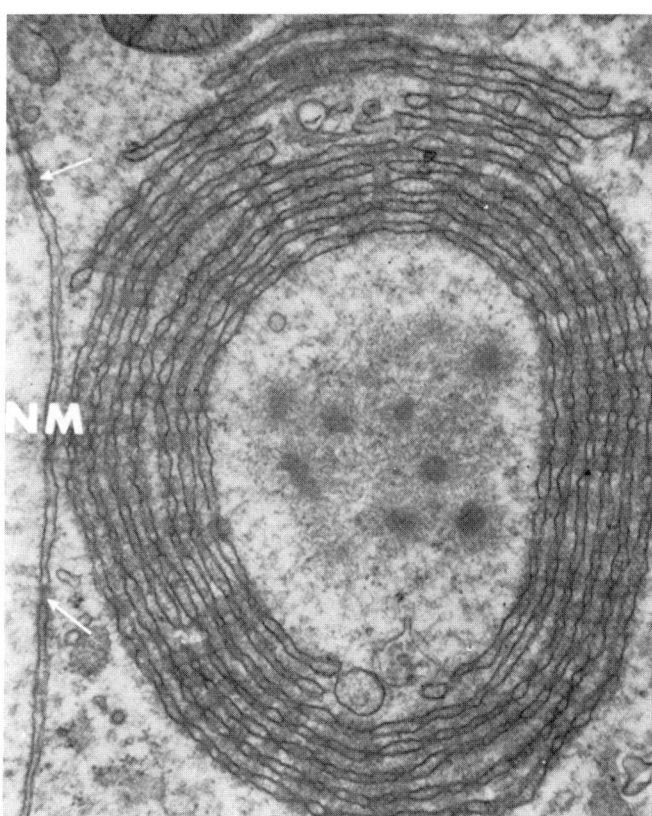

FIG. 15.13. A coiled stack of annulate lamellae from a primordial follicle. NM, nuclear membrane. (Reprinted by permission of Hertig, ref. 54.)

tion, the stigma is occluded by a mass of coagulated follicular fluid, fibrin, blood, and granulosa and connective tissue cells; it is eventually converted to scar tissue.[7] The specific components of the maturing follicle are considered in more detail.

OOCYTE AND ZONA PELLUCIDA

As the oocyte matures it triples in size and there is an increase in mitochondria, granular ER, free ribosomes, and Golgi, reflecting increased protein synthesis. The number of annulate lamellae, however, decrease.[6,41] The Golgi, which appear to be the source of dense, membrane-bound, 300–500-nm granules, are dispersed in aggregates under the plasma membrane (Fig. 15.17).[6] Surface microvilli are predominant and closely associated with the bordering granulosa cells (Fig. 15.17).

When the oocyte of the preantral follicle is 80 μm in diameter, it is encased by an eosinophilic, PAS-positive, homogeneous, acellular layer, the zona pellucida

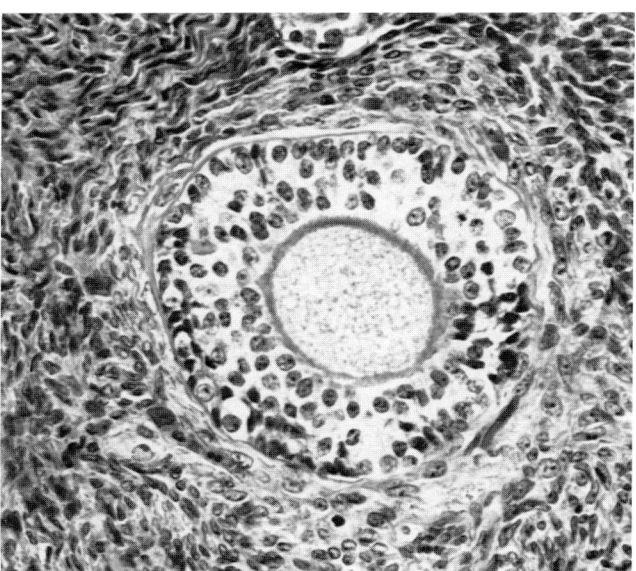

FIG. 15.14. Preantral follicle. Several layers of granulosa cells surround the oocyte. A theca interna layer is not yet apparent.

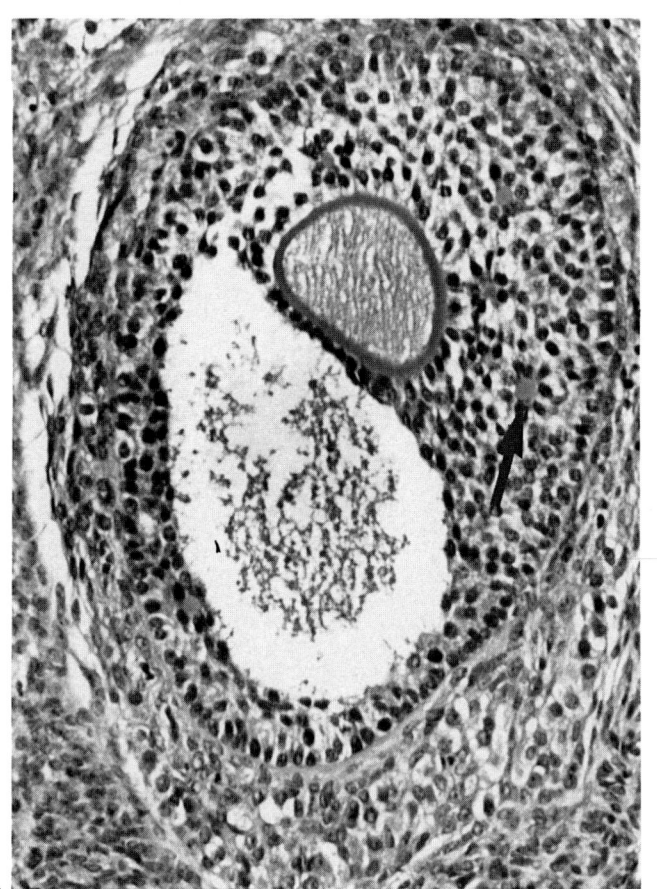

15.15

(Figs. 15.16–15.18). Its formation usually is attributed to the granulosa cells, but the oocyte also may play a role. At the end of its development, the zona pellucida is a 20–25-μm thick membrane consisting of fine filamentous material of medium electron density[6] rich in acid mucopolysaccharides and glycoprotein.[41]

During the early stages of follicular growth, the oocyte nucleus has an appearance similar to that seen in the primordial follicle. Soon before ovulation, the oocyte within the preovulatory follicle enters telophase of the first meiotic division. Chromosomal reduction occurs by migration of one-half the oocyte chromosomes into a portion of the oocyte cytoplasm that separates from the cell as the first polar body. The latter lies within the perivitelline space between the plasma membrane of the oocyte and the inner aspect of the zona pellucida (Fig. 15.18). After completion of the first meiotic division, the oocyte is now referred to as the *secondary oocyte*. Immediately after expulsion of the first

Fɪɢ. 15.15. **Antral follicle.** Note Call–Exner body (*arrow*) within the granulosa layer. A well-developed theca interna layer is now visible.

Fɪɢ. 15.16 a: **Graafian follicle with large antrum. b: Higher power view.** Note the cumulus oophorus containing the oocyte with its surrounding zona pellucida and corona radiata. (Reprinted by permission of Leeson and Leeson (1970) Histology, Philadelphia, Saunders.)

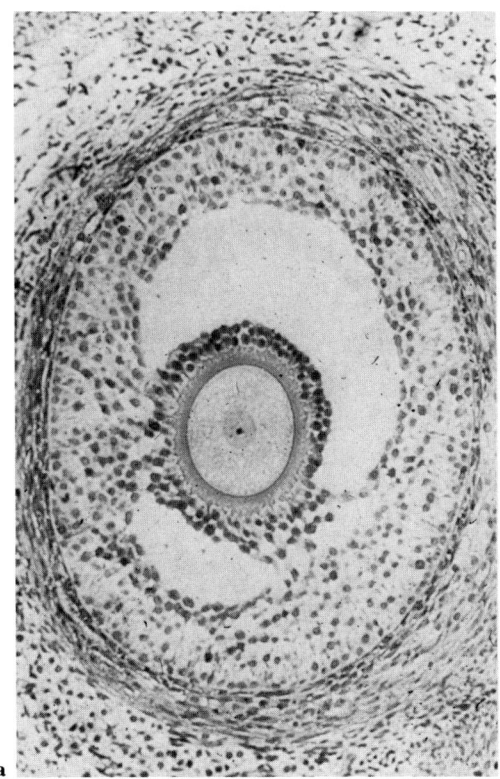

15.16a

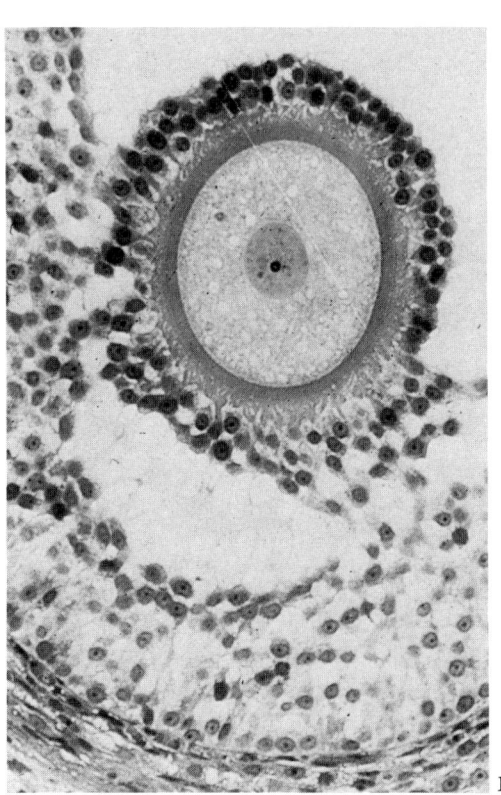

15.16b

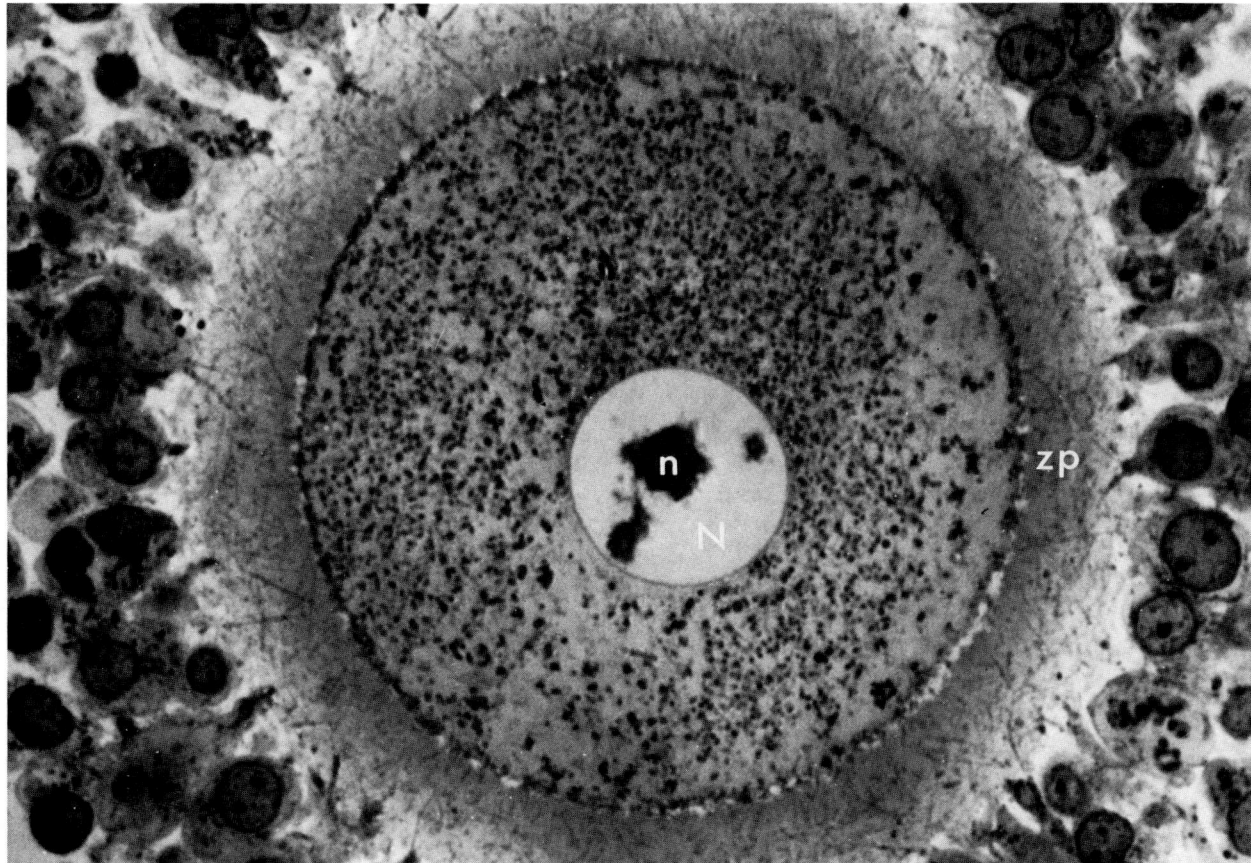

FIG. 15.17. Maturing oocyte. Note the uniform distribution of the organelles and the row of dense granules in the cytoplasm immediately subjacent to the plasma membrane of the oocyte. A continuous zona pellucida (*zp*) surrounds the oocyte and sepa-rates it from the granulosa cells. Numerous cytoplasmic processes of the granulosa cells are visible within the zone pellucida. N, nucleus; n, nucleolus. (Reprinted by permission of Baca and Zamboni, ref. 6.)

polar body, the secondary oocyte enters the second meiotic division, arresting at metaphase until fertilization occurs.

GRANULOSA CELLS

HISTOLOGY

Granulosa cells within maturing and mature follicles are polyhedral and measure 5–7 μm in diameter. Cells resting on the basement membrane are often columnar in shape. Granulosa cells have scant, pale, frothy cytoplasm, indistinct cell borders, and small, round to oval, hyperchromatic nuclei that typically lack nuclear grooves (Fig. 15.19a).[145] Until the onset of luteinization several hours before ovulation, cytoplasmic lipid is absent or sparse, and there is little histochemical evidence of steroidogenesis.[64] The cytoplasm of granulosa cells of primary, secondary, and mature follicles is immunoreactive for cytokeratin, vimentin, and desmoplakin.[11,31,92]

Mitotic figures usually are numerous in maturing follicles, but decrease immediately before ovulation. The granulosa cells typically surround small cavities, Call–Exner bodies (Fig. 15.15), that represent a distinctive feature of normal and neoplastic granulosa cells. Call–Exner bodies are delimited from the granulosa cells by a basal lamina, and contain a deeply eosinophilic, PAS-positive, filamentous material consisting of excess basal lamina.[15,41,124] Unlike the theca layers, the granulosa layer is avascular and devoid of a reticulum framework (Fig. 15.19b).

ULTRASTRUCTURE

Mitochondria with lamelliform cristae, granular ER, free ribosomes, and Golgi gradually increase within the granulosa cells of maturing follicles,[15] suggesting active protein synthesis. Histochemical and ultrastructural features indicative of steroid biosynthesis, such as abundant smooth ER and mitochondria with tubular cristae, are absent until shortly before ovulation.[33,40,65,91,126] The plasma membranes of the granulosa cells are connected by adherent junctions, gap junctions, and desmosomes.[6,31,39,41] The slender cytoplasmic extensions of the granulosa cells of the corona radiata that traverse the zona pellucida have gap

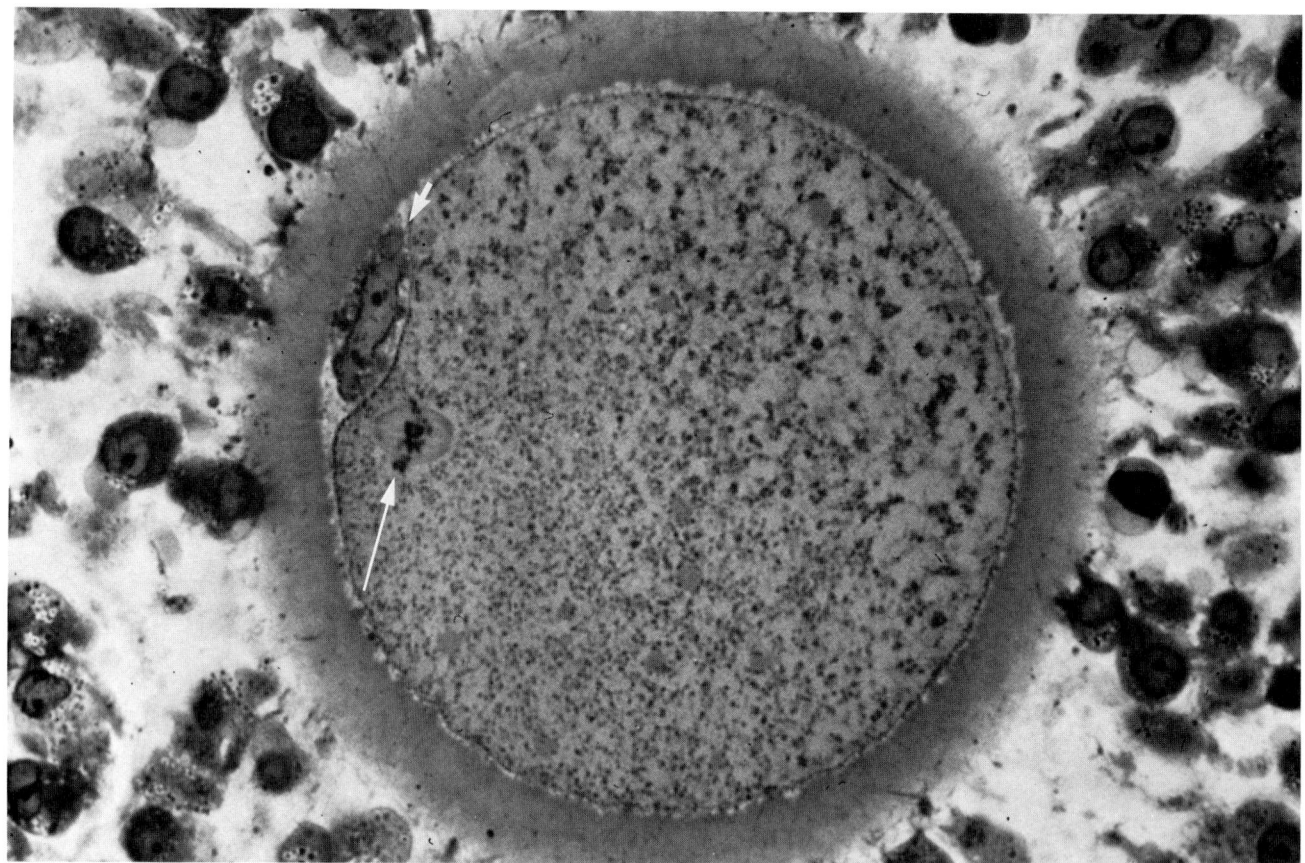

FIG. 15.18. Oocyte shortly after separation of the first polar body. The first polar body (*short arrow*) sits in the perivitelline space. The posttelophasic chromosomes are arranged on the equatorial plate of the meiotic spindle (*long arrow*). (Reprinted by permission of Baca and Zamboni, ref. 6.)

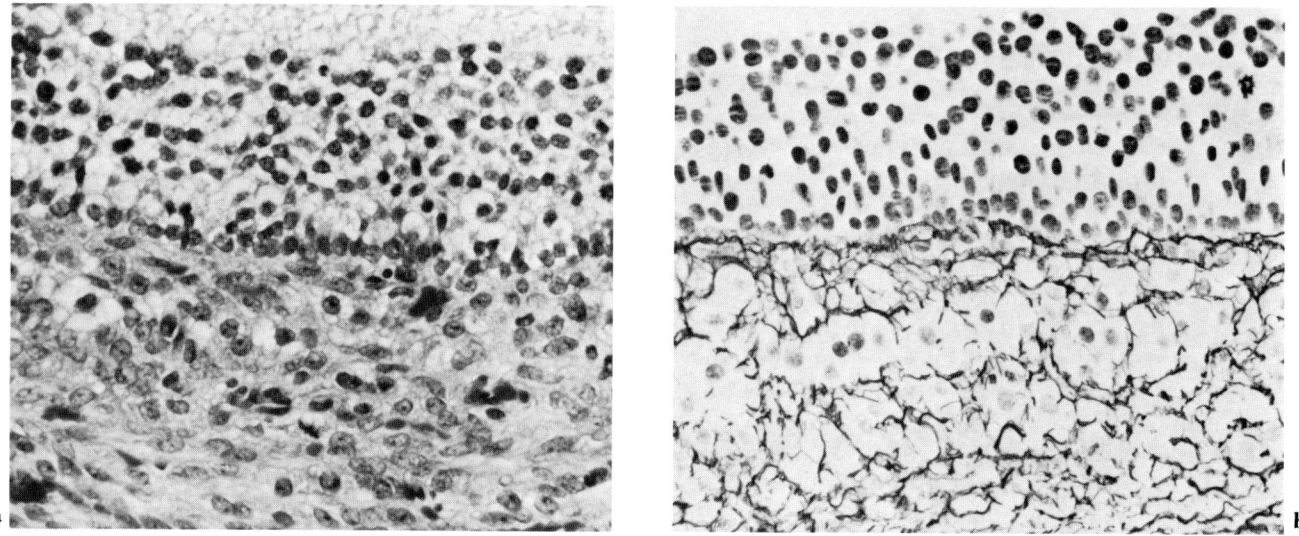

FIG. 15.19. Lining of mature follicle. a: The granulosa layer is surrounded by an outer layer of luteinized theca interna cells. **b:** A reticulin stain reveals a reticulum network in the theca interna layer but an absence of reticulin in the granulosa layer.

junctions and puncta adherentia with the plasma membrane of the oocyte (Fig. 15.17).[6,31,41]

Theca Cells

In contrast to granulosa cells, theca cells differentiate continuously from the stromal cells at the periphery of developing follicles, a process beginning in fetal life and ending after the menopause.[124] The thecal component of the antral follicle is characterized by a well-developed theca interna and a less well defined theca externa.

Histology

The theca interna layer is three or four cells thick and lies external to the granulosa layer from which it is separated by a basement membrane. Unlike the granulosa cells, the theca interna cells typically have a luteinized or partially luteinized appearance and have steroidogenic histochemical features.[33,40,65,124] The theca interna of maturing follicles is particularly prominent during pregnancy. The cells are round to polygonal and 12–20 μm in diameter. Their cytoplasm is abundant, eosinophilic to clear, and vacuolated with variable amounts of lipid. The nucleus is centrally located, round, and vesicular with a single, prominent nucleolus (Fig. 15.19a). Theca cells, like other ovarian stromal cells, are immunoreactive for vimentin but not cytokeratin.[11] Mitotic figures typically are present within the theca cells of maturing follicles. Occasional darkly eosinophilic, stellate "K" cells may be seen in the mature follicle within the theca interna, but these cells are more characteristic of the corpus luteum (see page 576).[145] The theca interna layer contains a rich vascular plexus consisting of dilated capillaries, as well as a dense reticulum that surrounds each cell (Fig. 15.19b).

The theca externa is an ill-defined layer of variable thickness that surrounds the theca interna and merges almost imperceptibly with the adjacent ovarian stroma. It is composed of circumferential collagen bundles, blood and lymphatic vessels, and plump, spindle stromal cells that lack steroidogenic histochemical features.[44] Some of the spindle cells are immunoreactive for actin.[32] The spindle cells typically are highly mitotic and may be misinterpreted as tumor cells, such as those of a fibrosarcoma, when only the theca externa edge of the follicle is seen in a microscopic section.

Ultrastructure

Theca interna cells contain steroidogenic organelles, similar to those within granulosa-lutein cells (see page 577). The theca externa cells, some of which exhibit smooth muscle differentiation, lack such organelles.[102]

Hormone Synthesis

The initiation of folliculogenesis and early preantral follicular development are independent of gonadotropin influence, whereas the later stages of follicular maturation are under gonadotropin control. As a small antral follicle develops into a preovulatory follicle, the sequence of endocrine events within its antral fluid differs from most, if not all, other antral follicles in the same ovary.[84,85] The early stages of this development are reflected by increasing concentrations of follicle-stimulating hormone (FSH) receptors and intrafollicular FSH within the preovulatory follicle.[39,84,85,129] There is a concomitant increase in estradiol (E$_2$) receptors within the granulosa cells and the E$_2$ levels within the follicular fluid. The latter reach peak concentrations (10,000 times the circulating level) during the mid- to late proliferative phase when plasma FSH falls to a basal level.[39,84,85] At this stage the preovulatory follicle is self-sustaining, continuing to mature under the influence of intrafollicular FSH and E$_2$.[86] During the late proliferative phase, plasma luteinizing hormone (LH) rises and LH receptors become apparent within the granulosa cells of the preovulatory follicle, but not other follicles.[129] In contrast, LH receptors are present within the theca cells of all follicles throughout the follicular phase.[129]

Whereas circulating E$_2$ is likely derived from both the granulosa cells and the LH-stimulated theca cells, intrafollicular E$_2$ is derived almost exclusively from the granulosa cells by both de novo synthesis and by FSH-dependent aromatization of theca-derived androstenedione.[86,87] Aromatase activity is highest in the preovulatory follicle, thereby maintaining a high E$_2$-androstenedione ratio.[57,84,85] In contrast, other follicles that will undergo atresia are FSH deficient and aromatase deficient and have a low E$_2$-androstenedione ratio within their intrafollicular fluid (see page 583). Granulosa and theca LH receptors increase gradually throughout follicular development, possible under the control of FSH, reaching peak concentrations just before ovulation.[39,84,85] Simultaneously, high estrogen levels initiate a preovulatory surge of plasma LH,[106,147] which induces luteinization of the granulosa cells, an increase in intrafollicular progesterone (P) concentration, and a small preovulatory rise in circulating P.[42,84,85] The rising plasma P and peaking estrogen levels further augment the LH surge, initiate a smaller increase in FSH, and trigger ovulation. Ovulation occurs 36–38 hours after the onset of the LH surge, 24–36 hours after the E$_2$ peak, and 10–12 hours after the LH peak.[42]

The ovarian follicles also produce nonsteroidal hormones. Inhibin, a glycoprotein synthesized by the granulosa cells, is secreted into the follicular fluid and ovarian venous effluent in amounts that correlate with steroid levels.[42,135,136] Although inhibin secretion is predominantly under the control of LH,[82] it reduces, by negative feedback, FSH secretion from the hypothalamic–pituitary unit. Granulosa, theca, and stromal cells are immunoreactive for renin and angiotensin II,[104] and high concentrations of prorenin are present within the fluid of mature follicles.[127] The function, if any, of the renin-angiotensin system within the ovary currently is unknown.

Corpus Luteum of Menstruation

DATING THE CORPUS LUTEUM

After ovulation on the 14th day of the typical 28-day menstrual cycle, and in the absence of fertilization, the collapsed ovulatory follicle becomes the corpus luteum of menstruation (CLM). When mature, the CLM is a 1.5- to 2.0-cm, round, yellow structure with a festooned contour and a cystic center filled with a gray, focally hemorrhagic coagulum (Figs. 15.20, 15.21). During the 14 days after ovulation, the CLM undergoes an orderly sequence of histologic changes that allow an approximate estimation of its age. Corner has described these stages in detail, using endometrial histology and menstrual data to establish the age of the CLM.[25,140] A subsequent study, using Corner's criteria, correlated the histologic date of the CLM with the interval between the LH peak and the biopsy of the CLM.[28] It was concluded that dating of the CLM was unreliable and therefore not useful in the retrospective timing of ovulation.

HISTOLOGY

The luteinized granulosa cells of the mature CLM are large (30–35 μm is diameter), polygonal cells with abundant, pale eosinophilic cytoplasm that may contain numerous small lipid droplets (Fig. 15.22a).[44] The spherical nu-

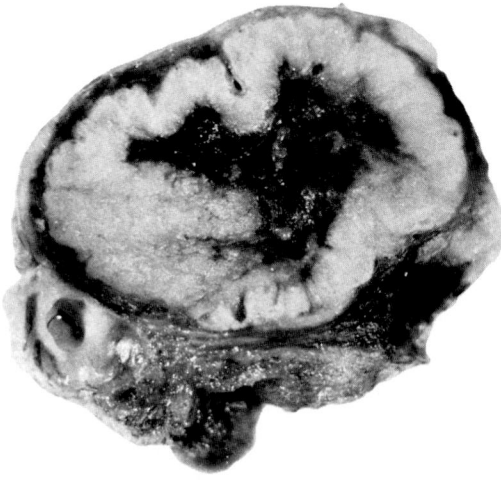

FIG. 15.20. Mature corpus luteum of menstruation. A yellow convoluted border surrounds a central hemmorrhagic coagulum.

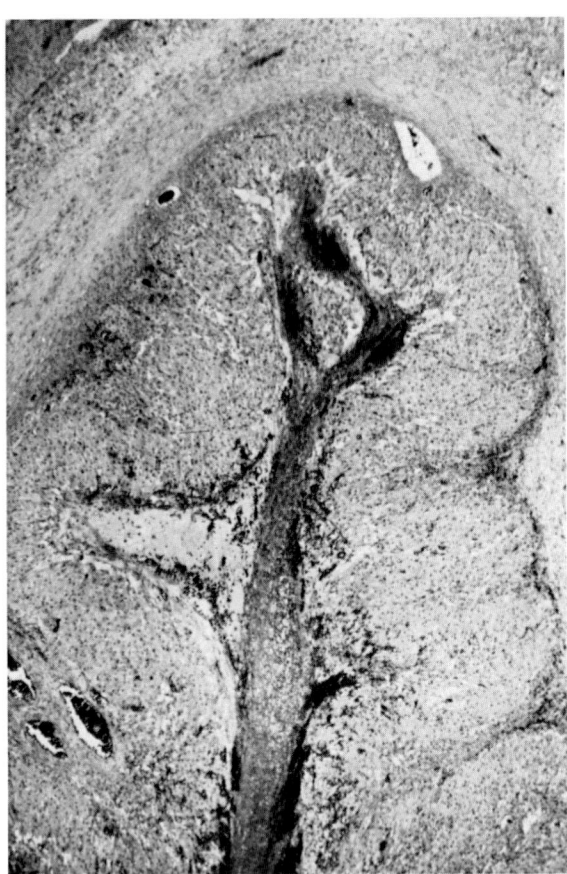

FIG. 15.21. Mature corpus luteum of menstruation. Festooned lining composed of granulosa–lutein cells surrounds a central cavity.

cleus contains one or two large nucleoli.[44] The histochemical features of these cells varies with the age of the CLM, but generally are typical of steroidogenic cells.[33,40,146] The cytoplasm of luteinized granulosa cells contains vimentin, but in contrast to granulosa cells of maturing and mature follicles, contains little or no cytokeratin.[31]

The theca interna forms an irregular and often interrupted layer several cells thick around the circumference of the CLM as well as ensheathing the vascular septa that extend into its center (Fig. 15.22).[44] When these septa are cut in cross-section, triangular-shaped nests of theca cells appear at intervals throughout the granulosa layer. In all but the earliest stages of the CLM, the theca lutein cells are approximately half the size of granulosa–lutein cells. They contain a round to oval nucleus with a single prominent nucleolus. Their less abundant, more darkly staining cytoplasm contains lipid droplets that usually are larger than those in granulosa–lutein cells.

A third type of cell, so-called K cells, that are present in small numbers within the theca interna of the mature follicle are more numerous within the granulosa layer of the early CLM.[1,97,98,145] K cells persist until menstruation, at

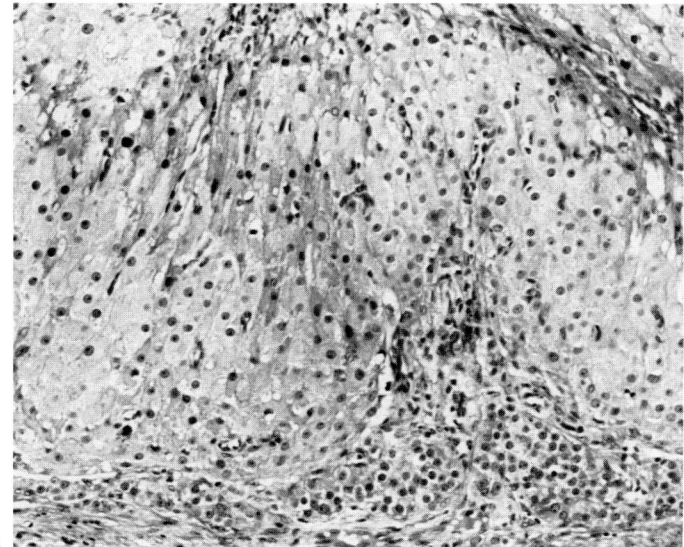

a

b

FIG. 15.22. Mature corpus luteum of menstruation. a: The lining is composed of a thick layer of large granulosa–lutein cells and an outer, thinner layer of smaller theca–lutein cells. **b:** A reticulin stain shows a dense reticulum network in the theca interna and a beginning reticulum network, predominantly perivascular, within the granulosa–lutein layer.

which time they degenerate. They are characterized by a stellate shape, a deeply eosinophilic cytoplasm, and an irregular, hyperchromatic or pyknotic nucleus (Fig. 15.23). Their cytoplasm is uniformly sudanophilic because of the presence of phospholipid.[145] K cells lack steroidogenic histochemical patterns and recently have been shown to be T lymphocytes.[51]

During the maturation of the CLM, capillaries from the theca interna penetrate the granulosa layer and reach the central cavity. Fibroblasts that accompany the vessels form an increasingly dense reticulum within the granulosa layer and the fibrous layer lining the central cavity (Fig. 15.22b).[83]

If fertilization does not occur, involutional changes begin on postovulatory days 8 or 9.[25] The granulosa–lutein cells decrease in size, develop pyknotic nuclei, and accumulate abundant cytoplasmic lipid (Fig. 15.24). There is a decrease in histochemical staining of enzymes associated with steroid biosynthesis and an increase in hydrolytic enzymes.[33] Eventually the cells undergo dissolution and are phagocytosed.[1] Over a period of several months there is progressive fibrosis and shrinkage of the corpus luteum with conversion to a corpus albicans (see page 581).[83]

ULTRASTRUCTURE

At the ultrastructural level, luteinization is characterized by a gradual increase in steroidogenic organelles, specifically smooth ER and abundant mitochondria with tubular cristae (Fig. 15.25).[1,26,44,47] The smooth ER exhibits a

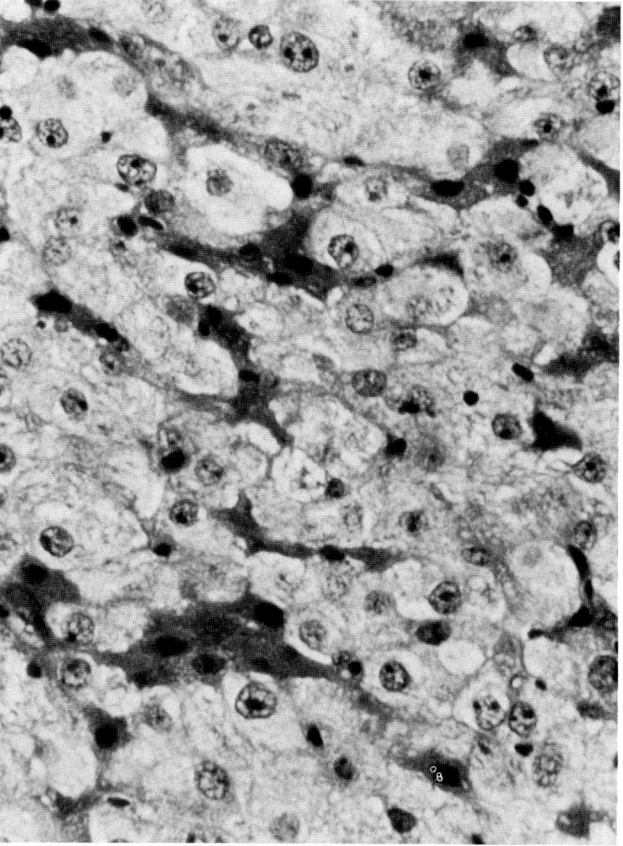

FIG. 15.23. Mature corpus luteum of menstruation. Darkly staining K cells are seen interspersed between granulosa–lutein cells.

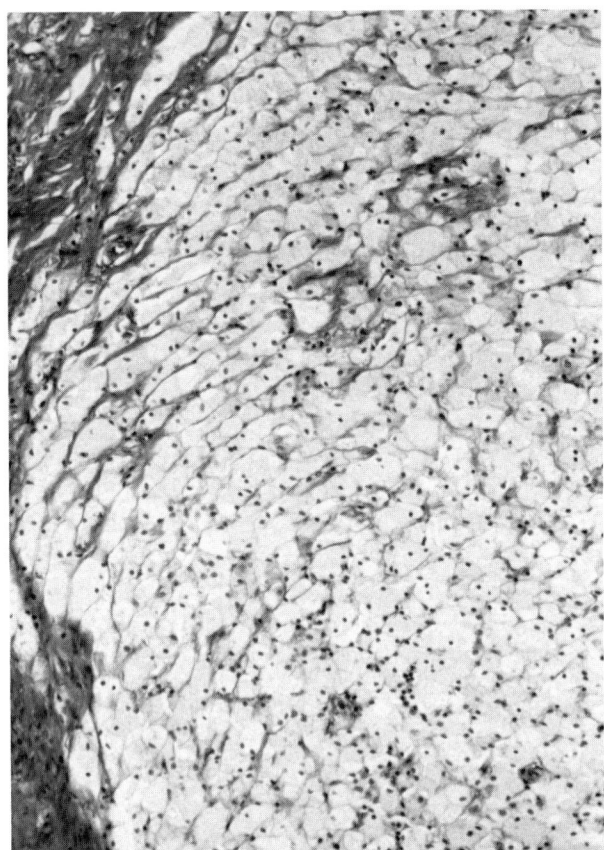

FIG. 15.24. Degenerating corpus luteum of menstruation.
Granulosa–lutein cells have pyknotic nuclei and abundant cytoplasmic lipid.

characteristic regional modification in the form of highly
folded, radiating, tubular cisternae that interdigitate and
communicate with adjacent cisternae.[26] Dispersed and
perinuclear Golgi, free and bound ribosomes, lipid droplets, and lipofuschin pigment also are seen (Fig.
15.25).[1,26,44,47] The cells are separated by a narrow space
of variable width, but occasionally the outer leaflets of their
plasma membranes become closely apposed and reinforced by desmosomal and pentalaminar tight junctional
complexes.[1,26,44] Most cells have a free surface that borders on a broad pericapillary space from which they are
separated by an interrupted basal lamina.[44] Many irregular
microvillous cytoplasmic extensions project into these pericapillary, as well as the intercellular, spaces (Fig.
15.25).[1,26,41,44] Occasional interdigitation of these microvilli has been noted between adjacent cells to form
intercellular channels.[26] Underlying the microvilli is a narrow zone of cytoplasm filled with a network of filaments
that also extend into the microvilli.[44]

Theca–lutein cells are similar ultrastructurally to granulosa–lutein cells except for the presence of localized perinuclear Golgi and the absence of folded-membrane complexes, microvilli, and a network of fine filaments.[26,44] The
theca externa layer of the CLM does not differ significantly
from that of the mature follicle (see page 575). K cells
have irregular nuclear membranes, vesicular ER, and pleomorphic mitochondria.[1] They lack ultrastructural evidence
of active steroidogenic activity.

The lutein cells of the degenerating CLM exhibit disorganization and fragmentation of the smooth ER, alterations of the mitochondria, and an increase in cytolyso-
somes.[41] Lipid droplets are increased and irregular in size
and show increased osmiophilia.[1]

HORMONE SYNTHESIS

The formation and function of the CLM are under the
control of LH, reflected by the high content of LH receptors within the granulosa–lutein cells.[42] FSH receptors also
have been identified in the early corpus luteum, although
the role of FSH in luteal function is unknown.[129] Although
P is the major steroid hormone formed in vivo and in vitro
by the CLM, it also synthesizes, both in vitro and in vivo,
estrone and E_2, as well as androgens, predominantly androstenedione.[75] In vitro P and estrogen synthesis are
stimulated by both hCG and LH.[118]

After ovulation, LH, FSH, and E_2 levels fall, but the LH
concentration is sufficient to maintain the CLM, producing a midluteal peak in P and E_2 concentrations. If fertilization does not occur, the increased levels of P and E_2
result in a fall of LH and FSH to basal levels, a reduction in
LH and FSH receptors within the CLM, and a marked
decline in P and E_2 synthesis after the 22nd day of the
cycle.[19,39,42,114] These changes are reflected by morphologic involution of the CLM and the onset of menses.
Luteolysis appears to be estrogen related, possibly secondary to an estrogen-induced reduction in LH receptors or
by enhancement of the luteolytic action of prostaglandins
synthesized by the CLM.[42,139] A nonsteroidal LH-receptor
binding inhibitor, which increases in concentration during
the luteal phase, also may play a role.[42] Epidermal growth
factor receptors also have been identified within the CLM,
but their physiological significance is unknown.[5]

Corpus Luteum of Pregnancy

GROSS APPEARANCE AND HISTOLOGY

On gross inspection, the corpus luteum of pregnancy
(CLP) may be indistinguishable from the CLM, but it is
usually larger and yellower, compared with the orange-
yellow of the late CLM.[53] The larger size, which may
account for up to one-half of the ovarian volume, is due
primarily to the presence of a central cystic cavity filled
with fluid or a coagulum composed of fibrin and blood
(Fig. 15.26).[98,132,141] When the cavity is large, typically in
early pregnancy, the wall of the CLP may lose its convolutions, becoming stretched and thinned to the extent that it

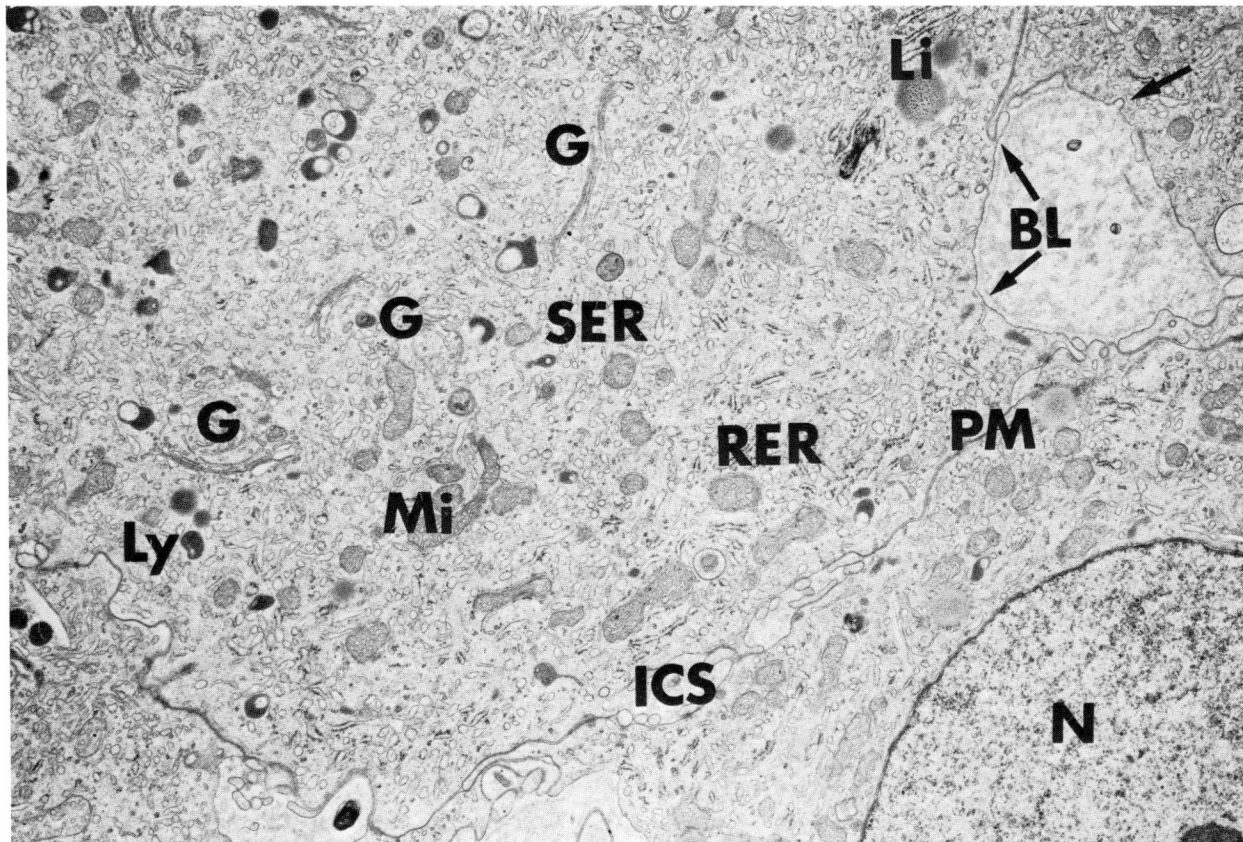

FIG. 15.25. **Electron micrograph of granulosa–lutein cells of a mature corpus luteum of menstruation.** Note abundant smooth endoplasmic reticulum (*SER*), mitochondria (*Mi*), Golgi (*G*), rough endoplasmic reticulum (*RER*), lipid droplets (*Li*), intercellular space (*ICS*), nucleus (*N*), lysosomes (*Ly*), plasma membrane (*PM*), micropinocytotic vesicles (*arrows*), and basal lamina (*BL*). (Courtesy of Dr. T. Okagaki. Reprinted by permission of Ferenczy and Richart, ref. 41. Copyright John Wiley & Sons, Inc., 1974.)

may consist focally of only fibrous tissue.[98] Obliteration of the cavity usually begins by the fifth month and typically is completed by term.[98] The CLP thus gradually decreases in size, and by the last trimester may be as small or smaller than the CLM.[98] During the puerperium, the CLP undergoes involution and conversion to a corpus albicans.

GRANULOSA CELLS

The first morphologic evidence within the corpus luteum that conception has occurred is the absence of the regressive changes that normally appear in the CLM on the 8th or 9th days. Instead, the granulosa–lutein cells enlarge, reaching their maximum size (50–60 μm in diameter) by 8–9 weeks' gestation. They become round or polyhedral and contain abundant eosinophilic cytoplasm, round to oval vesicular nuclei, and one or two prominent nucleoli (Fig. 15.27a).[98] They typically have polyploid levels of DNA.[131]

The granulosa cells of the early CLP have cytoplasmic vacuoles that intimally are minute but eventually increase

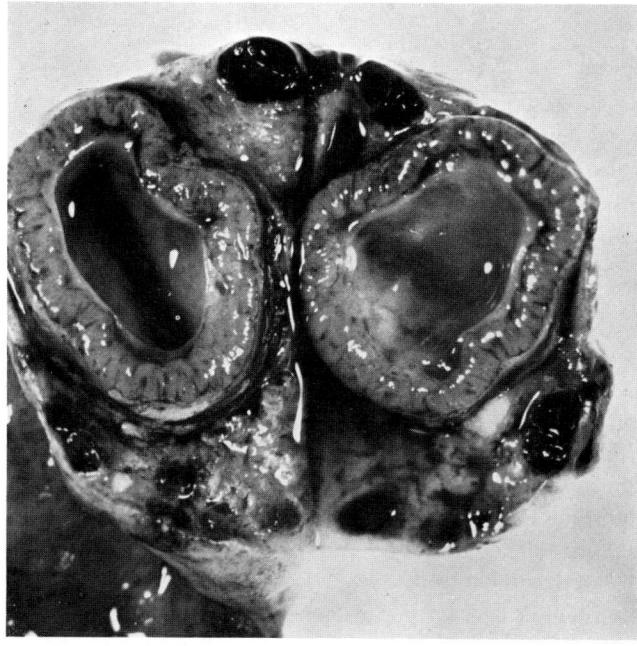

FIG. 15.26. **Cystic corpus luteum of pregnancy.** Note the convoluted lining, which was yellow.

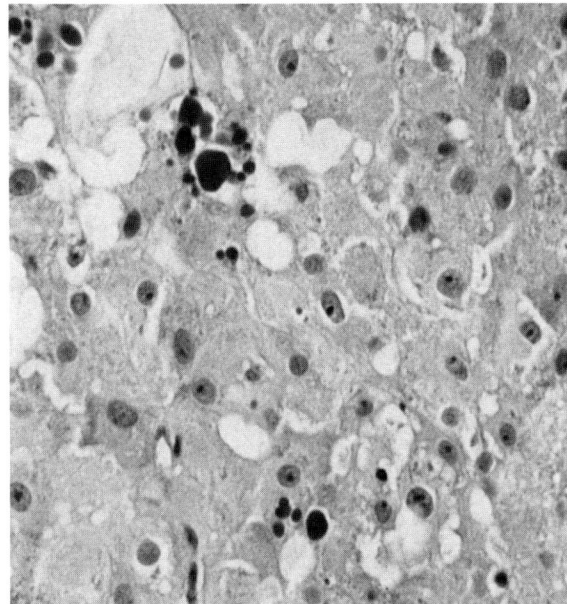

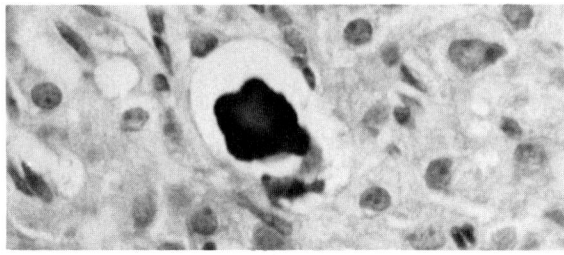

Fig. 15.27. **Corpus luteum of pregnancy. a:** Note granulosa–lutein cells with large irregular vacuoles and numerous, variably sized, darkly staining hyaline bodies. **b:** Focal calcification within a late corpus luteum of pregnancy.

in size to occupy almost the entire cell, often with displacement and flattening of the nucleus (Fig. 15.27a). The vacuoles tend to diminish in number and size as gestation progresses, and typically disappear after the 4th month.[98] Fine, diffusely scattered, cytoplasmic lipid droplets also are seen commonly within the cells, particularly in early CLP. With increasing age of the CLP, the droplets become fewer and larger.[98]

Eosinophilic colloid or hyaline droplets within the granulosa cells of a CLP are almost diagnostic of pregnancy, but can be seen rarely within a CLM.[98] They can be identified as early as 15 days after ovulation.[124] These inclusions initially appear as small, round, or irregular, often multiple, droplets but eventually enlarge, possibly by fusion of smaller droplets, into one or several large bodies that may fill the entire cell (Fig. 15.27a). They become more numerous as gestation progresses,[141] although by term their numbers decrease as they undergo calcification, a process that continues into the puerperium (Fig. 15.27b).[98,141] It is likely that these calcified bodies

eventually are resorbed, as they are not a feature of corpora albicantia.[98]

K cells, identical to those described within CLM (see page 576), are typically found in the granulosa layer of the early CLP. They are most numerous in the 2nd, 3rd, and 4th months of gestation, after which time they are rarely encountered.[97,98,141]

THECA CELLS

The theca interna is thickest in the early CLP, at which time it resembles its counterpart in the CLM. In the CLP, the theca cells are polyhedral or round and approximately one-fourth the size of the granulosa–lutein cells. Their cytoplasm is darker and more granular than that of the granulosa cells and is typically nonvacuolated. Their nuclei are central, round, and more hyperchromatic than those of the granulosa cells; one or two prominent nucleoli usually are present.[98] The characteristic colloid inclusions seen within the granulosa cells are absent or rare within the theca cells.[98] Occasional K cells may be seen in early pregnancy, but in smaller numbers than in the granulosa layer.[141,145] After the 4th month, the theca interna and its septa become thinner as the theca cells become smaller and fewer in number. Their nuclei become darker, more irregular, and oblong to spindle in shape, resembling fibroblasts.[141] By term, the theca interna layer has almost completely disappeared.[55,98] The theca externa layer may be more edematous and vascular than that of the CLM,[98] or in other examples, inapparent.[141]

CONNECTIVE TISSUE

As in the mature CLM, the central cystic cavity typically is lined by a layer of fibrous tissue, composed of variable numbers of fibroblasts, collagen, reticulin fibers, and blood vessels.[98] Its thickness is highly variable, not only within the same CLP, but also from one CLP to another and at different times in pregnancy.[141] As noted, in some CLP with large cystic cavities, the granulosa layer is focally absent, and its wall is formed entirely by a fibrous layer. As gestation advances, the central cyst or coagulum eventually is obliterated by connective tissue, which may be focally hyalinized and calcified.[97]

Reticulin staining reveals a pattern similar to that of the mature CLM, that is, a dense pattern within the theca interna and inner fibrous layer, and a sparser framework within the granulosa layer.[98] In the early CLP, many, often large, vessels are present in the theca externa and interna, which give origin to smaller vessels that penetrate the granulosa and inner fibrous layers.[98] In the late CLP, the vessels develop sclerotic walls with luminal narrowing or obliteration.[98,141] The amount of connective tissue around the vessels increases in proportion to the decreasing vascularization and regression of the theca interna layer.[141]

ULTRASTRUCTURE

The ultrastructural appearance of the CLP is similar to that of the CLM, and remains intact throughout pregnancy despite a reduction in its metabolic activity.[2,48,107] The increased cell volume of the granulosa cells in the CLP is reflected by increased smooth ER with many folded-membrane complexes. There also is an increase in rough ER, localized in stacks, as well as distinctive concentric whorls not usually seen in the CLM.[26,48] Electron-dense, 150–200-nm, membrane-bound granules are closely associated with the cisternae of the rough ER. Mitochondria, including large spherical mitochondria not seen in the CLM, typically are highly variable in size, shape, and internal structure.[26,48] The colloid or hyaline inclusions consist of homogeneous electron-opaque material that occasionally surrounds needle-shaped crystals (Fig. 15.28). They typically have no relationship to any organelle, although smaller hyaline bodies may be surrounded by rough ER.

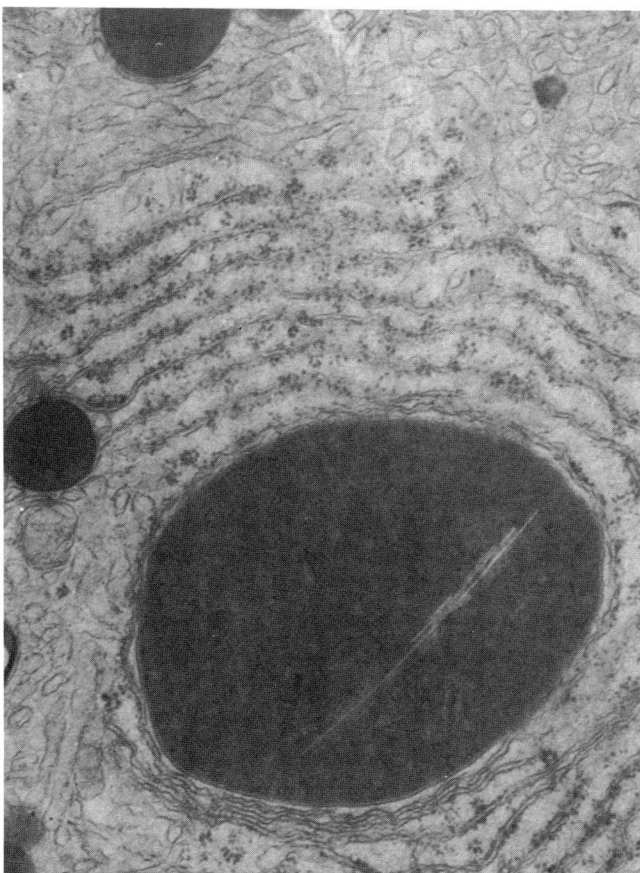

FIG. 15.28. **Hyaline bodies within a lutein cell from a corpus luteum of pregnancy.** The structures consist of homogeneous, electron-opaque material. Note the needle-shaped cleft within the largest hyaline body. ×22,000. (Reprinted by permission of Adams, Hertig, ref. 2. Reproduced from The Journal of Cell Biology, 1969, 41:716 by copyright permission of The Rockefeller University Press.)

The vacuoles seen by light microscopy are lined by attenuated microvilli and contain an electron-translucent material.[2] Unlike the CLM, extensive bundles of microfilaments typically are encountered throughout the cytoplasm in most lutein cells, and become more prominent as pregnancy progresses.[2,48] Collagen fibrils are encountered more frequently in the intercellular and perivascular spaces of the term CLP compared with the CLM.[48]

HORMONE SYNTHESIS

After fertilization, placental hCG stimulates P production by the granulosa–lutein cells. P concentration within the postovulatory corpus luteum increases sixfold, whereas the E_2 level drops to 10% of that within the preovulatory follicle.[84,85] HCG alone cannot maintain P secretion from the CLP for more than a few days, and the regulation of P secretion beyond that time is unknown.[27] P production by the CLP begins to decline by the end of the second month of gestation as the production of P is largely assumed by the placenta. However, in vivo and in vitro studies indicate that the CLP continues to produce P throughout the remainder of gestation, albeit in reduced amounts, consistent with the maintenance of its structural integrity until term.[2,48,75,93,144] It is not known if the P derived from the CLP has a biological role during this period or is redundant because of the massive P production by the placenta.[143] There is a rapid decline in function during the puerperium, reflecting falling hCG levels during this period.

Relaxin, a polypeptide hormone, is another substance produced during gestation and the puerperium by the CLP, probably under the control of hCG.[113,122,142,143] The concentration of relaxin in ovarian vein plasma during pregnancy correlates with P levels. The placenta and uterus also have been suggested as additional, but less important, sources for this hormone. Its reported actions include cervical dilatation and softening, inhibition of uterine contractions, and relaxation of the pubic symphysis and other pelvic joints.[113,122,142,143] Immunoreactivity for renin and angiotensin II, similar to that noted within the preovulatory follicle (see above), has been demonstrated with the CLP,[104] consistent with the observation that prorenin, likely of ovarian origin, increases tenfold in pregnant women soon after conception.[127]

Corpus Albicans

The regressing CLM is invaded by connective tissue that gradually converts it to a scar, the corpus albicans. The degenerating corpus luteum and the young corpus albicans may contain macrophages laden with ceroid and hemosiderin pigment.[115] The mature corpus albicans is well-circumscribed, has convoluted borders, and is composed almost entirely of densely packed collagen fibers with occasional admixed fibroblasts (Fig. 15.29). Most corpora albi-

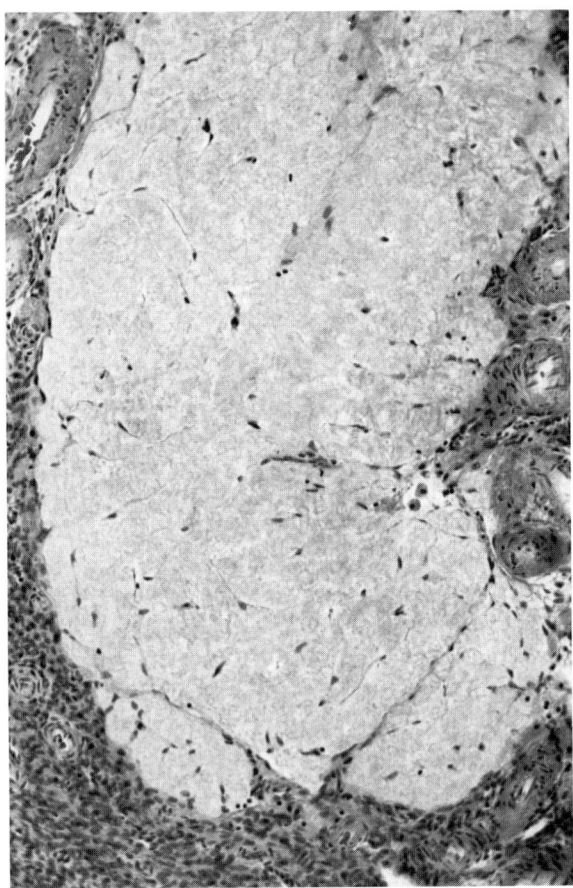

FIG. 15.29. **Corpus albicans.** Occasional fibroblasts are scattered throughout dense fibrous tissue.

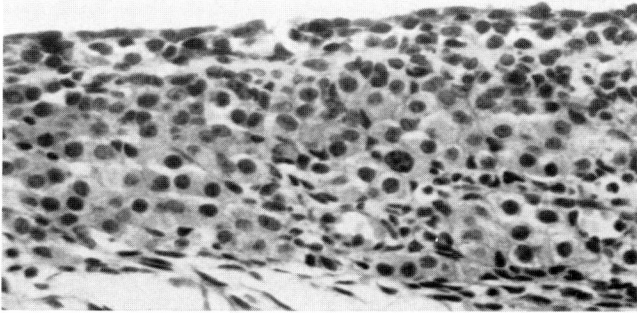

FIG. 15.30. **Lining of atretic cystic follicle.** The inner layer, composed of small granulosa cells, is thin and partially exfoliated. The outer, thicker theca interna layer exhibits prominent luteinization.

cantia eventually are resorbed and replaced by ovarian stroma.[64,124] Persistent corpora albicantia typically are found in the medulla of postmenopausal women, suggesting that this resorption process decelerates or terminates before the menopause.

Atretic Follicles

HISTOLOGY

Of the original 400,000 primordial follicles present at birth, approximately 400 mature to the point of ovulation. The remaining 99.9% undergo atresia, a process that begins before birth and continues throughout reproductive life, but is more intense immediately after birth and during puberty and pregnancy.[20,34,46,80,98] Factors that initiate atresia and determine which follicles ultimately will undergo atresia are unknown.

The atretic process varies with the stage of follicular maturation that has been reached. Atresia of early follicles (primordial and preantral) begins with degeneration of the oocyte manifested by chromatin condensation, pyknosis, and fragmentation, as well as cytoplasmic vacuolation. De-

generation of the granulosa cells soon follows and the follicle completely disappears. In contrast, atresia of follicles that have reached the antral stage of development is more complex and variable, but ultimately leads to obliterative atresia and the formation of a scar, the corpus fibrosum (corpus atreticum).[15] The earliest evidence of this process is a decrease in mitotic activity and in the number of granulosa cells, resulting in a thinning and focal exfoliation of the granulosa layer. Some follicles may persist for an indefinite period of time at this stage as atretic cystic follicles (Fig. 15.30). Ultimately, however, atretic follicles are invaded by vascular connective tissue, which eventually fills the central cavity (Fig. 15.31). The oocyte may persist for an indefinite period of time but eventually degenerates.[15] Concurrent with these changes, the basement membrane between the granulosa and theca interna layers becomes transformed into a thick, wavy, eosinophilic, hyalinized band, the *glassy membrane* (Figs. 15.31, 15.32). The theca interna typically persists, often with prominent luteinization, until the late stages of atresia, at which time cords and nests of theca cells become surrounded by connective tissue (Fig. 15.32).

During pregnancy, luteinization of both theca and granulosa layers is particularly striking in atretic follicles.[98] Microscopic, often multifocal, proliferations of nonluteinized granulosa cells, potentially mimicking small granulosa cell tumors, are encountered most commonly within the centers of atretic follicles during pregnancy (Fig. 15.33).[23] Rarely, the proliferating cells are luteinized granulosa cells or lipid-rich cells resembling Sertoli cells.[23] Their microscopic size, multifocality, and confinement to atretic follicles suggest that these proliferations are a response to the hormonal milieu of pregnancy rather than small neoplasms.[23] Continued shrinkage and hyalinization produces the corpus fibrosum, a small scar consisting of a wavy strand of hyaline tissue (Fig. 15.34). Like corpora albicantia, most corpora fibrosa are resorbed.

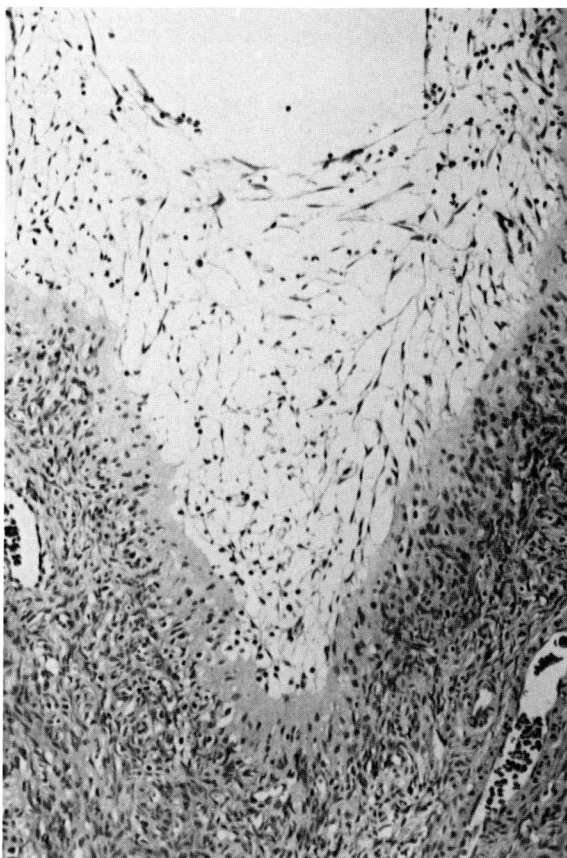

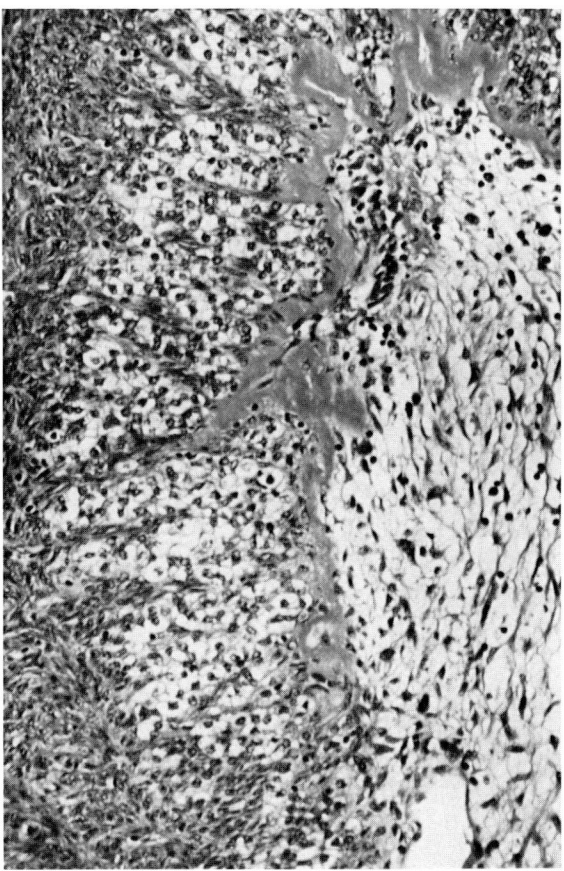

Fig. 15.31. Atretic cystic follicle undergoing obliterative atresia. Loose connective tissue is replacing the central cavity. The wavy basement membrane (glassy membrane) is thickened and hyalinized.

Fig. 15.32. Late stage of obliterative atresia. The thickened basement membrane separates the central fibrous tissue from the prominent luteinized theca interna layer.

HORMONE SYNTHESIS

In contrast to preovulatory follicles, the microenvironment of follicles undergoing atresia is predominantly androgenic, with high concentrations of intrafollicular androstenedione and low concentrations of FSH and E_2.[16,84,85,88,100] As noted, these follicles are deficient in granulosa cells, and the residual granulosa cells do not respond to FSH in vitro[88]; both FSH and LH receptors are lower than in nonatretic follicles.[129] Oocytes from atretic follicles are unable to complete the first meiotic division.[88] It is likely that an androgenic intrafollicular milieu is the major factor that halts follicular growth and initiates follicular atresia.

Hilus Cells

HISTOLOGY

Ovarian hilus cells, morphologically identical to testicular Leydig cells (with the exception of a female chromatin pattern), are present during fetal life but are not seen during childhood. They reappear at puberty and are demonstrable in virtually all postmenopausal women.[133,134] Their number and location are highly variable. They are more numerous during pregnancy, with increasing age after the menopause, and with increasing degrees of ovarian stromal proliferation and stromal luteinization.[17] Hilus cell hyperplasia is discussed in Chapter 16, Nonneoplastic Lesions of the Ovary.

Hilus cell aggregates of variable size and shape typically are found in the ovarian hilus and adjacent mesovarium (Fig. 15.35). They are more numerous in the lateral and medial poles of the hilus and near the junction of the ovarian ligament with the ovary, typically lying close to the junction of the hilus with the medullary stroma.[133] The hilus cells characteristically ensheath, or less commonly lie within, nonmedullated nerves (Fig. 15.36), and occasionally surround the rete ovarii. Hilus cells and their associated nerves frequently are juxtaposed to large hilar venous and lymphatic sinusoids, and may form nodular protrusions into their lumina.[133] Nests also may be seen within the ovarian stroma near the hilus, a finding probably

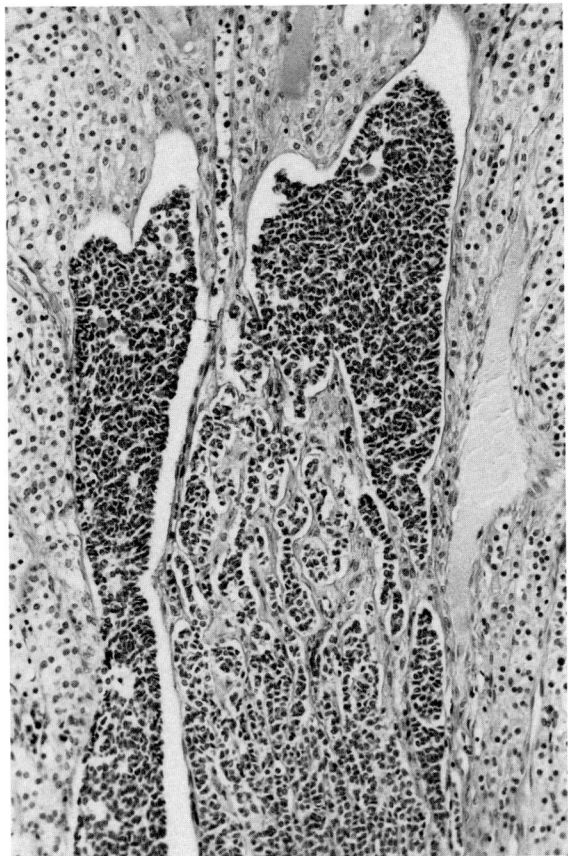

FIG. 15.33. Granulosa cell proliferation of pregnancy mimicking a small granulosa cell tumor. The proliferation is within the center of an atretic follicle, and is surrounded by the luteinized cells of the theca interna. (Reprinted by permission of Clement PB (1993) Tumor-like lesions of the ovary associated with pregnancy. Int J Gynecol Pathol 12: 108–115.)

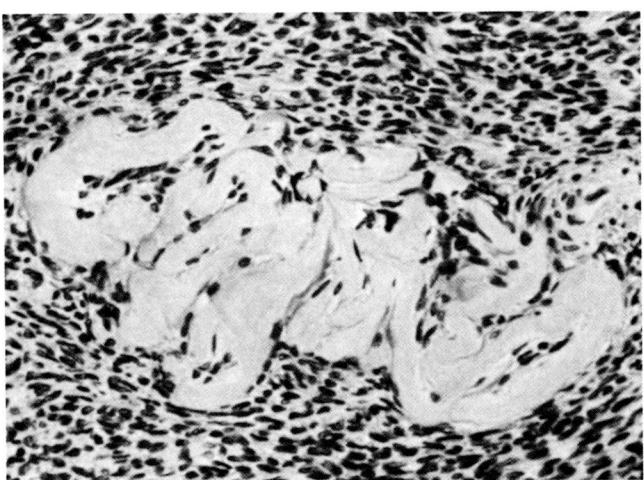

FIG. 15.34. Corpus fibrosum. The structure consists of a wavy hyalinized band.

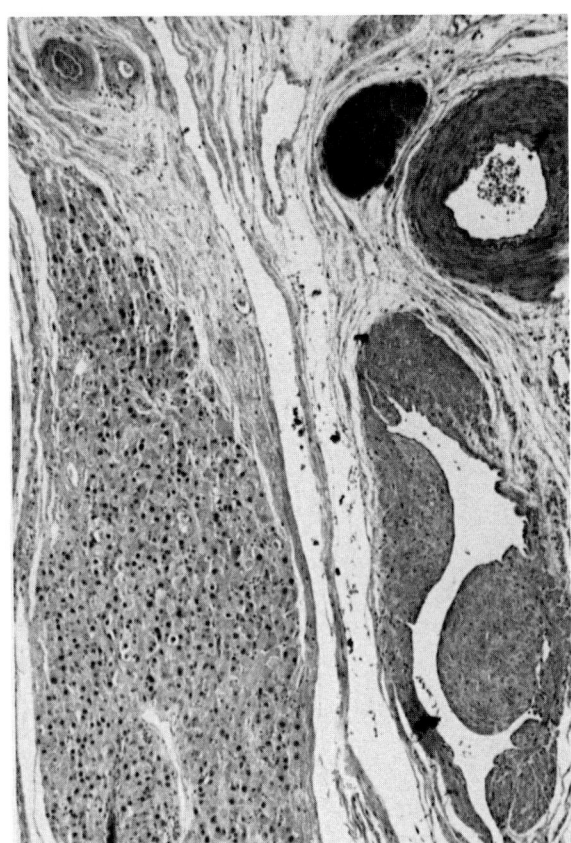

FIG. 15.35. Hilus cells. A nest of hilus cells lies adjacent to large vessels within the ovarian hilus.

caused by irregularities in the junction between the hilus and medulla and, rarely, as previously noted, within the ovarian stroma away from the hilus (stromal Leydig cells) (see Chapter 16). Ectopic hilus cells also may be encountered rarely in the perisalpinx and fimbrial endosalpinx.[59]

Hilus cell nests are unencapsulated, typically lying within loose connective tissue, or rarely ovarian-type stroma, within the hilus.[148] The cells are 15–25 μm in diameter, round to elongated, with abundant eosinophilic cytoplasm and a spherical vesicular nucleus that contains one or two prominent nucleoli (Fig. 15.37). Rare multinucleated cells may be seen. Those found incidentally in normal postmenopausal women do not exhibit mitotic activity in contrast to hyperplastic or neoplastic hilus cells. Hilus cells contain specific crystals of Reinke, which are homogeneous, eosinophilic, nonrefractile, rod-shaped structures, 10–35 μm in length, with blunt, but occasionally tapered, ends (Fig. 15.37, *inset*). The crystals typically lie in a parallel or stacked arrangement within a cell, and often are surrounded by a clear halo; occasionally they appear to be extending through or overlying cell membranes. The crystals typically are distributed unevenly and present in only a minority of cells; frequently they may not be demonstrable.[63] Their visualization may be facilitated

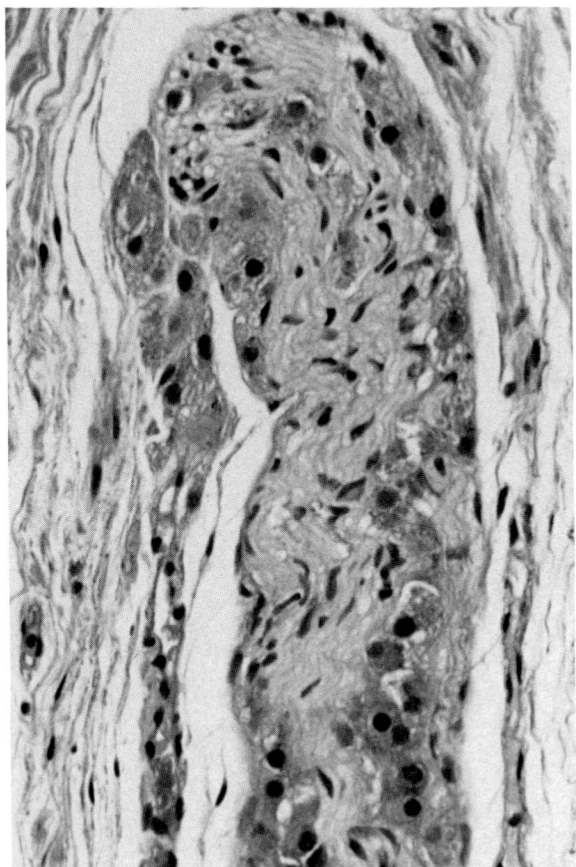

FIG. 15.36. Hilus cells. The cells ensheathe and lie within a nonmedullated nerve.

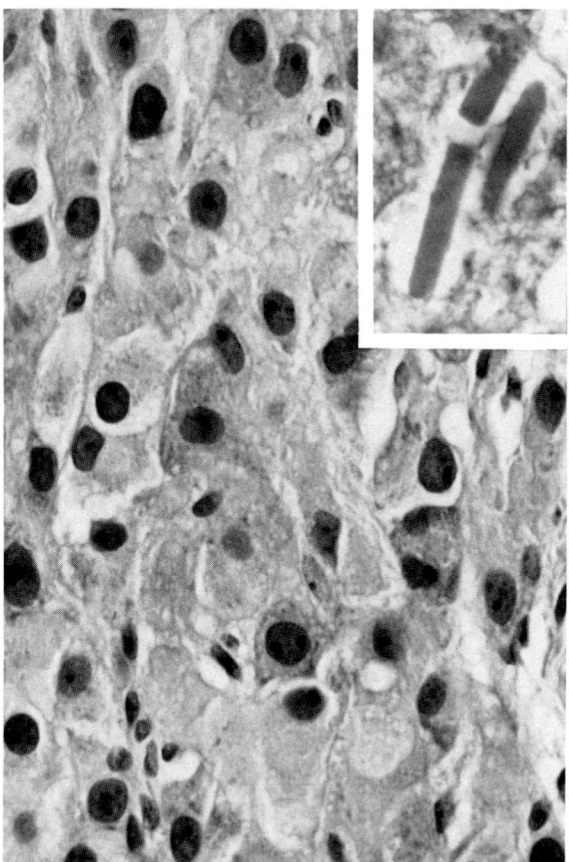

FIG. 15.37. Hilus cells. Note lipochrome pigment granules and Reinke crystals (*inset*).

by the use of Masson's trichrome and iron hematoxylin methods, which stain them magenta and black, respectively. Additionally, the crystals fluoresce yellow when H&E-stained sections are viewed by ultraviolet light.[123] Spherical or ellipsoidal, eosinophilic, hyaline structures, which probably represent precursors of crystals, can be identified in hilus cells, often in greater numbers than crystals. The cytoplasm also may contain perinuclear eosinophilic granules, peripheral lipid vacuoles, and golden brown lipochrome pigment (Fig. 15.37). Delicate collagen fibrils typically surround each cell. Typically admixed with the hilus cells are fibroblasts and cells intermediate in appearance between the two cell types.[72] The hilus cells and intermediate cells have intimate attachments to nerves, including true synaptic connection (see below). Hilus cells should be distinguished from adrenocortical rests (see Chapter 16).

ULTRASTRUCTURE

Hilus cells contain prominent smooth endoplasmic reticulum, mitochondria with tubular cristae, well developed Golgi, large lysosomes, and osmiophilic lipid inclusions.[72]

Reinke crystals have a true crystalline structure composed of dense, parallel hexagonal microtubules with a mean thickness of 12 nm separated by clear spaces 15 nm wide, producing a "woven fabric" appearance (Fig. 15.38).[41,72] They are formed by progressive association of precrystalline units each of which is composed of bundles of four or five parallel filaments (Fig. 15.39).[72] Hilus cells typically are admixed with fibroblasts and cells intermediate in ultrastructural appearance between the two cell types.[72] Hilus cells and, more commonly, the intermediate cells, have intimate attachments to nerves in the form of simple membranous contacts, invaginations of axon terminals into hilus cells, or surface membrane thickenings resembling a true synapse (Fig. 15.40).[72] These findings suggest that hilus cells most likely originate from hilar fibroblasts, possibly under the inductive influence of hilar nerves.[72,126]

HORMONE SYNTHESIS

The light and electron microscopic morphology and enzyme content of hilus cells are those of steroid hormone–producing cells. In addition, their cytoplasm is immunore-

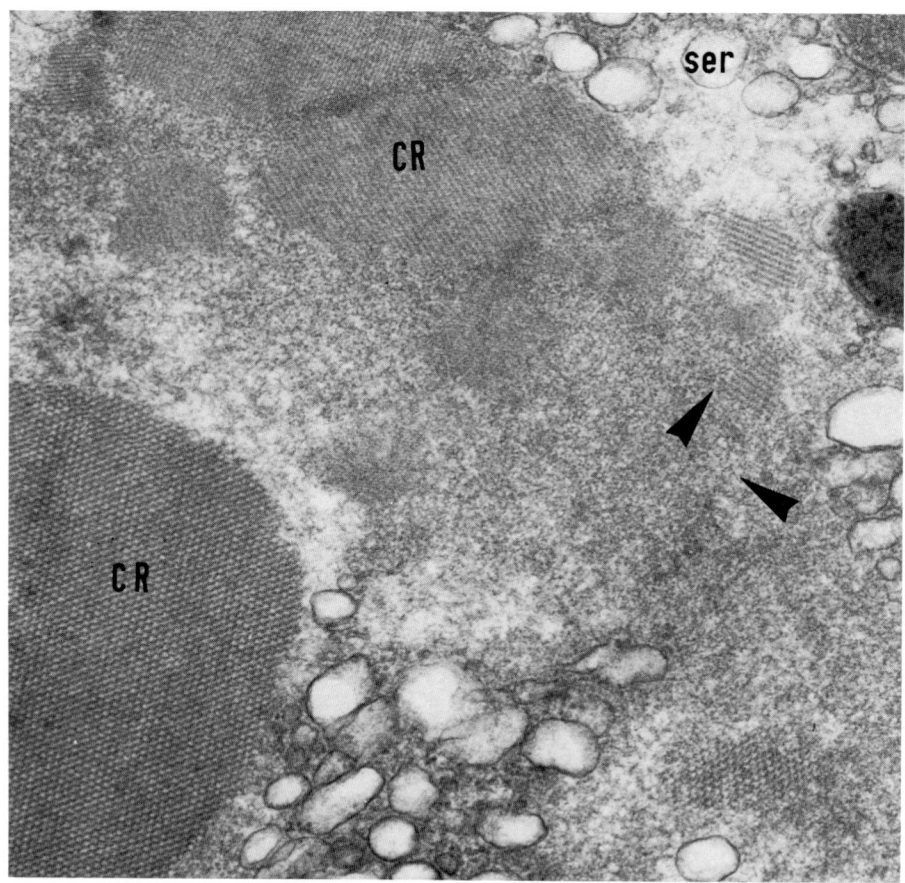

Fɪɢ. 15.38. **Reinke crystals with hexagonal internal pattern (CR).** The crystals are formed by association of precrystalline units (*arrows*). ser, smooth endoplasmic reticulum. ×25,000. (From Laffargue et al., ref. 72. Reprinted by permission of W. B. Saunders Co.)

active for testosterone binding sites.[4] To what extent hilus cells contribute to the steroid hormone pool in normal women, however, is unknown.[83,124,126] In vitro incubation studies indicate that the major steroid produced by ovarian hilus cells is androstenedione, which is produced in greater amounts than that elaborated from ovarian stroma.[36] Lesser amounts of E_2 and P also are produced in vitro. Hilus cells are responsive in vivo to both exogenous and endogenous hCG stimulation in vivo.[134]

Rete Ovarii

The rete ovarii, the ovarian analogue of the rete testis, is present in the hilus of all ovaries. It consists of a network of solid cords, irregular clefts, tubules, cysts, and intraluminal papillae lined by a single layer of flat to cuboidal epithelial cells (Fig. 15.41).[124] Characteristically, the rete is surrounded by a cuff of spindle-cell stroma morphologically similar to, but separate from, the ovarian stroma.

The cytoplasm of cells of the rete is immunoreactive for cytokeratin, vimentin, and desmoplakin.[11,31] Ultrastructural examination has revealed two types of cells, one ciliated and the other nonciliated with apical microvilli.[18,31]

The cytoplasm contains many mitochondria, a moderate amount of rough ER, many free polyribosomes, and some glycogen. Numerous desmosomes with associated tonofilament bundles connect adjacent cells. The basal lamina is well defined.

The rete is juxtaposed and may communicate with mesonephric tubules within the mesovarium.[43] Occasional hilar cysts originate from the rete (see Chapter 16) and small tumor-like proliferations of the rete have been referred to as *rete adenomas*.[43]

Fɪɢ. 15.39. **Aggregation of cytoplasmic precrystalline inclusions (*between arrows*).** ser, smooth endoplasmic reticulum. ×15,700. (From Laffargue et al., ref. 72. Reprinted by permission of W. B. Saunders Co.)

Fɪɢ. 15.40. **Axon relationships with a hilus cell.** Ax, axon terminal; HC, hilus cell; *large arrows*, synaptic membrane-like thickenings; *small arrow*, nonorientated filamentous material; nf, neurofilament; nt, neurotubules; sy, synapse between two axon terminals with parallel intersynaptic filaments; m, mitochondria. ×91,500. (From Laffargue et al., ref. 72. Reprinted by permission of W. B. Saunders Co.)

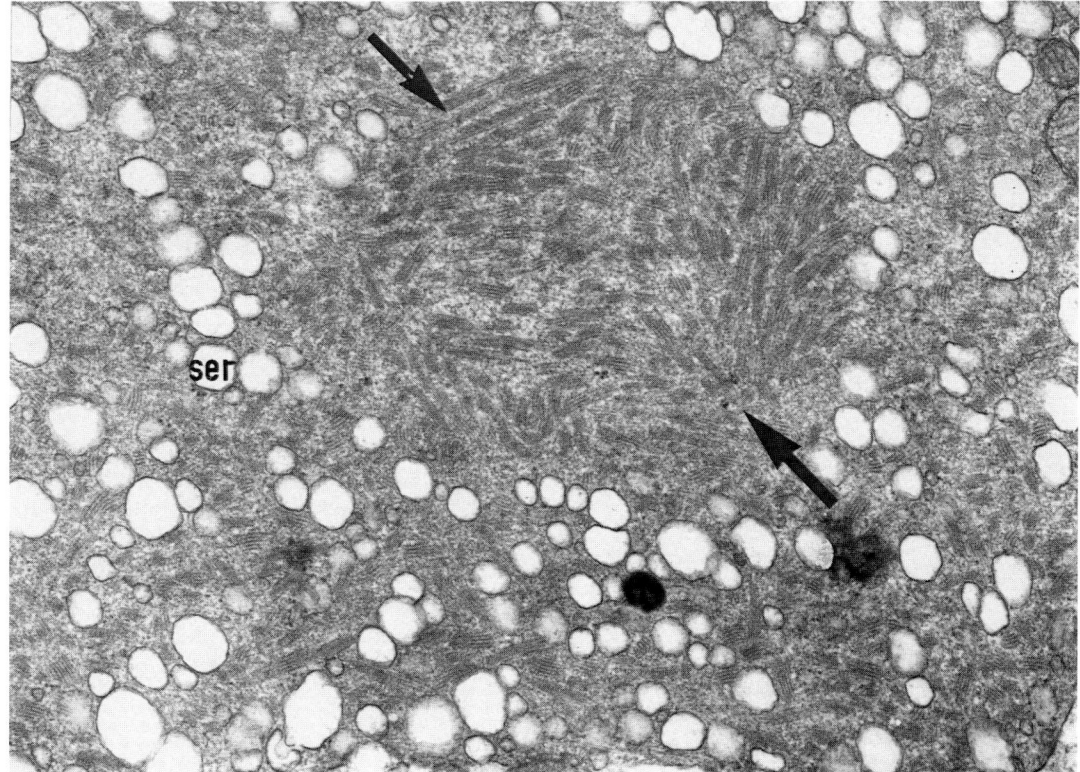

15.39

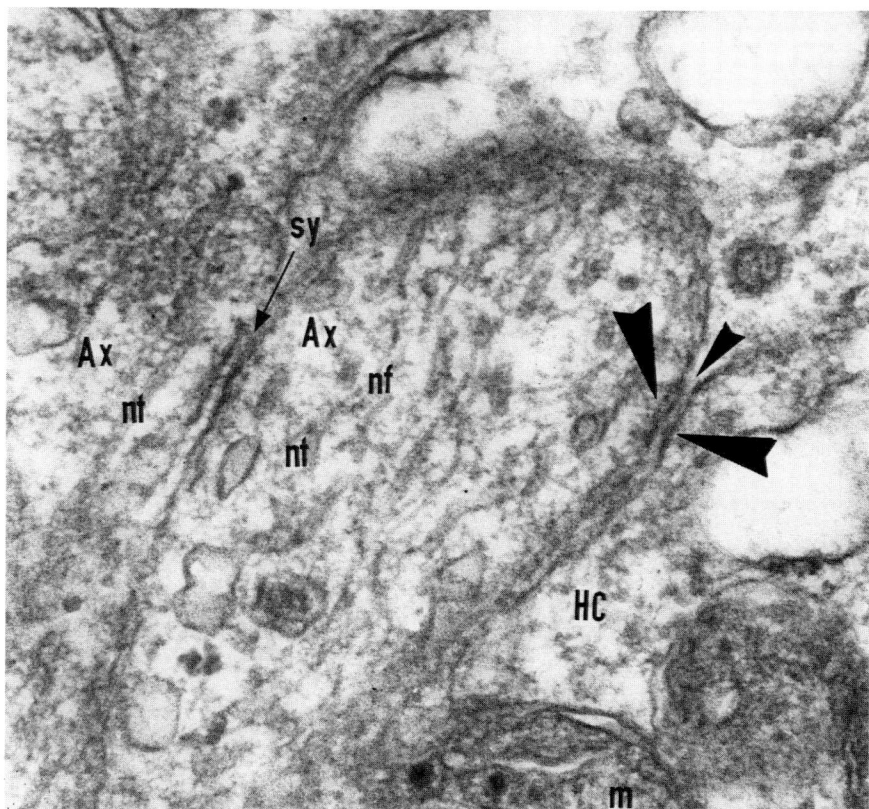

15.40

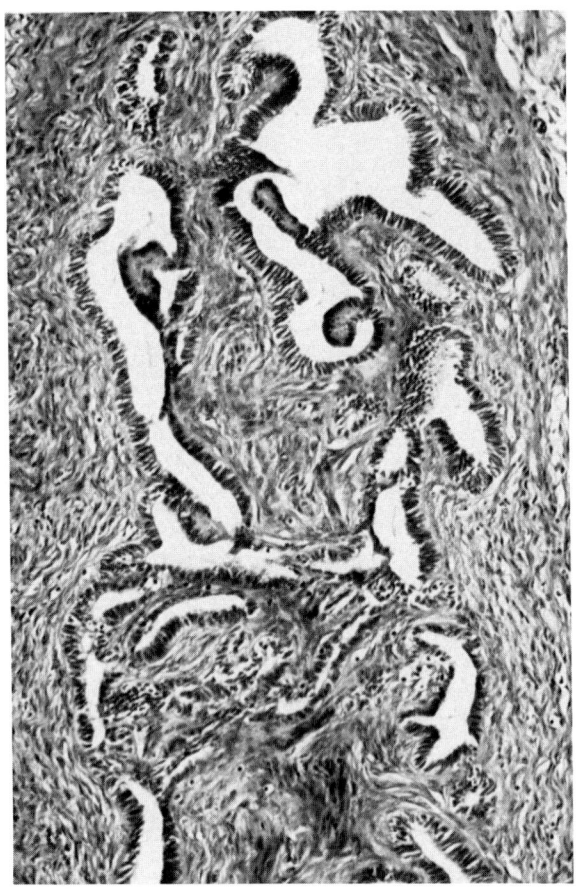

FIG. 15.41. **Rete ovarii.** Clefts and tubules, some with intraluminal papillae, are lined by a single layer of columnar epithelial cells.

The Ovary in Childhood

GROSS ANATOMY

The ovary in the newborn lies above the true pelvis. It is a tan, elongated, and flattened structure that may have a lobulated appearance with irregular edges (Fig. 15.42).[112]

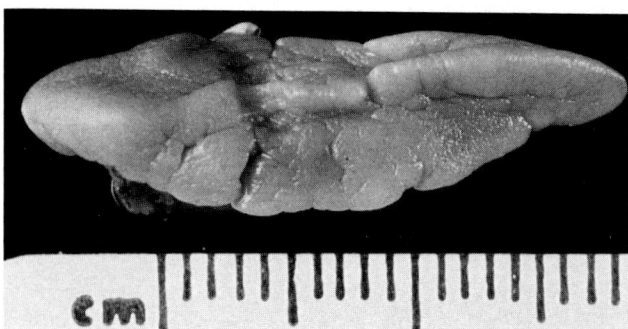

FIG. 15.42. **Ovary of newborn.** Note elongated shape and irregular edges.

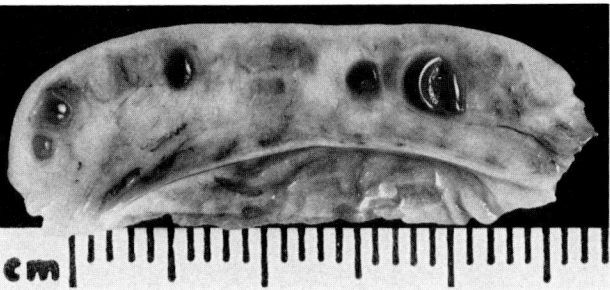

FIG. 15.43. **Ovary of 14-year-old girl (*cut surface*).** Note multiple cystic follicles within cortex.

Its approximate dimensions are 1.3 cm × 0.5 cm × 0.3 cm, and its weight is less than 0.3 g.[112,124,137] The ovary enlarges, increases in weight 30-fold, and changes in shape throughout infancy and childhood, and is fully developed and lies within the true pelvis by puberty.[112,124,137] During the first few months of life and at puberty the ovary may contain prominent cystic follicles, an appearance that should not be misinterpreted as polycystic ovary disease (Figure 15.43).

HISTOLOGY

At the time of birth, the ovarian cortex is filled with many closely packed primordial follicles (Figs. 15.44, 15.45). Some primordial follicles contain two or rarely more

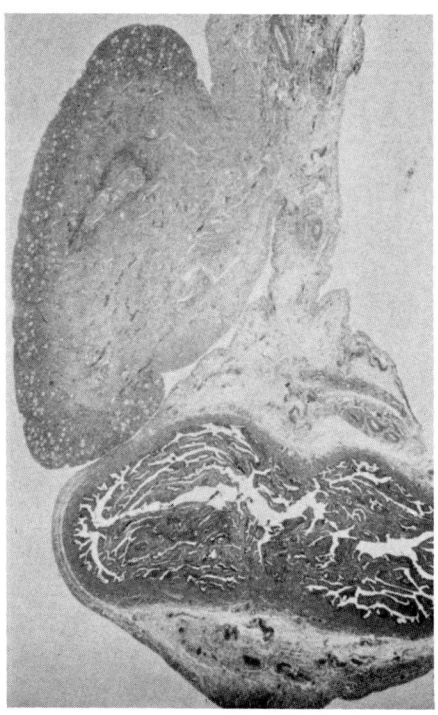

FIG. 15.44. **Ovary and fallopian tube of newborn in cross-section.** Ovarian cortex is packed with primordial follicles.

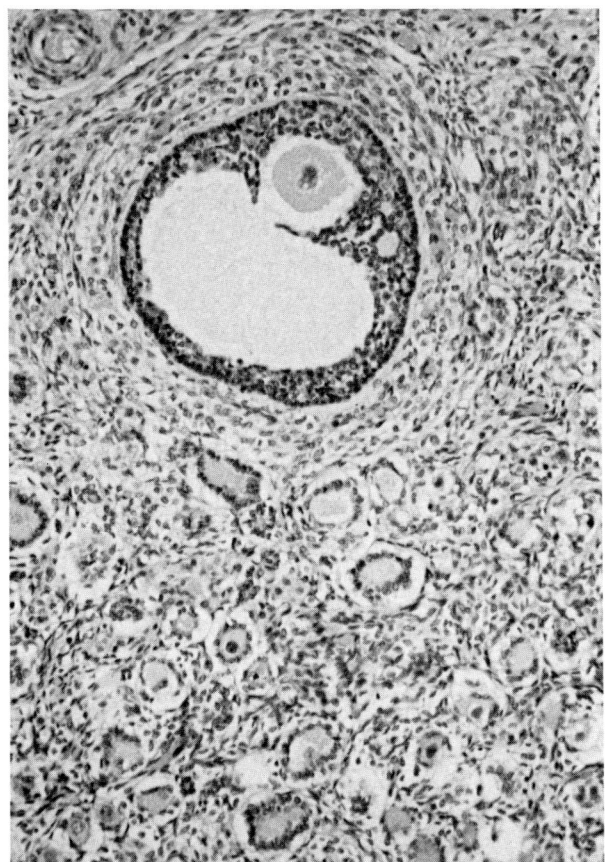

FIG. 15.45. Ovary of newborn. Note closely packed primordial follicles and antral follicle.

oocytes.[79,137] Follicle-derived structures resembling small sex cord tumors with annular tubules or, if germ cells are present, gonadoblastomas, may occur in normal ovaries from fetuses and children; they probably are a result of aberrant folliculogenesis.[69,79,121] Follicular maturation and atresia occur prenatally and throughout childhood, becoming more prominent after the age of six years.[29,58,90,100,109,137] Deceleration or arrest of folliculogenesis may occur in prepubertal patients with chronic illnesses, Down syndrome, and in those exposed to cytotoxic drugs or irradiation.[109] Follicular maturation is identical to that occurring in premenopausal women except that it does not proceed beyond antral follicles measuring 5 mm in diameter (Fig. 15.45). Because ovulation does not occur, corpora lutea and corpora albicantia are absent in the prepubertal ovary, and all maturing follicles undergo atresia in a manner identical to that occurring in adults. Prominent luteinization of the theca interna layer also may be seen in this age group.[70] By puberty, atresia has depleted more than 90% of the approximately 400,000 primordial follicles that were present at birth. This depletion and the concomitant increase in the amount of ovarian stroma results in the sparser distribution of the primordial follicles in the pubertal girl and young adult compared with that in childhood.

Adolescent prepubertal ovaries, in addition to prominent cystic follicles with luteinization of the theca interna, may exhibit focal fibrosis of the superficial cortex, further enhancing their resemblance to the ovaries of polycystic ovary disease.[90] This sclerocystic appearance is consistent with the conclusion that such changes are not specific for polycystic ovary disease but are a reflection of chronic anovulation (see Chapter 16, Nonneoplasic Lesions of the Ovary). As previously noted (see page 583), hilus cells are demonstrable during fetal life, but are not seen during infancy and childhood, reappearing at puberty.

HORMONE SYNTHESIS

Levels of gonadotropins and sex steroids, largely of placental origin, decline rapidly during the first few days of life. As a result, a rise in FSH and LH levels, paralleled by an elevation in follicle-derived estradiol (E_2), begins on the fifth day.[74] All three hormones reach peak levels at 3 to 4 months of age and then decline to low levels by the age of 2 years because of increasing sensitivity of the hypothalamic–pituitary unit to negative feedback by E_2. Low levels of gonadotropins are maintained until 6 to 8 years of age but are sufficient to maintain the growing ovary and stimulate continuous follicular development and atresia.[74,108] Only minimal quantities of E_2 are produced during this period. The onset of adrenal androgen secretion (adrenarche) at the age of 6 or 7 years usually precedes and may promote activation of the hypothalamic gonadostat.[74] As a result, there is a reduction in hypothalamic–pituitary sensitivity to negative feedback by estrogen, and FSH and LH levels progressively increase until menarche. They stimulate the increased production of follicular estrogens that are responsible for the development of secondary sexual characteristics at puberty.

The Ovary in the Menopause

GROSS ANATOMY

After the menopause, the ovaries typically shrink to a size approximately one-half that seen in the reproductive era. Their size varies considerably, however, depending on their content of ovarian stromal cells and the number of unresorbed corpora albicantia.[124] Most postmenopausal ovaries have a shrunken, gyriform, external appearance (Fig. 15.46) whereas some are smooth and uniform.[124] They are firm and have a predominantly solid, pale cut surface, although occasional inclusion cysts may be discernible within the cortex. Corpora albicantia typically are visible within the medulla as small white scars. Thick-

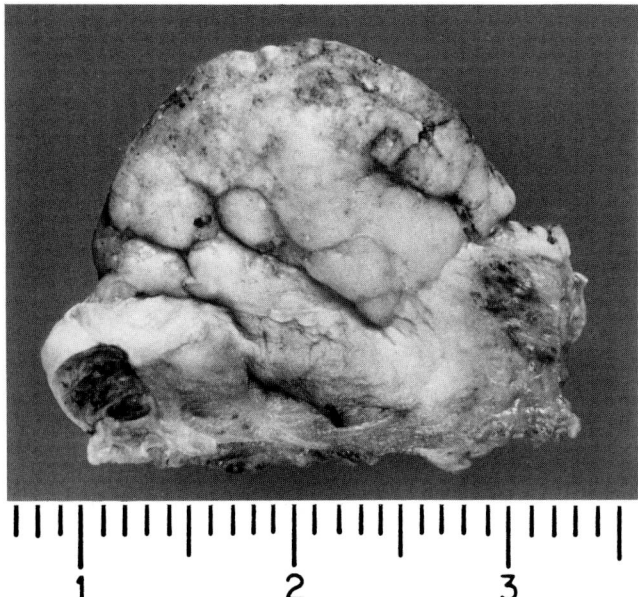

FIG. 15.46. Ovary of postmenopausal woman. Note the markedly irregular cortical surface.

walled blood vessels may be appreciable within the medulla and hilus.

HISTOLOGY

The characteristic feature of the postmenopausal ovary is the absence of primordial follicles and, consequently, an absence of maturing follicles, corpora lutea, and atretic follicles. Occasional primordial follicles, however, may persist for several years after cessation of menses, accounting for sporadic ovulation and postmenopausal bleeding in some women. After this period, the only follicle-derived structures typically encountered are occasional unresorbed corpora fibrosa and corpora albicantia, the latter typically within the medulla (Fig. 15.47).

Although the ovarian stroma typically increases in volume from the fourth to the seventh decades,[130] the ovarian stroma in postmenopausal women has a wide spectrum of appearances.[17,78,130] At one extreme is stromal atrophy manifested by a thin cortex and minimal amounts of medullary stroma (Fig. 15.47). In these women, the stroma becomes less cellular because of an increase in intercellular collagen and its cells have smaller, darker, more inactive-appearing nuclei (Fig. 15.48). At the other extreme, there is marked stromal proliferation warranting the designation *stromal hyperplasia* to connote a pathological process (see Chapter 16, Nonneoplastic Lesions of the Ovary). Most postmenopausal women, however, exhibit varying degrees of nodular or diffuse proliferation of cortical and medullary stromal cells that lie between these two extremes. Ovarian stromal changes that can be considered normal aging phenomena include occasional luteinized

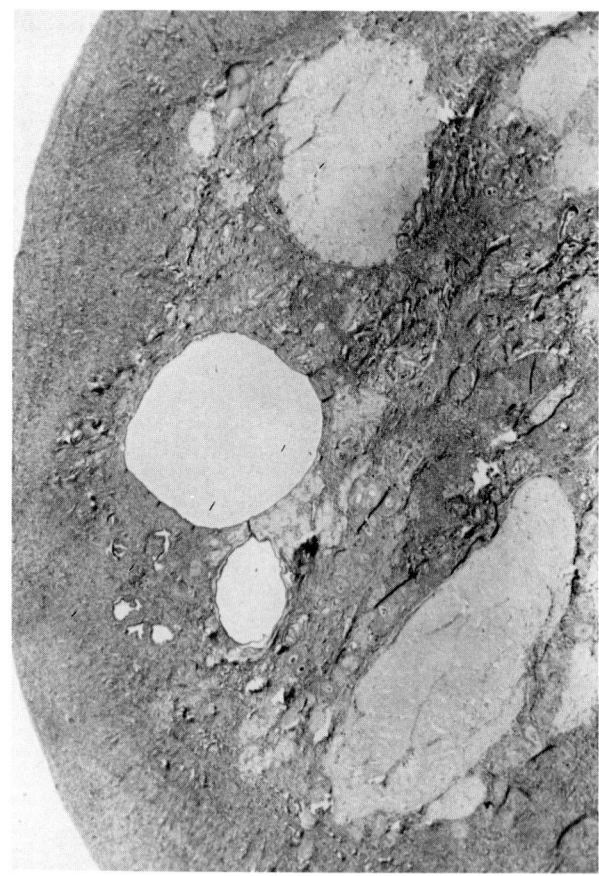

FIG. 15.47. Ovary of postmenopausal woman. Note the thin cortex devoid of follicular structures. Two inclusion cysts are present at the corticomedullary junction. Multiple corpora albicantia occupy the medulla.

stromal cells (see page 565), irregular areas of dense cortical stromal fibrosis,[17] cortical "granulomas" (see Chapter 16), spherical, cloud-like, hyaline scars (see Chapter 16), and surface papillary stromal proliferations (see Chapter 16). Less commonly, focal decidual transformation of the ovarian stroma may be seen in otherwise normal ovaries from postmenopausal women (see Chapter 16).

Other common changes within the ovaries of postmenopausal women include surface epithelial inclusion glands and cysts within the cortex and mild degrees of hilus cell hyperplasia (see Chapter 16). After the menopause, the medullary blood vessels exhibit a greater tortuosity, appearing more numerous and closely packed, and should not be mistaken for a hemangioma. Many of the same vessels and smaller vessels within the cortex have thickened walls and narrow lumina because of deposition of a hyaline, amyloid-like material.

HORMONE SYNTHESIS

With cessation of follicular activity at the time of the menopause, the ovarian stroma becomes, together with the ad-

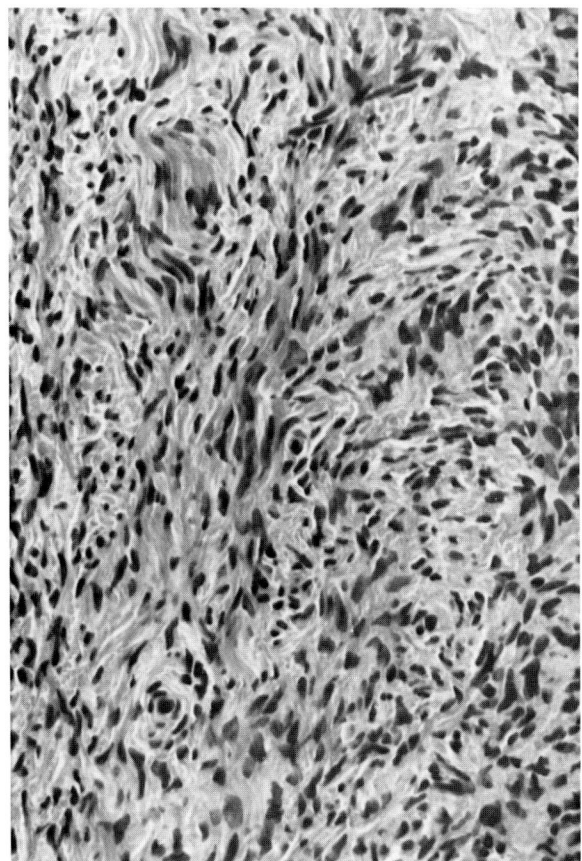

FIG. 15.48. **Ovarian stroma in postmenopausal woman.** Note the spindle-shaped cells with thin, darkly staining nuclei and abundant intercellular collagen.

renal glands, the major source of androgens. Testosterone is the major androgen secreted by the ovarian stroma in postmenopausal women.[3,138] Smaller amounts of androstenedione also are produced[21,36,66,67,77,81,111,138] but approximately 80% of the circulating levels of this hormone in postmenopausal women is of adrenal origin.[21] Despite a cessation of follicular synthesis of E_2 in postmenopausal women, small amounts of this hormone are present in the circulation, probably derived from the adrenal glands, by peripheral conversion of estrone,[21,76,116] and from the ovarian stroma itself.[3,77] Estrone, however, becomes the major circulating estrogen after the menopause. Estrone in postmenopausal women is derived predominantly from the peripheral aromatization of androstenedione that occurs in fat, muscle, liver, kidney, brain, and adrenals.[21,50,77] Increased aromatization in postmenopausal women, likely due to high endogenous LH levels in these women, leads to a twofold increase in the daily production rate of estrone compared with that in premenopausal women; aromatization also is higher in obese women. In some postmenopausal women, sufficient estrogen may be elaborated by this mechanism to prevent the clinical manifestations of estrogen withdrawal and to play a role in the genesis of endometrial carcinoma.[21,130] Indeed, an association between the degree of stromal proliferation and postmenopausal endometrial adenocarcinoma has been noted.[130] The variations that exist in the ovarian steroid hormone output from one postmenopausal woman to another may correspond to similar variations in the morphologic appearance of the stroma in this age group, although no correlative functional and structural studies have been performed.

References

1. Adams EC, Hertig AT (1969) Studies on the human corpus luteum. I. Observations on the ultrastructure of development and regression of the luteal cells during the menstrual cycle. J Cell Biol 41:696–715
2. Adams EC, Hertig AT (1969) Studies on the human corpus luteum. II. Observations on the ultrastructure of luteal cells during pregnancy. J Cell Biol 41:716–735
3. Aiman J, Fornery JP, Parker R Jr (1986) Secretion of androgens and estrogens by normal and neoplastic ovaries in postmenopausal women. Obstet Gynecol 68:1–5
4. Al-Timimi A, Buckley CH, Fox H (1985) An immunohistochemical study of the incidence and significance of sex steroid hormone binding sites in normal and neoplastic human ovarian tissue. Int J Gynecol Pathol 4:24–41
5. Ayyagari RR, Khan-Dawood FS (1987) Human corpus luteum: Presence of epidermal growth factor receptors and binding characteristics. Am J Obstet Gynecol 156:942–946
6. Baca M, Zamboni L (1967) The fine structure of the human follicular oocyte. J Ultrastruct Res 19:354–381
7. Balboni GC (1983) Structural changes: Ovulation and luteal phase. In: Serra GB (ed) The Ovary. New York, Raven Press, pp 123–141
8. Barad DH, Ryan KJ, Elkind-Hirsch K, Makris A (1988) Immunoreactive substance P in the human ovary. Am J Obstet Gynecol 159:242–246
9. Barbieri RL, Makris A, Randall RW, et al (1986) Insulin stimulates androgen accumulation in incubations of ovarian stroma obtained from women with hyperandrogenism. J Clin Endocrinol Metab 62:904–910
10. Bassis ML (1956) Pseudodeciduosis. Am J Obstet Gynecol 72:1029–1037
11. Benjamin E, Law S, Bobrow LG (1987) Intermediate filaments cytokeratin and vimentin in ovarian sex cord-stromal tumours with correlative studies in adult and fetal ovaries. J Pathol 152:253–263
12. Bersch W, Alexy E, Heuser HP, Staemmler HJ (1973) Ectopic decidua formation in the ovary (so-called deciduoma). Virch Archiv A (Pathol Anat) 360:173–177
13. Blaustein A (1984) Peritoneal mesothelium and ovarian surface epithelial cells—shared characteristics. Int J Gynecol Pathol 3:361–375
14. Blaustein A, Lee H (1979) Surface cells of the ovary and pelvic peritoneum: A histochemical and ultrastructural comparison. Gynecol Oncol 8:34–43
15. Bloom W, Fawcett DW (1975) A Textbook of Histology. Tenth Edition. Philadelphia, W. B. Saunders Co.

16. Bomsel-Helmreich O, Gougeon A, Thebault A, et al (1979) Healthy and atretic human follicles in the preovulatory phase: differences in evolution of follicular morphology and steroid content of follicular fluid. J Clin Endocrinol Metab 48:686–694

17. Boss JH, Scully RE, Wegner KH, Cohen RB (1965) Structural variations in the adult ovary—clinical significance. Obstet Gynecol 25:747–763

18. Bransilver BR, Ferenczy A, Richart RM (1974) Brenner tumors and Walthard cell nests. Arch Pathol Lab Med 98:76–86

19. Centola GM (1983) Structural changes: Follicular development and hormonal requirements. In: Serra GB (ed). The Ovary. New York, Raven Press, pp 95–111

20. Centola GM (1983) Structural changes: Atresia. In: Serra GB (ed) The Ovary. New York, Raven Press, pp 113–122

21. Chang RJ, Judd HL (1981) The ovary after menopause. Clin Obstet Gynaecol 24:181–191

22. Charpin C, Bhan AZ, Zurawski VR Jr, Scully RE (1982) Carcinoembryonic antigen (CEA) and carbohydrate determinant 19-9 (CA 19-9) localization in 121 primary and metastatic ovarian tumors: An immunohistochemical study with the use of monoclonal antibodies. Int J Gynecol Pathol 1:231–245

23. Clement PB, Young RH, Scully RE (1988) Ovarian granulosa cell proliferations of pregnancy: A report of nine cases. Hum Pathol 19:657–662

24. Cordon-Cardo C, Mattes MJ, Melamed MR, et al (1985) Immunopathologic analysis of a panel of mouse monoclonal antibodies reacting with human ovarian carcinomas and other human tumors. Int J Gynecol Pathol 4:121–130

25. Corner GW Jr (1956) The histological dating of the human corpus luteum of menstruation. Am J Anat 98:377–401

26. Crisp TM, Dessouky DA, Denys FR (1970) The fine structure of the human corpus luteum of early pregnancy and during the progestational phase of the menstrual cycle. Am J Anat 127:37–70

27. Crowley WF (1986) Progesterone antagonism. N Engl J Med 315:1607–1608

28. Croxatto, H., Ortiz M, Croxatto HB (1980) Correlation between histologic dating of human corpus luteum and the luteinizing hormone peak-biopsy interval. Am J Obstet Gynecol 136:667–670

29. Curtis EM (1962) Normal ovarian histology in infancy and childhood. Obstet Gynecol 19:444–454

30. Czernobilsky B, Moll R, Franke WW, et al (1984) Intermediate filaments of normal and neoplastic tissues of the female genital tract with emphasis on problems of differential tumor diagnosis. Pathol Res Pract 179:31–37

31. Czernobilsky B, Moll R, Levy R, Franke WW (1985) Coexpression of cytokeratin and vimentin filaments in mesothelial, granulosa and rete ovarii cells of the human ovary. Eur J Cell Biol 37:175–190

32. Czernobilsky B, Shezen E, Lifschitz-Mercer B, et al (1989) Alpha smooth muscle actin (alpha-SM actin) in normal human ovaries, in ovarian stromal hyperplasia and in ovarian neoplasms. Virchows Arch [B] 57:55–61

33. Deane HW, Lobel BL, Romney SL (1962) Enzymic histochemistry of normal human ovaries of the menstrual cycle, pregnancy, and the early puerperium. Am J Obstet Gynecol 83:281–294

34. Dekel N, David MP, Yedwab GA, Kraicer PF (1977) Follicular development during late pregnancy. Int J Fertil 22:24–29

35. Dennefors BL, Janson PO, Knutsson F, Hamberger L (1980) Steroid production and responsiveness to gonadotropin in isolated stromal tissue of human postmenopausal ovaries. Am J Obstet Gynecol 136:997–1002

36. Dennefors BL, Janson PO, Hamberger L, Knutsson F (1982) Hilus cells from human postmenopausal ovaries: gonadotrophin sensitivity, steroid and cyclic AMP production. Acta Obstet Gynecol Scand 61:413–416

37. Dyer CA, Erickson GF (1985) Norepinephrine amplifies human chorionic gonadotropin-stimulated androgen biosynthesis by ovarian theca-interstitial cells. Endocrinology 116:1645–1652

38. Eichner E, Bove ER (1954) In vivo studies on the lymphatic drainage of the human ovary. Obstet Gynecol 3:287–297

39. Erickson GF (1978) Normal ovarian function. Clin Obstet Gynecol 21:31–52

40. Feinberg R, Cohen RB (1965) A comparative histochemical study of the ovarian stromal lipid band, stromal theca cell, and normal ovarian follicular apparatus. Am J Obstet Gynecol 92:958–969

41. Ferenczy A, Richart RM (1974) Female reproductive system: Dynamics of scan and transmission electron microscopy. New York, Wiley & Sons.

42. Futterweit W (1985) In: Polycystic Ovarian Disease. Clinical Perspectives in Obstetrics and Gynecology. New York, Springer–Verlag.

43. Gardner GH, Greene RR, Peckham B (1957) Tumors of the broad ligament. Am J Obstet Gynecol 73:536–555

44. Gillim SW, Christensen AK, McLennan CE (1969) Fine structure of the human menstrual corpus luteum at its stage of maximum secretory activity. Am J Anat 126:409–428

45. Gougeon A (1981) Frequent occurrence of multiovular follicles and multinuclear oocytes in the adult human ovary. Fertil Steril 35:417–422

46. Govan ADT (1970) Ovarian follicular activity in late pregnancy. J Endocrinol 48:235–241

47. Green JA, Maqueo M (1965) Ultrastructure of the human ovary. I. The luteal cell during the menstrual cycle. Am J Obstet Gynecol 92:946–957

48. Green JA, Garcilazo JA, Maqueo M (1967) Ultrastructure of the human ovary. II. The luteal cell at term. Am J Obstet Gynecol 99:855–863

49. Greenblatt RB, Colle ML, Mahesh VB (1976) Ovarian and adrenal steroid production in the postmenopausal woman. Obstet Gynecol 47:383–387

50. Grodin JM, Siiteri PK, MacDonald PC (1973) Source of estrogen production in postmenopausal women. J Clin Endocrinol Metab 36:207–214

51. Hameed A, Fox WM, Kurman RJ, et al. (1993) Perforin expression in cell mediated luteolysis: Evidence for highly selective recruitment of CD8[+] T-lymphocytes in vivo (unpublished data)

52. Herr JC, Heidger PM Jr, Scott JR, et al (1978) Decidual cells in the human ovary at term. I. Incidence, gross anatomy and ultrastructural features of merocrine secretion. Am J Anat 152:7–28

53. Hertig AT (1964) Gestational hyperplasia of endometrium. A morphologic correlation of ova, endometrium, and cor-

pora lutea during early pregnancy. Lab Invest 13:1153–1191

54. Hertig AT (1968) The primary human oocyte: Some observations on the fine structure of Balbiani's vitelline body and the origin of the annulate lamellae. Am J Anat 122:107–138

55. Hertig AT, Adams EC (1967) Studies on the human oocyte and its follicle. I. Ultrastructural and histochemical observations on the primordial follicle stage. J Cell Biol 34:647–675

56. Hidvegi D, Cibils LA, Sorensen K, Hidvegi I (1982) Ultrastructural and histochemical observations of neuroendocrine granules in nonneoplastic ovaries. Am J Obstet Gynecol 143:590–594

57. Hillier SG (1987) Intrafollicular paracrine function of ovarian androgen. J Steroid Biochem 27:351–357

58. Himelstein-Braw R, Byskov AG, Peters H, Faber M (1976) Follicular atresia in the infant human ovary. J Reprod Fertil 46:55–59

59. Honore LH, O'Hara KE (1979) Ovarian hilus cell heterotopia. Obstet Gynecol 53:461–464

60. Isola J, Kallioniemi O, Korte J, et al (1990) Steroid receptors and Ki-67 reactivity in ovarian cancer and in normal ovary: Correlation with DNA flow cytometry, biochemical receptor assay, and patient survival. J Pathol 162:295–301

61. Israel SL, Rubenstone A, Meranze DR (1954) The ovary at term. I. Decidua-like reaction and surface cell proliferation. Obstet Gynecol 3:399–407

62. Jacobowitz D, Wallach EE (1967) Histochemical and chemical studies of the autonomic innervation of the ovary. Endocrinology 81:1132–1139

63. Janko AB, Sandberg EC (1970) Histochemical evidence for the protein nature of the Reinke crystalloid. Obstet Gynecol 35:493–503

64. Joel RV, Foraker AG (1960) Fate of the corpus albicans: A morphological approach. Am J Obstet Gynecol 80:314–316

65. Jones GES, Goldberg B, Woodruff JD (1968) Histochemistry as a guide for interpretation of cell function. Am J Obstet Gynecol 100:76–83

66. Judd HL, Judd GE, Lucas WE, Yen SSC (1974) Endocrine function of the postmenopausal ovary: Concentration of androgens and estrogens in ovarian and peripheral vein blood. J Clin Endocrinol Metab 39:1020–1024

67. Judd HL, Lucas WE, Yen SSC (1974) Effect of oophorectomy on circulating testosterone and androstenedione levels in patients with endometrial carcinoma. Am J Obstet Gynecol 118:793–798

68. Kabawat SE, Bast RC Jr, Bhan AK, et al (1983) Tissue distribution of coelomic-epithelium-related antigen recognized by the monoclonal antibody OC125. Int J Gynecol Pathol 2:275–285

69. Kedzia H (1983) Gonadoblastoma: Structures and background of development. Am J Obstet Gynecol 147:81–85

70. Kraus FT, Neubecker RD (1962) Luteinization of the ovarian theca in infants and children. Am J Clin Pathol 37:389–397

71. Laffargue P, Adechy-Benkoel L, Valette C (1968) Ultrastructure du stroma ovarien. Ann Anat Pathol 13:381–401

72. Laffargue P, Benkoel L, Laffargue F, et al (1978) Ultrastructural and enzyme histochemical study of ovarian hilar cells in women and their relationships with sympathetic nerves. Hum Pathol 9:649–659

73. Lastarria D, Sachdev RK, Babury RA, et al (1990) Immunohistochemical analysis for desmin in normal and neoplastic ovarian stromal tissue. Arch Pathol Lab Med 114:502–505

74. Lee PA (1983) Ovarian function from conception to puberty: Physiology and disorders. In: Serra GB (ed) The Ovary. New York, Raven Press, pp 177–189

75. LeMaire WJ, Rice BF, Savard K (1968) Steroid hormone formation in the human ovary: V. Synthesis of progesterone in vitro in corpora lutea during the reproductive cycle. J Clin Endocrinol Metab 28:1249–1256

76. Longcope C (1971) Metabolic clearance and blood production rates of estrogens in postmenopausal women. Am J Obstet Gynecol 111:778–781

77. Longcope C, Hunter R, Franz C (1980) Steroid secretion by the postmenopausal ovary. Am J Obstet Gynecol 138:564–568

78. Loubet R, Loubet A, Leboutet M-J (1984) The ovarian stroma after the menopause: Activity and ageing. In: de Brux J, Gautray J-P (eds) Clinical Pathology of the Ovary. Boston, MTP Press Ltd, pp 119–141

79. Manivel JC, Dehner LP, Burke B (1988) Ovarian tumorlike structures, biovular follicles, and binucleated oocytes in children: Their frequency and possible pathologic significance. Pediatr Pathol 8:283–292

80. Maqueo M, Goldzieher JW (1966) Hormone-induced alterations of ovarian morphology. Fertil Steril 17:676–683

81. Mattingly RF, Huang WY (1969) Steroidogenesis of the menopause and postmenopausal ovary. Am J Obstet Gynecol 103:679–693

82. McLachlan RI, Cohen NL, Vale WW, et al (1989) The importance of luteinizing hormone in the control of inhibin and progesterone secretion by the human corpus luteum. J Clin Endocrinol Metab 68:1078–1085

83. McKay DG, Pinkerton JHM, Hertig AT, Danziger S (1961) The adult human ovary: A histochemical study. Obstet Gynecol 18:13–39

84. McNatty KP (1978) Follicular determinants of corpus luteum function in the human ovary. In: Channing CP, Marsh JM, Sadler WA (eds). Ovarian Follicular and Corpus Luteum Function. Advances in Experimental Medicine and Biology, Vol 112. New York, Plenum Press.

85. McNatty KP (1978) Cyclic changes in antral fluid hormone concentrations in humans. Clin Endocrinol Metab 7:577–600

86. McNatty KP, Makris A, DeGrazia C et al (1979) The production of progesterone, androgens, and estrogens by granulosa cells, thecal tissue, and stromal tissue from human ovaries in vitro. J Clin Endocrinol Metab 49:687–699

87. McNatty KP, Makris A, DeGrazia C, et al (1979) The production of progesterone, androgens, and estrogens by human granulosa cells in vitro and in vivo. J Steroid Biochem 11:775–799

88. McNatty KP, Smith DM, Makris A, et al (1979) The microenvironment of the human antral follicle: interrelationships among the steroid levels in antral fluid, the population of granulosa cells, and the status of the oocyte in vivo and in vitro. J Clin Endocrinol Metab 49:851–860

89. McNatty KP, Smith DM, Makris A, et al (1980) The intraovarian sites of androgen and estrogen formation in women

with normal and hyperandrogenic ovaries as judged by in vitro experiments. J Clin Endocrinol Metab 50:755–763

90. Merrill JA (1963) The morphology of the prepubertal ovary: Relationship to the polycystic ovary syndrome. South Med J 56:225–231

91. Mestwardt W, Muller O, Brandau H (1978) Structural analysis of granulosa cells from human ovaries in correlation with function. In: Channing CP, Marsh JM, Sadler WA (eds) Ovarian Follicular and Corpus Luteum Function. Advances in Experimental Medicine and Biology, Vol 112, New York, Plenum Press

92. Miettinen M, Lehto V, Virtanen I (1983) Expression of intermediate filaments in normal ovaries and ovarian epithelial, sex cord-stromal, and germinal tumors. Int J Gynecol Pathol 2:64–71

93. Mikhail G, Allen WM (1967) Ovarian function in human pregnancy. Am J Obstet Gynecol 99:308–312

94. Mohsin S (1979) The sympathetic innervation of the mammalian ovary. A review of pharmacological and histochemical studies. Clin Exp Pharm Phys 6:335–354

95. Nagamani M, Hannigan EV, Van Dinh T, Stuart CA (1988) Hyperinsulinemia and stromal luteinization of the ovaries in postmenopausal women with endometrial cancer. J Clin Endocrinol Metab 67:144–148

96. Nakano R, Shima K, Yamoto M, et al (1989) Binding sites for gonadotropins in human postmenopausal ovaries. Obstet Gynecol 73:196–200

97. Nelson WW, Greene RR (1953) The human ovary in pregnancy. Int Abs Surg 97:1–23

98. Nelson WW, Greene RR (1958) Some observations on the histology of the human ovary during pregnancy. Am J Obstet Gynecol 76:66–89

99. Neunteufel W, Breitenecker G (1989) Tissue expression of CA 125 in benign and malignant lesions of ovary and fallopian tube: A comparison with CA 19-9 and CEA. Gynecol Oncol 32:297–302

100. Nicosia SV (1983) Morphological changes of the human ovary throughout life. In: Serra GB (ed) The Ovary. New York, Raven Press, pp 57–81

101. Nouwen EJ, Hendrix PG, Eerdekens MW, De Broe ME (1987) Tumor markers in the human ovary and its neoplasms. A comparative immunohistochemical study. Am J Pathol 126:230–242

102. Okamura H, Virutamasen P, Wright KH, Wallach EE (1972) Ovarian smooth muscle in the human being, rabbit, and cat. Am J Obstet Gynecol 112:183–191

103. Owman C, Rosengren E, Sjoberg N (1967) Adrenergic innervation of the human female reproductive organs: A histochemical and chemical investigation. Obstet Gynecol 30:763–773

104. Palumbo A, Jones C, Lightman A, et al (1989) Immunohistochemical localization of renin and angiotensin II in human ovaries. Am J Obstet Gynecol 160:8–14

105. Papadaki L, Beilby JOW (1971) The fine structure of the surface epithelium of the human ovary. J Cell Sci 8:445–465

106. Pauerstein CJ, Eddy CA, Croxatto HD, et al (1978) Temporal relationships of estrogen, progesterone, and luteinizing hormone levels to ovulation in women and infrahuman primates. Am J Obstet Gynecol 130:876–886

107. Pedersen PH, Larsen JF (1968) The ultrastructure of the human granulosal lutein cell of the first trimester of gestation. Acta Endocrinol 58:481–496

108. Pennington GW (1974) The reproductive endocrinology of childhood and adolescence. Clin Obstet Gynaecol 1:509–531

109. Peters H, Himelstein-Braw R, Faber M (1976) The normal development of the ovary in childhood. Acta Endocrinol 82:617–630

110. Plentl AA, Friedman EA (1971) Lymphatic System of the Female Genitalia. Philadelphia, W.B. Saunders

111. Plotz EJ, Wiener M, Stein AA, Hahn BD (1967) Enzymatic activities related to steroidogenesis in postmenopausal ovaries of patients with and without endometrial carcinoma. Am J Obstet Gynecol 99:182–197

112. Pryse-Davies J (1974) The development, structure and function of the female pelvic organs in childhood. Clin Obstet Gynaecol 1:483–508

113. Quagliarello J, Goldsmith L, Steinetz B, et al (1980) Induction of relaxin secretion in nonpregnant women by human chorionic gonadotropin. J Clin Endocrinol Metab 51:74–77

114. Rao CV (1982) Receptors for gonadotropins in human ovaries. Recent Advances in Fertility Research, Part A: Developments in Reproductive Endocrinology 123–135

115. Reagan JW (1950) Ceroid pigment in the human ovary. Am J Obstet Gynecol 59:433–436

116. Reed MJ, Beranek PA, Ghilchik MW, James VHT (1985) Conversion of estrone to estradiol and estradiol to estrone in postmenopausal women. Obstet Gynecol 66:361–365

117. Reeves G (1971) Specific stroma in the cortex and medulla of the ovary. Cell types and vascular supply in relation to follicular apparatus and ovulation. Obstet Gynecol 37:832–844

118. Rice BF, Hammerstein J, Savard K (1964) Steroid hormone formation in the human ovary: II. Action of gonadotropins in vitro in the corpus luteum. J Clin Endocrinol 24:606–615

119. Rice BF, Savard K (1966) Steroid hormone formation in the human ovary: IV. Ovarian stromal compartment; formation of radioactive steroids from acetate-1-^{14}C and action of gonadotropins. J Clin Endocrinol 26:593–609

120. Rodriguez GC, Berchuk A, Whitaker RS, et al (1991) Epidermal growth factor receptor expression in normal ovarian epithelium and ovarian cancer. II. Relationship between receptor expression and response to epidermal growth factor. Am J Obstet Gynecol 164:745–750

121. Safneck JR, DeSa DJ (1986) Structures mimicking sex cord-stromal tumours and gonadoblastomas in the ovaries of normal infants and children. Histopathology 10:909–920

122. Schmidt CL, Black VH, Sarosi P, Weiss G (1986) Progesterone and relaxin secretion in relation to the ultrastructure of human luteal cells in culture: Effects of human chorionic gonadotropin. Am J Obstet Gynecol 155:1209–1219

123. Schmidt WA (1986) Eosin-induced fluorescence of Reinke crystals. Int J Gynecol Pathol 5:88–89

124. Scully RE (1979) Tumors of the ovary and maldeveloped gonads. In: Atlas of Tumor Pathology, Second Series, Fascicle 16. Armed Forces Institute of Pathology, Washington, D.C.

125. Scully RE (1981) Smooth-muscle differentiation in genital tract disorders. (Editorial) Arch Pathol Lab Med 105:505–507

126. Scully RE, Cohen RB (1964) Oxidative-enzyme activity in normal and pathologic human ovaries. Obstet Gynecol 24:667–681

127. Sealey JE, Glorioso N, Itskovitz J, Laragh JH (1986) Prorenin as a reproductive hormone. New form of the renin system. Am J Med 81:1041–1046

128. Shaw JA, Dabbs DJ, Geisinger KR (1992) Sclerosing stromal tumor of the ovary: An ultrastructural and immunohistochemical analysis with histogenetic considerations. Ultrastr Pathol 16:363–377

129. Shima K, Kitayama S, Nakano R (1987) Gonadotropin binding sites in human ovarian follicles and corpora lutea during the menstrual cycle. Obstet Gynecol 69:800–806

130. Snowden JA, Harkin PJR, Thornton JG, Wells M (1989) Morphometric assessment of ovarian stromal proliferation—a clinicopathological study. Histopathology 14:369–379

131. Stangel JJ, Richart RM, Okagaki T, Cottral G (1970) Nuclear DNA content of luteinized cells of the human ovary. Am J Obstet Gynecol 108:543–549

132. Starup J, Visfeldt J (1974) Ovarian morphology in early and late human pregnancy. Acta Obstet Gynecol Scand 53:211–218

133. Sternberg WH (1949) The morphology, androgenic function, hyperplasia, and tumors of the human ovarian hilus cells. Am J Pathol 25:493–521

134. Sternberg WH, Segaloff A, Gaskill CJ (1953) Influence of chorionic gonadotropin on human ovarian hilus cells (Leydig-like cells). J Clin Endocrinol Metab 13:139–153

135. Tanabe K, Gagliano P, Channing CP, et al (1983) Levels of inhibin-F activity and steroids in human follicular fluid from normal women and women with polycystic ovarian disease. J Clin Endocrinol Metab 57:24–31

136. Tsonis CG, Messinis IE, Templeton AA, et al (1988) Gonadotropic stimulation of inhibin secretion by the human ovary during the follicular and early luteal phase of the cycle. J Clin Endocrinol Metab 66:915–921

137. Valdes-Dapena MA (1967) The normal ovary of childhood. Ann NY Acad Sci 142:597–613

138. Vermeulen A (1976) The hormonal activity of the postmenopausal ovary. J Clin Endocrinol Metab 42:247–253

139. Vijayakumar R, Walters WAW (1987) Ovarian stromal and luteal tissue prostaglandins, 17beta-estradiol, and progesterone in relation to the phases of the menstrual cycle in women. Am J Obstet Gynecol 156:947–951

140. Visfeldt J, Starup J (1974) Dating of the human corpus luteum of menstruation using histological parameters. Acta Pathol Microbiol Scand A 82:137–144

141. Visfeldt J, Starup J (1975) Histology of the human corpus luteum of early and late pregnancy. Acta Pathol Microbiol Scand A 83:669–677

142. Weiss G, O'Byrne EM, Steinetz BG (1976) Relaxin: A product of the human corpus luteum of pregnancy. Science 194:948–949

143. Weiss G, O'Byrne Em, Hochman JA, Goldsmith LT, Rifkin I, Steinetz BG (1977) Secretion of progesterone and relaxin by the human corpus luteum at midpregnancy and at term. Obstet Gynecol 50:679–681

144. Weiss G, Rifkin I (1975) Progesterone and estrogen secretion by puerperal human ovaries. Obstet Gynecol 46:557–559

145. White RF, Hertig AT, Rock J, Adams E (1951) Histological and histochemical observations on the corpus luteum of human pregnancy with special reference to corpora lutea associated with early normal and abnormal ova. Contrib Embryol 34:55–74

146. Wiley CA, Esterly JR (1976) Observations on the human corpus luteum: Histochemical changes during development and involution. Am J Obstet Gynecol 125:514–519

147. Yussman MA, Taymor ML (1970) Serum levels of follicle stimulating hormone and luteinizing hormone and of plasma progesterone related to ovulation by corpus luteum biopsy. J Clin Endocrinol 30:396–399

148. Zhang J, Young RH, Arseneau J, Scully RE (1982) Ovarian stromal tumors containing lutein or Leydig cells (luteinized thecomas and stromal Leydig cell tumors)—a clinicopathological analysis of fifty cases. Int J Gynecol Pathol 1:270–285

16

Nonneoplastic Lesions of the Ovary

Philip B. Clement, M.D.

Nonneoplastic lesions of the ovary frequently form a pelvic mass and often are associated with abnormal hormonal manifestations, so they may mimic an ovarian neoplasm on clinical examination, at operation, and on pathological examination. Many occur in the reproductive years and may be associated with infertility. Their proper recognition is, therefore, important to allow appropriate, usually conservative therapy, thereby avoiding unnecessary oophorectomy.

Congenital Lesions

Absent Ovary

In phenotypic females, absence of both ovaries usually is associated with an abnormal karyotype and a syndrome of gonadal dysgenesis (see Chapter 1, Embryology of the Female Genital Tract and Disorders of Abnormal Sexual

Development). In such cases, bilateral streak gonads or a unilateral streak gonad and contralateral intraabdominal testes usually are found. However, rare cases of truly agonadal individuals have been reported, usually with a karyotype that is 46XY, but rarely, 46XX.[352,354] Rare patients with ataxia telangiectasia have had no evidence of ovarian tissue at laparotomy.[57]

Rarely, one ovary may be absent in an otherwise normal woman, usually representing an incidental finding at operation or postmortem examination. Associated findings frequently include agenesis or malformation of the ipsilateral fallopian tube, round ligament, kidney, or ureter, alone or in various combinations.[65,299,504] The differential diagnosis includes (1) ectopic ovary, which may lie at the level of the liver, close to the kidney,[410] within the omentum,[352] or within an inguinal hernia,[63] and (2) adnexal torsion with atrophy or autoamputation (see page 631).

Lobulated, Accessory, and Supernumerary Ovary

Examples of lobulated, accessory, and supernumerary ovary are among the rarest of gynecological abnormalities. A lobulated ovary is a normally situated ovary divided by one or several fissures into two or more lobes.[481] The lobes may be completely separate or connected by fibrous tissue or ovarian stroma; rarely both ovaries may be affected. A closely related anomaly is an accessory ovary, a structure containing normal ovarian tissue located in the vicinity of a normal, eutopic ovary with which it has a direct or ligamentous attachment.[119,157,481] A supernumerary ovary is a similar structure but located at some distance from, and not connected to, a eutopic ovary.[110,179,250,256,364] It may be pelvic, attached to the uterus, bladder, or pelvic walls, or retroperitoneal, within the omentum, periaortic area, or mesentery.[410,481] In most cases, the accessory or supernumerary ovary is less than 1 cm in size, and smaller examples may go unrecognized at operation or autopsy.[119,481] They are multiple and bilateral in some cases.[157,179] The ectopic ovarian tissue possesses the functional potential, as evidenced by persistent menses after bilateral oophorectomy,[240] as well as the pathological potential of normal ovaries.[157,187,302] The presence of a supernumerary ovary therefore is one histogenetic mechanism for ovarian-type tumors in extraovarian sites. This derivation is even more likely for nonepithelial tumors, such as granulosa–theca tumor within the broad ligament,[161] which are unlikely to have a mesothelial or secondary mullerian origin (see Chapter 17, Diseases of the Peritoneum).

Embryologically, lobulated and accessory ovary are closely related. The former results from lobulation of the ovarian anlage, whereas the latter presumably develops from a slightly separated part of the otherwise normally developing and migrating ovarian anlage. Pathogenetic theories for supernumerary ovary include aberrant migration of part of the gonadal ridge after incorporation of the germ cells, or alternatively, arrest of some of the migrating germ cells in an ectopic location with inductive transformation of the surrounding tissue into ovarian stroma.[364] As many as one-third of patients with lobulated ovaries, accessory ovary, and supernumerary ovary have other congenital genitourinary abnormalities.

Ovarian Remnant Syndrome

Ectopic, accessory, and supernumerary ovary should be distinguished from examples of the *ovarian remnant syndrome* (ORS) or *ovarian implant syndrome*.[221,320,350,357,438,453,487,503] Patients with the ORS typically have a history of bilateral oophorectomy complicated by extensive periovarian adhesions, the latter usually a result of a prior pelvic operation, endometriosis, pelvic inflammatory disease, inflammatory bowel disease, or combinations thereof. Clues to the diagnosis in patients who had bilateral oophorectomy are premenopausal follicle-stimulating hormone (FSH) and luteinizing hormone (LH) levels,[438] an absence of menopausal symptoms, and a lack of atrophic changes on cervicovaginal smears. Within weeks to months but occasionally years after oophorectomy, patients with the ORS usually present with chronic or cyclic pelvic pain and a palpable pelvic mass. Ultrasonography or computed tomography (CT) scanning may aid preoperative detection of nonpalpable symptomatic remnants,[357] and stimulation of the residual ovarian tissue with clomiphene citrate therapy can facilitate their intraoperative localization.[221] Laparotomy typically reveals a 3 to 4-cm cystic mass, covered by dense adhesions, on the pelvic side wall[438] or, less commonly, the mesentery[350]; bilateral ovarian remnants rarely have been encountered.[438] Obstruction or compression of the ureter,[357,503] the colon,[350,357] or the bladder[320] have been encountered. In a unique case, an ovarian remnant formed an intussusceptum in the small intestine with secondary obstruction.[487] Pathological examination usually reveals one or several follicular or corpus luteum cysts within a remnant of ovarian tissue (Fig. 16.1), but endometriosis, benign neoplasms, or normal ovarian tissue also have been found. Excision of the remnants may be difficult and require multiple operations.[357]

Adrenal Cortical Rests

Although accessory adrenal cortical tissue frequently is observed within the wall of the fallopian tube and the broad ligament, it is an extremely rare finding in the ovary.[454] The adrenal rests are typically yellow, spherical, encapsulated nodules several millimeters in size (Fig. 16.2). Adrenal cortical ectopia in these sites can be explained by the close proximity of the anlage of the adrenal cortex to the gonadal ridge during embryonic development. Ovarian adrenal cortical rests may be the origin of occasional steroid cell tumors of the ovary that resemble adrenal cortical tissue in both their histologic appearance and endocrine manifestations.[410]

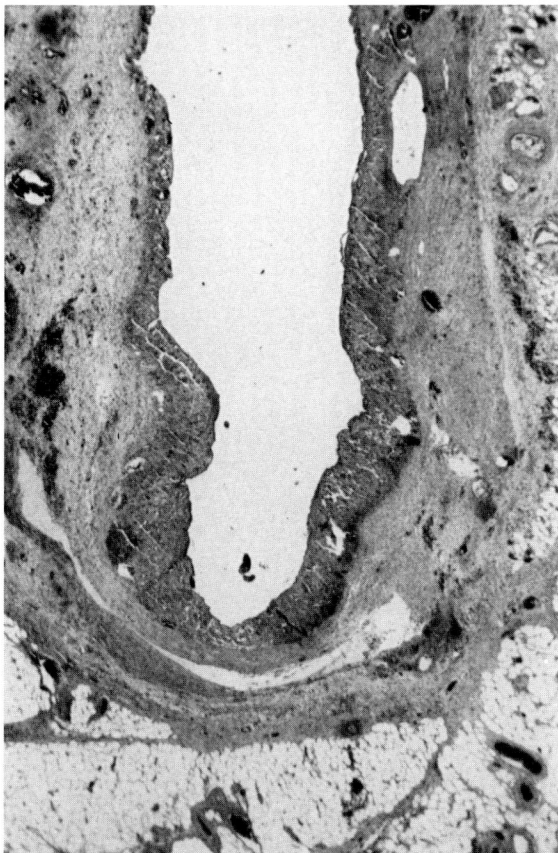

FIG. 16.1. **Ovarian remnant syndrome**. A corpus luteum cyst is surrounded by congested fibroadipose tissue.

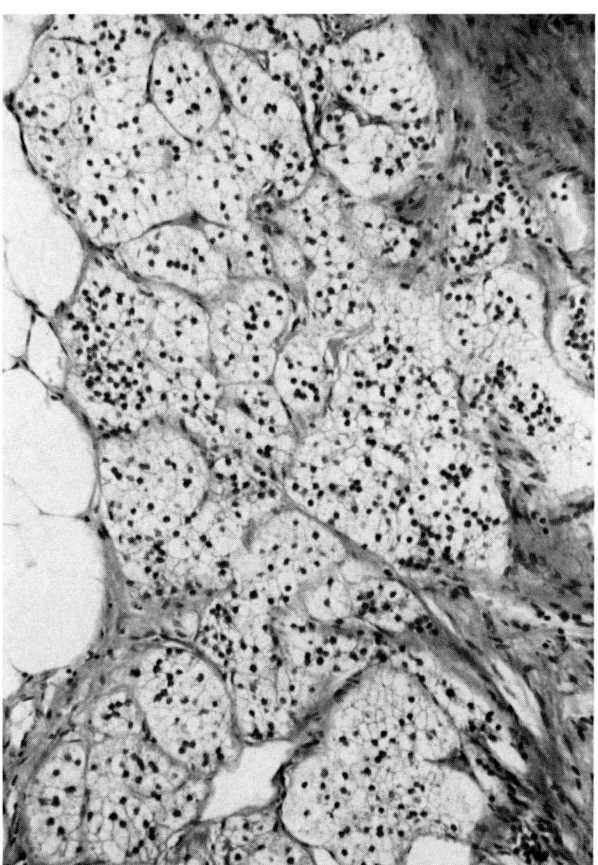

FIG. 16.2. **Adrenal cortical rest within mesovarium**. Nests of cells with foamy cytoplasm are separated by a scanty fibrous stroma.

Uterus-like Ovarian Mass

The three reported examples of a uterus-like ovarian mass have been characterized by a central cavity lined by endometrial tissue and surrounded by a thick, smooth muscle wall.[108,365,369] In one case, there was a contiguous endometrioid adenocarcinoma.[369] Although the lesions can be explained on the basis of an ovarian endometriotic cyst with smooth muscle metaplasia of its stromal component (*endomyometriosis*; see Chapter 17, Diseases of the Peritoneum), a congenital malformation of the ipsilateral müllerian duct has been suggested as a more likely origin.[365,381] This interpretation is supported by the presence of congenital abnormalities of the urinary tract in two of the reported cases. In the third case, however, residual ovarian parenchyma was identified at the periphery of the mass.[369]

Splenic–Gonadal Fusion

Splenic–gonadal fusion (Fig. 16.3) is an extremely rare anomaly resulting from fusion of the analage of both organs during embryonic development. The male/female ra-

tio is 9:1. Three examples have been described in newborn female infants, two of which were associated with partially undescended ovaries, as well as other, multiple congenital anomalies.[366] All three cases were of the continuous type in which a cord-like structure connected the spleen to the left ovary or surrounding structures. In one of these cases, several intraovarian splenic nodules were found. An additional case has been described in a woman who was found to have a septate uterus and a cluster of splenic nodules surrounding the otherwise normal left ovary.[10] The differential diagnosis in the latter case would include traumatic splenosis, but in such cases there usually is a history of trauma and the nodules of splenic tissue are more widely dispersed throughout the peritoneal cavity (see Chapter 17, Diseases of the Peritoneum).

Inflammatory Disorders

Infectious Diseases

Pelvic inflammatory disease (PID) of bacterial origin accounts for most ovarian infections in the western world.

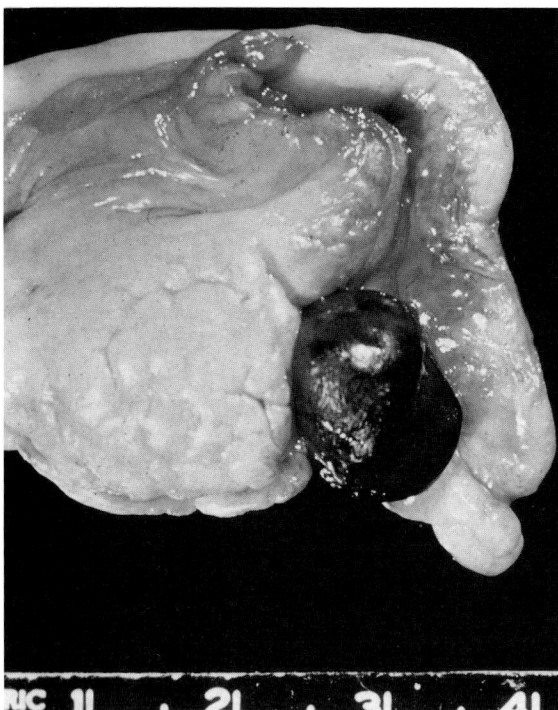

FIG. 16.3. Splenic–gonadal fusion. A nodule of splenic tissue is contiguous with the surface of the ovary.

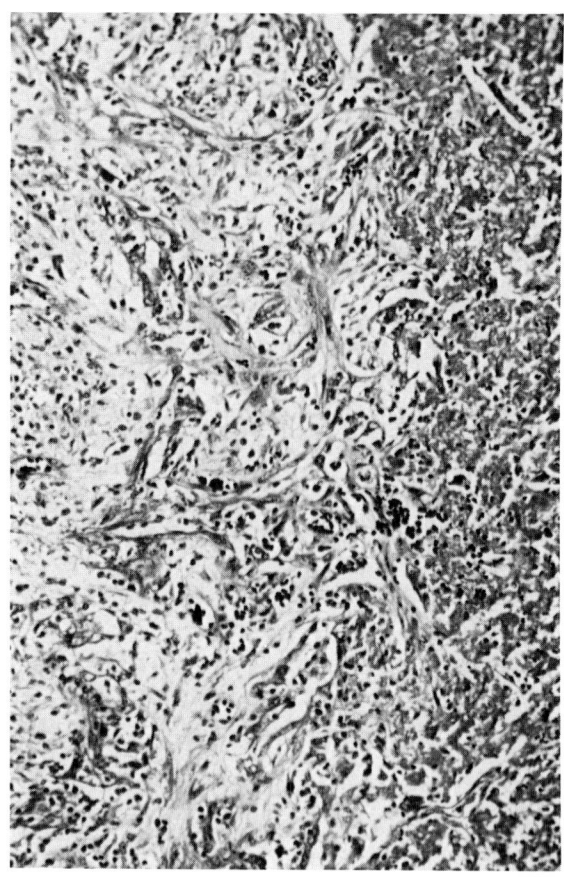

FIG. 16.4. Tuboovarian abscess. Lining consists of inflammatory debris with subjacent granulation tissue.

Although some studies have indicated that the presence of an intrauterine device (IUD) increases the risk of infection, other studies have shown that when the number of sexual partners are controlled for, IUDs do not increase the risk of PID.[131,225] Ovarian involvement in PID is almost always secondary to salpingitis, and typically takes the form of a tuboovarian abscess (Fig. 16.4), which usually is bilateral. The symptoms typically are abdominal or pelvic pain, and less consistently, fever, vaginal discharge or bleeding, and urinary symptoms.[253] An adnexal mass is palpable, demonstrable with imaging techniques, or visible at laparoscopy. A history of PID is present in only one-third to one-half of patients, suggesting that subclinical infections are common.[253] A mixed flora with a preponderance of anaerobic organisms typically is recovered from the contents of the abscess.[130,253] With resolution, the only sequela may be tuboovarian fibrous adhesions, but occasionally a healed abscess becomes a tuboovarian cyst.

A unilateral or bilateral ovarian abscess without tubal involvement is much rarer than a tuboovarian abscess. The former usually is secondary to direct or lymphatic spread of organisms from a nongynecologic pelvic inflammatory process, such as diverticulitis, appendicitis, inflammatory bowel disease, postoperative pelvic infection, or, rarely, from a blood-borne infection.[480,490] The external ovarian surface in such cases often is unremarkable, and the process may not be apparent until the organ is sectioned

(Fig. 16.5). Uncommonly, rupture of an ovarian or tuboovarian abscess leads to secondary peritonitis[94,304,351] or, rarely, fistulas involving the colon,[425] bladder,[267] or vagina.[13,90]

Milder, chronic, or recurrent forms of ovarian involvement by PID may take the form of a chronic perioophoritis, with periovarian and tuboovarian adhesions that may completely surround the ovary. Sclerocystic ovarian changes have been described in such cases.[367] Rarely a chronic ovarian abscess may result in a solid tumor-like mass, variably designated *ovarian xanthogranuloma*[308] or *xanthogranulomatous oophoritis*.[347] Both of the reported examples of this lesion occurred in patients with recurrent PID. The involved ovary in each case was replaced by a well-circumscribed, solid, yellow, lobulated mass, 4 cm and 8 cm in diameter, respectively, that consisted of foamy histiocytes admixed with multinucleated giant cells, plasma cells, fibroblasts, neutrophils, and foci of necrosis (Fig. 16.6). No organisms were demonstrable with special stains. Several additional examples of pseudotumorous xanthogranulomatous inflammation with a more diffuse involvement of the adnexa have been described.[247,251,418]

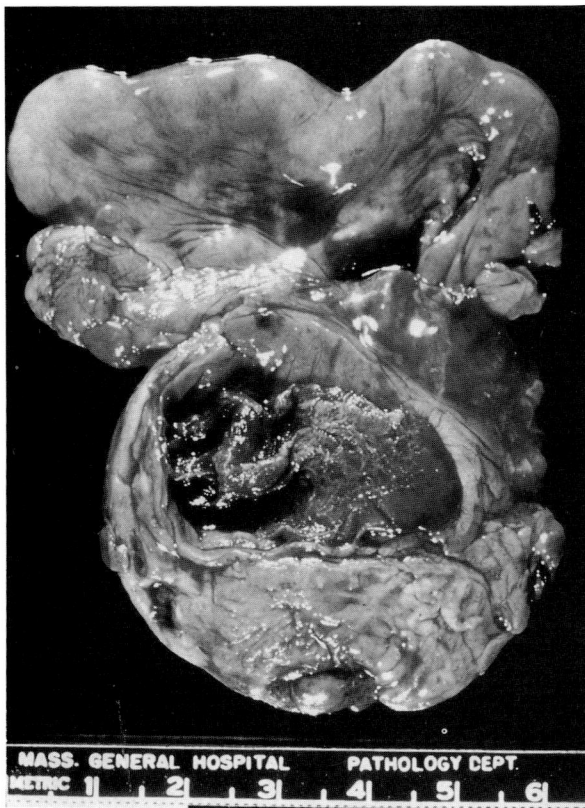

FIG. 16.5. **Ovarian abscess, sectioned surface**. Note the normal fallopian tube.

Actinomycosis

Pelvic actinomyces infection is uncommon and usually represents a complication of an IUD, although most cases of IUD-related PID probably are nonactinomycotic.* Almost 85% of cases have occurred in women who have had an IUD in place for 3 or more years,[404] and the infection may be more common in women using plastic, rather than copper, IUDs.[227] There is a high likelihood of subsequent sterility.[404]

The adnexal involvement usually is unilateral, with destructive, often multiple, abscesses involving the ovary (Fig. 16.7) and fallopian tube (see Chapter 14, Diseases of the Fallopian Tube). Rarely the characteristic actinomycotic (sulfur) granules may be grossly visible within the abscess cavities. Microscopic examination reveals a characteristic but nonspecific inflammatory response composed predominantly of neutrophils and foamy histiocytes that may be admixed with lesser numbers of lymphocytes and plasma cells. A specific diagnosis can be made only by finding the granules within the inflammatory exudate, but

*Refs. 46,227,253,272,294,402,404,405.

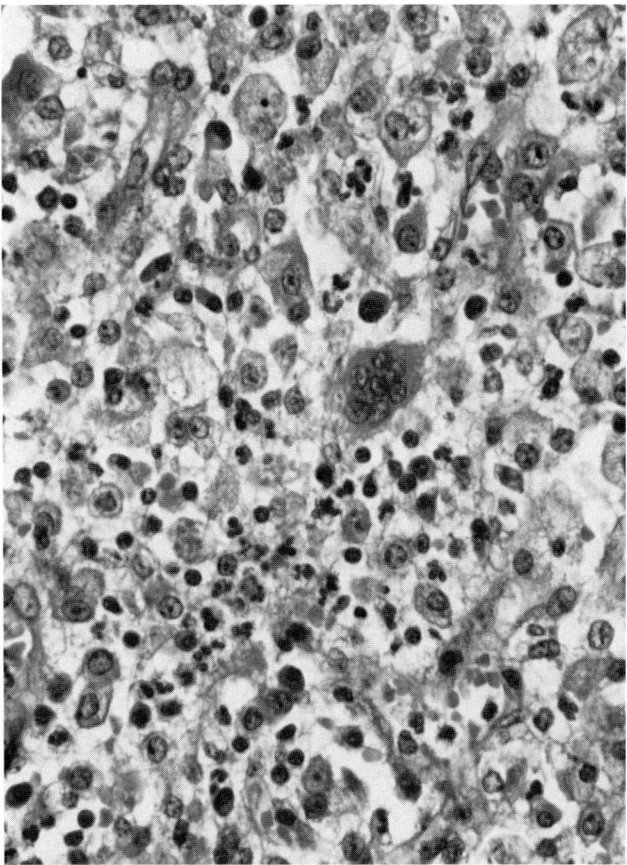

FIG. 16.6. **Xanthogranuloma of ovary**. Inflammatory reaction consists predominantly of foamy histiocytes, some of which are multinucleated. (Reprinted by permission of Pace et al., ref. 347.)

numerous blocks may be necessary to demonstrate their presence.[294] The granules are composed of circumscribed masses of basophilic, gram-positive, argyrophilic bacteria growing as branching filaments with a characteristic radial

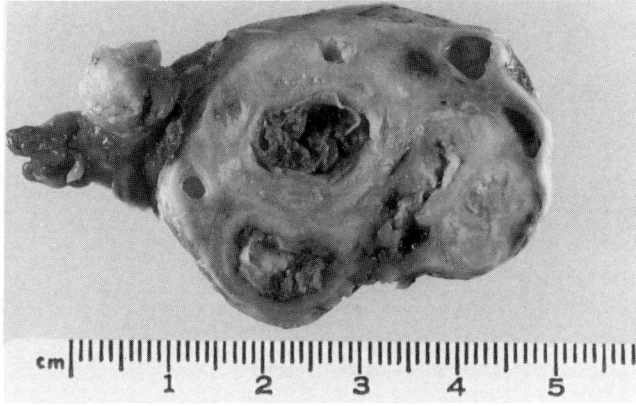

FIG. 16.7. **Actinomycosis of ovary**. The ovary is enlarged by many confluent abscesses. (Reprinted by permission of Schmidt et al., ref. 405.)

or palisading pattern at the periphery of the granule (Fig. 16.8). A fluorescent antibody stain may facilitate detection of the organisms.[358] A diagnosis of actinomycosis may be made before salpingo-oophorectomy in some cases by finding the granules within endometrial curettings and Papanicolaou cervicovaginal smears. In one study, almost 90% of patients with actinomyces demonstrated by the latter method were found to have a tuboovarian abscess.[71,227]

Tuberculosis

Tuberculous oophoritis is uncommon and usually secondary to extension from the more frequently involved fallopian tubes (see Chapter 14). Whereas the fallopian tubes are almost always involved in tuberculosis of the female genital tract, the ovarian parenchyma is involved in only 10% of cases.[338] On macroscopic inspection, the ovaries typically are surrounded by ampullary adhesions. Grossly visible caseous ovarian lesions are rare. On histological examination, ovarian parenchymal tuberculosis typically is confined to the cortex. In cases accompanied by ovarian

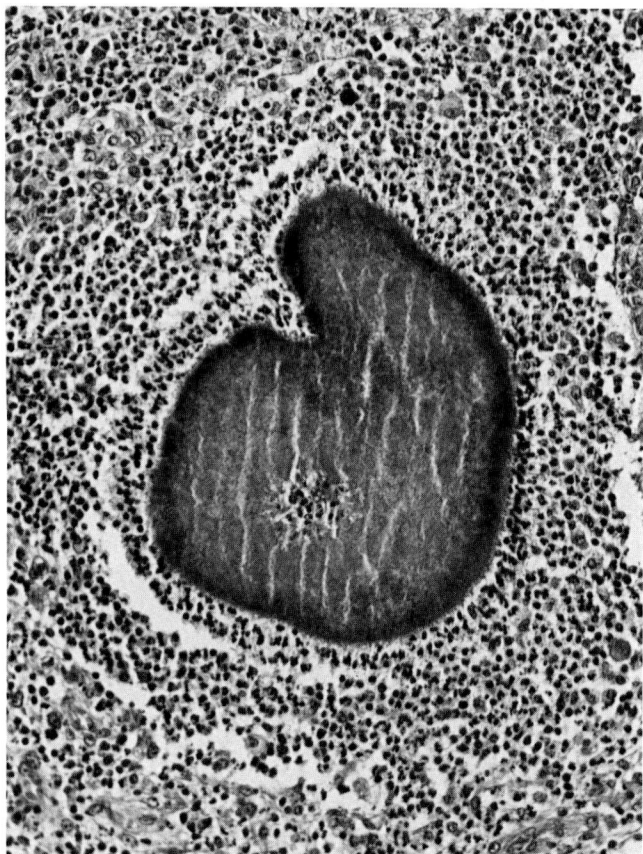

FIG. 16.8. Actinomycosis of ovary. A colony of actinomyces (sulfur granule) is surrounded by a purulent exudate. (Reprinted by permission of the Armed Forces Institute of Pathology, Neg. No. 74-13508.)

enlargement, granulomas involving the surrounding peritoneum may simulate metastatic ovarian cancer at the time of operation.[338,451]

Malacoplakia

Of approximately 25 reported cases of gynecological malacoplakia, only 3 examples have been described in the ovary.[5,81,237] Friable, yellow, focally hemorrhagic, and necrotic masses involved one or both ovaries and ipsilateral fallopian tube. In one case, the process also involved contiguous portions of small and large bowel, simulating a malignant ovarian tumor at operation.[237] Histological examination revealed the typical features of malacoplakia. Organisms including *Escherichia coli* and *Streptococcus faecalis* were demonstrated by culture in only one of the cases.[237]

Leprosy

Although leprosy rarely involves the female genital tract, the ovary is the most commonly involved gynecologic site.[59] In one well-documented case, microscopic examination of the grossly normal ovaries revealed many vacuolated histiocytes within the ovarian stroma. *Mycobacterium leprae* were demonstrated in these cells with an acid-fast stain. In chronic forms of leprous oophoritis, a chronic inflammatory cell infiltrate and fibrosis are seen, and bacilli usually are demonstrable.

Syphilis

For unknown reasons, syphilitic involvement of the ovary is very rare. Luetic oophoritis has been described in congenital, secondary, and tertiary forms of the disease. The pathology of these various stags is similar to that in extraovarian sites.[270]

Parasitic Infections

Parasitic infestations of the ovary are extremely rare in most parts of the world. Ovarian schistosomiasis, however, is relatively common in endemic areas, and the fallopian tube usually is involved simultaneously.[17,22,277,461] The patients typically have lower abdominal pain, a pelvic mass, and, occasionally, irregular menses and infertility. The typical operative findings are an enlarged tube and ovary, numerous adhesions, and scattered peritoneal nodules, potentially simulating a malignant tumor. On histological examination, a granulomatous inflammatory response, often containing eosinophils, surrounds the schistosoma eggs. Dense fibrosis frequently is seen in the later stages of the disease.

Ovarian involvement by *Enterobius vermicularis* usually is an incidental operative finding on the ovarian surface or, rarely, deeper within the ovary.[37,148,233,255,296,427] In several cases, there has been simultaneous involvement of the pelvic peritoneum, simulating a metastatic tumor.[148] The granulomas, which may include eosinophils and foci of caseous necrosis, surround the adult female worms and ova.[296,427] The worms probably reach the peritoneal cavity by migration from the perineum through the lumen of the uterus and fallopian tubes.

Rare cases of ovarian echinococcosis have been described.[20,182] In one of them, a 12-cm diameter, typical hydatid cyst involved the ovary.

Viral Infections

Oophoritis secondary to cytomegalovirus (CMV) has been described as an incidental finding at autopsy in five immunosuppressed patients.[133,450,488] In at least four of them, the ovarian involvement was part of a generalized infection. On macroscopic examination, the ovaries were of normal size but contained foci of superficial cortical hemorrhagic necrosis 1 to 2 mm in diameter[450]; in one case, there were white papillary projections from the cortical surface.[488] Microscopic examination revealed foci of coagulative necrosis, with variable numbers of neutrophils, nuclear debris, and hemorrhage. In the surrounding stroma, lymphocytes, plasma cells, and vascular dilatation were present. Ovarian stromal and endothelial cells, even at a distance from the necrotic foci, contained typical intranuclear and occasional intracytoplasmic inclusion bodies (Fig. 16.9). Immunohistochemical staining for CMV may facilitate the diagnosis in some cases,[488] and intranuclear and intracytoplasmic herpes-type viral particles have been found on ultrastructural examination. An additional example of cytomegaloviral oophoritis has been described in which the infection appeared confined to an ovarian thecoma.[263]

Mumps oophoritis as a clinical entity occurs much less commonly than mumps orchitis, with clinical evidence of the lesion in 5% of females with mumps. The pathology of the acute stage has not been well described.[14] It is postulated that germ cell depletion secondary to mumps oophoritis may result in premature menopause and possibly an increased risk of ovarian cancer.[9,109,314]

In view of the frequency of human papilloma virus (HPV) infection in the lower female genital tract, it is perhaps surprising that histologically documented examples of HPV infection of the ovary have not been described. Lai et al., however, recently have found HPV-16 or HPV-18 DNA sequences by the polymerase chain reaction (PCR) in 5 of 10 histologically normal ovaries.[252]

Fungal Infections

Fungal infections of the ovary are extremely rare, even in patients with disseminated mycoses. Three examples of

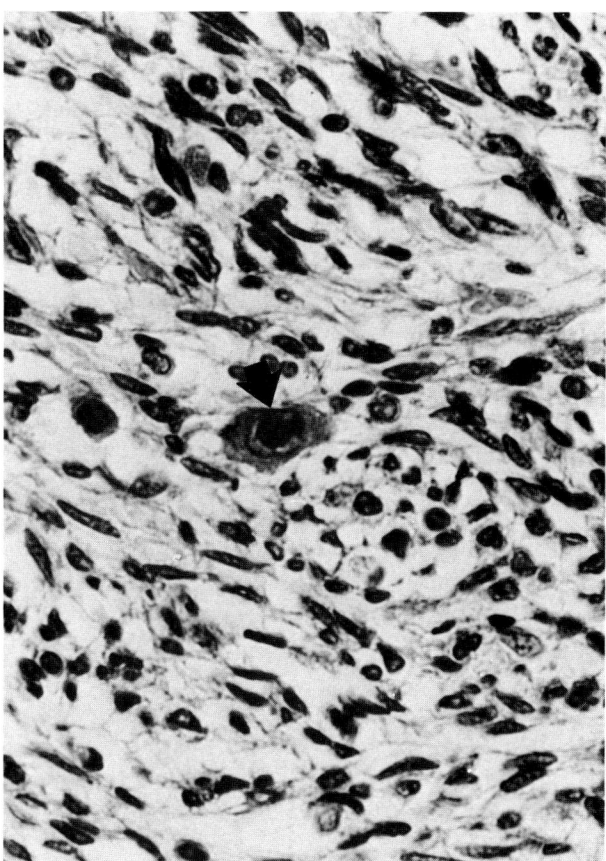

FIG. 16.9. **Cytomegalovirus infection of ovary.** Ovarian stromal cell contains an intranuclear inclusion (*arrow*). (Reprinted by permission of Subietas et al., ref. 450.)

tuboovarian abscess, as part of PID caused by *Blastomyces dermatitidis*, have been reported.[136,181,321] In one case the tuboovarian abscesses were bilateral and associated with miliary nodules involving the pelvic peritoneum.[181] Two of the cases probably were secondary to hematogenous spread from the lungs, whereas the third was sexually transmitted.

Of 11 patients with coccidioidomycosis of the upper female genital tract, 7 had tuboovarian and peritoneal involvement; 2 of the 7 had concomitant coccidioidal endometritis.[75] One case of adnexal involvement by *Aspergillus* has been reported in an IUD user.[242] Rupture of the tuboovarian abscess led to generalized peritonitis.

Noninfectious Inflammatory Disorders

A variety of noninfectious, typically granulomatous, inflammatory disorders may involve the ovary. In addition, granulomas may be seen rarely in autoimmune oophoritis (see page 629).

Foreign-body Granulomas

A variety of foreign materials may evoke a granulomatous reaction on the ovarian and peritoneal surfaces, potentially mimicking a malignant tumor at operation. Examples include a lipogranulomatous reaction to hysterosalpingographic contrast material,[458] as well as a foreign body reaction to crystalline material such as talc[316] or keratin (Fig. 16.10) from cystic tetratomas and the squamous elements of endometrial and ovarian endometrioid adenocarcinomas (peritoneal and ovarian keratin granulomas are discussed in more detail in Chapter 17, Diseases of the Peritoneum). A foreign-body reaction also occurs in response to starch granules from surgical gloves,[336,349] starch-containing douche fluid,[193] or lubricants.[400] Rarely, the starch granlomas are of the tuberculoid type, with or without caseous necrosis, rather than of foreign-body type, potentially mimicking tuberculosis on microscopic examination.[336] Finally granulomatous oophoritis has been en-countered rarely in response to bowel contents secondary to a coloovarian fistula.[40,165,287]

Isolated Palisading Granulomas

Isolated palisading granulomas of uncertain pathogenesis have been encountered in the ovary, typically as an incidental microscopic finding.[8,189,232,492] Of eight such cases, five patients had had an operative procedure performed on the same ovary 6 months to 12 years earlier. The granulomas typically are multiple and occasionally bilateral. Central zones of fibrinoid necrosis or hyalinization usually are surrounded by palisading, sometimes multinucleated, histiocytes and variable numbers of other inflammatory cells including lymphocytes, plasma cells, and eosinophils, and in some, a fibrous pseudocapsule (Fig. 16.11). The differential diagnosis of these granulomas includes the other ovarian granulomas discussed in this chapter, as well as

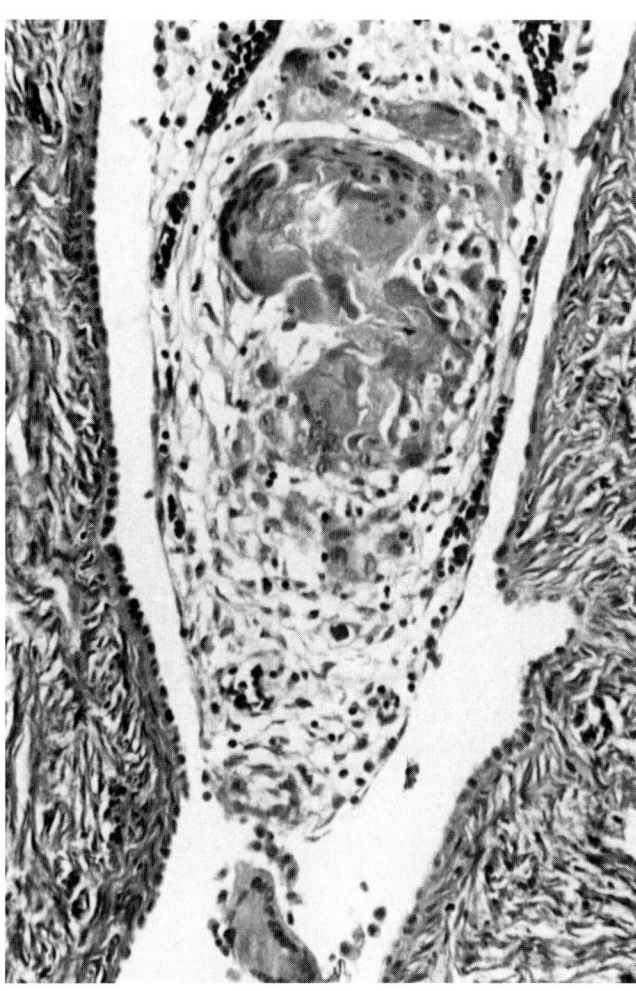

FIG. 16.10. **Foreign body reaction to keratin implants on ovarian serosal surface**. There was a coexistent endometrial adenoacanthoma confined to the uterus.

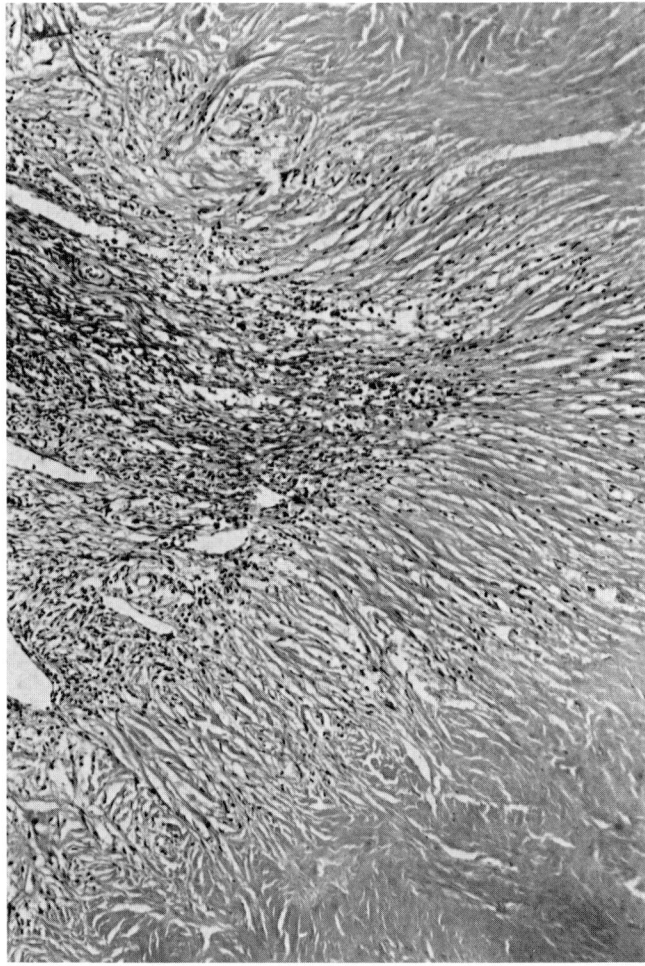

FIG. 16.11. **Isolated palisading granuloma of ovary**. (Reprinted by permission of Herbold et al., ref. 189.)

necrotic pseudoxanthomatous nodules of endometriosis (see Chapter 17).

Granulomas Secondary to Systemic Diseases

Four cases of ovarian involvement by sarcoidosis have been reported.[80,431,482,493] The sarcoid granulomas were an incidental histological finding in each case. The three patients reported in detail had systemic sarcoidosis, as well as involvement of other gynecological sites or para-aortic lymph nodes. Crohn's disease also may be a rare cause of granulomatous oophoritis, usually by direct extension of the inflammatory process from the bowel.[67,197,494] The ipsilateral fallopian tube also is usually involved.

Cortical Granulomas

Cortical granulomas are common, incidental, microscopic findings within the ovarian cortex. The granulomas are spherical, well-circumscribed, 100–500 μm in diameter, and are composed of spindle cells, epithelioid cells, lymphocytes, and in some, multinucleated giant cells; occasional anisotropic fat crystals also may be seen (Fig. 16.12A).[48,60,201,202,316,380,498] Hughesdon suggests that the granulomas become fibrotic with time, accounting for at least some of the spherical, cloud-like, hyaline scars commonly encountered in the cortical stroma of post-

menopausal women.[201,202] These scars resemble corpora fibrosa, but usually are distinguishable from the latter by their more superficial location within the cortex, greater cellularity, weaker eosinophilia, and the presence of a reticulin framework (Fig. 16.12B).[202] It also has been suggested that hyaline scars may represent foci of atropic endometrial stromatosis, luteinized stromal cells, or ectopic decidua.[201,202]

The frequency of cortical granulomas appears to be related to age. They are not usually encountered before the age of 30 years, but Hughesdon found active lesions in 40% of women over the age of 40 years; the number of lesions per cross-section of ovary increased in successive decades.[202] The clinical significance, if any, of cortical granulomas is unknown. Possible associations with ovarian stromal hyperplasia, endometrial carcinoma, or both have been suggested but not demonstrated consistently.[202,380,498]

Surface Proliferative Lesions

Surface Epithelial Inclusion Glands and Cysts

Surface epithelial inclusion (SEI) glands and their cystic counterparts, SEI cysts, arise from cortical invaginations of the ovarian surface epithelium that have lost their connec-

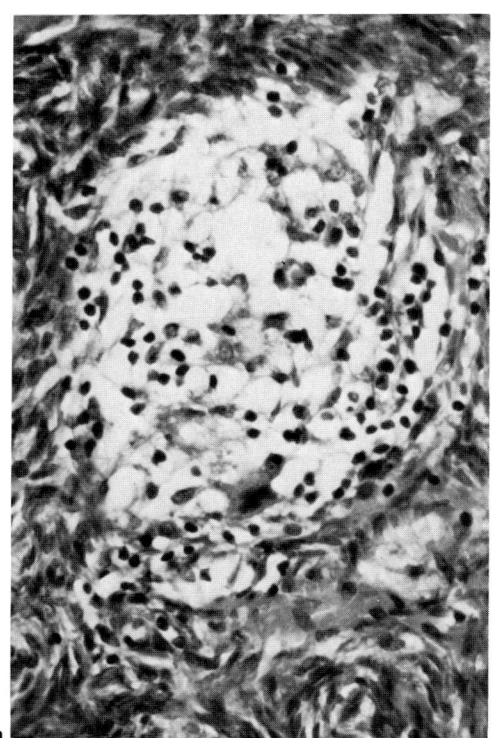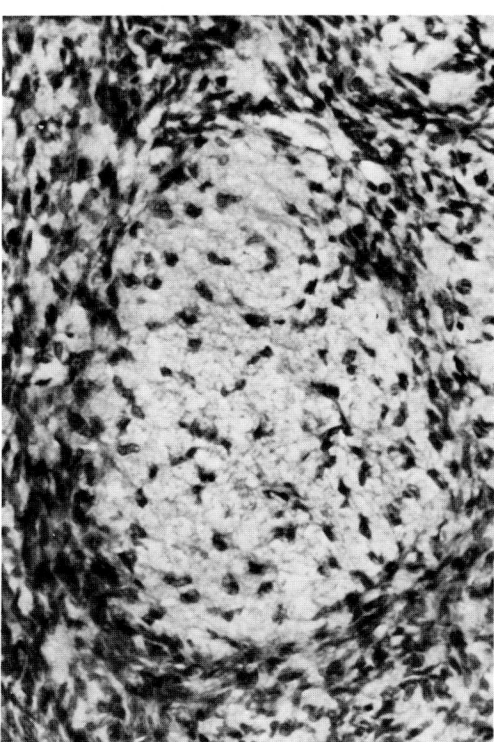

Fig. 16.12. a: **Cortical granuloma**. Circumscribed collection of lymphocytes, spindle cells, and occasional multinucleated giant cells lie within the ovarian stroma. b: **Hyaline scar**. The circumscribed nodule consists of collagen and spindle cells.

tion with the surface. Although most numerous in post-menopausal women, SEI glands and cysts can be found on thorough examination of ovaries from females of all ages, including fetuses, infants, and adolescents.[52,54]

SEI cysts, which may reach 1 cm in diameter, may be visible on gross inspection of the ovary, although most SEI glands and cysts are appreciable only on microscopic examination. They usually are multiple, scattered singly or in small clusters throughout the superficial cortex (Fig. 16.13); less commonly, they extend into the deeper cortical or medullary stroma. SEI glands and cysts typically are lined by a single layer of columnar epithelium. In post-menopasual patients, the epithelium is usually tubal, that is, endosalpingeal, in type. In such cases, psammoma bodies may be seen within the cysts, the adjacent stroma (Fig. 16.13), and rarely, within cervicovaginal Papanico-laou smears.[275] Less commonly, the lining of the glands and cysts consists of a single layer of endometrioid or endocervical columnar epithelium.[318,472] An Arias–Stella–like reaction has been described within SEI glands in pregnant patients.[54] Occasionally in adults, and typically in fetal and premenarcheal ovaries, the glands and cysts have a nonspecific, flat, cuboidal, or columnar lining. One study found that hyperplastic and metaplastic changes within SEI glands are more common in women with polycystic

ovary disease or endometrial carcinoma, suggesting a possible hormonal basis for these changes.[374]

SEI glands and cysts likely are the site of origin for most common epithelial tumors of the ovary.[410] A recent study found that patients with ovarian carcinoma had an increased number of SEI cysts in the contralateral ovary compared with controls.[308a] Additional support for this hypothesis is provided by the occasional presence of dysplastic changes within their linings[413] as well as immunoreactivity for a variety of ovarian epithelial tumor markers, including CA 125, CA 19-9, CEA, hCG, placental lactogen, α-2-glycoprotein, β-1-glycoprotein, placental alkaline phosphatase, and human milk fat globule protein.[53,85,99,218,340,341]

Mesothelial Proliferations

Proliferation of mesothelial cells on the ovarian surface, within periovarian fibrous adhesions or elsewhere on the pelvic peritoneum, usually is a response to pelvic inflammation (see Chapter 17, Diseases of the Peritoneum). Florid examples may be associated with complex glandular and papillary proliferations of mesothelial cells that may exhibit mild to moderate atypia (Fig. 16.14). Such a process may simulate a metastic carcinoma or primary serous surface carcinoma.

Surface Stromal Proliferations

Nodular and papillary stromal projections from the ovarian surface are a common incidental microscopic finding in women of late reproductive and postmenopausal age. These projections are composed of ovarian stroma exhibiting varying degrees of hyalinization covered by a single layer of surface epithelium (Fig. 16.15). Detachment of these structures may give rise to "collagen balls" occasionally found in peritoneal washings.[495]

Nonneoplastic Lesions of the Follicular and Stromal Elements

This section deals with the wide spectrum of nonneoplastic lesions that arise from the ovarian follicles and stroma. Many of them are secondary to ovarian stimulation by pituitary or chorionic gonadotropins and may be associated with excessive production of estrogens, androgens, or both. Although most nonneoplastic proliferations of Leydig cells are not of stromal origin, these lesions are discussed most conveniently in this section.

Solitary Cysts of Follicular Origin

Solitary (or occasionally a few) cysts of follicular origin should be distinguished from disorders characterized by multiple bilateral follicular cysts.

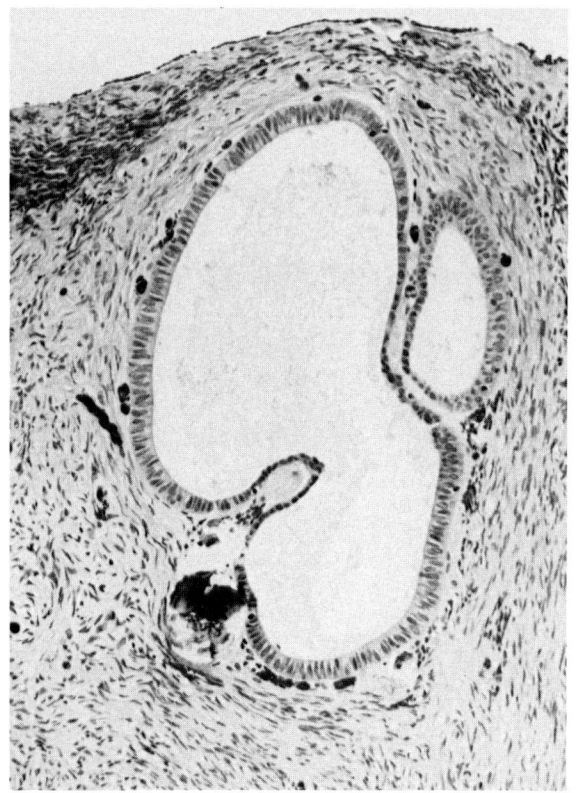

Fig. 16.13. Epithelial inclusion cyst. Cyst beneath ovarian surface epithelium is lined by a single layer of columnar cells. A psammoma body is present within the adjacent stroma.

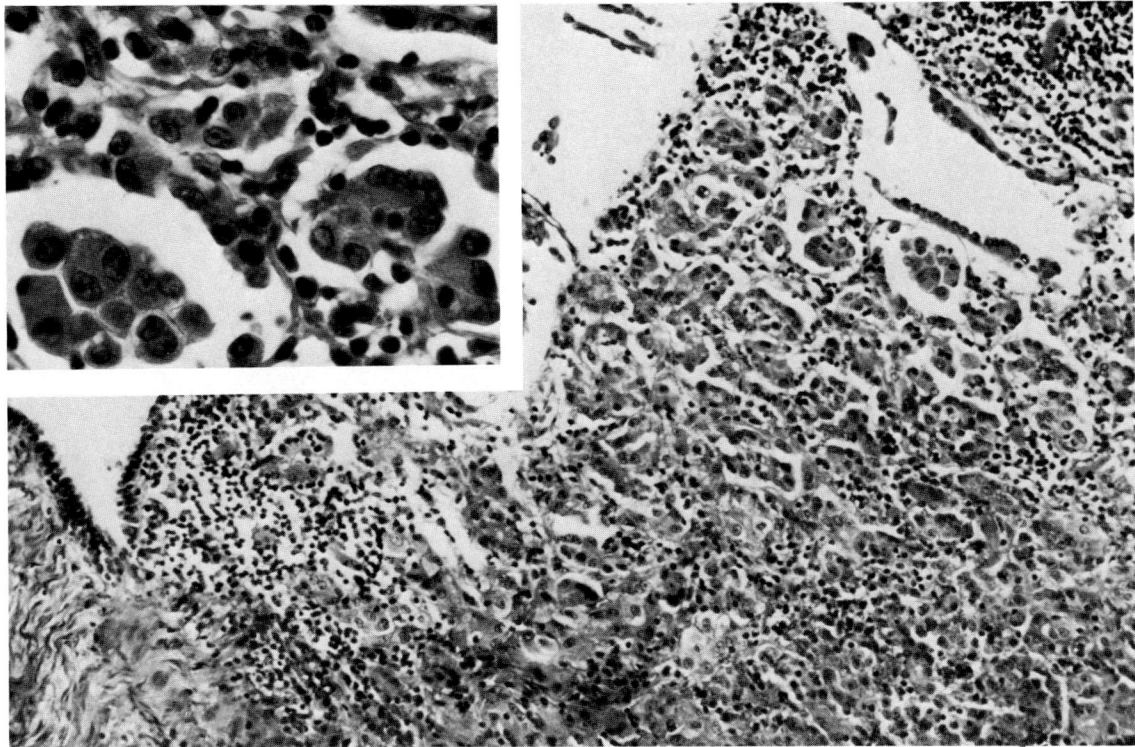

FIG. 16.14. Mesothelial proliferation on ovarian surface. Mesothelial cells, growing in papillary pattern, are admixed with lymphocytes. The mesothelial cells exhibit mild nuclear pleomorphism and multinucleation (*inset*).

Follicle and Corpus Luteum Cysts

CLINICAL FEATURES

Solitary follicular cysts (FCs) are common, occurring during fetal life,[254,300] in newborns,[62,69] throughout childhood,[3] in the reproductive era,[359] and rarely after the onset of the menopause.[447,449] Postpubertal patients with cystic fibrosis may be predisposed to the development of solitary FCs.[419] Corpus luteum cysts (CLCs) occur during the reproductive era but rarely follow sporadic ovulation in a postmenopausal woman.[410]

The proportion of FCs and CLCs associated with clinical manifestations is unknown because many are discovered incidentally by pelvic ultrasonography, laparoscopy, or laparotomy. Patients with clinically evident FCs and CLCs typically have either a palpable adnexal mass or manifestations related to increased estrogen production, such as sexual precocity or pseudoprecocity,° menstrual disturbances,[359] or endometrial hyperplasia.[447] As noted earlier, a CLC is the most common finding in the ovarian remnant syndrome. An uncommon clinical presentation of FCs and CLCs is rupture with hemoperitoneum,[147,180] a

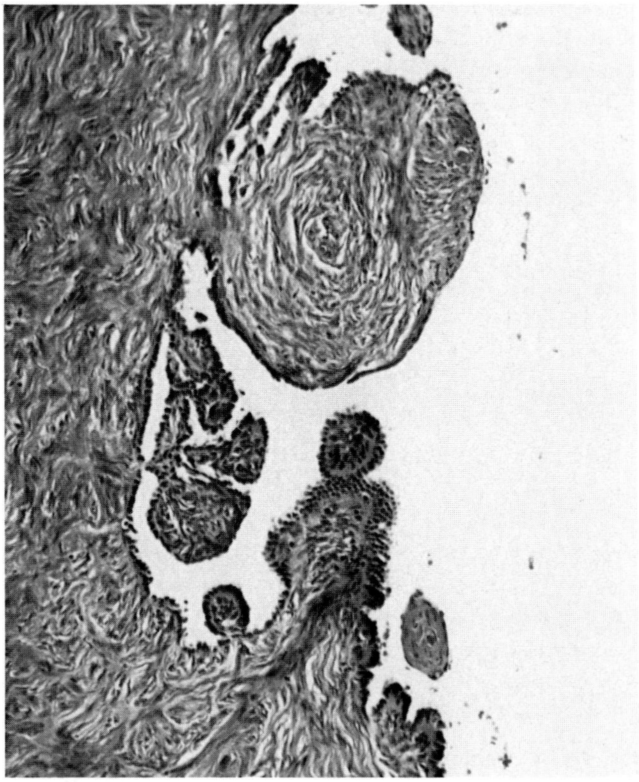

°Refs. 95,113,241,281,311,317,363,449,485.

FIG. 16.15. Ovarian surface stromal proliferation. Papillary and nodular stromal proliferation involves ovarian surface.

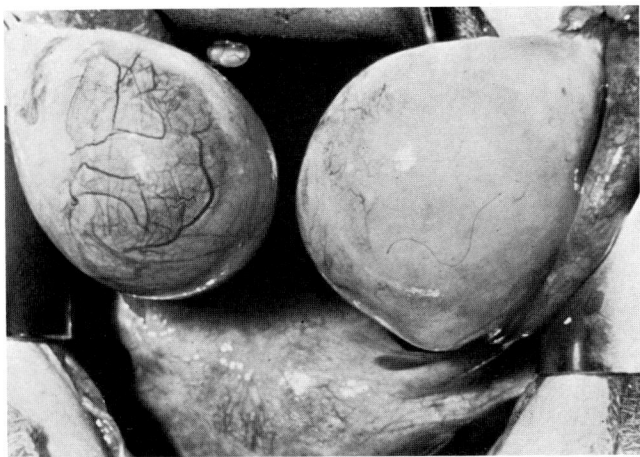

FIG. 16.16. Solitary follicle cyst within each ovary. (Reprinted by permission of The New England Journal of Medicine, 292; 199–203, 1975)

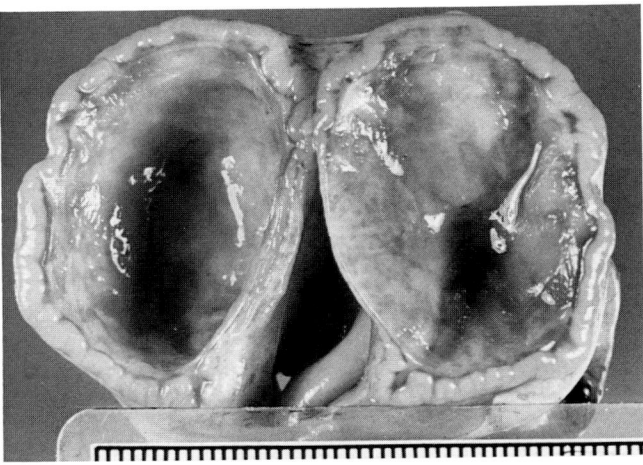

FIG. 16.17. Corpus luteum cyst. Note the convoluted lining, which was yellow.

complication more likely to occur in patients receiving anticoagulant therapy[257,355,356,416] or with bleeding diatheses.[406,478]

GROSS FINDINGS

Solitary FCs and CLCs are thin-walled and unilocular, ranging from 3 to 8 cm in diameter, although larger examples occur rarely (Fig. 16.16).[3,55,62,69] CLCs usually are distinguishable by the presence of a convoluted yellow lining (Fig. 16.17). Contents of FCs and CLCs vary from serous or serosanguinous fluid to clotted blood.

MICROSCOPIC FINDINGS

FCs are lined by an inner layer of granulosa cells and an outer layer of theca interna cells (Fig. 16.18). The cells in either layer may be luteinized. Distinction between the two layers can be facilitated by a reticulin stain, which reveals dense reticulum surrounding the theca cells but sparse or absent reticulum in the granulosa layer (Fig. 16.16). CLCs exhibit a convoluted lining composed of large luteinized granulosa cells and smaller luteinized theca interna cells, with a prominent innermost layer of connective tissue (Fig. 16.19). CLCs associated with pregnancy typically have characteristic hyaline bodies and cal-

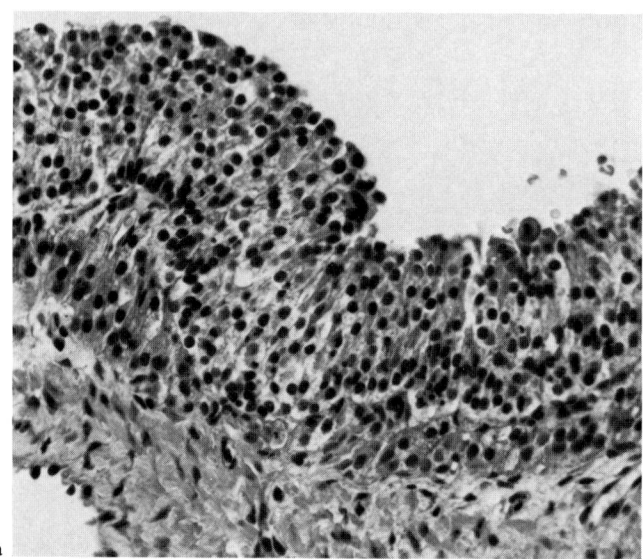

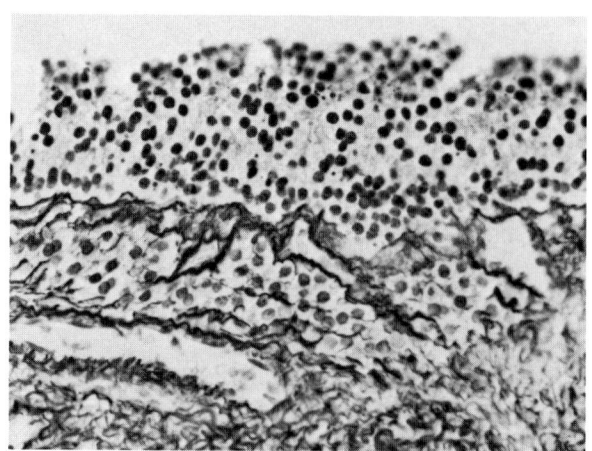

FIG. 16.18. Follicle cyst. a: Lining consists of an inner layer of granulosa cells and an outer layer of theca interna cells. **b:** Distinction between the two layers is enhanced with reticulin stain, showing reticulum network within the theca interna layer and an absence of reticulin within the granulosa layer. (Reprinted by permission of Clement (1985) In: Contemporary Issues in Surgical Pathology, Vol 6. Roth, Czernobilsky (eds). New York, Churchill Livingstone.)

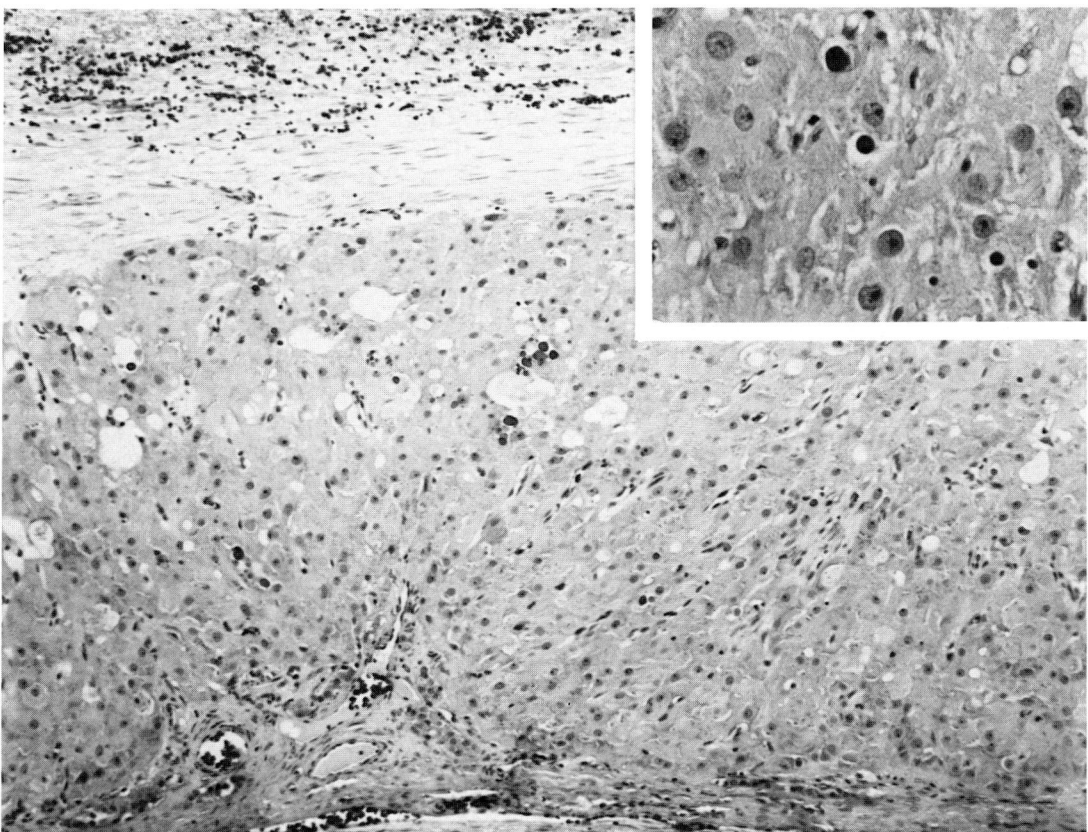

Fig. 16.19. Corpus luteum cyst of pregnancy. The cyst has an inner lining of connective tissue and an outer layer of large luteinized granulosa cells, some of which contain hyaline bodies (*inset*).

cific foci within the granulosa cells (Fig. 16.19, *inset*). Focal infarction of a CLC, possibly secondary to inadequate human chorionic gonadotropin (hCG) production, has been encountered in association with tubal pregnancy.[464] Involutional fibrosis of FCs and CLCs usually leads to the formation of corpora fibrosa and corpora albicantia, respectively; rarely, the latter may be cystic.

Pathogenesis

The pathogenesis of most FCs probably is related to abnormalities in the release of anterior pituitary gonadotropins. These cysts may be multiple, recurrent, and accompanied by corpora lutea, and therefore the possibility of pregnancy.[284,317] Other FCs appear to be autonomous and do not recur after removal.[363] Girls with McCune–Albright syndrome and precocious puberty secondary to an FC may have elevated levels of gonadotropins, whereas in others it appears to be mediated by a gonadotropin-independent mechanism.[95,114,284,486] FCs and CLCs also may occur secondary to treatment with low-dose phasic oral contraceptives[77] and gonadotropin-releasing hormone (GnRH) analogues.[41]

Clinical Behavior and Treatment

Most cases of FC and CLC regress spontaneously within 2 months. Thus, observation of small (<6 cm) ovarian cysts in women of reproductive age is justifiable for this period. The regression in some cases can be accelerated by administration of a high-dose, combined estrogen–progestogen preparation.[433] Persistence of a cyst suggests that it is neoplastic, and in these cases laparotomy or laparoscopy is necessary.

Large Solitary Luteinized Follicle Cyst of Pregnancy and Puerperium

A rare type of solitary FC with distinctive clinical and pathological features occurs during pregnancy and the puerperium, and presumably is related to hCG stimulation.[91,184,243] Patients present with a palpable adnexal mass or are found to have a unilateral ovarian cyst at cesarean section. None have exhibited clinical evidence of an endocrine disturbance. On gross inspection, the cyst resembles a typical FC except for its large size (median diameter 25 cm). On microscopic examination, one to many layers of luteinized cells with clear to eosinophilic cytoplasm line

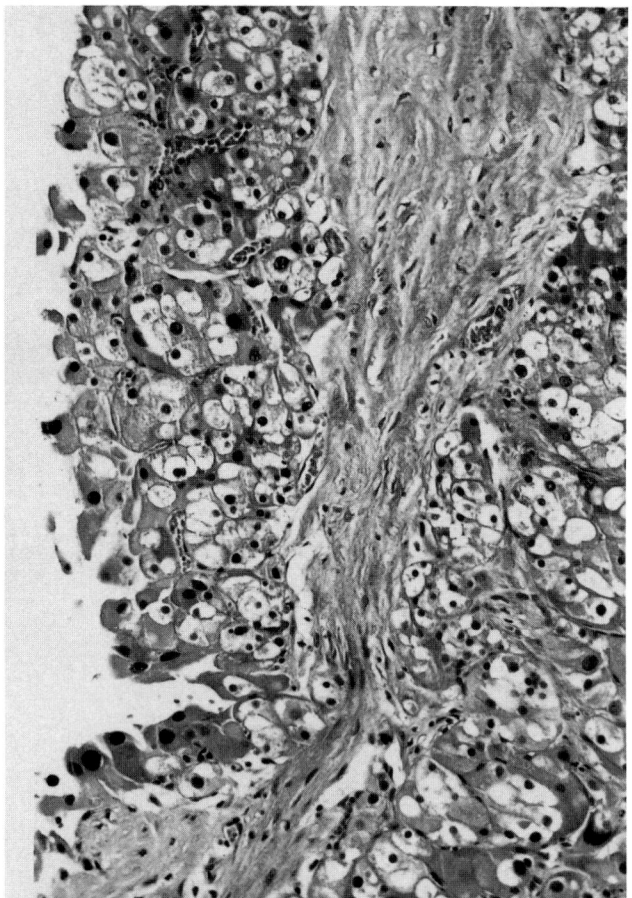

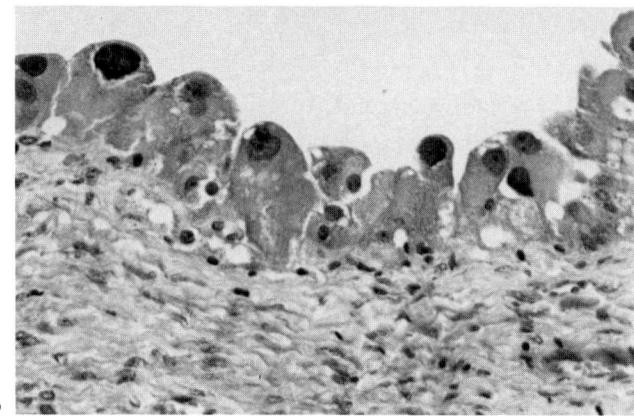

FIG. 16.20. Large solitary luteinized follicle cyst of pregnancy and puerperium. a: Luteinized cells with abundant (eosinophilic) to clear cytoplasm line cyst (*left*) and lie within its fibrous wall (*right*). Note focal nuclear atypicality. **b:** Higher power view of lining cells showing marked nuclear hyperchromasia and atypicality. (Fig. 20a reprinted with permission from Clement et al (1989) Nontrophoblastic pathology of the female genital tract and peritoneum associated with pregnancy. Semin Diagn Pathol 6: 372–406.)

the cyst. There is no separation into granulosa and theca layers, and similar cells may be found within the connective tissue wall of the cyst (Fig. 16.20a). The luteinized

cells typically exhibit focal marked nuclear pleomorphism and hyperchromatism (Fig. 16.20). Other cytological features of malignancy are absent, and the atypical changes most likely are degenerative in nature.

DIFFERENTIAL DIAGNOSIS OF SOLITARY FOLLICLE CYSTS

Solitary cysts of follicular origin should be distinguished from other solitary, unilocular ovarian cysts. Cysts otherwise identical to FCs and CLCs but less than 2.5 cm in diameter generally are regarded as physiological, that is, cystic follicles and cystic corpora lutea, respectively. Simple cysts have an absent lining or one composed of a layer of nonspecific cuboidal or flattened cells. Most probably are of follicular or surface epithelial origin.

Cysts of surface epithelial origin that usually are small, incidental microscopic findings are designated inclusion cysts (see page 605). Otherwise similar cysts measuring more than 1 cm are considered neoplastic and designated serous, endometrioid, or mucinous cystadenoma depending on the nature of their lining (see Chapter 18, Surface Epithelial–Stromal Tumors of the Ovary). Epidermoid cysts are those lined exclusively by mature squamous epithelium, and are considered either monodermal teratomas or of surface epithelial origin.[337,501] The finding of Walthard nests in the walls of some of these cysts favor the latter origin in at least some cases.[501] Endometriotic cysts are readily distinguishable by their characteristic lining of endometrial epithelium and stroma and pigmented histiocytes within their walls (see Chapter 17, Diseases of the Peritoneum).

Solitary FCs also should be distinguished from those of rete origin, which are located within the hilus.[392] In one series, the cysts had a mean diameter of 8.7 cm (range, 1–24 cm); most were unilocular, although several multilocular cysts also were encountered.[392] Rete cysts typically are lined by a single layer of nonciliated epithelium that varies from flat to cuboidal to columnar. Aside from their hilar location, clues to the origin of the cysts are an irregular contour of their inner surface with small crevice-like outpouchings and a fibromuscular wall that often contains hyperplastic hilus cells.

Differentiating large FCs from unilocular cystic granulosa cell tumors may be difficult (see Chapter 19, Sex Cord–Stromal, Steroid Cell, and Other Ovarian Tumors with Endocrine, Paraendocrine, and Paraneoplastic Manifestations). The latter usually are considerably larger and are lined by several layers of granulosa cells that form Call–Exner bodies; luteinization of the granulosa cells is unusual.

Multiple Cysts of Follicular Origin

This section considers disorders characterized by the presence of multiple cysts of follicular origin excluding polycystic ovary disease (see page 613).

HYPERREACTIO LUTEINALIS

Hyperreactio luteinalis (HL) is characterized by ovarian enlargement due to the presence of multiple luteinized follicle cysts secondary to hCG stimulation.[79,167,188,312,397,473,483]

CLINICAL FEATURES

HL occurs most commonly with disorders resulting in high levels of hCG, such as hydatidiform moles, choriocarcinoma, and fetal hydrops, usually secondary to Rh sensitization but rarely of nonimmunologic type,[186] and multiple gestations.[79,167] Sixty percent of cases unassociated with gestational trophoblastic disease (GTD), however, have accompanied a singleton pregnancy.[473] The frequency of HL in women with GTD ranges from 10% to 50%, depending on whether it is detected by clinical examination or sonography.[398] The presence of HL in these patients may indicate an increased risk for persistent or metastatic GTD (see Chapter 26, Immunohistochemistry).[111,238,312,315] Rarely, HL has been preceded by polycystic ovary syndrome.[42]

HL can be detected as a pelvic mass during any trimester, at cesarean section, or, rarely, immediately postpartum[79] or later in the puerperium.[32] Symptoms usually are absent, but hemorrhage into the cysts may cause abdominal pain. Rarely, the involved ovary undergoes torsion or rupture, sometimes with intraabdominal bleeding, which may be fatal. In contrast to patients with the ovarian hyperstimulation syndrome (see below), ascites is rare.[473] In patients with HL accompanying GTD, cystic ovarian enlargement is detected at the time of the diagnostic curettage or during the postoperative follow-up period.[315,360] In approximately 15% of cases unassociated with trophoblastic disease, there has been virilization of the patient but not the female infant.[42,188,216] Elevated plasma testosterone levels have been found in these patients as well as nonvirilized patients with trophoblastic disorders, with the levels proportional to the degree of ovarian enlargement.[397]

PATHOLOGIC FINDINGS

On macroscopic examination, multiple, usually bilateral, thin-walled cysts cause moderate to massive ovarian enlargement (up to 26 cm) (Fig. 16.21). The cysts are filled with clear or hemorrhagic fluid. Microscopic examination reveals FCs with prominent luteinization of the theca interna cells and, in some cases, the granulosa cells (Fig. 16.22). There usually is marked edema of the theca layer and the intervening stroma; the latter frequently contains luteinized stromal cells.

PATHOGENESIS

Because HL occasionally occurs in patients with otherwise normal pregnancies and normal hCG levels, and because HL does not occur in all women with high hCG levels,

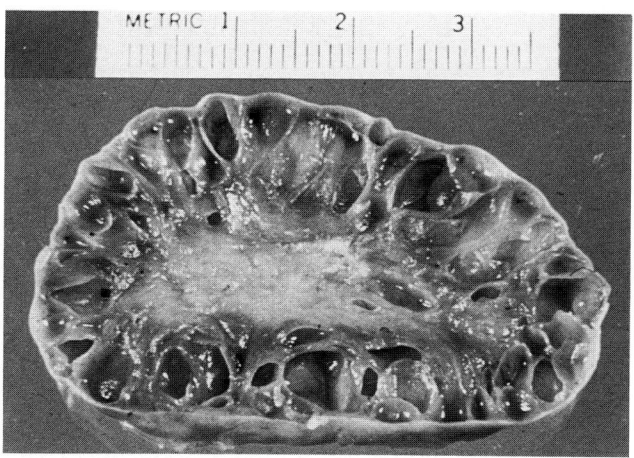

FIG. 16.21. **Hyperreactio luteinalis.** Multiple thin-walled follicle cysts are present within the cortex. (Courtesy of Dr. R.E. Scully. Reprinted by permission of Clement (1985) In: Contemporary Issues in Surgical Pathology, Vol 6. Roth, Czernobilsky (eds). New York, Churchill Livingstone.)

factors other than the latter likely play a role in the pathogenesis of HL. An increased ovarian sensitivity to hCG in patients with the disorder has been suggested.[64] One study found elevated levels of other hormones, specifically progesterone, prolactin, and estradiol, in patients with HL and GTD, possibly implicating these hormones in the pathogenesis or maintenance of HL.[346]

CLINICAL BEHAVIOR AND TREATMENT

The cysts of HL typically involute during the puerperium, but occasionally regression is not complete until 6 months postpartum.[274] Exceptional cases regress spontaneously during pregnancy.[259] In cases associated with trophoblastic disease, gradual regression typically occurs 2–12 weeks after uterine evacuation,[315] but occasionally the cysts persist for months or continue to enlarge even after the hCG level has returned to normal.[312,360] Operative treatment of HL is needed only to remove infarcted tissue, control hemorrhage, or reduce ovarian size in order to diminish androgen production in virilized patients.[79] Rarely, HL recurs in subsequent pregnancies.[129,420]

Ovarian Hyperstimulation Syndrome

An iatrogenic form of HL, the ovarian hyperstimulation syndrome (OHS) occurs in a variable proportion of women undergoing ovulation induction, typically after the administration of FSH followed by hCG, or rarely clomiphene alone.[89,183,293,401,463,483] The frequency of OHS has varied widely in the literature, although it has been suggested that some degree of the syndrome exists in all patients undergoing ovulation induction.[172] Mild OHS has been documented ultrasonographically in as many as 65% of such

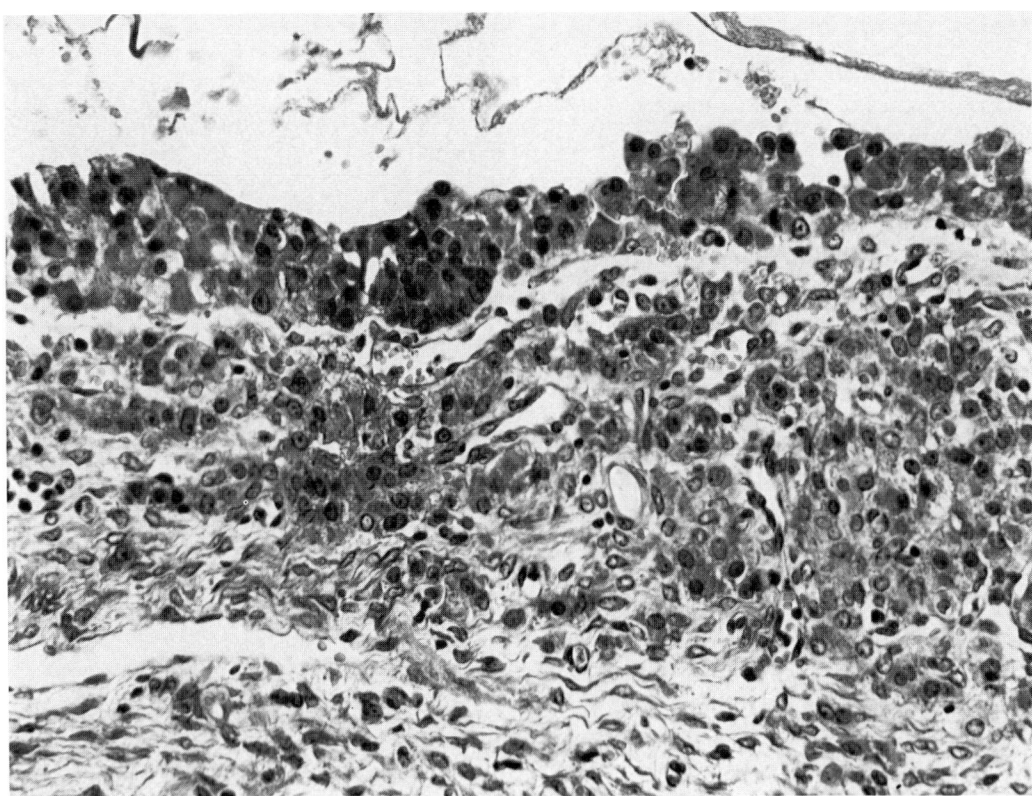

FIG. 16.22. **Hyperreactio luteinalis.** The cyst lining consists of granulosa and theca layers, both of which exhibit marked luteinization. (Reprinted by permission of Clement (1985) In: Contem- porary Issues in Surgical Pathology, Vol 6. Roth, Czernobilsky (eds). New York, Churchill Livingstone.)

women.[293] OHS occurs only after ovulation, is more severe in patients who conceive, and is particularly prone to occur if the ovaries were polycystic before the institution of therapy. Several cases of spontaneous OHS unassociated with ovulation induction have been reported.[382,387,505] Two such patients, one with antecedent polycystic ovary disease, had otherwise normal pregnancies[382,505]; one non-pregnant patient with spontaneous OHS had severe hypothyroidism.[387]

In severe cases, the ovaries become massively enlarged, and ascites, sometimes with hydrothorax, so-called acute Meigs' syndrome, develops because of increased serosal permeability. Elevation of serum estrogens, progesterone, and testosterone typically occurs.[183,401,408] Hemoconcentration with secondary oliguria and thromboembolic phenomena is a life-threatening complication. Elevated serum levels of renin, aldosterone, and antidiuretic hormone may occur in such patients.[183] There usually is a response to conservative therapy, and operative intervention is necessary only in the rare instance of cyst torsion or rupture. The cysts usually regress within 6 weeks. Pathological examination of the ovaries reveals changes identical to those seen in HL, with the additional finding of one or more corpora lutea. Careful selection of patients and regulation of drug dosage by monitoring estrogen levels and ovarian size have reduced the frequency of OHS. The frequency of OHS in women with multiple ovulations undergoing in vitro fertilization is not abnormally high, despite estrogen levels that exceed the "safe" range. Aspiration of the multiple follicles may help prevent the development of the syndrome in some of these cases.[153,172]

Juvenile Hypothyroidism

Depending on the method of detection, as many as 75% of girls with juvenile hypothyroidism have multicystic ovaries.[34,135,262,378,424,467,499] Rarely, the ovarian enlargement may be the presenting sign leading to a diagnosis of hypothyroidism.[262,378] The clinical features, in addition to the ovarian enlargement and manifestations of hypothyroidism, include varying degrees of sexual precocity in more than half the patients, and galactorrhea. The sexual precocity and galactorrhea appear to be due to increased secretion of pituitary gonadotropins and prolactin, respectively.[34,262] Pathological examination, which has been performed in only a few cases, has revealed FCs, some with luteinization of the theca interna layer.[424,467,499] In two cases, a depletion of primordial follicles also was noted. Treatment with thyroxin has resulted in regression of the hypothyroidism, the ovarian cysts, and sexual precocity, and a decline in the elevated gonadotropin and prolactin levels.

Prematurity

Multiple, bilateral FCs associated with estradiol production have been described in infants born before the 30th week of gestation.[414] The cysts, which are secondary to elevated levels of FSH and LH, appear at a postconception age that slightly precedes the expected time of delivery. It is postulated that marked prematurity is associated with relative insensitivity of the hypothalamus and anterior pituitary to negative feedback by estradiol.[414]

17-Hydroxylase Deficiency

Congenital deficiency of 17-hydroxylase, an enzyme required for both cortisol and estrogen synthesis, results in low estrogen levels and secondarily elevated levels of FSH and LH. The rare patients with this disorder have congenital adrenal hyperplasia, hypokalemia, hypertension, primary amenorrhea, absence of sexual maturation, and ovarian enlargement due to multiple, bilateral FCs.[278]

Polycystic Ovary Disease

Polycystic ovary disease (PCO) is characterized by inappropriate gonadotropin secretion, hyperandrogenemia, increased peripheral conversion of androgens to estrogens, chronic anovulation, and sclerocystic ovaries. The current clinical spectrum of PCO is broader than that initially defined by Stein and Leventhal in 1935, and as will be discussed, PCO is likely a result of a variety of disorders that lead to abnormal gonadotropin secretion and the other changes noted above. Stromal hyperthecosis (see page 615) is a closely related disorder that overlaps both clinically and pathologically with PCO.

Clinical Features

PCO has been estimated to involve 3.5–7.0% of the female population.[156] The affected patients typically are in their third decade with a history of premenarcheal obesity, secondary amenorrhea or oligomenorrhea, infertility, and hirsutism.[49,156,173,500] These features may occur alone or in any combination. Frank virilization, that is, clitoromegaly, deep voice, temporal baldness, male habitus, is rare, and if of sudden onset, suggests stromal hyperthecosis or a virilizing ovarian tumor. The ovaries in PCO may or may not be palpably enlarged. Pelvic ultrasonography may be useful in establishing the diagnosis.

PCO can be familial and may be the most common endocrinopathy causing familial hirsutism.[156] A genetic basis for the disease therefore may exist in some patients, although its frequency is unknown.[156] In one study of fa-

milial PCO, approximately one-half of the sisters of patients with PCO were similarly affected, consistent with an autosomal dominant mode of inheritance.[97] Other studies have suggested an X-linked transmission.[156]

Manifestations of unopposed estrogenic stimulation including menometrorrhagia, endometrial hyperplasia, and endometrial carcinoma occur in a significant proportion of patients. The tumors typically occur in obese patients under the age of 40 years. Conversely, up to one-quarter of patients with endometrial carcinoma under 40 years of age have PCO.[156] The tumors are almost always well-differentiated adenocarcinomas that do not invade the myometrium or invade the latter only superficially.[103,139,141,158,213,370] The carcinomas are rarely, if ever, fatal, and many are reversible with progesterone therapy or by ovulation induction. A wide variety of extrauterine tumors also have been described in patients with PCO, but their association probably is coincidental.[103]

Hyperprolactinemia is present in approximately 25% and galactorrhea in 13% of patients with PCO.[100,155,156] Some hyperprolactinemic patients have pituitary adenomas, and therefore tomographic scanning of the sella may be necessary.[155,156,432] Some patients with PCO have the HAIR-AN syndrome of hyperandrogenism (HA), insulin resistance (IR), and acanthosis nigricans (AN), a syndrome discussed in the section dealing with stromal hyperthecosis (see page 615).[70,83,124,142,164,422,457]

Gross Findings

Both ovaries or, rarely, only one,[156] are typically rounded and two to five times normal size; in one recent study, the ovarian volume in patients with PCO was three times that of control subjects.[273] Occasionally, however, the ovaries may be of normal size. Superficial cortical cysts usually are visible beneath the white ovarian surface. Examination of the sectioned ovarian surface reveals a thickened, white, superficial cortex and numerous subjacent cysts, typically less than 1 cm in diameter (Fig. 16.23). There usually is a central zone of stroma with few or no stigmata of ovulation (i.e., corpora lutea or albicantia).[49,156,174]

Microscopic Findings

The superficial cortex is fibrotic and hypocellular, resembling a capsule (Fig. 16.24), and may contain prominent thick-walled blood vessels.[173,174,203] Tongues of similarly fibrotic stroma may extend from the superficial cortex into the deeper cortex and medulla.[203] The cysts are atretic cystic follicles and have an inner lining of several layers of nonluteinized granulosa cells that may be focally exfoliated.[173] An outer layer of luteinized theca interna cells (Fig. 16.25) is sometimes referred to as "follicular hyperthecosis," but cystic follicles in women with PCO differ from those in normal women only in their increased num-

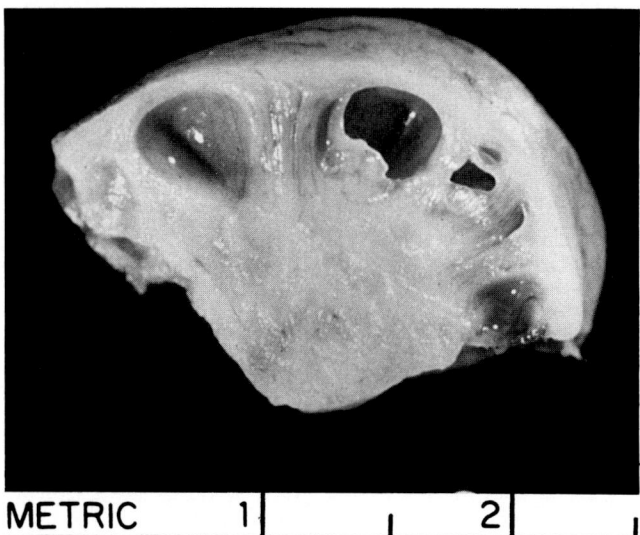

Fig. 16.23. Polycystic ovary disease. Superficial cortical fibrosis and multiple cystic follicles are present. (Courtesy of Dr. R.E. Scully. Reprinted by permission of Clement (1985) In: Contemporary Issues in Surgical Pathology, Vol 6. Roth, Czernobilsky (eds). New York, Churchill Livingstone.)

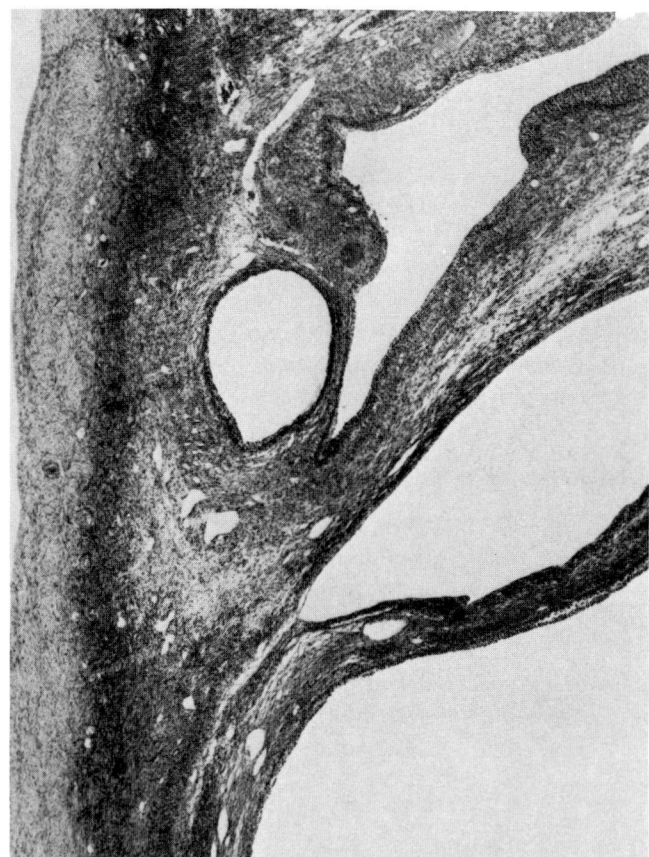

Fig. 16.24. Polycystic ovary disease. Multiple cystic follicles lie beneath the superficially fibrotic cortex. (Reprinted by permission of Clement (1985) In: Contemporary Issues in Surgical Pathology, Vol. 6. Roth, Czernobilsky (eds). New York, Churchill Livingstone.)

ber.[174,273] Maturing follicles up to mid-antral stage and atretic follicles exhibiting prominent luteinization of the theca interna may be twice as numerous as in normal ovaries.[156,173,203] Primordial follicles are normal in number and appearance.[173,203] As noted, stigmata of prior ovulation typically are absent, but corpora lutea have been described in as many as 30% of otherwise typical cases of PCO.[174,203] The deeper cortical and medullary stroma may have up to a five-fold increase in volume. The stroma may contain luteinized stromal cells and foci of smooth muscle.[203] Nests of ovarian hilus (Leydig) cells may be more numerous in patients with PCO than in age-matched controls.[203]

Pathophysiology

The pathophysiology of PCO is complex, and although the initiating factor(s) are not yet completely understood, the characteristic endocrine disturbances of PCO, once established, likely are self-perpetuating. A cardinal finding is a tonic elevation of the serum level of LH.[49,156,500] LH stimulates the follicular theca interna cells to produce androstenedione, which is converted peripherally, primarily within adipose tissue, to estrone (E_1),[50] and to a lesser extent, testosterone. The plasma levels of the latter usually are high normal or only slightly elevated in contrast to patients with stromal hyperthecosis (see below).[49,500] Estradiol (E_2) levels remain normal or low normal, resulting in an elevated E_1/E_2 ratio.[156] Elevated E_1 levels, and in some patients an increased secretion of inhibin-F, a nonsteroidal peptide produced by granulosa cells,[456] inhibit secretion of FSH. An elevated LH/FSH ratio thus is a characteristic finding in PCO. The increased circulating estrogens likely increase the secretion of luteinizing hormone releasing factor (LHRF) and enhance the sensitivity of pituitary LH-producing cells to LHRF.[49,500] Ovarian estrogen production in PCO is markedly diminished as reflected by almost undetectable estrogens in the follicular fluid and ovarian tissue, probably because of inactivity of the FSH-dependent aromatase system within the granulosa cells.[128,156,298,491] Inadequate intrafollicular estrogen synthesis, increased intrafollicular androgens, and an elevated LH/FSH ratio result in cessation of follicle growth at the mid-antral stage, anovulation, and sclerocystic ovaries.

A number of disorders resulting in hyperestronemia and altered gonadotropin secretion potentially play a role in initiating or perpetuating PCO[295]:

Obesity. As noted above, the conversion of androstenedione to E_1 occurs predominantly in adipose tissue, and the extent of the conversion correlates with the amount of adipose tissue.[35,96,156,295] Similarly, weight reduction in obese women is associated with a reduction in serum androgen and estrone levels.[35,295] Hyperestronemia, and as

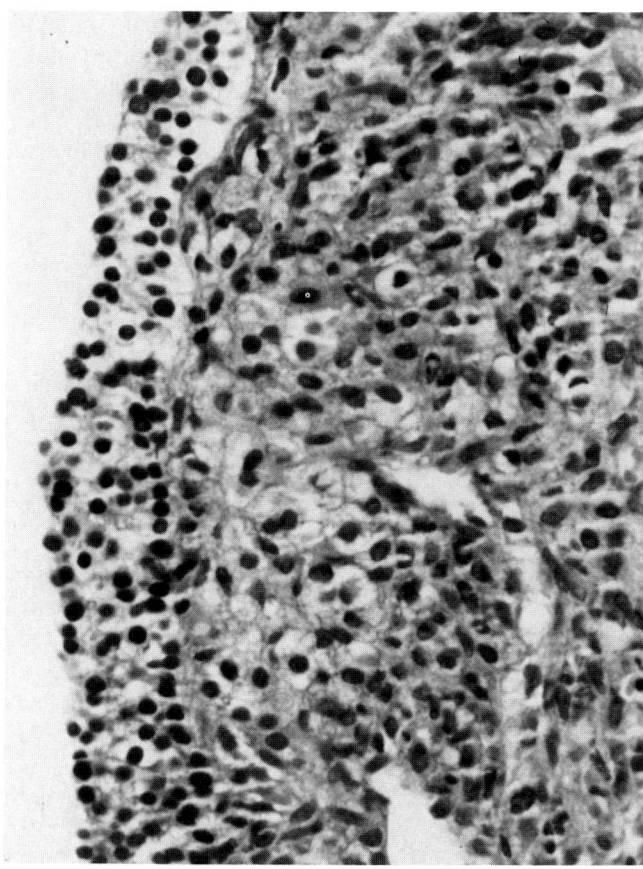

FIG. 16.25. **Polycystic ovary disease.** A cystic follicle is lined by nonluteinized granulosa cells and an outer, thicker layer of luteinized theca interna cells. (Reprinted by permission of Clement (1985) In: Contemporary Issues in Surgical Pathology, Vol 6. Roth, Czernobilsky (eds). New York, Churchill Livingstone.)

discussed below, hyperinsulinemia, therefore are two obesity-related factors that may play a role in the pathogenesis of PCO.

Adrenal Androgen Excess. The adrenal contribution to the androgen pool is increased in many patients with PCO, as manifested by an elevated level of the adrenal androgen dehydroepiandrosterone sulphate (DHES) and abnormal adrenal androgen responses to adrenocorticotropic hormone (ACTH) and metapyrone.* The increased adrenal androgens can lead to hyperestronemia and, consequently, an elevated LH/FSH ratio. Dexamethasone treatment can correct the abnormal LH/FSH ratio in some patients with PCO, resulting in resumption of ovulation.[295] Although some investigators believe that the adrenal abnormalities are a primary disturbance, others have concluded that they are secondary to the hormonal milieu of PCO.[123]

---

*Refs. 19,156,177,249,264,265,269,299,306,500.

Hyperinsulinemia. Insulin resistance and hyperinsulinemia have been noted in obese and nonobese women with PCO.[70,83,295,333,352] As discussed later (see HAIR-AN syndrome), insulin stimulates androgen secretion from the ovarian stroma. Hyperinsulinemia thus potentially leads to increased levels of circulating androgens (and by peripheral conversion, estrone) in patients with PCO. The resultant hyperandrogenism may in turn increase insulin resistance.[322]

Hyperprolactinemia. The hyperprolactinemia occasionally present in PCO may be due to a pituitary adenoma, but in other cases may be related to a hyperplasia of prolactin-secreting cells induced by the hyperestronemia in these patients.[155,156,295,500] The hyperprolactinemia, either through a direct effect on gonadotropin-secreting cells or indirectly through other mechanisms (such as decreased dopaminergic tone), may result in an elevated LFH/FSH ratio.[295] Prolactin also may increase DHES secretion from the adrenal gland. In some patients, treatment with bromocriptine reverses the hyperprolactinemia, lowers androgen levels, and in some patients restores ovulatory cycles.[295]

DIFFERENTIAL DIAGNOSIS

The differential diagnosis includes a wide variety of other disorders that result in abnormal gonadotropin release, chronic anovulation, and sclerocystic ovaries. Sclerocystic ovaries are a nonspecific morphologic expression of chronic anovulation in the premenopausal patient, and can accompany (1) adrenal lesions, such as Cushing's syndrome, congenital adrenal hyperplasia, and virilizing adrenal tumors, (2) primary hypothalamic–pituitary disorders, and (3) ovarian lesions that produce excessive quantities of estrogens or androgens, including sex cord–stromal tumors, steroid cell tumors, and such nonneoplastic lesions as Leydig cell hyperplasia and stromal hyperthecosis. As previously noted, the latter overlaps both clinically and pathologically with PCO, and the two disorders may represent opposite poles of a single disease spectrum.[282,283] Sclerocystic ovaries also have been described in patients with autoimmune oophoritis (see page 629),[26] after long-term use of oral contraceptives,[361,394] in association with periovarian adhesions,[367] after long-term androgen therapy in female to male transsexuals,[348] and as a normal finding in prepubertal subjects.[303]

Stromal Hyperplasia and Stromal Hyperthecosis

Stromal hyperplasia (SH) is characterized by varying degrees of nonneoplastic proliferation of the ovarian stromal cells. Stromal hyperthecosis (HT) refers to the presence of luteinized stromal cells at a distance from the follicles; it is usually accompanied by at least a moderate degree of SH.

CLINICAL FEATURES

The clinical manifestations are variable. Moderate to severe SH is most commonly encountered in patients in their sixth and seventh decades, and has been documented in more than one-third of autopsied patients in this age group.[60,430] Similar degrees of SH are found less commonly in patients in the eighth decade (18% of patients in one study[60]), suggesting that it may be a reversible process.[60,430] A strong negative association with parity was found in one study.[430] SH of moderate to severe degree may be associated with androgen hypersecretion[60] and endometrial carcinoma.[430] Obesity, hypertension, and glucose intolerance also are seen more frequently in patients with SH.[60]

HT is most frequent in patients in the sixth to ninth decades. Some familial cases of HT have been reported,[169,217] and one case of HT has been described in a patient with acromegaly.[326] The process has been documented in one-third of autopsied patients over the age of 55 years, and it has been suggested that exhaustive microscopic sampling may reveal that rare luteinized stromal cells are a normal finding in postmenopausal patients (see Chapter 15, Anatomy and Histology of the Ovary).[60] In this age group, HT usually is mild and of doubtful clinical significance.[60] Clinically florid examples of HT are more common in patients in the younger reproductive age group, although rare cases occur in adolescents and postmenopausal patients.[66,258,276,342,479] These patients are characteristically virilized, obese, hypertensive, hyperinsulinemic, and have a broad range of circulating glucose patterns. Less commonly, the clinical findings are more characteristic of PCO.[33,282,283] In some patients with HT, estrogenic, rather than androgenic, manifestations predominate, typically manifested by the presence of endometrial hyperplasia or even well-differentiated adenocarcinoma.° Conversely, women with endometrial hyperplasia or carcinoma in some studies have had a high frequency of HT on microscopic examination of their ovaries.[324,399] One patient with HT had pseudosarcomatous changes in the endometrial stroma and foci of ectopic decidua within the ovaries,[371] findings suggesting progesterone production by the ovarian stroma. HT-related virilization has been present in two cases of placental site trophoblastic tumor, and in one case it was the presenting manifestation of the tumor.[325,331]

GROSS FINDINGS

SH and HT are almost invariably bilateral, and may be associated with ovaries of normal size or those up to 7 cm in maximum dimension, thus potentially mimicking an ovarian neoplasm.[60,276,410] Examination of the cut surface

°Refs. 1,143,228,276,283,324,399,430,437.

reveals parenchymal replacement by homogeneous, firm, white to yellow tissue (Fig. 16.26).[60,326] In cases of nodular hyperthecosis, multiple yellow nodules may be appreciable macroscopically.[258,410] In premenopausal patients, sclerocystic changes similar to those seen in PCO also may be present.[137,203,282,283,327]

MICROSCOPIC FINDINGS

A varying degree of nodular or diffuse cortical and medullary proliferation of ovarian stromal cells is present (Fig. 16.27). A mild degree of SH cannot be distinguished reliably from the normal appearance (see Chapter 15).[60] The stromal cells in SH are plumper than the normal postmenopausal ovarian stromal cell, and have oval to fusiform, vesicular nuclei and, frequently, cytoplasmic lipid.[410] The luteinized stromal cells of HT are more common in the medulla but also may be present in the cortex. They appear as small clusters or nodules of polygonal cells with abundant eosinophilic to vacuolated cytoplasm containing variable amounts of lipid (Fig. 16.28).[60,143,410] The round nucleus of the luteinized cells typically has a central small nucleolus. In cases of HT accompanying the HAIR-AN syndrome (see below), edema and fibrosis of the ovarian stroma, rather than SH, frequently is a prominent change.[290]

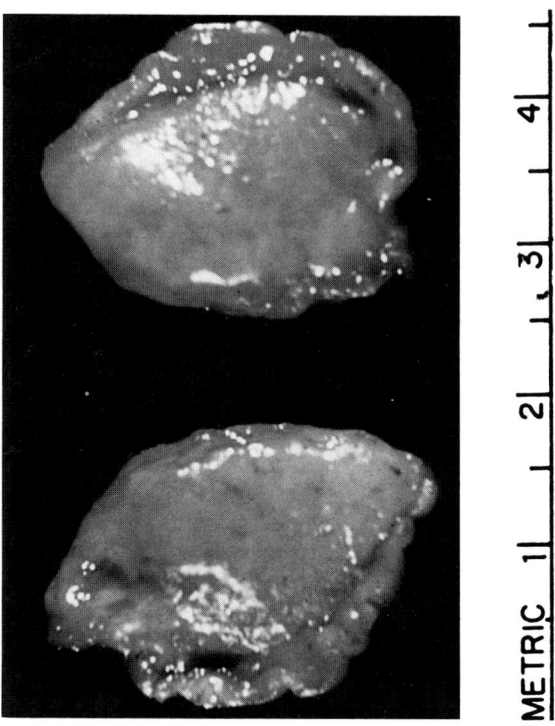

FIG. 16.26. Stromal hyperplasia and hyperthecosis. The ovaries are involved by a solid, homogeneous proliferation that had a yellow color in the unfixed state. (Courtesy of R.E. Scully, M.D., Boston, MA.)

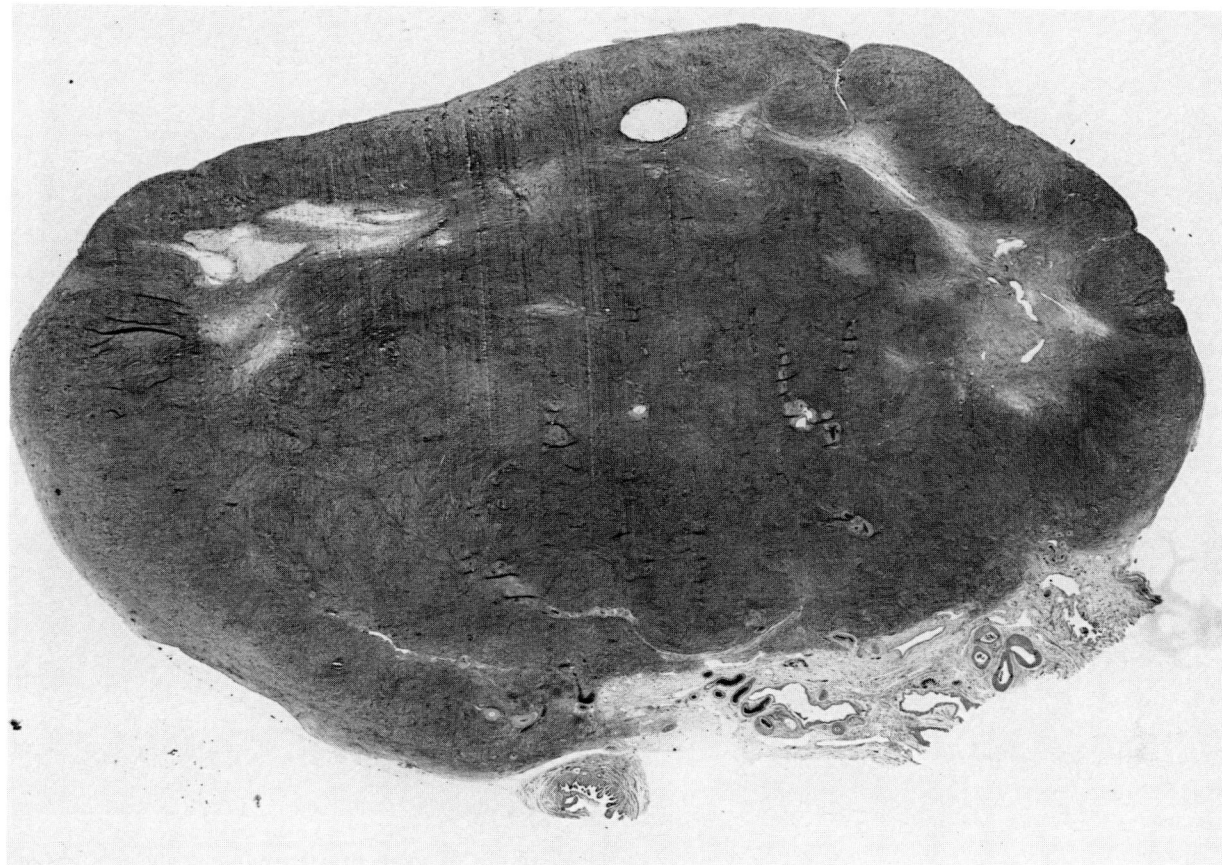

FIG. 16.27. **Stromal hyperplasia.** A diffuse proliferation of ovarian stromal cells within the cortex and medulla is seen. (Reprinted by permission of Clement (1985) In: Contemporary Issues in Surgical Pathology, Vol 6. Roth, Czernobilsky (eds). New York, Churchill Livingstone.)

Histochemical analyses have shown that luteinized stromal cells have oxidative activity similar to those of theca interna cells.[144,412] The luteinized cells were immunoreactive for cytochrome P-450$_{17\alpha}$, which catalyzes androgen synthesis, in approximately 50% of the cases in one series.[399] Luteinized stromal cells also have been shown to be immunoreactive for testosterone, estradiol, and FSH.[276,324]

Other ovarian findings occasionally encountered in HT include an increased number of atretic follicles,[342] small stromal nodules of metaplastic smooth muscle,[411] Leydig cell hyperplasia,[60,445] Leydig cell tumors,[224,384,445] stromal luteomas,[409] and thecomas.[444,508] SH in the absence of HT also has been associated with thecomas.[385,444,508] Some cases of HT may be associated with massive ovarian edema (see page 619).

PATHOPHYSIOLOGY

In vitro and in vivo studies have shown that ovaries with SH secrete larger amounts of androstenedione, estrone, and estradiol than nonhyperplastic ovaries.[117,271] Similar studies using ovarian tissue from patients with HT[329] as well as in vivo

studies in these patients have shown, respectively, markedly increased production rates and serum levels of ovarian testosterone, dihydrotestosterone, and androstenedione, usually in the male range.[1,6,33,137,138,223,276,326] One in vitro study suggested that the abnormal androgen production is due to an increase in the volume of the ovarian stroma rather than to a biochemical defect in the latter.[38] As in PCO, the predominant estrogen in patients with SH and HT is estrone, derived predominantly from peripheral aromatization of ovarian androgens, resulting in an increased estrone/estradiol ratio.[326,399]

Unlike patients with PCO, most premenopausal patients with HT have normal gonadotropin levels.[217,326] That gonadotropins may play a role in SH and HT, however, is suggested by (1) elevated LH levels in occasional premenopausal with HT and postmenopausal patients with SH and HT,[169,223] (2) immunoreactivity for FSH and LH within ovarian stromal cells,[332] (3) in vitro incubation studies showing that FSH and LH stimulate proliferation of the ovarian stroma of pre- and postmenopausal women,[430] (3) studies showing that androgen production by the ovarian stromal cells in patients with and without HT is enhanced by LH,[29,117,329] (4) the often prominent stromal luteiniza-

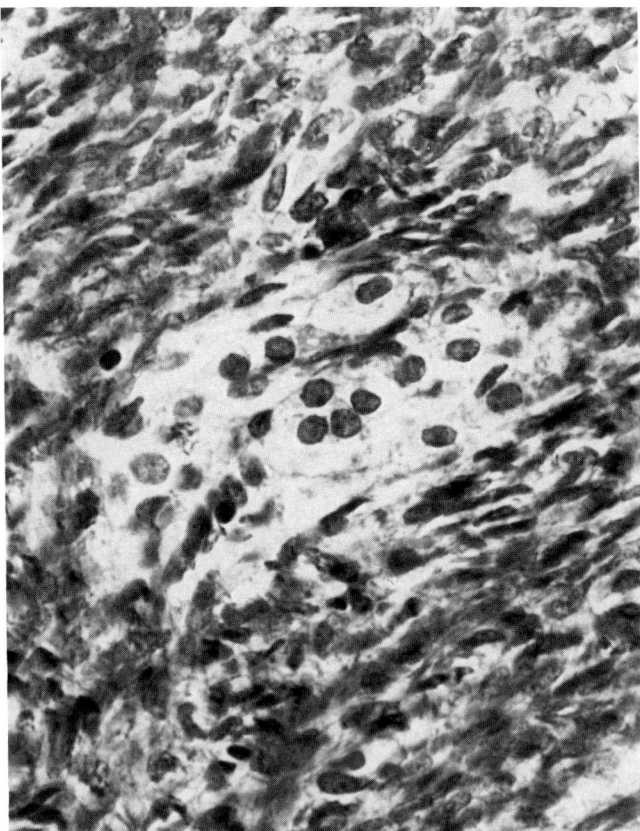

FIG. 16.28. **Stromal hyperthecosis.** A nest of luteinized stromal cells is present within the ovarian stroma. (Reprinted by permission of Clement (1985) In: Contemporary Issues in Surgical Pathology, Vol 6. Roth, Czernobilsky (eds). New York, Churchill Livingstone.)

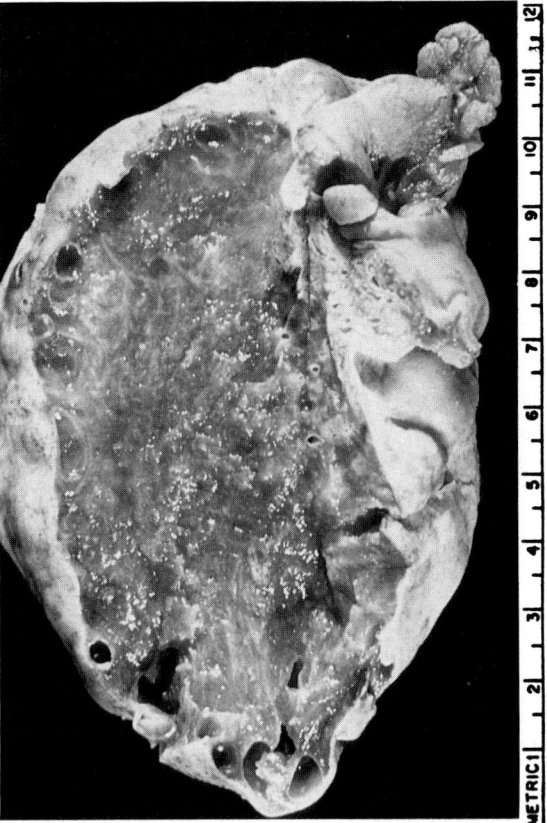

FIG. 16.29. **Massive ovarian edema.** The ovary is enlarged and markedly edematous. (Courtesy of Dr. R.E. Scully. Reprinted by permission of Clement (1985) In: Contemporary Issues in Surgical Pathology, Vol 6. Roth, Czernobilsky (eds). New York, Churchill Livingstone.)

tion during pregnancy, (5) cases of symptomatic HT complicating pregnancy[379] and trophoblastic disease,[325,331] and (6) the increase in pituitary amphophils in some cases of severe HT.[73,276] As noted above, insulin resistance and hyperinsulinemia occur in as many as 90% of patients with HT, and likely play a role in the pathogenesis of the stromal luteinization in these patients (see HAIR-AN Syndrome).[330]

DIFFERENTIAL DIAGNOSIS

The differential diagnosis of HT includes other nonneoplastic and neoplastic solid proliferations of luteinized cells, most of which also are virilizing. The nonneoplastic category includes pregnancy luteoma and Leydig cell hyperplasia (discussed elsewhere in this chapter) and the neoplasms include luteinized thecoma and steroid cell tumors (see Chapter 19, Sex Cord–Stromal, Steroid Cell, and Other Ovarian Tumors with Endocrine, Paraendocrine, and Paraneoplastic Manifestations). These neoplasms, in contrast to HT, almost always are unilateral and typically form distinct tumors or nodules appreciable on gross examination. Luteinized stromal cells, histologically similar to those present in HT, also may be encountered within the nonneoplastic stroma of a wide variety of benign and malignant ovarian tumors, including primary surface epithelial and germ cell tumors as well as metastatic tumors, that is, "tumors with functioning stroma" (see Chapter 19).

CLINICAL BEHAVIOR AND TREATMENT

In contrast to patients with PCO, those with HT usually exhibit little or no response to clomiphene treatment and often only a transient response to wedge resection.[137,217,223,327] Many patients require bilateral oophorectomy to halt progressive virilization. Such treatment also may result in the disappearance of hypertension and abnormalities in glucose tolerance.[66,283] More recently, successful treatment of HT has been achieved with gonadotropin-releasing hormone (GnRH) agonists.[439]

HAIR-AN Syndrome

In addition to the common occurrence of insulin resistance and hyperinsulinemia in patients with HT, some patients with HT have HAIR-AN syndrome, a syndrome that has been estimated to be present in as many as 5% of all women with hyperandrogenism.[15,28,30,124,285] The syndrome consists of hyperandrogenism (HA), typically of early, sometimes premenarcheal, onset, insulin resistance (IR), and acanthosis nigricans (AN).[30] Striking degrees of masculinization are present in some patients with HAIR-AN syndrome and may be disproportionate to the degree of hyperandrogenism.[124] Some patients have a normal glucose tolerance whereas others have symptomatic diabetes.[219]

The syndrome has been described most frequently in patients with PCO, although it appears likely that most, if not all, such patients also have HT.[124,290] Unusual histological findings in patients with HT and HAIR-AN syndrome have included prominent follicular atresia, many degenerating oocytes, medullary stromal fibrosis, and numerous small nests of granulosa cells forming Call–Exner bodies.[285] Dermoid cysts[206] and stromal luteoma[168] have been rarely described in patients with HAIR-AN syndrome in association with HT, sclerocystic ovaries, or both.

The typical laboratory findings include hyperinsulinemia and increased production rates and elevated serum levels of testosterone and androstenedione.[28,124,164,423] In some patients, the severity of the insulin resistance is proportional to the testosterone elevation.[28,70] Proposed mechanisms of insulin resistance have included a decreased number or functional capacity of insulin receptors, which may be associated with obesity, or in other cases, genetic alterations in the structure of the receptors (type A), anti-insulin receptor antibodies that decrease insulin receptor affinity for insulin and that often are associated with autoimmune diseases (type B), and postreceptor defects in insulin action or clearance (type C).[27,31,142,149,219,309,310,457]

Recent studies have demonstrated that (1) there is a 50–250-fold increase in testosterone production from the ovarian stroma in women with the syndrome compared with normal ovaries,[298] (2) in some women with hyperandrogenism and insulin resistance, a glucose load can produce an acute rise in circulating androgens,[429] (3) insulin can stimulate the accumulation of androstenedione and testosterone in cultures of ovarian stromal cells in women with and without hyperandrogenism,[29,30,329] and (4) insulin and insulin-like growth factor I receptors are present in the ovarian stromal cells, the insulin-like growth factor possibly mediating the androgenic effects of insulin.[324,328,362] Additionally, insulin may enhance LH secretion from the pituitary[2] and act synergistically with LH in stimulating the ovarian stromal cells.

On the basis of these and other findings, it has been postulated that the primary defect in HAIR-AN syndrome is insulin resistance leading to hyperinsulinemia and the other findings in the syndrome.[28] Thus, any cause of insulin resistance leading to hyperinsulinemia can produce HAIR-AN syndrome. The hyperandrogenism itself may increase the severity of the insulin resistance, and thus a self-perpetuating cycle that increases in severity may result.[30] The acanthosis nigricans probably is an epiphenomenon secondary to the hyperandrogenism, hyperinsulinemia, or both.[28]

Bilateral oophorectomy in patients with HAIR-AN syndrome decreases the hyperandrogenism but usually does not ameliorate the insulin resistance.[28,206,285,330] Gonadotropin suppression with oral contraceptives has been successful in decreasing ovarian androgen production in some patients.[28] Marked improvement of the acanthosis nigricans may follow correction of the hyperandrogenism.[168]

Massive Ovarian Edema and Ovarian Fibromatosis

Tumor-like enlargement of one, or occasionally both, ovaries secondary to an accumulation of edema fluid within the ovarian stroma is referred to as *massive ovarian edema*. Approximately 60 cases of this disorder have been reported.° A lesion designated *ovarian fibromatosis* by Young and Scully,[502] characterized by diffuse ovarian fibrosis, is closely related to massive edema and therefore is considered in this section.

CLINICAL FEATURES

Patients with massive edema are typically young, with a mean age of 21 years (range 6–37 years) and have abdominal or pelvic pain, menstrual irregularities, and abdominal distension. The pain may be of several years' duration[74] or have a sudden onset and mimic the pain of acute appendicitis. In approximately 20% of patients, androgenic manifestations are present. Of these, two-thirds are masculinized, and the rest exhibit only hirsutism.[468,502] The androgenic manifestations nearly always have been associated with the presence of lutein cells. Serum testosterone has been elevated in some cases. Only one patient has exhibited estrogenic manifestations, manifested by precocious puberty.[386] Pelvic examination typically reveals a palpable adnexal mass, which in 70% of cases has been right-sided. In approximately one-half of patients, there is evidence of partial or complete torsion of the involved ovary and in one patient, the contralateral ovary had a twisted pedicle and was infarcted.[220] Intraperitoneal fluid usually is not present, although rare patients have had an associated Meigs' syndrome.[154]

Patients with ovarian fibromatosis have ranged in age from 13 to 39 years, with an average of 25 years.[502] Clinical manifestations include menstrual abnormalities, abdomi-

---

° Refs. 74,88,154,222,229,386,466,502.

nal pain, and, less commonly, hirsutism or virilization. Most patients have a palpable adnexal mass. Occasionally, the ovarian enlargement is an incidental finding late in pregnancy or during cesarean section. In some cases, the involved ovary was found twisted on its pedicle at the time of operation. The endocrine manifestations, including, in several cases, infertility, disappear after oophorectomy, indicating that the lesion produces steroid hormones.

GROSS FINDINGS

The involved ovary in massive edema is enlarged, soft, and fluctuant, ranging from 5.5 to 35 cm in maximum dimension (mean, 11.5 cm). The heaviest ovary has weighed 2400 g.[502] The ovary has a shiny, white, smooth exterior, and a cut surface that is solid, tan, homogeneous, and gelatinous, exuding a watery fluid (Fig. 16.29). The most superficial cortex is white and fibrotic, resembling a capsule. Occasional superficial FCs may be present. The ipsilateral fallopian tube also may be edematous.

In ovarian fibromatosis, there usually is complete or almost complete ovarian involvement by a fibromatous process.[502] The ovaries are 6–12 cm in maximumn dimension, and have external surfaces that are white and typically smooth or lobulated. The cut surfaces are firm, white, and solid, although residual cystic follicles surrounded by the fibrous tissue are present in one-third of cases (Fig. 16.30).

MICROSCOPIC FINDINGS

The striking finding on low magnification in massive edema is marked, diffuse, stromal edema that separates and sometimes involves the follicular structures, but typically spares the superficial cortex (Fig. 16.31). The latter

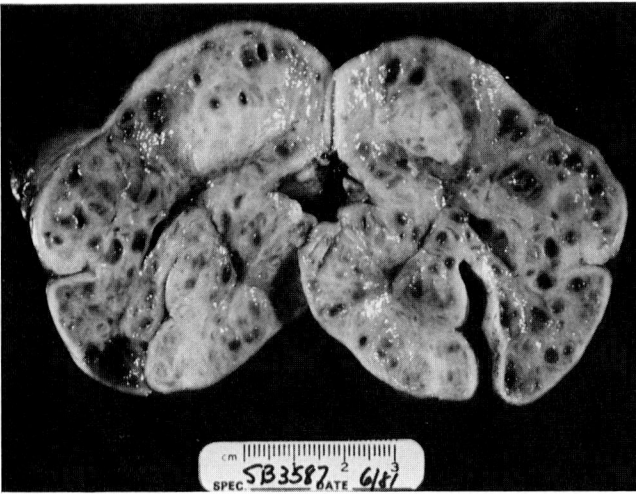

FIG. 16.30. **Ovarian fibromatosis.** The ovary is enlarged by a diffuse fibrous proliferation that surrounds multiple cystic follicles. (Courtesy of Young and Scully, ref. 502.)

usually is thickened and fibrotic. Higher magnification reveals spindle-shaped ovarian stromal cells separated by abundant pale-staining fluid that focally may create a microcystic appearance.[502] In nonedematous areas, the stroma has the appearance of normal stroma, hyperplastic stroma, or ovarian fibromatosis.[502] In approximately 40% of cases, foci of luteinized cells are present (Fig. 16.32). Associated nonspecific findings include vascular and lymphatic dilatation within the ovary and occasionally the mesosalpinx, rare foci of necrosis, as well as extravasated erythrocytes, hemosiderin-laden macrophages, and mast cells.[386,502] The contralateral ovary is normal in more than 75% of cases; in the rest, it is enlarged and edematous, or is nonedematous but altered by stromal hyperthecosis or sclerocystic changes.[460,466,502]

Ovarian fibromatosis is characterized by a proliferation of collagen-producing spindle cells that typically surround normal follicular structures and thicken the superficial cortex (Fig. 16.33).[502] The process varies from moderately cellular fascicles of spindle cells with a focal storiform pattern to relatively acellular bands of dense collagen. Small foci of uninvolved ovarian stroma usually are present. In rare cases, luteinized cells are seen within the lesion or the adjacent nonfibrotic stroma. Minor foci of stromal edema and microscopic foci of sex cord elements within the fibromatous tissue, alone or in combination, have been encountered in occasional cases.[76,502] Occasionally the process is bilateral.

PATHOGENESIS

The pathogenesis of massive edema is thought to be intermittent torsion of the ovary on its pedicle, causing partial obstruction of venous and lymphatic drainage. Torsion is observed in half the cases of massive edema, and a few cases have been reported in association with obstruction of ovarian lymphatics secondary to metastatic carcinoma within pelvic and para-aortic lymph nodes.[502] Luteinization of the ovarian stromal cells is considered a secondary phenomenon, possibly caused by an hCG-like substance within the edema fluid.[220,443]

In at least some cases, the massive edema likely occurs in an ovary with an underlying stromal proliferation, either fibromatosis or stromal hyperthecosis, that enlarges the ovary, promoting torsion with subsequent edema.[74,502] This interpretation is supported by the clinical similarities and pathological overlap between massive edema and ovarian fibromatosis. Young and Scully suggest that massive edema is simply ovarian fibromatosis following torsion and accumulation of edema fluid.[502] Similarly, some examples of massive edema in which luteinized stromal cells are present in the same ovary and in the contralateral, edematous, or nonedematous ovary may represent cases of stromal hyperthecosis in which one or both ovaries have undergone torsion.

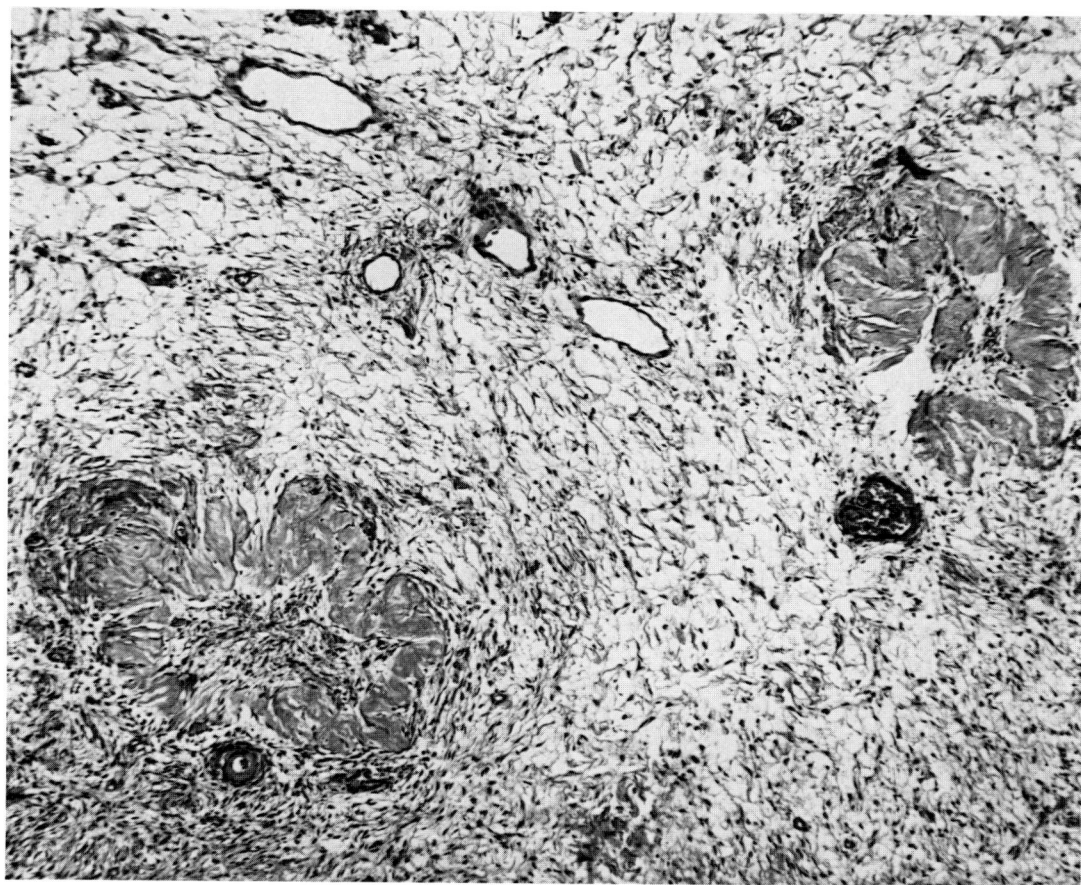

FIG. 16.31. Massive ovarian edema. The edematous ovarian stroma separates several corpora fibrosa. (Reprinted by permission of Clement (1985) In: Contemporary Issues in Surgical Pathology, Vol 6. Roth, Czernobilsky (eds). New York, Churchill Livingstone.)

DIFFERENTIAL DIAGNOSIS

The differential diagnosis of massive edema includes ovarian neoplasms, which may exhibit an edematous or myxoid appearance, most commonly fibroma, but also sclerosing stromal tumor,[82] Krukenberg tumor, and the rare ovarian myxoma.[127] Massive edema and fibromatosis are distinguished from a neoplasm by the presence of follicular derivatives visible on both macroscopic and microscopic examination. A neoplasm may be surrounded by a rim of normal ovarian tissue in contrast to massive edema and fibromatosis, which usually diffusely involve the ovarian tissue. Additionally, ovarian fibromas occur in an older age group and are hormonally inactive.

CLINICAL BEHAVIOR AND TREATMENT

Although most of the reported patients with massive edema have been treated by oophorectomy, the condition should be managed conservatively, especially if the patient is young.[460] After an intraoperative frozen section of a wedge biopsy to exclude a neoplasm, an ovarian suspension procedure should be performed, with fixation of the involved ovary.[460]

Pregnancy Luteoma

Pregnancy luteoma is a distinctive, nonneoplastic lesion of pregnancy characterized by solid proliferations of luteinized cells resulting in tumor-like ovarian enlargement. Approximately 100 cases have been described.[160,339,376,442,443,459]

CLINICAL FEATURES

The patients usually are in their third or fourth decades, are multiparous in 80% of the cases, and black in 80% of the cases. Most patients are asymptomatic, and the ovarian enlargement is discovered incidentally at cesarean section or postpartum tubal ligation. Rarely, a pelvic mass is palpable or causes obstruction of the birth canal. In approximately 25% of cases, hirsutism or virilization appear or worsen during the latter half of pregnancy; two-thirds of female infants born to virilized mothers also are virilized,

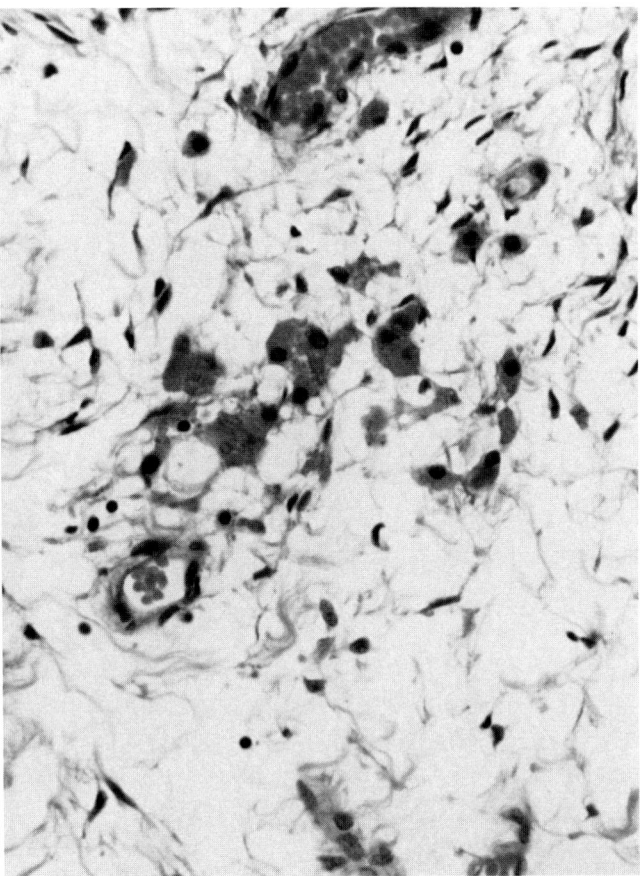

FIG. 16.32. **Massive ovarian edema with luteinized stromal cells.** (Reprinted by permission of Clement (1985) In: Contemporary Issues in Surgical Pathology, Vol 6. Roth, Czernobilsky (eds). New York, Churchill Livingstone.)

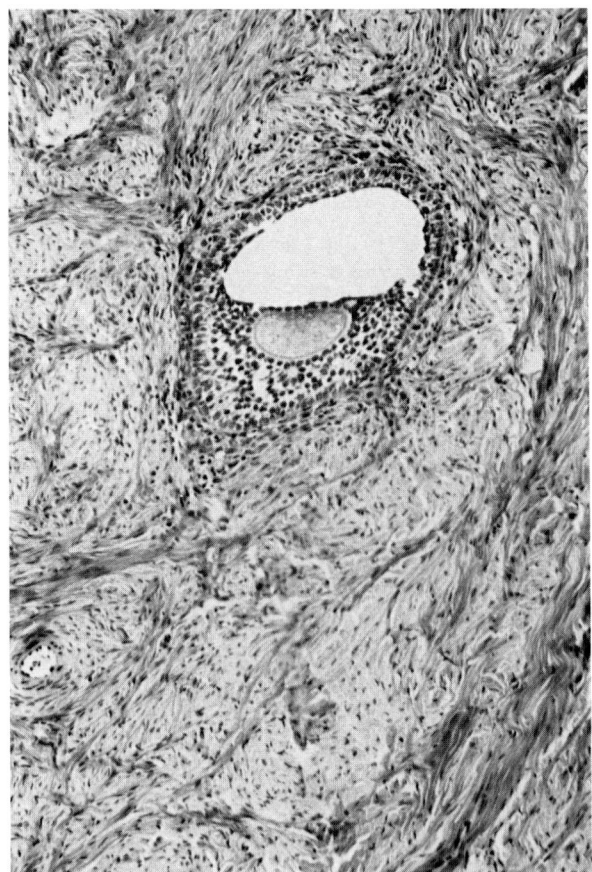

FIG. 16.33. **Ovarian fibromatosis.** Fibrotic ovarian stroma surrounds an antral follicle.

manifested by clitoromegaly and labial fusion.[160,470] Regression of the lesions usually begins within days after delivery and is complete within several weeks. In rare cases, pregnancy luteomas occur in consecutive pregnancies.[160,230] The diagnosis is made by excisional biopsy and frozen section examination of one nodule.

Plasma testosterone[323,470,497,506] and other androgens[506] may reach levels 70 times above normal in virilized patients. Elevated testosterone also has been demonstrated in nonvirilized patients.[323] The hormone levels decrease rapidly after delivery, usually normalizing within 2 weeks postpartum. Besides the high circulating levels of testosterone, virilization of the mother may be due to a decrease in testerone-binding proteins with a resultant increase in the biologically active unbound fraction.[470,497] Androgen levels in the infants may be increased but usually are lower than maternal levels[470] or normal.[323] Since the placenta aromatizes androgens to estrogens, virilization of female infants is unusual, and may reflect defective aromatization or an androgen load that exceeds the aromatization capacity of the placenta.[188,323]

GROSS FINDINGS

Solid, fleshy, circumscribed, red, brown, or gray nodules ranging up to 20 cm in diameter (mean, 6.6 cm) occupy the ovarian parenchyma (Fig. 16.34).[339] Hemorrhagic foci are common. The lesions are bilateral in at least one-third of the cases and multiple in almost half of them.[410] A separate corpus luteum of pregnancy also may be visible. Postpartum involution of the lesions results in infarct-like necrosis, and eventually, brown, puckered scars.[410]

MICROSCOPIC FINDINGS

The lesions are composed of sharply circumscribed, rounded masses of cells (Fig. 16.35), that also are arranged occasionally in a trabecular or follicular pattern, the latter associated with spaces containing colloid-like material (Fig. 16.36a). The cells are intermediate in size between the luteinized granulosa cells and luteinized theca cells of adjacent follicles, having abundant eosinophilic cytoplasm that contains little or no stainable lipid (Fig. 16.36b). Al-

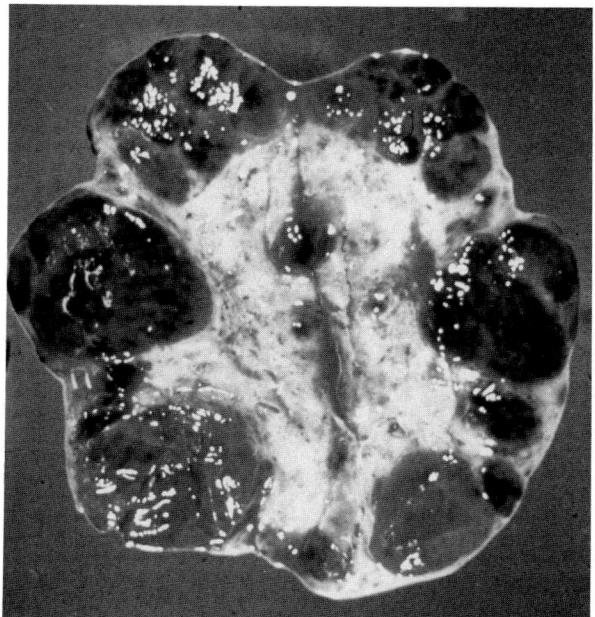

FIG. 16.34. Pregnancy luteoma. Multiple, solid, circumscribed, focally hemorrhagic nodules replace the normal parenchyma. (Reproduced by permission of Malinak and Miller (1965). Am J Obstet Gynecol 91:251–259.)

though nuclear atypism is minimal, the nuclei usually are somewhat larger, more pleomorphic, and hyperchromatic than the adjacent luteinized stromal cells; nucleoli may be prominent.[339] Mitotic figures usually are present, with an average of 2 or 3 per 10 high-power fields (HPFs) (range, 0–7 mitotic figures/10 HPFs), and occasional mitotic figures may be atypical.[339,442] Small numbers of intracellular colloid droplets similar to those seen in corpora lutea of pregnancy may be present in rare cases. The stroma between the cells is scant, and reticulin fibrils surround groups of cells in an organoid pattern. Ultrastructural examination has shown the characteristic features of steroid-producing cells.[159] Occasional pregnancy luteomas that have been examined several weeks postpartum are composed of degenerating lipid-filled luteoma cells with pyknotic nuclei, accompanied by an inflammatory cell infiltrate and fibrosis.[410,443]

PATHOGENESIS

Pregnancy luteomas most likely arise from hCG-induced proliferations of luteinized ovarian stromal cells,[442] a conclusion favored by in vitro incubation studies that have shown that luteoma cells resemble ovarian stromal cells in their steroidogenic capacity.[345,377] Some authors, however,

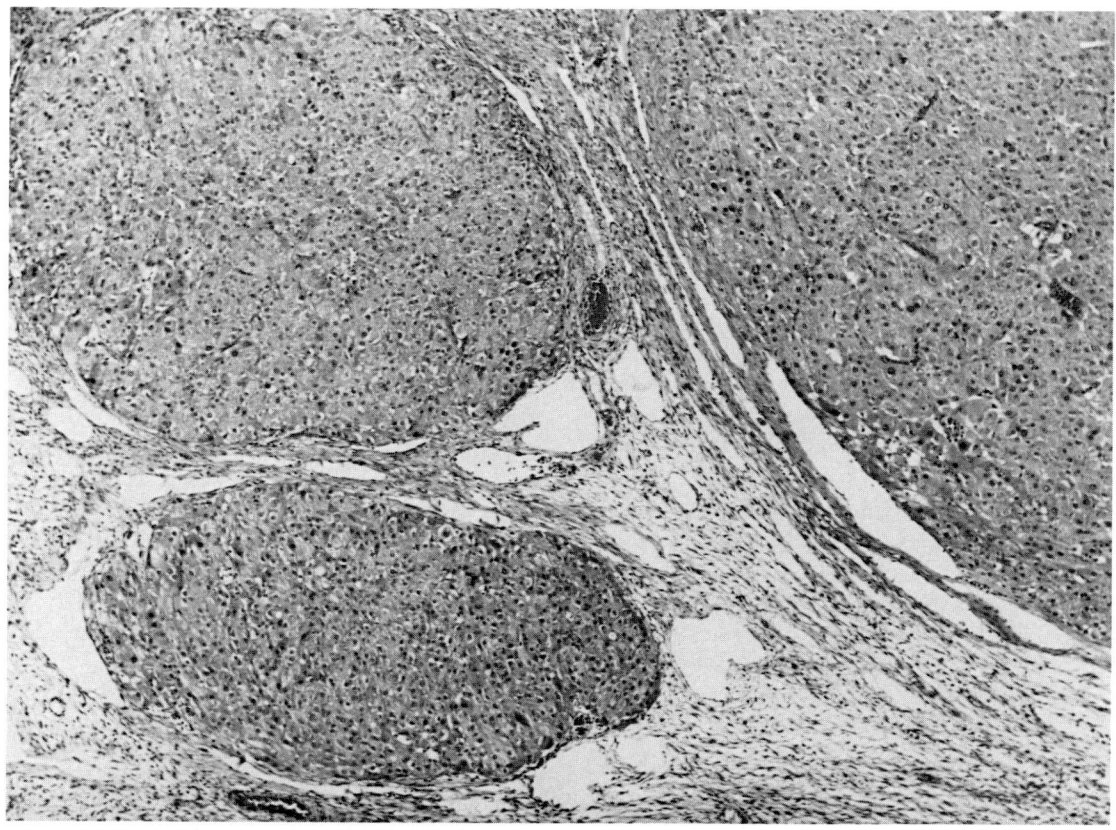

FIG. 16.35. Pregnancy luteoma. Three solid nodules of luteinized cells are present. (Reprinted by permission of Clement (1985) In: Contemporary Issues in Surgical Pathology, Vol 6. Roth, Czernobilsky (eds). New York, Churchill Livingstone.)

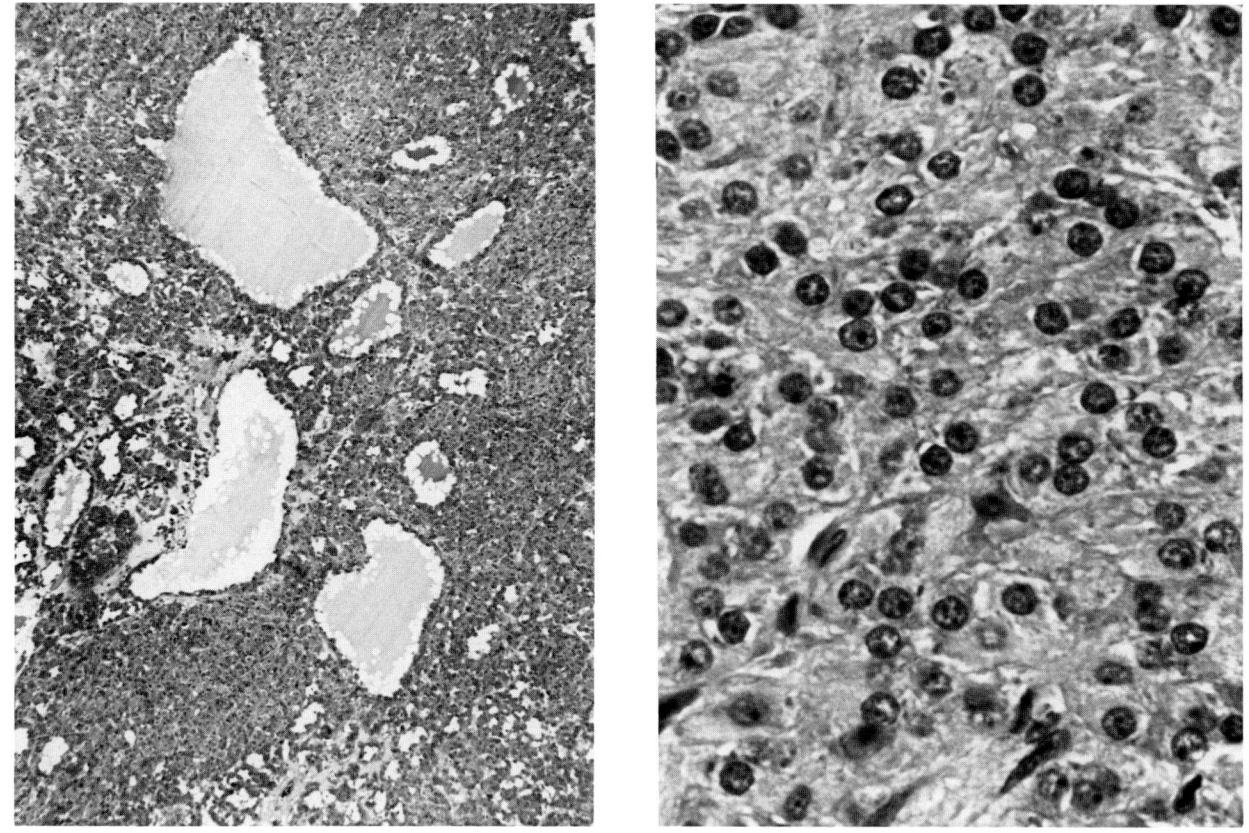

FIG. 16.36. **Pregnancy luteoma. a:** Follicular pattern. **b:** Solid growth pattern of polygonal luteinized cells.

have favored origin from luteinized follicular granulosa and theca cells.[339] The exclusive occurrence of the lesion in pregnancy suggests a role for hCG in its pathogenesis, and augmentation of steroidogenesis by pregnancy luteomas in response to hCG, both in vitro[377] and in vivo,[459] supports this interpretation. However, the rarity of pregnancy luteomas in association with gestational trophoblastic disease, which typically is accompanied by very high levels of hCG, and the almost exclusive recognition of the lesions during the third trimester when hCG levels are lower than earlier in pregnancy, indicate that hCG is not the only factor in their development. The occasional history of hirsutism, sometimes familial, antedating the pregnancy suggests that a preexistent endocrinopathy, such as stromal hyperthecosis or PCO, may predispose to the development of the lesion in some patients.[410]

DIFFERENTIAL DIAGNOSIS

Although a number of lesions composed of luteinized cells occurring during pregnancy may resemble a pregnancy luteoma on microscopic examination, the typical gross appearance of the pregnancy luteoma readily distinguishes it from a large solitary luteinized follicle cyst of pregnancy

and puerperium, hyperreactio luteinalis, and corpus luteum of pregnancy. Solid primary neoplasms composed partially or entirely of luteinized cells such as granulosa tumors, thecomas, and steroid cell tumors may occur during pregnancy and enter the differential diagnosis. Such tumors almost always will be unilateral and solitary compared with the more frequent bilaterality and multinodularity of the pregnancy luteoma. The partly luteinized group, that is, luteinized granulosa cell tumors and luteinized thecomas, will always contain more typical nonluteinized foci and usually have denser reticulum patterns and more abundant intracellular lipid than seen in pregnancy luteoma. Entirely luteinized tumors belonging to the steroid cell category may closely resemble pregnancy luteoma histologically. Features favoring a steroid cell neoplasm include a dense reticulum pattern, intracellular lipid, lipochrome pigment, and in Leydig cell tumors, a hilar location and the presence of Reinke crystals (see Chapter 19, Sex Cord–Stromal, Steroid Cell, and Other Ovarian Tumors with Endocrine, Paraendocrine, and Paraneoplastic Manifestations). Differentiation of a solitary pregnancy luteoma from a lipid-poor steroid cell tumor may be impossible, but such a lesion in a pregnant woman generally is considered a pregnancy luteoma until proven otherwise.

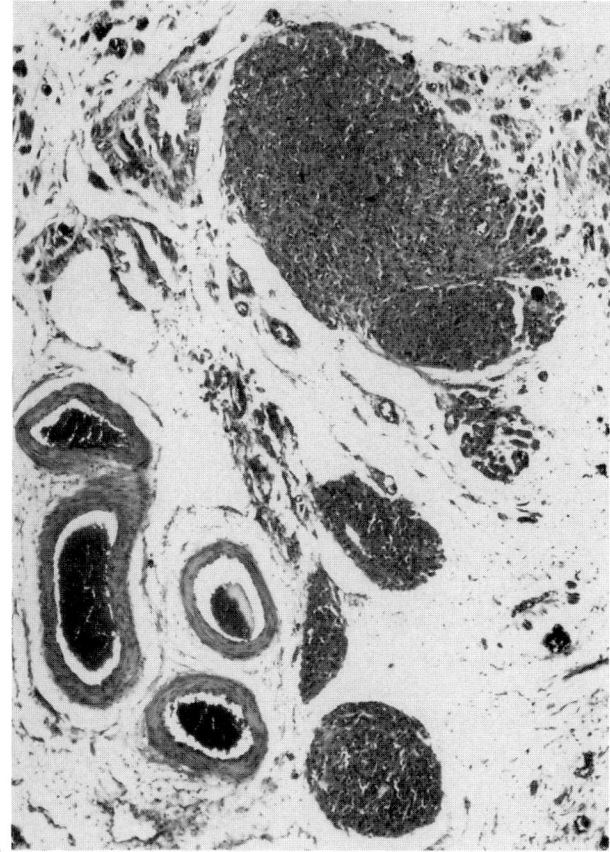 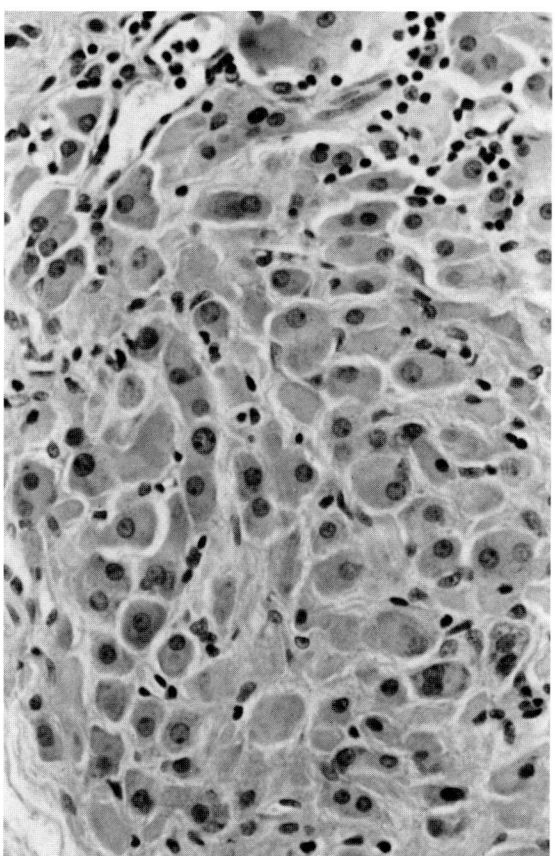

Fɪɢ. 16.37. **Leydig cell hyperplasia. a:** Nodular proliferation of hilar Leydig cells. **b:** There is mild nuclear pleomorphism and occasional multinucleated cells are present. No crystals are seen in this field.

CLINICAL BEHAVIOR AND TREATMENT

Since the pregnancy luteoma is a benign, self-limited condition, no treatment is required.

Leydig Cell Hyperplasia

Leydig cells typically occur in the ovarian hilus, where they are also referred to as hilus cells, and can be found in virtually all adult ovaries, typically intermingled with nonmyelinated nerves (see Chapter 15, Anatomy and Histology of the Ovary). Rarely, Leydig cells occur in nonhilar locations, either within the ovarian stroma or in extraovarian sites, such as the lamina propria or adventitia of the fallopian tube.[198,260]

Hilar Leydig Cell Hyperplasia

On histological examination hilar Leydig cell hyperplasia is characterized by an increased number of cells in a nodular or diffuse arrangement, increased cell size, the presence of mitotic figures, cellular and nuclear pleomorphism, hyperchromasia, and multinucleation (Fig. 16.37).[446] Mild hyperplasia, usually unassociated with clinical endocrine disturbance, is found commonly in postmenopausal women.[410]

More severe degrees of hyperplasia, often associated with virilization, may occur in younger women, sometimes during pregnancy.[115,301,440,446] In some cases, elevated serum testosterone levels have been documented.[301]

Hilar Leydig cell hyperplasia may be associated with other ovarian lesions, including stromal hyperplasia, stromal hyperthecosis, stromal Leydig cell hyperplasia, and hilar Leydig cell neoplasia.[115,440,441,445] One case of hilus cell hyperplasia has been associated with the gonadotropin-resistant ovary syndrome.[301]

Stromal Leydig Cell Hyperplasia

Reinke crystal-containing Leydig cells rarely occur within the ovarian stroma, from which they are probably derived (Fig. 16.38). Such cells may represent a focal microscopic finding in ovaries exhibiting otherwise typical stromal hyperthecosis.[58,445] In one such case, there also was bilateral hilar Leydig cell hyperplasia and bilateral hilar Leydig cell tumors.[445] Stromal Leydig cells are likely the origin of the rare Leydig cell tumors encountered within the ovarian stroma (see Chapter 19). Stromal Leydig cells also have been encountered rarely within the nonneoplastic stroma

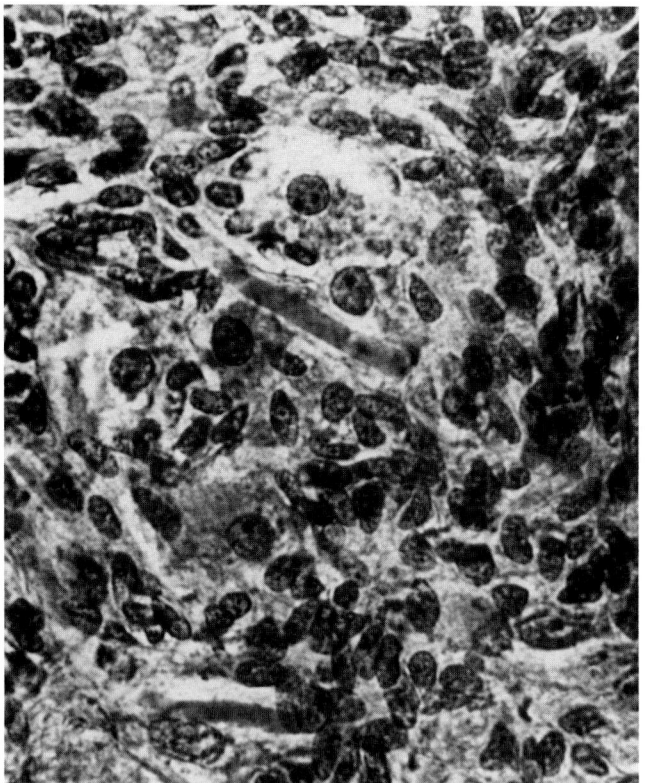

FIG. 16.38. **Stromal Leydig cells.** Occasional crystal-containing Leydig cells are present within the ovarian stroma. (Reprinted by permission of Sternberg and Roth, ref. 445.)

of a variety of ovarian neoplasms, including mucinous and serous cystadenomas, Brenner tumors, struma ovarii, and strumal carcinoid tumors.[393,443]

Ovarian Stromal Metaplasias Including Decidual Reaction

The ovarian stromal cell has the potential to differentiate, presumably by a process of metaplasia, into a variety of other mesenchymal cell types, most commonly decidua, but rarely smooth muscle, fat, and bone.

Ovarian Decidual Reaction

An ectopic decidual reaction may be encountered within the ovarian stroma as an isolated finding or as part of a more widespread decidual transformation of the subperitoneal pelvic mesenchyme (see Chapter 17, Diseases of the Peritoneum).[43,190,191,212,375,436] The decidual foci may be visible on macroscopic examination as small, soft, reddish subserosal nodules, ridges, or patches that tend to bleed easily on contact.[191,212,436] More frequently, however, the decidua is an incidental finding on microscopic examination. The process typically involves the stroma of the superficial cortex beneath the ovarian surface epithe-

lium (Fig. 16.39). The decidualized cells occur singly, as small nodules, or confluent sheets, and may form small polypoid projections from the ovarian surface.[191,212] The cells are indistinguishable from eutopic decidua on light microscopic examination, and have a similar ultrastructure.[191] Cells transitional in appearance between spindle-shaped ovarian stromal cells and fully decidualized cells usually are present. In some cases, ultrastructural examination has revealed cells exhibiting smooth muscle differentiation and intercellular collagen fibrils.[190] A rich vascular network of distended capillaries and a sprinkling of lymphocytes typically are found within the decidual foci. Florid examples, particularly if the decidual cells show focal cytological atypia, can simulate metastatic carcinoma on histological examination.[43] Degenerative changes within the decidua typically are seen postpartum.

As in other sites of the secondary müllerian system, an ovarian decidual reaction usually represents a response of the indigenous stromal cells to high circulating or local levels of estrogen and progesterone.[60] The process is seen most commonly during pregnancy, occurring as early as the ninth week of gestation, and by term is a finding present in virtually all ovaries.[43,191,212,436] Less commonly,

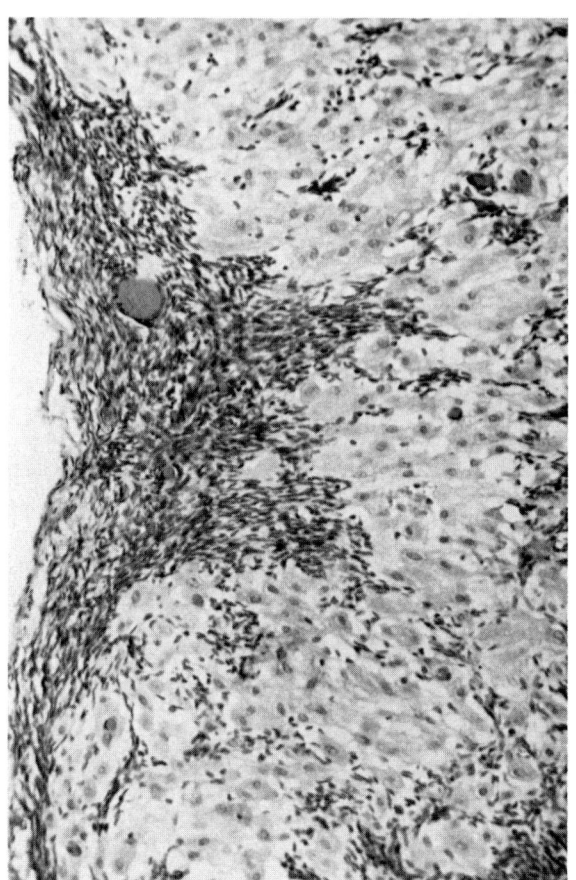

FIG. 16.39. **Ovarian decidual reaction.** Sheets of decidual cells replace the normal ovarian stroma.

the decidua is associated with trophoblastic disease, in patients treated with progestagens, in the vicinity of a corpus luteum, and in association with hormonally active neoplastic and nonneoplastic lesions of the ovaries and adrenal glands.[60,343,410] Prior ovarian radiation may be a predisposing factor by increasing the sensitivity of the stromal cells to the hormonal stimulation.[343] Occasionally foci of ectopic decidua may occur within the ovaries of pre- and postmenopausal women with no obvious cause.[343]

Rare Ovarian Stromal Metaplasias

Foci of metaplastic smooth muscle (Fig. 16.40a) may be encountered rarely in the ovarian stroma of otherwise normal ovaries, in association with stromal hyperthecosis or sclerocystic changes, or within the walls of ovarian cysts of various types.[203,411] Foci of mature fat have been described as a rare incidental histological finding within the superficial ovarian stroma in obese, but otherwise normal, women (Fig. 16.40b).[185,199] Heterotopic bone formation in the ovary in the absence of an ovarian neoplasm also is unusual, typically occurring within periovarian adhesions or the walls of endometriotic cysts but rarely within otherwise normal ovaries.[163,421] Although not a metaplasia, a case of multifocal psammomatous calcification of the ovarian stroma has been described within otherwise normal ovaries.[92]

Disorders of Ovarian Failure

Premature ovarian failure (POF) or premature menopause is a result of a variety of disorders that lead to the onset of amenorrhea and infertility before the age of 35 years, or according to others, 40 years.[7,11,56,101,105,372,373,391,434,462,465] POF is uncommon, accounting for only 4–10% of patients with secondary amenorrhea.[389,391] The ovarian failure usually is permanent, but occasionally it is reversible, at least temporarily, as manifested by subsequent ovulation and even conception.[12,344,373]

Patients with POF typically have a 46XX karyotype, normal secondary sexual characteristics, and secondary amenorrhea, although rarely prepubertal ovarian failure causes primary amenorrhea or oligomenorrhea and incompletely developed secondary sexual features. POF, therefore, probably represents a continuum in which individuals may be affected at any age before the expected age of menopause.[373] In contrast to patients with POF, patients with gonadal dysgenesis (see Chapter 1, Embryology of the Female Genital Tract and Disorders of Abnormal Sexual Development) usually have an abnormal karyotype, streak gonads or abdominal testes, primary amenorrhea, ambiguous internal and external genitalia, and somatic abnormalities.

The absence or decline in follicular activity in patients with POF typically results in low serum estrogen levels, often accompanied by estrogen withdrawal symptoms. Because of the failure of negative feedback, the low estrogen levels lead to elevated levels of pituitary gonadotropins, a feature that differentiates POF from central causes of amenorrhea related to hypothalamic or pituitary dysfunction.[391]

If the evaluation of a patient with hypergonadotropic POF is to include microscopic examination of ovarian tissue, the latter should be obtained by bilateral wedge biopsies at the time of laparotomy.[373] Although three histologi-

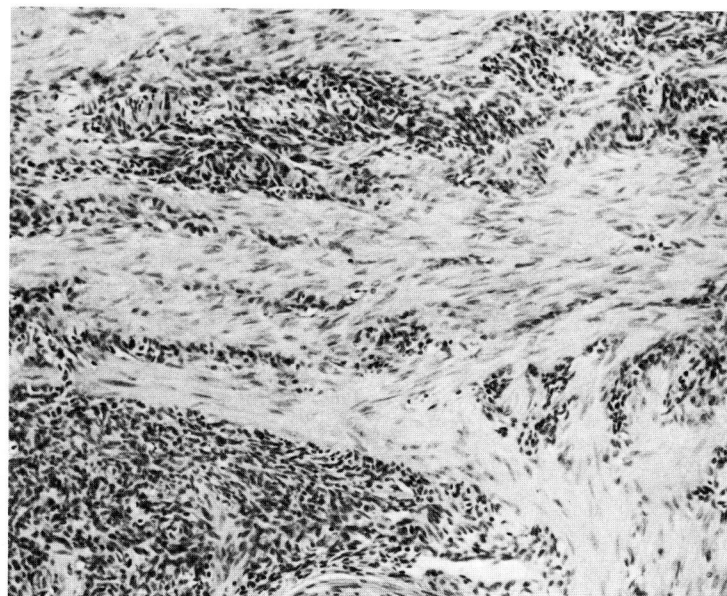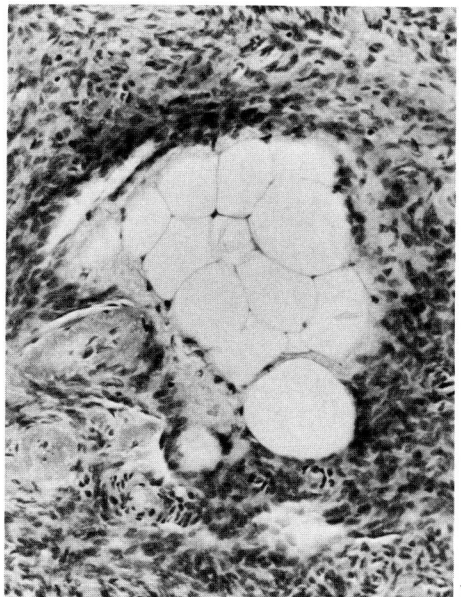

FIG. 16.40. Ovarian stromal metaplasia. a: Foci of smooth muscle are separated by ovarian stromal cells. **b:** A focus of adipose tissue lies within the ovarian stroma.

cal patterns have been recognized, specifically premature follicular depletion (true premature menopause), resistant ovary syndrome, and autoimmune oophoritis, it is not known with certainty if each represents a distinct disorder or a nonspecific morphologic manifestation of a number of different disorders.[391]

Premature Follicular Depletion

Premature follicular depletion is characterized by ovaries that typically are small on gross inspection, resembling streak gonads. On microscopic examination, there is premature follicular depletion, with the ovaries resembling normal peri- or postmenopausal ovaries with complete, or nearly complete, absence of primordial and developing follicles (Fig. 16.41).[56,236,391,507] Follicles in varying stages of atresia and stigmata of prior ovulation typically are present and exclude a streak gonad.

Postulated pathogenetic mechanisms include a decreased number of ovarian germ cells at birth, acceleration of normal follicular atresia, or prepubertal or postpubertal destruction of germ cells.[389] With respect to the latter, there is strong evidence, including the presence of antiovarian antibodies, autoimmune disorders, or both, implicating immune factors in a substantial proportion of women with POF. As some or all of these cases likely represent an end stage of autoimmune oophoritis, they are considered further in that section (see below).[390,391] Additionally, postnatal destruction of germ cells may be caused by cyto-

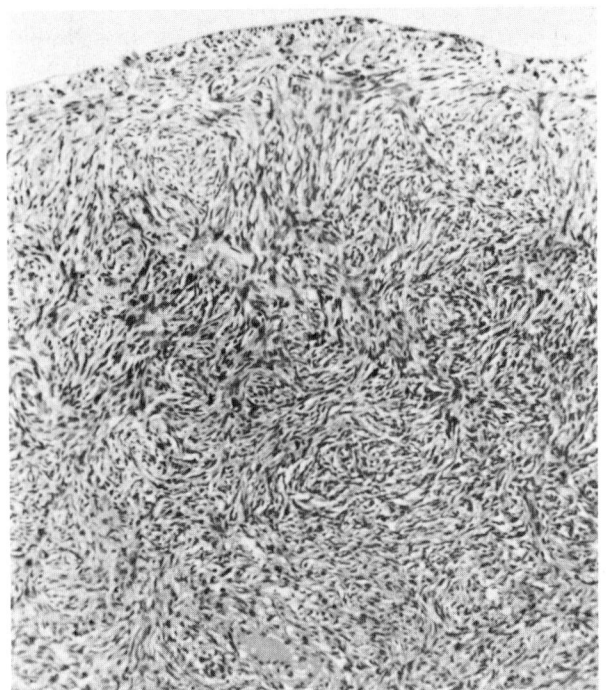

Fig. 16.41. Premature follicular depletion. No primordial or maturing follicles are present within the stroma.

toxic drugs (see page 631), radiation (see page 632), and mumps oophoritis (see page 603). Because mumps oophoritis probably is clinically occult in most cases, it may be a more frequent cause of premature menopause, including familial cases, than is generally suspected.[9,314]

The occurrence of familial cases of POF, in a pattern consistent with an autosomal dominant mode of inheritance,[106,292,428] implicates genetic factors in some cases. Occasional patients with an otherwise typical presentation have had chrosomal abnormalities, usually 47XXX, pure or mosaic, but occasionally 45XO/46XX.[56,389,471] In some familial cases, the affected women were 46XX but had an interstitial deletion of the long arm of the X chromosome.[245] Some authors, however, exclude cases with chromosomal abnormalities from the category of POF so that it includes only "chromosomally competent" patients.[13]

The presence of galactosemia in some patients with POF suggests that it may play a pathogenetic role. Approximately two-thirds of females with galactosemia in one study had POF.[226] In many such patients dietary treatment of galactosemia had been delayed. One galactosemic patient with POF had the pattern of the resistant ovary syndrome (see below) on ovarian biopsy, but in a series of galactosemic patients who were not biopsied, some patients had severely atrophic ovaries, suggesting premature follicular depletion.[202] Similarly, experimental studies indicate that galactose or its metabolites may interfere with normal prenatal oogenesis.[87]

Depletion of primordial follicles has been described in several women with ataxia telangiectasia, which may be related to their severe immunosuppression or to their athymic state.[61,152,307] Athymic mice have been shown to have low neonatal gonadotropin levels, an abnormality that is believed to result in disorganized folliculogenesis and premature follicular depletion observed in these animals. The existence of a thymic–ovarian–pituitary–hypothalamic axis also has been suggested to be present in human females.[152]

Resistant Ovary Syndrome

Resistant ovary syndrome, a rare syndrome, also known as Savage syndrome, is found in approximately 20% of patients with POF and is characterized by primary or secondary amenorrhea, endogenous hypergonadotropinemia, and resistance to exogenous gonadotropins, often in massive doses.° The resistance to endogenous and exogenous gonadotropins may be relative or absolute, episodic or chronic.

The ovaries typically have a normal prepubertal or adult appearance on macroscopic inspection. Microscopic examination reveals an appropriate number of normal-appearing primordial follicles, but a complete, or nearly complete, absence of developing follicles. Atretic follicles and stigmata of prior ovulation may be present. In occasional patients, the space normally occupied by the ovum in some of the atretic follicles contains calcified material.[47,171] In another case, numerous abnormal preantral follicles were found that contained multiple nodules of basement membrane material.[289] A histological pattern similar to that in the resistant ovary syndrome occurs in morbid obesity,[146] Cushing's syndrome,[204] and hypogonadotropic ovarian failure secondary to hypothalamic–pituitary dysfunction.[383]

The pathogenesis of this disorder is not yet established, but a possible deficiency of FSH and LH receptors within the ovary, the presence of antibodies to these receptors, or a postreceptor defect have been postulated.[239,455] An IgG-like substance that alters FSH receptors and thereby impairs binding of this hormone was present in the serum of several patients with associated myasthenia gravis.[86,132,246] In another patient with the resistant ovary syndrome, lupus erythematosus appeared while the ovarian failure was evolving, and a serum antibody specific for the FSH receptor was found.[289] In another study, circulating autoimmune antibodies to thyroglobulin and smooth muscle were found in some patients.[391] As noted above, one patient with resistant ovary syndrome had galactosemia.[391]

Autoimmune Oophoritis

CLINICAL AND PATHOGENETIC FEATURES

Approximately 25 cases of autoimmune oophoritis have been documented pathologically.° The patients, who have ranged in age from 17 to 48 years (mean, 31 years), typically present with oligomenorrhea or amenorrhea, or symptoms relating to multiple follicular cysts, including pelvic pain, adnexal torsion, and estrogenic manifestations, such as abnormal bleeding, and in one case, endometrial adenocarcinoma.[26,51,268] Most patients have steroid cell antibodies in their sera; Addison's disease, Hashimoto's thyroiditis, or both, also have been present in some cases.[26] The Addison's disease may arise at the same time or subsequent to the ovarian failure, and is associated in at least some cases with a lymphocytic adrenalitis. The steroid cell antibodies, which are rare in the general population, belong to a group of antibodies reactive with a range of antigens in steroid-producing cells.[207] They are typically reactive against adrenal cortex, but in some cases also to theca interna, corpus luteum, thyroid epithelium and thyroglobulin, parathyroid cells, gastric parietal cells, and thymocytes, alone or in combination.† The antiovarian antibodies are cross-reactive with antigens in the adrenal cortex,[207,209–211] are cytotoxic to human granulosa cells in

tissue culture,[297] and have been localized by immunohistochemical methods to granulosa cells and oocytes.

There also is evidence supporting a role for cell-mediated immune mechanisms in the pathogenesis of autoimmune oophoritis. These include clinical studies,[126,368] in vitro assays,[126] and experimental murine models.[205,395] Recent studies have shown expression of major histocompatibility class II antigens by granulosa cells in autoimmune oophoritis, a phenomenon inducible by interferon gamma, a product of activated T cells.[194] Additionally, there have been reports of occasional patients with POF, including some with documented autoimmune oophoritis, in whom menses and ovulation resumed after administration of corticosteroids.[107,140,368] All of the foregoing observations suggest that a complex immune process with an interplay of humoral and cellular mechanisms is involved in the pathogenesis of autoimmune oophoritis.[415]

Autoimmune oophoritis is almost certainly more common than the small number of histologically documented cases would suggest. In two studies of women of POF who were not biopsied or in whom a biopsy revealed an afollicular pattern, two-thirds[353] and 90%[305] of patients, respectively, had some evidence of autoimmune phenomena with immunologic testing. In a third study, some women with POF had a decreased ratio of inducer/helper lymphocytes to suppressor/cytotoxic lymphocytes, as well as a decreased concentration of serum IgA, suggesting a mild suppression of immune competence.[152] Similarly, as many as one-half of patients with POF in some series have or subsequently develop one or more associated autoimmune disorders; an average figure calculated from the literature since 1980 is 20%.[248] Addison's disease or thyroid disease (Hashimoto's thyroiditis, Grave's disease) are the most common of these disorders, and typically are accompanied or preceded by the presence of steroid cell antibodies.[4,11,102,208,209] Conversely, as may as 25% of patients with idiopathic Addison's disease may have POF,[209] the latter usually preceding the former by several, but occasionally many years.[248] Other autoimmune diseases that occur less commonly in these patients include rheumatoid arthritis, hypoparathyroidism, myasthenia gravis, diabetes mellitus, atrophic gastritis, pernicious anemia, hemolytic anemia, idiopathic thrombocytopenia purpura, alopecia, vitiligo, and sicca syndrome.° POF occurs frequently in patients with two or more such diseases (polyglandular endocrinopathy).[248]

Additionally, a subgroup of patients with POF have chronic mucocutaneous candidiasis or chronic vaginal candidiasis, suggesting a defect in T-cell function, possibly secondary to circulating antibodies against T lymphocytes demonstrable in some of these patients.[291] Patients with

---

°Refs. 26,51,104,151,170,207,211,268,288,368,391,415,496
†Refs. 16,18,93,112,211,390,391,469,489.

°Refs. 11,16,18,93,102,126,209,211,390,469,489.

these two types of candidiasis also frequently have anti-*Candida*, antithymocyte, and antiovarian antibodies, suggesting a shared antigen on these cells.[291] A partial genetic basis is suggested by a family history of an autoimmune disease in 18% of patients in one study who had both POF and an autoimmune disease.[11] Similarly, a prevalence of certain human leukocyte (HLA) antigens has been found in some patients with autoimmune endocrine disease.[140,474] The foregoing findings suggest that a substantial proportion of patients with the histological pattern of premature follicular depletion likely represent an end stage of autoimmune oophoritis that is no longer recognizable on histological examination.

Gross Findings

On gross examination, the ovaries may be small or normal in size, but in one-third of cases one or both ovaries are enlarged by multiple follicular cysts.[26,51,268] The follicular cysts are more common in the earlier phases of the disease and are likely due to elevated pituitary gonadotropins.[51] Small ovaries presumably reflect a late or end stage of the disorder, after complete destruction of the follicles.[51]

Microscopic Findings

The cardinal feature on microscopic examination is a folliculotropic lymphoid infiltrate that affects developing follicles with a theca layer, corpora lutea, and atretic follicles (Fig. 16.42). The intensity of the inflammatory infiltrate increases with the degree of follicular maturation. The theca interna layer typically is infiltrated more intensely than the granulosa layer and may be focally destroyed; the granulosa layer may be focally disrupted with sloughing of granulosa cells. The inflammatory infiltrate consists predominantly of lymphocytes and plasma cells, but eosinophils, histiocytes, and rarely, sarcoid-like granulomas also are present, or even predominate.[26] Primordial follicles typically are present but uninvolved.[26] Additionally, perivascular and perineural lymphoid infiltrates may be found in the hilus, and in some such cases, there has been an absence of Leydig cells, suggesting destruction of the latter by the inflammatory process.[170,288] Nonspecific findings have included the presence of abnormal "dysplastic" follicles,[26] follicle cysts (as noted above), and superficial cortical fibrosis.[26] Immunophenotyping of the inflammatory infiltrate has revealed, variously, B and T lymphocytes, polyclonal plasma cells, macrophages, and natural killer cells.[151,170,268,415]

Vascular Lesions

Ovarian Hemorrhage

Rupture of the normal corpus luteum or a corpus luteum cyst occasionally may result in hemorrhage and, rarely, fatal he-

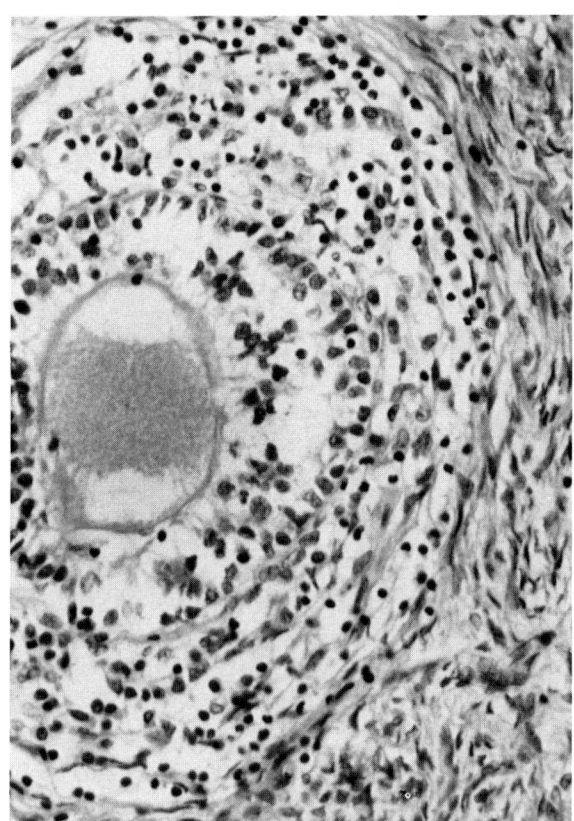

Fig. 16.42. Autoimmune oophoritis. A maturing follicle is infiltrated by mononuclear inflammatory cells.

moperitoneum. Although hemorrhage may occur in otherwise normal women, it is observed more often in women receiving anticoagulant therapy (Figure 16.43).[180,355,416] The right ovary is the source of the hemorrhage in almost two-thirds of patients, and the clinical manifestations frequently resemble acute appendicitis.[180]

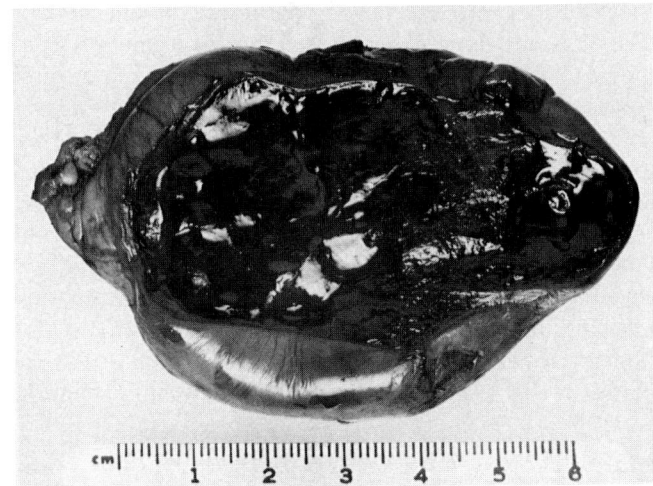

Fig. 16.43. Ovarian hemorrhage. Ovary from a patient being treated with anticoagulation therapy is replaced by a large hematoma.

Ovarian Torsion

Ovarian or adnexal torsion most frequently is a complication of an underlying ovarian lesion, usually a nonneoplastic cyst, abscess, or benign tumor, but rarely a malignant neoplasm.[21,116] Less commonly, torsion of a normal ovary may occur, especially in infants or children[134,176,407] but also in adults.[192] The etiology of the torsion in females with normal adnexa is not known, but an unusual degree of adnexal mobility has been noted in children at postmortem examination.[407] Bilateral adnexal torsion, synchronous or asynchronous, has been rarely reported.[125]

The patients present with clinical findings similar to those of acute appendicitis or recurrent episodes of abdominal pain and, occasionally, a palpable adnexal mass. Laparotomy reveals a swollen, hemorrhagic, and in some cases infarcted, tuboovarian mass twisted on its pedicle. In rare cases the torsion and infarction may be asymptomatic.[21,44,45,335] In such cases autoamputation can result in a separate, occasionally calcified, mass lying free or attached to adjacent structures in the peritoneal cavity. The differential diagnosis in such cases, as noted earlier, is with congenital unilateral absence of the ovary and tube.

Ovarian Vein Thrombophlebitis

Ovarian vein thrombosis or thrombophlebitis is an uncommon but potentially fatal disorder that most often occurs postpartum, but may follow pelvic operations or pelvic trauma or complicate other pelvic disorders such as pelvic inflammatory disease.[122,319] Patients usually present with fever and lower abdominal pain and an abdominal mass, almost always on the right side. The clinical picture may simulate acute appendicitis. The marked right-sided predominance in the puerperal cases is explained on the basis of retrograde venous flow in the left ovarian vein during the puerperium, protecting that side from bacterial spread from the uterus[319] or, as documented in one case, amniotic fluid embolism.[231] Sonography, computed tomographic scanning, and magnetic resonance imaging studies may be useful in establishing the diagnosis preoperatively.[24,68,234]

At operation, the involved ovarian vein is markedly enlarged and the thrombus usually extends to the inferior vena cava on the right or to the renal vein on the left.[23] Rarely one or both of the latter structures also are thrombosed.[23] There is marked edema and inflammation of the surrounding retroperitoneal tissues. The ipsilateral ovary usually is congested but not infarcted, although asymptomatic bilateral ovarian infarction in a postpartum patient secondary to massive pelvic venous thrombosis has been reported.[162] Some cases may be associated with the ovarian vein syndrome (see next section).

Rare Vascular Lesions

Giant cell arteritis rarely can involve the female genital tract, including the ovaries.[39,280] The patients are almost invariably postmenopausal. Most patients with ovarian involvement have had systemic manifestations, such as a history of polymyagia rheumatica or temporal arteritis, an elevated erythrocyte sedimentation rate (ESR), or both. Less commonly, the arteritis is an incidental microscopic finding in an asymptomatic patient. Treatment probably is unnecessary in this group of patients, but they should be followed carefully, including repeated determinations of the ESR.[39,280] Rare examples of systemic polyarteritis nodosa with ovarian involvement also have been reported.[266]

A rare cause of retroperitoneal hemorrhage is rupture of an ovarian artery or vein, typically during pregnancy or the puerperium.[72,166,178,214] In some cases, the rupture represents a complication of an aneurysm of the ovarian artery.[72,214]

Varicosities of the ovarian vein, almost always on the right side, may occur in pregnant or parous women and cause ipsilateral ureteric compression and pyelonephritis, constituting the so-called ovarian vein syndrome.[200] Ovarian arteriovenous fistulas have been reported as a rare complication of gynecological surgery.[452]

Ovarian Changes Secondary to Metabolic Diseases

Amyloidosis rarely may involve the ovaries, typically representing an incidental histological finding in patients with systemic amyloidosis (Fig. 16.44).[98] There has been a single case of tumorous amyloidosis confined to the ovary that was associated with endometriosis in that site.[396]

Rare cases of ovarian enlargement secondary to involvement by systemic storage disorders (lipidoses, mucopolysaccharides) have been reported.[120,476] In such cases, the stored material typically is within macrophages, allowing histological distinction from a steroid cell tumor and from foci of mature adipose tissue within the ovarian stroma. An autopsy study in patients with diabetes mellitus revealed atrophic and fibrotic changes in the ovaries more frequently than in ovaries from control patients, although the differences were not statistically significant.[150]

In contrast to frequent testicular involvement in hemochromatosis in which hemosiderin is typically seen within walls of testicular blood vessels,[286] pathological changes in the ovary secondary to this disorder appear to be rare or nonexistent.

Ovarian Changes Secondary to Cytotoxic Drugs and Radiation

Cytotoxic Drugs

Cytotoxic drugs may cause a variety of histological changes in the ovaries of prepubertal and postpubertal patients, including focal or diffuse cortical fibrosis, impaired follicu-

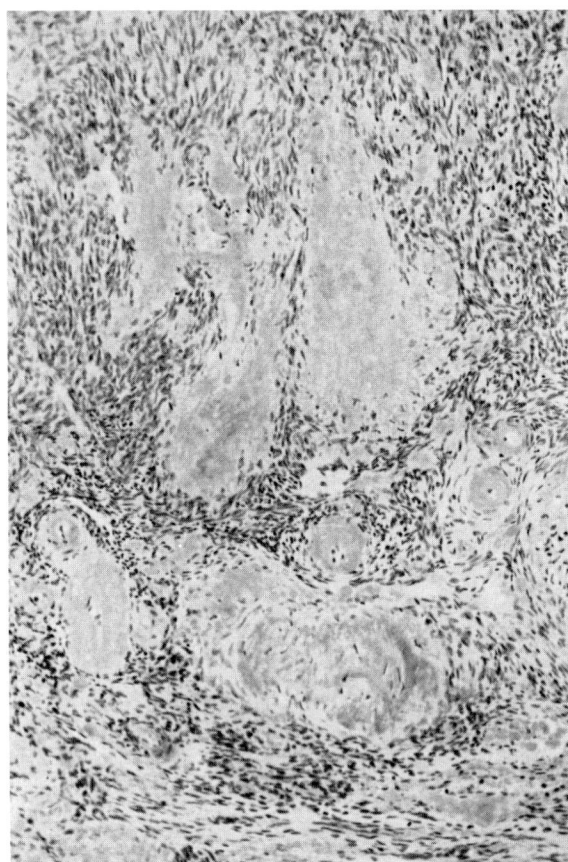

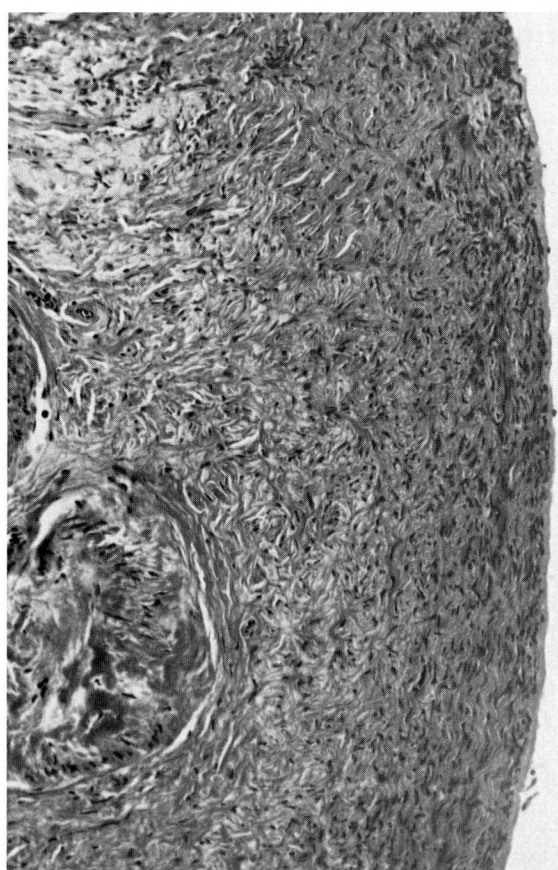

FIG. 16.44. **Ovarian amyloidosis.** Amyloid involves the ovarian stroma and vessels.

FIG. 16.45. **Radiation changes.** The ovarian stroma is fibrotic, and blood vessels are hyalinized.

lar maturation, and a reduction or depletion in follicle numbers.[195,196,244,279,313,334,475,477] Some studies have shown a direct correlation between the severity of these changes and the duration of the chemotherapy, the number of drugs, and malnourishment of the patients.[196,334] These morphologic findings are consistent with clinical observations of diminished ovarian endocrine function or ovarian failure in some of these patients.[36,84,313,403,426,475,484]

The risk of ovarian failure appears to be greater in patients in whom treatment is begun after the age of 25 years.[36,403] In rare cases, the ovarian failure has reversed after cessation of the therapy.[426,475]

Radiation

The ovary is among the most radiosensitive of organs. Relatively low doses of radiation (500–600 R) to the ovaries cause complete or nearly complete disappearance of primordial and developing follicles, fibrosis of the ovarian stroma, and vascular sclerosis in more than 90% of patients (Fig. 16.45).[25,145,175,195,388] Follow-up studies of both children and adults who received pelvic radiation have shown that ovarian failure occurs in most such pa-

tients.[121,195,417,448] The ovarian stroma appears to be more radioresistant than the follicles and may continue to secrete androgens after radiation.[215]

References

1. Abraham GE, Buster JE (1976) Peripheral and ovarian steroids in ovarian hyperthecosis. Obstet Gynecol 47: 581–586

2. Adashi EY, Hsueh AJW, Yen SSC (1981) Insulin enhancement of luteinizing hormone and follicle-stimulating hormone release by cultured pituitary cells. Endocrinology 108: 1441–1449

3. Adelman S, Benson CD, Hertzler JH (1975) Surgical lesions of the ovary in infancy and childhood. Surg Gynecol Obstet 141: 219–222

4. Ahonen P, Miettinen A, Perheentupa J (1987) Adrenal and steroidal cell antibodies in patients with autoimmune polyglandular disease type I and risk of adrenocortical and ovarian failure. J Clin Endocrinol Metab 64: 494–500

5. Aikat BK, Radhakrishnan VV, Rao MS (1973) Malakoplakia–a report of two cases with review of the literature. Ind J Path Bact 16: 64–70

6. Aiman J, Edman CD, Worley RJ, et al (1978) Androgen

and estrogen formation in women with ovarian hyperthecosis. Obstet Gynecol 51: 1–19

7. Aiman J, Smentek C (1985) Premature ovarian failure. Obstet Gynecol 66: 9–14

8. Al Dawoud A, Yates R, Foulis AK (1991) Postoperative necrotizing granulomas in the ovary. J Clin Pathol 44: 524–525

9. Aleem FA (1981) Familial 46,XX gonadal dysgenesis. Fertil Steril 35: 317–320

10. Almenoff IA (1966) Splenic-gonadal fusion. N Y State J Med 66:1679–1691.

11. Alper MM, Garner PR (1985) Premature ovarian failure: Its relationship to autoimmune disease. Obstet Gynecol 66: 27–30

12. Alper MM, Jolly EE, Garner PR (1986) Pregnancies after premature ovarian failure. Obstet Gynecol 67: 59S–62S

13. Altman LC (1972) Ovarian abscess and vaginal fistula. Obstet Gynecol 40: 321–322

14. Andreoli C, Vischi F (1961) Parotitis and ovaritis. Panminerva Med 3: 358–361

15. Annos T, Taymor ML (1981) Ovarian pathology associated with insulin resistance and acanthosis nigricans. Obstet Gynecol 58: 662–664

16. Appel GB, Holub DA (1976) The syndrome of multiple endocrine gland insufficiency. Am J Med 61: 129–133

17. Arean VM (1956) Manson's schistosomiasis of the female genital tract. Am J Obstet Gynecol 72: 1038–1053

18. Ayala A, Canales ES, Karchmer S, et al (1979) Premature ovarian failure and hypothyroidism associated with sicca syndrome. Obstet Gynecol 53: 98S–101S

19. Ayers JWT (1982) Differential response to adrenocorticotropin hormone stimulation in polycystic ovarian disease with high and low dehydroepiandrosterone sulfate levels. Fertil Steril 37: 645–649

20. Azhar H (1977) Primary echinococcal infection of the ovary. Br J Obstet Gynaecol 84: 633

21. Azoury RS, Chehab RM, Mufarrij IK (1980) The twisted adnexa. A clinical pathological review. Diagn Gynecol Obstet 2: 185–191

22. Bahary CM, Ovadia Y, Neri A (1967) Schistosoma mansoni of the ovary. Am J Obstet Gynecol 98: 290–292

23. Bahnson RR, Wendel EF, Vogelzang RL (1985) Renal vein thrombosis following puerperal ovarian vein thrombophlebitis. Am J Obstet Gynecol 152: 290–291

24. Baka JJ, Lev-Toaff AS, Friedman AC, et al (1989) Ovarian vein thrombosis with atypical presentation: Role of sonography and duplex doppler. Obstet Gynecol 73: 887–889

25. Baker TG (1971) Radiosensitivity of mammalian oocytes with particular reference to the human female. Am J Obstet Gynecol 110: 746–761

26. Bannatyne P, Russell P, Shearman RP (1990) Autoimmune oophoritis: A clinicopathologic assessment of 12 case. Int J Gynecol Pathol 9: 191–207

27. Bar RS, Muggeo M, Kahn CR, et al (1980) Characterization of insulin receptors in patients with the syndromes of insulin resistance and acanthosis nigricans. Diabetologia 18: 209

28. Barbieri RL, Makris A, Ryan KJ (1984) Insulin stimulates androgen accumulation in incubations of human ovarian stroma and theca. Obstet Gynecol 64: 73S–80S

29. Barbieri RL, Makris A, Randall RW, et al (1986) Insulin stimulates androgen accumulation in incubations of ovarian stroma obtained from women with hyperandrogenism. J Clin Endocrinol Metab 62: 904–910

30. Barbieri RL, Ryan KJ (1983) Hyperandrogenism, insulin resistance, and acanthosis nigricans syndrome: A common endocrinopathy with distinct pathophysiologic features. Am J Obstet Gynecol 147: 90–101

31. Barbieri RL, Smith S, Ryan KJ (1988) The role of hyperinsulinemia in the pathogenesis of ovarian hyperandrogenism. Fertil Steril 50: 197–212

32. Barclay DL, Leverich EB, Kemmerly JR (1969) Hyperreactio luteinalis: Postpartum persistence. Am J Obstet Gynecol 105: 642–644

33. Bardin CW, Lipsett MB, Edgcomb JH, Marshall JR (1967) Studies of testosterone metabolism in a patient with masculinization due to stromal hyperthecosis. N Engl J Med 277: 399–402

34. Barnes ND, Hayles AB, Ryan RJ (1973) Sexual maturation in juvenile hypothyroidism. Mayo Clin Proc 48: 849–856

35. Bates GW, Whitworth NS (1982) Effect of body weight reduction on plasma androgens in obese, infertile women. Fertil Steril 38: 406–409

36. Beard MEJ, Conder JL, Clark VA (1984) Ovarian failure following cytotoxic therapy. NZ Med J 97: 759–762

37. Beckman EN, Holland JB (1981) Ovarian enterobiasis—a proposed pathogenesis. Am J Trop Hyg 30:74–76

38. Belisle S, Lehoux J-G, Benard B, Ainmelk Y (1981) Ovarian hyperthecosis: In vivo and in vitro correlations of the androgen profile. Obstet Gynecol 57: 70S–75S

39. Bell DA, Mondschein M, Scully RE (1986) Giant cell arteritis of the female genital tract. A report of three cases. Am J Surg Pathol 10: 696–701

40. Benirschke K, Bonin ML, Rost T (1984) Plant material in ovary following barium enema. (Letter) Arch Pathol Lab Med 108: 359–360

41. Ben-Rafael Z, Bider D, Menashe Y, et al (1990) Follicular and luteal cysts after treatment with gonadotropin-releasing hormone analogue for in vitro fertilization. Fertil Steril 53: 1091–1094

42. Berger NG, Repke JT, Woodruff JD (1984) Markedly elevated serum testosterone in pregnancy without fetal virilization. Obstet Gynecol 63: 260–262

43. Bersch W, Alexy E, Heuser HP, Staemmler HJ (1973) Ectopic decidua formation in the ovary (so-called deciduoma). Virch Archiv A (Pathol Anat) 360: 173–177

44. Best CL, Feldman DB, Sobenes JR, Sueldo CE (1991) Unexplained displacement of ipsilateral ovary and fallopian tube. Obstet Gynecol 78: 558–560

45. Beyth Y, Bar-On E (1984) Tuboovarian autoamputation and infertility. Fertil Steril 42: 932–934

46. Bhagavan BS, Gupta PK (1978) Genital actinomycosis and intrauterine contraceptive devices. Hum Pathol 9: 567–578

47. Biberoglu KO, Damewood MD, Parmley T, Rock JA (1988) Insensitive ovary syndrome with a unique process of follicular degeneration. Fertil Steril 49: 367–369

48. Bigelow B (1958) Comparison of ovarian and endometrial morphology spanning the menopause. Obstet Gynecol 11: 487–513

49. Biggs JSG (1981) Polycystic ovarian disease—current concepts. Aust NZ J Obstet Gynaecol 21: 26–36

50. Biggs JSG, Thomas FJ (1981) Sites of steroid production in the polycystic ovary. Br J Obstet Gynaecol 88: 42–46

51. Biscotti CV, Hart WR, Lucas JG (1989) Cystic ovarian enlargement resulting from autoimmune oophoritis. Obstet Gynecol 74: 492–495

52. Blaustein A (1981) Surface cells and inclusion cysts in fetal ovaries. Gynecol Oncol 12: 222–233

53. Blaustein A, Kaganowicz A, Wells J (1982) Tumor markers in inclusion cysts of the ovary. Cancer 49: 722–726

54. Blaustein A, Kantius M, Kaganowicz A, et al (1982) Inclusions in ovaries of females aged day 1–30 years. Int J Gynecol Pathol 1: 145–153

55. Bloomfield RD, Suarez JR, Malangit AC (1979) Giant theca–lutein cyst. Am J Obstet Gynecol 133: 459–460

56. Board JA, Redwine FO, Moncure CW, et al (1979) Identification of differing etiologies of clinically diagnosed premature menopause. Am J Obstet Gynecol 134: 936–944

57. Boder E, Sedgwick RP (1958) Ataxia-telangiectasia. A familial syndrome of progressive cerebellar ataxia, oculocutaneous telangiectasia and frequent pulmonary infection. Pediatr 21: 526–554

58. Bohm J, Roder-Weber M, Hofler H, Kolben M (1991) Bilateral stromal Leydig cell tumour of the ovary. Case report and literature review. Path Res Pract 187: 348–352

59. Bonar BE, Rabson AS (1957) Gynecological aspects of leprosy. Obstet Gynecol 9: 33–43

60. Boss JH, Scully RE, Wegner KH, Cohen RB (1965) Structural variations in the adult ovary—clinical significance. Obstet Gynecol 25: 747–763

61. Bowden DH, Danis PG, Sommers SC (1963) Ataxia-telangiectasia. A case with lesions of ovaries and adenohypophysis. J Neuropathol Exp Neurol 22: 549–554

62. Bower R, Dehner LP, Ternberg JL (1974) Bilateral ovarian cysts in the newborn. A triad of neonatal abdominal masses, polyhydramnios, and maternal diabetes mellitus. A J Dig Dis 128: 731–733

63. Bradshaw KD, Carr BR (1986) Ovarian and tubal inguinal hernia. Obstet Gynecol 68: 50S–51S

64. Bradshaw KD, Santos-Ramos R, Rawlins SC, et al (1986) Endocrine studies in a pregnancy complicated by ovarian theca lutein cysts and hyperreactio luteinalis. Obstet Gynecol 67: 66S–69S

65. Bradley B, Gleicher N (1980) Grand multiparity associated with unilateral renal, ovarian, and mullerian agenesis. Mt Sinai J Med 47: 418–422

66. Braithwaite SS, Erkman-Balis B, Avila TD (1978) Postmenopausal virilization due to ovarian stromal hyperthecosis. J Clin Endocrinol Metab 46: 295–300

67. Brooks JJ, Wheeler JE (1977) Granulomatous salpingitis secondary to Crohn's disease. Obstet Gynecol 49: 31S–37S

68. Brown CEL, Lowe TW, Cunningham FG, Weinreb JC (1986) Puerperal pelvic thrombophlebitis: Impact on diagnosis and treatment using x-ray computed tomography and magnetic resonance imaging. Obstet Gynecol 68: 789–794

69. Brune WH, Pulaski EJ, Shuey HE (1957) Giant ovarian cyst. Report of a case in a premature infant. N Engl J Med 257: 876–878

70. Burghen GA, Givens JR, Kitabchi AE (1980) Correlation of hyperandrogenism with hyperinsulinemia in polycystic ovarian disease. J Clin Endocrinol Metab 50: 113–116

71. Burkman R, Schlesselman S, McCaffrey L, et al (1982) The relationship of genital tract actinomycetes and the development of pelvic inflammatory disease. Am J Obstet Gynecol 143: 585–589

72. Burnett RA, Carfrae DC (1976) Spontaneous rupture of ovarian artery aneurysm in the puerperium. Two case reports and a review of the literature. Br J Obstet Gynaecol 83: 744–750

73. Burt AS (1954) The human hypophysis in ovarian stromal hyperplasia and pregnancy. Cancer 7: 1227–1234

74. Bychkov V, Kijek M (1987) Massive ovarian edema. Four cases and some pathogenetic considerations. Acta Obstet Gynecol Scand 66: 397–399

75. Bylund DJ, Nanfro JJ, Marsh WL Jr (1986) Coccidiooidomycosis of the female genital tract. Arch Pathol Lab Med 110: 232–235

76. Byrne P, Vella EJ, Rollason T, Frampton J (1989) Ovarian fibromatosis with minor sex cord elements. Case report. Br J Obstet Gynaecol 96: 245–248

77. Caillouette JC, Koehler AL (1987) Phasic contraceptive pills and functional ovarian cysts. Am J Obstet Gynecol 156: 1538–1542

78. Campenhout JV, Vauclair R, Maraghi K (1972) Gonadotropin-resistant ovaries in primary amenorrhea. Obstet Gynecol 40: 6–12

79. Caspi E, Schreyer P, Bukovsky J (1973) Ovarian lutein cysts in pregnancy. Obstet Gynecol 42: 388–398

80. Chalvardjian A (1978) Sarcoidosis of the female genital tract. Am J Obstet Gynecol 132: 78–80

81. Chalvardjian A, Picard L, Shaw R, et al (1980) Malacoplakia of the female genital tract. Am J Obstet Gynecol 138: 391–394

82. Chalvardjian A, Scully RE (1973) Sclerosing stromal tumors of the ovary. Cancer 31: 664–670

83. Chang RJ, Nakamura RM, Judd HL, Kaplan SA (1983) Insulin resistance in nonobese patients with polycystic ovarian disease. J Clin Endocrinol Metab 57:356–359

84. Chapman RM (1983) Gonadal injury resulting from chemotherapy. Am J Indust Med 4: 149–161

85. Charpin C, Bhan AK, Zurawski VR Jr, Scully RE (1982) Carcinoembryonic antigen (CEA) and carbohydrate determinant 19-9 (CA 19-9) localization in 121 primary and metastatic ovarian tumors: An immunohistochemical study with the use of monoclonal antibodies. Int J Gynecol Pathol 1: 231–245

86. Charreau EH, Chiauzzi V, Cigorraga S, et al (1982) Immunoglobulin anti FSH receptor in the resistant ovary syndrome. Rec Adv Fertil Res Part A: 111–121

87. Chen YT, Mattison DR, Schulman JD (1981) Hypogonadism and galactosemia. (Letter) N Engl J Med 305:464

88. Chervenak FA, Castadot MJ, Wiederman J, Sedlis A (1980) Massive ovarian edema: Review of world literature and report of two cases. Obstet Gynecol Surv 35: 677–684

89. Chow KK, Choo HT (1984) Ovarian hyperstimulation syndrome with clomiphene citrate. Case report. Br J Obstet Gynaecol 91: 1051–1052

90. Claman P, Dover M, Saginur R, et al (1991) Spontaneous ovarian-to-vaginal fistula: A case report. Am J Obstet Gynecol 164: 71–72

91. Clement PB, Scully RE (1980) Large solitary luteinized

follicle cyst of pregnancy and puerperium. Am J Surg Pathol 4: 431–438

92. Clement PB, Cooney TP (1992) Idiopathic multifocal calcification of the ovarian stroma. Arch Pathol Lab Med 116: 204–205

93. Collen RJ, Lippe BM, Kaplan SA (1979) Primary ovarian failure, juvenile rheumatoid arthritis, and vitiligo. Am J Dis Child 133: 598–600

94. Collins CG, Nix FG, Cerha HT (1956) Ruptured tuboovarian abscess. Am J Obstet Gynecol 72: 820–829

95. Comite F, Shawker TH, Pescovitz OH, et al (1984) Cyclical ovarian function resistent to treatment with an analogue of luteinizing hormone releasing hormone in McCune-Albright syndrome. N Engl J Med 311: 1032–1036

96. Coney P (1984) Polycystic ovarian disease: Current concepts of pathophysiology and therapy. Fertil Steril 42: 667–682

97. Cooper HE, Spellacy WN, Prem KA, Cohen WD (1968) Hereditary factors in the Stein–Leventhal syndrome. Am J Obstet Gynecol 100: 371–387

98. Copeland W Jr, Hawley PC, Teteris NJ (1985) Gynecologic amyloidosis. Am J Obstet Gynecol 153: 555–556

99. Cordon-Cardo C, Mattes MJ, Melamed MR, et al (1985) Immunopathologic analysis of a panel of mouse monoclonal antibodies reacting with human ovarian carcinomas and other human tumors. Int J Gynecol Pathol 4: 121–130

100. Corenblum B, Taylor PJ (1982) The hyperprolactinemic polycystic ovary syndrome may not be a distinct entity. Fertil Steril 38: 549–552

101. Coulam CB (1982) Premature gonadal failure. Fertil Steril 38: 645–655

102. Coulam CB (1983) The prevalence of autoimmune disorders among patients with primary ovarian failure. Am J Reprod Immunol 4: 63–66

103. Coulam CB, Annegers JF, Kranz JS (1983) Chronic anovulation syndrome and associated neoplasia. Obstet Gynecol 61: 403–407

104. Coulam CB, Kempers RD, Randall RV (1981) Premature ovarian failure: Evidence for autoimmune function. Fertil Steril 36: 238–240

105. Coulam CB, Ryan RJ (1979) Premature menopause I. Etiology. Am J Obstet Gynecol 133: 639–643

106. Coulam CB, Stringfellow S, Hoefnagel D (1983) Evidence for a genetic factor in the etiology of premature ovarian failure. Fertil Steril 40: 693–695

107. Cowchock FS, McCabe JL, Montgomery BB (1988) Pregnancy after corticosteroid administration in premature ovarian failure (polyglandular endocrinopathy syndrome). Am J Obstet Gynecol 158: 118–119

108. Cozzutto C (1981) Uterus-like mass replacing ovary. Arch Pathol Lab Med 105: 508–511

109. Cramer DW, Welch WR, Cassells S, Scully RE (1983) Mumps, menarche, menopause, and ovarian cancer. Am J Obstet Gynecol 147: 1–6

110. Cruikshank SH, Van Drie DM (1982) Supernumerary ovaries: Update and review. Obstet Gynecol 60: 126–129

111. Curry SL, Hammond CB, Tyrey L, et al (1975) Hydatidiform mole. Diagnosis, management, and long-term followup of 347 patients. Obstet Gynecol 45: 1–8

112. Damewood MD, Zacur HA, Hoffman GJ, Rock JA (1986) Circulating antiovarian antibodies in premature ovarian failure. Obstet Gynecol 68: 850–854

113. Danon M, Robboy SJ, Kim S, et al. (1975) Cushing syndrome, sexual precocity and polyostotic fibrous dysplasia (Albright syndrome) in infancy. J Pediatr 87: 917–921

114. D'Armiento M, Reda G, Camagna A, Tardella L (1983) McCune-Albright syndrome: Evidence for autonomous multiendocrine function. J Pediatr 102: 584–586

115. Davidson BJ, Waisman J, Judd HL (1981) Longstanding virilism in a woman with hyperplasia and neoplasia of ovarian lipidic cells. Obstet Gynecol 58: 753–759

116. Demopoulos RI, Bigelow B, Vasa U (1978) Infarcted uterine adnexa. Associated pathology. N Y State J Med 78: 2027–2029.

117. Dennefors BL, Janson PO, Knutson F, Hamberger L (1980) Steroid production and responsiveness to gonadotropin in isolated stromal tissue of human postmenopausal ovaries. Am J Obstet Gynecol 136: 997–1002

118. Dewhurst CJ, de Koos EB, Ferreira HP (1975) The resistant ovary syndrome. Br J Obstet Gynaecol 82: 341–345

119. Dillon WP, Dewey M (1981) A case of accessory ovary. Obstet Gynecol 58: 660–661

120. Dincsoy HP, Rolfes DB, McGraw CA, Schubert WK (1984) Cholesterol ester shortage disease and mesenteric lipodystrophy. Am J Clin Pathol 81: 263–269

121. Doll R, Smith PG (1968) The long-term effects of X irradiation in patients treated for metropathia haemorrhagica. Br J Radiol 41: 362–368

122. Duff P, Gibbs RF (1983) Pelvic vein thrombophlebitis: Diagnostic dilemma and therapeutic challenge. Obstet Gynecol Surv 38: 365–373

123. Dunaif A, Futterweit W (1988) Polycystic ovary syndrome. (Letter) N Engl J Med 319: 584

124. Dunaif A, Hoffman AR, Scully RE, et al (1985) Clinical, biochemical, and ovarian morphologic features in women with acanthosis nigricans and masculinization. Obstet Gynecol 66: 545–552

125. Dunnihoo DR, Wolff J (1984) Bilateral torsion of the adnexa: A case report and a review of the world literature. Obstet Gynecol 64: 55S–59S

126. Edmonds M, Lamki L, Killinger DW, Volpe R (1973) Autoimmune thyroiditis, adrenalitis and oophoritis. Am J Med 54: 782–787

127. Eichhorn JH, Scully RE (1991) Ovarian myxoma: Clinicopathologic and immunocytologic analysis of five cases and a review of the literature. Int J Gynecol Pathol 10: 156–169

128. Erickson GF, Hsueh AJW, Quigley ME, et al (1979) Functional studies of aromatase activity in human granulosa cells from normal and polycystic ovaries. J Clin Endocrinol Metab 49: 514–519

129. Erkkola R, Seppala P, Klemi PJ (1985) Virilization during pregnancy due to bilateral hyperthecosis. Horm Res 21: 83–87

130. Eschenbach DA (1980) Epidemiology and diagnosis of acute pelvic inflammatory disease. Obstet Gynecol 55: 142S–152S

131. Eschenbach DA, Harnisch JP, Holmes KK (1977) Pathogenesis of acute pelvic inflammatory disease: Role of contraception and other risk factors. Am J Obstet Gynecol 128: 838–850

132. Escobar ME, Cigorraga SB, Chiauzzi VA, et al (1982) Development of gonadotropin resistant ovary syndrome in myasthenia gravis: Suggestion of similar autoimmune mechanisms. Acta Endocrinol 99: 431–436

133. Evans DJ, Lampert IA (1978) Ovarian involvement by cytomegalovirus. (Letter) Hum Pathol 9:122

134. Evans JP (1978) Torsion of the normal uterine adnexa in premenarcheal girls. J Pediatr Surg 13: 195–196

135. Evers JLH, Rolland R (1981) Primary hypothyroidism and ovarian activity: Evidence for an overlap in the synthesis of pituitary glycoproteins. Case report. Br J Obstet Gynaecol 88: 195–202

136. Farber ER, Leahy MS, Meadows TR (1968) Endometrial Blastomycosis acquired by sexual contact. Obstet Gynecol 32: 195–199

137. Farber M, Daoust PR, Rogers J (1974) Hyperthecosis syndrome. Obstet Gynecol 44: 35–41

138. Farber M, Madanes A, O'Brian D, et al (1981) Asymmetric hyperthecosis ovarii. Obstet Gynecol 57: 521–525

139. Farhi DC, Nosanchuk J, Silverberg SG (1986) Endometrial adenocarcinoma in women under 25 years of age. Obstet Gynecol 68: 741–745

140. Farid NR, Bear JC (1981) The human major histocompatibility complex and endocrine disease. Endocr Rev 2: 50–86

141. Fechner RE, Kaufman RH (1974) Endometrial adenocarcinoma in Stein–Leventhal syndrome. Cancer 34: 444–452

142. Ferrannini E, Muggeo M, Navalesi R, Pilo A (1982) Impaired insulin degradation in a patient with insulin resistance and acanthosis nigricans. Am J Med 73: 148–154

143. Fienberg R (1969) The stromal theca cell and postmenopausal endometrial adenocarcinoma. Cancer 24: 32–38

144. Feinberg R, Cohen RB (1966) Oxidative enzymes in luteinization. Obstet Gynecol 28: 406–415

145. Fisher B, Cheung AYC (1984) Delayed effect of radiation therapy with or without chemotherapy on ovarian function in women with Hodgkin's disease. Acta Radiol Oncol 23: 43–48

146. Fisher ER, Gregorio R, Stephan T, et al (1974) Ovarian changes in women with morbid obesity. Obstet Gynecol 44: 839–844

147. Fitzgerald JA, Berrigan MV (1959) Accurate diagnosis of "ovarian vascular accidents." Review of 32 instances, with clinical conclusions. Obstet Gynecol 13: 175–180

148. FitzGerald TB, Mainwaring AR, Ahmed A (1974) Pelvic peritoneal oxyuriasis similating metastatic carcinoma. A case report. Br J Obstet Gynaecol 81: 248–250

149. Flier JS, Kahn CR, Roth J (1979) Receptors, antireceptor antibodies and mechanisms of insulin resistance. N Engl J Med 300: 413–419

150. Fraley DS, Totten RS (1968) An autopsy study of endocrine organ changes in diabetes mellitus. Metabolism 17: 896–900

151. Friedman CI, Gurgen-Varol F, Lucas J, Neff J (1987) Persistent progesterone production associated with autoimmune oophoritis. J Reprod Med 32: 293–296

152. Friedman CI, Neff J, Kim MH (1984) Immunologic parameters in premature follicular depletion: T and B lymphocytes, T-cell subpopulations, cutaneous reactivity, and serum immunoglobulin concentrations. Diagn Immunol 2: 48–52

153. Friedman CI, Schmidt GE, Chang FE, Kim MH (1984) Severe ovarian hyperstimulation following follicular aspiration. Am J Obstet Gynecol 150: 436–437

154. Fukuda O, Munemura M, Tohya T, et al (1984) Massive edema of the ovary associated with hydrothorax and ascites. Gynecol Oncol 17: 231–237

155. Futterweit W (1983) Pituitary tumors and polycystic ovarian disease. Obstet Gynecol 62:74S–79S

156. Futterweit W (1985) Polycystic Ovarian Disease. Clinical Perspectives in Obstetrics and Gynecology. Springer Verlag, New York.

157. Gabbay-Moore M, Ovadia Y, Neri A (1982) Accessory ovary with bilateral dermoid cysts. Eur J Obstet Gynecol Reprod Biol 14: 171–173

158. Gallup DG, Stock RJ (1984) Adenocarcinoma of the endometrium in women 40 years of age or younger. Obstet Gynecol 64: 417–419

159. Garcia-Bunuel R, Berek JS, Woodruff JD (1975) Luteomas of pregnancy. Obstet Gynecol 45: 407–414

160. Garcia-Bunuel R, Brandes D (1976) Luteoma of pregnancy: Ultrastructural features. Hum Pathol7: 205–214

161. Gardner GH, Greene RR, Peckham B (1957) Tumors of the broad ligament. Am J Obstet Gynecol 73: 536–555

162. Gardstein HF Jr, Ferenczy A, Richart RM (1973) Asymptomatic bilateral ovarian infarction and venous thrombosis. Am J Obstet Gynecol 116: 1164–1166

163. Gerbie AB, Greene RR, Reis RA (1958) Heteroplastic bone and cartilage in the female genital tract. Obstet Gynecol 11: 573–578

164. Gibson M, Schiff I, Tulchinsky D, Ryan KJ (1980) Characterization of hyperandrogenism with insulin-resistant diabetes type A. Fertil Steril 33: 501–505

165. Gilks CB, Clement PB (1987) Colo-ovarian fistula: A report of two cases. Obstet Gynecol 69: 533–537

166. Ginsburg KA, Valdes C, Schnider G (1987) Spontaneous utero-ovarian vessel rupture during pregnancy: Three case reports and a review of the literature. Obstet Gynecol 69: 474–476

167. Girouard DP, Barclay DL, Collins CG (1964) Hyperreactio luteinalis. Review of the literature and report of 2 cases. Obstet Gynecol 23:513–525

168. Givens JR, Kerber IJ, Wiser WL, et al (1974) Remission of acanthosis nigricans associated with polycystic ovarian disease and a stromal luteoma. J Clin Endocrinol Metab 38:347–355

169. Givens JR, Wiser WL, Coleman SA, et al (1971) Familial ovarian hyperthecosis: A study of two families. Am J Obstet Gynecol 110:959–972

170. Gloor E, Hurlimann J (1984) Autoimmune oophoritis. Am J Clin Pathol 81: 105–109

171. Gloor E, Juillard E, Curchod A, Legeret J (1982) Ovarian hypoplasia with follicular calcifications. Am J Clin Pathol 78: 857–860

172. Golan A, Ron-El R, Herman A, et al (1989) Ovarian hyperstimulation syndrome: An update review. Obstet Gynecol Surv 44: 430–440

173. Goldzieher JW, Green JA (1962) The polycystic ovary. I. Clinical and histologic features. J Clin Endocrinol Metab 22: 325–338

174. Green JA, Goldzieher JW (1965) The polycystic ovary. IV.

Light and electron microscope studies. Am J Obstet Gynecol 91: 173–181

175. Gronroos M, Klemi P, Piiroinen O, et al (1982) Ovarian function during and after curative intracavitary high dose-rate irradiation: Steroidal output and morphology. Eur J Gynecol Reprod Biol 14: 13–21

176. Grosfeld JL (1969) Torsion of the normal ovary in the first two years of life. Am J Surg 117: 726–727

177. Gross MD, Wortsman J, Shapiro B, et al (1986) Scintographic evidence of adrenal cortical dysfunction in the polycystic ovary syndrome. J Clin Endocrinol Metab 62: 197–201

178. Hager WD (1978) Ruptured utero-ovarian vein syndrome: A case report. Am J Obstet Gynecol 131: 697–698

179. Hahn-Pedersen J, Larsen PM (1984) Supernumerary ovary. Acta Obstet Gynecol Scand 63: 365–366

180. Hallatt JG, Steele CH Jr, Snyder M (1984) Ruptured corpus luteum with hemoperitoneum: A study of 173 surgical cases. Am J Obstet Gynecol 149: 5–9

181. Hamblen EC, Baker RD, Martin DS (1935) Blastomycosis of the female reproductive tract with report of a case. Am J Obstet Gynecol 30: 345–356

182. Hangval H, Habibi H, Moshref A, Rahimi A (1979) Case report of an ovarian hydatid cyst. J Trop Med Hyg 82: 34–35

183. Haning RV Jr, Strawn EY, Holten WE (1985) Pathophysiology of the ovarian hyperstimulation syndrome. Obstet Gynecol 66: 220–224

184. Harper SL, Tiltman AJ (1991) Non-neoplastic ovarian cysts with ectopic pregnancy. Int J Gynecol Pathol 10: 372–379

185. Hart WR, Abell MR (1970) Adipose prosoplasia of ovary. Am J Obstet Gynecol 106: 929–930

186. Hatjis CG (1985) Nonimmunologic fetal hydrops associated with hyperreactio luteinalis. Obstet Gynecol 65: 11S–13S

187. Heller DS, Harpaz N, Breakstone B (1990) Neoplasms arising in ectopic ovaries: A case of Brenner tumor in an accessory ovary. Int J Gynecol Pathol 9: 185–189

188. Hensleigh PA, Woodruff JD (1978) Differential maternal-fetal response to androgenizing luteoma or hyperreactio luteinalis. Obstet Gynecol Surv 33: 262–271

189. Herbold DR, Frable WJ, Kraus FT (1984) Isolated noninfectious granuloma of the ovary. Int J Gynecol Pathol 2: 380–391

190. Herr JC, Heidger PM Jr, Scott JR, Anderson JW, Curet LB, Mossman HW (1978) Decidual cells in the human ovary at term. I. Incidence, gross anatomy and ultrastructural features of merocrine secretion. Am J Anat 152: 7–28

191. Herr JC, Platz CE, Heidger PM Jr, Curet LB (1979) Smooth muscle within ovarian decidual nodules: A link to leiomyomatosis peritonealis disseminata? Obstet Gynecol 53: 451–456

192. Hibbard LT (1985) Adnexal torsion. Am J Obstet Gynecol 152: 456–461

193. Hidvegi D, Hidvegi I, Barrett J (1978) Douche-induced pelvic peritoneal starch granuloma. Obstet Gynecol 52: 15S–18S

194. Hill JA, Welch WR, Faris HMP, Anderson DJ (1990) Induction of class II major histocompatibility complex antigen expression in human granulosa cells by interferon gamma: A potential mechanism contributing to autoimmune ovarian failure. Am J Obstet Gynecol 162: 534–540

195. Himelstein-Braw R, Peters H, Faber M (1977) Influence of irradiation and chemotherapy on the ovaries of children with abdominal tumours. Br J Cancer 36:269–275

196. Himelstein-Braw R, Peters H, Faber M (1978) Morphological study of the ovaries of leukaemic children. Br J Cancer 38: 82–87

197. Honore LH (1981) Combined suppurative and noncaseating granulomatous oophoritis associated with distal ileitis (Crohn's disease). Eur J Obstet Gynaecol Reprod Biol 12: 91–94

198. Honore LH, O'Hara KE (1979) Ovarian hilus cell heterotopia. Obstet Gynecol 53: 461–464

199. Honore LH, O'Hara KE (1980) Subcapsular adipocytic infiltration of the human ovary: A clinicopathological study of eight cases. Eur J Obstet Gynaecol Reprod Biol 10: 13–20

200. Hubmer G (1978) The ovarian vein syndrome. Eur Urol 4: 263–268

201. Hughesdon PE (1972) The origin and development of benign stromatosis of the ovary. Br J Obstet Gynaecol 79: 348–359

202. Hughesdon PE (1976) The endometrial identity of benign stromatosis of the ovary and its relation to other forms of endometriosis. J Pathol 119: 201–209

203. Hughesdon PE (1982) Morphology and morphogenesis of the Stein-Leventhal ovary and of so-called "hyperthecosis." Obstet Gynecol Surv 37: 59–77

204. Iannaccone A, Gabrilove JL, Sohval AR, Soffer LJ (1959) The ovaries in Cushing's syndrome. N Engl J Med 261: 775–780

205. Ikeda H, Taguchi O, Takahashi T, et al (1988) L3T4 effector cells in multiple organ localized autoimmune disease in nude mice grafted with embronic rat thymus. J Exp Med 168: 2397–2492

206. Imperato-McGinley J, Peterson RE, Sturla E, et al (1978) Primary amenorrhea associated with hirsutism, acanthosis nigricans, dermoid cysts of the ovaries and a new type of insulin resistance. Am J Med 65: 389–395

207. Irvine WJ (1980) Autoimmunity in endocrine disease. Rec Prog Horm Res 36: 509–556

208. Irvine WJ, Barnes EW (1974) Addison's disease and autoimmune ovarian failure. J Reprod Fertil 21(suppl): 1–31

209. Irvine WJ, Barnes EW (1975) Addison's disease, ovarian failure and hypoparathyroidism. Clin Endocrinol Metab 4: 379–434

210. Irvine WJ, Chan MMW, Scarth L (1969) The further characterization of autoantibodies reactive with extra-adrenal steroid-producing cells in patients with adrenal disorders. Clin Exp Immunol 4: 489–503

211. Irvine WJ, Chan MMW, Scarth L, et al (1968) Immunological aspects of premature ovarian failure associated with idiopathic Addison's disease. Lancet 2: 883–887

212. Israel SL, Rubenstone A, Meranze DR (1954) The ovary at term. I. Decidua-like reaction and surface cell proliferation. Obstet Gynecol 3: 399–407

213. Jafari K, Javaheri G, Ruiz G (1978) Endometrial adenocarcinoma and the Stein–Leventhal syndrome. Obstet Gynecol 51: 97–100

214. Jafari K, Saleh I (1977) Postpartum spontaneous rupture of ovarian artery aneurysm. Obstet Gynecol 49: 493–494

215. Janson PO, Janssson I, Skryten A, et al (1981) Ovarian endocrine function in young women undergoing radiotherapy for carcinoma of the cervix. Gynecol Oncol 11: 218–223

216. Judd HL, Benirschke K, DeVane G, et al (1973) Maternal virilization developing during a twin pregnancy. N Engl J Med 288: 118–122

217. Judd HL, Scully RE, Herbst AL, et al (1973) Familial hyperthecosis: comparison of endocrinologic and histologic findings with polycystic ovarian disease. Am J Obstet Gynecol 117: 976–982

218. Kabawat SE, Bast RC Jr, Bhan AK, et al (1983) Tissue distribution of a coelomic-epithelium-related antigen recognized by the monoclonal antibody OC125. Int J Gynecol Pathol 2: 275–285

219. Kahn CR, Flier JS, Bar RS, et al (1976) The syndromes of insulin resistance and acanthosis nigricans: Insulin-receptor disorders in man. N Engl J Med 294: 739–745

220. Kalstone CE, Jaffe RB, Abell MR (1969) Massive edema of the ovary simulating fibroma. Obstet Gynecol 34: 564–571

221. Kaminski PF, Sorosky JI, Mandell MJ, et al (1990) Clomiphene citrate stimulation as an adjunct in locating ovarian tissue in ovarian remnant syndrome. Obstet Gynecol 76: 924–926

222. Kanbour AI, Salazar H, Tobon H (1979) Massive ovarian edema. A nonneoplastic pelvic mass of young women. Arch Pathol Lab Med 103: 42–45

223. Karam K, Hajj S (1979) Hyperthecosis syndrome. Acta Obstet Gynecol Scand 58: 73–79

224. Katz M, Hamilton SM, Albertyn L, et al (1977) Virilization with diffuse involvement of ovarian androgen secreting cells. Obstet Gynecol 50: 623–627

225. Kaufman DW, Shapiro S, Rosenberg L, et al (1980) Intrauterine contraceptive device use and pelvic inflammatory disease. Am J Obstet Gynecol 136: 159–162

226. Kaufman FR, Kogut MD, Donnell GN, et al (1981) Hypergonadotropic hypogonadism in female patients with galactosemia. N Engl J Med 304: 994–998

227. Keebler C, Chatwani A, Schwartz R (1983) Actinomycosis infection associated with intrauterine contraceptive devices. Am J Obstet Gynecol 145: 596–599

228. Kemmann E, Orenstein D, Smith C, et al (1980) Estrogenization in women with postmenopausal ovarian hyperthecosis. Int J Obstet Gynecol 18: 188–191

229. Kent BK (1956) Ectopic pregnancy in a congenitally defective tube with absence of the ipsilateral ovary. Am J Obstet Gynecol 72: 1150–1151

230. Kerber IJ, Bell JS, Camacho AM, Fish SA (1969) Luteoma of pregnancy: Recurrent or persistent? South Med J 62: 1343–1348

231. Kern SB, Duff P (1981) Localized amniotic fluid embolism presenting as ovarian vein thrombosis and refractory postoperative fever. Am J Clin Pathol 76: 476–480

232. Kernohan NM, Best PV, Jandial V, Kitchener HC (1991) Palisading granuloma of the ovary. Histopathology 19: 279–280

233. Khan JS, Steele RJC, Stewart D (1981) Enterobius vermicularis infestation of the female genital tract causing generalized peritonitis. Case report. Br J Obstet Gynaecol 88: 681–683

234. Khurana BK, Rao J, Friedman SA, Cho KC (1988) Computed tomographic features of puerperal ovarian vein thrombosis. Am J Obstet Gynecol 159: 905–908

235. Kim MH (1974) "Gonadotropin-resistant ovaries" syndrome in association with secondary amenorrhea. Am J Obstet Gynecol 120: 257–263

236. Kinch RAH, Plunkett ER, Smout MS, Carr DH (1965) Primary ovarian failure. A clinicopathological and cytogenetic study. Am J Obstet Gynecol 91: 630–641

237. Klempner LB, Giglio PG, Niebles A (1987) Malacoplakia of the ovary. Obstet Gynecol 69: 537–540

238. Kohorn EI (1983) Theca lutein ovarian cyst may be pathognomonic for trophoblastic neoplasia. Obstet Gynecol 62: 80S–81S

239. Koninckx PR, Brosens IA (1977) The "gonadotropin-resistant ovary" syndrome as a cause of secondary amenorrhea and infertility. Fertil Steril 28: 926–931

240. Kosasa TS, Griffiths CT, Shane JM, Leventhal JM, Naftolin F (1976) Diagnosis of a supernumerary ovary with human chorionic gonadotropin. Obstet Gynecol 47: 236–238

241. Kosloske AM, Goldthorn JF, Kaufman E, Hayek A (1984) Treatment of precocious pseudopuberty associated with follicular cysts of the ovary. Am J Dis Child 138: 147–149

242. Kostelnik FV, Fremount HN (1976) Mycotic tubo-ovarian abscess associated with the intrauterine device. Am J Obstet Gynecol 125: 272–274

243. Kott MM, Schmidt WA (1981) Massive postpartum corpus luteum cyst: A case report. Hum Pathol 12: 468–470

244. Kuhajda FP, Haupt HM, Moore GW, Hutchins GM (1982) Gonadal morphology in patients receiving chemotherapy for leukemia. Am J Med 72: 759–767

245. Krauss CM, Turksoy N, Atkins L, et al (1987) Familial premature ovarian failure due to an interstitial deletion of the long arm of the X chromosome. N Engl J Med 317: 125–131

246. Kuki S, Morgan RL, Tucci JR (1981) Myasthenia gravis and premature ovarian failure. Arch Intern Med 141: 1230–1232

247. Kunakemakorn P, Ontai G, Balin H (1976) Pelvic inflammatory pseudotumor: A case report. Am J Obstet Gynecol 126: 286–287

248. LaBarbera AR, Miller MM, Ober C, Rebar RW (1988) Autoimmune etiology in premature ovarian failure. Am J Reprod Immunol Microbiol 16: 115–122

249. Lachelin GCL, Barnett M, Hopper BR, et al (1979) Adrenal function in normal women and women with the polycystic ovary syndrome. J Clin Endocrinol Metab 49: 892–898

250. Lachman MF, Berman MM (1991) The ectopic ovary. A case report and review of the literature. Arch Pathol Lab Med 115: 233–235

251. Ladefoged C, Lorentzen M (1988) Xanthogranulomatous inflammation of the female genital tract. Histopathology 13: 541–551

252. Lai C, Hsueh S, Lin C, et al (1992) Human papillomavirus in benign and malignant ovarian and endometrial tissues. Int J Gynecol Pathol 11: 210–215

253. Landers DV, Sweet RL (1985) Current trends in the diagnosis and treatment of tuboovarian abscess. Am J Obstet Gynecol 151: 1098–1110

254. Landrum B, Ogburn PL Jr, et al (1986) Intrauterine aspiration of a large fetal ovarian cyst. Obstet Gynecol 68: 11S–14S

255. Lansman HH, Lapin A, Blaustein A (1960) Pelvic oxyuris granuloma associated with endometriosis. Am J Obstet Gynecol 79: 1178–1180

256. Lee B, Gore BZ (1984) A case of supernumerary ovary. Obstet Gynecol 63: 738–740

257. Lee RA, Kazmier FJ (1977) Ovarian hematoma complicating anticoagulant therapy. Mayo Clin Proc 52: 19–23

258. Leedman PJ, Bierre AR, Martin FIR (1989) Virilizing nodular ovarian stromal hyperthecosis, diabetes mellitus and insulin resistance in a postmenopausal woman. Case report. Br J Obstet Gynaecol 96: 1095–1098

259. Levine SC, Huffaker J, Jacobson JB, et al (1982) Second-trimester spontaneous regression of theca lutein cysts. Obstet Gynecol 60: 124–126

260. Lewis JD (1964) Hilus-cell hyperplasia in ovaries and tubes. Obstet Gynecol 24: 728–731

261. Lim HT, Meinders AE, de Haan LD, Bronkhorst FB (1984) Anovulation presumably due to the gonadotropin-resistant ovary syndrome. Eur J Obstet Gynecol Reprod Biol 16: 327–337

262. Lindsay AN, Voorhess ML, MacGillivray MH (1983) Multicystic ovaries in primary hypothyroidism. Obstet Gynecol 61: 433

263. LiVolsi VA, Merino MJ (1979) Cytomegalovirus infection of ovarian thecoma. (Letter) Arch Pathol Lab Med 103: 653–654

264. Lobo RA (1991) Hirsuitism in polycystic ovary syndrome: Current concepts. Clin Obstet Gynecol 34: 817–826

265. Lobo RA, Goebelsmann U (1981) Evidence for reduced 3beta-ol-hydroxysteroid dehydrogenase activity in some hirsute women thought to have polycystic ovary syndrome. J Clin Endocrinol Metab 53: 394–400

266. Lombard CM, Moore MH, Seifer DB (1986) Diagnosis of systemic polyarteritis nodosa following total abdominal hysterectomy and bilateral salpingo-oophorectomy: A case report. Int J Gynecol Pathol 5: 63–68

267. London AM, Burkman RT (1979) Tuboovarian abscess with associated rupture with fistula formation into the urinary bladder. Am J Obstet Gynecol 135: 1113–1114

268. Lonsdale RN, Roberts PF, Trowell JE (1991) Autoimmune oophoritis associated with polycystic ovaries. Histopathology 19: 77–81

269. Loughlin T, Cunningham S, Moore A, et al (1986) Adrenal abnormalities in polycystic ovary syndrome. J Clin Endocrinol Metab 62: 142–147

270. Lubarsch O, Henke F (1937) Handbuch der Speziellen Pathologischen Anatomie und Histologie. Dritter Teil. Die Krankheiten des Eierstockes. Springer, Berlin.

271. Lucisano A, Russo N, Acampora MG, et al (1986) Ovarian and peripheral androgen and oestrogen levels in postmenopausal women: Correlations with ovarian histology. Maturitas 8: 57–65

272. Luff RD, Gupta PK, Spence MR, Frost JK (1978) Pelvic actinomycosis and the intrauterine contraceptive device. Am J Clin Pathol 69: 581–586

273. Lunde O, Hoel PS, Sandvik L (1988) Ovarian morphology in patients with polycystic ovaries and in an age-matched reference material. Gynecol Obstet Invest 25: 192–201

274. Lupien C, Wagar H, Sauerbrei EE (1984) Delayed regression of huge theca lutein cysts monitored by serial sonograms and B-HCG levels. J Can Assoc Rad 35: 70–72

275. Luzzatto R, Brucker N (1981) Benign inclusion cysts of the ovary associated with psammoma bodies in vaginal smears. Acta Cytol 25: 282–284

276. Madeido G, Tieu TM, Aiman J (1985) Atypical ovarian hyperthecosis in a virilized postmenopausal woman. Am J Clin Pathol 83: 101–107

277. Mahmood K (1975) Granulomatous oophoritis due to Schistosoma mansoni. Am J Obstet Gynecol 123: 919–920

278. Mallin SR (1969) Congenital adrenal hyperplasia secondary to 17-hydroxylase deficiency. Two sisters with amenorrhea, hypokalemia, hypertension, and cystic ovaries. Ann Intern Med 70: 69–75

279. Marcello MF, Nuciforo G, Romeo R, et al (1990) Structural and ultrastructural study of the ovary in childhood leukemia after successful treatment. Cancer 66: 2099–2104

280. Marrogi AJ, Gersell DJ, Kraus FT (1991) Localized asymptomatic giant cell arteritis of the female genital tract. Int J Gynecol Pathol 10: 51–58

281. Massachusetts General Hospital Case Records (1957) Case 43461. Follicle cyst with sexual precocity. N Engl J Med 257: 987–992

282. Massachusetts General Hospital Case Recrods (1972) Case 49-1972. Hyperthecosis of ovaries. N Engl J Med 287: 1192–1195

283. Massachusetts General Hospital Case Records (1974) Case 12-1974. Stromal hyperthecosis of ovaries. N Engl J Med 290: 730–736

284. Massachusetts General Hospital Case Records (1975) Case 4-1975. Luteinized follicle cysts of ovary, bilateral. Albright's syndrome. N Engl J Med 292: 199–203

285. Massachusetts General Hospital Case Records (1982) Case 25-1982. Ovarian stromal hyperthecosis. Acanthosis nigricans. N Engl J Med 306: 1537–1544

286. Massachusetts General Hospital Case Records (1983) Case 25-1983. Hemochromatosis, involving liver and testes, with hypogonadotropic hypogonadism. N Engl J Med 308: 1521–1529

287. Massachusetts General Hospital Case Records (1988) Case 13-1988. Diverticulitis, sigmoid colon, with colo-ovarian fistula formation and left ovarian abscess. N Engl J Med 318: 835–842

288. Massachusetts General Hospital Case Records (1987) Case 46-1987. Autoimmune oophoritis with primary ovarian failure. N Engl J Med 317: 1270–1278

289. Massachusetts General Hospital Case Records (1986) Case 46-1986. Resistant-ovary syndrome, with hyalization of preantral follicles. N Engl J Med 315: 1336–1344

290. Massachusetts General Hospital Case Records (1988) Case 22-1988. Ovarian stromal hyperthecosis, with virilization, insulin resistance, and acanthosis nigricans. N Engl J Med 318: 1449–1457

291. Mathur S, Melchers JT III, Ades EW, et al (1980) Anti-ovarian and anti-lymphocyte antibodies in patients with chronic vaginal candidiasis. J Reprod Immunol 2: 247–262

292. Mattison DR, Evans MI, Schwimmer WB, et al (1984) Familial premature ovarian failure. Am J Hum Genet 36: 1341–1348

293. McArdle C, Seibel M, Hann LE, et al (1983) The diagnosis of ovarian hyperstimulation (OHS): The impact of ultrasound. Fertil Steril 39: 464–467

294. McCormick JF, Scorgie RDF (1977) Unilateral tubo-ovarian actinomycosis in the presence of an intrauterine device. Am J Clin Pathol 68: 622–626

295. McKenna TJ (1988) Pathogenesis and treatment of polycystic ovary syndrome. N Engl J Med 318: 558–562

296. McMahon JN, Connolly CE, Long SV, Meehan FB (1984) Enterobius granulomas of the uterus, ovary and pelvic peritoneum. Two case reports. Br J Obstet Gynaecol 91: 289–290

297. McNatty KP, Short RV, Barnes EW, Irvine WJ (1975) The cytotoxic effect of serum from patients with Addison's disease and autoimmune ovarian failure on human granulosa cells in culture. Clin Exp Immunol 22: 378–384

298. McNatty KP, Smith DM, Makris A, et al (1980) The intra-ovarian sites of androgen and estrogen formation in women with normal and hyperandrogenic ovaries as judged by in vitro experiments. J Clin Endocrinol Metab 50: 755–763

299. Mechanick JI, Futterweit W (1984) Hypothesis: Aberrant puberty and the Stein–Leventhal syndrome. Int J Fertil 29: 35–38

300. Meizner I, Levy A, Katz M, et al (1991) Fetal ovarian cysts: Prenatal ultrasonographic detection and postnatal evaluation and treatment. Am J Obstet Gynecol 164: 874–878

301. Meldrum DR, Frumar AM, Shamonki IM, et al (1980) Ovarian and adrenal steroidogenesis in a virilized patient with gonadotropin-resistant ovaries and hilus cell hyperplasia. Obstet Gynecol 56: 216–221

302. Mercer LJ, Toub DB, Cibils LA (1987) Tumors originating in supernumerary ovaries. A report of two cases. J Reprod Med 2: 932–934

303. Merrill JA (1963) The morphology of the prepubertal ovary: relationship to the polycystic ovary syndrome. Southern Med J 56: 225–231

304. Mickal A, Sellmann AH, Beebe JL (1968) Ruptured tuboovarian abscess. Am J Obstet Gynecol 100: 432–436

305. Mignot MH, Schoemaker J, Kleingeld M, et al (1989) Premature ovarian failure. I: The association with autoimmunity. Eur J Obstet Gynecol Reprod Biol 30: 59–66

306. Milewicz A, Silber D, Mielecki T (1983) The origin of androgen synthesis in polycystic ovary syndrome. Obstet Gynecol 62: 601–604

307. Miller ME, Chatten J (1967) Ovarian changes in ataxia telangiectasia. Acta Paediatr Scand 56: 559–561

308. Minkowitz S, Friedman F, Henninger G (1965) Xanthogranuloma of the ovary. Arch Pathol 80: 209–213

308a. Mittal KR, Zeleniuch-Jacquotte A, Cooper JL, Demopoulos RI (1993) Contralateral ovary in unilateral ovarian carcinoma: A search for preneoplastic lesions. Int J Gynecol Pathol 12: 59–63

309. Moller DE, Flier JS (1988) Detection of an alteration in the insulin-receptor gene in a patient with insulin resistance, acanthosis nigricans, and the polycystic ovary syndrome (type A insulin resistance). N Engl J Med 319: 1526–1529

310. Moller DE, Flier JS (1991) Insulin resistance—mechanisms, syndromes, and implications. N Engl J Med 325: 938–948

311. Monteleone JA, Monteleone PL, Danis RK (1973) Pseudoprecocious puberty associated with isolated follicle cyst of the ovary. J Pediatr Surg 8: 949–950

312. Montz FJ, Schlaerth JB, Morrow CP (1988) The natural history of theca lutein cysts. Obstet Gynecol 72: 247–251

313. Morgenfeld MC, Goldberg V, Parisier H, et al (1972) Ovarian lesions due to cytostatic agents during the treatment of Hodgkin's disease. Surg Gynecol Obstet 134: 826–828

314. Morrison JC, Givens JR, Wiser WL, Fish SA (1975) Mumps oophoritis: A cause of premature menopause. Fertil Steril 26: 655–659

315. Morrow CP, Kletzky OA, Disaia PJ, et al (1977) Clinical and laboratory correlates of molar pregnancy and trophoblastic disease. Am J Obstet Gynecol 128: 424–430

316. Mostafa SAM, Bargeron CB, Flower RW, et al (1985) Foreign body granulomas in normal ovaries. Obstet Gynecol 66: 701–702

317. Muechler EK, Florack AJ, Cary D, Kapakis M (1982) Isosexual precocious puberty with luteinized follicular cyst. NY State J Med 82: 1353–1356

318. Mulligan RM (1976) A survey of epithelial inclusions in the ovarian cortex of 470 patients. J Surg Oncol 8: 61–66

319. Munslick RA, Gillanders LA (1981) A review of the syndrome of puerperal ovarian vein thrombophlebitis. Obstet Gynecol Surv 36: 57–66

320. Muram D, Drouin P (1982) Ovarian remnant syndrome. Can Med Assoc J 127: 399–400

321. Murray JJ, Clark CA, Lands RH, Heim CR, Burnett LS (1985) Reactivation Blastomycosis presenting as a tuboovarian abscess. Obstet Gynecol 64: 828–830

322. Nader S (1991) Polycystic ovary syndrome and the androgen-insulin link. Am J Obstet Gynecol 165: 346–348

323. Nagamani M, Gomez LG, Garza J (1982) In vivo steroid studies in luteoma of pregnancy. Obstet Gynecol 59: 105S–111S

324. Nagamani M, Hannigan EV, Van Dinh T, Stuart CA (1988) Hyperinsulinemia and stromal luteinization of the ovaries in postmenopausal women with endometrial cancer. J Clin Endocrinol Metab 67: 144–148

325. Nagamani H, Kaspar HG, Van Dinh T, et al (1990) Hyperthecosis of the ovaries in a woman with a placental site trophoblastic tumor. Obstet Gynecol 76: 931–935

326. Nagamani M, Lingold JC, Gomez JR (1980) Hyperthecosis of the ovaries in acromegaly. Obstet Gynecol 56: 258–262

327. Nagamani M, Lingold JC, Gomez JR, Garza JR (1981) Clinical and hormonal studies in hyperthecosis of the ovaries. Fertil Steril 36: 326–332

328. Nagamani M, Stuart CA (1990) Specific binding sites for insulin-like growth factor I in the ovarian stroma of women with polycystic ovarian disease and stromal hyperthecosis. Am J Obstet Gynecol 163: 1992–1997

329. Nagamani M, Stuart CA, Doherty MG (1992) Increased steroid production by the ovarian stromal tissue of postmenopausal women with endometrial cancer. J Clin Endocrinol Metab 74: 172–176

330. Nagamani M, Van Dinh T, Kelver ME (1986) Hyperinsulinemia in hyperthecosis of the ovaries. Am J Obstet Gynecol 154: 384–389

331. Nagelberg SB, Rosen SW (1985) Clinical and laboratory investigation of a virilized woman with placental-site trophoblastic tumor. Obstet Gynecol 65: 527–534

332. Nakano R, Shima K, Yamoto M, et al (1989) Binding sites for gonadotropins in human postmenopausal ovaries. Obstet Gynecol 73: 196–200

333. Nestler JE, Clore JN, Blackard WG (1989) The central role of obesity (hyperinsulinemia) in the pathogenesis of the polycystic ovary syndrome. Am J Obstet Gynecol 161: 1095–1097

334. Nicosia SV, Matus-Ridley M, Meadows AT (1985) Gonadal effects of cancer therapy in girls. Cancer 55: 2364–2372

335. Nissen ED, Kent DR, Nissen SE, Feldman BM (1977) Unilateral tuboovarian autoamputation. J Reprod Med 19: 151–153

336. Nissim F, Ashkenazy M, Borenstein R, Czernobilsky B (1981) Tuberculoid cornstarch granulomas with caseous necrosis. A diagnostic challenge. Arch Pathol Lab Med 105: 86–88

337. Nogales FF, Silverberg SG (1976) Epidermoid cysts of the ovary: A report of five case with histogenetic considerations and ultrastructural findings. Am J Obstet Gynecol 124: 523–528

338. Nogales-Ortiz F, Taracon I, Nogales FF (1979) The pathology of female genital tract tuberculosis. Obstet Gynecol 53: 422–428

339. Norris HJ, Taylor HB (1967) Nodular theca-lutein hyperplasia of pregnancy (so-called "pregnancy luteoma"). A clinical and pathologic study of 15 cases. Am J Clin Pathol 47: 557–566

340. Nouwen EJ, Pollet DE, Schelstraete JB, et al (1985) Human placental alkaline phosphatase in benign and malignant ovarian neoplasia. Cancer Res 45: 892–902

341. Nouwen EJ, Hendrix PG, Eerdekens MW, De Broe ME (1987) Tumor markers in the human ovary and its neoplasms. A comparative immunohistochemical study. Am J Pathol 126: 230–242

342. Nuovo GJ (1989) Virilizing stromal thecosis of the ovary associated with multiple corpora atretica. Am J Clin Pathol 92: 505–508

343. Ober WB, Grady HG, Schoenbucher AK (1957) Ectopic ovarian decidua without pregnancy. Am J Pathol 33: 199–217

344. Ohsawa M, Wu M, Masahashi T, et al (1985) Cyclic therapy resulted in pregnancy in premature ovarian failure. Obstet Gynecol 66: 64S–67S

345. O'Malley BW, Lipsett MB, Jackson MA (1967) Steroid content and synthesis in a virilizing luteoma. J Clin Endocrinol Metab 27: 311–319

346. Osathanondh R, Berkowitz RS, de Cholnoky C, et al (1986) Hormonal measurements in patients with theca lutein cysts and gestational trophoblastic disease. J Reprod Med 31: 179–183

347. Pace EH, Voet EH, Melancon JT (1984) Xanthogranulomatous oophoritis: An inflammatory pseudotumor of the ovary. Int J Gynecol Pathol 3: 398–402

348. Pache TD, Chadha S, Goorens LJG, et al (1991) Ovarian morphology in long-term androgen-treated female to male transsexuals. A human model for the study of polycystic ovary syndrome? Histopathology 19: 445–452

349. Paine CG, Smith P (1957) Starch granulomata. J Clin Pathol 10: 51–55

350. Payan HM, Gilbert EF (1987) Mesenteric cyst-ovarian implant syndrome. Arch Pathol Lab Med 111: 282–284

351. Pedowitz P, Bloomfield RD (1964) Ruptured adnexal abscess (tubo-ovarian) with generalized peritonitis. Am J Obstet Gynecol 88: 721–729

352. Peer E, Peretz BA, Makler A, Paldi E (1981) Bilateral adnexal agenesis with an ectopic ovary—case report and review of the literature. Eur J Obstet Gynec Reprod Biol 12: 37–42

353. Pekonen F, Seigberg R, Makinen T, et al (1986) Immunological disturbances in patients with premature ovarian failure. Clin Endocrinol 25: 1–6

354. Penney LL, Betz G (1977) Agonadism. Case report and review. Am J Obstet Gynecol 127: 299–301

355. Perlman JA, Barnes AB, Demirjian Z (1977) Corpus luteum hemorrhages complication chronic anticoagulation. Obstet Gynecol 49: 20S–21S

356. Peters WA, Thiagarajah S, Thornton WN Jr (1979) Ovarian hemorrhage in patients receiving anticoagulant therapy. J Reprod Med 22: 82–86

357. Pettit PD, Lee RA (1988) Ovarian remnant syndrome: Diagnostic dilemma and surgical challenge. Obstet Gynecol 71: 580–583

358. Pine L, Curtis EM, Brown JM (1985) Actinomyces and the intrauterine contraceptive device: Aspects of the fluorescent antibody stain. Am J Obstet Gynecol 152: 287–290

359. Piver MS, Williams LJ, Marcuse PM (1970) Influence of luteal cysts on menstrual function. Obstet Gynecol 35: 740–751

360. Planner RS, Abell DA, Barbaro CA, Beischer NA (1982) Massive enlargement of the ovaries after evacuation of hydatidiform moles. Aust NZ J Obstet Gynaec 22: 96–100

361. Plate WP (1967) Ovarian changes after long-term oral contraception. Acta Endocrinol 55: 71–77

362. Poretsky L, Smith D, Seibel M, Pazionos A, Moses AC, Flier JS (1984) Specific insulin binding sites in human ovary. J Clin Endocrinol Metab 59: 809–811

363. Pray LG (1951) Sexual precocity in females: Report of 2 cases, with arrest of precocity in the McCune-Albright syndrome after removal of cystic ovary. Pediatrics 8: 684–692

364. Printz JL, Choate JW, Townes PL, Harper RC (1973) The embryology of supernumerary ovaries. Obstet Gynecol 41: 246–252

365. Pueblitz-Peredo S, Luevano-Flores E, Rincon-Taracena R, Ochoa-Carrillo FJ (1985) Uteruslike mass of the ovary: Endomyometriosis or congenital malformation? A case with a discussion of histogenesis. Arch Pathol Lab Med 109: 361–364

366. Putschar WGJ, Manion WC (1956) Splenic-gonadal fusion. Am J Pathol 32: 15–33

367. Quan A, Charles D, Craig JM (1963) Histologic and functional consequences of periovarian adhesions. Obstet Gynecol 22: 96–101

368. Rabinowe SL, Berger MJ, Welch WR, Dluhy RG (1986) Lymphocyte dysfunction in autoimmune oophoritis. Resumption of menses with corticosteroids. Am J Med 81: 347–350

369. Rahilly MA, Al-Nafussi A (1991) Uterus-like mass of the ovary associated with endometrioid carcinoma. Histopathology 18: 549–551

370. Ramzy I, Nisker JA (1979) Histologic study of ovaries from young women with endometrial adenocarcinoma. Am J Clin Pathol 71: 253–256

371. Ravinsky E (1984) Ovarian hyperthecosis associated with pseudosarcomatous changes in the endometrial stroma. Am J Surg Pathol 8: 939–943

372. Rebar RW (1982) Hypergonadotropic amenorrhea and premature ovarian failure. A review. J Reprod Med 27: 179–186

373. Rebar RW, Erickson GF, Yen SSC (1982) Idiopathic premature ovarian failure: clinical and endocrine characteristics. Fertil Steril 37: 35–41

374. Resta L, Scordari MD, Colucci GA, et al (1989) Morphological changes of the ovarian surface epithelium in ovarian polycystic disease or endometrial carcinoma and a control group. Eur J Gynaecol Oncol 10: 39–41

375. Rewell RE (1972) Extra-uterine decidua. J Pathol 105: 219–222

376. Rice BF, Barclay DL, Sternberg WH (1969) Luteoma of pregnancy. Am J Obstet Gynecol 104: 871–878

377. Rice BF, Savard K (1966) Steroid hormone formation in the human ovary: IV. Ovarian stromal compartment; formation of radioactive steroids from acetate-1-^{14}C and action of gonadotropins. J Clin Endocrinol 26: 593–609

378. Riddlesberger MM Jr, Kuhn JP, Munschauer RW (1981) The association of juvenile hypothyroidism and cystic ovaries. Radiology 139: 77–80

379. Rivera-Alsina ME, DeSanctis VM, Schmidt WA (1987) Bilateral ovarian thecosis and virilization in pregnancy. A case report. J Reprod Med 32: 873–878

380. Roddick JW Jr, Greene RR (1957) Relation of ovarian stromal hyperplasia to endometrial carcinoma. Am J Obstet Gynecol 73: 843–852

381. Rosai J (1982) Uterus-like mass replacing ovary. (Letter) Arch Pathol Lab Med 106: 364–365

382. Rosen GF, Lew MW (1991) Severe ovarian hyperstimulation in a spontaneous singleton pregnancy. Am J Obstet Gynecol 165: 1312–1313

383. Ross GT (1976) Hormones and preantral follicle growth in women. May Clin Proc 51: 617–620

384. Roth LM, Sternberg WH (1973) Ovarian stromal tumors containing Leydig cells. II. Pure Leydig cell tumor, nonhilar type. Cancer 32: 952–960

385. Roth LM, Sternberg WH (1983) Partly luteinized theca cell tumor of the ovary. Cancer 51: 1697–1704

386. Roth LM, Deaton RL, Sternberg WH (1979) Massive ovarian edema. A clinicopathologic study of five cases including ultrastructural observations and review of the literature. Am J Surg Pathol 3: 11–21

387. Rotmensch S, Scommenga A (1989) Spontaneous ovarian hyperstimulation syndrome associated with hypothyroidism. Am J Obstet Gynecol 160: 1220–1222

388. Rubin P, Casarett GW (1968) Clinical Radiation Pathology, Vol I. Philadelphia, W. B. Saunders.

389. Ruehsen MDM, Blizzard RM, Garcia-Bunuel R, Jones GS (1972) Autoimmunity and ovarian failure. Am J Obstet Gynecol 112: 693–703

390. Ruehsen MDM, Jones GS (1967) Premature ovarian failure. Fertil Steril 18: 440–461

391. Russell P, Bannatyne P, Shearman RP, Fraser IS, Corbett P (1982) Premature hypergonadotropic ovarian failure: Clinicopathological study of 19 cases. Int J Gynecol Pathol 1: 185–201

392. Rutgers JL, Scully RE (1988) Cysts (cystadenomas) and tumors of the rete ovarii. Int J Gynecol Pathol 7: 330–342

393. Rutgers JL, Scully RE (1986) Functioning ovarian tumors with peripheral steroid cell proliferation: A report of twenty-four cases. Int J Gynecol Pathol 5: 319–337

394. Ryan GM, Craig J, Reid DE (1964) Histology of the uterus and ovaries after long-term cyclic norethynodrel therapy. Am J Obstet Gynecol 90: 715–725

395. Sakaguchi S, Sakaguchi N (1989) Organ-specific autoimmune disease induced in mice by elimination of T cell subsets. V. Neonatal administration of cyclosporin A causes autoimmune disease. J Immunol 142: 471–480

396. Salomonowitz E (1980) Tumorformige Amyloidose des Ovars. Geburtsh u Frauenheilk 40: 644–647

397. Samaan NA, Smith JP, Rutledge FN, Barcellona JM (1972) Plasma testosterone levels in trophoblastic disease and the effects of oophorectomy and chemotherapy. J Clin Endocrinol Metab 34: 558–561

398. Santos-Ramos R, Forney JP, Schwarz BE (1980) Sonographic findings and clinical correlations in molar pregnancy. Obstet Gynecol 56: 186–192

399. Sasano H, Fukunaga M, Rojas M, Silverberg SG (1989) Hyperthecosis of the ovary. Clinicopathologic study of 19 cases with immunohistochemical analysis of steroidogenic enzymes. Int J Gynecol Pathol 8: 311–320

400. Saxen L, Kassinen A, Saxen E (1963) Peritoneal foreign-body reaction caused by condom emulsion. Lancet 1: 1295–1296

401. Schenker JG, Weinstein D (1978) Ovarian hyperstimulation syndrome: A current survey. Fertil Steril 30: 255–268

402. Schiffer MA, Elguezabal A, Sultana M, Allen AC (1975) Actinomycosis infections associated with intrauterine contraceptive devices. Obstet Gynecol 45: 67–72

403. Schilsky RL, Sherins RJ, Hubbard SM, et al (1981) Long-term follow-up of ovarian function in women treated with MOPP chemotherapy for Hodgkin's disease. Am J Med 71: 552–556

404. Schmidt WA (1982) IUDs, inflammation, and infection: Assessment after two decades of IUD use. Hum Pathol 13: 878–881

405. Schmidt WA, Bedrossian CWM, Ali V, et al (1980) Actinomycosis and intrauterine contraceptive devices. Diag Gynecol Obstet 2: 165–177

406. Schneider D, Bukovsky I, Kaufman S, et al (1981) Severe ovarian hemorrhage in congenital afibrinogenemia. Acta Obstet Gynecol Scand 60: 431

407. Schultz LR, Lewton WA Jr, Clatworthy HW Jr (1963) Torsion of previously normal tube and ovary in children. N Engl J Med 268: 343–346

408. Schumert Z, Spitz I, Diamant Y, et al (1975) Elevation of serum testosterone in ovarian hyperstimulation syndrome. J Clin Endocrinol Metab 40: 889–892

409. Scully RE (1964) Stromal luteoma of the ovary. Cancer 17: 769–778

410. Scully RE (1979) Tumors of the ovary and maldeveloped

gonads. In: Atlas of Tumor Pathology, Second Series, Fascicle 16. Armed Forces Institute of Pathology, Washington, D.C.

411. Scully RE (1981) Smooth-muscle differentiation in genital tract disorders. (Editorial) Arch Pathol Lab Med 105: 505–507

412. Scully RE, Cohen RB (1964) Oxidative-enzyme activity in normal and pathologic human ovaries. Obstet Gynecol 24: 667–681

413. Scully RE (1986) Ovary. In: Henson DE, Albores-Saavedra J (eds) The Pathology of Incipient Neoplasia. Philadelphia, W. B. Saunders, pp 279–293

414. Sedin G, Bergquist C, Lindgren PG (1985) Ovarian hyperstimulation syndrome in preterm infants. Pediatr Res 19: 548–551

415. Sedmak DD, Hart WR, Tubbs RR (1987) Autoimmune oophoritis: A histopathologic study of involved ovaries with immunologic characterization of the mononuclear cell infiltrate. Int J Gynecol Pathol 6: 73–81

416. Semchyshyn S, Zuspan FP (1978) Ovarian hemorrhage due to anticoagulants. Am J Obstet Gynecol 131: 837–844

417. Shalet SM, Beardwell CG, Morris Jones PH, et al (1976) Ovarian failure following abdominal irradiation in childhood. Br J Cancer 33: 655–658

418. Shalev E, Zuckerman H, Rizescu I (1982) Pelvic inflammatory pseudotumor (xanthogranuloma). Acta Obstet Gynecol Scand 61: 285–286

419. Shawker TH, Hubbard VS, Reichert CM, Guerreiro de Matos OM (1983) Cystic ovaries in cystic fibrosis: an ultrasound and autopsy study. J Ultrasound Med 2: 439–444

420. Shettles LB (1963) Recurrent theca lutein cysts. Obstet Gynecol 21: 339–342

421. Shipton EA, Meares SD (1965) Heterotopic bone formation in the ovary. Aust NZ J Obstet Gynaecol 5: 100–102

422. Shoupe D, Kumar DD, Lobo RA (1983) Insulin resistance in polycystic ovary syndrome. Am J Obstet Gynecol 147: 588–592

423. Shoupe D, Lobo RA (1984) The influence of androgens on insulin resistance. Fertil Steril 41: 385–388

424. Silver HK (1958) Juvenile hypothyroidism with precocious sexual development. J Endocrinol Metab 18: 886–891

425. Simstein NL (1981) Colo-tubo-ovarian fistula as complication of pelvic inflammatory disease. South J Med 74: 512–513

426. Siris ES, Leventhal BG, Vaitukaitis JL (1976) Effects of childhood leukemia and chemotherapy on puberty and reproductive function in girls. N Engl J Med 294: 1143–1146

427. Sjovall A, Akerman M (1968) Peritoneal granulomas in women due to the presence of Enterobius S. Oxyuris vermicularis. Acta Obstet Gynecol Scand 47: 361–373

428. Smith A, Fraser IS, Noel M (1979) Three siblings with premature gonadal failure. Fertil Steril 32: 528–530

429. Smith S, Ravnikar VA, Barbieri RL (1987) Androgen and insulin response to an oral glucose challenge in hyperandrogenic women. Fertil Steril 48: 72–77

430. Snowden JA, Harkin PJR, Thornton JG, Wells M (1989) Morphometric assessment of ovarian stromal proliferation—a clinicopathological study. Histopathology 14: 369

431. Sommers SC (1983) Female genital tract granulomas. In: Ioachim HL (ed): Pathology of Granulomas. New York, Raven Press, pp 395–409

432. Sommers SC, Wadman PJ (1956) Pathogenesis of polycystic ovaries. Am J Obstet Gynecol 72: 160–169

433. Spanos WJ (1973) Preoperative hormonal therapy of cystic adnexal masses. Am J Obstet Gynecol 116: 551–554

434. Starup J, Sele V (1973) Premature ovarian failure. Acta Obstet Gynecol Scand 52: 259 268

435. Starup J, Sele V, Henriksen B (1971) Amenorrhea associated with increased production of gonadotropins and a morphologically normal ovarian follicular apparatus. Acta Endocrinol 66: 248–256

436. Starup J, Visfeldt J (1974) Ovarian morphology in early and late human pregnancy. Acta Obstet Gynecol Scand 53: 211–218

437. Stearns HC, Sneeden VD, Fearl JD (1974) A clinical and pathologic review of ovarian stromal hyperplasia and its possible relationship to common diseases of the female reproductive system. Am J Obstet Gynecol 119: 375–381

438. Steege JF (1987) Ovarian remnant syndrome. Obstet Gynecol 70: 64–67

439. Steingold KA, Judd HL, Nieberg RK, et al (1986) Treatment of severe androgen excess due to ovarian hyperthecosis with a long-acting gonadotropin-releasing hormone agonist. Am J Obstet Gynecol 154: 1241–1248

440. Sternberg WH (1949) The morphology, androgenic function, hyperplasia, and tumours of the human ovarian hilus cells. Am J Pathol 25: 493–521

441. Sternberg WH (1955) Association of masculinizing ovarian hilus cell tumors, ovarian stromal hyperplasia, and lutein-like cell proliferation (abstr). Am J Pathol 31: 571

442. Sternberg WH, Barclay DL (1966) Luteoma of pregnancy. Am J Obstet Gynecol 95: 165–181

443. Sternberg WH, Dhurandhar HN (1977) Functional ovarian tumors of stromal and sex cord origin. Human Pathol 8: 565–582

444. Sternberg WH, Gaskill CJ (1950) Theca-cell tumors: With a report of twelve new cases and observations on the possible etiologic role of ovarian stromal hyperplasia. Am J Obstet Gynecol 59: 575–587

445. Sternberg WH, Roth LM (1973) Ovarian stromal tumors containing Leydig cells. I. Stromal–Leydig cell tumor and non-neoplastic transformation of ovarian stroma to Leydig cells. Cancer 32: 940–951

446. Sternberg WH, Segaloff A, Gaskill CJ (1953) Influence of chorionic gonadotropin on human ovarian hilus cells (Leydig-like cells). J Clin Endocrinol Metab 13: 139–153

447. Stevens ML, Plotka ED (1977) Functional lutein cyst in a postmenopausal women. Obstet Gynecol 50: 27s–29s

448. Stillman RJ, Schinfeld JS, Schiff I, et al (1981) Ovarian failure in long-term survivors of childhood malignancy. Am J Obstet Gynecol 139: 62–66

449. Strickler RC, Kelly RW, Askin FB (1984) Postmenopausal ovarian follicle cyst: An unusual cause of estrogen excess. Int J Gynecol Pathol 3: 318–322

450. Subietas A, Deppisch LM, Astarloa J (1977). Cytomegalovirus oophoritis: Ovarian cortical necrosis. Hum Pathol 8: 285–292

451. Sutherland AM (1982) Postmenopausal tuberculosis of the female genital tract. Obstet Gynecol 59: 54s–57s

452. Swenson WM, Tolstedt GE, Ramos P, Peters C (1978)

Ovarian arteriovenous fistula. An unusual cause of abdominal pain. Obstet Gynecol 51: 62S–63S

453. Symmonds RE, Pettit PDM (1979) Ovarian remnant syndrome. Obstet Gynecol 54: 174–177

454. Symonds DA, Driscoll SG (1973) An adrenal cortical rest within the fetal ovary: Report of a case. Am J Clin Pathol 60: 562–564

455. Talbert LM, Raj MHG, Hammond MG, Greer T (1984) Endocrine and immunologic studies in a patient with resistant ovary syndrome. Fertil Steril 42: 741–744

456. Tanabe K, Gagliano P, Channing CP, et al (1983) Levels of inhibin-F activity and steroids in human follicular fluid from normal women and women with polycystic ovarian disease. J Clin Endocrinol Metab 57: 24–31

457. Taylor SI, Dons RF, Hernandez E, et al (1982) Insulin resistance associated with androgen excess in women with autoantibodies to the insulin receptor. Ann Intern Med 97: 851–855

458. Teilum G, Madsen V (1950) Endometriosis ovarii et peritonaei caused by hysterosalpingography. Br J Obstet Gynaecol 57: 10–16

459. Thomas E, Mestman J, Henneman C, et al (1972) Bilateral luteomas of pregnancy with virilization. Obstet Gynecol 39: 577–584

460. Thorp JM Jr, Wells SR, Droegemueller W (1990) Ovarian suspension in massive ovarian edema. Obstet Gynecol 76: 912–914

461. Tiboldi T (1975) Involvement of human and primate ovaries in schistosomiasis. A review of the literature. Ann Soc Belge Med Trop 58: 9–20

462. Tulandi T, Kinch RAH (1981) Premature ovarian failure. Obstet Gynecol Surv 36: 521–527

463. Tulandi T, McInnes RA, Arronet GH (1984) Ovarian hyperstimulation syndrome following ovulation induction with human menopausal gonadotropin. Int J Fertil 29: 113–117

464. Turksoy RN, Safaii H, Kappy KA, et al (1978) Infarction of corpora lutei associated with intrauterine and extrauterine pregnancy. J Reprod Med 21: 102–106

465. Vaidya RA, Aloorkar SD, Rege NR, et al (1977) Premature ovarian failure. J Reprod Med 19: 348–352

466. VanWingen T, Upton RT, Cloherty MG, et al (1984) Bilateral massive edema. A case report. J Reprod Med 29: 875–877

467. Van Wyk JJ, Grumbach MM (1960) Syndrome of precocious menstruation and galactorrhea in juvenile hypothyroidism: An example of hormonal overlap in pituitary feedback. J Pediatr 57: 416–435

468. Vasquez SB, Sotos JF, Kim MH (1982) Massive edema of the ovary and virilization. Obstet Gynecol 59: 95s–99s

469. Vazquez AM, Kenny FM (1973) Ovarian failure and antiovarian antibodies in association with hypoparathyroidism, moniliasis, and Addison's and Hashimoto's diseases. Obstet Gynecol 41: 414–418

470. Verkauf BS, Reiter EO, Hernandez L, Burns SA (1977) Virilization of mother and fetus associated with luteoma of pregnancy: A case report with endocrinologic studies. Am J Obstet Gynecol 129: 274–280

471. Villanueva AL, Rebar RW (1983) Triple-X syndrome and premature ovarian failure. Obstet Gynecol 62: 70S–73S

472. von Numers C (1965) Observations on metaplastic changes in the germinal epithelium of the ovary and on the aetiology of ovarian endometriosis. Acta Obstet Gynecol Scand 44: 107–116

473. Wajda KJ, Marsh WL Jr (1989) Hyperreactio luteinalis. Benign disorder masquerading as an ovarian neoplasm. Arch Pathol Lab Med 113: 921–925

474. Walfish PG, Gottesman IS, Shewchuk AB, et al (1983) Association of premature ovarian failure with HLA antigens. Tissue Antigens 21: 168–169

475. Warne GL, Fairley KF, Hobbs JB, Martin FIR (1973) Cyclophosphamide-induced ovarian failure. N Engl J Med 289: 1159–1162

476. Wassman ER, Johnson K, Shapiro LJ, et al (1982) Postmortem findings in the Hurler–Scheie syndrome (mucopolysaccharidosis I-H/S). Birth Defects: Original Article Series 18 (3B): 13–18

477. Waxman JHX, Terry YA, Wrigley PFM, et al (1982) Gonadal function in Hodgkin's disease: long-term follow-up of chemotherapy. Br Med J 285: 1612–1613

478. Weinstein D, Rabinowitz R, Malach D, et al (1983) Ovarian hemorrhage in women with Von Willebrand's disease. A report of two cases. J Reprod Med 28: 500–502

479. Wentz AC, Gutai JP, Jones GS, Migeon CJ (1976) Ovarian hyperthecosis in an adolescent patient. J Pediatr 88: 488–493

480. Wetchler SJ, Dunn LJ (1985) Ovarian abscess. Report of a case and a review of the literature. Obstet Gynecol Surv 40: 476–485

481. Wharton LR (1959) Two cases of supernumerary ovary and one of accessory ovary, with an analysis of previously reported cases. Am J Obstet Gynecol 78: 1101–1119

482. White A, Flaris N, Elmer D, et al (1990) Coexistence of mucinous cystadenoma of the ovary and ovarian sarcoidosis. Am J Obstet Gynecol 162: 1284–1285

483. White CA, Bradbury JT (1965) Ovarian theca lutein cysts. Experimental formation in women prior to repeat cesarean section. Am J Obstet Gynecol 92: 973–980

484. Whitehead E, Shalet SM, Blackledge G, et al (1983) The effect of combination chemotherapy on ovarian function in women treated for Hodgkin's disease. Cancer 52: 988–993

485. Wieland RG, Bendezu R, Hallberg MC, et al (1976) Hormonal evaluation of premature menarche produced by a follicular cyst. Am J Obstet Gynecol 126: 731–733

486. Wierman ME, Beardsworth DE, Mansfield MJ, et al (1985) Puberty without gonadotropins. A unique mechanism of sexual development. N Engl J Med 312: 65–72

487. Wilder JR, Barnes WA (1953) Obstruction of the small intestine by corpus luteum cyst. Report of a case. JAMA 151: 730–732

488. Williams DJ, Connor P, Ironside JW (1990) Pre-menopausal cytomegalovirus oophoritis. Histopathology 16: 405–407

489. Williamson HO, Phansey SA, Mathur RS, et al (1980) Myasthenia gravis, premature menopause, and thyroid autoimmunity. Am J Obstet Gynecol 137: 893–901

490. Willson JB, Black JR III (1964) Ovarian abscess. Am J Obstet Gynecol 90: 34–43

491. Wilson EA, Erickson GF, Zarutski P, et al (1979) Endocrine studies of normal and polycystic ovarian tissues in vitro. Am J Obstet Gynecol 134: 56–63

492. Wilson GE, Haboubi NY, McWilliam LJ, Hirsch PJ (1990) Postoperative necrotizing granulomata in the cervix and ovary. (Letter) J Clin Pathol 43: 1037–1038

493. Winslow RC, Funkhouser JW (1968) Sarcoidosis of the female reproductive organs. Report of a case. Obstet Gynecol 32: 285–289

494. Wlodarski FM, Trainer TD (1975) Granulomatous oophoritis and salpingitis associated with Crohn's disease of the appendix. Am J Obstet Gynecol 122: 527–528

495. Wojcik EM, Naylor B (1992) "Collagen balls" in peritoneal washings. Acta Cytol 46: 466–470

496. Wolfe CDA, Stirling RW (1988) Premature menopause associated with autoimmune oophoritis. Case report. Br J Obstet Gynaecol 95: 63–632

497. Wolff E, Glasser M, Gordon GG, et al (1973) Virilizing luteoma of pregnancy. Am J Med 54: 229–233

498. Woll E, Hertig AT, Smith GVS, Johnson LC (1948) The ovary in endometrial carcinoma. Am J Obstet Gynecol 56: 617–633

499. Wood LC, Olichney M, Locke H, et al (1965) Syndrome of juvenile hypothyroidism associated with advanced sexual development: Report of two new cases and comment on the management of an associated ovarian mass. J Clin Endocrinol Metab 25: 1289–1295

500. Yen SSC (1980) The polycystic ovary syndrome. Clin Endocrinol 12: 177–207

501. Young RH, Prat J, Scully RE (1980) Epidermoid cyst of the ovary. A report of three cases with comments on histogenesis. Am J Clin Pathol 73: 272–276

502. Young RH, Scully RE (1984) Fibromatosis and massive edema of the ovary, possibly related entites: A report of 14 cases of fibromatosis and 11 cases of massive edema. Int J Gynecol Pathol 3: 153–178

503. Zaitoon MM (1987) Ureteral obstruction secondary to retained ovarian remnants: A case report and review of the literature. J Urol 137: 973–974

504. Zaitoon MM, Florentin H (1982) Crossed renal extopia with unilateral agenesis of fallopian tube and ovary. J Urol 128: 111

505. Zalel Y, Caspi B, Ben-Hur H, et al (1992) Spontaneous ovarian hyperstimulation syndrome concomitant with spontaneous pregnancy in a woman with polycystic ovary disease. Am J Obstet Gynecol 167: 122–124

506. Zander J, Mickan H, Holzmann K, Lohe KJ (1978) Androluteoma syndrome of pregnancy. Am J Obstet Gynecol 130: 170–177

507. Zarate A, Karchmer S, Gomez E, Castelazo-Ayala L (1970) Premature menopause. A clinical, histologic, and cytogenetic study. Am J Obstet Gynecol 106: 110–114

508. Zhang J, Young RH, Arseneau J, Scully RE (1982) Ovarian stromal tumors containing lutein or Leydig cells (luteinized thecomas and stromal Leydig cell tumors)—a clinicopathological analysis of fifty cases. Int J Gynecol Pathol 1: 270–285

17

Diseases of the Peritoneum

Philip B. Clement, M.D.

This chapter considers the wide range of nonneoplastic and neoplastic lesions that involve the peritoneum, and in some cases the retroperitoneal lymph nodes, of females. The first half of the chapter deals with inflammatory lesions, tumor-like lesions (including mesothelial hyperplasia), mesothelial neoplasms, miscellaneous primary tumors, and metastatic tumors. The second half of the chapter is devoted to a large group of lesions that share a potential origin from the secondary müllerian system, the prototypical example of which is endometriosis.

Inflammatory Lesions

Acute Peritonitis

Acute diffuse peritonitis, characterized by a serosal fibrinopurulent exudate, is most commonly associated with a perforated viscus, and usually is bacterial or chemical (bile or gastric or pancreatic juice) in origin. The lipases in pancreatic juice also typically produce fat necrosis. Spontaneous bacterial peritonitis occurs most often in children and in adults who are immunocompromised or have cirrhosis of the liver.[529,565] Rare infectious causes of acute peritonitis include candida,[27] actinomycetes,[577] and amebae.[266] Recurrent attacks of acute peritonitis are an almost constant feature of familial Mediterranean fever (recurrent polyserositis; periodic disease).[507] Localized acute peritonitis may be associated with infection (or infarction) of specific organs, as in pelvic inflammatory disease.

Granulomatous Peritonitis

A variety of infectious and noninfectious agents can cause granulomatous peritonitis. The peritoneum may be studded with nodules, which can mimic disseminated tumor at operation. The diagnosis rests on the histological, and in some cases, microbiological, identification of the causative agent.

INFECTIOUS

Tuberculous peritonitis may be secondary to spread from a focus within the abdominopelvic cavity or be a manifestation of miliary spread.[26,207] The granulomas are characterized by caseous necrosis and Langhans'-type giant cells; mycobacteria may be demonstrated by acid-fast stains or immunofluorescence methods. Rarely, granulomatous peritonitis is a complication of fungal infections, including histoplasmosis,[432] coccidioidomycosis,[465] and cryptococcosis,[560] and parasitic infestations, including schistosomiasis,[46] oxyuriasis,[122,503] echinococcosis,[577] ascariasis,[431] and strongyloidiasis.[319]

NONINFECTIOUS

Foreign material, typically recognizable on histological examination, can elicit a granulomatous reaction on the peritoneum. Starch granules from surgical gloves,[105,231,242] douche fluid,[225] and lubricants[466] typically incite a granulomatous and fibrosing peritonitis; in occasional cases the inflammatory reaction may be of tuberculoid type with caseous necrosis.[380] The periodic acid-Schiff (PAS)-positive starch granules exhibit a characteristic Maltese-cross configuration under polarized light. Talc was once an important cause of granulomatous and fibrosing peritonitis because of its use as a lubricant on surgical gloves,[150,414] and talc-induced peritonitis has been described more recently in drug abusers.[73] Other iatrogenic causes of granulomatous peritonitis include cellulose and cotton fibers from surgical pads and drapes,[189,252,540] microcrystalline collagen hemostat (Avitene),[397] and oily materials, such as hysterosalpingographic contrast medium, mineral oil, and paraffin.[339,383,532] The last three substances are associated with a lipogranulomatous reaction.

Escaped bowel contents, including vegetable matter, food-derived starch,[125] and barium sulphate,[272] can produce a peritoneal foreign-body reaction. Sebaceous material and keratin from ruptured dermoid cysts typically evoke an intense granulomatous, lipogranulomatous, and fibrosing peritoneal inflammatory reaction that may mimic a neoplasm at operation.[516,521,562] Meconium, containing lanugo hair, squamous cells, keratin, bile, and pancreatic and intestinal secretions, produces a granulomatous peritonitis; calcification also may be prominent.[171,224,538] In boys, the process may involve the tunica vaginalis and result in a tumor-like scrotal mass.[166] Granulomatous inflammation to keratin derived from uterine and ovarian adenoacanthomas is discussed below (see Tumor-like Lesions). Chronic bile peritonitis may be associated with granulomatous inflammation and fibrosis; cholesterol crystals and bile pigment may be identifiable within giant cells. Granulomatous peritonitis also has been described secondary to Crohn's disease,[123] sarcoidosis,[543,582] and Whipple's disease.[244] Necrotizing peritoneal granulomas recently have been described following diathermy ablation of endometriosis.[94]

Peritoneal Fibrosis

Reactive peritoneal fibrosis, often accompanied by fibrous adhesions, is a common sequela of prior peritoneal inflammation, and a frequent complication of a surgical procedure.[564] In occasional cases, it may be difficult to differentiate between markedly reactive peritoneal fibrosis and a desmoplastic mesothelioma, particularly in a small biopsy specimen.[348] Features favoring a diagnosis of mesothelioma include nuclear atypia, necrosis, organized patterns of collagen deposition (fascicular, storiform), and infiltration of adjacent tissues.[348]

Localized hyaline plaques are a common incidental finding on the splenic capsule, and probably are related to splenic congestion.[558] Nonspecific fibrous thickening of the peritoneum has been described as a histological finding in patients with hepatic cirrhosis and ascites.[59] In contrast, the designation "sclerosing peritonitis" has been applied to a clinically significant, potentially fatal lesion that represents a reactive hyperplasia of the submesothelial mesenchymal cells to a variety of stimuli. The first description, by Concato,[106] was that of pearly white thickening of the visceral peritoneum, either as discrete plaques or continuous sheets involving the hepatic, splenic, and diaphragmatic peritoneum. The process often encases the small bowel ("abdominal cocoon"), causing bowel obstruction. Sclerosing peritonitis occurs in an idiopathic form, which most frequently, but not invariably, affects adolescent girls in tropical countries.[131,165,310a] Known causes include practolol therapy,[338] chronic ambulatory peritoneal dialysis,[51,556] the use of a peritoneovenous (LeVeen) shunt,[66] bacterial or mycobacterial infection, sarcoidosis,[380a] the carcinoid syndrome, familial Mediterranean fever, and fibrogenic foreign materials as seen in drug users. We have encountered six cases of sclerosing peritonitis associated with luteinized thecomas of the ovary[103a] (Fig. 17.1). Sclerosing peritonitis should be distinguished from the rarer "peritoneal encapsulation," a congenital malformation in which an accessory peritoneal membrane encases

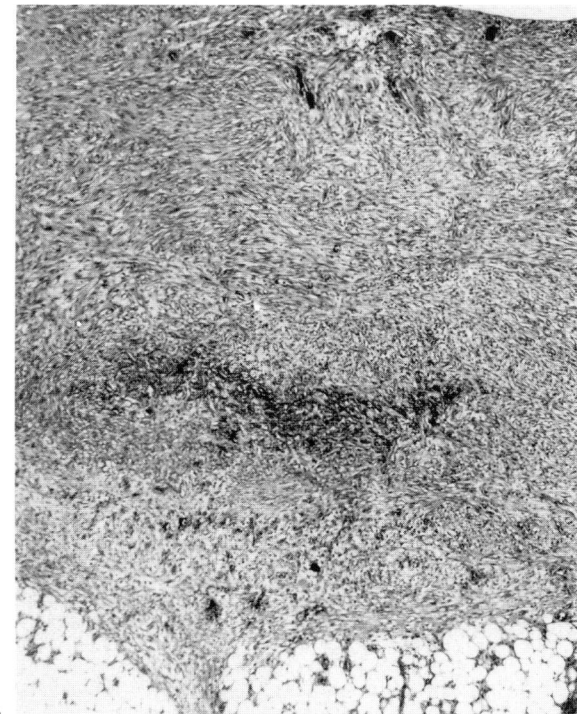

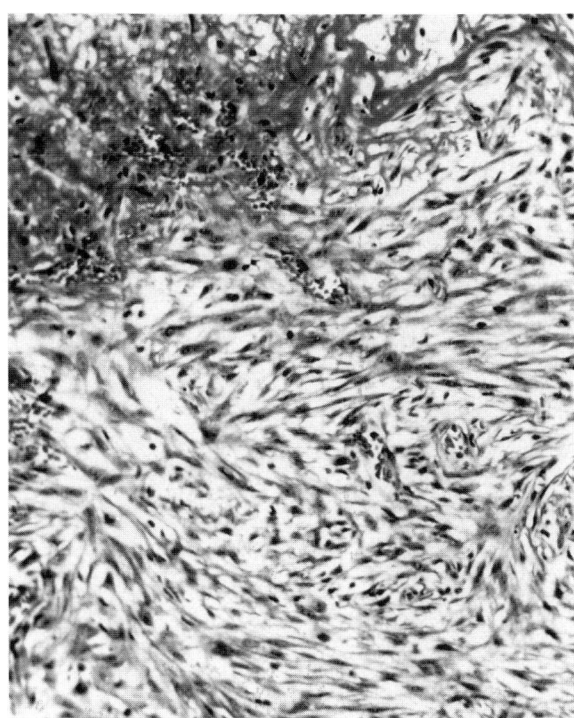

FIG. 17.1. **Sclerosing peritonitis associated with bilateral luteinized thecomas of the ovary. a:** Low-power view of omentum showing involvement of its surface by a layer of cellular fibrous tissue. **b:** Higher-power view showing fibrin *(top)*, plump fibroblasts, and a sprinkling of chronic inflammatory cells.

loops of small bowel in a sac-like structure.[467,497] The latter condition is largely asymptomatic, and usually found incidentally at laparotomy or autopsy. Confusion arises when the two terms are used interchangeably or even together, as in "encapsulating peritonitis."

Rare Types of Peritonitis

Eosinophilic peritonitis is seen rarely in cases of eosinophilic gastroenteritis and the hypereosinophilic syndrome.[4] Isolated cases of eosinophilic ascites have been associated with childhood atopy, peritoneal dialysis, vasculitis, lymphoma or metastatic carcinoma, and ruptured hydatid cysts.[4] Rare cases of peritonitis may be secondary to peritoneal involvement by collagen-vascular diseases, including systemic lupus erythematosus[358] and Degos' disease.[324]

Tumor-like Lesions

Mesothelial Hyperplasia

Hyperplasia of mesothelial cells is a common response to inflammation and chronic effusions (Figs. 17.2–17.4). Hyperplastic lesions may be noted at operation as solitary or multiple small nodules, but more commonly are incidental findings on microscopic examination.[129,169,216,348,350] Mesothelial hyperplasia often involves the adnexal areas in cases of chronic salpingitis and endometriosis,[280] and occasionally is encountered, particularly in the omentum, in association with ovarian tumors.[100] We also have seen cases in which mesothelial hyperplasia on the surface of the ovary or within the superficial ovarian stroma overlying a borderline epithelial tumor has been misinterpreted as invasive tumor (Fig. 17.4).[100] Mesothelial hyperplasia may be confined to a hernia sac, and in such cases may be caused by trauma or incarceration.[447]

In florid examples, solid, trabecular, tubular, papillary, or tubulopapillary patterns (Figs. 17.2–17.4) and limited degrees of extension of the mesothelial cells into the underlying tissues may be seen. The cells often are disposed focally in linear, sometimes parallel, thin layers, separated by fibrin or fibrous tissue (Fig. 17.4). The mesothelial cells may have cytoplasmic vacuoles containing acid mucin (predominantly hyaluronic acid) or, less commonly, exhibit marked cytoplasmic clearing.[348] Mild to moderate nuclear pleomorphism (Fig. 17.3), mitotic figures, and occasional multinucleated cells may be seen. Psammoma bodies are encountered in occasional cases and rarely, eosinophilic strap-shaped cells resembling rhabdomyoblasts have been described.[447]

The major differential diagnosis is with diffuse malignant mesothelioma (DMM). McCaughey and co-workers[129,348] have noted that the presence of grossly visible

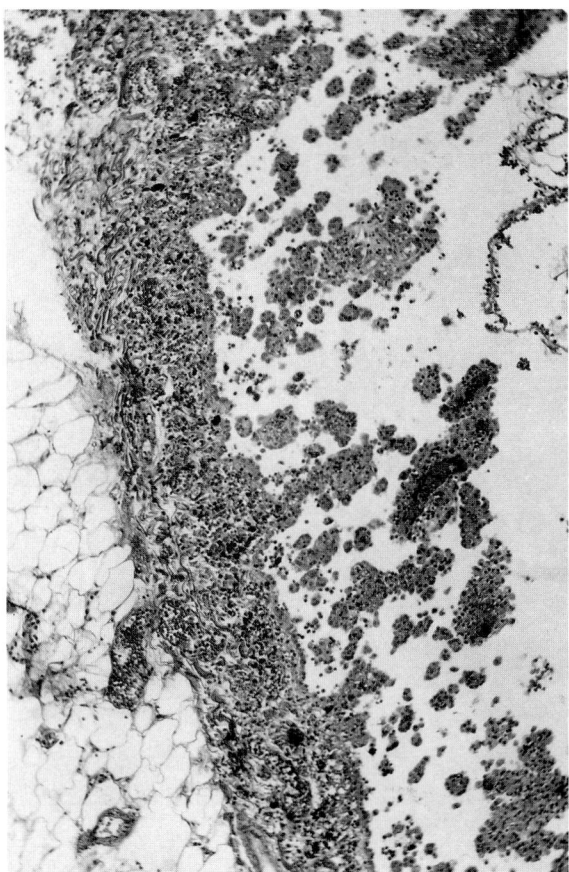

Fɪɢ. 17.2. Papillary mesothelial hyperplasia. (Reprinted by permission of Daya and McCaughey, ref. 129.)

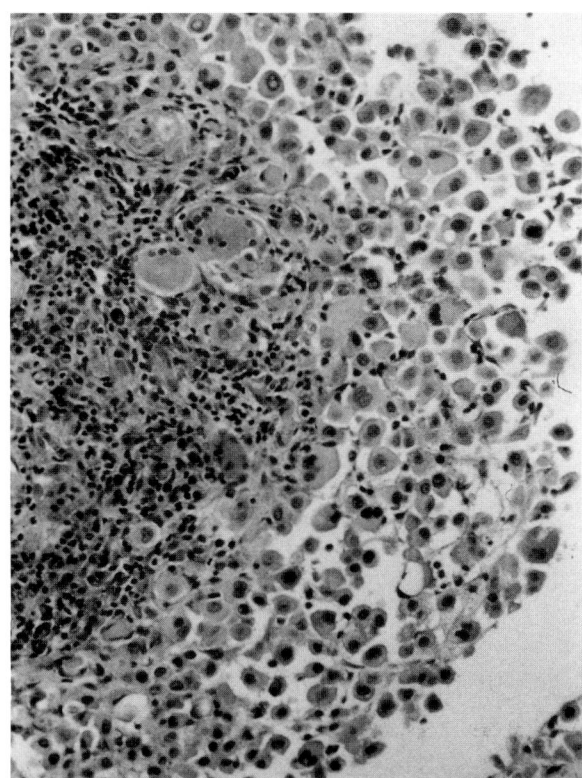

Fɪɢ. 17.3. Mesothelial hyperplasia with moderate nuclear atypia. (Reprinted by permission of Daya and McCaughey, ref. 129.)

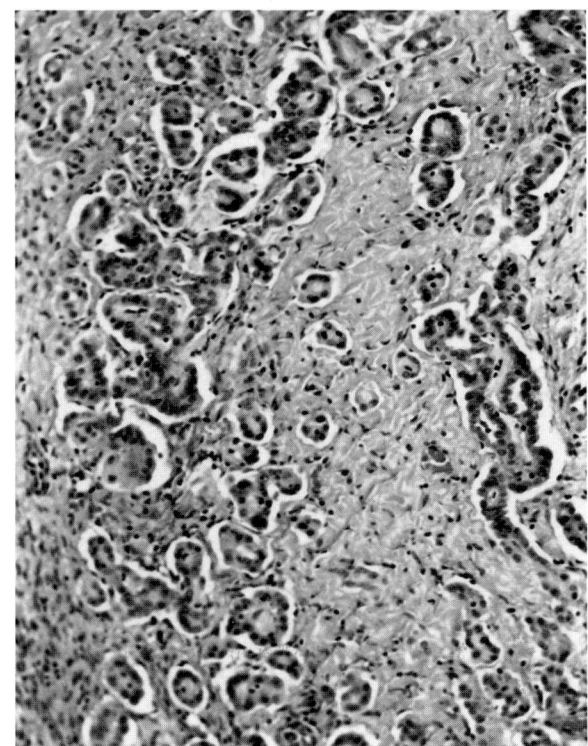

Fɪɢ. 17.4. Florid mesothelial hyperplasia in wall of borderline mucinous tumor of the ovary. The mesothelial proliferation was initially misdiagnosed as stromal invasion (Reprinted by permission of Clement and Young, ref. 100.)

nodules, necrosis, conspicuous large cytoplasmic vacuoles, marked nuclear pleomorphism, and deep infiltration favor DMM over mesothelial hyperplasia. Some of these features, however, such as marked nuclear atypia, are not always present or may be present only focally within a DMM. Special techniques may facilitate the differential diagnosis. Immunoreactivity for p53[259a] and intense cytoplasmic immunoreactivity for epithelial membrane antigen[569] are characteristic of the cells of DMM but not hyperplastic mesothelial cells. Morphometry has shown that reactive mesothelial cells generally have smaller nuclei than the cells of a DMM,[297] and there are more nucleolar organizer regions in malignant mesothelial cells than in reactive ones.[18,509] Despite these differential features, in occasional cases the distinction between a hyperplastic and malignant mesothelial lesion may be difficult or impossible, particularly in a biopsy specimen. If the lesion in question is a DMM, follow-up usually reveals its nature within several months because of its typically rapid growth.[348] In contrast, an atypical mesothelial proliferation occasionally persists for years without an apparent cause.[348] An apparently benign, otherwise typical mesothelial proliferation, however, occasionally precedes the appearance of a DMM.[348,438]

The differential diagnosis of mesothelial hyperplasia also includes borderline serous tumors of primary peritoneal or ovarian origin. Grossly visible ovarian or peritoneal tumor, columnar cells with or without cilia, the presence of intracellular or extracellular neutral mucin, and large numbers of psammoma bodies all favor a serous tumor. Immunohistochemical markers for epithelial differentiation (see section on DMM) also may be of value in the differential diagnosis.[335]

Peritoneal Inclusion Cysts

Peritoneal inclusion cysts typically occur in the peritoneal cavity of women in the reproductive age group.° Rarely they occur in men and in the pleural cavity.[47,289,350,498] Some are incidental findings at laparotomy in the form of single or multiple, small, thin-walled, translucent, unilocular cysts that may be attached or lie free in the peritoneal cavity. Occasionally they may involve the round ligament simulating an inguinal hernia.[220] The cysts have a smooth lining, contents that vary from yellow and watery to gelatinous. Microscopically, they are characterized by a single layer of flattened, benign-appearing mesothelial cells. Although most of these unilocular mesothelial cysts probably are reactive in origin, some of those located in the mesocolon, mesentery of the small intestine, retroperitoneum, and splenic capsule may be developmental.[448]

Multilocular cystic masses that may be up to 20 cm in diameter (Fig. 17.5) and that are lined by mesothelial cells are referred to as *multilocular peritoneal inclusion cysts* (MPICs), "benign cystic mesotheliomas", "inflammatory cysts of the peritoneum", or "postoperative peritoneal cysts".† MPICs usually are associated with clinical manifestations, most commonly lower abdominal pain, a palpable mass, or both. They usually adhere to pelvic organs and may simulate a cystic ovarian tumor on clinical examination, at laparotomy,[354] or even on pathological examination[259]; the upper abdominal cavity, the retroperitoneum, or hernia sacs also may be involved.[448] Unlike the smaller unilocular cysts, the septa and walls of MPICs may contain considerable amounts of fibrous tissue. Their contents may resemble those of the unilocular cysts or be serosanguinous or bloody.

On microscopic examination, MPICs typically are lined by a single layer of flat to cuboidal, occasionally hobnail-shaped, mesothelial cells with generally bland nuclear features (Fig. 17.6), although a degree of reactive atypia is not infrequent. The lining cells occasionally form small papillae and cribriform patterns or undergo squamous metapla-

---

°Refs. 71,145,268,354,355,364,372,448,472,567.
†Refs. 71,145,268,354,355,364,372,448,472,567.

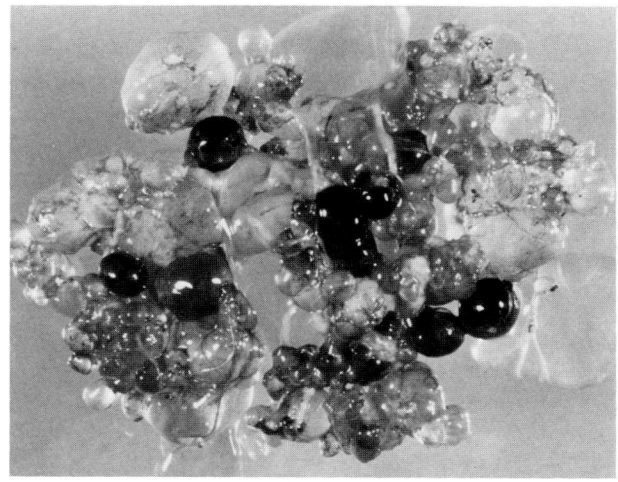

FIG. 17.5. **Peritoneal inclusion cyst.** Multilocular cystic masses consist of thin-walled cysts with a smooth lining. (Reprinted by permission of the Cleveland Clinic Foundation from Miles JM, Hart WR, McMahon JT (1986) Cystic mesothelioma of the peritoneum. Cleve Clin Q 53: 109–114.)

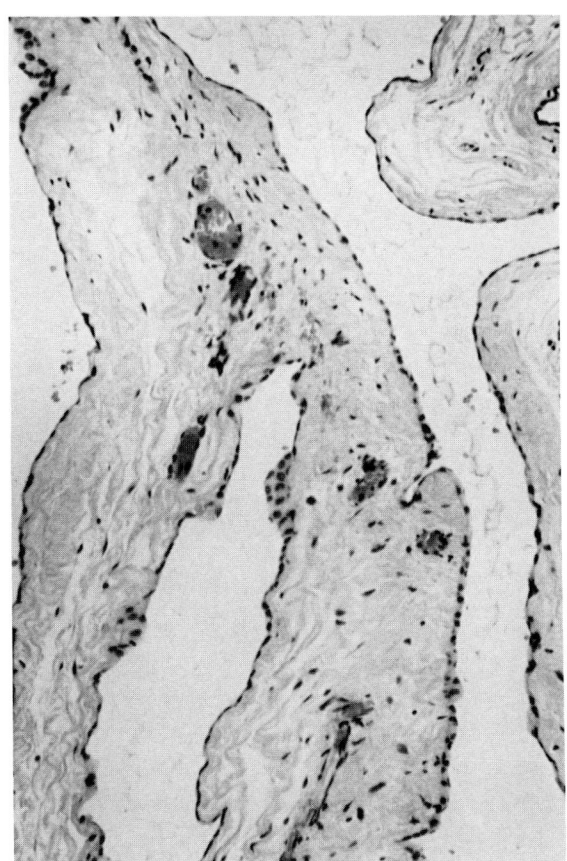

FIG. 17.6. **Peritoneal inclusion cyst.** Cystic spaces are lined by a single layer of flat mesothelial cells and are separated by thin fibrous septa.

sia.[448,567] In some cases, mural proliferations of typical or atypical mesothelial cells arranged singly, as gland-like structures or nests (Fig. 17.7), or in patterns resembling those in adenomatoid tumors, may be encountered.[354,448,567] Occasional vacuolated mesothelial cells in the stroma may simulate signet-ring cells.[448] The septa typically consist of a loose, fibrovascular connective tissue with a sparse inflammatory infiltrate. In some cases, marked acute and chronic inflammation, abundant fibrin, broad bands of granulation and fibrous tissue, and evidence of recent and remote hemorrhage are present in the cyst walls.

A history of a prior abdominal operation, pelvic inflammatory disease, endometriosis, or combinations thereof was present in 84% of patients in one series,[448] suggesting a role for inflammation in the pathogenesis of the

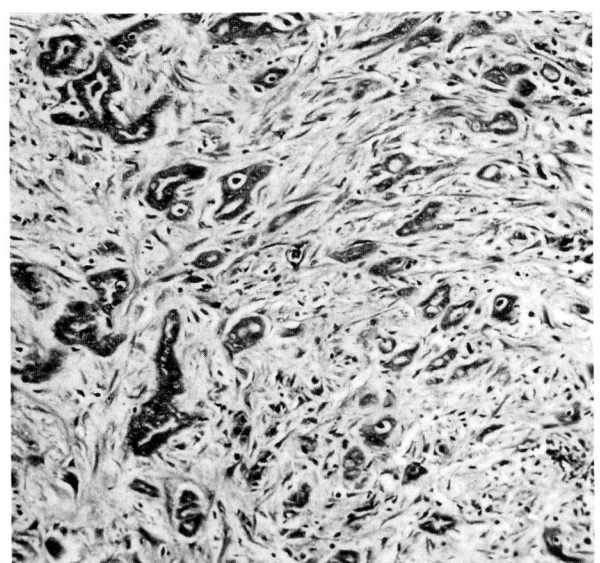

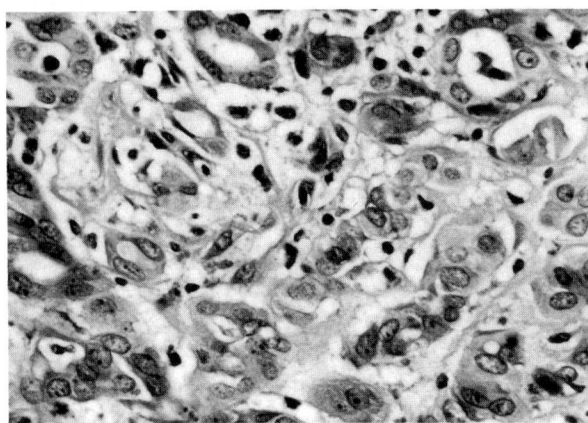

Fig. 17.7. Multilocular peritoneal inclusion cyst with mural mesothelial proliferation. a: Gland-like arrangements within a reactive fibrous stroma create an infiltrative pattern. **b:** Higher-power view showing benign appearing mesothelial cells forming small nests, cords, and lining small tubules.

cysts.[132,205,311,354,448,567] An inflammatory pathogenesis also is supported by the occurrence of cases in which the dividing line between florid adhesions associated with inflammation and a MPIC may be difficult. With one exception,[289] there has been no association with asbestos exposure. Follow-up examinations have not disclosed malignant behavior in cases that we consider MPICs, but in as many as one-half of these, the lesions have recurred from months to many years postoperatively.[448] It is likely, however, that at least some of these "recurrences" are the result of newly formed postoperative adhesions. For these reasons (while accepting that low-grade cystic mesotheliomas occur rarely, see below), we prefer the designation *multilocular peritoneal inclusion cyst* to "benign cystic mesothelioma" for such lesions, until there is convincing evidence for their neoplastic nature.

Aside from the contentious problem of their distinction from "true" cystic mesotheliomas (see below), MPICs are confused most often with multilocular cystic lymphangiomas.[71] In contrast to MPICs, the latter typically occur in children, more frequently in boys. In addition, they usually are extrapelvic, being almost always localized to the mesentery of the small intestine, omentum, mesocolon, or retroperitoneum. Their contents may be chylous, and on histological examination lymphoid aggregates and smooth muscle, which are rare findings in MPICs, typically are present within their walls. In problematic cases, immunohistochemical stains are useful in distinguishing endothelial from mesothelial cells. Another lesion that merits consideration in the differential diagnosis of MPICs is the rare multicystic adenomatoid tumor.[44,250] In contrast to MPICs, the latter typically involve the myometrium, contain foci of typical adenomatoid tumor, and lack prominent numbers of inflammatory cells. A detailed discussion of other lesions in the differential diagnosis of MPICs has been presented elsewhere.[448]

Splenosis

Splenosis, which results from implantation of splenic tissue, typically is an incidental finding at laparotomy or autopsy months to years after splenectomy for traumatic splenic rupture.[71a,163,394,561] A few to innumerable red-blue, peritoneal nodules, ranging from punctate to 7 cm in diameter, are scattered widely throughout the abdominal, and less commonly the pelvic, cavity. The intraoperative appearance may mimic endometriosis, benign or malignant vascular tumors, or metastatic cancer.

Trophoblastic Implants

Implants of trophoblast on the pelvic or omental peritoneum may complicate the operative treatment of tubal pregnancy.[72,436,536] The implants are more likely to occur in cases managed by laparoscopy (1.9% of cases) than those managed by laparotomy (0.6% of cases), and are more likely to occur after salpingotomy than salpingectomy.[72] The clinical presentation in such cases includes an initial decline in the serum human chorionic gonadotropin (hCG) level after removal of the ectopic pregnancy, followed by a rising level, abdominal pain, and in some cases, intraabdominal hemorrhage.[72] Microscopic examination of the implants reveals viable trophoblastic tissue that may include chorionic villi.

Melanosis

The four reported cases of melanosis, or melanotic pigmentation of the peritoneum, have all been associated with ovarian dermoid cysts; in two cases, the cysts had ruptured preoperatively.[5,174,309,462a] At laparotomy, focal or diffuse, tan to black, peritoneal staining or similarly pigmented, tumor-like nodules are encountered within the pelvis and in the omentum. Some of the cysts within the ovarian tumors exhibit pigmentation of their contents and lining. On histological examination, the ovarian and peritoneal pigmentation consists of melanin-laden histiocytes within a fibrous stroma. In at least three of the reported cases and in a fourth case we have encountered, gastric mucosa was prominent within an otherwise typical dermoid cyst. No obvious source for the pigment could be identified in any of the cases. These cases of benign peritoneal melanosis should be distinguished from metastatic malignant melanoma, a distinction that is straightforward because of the bland nuclear features and mitotic inactivity of the pigmented histiocytes.

Peritoneal Keratin Granulomas

Peritoneal granulomas that form in response to implants of keratin derived from neoplasms of the female reproductive tract may be confused with metastatic tumor.[85,285] The tumors most commonly are endometrioid carcinomas with squamous differentiation originating in the endometrium (see Chapter 12, Endometrial Carcinoma) or ovary or, rarely, squamous cell carcinomas of the cervix or atypical polypoid adenomyomas of the uterus.[85,285] The granulomas consist of laminated deposits of keratin, sometimes with ghost squamous cells, surrounded by foreign-body giant cells and fibrous tissue (see Chapter 16, Non-neoplastic Lesions of the Ovary, Fig. 16.10). Follow-up data on these patients suggest that the granulomas have no prognostic significance, although they should be sampled thoroughly by the gynecologist and carefully examined microscopically to exclude the presence of viable tumor. The differential diagnosis includes peritoneal granulomas in response to keratin derived from other sources, as discussed earlier in this chapter.

Infarcted Appendix Epiploica

Appendices epiploicae may undergo torsion and infarction.[153,155] Subsequent calcification can result in a hard, tumor-like mass that may be found attached or loose in the peritoneal cavity. In the late stages, these structures typically are composed of layers of hyalinized connective tissue surrounding a central necrotic and calcified zone in which infarcted adipose tissue usually is recognizable.

Mesothelial Neoplasms

Localized Fibrous Tumor

Localized fibrous tumors of the type that involve the pleura are extremely rare in the peritoneal cavity.[587] Although once referred to as "fibrous mesotheliomas," they are now generally considered to originate from submesothelial fibroblasts. Their clinical and pathological features are similar to their pleural counterparts.

Adenomatoid Tumor

This benign tumor of mesothelial origin rarely arises from extragenital peritoneum, such as the omentum[215] or mesentery,[114] but is encountered much more commonly within the fallopian tube and myometrium (see Chapters 13, Mesenchymal Tumors of the Uterus, and Chapter 14, Diseases of the Fallopian Tube), and in the male, the epididymis.

Well-differentiated Papillary Mesothelioma

Well-differentiated papillary mesotheliomas (WDPMs) of the peritoneum are uncommon lesions; approximately 35 cases have been reported in detail,[33,128,190] including 22 in a recently published series by Daya and McCaughey.[128] Seventy-five percent of the cases have occurred in women, who usually are of reproductive age; occasional patients are postmenopausal. WDPMs usually are an incidental finding at operation but rare cases have been associated with abdominal pain or ascites. Occasional patients, including two who were sisters, have had possible exposure to asbestos.[128]

At laparotomy and on gross examination, WDPMs may be solitary but usually are multiple, and appear as gray to white, firm, papillary, or nodular lesions measuring <2 cm in diameter. The omental and pelvic peritoneum typically are involved[128]; several examples also have been encountered on the gastric, intestinal, or mesenteric peritoneum.[190] Microscopic examination reveals fibrous papillae covered by a single layer of flattened to cuboidal mesothelial cells (Fig. 17.8) with occasional basal vacuoles; the nuclear features are bland and mitotic figures are rare or absent. Less commonly, the mesothelial cells are arranged in a tubulopapillary pattern, branching cords, or

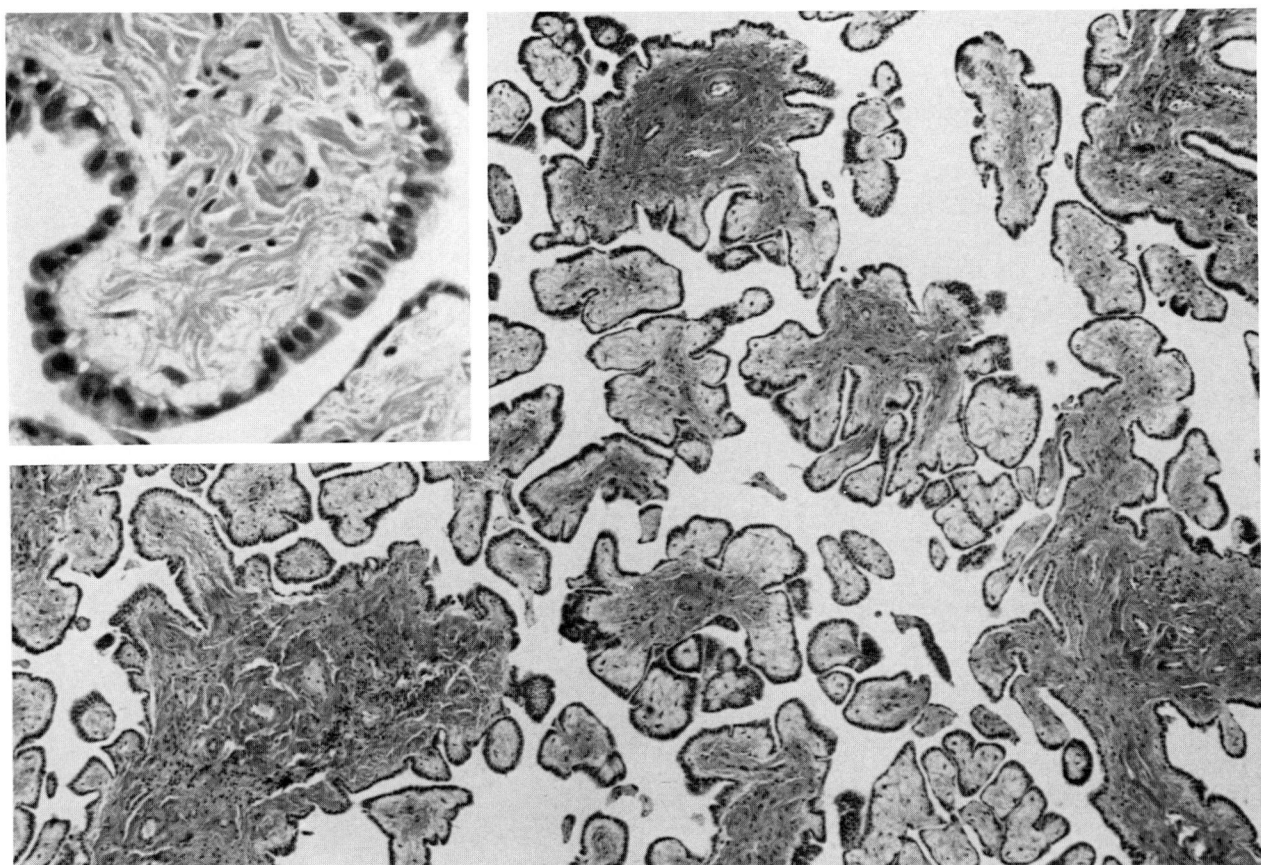

Fig. 17.8. Well-differentiated papillary mesothelioma. Fibrous papillae are lined by a single layer of uniform, flat to cuboidal, mesothelial cells (*inset*).

solid sheets.[128] The stroma of some tumors may be extensively fibrotic, and psammoma bodies are encountered in occasional cases. When multiple lesions are present, they should each be sampled histologically as lesions with the appearance of a WDPM may rarely be associated with others that have the appearance of malignant mesothelioma. The diagnosis of WDPM should be reserved strictly for tumors with bland nuclear features.

With the exception of one case that appeared to evolve into a diffuse malignant mesothelioma,[64] follow-up studies suggest that most WDPMs are benign. Occasional examples, however, have persisted for as many as 29 years.[128] In addition, several patients with WDPM have died, although it is possible that the adjuvant therapy used in such cases was a contributory factor.[128] Daya and McCaughey therefore suggest that adjuvant therapy be withheld from patients with WDPM unless there is clear evidence of progression.[128]

Low-grade Cystic Mesothelioma

Although we believe that most multilocular cystic mesothelial lesions are MPICs, we have seen very rare cases of what appear to be bona fide multicystic mesotheliomas.

In contrast to MPICs, the cysts are lined, at least focally, by markedly atypical mesothelial cells (Fig. 17.9), and the tumors may contain areas of conventional malignant mesothelioma on histological examination.[133]

Diffuse Malignant Mesothelioma

CLINICAL FEATURES

Diffuse malignant mesotheliomas (DMMs) of the peritoneal cavity are much less common than similar tumors in the pleural cavity, and account for only 10–20% of all mesotheliomas.[12,258,262,409,413] These tumors are particularly rare in women, in whom most malignant papillary neoplasms of the peritoneum are extraovarian papillary serous carcinomas (see Lesions of the Secondary Müllerian System).

More than 90% of the patients with DMM are middle-aged or elderly men. Several recent studies, however, have noted the occasional occurrence of DMMs of the peritoneum in young adults[261] and children.[38,178,527] The patients typically present with nonspecific manifestations, including abdominal discomfort and distension, digestive disturbances, and weight loss. Ascites is present in most cases, and cytologic examination of the ascitic fluid may be

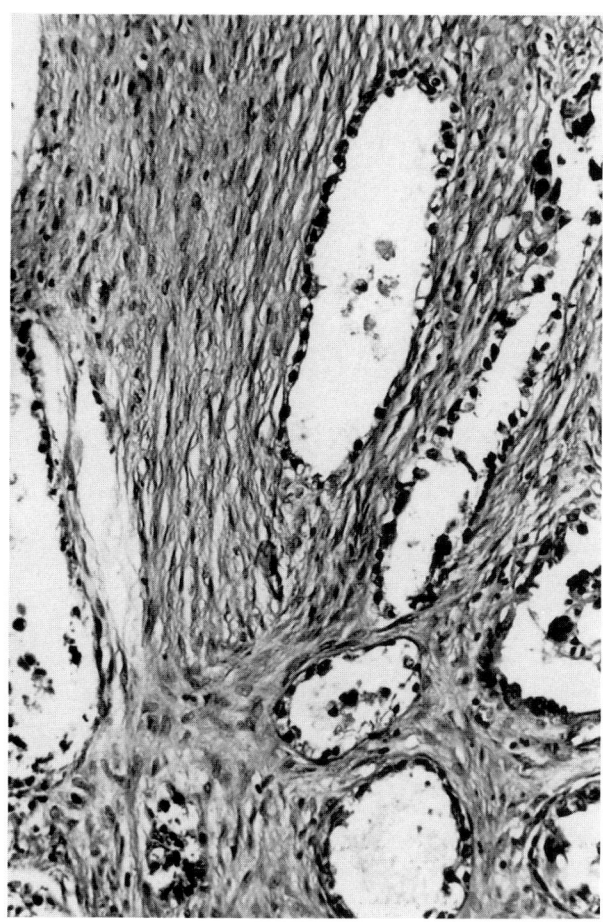

Fig. 17.9. Low-grade cystic mesothelioma. Small cysts are lined by mesothelial cells with hyperchromatic, pleomorphic nuclei. (Reprinted by permission of Thor et al., Pathology of the fallopian tube, broad ligament, peritoneum, and pelvic soft tissues. Hum Pathol (1991) 22:856–867.)

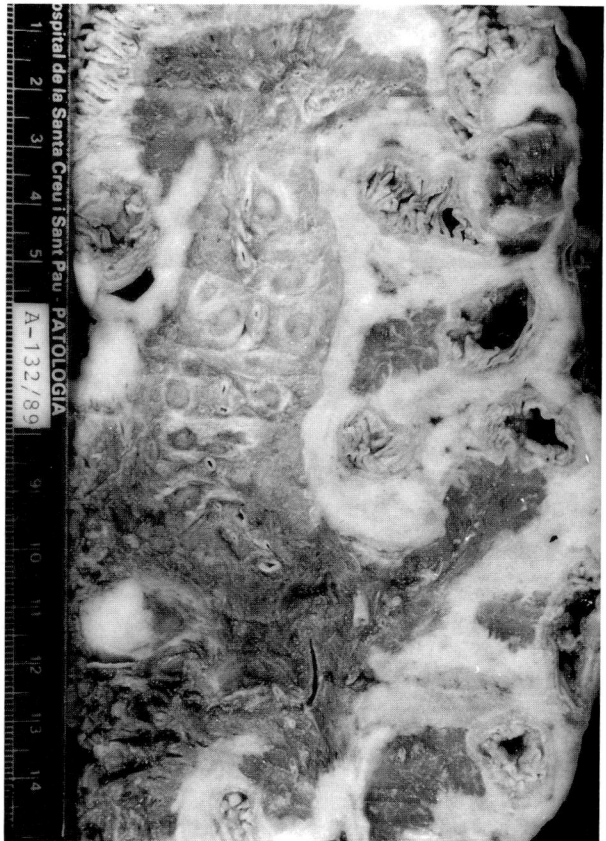

Fig. 17.10. Diffuse malignant mesothelioma encasing loops of bowel. (Courtesy of Dr. J. Prat, Barcelona, Spain.)

diagnostic of DMM in some cases.[12] The diagnosis, however, usually requires laparotomy or laparoscopy and biopsy.[409] Peritoneal DMMs rarely may present within a hernia or hydrocele sac,[12] as a retroperitoneal, umbilical, intestinal, or pelvic tumor,[12,84,173,345] or as cervical or inguinal lymphadenopathy.[524]

More than 80% of the patients in one large series had a history of asbestos exposure,[262] and occasional cases are a late complication of abdominal irradiation.[186] Rare DMMs have been preceded by recurrent peritonitis and atypical mesothelial hyperplasia.[348,438] Most patients survive less than a year after diagnosis, although there are occasional long-term survivors.[12,55,178,382,409] More recently, intensive chemotherapy of patients with early tumors has resulted in improved survival.[10]

Pathological Findings

At laparotomy, the visceral and parietal peritoneum are diffusely thickened or extensively involved by nodules and

plaques. The viscera often are encased by tumor (Fig. 17.10) and may be invaded, although local invasion and metastases to lymph nodes, liver, lungs, and pleura are less frequent than in association with carcinomas with comparable degrees of peritoneal involvement.[262] Significant degrees of invasion or metastatic involvement of abdominal viscera, however, may be encountered at autopsy, such as transmural invasion of bowel wall or massive replacement of the pancreas.[262]

The typical histological features (Fig. 17.11) are identical to DMMs involving the pleura, except for a possibly lower frequency of purely sarcomatoid tumors.[262] Rare tumors with an exclusively sheet-like pattern composed of polygonal cells with abundant eosinophilic cytoplasm (Fig. 17.12) may be confused with an ectopic decidual reaction (see page 684).[527] Occasional peritoneal DMMs may contain a prominent inflammatory infiltrate, which may include a dense lymphocytic infiltrate with granulomas[38] or many foamy, lipid-rich histiocytes.[288] The immunohistochemical (see next section) and ultrastructural features° of peritoneal DMMs are similar to their pleural counterparts.

°Refs. 38,173,178,345,409,413,527.

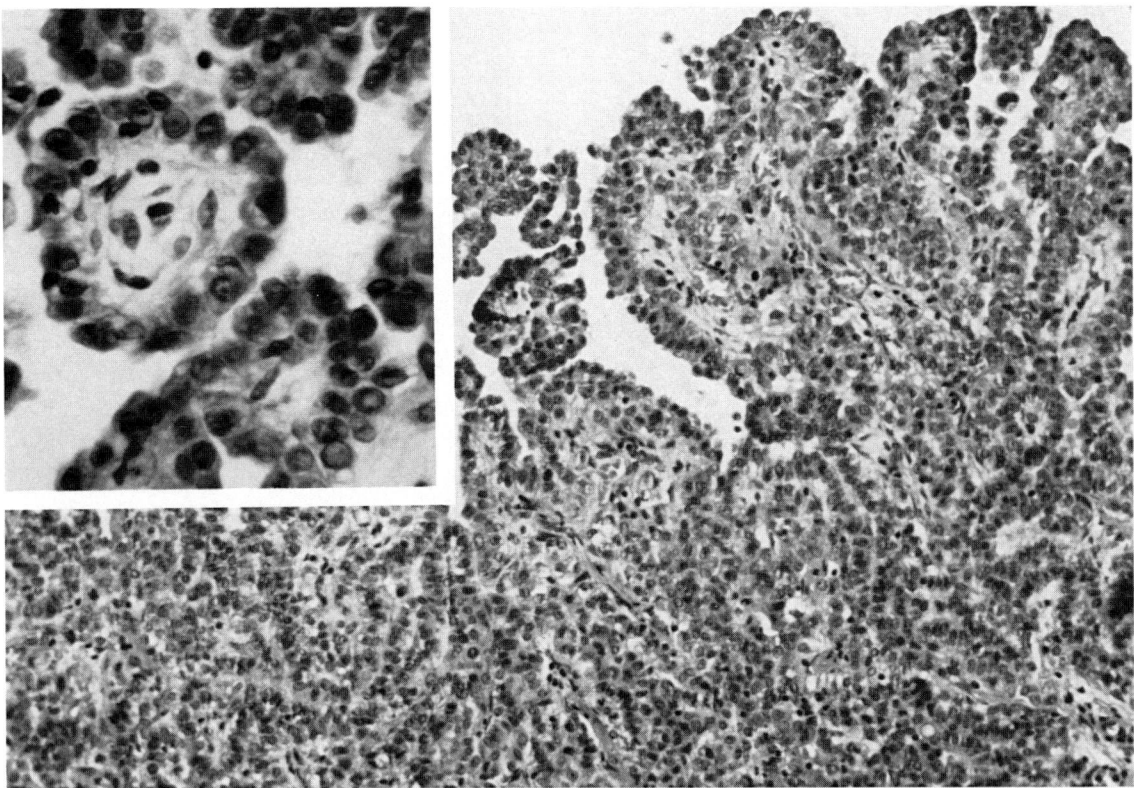

FIG. 17.11. Diffuse malignant mesothelioma. Atypical mesothelial cells (*inset*) are arranged in tubulopapillary and solid patterns.

DIFFERENTIAL DIAGNOSIS

The differential diagnosis of DMM with atypical mesothelial hyperplasia has been previously discussed (see Mesothelial Hyperplasia). The other frequently problematic lesion in the differential diagnosis is adenocarcinoma with diffuse peritoneal involvement, including metastatic adenocarcinomas and adenocarcinomas of primary peritoneal origin (see Lesions of the Secondary Müllerian System). Certain patterns of DMM, such as the biphasic and the sarcomatoid, particularly when considered in conjunction with the gross characteristics of the tumor, are almost diagnostic. Tumors with a tubulopapillary pattern may present a greater problem, but such a pattern may be distinctive, particularly when the lesional cells are characteristic of mesothelial cells, that is, polygonal cells with moderate amounts of eosinophilic cytoplasm. The presence of columnar cells favors a diagnosis of adenocarcinoma. Most of the primary peritoneal adenocarcinomas are of papillary serous type and are indistinguishable from primary ovarian serous carcinomas. In contrast to most DMMs, serous carcinomas frequently contain cells with bizarre nuclear features and many psammoma bodies.

Histochemical and immunohistochemical stains may be helpful in the differential diagnosis with adenocarcinoma. DMMs are characterized by an absence of neutral mucins (in contrast to adenocarcinomas) and the presence of acid mucin (predominantly hyaluronic acid) within vacuoles, appreciable as alcian blue–positive, digested periodic acid-Schiff (DPAS)–negative, hyaluronidase-sensitive material.[349] It should be remembered, however, that hyaluronic acid may leach from formalin-fixed tumors, resulting in false-negative staining. Also, the cell borders and stroma of DMMs may be intensely DPAS-positive and occasional DMMs may contain small DPAS-positive cytoplasmic granules.[349] Immunoreactivity for both cytokeratin (including sarcomatous DMMs) and vimentin, and negative staining for a variety of epithelial antigens [carcinoembryonic antigen (CEA), B72.3, Leu-M1, LN1, Ca19-9, beta$_1$ pregnancy-specific glycoprotein, S-100 protein, CA-125, 44-3A6, Ber-EP4, AUA1, BCA-225, secretory component, placental alkaline phosphatase] favor a diagnosis of DMM over carcinoma.* Reactivity for at least two epithelial markers (especially CEA, B72.3, Leu M1, S-100, Ber-EP4) is especially useful in excluding DMM.[188,571] Epithelial membrane antigen (EMA) and human milk–fat globule protein appear to be unreliable in distinguishing between adenocarcinoma and mesothelioma.[393] Similarly, a significant proportion of both mesotheliomas and adenocarcino-

---

*Refs. 19,45,49,90,91,139,175,184,230,290,303,326,327,333,346, 349,388,389,393,441,490,491,499,509,510,526,544,559,571,573.

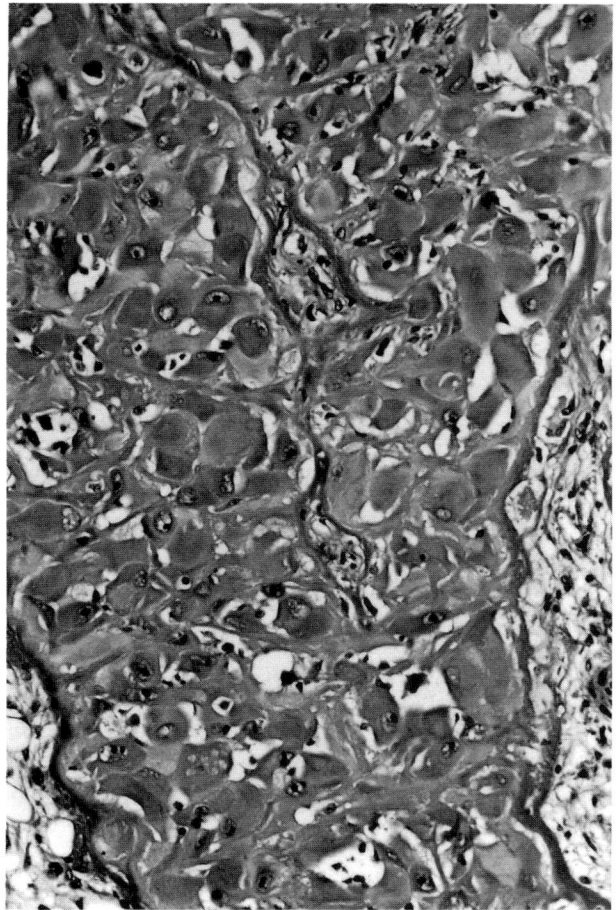

FIG. 17.12. **Diffuse malignant mesothelioma of the peritoneum.** The tumor had an exclusively solid growth pattern composed of cells with abundant cytoplasm that was eosinophilic.

mas were immunoreactive for neuron-specific enolase and Leu-7 in one study.[346] Bollinger et al.[49] have suggested that two profiles (S-100 and B72.3 positivity; S-100 and PLAP positivity) are seen in most serous adenocarcinomas but are absent in DMMs. It should be stressed that no single immunohistochemical stain is diagnostic in the separation of DMM from adenocarcinoma, and the results of a panel of antibodies should be interpreted in conjunction with the H&E and mucin stains. Occasional DMMs, for example, may be immunoreactive for CEA and Leu-M1, reflecting a high content of hyaluronic acid,[441] and in one recent series, 10% of DMMs exhibited a granular pattern of CEA immunoreactivity.[517] A recently developed antimesothelial cell antibody may prove useful in distinguishing DMM from metastatic adenocarcinoma; however, primary peritoneal serous carcinomas also are immunoreactive with this antibody.[139] A preliminary study also indicates that a biotinylated probe specific for hyaluronate is highly predictive of DMM.[19]

A final consideration in the differential diagnosis is the distinction of DMMs composed of sheets of polygonal cells

with abundant eosinophilic cytoplasm from ectopic decidua.[527] A variety of features, including prominent nucleoli, mitotic activity, immunoreactivity of the tumor cells for cytokeratin, and ultrastructural findings, facilitate the diagnosis.

Miscellaneous Primary Tumors

Intraabdominal Desmoplastic Small Round Cell Tumor

Approximately 50 examples of this tumor have been described since the initial report by Gerald and Rosai in 1989.° The tumor is of uncertain histogenesis, but it has been suggested that it may ultimately prove to be a primitive tumor of mesothelial origin ("mesothelioblastoma").[180] These tumors have a strong male predilection (M:F ratio 4:1) and are most common in adolescents and young adults (mean age 17 years). The patients typically present with abdominal distension, pain, and a palpable abdominal, pelvic, or scrotal mass, sometimes in association with ascites. Laparotomy typically discloses a variably sized but usually large, intraabdominal mass associated with smaller peritoneal "implants" of similar appearance.[180] Any portion of the peritoneal cavity, or less commonly the retroperitoneum, may be affected; the tumor frequently is confined to the pelvis. In men, there may be significant involvement of the tunica vaginalis,[488] and in women, the ovaries, in some cases mimicking a primary ovarian tumor.[588]

On gross examination, the outer aspect of the tumors, which may reach 40 cm in diameter, is smooth or bosselated, and the neoplastic tissue is firm to hard and graywhite, with foci of myxoid change and necrosis. Direct invasion of intraabdominal or pelvic viscera has been noted in occasional cases.[180,588] On microscopic examination, sharply circumscribed aggregates of small epithelioid cells are delimited by a cellular desmoplastic stroma (Fig. 17.13a). The aggregates vary in size and shape from tiny clusters and slender trabeculae to rounded or irregularly shaped islands that often coalesce. Rosette-like or gland-like spaces may be present in some cases. Peripheral palisading of basaloid cells in some of the nests is a common feature. Central necrosis with or without calcification, or occasional spaces containing eosinophilic fluid, may be present in some of the larger islands. The tumor cells typically are uniform with scanty cytoplasm (Fig. 17.13b), although tumor cells with eosinophilic cytoplasmic "inclusions" and an eccentric nucleus, resulting in a rhabdoid appearance, frequently are also present.[180] The tumor

°Refs. 87,180,181,192,308,384,389,416,488,489,550,588.

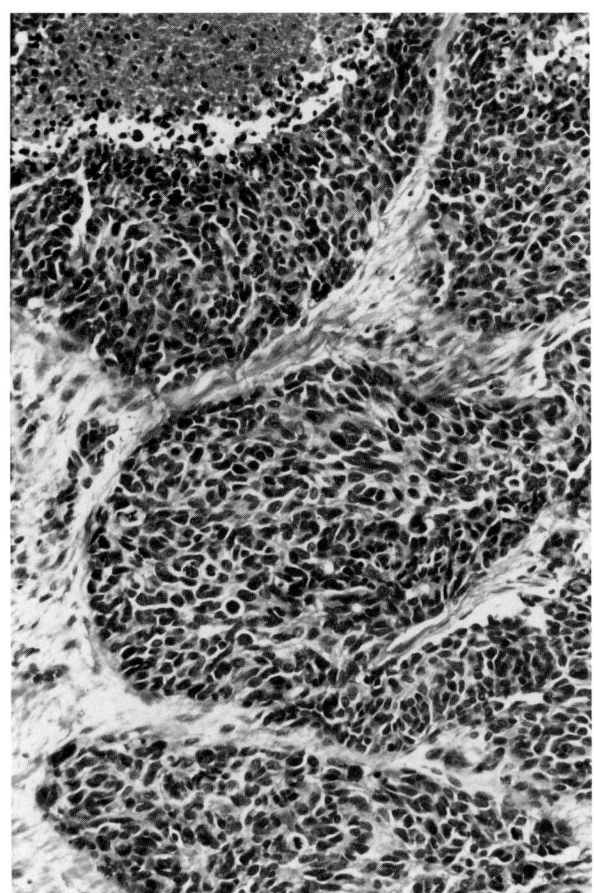

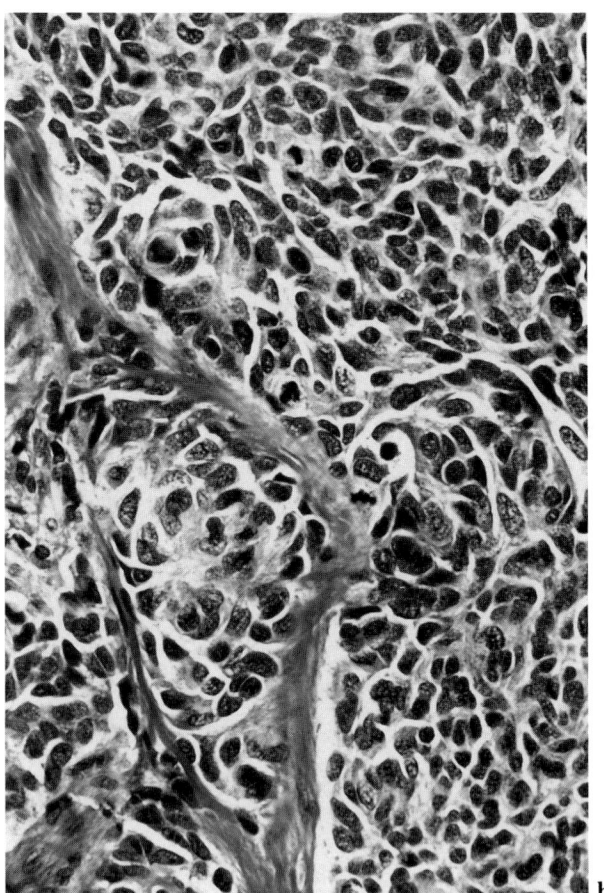

Fig. 17.13. Intraabdominal desmoplastic small round cell tumor. a: The cellular nests of tumor are sharply circumscribed and separated by a fibrous stroma. Focal necrosis of the tumor is seen in the upper left. **b:** The tumor cells have scant cytoplasm and malignant nuclear features.

cells have indistinct cell borders and small to medium-sized, round, oval, or spindle-shaped hyperchromatic nuclei with clumped chromatin. The nucleoli usually are inapparent but one or more small nucleoli may be visible in some cells. Mitotic figures and single necrotic cells are numerous.

Features noted in occasional cases have included a biphasic pattern because of a population of cells with more abundant cytoplasm admixed with the typical population of small cells (Fig. 17.14), definite tubules and glands (sometimes with luminal mucin), signet-ring–like cells, and minor foci of pleomorphic tumor cells.[180,588] The stroma frequently contains blood vessels with prominent endothelial and perithelial cells.[180] Invasion of vascular spaces, especially lymphatics, is a common feature; lymph nodes occasionally are involved by tumor.

Special techniques, especially immunohistochemistry, indicate simultaneous multidirectional phenotypical expression within the tumor, including immunoreactivity for epithelial (low molecular weight cytokeratins, EMA), neural/neuroendocrine (NSE, Leu-7), and muscle

(desmin) markers, as well as vimentin.[180] Desmin and vimentin immunoreactivity typically is paranuclear and globular, and is particularly intense in cells with a rhabdoid appearance. Immunoreactivity for other antigens has been noted in rare cases, including Leu-M1, S-100, B72.3, human milk–fat globule, actin (muscle and smooth muscle), desmoplakin, chromogranin, and synaptophysin. The stroma typically is immunoreactive for vimentin and muscle-specific actin. Ultrastructural variability suggests a range of differentiation in these tumors. Cell junctions have varied from scant and primitive to more prominent ones including intermediate, desmosomal, and tight types. Paranuclear intermediate cytoplasmic filaments and basal lamina surrounding the nests of tumor have been prominent features in most of the cases. Intraluminal microvillus-like structures, polar cell processes, microtubules, lipid droplets, glycogen, and dense-core granules have been encountered in some cases.

These tumors should be distinguished from other malignant small cell tumors that may involve the peritoneum; this differential diagnosis is detailed elsewhere.[180] The

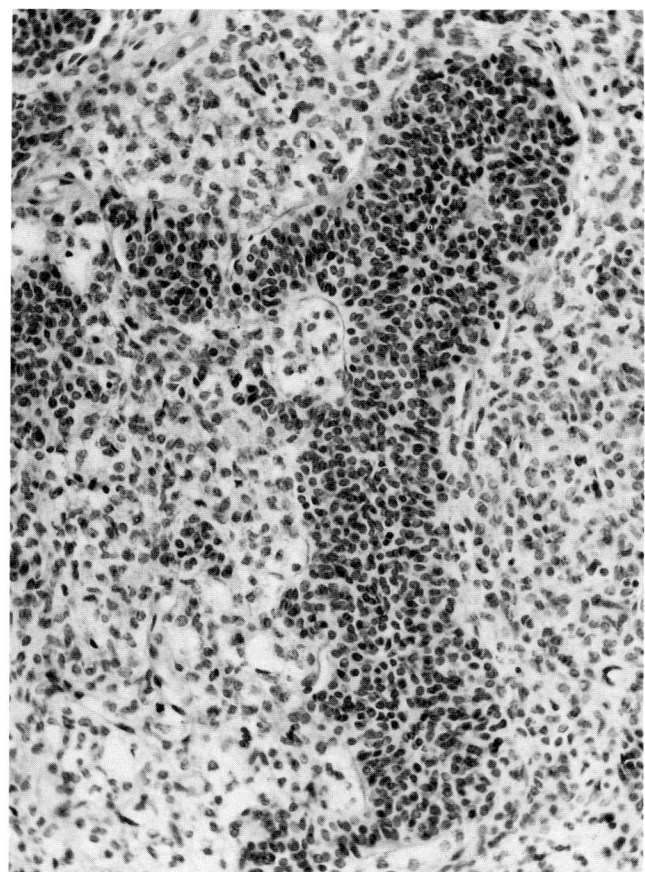

FIG. 17.14. Intraabdominal desmoplastic small round cell tumor. A nest of small cells is surrounded by cells with moderate amounts of pale cytoplasm.

characteristic age of the patient, the distribution of the tumor, and its typical microscopic and immunohistochemical features should facilitate the diagnosis in most cases.

The treatment of the tumors usually has consisted of debulking and postoperative chemotherapy, irradiation, or both. The tumor is highly aggressive, with more than 90% of patients dying from tumor progression. In many cases, there has been an initial partial response to chemotherapy followed by uncontrollable tumor relapse. Even in advanced stages, the bulk of the tumor tends to remain within the peritoneal cavity; extraabdominal metastases, however, have occurred in occasional patients.[180]

Inflammatory Myofibroblastic Tumor

Day et al. reviewed the features of seven cases of abdominal "inflammatory pseudotumor,"[127] a lesion that also has been referred to as "plasma cell granuloma" or, more recently, "inflammatory myofibroblastic tumor."[408] The abdominal lesions are encountered typically in patients younger than 20 years who present with a mass, fever, growth failure or weight loss, hypochromic anemia, throm-

bocytosis, and polyclonal hypergammaglobulinemia.[127] Laparotomy typically reveals a solid mesenteric mass that on microscopic examination consists of myofibroblastic spindle cells, mature plasma cells, and small lymphocytes. All of the patients have had an uneventful postoperative course with disappearance of the clinical manifestations.

Omental-mesenteric Myxoid Hamartoma

This designation was applied by Gonzalez-Crussi et al.[193] to a lesion in infants characterized by multiple omental and mesenteric nodules composed of plump mesenchymal cells in a myxoid, vascularized stroma. The diagnosis of the referring pathologists usually was that of some type of sarcoma, but the follow-up was uneventful. The lesions may be hamartomatous.

Metastatic Tumors

Peritoneal involvement by metastatic tumor typically is a result of seeding from a primary tumor arising within the abdomen or pelvis, most commonly the ovary. Peritoneal serous tumors in which the ovaries are normal or only minimally involved may arise directly from the peritoneum (see Lesions of the Secondary Müllerian System) or rarely are metastatic from a serous papillary carcinoma of the endometrium or fallopian tube. Other tumors that may be associated with peritoneal seeding include carcinomas of the breast[356] and gastrointestinal tract, especially the colon and stomach, and the pancreas. In such cases, the metastatic tumor may take the form of signet-ring cells scattered widely in a fibrous stroma. Occasionally the signet-ring cells can have relatively bland nuclear features, resulting in a deceptively benign appearance.

Peritoneal extension of a mucinous neoplasm, usually from the appendix or ovary, may be accompanied by pseudomyxoma peritonei.° Histological examination discloses large pools of mucin surrounded by or associated with well-differentiated mucinous epithelium of intestinal type (Fig. 17.15), although in some cases the epithelium may be scanty or even absent. Accordingly, if pseudomyxoma is suspected from the intraoperative apperance, extensive histological sampling should be performed before the diagnosis is excluded. The collections of mucin typically elicit a proliferation of dense, often hyalinized, fibrous stroma. Pseudomyxoma peritonei most commonly is associated with a mucinous ovarian tumor, typically of borderline malignancy or, less commonly, carcinoma (see Chapter 18, Surface Epithelial–Stromal Tumors of the Ovary). An appendiceal lesion also is usually present in such cases, typically a low-grade adenocarcinoma similar in

---

°Refs. 67,82,226,317,421,589.

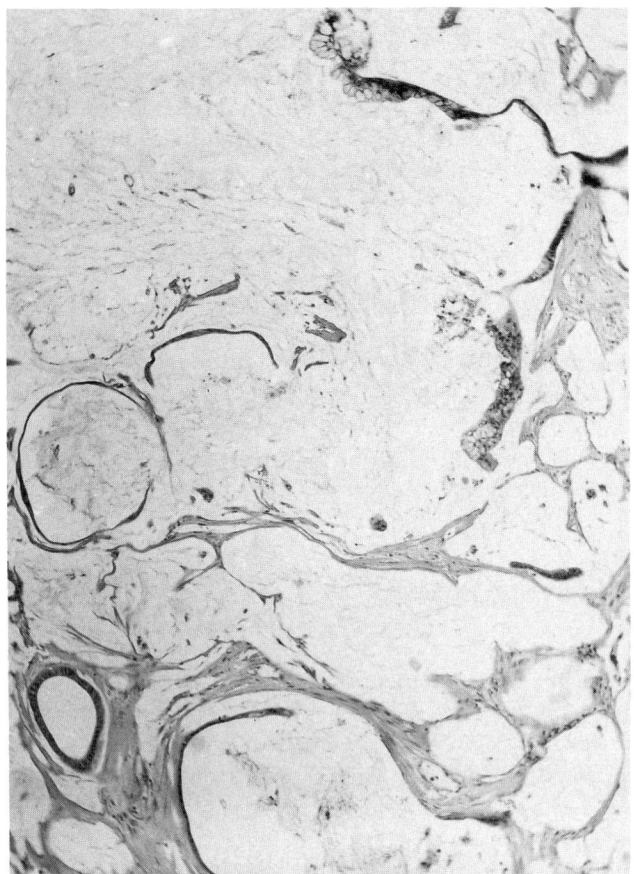

FIG. 17.15. **Pseudomyxoma peritonei.** Large pools of mucin are surrounded by hyalinized fibrous tissue.

appearance to the ovarian tumor.[589] It may be difficult or impossible to determine if the appendiceal and ovarian tumors are independent lesions, or if the latter is metastatic from the former. Indeed, two recent large studies reached different conclusions regarding the origin of the ovarian tumors in such cases. In one of the studies, it was concluded that when mucinous appendiceal and ovarian tumors coexist, the latter usually are metastatic from an appendiceal primary tumor.[589] Evidence supporting this interpretation included the typical synchronous presentation of the ovarian and appendiceal tumors, their histological similarity, the frequency of bilaterality of the ovarian tumors (one-third of cases), the predominance of right-sided ovarian involvement, and the usual presence of mucin and atypical mucinous cells on the ovarian surfaces. In contrast, the conclusions of the other study favored an independent origin for the appendiceal and ovarian tumors, and that the peritoneal lesions also may be part of a multifocal neoplastic process.[486a] The finding of acellular mucin dissecting through the ovarian stroma ("pseudomyxoma ovarii")[362] was a frequent finding in both series.[486a,589] Careful examination of the appendix is important, there-

fore, in all cases of ovarian tumors associated with pseudomyxoma peritonei. Pseudomyxoma peritonei rarely is associated with other mucin-secreting tumors, including carcinomas of the stomach, colon, pancreas, gallbladder, uterine corpus, and urachus.[82,589] Pseudomyxoma peritonei should be distinguished from localized collections of acellular mucin surrounding a ruptured mucinous ovarian tumor or an appendiceal mucocele. These mucin collections are associated with a self-limiting inflammatory reaction and fibrosis.

Lesions of the Secondary Müllerian System

These peritoneal lesions are characterized by müllerian differentiation on microscopic examination and share an origin from the so-called secondary müllerian system, that is, the pelvic and lower abdominal mesothelium and the subjacent mesenchyme of females.[307] The müllerian potential of this layer is consistent with its close embryonic relation to the primary müllerian system (the müllerian ducts) that arises by invagination of the coelomic epithelium. Displacement of coelomic epithelium and subcoelomic mesenchyme during embryonic development could account for the presence of identical lesions within pelvic and abdominal lymph nodes. The origin of many of these lesions, however, is controversial, and other proposed histogenic mechanisms also are discussed.

Lesions of the secondary müllerian system include those containing endometrioid, serous, and mucinous epithelium, simulating normal or neoplastic endometrial, tubal, and endocervical epithelium. The metaplastic potential of the pelvic peritoneum also includes differentiation toward cells of transitional (urothelial) type, exemplified most commonly by Walthard nests. Proliferation of the subjacent mesenchyme may accompany epithelial differentiation of the mesothelium or may give rise to a variety of pure mesenchymal lesions composed of endometrial stromal-type cells, decidua, or smooth muscle.

Endometriosis

Endometriosis is defined as the presence of endometrial tissue outside the endometrium and myometrium. Usually both epithelium and stroma are seen, but occasionally the diagnosis of endometriosis can be made when only one component is present, as discussed below.

Endometriosis can involve a variety of locations both within and outside of the peritoneal cavity. These sites are summarized below.

Common
Ovaries
Uterine ligaments (uterosacral, round, broad)

Rectovaginal septum

Cul-de-sac

Peritoneum of uterus, tubes, rectosigmoid, ureter, and
bladder

Less Common

Large bowel, small bowel, appendix

Mucosa of cervix, vagina, and fallopian tubes

Skin (scars, umbilicus, vulva, perineum, inguinal region)

Ureter, bladder

Omentum, pelvic lymph nodes

Inguinal (noncutaneous)

Rare

Lungs, pleura

Soft tissues, breast

Bone

Upper abdominal peritoneum

Stomach, pancreas, liver

Kidney, urethra, prostate, paratesticular

Sciatic nerve, subarachnoid space, brain

ETIOLOGY AND PATHOGENESIS

Two theories have been proposed for the pathogenesis of
endometriosis: (1) metastases of endometrial tissue to its
ectopic location (metastatic theory), and (2) metaplastic
development of endometrial tissue at the ectopic site
(metaplastic theory). The metastatic theory explains most
cases, but a metaplastic origin likely accounts for occasional cases in which metastatic spread of endometrial tissue is unlikely or impossible (see below).

METASTATIC THEORY

Menstrual Implantation. Sampson proposed that endometriosis was caused by reflux of endometrial tissue
through the fallopian tubes by a process of retrograde
menstruation, with subsequent implantation and growth
on peritoneal surfaces.[464] Implantation of menstrual endometrium also has been proposed to explain endometriosis within surgical scars, on traumatized cervical and vaginal mucosa, and within perineal and vulvar scars after
vaginal delivery.[177,482] Passage of refluxed menstrual endometrium from the peritoneal cavity through diaphragmatic defects, diaphragmatic lymphatics, or both may explain pleural endometriosis.

Observations supporting the menstrual implantation hypothesis include (1) endometriotic lesions are most common in areas closest to the tubal ostia and occur in a
distribution that appears dependent on gravity and uterine
position,[246,256] (2) retrograde menstruation through the
fallopian tubes is a common physiologic process, occurring
in 90% of menstruating women with patent tubes,[48,212] (3)
endometriosis is more common in women with early menarche, heavy menstrual flow, long menstrual flow (>7

days), and frequent menses (cycle <27 days),[115] (4) menstrual endometrium is viable, capable of growth in tissue
culture[273] and after subcutaneous injection,[439] (5) endometriosis is more frequent in women with congenital obstruction to menstrual flow,[217,238,387] and (6) endometriosis may follow uteropelvic or uteroabdominal wall fistulas
in experimental animals[483,534] and humans.[525]

Intraoperative Implantation. Although endometriosis in
some scars may be a result of menstrual implantation,
endometriosis within scars after uterine operations may be
secondary to intraoperative implantation of endometrial
tissue.[80,513] Supporting this theory is the greater frequency
of scar endometriosis after abdominal hysterotomy than
after cesarean section in some studies, consistent with the
greater viability of transplanted early-pregnancy endometrium compared with late-pregnancy endometrium.[482]
Also, the occurrence of endometriosis within an episiotomy scar is much higher if uterine curettage is performed
immediately after delivery than in patients without postde-
livery curettage.[401]

Lymphatic and Vascular Spread. The presence of endometriosis in distant sites (e.g., lungs, extremities, brain) is
explained most easily by hematogenous spread from the
uterus.[463] Similarly, it has been proposed that endometriosis within lymph nodes is a result of lymphatic spread.[254]
Evidence supporting the origin of endometriosis from lymphatic or hematogenous spread includes (1) the presence
of normal endometrial tissue within endothelium-lined
spaces as an incidental histological finding within the myometrium,[254,463] (2) the presence of intraluminal vascular
involvement in rare endometriotic lesions,[1,583] (3) the
presence of intravascular or perivascular trophoblastic tissue and "decidua"* as an incidental microscopic finding
within the lungs of pregnant patients,[318] (4) the occurrence
of pulmonary endometriosis almost exclusively in women
who have had prior uterine operations that could predispose to the embolisation of endometrial tissue (see page
677), (5) the experimental production of pulmonary
endometriosis by intravenous injection of endometrial
tissue in rabbits,[228] and (6) the observations that tumor
cells, blood, dye, and radiographic material can migrate
from the pelvis to the umbilicus by retrograde lymphatic
flow.[481]

METAPLASTIC THEORY

The origin of pelvic endometriosis by a process of metaplasia from the pelvic peritoneum is consistent with the puta-

---

*By current criteria, these intrapulmonary foci of "decidua" prob-
ably would be interpreted as foci of intermediate trophoblast.[295,296]

tive müllerian potential of this tissue which, as noted earlier, has been referred to as the *secondary müllerian system*.[307] Evidence for the metaplastic theory includes (1) the demonstration of endometriosis in women in whom metastasis of normally situated endometrium could not occur or is highly unlikely, such as those with Turner's syndrome and pure gonadal dysgenesis who are amenorrheic and have hypoplastic uteri,[42,143,151,406] and in males (see page 678), (2) the experimental induction of peritoneal endometriosis adjacent to millipore filters that contain endometrial tissue but that prevent cellular transfer,[357] (3) the observation that autologous endometrial implants in rabbits degenerate but are associated with the subsequent development of endometriosis in adjacent tissues,[316] and (4) the juxtaposition of endometriosis with other putative metaplastic lesions of the peritoneum, such as diffuse peritoneal leiomyomatosis (see page 685).[32,265,293]

OTHER ETIOLOGIC FACTORS

Endometriosis is an idiopathic disease in most patients and why only a minority of women are affected despite the common occurrence of retrograde menstruation is unknown. Some potential etiologic factors have been discussed (congenital obstruction, iatrogenic implantation); others are summarized in the following section.

Genetic Factors. Several studies concluded that the prevalence of endometriosis is greater in mothers and sisters of women with endometriosis than in the mothers and sisters of their husbands.[299,334,426,501] Lamb et al.[299] calculated the overall risk for first-degree relatives to be 4.9%. Genetic studies suggest a polygenic mode of inheritance (influenced by several different genes) or one that is multifactorial (a result of interaction between genetic and environmental factors). In opposition to the foregoing, Houston et al.[236] concluded that there were methodological flaws in three of the studies,[299,426,501] and that an inherited tendency to endometriosis has not been substantiated.

Hormonal Factors. Because endometriosis occurs almost exclusively in women during the reproductive age, hormonal factors may play an etiologic role. The rare examples of endometriosis in phenotypic women with gonadal dysgenesis and in men usually have been associated with the use of exogenous estrogens.° Also, it has been shown that maintenance of autologous peritoneal transplants of endometrium in monkeys requires either estradiol, progesterone, or both.[135,484] Similarly, smoking and exercise, which are inversely correlated with endogenous estrogen

levels, appear to be protective factors for the development of endometriosis.[115]

It has been suggested that the progestational milieu of pregnancy may inhibit the development of endometriosis. Many studies have indicated that endometriosis is more likely to occur in women who have delayed pregnancy and is less common in multiparous women.[134,434] Similarly, one study found that patients with endometriosis were much less likely to have used oral contraceptives than similar patients without endometriosis.[487]

Recently, some studies have found an increased frequency of the luteinized unruptured follicle syndrome (LUFS) in patients with endometriosis.[81,138,140,141] In normal women, the ruptured corpus luteum releases its progesterone-rich fluid into the peritoneal cavity. It has been postulated that this fluid may inhibit implantation and growth of refluxed endometrial fragments at the time of menstruation.[291] In patients with the LUFS, a corpus luteum is formed, but rupture and fluid release does not occur, resulting in lowered luteal phase levels of progesterone in the peritoneal fluid.[140,291] This local hormonal imbalance may be critical in allowing endometrial cells to implant on the peritoneum.[291] Other studies, however, have shown no difference in the luteal phase peritoneal fluid hormone values in women with and without endometriosis.

Immune Factors. One study has demonstrated a reduced T-lymphocyte–mediated cytotoxicity to autologous endometrial cells and a decreased lymphocyte stimulation response to autologous endometrial antigens in patients with endometriosis.[514] The degree of the depressed cellular immunity was directly proportional to the severity of the disease. The authors of this study suggested that certain cell-mediated immune mechanisms that may be operative in limiting the growth of endometriotic tissue may be impaired in patients with endometriosis. Another study has suggested that the growth of endometriotic implants may be stimulated by activated macrophages.[210]

EPIDEMIOLOGY

The highest risk of the disease traditionally has been considered to be in the upper socioeconomic levels of developed societies, especially among women who delay pregnancy, although, according to Houston, these associations have not been proved statistically.[236] Although endometriosis was once considered to be more common in Caucasians, recent studies showing a similar frequency of the disease in Asians[368] and blacks[76] cast doubt on this view.

The true prevalence of endometriosis is unknown because many patients are asymptomatic; estimates for the prevalence of the disease in women of reproductive age are 1–7%,[22] 10%,[568] and 10–15%.[115,359] Prevalence figures, however, have varied widely, depending on the population studied and the method of diagnosis (clinical, operative, or

---

°Refs. 29,42,143,151,342,406,475,591.

pathological). Similarly, a study of the incidence rates of pelvic endometriosis in white women of reproductive age in Rochester, Minnesota, found that the overall incidence of the disease more than doubled (from 108.8 to 246.9 cases per 100,000 person-years) as the definition of a case was extended from histologically confirmed cases to clinically and surgically diagnosed cases.[235]

More than 80% of affected patients are in the reproductive age group. In one study, the age-specific incidence rates increased in successive age groups through age 44 years and then declined for women aged 45 to 49 years.[235] Less than 5% of cases occur in postmenopausal women, and in these patients the disease frequently is not diagnosed premenopausally.[274] Endometriosis can be clinically significant in this age group, with 20–30% of affected patients requiring operative management.[274,420] In some postmenopausal patients with endometriosis, an association with obesity and endometrial carcinoma has been noted, suggesting that hyperestrinism may play a role, but in other series, most patients have had no obvious exogenous or endogenous source of estrogen.[222,274] Almost 10% of patients with endometriosis are adolescents.[77] In three studies endometriosis was found at laparoscopy in approximately 50% of teenage patients with dysmenorrhea or chronic pelvic pain.[60,77,191] In some studies, adolescents with endometriosis have a particularly high frequency of a congenital obstruction to menstrual flow.[238,469]

CLINICAL FEATURES

SYMPTOMS AND SIGNS

The recurrent cyclic menstrual, inflammatory, and fibrotic changes within endometriotic lesions likely are responsible for most of the symptomatology of endometriosis, although there often is no direct relationship between the extent of the disease and the severity of the symptoms.[77,427] One study, however, found that deeper implants were more likely to be associated with pain than superficial lesions.[110] Hormonal responsiveness of the lesions as judged histologically also does not correlate with symptoms,[443] and microscopic examination of symptomatic endometriosis in postmenopausal patients typically reveals atrophic changes.[274] Age generally does not appear to affect disease severity in most studies.[236] An exception to the foregoing is one study in which women 26 to 52 years of age had less extensive disease than women 16 to 25 years of age.[434] A higher frequency of nulliparity in the younger women appeared to account for part of this difference.[236]

The typical symptoms that are attributed to pelvic endometriosis are acquired dysmenorrhea, lower abdominal, pelvic, and back pain, dyspareunia, irregular bleeding, and infertility.[136,375] Infertility is present in up to 30% of women with endometriosis, although the putative association between mild endometriosis and infertility has recently been challenged.[69,523] The subject of endometriosis-related infertility has been reviewed elsewhere,[206,359,375,523] and is not considered in detail here. Potential pathogenetic factors include tubal factors (adhesions, luminal obstruction), ovarian factors (anovulation, luteal phase dysfunction, LUFS), immune factors (antiendometrial antibodies), peritoneal factors (increased prostaglandins, increased macrophages), and an increased risk of spontaneous abortion.

Pelvic examination may reveal tender nodules in the cul-de-sac and uterosacral ligaments, tender, semifixed, cystic ovaries, and a fixed, retroverted uterus.[287,375,427] The rectovaginal septum also may be tender and indurated. The endometriotic lesions frequently enlarge and become more painful during menses. The clinical manifestations also vary according to the site of the endometriosis, as is discussed later in this chapter. As the clinical manifestations of endometriosis frequently are nonspecific, vary widely between patients, and may be absent in a high proportion of patients, a definitive diagnosis requires direct visualization by laparoscopy (or laparotomy) and, ideally, biopsy.[137,443]

LAPAROSCOPIC FINDINGS

A number of recent studies have stressed that endometriotic foci, especially early ones, frequently are nonpigmented and may have a wide variety of laparoscopic appearances, including clear, white, and red lesions.[253,341,433,519,520,552] Sequential laparoscopic examinations indicate that nonpigmented endometriotic implants eventually evolve into the typical pigmented lesions.[253] Even in patients with laparoscopically typical disease, biopsy may yield only nondiagnostic tissue and, thus, in the opinion of some authors, diagnosis and treatment should not always depend on histological confirmation.[79,375] Laparoscopically detectable defects or "pockets" involving the pelvic peritoneum frequently are associated with, and likely caused by, endometriosis.[78,435] In one study, 79% of women with pelvic peritoneal defects had endometriosis,[78] and in another, the endometriotic foci often were located along the edges of the defects.[435] Conversely, 18–28% of women with endometriosis in the two studies had peritoneal defects.

SERUM MARKERS

Levels of CA-125 may be elevated in the serum and peritoneal fluid of patients with endometriosis.[23,126,156,157,412] The concentrations of serum CA-125 correlate with both the severity and the clinical course of the disease. The serum test has low sensitivity, however, and is not appropriate for general screening purposes.[412] In contrast, CA-

125 levels have acceptable sensitivities and very high specificities in populations with a relatively high prevalence of the disease, and are useful in monitoring response to treatment.[412]

Antiendometrial antibodies have been found in 35%,[276] 74%,[88] and 83%[574] of women with laparoscopically confirmed endometriosis in three different studies. In one of the latter, the antibody titers in women who had had a good response to hormonal treatment were lower than in those with untreated endometriosis or in whom there had been a poor response to treatment.[88] In another of these studies, sequential determination of antibody levels showed that they were lowered by hormonal treatment.[277]

Telimaa et al. have found that endometriotic foci contribute to the circulating level of PP14, an endometrial protein synthesized by secretory endometria.[533] The PP14 levels correlated with the severity of the endometriosis and declined after surgical or hormonal treatment.

EFFECTS OF PREGNANCY

Although rare cases of endometriosis undergo permanent regression during pregnancy, the ameliorative effect of pregnancy noted in many cases of endometriosis is only temporary.[347,557] The behavior of endometriosis during pregnancy is extremely variable among different patients and between one pregnancy and another in the same patient.[347] During pregnancy, visible endometriotic lesions frequently undergo initial enlargement, with occasional ulceration and bleeding, followed by shrinkage. In most sites, there is a decrease in the associated pain.[347]

A rare complication of endometriosis during pregnancy is intrapartum or postpartum rupture of the lesion, most probably caused by a softening of the lesion secondary to stromal decidualization, pressure from the expanding uterus, or both. Rupture occurs most frequently in the ovaries or bowel, typically resulting in perforation and an acute abdomen.[9,164,449] Rarely, hemoperitoneum, sometimes fatal, is caused by hemorrhage from decidualized endometriotic lesions at term.[444]

RARE COMPLICATIONS

Massive, sometimes serosanguinous, ascites occurs in patients with pelvic endometriosis; a right pleural effusion also is present in one-third of such patients.[86,211,249,257] Seventy percent of the reported cases of this complication have occurred in black women, suggesting a possible racial predilection.[211] If one or both ovaries are involved, the findings at surgery may simulate those of an ovarian carcinoma. The pathogenesis of the ascites is not clear. Possible sources include production by endometriotic cysts, irritated peritoneal mesothelial cells, or the ovarian serosa (Meigs-like syndrome). The ascites typically responds to danazol treatment.[249] Other rare complications include hemorrhage from an endometriotic focus[238,425] and spontaneous rupture of ovarian endometriotic cysts, resulting in an acute abdomen.[222,417]

GROSS FINDINGS

Depending on their duration and their superficial or deep location in relation to the peritoneal surface, endometriotic foci may appear as punctate, red, blue, brown, or white spots or patches with either a slightly raised or puckered surface (Fig. 17.16).[136,170,253] Ecchymotic or brown areas sometimes have been described as "powder burns." The endometriotic foci frequently are associated with dense fibrous adhesions. The lesions may form nodules or cysts, or both. Rarely, pelvic peritoneal endometriosis may present as multiple, polypoid masses of soft gray tissue that fill the pelvis, simulating a malignant tumor.[70,374,486]

Endometriotic cysts (endometriomas) most commonly involve the ovaries, where they may partially or almost

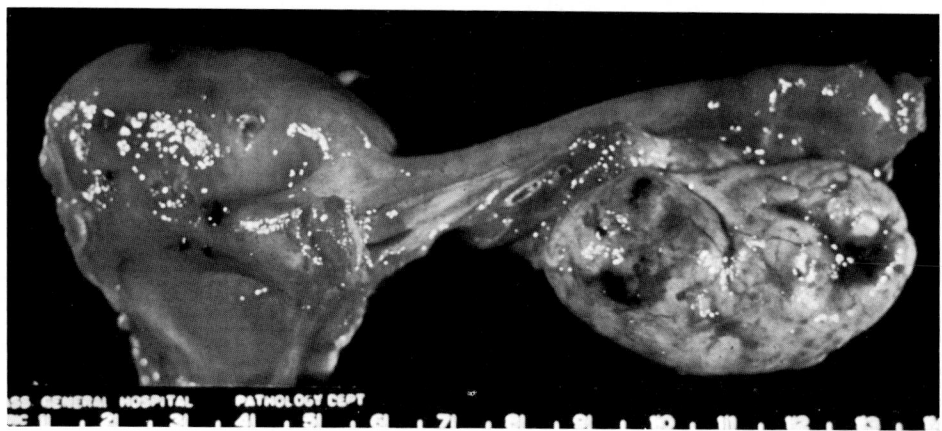

FIG. 17.16. Endometriosis of uterine serosa and ovary. Multiple, hemorrhagic lesions involve the serosal surfaces. (Courtesy of Dr. R. E. Scully, Boston, MA.)

completely replace the normal tissue; bilateral involvement occurs in one-third to one-half of the cases.[137,148] The cysts rarely exceed 15 cm in diameter; larger examples are more likely to harbor a neoplasm. Endometriotic cysts commonly are covered by dense fibrous adhesions, which may result in fixation to adjacent structures. The cyst walls usually are thick and fibrotic, with a smooth or shaggy, brown to yellow lining (Fig. 17.17). The cyst contents typically consist of altered, semifluid or inspissated, chocolate-colored material; rarely, the cyst is filled with watery fluid. Any solid areas in the cyst wall or intraluminal polypoid projections should be sampled histologically because a malignant tumor may arise from the epithelial or stromal component of the cyst.

MICROSCOPIC FINDINGS

The appearance of endometriotic tissue varies with the extent of its response to the normal hormonal fluctuations of the menstrual cycle and the duration of the process (Figs. 17.18–17.20). When the appearance of simultaneous samples of eutopic endometrium and endometriotic foci is compared, the latter exhibit cyclic changes in from 44% to 80% of the cases, and there is considerable variability in glandular morphology.[36,361] When more than one endometriotic focus is examined in the same patient, the appearance of the specimens does not differ significantly from one to another.[36] In most menopausal patients with endometriosis, the endometriotic tissue is atrophic with glands that occasionally are cystic and are lined by flattened epithelial cells surrounded by a dense fibrotic stroma (Fig. 17.21); the appearance is similar to that of simple or cystic atrophy of the endometrium.[274] In a mi-

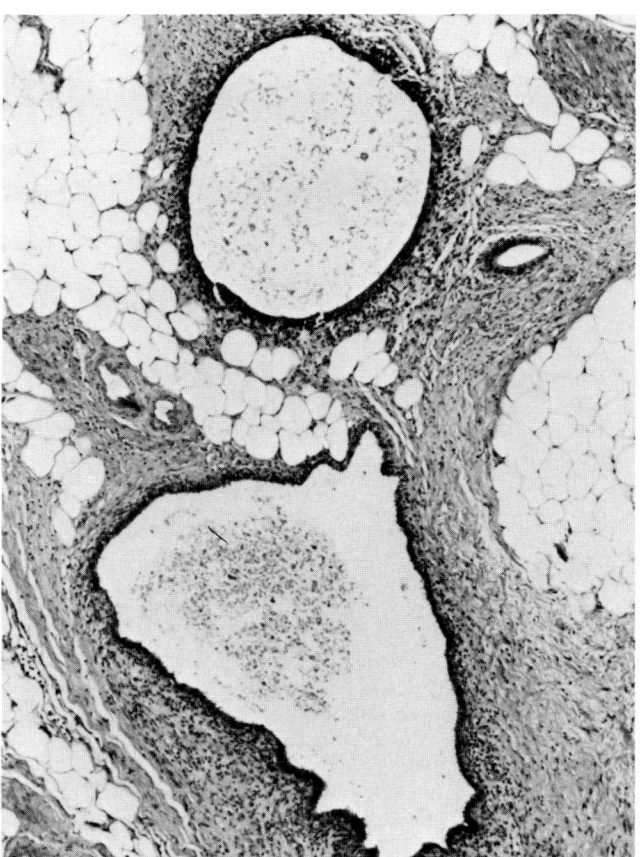

FIG. 17.18. Endometriosis of cul-de-sac. Cystic endometrial glands with a cuff of endometrial stroma are surrounded by fibrous and adipose tissue.

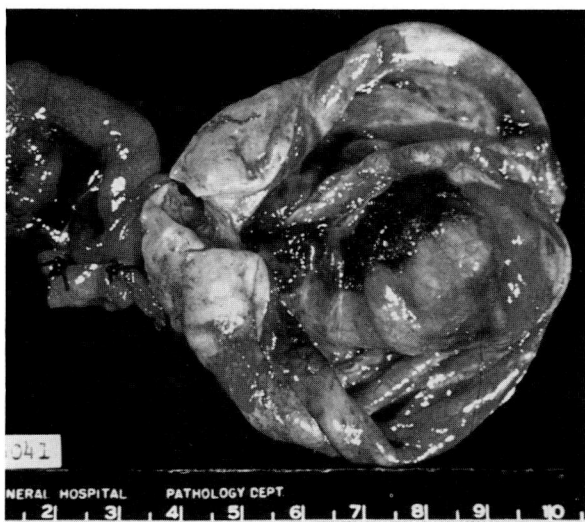

FIG. 17.17. Endometriotic cyst of ovary. The cyst has been opened to reveal a focally hemorrhagic lining. (Courtesy of Dr. R. E. Scully, Boston, MA.)

nority of cases, however, the endometriotic tissue has an active appearance, with or without the metaplastic and hyperplastic changes that are present more commonly in premenopausal women (see below).

Menstruation into endometriotic foci results in hemorrhage within the stroma and glandular lumens, as well as in a secondary inflammatory response consisting predominantly of a diffuse infiltration of histiocytes. The latter typically convert the extravasated red blood cells into glycolipid and granular brown pigment, becoming so-called pseudoxanthoma cells (Fig. 17.22).[96,101] Most of the pigment is hemofuscin, and hemosiderin typically is present to a much lesser extent.[96,101] The amount of pigment in an endometriotic lesion appears to increase with its age, and early lesions frequently are nonpigmented.[253] Variable numbers of lymphocytes and smaller numbers of other inflammatory cells may be present. Large numbers of neutrophils with microabscess formation should raise the possibility of secondary bacterial infection.[320,470]

The epithelial and stromal lining of an endometriotic cyst frequently becomes attenuated, and the former may be reduced to a single layer of cuboidal cells that may

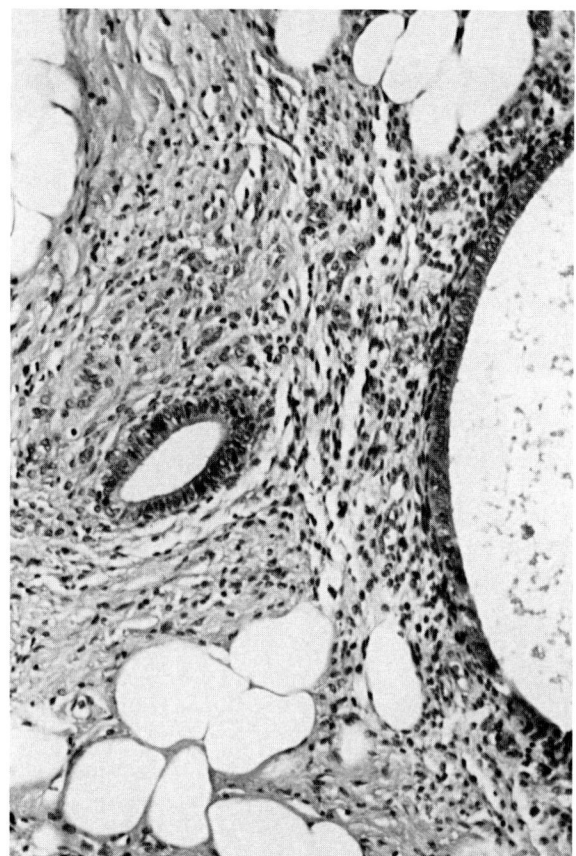

Fig. 17.19. Endometriosis of cul-de-sac (higher magnification of Fig. 17.18). Endometriotic glands are lined by inactive epithelium and surrounded by a thin rim of endometrial stroma.

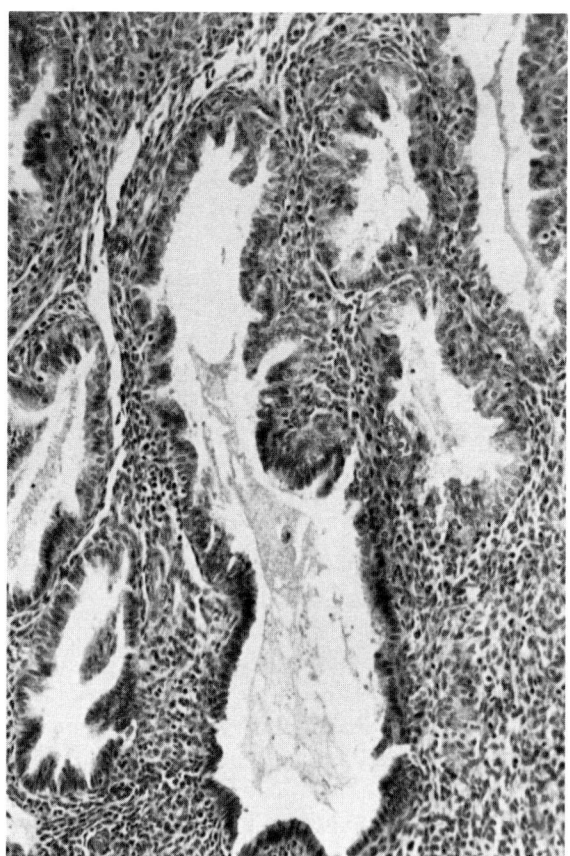

Fig. 17.20. Irregular secretory changes within a focus of endometriosis. The progestational response is less pronounced in the glandular epithelium at the bottom of the figure.

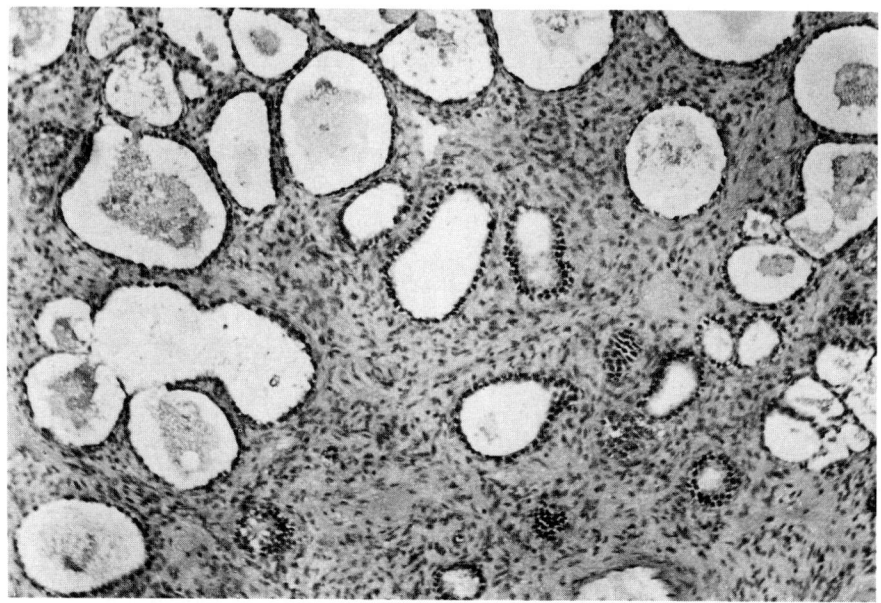

Fig. 17.21. Endometriosis in a postmenopausal woman. The glands are cystic, atrophic, and separated by a fibrous stroma. (Reprinted by permission of Clement, ref. 96.)

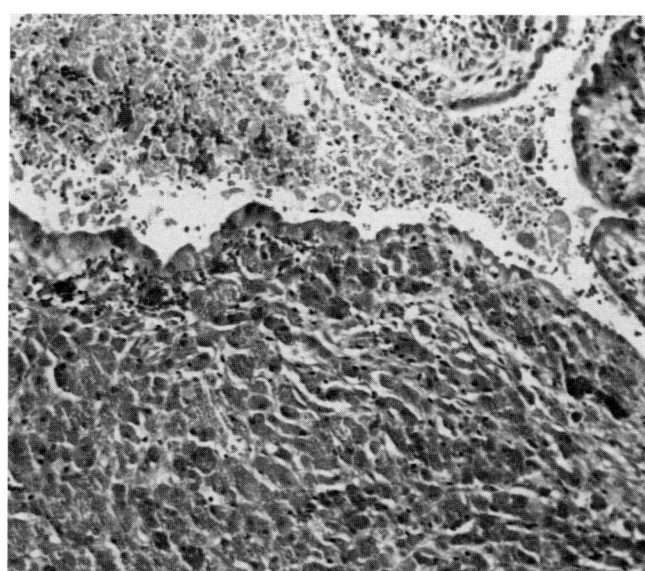

FIG. 17.22. **Lining of ovarian endometriotic cyst.** The lining consists of endometrial surface epithelium and numerous pigment-laden histiocytes within the subjacent stroma. Menstrual debris is present within the cyst lumen.

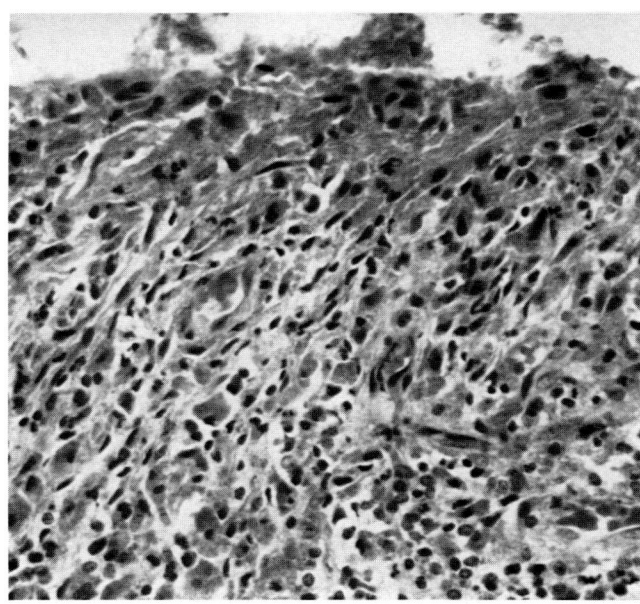

FIG. 17.23. **Lining of ovarian endometriotic cyst.** In this field, the lining consists only of fibrotic granulation tissue and pigment-laden histiocytes (presumptive endometriosis).

retain some endometrial characteristics but that often are devoid of specific features.[170] In such circumstances, recognition of the cyst as endometriotic may be possible only if a rim of subjacent endometrial stroma persists. Commonly, the cyst lining of endometrial epithelium and stroma is lost completely and replaced by granulation tissue, dense fibrous tissue, and variable numbers of pseudoxanthoma cells (presumptive endometriosis) (Fig. 17.23). In some cases, the epithelial cells lining the cyst may be large and cuboidal with abundant eosinophilic cytoplasm and large atypical nuclei (Fig. 17.24).[96,117,458,459] The significance of such nuclear atypia is unclear. Although it may be reactive, cells with these features may merge with clear cell adenocarcinomas and borderline mucinous neoplasms of mullerian type.[458,459] Occasionally ovarian and extraovarian endometriosis takes the form of "necrotic pseudoxanthomatous nodules" characterized by a central zone of necrosis surrounded by pseudoxanthoma cells, often in a palisaded arrangement, hyalinized fibrous tissue, or both (Fig. 17.25); typical endometriotic glands and stroma may be sparse or absent.[101]

Endometriosis that involves smooth muscle in the uterine ligaments or the walls of hollow viscera typically is associated with a striking proliferation of the smooth muscle, creating an appearance similar to that of adenomyosis.[96,486] The endometriotic stroma itself also may undergo smooth muscle metaplasia, which is encountered most often within the walls of ovarian endometriotic cysts, but

occasionally elsewhere.° Extensive amounts of smooth muscle within the endometriotic stroma can result in "endomyometriosis" or uterus-like masses, which have been described within an obturator lymph node (Fig. 17.26),[445] the ovary,[113,419,423] the small bowel,[407] the broad ligament,[75] and the lumbosacral region,[294] and in males, in the scrotum.[591] In some cases, a uterus-like mass in the region of the ovary may represent a congenital malformation rather than an unusual manifestation of endometriosis.[446]

Rare cases of endometriosis are characterized by an absence or rarity of glands, so-called stromal endometriosis[103]; it should be noted, however, that the same term has been used in the older literature to refer to what is now designated low-grade endometrial stromal sarcoma. Stromal endometriosis is encountered most commonly in the ovary, where it is typically an incidental microscopic finding within the ovarian stroma ("benign stromatosis").[239] There usually is no associated pelvic endometriosis, and the process likely represents a metaplastic response of the ovarian stromal cells. We also have encountered a disproportionate number of cases of stromal endometriosis within the uterine cervix (see below).[103]

Metaplastic changes similar to those occurring in eutopic endometrial glands have been described in endometriotic glands. These include tubal (ciliated),[117,306,307]

°Refs. 75,113,294,353,419,423,445,485.

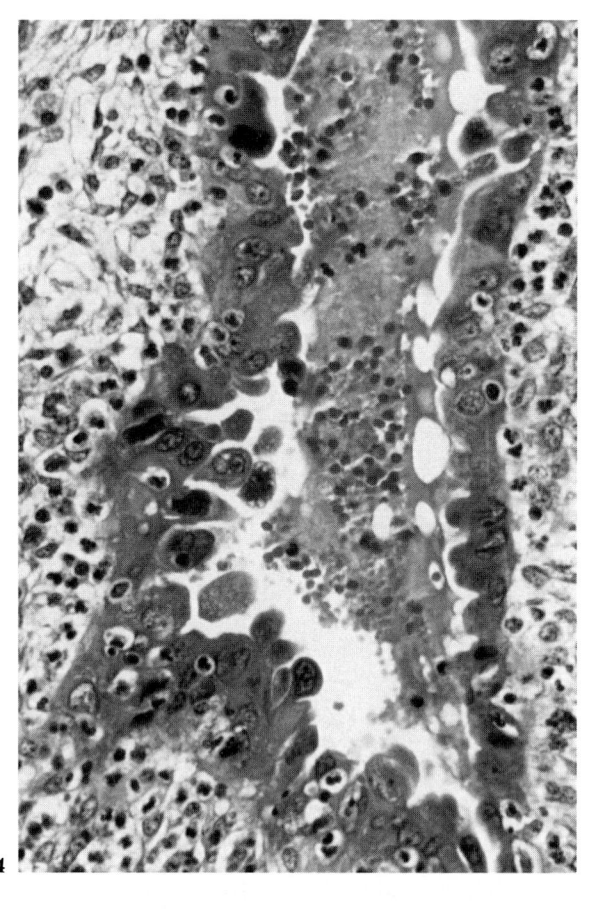

17.24

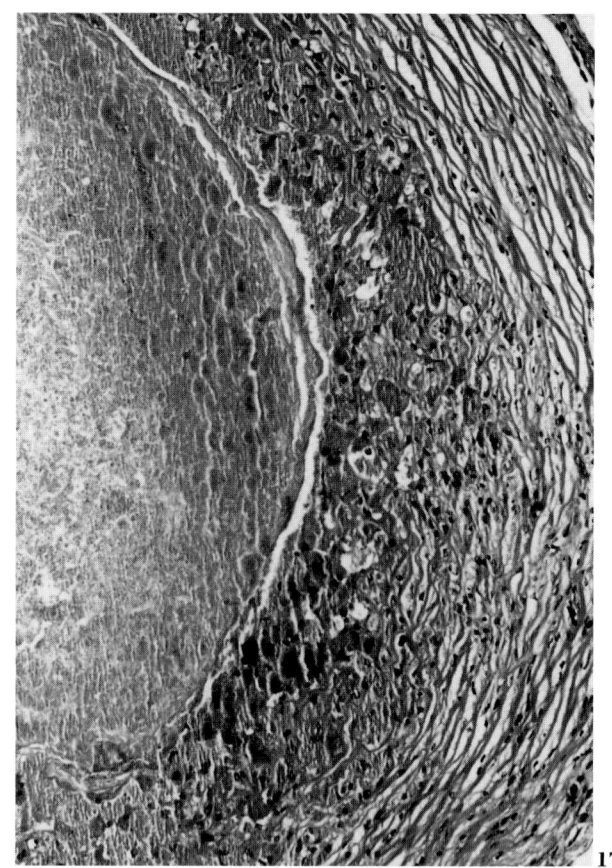

17.25

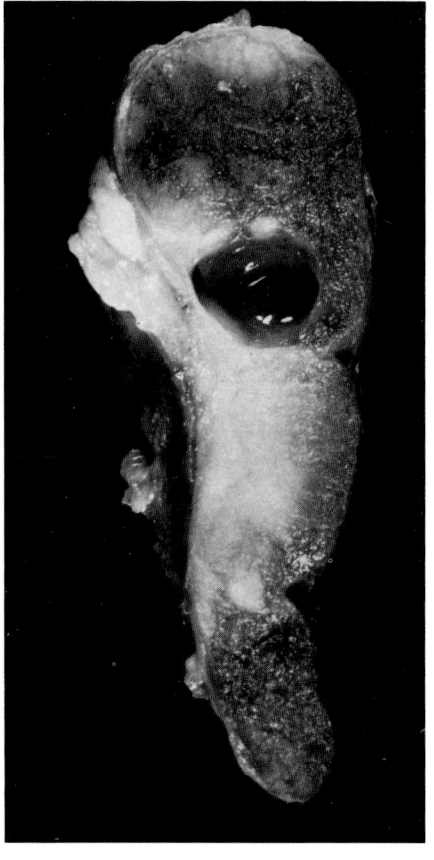

17.26a

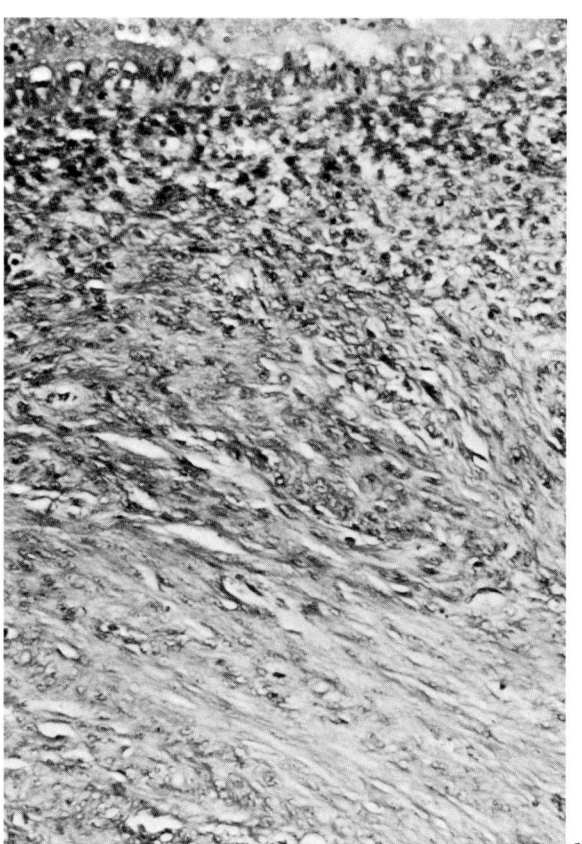

17.26b

hobnail,[117] and rarely, squamous[554] (Fig. 17.27a) and mucinous metaplasia (Fig. 17.27b); the latter may be characterized by the presence of endocervical-type cells or, less often, goblet cells.[312,590] Rarely, endometriotic stroma may exhibit a myxoid appearance, or focal ossification and calcification.[182,494] Perineural[450] and vascular invasion[1,583] have been reported rarely in otherwise typical, benign endometriotic lesions.

A variety of hyperplastic and atypically hyperplastic changes similar to those occurring in the endometrium have been described in endometriotic glands, sometimes related to an endogenous or exogenous estrogenic stimulus (Fig. 17.28),[74,117,200,264,429,586] or more recently, secondary to tamoxifen therapy.[58] It is logical to conclude that such atypical changes have a malignant potential similar to those in the endometrium, although there is little evidence on which to base such a conclusion. Rare cases of hyperplastic endometriosis, however, have preceded the development of an adenocarcinoma in the same area[74,200,369,586] or have co-existed with carcinoma in the same specimen.[298]

Endometriotic tissue also may exhibit progestational changes (Fig. 17.29), especially during pregnancy or progestin therapy.[286] In such cases, examination reveals a decidual reaction with atrophy of the endometrial glands, which are small and lined by cuboidal or flattened epithelial cells (Fig. 17.29a). In pregnancy the glands rarely exhibit an Arias–Stella reaction (Fig. 17.29b), optically clear nuclei, or both.[370,506] Necrosis of the decidual cells, foci of marked stromal edema, and infiltration by lymphocytes are additional findings in patients receiving progestational agents.[286] Inactive or atrophic changes similar to those that are seen typically in the endometriotic foci of postmenopausal patients may be present in premenopausal patients treated with oral contraceptives,[155] danazol,[402,477] antiprogesterone steroids (gestrinone),[109,111,270,379] and some progestins.[111] In one study, one-third of the endometriotic foci disappeared or were replaced by fibrous tissue after danazol therapy.[477]

Associated Lesions and Differential Diagnosis

Microscopic examination of the fallopian tubes in patients with endometriosis has revealed nonspecific chronic salp-

◁

FIG. 17.24. **Lining of ovarian endometriotic cyst.** The surface epithelial cells show striking nuclear atypia.

FIG. 17.25. **Necrotic pseudoxanthomatous nodule of endometriosis.** A central area of necrosis is surrounded by pseudoxanthoma cells and an outer zone of fibrous tissue.

FIG. 17.26. **Smooth muscle metaplasia in endometriosis (endomyometriosis of obturator lymph node). a:** The cut surface of the lymph node is focally replaced by solid, pale tissue that partially surrounds a cystic space. (Reprinted from Arch Pathol Lab Med (1981), 105:556–557. Copyright 1981. American Medical Association.) **b:** The cyst is lined by endometrial epithelium, a thin rim of endometrial stroma, and a thick layer of smooth muscle. (Courtesy of Dr. E. Bossen.)

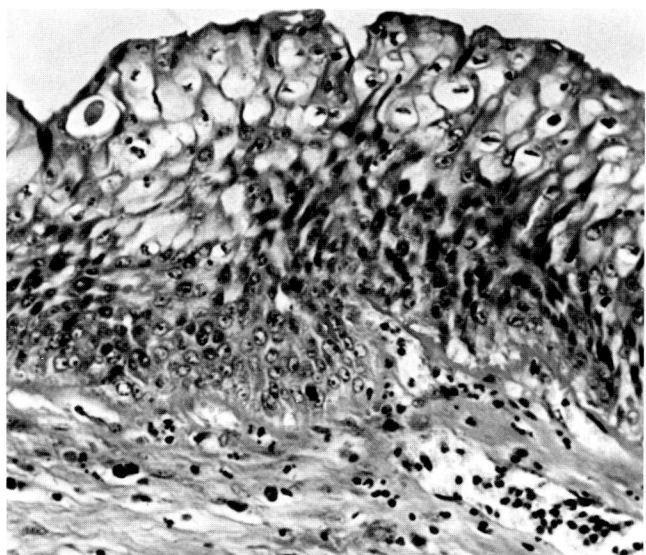
a

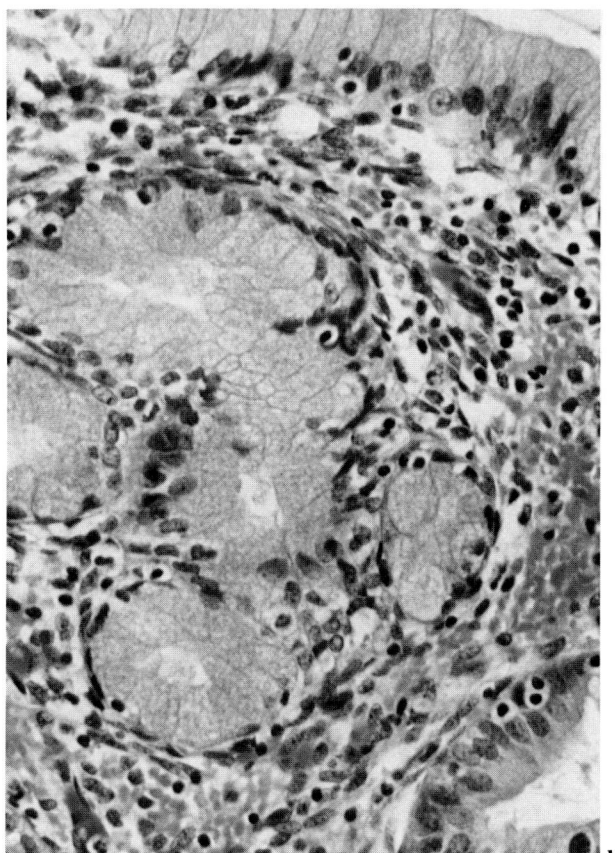
b

FIG. 17.27. **Glandular metaplasia in endometriosis. a:** Squamous metaplasia in the lining of an endometriotic cyst. **b:** Mucinous metaplasia of endometriotic glands.

ingitis in as many as one-third of cases.[118] A less common lesion, so-called pseudoxanthomatous salpingitis or pseudoxanthomatous salpingiosis, characterized by infiltration of the tubal mucosa by pseudoxanthoma cells, is associated almost always with pelvic endometriosis.[96,101,118,486b]

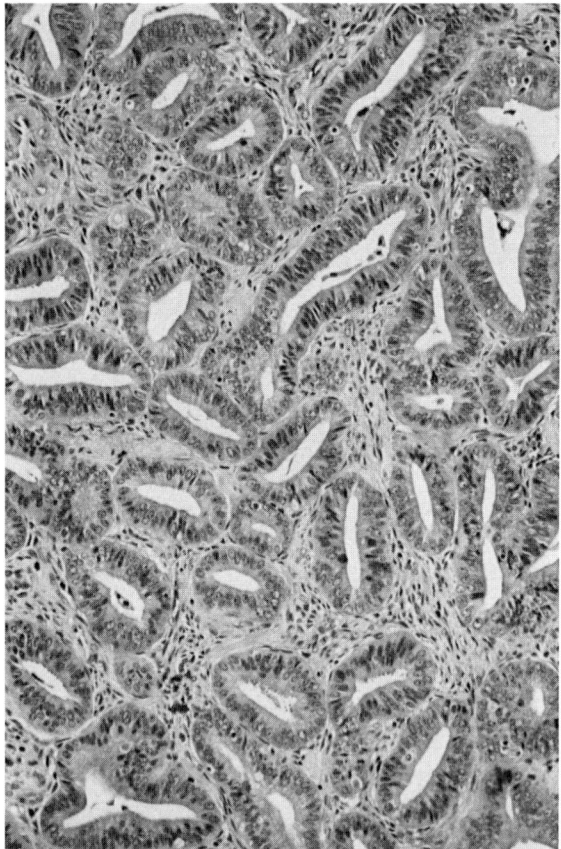

Fig. 17.28. Hyperplasia within endometriosis. Endometriotic glands exhibit architectural and cytologic atypia. Endometrioid carcinoma was found elsewhere in the specimen (see Fig. 17.40).

Rare examples of endometriosis have been encountered in intimate association with foci of peritoneal leiomyomatosis,[234,265,293] glial implants of ovarian teratomas,[7,25,147] and nodules of splenosis.[502] Liesegang rings rarely may be found within foci of endometriosis.[102,476] Endometriosis also may be accompanied by, and should be distinguished from, endosalpingiosis, which is characterized by glands lined by benign tubal-type epithelium, unassociated with endometrial stroma (see page 680).

Necrotic pseudoxanthomatous nodules should be distinguished from other ovarian and peritoneal necrotic nodules, such as infectious granulomas and isolated palisading granulomas of the ovary (see Chapter 16, Nonneoplastic Lesions of the Ovary) and as noted earlier, peritoneal granulomas related to diathermy.[94] Such lesions, in addition to having characteristic features, lack the numerous pseudoxanthoma cells that are typical of endometriotic lesions.

Rare low-grade endometrial stromal sarcomas (ESSs) contain numerous benign-appearing or atypical endometrial glands, to the extent that confusion with endometriosis may occur.[98] Indeed, it is likely that at least some cases referred to as "aggressive endometriosis" are examples of ESS with prominent glandular differentiation.[98] These tumors, however, in contrast to typical endometriosis, contain foci of more typical ESS devoid of glands, and in some cases, prominent mitotic activity of the stromal cells, sexcord–like elements, and prominent vascular invasion.

Ultrastructural, Histochemical, and Steroid Receptor Findings

Endometriotic glands typically exhibit ultrastructural features that represent a response, but an incomplete one, to the prevailing hormonal milieu of the particular phase of the menstrual cycle.[478–480] In one study, 25% of the endometriotic foci contained glands that were poorly differentiated and showed no hormonal response ultrastructurally.[480] In the remaining foci, as the proliferative phase progressed, there was an increase in Golgi, mitochondria, rough endoplasmic reticulum, and secretory vesicles, with a further increase in secretory vesicles and intraluminal secretion during the secretory phase. In contrast to eutopic glands, however, it usually was not possible to date the glands precisely within the secretory phase because of marked interglandular and intraglandular variability and the absence of specific ultrastructural characteristics (giant mitochondria, nuclear channel systems[233]) that occur in the normal endometrium after ovulation. Ultrastructural examination of endometriotic tissue after danazol treatment shows either arrest of the endometriotic glandular epithelium in the early proliferative phase or disorganization of the epithelial cells with atrophic changes, including vacuolization of organelles, especially mitochondria.[477,479] Additional ultrastructural findings secondary to danazol include deep nuclear indentations of the epithelial cells and large numbers of membrane-bound granules filled with a fine fibrillar material within the cytoplasm.[402]

Histochemical studies comparing enzyme profiles of alkaline phosphatase, acid phosphatase, and oxidative enzymes between normal endometrium and endometriotic foci have shown similar but not identical staining reactions in the two sites.[415] One study has shown that the normal increase in 17β-hydroxysteroid dehydrogenase present in eutopic endometrium during the secretory phase and in response to danazol is absent in endometriotic foci.[553]

Estrogen (ER) and progesterone receptors (PR) are present in endometriotic glands and stroma but usually in lower concentrations than in eutopic endometrium.[34,37,61,251,271,329,528] In a variable number of cases, one or both receptors are absent.[37] In addition, the normal variation in the quantity of both receptors exhibited by eutopic endometrium during the menstrual cycle is diminished or absent within foci of endometriosis.[35,198,315,553] Differences in receptor concentrations between eutopic endometrium and endometriotic epithelium in response to danazol also has been noted.[271,553] No correlation has been found between receptor levels and

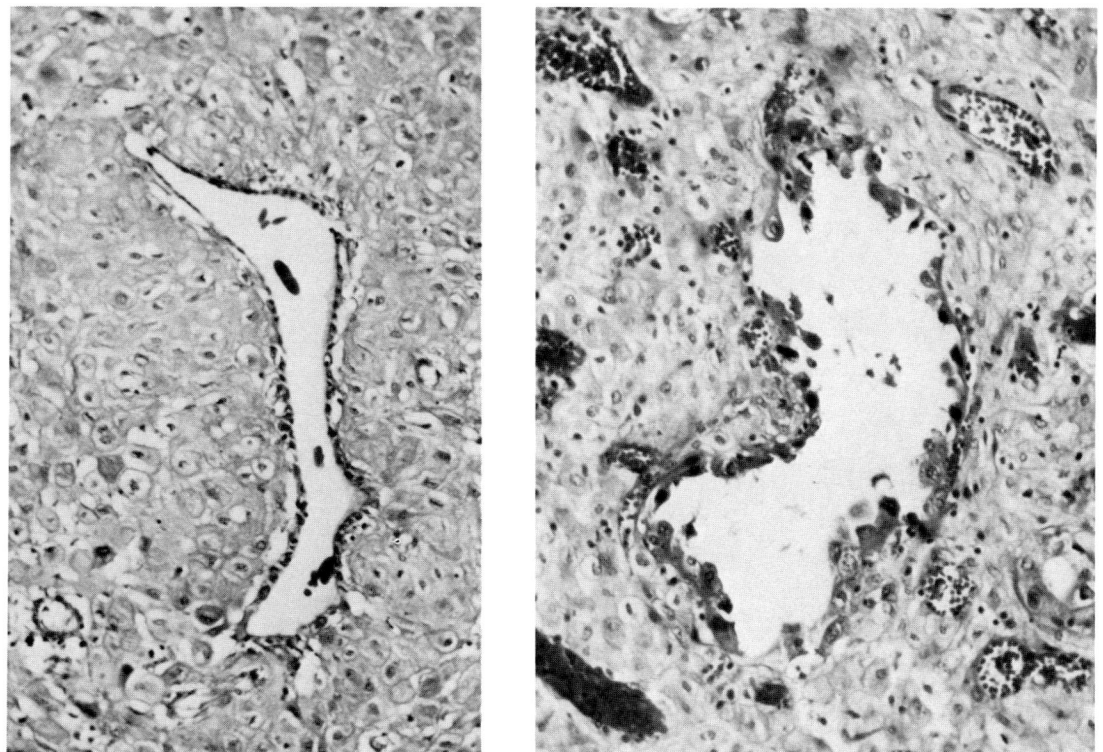

FIG. 17.29. Pregnancy-induced changes within endometriosis. a: The endometriotic gland is atrophic, and the stroma exhibits marked decidual transformation. **b:** The endometriotic gland exhibits an Arias–Stella reaction. The stroma is decidualized.

severity of symptoms. It also has been found that endometriotic implants, in contrast to eutopic luteal phase endometrium, do not secrete measurable quantities of prolactin.[214]

In summary, the findings of these studies are consistent with the incomplete and variable hormonal response of endometriotic foci observed on microscopic examination. They indicate a greater degree of autonomy of endometriotic tissue from the mechanisms controlling eutopic endometrium and may explain the failure of hormonal therapy in some patients.[360]

CLINICOPATHOLOGICAL FEATURES OF ENDOMETRIOSIS IN UNUSUAL AND RARE SITES

CERVICAL AND VAGINAL ENDOMETRIOSIS

Superficial endometriosis of the uterine cervix is more common than is generally appreciated.° It was documented in 2.4% of patients attending a colposcopic clinic in one study,[551] but may occur in as many as 15% of patients who have had extensive cervical trauma, such as electrocautery.[177] The condition may be an incidental finding in an asymptomatic patient or be associated with pre-

menstrual or postcoital spotting or menorrhagia. The solitary or multiple lesions typically involve the ectocervix; endocervical lesions have been described only rarely.[581] The endometriotic foci appear as friable, ecchymotic streaks, patches, nodules, or cysts measuring from 1 mm to 2 cm in diameter. Rare lesions have been puckered secondary to fibrosis within the lesion or papillary, simulating a carcioma.[581] Almost without exception, the endometriotic foci involve areas of prior trauma, and in patients who have had a cone biopsy[245] or extensive cautery, the entire transformation zone may be involved. Before menses, the lesions typically enlarge and change from bright red to blue; during menses they may rupture, leaving an irregular ulcer. On histological examination, the endometriotic focus usually is confined to the superficial lamina propria (Fig. 17.30). As previously noted, only endometrial stroma is found in occasional cases, even after serial sectioning (Fig. 17.31).[52,103] Because a punch biopsy may yield nondiagnostic tissue because of the frequently small size of the lesion, tissue crushing, and fragmentation, aspiration cytology may be useful in establishing the diagnosis.[551] The predilection for sites of trauma and the usual absence of associated pelvic endometriosis suggest implantation as the most likely pathogenetic mechanism.

In contrast to superficial cervical endometriosis, deep cervical endometriosis usually is an extension of cul-de-sac involvement in association with more widespread pelvic

---

°Refs. 52,103,177,247,385,551,576,581.

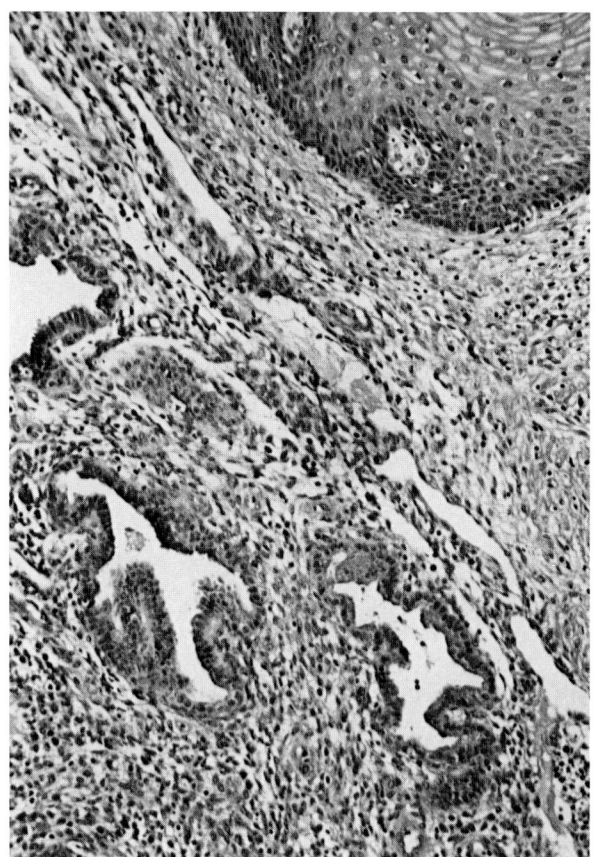

FIG. 17.30. Superficial cervical endometriosis. Endometrial glands (exhibiting secretory changes) and surrounding stroma lie beneath squamous epithelium.

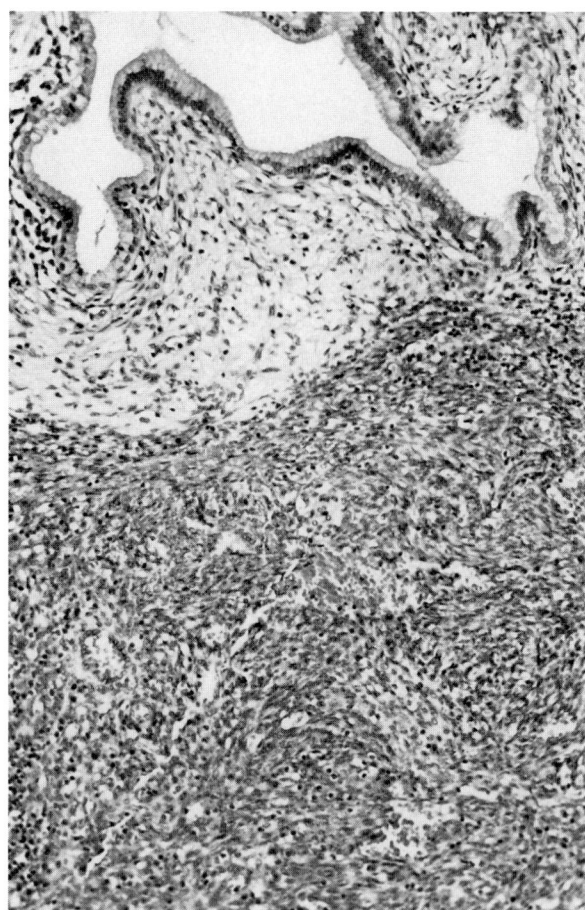

FIG. 17.31. Stromal endometriosis of uterine cervix. A cellular sheet of endometriotic stroma lies adjacent to an endocervical gland. (Reprinted by permission of Clement, ref. 96.)

endometriosis. It may be palpable as deep, firm nodules or cysts in the posterior wall of the cervix.[177,385,581] The diagnosis is made by biopsy or pathological examination of the hysterectomy specimen. The differential diagnosis includes downgrowth of adenomyosis from the uterine corpus.

Superficial vaginal endometriosis, which typically involves the vault, is rarer than cervical endometriosis, but is similar to the latter macroscopically, in its predilection for involving sites of prior trauma and in its lack of associated pelvic endometriosis.[177] Deep vaginal endometriosis is more common, is typically associated with pelvic endometriosis, and appears as nodular or polypoid masses involving the posterior vaginal fornix.[177,385] The differential diagnosis of vaginal endometriosis, particularly of the superficial type, includes vaginal adenosis of the tuboendometrial variety; the latter, however, lacks endometrial stroma and the characteristic inflammatory response of endometriosis. Endometriosis of the vulva is discussed in a subsequent section (see Cutaneous Endometriosis).

TUBAL ENDOMETRIOSIS

The term *endometriosis* has been applied to at least three different, unrelated lesions of the fallopian tube. The most common type is serosal or subserosal endometriosis, typically associated with endometriosis elsewhere in the pelvis; the myosalpinx usually is not involved.[492]

Endometrial tissue may extend directly from the uterine cornu and replace the mucosa of the interstitial and isthmic portions of the tube in as many as 25% and 10% of women in the general population, respectively.[321,453] This finding is considered to represent a normal morphologic variation, although in some cases the ectopic endometrial tissue may give rise to intratubal polyps.[124] In occasional cases, the endometrial tissue may occlude the tubal lumen, that is, *intraluminal endometriosis* or *endometrial colonization* (Fig. 17.32); involvement may be bilateral.[92,130,167,331] Colonization typically is unassociated with endometriosis elsewhere. The disorder accounts for 15–20% of tubal-related infertility; it also may be associated with tubal pregnancy.

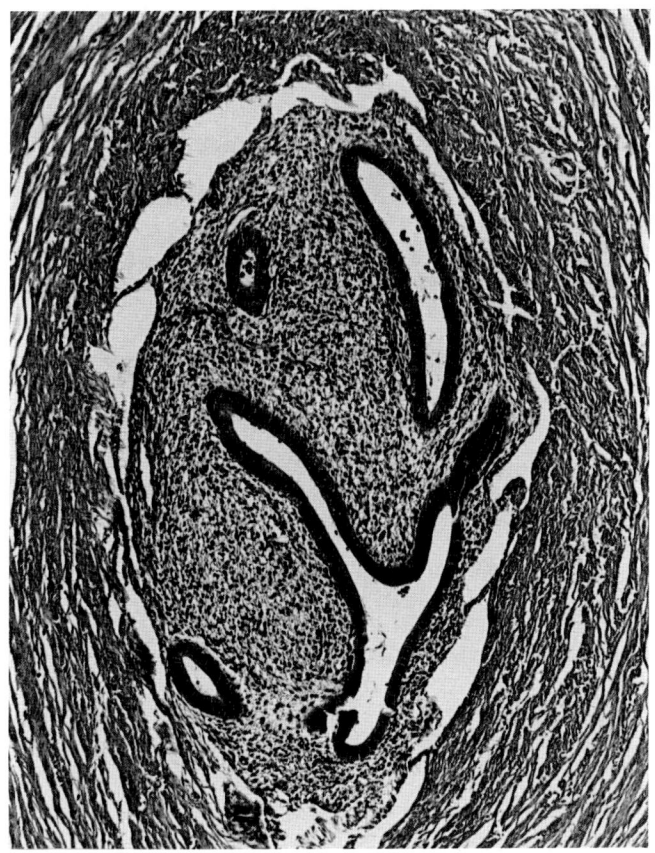

FIG. 17.32. Endometriosis (colonization) of the fallopian tube. The tubal lumen is occluded by endometrial glands and stroma. Spaces at the junction of endometrial tissue and myosalpinx represent dilated lymphatic channels.

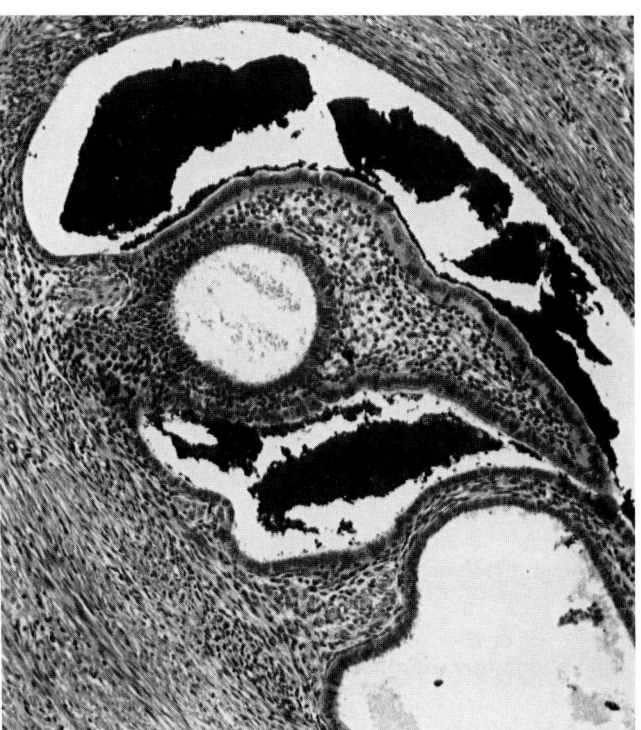

FIG. 17.33. Postsalpingectomy endometriosis of the fallopian tube. After removal, the lumen of the specimen has been injected with India ink. Endometrial glands and stroma are surrounded by smooth muscle of the myosalpinx. The lumens of the endometrial glands contain India ink (From Rock JA, Parmley TH, King TM, Laufe LE, Su BC (1981) Endometriosis and the development of tuboperitoneal fistulas after tubal ligation. Fertil Steril 35: 16. Reproduced by permission of the publisher, The American Fertility Society.)

The third type of endometriosis involving the fallopian tube has been designated *postsalpingectomy endometriosis*. It occurs in the tip of the proximal tubal stump, typically 1 to 4 years after tubal ligation.[442,518] It is closely related to, and may be associated with, salpingitis isthmica nodosa. The lesion is analogous to uterine adenomyosis, consisting of endometrial glands and stroma extending from the endosalpinx into the myosalpinx, and frequently to the serosal surface. Hysterosalpingography or India ink injection of the specimen may show tuboperitoneal fistulous tracts (Fig. 17.33); postligation pregnancies are a rare complication. Postsalpingectomy endometriosis has been documented in 20–50% of tubes examined after ligation. The frequency of this complication is increased with the electrocautery method of ligation, with short proximal stumps, and with increasing postligation intervals.

INTESTINAL ENDOMETRIOSIS

Intestinal involvement has been documented in as many as 37% of patients with endometriosis undergoing laparot-

omy.[579] Macafee and Greer,[330] however, in their review of the literature before 1960 calculated an average frequency of 12%, a figure similar to that in several recent studies.[201] In most such cases, the involvement is confined to the serosa or subserosa and is unassociated with clinical manifestations referable to the intestinal tract. In contrast, from 0.7% to 2.5% of patients with endometriosis require bowel resection for symptomatic lesions.[201,330,418] In some series, as many as half of the patients with symptomatic intestinal endometriosis have no extraintestinal involvement; the endometriotic nature of the intestinal lesions in such cases is more likely to be unrecognized preoperatively or at the time of laparotomy.[330] Misdiagnosis also is common in postmenopausal patients because of a decreased index of suspicion, even though it has been shown that the intestine is one of the more common sites of clinically significant endometriosis in this age group.[222,274,330] Similarly, Macafee and Greer found that 7% of patients with symptomatic intestinal endometriosis were postmenopausal.[330]

Intestinal sites of involvement include, in descending order of frequency, the rectum and sigmoid, the appendix, the terminal ileum, the cecum, and other parts of the large and small bowel, including Meckel's diverticulum.[96,563] In one large study,[418] 15% of patients had more than one site of involvement. The presenting symptoms include, alone or in combination, acute or chronic abdominal pain, diarrhea, constipation, hematochezia, and decrease in stool caliber. Although the frequent catamenial nature of the symptoms may suggest the correct diagnosis, the clinical presentation can mimic acute appendicitis, bowel obstruction caused by adhesions or a hernia, a neoplasm, or even inflammatory bowel disease. Endoscopic and radiographic studies typically demonstrate an extramucosal stenosing lesion; endoscopic biopsies usually are of no diagnostic value.

Endometriosis of the rectosigmoid area usually is a solitary lesion, involving a segment several centimeters in length, whereas ileal involvement frequently is multifocal and may involve segments of bowel up to 45 cm in length.[96,152,322,340,511] On gross examination, the segment of bowel is indurated and often angulated by an ill-defined, usually noncircumferential mass; the serosal surface may be puckered and covered by adhesions. Sectioning typically reveals a firm, gray-white, solid, mural mass, the bulk of which represents markedly thickened muscularis propria; the latter often has a radiating fan-like appearance (Fig. 17.34). Small cystic spaces containing altered blood may be seen but are uncommon. In contrast to a primary adenocarcinoma, the overlying mucosa usually is intact, a feature difficult to reconcile with the high frequency of symptomatic bleeding in some series of patients.[222] Rare cases of polypoid mucosal involvement, however, may groosly mimic an adenocarcinoma.[31,159] On microscopic examination, islands of endometriotic tissue typically are scattered throughout the hyperplastic muscularis propria (Fig. 17.35), with or without involvement of other layers.

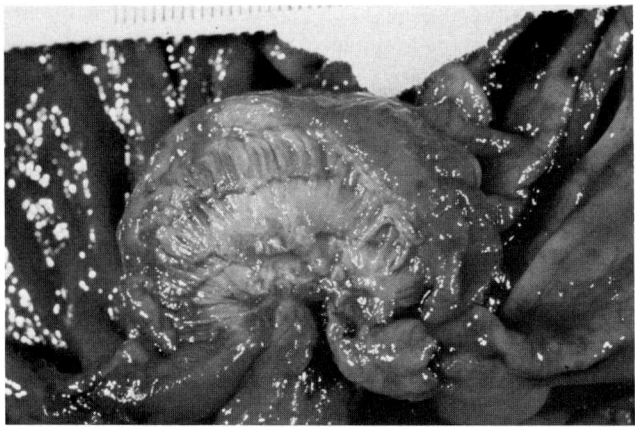

FIG. 17.34. **Colonic endometriosis (cut surface).** There is marked mural thickening and fibrosis. The serosal surface is retracted, and the overlying mucosa is intact. (Courtesy of Dr. R. D. Croom.)

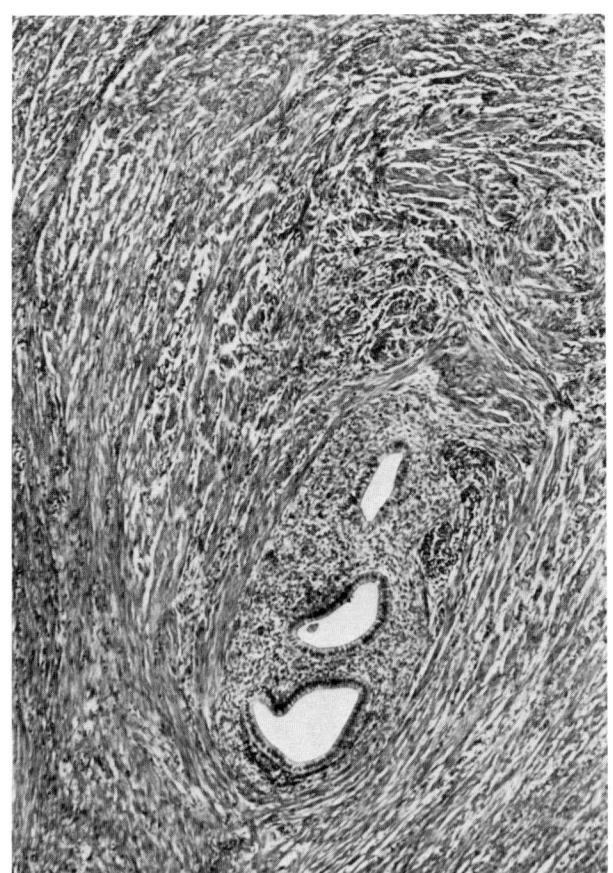

FIG. 17.35. **Intestinal endometriosis.** The endometriotic tissue within the muscularis propria is surrounded by markedly hyperplastic smooth muscle.

A complication of intestinal endometriosis is perforation, which typically is associated with pregnancy; a marked decidual reaction typically is seen with the endometriotic stroma in such cases.[164,376] Other complications include volvulus,[322] intussusception,[336,396] acute appendicitis,[376] appendiceal mucocoele,[218] intramural hematoma,[584] and the development of a malignant neoplasm.[56,301,374]

URINARY TRACT ENDOMETRIOSIS

Urinary tract involvement has been documented at laparotomy in from 16% to 20% of patients with endometriosis.[434,579] In most of these cases, the endometriosis is found on the serosa of the urinary bladder or that overlying the ureter and is without local clinical manifestations. Similarly, high-volume intravenous urography has demonstrated subtle, clinically insignificant abnormalities in almost 16% of women with proven pelvic endometriosis before therapy.[344] In contrast, only 0.5–1% of patients with endometriosis have clinically significant urinary tract involvement; approximately 30% of such patients ultimately require nephrectomy for a hydronephrotic or nonfunctioning kidney.[282] The vast majority of the more than 300 reported cases of urinary tract endometriosis have involved the urinary bladder or the ureters (with approximately equal frequency); the kidneys (10 cases) and the urethra (2 cases) are involved much less commonly. Urinary tract involvement usually is associated with endometriosis elsewhere in the pelvis, although the symptoms relating to the urinary tract may be the initial or sole manifestations of the disease in such patients.[512] In some series, however, as many as half of the patients with ureteral involvement have disease restricted to the ureter and the adjacent uterosacral ligament.[260,373] Patients with renal endometriosis typically do not have endometriosis elsewhere, suggesting an embolic, likely blood-borne, origin.

From one-third to one-half of the affected patients are over 40 years of age and almost 5% of the patients are postmenopausal, some of whom had received estrogen replacement therapy.[96,264,429] A preoperative diagnosis may be suspected by the catamenial nature of the symptoms, which include suprapubic or flank pain, frequency, urgency, dysuria, and hematuria; chills and fever secondary to a urinary tract infection have been the presenting symptoms in occasional cases. A tender suprapubic or flank mass may be palpable. Many patients, however, particularly those with ureteric involvement, have nonspecific manifestations or present with a silent obstructive uropathy, occasionally complicated by hypertension, renal failure (in cases of bilateral involvement), or both.[3,260,304,373,512] In patients with bladder involvement, urography may reveal a filling defect; a stricture in the lower ureter with hydroureter and hydronephrosis or a nonfunctioning kidney is the typical urographic finding in those with ureteral involvement. Endoscopy may be confirmatory of vesical or even ureteral involvement, and the lesions may exhibit catamenial enlargement, darkening, and bleeding. Endoscopy and biopsy, however, often are nondiagnostic.[3,512]

Symptomatic endometriosis of the bladder is almost always a result of mural involvement, and the lesions typically are located on the trigone, the floor of the bladder, or low on the posterior wall.[512] Involvement rarely is confined to the lateral walls, the dome, or the ureterovesical junction.[3,512] Gross examination typically reveals a solitary, blue, red, gray, or brown multicystic mass that thickens the wall and sometimes projects into the bladder lumen (Fig. 17.36); the lesions have ranged from several millimeters to 14 cm in diameter. The mucosa usually is intact, but occasionally may be ulcerated and bleeding, particularly during menses.[512] Histological examination reveals fibrosis and proliferation of the muscularis around the foci of endometriosis; the lamina propria also was involved in 60% of the cases in one study.[512] Obstruction of both ureteric orifices, vesicolic fistula, and malignant transformation have been rare complications.[3]

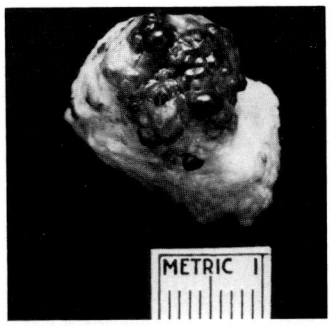

FIG. 17.36. Endometriosis of the bladder. The mucosal surface is replaced by a hemorrhagic, nodular lesion. (Reprinted by permission of Surgery, Gynecology & Obstetrics, ref. 512.)

With rare exceptions, endometriosis of the ureter is confined to its lower one-third, usually involving a segment less than 2 cm in length that lies 2 to 5 cm from the ureterovesical junction; involvement has been bilateral in approximately 10% of the cases.[96,300,328,504,512] Ureteral endometriosis traditionally has been divided into extrinsic and intrinsic forms, although this distinction has not been possible in many of the reported cases because the affected segment of the ureter was not removed and examined histologically. Also, it is likely that at least some intrinsic cases initially were extrinsic in type. In the latter, endometriosis of the uterosacral ligament or ureteral adventitia causes ureteral luminal narrowing by compression, fibrosis, or both; in some such cases, there is transmural scarring of the ureter.[512] Intrinsic involvement is characterized by endometriotic tissue within a typically hyperplastic and fibrotic muscularis; in some cases the lamina propria also is involved. Mucosal involvement rarely takes the form of a polypoid mass projecting into the lumen (Fig. 17.37).[264,374,512]

On gross examination, endometriosis of the kidney typically is a solitary, well-circumscribed, hemorrhagic, solid and cystic mass that focally replaces the renal parenchyma; the lesions in the 10 reported cases have measured from 1.5 cm to 13 cm in diameter.[28,96] In occasional cases, polypoid masses have projected into the renal pelvis. Foci of smooth muscle have been found admixed with the endometriotic tissue on microscopic examination in some of the cases.

Only two cases of urethral endometriosis have been described. In one, a caruncle-like nodule projected from the urethral orifice in a 38-year-old woman with dysuria.[194] In the other, a 24-year-old woman with dysuria and dyspareunia was found to have endometriosis in the wall of a large urethral diverticulum.[395]

CUTANEOUS ENDOMETRIOSIS

Most of the reported cases of cutaneous endometriosis have occurred within surgical scars[80,305,312,513,580] or,

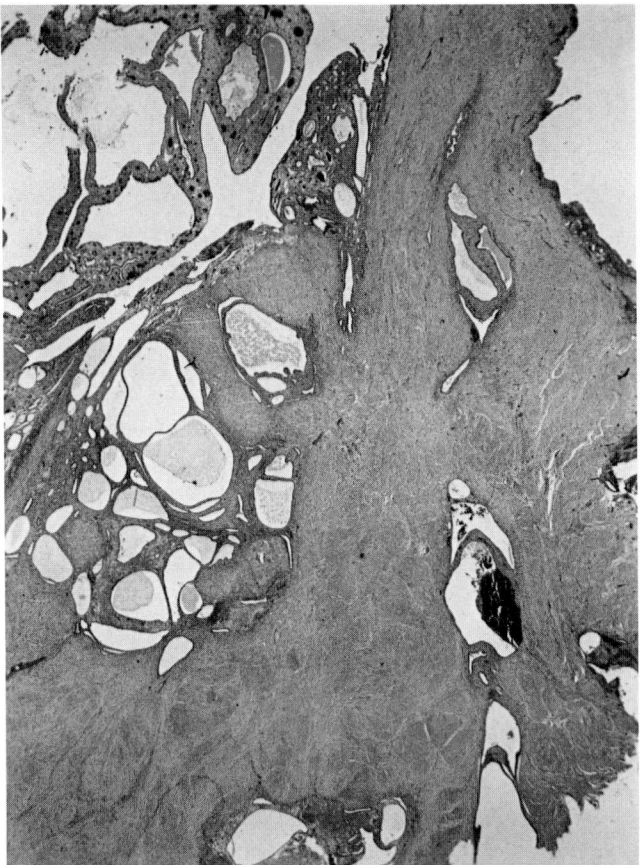

FIG. 17.37. Polypoid endometriosis of the ureter. The endometriosis involves the wall of the ureter and forms a polypoid mass projecting into its lumen (*top left*). (Reprinted by permission of Mostoufizadeh and Scully, ref. 374.)

rarely, within needle tracts[269]; the remainder are spontaneous. Both types are associated with pelvic endometriosis in only a minority of cases.[80,513] As scar-related endometriosis typically occurs after operations on the uterus or fallopian tubes, the site most commonly involved is the lower abdominal wall; the umbilicus is involved less commonly.[513] Similarly, most cases of endometriosis of the lower vagina, vulva, Bartholin's gland, perineum, and perianal region involve areas of obstetrical or surgical truma, most commonly episiotomy scars.* Scar-related cases occur less commonly after nongynecological procedures, such as an appendectomy or inguinal hernia repair.[513] Spontaneous cutaneous endometriosis typically involves the umbilicus[363,481,513,539] and, less commonly, the inguinal[513] and perianal regions.[367]

The most common symptoms are those relating to a cutaneous mass or nodule that, in the scar-related cases, appears weeks to years after surgery; the average postoper-

*Refs. 80,146,177,196,343,385,401,513.

ative interval in one study was 30 months.[513] A catamenial increase in size and tenderness and, occasionally, bleeding from the lesion, suggest the diagnosis. Patients with perianal lesions may have involvement of the external sphincter producing anorectal pain and irritation simulating an anal fistula, abscess, or thrombosed hemorrhoid. Umbilical endometriosis may simulate an umbilical hernia on physical examination.[363] The lesions occasionally recur after excision.[513]

On clinical examination, the lesions are firm, solitary nodules varying from a few millimeters to 6 cm in diameter (Fig. 17.38). They range from pink to brown to blue-black, depending on the age of the lesion and the depth within the skin.[513] The cut surface of the scar-related lesions typically is gray-white, with or without focal areas of recent or old hemorrhage.[80] On microscopic examination, the endometriosis may involve the dermis (Fig. 17.39), the subcutis, or both,[513] and in occasional cases, underlying skeletal muscle.[218,227] There typically is no continuity between the cutaneous and peritoneal lesions in patients with associated pelvic endometriosis.[513]

The association of abdominal scar-related endometriosis and episiotomy scar-related endometriosis with uterine operations and episiotomies, respectively, suggests implantation of endometrial tissue as the most likely pathogenesis. The risk of implantation appears to be much higher after hysterotomy than after cesarean section or vaginal delivery, suggesting that the decidua of late pregnancy has a reduced ability to implant.[482] When curettage is performed immediately after vaginal term delivery, however, the frequency of endometriosis in the episiotomy scar becomes much higher.[401] In nonpregnant patients, implantation of endometrium during endometrial curettage or spontaneous implantation of menstrual endometrium also has been implicated in occasional cases of scar-related endometrio-

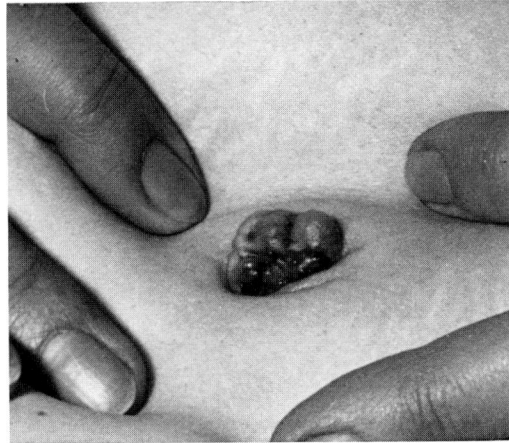

FIG. 17.38. Cutaneous endometriosis. A hemorrhagic, polypoid mass involves the umbilicus. (Reprinted by permission of Steck and Helwig, ref. 513.)

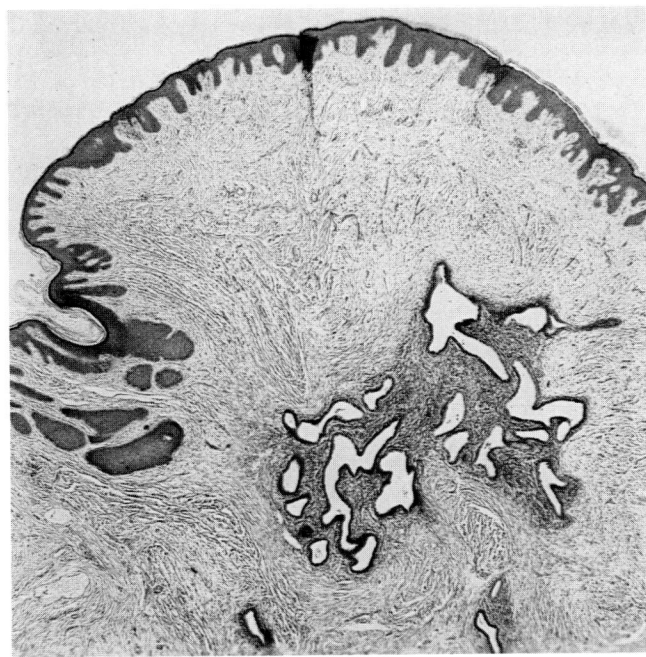

FIG. 17.39. Cutaneous endometriosis. Endometriotic foci are present within the dermis. (Reprinted by permission of Steck and Helwig, ref. 513.)

sis.[146] Scott et al.[481] have demonstrated lymphatics between the pelvis and umbilicus that may explain cases of spontaneous endometriosis in the latter site.

INGUINAL ENDOMETRIOSIS

Noncutaneous inguinal endometriosis, secondary to involvement of the extraperitoneal portion of the round ligament, occurs in approximately 0.4% of patients with endometriosis.[68,95,403] The usual presentation is that of a painful, typically right-sided, hernia-like inguinal mass, with catamenial exacerbation in some cases. In approximately one-third of the reported cases, an inguinal hernia also was present.[95] The lesion can impinge on the pubic tubercle and mimic arthritis, bursitis, or tendinitis.[403] Rarely, endometriosis in the inguinal region also has been described in inguinal or femoral hernia sacs or the canal of Nuck.[422,430] In one case of femoral hernial involvement, the adventitia of the femoral vein was involved and its lumen was thrombosed.[430]

ENDOMETRIOSIS OF LYMPH NODES

Lymph node involvement by endometriosis is uncommon, and many examples reported as such, particularly in the older literature, represent lymph nodes involved by benign müllerian (usually endosalpingiotic) glands devoid of an endometrial stromal component.[11] By performing "selective lymphadenectomies," Javert found that 12% of pa-

tients with pelvic endometriosis, adenomyosis, or both had endometriosis of pelvic lymph nodes.[255] The involved lymph nodes may be enlarged visibly or palpably at operation. On microscopic examination, in contrast to glandular inclusions, endometriotic foci are characterized by a more central location within the node, an endometrial stromal component, and the frequent presence of erythrocytes and pseudoxanthoma cells.[255] Endosalpingiosis and endometriosis may co-exist, however, in the same lymph node.[255] As in other sites, decidual transformation of the endometriotic stroma has been encountered during pregnancy.[454] As previously noted, a unique case of intranodal endometriosis was characterized by an extensive smooth muscle component (see Fig. 17.26).[445]

PLEUROPULMONARY ENDOMETRIOSIS

Pathologically documented cases of endometriosis involving the lungs or pleura are rare. Some reported examples interpreted as pulmonary endometriosis have taken the form of microscopic foci of "decidua" found at autopsy in pregnant or recently pregnant women.[318] Such lesions would be interpreted almost certainly by current criteria as foci of embolic intermediate trophoblast.[295,296] Many other cases of purported pleuropulmonary endometriosis have been diagnosed solely on the basis of clinical manifestations or in conjunction with nonspecific histological or cytological findings. This discussion is based on the 28 pathologically documented cases of thoracic endometriosis in the literature, 17 of which were pleural and 11 of which were parenchymal.[17,96,168,302,318,391,575]

The clinical manifestations of pleural endometriosis differ from those associated with parenchymal involvement. In the former, the characteristic presentation is one of repeated episodes of catamenial pneumothorax, typically on the right side. Less common presentations include recurrent right-sided, typically hemorrhagic effusions, hemoptysis, and catamenial periscapular pain. Co-existent intraabdominal endometriosis has been demonstrated in approximately one-third of cases, although in another one-third of cases, its presence or absence was not confirmed. In contrast, patients with parenchymal endometriosis typically present with catamenial hemoptysis; other patients are asymptomatic and the lesion is an incidental radiographic finding. Only one patient has had documented peritoneal endometriosis, although in most patients, the peritoneum has not been visualized. With rare exceptions, patients with parenchymal endometriosis have had prior uterine operations.

Pleural endometriosis is confined almost invariably to the right side; one case with bilateral involvement has been reported.[575] The lesions typically are multiple, dark red or blue nodules or cysts on the diaphragmatic pleura; parietal, visceral, and pericardial pleural surfaces also are affected less commonly. Associated pathological changes have included diaphragmatic fenestrations in 50% of the cases and, occasionally, pleural blebs. Parenchymal endometriotic lesions typically are solitary, tan to gray, focally hemorrhagic nodules or thin-walled cysts measuring up to 6 cm in diameter. Several lesions have been subpleural or have involved bronchial walls and lumina. Parenchymal lesions lack the almost exclusively right-sided location of pleural endometriosis; one case had a bilateral miliary distribution.[318] In additional contrast to pleural lesions, associated diaphragmatic fenestrations have not been described.

The clinicopathological differences between pleural and parenchymal endometriosis of the lung suggest that they differ in their histogenesis. The distribution of the parenchymal lesions and their strong association with prior uterine trauma strongly suggest an embolic origin. In contrast, most if not all pleural lesions are likely a result of passage of endometriotic tissue from the peritoneal cavity through diaphragmatic defects or diaphragmatic lymphatics, consistent with the right-sided predominance of both structures. The catamenial pneumothorax in these patients, and in those with catamenial pneumothorax unassociated with pleural endometriosis, may be related to the diaphragmatic defects that allow passage of air from the peritoneal into the pleural cavity. The escape of air from defects in the visceral pleura produced by the endometriotic lesions or from preexistent blebs is another possible explanation for the pneumothorax in these patients. It has been suggested that prostaglandins produced by eutopic endometrium or endometriotic tissue at the time of the menses may predispose to alveolar rupture.

Soft Tissue and Skeletal Endometriosis

Rarely, typical endometriomas have occurred in skeletal muscle or deep soft tissues in distant sites. The presentation usually is that of a mass associated with catamenial pain, tenderness, and enlargement. The involved sites have included the trapezius,[179] extensor carpi radialis,[378] thumb,[204] biceps femoris,[183] thigh,[187] and the knee.[400] A case of endomyometriosis interpreted as a choristoma has been described in the lumbosacral soft tissues attached to the dura in a patient with spina bifida.[294] A unique endometrioma occurred in the breast of a patient with a 2-year history of catamenial bloody nipple discharge.[371] Rare pelvic endometriotic cysts have eroded lumbar vertebrae causing catamenial lumbar pain.[119,162]

Upper Abdominal Endometriosis

Endometriotic implants occasionally may occur on the omentum; omental endometriosis was only one-eighth as common as omental endosalpingiosis in one study.[593] Rarely, endometriotic implants may involve the peritoneal surfaces of the liver[243] or diaphragm.[381] As with pleural diaphragmatic involvement, implants on the peritonal side

of the diaphragm occasionally have been associated with diaphragmatic defects and catamenial pneumothorax. Rare endometriomas of the epigastrium,[404] the tail of the pancreas,[197,337] and the liver parenchyma[161,199,452] have been reported.

Endometriosis of the Nervous System

Approximately 20 cases of endometriosis of the sciatic nerve sheath at the level of the sciatic notch have been described, typically associated with catamenial sciatica.[542] Some cases have been associated with a visible peritoneal evagination attached to the involved portion of the nerve ("pocket sign"). A case of subarachnoid endometriosis of the lumbar spinal cord caused catamenial radicular pain and recurrent subarachnoid hemorrhage.[323] In another case, a cerebral endometrioma was discovered in the parietal lobe of a patient who had a 3-year history of episodic headaches that culminated in a generalized seizure.[537]

Endometriosis in Men

Rare examples of endometriosis have been described in men receiving long-term estrogen therapy for prostatic carcinoma. With the exception of one case involving the abdominal wall,[342] the sites of involvement have been confined to the genitourinary tract, specifically the urinary bladder (three cases),[96,475] prostate (one case),[29] and paratesticular region (two cases).[591] As previously noted, the two paratesticular lesions were endomyometriotic in composition.[591]

Neoplasms Arising from Endometriosis

A malignant tumor has been documented to arise in from 0.3% to 0.8% of cases of ovarian endometriosis, but the exact frequency of cancer originating in pelvic endometriosis is unknown.[56,221,374] Approximately 75% of tumors complicating endometriosis arise within the ovary. The most common extraovarian site is the rectovaginal septum; less frequent sites include the vagina, colon and rectum, urinary bladder, and other sites in the pelvis and abdomen. In some cases, the tumors have been preceded by prolonged unopposed estrogen replacement therapy.[56,437]

Endometrioid carcinoma (Fig. 17.40) is the most common tumor arising within endometriosis, accounting for almost 70% of such cases.[221] Direct origin of endometrioid carcinoma from endometriotic tissue has been demonstrated in as many as 24% of cases in some series.[374] At least 90% of the carcinomas arising from extraovarian endometriosis have been of endometrioid type.[56,221,374] Rarely, endometrioid tumors arising in ovarian and extraovarian endometriosis may exhibit a benign or borderline adenofibromatous pattern.[200,486]

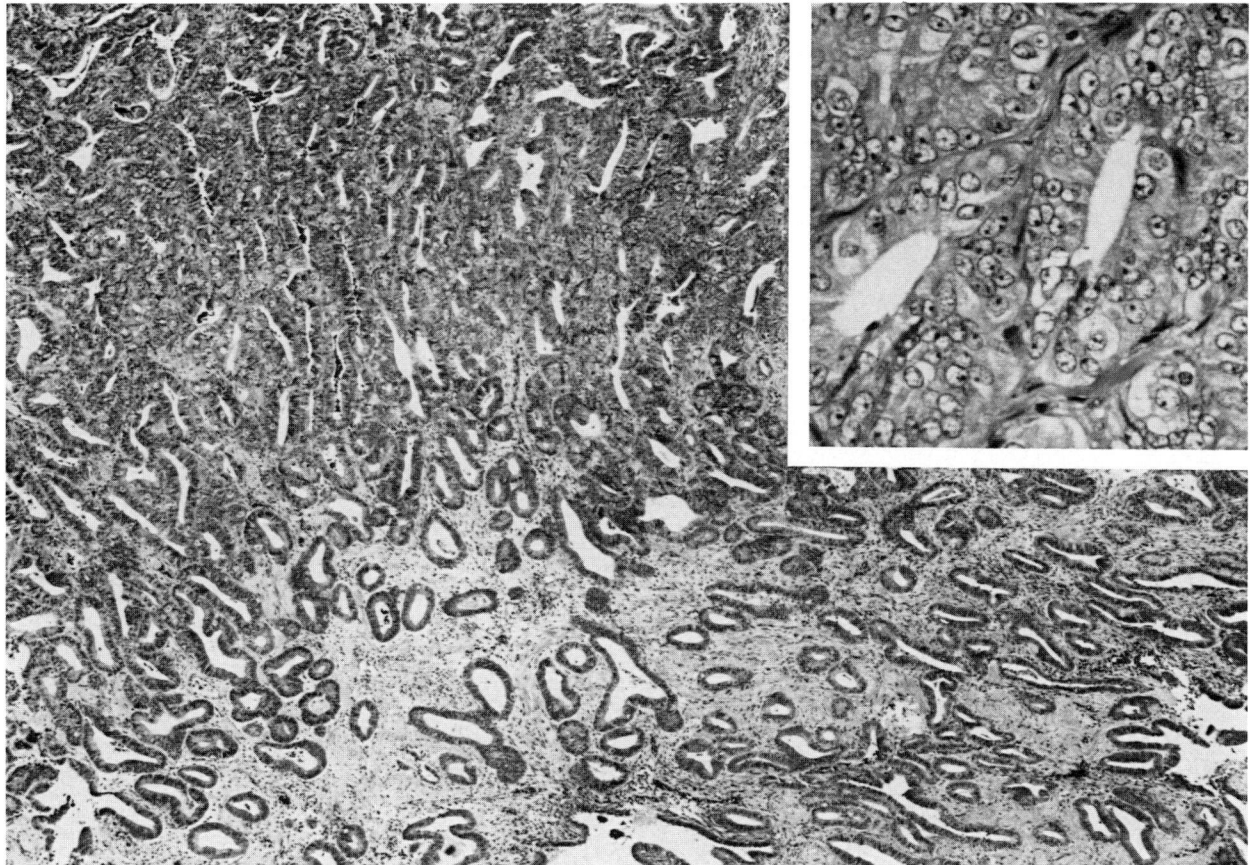

FIG. 17.40. Endometrioid carcinoma arising within endometriosis. Benign endometriotic glands and stroma merge with the carcinomatous glands. *Inset:* High-power view of carcinomatous glands.

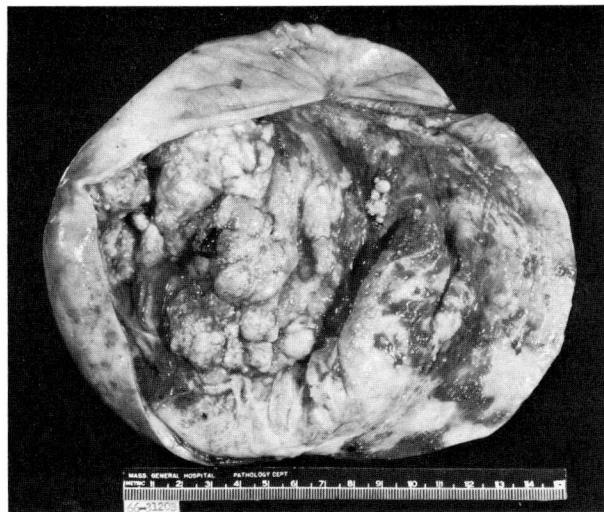

FIG. 17.41. Clear cell carcinoma arising within an endometriotic cyst. Fleshy pale tumor nodules protrude into the cyst lumen. (Reprinted by permission of Scully et al., ref. 486.)

Clear cell carcinoma (Figs. 17.41, 17.42) is the second most common tumor originating in endometriosis, accounting for approximately 14% of such cases.[221] In some studies, the frequency of endometriosis co-existing with clear cell carcinoma of the ovary is even higher than with endometrioid carcinoma; pelvic endometriosis has been reported in 24–49% of cases of ovarian clear cell carcinoma.[455] A few examples of clear cell carcinoma arising within extraovarian endometriosis also have been described.[6,200,227]

Rare epithelial tumors of other types arising from endometriosis include ovarian serous cystadenomas of low malignant potential,[202] benign and malignant mucinous tumors,[458,459,486] and squamous cell carcinomas.[313,377] ESSs and malignant mesodermal mixed tumors may originate in ovarian and extraovarian endometriosis.[89,107,495,590] In one study, 60% of ESSs apparently arising within the ovary were associated with ovarian endometriosis.[590] Vaginal endometriosis was the probable origin of one extrauterine pelvic adenosarcoma.[332] Two examples of yolk sac tumor have arisen in

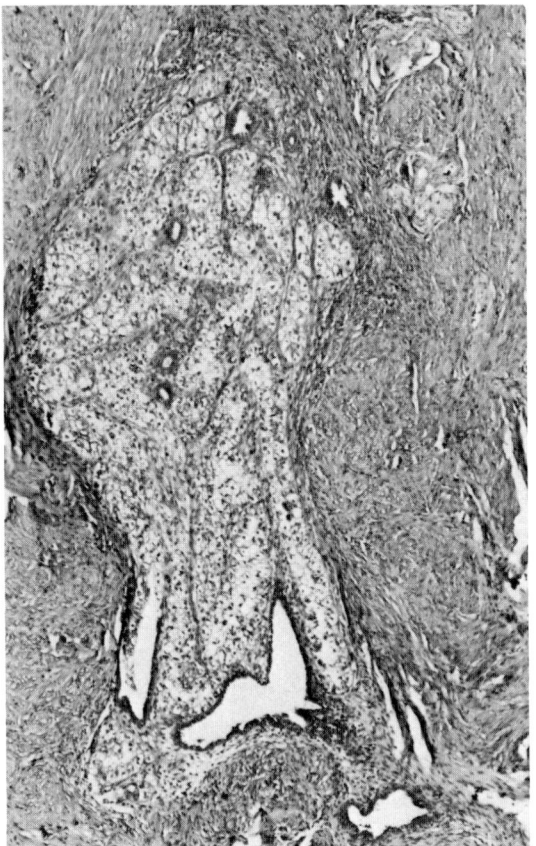

Fig. 17.42. Clear cell carcinoma arising within endometriosis. Benign endometriotic glands and stroma (*bottom*) merge with clear cell carcinoma. (Courtesy of Dr. A. B. P. Ng.)

association with endometriosis[301,460] and in one unique case, a sex cord tumor with annular tubules was intimately associated with endometriosis of the tubal serosa.[203]

Peritoneal Endometrioid Lesions Other than Endometriosis

Benign glands lined by endometrial epithelium (but lacking endometrial stroma) with the peritoneal distribution of endosalpingiosis occasionally occur.[307] Some may represent foci of endometriosis in which the stromal component has undergone atrophy. Benign endometrioid peritoneal "implants" lacking an endometrial stromal component also have been reported in association with a borderline ovarian endometrioid tumor.[455] The peritoneal lesions were interpreted as having arisen directly from the peritoneum.

A variety of extrauterine, extraovarian, pelvic, or retroperitoneal neoplasms of endometrioid type occur in the absence of demonstrable endometriosis. These tumors generally have been considered to arise directly from the mesothelium or submesothelial stroma. They have included endometrioid cystadenofibroma[208,390] and cystadenocarcinoma,[93] endometrioid stromal sarcoma,[547] homologous and heterologous types of malignant mesodermal mixed tumor,[176,508] and mesodermal adenosarcoma.[24,97,281,457]

Peritoneal Serous Lesions

Endosalpingiosis

CLINICAL FEATURES

Endosalpingiosis typically refers to the presence of histologically benign glands lined by tubal-type epithelium involving the peritoneum and subperitoneal tissues; the term also may be used to refer to similar glands within retroperitoneal lymph nodes (see page 685). This disorder occurs almost exclusively in women, typically during the reproductive era, with a mean age of 29.7 years in one study,[593] although occasional cases have been described in postmenopausal women. Endosalpingiosis is almost always an incidental finding either at the time of operation or more commonly on microscopic examination. Zinsser and Wheeler found endosalpingiosis in 12.5% of surgically removed omenta in a retrospective study, but this figure doubled when omenta were examined more thoroughly in a prospective study.[593] Endosalpingiosis may be detected as multiple fine pelvic calcifications on x-ray examination[546] or as psammoma bodies within cul-de-sac fluid,[232,279] peritoneal washings,[496,504a,505] the lumen of the fallopian tube,[209] or cervical Papanicolaou smears.[209,278,546]

An origin from mesothelium (the secondary müllerian system) is favored by most investigators, but the association of endosalpingiosis with chronic salpingitis implicates implantation of sloughed tubal epithelium as a possible histogenetic mechanism.[593] A similar association with serous tumors of borderline malignancy suggests that some endosalpingiotic foci may represent tumor implants that have undergone maturation.[352] Endosalpingiosis in the absence of residual tumor at the time of second-look laparotomy in patients with ovarian epithelial neoplasms does not justify additional treatment.[108]

PATHOLOGICAL FINDINGS

Endosalpingiosis is encountered most commonly on the pelvic peritoneum covering the uterus, fallopian tubes, ovaries, and cul-de-sac.[57,62,83,232,351,505,546] Less frequent sites include the pelvic parietal peritoneum,[62] omentum,[351,546,593] bladder,[83] and bowel serosa,[65,83,120] para-aortic area,[493] and skin, including laparotomy scars.[142] Endosalpingiosis usually is inapparent at the time of operation or on gross inspection of the involved tissues, but may be visible as multiple, punctate (1–2 mm), white to yellow, opaque or translucent, fluid-filled cysts that impart a vesicular or granular appearance to the involved surface; rarely, larger cysts up to 1 cm in diameter may be seen.[57,62,83,232]

Microscopic examination reveals multiple, simple glands, often cystically dilated and lined by a single layer of epithelium resembling that of the normal fallopian tube

(Figs. 17.43, 17.44). The glands frequently are surrounded by a loose or dense connective tissue stroma that may contain a sparse mononuclear inflammatory cell infiltrate. The glands may exhibit irregular contours, crowding, and intraluminal stromal papillae.[279] The three cell types of the normal fallopian tube epithelium are found in varying numbers: pale ciliated cells, secretory cells, and dark rod-like, intercalated or "peg" cells.[62,546,593] The cells have prominent luminal margins, distinct borders, and basal nuclei. Focal cellular pseudostratification may be present. The nuclei have fine chromatin and delicate nuclear membranes, and typically lack significant atypia or mitotic activity.[593] Psammoma bodies frequently are present within the lumens or in the adjacent stroma, and in occasional cases, large numbers of psammoma bodies embedded in subserosal connective tissue may be a striking finding. Endosalpingiotic glands rarely may extend into the underlying tissues to a limited degree.[65] Staining with the PAS method reveals a basement membrane surrounding each gland, and PAS-positive, diastase-resistant material in the apices of the lining cells and within the glandular lumens.[593] Estrogen and progesterone receptors have been identified immunohistochemically within the cells.[410]

The term *atypical endosalpingiosis* has been applied to endosalpingiotic lesions in which there is cellular stratification, including cellular buds, cribriform patterns, and varying degrees of cellular atypia, occurring in the absence of a

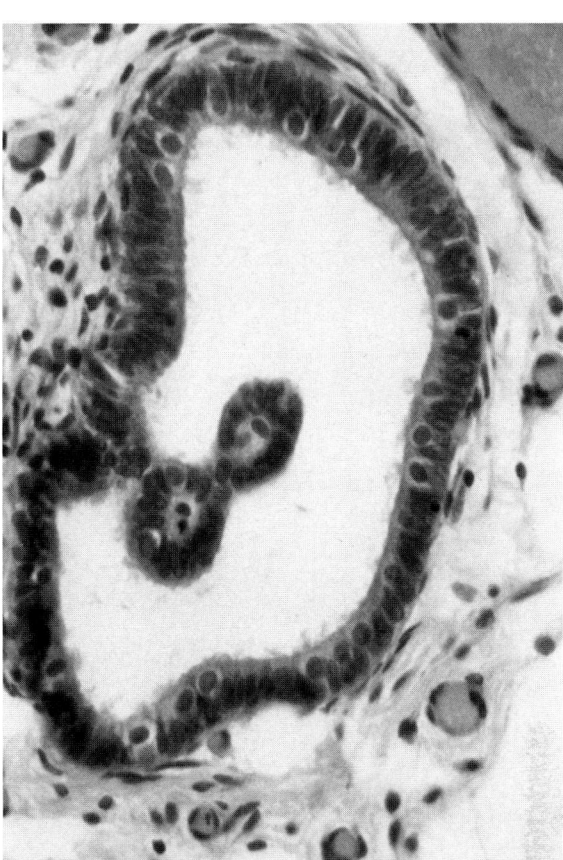

Fig. 17.44. Endosalpingiosis. A gland within the omentum is lined by benign endosalpingeal epithelium composed of multiple cell types.

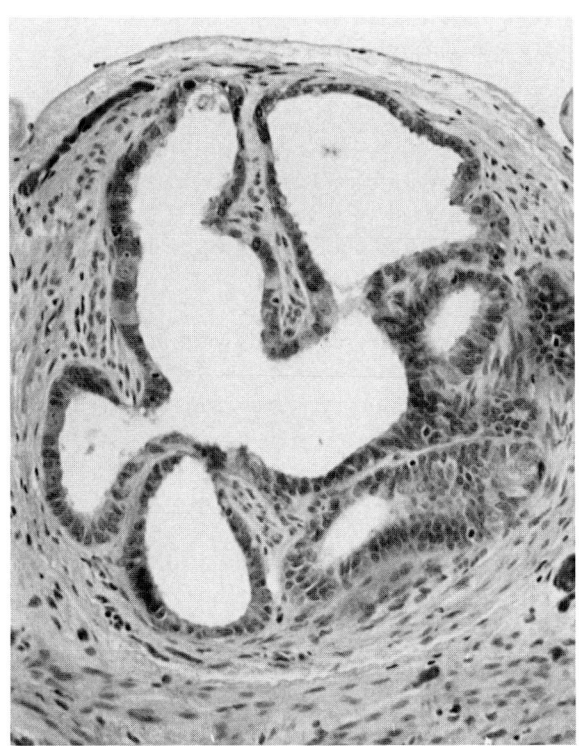

Fig. 17.43. Endosalpingiosis. Complex glandular structure lies beneath uterine serosa. Glands are lined by a single layer of benign endosalpingeal epithelium.

serous tumor of borderline malignancy. Such lesions merge histologically with peritoneal serous tumors of borderline malignancy (see next section). Bell and Scully use the latter term if the "lesions composed of tubal-type epithelium exhibit papillarity, tufting, or detachment of cell clusters . . . even when they arise on a background of endosalpingiosis."[30] Endosalpingiotic glands should be differentiated from mesonephric remnants, which are common incidental microscopic findings in the region of the fallopian tube. Mesonephric tubules typically are located more deeply than endosalpingiosis and characteristically have a collar of smooth muscle under the epithelial lining, which is typically a single layer of nonciliated, low columnar to cuboidal cells.[53]

Extraovarian Serous Tumors

The full spectrum of serous neoplasms arising within the ovary also may arise directly from the extraovarian peritoneum. These tumors are considered here only briefly because their clinicopathological features closely resemble those of their ovarian counterparts.

Occasional tumors resembling ovarian serous borderline tumors are characterized by widespread extraovarian peri-

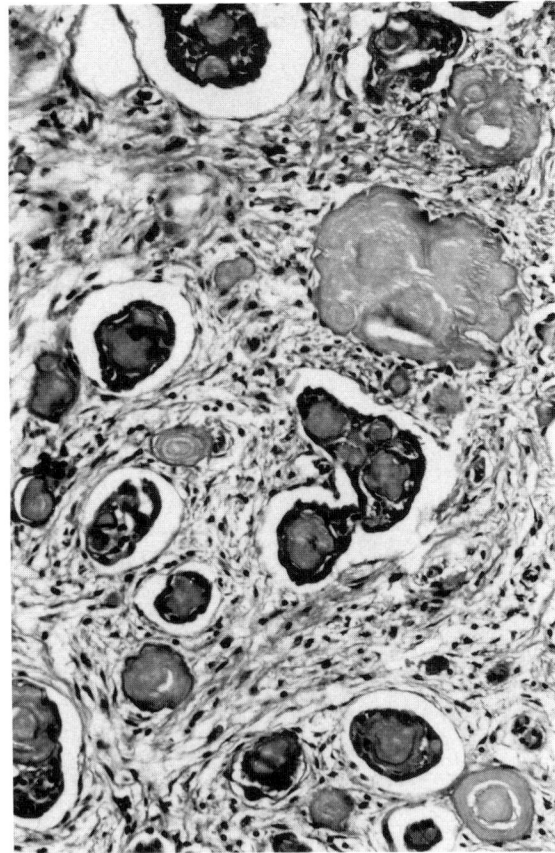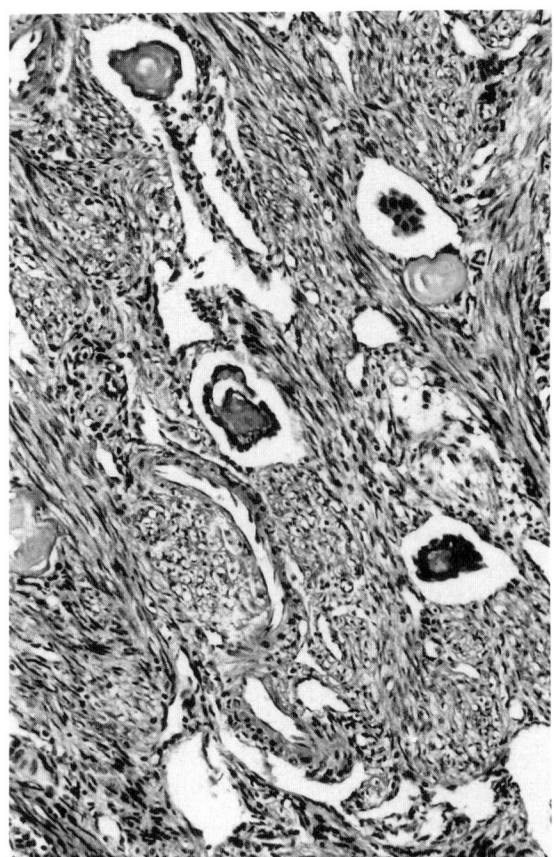

FIG. 17.45. Peritoneal psammocarcinoma. a: Numerous psammoma bodies, some of which are surrounded by a thin rim of neoplastic epithelial cells, lie within a demoplastic stroma. **b:** Tumor invades myometrial lymphatics. The patient was alive with no evidence of recurrent tumor 8 years after total abdominal hystrectomy and bilateral salpingo-oophorectomy. No adjuvant therapy was administered postoperatively.

toneal involvement and normal-sized ovaries that are free of disease or that have serosal involvement similar to that involving the extraovarian peritoneum.[30,43] The most common presenting features in patients with these tumors, who are typically under the age of 35 years (range, 16–67), are infertility and chronic pelvic or abdominal pain. Many cases, however, are discovered incidentally at laparotomy for other conditions. At operation, focal or diffuse miliary granules, fibrous adhesions, or both involve the pelvic peritoneum and omentum and, less commonly, the abdominal peritoneum. Microscopic examination reveals superficial tumor that resembles noninvasive epithelial or desmoplastic implants of borderline serous tumors of ovarian origin. Co-existent endosalpingiosis has been found in 85% of cases.[30,43] Similar tumors characterized by low-grade nuclear features, psammoma bodies in most of the tumor nests and, in contrast to borderline tumors, invasion of the underlying tissues and their lymphatics, have been referred to as *psammocarcinomas* (Fig. 17.45).[185,352] Both primary peritoneal serous borderline tumors and psammocarcinomas may persist or recur in a minority of cases, but they typically are indolent tumors associated with a highly favorable long-term prognosis.[30,43,185,352] Visible lesions should be resected as completely as possible, with preservation of the uterus and ovaries in young patients. Adjuvant treatment is not necessary.

Occasionally serous carcinomas with invasive properties and higher grade nuclear features than those associated with psammocarcinoma arise from the pelvic peritoneum, so-called serous surface papillary carcinomas or serous papillary carcinomas of the peritoneum.[*] In some cases, the ovaries also are involved by small surface "implants," but retain their normal size and shape. Some tumors have occurred in women who have had bilateral oophorectomy performed as prophylactic treatment for familial ovarian cancer.[541] The typical intraoperative appearance of a primary peritoneal serous carcinoma, with widespread peritoneal tumor associated with ovaries of normal size, may

---

[*]Refs. 8,16,121,160,172,195,229,263,284,314,366,424,428,461,541, 545,570,572.

mimic that of a diffuse malignant mesothelioma or perito-neal carcinomatosis associated with an unknown primary tumor. Primary peritoneal serous carcinomas resemble their ovarian counterparts on microscopic and immunohis-tochemical examination; their distinction from malignant mesothelioma has been previously discussed. These tu-mors have a prognosis similar to that of high-stage serous carcinomas of obvious ovarian origin.

Rare extraovarian serous tumors take the form of local-ized, typically cystic masses, usually within the broad liga-ment and, less commonly, within the retroperitoneum. Serous papillary cystadenomas and adenofibromas, serous borderline tumors, and serous carcinomas have been de-scribed in these sites.[14,15,515,548]

Peritoneal Mucinous Lesions

Benign glands of endocervical type involving the perito-neum, so-called endocervicosis, are rare, but examples in-volving the posterior uterine serosa, cul-de-sac, and the urinary bladder have been documented.[99,307] In the last site, the lesions formed tumor-like masses that involved the posterior wall or posterior dome of the bladder in women of reproductive age. On microscopic examination, benign endocervical-type glands were located predomi-nantly within the smooth muscle of the muscularis propria (Fig. 17.46).[99] In several cases, the infiltrative pattern of the glands, mild epithelial atypia, and a reactive periglan-dular stroma, alone or in combination, resulted in an initial misdiagnosis of well-differentiated adenocarcinoma.

Ovarian-type mucinous neoplasms, in the absence of a primary tumor within the ovary, have been described in extraovarian sites, typically in the retroperitoneum (Fig. 17.47)[21,144,307,398,405,578]; a single case has been described in the inguinal region.[522] These tumors form large cystic masses, which on histological examination resemble ova-rian mucinous cystadenomas, borderline tumors, or cyst-adenocarcinomas (Fig. 17.48); some contain ovarian-type stroma in their walls. Although it is possible that some of these tumors originate within a supernumerary ovary, the great rarity of the latter, the absence of follicles or their derivatives within the ovarian-like stroma, and the rare occurrence of similar tumors in men strongly support a peritoneal origin. Recently, it has been suggested that in some cases of pseudomyxoma peritonei associated with ovarian and appendiceal mucinous tumors, the peritoneal lesions may arise directly from the peritoneum as part of a multifocal neoplastic process.[486a]

Peritoneal Transitional, Squamous, and Clear Cell Lesions

Nests of transitional (urothelial) epithelium referred to as Walthard nests are commonly present on the pelvic perito-neum in women of all ages, typically involving the serosal

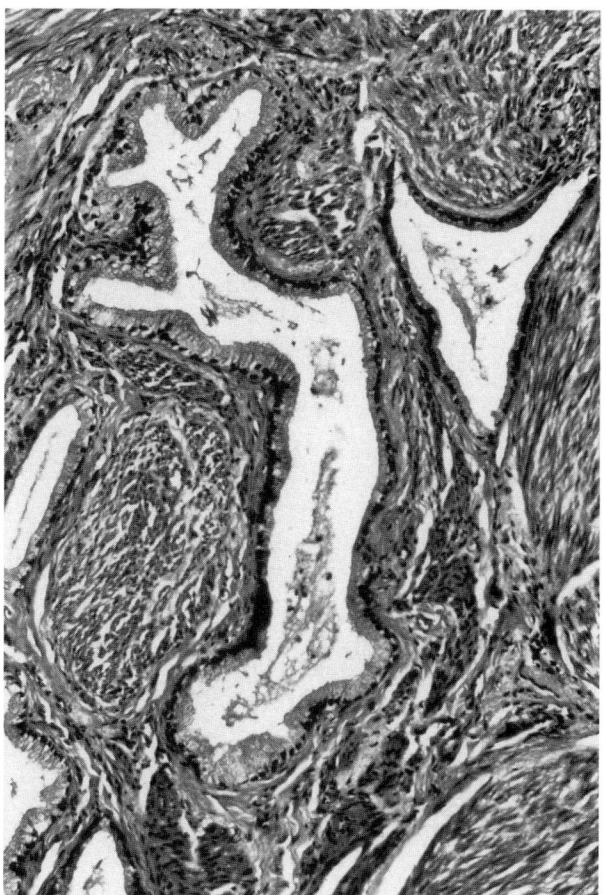

FIG. 17.46. **Endocervicosis of urinary bladder.** Benign en-docervical-type glands lie within the muscularis propria.

surfaces of the fallopian tubes (Figs. 17.49, 17.50), meso-salpinx, and mesovarium.[54,451,535] Walthard nests are un-common on the ovarian surface, but may be seen in the hilus, probably originating from the peritoneum of the mesovarium; they are most common on the tubal serosa

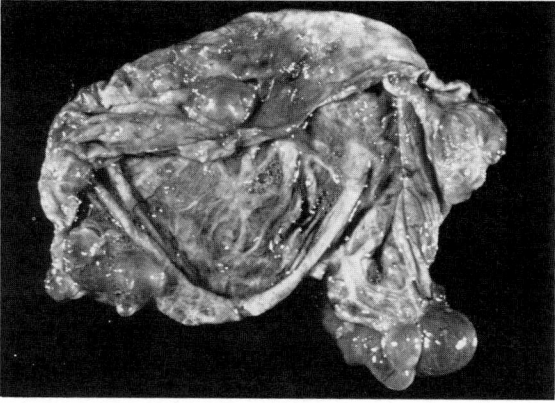

FIG. 17.47. **Retroperitoneal mucinous tumor.** The specimen has been opened to reveal multiple locules with mucinous con-tents. (Courtesy of Dr. R. E. Scully, Boston, MA.)

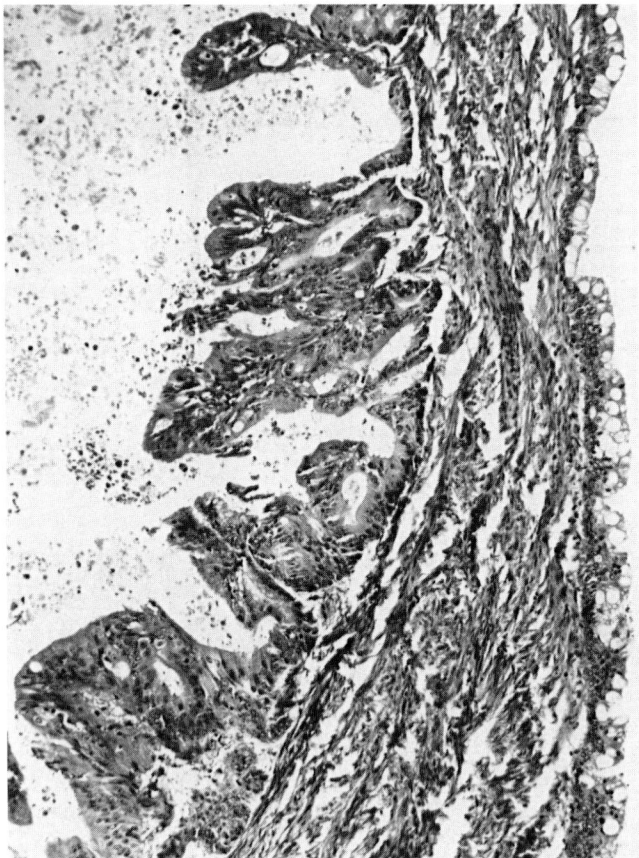

FIG. 17.48. Retroperitoneal mucinous cystadenocarcinoma. Cysts lined by papillary formations composed of atypical mucinous cells. (Reprinted by permission of The American College of Obstetricians and Gynecologists. Roth LM, Ehrlich CE (1977) Mucinous cystadenocarcinoma of the retroperitoneum. Obstet Gynecol 59:486–488.)

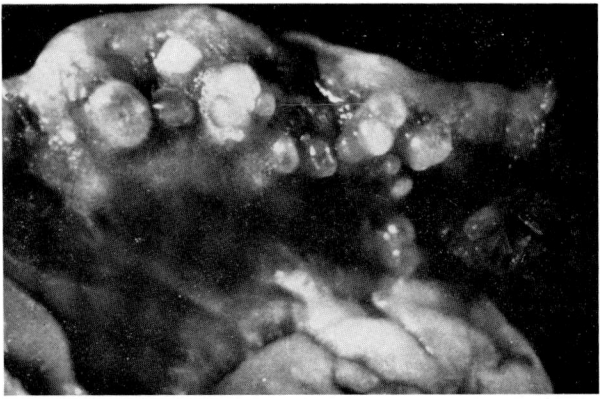

FIG. 17.49. Walthard nests. Multiple small cysts cover the serosa of fallopian tube and mesosalpinx. (From Teoh TB (1953) The structure and development of Walthard nests. J Pathol 66: 433–439. Copyright 1953 by John Wiley & Sons, Ltd. Reprinted by permission of John Wiley & Sons, Ltd.)

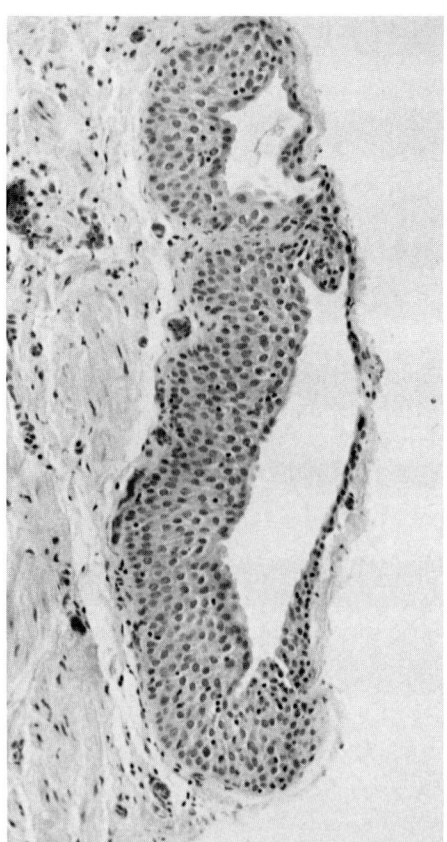

FIG. 17.50. Walthard nests on fallopian tube serosa. Nests with central cystic spaces are formed by benign transitional-type cells.

(see Chapter 14, Diseases of the Fallopian Tube). Rare extraovarian Brenner tumors have been encountered, most commonly in the broad ligament.[213] In contrast to Walthard nests, squamous metaplasia of the peritoneum is rare; one such case recently has been described.[468] Two clear cell carcinomas of apparent peritoneal origin recently have been reported. One was a localized mass within the sigmoid mesocolon[154] whereas the other diffusely involved the peritoneum[310]; no endometriosis was identified in either case.

Subperitoneal Mesenchymal Lesions

Ectopic Decidua

CLINICAL AND OPERATIVE FINDINGS

An ectopic decidual reaction similar to that seen in the lamina propria of the fallopian tube, cervix, and vagina also may be seen within the submesothelial stroma of the peritoneal cavity.* Frequent sites of ectopic decidua include

---

*Refs. 39,40,219,223,240,248,386,392,462,592.

the submesothelial stroma of the fallopian tubes, uterus and uterine ligaments, appendix and omentum, and within pelvic adhesions. Rare sites have included the serosal surfaces of the diaphragm, liver, and spleen,[219,392] and the renal pelvis.[40]

Submesothelial decidua typically is an incidental microscopic finding, but florid lesions may be visible at the time of cesarean section or postpartum tubal ligation as multiple, gray to white, focally hemorrhagic nodules or plaques studding the peritoneal surfaces and simulating a malignant tumor.[392] Several cases have been associated with massive, occasionally fatal, intraperitoneal hemorrhage during the third trimester, labor, or the puerperium.[240,462] Other rare clinical presentations include abdominal pain, which may simulate that of appendicitis, and hydronephrosis and hematuria secondary to renal pelvic involvement.[40,240]

MICROSCOPIC FINDINGS

Microscopic examination discloses submesothelial decidual cells disposed individually or arranged in nodules or plaques (Fig. 17.51). Smooth muscle cells, probably derived from submesothelial myofibroblasts,[223] may be admixed. The decidual foci typically are vascular and contain a sprinkling of lymphocytes. Focal hemorrhagic necrosis and varying degrees of nuclear pleomorphism and hyperchromasia of the decidual cells may suggest a tumor such as a malignant mesothelioma,[527] but their bland appearance and mitotic inactivity militate against such a diagnosis. We have seen several cases of an omental decidual reaction in which most of the decidual cells exhibited striking vacuolization with basophilic mucin and an eccentric location of the nucleus. The appearance of the cells raised the possi-

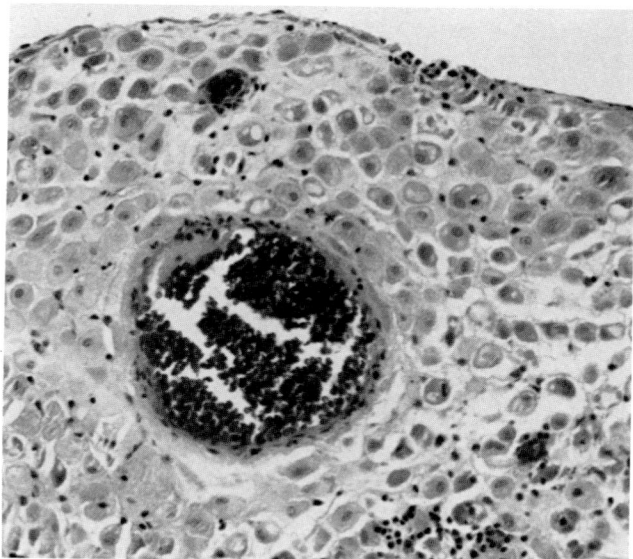

FIG. 17.51. Ectopic decidua beneath pelvic peritoneum. Note marked vascularity.

bility of metastatic signet-ring cell carcinoma, but in contrast to the cells of the latter, the vacuoles within the decidual cells contain acid, rather than neutral, mucin, and their cytoplasm would lack immunoreactivity for cytokeratin.

Leiomyomatosis

Disseminated peritoneal leiomyomatosis is a rare disorder characterized by the presence of multiple submesothelial nodules of cytologically benign smooth muscle, frequently associated with uterine leiomyomas and rarely ovarian leiomyomas.° The nodules generally are considered to arise from multipotential submesothelial mesenchymal cells. This disorder is discussed elsewhere (see Chapter 13, Mesenchymal Tumors of the Uterus).

Retroperitoneal Lymph Node Lesions
Benign Glands of Müllerian Type

CLINICAL FEATURES

Benign glands of müllerian type are most commonly encountered within pelvic and para-aortic lymph nodes of women,† and less often in inguinal and femoral lymph nodes.[471,500] Because these glands are almost always incidental microscopic findings in lymph nodes removed in cases of pelvic carcinoma, their reported frequency, which has varied from 2% to 41%, depends on the number of lymph nodes removed and the extent of the histological sampling. Almost all of the patients have been adults, although rare examples have been reported in children.[493] In men, the presence of similar glands have been recorded rarely within lymph nodes in the pelvis and abdomen[241,531] and mediastinum.[325] Although typically without clinical or intraoperative manifestations, rare examples of lymph nodes containing müllerian-type glands have been associated with a false-positive lymphangiogram,[473] ureteral obstruction secondary to lymph node enlargement,[566] or visible enlargement at the time of operation.[275]

In a number of patients, intranodal glandular inclusions have been accompanied by endosalpingiosis of the peritoneum,[83,493] salpingitis isthmica nodosa, or acute and chronic salpingitis.[275,283,493] Other patients have had coexistent ovarian serous tumors, which have been benign, borderline tumors, or carcinomas.[149,473]

PATHOLOGICAL FINDINGS

On gross examination, the glands usually are not apparent, although rarely they are recognizable as cysts measuring up to a few millimeters in diameter.[158,566] The glands typically

---

°Refs. 223,234,265,293,399,411,530,549.
†Refs. 83,149,267,283,456,474,493.

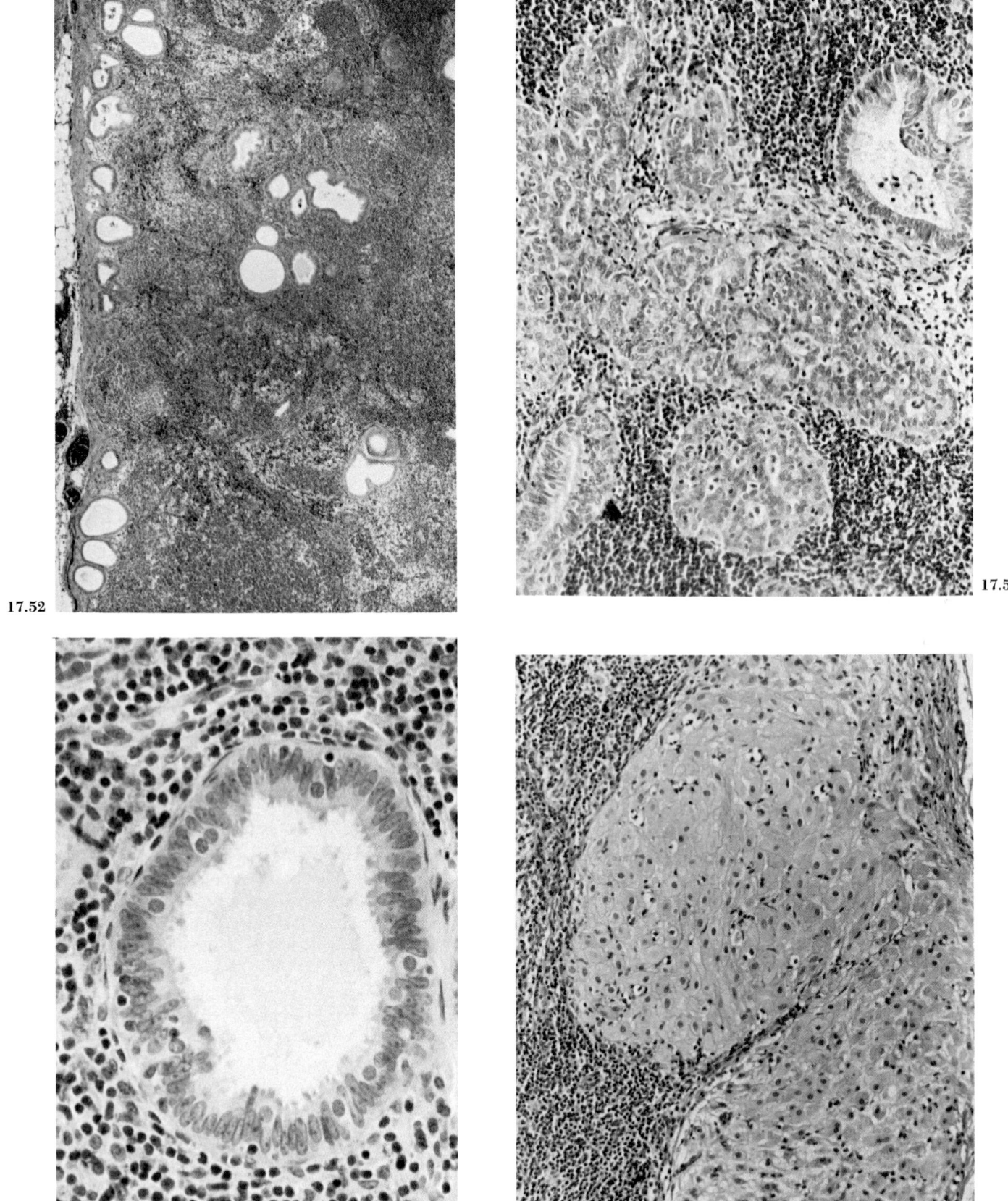

17.52

17.53

17.54

17.55

are located in the periphery of the node, most commonly within its capsule or between the lymphoid follicles in the superficial cortex (Fig. 17.52); rarely they lie free within the subcapsular sinuses.[283] In florid cases, they can be distributed diffusely throughout the lymph node.[275,283] Intraglandular or periglandular psammoma bodies commonly are present. Intranodal glands may be surrounded by a thin rim of fibrous tissue or abut directly on the surrounding lymphoid cells.

The glands may be round and cystically dilated or exhibit an irregular contour because of infolding. They are lined most commonly by a single layer of cuboidal to columnar tubal-type epithelium, with an admixture of ciliated, secretory, and intercalated cell types (Fig. 17.53). With special stains, mucin can be demonstrated in the apical portion of the secretory cells and within the gland spaces.[267,275] Acute and chronic inflammatory cells may be present within the lumina. The cells have a benign appearance with regular, basally oriented or pseudostratified, oval to round nuclei, fine nuclear chromatin, and occasional small nucleoli; mitotic figures typically are absent. In rare cases, the cells can exhibit varying degrees of atypia and stratification; the latter can produce an intraglandular cribriform pattern or luminal obliteration by sheets of cells (Fig. 17.54).[83,149,275]

Examples of intranodal glandular inclusions lined by benign endometrioid epithelium,[307,456] mucinous epithelium of endocervical[20,158,456] or goblet-cell type,[531] or metaplastic squamous epithelium[365,471] have been reported. Rarely endometriotic stroma is present around the glands, warranting a diagnosis of endometriosis.

Differential Diagnosis

In most cases the distinction between glandular inclusions and metastatic adenocarcinoma is not difficult unless a primary ovarian serous tumor of low malignant potential is present, in which case the distinction may be difficult or impossible. Features favoring a benign diagnosis include a capsular or interfollicular location of the glands, lining cells of multiple types including ciliated forms, a lack of significant cellular atypia and mitotic activity, periglandular base-

---

FIG. 17.52. **Endosalpingiotic glands within pelvic lymph node.** The glands are located within and immediately beneath the node capsule as well as deeper within the node.

FIG. 17.53. **Endosalpingiotic gland within pelvic lymph node.** The gland is lined by benign cells of multiple types, including ciliated cells.

FIG. 17.54. **Atypical endosalpingiotic glands within pelvic lymph node.** Some of the glands exhibit luminal obliteration by cells growing in solid and cribriform patterns. (Reprinted by permission of Chen, ref. 83.)

FIG. 17.55. **Ectopic decidua within pelvic lymph node.** The nodal architecture is focally replaced by sheets of decidualized cells. (Reprinted by permission of Mills, ref. 365.)

ment membranes, and an absence of a desmoplastic stromal reaction. Complicating the differential diagnosis is the very rare development of borderline or frankly malignant change in müllerian glandular inclusions in lymph nodes.[149,292] Similarly, intranodal nests of benign squamous epithelium should not be mistaken for metastatic squamous cell carcinoma.[365] Features favoring a benign diagnosis include bland cytological features, mitotic inactivity, and in some cases, an origin within benign glands.

Ectopic Decidua

Ectopic decidua, unassociated with endometriosis, has been described as a rare, incidental microscopic finding in para-aortic and pelvic lymph nodes, usually removed as part of a radical hysterectomy for carcinoma of the cervix in pregnant patients.[13,63,104,112,365,585,592] A subserosal ectopic decidual reaction may be present elsewhere in the pelvis.[112] In some cases, the decidual tissue has been recognized on careful gross examination as tiny, gray, subcapsular nodules.[112] On microscopic examination, the decidual nests typically occupy the subcapsular sinus and superficial cortex (Fig. 17.55), although more central parts of the lymph node also may be involved. The cells appear benign, but may contain occasional bizarre, hyperchromatic nuclei, mimicking metastatic squamous cell carcinoma.[112] The absence of mitotic activity, keratinization, and stromal desmoplasia should facilitate the diagnosis. Metastatic squamous cell carcinoma, however, may be present in the same node.[104]

Leiomyomatosis

Rare cases of lymph node involvement by mitotically inactive, cytologically benign smooth muscle have been described (Fig. 17.56).[2,50,116,234,237,346a,440] Most patients have had concurrent typical uterine leiomyomas or, less commonly, disseminated peritoneal leiomyomatosis,[237] or similar nodules within the lungs.[50,116] In pregnant patients, the process may merge with intranodal decidua.[237] The possible histogenesis of the lesion includes an origin from entrapped subcoelomic mesenchyme,[440] myofibroblastic organization of intranodal decidua,[237] and lymphatic spread from uterine leiomyomas.[2,50] The presence of benign-appearing smooth muscle in a lymph node also should bring into consideration the diagnosis of lymphangioleiomyomatosis.[41] There is usually, but not invariably, an association with pulmonary involvement. Benign intranodal smooth muscle also should be distinguished from metastatic well-differentiated leiomyosarcoma of uterine origin. Patients with the latter usually have a large uterine mass and on histological examination the intranodal tumor is cellular and exhibits evidence of cellular atypicality and mitotic activity.

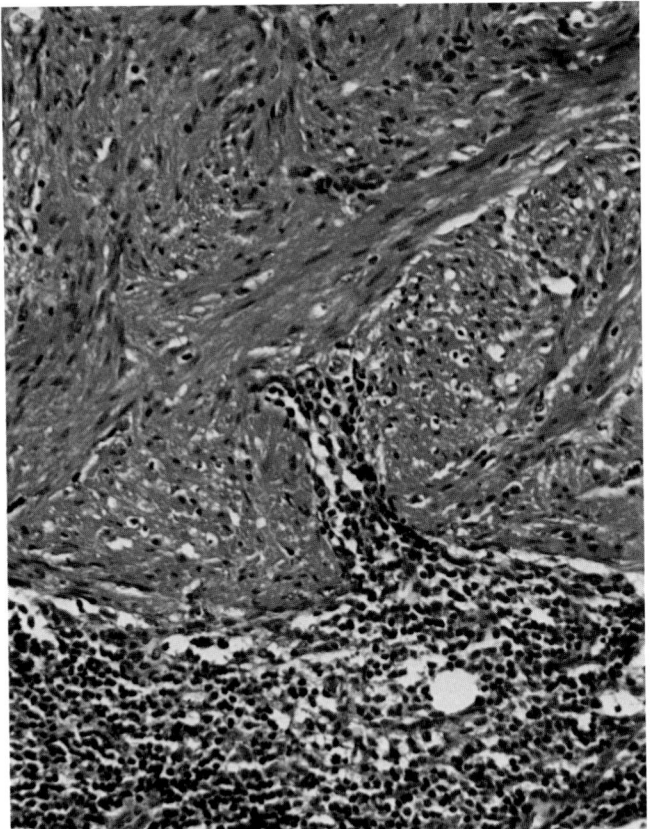

FIG. 17.56. **Benign smooth muscle within pelvic lymph node.** (Reprinted by permission of Abell and Littler, ref. 2.)

References

1. Abdel-Shahid RB, Beresford JM, Curry RH (1974) Endometriosis of the ureter with vascular involvement. Obstet Gynecol 43: 113–117
2. Abell MR, Littler ER (1975) Benign metastasizing uterine leiomyoma. Multiple lymph nodal metastases. Cancer 36: 2206–2213
3. Abeshouse BS, Abeshouse G (1960) Endometriosis of the urinary tract: A review of the literature and a report of four cases of vesical endometriosis. J Int Coll Surg 34: 43–63
4. Adams HW, Mainz DL (1977) Eosinophilic ascites. A case report and review of the literature. Digest Dis 22: 40–42
5. Afonso JF, Martin GM, Nisco FS, et al (1962) Melanogenic ovarian tumors. Am J Obstet Gynecol 84: 667–676
6. Ahn GH, Scully RE (1991) Clear cell carcinoma of the inguinal region arising from endometriosis. Cancer 67: 116–120
7. Albukerk JN, Berlin M, Palladino VC, et al (1979) Endometriosis in peritoneal gliomatosis. (Letter) Arch Pathol Lab Med 103: 98–99
8. Altaras MM, Aviram R, Cohen I, et al (1991) Primary peritoneal papillary serous adenocarcinoma: Clinical and management aspects. Gynecol Oncol 40: 230–236
9. Anderson M, Edmond RM (1974) Rupture of an endometriotic cyst in late pregnancy. Br J Obstet Gynaecol 81: 907–908
10. Antman KH, Klegar KL, Pomfret EA, et al (1985) Early peritoneal mesothelioma: A treatable malignancy. Lancet 2: 977–981
11. Aoki M (1967) Endometriosis of the pelvic lymph nodes. Acta Pathol Jpn 17: 217–234
12. Asensio JA, Goldblatt P, Thomford NR (1990) Primary malignant peritoneal mesothelioma. A report of seven cases and a review of the literature. Arch Surg 125: 1477–1481
13. Ashraf M, Boyd CB, Beresford WA (1984) Ectopic decidual reaction in para-aortic and pelvic lymph nodes in the presence of cervical squamous cell carcinoma during pregnancy. J Surg Oncol 26: 6–8
14. Aslani M, Scully RE (1989) Primary carcinoma of the broad ligament. Report of four cases and review of the literature. Cancer 64: 1540–1545
15. Aslani M, Ahn G, Scully RE (1988) Serous papillary cystadenoma of borderline malignancy of broad ligament. Int J Gynecol Pathol 7: 131–138
16. August CZ, Murad TM, Newton M (1985) Multiple focal extraovarian serous carcinoma. Int J Gynecol Pathol 4: 11–23
17. Austin MB, Frierson HF Jr, Fechner RE, Callicot JH Jr (1988) Endometrioma of the lung presenting as hemoptysis and a large pulmonary mass. Surg Pathol 1: 165–169
18. Ayres JG, Crocker JG, Skilbeck NQ (1988) Differentiation of malignant from normal and reactive mesothelial cells by the argyrophil technique for nucleolar organiser region associated proteins. Thorax 43: 366–370
19. Azumi N, Underhill CB, Kagan E, Sheibani K (1992) A novel biotinylated probe specific for hyaluronate: Its diagnostic value in diffuse malignant mesothelioma. Am J Surg Pathol 16: 116–121
20. Baird DB, Reddick RL (1991) Extraovarian mucinous metaplasia in a patient with bilateral mucinous borderline ovarian tumors: A case report. Int J Gynecol Pathol 10: 96–103
21. Banerjee R, Gough J (1988) Cystic mucinous tumours of the mesentery and retroperitoneum: Report of three cases. Histopathology 12: 527–532
22. Barbieri RL (1990) Etiology and epidemiology of endometriosis. Am J Obstet Gynecol 162: 565–567
23. Barbieri RL, Niloff JM, Bast RC Jr, et al (1986) Elevated serum concentrations of CA-125 in patients with advanced endometriosis. Fertil Steril 45: 630–634
24. Bard ES, Bard DS, Vargas-Cortes F (1978) Extrauterine mullerian adenosarcoma: A clinicopathologic report of a case with distant metastases and review of the literature. Gynecol Oncol 6: 261–274
25. Bassler R, Theele CH, Labach H (1982) Nodular and tumor-like gliomatosis peritonei with endometriosis caused by a mature ovarian teratoma. Path Res Pract 175: 392–403
26. Bastani B, Shariatzadeh MR, Dehdashti F (1985) Tuberculous peritonitis. Report of 30 cases and review of the literature. Q J Med 56: 549–557
27. Bayer AS, Blumenkrantz MJ, Montgomerie JZ, et al (1976) Candida peritonitis. Report of 22 cases and review of the English literature. Am J Med 61: 832–840
28. Bazaz-Malik G, Saraf V, Rana BS (1980) Endometrioma of the kidney: Case report. J Urol 123: 422–423
29. Beckman EN, Leonard GL, Pintado SO, Sternberg WH

(1985) Endometriosis of the prostate. Am J Surg Pathol 9: 374–379

30. Bell DA, Scully RE (1990) Serous borderline tumors of the peritoneum. Am J Surg Pathol 14: 230–239

31. Benz EJ, Dockerty MB, Dixon CF (1952) Polypoid endometrioma of colon: Report of a case in which unusual pathologic features were present. Proc Mayo Clin 27: 201–208

32. Bergen S, Owen J, Snider WR, Lim YC (1981) Disseminated adenomyomas of the abdominal and pelvic cavities. Am Surg 47: 232–235

33. Bergholz M, Altmannsberger M, Schauer A (1981) Benign mesothelioma of the cul-de-sac. A tumor with misleading histologic pattern in an unusual location. Gynecol Oncol 11: 393–395

34. Bergqvist A, Carlstrom K, Jeppsson S, Ljungberg O (1984) Histochemical localization of specific estrogen and progesterone binding in human endometrium and endometriotic tissue. A preliminary report. Acta Obstet Gynecol Scand 123(suppl): 15–18

35. Bergqvist A, Jeppsson S, Ljungberg O (1985) Histochemical demonstration of estrogen and progesterone binding in endometriotic tissue and in uterine endometrium. J Histochem Cytochem 33: 155–161

36. Bergqvist A, Ljungberg O, Myhre E (1984) Human endometrium and endometriotic tissue obtained simultaneously: A comparative histological study. Int J Gynecol Pathol 3: 135–145

37. Bergqvist A, Rannevik G, Thorell J (1981) Estrogen and progesterone cytosol receptor concentration in endometriotic tissue and intrauterine endometrium. Acta Obstet Gynecol Scand 101(suppl): 53–58

38. Berry PJ, Favara BE, Odom LF (1986) Malignant peritoneal mesothelioma in a child. Pediatr Pathol 5: 397–409

39. Bersch W, Alexy E, Heuser HP, Staemmler HJ (1973) Ectopic decidua formation in the ovary. Virch Arch A Path 360: 173–177

40. Bettinger HF (1947) Ectopic decidua in renal pelvis. J Pathol Bact 5: 686–687

41. Bhattacharyya AK, Balogh K (1985) Retroperitoneal lymphangioleiomyomatosis. A 36-year benign course in a postmenopausal woman. Cancer 56: 1144–1146

42. Binns BA, Banerjee R (1983) Endometriosis with Turner's syndrome treated with cyclic oestrogen/progesterone. Case report. Br J Obstet Gynaecol 90: 581–582

43. Biscotti CV, Hart WR (1992) Peritoneal serous micropapillomatosis of low malignant potential (serous borderline tumors of the peritoneum). A clinicopathologic study of 17 cases. Am J Surg Pathol 16: 467–475

44. Bisset DL, Morris JA, Fox H (1988) Giant cystic adenomatoid tumor (mesothelioma) of the uterus. Histopathol 12: 555–558

45. Blobel GA, Moll R, Franke WW, et al (1985) The intermediate filament cytoskeleton of mesotheliomas and its diagnostic significance. Am J Pathol 121: 235–247

46. Blumberg H, Srinivasan K, Parnes IH (1966) Peritoneal schistosomiasis simulating carcinoma. NY State J Med 66: 758–761

47. Blumberg NA, Murrary JF (1981) Multicystic peritoneal mesothelioma. S Afr Med J 59: 85–86

48. Blumenkrantz MJ, Gallagher N, Bashore RA, Tenckhoff H (1981) Retrograde menstruation in women undergoing chronic peritoneal dialysis. Obstet Gynecol 57: 667–670

49. Bollinger DJ, Wick MR, Dehner LP, et al (1989) Peritoneal malignant mesothelioma versus serous papillary adenocarcinoma. A histochemical and immunohistochemical comparison. Am J Surg Pathol 13: 659–670

50. Boyce CR, Buddhdev HN (1973) Pregnancy complicated by metastasizing leiomyoma of the uterus. Obstet Gynecol 42: 252–258

51. Bradley JA, McWhinnie DL, Hamilton DNH (1983) Sclerosing obstructive peritonitis after continuous ambulatory peritoneal dialysis. Lancet 2: 113–114

52. Branscomb L (1960) Habitual premenstrual spotting following electrocauterization of the cervix: A newly observed phenomenon. Am J Obstet Gynecol 79: 16–23

53. Bransilver BR, Ferenczy A, Richart RM (1973) Female genital tract remnants. An ultrastructural comparison of hydatid of Morgagni and mesonephric ducts and tubules. Arch Pathol Lab Med 96: 255–261

54. Bransilver BR, Ferenczy A, Richart RM (1974) Brenner tumors and Walthard cell nests. Arch Pathol Lab Med 98: 76–86

55. Brenner J, Sordillo PP, Magill GB (1981) Seventeen year survival in a patient with malignant peritoneal mesothelioma. Clin Oncol 7: 249–251

56. Brooks JJ, Wheeler JE (1977) Malignancy arising in extragonadal endometriosis. A case report and summary of the world literature. Cancer 40: 3065–3073

57. Bryce RL, Barbatis C, Charnock M (1982) Endosalpingiosis in pregnancy. Case report. Br J Obstet Gynaecol 89: 166–168

58. Buckley CH (1990) Tamoxifen and endometriosis. Case report. Br J Obstet Gynaecol 97: 645–646

59. Buhac I, Jarmolych J (1978) Histology of the intestinal peritoneum in patients with cirrhosis of the liver and ascites. Digest Dis 23: 417–422

60. Bullock JL, Massey FM, Gambrell RD (1974) Symptomatic endometriosis in teen-agers. A reappraisal. Obstet Gynecol 43: 896–900

61. Bur ME, Greene GL, Press MF (1987) Estrogen receptor localization in formalin-fixed, paraffin-embedded endometrium and endometriotic tissues. Int J Gynecol Pathol 6: 140–151

62. Burmeister RE, Fechner RE, Franklin RR (1969) Endosalpingiosis of the peritoneum. Obstet Gynecol 34: 310–318

63. Burnett RA, Millan D (1986) Decidual change in pelvic lymph nodes: A source of possible diagnostic error. Histopathology 1089–1092

64. Burrig K, Pfitzer P, Hort W (1990) Well-differentiated papillary mesothelioma of the peritoneum: A borderline mesothelioma. Virch Arch Pathol Anat 417: 443–447

65. Cajigas A, Axiotis CA (1990) Endosalpingiosis of the vermiform appendix. Int J Gynecol Pathol 9: 291–295

66. Cambria RP, Shamberger RC (1984) Small bowel obstruction caused by the abdominal cocoon syndrome: Possible association with the LeVeen shunt. Surgery 95: 501–503

67. Campbell JS, Lou P, Ferguson JP, et al (1973) Pseudomyxoma peritonei et ovarii with occult neoplasms of appendix. Obstet Gynecol 42: 897–902

68. Candiani GB, Vercellini P, Fedele L, et al (1991) Inguinal

endometriosis: Pathogenetic and clinical implications. Obstet Gynecol 78: 191–194

69. Candiani GB, Vercellini P, Fedele L, et al (1991) Mild endometriosis and infertility: A critical review of epidemiologic data, diagnostic pitfalls, and classification limits. Obstet Gynecol Surv 46: 374–381

70. Cantor JO, Fenoglio CM, Richart RM (1979) A case of extensive abdominal endometriosis. Am J Obstet Gynecol 134: 846–847

71. Carpenter HA, Lancaster JR, Lee RA (1982) Multilocular cysts of the peritoneum. Mayo Clin Proc 57: 634–638

71a. Carr NJ, Turk EP (1992) The histological features of splenosis. Histopathology 21: 549–553

72. Cartwright PS (1991) Peritoneal trophoblastic implants after surgical management of tubal pregnancy. J Reprod Med 36: 523–524

73. Castelli MJ, Armin A, Husain A, et al (1985) Fibrosing peritonitis in a drug abuser. Arch Pathol Lab Med 109: 767–769

74. Chalas E, Chumas J, Barbieri R, Mann WJ (1991) Nucleolar organizer regions in endometriosis, atypical endometriosis, and clear cell and endometrioid carcinomas. Gynecol Oncol 40: 26–263

75. Chalmers JA (1961) Mulleroma—a rare cause of dysmenorrhoea. Br J Obstet Gynaecol 68: 762–764

76. Chatman DL (1976) Endometriosis and the black woman. J Reprod Med 16: 303–306

77. Chatman DL, Ward AB (1982) Endometriosis in adolescents. J Reprod Med 27: 156–160

78. Chatman DL, Zbella EA (1986) Pelvic peritoneal defects and endometriosis: Further observations. Fertil Steril 46: 711–714

79. Chatman DL, Zbella EA (1987) Biopsy in laparoscopically diagnosed endometriosis. J Reprod Med 32: 855–857

80. Chatterjee SK (1980) Scar endometriosis: A clinicopathologic study of 17 cases. Obstet Gynecol 56: 81–84

81. Cheesman KL, Cheesman SD, Chatterton RT Jr, Cohen MR (1983) Alterations in progesterone metabolism and luteal function in infertile women with endometriosis. Fertil Steril 40: 590–595

82. Chejfec G, Rieker WJ, Jablokow VR, et al (1986) Pseudomyxoma peritonei associated with colloid carcinoma of the pancreas. Gastroenterology 90: 202–205

83. Chen KTK (1981) Benign glandular inclusions of the peritoneum and periaortic lymph nodes. Diagn Gynecol Obstet 3: 265–268

84. Chen KTK (1991) Malignant mesothelioma presenting as Sister Joseph's nodule. Am J Dermatopathol 13: 300–303

85. Chen KTK, Kostich ND, Rosai J (1978) Peritoneal foreign body granulomas to keratin in uterine adenocarcinoma. Arch Pathol Lab Med 102: 174–177

86. Chervenak FA, Greenlee RM, Lewenstein L, Tovell HMM (1981) Massive ascites associated with endometriosis. Obstet Gynecol 57: 379–381

87. Cheung NYA, Khoo US, Chan KW (1992) Intra-abdominal desmoplastic small round-cell tumour. Histopathology 20: 531–534

88. Chihal HJ, Mathur S, Holtz GL, Williamson HO (1986) An endometrial antibody assay in the clinical diagnosis and management of endometriosis. Fertil Steril 46: 408–411

89. Chumas JC, Thanning L, Mann WJ (1986) Malignant mixed mullerian tumor arising in extragenital endometriosis: Report of a case and review of the literature. Gynecol Oncol 23: 227–233

90. Churg A (1985) Immunohistochemical staining for vimentin and keratin in malignant mesothelioma. Am J Surg Pathol 9: 360–365

91. Cibas ES, Corson JM, Pinkus GS (1987) The distinction of adenocarcinoma from malignant mesothelioma in cell blocks of effusions. Hum Pathol 18: 67–74

92. Cioltei A, Tasca L, Titiriga L, Maakaron G, Calciu V (1979) Nodular salpingitis and tubal endometriosis. I. Comparative clinical study. Acta Eur Fertil 10: 135–141

93. Clark JE, Wood H, Jaffurs WJ, et al (1979) Endometrioid-type cystadenocarcinoma arising in the mesosalpinx. Obstet Gynecol 54: 656–658

94. Clarke TJ, Simpson RHW (1990) Necrotizing granulomas of peritoneum following diathermy ablation of endometriosis. Histopathology 16: 400–402

95. Clausen I, Nielsen KT (1987) Endometriosis in the groin. Int J Gynaecol Obstet 25: 469–471

96. Clement PB (1990) Pathology of endometriosis. Pathol Annu 25(1): 245–295

97. Clement PB, Scully RE (1978) Extrauterine mesodermal (mullerian) adenosarcoma. A clinicopathologic analysis of five cases. Am J Clin Pathol 69: 276–283

98. Clement PB, Scully RE (1992) Endometrial stroma sarcomas of the uterus with extensive endometrioid glandular differentiation. A report of three cases that caused problems in differential diagnosis. Int J Gynecol Pathol 11: 163–173

99. Clement PB, Young RH (1992) Endocervicosis of the urinary bladder: A report of six cases of a benign mullerian lesion that may mimic adenocarcinoma. Am J Surg Pathol 16: 533–542

100. Clement PB, Young RH (1993) Florid mesothelial hyperplasia associated with ovarian tumors: A possible source of error in tumor diagnosis and staging. Int J Gynecol Pathol 12: 51–58

101. Clement PB, Young RH, Scully RE (1988) Necrotic pseudoxanthomatous nodules of the ovary and peritoneum in endometriosis. Am J Surg Pathol 12: 390–397

102. Clement PB, Young RH, Scully RE (1989) Liesegang rings in endometriosis. A report of three cases. Int J Gynecol Pathol 8: 271–276

103. Clement PB, Young RH, Scully RE (1990) Stromal endometriosis of the uterine cervix. A variant of endometriosis that may simulate a sarcoma. Am J Surg Pathol 14: 449–455

103a. Clement PB, Young RH, Hanna W, Scully RE (1994) Sclerosing peritonitis associated with lutenized thecomas of the ovary. Am J Surg Pathol 18:1–13

104. Cobb CJ (1988) Ectopic decidua and metastatic squamous carcinoma: Presentation in a single pelvic lymph node. J Surg Oncol 38: 126–129

105. Coder DM, Olander GA (1972) Granulomatous peritonitis caused by starch glove powder. Arch Surg 105: 83–86

106. Concato L (1881) Sulla poliomenorrhea scrofolosa o tisi delle sierose. Gior Intern Sc Med 3: 1037–1053

107. Cooper P (1978) Mixed mesodermal tumour and clear cell

carcinoma arising in ovarian endometriosis. Cancer 42: 2827–2831

108. Copeland LJ, Silva EG, Gershenson DM, et al (1988) The significance of mullerian inclusions found at second-look laparotomy in patients with epithelial ovarian neoplasms. Obstet Gynecol 71: 763–770

109. Cornillie FJ, Brosens A, Vasquez G, Riphagen I (1986) Histologic and ultrastructural changes in human endometriotic implants treated with the antiprogesterone steroid ethylnorgestrienone (gestrinone) during 2 months. Int J Gynecol Pathol 5: 95–109

110. Cornillie FJ, Oosterlynck D, Lauweryns JM, Koninckx PR (1990) Deeply infiltrating pelvic endometriosis: Histology and clinical significance. Fertil Steril 53: 978–983

111. Cornillie FJ, Puttemans P, Brosens IA (1987) Histology and ultrastructure of human endometriotic tissues treated with dydrogesterone (duphaston). Eur J Obstet Reprod Biol 26: 39–55

112. Covell LM, Disciullo AJ, Knapp RC (1977) Decidual change in pelvic lymph nodes in the presence of cervical squamous cell carcinoma during pregnancy. Am J Obstet Gynecol 127: 674–676

113. Cozzutto C (1981) Uterus-like mass replacing ovary. Report of a new entity. Arch Pathol Lab Med 105: 508–511

114. Craig JR, Hart WR (1979) Extragenital adenomatoid tumor. Evidence for the mesothelial theory of origin. Cancer 433: 1678–1679

115. Cramer DW, Wilson E, Stillman RJ, et al (1986) The relation of endometriosis to menstrual characteristics, smoking, and exercise. JAMA 255: 1904–1908

116. Cramer SF, Meyer JS, Kraner JF, et al (1980) Metastasizing leiomyoma of the uterus. S-phase fraction, estrogen receptor, and ultrastructure. Cancer 45: 932–937

117. Czernobilsky B, Morris WJ (1979) A histologic study of ovarian endometriosis with emphasis on hyperplastic and atypical changes. Obstet Gynecol 53: 318–323

118. Czernobilsky B, Silverstein A (1978) Salpingitis and ovarian endometriosis. Fertil Steril 30: 45–49

119. d'Anglejan G, Goutallier, de Lara AC, Ryckewaert A (1970) Radiculalgie par endometriose pelvienne avec lesions osseuses. Rev Rhuma 37: 251–253

120. Dallenbach-Hellweg G (1987) Atypical endosalpingiosis: A case report with consideration of the differential diagnosis of glandular subperitoneal inclusions. Path Res Pract 182: 180–182

121. Dalrymple JC, Bannatyne P, Russell P, et al (1989) Extraovarian peritoneal serous papillary carcinoma. A clinicopathologic study of 31 cases. Cancer 64: 110–115

122. Dalrymple JC, Hunter JC, Ferrier A, et al (1986) Disseminated intraperitoneal oxyuris granulomas. Aust NZ J Obstet Gynaecol 26: 90–91

123. Daum F, Boley SJ, Cohen MI (1974) Miliary Crohn's disease. Gastroenterology 67: 527–530

124. David MP, Ben-Zwi D, Langer L (1981) Tubal intramural polyps and their relationship to infertility. Fertil Steril 35: 526–531

125. Davies JD, Ansell ID (1983) Food-starch granulomatous peritonitis. J Clin Pathol 36: 435–438

126. Dawood MY, Khan-Dawood FS, Ramos J (1988) Plasma and peritoneal fluid levels of CA 125 in women with endometriosis. Am J Obstet Gynecol 159: 1526–1531

127. Day DL, Sane S, Dehner LP (1986) Inflammatory pseudotumor of the mesentery and small intestine. Pediatr Radiol 16: 210–215

128. Daya D, McCaughey WTE (1990) Well-differentiated papillary mesothelioma of the peritoneum. A clinicopathologic study of 22 cases. Cancer 65: 292–296

129. Daya D, McCaughey WTE (1991) Pathology of the peritoneum: A review of selected topics. Semin Diagn Pathol 8: 277–289

130. De Brux J (1975) The contribution of pathological anatomy to the diagnosis and prognosis of different forms of tubal sterility. Acta Eur Fertil 6: 185–195

131. Dehn TCB, Lucas MG, Wood RFM (1985) Idiopathic sclerosing peritonitis. Postgrad Med J 61: 841–842

132. Demopoulos RI, Kahn MA, Feiner HD (1986) Epidemiology of cystic mesotheliomas. Int J Gynecol Pathol 5: 379–381

133. DeStephano DB, Wesley JR, Heidelberger KP, Hutchison RJ, Blane CE, Coran AG (1985) Primitive cystic hepatic neoplasm of infancy with mesothelial differentiation: Report of a case. Pediatr Pathol 4: 291–302

134. Devereux WP (1963) Endometriosis: Long-term observation, with particular reference to incidence in pregnancy. Obstet Gynecol 22: 444–450

135. Dizerega GS, Barber DL, Hodgen GD (1980) Endometriosis: Role of ovarian steroids in initiation, maintenance, and suppression. Fertil Steril 33: 649–653

136. Dmowski WP (1984) Pitfalls in clinical, laparoscopic and histologic diagnosis of endometriosis. Acta Obstet Gynecol Scand 123(suppl): 61–66

137. Dmowski WP, Radwanska E (1984) Current concepts on pathology, histogenesis and etiology of endometriosis. Acta Obstet Gynecol Scand 123(suppl): 29–33

138. Dmowski WP, Rao R, Scommegna A (1980) The luteinized unruptured follicle syndrome and endometriosis. Fertil Steril 33: 30–34

139. Donna A, Betta P, Jones JSP (1989) Verification of the histologic diagnosis of malignant mesothelioma in relation to the binding of an antimesothelial cell antibody. Cancer 63: 1331–1336

140. Donnez J, Langerock S, Thomas K (1983) Peritoneal fluid volume, 17beta-estradiol and progesterone concentrations in women with endometriosis and/or luteinized unruptured follicle syndrome. Gynecol Obstet Invest 16: 210–220

141. Donnez J, Thomas K (1982) Influence of the luteinized unruptured follicle syndrome in fertile women and in women with endometriosis. Eur J Obstet Gynecol Reprod Biol 14: 187–190

142. Dore N, Landry M, Cadotte M, et al (1980) Cutaneous endosalpingiosis. Arch Dermatol 116: 909–912

143. Doty DW, Gruber JS, Wolf GC, Winslow RC (1980) 46 XY pure gonadal dysgenesis: Report of 2 unusual cases. Obstet Gynecol 55: 61S–63S

144. Douglas GW, Kastin AJ, Huntington RW Jr (1965) Carcinoma arising in a retroperitoneal mullerian cyst, with widespread metastasis during pregnancy. Am J Obstet Gynecol 91: 210–216

145. Dumke K, Schnoy N, Specht G, et al (1983) Comparative light and electron microscopic studies of cystic and papillary tumors of the peritoneum. Virch Arch A 399: 25–39

146. Duson CK, Zelenik JS (1954) Vulvar endometriosis. Obstet Gynecol 3: 76–79

147. Dworak O, Knopfle G, Varchmin-Schultheiss K, Meyer G (1988) Gliomatosis peritonei with endometriosis externa. Gynecol Oncol 29: 263

148. Egger H, Weigmann P (1982) Clinical and surgical aspects of ovarian endometriotic cysts. Arch Gynecol 233: 37–45

149. Ehrmann RL, Federschneider JM, Knapp RC (1980) Distinguishing lymph node metastases from benign glandular inclusions in low-grade ovarian carcinoma. Am J Obstet Gynecol 136: 737–746

150. Eiseman B, Seelig MG, Womack NA (1947) Talcum powder granuloma: A frequent and serious postoperative complication. Ann Surg 126: 820–832

151. El-Mahgoub S, Yassen S (1980) A positive proof for the theory of coelomic metaplasia. Am J Obstet Gynecol 137: 137–140

152. Elliott GB, Christensen RM, Elliott KA (1970) Invasive endometriosis of the intestine: Report of 21 cases. Can J Surg 13: 387–395

153. Elliott GB, Freigang B (1962) Aseptic necrosis, calcification and separation of appendices epiploicae. Ann Surg 155: 501–505

154. Evans H, Yates WA, Palmer WE, et al (1990) Clear cell carcinoma of the sigmoid mesocolon: A tumor of the secondary mullerian system. Am J Obstet Gynecol 162: 161–163

155. Fechner RE (1971) The surgical pathology of the reproductive system and breast during oral contraceptive therapy. In: Sommers SC, Rosen PR (eds). Pathology Annual. New York, Appleton-Century Crofts, pp 299–319

156. Fedele L, Arcaini L, Vercellini P, et al (1988) Serum CA 125 measurements in the diagnosis of endometriosis recurrence. Obstet Gynecol 72: 19–22

157. Fedele L, Vercellini P, Arcaini L, et al (1988) CA 125 in serum, peritoneal fluid, active lesions, and endometrium of patients with endometriosis. Am J Obstet Gynecol 158: 166–170

158. Ferguson BR, Bennington JL, Haber SL (1969) Histochemistry of mucosubstances and histology of mixed mullerian pelvic lymph node glandular inclusions. Evidence for histogenesis by mullerian metaplasia of coelomic epithelium. Obstet Gynecol 33: 617–625

159. Ferraro LR, Hetz H, Carter H (1956) Malignant endometriosis. Pelvic endometriosis complicated by polypoid endometrioma of the colon and endometriotic sarcoma: Report of a case and review of the literature. Obstet Gynecol 7: 32–39

160. Feuer GA, Shevchuk M, Calanog A (1989) Normal-sized ovary carcinoma syndrome. Obstet Gynecol 73: 786–792

161. Finkel L, Marchevsky A, Cohen B (1986) Endometrial cyst of the liver. Am J Gastroenterol 81: 576–578

162. Fischer S (1953) Seltene lokalisation einer endometriosis externa extraperitonealis. Geburtsch Frauenh 13: 240–243

163. Fleming CR, Dickson ER, Harrison EG Jr (1976) Splenosis: Autotransplantation of splenic tissue. Am J Med 61: 414–419

164. Floberg J, Backdahl M, Silfersward C, Thomassen PA (1984) Postpartum perforation of the colon due to endometriosis. Acta Obstet Gynecol Scand 63: 183–184

165. Foo KT, Ng KC, Rauff A, et al (1978) Unusual small intestinal obstruction in adolescent girls: the abdominal cocoon. Br J Surg 65: 427–430

166. Forouhar F (1982) Meconium peritonitis. Pathology, evolution, and diagnosis. Am J Clin Pathol 78: 208–213

167. Fortier KJ, Haney AF (1985) The pathologic spectrum of uterotubal junction obstruction. Obstet Gynecol 65: 93–98

168. Foster DC, Stern JL, Buscema J, et al (1981) Pleural and parenchymal pulmonary endometriosis. Obstet Gynecol 58: 552–556

169. Foyle A, Al-Jabi M, McCaughey WTE (1981) Papillary peritoneal tumors in women. Am J Surg Pathol 5: 241–249

170. Fox H, Buckley CH (1984) Current concepts of endometriosis. Clin Obstet Gynaecol 11: 279–287

171. Freedman SI, Ang EP, Herz MG, et al (1982) Meconium granulomas in post-cesarean section patients. Obstet Gynecol 59: 383–385

172. Fromm G, Gershenson DM, Silva EG (1990) Papillary serous carcinoma of the peritoneum. Obstet Gynecol 75: 89–95

173. Fukayama M, Takizawa T, Koike M, et al (1987) Malignant peritoneal mesothelioma as a pelvic mass. Acta Pathol Jpn 37: 1149–1156

174. Fukushima M, Sharpe L, Okagaki T (1984) Peritoneal melanosis secondary to a benign dermoid cyst of the ovary: A case report with ultrastructural study. Int J Gynec Pathol 2: 403–409

175. Gaffey MJ, Mills SE, Swanson PE, et al (1992) Immunoreactivity for BER-EP4 in adenocarcinomas, adenomatoid tumors, and malignant mesotheliomas. Am J Surg Pathol 16: 593–599

176. Garde JR, Jones MA, McAfee R, Tarraza HM (1991) Extragenital malignant mixed mullerian tumor: Review of the literature. Gynecol Oncol 43: 186–190

177. Gardner HL (1966) Cervical and vaginal endometriosis. Clin Obstet Gynecol 9: 358–372

178. Geary WA, Mills SE, Frierson HF, Pope TL (1991) Malignant peritoneal mesothelioma in childhood with long-term survival. Am J Clin Pathol 95: 493–498

179. Gennari L, Luciani L (1965) A case of endometriosis of the trapezius muscle. Tumori 51: 361–366

180. Gerald WL, Miller HK, Battifora H, et al (1991) Intraabdominal desmoplastic small round cell tumor. Am J Surg Pathol 15: 499–513

181. Gerald WL, Rosai J (1989) Desmoplastic small cell tumor with divergent differentiation. Pediatr Pathol 9: 177–183

182. Gerbie AB, Greene RR, Reis RA (1958) Heteroplastic bone and cartilage in the female genital tract. Obstet Gynecol 11: 573–578

183. Giangarra C, Gallo G, Newman R, Dorfman H (1987) Endometriosis in the biceps femoris. J Bone Joint Surg 69A: 290–292

184. Gibbs AR, Harach R, Wagner JC, et al (1985) Comparison of tumour markers in malignant mesothelioma and pulmonary adenocarcinoma. Thorax 40: 91–95

185. Gilks CB, Bell DA, Scully RE (1990) Serous psammocarcinoma of the ovary and peritoneum. Int J Gynecol Pathol 9: 110–121

186. Gilks B, Hegedus C, Freeman H, et al (1988) Malignant

peritoneal mesothelioma after remote abdominal radiation. Cancer 61: 2019–2021

187. Gitelis S, Petasnick JP, Turner DA, et al (1985) Endometriosis simulating a soft tissue tumor of the thigh: CT and MR evaluation. J Comp Assist Tomogr 9: 573–576

188. Gitsch G, Tabery U, Feigl W, Breitnecker G (1992) The differential diagnosis of primary peritoneal papillary tumors. Arch Gynecol Obstet 251: 139–144

189. Godleski JJ, Gabriel KL (1981) Peritoneal responses to implanted fabrics used in operating rooms. Surgery 90: 828–834

190. Goepel JR (1981) Benign papillary mesothelioma of peritoneum: A histological, histochemical and ultrastructural study of six cases. Histopathology 5: 21–30

191. Goldstein DP, deCholnoky C, Emans SJ, Leventhal JM (1980) Laparoscopy in the diagnosis and management of pelvic pain in adolescents. J Reprod Med 24: 251–256

192. Gonzalez-Crussi F, Crawford SE, Sun CJ (1990) Intraabdominal desmoplastic small-cell tumors with divergent differentiation. Observations on three cases of childhood. Am J Surg Pathol 14: 633–642

193. Gonzalez-Crussi F, deMello DE, Sotelo-Avila C (1983) Omental-mesenteric myxoid hamartomas. Am J Surg Pathol 7: 567–578

194. Goodall JR (1944) Urinary complications of pelvic endometriosis. Ann Surg 120: 891–900

195. Gooneratne S, Sassone M, Blaustein A, et al (1982) Serous surface papillary carcinoma of the ovary: a clinicopathologic study of 16 cases. Int J Gynecol Pathol 1: 258–269

196. Gordon PH, Schottler JL, Balcos EG, Goldberg SM (1976) Perianal endometrioma. Report of five cases. Dis Colon Rectum 19: 260–265

197. Goswami AK, Sharma SK, Tandon SP, et al (1986) Pancreatic endometriosis presenting as a hypovascular renal mass. J Urol 135: 112–113

198. Gould SF, Shannon JM, Cunha GR (1983) Nuclear estrogen binding sites in human endometriosis. Fertil Steril 39: 520–525

199. Grabb A, Carr L, Goodman JD, et al (1986) Hepatic endometriosis. JCU 14: 478–480

200. Granai CO, Walters MD, Safaii H, et al (1984) Malignant transformation of vaginal endometriosis. Obstet Gynecol 64: 592–595

201. Gray LA (1966) The management of endometriosis involving the bowel. Clin Obstet Gynecol 9: 309–330

202. Gray LA, Barnes ML (1965) Relation of endometriosis to ovarian carcinoma. Am Surg 31: 798–806

203. Griffith LM, Carcangiu M (1991) Sex cord tumor with annular tubules associated with endometriosis of the fallopian tube. Am J Clin Pathol 96: 259–262

204. Gupta SD (1985) Endometriosis of the thumb. J Ind Med Assoc 83: 122–123

205. Gussman D, Thickman D, Wheeler JE (1986) Postoperative peritoneal cysts. Obstet Gynecol 68: 53S–55S

206. Guzick DS (1989) Clinical epidemiology of endometriosis and infertility. Obstet Gynecol Clin North Am 16: 43–59

207. Haddad FS, Ghossain A, Sawaya E, et al (1987) Abdominal tuberculosis. Dis Colon Rectum 30: 724–735

208. Hafiz MA, Toker C (1986) Multicentric ovarian and extraovarian cystadenofibroma. Obstet Gynecol 68: 94S–98S

209. Hallman KB, Nahhas WA, Connolly PJ (1991) Endosalpingiosis as a source of psammoma bodies in a Papanicolaou smear. A case report. J Reprod Med 36: 675–678

210. Halme J, Becker S, Haskill S (1987) Altered maturation and function of peritoneal macrophages: Possible role in pathogenesis of endometriosis. Am J Obstet Gynecol 156:783–789

211. Halme J, Chafe W, Currie JL (1985) Endometriosis with massive ascites. Obstet Gynecol 65: 591–592

212. Halme J, Hammond MG, Hulka JF, et al (1984) Retrograde menstruation in healthy women and in patients with endometriosis. Obstet Gynecol 64: 151–154

213. Hampton HL, Huffman HT, Meeks GR (1992) Extraovarian Brenner tumor. Obstet Gynecol 79: 844–846

214. Haney AF, Handwerger S, Weinberg JB (1984) Peritoneal fluid prolactin in infertile women with endometriosis: Lack of evidence of secretory activity by endometrial implants. Fertil Steril 42: 935–938

215. Hanrahan JB (1963) A combined papillary mesothelioma and adenomatoid tumor of the omentum. Report of a case. Cancer 16: 1497–1500

216. Hansen RM, Caya JG, Clowry LJ Jr, et al (1984) Benign mesothelial proliferation with effusion. Clinicopathologic entity that may mimic malignancy. Am J Med 77: 887–892

217. Hanton EM, Malkasian GD Jr, Dockerty MB, Pratt JH (1966) Endometriosis associated with complete or partial obstruction of menstrual egress. Report of 7 cases. Obstet Gynecol 28: 626–629

218. Hapke MR, Bigelow B (1977) Mucocele of the appendix secondary to obstruction by endometriosis. Hum Pathol 8: 585–589

219. Harbitz HF (1936) Ectopic decidua. Acta Path Microbiol Scand 26(suppl): 16–20

220. Harper GB Jr, Awbrey BJ, Thomas CG Jr, et al (1986) Mesothelial cysts of the round ligament simulating inguinal hernia. Report of four cases and review of the literature. Am J Surg 151: 515–517

221. Heaps JM, Nieberg RK, Berek JS (1990) Malignant neoplasms arising in endometriosis. Obstet Gynecol 75: 1023–1028

222. Henriksen E (1955) Endometriosis. Am J Surg 90: 331–337

223. Herr JC, Platz CE, Heidger PM Jr, et al (1979) Smooth muscle within ovarian decidual nodules: a link to leiomyomatosis peritonealis disseminata? Obstet Gynecol 53: 451–456

224. Herz MG, Stanley WD, Toot PJ, et al (1982) Symptomatic maternal intraperitoneal meconium granulomata. Report of two cases. Diagn Gynecol Obstet 4: 147–149

225. Hedvegi D, Hedvegi I, Barrett J (1978) Douche-induced pelvic peritoneal starch granuloma. Obstet Gynecol 52: 15S–18S

226. Higa E, Rosai J, Pizzimbono CA, et al (1973) Mucosal hyperplasia, mucinous cystadenoma, and mucinous cystadenocarcinoma of the appendix. A re-evaluation of appendiceal "mucocele." Cancer 32: 1525–1541

227. Hitti IF, Glasberg SS, Lubicz S (1990) Clear cell carcinoma arising in extraovarian endometriosis: Report of three cases and review of the literature. Gynecol Oncol 39: 314–320

228. Hobbs JE, Bortnick AR (1940) Endometriosis of the lungs. An experimental and clinical study. Am J Obstet Gynecol 40: 832–843

229. Hochster H, Wernz JC, Muggia FM (1984) Intra-abdominal carcinomatosis with histologically normal ovaries. Cancer Treatment Rep 68: 921–922

230. Holden J, Churg A (1984) Immunohistochemical staining for keratin and carcinoembryonic antigen in the diagnosis of malignant mesothelioma. Am J Surg Pathol 8: 277–279

231. Holmes EC, Eggleston JC (1972) Starch granulomatous peritonitis. Surgery 71: 85–90

232. Holmes MD, Levin HS, Ballard LA (1981) Endosalpingiosis. Cleve Clin Q 48: 345–352

233. Horbelt DV, Roberts DK, Walker N, Delmore JE (1986) Nucleolar canalicular structure in extrauterine endometriosis. Hum Pathol 17: 924

234. Horie A, Ishii N, Matsumoto M, et al (1984) Leiomyomatosis in the pelvic lymph node and peritoneum. Acta Pathol Jpn 34: 813–819

235. Houston DE, Noller KL, Melton J, et al (1987) Incidence of pelvic endometriosis in Rochester, Minnesota, 1970–1979. Am J Epidemiol 125: 959–969

236. Houston DE, Noller KL, Melton J III, Selwyn BJ (1988) The epidemiology of pelvic endometriosis. Clin Obstet Gynecol 31: 787–800

237. Hsu YK, Rosenshein NB, Parmley TH, et al (1981) Leiomyomatosis in pelvic lymph nodes. Obstet Gynecol 57: 91S–93S

238. Huffman JW (1981) Endometriosis in young teen-age girls. Pediatr Annu 10: 501–506

239. Hughesdon PE (1976) The endometrial identity of benign stromatosis of the ovary and its relation to other forms of endometriosis. J Pathol 119: 201–209

240. Hulme-Moir I, Ross MS (1969) A case of early postpartum abdominal pain due to hemorrhagic deciduosis peritonei. Br J Obstet Gynaecol 76: 746–749

241. Huntrakoon M (1985) Benign glandular inclusions in the abdominal lymph nodes of a man. Hum Pathol 16: 644–646

242. Ignatius JA, Hartmann WH (1972) The glove starch peritonitis syndrome. Ann Surg 175: 338–397

243. Irani S, Atkinson L, Cabaniss C, Danovitch SH (1976) Pleuroperitoneal endometriosis. Obstet Gynecol 47: 72S–74S

244. Isenberg JI, Gilbert SB, Pitcher JL (1971) Ascites with peritoneal involvement in Whipple's disease. Gastroenterology 60: 305–310

245. Ismail SM (1991) Cone biopsy causes cervical endometriosis and tubo-endometrioid metaplasia. Histopathology 18: 107–114

246. Ishimaru T, Masuzaki H (1991) Peritoneal endometriosis: Endometrial tissue implantation as its primary etiologic mechanism. Am J Obstet Gynecol 165: 210–214

247. Ismail SM (1991) Cone biopsy causes cervical endometriosis and tubo-endometrioid metaplasia. Histopathology 18: 107–114

248. Israel SL, Rubenstone A, Meranze DR (1954) The ovary at term I. Decidua-like reaction and surface cell proliferation. Obstet Gynecol 3: 399–407

249. Iwasaka T, Okuma Y, Yoshimura T, et al (1985) Endometriosis associated with ascites. Obstet Gynecol 66: 72S–75S

250. Iwasaki I, Yu TJ, Tamaru J, Asanuma K (1985) A cystic adenomatoid tumor of the uterus simulating lymphangioma grossly. Acta Pathol Jpn 35: 989–993

251. Janne O, Kauppila A, Kokko E, et al (1981) Estrogen and progestin receptors in endometriosis lesions: Comparison with endometrial tissue. Am J Obstet Gynecol 141: 562–566

252. Janoff K, Wayne R, Huntwork B, et al (1984) Foreign body reactions secondary to cellulose lint fibers. Am J Surg 147: 598–600

253. Jansen RPS, Russell P (1986) Nonpigmented endometriosis: Clinical, laparoscopic, and pathologic definition. Am J Obstet Gynecol 155: 1154–1159

254. Javert CT (1951) Observations on the pathology and spread of endometriosis based on the theory of benign metastasis. Am J Obstet Gynecol 62: 477–487

255. Javert CT (1952) The spread of benign and malignant endometrium in the lymphatic system with a note on coexisting vascular involvement. Am J Obstet Gynecol 64: 780–806

256. Jenkins S, Olive DL, Haney AF (1986) Endometriosis: Pathogenetic implications of the anatomic distribution. Obstet Gynecol 67: 335–338

257. Jenks JE, Artman LE, Hoskins WJ, Miremadi AK (1984) Endometriosis with ascites. Obstet Gynecol 63: 75S–77S

258. Jones DEC, Silver D (1979) Peritoneal mesotheliomas. Surgery 86: 556–560

259. Jones EG, Donovan AJ (1965) Adenomatoid tumor of the ovary versus mesothelial reaction. Am J Obstet Gynecol 92: 694–698

259a. Kafiri G, Thomas DM, Shepherd NA, et al (1992) p53 expression is common in malignant mesotheliomas. Histopathology 21: 331–334

260. Kane C, Drouin P (1985) Obstructive uropathy associated with endometriosis. Am J Obstet Gynecol 151: 207–211

261. Kane MJ, Chahinian AP, Holland JF (1990) Malignant mesothelioma in young adults. Cancer 65: 1449–1455

262. Kannerstein M, Churg J (1977) Peritoneal mesothelioma. Hum Pathol 8: 83–94

263. Kannerstein M, Churg J, McCaughey WTE, Hill DP (1977) Papillary tumors of the peritoneum in women: Mesothelioma or papillary carcinoma. Am J Obstet Gynecol 127: 306–314

264. Kapadia SB, Russak RR, O'Donnell WF, et al (1984) Postmenopausal ureteral endometriosis with atypical adenomatous hyperplasia following hysterectomy, bilateral oophorectomy, and long-term estrogen therapy. Obstet Gynecol 64: 60S–63S

265. Kaplan C, Benirschke K, Johnson KC (1980) Leiomyomatosis peritonealis disseminata with endometrium. Obstet Gynecol 55: 119–122

266. Kapoor OP, Nathwani BN, Joshi VR (1972) Amoebic peritonitis. A study of 73 cases. J Trop Med Hyg 1972;75: 11–15

267. Karp LA, Czernobilsky B (1969) Glandular inclusions in pelvic and abdominal para-aortic lymph nodes. Am J Clin Pathol 52: 212–218

268. Katsube Y, Mukai K, Silverberg SG (1982) Cystic mesothelioma of the peritoneum. A report of five cases and review of the literature. Cancer 50: 1615–1622

269. Kaunitz A, Di Sant'Agnese PA (1979) Needle tract endometriosis: An unusual complication of amniocentesis. Obstet Gynecol 54: 753–755

270. Kauppila A, Isomaa V, Ronnberg L, et al (1985) Effect of gestrinone in endometriosis tissue and endometrium. Fertil Steril 44: 466

271. Kauppila A, Vierikko P, Isotalo H, et al (1984) Cytosol estrogen and progestin receptor concentrations and 17-beta-hydroxysteroid dehydrogenase activities in the endometrium and endometriotic tissue. Effects of hormonal stimulation. Acta Obstet Gynecol Scand 123(suppl): 45–49

272. Kay S (1954) Tissue reaction to barium sulfate contrast medium. Arch Pathol 57: 279–284

273. Keettel WC, Stein RJ (1951) The viability of the cast-off menstrual endometrium. Am J Obstet Gynecol 61: 440–442

274. Kempers RD, Dockerty MB, Hunt AB, et al (1960) Significant postmenopausal endometriosis. Surg Gynecol Obstet 111: 348–356

275. Kempson RL (1978) Consultation case. Am J Surg Pathol 2: 321–325

276. Kennedy SH, Sargent IL, Starkey PM, et al (1990) Localization of anti-endometrial antibody binding in women with endometriosis using a double-labelling immunohistochemical method. Br J Obstet Gynaecol 97: 671–674

277. Kennedy SH, Starkey PM, Sargent IL, et al (1990) Antiendometrial antibodies in endometriosis measured by an enzyme-linked immunosorbent assay before and after treatment with danazol and nafarelin. Obstet Gynecol 75: 914–918

278. Kern SB (1991) Prevalence of psammoma bodies in Papanicolaou-stained cervicovaginal smears. Acta Cytol 35: 81–88

279. Kern WH (1969) Benign papillary structures with psammoma bodies in culdocentesis fluid. Acta Cytol 13: 178–180

280. Kerner H, Gaton E, Czernobilsky B (1981) Unusual ovarian, tubal and pelvic mesothelial inclusions in patients with endometriosis. Histopathology 5: 277–282

281. Kerner H, Lichtig C, Beck D (1989) Extrauterine mullerian adenosarcoma of the peritoneal mesothelium: A clinicopathologic and electron microscopic study. Obstet Gynecol 73: 510–513

282. Kerr WS (1966) Endometriosis involving urinary tract. Clin Obstet Gynecol 9: 331–357

283. Kheir SM, Mann WJ, Wilkerson JA (1981) Glandular inclusions in lymph nodes. The problem of extensive involvement and relationship to salpingitis. Am J Surg Pathol 5: 353–359

284. Khoury N, Raju U, Crissman JD, Zarbo RJ, Greenawald KA (1990) A comparative immunohistochemical study of peritoneal and ovarian serous tumors, and mesotheliomas. Hum Pathol 21: 811–819

285. Kim K, Scully RE (1990) Peritoneal keratin granulomas with carcinomas of endometrium and ovary and atypical polypoid adenomyoma of endometrium. Am J Surg Pathol 14: 925–932

286. Kistner RW (1966) Current status of the hormonal treatment of endometriosis. Clin Obstet Gynecol 9: 271–292

287. Kistner RW (1979) Endometriosis and infertility. Clin Obstet Gynecol 22: 101–119

288. Kitazawa M, Kaneko H, Toshima M, et al (1984) Malignant peritoneal mesothelioma with massive foamy cells. Acta Pathol Jpn 34: 687–692

289. Kjellevold K, Nesland JM, Holm R, et al (1986) Multicystic peritoneal mesothelioma. Pathol Res Pract 181: 767–771

290. Kondi-Paphitis A, Addis BJ (1986) Secretory component in pulmonary adenocarcinoma and mesothelioma. Histopathology 10: 1279–1287

291. Koninckx PR, Ide P, Vandenbroucke W, Brosens IA (1980) New aspects of the pathophysiology of endometriosis and associated infertility. J Reprod Med 24: 257–260

292. Koss LG (1963) Miniature adenocanthoma arising in an obturator lymph node. Report of a case. Cancer 16: 1369–1372

293. Kuo T, London SN, Dinh TV (1980) Endometriosis occurring in leiomyomatosis peritonealis disseminata. Ultrastructural study and histogenetic consideration. Am J Surg Pathol 4: 197–204

294. Kurman RJ, Funk RL, Kirshenbaum AH (1969) Spina bifida with associated choristoma of mullerian origin. J Pathol 99: 324–327

295. Kurman RJ, Main CS, Chen H (1984) Intermediate trophoblast: A distinctive form of trophoblast with specific morphological, biochemical and functional features. Placenta 5: 349–370

296. Kurman RJ, Young RH, Norris HJ, Main CS, Lawrence WD, Scully RE (1984) Immunocytochemical localization of placental lactogen and chorionic gonadotropin in the normal placenta and trophoblastic tumors, with emphasis on intermediate trophoblast and the placental site trophoblastic tumor. Int J Gynecol Pathol 3: 101–121

297. Kwee WS, Veldhuizen RW, Golding RP, et al (1982) Histologic distinction between malignant mesothelioma, benign pleural lesion and carcinoma metastasis. Virch Arch [A] 397: 287–299

298. LaGrenade A, Silverberg SG (1988) Ovarian tumors associated with atypical endometriosis. Hum Pathol 19: 1080–1084

299. Lamb K, Hoffmann RG, Nichols TR (1986) Family trait analysis: A case-control study of 43 women with endometriosis and their best friends. Am J Obstet Gynecol 154: 596–601

300. Langmade CF (1975) Pelvic endometriosis and ureteral obstruction. Am J Obstet Gynecol 122: 463–469

301. Lankerani MR, Aubrey RW, Reid JD (1982) Endometriosis of the colon with mixed "germ cell" tumor. Am J Clin Pathol 78: 555–559

302. Lattes R, Shepard F, Tovell H, Wylie R (1956) A clinical and pathological study of endometriosis of the lung. Surg Gynecol Obstet 103: 552–558

303. Latza U, Niedobitek G, Schwarting R, et al (1990) Ber-EP4: New monoclonal antibody which distinguishes epithelia from mesothelia. J Clin Pathol 43: 213–219

304. Laube DW, Calderwood GW, Benda JA (1985) Endometriosis causing ureteral obstruction. Obstet Gynecol 65: 69S–71S

305. Lauchlan SC (1965) Two types of mullerian epithelium in an abdominal scar. Am J Obstet Gynecol 93: 89–90

306. Lauchlan SC (1966) The cytology of endometriosis. Am J Obstet Gynecol 94: 533–535

307. Lauchlan SC (1972) The secondary mullerian system. Obstet Gynecol Surv 27: 133–146

308. Layfield LJ, Lenarsky C (1991) Desmoplastic small cell tumors of the peritoneum coexpressing mesenchymal and epithelial markers. Am J Clin Pathol 96: 536–543

309. Lee D, Pontifex AH (1975) Melanosis peritonei. Am J Obstet Gynecol 122: 526–527

310. Lee KR, Verma U, Belinson J (1991) Primary clear cell carcinoma of the peritoneum. Gynecol Oncol 41: 259–262

310a. Lee RG: Sclerosing peritonitis (1989) Digest Dis Sci 34: 1473–1476

311. Lees RF, Feldman PS, Brenbridge NAG, et al (1978) Inflammatory cysts of the pelvic peritoneum. Am J Roentgenol 131: 633–636

312. Leiman G, Naylor G (1985) Mucinous metaplasia in scar endometriosis. Diagnosis by aspiration cytology. Diagn Cytopathol 1: 153–156

313. Lele SB, Piver S, Barlow JJ, et al (1978) Squamous cell carcinoma arising in ovarian endometriosis. Gynecol Oncol 6: 290–293

314. Lele SB, Piver MS, Matharu J, Tsukada Y (1988) Peritoneal papillary carcinoma. Gynecol Oncol 31: 315–320

315. Lessey BA, Metzger DA, Haney AF, McCarty KS Jr (1989) Immunohistochemical analysis of estrogen and progesterone receptors in endometriosis: Comparison with normal endometrium during the menstrual cycle and the effect of medical therapy. Fertil Steril 51: 409–415

316. Levander G, Normann P (1955) The pathogenesis of endometriosis. An experimental study. Acta Obstet Gynecol Scand 34: 366–398

317. Limber GK, King RE, Silverberg SG (1973) Pseudomyxoma peritonei: A report of ten cases. Ann Surg 178: 587–593

318. Lindenberg K, Schmid J, Ruttner J, et al (1975) Endometriosis of the lung. Arch Gynecol 218: 219–226

319. Lintermans JP (1975) Fatal peritonitis, an unusual complication of strongyloides stercoralis infestation. Clin Ped 14: 974–975

320. Lipscomb GH, Ling FW, Photopulos GJ (1991) Ovarian abscess arising within an endometrioma. Obstet Gynecol 78: 951–954

321. Lisa JR, Gioia JD, Rubin IC (1954) Observations on the interstitial portion of the fallopian tube. Surg Gynecol Obstet 99: 159–169

322. LiVolsi VA, Perzin KH (1974) Endometriosis of the small intestine, producing intestinal obstruction or simulating neoplasm. Am J Digest Dis 19: 100–108

323. Lombardo L, Mateos JH, Barroeta FF (1968) Subarachnoid hemorrhage due to endometriosis of the spinal canal. Neurol 18: 423–426

324. Lomholt G, Hjorth N, Fischermann K (1968) Lethal peritonitis from Degos' disease (malign and atrophic papulosis). Acta Chir Scand 134: 495–501

325. Longo S (1976) Benign lymph node inclusions. Hum Pathol 7: 349–354

326. Loosli H, Hurlimann J (1984) Immunohistological study of malignant diffuse mesotheliomas of the pleura. Histopathology 8: 793–803

327. Loy TS, Diaz-Arias AA, Bickel JT (1990) Value of BCA-225 in the cytologic diagnosis of malignant effusions: An immunocytochemical study of 197 cases. Mod Pathol 3: 294–297

328. Lucero SP, Wise HA, Kirsh G, et al (1988) Ureteric obstruction secondary to endometriosis: Report of three cases with review of the literature. Br J Urol 61: 201–204

329. Lyndrup J, Thorpe S, Glenthoj A, et al (1987) Altered progesterone/estrogen receptor ratios in endometriosis. Acta Obstet Gynecol Scand 66: 625–629

330. Macafee CHG, Greer HLH (1960) Intestinal endometriosis. Br J Obstet Gynecol 67: 539–555

331. Madelenat P, De Brux J, Palmer R (1977) L'etiologie des obstructions tubaires proximales et son role dans le pronostic des implantations. Gynecologie 28: 47–53

332. Mahoney AD, Waisman J, Zeldis LJ (1977) Adenomyoma. A precursor of extrauterine mullerian adenosarcoma? Arch Pathol Lab Med 101: 579–584

333. Mainguene C, Aillet G, Kremer M, et al (1986) Immunohistochemical study of ovarian tumors using the OC 125 monoclonal antibody as a basis for potential in vivo and in vitro applications. J Nucl Med Allied Sci 30: 19–22

334. Malinak LR, Buttram VC, Elias S, Simpson JL (1980) Heritable aspects of endometriosis. II. Clinical characteristics of familial endometriosis. Am J Obstet Gynecol 137: 332–337

335. Manivel JC, Wick MR, Coffin MC, Dehner LP (1989) Immunohistochemistry in the differential diagnosis in the second-look operation for ovarian carcinomas. Int J Gynecol Pathol 8: 103–113

336. Mann WJ, Fromowitz F, Saychek T, Madariaga JR, Chalas E (1984) Endometriosis associated with appendiceal intussusception. A report of two cases. J Reprod Med 29: 625–629

337. Marchevsky AM, Zimmerman MJ, Aufses Jr AH, Weiss H (1984) Endometrial cyst of the pancreas. Gastroenterology 86: 1589–1591

338. Marshall AJ, Baddeley H, Barritt DW, et al (1977) Practolol peritonitis. A study of 16 cases and a survey of small bowel function in patients taking beta adrenergic blockers. Q J Med 46: 135–149

339. Marshall SF, Forse RA (1952) Peritoneal adhesions: Report of a case of paraffinoma. Surg Clin North Am 32: 903–908

340. Martimbeau PW, Pratt JH, Gaffey TA (1975) Small-bowel obstruction secondary to endometriosis. Mayo Clinic Proc 50: 239–243

341. Martin DC, Hubert GD, Vander Zwaag R, El-Zeky FA (1989) Laparoscopic appearances of peritoneal endometriosis. Fertil Steril 51: 63–67

342. Martin JD Jr, Hauck AE (1985) Endometriosis in the male. Am Surg 51: 426–430

343. Matseoane S, Harris T, Moscowitz E (1987) Isolated endometriosis in a Bartholin gland. NY State J Med 87: 575–576

344. Maxson WS, Pittaway DE, Hill GA, et al (1986) Ureteral abnormalities in women with endometriosis. Fertil Steril 46: 1159–1161

345. Mayall FG, Gibbs AR (1991) Malignant peritoneal mesothelioma giving rise to multiple intestinal polyps. Histopathology 18: 480–482

346. Mayall FG, Jasani B, Gibbs AR (1991) Immunohistochem-

ical positivity for neuron-specific enolase and Leu-7 in malignant mesotheliomas. J Pathol 165: 325–328

346a. Mazzoleni G, Salerno A, Santini D, et al (1992) Leiomyomatosis in pelvic lymph nodes. Histopathology 21: 588–589

347. McArthur JW, Ulfelder H (1965) The effect of pregnancy upon endometriosis. Obstet Gynecol Surv 20: 709–733

348. McCaughey WTE, Al-Jabi M (1986) Differentiation of serosal hyperplasia and neoplasia in biopsies. Pathol Annu 21(1): 271–292

349. McCaughey WTE, Colby TV, Battifora H, et al (1991) Diagnosis of diffuse malignant mesothelioma: Experience of a US/Canadian mesothelioma panel. Mod Pathol 4: 342–353

350. McCaughey WTE, Kannerstein M, Churg J (1985) Tumors and pseudotumors of the serous membranes. Atlas of Tumor Pathology, Armed Forces Institute of Pathology, series 2, fascicle 20

351. McCaughey WTE, Schryer MJP, Lin X, et al (1986) Extraovarian pelvic serous tumor with marked calcification. Arch Pathol Lab Med 110: 78–80

352. McCaughey WTE, Kirk ME, Lester W, et al (1984) Peritoneal epithelial lesions associated with proliferative serous tumours of the ovary. Histopathology 8: 195–208

353. McDougal RA, Roth LM (1986) Ovarian adenomyoma associated with an endometriotic cyst. South Med J 79: 640–642

354. McFadden DE, Clement PB (1986) Peritoneal inclusion cysts with mural mesothelial proliferation. A clinicopathological analysis of six cases. Am J Surg Pathol 10: 844–854

355. Mennemeyer R, Smith M (1979) Multicystic, peritoneal mesothelioma. A report with electron microscopy of a case mimicking intra-abdominal cystic hygroma (lymphangioma). Cancer 44: 692–698

356. Merino MJ, Livolsi VA (1981) Signet ring carcinoma of the female breast: A clinicopathologic analysis of 24 cases. Cancer 48: 1830–1837

357. Merrill JA (1963) Experimental induction of endometriosis across millipore filters. Surg Forum 14: 399–401

358. Metzger AL, Coyne M, Lee S, et al (1974) In vivo LE cell formation in peritonitis due to systemic lupus erythematosus. J Rheumatol 1: 130–133

359. Metzger DA, Haney AF (1988) Endometriosis: Etiology and pathophysiology of infertility. Clin Obstet Gynecol 31: 801–812

360. Metzger DA, Lessey BA, Soper JT, et al (1991) Hormone-resistant endometriosis following total abdominal hysterectomy and bilateral salpingo-oophorectomy: Correlation with histology and steroid receptor content. Obstet Gynecol 78: 946–950

361. Metzger DA, Olive DL, Haney AF (1988) Limited hormonal responsiveness of ectopic endometrium: Histologic correlation with intrauterine endometrium. Hum Pathol 1417–1424

362. Michael H, Sutton G, Roth LM (1987) Ovarian carcinoma with extracellular mucin production: Reassessment of "pseudomyxoma ovarii et peritonei." Int J Gynecol Pathol 6: 298–312

363. Michowitz M, Baratz M, Stavorovsky M (1983) Endometriosis of the umbilicus. Dermatologica 167: 326–330

364. Miles JM, Hart WR, McMahon JT (1986) Cystic mesothelioma of the peritoneum. Report of a case with multiple recurrences and review of the literature. Cleve Clin Q 53: 109–114

365. Mills SE (1983) Decidua and squamous metaplasia in abdominopelvic lymph nodes. Int J Gynecol Pathol 2: 209–215

366. Mills SE, Andersen WA, Fechner RE, Austin MB (1988) Serous surface papillary carcinoma. A clinicopathologic study of 10 cases and comparison with stage III–IV ovarian serous carcinoma. Am J Surg Pathol 12: 827–834

367. Minvielle UL, de la Cruz JV (1968) Endometriosis of the anal canal: Presentation of a case. Dis Col Rect 11: 32–35

368. Miyazawa K (1976) Incidence of endometriosis among Japanese women. Obstet Gynecol 48: 407–409

369. Moll UM, Chumas JC, Chalas E, Mann WJ (1990) Ovarian carcinoma arising in atypical endometriosis. Obstet Gynecol 75: 537–539

370. Moller NE (1959) The Arias–Stella phenomenon in endometriosis. Acta Obstet Gynecol Scand 38: 271–274

371. Moloshok AA, Ivanko AI (1984) Endometriosis of the breast (an observation). Vopr Onkol 30: 88–89

372. Moor JH Jr, Crum CP, Chandler JG, Feldman PS (1980) Benign cystic mesothelioma. Cancer 45: 2395–2399

373. Moore JG, Hibbard LT, Growdon WA, Schifrin BS (1979) Urinary tract endometriosis: enigmas in diagnosis and management. Am J Obstet Gynecol 134: 162–172

374. Mostoufizadeh M, Scully RE (1980) Malignant tumors arising in endometriosis. Clin Obstet Gynecol 23: 951–963

375. Muse K (1988) Clinical manifestations and classification of endometriosis. Clin Obstet Gynecol 31: 813–822

376. Nakatani Y, Hara M, Misugi K, Korehisa H (1987) Appendiceal endometriosis in pregnancy: Report of a case with perforation and review of the literature. Acta Pathol Jpn 37: 1685–1690

377. Naresh KN, Ahuja VK, Rao CR, et al (1991) Squamous cell carcinoma arising in endometriosis of the ovary. J Clin Pathol 44: 958–959

378. Navratil E, Kramer A (1936) Endometriose in der armmuskulatur. Klin Wchnschr 15: 1765–1770

379. Nisolle-Pochet M, Casanas-Roux F, Donnez J (1988) Histologic study of ovarian endometriosis after hormonal therapy. Fertil Steril 49: 423

380. Nissim F, Ashkenazy M, Borenstein R, et al (1981) Tuberculoid cornstarch granulomas with caseous necrosis. Arch Pathol Lab Med 105: 86–88

380a. Ngo Y, Messing B, Marteau P, et al (1992) Peritoneal sarcoidosis: An unrecognized cause of sclerosing peritonitis. Digest Dis Sci 37: 1776–1780

381. Norenberg DD, Gundersen JH, Janis JF, Gundersen AL (1977) Early pregnancy on the diaphragm with endometriosis. Obstet Gynecol 49: 620–622

382. Norman PE, Whitaker D (1989) Nine-year survival in a case of untreated peritoneal mesothelioma. Med J Austral 150: 43–44

383. Norris JC, Davison TC (1934) Peritoneal reaction to liquid petrolatum. JAMA 103: 1846–1847

384. Norton J, Monaghan P, Carter RL (1991) Intra-abdominal desmoplastic small cell tumour with divergent differentiation. Histopathology 19: 560–562

385. Novak ER, Hoge AF (1958) Endometriosis of the lower genital tract. Obstet Gynecol 12: 687–693

386. Ober WB, Grady HG, Schoenbucher AK (1957) Ectopic ovarian decidua without pregnancy. Am J Pathol 33: 199–214

387. Olive DL, Henderson DY (1987) Endometriosis and mullerian anomalies. Obstet Gynecol 69: 412–415

388. Ordonez NG (1989) The immunohistochemical diagnosis of mesothelioma. Differentiation of mesothelioma and lung adenocarcinoma. Am J Surg Pathol 13: 276–291

389. Ordonez NG, Zirkin R, Bloom RE (1989) Malignant small-cell epithelial tumor of the peritoneum coexpressing mesenchymal-type intermediate filaments. Am J Surg Pathol 13: 413–421

390. Ortega I, Nogales F, Gonzalez-Campora R, et al (1982) Extragenital endometrioid cystadenofibroma. Acta Obstet Gynecol Scand 61: 283–284

391. Oses AV, Rodriguez EH, Garcia JLS, et al (1982) Catamenial pneumothorax with pleural endometriosis and hemoptysis. Diagn Gynecol Obstet 4: 295–299

392. O'Sullivan D, Heffernan CK (1960) Deciduosis peritonei in pregnancy. Report of two cases. Br J Obstet Gynaecol 67: 1013–1016

393. Otis CN, Carter D, Cole S, Battifora H (1987) Immunohistochemical evaluation of pleural mesothelioma and pulmonary adenocarcinoma. A bi-institutional study of 47 cases. Am J Surg Pathol 11: 445–456

394. Overton TH (1982) Splenosis: A cause of pelvic pain. Am J Obstet Gynecol 143: 969–970

395. Palagiri A (1978) Urethral diverticulum with endometriosis. Urology 11: 271–272

396. Panganiban W, Cornog JL (1972) Endometriosis of the intestines and vermiform appendix. Dis Colon Rectum 15: 253–260

397. Park SA, Giannattasio C, Tancer ML (1981) Foreign body reaction to the intraperitoneal use of avitene. Obstet Gynecol 58: 664–668

398. Park U, Han KC, Chang HK, Huh MH (1991) A primary mucinous cystadenocarcinoma of the retroperitoneum. Gynecol Oncol 42: 64–67

399. Parmley TH, Woodruff JD, Winn K et al (1975) Histogenesis of leiomyomatosis peritonealis disseminata (disseminated fibrosing deciduosis). Obstet Gynecol 46: 511–227

400. Patel VC, Samuels H, Abeles E, Hirjibehedin PE (1982) Endometriosis of the knee. A case report. Clin Orthop 171: 140–144

401. Paull T, Tedeschi LG (1972) Perineal endometriosis at the site of episiotomy scar. Obstet Gynecol 40: 28–34

402. Pedersen H, Rank F (1984) Morphology of endometriosis before and during treatment with danazol. Acta Obstet Gynecol Scand 123(suppl): 13–14

403. Pellegrini VD Jr, Pasternak HS, Macaulay WP (1981) Endometrioma of the pubis: A differential in the diagnosis of hip pain. A report of two cases. J Bone Joint Surg 63A: 1333–1334

404. Pelzer SG (1954) Cystic endometriosis of the epigastrium. J Int Coll Surg 21: 528–531

405. Pennell TC, Gusdon JP Jr (1989) Retroperitoneal mucinous cystadenoma. Am J Obstet Gynecol 160: 1229–1231

406. Peress MR, Sosnowski JR, Mathur RS, Williamson HO (1982) Pelvic endometriosis and Turner's syndrome. Am J Obstet Gynecol 144: 474–476

407. Peterson CJ, Strickler JG, Gonzalez R, Dehner LP (1990) Uterus-like mass of the small intestine. Heterotopia or monodermal teratoma? Am J Surg Pathol 14: 390–394

408. Pettinato G, Manivel JC, De Rosa N, Dehner LP (1990) Inflammatory myofibroblastic tumor (plasma cell granuloma). Clinicopathologic study of 20 cases with immunohistochemical and ultrastructural observations. Am J Clin Pathol 94: 538–546

409. Piccigallo E, Jeffers LJ, Reddy R, et al (1988) Malignant peritoneal mesothelioma. A clinical and laparoscopic study of ten cases. Digest Dis Sci 33: 633–639

410. Pickartz H (1991) Tumor-like lesions of the secondary mullerian system: Immunohistochemical investigations and differential diagnosis. APMIS 23(suppl): 146–151

411. Pieslor PC, Orenstein JM, Hogan DL, et al (1979) Ultrastructure of myofibroblasts and decidualized cells in leiomyomatosis peritonealis disseminata. Am J Clin Pathol 72: 875–882

412. Pittaway DE (1989) CA-125 in women with endometriosis. Obstet Gynecol Clin North Am 16: 237–252

413. Plaus WJ (1988) Peritoneal mesothelioma. Arch Surg 123: 763–766

414. Postlethwait RW, Howard HL, Schanher PW, et al (1949) Comparison of tissue reaction to talc and modified starch glove powder. Surgery 25: 22–29

415. Prakash S, Ulfelder H, Cohen RB (1965) Enzyme-histochemical observations on endometriosis. Am J Obstet Gynecol 91: 990–997

416. Prat J, Matias-Guiu X, Algaba F (1992) Desmoplastic small round-cell tumor. (Letter) Am J Surg Pathol 16: 306–308

417. Pratt JH, Shamblin WR (1970) Spontaneous rupture of endometrial cysts of the ovary presenting as an acute abdominal emergency. Am J Obstet Gynecol 108: 56–62

418. Prystowsky JB, Stryker SJ, Ujiki GT, Poticha SM (1988) Gastrointestinal endometriosis. Incidence and indications for resection. Arch Surg 123: 855–858

419. Pueblitz-Peredo S, Luevano-Flores E, Rincon-Taracena R, Ochoa-Carrillo FJ (1985) Uteruslike mass of the ovary: Endomyometriosis or congenital malformation? A case with a discussion of histogenesis. Arch Pathol Lab Med 109: 361–364

420. Punnonen R, Klemi PJ, Nikkanen V (1980) Postmenopausal endometriosis. Eur J Obstet Gynec Reprod Biol 11: 195–200

421. Qizilbash AH (1975) Mucoceles of the appendix. Their relationship to hyperplastic polyps, mucinous cystadenomas, and cystadenocarcinomas. Arch Pathol 99: 548–555

422. Quagliarello J, Coppa G, Bigelow B (1985) Isolated endometriosis in an inguinal hernia. Am J Obstet Gynecol 152: 688–689

423. Rahilly MA, Al-Nafusi A (1991) Uterus-like mass of the ovary associated with endometrioid carcinoma. Histopathology 18: 549–551

424. Raju U, Fine G, Greenawald KA, Ohorodnik JM (1989) Primary papillary serous neoplasia of the peritoneum: A clinicopathologic and ultrastructural study of eight cases. Hum Pathol 20: 426–436

425. Ranney B (1970) Endometriosis: II. Emergency operations due to hemoperitoneum. Obstet Gynecol 36: 437–442

426. Ranney B (1971) Endometriosis: IV. Hereditary tendency. Obstet Gynecol 37: 734–737

427. Ranney B (1980) Endometriosis: pathogenesis, symptoms and findings. Clin Obstet Gynecol 23: 865–874

428. Ransom DT, Shreyaskumar RP, Keeney GL, et al (1990) Papillary serous carcinoma of the peritoneum. A review of 33 cases treated with platin-based chemotherapy Cancer 66: 1091–1094

429. Ray J, Conger M, Ireland K (1985) Ureteral obstruction in postmenopausal woman with endometriosis. Urology 26: 577–578

430. Recalde AL, Majmudar B (1977) Endometriosis involving the femoral vein. South Med J 70: 69–74

431. Reddy CRRM, Venkateswar Rao D, Sarma ENB et al (1975) Granulomatous peritonitis due to Ascaris lumbricoides and its ova. J Trop Med Hyg 78: 146–149

432. Reddy P, Gorelick DF, Brasher CA, et al (1970) Progressive disseminated histoplasmosis as seen in adults. Am J Med 48: 629–636

433. Redwine DB (1987) Age-related evolution in color appearance of endometriosis. Fertil Steril 48: 1062–1063

434. Redwine DB (1987) The distribution of endometriosis in the pelvis by age groups and fertility. Fertil Steril 47: 173–175

435. Redwine DB (1989) Peritoneal pockets and endometriosis. Confirmation of an important relationship, with further observations. J Reprod Med 34: 270–272

436. Reich H, De Caprio J, McGlynn F, et al (1989) Peritoneal trophoblastic tissue implants after laparoscopic treatment of tubal ectopic pregnancy. Fertil Steril 52: 337

437. Reimnitz C, Brand E, Nieberg RK, et al (1988) Malignancy arising in endometrosis associated with unopposed estrogen replacement. Obstet Gynecol 71: 444–447

438. Riddel RH, Goodman MJ, Moossa AR (1981) Peritoneal malignant mesothelioma in a patient with recurrent peritonitis. Cancer 48: 134–139

439. Ridley JH, Edwards IK (1958) Experimental endometriosis in the human. Am J Obstet Gynecol 76: 783–790

440. Rigaud C, Bogomoletz WV (1983) Leiomyomatosis in pelvic lymph node. (Letter) Arch Pathol Lab Med 107: 153–154

441. Robb JA (1989) Mesothelioma versus adenocarcinoma: False-positive CEA and Leu-M1 staining due to hyaluronic acid. (Letter) Hum Pathol 20: 400

442. Rock JA, Parmley TH, King TM, et al (1981) Endometriosis and the development of tuboperitoneal fistulas after tubal ligation. Fertil Steril 35: 16–20

443. Roddick JW, Conkey G, Jacobs EJ (1960) The hormonal response of endometrium in endometriotic implants and its relationship to symptomatology. Am J Obstet Gynecol 79: 1173–1177

444. Rogers WS, Seckinger DL (1965) Decidual tissue as a cause of intraabdominal hemorrhage during labor. Obstet Gynecol 25: 391–397

445. Rohlfing MB, Kao KJ, Woodard BH (1981) Endomyometriosis: Possible association with leiomyomatosis disseminata and endometriosis. (Letter) Arch Pathol Lab Med 105: 556–557

446. Rosai J (1982) Uteruslike mass replacing ovary. (Letter) Arch Pathol Lab Med 106: 364

447. Rosai J, Dehner LP (1975) Nodular mesothelial hyperplasia in hernia sacs. A benign reactive condition stimulating a neoplastic process. Cancer 35: 165–175

448. Ross MJ, Welch WR, Scully RE (1989) Multilocular peritoneal inclusion cysts (so-called cystic mesotheliomas). Cancer 64: 1336–1346

449. Rossman F, D'Ablaing III G, Marrs RP (1983) Pregnancy complicated by ruptured endometrioma. Obstet Gynecol 62: 519–521

450. Roth LM (1973) Endometriosis with perineural involvement. Am J Clin Pathol 59: 807–809

451. Roth LM (1974) The Brenner tumor and the Walthard cell nest. An electron microscopic study. Lab Invest 31: 15–23

452. Rovati V, Faleschini E, Vercellini P, et al (1990) Endometrioma of the liver. Am J Obstet Gynecol 163: 1490–1492

453. Rubin IC, Lisa JR, Trinidad S (1956) Further observations on ectopic endometrium of the fallopian tube. Surg Gynecol Obstet 103: 469–474

454. Russell HB (1945) Decidual reaction of endometrium ectopic in an abdominal lymph node. Surg Gynecol Obstet 81: 218–220

455. Russell P (1979) The pathological assessment of ovarian neoplasms. II. The proliferating 'epithelial' tumours. Pathology 11: 251–282

456. Russell P, Laverty CR (1980) Benign 'mullerian' rests in pelvic lymph node. Pathology 12: 129–130

457. Russell P, Slavutin L, Laverty CR, et al (1979) Extrauterine mesodermal (müllerian) adenosarcoma. A case report. Pathology 11: 557–560

458. Rutgers JL, Scully RE (1988) Ovarian mullerian mucinous papillary cystadenomas of borderline malignancy. A clinicopathological analysis. Cancer 61: 340–348

459. Rutgers JL, Scully RE (1988) Ovarian mixed-epithelial papillary cystadenomas of borderline malignancy of mullerian type. A clinicopathological analysis. Cancer 61: 546–554

460. Rutgers JL, Young RH, Scully RE (1987) Ovarian yolk sac tumor arising from an endometrioid carcinoma. Hum Pathol 18: 1296–1299

461. Rutledge ML, Silva EG, McLemore D, El-Naggar A (1989) Serous surface carcinoma of the ovary and peritoneum. A flow cytometric study. Pathol Annu 24(2): 227–235

462. Sabatelle R, Winger E (1973) Postpartum intraabdominal hemorrhage caused by ectopic deciduosis. Obstet Gynecol 41: 873–875

462a. Sahin AA, Ro JY, Chen J, Ayala AG (1990) Spindle cell nodule and peptic ulcer arising in a fully developed gastric wall in a mature cystic teratoma. Arch Pathol Lab Med 114:529–531

463. Sampson JA (1927) Metastatic or embolic endometriosis, due to the menstrual dissemination of endometrial tissue into the venous circulation. Am J Pathol 3: 93–109

464. Sampson JA (1940) The development of the implantation theory for the origin of peritoneal endometriosis. Am J Obstet Gynecol 40: 549–557

465. Saw EC, Shields SJ, Comer TP, et al (1974) Granulomatous peritonitis due to coccidioides immitis. Arch Surg 108: 369–371

466. Saxen L, Kassinen A, Saxen E (1963) Peritoneal foreign-body reaction caused by condom emulsion. Lancet 1: 1295–1296

467. Sayfan J, Adam YG, Reif R (1979) Peritoneal encapsulation in childhood. Case report, embryologic analysis, and review of literature. Am J Surg 138: 725–727

468. Schatz JE, Colgan TJ (1991) Squamous metaplasia of the peritoneum. Arch Pathol Lab Med 115: 397–398

469. Schifrin BS, Erez S, Moore JG (1973) Teen-age endometriosis. Am J Obstet Gynecol 116: 973–980

470. Schmidt CL, Demopoulos RI, Weiss G (1981) Infected endometriotic cysts: Clinical characterization and pathogenesis. Fertil Steril 36: 27–30

471. Schneider V (1980) Benign glandular lymph node inclusions. Diagn Gynecol Obstet 2: 313–320

472. Schneider V, Partridge JR, Gutierrez F, et al (1983) Benign cystic mesothelioma involving the female genital tract: Report of four cases. Am J Obstet Gynecol 145: 355–359

473. Schneider V, Walsh JW, Goplerud DR (1980) Benign glandular inclusions in para-aortic lymph nodes: a cause for false positive lymphangiography. Am J Obstet Gynecol 138: 350–352

474. Schnurr RC, Delgado G, Chun B (1978) Benign glandular inclusions in para-aortic lymph nodes in women undergoing lymphadenectomies. Am J Obstet Gynecol 130: 813–816

475. Schrodt GR, Alcorn MO, Ibanez J (1980) Endometriosis of the male urinary system: A case report. J Urol 124: 722–723

476. Schwartz DA, Bellin HJ (1991) Liesegang rings developing within intraperitoneal endometriotic implants. A case report. J Reprod Med 36: 403–406

477. Schweppe KW, Dmowski WP, Wynn RM (1981) Ultrastructural changes in endometriotic tissue during danazol treatment. Fertil Steril 36: 20–26

478. Schweppe KW, Wynn RM (1981) Ultrastructural changes in endometriotic implants during the menstrual cycle. Obstet Gynecol 58: 465–473

479. Schweppe KW, Wynn RM (1984) Endocrine dependency of endometriosis: An ultrastructural study. Eur J Obstet Gynecol Reprod Biol 17: 193–208

480. Schweppe KW, Wynn RM, Beller FK (1984) Ultrastructural comparison of endometriotic implants and ectopic endometrium. Am J Obstet Gynecol 148: 1024–1037

481. Scott RB, Nowak RJ, Tindale RM (1958) Umbilical endometriosis and the Cullen sign. A study of lymphatic transport from pelvis to the umbilicus in monkeys. Obstet Gynecol 11: 556–563

482. Scott RB, Te Linde RW, Wharton LR (1953) Further studies on experimental endometriosis. Am J Obstet Gynecol 66: 1082–1103

483. Scott RB, Te Linde RW (1954) Clinical external endometriosis. Probable viability of menstrually shed fragments of endometrium. Obstet Gynecol 4: 502–510

484. Scott RB, Wharton LR (1957) The effect of estrone and progesterone on the growth of experimental endometriosis in rhesus monkeys. Am J Obstet Gynecol 74: 852–865

485. Scully RE (1981) Smooth-muscle differentiation in genital tract disorders. (Editorial) Arch Pathol Lab Med 105: 505–507

486. Scully RE, Richardson GS, Barlow JF (1966) The development of malignancy in endometriosis. Clin Obstet Gynecol 9: 384–411

486a. Seidman JD, Elsayed AM, Sobin LH, Tavassoli FA (1993) Association of mucinous tumors of the ovary and appendix. A clinicopathologic study of 25 cases. Am J Surg Pathol 17: 22–34

486b. Seidman JD, Oberer S, Bitterman P, Aisner SC (1993) Pathogenesis of pseudoxanthomatous salpingiosis. Mod Pathol 6: 53–55

487. Sensky TE, Liu DTY (1980) Endometriosis: Associations with menorrhagia, infertility and oral contraceptives. Int J Gynaecol Obstet 17: 573–576

488. Sesterhenn WL, Davis CJ, Mostofi EK (1987) Undifferentiated malignant epithelial tumors involving serosal surfaces of scrotum and abdomen in young males. J Urol 137: 214a (abstr)

489. Setrakian S, Gupta PK, Heald J, Brooks JJ (1992) Intraabdominal desmoplastic small round cell tumor. Report of a case diagnosed by fine needle aspiration cytology. Acta Cytol 36: 373–376

490. Sheibani K, Esteban JM, Bailey A, et al (1992) Immunopathologic and molecular studies as an aid to the diagnosis of malignant mesothelioma. Hum Pathol 23: 107–116

491. Sheibani K, Shin SS, Kezirian J, Weiss LM (1991) Ber-EP4 antibody as a discriminant in the differential diagnosis of malignant mesothelioma versus adenocarcinoma. Am J Surg Pathol 15: 779–784

492. Sheldon RS, Wilson RB, Dockerty MB (1967) Serosal endometriosis of fallopian tubes. Am J Obstet Gynecol 99: 882–884

493. Shen SC, Bansal M, Purrazzella R, et al (1983) Benign glandular inclusions in lymph nodes, endosalpingiosis, and salpingitis isthmica nodosa in a young girl with clear cell adenocarcinoma of the cervix. Am J Surg Pathol 7: 293–300

494. Shipton EA, Meares SD (1965) Heterotopic bone formation in the ovary. Aust NZ J Obstet Gynaecol 5: 100–102

495. Shiraki M, Otis CN, Powell JL (1991) Endometrial stromal sarcoma arising from ovarian and extraovarian endometriosis—report of two cases and review of the literature. Surg Pathol 4: 333–343

496. Sidaway MK, Silverberg SG (1987) Endosalpingiosis in female peritoneal washings: A diagnostic pitfall. Int J Gynecol Pathol 6: 340–346

497. Sieck JO, Cowgill R, Larkworthy W (1983) Peritoneal encapsulation and abdominal cocoon. Case report and review of the literature. Gastroenterology 84: 1597–1601

498. Sienkowski I, Russell AJ, Dilly SA, et al (1986) Peritoneal cystic mesothelioma: An electron microscopic and immunohistochemical study of two male patients. J Clin Pathol 39: 440–445

499. Silcocks PB, Herbert A, Wright DH (1986) Evaluation of PAS-diastase and carcinoembryonic antigen staining in the differential diagnosis of malignant mesothelioma and papillary serous carcinma of the ovary. J Pathol 149: 133–141

500. Silton RM (1979) More glandular inclusions. (Letter) Am J Surg Pathol 3: 285–286

501. Simpson JL, Elias S, Malinak LR, Buttram VC (1980) Heritable aspects of endometriosis. I. Genetic studies. Am J Obstet Gynecol 137: 327–331

502. Sinder C, Dochat GR, Wentsler NE (1965) Splenoendometriosis. Am J Obstet Gynecol 92: 883–884

503. Sjovall A, Akerman M (1968) Peritoneal granulomas in women due to the presence of enterobius S. oxyuris vermicularis. Acta Obstet Gynecol Scand 47: 361–372

504. Slutsky JN, Callahan D (1983) Endometriosis of the ureter can present as renal failure: A case report and review of endometriosis affecting the ureters. J Urol 130: 336–337

504a. Sneige N, Fanning CV (1992) Peritoneal washing cytology in women: Diagnostic pitfalls and clues for correct diagnosis. Diagn Cytopathol 8: 632–642

505. Sneige M, Fernandez T, Copeland LJ, et al (1986) Mullerian inclusions in peritoneal washings. Acta Cytol 30: 271–276

506. Sobel HJ, Marquet E, Schwarz R, Mazur MT (1984) Optically clear endometrial nuclei. Ultrast Pathol 6: 229–231

507. Sohar E, Gafni J, Pras M, et al (1967) Familial Mediterranean fever. A survey of 470 cases and review of the literature. Am J Med 43: 227–253

508. Solis OG, Bui HX, Malfetano JH, Ross JS (1991) Extragenital primary mixed malignant mesodermal tumor. Gynecol Oncol 43: 182–185

509. Soosay GN, Griffiths M, Papadaki L, et al (1991) The differential diagnosis of epithelial-type mesothelioma from adenocarcinoma and reactive mesothelial proliferation. J Pathol 163: 299–305

510. Spagnolo D, Whitaker D, Carrello S, et al (1991) The use of monoclonal antibody 44-3A6 in cell blocks in the diagnosis of lung carcinoma, carcinomas metastatic to lung and pleura, and pleural malignant mesothelioma. Am J Clin Pathol 95: 322–329

511. Stahl C, Grimes EM (1987) Endometriosis of the small bowel. Case reports and review of the literature. Obstet Gynecol Rev 42: 131–136

512. Stanley KE, Utz DC, Dockerty MB (1965) Clinically significant endometriosis of the urinary tract. Surg Gynecol Obstet 120: 491–498

513. Steck WD, Helwig EB (1966) Cutaneous endometriosis. Clin Obstet Gynecol 9: 373–383

514. Steele RW, Dmowski WP, Marmer DJ (1984) Immunologic aspects of human endometriosis. Am J Reprod Immunol 6: 33–36

515. Steinberg L, Rothman D, Drey NW (1970) Mullerian cyst of the retroperitoneum. Am J Obstet Gynecol 107: 963–964

516. Stern JL, Buscema J, Rosenshein NB, et al (1981) Spontaneous rupture of benign cystic teratomas. Obstet Gynecol 57: 365–366

517. Stirling JW, Henderson DW, Spagnolo DV, Whitaker D (1990) Unusual granular reactivity for carcinoembryonic antigen in malignant mesothelioma. (Letter) Hum Pathol 21: 678–679

518. Stock RJ (1982) Poltsalpingectomy endometriosis: A reassessment. Obstet Gynecol 60: 560–570

519. Stripling MC, Martin DC, Chatman DL, et al (1988) Subtle appearance of pelvic endometriosis. Fertil Steril 49: 427–431

520. Stripling MC, Martin DC, Poston WM (1988) Does endometriosis have a typical appearance? J Reprod Med 33: 879–884

521. Stuart GCE, Smith JP (1983) Ruptured benign cystic teratomas mimicking gynecologic malignancy. Gynecol Oncol 16: 139–143

522. Sun CJ, Toker C, Masi JD, et al (1979) Primary low grade adenocarcinoma occurring in the inguinal region. Cancer 44: 340–345

523. Surrey ES, Halme J (1989) Endometriosis as a cause of infertility. Obstet Gynecol Clin North Am 16: 79–91

524. Sussman J, Rosai J (1990) Lymph node metastasis as the initial manifestation of malignant mesothelioma. Report of six cases. Am J Surg Pathol 14: 818–828

525. Szlachter NB, Moskowitz J, Bigelow B, Weiss G (1980) Iatrogenic endometriosis: substantiation of the Sampson hypothesis. Obstet Gynecol 55: 52S–53S

526. Szpak CA, Soper JT, Thor A, et al (1989) Detection of adenocarcinoma in peritoneal washings by staining with monoclonal antibody B72.3. Acta Cytol 33: 205–214

527. Talerman A, Montero JR, Chilcote RR, Okagaki T (1985) Diffuse malignant peritoneal mesothelioma in a 13-year-old girl. Report of a case and review of the literature. Am J Surg Pathol 9: 73–80

528. Tamaya T, Motoyama T, Ohono Y, Ide N, Tsurusaki T, Okada H (1979) Steroid receptor levels and histology of endometriosis and adenomyosis. Fertil Steril 31: 396–400

529. Targan SR, Chow AW, Guze LB (1977) Role of anaerobic bacteria in spontaneous peritonitis of cirrhosis. Report of two cases and review of the literature. Am J Med 62: 397–403

530. Tavassoli FA, Norris HJ (1982) Peritoneal leiomyomatosis (leiomyomatosis peritonealis disseminata): A clinicopathologic study of 20 cases with ultrastructural observations. Int J Gynecol Pathol 1: 59–74

531. Tazelaar HD, Vareska G (1986) Benign glandular inclusions. Hum Pathol 17: 100–101

532. Teilum G, Madsen V (1950) Endometriosis ovarii et peritonaei caused by hysterosalpingography. Br J Obstet Gynaecol 57: 10–16

533. Telimaa S, Kauppila A, Ronnberg L, et al (1989) Elevated serum levels of endometrial secretory protein PP14 in patients with advanced endometriosis. Am J Obstet Gynecol 161: 866–871

534. Te Linde RW, Scott RB (1950) Experimental endometriosis. Am J Obstet Gynecol 60: 1147–1173

535. Teoh TB (1953) The structure and development of Walthard nests. J Pathol 66: 433–439

536. Thatcher SS, Grainger DA, True LD, DeCherney AH (1989) Pelvic trophoblastic implants after laparoscopic removal of a tubal pregnancy. Obstet Gynecol 74: 514–515

537. Thibodeau LL, Prioleau GR, Manuelidis EE, et al (1987) Cerebral endometriosis. J Neurosurg 66: 609–610

538. Tibboel D, Gaillard JLJ, Molenaar JC (1986) The importance of mesenteric vascular insufficiency in meconium peritonitis. Hum Pathol 17: 411–416

539. Tidman MJ, MacDonald DM (1988) Cutaneous endometriosis: A histopathologic study. J Am Acad Dermatol 18: 373–377

540. Tinker MA, Burdman D, Deysine M, et al (1974) Granulomatous peritonitis due to cellulose fibers from disposable surgical fabrics. Ann Surg 180: 831–835

541. Tobacman JK, Tucker MA, Kase R, Greene MH, Costa J,

Fraumeni JF Jr (1982) Intra-abdominal carcinomatosis after prophylactic oophorectomy in ovarian-cancer-prone families. Lancet 2: 795–797

542. Torkelson SJ, Lee RA, Hildahl DB (1988) Endometriosis of the sciatic nerve: A report of two cases and a review of the literature. Obstet Gynecol 71: 473

543. Trimble EL, Saigo PE, Freeberg GW, Rubin SC, Hoskins WJ (1991) Peritoneal sarcoidosis and elevated CA 125. Obstet Gynecol 78: 976–977

544. Tron V, Wright JL, Churg A (1987) Carcinoembryonic antigen and milk-fat globule protein staining of malignant mesothelioma and adenocarcinoma of the lung. Arch Pathol Lab Med 111: 291–293

545. Truong LD, Maccato ML, Awalt H, et al (1990) Serous surface carcinoma of the peritoneum: A clinicopathologic study of 22 cases. Hum Pathol 21: 99–110

546. Tutschka BG, Lauchlan SC (1980) Endosalpingiosis. Obstet Gynecol 55: 57S–60S

547. Ulbright TM, Kraus FT (1981) Endometrial stromal tumors of extra-uterine tissue. Am J Clin Pathol 76: 371–377

548. Ulbright TM, Morley DJ, Roth LM, et al (1983) Papillary serous carcinoma of the retroperitoneum. Am J Clin Pathol 79: 633–637

549. Valente PT (1984) Leiomyomatosis peritonealis disseminata. A report of two cases and review of the literature. Arch Pathol Lab Med 108: 669–672

550. Variend S, Gerrard M, Norris PD, Goepel JR (1991) Intra-abdominal neuroectodermal tumour of childhood with divergent differentiation. Histopathology 18: 45–51

551. Veiga-Ferreira MM, Leiman G, Dunbar F, Margolius KA (1987) Cervical endometriosis: Facilitated diagnosis by fine needle aspiration cytologic testing. Am J Obstet Gynecol 157: 849–856

552. Vernon MW, Beard JS, Graves K, Wilson EA (1986) Classification of endometriotic implants by morphologic appearance and capacity to synthesize prostaglandin F. Fertil Steril 46:801–806

553. Vierikko P, Kauppila A, Ronnberg L, Vihko R (1985) Steroidal regulation of endometriosis tissue: Lack of induction of 17-beta-hydroxysteroid dehydrogenase activity by progesterone, medroxyprogesterone acetate, or danazol. Fertil Steril 43: 218–224

554. von Numers C (1965) Observations on metaplastic changes in the germinal epithelium of the ovary and on the aetiology of ovarian endometriosis. Acta Obstet Gynecol Scand 44: 107–116

555. Vuong PN, Guyot H, Moulin G, et al (1990) Pseudotumoral organization of a twisted epiploic fringe or 'hard-boiled egg' in the peritoneal cavity. Arch Pathol Lab Med 114: 531–533

556. Wallace S, Sabto J, Pedersen J, Gurr FW (1992) Peritoneal sclerosis in CAPD. Pathology 24: 4 (abstr)

557. Walton LA (1977) A reexamination of endometriosis after pregnancy. J Reprod Med 19: 341–344

558. Wanless IR, Bernier V (1983) Fibrous thickening of the splenic capsule. Arch Pathol Lab Med 107: 595–599

559. Warnock ML, Stoloff A, Thor A (1988) Differentiation of adenocarcinoma of the lung from mesothelioma. Periodic acid-Schiff, monoclonal antibodies B72.3, and Leu M1. Am J Pathol 133: 30–38

560. Watson NE Jr, Johnson AH (1973) Cryptococcal peritonitis. Southern Med J 66: 387–388

561. Watson WJ, Sundwall DA, Benson WL (1982) Splenosis mimicking endometriosis. Obstet Gynecol 59: 51S–53S

562. Waxman M, Boyce JG (1976) Intraperitoneal rupture of benign cystic ovarian teratoma. Obstet Gynecol 48: 9S–13S

563. Weed JC, Ray JE (1987) Endometriosis of the bowel. Obstet Gynecol 69: 727–730

564. Weibel MA, Majno G (1973) Peritoneal adhesions and their relation to abdominal surgery. Am J Surg 126: 345–353

565. Weinstein MP, Iannini PB, Stratton CW, et al (1978) Spontaneous bacterial peritonitis. A review of 28 cases with emphasis on improved survival and factors influencing prognosis. Am J Med 64: 592–598

566. Weir JH, Janovski NA (1963) Paramesonephric lymph-node inclusions—a cause of obstructive uropathy. Obstet Gynecol 21: 363–367

567. Weiss SW, Tavassoli FA (1988) Multicystic mesothelioma: An analysis of pathologic findings and biologic behavior in 37 cases. Am J Surg Pathol 12: 737–746

568. Wheeler JM (1989) Epidemiology of endometriosis-associated infertility. J Reprod Med 34: 41–46

569. Whitaker D, Shilkin KB (1984) Diagnosis of pleural malignant mesothelioma in life—a practical approach. J Pathol 143: 147–175

570. White PF, Merino MJ, Barwick KW (1985) Serous surface papillary carcinoma of the ovary: A clinical, pathologic, ultrastructural, and immunohistochemical study of 11 cases. Pathol Annu 20(1): 403–418

571. Wick MR, Loy T, Mills SE, et al (1990) Malignant epithelioid pleural mesothelioma versus peripheral pulmonary adenocarcinoma: A histochemical, ultrastructural, and immunohistologic study of 103 cases. Hum Pathol 21: 759–766

572. Wick MR, Mills SE, Dehner LP, et al (1989) Serous papillary carcinomas arising from the peritoneum and ovaries. A clinicopathologic and immunohistochemical comparison. Int J Gynecol Pathol 8: 179–188

573. Wick MR, Mills SE, Swanson PE (1990) Expression of "myelomonocytic" antigens in mesotheliomas and adenocarcinomas involving the serosal surfaces. Am J Clin Pathol 94: 18–26

574. Wild RA, Hirisave V, Podczaski ES, et al (1991) Autoantibodies associated with endometriosis: Can their detection predict presence of the disease? Obstet Gynecol 77: 927–931

575. Wilhelm JL, Scommegna A (1977) Catamenial pneumothorax. Bilateral occurrence while on suppressive therapy. Obstet Gynecol 50: 227–231

576. Williams GA (1969) Endometriosis of the cervix uteri—a common disease. Am J Obstet Gynecol 80: 734–741

577. Williams GT (1987) The peritoneum. In: Morson BC (ed) Alimentary Tract. Systemic Pathology, Vol 3. New York, Churchill Livingstone, pp 417–450

578. Williams PP, Gall SA, Prem KA (1971) Ectopic mucinous cystadenoma. A case report. Obstet Gynecol 38: 831–837

579. Williams TJ, Pratt JH (1977) Endometriosis in 1,000 consecutive celiotomies: Incidence and management. Am J Obstet Gynecol 129: 245–250

580. Wolf GC, Singh KB (1989) Cesarean scar endometriosis: A review. Obstet Gynecol Surv 44: 89–95

581. Wolfe SA, Mackles A, Greene HJ (1961) Endometriosis of the cervix. Am J Obstet Gynecol 8: 111–123

582. Wong M, Rosen SW (1962) Ascites in sarcoidosis due to peritoneal involvement. Ann Intern Med 57: 277–280

583. Wurster KH, Leu HJ (1972) Zur frage der hamatogenen Ausbreitung der Endometriose. Geburtsh Frauenheilk 32: 983–986

584. Wynn TE (1971) Endometriosis of the sigmoid colon. Massive intramural hematoma. Arch Pathol Lab Med 92: 24–27

585. Yoonessi M, Satchindanand SK, Ortinez CG, et al (1982) Benign glandular elements and decidual reaction in retroperitoneal lymph nodes. J Surg Oncol 19: 81–86

586. Young EE, Gamble CN (1969) Primary adenocarcinoma of the rectovaginal septum arising from endometriosis. Report of a case. Cancer 24: 597–601

587. Young RH, Clement PB, McCaughey ET (1990) Solitary fibrous tumors ("fibrous mesotheliomas") of the peritoneum: A report of three cases. Arch Pathol Lab Med 114: 493–495

588. Young RH, Eichhorn JH, Dickersin GR, Scully RE (1992) Ovarian involvement by the intra-abdominal desmoplastic small round cell tumor with divergent differentiation: A report of three cases. Hum Pathol 23: 454–464

589. Young RH, Gilks CB, Scully RE (1991) Mucinous tumors of the appendix associated with mucinous tumors of the ovary and pseudomyxoma peritonei. A clinicopathological analysis of 22 cases supporting an origin in the appendix. Am J Surg Pathol 15: 415–429

590. Young RH, Prat J, Scully RE (1984) Endometrioid stromal sarcomas of the ovary. A clinicopathologic analysis of 23 cases. Cancer 53: 1143–1155

591. Young RH, Scully RE (1986) Testicular and paratesticular tumors and tumor-like lesions of ovarian common epithelial and mullerian types. A report of four cases and review of the literature. Am J Clin Pathol 86: 146–152

592. Zaytsev P, Taxy JB (1987) Pregnancy-associated ectopic decidua. Am J Surg Pathol 11: 526–530

593. Zinsser KR, Wheeler JE (1982) Endosalpingiosis in the omentum. A study of autopsy and surgical material. Am J Surg Pathol 6: 109–117

Surface Epithelial–Stromal Tumors of the Ovary

Peter Russell, M.D., B.Sc. (Med.), F.R.C.P.A.

Classification

The ovaries do not arise from the müllerian ducts, yet they are commonly the site of a range of neoplasms seen elsewhere in the müllerian duct derivatives. These loosely associated, principally epithelial, neoplasms are generally accepted as originating from the surface epithelium (modified mesothelium) and subjacent stroma of the ovaries. In the second version of the World Health Organization (WHO) classification of ovarian tumors, these neoplasms are designated as *surface epithelial–stromal tumors*. The epithelial elements resemble those within tumors found in the fallopian tubes, uterus, cervix, and upper vagina. Transitional cell (formerly Brenner) tumors, as well as those mucinous tumors of "intestinal" differentiation, are retained in a classification of best fit. For practical reasons, pure müllerian mesenchymal tumors are noted briefly in this chapter, completing the spectrum that traditionally has encompassed endometrioid stromal sarcomas and malignant mixed müllerian tumors. Their approximate relative frequencies are shown in Table 18.1.

Five broad epithelial categories of tumors exist in this group, based on epithelial differentiation (serous, muci-

Table 18.1. Approximate relative (%) frequencies of surface epithelial–stromal tumors

| | Noninvasive | | | |
	Benign %	Atypically proliferating %	Invasive carcinomas %	Total %
Serous	23	7	16	46
Mucinous	29.5	5	2	36.5
Endometrioid	Rare	1.5	6	7.5
Mesenchymal and mixed	Rare	Rare	0.7	0.7
Clear cell	Rare	Rare	3	3
Transitional (Brenner)	2	Rare	Rare	2
Squamous[a]	Rare	—	Rare	Rare
Mixed epithelial	1.5	0.5	0.5	2.5
Undifferentiated carcinomas	—	—	1.5	1.5
Unclassified epithelial	Rare	Rare	0.3	0.3
Total	56.0	14.0	30.0	100.0

[a] Squamous cell neoplasms of nonteratomatous origin.

nous, endometrioid, clear cell, and transitional or Brenner). Mixed or intermediate patterns are common at both architectural and cellular levels. This is not because of serendipitous or random post-transformation differentiation. Considering them as a single (müllerian) neoplastic spectrum has led to blurring of what are, in all probability, well-defined and distinct neoplastic entities, with their own patterns of metastasis, pathological correlates, therapeutic responses, and clinical outcomes. For example, virtually all primary mucinous ovarian carcinomas are of "intestinal" rather than endocervical (müllerian) type. Malignant Brenner tumors/transitional cell carcinomas share much in common with carcinomas of the urinary tract. There is strong circumstantial evidence to support the proposition that it is probably serosal inclusions, surface proliferations, metaplasias, or heterotopias that manifest the müllerian potential of the surface "epithelium" of the ovaries. Accordingly, it is this process that dictates the relative frequency and histological range of some of the epithelial and related mesenchymal tumors seen in the ovaries as well as in other sites in the female pelvis and abdomen, such as the broad ligaments.[198] The most common and important of these surface proliferations are serous (endosalpingiosis) and endometrioid (endometriosis) in type.[149] It is less clear whether such a concept extends to the mesenchymal and nonmüllerian (e.g., transitional and mucinous) epithelial neoplasms. Tumors homologous to those noted above have been reported rarely in testicular and paratesticular tissues in men.[15,289]

The spectrum of proliferative change these tumors exhibit is divided arbitrarily into three categories according to recommendations of both the International Federation of Gynecology and Obstetrics (FIGO) and WHO. The surface epithelial–stromal ovarian tumors are thus subgrouped into benign, atypically proliferating ("borderline," "of low malignant potential") and malignant categories. The intermediate group of atypically proliferating tumors are defined as exhibiting greater cellular proliferation than that encountered in the benign form of the same type of tumor, but showing no destructive invasion of the stromal component.[230] The criteria that are currently advocated to distinguish these atypically proliferating tumors from their strictly benign counterparts are ill-defined at best. A tumor qualifies for inclusion in the intermediate group if any two of the following criteria are present to a *significant* degree[207]:

1. *epithelial budding:* epithelial cell proliferation, usually in the form of small papillae but without connective tissue cores, and with a tendency for single cells or cell clusters to detach into the cyst lumen
2. *multilayering of epithelium:* stratification of epithelial cells covering papillae or lining glandular spaces or the presence of solid morules of cells where a single layered epithelium is usual in the corresponding benign tumor
3. *mitotic activity:* an increase over the very low mitotic activity of benign tumors or, in the case of mucinous tumors, an alteration in distribution of mitoses
4. *nuclear atypia:* an increase in nuclear/cytoplasmic ratio, alterations in nuclear chromatin pattern, abnormalities of size, shape, and number of nucleoli.

These criteria are not uniformly applicable to all surface epithelial–stromal ovarian tumors. For example, the first two are more important in serous tumors whereas the last two are applied more easily to mucinous lesions. Although there are no published quantitative parameters to define the boundary between benign and atypically proliferating tumors, it is suggested that 10% of the available histological material showing proliferation is a reasonable minimum.

The original reason for delineating the so-called borderline or low malignant potential group of ovarian epithelial tumors was to explain the remarkably good prognosis in women with serous ovarian tumors showing pathological features suggesting malignancy[260,261] and evidence, at laparotomy, of apparent widespread metastases. It is a valid contention, although not yet proved fact, that most extraovarian manifestations of these neoplasms result from widespread multifocal in situ neoplasia arising from peritoneal serous inclusions (endosalpingiosis) and corresponding to part of the same neoplastic spectrum that has been delineated in the ovaries.[149,210] Consequently, the general term, *atypically proliferating surface epithelial–stromal tumor,*[221] which carries the connotation of "atypical hyperplasia," "premalignant atypia," "adenocarcinoma in situ" or "ovarian intraepithelial neoplasia"[287] superimposed on a benign epithelial tumor is preferable to "of low malignant potential" or "of borderline malignancy."[231,299] Pathological discussion of individual tumors in the following sections reflects this approach, grouping tumors that histologically show atypical proliferation into a noninvasive (?preinvasive) category with benign tumors as one would do for tumors of the other major organ systems of the body.

The critical point of discrimination in this neoplastic continuum, therefore, is between atypically proliferating tumors and frank carcinomas as defined by the presence or absence of destructive stromal invasion. Genuine destructive invasion must be distinguished from the plethora of patterns generated by pseudoinvasion or benign intrusion of the stromal component in cystic tumors and the increasingly complex proliferative pattern of glands in solid (adenofibromatous) tumors. The problem is least difficult in serous tumors and greater in mucinous and endometrioid lesions, although destructive invasion, an ill-defined concept, is not even constant in cases of serous carcinoma. This is a perceptual rather than a conceptual difficulty and, in well-differentiated tumors, many sections may be necessary to appreciate the focal alterations that herald the progression to invasive carcinoma. Pathologists should pay particular attention to the following histological features in identifying areas of invasion:

1. in mostly cystic tumors (e.g., serous and mucinous) changes in architectural contour at the epithelial/stromal interface of the tumor from broad front to tentacular with polymorphic epithelial structures projecting into the stroma; in mainly adenofibromatous tumors (e.g., endometrioid and clear cell) a haphazard arrangement of irregular-sized and -shaped glandular structures. Such changes represent a true qualitative change in the orientation of epithelial elements to each other. By contrast, within atypically proliferating tumors, there is merely a relative increase of epithelial elements (crowding or complexity) but within an architectural configuration similar to that seen in the equivalent benign tumor

2. alteration in the character of the tumor stroma from hypercellular, fibrous, or hyalinized stroma to reactive immature stroma with dilated thin-walled sinusoidal vessels, resembling reparative granulation tissue, so-called desmoplasia

3. inflammatory cell infiltrates, although more frequently present in frank carcinomas, are poor discriminators of stromal invasion.

General Features

Surface epithelial–stromal tumors of the ovaries account for about 60% of all ovarian neoplasms and 80–90% of primary ovarian malignancies.[130,143] They rarely occur before puberty, and in this age group most are benign or atypically proliferating tumors.[168] The mean age of patients with benign epithelial tumors is 45 years and 50 years for those with atypically proliferating neoplasms. Malignant (frankly invasive) epithelial tumors are uncommon under 40 years of age. Most occur in the peri- and postmenopausal age group (mean age, 55 years), a pattern similar to that for breast and endometrial carcinomas. A variety of risk factors have been delineated, including environmental and genetic factors and events of reproductive life. These are addressed in the excellent reviews of Smith and Oi,[245] Heintz et al.,[113] and the Collaborative Ovarian Cancer group.[106,277–279]

Müllerian epithelial and mesenchymal ovarian tumors do not produce specific symptoms. As they grow, local symptoms relating to size and weight such as urinary frequency, constipation, and a sense of pelvic "heaviness" may be experienced. Larger or more rapidly growing tumors present with pelvic or lower abdominal pain or swelling in one-half of cases, abnormal uterine bleeding in one-third, gastrointestinal symptoms (such as dyspepsia, nausea, cramps, diarrhea) in 20%, and weight loss and urinary symptoms slightly less frequently. Acute abdominal symptoms caused by rupture, torsion, or hemorrhage are uncommon with benign and rare with malignant tumors. In addition, a plethora of unusual paraneoplastic syndromes occasionally may draw the clinician's attention to the ovarian mass.[212]

Principles of Staging and Management

The diagnosis and characterization of ovarian tumors ultimately depends on histological examination of tissue specimens. FIGO staging (Table 18.2) of the atypically proliferating and invasive malignant tumors is based on clinical and laparotomy findings. This includes the final histological typing and grading as well as cytological evaluation of peritoneal washings or ascitic fluid. Assessment of tumor tissue removed at laparotomy for DNA ploidy and cell cycle studies,[93,196] estrogen and progesterone receptor levels,[228] and tumor markers[45,123] offer additional prognostic data and the pathologist should be aware of the requirements of these techniques. It has been standard practice for some time to remove the omentum as part of both staging and primary therapy of ovarian epithelial tumors. More recently, excision of peritoneal lesions and biopsy of subdiaphragmatic tissue, pelvic peritoneum, and retroperitoneal lymph nodes have been added to the surgical staging procedures.[52] The pelvic and/or para-aortic lymph nodes contain tumor metastases in about 25% of carcinomas in Stage I, 50% in Stage II, and 75% in Stages III and IV.[40]

Primary management of surface epithelial–stromal ovarian tumors is surgical removal. This is adequate for benign tumors and most atypically proliferating neoplasms.[47,53] Intraoperative frozen section plays a crucial role in our institution in the exclusion of invasive carcinoma when preservation of fertility is desirable and conservative sur-

Table 18.2. 1988 protocol of FIGO staging of surface epithelial–stromal tumors,[10] based on clinical examination and surgical exploration

Stage I: Growth limited to the ovaries
   Stage Ia: Growth limited to one ovary; no ascites
      1. No tumor on the external surface; capsule intact
      2. Tumor present on external surface and/or capsule ruptured
   Stage Ib: Growth limited to both ovaries; no ascites
      1. No tumor on the external surface; capsules intact
      2. Tumor present on external surface and/or capsule(s) ruptured
   Stage Ic: Tumor either Stage Ia or Stage Ib, but with ascites [a] present or positive peritoneal washings
Stage II: Growth involving one or both ovaries with pelvic extension
   Stage IIa: Extension and/or metastases to uterus and/or tubes
   Stage IIb: Extension to other pelvic tissues
   Stage IIc: Tumor either Stage IIa or Stage IIb, but with ascites[a] present or positive peritoneal washings
Stage III: Growth involving one or both ovaries with intraperitoneal metastases outside the pelvis and/or positive retroperitoneal nodes
   Tumor limited to the true pelvis with histologically proved malignant extension to small bowel or omentum
Stage IV: Growth involving one or both ovaries with distant metastases
   If pleural effusion is present, there must be positive cytology to allot a case to Stage IV
   Parenchymal liver metastases equals Stage IV
Special category: Unexplored cases that are thought to be ovarian carcinoma

[a] Ascites is peritoneal effusion, which in the opinion of the surgeon is pathological and/or clearly exceeds normal amounts.
Final histology after surgery is to be considered in the staging, as well as cytology as far as effusions are concerned.
FIGO, International Federation of Gynecology and Obstetrics.

gery is planned. The proper place of radiotherapy in the management of ovarian cancer has not been established, and multiagent adjuvant chemotherapy is the preferred therapy for most müllerian ovarian carcinomas. These neoplasms are more aggressive than sex cord–stromal tumors and less amenable to therapy than malignant germ cell tumors. During the follow-up of a patient being treated for ovarian carcinoma, histological or cytological analysis of recurrent disease may be sought from tissue specimens obtained at a so-called second-look laparotomy. Familiarity with the vagaries of this determination is desirable.[59,187,192] Autopsy examination is all too frequently the final exposure of the pathologist to the patient with ovarian carcinoma and adherence to a full standard autopsy protocol can still yield useful information.[81]

Serous Tumors

Benign Serous Tumors

GENERAL FEATURES

Benign serous tumors are common, accounting for about one-quarter of all benign ovarian neoplasms and 50–70% of all ovarian serous tumors. Although encountered at any age, they show a peak incidence in the fourth and fifth decades. They are bilateral in 12–20% of all cases,[63,207,230] but more so in elderly patients. Apparently unilateral tumors may be associated with very small or indeed microscopic cortical adenofibromas in the contralateral ovary. Rarely, benign tumors are associated with extraovarian epithelial inclusions of serous type.[30,207]

GROSS FINDINGS

Three basic patterns are encountered: cystic, papillary, and adenofibromatous. Cysts are filled with clear watery (serous) fluid, occasionally thin mucoid material, and only rarely the thick mucus more typical of mucinous tumors. External surfaces of the thin-walled cysts are smooth and glistening, often with a marked vascular pattern. Most cystic tumors are unilocular but multilocular forms occur, and they vary in size up to 30 cm in diameter (mean, 10 cm). Small papillary projections arising from the ovarian surface and serosal inclusion cysts are common, so it is suggested that serous neoplasms be diagnosed only if the tumor is greater than 1 cm in diameter. Cyst linings are either entirely flat or have focal, grossly visible coarse papillary projections (Fig. 18.1). Such papillary excrescences rarely cover the entire inner surface of benign serous cysts. Whenever this occurs, differentiation from an atypically proliferating tumor is difficult. The presence of coarse, less friable, and more gelatinous or fibrous papillae suggests a benign tumor (Fig. 18.2). Papillary structures may also be present on the external surface of the cyst. The third (adenofibromatous) variant is a solid neoplasm composed of tough, rubbery fibrous tissue (Fig. 18.3) with interspersed glandular spaces of various sizes. All variations in gross appearances are due to the relative prominence, in a given lesion, between these three growth patterns.

MICROSCOPIC FINDINGS

The dominant architectural and cellular features of these tumors are due to the tendency of the epithelium to display fine papillary structures and for the epithelial cells to re-

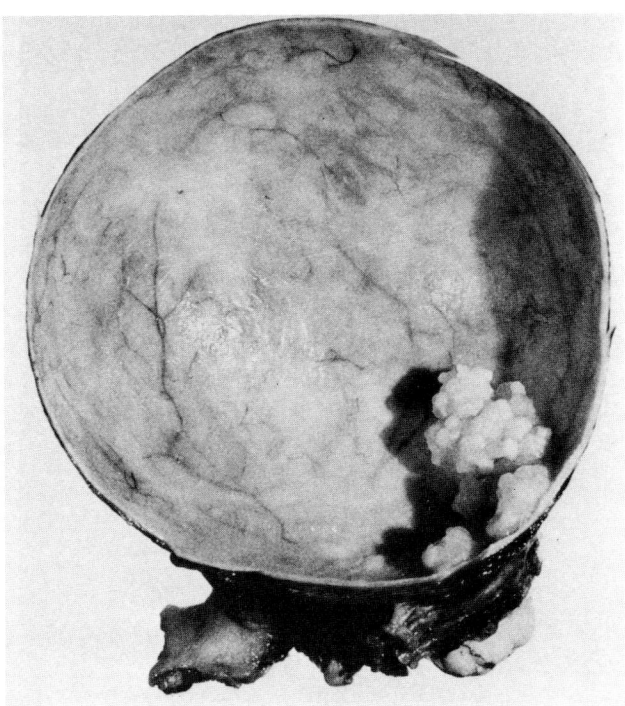

FIG. 18.1. **Benign cystic serous tumor.** A small papillary component is present within the lumen.

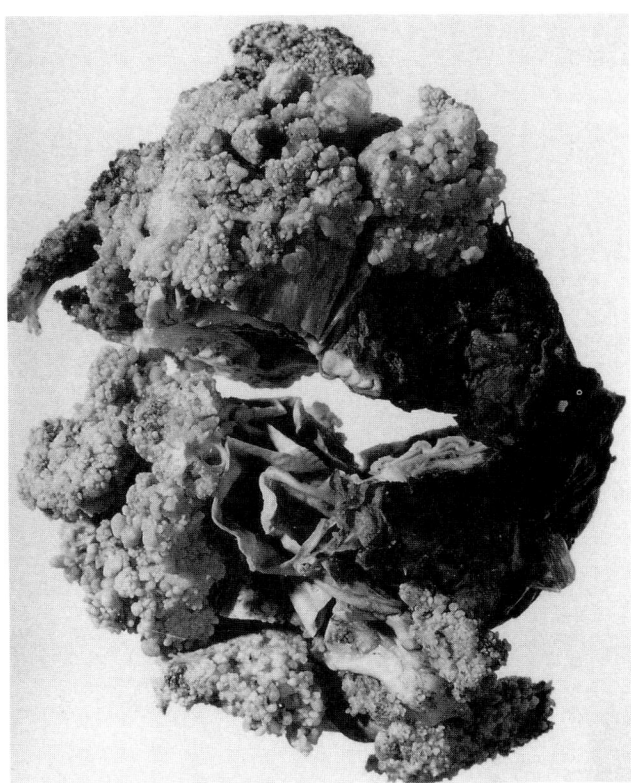

FIG. 18.2. **Benign serous surface papilloma.** Coarse gelatinous papillae are present on the surface.

semble those of the native fallopian tube mucosa. Less commonly, the epithelium resembles the cuboidal surface epithelium of the ovaries. Some cells produce mucin, which is mostly extracellular; the apical cell border shows diastase resistant periodic acid-Schiff (PAS) and mucicarmine-positive glycocalyx. Obvious intracellular mucin should suggest a diagnosis other than ovarian serous tumor.

Architecturally, these tumors are composed of relatively thin-walled cysts (Fig. 18.4), papillary structures (Fig. 18.5), or glandular spaces embedded in fibrous stroma (Fig. 18.6)—often a combination of these patterns. A complex papillary pattern is within the accepted spectrum (Fig. 18.7). Epithelium lining cysts and papillae is often a single layer of regular flattened to cuboidal cells with uniform basal nuclei, or is pseudostratified and tubal in type, with the characteristic elongated (secretory cell) or rounded (ciliated cell) nuclei. This epithelium may show morphologic changes analogous to those of the endosalpingeal mucosa during different phases of the menstrual cycle, including secretory change with tall columnar vacuolated or even clear cells. Secretory and ciliated cells may occur in patches and height difference between these two cell types may be quite marked and cause unevenness of the free epithelial border (Fig. 18.8). This should not be mistaken for atypical proliferation. In large cysts the epithelium may become attenuated because of pressure. Mitoses are rarely seen and nuclear atypia is absent. Rounded

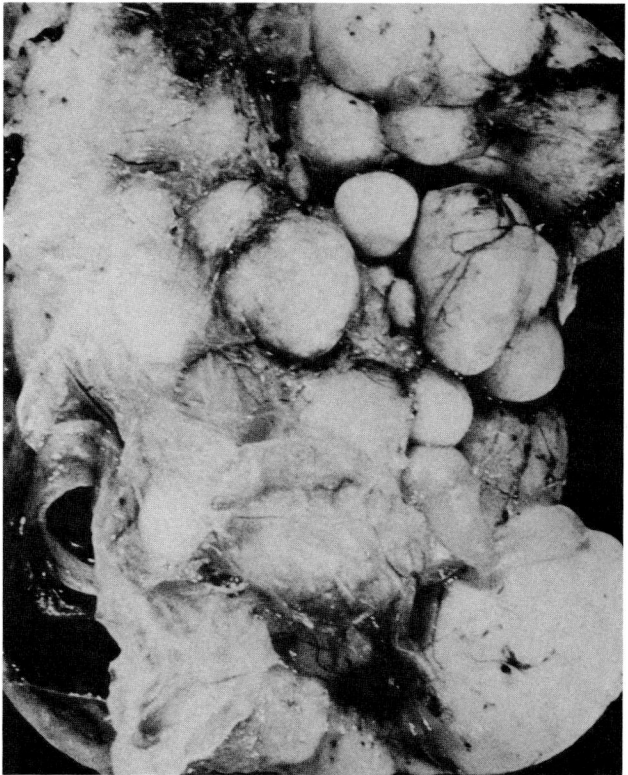

FIG. 18.3. **Benign serous adenofibroma.** The tumor has a complex bosselated surface.

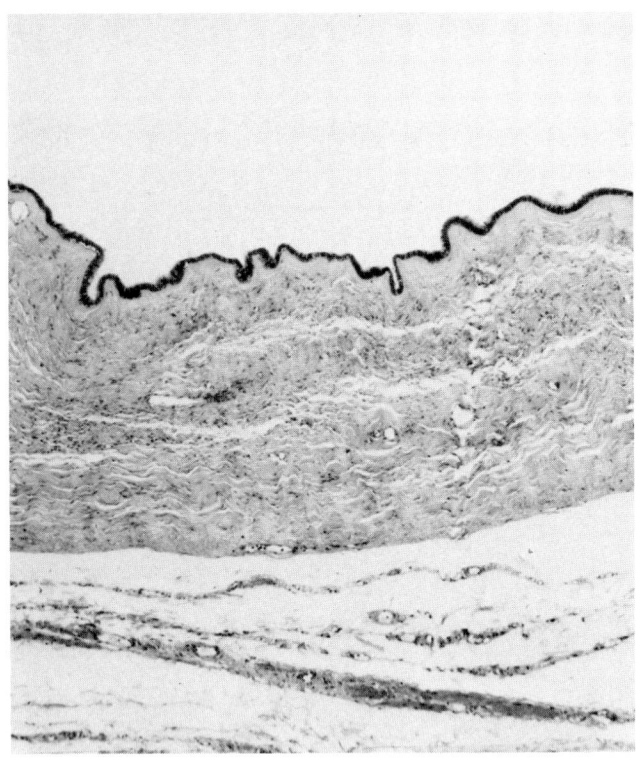

FIG. 18.4. **Benign serous cyst.** A single-layered epithelium covers a dense fibrous tissue wall.

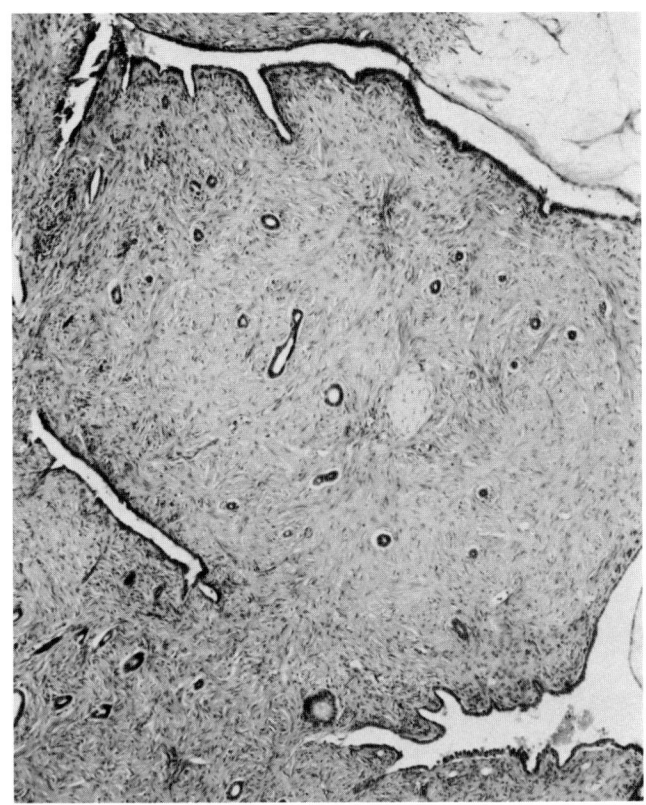

FIG. 18.6. **Benign serous adenofibroma.** Small slit-like or gland-like spaces lie in dense ovarian stroma.

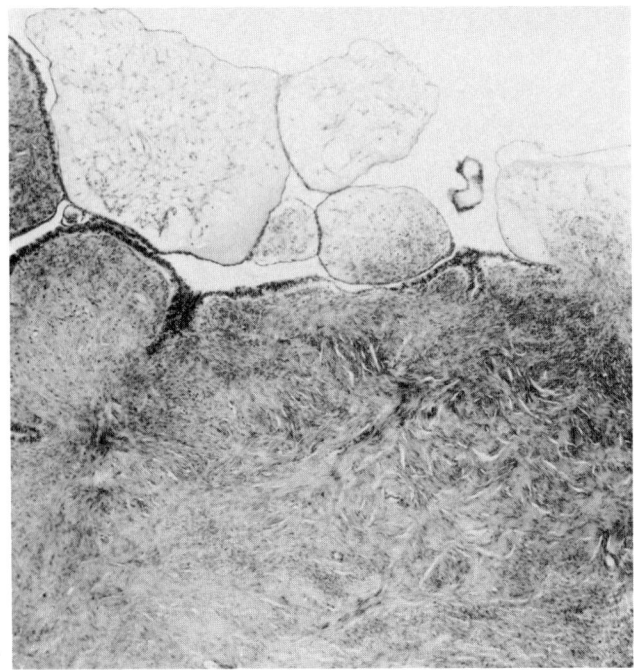

18.5a

FIG. 18.5a. **Benign papillary serous tumor.** Papillary excrescences may (**a**) line large cysts or (**b**) fill smaller cyst-like spaces. Psammoma bodies are prominent in the latter.

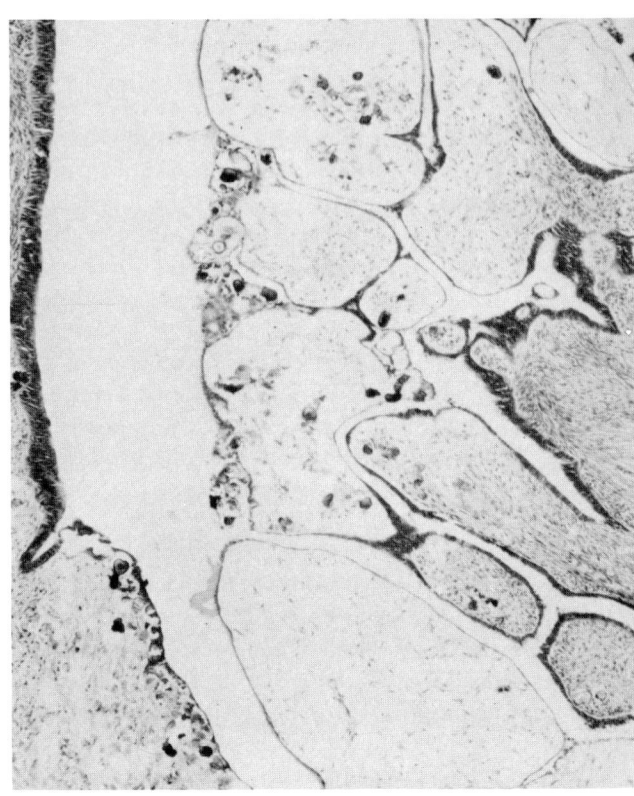

18.5b

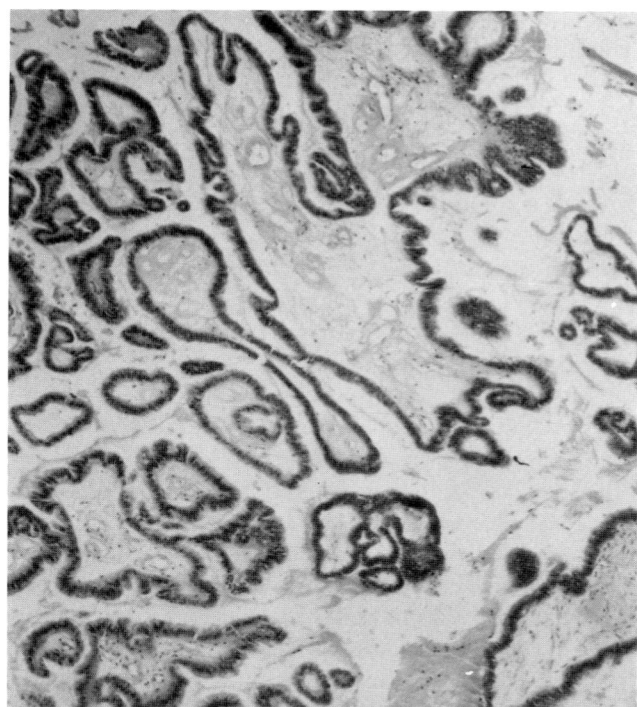

FIG. 18.7. Benign papillary serous cystadenoma. The tumor has a complex papillary pattern. The single layer of cells distinguishes such areas from atypical epithelial proliferation.

microscopic calcifications, psammoma bodies, are presentin the stroma of about 15% of benign serous tumors (Fig. 18.5b), but they are not specific diagnostic features because they can be found occasionally in nonneoplastic fallopian tube mucosa as well as other müllerian and non-müllerian tumors.

Tumor stroma varies from highly cellular and fibrous to almost acellular hyalinized tissue with marked stromal edema a common finding. There is typically a narrow, acellular zone between the epithelial cells and cellular fibrous stroma of the papillae or cyst wall that is thought to be analogous to a similar zone in the cortex of normal ovaries.[65] Granular eosinophilic pseudoxanthoma cells beneath the epithelium are a common finding (Fig. 18.9), and when prominent may produce *ceroid granulomas.*[6] The light brown pigment such cells contain is ceroid (lipofuscin), not hemosiderin, and these changes should not be misinterpreted as endometriosis. Stromal fatty degeneration has been noted in cyst walls.

Benign serosal inclusions (endosalpingiosis) that are found occasionally on the surface of the pelvic viscera or omentum in association with benign tumors exhibit the same epithelial characteristics as the ovarian tumors (Fig. 18.10), including papilla formation and psammoma bodies. They have no prognostic significance for the patient.

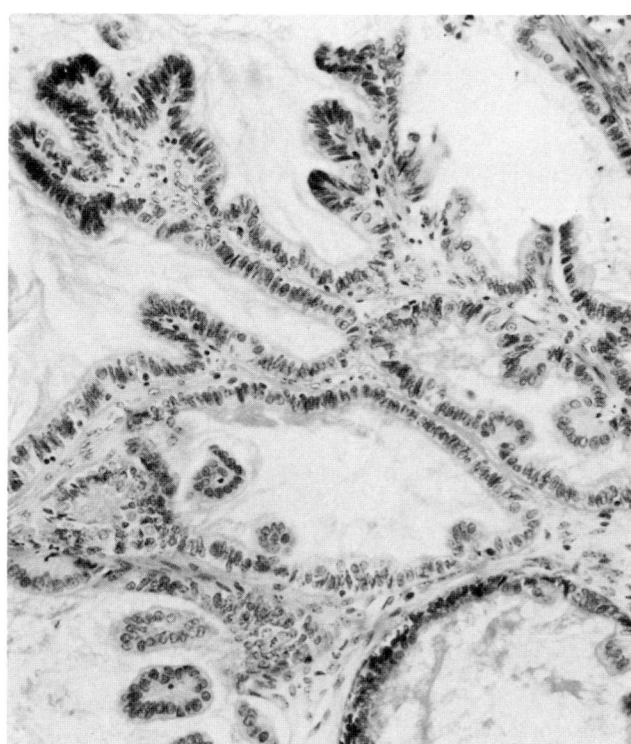

FIG. 18.8. Benign papillary serous cystadenoma. Epithelium is tubal in type with patches of secretory and ciliated cells. The latter form small, fan-like projections.

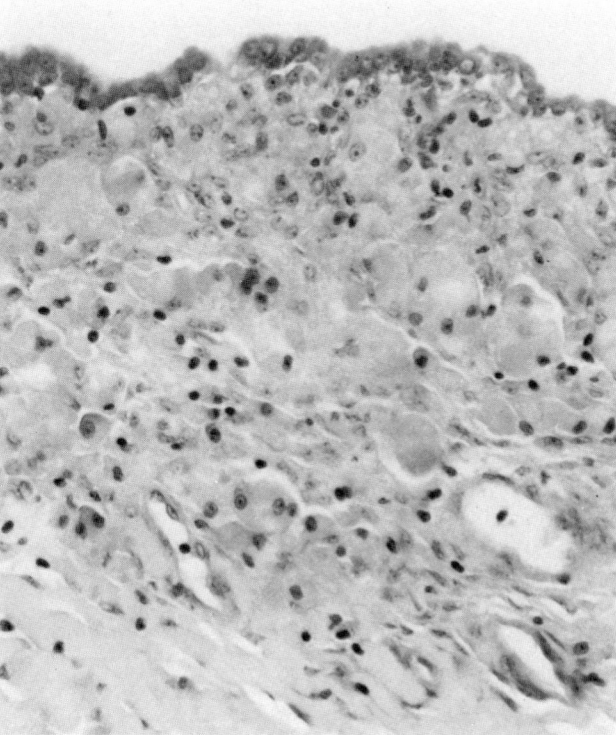

FIG. 18.9. Benign serous cystadenoma. Pseudoxanthomatous area beneath otherwise typical serous epithelium. These large foamy cells contain ceroid pigment.

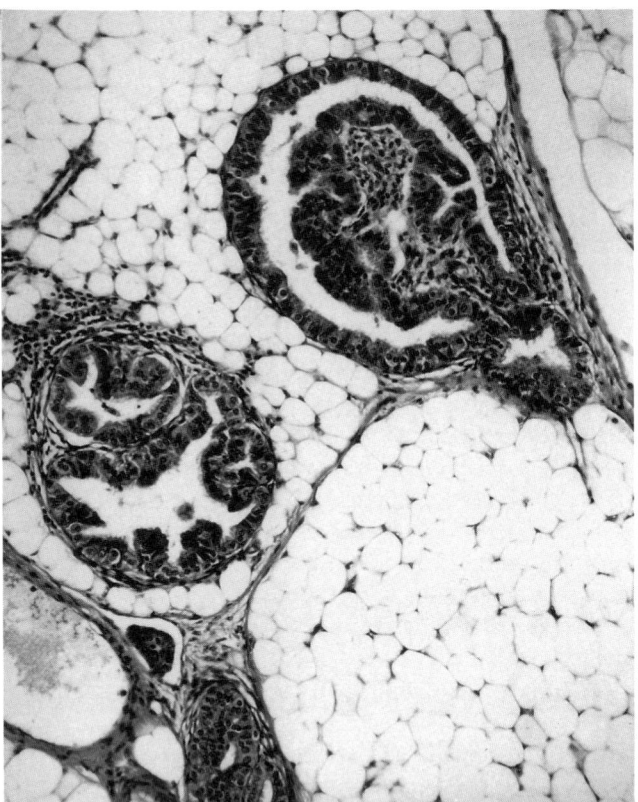

Fig. 18.10. Endosalpingiosis. One of multiple benign peritoneal lesions (endosalpingiosis) associated with a benign serous tumor.

ULTRASTRUCTURAL FINDINGS

Epithelial lining cells of benign serous tumors have uniform oval nuclei, with only mild irregularities of the nuclear envelope and relatively homogeneous central but peripherally condensed chromatin (Fig. 18.11). Microvilli, cilia, and crossed-striated ciliary rootlets are present along the luminal border of the cells (Fig. 18.12). Interdigitations are prominent and abundant, as are supranuclear mitochondria.[102]

CLINICAL BEHAVIOR AND TREATMENT

Removal of the tumor is curative. If unilateral salpingo-oophorectomy is performed, there is a small risk of a second tumor arising in the residual ovary but this will generally also be benign.

Atypically Proliferating Serous Tumors

GENERAL FEATURES

Between 10% and 15% of ovarian serous tumors fall into this category. Their peak age of incidence, at 45 to 50

years, is slightly greater than that for benign serous tumors. They are bilateral in one-quarter to one-third of all cases, although some of these only on the basis of microscopic lesions in the contralateral ovary. Examples of atypically proliferating serous lesions in the pelvic and abdominal peritoneum in the absence of a co-existent ovarian tumor have been recorded[28,30,33] as well as rare cases in the broad ligaments.[11,49]

In between 20% and 40% of patients, the ovarian tumors are associated with small papillary or cystic serous epithelial lesions beneath the surface of pelvic viscera or the omentum or in pelvic lymph nodes. The presence of these often widely distributed peritoneal lesions is usually (70–80%) associated with a nonprogressive clinical course, thus inviting an alternative interpretation of their significance other than straightforward metastases or "implants." Generally, they have the same epithelial characteristics as the dominant ovarian mass, including papillae and psammoma bodies, but lack much of a stromal component.

Controversy and active debate still accompany interpretation of their pathogenesis and significance. On the one hand, for example, such peritoneal epithelial lesions are accepted as having arisen in situ when morphologically benign (termed *endosalpingiosis*) or when accompanying benign serous tumors. On the other hand, widespread invasive deposits associated with frankly malignant ovarian serous tumors are most likely metastases, although the possibility exists that many such deposits also arise outside the ovaries.[211] Between these two biological extremes, there is uncertainty regarding the origin and nature of the peritoneal lesions when found associated with ovarian atypically proliferating serous tumors, termed *implants* rather than metastases. The extraovarian lesions may be histologically benign or show proliferative changes up to and including locally invasive well-differentiated serous carcinoma, despite stromal invasion being absent, by definition, from the ovarian tumor.[154,211]

GROSS FINDINGS

Atypically proliferating serous tumors have gross features similar to benign serous tumors but tend to have finer, more friable, and more exuberant papillary projections. Papillae may be present on the external surface of the cysts (Fig. 18.13) in as many as 70% of cases.[154] The importance of this finding in explaining the extraovarian lesions or "implants" is currently unsettled.[233] The adenofibromatous variant of atypically proliferating serous tumors is a solid neoplasm composed of tough, rubbery fibrous tissue interspersed with glandular spaces of various sizes.

MICROSCOPIC FINDINGS

Escalation in the severity of atypical serous epithelial proliferation is manifested by increasing prominence and

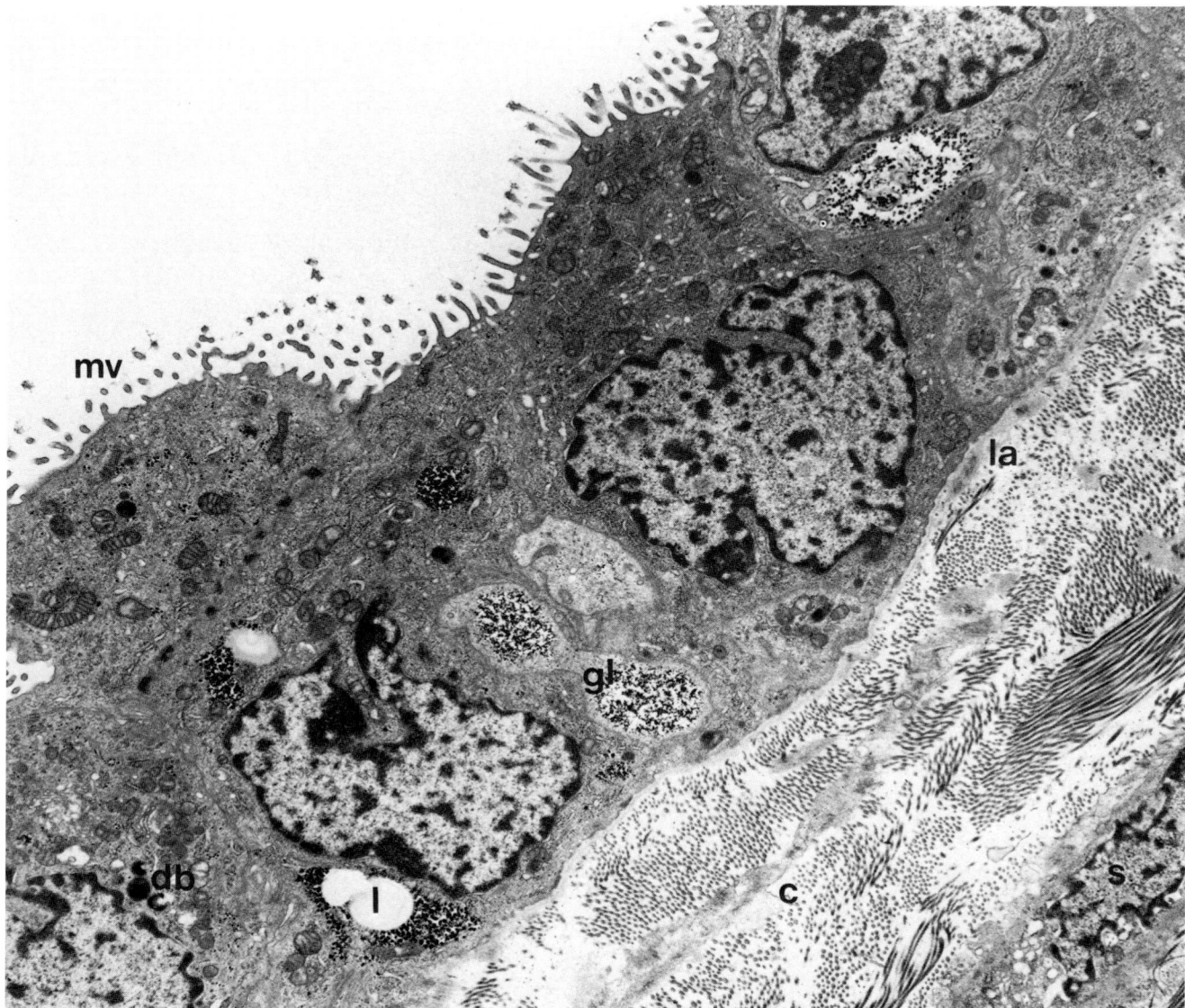

Fig. 18.11. Serous cystadenofibroma. Lumen lined by nonciliated cells, separated by a basal lamina (*la*) from dense stroma containing collagen (*c*) and a stromal cell (*s*). The cytoplasmic organelles of epithelial cells include characteristic patches of glycogen (*gl*) sometimes associated with lipid droplets (*l*), and occasional dense bodies (*db*) of uncertain nature, possibly either lysosomal or secretory. Microvilli (*mv*) present at luminal surface. ×7000. (Courtesy of Dr. E. J. Wills, Royal Prince Alfred Hospital, Sydney, Australia.)

complexity of the papillae lining most cystic spaces. The epithelium covering these papillary excrescences also shows a variable distribution and/or severity of proliferative features noted in the introductory section. These proliferative changes run *pari passu*, but for serous epithelial tumors the two most easily quantifiable are stratification of the epithelial lining of papillae and epithelial budding or tufting, ranging from barely above benign (so-called serous cystadenomas with focal proliferative activity[131]) to in situ malignancy (Figs. 18.14–18.16). Although clinical follow-up studies suggest that "microinvasion" is not associated with adverse consequences for the patient, this subject is dealt with in the section on malignant serous tumors.

Nuclei resemble those described in benign tumors or are more hyperchromatic and rounded in proliferating areas, with obvious although not prominent nucleoli. Mitoses uncommonly exceed 4 mitotic figures (MF)/10 high power fields (HPF),[131,208] and bizarre nuclei and tumor giant cells are not seen. Focal secretory changes may be seen as well as extracellular mucin and rare squamoid morules. Attenuation of epithelial cells so as to resemble mesothelium occasionally is seen (Fig. 18.17). Hobnail-type cells

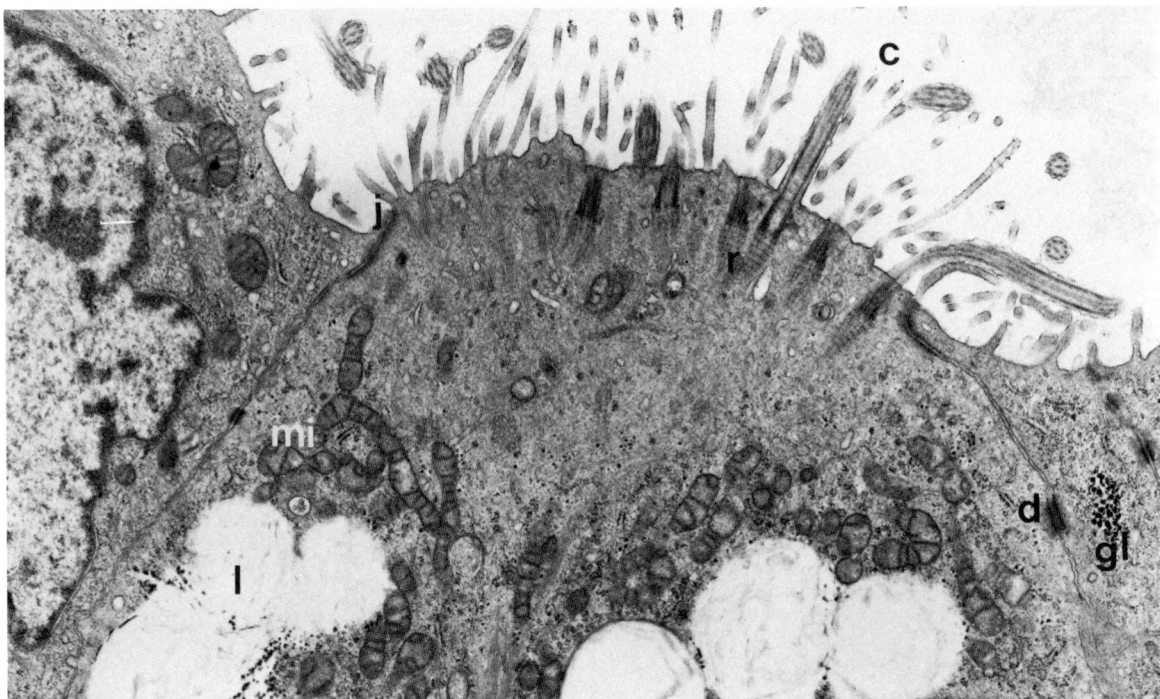

FIG. 18.12. Serous cystadenofibroma. Detail of apical portion of ciliated cell showing mixture of microvilli and cilia (*c*) with well-developed cytoplasmic rootlets (*r*). Desmosomes (*d*) and apical junction complexes (*j*) are seen at the lateral aspects of the cells. Mitochondria (*mi*), lipid droplets (*l*) and glycogen particles (*gl*) also present. ×15,000. (Courtesy of Dr. E. J. Wills, Royal Prince Alfred Hospital, Sydney, Australia.)

and ciliated cells (sometimes with abundant eosinophilic cytoplasm) may be encountered. Psammoma bodies are present in up to 50% of these tumors and mild scatterings of lymphocytes are seen in about 25% of these tumors. Epithelial proliferation in adenofibromatous serous tumors is a rare variation that is difficult to assess with regard to the presence or absence of stromal invasion. Extremely rare examples of "sarcoma-like" mural nodules, similar to those better defined in association with mucinous tumors (see below), have been reported in the walls of atypically proliferating serous tumors.[76]

The epithelial lesions in omentum and on pelvic/abdominal viscera often are found on or beneath the surface mesothelium and exhibit many of the cellular characteristics seen in the associated ovarian tumor, including papilla formation and psammoma bodies. Most of these are either morphologically benign or atypically proliferating but well circumscribed and without architectural features, thus suggesting local invasion (Fig. 18.19a). It is my view that such lesions always arise in situ as a manifestation of multifocal tumorigenesis.

Some extraovarian lesions are associated with irregular glandular structures in immature, desmoplastic, or inflamed stroma, and these represent a most crucial but difficult differential diagnostic problem. Closer examination of some of these lesions suggests locally invasive well-differentiated serous carcinoma (Fig. 18.18), and such lesions are characterized not only by desmoplastic stroma that surrounds the tumor cells, but also a clear pattern of tentacular invasion of the subjacent tissue and cellular features of malignancy. Therefore, they exhibit a capacity for invasion absent, by definition, from the associated ovarian tumor and such a capacity argues strongly in favor of their independence or autochthonous origin (multifocal tumorigenesis). Others show relatively bland cellular components (comprising single cells, small groups, or clusters or even large papillary fragments[212]) in desmoplastic reactive granulation tissue that is confined to the surface of the intraperitoneal structures or in peritoneal adhesions and do not invade the underlying tissues (Fig. 18.19b). These latter lesions, I believe, are the *only* lesions that are true "implants" and it is likely that they are the "implants" associated with tumors exhibiting a surface epithelial papillary component.[233] The significance of identifying the various noninvasive or "pseudoinvasive" lesions lies in the banal clinical course these particular patients pursue despite apparent widespread "metastatic malignant" disease.[31,98,154,211]

In peritoneal washings, tumor cells will be aggregated into small or large cohesive papillary fragments with smooth borders. Cells are small and uniform with high N/C ratios of >1:2 and nuclei have inconspicuous nucleoli.[121]

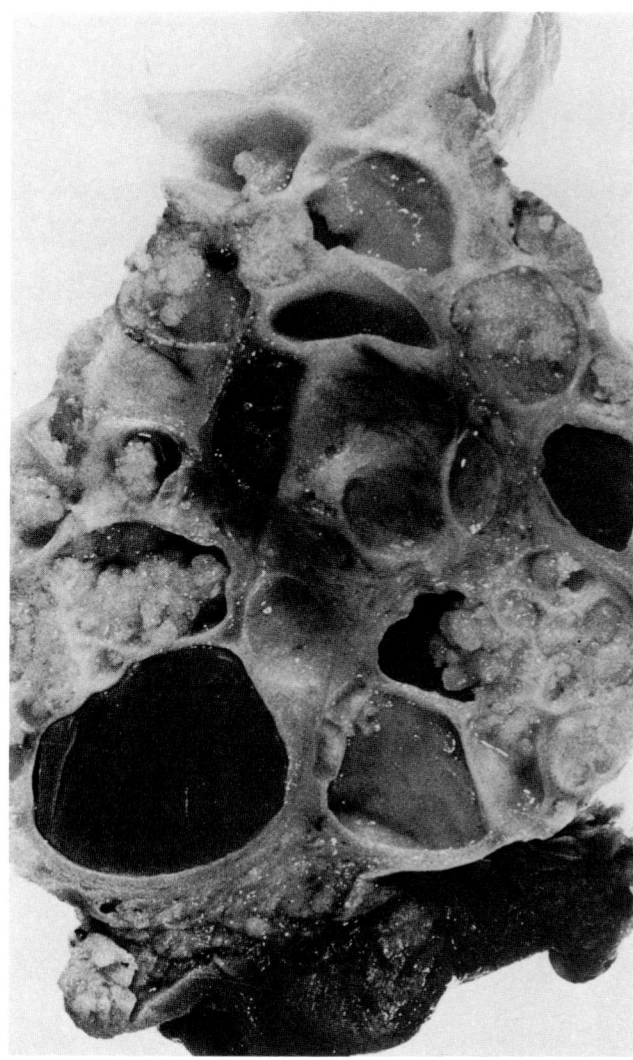

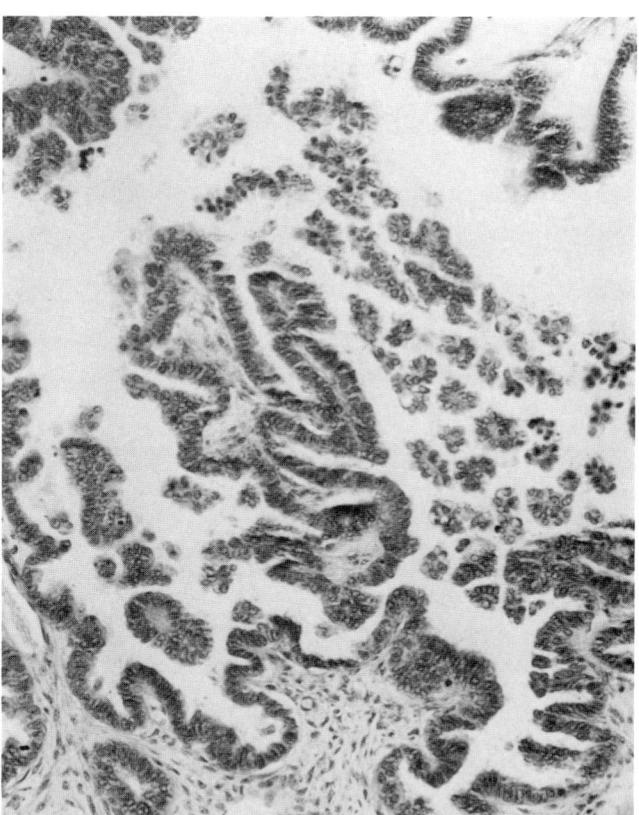

18.14a

FIG. 18.13. Multilocular atypically proliferating serous tumor. The tumor has a prominent surface and intracystic papillary component.

ULTRASTRUCTURAL FINDINGS

Atypical serous cells show marked nuclear infolding similar to that seen in serous carcinomas, with cilia.[102] Interdigitations are less obvious than in benign serous tumors.

CLINICAL BEHAVIOR AND TREATMENT

Five-year survival for all patients with atypically proliferating serous tumors is 90–95%, whereas 10-year survival is 75–90%.[100,131,159,175,213] For practical purposes, patients with tumor confined to the ovaries, that is, patients without extraova-

---

⊳

FIG. 18.14. Atypically proliferating serous tumor. There is mild epithelial proliferation: **a:** papillary cystadenoma; **b:** adenofibroma.

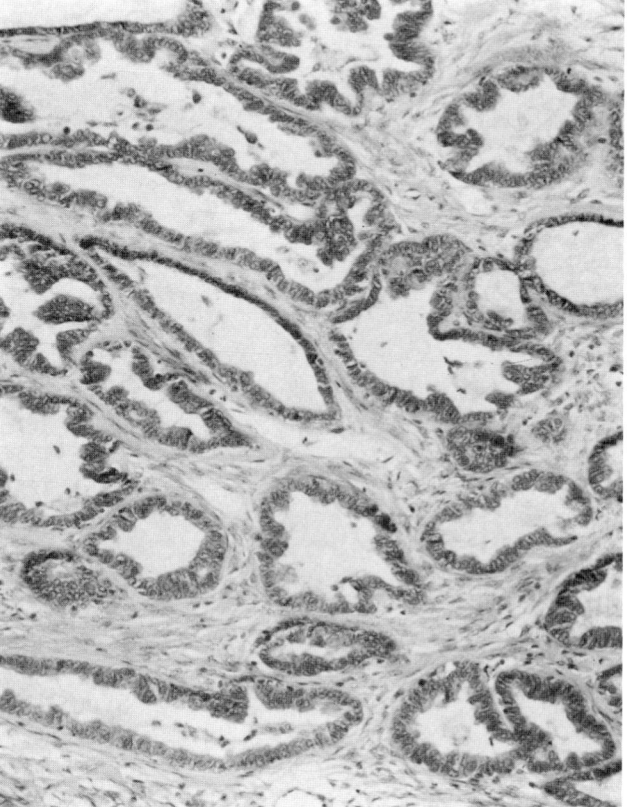

18.14b

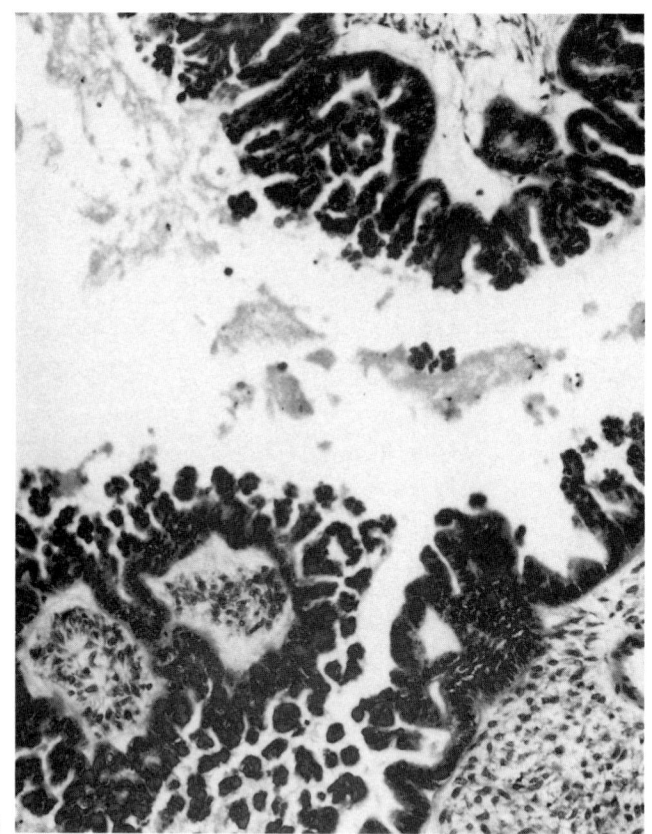

18.15

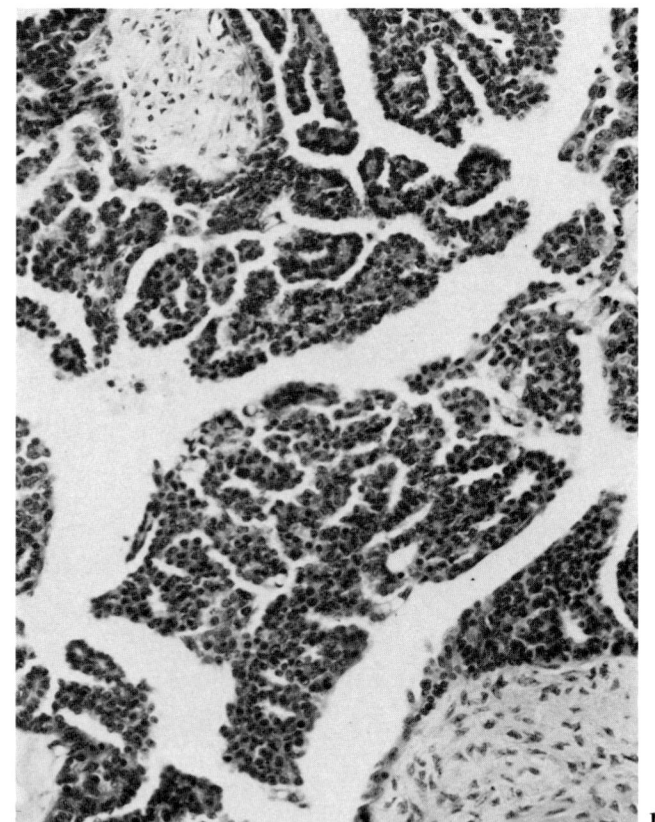

18.16

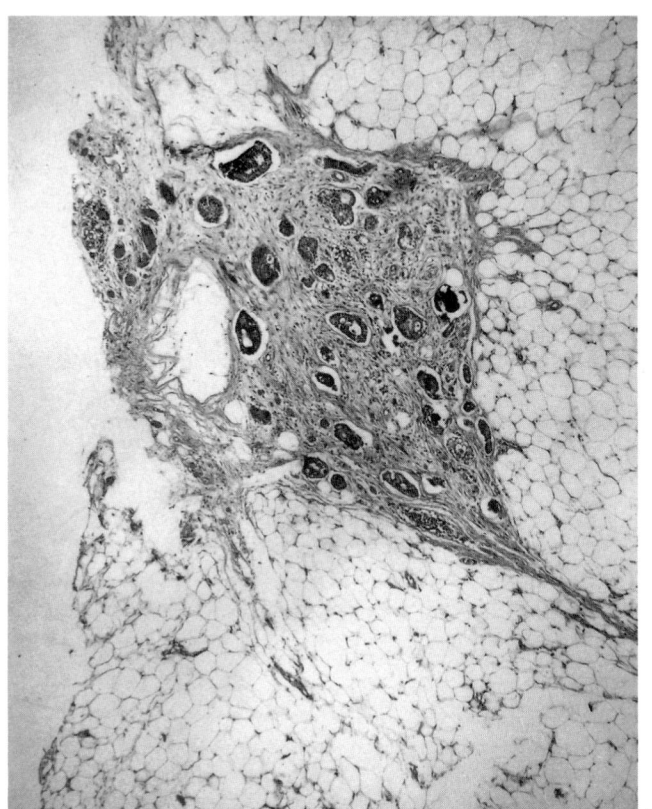

18.17

18.18

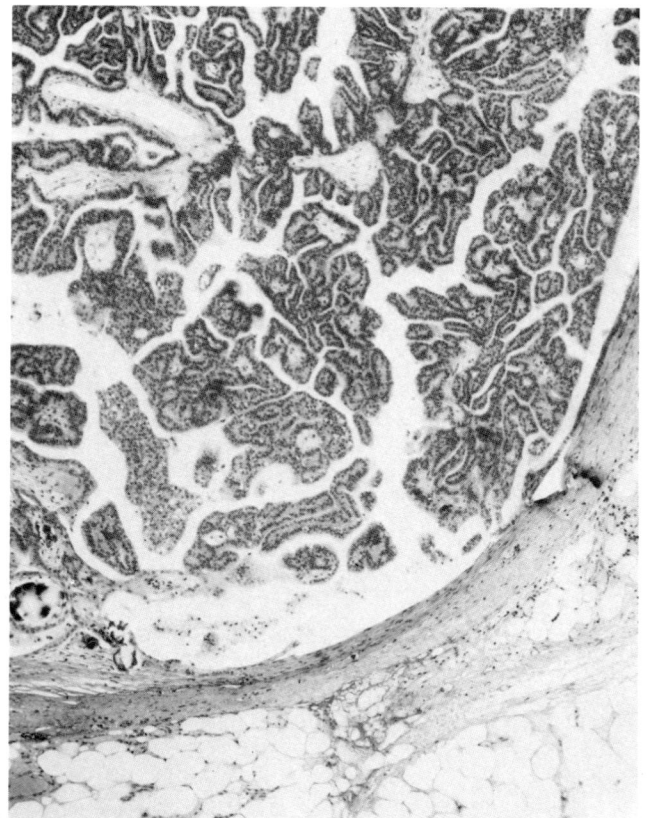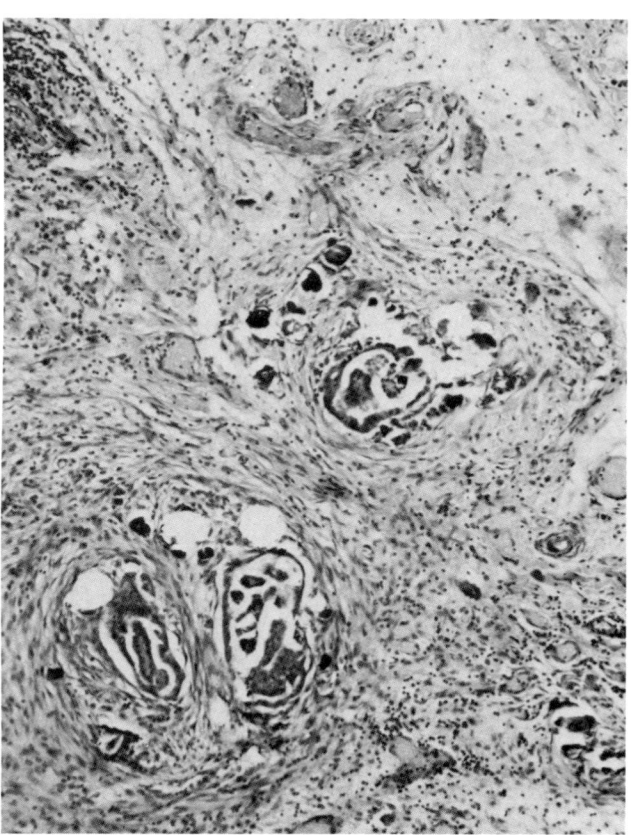

a　　　　　　　　　　　　　　　　　　　　　　　　　　　　　　b

Fig. 18.19. Noninvasive "implants." These lesions often are associated with atypically proliferating serous tumors of ovaries. **a:** epithelial; **b:** desmoplastic.

rian lesions or "positive" peritoneal washings at *thorough* staging laparotomy can all be expected to survive without recurrence.[146,287] This is an important precondition as immediate reexploration by a gynecological oncology team can be expected to upstage at least 30% of patients with apparent Stage I disease treated initially in a "general" unit.[246]

Treatment should aim at surgical excision of the tumor. Unilateral salpingo-oophorectomy is considered sufficient in a young woman if the neoplasm is confined to one ovary, at a thorough staging laparotomy. Occasionally, a conserva-

◁——————————————————————

Fig. 18.15. **Atypically proliferating serous tumor.** There is moderate epithelial proliferation.
Fig. 18.16. **Atypically proliferating serous tumor.** There is marked epithelial proliferation.
Fig. 18.17. **Atypically proliferating serous cystadenoma.** There is mesothelial-like attenuation of the epithelium. Similar changes may be seen in invasive serous carcinomas.
Fig. 18.18. **Invasive "implants."** These lesions may be associated with an atypically proliferating serous tumor of ovary (i.e., simultaneous extraovarian well-differentiated carcinoma). Note position of lesion beneath peritoneal surface and desmoplasia around the invasive focus.

tive approach in young women with bilateral disease is justified, namely, resection of the ovarian masses with conservation of as much ovarian tissue as possible[152] and close clinical follow-up until after childbearing, at which time, pelvic clearance may be considered. In other cases of bilateral involvement, older patients, or peritoneal spread, total hysterectomy, bilateral salpingo-oophorectomy, and omentectomy are appropriate.

For patients with extraovarian (peritoneal) disease, the clinical outlook is determined by the anatomical distribution of lesions and, more importantly, by their histology. There is considerable variation in histological features of individual peritoneal lesions and extensive sampling and careful examination of these tumor foci is mandatory. About 30–40% of patients in this category ultimately succumb to progressive disease, "benign" complications (e.g., bowel obstruction), or side effects of therapy.[146] Our experience[210,213] and that of others[24,31,154] suggests that those "implants" showing patterns of locally invasive carcinoma appear most likely to reflect unfavorably on the clinical outcome for the patient, although this is by no means universally accepted.[100,162] It is our practice to regard such cases as low-grade serous carcinoma and to treat them accordingly.[211] Extraovarian lesions, which are benign or atypically proliferating but noninvasive, are noted and careful clinical follow-up is recommended. The same principles apply to the rarely encountered cases of extraovarian serous neoplasia, which, with minimal or no ovarian involvement, show similar atypical proliferation.[28,30,33]

Recurrences may develop up to 20 to 50 years postoperatively, for which reason it is difficult to define the precise role, if any, for second-look laparotomy. Postoperative adjuvant chemotherapy may be considered in Stage II–IV cases on the understanding that the long-term risks of such treatment may outweigh equivocal results of chemotherapy,[31,36,47,100,141,146] and that randomized prospective trials have not been conducted for establishing the efficacy of such treatment.

Malignant Serous Tumors

GENERAL FEATURES

Malignant serous tumors are common tumors, accounting for approximately 40–50% of malignant ovarian neoplasms. They are bilateral in about two-thirds of all cases (one-third in Stage I) and occur most frequently between 45 and 65 years of age.

In 80–85% of cases, they are widely disseminated at the time of diagnosis. Inasmuch as stage for stage and grade for grade there appears little difference in prognosis between the histological subtypes of ovarian epithelial cancer,[72] the most likely explanation for this dissemination at diagnosis is that these neoplasms often commence as bilateral tumors and/or widespread multifocal neoplasia.[18,184] Indeed, probably about 10% of all cases of widespread (Stage III or IV) intraperitoneal carcinoma of serous papillary type are associated with ovaries that are completely normal or at most minimally involved (Fig. III.2[209]), or have been previously removed.[51] Such tumors have been termed *extraovarian papillary serous carcinomas* by Foyle et al.[92] and probably arise from peritoneal lesions analogous to the "implants" or serosal inclusions of histologically less aggressive serous tumors.°

GROSS FINDINGS

Size of invasive serous carcinomas ranges from microscopic to 20 cm or so in diameter. Well-differentiated carcinomas are mostly cystic, multilocular tumors with soft, friable, papillae partly or mostly filling the cavities and containing usually turbid or bloody fluid. External surfaces may be smooth or bosselated and sometimes include surface papillae. Tumor adhesions to surrounding organs are common and care should be taken to ensure sampling of

---

°Refs.   13,70,92,94,103,126,150,155,164,194,209,214,221,264,265, 269,276

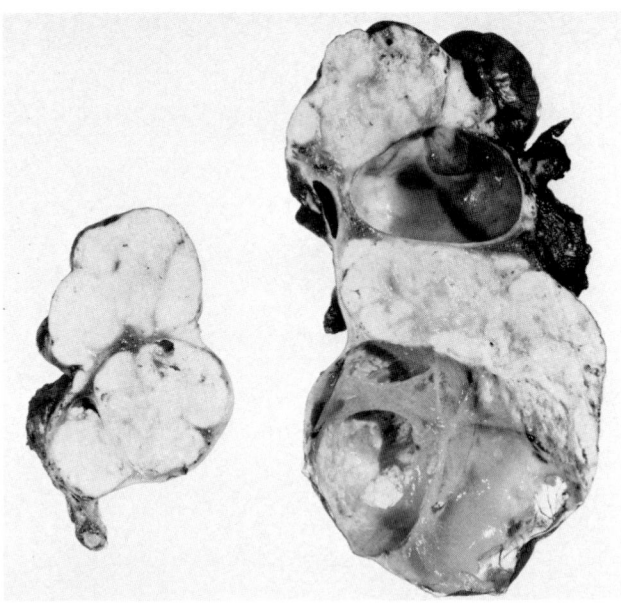

FIG. 18.20. Bilateral serous carcinomas. The tumors are partly solid with bosselated external contours and solid nodules of friable and partly necrotic tumor in the cut surfaces.

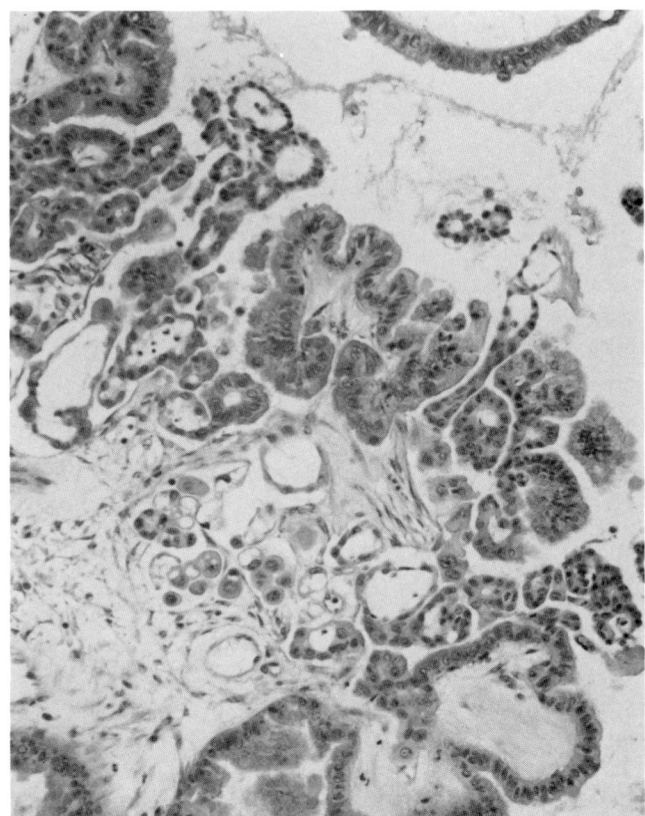

FIG. 18.21. Atypically proliferating serous tumor. Focus of microinvasion.

these areas as part of tumor assessment in Stage I–II cases. Less well-differentiated serous carcinomas (Fig. 18.20) contain solid areas of friable pink to gray tissue with less obvious papillae. Nonspecific features such as necrosis and hemorrhage often are present.

MICROSCOPIC FINDINGS

Microinvasion ought to represent a definable stage in the adenoma–carcinoma sequence for ovarian epithelial–stromal tumors, a transition between atypically proliferating but noninvasive tumors and frankly invasive cancers (Fig. 18.21). Interpretation of such findings is still controversial, however, and the few cases reported to date appear to indicate no adverse consequences for the patients.[29,259] These foci are recognizable not only by the hallmarks of invasion—disorganized architecture and stromal desmoplasia—but also by changes in the appearance of the invading cells. They tend to become enlarged, with abundant eosinophilic cytoplasm, and often are single cells rather than cohesive groups. They may even appear to lie within lymphatic-like spaces. Serous carcinomas tend to be uniform, varying little from area to area; it is relatively uncommon to find a conjunction of poorly differentiated and well-differentiated serous carcinoma. Grading is increas-

ingly being recognized as a significant correlate of prognosis,[75] and of all ovarian müllerian-type carcinomas, serous tumors most readily present a gradable spectrum.[209]

In well-differentiated serous carcinomas, the papillary structures are clearly formed (Fig. 18.22), with immature connective tissue stromal cores. The papillae grow into cystic spaces or onto the peritoneal surface of the tumor. They also are prominent in the cellular, immature stroma of fibrous or solid portions of tumor, and occasionally may appear to be in lymphatic spaces (Fig. 18.23). Psammoma bodies occur in 60–70% of well-differentiated serous carcinomas and occasionally are very prominent (Fig. 18.24), producing so-called psammomatous carcinomas.[101] These are relatively indolent carcinomas but care nevertheless should be taken to identify clearly cytological features of malignancy in the tumor cells that are obscured by the massive overburden of calcispherules. An extreme example of this phenomenon may explain the unique "complete psammomatous degeneration" of a 23-cm ovarian mass described by Schneider et al.[227] Spicules of new bone of dystrophic origin have been reported rarely in the stroma.[20,35] Rare histological variants are malignant adenofibromas (Fig. 18.25) in which epithelial but not fibrous elements are malignant; this pattern may be seen focally in otherwise typical serous carcinomas. Occasionally, acute

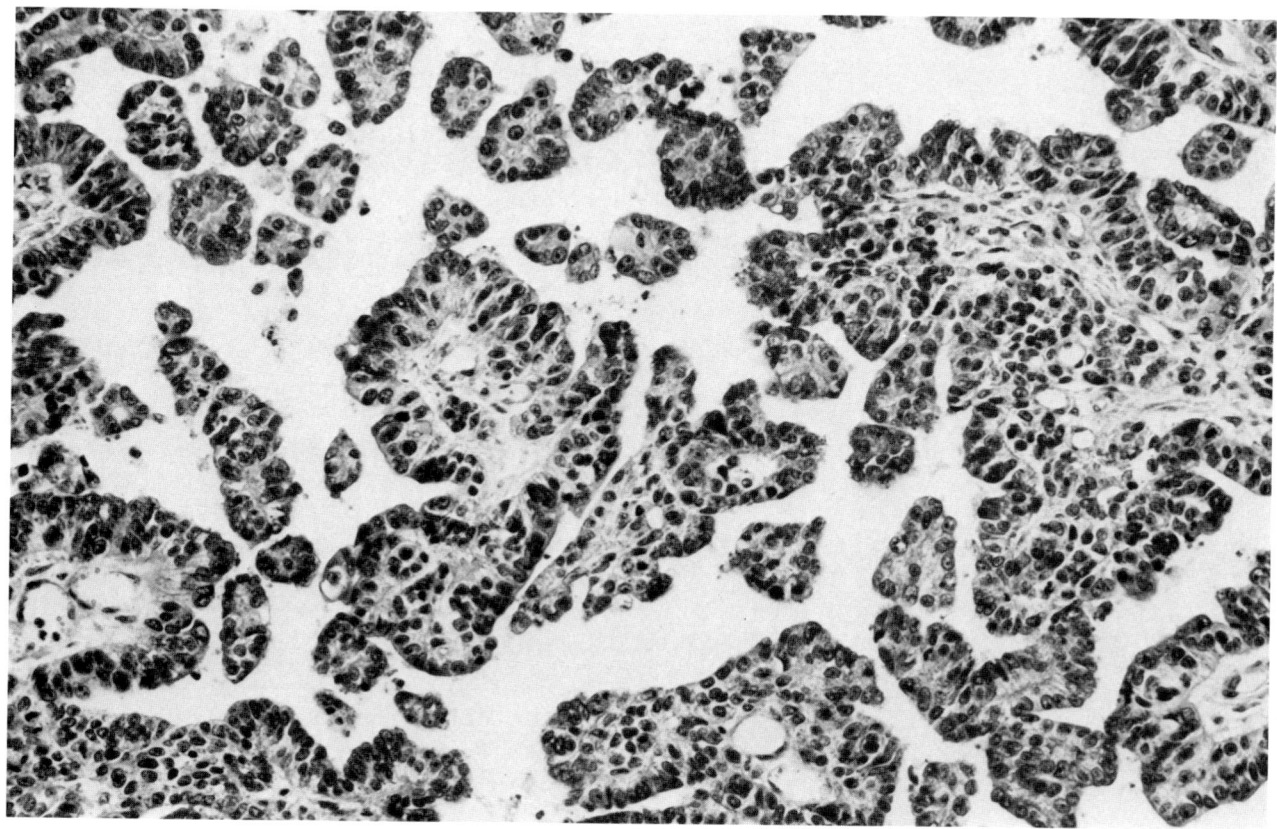

FIG. 18.22. **Well-differentiated serous carcinoma.** The tumor has a papillary pattern.

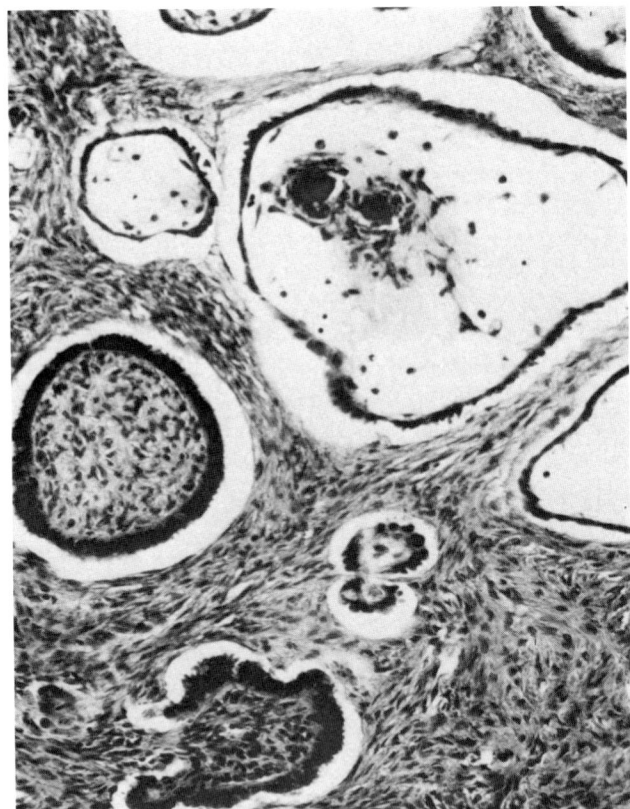

18.23

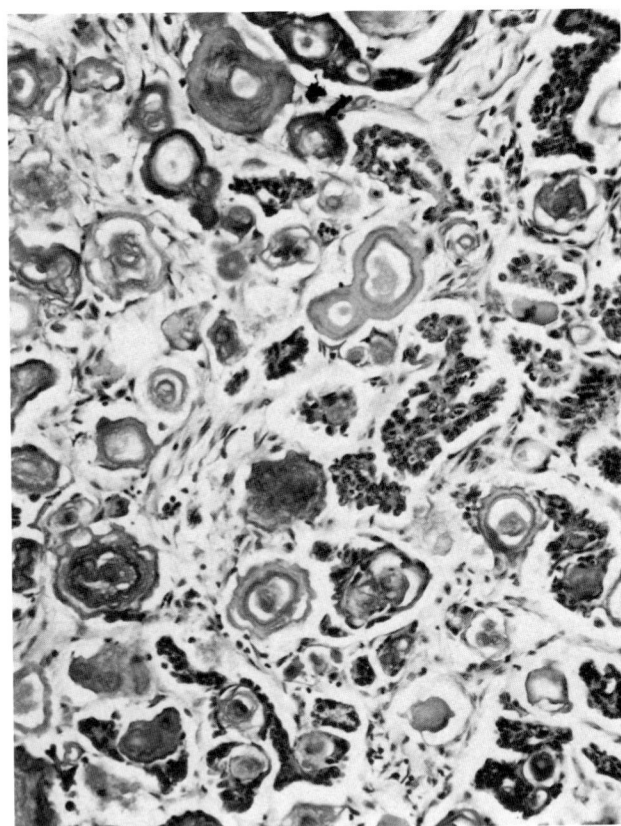

18.24

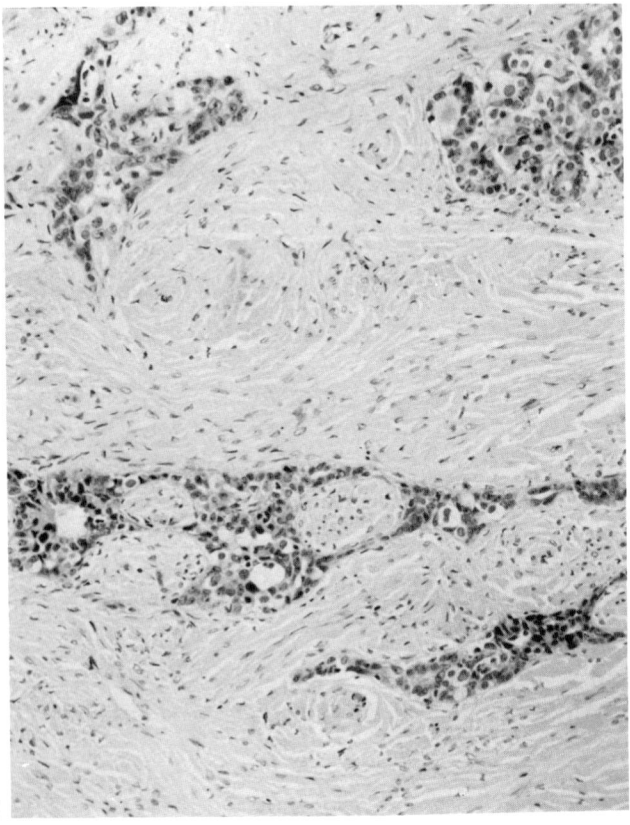

18.25

inflammatory cell infiltrates, unassociated with foci of necrosis, are seen in relation to the epithelium,[212] although not as frequently as in mucinous tumors. In my experience, these changes are almost always incidental findings in tumors from patients who do not exhibit systemic signs of infection.

Moderately differentiated serous carcinomas exhibit papillae that are finer and more crowded. A frequently encountered and quite characteristic pattern to recognize is lace-like (Fig. 18.26), which may only be focal but often predominates, and is due to a very fine micropapillary arrangement of the cells that grow centripetally and subsequently bridge or partially coalesce. The slit-like spaces created between these micropapillae tend to be uniform in size and oriented radially. Cells are small and uniform. Other less frequently seen variants are illustrated in Figures 18.27 and 18.28. It should be remembered that glandular patterns do not exclude serous carcinoma and the discrimination between poorly differentiated endo-

---

FIG. 18.23. **Well-differentiated serous carcinoma.** The papillae appear to be in dilated lymphatic spaces.

FIG. 18.24. **Psammomatous carcinoma.** Malignant epithelial criteria should still be evident to establish the diagnosis.

FIG. 18.25. **Malignant serous adenofibroma.** Irregular cords of malignant cells in dense ovarian stroma.

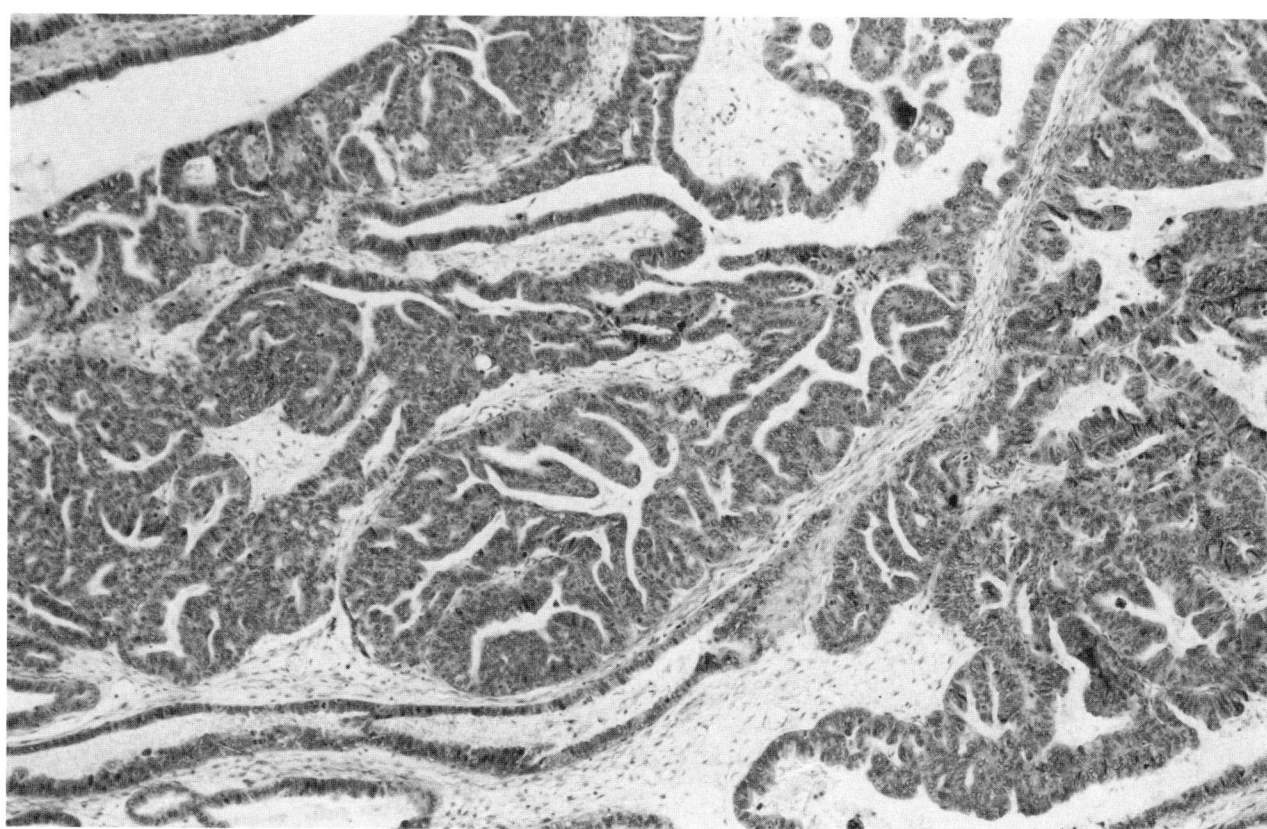

18.26

metrioid carcinoma and serous carcinoma with a predominantly microglandular pattern usually is difficult and sometimes impossible. Psammoma bodies occur in 20–30% of cases. Secretory activity also may be present (Fig. 18.29), and foci of squamous differentiation have been reported rarely.[272]

In poorly differentiated serous carcinomas, micropapillary patterns as described above are largely obliterated and tumors are made up of solid sheets of small, uniform, dark cells that often are slightly spindled (Fig. 18.30). The cells at the margins of these small cell masses are not palisaded as occurs in granulosa cell tumors, and only rarely produce microglandular aggregates as occur in endometrioid carcinomas. A further histological feature, which also is seen often in better differentiated serous carcinomas, is the presence of occasional bizarre mononuclear giant cells (Fig. 18.31) or syncytial-like aggregates. It has been suggested that these syncytial-like cells are responsible for aberrant gonadotrophin secretion associated with some serous carcinomas,[108] but immunohistochemical confirmation of this has not been my experience. These may be the

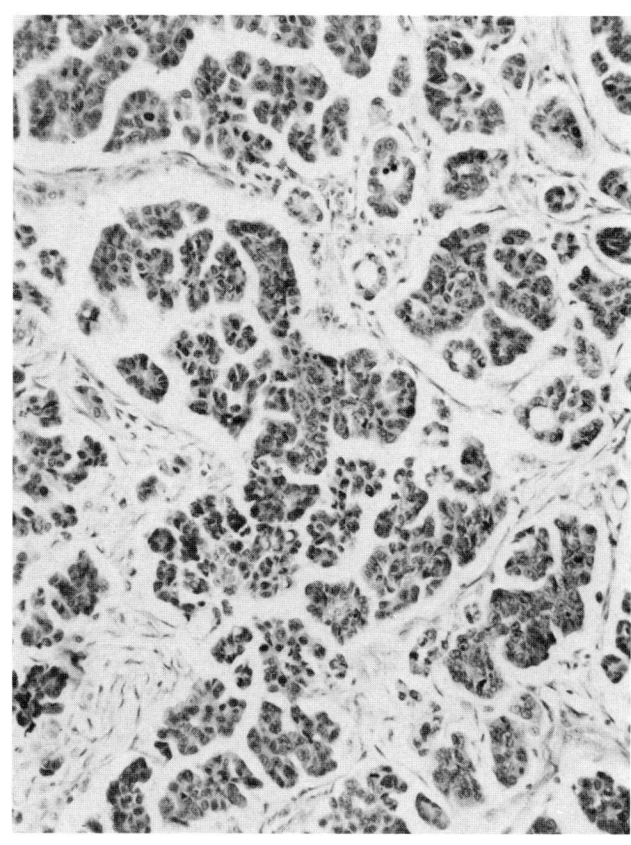

18.27

FIG. 18.26. **Moderately differentiated serous carcinoma.** The intracystic papillary growth has a "lacy" pattern characteristic of many of these tumors.

FIG. 18.27. **Serous carcinoma.** The tumor has a finely micropapillary pattern.

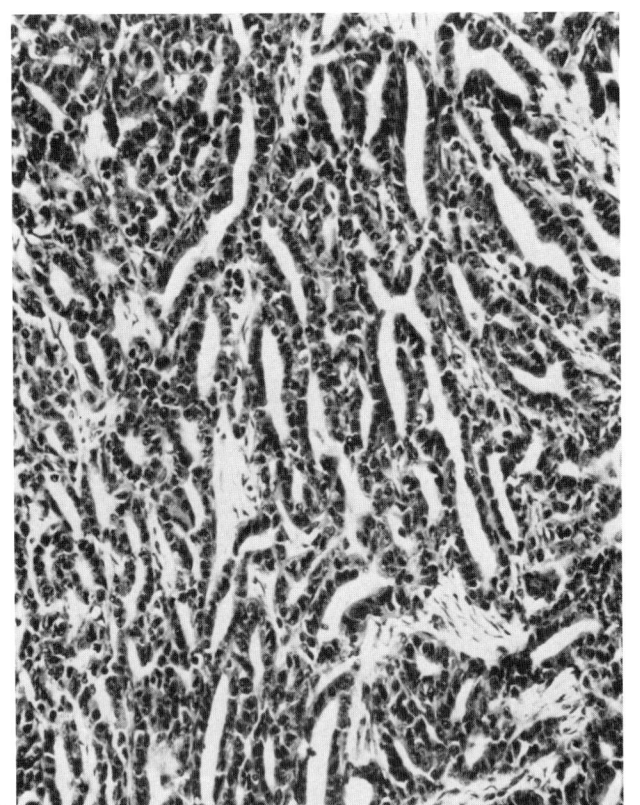

18.28

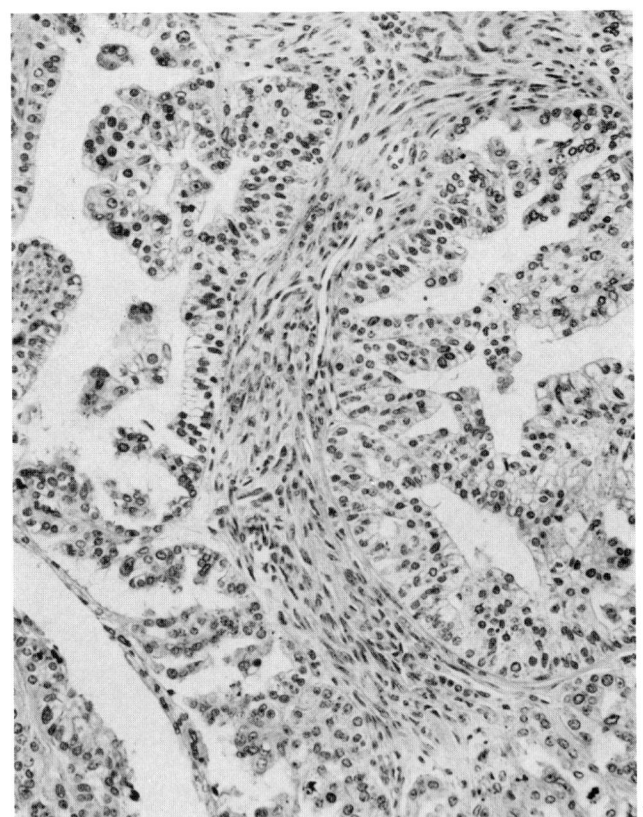

18.29

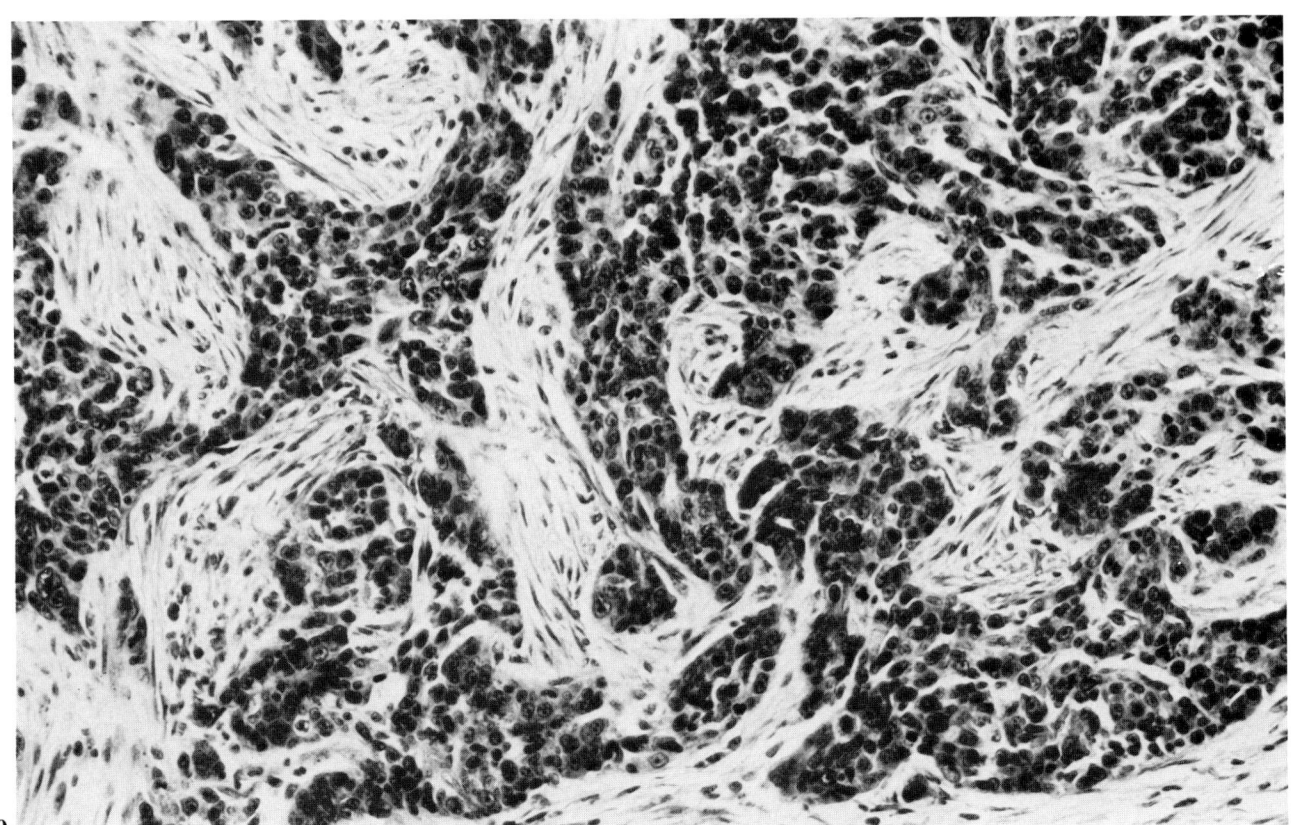

18.30

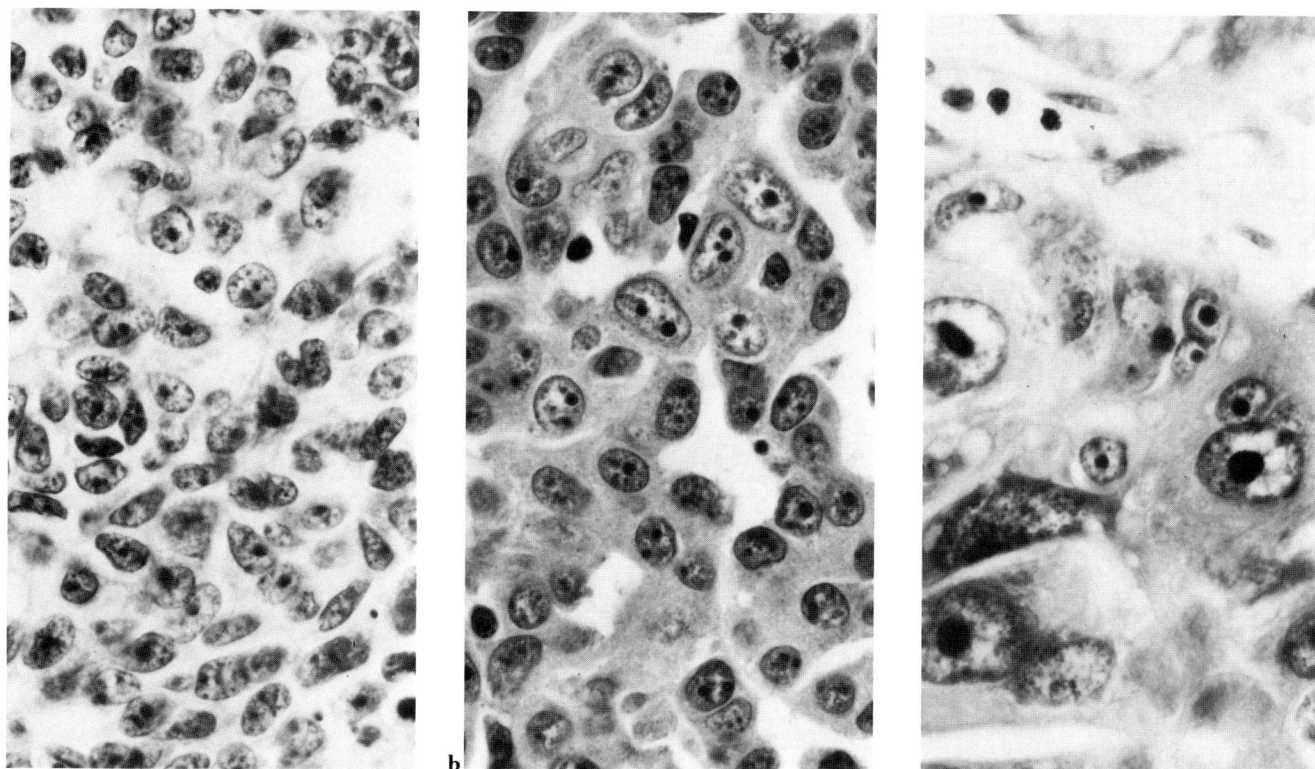

FIG. 18.31. **Poorly differentiated serous carcinoma.** High power of common cellular variants. **a:** Small cells with scanty cytoplasm. **b:** Larger cells with moderate amphophilic cytoplasm. **c:** Bizarre mononuclear or syncytial-like giant cells.

only features suggestive of serous neoplasia in otherwise undifferentiated carcinomas. Mitoses usually are very numerous and tumor necrosis often is pronounced.

IMMUNOHISTOCHEMICAL AND ULTRASTRUCTURAL FINDINGS

A plethora of immunohistochemical tumor markers such as alpha-amylases,[39,273] NS19-9 and OC-125,[123] CEA, S-100 protein, Leu-M1, B72.3,[280] and even GFAP[165] are all variously useful in typing the cells (see Chapter 26, Immunohistochemistry).

Ultrastructural characteristics of malignant serous epithelium include marked nuclear irregularity, diminished cell membrane interdigitation, and numerous dense bodies (Fig. 18.32). Ferenczy and Richart[88] described both endometrial and endocervical-type cells in the well-differentiated tumors. These authors postulate that the latter are the source of the occasional mucin production seen in these neoplasms. Ciliated cells are rare in serous carcinomas.[139]

CLINICAL BEHAVIOR AND TREATMENT

Total hysterectomy with bilateral adnexectomy and omentectomy are part of a full staging laparotomy that also includes biopsies of peritoneum, para-aortic, and pelvic nodes and peritoneal "washings" for cytological assessment. Accurate staging is vital, such procedures "upstaging" more than one-third of cases apparently confined to the pelvis. If complete surgical removal is not possible, cytoreductive surgery is advocated before adjuvant therapy. Postoperative radiation has an ill-defined place in the management of localized residual disease (usually Stage IIb) and combination chemotherapy has been shown to be of value in *all* stages if added to surgical treatment.[169,258] Management of patients with primary extraovarian (peritoneal) serous carcinoma is along similar lines, with most recent studies showing no differences in clinical outcome from those associated with an ovarian tumor.[70,94,194]

◁ ──────────────────────────────

FIG. 18.28. **Serous carcinoma.** A more glandular pattern with elongate or slit-like glands. Contrast with the typical microglandular pattern of endometrioid carcinoma, Fig. 18.69.

FIG. 18.29. **Moderately differentiated serous carcinoma.** The tumor displays prominent secretory activity—clear or vacuolated cytoplasm.

FIG. 18.30. **Poorly differentiated serous carcinoma.** Sheets and cords of small "dark" cells with high N/C ratio. Note some spindling and lack of peripheral palisading.

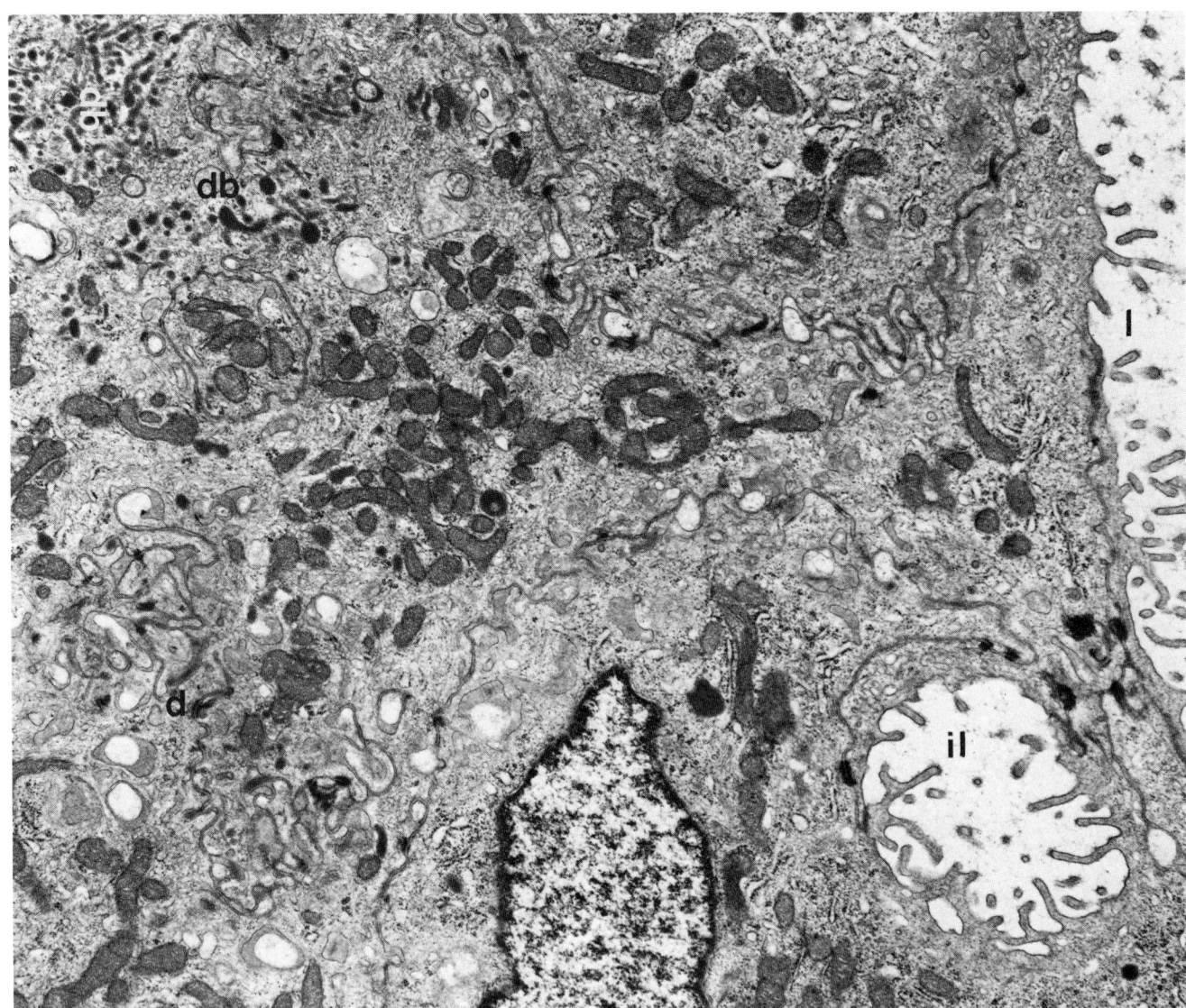

FIG. 18.32. Serous carcinoma. Solid area showing, at right, an abortive glandular lumen (*l*) and an intracellular lumen (*il*) each lined by branched microvilli with a glycocalyx coat. Desmosomes (*d*) are associated with convoluted plasma membranes at lower left. Cytoplasmic organisation differs little from benign serous tumors (see Figs. 18.11, 18.12) but dense bodies (*db*) are more numerous. ×12,000. (Courtesy of Dr. E. J. Wills, Royal Prince Alfred Hospital, Sydney, Australia.)

Mucinous Tumors

Benign Mucinous Tumors

GENERAL FEATURES

Although the origin of ovarian mucinous neoplasms is still controversial, evidence points to diverse origins. This conclusion is based on their association with cystic teratomas in about 5% of cases, including rare atypically proliferating mucinous tumors,[118] occasional concurrence with appendiceal mucoceles and/or pseudomyxoma peritonei, and the demonstration of intestinal-type mucins in many of these tumors. In addition, rare mucinous tumors are associated with Sertoli–Leydig cell, granulosa cell,[193] and carcinoid tumors.[281] Paradoxically, many mucinous ovarian tumors of intestinal type[291] are associated with müllerian-type adenocarcinomas of the endocervix.

Benign mucinous cysts and cystadenomas comprise 20–25% of all benign ovarian neoplasms and 75–85% of all ovarian mucinous tumors. They occur most often during the third to fifth decades, although they may be encountered in very young women and rarely in children. They are bilateral in only about 2–3% of cases. Their frequent large size and common occurrence in pregnancy contribute to these tumors being disproportionately represented among ovarian masses associated with acute torsion.

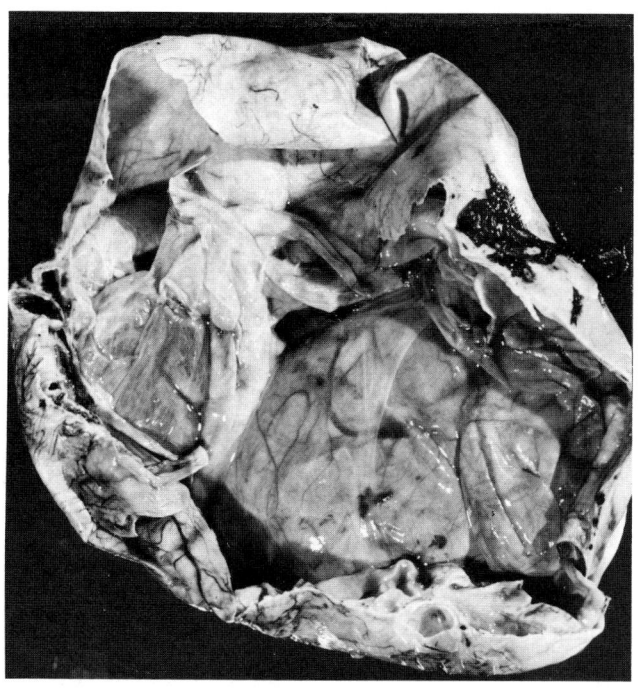

FIG. 18.33. Mucinous cystadenoma. The multilocular tumor has thick-walled cysts.

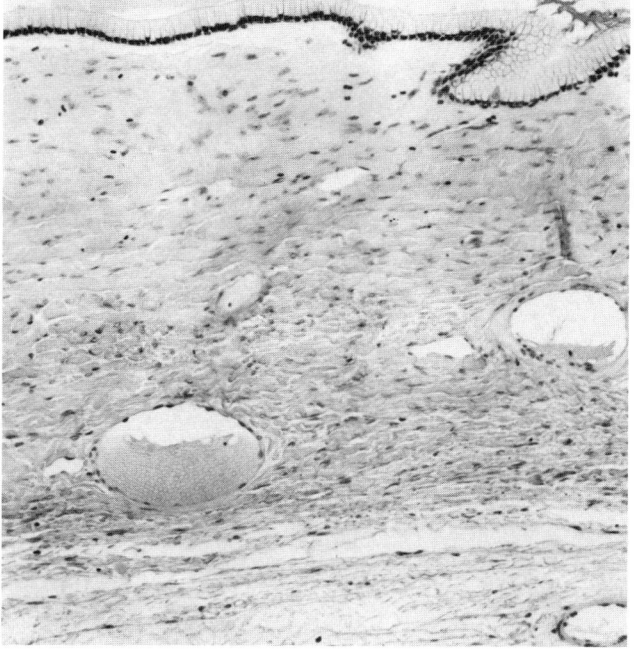

FIG. 18.34. Mucinous cystadenoma. Typical "picket-fence" epithelium and a thick fibrous wall are present.

GROSS FINDINGS

They are typically multiloculated, cystic tumors measuring up to 50 cm in diameter; rare gigantic lesions weighing more than 100 kg have been documented. The serosal surface of the usually thick outer wall is smooth and opaque. Cysts contain a thick, tenacious mucinous material—occasionally somewhat more watery in consistency. Locules usually are small and multiple. (Fig. 18.33), but tumors may be parvilocular, or even a large simple cyst. Fibrous stroma varies in prominence but usually is inconspicuous. Mucinous adenofibromas are uncommon neoplasms.[25]

MICROSCOPIC FINDINGS

The characteristic epithelium of benign mucinous tumors is a single layer of uniform tall columnar cells with clear, homogeneous cytoplasm and small, basal, hyperchromatic nuclei. Most cells contain abundant diastase-resistant PAS-positive, and mucicarmine-positive neutral mucins. Histologically and ultrastructurally as well as immunohistochemically, the mucin-filled cells are *endocervical-like* (müllerian) or of *intestinal type*[71,85–87,147,182]; this dichotomy is reflected in the WHO histological classification of ovarian tumors. Benign mucinous tumors are divided approximately equally among those showing endocervical-like and intestinal epithelial differentiation. In tumors of mixed or predominantly intestinal epithelial differentiation, goblet cells are common; argentaffin or argyrophil

cells often are seen[1,135,138,153,225] and Paneth cells very occasionally are present. An apparently unique case of a benign mucinous tumor has been reported showing atypia of the epithelium resembling the Arias-Stella reaction of gestational endometrium.[250]

Tumor architecture reflects the size and number of the cysts and the relative prominence of the intervening stroma. At the lower end of the spectrum there are simple mucinous cysts (Fig. 18.34) with thick, collagenous, acellular outer walls (sometimes showing large spicules of dystrophic calcification). More complex arrangements are due to multiple locules of similar size (Fig. 18.35) or to the peripheral proliferation of small acini or "daughter-cysts," giving a pseudoinvasive pattern. These latter, in some ways, represent the growing edge of the tumor and mitotic activity is seen here (Fig. 18.36). This alone should not be interpreted as evidence of atypical epithelial proliferation. These areas may also exhibit crypt-like epithelial structures with mitoses at the base of the crypts. These proliferating cells show some diminution of intracellular mucins and cytoplasmic basophilia similar to the generative zones at the crypt bases in normal colonic mucosa. Quite complex papillary areas (Fig. 18.37), foci of squamous metaplasia, simple fronding, or crypt formation (Fig. 18.38) also may be observed. Tension of accumulated secretion within cysts leads to attenuation of the epithelium. This may proceed to breakdown in its integrity with leakage of the mucin into the surrounding stroma. Under such circumstances the mucin elicits focal stromal reactions varying

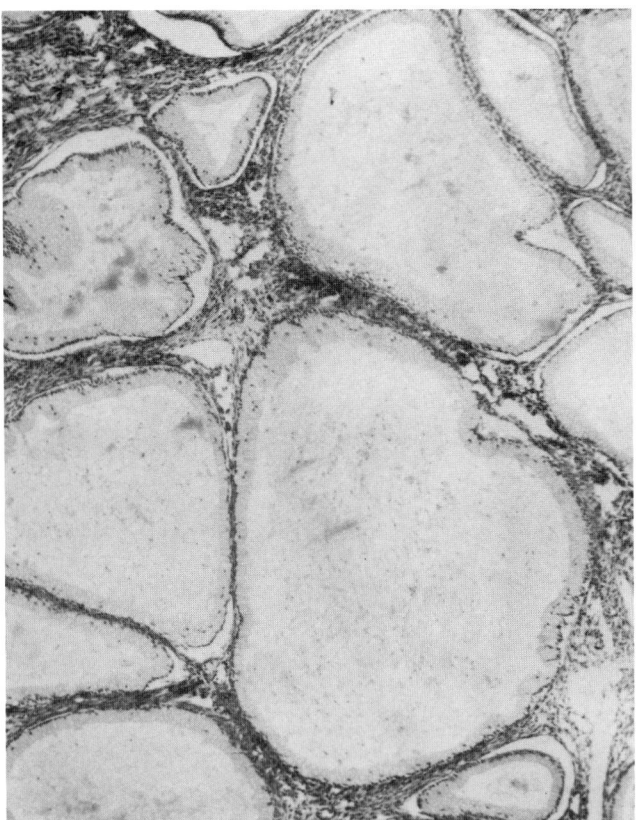

18.35

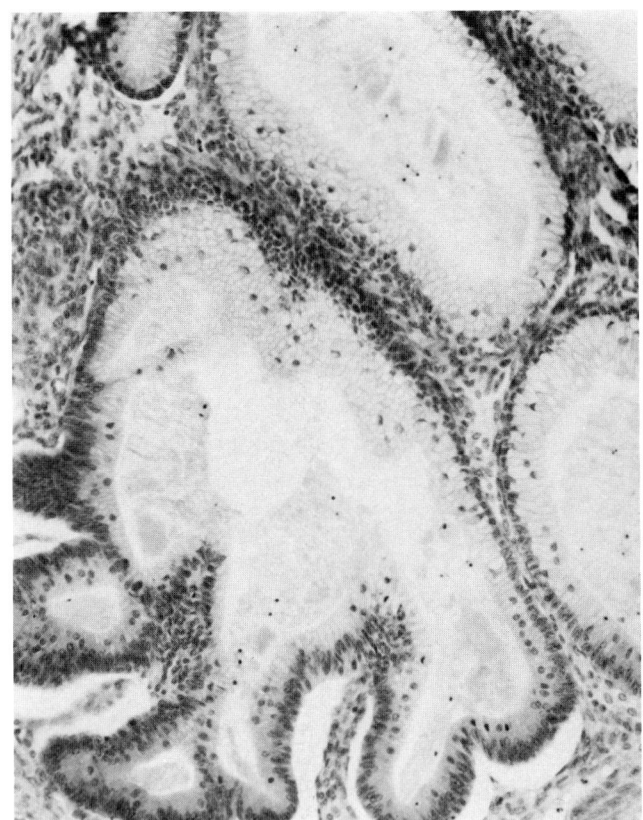

18.36

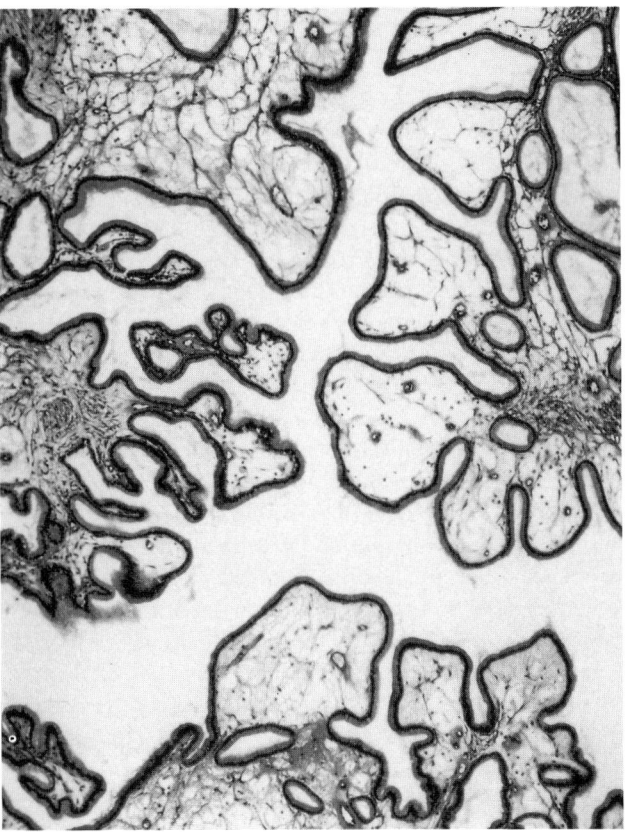

from very little in "pseudomyxoma ovarii" (see below) to quite florid foreign body histiocytic responses. Acute inflammatory cells may selectively infiltrate the epithelium and adjacent luminal mucin without necessarily indicating infection. Such infiltrates, which may be quite marked yet very focal, are almost always incidental findings in the tumors of afebrile patients.

Tumor stroma is fibrocollagenous and the cellularity, although variable, rarely approaches that of the ovarian-like stroma of serous tumors. Stromal cellularity may be increased in the vicinity of the epithelium and in this zone lutein-like cells are seen in 25% of cases. Rare benign tumors may show definite Leydig cells (with Reinke crystals) in the adjacent stroma without altering the diagnosis.[77,185,212,217] Smooth muscle is noted sometimes in the

---

FIG. 18.35. **Mucinous cystadenoma.** The tumor has a multi-locular pattern.

FIG. 18.36. **Mucinous cystadenoma.** There is apparent maturation of the intestinal-type epithelium from the outer tumor margin (*bottom*: mitoses and decreased intracellular mucin) toward the tumor center (*top*: with mature epithelium, goblet cells and no mitoses).

FIG. 18.37. **Papillary mucinous cystadenoma.** A coarse papillary pattern is associated with a single-layered tall columnar mucinous epithelium of endocervical type.

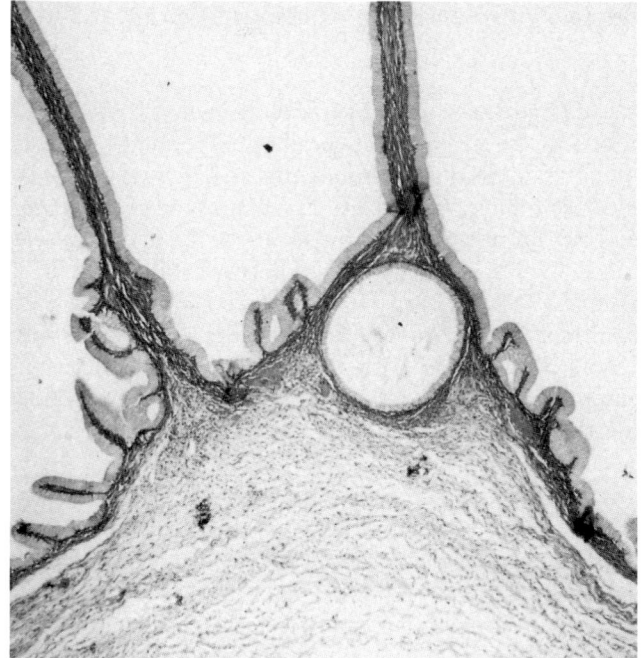

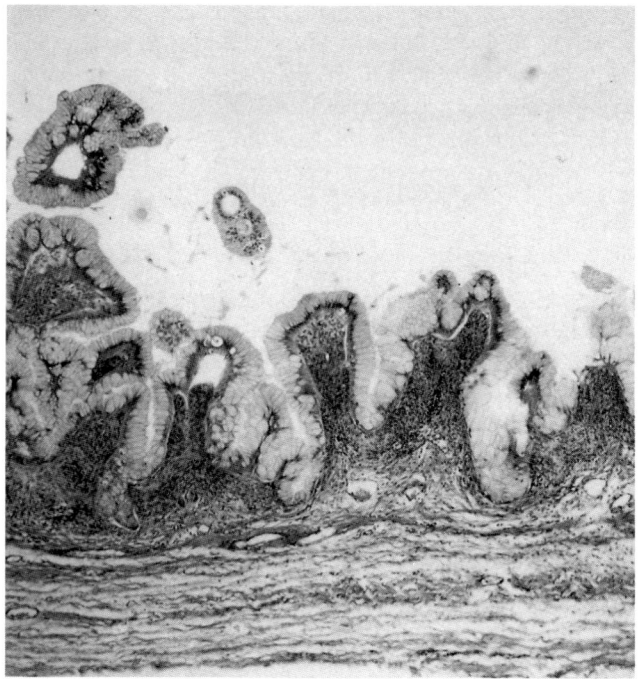

FIG. 18.38. Mucinous cystadenomas. a: Simple epithelial fronding is present. b: Crypt formation in the absence of atypia or mitotic activity.

stroma running parallel to the cyst linings,[230] but never as prominently as in the rare cysts of the rete ovarii. Occasionally, prominent stroma between locules (Fig. 18.39) gives rise to patterns of adenofibroma.[25]

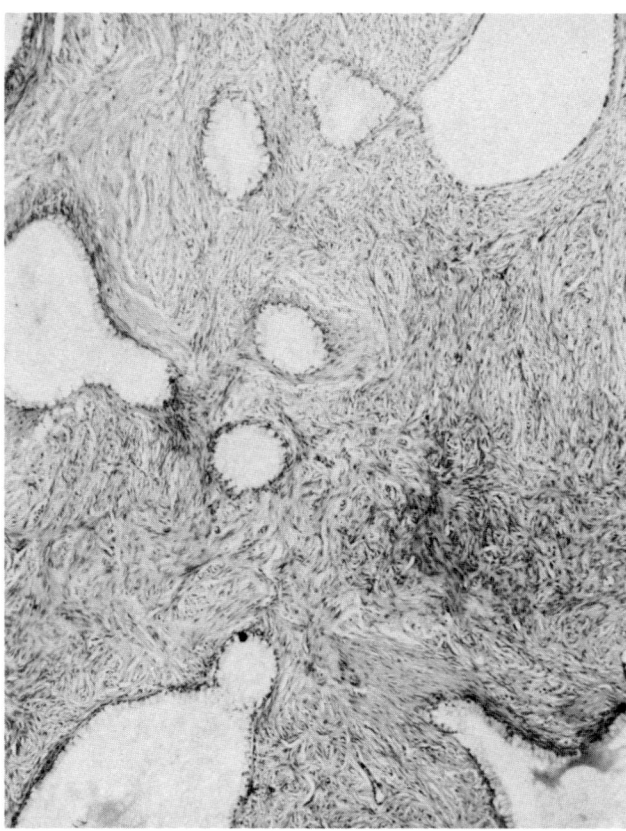

FIG. 18.39. Mucinous adenofibroma. Cysts lined by mucinous epithelium in dense fibrocollagenous stroma.

ULTRASTRUCTURAL FINDINGS

As noted above, studies have shown two types of mucinous cells in these tumors.[85,86,147] Mostly, the epithelium resembles that of the endocervix. Columnar cells have irregular, short, apical microvilli. Much of the supranuclear cytoplasm is filled with round to oval mucin droplets (Fig. 18.40). There is a well-developed supranuclear Golgi. Basal mitochondria are small and a variable amount of rough endoplasmic reticulum is present but there is no smooth endoplasmic reticulum. Lysosomes and glycogen are absent. In the remainder of tumors, the epithelium is of mixed endocervical and intestinal type (Fig. 18.41). The latter may show argentaffin/argyrophil cells. Fenoglio et al.[86] do not consider the mixture of these cells as evidence to dispute the surface epithelial origin of such neoplasms.

CLINICAL BEHAVIOR AND TREATMENT

Removal of the involved ovary is adequate therapy, provided the opposite ovary is examined carefully to rule out bilaterality. The appendix should be inspected for the presence of an associated mucocele.

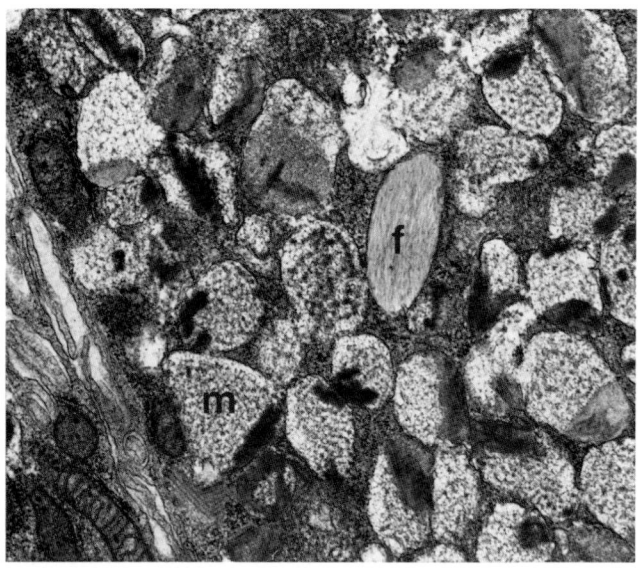

FIG. 18.40. Benign mucinous tumor. Detail showing pleomorphic mucin granules (*m*). The fibrillogranular body (*f*) is thought to be an unusual form of the mucin storage granule. ×20,000. (Courtesy of Dr. E. J. Wills, Royal Prince Alfred Hospital, Sydney, Australia.)

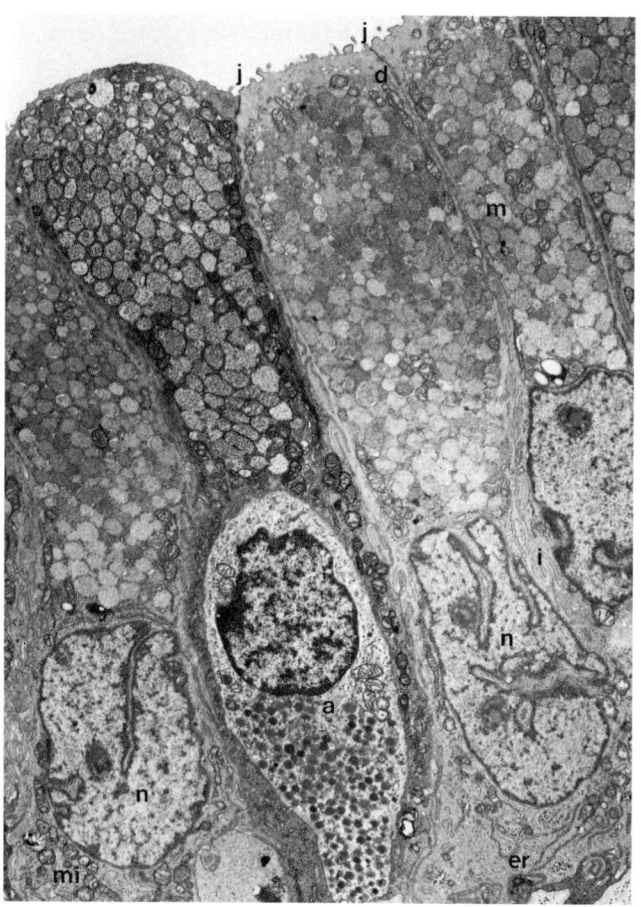

FIG. 18.41. Mucinous cystadenoma. Principal cells have a basal lobulated nucleus (*n*) and supranuclear cytoplasm is occupied mostly by mucin granules (*m*). Endoplasmic reticulum (*er*), mitochondria (*mi*,) and other cytoplasmic organelles are predominantly basal in position. The lateral plasma membranes show complex interdigitations (*i*), desmosomes (*d*), and junction complexes at the luminal border (*j*). An argentaffin cell (*a*) with basal secretory granules is also present. ×7000. (Courtesy of Dr. E. J. Wills, Royal Prince Alfred Hospital, Sydney, Australia.)

Atypically Proliferating Mucinous Tumors

GENERAL FEATURES

In two large series[109,207] 14% of all mucinous tumors were placed in the group of atypically proliferating mucinous tumors, significantly outnumbering frankly invasive mucinous carcinomas. They have a peak prevalence in women in their 30s and are bilateral in 6–8% of intestinal-type tumors of 40% of müllerian or endocervical-like tumors.[218] About 15% of each type are associated with extraovarian manifestations or spread; however, the endocervical-like tumors are associated with benign subperitoneal inclusions ("implants") and the intestinal-type tumors with pseudomyxoma peritonei (see below).

GROSS FINDINGS

These neoplasms do not differ grossly from their benign counterparts, being multilocular, cystic lesions with a smooth outer surface and an average diameter of 15 to 20 cm. There is a tendency to finer honeycombing of the cut surface in higher grade intestinal-type atypically proliferating mucinous tumors (Fig. 18.42), but this may be only focal. The müllerian tumor subgroup tends to be parvilocular, to have papillary projections in the cyst spaces, and to be associated with pelvic endometriosis in about 30% of cases.[218] Capsular thickening, necrosis, and hemorrhage are uncommon.

MICROSCOPIC FINDINGS

Architecturally, atypically proliferating mucinous tumors differ from their benign counterparts only in the exuberant growth of epithelium at the relative expense of stroma. Glandular buds and a microscopic filigree pattern similar to the tufting of atypically proliferating serous tumors are typical (Fig. 18.43). With increasing epithelial proliferation, a more complex glandular/papillary pattern emerges (Fig. 18.44) with multilayering and luminal reduplication (Fig. 18.45). Such changes commonly are focal and are likely to vary considerably from area to area in the same tumor. It is common to find all grades of proliferation as well as benign epithelium in the same field. Extensive

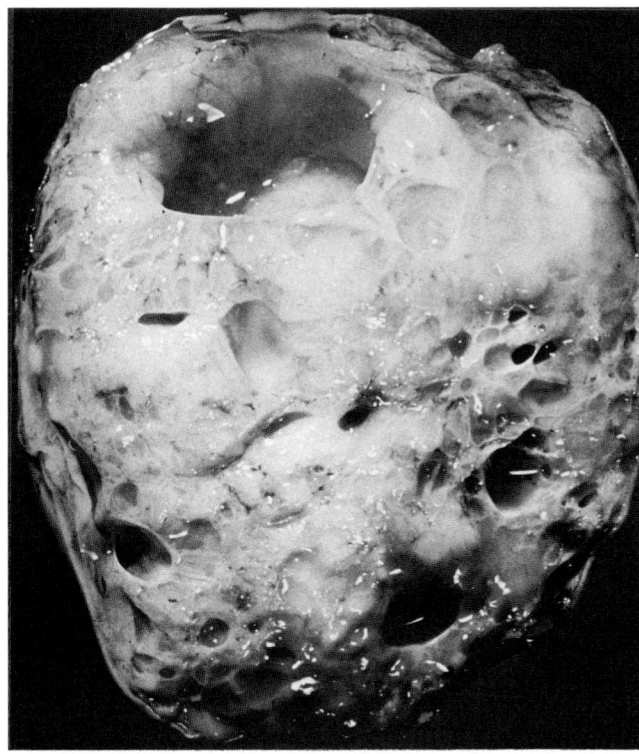

Fig. 18.42. Atypically proliferating mucinous tumor. The tumor is multilocular with a fine sieve-like cut surface.

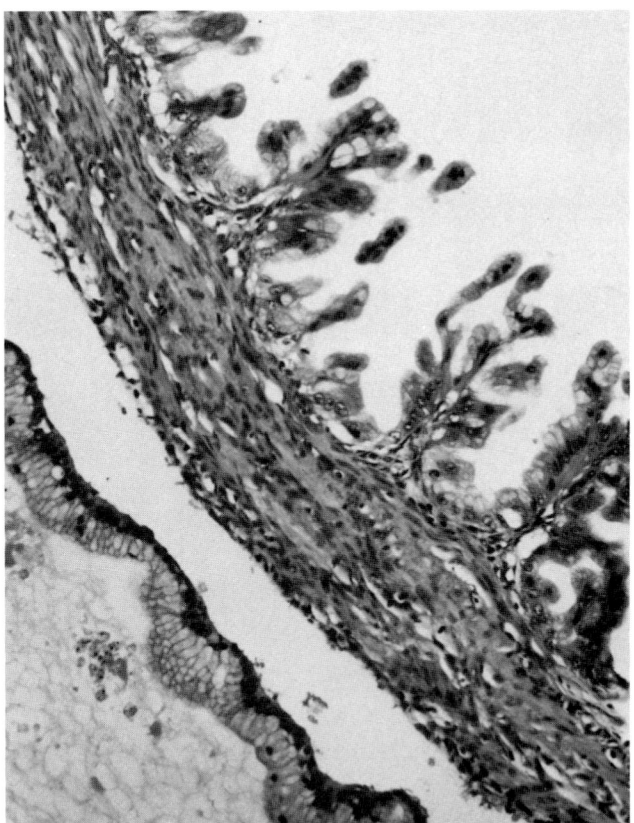

Fig. 18.43. Atypically proliferating mucinous tumor. Mild epithelial proliferation with tufting and bridging and mild nuclear atypia. Benign epithelium is seen at lower left.

sampling in thus vital in the assessment of such neoplasms. In 85% of tumors, the epithelium is recognizably intestinal in character with goblet cells present.[255] Variable cellular atypia, irregular, hyperchromatic nuclei with large nucleoli, decreased cytoplasmic mucin, and increased mitotic activity are evident. Neuroendocrine cells may be shown immunohistochemically in many such tumors.[225]

In 15% (particularly with a papillary pattern of growth), müllerian endocervical-like features are exclusively present.[218] These latter tumors frequently are associated with an acute inflammatory cell infiltrate, within the epithelium itself and the luminal mucin (Fig. 18.44). Rutgers and Scully[218] have described so-called "implants" similar to those associated with serous tumors, and seen with atypically proliferating mucinous tumors of müllerian or endocervical type. Mucinous "metaplastic" lesions have been described in the fallopian tube mucosa,[291] endometrium, and pelvic lymph nodes.[16]

Although capsular or stromal invasion is definitionally absent, they often are more difficult to exclude than in atypically proliferating serous tumors because of the irregular "centrifugal" glandular budding characteristic of many mucinous tumors. This should be differentiated from genuine microinvasion (see section of Malignant Mucinous Tumors). Attempts have been made to optimize the discrimination between atypically proliferating and frankly malignant mucinous tumors by adding histological criteria

that, in the absence of obvious stromal invasion, nevertheless predict progressive disease. Hart and Norris[109] reported a malignant course in occasional atypically proliferating mucinous tumors that exhibited epithelial multilayering of four or more cells thick and "large sheets of glands with back-to-back arrangement and no intervening stroma." Figure 18.46 demonstrates that watershed between noninvasive atypically proliferating and malignant as suggested by these authors. Since then, Hart has suggested extra criteria be considered as indicative of mucinous carcinoma[107] and many series of atypically proliferating mucinous tumors have used either the Hart and Norris criteria or the original FIGO/WHO criteria.° Comparing data from these series for Stage I cases reveals no statistically significant discriminatory value in the Hart and Norris criteria[211] versus the FIGO/WHO criteria. There appears to be about a 2–4% risk of recurrence and/or tumor-associated death irrespective of inclusion or exclusion of such cases (Table 18.3).

°Refs. 19,36,46,91,141,173,213,252,257.

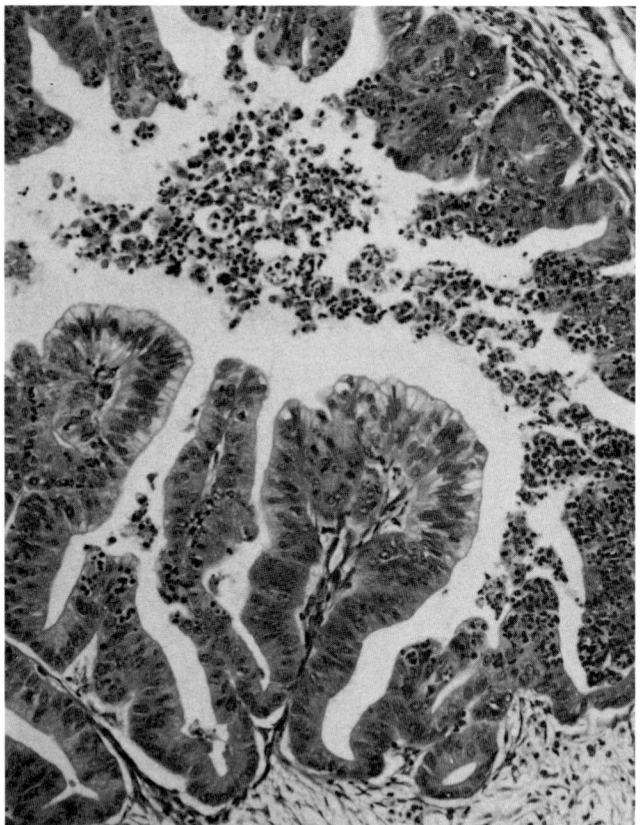

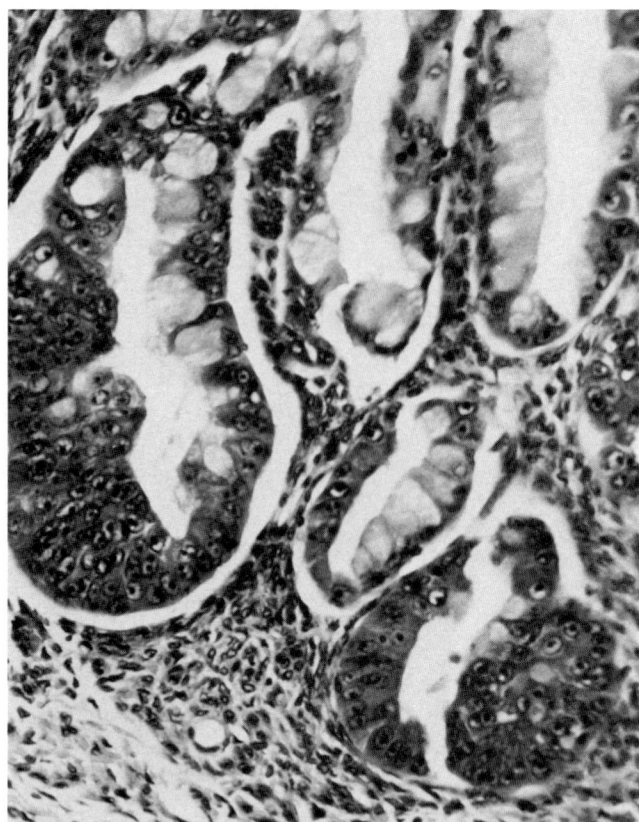

FIG. 18.44. Atypically proliferating mucinous tumor. The tumor has endocervical-like features. Moderate epithelial proliferation and nuclear atypia. The acute inflammatory infiltrate is degenerative in origin.

FIG. 18.45. Atypically proliferating mucinous tumor. There is marked epithelial proliferation and atypia. Note intestinal type differentiation.

In the stroma of these neoplasms, a foreign body–type giant cell reaction sometimes is present in relation to focal mucin spillage from ruptured or degenerating cysts or glands (Fig. 18.47). This may or may not be a clue to the genesis of a small number of reported cases of osteoclastoma-like giant cell (sarcoma-like) nodules (Fig. 18.48) in ovarian mucinous tumors. Such mucinous tumors are rarely benign—most are atypically proliferating or frankly malignant.[188] These tumors have shown one or more discrete hemorrhagic mural nodules with pushing margins, containing a heterogeneous population of benign osteoclast-like giant cells, mixed reactive mononuclear inflammatory cells, and bizarre mononuclear tumor giant cells (Fig. 18.49). The latter show atypical mitoses and ultrastructural and immunohistochemical evidence of epithelial differentiation.[66,133,174,216] The nature of the lesions is uncertain, but they do not appear to alter the behavior of the associated mucinous tumor.[24] They must be distinguished from true sarcomas,[38,189,266] anaplastic carcinomas,[48,95,112,190,248,285] or even carcinosarcomas[253] occurring as mural nodules in association with mucinous tumors and carrying a much worse clinical prognosis.

Pseudomyxoma peritonei is by far the most common extraovarian manifestation of those 15% or so of atypically proliferating mucinous tumors that present with apparent spread beyond the ovaries and is exclusively associated with the intestinal variant of such tumors. Theories of genesis include gross rupture of the cysts but pseudomyxoma, when present at the time of initial surgery, does not correlate with an obvious rupture, and likewise does not seem to follow accidental rupture during surgical removal.[180] The associated ovarian neoplasms are bilateral in one-third to two-thirds of cases,[41,294] often with an appendiceal mucocele also present, and always seem to show *pseudomyxoma ovarii*, an insidious penetration of tumor stroma by pools and tracts of mucin (Fig. 18.50). This is apparently due to breakdown of the cyst epithelium with little or no cellular reaction to the mucins released, and points to the probable mode of genesis of generalized disease, although it is not known whether mucin and cells disseminate or whether mucin alone can induce a metaplasia of the peritoneum.[223] Pseudomyxoma may be associated with intestinal-type mucinous ovarian neoplasms of any type (i.e., benign, atypically proliferating, or malig-

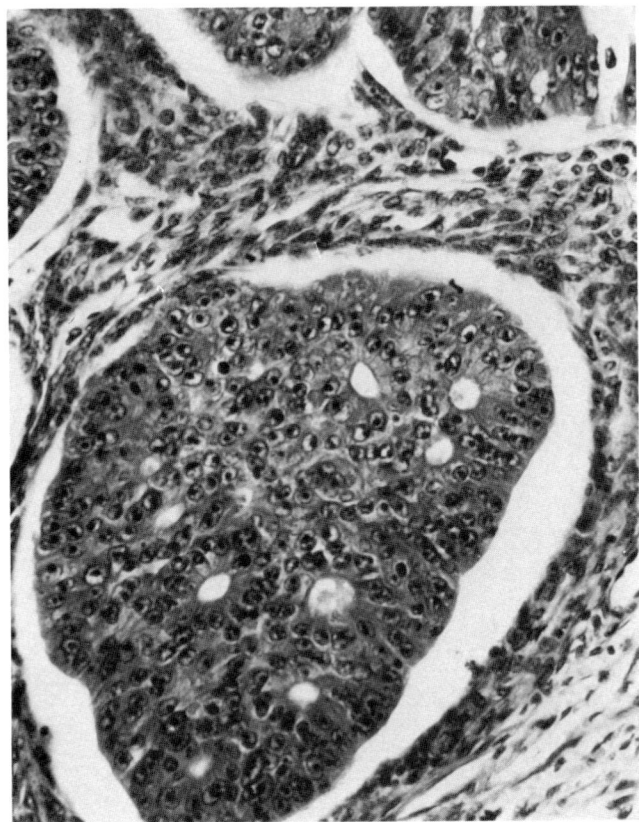

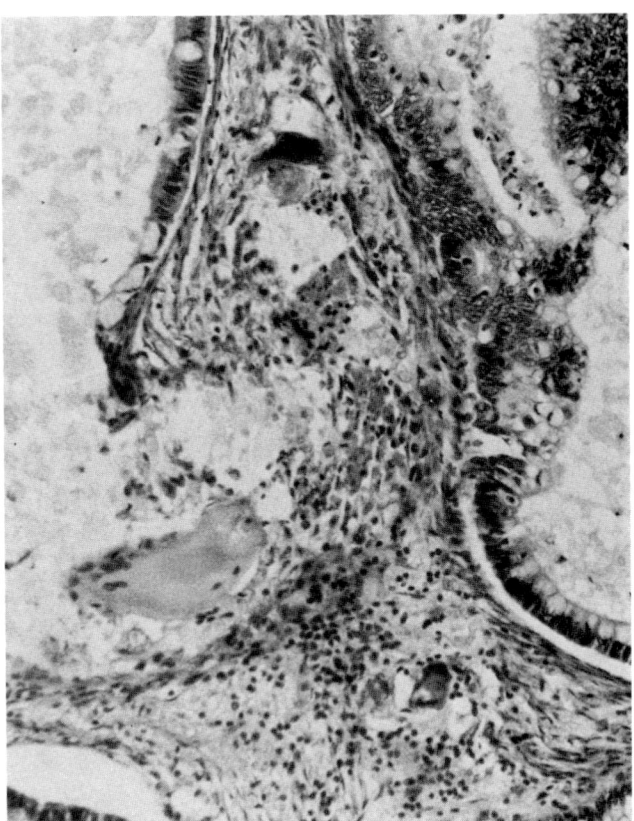

Fig. 18.46. **Atypically proliferating mucinous tumor.** There is marked epithelial atypia, multilayering, and cribriform nests but no destructive stromal invasion.

Fig. 18.47. **Mucinous cystadenoma.** The tumor contains intestinal-type epithelium. There are focal breaches in the integrity of the glands/cysts and a prominent giant-cell reaction.

nant). The presence of pseudomyxoma ovarii does not indicate malignant stromal invasion and tumors showing it should not be categorized automatically as carcinomas.[208] Similar findings can be observed in appendiceal cystadenomas that may or may not progress to generalized pseudomyxoma.[116] The frequent, but far from invariable,[124] association of cytologically similar tumors in the appendix and ovaries has led some investigators to propose that the appendiceal lesions are the initial site of neoplastic transformation and that the ovarian masses are most likely

metastatic in nature.[294] The concept of independent primary neoplasms is favored by others.[235]

ULTRASTRUCTURAL FINDINGS

The proliferating cells are stratified with some loss of polarity. Common cell types are immature colonic-type absorptive cells with numerous supranuclear mitochondria, extensive Golgi, and rough endoplasmic reticulum. Long apical microvilli are present and covered by thick glycocalyx.[87] Other cell types present are endocervical and colonic-type secretory cells, goblet cells, and argentaffin cells.[138]

CLINICAL BEHAVIOR AND TREATMENT

About 2–4% of patients with atypically proliferating mucinous tumors apparently confined to the ovaries at staging laparotomy will develop tumor recurrence or metastatic disease.[211] These often are patients who have had removal of the tumor only, and the first recurrence usually is in the contralateral ovary or elsewhere in the pelvis. Close clinical follow-up is justifiable in young women, desirous of retained fertility, with a neoplasm of this type confined to one ovary. Pelvic clearance is recommended when child-

Table 18.3. Analysis of clinical outcome of patients with FIGO Stage I atypically proliferating mucinous as defined by FIGO/WHO criteria[19,141,173,213,257] and by Hart and Norris criteria[36,46,109]

FIGO/WHO criteria			Hart and Norris criteria		
Total cases	Clinical recurrences	Fatal outcome	Total cases	Clinical recurrences	Fatal outcome
148	4	2	148	7	5

Modified from Russell, ref. 211.
FIGO, International Federation of Gynaecologists and Obstetricians; WHO, World Health Organization.

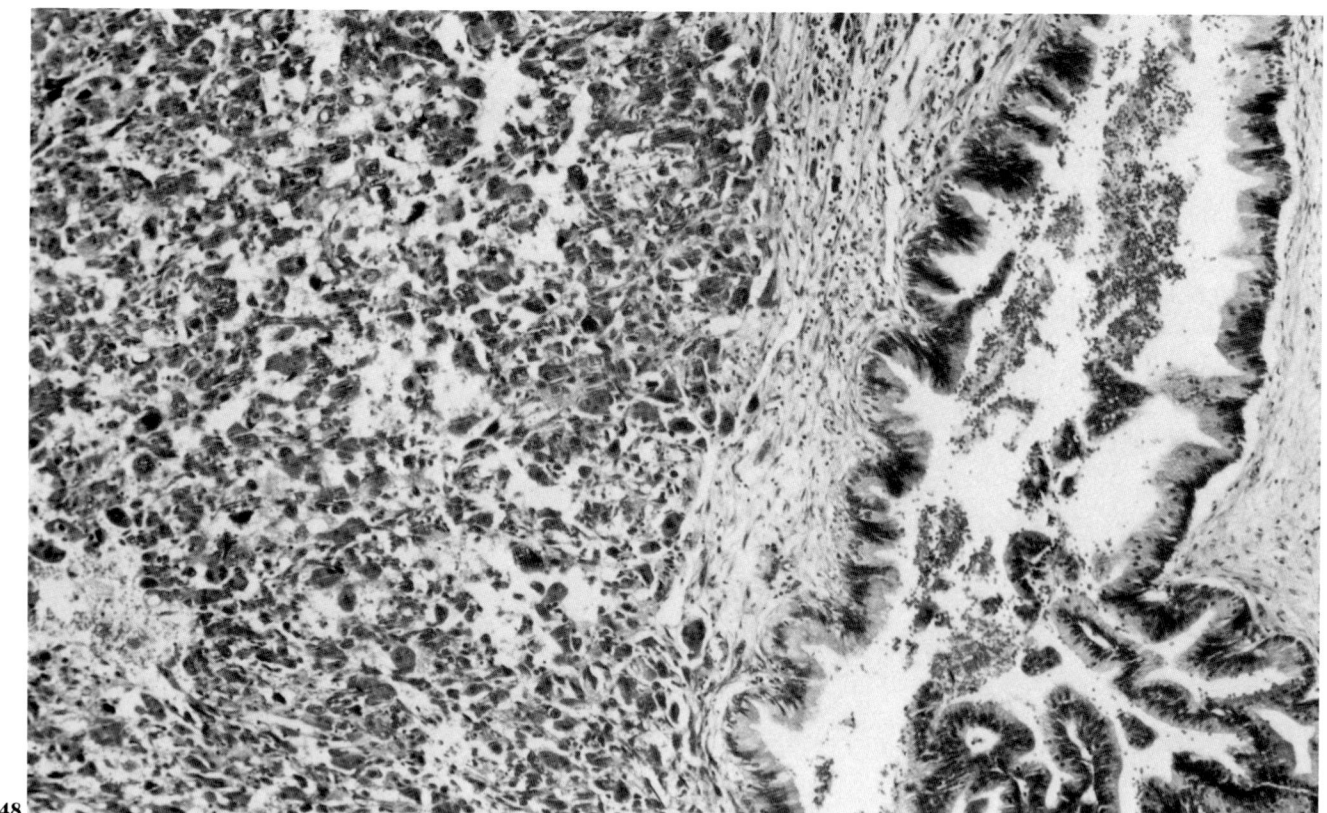

18.48

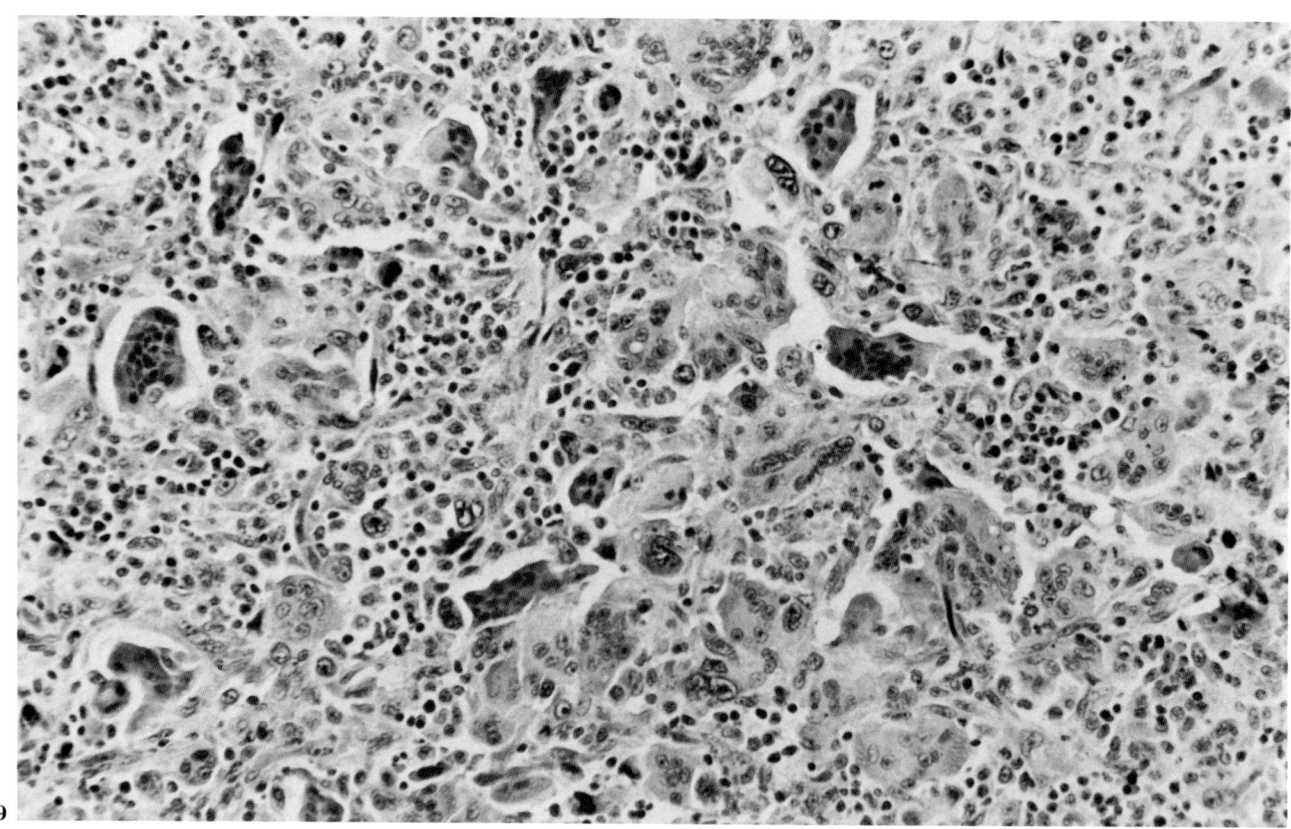

18.49

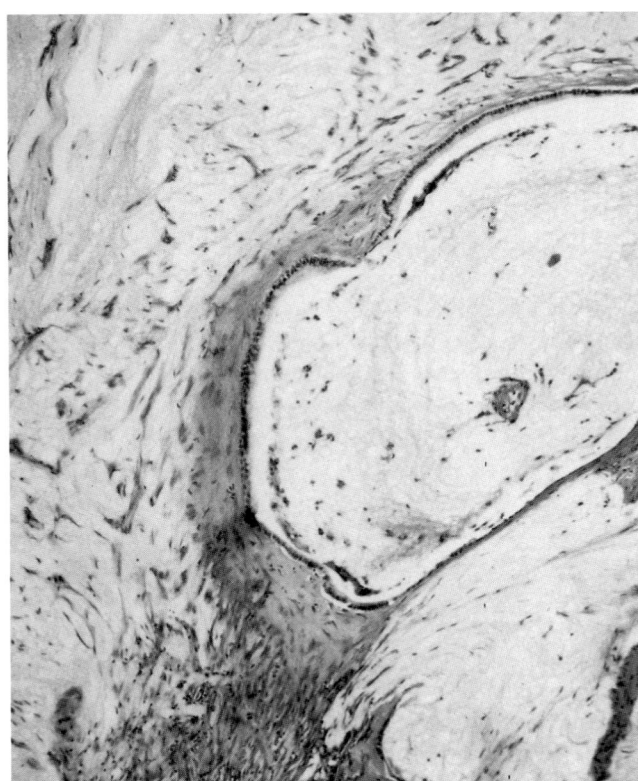

FIG. 18.50. Pseudomyxoma ovarii. A pattern within the benign ovarian mucinous tumor of a patient with widespread pseudomyxoma peritonei.

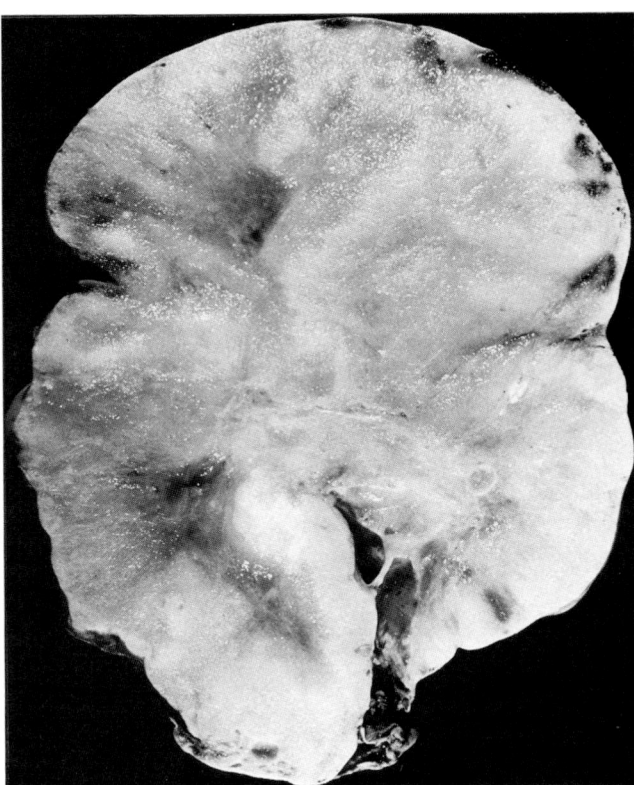

FIG. 18.51. Mucinous carcinoma. The tumor is usually solid without any appreciable cystic component. The cut surface has a glistening "mucoid" appearance.

bearing is completed. Hysterectomy and bilateral adnexectomy are suggested in all other cases.

For the rare patient with endocervical-like tumors and extraovarian lesions of focal type ("implants" as described by Rutgers and Scully[218]), careful examination of these lesions is mandatory. To date, these have not shown destructive stromal invasion, and clinical follow-up of the patient appears adequate. For patients with pseudomyxoma peritonei, a more favorable prognosis has been suggested for those cases in which tumors cells are not demonstrable in the masses of peritoneal mucin. Although this is a crude grading measure, it should be undertaken in each case.[116,294] Standard protocols of cytoreductive surgery at initial presentation and repeated palliative debulking, mucolytic agents, chemotherapy, and/or radiotherapy have modified little the natural history of the condition. Two-thirds of patients with pseudomyxoma peritonei survive 5 years and approximately 50% survive 10 years.[44]

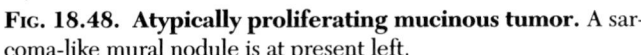

FIG. 18.48. Atypically proliferating mucinous tumor. A sarcoma-like mural nodule is at present left.
FIG. 18.49. Sarcoma-like mural nodule. There is a mixture of benign osteoclast-like and bizarre malignant giant cells (of epithelial origin) set in a chronic inflammatory background.

Malignant Mucinous Tumors

GENERAL FEATURES

Mucinous carcinomas represent 5–10% of malignant primary ovarian neoplasms and a similar percentage of all ovarian mucinous tumors. They occur mostly in patients in their fourth to seventh decades. Although 15–20% are bilateral, only 5% show extension beyond the ovaries at the time of laparotomy.

GROSS FINDINGS

The frank mucinous carcinomas tend to be cystic, multiloculated neoplasms usually measuring 15 to 30 cm in diameter. Solid areas and luminal nodules are more common than in atypically proliferating tumors, as are hemorrhage and necrosis. Infrequently, tumors are mainly or entirely solid (Fig. 18.51), with a soft mucoid consistency to the cut surface.

MICROSCOPIC FINDINGS

More commonly than in the equivalent serous tumors, microinvasion is an observable phenomenon in malignant mucinous tumors (Fig. 18.52). It is characterized by iso-

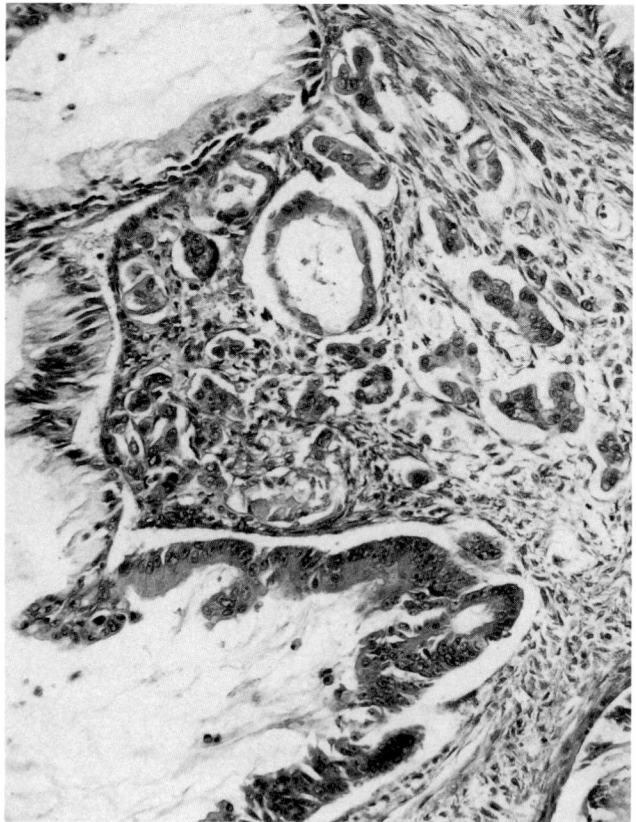

FIG. 18.52. **Microinvasive mucinous carcinoma.** Note both apparently benign mucinous epithelium (*top left*) and proliferating or in situ atypical epithelium (*lower*) adjacent to invasive focus.

lated foci of disordered growth of small irregular glandular acini or single cells in immature desmoplastic stroma. The invading cells frequently are ballooned by eosinophilic cytoplasm, but nuclear features do not differ significantly from those in the nearby in situ areas. Whether such stromal invasion represents the only valid, or even the most important, distinction between apparently in situ atypically proliferating and frankly invasive tumor groups is yet to be settled, and many frank mucinous carcinomas show focal atypical but in situ proliferation and even benign areas.

Invasive well-differentiated mucinous carcinomas resemble mucin-secreting adenocarcinomas of colonic origin and their architecture varies with the amount of mucin produced, cellular differentiation, and prominence of stroma. Solid tumors with a predominant fibrous stromal component (malignant adenofibromas) cause great difficulty in determining the presence of destructive stromal invasion. Subtle irregularities in gland contour and irregular budding may be the sole features (Fig. 18.53), as little if any change in the character of the stroma is seen in these areas.

Moderately differentiated mucinous carcinomas are more straightforward in this regard (Fig. 18.54). Pseudomyxomatous patterns in mucin-secreting carcinomas (Fig. 18.55) characterized by a minor cellular component in large pools of mucin, analogous to colloid carcinoma of colon, sometimes are seen. Pseudomyxoma peritonei associated with such carcinomas demonstrates the same degree of cellular atypia as the "primary" ovarian tumor.

Differention between primary mucinous ovarian carcinomas and metastases from occult colonic carcinomas masquerading as primary ovarian neoplasms can be difficult; in my experience, colonic metastases are encountered more frequently and should be excluded as far as practicable each time (see Chapter 22, Metastatic Tumors of the Ovary). The clinical setting, especially the presence of widespread intraperitoneal disease, must be taken into account and the pathologist has to accept that in some cases it is impossible, on histological grounds alone, to make this distinction. The frequency with which colonic metastases produce a cribriform or "garland" pattern of surviving glands around central areas of necrosis also should alert pathologists to this possibility.[148]

Poorly differentiated mucinous carcinomas show small clusters or single infiltrating cells embedded in dense reactive ovarian stroma (Fig. 18.56). Typical signet-ring cells often are present, containing intracellular mucin, and the lesion may in parts resemble a Krukenberg tumor. Indeed, rare instances have been reported of so-called primary Krukenberg tumor of the ovaries.[122]

IMMUNOCHEMICAL AND ULTRASTRUCTURAL FINDINGS

The discrimination between poorly differentiated primary müllerian carcinomas of serous or endometrioid types and mucinous carcinomas rests largely on demonstrating intracellular mucins histochemically or ultrastructurally. Immonohistochemically, CEA and NS19-9 are expressed in nearly all mucinous carcinomas, but only about 30% of endometrioid carcinomas and some serous tumors. OC-125, on the other hand, is identifiable in virtually all serous carcinomas and more than 50% of endometrioid tumors but is present only occasionally in mucinous carcinomas.

Studies of mucinous carcinomas have revealed cells similar to those in mucin-secreting intestinal adenocarcinoma.[87]

_____ ▷

FIG. 18.53. **Well-differentiated mucinous carcinoma.** Irregular-shaped and budding glands embedded in dense stroma. Other stromal signs of invasion, immaturity and inflammation, are absent.

FIG. 18.54. **Moderately differentiated mucinous carcinoma.** Cords and "crescents" of atypical cells with much intra- and extracellular mucin.

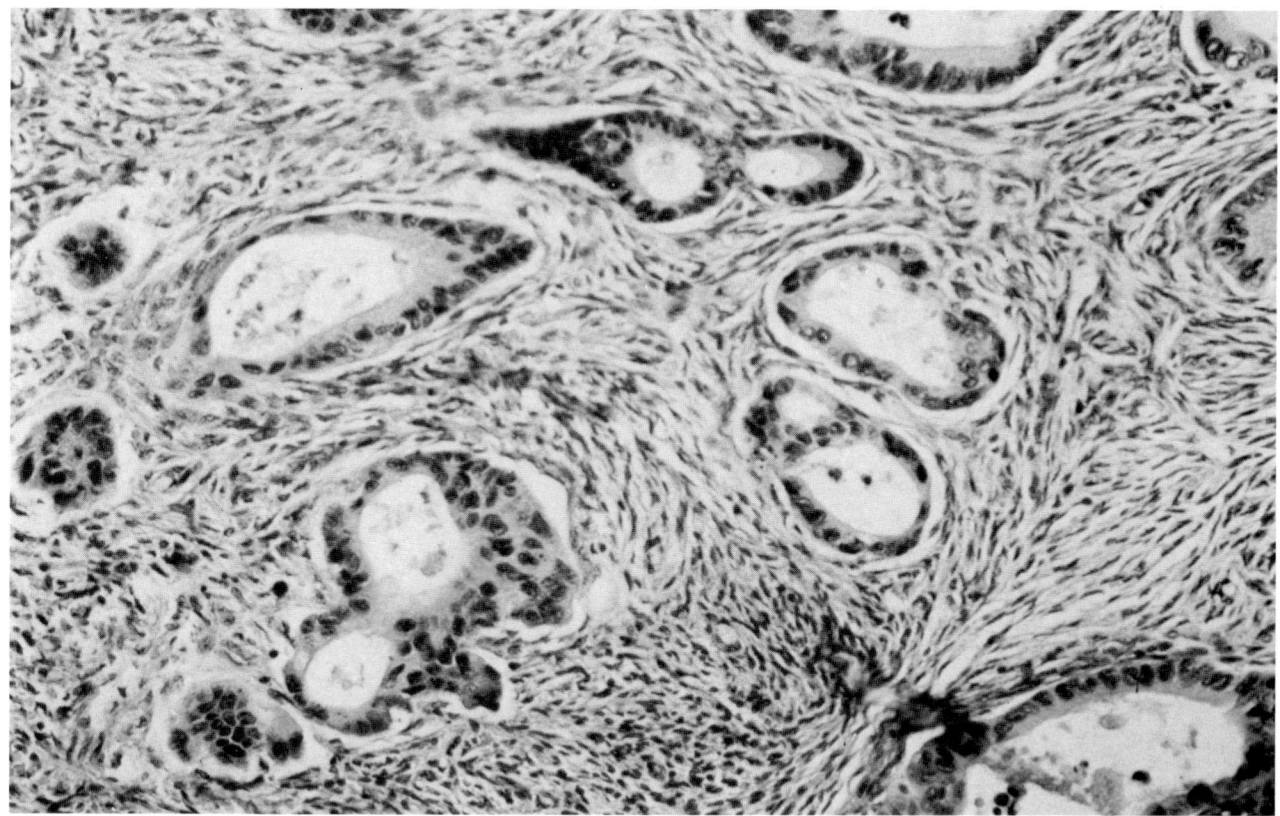

18.53

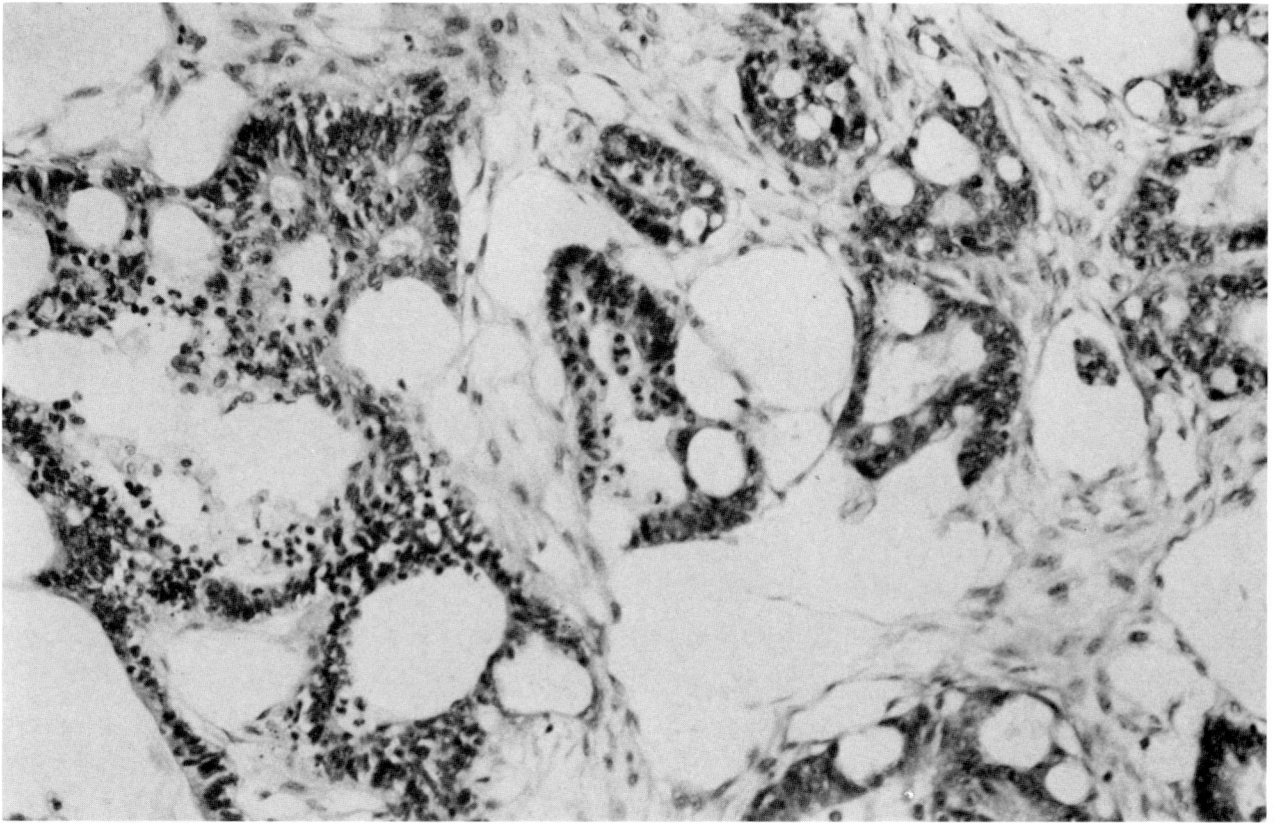

18.54

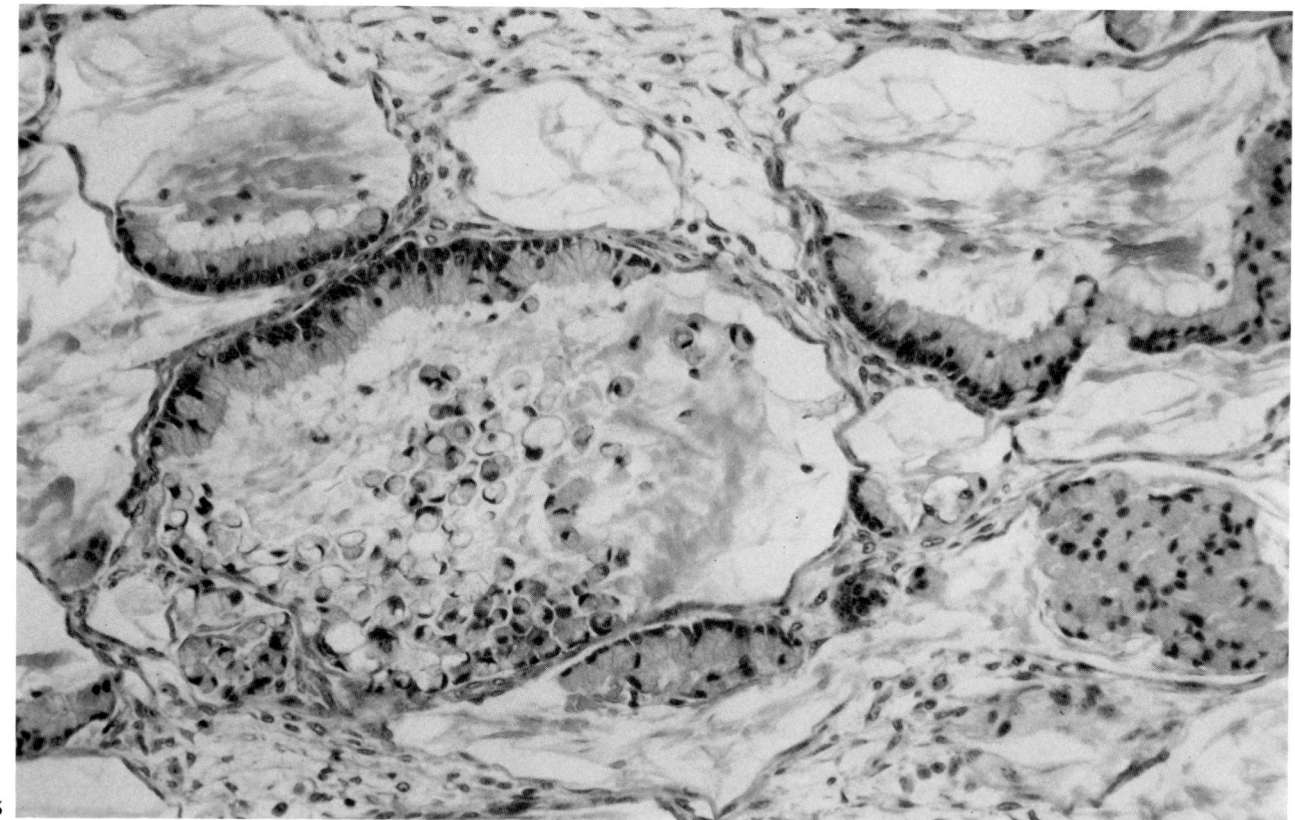

18.55

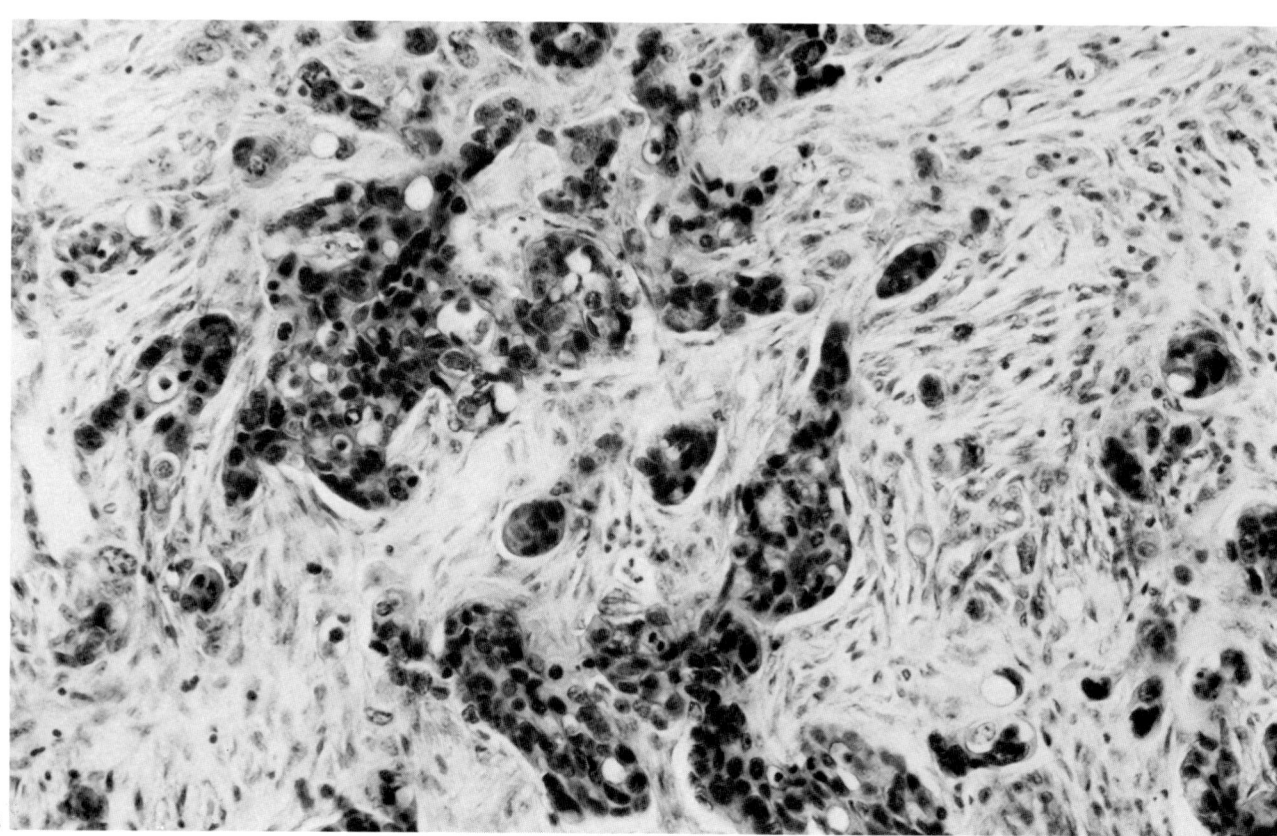

18.56

CLINICAL BEHAVIOR AND TREATMENT

The overall 5-year survival rate for all patients with mucinous carcinoma is about 40% whereas that for Stage I tumors is 66% at 5 years and 59% at 10 years.[109] The surgical management of Stage I is hysterectomy with bilateral adnexectomy and omentectomy, which can be followed by chemotherapy. The pattern of metastasis of mucinous carcinomas differs from that of serous carcinomas in that late extraperitoneal recurrences, particularly to the lungs, and characteristic, whereas with serous carcinomas, deaths tend to occur early and mostly from intraperitoneal disease.

Endometrioid Tumors

Ovarian endometrioid tumors are defined by "the presence of epithelial elements, stromal elements, or a combination of the two, that resemble closely the components of typical tumors of the endometrium."[230] By definition they are homologues of *all* neoplasms arising in the endometrium; however, in practice this spectrum of tumors is restricted to only the more commonly occurring variants. By convention rather than rational argument, tumors containing malignant stromal elements, that is, pure and mixed müllerian sarcomas, adenosarcomas and malignant mixed müllerian tumors are included in this group. Although they are müllerian in differentiation, these latter need not be regarded necessarily as specifically endometrioid, and in this chapter are dealt with separately in the next section.

Benign Endometrioid Tumors

GENERAL FEATURES

Single case reports represent most of the recorded experience with benign endometrioid tumors. This rarity may be explained partly by failure to recognize endometrioid epithelial differentiation in indolent tumors.[119] Twelve cases reported by Kao and Norris[129] confirm previous limited impressions that they are predominantly unilateral cystadenofibromas occurring in older women with a median age of 57 years. An architecturally and cytologically benign ovarian endometrioid adenofibroma, associated with omental lesions, has been described as malignant on the

basis of "metastatic disease" alone,[96] whereas an extra-ovarian endometrioid cystadenofibroma from the posterior wall of the uterus has been reported.[181]

GROSS FINDINGS

Mean diameter of benign endometrioid tumors is about 10 cm. The external surface is smooth and the cut surface densely fibrous, with a honeycomb appearance composed of multiple variously sized cysts. The latter contain clear or straw-colored fluid. Scully et al.[232] described a solitary example of a polypoid nodule arising within an endometriotic cyst.

MICROSCOPIC FINDINGS

Benign endometrioid tumors are histologically adenofibromas or cystadenofibromas. Epithelial elements are arranged in branching tubular glands and cystic spaces (Fig. 18.57). The tumor cells tend to resemble those of proliferative endometrium (Fig. 18.58), being tall columnar with basophilic to amphophilic cytoplasm and elongated nuclei with relatively coarse chromatin and small but obvious nucleoli, or of inactive endometrium with uniform, elongated, dark nuclei and scanty cytoplasm. Staining by diastase-PAS and mucicarmine reveals some extracellular mucin plus some staining of the glycocalyx at the luminal border of the cells. Mitoses are rarely seen, in contrast to nonneoplastic proliferative endometrium (e.g., endometriosis). Secretory changes similar to those seen in postovulatory endometrium are frequently seen in well-differentiated tumors and squamoid elements also are often noted.[90,233] The fibrovascular stroma resembles that of endometrial polyps or, less often, ovarian cortex. The absence of typical endometrial type stroma and no evidence of recurrent local hemorrhage further assists in differentiating these lesions from endometriosis.

CLINICAL BEHAVIOR AND TREATMENT

Local removal is considered adequate management, although it should be noted that of the 12 or so reported cases one has recurred after apparent incomplete removal and a second was associated with benign omental "implants."

Atypically Proliferating Endometrioid Tumors

GENERAL FEATURES

Endometrioid tumors that exhibit only those changes of low-grade atypical proliferation are described rarely in the literature. This may be partly because of genuine rarity, although criteria for defining atypically proliferating endometrioid tumors are certainly less well established than

◁ ────────────────────────────

FIG. 18.55. **Moderately differentiated mucinous carcinoma.** There are large pools of mucin in the stroma (malignant pseudomyxoma), nests of tumor cells and signet-ring cells (same tumor as Fig. 18.51).

FIG. 18.56. **Poorly differentiated mucinous carcinoma.** Abortive acini and signet-ring cells are present.

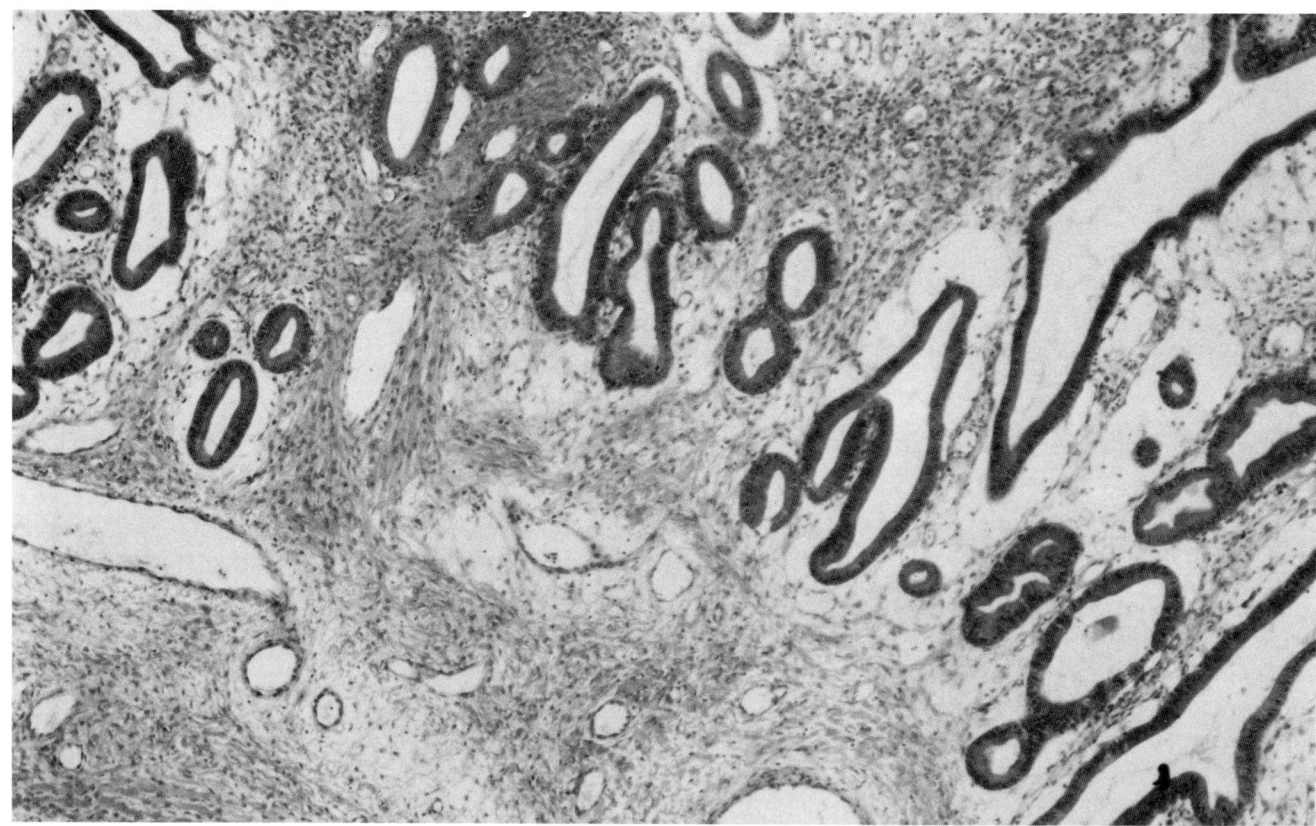

Fig. 18.57. Endometrioid adenofibroma. Simple tubular and cystic glands with focal branching are surrounded by fibrous stroma.

for their serous or mucinous counterparts, particularly the line dividing them from invasive endometrioid carcinomas.[91] They comprise about 20% of endometrioid neoplasms in our material[207] and have a mean age at presentation of 50 to 55 years. The common presenting symptoms are abnormal vaginal bleeding, abdominal pain, and/or mass. They may be associated with synchronous or metachronous hyperplasia or adenocarcinoma of the uterine endometrium.[27,208]

GROSS FINDINGS

There appear to be two macroscopically distinct patterns. The more frequently encountered are unilateral adenofibromas or cystadenofibromas with features similar to those of the benign lesions noted above.[27,127,203,208,247]

Even less often the solid areas are softer in consistency and the cut surface (Fig. 18.59) features hemorrhage or necrosis. Papillary areas also may be noted. These tend to be the tumors with high-grade epithelial proliferation and grossly resemble frankly invasive endometrioid carcinomas.[208]

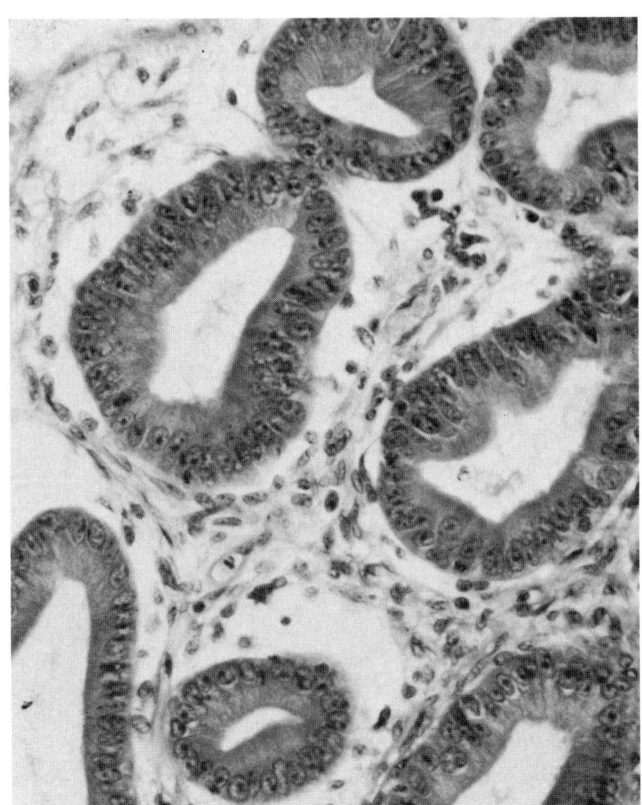

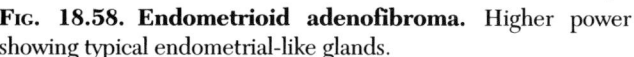

Fig. 18.58. Endometrioid adenofibroma. Higher power showing typical endometrial-like glands.

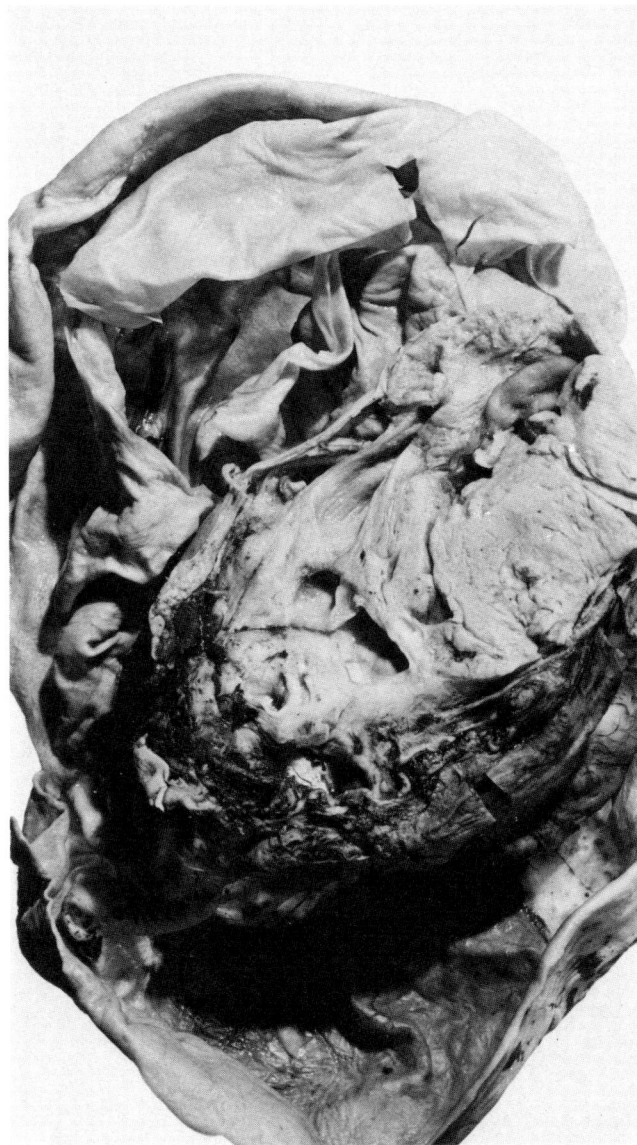

FIG. 18.59. Atypically proliferating endometrioid tumor. Thick-walled multilocular cyst with a single, firm, fibrous intraluminal nodule.

MICROSOPIC FINDINGS

Low-grade atypically proliferating endometrioid tumors are characterized by crowded endometrial-like glands and cystic spaces in stroma, which is ovarian in type or is hyaline/collagenous (Fig. 18.60). Smooth muscle and stromal luteinization may both be seen focally. Glands are oriented randomly and cytologically show nuclear crowding and mild to moderate atypia and epithelial stratification with tufting and bridging (Fig. 18.61). This stratification is stressed as being a critical feature differentiating atypically proliferating from benign endometrioid cystadenofibro-

mas.[127,203] Tumors showing such characteristics are termed *atypical endometrioid adenofibromas* by Bell and Scully[27] or *proliferative endometrioid tumors.*[177,247] Mitoses range up to 4 MF/10 HPF but are rarely atypical.

High-grade atypically proliferating endometrioid tumors show less obvious stroma and more exuberant intracystic papillary and glandular epithelial proliferation (Fig. 18.62). Except for the tendency to display a papillary architecture, they resemble the various patterns of complex atypical endometrial hyperplasia. There may be back-to-back glandular arrangements[27,208] giving a smooth, well-defined interface between the mature acellular stroma and the intracystic epithelial compartment, with an almost total lack of chronic inflammatory cell infiltrates. In my view, and that of others,[27,177,247] this is a defensible upper limit for noninvasive but atypically proliferating endometrioid neoplasia. Occasional tumors show foci of microinvasion[177,247] characterized by haphazard stromal infiltration by nests and cords of malignant epithelial cells. Limited experience with such tumors precludes any sensible assessment of this change but there appear to be no adverse consequences for the patients.[177] Benign squamous metaplasia is present in 35–50% of all cases (Fig. 18.63).

CLINICAL BEHAVIOR AND TREATMENT

Despite lack of unanimity as to histological definition, there appears consensus as to their excellent prognosis. Some are associated with endometrial hyperplasia or carcinoma and rarely with extraovarian manifestations.[129,208,247] Two patients developed endometrioid carcinomas in contralateral ovaries after unilateral adnexectomy.[27,213] The recommended treatment therefore is diagnostic curettage to assess endometrial status, peritoneal washings, and biopsies followed by total hysterectomy and bilateral adnexectomy.[213] Conservation of reproductive function may be considered in a young woman.

Malignant Endometrioid Tumors

GENERAL FEATURES

Approximately 80% of ovarian endometrioid tumors are frankly malignant. Endometrioid carcinomas are the second most frequently encountered malignant ovarian epithelial tumor, accounting for 20–25% of all ovarian carcinomas, yet are frequently misdiagnosed.[267] Some series, particularly European, place this relative incidence as high as 30% or more.[90]

They are bilateral in 28% of cases overall. Endometrioid carcinomas are confined to the ovaries and adjacent pelvic structures in most patients and in such instances only 13% are bilateral. They occur most frequently in the fifth and sixth decades but not infrequently in older women. Many

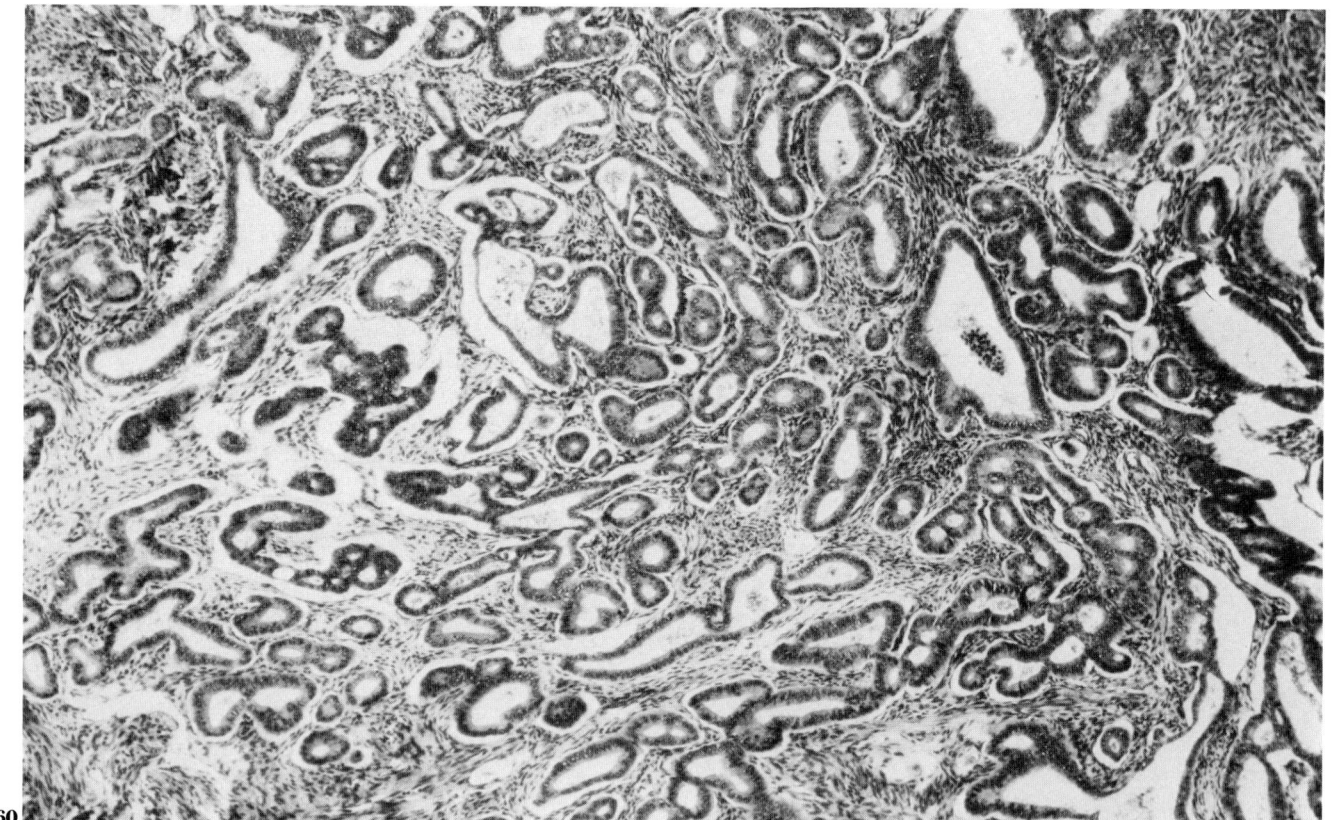

18.60

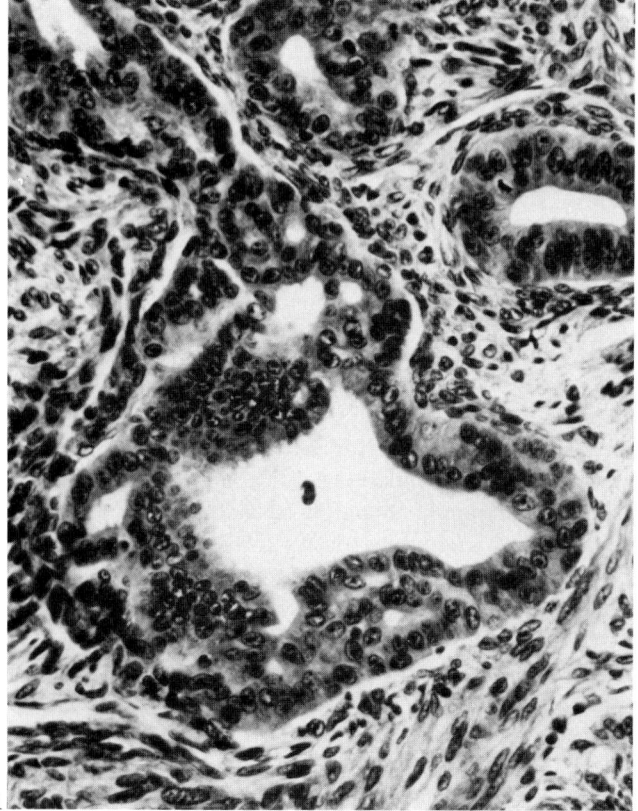

18.61

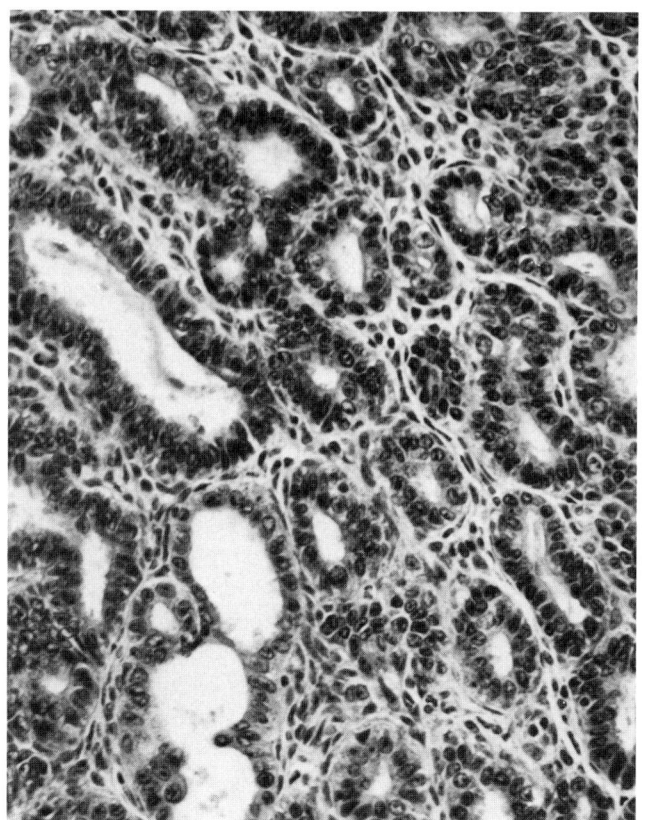

18.62

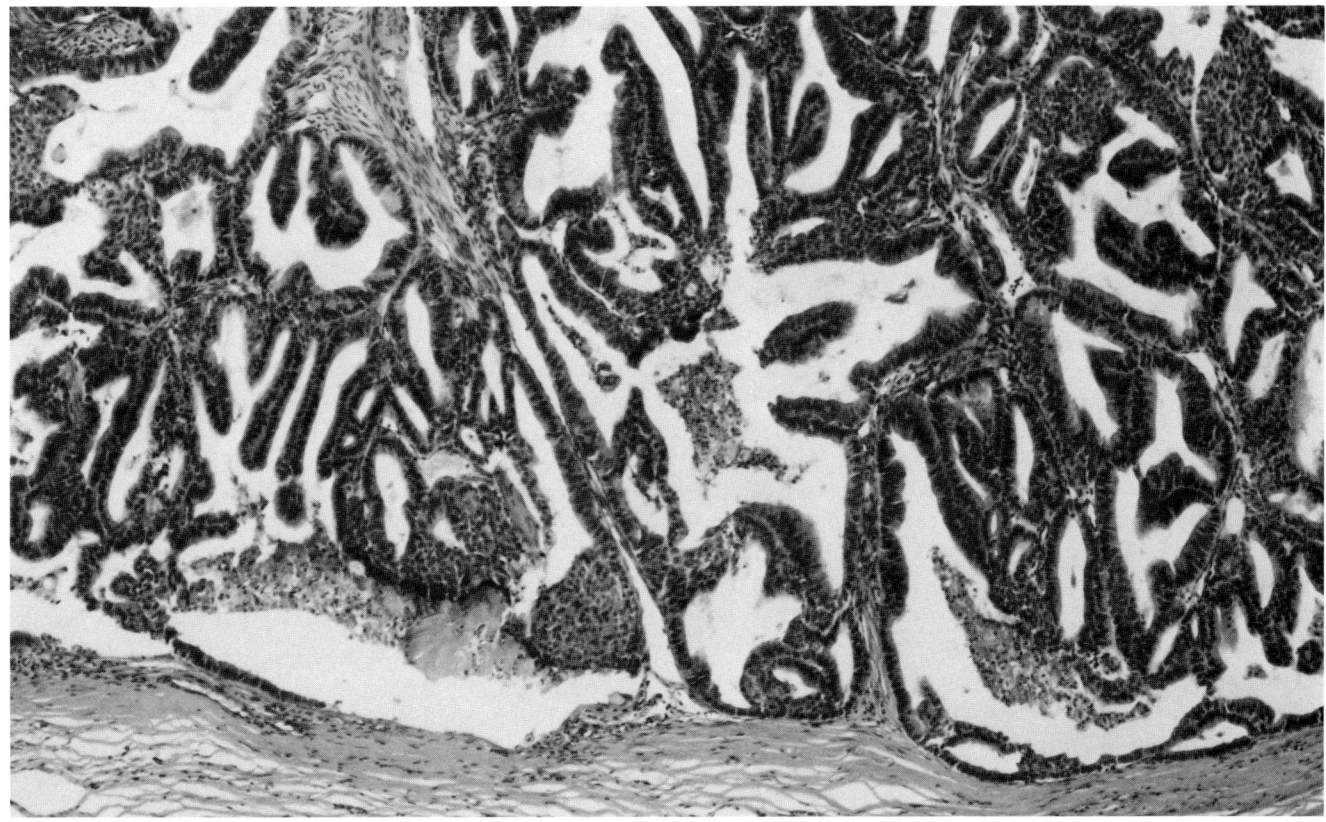

FIG. 18.63. Atypically proliferating endometrioid tumor. There is marked epithelial proliferation (back-to-back arrangement of glands) and prominent squamous metaplasia, but smooth epithelial–stromal interface.

endometrioid carcinomas are thought to derive from the modified surface epithelium of the ovaries without the interposition of preexisting endometriosis. Interestingly, up to 31% of such tumors are associated with endometriosis in the same ovary or elsewhere in the pelvis.[37,207] Those carcinomas that can be shown to arise within an endometriotic cyst, on the other hand, present in women younger than the average by 10 or more years.[171] About 20–25% of these carcinomas are associated with a histologically similar lesion in the endometrium[263]; the latter usually are regarded as independent autochthonous neoplasms, although metastasis from one site to the other is theoretically difficult to exclude in some cases.[84,298] Rare

◁————————————————

FIG. 18.60. Atypically proliferating endometrioid adenofibroma. Irregularly branching and budding glands in fibrous stroma.

FIG. 18.61. Atypically proliferating endometrioid adenofibroma. Higher power showing glands with mild nuclear atypia as well as atypical proliferation—bridging and stratification. Contrast with Figure 18.58.

FIG. 18.62. Atypically proliferating endometrioid tumor. There is a moderate degree of atypical grandular proliferation.

instances have been observed of synchronous or metachronous endometrioid carcinomas of the ovaries and cervix,[125] and occasional primary extraovarian endometrioid carcinomas have been noted.[119]

It has been estimated that endometrial adenocarcinomas account for up to one-third of tumors metastatic to the ovaries. Endometrial stromal sarcomas and malignant mixed müllerian tumors occasionally also metastasize to the ovaries.[161,269] Ovarian tumors have been found at autopsy in 34–47% of women with endometrial carcinoma[115] and in 2–12% of women undergoing surgery for endometrial malignancy.[9,14,230] Survival studies of patients with simultaneous or metachronous uterine and ovarian carcinomas suggest that, on the balance of probabilities, most of them do not represent metastases from one site to the other but rather independent primary lesions, arising in response to the same carcinogenic influences.[84,183,209,230,284] This is in accord with the developing concept of multifocal tumorigenesis in the upper genital tract, ovaries, and pelvic peritoneum.[214] This possibility is important to consider because of the implications for treatment. Most simultaneous tumors are of similar histological type—predominantly endometrioid.[54,161,230,269,293] A similar but rarer problem exists with simultaneous endometrioid carcinomas in the ovaries and cervix.[125] In many cases, the endometrial adenocarcinoma arises against a background of atypical hyperplasia. Likewise, careful and extensive examination of the ovarian tumor will reveal, in many cases, areas of co-existing benign or atypically proliferating endometrioid tumor or an origin in an endometriotic cyst, indicating an in situ genesis.

GROSS FINDINGS

Endometrioid carcinomas are primarily cystic and most measure 12 to 20 cm in diameter. The external surfaces more frequently are smooth than bosselated. On section, cysts contain friable soft masses or papillae as well as blood-stained fluid (Fig. 18.64). Less commonly, the neoplasms are completely solid with widespread necrosis and hemorrhage. Mucus sometimes may be noted in the cysts, erroneously suggesting mucinous carcinoma. Tumors arising in an endometriotic cyst tend to exhibit exophytic polypoid masses rather than mural nodules and if there is endometriosis in the adjacent uninvolved portion of ovary, the characteristic features of these nonneoplastic lesions also will be present.

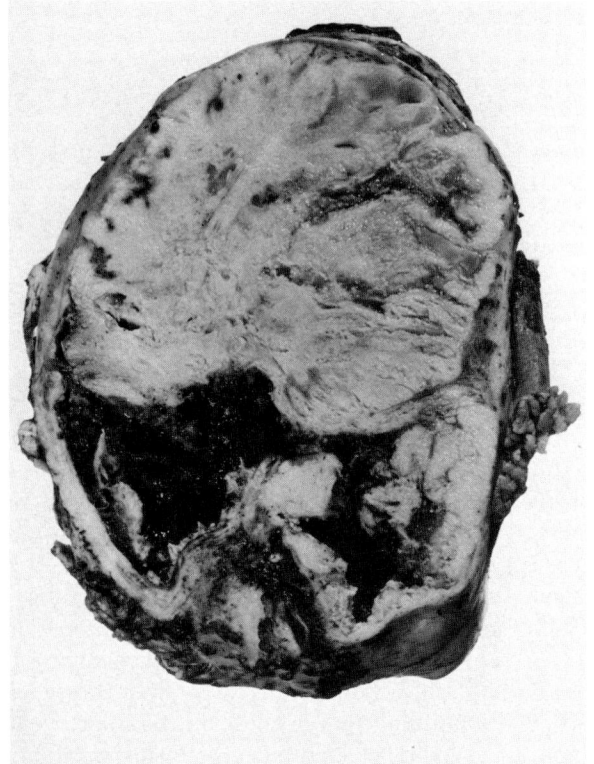

FIG. 18.64. **Endometrioid carcinoma.** Epithelial nodules protrude into the ragged cystic cavities, which also contain altered blood.

MICROSCOPIC FINDINGS

All carcinoma subtypes documented in the uterine corpus also have been identified in the ovaries, including typical adenocarcinomas (Fig. 18.65), adenocarcinomas with benign (Fig. 18.66) and malignant (Fig. 18.67) squamous differentiation, glycogen-rich adenocarcinoma, so-called secretory adenocarcinomas (Fig. 18.68), and, of course, papillary serous and clear cell carcinomas, which are excluded by convention from this group and discussed separately. By definition, these tumors closely resemble their uterine counterparts although some differences exist. The tendency for cystic ovarian tumors to be accompanied by a coarse papillary pattern of growth is encountered more often than in the exophytic luminal component of uterine tumors.

Well-differentiated endometrioid adenocarcinomas account for most cases and also are overly represented among tumors seen to arise from endometriotic cysts. They have a glandular growth pattern with irregular budding and luminal reduplication (Fig. 18.65). Glandular buds have smooth, rounded contours, with tall columnar pseudostratified or multilayered epithelium. Mitoses range up to 5 MF/10 HPF. Cellular debris occasionally is present within gland-like spaces accompanied by reactive histiocytic giant cells.[212] This response is dissimilar, however, to that associated with ovarian mucinous tumors (Fig. 18.47). Squamous differentiation is seen in about 30% and usually is cytologically benign—varying in prominence from small morules to large confluent sheets connecting the malignant glands (Fig. 18.66). If the squamous epithelium is in direct contact with the stroma, and particularly if it is degenerative, a foreign body giant cell reaction may be induced. Infrequently, the squamous epithelium appears malignant and may be either intimately admixed with the adenocarcinoma[230] or separate from the glandular elements, producing a distinct area of invasive squamous cell carcinoma.

Tumor stroma is ovarian in type or is nonspecific and fibroblastic in appearance. Occasional well-differentiated endometrioid carcinomas with prominent fibrous stroma have been described,[203] usually with obvious benign squamous metaplasia. Stromal invasion in such tumors is difficult to document and inferred only by the extent, complexity, and irregularity of the epithelial component and the immature desmoplastic nature of the stroma.[27]

Secretory patterns are seen focally in approximately one-third of endometrioid ovarian carcinomas (Fig. 18.68) and are to be distinguished from clear cell carcinoma; the cells remain tall columnar and show supranuclear and/or subnuclear vacuoles (rather than diffuse cytoplasmic clearing around eccentric nuclei producing large, pavement-like clear cells). Hobnail cells are not seen. Papillary areas are common, the papillae being broad, blunt structures with obvious connective tissue cores. They differ markedly

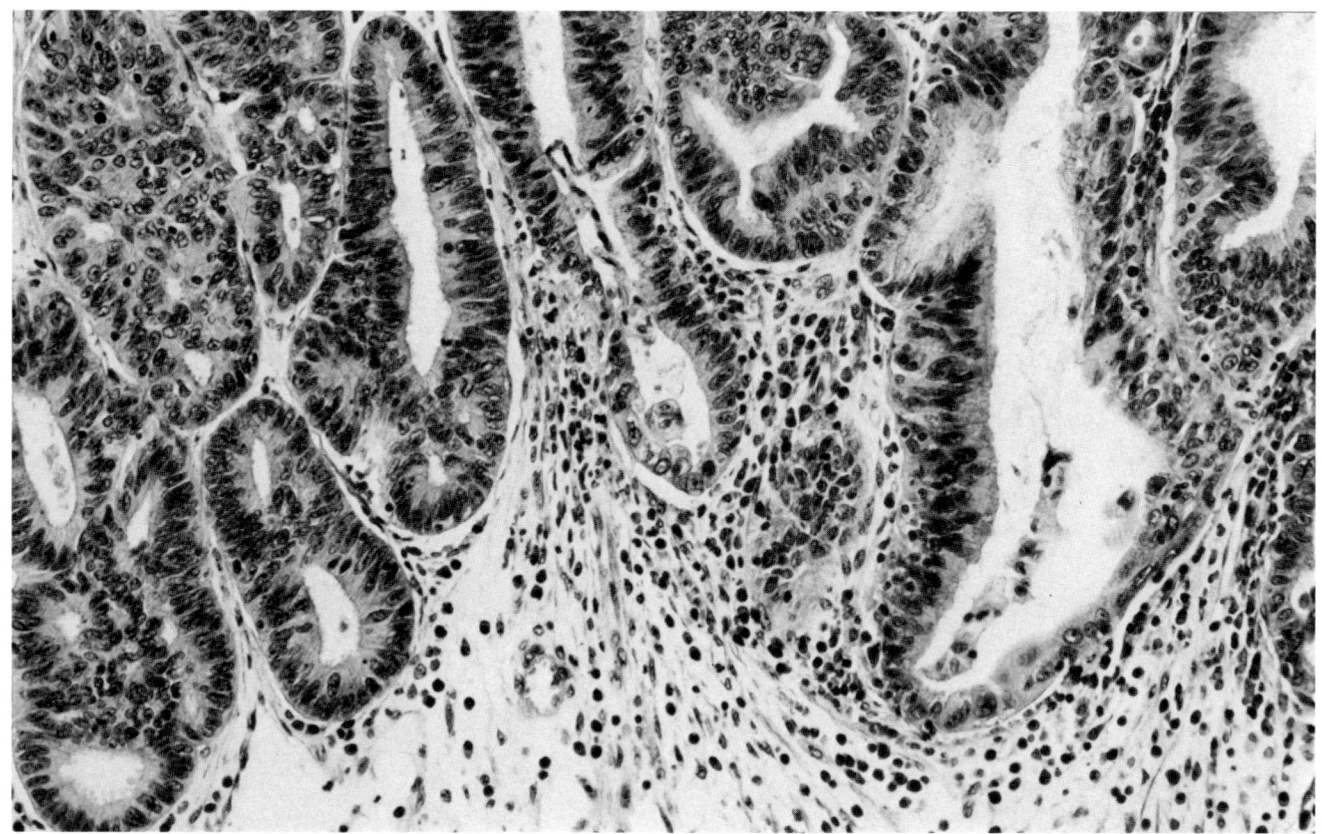

18.65

from the usually fine micropapillae of serous carcinoma; psammoma bodies also can be present occasionally but are never prominent. Extracellular mucin also is sometimes focally prominent and may give rise to difficulty in differentiating endometrioid from mucinous cancers. Mucin stains (diastase-PAS, mucicarmine, alcian blue), however, show only apical staining of the glycocalyx in typical endometrioid tumor cells. On the other hand, many cells with abundant intracellular mucin, goblet cells, pseudomyxoma ovarii, and/or "mucoid degeneration" suggest mucinous differentiation.

Moderately differentiated endometrioid adenocarcinomas show complex glandular and microglandular patterns. Epithelial multilayering is less prominent (Fig. 18.69) but pleomorphism, mitotic activity (up to 1 MF/HPF), and nuclear atypia are all increased and tumor giant cells may be seen. Necrosis and hemorrhage also are more obvious. Secretory change and squamous differentiation are noted about as frequently as in well-differentiated tumors, but

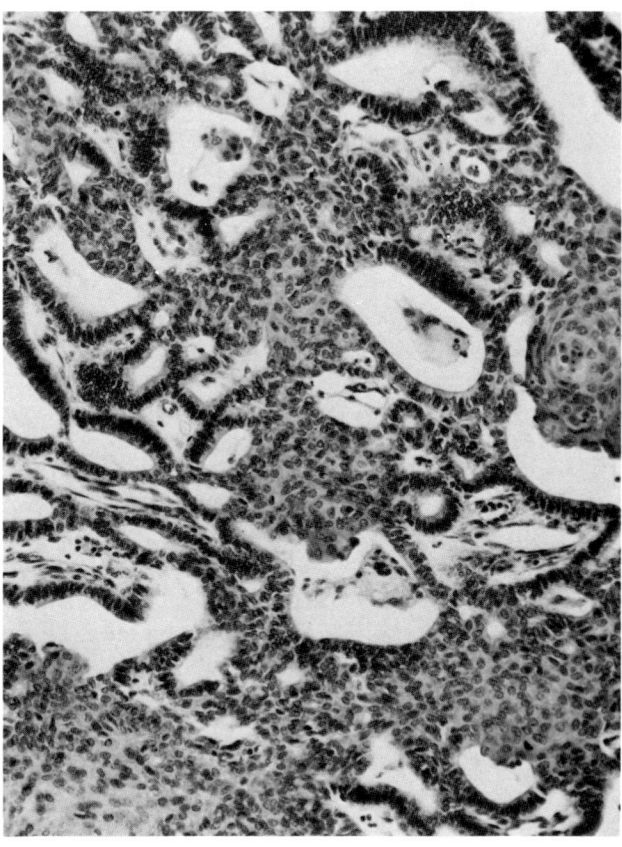

18.66

FIG. 18.65. **Well-differentiated endometrioid carcinoma.** Commonly observed pattern with malignant glands showing smooth growth rounded contours.
FIG. 18.66. **Endometrioid carcinoma.** There is prominent benign squamous metaplasia (adenoacanthoma).

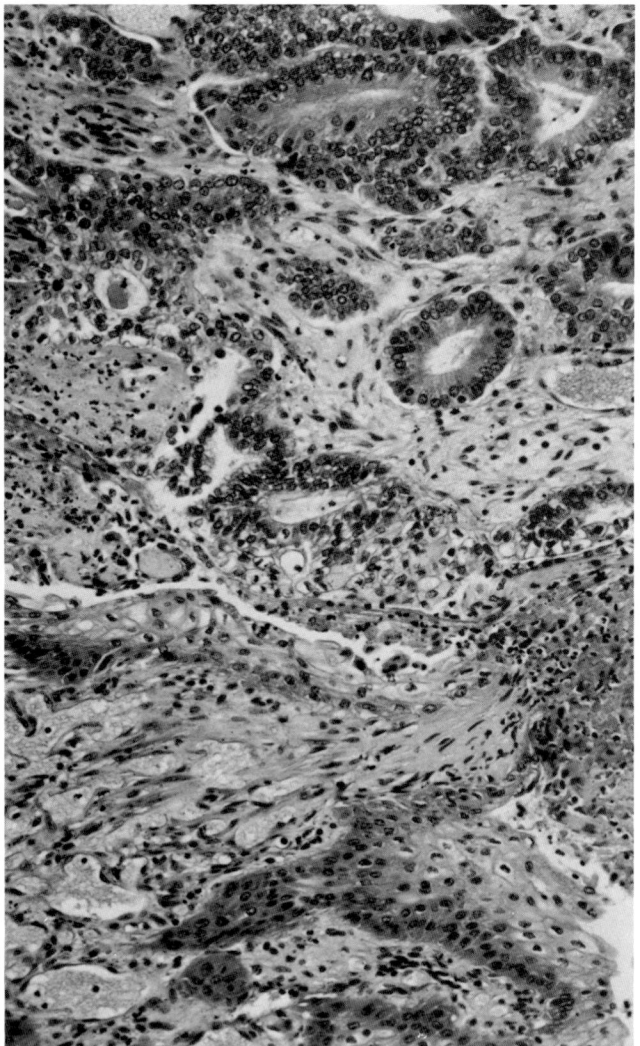

Fig. 18.67. Adenosquamous carcinoma. An invasive squamous (*bottom*) and glandular (*top*) component is present.

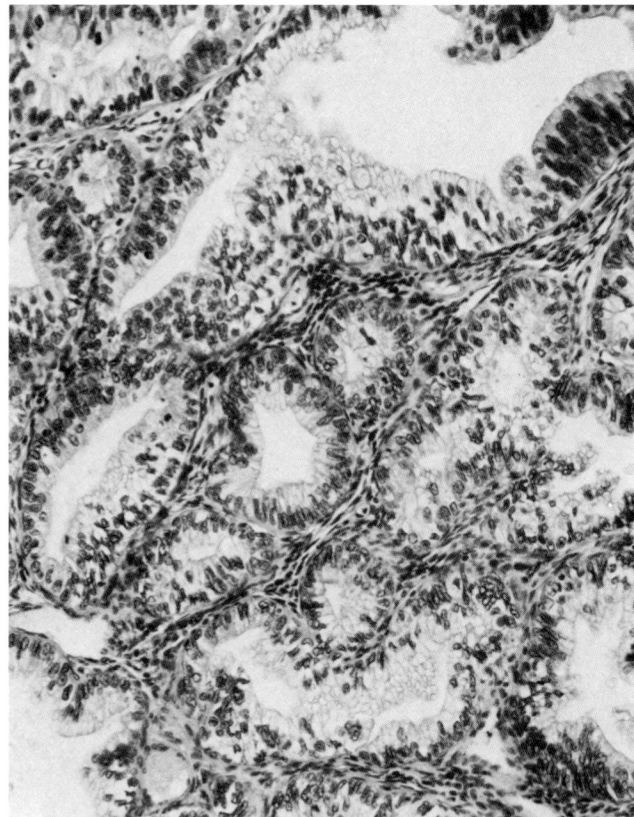

Fig. 18.68. Well-differentiated endometrioid carcinoma. Tall columnar cells with supranuclear vacuoles, so-called secretory adenocarcinoma.

the squamous component in such tumors appears more likely to be malignant.

Poorly differentiated endometrioid carcinomas have a mainly solid pattern with residual microglandular areas (Fig. 18.70), the latter as either separate foci or producing a peripheral cuff about islands of solid undifferentiated carcinoma. This latter point is the basis of distinction from poorly differentiated serous carcinomas on the one hand and from undifferentiated carcinomas on the other. The glandular spaces often seen in serous carcinomas tend to be elongated or slit-like. There are no clear criteria on how much gland formation is required to exclude a given tumor from the WHO undifferentiated category; some would suggest that, by convention, the term *endometrioid carcinoma* be reserved for those tumors with significant tubular or microglandular differentiation.[229] Mitotic activity ranges up to 5 MF/HPF or more but squamous or secre-

tory change are rarely noted. Hemorrhage and necrosis are widespread.

Differential Diagnosis

Occasional endometrioid tumors superficially resemble sex cord–stromal tumors[206,296] because of microglandular areas simulating Call–Exner bodies in granulosa cell tumors (Fig. 18.71) or trabecular/tubular areas in Sertoli cell tumors (Fig. 18.72). Troublesome but important histological differentiations can be compounded further by the presence of luteinized stromal cells which, if present, may be mistaken for Leydig cells. The correct identification of endometrioid carcinomas in these cases should be assisted by their much greater cellular pleomorphism and mitotic activity, obvious true gland formation in parts of the tumor, and squamous differentiation. Immunohistochemical pres-

──────────────────────────────────── ▷

Fig. 18.69. Moderately differentiated endometrioid carcinoma. The tumor displays the typical microglandular pattern and luminal debris (*left*).

Fig. 18.70. Poorly differentiated endometrioid carcinoma. Solid carcinoma with prominent necrosis but still an identifiable microglandular pattern.

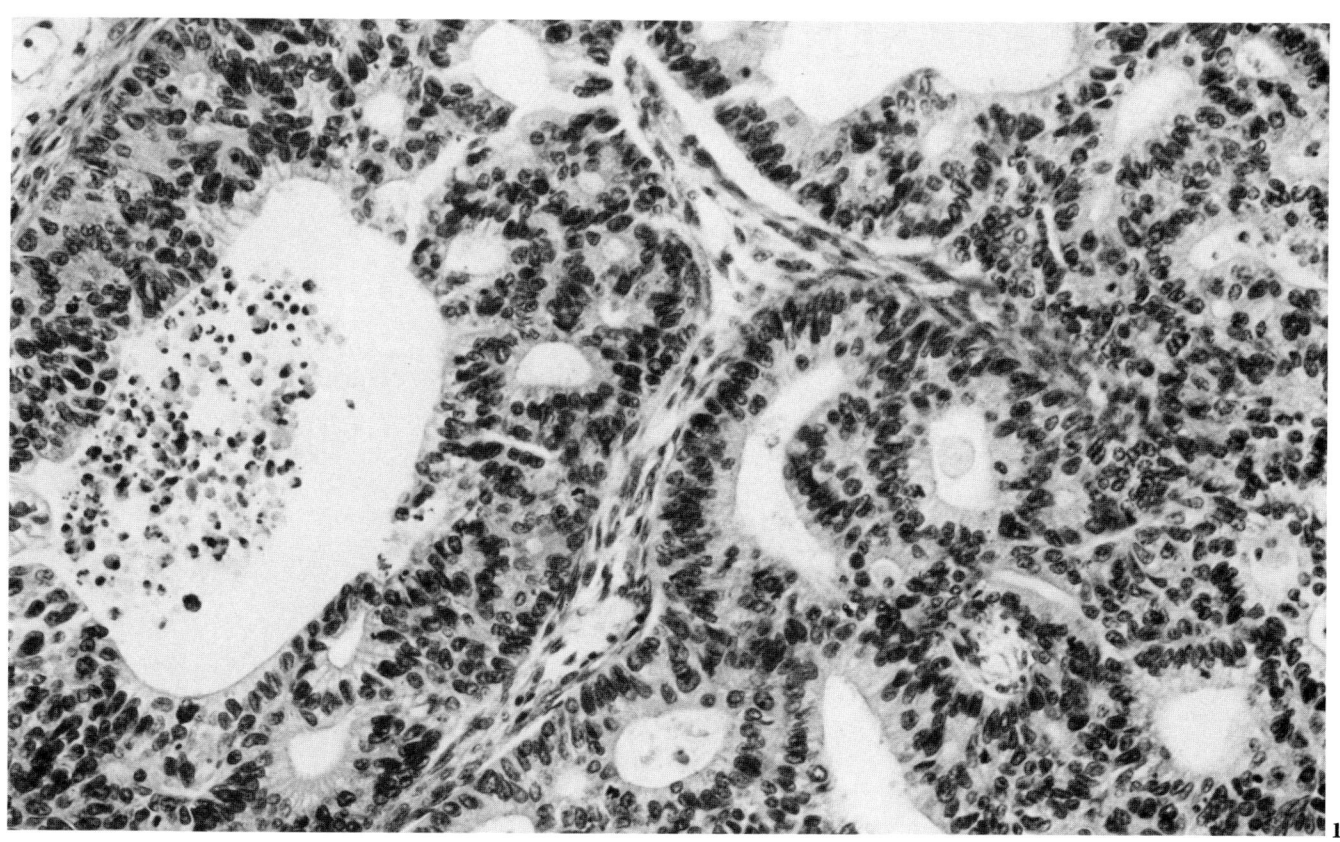

18.69

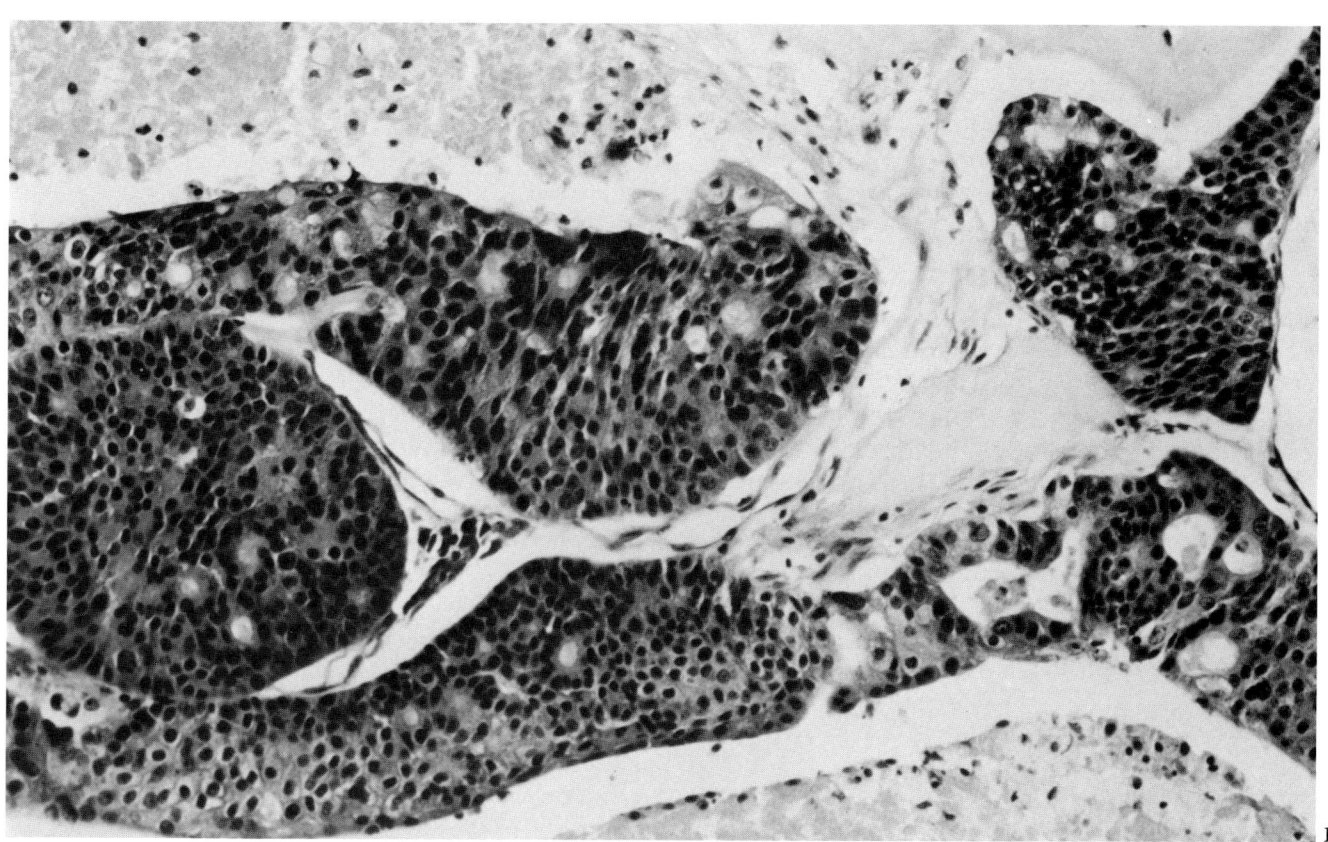

18.70

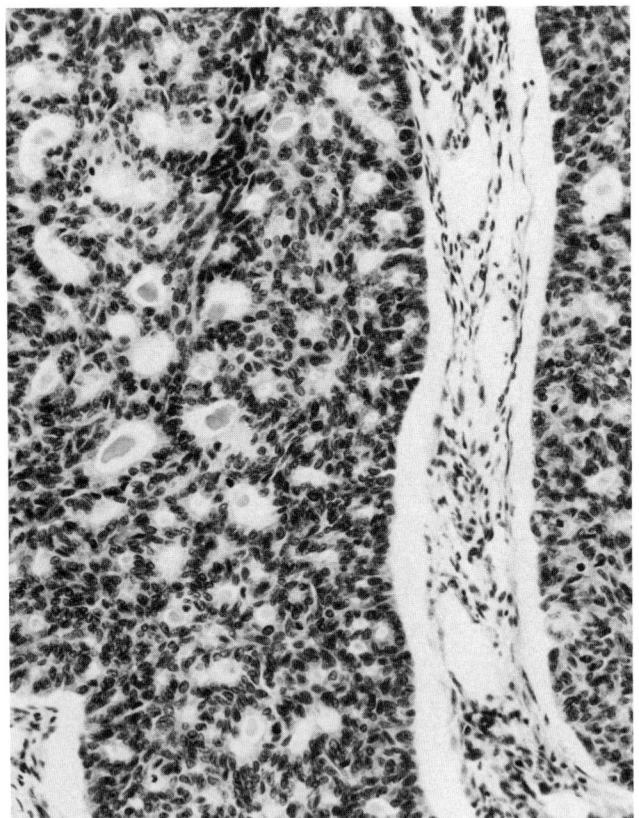

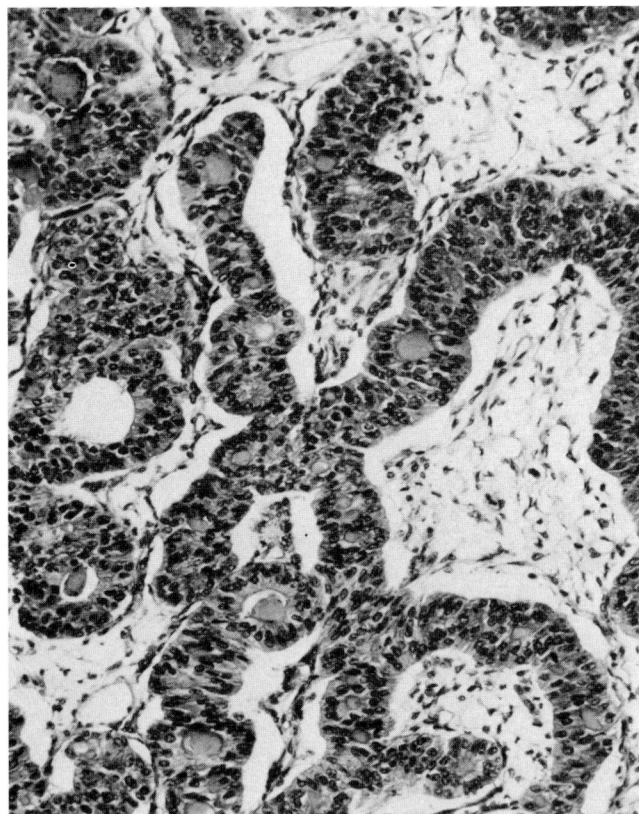

Fig. 18.71. Endometrioid carcinoma. The tumor has a solid pattern resembling microfollicular variant of granulosa cell tumor.

Fig. 18.72. Endometrioid carcinoma. The tumor has a tubular pattern resembling Sertoli cell tumor.

ence of EMA and OM-1[3] may further assist. Conversely, rare examples of yolk sac tumor may mimic moderately differentiated endometrioid adenocarcinoma, particularly those with secretory activity.[57] These tumors will characteristically occur in young women and are associated with raised serum alpha-fetoprotein (AFP) levels. In many cases of colonic adenocarcinoma metastatic to one or both ovaries, the metastases resemble primary mucinous ovarian tumors, but others are non–mucin-producing with cribriform glandular arrangements masquerading as endometrioid adenocarcinomas.[150] Features that suggest metastatic colonic adenocarcinoma are bilaterality, low power architectural patterns that appear to be due to the coalescence of multiple tumor deposits, infiltration of residual ovarian structures, garland and cribriform epithelial patterns around central necrosis, segmental destruction of glands, absence of squamous metaplasia, and strong positive immunohistochemical staining for CEA.

Immunohistochemical and Ultrastructural Findings

Immunohistochemical staining reveals similar differential patterns as exist between mucinous and serous tumors

(q.v.); a greater percentage of endometrioid tumors (71%) show co-expression of vimentin and cytokeratin intermediate filaments than other histological types.[69] Up to one-half of ovarian endometrioid carcinomas contain argyrophil cells without otherwise altering their classification.[136,268]

Electron microscopic studies have stressed the similarity between ovarian endometrioid carcinomas and tumors of the uterine corpus[250] with most tumor cells resembling preovulatory phase endometrial glandular cells and the glycogen-containing cells of the "secretory" carcinomas resembling postovulatory or secretory phase endometrial epithelium. Cummins et al.[62] have described the tumor cells as having apical microvilli and lateral desmosomes. Many cells contain apical mucus droplets and the secretory cells exhibit amorphous glycogen masses. Variable rough endoplasmic reticulum, moderate free ribosomes, and numerous Golgi bodies and lysosomes are characteristic. The nuclei vary in size with prominent nucleoli, often with a loose "mesh-basket" appearance (Fig. 18.73) and fibrillary nuclear bodies. Argyrophilic granules noted histochemically prove, ultrastructurally, to be mucin in the superficial cytoplasm, whereas the basal and diffuse cytoplasmic granules probably are neurosecretory in type.

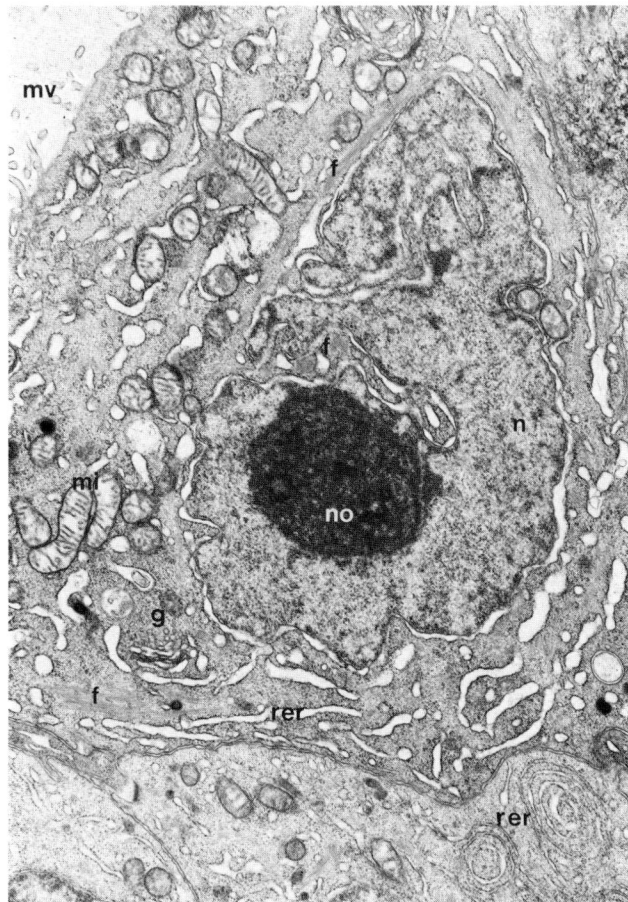

FIG. 18.73. Endometrioid carcinoma. Large "basket weave" nucleolus (*no*) is seen within the irregular nucleus (*n*). Cytoplasm contains conspicuous microfilaments (*f*) that are mostly perinuclear in location, as well as prominent rough-surfaced endoplasmic reticulum (*rer*), mitochondria (*mi*), and large Golgi zones (*g*). Microvilli (*mv*) line the lumen. ×20,000. (Courtesy of Dr. E. J. Wills, Royal Prince Alfred Hospital, Sydney, Australia.)

CLINICAL BEHAVIOR AND TREATMENT

Endometrioid ovarian carcinomas generally are regarded as having an overall better prognosis than either mucinous or serous carcinomas. It is relevant to observe that a high proportion of reported endometrioid carcinomas are well differentiated—partly because of a reluctance to diagnose less well-differentiated tumors as being specifically of endometrioid type[90] and perhaps equally a tendency to incorrectly categorize well-differentiated noninvasive tumors as carcinomas rather than as atypically proliferating tumors[209]; this may introduce a significant bias into survival statistics. Twenty-five percent of tumors are diagnosed at Stage I, 20% Stage II, and 55% are Stages III–IV. Two large series[37,68] reported overall 5-year survival figure of 40–52%. FIGO Stage correlates strongly with 5-year patient survival: 80% for Stage I, 62% for Stage II, and 21% for Stage III–IV.[263]

Optimum therapy for patients with Stage I tumors is total hysterectomy, bilateral adnexectomy, and thorough staging. More advanced tumors require surgical management along lines suggested for serous carcinomas and postoperative chemotherapy of either single-agent or combination types.[142]

Müllerian Mesenchymal and Mixed Tumors

Müllerian mesenchymal and mixed tumors are uncommon in the ovaries. They are characterized by the presence of neoplastic stromal or mesenchymal cells exhibiting varying degrees of proliferation and malignant potential (mitotic activity, tissue or vascular space invasion, metastasis). The patterns of mesenchymal differentiation are those of the more frequently observed uterine counterparts. Rarely, these tumors may occur beneath the pelvic and abdominal peritoneum or within the omentum, presumably from the same cells that give rise to endometriosis and endosalpingiosis. Many also contain neoplastic epithelial elements, which may be benign or malignant.

Smooth Muscle Tumors and Tumor-like Conditions

Ovarian tumors exclusively of smooth muscle differentiation are encountered rarely but should be considered part of the spectrum of müllerian-differentiated tumors, as in the uterus. The rare *peritoneal leiomyomatosis* affects the ovaries in about 25% of patients. *Benign leiomyomas* occur in ovaries of premenopausal women (Fig. 18.74) and require differentiation from the far more commonly encountered ovarian fibromas whereas leiomyosarcomas also have been reported in ovaries of elderly women. Details of these lesions are given in Chapter 21, Nonspecific Tumors of the Ovary, Including Mesenchymal Tumors and Malignant Lymphoma.

Adenosarcomas

GENERAL FEATURES

These rare lesions contain both epithelial and mesenchymal elements. They differ from the malignant mesodermal mixed tumors described below in that the epithelial component is benign and from adenofibromas in that the stroma is hypercellular and often frankly sarcomatous. The term *adenosarcoma* was used first by Clement and Scully[55] to describe such tumors in the uterus and has since been applied to ovarian and adnexal tumors.[56,128,215] These tumors are unilateral and almost always are confined to the ovaries at laparotomy. The mean age for patients with this tumor is 50 years.

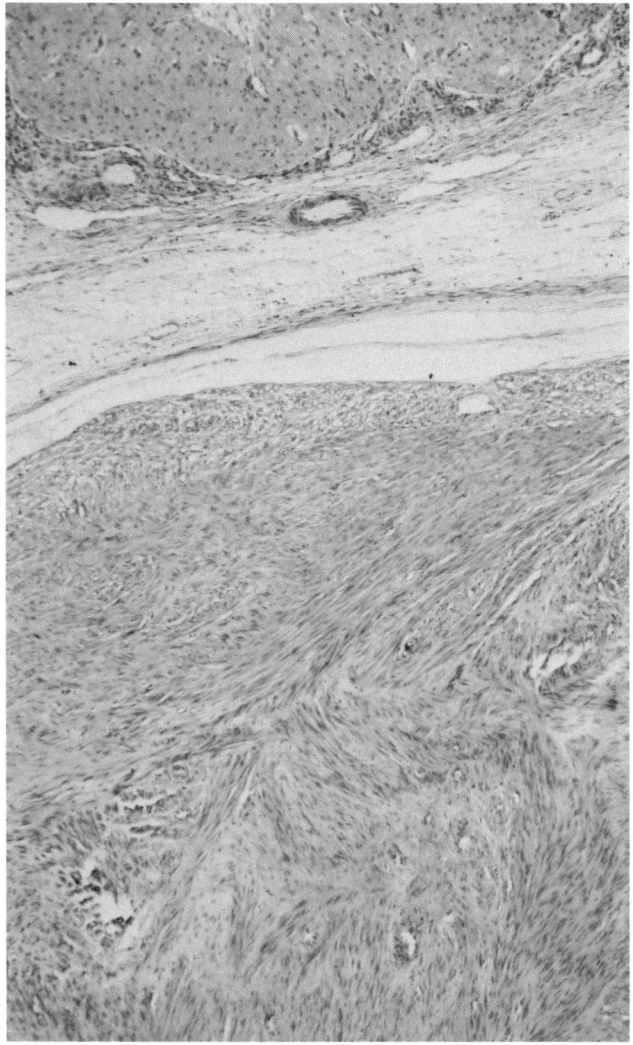

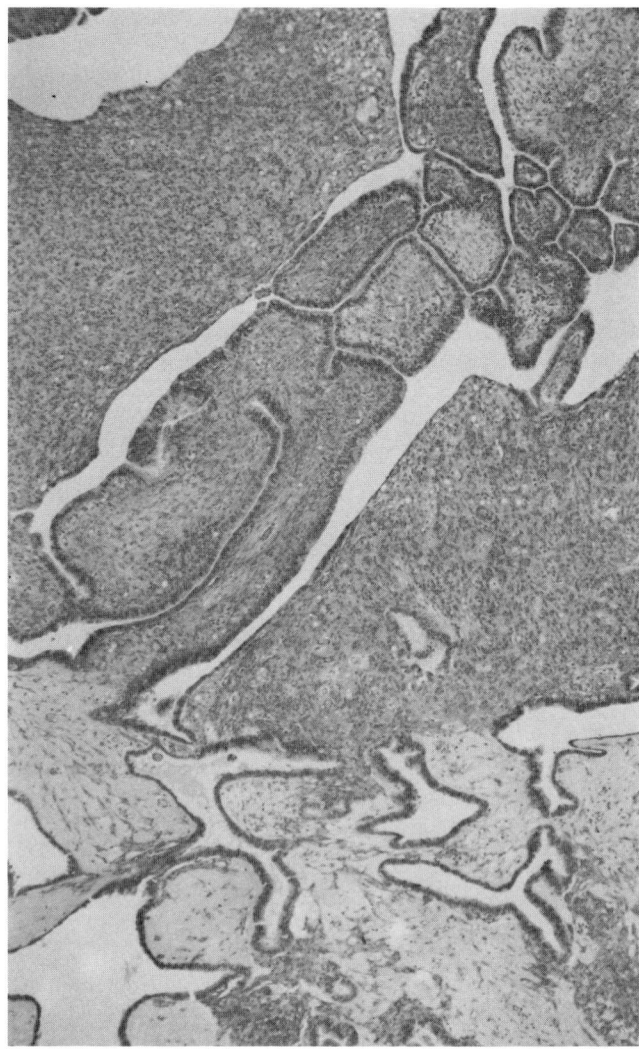

FIG. 18.74. Leiomyoma. The tumor is arising in the ovary and has a well-circumscribed margin abutting adjacent ovarian stroma and a corpus luteum (*top*).

FIG. 18.75. Adenosarcoma. Low power showing coarse papillary pattern and hypercellular stroma.

GROSS FINDINGS

Adenosarcomas average about 10 cm in diameter, some with smooth external contours and others with a surface papillary component. Cut surfaces are spongy and multicystic with intervening tough fibrous tissue. Cysts are filled with clear or yellowish fluid. Focal hemorrhage may be present in larger tumors.

MICROSCOPIC FINDINGS

Adenosarcomas show an epithelial component that usually is endometrial in type and lines clefts or cystic spaces. Less often they exhibit a serous papillary pattern (Fig. 18.75).

Epithelial patterns are bland, although pseudostratification sometimes is present. The stroma is most cellular immediately adjacent to the epithelium but varies greatly within each tumor. Stromal cell nuclei are more pleomorphic than in benign adenofibromas (Fig. 18.76), and mitoses are increased up to 5 MF/10 HPF in tumors subcategorized as *cellular adenofibromas* and 2 to 25 MF/10 HPF in those designated as *adenosarcoma* by Kao and Norris.[128]

ULTRASTRUCTURAL FINDINGS

A single case of ovarian adenosarcoma examined ultrastructurally has shown features weakly supporting the ovarian stromal rather than endometrial nature of the lesion.

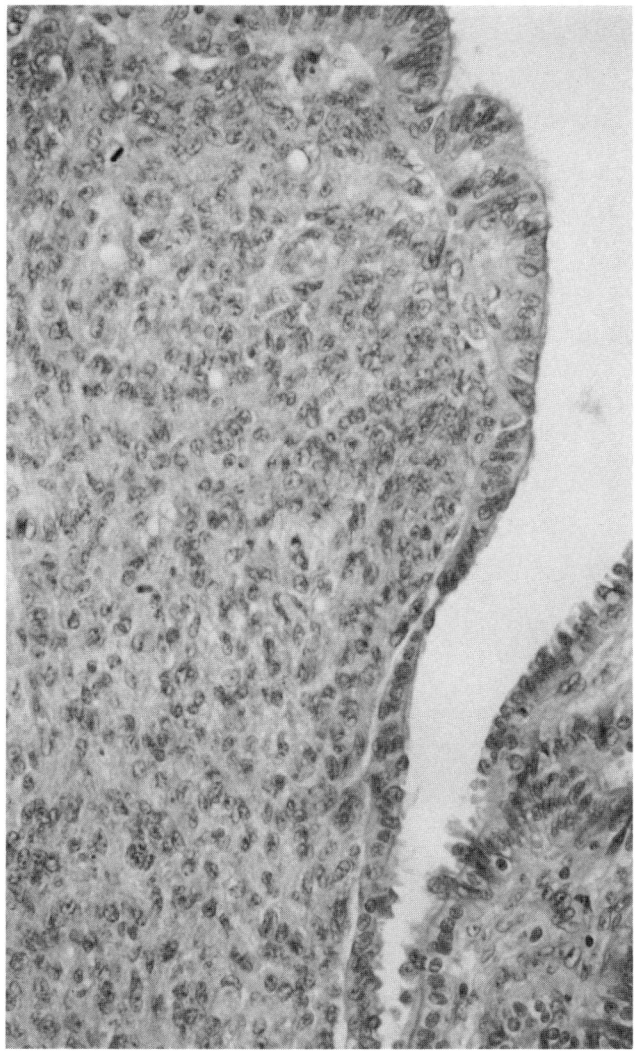

FIG. 18.76. Adenosarcoma. Benign serous epithelium and atypical hypercellular stroma.

CLINICAL BEHAVIOR AND TREATMENT

Adenosarcomas can be expected to recur or metastasize locally, and few behave as benign tumors. Large tumors may be difficult to remove completely. Total hysterectomy and bilateral adnexectomy has been employed, followed by cytotoxic[128] or radiation therapy,[215] to control recurrent disease.

Malignant Mixed Mesodermal (Müllerian) Tumors (Carcinosarcomas)

GENERAL FEATURES

These uncommon tumors account for less than 1% of malignant ovarian neoplasms and contain epithelial and mesenchymal elements, both of which are histologically malignant. The mesenchymal elements may differentiate toward tissues "homologous" to the female genital tract such as endometrial stroma, fibrous tissue, or smooth muscle, or to "heterologous" tissues foreign to the female genital tract such as bone, cartilage, fat, and skeletal muscle. Of the 300 or so cases in the English literature,[43,79,80,170,186] one-third fall into the homologous group. Barwick and LiVolsi[22] observed that all sarcomas, except fibrosarcoma, are heterologous to the ovaries and that there is no justification for this distinction, although some studies suggest a reduced median survival of the heterologous group.[73,79] They are reported almost exclusively in postmenopausal women, who often are nulliparous, with a mean age of 65 years; they are bilateral in only 10% of cases.

GROSS FINDINGS

These neoplasms are large, averaging 15 to 20 cm in diameter with bosselated serosal surfaces showing prominent vessels and focal hemorrhage. Cut surfaces are characterized by yellow to brown, friable, fleshy nodules, showing obvious hemorrhage and necrosis. A variable cystic component usually contains polypoid excrescences and blood-stained fluid. Heterologous tumors may contain cartilage or bony areas.

MICROSCOPIC FINDINGS

Epithelial elements, in my experience and in some reported series,[75] most frequently are serous (Fig. 18.77), followed by endometrioid (Fig. 18.78), mucinous, clear cell, or squamous. Other investigators have found endometrioid differentiation to be the most common.[80,170] If the epithelium is exclusively mucinous, the problem arises of differentiating such neoplasms (Fig. 18.79) from mucinous tumors with mural nodules (see previous section, Figs. 18.48, 18.49).

Areas may be encountered composed entirely of carcinoma or sarcoma, but there usually is a complex mixture of epithelial and malignant stromal elements, particularly if the latter comprises undifferentiated mesenchyme (Fig. 18.77). Reticulin stains and immunohistochemical stains for epithelial membrane antigen (EMA) and various keratin intermediate filaments accentuate the differentiation of otherwise undifferentiated carcinoma from sarcoma. Sarcomatous elements are mostly hypercellular sheets of small hyperchromatic round to spindle cells with a high mitotic rate (Figs. 18.78, 18.79). Pleomorphic and bizarre giant cells are common, as are cells with hyaline cytoplasmic droplets.[230] In routine sections, chondrosarcoma is the most frequently encountered heterologous stromal element (Fig. 18.80); less often are malignant osteoid (Fig. 18.81) and skeletal muscle. Use of immunohistochemical techniques to identify myoglobin[172] and desmin suggests that rhabdomyoblasts are more common than has been previously reported.[73] Rarely, bizarre malig-

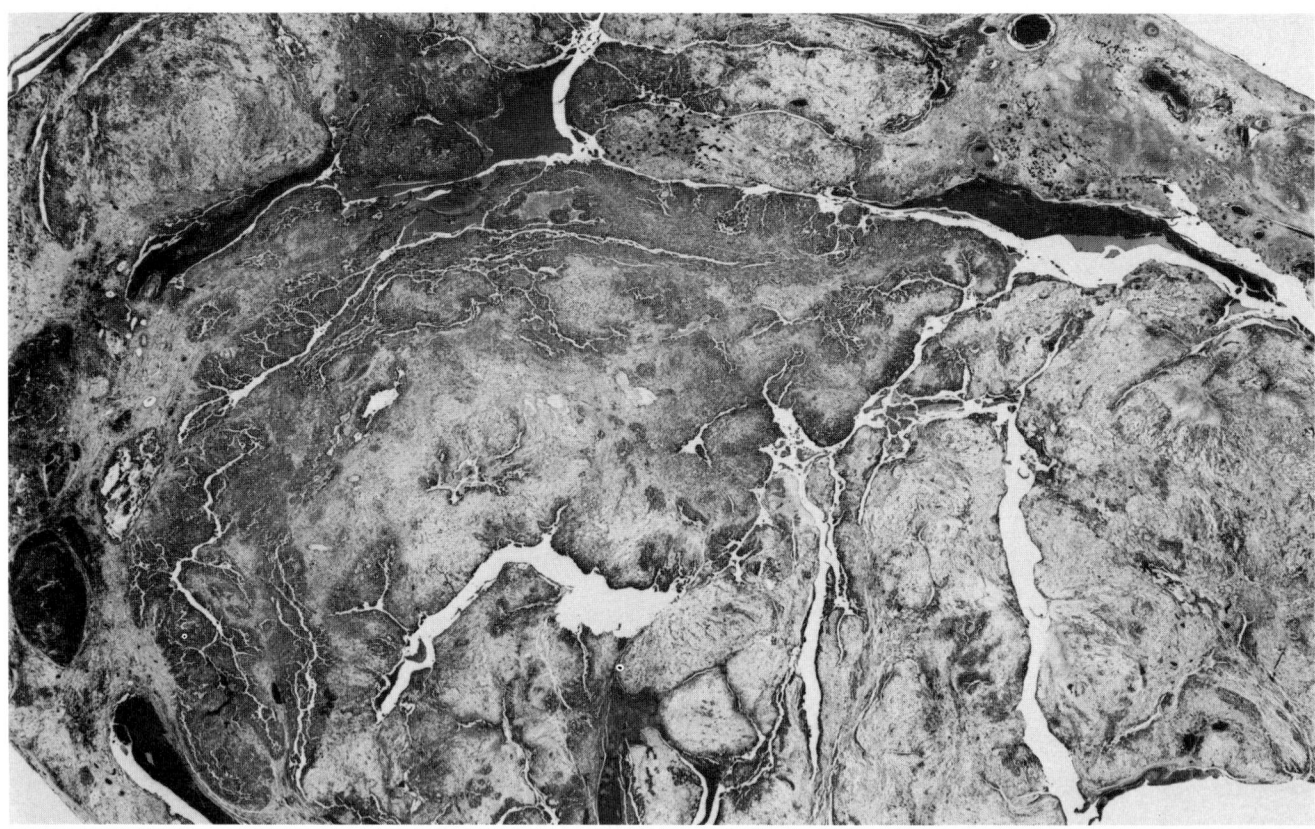

FIG. 18.77. Homologous malignant mixed müllerian tumor. There is a variegated appearance occasioned by a complex admixture of epithelial and stromal elements. The fine slit-like spaces (*center-left*) suggest serous epithelial differentiation. Pale myxoid stroma is noted to right.

nant lipoblasts are encountered,[74,79] as may be trophoblastic differentiation.[21]

Differentiation of these tumors from immature teratomas is based on clinical and histological features. Immature teratomas occur in young women (rarely over 40 years). Histologically, teratomas show some orderly arrangement of immature stromal and epithelial tissues with ectodermal, particularly neuroectoderm, and endodermal, typically intestinal or respiratory, as well as elements of mesodermal origin being present. Malignant mixed mesodermal tumors show greater disorganization of malignant adult tissues, with ectodermal and endodermal derivatives conspicuously absent. An apparently unique tumor so-called *teratoid carcinosarcoma* has been described[83] recently showing architectural and cellular features intermediate between immature teratoma and carcinosarcoma.

CLINICAL BEHAVIOR AND TREATMENT

More than 85% of patients exhibit extraovarian spread at diagnosis, and it is generally the sarcomatous components that have spread early to omentum, pelvic organs, and liver.[80] The progression of these tumors is rapid; only one-quarter of patients survive 2 years and examples of long-term survival are anecdotal, although individual small series give some promise for combination radiotherapy and chemotherapy.[43] Surgical management is similar to that detailed for the epithelial tumors.

Stromal Sarcomas

GENERAL FEATURES

There are occasional reports of primary ovarian sarcomas of endometrioid type, although clear interpretation of instances with co-existent or sequential involvement of both uterus and ovaries is seldom given.[297] Such tumors are mostly low-grade endometrioid stromal sarcomas (endolymphatic stromal myosis or *stromatosis*[237]). Less frequently, they are high-grade endometrioid stromal sarcomas. Most of the low-grade sarcomas are thought to arise in preexisting endometriosis, which is found in association with the tumors in 50–85% of cases.[230,243,297] They often are bilateral and widespread within the abdomen at the time of diagnosis and present clinically in women in their fifth and sixth decades.

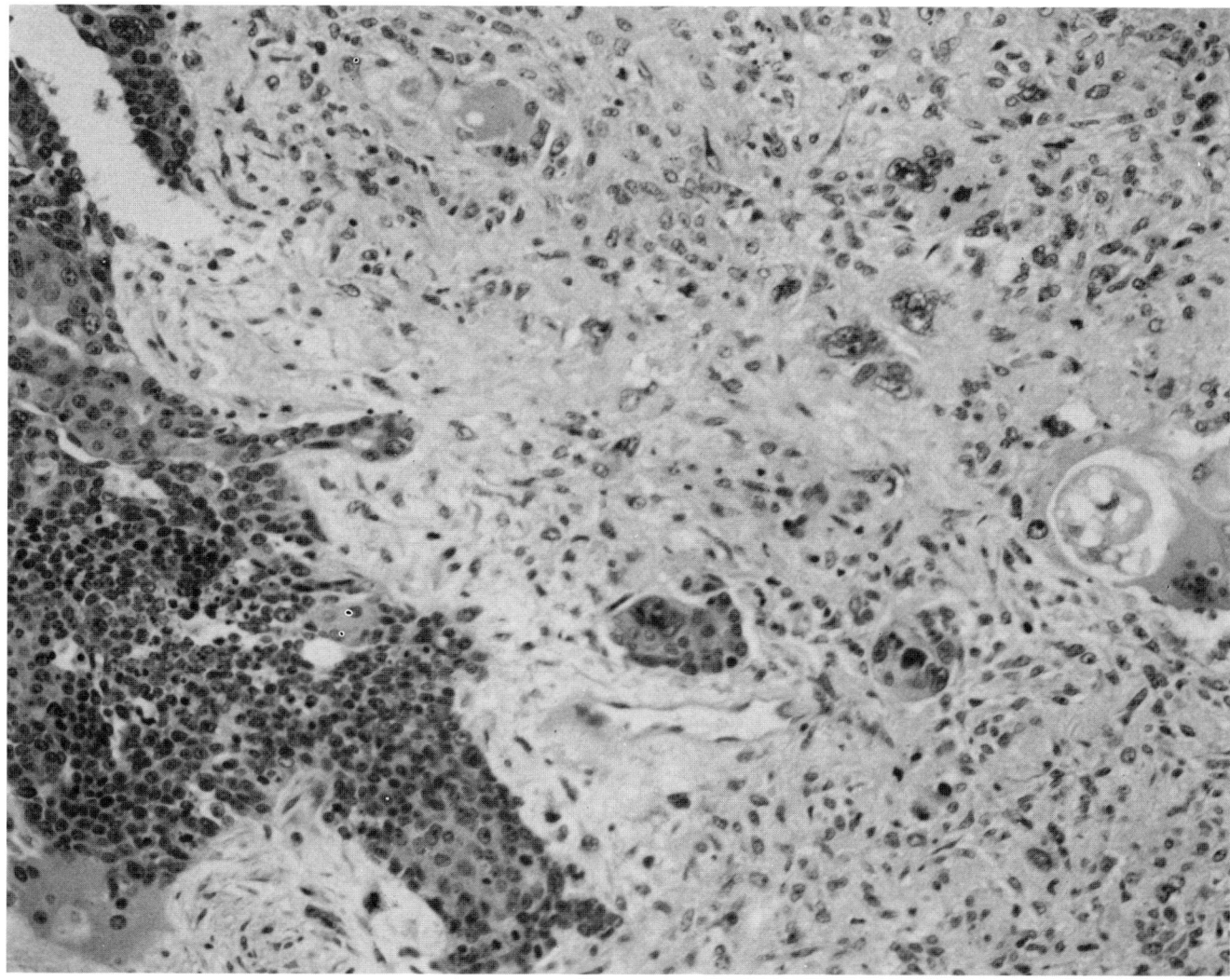

FIG. 18.78. **Homologous malignant mixed müllerian tumor.** A poorly differentiated endometrioid carcinoma is admixed with high-grade sarcoma. Cellular pleomorphism is prominent in both components.

GROSS FINDINGS

Low-grade endometrioid stromal sarcomas tend to appear as ill-defined and homogeneous ovarian enlargement with extension into adjacent tissues. Less commonly, they appear as multinodular fleshy tumors. A cystic component occasionally may be prominent. Focal intracystic hemorrhage may indicate endometriosis.

High-grade stromal sarcomas usually are discrete, white, fleshy ovarian masses averaging 10 cm in diameter, with prominent necrosis and evidence of local invasion.

MICROSCOPIC FINDINGS

Endometrioid stromal sarcomas, either low or high grade, show changes similar to those seen in the more familiar uterine tumors. Most often they are composed of closely packed sheets of small, round to oval, cells that often are

whorled around a fine meshwork of small arteriolar vessels. In low-grade tumors nuclei are bland, round to oval, with inapparent nucleoli; mitoses are infrequent and always normal; cytoplasm is scant. Reticulin fibers invest individual cells and accentuate the vascularity. Tongues of apparently intravascular tumor growth also may be present (Fig. 18.82).

A second distinct architectural pattern is created by the deposition of intercellular hyaline material that may be focally prominent, and that separates clusters of small tumor cells (Fig. 18.83). Thick-walled cleft-like vascular spaces are evident in this variant. Storiform patterns sometimes are seen, as are less cellular areas more closely resembling those of ovarian fibromas.[297] Nuclear atypia is seen in high-grade tumors with mitoses well above 10 MF/10 HPF (Fig. 18.84). An important differential diagnosis is malignant melanoma metastatic to the ovaries which, in one of its many guises, may produce sheets of

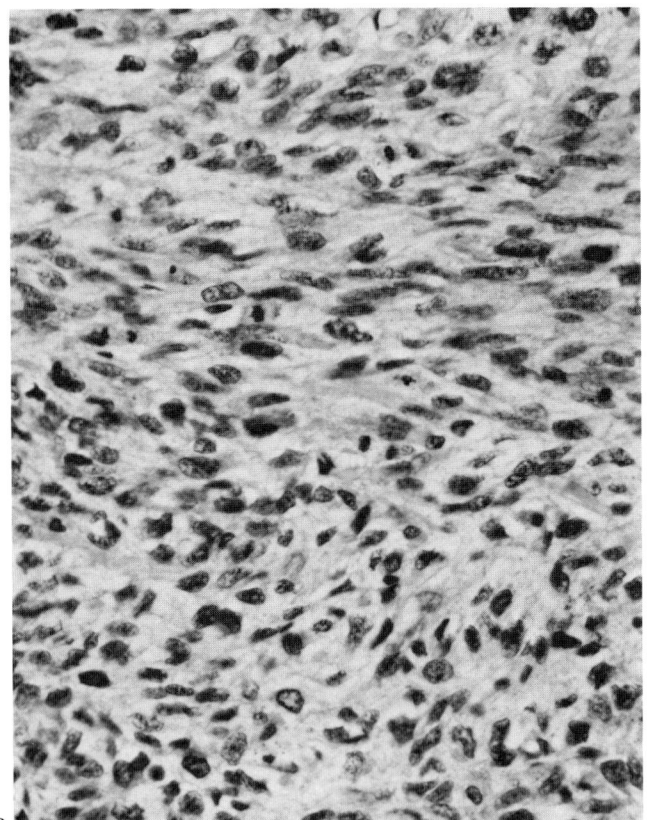

18.79

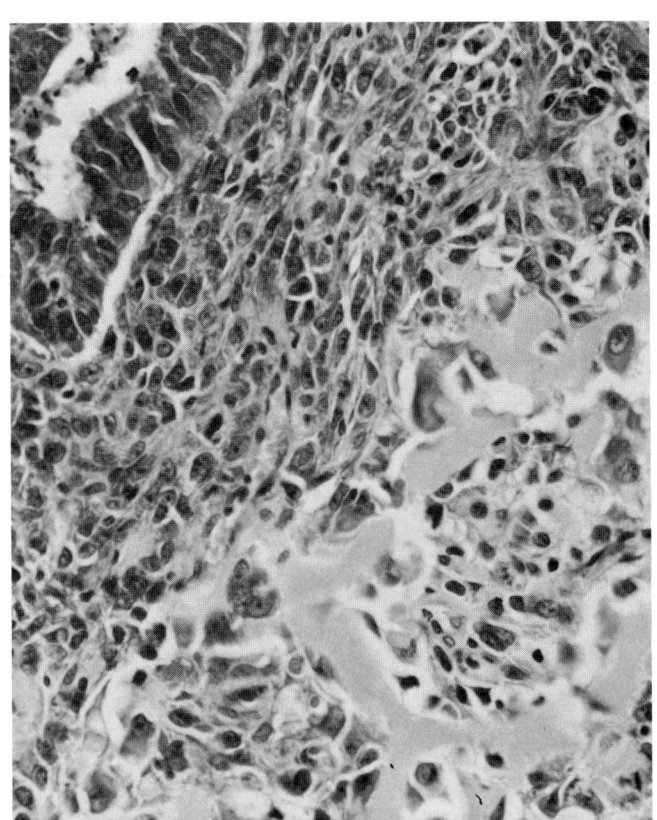

18.81

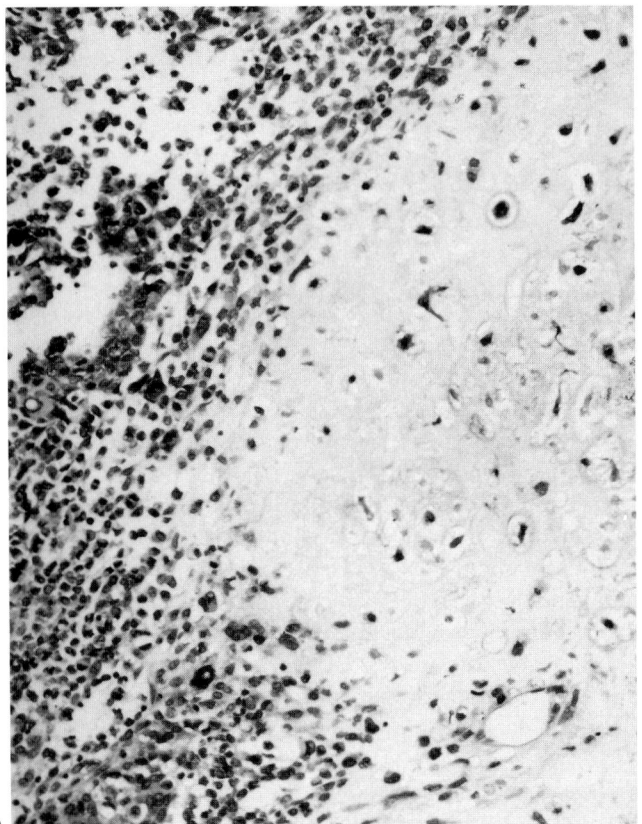

18.80

uniform, spindled, sarcoma-like cells in routine sections.[89,293] However, even in the absence of pigment, immunohistochemical stains for S-100 protein, NKI/C-3, and/or HMB-45 should confirm this diagnosis (see Chapter 22, Metastatic Tumors of the Ovary).

CLINICAL BEHAVIOR AND TREATMENT

The clinical behavior and treatment of ovarian stromal sarcomas is similar to their counterparts arising in the uterus.

Clear Cell Tumors

Benign Clear Cell Tumors

GENERAL FEATURES

Clear cell tumors show a similar proliferative spectrum to other common epithelial tumors,[236] but benign lesions are

---

FIG. 18.79. **Malignant mixed müllerian tumor.** A sarcomatous area shows some features of smooth muscle differentiation.
FIG. 18.80. **Heterologous malignant mixed müllerian tumor.** This is an area composed of malignant cartilage.
FIG. 18.81. **Heterologous malignant mixed müllerian tumor.** Small, discrete foci of malignant osteoid are present. The nearby (*top left*) epithelium is endometrioid in type.

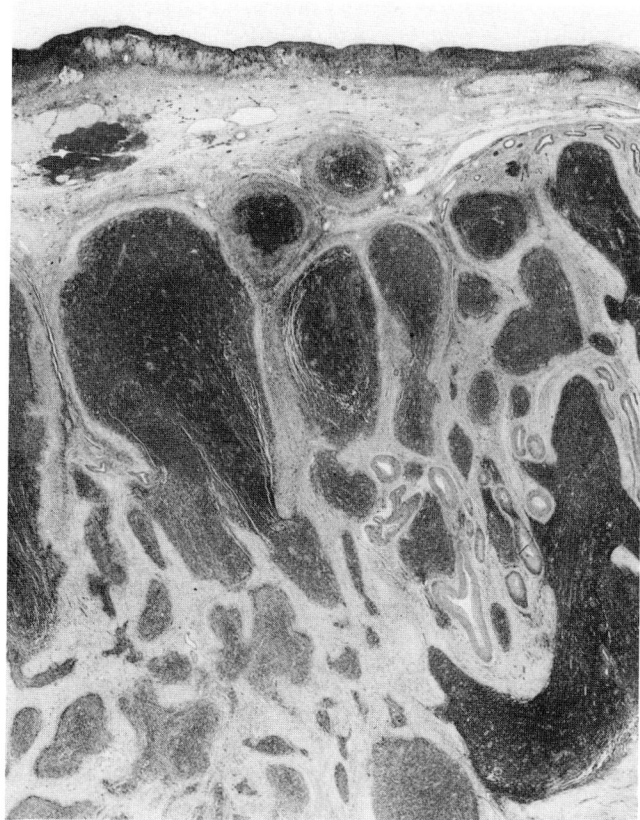

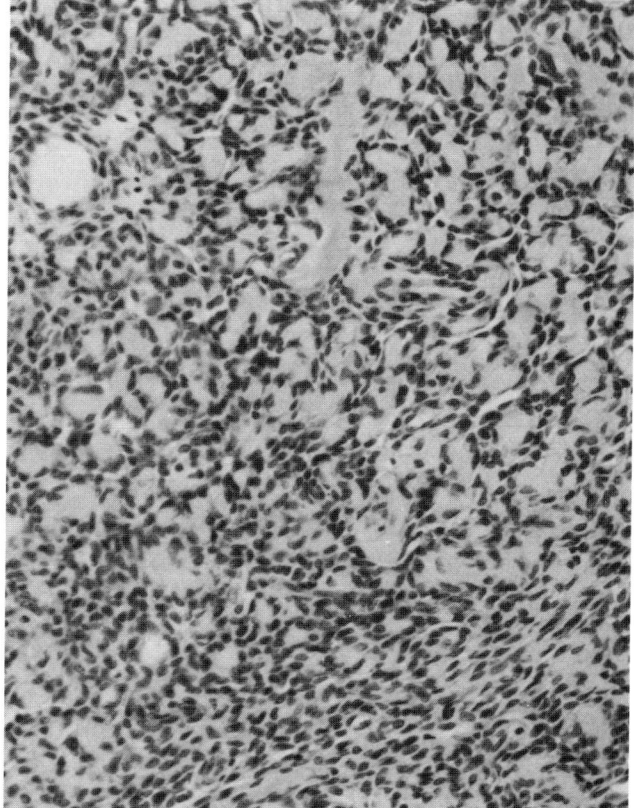

FIG. 18.83. Low-grade endometrioid stromal sarcoma. Prominent deposition of intercellular hyaline material.

only rarely reported. There are approximately 12 in the English literature.[8,26,111,129,205] The mean age is 45 years. One case was bilateral.

GROSS FINDINGS

Clear cell adenofibromas have a median diameter of 12 cm. Smooth, somewhat lobulated external surfaces without adhesions are typical. The cut surfaces display a fine honeycomb appearance with minute cysts embedded in firm rubbery stroma. Cyst fluid is clear and watery.

MICROSCOPIC FINDINGS

Architecturally, adenofibromas are characterized by tubular spaces in a compact, fibrocollagenous stroma, which often is more cellular in the immediate vicinity of the epithelial elements (Fig. 18.85). Epithelial spaces are lined

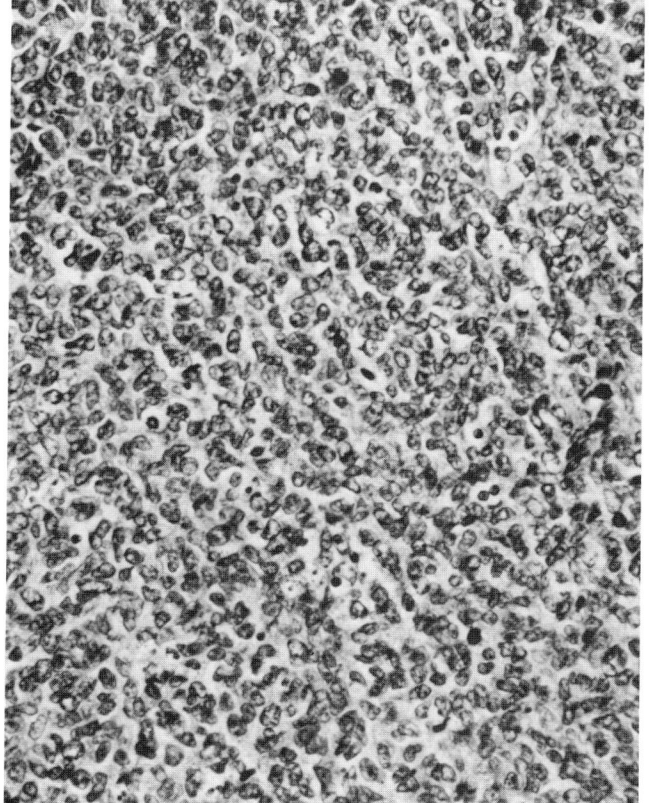

◁————————————————

FIG. 18.82. Low-grade endometrioid stromal sarcoma. a: Slug-like processes of hypercellular tumor infiltrating the ovarian medulla. **b:** Higher power showing the extreme hypercellularity but negligible atypia or mitotic activity.

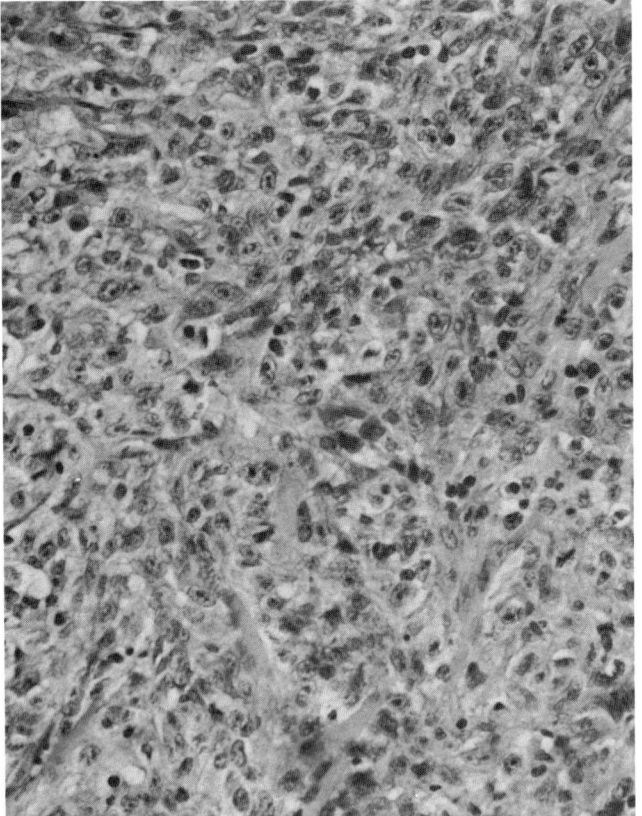

FIG. 18.84. High-grade endometrioid stromal sarcoma. Area showing pleomorphic tumor cells and mitoses.

by one or two layers of peg-like hobnail cells with little cytoplasm and large nuclei that bulge toward the lumens of cystic spaces. Large polyhedral clear cells that resemble to some extent those found in the Arias–Stella reaction or less commonly "indifferent" cuboidal cells, with eosinophilic granular cytoplasm, also occur (Fig. 18.86). Nuclei tend to be regular in size and shape. Atypia, if present, is only mild and focal, and mitoses are rarely encountered. Solid sheets of clear cells and luminal tufting are absent. Cells contain intracytoplasmic glycogen. Mucicarmine- and diastase-resistant PAS-stained material is sometimes present at the apical cell borders and commonly in the luminal secretions[178]; immunohistochemically, cells stain for cytokeratins and focally for OC-125, but rarely for CEA.[105]

CLINICAL BEHAVIOR AND TREATMENT

There are benign tumors that are cured by oophorectomy.

Atypically Proliferating Clear Cell Tumors

GENERAL FEATURES

About 30 atypically proliferating clear cell tumors without destructive stromal invasion have been described.[26,205,208]

Just where the parvilocular tumors of Schiller et al.[226] fit into this tumor spectrum is not settled. Fox and Langley[90] regard them as benign and certainly some merge with those described by Kao and Norris[131] (Figs. 18.85, 18.86). On the other hand, some show epithelial atypia and mitotic activity, arguably sufficient to substantiate designating them as atypically proliferating or "of low malignant potential."[205] Similar areas may be seen in otherwise typical clear cell carcinomas; this is suggested by Scully[230] as further support for such a proposition.

In our material, atypically proliferating clear cell tumors occur in patients of a similar age to those with benign clear cell tumors, although patients reported by Roth et al.[205] and of Bell and Scully[26] have mean ages in the seventh decade, that is, significantly older than with either benign or frankly malignant clear cell tumors.

GROSS FINDINGS

Atypically proliferating clear cell tumors vary up to 23 cm in diameter (mean diameter, 15 cm) and have smooth external surfaces. Grossly, they are unilateral adenofibromas with abundant stroma and cystic spaces of various sizes filled with clear, watery fluid. Softer, fleshier areas denote higher grade epithelial proliferation.

MICROSCOPIC FINDINGS

These tumors have a nonspecific fibrocollagenous to ovarian-type stroma. The cell types lining the cystic spaces are similar to those in benign tumors, and indeed it is the norm for such tumors also to contain focal areas of typical benign clear cell adenofibroma. Nuclear atypia, epithelial budding (Fig. 18.87), and mitoses (up to 3 MF/10 HPF[208]) are present. Papillary structures are rarely seen (Fig. 18.88). Epithelial proliferation may produce solid morules of clear cells and here, in the absence of destructive stromal invasion (Fig. 18.89), the separation from potentially metastatic clear cell carcinoma has not been clarified. As with other surface epithelial–stromal tumors, it is suggested that if the stromal—epithelial interface is smooth and the stroma itself is "inactive" or "mature," without an inflammatory infiltrate, a diagnosis of noninvasive (atypically proliferating) tumor is favored and conservative management for the patient is recommended.

CLINICAL BEHAVIOR AND TREATMENT

Extraovarian lesions have not been reported with atypically proliferating clear cell tumors and only one case of possible distant (lung) metastasis has been noted.[26] As most cases are in older patients, total hysterectomy and bilateral adnexectomy with careful follow-up are suggested as adequate therapy.

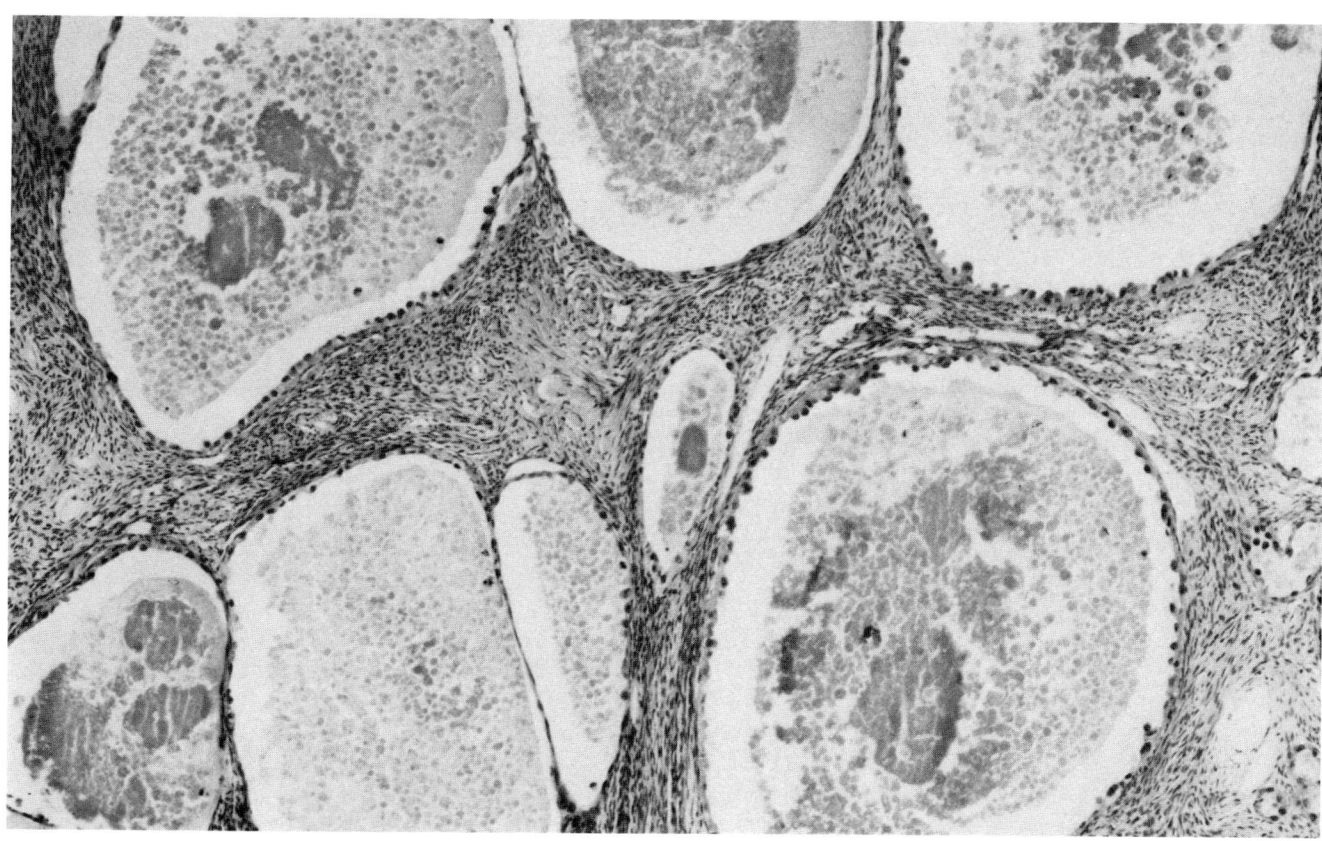

18.85

Malignant Clear Cell Tumors

General Features

The vast majority of clear cell tumors are frankly invasive clear cell carcinomas[60,197,229,230] and these constitute 5–10% of all malignant ovarian epithelial–stromal tumors. Typically, they occur in patients in the fifth to seventh decades, with a peak age of 52 years.[133] Two-thirds of women are nulliparous.[166] Symptoms at presentation usually relate to an enlarging abdominal mass, but such tumors are well documented to be associated with paraneoplastic hypercalcaemia.[212] Clear cell carcinomas have a great frequency of associated pelvic endometriosis (50–70%) and 25% arise from the lining of endometriotic cysts. Mixed clear cell/endometrioid and clear cell/serous carcinomas occur both within the ovaries and uterus. These observations suggest that clear cell carcinomas represent merely histological variants of endometrioid and serous carcinomas.[238] At operation, up to 60% of tumors are in FIGO Stage I and, of these cases, only 4% are bilateral (overall bilaterality rate of 15–20%).

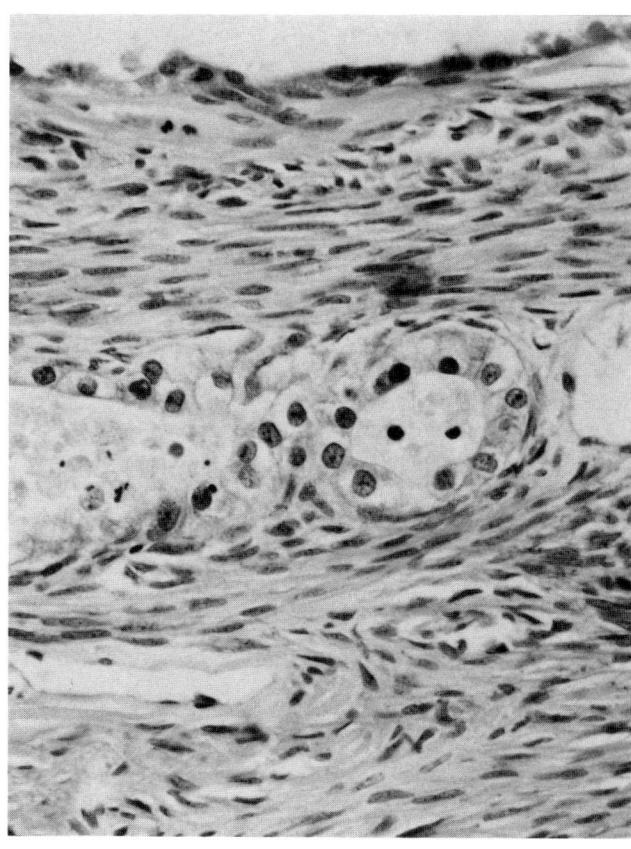

18.86

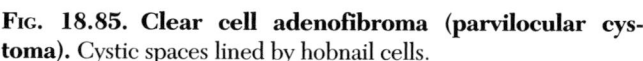

Fig. 18.85. Clear cell adenofibroma (parvilocular cystoma). Cystic spaces lined by hobnail cells.
Fig. 18.86. Clear cell adenofibroma. Tubules in center of field and lining of cyst (top).

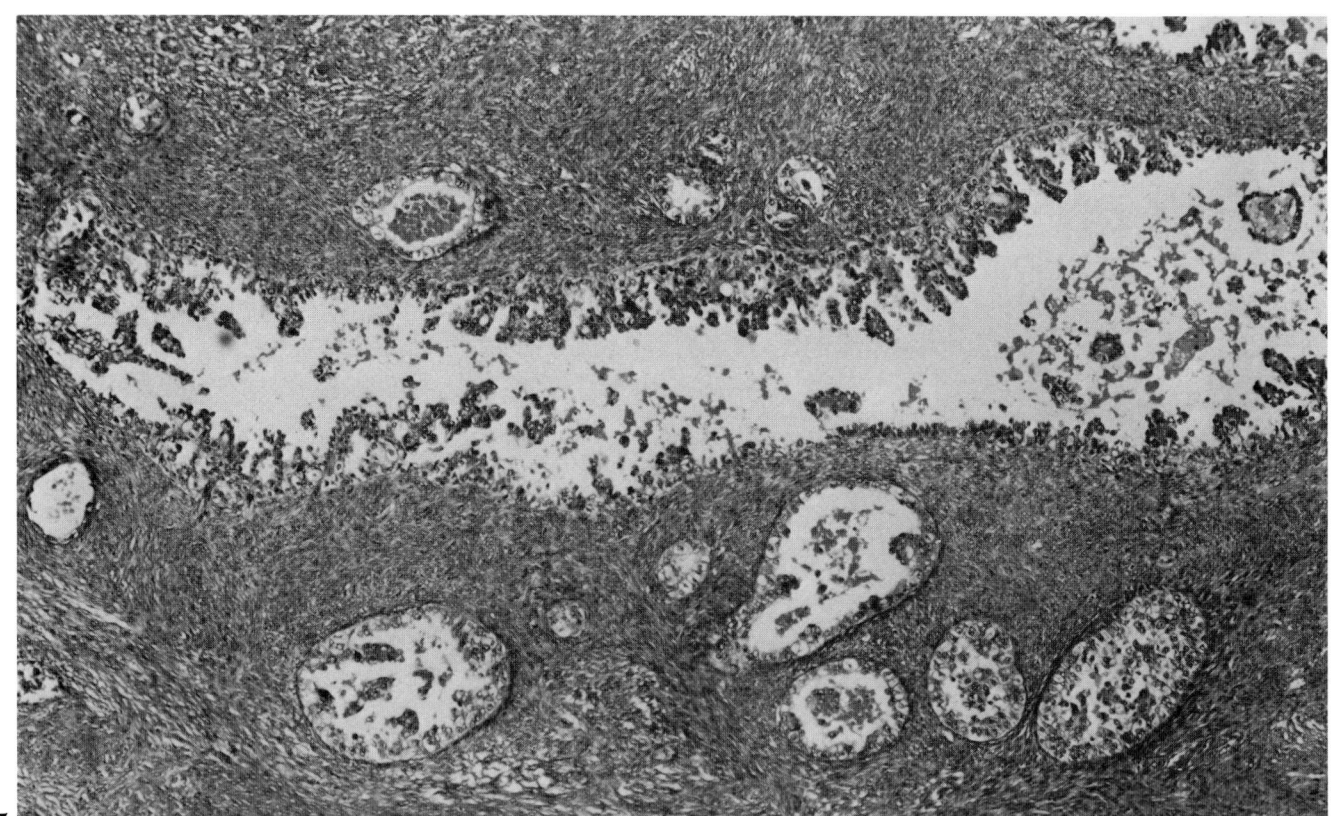

18.87

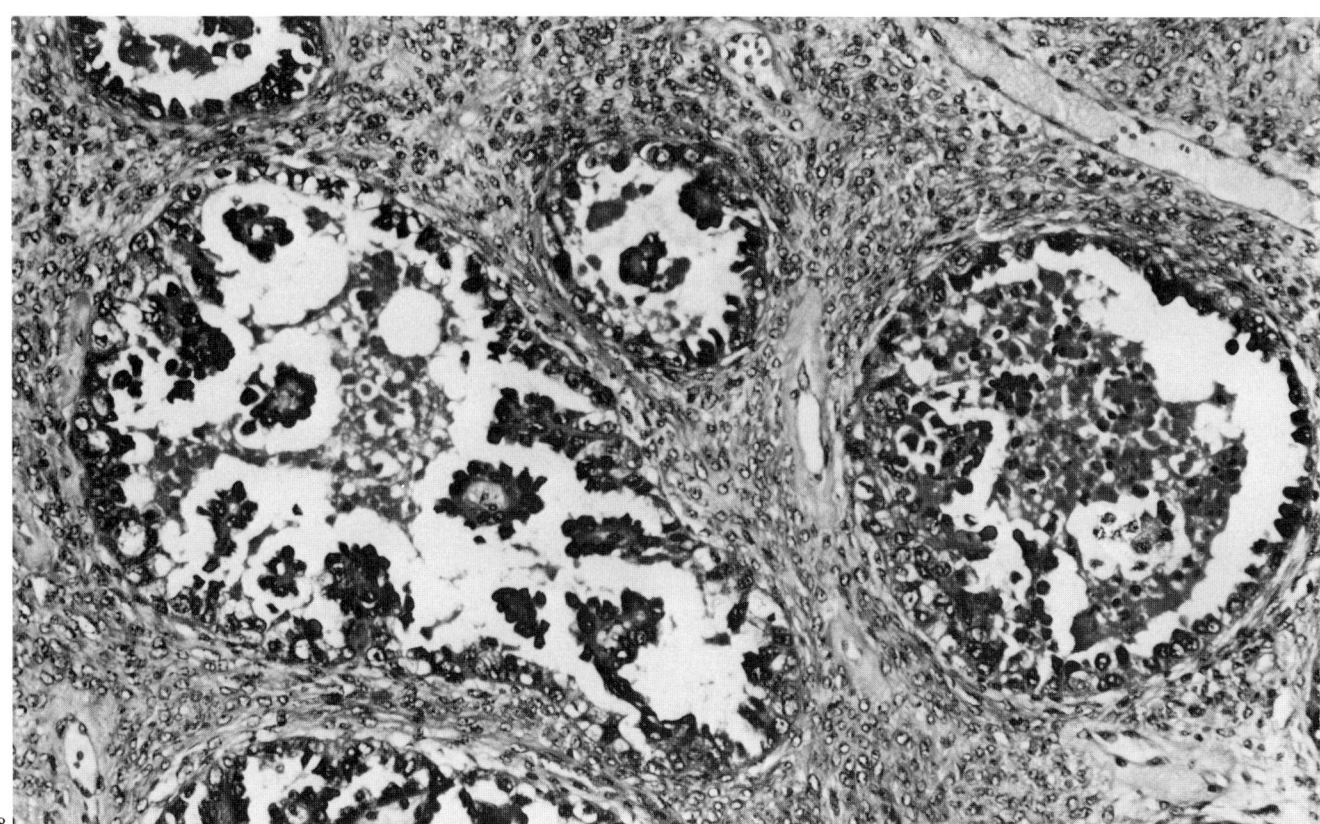

18.88

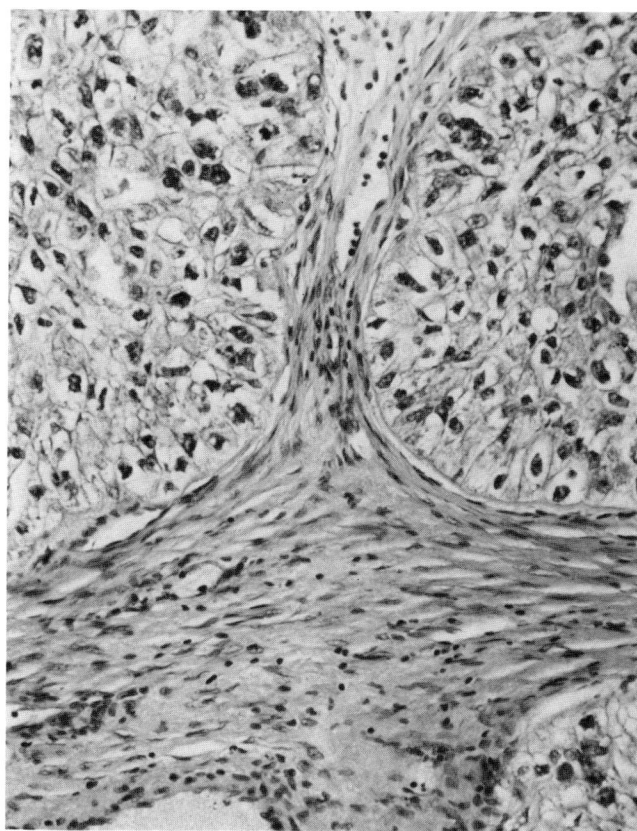

FIG. 18.89. **Atypically proliferating clear cell tumor.** The tumor is high grade, with solid nests of clear cells and a smooth epithelial–stromal interface.

GROSS FINDINGS

Clear cell carcinomas range in size up to 30 cm with a mean diameter of about 15 cm. Surface adhesions are common, but in most cases these prove to be inflammatory and do not indicate extraovarian extension. The cut surface typically reveals a thick-walled unilocular cyst into which project several yellow, beige, fleshy nodules (Fig. 18.90) with focal necrosis and hemorrhage. Slightly less frequently, the tumors are multilocular with cysts containing either watery or mucinous fluid. Rarely the tumors are solid and fibrous.

MICROSCOPIC FINDINGS

There are several described architectural patterns, any one or more of which may be identified in an individual tumor.

◁————————————————————————

FIG. 18.87. **Atypically proliferating clear cell adenofibroma.** The tumor is low grade. Tubules are well circumscribed, in typical ovarian stroma, yet show budding and micropapillary formation.

FIG. 18.88. **Atypically proliferating clear cell tumor.** Higher power showing glomerulus-like structures because of epithelial budding.

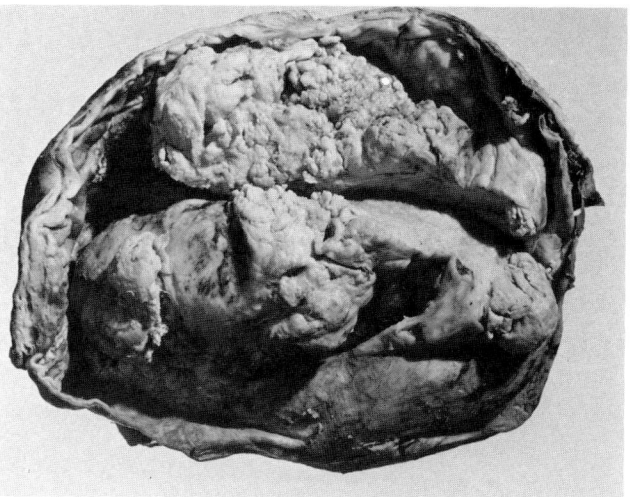

FIG. 18.90. **Clear cell carcinoma.** Cut surface with large solid tumor nodules protruding into the cyst lumen.

A common pattern is created by small to large sheets of polyhedral clear cells separated by delicate fibrovascular septa (Fig. 18.91). The tumor cells have distinct cell borders and eccentric, rounded, or slightly angular nuclei, often with prominent nucleoli. Mitoses are infrequent, tending not to be as numerous as in other primary epithelial carcinomas, and averaging fewer than 10 MF/10 HPF.[132,212] The cytoplasm is distended by abundant glycogen, but not mucin, and may contain variable amounts of fat.[178] Cells with eosinophilic granular cytoplasm may be mixed with typical clear cells.

The second major pattern is tubulopapillary (Fig. 18.92). Papillae are approximately the same size as seen in well-differentiated serous carcinomas and may be simple or complex. Cores of the papillae are composed of delicate immature mesenchymal tissue—occasionally hyalinized. Tubules and cystic structures also may be complex and often are separated by fibrous or hyaline stroma. Tubules and papillae are lined by typical clear, hobnail, or eosinophilic cells, or by columnar secretory cells. The latter have well-defined vacuoles (so-called vacuolated cells of Czernobilsky et al.[67]) that also are seen in secretory serous (Fig. 18.29) or endometrioid carcinomas (Fig. 18.68). When numerous, these tall, columnar secretory cells account for blurring of the distinction between clear cell carcinoma on the one hand and both serous and endometrioid carcinomas on the other and are part of the interface in carcinomas of mixed epithelial differentiation. Therefore, the diagnosis of clear cell carcinoma is predicated on the presence of typical pavement-like clear or eosinophilic cells or hobnail cells.

Other appearances, because of eosinophilic granular cells scattered singly among typical clear cells (Fig. 18.93) or forming small clusters to give an organoid appearance to the tumor (Fig. 18.94), as well as the so-called oxyphilic clear cell carcinoma of Young and Scully,[290] are less fre-

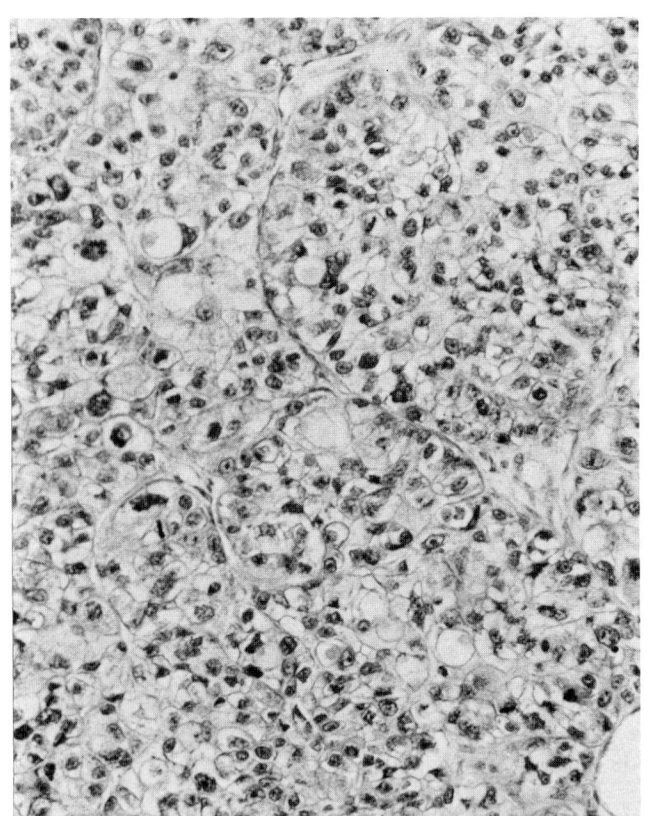

18.91a

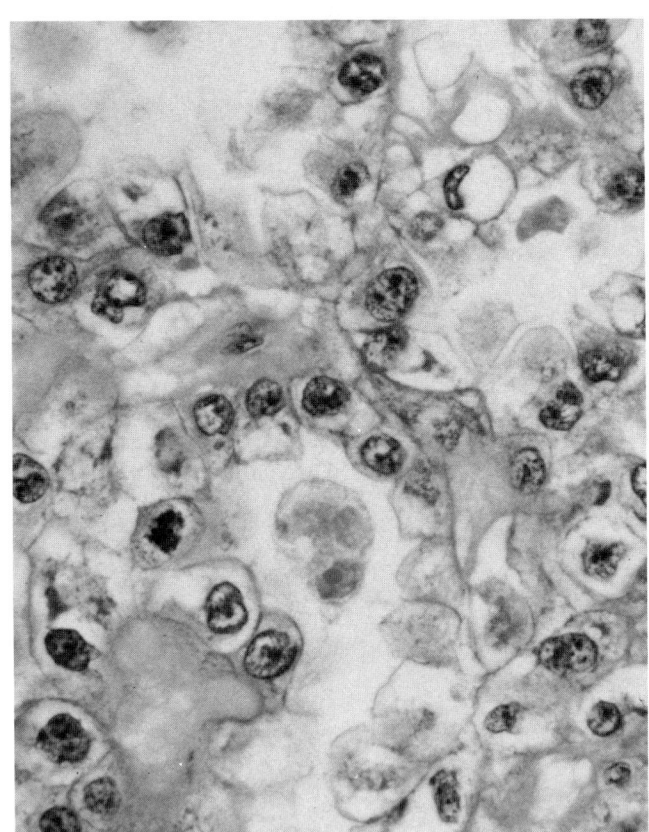

18.91b

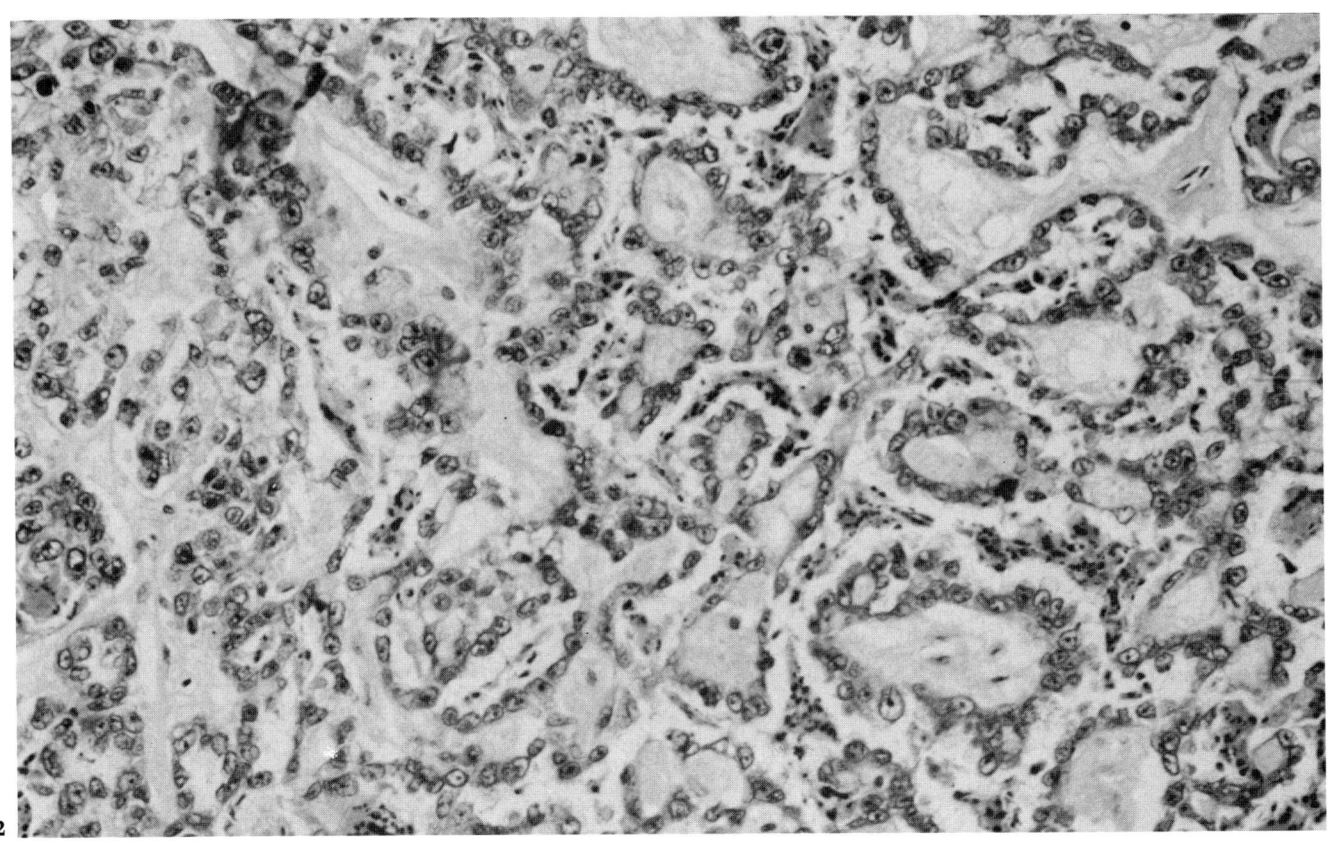

18.92

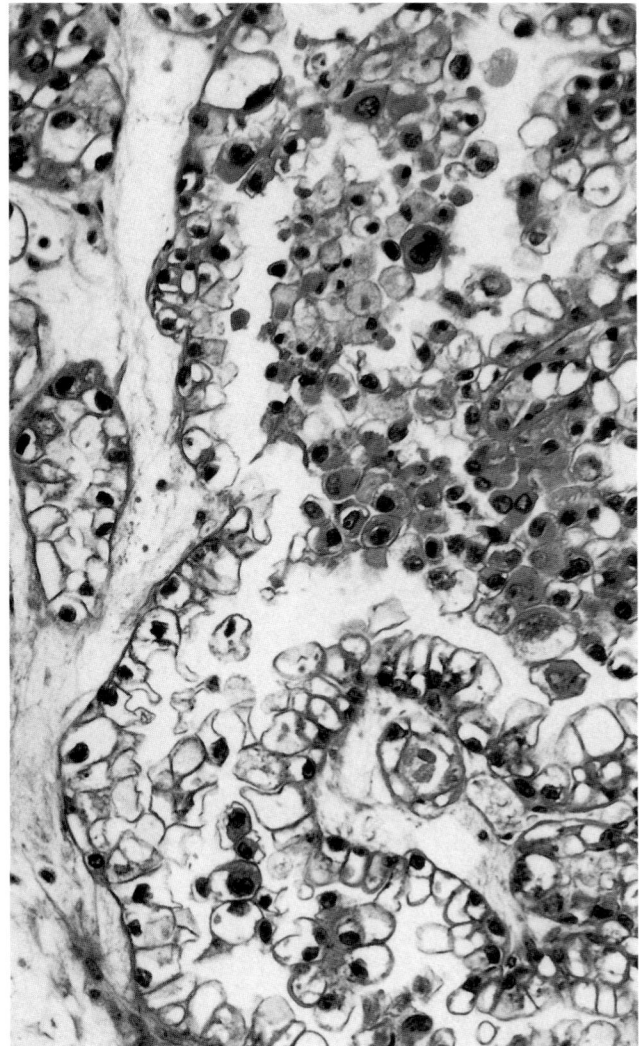

FIG. 18.93. **Clear cell carcinoma.** Most of the cells are clear but there also are clusters of cells with eosinophilic cytoplasm.

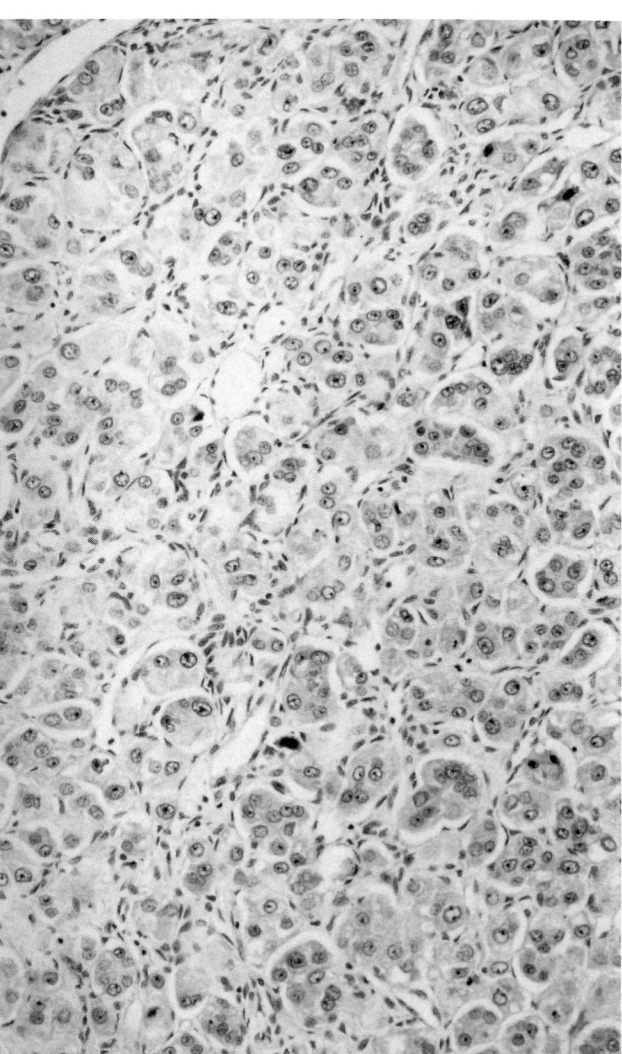

FIG. 18.94. **Clear cell carcinoma.** Eosinophilic cells in an organoid arrangement resembling a lipid cell tumor.

quently seen. Degenerative changes in these eosinophilic granular cells may be extreme and bizarre cell forms result. Clear cells with coalescent vacuoles containing "targetoid" eosinophilic PAS-positive globules (Fig. 18.95) represent another cellular variation. An uncommonly encountered but important pattern shows small groups of acini of these eosinophilic or clear cells set in loose edematous or hyalinized stroma (Fig. 18.96). Such areas may suggest Kruken-

FIG. 18.91. **Clear cell carcinoma. a:** Solid pattern with sheets of polyhedral clear cells and delicate connective tissue septa. **b:** Higher power showing nuclear detail. Mitoses are relatively infrequent.
FIG. 18.92. **Clear cell carcinoma.** Predominantly tubulopapillary pattern with prominent hobnail cells and somewhat hyalinized stroma.

berg tumor,[212] particularly if otherwise typical clear cell carcinoma patterns are not readily seen elsewhere in the sections.

Rare cases of entirely solid tumor have been observed (Fig. 18.97). There is no obvious destructive stromal invasion, yet the appearance differs significantly from the parvilocular pattern of atypically proliferating clear cell tumors. It is arguable whether such tumors are truly malignant adenofibromas. Except in these so-called malignant adenofibromas, the tumor stroma rarely resembles ovarian cortex and does not exhibit the periglandular hypercellularity of the benign and atypically proliferating clear cell tumors. Luteinized stromal cells are only occasionally noted. Microcalcification is seen in up to 50% of cases,[132] but rarely exceeds occasional psammoma bodies. Necrosis, hemorrhage, and stromal lymphocytic infiltrates are variable. The common systems of architectural and

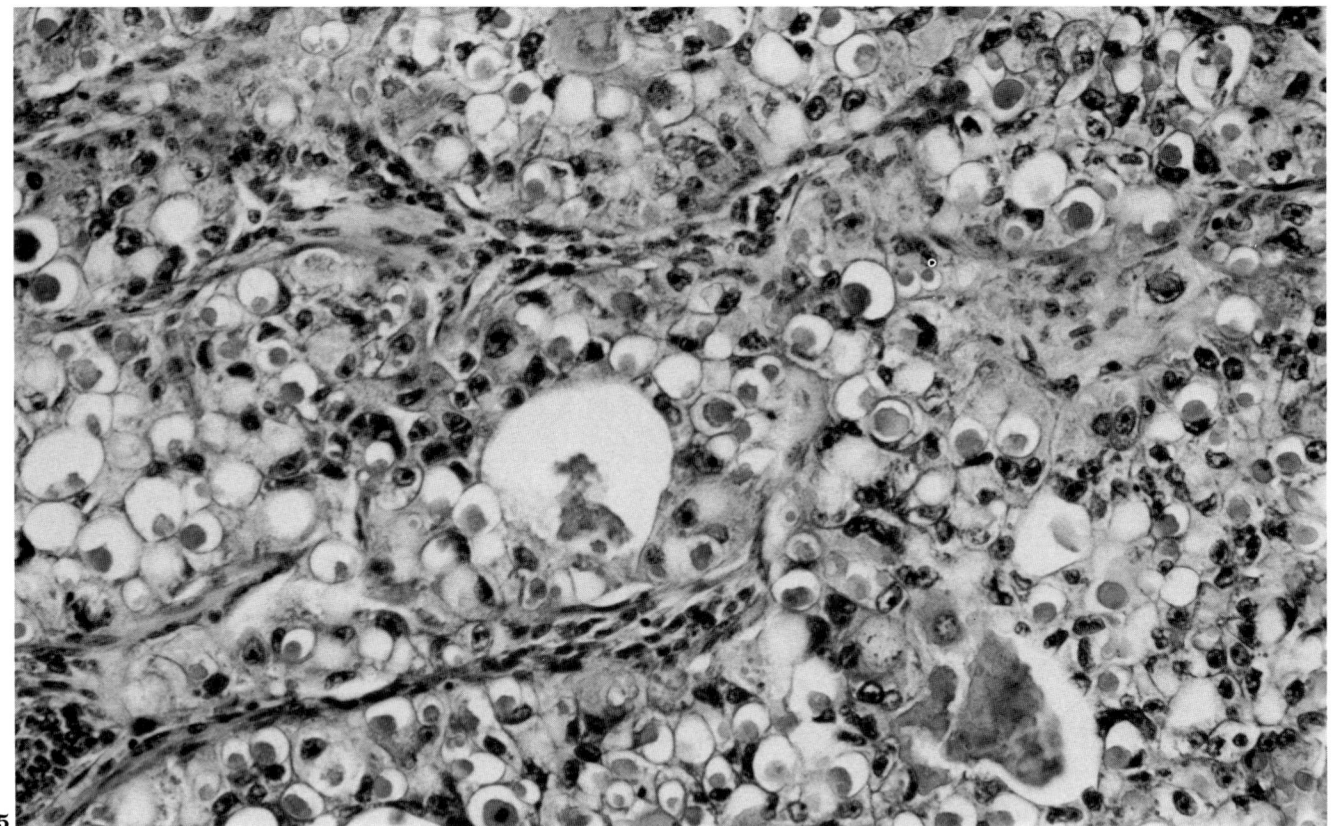

18.95

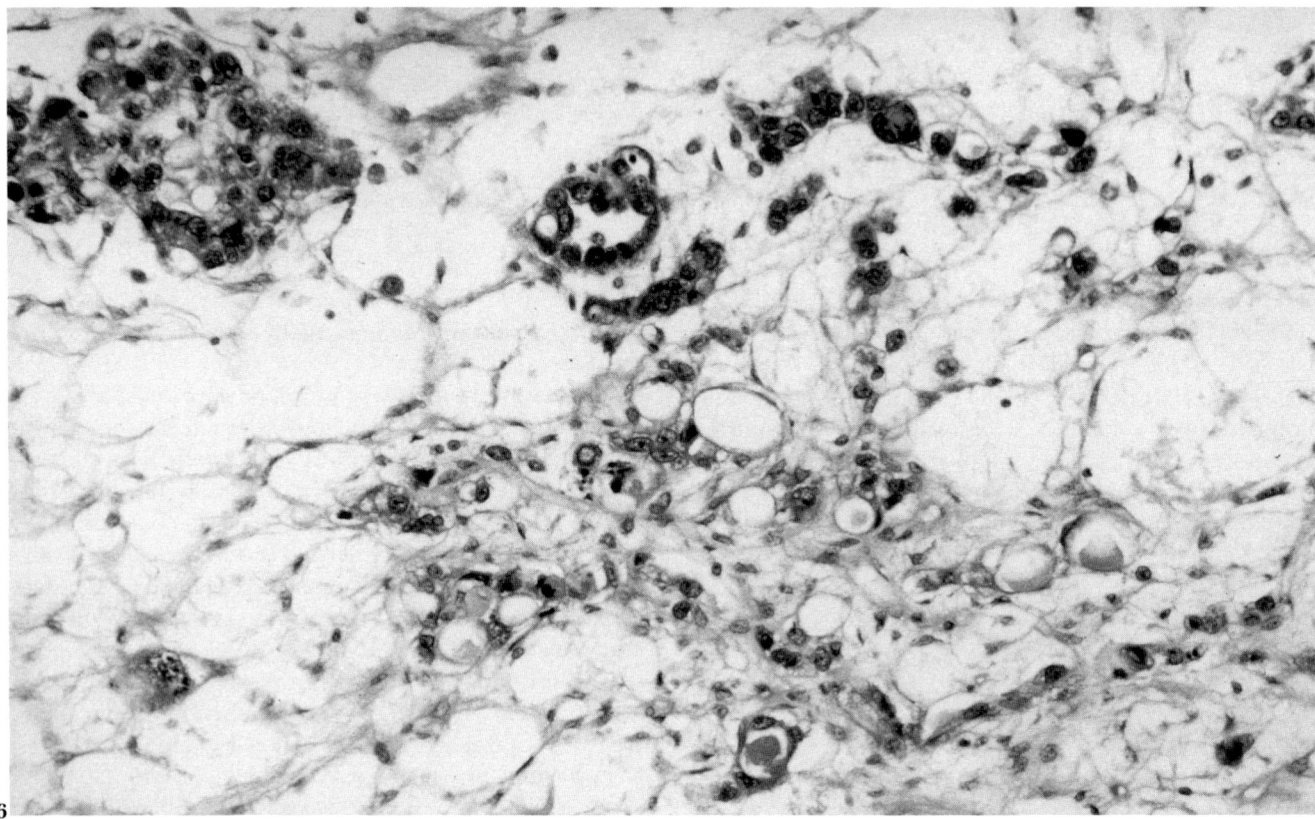

18.96

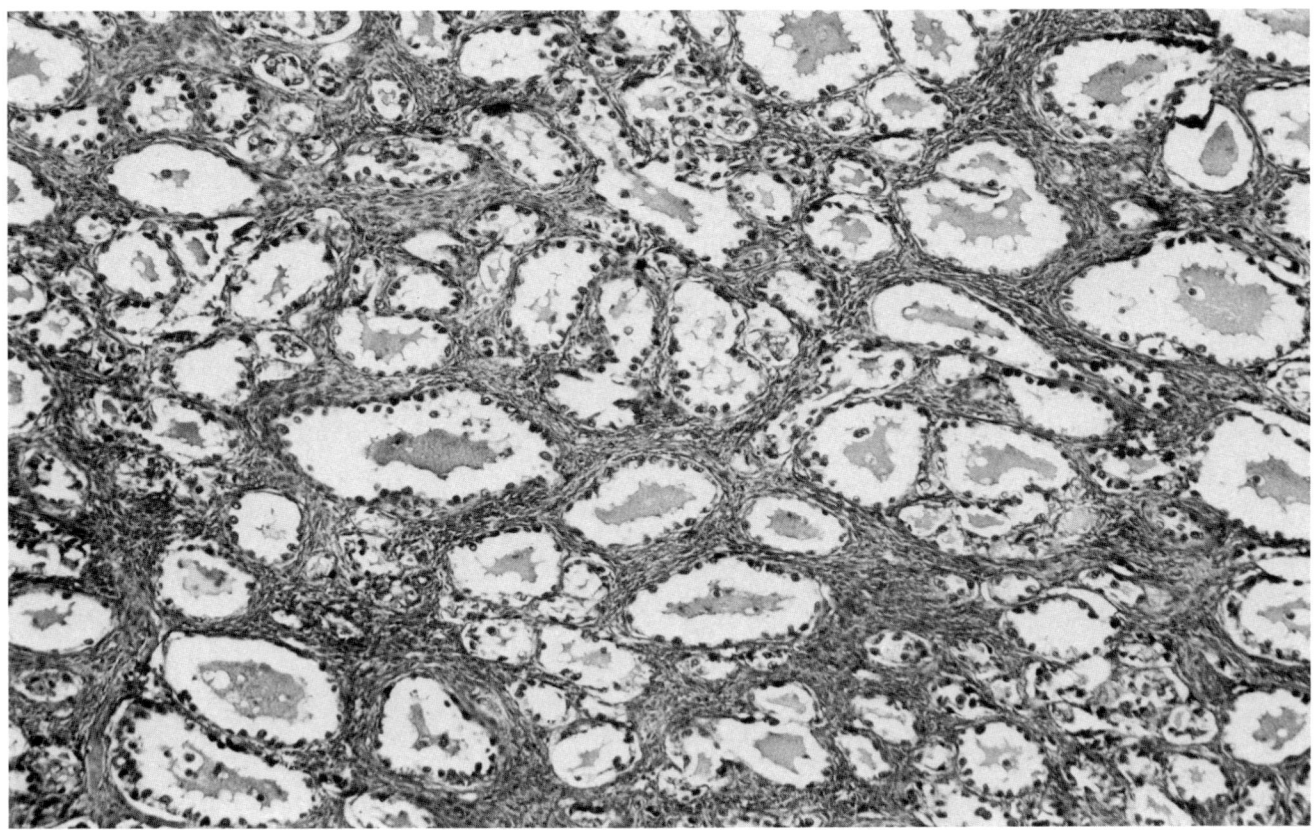

Fig. 18.97. Clear cell carcinoma. This tumor may qualify as a malignant clear cell adenofibroma. Contrast with benign lesion (Fig. 18.85).

cytological grading do not correlate well with prognosis, and grading of clear cell carcinomas is not routinely performed.

Differential Diagnosis

Yolk sac tumors may be mistaken for clear cell carcinomas; they typically occur at a much younger age and are always associated with raised serum AFP levels, this tumor-associated antigen (as well as alpha-1-antitrypsin) being demonstrable immunohistochemically within tumor cells of the former but not the targetoid cells of the latter.[140] The papillary structures of clear cell carcinomas are more complex than those seen in the "festoon" pattern of yolk sac tumors and may be distinguished by both the character of the epithelial lining cells as well as the absence of typical Schiller–Duval bodies.

Ultrastructural Findings

Clear cells typically are polyhedral with well-defined basal lamina. The nuclei vary from rounded to convoluted and usually with prominent nucleoli: these nucleoli do not show the "mesh-basket" or "nucleolar channel systems" seen in endometrioid carcinomas.[179] Cytoplasm usually is packed with glycogen granules (Fig. 18.98) obscuring other organelles, whereas other cells show abundant rough endoplasmic reticulum, small rounded basal mitochondria, Golgi apparatus, and free ribosomes. Infrequent lipid droplets, lipid lysosome complexes, and characteristic dense bodies (Fig. 18.99) are noted. Intracellular mucin is rarely present. The hobnail cells also show a thick basal lamina and lateral desmosomes. The nuclei project into the tubular lumen, which may contain lysosomal debris. The apical cell surfaces exhibit short, stubby microvilli.

◁

Fig. 18.95. Clear cell carcinoma. Vacuolated cells containing "targetoid" amorphous inclusions.

Fig. 18.96. Clear cell carcinoma. Loose edematous stroma with small clusters of epithelial cells. Mucin stains, which would show absence of intracellular mucins, readily distinguish this from mucinous carcinoma (primary or metastatic).

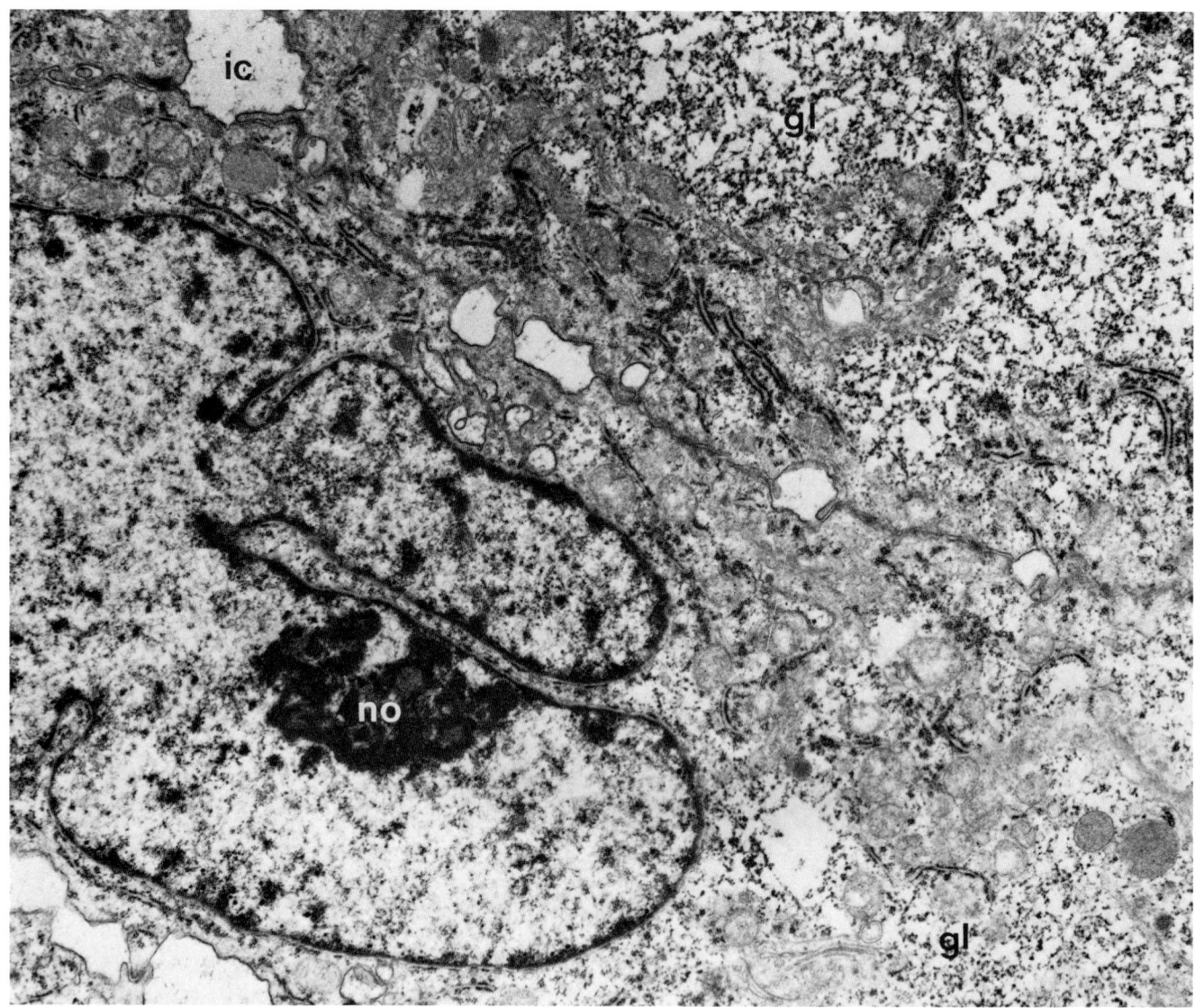

Fig. 18.98. Clear cell carcinoma. Cytoplasm is occupied by abundant glycogen (*gl*), which produces the histological clear cell appearance. Irregularly shaped nucleus contains a prominent nucleolus (*no*). Adjoining cells are closely apposed except where there are focal dilatations of the intercellular space (*ic*). ×15,000. (Courtesy of Dr. E. J. Wills, Royal Prince Alfred Hospital, Sydney, Australia.)

Clinical Behavior and Treatment

The most sensitive indicator of clinical outcome is the FIGO stage at laparotomy. Overall, the survival at 5 years with Stage I clear cell carcinoma is about 80–90%,[37,238] although surgical rupture and/or positive peritoneal washings mitigate strongly against survival in Stage I.[132,166] In Stage Ia disease in a young woman, unilateral adnexectomy may be considered as this conservative surgery does not appear to affect survival adversely.[197] The 5-year survival for Stage II disease is only 17% according to one large series[197] and those cases with extrapelvic extension do uniformly poorly despite various adjuvant regimes.[90]

Transitional Cell (Brenner) Tumors

Benign Transitional Cell Tumors

General Features

In the WHO classification, the preferred generic term for this group of neoplasms is now *transitional cell*, although it is conceded that continued use of the eponymous *Brenner tumor* has some merit in malignant lesions, given their histological diversity. Most ovarian transitional cell tumors are derived from the surface epithelium, which undergoes

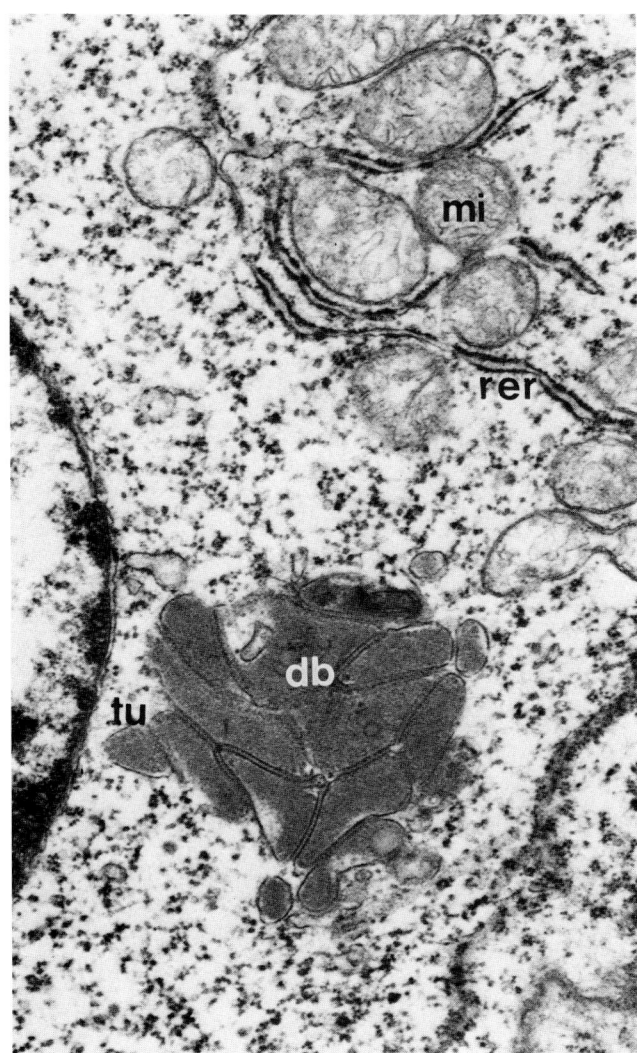

FIG. 18.99. **Clear cell carcinoma.** Detail of the tumor cell illustrating cytoplasmic dense bodies (*db*) of polygonal form interconnected by tubules (*tu*). These bodies are characteristic of clear cell carcinoma and are thought to be lysosomal in nature. Mitochondria (*mi*) are clustered together. The rough-surfaced endoplasmic reticulum (*rer*) is often more abundant than here and forms stacked cisternae. ×30,000. (Courtesy of Dr. E. J. Wills, Royal Prince Alfred Hospital, Sydney, Australia.)

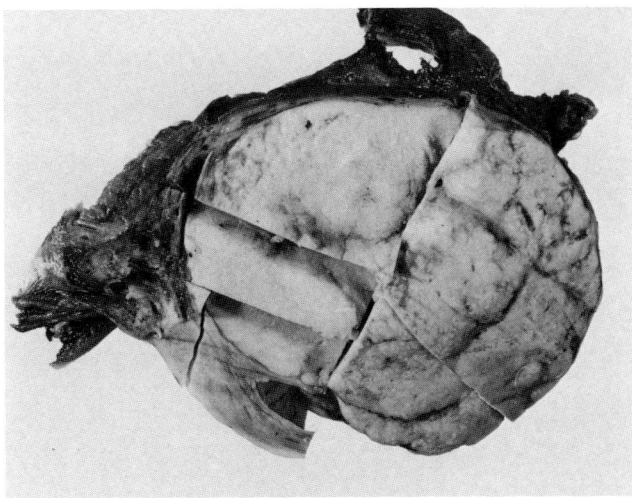

FIG. 18.100. **Benign transitional cell tumor.** The tumor measures 5 cm and has a faintly lobulated cut surface.

metaplasia to form the typical urothelial-like components. Their cellular features are similar to those of Walthard nests, which are epithelial inclusions found most commonly beneath the serosa of the fallopian tubes but also occasionally in the hilar regions of the ovaries. This, along with a frequent mixture of transitional with other epithelial elements (i.e., endocervical-type mucinous, or serous), prompts grouping of transitional cell tumors with other surface epithelial–stromal tumors in this chapter. *Urothelial* is the term used most frequently to characterize Brenner epithelium and cytologically there are similarities with the lining cells of the urinary tract.[224,234] Foci of metaplastic transitional cell epithelium at various sites in müllerian duct derivatives, rarely fallopian tube mucosa, but relatively commonly the ecto and endocervix, support the view of Woodruff[97,283] that benign transitional cell epithelium and the epithelia of müllerian type are more interrelated than has thus far been claimed.

Transitional cell tumors constitute 1–2% of all primary ovarian tumors (Table 18.1) and the vast majority are benign. Most are either microscopic or, if larger, are discovered incidentally at laparotomy for unrelated pelvic pathology. Patients are mostly in their fourth to eighth decades (mean age, 50 years). Six percent to 7% of tumors are bilateral; unilateral lesions are more common in the left ovary.[242] Rare examples have been reported in ectopic (accessory) ovaries.[114]

GROSS FINDINGS

Occasional very large benign transitional cell tumors have been reported, but few exceed 10 cm and most are smaller than 2 cm across. Most are well-circumscribed, firm, rubbery tumors with a smooth or slightly bosselated serosal surface. Less commonly they may have a significant cystic component. The cut surfaces are whorled or sometimes faintly lobulated (Fig. 18.100) and usually gray, white, or yellow. Flecks of calcification sometimes are noted. Smaller tumors usually are identified as cortical in position, but hilar lesions occasionally may be seen.

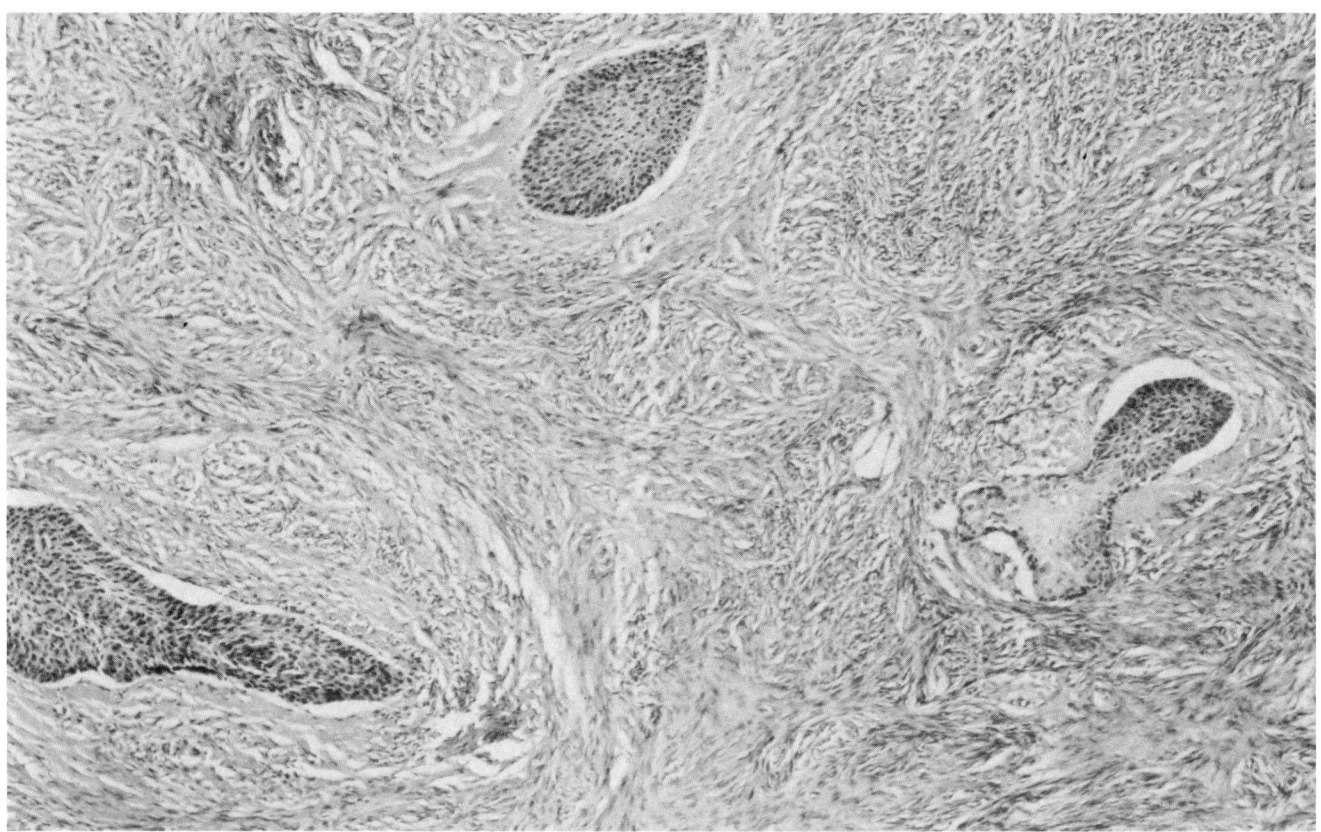

Fig. 18.101. Benign transitional cell adenofibroma (Brenner tumor). Circumscribed epithelial nests embedded in fibromatous stroma.

Microscopic Findings

Architecturally, there are sharply demarcated epithelial nests in a fibrous stroma (Fig. 18.101), the former varying from tumor to tumor in size as well as in prominence. The epithelial cells are round to polygonal with defined cell borders and eosinophilic to clear cytoplasm. The oval nuclei have obvious nucleoli and often exhibit longitudinal grooves, the so-called coffee-bean appearance (Fig. 18.102). This latter feature is not always prominent and additionally is far from diagnostic, being noted in some other cell types of "epithelial–stromal" and "sex cord" derivation. Nuclear atypia is rare and mitoses infrequent (fewer than 1 MF/10 HPF). Histochemically, these cells contain abundant diffuse glycogen, acidic sialomucins at their apical borders, and both sialomucins and neutral mucins in luminal secretions. Immunohistochemical demonstration of various cytokeratin intermediate filaments is well documented.[151] Argyrophil cells, which regularly exhibit serotonin, chromogranin, and neurone-specific enolase, are present among the epithelial cells in many tumors.[3,224]

Cell nests often become cystic and these microcysts contain eosinophilic debris or mucin. They usually are lined by transitional cells or, less commonly, endocervical-type mucinous or, rarely, ciliated cells. Cystic change may be more prominent, to the extent of being visible grossly. Such cysts are lined by transitional cell epithelium or by metaplastic mucinous epithelium (Fig. 18.103). Roth et al.[201,205] have designated these tumors as *metaplastic Brenner tumors;* an equally justifiable approach would be to classify them among tumors of mixed epithelial differentiation, provided at least 10% of the tumor is represented by the minor epithelial element (see below). The other extreme end of this spectrum is for a small transitional cell tumor nodule to be found in the wall of an otherwise typical benign mucinous cystadenoma.

The tumor stroma is composed of spindled cells and differs little from that of other epithelial–stromal adenofibromas. Cellularity varies inversely with collagen formation and hyalinization. The latter usually occurs around, or adjacent to, epithelial nests. Spiculate dystrophic calcification is present in 50% of benign transitional cell tumors[207] and frequently is present in the hyalinized areas (Fig. 18.104). Focal ossification and marked stromal edema[212] rarely may be noted. Stromal luteinization is present in 10–15% of tumors, occasionally prominent enough to appear thecoma-like. Rare reports claim to show malignant stroma but documentation is not conclusive.[17,23]

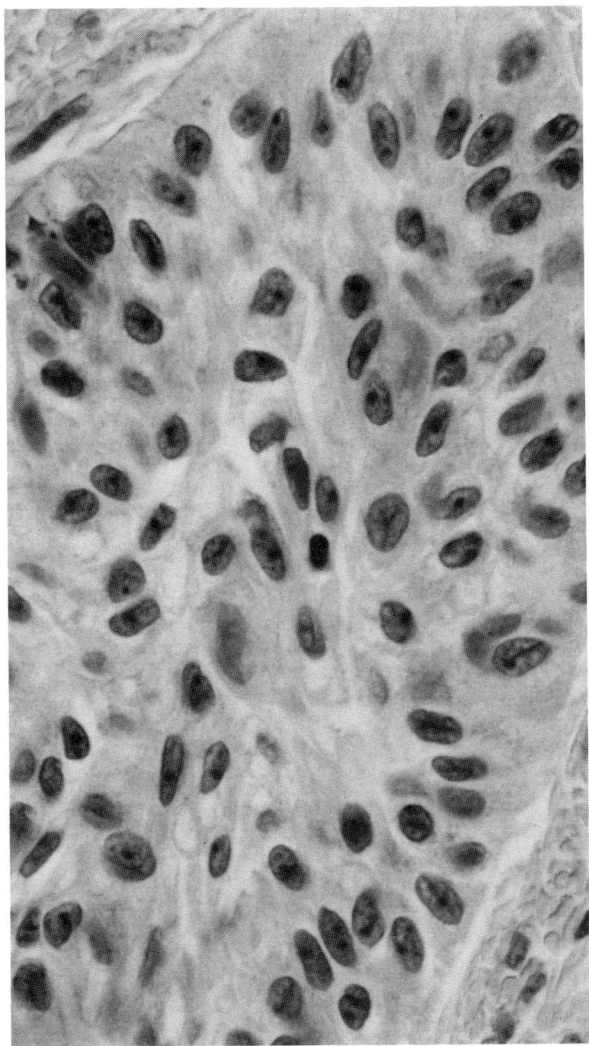

FIG. 18.102. **Benign transitional cell adenofibroma (Brenner tumor).** High power of transitional cell epithelial nests, showing occasional "coffee bean" nuclei.

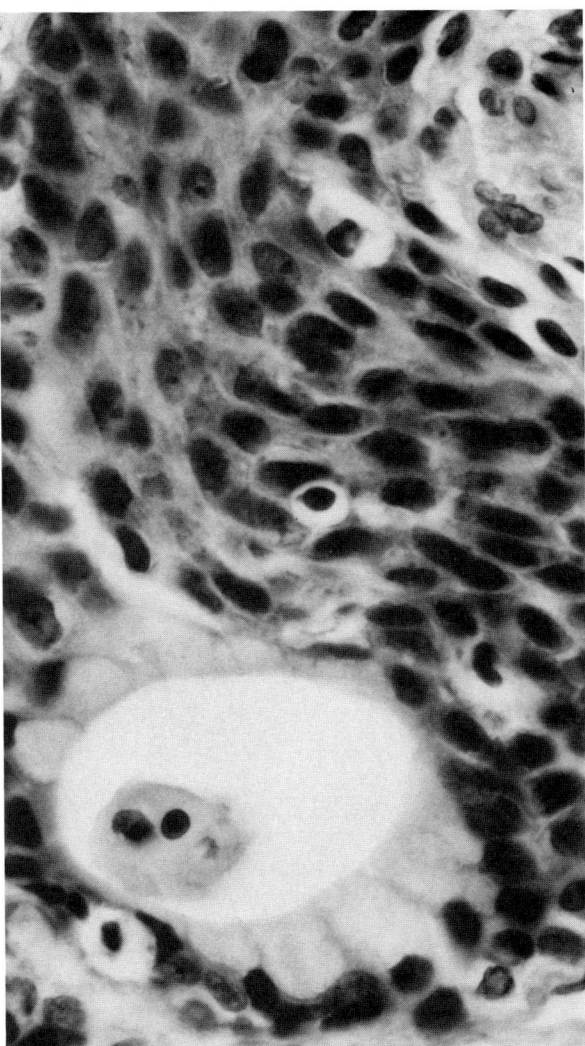

FIG. 18.103. **Benign transitional cell tumor (Brenner tumor).** High power of transitional cell epithelial nests, showing mucinous cells lining microcysts.

ULTRASTRUCTURAL FINDINGS

Ultrastructural studies[61,224,244] show large polyhedral cells from which project villiform cytoplasmic processes into wide intercellular spaces. These processes are not connected by desmosomes, although such junctions are noted elsewhere at interdigitating cell junctions. Mitochondria, free ribosomes, lysosomes, and glycogen are abundant but Golgi bodies and granular endoplasmic reticulum are inconspicuous. Nuclei are ovoid and often deeply grooved. They have fine, evenly dispersed chromatin and prominent nucleoli.

CLINICAL BEHAVIOR AND TREATMENT

Benign transitional cell tumors are treated by local excision, which is curative.

Atypically Proliferating Transitional Cell Tumors

GENERAL FEATURES

These were first described in 1971[200] and have been referred to either as *proliferating*[163,200,283] or *borderline*.[104] Roth has since expanded the spectrum by referring to *proliferating* and *metaplastic* Brenner tumors as well as those *of low malignant potential*.[201,270]

These rare neoplasms appear to occur at an older age than benign transitional cell tumors (mean age, 60 years) and, being larger tumors, tend to present with symptoms referable to the ovarian mass. Occasional examples of atypically proliferating transitional cell tumors are associated with synchronous or metachronous transitional cell carcinomas in the urinary bladder.[58,145,254]

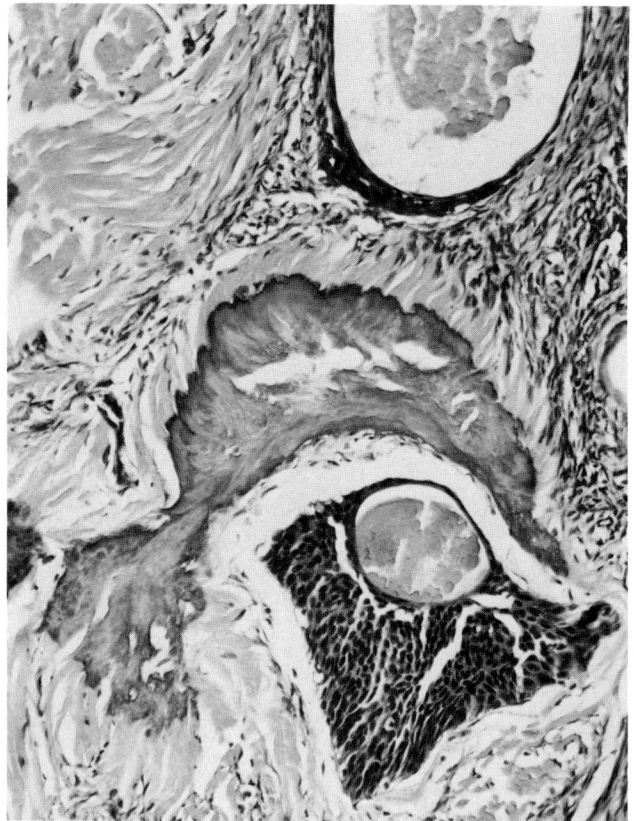

FIG. 18.104. Benign transitional cell tumor. There is stromal hyalinization and dystrophic calcification.

GROSS FINDINGS

They are typically unilateral, multilocular cysts measuring 10 to 25 cm in diameter, but may be bilateral. Friable, papillary, or polypoid masses project into the cyst lumens, contrasting with the tough fibrous consistency of benign transitional cell tumor, which is usually noted nearby (Fig. 18.105). Rare examples have shown a surface papillary component.

MICROSCOPIC FINDINGS

The soft, coarsely papillary elements in the tumors, as well as cysts, are lined by multilayered epithelium (Fig. 18.106). This appearance has been likened to that of low-grade transitional cell carcinomas of the bladder[201] and squamous carcinoma in situ of the cervix.[283] In deeper portions of the proliferative nodules, papillary patterns merge with those of closely packed sheets of transitional cell epithelium with little intervening stroma. Adjacent zones of typical benign transitional cell tumor are seen in almost all cases. Cellular details do not differ significantly from those described for benign transitional cell tumors, with prominent nucleoli and nuclear grooves. Mitoses are present (up to 1 MF/10 HPF) but there is, by definition, no

stromal invasion (Fig. 18.107). Endocervical-type mucin-secreting cells, ciliated cells, and squamous cells sometimes line microcysts, as in benign tumors. Stromal luteinization of the stroma occasionally is noted.[99,163] Focal necrosis is uncommonly observed.

CLINICAL BEHAVIOR AND TREATMENT

More than 50 atypically proliferating transitional cell tumors have been reported,* and only one has recurred locally.[157] All the others have pursued an entirely benign course. The case of Pratt-Thomas et al.[191] documenting liver metastases has been reviewed and reinterpreted as an example of a frankly malignant transitional cell tumor.[64]

Therefore, conservative treatment consisting of total hysterectomy with bilateral adnexectomy is appropriate and, in a younger patient, unilateral adnexectomy would appear adequate.

Malignant Transitional Cell Tumors

GENERAL FEATURES

These are rare tumors and it is hard to establish their true prevalence. Using current WHO criteria, many earlier reported cases are indeed atypically proliferating rather than frankly malignant neoplasms. It is recommended that a careful search, in suspected cases of transitional cell carcinoma, be made for areas of typical benign or atypically proliferating transitional cell tumor.[199,230] Austin and Norris[13] and others[195,204] have nominally distinguished between transitional cell carcinomas of the ovaries, without associated benign transitional cell elements, and malignant Brenner tumors in which benign transitional cell areas are present. Although the confusion in terminology is acknowledged, these investigators noted significant differences between the two tumor subgroups in both their histological features and clinical course. On the other hand, if mucinous or serous carcinomas are found in association with benign transitional cell tumor they should be so classified[199] and not categorized as malignant Brenner tumors. Likewise, carcinomas of apparent mixed epithelial differentiation should be assessed carefully and placed into this category. Applying such restrictions, many cases in the literature are not acceptable; a residuum of about 100 examples remains.[13,199,222,283,240]

The mean age at presentation of patients with malignant Brenner tumors/transitional cell carcinomas is about 55 years. Abdominal pain and swelling are the common presenting symptoms with abnormal uterine bleeding occurring in 20% of cases. About 15% of patients have associated endometrial hyperplasia[90] and occasional tumors appear to be estrogen-secreting.[144]

---

*Refs. 50,99,104,137,157,163,200,201,208,283.

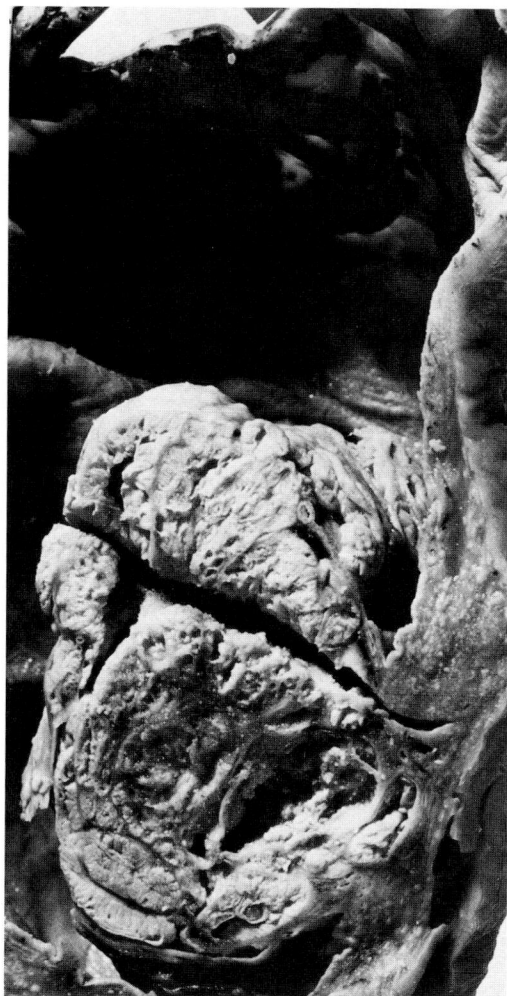

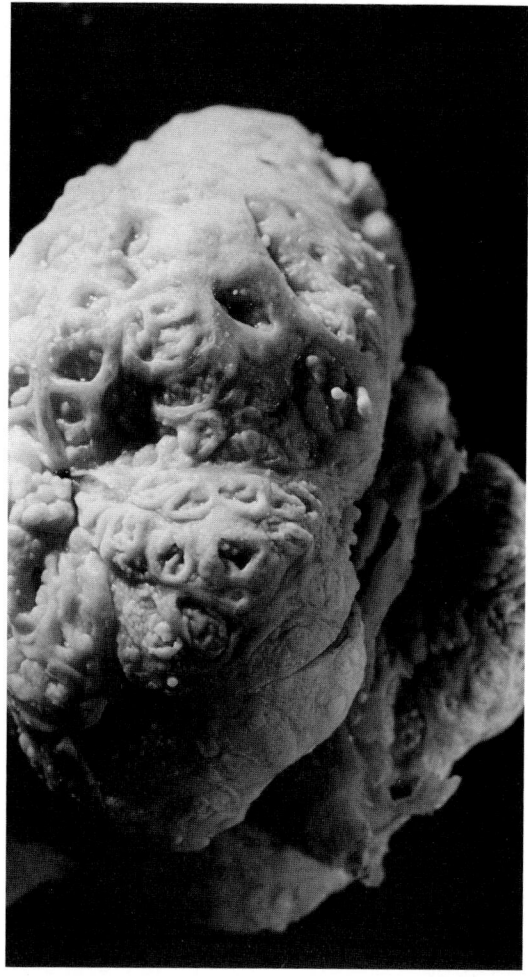

FIG. 18.105. **Atypically proliferating transitional cell tumor. a:** Nodular mass projecting into lumen of a thick-walled cyst. Stippled fibrous tissue, below the nodule, in the cyst wall is an area of benign transitional tumor. **b:** Closer view of surface of large luminal nodule.

GROSS FINDINGS

Malignant transitional cell tumors usually are partly cystic and vary in diameter between 10 and 30 cm (mean, 20 cm). They are rarely bilateral.[110] Cystic spaces frequently have a ragged lining and exhibit friable, polypoid mural nodules. Cyst fluid is watery or mucinous in consistency. Areas of hemorrhage and necrosis may be prominent and 50% have foci of gritty calcification. Fibrous tumors grossly indistinguishable from benign transitional cell tumors are less frequently found.

MICROSCOPIC FINDINGS

Malignant transitional cell tumors typically show heterogeneous solid epithelial growth with little intervening stroma (Fig. 18.108). Cysts are lined by multilayered epithelium, frequently thrown into thick blunt papillary folds with fibrovascular connective tissue cores. Cells have hyperchromatic, pleomorphic nuclei and mitotic figures are numerous. Occasional bizarre giant cells are encountered. Similar features are present in the underlying sheets of usually transitional-like cells. Squamoid areas (Fig. 18.109) or attempts at glandular differentiation (Fig. 18.110) are common. Discrete nests of carcinoma cells may undergo central necrosis giving rise to a "comedo carcinoma" pattern. Sparse intervening stroma is immature and contains a variable inflammatory infiltrate. Focal necrosis is present in most tumors, as is spiculate dystrophic calcification.[13]

Less often, the stromal component is more prominent and the tumor architecture more closely resembles that of a malignant adenofibroma.[205] Epithelial nests show cytological evidence of malignancy but, as in other malignant epithelial adenofibromas, the demonstration of clear-cut stromal invasion required for the diagnosis of frank malignancy is subjective and may require extensive sampling.

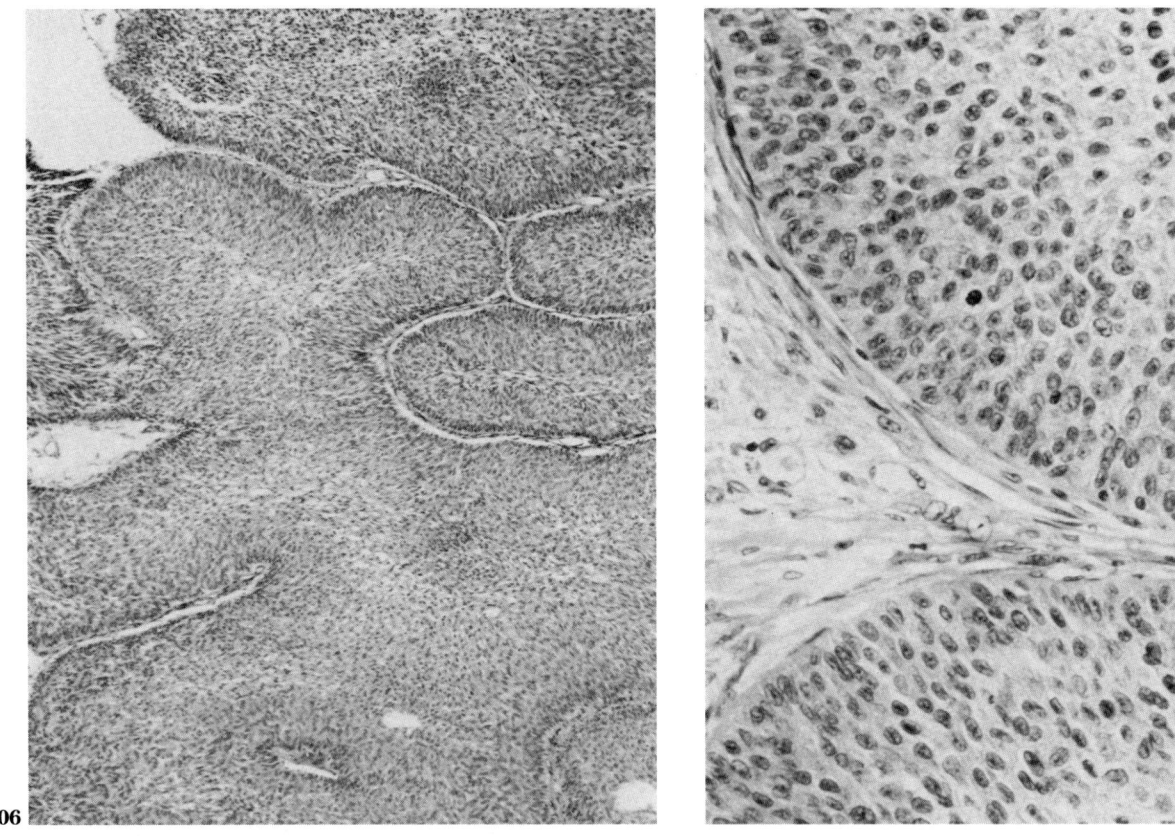

18.106

18.107

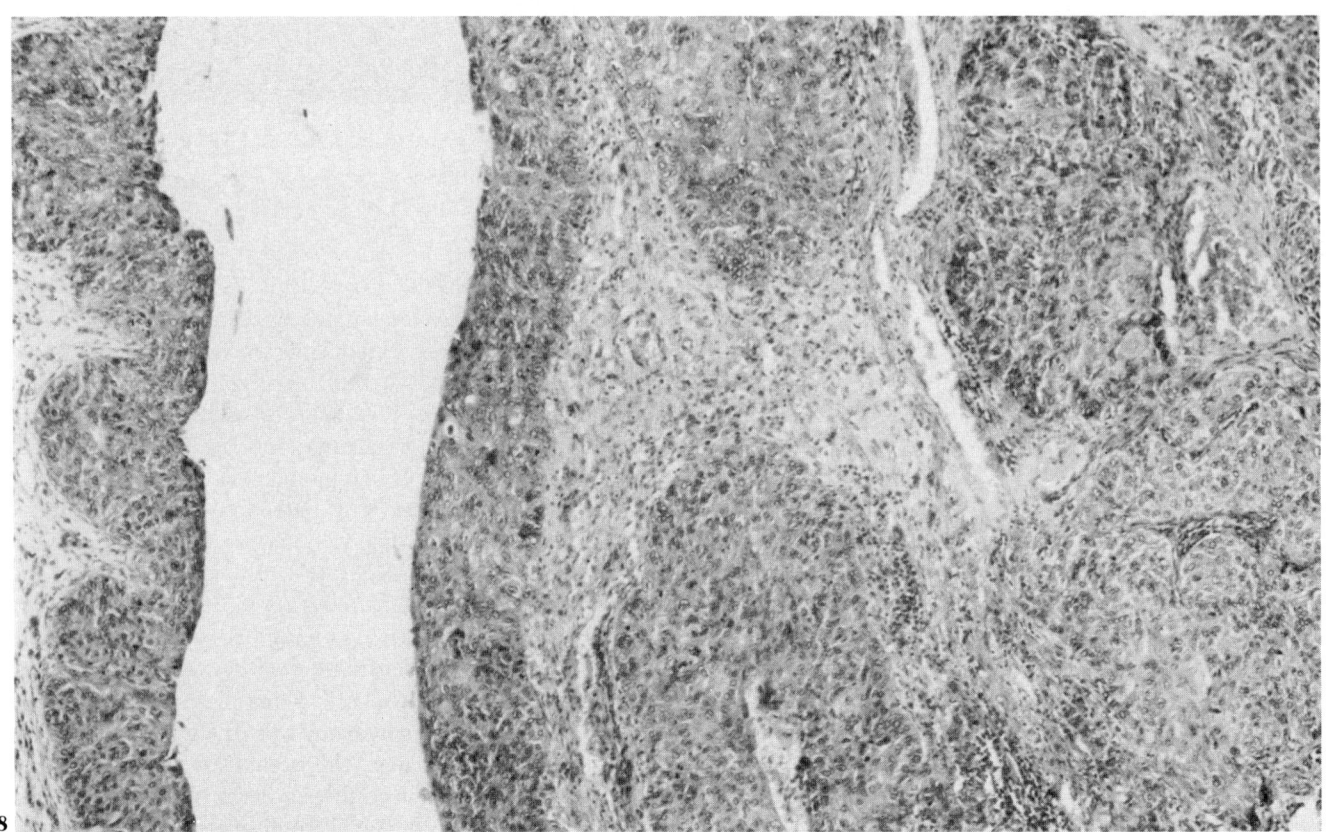

18.108

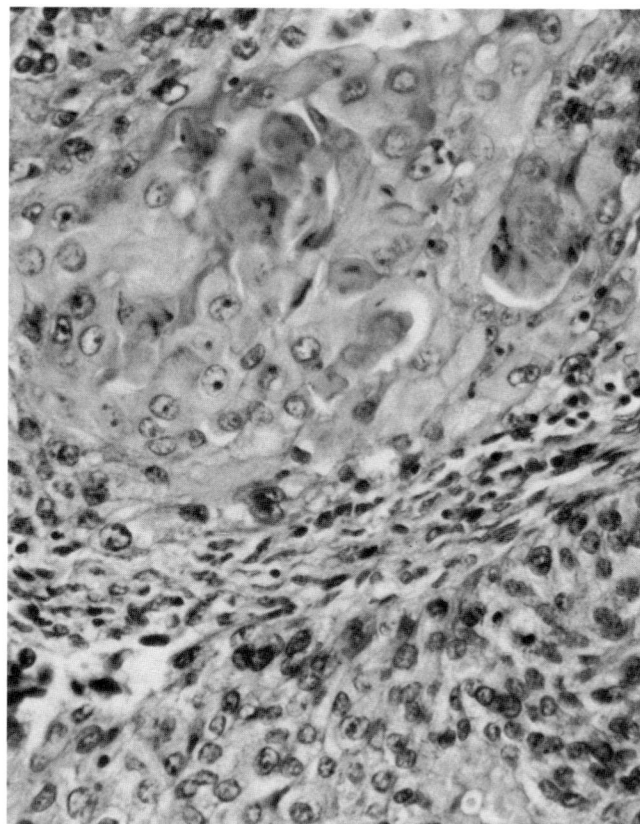

FIG. 18.109. **Malignant transitional cell tumor.** Squamous areas are present in this field.

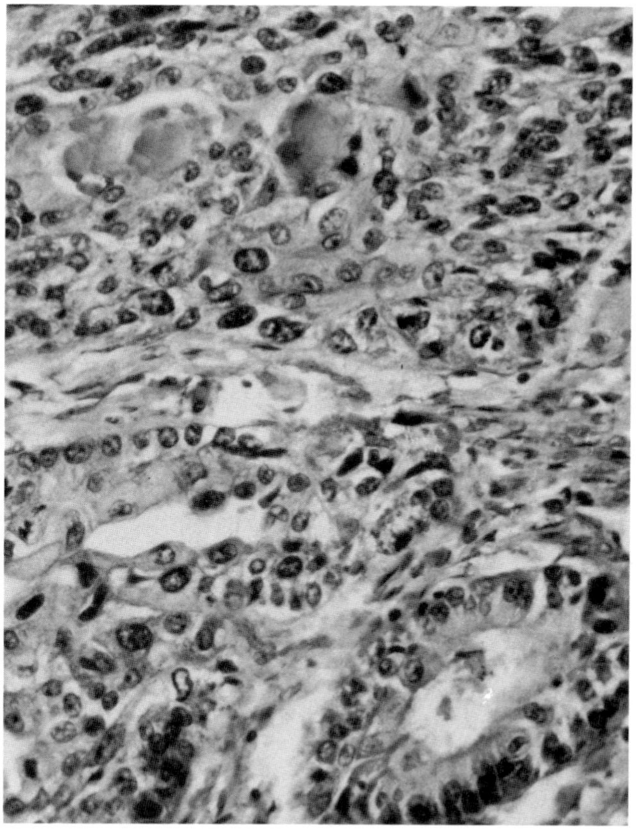

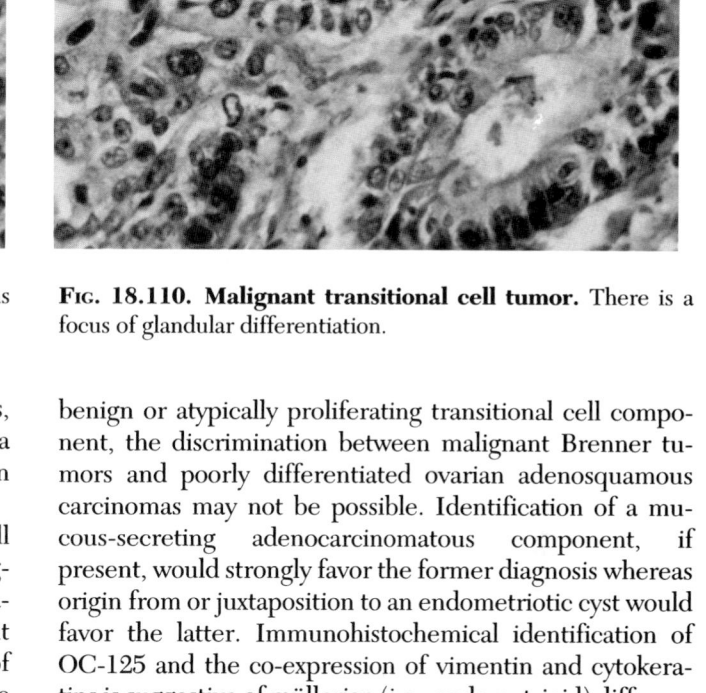

FIG. 18.110. **Malignant transitional cell tumor.** There is a focus of glandular differentiation.

Irregularity, branching, and confluence of epithelial nests, depletion of stroma by crowded epithelial masses, and a desmoplastic stromal reaction[199] are helpful features in making the distinction.

Foci of benign or atypically proliferating transitional cell tumor occur in association with more than 50% of malignant tumors in this group. As noted above, some investigators[13,199] regard their presence as definitional of malignant Brenner tumor and, in their absence, make a diagnosis of transitional cell carcinoma. Austin and Norris[13] describe small areas of squamous or glandular differentiation in more than one-third of their cases of transitional cell carcinoma; dystrophic calcification is conspicuously absent and mitoses numerous (average about 3 MF/HPF). Without a

⊲─────────────────────

FIG. 18.106. **Atypically proliferating transitional cell tumor.** Solid sheets of epithelial cells separated by sparse intervening stroma.

FIG. 18.107. **Atypically proliferating transitional cell tumor.** Smooth epithelial–stromal interface with typical transitional cells and occasional mitoses, but no invasion.

FIG. 18.108. **Malignant transitional cell tumor.** Cysts lined by malignant transitional epithelium with areas of solid carcinoma.

benign or atypically proliferating transitional cell component, the discrimination between malignant Brenner tumors and poorly differentiated ovarian adenosquamous carcinomas may not be possible. Identification of a mucous-secreting adenocarcinomatous component, if present, would strongly favor the former diagnosis whereas origin from or juxtaposition to an endometriotic cyst would favor the latter. Immunohistochemical identification of OC-125 and the co-expression of vimentin and cytokeratins is suggestive of müllerian (i.e., endometrioid) differentiation in this specific context. Discriminating primary transitional cell carcinomas of ovary from metastatic transitional cell carcinomas of urinary tract origin is heavily dependent on clinical features.[292]

CLINICAL BEHAVIOR AND TREATMENT

Major behavioral differences exist between ovarian transitional cell carcinomas, as defined above, and malignant Brenner tumors. Transitional cell carcinomas are far more frequently in advanced stage at presentation (70–100% in the former vs. 10–20% in the latter) and regularly pursue a more aggressive clinical course.[13,240,292] Furthermore, there is a greatly increased likelihood of complete response to chemotherapy of transitional cell (83%) versus nontransitional cell (33%) malignancies of the ovaries.[13,240]

Treatment consists of total hysterectomy with bilateral adnexectomy and omentectomy at a thorough staging laparotomy, and postoperative adjuvant chemotherapy.[195]

Nonteratomatous Tumors of Squamous Differentiation

Subcortical and Hilar Epidermoid Cysts

Subcortical and hilar epidermoid cysts are rare cysts that are lined by stratified squamous epithelium, unaccompanied by skin appendages or other teratomatous elements. They usually are small cysts incidentally found at laparotomy, although the largest reported example (5 cm in diameter) was associated with abdominal symptoms.[42] Lesions are located in the hilus, medulla, or cortex of the ovary and are filled with yellow creamy material. Although previously thought to be most often of teratomatous origin, they are now classified among the epithelial–stromal tumors in the revised WHO classification, and other histogenetic possibilities have been accepted such as squamous metaplasia of endometriotic cysts,[156] rete ovarii,[167] mesonephric tubules,[275] or coelomically derived epithelium.[42,176,295] Within the walls of some cysts are nests of epithelial cells resembling those of Walthard nests or transitional cell tumors, perhaps supporting a coelomic origin.[176,295] It is likely that not all cysts have a common histogenesis and that the origins may vary according to location.

Squamous Cell Carcinomas

Rare examples of squamous carcinoma in situ,[34] squamous carcinoma in situ with microinvasion,[286] or frank carcinoma[32,158,239,262] have been reported. In the last instance it is even more difficult to exclude origin in a teratoma that may have been overgrown by malignant tumor growth. Other histogeneses, such as adenosquamous carcinoma or malignant Brenner tumor, should be excluded histologically by identifying appropriate epithelial differentiation. In three ovarian pure squamous carcinomas (two in situ, one in situ and invasive), Scully[230] observed that two of these patients had autochthonous squamous carcinoma in situ of the uterine cervix. Genadry et al.[97] reported a similar case and suggested a field change to an as yet unknown carcinogen.

The histological features of these tumors include an ovarian cyst lined by atypical squamous epithelium with or without solid areas of infiltrating squamous carcinoma (Fig. 18.111).

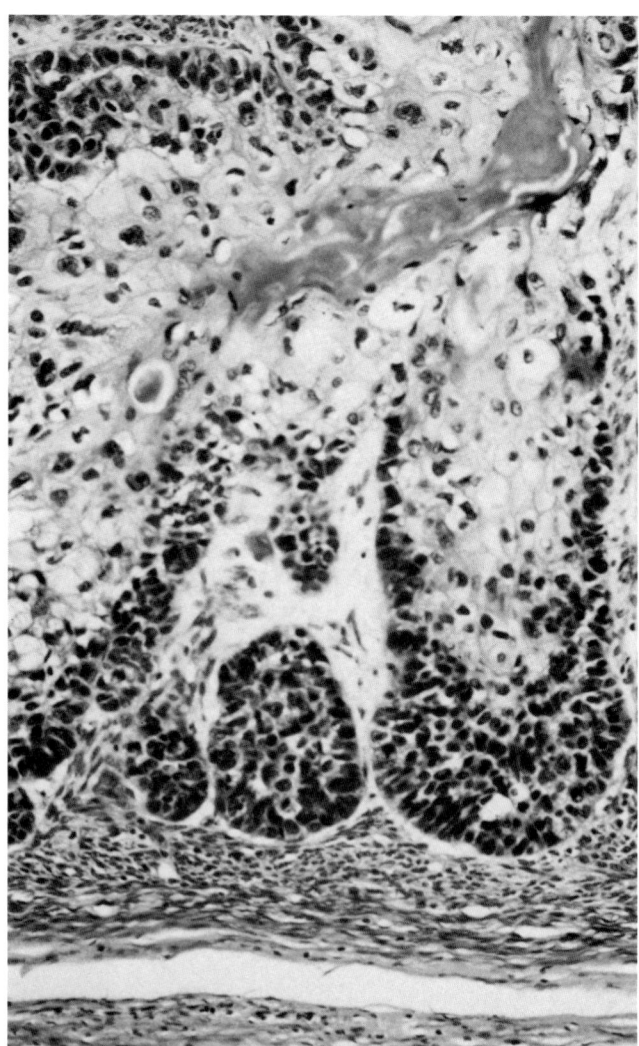

Fig. 18.111. Nonteratomatous epidermoid tumor. In this field there is an infiltrating squamous carcinoma.

Mixed Epithelial Tumors

GENERAL FEATURES

Mixed epithelial tumors are defined as exhibiting two or more of the epithelial elements described in the preceding sections of this chapter, present in variable proportions, intimately mixed or in discrete areas. Like the pure neo-

Fig. 18.112. Mixed serous and mucinous cystadenoma. An intimate mixture of tall columnar mucin-secreting cells and typical tubal-type pseudostratified epithelium.
Fig. 18.113. Atypically proliferating endometrioid and serous tumor. The latter component (*right*) is architecturally benign, whereas the endometrioid area shows complex glandular hyperplasia.

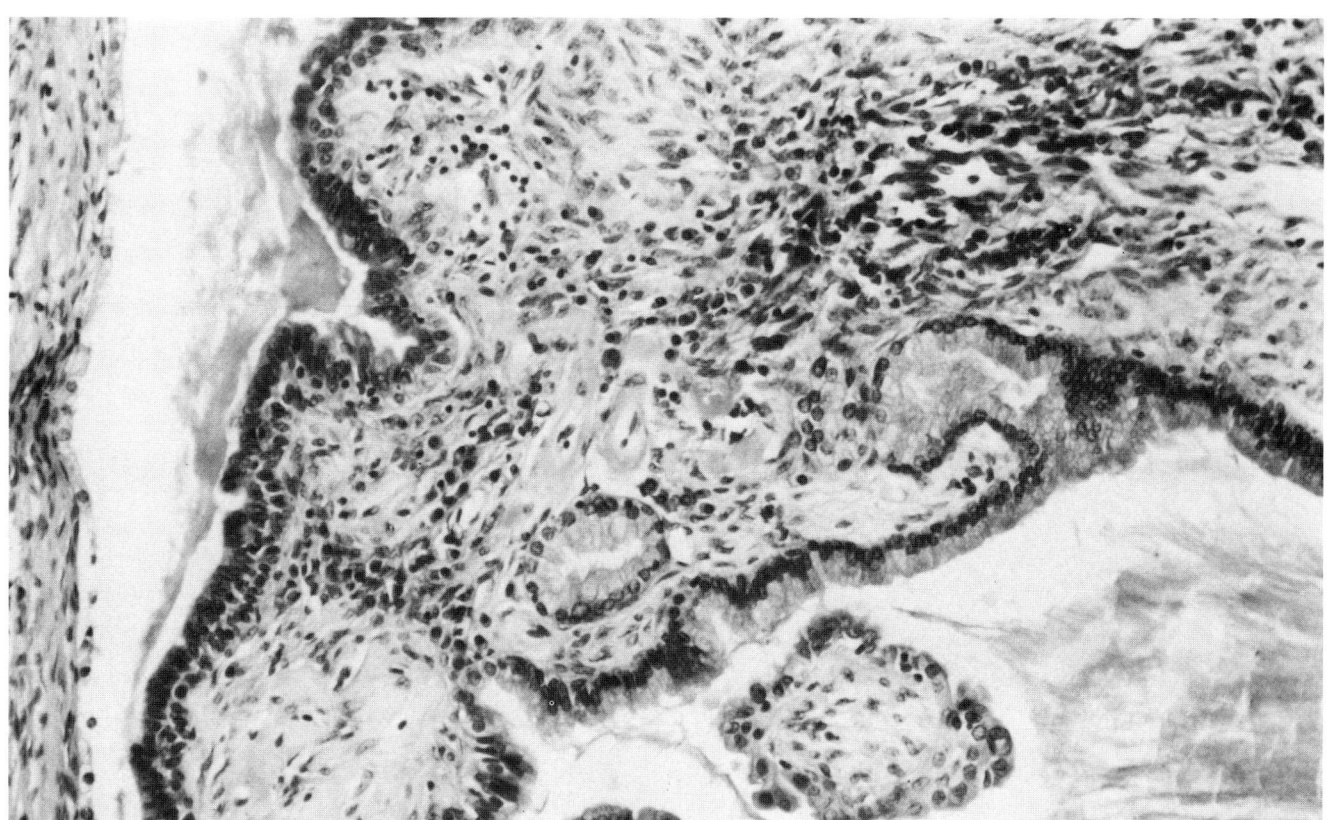

18.112

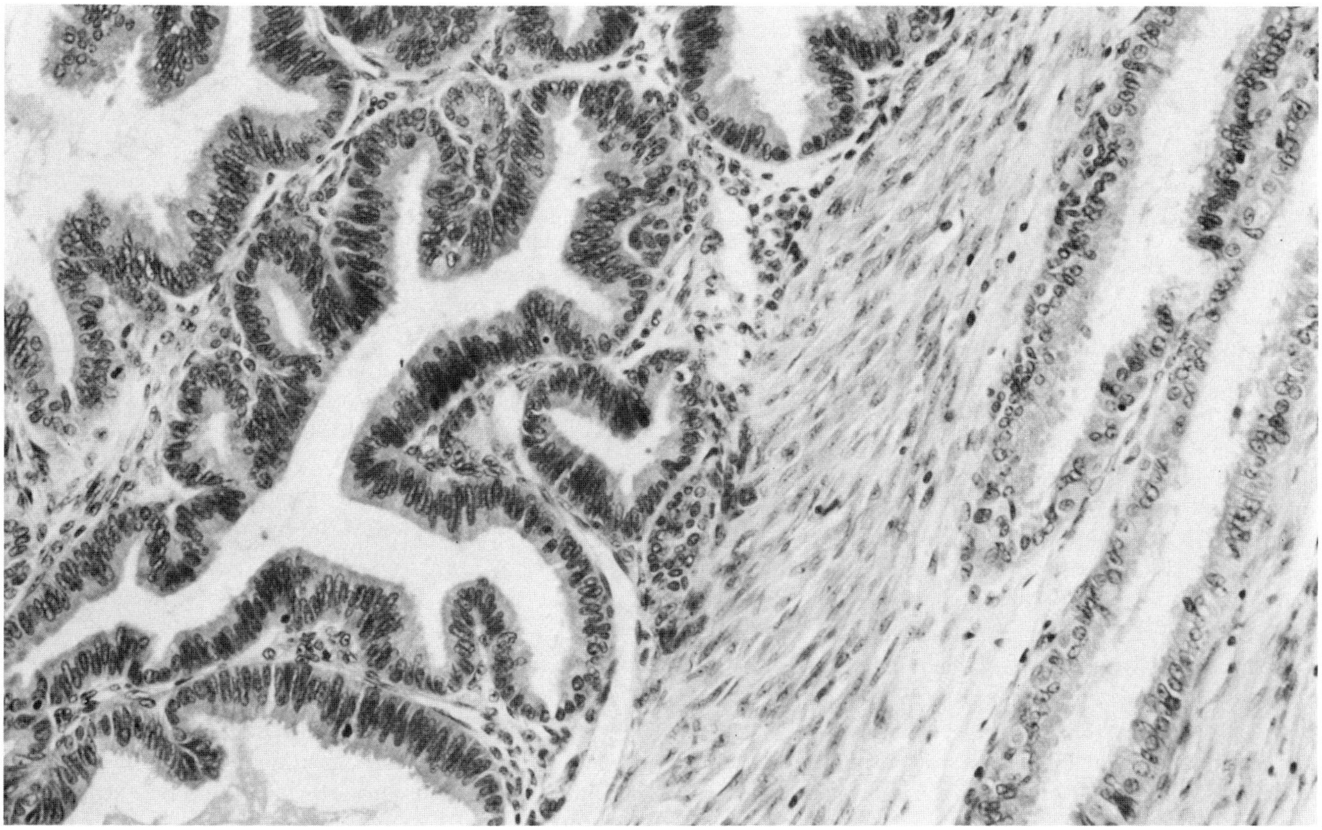

18.113

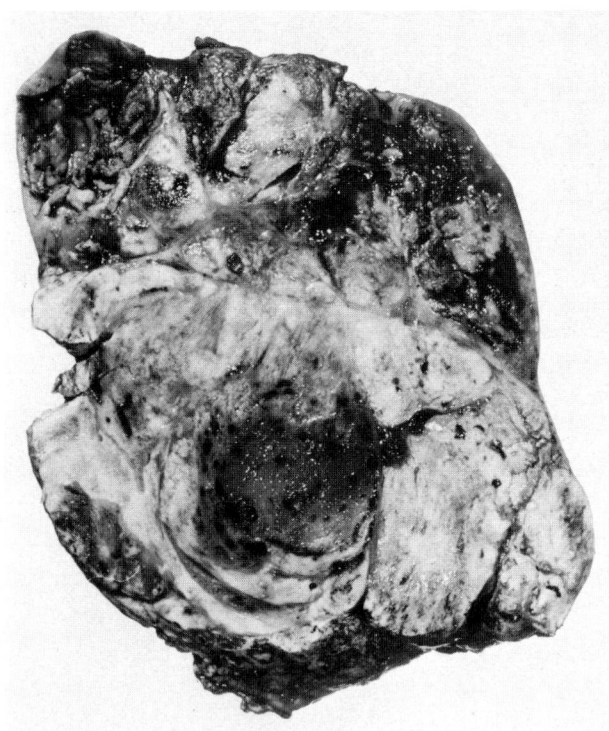

Fig. 18.114. **Solid undifferentiated carcinoma.** There is obvious necrosis and hemorrhage.

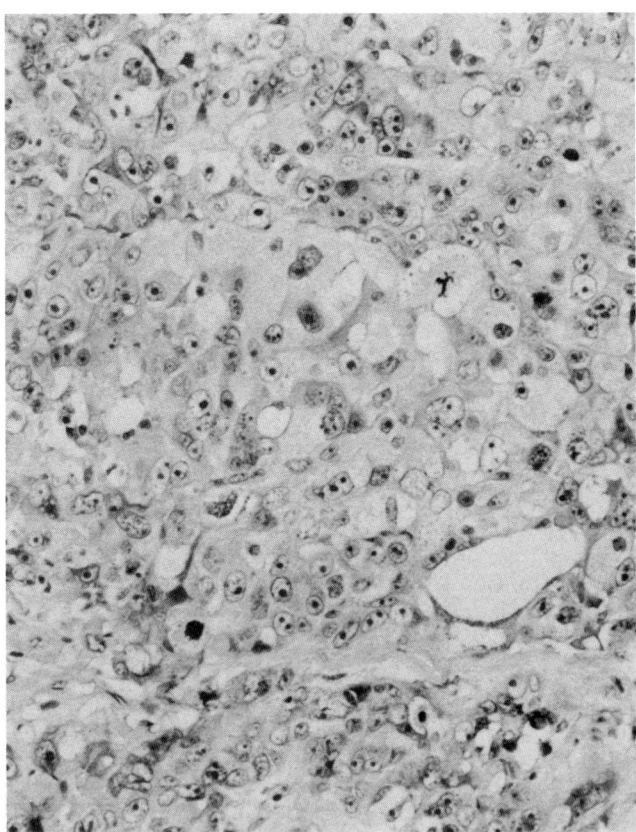

Fig. 18.115. **Undifferentiated carcinoma.** The tumor is composed of large anaplastic cells.

plasms, they display the full proliferative spectrum from benign to invasive carcinoma. Their origin most likely results from biphasic or multiphasic differentiation. Carcinomas of mixed differentiation are not uncommon elsewhere in the female genital tract, expressing much the same spectrum as is observed in the ovaries.

By convention, minor components (isolated fields or cellular aggregates) of a second or third epithelial tissue type should be disregarded for the purposes of classification[207,236] and such neoplasms should be categorized according to the differentiation of the dominant epithelial element. Examples of this include typical endometrioid carcinomas with focal areas of ciliated cells, the latter not qualifying as significant serous differentiation, or transitional cell tumors with occasional microcysts lined by mucinous epithelium. Similarly, mucinous carcinomas arising in association with benign transitional cell tumors should be classified as mixed epithelial carcinomas rather than malignant Brenner tumors. The arbitrary minimum criterion adopted here for inclusion in this category is 10% representation of the minor epithelial elements in the tissue sections.[207,231] This results in about 2–3% of benign epithelial–stromal tumors, a similar percentage of those showing atypical proliferation and 1–2% of invasive carcinomas being categorized as mixed (Table 18.1).

Their diagnosis may be difficult in poorly differentiated carcinomas where lack of epithelial differentiation compromises assessment, and also in benign examples in which

intermediate or "indifferent" epithelial elements may be present. Epithelial combinations reflect the approximate relative frequencies with which the various "pure" types occur. Of benign mixed epithelial tumors, serous/mucinous and mucinous/transitional cell are the most commonly observed associations (Fig. 18.112). Roth et al.[201] proposed that mixed transitional cell/mucinous tumors be classified as metaplastic Brenner tumors. Atypically proliferating mixed epithelial tumors are rare and show various combinations of serous, mucinous, and/or endometrioid epithelia (Fig. 18.113). Not all epithelial elements need be proliferating to categorize a tumor as such.[7] Of malignant mixed epithelial tumors, serous/endometrioid and endometrioid/clear cell are the most easily identified patterns.

CLINICAL BEHAVIOR AND TREATMENT

These tumors appear to behave similarly to the pure counterpart of their dominant epithelial element, both with respect to patterns of pathogenesis and clinical course. A predominantly serous tumor is likely to have extraovarian manifestations at laparotomy and a predominantly endo-

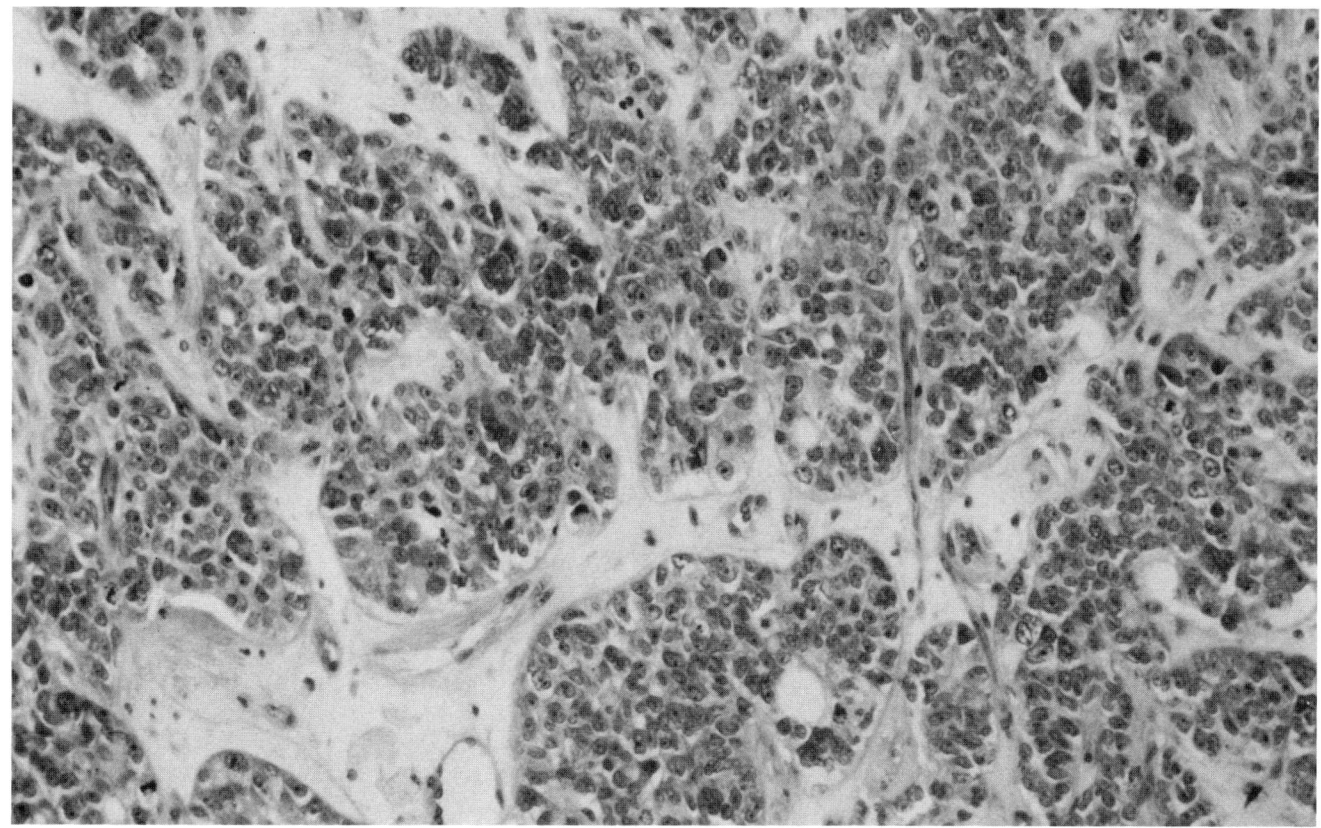

Fig. 18.116. Undifferentiated carcinoma. The tumor is composed of small cells possibly of serous type.

metrioid tumor often is associated with pelvic endometriosis.[37,207–209,219] Regimes of management, although not specifically delineated, would be similar to those outlined for other surface epithelial–stromal tumors of equivalent stage and grade.

Undifferentiated Carcinomas

GENERAL FEATURES

The current WHO definition of undifferentiated carcinoma permits inclusion of tumors with occasional endometrial-like glands, psammoma bodies, and droplets or pools of mucin. However, in my view, this is probably undesirable, and neoplasms placed into the "undifferentiated" category should show no readily identifiable features of any of the müllerian-differentiated tumors described in the preceding sections of this chapter. Only rare tumors, therefore, are truly "poorly differentiated mullerian epithelial malignancies not otherwise classifiable." The concept of "minimal differentiation" is impossible to quantify and precludes any real reproducibility in separating such carcinomas from poorly differentiated serous, endometrioid, or transitional cell carcinomas. This is manifested in the great disparity in their reported frequency of 5–15% of all primary ovarian malignancies.[12,229,241]

The only truly undifferentiated carcinomas are unilateral tumors in young women (and often associated with hypercalcaemia) and the exceedingly rare primary undifferentiated small cell carcinoma (neuroendocrine or "oat cell" carcinoma). The former are not currently regarded as of surface epithelial–stromal type and are discussed in Chapter 19, Sex Cord–Stromal, Steroid Cell, and Other Ovarian Tumors with Endocrine, Paraendocrine, and Paraneoplastic Manifestations. The latter are most probably of endometrioid derivation.

The mean age of patients with undifferentiated carcinomas is 55 years. They are bilateral in 50% of cases and disseminated at laparotomy in more than 80% of cases.[241]

GROSS FINDINGS

No distinctive gross features are present. They are large, mostly solid masses often showing widespread hemorrhage and necrosis (Fig. 18.114). Surface adhesions and rupture of the capsule are often seen. Less commonly they may be partly cystic, usually with hemorrhage into the cysts.

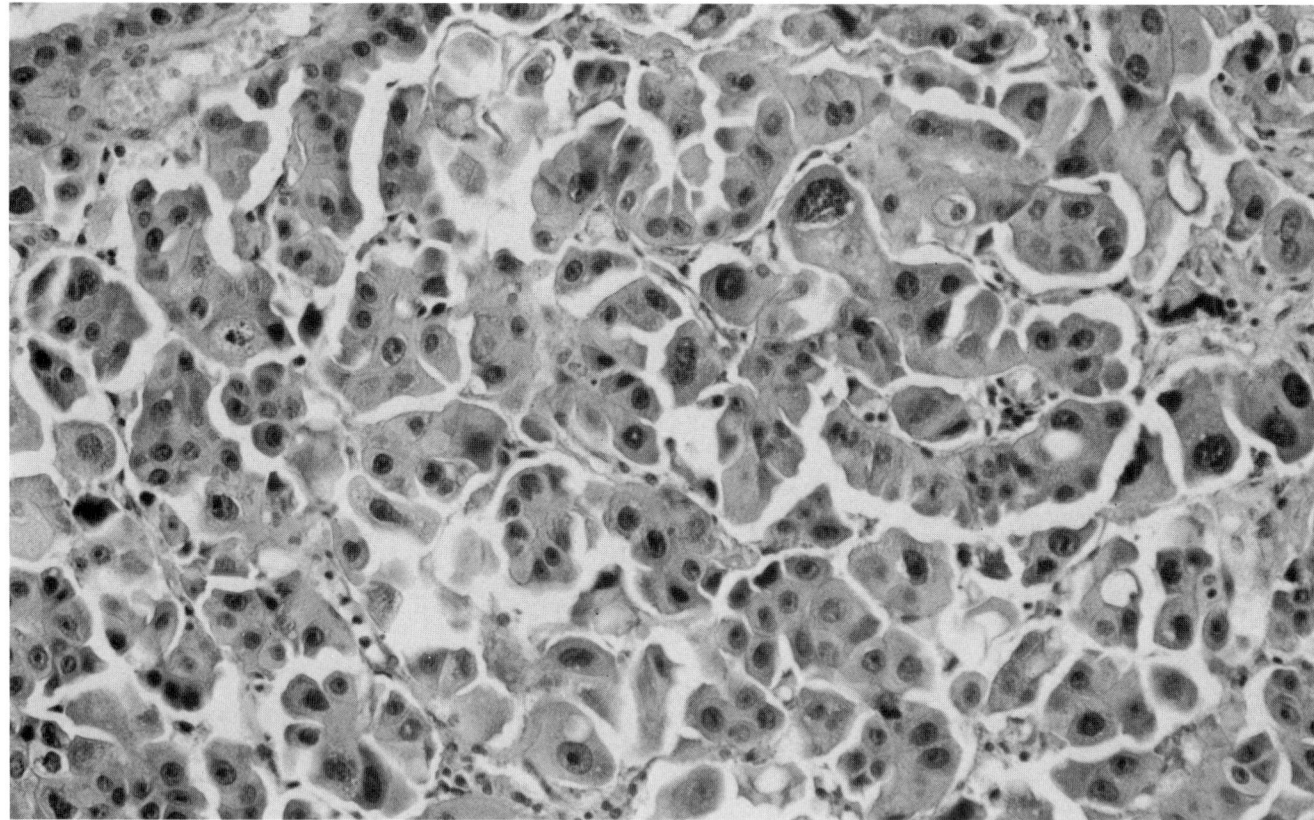

FIG. 18.117. Giant cell undifferentiated carcinoma. Pleomorphic giant cells with eosinophilic cytoplasm, possibly of clear cell type.

MICROSCOPIC FINDINGS

Many morphologic patterns are observed, based on variation in cell size and relative prominence of the stroma. The epithelial nature of the cells is confirmed by the sparseness of the reticulin fibers and immunohistochemical staining for epithelial cell markers (e.g., EMA, cytokeratins, OC-125, or B72.3).

Many such tumors are composed of solid sheets of anaplastic epithelial cells (Fig. 18.115), which may have a vaguely squamoid or transitional appearance. Alternatively, cell size and shape may suggest poorly differentiated serous (Fig. 18.116) or endometrioid carcinomas and it is likely that most undifferentiated carcinomas probably are at the end of one or another of these neoplastic spectra.[63,230] Bizarre eosinophilic mononuclear giant cells are not infrequently encountered in otherwise typical clear cell carcinomas; undifferentiated epithelial malignancies composed predominantly or exclusively of such cells (Fig. 18.117) may well be of clear cell derivation. Nuclear pleomorphism and the absence of coarse cytoplasmic granularity would distinguish these carcinomas from the recently described ovarian oncocytomas (see below).

Other examples have more prominent stroma between nests and cords of undifferentiated carcinoma cells.

Stroma generally is immature but may be quite desmoplastic and often contains a variable inflammatory infiltrate, usually lymphoplasmacytic but occasionally with many eosinophils.

CLINICAL BEHAVIOR AND TREATMENT

Prognosis is poor, with Silva et al.[241] giving a 5-year survival rate of only 11%. Treatment is along lines advocated for other epithelial carcinomas.

Unclassified Epithelial Tumors

The epithelial component of occasional tumors, not necessarily undifferentiated carcinomas, have features insufficiently characteristic to allow classification into one or another of the previously described groups. Tumors with epithelial features intermediate between serous and endometrioid differentiation can be extremely difficult to interpret and such neoplasms account for many examples in this category. This difficulty is present at both ends of the neoplastic spectrum, in adenofibromas with ill-defined epithelial components as well as carcinomas.

So-called ovarian oncocytomas would be placed into this category. The first of two reported cases,[256] occurring in a 39-year-old woman, was morphologically a well-differentiated adenocarcinoma with a papillary pattern of growth. The second tumor,[288] occurring in a 22-year-old woman, had a solid pattern of growth histologically. Both tumors were composed uniformly of typical oncocytes with small, round, uniform vesicular nuclei and abundant eosinophilic granular cytoplasm that ultrastructurally was filled with mitochondria. Neither tumor has pursued a malignant course.

Other rare epithelial tumors of uncertain histogenesis such as the so-called hepatoid carcinomas[120,160] and small cell undifferentiated carcinoma associated with hypercalcaemia[4,78] and tumors of rete[220] or Wolffian origin are discussed in Chapter 19, Sex Cord–Stromal, Steroid Cell, and Other Ovarian Tumors with Endocrine, Paraendocrine, and Paraneoplastic Manifestations.

References

1. Aguirre P, Daval Y, Scully RE, de Lellis RA (1984) Mucinous tumors of the ovary with argyrophil cells. An immunohistochemical analysis. Am J Surg Pathol 8: 345–356
2. Aguirre P, Scully RE, Wolfe HJ, de Lellis RA (1986) Argyrophil cells in Brenner tumors. Histochemical and immunohistochemical analysis. Int J Gynecol Pathol 5: 223–234
3. Aguirre P, Thor AD, Scully RE (1989) Ovarian endometrioid carcinomas resembling sex-cord stromal tumors. An immunohistochemical study. Int J Gynecol Pathol 8: 364–373
4. Aguirre P, Thor AD, Scully RE (1989) Ovarian small cell carcinoma: Histogenetic considerations based on immunohistochemical and other findings. Am J Clin Pathol 92: 140–149
5. Alenghat E, Okagaki T, Talerman A (1986) Primary mucinous carcinoid tumor of the ovary. Cancer 58: 777–783
6. Amazon K, Rywlin AM (1980) Ceroid granulomas in a tubo-ovarian cyst. South Med J 73: 1067–1070
7. Anderson MC (1972) Endometrioid tumor of the ovary with mucinous and serous components. Am J Obstet Gynecol 113: 686–690
8. Anderson MC, Langley FA (1970) Mesonephroid tumours of the ovary. J Clin Pathol 23: 210–218
9. Annegers JF, Malkasian GD (1981) Patterns of other neoplasia in patients with endometrial carcinoma. Cancer 48: 856–859
10. Pettersson F (ed) (1988) Annual Report on Gynecologic Cancer of FIGO, Vol 20. Stockholm, Panorama Press
11. Aslani M, Ahn G-W, Scully RE (1988) Serous papillary cystadenoma of borderline malignancy of broad ligament. A report of 25 cases. Int J Gynecol Pathol 7: 131–138
12. Aure JC, Hoeg K, Kolstad P (1971) Clinical and histologic studies of ovarian carcinoma. Long term follow-up of 990 cases. Obstet Gynecol 37: 1–9
13. Austin RM, Norris HJ (1987) Malignant Brenner tumors and transitional cell carcinoma of the ovary. Int J Gynecol Pathol 6: 29–39

14. Axelrod JH, Fruchter R, Boyce JG (1984) Multiple primaries among gynecologic malignancies. Gynecol Oncol 18: 359–372
15. Axiotis CA (1988) Intratesticular serous papillary cystadenoma of low malignant potential: An ultrastructural and immunohistochemical study suggesting müllerian differentiation. Am J Surg Pathol 12: 56–63
16. Baird DB, Reddick RL (1991) Extraovarian mucinous metaplasia in a patient with bilateral mucinous borderline ovarian tumors: A case report. Int J Gynecol Pathol 10: 96–103
17. Bamforth J, Dempster KR, Garland GW (1956) Brenner tumour of the ovary. A report of 2 cases presenting unusual features. J Obstet Gynaecol Br Emp 63: 344–348
18. Bannatyne PM, Russell P (1981) Early adenocarcinoma of the fallopian tubes. A case for multifocal tumorigenesis. Diagn Gynecol Obstet 3: 49–60
19. Barnhill D, Heller P, Brzozowski P, Advani H, Gallup D, Park R (1985) Epithelial ovarian carcinoma of low malignant potential. Obstet Gynecol 65: 53–59
20. Barua R, Cox LW (1982) Occurrence of bone in serous cystadenocarcinoma of the ovary. Aust NZ J Obstet Gynaecol 22: 183–186
21. Barua R, Richmond D (1988) Trophoblastic differentiation in a malignant mixed mesodermal tumor of the ovary. Hum Pathol 19: 1235–1236
22. Barwick KW, LiVolsi VA (1980) Malignant mixed mesodermal tumors of the ovary. A clinicopathologic assessment of 12 cases. Am J Surg Pathol 4: 37–42
23. Behrens H (1953) Ein Brennertumorahnliches Sarkom des Ovars. Arch Geschwulstforschung 5: 212–215
24. Bell DA (1991) Ovarian surface epithelial-stromal tumors. Hum Pathol 22: 750–762
25. Bell DA (1991) Mucinous adenofibromas of the ovary. A report of 10 cases. Am J Surg Pathol 15: 227–232
26. Bell DA, Scully RE (1985) Benign and borderline clear cell adenofibromas of the ovary. Cancer 56: 2911–2931
27. Bell DA, Scully RE (1985) Atypical and borderline endometrioid adenofibromas of the ovary. Am J Surg Pathol 9: 205–214
28. Bell DA, Scully RE (1989) Benign and borderline serous lesions of the peritoneum in women. Pathol Annu 24(pt 2): 1–21
29. Bell DA, Scully RE (1990) Ovarian serous borderline tumors with stromal microinvasion. A report of 21 cases. Hum Pathol 21: 397–403
30. Bell DA, Scully RE (1990) Serous borderline tumors of the peritoneum. Am J Surg Pathol 14: 230–239
31. Bell DA, Weinstock MA, Scully RE (1988) Peritoneal implants of ovarian serous borderline tumors: Histologic features and prognosis. Cancer 62: 2212–2222
32. Ben-Baruch G, Menashe Y, Herczeg E, Menczer J (1988) Pure primary ovarian squamous cell carcinoma. Gynecol Oncol 29: 257–262
33. Biscotti CV, Hart WR (1992) Peritoneal serous micropapillomatosis of low malignant potential (serous borderline tumors of the peritoneum). Am J Surg Pathol 16: 467–475
34. Black WC, Benitez RE (1964) Nonteratomatous squamous cell carcinoma in-situ of the ovary. Obstet Gynecol 24: 865–868

35. Bosscher J, Barnhill D, O'Connor D, Doering D, Nash J, Park R (1990) Osseous metaplasia in ovarian papillary serous cystadenocarcinoma. Gynecol Oncol 39: 228–231

36. Bostwick DG, Tazelaar HD, Ballon SC, Hendrickson MR, Kempson RL (1986) Ovarian epithelial tumors of borderline malignancy. A clinical and pathologic study of 109 cases. Cancer 58: 2052–2065

37. Brescia RJ, Dubin N, Demopoulos RI (1989) Endometrioid and clear cell carcinoma of the ovary. Factors affecting survival. Int J Gynecol Pathol 8: 132–138

38. Bruijn JA, Smit VTHBM, Que D-Q, Fleuren GJ (1987) Immunohistology of a sarcomatous mural nodule in an ovarian mucinous cystadenocarcinoma. Int J Gynecol Pathol 6: 287–293

39. Bruns DE, Mills SE, Savory J (1982) Amylase in fallopian tube and serous ovarian neoplasms. Immunohistochemical localization. Arch Pathol Lab Med 106: 17–20

40. Burghardt E, Girardi F, Lahousen M, Tamussino K, Stettner H (1991) Patterns of pelvic and paraaortic lymph node involvement in ovarian cancer. Gynecol Oncol 40: 103–106

41. Campbell JS, Lou P, Ferguson JP, Kemeny T, Mitton DM, Allen N (1973) Pseudomyxoma peritonei et ovarii with occult neoplasms of appendix. Obstet Gynecol 42: 897–902

42. Carinelli SG, Senzani FM (1985) Cisti epidermoide dell' ovario. Ann Ostet Ginecol Med Perinatol 106: 43–47

43. Carlson JA Jr, Edwards C, Wharton JT, Gallager HS, Delclos L, Rutledge F (1983) Mixed mesodermal sarcoma of the ovary. Treatment with combination radiation therapy and chemotherapy. Cancer 52: 1473–1477

44. Carter J, Carson LF, Moradi MM, Adcock LA, Twiggs LB (1991) Pseudomyxoma peritonei: A review. Int J Gynecol Cancer 1: 243–247

45. Casper S, van Nagell JR, Powell DF, et al (1984) Immunohistochemical localization of tumor markers in epithelial ovarian cancer. Am J Obstet Gynecol 149: 154–158

46. Chaitin BA, Gershenson DM, Evans HL (1985) Mucinous tumors of the ovary: A clinicopathologic study of 70 cases. Cancer 55: 1958–1962

47. Chambers JT, Merino MJ, Kohorn EJ, Schwartz PE (1988) Borderline ovarian tumors. Am J Obstet Gynecol 159: 1088–1094

48. Chan Y-F, Ho HC, Yau SM, Ma L (1989) Ovarian mucinous tumor with mural nodules of anaplastic carcinoma. Gynecol Oncol 35: 112–119

49. Chandraratnam E, Leong AS-Y (1983) Papillary serous cystadenoma of borderline malignancy arising in a parovarian paramesonephric cyst. Light microscopic and ultrastructural observations. Histopathology 7: 601–611

50. Chang SH, Roberts JM, Homesley HD (1977) Proliferating Brenner tumor. Obstet Gynecol 49: 489–493

51. Chen KTK, Schooley JL, Flam MS (1985) Peritoneal carcinomatosis after prophylactic oophorectomy in familial ovarian cancer syndrome. Obstet Gynecol 66: 93s–94s

52. Chen SS, Lee L (1984) Prognostic significance of morphology of tumor and retroperitoneal lymph nodes in epithelial carcinoma of the ovary. Gynecol Oncol 18: 87–93

53. Chien RT, Rettenmaier MA, Micha JP, di Saia PJ (1989) Ovarian epithelial tumors of low malignant potential. Surg Gynecol Obstet 169: 143–146

54. Choo YC, Naylor B (1982) Multiple primary neoplasms of the ovary and uterus. Int J Gynaecol Obstet 20: 327–334

55. Clement PB, Scully RE (1974) Mullerian adenosarcoma of the uterus. A clinicopathologic analysis of ten cases of a distinctive type of mullerian mixed tumor. Cancer 34: 1138–1149

56. Clement PB, Scully RE (1978) Extrauterine mesodermal (müllerian) adenosarcoma. Am J Clin Pathol 69: 276–283

57. Clement PB, Young RH, Scully RE (1987) Endometrioid-like variant of ovarian yolk sac tumor. A clinicopathological analysis of eight cases. Am J Surg Pathol 11: 767–778

58. Colgan TJ, Norris HJ (1983) Ovarian epithelial tumors of low malignant potential: A review. Int J Gynecol Pathol 2: 367–382

59. Copeland LJ, Gershenson DM, Wharton JT, et al (1985) Microscopic disease at second-look laparotomy in advanced ovarian disease. Cancer 55: 472–478

60. Crozier MA, Copeland LJ, Silva EG, Gershenson DM, Stringer CA (1989) Clear cell carcinoma of the ovary: A study of 59 cases. Gynecol Oncol 35: 199–203

61. Cummins PA, Fox H, Langley FA (1973) An ultrastructural study of the nature and origin of the Brenner tumour of the ovary. J Pathol 110: 167–176

62. Cummins PA, Fox H, Langley FA (1974) An electronmicroscopic study of the endometrioid adenocarcinoma of the ovary and a comparison of its fine structure with that of normal endometrium and of adenocarcinoma of the endometrium. J Pathol 113: 165–173

63. Czernobilsky B (1977) Primary epithelial tumors of the ovary. In Blaustein A (ed) Pathology of the Female Genital Tract, Chapter 24. New York, Springer-Verlag, pp 453–504

64. Czernobilsky B (1985) Common epithelial tumors of the ovary. In: Roth LM, Czernobilsky B (eds) Tumors and Tumorlike Conditions of the Ovary. New York, Churchill Livingstone, pp 11–43

65. Czernobilsky B, Borenstein R, Lancet M (1974) Cystadenofibroma of the ovary. A clinicopathologic study of 34 cases and comparison with serous cystadenoma. Cancer 34: 1971–1981

66. Czernobilsky B, Dgani R, Roth L (1983) Ovarian mucinous cystadenocarcinoma with mural nodule of carcinomatous derivation. A light and electron microscopic study. Cancer 51: 141–148

67. Czernobilsky B, Silverman BB, Enterline HT (1970) Clear-cell carcinoma of the ovary. Cancer 25: 762–772

68. Czernobilsky B, Silverman BB, Mikuta JJ (1970) Endometrioid carcinoma of the ovary. A clinicopathologic study of 75 cases. Cancer 26: 1141–1152

69. Dabbs DJ, Geisinger KR (1988) Common epithelial ovarian tumors. Immunohistochemical intermediate filament profiles. Cancer 62: 368–374

70. Dalrymple JC, Bannatyne P, Russel P, et al (1989) Extraovarian peritoneal serous papillary carcinoma. A clinicopathologic study of 31 cases. Cancer 64: 110–115

71. de Boer WGRM, Ma J, Nayman J (1981) Intestine associated antigens in ovarian tumours: An immunohistological study. Pathology 13: 547–555

72. Decker DG, Mussey ME, Williams TJ, Taylor WF (1973) Grading of gynecological malignancy: Epithelial ovarian

cancer. In: Seventh National Cancer Conference Proceedings, Philadelphia, JB Lippincott, pp 223–231

73. Dehner LP, Norris HJ, Taylor HB (1971) Carcinosarcomas and mixed mesodermal tumors of the ovary. Cancer 27: 207–216

74. Deligdisch L, Plaxe S, Cohen CJ (1988) Extrauterine pelvic malignant mixed mesodermal tumors. A study of 10 cases with immunohistochemistry. Int J Gynecol Pathol 7: 361–372

75. Dembo AJ, Bush RS, Brown TC (1982) Clinicopathological correlates in ovarian cancer. Bull Cancer (Paris) 69: 239–247

76. de Rosa G, Donofrio V, de Rosa N, Fulciniti F, Zeppa P (1991) Ovarian serous tumor with mural nodules of carcinomatous derivation (sarcomatoid carcinoma): Report of a case. Int J Gynecol Pathol 10: 311–318

77. Detre Z, Foldes E (1984) Mucinous cystadenocarcinoma of ovary with Leydig cell hyperplasia. Pathol Res Pract 178: 400–402

78. Dickersin GR, Kline IW, Scully RE (1982) Small cell carcinoma of the ovary with hypercalcemia: A report of eleven cases. Cancer 49: 188–197

79. Dictor M (1985) Malignant mixed mesodermal tumor of the ovary: A report of 22 cases. Obstet Gynecol 65: 720–724

80. Dinh TV, Slavin RE, Bhagavan BS, Hannigan EV, Tiamson EM, Yandell RB (1988) Mixed mesodermal tumors of the ovary. A clinicopathologic study of 14 cases. Obstet Gynecol 72: 409–412

81. Dvoretsky P, Richards K, Angel C, et al (1987) An autopsy study of 100 women with ovarian cancer (abstr). Lab Invest 56: 21a

82. Ehrmann RL, Federschneider JM, Knapp RC (1980) Distinguishing lymph node metastases from benign glandular inclusions in low-grade ovarian carcinoma. Am J Obstet Gynecol 136: 737–746

83. Ehrmann RL, Weidner N, Welch WR, Gleiberman I (1990) Malignant mixed müllerian tumor of the ovary with prominent neuroectodermal differentiation (teratoid carcinosarcoma). Int J Gynecol Pathol 9: 272–282

84. Eifel P, Hendrickson M, Ross J, Ballon S, Martinez A, Kempson R (1982) Simultaneous presentation of carcinoma involving the ovary and the uterine corpus. Cancer 50: 163–170

85. Fenoglio CM, Cottral GA, Ferenczy A, Richart RM (1976) Mucinous tumors of the ovary. III: Histochemical studies. Gynecol Oncol 4: 151–157

86. Fenoglio CM, Ferenczy A, Richart RM (1975) Mucinous tumors of the ovary. Ultrastructural studies of mucinous cystadenomas with histogenetic considerations. Cancer 36: 1709–1722

87. Fenoglio CM, Ferenczy A, Richart RM (1976) Mucinous tumors of the ovary. II: Ultrastructural features of mucinous cystadenocarcinomas. Am J Obstet Gynecol 125: 990–999

88. Ferenczy A, Richart RM (1974) The Female Reproductive System. Dynamics of Scan and Transmission Electron Microscopy. New York, Wiley, pp 287–309

89. Fitzgibbons PL, Martin SE, Simmons TJ (1987) Malignant melanoma metastatic to the ovary. Am J Surg Pathol 11: 959–964

90. Fox H, Langley FA (1976) Tumours of the ovary. London, Heinemann, pp 74–118

91. Fox H, Anderson MC, Beilby JOW, et al (1983) Ovarian epithelial tumours of borderline malignancy: Pathological features and current status. Br J Obstet Gynaecol 90: 743–750

92. Foyle A, Al-Jabi M, McCaughey WTE (1981) Papillary peritoneal tumors in women. Am J Surg Pathol 5: 241–249

93. Friedlander ML, Hedley DW, Taylor IW, Russell P, Coates AS, Tattersall MHN (1984) Influence of cellular DNA content on survival in advanced ovarian cancer. Cancer Res 44: 397–400

94. Fromm G-L, Gershenson DM, Silva EG (1990) Papillary serous carcinoma of the peritoneum. Obstet Gynecol 75: 89–95

95. Fujii S, Konishi I, Kobayashi F, Okamura H, Yamabe H, Mori T (1985) Sarcoma-like mural nodules combined with a microfocus of anaplastic carcinoma in mucinous ovarian tumor. Gynecol Oncol 20: 219–233

96. Gaing AA, Kimble CC, Belmonte AH, Agustin E, Tchertkoff V (1988) Invasive ovarian endometrioid adenofibroma with omental implants and collision with endometrial adenocarcinoma. Obstet Gynecol 71: 440–444

97. Genadry R, Parmley T, Woodruff JD (1979) Simultaneous malignant squamous metaplasia of the cervix and ovary. Gynecol Oncol 8: 87–91

98. Genadry R, Poliakoff S, Rotmensch J, Rosenhein NB, Parmley TH, Woodruff JD (1981) Primary papillary peritoneal neoplasia. Obstet Gynecol 58: 730–734

99. Genton CY (1984) An unusual tumor of the ovary. Pathol Res Pract 179: 110–112

100. Gershenson DM, Silva EG (1990) Serous ovarian tumors of low malignant potential with peritoneal implants. Cancer 65: 578–585

101. Gilks CB, Bell DA, Scully RE (1990) Serous psammocarcinoma of the ovary and peritoneum. Int J Gynecol Pathol 9: 110–121

102. Gondos B (1971) Electron microscopic study of papillary serous tumors of the ovary. Cancer 27: 1455–1464

103. Gooneratne S, Sassone M, Blaustein A, Talerman A (1982) Serous surface papillary carcinoma. A clinicopathologic study of 16 cases. Int J Gynecol Pathol 1: 258–269

104. Hallgrimsson J, Scully RE (1972) Borderline and malignant Brenner tumours of the ovary. A report of 15 cases. Acta Pathol Microbiol Immunol Scand (A) 80 (suppl 233): 56–66

105. Hammond RH, Bates TD, Clarke DG, et al (1991) The immunoperoxidase localisation of tumour markers in ovarian cancer: The value of CEA, EMA, cytokeratin and DD9. Br J Obstet Gynaecol 98: 73–83

106. Harris R, Whittemore AS, Itnyre J (1992) Characteristics relating to ovarian cancer risk: Collaborative analysis of 12 US case-control studies. III: Epithelial tumors of low malignant potential in white women. Am J Epidemiol 136: 1204–1211

107. Hart WR (1977) Ovarian epithelial tumors of borderline malignancy (carcinomas of low malignant potential). Hum Pathol 8: 541–549

108. Hart WR (1981) Pathology of malignant and borderline epithelial tumours of ovary. In: Coppleson M (ed) Gynecologic Oncology, Chapter 49. Edinburgh, Churchill Livingstone, pp 633–654

109. Hart WR, Norris HJ (1973) Borderline and malignant mucinous tumors of the ovary. Cancer 31: 1031–1045

110. Hayden MT (1981) Bilateral malignant Brenner tumor. Report of a case with ultrastructural study. Hum Pathol 12: 89–92

111. Hayes D (1972) Mesonephroid tumours of the ovary. J Obstet Gynaecol Br Commow 79: 728–736

112. Hayman JA, Ostor AG (1985) Ovarian mucinous tumour with a focus of anaplastic carcinoma: A case report. Pathology 17: 591–593

113. Heintz PM, Hacker NF, Lagasse LD (1985) Epidemiology and etiology of ovarian cancer: A review. Obstet Gynecol 66: 127–135

114. Heller DS, Harpaz N, Breakstone B (1990) Neoplasms arising in ectopic ovaries: A case of Brenner tumor in an accessory ovary. Int J Gynecol Pathol 9: 185–189

115. Henriksen E (1975) The lymphatic dissemination in endometrial carcinoma. A study of 188 necropsies. Am J Obstet Gynecol 123: 570–576

116. Higa E, Rosai J, Pizzimbono CA, Wise L (1973) Mucosal hyperplasia, mucinous cystadenoma, and mucinous cystadenocarcinoma of the appendix. Cancer 32: 1525–1541

117. Hughesdon PE (1984) Benign endometrioid tumours of the ovary and the müllerian concept of ovarian epithelial tumours. Histopathology 8: 977–990

118. Hunter V, Barnhill D, Jadwin D, Crooks L (1988) Ovarian mucinous cystadenocarcinoma of low malignant potential associated with a mature cystic teratoma. Gynecol Oncol 29: 250–254

119. Hyman MP (1977) Extraovarian endometrioid carcinoma. Am J Clin Pathol 68: 522–526

120. Ishikura H, Scully E (1987) Hepatoid carcinoma of the ovary. A newly described tumor. Cancer 60: 2775–2784

121. Johnson TL, Kumar NB, Hopkins M, Hughes JD (1988) Cytological features of ovarian tumors of low malignant potential. Acta Cytol 32: 513–518

122. Joshi VV (1968) Primary Krukenberg tumor of the ovary. Review of the literature and a case report. Cancer 22: 1199–1207

123. Kabawat SE, Bast RC, Welch WR, Knapp RC, Colvin RB (1983) Immunopathologic characterization of a monoclonal antibody that recognizes common surface antigens of human ovarian tumors of serous, endometrioid and clear cell types. Am J Clin Pathol 79: 98–104

124. Kahn MA, Demopoulos RI (1992) Mucinous ovarian tumors with pseudomyxoma peritonei: A clinicopathological study. Int J Gynecol Pathol 11: 15–23

125. Kaminski PF, Norris HJ (1984) Coexistence of ovarian neoplasms and endocervical adenocarcinoma. Obstet Gynecol 64: 553–556

126. Kannerstein M, Churg J, McCaughey WTE, Hill DP (1977) Papillary tumors of the peritoneum in women: Mesothelioma or papillary carcinoma. Am J Obstet Gynecol 127: 306–314

127. Kao GF, Norris HJ (1978) Cystadenofibroma of the ovary with epithelial atypism. Am J Surg Pathol 2: 357–363

128. Kao GF, Norris HJ (1978) Benign and low grade variants of mixed mesodermal tumor (adenosarcoma) of the ovary and adnexal region. Cancer 42: 1314–1324

129. Kao GF, Norris HJ (1979) Unusual cystadenofibromas: Endometrioid, mucinous and clear cell types. Obstet Gynecol 54: 729–736

130. Katsube Y, Berg JW, Silverberg SG (1982) Epidemiologic pathology of ovarian tumors. Int J Gynecol Pathol 1: 3–16

131. Katzenstein A-LA, Mazur MT, Morgan TE, Kao M-S (1978) Proliferative serous tumors of the ovary. Histologic features and prognosis. Am J Surg Pathol 2: 339–355

132. Kennedy AW, Biscotti CV, Hart WR, Webster KD (1989) Ovarian clear cell adenocarcinoma. Gynecol Oncol 32: 342–349

133. Kessler E, Halpern M, Koren R, Dekel A, Goldman J (1990) Sarcoma-like mural nodules with foci of anaplastic carcinoma in ovarian mucinous tumor: Clinical, histological, and immunohistochemical study of a case and review of the literature. Surg Pathol 3: 211–219

134. Khalifa MA, Sesterhenn IA (1990) Tumor markers of epithelial ovarian neoplasms. Int J Gynecol Pathol 9: 217–230

135. Klemi PJ (1978) Pathology of mucinous ovarian cystadenomas. I: Argyrophil and argentaffin cells and epithelial mucosubstances. Acta Pathol Microbiol Scand A 86: 465–470

136. Klemi PJ, Gronroos M (1979) Endometrioid carcinoma of the ovary. A clinicopathologic, histochemical and electron microscopic study. Obstet Gynecol 53: 572–579

137. Klemi PJ, Nevalainen TJ (1977) Ultrastructure of the benign and borderline Brenner tumors. Acta Pathol Microbiol Scand (A) 85: 826–835

138. Klemi PJ, Nevalainen TJ (1978) Pathology of mucinous ovarian cystadenomas. II: Ultrastructural findings. Acta Pathol Microbiol Scand A 86: 471–481

139. Klemi PJ, Nevalainen TJ (1978) Ultrastructural and histochemical observations on serous ovarian cystadenomas. Acta Pathol Microbiol Scand A 86: 303–312

140. Klemi PJ, Meurman L, Gronroos M, Talerman A (1982) Clear cell (mesonephroid) tumors of the ovary with characteristics resembling endodermal sinus tumor. Int J Gynecol Pathol 1: 95–100

141. Kliman L, Rome RM, Fortune DW (1986) Low malignant potential tumors of the ovary: A study of 76 cases. Obstet Gynecol 68: 338–344

142. Kline RC, Wharton JT, Atkinson EN, Burke TW, Gershenson DM, Edwards CL (1990) Endometrioid carcinoma of the ovary: Retrospective review of 145 cases. Gynecol Oncol 39: 337–346

143. Koonings PP, Campbell AC, Mishell DR, Grimes DA (1989) Relative frequency of primary ovarian neoplasms: A 10-year review. Obstet Gynecol 74: 921–926

144. Kuhnel R, Rao BR, Stolk JG, van Kessel H, Seldenrijk CA, Willig AP (1987) Estrogen synthesizing rare malignant Brenner tumor of the ovary with the presence of progesterone and androgen receptors in the absence of estrogen receptors. Gynecol Oncol 26: 263–269

145. Kunze E, Schauer A, Schmitt M (1983) Histology and histogenesis of two different types of inverted urothelial papillomas. Cancer 51: 348–358

146. Kurman RJ, Trimble CL (1993) The behavior of serous tumors of low malignant potential: Are they ever malignant? Int J Gynecol Pathol 12: 120–127

147. Langley FA, Cummins PA, Fox H (1972) An ultrastructural study of mucin secreting epithelia in ovarian neoplasms. Acta Pathol Microbiol Scand A 80 (suppl 233): 76–86

148. Lash RH, Hart WR (1987) Intestinal adenocarcinomas met-

astatic to the ovaries. A clinicopathologic evaluation of 22 cases. Am J Surg Pathol 11: 114–121

149. Lauchlan SC (1990) Non-invasive ovarian carcinoma. Int J Gynecol Pathol 9: 158–169

150. Lele SB, Piver MS, Matharu J, Tsukada Y (1988) Peritoneal papillary carcinoma. Gynecol Oncol 31: 315–320

151. Lifschitz-Mercer B, Czernobilsky B, Shezen E, Dgani R, Leitner O, Geiger B (1988) Selective expression of cytokeratin polypeptides in various epithelia of human Brenner tumor. Hum Pathol 19: 640–650

152. Lim-Tam S, Cajigas HE, Scully RE (1988) Ovarian cystectomy for serous borderline tumors: A follow-up study of 35 cass. Obstet Gynecol 72: 775–780

153. Louwerens JK, Schaberg A, Bosman FT (1983) Neuroendocrine cells in cystic mucinous tumors of the ovary. Histopathology 7: 389–398

154. McCaughey WTE, Kirk ME, Lester W, Dardick I (1984) Peritoneal epithelial lesions associated with proliferative serous tumours of ovary. Histopathology 8: 195–208

155. McCaughey WTE, Schryer MJP, Lin X-S, Al-Jabi M (1986) Extraovarian pelvic serous tumor with marked calcification. Arch Pathol Lab Med 110: 78–80

156. McCullough K, Froats E, Falk H (1946) Epidermoid cyst arising in an endometrial cyst of the ovary. Arch Pathol 41: 335–337

157. McKenna H, Ansford A (1976) Malignant Brenner tumour. Aust NZ J Obstet Gynaecol 16: 244–248

158. Macko MB, Johnson LA (1983) Primary squamous ovarian carcinoma. A case report and review of the literature. Cancer 52: 1117–1119

159. Massad LS Jr, Hunter VJ, Szpak CA, Clarke-Pearson DL, Creasman WT (1991) Epithelial ovarian tumors of low malignant potential. Obstet Gynecol 78: 1027–1032

160. Matsuta M, Ishikura H, Murakami K, Kagabu T, Nishiya I (1991) Hepatoid carcinoma of the ovary: A case report. Int J Gynecol Pathol 10: 302–310

161. Mazur MT, Hsueh S, Gersell DJ (1984) Metastases to the female genital tract: Analysis of 325 cases. Cancer 53: 1978–1984

162. Michael H, Roth LM (1986) Invasive and non-invasive implants in ovarian serous tumors of low malignant potential. Cancer 57: 1240–1247

163. Miles PA, Norris HJ (1972) Proliferative and malignant Brenner tumors of the ovary. Cancer 30: 174–186

164. Mills SE, Anderson WA, Fechner RE, Austin MB (1988) Serous surface papillary carcinoma. A clinicopathologic study of 10 cases and comparison with Stage III–IV ovarian serous carcinoma. Am J Surg Pathol 12: 827–834

165. Moll R, Pitz S, Levy R, Weikel W, Franke WW, Czernobilsky B (1991) Complexity of expression of intermediate filament proteins, including glial filament protein, in endometrial and ovarian adenocarcinoma. Hum Pathol 22: 989–1001

166. Montag AG, Jenison EL, Griffiths CT, Welch WR, Lavin PT, Knapp RC (1989) Ovarian clear cell carcinoma: A clinicopathologic analysis of 44 cases. Int J Gynecol Pathol 8: 85–96

167. More JRS (1967) Epidermoid cyst of the ovary. Gynaecol Invest 164: 240–248

168. Morris HB, La Vecchia C, Draper GJ (1984) Malignant epithelial tumors of the ovary in childhood: A clinicopathological study of 13 cases in Great Britain 1962–1978. Gynecol Oncol 19: 290–297

169. Morrow CP (1981) Malignant and borderline epithelial tumors of ovary: Clinical features, staging, diagnosis, intraoperative assessment and review of management. In: Coppleson M (ed) Gynecologic Oncology, Chapter 50. Edinburgh, Churchill Livingstone, pp 655–679

170. Morrow CP, d'Ablaing G, Brady LW, Blessing JA, Hreshchyshyn MM (1984) A clinical and pathologic study of 30 cases of malignant mixed mullerian epithelial and mesenchymal ovarian tumors: A Gynecologic Oncology Group study. Gynecol Oncol 18: 278–292

171. Mostoufizadeh M, Scully RE (1980) Malignant tumors arising in endometriosis. Clin Obstet Gynecol 23: 951–963

172. Mukai K, Varela-Duran J, Nochomovitz LE (1980) The rhabdomyoblast in mixed mullerian tumors of the uterus and ovary: An immunohistochemical study of myoglobin in 25 cases. Am J Clin Pathol 74: 101–104

173. Nation JG, Krepart GV (1986) Ovarian carcinomas of low malignant potential: Staging and treatment. Am J Obstet Gynecol 154: 290–293

174. Nichols GE, Mills SE, Ulbright TM, Czernobilsky B, Roth LM (1991) Spindle cell mural nodules in cystic ovarian mucinous tumors. A clinicopathologic and immunohistochemical study of five cases. Am J Surg Pathol 15: 1055–1062

175. Nikrui N (1981) Survey of clinical behaviour of patients with borderline epithelial tumors of the ovary. Gynecol Oncol 12: 107–119

176. Nogales FF Jr, Silverberg SG (1976) Epidermoid cysts of the ovary. A report of five cases with histogenetic and ultrastructural findings. Obstet Gynecol 124: 523–528

177. Norris HJ (1993) Proliferative endometrioid tumors and endometrioid tumors of low malignant potential. Int J Gynecol Pathol 12: 134–140

178. Norris HJ, Robinowitz (1971) Ovarian adenocarcinoma of mesonephric type. Cancer 28: 1074–1081

179. Okagaki T, Richart RM (1970) Mesonephroma ovarii (hypernephroid carcinoma). Light microscopic and ultrastructural study of a case. Cancer 26: 453–461

180. Osborn LC (1973) Pseudomyxoma peritonei. Report of seven cases. Gynecol Oncol 1: 195–202

181. Ortega I, Nogales F, Gonzalez-Campora R, Matilla A, Galera H (1982) Extragenital endometrioid cystadenofibroma. Acta Obstet Gynecol Scand 61: 283–284

182. Pant KD, Fenoglio-Preiser CM, Berry COA, et al (1986) COTA (colon-ovarian tumor antigen). An immunohistochemical study. Am J Clin Pathol 86: 1–9

183. Parker RT, Currie JL (1981) Metastatic tumors of the ovary. In: Coppleson M (ed) Gynecologic Oncology. Edinburgh, Churchill Livingstone, pp 731–742

184. Parmley TH, Woodruff JD (1974) The ovarian mesothelioma. Am J Obstet Gynecol 120: 234–241

185. Pascal RR, Grecco LA (1988) Mucinous cystadenoma of the ovary with stromal luteinisation and hilar cell hyperplasia during pregnancy. Hum Pathol 19: 179–180

186. Pfeiffer P, Hardt-Madsen M, Rex S, Holund B, Bertelsen K (1991) Malignant mixed mullerian tumors of the ovary: Report of 13 cases. Acta Obstet Gynecol Scand 70: 79–84

187. Podratz KC, Malkasian GD, Hilton JF, Harris EA, Gaffey TA (1985) Second-look laparotomy in ovarian cancer: Evaluation of pathologic variables. Am J Obstet Gynecol 152: 230–238

188. Prat J, Scully RE (1979) Ovarian mucinous tumors with sarcoma-like mural nodules. A report of seven cases. Cancer 44: 1332–1344

189. Prat J, Scully RE (1979) Sarcomas in ovarian mucinous tumors. A report of two cases. Cancer 44: 1321–1325

190. Prat J, Young RH, Scully RE (1982) Ovarian mucinous tumor with foci of anaplastic carcinoma. Cancer 50: 300–304

191. Pratt-Thomas HR, Kreutner A Jr, Underwood PB, Dowdeswell RH (1976) Proliferative and malignant Brenner tumors of the ovary. Report of 2 cases, one with Meig's syndrome, review of the literature and ultrastructural comparisons. Gynecol Oncol 4: 176–193

192. Pretorius RG, Lee KR, Papillo J, Baker S, Belinson J (1986) False-negative peritoneal cytology in metastatic ovarian carcinoma. Obstet Gynecol 68: 619–623

193. Price A, Russell P, Elliott P, Bannatyne P (1990) Composite mucinous and granulosa cell tumor of ovary: Case report of a unique neoplasm. Int J Gynecol Pathol 9: 372–378

194. Ransom DT, Patel SR, Keeney GL, Malkasian GD, Edmondson JH (1990) Papillary serous carcinoma of the peritoneum. A review of 33 cases treated with platin-based chemotherapy. Cancer 66: 1091–1094

195. Robey SS, Silva EG, Gershenson DM, McLemore D, El-Naggar A, Ordonez N G (1989) Transitional cell carcinoma in high-grade high stage ovarian carcinoma. An indication of favourable response to chemotherapy. Cancer 63: 839–847

196. Rodenburg CJ, Cornelisse CJ, Heintz PAM, Hermans J, Fleuren GJ (1987) Tumor ploidy as a prognostic factor in advanced ovarian cancer. Cancer 59: 317–323

197. Rogers LW, Julian CG, Woodruff JD (1972) Mesonephroid carcinoma of the ovary. A study of 95 cases from the Emil Novak Tumor Registry. Gynecol Oncol 1: 76–89

198. Rojansky N, Ophir E, Sharony A, Spira H, Suprun H (1985) Broad ligament adenocarcinoma—its origin and clinical behavior. A literature review and report of a case. Obstet Gynecol Surv 40: 665–671

199. Roth LM, Czernobilsky B (1985) Ovarian Brenner tumors. II: Malignant. Cancer 56: 592–601

200. Roth LM, Sternberg WH (1971) Proliferating Brenner tumors. Cancer 27: 687–693

201. Roth LM, Dallenbach-Hellweg G, Czernobilsky B (1985) Ovarian Brenner tumors. I: Metaplastic, proliferating and of low malignant potential. Cancer 56: 582–591

202. Roth LM, Cleary RE, Rosenfield RL (1974) Sertoli–Leydig cell tumor of the ovary, with an associated mucinous cystadenoma: An ultrastructural and endocrine study. Lab Invest 31: 648–657

203. Roth LM, Czernobilsky B, Langley FA (1981) Ovarian endometrioid adenofibromatous and cystadenofibromatous tumors: Benign, proliferating and malignant. Cancer 48: 1838–1845

204. Roth LM, Gershell DJ, Ulbright TM (1993) Ovarian Brenner tumors and transitional cell carcinoma: Recent developments. Int J Gynecol Pathol 12: 128–133

205. Roth LM, Langley FA, Fox H, Wheeler JE, Czernobilsky B (1984) Ovarian clear cell adenofibromatous tumors: Benign, of low malignant potential, and associated with invasive clear cell carcinoma. Cancer 53: 1156–1163

206. Roth LM, Liban E, Czernobilsky B (1982) Ovarian endometrioid tumors mimicking Sertoli and Sertoli–Leydig cell tumors. Sertoliform variant of endometrioid carcinoma. Cancer 50: 1322–1331

207. Russell P (1979) The pathological assessment of ovarian neoplasms. I: Introduction to the common "epithelial" tumours and analysis of benign "epithelial" tumours. Pathology 11: 5–26

208. Russell P (1979) The pathological assessment of ovarian neoplasms. II: The proliferating "epithelial" tumours. Pathology 11: 251–282

209. Russell P (1979) The pathological assessment of ovarian neoplasms. III: The malignant "epithelial" tumours. Pathology 11: 493–532

210. Russell P (1984) Borderline epithelial tumours of the ovary: A conceptual dilemma. Clin Obstet Gynaecol 11: 259–277

211. Russell P (1992) Ovarian epithelial tumours with atypical proliferation. In: Lowe D, Fox H (eds) Advances in Gynaecological Pathology. Edinburgh, Churchill Livingstone, pp 299–320

212. Russell P, Bannatyne PM (1989) Surgical Pathology of the Ovaries. Edinburgh, Churchill Livingstone, pp 189–314

213. Russell P, Merkur (1979) Proliferating ovarian "epithelial" tumours: A clinicopathological analysis of 144 cases. Aust NZ J Obstet Gynaecol 19: 45–51

214. Russell P, Bannatyne PM, Solomon HJ, Stoddard LD, Tattersall MHN (1985) Multifocal tumorigenesis in the upper female genital tract—implications for staging and management. Int J Gynecol Pathol 4: 192–210

215. Russell P, Slavutin L, Laverty CR, Cooper-Booth J (1979) Extrauterine mesodermal (Müllerian) adenosarcoma. A case report. Pathology 11: 557–560

216. Russell P, Wills EJ, Schweitzer P, Bannatyne PM (1981) Mucinous ovarian tumors with giant cell mural nodules. Diagn Gynecol Obstet 3: 233–249

217. Rutgers JL, Scully RE (1986) Functioning ovarian tumors with peripheral steroid cell proliferation: A report of twenty-four cases. Int J Gynecol Pathol 5: 319–337

218. Rutgers JL, Scully RE (1988) Ovarian mullerian mucinous papillary cystadenomas of borderline malignancy. A clinicopathologic analysis. Cancer 61: 340–348

219. Rutgers JL, Scully RE (1988) Ovarian mixed-epithelial papillary cystadenomas of borderline malignancy. A clinicopathologic analysis. Cancer 61: 546–554

220. Rutgers JL, Scully RE (1988) Cysts (cystadenomas) and tumors of the rete ovarii. Int J Gynecol Pathol 7: 330–342

221. Rutledge ML, Silva EG, McLemore D, El-Naggar A (1989) Surface serous carcinoma of the ovary and peritoneum. A flow cytometric study. Pathol Annu 24 (part 2): 227–236

222. Rybak BJ, Ober WB, Bernacki EG (1981) Malignant Brenner tumor of the ovary. Diagn Gynecol Obstet 3: 61–74

223. Sandenbergh HA, Woodruff JD (1977) Histogenesis of pseudomyxoma peritonei. Review of nine cases. Obstet Gynecol 49: 339–345

224. Santini P, Gelli MC, Mazzoleni G, et al Brenner tumor of the ovary: A correlative histologic, histochemical, immunohistochemical and ultrastructural investigation. Hum Pathol 20: 787–795

225. Sasaki E, Sasano N, Kimura N, Andoh N, Yajima A (1989) Demonstration of neuroendocrine cells in ovarian mucinous tumors. Int J Gynecol Pathol 8: 189–200

226. Schiller W, Rilke F, Degna AT (1957) Parvilocular ovarian cystomas. Obstet Gynecol 10: 28–33

227. Schneider J, Gonzalez-Rodilla I, Eizaguirre MJ, Garcia-Satue E (1985) Complete psammomatous degeneration of the ovary. Case report. Br J Obstet Gynaecol 92: 419–422

228. Schwartz PE, Merino MJ, LiVolsi VA, Lawrence R, MacLusky N, Eisenfeld A (1985) Histopathologic correlations of estrogen and progestin receptor protein in epithelial ovarian carcinomas. Obstet Gynecol 66: 428–433

229. Scully RE (1977) Ovarian tumors. A review. Am J Pathol 87: 686–720

230. Scully RE (1979) Tumors of the ovary and maldeveloped gonads (AFIP Fascicle 16, Second Series). Armed Forces Institute of Pathology, Washington, D.C., pp 53–151

231. Scully RE (1982) Common epithelial tumors of borderline malignancy (carcinomas of low malignant potential). Bull Cancer (Paris) 69: 228–238

232. Scully RE, Richardson GS, Barlow JF (1966) The development of malignancy in endometriosis. Clin Obstet Gynecol 9: 384–411

233. Segal GH, Hart WR (1992) Ovarian serous tumors of low malignant potential (serous borderline tumors). The relationship of exophytic surface tumor to peritoneal "implants." Am J Surg Pathol 16: 577–581

234. Seldenrijk CA, Willig AP, Baak JPA, et al (1986) Malignant Brenner tumor: A histologic, morphometrical, immunohistochemical and ultrastructural study. Cancer 58: 754–760

235. Seidman JD, Elsayad AM, Sobin LH, Tavassoli FA (1993) Association of mucinous tumors of the ovary and appendix. Am J Surg Pathol 17: 22–34

236. Serov SF, Scully RE, Sobin LH (1973) Histological typing of ovarian tumours (International histological classification of tumours No. 9). World Health Organization, Geneva, pp 17–54

237. Shakfeh SM, Woodruff JD (1987) Primary ovarian sarcomas: Report of 46 cases and review of the literature. Obstet Gynecol Surv 42: 331–349

238. Shevchuk MM, Winkler-Monsanto B, Fenoglio CM, Richart RM (1981) Clear cell carcinoma of the ovary: A clinicopathologic study with review of the literature. Cancer 47: 1344–1351

239. Shingleton HM, Middleton FF, Gore H (1974) Squamous cell carcinoma of the ovary. Am J Obstet Gynecol 120: 556–560

240. Silva EG, Robey-Cafferty SS, Smith TL, Gershenson DM (1990) Ovarian carcinomas with transitional cell carcinoma patterns. Am J Clin Pathol 93: 457–465

241. Silva EG, Tornos C, Bailey MA, Morris M (1991) Undifferentiated carcinoma of the ovary. Arch Pathol Lab Med 115: 377–381

242. Silverberg SG (1971) Brenner tumor of the ovary. A clinicopathologic study of 60 tumors in 54 women. Cancer 28: 588–596

243. Silverberg SG, Fernandez FN (1981) Endolymphatic stromal myosis of the ovary. A report of three cases and literature review. Gynecol Oncol 12: 129–138

244. Silverberg SG, Wilson MA (1972) Ultrastructure of the Brenner tumor. Am J Obstet Gynecol 112: 91–100

245. Smith LH, Oi RH (1984) Detection of malignant ovarian neoplasms: A review of the literature. I. Detection of the patient at risk: Clinical, radiological and cytological detection. Obstet Gynecol Surv 39: 313–328

246. Snider DD, Stuart GCE, Nation JG, Robertson DI (1991) Evaluation of surgical staging in Stage 1 low malignant potential ovarian tumors. Gynecol Oncol 40: 129–132

247. Snyder RR, Norris HJ, Tavassoli F (1988) Endometrioid proliferative and low malignant potential tumors of the ovary. A clinicopathologic study of 46 cases. Am J Surg Pathol 12: 661–671

248. Sondergaard G, Kaspersen P (1991) Ovarian and extraovarian mucinous tumors with solid mural nodules. Int J Gynecol Pathol 10: 145–155

249. Sorbe B, Frankendal B, Veress B (1982) Importance of histologic grading in the prognosis of epithelial ovarian carcinoma. Obstet Gynecol 59: 576–582

250. Spaun E, Toft B (1986) Epithelial atypia in ovarian mucinous cystadenoma during the puerperium. Acta Obstet Gynecol Scand 65: 505–506

251. Stenback F, Kauppila A (1981) Endometrioid ovarian tumors: Morphology and relation to other endometrial lesions. Gynecol Obstet Invest 12: 57–70

252. Sumithran E, Susil BJ, Looi L-M (1988) The prognostic significance of grading in borderline mucinous tumors of the ovary. Hum Pathol 19: 15–18

253. Suurmeijer AJH (1991) Carcinosarcoma-like mural nodule in an ovarian mucinous tumour. Histopathology 18: 268–271

254. Svenes KB, Eide J (1984) Proliferative Brenner tumor or ovarian metastases? A case report. Cancer 53: 2692–2697

255. Szymanska K, Szamborski J, Miechowiecka N, Czerwinski W (1983) Malignant transformation of mucinous ovarian cystadenomas of intestinal type. Histopathology 7: 497–509

256. Takeda A, Matsuyama M, Sugimoto Y, et al (1983) Oncocytic adenocarcinoma of the ovary. Virch Arch A 399: 345–353

257. Tasker M, Langley FA (1985) The outlook for women with borderline epithelial tumours of the ovary. Br J Obstet Gynaecol 92: 969–973

258. Tattersall MHN (1981) Pharmacology and selection of cytotoxic drugs. In: Coppleson M (ed) Gynecologic Oncology, Chapter 9, Edinburgh, Churchill Livingstone, pp 121–138

259. Tavassoli FA (1988) Serous tumor of low malignant potential with early stromal invasion (serous LMP with microinvasion). Mod Pathol 1: 407–414

260. Taylor HC Jr (1929) Malignant and semimalignant tumors of the ovary. Surg Gynecol Obstet 48: 204–230

261. Taylor HC Jr (1959) Studies in the clinical and biological evolution of adenocarcinoma of the ovary. J Obstet Gynaecol Br Commonw 66: 827–842

262. Tetu B, Silva EG, Gershenson DM (1987) Squamous cell carcinoma of the ovary. Arch Pathol Lab Med 111: 864–866

263. Tidy J, Mason WP (1988) Endometrioid carcinoma of the ovary: A retrospective study. Br J Obstet Gynaecol 95: 1165–1169

264. Tobacman JK, Greene MH, Tucker MA, Costa J, Kase R, Fraumeni JF Jr (1982) Intra-abdominal carcinomatosis after prophylactic oophorectomy in ovarian cancer-prone families. Lancet 2: 795–797

265. Truong LD, Maccato ML, Awalt H, Cagle PT, Schwartz MR, Kaplan AL (1990) Serous surface carcinoma of the

peritoneum. A clinicopathologic study of 22 cases. Hum Pathol 21: 99–110

266. Tsujimura T, Kawano K (1992) Rhabdomyosarcoma coexistent with ovarian mucinous cystadenocarcinoma: A case report. Int J Gynecol Pathol 11: 58–62

267. Tyler CW Jr, Lee NC, Robboy SJ, et al (1991) The diagnosis of ovarian cancer by pathologists: How often do diagnoses by contributing pathologists agree with a panel of gynecologic pathologiss? Am J Obstet Gynecol 164: 65–70

268. Ueda G, Yamasaki M, Inoue M, et al (1984) Argyrophil cells in the endometrioid carcinoma of the ovary. Cancer 54: 1569–1573

269. Ulbright TM, Roth LM (1985) Metastatic and independent cancers of the endometrium and ovary. A clinicopathologic study of 34 cases. Hum Pathol 16: 28–34

270. Ulbright TM, Roth LM (1985) Common epithelial tumors of the ovary: Proliferating and of low malignant potential. Semin Diagn Pathol 2: 2–15

271. Ulbright TM, Mosley DJ, Roth LM, Berkow RL (1983) Papillary serous carcinoma of the retroperitoneum. Am J Clin Pathol 79: 633–637

272. Ulbright TM, Roth LM, Sutton GP (1990) Papillary serous carcinoma of the ovary with squamous differentiation. Int J Gynecol Pathol 9: 86–94

273. van Kley H, Cramer S, Bruns DE (1981) Serous ovarian neoplastic amylase (SONA): A potentially useful marker for serous ovarian tumours. Cancer 48: 1444–1449

274. Waxman M, Damjanov I, Alpert L, Sardinsky T (1981) Composite mucinous ovarian neoplasms associated with Sertoli-Leydig and carcinoid tumors. Cancer 47: 2044–2052

275. Wheeler DA, Turkel SB, Pettross CW (1984) Ovarian hilar epidermoid cysts. Case reports. Br J Obstet Gynaecol 91: 819–820

276. White PF, Merino MJ, Barwick KW (1985) Serous surface papillary carcinoma of the ovary: A clinical, pathologic, ultrastructural, and immunohistochemical study of 11 cases. Pathol Annu 20: 403–418

277. Whittemore AS, Harris R, Itnyre J, Halpern J (1992) Characteristics relating to ovarian cancer risk: Collaborative analysis of 12 US case-control studies. I: Methods. Am J Epidemiol 136: 1175–1183

278. Whittemore AS, Harris R, Intyre J (1992) Characteristics relating to ovarian cancer risk: Collaborative analysis of 12 US case-control studies. II: Invasive epithelial ovarian cancer in white women. Am J Epidemiol 136: 1184–1203

279. Whittemore AS, Harris R, Intyre J (1992) Characteristics relating to ovarian cancer risk: Collaborative analysis of 12 US case-control studies. IV: The pathogenesis of epithelial ovarian cancer. Am J Epidemiol 136: 1212–1220

280. Wick MR, Mills SE, Dehner LP, Bollinger DJ, Fechner RE (1989) Serous papillary carcinomas arising from the peritoneum and ovaries. A clinicopathologic and immunohistochemical comparison. Int J Gynecol Pathol 8: 179–188

281. Wolpert HR, Fuller AF, Bell DA (1989) Primary mucinous carcinoid tumor of the ovary. A case report. Int J Gynecol Pathol 8: 156–162

282. Woodruff JD (1981) Proliferating and malignant Brenner tumors. Review of 47 cases. Am J Obstet Gynecol 141: 118–125

283. Woodruff JD, Dietrich D, Genadry R, Parmley TH (1981)

Proliferative and malignant Brenner tumors. Review of 47 cases. Am J Obstet Gynecol 141: 118–125

284. Woodruff JD, Solomon D, Sullivant H (1985) Multifocal disease in the upper genital tract. Obstet Gynecol 65: 695–698

285. Yamana K, Kinoshita T, Nakano R, Morimatsu M, Nakashima T (1984) Anaplastic giant cell tumor with mucinous cystadenocarcinoma of the ovary. Acta Pathol Jpn 34: 399–402

286. Yetman TJ, Dudzinski MR (1989) Primary squamous carcinoma of the ovary: A case report and review of the literature. Gynecol Oncol 34: 240–243

287. Yoonessi M, Crickard K, Celik C, Yoonessi S (1988) Borderline epithelial tumors of the ovary. Ovarian intraepithelial neoplasia. Obstet Gynecol Surv 43: 435–444

288. Yoshida Y, Tenzaki T, Ishiguro T, Kawanami D, Ohshima M (1984) Oncocytoma of the ovary: Light and electron microscopic study. Gynecol Oncol 18: 109–114

289. Young RH, Scully RE (1986) Testicular and paratesticular tumors and tumor-like lesions of ovarian common epithelial and Mullerian types. A report of four cases and review of the literature. Am J Clin Pathol 86: 146–152

290. Young RH, Scully RE (1987) Oxyphilic clear cell carcinoma of the ovary. Report of nine cases. Am J Surg Pathol 11: 661–667

291. Young RH, Scully RE (1988) Mucinous ovarian tumors associated with mucinous adenocarcinomas of the cervix. A clinicopathological analysis of 16 cases. Int J Gynecol Pathol 7: 99–111

292. Young RH, Scully RE (1988) Urothelial and ovarian carcinomas of identical cell types: Problems in interpretation. A report of three cases and review of the literature. Int J Gynecol Pathol 7: 197–211

293. Young RH, Scully RE (1991) Malignant melanoma metastatic to the ovary. A clinicopathologic analysis of 20 cases. Am J Surg Pathol 15: 849–860

294. Young RH, Gilks CB, Scully RE (1991) Mucinous tumors of the appendix associated with mucinous tumors of the ovary and pseudomyxoma peritonei. A clinicopathological analysis of 22 cases supporting an origin in the appendix. Am J Surg Pathol 15: 415–429

295. Young RH, Prat J, Scully RE (1980) Epidermoid cysts of the ovary. A report of three cases with comments on histogenesis. Am J Clin Pathol 73: 272–276

296. Young RH, Prat J, Scully RE (1982) Ovarian endometrioid carcinomas resembling sex cord-stromal tumors. A clinicopathological analysis of 13 cases. Am J Surg Pathol 6: 513–522

297. Young RH, Prat J, Scully RE (1984) Endometrioid stromal sarcomas of the ovary. A clinicopathologic analysis of 23 cases. Cancer 53: 1143–1155

298. Zaino RJ, Unger ER, Whitney C (1984) Synchronous carcinomas of the uterine corpus and ovary. Gynecol Oncol 19: 329–335

299. Zaloudek C, Kurman RJ (1983) Recent advances in the pathology of ovarian cancer. Clin Obstet Gynaecol 10: 155–185

300. Zinsser KR, Wheeler JE (1982) Endosalpingiosis in the omentum. A study of autopsy and surgical material. Am J Surg Pathol 6: 109–116

19

Sex Cord–Stromal, Steroid Cell, and Other Ovarian Tumors with Endocrine, Paraendocrine, and Paraneoplastic Manifestations

Robert H. Young, M.D., F.R.C. Path., and Robert E. Scully, M.D.

Sex Cord–Stromal Tumors

This category of ovarian neoplasms includes all those that contain granulosa cells, theca cells, and their luteinized derivatives; Sertoli cells; Leydig cells; and fibroblasts of gonadal stromal origin, singly or in various combinations and in varying degrees of differentiation.[364,369,462,466,467,468] The generic terms that have been applied most widely to these tumors reflect differing views of gonadal embryology. Those who believe that all the above cell types are derived from the mesenchyme or "specialized stroma" of the genital ridge have proposed the terms "mesenchymomas"[68] and "gonadal stromal tumors" for these neoplasms.[301,305] In contrast, others, recognizing that many embryologists favor the participation of coelomic and mesonephric epithelium in the formation of the sex cords, which are the proximal precursors of granulosa cells and Sertoli cells, favor the terms *sex cord–mesenchyme tumors*[286,366] and *sex cord–stromal tumors*.[378]

In the developing testis the sex cords are clearly distinguishable by the fifth week of embryonic life as slender columns of primitive Sertoli cells, but similar cords, at least in the sense of thin columns, are not encountered in the developing ovary; instead, packets of small pregranulosa cells enveloping germ cells become evident later in embryonic life. For that reason, the term "sex cords" has been criticized as inaccurate to describe the progenitors of granulosa cells. Nevertheless, the long-established usage of this designation by embryologists and the lack of a better term justify its retention. The term *sex cord–stromal tumors*, which has been adopted by the World Health Organization (WHO),[378] has the advantage of acknowledging the presence of neoplasms in this general category of derivatives of either or both the sex cords and the stroma. The components derived from the sex cords (granulosa and Sertoli cells) typically are arranged in epithelial configurations, whereas those derived from the stroma have the appearance of cellular gonadal stroma or its specialized derivatives, the theca and Leydig cells.

Most sex cord–stromal tumors (granulosa–stromal cell tumors) are composed of ovarian cell types but some (Sertoli–stromal cell tumors) contain cells of only testicular type; occasionally cells and patterns of growth characteristic of both gonads are present in single tumors (gynandroblastomas). When the neoplastic cells are immature and their appearance is intermediate between those of testicular and ovarian cell types, or when the architectural patterns of the tumor are not specific for either the testis or ovary, it may be impossible to determine whether the tumor belongs in the granulosa–stromal or Sertoli–stromal cell category; in such cases the term *sex cord–stromal tumor, unclassified* is used. The classification of sex cord–stromal tumors used in this chapter is essentially similar that of the WHO (Table 19.1).

Sex cord–stromal tumors account for approximately 8% of all ovarian tumors,[41,155,222,451] with fibromas, which are not associated with endocrine manifestations, accounting for approximately half the cases. Most of the other tumors in this category are granulosa cell tumors, which are neoplasms of a low grade of malignancy.[47–49,145,301,387,397]

Granulosa–Stromal Cell Tumors

This category includes all ovarian tumors composed of granulosa cells, theca cells, and fibroblasts, singly or in any combination and in varying degrees of differentiation. Granulosa cell tumors that occur typically in middle-aged and older women differ in several important respects from those that usually arise in children and young adults and these two subtypes, which are referred to as *adult* and *juvenile* granulosa cell tumors, are discussed separately.

Tumors in the thecoma–fibroma group are composed exclusively or almost exclusively of theca cells, fibroblasts of ovarian stromal origin, or both. The presence of occasional small nests of granulosa cells or occasional tubules lined by Sertoli cells does not exclude tumors from this

Table 19.1. Classification of sex cord–stromal tumors

Granulosa–stromal cell tumors
Granulosa cell tumor
Adult type
Juvenile type
Tumors in the thecoma–fibroma group
Thecoma
Typical
Luteinized
Fibroma–fibrosarcoma
Fibroma
Cellular fibroma
Fibrosarcoma
Stromal tumors with minor sex cord elements
Sclerosing stromal tumor
Unclassified
Sertoli–stromal cell tumors
Sertoli cell tumor
Leydig cell tumor
Sertoli–Leydig cell tumors
Well differentiated
Of intermediate differentiation
Poorly differentiated
With heterologous elements
Retiform
Mixed
Other types of sex cord–stromal tumors
Gynandroblastoma
Sex cord tumor with annular tubules
Unclassified

category; such tumors have been referred to as fibromas or thecomas with minor sex cord elements.[462]

Adult Granulosa Cell Tumor

Clinical Features

Adult granulosa cell tumors[47–49,145,301,387,397] account for approximately 1–2% of all ovarian tumors and 95% of all granulosa cell tumors. They occur more often in postmenopausal than premenopausal women, with a peak incidence between 50 and 55 years of age. They are the most common clinically estrogenic ovarian tumors but the precise proportion of adult granulosa cell tumors that secrete hormones is difficult to establish because a specimen of endometrium to evaluate the effects of estrogenic stimulation often is unavailable. The typical endometrial alteration associated with functioning tumors in this category is simple hyperplasia, usually exhibiting some degree of precancerous atypicality.[174] Carcinoma of the endometrium, which almost always is well differentiated, has been reported in from slightly less than 5% to slightly more than 25% of the cases; the wide variation in these figures is attributable, at least in part, to differing views of the dividing line between complex atypical hyperplasia and grade 1 adenocarcinoma. If strict criteria for the diagnosis of carcinoma are used and if all patients with a granulosa cell tumor, not just those who have had an endometrial curettage or hysterectomy, are considered, the best estimate for the frequency of associated endometrial carcinoma is under 5%.[397]

The endometrial changes associated with adult granulosa cell tumors are manifested clinically in women in the reproductive age group by metropathia hemorrhagica, which is characterized by irregular, excessive uterine bleeding, but amenorrhea, lasting from months to years, may precede the abnormal bleeding or may be the only hormonal manifestation at the time of presentation.[132,397] Postmenopausal bleeding is the most common endocrine symptom in older women, in whom carcinoma of the endometrium is encountered about twice as often as in younger patients.[174] Occasionally, swelling and tenderness of the breasts are prominent symptoms. Elevated levels of estrogens have been reported in the blood and urine,[419] and vaginal cytological smears typically show increased maturation of squamous epithelial cells.[211] Alterations resembling those seen in a secretory endometrium have been observed rarely in association with granulosa cell tumors, suggesting the possibility of a significant production of progesterone[455a] as well as estrogen by the neoplasm.

Rarely, androgenic changes are the sole endocrine manifestation of an adult granulosa cell tumor; 22 androgen-secreting tumors have been reported.[173,208,292,302] Most of the patients have been frankly virilized but some have been only hirsute. The tumors in these 22 cases have been solid or solid and cystic in 12 cases, and cystic in 10. The cysts typically are thin-walled and may be single or multiple, resembling serous cystadenomas.[292,302] Since granulosa cell tumors in general are composed exclusively of thin-walled cysts in only 3% of the cases,[380] the almost 50% frequency of a cystic gross appearance of tumors associated with androgenic manifestations is of great interest. From another viewpoint, 17% of granulosa cell tumors composed of thin-walled cysts seen in consultation by one of us (RES) have been androgenic in contrast to only 1.5% of solid or solid and cystic granulosa cell tumors. The nature of the association of androgen production with the formation of thin-walled cysts remains an enigma.

Gross Findings

Adult granulosa cell tumors vary in size from those that are too small to be felt on pelvic examination (10–15%)[134] to very large masses that distend the abdomen. One of the largest recorded tumors weighed 15.4 kg[121]; the average diameter is approximately 12 cm. At operation the tumor may appear predominantly solid or predominantly cystic, and is unilateral in more than 95% of the cases. Sectioning a solid tumor reveals a gray-white or yellow color, depend-

ing on its lipid content, and a soft or firm consistency, depending on its relative content of neoplastic cells and fibrothecomatous stroma. Hemorrhage, which may be massive, is common. Most characteristically, however, the tumor is predominantly cystic, with numerous compartments that are typically filled with fluid or clotted blood and separated by solid tissue (Fig. 19.1). An interesting clinical corollary of the hemorrhage in both solid and solid and cystic granulosa cell tumors is the presentation in 10–12% of them with an acute abdominal disorder caused by rupture and hemoperitoneum.[47–49,397] The occasional tumor that is a multilocular or unilocular cyst (Fig. 19.2) typically has a smooth lining.

Microscopic Findings

Microscopic examination of an adult granulosa cell tumor reveals only granulosa cells or, more often, an additional component of theca cells, fibroblasts, or both; in some cases, the latter cell types predominate. The granulosa cells grow in a wide variety of patterns, which are commonly admixed (Figs. 19.3–19.9). The better differentiated tumors typically have microfollicular, macrofollicular, insular, trabecular, solid-tubular, and rarely hollow-tubular patterns (Figs. 19.3–19.6). The microfollicular pattern is characterized by the presence of numerous small cavities simulating the Call–Exner bodies of the developing graafian follicle (Figs. 19.4, 19.10). These cavities may contain eosinophilic fluid and often one or a few degenerating nuclei (Fig. 19.10), hyalinized basement membrane material, or rarely basophilic fluid. The microfollicles are separated typically by well-differentiated granulosa cells

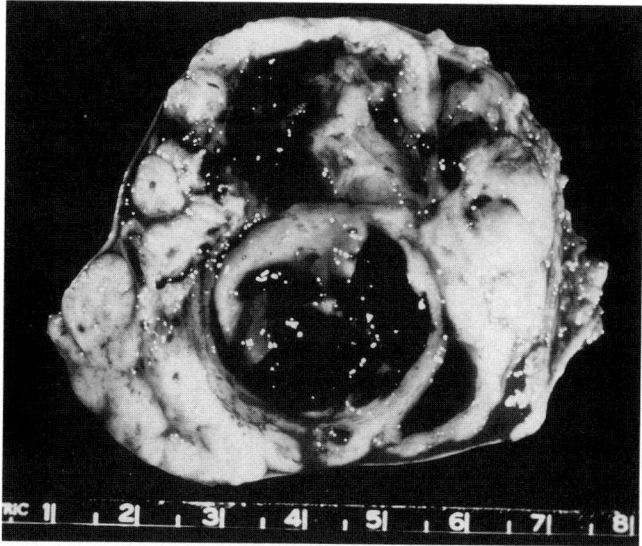

Fig. 19.1. Granulosa cell tumor. The sectioned surface of the neoplasm is solid and cystic with the cysts containing clotted blood. (Reprinted by permission of ref. 461.)

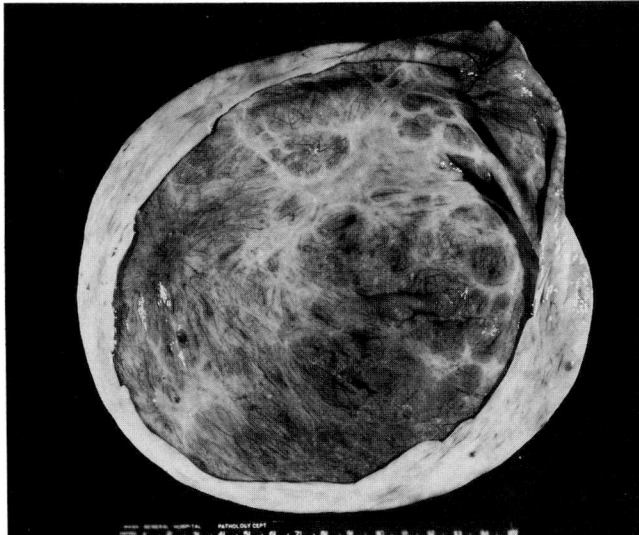

Fig. 19.2. Granulosa cell tumor. The neoplasm is a unilocular cyst with a smooth inner lining. (Reprinted by permission of ref. 292.)

that contain scanty cytoplasm and pale, angular or oval, often grooved nuclei (Fig. 19.11) arranged haphazardly in relation to one another and to the follicles (Fig. 19.4). The macrofollicular pattern of the granulosa cell tumor (Fig. 19.5) is characterized by cysts lined by well-differentiated granulosa cells, beneath which theca cells usually are present.

The trabecular (Fig. 19.6) and insular forms of granulosa cell tumors are characterized by bands and islands of gran-

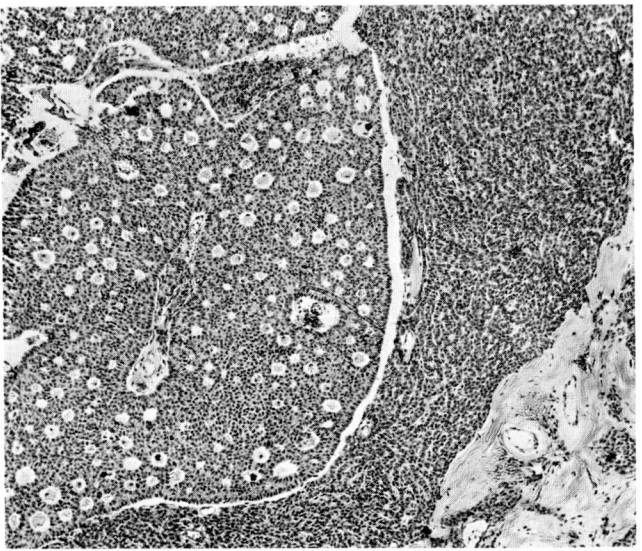

Fig. 19.3. Granulosa cell tumor. Microfollicular pattern is present (*left*), and watered-silk pattern (*right*). (Reprinted by permission of Morris and Scully, ref. 286.)

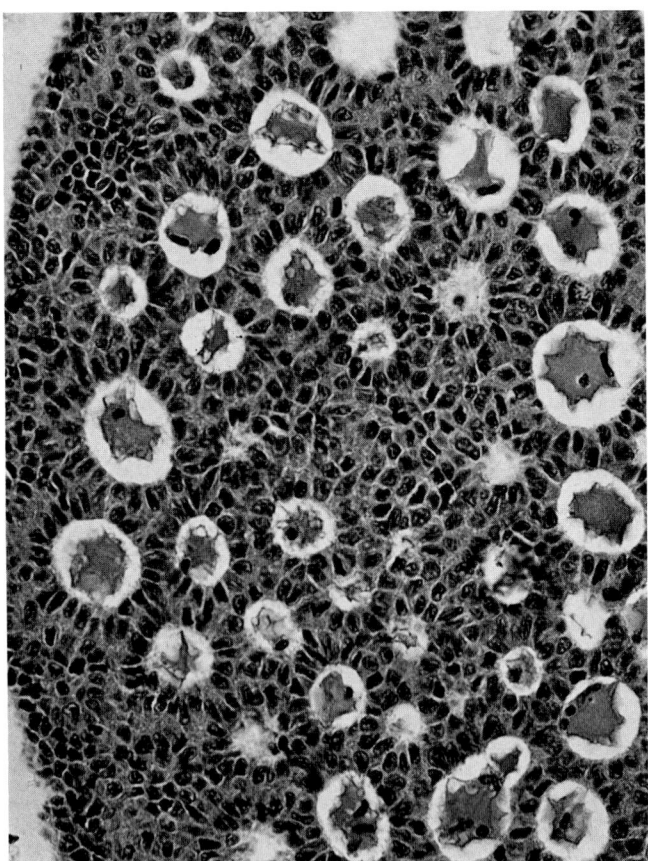

Fig. 19.4. Granulosa cell tumor, microfollicular pattern. Call–Exner bodies are surrounded by granulosa cells with angular nuclei in haphazard arrangement. (Reprinted by permission of Scully and Morris (1957) Functioning ovarian tumors. In: Meigs JV, Sturgis SH (eds) Progress in Gynecology, Vol. 3, New York, Grune & Stratton, pp 20–34).

ulosa cells separated by a fibromatous or thecomatous stroma. In the solid tubular pattern the tubules may be uniformly cellular or contain peripheral nuclei and central masses of cytoplasm; occasionally a few hollow tubules or gland-like structures are encountered. The various tubular patterns encountered in granulosa cell tumors are indistinguishable from those of well-differentiated Sertoli cell tumors; their presence is ignored as a diagnostic criterion unless they account for a significant portions of the tumor (10% or more); in such cases a diagnosis of mixed granulosa cell and Sertoli cell tumor, or gynandroblastoma, is warranted.

The less well-differentiated forms of granulosa cell tumor typically have a watered silk (moiré silk) (Fig. 19.3), gyriform (Fig. 19.7), or diffuse (sarcomatoid) pattern (Fig. 19.8), alone or in combination. The first two patterns are manifested by undulating or zigzag rows of granulosa cells, generally in single file, whereas the diffuse pattern is characterized by a monotonous cellular growth. In some

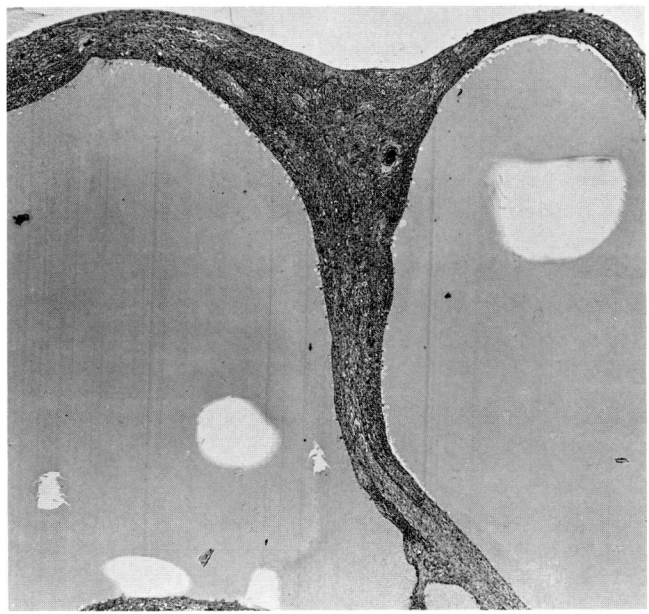

FIG. 19.5. Granulosa cell tumor, macrofollicular pattern. (Reprinted by permission from Case Records of the Massachusetts General Hospital, (Case 89-1961) N Engl J Med 265: 1213, 1961.)

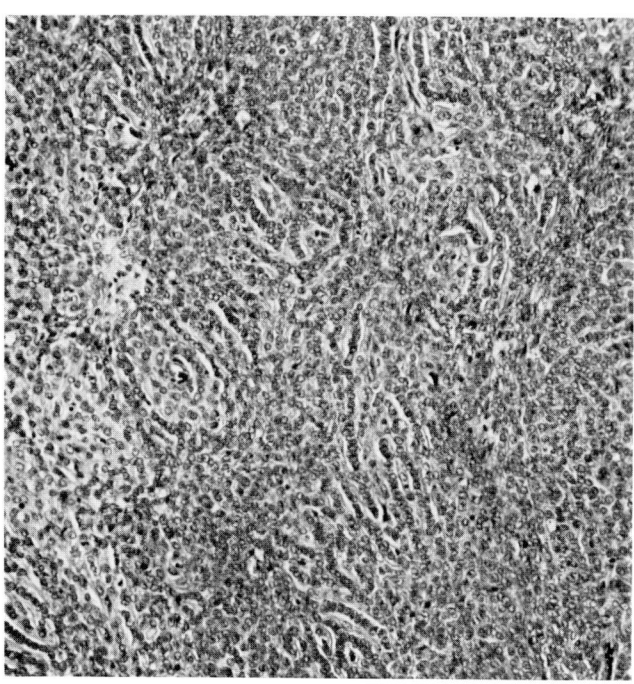

FIG. 19.7. Granulosa cell tumor, gyriform pattern.

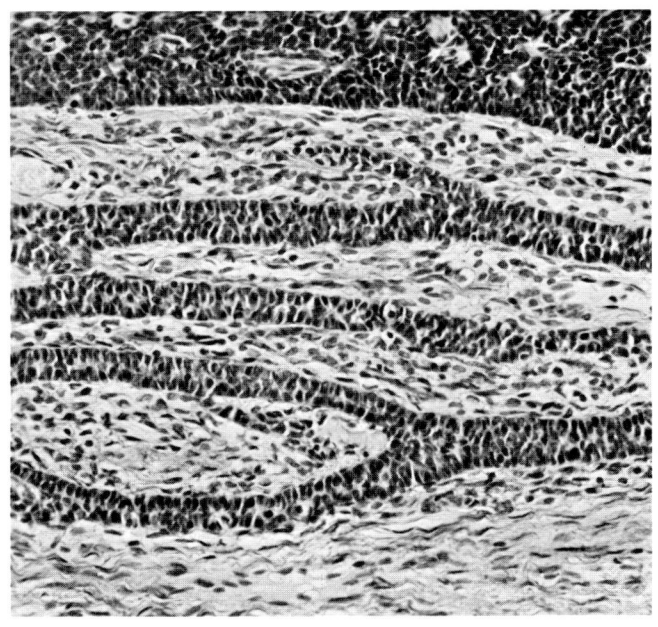

FIG. 19.6. Granulosa cell tumor, trabecular pattern. (Reprinted by permission of Serov, Scully, and Sobin, ref. 378.)

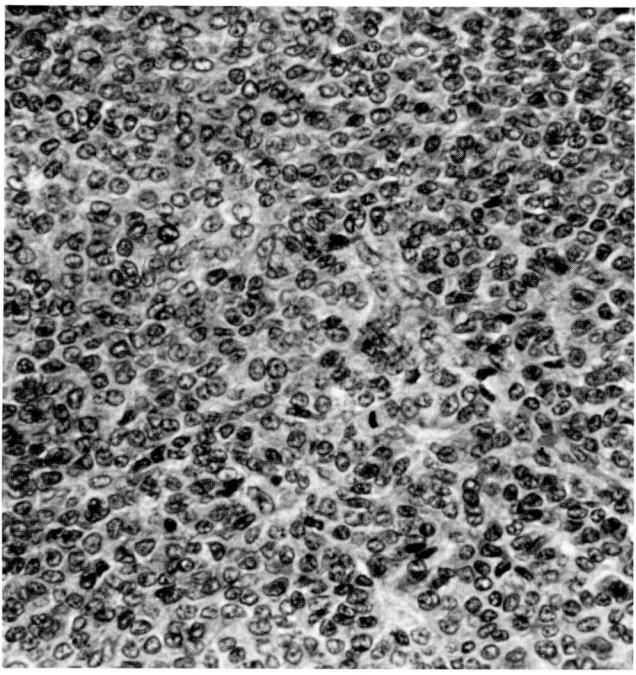

FIG. 19.8. Granulosa cell tumor, diffuse pattern. The nuclei are pale and oval. (Reprinted by permission from Case Records of the Massachusetts General Hospital, (Case 45292) N Engl J Med 261: 146, 1959.)

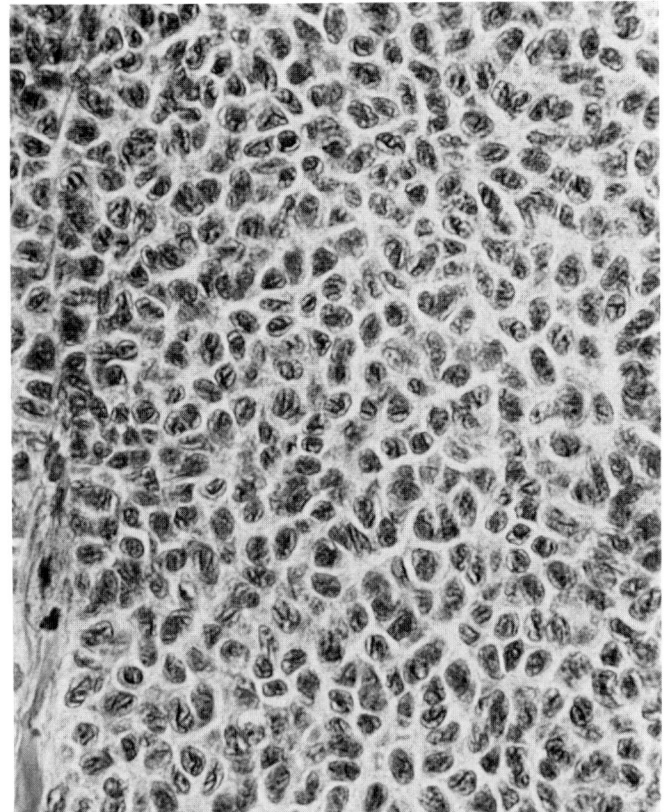

19.9

granulosa cell tumors, the neoplastic cells contain abundant dense or vacuolated cytoplasm (Fig. 19.12), approaching, to varying degrees, the appearance of the granulosa cells of the corpus luteum; in such cases the term *luteinized granulosa cell tumor* is appropriate.[455a]

Very rarely a granulosa cell tumor undergoes sarcomatous transformation[405] or transforms into an anaplastic carcinoma (personal observations). One granulosa cell tumor was intimately associated with a mucinous cystic tumor[326] and another contained liver cells.[300]

The nuclear features of a granulosa cell tumor are characteristic and although the diagnosis usually is apparent, or

---

Fig. 19.9. Granulosa cell tumor. The nuclei are pale and have prominent grooves. (Reprinted by permission of Young and Scully (1985) Ovarian sex cord-stromal and steroid cell tumors. In: Roth LM, Czernobilsky B (eds) Tumors and tumor-like conditions of the ovary, Contemporary Issues in Surgical Pathology, Vol. 6, New York, Churchill Livingstone.)

Fig. 19.10. Granulosa cell tumor. A Call–Exner body contains cellular fragments and amorphous debris. The surrounding cells show prominent microvilli and junctional complexes. ×12,000. (Reprinted by permission of Gondos and Monroe, ref. 164.)

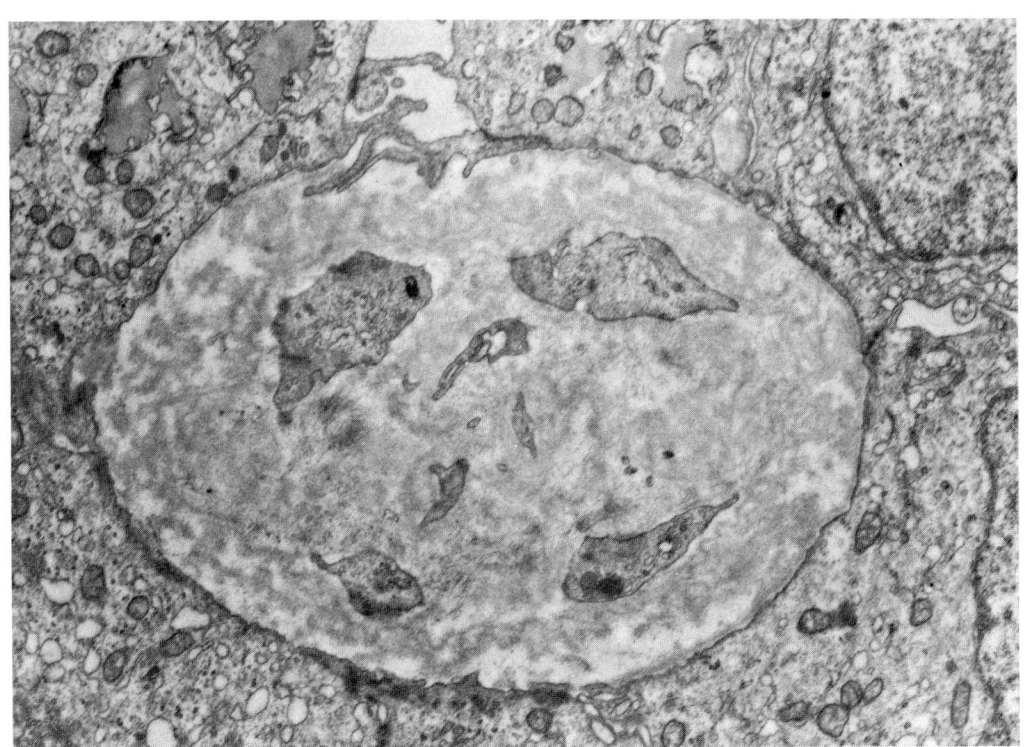

19.10

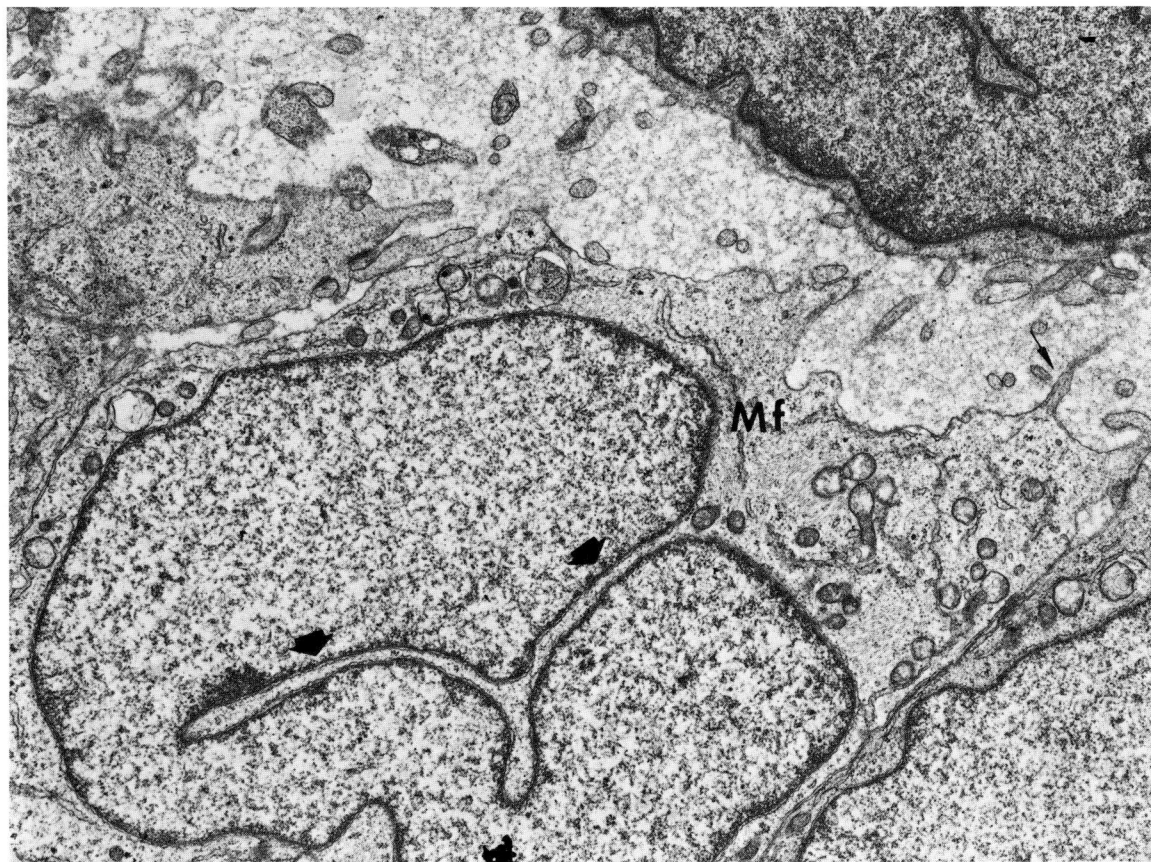

FIG. 19.11. Granulosa cell tumor. The deep indentation of the nuclear membranes (*large arrows*) corresponds to the nuclear wrinkling on light microscopic examination. The sparse cytoplasm contains clusters of small mitochondria and numerous microfibrils (*MF*). The plasma membrane has hair-like microvillous processes (*small arrow*) projecting into the intercellular space. ×8000. (Courtesy of Dr. A. Ferenczy, Montreal, Canada. Reprinted by permission of Scully, ref. 369.)

at least suggested, on the basis of low-power features, the diagnosis must be confirmed by appropriate supportive cytological features on high power, specifically pale, relatively uniform nuclei, at least some of which contain nuclear grooves (Fig. 19.9). The prominence of the latter varies from one neoplasm to the next. Sometimes they are seen in virtually every nucleus whereas in other cases they are seen only occasionally. In cases of the latter type the characteristic nuclear pallor is still usually seen. An exception to the characteristic nuclear features just described is seen in approximately 2% of granulosa cell tumors that contain bizarre, enlarged hyperchromatic nuclei, including multinucleated forms (Fig. 19.13). Cells with these nuclear features typically are a focal finding but rarely are conspicuous and may overshadow more characteristic foci, which can be overlooked if not carefully sought.

The mitotic rate in granulosa cell tumors is variable but usually not pronounced. If numerous mitoses are found the diagnosis of granulosa cell tumor should be made with caution. In one large series[396] 49% of the tumors had less than 1 mitotic figure (MF) per 10 high power fields (HPF), 27% had 1 to 2 MF/10 HPF, 15% had 3 to 5 MF/10 HPF, and 9% had 6 or more MF/10 HPF.

The presence of theca cells in varying quantities in most granulosa cell tumors has led to the occasional usage of the term *granulosa–theca cell tumor*. Although this designation accurately describes the cellular content of many of these neoplasms, the term *granulosa cell tumor* is more widely accepted for tumors containing both cell types. One reason for this preference is the probability that the presence of theca cells in some cases reflects a response of the ovarian stroma to the growth of granulosa cells rather than the co-existence of a second neoplastic cell component. Evidence favoring such an interpretation includes the nonspecific presence of theca-like cells in a variety of ovarian tumors, both benign and malignant and both primary and metastatic, and the observation that theca cells usually are absent in granulosa cell tumors that have extended beyond

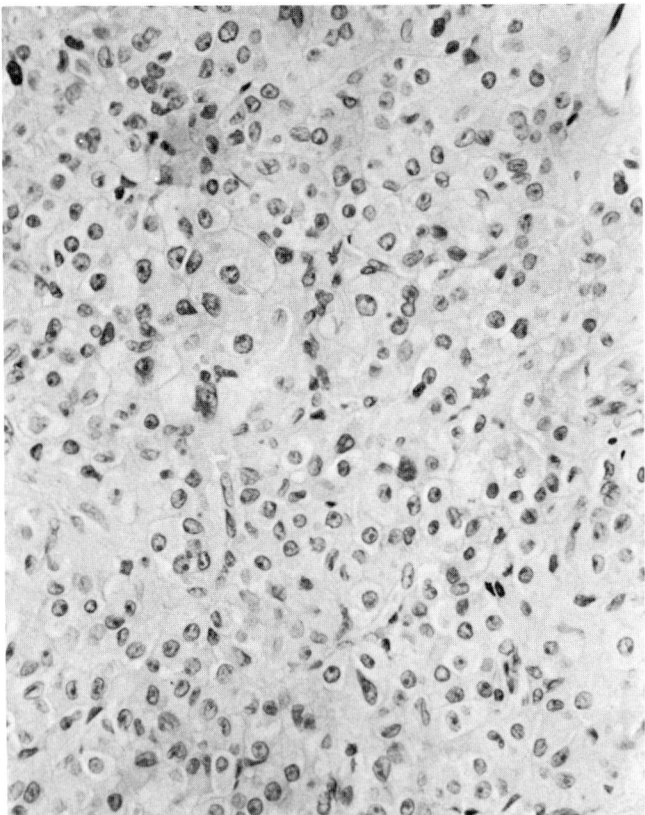

FIG. 19.12. **Granulosa cell tumor, luteinized.** The tumor cells have abundant cytoplasm.

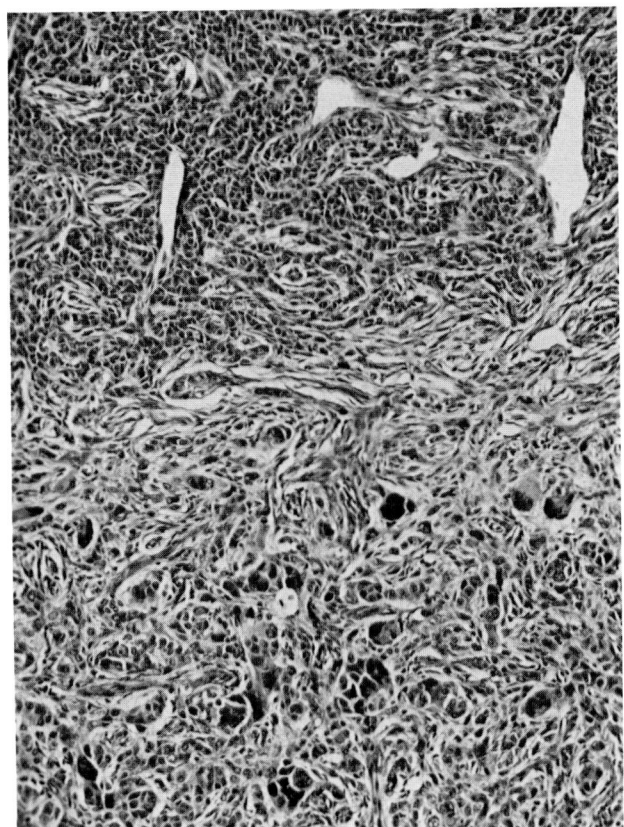

FIG. 19.13. **Typical granulosa cell tumor.** The tumor (*top*) is adjacent to area with bizarre nuclei (*bottom*). (Reprinted by permission of Young and Scully, ref. 463.)

the ovary.[135] It is possible, however, that some tumors in which the theca cell element is prominent or even greatly preponderant are truly mixed neoplasms.

The theca cells in granulosa cell tumors may resemble theca externa or theca interna cells and may be luteinized. In some tumors, particularly those with a diffuse pattern, differentiation of granulosa and theca cells with routine staining may be difficult or impossible. In such cases a reticulum stain may be helpful. Just as in a developing graafian follicle, so in a granulosa cell tumor the fibrils typically invest theca cells individually. In contrast, the granulosa cell layer of a follicle contains no fibrils, and in a granulosa cell tumor the reticulum usually is sparse, being typically confined to perivascular zones (Fig. 19.14). In occasional tumors an intermediate pattern of fibril distribution is present and the reticulum stain is not useful in the differentiation of the two cell types.

The presence of blood-filled cysts in many granulosa cell tumors results in the frequent presence in the tumors of related changes that are nonspecific but in the context of other typical features of granulosa cell tumors are at the same time quite characteristic. For example, the cysts often are lined by fibrous tissue associated with evidence of old and recent hemorrhage that is sometimes conspicuous.

Several histochemical reactions that are characteristic of steroid hormone-producing cells, particularly those that demonstrate various types of lipid content or oxidative enzyme activity, usually are positive in the theca cells and negative or only weakly positive in the granulosa cells of a tumor containing both cell types.[163,266,267,372,450] This finding, as well as ultrastructural observations,[141,150,158,164] have led some observers to conclude that the theca cell component of granulosa cell tumors produces the hormones responsible for estrogenic manifestations. Additional evidence in favor of this conclusion is the observation that granulosa cell tumors that recur outside ovarian tissue and lack theca cells typically are not obviously estrogenic. In some cases, however, histochemical and other evidence[150,250] has suggested a role for the granulosa cells in estrogen secretion. Likewise, Kurman et al.[238] have demonstrated immunohistochemically the presence of a variety of steroid hormones in granulosa cells; whether these findings reflect production, storage, or binding of these hormones, however, has not been established. Possibly the theca cells in granulosa cell tumors produce androgens, and aromatase in the granulosa cells converts these hormones to estrogens according to the two-cell theory of estrogen production by the normal graafian follicle.[23,123]

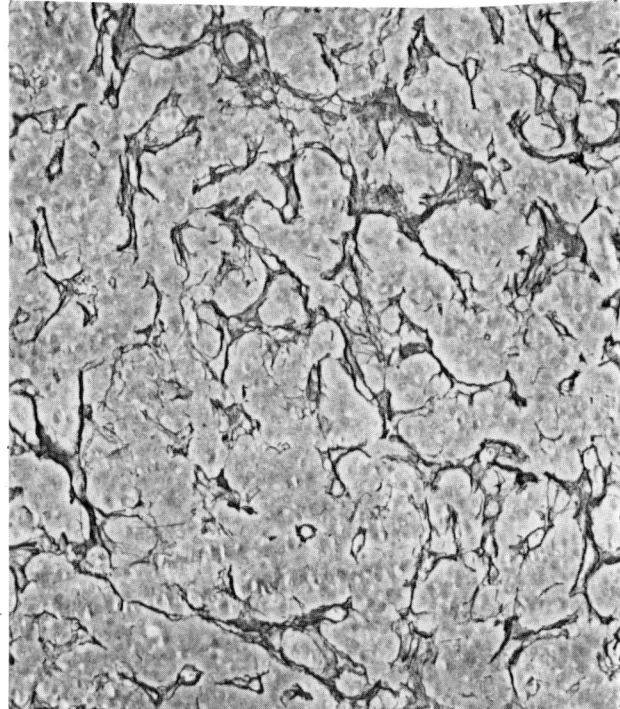

FIG. 19.14. Granulosa cell tumor (reticulum stain.) Reticulum surrounds aggregates of granulosa cells. Contrast with Fig. 19.22.

DIFFERENTIAL DIAGNOSIS

The misinterpretation of an undifferentiated carcinoma as an adult granulosa cell tumor (AGCT) with a diffuse pattern is one of the most frequent errors in ovarian tumor pathology. If the clinical course of the patient is atypically malignant for an AGCT, the possibility of such a misdiagnosis must be considered. The single best criterion for distinguishing these two tumors is the appearance of the nuclei, which are typically uniform, pale, and often grooved in AGCT (Figs. 19.8, 19.9) and are hyperchromatic, usually of unequal size and shape, and rarely grooved in undifferentiated carcinomas; atypical mitotic figures often are found in the latter as well. Other features helpful in the differential diagnosis are summarized in Table 19.2. The highly malignant small cell carcinoma, which usually is associated with hypercalcemia,[116] also may be misdiagnosed as an AGCT. The differential features of these tumors are presented in Table 19.3. The most helpful features are the much higher mitotic rate of the small cell carcinoma and the lack in that tumor of the typical cytological features of the AGCT. A diffuse AGCT occasionally is confused with a primary endometrioid stromal sarcoma[459] or metastatic endometrial stromal sarcoma of the ovary[471] but a variety of features, including the frequent high stage and bilaterality of the latter tumors, the characteristic pattern of growth in extraovarian sites of

Table 19.2. Granulosa cell tumor versus undifferentiated carcinoma and poorly differentiated adenocarcinoma

Granulosa cell tumor	Carcinoma
Bilateral—less than 5%	Bilateral >25%
Stage I in 90% of cases	Stage III or IV in most cases
Nuclei round to angular, pale, and commonly grooved[a]	Nuclei hyperchromatic, often bizarre with atypical mitoses
Mucin occasionally in follicles (mainly in juvenile type)	Intracellular droplets or extracellular pools of mucin, psammoma bodies, or glands may be present
Good prognosis	Poor prognosis
Indolent course, when clinically malignant[b]	Rapid course

[a] Exception—dark, ungrooved nuclei of juvenile granulosa cell tumor.
[b] Exception—rare juvenile granulosa cell tumors.

spread, their typical content of numerous arterioles, and their rich reticulum content aid in this differential diagnosis. In this, as in other problems in the diagnosis of granulosa cell and other sex cord–stromal tumors, extensive sampling of the specimen often is helpful as is an appreciation of the rarity of bilaterality and extraovarian spread at presentation in cases of sex cord–stromal tumors.

AGCTs may be difficult to distinguish from pure stromal tumors such as cellular thecomas, fibromas, and fibrosarcomas. Reticulum stains may show abundant intercellular fibrils in these tumors, unlike the scant reticulum of AGCTs. In some cases the pattern of fibrils is intermediate between an AGCT and a typical thecoma, and in such cases, the differential diagnosis may be difficult or impossible. The almost exclusive spindle cell nature of the cells in fibromas and fibrosarcomas is rarely seen in an AGCT.

Occasionally the distinction of a unilocular or multilocular macrofollicular AGCT from one or more follicular cysts may be troublesome. This is particularly likely if the patient is pregnant or in the puerperium because a large solitary luteinized follicle cyst of pregnancy and the puerperium[95] is indistinguishable grossly from a unilocular cystic AGCT. The large luteinized cells of the former, some of which contain large bizarre nuclei, differ from those of a unilocular AGCT, which are rarely uniformly luteinized and rarely contain bizarre nuclei.

Endometrioid carcinomas occasionally are misdiagnosed as AGCT when the former have small acini imparting a microfollicular pattern. In addition, some endometrioid carcinomas have an insular pattern that on low power may suggest the diagnosis of an insular AGCT.[457] In most of these cases the cytological features in an endometrioid carcinoma differ from those of an AGCT, although there are rare cases in which the former tumors have pale nuclei that on cytological grounds are consistent with a diagnosis of AGCT. In our experience a combination of at least focal cytological differences, and the presence in endometrioid tumors that are well sampled of other foci incompatible

Table 19.3. Granulosa cell tumors versus small cell carcinoma

Juvenile GCT	*Adult GCT*	*Small cell CA*
Mostly before age 30 yrs	All ages, but mostly postmenopausal	Always premenopausal
Rarely malignant	Indolent course if malignant	Highly malignant
No hypercalcemia	No hypercalcemia	Hypercalcemia common
Usually estrogenic	Usually estrogenic	Never estrogenic
Thecomatous component common	Fibrothecomatous component common	Stroma scanty and non specific
Cytoplasm usually abundant	Cytoplasm usually scanty	Cytoplasm usually scanty, but may be abundant
Nuclei dark, ungrooved, and often pleomorphic	Nuclei pale and often grooved	Nuclei dark and uniform
Mitoses usually numerous	Mitoses variable	Mitoses numerous

GCT, granulosa cell tumor; CA, carcinoma.

with the diagnosis of an AGCT, such as squamous foci, establish the diagnosis.

The rare AGCT in which the cells are extensively luteinized (Fig. 19.12) may superficially resemble a steroid cell tumor. The focal presence of areas with the architectural and cytological features of an AGCT usually facilitates the diagnosis in these cases. AGCTs should be distinguished from the small proliferations of granulosa cells within atretic follicles that are typically an incidental finding within the ovaries of pregnant women.[97]

It is important to distinguish the Call–Exner bodies of AGCTs from the acini of carcinoid (Table 19.4) and from the hyaline bodies that are seen in gonadoblastomas[368] and sex cord tumors with annular tubules.[367,478] The acini of carcinoids often contain dense eosinophilic secretion that is sometimes calcified: the latter is not a feature of AGCT. The nuclei of carcinoids, which have coarse chromatin, contrast with the pale nuclei of AGCT. The hyaline bodies of gonadoblastomas and sex cord tumors with annular tubules typically are larger than Call–Exner bodies. Some-

Table 19.4. Granulosa cell tumor versus carcinoid

Granulosa cell tumor	*Insular carcinoid*
Variety of patterns	Islands, round acini, solid tubules, and ribbons
Call–Exner bodies, ill-defined, with watery to dense eosinophilic content, occasionally pyknotic nuclei	Acini sharply outlined with dense content, sometimes calcified
Nuclei round to angular, pale, often grooved, haphazardly oriented	Nuclei round with coarse chromatin and regular orientation
Thecomatous stroma common, at least focally	Fibromatous or hyalinized stroma, may be focally luteinized
Usually uninodular and almost always unilateral—no teratomatous elements	Often multinodular and almost always bilateral if metastatic; always unilateral and usually associated with other teratomatous elements if primary
Cells nonargentaffin; may contain fine argyrophilic granules	Cells usually argentaffin— almost always argyrophilic

times the hyaline bodies can be observed to be continuous with hyaline thickenings of the basement membrane along the periphery of the tumor cell nests; these bodies also undergo calcification.

The AGCT may be confused with two types of metastatic tumors, metastatic malignant melanoma[460] and metastatic breast carcinoma (see Chapter 22, Metastatic Tumors of the Ovary). Metastatic melanomas may have cells with scant cytoplasm that grow diffusely, imparting a low-power appearance that may mimic closely that of an AGCT. Patterns of growth incompatible with a diagnosis of AGCT usually are found when a tumor is thoroughly sampled and the finding of melanin pigment or immunohistochemical stains may be helpful in problematic cases. Metastatic breast carcinoma sometimes also has a diffuse growth of cells with scant cytoplasm, particularly in cases of lobular carcinoma. The history often is helpful in these cases because breast carcinoma rarely presents with an ovarian metastasis. In cases in which a breast cancer is not known of in the patient, it is only the presence of focal patterns more suggestive of breast cancer than a granulosa cell tumor, and a lack of the typical cytological features of granulosa cell tumor that will alert the pathologist to the possible correct diagnosis. In both this situation and that of metastatic melanoma, the ovarian metastatic tumors are much more frequently bilateral than is the AGCT.

CLINICAL BEHAVIOR AND TREATMENT

After the removal of a granulosa cell tumor, the manifestations of hyperestrinism typically regress. If the uterus has been conserved in a young woman, estrogen withdrawal bleeding usually occurs in 1 or 2 days and regular menses ensue shortly thereafter. Granulosa cell tumors of all patterns have a malignant potential, with a capacity to extend beyond the ovary or recur after apparently successful removal. Spread is largely within the pelvis and lower abdomen; distant metastases are rare, but have been reported in many sites.[260,407] Although recurrences may appear within 5 years, they often are not evident until a much longer postoperative interval has elapsed, and numerous cases have been reported in which the tumor has reappeared two or even three or more decades after the initial therapy. The 10-year survival figures that have been recorded in the literature have varied widely from under 60% to more than 90%, and progressive declines in survival have been documented after longer follow-up periods.°

The optimal treatment of a granulosa cell tumor in menopausal or postmenopausal women is total hysterectomy with bilateral salpingo-oophorectomy. In younger women, in whom the preservation of fertility is an important consideration, however, removal of only the tumor and the adjacent fallopian tube is justifiable if spread beyond the ovary is not demonstrable and examination of the contralateral ovary shows no suggestion of involvement. Recurrence usually is fatal, but some recurrent tumors have been treated successfully by reoperation, radiation therapy, or a combination thereof.[219,362,386] Too little information is available on the chemotherapy of granulosa cell tumors to evaluate the comparative merits of various agents, but several of them have been used with varying degrees of success.†

Ninety percent of granulosa cell tumors are stage I[47–49,397] and these tumors have a considerably better prognosis than higher stage tumors, as shown by an 86% versus a 49% relative survival at 10 years, respectively, in one large series[397] and a 96% versus a 26% survival in another.[49] Rupture also adversely affects the outlook, with an 86% relative 25-year survival of patients with intact stage I tumors compared with only 60% survival of those with ruptured tumors that are otherwise in the same stage.[49]

The size of granulosa cell tumors also has been related to their prognosis. In one series all the patients with tumors 5 cm or less in diameter survived 10 years, but only 57% of those with tumors 6 to 15 cm in diameter and 53% of those with even larger tumors survived for that period of time.[145] Another investigation reported a 73% crude overall survival of patients with tumors under 5 cm in diameter, a 63% survival of those with tumors between 5 and 15 cm, and a 34% survival of those with a tumor over 15 cm in diameter.[397] In a final series stage I tumors 5 cm or less in diameter were associated with a 100% relative 10-year survival in contrast to a 92% survival of patients with larger stage I tumors.[49] The last series is the only one in which the survival rate was corrected for stage and on that basis the improvement in prognosis for the smaller stage I tumors was not statistically significant. Therefore, a relationship between tumor size and prognosis independent of stage has not been clearly established.

Attempts to correlate the histological pattern and the degrees of nuclear atypia and mitotic activity with prognosis have met with varying success. Kottmeier[231] reported a significantly better prognosis if the tumor was well differentiated (with a follicular or "cylindromatous" pattern)

than if it was more poorly differentiated ("sarcomatoid"). This difference was reflected in 5-year survival figures of 87% and 64%, respectively, but was more obtrusive in the figures for 10 years, which were 82% versus 29%. The latter figures emphasize that long follow-up is necessary before survival data for any series of granulosa cell tumors become meaningful. Several other investigators have failed to confirm the prognostic importance of pattern alone in granulosa cell tumors.[49,145,301,387,397]

The degree of nuclear atypicality within granulosa cell tumors also has been correlated with their prognosis. In one study the 5-year survival of patients whose tumors showed no atypia was 92% compared with 80% for those with slight atypicality and 30% for those with moderate atypicality.[397] In another study there was an 80% relative 25-year survival in cases with grade 1 nuclear atypicality in contrast to only a 60% survival in those with grade 2 atypia.[49] In both of these studies nuclear atypicality was the most reliable prognostic index in cases of stage I tumors; for higher stage tumors nuclear atypicality and mitotic rate were of similar significance. With regard to the relation of nuclear atypicality to prognosis, it should be noted that assessment of its degree is somewhat subjective. Also, as noted earlier, approximately 2% of granulosa cell tumors contain mononucleate and multinucleate cells with large, bizarre, hyperchromatic nuclei (Fig. 19.13), the presence of which has not been shown to worsen the prognosis. These nuclear changes, which resemble those seen in the uterine leiomyoma with bizarre nuclei, also are encountered in occasional Sertoli–Leydig cell tumors and thecomas, and probably are degenerative. In a study of eight granulosa cell tumors, seven Sertoli–Leydig cell tumors and two thecomas with bizarre nuclei, follow-up was obtained on 11 patients, all of whom were alive without evidence of disease from 3 to 21 years postoperatively.[463]

The mitotic activity of granulosa cell tumors also has been correlated with their prognosis. In one study there was a 70% 10-year survival associated with tumors that had 2 or fewer MF/10 HPF compared with only a 37% survival for those with three or more.[397] In another investigation[145] tumors with many mitotic figures were associated with a worse prognosis than those with few, but most of the tumors with high mitotic rates also were at a higher stage than those with low mitotic rates, and differences in mitotic rate did not have a statistically significant effect on the prognosis of stage I tumors.

Juvenile Granulosa Cell Tumor

Clinical Features

Somewhat under 5% of granulosa cell tumors are diagnosed before the age of normal puberty. The great majority of these tumors as well as many granulosa cell tumors in young adults differ histologically from adult granulosa cell tumors (Table 19.5), and the designation *juvenile* has been

---

°Refs. 20,47–49,66,68,118,132,145,261,301,387.
†Refs. 120,207,248,256,295,362,388.

Table 19.5. Adult versus juvenile granulosa cell tumor

Adult GCT	Juvenile GCT
Less than 1% prepubertal	50% prepubertal
Usual after 30 yrs	Rare after 30 yrs
Mature follicles and Call–Exner bodies common	Immature follicles with mucin content; Call–Exner bodies rare
Nuclei pale, angular, commonly grooved	Nuclei darker, round, rarely grooved
Luteinization infrequent	Luteinization frequent

GCT, granulosa cell tumor.

selected for such tumors because 97% of them occur in the first three decades.[454] Approximately 80% of juvenile granulosa cell tumors (JGCTs) occurring in children result in isosexual precocity,[454] accounting for 10% of cases of that syndrome in the female.[205,213,299] More common forms of isosexual precocity are those of central origin, with premature release of gondadotropins from the anterior pituitary gland and those due to apparently autonomous formation of one or more follicle cysts. The precocity caused by granulosa cell tumors is more specifically designated *pseudoprecocity* because there is no associated ovulation or progesterone production, precluding the possibility of pregnancy, which exists, in contrast, in cases of true sexual precocity. Typically, pseudoprecocity is heralded by development of the breasts, followed by the appearance of pubic and axillary hair, stimulation and enlargement of the external and internal secondary sex organs, irregular uterine bleeding, and a whitish vaginal discharge, believed to originate in the stimulated endocervical glands. Somatic and skeletal development typically are accelerated as well. Androgenic manifestations such as clitoromegaly occasionally occur.[45,454]

When it occurs after puberty the JGCT usually presents with abdominal pain or swelling, sometimes associated with menstrual irregularities or amenorrhea. Approximately 6% of all the patients present with acute abdominal symptoms because of rupture of the tumor and hemoperitoneum.[454] One tumor was associated with ascites and acute respiratory distress.[203] An interesting clinical association of the JGCT has been its association with Ollier's disease (enchondromatosis) in 10 patients,[171,403,416,441,442,454] and with Maffucci's syndrome (enchondromatosis and hemangiomatosis) in an additional four patients.[241,245,417,454]

The JGCT is bilateral in only about 2% of the cases.[303,330,454] It appears ruptured at operation in approximately 10% of the cases, and ascites is present in a similar percentage. Spread beyond the ovary is unusual; in our series only 2% of the tumors were stage II[454] and we have seen one case in which the tumor was stage III on the basis of omental spread. The diameter of the tumor has ranged from 3.0 cm to 32.0 cm, with an average of 12.5 cm. Because of a usual moderate to large size of the tumor, an adnexal mass is almost always detectable clinically. Rarely,

however, a mass has not been palpable preoperatively even on bimanual rectal examination.[82]

Gross Findings

The range of gross appearances of the JGCT is similar to that of an adult form. Like the latter, the single most common presentation is as a solid and cystic neoplasm, in which the cysts may contain hemorrhagic fluid (Fig. 19.15). Uniformly solid and uniformly cystic neoplasms also are encountered; the latter may be multilocular or, rarely, unilocular. The solid component typically is yellow-tan or gray, and occasionally exhibits extensive necrosis, hemorrhage, or both.

Microscopic Findings

Microscopic examination typically reveals a solid cellular neoplasm, with focal follicle formation (Figs. 19.16, 19.17), but the tumor also may be uniformly solid or uniformly follicular. In the solid areas the neoplastic cells may be arranged diffusely or divided into nodules by fibrous septa; occasionally small clusters of tumor cells are present in a fibrous stroma. In the solid foci the granulosa cells usually predominate but often there is an admixture of theca cells and in some areas the latter may predominate. Occasionally, the granulosa cells and theca cells are admixed in a haphazard fashion. In such cases reticulum stains may aid in their differentiation. Foci resembling typical thecoma with hyaline bands are encountered rarely, but usually are minor in extent. Rarely, areas of sclerosis and calcification are seen.

The follicles usually vary in size and shape (Fig. 19.16) but may be regular and round to oval (Fig. 19.17). They

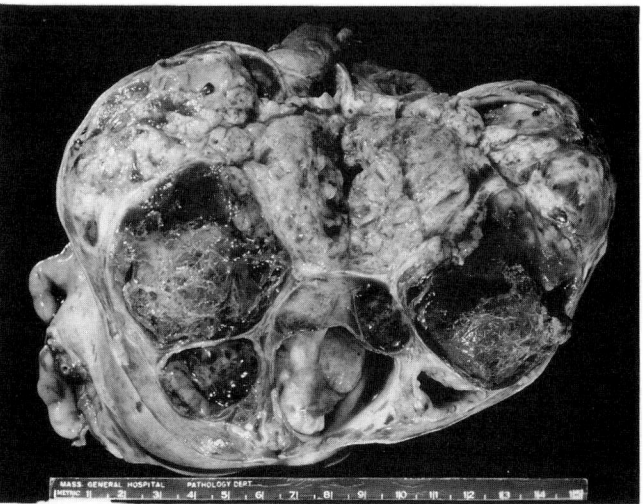

Fig. 19.15. Juvenile granulosa cell tumor. The sectioned surface of the neoplasm is solid and cystic. Clotted blood is present in most of the cysts.

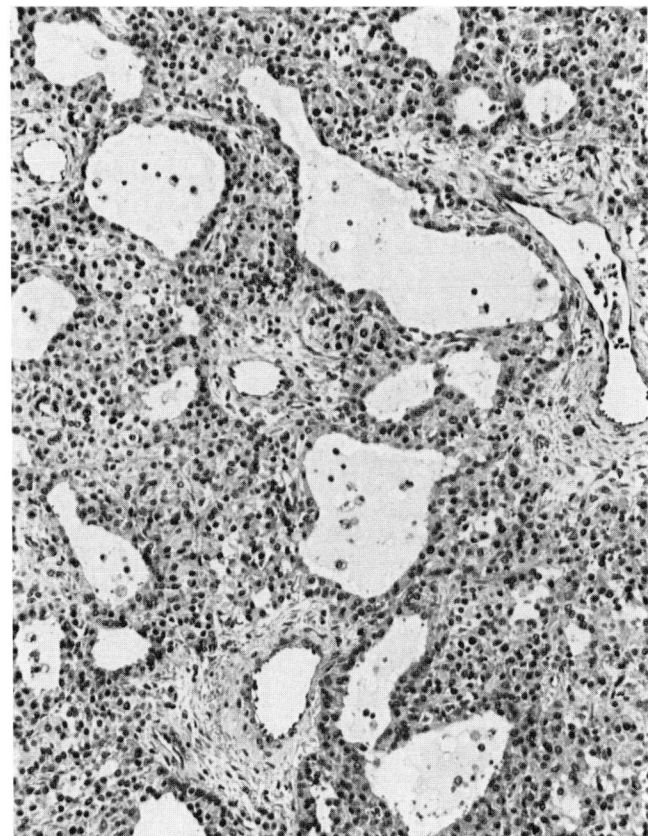

FIG. 19.16. Juvenile granulosa cell tumor. Follicles of vary-ing sizes and shapes are separated by cellular areas. (Reprinted by permission of Young, Dickersin, and Scully, ref. 454.)

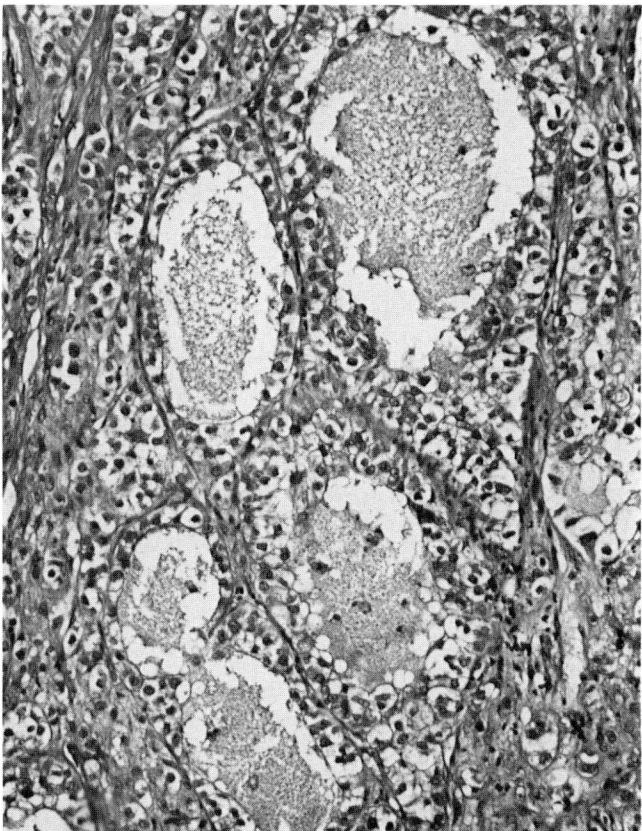

FIG. 19.17. Juvenile granulosa cell tumor. Round to oval follicles lined by cells with abundant pale cytoplasm enclose se-cretion that was basophilic. (Reprinted by permission of Young and Scully, ref. 461.)

generally do not reach the large size of the follicles in the macrofollicular form of the AGCT. Their lumens contain eosinophilic or basophilic secretion, which stains with mu-cicarmine in approximately two-thirds of the cases.[454] Granulosa cells of varying layers of thickness line the folli-cles and occasionally are surrounded by mantles of theca cells. More often, however, the granulosa cells lining the follicles blend into the intervening diffusely cellular areas. Rarely, the lining cells resemble hobnail cells.

The two characteristic cytological features of the neo-plastic granulosa cells that distinguish them from those of the AGCT are their generally rounded, hyperchromatic nuclei, which lack grooves in most cases, and their fre-quent abundant content of eosinophilic (luteinized) cyto-plasm (Fig. 19.18). The theca-cell element of the tumors usually is also luteinized, and lipid stains typically disclose moderate to large amounts of fat within the cytoplasm of both cellular components. The theca cells are more often spindle-shaped than the granulosa cells and, like the latter, usually contain hyperchromatic nuclei. In rare JGCTs small foci more characteristic of the AGCT are encoun-tered.

Nuclear atypicality in JGCTs varies from minimal to marked. In approximately 13% of the cases severe degrees

are present (Fig. 19.19). The mitotic rate also varies greatly but is generally higher than that seen in AGCTs.[397] In our series of JGCTs[454] the average count was 7 MF/10 HPF and in the series from the Armed Forces Institute of Pa-thology[476] it was 5.5 MF/10 HPF.

DIFFERENTIAL DIAGNOSIS

The differential diagnosis of the JGCT includes the AGCT and a wide variety of other neoplasms. The follicles of the JGCT are more irregular in size and shape than those of an AGCT and its cells are more extensively luteinized with nuclei that are typically round and more hyperchromatic, and lack nuclear grooves. (Table 19.5). The mucicarmino-philic, often basophilic follicular content in the JGCT also differs from the eosinophilic fluid often accompanied by degenerating nuclei or basement-membrane material that are usually present in the microfollicles of AGCTs.

The JGCT often is misdiagnosed as a malignant germ cell tumor. The latter are more common in young females than the JGCT and may be associated with human chori-onic gonadotropin (hCG)–induced isosexual pseudopre-cocity. The nuclei of the JGCT are not as primitive-appear-ing as those of either a yolk sac tumor or an embryonal

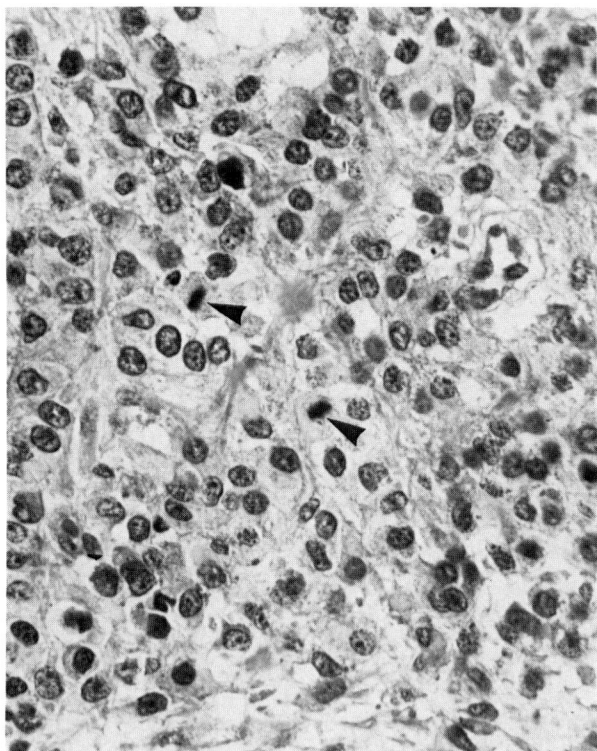

Fig. 19.18. Juvenile granulosa cell tumor. The cells have abundant cytoplasm; their nuclei are hyperchromatic, lack grooves, and exhibit mitotic activity (*arrows*). (Reprinted by permission of Young and Scully (1985) Ovarian sex cord–stromal and steroid cell tumors. In: Roth LM, Czernobilsky B (eds) Tumors and Tumor-like Conditions of the Ovary, Contemporary Issues in Surgical Pathology, Vol. 6, New York, Churchill Livingstone.)

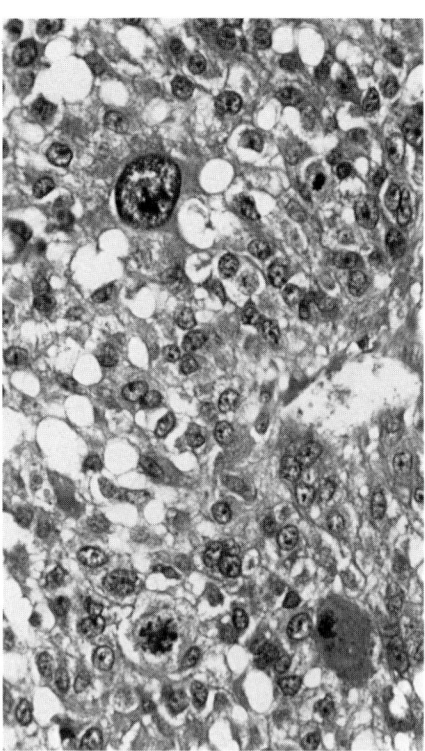

Fig. 19.19. Juvenile granulosa cell tumor. Marked nuclear atypicality and an abnormal mitotic figure are visible. This tumor was clinically malignant. (Reprinted by permission of Young and Scully, ref. 461.)

carcinoma and the follicular pattern of the JGCT is not a feature of either germ cell tumor, although the cysts of the polyvesicular variant of yolk sac tumor can superficially resemble the follicles of a JGCT in rare cases. Immunohistochemical demonstration of hCG in embryonal carcinomas and of alpha-fetoprotein in yolk sac tumors may be helpful in difficult cases.

The JGCT is sometimes misinterpreted as a thecoma because of the occasional absence or rarity of follicles, the typically abundant cytoplasm of the neoplastic cells, and the occasional predominance of theca cells. Thorough sampling to demonstrate follicles and the performance of reticulum stains to establish the granulosa cell nature of at least some of the tumor cells are important diagnostically. Also, thecomas rarely exhibit significant mitotic activity, rarely occur before 30 years of age, and are exceptionally rare in children. A focally diffuse pattern in a luteinized JGCT may suggest the diagnosis of a steroid (lipid) cell tumor but the uniformity of the pattern and cytological features of the latter tumor would be unusual for a JGCT, which almost always contains more diagnostic areas. The pregnancy luteoma rarely contains rounded follicle-like

spaces and may suggest a luteinized JGCT but, like the steroid cell tumor, its cells are uniform in appearance and it is multiple and bilateral in one-half and one-third of the cases, respectively.

The common epithelial tumors with which a JGCT may be confused are clear cell, undifferentiated, and transitional cell carcinomas. The tubulocystic variant of the clear cell carcinoma is rarely suggested when follicles in a JGCT are lined by cells resembling hobnail cells and JGCTs with high-grade nuclear atypia may suggest an undifferentiated carcinoma. Transitional cell carcinoma is mimicked in rare cases in which a cystic JGCT contains pseudopapillae lined by uniform granulosa cells. The young age of the patient and the presence of follicles and of focal areas typical of a JGCT should help indicate the correct diagnosis in these cases.

The JGCT may be confused with a small cell carcinoma of hypercalcemic type (Table 19.3) because both neoplasms contain follicles and both are characteristically found in young patients. In the typical case of small cell carcinoma the presence of cells with scanty cytoplasm is in marked contrast to the JGCT, in which the tumors almost without exception have cells with appreciable to abundant cytoplasm. The follicles in the small cell carcinoma rarely contain the basophilic secretion that is seen in many

JGCTs. Although the JGCT characteristically has easily found mitotic figures, mitoses are in general much more numerous in the small cell carcinoma. Particular difficulty may be caused by cases of small cell carcinoma in which the tumor cells have abundant eosinophilic cytoplasm. Even in these cases, the tumors usually can be distinguished because the small cell carcinomas have a much more disorderly growth than seen in the JGCT. Additionally, the large cells seen in cases of small cell carcinoma often have a rather distinctive dense, globular cytoplasm, a feature only occasionally seen in the JGCT.

The only metastatic tumor that we have seen confused with a JGCT is metastatic malignant melanoma.[246,460] This is because some malignant melanomas, like many metastatic tumors, contain follicle-like spaces and this metastatic tumor frequently has cells with abundant eosinophilic cytoplasm. This may result in a striking simulation of the solid and follicular pattern of a JGCT. It is helpful clinically that metastatic malignant melanoma is very rare in the first two decades, when approximately 80% of JGCTs are encountered. The clinical history will, of course, be helpful in many cases but as the history of malignant melanoma may be remote, or the primary tumor may have regressed, the possibility of malignant melanoma should be considered when entertaining the diagnosis of JGCT in a patient over 20 years of age. The likelihood of this diagnosis will be heightened if the ovarian tumor is bilateral. Other features of metastatic melanoma discussed in Chapter 22 also may be helpful.

Clinical Behavior and Treatment

Although the JGCT usually appears less well differentiated than the adult type, follow-up data in our series of 125 cases and in the series of others[242,344,440,476] indicate a high cure rate. In contrast to AGCTs, which often recur late, all the clinically malignant juvenile tumors have reappeared within 3 years and several have had a rapid course.[411,454]

In our series the feature of greatest prognostic significance was the stage of the tumor.[454] Only 2 of the 80 stage I tumors for which follow-up information was available were clinically malignant. Rupture did not have an adverse effect on prognosis. Two of the 10 stage IC tumors were malignant; in one of them malignant cells were present on cytological examination of the ascitic fluid. All three stage II tumors were fatal. Although both the mitotic rate and the degree of nuclear atypicality correlated with the prognosis when tumors of all stages were considered, no such correlation was evident when only stage I tumors were evaluated. In conclusion, despite the frequent presence of disquieting features such as severe nuclear atypicality and very high mitotic rates, a JGCT that is confined to the ovary appears to have an excellent prognosis.

In view of the rarity of bilateral ovarian involvement, and their excellent prognosis, stage 1A granulosa cell tumors

can be treated by a unilateral salpingo-oophorectomy. Little experience has accumulated on the role of radiation therapy and chemotherapy in the management of persistent or recurrent tumor, but isolated examples of the efficacy of these modes of therapy have been recorded.[454]

Thecoma

Thecomas can be divided into typical[31,156] and luteinized[200,347,479] forms. The typical thecoma is composed of swollen lipid-laden stromal cells resembling theca cells; varying numbers of fibroblasts usually are present as well. Although differing criteria for the microscopic separation of thecoma and fibroma have resulted in varying estimates of the frequency of these tumors, thecomas are approximately one-third as common as granulosa cell tumors if one includes in the former category only those tumors containing moderate to abundant lipid or those tumors associated with evidence of estrogen secretion. The thecoma occurs at an older average age than the granulosa cell tumor, being very rare before puberty and uncommon before the age of 30 years. In a recent large series 84% of the patients were postmenopausal, with a mean age of 59 years; only 10% of the patients were under 30 years of age.[50] In the same series 60% of the postmenopausal women presented because of uterine bleeding and 21% of the patients had endometrial carcinoma.

Thecomas range in size from small, impalpable tumors to large, solid masses, most of which are 5 to 10 cm in diameter.[31,156] Sectioning typically discloses a solid yellow mass (Fig. 19.20), but in some cases the tumor is white with only focal tinges of yellow; cystic change and foci of hemorrhage and necrosis occur occasionally. Microscopic examination reveals masses of cells, most of which are

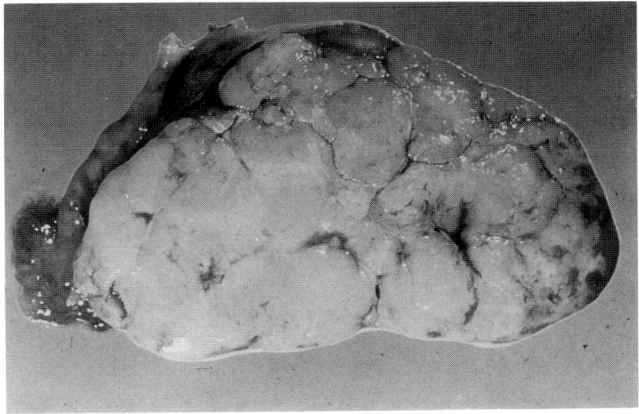

Fig. 19.20. Thecoma. The sectioned surface of the neoplasm is uniformly solid and lobulated. The tumor was yellow in the fresh state.

ill-defined and oval or rounded; the cytoplasm usually is abundant, pale, and vacuolated, containing moderate to abundant amounts of lipid (Fig. 19.21). In occasional cellular thecomas the cytoplasm is less conspicuous. The nuclei vary from round to spindle-shaped and exhibit little or no atypia; mitoses are absent or infrequent. Hyaline plaques often are conspicuous (Fig. 19.21). In thecomas, in contrast to granulosa cell tumors, reticulum fibrils typically surround individual tumor cells (Fig. 19.22).

Typical thecomas are unilateral in 97% of the cases and are almost never malignant. A number of tumors have been reported as "malignant thecomas," but some of these tumors are better interpreted as endocrinologically inactive fibrosarcomas or diffuse granulosa cell tumors.[448] In cases in which the preservation of fertility is important, a thecoma can be treated adequately by oophorectomy. Total hysterectomy with bilateral salpingo-oophorectomy is indicated, however, in most patients who are menopausal or postmenopausal.

Tumors that are predominantly fibromatous or thecomatous but also contain collections of steroid-type cells resembling luteinized theca and luteinized stromal cells have been called *luteinized thecomas* (Fig. 19.23). In our

series of 46 cases of these tumors, half of them were estrogenic, 39% were nonfunctioning, and 11% were androgenic.[479] Two of the four patients with tumors of this type described by Roth and Sternberg[347] also were virilized. This relatively high frequency of masculinization contrasts with its great rarity in association with nonluteinized thecomas. Luteinized thecomas also occur in a younger age group than typical thecomas; although they are most frequent in postmenopausal women, 30% of them have occurred in patients under 30 years of age. When, on rare occasions, crystals of Reinke are identified in the steroid-type cells (Fig. 19.24),[363] the term *stromal Leydig cell tumor* is appropriate.[51,315,400,479] Approximately half these tumors have been virilizing.

Rare luteinized thecomas, some of which have exhibited prominent mitotic activity and most of which have occurred in young women and have been bilateral, have been associated with an unusual fibromatous process on the peritoneum (see Chapter 17, Disease of the Peritoneum). Follow-up to date has suggested that the peritoneal process is reactive rather than neoplastic.[97a]

Fibroma

This tumor, which is composed of spindle cells forming variable amounts of collagen, accounts for 4% of all ovarian tumors. It occurs at all ages,[210] but is most frequent during middle age, with an average age of 48 years; fewer than 10% of the cases are encountered under the age of 30 years.[58,218,287,434] The fibroma is not associated with ste-

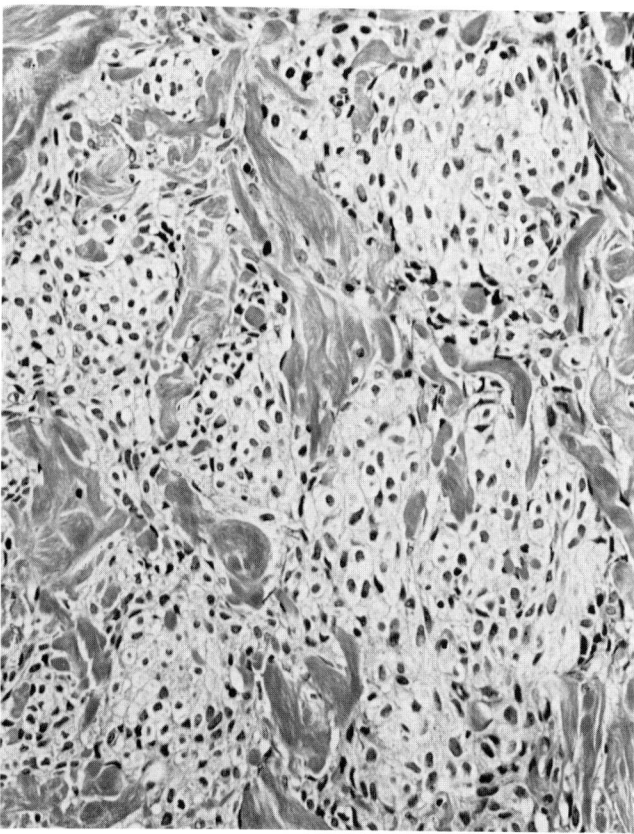

FIG. 19.21. **Thecoma.** The tumor cells have abundant pale cytoplasm. Hyaline plaques are conspicuous. (Reprinted by permission of Young and Scully, ref. 466.)

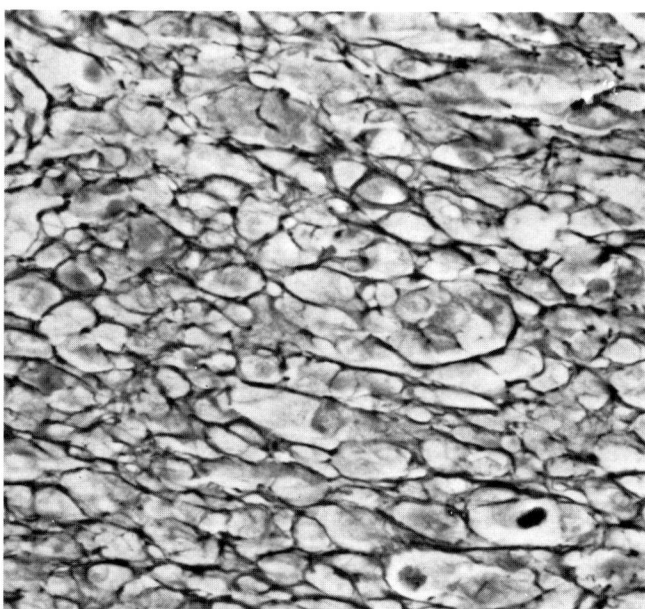

FIG. 19.22. **Thecoma (reticulum stain).** Contrast with reticulum pattern of granulosa cell tumor in Fig. 19.14. (Reprinted by permission of Serov, Scully, and Sobin, ref. 378.)

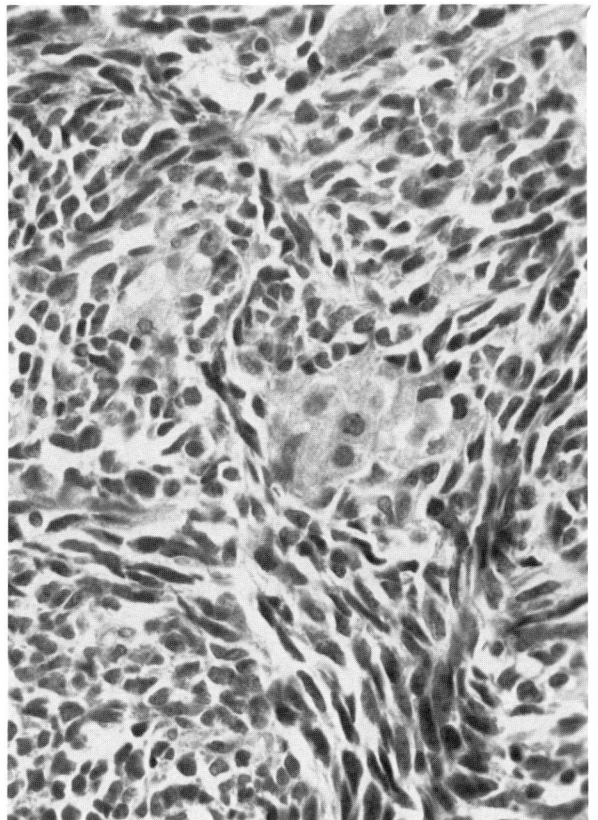

FIG. 19.23. Luteinized thecoma. Luteinized cells are present within a fibromatous background. (Reprinted by permission of Young and Scully, ref. 462.)

roid hormone production but may be accompanied by two unusual clinical syndromes, Meigs' syndrome[272] and the basal cell nevus syndrome (Gorlin's syndrome).[42,65,166,167,332] The former, which complicates about 1% of ovarian fibromas, is defined as ascites and pleural effusion accompanying a fibrous ovarian tumor, usually a fibroma, and disappearing after the removal of the tumor. Ascites alone is present in association with 10–15% of ovarian fibromas larger than 10 cm in diameter.[357] The most widely accepted explanation of Meigs' syndrome is seepage of fluid from the tumor through its serosal surface into the peritoneal cavity, with subsequent passage into one or both pleural cavities either via lymphatics or through a communication between the abdominal and pleural cavity, such as the foramen of Bochdalek.[272]

The hereditary basal cell nevus syndrome is characterized by one or more of the following findings: basal cell carcinomas appearing early in life, keratocysts of the jaw, calcification of the dura, mesenteric cysts, and other less common abnormalities,[165–167,350] as well as ovarian fibromas, which typically are bilateral, multinodular, and calcified (Fig. 19.25).[79] A case of fibrosarcoma of the ovary in a child with the basal cell nevus syndrome has been reported.[232]

Fibromas range in size from microscopic to very large.[122] Very small tumors are not uncommon, and their occurrence probably accounts for the high frequency of such tumors in some series of ovarian neoplasms. For statistical purposes a fibromatous nodule less than 3 cm in diameter should not be considered a true neoplasm. Sectioning of fibromas typically reveals hard, flat, chalky white surfaces that have a whorled appearance. Areas of edema, occasionally with cyst formation, are relatively common (Fig. 19.26). Focal or diffuse calcification and bilaterality

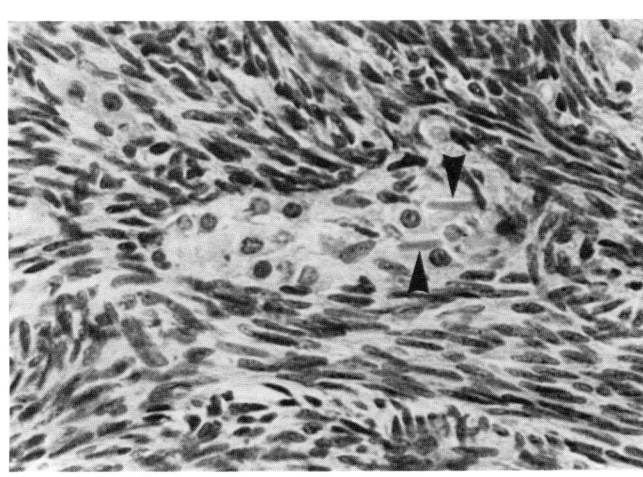

FIG. 19.24. Stromal–Leydig cell tumor. Crystalloids of Reinke (*arrows*) are present within steroid type cells. (Reprinted by permission of Scully, ref. 363.)

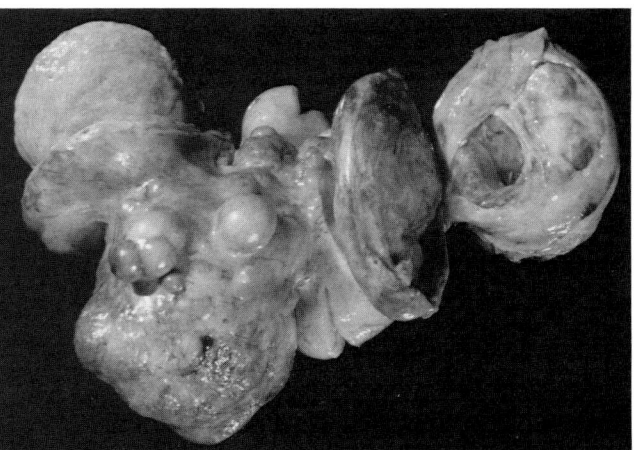

FIG. 19.25. Multinodular Fibroma. The tumor is partly sectioned. The patient had basal cell nevus syndrome. (Reprinted by permission from Case Records of the Massachusetts General Hospital (Case 14-1976); ref. 79.)

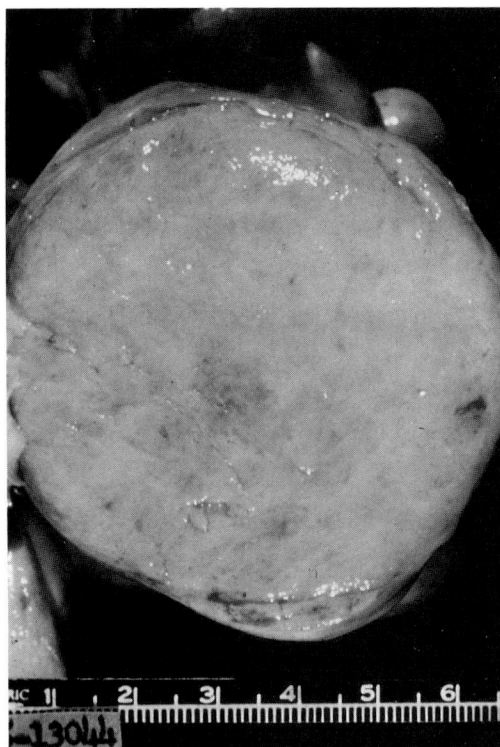

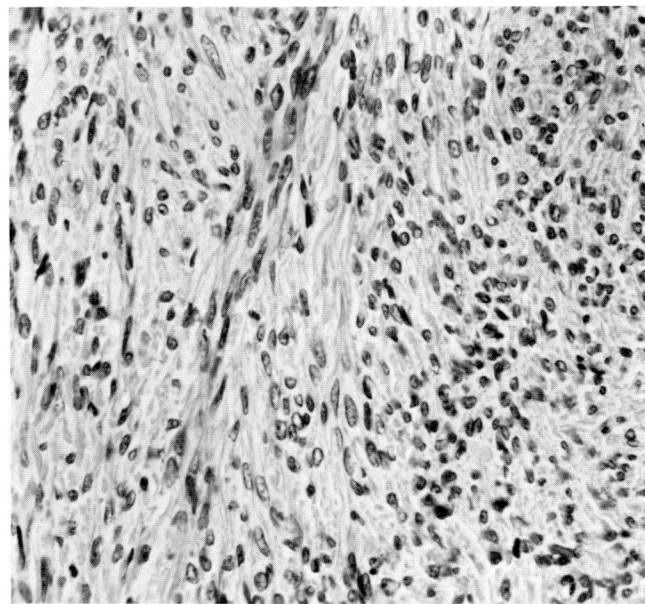

FIG. 19.28. Fibroma. The cells have small, spindle-shaped nuclei lacking atypia or mitotic activity. (Reprinted by permission of Serov, Scully, and Sobin, ref. 378.)

FIG. 19.26. Fibroma. The sectioned surface of the neoplasm is solid. In the fresh state the neoplasm was white and slightly edematous.

are each observed in fewer than 10% of the cases[393] but, as mentioned above, these features are characteristic of the fibromas associated with the basal cell nevus syndrome. Microscopic examination reveals intersecting bundles of spindle cells producing collagen; a storiform pattern often is encountered (Figs. 19.27, 19.28). The presence of bands of hyalinized fibrous tissue is not uncommon. Many tumors

show varying degrees of intercellular edema (Fig. 19.29), which may have a myxoid appearance.[357] The cytoplasm of the neoplastic cells may contain small quantities of lipid. In rare tumors the cytoplasm contains small red granules reminiscent of hyaline bodies, probably representing a degenerative phenomenon. As previously mentioned, an occasional fibroma contains a minor component of sex cord elements (Fig. 19.30).

The fibroma must be distinguished from several nonneoplastic ovarian processes, specifically massive edema, fibromatosis, and stromal hyperplasia. The first two disorders usually are unilateral but may be bilateral, and are

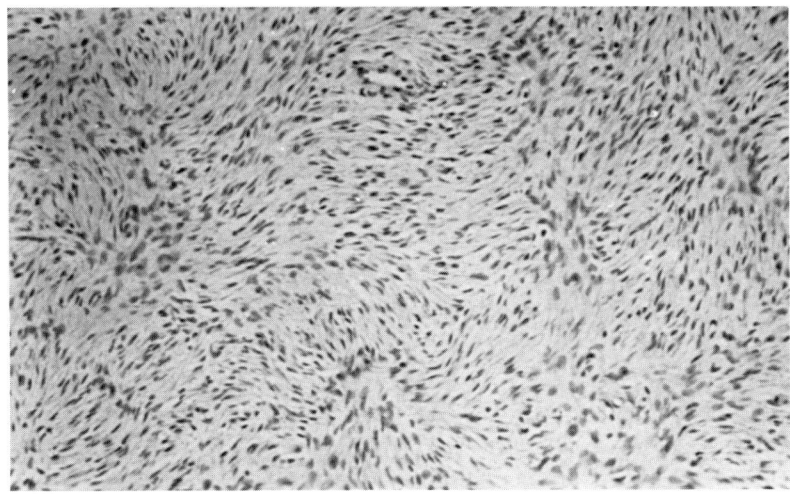

FIG. 19.27. Fibroma. The tumor has a storiform pattern.

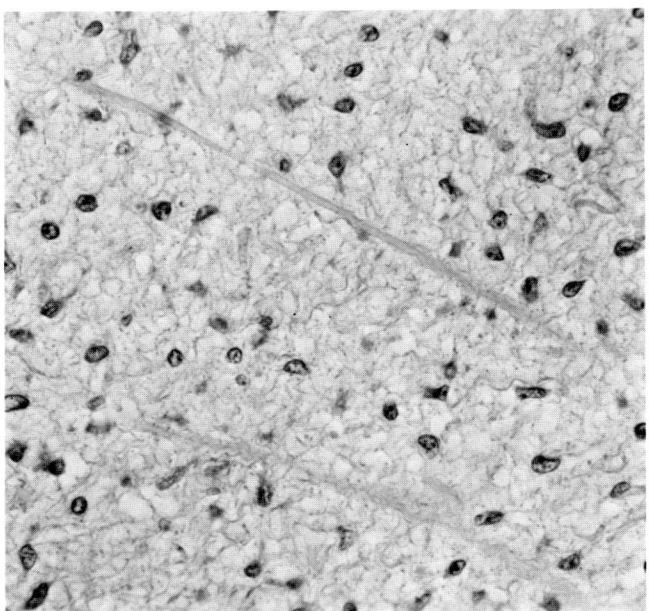

FIG. 19.29. Edematous fibroma. (Reprinted by permission of Serov, Scully, and Sobin, ref. 378.)

characterized by proliferation of ovarian stromal cells with marked intercellular edema and the production of abundant dense collagen, respectively.[467] Unlike fibromas, which almost always displace follicles, corpora lutea, and corpora albicantia, massive edema and fibromatosis encompass these structures. Stromal hyperplasia, in contrast to the ovarian fibroma, is bilateral and is characterized by a multinodular or diffuse proliferation of closely packed, small stromal cells with minimal collagen formation.[57]

Ovarian fibromas are almost always benign, but cellular forms containing an average of 1 to 3 MF/10 HPF and showing no more than slight nuclear atypicality are of low malignant potential (Fig. 19.31), occasionally recurring, particularly if they are adherent or have ruptured.[324] Very rarely, fibromas without any atypical features are associated with peritoneal implants.[249,461] Tumors with an average of 4 or more MF/10 HPF and significant nuclear atypicality are almost always associated with a malignant course and warrant the designation *fibrosarcoma*.[92,324]

Sclerosing Stromal Tumor

This tumor differs from the fibroma and the thecoma both clinically and pathologically. Whereas the latter tumors are uncommon in the first three decades, more than 80% of sclerosing stromal tumors have been encountered during the second and third decades, with an average age at diag-

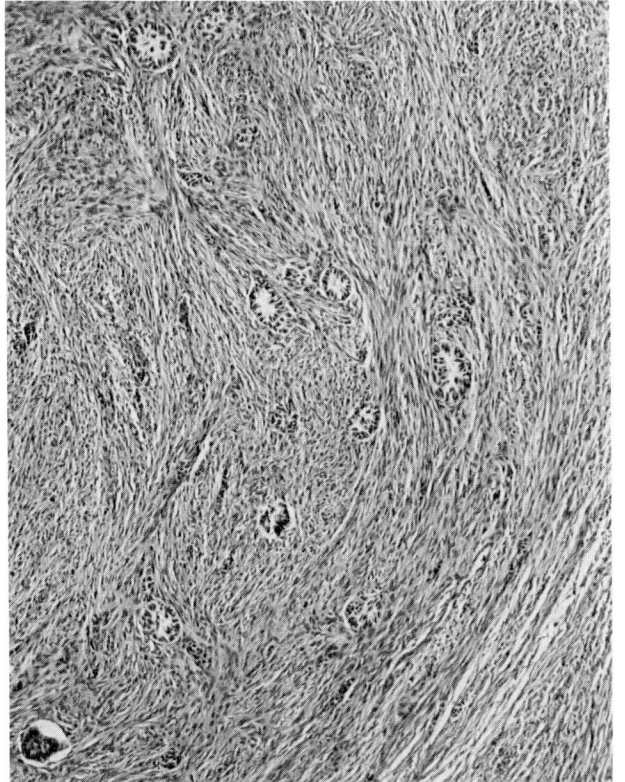

FIG. 19.30. Fibroma with minor sex-cord elements. Sertoliform tubules are scattered within a fibromatous tumor. (Reprinted by permission of Young and Scully, ref. 462.)

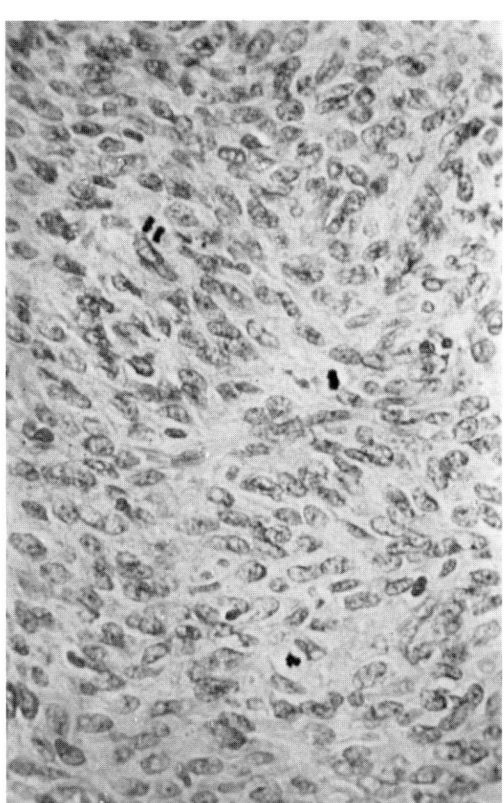

FIG. 19.31. Cellular fibroma. Note mitotic figures.

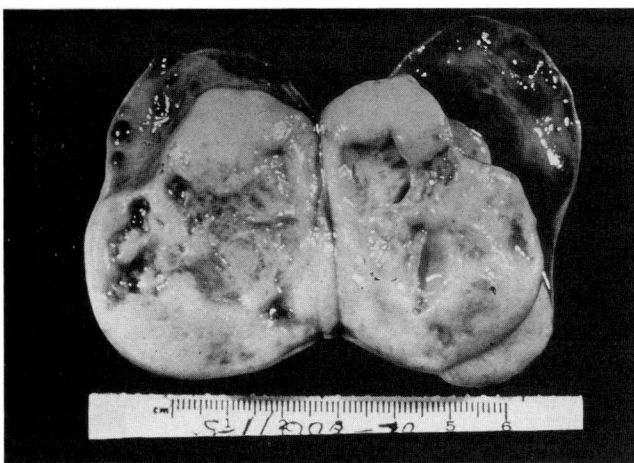

FIG. 19.32. **Sclerosing stroma tumor.** The sectioned surface of the neoplasm is solid and cystic. The solid tissue was white to focally tan.

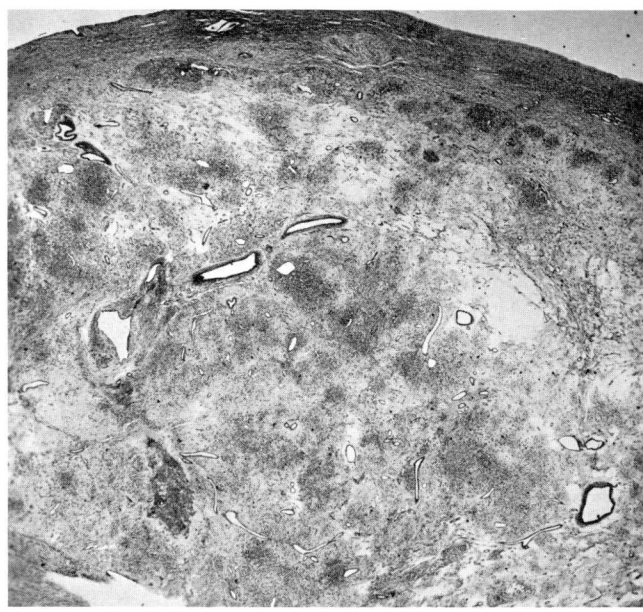

FIG. 19.33. **Sclerosing stromal tumor.** Cellular pseudolobules are separated by edematous hypocellular tumor. (Reprinted by permission of Chalvardjian and Scully, ref. 88.)

nosis of 27 years.[461] In contrast to the thecoma, the sclerosing stromal tumor has been associated with evidence of estrogen secretion in only a few cases[154,418]; in two cases there was evidence of both estrogen and androgen production[108,479] and in three only androgenic manifestations were present.[84,262,331] One of the tumors in the last group that occurred in a pregnant patient was associated with virilization.[84] Another neoplasm was associated with endometrial adenocarcinoma.[223] All sclerosing stromal tumors encountered to date have been benign.°

Gross examination typically reveals a unilateral, discrete, sharply demarcated mass; the neoplasm is rarely bilateral.[204] Its sectioned surface is solid and white but often shows areas of edema and cyst formation and foci of yellow discoloration (Fig. 19.32). A rare specimen presents as a unilocular cyst.[197,429] Microscopic examination discloses a number of distinctive features: a pseudolobular pattern (Fig. 19.33), in which cellular nodules are separated by less cellular areas of densely collagenous or edematous connective tissue; sclerosis within the nodules; prominent thin-walled vessels in some of the nodules (Fig. 19.34); and a disorganized admixture of fibroblasts and rounded, vacuolated cells within the nodules (Fig. 19.35). Occasionally, the vacuolated cells have a signet-cell appearance, creating some confusion with the signet cells of a Krukenberg tumor, but the former cells contain lipid instead of mucin. The lipid-laden cells appear to be inactive or weakly active lutein cells; in the rare functioning tumors the lutein cells resemble more closely those encountered in a luteinized thecoma. Although overlap exists between fibromas, thecomas, sclerosing stromal tumors, and even steroid cell tumors, the presence of various distinctive features of

these four tumors, which are presented in Table 19.6, almost always allows a specific diagnosis.

Unclassified Tumors

Rare tumors in the intermediate zone between fibromas and thecomas are impossible to classify more specifically. Such tumors are made up of cells having some but not all the features of theca cells, containing small to moderate amounts of lipid, and being associated with equivocal evidence of estrogen secretion.

In 1976 Ramzy[333] described an unusual ovarian tumor, which he designated signet-ring stromal tumor, from a 28-year-old woman. Microscopic examination disclosed signet-ring cells that failed to stain for lipid or mucin. Reticulum stains suggested that the neoplastic cells were mesenchymal in origin. No additional examples of this entity have been reported, but we have seen one such tumor from a 34-year-old woman. The nature of the tumor and its vacuoles remains unclear.

Sertoli–Stromal Cell Tumors (Androblastomas)

Sertoli–stromal cell tumors contain Sertoli cells, Leydig cells, fibroblasts, or all of these cells, in varying proportions and varying degrees of differentiation. Because the less well-differentiated neoplasms within this category may recapitulate the development of the testis, the terms *androblastomas* and *arrhenoblastomas* have been used as synonyms. However, the connotation of masculinization associated with the latter designations is misleading be-

---

°Refs. 88,108,154,197,262,331,352,379,404,418,432,475.

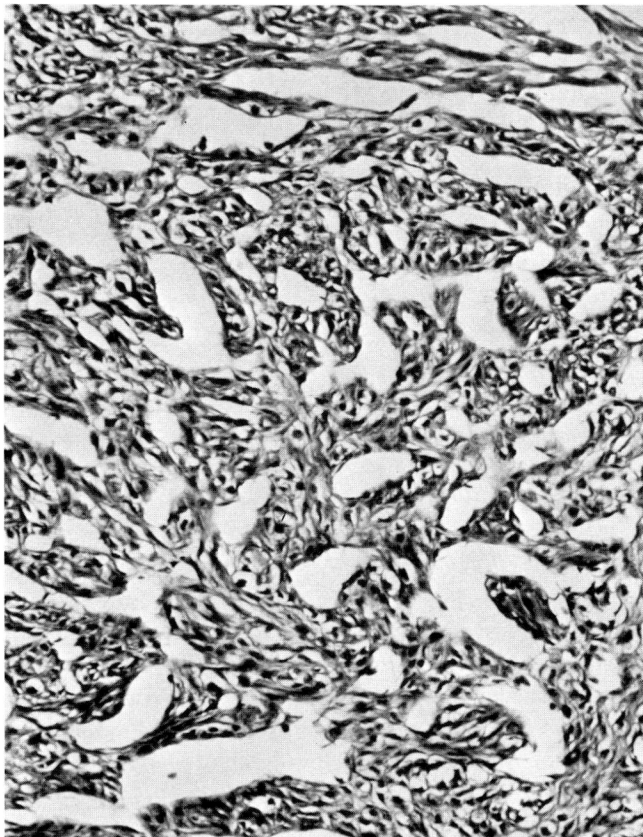

FIG. 19.34. **Sclerosing stromal tumor.** Pseudolobule is richly vascularized. (Reprinted by permission of Chalvardjian and Scully, ref. 88.)

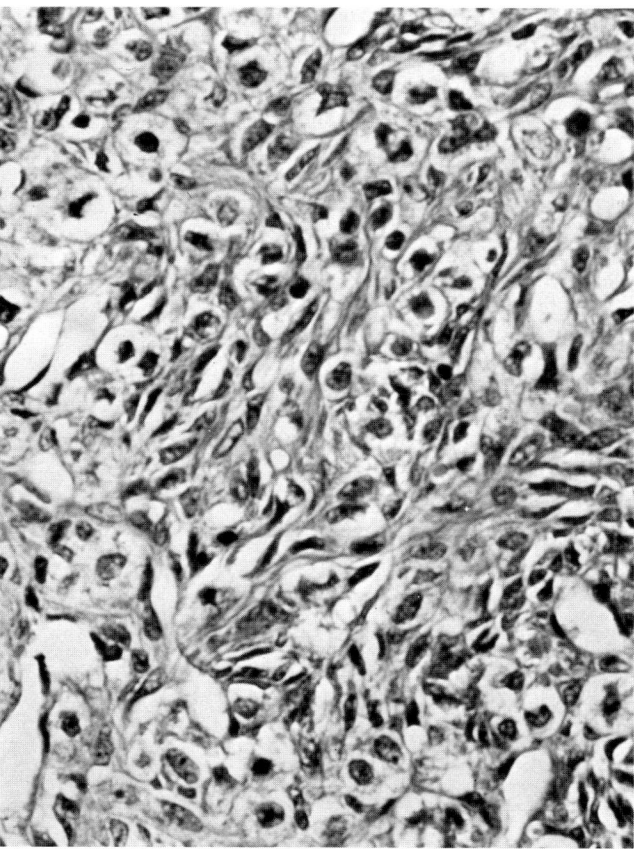

FIG. 19.35. **Sclerosing stromal tumor.** Spindle cells are mixed with large rounded vacuolated cells. (Reprinted by permission of Chalvardjian and Scully, ref. 88.)

cause many tumors in this category have no endocrine manifestations and a few are estrogenic or progestagenic. Nevertheless, the WHO has selected *androblastomas* as an alternative term for these tumors.[378] Other tumors within this group are pure Sertoli cell tumors, pure Leydig cell tumors, and stromal Leydig cell tumors; the latter already have been mentioned in the discussion of luteinized thecomas, and pure Leydig cell tumors are considered in the section on steroid cell tumors.

Sertoli Cell Tumors

Sertoli cell tumors account for approximately 4% of Sertoli–stromal cell tumors.[420,422–424,465] They are characterized by a predominant pattern of hollow (Fig. 19.36) or solid tubules (Figs. 19.37, 19.38), usually dispersed within a fibrous stroma that contains no Leydig cells or very few of them. When the Sertoli cells contain abundant cytoplasmic lipid (Figs. 19.37, 19.38), the term *lipid-rich Sertoli cell tumor* is appropriate. This tumor had been interpreted initially as a lipid-rich granulosa cell tumor and designated folliculome lipidique.[91] Occasional Sertoli cell tumors have

cells with abundant eosinophilic cytoplasm.[141a] Seven Sertoli cell tumors, most or all of which appear to have been of the lipid-rich type, have resulted in isosexual pseudoprecocity. Two of these tumors were from patients with Peutz-Jeghers syndrome.[391,465] One Sertoli cell tumor was associated with progesterone as well as estrogen production.[431] All the Sertoli cell tumors reported to date have been unilateral and stage I. They have averaged approximately 9 cm in diameter and typically formed lobulated, solid, yellow or brown masses. Microscopic examination usually discloses little if any nuclear atypia or mitotic activity, and the prognosis is excellent. Rare tumors exhibiting moderate degrees of nuclear atypicality occur, however, and we have seen one example in a sexually precocious child that was focally poorly differentiated, metastasized distantly, and was rapidly fatal.[465]

Sertoli–Leydig Cell Tumors

Sertoli–Leydig cell tumors account for less than 0.5% of all ovarian tumors but are among the most interesting from both pathological and clinical viewpoints.[157,306,310,342,477]

Table 19.6. Sclerosing versus other stromal tumors and steroid cell tumors

	Sclerosing stromal tumor	Fibroma	Thecoma	Steroid cell tumor
Age	80% under 30 yrs		10% under 30 yrs	25% under 30 yrs
Function	Almost always absent	Absent	Typically estrogenic[a]	Typically androgenic
Gross variegation	Yes	No	No	No
Pseudolobulation	Yes	Rare	Rare	No
Prominent ectatic vessels	Yes	Rare	Rare	Rare
Two cell types	Yes	No	Only in luteinized form	No
Hyaline plaques	No	Common	Common	No
Behavior	Benign	Almost always benign	Almost always benign	Often malignant

[a] Luteinized form androgenic in 11% cases.

They have been divided into six subtypes by the WHO: well differentiated, of intermediate differentiation, poorly differentiated, with heterologous elements, retiform, and mixed. Sertoli–Leydig cell tumors occur in all age groups but are encountered most often in young women. In our series of more than 200 cases, the average age was 25 years; 75% of the patients were 30 years of age or younger and only 9.5% were over 50 years of age.[473] The average age in the two other large series was 24 and 24.5 years.[342,477] The well-differentiated tumors[472] occur on an average a decade later, and retiform tumors,[464] a decade earlier than other Sertoli–Leydig cell tumors. Tumors with a retiform pattern are more common in the first decade than any other subtype.

CLINICAL FEATURES

Although the most striking mode of presentation of Sertoli–Leydig cell tumors is virilization, it develops in only about one-third of the cases.[473] In such cases a patient who has been having normal menstrual periods typically begins to have oligomenorrhea, followed within a few months by

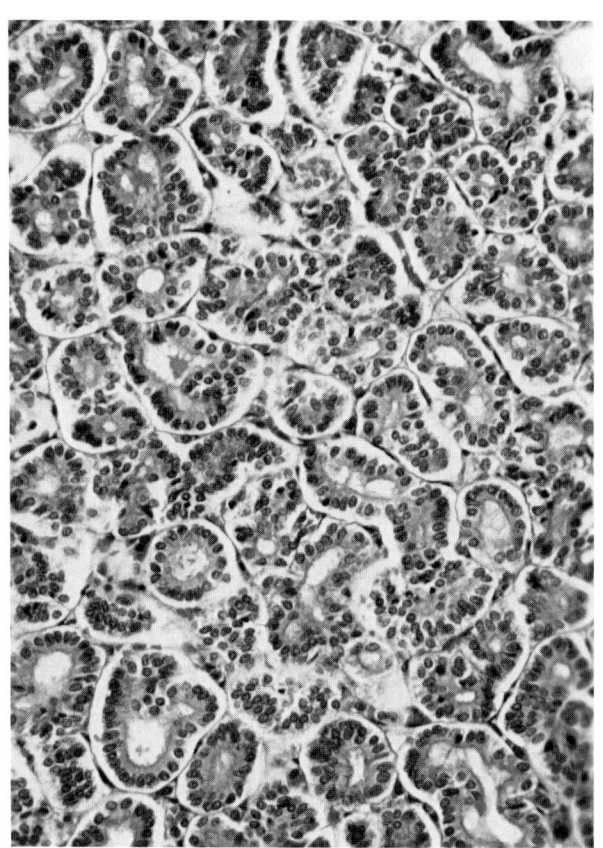

Fig. 19.36. Sertoli cell tumor. Closely packed hollow tubules lined by well-differentiated cuboidal to columnar epithelial cells. (Reprinted by permission of Young and Scully, ref. 465.)

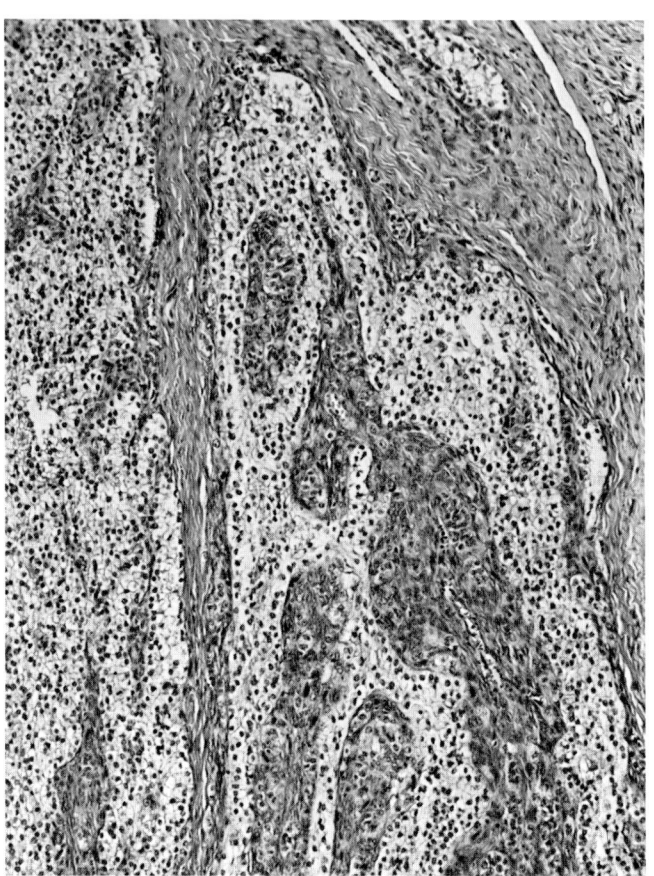

Fig. 19.37. Sertoli cell tumor, lipid rich. (Reprinted by permission of Serov, Scully, and Sobin, ref. 378.)

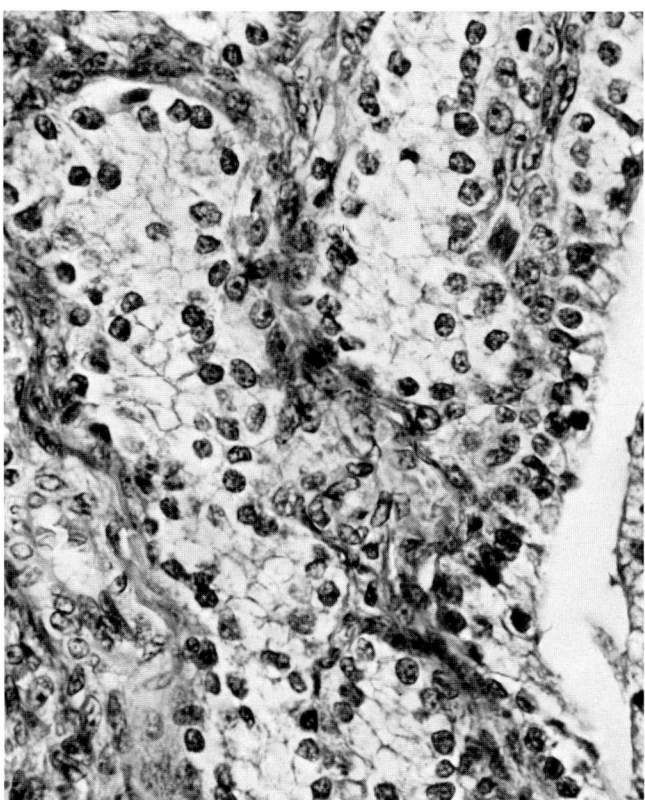

FIG. 19.38. **Sertoli cell tumor, lipid rich.** (Reprinted by permission of Serov, Scully, and Sobin, ref. 378.)

amenorrhea. There is a concomitant loss of female secondary sex characteristics, with atrophy of the breasts and disappearance of normal bodily contours. Progressive masculinization is heralded by acne, with hirsutism, temporal balding, deepening of the voice, and enlargement of the clitoris following in its wake. The androgen secretion by the tumor also may result in erythrocytosis. Although two studies[310,342] reported an increased frequency of androgenic changes in association with less well-differentiated tumors, there was no significant difference in the frequency of these manifestations among the various subtypes in our series except that it was lower with tumors containing heterologous elements and lowest with tumors having a prominent retiform component.[473]

Plasma levels of testosterone, androstenedione, and other androgens, alone or in combination, may be elevated in patients with Sertoli–Leydig cell tumors.[313,329] The urinary 17-ketosteroid values usually are normal or only slightly raised, although occasionally a high level has been recorded. These findings are in contrast to those associated with virilizing adrenal tumors, which often are accompanied by high urinary levels of 17-ketosteroids.[160] The values for plasma androgens and urinary 17-ketosteroids are not reliable, however, in the differentiation of ovarian and adrenal virilizing tumors because the latter often are associated with elevated testosterone and normal urinary 17-ketosteroid levels.[5] Also, tests involving attempted stimulation by tropic hormones and suppression by gonadal and adrenocortical steroids have not proved decisive in differentiating these tumors.[216] Approximately 20 Sertoli–Leydig cell tumors associated with elevated plasma levels of alpha-fetoprotein have been reported,[38,93,151,257,414,427] but values as high as those accompanying yolk sac tumors are rare.[414,456] Rare tumors have arisen in patients with a chromosomal abnormality.[162]

Approximately 50% of patients with Sertoli–Leydig cell tumors have no endocrine manifestations, and usually complain of abdominal swelling or pain.[473] Occasional tumors have been associated with various estrogenic syndromes, including irregular menses, menorrhagia or menometrorrhagia in women in the reproductive age group, and postmenopausal bleeding in older women.[115,473] No well documented case of a Sertoli–Leydig cell tumor associated with isosexual precocity has been reported.

At laparotomy almost all Sertoli–Leydig cell tumors are unilateral; in our series only 1.5% were bilateral.[473] Rare tumors are asynchronously bilateral.[289] The tumors are stage Iai in about 80% of the cases; in 12% the tumor has either ruptured or involved the external surface of the ovary and in 4% ascites is present. Only about 2.5% of the tumors have spread beyond the ovary, usually within the pelvis and rarely into the upper abdomen. All the well-differentiated tumors in our series were stage Ia; the poorly differentiated tumors more often were ruptured or presented at a higher stage than the tumors of intermediate differentiation.

Pathologic Findings

Sertoli–Leydig cell tumors vary as greatly in their gross appearance as granulosa cell tumors and these neoplasms cannot be distinguished on gross examination alone. There are, however, a few general differences. Sertoli–Leydig cell tumors contain blood-filled cysts less often than granulosa cell tumors and, unlike the latter, almost never have the appearance of a unilocular thin-walled cyst. Sertoli–Leydig cell tumors vary in size from microscopic to huge masses but most are between 5 and 15 (average 13.5) cm in diameter (Fig. 19.39). Poorly differentiated tumors including those with mesenchymal heterologous elements tend to be larger than those of better differentiation and contain areas of hemorrhage and necrosis more frequently (Fig. 19.40). Tumors with heterologous or retiform components are cystic more often than tumors without these elements. The heterologous tumors occasionally simulate mucinous cystic tumors on gross examination (Fig. 19.41) and retiform tumors may contain large, edematous papillae, resembling serous papillary tumors (Fig. 19.42).

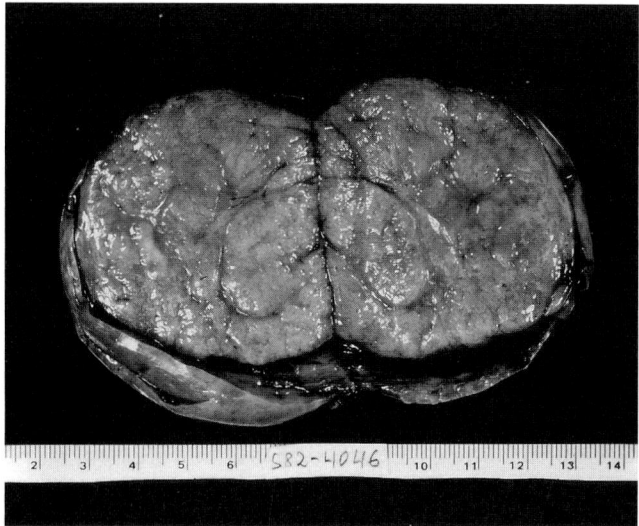

Fig. 19.39. Sertoli–Leydig cell tumor. The sectioned surface of the neoplasm is solid and lobulated. The neoplasm was yellow in the fresh state.

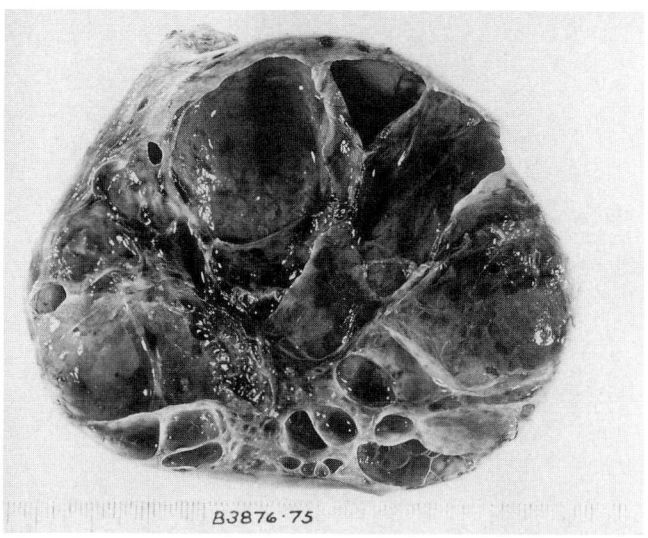

Fig. 19.41. Sertoli–Leydig cell tumor with mucinous heterologous elements. The sectioned surface of the tumor displays a multiloculated cystic neoplasm. (Reproduced by permission of Young et al., ref. 458.)

Well-differentiated Sertoli–Leydig Cell Tumor

These tumors are characterized by a predominantly tubular pattern (Fig. 19.43).[472] On low-power examination a nodular architecture often is conspicuous, with fibrous bands separating lobules composed of hollow or less often solid tubules; in some tumors tubules of both types are present. The hollow tubules typically are round to oval and small, but may be cystically dilated, and some of them resemble the tubular glands of a well-differentiated endometrioid adenocarcinoma.[109] The lumens usually are

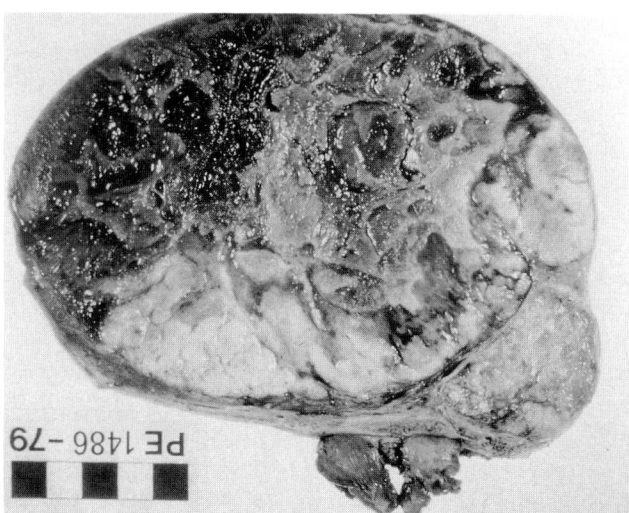

Fig. 19.40. Sertoli–Leydig cell tumor with mesenchymal heterologous elements. The sectioned surface of the tumor exhibits extensive areas of hemorrhage and necrosis. (Reproduced by permission of Prat et al., ref. 325.)

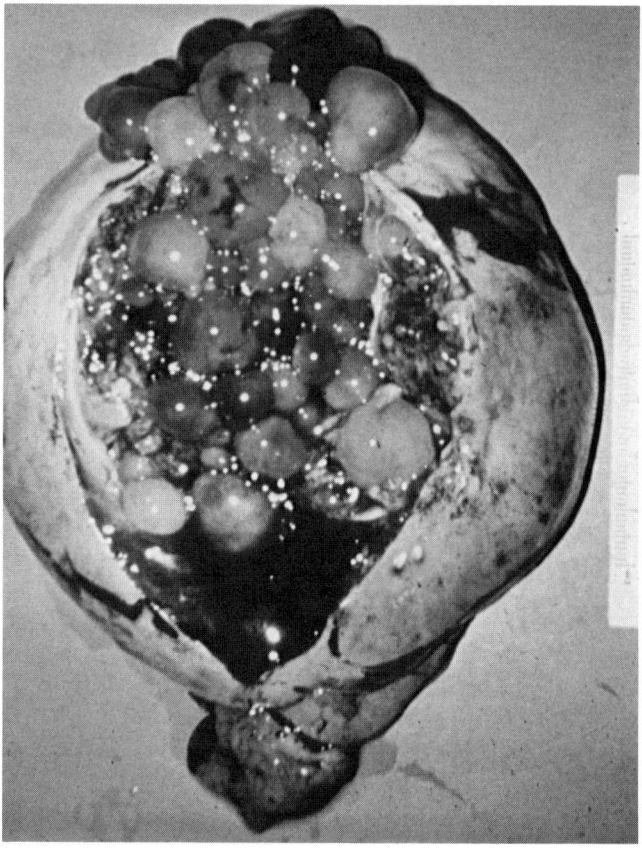

Fig. 19.42. Sertoli–Leydig cell tumor with retiform pattern. Edematous polypoid structures project into lumen of cystic neoplasm. (Reprinted by permission of Young and Scully, ref. 464.)

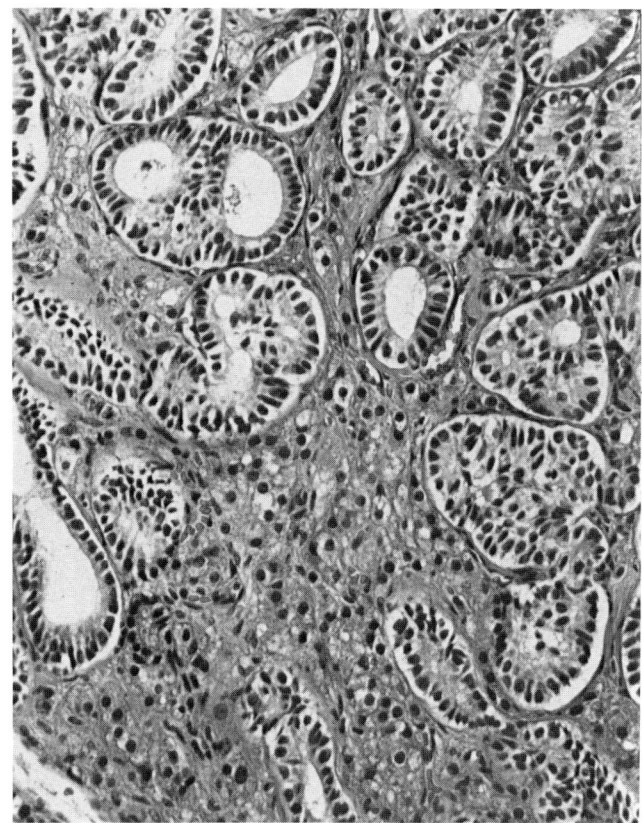

FIG. 19.43. Sertoli–Leydig cell tumor, well-differentiated. Hollow tubules separated by Leydig cells in intervening stroma. (Reprinted by permission of Young and Scully, ref. 472.)

devoid of conspicuous secretion but in some cases eosinophilic fluid, which is occasionally mucicarminophilic, is present. The solid tubules typically are elongated but may be round or oval, and occasionally resemble prepubertal or atrophic testicular tubules. The tubules contain cuboidal to columnar epithelial cells with round or oblong nuclei without prominent nucleoli. Nuclear atypicality usually is absent or minimal and mitotic figures are rare. The cells lining the hollow tubules and filling the solid tubules typically contain moderate amounts of dense cytoplasm but in some cases varying numbers of them have abundant pale cytoplasm rich in lipid. The stromal component consists of bands of mature fibrous tissue containing variable but usually conspicuous numbers of Leydig cells. These cells may contain abundant lipochrome pigment; in our series crystals of Reinke were identified in some of the Leydig cells in approximately 20% of the cases (Fig. 19.44).[472]

SERTOLI–LEYDIG CELL TUMORS OF INTERMEDIATE AND POOR DIFFERENTIATION

These tumors form a continuum characterized by a variety of patterns and combinations of cell types. Some tumors exhibit intermediate differentiation in some areas and poor differentiation in others and, less commonly, tumors of intermediate differentiation contain well differentiated foci. Either the Sertoli cells or Leydig cells or both may exhibit varying degrees of immaturity. In the tumors of intermediate differentiation, immature Sertoli cells with

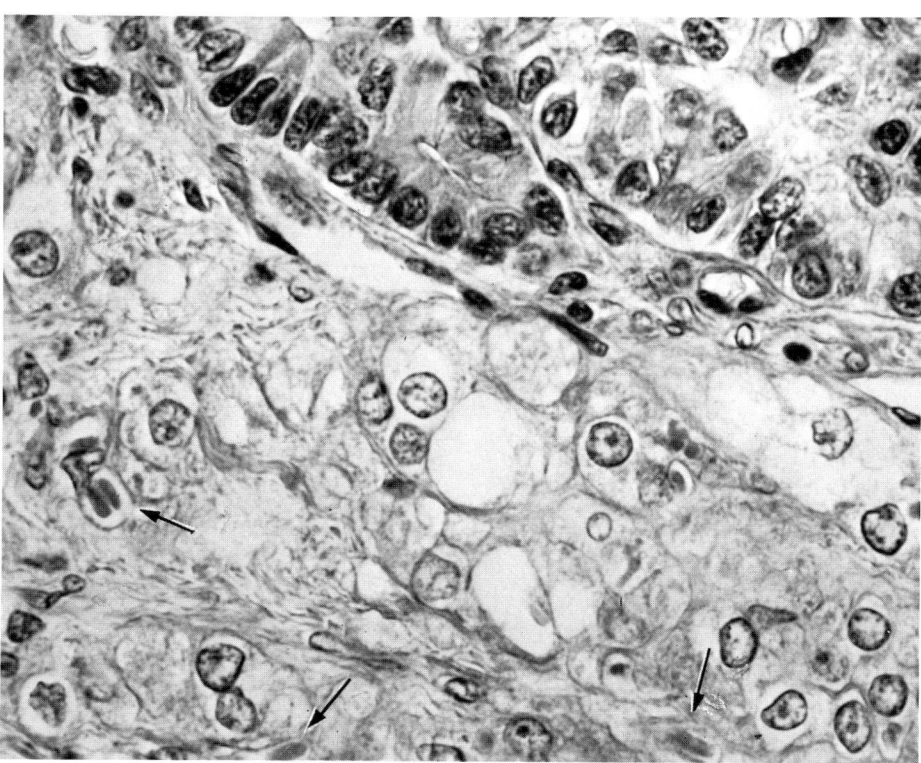

FIG. 19.44. Sertoli–Leydig cell tumor, well-differentiated. *Arrows* point to crystals of Reinke. (Reprinted by permission of Scully, ref. 475.)

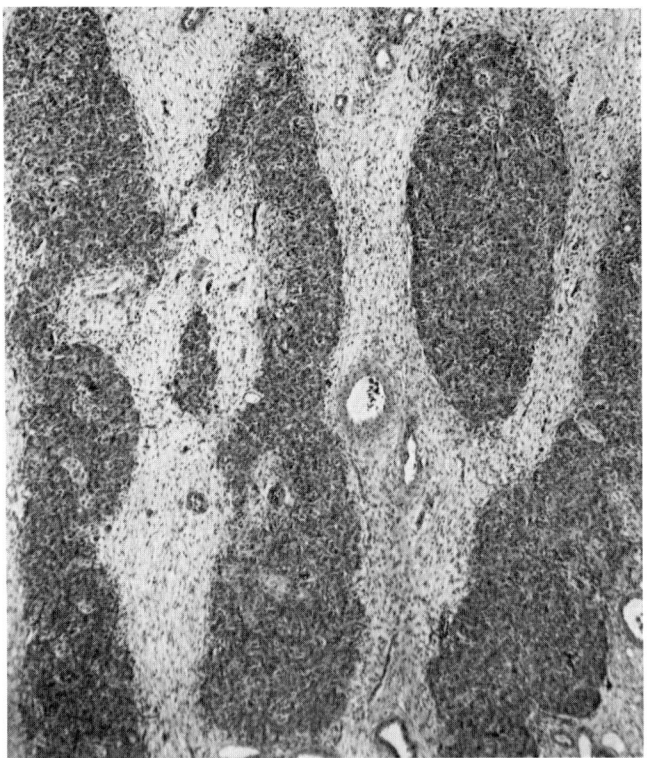

FIG. 19.45. Sertoli–Leydig cell tumor of intermediate differentiation. Cellular lobules are intersected by slightly edematous stromal component. (Reprinted by permission of Young and Scully, ref. 473.)

small, round, oval, or angular nuclei are arranged typically in ill-defined masses, often creating a lobulated appearance on low power (Fig. 19.45); solid and hollow tubules (Fig. 19.46), nests, thin cords resembling the sex cords of the embryonic testis (Fig. 19.47), and broad columns of Sertoli cells (Fig. 19.48) often are present. Cysts containing eosinophilic secretion may create a thyroid-like appearance and follicle-like spaces are encountered rarely. The Sertoli cells, or the Leydig cells, may have bizarre nuclei similar to those seen in some granulosa cell tumors.[463] The Sertoli cell aggregates are separated by a stromal component that ranges from fibromatous to densely cellular to edematous, and typically contain clusters of well-differentiated Leydig cells. Occasionally, part or all of the stromal component is made up of immature, cellular mesenchymal tissue resembling a nonspecific sarcoma. The Sertoli and Leydig cell elements, singly or together, may contain varying and sometimes large amounts of lipid in the form of small or large droplets (Fig. 19.49). Poorly differentiated Sertoli–Leydig cell tumors originally were classified as sarcomatoid because, aside from the presence of specifically diagnostic elements, they resemble fibrosarcomas (Fig. 19.50); however, they often have a diffuse pattern that is not clearly recognizable as that of a fibrosarcoma.

Retiform Sertoli–Leydig Cell Tumor

Fifteen percent of Sertoli-Leydig cell tumors are composed usually partially but occasionally entirely of tubular structures arranged in a pattern resembling that of the rete testis.[345,366,413,464] So far a retiform pattern has been encountered only in tumors that are otherwise intermediate, poorly differentiated, or heterologous. Microscopic examination reveals a network of irregularly branching, elongated, narrow, often slit-like tubules and cysts, into which papillae or polypoid structures may project (Fig. 19.51). The tubules and cysts may contain eosinophilic secretion. They are lined by epithelial cells that exhibit varying degrees of stratification and nuclear atypicality. The papillae and polyps are of three types. Most commonly they are small and rounded or blunt, often containing hyalinized cores (Fig. 19.52). Sometimes they are large and bulbous, containing edematous cores. Finally, in some cases they are delicate and branch extensively and may be lined by stratified cells, simulating the papillae of a serous tumor of borderline or invasive type (Fig. 19.53). A common finding in the retiform Sertoli–Leydig cell tumor is the presence of columns or ribbons of immature Sertoli cells. The stroma within a retiform area may be hyalinized or edematous, moderately cellular or densely cellular, and immature.

HETEROLOGOUS SERTOLI–LEYDIG CELL TUMOR

Heterologous elements occur in approximately 20% of the Sertoli–Leydig cell tumors, most of which are otherwise of intermediate differentiation, but some of which are poorly differentiated.[22,325,458] In our series of more than 200 tumors, 18% contained glands and cysts lined by moderately to well-differentiated gastric-type or intestinal-type epithelium (Fig. 19.54). Intestinal-type epithelium at times may contain goblet cells, argentaffin cells, and rarely Paneth cells. Sixteen percent of the heterologous Sertoli–Leydig cell tumors had one or a few microscopic foci of carcinoid tumor (Fig. 19.55).[447,458] Stromal heterologous elements, encountered in 5% of all Sertoli–Leydig cell tumors,[172,201,325] include islands of cartilage arising on a sarcomatous background, areas of embryonal rhabdomyosar-

---

▷

FIG. 19.46. Sertoli–Leydig cell tumor of intermediate differentiation. The tubules in this neoplasm resemble those of an endometrioid tumor.

FIG. 19.47. Sertoli–Leydig cell tumor of intermediate differentiation. Cords of immature Sertoli cells and clusters of Leydig cells with abundant cytoplasm. (Reprinted by permission of Young and Scully, ref. 464.)

FIG. 19.48. Sertoli–Leydig cell tumor of intermediate differention. Anastomosing columns of immature Sertoli cells. (Reprinted by permission of Young and Scully, ref. 473.)

FIG. 19.49. Sertoli–Leydig cell tumor of intermediate differentiation. Nests of Leydig cells with large lipid vacuoles. (Reprinted by permission of Young and Scully, ref. 473.)

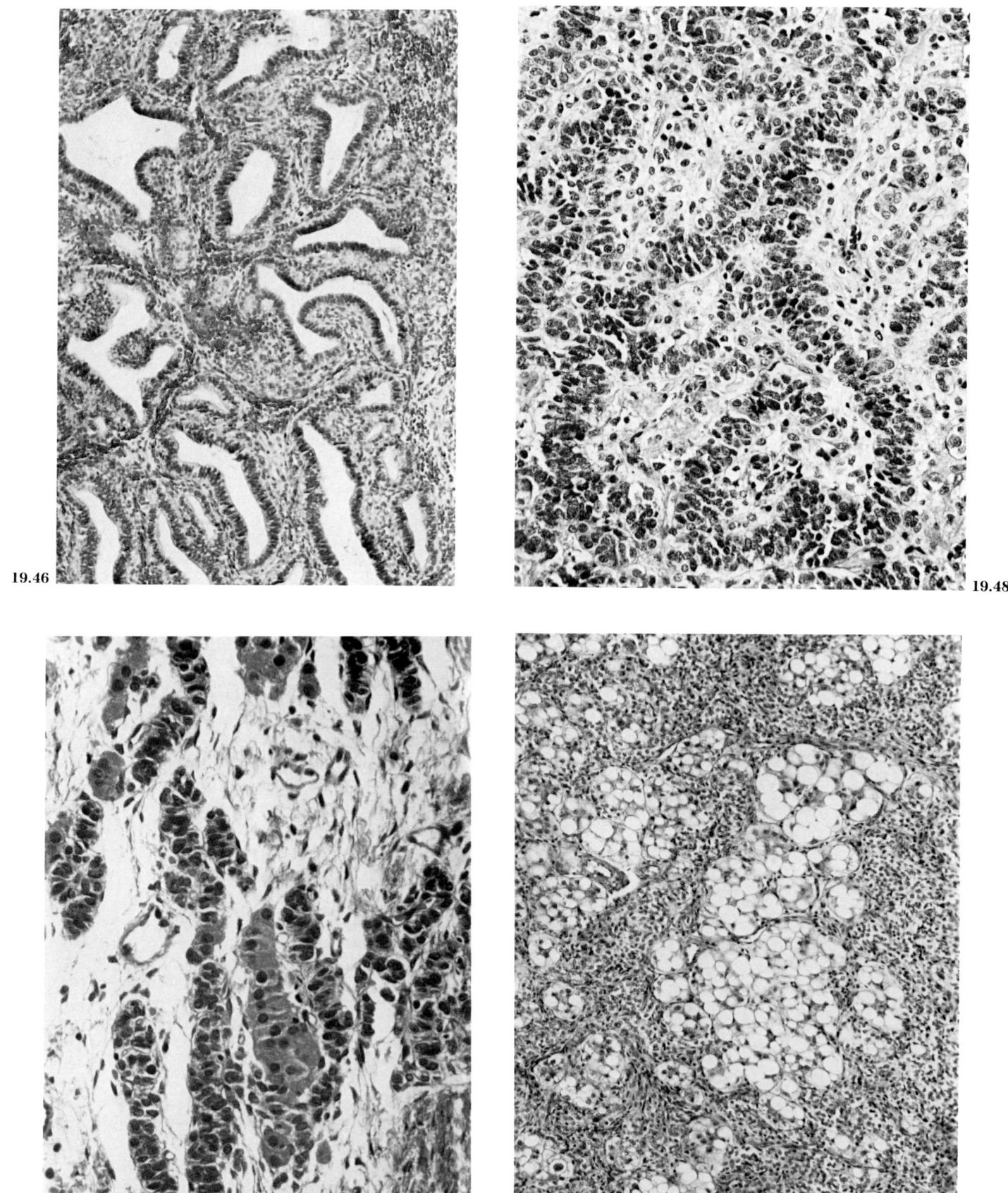

19.46

19.47

19.48

19.49

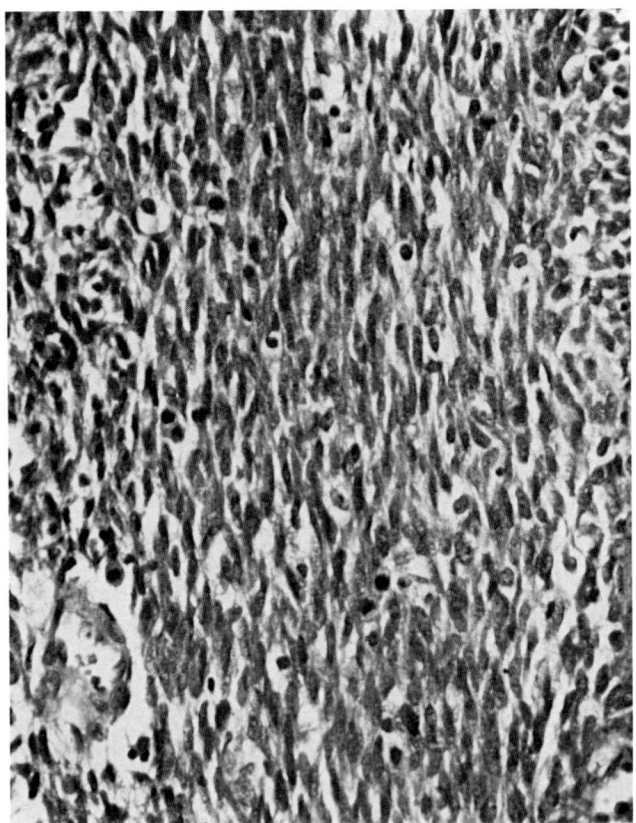

FIG. 19.50. Sertoli–Leydig cell tumor, poorly differentiated. The tumor cells are spindle-shaped and exhibit nuclear
atypia and mitotic activity. ×400. (Reprinted by permission of
Young and Scully, ref. 473.)

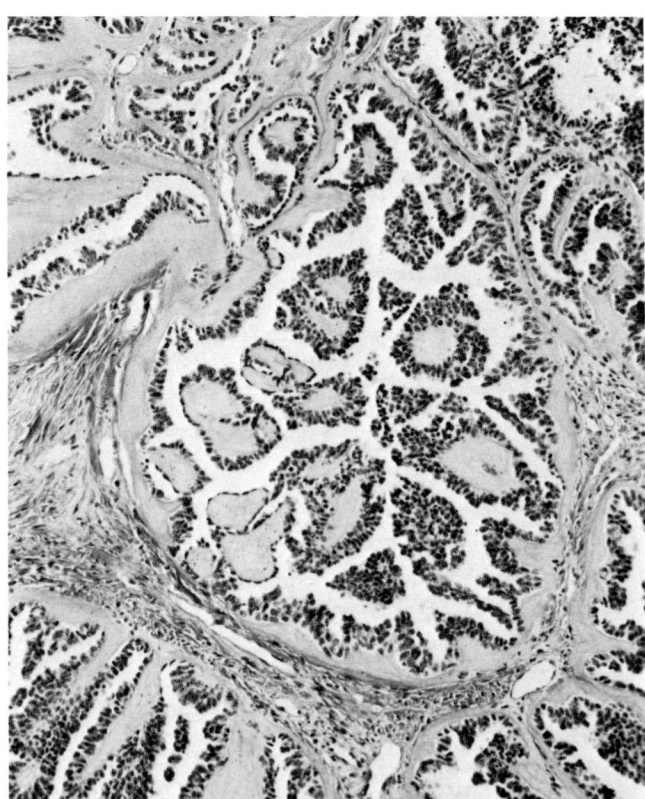

FIG. 19.52. Sertoli–Leydig cell tumor with retiform pattern. The papillae have prominent hyalinized cores and are lined
by stratified epithelial cells. (Reprinted by permission of Young
and Scully (1985) Ovarian sex cord-stromal and steroid cell tumors. In: Roth LM, Czernobilsky B (eds) Tumors and Tumor-
like Conditions of the Ovary. Contemporary Issues in Surgical
Pathology, Vol. 6. New York: Churchill Livingstone.)

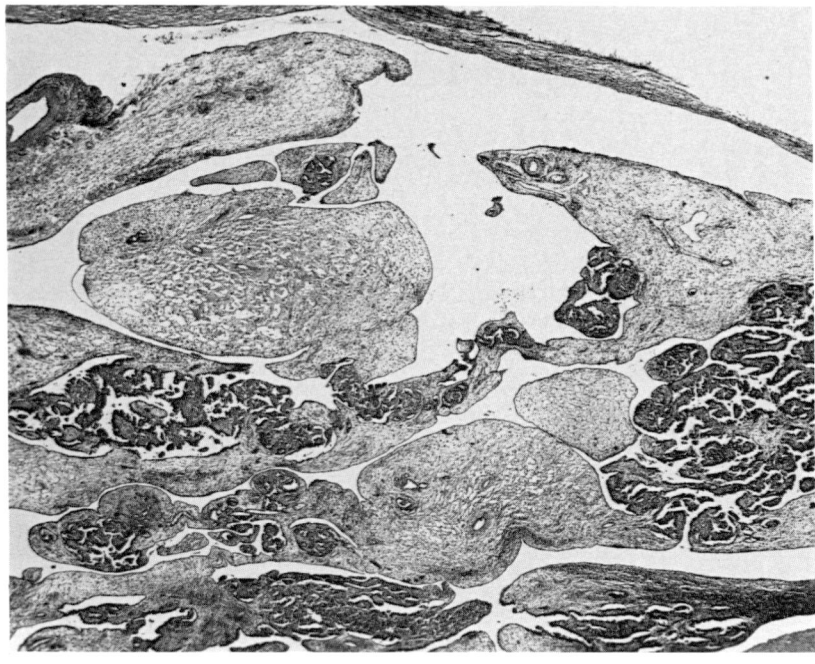

FIG. 19.51. Sertoli–Leydig cell tumor with
retiform pattern. Large edematous polypoid
structures and many small papillae. (Reprinted
by permission of Young and Scully, ref. 464.)

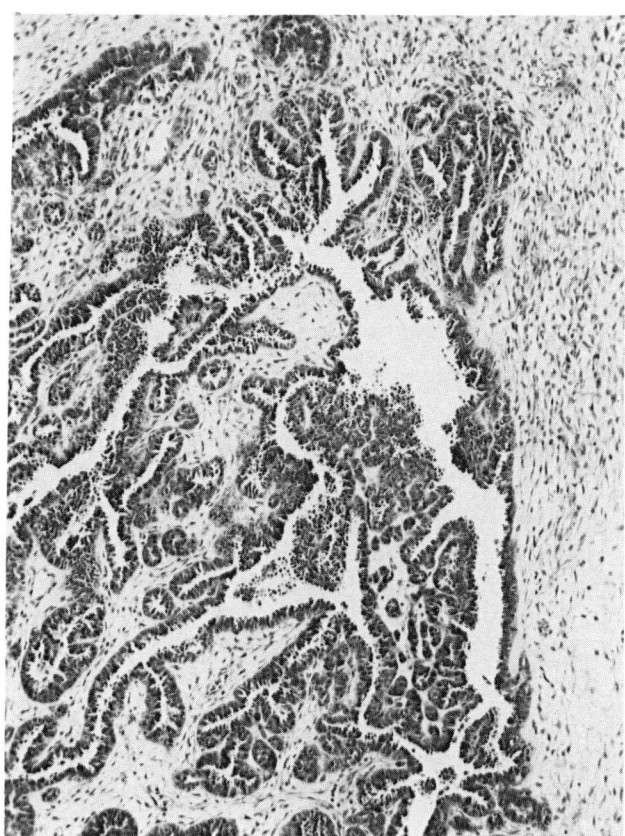

FIG. 19.53. Sertoli–Leydig cell tumor with retiform pattern. A complex papillary pattern simulates a serous papillary adenocarcinoma.

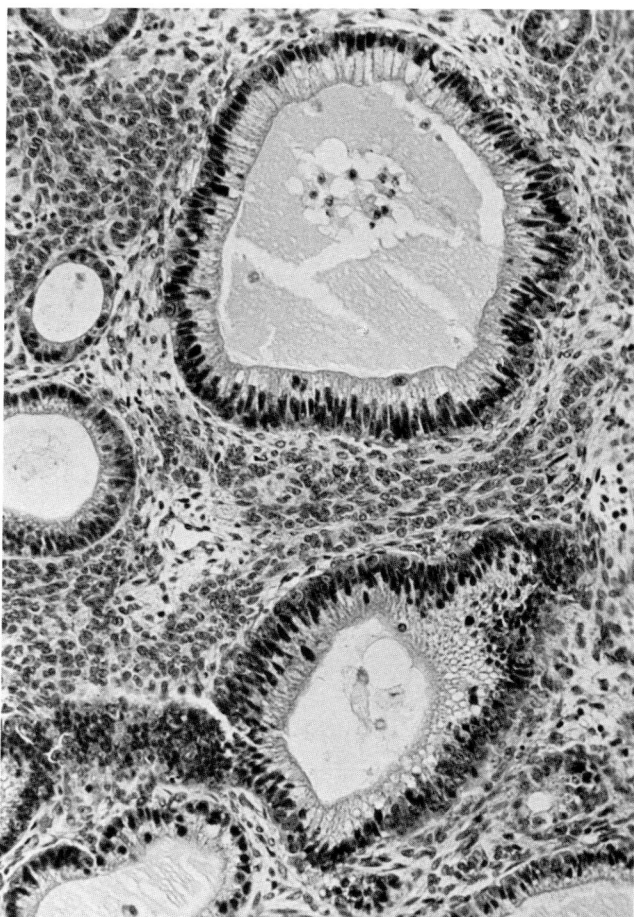

FIG. 19.54. Sertoli–Leydig cell tumor with heterologous elements. Mucinous glands are separated by intermediate form of tumor. (Reprinted by permission of Serov, Scully, and Sobin, ref. 378.)

coma, or both (Fig. 19.56). We also have seen one heterologous tumor that contained cells resembling hepatocytes,[456] one containing retinal tissue, and another with neuroblastoma, in a recurrent tumor.[325] Despite the variety of unexpected tissues in heterologous Sertoli–Leydig cell tumors, it appears unlikely that such neoplasms are of germ cell origin[334] inasmuch as neither Sertoli nor Leydig cells have ever been identified in gonadal tumors clearly recognizable as teratomas.

DIFFERENTIAL DIAGNOSIS

Because of their many patterns, Sertoli–stromal cell tumors often are difficult to differentiate from tumors outside the sex cord–stromal category as well as from granulosa cell tumors. The small hollow tubular structures, solid tubular aggregates, and cords that occasionally are seen in endometrioid carcinomas may closely mimic structures characteristically encountered in Sertoli and Sertoli–Leydig cell tumors.[343,457] Endometrioid carcinomas also may contain luteinized stromal cells that resemble Leydig cells, creating an even greater problem in differentiation. At least some of the glands of endometrioid carcinomas, however, usually are larger than the tubules of Sertoli–Leydig

cell tumors and are lined by epithelium that is less well differentiated. In addition, mucin secretion, areas of squamous differentiation, which range from nests of uniform immature spindle-shaped epithelial cells to morules to keratinizing foci, and an adenofibromatous component of common epithelial type are present in most endometrioid carcinomas, facilitating their diagnosis. Clinical features, such as the much older age of the patient and the absence of androgenic manifestations, support the diagnosis of endometrioid carcinoma,[457] but it must be emphasized that endometrioid carcinomas occasionally have a functioning stroma, which sometimes is manifested clinically by estrogenic changes and rarely by virilization. Immunohistochemical staining for epithelial membrane antigen may be helpful in difficult cases because it is almost always positive in cases of endometrioid carcinoma and only rarely positive in a few cells within a Sertoli–Leydig cell tumor.[7] Sertoli–Leydig cell tumors may be simulated by primary or metastatic endometrioid stromal sarco-

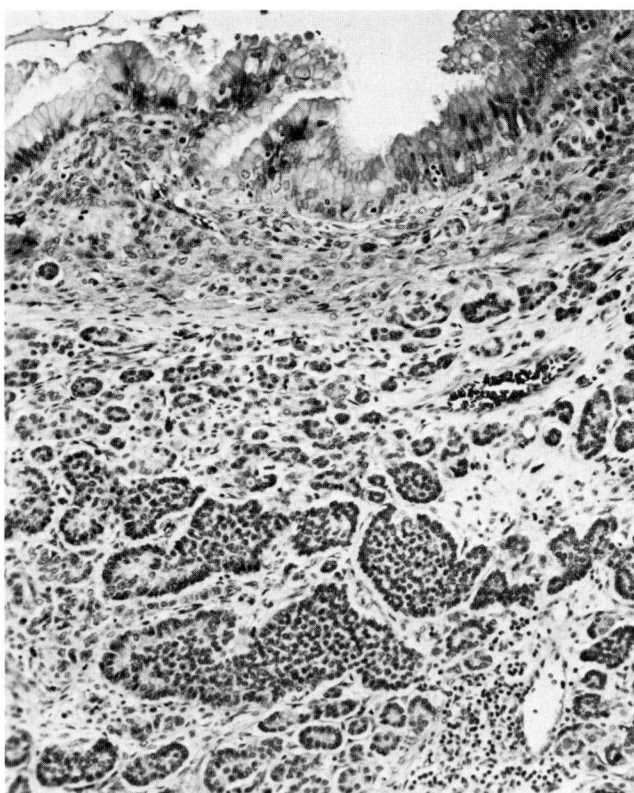

FIG. 19.55. Sertoli–Leydig cell tumor with heterologous elements. Insular carcinoid adjacent to mucinous epithelium.

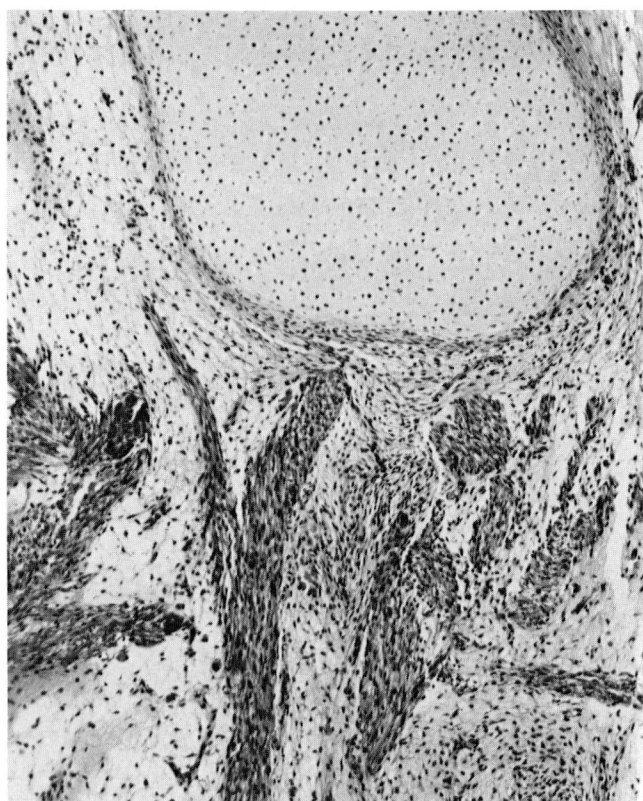

FIG. 19.56. Sertoli–Leydig cell tumor with heterologous elements. Nodule of fetal type cartilage and bundles of strap cells. (Reprinted by permission of Prat, Young, and Scully, ref. 325.)

mas.[459,471] Criteria that are applicable in the differential diagnosis of these tumors with granulosa cell tumors also are helpful in this situation.

The tubular Krukenberg tumor may mimic a Sertoli–Leydig cell tumor especially if luteinization of the stroma is present[64]; further confusion arises in the rare case in which the former tumor is associated with virilization. Tubular Krukenberg tumors have been reported to be bilateral, however, in 50% of the cases and contain markedly atypical cells, including signet-ring cells that contain mucin, easily demonstrable by special stains.[64]

Carcinoid tumors, especially those of the trabecular type, may be confused with Sertoli–Leydig cell tumors of intermediate differentiation. The ribbons of the former, however, are longer, thicker, and more uniformly distributed than the sex cord–like formations of the latter. Also, rare carcinoid tumors with a solid tubular pattern[461] can be difficult to distinguish from well-differentiated Sertoli cell tumors. Examination of the stroma of carcinoid tumors may be helpful in the differential diagnosis. It is typically less cellular and more fibromatous than that of Sertoli–Leydig cell tumors and does not contain Leydig cells. The most specific diagnostic criterion is the presence of argyrophil granules in almost all carcinoid tumors and of argen-

taffin granules in many of them; in contrast, only heterologous Sertoli–Leydig cell tumors with glands and cysts lined by gastrointestinal-type epithelium contain such granules. Finally, primary carcinoid tumors are associated with teratomatous elements in 70% of the cases[335–337] and metastatic carcinoids are almost always bilateral and usually are associated with obvious primary tumor of the intestine and metastases elsewhere in the abdomen (see Chapter 22, Metastatic Tumors of the Ovary).

The tubules seen in ovarian wolffian tumors (see Chapter 21, Nonspecific Tumors of the Ovary, Including Mesenchymal Tumors and Malignant Lymphoma) may be indistinguishable from those seen in Sertoli and Sertoli–Leydig cell tumors but are virtually always accompanied by other patterns that exclude the diagnosis of a sex cord–stromal tumor.

The retiform variant of Sertoli–Leydig cell tumor causes specific problems in differential diagnosis. The most common misdiagnosis is yolk sac tumor, which is suggested clinically by the young age of the patient and pathologically by the presence of papillae within cystic spaces. The occurrence of androgenic manifestations with about one-quarter of cases of retiform Sertoli–Leydig cell tumor, however, contrasts with the rare occurrence of such changes in cases of yolk sac tumor, attributable to a functioning stroma.[402] On gross examination, the retiform tumors generally appear less malignant than yolk sac tumors and microscopic examination reveals less primitive-appearing cells. The presence of other distinctive patterns of either tumor and positive immunohistochemical staining for alpha-fetoprotein in the yolk sac tumor almost always facilitate the diagnosis. A greater problem in the differential diagnosis of retiform Sertoli–Leydig cell tumors arises because of their characteristic papillary patterns and the frequent presence of cellular stratification on the papillae, particularly if those features predominate in the specimen. Under such circumstances, a misdiagnosis of a serous cystadenoma of borderline malignancy or a serous or endometrioid carcinoma occasionally is made. A variety of clinical and pathological features, including the young age of the patient, the association with virilization, and the presence of other more easily recognizable patterns of Sertoli–Leydig cell tumor are helpful clues to the correct diagnosis. Finally, the juxtaposition of epithelial and immature mesenchymal elements in some retiform tumors has caused confusion with a malignant mesodermal mixed tumor, but the features outlined above also serve to exclude the latter diagnosis.

Because occasional sex cord–stromal tumors have a morphologic appearance intermediate between granulosa cell tumors and Sertoli–Leydig cell tumors or exhibit features of both tumors, it is sometimes difficult to decide whether a given tumor should be placed in the granulosa, Sertoli–Leydig cell, or mixed category. Major criteria that help to differentiate granulosa cell tumors and Sertoli–Leydig cell tumors are listed in Table 19.7.

Table 19.7. Adult granulosa cell tumor versus Sertoli–Leydig cell tumor

Granulosa cell tumor	Sertoli–Leydig cell tumor
All age groups, mostly postmenopausal	Mainly young women
Usually estrogenic, rarely androgenic	Usually androgenic occasionally estrogenic
Microfollicular, macrofollicular, trabecular, insular, and diffuse patterns	Hollow or solid tubules, cords, diffuse patterns
Granulosa cells usually mature with pale, often grooved nuclei	Sertoli cells often immature
Fibrothecomatous component common	Fibromatous component uncommon; mesenchyme often immature and cellular
Steroid-type cells (lutein cells) usually not prominent and uncommonly clustered	Steroid-type cells (Leydig cells) tend to cluster; rarely contain crystals of Reinke
Heterologous elements absent	Heterologous elements in 20% of cases
Retiform elements absent	Retiform elements in 15% of cases

CLINICAL BEHAVIOR AND TREATMENT

After the removal of a virilizing Sertoli–Leydig cell tumor, normal menses characteristically resume in about 4 weeks. The excessive hair usually diminishes to some extent. Clitoromegaly and deepening of the voice are less apt to regress. The prognosis in cases of Sertoli–Leydig cell tumor is closely related to its stage and degree of differentiation. The rare tumors that present at a stage higher than I have a poor prognosis, with a mortality rate of 100% in our series of cases.[473] The survival rates of patients with stage I tumors correlate with the degree of differentiation. In our series none of the well-differentiated tumors, 11% of those of intermediate differentiation, 59% of the poorly differentiated tumors, and 19% of those with heterologous elements were clinically malignant. The homologous component of the tumor was poorly differentiated in all eight clinically malignant tumors in the heterologous category and in seven of them the heterologous elements included skeletal muscle, cartilage, or both. Earlier studies in the literature failed to establish a relation between the degree of differentiation of Sertoli–Leydig cell tumors and their prognosis,[306,310] but later investigations have supported the findings in our series. The only clinically malignant tumor in the series of Roth et al.[342] was poorly differentiated, and 4 of the 20 poorly differentiated tumors reported by Zaloudek and Norris[477] were malignant in contrast to only 1 of the 44 tumors of intermediate differentiation and none of the 7 well-differentiated tumors. In our series there also was evidence that the presence of a retiform pattern had an adverse effect on the prognosis; 25% of stage I tumors of intermediate differentiation with a retiform component were malignant as opposed to 10% of those with no retiform component.[473] It is noteworthy that the only stage III tumor of intermediate differentiation in our series had an almost completely retiform pattern, and we have seen an additional Sertoli–Leydig cell tumor with a predominantly retiform pattern that was stage III. Rupture also adversely affected the outcome of stage I tumors. Thirty percent of the tumors of intermediate differentiation that had ruptured were clinically malignant, in contrast to only 7% of those that were intact; in the poorly differentiated category 86% of the ruptured tumors were malignant compared with 45% of those that had not ruptured.

In contrast to granulosa cell tumors, which often recur many years after primary therapy, Sertoli–Leydig cell tumors typically reappear relatively early. Sixty-six percent of the malignant tumors in our series recurred within 1 year and only 6.6% recurred after 5 years.[473] The recurrent tumor usually is confined to the pelvis and abdomen but distant metastases to the lung, scalp, and supraclavicular lymph nodes have been reported. Three of the patients in our series had parenchymal liver metastases.

The treatment of a patient with Sertoli–Leydig cell tumor depends on her age, the stage of her tumor, the presence or absence of rupture, and the degree of differentiation. In young women the low frequency of bilaterality justifies the performance of a unilateral salpingo-oophorectomy if the tumor is stage IA and preservation of fertility is desired. More aggressive surgical therapy and adjuvant therapy are indicated for tumors higher than stage I. Adjuvant therapy also may be advisable for stage I tumors that are poorly differentiated, contain mesenchymal heterologous elements, or are ruptured tumors of intermediate differentiation. Experience with the nonsurgical therapy of Sertoli–Leydig cell tumors is relatively limited. Radiation therapy, combination chemotherapy, or both seem to have been of benefit in occasional reported cases.[326,473]

Other Types of Sex Cord–Stromal Tumors

Gynandroblastoma

Gynandroblastoma, an extremely rare tumor,[17,87,131,294,304] has been greatly overdiagnosed. According to the WHO, the term should be used only if well-differentiated ovarian and testicular-type cells are clearly recognizable within the neoplasm (Fig. 19.57). Since small foci of ovarian cell types often are encountered in well-sampled, otherwise typical Sertoli–Leydig cell tumors and conversely, testicular cell types are demonstrable focally in occasional granulosa–stromal cell tumors, the diagnosis of gynandroblastoma should be restricted to the very rare tumors that contain significant components of both forms of neoplasia. According to our criteria, the minor component should account for at least 10% of a tumor in the sex cord–stromal category to warrant a diagnosis of gynandroblastoma. The nature of the hormones secreted by a sex cord–stromal tumor should not, of course, determine its morphologic diagnosis in view of the proven capacity of tumors of testicular cell types to secrete estrogens and of those of ovarian cell types to produce androgens.

Sex Cord Tumor with Annular Tubules

The sex cord tumor with annular tubules (Figs. 19.58–19.61), which originally was included within the WHO category of "sex cord–stromal tumors, unclassified" (see below), has been established as a distinctive entity.[367,474] It is characterized basically by the presence of simple and complex annular tubules (Figs. 19.59, 19.61). The simple tubules have the shape of a ring, with the nucleus oriented peripherally and around a central hyalinized body composed of basement membrane material; an intervening anuclear cytoplasmic zone forms the major component of the ring. The much more numerous complex tubules are rounded structures made up of intercommunicating rings revolving around multiple hyaline bodies. Tumors containing annular tubules have been interpreted as Sertoli cell tumors by some observers[420] and granulosa cell tumors by

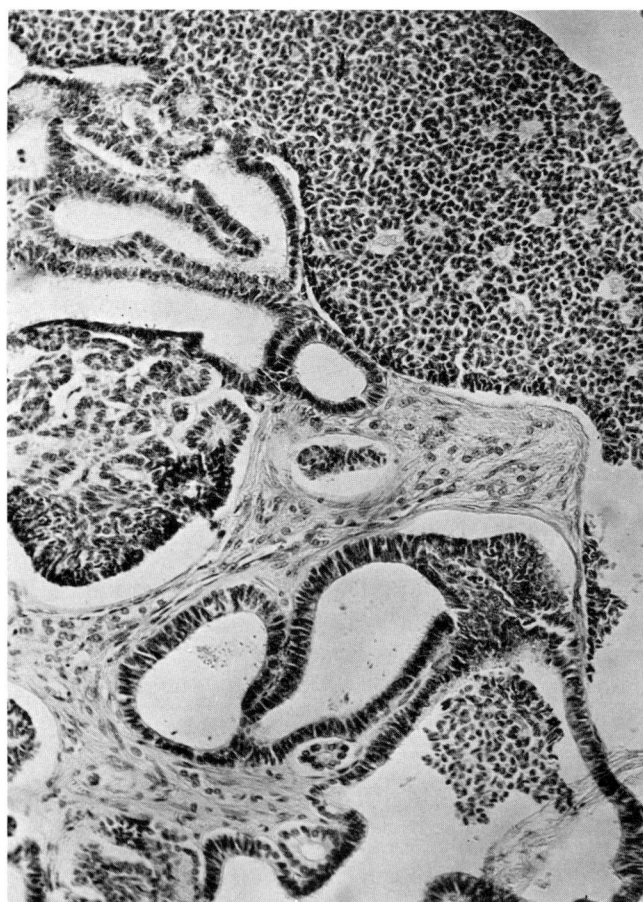

FIG. 19.57. **Gynandroblastoma.** (Reprinted by permission of Scully, ref. 364.)

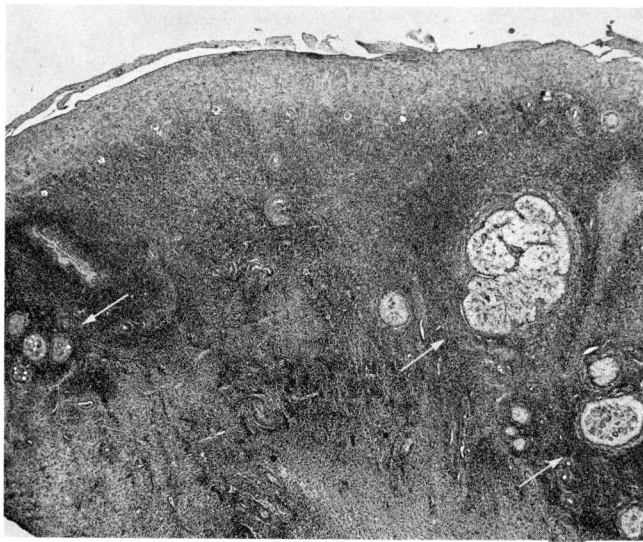

FIG. 19.58. **Sex cord tumor with annular tubules.** Multicentric foci are present within ovary from patient with Peutz–Jeghers syndrome. (Reprinted by permission of Scully, ref. 367.)

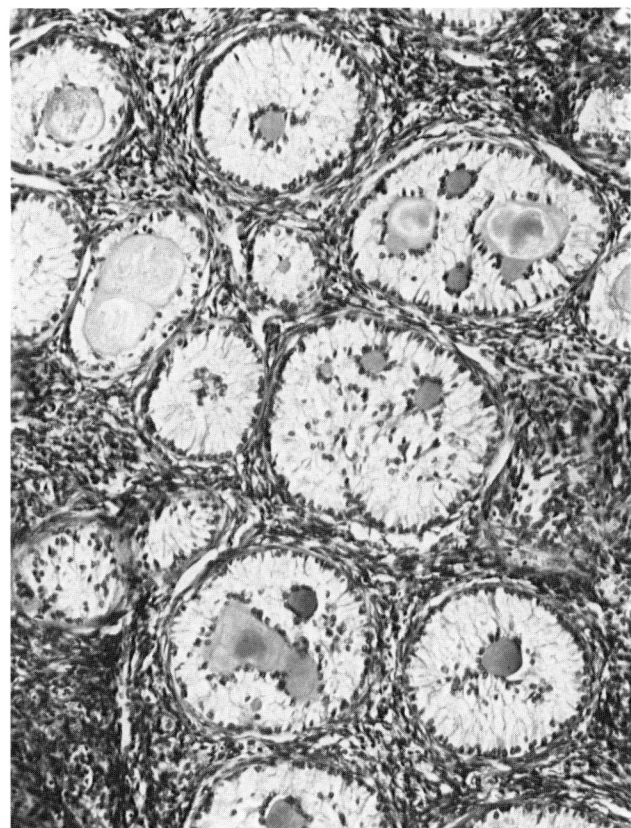

FIG. 19.59. **Sex cord tumor with annular tubules.** Simple and complex annular tubules encircle hyaline material.

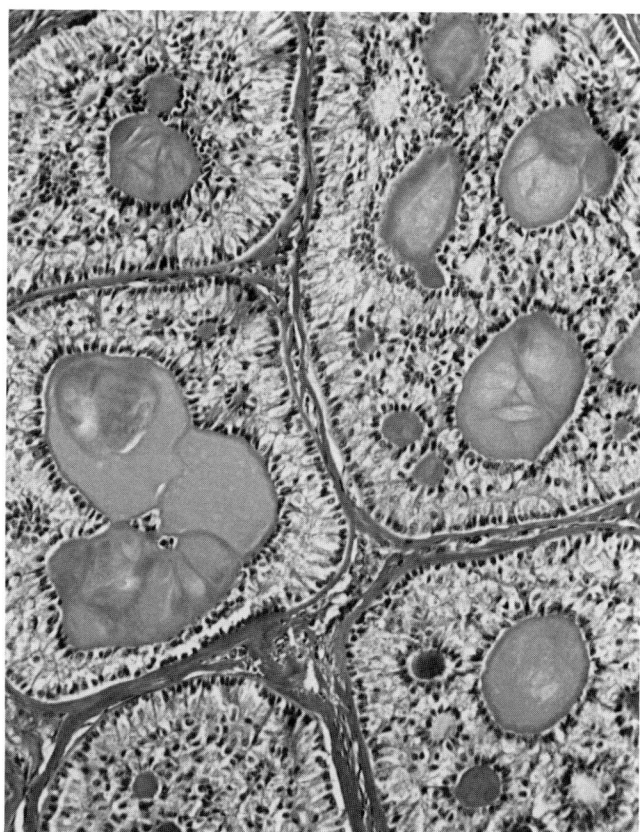

FIG. 19.61. **Sex cord tumor with annular tubules.** There was no evidence of Peutz–Jeghers syndrome in the patient with this neoplasm. ×160.

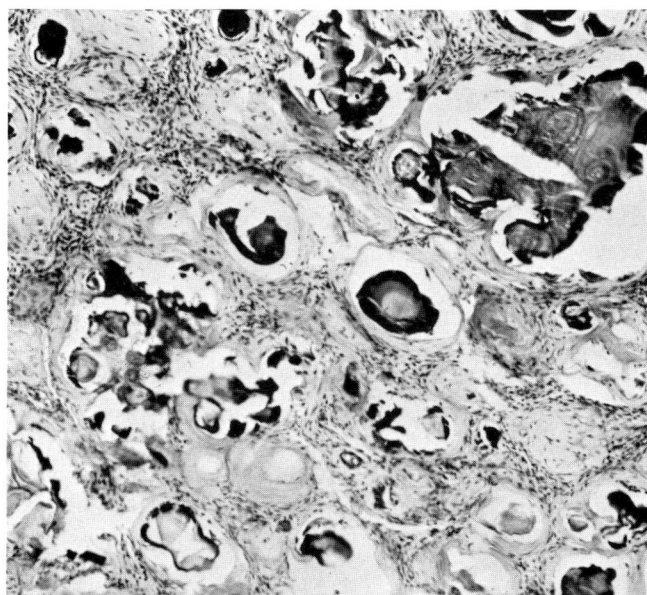

FIG. 19.60. **Sex cord tumor with annular tubules.** Extensive calcification of the epithelial nests has occurred in this tumor from a patient with Peutz–Jeghers syndrome.

others,[181] but the pattern of growth has features intermediate between these two tumors and focal differentiation into both typical Sertoli cell tumor with elongated tubules and typical granulosa cell tumor with Call–Exner bodies is seen in some of the cases. Sertoli-type cells have been identified ultrastructurally by the demonstration of Charcot–Bottcher filament bundles (Fig. 19.62),[9,25,420] which are considered specific cytoplasmic inclusions of Sertoli cells. A study of small tumors of this type suggests an origin in the ovarian cortex from the granulosa cells of follicles. Other evidence of such an origin is the well-known tubular differentiation of follicles that occurs in the canine ovary, and the occasional observation of tubular differentiation in graafian follicles during pregnancy.

Sex cord tumors with annular tubules vary both clinically and pathologically, depending on whether or not the patient has Puetz–Jeghers syndrome[37,90,142,474] (mucocutaneous melanin pigmentation, gastrointestinal hamartomatous polyposis, and occasionally carcinomas of the gastric intestinal tract and adenoma malignum of the cervix)[265] (Table 19.8). Almost all female patients with this syndrome whose ovaries have been examined microscopically have

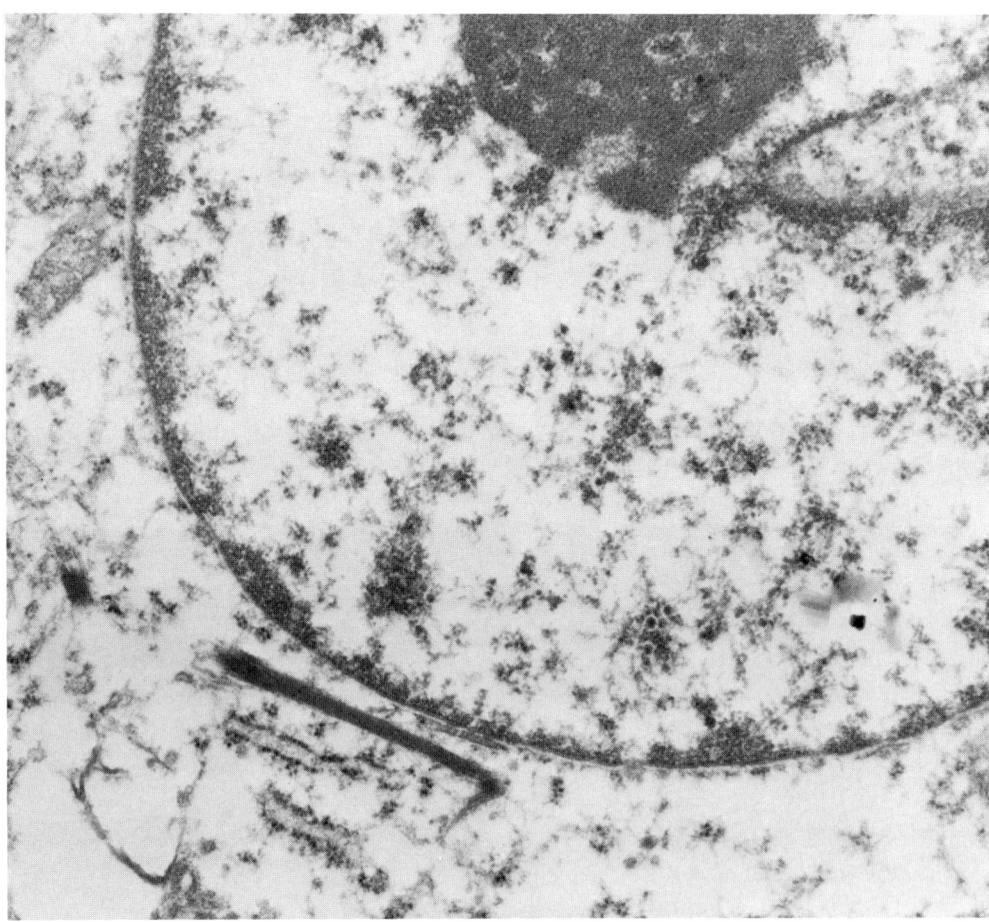

Fig. 19.62. Charcot–Bottcher filament in characteristic paranuclear location. ×27,300. (Reprinted by permission of Tavassoli and Norris, ref. 420.)

had sex cord tumorlets with annular tubules, which have been multifocal (Fig. 19.58) and bilateral in at least two-thirds of the cases; the largest reported lesion in a patient with this syndrome was 3 cm in diameter. Focal calcification has been seen in more than half the cases (Fig. 19.60). In almost all the patients the lesions have been incidental findings in ovaries removed for other reasons. All the tumorlets associated with Peutz–Jeghers syndrome have been benign, warranting conservative treatment.

Table 19.8. Sex cord tumor with annular tubules with and without Peutz–Jeghers syndrome

	With (%)	*Without (%)*
Bilateral	62	5
Grossly visible	27	75
Size	3 cm or less	Usually large
Multifocal	82	6
Calcification	62	12
Clinically malignant	0	20[a]
Adenoma malignum cervix	15	4

[a] Only grossly visible tumors used in this evaluation.

In patients without Peutz–Jeghers syndrome (Fig. 19.61), in contrast, the tumors are almost always unilateral and usually form palpable masses. Transitions to typical granulosa cell tumor are much more common than in tumorlets associated with Peutz–Jeghers syndrome. Forty percent of the patients have had manifestations of estrogen secretion; progesterone secretion, which may be associated with decidual change of the endometrium, is relatively common. At least one-fifth of the tumors have been clinically malignant, with a characteristic spread via the lymphatic system. Recurrences often are late. In one remarkable case multiple recurrences occurred, mostly within regional and distal lymph nodes over a period of 24 years, with each recurrent tumor removed surgically. In that case the tumor produced large amounts of müllerian-inhibiting substance as well as progesterone, both of which were found useful as tumor markers in the serum in monitoring the course of the patient.[175]

Four other ovarian tumors from girls with Peutz–Jeghers syndrome have caused sexual precocity. Two of them, occurring in sisters, had the features of Sertoli cell tumors with lipid storage,[391] whereas the other two had microscopic findings that were unique in our experience, including diffuse areas, tubular differentiation, microcysts and papillae, and the presence of two distinctive cell types, one containing abundant eosinophilic cytoplasm and the other, scanty cytoplasm (Figs. 19.63, 19.64).[453] All four tumors appeared to be clinically benign. The occurrence of these unusual neoplasms in association with Peutz–Jeghers syndrome suggested an association.

Sex Cord–Stromal Tumors, Unclassified

Sex cord–stromal tumors, unclassified, is an ill-defined group of tumors that accounts for less than 10% of those in the sex cord–stromal category. This group includes neoplasms in which a predominant pattern of testicular or ovarian differentiation is not clearly recognizable. The boundary lines between these tumors and those of both ovarian and testicular cell types are vague because interpretations of intermediate patterns of growth and closely similar cell types inevitably are subjective.

Talerman and his associates[415] have described a group of sex cord–stromal tumors containing diffuse fibrothecoma-

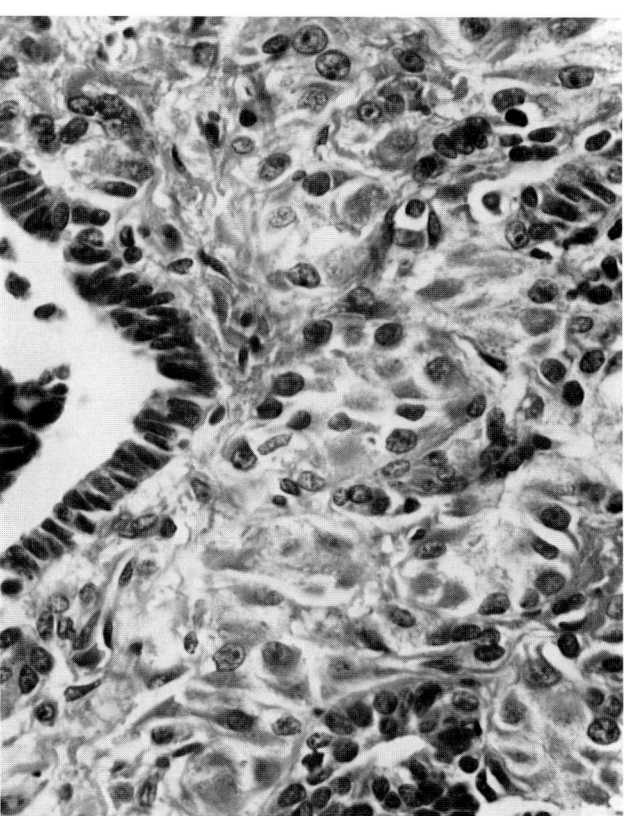

FIG. 19.64. **Ovarian sex cord tumor from patient with sexual precocity and Peutz–Jeghers syndrome.** Tubules separated by cells with abundant cytoplasm and vesicular nuclei. (Reprinted by permission of Young, Dickersin, Scully, ref. 453.)

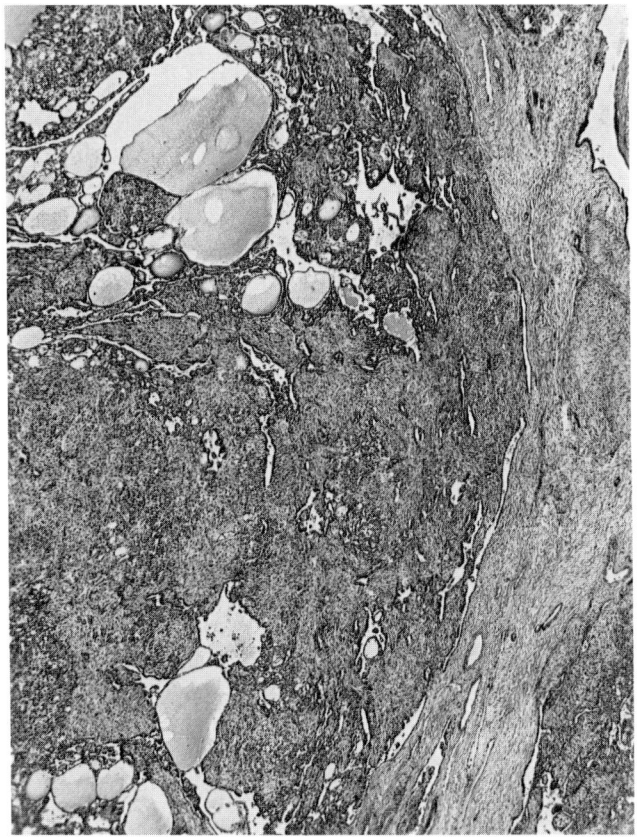

FIG. 19.63. **Ovarian sex cord tumor from patient with sexual precocity and Peutz–Jeghers syndrome.** Solid areas interrupted by cysts of varying sizes. (Reprinted by permission of Young, Dickersin, and Scully, ref. 453.)

tous and/or granulosa cell–like proliferation as well as areas of tubular differentiation in most of the cases. These authors have interpreted these tumors, which differ in appearance from usual forms of Sertoli–Leydig cell tumor, as diffuse nonlobular androblastomas, but in our opinion it is more appropriate to place them in the unclassified sex cord–stromal category.

Sex Cord–Stromal Tumors During Pregnancy

Sex cord–stromal tumors may be particularly difficult to subclassify when they occur in pregnant patients[455] because of alterations of their usual clinical and pathological features. Their diagnosis is rarely suggested clinically because estrogenic manifestations are not recognizable during pregnancy, and androgenic manifestations are rare, possibly because of the ability of the placenta to aromatize androgens to estrogens. Indeed, virilization of a pregnant patient is much more likely to be caused by a nonneoplastic lesion such as the pregnancy luteoma and hyperreactio luteinalis or to a tumor with functioning stroma than to a sex cord–stromal tumor.

In one study, 17% of 36 sex cord–stromal tumors that were removed during pregnancy were placed in the unclassified group, and many of those that were classified in the granulosa cell or Sertoli–Leydig cell category had large areas with an indifferent appearance.[455] The features that led to difficulty in classification were the presence of prominent intercellular edema, increased luteinization in the granulosa cell tumors, and marked degrees of Leydig cell maturation in one-third of the Sertoli–Leydig cell tumors. All of these changes, which were most common in tumors removed during the third trimester, tended to obscure the underlying architecture. The behavior of sex cord–stromal tumors during pregnancy appeared to be similar to that of tumors of similar type unassociated with pregnancy on the basis of limited follow-up of the 36 cases.

IMMUNOHISTOCHEMISTRY OF SEX CORD–STROMAL TUMORS

Kurman and his associates[236–238] have demonstrated immunohistochemically a variety of steroid hormones, including estrogens, androgens, and progesterone in the granulosa, theca, Sertoli, and Leydig cells of sex cord–stromal tumors. It is not clear, however, whether their presence reflects secretion or binding of these hormones to cellular receptors. Sasano and others[358,359] have used antibodies to demonstrate immunohistochemically many of the enzymes that are involved in the conversion of cholesterol to various steroid hormones, helping to pinpoint their site of origin in the cells of sex cord–stromal tumors.

Immunohistochemical techniques occasionally are of help in the differential diagnosis of sex cord–stromal tumors,[105,274,277,278] particularly in their distinction from epithelial–stromal cancers. Although both granulosa cells and Sertoli cells initially were thought to be positive for vimentin[147] and negative for keratin, it has since been demonstrated that both cell types in neoplasms are commonly positive for various cytokeratins.[39,86] Epithelial membrane antigen, however, can be demonstrated in the great majority of the epithelial cancers, but has not been shown to be stainable in granulosa cell tumors, and is present immunohistochemically in only rare cells in Sertoli cell tumors. S-100 protein can be demonstrated immunohistochemically in approximately one-third of both adult and juvenile granulosa cell tumors[8] but has not yet been demonstrated in the small number of Sertoli cell tumors studied.

It is of interest that one sex cord tumor with annular tubules has been shown to be positive immunohistochemically for müllerian-inhibiting substance[175]; its presence has not been tested for as yet in other types of ovarian tumors.

The argyrophil cells of mucinous and carcinoid components of heterologous Sertoli–Leydig cell tumors have reacted for serotonin and one or more polypeptide hormones on immunohistochemical examination.[371] In one Sertoli–Leydig cell tumor associated with elevated levels of alpha-fetoprotein in the serum, immunohistochemical staining for this antigen was localized in cells resembling liver cells within the tumor[456]; in other cases there was staining of the Sertoli–Leydig cell component of the neoplasm.[93,257,427]

Steroid Cell Tumors

The terms *lipid cell tumor* and *lipoid cell tumor* have been applied to ovarian neoplasms composed entirely of cells resembling typical steroid hormone–secreting cells, that is, lutein cells, Leydig cells, and adrenal cortical cells.[421] These terms are nonspecific and inaccurate, however, since up to 25% of tumors in this category contain little or no lipid. Several years ago one of us proposed the term *steroid cell tumors* for these neoplasms, because it reflects both the morphologic features of the neoplastic cells and their propensity to secrete steroid hormones.[369] These tumors, which account for approximately 0.1% of ovarian tumors, have been subdivided into two subtypes according to their cell of origin and a third subtype whose specific cell lineage is unknown (Table 19.9). The features of the various subtypes of steroid cell tumors are contrasted in (Table 19.10).

Stromal Luteoma

The stromal luteoma accounts for approximately 25% of steroid cell tumors. This designation[365] is applied to small steroid cell tumors that lie within the ovarian stroma (Fig. 19.65) and therefore are presumed to arise from it. Such an origin is supported by the capacity of the ovarian stroma to differentiate into lutein cells in the nonneoplastic disorder designated *stromal hyperthecosis*.[400] Adrenal rest cells and Leydig cells, the other possible sources of tumors of this type, on the other hand, have been identified within the ovarian stroma on only extremely rare occasions. The diagnosis of stromal luteoma is supported in approximately 90% of the cases by the finding of stromal hyperthecosis elsewhere in the same or contralateral ovary. In some cases of the latter disorders the nests of lutein cells may form nodules (nodular hyperthecosis); the dividing line between a large hyperthecotic nodule and a stromal luteoma is arbitrary; we reserve the former designation for large nodular foci of microscopic size and the latter for nodules that are grossly visible.

Table 19.9. Steroid cell tumors

Stromal luteoma
Leydig cell tumors
Hilus cell tumor
Leydig cell tumor, nonhilar type
Steroid cell tumor, not otherwise specified

Table 19.10. Clinical and pathological features of steroid cell tumors

	Stromal luteoma	*C+ Hilus cell tumor*	*C− Hilus cell tumor*	*Steroid cell tumor nos.*
No. of cases	25	12	9	63
Age range (mean)	28–74 (58)	32–75 (57)	34–82 (61)	2–80 (43)
Virilization/hirsutism	12%	83%	33%	52%
Estrogenic manifestations	60%	0	44%	8%
Duration of androgenic manifestations	1.5–5 yrs	2–20 yrs	1–24 yrs	0.5–30 yrs
No endocrine abnormality	20%	17%	23%	27%
Cushing's syndrome	0	0	0	0
Diameter cm (mean)	1.3	2.4	1.8	8.4
Stromal hyperthecosis	92%	42%	67%	23%
Endometrial hyperplasia or carcinoma	88%	8%	33%	24%

C, Reinke crystal.
From Paraskevas and Scully, ref. 317.

Stromal luteomas are almost always under 3 cm in diameter and, with rare exceptions, are unilateral.[184] They are well circumscribed, solid, and usually gray-white or yellow, but one-third of them have red or brown areas.

Microscopic examination of a stromal luteoma reveals a more or less rounded nodule of cells of lutein type, which generally contain relatively little lipid. Intracytoplasmic lipochrome pigment may be conspicuous. The nuclei are small and round with a single prominent nucleoli. Mitoses generally are rare. The cells may be arranged diffusely or in small nests or cords and are more or less completely surrounded by ovarian stroma. One confusing feature, seen in about 20% of the cases, is focal degeneration, with the formation of irregular spaces that may stimulate glands or vessels (Fig. 19.66).[184] These spaces may contain, or be surrounded by, lipid-laden cells and chronic inflammatory cells and may be associated with fibrosis. In some cases they contain red blood cells. Some steroid cell tumors in the "not otherwise specified" category may be overgrown stromal luteomas, but the specific diagnosis cannot be made with certainty when the tumor is no longer confined to the ovarian stroma.

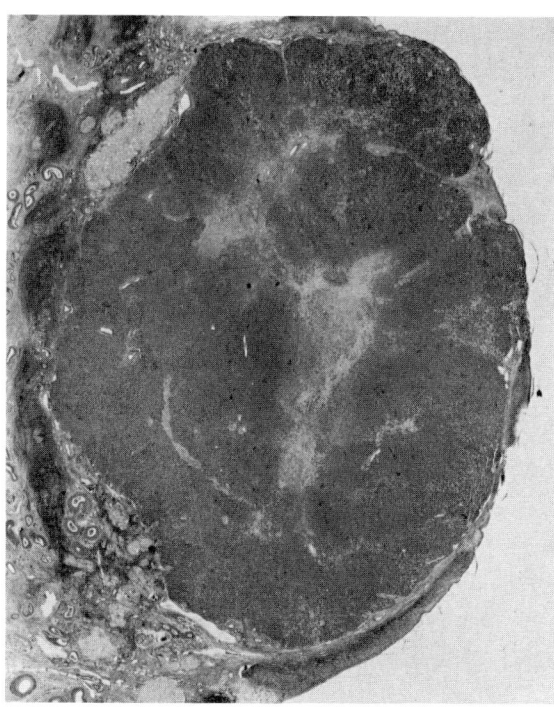

Fig. 19.65. Stromal luteoma. The tumors partly surrounded by ovarian stroma.

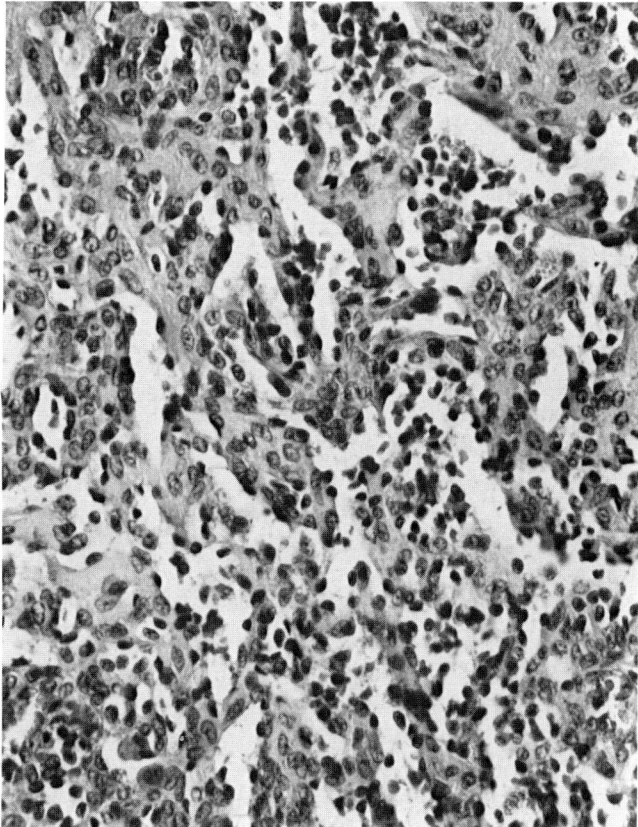

Fig. 19.66. Stromal luteoma. Degenerative changes have produced irregular spaces.

Eighty percent of stromal luteomas occur in postmenopausal women.[184] The initial symptom in 60% of the cases is abnormal vaginal bleeding probably related to hyperestrinism, although whether the tumor secretes estrogen directly or secretes an androgen that is converted peripherally to an estrogen is unknown. Androgenic manifestations are present in only 12% of the cases. This profile of hormonal function is the opposite of that associated with other categories of steroid cell tumor, which usually are androgenic and only occasionally estrogenic. Underlying stromal hyperthecosis may contribute to the clinical picture in some cases, particularly those in which there is a long history of hormonal disturbance. At least one stromal luteoma was associated with the insulin resistance–acanthosis nigricans–hyperandrogenism syndrome,[161] in which the ovaries are polycystic with stromal hyperthecosis.[124] All of the reported tumors have been benign, as expected because of their small size and generally bland cytological features.

Leydig Cell Tumors

A Leydig cell nature of a steroid cell tumor (Figs. 19.58–19.60) can be proved only by the identification of the more or less specific crystals of Reinke in the cytoplasm of the neoplastic cells on either light microscopic (Fig. 19.59) or electron microscopic (Fig. 19.60) examination.° Since only 35–40% of Leydig cell tumors of the testis contain crystals of Reinke on light microscopic examination[227] and Leydig cells cannot be differentiated from lutein cells or adrenal cortical cells in the absence of these inclusions, it is probable that a number of unclassified steroid cell tumors are Leydig cell tumors that cannot be identified specifically as such.

Ovarian Leydig cell tumors have been divided into two subtypes by Roth and Sternberg,[346] the *hilus cell tumor* and the *Leydig cell tumor, nonhilar type*. The former, which are much more common, originate in the ovarian hilus from hilar Leydig cells, which have been identified in 80–85% of adult ovaries, usually lying in relation to nonmedullated nerve fibers.[398]

Hilus cell tumors, which account for approximately 20% of steroid cell tumors,[317] occur at an average age of 58 years and cause hirsutism or virilization in three-quarter of the cases[126]; rarely they are associated with estrogenic manifestations.[198,202] The androgenic changes typically have a less abrupt onset and are milder than those associated with Sertoli–Leydig cell tumors. They sometimes have been present for many years.[110] The urinary 17-ketosteroid levels usually are normal or only slightly elevated because these tumors produce predominantly the potent androgen, testosterone, which is not a 17-ketosteroid, in-

stead of the weaker androgens, androstenedione and dehydroepiandrosterone, elevations of which are typically associated with high values of urinary 17-ketosteroids. Hilus cell tumors occasionally are palpable preoperatively. They are rarely bilateral.[32] Almost all the hilus cell tumors recorded in the literature have been benign; only one case of malignant hilus cell tumor merits serious consideration, but the presence of crystals of Reinke in the neoplastic cells in that case was not convincingly documented in the illustrations.[127]

Hilus cell tumors usually are reddish brown to yellow, are centered in the hilar region, and rarely are large (Fig. 19.67) (mean diameter 2.4 cm).[317] Microscopic examination typically reveals a circumscribed mass of steroid cells with abundant eosinophilic cytoplasm and little intracellular lipid; cytoplasmic lipochrome pigment may be abundant. The cells usually are distributed diffusely but occasionally their nuclei cluster and are separated by nucleus-free eosinophilic zones (Fig. 19.68); this pattern is highly suggestive of a hilus cell tumor even in the absence of crystals of Reinke. In some tumors the presence of a prominent fibrous stroma imparts a nodular appearance. An unusual feature in one-third of the cases is fibrinoid replacement of the walls of moderate-sized vessels unaccompanied by inflammatory cell infiltration.[317] Degenerative spaces similar to those seen in stromal luteomas may be present. The tumor cells typically contain abundant granular eosinophilic cytoplasm; occasional cells have spongy cytoplasm, indicating the presence of lipid. Cytoplasmic lipochrome pigment, which usually is sparse, is present in most cases. The typically round nuclei often are hyperchromatic and contain single small nucleoli, there may be slight to moderate variation in nuclear size and shape, and occasionally bizarre nuclei and multinucleated cells are encountered. Rare mitotic figures occasionally are present. Pseudoinclusions of cytoplasm into the nucleus

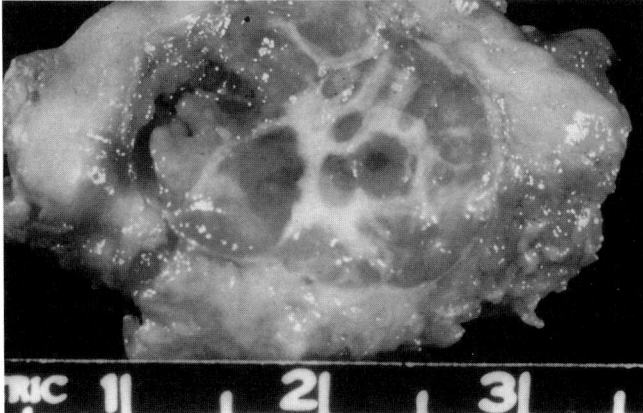

FIG. 19.67. Hilus cell tumor. A dark mass lobulated by septa occupies the center of the sectioned surface of the ovary. (Reproduced by permission of Scully, ref. 369.)

°Refs. 14,16,52,61,198,291,307,317,353,354,361,399.

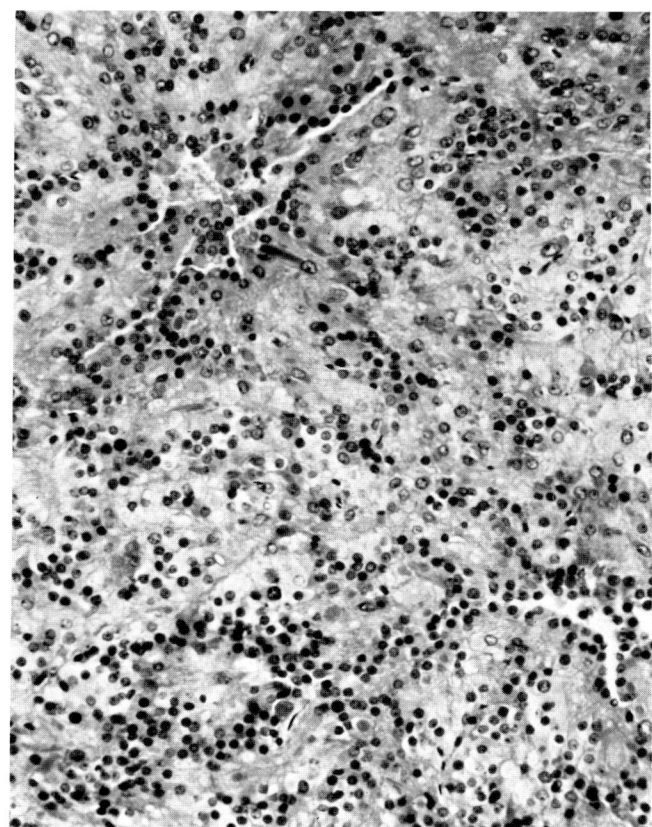

FIG. 19.68. **Hilus cell tumor.** (Reprinted by permission of Scully, ref. 369.)

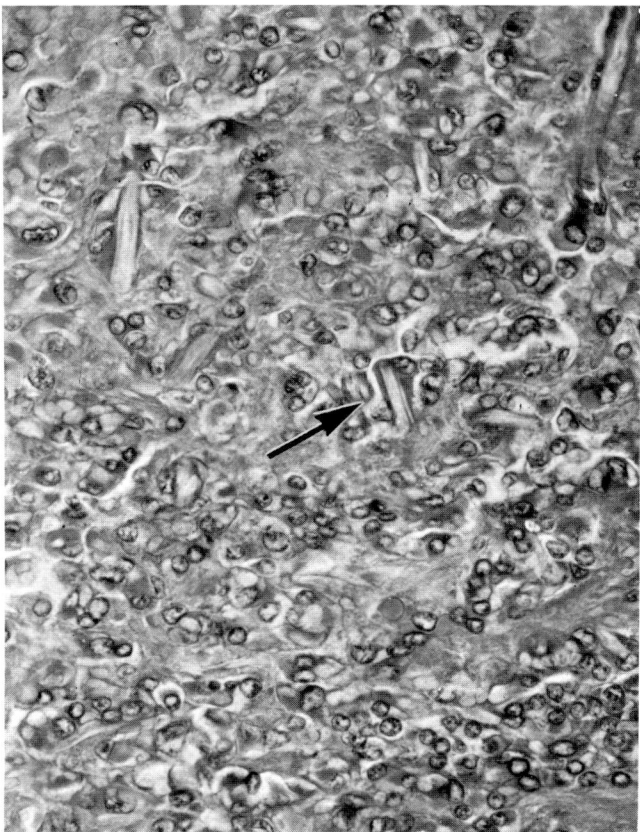

FIG. 19.69. **Hilus cell tumor.** *Arrow* points to crystals of Reinke. (Reprinted by permission of Morris and Scully, ref. 286.)

may be seen. Elongated eosinophilic Reinke crystals of varying sizes are present in varying numbers in the cytoplasm (Fig. 19.69) or sometimes in the nucleus, but often are found only after prolonged search. The diagnosis of hilus cell tumor is favored if a crystal-free steroid cell tumor located in the hilus has a background of hilus cell hyperplasia, is associated with nonmedullated nerve fibers, has fibrinoid necrosis of blood vessel walls, or shows nuclear clustering with intervening nucleus-free zones. On electron microscopic examination crystals of Reinke typically are needle-shaped when cut longitudinally, and hexagonal when cut in cross-section (Fig. 19.70). The interior of the crystal has a cross-hatched appearance. Intracytoplasmic eosinophilic spheres, which may be crystal precursors, also are typically present, but are not specific for hilus cell tumors. Stromal hyperthecosis, hilus cell hyperplasia, or both are associated findings in occasional cases.

The *Leydig cell tumor of nonhilar type* is thought to arise directly from ovarian stromal cells. Only four examples of this tumor have been reported[346] and except for their location, their clinical and pathological features have not differed from those of hilus cell tumors. An ovarian stromal cell derivation of these tumors is supported by the very rare finding of Leydig cells containing crystals in the steroid-cell nests of ovaries that otherwise have the typical appearance of stromal hyperthecosis.[400] In some cases in which a Leydig cell tumor is in equal contact with ovarian stroma and hilar stroma, it may be impossible to determine whether it is of the hilar or nonhilar type.

Steroid Cell Tumor, Not Otherwise Specified

Steroid cell tumors, not otherwise specified (NOS), which account for approximately 60% of steroid cell tumors, in all probability are large stromal luteomas or Leydig cell tumors but because they lack crystals of Reinke and their topographic features have been obliterated, they cannot be identified specifically as either type of tumor. These tumors occur at any age but typically at a younger age (mean 43 years) than other types of steroid cell tumor, and in contrast to the latter occasionally occur before puberty. Steroid cell tumors NOS are associated with androgenic changes, which may be of many years duration, in approximately half the cases, estrogenic changes including rare examples of isosexual pseudoprecocity[71] in approximately 10% of the cases, and occasionally progestagenic changes.[55] Four tumors have secreted cortisol and caused Cushing's syndrome,[4,261,469] and occasional others have

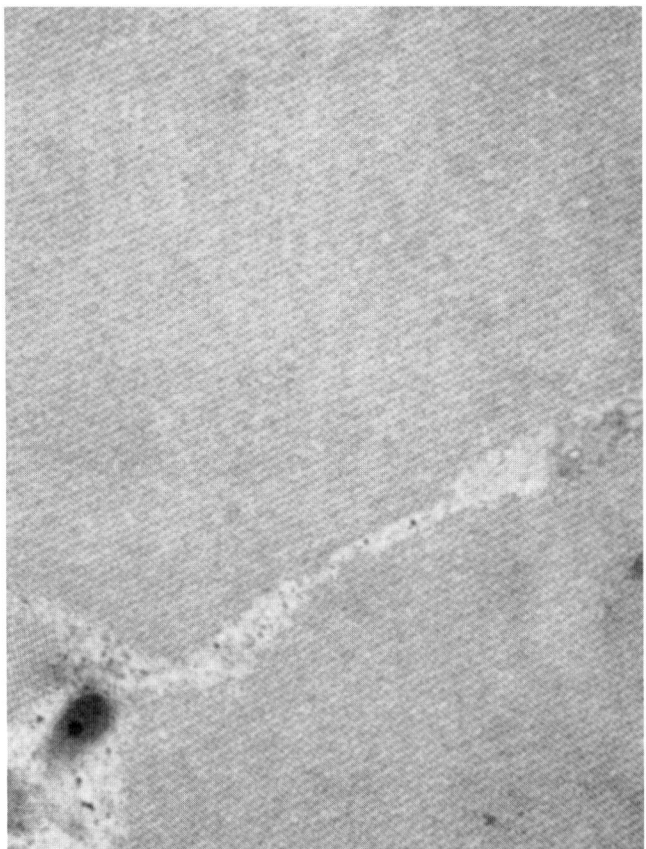

FIG. 19.70. Hilus cell tumor. Reinke crystal is composed of protein-containing, tightly-apposed 300 Å–wide hexagonal microtubular units. (Courtesy of Dr. A. Ferenczy, Montreal, Canada. Reprinted by permission of Scully, ref. 369.)

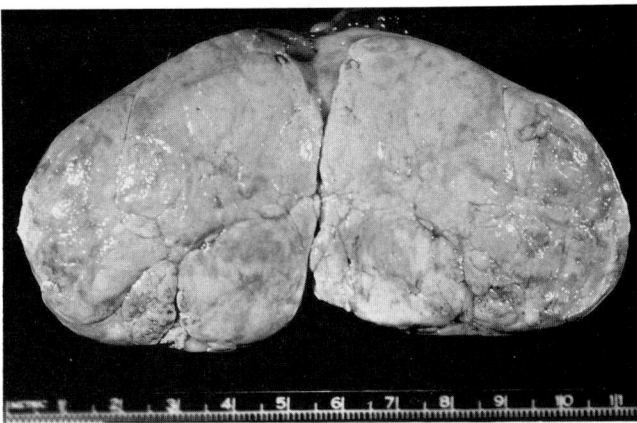

FIG. 19.71. Sertoid cell tumor, not otherwise specified. The sectioned surface of the tumor is uniformly solid and focally lobulated. The neoplasm was bright orange in the fresh state and was from a young girl who was virilized.

been accompanied by elevated cortisol levels in the absence of clinical manifestations of the syndrome, and one secreted aldosterone.[234] Rare tumors have been associated with hypercalcemia, erythrocytosis, or ascites. The remaining cases have not been accompanied by endocrine or paraendocrine manifestations. Hormone studies performed in patients with androgenic changes, Cushing's syndrome, or both typically show elevated urinary levels of 17-ketosteroids and 17-hydroxycorticosteroids as well as increased serum levels of testosterone and androstenedione. The tumors that resulted in Cushing's syndrome were associated with elevated levels of free cortisol in the blood or urine.

GROSS FINDINGS

The tumors typically are solid and well circumscribed (Fig. 19.71), occasionally are lobulated, and have a mean diameter of 8.4 cm; only about 5% of them are bilateral.[183] The sectioned surfaces typically are yellow or orange if large amounts of intracytoplasmic lipid are present, red to brown if the cells are lipid-poor, or dark brown to black if large quantities of intracytoplasmic lipochrome pigment are present. Necrosis, hemorrhage, and cystic degeneration occasionally are observed.

MICROSCOPIC FINDINGS

On microscopic examination, the cells typically are arranged diffusely (Fig. 19.72), but occasionally they grow in large aggregates, small nests (Fig. 19.73), irregular clusters, thin cords, or columns. The stroma is inconspicuous in most cases but in approximately 15% of them it is relatively prominent. A minor fibromatous component may be seen, indicating, as suggested by Hughesdon,[200] that steroid cell tumors may be completely luteinized thecomas. Rarely the stroma is edematous or myxoid, with tumor cells loosely dispersed within it and, exceptionally, it exhibits calcification and even psammoma body formation. Necrosis and hemorrhage may be prominent, particularly in tumors that have significant cytological atypia.

The polygonal to rounded tumor cells have distinct cell borders, central nuclei, and moderate to abundant amounts of cytoplasm that varies from eosinophilic and granular (lipid-free or lipid-poor) to vacuolated and spongy (lipid-rich) (Figs. 19.72, 19.73); lipid was present in 75% of the tumors in one series.[183] Steroid cell tumors NOS have lipid-rich cytoplasm more often than other subtypes of steroid cell tumor. Rarely, cells with large fat droplets have a signet-ring appearance. Intracytoplasmic lipochrome pigment has been found in 40% of the cases. In 60% of the cases in the largest published series, nuclear atypia was absent or slight, and mitotic activity was low (less than 2 MF/10 HPFs).[183] In the remaining cases, grade 1 to 3 nuclear atypia, usually associated with an increase in mitotic activity (up to 15 MFs/10 HPFs), was present (Fig. 19.73).

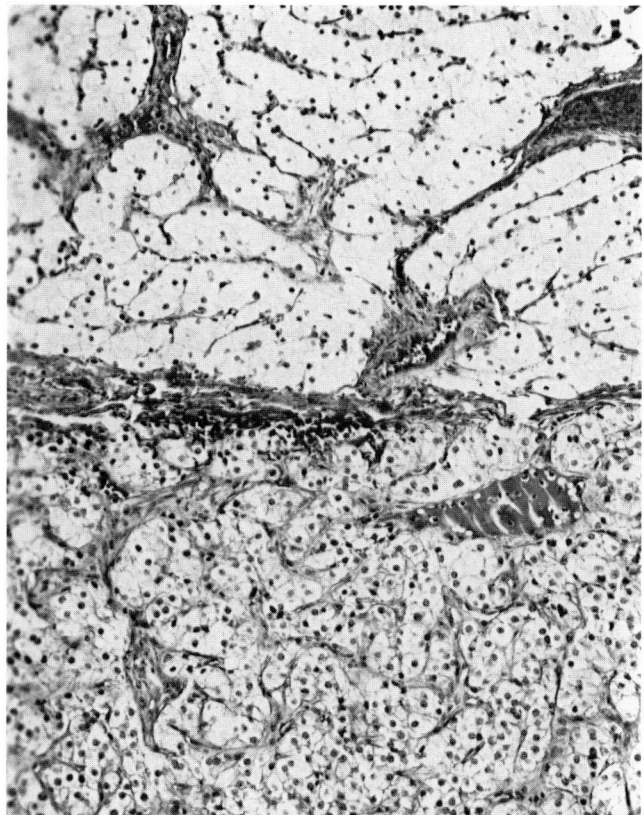

FIG. 19.72. Steroid cell tumor, not otherwise specified. Cells at the top have abundant pale cytoplasm whereas those at the bottom have less abundant cytoplasm. (Reprinted by permission of Young and Scully (1985). Ovarian sex cord-stromal and steroid cell tumors. In: Roth LM, Czernobilsky B (eds) Tumors and Tumor-like Conditions of the Ovary, Contemporary Issues in Surgical Pathology, Vol. 6. New York, Churchill Livingstone.)

As mentioned above, tumors in this category are thought to arise from the ovarian stroma or hilus cells. The striking resemblance of many of these tumors to adrenal cortical tumors has suggested, however, the possibility that some of them arise from adrenal cortical rests. Although such rests are extremely rare within the ovary,[408] they have been identified on careful search in the broad ligament and occasionally in the ovarian hilus in about one-quarter of women.[133] In a few patients with steroid cell tumors the responses of elevated levels of urinary 17-ketosteroids and 17-hydroxycorticosteroids to adrenocorticotropic hormone (ACTH) stimulation and dexamethasone suppression have been more suggestive of an origin from cells of adrenal cortical than gonadal type, but such responses are not diagnostic.[225,425] The strongest evidence that rare steroid cell tumors arise from adrenal cortical rests is their association with either the adrenogenital syndrome[290] or Cushing's syndrome.[469] Despite this, the confinement of these tumors to the ovary on gross and microscopic examination

strongly supports an atypical production of adrenal cortical hormones by gonadal cells rather an ectopic adrenal cortical tumor.

CLINICAL BEHAVIOR AND TREATMENT

In 20% of the cases, extraovarian spread of tumor is present at the time of operation; three of the four patients with Cushing's disease (Fig. 19.73) had extensive intraabdominal spread of tumor.[469] In the two largest series in the literature, the proportion of tumors that were clinically malignant was 25% and 43%[183,421]; rare tumors have recurred as many as 19 years postoperatively. Patients with clinically malignant tumors were on average 16 years older than patients with benign tumors in one series; no malignant steroid cell tumors have been reported in patients in the first two decades.

The best pathological correlates with malignant behavior in one series[183] were: 2 or more MF/10 HPFs (92% malignant); necrosis (86% malignant); a diameter of ≥ 7 cm (78% malignant); hemorrhage (77% malignant); and grade 2 or 3 nuclear atypia (64% malignant); occasional tumors that appear cytologically benign, however, may be malignant. The metastatic tumor appears similar to the primary tumor in some cases but more poorly differentiated in others.

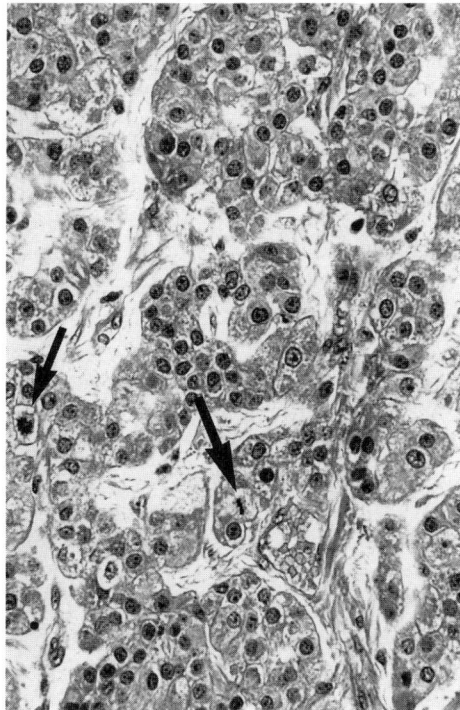

FIG. 19.73. Steroid cell tumor, not otherwise specified. This tumor, which was from a patient with Cushing's syndrome, exhibited prominent mitotic activity (*arrows*). (Reproduced by permission of Clement et al., ref. 96.)

DIFFERENTIAL DIAGNOSIS OF STEROID CELL TUMORS

Stromal luteomas and Leydig cell tumors usually do not pose great diagnostic difficulty for the pathologist because of their characteristic locations and obvious composition of steroid-type cells, which contain crystals of Reinke in the Leydig cell tumor. The extensive formation of spaces in occasional tumors in these categories, however, may cause confusion with an adenocarcinoma and more often with a vascular tumor. Awareness of this degenerative phenomenon and its association with cellular debris, inflammatory cell infiltration, and fibrosis, as well as the finding of typical areas elsewhere in the specimen, particularly at the periphery, should facilitate the diagnosis.

Steroid cell tumors in the NOS category vary more widely in appearance than the stromal luteoma and Leydig cell tumor both architecturally and cytologically and are accordingly the cause of greater diagnostic difficulty. The tumors that may enter the differential diagnosis include extensively luteinized granulosa cell tumors and thecomas, lipid-rich Sertoli cell tumors, clear cell carcinomas, particularly those of the oxyphil type, rare oxyphilic endometrioid carcinomas, hepatoid yolk sac tumors and hepatoid carcinomas, endocrine tumors such as oxyphilic struma ovarii, pituitary-type tumors and paragangliomas (pheochromocytoma), metastatic renal cell carcinomas, adrenocortical carcinomas, hepatocellular carcinomas, other metastatic tumors with oxyphilic appearance, and primary and metastatic melanomas. The presence of characteristic nonluteinized cells in both luteinized granulosa cell tumors and thecomas, as well as the typical cytological features and patterns of these neoplasms, and the finding of abundant reticulum in thecomas are of help in the identification of these tumors. The recognition of areas with a solid tubular pattern helps distinguish a usually estrogenic lipid-rich Sertoli cell tumor with a predominant diffuse pattern from a typically androgenic steroid cell tumor. In contrast to steroid cell tumors, the clear cells of clear cell carcinomas and metastatic renal cell carcinomas have glycogen-rich cytoplasm and eccentric nuclei. Also, the presence of tubular, glandular, and papillary patterns, which are inconsistent with a steroid cell tumor, generally facilitate the differential diagnosis. Radiologic studies to rule out a renal cell carcinoma may be additionally helpful. Oxyphilic clear cell carcinomas and endometrioid carcinomas, and hepatoid yolk sac tumors and hepatoid carcinomas are all characterized by neoplastic cells with abundant eosinophilic cytoplasm. The first two tumors generally exhibit epithelial patterns, may contain glandular lumens, and are almost always accompanied by more easily recognized patterns. The oxyphilic clear cell carcinoma is almost always accompanied by a variable component of clear and hobnail cells not seen in steroid cell tumors. The hepatoid tumors also have epithelial patterns and may contain glandular lumens; they are characterized by immunohistochemical staining for alpha-fetoprotein. We are not aware of any cases of adrenocortical carcinoma that have presented in the form

of a metastatic mass involving the ovary, but the possibility exists. Primary and metastatic melanomas can simulate steroid cell tumors if melanotic, and if they are pigmented the pigment granules may be confused with the lipochrome granules of a steroid cell tumor. Melanomas generally have more malignant nuclear features than steroid cell tumors. Special staining, including staining for S-100 protein and HMB-45, may be helpful in difficult cases. An association with other teratomatous elements and the presence of colloid and immunohistochemical staining for thyroglobulin should enable one to distinguish an oxyphil struma from a steroid cell tumor NOS. A rare pituitary-type tumor containing cells with abundant eosinophilic cytoplasm that arose in a wall of a dermoid cyst secreted ACTH and caused Cushing's syndrome.[27] Such a tumor might be confused with a steroid cell tumor. In that case, immunohistochemical staining for ACTH and several other pituitary hormones was positive. Finally, we have seen a case of apparently primary pheochromocytoma of the ovary in which the diagnosis of a steroid cell tumor was a consideration and rare other examples of this tumor have been primary in the ovary.[137] In our case immunohistochemical staining of the tumor cells for chromogranin was helpful in establishing the diagnosis. Electron microscopic examination of most of the neoplasms that simulate steroid cell tumors should disclose strikingly different features. Finally, the presence or absence of endocrine manifestations and their nature may be important clinical clues to the diagnosis.

Pregnancy luteomas, which are hyperplastic nodules composed of lutein cells that develop during pregnancy, may form large masses that resemble steroid cell tumors grossly and microscopically (see Chapter 16, Nonneoplastic Lesions of the Ovary). As with the latter, they also may be virilizing (in about one-quarter of the cases). Unlike steroid cell tumors, however, approximately one-third of pregnancy luteomas are bilateral and approximately one-half are multiple. Microscopic examination reveals masses of cells with abundant eosinophilic cytoplasm containing little or no lipid; mitotic figures may be numerous, sometimes up to 2 or 3/10 HPF. In contrast, a steroid cell tumor with minimal cytological atypia that resembles a pregnancy luteoma usually contains only rare mitotic figures. Although it may be impossible to distinguish a lipid-poor or lipid-free steroid cell tumor from a solitary pregnancy luteoma, a lesion encountered during the third trimester of pregnancy is presumed to be a solitary pregnancy luteoma unless clear-cut evidence indicates otherwise.

Other Ovarian Tumors with Endocrine Function

Ovarian Tumors with Functioning Stroma

A wide variety of ovarian tumors other than those in the sex cord–stromal and steroid cell categories may be hormon-

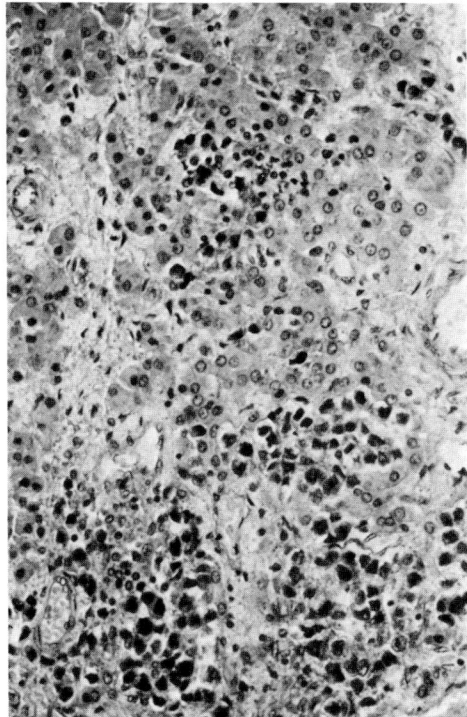

FIG. 19.74. Dysgerminoma with syncytiotrophoblast cells. Degenerating dysgerminoma cells are separated by steroid-type cells with pale nuclei and abundant dense cytoplasm in the peripheral portion of the tumor.

ally active as a result of steroid hormone production by stromal cells within or adjacent to the tumor (Figs 19.74–19.77). These tumors, which have been designated *ovarian tumors with functioning stroma*,[374] may be benign or malignant and, if in the latter category, primary or metastatic. Almost every ovarian tumor has been reported to be associated with stromal hormone production but, as discussed below, this phenomenon is seen much more often with some neoplasms than others.

Ovarian tumors with functioning stroma are associated infrequently with overt endocrine manifestations but commonly accompanied by subclinical elevations of steroid hormone values.[340,341] In one early investigation,[348] 39% of postmenopausal women with ovarian cancer were reported to have increased cornification of their cervical and vaginal squamous cells on cytological smears. In a more recent study, Rome et al.,[340] demonstrated a 50% frequency of elevation of total urinary estrogens in patients with surface epithelial–stromal tumors or metastatic carcinomas in the ovary. Aiman et al.[11] found that 4 of 11 premenopausal women with benign and malignant epithelial and germ cell tumors had increased testosterone, androstenedione, or both in their peripheral or ovarian venous blood. The stromal cells responsible for the hormone secretion in ovarian tumors with functioning stroma typically resemble lutein or Leydig cells and have been referred to as *luteinized stromal cells*. These cells almost

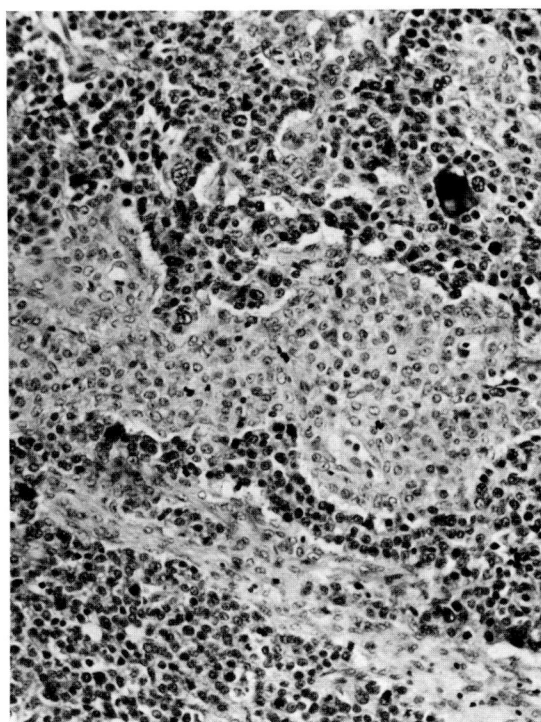

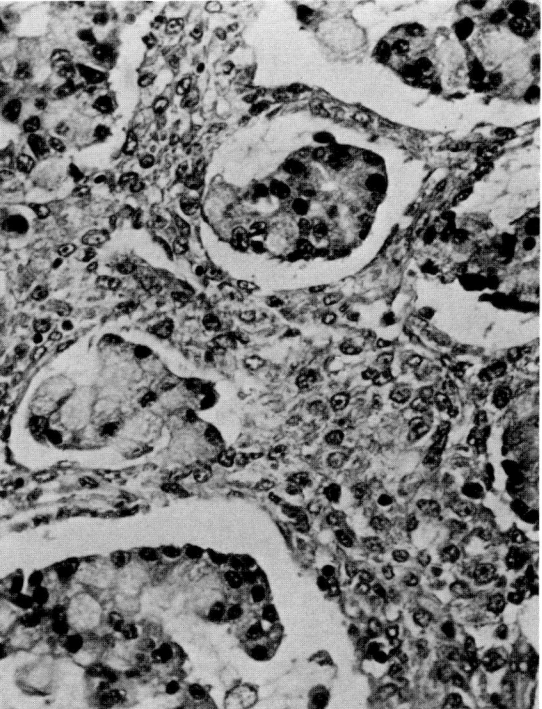

FIG. 19.75. Krukenberg tumor with luteinization of stroma. In the left frame cords of carcinoma cells are separated by masses of luteinized cells. In the right frame clusters of mucin-filled cells are separated by luteinized stromal cells. This tumor was associated with virilization and decidual change of the endometrium. (Reprinted by permission of Scully and Richardson, ref. 375.)

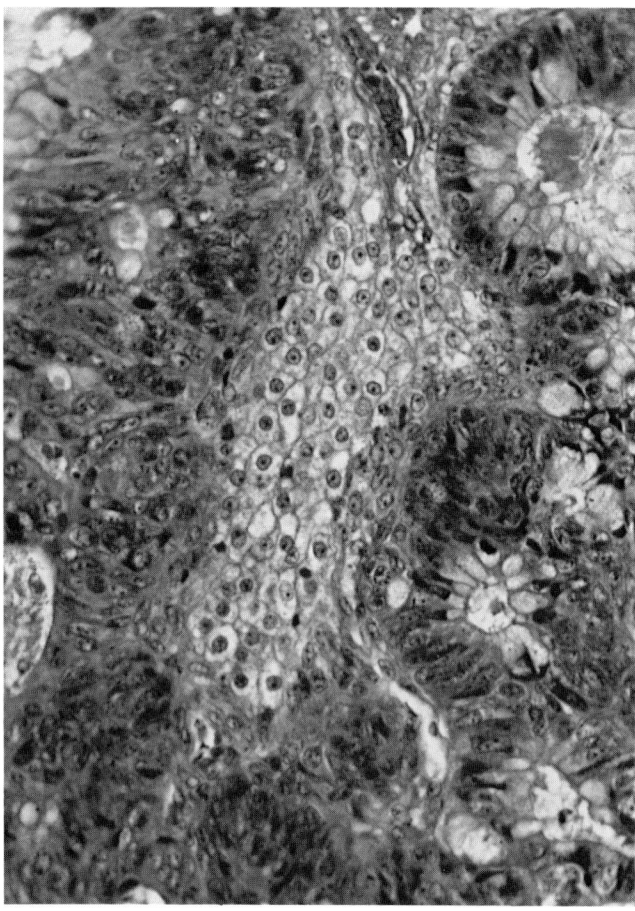

Fig. 19.76. Metastatic adenocarcinoma from colon. The neoplastic glands are separated by vacuolated luteinized stromal cells. (Reprinted by permission of Scully and Richardson, ref. 375.)

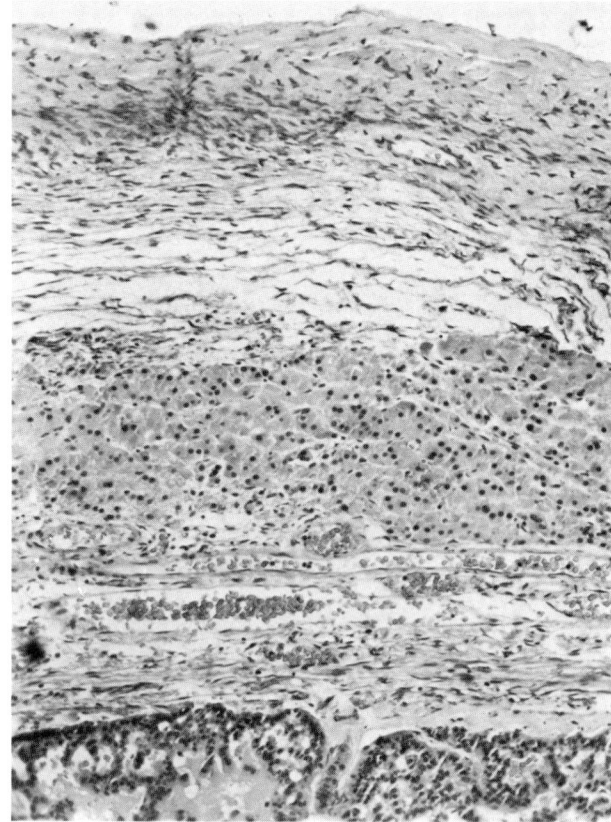

Fig. 19.77. Strumal carcinoid. There is a peripheral band of steroid-type cells.

always lie within the tumor singly, diffusely, or in clusters (Figs. 19.74–19.76), but rarely they are mainly distributed just outside the tumor, sometimes forming a peripheral band (Fig 19.77).[349] Exceptionally, crystals of Reinke can be identified in the lutein-like cells, warranting their interpretation as Leydig cells. It must be emphasized, however, that steroid-type cells may be prominent in the absence of clinical evidence of hormone overproduction and, conversely, evidence of function may exist in the absence of fully developed cells of steroid type.

Ovarian tumors with functioning stroma can be divided into three major categories.[370] In the first two categories, germ cell tumors that contain syncytiotrophoblast cells and tumors in pregnant patients, the luteinized stromal cells probably develop as a result of stimulation by hCG. The cause of the stromal alteration in the third (idiopathic) group, which accounts for most of the cases, is unclear, but ectopic production of hCG or some other stromal stimulant by the neoplastic cells may be responsible.

Germ Cell Tumors Containing Syncytiotrophoblast Cells

Two dysgerminomas with syncytiotrophoblast cells have been associated with luteinization of the stroma (Fig. 19.74) and endocrine manifestations; one was accompanied by isosexual precocity[435] and the other by postpubertal virilization.[77]

Germ cell tumors that produce hCG, including dysgerminomas with syncytiotrophoblast giant cells,[221,478] choriocarcinomas, embryonal carcinomas, and polyembryomas[35] and mixed primitive germ cell tumors,[377] also may cause manifestations of steroid hormone secretion[56,239,240] as a result of hCG stimulation of the ovary contralateral to the tumor to form luteinized follicles that secrete steroid hormones.[188,239,240,377]

Tumors with Functioning Stroma Occurring During Pregnancy

Although it is logical to speculate that ovarian tumors with functioning stroma in pregnant patients may secrete estrogens, this possibility has not been investigated by hormone assay, and clinical manifestation of estrogen excess are not expected to be present during gestation. In contrast, 23 examples of virilization caused by ovarian tumors with functioning stroma during pregnancy have been reported. These tumors have included 11 Krukenberg tumors,[°] seven mucinous cystic tumors,[60,89,303,322,355,364,444] two Brenner tumors,[44,180,273,286] and single examples of serous cystadenoma,[138] endodermal sinus tumor,[364] and dermoid cyst.[76] The onset of the virilization in these patients has ranged from the third to the ninth month of gestation. The endocrine status of the offspring is known in 10 cases; the child was a normal male in three, a normal female in two, and a virilized female in five cases.

Idiopathic Group

Whereas ovarian tumors with functioning stroma in the first two categories are encountered in young girls, patients with tumors in the idiopathic group usually are postmenopausal, reflecting the higher prevalence of ovarian tumors, both primary and metastatic, and possibly the higher levels of circulating luteinizing hormone in this age group. A wide variety of ovarian tumors has been associated with an idiopathic functioning stroma but its frequency has varied from one type of neoplasm to another.[†]

Mucinous tumors often contain functioning stroma, resulting in either estrogenic or androgenic manifestations. In one series,[128] approximately one-quarter of both mucinous cystadenomas and cystadenocarcinomas were accompanied by evidence of an "active endometrium" in postmenopausal women. In another study approximately two-thirds of patients with mucinous tumors of various types had elevated total estrogen levels in the urine.[340] Five mucinous tumors have been responsible for virilization of nonpregnant patients.[15,46,102,106,153]

Occasional cases of endometrioid carcinoma have been reported to be associated with endometrial hyperplasia in postmenopausal women,[199,374,458] and in one case virilization and breast secretion developed.[374] We have seen a well-differentiated endometrioid carcinoma from a patient with an elevated serum testosterone level and the recent development of hirsutism.[371] Rome et al.[340] found that urinary estrogen levels were elevated in five of six patients with endometrioid carcinoma, indicating that these tumors may be associated with function more often than had been realized. Clear cell carcinomas have been accompanied only exceptionally by endometrial hyperplasia,[199] and Rome et al.[340] found that the urinary estrogens were normal in all four of their patients with tumors of this type. Serous tumors also have been associated only rarely with evidence of hyperestrinism[128,144,270] or hyperandrogenism.[138,311,316] Two of three patients with undifferenti-

ated carcinoma of the ovary studied by Rome et al.[340] had elevated urinary total estrogen excretion. Brenner tumors have been accompanied by endometrial hyperplasia in 10–16% of the cases.[19,30,214,385,428] In one case[177] Leydig cells were identified in the stroma. One estrogenic Brenner tumor was malignant.[233] Four Brenner tumors have been associated with virilization.[44,114,180,273] These studies indicate that all types of common epithelial tumor may be associated with stromal activation but that endocrine manifestations are seen with significant frequency only in patients with mucinous tumors.

Germ cell tumors of various types lacking trophoblastic cells have been associated rarely with stromal luteinization and evidence of steroid hormone secretion in the absence of pregnancy.[188] The germ cell tumors within the idiopathic category that have been accompanied by androgenic or estrogenic manifestations have included a variety of subtypes such as dermoid cyst,[12] struma ovarii,[449] carcinoid tumors,[117,335,336] embryonal carcinoma,[1] and yolk sac tumor.[2,323,402]

The steroid cells that are stimulated in cases of germ cell tumor are peripheral (Fig. 19.77) rather than within the tumor in many, if not most, of the cases.[349] Solid mature teratomas and immature teratomas have not been accompanied by evidence of steroid hormone production to the best of our knowledge. The lesions associated with peripheral steroid cell formation in the series of Rutgers and Scully[349] describing this phenomenon were struma ovarii (nine cases), strumal or trabecular carcinoids (four cases), rete cysts (four cases), mucinous cystadenomas (three cases), dermoid cysts (two cases), and single examples of dysgerminoma with syncytiotrophoblast giant cells and metastatic carcinoid. In three of the cases, all strumas, a yellow color was appreciated grossly at the periphery or on the surface of the tumor.

The steroid cells that develop adjacent to ovarian tumors rather than within them are of three types: lutein cells within adjacent ovarian stroma, Leydig cells within ovarian stroma, and hilus cells, which are present only along the hilar border of the tumor. The number of cases in each of these three categories in the series of Rutgers and Scully[349] were 14, 2, and 8, respectively. The tumors with hilus cell hyperplasia were typically large with an average greatest diameter of 18 cm. The lutein cells and stromal Leydig cells were located predominantly or exclusively in the cortex or medulla peripheral to the tumor and were arranged singly and in nests forming a discontinuous band up to 2 mm in thickness. The hilus cells were arranged singly and in small nests forming discontinuous bands in the walls of the cysts in which they arose. Lutein cell formation is accompanied most often by estrogenic manifestations, whereas stromal Leydig formation and hilar Leydig cell hyperplasia are associated most often with androgenic changes. Other examples of this phenomenon reported have been two additional rete cysts with peripheral hilus

---

°Refs. 36,101,143,146,355,384,444,445.
†Refs. 11,28,73,135,185,186,209,226,228,252–254,348.

cell hyperplasia,[34,339] a fibroma with peripheral stromal Leydig cell proliferation,[229] and a leiomyoma with peripheral hilus cell hyperplasia[318]; all four cases were associated with virilization.

Metastatic carcinomas that contain mucinous cells, like primary mucinous tumors of the ovary, frequently are associated with luteinization of the stroma (Figs. 19.75, 19.76) and in a significant proportion of cases with clinical evidence of elevated steroid hormone levels. Scully and Richardson[375] found clinical evidence of excess estrogens as manifested by irregular premenopausal bleeding or postmenopausal bleeding in one-quarter of patients with metastatic adenocarcinoma from the large intestine and stomach. One metastatic adenocarcinoma from the colon was responsible for masculinization[375] and another for both androgenic and estrogenic changes.[78] Eight Krukenberg tumors from nonpregnant patients have been associated with virilization (Fig. 19.73). Most of these tumors were of gastric origin[36,143,149,355,445,446] but one arose in the breast[394] and another, a tubular Krukenberg tumor, in the appendix.[64] One Krukenberg tumor of gastric origin and a metastatic adenocarcinoma of colonic origin have been associated with decidual changes in the endometrium in addition to virilization.[63,309] An additional metastatic colonic adenocarcinoma was associated with progesterone production.[212] Other metastatic tumors are associated much less often with stromal luteinization. One postmenopausal woman was virilized as a result of luteinization caused by bilateral metastatic lobular carcinoma of the breast.[74] As mentioned above, one metastatic colonic carcinoid was associated with peripheral stromal luteinization.[349] Finally, in one case of malignant lymphoma there was stromal luteinization associated with secondary amenorrhea.[279]

Thyroid Hyperfunction Associated with Ovarian Tumors

Although strumas and strumal carcinoids of the ovary have been demonstrated by immunohistochemical staining to contain thyroglobulin, triiodothyronine, and thyroxine[182,235,392,409] and, therefore, probably produce thyroid hormones at subclinical levels in many cases, clinical evidence suggestive of hyperthyroidism is present in only 25% of the cases,[224,298] and florid thyrotoxicosis in only about 5%.[259] Factors that make it difficult to determine accurately the frequency of hyperthyroidism in patients with struma ovarii include variable criteria for the amount of thyroid tissue required for a diagnosis of struma; the observation that approximately one-sixth of patients with struma ovarii have concomitant enlargement of the thyroid gland,[259] and a lack of confirmation of the hyperthyroidism by modern laboratory tests in most of the reported cases.

In some patients with clinical or laboratory evidence of hyperthyroidism, the preoperative diagnosis of hyperfunc-

tioning struma ovarii has been established by high [195]I uptake in the pelvis with low radioiodine uptake in the neck.[62,258,452] Other cases of struma-associated hyperthyroidism have not been recognized until the symptoms regressed after removal of an ovarian tumor. In some of these cases, a prior thyroidectomy had had no effect on the hyperthyroidism. Occasionally, oophorectomy for struma may precipitate compensatory enlargement of the thyroid gland, increased uptake of radioactive iodine by the thyroid gland, or an episode of thyrotoxicosis.[259,298] Similarly, torsion of an ovary containing a struma precipitated striking hyperthyroxinemia in a pregnant patient.[235]

A microscopic comparison of strumas associated with hyperthyroidism and those without this disorder has shown no significant differences.[224] However, in one study, a correlation was noted between the presence of thyrotoxicity and the size of the struma; evidence of hyperthyroidism was rare in cases of struma in which the tumor was less than 3 cm in diameter. Eight percent of strumal carcinoids (see Chapter 20, Germ Cell Tumors of the Ovary) in one study have been accompanied by evidence of hypersecretion of thyroid hormone in the form of postoperative thyroid storm or hypothyroidism,[336] and thyroglobulin has been demonstrated in the colloid within tumors of this type.[169,390,436]

Ovarian Tumors Associated with the Carcinoid Syndrome

Of the four major categories of primary carcinoid tumor of the ovary (see Chapter 20), insular, trabecular, strumal, and mucinous, one-third of the insular tumors[335] and a single example of strumal carcinoid[437] have been associated with the carcinoid syndrome. In the largest series of metastatic carcinoids involving the ovary, 40% of the tumors were associated with the carcinoid syndrome.[338] The volume of the carcinoid is an important factor determining the presence or absence of the syndrome. In the largest study of insular carcinoids in the literature, no patient had the syndrome whose carcinoid formed only a small portion of a teratoma, whereas patients with carcinoid tumors (pure or associated with teratoma) between 4 and 7 cm in diameter had the syndrome in one-half of the cases, and those with larger tumors had it in two-thirds of the cases.[335] The case of a 74-year-old woman with the carcinoid syndrome attributable to an ovarian tumor that resembled an atypical carcinoid with areas of neuroendocrine (oat cell) carcinoma was reported by Brown and Lane in 1965.[61] That patient also was virilized and had Cushing's syndrome. Although no immunohistochemical staining was performed in that case, the authors concluded that the tumor was elaborating both serotonin and ACTH.

The carcinoid syndrome typically occurs in the absence of hepatic or other metastases in cases of ovarian carcinoid, because the hormonal effluent of the tumor enters the

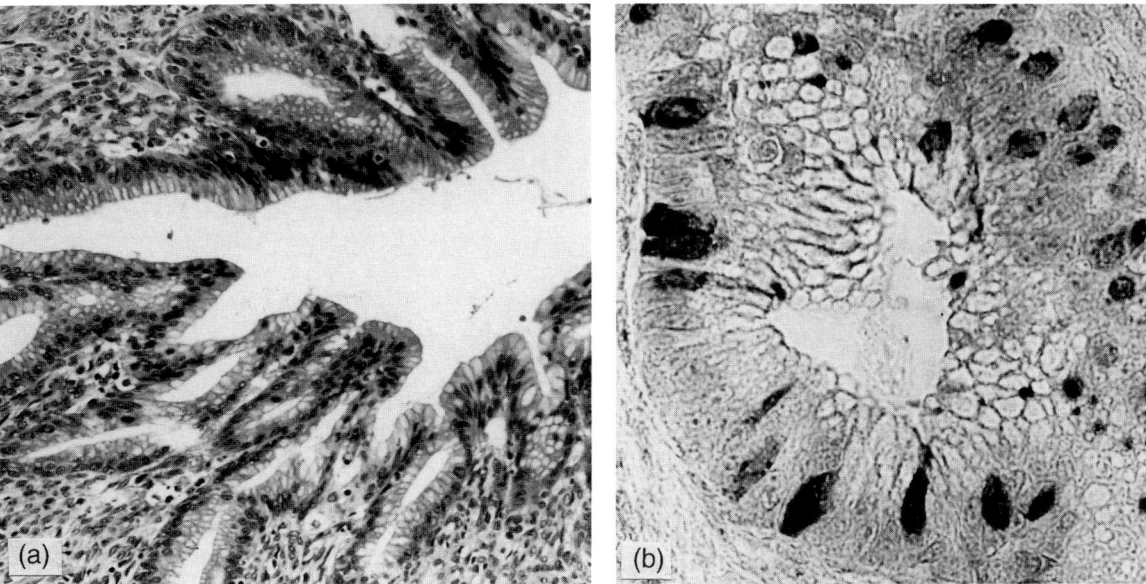

FIG. 19.78. Mucinous cystic tumor of borderline malignancy that was associated with the Zollinger–Ellison syndrome. In the right panel some of the neoplastic cells are immunoreactive for gastrin. (Reproduced with permission from Clement et al., ref. 96.)

systemic circulation directly, bypassing the portal venous system and avoiding inactivation in the liver. The carcinoid syndrome caused by a primary ovarian carcinoid therefore is usually curable if the tumor is confined to the ovary and irreversible damage to cardiac valves has not occurred. However, in the series of insular carcinoid tumors cited above, fatal recurrences of tumor developed in two of the 48 patients. In another patient, progressive tricuspid valve damage led to cardiac decompensation despite removal of the ovarian tumor.[335]

Ovarian Tumors Associated with Zollinger–Ellison Syndrome

Ten mucinous tumors (two cystademomas, five borderline tumors, and three cystadenocarcinomas) have caused the Zollinger–Ellison syndrome.° Most of the tumors were large, with a maximum dimension of 12 to 35 cm (mean, 21.5 cm) and a weight of 700 to 7000 g (median, 1100g). Gastrin-containing cells were identified immunohistochemically within the cyst lining in all nine of the cases in which staining was performed (Fig. 19.78); in six cases, gastrin was demonstrated within the cyst fluid. The clinical manifestations of Zollinger–Ellison syndrome, including elevated serum gastrin levels, disappeared after removal of the ovarian tumor in each case.

The association between ovarian mucinous tumors and Zollinger–Ellison syndrome is consistent with the frequent finding of neuroendocrine intestinal-type cells within mucinous tumors. A number of studies have shown that all categories of mucinous tumors (benign, borderline, and malignant) commonly contain argyrophil and hormone-immunoreactive cells, although in most of the studies, these cells have been found most frequently in mucinous borderline tumors.[6] The argyrophilic cells often are immunoreactive for serotonin and a variety of polypeptide hormones. The most commonly identified of the latter have been corticotropin, gastrin, somatostatin, glucagon, secretion, and pancreatic polypeptide; in many cases, the tumors have been immunoreactive for multiple hormones.

Ovarian Tumors with Paraendocrine Disorders

A variety of paraendocrine disorders have been described in association with numerous types of ovarian tumor, some manifested by signs and symptoms of a well-known endocrine disease and others by subclinical laboratory abnormalities, indicating ectopic production of hormones or hormone-like substances by the tumor cells. In some of these cases the hormone being produced has been identified whereas in others, such as in cases of hypercalcemia, the mechanism of the disorder remains unclear. In all the cases included within this category of neoplasms, successful therapy of the tumor has led to disappearance of the paraendocrine state.

°Refs. 53,54,64,98,152,162,186,192,217,264,284,327.

Hypercalcemia, Including Small Cell Carcinoma

One hundred four ovarian tumors have been reported to be associated with paraendocrine hypercalcemia.[455b] They have not been accompanied by recognizable clinical manifestations of hypercalcemia in most of the cases.° Fifty-nine percent of the tumors have been a distinctive type of small cell carcinoma; the remainder have included clear cell carcinomas (19 cases), serous carcinomas (6 cases), squamous cell carcinoma arising in a dermoid cyst (6 cases), dysgerminoma (6 cases), and miscellaneous other neoplasms (5 cases).

The mechanism of the hypercalcemia associated with ovarian cancers is unknown. Attempts to demonstrate parathormone (PTH) within the tumor cells have been unsuccessful with rare exceptions, and in several cases in which PTH has been measured in the serum, the level was normal. Recent evidence has implicated PTH-related peptide (PTHRP). Two hypercalcemic clear cell carcinomas of the ovary were associated with elevated serum levels of PTHRP,[193,308] in another PTHRP was detected by radioimmunoassay,[148] and two other hypercalcemic ovarian tumors (one a small cell carcinoma) were immunoreactive for PTHRP.[67] Because of the binding of PTHRP to a receptor common for PTH and PTHRP, the secretion of PTHRP by a neoplasm may produce the biochemical features of hyperparathyroidism. In one case[193] the patient also had abnormally high serum concentrations of 1.25-dihydroxyvitamin D (1.25-DHD) and increased intestinal calcium absorption. Tumor removal was followed by normalization of the serum calcium, PTHRP, and 1.25-DHD levels, suggesting an intestinal contribution to the maintenance of the hypercalcemia in this patient.

The *small cell carcinoma* that is often associated with hypercalcemia was first described by Dickersin and his colleagues in 1981 (Figs. 19.68, 19.69).[116] This tumor, of which we have now seen 150 examples,[455b] is, in our experience, the most common form of undifferentiated carcinoma of the ovary in females under 40 years of age and has been accompanied by elevated levels of calcium in 62% of the cases in which it has been measured. The age of the patients has ranged from 9 to 44 (average 24) years. The presenting symptoms usually are abdominal pain and swelling.

At laparotomy almost all the tumors have been unilateral; spread beyond the ovary has occurred in approximately one-quarter of the cases. Gross examination reveals fleshy white to pale tan masses, often containing large areas of hemorrhage and necrosis (Fig. 19.79). The most common microscopic appearance is a diffuse arrangement of closely packed epithelial cells interrupted focally in most cases by distinctive follicle-like structures containing eosinophilic fluid (Fig. 19.80). The neoplastic cells typi-

---

°Refs. 1,3,13,72,116,140,142a,195,215,255,328,376,401,410,438.

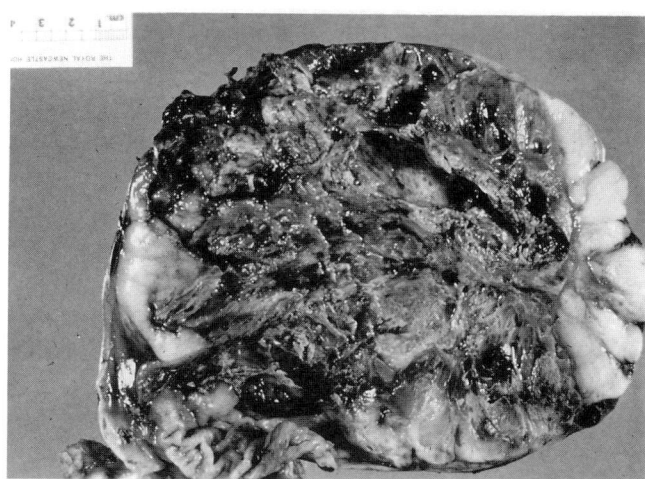

FIG. 19.79. Small cell carcinoma, hypercalcemic type. The sectioned surface of the neoplasm exhibits massive hemorrhage and necrosis. Viable lobulated tumor that was creamy white is still visible at the periphery.

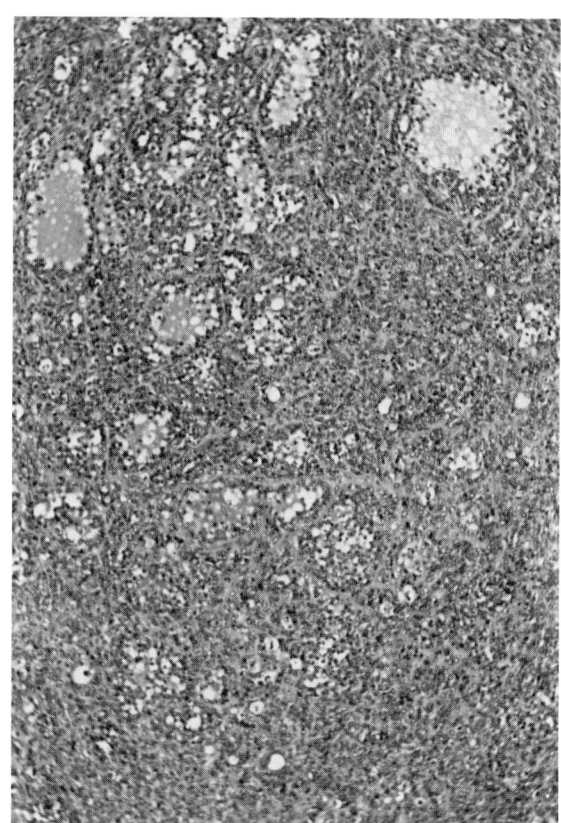

FIG. 19.80. Small cell carcinoma. Many small follicles are present within an otherwise densely cellular neoplasm.

cally have scanty cytoplasm and small nuclei that typically contain single small nucleoli; mitotic figures are numerous (Fig. 19.81). The tumor cells also grow in nests, cords, and irregular groups. In about 50% of the tumors large cells with abundant eosinophilic cytoplasm resembling to varying extents lutein cells have been present focally (Fig. 19.82); rarely, these cells predominate. The stroma is generally relatively scanty and consists of nonspecific fibrous tissue.

Special staining and immunohistochemical[8] and ultrastructural[269] examination have not revealed any features that identify the specific cell type of this epithelial tumor; rare dense-core granules have been reported to be present in the literature, but we have not observed them ultrastructurally in our cases.[373] They also were absent in one major series.[269] Flow cytometry on paraffin-embedded material typically shows that the cells are diploid.[130] The age distribution and the characteristic presence of uniform small cells and follicle formation suggest a sex cord derivation, but transitions to recognizable forms of sex cord tumors have not been observed. No unquestionable teratomatous elements have been found, but in 10% of the cases occasional glands lined by mature mucinous epithelium, signet cells, or highly atypical cells containing mucin have been

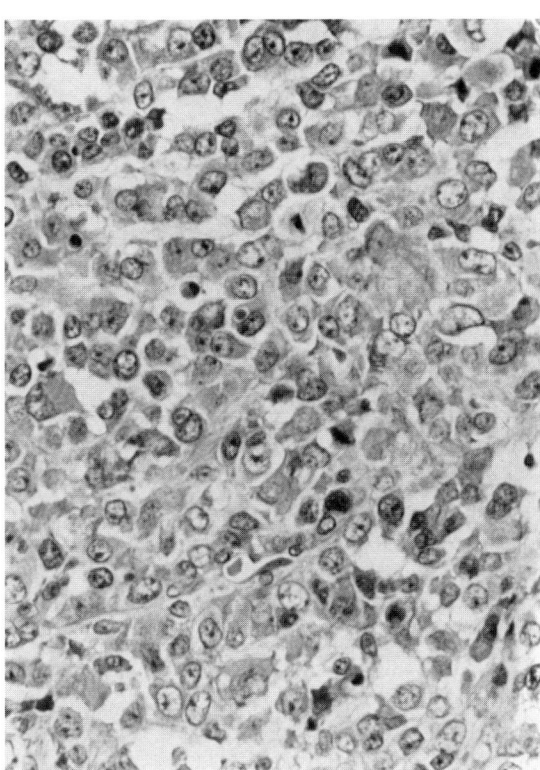

FIG. 19.82. **Small cell carcinoma.** Focal area is composed of large cells with abundant dense cytoplasm.

present. Unfortunately, this finding does not establish the origin of the tumor since mucinous epithelium may be seen in surface epithelial tumors, germ cell neoplasm, and Sertoli–Leydig cell tumors.

The small cell carcinoma often is confused with a granulosa cell tumor of either adult or juvenile type. The features of these three types of tumor are contrasted in Table 19.3. Diffuse small cell carcinomas also may resemble malignant lymphomas, particularly on low-power examination, but adequate sampling reveals patterns of growth that indicate the epithelial nature of the tumor; also, the cytological features of the neoplastic cells are incompatible with any form of malignant lymphoma. Exceptionally, the differential diagnosis of a small cell carcinoma includes other small cell malignant tumors of the ovary, including several metastatic tumors such as metastatic melanoma[406,460] and metastatic small cell sarcomas[470] (see Chapter 22, Metastatic Tumors of the Ovary). The small cell carcinoma has a poor prognosis even when stage I and no form of adjuvant therapy is of proven benefit.

Cushing's Syndrome

Four cases of clinically typical and biochemically documented Cushing's syndrome have been caused by cortisol production by a steroid cell tumor. Three of the tumors

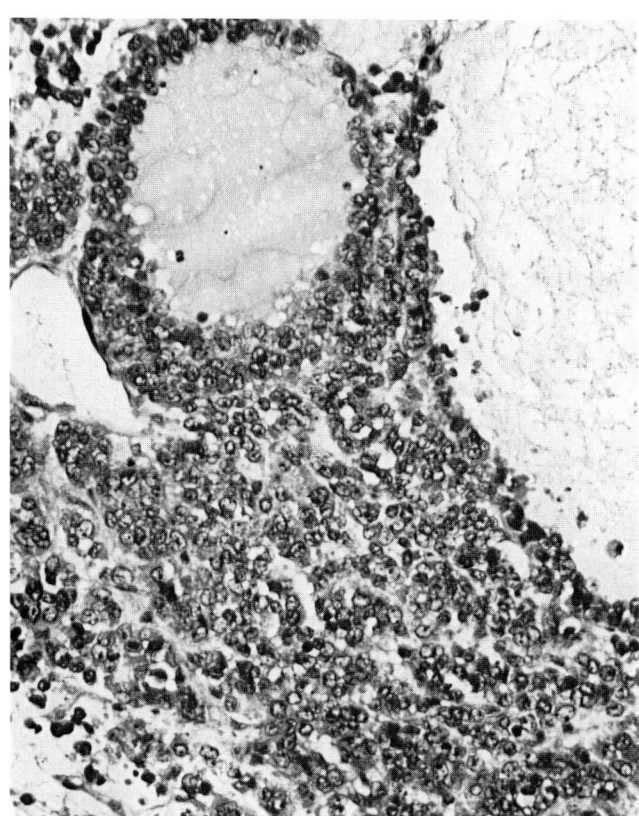

FIG. 19.81. **Small cell carcinoma.** Follicle-like structures lined by and surrounded by small cells with scanty cytoplasm and hyperchromatic nuclei.

occurred in adults and had metastasized within the abdomen at the time of presentation.[261,470] In contrast to clinically benign steroid cell tumors, the ovarian tumors in these cases had significantly atypical cytological features. The patients died from tumor progression 6 to 17 months postoperatively. The fourth case occurred in a 2-year-old girl who also had isosexual precocious pseudopuberty.[4]

Rarely, primary ovarian tumors other than those of steroid cell type have been associated with Cushing's syndrome, probably in most cases on the basis of ectopic production of corticotropin or corticotropin-releasing factor. These cases have included tumors interpreted as a poorly differentiated adenocarcinoma,[319] a malignant Sertoli cell tumor,[297] a trabecular carcinoid (in which the tumor cells were immunoreactive for corticotropin),[96] and a tumor that resembled an atypical carcinoid and small cell carcinoma of the lung.[61] Finally, two cases have been described in which anterior pituitary tissue within a dermoid cyst caused Cushing's syndrome. In one of these cases, it was not clear whether the pituitary tissue was neoplastic or hyperplastic, but in the other case there was a chromophobe adenoma in which the neoplastic cells were immunoreactive for corticotropin.[27]

Human Chorionic Gonadotropin Secretion

Ectopic hCG production was reported by Civantos and Rywlin in three women with serous papillary or mucinous adenocarcinomas of the ovary.[94] All the patients had elevated urinary hCG levels ranging from 1000 to 25,000 I.U. per 24 hours. Each of the tumors contained poorly differentiated areas with cells resembling syncytiotrophoblast cells; these cells were positive for hCG on immunofluorescence. In one of these cases the contralateral ovary contained numerous lutein cells, and a decidual reaction was present in the endometrium; the patient in that case had vaginal bleeding but no endocrine effects were present in the other two patients. Recently, Kobayashi et al.[218] reported a case of an ovarian clear cell carcinoma in a patient who presented with postmenopausal bleeding. Elevated serum concentrations of hCG and estradiol were found and the tumor cells were immunoreactive for both hormones. No syncytiotrophoblastic differentiation was found within the tumor. Vaitukaitis[439] reported that 10 of 28 ovarian tumors of various types were associated with the presence of immunoreactive hCG in the plasma and Samaan and associates[356] found the beta subunit of hCG in the plasma of 41% of women with common epithelial carcinomas. Immunohistochemical staining of common epithelial tumors for hCG has yielded varying results.[85,139,281] One group[281] found an approximately 40% frequency of staining, with no significant differences among benign, borderline, and invasive tumors whereas another group[138] found only a 10% frequency of staining of carcinomas and no staining of benign tumors. Because of its presence in a wide variety of tumors, including one granulosa cell tu-

mor,[139] immunohistochemical identification of hCG is of relatively little help in differential diagnosis. Matias-Guiu and Prat[263] conducted the most extensive immunohistochemical investigation of hCG in ovarian tumors, using single polyclonal antibodies to the whole hormone and its beta subunit and four monoclonal antibodies to the whole hormone, its beta subunit, and two regions of the carboxyl terminal of the beta subunit. Correlating positive staining results with the presence or absence of an "active" stroma of the tumor (luteinization and/or "condensation"), these authors found that the epithelial cells of 41% of the tumors with active stroma reacted with the polyclonal antibodies and 62% with the monoclonal antibodies; the corresponding figures for the epithelial cells of the tumor with an inactive stroma were 14% and 37%, respectively.

Hypoglycemia

Five cases have been reported in which an ovarian neoplasm has been associated with hypoglycemia.[275] The tumors have been a serous cystadenocarcinoma, a dysgerminoma, a fibroma, a malignant schwannoma, and a carcinoid tumor with a mixed insular and trabecular pattern.[276,285,312,381,395] In the case of the malignant schwannoma, insulin and proinsulin were recovered from the tumor tissue[381] and the cells of the carcinoid tumor were immunoreactive for insulin. Both tumors contained dense-core granules on ultrastructural examination.

Renin and Aldosterone Secretion

Eleven cases of hypertension related to hormone secretion by an ovarian tumor have been reported. In six cases, the hypertension was associated with a renin-secreting tumor, hyperreninism, and secondary hyperaldosteronism.[10,18,26,190,230,426] In three cases, an aldosterone-secreting ovarian tumor resulted in primary hyperaldosteronism associated with low or normal plasma renin levels.[206,234,430] Elevated aldosterone levels were present in a tenth case (but plasma renin levels were not measured),[129] and in the eleventh case, reported in 1966, neither renin nor aldosterone levels were determined.[288] In three cases, the tumor also elaborated steroid hormones, as manifested by isosexual pseudoprecocity in two cases[129,288] and elevated serum levels of estradiol and testosterone in a third.[430]

Seven of the ovarian tumors were interpreted as sex cord-stromal tumors and two as steroid cell tumors. Three tumors in the first category were well-differentiated Sertoli cell tumors, whereas the other four had an appearance that was too nonspecific or poorly differentiated to subclassify. One of these last four tumors occurred in a woman with Peutz–Jeghers syndrome and was benign, whereas the other three were clinically malignant and two were fatal. One of the "steroid cell" tumors occurred in a 7-year-old girl and had a prominent follicular pattern, more in keeping with a diagnosis of JGCT. The final two tumors were a leiomyosarcoma and a mucinous adenocarcinoma. Immunohistochemical staining in three of the sex cord–stromal tumors and the leiomyosarcoma showed cells containing immunoreactive renin or prorenin.[10,18,230,426]

Prolactin Secretion

Two ovarian dermoid cysts have been associated with the elaboration of prolactin.[220,314] The patients were both in the reproductive age group. In one case, the dermoid cyst contained a 2.5-cm tumor composed of small rounded nests of epithelial cells, some of which surrounded lumens filled with colloid-like material (Fig. 19.83). The cells had scanty cytoplasm and small, round, uniform, mitotically inactive nuclei. Most of the tumor cells were strongly immunoreactive for prolactin (Fig. 19.83). In the other case pathological examination of an otherwise typical dermoid cyst disclosed a 1-mm focus of pituitary tissue composed of large polygonal cells with abundant eosinophilic cytoplasm that was immunoreactive for prolactin.

Ovarian Tumors Associated with Paraneoplastic Syndromes

Nervous System Disorders

Ovarian cancer is among the most common malignant tumor associated with nervous system disorders; in one series the frequency of such disorders was 16%.[103] A variety of

lesions affecting both the gray matter and white matter of the cerebrum, cerebellum, and spinal cord, the peripheral nerves, and the myoneural junction, accompanied by myasthenia gravis, may occur.[59,187,433] Paraneoplastic subacute cerebellar degeneration (SCD) is one of the most common lesions, with ovarian cancer accounting for 16% of the cases in one series[187] and 37% in another.[178] The cerebellar manifestations usually antedate recognition of the cancer and typically there is no improvement after removal of the tumor.[176] In one recently reported case manifestations of the cerebellar degeneration partially regressed after plasmapheresis.[99] The pathogenesis of SCD in these cases appears to be related to the presence of circulating anti-Purkinje cell antibodies that have been shown to react with antigens in the tumor.[170,178,268] The presence of such antibodies appears to be much more common in patients with SCD and gynecological or breast cancer than in patients with SCD and other types of carcinoma. In a study of 19 women with a gynecological carcinoma, SCD, and anti-Purkinje cell antibodies, 14 of the tumors were primary in the ovary.[191] In several cases, the presence of the antibodies was the only initial evidence of the carcinoma. Limbic encephalitis also has been associated with ovarian carcinoma,[83] and necrotizing myelopathy, a rare paraneoplastic complication of cancer, accompanied an ovarian adenosquamous carcinoma in one patient.[80]

Connective Tissue Disorders

The connective tissue disorder most commonly associated with ovarian cancer is dermatomyositis.[33,70,412,443] In one

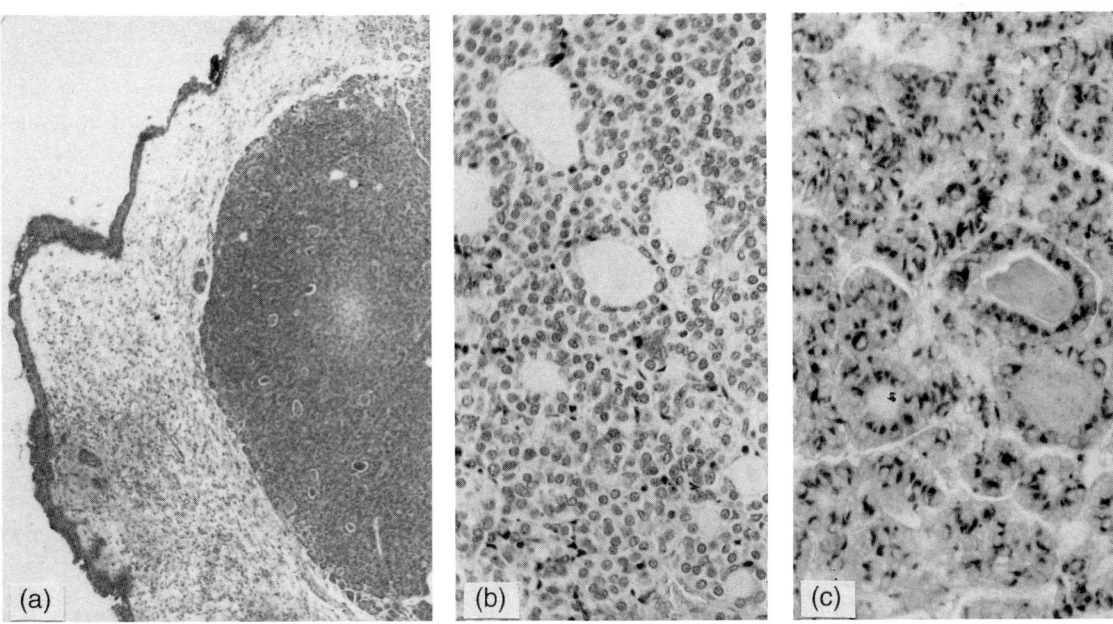

FIG. 19.83. Prolactinoma within ovarian dermoid cyst. a: A nodule of tumor is present beneath the squamous epithelial lining of the dermoid cyst. **b:** The tumor is composed of epithelial cells with scanty cytoplasm and small round uniform nuclei, some of which surround lumens filled with colloid-like material. **c:** Most of the tumor cells are strongly immunoreactive for prolactin. (Reproduced by permission of Clement et al., ref. 96.)

review of 25 cases of this disease in women, 5 were found to have malignant tumors, 3 of which were ovarian carcinomas.[360] In another study of 10 patients with dermatomyositis or polymyositis and a malignant tumor of the female genital tract, 5 had ovarian cancer.[443] Mordel et al.,[283] in a recent review of 30 literature cases of ovarian tumors associated with dermatomyositis, found that all of the histologically verified tumors were adenocarcinomas (most commonly high-grade serous carcinomas), and with one exception were stage III or IV. One dysgerminoma has been associated with dermatomyositis.[392]

Medsger and his associates[271] described six patients with ovarian carcinoma in whom polyarthritis and palmar fasciitis preceded the diagnosis of carcinoma by 5 to 25 months. The arthritic symptoms were similar to those of rheumatoid arthritis. Four of the ovarian tumors were endometrioid carcinomas, one, a serous carcinoma and one, an undifferentiated carcinoma. An additional example of this syndrome associated with serous carcinoma was subsequently described.[382] One woman with ovarian carcinoma had hypertrophic pulmonary osteoarthropathy[251] and occasional patients have had rheumatoid arthritis, scleroderma, or systemic lupus erythematosus.[40,69,125,251]

Cutaneous Disorders

A variety of cutaneous lesions have been described in association with ovarian tumors.[136,389] Acanthosis nigricans occurs in some, typically young, women in association with polycystic ovary disease (POD), stromal hyperthecosis, or combinations thereof,[124] representing a component of the so-called HAIR-AN syndrome (hyperandrogenemia, insulin resistance, and acanthosis nigricans). In one such case, bilateral wedge resections of the ovaries showed a stromal luteoma in addition to the typical findings of PCOD.[161] Four cases of so-called malignant acanthosis nigricans have been cases of ovarian carcinoma.[104,119] The sign of Leser-Trelat, the sudden onset and rapid increase in size of numerous seborrheic keratoses in association with an occult cancer, considered by some a variant of "malignant" acanthosis nigricans, has been associated with ovarian cancer in one case.[194] Rarely, ovarian carcinomas have occurred in patients with Muir–Torre syndrome.[100,168]

Nephrotic Syndrome

Five to 10% of cases of the nephrotic syndrome have a paraneoplastic background, although the causative tumors in such cases are located only rarely in the female genital tract. In 1966, Lee et al.[244] documented the presence of the nephrotic syndrome and membranous glomerulopathy in two patients with ovarian tumors (one "adenocarcinoma," one dermoid cyst). However, it was not established in either case that the two lesions were more than coincidental. More recently, Hoyt and Hamilton[196] described a 65-year-old woman who was found to have the nephrotic syndrome 8 months before the detection of a stage IV poorly differentiated serous carcinoma of the ovary. A renal biopsy showed membranous glomerulopathy. The proteinuria markedly diminished after debulking of the tumor, and after 10 months of combination chemotherapy the proteinuria had disappeared and there was no evidence of tumor at a second-look laparotomy.

Hematologic Disorders

Approximately 30 ovarian tumors have been reported to be associated with autoimmune hemolytic anemia, which is usually Coombs-positive.[75] Most of these tumors have been dermoid cysts[29,43,75,112,320] but occasional examples of carcinoma[75] and a single case of granulosa cell tumor also have been reported.[111] In the last case the patient also had splenic angiomas. In many cases corticosteroid therapy, splenectomy, or both have resulted in little or no improvement but removal of the ovarian tumor has produced a rapid remission of the hemolytic disorder. Payne and co-workers[320] have listed several mechanisms proposed to explain the relation of the dermoid cyst to the anemia: (1) liberation by the tumor of a substance that alters the surface of red cells, making them antigenic to the host, (2) stimulation of production of an antibody that cross-reacts with the red cells by an antigen in the wall or lumen of the cyst, and (3) direct production of a red cell antibody by the tumor. Support for the last theory is provided by the finding of immunoglobulin in the cyst fluid in several cases.[320]

Ovarian tumors are commonly associated with laboratory evidence of disseminated intravascular coagulation (DIC), but clinical manifestations of this disorder are uncommon.[321] In one study[24] 72%, and in another,[21] 94% of women with ovarian cancer had fibrin degradation products in their serum. In their review of cases of clinically evident DIC, however, Sack and associates[351] cited seven that were associated with ovarian cancer; at least three other cases have been reported subsequently.[81,113,383] Ovarian tumors also have been associated with migratory thrombophlebitis (Trousseau's syndrome). Nonbacterial thrombotic endocarditis also has been recorded as a complication of ovarian cancer,[113] as has microangiopathic hemolytic anemia.[321]

Excluding cases of mild erythrocytosis that may accompany androgenic ovarian tumors, paraneoplastic erythrocytosis is associated only rarely with ovarian tumors.[179] In a series of 340 cases of paraneoplastic erythrocytosis collected from the literature, ovarian tumors accounted for 2% of the cases; the histological types of tumors were not specified.[180] Examples of erythropoetin-secreting ovarian tumors have included a dermoid cyst and a steroid cell tumor.[159,282] Other hematologic abnormalities that have been described rarely in association with ovarian tumors include nonthrombocytopenic purpura (associated with a mucinous cystadenoma),[107] granulocytosis (clear cell carcinoma),[410] thrombocytosis (serous carcinoma),[40] thrombocytopenia (hemangioma, adenofibroma),[243,280,446] and pancytopenia (granulosa cell tumor).[293]

References

1. Abeler V, Kjorstad KE, Nesland JM (1988) Small cell carcinoma of the ovary. A report of six cases. Int J Gynecol Pathol 7: 315–329

2. Abell MR (1968) Undifferentiated malignant germ cell neoplasm (embyonal carcinoma) of the ovary with stromal luteinization. Am J Obstet Gynecol 101: 570–572

3. Abouav J, Berkowitz SB, Kolb FO (1959) Reversible hypercalcemia in masculinizing hypernephroid tumor of the ovary. Report of a case. N Engl J Med 260: 1057–1062

4. Adeyemi SD, Grange AO, Giwa-Osagie OF, et al (1986) Adrenal rest tumor of the ovary associated with isosexual precocious pseudopuberty and cushingoid features. Eur J Pediatr 145: 236–238

5. Aguirre P, Scully RE (1983) Testosterone-secreting adrenal ganglioneuroma containing Leydig cells. Am J Surg Pathol 7: 699

6. Aguirre P, Scully RE, Delellis RA (1986) Ovarian heterologous Sertoli-Leydig cell tumors with gastrointestinal-type epithelium. An immunohsitochemical analysis. Arch Pathol Lab Med 110: 528–533.

7. Aguirre P, Thor AD, Scully RE (1989) Ovarian endometrioid carcinomas resembling sex cord-stromal tumors: An immunohistological study. Int J Gynecol Pathol 8: 364–373

8. Aguirre P, Thor AD, Scully RE (1989) Ovarian small cell carcinoma—histogenetic considerations based on immunohistochemical and other findings. Am J Clin Pathol 92: 140–149

9. Ahn GH, Chi JG, Lee SK (1986) Ovarian sex cord tumor with annular tubules. Cancer 57: 1066–1073

10. Aiba M, Hirayama A, Sakurada M, Naruse K, Ishikawa C, Aiba S (1990) Spironolactone rod-like structure in renin-producing Sertoli cell tumor of the ovary. Surg Pathol 3: 143–149

11. Aiman J, Forney JP, Parker CR (1986) Androgen and estrogen secretion by normal and neoplastic ovaries in premenopausal women. Obstet Gynecol 68: 327–332

12. Aiman J, Nalick RH, Jacobs A, et al (1977) The origin of androgen and estrogen in a virilized postmenopausal woman with bilateral benign cystic teratomas. Obstet Gynecol 49: 695–704

13. Allan SG, Lockhart SP, Leonard RCF, Smyth JF (1984) Paraneoplastic hypercalcemia in ovarian carcinoma. Br Med J 288: 1714–1715

14. Allander E, Wagermark J (1969) Leydig cell tumors of the ovary. Report of three cases. Acta Obstet Gynecol Scand 48: 433

15. Alvarez RD, Varner RE (1987) Hyperandrogenic state associated with a mucinous cystadenoma. Obstet Gynecol 69: 507–510

16. Anderson MC (1972) Hilar cell tumour of the ovary. J Clin Pathol 25: 106

17. Anderson MC, Rees DA (1975) Gynandroblastoma of the ovary. Br J Obstet Gynaecol 82: 68

18. Anderson PW, Macaulay L, Do YS, et al (1989) Extrarenal renin-secreting tumors: Insights into hypertension and ovarian renin production. Medicine 68: 257–268

19. Andujar JJ, Enloe GR, Swift WB (1947) Brenner tumor of the ovary; 2 cases associated with postmenopausal endometrial changes. Texas J Med 43: 70–75

20. Anikwue C, Dawood MY, Kramer E (1979) Granulosa and theca cell tumors. Obstet Gynecol 51:214–220

21. Anstey JT, Blythe JG (1972) Fibrin degradation products and the diagnosis of ovarian carcinoma. Obstet Gynecol 52: 605–608

22. Arai N, Misugi K, Kamiya T, Shima S (1988) An ovarian Sertoli–Leydig cell tumor with heterologous mucinous gland and NSE-immunoreactive-cell. Arch Gynecol Obstet 243: 55–60

23. Armstrong DT, Papkoff H (1976) Stimulation of aromatization by endogenous and exogenous androgens in ovaries of hypophysectomized rats in vivo by FSH. Endocrinology 99: 1144–1151

24. Astedt B, Svanberg L, Nilsson IM (1971) Fibrin degradation products and ovarian tumours. Br Med J 4: 458–459

25. Astengo-Osuna C (1984) Ovarian sex-cord tumor with annular tubules. Case report with ultrastructural findings. Cancer 54: 1070–1075

26. Atlas SA, Sherman RL, Pasmantier MW, et al (1982) Response of active and inactive renins, aldosterone and blood pressure to chemotherapy in a patient with a possible renin-secreting ovarian carcinoma. Clin Res 30: 333A (abstr)

27. Axiotis CA, Lippes HA, Merino MJ, deLanerolle NC, Stewart AF, Kinder B (1987) Corticotroph cell pituitary adenoma within an ovarian teratoma. A new cause of Cushing's syndrome. Am J Surg Pathol 11: 218–224

28. Backstrom T, Mahlck C, Kjellgren O (1983) Progesterone as a possible tumor marker for "nonendocrine" ovarian malignant tumors. Gynecol Oncol 16:129–138

29. Baker LRI, Brain MC, Azzopardi JG, Worlledge SM (1968) Autoimmune haemolytic anaemic associated with ovarian dermoid cyst. J Clin Pathol 21: 626

30. Balasa RW, Adcock LL, Prem KA, Dehner LP (1977) The Brenner tumor. Obstet Gynecol 50: 120–128

31. Banner EA, Dockerty MB (1945) Theca cell tumors of the ovary. A clinical and pathological study of twenty-three cases (including thirteen new cases) with a review. Surg Gynecol Obstet 81: 234–242

32. Baramki TA, Leddy AL, Woodruff JD (1983) Bilateral hilus cell tumors of the ovary. Obstet Gynecol 62: 128–131

33. Barnes BE (1976) Dermatomyositis and malignancy. A review of the literature. Ann Intern Med 84: 68–76

34. Beauchamp PJ, Hughes RS, Schmidt WA (1989) Virilizing serous cystadenoma. Obstet Gynecol 73: 513–517

35. Beck JS, Fulman HF, Lee ST (1969) Solid malignant ovarian teratoma with 'embryoid bodies' and trophoblastic differentiation. J Pathol 99: 67–73

36. Bell RJM (1977) Fetal virilisation due to maternal Krukenberg tumour. Lancet 1: 1162–1163

37. Benagiano G, Bigotti G, Buzzi M, et al (1988) Endocrine and morphological study of case of ovarian sex-cord tumor

with annular tubules in a woman with Peutz–Jeghers syndrome. Int J Gynecol Obstet 26: 441–452

38. Benfield GFA, Tapper-Jones L, Stout TV (1982) Androblastoma and raised serum alpha-fetoprotein with familial multinodular goitre. Case report. Br J Obstet Gynaecol 89: 323

39. Benjamin E, Law S, Bobrow LG (1987) Intermediate filament cytokeratin and vimentin in ovarian sex cord-stromal tumors with correlative studies in adult and fetal ovaries. J Pathol 152: 253–263

40. Bennett RM, Ginsberg MH, Thomsen S (1976) Carcinomatous polyarthritis. Arthritis Rheum 19: 953–959

41. Bennington JL, Ferguson BR, Haber SL (1968) Incidence and relative frequency of benign and malignant ovarian neoplasms. Obstet Gynecol 32: 627–732

42. Berlin NI, Van Scott EJ, Clendenning WE, et al (1966) Basal cell nevus syndrome. Ann Intern Med 64: 403

43. Bernstein D, Naor S, Rikover M, Menahem H (1974) Hemolytic anemia related to ovarian tumor. Obstet Gynecol 43: 276–280

44. Besch PK, Byron RC, Barry RD, et al (1963) Testosterone synthesis by a Brenner tumor. Part II. In vitro biosynthetic steroid conversion of a Brenner tumor. Am J Obstet Gynecol 86: 1021–1026

45. Betta P, Bellingeri D (1985) Androgenic juvenile granulosa cell tumor. Case report. Eur J Gynaecol Oncol 6: 71–74

46. Bettinger JF, Jacobs H (1946) A contribution to the problem of masculinization. Med J Aust 1: 10–13

47. Bjorkholm E (1980) Granulosa cell tumors: A comparison of survival in patients and matched controls. Am J Obstet Gynecol 138: 329–331

48. Bjorkholm E, Pettersson F (1980) Granulosa-cell and theca-cell tumors. The clinical picture and long term outcome for the Radiumhemmet series. Acta Obstet Gynec Scand 59: 361

49. Bjorkholm E, Silfversward C (1981) Prognostic factors in granulosa cell tumors. Gynecol Oncol 11: 261

50. Bjorkholm E, Silfversward C (1980) Theca-cell tumors. Clinical features and prognosis. Acta Radiol Oncol Radiat Phys Biol 19: 241

51. Bohm J, Roder-Weber M, Hofler H (1991) Bilateral stromal Leydig cell tumor of the ovary. Case report and literature review. Path Res Pract 187: 348–352

52. Boivin Y, Richart RM (1965) Hilus cell tumors of the ovary. A review with a report of 3 new cases. Cancer 18: 231

53. Boixeda D, Roman AL, Pascasio JM, et al (1990) Zollinger-Ellison syndrome due to gastrin-secreting ovarian cystadenocarcinoma. Case report. Acta Chir Scand 156: 409–410

54. Bollen ECM, Lamers CBHW, Jansen JMBJ, et al (1981) Zollinger-Ellison syndrome due to a gastrin-producing ovarian cystadenocarcinoma. Br J Surg 68: 776–777

55. Bonaventura LM, Judd H, Roth LM, Cleary RE (1978) Androgen, estrogen, and progesterone production by a lipid cell tumor of the ovary. Am J Obstet Gynecol 131: 403

56. Borushek S, Berger I, Echt C. Gold JJ (1965) Functioning malignant germ cell tumor of the ovary in a 4?-year-old girl. Cancer 18: 1485–1488

57. Boss JH, Scully RE, Wegner KH, Cohen RB (1965) Structural variations in the adult ovary—clinical significance. Obstet Gynecol 25: 747–764

58. Bower JF, Erickson ER (1967) Bilateral ovarian fibromas in a 5-year-old. Am J Obstet Gynecol 99: 880

59. Brain Lord (1963) The neurological complications of neoplasms. Lancet 1: 179–184

60. Bronstein R, Hardouin G, Henrion R (1972) Kyste mucoide virilisant au cours de la grossesse. J Gynecol Obstet Biol Reprod 1: 891–899

61. Brown H, Lane M (1965) Cushing's and malignant carcinoid syndromes from ovarian neoplasm. Arch Intern Med 115: 490–494

62. Brown WW, Shetty KR, Rosenfeld PS (1973) Hyperthyroidism due to struma ovarii: Demonstration by radioiodine scan. Acta Endocrinol 73: 266–272

63. Bruno MS, Ober WB (1959) Clincopathologic Conference. N Y State J Med 59: 4001–4007

64. Bullon A, Arseneau J, Prat J, Young RH, Scully RE (1981) Tubular Krukenberg tumor. A problem in histopathologic diagnosis. Am J Surg Pathol 5: 225–232

65. Burket RL, Rauh JL (1976) Gorlin's syndrome: Ovarian fibromas at adolescence. Obstet Gynecol 47: 43s–44s

66. Burslem RW, Langley FA, Woodcock AS (1954) A clincopathological sutdy of oestrogenic ovarian tumors. Cancer 7: 552

67. Burton PBJ, Knight DE, Quirke P, et al (1990) Parathyroid hormone related peptide in ovarian carcinoma. J Clin Pathol 43: 784

68. Busby T, Anderson GW (1954) Feminizing mesenchymomas of the ovary. Am J Obstet Gynecol 68: 1391

69. Calabro JJ (1967) Cancer and arthritis. Arthritis Rheum 10: 553–567

70. Callen JP (1986) Dermatomyositis and female malignancy. J Surg Oncol 32: 121–124

71. Campbell PE, Danks DM (1963) Pseudoprecocity in an infant due to a luteoma of the ovary. Arch Dis Child 38: 519

72. Cannon PM, Smart CR, Wilson ML, Edwards CB (1975) Hypercalcemia with ovarian granulosa cell carcinoma. Rocky Mountain Med J 72: 72–74

73. Carlstrom K, Lagrelius A, von Schoultz B (1985) Serum levels of dehydroepiandrosterone sulphage and total estrone in postmenopausal women with special regard to 'non-endocrine' ovarian carcinoma. Acta Obstet Gynecol Scand 64: 267–268

74. Caron P, Roche H, Gorguet B, Martel P, Bennet A, Carton M (1990) Mammary ovarian metastases with stroma cell hyperplasia and postmenopausal virilization. Cancer 66: 1221–1224

75. Carreras Vescio LA, Toblli JE, Rey JA, Assaf ME, De Maria HE, Marletta J (1983) Autoimmune hemolytic anemia associated with an ovarian neoplasm. Medicina 43: 415–424

76. Case Records of the Massachusetts General Hospital (1970) Case 13-1970. N Engl J Med 282: 676–681

77. Case Records of the Massachusetts General Hospital (1972) Case 11-1972. N Engl J Med 286: 594–600

78. Case Records of the Massachusetts General Hospital (1975) Case 10, 1975. N Engl J Med 292: 521

79. Case Records of the Massachusetts General Hospital (1976) Case 14, 1976. N Engl J Med 294: 772

80. Case Records of the Massachusetts General Hospital (1976) Case 26-1976. N Engl J Med 294: 1447–1454

81. Case Records of the Massachusetts General Hospital (1978) Case 13, 1978. N Engl J Med 298: 786–792

82. Case Records of the Massachusetts General Hospital (1983) Case 21-1983. N Engl J Med 308: 1279–1284

83. Case Records of the Massachusetts General Hospital (1985) Case 30-1985. N Engl J Med 313: 249–257.

84. Cashell AW, Cohen ML (1991) Masculinizing sclerosing stromal tumor of the ovary during pregnancy. Gynecol Oncol 43: 281–285

85. Casper S, van Nagell JR, Powell DF, et al (1981) Immuno-histochemical localization of tumor markers in epithelial ovarian cancer. Am J Obstet Gynecol 149: 154–158

86. Chadha S, van der Kwast TH (1989) Immunohistochemistry of ovarian granulosa cell tumors. The value of tissue specific proteins and tumor markers. Virchows Arch (A) 414: 439–445

87. Chalvardjian A, Derzko C (1982) Gynandroblastoma. Its ultrastructure. Cancer 50: 710

88. Chalvardjian A, Scully RE (1973) Sclerosing stromal tumors of the ovary. Cancer 31: 664

89. Chan LKC, Prathap K (1970) Virilization in pregnancy associated with an ovarian mucinous cystadenoma. Am J Obstet Gynecol 108: 946–949

90. Chen KTK (1986) Female genital tract tumors in Peutz-Jeghers syndrome. Hum Pathol 17: 858–861

91. Christian E (1910) Un Cas d'epitheliome a granulations de luteine d'origine probablement ovarienne. Soc Anat Ann 12: 639–641

92. Christman JE, Ballon SC (1990) Ovarian fibrosarcoma associated with Maffucci's syndrome. Gynecol Oncol 37: 290–291

93. Chumas JC, Rosenwaks Z, Mann WJ, Finkel G, Pastore J (1984) Sertoli-Leydig cell tumor of the ovary producing alpha-fetoprotein. Int J Gynecol Pathol 3: 213–219

94. Civantos F, Rywlin AM (1972) Carcinomas with trophoblastic differentiation and secretion of chroionic gonadotrophins. Cancer 29: 789–798

95. Clement PB, Scully RE (1980) Large solitary luteinized follicle cyst of pregnancy and puerperium. A clinicopathological analysis of eight cases. Am J Surg Pathol 4: 431–438

96. Clement PB, Young RH, Scully RE (1991) Clinical syndromes associated with tumors of the female genital tract. Semin Diagn Pathol 8: 204–233

97. Clement PB, Young RH, Scully RE (1988) Ovarian granulosa cell proliferations of pregnancy: A report of nine cases. Hum Pathol 19: 657–662

97a. Clement PB, Young RH, Hanna W, Scully RE (1994) Sclerosing peritonitis associated with lutenized thecomas of the ovary. A clinicopathological analysis of six cases. Am J Surg Pathol 18: 1–13

98. Cocco AE, Conway SJ (1975) Zollinger–Ellison syndrome associated with ovarian mucinous cystadenocarcinoma. N Engl J Med 293: 485–486

99. Cocconi G, Ceci G, Juvarra G, et al (1985) Successful treatment of subacute cerebellar degeneration in ovarian carcinoma with plasmapheresis. A case report. Cancer 56: 2318–1320

100. Cohen PR, Kohn SR, Kurzrock R (1991) Association of sebaceous gland tumors and internal malignancy: The Muir-Torre syndrome. Am J Med 90: 606–613

101. Connor TB, Ganis FM, Levin HS, Migeon CJ, Martin LG (1968) Gonadotropin-dependent Krukenberg tumor causing virilization during pregnancy. J Clin Endocrinol Metab 28: 198–214

102. Cotton DH, Hanson FW, Oi RH (1981) A mucinous cystadenoma associated with testosterone production. J Reprod Med 26: 276–278

103. Croft PB, Wilkinson M (1965) The incidence of carcinomatous neuromyopathy in patients with various types of carcinoma. Brain 88: 427–434

104. Curth HO, Hilberg AW, Machacek GF (1962) The site and histology of the cancer associated with malignant acanthosis nigricans. Cancer 15: 364–382

105. Czernobilsky B (1984) Immunohistochemistry of normal tissues of the female genital tract. Presentation at XVth International Congress of International Academy of Pathology, Miami Beach, FL

106. DaCosta CC (1938) Tumor masculinizante. Rev Gynecol Obstet 2: 3–9

107. Dales M (1965) Purpura associated with ovarian tumor. Br Med J 1: 127

108. Damjanov I, Drobnjak P, Grizelj V, Longhino N (1975) Sclerosing stromal tumor of the ovary. A hormonal and ultrastructural analysis. Obstet Gynecol 45: 675–679

109. Dardi LE, Miller AW, Gould VE (1982) Sertoli-Leydig cell tumor with endometrioid differentiation. Case report and discussion of histogenesis. Diagn Gynecol Obstet 4: 227–234

110. Davidson BJ, Waisman J, Judd HL (1981) Long-standing virilism in a woman with hyperplasia and neoplasia of ovarian lipidic cells. Obstet Gynecol 58: 753–759

111. Dawson MA, Talbert W, Yarbro JW (1971) Hemolytic anemia associated with an ovarian tumor. Am J Med 50: 552

112. DeBruyere M, Sokal G, Devoitille JM, Fauchet-Dutrieux MC, De Spa V (1971) Autoimmune haemolytic anaemia and ovarian tumour. Br J Haemat 20: 83

113. Delgado G, Smith JP (1975) Gynecological malignancy associated with non-bacterial thrombotic endocarditis (NBTE). Gynecol Oncol 3: 205–209

114. de Lima GR, de Lima OA, Baracat EC, Vasserman J, Burnier M (1989) Virilizing Brenner tumor of the ovary: Case report. Obstet Gynecol 73: 895–898

115. DeTorres EF (1974) Feminization in tumors of Sertoli-Leydig cells. Acta Cytol 18: 187

116. Dickersin GR, Kline IW, Scully RE (1982) Small cell carcinoma of the ovary with hypercalcemia. A report of eleven cases. Cancer 49: 188

117. Dikman SH, Toker C (1971) Strumal carcinoid of the ovary with masculinization. Cancer 27: 925–930

118. Diddle AW (1951) Granulosa- and theca-cell ovarian tumors: Prognosis. Cancer 15: 215–228

119. Dingley ER, Marten RH (1957) Adenocarcinoma of the ovary presenting as acanthosis nigricans. J Obstet Gynaecol Br Commonw 64: 898–900

120. Disaia PJ, Saltz A, Kagan AR, Rich W (1978) A temporary response of recurrent granulosa cell tumor to adriamycin. Obstet Gynecol 52: 355

121. Dockerty MB, MacCarty WC (1939) Granulosa cell tumors; with the report of a 34-lb specimen and a review. Am J Obstet Gynecol 37: 425

122. Dockerty MB, Masson JC (1944) Ovarian fibromas: A clinical and pathologic study of two hundred and eighty-three cases. Am J Obstet Gynecol 47: 741

123. Dorrington JH, Moon YS, Armstrong DT (1975) Estradiol-17B biosynthesis in cultured granulosa cells from hypophysectomized immature rats: Stimulation by FSH. Endocrinology 97: 1328–1331

124. Dunaif A, Hoffman AR, Scully RE, et al (1985) Clinical, biochemical, and ovarian morphologic features in women with acanthosis nigricans and masculinization. Obstet Gynecol 66: 545–552

125. Duncan SC, Winkelmann RK (1979) Cancer and scleroderma. Arch Dermatol 115: 950–955

126. Dunnihoo DR, Grieme DL, Woolf RB (1966) Hilar-cell tumors of the ovary. Report of 2 new cases and a review of the world literature. Obstet Gynecol 27: 703

127. Echt CR, Hadd HE (1968) Androgen excretion patterns in a patient with a metastatic hilus cell tumor of the ovary. Am J Obstet Gynecol 100: 1055

128. Eddie DAS (1967) Hormonal activity with ovarian tumours. J Obstet Gynaecol Br Commonw 74: 283–285

129. Ehrlich EN, Dominguez OV, Samuels LT, Lynch D, Oberhelman H, Warner NE (1963) Aldosteronism and precocious puberty due to an ovarian androblastoma (Sertoli cell tumor). J Clin Endocrinol Metab 23: 358–367

130. Eichhorn JH, Bell DA, Young RH, et al (1992) DNA content and proliferative activity in ovarian small cell carcinomas of the hypercalcemic type. Implications for diagnosis, prognosis and histogenesis. Am J Clin Pathol 98: 579–586

131. Emig OR, Hertig AT, Rowe FJ (1959) Gynandroblastoma of the ovary. Review and report of a case. Obstet Gynecol 13: 135

132. Evans AT, Gaffey TA, Malkasian GD Jr, Annegers JF (1980) Clinicopathologic review of 118 granulosa and 82 theca cell tumors. Obstet Gynecol 55: 231

133. Falls JL (1955) Accessory adrenal cortex in the broad ligament. Incidence and functional significance. Cancer 8: 143

134. Fathalla MF (1967) The occurrence of granulosa and theca tumors in clinically normal ovaries. A study of 25 cases. J Obstet Gynaecol Br Commonw 74: 279

135. Fathalla MF (1968) The role of the ovarian stroma in hormone production by ovarian tumors. J Obstet Gynaecol Br Commonw 75: 78–83

136. Fathizadeh A, Medenica MM, Soltani K, et al (1982) Aggressive keratoacanthoma and internal malignant neoplasm. Arch Dermatol 118: 112–114

137. Fawcett FJ, Kimbell NKB (1971) Phaeochromocytoma of the ovary. J Obstet Gynaecol Br Commonw 78: 458–459

138. Fayez JA, Bunch TR, Miller GL (1974) Virilization in pregnancy associated with an ovarian serous cystadenoma. Am J Obstet Gynecol 120: 341–346

139. Fenoglio CM, Hayata T, Crum CP, Richart RM (1982) The expression of human chorionic gonadotrophin in the female genital tract. Localization by the immunoperoxidase technique. Diagn Gynecol Obstet 4: 94–97

140. Ferenczy A, Okagaki T, Richart RM (1971) Para-endocrine hypercalcemia in ovarian neoplasms. Report of mesonephroma with hypercalcemia and review of literature. Cancer 27: 427–433

141. Ferenczy A, Richart RM (1974) Female reproductive system: Dynamics of scan and transmission electron microscopy. New York, John Wiley & Sons

141a. Ferry JA, Young RH, Engel G, Scully RE (in press) Oxyphilic sertoli cell tumor of the ovary: A report of three cases, two in patients with the Peutz-Jeghers Syndrome. Int J Gynecol Pathol

142. Fetissof F, Berger G, Dubois MP, et al (1985) Female genital tract and Peutz-Jeghers syndrome: An immunohistochemical study. Int J Gynecol Pathol 4: 219–229

142a. Fleischhacker DS, Young RH (in press) Dysgerminoma of the ovary associated with hypercalcemia. Gynecol Oncol

143. Forest MG, Orgiazzi J, Tranchant D, Mornex R, Bertrand J (1978) Approach to the mechanism of androgen overproduction in a case of Krukenberg tumor responsible for virilization during pregnancy. J Clin Endocrinol Metab 47: 428–434

145. Fox H (1965) Estrogenic activity of the serous cystadenoma of the ovary. Cancer 18: 1041–1047

144. Fox H, Agrawal K, Langley FA (1975) A clinicopathological study of 92 cases of granulosa cell tumor of the ovary with special reference to the factors influencing prognosis. Cancer 35: 231

145. Fox LP, Stamm WJ (1965) Krukenberg tumor complicating pregnancy. Report of a case with androgenic activity. Am J Obstet Gynecol 92: 702–710

147. Franke WW, Grund C, Schmid E (1979) Intermediate-sized filaments in Sertoli are of vimentin-type. Eur J Cell Biol 19: 269–275

148. Fujino T, Watanabe T, Yamaguchi K, et al (1992) The development of hypercalcemia in a patient with an ovarian tumor producing parathyroid hormone-related protein. Cancer 70: 2845–2850

149. Fung MFK, Vadas G, Lotocki R, Heywood M, Krepart G (1991) Tubular Krukenberg tumor in pregnancy with virilization. Gynecol Oncol 41: 81–84

150. Gaffney EF, Majmudar B, Hertzler GL, Zane R, Furlong B, Breding E (1983) Ovarian granulosa cell tumors—immunohistochemical localization of estradiol and ultrastructure, with functional correlations. Obstet Gynecol 61: 311–318

151. Gagnon S, Tetu B, Silva EG, McCaughey WTE (1989) Frequency of α-fetoprotein production by Sertoli-Leydig cell tumors of the ovary: an immunohistochemical study of eight cases. Mod Pathol 2: 63–67

152. Garcia-Villaneuva M, Figuerola NB, del Arbol LR, Ortiz MJH (1990) Zollinger–Ellison syndrome due to a borderline mucinous cystadenoma of the ovary. Obstet Gynecol 75: 549–551

153. Garneau R, Cabanne F (1968) Dysembryome ovarien de type enteroide et bilio-Berger. A propos d'une observation. Ann Anat Pathol 13: 423–432

154. Gee DC, Russell P (1979) Sclerosing stromal tumours of the ovary. Histopathology 3: 367–376

155. Gee DC, Russell P (1981) The pathological assessment of ovarian neoplasms. IV: The sex cord stromal tumors. Pathology 13: 235–255

156. Geist SH, Gaines JA (1938) Theca cell tumors. Am J Obstet Gynecol 35: 39–51

157. Genton CY (1980) Ovarian Sertoli–Leydig cell tumors. A clinical, pathological and ultrastructural study with particular reference to the histogenesis of these tumors. Arch Gynecol 230: 49–75

158. Genton CY (1980) Some observations on the fine structure of human granulosa cell tumors. Virchows Arch A Path Anat Histol 387: 353–369

159. Ghio R, Haupt E, Ratti M, Boccaccio P (1981) Erythrocytosis associated with a dermoid cyst of the ovary and erythropoietic activity of the tumour fluid. Scand J Haematol 27: 70–74

160. Givens JR (1976) Hirsutism and hyperandrogenism. Adv Intern Med 21: 221–247

161. Givens JR, Kerber IJ, Wiser WL, Anderson RW, Coleman SA, Fish SA (1974) Remission of acanthosis nigricans associated with polycystic ovarian disease and a stromal luteoma. J Clin Endocrinol Metab 38: 347

162. Glaser D, Nienhaus H, Kohler R, Walther G, Pawlowitzki IH (1988) A sex cord stromal tumour in a woman with XO/XX/XXX-mosaicism. Arch Gynecol Obstet 243: 115–118

163. Goldberg B, Seegar Jones GE, Woodruff JD (1963) A histochemical study of steroid 3β-ol dehydrogenase activity in some steroid-producing tumors. Am J Obstet Gynecol 86: 1003–1014

164. Gondos B, Monroe SA (1971) Cystic granulosa cell tumor with massive hemoperitoneum. Light and electron microscopic study. Obstet Gynecol 38: 683–689

165. Gorlin RJ (1987) Nevoid basal-cell carcinoma syndrome. Medicine 66: 98–113

166. Gorlin RJ, Sedano HO (1971) The multiple nevoid basal cell carcinoma syndrome revisited. Birth Defects 7: 140

167. Gorlin RJ, Vickers RA, Kelln E, Williamson JJ (1965) The multiple basal cell nevi syndrome. Cancer 18: 89

168. Graham R, McKee P, McGibbon D, et al (1985) Torre-Muir syndrome. An association with isolated sebaceous carcinoma. Cancer 55:2868–2873

169. Greco MA, LiVolsi VA, Pertschuk KP, Bigelow B (1979) Strumal carcinoid of the ovary. An analysis of its components. Cancer 43: 1380–1388

170. Greenlee JE, Brashear HR (1983) Antibodies to cerebellar Purkinje cells in patients with paraneoplastic cerebellar degeneration and ovarian carcinoma. Ann Neurol 14: 609–613

171. Grenet P, Badoual J, Gallet JP, et al (1972) Dyschondroplasie et tumeur de l'ovaire. Ann Pediatr (Paris) 19: 759–764

172. Guerard MJ, Ferenczy A, Arguelles MA (1982) Ovarian Sertoli-Leydig cell tumor with rhabdomyosarcoma: An ultrastructural study. Ultrastruct Pathol 3: 347

173. Guintoli RL, Celebre JA, Wu CH, Wheeler JE, Mikuta JJ (1976) Androgenic function of a granulosa cell tumor. Obstet Gynecol 47: 77

174. Gusberg SB, Kardon P (1967) Proliferative endometrial response to theca–granulosa cell tumors. Am J Obstet Gynecol 111: 633

175. Gustafson ML, Lee MM, Scully RE, et al (1992) Mullerian inhibiting substance as a marker for ovarian sex-cord tumor. N Engl J Med 326: 466–471

176. Hall DJ, Dyer ML, Parker JC (1985) Ovarian cancer complicated by cerebellar degeneration: A paraneoplastic syndrome. Gynecol Oncol 21: 240–246

177. Hameed H (1972) Brenner tumor of the ovary with Leydig cell hyperplasia. A histologic and ultrastructural study. Cancer 30: 945–952

178. Hammack JE, Kimmel DW, O'Neill BP, et al (1990) Paraneoplastic cerebellar degeneration: A clinical comparison of patients with and without Purkinje cell cytoplasmic antibodies. Mayo Clin Proc 65: 1423–1431

179. Hammond D, Winnick S (1974) Paraneoplastic erythrocytosis and ectopic erythropoietins. Ann NY Acad Sci 230: 219–227

180. Hamwi GJ, Byron RC, Besch PK, Vorys N, Teteris NJ, Ullery JC (1963) Testosterone synthesis by a Brenner tumor. Part I. Clinical evidence of masculinization during pregnancy. Am J Obstet Gynecol 86: 1015–1020

181. Hart WR, Kumar N, Crissman JD (1980) Ovarian neoplasms resembling sex cord tumors with annular tubules. Cancer 45: 2352–2363

182. Hasleton PS, Kelehan P, Whittaker JS, Burslen RW, Turner L (1978) Benign and malignant struma ovarii. Arch Pathol Lab Med 102: 180–184

183. Hayes MC, Scully RE (1987) Ovarian steroid cell tumor (not otherwise specified): A clinicopathological analysis of 63 cases. Am J Surg Pathol 11: 835–845

184. Hayes MC, Scully RE (1987) Stromal luteoma of the ovary: A clinico-pathological analysis of 25 cases. Int J Gynecol Pathol 6: 313–321

185. Heinonen PK, Koivula T, Pystynen P (1989) Elevated progesterone levels in serum and ovarian venous blood in patients with ovarian tumors. Acta Obstet Gynecol Scand 64: 649–652

186. Heinonen PK, Koivula T, Rajaniemi H, et al (1986) Peripheral and ovarian venous concentrations of steroid and gonadotropin hormones in postmenopausal women with epithelial ovarian tumors. Gynecol Oncol 25: 1–10

187. Henson RA, Urich H (1982) Cancer and the nervous system: The neurological manifestations of systemic malignant disease. Boston, Blackwell Scientific Publications

188. Herrington JB, Scully RE (1983) Endocrine aspects of germ cell tumors. In: Damjanov I, Knowles B and Solter D (eds) The Human Teratomas. New York, The Humana Press

189. Herruzo, Redondo E, De Avila IP, et al (1990) Ovarian sex cord tumor with annular tubules and Peutz-Jeghers syndrome. Eur J Gynaecol Oncol 11: 141–144

190. Herve JP, Leroy JP, Gentric-Tilly A, et al (1989) Hypertension arterielle secondaire a une tumeur a renine d'origine ovarienne. Presse Med 18: 2021–2022

191. Hetzel DJ, Stanhope R, O'Neill BP, et al (1990) Gynecologic cancer in patients with subacute cerebellar degeneration predicted by anti-Purkinje cell antibodies and limited in metastatic volume. Mayo Clin Proc 65: 1558–1563

192. Heyd J, Livni N, Herbert D, Mor-Yosef S, Glaser B (1989) Gastrin-producing ovarian cystadenocarcinoma: Sensitivity to secretin and SMS 201-995. Gastroenterology 97: 464–467

193. Hoekman K, Tjandra Y, Papapoulos SE (1991) The role of 1,25-dihydroxyvitamin D in the maintenance of hypercalcemia in a patient with an ovarian carcinoma producing parathyroid hormone-related protein. Cancer 68: 642–647

194. Holguin T, Padilla RS, Ampuero F (1986) Ovarian adenocarcinoma presenting with the sign of Leser–Trelat. Gynecol Oncol 25: 128–132

195. Holtz G, Johnson TR Jr, Schrock ME (1979) Paraneoplastic hypercalcemia in ovarian tumors. Obstet Gynecol 54: 483–487

196. Hoyt RE, Hamilton JF (1987) Ovarian cancer associated with the nephrotic syndrome. Obstet Gynecol 70: 513–514

197. Hsu C, Ma L, Mak L (1983) Sclerosing stromal tumor of the ovary: Case report and review of the literature. Int J Gynecol Pathol 2: 192–200

198. Huang TY, Holaday WJ (1970) An ovarian hilus cell tumor associated with endometrial carcinoma: Report of a case. Am J Clin Pathol 54: 147

199. Hughesdon PE (1958) Thecal and allied reactions in epithelial ovarian tumours. J Obstet Gynaecol Br Commonw 65: 702–709

200. Hughesdon PE (1983) Lipid cell thecomas of the ovary. Histopathology 7: 681–692

201. Hughesdon PE, Fraser IT (1953) Arrhenoblastoma of ovary. Case report and historical review. Acta Obstet Gynecol Scand (suppl 4)32: 1

202. Ichinohasama R, Teshima S, Kishi K, et al (1989) Leydig cell tumor of the ovary associated with endometrial carcinoma and containing 17 beta-hydroxysteroid dehydrogenase. Int J Gynecol Pathol 8: 64–71

203. Imai A, Furui T, Shimokawa K, Tamaya T (1992) Juvenile granulosa cell tumor in a 2-year-old infant: Report of a case complicated with ascites and acute respiratory distress. Gynecol Oncol 46: 397–400

204. Ismail SM, Walker SM (1990) Bilateral virilizing sclerosing stromal tumours of the ovary in a pregnant woman with Gorlin's syndrome: Implications for pathogenesis of ovarian stromal neoplasms. Histopathology 17: 159–163

205. Iturzaeta N, Kenny FM, Sieber W (1967) Precocious pseudopuberty due to granulosa cell tumor in three girls. Am J Dis Child 114: 39

206. Jackson B, Valentine R, Wagner G (1986) Primary aldosteronism due to a malignant ovarian tumour. Aust NZ J Med 16: 69–71

207. Jacobs AJ, Deppe G, Cohen CJ (1982) Combination chemotherapy of ovarian granulosa cell tumor with CIS-platinum and doxorubicin. Gynecol Oncol 14: 294

208. Jarabak J, Talerman A (1983) Virilization due to a metastasizing granulosa cell tumor. Int J Gynecol Pathol 2: 316–324

209. Jeppsson S, Karlsson S, Kullander S (1986) Gonadal steroids, gonadotropins and endometrial histology in postmenopausal women with malignant ovarian tumors. Acta Obstet Gynecol Scand 65: 207–210

210. Johnson AD, Herbert AA, Esterly NB (1986) Nevoid basal cell carcinoma syndrome. Bilateral ovarian fibromas in a 3½-year-old girl. J Am Acad Dermatol 14: 371–374

211. Johnston WW, Goldston WR, Montgomery MS (1971) Clinicopathologic studies in feminizing tumors of the ovary. III. The role of genital cytology. Acta Cytol 15: 334

212. Jolles CJ, Beeson JH, Abbott T (1985) Progesterone production in adenocarcinoma of the colon metastatic to the ovaries. Obstet Gynecol 65: 853–857

213. Jolly H (1955) Sexual Precocity. A personal study of 69 patients. American Lecture Series, Springfield, IL, Charles C Thomas

214. Jorgensen EO, Dockerty MB, Wilson RB (1970) Clinicopathologic study of 53 cases of Brenner tumors of the ovary. Am J Obstet Gynecol 108: 122–127

215. Josse RG, Wilson DR, Heersche JNM, Mills JRF, Murray TM (1981) Hypercalcemia with ovarian carcinoma: Evidence of a pathogenetic role for prostaglandins. Cancer 48: 1233–1241

216. Judd HL, Spore WW, Talner LB, Rigg LA, Yen SSC, Benirschke K (1974) Preoperative localization of a testosterone-secreting ovarian tumor by retrograde venous catheterization and selective sampling. Am J Obstet Gynecol 120: 91

217. Julkunen R, Partanen S, Salaspuro M (1983) Gastrin-producing ovarian mucinous cystadenoma. J Clin Gastroenterol 5: 67–70

218. Junaid TA, Nkposong EO, Kolawole TM (1972) Cutaneous meningiomas and an ovarian fibroma in a 3-year-old girl. J Pathol 108: 165

219. Kalavathi N (1971) Granulosa cell tumor—hormonal aspects and radiosensitivity. Clin Radiol 22: 524–527

220. Kallenberg GA, Pesce CM, Norman B, Ratner RE, Silverberg SG (1990) Ectopic hyperprolactinemia resulting from an ovarian teratoma. JAMA 263: 2472–2474

221. Kaplan C, Hawley R (1981) Dysgerminoma with giant cells. A case report with immunoperoxidase. Diagn Gynecol Obstet 3/4: 325–329

222. Katsube Y, Berg JM, Silverberg SG (1982) Epidemiologic pathology of ovarian tumors: A histopathologic review of primary ovarian neoplasms dia area, 1 July–31 December 1969 and 1 July–31 December 1979. Int J Gynecol Pathol 1: 3–16

223. Katsube Y, Iwaoki Y, Silverberg SG, Fujiwara A (1988) Sclerosing stromal tumor of the ovary associated with endometrial adenocarcinoma. A case report. Gynecol Oncol 29: 392–398

224. Kempers RD, Dockerty MB, Hoffman DL, et al (1970) Struma ovarii—ascitic, hyperthyroid, and asymptomatic syndromes. Ann Intern Med 72: 883–893

225. Kempson RL (1968) Ultrastructure of ovarian stromal cell tumors. Sertoli–Leydig cell tumor and lipid cell tumor. Arch Pathol 86: 492

226. Khalifa MA, Sesterhenn IA (1990) Tumor markers of epithelial ovarian neoplasms. Int J Gynecol Pathol 9: 217–230

227. Kim I, Young RH, Scully RE (1985) Leydig cell tumors of the testis. A clinicopathological analysis of 40 cases and review of the literature. Am J Surg Pathol 9: 177–192

228. Kobayashi M, Hamada H, Yamoto M, et al (1990) Ovarian clear-cell carcinoma producing estradiol and human chorionic gonadotropin. Acta Obstet Gynecol Scand 69: 183–185

229. Konishi I, Fujii S, Ishikawa Y, Suzuki A, Okamura H, Mori T (1986) Ovarian fibroma with Leydig cell hyperplasia of the adjacent stroma: A light and electron microscopic study. Int J Gynecol Pathol 5: 170–178

230. Korzets A, Nouriel H, Steiner Z, et al (1986) Resistant hypertension associated with a renin-producing ovarian Sertoli cell tumor. Am J Clin Pathol 85: 242–247

231. Kottmeier HL (1953) Carcinoma of the Female Genitalia. The Abraham Flexner Lectures, Series No. 11, Baltimore, Williams and Wilkins

232. Kraemer BB, Silva EG, Sneige N (1984) Fibrosarcoma of the ovary. A new component in the nevoid basal-cell carcinoma syndrome. Am J Surg Pathol 8: 231–236

233. Kuhnel R, Rao BR, Stolk JG, van Kessel H, Seldernrijk CA, Willig AP (1987) Estrogen synthesizing rare malignant Brenner tumor of the ovary with the presence of progesterone and androgen receptors in the absence of estrogen receptors. Gynecol Oncol 26: 263–269

234. Kulkarni JN, Mistry RC, Kamat MR, Chinoy R, Lotlikar RG (1990) Autonomous aldosterone-secreting ovarian tumor. Gynecol Oncol 37: 284–289

235. Kung AWC, Ma JTC, Wang C, et al (1990) Hyperthyroidism during pregnancy due to coexistence of struma ovarii and Graves' disease. Postgrad Med J 66: 132–133

236. Kurman RJ, Andrade D, Goebelsmann U, Taylor CR (1978) An immunohistochemical study of steroid localization in Sertoli–Leydig tumors of the ovary and testis. Cancer 42: 1772

237. Kurman RJ, Ganjei P, Nadjii M (1984) Contributions of immunocytochemistry to the diagnosis and study of ovarian neoplasms. Int J Gynecol Pathol 3: 3–26

238. Kurman RJ, Goebelsmann U, Taylor CR (1979) Steroid localization in granulosa–theca tumors of the ovary. Cancer 43: 2377

239. Kurman RJ, Norris HJ (1976) Malignant mixed germ cell tumors of the ovary. Obstet Gynecol 48: 579–589

240. Kurman RJ, Norris HJ (1976) Embryonal cell carcinoma of the ovary. A clinicopathologic entity distinct from endodermal sinus tumor resembling embryonal carcinoma of the adult testis. Cancer 38: 2420–2433

241. Kuzma JF, King JM (1948) Dyschondroplasia with hemangiomatosis (Maffucci's syndrome) and teratoid tumor of the ovary. Arch Pathol 46: 74

242. Lack EE, Perez-Atayde AR, Murthy ASK, Goldstein DP, Crigler JF, Vawter GF (1981) Granulosa theca cell tumors in premenarchal girls. A clinical and pathologic study of ten cases. Cancer 48: 1846

243. Lawhead RA, Copeland LJ, Edwards CL (1985) Bilateral ovarian hemangiomas associated with diffuse abdominopelvic hemangiomatosis. Obstet Gynecol 65: 597–599

244. Lee JC, Yamauchi H, Hopper J Jr (1966) The association of cancer and the nephrotic syndrome. Ann Intern Med 64: 41–57

245. Lewis RJ, Ketcham AS (1973) Maffucci's syndrome: Functional and neoplastic significance. Case report and review of the literature. J Bone Joint Surg 55-A: 1465

246. Listrom WB, Foucar CE (1990) Letter to the Editor. Am J Clin Pathol 94: 803–804

247. Long TT, Barton TK, Draffin R, Reeves WJ, McCarty KS (1980) Conservative management of the Zollinger–Ellison syndrome. Ectopic gastrin production by an ovarian cystadenoma. JAMA 243: 1837–1839

248. Lusch CJ, Mercurio TM, Runyeon WK (1978) Delayed recurrence and chemotherapy of a granulosa cell tumor. Obstet Gynecol 51: 505

249. Lyday RO (1952) Fibroma of the ovary with abdominal implants. Am J Surg 84: 737

250. MacAulay MA, Weliky I, Schulz RA (1967) Ultrastructure of a biosynthetically active granulosa cell tumor. Lab Invest 17: 562–570

251. MacKenzie AH, Scherbel AL (1963) Connective tissue syndromes associated with carcinoma. Geriatrics 18: 745–753

252. Mahlck C, Backstrom T, Kjellgren O (1986) Androstenedione production by malignant epithelial ovarian tumors. Gynecol Oncol 25: 217–222

253. Mahlck C, Backstrom T, Kjellgren O (1988) Plasma level of estradiol in patients with ovarian malignant tumors. Gynecol Oncol 30: 313–320

254. Mahlck C-G, Grankvist K, Kjellgren O, Backstrom T (1990) Human chorionic gonadotropin, follicle-stimulating hormone, and luteinizing hormone in patients with epithelial ovarian carcinoma. Gynecol Oncol 36: 219–225

255. Malfetano JH, Degnan E, Florentin R (1990) Para-endocrine hypercalcemia and ovarian small cell carcinoma. NY State J Med 90: 206–207

256. Malkasian GD Jr, Webb MJ, Jorgensen EO (1974) Observations on chemotherapy of granulosa cell carcinomas and malignant ovarian teratomas. Obstet Gynecol 44: 885

257. Mann WJ, Chumas J, Rosenwaks Z, Merrill JA, Davenport D (1986) Elevated serum alpha-fetoprotein associated with Sertoli-Leydig cell tumors of the ovary. Obstet Gynecol 67: 141–144

258. March DE, Desai AG, Park CH, et al (1988) Struma ovarii: Hyperthyroidism in a postmenopausal woman. J Nucl Med 29: 263–265

259. Marcus CC, Marcus SL (1961) Struma ovarii. A report of 7 cases and a review of the subject. Am J Obstet Gynecol 81: 752–762

260. Margolin KA, Pak HY, Esensten ML, Doroshow JH (1985) Hepatic metastasis in granulosa cell tumor of the ovary. Cancer 56: 691–695

261. Marieb HJ, Spangler S, Kashgarian M, Heiman A, Schwartz ML, Schwartz PE (1983) Cushing's syndrome secondary to ectopic cortisol production by an ovarian carcinoma. J Clin Endocrinol Metab 57: 737–740

262. Martinelli G, Govoni E, Pileri S, Grigioni FW, Doglioni C, Pelusi G (1983) Sclerosing stromal tumor of the ovary. Virchows Arch (Pathol Anat) 402: 155–161

263. Matias-Guiu X, Prat J (1990) Ovarian tumors with functioning stroma. An immunohistochemical study of 100 cases with human chorionic gonadotropin monoclonal and polyclonal antibodies. Cancer 65: 2001–2005

264. Matson PN, Mackem SM, Norton JA, Gardner JD, O'Dorisio TM, Jensen RT (1989) Ovarian carcinoma as a cause of Zollinger-Ellison syndrome. Natural history, secretory products, and response to provocative tests. Gastroenterology 97: 468–471

265. McGowan L, Young RH, Scully RE (1980) Peutz–Jeghers syndrome with adenoma malignum of cervix. A report of two cases. Gynecol Oncol 10: 125

266. McKay DG, Hertig AT, Hickey WF (1953) The histogenesis of granulosa and theca tumors of the human ovary. Obstet Gynecol 1: 125–136

267. McKay DG, Robinson D, Hertig AT (1949) Histochemical observations on granulosa cell tumors, thecomas, and fibromas of the ovary. Am J Obstet Gynecol 58: 625–639

268. McLellan R, Currie JL, Royal W, et al (1988) Ovarian carcinoma and paraneoplastic cerebellar degeneration. Obstet Gynecol 72: 922–924

269. McMahon JT, Hart WR (1988) Ultrastructural analysis of small cell carcinomas of the ovary. Am J Clin Pathol 90: 523–529

270. McNulty JR (1959) The ovarian serous cystadenofibroma. A report of 25 cases. Am J Obstet Gynecol 77: 1338–1344

271. Medsger TA, Dixon JA, Garwood VF (1982) Palmar fasciitis and polyarthritis associated with ovarian carcinoma. Ann Intern Med 96: 424–431

272. Meigs JV (1954) Fibroma of the ovary with ascites and hydrothorax. Meigs' syndrome. Am J Obstet Gynecol 67: 962

273. Meiling RL, Bouselis JG, Teteris NJ, Ullery JC, George OT (1963) Histochemical observations of a Brenner cell tumor with masculinization. Am J Obstet Gynecol 87: 463–470

274. Miettinen M, Talerman A, Wahlstrom T, Astengo-Osuna C, Virtanen I (1988) Cellular differentiation in ovarian sex-cord-stromal and germ-cell tumors studied with antibodies to intermediate filament proteins. Am J Surg Pathol 9: 640–651

275. Meyer-Hofmann G, Schwarzkopf H, Hartmann H (1960) Spontaneous hypoglycemia with extrapancreatic tumors. Dtsch Med Wochenschr 85: 2106–2108

276. Michael CA (1967) Pelvic fibroma causing recurrent attacks of hypoglycemia. J Obstet Gynaecol Br Commonw 74: 301–303

277. Miettinen M, Lehto V-P, Virtanen I (1983) Expression of intermediate filaments in normal ovaries and ovarian epithelial, sex cord–stromal, and germinal tumors. Int J Gynecol Pathol 2: 64–71

278. Miettinen M, Talerman A, Wahlstrom T, Astengo-Osuna C, Virtanen I (1985) Cellular differentiation in ovarian sex-cord–stromal and germ-cell tumors studied with antibodies to intermediate-filament proteins. Am J Surg Pathol 9: 640–651

279. Mittal KR, Blechman A, Greco MA, Alfonso F, Demopoulos R (1992) Lymphoma of ovary with stromal luteinization, presenting as secondary amenorrhea. Gynecol Oncol 45: 69–75

280. Miyauchi J, Yamazaki K, Kiso I, et al (1987) Bilateral ovarian hemangiomas associated with diffuse hemangioendotheliomatosis: A case report. Acta Pathol Jpn 37: 1347–1355

281. Mohabeer J, Buckley CH, Fox H (1983) An immunohistochemical study of the incidence and significance of human chorionic gonadotrophin synthesis by epithelial ovarian neoplasms. Gynecol Oncol 16: 78–84

282. Montag TW, Murphy RE, Belinson JL (1984) Virilizing malignant lipid cell tumor producing erythropoietin. Gynecol Oncol 19: 98–103

283. Mordel N, Margalioth EJ, Harats N, et al (1988) Concurrence of ovarian cancer and dermatomyositis. A report of two cases and literature review. J Reprod Med 33: 649–655

284. Morgan DR, Wells M, MacDonald RC, Johnston D (1985)

285. Morgello S, Schwartz E, Horwith M, et al (1988) Ectopic insulin production by a primary ovarian carcinoid. Cancer 61: 800–805

286. Morris J McL, Scully RE (1958) Endocrine Pathology of the Ovary. St. Louis, C.V. Mosby Co.

287. Morrison CW, Woodruff JD (1964) Fibrothecoma and associated ovarian stromal neoplasia. Obstet Gynecol 23: 344

288. Motlik K (1966) An estrogen-producing "yellow tumour" of the ovary associated with arterial hypertension. Endokrynol Pol 17: 525–539

289. Motlik K, Abrahamova J, Koutecky J, Horejsi J, Starka L (1987) Successive bilateral arrhenoblastoma. Path Res Pract 182: 453–584

290. Motlik K, Starka L (1973) Adrenocortical tumour of the ovary. (A case report with particular stress upon morphological and biochemical findings.) Neoplasma 20: 97

291. Motlik K, Stejskalova A, Stejskal J, Kobilkova J, Starka L (1988) Hilus cell tumors of the ovary. Cesk Pathol 24: 144–160

292. Nakashima N, Young RH, Scully RE (1984) Androgenic granulosa cell tumors of the ovary. A clinicopathological analysis of seventeen cases and review of the literature. Arch Pathol Lab Med 108: 786

293. Napoli VM, Wallach H (1976) Pancytopenia associated with a granulosa-cell tumor of the ovary. Report of a case. Am J Clin Pathol 65: 344–350

294. Neubecker RD, Breen JL (1962) Gynandroblastoma. A report of five cases with a discussion of the histogenesis and classification of ovarian tumors. Am J Clin Pathol 38: 60

295. Neville AJ, Gilchrist KW, Davis TE (1984) The chemotherapy of granulosa cell tumors of the ovary: Experience of the Wisconsin Clinical Cancer Center. Med Pediatr Oncol 12: 397–400

296. Nguyen KQ, Hurst CG, Pierson DL, et al (1983) Sweet's syndrome and ovarian carcinoma. Cutis 32: 152–154

297. Nichols J, Warren JC, Mantz FA (1962) ACTH-like excretion from carcinoma of the ovary. JAMA 182: 713–718

298. Nieminen U, Von Numers C, Widholm O (1963) Struma ovarii. Acta Obstet Gynecol Scand 42: 399–424

299. Niswander KR, Courey NG, Woodward T (1965) Precocious pseudopuberty caused by ovarian tumors. Obstet Gynecol 26: 381

300. Nogales FF, Concha A, Plata C, Ruiz-Avila I (1993) Granulosa cell tumor of the ovary with diffuse true hepatic differentiation simulating stromal luteinization. Am J Surg Pathol 17: 85–90

301. Norris HJ, Taylor HB (1968) Prognosis of granulosa-theca tumors of the ovary. Cancer 21: 255

302. Norris HJ, Taylor HB (1969) Virilization associated with cystic granulosa tumors. Obstet Gynecol 34: 629

303. Novak DJ, Lauchlan SC, McCawley JC, Faiman C (1970) Virilization during pregnancy. Case report and review of literature. Am J Med 49: 281–290

304. Novak ER (1967) Gynandroblastoma of the ovary. Review of 8 cases from the Ovarian Tumor Registry. Obstet Gynecol 30: 709

Zollinger–Ellison syndrome due to a gastrin secreting ovarian mucinous cystadenoma. Case report. Br J Obstet Gynaecol 92: 867–869

305. Novak ER, Kutchmeshgi J, Mupas RS, Woodruff JD, et al (1971) Feminizing gonadal stromal tumors. Obstet Gynecol 38: 701

306. Novak ER, Long JH (1965) Arrhenoblastoma of the ovary. A review of the Ovarian Tumor Registry. Am J Obstet Gynecol 92: 1082

307. Novak ER, Mattingly RF (1960) Hilus cell tumor of the ovary. Obstet Gynecol 15: 425

308. Nussbaum SR, Gas R, Arnold A (1990) Hypercalcemia and ectopic secretion of parathyroid hormone by an ovarian carcinoma with rearrangement of the gene for parathyroid hormone. N Engl J Med 323: 1324–1328

309. Ober WB, Pollak A, Gerstmann KE, Kupperman HS (1962) Krukenberg tumor with androgenic and progestational activity. Am J Obstet Gynecol 84: 739–744

310. O'Hern TM, Neubecker RD (1962) Arrhenoblastoma. Obstet Gynecol 19: 758

311. Okolo SO, Darley C, Melville HAH, Kirkham N (1990) Virilizing ovarian serous cystadenoma. Case report. Br J Obstet Gynecol 97: 269–271

312. O'Neill RT, Mikuta JJ (1970) Hypoglycemia associated with serous cystadenocarcinoma of the ovary. Obstet Gynecol 35: 287–289

313. Osborn RH, Yannone ME (1971) Plasma androgens in the normal and androgenic female. A review. Obstet Gynecol Surv 26: 195

314. Palmer PE, Bogojavlensky S, Bhan AK, Scully RE (1990) Prolactinoma in wall of ovarian dermoid cyst with hyperprolactinemia. Obstet Gynecol 75: 540–543

315. Paoletti M, Pridjian G, Okagaki T, Talerman A (1987) A stromal Leydig cell tumor of the ovary occurring in a pregnant 15-year-old girl. Ultrastructural findings. Cancer 60: 2806–2810

316. Plotz EJ, Wiener M, Stein AA (1966) Steroid synthesis in cystadenocarcinoma of the ovaries. Am J Obstet Gynecol 94: 189–194

317. Paraskevas M, Scully RE (1989) Hilus cell tumor of the ovary. A clinicopathological analysis of 12 Reinke crystal-positive and 9 crystal-negative cases. Int J Gynecol Pathol 8: 299–310

318. Parish JM, Lufkin EG, Lee RA, Gaffey TA (1984) Ovarian leiomyoma with hilus cell hyperplasia that caused virilization. Mayo Clinic Proc 59: 275–277

319. Parsons V, Rigby R (1958) Cushing's syndrome associated with adenocarcinoma of the ovary. Lancet 2: 992–994

320. Payne D, Muss HB, Homesley HD, Jobson VW, Baird FG (1981) Autoimmune hemolytic anemia and ovarian dermoid cysts: Case report and review of the literature. Cancer 48: 721–724

321. Pogliani EM, Fowst C, Maffe P, et al (1988) CNS metastasis in ovarian cancer with microangiopathic hemolytic anemia associated with diffuse intravascular coagulation. Tumor 74: 731–736

322. Post WD, Steele HD, Gorwill RH (1978) Mucinous cystadenoma and virilization during pregnancy. Can Med Assoc J 118: 952–953

323. Prat J, Bhan AK, Dickersin GR, Robboy SJ, Scully RE (1982) Hepatoid yolk sac tumor of the ovary (endodermal sinus tumor with hepatoid differentiation). A light micro-scopic, ultrastructural and immunohistochemical study of seven cases. Cancer 50: 2355–2368

324. Prat J, Scully RE (1981) Cellular fibromas and fibrosarcomas of the ovary: A comparative clinicopathologic analysis of seventeen cases. Cancer 47: 2663

325. Prat J, Young RH, Scully RE (1982) Ovarian Sertoli-Leydig cell tumors with heterologous elements. (ii) cartilage and skeletal muscle: A clinicopathologic analysis of twelve cases. Cancer 50: 2465

326. Price A, Russell P, Elliott P, Bannatyne P (1990) Composite mucinous and granulosa-cell tumor of ovary: Case report of a unique neoplasm. Int J Gynecol Pathol 9: 372–378

327. Primrose JN, Maloney M, Wells M, Bulgim O, Johnston D (1988) Gastrin-producing ovarian mucinous cystadenomas: A cause of the Zollinger–Ellison syndrome. Surgery 104: 830–833

328. Pruett KM, Gordon AN, Estrada R, et al (1988) Small-cell carcinoma of the ovary: An aggressive epithelial cancer occurring in young patients. Gynecol Oncol 29: 365–369

329. Prunty FTG. (1967) Hirsutism, virilism and apparent virilism and their gonadal relationship. Part I. J Endocrinol 38: 85

330. Pysher TJ, Hitch DC, Krous HF (1981) Bilateral juvenile granulosa cell tumors in a 4-month ody dysmorphic infant. A clinical, histologic, and ultrastructural study. Am J Surg Pathol 5: 789

331. Quinn MA, Oster AO, Fortune D, Hudson B (1981) Sclerosing stromal tumor of the ovary. Case report with endocrine studies. Br J Obstet Gynaecol 88: 555–558

332. Raggio M, Kaplan AL, Harberg JF (1983) Recurrent ovarian fibromas with basal cell nevus syndrome (Gorlin syndrome). Obstet Gynecol 61: 95s–96s

333. Ramzy I (1976) Signet-ring stromal tumor of ovary. Histochemical, light, and electron microscopic study. Cancer 38: 166–172

334. Reddick RL, Walton LA (1982) Sertoli-Leydig cell tumor of the ovary with teratomatous differentiation. Cancer 50: 1171–1176

335. Robboy SJ, Norris HJ, Scully RE (1975) Insular carcinoid primary in the ovary. A clinicopathologic analysis of 48 cases. Cancer 36: 404–418

336. Robboy SJ, Scully RE (1980) Strumal carcinoid of the ovary. Cancer 46: 2019–2034

337. Robboy SJ, Scully RE, Norris HJ (1977) Primary trabecular carcinoid of the ovary. Obstet Gynecol 49: 202–207

338. Robboy SJ, Scully RE, Norris HJ (1974) Carcinoid metastatic to the ovary. A clinicopathologic analysis of 35 cases. Cancer 33: 798–811

339. Robinson B, Eckstein R, Stiel JN, Payne WH, Kemp J (1988) An ovarian cyst associated with virilization. Aust NZ J Med 18: 161–163

340. Rome RM, Fortune DW, Quinn MA, Brown JB (1981) Functioning ovarian tumors in postmenopausal women. Obstet Gynecol 57: 705–710

341. Rome RM, Laverty CR, Brown JB (1973) Ovarian tumours in postmenopausal women. Clinicopathological features and hormonal studies. J Obstet Gynaecol Br Commonw 80: 984–991

342. Roth LM, Anderson MC, Govan ADT, Langley FA, Gow-

ing NFC, Woodcock AS (1981) Sertoli-Leydig cell tumors. A cliniclpathologic study of 34 cases. Cancer 48: 187

343. Roth LM, Liban E, Czernobilsky B (1982) Ovarian endometrioid tumors mimicking Sertoli and Sertoli-Leydig cell tumors. Sertoliform variant of endometrioid carcinoma. Cancer 50: 1322

344. Roth LM, Nicholas TR, Ehrlich CE (1979) Juvenile granulosa cell tumor. A clinicopathologic study of three cases with ultrastructural observations. Cancer 44: 2194

345. Roth LM, Slayton RE, Brady LW, Blesdsing JA, Johnson G (1985) Retiform differentiation in ovarian Sertoli–Leydig cell tumors. A clinicopathologic study of six cases from a gynecologic oncology study group. Cancer 55: 1093

346. Roth LM, Sternberg WH (1973) Ovarian stromal tumors containing Leydig cells. II. Pure Leydig cell tumor, nonhilar type. Cancer 32: 952

347. Roth LM, Sternberg WH (1983) Partly luteinized theca cell tumor of the ovary. Cancer 51: 1697

348. Rubin DK, Frost JF (1963) The cytologic detection of ovarian cancer. Acta Cytol 7: 191–195

349. Rutgers J, Scully RE (1986) Functioning ovarian tumors with peripheral steroid cell proliferation: A report of twenty-four cases. Int J Gynecol Pathol 5: 319–337

350. Ryan DE, Burkes EJ Jr (1973) The multiple basal-cell nevus syndrome in a Negro family. Oral Surg 36: 831–840

351. Sack GH, Levin J, Bell WR (1977) Trousseau's syndrome and other manifestations of chronic disseminated coagulopathy in patients with neoplasms: Clinical, pathophysiologic and therapeutic features. Medicine 56: 1–37

352. Saitoh A, Tsutsumi Y, Osamura RY, Watanabe K (1989) Sclerosing stromal tumor of the ovary. Immunohistochemical and electron-microscopic demonstration of smooth-muscle differentiation. Arch Pathol Lab Med 113: 372–376

353. Salm R (1967) Pure and mixed hilus cell tumors of ovary. Ann Roy Coll Surg Engl 41: 344

354. Salm R (1974) Ovarian hilus-cell tumors: their varying presentations. J Pathol 113: 117

355. Salomon-Bernard Y, Thibaud E, Vignal J, Musset R (1975) Tumeurs a Stroma Fonctionnel. In: Cabanne F (ed) Tumeurs de l'ovaire, Chapter II. Paris, Masson et Cie, pp 309

356. Samaan NA, Smith JP, Rutledge FN, Schultz PN (1976) The significance of measurement of human placental lactogen, human chorionic gonadotropin, and carcinoembryonic antigen in patients with ovarian carcinoma. Am J Obstet Gynecol 126: 186–189

357. Samanth KK, Black WC (1970) Benign ovarian stromal tumors associated with free peritoneal fluid. Am J Obstet Gynecol 107: 538

358. Sasano H, Sasano N (1989) What's new in the localization of sex steroids in the human ovary and its tumors? Pathol Res Pract 185: 942–948

359. Sasano H, Okamoto M, Mason JI, et al (1989) Immunohistochemical studies of steroidogenic enzymes (aromatase, 17-hydroxylase and cholesterol side-chain cleavage cytochromes P-450) in sex cord-stromal tumors of the ovary. Hum Pathol 20: 452–457

360. Scaling ST, Kaufman RH, Patten BM (1979) Dermatomyositis and female malignancy. Obstet Gynecol 54: 474–477

361. Schnoy N (1982) Ultrastructure of a virilizing ovarian Leydig-cell tumor. Virchows Arch (Pathol Anat) 397: 17

362. Schwartz PE, Smith JP (1976) Treatment of ovarian stromal tumors. Am J Obstet Gynecol 125: 402

363. Scully RE (1953) An unusual ovarian tumor containing Leydig cells but associated with endometrial hyperplasia, in a postmenopausal woman. J Clin Endocrinol Metab 13: 1254–1263

364. Scully RE (1962) Androgenic lesions of the ovary. In: Grady HG, Smith DE (eds) The Ovary, Chapter 9, International Academy of Pathology Monograph No. 3. Baltimore, Williams and Wilkins, pp 143

365. Scully RE (1964) Stromal luteoma of the ovary. A distinctive type of lipoid-cell tumor. Cancer 17: 769

366. Scully RE (1968) Sex cord-mesenchyme tumours. Pathologic classification and its relation to prognosis and treatment. In: Junqueira, AC, Gentil F (eds) Ovarian Cancer, IUCC Monograph Series, Vol II. Heidelberg, Springer-Verlag, pp 40–56

367. Scully RE (1970) Sex cord tumor with annular tubules. A distinctive ovarian tumor of the Peutz–Jeghers syndrome. Cancer 25: 1107

368. Scully RE (1970) Gonadoblastoma. A review of 74 cases. Cancer 25: 1340

369. Scully RE (1979) Tumors of the Ovary and Maldeveloped Gonads. In Atlas of Tumor Pathology, 2nd series, Fascicle No. 16, Armed Forces Institute of Pathology, Washington DC

370. Scully RE (1987) Ovarian tumors with functioning stroma. In: Fox H (ed) Haines and Taylor's Gynaecological and Obstetrical Pathology, 3rd ed. Edinburgh, Churchill Livingstone, pp 724–736

371. Scully RE, Aguirre P, DeLellis RA (1984) Argyrophilia, serotonin, and peptide hormones in the female genital tract and its tumors. Int J Gynecol Pathol 3: 51–70

372. Scully RE, Cohen RB (1964) Oxidative-enzyme activity in normal and pathologic human ovaries. Obstet Gynecol 24: 667–681

373. Scully RE, Dickerson GR (1989) Letter to the editor. Int J Gynecol Pathol 8: 196

374. Scully RE, Morris JMcL (1957) Functioning ovarian tumors. In: Meigs J, Sturgis SH (eds) Progress in Gynecology III, Chapter 2. New York, Grune and Stratton, pp 20

375. Scully RE, Richardson GS (1961) Luteinization of the stroma of metastatic cancer involving the ovary and its endocrine significance. Cancer 14: 827–840

376. Senekjian EK, Weiser PA, Talerman A, et al (1989) Vinblastine, cisplatin, cyclophosphamide, bleomycin, doxorubicin, and etoposide in the treatment of small cell carcinoma of the ovary. Cancer 64: 1183–1187

377. Serment HL, Laffargue P, Piana L, Blanc B (1970) Ovarian hormone tumors of female children. Int J Gynaecol Obstet 8: 409

378. Serov SF, Scully RE, Sobin LH (1973) International Histological Classification of Tumours, No. 9. Histological Typing of Ovarian Tumours. Geneva, World Health Organization

379. Shah KH, Steele HD (1981) Sclerosing stromal tumor of the ovary. A case report and further observations. Diagn Gynecol Obstet 3: 155–159

380. Sher J, Marsh M (1963) Multilocular cystic granulosa cell tumor. Am J Clin Pathol 40: 72

381. Shetty MR, Boghossian HM, Duffell D, Freel R, Gonzalez JC (1982) Tumor induced hypoglycemia. A result of ectopic insulin production. Cancer 49: 1920–1923

382. Shiel WC, Prete PE, Jason M, Andrews BS (1985) Palmar fasciitis and arthritis with ovarian and non-ovarian carcinomas. New syndrome. Am J Med 79: 640–644

383. Siegman-Igra Y, Flatau E, Deligdish L (1977) Chronic diffuse intravascular coagulation (DIC) in nonmetastatic ovarian cancer. Report of a case and review of the literature. Gynecol Oncol 5: 92–100

384. Silva PD, Porto M, Moyer DL, Lobo RA (1988) Clinical and ultrastructural findings of an androgenizing Krukenberg tumor in pregnancy. Obstet Gynecol 71: 432–434

385. Silverberg SG (1971) Brenner tumor of the ovary: A clinicopathologic study of 60 tumors in 54 women. Cancer 28: 588–596

386. Simmons RL, Sciarra JJ (1967) Treatment of late recurrent granulosa cell tumors of the ovary. Surg Gynecol Obstet 124: 65

387. Sjostedt S, Wahlen T (1961) Prognosis of granulosa cell tumors. Acta Obstet Gynecol Scand 40: 1

388. Smith JP, Rutledge F (1970) Chemotherapy in the treatment of cancer of the ovary. Am J Obstet Gynecol 107: 691

389. Snider BL, Benjamin DR (1981) Eruptive keratoacanthoma with an internal malignant neoplasm. Arch Dermatol 117: 788–790

390. Snyder RR, Tavassoli FA (1986) Ovarian strumal carcinoid: Immunohistochemical, ultrastructural, and clinicopathologic observations. Int J Gynecol Pathol 5: 187–201

391. Solh HM, Azoury RS, Najjar SS (1983) Peutz–Jeghers syndrome associated with precocious puberty. J Pediatr 103: 593–595

392. Solomon SD, Maurer KH (1983) Association of dermatomyositis and dysgerminoma in a 16-year-old patient. Arthritis Rheum 26: 572–573

393. Sotto LSJ, Postoloff AV, Carr F (1956) A case of calcified ovarian fibroma with ossification. Am J Obstet Gynecol 71: 1355

394. Spadoni LR, Lindberg MC, Mottet NK, Herman WL (1965) Virilization coexisting with Krukenberg tumor during pregnancy. Am J Obstet Gynecol 92: 981–991

395. Srivastava KP (1976) Hypoglycemia associated with nonpancreatic mesenchymal tumors. Int Surg 61: 282–286

396. Stagno PA, Petras RE, Hart WR (1987) Strumal carcinoids of the ovary. An immunohistologic and ultrastructural study. Arch Pathol Lab Med 111: 440–446

397. Stenwig JT, Hazekamp JT, Beecham JB (1979) Granulosa cell tumors of the ovary. A clinicopathological study of 118 cases with long-term follow-up. Gynecol Oncol 7: 136

398. Sternberg WH (1949) The morphology, endocrine function, hyperplasia and tumors of the human ovarian hilus cells. Am J Pathol 25: 493

399. Sternberg WH, Dhurandhar HN (1977) Functional ovarian tumors of stromal and sex cord origin. Hum Pathol 8: 565

400. Sternberg WH, Roth LM (1973) Ovarian stromal tumors containing Leydig cells. 1. Stromal-Leydig cell tumor and

non-neoplastic transformation of ovarian stroma to Leydig cells. Cancer 32: 940

401. Stewart AF, Romero R, Schwartz PE, Kohorn EI, Broadus AE (1982) Hypercalcemia associated with gynecologic malignancies. Biochemical characterization. Cancer 49: 2389–2394

402. Stewart KR, Casey MJ, Gondos B (1981) Endodermal sinus tumor of the ovary with virilization. Light and electronmicroscopy study. Am J Surg Pathol 5: 385–391

403. Sugiyama M, Kohmoto Y, Miyoshi T, et al (1983) In vivo and vitro steroid biosynthesis by ovarian juvenile granulosa cell tumor of a girl with Ollier's disease. Acta Gynaecol Jpn 35: 2185

404. Suit PF, Hart WR (1988) Sclerosing stromal tumor of the ovary. An ultrastructural study and review of the literature to evaluate hormonal function. Cleve Clin J Med 55: 189–194

405. Susil BJ, Sumithran E (1987) Sarcomatous change in granulosa cell tumor. Hum Pathol 18: 397–399

406. Swanson PE, Dehner LP (1990) Letter to the Editor. Am J Clin Pathol 94: 805

407. Sweeney EC, Lee G (1979) Granulosa cell tumour of the ovary metastasizing to the heart: A light and electron microscopic study. Ir J Med Sci 148: 11–12

408. Symonds DA, Driscoll SG (1973) An adrenal cortical rest within the fetal ovary. Report of a case. Am J Clin Pathol 60: 562

409. Synder RR, Tavassoli FA (1986) Ovarian strumal carcinoid. Immunohistochemical, ultrastructural, and clinicopathologic observations. Int J Gynecol Pathol 5: 187–201

410. Takeda A, Suzumori K, Sugimoto Y, et al (1984) Clear cell carcinoma of the ovary with colony-stimulating-factor production. Occurrence of marked granulocytosis in a patient and nude mice. Cancer 54: 1019–1023

411. Takeuchi H, Hamada H, Sodemoto Y, Ushigome S (1983) Juvenile granulosa cell tumor with rapid distant metastases. Acta Pathol Jpn 33: 537

412. Talbott JH (1977) Acute dermatomyositis-polymyositis and malignancy. Semin Arthritis Rheum 6: 305–360

413. Talerman A (1987) Ovarian Sertoli-Leydig cell tumor (androblastoma) with retiform pattern: A clinicopathologic study. Cancer 60: 3056–3064

414. Talerman A, Haije WG (1985) Letter to the Editor. Int J Gynecol Pathol 4: 171–172

415. Talerman A, Hughesdon PE, Anderson MC (1982) Diffuse nonlobular ovarian androblastoma usually associated with feminization. Int J Gynecol Pathol 1: 155–171

416. Tamini HK, Bolen J (1984) Enchondromatosis (Ollier's disease) and ovarian juvenile granulosa cell tumor. Cancer 53: 1605–1608

417. Tanaka Y, Sasaki Y, Nishihira H, Izawa T, Nishi T (1992) Ovarian juvenile granulosa cell tumor associated with Maffucci's syndrome. Am J Clin Pathol 97: 523–527

418. Tang M, Liu T (1982) Ovarian sclerosing stromal tumors. Clinicopathologic study of 10 cases. Chinese Med J 95: 186–190

419. Targett CS (1974) Estrogen excretion in a case of theca-granulosa cell tumor. Am J Obstet Gynecol 119: 859

420. Tavassoli FA, Norris HJ (1980) Sertoli tumors of the ovary. A clinicopathologic study of 28 cases with ultrastructural observations. Cancer 46: 2282

421. Taylor HB, Norris HJ (1967) Lipid cell tumors of the ovary. Cancer 20: 1953

422. Teilum G (1958) Classification of testicular and ovarian androblastoma and Sertoli cell tumors. Cancer 11: 769

423. Teilum G (1949) Homologous ovarian and testicular tumors. III. Estrogen producing Sertoli cell tumors (androblastoma tubulare lipoides) of the human testis and ovary. J Clin Endocrinol 9: 301

424. Teilum G (1971) Special Tumors of Ovary and Testis. Comparative Pathology and Histological Identification. Philadelphia, JB Lippincott

425. Teter J, Bulski T, Wasilewska B (1962) A virilizing adrenal rest tumor of the ovary with postmenopausal uterine hypertrophy. Bull Pol Med Sci Hist 5: 144

426. Tetu B, Lebel M, Camilleri J (1988) Renin-producing ovarian tumor. A case report with immunohistochemical and electron-microscopic study. Am J Surg Pathol 12: 634–640

427. Tetu B, Ordonez NG, Silva EG (1986) Sertoli-Leydig cell tumor of the ovary with alpha-fetoprotein production. Arch Pathol Lab Med 110: 65–68

428. Tighe JR (1961) Brenner tumours of the ovary: A clinicopathological study. J Obstet Gynaecol Brit Commonw 68: 292–296

429. Tiltman AJ (1985) Sclerosing stromal tumor of the ovary: Demonstration of Ligandin in three cases. Int J Gynecol Pathol 4: 362–369

430. Todesco S, Terribile V, Borsatti A, et al (1975) Primary aldosteronism due to a malignant ovarian tumor. J Clin Endocrinol Metab 41: 809–819

431. Tracy SL, Askin FB, Reddick RL, Jackson B, Kurman RJ (1985) Progesterone secreting Sertoli cell tumor of the ovary. Gynecol Oncol 22: 85–96

432. Tsukamoto N, Nakamura M, Ishikawa H (1976) Sclerosing stromal tumor of the ovary. Gynecol Oncol 4: 335–339

433. Tyler HR (1974) Paraneoplastic syndromes of nerve, muscle, and neuromuscular junction. Ann NY Acad Sci 230: 348–357

434. Tytle T, Rosin D (1984) Bilateral calcified ovarian fibromas. South Med J 77: 1178–1180

435. Ueda G, Nobuaki H, Hayakawa K, et al (1972) Clinical histochemical and biochemical studies of an ovarian dysgerminoma with trophoblasts and Leydig cells. Am J Obstet Gynecol 114: 748–754

436. Ueda G, Sato Y, Yamasaki M, et al (1978) Strumal carcinoid of the ovary. Histological, ultrastructural and immunohistological studies with anti-human thyroglobulin. Gynecol Oncol 6: 411–419

437. Ulbright TM, Roth LM, Ehrlich CE (1982) Ovarian strumal carcinoid. An immunocytochemical and ultrastructural study of two cases. Am J Clin Path 77: 622–631

438. Ulbright TM, Roth LM, Stehman FB, Talerman A, Senekjian EK (1987) Poorly differentiated (small cell) carcinoma of the ovary in young women: Evidence supporting a germ cell origin. Hum Pathol 18: 175–184

439. Vaitukaitis JL (1974) Human chorionic gonadotropin as a tumor marker. Ann Clin Lab Sci 4: 276–280

440. Vassal G, Flamant F, Caillaud JM, et al (1988) Juvenile granulosa cell tumor of the ovary in children: A clinical study of 15 cases. J Clin Oncol 6: 990–995

441. Vaz RM, Turner C (1986) Ollier disease (Enchondromatosis) associated with ovarian juvenile granulosa cell tumor and precocious puberty. J Pediatr 108: 945–947

442. Velasco-Oses A, Alonso-Alvaro A, Blanco-Pozo A, et al (1988) Ollier's disease associated with ovarian juvenile granulosa cell tumor. Cancer 62: 222–225

443. Verducci MA, Malkasian GD, Friedman SJ, Winkelmann RK (1984) Gynecologic carcinoma associated with dermatomyositis-polymyositis. Obstet Gynecol 64: 695–698

444. Verhoeven ATM, Mastboom JL, Van Leusden HAIM, Van Der Velden WHM (1973) Virilization in pregnancy coexisting with an (ovarian) mucinous cystadenoma: A case report and review of virilizing ovarian tumors in pregnancy. Obstet Gynec Surv 28: 597–622

445. Vicens E, Martinez-Mora J, Potau N, Sans M, Boix-Ochoa J (1980) Masculinization of a female fetus by Krukenberg tumor during pregnancy. J Pediatr Surg 15: 188–190

446. von dem Borne AEGK, van Oers RHJ, Wiersinga WM, et al (1990) Complete remission of autoimmune thrombocytopenia after extirpation of a benign adenofibroma of the ovary. Br J Rheumatol 74: 119–120

447. Waxman M, Damjanov I, Alpert L, Sardinsky T (1981) Composite mucinous ovarian neoplasms associated with Sertoli-Leydig and carcinoid tumors. Cancer 47: 2044

448. Waxman M, Vuletin JC, Urcuyo R, Belling CG (1979) Ovarian low-grade stromal sarcoma with thecomatous features. A critical reappraisal of the so-called "malignant thecoma." Cancer 44: 2206

449. Woodruff JD, Rauh JT, Markley RL (1966) Ovarian struma. Obstet Gynecol 27: 194–201

450. Woodruff JD, Williams TJ, Goldberg B, Lawterbach M, Preece E (1973) Hormonal activity of the common ovarian neoplasms. Am J Obstet Gynecol 87: 679–695.

451. Yaker A, Benirschke K (1975) A ten year study of ovarian tumors. Virchows Arch A Path Anat Histol 366: 275–286

452. Yeh E, Meade RC, Ruetz PP (1973) Radionuclide study of struma ovarii. J Nucl Med 14: 118–121

453. Young RH, Dickersin GR, Scully RE (1983) A distinctive ovarian sex cord–stromal tumor causing sexual precocity in the Peutz–Jeghers syndrome. Am J Surg Pathol 7: 223

454. Young RH, Dickersin GR, Scully RE (1984) Juvenile granulosa cell tumor of the ovary. A clinicopathologic analysis of 125 cases. Am J Surg Pathol 8: 575

455. Young RH, Dudley AG, Scully RE (1984) Granulosa cell, Sertoli-Leydig cell and unclassified sex cord-stromal tumors associated with pregnancy. A clinicopathological analysis of thirty-six cases. Gynecol Oncol 18: 181

455a. Young RH, Oliva E, Scully RE (in press) Lutenized adult granulosa cell tumors of the ovary: A report of four cases. Int J Gynecol Pathol

455b. Young RH, Oliva E, Scully RE Small cell carcinoma of the ovary, hypercalcemia type. A clinico pathological analysis of 150 cases. Submitted

456. Young RH, Perez-Atayde AR, Scully RE (1984) Ovarian Sertoli-Leydig cell tumor with retiform and heterologous components. Report of a case with hepatocytic differentiation and elevated serum alpha-fetoprotein. Am J Surg Pathol 8: 709

457. Young RH, Prat J, Scully RE (1982) Ovarian endometrioid carcinomas resembling sex cord-stromal tumors. A clinico-

pathological analysis of 13 cases. Am J Surg Pathol 6: 513–522

458. Young RH, Prat J, Scully RE (1982) Ovarian Sertoli-Leydig cell tumors with heterologous elements. (i) Gastrointestinal epithelium and carcinoid: A clinicopathologic analysis of thirty-six cases. Cancer 50: 2448–2456

459. Young RH, Prat J, Scully RE (1983) Endometrioid stromal sarcomas of the ovary. A clinicopathological analysis of twenty-three cases. Cancer 53: 1143

460. Young RH, Scully RE (1991) Malignant melanoma metastatic to the ovary. A clinicopathologic analysis of 20 cases. Am J Surg Pathol 15: 849–860

461. Young RH, Scully RE (1992) Ovarian sex cord–stromal tumors. Recent progress. Int J Gynecol Pathol 1: 101

462. Young RH, Scully RE (1983) Ovarian stromal tumors with minor sex cord elements: A report of seven cases. Int J Gynecol Pathol 2: 227

463. Young RH, Scully RE (1983) Ovarian sex cord-stromal tumors with bizarre nuclei. A clinicopathologic analysis of seventeen cases. Int J Gynecol Pathol 1: 325

464. Young RH, Scully RE (1983) Ovarian Sertoli-Leydig cell tumors with a retiform pattern: A problem in histopathologic diagnosis. A report of 25 cases. Am J Surg Pathol 77: 755

465. Young RH, Scully RE (1984) Ovarian Sertoli cell tumors. A report of ten cases. Int J Gynecol Pathol 2: 349

466. Young RH, Scully RE (1984) Ovarian sex cord-stromal tumors: Recent advances and current status. Clin Obstet Gynecol 11: 93

467. Young RH, Scully RE (1984) Fibromatosis and massive edema of the ovary, possibly related entities. A report of 14 cases of fibromatosis and 11 cases of massive edema. Int J Gynecol Pathol 3: 153

468. Young RH, Scully RE (1988) Ovarian sex cord-stromal tumors: Problems in differential diagnosis. Pathol Annu 23(PT I): 237–296

469. Young RH, Scully RE (1987) Ovarian steroid cell tumors associated with Cushing's syndrome. A report of three cases. Int J Gynecol Pathol 6: 40–48

470. Young RH, Scully RE (1989) Alveolar rhabdomyosarcoma metastatic to the ovary. A report of two cases and discussion of the differential diagnosis of small cell malignant tumors of the ovary. Cancer 64: 899–904

471. Young RH, Scully RE (1990) Sarcomas metastatic to the ovary. A report of 21 cases. Int J Gynecol Pathol 9: 231–252

472. Young RH, Scully RE (1984) Well-differentiated ovarian Sertoli–Leydig cell tumors. A clinicopathological analysis of 23 cases. Int J Gynecol Pathol 3: 277

473. Young RH, Scully RE (1985) Ovarian Sertoli-Leydig cell tumors. A clinicopathological analysis of 207 cases. Am J Surg Pathol 9: 543–569

474. Young RH, Welch WR, Dickersin GR, Scully RE (1982) Ovarian sex cord tumor with annular tubules: Review of 74 cases including 27 with Peutz–Jeghers syndrome and 4 with adenoma malignum of the cervix. Cancer 50: 1384

475. Yuen BH, Robertson I, Clement PB, Mincey EK (1982) Sclerosing stromal tumor of the ovary. Obstet Gynecol 60: 252–256

476. Zaloudek C, Norris HJ (1982) Granulosa tumors of the ovary in children. A clinical and pathologic study of 32 cases. Am J Surg Pathol 6: 503

477. Zaloudek C, Norris HJ (1984) Sertoli-Leydig tumors of the ovary. A clinicopathologic study of 64 intermediate and poorly differentiated neoplasms. Am J Surg Pathol 8: 405–418

478. Zaloudek CJ, Tavassoli FA, Norris HJ (1981) Dysgerminoma with syncytiotrophoblastic giant cells. A histologically and clinically distinctive subtype of dysgerminoma. Am J Surg Pathol 5: 361–367

479. Zhang J, Young RH, Arseneau J, Scully RE (1982) Ovarian stromal tumors containing lutein or Leydig cells (luteinized thecomas and stromal Leydig cell tumors). A clinicopathological analysis of fifty cases. Int J Gynecol Pathol 1: 270

20

Germ Cell Tumors of the Ovary

Aleksander Talerman, M.D., Ph.D., F.R.C. Path.

Germ cell tumors are composed of a number of histologically different tumor types derived from the primitive germ cells of the embryonic gonad. The concept of germ cell tumors as a specific group of gonadal neoplasms has evolved in the last five decades. It is based on (1) the common histogenesis of these neoplasms, (2) the relatively frequent presence of histologically different neoplastic elements within the same tumor mass, and (3) the presence of histologically similar neoplasms in extragonadal locations along the line of migration of the primitive germ cells from the wall of the yolk sac to the gonadal ridge,[384] as well as on the remarkable homology between the various tumors in the male and the female. In no other group of gonadal neoplasms is this homology better illustrated. Although the strong morphologic resemblance between the testicular seminoma and its ovarian counterpart, the dysgerminoma, was noted soon after these neoplasms were first described, for a long time there was no agreement as to their histogenesis. Nevertheless, these were the first neoplasms to become accepted as originating from germ cells. It was not until the studies by Teilum[339,340] on the homology of ovarian and testicular neoplasms, the studies by Friedman and Moore[95] and Dixon and Moore[76] on testicular tumors, and those by Friedman[94] on related extragonadal neoplasms that the germ cell origin of other neoplasms belonging to this group was suggested. These views were supported by the embryologic studies of Witschi[384] and Gillman,[107] and later by the experimental work of Stevens[305–307] and Pierce et al.[238,239,241,244] on germ cell tumors in rodents.

Although occasional unusual neoplasms composed of germ cells and sex cord derivatives had been noted previously,[194,276] it was not until Scully's detailed description of gonadoblastoma[276] that these neoplasms were recognized. More recently, another neoplasm composed of germ cells and sex cord derivatives, the mixed germ cell–sex cord stroma tumor, has been described in detail.[313,314] This chapter, therefore, is devoted not only to neoplasms of germ cell origin but also to those composed of germ cells and sex cord derivatives.

Histogenesis

The histogenesis and interrelationships of the various types of germ cell neoplasms, as suggested by Teilum,[344] are shown in Fig. 20.1.

According to Teilum,[344] dysgerminoma (seminoma) is a primitive germ cell neoplasm that has not acquired the potential for further differentiation. Embryonal carcinoma is regarded as a conceptual as well as a morphologic entity and represents a germ cell neoplasm composed of multipotential cells that are capable of further differentiation. This can take place in an embryonal or somatic direction, resulting in teratomatous neoplasms showing various degrees of maturity, or in an extraembryonal direction along either of two pathways: vitelline, differentiating toward yolk sac (endodermal sinus) tumor, or trophoblastic, differentiating toward a choriocarcinoma. The process of differentiation is

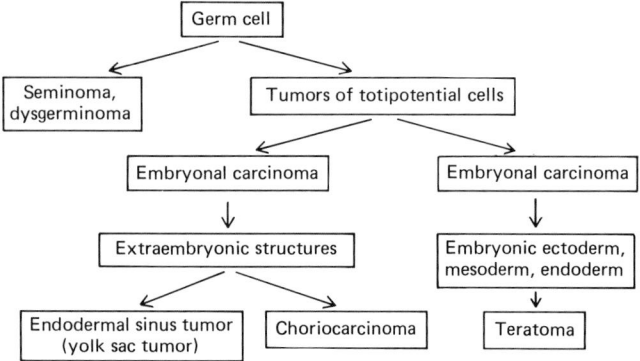

FIG. 20.1. **The histogenesis and interrelationship of tumors of germ cell origin.** (Modified from Teilum, ref. 344.)

dynamic and, therefore, the resulting neoplasms may be composed of different elements showing various stages of development. Although according to this view[344] dysgerminoma is considered incapable of further differentiation, recent immunocytochemical evidence indicates that some seminoma or dysgerminoma cells can differentiate into embryonal carcinoma and further. Although the great majority of seminoma or dysgerminoma cells are cytokeratin-negative, whereas embryonal carcinoma, endodermal sinus tumor, and choriocarcinoma are composed entirely of cytokeratin-positive cells,[25,200,201] some seminomas and dysgerminomas contain cytokeratin-positive cells.[200] The intimate admixture of dysgerminoma cells with other neoplastic germ cell elements seen in some germ cell tumors also supports this view.[141,316,365]

Classification

A number of classifications of germ cell neoplasms of the ovary have been proposed over the years,* each one becoming progressively more detailed. Some years ago, a panel of pathologists was established under the auspices of the World Health Organization (WHO) to formulate a histological classification of ovarian neoplasms to be used throughout the world. The classification[289] divides the germ cell tumors into a number of groups and also includes neoplasms composed of germ cells and sex cord–stromal derivatives. Recently, the WHO classification of ovarian neoplasms has been modified based on advances in our understanding of the pathology of ovarian neoplasms that have taken place during the last two decades (Table 20.1).[284]

There are several changes in the new classification. The main change is the use of the term *yolk sac tumor* instead of the more specific term *endodermal sinus tumor*. The latter term is retained as a synonym. The yolk sac tumor category has been expanded to include the polyvesicular vitelline, hepatoid, and glandular subtypes, which unlike other patterns of differentiation in yolk sac tumors can occur in pure form and thus pose diagnostic problems. The new classification also expands the category of *teratoma*, especially the group of monodermal teratomas to include some newly described entities. The tumors composed of germ cells and the sex cord–stromal derivatives are divided into two categories, gonadoblastoma and mixed germ cell–sex cord stromal tumor; each of these is subclassified to include those tumors associated with dysgerminoma or other germ cell tumors.

_____

*Refs. 127,143,277–279,342,345.

Table 20.1. WHO classification of germ cell tumors of the ovary

Germ cell tumors
Dysgerminoma
Variant—with syncytiotrophoblastic cells
Yolk sac tumor (endodermal sinus tumor)
Variants
Polyvesicular vitelline tumor
Hepatoid
Glandular
Embryonal carcinoma
Polyembryoma
Choriocarcinoma
Teratomas
Immature
Mature
Solid
Cystic (dermoid cyst)
With secondary tumor formation (specify type)
Fetiform (homunculus)
Monodermal and highly specialized
Struma ovarii
Variant—with thyroid tumor (specify type)
Carcinoid
Insular
Trabecular
Strumal carcinoid
Mucinous carcinoid
Neuroectodermal tumors
Sebaceous tumors
Others
Mixed (specify type)
Mixed forms (tumors composed of two or more of the above pure types)
Tumors composed of germ cells and sex cord–stromal derivatives
Gonadoblastoma
Variant—with dysgerminoma or other germ cell tumor
Germ cell–sex cord–stromal tumor
Variant—with dysgerminoma or other germ cell tumor

WHO, World Health Organization.

Cytogenetic Aspects

The great majority of ovarian germ cell tumors are mature cystic teratomas that are diploid, have a normal 46,XX karyotype, and have been considered to originate from germ cells after the first meiotic division.[174] This is unlike testicular germ cell tumors, which are nearly always malignant, aneuploid, have a higher than normal chromosome complement,[14] and are considered to originate before the first meiotic division.[229] Recent studies[211,228] using new and more advanced banding techniques have demonstrated diverse modes of origin of mature cystic teratoma. Although most ovarian mature cystic teratomas originate from germ cells after the first meiotic division, it has been demonstrated conclusively that some originate before this event.[211,228] This also applies to immature ovarian teratomas, which tend to be aneuploid, resembling their testicular counterparts. The demonstration of a small isochromo-

some, i(12p), as a specific abnormality and therefore a possible chromosomal marker for testicular germ cell tumors, especially seminoma,[15,105] has been extended to some ovarian germ cell neoplasms. The presence of this chromosome has been noted in two dysgerminomas.[16,146] Neither mature cystic teratoma,[228] immature cystic teratoma,[115] or mixed germ cell tumors and their metastases[106] have demonstrated this abnormality.

Clinical and Pathological Features of Germ Cell Tumors

Germ cell tumors constitute the second largest group of ovarian neoplasms after the common epithelial tumors and comprise approximately 20% of all ovarian neoplasms in Europe and North America. In countries in Asia and Africa where the prevalence of common epithelial tumors is much lower, germ cell tumors constitute a much larger proportion of ovarian neoplasms. Germ cell tumors are encountered at all ages from infancy to old age but are seen most frequently from the first to the sixth decades. They also have been observed during fetal life. In children and adolescents, more than 60% of ovarian neoplasms are of germ cell origin, and one-third of them are malignant.[2,42,44,213] In adults, the great majority of germ cell tumors (95%) are benign and consist of mature cystic teratomas (dermoid cysts).

Dysgerminoma

GENERAL FEATURES

Although the term *dysgerminoma* was first introduced by Meyer[199] in 1931, ovarian neoplasms showing this histological pattern had been recognized earlier. Chenot[51] in 1911 was the first to note their occurrence and their similarity to the testicular seminoma described some years earlier.[52] In view of the strong resemblance to their testicular counterpart, the tumor was named *ovarian seminoma* by Masson,[193] and this became the most popular term until its replacement by *dysgerminoma*. It is still widely used in the French literature. The term *disgerminoma*, as originally suggested by Meyer,[199] and which later became *dysgerminoma*, has over the years gained almost universal acceptance.

Histogenesis

Dysgerminoma is composed entirely of germ cells that show morphologic, including ultrastructural[131,151,179,223] and histochemical[184,185] similarity to primordial germ cells. The cells of dysgerminoma are considered to be in an early and sexually indifferent stage of differentiation. They are arrested at a developmental stage at which they have not yet gained the ability for further differentiation.[344]

However, there is now evidence that occasional cells may acquire this ability and differentiate to embryonal carcinoma and further.[200] These cells are hormonally inert. An origin from the primordial germ cells that migrate to the ovary during early embryogenesis from their site of origin in the wall of the yolk sac[384] is the most widely accepted view of the histogenesis of dysgerminoma. It is supported by the occurrence of homologous neoplasms in the testis (seminoma) and along the route of migration of the primordial germ cells from the wall of the yolk sac to the primitive gonad, in the mediastinum, retroperitoneum, posterior abdominal wall, and parapineal and sacrococcygeal regions.[94,107]

The presence of sex chromatin bodies (Barr bodies) in the cells of dysgerminoma is a matter of controversy. Sex chromatin bodies were said to be present in the cells of a number of dysgerminomas by some investigators,[353] whereas others[13] could not identify them. The latter view is more in accordance with an origin from the primordial germ cells. The finding of twice the amount of DNA in the nuclei of dysgerminoma cells as compared with the nuclei of lymphocytes in all the cases studied[13,161] further supports the origin from primordial germ cells, which have the same amount of DNA in their nuclei (twice the amount present in normal diploid cells).

Genetic Aspects

When Meyer[199] described dysgerminoma, he observed that the tumor frequently occurred in hermaphrodites, pseudohermaphrodites, and patients with underdeveloped or malformed genitalia. In fact, 27 of 48 cases collected by Meyer[199] occurred in sexually abnormal patients, and this relationship was strongly emphasized. It is considered that most of these reports described patients with gonadal dysgenesis and dysgerminoma that had originated from a gonadoblastoma. Although subsequent authors supported Meyer's contention about the very close association between dysgerminoma and developmental and sexual abnormalities, later reports suggested that it is not as close as had been postulated. These later reports stated that most patients with dysgerminoma were normally developed females without any sexual abnormalities.[*] Most patients with dysgerminoma do not exhibit any menstrual abnormalities and are either capable of bearing or have actually borne children.[13,36,45,72] In a number of cases, the diagnosis has been made during pregnancy.[†] A number of patients have become pregnant and have had normal offspring after therapy.[13,36,45,100,373] Most recent reports emphasize the occurrence of dysgerminoma in normal female patients,[*] and some have even cast doubt on the relationship with developmental and sexual abnormalities.[13]

The common association of dysgerminoma with gonadoblastoma, a tumor that nearly always occurs in patients with dysgenetic gonads,[†] indicates that there is a relationship between dysgerminoma and genetic and somatosexual abnormalities (see Chapter 2, Abnormal Sexual Development).

Endocrine Aspects

In the great majority of cases, dysgerminoma is not associated with endocrine manifestations. Occasional cases have been described in which the tumor was associated with elevated urinary chorionic gonadotropins, positive pregnancy tests, or signs of precocious puberty, and these manifestations have disappeared after tumor excision. Although in these cases the tumor has been said to be a pure dysgerminoma,[122,205] the possibility of admixture with choriocarcinomatous elements that have not been detected, perhaps because of inadequate sampling, is the most likely explanation.[47,127,232,266]

The presence of choriocarcinoma in association with dysgerminoma is not frequent, but most of the reported series contain cases of this type.[139,232,266,331,354] Occasional cases of pure dysgerminoma, containing multinucleated syncytiotrophoblastic giant cells but lacking cytotrophoblastic elements, have been noted to be associated with gonadotropin production. Although some cases of dysgerminoma showing these histological appearances were recognized previously, evidence of gonadotropin production by the syncytiotrophoblastic giant cells was obtained more recently. This provides another possible explanation, apart from the presence of true choriocarcinomatous elements, for the occasional presence of endocrine activity in cases of dysgerminoma. However, there remains a small group of cases in which, despite a careful search, trophoblastic elements have not been found. In some of these cases, the dysgerminoma has been associated with an increase in luteinized stromal or Leydig-like cells and it is likely that these cells may be responsible for the feminizing side effects. These cells may be found within the stroma of the tumor, within the uninvolved ovarian stroma either in the vicinity of the tumor, or located at the periphery of the ovary.[260] These cells also may be responsible for the virilizing side effects observed in occasional cases of dysgerminoma.[367] Dysgerminoma associated with evidence of virilization is found mostly in association with gonadoblastoma in patients with pure or mixed gonadal dysgenesis.

°Refs. 13,36,47,93,203,217,232,262,285,293.
†Refs. 13,36,45,159,162,266,331,354.

°Refs. 13,36,45,72,139,331,354.
†Refs. 100,124,269,270,280,380.

Prevalence

Dysgerminoma is an uncommon tumor, accounting for 1–2% of primary ovarian neoplasms and for 3–5% of ovarian malignancies.[203,220,266] Although until 1950 only 427 cases had been recorded in the literature,[203] more than twice as many cases have been reported since and dysgerminoma is considered the most common malignant ovarian germ cell neoplasm occurring in pure form. The exact prevalence of dysgerminoma in different parts of the world is not known, since most cancer registry reports do not differentiate between the various types of ovarian neoplasms.[176] In some countries there are considerable regional variations.[29] Although most reports emanate from Europe and North America, dysgerminoma has been encountered in all parts of the world and in all races. A high prevalence has been reported in Japan[128] and in a study from Bombay, India.[144]

CLINICAL FEATURES

The tumor may occur at any age from infancy to old age; the reported cases range between the ages of 7 months[49] to 70 years,[203] but most cases occur in adolescence and early adult life.° Dysgerminoma occurs not infrequently before puberty[44] but is very rare after menopause.[72,278] Most cases occur in the second and third decades; nearly half the patients are under 20 years of age and 80% are under 30 years.† Therefore, dysgerminoma is one of the most common malignant ovarian neoplasms of childhood, adolescence, and early adult life.‡ Dysgerminoma has been reported in siblings[331] as well as in a mother and daughter.[139]

The symptomatology of dysgerminoma is not distinctive and is similar to that observed in patients with other solid ovarian neoplasms.§ The duration of symptoms is usually short; despite this, the tumor is often large, indicating a rapid growth.[36,266,331] The most common presenting symptoms are abdominal enlargement and presence of a mass in the lower abdomen, sometimes associated with abdominal pain that may be caused by torsion. Loss of weight may also be an accompanying symptom. In a number of cases, the tumor has been found incidentally; in these cases, the tumor is usually small. Sometimes the tumor may be detected during pregnancy.‖ In such cases it may be discovered as an incidental finding or may be obstructing labor.[266] Dysgerminoma is one of the two most common ovarian neoplasms observed in pregnancy—the other being serous cystadenoma.[127,162] The relatively common finding of dysgerminoma in pregnant patients is nonspecific and relates to the age of the patients.

Dysgerminoma may also be discovered incidentally in patients investigated for primary amenorrhea; in these cases it is not infrequently associated with gonadoblastoma.[268,269,282,380] Occasionally, menstrual and endocrine abnormalities may be the presenting symptom,[72] but this tends to be more common in patients with dysgerminoma combined with other neoplastic germ cell elements, especially choriocarcinoma. In children, precocious sexual development may occur.[2,39,43,260]

GROSS FINDINGS

Dysgerminoma usually is unilateral. It tends to occur more often in the right ovary,[203,266,285,331] which is affected in approximately 50% of cases, whereas the left is affected in 33–35% and bilateral involvement occurs in 10–17%.[36,117,203,266] More frequent bilateral involvement has been reported in some series[221,232,331] and less frequent in others.[13,36,72,195] A much higher frequency of bilateral tumors is observed in patients with dysgerminoma associated with gonadoblastoma, the dysgerminoma arising from and overgrowing the gonadoblastoma.° Thus, inclusion of such cases tends to increase the prevalence of bilaterality.

Pure dysgerminomas are solid tumors that are round, oval, or lobulated, with a smooth, gray-white, slightly glistening fibrous capsule. They vary in size from a few centimeters in diameter to large masses measuring 50 cm across,[13,44] which fill the pelvic and abdominal cavities. Tumors heavier than 5 kg have been described.[203] Compressed ovarian tissue may be seen surrounding small tumors, but in large tumors it is not discernible. The capsule is usually intact but may be ruptured, especially in large tumors. This may lead to the formation of adhesions between the tumor and the surrounding structures. The consistency of dysgerminoma varies from firm and rubbery in small and medium-sized tumors to soft in the large ones. On cut surface (Fig. 20.2), the tumor is solid and varies from gray-pink to light tan. Red, brown, or yellow discoloration caused by hemorrhage or necrosis is also seen, especially in large tumors. This may sometimes lead to the formation of small cysts, but cystic areas are seen only occasionally in pure dysgerminoma. The presence of cystic areas suggests the possibility that other neoplastic elements may be present. In view of the important prognostic implications concerning the presence of other neoplastic germ cell elements, extensive and judicious sampling of different parts of the tumor, especially of the less typical areas, is recommended.

°Refs. 4,13,36,47,72,93,117,128,145,159,162,203,216,217,232, 262,278,285,331,374.
†Refs. 13,36,45,117,128,203,266,331,354,374.
‡Refs. 4,13,36,47,93,117,128,162,203,213,266,374.
§Refs. 13,36,72,117,203,266,374.
‖Refs. 13,72,162,232,266,331,354.

°Refs. 101,124,269,270,280,312.

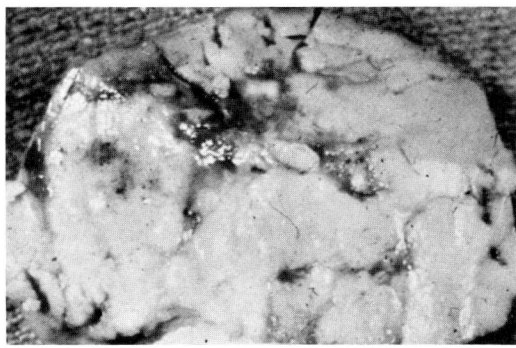

FIG. 20.2. Dysgerminoma. The cut surface is solid. There is some hemorrhage present.

MICROSCOPIC FINDINGS

Dysgerminoma exhibits a distinctive histological appearance. It is histologically identical to seminoma of the testis. It is composed of aggregates, islands, or strands of large uniform cells surrounded by varying amounts of connective tissue stroma containing lymphocytes (Figs. 20.3, 20.4). The cells are large and measure from 15 to 25 μm across. They are oval or round and usually have distinguishable cytoplasmic borders (Fig. 20.5). In well-fixed material, the cell boundaries are well-defined. The cells contain an ample amount of pale, slightly granular eosinophilic or clear cytoplasm. The centrally located vesicular nucleus is large, occupying nearly half the cell. The nucleus is oval or round, has a sharp nuclear membrane with unevenly dispersed finely granular chromatin, and contains usually one, but sometimes two, prominent eosinophilic nucleoli. Some variation in the size of the cells and nuclei and in the amount of nuclear chromatin is usually seen. Large or giant uninucleate tumor cells, which in all other respects resemble typical dysgerminoma cells, may be seen (Fig. 20.6). Mitotic activity is almost always detectable (Figs. 20.5, 20.6) and may vary from slight to brisk. This difference in mitotic activity may be observed not only in different tumors but also in different parts of the same tumor.

The cytoplasm of the tumor cells contains glycogen, which can be demonstrated with the periodic acid–Schiff (PAS) reaction, and this can be used as an aid in diagnosis. The amount of glycogen in tumor cells is variable, and glycogen is lost from the cytoplasm on prolonged fixation in formalin. In view of this, the PAS reaction may vary from strong to very weak. Most dysgerminoma cells do not show positive immunocytochemical staining for cytokeratin, although occasional cells may show a positive reaction.[200,201] In view of this, immunocytochemical staining for cytokeratin provides a useful diagnostic test that distinguishes between dysgerminoma and embryonal carcinoma or endo-

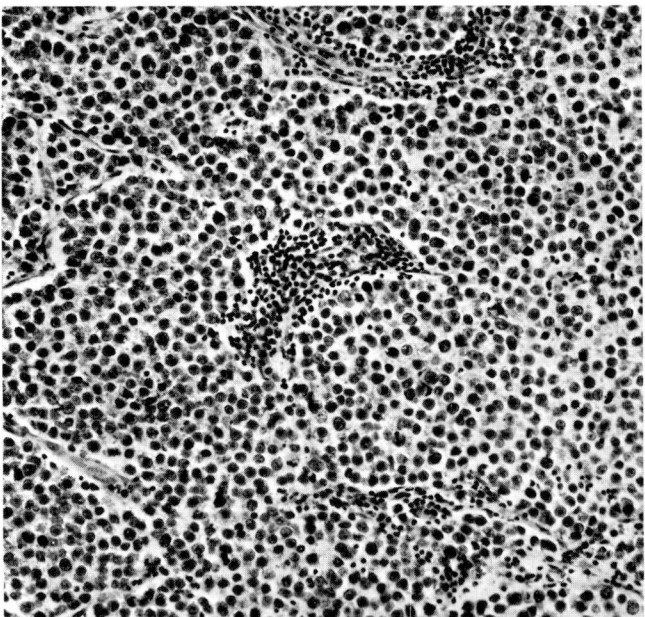

FIG. 20.3. Dysgerminoma. The tumor is composed of large aggregates of uniform cells surrounded by delicate strands of connective tissue containing lymphocytes.

dermal sinus tumor, which show a uniformly positive staining reaction for cytokeratin.[200,201]

Lipid can be demonstrated in the cytoplasm of the tumor cells in frozen tissue. The cells of dysgerminoma, like the primordial germ cells, show a positive alkaline phosphatase reaction beneath the cytoplasmic rim[184] and, in general, show similar histochemical reactions to those of primordial germ cells. An increased amount of DNA, double the amount present in normal somatic cells, has been observed in the nuclei of dysgerminoma using densitometry[13] and more sophisticated methods of DNA measurement.[161]

The stroma that surrounds the tumor cells is almost always infiltrated by lymphocytes. The lymphocytic infiltration may vary from slight to marked (Fig. 20.7). Occasionally, lymphoid follicles containing germinal centers may be seen. Plasma cells and eosinophils are not infrequently seen within the connective tissue stroma. Granulomatous reaction is also not infrequently seen; this manifests itself as collections of histiocytes surrounded by lymphocytes, plasma cells, and occasional giant cells of both the Langhans and foreign body types (Fig. 20.8). The lymphoreticular cell infiltrate recently has been studied immunocytochemically, and most of the cells were found to consist of T cells and macrophages. There were relatively few B cells, natural killer cells, and other types of lymphoreticular cells.[72] Similar findings were observed in

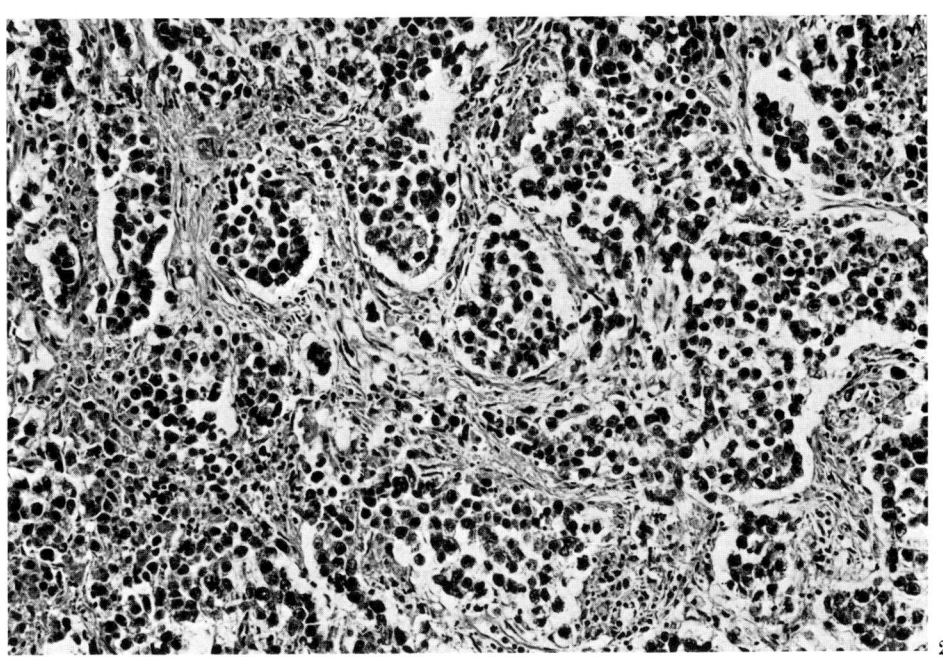

Fig. 20.4. **Dysgerminoma.** The tumor is composed of islands of tumor cells surrounded by connective tissue stroma containing lymphocytes.

Fig. 20.5. **Dysgerminoma.** Nests of dysgerminoma cells surrounded by a connective tissue septum infiltrated by lymphocytes. An abnormal mitosis is seen just below the *center*.

Fig. 20.6. **Dysgerminoma.** There is slight variation in size of the cells, a large uninucleate cell, and a mitosis in the center.

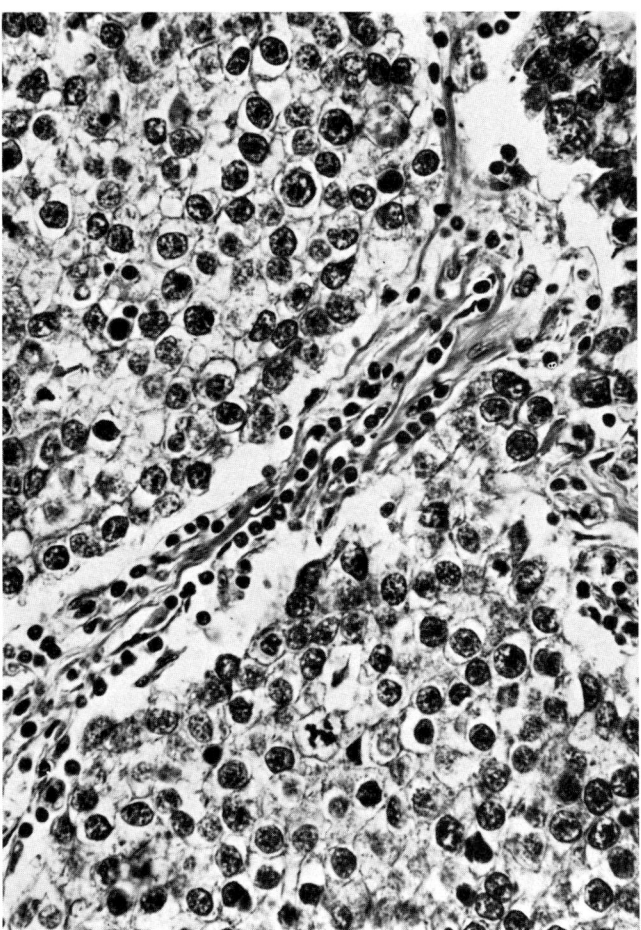

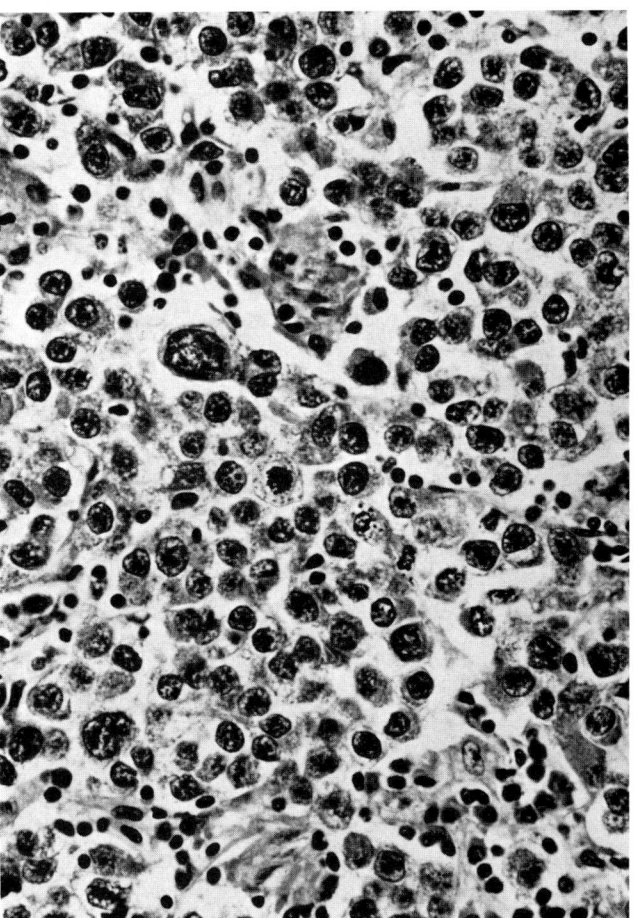

20.5

20.6

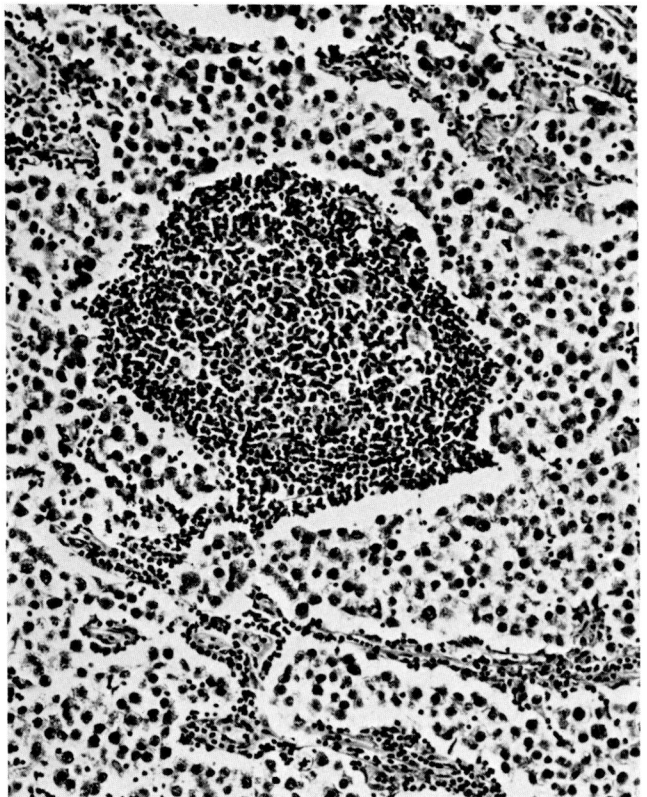

FIG. 20.7. **Dysgerminoma.** A large collection of lymphocytes and fine connective tissue septa surrounding the tumor cells are shown.

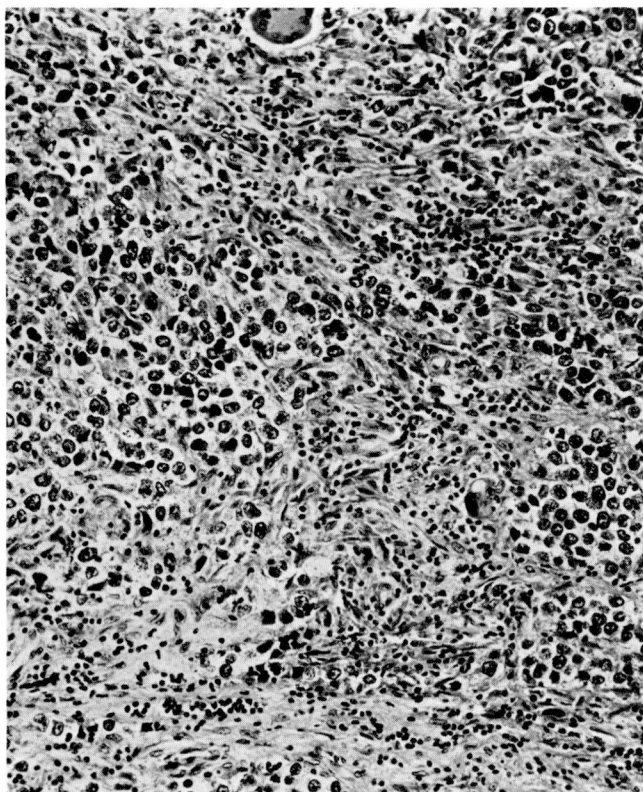

FIG. 20.8. **Dysgerminoma.** A granulomatous reaction with foreign body and Langhans giant cells is present.

testicular seminoma.[28] The connective tissue stroma shows considerable variation in its appearance. Depending on the amount of stroma, the tumor cells form large aggregates, smaller nests, islands, cords, or strands. The stroma varies from a fine, delicate fibrovascular network that can be loose and edematous to densely hyalinized. Occasionally, the amount of stroma may be very large, and this leads to wide separation of the nests of tumor cells (Fig. 20.4). At the opposite end of the spectrum, there are tumors that are cellular and contain only an imperceptible amount of stroma. There may be a considerable variation in the amount of stroma in various parts of the same tumor.

Foci of necrosis and hemorrhage are frequently found and may be of considerable size in large tumors or in tumors affected by torsion. Small foci of hyalinization may also be present, but large hyalinized areas sometimes observed in testicular seminoma are uncommon. Calcification is only occasionally seen in dysgerminoma. It occurs as small untidy spots or flecks of calcified material that are found in association with necrosis, hemorrhage, fibrosis, or hyalinization. Occasionally, relatively large, round, or ovoid calcified bodies are found, which may indicate the presence of a burnt-out gonadoblastoma[280] (Fig. 20.9).

In 6–8% of dysgerminomas, there are individual or collections of syncytiotrophoblastic giant cells that produce human chorionic gonadotropin (hCG). The presence of these cells is associated with elevation of serum hCG levels; hCG can also be demonstrated in tissue sections by immunoperoxidase techniques. The syncytiotrophoblastic giant cells may form large syncytial masses resembling the syncytiotrophoblast of a choriocarcinoma but they differ from the latter because there is no cytotrophoblast (Fig. 20.10). The syncytiotrophoblastic cells must also be differentiated from foreign body and Langhans giant cells and from uninucleate and multinucleate tumor giant cells, which are seen in some dysgerminomas. There is no evidence that dysgerminomas containing syncytiotrophoblastic giant cells are associated with worse prognosis.[392] The serum hCG level can be monitored as a tumor marker in the same way as in patients with gestational trophoblastic disease (see Chapter 24, Gestational Trophoblastic Disease) or with mixed germ cell tumors containing choriocarcinoma.

Pure dysgerminoma is not associated with elevated levels of serum alpha-fetoprotein (AFP).[330] The presence of elevated levels of AFP is an indication of presence of other neoplastic germ cell elements, virtually always yolk sac tumor (YST), either within the primary tumor or its metastases.

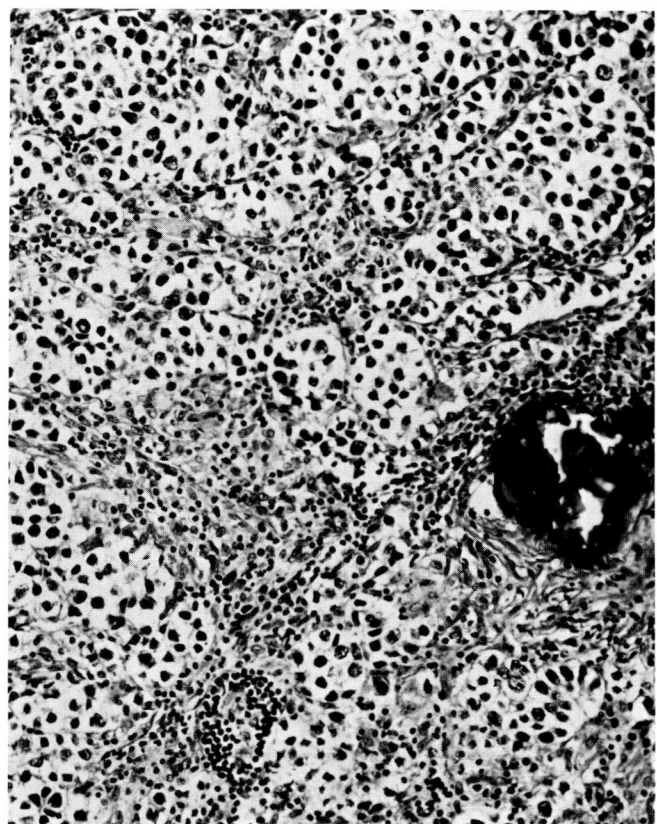

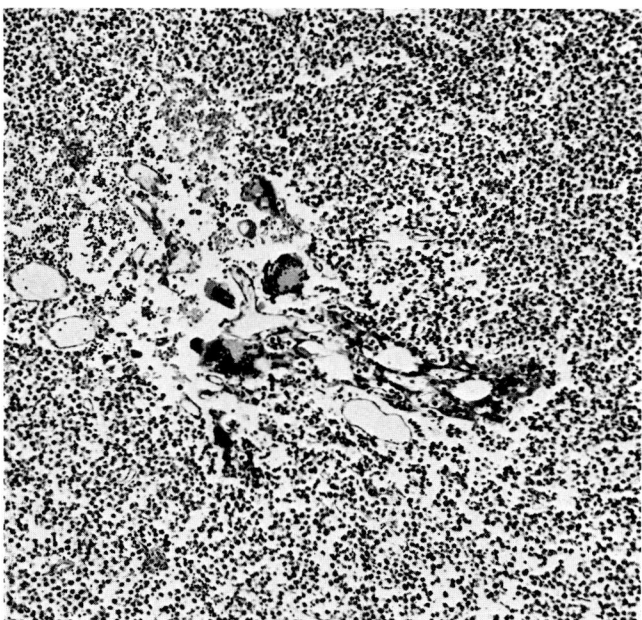

FIG. 20.10. **Dysgerminoma.** Collections of giant cells forming large syncytial masses resembling syncytiotrophoblast are present.

FIG. 20.9. **Dysgerminoma.** A large calcified concretion is present. Nests of gonadoblastoma were found in other parts of the tumor.

Immunocytochemical staining for placenta specific alkaline phosphatase (PLAP) has not been used and studied as extensively in ovarian dysgerminoma as in testicular seminomas,[141,168] but when applied PLAP stains dysgerminoma cells in the same way as testicular seminoma cells showing membrane-bound staining in most cells.[141] As PLAP also stains positively the tumor cells in other malignant germ cell tumors, it cannot be used to differentiate dysgerminoma from other malignant germ cell neoplasms.[141] It may be useful in differentiating dysgerminoma from non–germ cell malignancies that occasionally may resemble it like clear cell carcinoma, malignant lymphoma, granulosa cell tumor, and so forth.

The cells of dysgerminoma, when studied with the electron microscope,[65,131,151,179,223] have been found to resemble closely the cells of testicular seminoma[237] and germ cell neoplasms in other locations showing a similar histological pattern,[170,249] as well as normal maturing germ cells in the ovary.[126,185] Slight ultrastructural differences have been noted between individual germ cells present within a tumor, as well as between those present in the different tumors studied. It is likely that some of these differences

are related to the degree of differentiation and maturity of the tumor cells.

Dysgerminoma may be associated with other neoplastic germ cell elements. Recent studies indicate a greater frequency of these mixed tumors° as compared with earlier reports.[203] This is a result of a more detailed examination of the tumors and from a better recognition of the fact that germ cell tumors may be composed of histologically different neoplastic elements occurring in combination. For example, dysgerminoma may be combined with teratoma (Fig. 20.11), yolk sac tumor (Fig. 20.12), embryonal carcinoma, and choriocarcinoma. Some tumors may contain all these neoplastic germ cell elements. The association of dysgerminoma with gonadoblastoma is frequent, occurring in 50% of cases of gonadoblastoma.[280] Histologically, the other neoplastic germ cell elements may be intimately admixed with the dysgerminoma (Fig. 20.11) or may be found adjacent to the dysgerminoma and separated from it by a fibrous septum (Fig. 20.12).

CLINICAL BEHAVIOR

Dysgerminoma is a malignant neoplasm capable of metastatic and local spread. Despite its less aggressive behavior

---

°Refs. 44,90,139,148,166,232,266,331,354.

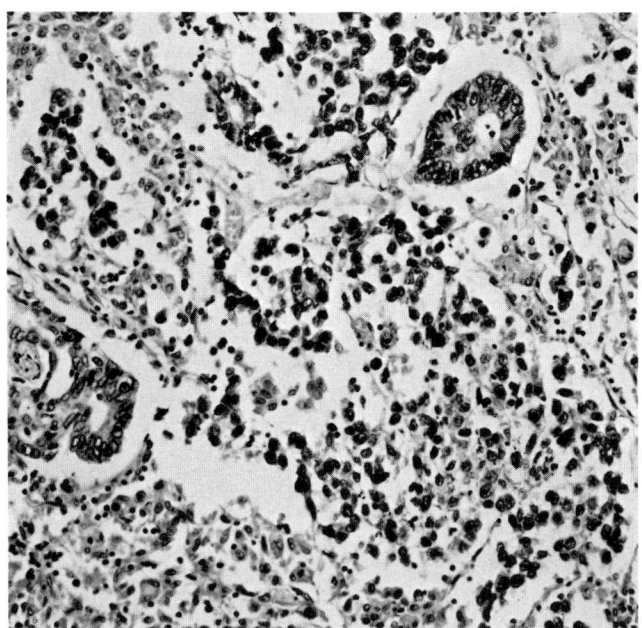

FIG. 20.11. Dysgerminoma intimately admixed with imma-ture teratoma. Note the primitive glandular epithelium of the teratoma. (Reprinted by permission of Talerman et al., ref. 333.)

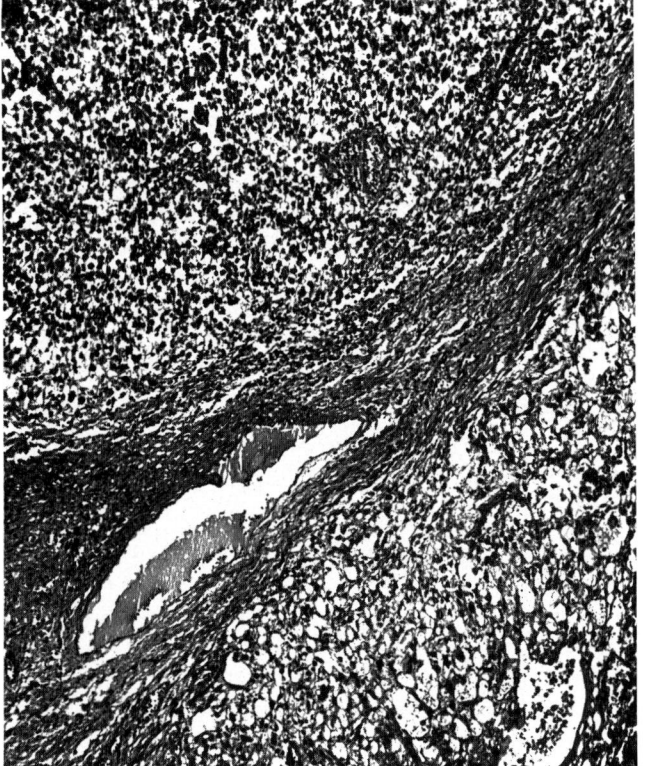

FIG. 20.12. Dysgerminoma admixed with yolk sac tumor. Note the fibrous septum separating the two elements.

and its marked radiosensitivity as compared with other malignant germ cell neoplasms, the malignant potential of dysgerminoma should not be minimized. Dysgerminoma is a rapidly growing neoplasm, but metastatic spread does not occur early in the course of the disease (although it is not possible to predict this in individual cases). When the tumor is small and freely mobile, its capsule is usually intact, but large tumors may be adherent to the surrounding structures or may rupture.[72,266] Rupture may occur either spontaneously or at operation. This leads to spillage of the tumor contents and peritoneal implantation, causing serious consequences.[72,266] Penetration of the ovarian surface by the tumor and formation of adhesions to surrounding structures may lead to direct extension by the tumor.

Metastatic spread occurs via the lymphatic system; the lymph nodes in the vicinity of the common iliac arteries and the terminal part of the abdominal aorta are first affected. Occasionally, there may be marked enlargement of these lymph nodes, with formation of large masses. Usually the enlargement is slight to moderate and can be detected by lymphangiography, computerized tomography (CT) scanning, or magnetic resonance imaging (MRI). In view of the superior results and fewer side effects with the last two methods, the use of lymphangiography, in this context, has been virtually abandoned in the developed countries. From the abdominal lymph nodes, the tumor spreads to the mediastinal and supraclavicular lymph nodes. Hematogenous spread to distant organs occurs later, and any organ may be affected, although involvement of the liver, lungs, and bones tends to be most common.* In cases of pure dysgerminoma, the metastases usually present a similar histological appearance to the primary tumor but, occasionally, tumors composed of pure dysgerminoma may be associated with metastases composed of other neoplastic germ cell elements. This metastatic pattern is observed much more commonly in combined tumors. It has been suggested that cellular tumors with small amounts of stroma, slight lymphocytic infiltration, and associated with cellular atypia and high mitotic activity tend to be more aggressive.[13,72] However, in view of the inconstancy of these findings—marked histological variations within the same tumor and its radiosensitivity—there is at present no good evidence that the behavior of an individual tumor can be assessed from its histological appearance.[85,266,331]

Recent studies describing therapeutic results failed to identify a group of patients with worse prognosis based on histology.[36,335] This does not apply to dysgerminomas admixed with other, more malignant germ cell elements; in these cases the outcome is less favorable.†

Dysgerminoma, like its testicular counterpart semi-

---

*Refs. 4,13,47,72,93,203,266.
†Refs. 44,72,90,148,159,166,232,266,331,354.

noma, is associated with elevated levels of serum lactic dehydrogenase (LDH) and its isoenzyme-1 (LDH-1). These substances can be used as tumor markers.[17,96,275,393] There is a good correlation between the volume of tumor tissue present and the serum levels of the enzymes.

It has been shown recently that patients with testicular seminoma have elevated levels of serum placental alkaline phosphatase (Regan isoenzyme) (PLAP), but so far serum PLAP has not come into use as a tumor marker.[168]

The prognosis of patients with pure dysgerminoma is now considered to be favorable. Although earlier reports indicated that the prognosis was poor and that the 5-year survival was only 27%,[87,203] more recent studies have reported a much better prognosis for pure dysgerminoma, with a 5-year survival of 75–90%.[*] At the same time, the 5-year survival of patients with unilateral encapsulated dysgerminoma has been reported in excess of 90%,[13,36,45,72,162,186,355] although patients who were treated by unilateral salpingo-oophorectomy had 18–52% recurrence rates. The recurrences were treated successfully with radiation therapy. The unfavorable prognostic parameters include presence of metastases at the time of diagnosis, presence of adhesions and spread into adjacent structures, bilaterality, and large size of the tumor.[†] It should be noted that none of these parameters is by itself considered to indicate a hopeless outcome, and many patients with these findings have been cured with radiotherapy. Some investigators consider patients younger than 20 years[45,72,195,232] as well as patients older than 40 years[45,195,232] to have a worse prognosis. Others[13,36,44,255] do not regard age as important in this connection.

There is general agreement that the presence of other neoplastic germ cell elements has an adverse effect on prognosis.[‡] Eighty percent of recurrences occur in the first 2 years after diagnosis,[232] and it has been reported that more than 75% occur in the first year.[45,72]

Treatment

Dysgerminoma, like its testicular counterpart the classic seminoma, is a highly radiosensitive tumor. Patients with bilateral or disseminated dysgerminoma, as well as patients with unilateral encapsulated tumors no longer desirous of having children, are treated by hysterectomy and bilateral salpingo-oophorectomy followed by radiation therapy to the abdominal and, in some centers, to the mediastinal lymph nodes.

For young women with unilateral encapsulated pure dysgerminoma, two different therapeutic approaches have

been advocated. One consists of unilateral oophorectomy, or salpingo-oophorectomy, wedge biopsy of the remaining ovary, and careful follow-up of the patient. The second approach advocates similar surgical therapy, but to decrease and prevent metastases and recurrences, radiotherapy is administered to the abdominal lymph nodes on the ipsilateral side while the remaining ovary is shielded. The advantages of the first approach are that fertility is preserved and there are no genetic hazards associated with administration of radiotherapy. There is evidence that the second approach tends to decrease the risk of metastases and recurrences,[36,45,162,331] but it is suggested by the advocates of conservative surgery without radiotherapy that this risk is not very serious, especially as the metastases or recurrence can be treated successfully by radiotherapy or combination chemotherapy when they develop.[4,13,47,72,104,186,278,335,354]

The conservative approach to the therapy of unilateral encapsulated dysgerminoma has been gaining wider acceptance over the years, and this approach is strongly recommended, but each individual case should be considered on its merits. It should be noted that before this mode of treatment can be considered, the opposite ovary must be normal, there should be no evidence of spread of the tumor in the abdominal cavity, and the abdominal and pelvic lymph nodes must be free from metastases on inspection, CT scanning, and lymphangiography. In addition, the patient must be chromatin positive and have a normal female 46XX karyotype.

In patients with widely disseminated metastases, administration of three to four cycles of combination chemotherapy comprising cis-diamino platinum, etopoxide (VP16), and bleomycin combination (BEP) has been successful in eradicating the disease.[104]

The treatment of patients with dysgerminoma occurring in dysgenetic gonads must be hysterectomy and bilateral salpingo-gonadectomy in view of the high risk of development of bilateral neoplasms in these patients and in view of the fact that the gonads are hormonally and functionally inactive (see Chapter 2, Abnormal Sexual Development). Therefore, determination of the karyotype of all patients with dysgerminoma, especially those with evidence of virilization or developmental and menstrual abnormalities, is strongly recommended. This is important in prepubertal patients, for in these patients other signs of abnormal function, such as primary amenorrhea, virilization, and absence of normal sexual development, are lacking. In patients who are sexually and genetically abnormal, the excision of the tumor is not associated with reversion to a normal state, and substitution hormonal therapy must be administered. Adequate treatment in these cases prevents development of a tumor in the opposite gonad or leads to the removal of a clinically inapparent lesion that may subsequently prove lethal.[97]

---

[*]Refs. 4,13,26,44,45,117,162,186,354,355.
[†]Refs. 44,45,72,117,162,232,331.
[‡]Refs 13,36,44,232,266,267,331,354.

Yolk Sac Tumor

GENERAL FEATURES

Histogenesis

Yolk sac tumor is a malignant germ cell neoplasm that is thought to arise from the undifferentiated and multipotential embryonal carcinoma by selective differentiation toward yolk sac or vitelline structures, in the same way as nongestational choriocarcinoma differentiates toward trophoblastic structures. The recognition and classification of yolk sac (endodermal sinus) tumor as a specific entity stems from the studies of Teilum, stretching over nearly three decades.[340,341,343,346] The concepts regarding the histogenesis of this neoplasm that he proposed have been supported by the experimental studies of the neoplastic rodent yolk sac by Pierce et al.[239,241,242,244]

In 1939 Schiller[272] described an ovarian neoplasm composed of clear and hobnail cells with a pattern that he designated a *mesonephroma* because of the presence of structures resembling immature glomeruli. Other investigators[152] were unable to demonstrate the mesonephric origin of this tumor and considered it an endothelioma of the ovary as suggested earlier.[274] In 1946, Teilum[340] demonstrated that the tumor described as mesonephroma[272,273] included two distinct neoplasms with different histogenesis, histological pattern, age distribution, and clinical behavior.[239,241,242,244] One of these tumors was highly malignant, occurred in young patients, was homologous with certain testicular neoplasms, and was of germ cell origin.[340] The other tumor was less aggressive, occurred in older women, and ultimately was shown by Scully to be of Müllerian-type origin. He designated this neoplasm *clear cell carcinoma.*[279]

In addition to the terms *mesonephroma*[77,272,273] and *endothelioma*,[152,274] yolk sac tumors have been designated as *embryonal carcinoma*[2,206] because of certain similarities to the embryonal carcinoma of the testis.[76] Although embryonal carcinoma showing the histological pattern resembling the typical embryonal carcinoma of the testis[76] is seen occasionally in ovarian tumors,[165] most ovarian tumors of this type show a distinctive pattern with differentiation toward yolk sac or vitelline structures[134,136,343,344,346] and should be termed *yolk sac tumor* or *endodermal sinus tumor.* These tumors differ from the undifferentiated embryonal carcinoma,[76] although they resemble closely the yolk sac tumor of both infantile[44,242,346] and adult testes.° It is now generally accepted that the term *embryonal carcinoma* should be used only to designate ovarian neoplasms showing the typical histological pattern of the embryonal carcinoma as described in testicular tumors.[76,165] It is notable that most true ovarian embryonal carcinomas

Table 20.2. Serum AFP in patients with ovarian germ cell tumors measured by radioimmunoassay[a]

	No. of cases	Serum AFP
Mixed germ cell tumors containing EST	39	Elevated
Pure EST	23	Elevated
Pure dysgerminoma	25	Normal
Dysgerminoma with syncytiotrophoblastic giant cells	4	Normal
Teratoma (immature and mature)	12	Normal
Teratoma (immature and mature) with dysgerminoma	8	Normal
Mature cystic teratoma (dermoid cyst)	15	Normal

[a] Unpublished data.
AFP, alpha-fetoprotein; EST, endodermal sinus tumor.

are combined with yolk sac tumor. The not infrequent combination of yolk sac tumor elements in ovarian tumors with other neoplastic germ cell elements° is one of the arguments in favor of the germ cell origin of this neoplasm. Yolk sac tumor, either pure or combined with other neoplastic germ cell elements, has been encountered in extragonadal locations where germ cell tumors are known to occur, in the mediastinum,[135,212,328,338,346] the sacrococcygeal region,[53,135,138,251,346] the pineal gland,[6,33,346] and the vagina.[138,346,369]

Alpha-fetoprotein (AFP), an alpha$_1$-globulin, was first identified as a specific constituent of normal human fetal serum by Bergstrand and Czar[31] in 1956. In the human embryo, serum AFP peaks at approximately 3000 mg/l at about 12 to 13 weeks of gestation. The level then decreases slowly until birth, when it is approximately 55 mg/l. After birth, AFP disappears rapidly from the serum, and 3 weeks after full-term delivery, it can be detected only in very small amounts (0–15 ng/ml) by radioimmunoassay or sensitive-enzyme immunoassays.

The sites of AFP synthesis in the human fetus and in other mammalian species have been studied by Gitlin et al.,[108–110] who demonstrated that during fetal life AFP is produced by the yolk sac, liver, and upper gastrointestinal tract. They also demonstrated that AFP synthesis commences in the yolk sac. In recent years there has been considerable interest in the histological aspects of germ cell neoplasms associated with elevated serum AFP, and it has been demonstrated that germ cell tumors in patients with elevated serum AFP either are composed entirely of or contain yolk sac tumor elements.† Table 20.2 shows the results of preoperative serum AFP determinations in patients with ovarian germ cell tumors. Elevation of serum AFP has not been observed in patients with pure

---

° Refs. 242,316,343,344,346,388.

° Refs. 34,44,134,148,166,206,267,328,329,346.
† Refs. 20,21,88,138,172,212,286,328–330,346,377.

dysgerminoma or seminoma of the testis,[296,322,328–330,346] mature cystic teratoma of the ovary,[20,322,330] immature teratoma of the ovary or testes, or pure gonadoblastoma.[322,328,330]

Although occasional Sertoli–Leydig cell tumors, especially those showing a retiform pattern,[319,389] may be associated with elevated levels of serum AFP,[55,319,323] this has not been observed in patients with other ovarian or testicular tumors that are not of germ cell origin.[322,328,330] Slightly elevated levels of serum AFP up to 60 ng/ml (upper limit of normal serum AFP, 20 ng/ml) have been observed in some cases of embryonal carcinoma of the testis.[328,330] Using immunofluorescent and immunoperoxidase techniques, AFP has been identified in the cells of yolk sac tumor and in the eosinophilic, PAS-positive, diastase-resistant globules present both inside and outside the tumor cells.[138,164,292,347] Large amounts of AFP have been extracted from tumor tissue in yolk sac tumors of the ovary and testis.[329,347,377] The results of these studies indicate that yolk sac tumor elements are associated with AFP synthesis. In view of the fact that normal yolk sac in the human and other mammalian species has been shown to be associated with AFP synthesis[110], it is reasonable to assume that the selective synthesis of AFP by yolk sac tumors provides further support to the view that yolk sac tumor develops as a result of differentiation of primitive malignant germ cell elements in the direction of yolk sac or vitelline structures.[138,164,322,330,348] The immunocytochemical localization of AFP in embryonal carcinoma and in areas of yolk sac tumor showing no morphologic evidence of yolk sac differentiation suggests that the biochemical manifestations of yolk sac differentiation, like AFP synthesis, precede morphologic differentiation.[141,165]

Prevalence

Although originally yolk sac tumor was considered very rare, it is being diagnosed with much greater frequency nowadays and is the second most common malignant ovarian germ cell neoplasm after dysgerminoma. Yolk sac tumor often occurs in pure form, but it is also a frequent component of mixed malignant germ cell tumors. More than 350 cases have been reported.[89,102,147,148,164,329] It is one of the most common malignant ovarian neoplasms of childhood, adolescence, and early adult life.

Although most reports deal with Caucasians, yolk sac tumor has been encountered in other races.* The reported age distribution of patients with yolk sac tumor ranges from 16 months[134] to 46 years,[138] but most patients have been under 30 years of age.† Yolk sac tumor is encoun-

tered most frequently in the second and third decades, followed by first and fourth, and is rare in women in the fifth decade. Yolk sac tumor of the ovary has been encountered in two postmenopausal patients, aged 57[46] and 67 years.[283] These cases are considered exceptional. Two cases of ovarian surface epithelial–stromal tumor associated with yolk sac tumor occurring in elderly patients have also been reported,[107,261] and another well-documented case is known to the author. Although the histogenesis of the yolk sac component of such tumors is uncertain, the likely explanation is that it originates from the surface epithelium by a process of neoplastic differentiation or transformation and therefore the histogenesis is totally different from that of germ cell neoplasms.[107,261]

CLINICAL FEATURES

The symptomatology is nonspecific. Most patients have symptoms of abdominal enlargement and pain and present with a lower abdominal or pelvic mass.* Occasionally, the symptoms are acute and severe and may lead to the diagnosis of acute appendicitis or a ruptured ectopic pregnancy.[27,147,148,164,206,267] This usually is caused by torsion of the tumor.[134,206,267] A number of cases have been encountered during pregnancy.[43,134,147,148,164,206] The presence of yolk sac tumor is not associated with endocrine symptoms,[44,134,206,267] although endocrine symptoms may be present if the tumor is combined with choriocarcinoma.[90,164,267] Such neoplasms are classified as mixed germ cell tumors. On clinical examination, a tumor mass is usually palpable and is frequently of considerable size.† Increased levels of AFP are found in sera of patients with yolk sac tumor,‡ and this is considered a useful diagnostic test for the presence of yolk sac tumor elements in the primary tumor, its metastases, and recurrences.

GROSS FINDINGS

Yolk sac tumors are almost always unilateral.§ Bilaterality typically is a manifestation of metastatic spread. Yolk sac tumor shows a certain predilection for the right ovary.[44,134,164,206,267] The tumor is usually large, varying in size from 3 to 30 cm in diameter, with most tumors measuring more than 10 cm.‖ It frequently weighs more than 500 g; tumors weighing 5 kg have been recorded.[147] The tumors are usually encapsulated round, oval, or globular; firm, smooth, or somewhat lobulated; and gray-yellow,

---

*Refs. 102,134,148,166,172,206.
†Refs. 102,134,148,166,206,267,328,346.

---

*Refs. 44,102,134,147,166,206,267.
†Refs. 27,44,102,134,147,148,164,206,267,329.
‡Refs. 20,21,102,138,212,286,329,348,377.
§Refs. 44,102,134,147,148,164,206,267,286,329,346.
‖Refs. 27,44,102,134,147,148,164,206,267,329.

with areas of hemorrhage and cystic or gelatinous changes (Fig. 20.13). The tumor may form adhesions to the surrounding structures and invade them. On sectioning, yolk sac tumors are mainly solid, but cystic spaces frequently are present. The fluid present in the cysts also may be gelatinous. Necrosis and hemorrhage and the presence of other neoplastic germ cell elements, especially teratoma, may alter the appearance of the tumor.

MICROSCOPIC FINDINGS

Yolk sac tumors exhibit a wide range of histological patterns that differ considerably from each other and, although all the different patterns are frequently observed in the same tumor, one or two may predominate. The following histological patterns may be observed in yolk sac tumor: (1) microcystic, (2) endodermal sinus, (3) solid, (4) alveolar–glandular, (5) polyvesicular vitelline, (6) myxomatous, (7) papillary, (8) macrocystic, (9) hepatoid, and (10) glandular or primitive endodermal (intestinal).

The polyvesicular vitelline, the hepatoid, and the primitive endodermal (intestinal) elements tend to occur in pure form, unassociated with other yolk sac tumor elements forming a yolk sac tumor exhibiting a single histological pattern. Although such tumors are rare, they pose considerable diagnostic difficulties. Because of this they have been classified as specific subtypes of yolk sac tumor in the revised WHO classification of ovarian neoplasms[284] (Table 20.1).

The first five histological patterns were described by Teilum[344,346] and were considered by him as the principal microscopic patterns of yolk sac tumor.

Microcystic (Fig. 20.14) and myxomatous (Fig. 20.15) patterns are composed of a loose vacuolated network with small cystic spaces or microcysts forming a honeycomb

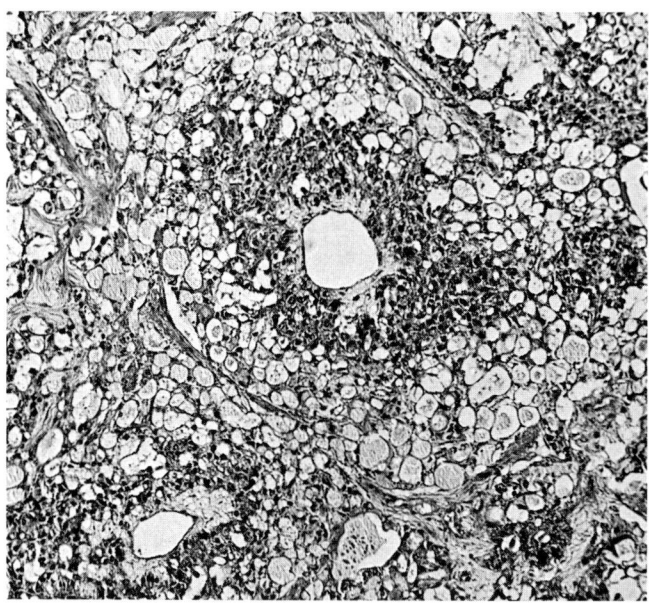

FIG. 20.14. Yolk sac tumor, microcystic pattern. A labyrinthine structure composed of tumor cells radiating around a blood vessel resembling a perivascular formation is seen in the *center*.

pattern. The microcysts are lined by flat, pleomorphic, mesothelial-like cells with large hyperchromatic or vesicular nuclei that show brisk mitotic activity. There is usually some variation in the size of the cysts (Fig. 20.14). In the underlying capillary spaces, hematopoiesis may be seen. The vacuolated network may contain pale, PAS-positive, mucinous material, forming small lakes or precipitates as

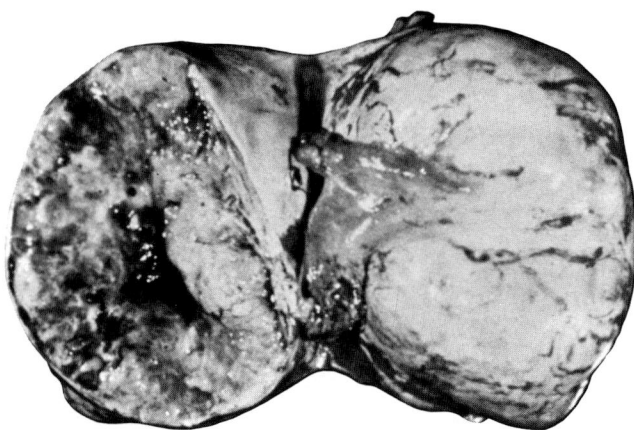

FIG. 20.13. Yolk sac tumor. It is oval shaped, encapsulated, with a central area of cystic degeneration. (Courtesy of R. Scully, M.D., Boston, MA.)

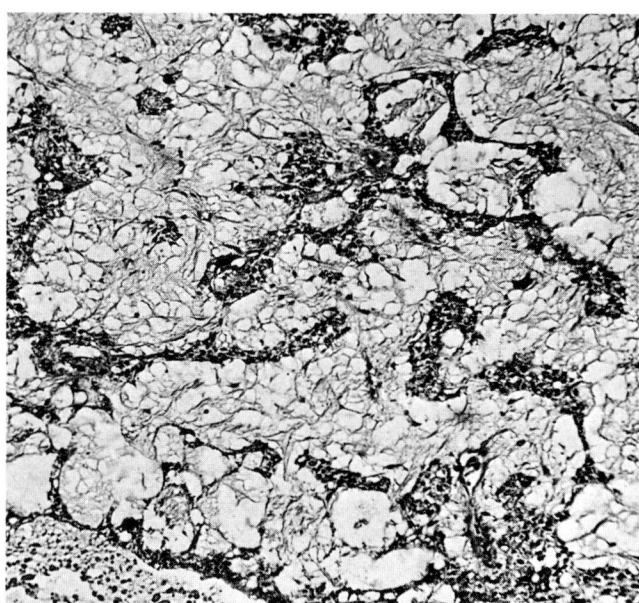

FIG. 20.15. Yolk sac tumor, myxomatous pattern. Small collections of epithelial-like cells forming strands or gland-like structures are seen within myxomatous tissue.

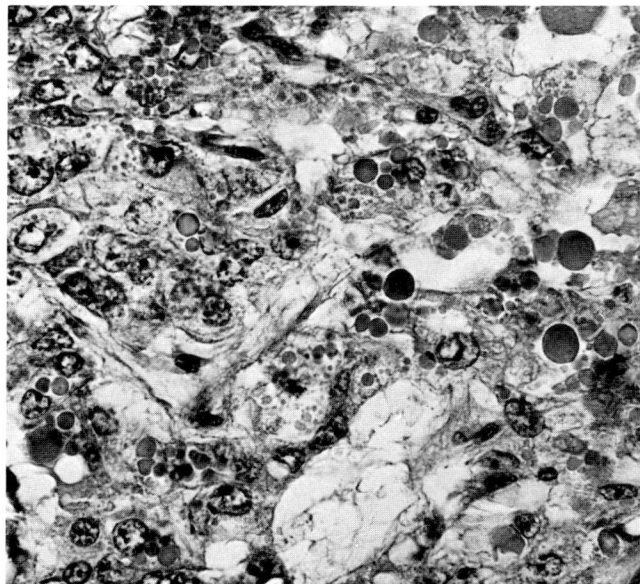

FIG. 20.16. Yolk sac tumor. Numerous round hyaline globules are present both inside and outside the cells. Larger precipitates of this material are seen at the *upper right*.

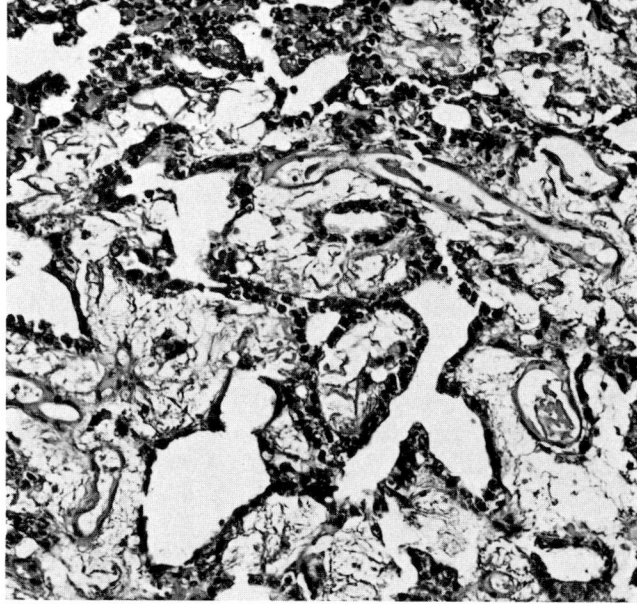

FIG. 20.18. Endodermal sinus tumor, myxomatous pattern. Numerous cavities and channels are present. Note hyaline material at *top left*.

well as small, round, brightly eosinophilic, PAS-positive, diastase-resistant globules or droplets. These globules are also found within the cytoplasm of the tumor cells (Fig. 20.16). Areas composed of fine, loose myxomatous tissue containing alveolar spaces (Fig. 20.17), occasional gland-

like structures lined by cuboidal epithelium (Fig. 20.18), and small cellular aggregates, often merging with the microcystic or other patterns, are also present (Fig. 20.19). The loose myxomatous pattern was considered to be analogous to the magma reticulare or the extraembryonic me-

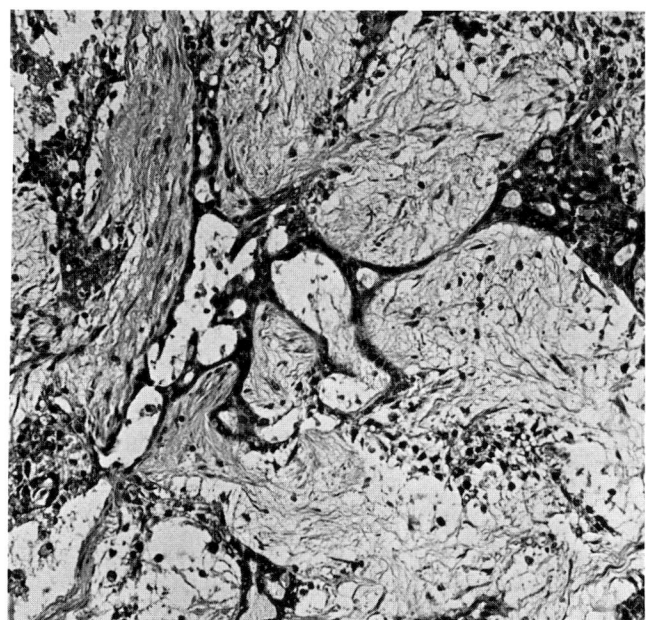

FIG. 20.17. Yolk sac tumor. The tumor is composed of myxomatous tissue containing glandular and alveolar spaces and channels.

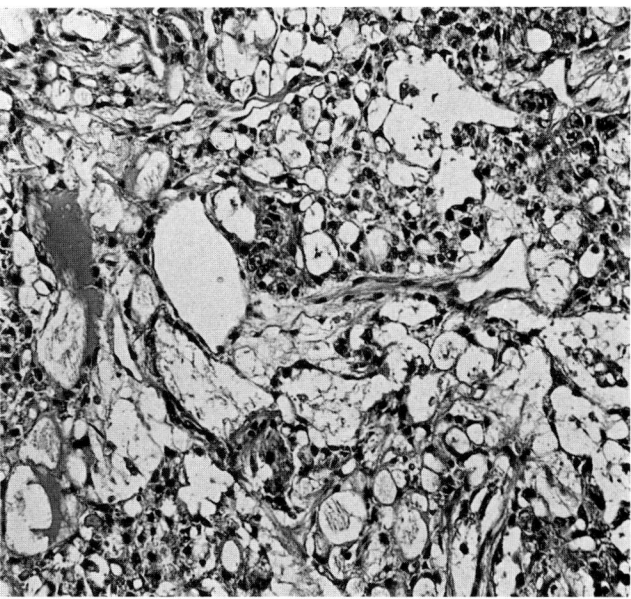

FIG. 20.19. Yolk sac tumor. Small cellular aggregates, microcysts, and myxomatous tissue are present. Mucinous material also is seen.

soderm of the exocoelom,[348] and the presence of this pattern led to the recognition of the mesoblastic nature of this tumor.[341] These two histological patterns should be considered as separate principal patterns.

Endodermal sinus pattern (Fig. 20.20) is composed of perivascular formations, consisting of a narrow band of connective tissue with a capillary blood vessel in the center and lined by a layer of cuboidal or low columnar embryonal epithelial-like cells. The cells have large, slightly vesicular nuclei, prominent nucleoli, and show mitotic activity. The surrounding capsular sinusoid space is lined by a single layer of flat cells with prominent hyperchromatic nuclei. These characteristic perivascular formations are said to recapitulate the so-called endodermal sinuses[343,344,346] that, although not conspicuous in the human placenta, are well-defined embryologic structures in the rat placenta.[78] These structures are also known as sinuses of Duval, Schiller–Duval bodies,[134,242] or glomerulus-like structures and resemble superficially immature renal glomeruli. When sectioned longitudinally, the perivascular structures consist of a central connective tissue core containing a longitudinal vessel surrounded by epithelial-like cells that often form small papillary formations projecting into the surrounding capsular sinusoid space. The presence of these perivascular formations or Schiller–Duval bodies can be considered diagnostic of yolk sac tumor, but in some tumors they may be poorly represented, somewhat atypical, or absent. Although the tumor should always be examined carefully and searched to identify these structures,

their absence does not preclude the diagnosis, if the appearances of the tumor are typical in all other respects. Apart from the presence of the perivascular structures, this pattern consists of a complicated labyrinth of communicating cavities and channels. In addition, there are papillary processes and blood vessels surrounded by narrow connective tissue cores and epithelial-like cells radiating into the surrounding stroma, resembling the typical perivascular formations but differing from them by the absence of the sinusoid space[346] (Fig. 20.14).

Solid pattern (Fig. 20.21) is composed of aggregates of small epithelial-like polygonal cells with clear cytoplasm and large vesicular or pyknotic nuclei with prominent nucleoli and exhibits brisk mitotic activity. The tumor cells in the solid aggregate may resemble dysgerminoma cells, but they usually show greater cellular and nuclear pleomorphism and presence of at least occasional microcysts (Fig. 20.21). The presence of the latter helps to differentiate between these two entities. The presence of other patterns of yolk sac tumor is also helpful in this respect, as is diffuse or focal staining for AFP and uniformly positive staining for cytokeratin (Fig. 20.22), which are observed in yolk sac tumor and not in dysgerminoma.

Alveolar-glandular pattern (Figs. 20.18, 20.23) is composed of alveolar, gland-like, or larger cystic spaces and cavities lined by flat or cuboidal epithelial-like cells with large, prominent nuclei and surrounded by myxomatous stroma or cellular aggregates. Some of these spaces may be lined by more than one layer of cells and sometimes the

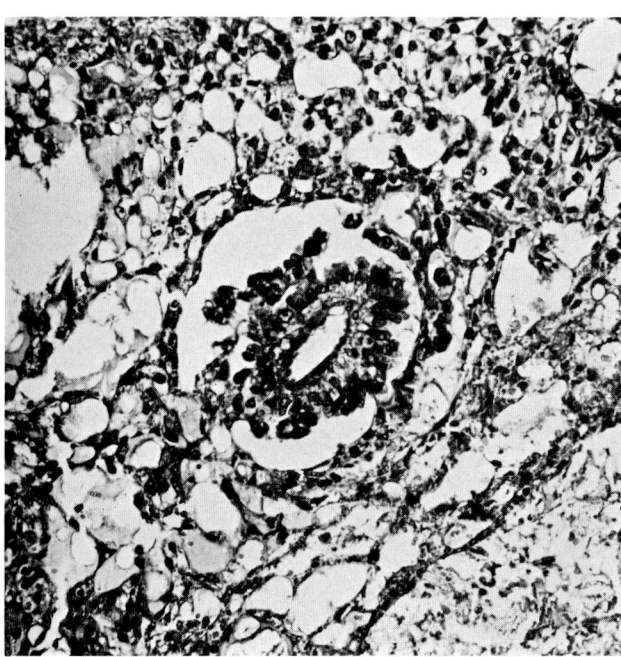

FIG. 20.20. Yolk sac tumor. A typical perivascular formation (Schiller–Duval body) is illustrated.

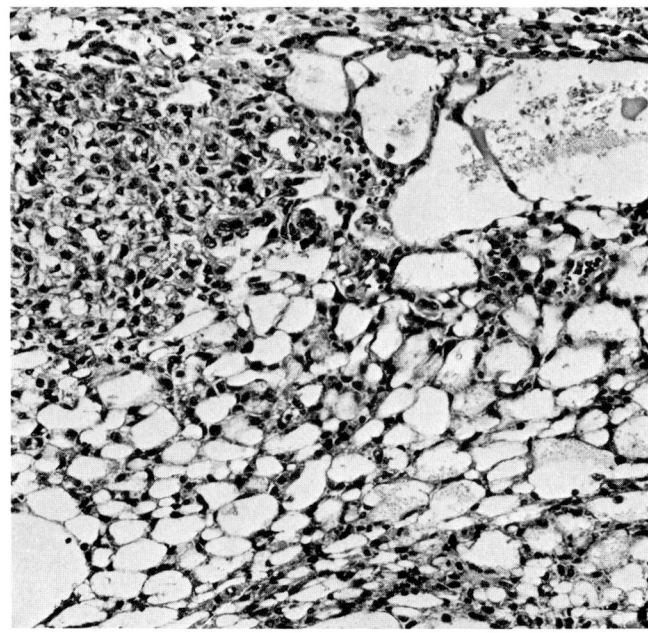

FIG. 20.21. Yolk sac tumor, solid and microcystic patterns. Some larger cysts (macrocysts) are seen at *top right*.

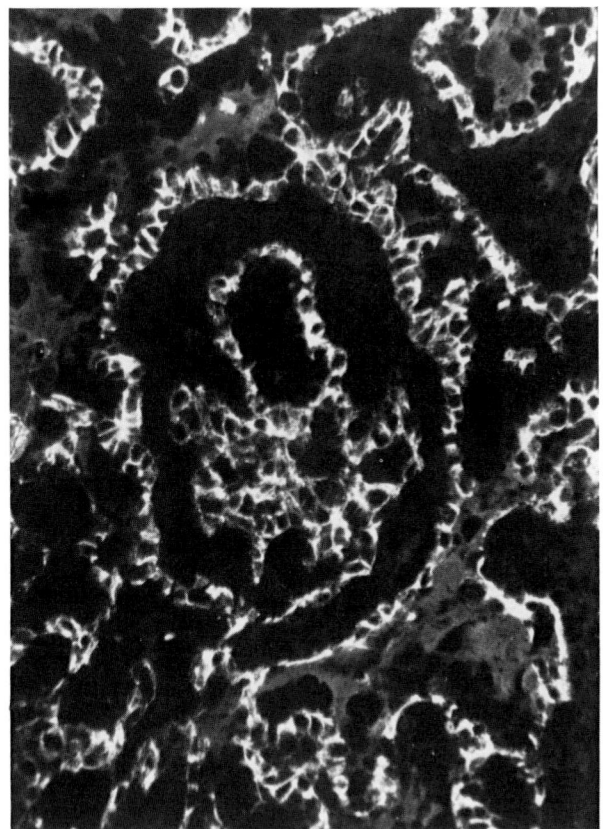

FIG. 20.22. Yolk sac tumor stained for low molecular weight cytokeratin. Note the uniformly positive staining of all the tumor cells. The intervening connective tissue cells are unstained.

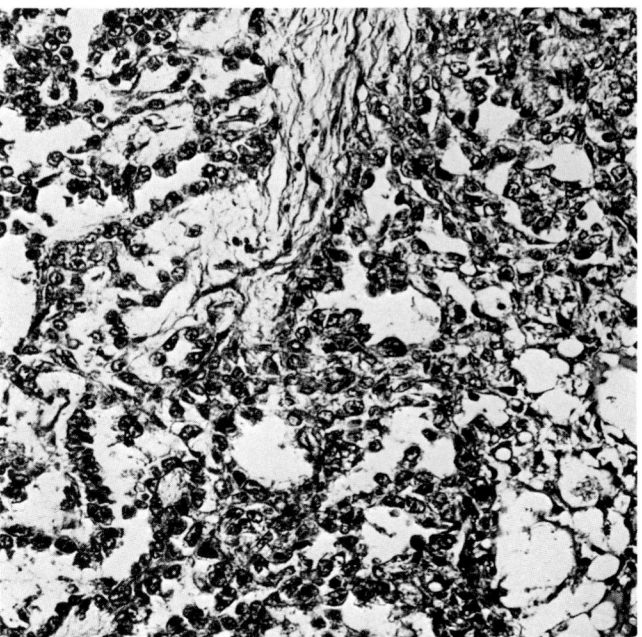

FIG. 20.23. Yolk sac tumor, glandular alveolar pattern. Note the alveoli lined by epithelial-like cells (*left and center*).

within the tumor cells or outside them; they may be numerous and prominent in some tumors (Fig. 20.16). The droplets may be observed in tumors exhibiting all the histological patterns described above, and their identification is a helpful diagnostic feature. However, their presence is not diagnostic of yolk sac tumor because they are observed

lining cells form small papillary projections protruding into the lumen. The layer of cells lining these spaces may be continuous with the lining of the perivascular sinusoid spaces.[343] Gland-like formations lined by columnar or cuboidal epithelial-like cells may be seen and in some tumors may be prominent and may form bizarre patterns (Fig. 20.18).

Polyvesicular vitelline pattern[209,344–346] is composed of numerous cysts or vesicles surrounded by compact connective tissue stroma (Figs. 20.24, 20.25). The vesicles are lined partly by columnar or cuboidal epithelial cells, frequently showing basal or paraluminal vacuolation, and partly by flat mesothelial-like cells (Fig. 20.25). The individual vesicles or cysts vary in size and shape. The wall of the cyst may show a constriction dividing the part lined by the mesothelial cells from that lined by the columnar or cuboidal epithelium (Fig. 20.25). This was considered to reflect the embryologic conversion of the primary yolk sac into the secondary yolk sac.[344–346] Occasionally, the whole tumor may exhibit the polyvesicular vitelline pattern; such tumors have been designated as *polyvesicular vitelline tumors*.[209,344–346]

The eosinophilic, hyaline droplets may be present either

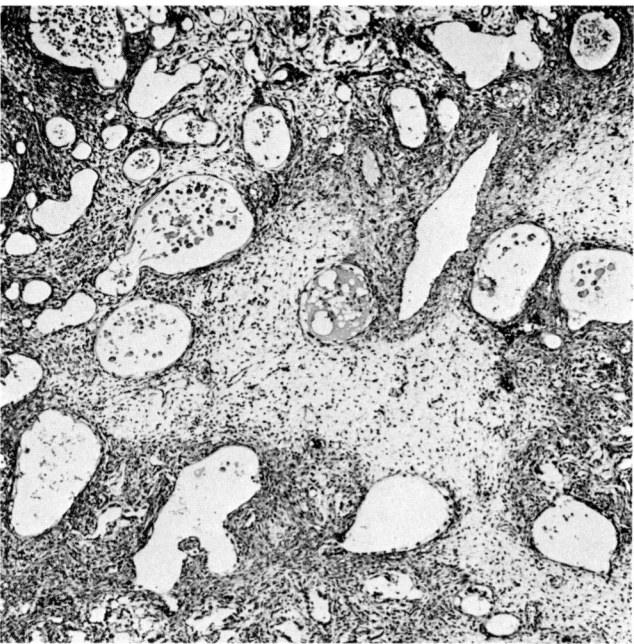

FIG. 20.24. Yolk sac tumor, polyvesicular vitelline pattern. The tumor is composed of numerous small vesicles surrounded by connective tissue.

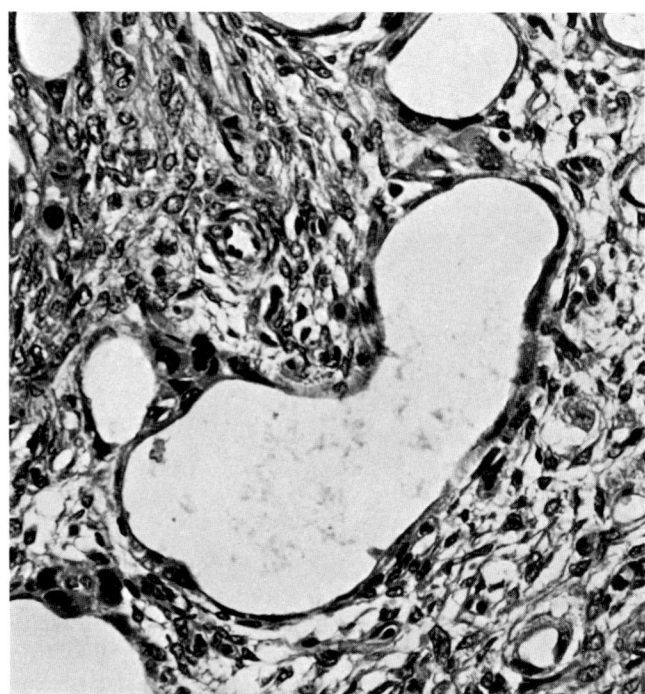

FIG. 20.25. Yolk sac tumor, polyvesicular vitelline pattern.
A typical vesicle surrounded by cellular stroma is shown.

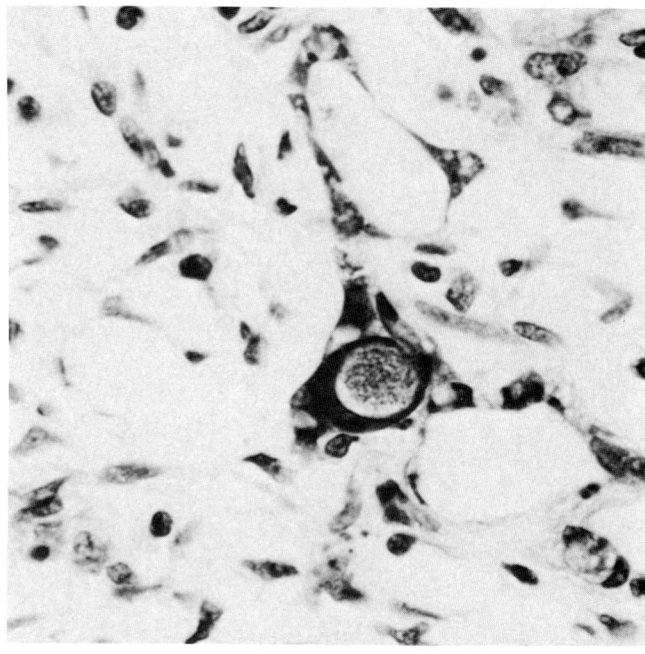

FIG. 20.26. Yolk sac tumor stained for AFP. The AFP forms a granular deposit within the cytoplasm of the large tumor cell (*center*).

in many malignant, often poorly differentiated neoplasms. The droplets are considered to be secreted by the tumor cells and accumulate within the cytoplasm. As the amount of secretion increases, the cell becomes distended and ruptures, discharging its contents into the surrounding tissue. Recently, the significance of these globules in yolk sac tumor has been enhanced further by demonstrating with immunofluorescent and immunoperoxidase techniques that some contain AFP[138,164,292,347] (Fig. 20.26). Other globules may contain alpha1-antitrypsin and other plasma proteins, such as transferrin.[224,292,360] The presence of hyaline, PAS-positive material forming bands or connective tissue cores surrounded by tumor cells is not an infrequent finding in yolk sac tumor; in some tumors, it may be a prominent feature, with the tumor cells resting on and surrounding the bands of hyaline material (Fig. 20.27). There may be an increased amount of the eosinophilic, PAS-positive globules described above in the vicinity of the hyaline bands, suggesting a relationship between them and a possibility of common origin.[344,346] The hyaline, PAS-positive material in yolk sac tumor has been found to be similar to the hyaline material produced by mouse teratocarcinoma during its conversion to the ascitic form, and this is considered to be a strong argument in favor of the yolk sac origin of the tumor.[238,239,242,244] The cells of yolk sac tumor, when examined with the electron microscope, resemble those of the normal human yolk sac.[115,138,209,210,346]

In addition to the five histological patterns described

above, five additional patterns merit consideration as specific patterns.

Myxomatous pattern (Fig. 20.15), which Teilum[344–346] combined with the microcystic, may be observed on its own or may predominate.

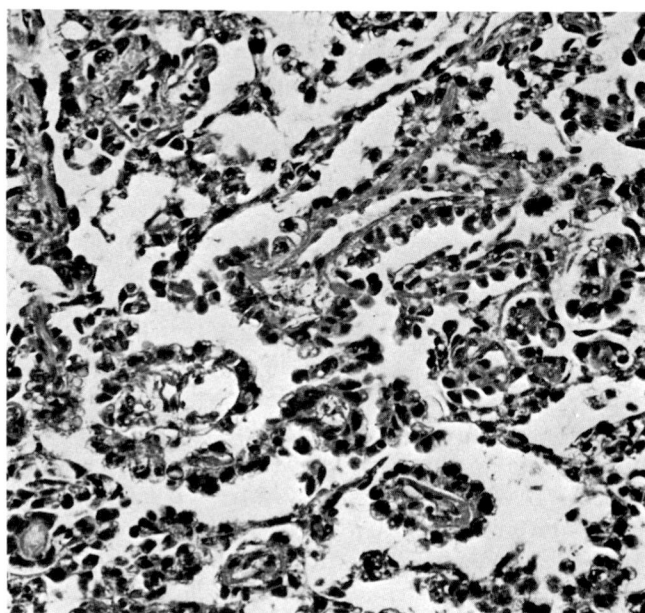

FIG. 20.27. Yolk sac tumor, papillary pattern. The papillae are composed of hyaline material lined by tumor cells.

Papillary pattern (Fig. 20.27) is composed of papillary structures consisting of connective tissue cores lined by epithelial-like cells showing a considerable degree of cellular and nuclear pleomorphism and mitotic activity. The connective tissue may show extensive hyalinization. This pattern may be the predominant pattern within a tumor.

Macrocystic pattern is observed when yolk sac tumor exhibits larger cysts in contrast to microcysts or alveolar spaces. In some tumors, this pattern may predominate.

Hepatoid pattern is composed of cells with eosinophilic, uniform, or granular cytoplasm, showing a solid pattern and considerable resemblance to hepatocytes. This pattern was considered by Teilum[344-346] as a variant of the solid pattern. Although such collections of hepatocyte-like cells are not infrequently observed in yolk sac tumors, tumors composed entirely or predominantly of such cells have been designated as *hepatoid yolk sac tumors*[246] or *yolk sac tumors with hepatoid pattern* (Fig. 20.28). These tumors are admixed only infrequently with other histological patterns of yolk sac tumor or other neoplastic germ cell elements, and this, together with the rarity of the tumor, may cause diagnostic problems. The presence of a solid ovarian tumor composed of hepatocyte-like cells surrounded by connective tissue and forming solid aggregates, cords, or clusters and associated with elevated serum AFP in a young patient would strongly favor a diagnosis of yolk sac tumor with a hepatoid pattern.

Grandular or primitive endodermal (intestinal) pattern, in which the tumor is composed entirely of primitive endodermal glands, is encountered occasionally[58,59] (Fig. 20.29). This pattern has been designated as *glandular (intestinal) yolk sac tumor.* The tumor in these cases is composed of nests or collections of primitive endodermal glands surrounded by connective tissue, which varies from loose and edematous to dense and hyalinized. The degree of differentiation varies from primitive to relatively well differentiated. The glands may contain inspissated secretion within the lumen, and the tumor may resemble a mucin-secreting adenocarcinoma. Ultrastructurally, the nuclei are large and show prominent nucleolonema, whereas the cytoplasm contains many ribosomes, rough endoplasmic reticulum, and mitochondria. Dense amorphous intracellular material is also present. Yolk sac tumors showing this pattern have been associated with very high levels of serum AFP.[59] The presence of primitive endodermal glandular tissue, lobular or nest-like pattern, and high levels of serum AFP differentiate this type of yolk sac tumor from mucinous tumors of the ovary. A variant of this pattern composed of primitive glands of various sizes lined by tall columnar or cuboid cells with clear cytoplasm re-

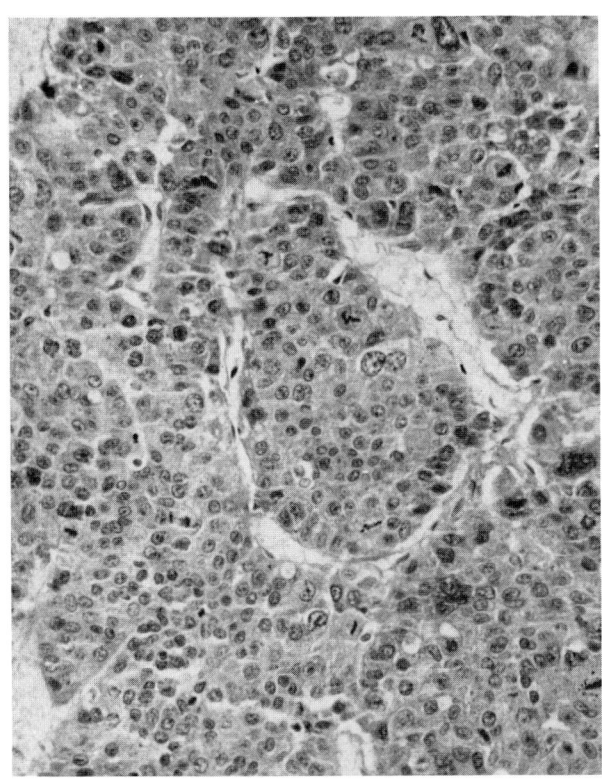

Fig. 20.28. Yolk sac tumor, hepatoid pattern. The tumor is composed of solid aggregates or cords of polygonal cells with even or granular eosinophilic cytoplasm resembling hepatocytes. Note the brisk mitotic activity.

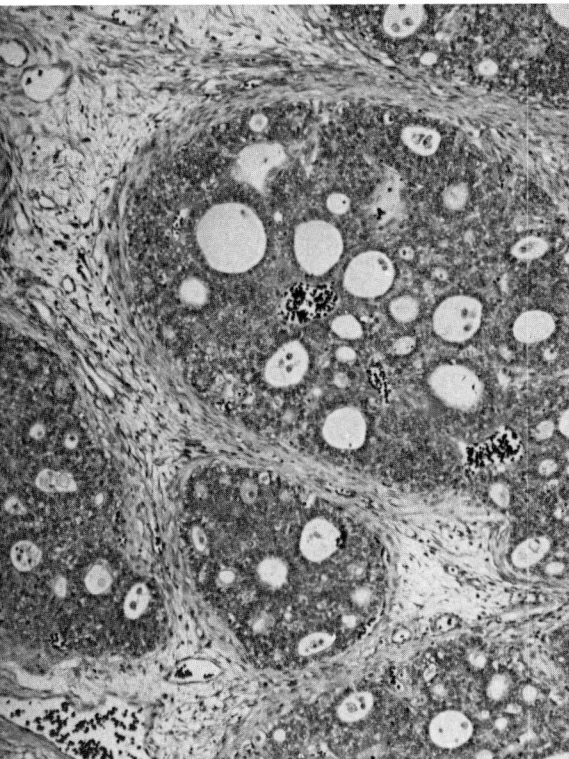

Fig. 20.29. Yolk sac tumor, the endodermal (intestinal) pattern. The tumor is composed of nests of primitive endodermal cells forming glands or solid aggregates, which are surrounded by connective tissue.

sembling secretory endometrial carcinoma, so-called endometrioid variant, has been described.[56]

DIFFERENTIAL DIAGNOSIS

Before it was recognized as a specific entity, yolk sac tumor was included with neoplasms composed of clear or parvilocular cells in the group of neoplasms of the ovary designated as mesonephroma,[272,273] or it was grouped together with embryonal carcinoma of the ovary.[2,44,206] It is with these two histogenetically different neoplasms that the yolk sac tumor may be confused. The clear cell tumors of the ovary show much more regular tubular patterns, lack the honeycomb network composed of microcysts, and have papillary frond-like projections that are often lined by clear or hobnail cells. The typical perivascular formations, endodermal sinuses, or Schiller–Duval bodies present in yolk sac tumor are absent. The epithelial cells lining the tubules are cuboidal with clear cytoplasm or are hobnail with nuclei bulging into the lumen. Areas composed of large polygonal cells with clear cytoplasm and small, dark, uniform, centrally situated nuclei resembling those of renal carcinoma are present. Since these cells line cystic spaces, they frequently proliferate in a papillary fashion or form solid aggregates. When the clear cell carcinoma is composed entirely of tubules or spaces, confusion may arise with the polyvesicular vitelline pattern. However, the epithelial lining is usually composed of the projecting hobnail cells and not of the two types of epithelia seen in the vesicles forming the polyvesicular vitelline pattern. The cystic spaces are more tubular and less vesicle-like. The clear cell tumors occur also in other parts of the female genital tract and usually occur in older patients.[206,218,346]

The embryonal carcinoma, which is uncommon in the ovary,° lacks the specific patterns observed in the yolk sac tumor. In its undifferentiated form, it is composed of aggregates of primitive embryonal cells. The tumor cells are frequently larger than those seen in the solid cellular aggregates in yolk sac tumor. The cytoplasm is more granular, there is more marked cellular and nuclear pleomorphism, and the nucleoli are more prominent. Even when the tumor is somewhat better differentiated, with the embryonal cells forming cords, tubules, or papillae and lining clefts or spaces, it still lacks the typical patterns associated with yolk sac tumor.

The cells of yolk sac tumor are uniformly cytokeratin positive[200,201] (Fig. 20.22). The presence of this feature as well as positive staining for AFP differentiates between yolk sac tumor showing solid pattern and dysgerminoma, with which it may be confused and which shows only occasional cytokeratin-positive cells. The cells of dysgerminoma are usually more uniform, lack microcysts, and are usually associated with lymphocytic and granulomatous reactions.

Yolk sac tumor, because of its cystic pattern and presence of numerous small blood vessels, has been confused with vascular tumors, but careful examination reveals that the pattern is more cystic and the absence of a true vascular pattern is confirmed by reticulum stains. It should be pointed out in this context that yolk sac tumor elements are sometimes intimately associated with immature vascular tissue in some mixed germ cell tumors and this may also contribute to the diagnostic problems. The presence of positive immunocytochemical staining for vimentin and for Factor VIII further confirms the presence of vascular tissue, whereas positive staining for cytokeratin (Fig. 20.22) favors yolk sac tumor.

Confusion may arise occasionally, with some Sertoli–Leydig cell tumors showing a retiform pattern.[319,389] The presence of more marked cellular and nuclear pleomorphism, brisk mitotic activity, the presence of other histological patterns observed in yolk sac tumor, and their absence in Sertoli–Leydig cell tumors aid in the differential diagnosis.

Occasionally confusion may arise with juvenile granulosa cell tumor when it presents with small vesicle-like collections of cells surrounded by connective tissue stroma that simulate the vesicles seen in polyvesicular vitelline yolk sac tumor. Presence of solid nests typical of juvenile granulosa cell tumor, absence of the various patterns of yolk sac tumor, and absence of immunocytochemical staining for AFP and a lack of elevated levels of serum AFP indicate that the tumor is a juvenile granulosa cell tumor.

CLINICAL BEHAVIOR

Yolk sac tumor of the ovary is a highly malignant neoplasm, metastasizing early and invading the surrounding structures and organs. Local invasion and intracoelomic spread frequently lead to extensive involvement of the abdominal cavity by tumor deposits. Yolk sac tumor metastasizes first via the lymphatic system to the para-aortic and common iliac lymph nodes and then to the mediastinal and supraclavicular lymph nodes. Hematogenous spread occurs later, with metastases found in the lungs, liver, and other organs. The tumor is aggressive locally, and spread beyond the ovary is observed in a number of patients at the time of operation.° Recurrences in the pelvis are frequent, even when the tumor and the affected adnexa have been excised completely.[134,147,164,206,329] They usually appear within a few weeks or months after excision of the primary tumor.

°Refs. 134,165,206,278,329,343–346.

°Refs. 44,102,147,148,164,206,278,329,346.

TREATMENT

Until recently, the treatment of patients with yolk sac tumor was disappointing. The treatment was primarily surgical,[°] since yolk sac tumor is not sensitive to radiation therapy.[27,267] Extensive surgery is not justified, since it does not improve prognosis.[134,147,164] The small number of long-term survivors treated this way in the past were mainly patients with tumors confined to the ovary, most of whom were treated by unilateral adnexectomy.[†] In recent years there has been marked improvement in prognosis with conservative surgery (unilateral salpingo-oophorectomy) and adjuvant multiagent combination chemotherapy.[‡] The combination chemotherapy originally used was dactinomycin, vincristine, and cyclophosphamide[98,103,297] or dactinomycin, 5-fluorouracil, and cyclophosphamide.[89,298] Although this therapy proved to be effective in many cases, the number of tumors that recurred was still high. The introduction of a combination of cis-platinum, bleomycin, and vinblastine, which has now been superseded by cisplatinum, etoposide (VP16), and bleomycin (BEP) combination, has been found to be much more effective and has produced remissions in patients with advanced stage disease and in patients in whom other combinations of multiagent chemotherapy have failed.[40,79,103,104,337] This combination chemotherapy has revolutionized the treatment of patients with yolk sac tumor. Complete cure for all stages is now more than 80%.[104] The occasional cases of pure hepatoid and glandular (primitive intestinal) yolk sac tumor show a less satisfactory response to combination chemotherapy and are therefore associated with worse prognosis.[56,59,246] It is of interest that the only tumor that was diploid in a series of 20 yolk sac tumors was a tumor of the pure glandular (primitive intestinal) type, whereas all the other tumors were aneuploid.[161]

Serum AFP determination is a useful diagnostic test in patients with yolk sac tumor. It is also of value in monitoring the results of therapy and for early detection of metastases and recurrences. It should be noted, however, that a normal result may not always indicate the absence of active disease but only the absence of the tumor element associated with AFP synthesis. Preoperatively, if the tumor contains yolk sac tumor elements, the AFP can be detected in the serum. AFP levels fall postoperatively and, if there are no metastases, reach normal levels within 4 to 6 weeks, depending on the preoperative serum AFP level. The use of serial serum AFP estimations for diagnosis, monitoring of therapy, and early detection of metastases and recurrences in patients with tumors containing yolk sac tumor elements is illustrated in Figures 20.30 through 20.33.

°Refs. 44,134,147,164,206,267,278,346.
†Refs. 44,134,147,148,164,206,278.
‡Refs. 40,79,89,98,104,265,297,298,329,337.

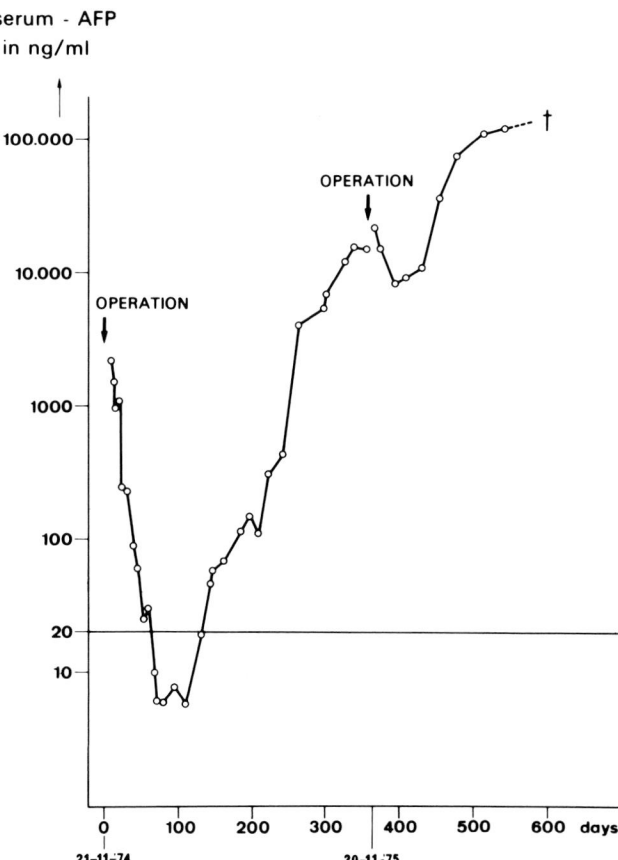

FIG. 20.30. Serial serum AFP determinations (logarithmic scale) during the course of disease in a 17-year-old patient with large ovarian mixed germ cell tumor containing endodermal sinus tumor. The first operation was hysterectomy and bilateral adnexectomy. VAC therapy was given postoperatively, and AFP returned to normal. Although clinically there was no evidence of disease, a sustained rise of AFP occurred and was the first indication of disease activity. Despite a second operation for excision of metastases and additional chemotherapy, the patient died. Upper limit of normal serum AFP (20 ng/ml) is indicated by line.

It has been shown by Gitlin and Pericelli[109] that, apart from AFP, normal human yolk sac synthesizes a number of other proteins, and their presence has been demonstrated by immunofluorescence within yolk sac tumor.[224,292,360] One of these proteins, alpha$_1$-antitrypsin, has been studied serially together with AFP in sera of a number of patients with yolk sac tumor.[327,360] Although it was found to be capable of monitoring disease activity, it was shown to be inferior to AFP in this respect.[327]

Human chorionic gonadotropin (hCG)[247,348] and its beta subunit (beta-hCG)[329] have been found to be normal in patients with yolk sac tumor. Carcinoembryonic antigen (CEA) has also been studied in patients with germ cell neoplasms and has been found to be of no value as a tumor marker in this group of patients.[333] Estrogen and progesterone receptors are not detected in yolk sac tumors.[160]

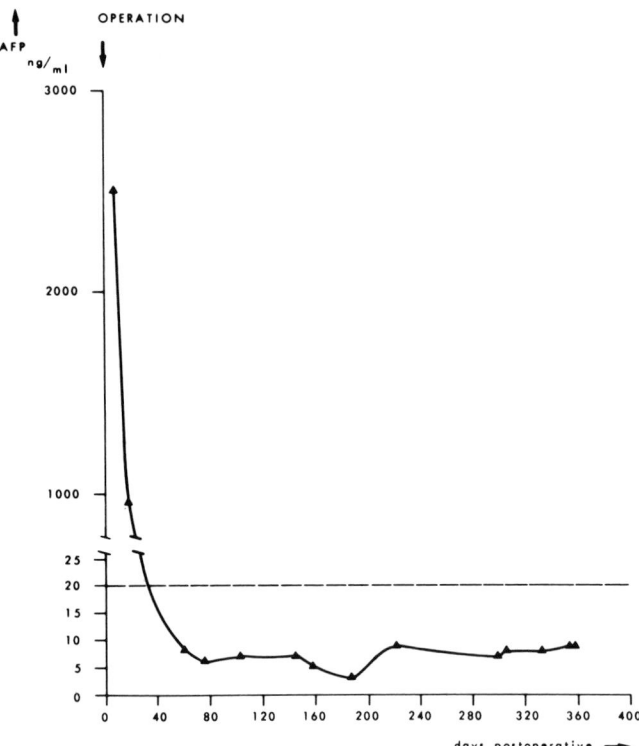

FIG. 20.31. **Serial serum AFP determinations.** A 26-year-old patient with pure ovarian endodermal sinus tumor treated surgically and with VAC chemotherapy. The patient is well and disease-free, and the AFP is normal 5 years after surgery.

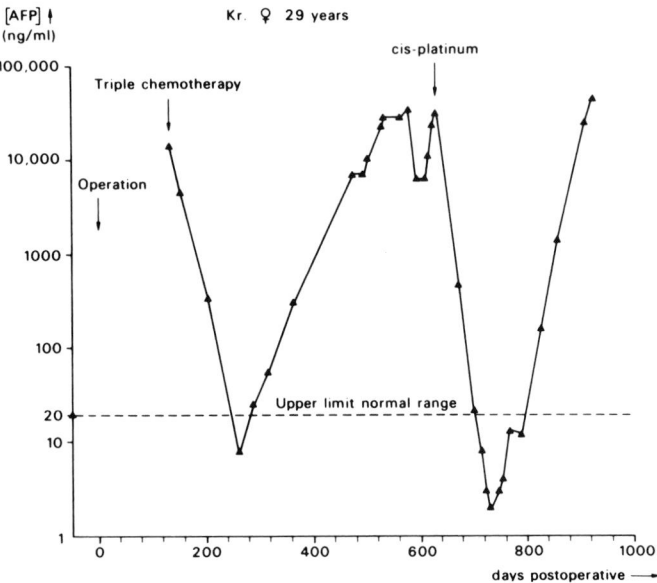

FIG. 20.32. **Serial serum AFP determinations (logarithmic scale).** A 29-year-old patient with pure ovarian endodermal sinus tumor showing the value of AFP in monitoring disease activity and response to chemotherapy during the course of the disease. The patient died with extensive metastatic disease and very high serum AFP.

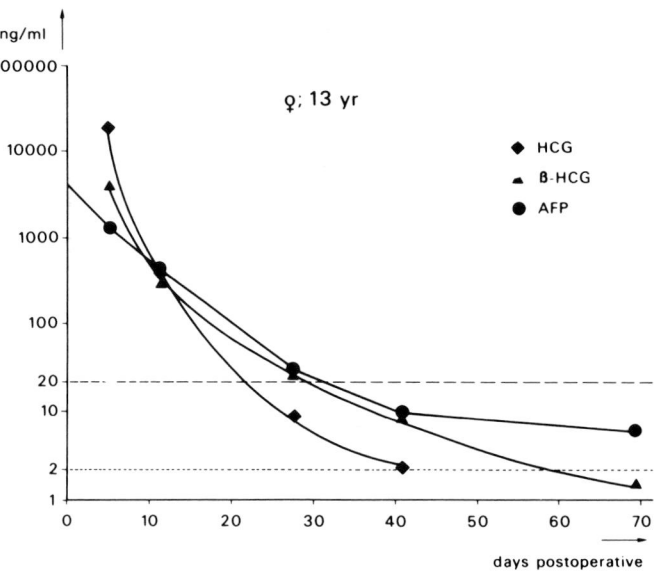

FIG. 20.33. **Serial serum AFP, hCG, and beta-hCG determinations (logarithmic scale).** A 13-year-old patient with ovarian mixed germ cell tumor composed of endodermal sinus tumor, choriocarcinoma, dysgerminoma, and teratoma. All the tumor markers have remained normal, and the patient is well and disease-free 4 years after one-sided adnexectomy. Upper limits of normal AFP, hCG, and beta-hCG are shown by large dashes (AFP) and small dashes (hCG and beta-hCG).

Embryonal Carcinoma

The term *embryonal carcinoma* in this text includes only ovarian neoplasms showing histological appearances resembling those observed in most embryonal carcinomas occurring in the testis of adults. Dixon and Moore[76] consider embryonal carcinoma as both a morphologic and a conceptual entity, and this interpretation is being followed. Embryonal carcinoma was considered to be the least-differentiated form of germ cell tumor, which may differentiate either toward somatic structures (teratomatous tumors of various degrees of differentiation) or toward extraembryonal structures, forming yolk sac or vitelline structures (yolk sac tumor) or trophoblastic structures (choriocarcinoma) (Fig. 20.1). Although ovarian embryonal carcinoma[88,165,329] shows similar appearances and is considered to be homologous with its testicular counterpart, it is uncommon both as a component of mixed germ cell tumors and even more so as a pure entity. However, tumors showing this histological pattern are relatively frequent in the testis. The reason for this difference is unknown.

Ovarian embryonal carcinoma is usually combined with other neoplastic germ cell elements, most frequently yolk sac tumor, and forms a part of a mixed germ cell tumor.[88,141,166,329] Only 15 cases of pure embryonal carci-

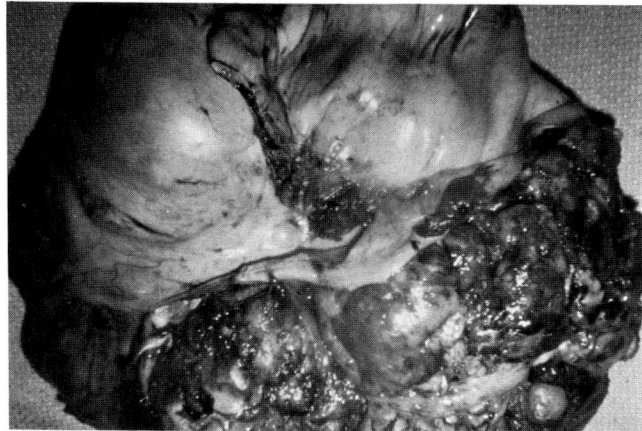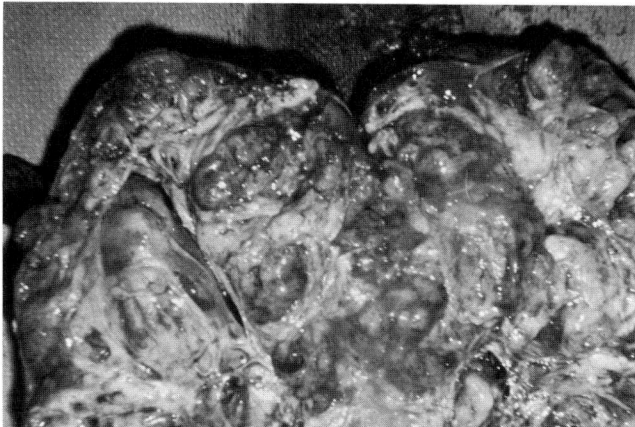

FIG. 20.34. **Embryonal carcinoma.** *Left:* A large lobular mass that is partially encapsulated. *Right:* The cut surface is red-gray to gray-white in color corresponding to areas of hemorrhage and necrosis.

noma of the ovary have been found in the archives of the Armed Forces Institute of Pathology, as compared with 71 cases of yolk sac tumor over the same period of time.[165] Embryonal carcinoma also has been observed in association with gonadoblastoma.[280,315]

CLINICAL FEATURES

The age incidence, clinical presentation, and findings are similar to those observed in patients with other malignant germ cell neoplasms, such as yolk sac tumor, immature teratoma, and dysgerminoma, with the tumor occurring in children and young adults.[88,165,329]

Embryonal carcinoma may produce AFP. In addition, when it contains syncytiotrophoblastic giant cells, as is often the case, or is combined with choriocarcinoma, it produces hCG and is associated with endocrine manifestations, such as isosexual precocious puberty in children and abnormal vaginal bleeding in adults.[165] A positive pregnancy test is found in almost all such patients.

GROSS FINDINGS

Since embryonal carcinoma usually is a component of mixed germ cell tumors, the appearances of the tumor vary according to the type and amount of the different components present. On sectioning, the embryonal carcinomatous component is solid, gray-white, and slightly granular, with foci of necrosis and hemorrhage in the larger tumors (Fig. 20.34).

MICROSCOPIC FINDINGS

In its most primitive and undifferentiated form, embryonal carcinoma is composed of solid aggregates of epithelial-like, medium to large, polygonal or ovoid cells containing an ample amount of somewhat pale eosinophilic granular

cytoplasm, with ill-defined cytoplasmic borders, frequently forming a syncytial arrangement (Fig. 20.35). The cells have a large, prominent, centrally situated, and somewhat irregular vesicular or hyperchromatic nucleus with a fine nuclear membrane and frequently more than one nucleolus. Mitotic activity is usually brisk, and abnormal mitoses are frequently seen. Cellular and nuclear pleomorphism is usually marked. Giant cells and multinucleated cells may be seen. In the slightly better differentiated tumors, the cells, apart from forming solid areas, also tend to line clefts and spaces and form papillae (Fig. 20.36). The cells appear more epithelial than those of the more undifferentiated

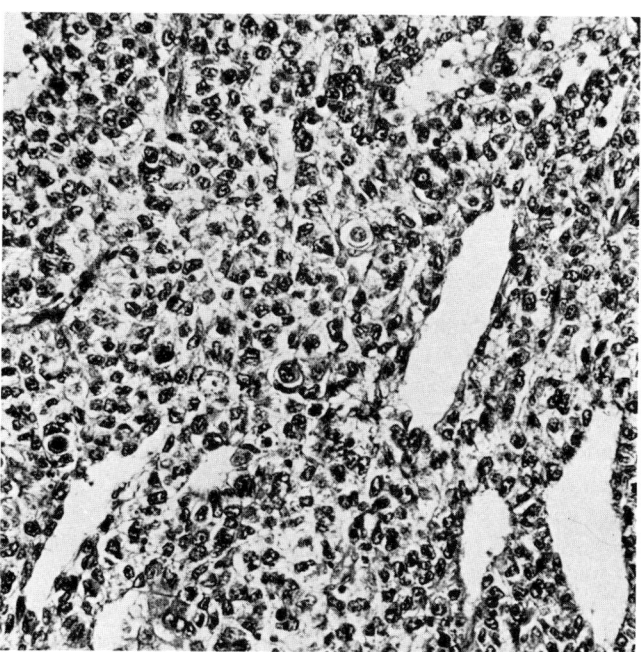

FIG. 20.35. **Embryonal carcinoma.** The tumor displays a solid pattern. The tumor was admixed with teratoma and endodermal sinus tumor.

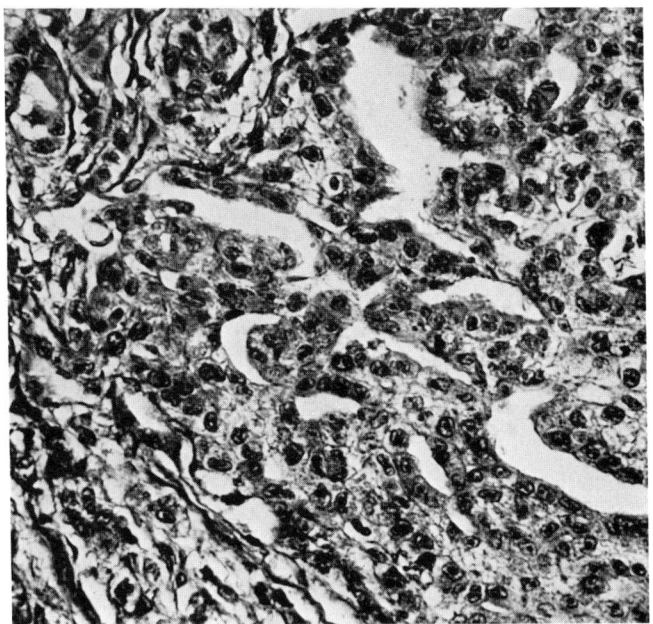

FIG. 20.36. Embryonal carcinoma. The tumor forms clefts and spaces. (Reprinted with permission from The American College of Obstetricians and Gynecologists. (Obstetrics and Gynecology, 43: 138, 1974).)

type, being more cuboidal or columnar in shape (Fig. 20.36). Although there is a suggestion of glandular differentiation, true gland formation is absent. The papillae are composed of solid collections of cells or may contain a cystic space or a small vessel surrounded by tumor cells. They must be differentiated from perivascular formations observed in yolk sac tumor. Very primitive mesenchymal tissue may be present in conjunction with the epithelial-like component. Syncytiotrophoblastic giant cells immediately adjacent to aggregates of embryonal carcinoma cells or lying isolated in the stroma are found very frequently. Foci of necrosis and hemorrhage are frequently seen.

DIFFERENTIAL DIAGNOSIS

Embryonal carcinoma may be present in the form of small solid aggregates or pseudoglandular or cleft-like formations surrounded by better differentiated malignant teratomatous elements showing somatic differentiation. It may co-exist with other neoplastic germ cell elements, such as yolk sac tumor, immature or mature teratoma, choriocarcinoma, polyembryoma, or dysgerminoma. Differentiation from dysgerminoma is important because of a totally different prognosis and response to treatment. It is usually the solid primitive type of embryonal carcinoma that is more likely to be confused with dysgerminoma, but the presence of clefts, alveoli, or cell-lined spaces militates against the diagnosis of dysgerminoma. The cells of embryonal carcinoma are usually larger and show much more marked cellular and nuclear pleomorphism. Mitotic activity is usually more prominent, and bizarre mitoses are more frequent. The nuclear membrane is less sharp and the nuclei are more irregular, larger, and usually contain more than one dark hyperchromatic nucleolus, in contrast with the rounded, prominent, usually single, and frequently eosinophilic nucleolus of dysgerminoma. The presence of connective tissue stroma infiltrated by lymphocytes and at times a granulomatous reaction is a prominent feature of dysgerminoma. These features usually are absent in embryonal carcinoma.

Cells of embryonal carcinoma stain positively for cytokeratin, whereas most dysgerminoma cells are negative. In addition, most embryonal carcinoma cells show at least some positive staining for AFP, whereas dysgerminoma cells are invariably negative. Immunocytochemical localization of AFP and cytokeratin provides a useful method for differentiating between these two neoplasms.[25,200,201]

CLINICAL BEHAVIOR AND TREATMENT

Embryonal carcinoma of the ovary, as its testicular counterpart, is a highly malignant neoplasm. It is aggressive locally, spreads extensively in the abdominal cavity, and metastasizes early. The metastatic spread is similar to that observed with other germ cell neoplasms, taking place first via the lymphatic system and later by hematogenous spread. The primary treatment of embryonal carcinoma is surgical. Since the tumors are usually unilateral, conservative treatment is advocated if the tumor is localized to the ovary. Embryonal carcinoma is not radiosensitive. The prognosis in the past has been unfavorable, but introduction of the various forms of combination chemotherapy effective in the treatment of malignant germ cell tumors has led to marked improvement resulting in a complete cure in most patients. The response to combination chemotherapy using bleomycin, vinblastine, and *cis*platin or, preferably, *cis*platin, etoposide (VP 16), and bleomycin[104] is similar to that observed in patients with embryonal carcinoma of the testis.[11,79,112,265,300]

Polyembryoma

GENERAL FEATURES

Polyembryoma is a rare ovarian germ cell neoplasm composed of numerous embryoid bodies resembling morphologically normal presomite embryos. Similar homologous neoplasms occur more frequently in the human testis,[26,84,85,346] although pure polyembryoma is very rare. Less than a dozen cases of ovarian polyembryoma have been recorded.[26,156,311] In all these cases the polyembryoma was associated with other neoplastic germ cell elements, mainly immature or mature teratoma.[26,156,294,311] All these tumors occurred in young patients or in patients in the reproductive age group.[26,156,236,294,311] The oldest patient was 38 years old.[294] The clinical findings are similar to those observed in patients with other malignant germ cell neoplasms of the ovary.

Histogenesis

There are conflicting views of the origin of embryoid bodies. It has been suggested that they arise by parthenogenic development from primitive germ cells present in a malignant teratoma.[191,236,294] Other investigators question this view as well as the entire concept that embryoid bodies bear a close similarity to early human embryos, since embryoid bodies never appear to develop beyond the 18-day stage.[26,345,346] They consider that embryoid bodies probably develop transiently by bizarre differentiation, possibly in response to local release of organizers in malignant teratomas of the gonads. Another view that has been advanced accepts the morphologic similarities between the early embryo and the embryoid bodies but disputes their parthenogenic origin.[84,239,240,305,306] It maintains that embryoid bodies are formed after initiation of teratogenesis, most likely from multipotential malignant embryonal cells present in a tumor and not directly from germ cells.[307] This is supported by the observations of the development of embryoid bodies from undifferentiated embryonal cells in strain-129 mice. The tumor, a teratoma that had been serially transplanted for many years, was considered to be devoid of germ cells.[239,240,305,306] These findings are in accordance with the view that embryoid bodies probably persist only transiently within the tumor, and while new embryoid bodies are being formed others lose their identity and their multipotential cells undergo further differentiation.[85] Although the origin and development of embryoid bodies are still a matter of dispute, the view that they originate from multipotential malignant embryonal cells, which is supported by experimental observations,[239,240,305,306] is most favored at present.

GROSS FINDINGS

Polyembryoma is usually unilateral. Macroscopically, the tumor resembles other malignant germ cell tumors, varying in size from relatively small (9.5 cm in longest diameter)[26] to tumors filling almost the whole abdominal cavity and invading the surrounding structures.[294] The tumor is usually solid and contains hemorrhagic and necrotic areas.

MICROSCOPIC FINDINGS

Polyembryoma is composed of numerous embryoid bodies, and the better differentiated ones are composed of an embryonic disk, amniotic cavity, and yolk sac surrounded by primitive extraembryonic mesenchyme (Fig. 20.37). Sometimes trophoblastic differentiation may be seen in the vicinity of the embryoid body. When the embryoid bodies are less well formed, they are composed of a medullary

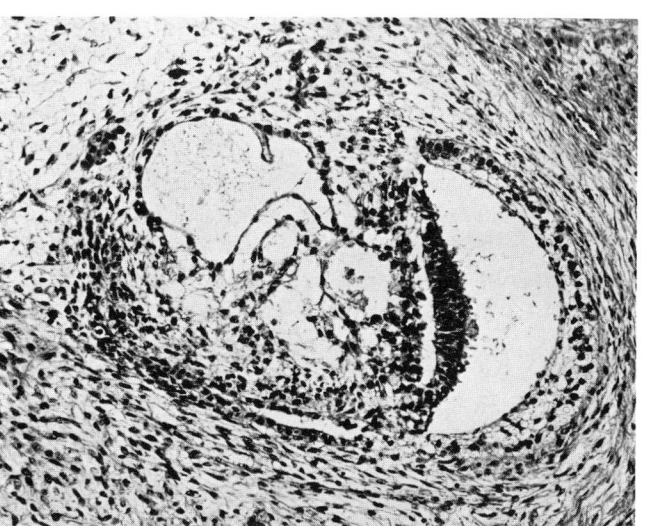

FIG. 20.37. **Polyembryoma.** Embryoid body showing amniotic cavity (*right*), embryonic disk (*center*), and atypical yolk sac (*left*).

plate and amnion associated with a blastocystic space or with extraembryonic mesenchyme. They may have two or more amniotic cavities and share a single yolk sac cavity or vice versa. There may be a considerable disproportion between the two cavities, and the cavities may be malformed. There may be considerable variation in size between the different embryoid bodies; some may be more primitive and others appear to be better developed. Some embryoid bodies may be malformed and show bizarre appearances (Fig. 20.38). None of the embryoid bodies appear to have developed beyond the 18-day stage. The embryonic disk of a typical embryoid body is lined on one side by cuboidal epithelial cells of uniform size, resembling endoderm, and on the other by tall columnar epithelium, resembling ectoderm. The latter merges with low cuboidal epithelium lining the rest of the cavity, which resembles the amnion.

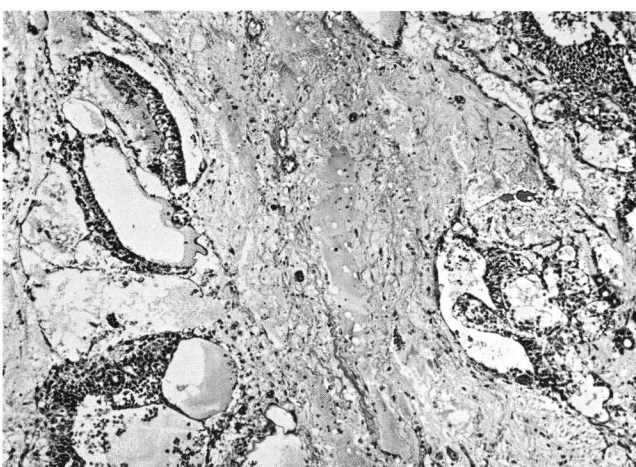

FIG. 20.38. **Polyembryoma.** Embryoid bodies showing bizarre appearances.

The cavity resembling the yolk sac is on the opposite side of the embryonic disk from the amnion (Fig. 20.37). The embryoid bodies are surrounded by extraembryonic mesenchyme, which is composed of either closely or more loosely packed spindle-shaped cells of regular appearance (Fig. 20.37) and showing occasional mitotic figures. Loose myxomatous areas may be present (Fig. 20.38).

Occasionally, embryoid bodies in earlier developmental stages, mainly the blastocyst and morula stage, form numerous round or oval structures. In some tumors this pattern may predominate, although occasional fully developed embryoid bodies may be seen.[156] Teratomatous structures in various stages of differentiation are frequently seen interspersed among the embryoid bodies. In one reported case,[26] hCG and human placental lactogen were demonstrated within syncytiotrophoblastic cells that were present in the vicinity of the embryoid bodies. Cytotrophoblastic cells were not identified in this tumor. In another reported case, there was elevation of serum AFP and hCG. AFP was demonstrated by immunoperoxidase within the cells lining the yolk sac cavities and hCG within the syncytiotrophoblastic giant cells that were present in the vicinity of the embryoid bodies.[311]

CLINICAL BEHAVIOR AND TREATMENT

Polyembryoma is a highly malignant germ cell neoplasm. In most cases, it has been associated with invasion of adjacent structures and extensive metastases, which were mainly confined to the abdominal cavity.[294]

The primary treatment of polyembryoma is surgical, and since the tumor is usually unilateral unless there is spread beyond the ovary, excision of the tumor and the adjoining adnexa is the treatment of choice. The tumor is not sensitive to radiotherapy, but responds to the combination chemotherapy used in treatment of malignant germ cell tumors.[104,311]

One patient with a relatively small mobile tumor, absence of capsular penetration, and no evidence of metastases has survived more than 5 years.[26] Another patient is alive and free of disease for more than 12 years after excision of the affected adnexa and excision of intraabdominal metastases composed of grade 1 immature teratoma.[156] A third patient is well and disease-free 6 months after diagnosis.[311] Before the introduction of effective combination chemotherapy, most patients with polyembryoma died of their disease.

Choriocarcinoma

GENERAL FEATURES

Pure ovarian choriocarcinoma of germ cell origin is a rare neoplasm,[140,368] and even the presence of choriocarcinomatous elements admixed with other neoplastic germ cell elements is rare.[85] In most cases, the tumor is admixed with other neoplastic germ cell elements, and their presence is diagnostic of nongestational choriocarcinoma, except for the remote possibility of the tumor being a gestational choriocarcinoma metastatic to an ovarian germ cell tumor. The presence of other neoplastic germ cell elements is a particularly helpful diagnostic feature in postmenarchal patients, in whom exclusion of gestational origin of the tumor may be difficult. In view of this, nongestational choriocarcinoma may be diagnosed with confidence in postmenarchal patients and not only in young children, as had been considered earlier.[222] At least 50 cases of ovarian germ cell tumors containing choriocarcinoma have been reported.* The tumor occurs in children and young adults. Its occurrence in children has been emphasized; in some series, 50% of cases occurred in children who had not reached puberty.[192] This high frequency in children may result from the previous reluctance of making the diagnosis in adults.

Histogenesis

Choriocarcinoma of the ovary may originate in three different ways: (1) as a primary gestational choriocarcinoma associated with ovarian pregnancy, (2) as metastatic choriocarcinoma from a primary gestational choriocarcinoma arising in other parts of the genital tract, mainly the uterus, and (3) as a germ cell tumor differentiating in the direction of trophoblastic structures, usually admixed with other neoplastic germ cell elements. In each case it is important to ascertain the mode of origin of the tumor because this has important therapeutic and prognostic implications. Alternatively, choriocarcinoma of the ovary may be divided into two broad groups: (1) gestational choriocarcinoma encompassing the first two groups mentioned above and (2) nongestational choriocarcinoma, a germ cell tumor differentiating toward trophoblastic structures. As this chapter deals solely with germ cell tumors, only the nongestational choriocarcinoma is discussed here.

CLINICAL FEATURES

The clinical findings in patients with ovarian nongestational choriocarcinoma are similar to those observed in patients with other malignant ovarian germ cell neoplasms, except that they may be modified by the endocrine activity of the tumor, which secretes hCG. This is particularly noticeable in prepubertal children who show evidence of isosexual precocious puberty, with mammary development, growth of pubic and axillary hair, and uterine bleeding. Adult patients may have signs of ectopic pregnancy.

---

*Refs. 39,70,90,140,169,192,222,267,361.

Because the nongestational choriocarcinoma, like its gestational counterpart, is associated with increased production of hCG, determination of urinary or plasma hCG is a useful diagnostic test. Serum hCG levels are also useful in monitoring the response to therapy, as well as in detecting metastases and recurrences containing choriocarcinomatous tissue. It should be noted that normal levels of hCG do not exclude the presence of metastases or recurrences composed of other neoplastic germ cell elements. Table 20.3 shows the results of preoperative serum hCG and beta-hCG determinations in patients with ovarian germ cell tumors.

GROSS FINDINGS

The tumor typically is large, unilateral, solid, gray-white, and hemorrhagic. Necrosis may be evident. Since most of these tumors are composed of a combination of neoplastic germ cell elements, the appearances tend to vary according to the elements present in the tumor.

MICROSCOPIC FINDINGS

Choriocarcinoma is composed of two types of cells, cytotrophoblast and syncytiotrophoblast (Fig. 20.39). The cytotrophoblast is composed of medium-sized polygonal, round, or oval cells with clear cytoplasm and sharp borders. Some cells have centrally situated, small, round, and hyperchromatic nuclei whereas others have larger vesicular nuclei containing nucleoli and showing brisk mitotic activity. The syncytiotrophoblast is composed of large basophilic, vacuolated cells with irregular outlines, and although frequently elongated, they may vary in shape. These cells contain multiple hyperchromatic nuclei, varying in shape and size. The cytotrophoblastic cells are usually disposed centrally within a tumor mass and are partly or completely surrounded by irregular collections or layers

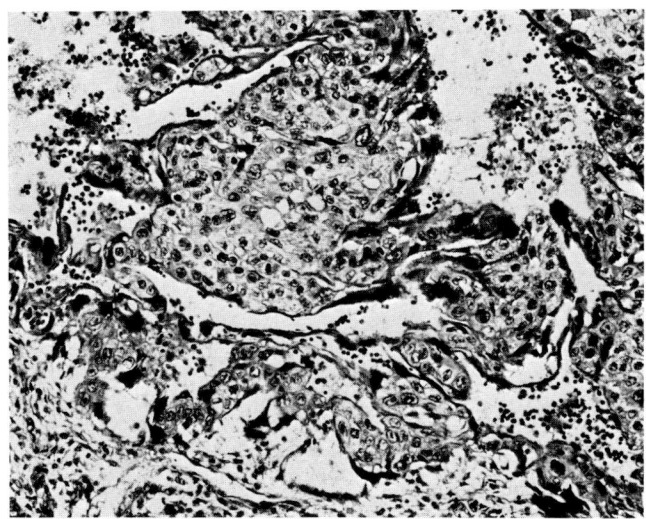

FIG. 20.39. Choriocarcinoma. Cytotrophoblast composed of medium-sized cells, situated centrally, and syncytiotrophoblast composed of very large multinucleated cells, situated peripherally are present.

of the syncytiotrophoblastic cells (Fig. 20.39). There is a considerable variation in the pattern and in the ratio of the two components in different parts of the same tumor and in different tumors. The tumor cells form solid aggregates, nearly always associated with hemorrhage and necrosis. At times the tumor is limited to the periphery of the hemorrhagic mass. When the tumor is combined with other germ cell elements, the choriocarcinoma may form small nodules associated with hemorrhage and surrounded by other germ cell elements. The presence of other germ cell elements within the tumor is a frequent finding.

It appears that the cytotrophoblast is the more primitive element, and the syncytiotrophoblast is formed from it either directly or indirectly. The syncytiotrophoblast is the differentiated, nondividing, hormone-secreting component. These findings are supported by electron microscopic and immunohistochemical studies[240,243] (Fig. 20.40).

CLINICAL BEHAVIOR AND TREATMENT

Nongestational choriocarcinoma of the ovary is a highly malignant germ cell neoplasm. It invades adjacent structures, spreads widely throughout the abdominal cavity, and metastasizes via both the lymphatics and the blood vessels. Although gestational choriocarcinoma tends to spread primarily via the bloodstream, nongestational choriocarcinoma shows lymphatic and intraabdominal spread and hematogenous spread may not be so marked.

Until the introduction of effective combination chemotherapy the prognosis of patients with choriocarcinoma was distinctly unfavorable but was somewhat better than of

Table 20.3. Serum hCG and beta-hCG in ovarian germ cell tumors measured by radioimmunoassay[a]

	No. of cases	Serum hCG
Mixed germ cell tumors containing choriocarcinoma	8	Elevated
Mixed germ cell tumors containing EST	26	Normal
Pure EST	15	Normal
Pure dysgerminoma	18	Normal
Dysgerminoma with syncytiotrophoblastic giant cells	3	Elevated
Teratoma (immature and mature)	8	Normal
Teratoma (immature and mature) and dysgerminoma	7	Normal
Mature cystic teratoma (dermoid cyst)	11	Normal

[a] Unpublished data.
hCG, human chorionic gonadotropin; EST, endodermal sinus tumor.

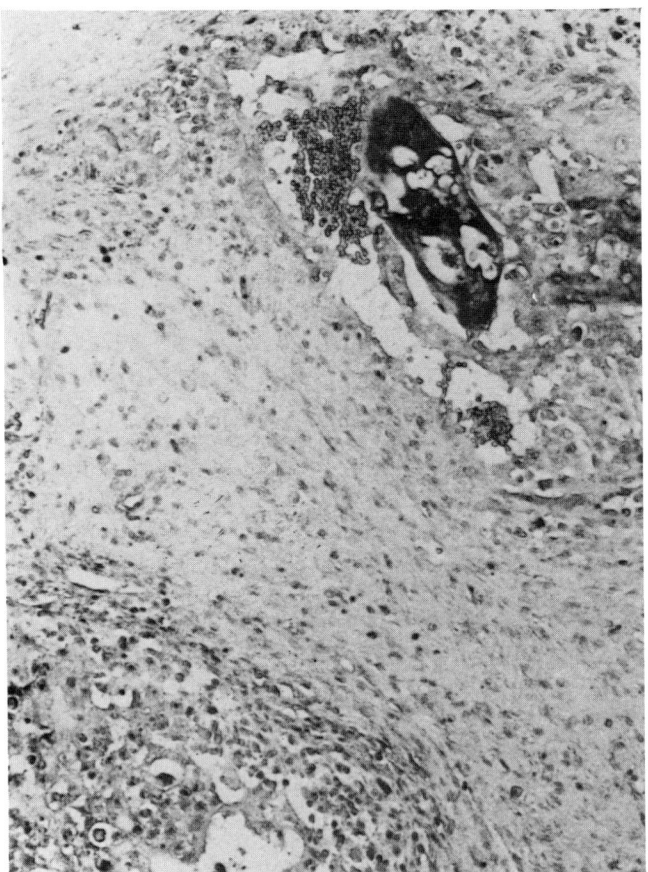

FIG. 20.40. Mixed germ cell tumor containing choriocarcinoma. The syncytiotrophoblastic element of the latter shows strong positive staining for beta-hCG. The cytotrophoblast is negative. Note the hemorrhage that usually is associated with this tumor.

patients with yolk sac tumor.[70,148,171,278,346] In one large series there were 4 survivors out of 12 patients with tumors containing choriocarcinoma as compared with 5 out of 35 patients with tumors containing yolk sac tumor.[148] More recently, the treatment has been revolutionized by the introduction of combination chemotherapy containing *cis*-platin with marked improvement in prognosis and survival. *Ci*splatin, etoposide (VP 16), and bleomycin currently is the most favored combination.[40,103,104,112,337,375]

Teratoma

The origin of teratomas has been a matter of interest, speculation, and dispute for centuries.[37] The parthenogenic theory, which suggests an origin from the primordial germ cell is now the most widely accepted. Two other theories, one suggesting an origin from blastomeres segregated at an early stage of embryonic development and the second suggesting an origin from embryonal rests, have few adherents nowadays.[85,220] Support for the germ cell

theory has come from the anatomic distribution of the tumors, which occur along the line of migration of the primordial germ cells from the yolk sac to the primitive gonad, and from the fact that the tumors occur most commonly during the years of reproductive activity. Support also comes from animal experiments in which cystic teratomas can be produced only during the period of reproductive activity of the gonad, as in roosters injected with zinc and copper salts,[19,49] and from the nuclear sexing and karyotyping of teratomas. It has been shown that cells of ovarian teratomas are always chromatin-positive, unlike the cells of testicular teratomas, which may be chromatin-negative, chromatin-positive, or mixed.[353] The karyotypes of all benign ovarian teratomas studied have been found to be 46XX.[62,99,175,252] Further support for the germ cell theory of origin has come from the work of Linder et al.[173–175] They studied the histogenesis of mature cystic teratoma of the ovary using both cytogenetic techniques and the electrophoretic variants of four enzymes in normal as well as in tumor cells. They demonstrated that these tumors are of germ cell origin and arise from a single germ cell after the first meiotic division.[175] Recent studies using more advanced cytogenetic techniques further confirm these observations. Although most mature cystic teratomas arise in this manner, some arise before the first meiotic division.[211,228]

The classification of ovarian teratomas is shown in Table 20.1. Briefly, they are divided into three main groups: (1) immature teratomas, (2) mature teratomas, and (3) monodermal and highly specialized teratomas. Most cases (99%) are mature cystic teratomas also known as dermoids.*

Immature Teratoma

Immature teratomas are composed of tissues derived from the three germ layers—ectoderm, mesoderm, and endoderm—and, in contrast to the much more common mature teratoma, they contain immature or embryonal structures. Mature tissues are frequently present and sometimes may predominate. In these cases, the tumor should be differentiated from a mature teratoma with malignant transformation. The presence of immature or embryonal elements as opposed to the neoplastic transformation of mature tissues differentiates between these two types of neoplasm.

CLINICAL FEATURES

The immature teratoma of the ovary is an uncommon tumor, comprising less than 1% of teratomas of the ovary.[43,50,188,219,386] In contrast with the mature cystic teratoma, which is encountered most frequently during the reproductive years but occurs at all ages, the immature

---

*Refs. 85,127,143,216,220,277–279,289,345,386.

teratoma has a specific age incidence, occurring most commonly in the first two decades of life and being almost unknown after the menopause.[43,44,188,386] In view of this, teratomas occurring in childhood, adolescence, and early adult life should always be examined carefully and thoroughly sampled.

The tumor is usually asymptomatic until it reaches a considerable size. It tends to grow rapidly and may manifest itself as a pelvic or lower abdominal mass. It may cause pressure symptoms, abdominal heaviness, or dull pain, or it may undergo torsion, causing acute abdominal pain.

GROSS FINDINGS

The tumor is usually unilateral,[43,44,50,219,220,382,386] but may co-exist with a benign cystic teratoma in the opposite ovary.[383] The tumors are usually large, varying in size from 9 to 28 cm in the largest dimension.[44] They may form a round, oval, or lobulated soft or firm mass (Fig. 20.41). The tumor is often prone to perforate its capsule, which is not always well defined.[43,44,383] It tends to form adhesions to the surrounding structures and to invade locally.[43,44] The tumor is predominantly solid but frequently contains cystic structures.[43,44,50,188,383] Occasionally, it may be predominantly cystic, with solid areas present in the cyst wall.[44,181,356] The cut surface is usually variegated, trabeculated, and lobulated, varying in color from gray to dark brown. Occasionally, foci of cartilage or bone may be recognizable and hair may be present. The cystic areas are usually filled with serous or mucinous fluid, colloid, or fatty material.

MICROSCOPIC FINDINGS

The tumor is composed of a variety of immature and mature tissues derived from the three germ layers. Occasionally, the tumor may be composed of a small number of tissues, although usually derivatives of all the three germ

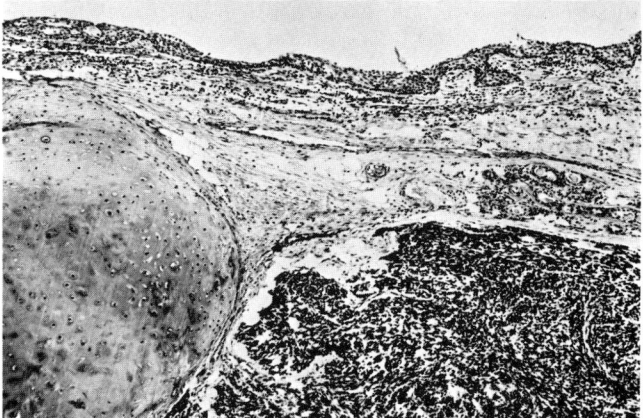

FIG. 20.42. Immature teratoma. Both solid and cystic areas are shown. The tumor was mainly composed of neuroblastic tissue (*right*). Note the squamous epithelium, adnexal glands, and cartilage.

layers are present. Ectoderm is usually represented by neural tissue. Glia, ganglion cells, neuroblastic tissue (Fig. 20.42), neuroepithelium, nerve trunks, and ocular structures are often represented. Skin elements (Fig. 20.42), including pilosebaceous units, sweat glands, and hair, are not infrequently present. Mesodermal elements include fibrous connective tissue, cartilage (Fig. 20.42), bone, muscle, usually smooth but occasionally striated, lymphoid tissue, and undifferentiated embryonic mesenchyme. Endodermal elements are usually represented by tubules lined by columnar, sometimes ciliated, epithelium. Occasionally, gastrointestinal or bronchial epithelium may be present. All these tissues, which may be in stages of maturity varying from embryonic to mature, are scattered haphazardly throughout the tumor and so differ from the orderly organoid arrangement seen in a mature teratoma. In cases in which the tumor is composed mainly of mature tissues, differentiation from mature teratoma may be difficult, and patients have been diagnosed as having a benign lesion only to return within a short time with recurrence. In a number of such cases, review of the material taken from the original tumor has revealed immature elements. Therefore, careful examination and thorough sampling of the tumor are strongly recommended. Immature teratoma may be combined with other neoplastic germ cell elements, such as yolk sac tumor, dysgerminoma, embryonal carcinoma, choriocarcinoma, and polyembryoma. It can therefore form a part of a malignant germ cell tumor composed of two or more neoplastic germ cell elements (mixed germ cell tumor). Immature teratoma has been reported to develop from the germ cell element of gonadoblastoma.[280]

DIFFERENTIAL DIAGNOSIS

Immature solid teratoma must be differentiated from the malignant mixed müllerian (mesodermal) tumor, which

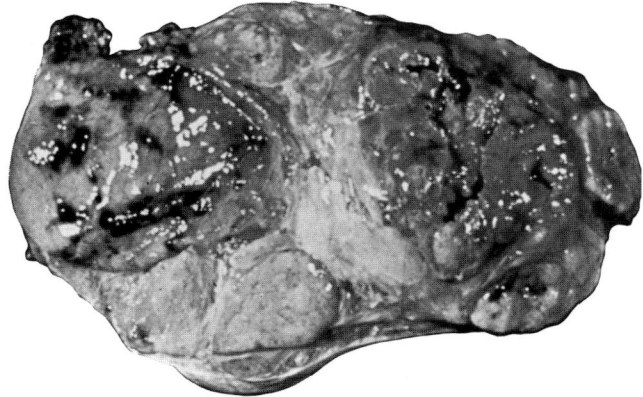

FIG. 20.41. Immature teratoma. A large lobulated, firm to soft tumor mass with areas of hemorrhage and necrosis.

although occurring most frequently in the uterus, also occurs in the ovary. Malignant mixed müllerian (mesodermal) tumor is composed of derivatives of müllerian mesoderm, a primitive structure that gives rise both to the stroma and epithelium of the endometrium. The monodermal origin of malignant mixed müllerian (mesodermal) tumor distinguishes it from teratoma.[336] Malignant mixed müllerian (mesodermal) tumor occurs most frequently in postmenopausal women between the ages of 50 and 70 years and, unlike solid immature teratoma, occurs only occasionally in younger patients. The tumor is composed of sarcomatous and carcinomatous tissue. The carcinoma is invariably an adenocarcinoma, squamous cell carcinoma, or adenosquamous carcinoma, and the sarcomatous elements may be composed of a wide variety of tissues, including leiomyosarcoma, chondrosarcoma, rhabdomyosarcoma, fibrosarcoma, undifferentiated sarcomatous tissue, and myxomatous tissue. Derivatives of the three germ layers are absent in malignant mixed müllerian (mesodermal) tumor; neuroectodermal derivatives, prominent in solid immature teratoma, are seen only exceptionally. Malignant mixed müllerian (mesodermal) tumor does not exhibit the great variety of tissues present in teratoma, and the tissues present in malignant mixed müllerian (mesodermal) tumor generally form more typical sarcomatous or carcinomatous patterns (see Chapter 13, Mesenchymal Tumors of Uterus).

CLINICAL BEHAVIOR AND TREATMENT

Immature teratoma is a malignant neoplasm that usually grows rapidly, penetrates its capsule, and forms adhesions to the surrounding structures. It spreads throughout the peritoneal cavity by implantation. It metastasizes first to the retroperitoneal, para-aortic, and more distant lymph nodes and later to the lungs, liver, and other organs. Peritoneal implants and metastases are not infrequently present at operation for the removal of the primary tumor.[43,44,383] Excision of the tumor is usually followed by a local recurrence, which occurs within a few weeks or months. Recurrences usually occur within the first year after the primary treatment, and patients free from recurrence for 12 to 18 months survive.[43,44] Rupture of the tumor with spillage of the contents during operation is not infrequent and tends to be associated with less favorable outcome. The metastases and peritoneal implants may be composed of different tissues, and thus their teratomatous nature is readily apparent, but they may also be composed of a single tissue. The histological appearances of the metastases and of the peritoneal implants may or may not reflect the appearances of the primary tumor.

In the past treatment has been unsatisfactory and prognosis was poor, with less than 20% of patients surviving 5 years after the operation.[43,50,188] Better results have been claimed in cases in which the only immature element was

neurogenic.[188,386] It has been noted that there is a good correlation between the histological appearances of the tumor and prognosis.[215,356] Very immature and poorly differentiated tumors have been found to be associated with worse prognosis, whereas a more favorable outcome has been observed in patients with more mature and better differentiated tumors.[215,356,383]

A histological grading has been proposed and it is of value for predicting prognosis and planning treatment. This grading[356] is based on the relative amounts of immature and mature tissues, the degree of differentiation, and the mitotic activity within the immature components. The most common immature element present and the one that is evaluated most often in grading is primitive neuroepithelium. The grading is as follows:

Grade 0   All tissues mature; no mitotic activity
Grade 1   Minor foci of abnormally cellular or immature tissue mixed with mature elements; slight mitotic activity
Grade 2   Moderate quantities of immature tissue mixed with mature elements; moderate mitotic activity
Grade 3   Large quantities of immature tissue present; high mitotic activity

This grading system has been accepted by most investigators[43,44,356] and its use is strongly recommended. Recently, Norris[214] proposed that immature teratomas should be divided into two grades, those with a slight degree of immaturity (Grade 1), which are not treated with combination chemotherapy, and those with a more marked degree of immaturity (Grades 2 and 3), which are treated. It was demonstrated that whereas there was considerable inter- and intraobserver disagreement when a large series of immature teratomas were being graded into three grades, this was markedly decreased when a two-grade system was used. The study further confirmed the good correlation between the grade of the tumor and its behavior.

The recommended treatment for patients with grade 1 (low grade) immature teratoma confined to one ovary is unilateral salpingo-oophorectomy. For grade 2 and 3 (high grade) tumors adjuvant chemotherapy is given. More extensive surgery is necessary if tumor extends beyond the ovary.[43,278,283,286] Current combination therapy is either vincristine, dactinomycin, and cyclophosphamide (VAC), vinblastine, bleomycin, and cisplatin (VBP), or cisplatin, etoposide (VP 16), and bleomycin (BEP) regimens. Therapy with VAC has been the treatment of choice[103,215,297,298,337] because the results obtained were considered to be similar to those with VBP or BEP regimens, and the latter are more toxic. There is evidence that the recurrence rate with BEP is less than with VAC regimen and in patients with metastatic disease the cisplatin-containing regimens are the treatment of choice, especially as the more recently introduced BEP regimen is less toxic than the VBP.[104]

Mature Solid Teratoma

GENERAL FEATURES

Solid mature teratoma is an uncommon ovarian teratoma. The age incidence is similar to that of solid immature teratoma, the tumor occurring mainly in children and young adults.[233,356,386] Most solid ovarian teratomas are composed at least partly of immature tissues and therefore are considered to be malignant. The occasional cases of solid ovarian teratoma composed entirely of mature tissues have usually been included in this group and thus misinterpreted as malignant. At the same time, this practice has improved the survival statistics, which were generally very poor in patients with immature ovarian teratoma. Solid mature teratoma is composed entirely of mature tissues derived from the three germ layers. Rigid diagnostic criteria must be adhered to, and the examination and sampling of the tumor must be thorough, since inclusion of cases with immature elements completely changes the prognosis of this neoplasm, which otherwise is excellent.[220,233,356,383,386] Neurogenic elements, which are one of the most common tissues present in this tumor, often may be the cause of difficulties.[278] The presence of immature neural elements immediately excludes the tumor from this group, as by definition only tumors composed entirely of mature tissues may be included.

GROSS FINDINGS

The tumors are usually large, do not show any specific features, and show similar appearance to most solid teratomas, which are composed of immature tissues. They grow slowly in comparison with immature solid teratoma, but since they are usually discovered after they have reached a considerable size, this feature is of little help in diagnosis. In all reported cases of solid mature teratoma, the tumor has been unilateral.[219,233,356,383,386]

MICROSCOPIC FINDINGS

The tumor is composed of a variety of tissues derived from the three germ layers and arranged in an orderly manner resembling the much more common mature cystic teratoma, except that the neoplasm is solid or at least predominantly solid. The tumor is composed entirely of mature tissues (Figs. 20.43, 20.44). Sometimes neurogenic elements may predominate (Fig. 20.44).

Occasionally, solid mature teratoma may be associated with peritoneal implants composed entirely of mature glial tissue (Fig. 20.45). Despite extensive peritoneal disease and irrespective of the mode of therapy employed, the prognosis is excellent.[253] Presence of peritoneal implants composed entirely of mature glial tissue occasionally may be observed in patients with immature solid teratoma and

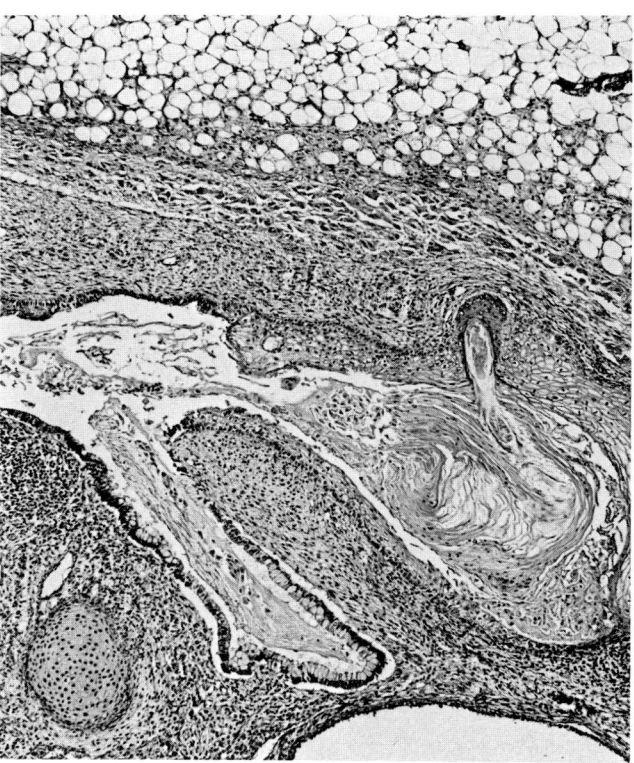

FIG. 20.43. Mature solid teratoma. The tumor is composed of squamous and glandular epithelium, adipose and fibrous tissue, and cartilage.

with mature cystic teratoma. The prognosis is likewise excellent.[207,253]

CLINICAL BEHAVIOR AND TREATMENT

Since the tumor is unilateral, oophorectomy or unilateral adnexectomy is the treatment of choice, resulting in a complete cure.[233,356,383,386]

Mature Cystic Teratoma

GENERAL FEATURES

Mature cystic teratoma of the ovary, or dermoid cyst, has been known since antiquity. The tumor is composed of well-differentiated derivatives of the three germ layers—ectoderm, mesoderm, and endoderm—with ectodermal elements predominating. In its pure form, mature cystic teratoma is always benign, but occasionally it may undergo malignant change in one of its elements. It may also form a part of a germ cell neoplasm composed of a number of different neoplastic germ cell elements (mixed germ cell tumor).

CLINICAL FEATURES

Mature cystic teratoma is the most common type of ovarian teratoma and the most common type of ovarian germ cell

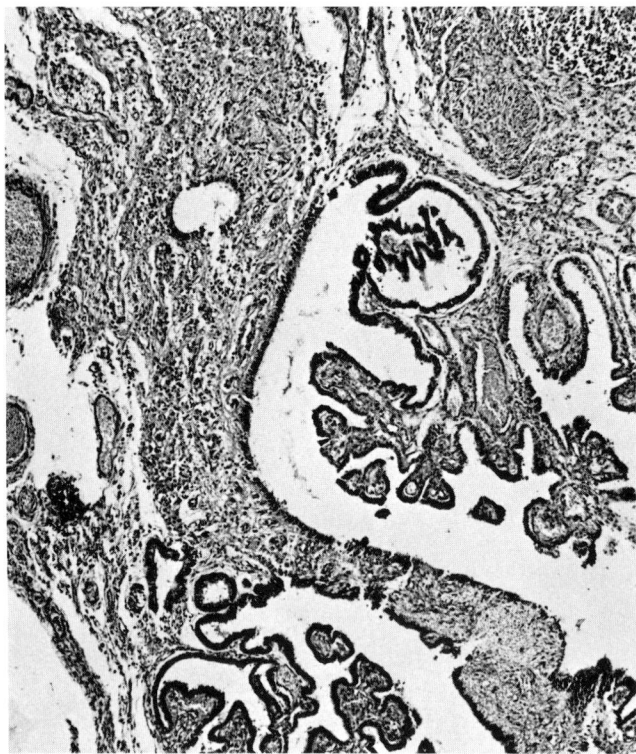

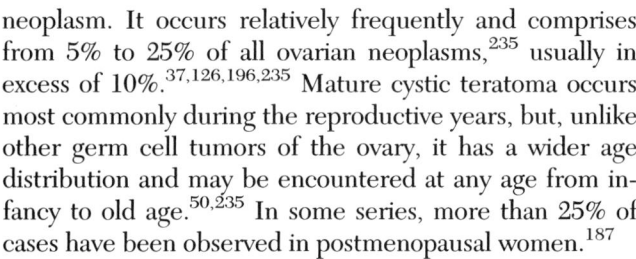

Fig. 20.44. **Mature solid teratoma.** The tumor is composed of mature neural tissue and choroid plexus.

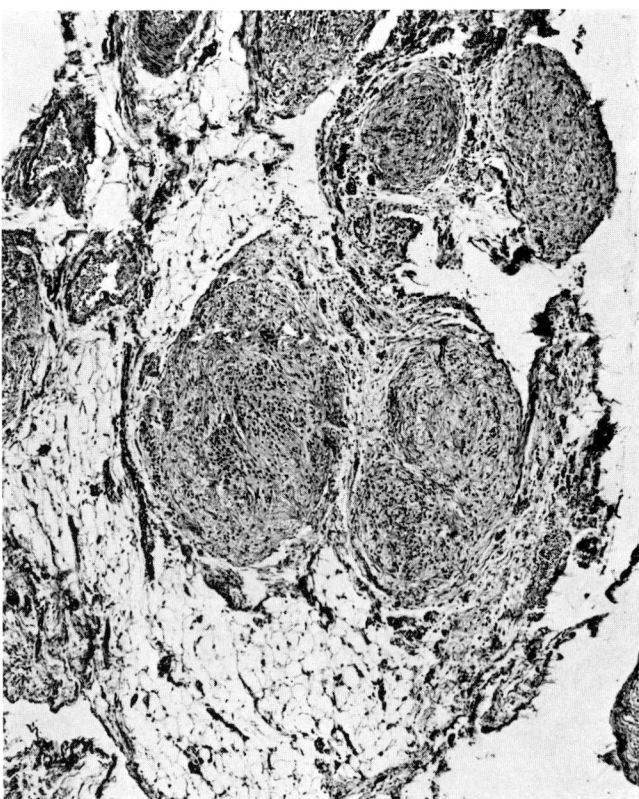

Fig. 20.45. **Mature solid teratoma.** Mature glial implants on omentum.

neoplasm. It occurs relatively frequently and comprises from 5% to 25% of all ovarian neoplasms,[235] usually in excess of 10%.[37,126,196,235] Mature cystic teratoma occurs most commonly during the reproductive years, but, unlike other germ cell tumors of the ovary, it has a wider age distribution and may be encountered at any age from infancy to old age.[50,235] In some series, more than 25% of cases have been observed in postmenopausal women.[187]

Mature cystic teratoma is often discovered as an incidental finding on physical examination, radiologic examination, or at abdominal operation performed for other indications. When symptoms are present, they are usually abdominal pain (47.6%), abdominal mass or swelling (15.4%), and abnormal uterine bleeding (15.1%).[235] The abdominal pain is usually constant, slight, or moderate but, in a number of cases, may be severe and acute because of torsion or rupture of the tumor. This tends to occur more commonly when the tumor is large. The abnormal uterine bleeding and its relief after excision of the tumor suggests hormone synthesis by the tumor but histologic examination has failed to reveal any explanation for the endocrine function.[187] Decreased fertility has been observed in patients with mature cystic teratoma of the ovary,[37,126] but in most cases there is no satisfactory explanation. In 10% of cases, the tumor is diagnosed during pregnancy.[50] Mature cystic

teratoma has been diagnosed radiologically because of the presence of teeth, bone, and cartilage[187,235] (Fig. 20.46).

Gross Findings

Mature cystic teratoma does not have a predilection for either ovary; 8–15% of cases are bilateral.[235] The tumor varies in size from very small (0.5 cm across) to large (measuring more than 40 cm) and weighing several kilograms. Approximately 60% of mature cystic teratomas measure from 5 to 10 cm across, and more than 90% measure less than 15 cm across.[235] The tumor is round, oval, or globular, with a smooth, gray-white, glistening surface (Fig. 20.46). It is usually freely mobile but occasionally may form adhesions to the surrounding structures, especially if there has been leakage of the contents. On palpation, the tumor is soft and fluctuant, with firm or hard areas. This is usually observed immediately after its removal, since at room temperature the tumor tends to solidify. The contents of the tumor are liquid at temperatures above 34°C and become solid at temperatures below 25°C.[37] The cut surface of the tumor reveals a cavity filled with fatty material and hair surrounded by a firm capsule of varying thickness. The fatty material is similar to normal sebum.[372] The tumor is usually unilocular but may be

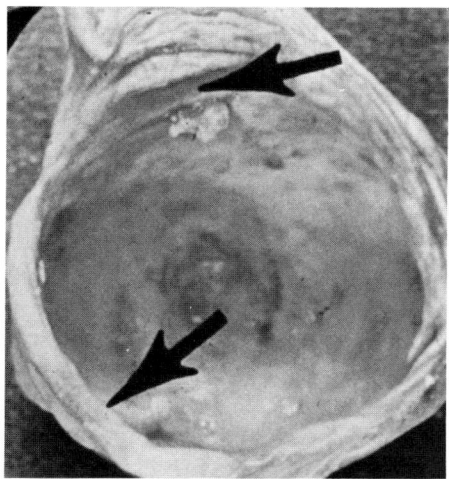 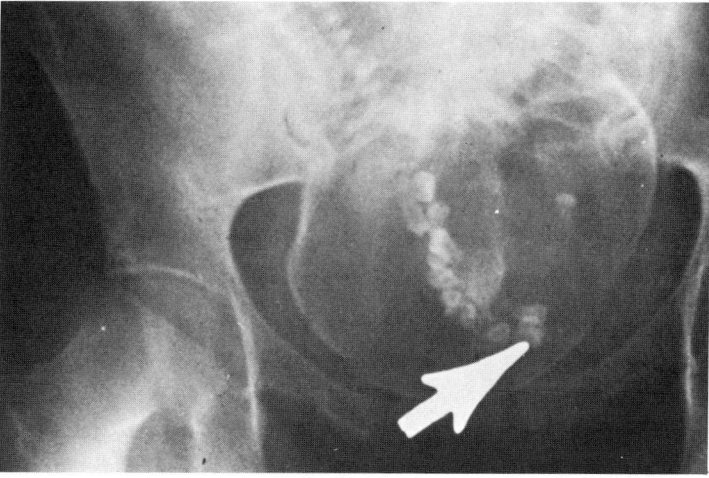

Fig. 20.46. Mature cystic teratoma. *Left:* Well-encapsulated spherical cystic mass. *Arrows* point to teeth. *Right:* Tumor produced dystocia and was diagnosed by pelvimetry. A row of teeth is seen at *arrow tip*. (Courtesy of A. Blaustein, M.D.)

multilocular. Several tumors may be present in the same ovary. Arising from the cyst wall and projecting into the cavity is a protuberance that may vary in size from a small nodule to a rounded elevated mass. It is usually single but may be multiple. It is frequently solid but may be partly cystic. This protuberance has been variously termed *dermoid mamilla, dermoid protuberance, Rokitansky protuberance, embryonic node,* or *dermoid nipple.* The hair present in the tumor arises from this protuberance, and when bone or teeth are present they tend to be located within this area, which is composed of a variety of different tissues and is one of the sites that should always be carefully sampled. Mature cystic teratomas contain macroscopically recognizable and well-formed teeth in 31% of cases.[37] Phalanges, long and other bones, parts of the rib cage, loops of intestine, and even fetus-like structures are occasionally encountered.[1,18,371]

MICROSCOPIC FINDINGS

The outer side of the cyst wall is composed of ovarian stroma that may often be hyalinized, making its recognition difficult. The cavity of the cyst is lined mainly by skin, and in small tumors cutaneous structures may form the entire lining. The skin is composed of keratinized squamous epithelium (Figs. 20.47, 20.48) and usually contains abundant sebaceous and sweat glands (Fig. 20.47). Hair and other dermal appendages are usually present. Occasionally, the cyst wall may be lined by bronchial or gastrointestinal epithelium or epithelium of columnar or cuboidal type. The squamous epithelium may be present only in the region of the dermoid protuberance. Sometimes, there may be loss of the lining epithelium caused by desquamation, and this may be associated with a foreign body giant cell reaction. The latter may be seen in other parts of the tumor

as a reaction to the contents of the tumor. Foreign body giant cell reaction may also be seen when the contents of the tumor are spilled, leading to the formation of adhesions. The area around the dermoid protuberance may contain a large variety of tissues derived from the three

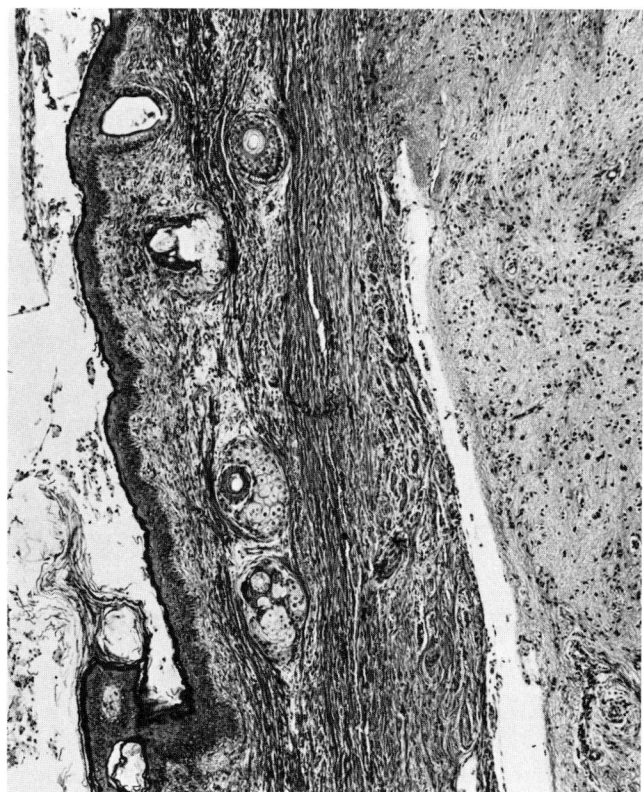

Fig. 20.47. Mature cystic teratoma. The lining of the cyst is composed of skin with its appendages. Mature neural tissue is seen beneath the cutaneous structures.

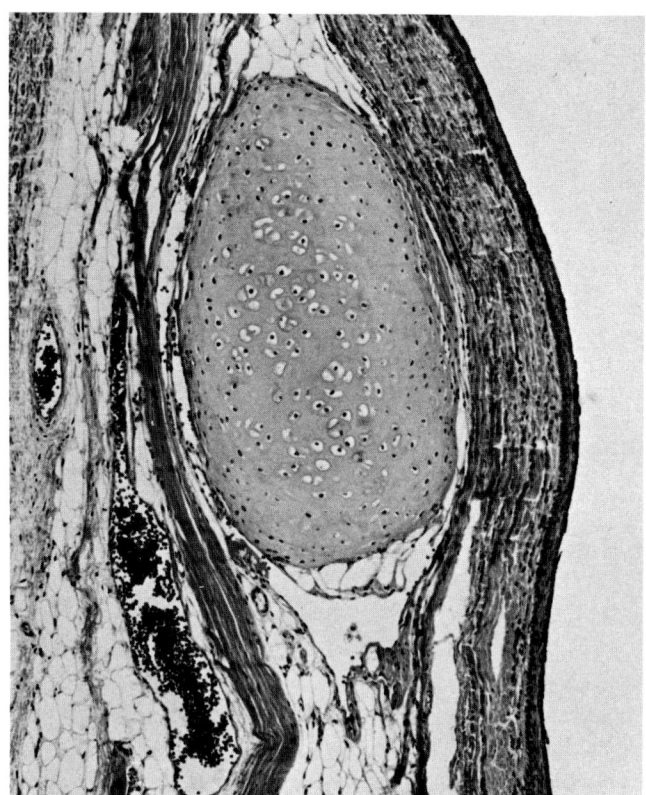

FIG. 20.48. **Mature cystic teratoma.** The tumor is lined by squamous epithelium and containing cartilage, muscle, and fatty tissue.

germ layers. Ectodermal tissue, represented by squamous epithelium and other skin derivatives, is usually most abundant. Brain tissue, glia, neural tissue, retina, choroid plexus, and ganglia may also be encountered. Mesodermal tissue is represented by bone, cartilage (Fig. 20.48), smooth muscle, and fibrous and fatty tissue. Endodermal tissue is represented by gastrointestinal and bronchial epithelium and glands, thyroid, and salivary gland tissue. In a careful study of 100 cases, ectodermal structures were found in 100%, mesodermal in 93%, and endodermal in 71% of cases.[37] The various tissues present in mature cystic teratoma show an orderly organoid arrangement forming cutaneous, bronchial, and gastrointestinal tissues, as well as bone and other structures. Although these tissues may be scattered diffusely, they do not exhibit the disorderly haphazard arrangement that is observed in immature teratoma.

With the exception of thyroid tissue, the presence of endocrine tissue of other types is distinctly uncommon in mature cystic teratoma, but pituitary, adrenal, and parathyroid tissue have been documented. Occasionally functioning endocrine tissue, forming an adenoma, may be found in a mature cystic teratoma.

Mature cystic teratoma must be differentiated from the rare cases of fetus in fetu, considered most likely to be caused by an inclusion of a monozygotic diamniotic twin.

Fetus in fetu can be distinguished from a teratoma by its location in the retroperitoneal space, presence of vertebral organization with formation of limb buds, and a well-developed organ system. Fetus in fetu shows better organization than the most differentiated teratomas.[120,178] Like mature cystic teratoma, fetus in fetu is a benign lesion.

CLINICAL BEHAVIOR

Mature cystic teratoma of the ovary may be associated with various complications. In view of the fact that in many of these cases the condition is amenable to cure, their recognition is of considerable importance. These complications include (1) torsion, (2) rupture, (3) infection, (4) hemolytic anemia, and (5) development of malignancy.

Torsion is the most frequent complication,[50,225,235] occurring in 16.1% of cases in one large series.[235] This complication tends to be more common during pregnancy and puerperium.[187,235] Mature cystic teratoma is said to comprise from 22% to 40% of ovarian tumors in pregnancy, and from 0.8% to 12.8% of reported cases of mature cystic teratoma have occurred in pregnancy.[50,235] The fact that these tumors, when they occur during pregnancy, are more liable to be associated with this complication is of considerable importance. Torsion is also more common in children and younger patients.[225,235] The patients usually have severe acute abdominal pain, and the condition is an acute abdominal emergency. Excision of the affected ovary or salpingo-oophorectomy is the treatment of choice.

Torsion tends to predispose to rupture of the tumor. Rupture of mature cystic teratoma is an uncommon complication, occurring in approximately 1% of cases.[187,235] It is much more common during pregnancy and may manifest itself during labor.[187,235] The immediate result of the rupture may be shock or hemorrhage, especially during pregnancy or labor, but the prognosis even in these cases is usually favorable. Rupture of the tumor into the peritoneal cavity may be followed by chemical peritonitis caused by the spillage of the contents of the tumor. It produces a marked granulomatous reaction and leads to the formation of dense adhesions throughout the peritoneal cavity. Rupture of the tumor occasionally may be followed by the development of glial implants on the peritoneum. This occurs when the tumor contains mature neuroglial elements, and spillage leads to deposition of numerous small nodules composed of mature glia in the peritoneal cavity. Despite the wide dissemination of these deposits throughout the peritoneal cavity, the prognosis is favorable, and simple surgical excision of the primary tumor is considered to be adequate therapy.[253] Mature cystic teratoma may rupture not only into the peritoneal cavity but also into adjacent organs, usually the bladder or the rectum. More than 30 such cases have been reported.[66]

Infection is an uncommon complication and occurs in approximately 1% of cases.[187] The infecting organism is usually a coliform, but *Salmonella* infection causing typhoid fever has also been reported.[129]

Autoimmune hemolytic anemia has been noted occasionally in patients with teratoma of the ovary, mainly mature cystic teratoma. Excision of the tumor in these cases resulted in the disappearance of the anemia and a complete cure.[23,32,67,68,231] Nineteen cases of mature cystic teratoma and seven other cystic ovarian tumors associated with this complication have been reported.[32,231] The patients have symptoms and signs of progressive anemia, which may be moderate or severe. It is accompanied by reticulocytosis, spherocytosis, and increased osmotic fragility. Normoblasts may be present in the peripheral blood. The indirect serum bilirubin is elevated, and the direct antiglobulin test (Coombs test) is positive, indicating the presence of autoantibodies that react with the patient's red blood cells. The platelets are normal in number. The spleen may be palpable but is only slightly enlarged. Steroids are only transiently effective in treating the disease, and splenectomy has no effect on the progress of the disease.[32,231] Excision of the ovarian tumor leads to the permanent disappearance of the anemia.[32,67,68,231] The following possible pathogenetic mechanisms have been suggested[32]:

1. presence in the tumor of substances that are antigenically different from the host and that stimulate the production by the host of antibodies, which cross-react with her own red blood cells
2. antibody production by the tumor directed specifically against the host's red blood cells resembling the graft-versus-host reaction
3. coating of red blood cells with products secreted by the tumor, resulting in changed red blood cell antigenicity.

In view of this, pelvic and radiologic examination is indicated in a young woman with autoimmune hemolytic anemia that does not respond to steroid treatment, as it may help to detect an ovarian teratoma and prevent an unnecessary splenectomy.[67,231,278]

TREATMENT

The treatment of choice for an uncomplicated mature cystic teratoma in young patients is excision of the cyst with conservation of a part of the ovary if possible. This treatment usually results in a complete cure. Local recurrences after conservative treatment for mature cystic teratoma are uncommon and occur in less than 1% of cases.[81]

Mature Cystic Teratoma (Dermoid Cyst) with Malignant Transformation

GENERAL FEATURES

Malignant transformation is an uncommon complication of mature cystic teratoma. It occurs in approximately 2% of

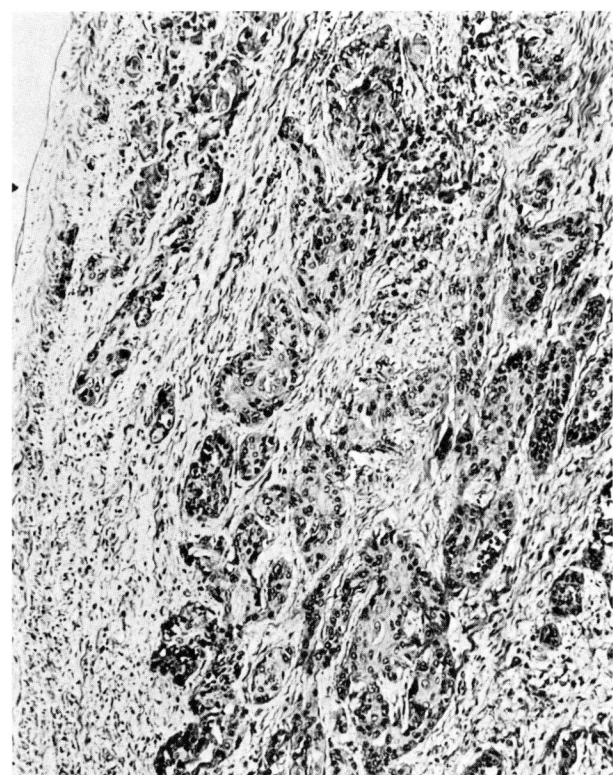

FIG. 20.49. **Squamous cell carcinoma arising in a mature cystic teratoma.** Surface of the ovary is seen at *top left*.

cases,[57,163,187,234,235,303] although in one report the frequency was almost 4%.[226] The age of patients with this complication as reported in the literature ranges from 19 to 88 years,[235] but this tumor usually is observed in postmenopausal patients.[*]

Clinically, this tumor cannot be readily differentiated from an uncomplicated mature cystic teratoma or other ovarian tumor, although evidence of its rapid growth, pain, loss of weight, and other systemic symptoms suggest the presence of a malignant tumor. Sometimes, the tumor may be found as an incidental observation. We have encountered, at autopsy, a large mature cystic teratoma containing a squamous cell carcinoma (Fig. 20.49) in a 56-year-old woman.

GROSS FINDINGS

The tumor is frequently larger than an average mature cystic teratoma.[50,163,303] It may exhibit a more solid appearance, but differentiation cannot be made on gross examination. Malignant transformation in mature cystic teratoma tends to occur in patients with unilateral tumors.[16,234,235]

---

*Refs. 57,153,163,187,226,234,235,303.

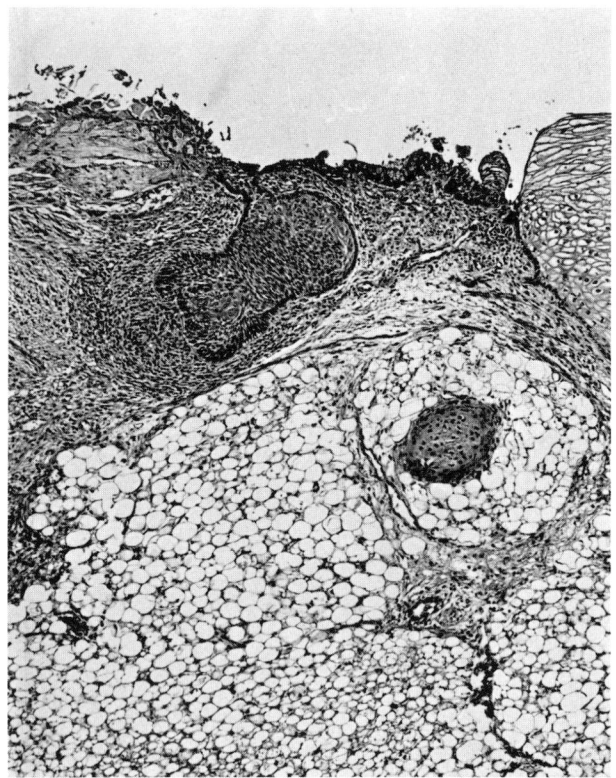

Fig. 20.50. Basal cell carcinoma arising in a mature cystic teratoma.

Microscopic Findings

The tumor exhibits malignant transformation in one of its constituent tissues, most frequently the squamous epithelium (Fig. 20.49), with formation of a typical squamous cell carcinoma.[50,57,163,226,234,303] Any of the tissues present in a mature cystic teratoma may undergo malignant transformation, and a variety of malignant tumors have been reported, including carcinoid tumor, thyroid carcinoma, basal cell carcinoma (Fig. 20.50), adenocarcinoma of the intestinal epithelium, malignant melanoma, leiomyosarcoma, and chondrosarcoma.* The malignant element invades other parts of the tumor and its wall (Fig. 20.49), which it tends to perforate. Invariably, only one tissue element becomes malignant, and the presence of many different malignant elements indicates that the tumor is an immature teratoma and not a mature cystic teratoma that has undergone malignant transformation.

Clinical Behavior and Treatment

The mode of spread of the malignant tumor differs from that observed in other tumors of germ cell origin. The

---

*Refs. 57,85,153,187,190,234,235,303,363,382.

tumor spreads by direct invasion and peritoneal implantation and generally does not metastasize to the lymph nodes.[163,234] Extensive local invasion and absence of lymph node involvement usually is observed at laparotomy.[226,303] Hematogenous dissemination is uncommon.

The prognosis of patients with mature cystic teratoma with malignant transformation is unfavorable.[57,163,226,234,235,303] There are only 15–30.8% 5-year survivors.[163,234,235] Better prognosis has been reported when the malignant element is a squamous cell carcinoma confined to the ovary and is excised without spillage of the contents. In such cases the 5-year survival is 63%.[234] Although previous reports have indicated that there have been no 5-year survivors when the malignant element was an adenocarcinoma or a sarcoma, Ueda et al[363] recently reported a case of a patient with an adenocarcinoma arising in a mature cystic teratoma, who has survived for more than 15 years. The authors also cite a number of other cases, but include thyroid and sebaceous carcinomas, which are usually considered separate entities. The present author has seen a patient with an intestinal-type adenocarcinoma arising in a mature cystic teratoma, who has survived for more than 5 years. The outlook with this type of neoplasm may not be as dismal as previously believed, especially if there is no evidence of metastases at presentation.

Treatment is hysterectomy and bilateral adnexectomy.[163,303] Since the tumors are usually unilateral, however, in cases where there is no penetration of the capsule and no involvement of the adjacent structures, a more conservative surgical procedure may be just as effective. However, since malignant transformation of a mature cystic teratoma almost always occurs in postmenopausal women, total abdominal hysterectomy and bilateral salpingo-oophorectomy is the treatment of choice. If the tumor has spread beyond the confines of the ovary and there is involvement of the adjacent structures, a more radical procedure with resection of the tumor and the involved structures or viscera is advocated.[226] Response to radiation and chemotherapy is unsatisfactory.[163,226]

Struma Ovarii

General Features

Thyroid tissue is a relatively frequent constituent of mature cystic teratoma and has been demonstrated in 5–20% of cases.[278,279] Struma ovarii is considered a one-sided development of a teratoma, in which the thyroid tissue has overgrown all other tissues, or one in which only the thyroid tissue has developed. The term *struma ovarii* should be reserved only for tumors composed either entirely or predominantly of thyroid tissue or for those in which thyroid tissue can be recognized macroscopically.

CLINICAL FEATURES

Struma ovarii is uncommon; it comprises 2.7% of ovarian teratomas.[121] The age distribution of patients with struma ovarii is generally the same as that of patients with mature cystic teratoma and ranges from 6 to 74 years. Most patients are in the reproductive years.[64,208,295,385,387] There are usually no specific symptoms; the clinical findings are similar to those observed in patients with mature cystic teratoma. The only differences are that in some cases struma ovarii is associated with enlargement of the thyroid gland, and in other cases there is clinical evidence that the struma ovarii is responsible for the development of thyrotoxicosis, although this has not been confirmed preoperatively by laboratory tests.[208,278,295,387] Some cases of thyrotoxicosis have been associated with struma ovarii, which has also shown evidence of thyroid hyperactivity.[121,263] The ectopic thyroid tissue present within struma ovarii, therefore, may be the subject of the same physiological and pathological changes as the thyroid gland.[80,245,295]

GROSS FINDINGS

Struma ovarii usually is unilateral.[64,208,387] In one report, the contralateral ovary also contained a teratoma and this tumor contained thyroid tissue in some of the cases.[295] Struma ovarii is often associated with mature cystic teratomas and rarely with a cystadenoma.[208,295,387]

Struma ovarii varies in size but usually measures less than 10 cm in diameter. It tends to be larger if it is associated with other elements. The surface is usually smooth and, before sectioning, the tumor shows similar appearances to mature cystic teratoma. Occasionally, adhesions may be present. The cut surface of the tumor may be composed entirely of light tan, glistening thyroid (Fig. 20.51) tissue or may consist of thyroid tissue associated with other tissues. Hemorrhage, necrosis, and foci of fibro-

sis may be present. Solid tumors with small amounts of colloid appear less glistening and more fleshy.

MICROSCOPIC FINDINGS

The tumor is composed of mature thyroid tissue consisting of acini of various sizes, lined by a single layer of columnar or flattened epithelium (Fig. 20.52). The acini contain eosinophilic, PAS-positive colloid. The intensity of the staining may vary. There may be a considerable variation in the size of the acini, which may be large, containing a large amount of colloid, or may be small. Thyroglobulin can be identified in the epithelial cells by immunohistochemistry. Occasionally, the lining of the acini may be columnar, containing small papillary projections not unlike those seen in hyperactive thyroid gland. Sometimes the appearances may resemble a nodular adenomatous goiter. Adenoma-like lesions may also be observed. Struma ovarii showing appearances suggestive of Hashimoto's thyroiditis has also been reported.[82]

CLINICAL BEHAVIOR AND TREATMENT

Most cases of struma ovarii are benign and can be treated by excision of the ovary or by unilateral salpingo-oophorectomy. In a small number of cases, there are complications, the most important being the development of malignancy and the presence of ascites or ascites associated with pleu-

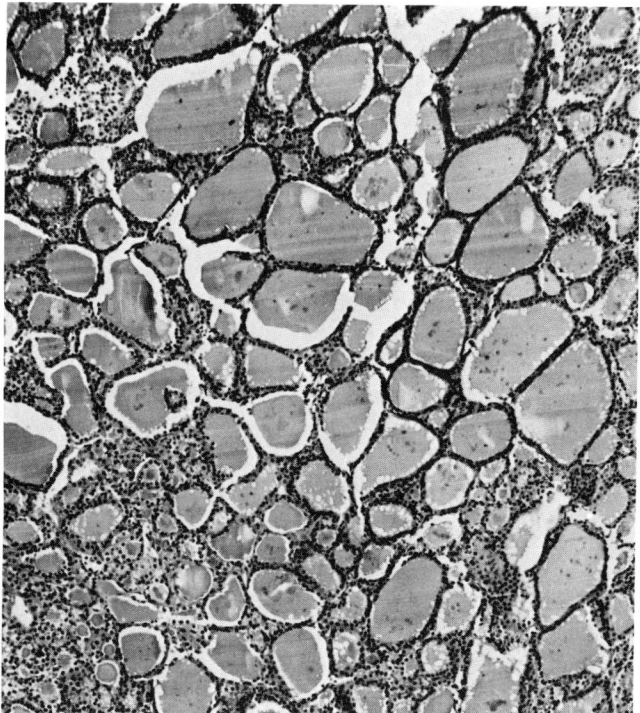

FIG. 20.52. **Struma ovarii.** The tumor is composed of normal thyroid tissue.

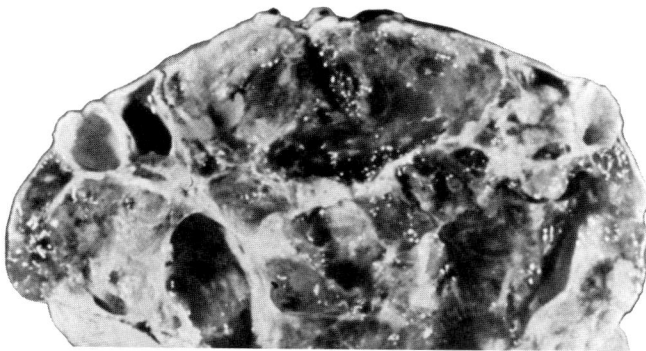

FIG. 20.51. **Struma ovarii.** The cut surface shows compartments of amber-colored thyroid tissue separated by thick fibrous septae. (Courtesy of B. Bigelow, M.D., New York, NY.)

ral effusion producing a pseudo-Meigs' syndrome.[150,278] Ascites may be found in 17% of cases of struma ovarii, and its presence does not indicate that the tumor is malignant.[295] The cause of the ascites and pleural effusion has not been fully elucidated. In most reported cases, excision of the tumor led to complete remission.[278]

Malignant change in struma ovarii is uncommon. In a number of reported cases, the diagnosis was based on the histology of the tumor, and there were no metastases or other features of malignancy. The diagnosis of malignancy is difficult in such cases. The tumor must be extensively sampled. The criteria for malignancy in struma ovarii are the same as those for thyroid tumors. This applies mainly to the tumors showing a follicular pattern, as papillary carcinomas occurring in struma ovarii are much easier to diagnose.

A number of reported cases of malignant struma ovarii were examples of strumal carcinoid.[278,279] Only 17 of 45 reported cases of malignant struma ovarii were associated with metastases.[114,208,278,279,387] Malignant struma ovarii often shows a follicular pattern, but papillary carcinoma is not infrequent. We have encountered a 26-year-old patient with a mature cystic teratoma containing thyroid tissue and a typical well-differentiated papillary adenocarcinoma of the thyroid (Fig. 20.53), which was associated with metastases in the para-aortic lymph nodes. The patient was

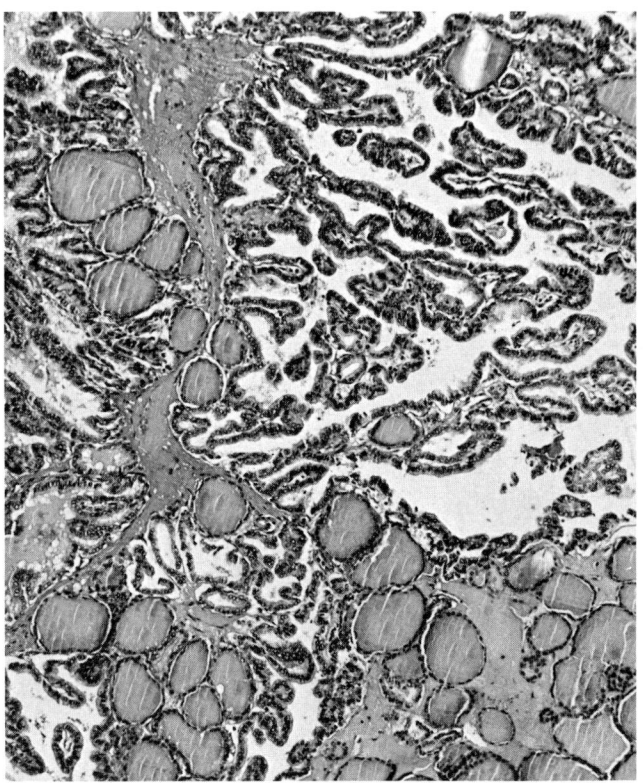

FIG. 20.53. Papillary thyroid carcinoma in mature cystic teratoma.

well and symptom-free 3½ years after excision of the tumor followed by laparotomy and dissection of the para-aortic lymph nodes, as well as a course of radiation therapy. There was no evidence of metastases elsewhere. In three other cases of papillary carcinoma developing in struma ovarii known to the author, the patients were cured by the excision of the affected adnexa, although in a fourth case the patient died with extensive metastatic disease.

Malignant struma ovarii may involve the peritoneum. The tumor deposits, which are composed of malignant thyroid tissue, should not be confused with deposits of benign thyroid tissue representing peritoneal spread of nonmalignant struma ovarii (see below, benign strumosis).[278,279] Occasionally, the distinction between these entities may pose considerable difficulties, especially when the malignant neoplasm is of the well-differentiated follicular type. Other routes of spread are via the lymphatics to the para-aortic and other lymph nodes and via the bloodstream to the lungs and bones. The prognosis in cases unassociated with metastases is generally good, but when metastases are present, it is less favorable. Treatment consists of surgery and administration of radioactive iodine (^{131}I) and other agents used in the treatment of thyroid malignancy, including radiation therapy.

Occasionally, struma ovarii may be associated with extraovarian extension caused either by rupture of the tumor or by local spread. In such cases, the peritoneal cavity contains tumor deposits, which may be numerous and are composed of mature thyroid tissue. The condition is benign and is termed *benign strumosis*.[278,279] It is only rarely associated with untoward side effects, which are mainly due to the formation of adhesions. Benign strumosis may be treated by excision of the tumor deposits or by administration of radioactive iodine (^{131}I).

Carcinoid

Carcinoid tumors of the ovary may be primary or metastatic. Primary carcinoids are subdivided into four categories: (1) insular or islet, (2) trabecular, (3) mucinous, and (4) mixed (composed of any combination of the three pure types). The latter are rare and usually are associated with a mature cystic teratoma. Thus far all have behaved in a benign fashion.

Of the metastatic carcinoids, the insular carcinoid tumor is the most common, followed by the trabecular and mucinous types. The metastatic carcinoid tumors of the ovary are discussed in Chapter 22, Metastatic Tumors of the Ovary.

Insular or Islet Carcinoid

GENERAL FEATURES

Insular carcinoid tumor, considered to be of mid-gut derivation, is the most common type of primary ovarian carcinoid tumor. It usually arises in association with gastrointestinal or respiratory epithelium present in a mature cystic teratoma. It may also be observed within a solid teratoma, a mucinous tumor, in association with a Sertoli–Leydig cell tumor,[391] or may occur in a pure form.[255,278,282,318,358] The latter is considered to arise either as a one-sided development of a teratoma or from enterochromaffin cells present within the ovary. The former is considered more likely. Approximately 40% of ovarian insular carcinoids occur in pure form; the remaining 60% are combined.[318]

CLINICAL FEATURES

More than 70 cases of primary ovarian insular carcinoid tumors have been reported.[255] The author is aware of an even greater number of unreported cases. The age of patients ranges from 31 to 79 years, but most patients are either postmenopausal or perimenopausal.[255,282] One-third of the reported cases have been associated with the typical carcinoid syndrome, despite the absence of metastases.[248,255] This is in contrast with intestinal carcinoids, which are associated with the syndrome only when there is metastatic spread to the liver. One reason for this difference is that the blood flow from the ovary goes directly into the systemic circulation and does not pass through the liver, which inactivates the serotonin produced by the tumor. The presence or absence of symptoms of carcinoid syndrome is also dependent on the number of secreting tumor cells. Functioning ovarian carcinoid tumors have all measured approximately 10 cm in diameter (with only one exception[268]), whereas intestinal carcinoids are usually smaller. Thus, there is a good correlation between the size of the tumor and the presence of carcinoid syndrome. The excision of the tumor is associated with rapid remission of the symptoms, disappearance of 5-hydroxyindole acetic acid (5-HIAA) from the urine,[255] and marked decrease of serum serotonin. Determination of serum serotonin and urinary 5-HIAA may be used to monitor disease activity and response to therapy. If the tumor is nonfunctioning, there is no specific presentation.

GROSS FINDINGS

The tumor shows similar appearances to those of mature cystic teratoma within which it is usually found. The same applies if the tumor is associated with a solid teratoma or a mucinous tumor. If the carcinoid is not associated with other tissue elements, the tumor is solid. The carcinoid may vary in size from microscopic to 20 cm in longest diameter and is solid and homogeneous (Fig. 20.54). Its color may vary from light brown to yellow or pale gray. Primary ovarian carcinoids practically always are unilateral, although they may be associated with a benign cystic teratoma in the contralateral ovary.

MICROSCOPIC FINDINGS

The primary ovarian carcinoid usually shows the typical appearance associated with midgut carcinoids.[255,379] The tumor is composed of collections of small acini and solid nests of uniform polygonal cells with ample amounts of cytoplasm and round or oval, centrally located hyperchromatic nuclei (Fig. 20.55). Mitotic activity is low. The cytoplasm is basophilic or amphophilic and may contain red, brown, or orange argentaffin (Fig. 20.56) or argyrophil granules, which are demonstrated in the great majority of cases of primary ovarian carcinoids.[255] Ultrastructurally, the cells of the ovarian insular carcinoid show similar appearances to those of insular carcinoid tumors from other locations[318,358] and show abundant neurosecretory granules, which exhibit marked variation in size and shape, being round, oval, or elongated. Serotonin may be demonstrated within the cytoplasm of the tumor cells by immunoperoxidase techniques.[301] Demonstration of positive Chromogranin A staining immunocytochemically further

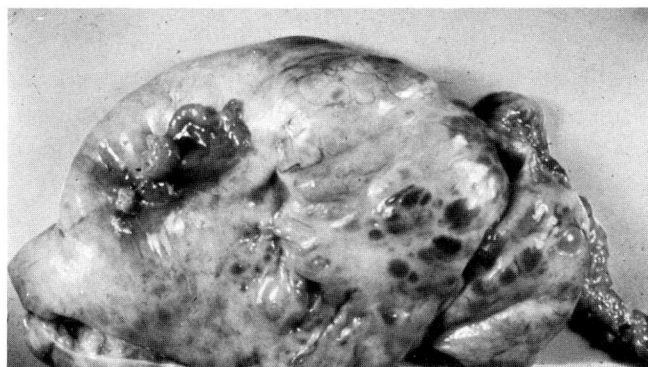
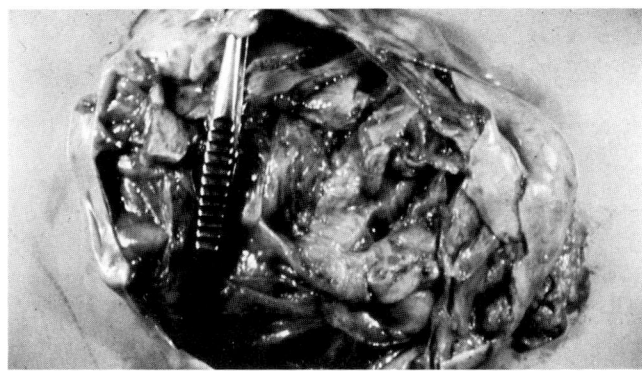

FIG. 20.54. Primary carcinoid. *Left:* It is oval-shaped and encapsulated. *Right:* The cut surface is yellow to brown and largely cystic. (Courtesy of B. Bigelow, M.D., New York, NY.)

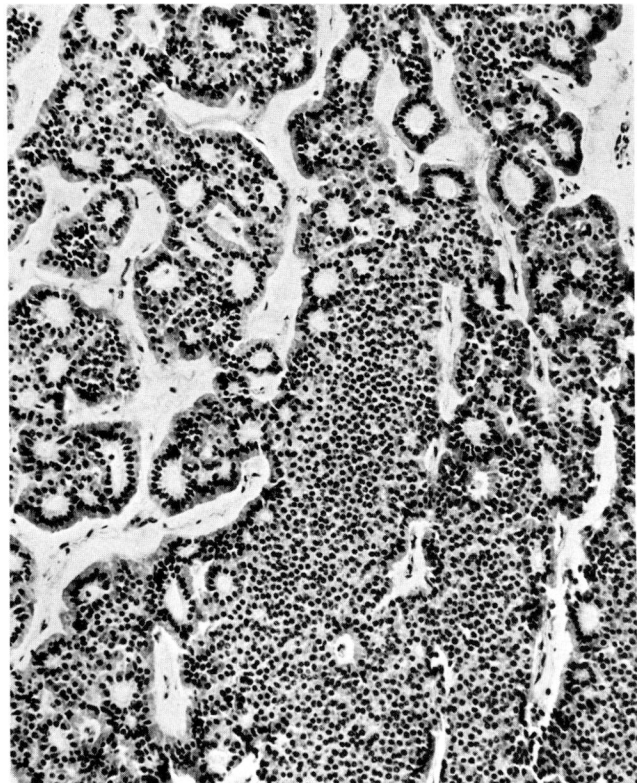

Fig. 20.55. Primary ovarian carcinoid. The typical solid and acinar patterns of midgut carcinoid are shown.

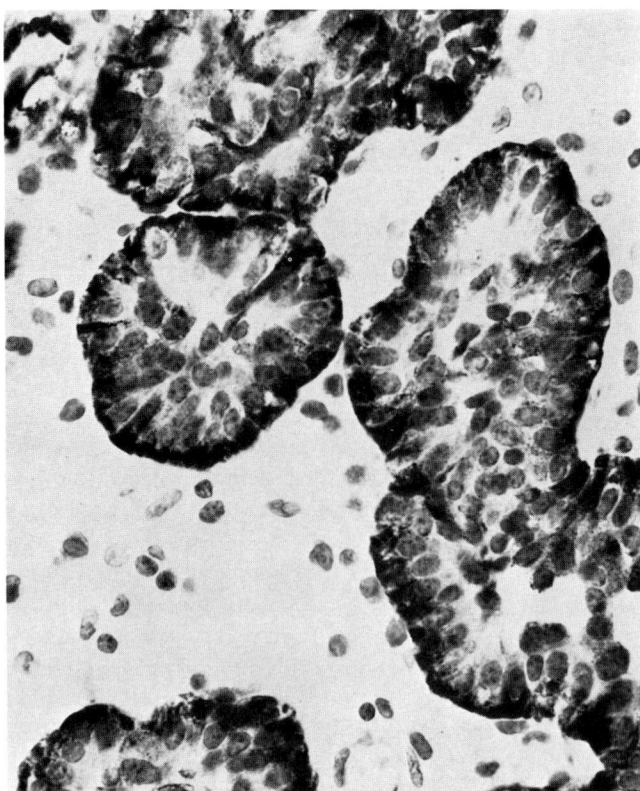

Fig. 20.56. Ovarian carcinoid. The tumor cells contain numerous argentaffin granules stained black.

supports the diagnosis, and has become the method of choice to confirm the diagnosis.

Occasionally, other neurohormonal peptides may also be demonstrated within the cytoplasm of the tumor cells, but their finding is much less frequent than in trabecular or strumal carcinoids.[301] The connective tissue surrounding the tumor nests is frequently dense and hyalinized because the fibrogenic effect of the serotonin produced by the tumor.

DIFFERENTIAL DIAGNOSIS

Primary carcinoid of the ovary must be differentiated from metastatic carcinoid of the ovary, which is usually of gastrointestinal origin. Metastatic carcinoids nearly always affect both ovaries,[256,290] unlike primary ovarian carcinoid, which is unilateral.[255] Macroscopically, the metastatic carcinoid is composed of tumor nodules, whereas primary ovarian carcinoid forms a single homogeneous mass. Other teratomatous elements associated with an ovarian carcinoid, confirm that it is primary.[255]

Primary ovarian carcinoid sometimes may be confused with Brenner tumor, but the appearances of the cell nests and the grooved coffee-bean nuclei of the cells of Brenner tumor are against the diagnosis of a carcinoid, whereas the typical small acinar pattern and the presence of argyrophil- and argentaffin-positive cells, as well as positive Chromogranin A staining are in favor of a carcinoid.

Confusion with granulosa cell tumor may also arise because Call–Exner bodies may be confused with carcinoid acini, but the cells of the carcinoid tumor usually show an acinar pattern and contain more cytoplasm and argentaffin granules.[255,358] Cystic areas that may be present in a granulosa cell tumor are nearly always absent in a carcinoid.

Occasionally, ovarian carcinoid may be confused with a Krukenberg tumor, but the latter is usually bilateral and larger. The cells of Krukenberg tumor tend to merge with the stroma, are larger, and show greater pleomorphism, a signet-ring appearance, and more brisk mitotic activity. An acinar pattern is less evident. Demonstration of argyrophil and argentaffin granules, which can be detected in most ovarian carcinoids, confirms the diagnosis. Although these granules may be observed in some cells in Krukenberg tumors, they are much more numerous in ovarian carcinoids. These granules can be identified even more easily with the aid of the electron microscope, manifesting themselves as numerous pleomorphic neurosecretory granules present within the cytoplasm.[255,290,318,358] Chromogranin A stains further enhance their presence.

Clinical Behavior and Treatment

Although insular carcinoid tumors of the ovary are considered to be malignant, they are slow growing and are associated only occasionally with metastases. Metastasis has been observed in only five patients, and four of these patients died with metastatic disease.[90,255,282,287] In occasional patients, features of carcinoid syndrome, such as tricuspid incompetence resulting in right-sided heart failure, may progress after the excision of the tumor and lead to the death of the patient. This has been observed in two cases.[255] In the great majority of patients with the carcinoid syndrome, the symptoms and signs of the syndrome observed preoperatively disappear or regress during the postoperative period.[255]

Since nearly all patients with this tumor are postmenopausal or perimenopausal, bilateral salpingo-oophorectomy and hysterectomy is the treatment of choice. Surgical excision of foci of extraovarian spread or of metastases if present is indicated. The tumor does not respond to radiation therapy, and there is at present little experience with chemotherapy. Estimation of serum serotonin and 5-HIAA in the urine may be used to monitor the progress of the disease.

Trabecular Carcinoid

General Features

Trabecular carcinoid includes carcinoid tumors of hindgut or foregut derivation. Primary trabecular or ribbon carcinoid usually arises in association with teratomatous elements,[257] but of four cases of trabecular carcinoid seen by the author, two were pure and not associated with teratomatous elements.[321]

Clinical Features

Trabecular carcinoid is rare; only 21 cases have been reported. The age varies from 24 to 74 years, with most patients being postmenopausal.[257,321] Trabecular carcinoid is a slowly growing neoplasm that can reach a large size. None of the known cases have been associated with the carcinoid syndrome. In three patients whose urine was examined immediately after the operation, 5-HIAA was normal.[257]

Gross Findings

The appearance of trabecular carcinoid depends on whether the tumor is associated with teratomatous elements or not. When associated with teratoma, the appearance is similar to that of a mature cystic teratoma. When the tumor is pure, it is a solid, firm to hard, round or oval mass with a smooth outline and tan to yellow on cross-section (Fig. 20.57). The tumors have always been unilat-

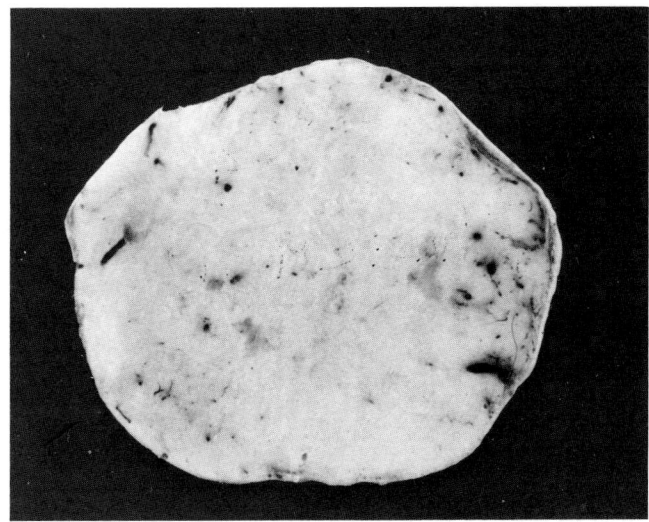

Fig. 20.57. **Pure trabecular carcinoid tumor of the ovary.** The cut surface is solid, uniform, and yellow. The outer surface is smooth.

eral[257,321] but occasionally have been associated with mature cystic teratoma in the opposite ovary.[257] In the reported cases, the tumors measured from 4 to 25 cm in the longest diameter.[257,321]

Microscopic Findings

The tumor is composed of long, usually wavy ribbons, cords, or parallel trabeculae surrounded by fibromatous connective tissue stroma that is usually dense (Fig. 20.58). The ribbons, cords, or trabeculae are composed of cells that are usually one but sometimes two cells thick (Fig. 20.58). The nuclei are elongated or ovoid and contain finely dispersed chromatin. The cytoplasm is abundant and often contains orange to red-brown granules, which usually stain with argyrophil and argentaffin stains. Ultrastructurally, the neurosecretory granules are round or oval and show slight variation in size,[257,290,318,324] and thus differ from those seen in insular carcinoids. Immunocytochemistry is positive for Chromogranin A and demonstrates a much wider range of neurohormonal polypeptides than insular carcinoids; these include serotonin, pancreatic polypeptide, glucagon, enkephalin, gastrin, vasoactive intestinal polypeptide, and calcitonin.[301]

Differential Diagnosis

Primary trabecular carcinoid must be distinguished from metastatic trabecular carcinoid, which is usually bilateral and frequently associated with metastases elsewhere. The presence of teratomatous elements, which are found frequently in the primary lesion, helps to distinguish the primary from a metastatic lesion. Trabecular carcinoid some-

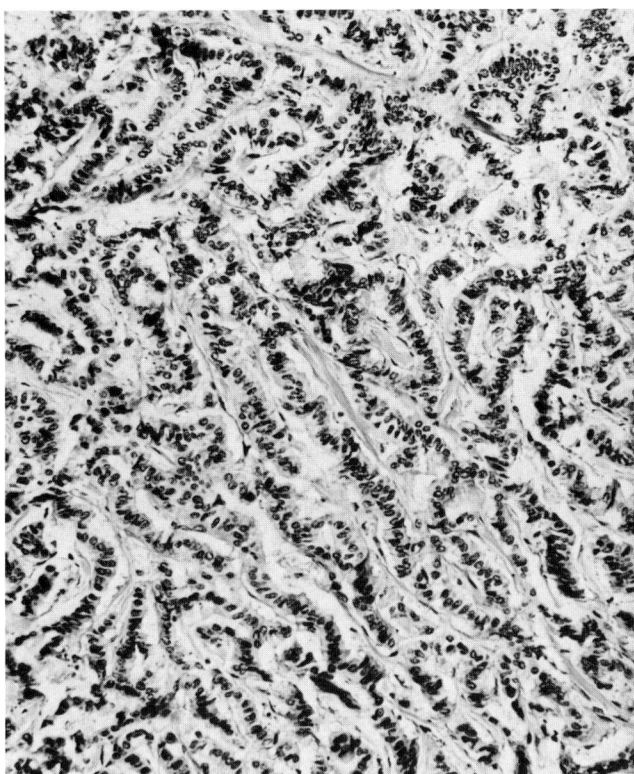

FIG. 20.58. Trabecular carcinoid. The tumor is composed of long ramifying cords of tumor cells surrounded by dense fibrous stroma.

times may exhibit an insular pattern in foci, but unless this is a major component the tumor need not be classified as a mixed carcinoid.

The presence of thyroid follicles indicates that the tumor is a struma ovarii and carcinoid (strumal carcinoid), and their presence must be excluded before a diagnosis of trabecular carcinoid is made. Occasionally, trabecular carcinoid must be distinguished from a Sertoli–Leydig cell tumor showing a cord-like pattern. In contrast to a Sertoli–Leydig tumor, trabecular carcinoid lacks tubules. The presence of argyrophil and argentaffin granules, positive Chromogranin A staining, and neurosecretory granules ultrastructurally confirm the diagnosis of carcinoid.

CLINICAL BEHAVIOR AND TREATMENT

The prognosis of patients with trabecular carcinoid of the ovary is favorable, since these tumors are not associated with metastases.[379] In one case, a peritoneal implant was found 2 years after bilateral salpingo-oophorectomy and hysterectomy.[257]

The optimal treatment is the excision of the affected adnexa, which results in a complete cure, but follow-up of the patient is advisable.

Mucinous Carcinoid

GENERAL FEATURES

Mucinous carcinoid is a relatively recently described variant of carcinoid tumor, which has been encountered mainly in the vermiform appendix[158,309,370] and occasionally has been observed in the ovary.[7,318] However, it should be noted that at least some of the tumors described as primary Krukenberg tumors of the ovary may have been examples of this entity. A number of cases of mucinous carcinoid tumor metastatic to the ovary have been reported.[130]

CLINICAL FEATURES

The age of patients ranges from 14 to 53 years. Mucinous carcinoid is usually observed in pure form but may be seen in association with mature cystic teratoma. The tumor is unilateral but may be associated with metastases in the contralateral ovary.[7,318]

GROSS FINDINGS

Macroscopically, the tumor is usually of considerable size, and most of the tumors have been more than 8 cm in the longest diameter. The tumor is gray-yellow, firm, and usually solid but may contain cystic areas.[7,318] Similar appearances are encountered when the tumor forms part of a mature cystic teratoma.

MICROSCOPIC FINDINGS

Microscopically, it is composed of numerous small glands or acini with very small lumens lined by uniform columnar or cuboid epithelium. The cells contain small round or oval nuclei or goblet cells distended with mucin (Fig. 20.59). Some cells may be disrupted by excessive distention with mucin. This may result in the formation of small pools of mucin within the glands or even in the obliteration of the gland with pools of mucinous material within the connective tissue (Fig. 20.60). The glands are surrounded by connective tissue, which may vary from loose and edematous to dense fibrous or hyalinized. Some of the glands or acini may be larger and occasionally may be cystic (Fig. 20.60). In some areas the tumor cells tend to invade the surrounding connective tissue, often assuming signet-ring appearance, and in these areas the tumor resembles a Krukenberg tumor. In some tumors, such appearances may predominate. The tumor cells may form large solid aggregates and show a less uniform appearance and more atypical features, with large hyperchromatic nuclei and brisk mitotic activity. The cytoplasm may exhibit orange-red granules and may even be bright red. Argyrophil and argentaffin granules are present and, in some tumors, may be

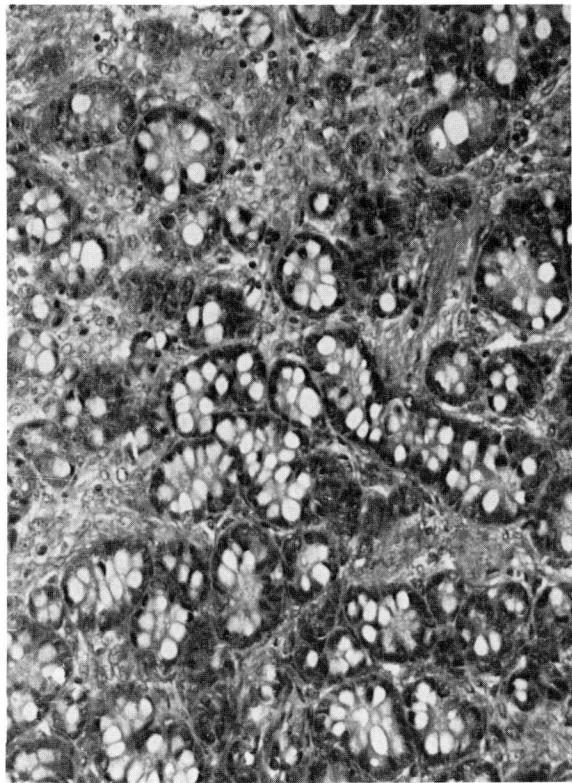

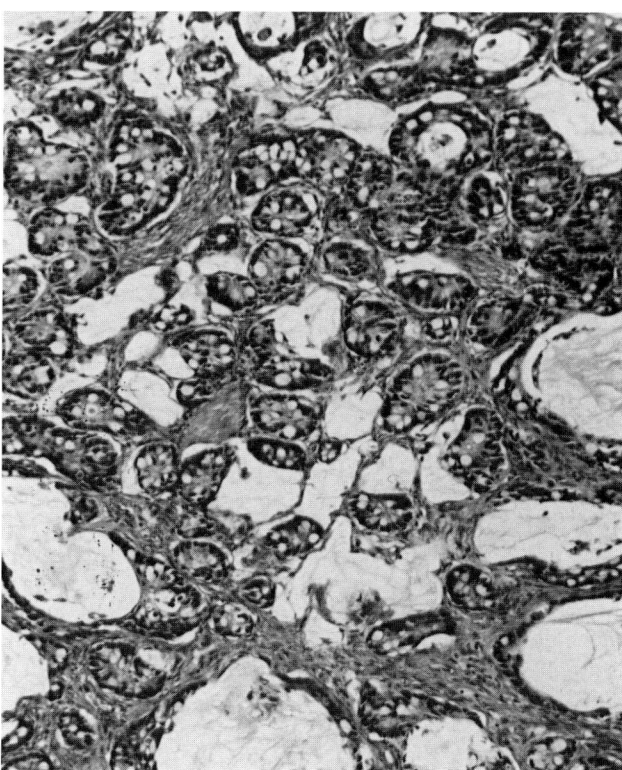

FIG. 20.59. **Mucinous carcinoid tumor.** The tumor is composed of numerous small glands and acini with imperceptible or very small lumens. Numerous goblet cells distended with mucin are present.

FIG. 20.60. **Mucinous carcinoid tumor.** The tumor is composed of small glands and acini. Many acini are disrupted by excessive distention with mucin, resulting in the formation of pools of mucin within the surrounding connective tissue. Larger glands distended with mucin also are present.

abundant, although in general they are seen less frequently than in other types of carcinoid tumors.[7,318,325]

Ultrastructurally, neurosecretory granules are present in some cells and absent in others. The tumor cells may contain both neurosecretory granules and mucinous material. Using immunocytochemical techniques, some of the tumor cells have been shown to contain serotonin and gastrin, and these substances may be present within the same tumor cell.[325] Other neurohormonal polypeptides such as pancreatic polypeptide and prolactin also have been detected in the tumor cells, but the range is narrower than that observed in trabecular carcinoids. CEA and low molecular weight cytokeratin also can be demonstrated within the cytoplasm of the tumor cells.

DIFFERENTIAL DIAGNOSIS

Primary mucinous carcinoid tumor of the ovary must be differentiated from its metastatic counterpart. The latter, in common with other types of carcinoid metastatic to the ovary, is nearly always bilateral and instead of forming a single tumor mass shows scattered tumor deposits involving ovarian tissue. Depending on their size, these deposits may form tumor nodules observed macroscopically or may be detectable only microscopically. Histologically, they may have appearances indistinguishable from the primary tumor.

Mucinous carcinoid must be distinguished from mucinous tumors of the ovary, especially when the carcinoid tumor is composed of large acini, shows increased mucin production, and exhibits a pleomorphic pattern. Occasionally, confusion may arise with well-differentiated endometrioid tumors of the ovary, which may resemble mucinous tumors.

Mucinous carcinoid must be distinguished from a Krukenberg tumor. The differentiation between these two entities may be difficult, especially if the mucinous carcinoid assumes a predominantly Krukenberg-like pattern or if the Krukenberg tumor contains numerous argentaffin and argyrophil granules. The presence of these granules as well as of the neurosecretory granules observed ultrastructurally cannot be used for differentiation between these two entities. Involvement of both ovaries and the presence of primary extraovarian signet-ring or mucinous adenocarcinoma are indicative of Krukenberg tumor.

CLINICAL BEHAVIOR AND TREATMENT

The primary mucinous carcinoid of the ovary behaves in a more aggressive manner than other types of primary ovarian carcinoid tumors.[7,318] This is similar to the behavior of mucinous carcinoid tumors of the vermiform appendix.[158,309,370] The tumor tends to spread mainly via the lymphatics, and metastases may be present at the time of initial laparotomy. Patients who do not exhibit metastatic disease at the time of diagnosis have much better prognosis compared with those who have metastases, however small, at the time of diagnosis.[7,318]

The treatment is surgical depending on the extent of the disease, but in postmenopausal patients, those with involvement of the contralateral ovary, and patients who do not want children, hysterectomy, bilateral salpingo-oophorectomy, and omentectomy, as well as excision of all the tumor deposits present, are indicated. Para-aortic lymph node dissection may be indicated, since metastatic tumor deposits may be present. Surgery may be followed by combination chemotherapy, including 5-fluorouracil, although the efficacy of this mode of therapy is not proved. Radiation therapy does not appear to be effective. Premenopausal patients with tumors localized to the ovary may be treated by unilateral salpingo-oophorectomy and carefully followed-up. Two such patients with pure mucinous carcinoid tumors and no evidence of metastases are well and disease-free for periods of 3 and 9 years, respectively, whereas two patients with similar tumors and intraabdominal metastases died of their disease within 2 years of diagnosis.

Strumal Carcinoid

GENERAL FEATURES

Strumal carcinoid is an uncommon ovarian tumor composed of thyroid tissue intimately admixed with carcinoid tumor, showing a ribbon or cord-like pattern. Other teratomatous elements are also present in most of the tumors.[254,279] It has become recognized as a separate entity only in recent years.[278,279,289] The histological pattern of struma ovarii, merging imperceptibly with carcinoid tumor that exhibits the ribbon-like pattern observed in hindgut carcinoids,[379] had been recognized previously.* However, it was usually interpreted as a carcinoma developing in a struma ovarii, although the resemblance to a carcinoid tumor was noted in some cases.[114,153]

CLINICAL FEATURES

More than 60 cases have been reported[254,299] and there are probably as many unreported cases. The age distribution is similar to struma ovarii, ranging from 21 to 77 years.[254,299] The tumor is usually not associated with any specific clinical findings. In one reported case it was associated with virilization.[74] Like hindgut carcinoids and unlike the primary ovarian insular carcinoid, strumal carcinoid is not as a rule associated with the carcinoid syndrome,[254,282,299] although this association has been described in a single case.[364]

GROSS FINDINGS

Macroscopically, this tumor, if pure, may be similar to struma ovarii or carcinoid. If the tumor is a part of a teratoma it manifests as a yellow nodule within the teratoma.[254,299]

MICROSCOPIC FINDINGS

Microscopically, the tumor is composed of thyroid follicles containing colloid that merge with ribbons of neoplastic cells usually set in dense fibrous tissue stroma similar to the trabecular carcinoid (Figs. 20.61, 20.62). The thyroid follicles are often small in size at the junction between the two

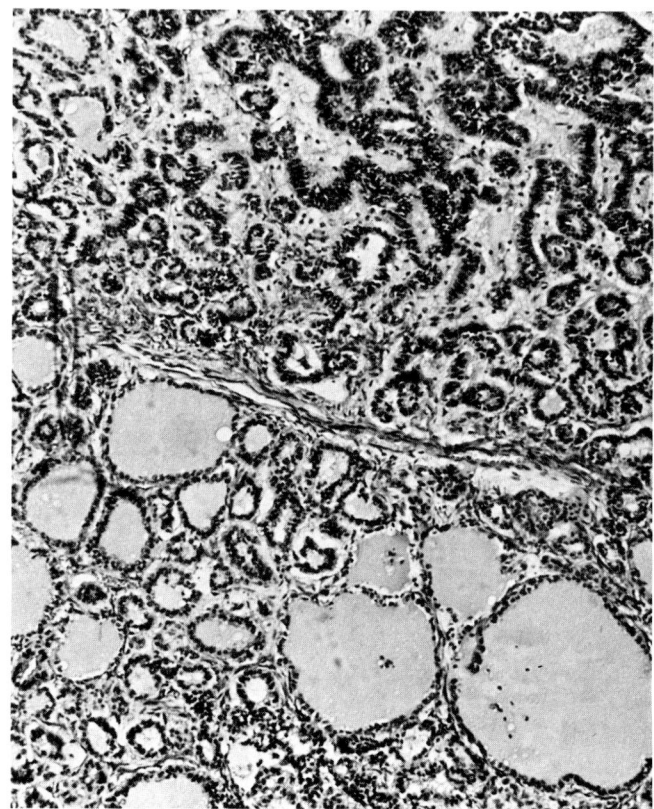

FIG. 20.61. Struma ovarii and carcinoid. The carcinoid forms long narrow cords and ribbons (*top*) merging with thyroid follicles (*bottom*).

---

*Refs. 114,132,153,245,385,387.

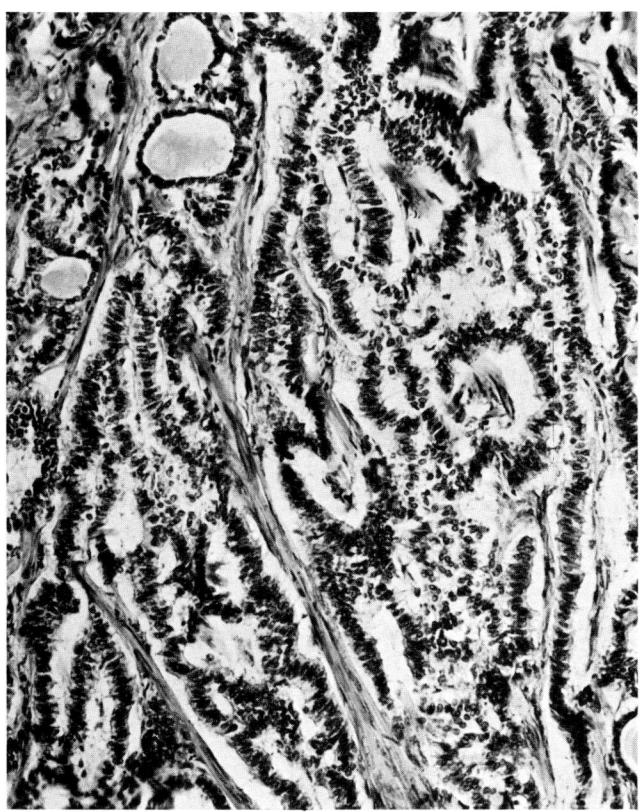

FIG. 20.62. **Struma ovarii and carcinoid.** The carcinoid is composed of columnar or cuboidal epithelial cells forming narrow winding cords and ribbons. Thyroid follicles also are seen.

types of tissue. The carcinoid is usually composed of long, winding or straight ribbons of columnar cells with elongated hyperchromatic nuclei (Fig. 20.60). It may also be composed of small islands of tumor cells surrounded by dense fibrous tissue stroma (Fig. 20.61). Slight mitotic activity is present in the carcinoid part of the lesion.

Argyrophil and argentaffin granules are identified in the carcinoid cells,[12,278,279,288,299,302] as well as in some cells lining the thyroid follicles both histochemically and immunohistochemically. Ultrastructural examination demonstrates neurosecretory granules in the carcinoid component and in some of the thyroid follicular cells.[299,302] In two tumors, amyloid deposits were identified and were verified both histochemically and ultrastructurally.[12,69] This ultrastructural similarity between the cells of medullary carcinoma of the thyroid and carcinoid tumors has been noted previously.[41,116] One case of medullary carcinoma of the thyroid has been associated with the carcinoid syndrome.[202] It has been considered by some investigators that the whole lesion represents a carcinoid tumor, and that the thyroid tissue is only thyroid-like and represents a carcinoid.[125,177,250] Other investigators have conclusively demonstrated thyroglobulin within the thyroid component

of the tumor, thus indicating its thyroid nature.[*] It is therefore considered that in verified cases of strumal carcinoid the tumor consists of thyroid tissue intimately admixed with a carcinoid. Strumal carcinoid should be distinguished from carcinoma of the thyroid arising in struma ovarii, with which it has often been confused. The latter has the typical appearances observed in carcinoma of the thyroid and usually exhibits the follicular or papillary pattern.

CLINICAL BEHAVIOR AND TREATMENT

Strumal carcinoid has been associated only once with metastases, and even in this case the patient was apparently cured by a combination of surgery and radiation therapy.[387] All other cases have followed a benign course.[254,282,299]

Monodermal Teratomas with Neuroectodermal Differentiation

During the past decade both malignant[5,157] and benign[357,366] monodermal teratomas with neuroectodermal differentiation have been described. The benign tumors consist of a cyst lined entirely by mature glial tissue[366] or by ependymal tissue.[357] The former has been described as a neurogenic cyst. It is important to recognize the benign nature of such tumors. The fact that the tumor is composed of mature neural tissue distinguishes it from its malignant counterparts.

The malignant tumors can be divided into malignant neuroectodermal tumor[5] and ependymoma.[71,157]

Malignant Neuroectodermal Tumor

Aguirre and Scully[5] described five ovarian tumors occurring in patients in the second decade that showed pure neuroectodermal differentiation characterized by histological patterns resembling those of glioblastoma, medulloblastoma, and neuroblastoma present alone or in combination. Small foci of more mature glia or ependyma, as well as small foci of mature teratoma, may also be seen in these tumors. Although tumors of this type may be confused with other ovarian tumors composed of small cells, special stains for neural tissue and immunocytochemical stains for glial fibrillary acidic protein (GFAP) and neurofilaments are helpful in reaching the correct diagnosis.

The tumors thus far reported occurred in patients in the second decade. They pursue an aggressive course and the prognosis is poor.[5]

---

*Refs. 118,254,288,299,302,362,364.

Ependymoma

Four cases of pure ovarian ependymoma representing one-sided development of a teratoma have been reported.[71,157] The patients were all in the third and fourth decades and presented with abdominal pain and a palpable abdominal mass. Three patients had intraabdominal metastases and in one case the tumor was confined to the ovary.

The tumors were cystic, containing fleshy mural nodules or papillary processes arising from the cyst wall. Microscopically they showed typical features of ependymoma arising in the central nervous system (Fig. 20.63). Perivascular pseudorosettes consisting of a blood vessel surrounded by tumor cells with long radiating processes and antipodally arranged nuclei characteristic of ependymoma were prominent. Central lumen (Homer Wright) rosettes were also seen (Fig. 20.63). Mitotic activity varied from 1 to 3 mitotic figures (MF) per 10 high power fields (HPF). Special stains for neural tissue and for GFAP are helpful in confirming the diagnosis.[157]

The prognosis of patients with this tumor is much more favorable than that of those with malignant neuroectodermal tumor; despite the presence of metastases on presentation in three of the four patients, only one of them succumbed to the disease.[157]

Monodermal Teratoma Composed of Vascular Tissue

Another type of monodermal teratoma is represented by neoplasms composed entirely or predominantly of immature vascular tissue. They occur in children and young adults, and the patients present with symptoms and signs suggestive of an ovarian tumor. The tumors may vary in size and are smooth, soft, solid, and gray-pink, but may be hemorrhagic. Microscopically they consist of collections of small vascular spaces lined by immature endothelial cells and surrounded by connective tissue, which varies from loose and edematous to dense and fibrous. The lining of the vascular spaces may be multilayered and the endothelial cells may form small projections bulging into the lumen. Small collections of endothelial cells, some forming abortive lumina and some devoid of a lumen, are also seen within the connective tissue and may predominate (Fig. 20.64). The endothelial cells show a considerable degree of cellular and nuclear pleomorphism, and mitotic activity is usually evident. Occasionally hematopoietic activity may be seen within some of the vascular spaces. When these tumors contain small teratomatous foci their nature is more readily apparent, but when they occur in pure form, especially when the endothelial cells form a more solid pattern with fewer obvious vascular spaces (Fig. 20.64), the nature of the lesion is more difficult to recognize. Occa-

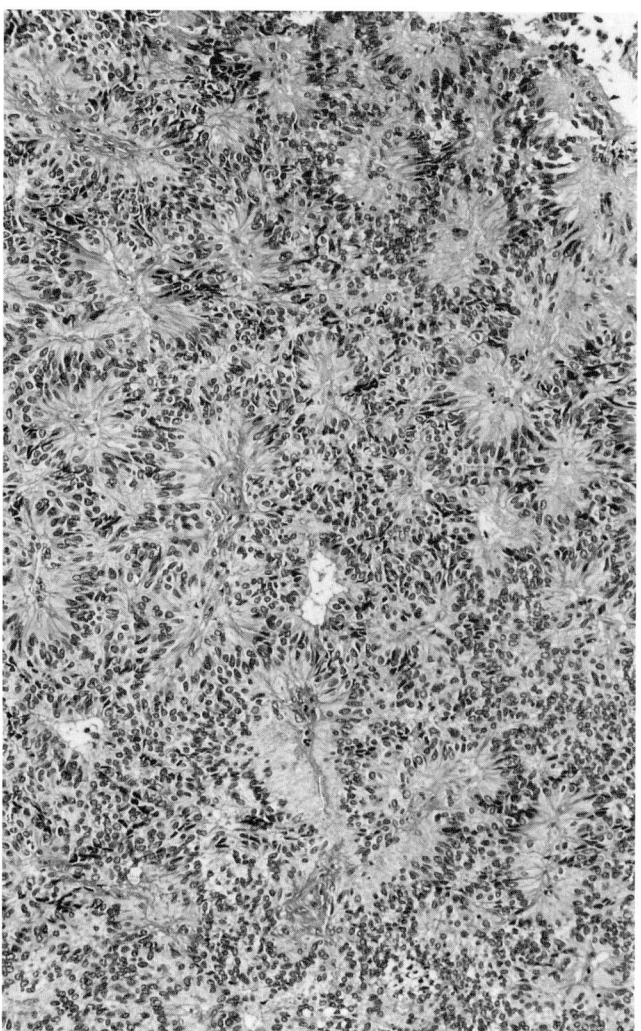

FIG. 20.63. Monodermal teratoma with ependymona. Homer Wright rosettes and perivascular pseudorosettes are present.

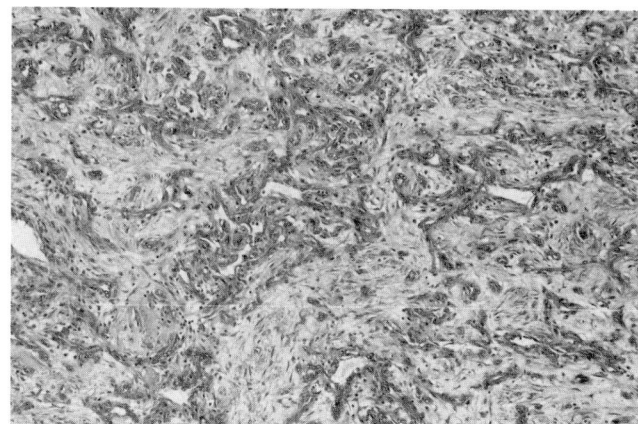

FIG. 20.64. Monodermal teratoma with vascular differentiation. The tumor is composed of immature vessels, including some forming cord-like structures either with small inconspicuous lumina, or devoid of a lumen.

sionally these tumors may be composed of immature pericytes and resemble a hemangiopericytoma. Further sectioning of the tumor, which may reveal a more typical vascular pattern, and immunocytochemical stains for Factor VIII and *Ulex Europaeus*, may be helpful in reaching the correct diagnosis. This is important because monodermal teratomas composed of immature vascular tissue or with a predominant vascular component behave on the whole in a less aggressive manner compared with high-grade immature teratomas and hemangioendothelial sarcomas of the ovary, with which they tend to be confused. As in most immature teratomas, the grade of the tumor is an important prognostic feature.

Monodermal Teratoma with Sebaceous Differentiation

Sebaceous tumors showing one-sided development of a teratoma or arising in mature cystic teratomas are rare and until a recent report describing five such tumors only three cases have been recorded in the literature.[54,308] Review of these eight cases shows an age range from 31 to 79 years at presentation, but most patients were older than 49 years. All presented with lower abdominal enlargement. The ovarian tumors found at laparotomy were all large, ranging from 10 to 35 cm. Three of the patients were found to have a mature cystic teratoma in the contralateral ovary. The tumors were mainly cystic. Partly solid yellow and tan masses protruded into the cysts. The latter contained necrotic or cheesy material.[54] Microscopically the tumors consisted of five cases of sebaceous adenomas, two cases of basal cell carcinomas with sebaceous differentiation, and a single sebaceous carcinoma[54] using the criteria proposed by Rulon and Helwig[259] for classifying cutaneous sebaceous neoplasms. The adenomas were all composed of nodules or lobules of proliferating normal sebaceous cells showing various degrees of maturity, with mature cells predominating. The basal cell carcinomas with sebaceous differentiation were composed of masses or nests of malignant basal cells containing collections of mature sebaceous cells. The sebaceous carcinoma was composed of sebaceous cells showing marked cellular and nuclear pleomorphism growing in an infiltrative pattern. The cells comprising the tumors had the typical appearance of sebaceous cells. Lipid stains were strongly positive in all the tumors confirming the diagnosis.[54]

The patients were treated either by excision of the affected adnexa or by hysterectomy and bilateral salpingo-oophorectomy. The outcome was favorable; only one tumor was known to have recurred.[54] The tumor, a basal cell carcinoma with sebaceous differentiation, recurred in the pelvis. Further follow-up was not available. All the other patients were well and disease-free for periods ranging from 1½ to 6 years postoperatively.[54] One patient had in addition to the sebaceous adenoma a squamous cell carcinoma arising in the same ovary and died as a result of disseminated disease 1 year after the diagnosis. The patient with sebaceous carcinoma was well and disease-free 6 years after diagnosis.[54]

Other Types of Monodermal Teratoma

Mucinous tumors of the ovary usually are described with the epithelial neoplasms and are considered to be derived from the surface epithelium of the ovary. They are generally not regarded as germ cell neoplasms. However, there is undoubtedly a considerable number of cases in which the tumor is of germ cell origin, forming a monodermal teratomatous neoplasm in which the mucinous element (of intestinal derivation) developed in a pure form or has overgrown all the other tissues in the same manner that the thyroid tissue in a pure struma ovarii has developed in a pure form or has overgrown all the other tissues. The presence of occasional teratomatous tumors composed mainly of mucinous (intestinal type) epithelium of endodermal derivation and only a small amount of other tumor elements, as well as a 5% association of mature cystic teratoma with mucinous cystadenoma, lends strong support to this mode of origin for at least some mucinous tumors. Mucinous epithelium resembling intestinal epithelium has been observed in association with struma ovarii and with strumal carcinoid. In these cases, it was the only other tissue element present. The mucinous epithelium frequently contains goblet cells and so shows greater resemblance to intestinal than to endocervical epithelium. In 21% of cases, the epithelium lining mucinous tumors of the ovary contains argyrophil and argentaffin granules.[91] In a number of cases, Paneth cells are also present.[278] These findings are considered to be a strong argument in favor of the derivation of at least some mucinous ovarian tumors from intestinal type of epithelium and their teratomatous (germ cell) origin. It is possible that studies of the type undertaken by Linder et al., using both chromosomal and isoenzyme techniques,[175] may help to clarify the origin of mucinous tumors of the ovary and confirm that some of these are of germ cell origin. Mucinous tumors of the ovary are discussed fully with tumors of epithelial derivation (see Chapter 18, Surface Epithelial–Stromal Tumors of the Ovary).

Other rare examples of monodermal teratomatous neoplasms observed in the ovary include the epidermoid cyst, which is lined by epidermis without appendages, the melanotic tumor, resembling the retinal anlage tumor,[123,154] and the possible benign cystic counterpart of the latter.[10] Monodermal teratomatous origin of some malignant connective tissue tumors is difficult to prove because of the occurrence of connective tissue neoplasms derived from normal ovarian tissue. Monodermal teratomatous origin of tumors derived from ectodermal or endodermal tissues is more easily acceptable, and there may be as yet undescribed tumors of this type.

Mixed Germ Cell Tumors

Mixed germ cell tumors are tumors composed of more than one neoplastic germ cell element, such as dysgerminoma combined with teratoma, yolk sac tumor, choriocarcinoma, embryonal carcinoma, or polyembryoma, as well as any other possible combination of these tumor types. This group includes only neoplasms composed entirely of neoplastic germ cell elements and does not include the gonadoblastoma and mixed germ cell–sex cord stromal tumor, which in addition to germ cells contains sex cord–stromal derivatives as an integral component. The relatively frequent finding of different neoplastic germ cell elements in gonadal tumors of germ cell origin is considered to be a strong argument in favor of the common histogenesis of this group of neoplasms. The various tumor elements present in these tumors may be intimately admixed (Fig. 20.11) or may form separate areas adjacent to each other and separated by fibrous septa (Fig. 20.12). Although many ovarian tumors belonging to this group are classified according to the predominant element present, it is emphasized that when these tumors are examined, all areas of varying appearance should be sampled carefully and thoroughly analyzed. All the neoplastic germ cell elements observed within the tumor, however small, should be reported and described and, if possible, their relative size estimated. The importance of this practice is by no means only academic, since the behavior and treatment of neoplasms belonging to this group vary considerably, and the presence of a small area composed of a more malignant element may alter the therapeutic approach and the prognosis. The presence of more malignant elements within a tumor is usually associated with a more aggressive behavior, and before the introduction of effective combination chemotherapy it was associated with an unsatisfactory response to therapy and a poor prognosis.[*] However, it should be noted that the clinical course in most patients with tumors composed of yolk sac tumor associated with dysgerminoma or other germ cell elements usually does not differ materially from that observed in patients with pure yolk sac tumor.[44,102–104,134,148,267] The different response to treatment and the different behavior of some cases of dysgerminoma described in the past may have been a result of the presence of other germ cell elements that were not identified. Although in the past mixed germ cell tumors were considered to be uncommon,[206] they tend to figure much more frequently in recent reports,[†] probably because of more careful and extensive examination of the tumor.

---

[*]Refs. 13,166,232,267,331,354.
[†]Refs. 13,43,44,88,102,134,166,206,212,267,329,331,354.

Clinical and Pathological Features of Tumors Composed of Germ Cells and Sex Cord–Stromal Derivatives

Gonadoblastoma

GENERAL FEATURES

In 1953, Scully[276] described two patients with a distinctive gonadal tumor, which he designated *gonadoblastoma*. The tumor was composed of germ cells and sex cord–stromal derivatives, resembling immature granulosa, and Sertoli cells. One of the tumors also contained stromal elements indistinguishable from lutein or Leydig cells. Both tumors occurred in phenotypic females who showed abnormal sexual development. The older patient who was postpubertal showed virilization and it was considered that the tumor was capable of steroid hormone secretion. The tumors were located at the site of normal ovaries, but normal ovarian tissue was not discernible and the exact nature of the gonads in which the tumors had originated could not be determined. Both patients had bilateral tumors that were partly overgrown by dysgerminoma. It was subsequently demonstrated that both patients were chromatin-negative. The tumor was designated *gonadoblastoma* because it appeared to recapitulate the development of the gonads and because it occurred in individuals with abnormal sexual development and in gonads, the nature of which could not be determined.[280]

The neoplastic nature of gonadoblastoma has been questioned because some lesions are very small and may undergo complete regression by hyalinization and calcification. Furthermore, when malignancy supervenes, it manifests itself as germ cell neoplasia despite the fact that gonadoblastoma is composed of two or three different cell types. When the tumor has metastasized, gonadoblastoma as such has never been observed in the metastases. Nevertheless, gonadoblastoma shows exactly the same pattern in the very small lesions[352] as in the large ones, including mitotic activity in the germ cell element and early overgrowth by dysgerminoma. The association with dysgerminoma is seen in 50% of cases[124,280] and with other more malignant germ cell neoplasms in an additional 10%.[280,314] In view of this, the concept that gonadoblastoma represents an in situ germ cell malignancy[280] is considered to be justified.

Genetic Aspects

Gonadoblastoma occurs almost entirely in patients with pure or mixed gonadal dysgenesis or in male pseudohermaphrodites (see Chapter 2, Embryology and Abnormal Sexual Development). Occasional patients are of short stature and may have other stigmata of Turner's syndrome.[269,291] Most patients are chromatin-negative; this has been observed in 89% of cases.[280] Nearly all patients with gonadoblastoma whose karyotype was recorded (96%) were found to have a Y chromosome.[269] Eight patients had 46 XX karyotype,[30,83,111,204,264,334] and four of these were fertile.[30,83,204,334] One patient had a 45 X/46 XX mosaicism.[230] The most frequently encountered karyotype was 46 XY, which was seen in half the cases; this was followed by 45 X/46 XY mosaicism, which was seen in a quarter of the cases. The remainder showed many different forms of mosaicism.[269] Six patients had morphologic abnormalities of the Y chromosome. Of 25 patients with gonadal dysgenesis and dysgerminoma, 96% had a Y chromosome. The karyotype was 46 XY in 60%, followed by 45 X/46 XY in 24%. The remainder showed various forms of mosaicism.[269] One patient had 45 X monosomy and Turner syndrome. All other patients with features of Turner syndrome had various forms of mosaicism containing a Y chromosome. The similarity between the distribution of the karyotypes in the gonadoblastoma group and patients with dysgerminoma and gonadal dysgenesis is striking, and 62% of the former group and 45% of the latter had clitoral hypertrophy.[269]

Family history of gonadal dysgenesis has been noted in at least 10 reports of patients with gonadoblastoma.[8,9,38,312] Evidence of gonadal dysgenesis affecting three generations of the family of a patient with gonadoblastoma was obtained in two instances.[8,24] Gonadoblastoma has been reported in one pair of twins[92] and in four pairs of siblings.[8,9,38,312] All these patients had 46 XY karyotype. It has been postulated that the mode of inheritance is either an X-linked recessive gene or an autosomal sex-linked mutant gene.[24,269,270,304]

Endocrine Aspects

The association of gonadoblastoma with certain endocrine abnormalities was noted in one of the two cases first reported.[276] In view of the fact that gonadoblastoma occurs almost entirely in patients with gonadal dysgenesis, the defective gonadal development present in these patients should not be confused with the presence of endocrine effects that are associated with the tumor and are not a result of the abnormal gonadal development. Although the virilization produced by the tumor may regress after the excision of the tumor, there is no further gonadal development and the gonadal abnormalities remain.

Although the exact source of the steroid hormone production was not originally known, the interstitial cells resembling Leydig or lutein cells were considered to be the most likely source of the androgens.[276] Further observations have shown that the presence of Leydig or lutein-like cells is not always associated with the presence of virilization, although they are encountered more frequently in tumors from virilized phenotypic female patients than in those from nonvirilized patients. The possibility that the tumor may secrete estrogens, as evidenced by complaints

of hot flushes and other menopausal symptoms after the excision of the tumor, has also been noted.[280] Originally, the evidence of hormone secretion was mainly clinical, usually evidenced by virilization occurring after puberty and manifesting itself as masculine body contour, hirsutism, and clitoromegaly. Slight elevation of the urinary 17-ketosteroid excretion was noted in some cases.[61,183] The gonadotropins, when estimated, were usually elevated.[349]

In recent years it has been shown that gonadoblastoma is capable of producing testosterone and estrogens from progesterone in vitro.[9,22,119,180,258] Evidence of testosterone secretion in vivo in patients with gonadal dysgenesis has been presented.[149,376] Androgen and estrogen formation from progesterone in vitro has been demonstrated in a streak gonad that did not contain any Leydig and lutein cells microscopically but from the description may have contained a small burned-out gonadoblastoma.[180] Although in vitro testosterone formation has been ascribed to the Leydig or lutein-like cells present in the gonadoblastoma,[22,258] the demonstration of steroid production by a streak gonad that did not contain Leydig or lutein cells indicates that the stromal tissue also has the capability of steroid synthesis.[180]

Despite all these advances in the study and understanding of the hormonal aspects of gonadoblastoma and dysgenetic gonads, considerable problems remain, the most important being why some patients become virilized and others do not. Although there is a relationship between the virilization of patients with gonadoblastoma and the presence of Leydig or lutein-like cells, this relationship is not constant. It may be that the reason is quantitative and that the amount of the steroid secretion may be inadequate to produce virilization because of a small cell mass. Another possible reason is that the steroid metabolic pathways may be different and that gonadoblastoma may produce different steroid hormones or different quantities of various steroid hormones. Some of these hormones may be metabolically nonfunctioning and therefore unassociated with endocrine side effects, whereas the metabolically active steroids may be associated with evidence and visible signs of endocrine activity.[180]

CLINICAL FEATURES

The exact prevalence of gonadoblastoma is not known. Although more than 200 cases have been reported, it is considered to be uncommon. Gonadoblastoma is usually seen in young patients, occurring most frequently in the second and somewhat less frequently in the third and first decades, in that order. With a few exceptions all the reported cases occurred in patients under 30 years of age. Gonadoblastoma is much more common in phenotypic females than in phenotypic males, the ratio being 4:1.[280]

Patients with gonadoblastoma usually have primary amenorrhea, virilization, or developmental abnormalities of the genitalia (see Chapter 2). The discovery of gonado-blastoma is made in the course of investigations of these conditions. Another mode of presentation is the presence of a gonadal tumor. The gonadoblastoma forms part of the tumor in these cases and is discovered on histological examination. Most patients with gonadoblastoma (80%) are phenotypic females, and the remainder are phenotypic males with cryptorchidism, hypospadias, and female internal secondary sex organs. Among the phenotypic females, 60% are virilized and the remainder are normal in appearance.[280] Most of the phenotypic female patients exhibit abnormal genital development, and breast development is often diminished even among the nonvirilized females. Although primary amenorrhea is a common presenting symptom among phenotypic females with gonadoblastoma, a few patients have episodes of spontaneous cyclical bleeding, but in most of these patients the episodes are sporadic and the bleeding scanty. Occasional patients menstruate normally.[280] The virilization present in phenotypic female patients with gonadoblastoma usually does not regress after excision of the tumor, although this has been seen in occasional cases, and in a few additional cases there was partial regression. Although most patients have gonadal dysgenesis, gonadoblastoma has been described in one patient who has had two normal pregnancies after the excision of a dysgerminoma containing a small focus of gonadoblastoma. This patient was chromatin-positive and had a 46 XX karyotype.[30]

Normal pregnancies have also been documented in a patient with a normal female 46 XX karyotype and gonadoblastoma occurring in a normal ovary,[204] in a true hermaphrodite with bilateral ovotestes, gonadoblastomas, and dysgerminomas,[334] and in a normal 46 XX female with one normal ovary and the other gonad overgrown by a large dysgerminoma originating in a gonadoblastoma.[83] Gonadoblastoma has been observed in seven true hermaphrodites, four of whom had 46 XX karyotype[182,322,334] and the other three 46 XY.[227,310] It was also seen in five males with normally descended testes,[133,320] some of whom fathered children subsequent to the excision of the testis bearing the lesion.

Gross Findings

Gonadoblastoma has been found more often in the right gonad than in the left and has been bilateral in 38% of cases.[280] Recent reports suggest an even higher frequency of bilateral involvement. Although many tumors are recognized on gross examination, in a number of cases the lesion is detected only on histological examination. This may be the case with bilateral tumors, only one of which may be recognized macroscopically. In most cases, the gonad of origin is indeterminate because it is overgrown by the tumor. When the nature of the gonad can be identified, it is usually a streak or a testis. The contralateral gonad in

these cases may be a streak or a testis, and the former is more likely to harbor a gonadoblastoma.[280] Occasionally gonadoblastoma has been found in otherwise normal ovaries.[111,204,247]

Pure gonadoblastoma varies in size from a microscopic lesion to 8 cm in diameter, with most tumors measuring a few centimeters. When gonadoblastoma becomes overgrown by dysgerminoma (Fig. 20.65) or other malignant germ cell elements, much larger tumors may be observed.[280,315] The macroscopic appearance of the tumor varies to some extent according to the presence of hyalinization and calcification, as well as overgrowth by dysgerminoma. Gonadoblastoma is a solid tumor and presents a smooth or slightly lobulated surface. It varies from soft and fleshy to firm and hard. It is speckled with calcific granules and may be almost completely calcified. Calcification has been recognized on gross examination in 45% of cases, and in more than 20% it has been detected radiologically.[280] The tumor varies in color from gray or yellow to brown, and on cross-section it appears to be somewhat granular.

Although the external sex organs in patients with gonadoblastoma present a wide variety of appearances ranging from normal to completely ambiguous, the secondary internal sex organs consist almost always of a uterus, which is hypoplastic in most cases, and two or occasionally one normal fallopian tube. This is also seen in the phenotypic males. Male secondary internal sex organs, such as the epididymis, vas deferens, and prostate, are found occasionally in the virilized phenotypic females and are always found in the phenotypic male pseudohermaphrodites.[280]

Microscopic Findings

Gonadoblastoma is composed of collections of cellular nests surrounded by connective tissue stroma (Fig. 20.66).

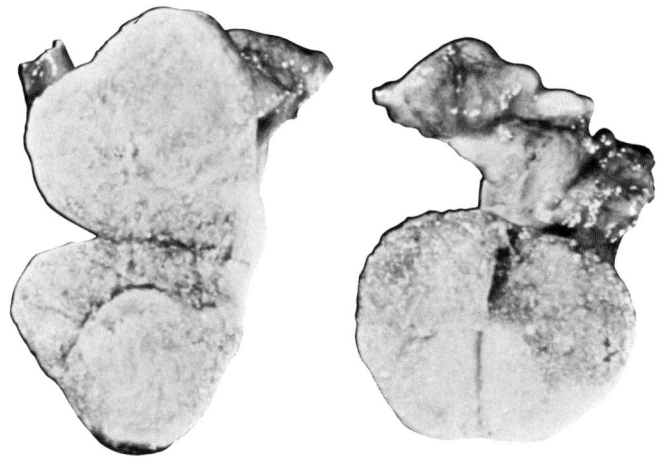

Fig. 20.65. **Gonadoblastoma with dysgerminoma.** The outer surface is smooth, the cut surface solid, granular, and yellow-brown in color. (Courtesy of R. Scully, M.D., Boston, MA.)

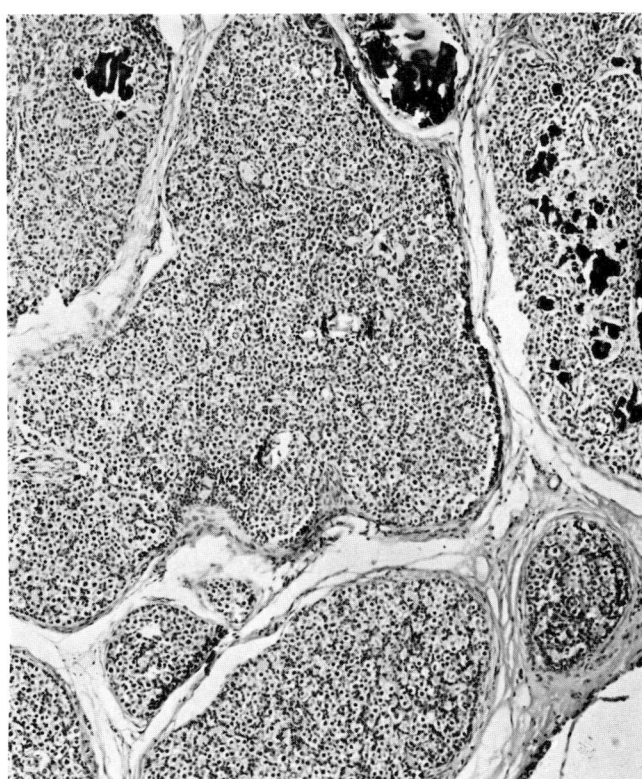

FIG. 20.66. **Gonadoblastoma.** Cellular nests surrounded by connective tissue stroma. Note foci of calcification (*heavy black areas*).

The nests are solid, usually small, and oval or round but occasionally may be larger and elongated. The cellular nests contain a mixture of germ cells and sex cord derivatives resembling immature Sertoli and granulosa cells (Fig. 20.67). The germ cells are large and round, with pale or slightly granular cytoplasm and large round vesicular nuclei, often with prominent nucleoli showing histological and ultrastructural appearances and histochemical reactions similar to the germ cells of dysgerminoma or seminoma. The germ cells show mitotic activity, which may be marked in some cases. They are intimately admixed with immature Sertoli and granulosa cells, which are smaller and epithelial-like. The latter are round or oval and have dark, oval or slightly elongated carrot-shaped nuclei. Mitotic activity is not seen in these cells. The immature Sertoli and granulosa cells are arranged within the cell nests in three typical patterns (Fig. 20.67): (1) along the periphery of the nests in a coronal pattern, (2) surrounding individual or collections of germ cells in the same way as the follicular epithelium surrounds the ovum of the primary follicle, or (3) surrounding small round spaces containing amorphous hyaline, eosinophilic, and PAS-positive material that resemble Call–Exner bodies.

The connective tissue stroma surrounding the cellular nests frequently contains collections of cells indistinguishable from Leydig cells or luteinized stromal cells (Fig. 20.68). There is considerable variation in the number of these cells from case to case; in some cases they are numerous, in others they are identified with difficulty.

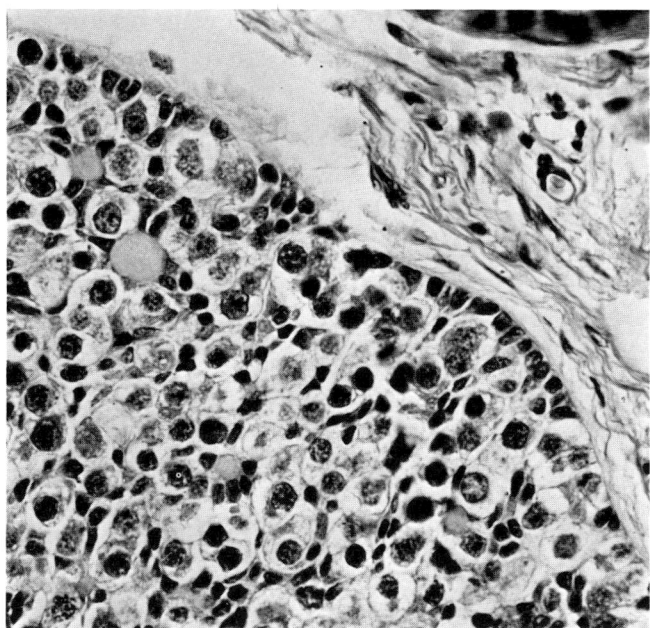

FIG. 20.67. **Gonadoblastoma.** A nest composed of large germ cells intimately admixed with smaller sex cord derivatives is present. Hyaline Call–Exner-like bodies also are seen.

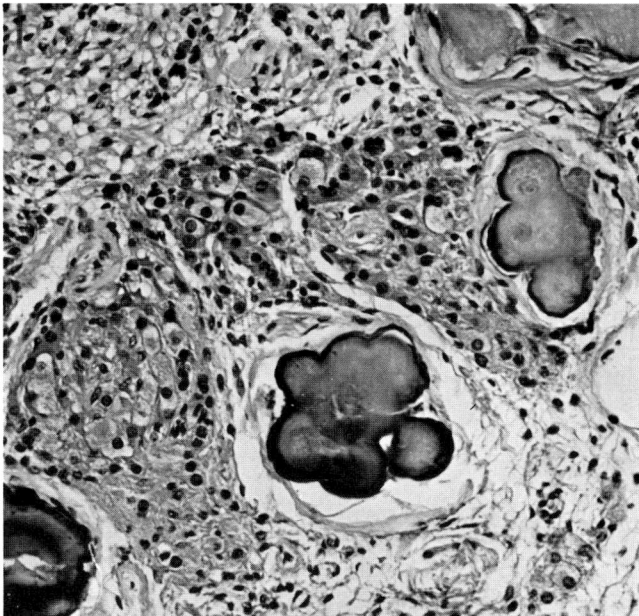

FIG. 20.68. **Gonadoblastoma.** Calcified nest surrounded by connective tissue containing numerous Leydig or lutein-like cells. Same case as in Fig. 20.65.

Although in many cases the cells are indistinguishable from Leydig cells and may contain lipochrome granules, Reinke crystals, which are specifically diagnostic of Leydig cells, have never been identified in their cytoplasm. The Leydig or lutein-like cells are identified in 66% of cases, and they are present nearly twice as frequently in older patients as in those 15 years of age or younger.[280] The presence of Leydig or lutein-like cells is not necessary for the diagnosis of gonadoblastoma. The connective tissue stroma surrounding the cellular nests may be scanty or abundant and may vary from dense and hyalinized to cellular, resembling ovarian stroma. These latter appearances are more common in tumors that either have arisen in or are suspected to originate in a gonadal streak.[280] Occasionally, the stroma may be loose and edematous. The basic composition of gonadoblastoma, consisting of the two cell types present within the cellular nests and with the Leydig or lutein-like cells present in the stroma, has been confirmed by electron microscopy.[65,101,131,137,180] Although there is agreement concerning the nature of the germ cells, the nature of the stromal cells is in dispute. They are considered by some to be Sertoli cells or their precursors,[180] whereas others consider them as primitive sex cord–stromal cells and are unable to differentiate them further.[65,131,280,317] The nature of the amorphous, hyaline, eosinophilic material forming Call–Exner-like bodies also is a matter of dispute. It is considered to be either of basement membrane origin[65,137,180] or composed of fibrillar material formed by the stromal cells before they undergo fragmentation and cell death.[131] The former view is supported by most investigators.

The basic histological appearance of gonadoblastoma may be altered by three processes: hyalinization, calcification, and overgrowth by dysgerminoma.[101,280,380] Hyalinization takes place by coalescence of the hyaline Call–Exner-like bodies within the nests and of the basement membrane–like band of similar material present around the nests. The hyaline material replaces the tumor cells, and the whole nest may be replaced. Calcification is a common feature (Figs. 20.66, and 20.68) and is seen microscopically in 81% of cases; it usually begins in the Call–Exner-like bodies with formation of small calcific spherules that are frequently laminated, resembling psammoma bodies (Fig. 20.68). The process continues with enlargement and fusion of the calcified bodies and calcification of the hyalinized material. This results in formation of a calcified mass embracing the whole nest. The process may extend to the stroma, which may also undergo hyalinization and calcification. In such cases, tumor cells become very scarce or absent, and the presence of smooth, rounded, calcified masses may be the only evidence that gonadoblastoma was present (Fig. 20.9). Although this finding is not considered to be diagnostic of gonadoblastoma—it has been called a *burned-out gonadoblastoma*[280,312]—it is a strong argument in favor of the diagnosis and indicates that a careful search for more viable areas of the tumor should be made.

Gonadoblastoma is frequently overgrown by dysgerminoma (Fig. 20.69). This is seen in 50% of cases.[280] The overgrowth of dysgerminoma may vary from the presence of a small collection of germ cells in the stroma outside the gonadoblastoma nests to massive overgrowth of the whole tumor, in which occasional nests of gonadoblastoma may be seen. The dysgerminoma in these cases shows the typical appearances of pure dysgerminoma or seminoma, histologically, histochemically, and ultrastructurally.[65,131,137]

It should be noted that when gonadoblastoma becomes overgrown by dysgerminoma, the germ cell component present within the gonadoblastoma nests shows marked proliferative activity and overgrows the sex cord elements. When gonadoblastoma undergoes regressive changes, they manifest first as a decrease in germ cells. Gonadoblastoma may also be associated with and overgrown by other more malignant germ cell neoplasms, such as immature teratoma, yolk sac tumor, embryonal carcinoma, and choriocarcinoma. This occurs in 10% of cases.[280,317] Although it has been postulated that gonadoblastoma may co-exist with mixed germ cell–sex cord stromal tumor, the only case describing such an association[35] is in reality a typical gonadoblastoma and not a combined tumor.

DIFFERENTIAL DIAGNOSIS

Gonadoblastoma, because of its distinctive histological appearance and its cellular composition, cannot be easily confused with any of the well-recognized gonadal neoplasms. The gonadal tumors with which confusion may

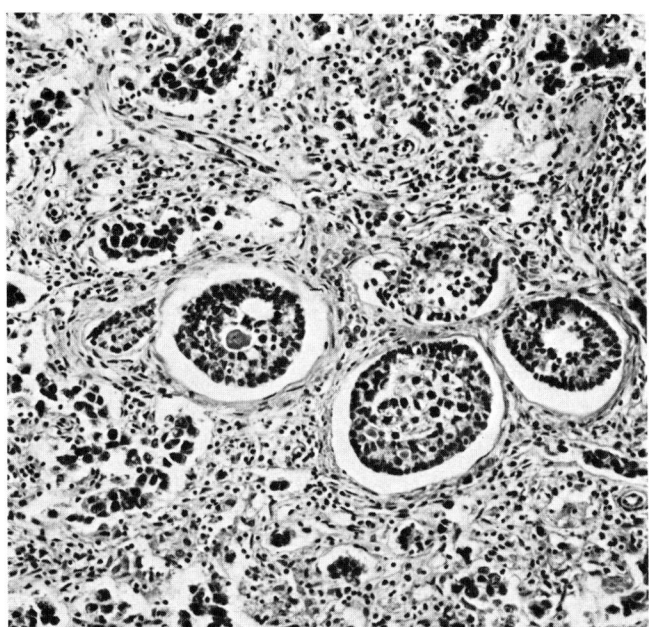

FIG. 20.69. **Gonadoblastoma nests surrounded by dysgerminoma.** (Reprinted with permission from The American College of Obstetricians and Gynecologists. (Obstetrics and Gynecology, 38: 416, 1971).)

arise are all newly recognized entities and may be related to it. Gonadoblastoma may be confused with the mixed germ cell–sex cord–stromal tumor,[313,314,326] which shares with gonadoblastoma the unique distinction of being composed of germ cells and sex cord–stromal derivatives. The mixed germ cell–sex cord–stromal tumor shows less uniform appearance, absence of nest-like pattern, absence of calcification and hyalinization, a more pronounced proliferative activity involving also the sex cord–stromal derivatives, the tendency to occur in normal gonads, and other genetic, endocrine, and somatic differences. The other lesion resembling gonadoblastoma is the ovarian sex cord tumor with annular tubules,[281,282] which is frequently found in patients with Peutz–Jeghers syndrome. This lesion, which is also frequently bilateral, is composed of tubules lined by Sertoli and granulosa-like cells, contains similar round, eosinophilic, and hyaline Call–Exner-like bodies, and tends to calcify in the same manner as gonadoblastoma. The basic difference from gonadoblastoma is the absence of germ cells (see Chapter 19, Sex Cord–Stromal, Steroid Cell, and Other Ovarian Tumors with Endocrine, Paraendocrine, and Paraneoplastic Manifestations).

CLINICAL BEHAVIOR AND TREATMENT

The prognosis of patients with pure gonadoblastoma is excellent, provided the tumor and the contralateral gonad, which may be harboring a macroscopically undetectable gonadoblastoma, are excised. When gonadoblastoma is associated with dysgerminoma, the prognosis is still very good. Metastases tend to occur later and more infrequently than in dysgerminoma arising de novo. All patients with gonadoblastoma and dysgerminoma with known follow-up, including the occasional cases with metastases,[2,124,271] are alive and well after treatment, with the exception of two patients who died with disseminated dysgerminoma.[124,351] The prognosis is different when gonadoblastoma is associated with more malignant germ cell neoplasms, such as embryonal carcinoma, yolk sac tumor, choriocarcinoma, and immature teratoma. In the past, none of these patients survived longer than 18 months.[315] More recently, the administration of combination chemotherapy used successfully in the treatment of malignant germ cell tumors has markedly improved this dismal prognosis, which with adequate treatment is now favorable.

Since gonadoblastoma occurs almost entirely in patients with dysgenetic gonads, which are not capable of normal function and because the gonadoblastoma may act as a source from which malignant germ cell neoplasms may originate,[269] there is general agreement that excision of the gonads is the treatment of choice.* This applies not only to a contralateral gonad that appears to be abnormal but also to a normal-appearing one. There is no complete agree-

---

*Refs. 101,124,270,280,317,351,380.

ment regarding whether the uterus should be excised together with the gonads. It has been considered that for psychologic reasons it should be left in situ so that periodic bleeding simulating menstruation can take place on estrogen–progesterone substitution therapy. However, since estrogen administration is associated with a risk of development of endometrial carcinoma,[63] excision of the uterus together with the gonads has been advocated.[270]

Mixed Germ Cell–Sex Cord–Stromal Tumor

GENERAL FEATURES

The descriptive term *mixed germ cell–sex cord–stromal tumor* originally was intended to embrace all the tumors composed of these cell types, including the gonadoblastoma. In view of the fact that the latter term is now so well established, the term *mixed germ cell–sex cord–stromal tumor* should be reserved for tumors composed of these cell types that exhibit distinctive histological appearances differing from those of gonadoblastoma.[313,314] This term is preferable to *Pflügerome*[48] or *epithelioma Pflügerien*[194] because these terms imply a possible origin from Pflüger's tubes (germ cell clusters in a granulosa cell envelope that are formed during gonadal embryogenesis and may persist into infancy). Since there is no good evidence for this mode of origin and there is some doubt as to the formation of Pflüger's tubes during human embryogenesis, the term *Pflügerome* is not considered to be satisfactory. The term *mixed germ cell tumor*[133] is considered to be unsatisfactory because it implies a tumor composed of a mixture of different types of germ cell elements without the presence of sex cord–stromal elements, and this term is used in this context in the classification of ovarian tumors proposed by the WHO ovarian tumor panel.[284,289]

Genetic Aspects

Nearly all female patients with this neoplasm have had genotype and karyotype determinations and have been found chromatin-positive and to have the normal female chromosome complement of 46XX. All the patients with this tumor showed normal somatosexual development. Therefore, there is no evidence that patients with this tumor have chromosomal abnormalities or gonadal dysgenesis.

Endocrine Aspects

Most patients with mixed germ cell–sex cord–stromal tumor do not exhibit any endocrine abnormalities as observed clinically. In most cases, tests of hormonal function have not been performed preoperatively. In cases in which they have been performed postoperatively, they have been found to be normal. In one case, the patient, an 8-year-old girl, exhibited signs of precocious pseudopuberty manifest-

ing as mammary development and menstrual bleeding for
3 years before the diagnosis of a large ovarian tumor.[326]
There was an increased urinary estrogen excretion. After
excision of the ovarian tumor, the uterine bleeding ceased
and the urinary estrogens became normal.[326] Isosexual
precocious pseudopuberty has been seen in nine other
patients in the first decade, including four infants under 1
year of age, who exhibited mammary development and
vaginal bleeding. The urinary estrogens were elevated, and
vaginal smears showed estrogen effect. After the excision
of the tumor, there was a complete return to normality.
There was no evidence of virilization in any of the patients.
These findings indicate that female patients with this neoplasm either do not have any associated endocrine abnormalities, or if these are present they manifest themselves as
feminization. One of the patients, who had a mixed germ
cell–sex cord–stromal tumor excised at the age of 10
years,[313] has developed normally and commenced menstruating at the age of 15 years. She is well and disease-free
12 years after excision of the tumor.

CLINICAL FEATURES

These neoplasms are rare, and only a few adequately documented cases have been recorded, although it is likely
that some cases may not have been recognized and have
been classified with tumors of germ cell origin or with sex
cord–stromal tumors. This is supported by the fact that
since this neoplasm has been recognized as a specific entity, additional well-documented and so far unreported
cases have been encountered. Tumors of this type have
been observed more frequently in normal phenotypic female patients but have also been encountered in normal
adult males. Most of the known cases in females were
encountered in children in the first decade. More than a
dozen cases occurred in infants under 1 year of
age.[75,314,317] In three cases, the tumor occurred in women
aged 26, 31, and 43, respectively, who had normal pregnancies. In the ovary the tumor is most common in the first
decade, followed by the second and third, and is uncommon thereafter. Therefore, the age distribution of patients
with this neoplasm differs from that of patients with gonadoblastoma.[317]

GROSS FINDINGS

The tumors encountered have been relatively large (Fig.
20.70), varying in size from 7.5 to 18 cm in diameter and
weighing from 100 to 1050 g. The tumor was found to be
unilateral in all except two patients, and the contralateral
gonad has always been described as a normal ovary. In
some cases in which excision or biopsy was performed, this
was confirmed on microscopic examination.

The tumor is usually round or oval, firm in consistency,
and surrounded by a smooth, slightly glistening gray or

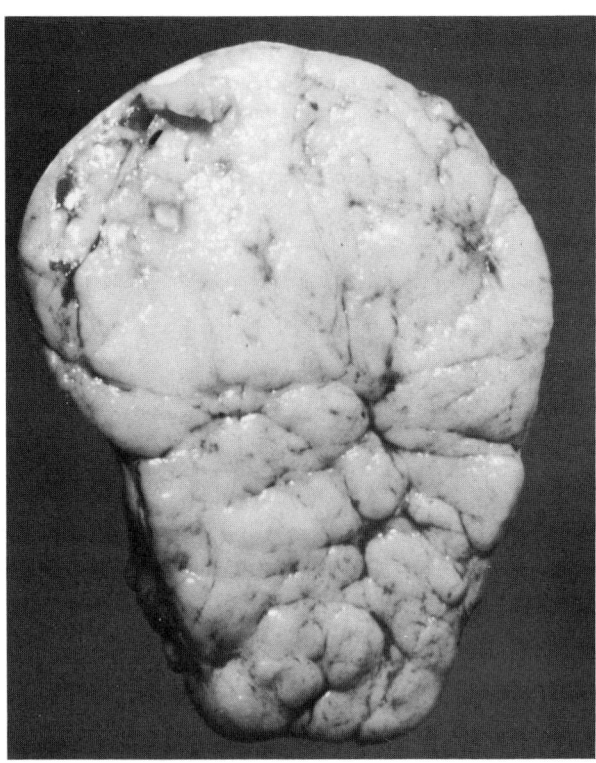

FIG. 20.70. **Mixed germ cell–sex cord–stromal tumor.** The
tumor is large, and the external surface is lobulated. The cut
surface is solid, bulging, uniform, and gray-yellow. (Courtesy H.
W. Oechler, M.D.)

gray-yellow capsule. In most cases the tumor was
solid[313,314] (Fig. 20.70), but in some cases it was partly
cystic.[326] The cut surface of the tumor is uniformly gray,
pink, or yellow to pale brown. Neither calcified areas nor
foci of necrosis have been observed on gross examination.
The fallopian tubes and the uterus have always been found
to be normal. There have been no abnormalities affecting
the external genitalia.

MICROSCOPIC FINDINGS

The tumor is composed of germ cells and sex cord derivatives, intimately admixed with each other. The tumor cells
form three different histological patterns, which in places
intermingle with each other.[313,314,317,326] One is composed
of long, narrow ramifying cords or trabeculae (Fig. 20.71),
which in places expand to form wider columns and larger
round or oval cellular aggregates surrounded by connective tissue stroma (Fig. 20.72). The second consists of tubular structures devoid of a lumen and surrounded by a
fine connective tissue network (Figs. 20.73, 20.74). In
some places, the tubular pattern is less obvious, and the
tumor forms small clusters or larger round or oval cellular
masses surrounded by connective tissue stroma. The latter
varies in amount and appearance and tends to be more

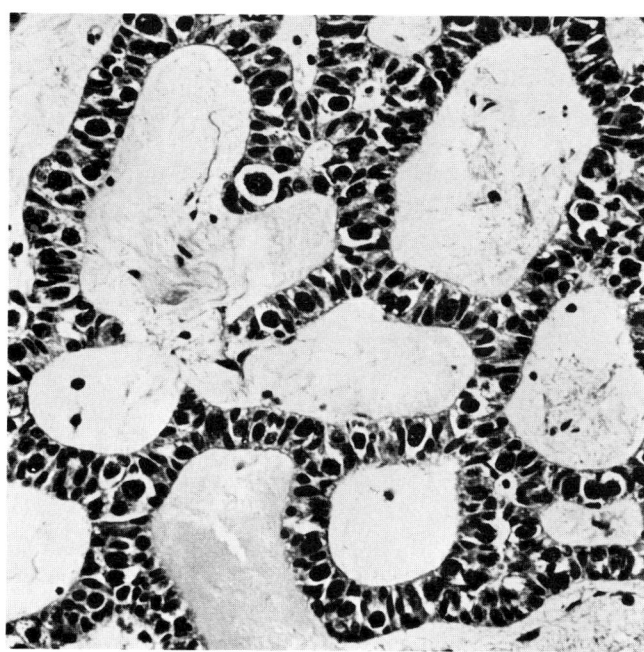

FIG. 20.71. **Mixed germ cell–sex cord–stromal tumor.** The neoplasm is composed of long ramifying cords. Note the large germ cells and smaller sex cord derivatives and the loose connective tissue stroma.

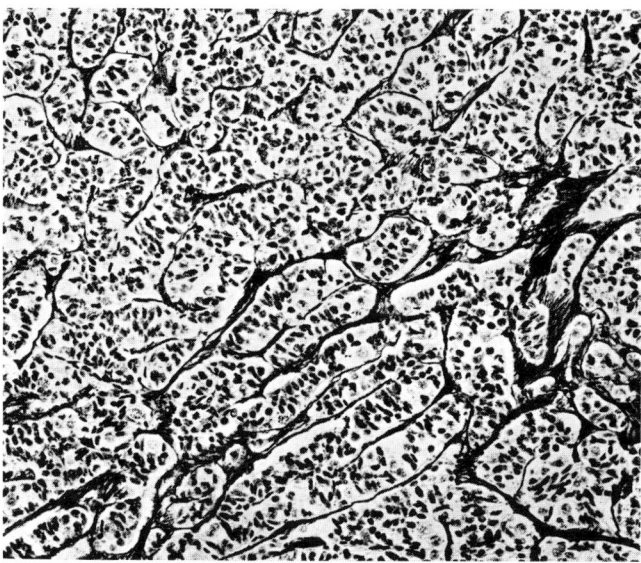

FIG. 20.73. **Mixed germ cell–sex cord–stromal tumor.** The neoplasm is composed of solid tubules surrounded by fine connective tissue septa. (Reprinted with permission from The American College of Obstetricians and Gynecologists. (Obstetrics and Gynecology, 40: 473, 1972).)

abundant in tumors showing mainly the cord-like or trabecular pattern (Fig. 20.71), whereas the tubular variety tends to be more cellular and contains less connective tissue (Figs. 20.73, 20.74). The stroma may vary from loose and edematous (Fig. 20.71) to dense fibrous and hyalinized (Fig. 20.72). The former is seen more often where the cord-like pattern is most prominent, whereas the latter surrounds the larger cellular aggregates. The third pattern

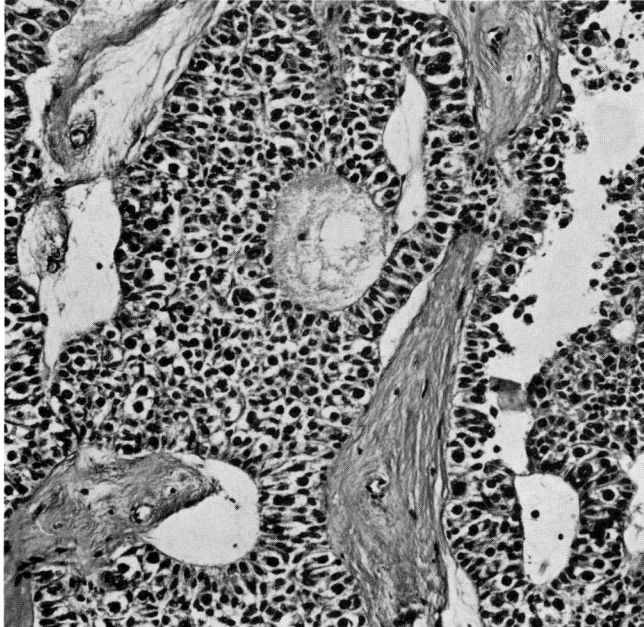

FIG. 20.72. **Mixed germ cell–sex cord–stromal tumor.** The neoplasm is composed of large cellular aggregates and more slender cords. Note the hyaline connective tissue stroma.

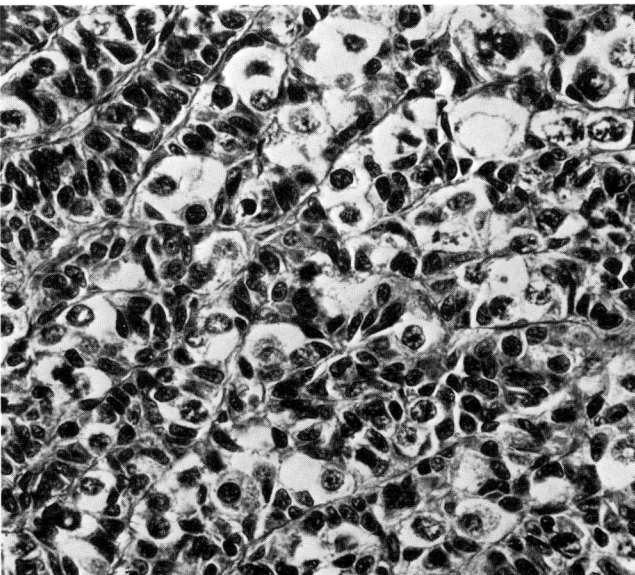

FIG. 20.74. **Mixed germ cell–sex cord–stromal tumor.** The tubular pattern is illustrated. Note large germ cells surrounded by sex cord–stromal cells. (Reprinted with permission from The American College of Obstetricians and Gynecologists. (Obstetrics and Gynecology, 40: 473, 1972).)

consists of scattered collections of germ cells surrounded by sex cord elements that may be very abundant. The germ cells admixed with sex cord derivatives may also be scattered individually and in small groups within connective tissue stroma.

Sometimes there may be a suggestion of an insular pattern with islands of various sizes surrounded by fine fibrovascular stroma coalescing and forming aggregates (Fig. 20.75), or occasionally being separated by large amounts of connective tissue and forming a more pronounced insular pattern. Admixture between the above-described patterns is often seen. The typical nest-like pattern present in gonadoblastoma is not observed. In one case, only a few small collections of Leydig or lutein-like cells were observed,[313] but in all the remaining cases these cells were not identified.

The two cellular elements present in the tumor, the germ cells and the sex cord derivatives, are intimately admixed. The sex cord derivatives are arranged peripherally in a single file, forming long rows at the periphery of the cords (Figs. 20.71, 20.76) or peripherally lining the tubular structures (Fig. 20.74) as well as surrounding individual or groups of germ cells within the small clusters or larger aggregates. The germ cells resemble those observed in dysgerminoma and gonadoblastoma in all respects, including histochemical reactions. In some cases, a number of the germ cells present in this tumor appear more mature than the germ cells observed in gonadoblastoma or dysgerminoma and tend to resemble primordial germ cells. In view of this, it is possible that they may represent a later stage in the maturation of the germ cell than that seen in gonadoblastoma or dysgerminoma. They show brisk mitotic activity (Fig. 20.76). The sex cord derivatives tend to resemble Sertoli cells more than granulosa cells. They show variable degrees of mitotic activity. The tumor does

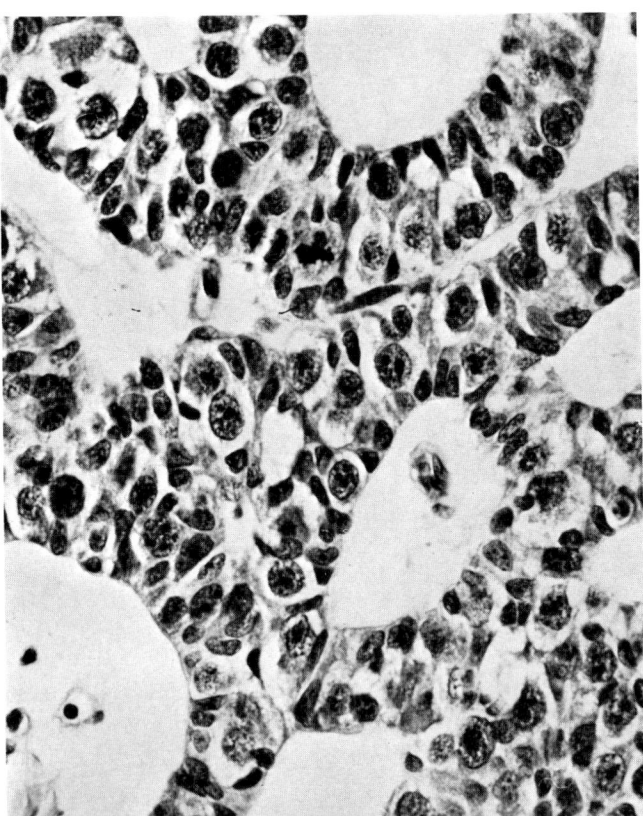

FIG. 20.76. **Mixed germ cell–sex cord–stromal tumor.** The cord-like pattern is shown. Tripolar mitosis is seen above *center.*

not show hyalinization, calcification, or the regressive changes observed in gonadoblastoma and appears to be actively proliferative. There is some variation in the cellular content in some parts of the tumor; in some areas there is a preponderance of germ cells, whereas in others the sex cord derivatives predominate. However, the intimate admixture of these two cell types is seen everywhere. Most tumors show a solid pattern, although occasional small clefts lined by sex cord elements may be present. In some tumors cystic spaces of varying size either lined by sex cord derivatives, flattened epithelial-like cells, or devoid of lining may be observed.[326,335,359] They closely resemble the cystic spaces observed in some retiform Sertoli–Leydig cells tumors[319,323,389] or cystic sex cord–stromal tumors. In occasional tumors this pattern may be pronounced and may suggest that the tumor contains epithelial cells, in addition to germ cells and sex cord derivatives.[335] It is considered that these cells are in fact sex cord derivatives and that the tumor in common with some sex cord tumors exhibits a retiform or cystic pattern, or both.

Normal ovarian tissue as evidenced by the presence of normal ovarian stroma and at least some primordial follicles has been identified in all cases, including a case in which it could not be identified in the original sections available.[313] In some cases, graafian follicles also are

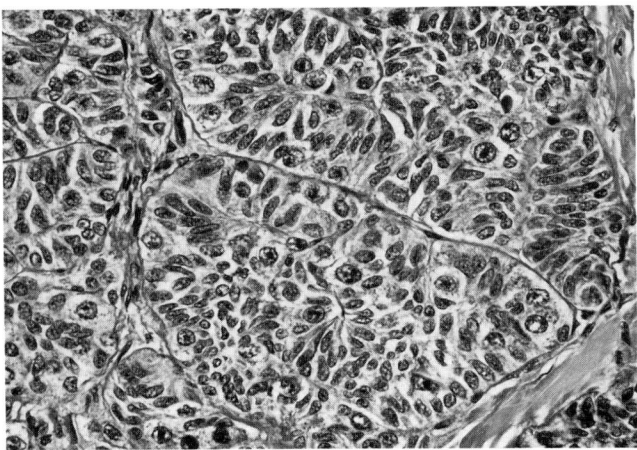

FIG. 20.75. **Mixed germ cell–sex cord–stromal tumor.** There is a suggestion of an insular pattern. The tumor islands are surrounded by fine fibrovascular connective tissue.

present.[314,326] In other cases, tumor deposits are found very close to the surface of the ovary.

DIFFERENTIAL DIAGNOSIS

Histologically, this tumor is most likely to be confused with gonadoblastoma. In contrast to gonadoblastoma, this tumor lacks the typical nest-like pattern, has greater proliferative activity of both the germ cell and sex cord component, lacks calcification, hyalinization, and in most cases Leydig or lutein-like cells. Macroscopically, the tumors are larger. The gonad of origin is a normal ovary, and there is no evidence of gonadal dysgenesis or any somatosexual abnormalities. The patients are chromatin-positive and have a normal female 46XX karyotype. There is no evidence of virilization, and if there are signs of abnormal endocrine activity, they manifest themselves as feminization.

Occasionally, if the germ cells are relatively scanty, the tumor may be confused with the sex cord–stromal tumors of the ovary, but the presence of germ cells should alert the observer to the true identity of the tumor. If the sex cord derivatives either are few in number, are missed, or are disregarded, the tumor may be included with the germ cell tumors, but the presence of sex cord elements intimately admixed with the germ cells should indicate its true identity. The presence of prominent clefts and cystic spaces, especially when the latter contain papillary projections, may cause confusion with Sertoli–Leydig cell tumors showing the retiform pattern or even with serous papillary tumors. The presence of germ cells admixed with sex cord derivatives indicates that the tumor is a mixed germ cell–sex cord–stromal tumor.

CLINICAL BEHAVIOR AND TREATMENT

The prognosis of patients with mixed germ cell–sex cord–stromal tumor of the ovary occurring in pure form is favorable. In the great majority of known cases when the tumor was confined to the ovary and not associated with other malignant neoplastic germ cell elements, there has been no recurrence or metastases after excision of the affected adnexa. The patients are well and disease-free for periods varying from 1 to 15 years.[326] Accordingly, after a unilateral salpingo-oophorectomy, careful examination of the abdomen and a biopsy of the contralateral ovary are recommended. After this procedure, the patient should have chromosome studies. If the karyotype is 46XX and if no other abnormalities are detected, further therapy is not necessary, although careful long-term follow-up is essential.

One well-documented case of metastasizing mixed germ cell–sex cord–stromal tumor occurring in an 8-year-old girl has been reported.[167] The metastases were found in the para-aortic lymph nodes and in the peritoneal cavity. The patient was well and disease-free 2 years after excision of the affected adnexa, para-aortic lymphadenectomy, excision of peritoneal metastases, and a course of cisplatin-based combination chemotherapy.[167]

In three patients in their 20s, one in her early 30s, and one in her early 40s, the mixed germ cell–sex cord–stromal tumor was associated with dysgerminoma. There was no evidence of metastases. The patients are well and disease-free from 2 to 7 years after one-sided adnexectomy and radiation therapy. In four children aged 5 to 16 years, the tumor was overgrown by other malignant germ cell elements, including choriocarcinoma and yolk sac tumor. In three of these cases, the tumor metastasized and resulted in the death of the patients. The metastases were composed of the malignant germ cell elements. One patient treated with cisplatinum-based chemotherapy is alive and well 5 years later. When the tumor is associated with the latter, the patient should be treated with the appropriate combination chemotherapy used in treatment of malignant nondysgerminomatous germ cell tumors. When the tumor is encountered in postmenarchal women there is an increased possibility that the tumor may not present in pure form, but may be associated with other neoplastic germ cell elements. In such cases appropriate therapy to treat the neoplastic germ cell elements in addition to excision of the affected adnexa is recommended.

References

1. Abbot TM, Herman WJ Jr, Scully RE (1984) Ovarian fetiform teratoma (homunculus) in a 9-year-old girl. Int J Gynecol Pathol 2: 392
2. Abell MR, Johnson VJ, Holtz F (1965) Ovarian neoplasms in childhood and adolescence. Part 1. Tumors of germ cell origin. Am J Obstet Gynecol 92: 1059
3. Abitol MM, Pomerance W, Mackles A (1959) Spontaneous intraperitoneal rupture of benign cystic teratomas. Review of literature and report of two cases. Obstet Gynecol 13: 198
4. Afridi MA, Vongtama V, Tsukada Y, Piver MS (1976) Dysgerminoma of the ovary. Radiation therapy for recurrence and metastases. Am J Obstet Gynecol 126: 190
5. Aguirre P, Scully RE (1982) Malignant neuroectodermal tumor of the ovary: A distinctive form of monodermal teratoma. Report of five cases. Am J Surg Pathol 6: 283
6. Albrechtsen R, Klee JG, Moller JE (1972) Primary intracranial germ cell tumours, including five cases of endodermal sinus tumour. Acta Pathol Microbiol Scand 233 [suppl 80A]:32
7. Alenghat E, Okagaki T, Talerman A (1986) Primary mucinous carcinoid tumor of the ovary. Cancer 58: 777
8. Allard S, Cadotte M, Boivin Y (1972) Dysgenesie gonadique pure familiale et gonadoblastome. L'Union Medicale du Canada 101: 448
9. Anderson CT Jr, Carlson IH (1975) Elevated plasma testosterone and gonadal tumors in two 46XY "sisters." Arch Pathol 99: 360

10. Anderson MC, McDicken IW (1971) Melanotic cyst of the ovary. J Obstet Gynaecol Br Commonw 78: 1047

11. Ansfield FJ, Korbitz BC, Davis HL, Ramirez G (1969) Triple drug therapy in testicular tumors. Cancer 24: 442

12. Arhelger RB, Kelly B (1974) Strumal carcinoid. Report of a case with electron microscopical observations. Arch Pathol 97: 323

13. Asadourian LA, Taylor HB (1969) Dysgerminoma. An analysis of 105 cases. Obstet Gynecol 33: 370

14. Atkin NB (1973) High chromosome numbers of seminomata and malignant teratomata of the testis: A review of data on 103 tumors. Br J Cancer 28: 275

15. Atkin NB, Baker MC (1983) i (12p): specific chromosomal marker in seminoma and malignant teratoma of the testis? Cancer Genet Cytogenet 10: 199

16. Atkin NB, Baker MC (1987) Abnormal chromosomes including small metacentrics in 14 ovarian cancers. Cancer Genet Cytogenet 26: 355

17. Awais GA (1983) Dysgerminoma and serum lactic dehydrogenase levels. Obstet Gynecol 61: 99

18. Azoury RS, Jubayli NW, Barakat BY (1973) Dermoid cyst of the ovary containing fetus-like structure. Obstet Gynecol 42: 887

19. Bagg HJ (1936) Experimental production of teratoma testis in a fowl. Am J Cancer 26: 69

20. Ballas M (1972) Yolk sac carcinoma of the ovary with alpha-fetoprotein in serum and ascitic fluid demonstrated by immunoosmophoresis. Am J Clin Pathol 57: 511

21. Ballas M (1974) The significance of alpha-fetoprotein in the serum of patients with malignant teratomas and related gonadal neoplasms. Am J Clin Lab Sci 4: 267

22. Bardin CW, Rosen S, Le Maire WJ, et al (1968) In vivo and in vitro studies of androgen metabolism in a patient with pure gonadal dysgenesis and Leydig cell hyperplasia. J Clin Endocrinol Metab 29: 1429

23. Barry KG, Crosby WH (1957) Autoimmune hemolytic anemia arrested by removal of ovarian teratoma: Review of the literature and report of a case. Ann Intern Med 47: 1002

24. Bartlett DJ, Grant JK, Pugh MA, Aherne W (1968) A familial feminizing syndrome. A family showing intersex characteristics with XY chromosomes in three female members. J Obstet Gynaecol Br Commonw 75: 199

25. Battifora H, Sheibani K, Tubbs RR, Kopinski MI, Sun TT (1984) Antikeratin antibodies in tumor diagnosis. Distinction between seminoma and embryonal carcinoma. Cancer 54: 843

26. Beck JS, Fulmer HF, Lee ST (1969) Solid malignant ovarian teratoma with "embryoid bodies" and trophoblastic differentiation. J Pathol 99: 67

27. Beilby JOW, Todd PJ (1974) Yolk sac tumour of the ovary. J Obstet Gynaecol Br Commonw 81: 90

28. Bell DA, Flotte TJ, Bhan AK (1987) Immunohistochemical characterization of seminoma and its inflammatory infiltrate. Hum Pathol 18: 511

29. Berg JW, Baylor SM (1973) The epidemiologic pathology of ovarian cancer. Hum Pathol 4: 537

30. Bergher de Bacalao E, Dominguez I (1969) Unilateral gonadoblastoma in a pregnant woman. Am J Obstet Gynecol 105: 1279

31. Bergstrand CG, Czar B (1956) Demonstration of a new protein fraction in serum from human fetus. Scand J Lab Invest 8: 174

32. Bernstein D, Naor S, Rikover M, Manahem H (1974) Hemolytic anemia related to ovarian tumor. Obstet Gynecol 43: 276

33. Bestle J (1968) Extragonadal endodermal sinus tumours originating in the region of the pineal gland. Acta Pathol Microbiol Scand 74: 214

34. Bettinger HF, Jacobs H (1948) Mesonephroma ovarii. Med J Aust 1: 100

35. Bhatena D, Haning RV Jr, Shapiro S, Hafez GR (1985) Coexistence of a gonadoblastoma and mixed germ cell–sex cord stroma tumor. Pathol Res Pract 180: 203

36. Bjorkholm E, Lundell M, Gyftodimos A, Silversward C (1990) Dysgerminoma. The Radiumhemmet series 1927–1984. Cancer 65: 38

37. Blackwell WJ, Dockerty MB, Masson JC, Mussey RD (1946) Dermoid cysts of the ovary: clinical and pathological significance. Am J Obstet Gynecol 51: 151

38. Boczkowski K, Teter J, Sternadel Z (1972) Sibship occurrence of XY gonadal dysgenesis with dysgerminoma. Am J Obstet Gynecol 113: 952

39. Borushek S, Berger I, Echt C, Gold JJ (1965) Functioning malignant germ cell tumor of the ovary in a 4½ year old girl. Cancer 18: 1485

40. Bradof JE, Hakes TB, Ochoa M, Golbey R (1982) Germ cell malignancies of the ovary. Treatment with vinblastine, actinomycin D, bleomycin and cisplatin containing chemotherapy combinations. Cancer 50: 1070

41. Braunstein H, Stephens CL, Gibson RL (1968) Secretory granules in medullary carcinoma of the thyroid. Electron microscopic demonstration. Arch Pathol 85: 306

42. Breen JL, Maxson WS (1977) Ovarian tumors in children and adolescents. Clin Obstet Gynecol 20: 607

43. Breen JL, Neubecker RD (1963) Malignant teratoma of the ovary. An analysis of 17 cases. Obstet Gynecol 21: 669

44. Breen JL, Neubecker RD (1967) Ovarian malignancy in children with special reference to the germ cell tumors. Ann NY Acad Sci 142: 658

45. Brody S (1961) Clinical aspects of dysgerminoma of the ovary. Acta Radiol (Stockh) 56: 209

46. Brown JR, Green JD (1976) Yolk sac carcinoma. South Med J 69: 728

47. Burkons DM, Hart WR (1978) Ovarian germinomas (dysgerminomas). Obstet Gynecol 51: 221

48. Cabanne F (1971) Gonadoblastomes et tumerus de l'ebauche gonadique. Ann Anat Pathol (Paris) 16: 387

49. Carleton RL, Friedman NB, Bomze EJ (1953) Experimental teratomas of testis. Cancer 6: 464

50. Caruso PA, Marsh MR, Minkowitz S, Karten G (1971) An intense clinicopathologic study of 305 teratomas of the ovary. Cancer 27: 343

51. Chenot M (1911) Contribution à l'étude des épithéliomas primitifs de l'ovaire. Thesis, Paris

52. Chevassu M (1906) Tumeurs du Testicule. Thesis, Steinhall Paris

53. Chretien PB, Milam JD, Foote FW, Miller TR (1970) Embryonal adenocarcinomas (a type of malignant teratoma) of the sacrococcygeal region. Clinical and pathologic aspects of 21 cases. Cancer 26: 522

54. Chumas JC, Scully RE (1991) Sebaceous tumors arising in ovarian dermoid cysts. Int J Gynecol Pathol 10: 356

55. Chumas JC, Rosenwaks Z, Mann JW, Finkel G, Pastore J (1984) Sertoli-Leydig cell tumor of the ovary producing alpha-fetoprotein. Int J Gynecol Pathol 3: 213

56. Clement PB, Young RH, Scully RE (1987) Endometrioid-like variant of ovarian yolk sac tumor. A clinicopathological analysis of eight cases. Am J Surg Pathol 11: 767

57. Climie AR, Heath LP (1968) Malignant degeneration of benign cystic teratoma of the ovary. Review of the literature and report of a chondrosarcoma and a carcinoid tumor. Cancer 22: 824

58. Cohen MB, Mulchahey KM, Molnar JJ (1986) Ovarian endodermal sinus tumor with intestinal differentiation. Cancer 57: 1580

59. Cohen MB, Friend DS, Molnar JJ, Talerman A (1987) Gonadal endodermal sinus (yolk sac) tumor with pure intestinal differentiation; a new histologic type. Pathol Res Pract 182: 609

60. Collins DH, Symington T (1965) Sertoli cell tumour. In: Collins DH, Pugh RCB (eds) The pathology of testicular tumours. Edinburgh and London, Livingstone Ltd., pp 52–61

61. Cooperman LR, Hamlin J, Elmer N (1968) Gonadoblastoma: A rare ovarian tumor with characteristic roentgen appearance. Radiology 90: 322

62. Corfman PA, Richart RM (1964) Chromosome number and morphology of benign cystic teratomas. N Engl J Med 271: 1241

63. Cutler BS, Forbes AP, Ingersoll FM, Scully RE (1972) Endometrial carcinoma after stilbestrol therapy in gonadal dysgenesis. N Engl J Med 287: 628

64. Dalgaard JB, Wetteland P (1956) Struma ovarii. A follow-up study of 20 cases. Acta Chir Scand 112: 1

65. Damjanov I, Drobnjak P, Grizelj V (1975) Ultrastructure of gonadoblastoma. Arch Pathol 99: 25

66. Dandia SD (1967) Rectovesical fistula following an ovarian dermoid with recurrent vesical calculus. A case report. J Urol 97: 85

67. Davidsohn I, Kovarik S, Stejskal R (1968) Immunological aspects. Influence of prognosis and treatment. In: Gentil F, Junqueira AC (eds) Ovarian Cancer U.I.C.C. Monograph Series, Vol 11. Berlin, Heidelberg, New York, Springer–Verlag, pp 105–121

68. Dawson MA, Wilimer T, Yarbro JW (1971) Hemolytic anemia associated with an ovarian tumor. Am J Med 50: 552

69. Dayal Y, Tashjian AH Jr, Wolfe HJ (1979) Immunocytochemical localization of calcitonin-producing cells in a strumal carcinoid with amyloid stroma. Cancer 43: 1331

70. De Haan QC (1965) Non-gestational choriocarcinoma of the ovary. Obstet Gynecol 26: 708

71. Dekmezian R, Sneige N, Ordonez NG (1986) Ovarian and omental ependymomas in peritoneal washings: cytologic and immunocytochemical features. Diagn Cytopathol 2: 62

72. De Lima FAO (1966) Disgerminoma do Ovario, contribucao para o seo estudo anatomo-clinico. Thesis, Sao Paulo, Brazil

73. Dietl J, Horny HP, Ruck P, Kaiserling E (1993) Dysgerminoma of the ovary. An immunohistochemical study of tumor-infiltrating lymphoreticular cells and tumor cells. Cancer 71: 2562

74. Dikman SH, Toker C (1971) Strumal carcinoid of the ovary with musculinization. Cancer 27: 925

75. Diligent E (1971) Gonadoblastomes et dysgenesies pseudogonadoblastiques. Thesis, Nancy, France

76. Dixon FJ, Moore RA (1952) Tumors of the male sex organs. Atlas of Tumor Pathology, Sect VIII, Fasc 31b and 32. Washington, D.C., Armed Forces Institute of Pathology

77. Duhig JT (1959) An unusual adenocarcinoma of the ovary. A case simulating Schiller's mesonephroma. Am J Obstet Gynecol 77: 201

78. Duval M (1891) Le placenta de rongeurs. J Anat Physiol (Paris) 27: 515

79. Einhorn LH, Donohue J (1977) Cisdiammine dichloroplatinum, vinblastine, and bleomycin combination chemotherapy in disseminated testicular cancer. Ann Intern Med 87: 293

80. Emge LA (1940) Functional and growth characteristics of struma ovarii. Am J Obstet Gynecol 40: 738

81. Engel T, Greeley AV, Sweeney WJ III (1965) Recurrent dermoid cysts of the ovary. Report of 2 cases. Obstet Gynecol 26: 757

82. Erez SE, Richart RM, Shettles LB (1965) Hashimoto's disease in a benign cystic teratoma of the ovary. Am J Obstet Gynecol 92: 273

83. Erhan Y, Toprak AS, Ozdemir N, Tiras B (1992) Gonadoblastoma and fertility. J Clin Pathol 45: 828

84. Evans RW (1957) Developmental stages of embryo-like bodies in teratoma testis. J Clin Pathol 10: 321

85. Evans RW (1966) Histological Appearances of Tumours, 2nd ed. Edinburgh and London, Livingstone

86. Ewing J (1940) Neoplastic Diseases, 4th ed. Philadelphia, W. B. Saunders, pp 641, 672

87. Felmus LB, Pedowitz P (1968) Clinical malignancy of endocrine tumors of the ovary and dysgerminoma. Obstet Gynecol 29: 344

88. Flamant F, Caillou B, Pejovic MH, et al (1978) Prognostic factors in malignant germ cell tumors of the ovary in children excluding pure dysgerminoma. Eur J Cancer 14: 901

89. Forney JP, Di Saia PJ, Morrow CP (1975) Endodermal sinus tumor. A report of two sustained remissions treated postoperatively with a combination of actinomycin D, 5-fluorouracil and cyclophosphamide. Obstet Gynecol 45: 186

90. Fox H, Langley FA (1976) Tumours of the Ovary. London, William Heinemann Medical Books

91. Fox H, Kazzaz B, Langley FA (1964) Argyrophil and argentaffin cells in the female genital tract and in ovarian mucinous cysts. J Pathol Bacteriol 88: 479

92. Frazier SD, Bashore RA, Mosier HD (1964) Gonadoblastoma associated with pure gonadal dysgenesis in monozygous twins. J Pediatr 64: 740

93. Freel JH, Cassir JF, Pierce VK, Woodruff J, Lewis JL Jr (1979) Dysgerminoma of the ovary. Cancer 43: 798

94. Friedman NB (1951) The comparative morphogenesis of extragenital and gonadal teratoid tumors. Cancer 4: 265

95. Friedman NB, Moore RA (1946) Tumors of the testis. A report of 922 cases. Mil Surgeon 99: 573

96. Fujii S, Konishi I, Suzuki A, Okamura H, Okazaki T, Mori T (1985) Analysis of serum lactic dehydrogenase levels and its isoenzymes in ovarian dysgerminoma. Gynecol Oncol 22: 65

97. Galager HS, Lewis RP (1973) Sequential gonadoblastoma and choriocarcinoma. Obstet Gynecol 41: 123

98. Gallion H, Van Nagell JR, Powell DF, Donaldson ES, Hanson M (1979) Therapy of endodermal sinus tumor of the ovary. Am J Obstet Gynecol 135: 447

99. Galton M, Benirschke K (1959) 46 chromosomes in an ovarian teratoma. Lancet 2: 761

100. Gans B, Bahary C, Levie B (1963) Ovarian regeneration and pregnancy following massive radiotherapy for dysgerminoma. Report of a case. Obstet Gynecol 22: 596

101. Garvin AJ, Pratt-Thomas HR, Spector M, Spicer SS, Williamson HO (1976) Gonadoblastoma: Histologic ultrastructural and histochemical observations in five cases. Am J Obstet Gynecol 125: 459

102. Gershenson DM, Del Junco G, Herson J, Rutledge FN (1983) Endodermal sinus tumor of the ovary. The M.D. Anderson experience. Obstet Gynecol 61: 194

103. Gershenson DM, Copeland LJ, Kavanagh JJ, et al (1985) Treatment of malignant nondysgerminomatous germ cell tumors of the ovary with vincristine, dactinomycin and cyclophosphamide. Cancer 56: 2756

104. Gershenson DM (1993) Update on malignant ovarian germ cell tumors. Cancer 71: 1581

105. Gibas Z, Prout FR Jr, Sandberg AA (1984) Malignant teratoma of the testis with an isochromosome No 12, i (12p), as the sole structural abnormality. J Urol 131: 762

106. Gibas Z, Talerman A, Faruqi S, Carlson J, Noumoff J (1993) Cytogenetic analysis of an immature teratoma of the ovary and its metastasis. Int J Gynecol Pathol 12: 276

107. Gillman J (1948) The development of the gonads in man with consideration of the role of fetal endocrines and the histogenesis of ovarian tumors. Contrib Embryol 32: 83

108. Gitlin D, Boesman M (1967) Sites of serum alpha-fetoprotein synthesis in the human and in the rat. J Clin Invest 46: 1010

109. Gitlin D, Pericelli A (1970) Synthesis of serum albumin, prealbumin, alpha-fetoprotein, alpha-1-antitrypsin and transferrin by the human yolk sac. Nature 228: 995

110. Gitlin D, Pericelli A, Gitlin G (1972) Synthesis of alpha-fetoprotein by liver, yolk sac and gastrointestinal tract of the human conceptus. Cancer Res 32: 979

111. Goldsmith CI, Hart WR (1975) Ataxia–telangiectasia with ovarian gonadoblastoma and contralateral dysgerminoma. Cancer 36: 1838

112. Goldstein DP, Piro JA (1972) Combination chemotherapy in the treatment of germ cell tumors containing choriocarcinoma. Surg Gynecol Obstet 134: 61

113. Gondos B, Bhiraleus P, Hobel CJ (1971) Ultrastructural observations on germ cells in human fetal ovaries. Am J Obstet Gynecol 110: 644

114. Gonzalez-Angulo A, Kaufman R, Braungardt CD, Chapman FC, Hinshaw AJ (1963) Adenocarcinoma of thyroid arising in struma ovarii (malignant struma ovarii). Report of two cases and review of the literature. Obstet Gynecol 21: 567

115. Gonzalez-Crussi F, Roth LM (1976) The human yolk sac and yolk sac carcinoma. Hum Pathol 7: 675

116. Gonzalez-Licea A, Hartman WH, Yardley JH (1968) Medullary carcinoma of the thyroid. Ultrastructural evidence of its origin from the parafollicular cell and its possible relation to carcinoid tumors. Am J Clin Pathol 49: 512

117. Gordon A, Lipton D, Woodruff JD (1981) Dysgerminoma: A review of 158 cases from the Emil Novak Ovarian Tumor Registry. Obstet Gynecol 58: 497

118. Greco MA, LiVolsi VA, Pertschuk LP, Bigelow B (1979) Strumal carcinoid of the ovary: An analysis of its components. Cancer 43: 1380

119. Griffiths K, Grant JK, Browning NCK, Whyte WG, Sharp JL (1966) Steroid synthesis in vitro by tumor tissue from dysgenetic gonad. J Endocrinol 34: 155

120. Grosfeld JL, Stepita DS, Nance WE, Palmer CG (1974) Fetus-in-fetu. An unusual cause for an abdominal mass in infancy. Ann Surg 180: 80

121. Gusberg SB, Danforth DN (1944) Clinical significance of struma ovarii. Am J Obstet Gynecol 48: 537

122. Hain AM (1949) An unusual case of precocious puberty associated with ovarian dysgerminoma. J Clin Endocrinol 9: 1349

123. Hameed K, Burslem MRG (1970) A melanotic ovarian neoplasm resembling the "retinal anlage" tumor. Cancer 25: 564

124. Hart WR, Burkons DM (1979) Germ cell neoplasms arising in gonadoblastomas. Cancer 34: 669

125. Hart WR, Regezi JA (1978) Strumal carcinoid of the ovary. Ultrastructural observations and long-term follow-up study. Am J Clin Pathol 69: 356

126. Hertig AT, Adams CE (1967) Studies on the human oocyte and its follicle. 1. Ultrastructural and histochemical observations on primordial follicle stage. J Cell Biol 34: 647

127. Hertig AT, Gore H (1961) Tumors of the female sex organs. Part 3. Tumors of the ovary and fallopian tube. Atlas of Tumor Pathology, Sec 9, Fasc 33. Washington, D.C., Armed Forces Institute of Pathology

128. Higuchi K, Kato T (1958) Dysgerminoma of the ovary. J Jpn Obstet Gynecol Soc 5: 206

129. Hingorani V, Narula RK, Bhalla S (1963) *Salmonella typhi* infection in an ovarian dermoid. Report of a case. Obstet Gynecol 22: 118

130. Hirschfield LS, Kahn LB, Winkler B, Bochner RZ, Gibstein AA (1985) Adenocarcinoid of the appendix presenting as bilateral Krukenberg's tumor of the ovaries. Arch Pathol Lab Med 109: 930

131. Hou-Jensen K, Kempson RL (1974) The ultrastructure of gonadoblastoma and dysgerminoma. Hum Pathol 5: 79

132. Hughesdon PE (1955) Two cases of struma ovarii showing the histogenesis of thyroid and thymus in ovarian teratoma. J Pathol Bacteriol 70: 35

133. Hughesdon PE, Kumarasamy T (1970) Mixed germ cell tumors (gonadoblastomas) in normal and dysgenetic gonads. Virch Arch [Pathol Anat] 349: 258

134. Huntington RW Jr, Bullock WK (1970) Yolk sac tumors of the ovary. Cancer 25: 1357

135. Huntington RW Jr, Bullock WK (1970) Yolk sac tumors of extragonadal origin. Cancer 25: 1368

136. Huntington RW Jr, Morgenstern NL, Sargent JA, Giem RN, Richards A, Hanford KC (1963) Germinal tumors exhibiting the endodermal sinus pattern of Teilum in young children. Cancer 16: 34

137. Ishida T, Tagatz GE, Okagaki T (1976) Gonadoblastoma. Ultrastructural evidence of testicular origin. Cancer 37: 1770

138. Itoh T, Shirai T, Naka A, Matsumoto S (1974) Yolk sac tumor and alpha-fetoprotein: Clinicopathological study of four cases. Gann 65: 215

139. Jackson SM (1967) Ovarian dysgerminoma. Br J Radiol 40: 459

140. Jacobs AJ, Newland JR, Green RK (1982) Pure choriocarcinoma of the ovary. Obstet Gynecol Surv 37: 603

141. Jacobsen GK, Talerman A (1989) Atlas of Germ Cell Tumors. Munksgaard, Copenhagen

142. Jacobsen GK, Braendstrup O, Talerman A (1991) Bilateral mixed germ cell-sex cord stroma tumour in a young adult woman. Case Report. Acta Pathol Microbiol Immunol Scand 23 (suppl): 132

143. Janovski NA, Paramanandhan TL (1973) Ovarian Tumors. Tumors and Tumor-like Conditions of the Ovaries, Fallopian Tubes and Ligaments of the Uterus. Stuttgart, Georg Thieme Verlag

144. Jatoi AF (1959) Dysgerminoma of the ovary (a study of 23 cases). J Postgrad Med 5: 22

145. Jedberg H (1949) Some clinical aspects of dysgerminoma ovarii. Acta Obstet Gynecol Scand 28: 194

146. Jenkyn DJ, McCartney AJ (1987) A chromosome study of three ovarian tumors. Cancer Genet Cytogenet 26: 327

147. Jimerson GK, Woodruff JD (1977) Ovarian extraembryonal teratoma: 1. Endodermal sinus tumor. Am J Obstet Gynecol 127: 73

148. Jimerson GK, Woodruff JD (1977) Ovarian extraembryonal teratoma: 2. Endodermal sinus tumor mixed with other germ cell tumors. Am J Obstet Gynecol 127: 302

149. Judd HL, Scully RE, Atkins L, Neer RM, Kliman B (1970) Pure gonadal dysgenesis with progressive hirsutism. N Engl J Med 282: 881

150. Kawahara H (1963) Struma ovarii with ascites and hydrothorax. Am J Obstet Gynecol 85: 85

151. Kay S, Silverberg SG, Schatzki PF (1972) Ultrastructure of an ovarian dysgerminoma. Report of a case featuring neurosecretory-type granules in stromal cells. Am J Clin Pathol 58: 458

152. Kazancigil TR, Laquer W, Ladewig P (1940) Papilloendothelioma of the ovary; report of three cases and discussion of Schiller's "mesonephroma ovarii." Am J Cancer 40: 199

153. Kelley RR, Scully RE (1961) Cancer developing in dermoid cysts of the ovary. A report of 8 cases including a carcinoid and a leiomyosarcoma. Cancer 14: 989

154. King ME, Mouradian JA, Micha JP, Chaganti RSK, Allen SL (1985) Immature teratoma of the ovary with predominant malignant retinal anlage tumor. A parthenogenetically derived tumor. Am J Surg Pathol 9: 221

155. King ME, DiGiovanni LM, Yung JF, Clarke-Pearson DL (1990) Immature teratoma of the ovary grade 3, with karyotype analysis. Int J Gynecol Pathol 9: 178

156. King ME, Hubbell MJ, Talerman A (1991) Mixed germ cell tumor of the ovary with prominent polyembryoma component. Int J Gynecol Pathol 10: 88

157. Kleiman GM, Young RH, Scully RE (1984) Ependymoma of the ovary: report of three cases. Hum Pathol 15: 632

158. Klein HZ (1974) Mucinous carcinoid tumor of the vermiform appendix. Cancer 33: 770

159. Koller O, Gjonnes H (1964) Dysgerminoma of the ovary. Acta Obstet Gynecol Scand 43: 268

160. Kommoss F, Franklin WA, Talerman A (1989) Estrogen and progesterone receptors in endodermal sinus (yolk sac) tumor. Evaluation of immunocytochemical and biochemical methods. J Reprod Med 34: 943

161. Kommoss F, Bibbo M, Talerman A (1990) Nuclear deoxyribonucleic acid content (ploidy) of endodermal sinus (yolk sac) tumor. Lab Invest 62: 223

162. Krepart G, Smith JP, Rutledge F, Declos L (1978) The treatment for dysgerminoma of the ovary. Cancer 41: 986

163. Krumerman MS, Chung A (1977) Squamous carcinoma arising in benign cystic teratoma of the ovary. Cancer 39: 1237

164. Kurman RJ, Norris HJ (1976) Endodermal sinus tumor of the ovary. A clinical and pathological analysis of 71 cases. Cancer 38: 2404

165. Kurman RJ, Norris HJ (1976) Embryonal carcinoma of the ovary. A clinicopathologic entity distinct from endodermal sinus tumor resembling embryonal carcinoma of the adult testis. Cancer 38: 2420

166. Kurman RJ, Norris HJ (1976) Malignant mixed germ cell tumors of the ovary. A clinical and pathological analysis of 30 cases. Obstet Gynecol 48: 579

167. Lacson AG, Gillis DA, Shawwa A (1988) Malignant mixed germ cell–sex cord stromal tumors of the ovary associated with isosexual precocious puberty. Cancer 61: 2122

168. Lange PH, Millan JL, Stigbrand T, Vessella RL, Ruoslahti E, Fishman WH (1982) Placental alkaline phosphatase as a tumor marker for seminoma. Cancer Res 42: 3244

169. Larson NE, Dockerty MB, Pratt JH (1958) Primary mixed choriocarcinoma and dysgerminoma of the ovary. Report of a case. Proc Mayo Clin 33: 341

170. Levine GD (1973) Primary thymic seminoma—a neoplasm ultrastructurally similar to testicular seminoma and distinct from epithelial thymoma. Cancer 31: 729

171. Liebert KI, Stent L (1960) Dysgerminoma of the ovary with chorionepithelioma. J Obstet Gynaecol Br Emp 77: 627

172. Lien L (1979) Determination of serum AFP for the diagnosis and treatment of ovarian endodermal sinus tumor. Zhonghua Fuchanke Zazhi 14: 22 (in Chinese)

173. Linder D (1969) Gene loss in human teratomas. Proc Natl Acad Sci USA 63: 699

174. Linder D, Power J (1970) Further evidence for postmeiotic origin of teratomas in the human female. Ann Hum Genet 34: 21

175. Linder D, McCaw BK, Hecht F (1975) Parthenogenic origin of benign ovarian teratoma. N Engl J Med 292: 63

176. Lingeman CH (1974) Etiology of cancer of the human ovary. A review. J Natl Cancer Inst 53: 1603

177. Livnat EJ, Scommegna A, Recant W, Jao W (1977) Ultrastructural observations of the so-called strumal carcinoid of the ovary. Arch Pathol Lab Med 101: 585

178. Lord JM (1956) Intra-abdominal foetus in fetu. J Pathol Bacteriol 72: 627

179. Lynn JA, Varon HH, Kingsley WB, Martin JH (1967) Ultrastructure and biochemical studies of estrogen-secreting capacity of a "non-functional" ovarian neoplasm (dysgerminoma). Am J Pathol 51: 639

180. Mackay AM, Pattigrew N, Symington T, Neville AM (1974) Tumors of dysgenetic gonads (gonadoblastoma). Ultrastructural and steroidogenic aspects. Cancer 34: 1108

181. McCullough CD, Hardart F (1963) Neuroblastomatous transformation in a benign cystic teratoma. Obstet Gynecol 21: 259

182. McDonough PG, Byrd JR, Tho PT, Otken L (1976) Gonadoblastoma in a true hermaphrodite with 46XX karyotype. Obstet Gynecol 47: 355

183. McDonough PG, Greenblatt RB, Byrd JR, Hastings EV (1967) Gonadoblastoma (gonocytoma III). Report of a case. Obstet Gynecol 29: 54

184. McKay DG, Hertig AT, Adams EC, Danziger S (1953) Histochemical observations on the germ cells of human embryos. Anat Rec 117: 201

185. McKay DG, Pinkerton JHM, Hertig AT, Danziger S (1961) The adult human ovary: A histochemical study. Obstet Gynecol 18: 13

186. Malkasian GD Jr, Symmonds RE (1964) Treatment of the unilateral encapsulated germinoma. Am J Obstet Gynecol 90: 379

187. Malkasian GD Jr, Dockerty MB, Symmonds RE (1967) Benign cystic teratomas. Obstet Gynecol 29: 719

188. Malkasian GD Jr, Symmonds RE, Dockerty MB (1965) Malignant ovarian teratomas. Report of 31 cases. Obstet Gynecol 25: 810

189. Malkasian GD Jr, Webb MJ, Jorgensen EO (1974) Observations on chemotherapy of granulosa cell carcinoma and malignant ovarian teratoma. Obstet Gynecol 44: 885

190. Marcial-Rojas RA, de Arellano RGA (1956) Malignant melanoma arising in a dermoid cyst of the ovary. Cancer 9: 523

191. Marin-Padilla M (1965) Origin, nature and significance of the "embryoids" of human teratomas. Virch Arch [Pathol Anat] 340: 105

192. Marrubini G (1949) Primary chorionepithelioma of the ovary. Report of two cases. Acta Obstet Gynecol Scand 28: 251

193. Masson P (1912) Seminomes ovariennes. Bull Soc Anat (Paris) 87: 402

194. Masson P (1923) Epitheliomas pflügeriens. In: Diagnostics de Laboratoire. Les Tumeurs. Paris, Maloine

195. Mathieu J, Planchu M (1950) Le prognostic et le traitement du seminome de l'ovaire. Les oestrogenes out-ils place dans le traitement du seminome en general? Lyon Chir 45: 76

196. Matz MH (1961) Benign cystic teratomas of the ovary. Obstet Gynecol Surv 16: 591

197. Mazur MT, Talbot WH Jr, Talerman A (1988) Endodermal sinus tumor and mucinous cystadenofibroma of the ovary. Occurrence in an 82-year-old woman. Cancer 62: 2011

198. Melicow MM, Uson AC (1959) Dysgenetic gonadomas and other gonadal neoplasms in intersex. Cancer 12: 552

199. Meyer R (1931) The pathology of some special ovarian tumors and their relation to sex characteristics. Am J Obstet Gynecol 22: 697

200. Miettinen M, Virtanen I, Talerman A (1985) Intermediate filament proteins in human testis and testicular germ-cell tumors. Am J Pathol 120: 402

201. Miettinen M, Talerman A, Wahlstrom T, Astengo-Osuna C, Virtanen I (1985) Cellular differentiation in ovarian sex cord–stromal and germ-cell tumors studied with antibodies to intermediate-filament proteins. Am J Surg Pathol 9: 640

202. Moertel CG, Beahrs OH, Woolner LB, Tyce GM (1965) "Malignant carcinoid syndrome" associated with noncarcinoid tumors. N Engl J Med 273: 244

203. Mueller CW, Topkins P, Lapp WA (1950) Dysgerminoma of the ovary. An analysis of 427 cases. Am J Obstet Gynecol 60: 153

204. Nakashima M, Nagasaka T, Fukata S, Oiwa N, Nara Y, Fukatsu T, Takeuchi J (1989) Ovarian gonadoblastoma with dysgerminoma in a woman with two normal children. Hum Pathol 20: 814

205. Neigus I (1952) Ovarian dysgerminoma with chorionepithelioma. Am J Obstet Gynecol 64: 422

206. Neubecker RD, Breen JL (1962) Embryonal carcinoma of the ovary. Cancer 15: 546

207. Nielsen SNJ, Scheithauer BW, Gaffey TA (1985) Gliomatosis peritonei. Cancer 56: 2499

208. Nieminen I, Von Numers C, Widholm O (1964) Struma ovarii. Acta Obstet Gynecol Scand 42: 399

209. Nogales FF Jr, Matilla A, Nogales-Ortiz F, Galera-Davidson HL (1978) Yolk sac tumors with pure and mixed polyvesicular vitelline patterns. Hum Pathol 9: 553

210. Nogales FF Jr, Silverberg SG, Bloustein PA, Martinez-Hernandez A, Pierce GB (1977) Yolk sac carcinoma (endodermal sinus tumor). Ultrastructure and histogenesis of gonadal and extragonadal tumors in comparison with normal human yolk sac. Cancer 39: 1462

211. Nomura K, Ohama K, Okamoto E, Fujiwara A (1983) Cytogenetic studies of multiple ovarian dermoid cysts in a single host. Acta Obstet Gynecol Jpn 35: 1938

212. Norgaard-Pedersen B, Albrechtsen R, Teilum G (1975) Serum alpha-fetoprotein as a marker for endodermal sinus tumor (yolk sac tumor), or a vitelline component of teratocarcinoma. Acta Pathol Microbiol Scand (A) 83: 573

213. Norris HJ, Jensen RD (1972) Relative frequency of ovarian neoplasms in children and adolescents. Cancer 30: 713

214. Norris HJ (1993) Personal communication

215. Norris HJ, Zirkin HJ, Benson WL (1976) Immature (malignant) teratoma of the ovary. A clinical and pathologic study of 58 cases. Cancer 37: 2359

216. Novak E (1952) Gynecologic and Obstetric Pathology, 3rd ed. Philadelphia, W. B. Saunders

217. Novak E, Gray LA (1938) Dysgerminoma of the ovary. Am J Obstet Gynecol 35: 925

218. Novak E, Woodruff JD, Novak ER (1954) Probable mesonephric origin of certain female genital tumors. Am J Obstet Gynecol 68: 1224

219. Novak ER (1948) Solid teratoma of the ovary, with report of five cases. Am J Obstet Gynecol 56: 300

220. Novak ER, Woodruff JD (1967) In: Novak ER (ed) Gynecologic and Obstetric Pathology, 6th ed. Philadelphia, W. B. Saunders, p 367

221. Nystrom C (1956) Dysgerminoma of the ovary. Acta Obstet Gynecol Scand 35: 385

222. Oliver HM, Horne EO (1948) Primary teratomatous chorionepithelioma of the ovary. Report of a case. N Engl J Med 239: 14

223. Overbeck L, Philipp E (1969) Die Ultrastruktur des Disgerminoms in Ovar. Zugleich ein Beitrag zur Histogenese des Tumors. Z Geburtschilfe Gynaekol 170: 125

224. Palmer PE, Safaii H, Wolfe HJ (1976) Alpha-1-antitrypsin and alpha-fetoprotein markers in endodermal sinus (yolk sac) tumors. Am J Clin Pathol 65: 575

225. Pantoja E, Noy MA, Axtmayer RW, Colon FE, Pelegrina I

(1975) Ovarian dermoids and their complications. Comprehensive historical review. Obstet Gynecol Surv 30: 1

226. Pantoja E, Rodriguez-Ibanez I, Axtmayer RW, Noy MA, Pelegrina I (1975) Complications of dermoid tumors of the ovary. Obstet Gynecol 45: 89

227. Park IJ, Pyeatte JC, Jones HW, Woodruff JD (1972) Gonadoblastoma in a true hermaphrodite with 46XY genotype. Obstet Gynecol 40: 466

228. Parrington JM, West LF, Povey S (1984) The origin of ovarian teratomas. J Med Genet 21: 4

229. Parrington JM, West LF, Povey S (1986) Chromosome changes in germ cell tumors. In: Jones WG, Milford Ward A, Anderson CK (eds) Germ Cell Tumors II. Oxford, Pergamon, pp 61–67

230. Patel SK, Prentice SA (1972) Gonadoblastoma—distinctive ovarian tumor. Arch Pathol 94: 165

231. Payne D, Muss HB, Homesley HD, Jobson VM, Baird FG (1981) Autoimmune hemolytic anemia and ovarian dermoid cysts. Case report and review of the literature. Cancer 48: 721

232. Pedowitz P, Felmus LB, Grayzel DM (1955) Dysgerminoma of the ovary. Prognosis and treatment. Am J Obstet Gynecol 70: 1284

233. Peterson WF (1956) Solid histologically benign teratomas of the ovary. A report of four cases and review of the literature. Am J Obstet Gynecol 72: 1094

234. Peterson WF (1957) Malignant degeneration of benign cystic teratomas of the ovary: A collective review of the literature. Obstet Gynecol Surv 12: 793

235. Peterson WF, Prevost EC, Edmunds FT, Huntley JM Jr, Morris FK (1955) Benign cystic teratomas of the ovary. A clinico-statistical study of 1007 cases with review of the literature. Am J Obstet Gynecol 70: 368

236. Peyron A (1939) Faits nouveaux relatifs à l'origine et à l'histogenese des embryomes. Bull Assoc Franc Cancer 28: 658

237. Pierce GB Jr (1966) Ultrastructure of human testicular tumors. Cancer 19: 1963

238. Pierce GB Jr, Dixon FJ (1959) Testicular teratomas. 1. Demonstration of teratogenesis by metamorphosis of multipotential cells. Cancer 12: 573

239. Pierce GB Jr, Dixon FJ (1959) Testicular teratomas. 2. Teratocarcinoma as ascitic tumor. Cancer 12: 584

240. Pierce GB Jr, Midgley AR (1963) The origin and function of human syncytiotrophoblastic giant cells. Am J Pathol 43: 153

241. Pierce GB Jr, Verney EL (1961) An in vitro and in vivo study of differentiation in teratocarcinomas. Cancer 14: 1017

242. Pierce GB Jr, Bullock WK, Huntington RW Jr (1970) Yolk sac tumors of the testis. Cancer 25: 644

243. Pierce GB Jr, Midgley AR, Beals TF (1962) An ultrastructural study of differentiation and maturation of trophoblast of the monkey. Lab Invest 13: 451

244. Pierce GB Jr, Midgley AR, Sri Ram J, Feldman JD (1964) Parietal yolk sac carcinoma. Clue to the histogenesis of Reichert's membrane of the mouse embryo. Am J Pathol 41: 549

245. Plaut A (1933) Ovarian struma: A morphologic, pharmacologic, and biologic examination. Am J Obstet Gynecol 25: 351

246. Prat J, Bhan AK, Dickersin GR, Robboy SJ, Scully RE (1982) Hepatoid yolk sac tumor of the ovary (endodermal sinus tumor with hepatoid differentiation). A light microscopic ultrastructural and immunohistochemical study of seven cases. Cancer 50: 2355

247. Pratt-Thomas HR, Cooper JM (1976) Gonadoblastoma with tubal pregnancy. Am J Clin Pathol 65: 121

248. Qizilbash AH, Trebilcock RG, Patterson MC, Lamont KG (1974) Functioning primary carcinoid tumor of the ovary. A light and electron microscopic study with review of the literature. Am J Clin Pathol 62: 629

249. Ramsey HJ (1965) Ultrastructure of a pineal tumor. Cancer 18: 1014

250. Ranchod M, Kempson RL, Dorgeloh JR (1976) Strumal carcinoid of the ovary. Cancer 37: 1913

251. Rao NR, Veliath GD, Srinivasan M (1964) An unusual case of sacrococcygeal mesonephroma (Schiller). Cancer 17: 1604

252. Rashad MH, Fathalla MF, Kerr MC (1966) Sex chromatin and chromosome analysis in ovarian teratomas. Am J Obstet Gynecol 96: 461

253. Robboy SJ, Scully RE (1970) Ovarian teratoma with glial implants on the peritoneum. An analysis of 12 cases. Hum Pathol 1: 643

254. Robboy SJ, Scully RE (1980) Strumal carcinoid of the ovary. An analysis of 50 cases of a distinctive tumor composed of thyroid tissue and carcinoid. Cancer 46: 2019

255. Robboy SJ, Norris HJ, Scully RE (1975) Insular carcinoid primary in the ovary—a clinicopathologic analysis of 48 cases. Cancer 36: 404

256. Robboy SJ, Scully RE, Norris HJ (1974) Carcinoid metastatic to the ovary. A clinicopathologic analysis of 35 cases. Cancer 33: 798

257. Robboy SJ, Scully RE, Norris HJ (1977) Primary trabecular carcinoid of the ovary. Obstet Gynecol 49: 202

258. Rose LI, Underwood RH, Williams GH, Pincus GS (1974) Pure gonadal dysgenesis. Studies of in vitro androgen metabolism. Am J Med 57: 957

259. Rulon DB, Helwig EB (1974) Cutaneous sebaceous neoplasms. Cancer 33: 82

260. Rutgers JL, Young RH, Scully RE (1987) Ovarian yolk sac tumor arising from endometrioid carcinoma. Hum Pathol 18: 1296

261. Rutgers JL, Scully RE (1986) Functioning ovarian tumors with peripheral steroid cell proliferation. A report of 24 cases. Int J Gynecol Pathol 5: 319

262. Sailer S (1940) Ovarian dysgerminoma. Am J Cancer 38: 473

263. Sailer S (1943) Struma ovarii. Am J Clin Pathol 13: 271

264. Salet J, de Gennes LJ, de Grouchy J, et al (1970) A propos d'un cas de gonadoblastome 46XX. Ann Endocrinol (Paris) 31: 927

265. Samuels ML, Lanzotti VJ, Holoye PY, Boyle LY, Smith TL, Johnson DE (1976) Combination chemotherapy of germinal cell tumors. Cancer Treat Rev 3: 185

266. Santesson L (1947) Clinical and pathological survey of ovarian tumours treated at the Radiumhemmet. 1. Dysgerminoma. Acta Radiol (Stockholm) 28: 643

267. Santesson L, Marrubini G (1957) Clinical and pathological survey of ovarian embryonal carcinomas, including so-

called "mesonephreomas" (Schiller) or "mesoblastomas" (Teilum) treated at the Radiumhemmet. Acta Obstet Gynecol Scand 36: 399

268. Saunders AM, Hertzman VO (1960) Malignant carcinoid teratoma of the ovary. Can Med Assoc J 83: 602

269. Schellhas HF (1974) Malignant potential of the dysgenetic gonad. Part 1. Obstet Gynecol 44: 298

270. Schellhas HF (1974) Malignant potential of the dysgenetic gonad. Part 2. Obstet Gynecol 44: 455

271. Schellhas HF, Trujillo JM, Rutledge FN, Cork A (1971) Germ cell tumors associated with XY gonadal dysgenesis. Am J Obstet Gynecol 109: 1197

272. Schiller W (1939) Mesonephroma ovarii. Am J Cancer 35: 1

273. Schiller W (1942) Histogenesis of ovarian mesonephroma. Arch Pathol 33: 443

274. Schmitz EF (1925) Malignant endothelioma of perithelioma type in the ovary. Am J Obstet Gynecol 9: 247

275. Schwartz PE, Morris JM (1988) Serum lactic dehydrogenase. A tumor marker for dysgerminoma. Obstet Gynecol 72: 511

276. Scully RE (1953) Gonadoblastoma. A gonadal tumor related to dysgerminoma (seminoma) and capable of sex hormone production. Cancer 6: 455

277. Scully RE (1963) Germ cell tumors of the ovary and Fallopian tube. In: Meigs JV, Sturgis SH (eds) Progress in Gynecology, Vol 4. New York, Grune and Stratton, pp 335–347

278. Scully RE (1970) Germ cell tumors of the ovary. In: Sturgis SH, Taymor ML (eds) Progress in Gynecology, Vol 5. New York, Grune and Stratton, pp 329–348

279. Scully RE (1970) Recent progress in ovarian cancer. Hum Pathol 1: 73

280. Scully RE (1970) Gonadoblastoma. Cancer 25: 1340

281. Scully RE (1970) Sex cord tumor with annular tubules. A distinctive ovarian tumor of the Peutz–Jeghers syndrome. Cancer 25: 1107

282. Scully RE (1979) Tumors of the ovary and maldeveloped gonads. In: Atlas of tumor pathology, 2nd series, Fasc 16. Washington, D.C., Armed Forces Institute of Pathology

283. Scully RE (1980) Personal communication

284. Scully RE, Fox H, Russell P, Saksela E, Sasano N, Sobin LH, Talerman A (in press) World Health Organization and International Society of Gynecological Pathologists classification of the tumors of the ovary, Fallopian tube and peritoneum. Heidelberg, Springer–Verlag

285. Seegar GE (1938) Ovarian dysgerminomas. Arch Surg 37: 697

286. Sell A, Sogaard H, Norgaard-Pedersen B (1976) Serum alpha-fetoprotein as a marker for the effects of postoperative radiation therapy and/or chemotherapy in 8 cases of ovarian endodermal sinus tumor. Int J Cancer 18: 574

287. Sens MA, Levenson TB, Metcalf JS (1982) A case of metastatic carcinoid arising in an ovarian teratoma. Cancer 49: 2541

288. Senterman MK, Cassidy PN, Fenoglio CM, Ferenczy A (1984) Histology, ultrastructure and immunocytochemistry of strumal carcinoid. A case report. Int J Gynecol Pathol 3: 232

289. Serov SF, Scully RE, Sobin LH (1973) Histological typing of ovarian tumors. International histological classification of tumors. No 9. Geneva, World Health Organization

290. Serratoni FT, Robboy SJ (1975) Ultrastructure of primary and metastatic ovarian carcinoids—analysis of 11 cases. Cancer 36: 157

291. Shah KD, Kaffe S, Gilbert F, Dolgin S, Gertner M (1988) Unilateral microscopic gonadoblastoma in a prepubertal Turner mosaic with Y chromosome material identified by restriction fragment analysis. Am J Clin Pathol 90: 622

292. Shirai T, Itoh T, Yoshiki T, Noro T, Tomino Y, Hayasaka T (1976) Immunofluorescent demonstration of alpha-fetoprotein, and other plasma proteins in yolk sac tumor. Cancer 38: 1661

293. Sjovall A (1943) Disgerminome des Ovariums. Acta Obstet Gynecol Scand 23: 585

294. Simard LC (1957) Polyembryonic embryoma of the ovary of parthenogenetic origin. Cancer 10: 215

295. Smith FG (1946) Pathology and physiology of struma ovarii. Arch Surg 53: 603

296. Smith JB, O'Neill RT (1971) Alpha-fetoprotein. Occurrence in germinal cell and liver malignancies. Am J Med 51: 767

297. Smith JP, Rutledge F (1975) Advances in chemotherapy for gynecologic cancer. Cancer 36: 669

298. Smith JP, Rutledge FN, Sutow WW (1963) Malignant gynecologic tumors in children. Current approaches to treatment. Am J Obstet Gynecol 116: 261

299. Snyder RR, Tavassoli FA (1986) Ovarian strumal carcinoid: Immunohistochemical, ultrastructural, and clinicopathologic observations. Int J Gynecol Pathol 5: 187

300. Solomon J, Steinfeld JL, Bateman JR (1967) Chemotherapy of germinal tumors. Cancer 26: 747

301. Sporrong B, Falkmer S, Robboy SJ, et al (1982) Neurohormonal peptides in ovarian carcinoids. An immunohistochemical study of 81 primary carcinoids and of intraovarian metastases from six midgut carcinoids. Cancer 49: 68

302. Stagno PA, Petras RE, Hart WR (1987) Strumal carcinoids of the ovary. An immunohistologic and ultrastructural study. Arch Pathol Lab Med 111:440

303. Stamp GWH, McConnell EM (1983) Malignancy arising in cystic ovarian teratomas. Br J Obstet Gynecol 90: 671

304. Sternberg WH, Barclay DL, Kloepfer HW (1968) Familial XY gonadal dysgenesis. N Engl J Med 278: 695

305. Stevens LC (1959) Embryology of testicular teratomas in strain 129 mice. J Natl Cancer Inst 23: 1249

306. Stevens LC (1960) Embryonic potency of embryoid bodies derived from a transplantable testicular teratoma of the mouse. Dev Biol 2: 285

307. Stevens LC (1962) The biology of teratomas including evidence indicating their origin from primordial germ cells. Ann Biol 1: 585

308. Strauss AF, Gates HS (1964) Giant sebaceous gland tumor of the ovary. Am J Clin Pathol 41: 78

309. Subbuswamy SG, Gibbs NM, Ross CF, Morson BC (1974) Goblet cell carcinoid of the appendix. Cancer 34: 338

310. Szokol M, Kondrai G, Papp Z (1977) Gonadal malignancy and 46XY karyotype in a true hermaphrodite. Obstet Gynecol 49: 358

311. Takeda A, Ishizuka T, Goto T, et al (1982) Polyembryoma of ovary producing alpha-fetoprotein and HCG. Immunoperoxidase and electron microscopic study. Cancer 49: 1878

312. Talerman A (1971) Gonadoblastoma and dysgerminoma in two siblings with dysgenetic gonads. Obstet Gynecol 38: 416

313. Talerman A (1972) A distinctive gonadal neoplasm related to gonadoblastoma. Cancer 30: 1219

314. Talerman A (1972) A mixed germ cell–sex cord stroma tumor in a normal female infant. Obstet Gynecol 40: 473

315. Talerman A (1974) Gonadoblastoma associated with embryonal carcinoma. Obstet Gynecol 43: 138

316. Talerman A (1975) The incidence of yolk sac tumor (endodermal sinus tumor) elements in germ cell tumors of the testis in adults. Cancer 36: 211

317. Talerman A (1980) The pathology of gonadal neoplasms composed of germ cells and sex cord stroma derivatives. Pathol Res Pract 170: 24

318. Talerman A (1984) Carcinoid tumors of the ovary. J Cancer Res Clin Oncol 107: 125

319. Talerman A (1987) Ovarian Sertoli–Leydig cell tumor (androblastoma) with retiform pattern. A clinicopathologic study. Cancer 60: 3056

320. Talerman A, Delemarre JFM (1975) Gonadoblastoma associated with embryonal carcinoma in an anatomically normal male. J Urol 113: 355

321. Talerman A, Evans MI (1982) Primary trabecular carcinoid tumor of the ovary. Cancer 50: 1407

322. Talerman A, Haije WG (1974) Alpha-fetoprotein and germ cell tumors. A possible role of yolk sac tumor in production of alpha-fetoprotein. Cancer 34: 1722

323. Talerman A, Haije WG (1985) Ovarian Sertoli cell tumor with retiform and heterologous elements. Am J Surg Pathol 9: 459

324. Talerman A, Okagaki T (1985) Ultrastructural features of primary trabecular carcinoid tumor of the ovary. Int J Gynecol Pathol 4: 153

325. Talerman A, Okagaki T (unpublished observations)

326. Talerman A, van der Harten JJ (1977) A mixed germ cell–sex cord stroma tumor of the ovary associated with isosexual precocious puberty in a normal female child. Cancer 40: 889

327. Talerman A, Haije WG, Baggerman L (1977) Alpha-1-antitrypsin (AAT) and alpha-foetoprotein (AFP) in sera of patients with germ cell neoplasms. Value as tumor markers in patients with endodermal sinus tumour (yolk sac tumour). Int J Cancer 19: 741

328. Talerman A, Haije WG, Baggerman L (1978) Histological patterns in germ cell neoplasms associated with raised serum alphafoetoprotein (AFP). Scand J Immunol 8 (suppl): 97

329. Talerman A, Haije WG, Baggerman L (1978) Serum alpha-fetoprotein in diagnosis and management of endodermal sinus (yolk sac) tumor and mixed germ cell tumor of the ovary. Cancer 41: 272

330. Talerman A, Haije WG, Baggerman L (1980) Serum alpha-fetoprotein (AFP) in patients with germ cell tumors of the gonads and extragonadal sites. Correlation between endodermal sinus (yolk sac) tumor and raised serum AFP. Cancer 46: 340

331. Talerman A, Huyzinga WT, Kuipers T (1973) Dysgerminoma. Clinicopathologic study of 22 cases. Obstet Gynecol 41: 137

332. Talerman A, Jarabak J, Amarose A (1981) Gonadoblastoma and dysgerminoma in a true hermaphrodite with 46,XX karyotype. Am J Obstet Gynecol 140: 175

333. Talerman A, van der Pompe WB, Haije WG, Baggerman L, Boekestein-Tjahjadi HM (1977) Alpha-fetoprotein and carcinoembryonic antigen in germ cell neoplasms. Br J Cancer 35: 288

334. Talerman A, Verp M, Senekjian E, Gilewski T, Vogelzang N (1990) True hermaphrodite with normal female 46,XX karyotype, bilateral gonadoblastomas and dysgerminomas and normal pregnancy. Cancer 66: 2668

335. Tavassoli FA (1983) A combined germ cell–gonadal stromal–epithelial tumor of the ovary. Am J Surg Pathol 7: 73

336. Taylor CW (1972) Müllerian mixed tumor. Acta Pathol Microbiol Scand 233 (suppl 80A): 48

337. Taylor MH, Depetrillo AD, Turner AR (1985) Vinblastine, bleomycin, and cisplatin in malignant germ cell tumors of the ovary. Cancer 56: 1341

338. Teilmann I, Kassis H, Pietra G (1967) Primary germ cell tumour of the anterior mediastium with features of endodermal sinus tumour (mesoblastoma vitellinum). Acta Pathol Microbiol Scand 70: 267

339. Teilum G (1944) Homologous tumours in ovary and testis: Contribution to classification of gonadal tumours. Acta Obstet Gynecol Scand 24: 480

340. Teilum G (1946) Gonocytoma; homologous ovarian and testicular tumours. 1. With discussion of "mesonephroma ovarii" (Schiller: Am J Cancer 1939). Acta Pathol Microbiol Scand 23: 242

341. Teilum G (1950) "mesonephroma ovarii" (Schiller) extraembryonic mesoblastoma of germ cell origin in ovary and testis. Acta Pathol Microbiol Scand 27: 249

342. Teilum G (1952) Classification of ovarian tumours. Acta Obstet Gynecol Scand 31: 292

343. Teilum G (1959) Endodermal sinus tumors of the ovary and testis. Comparative morphogenesis of the so-called mesonephroma ovarii (Schiller) and extraembryonic (yolk sac-allantoic) structures of the rat's placenta. Cancer 12: 1092

344. Teilum G (1965) Classification of endodermal sinus tumour (mesoblastoma vitellinum) and so-called embryonal carcinoma of the ovary. Acta Pathol Microbiol Scand 64: 407

345. Teilum G (1968) Tumours of germinal origin. In: Gentil F, Junqueira AC (eds) Ovarian Cancer, U.I.C.C. Monograph Series, Vol 11. Berlin, Heidelberg, New York, Springer–Verlag, pp 58–73

346. Teilum G (1976) Special Tumors of the Ovary and Testis. Comparative Histology and Identification, 2nd ed. Copenhagen, Munksgaard

347. Teilum G, Albrechtsen R, Norgaard-Pedersen B (1974) Immunofluorescent localization of alpha-fetoprotein synthesis in endodermal sinus tumor (yolk sac tumor). Acta Pathol Microbiol Scand 82A: 586

348. Teilum G, Albrechtsen R, Norgaard-Pedersen B (1975) The histogenetic–embryologic basis for reappearance of alpha-fetoprotein in endodermal sinus tumors and teratomas. Acta Pathol Microbiol Scand 83A: 80

349. Teter J (1960) A new concept of classification of gonadal tumors arising from germ cell (gonocytoma) and their histogenesis. Gynaecologia (Basel) 150: 84

350. Teter J (1962) A mixed form of feminizing germ cell tumor (gonocytoma II). Am J Obstet Gynecol 84: 722

351. Teter J (1970) Prognosis, malignancy and curability of the germ cell tumor occurring in dysgenetic gonads. Am J Obstet Gynecol 108: 894

352. Teter J, Boczkowski K (1967) Occurrence of tumors in dysgenetic gonads. Cancer 20: 1301

353. Theiss EA, Ashley DJB, Mostofi FK (1959) Nuclear sex of testicular tumors and some related ovarian and extragonadal neoplasms. Cancer 13: 323

354. Thoeny RH, Dockerty MB, Hunt AB, Childs DS Jr (1961) Study of ovarian dysgerminoma with emphasis on the role of radiation therapy. Surg Gynecol Obstet 113: 692

355. Thomas GM, Dembo AJ, Hacker NE, DePetrillo AD (1987) Current therapy for dysgerminoma of the ovary. Obstet Gynecol 70: 268

356. Thurlbeck WM, Scully RE (1960) Solid teratoma of the ovary. Cancer 13: 804

357. Tiltman AJ (1985) Ependymal cyst of the ovary. South Afr Med J 68: 424

358. Toker C (1969) Ovarian carcinoid. A light and electron microscopic study. Am J Obstet Gynecol 103: 1019

359. Tokuoka S, Aoki Y, Yokoyama T, Ishii T (1985) A mixed germ cell–sex cord stromal tumor of the ovary with retiform tubular structure. A case report. Int J Gynecol Pathol 4: 161

360. Tsuchida Y, Kaneko M, Yokomori K, et al (1978) Alpha-fetoprotein, prealbumin, albumin, alpha-1-antitrypsin, and transferrin as diagnostic and therapeutic markers for endodermal sinus tumors. J Pediatr Surg 13: 25

361. Turner HB, Douglas WM, Gladding TC (1964) Choriocarcinoma of the ovary. Obstet Gynecol 24: 918

362. Ueda G, Sato Y, Yamasaki M, et al (1978) Strumal carcinoid of the ovary. Histological, ultrastructural, and immunohistological studies with anti-human thyroglobulin. Gynecol Oncol 6: 411

363. Ueda G, Fujita M, Ogawa H, Sawada M, Inoue M, Tanizawa O (1993) Adenocarcinoma in a benign cystic teratoma of the ovary. Report of a case with a long survival period. Gynecol Oncol 48: 259

364. Ulbright TM, Roth LM, Erlich CE (1982) Ovarian strumal carcinoid. An immunocytochemical and ultrastructural study of two cases. Am J Clin Pathol 77: 622

365. Ulbright TM, Roth LM (1987) Recent developments in the pathology of germ cell tumors. Semin Diagn Pathol 4: 304

366. Ulirsch RC, Goldman RL (1982) An unusual teratoma of the ovary: neurogenic cyst with lactating breast tissue. Obstet Gynecol 60: 400

367. Uzisima H (1956) Ovarian dysgerminoma associated with virilization. Report of a case. Cancer 9: 736

368. Vance RP, Geisinger KR (1985) Pure nongestational choriocarcinoma of the ovary. Report of a case. Cancer 56: 2321

369. Vawter GF (1965) Carcinoma of the vagina in infancy. Cancer 18: 1479

370. Warkel RL, Cooper PH, Helwig EB (1978) Adenocarcinoid, a mucin-producing carcinoid of the appendix. Cancer 42: 2781

371. Weldon-Linne CM, Rushovich AM (1983) Benign ovarian cystic teratomas with homunculi. Obstet Gynecol 61: 88S

372. Wheatley VR (1957) Further observations on the nature of the dermoid cyst fat. J Invest Dermatol 29: 445

373. Whelton JA, Fallon RJ (1964) Successful pregnancy after surgery and supervoltage therapy for metastatic dysgerminoma. N Engl J Med 271: 145

374. Wider JA, O'Leary JA (1968) Dysgerminoma: A clinical review. Obstet Gynecol 31: 560

375. Wider JA, Marshall JR, Bardin CW, Lipsett MB, Rose GT (1969) Sustained remissions after chemotherapy for primary ovarian cancers containing choriocarcinoma. N Engl J Med 280: 1439

376. Wieland RG, Ekstrom B, Vorijs N (1968) $C_{19}O_2$ Steroid secretion by dysgenetic gonads. Obstet Gynecol 32: 643

377. Wilkinson EJ, Friedrich EG, Hosty TA (1973) Alpha-fetoprotein and endodermal sinus tumor of the ovary. Am J Obstet Gynecol 116: 711

378. Williams ED (1966) Histogenesis of medullary carcinoma of the thyroid. J Clin Pathol 19: 114

379. Williams ED, Sandler M (1963) Classification of carcinoid by embryologic grouping. Lancet 1: 238

380. Williamson HO, Underwood PB Jr, Kreutner A Jr, Rogers JF, Mathur RS, Pratt-Thomas HR (1976) Gonadoblastoma: Clinicopathologic correlation in six patients. Am J Obstet Gynecol 126: 579

381. Willis RA (1958) The borderland of embryology and pathology. London, Butterworths

382. Willis RA (1967) Pathology of Tumours, 4th ed. London, Butterworths

383. Wisniewski M, Deppisch LM (1973) Solid teratomas of the ovary. Cancer 32: 440

384. Witschi E (1948) Migration of the germ cells of human embryos from the yolk sac to the primitive gonadal folds. Contrib Embryol 32: 69

385. Woodruff JD, Markley RL (1957) Struma ovarii. Demonstration of both pathologic change and physiologic activity; report of four cases. Obstet Gynecol 9: 707

386. Woodruff JD, Protos P, Peterson WF (1968) Ovarian teratomas. Relationship of histologic and ontogenic factors to prognosis. Am J Obstet Gynecol 102: 702

387. Woodruff JD, Rauh JT, Markley RL (1966) Ovarian struma. Obstet Gynecol 27: 194

388. Wurster K, Hedinger C, Meienberg O (1972) Orchioblastomatous foci in testicular teratoma of adults. Virch Arch [Pathol Anat] 357: 231

389. Young RH, Scully RE (1983) Ovarian Sertoli–Leydig cell tumors with a retiform pattern. A problem in histopathologic diagnosis. A report of 25 cases. Am J Surg Pathol 7: 755

390. Young RH, Perez-Atayde AR, Scully RE (1984) Ovarian Sertoli–Leydig cell tumor with retiform and heterologous elements. Report of a case with hepatocytic differentiation and elevated serum alpha-fetoprotein. Am J Surg Pathol 8: 709

391. Young RH, Prat J, Scully RE (1982) Ovarian Sertoli–Leydig cell tumors with heterologous elements (1) gastrointestinal epithelium and carcinoid: A clinicopathologic analysis of thirty six cases. Cancer 50: 2448

392. Zaloudek C, Tavassoli FA, Norris HJ (1981) Dysgerminoma with syncytiotrophoblastic giant cells. A histologically and clinically distinctive subtype of dysgerminoma. Am J Surg Pathol 5: 361

393. Zondag HA (1964) Enzyme activity in dysgerminoma and seminoma. A study of lactic dehydrogenase isoenzymes in malignant diseases. Rhode Island Med J 47: 273

21

Nonspecific Tumors of the Ovary, Including Mesenchymal Tumors and Malignant Lymphoma

Aleksander Talerman, M.D., Ph.D., F.R.C. Path.

The tumors discussed in this chapter comprise a heterogeneous group of neoplasms that are not specific to the ovary. They are uncommon in this location, occurring much more frequently in other parts of the body. Consequently, whenever they are encountered in the ovary, these tumors pose difficult problems in diagnosis, histogenesis, behavior, and therapy for the pathologist and clinician. These neoplasms must be differentiated from primary ovarian neoplasms containing mesenchymal tissue, as well as from metastatic and disseminated neoplasms affecting the ovary. Thus, mesenchymal neoplasms nonspecific to the ovary must be differentiated primarily from teratomatous neoplasms containing large amounts of mature or immature mesenchymal elements and from the mixed müllerian (mesodermal) tumors (MMMT), composed of different malignant connective tissue elements. In contrast, the primary malignant lymphomas must be differentiated from the more common disseminated malignant lymphoma and leukemia, which not infrequently affect the ovary. These two different groups of neoplasms—the connective tissue neoplasms nonspecific to the ovary and malignant lymphoma of the ovary—although included under the same heading, are discussed separately because of their different nature, behavior, and histogenesis. In addition, the adenomatoid tumor, which is of mesothelial origin, the ovarian tumor of probable wolffian origin, ovarian neoplasms of neural origin, hepatoid carcinoma of the ovary, and small cell carcinoma of the ovary with pulmonary differentiation also are included.

Mesenchymal Tumors Nonspecific to the Ovary

Mesenchymal neoplasms nonspecific to the ovary include all primary ovarian neoplasms of connective tissue origin found in the ovary that are nonspecific to it but considered to originate from ovarian tissue, and not of teratomatous or surface epithelial (müllerian) origin. However, this mode of origin cannot be excluded in a number of cases. The neoplasms discussed here are composed of a single neoplastic mesenchymal element, either benign or malignant, in contrast to teratomatous or mixed müllerian tumors, which usually are composed of a number of tissue elements.

Some issues of classification and histogenesis may not be reconcilable in view of the possibility of one-sided differentiation of a teratoma or of a mixed müllerian tumor of the ovary. Thus, although some of these neoplasms can be shown to originate directly from ovarian tissue, a considerable number of cases are of indeterminate histogenesis and origin. Mesenchymal neoplasms nonspecific to the ovary can be benign or malignant, and are classified based on the tissue of origin.

Tumors of Fibrous Tissue Origin

Fibroma

Fibroma is the most common ovarian neoplasm of connective tissue origin and comprises 3–5% of ovarian neoplasms. An even higher frequency occurs when fibrosed thecomas are included in this category.

The histogenesis of ovarian fibroma is controversial. The neoplasm most likely arises from mesenchymal cells of the ovarian stroma, which differentiate in the fibroblastic direction. Some investigators postulate that it arises from a fibrosed thecoma or a Brenner tumor, whereas others believe that it originates from the connective tissue within the ovary, primarily within the ovarian cortex or in the walls of blood and lymphatic vessels. Although it can be difficult or even impossible to differentiate between fibroma and fibrosed thecoma, it is worthwhile to make the attempt.

Ovarian fibroma is bilateral in 4–8% of patients, and in 10% of patients, the tumors are multiple.[23] Ovarian fibroma usually is encountered in menopausal and postmenopausal women, but is seen at all ages. It is rare in children: fewer than 10 examples have been reported.[9,13,17,44,54,62,82]

Clinically, patients with ovarian fibroma frequently are asymptomatic, mainly because of the tumor's small size. When symptoms do occur, they manifest themselves as abdominal enlargement, urinary symptoms, and abdominal pain. Acute pain is associated with torsion of the tumor. Ascites is a relatively common associated finding and is seen in 50% of cases of fibromas measuring more than 5 cm in diameter. Ascites and hydrothorax (Meigs's syndrome) are seen in 1–3% of cases.[8,23,49] Excision of the tumor results in resolution of the ascites and hydrothorax. In one case,[67] the tumor was associated with hypoglycemia, which resolved after excision of the fibroma. An increased frequency of ovarian fibroma was noted in women with hereditary basal cell nevus (Gorlin) syndrome.[13,14,54,82] In these women the fibroma usually is bilateral[13,19,54,82] and may become malignant[54] or recur.[82]

Macroscopically, the tumors vary from small round nodules 1–2 cm in diameter to large masses weighing up to 13 kg.[49] The tumor usually forms a round or oval solid mass that is gray-white and firm in consistency. It sometimes may be bosselated or lobulated, but usually the external surface is smooth. The cut surface is uniformly white or gray-white, with a whorled pattern similar to that observed in leiomyoma. In large tumors, foci of hemorrhage or necrosis, sometimes resulting in cyst formation, may be seen.

Microscopically, the tumor is composed of short spindle-shaped cells having narrow or ovoid spindle-shaped nuclei. Mitotic activity is absent or very low. The cells form bundles frequently intersected by hyalinized tissue. Hyalinization and myxomatous change frequently are present. Calcification, edema, hemorrhage, and necrosis also may be seen. Fat is absent except in necrotic areas.

The absence of fat differentiates between a fibroma and a thecoma, but it cannot distinguish between a fibroma and a fibrosed thecoma. Thus, these two entities cannot always be distinguished satisfactorily. Massive edema of the ovary[50,111] and fibromatosis, which may be related to massive edema and usually affects the entire ovary, may resemble an edematous fibroma and must be differentiated from it (see Chapter 16, Nonneoplastic Lesions of the Ovary). Cellular fibroma of the ovary must be differentiated from fibrosarcoma. Although in well-differentiated examples of the latter the distinction may be difficult, the presence of mitotic activity tends to be the best distinguishing feature, and the presence of more than 4 mitoses/10 high power fields (HPF) places the tumor in the fibrosarcoma category.[54,84,92]

Fibroma of the ovary is a benign neoplasm, and the treatment of choice is excision of the affected ovary. This results in resolution of all symptoms. In the occasional patient, ovarian fibroma may be associated with implants in the peritoneum.[59] The presence of these implants should not be taken as evidence of malignancy. The prognosis in these, as in other cases of ovarian fibroma, is excellent.

Fibrosarcoma

Primary fibrosarcoma of the ovary is uncommon.[2,54,84,92] In a series of 283 ovarian tumors of fibrous tissue origin, there were four primary fibrosarcomas.[23] Although some fibrosarcomas of the ovary may have been classified as malignant thecomas and as spindle-cell sarcomas,[35] fully documented tumors of this type are uncommon, although they occur more frequently than do other pure primary sarcomas of the ovary. Fibrosarcoma usually is seen in menopausal and postmenopausal patients.[2,68,75] This tumor may arise de novo from ovarian stroma or may originate as a result of malignant change in a preexistent fibroma. Occasional cases have been observed in children.[1] In one case the tumor was associated with nevoid basal cell carcinoma syndrome.[54]

Macroscopically, fibrosarcoma of the ovary resembles

ovarian fibroma, but the tumor usually is larger and is more likely to be associated with hemorrhage and necrosis.[68,84]

Microscopically, ovarian fibrosarcoma shows typical appearances of fibrosarcoma seen in other locations and usually shows marked cellular pleomorphism and brisk mitotic activity.[68,84] The prognosis is generally poor, the tumor metastasizing early via the bloodstream to the lungs. Occasionally, the course of the disease is more protracted, with patients surviving up to 9 years from time of diagnosis.[2,54,68,74] Tumors showing less marked mitotic activity tend to be less aggressive.[54,84]

Myxoma

Primary myxoma of the ovary is a very rare neoplasm; only nine cases have been reported in the literature.[10,26,28,60,63] The patients were aged 14–45 years and in each case had an adnexal mass. The other adnexa was normal.[10,26,28,60,63] Macroscopically, the tumors measured from 5 to 22 cm in the greatest dimension.[28] They were encapsulated, gray-white, and soft. On cut section they were found to be partly cystic. Solid areas were slimy and mucinous, whereas the cystic spaces contained a viscous, glassy, gelatinous material. Microscopically, the tumors showed the typical appearances of myxoma as described by Stout.[100] They were composed of loose myxomatous stroma within which there were scattered stellate or spindle-shaped cells, some of which contained hyperchromatic nuclei. There was no nuclear pleomorphism and mitotic activity was absent. The tumors varied from poorly vascularized, containing only a few capillary blood vessels and showing absence of plexiform vessels, to tumors with prominent capillary vessels within the tumor, and larger vessels with muscular walls at its periphery. The myxomatous stroma stained positively with alcian blue stain and contained a network of fine reticulum fibers. Stains for fat are negative. In some areas, fibrosis is present. There are no other connective tissue elements, and the tumors have a homogeneous appearance. The tumor is immunoreactive for vimentin, and focally for actin, but negative for desmin, cytokeratins, vascular markers, S-100, and neurofilaments.[28] Most myxomas originate within connective tissue, and the origin of the tumor is still a matter of dispute.[26,28,100,108] The histogenesis of ovarian myxomas is unknown.

Although myxoma is a benign neoplasm, because of its viscous nature, it is difficult to excise completely and recurrences are not uncommon unless the entire adnexa bearing the tumor is excised.[26,100] All the patients treated by unilateral adnexectomy and for whom there is follow-up information are free of disease from 1 to 13 years.[28,60,63]

Myxoma must be differentiated from fibroma with myxoid degeneration, which contains normal fibrous tissue in some areas. Ovarian myxoma must be distinguished from massive edema of the ovary (see Chapter 16, Nonneoplastic Lesions of the Ovary).[50,111] The patients with massive edema usually are younger, and the lesion shows entrapment of follicular derivatives, which is not observed in ovarian myxoma. More importantly, myxoma must be differentiated from myxomatous liposarcoma, which contains fat, is more vascularized, and shows lipoblasts at least in some areas. It also must be differentiated from mucinous cystadenomas and carcinomas—either primary or metastatic—which contain epithelial cells, show absence of stellate and spindle-shaped cells, and may show glandular differentiation. Myxoma also should be distinguished from embryonal rhabdomyosarcoma. The latter tumor shows less of a uniform appearance, displays greater cellular and nuclear pleomorphism, and contains rhabdomyoblasts. In addition, embryonal rhabdomyosarcoma shows positive immunocytochemical staining for sarcomeric actin filaments and desmin. Ultrastructurally Z-band formation, glycogen granules, and thick filament ribosomal complexes are observed.

Tumors of Muscle Origin

Leiomyoma

Primary leiomyoma of the ovary is uncommon.[31,51,64,85] Approximately 50 cases are on record, but it is likely that many cases are not reported, especially when the tumor is small and is discovered incidentally. At least eight unreported cases are known to the author.

Primary ovarian leiomyoma probably originates from smooth muscle present in the walls of blood vessels in the cortical stroma, in the corpus luteum,[79] and in the ovarian ligaments at their point of attachment to the ovary; its precise histogenesis is uncertain, however. This tumor usually is found in menopausal and postmenopausal women but sometimes occurs in young women. The age of patients ranges from 20 to 65 years.[35,64,85] Clinically, many patients are asymptomatic, and the tumor is discovered incidentally. When symptoms are present, they are related to the presence of an adnexal mass, becoming manifest as abdominal swelling and abdominal pain. The latter may be acute, because of torsion. Ascites is rare, and hydrothorax has not been reported. The uterus usually contains leiomyomata.

Ovarian leiomyoma is unilateral, although a single case of large bilateral ovarian leiomyomas occuring in a 21-year-old woman has been reported.[51] Macroscopically the tumors are solid, firm, round or oval masses having a smooth surface. On cut section they have a white or gray-white solid whorled surface. Hemorrhage and necrosis may be evident, altering the appearance. Cyst formation caused by necrosis may occur, and calcification also may be present.

Microscopically, the tumor shows typical appearances of a leiomyoma, as observed in the uterus, the tumor being composed of smooth muscle cells that are uniformly spindle-shaped or elongated and contain elongated blunt-ended or cigar-shaped nuclei. Palisading of the nuclei may be present and may be prominent. Mitotic activity is absent or very low, and cellular and nuclear pleomorphism is not a feature. The tumor cells form bundles intersected by fibrous septa that may be wide and show marked hyalinization. Other degenerative changes seen in uterine leiomyomas also may be present. Connective tissue stains confirm the leiomyomatous nature of the tumor. In four tumors that I have studied this was further confirmed ultrastructurally. A well documented case of a large ovarian lipoleiomyoma occuring in a 63-year-old woman has been reported.[69] The tumor replaced nearly the entire ovary. The adipose tissue was found replacing and dissecting the smooth muscle within the tumor. There was no associated uterine leiomyomatosis.[69] Primary ovarian leiomyoma must be differentiated from pedunculated subserosal (parasitic) uterine leiomyoma, which has lost its attachment and instead has become attached to the ovary, from which it draws its blood supply.

Leiomyosarcoma

Primary leiomyosarcoma of the ovary is very rare. There are fewer than 15 cases reported in the literature. These tumors usually are found in postmenopausal women,[2,74] but may be seen in younger women.[3,85] The tumors usually are large and solid, and patients have symptoms and signs related to the presence of an abdominal or pelvic mass. The tumors are gray-yellow, soft, fleshy, and frequently associated with hemorrhage and necrosis. Microscopically, they differ from a leiomyoma by the presence of mitotic activity and cellular and nuclear pleomorphism (Figs. 21.1, 21.2). In well-differentiated tumors, the mitotic activity may be the only distinguishing feature from a cellular leiomyoma and is considered to be far more important in this respect than cellular and nuclear pleomorphism. Primary leiomyosarcoma of the ovary metastasizes via the bloodstream; the prognosis is generally unfavorable, although the use of combination chemotherapy may improve it. Primary leiomyosarcoma of the ovary must be distinguished from MMMTs containing a prominent leiomyosarcomatous component. Primary leiomyosarcoma also should be distinguished from immature teratomas with a prominent leiomyomatous tissue component. It also must be distinguished from metastatic leiomyosarcoma of uterine or other origin, as well as from poorly differentiated sarcomas and carcinosarcomas, both primary and metastatic to the ovary.

Rhabdomyoma

No well-documented case of ovarian rhabdomyoma has been recorded.

Rhabdomyosarcoma

Primary rhabdomyosarcoma of the ovary occurs rarely; only 12 well-documented cases have been reported in the

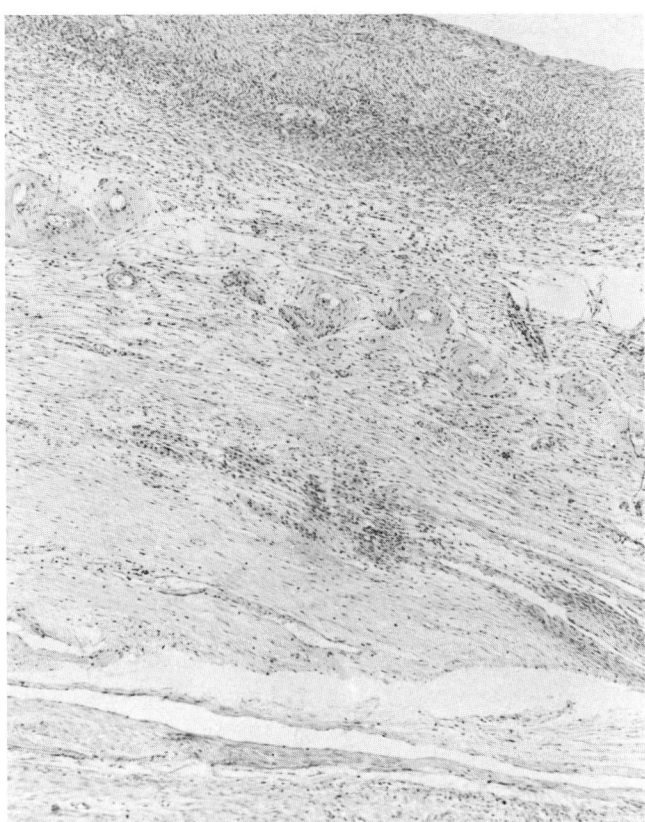

FIG. 21.1. **Primary ovarian leiomyosarcoma.** The tumor is seen beneath normal ovarian cortex (*top*).

literature, and 9 unreported cases are known to me. A careful review of the literature shows that some cases, such as the frequently quoted case reported by Sandison,[90] were not pure rhabdomyosarcomas but rather examples of MMMT or teratomas with a marked rhabdomyoblastic component. Therefore, before a diagnosis of primary ovarian rhabdomyosarcoma can be made, the tumor must be sampled carefully and extensively to exclude the presence of other neoplastic elements, the presence of which would preclude a diagnosis of a pure rhabdomyosarcoma of the ovary.

The histogenesis of primary rhabdomyosarcoma of the ovary is uncertain. These tumors may originate from the connective tissue of the ovary, as a one-sided development of teratoma, as a result of malignant transformation of a mature cystic teratoma with the malignant element overgrowing the tumor, or as a one-sided development of a MMMT.

The age of patients with ovarian rhabdomyosarcoma ranges from 2.5 to 84 years. The small number of cases makes it impossible to state whether there is a predilection for any particular age group, but, as with rhabdomyosarcomas occurring in other locations, the pleomorphic type occurs in older patients, whereas the embryonal and alveolar types occur in young women.[16] Patients with ovarian

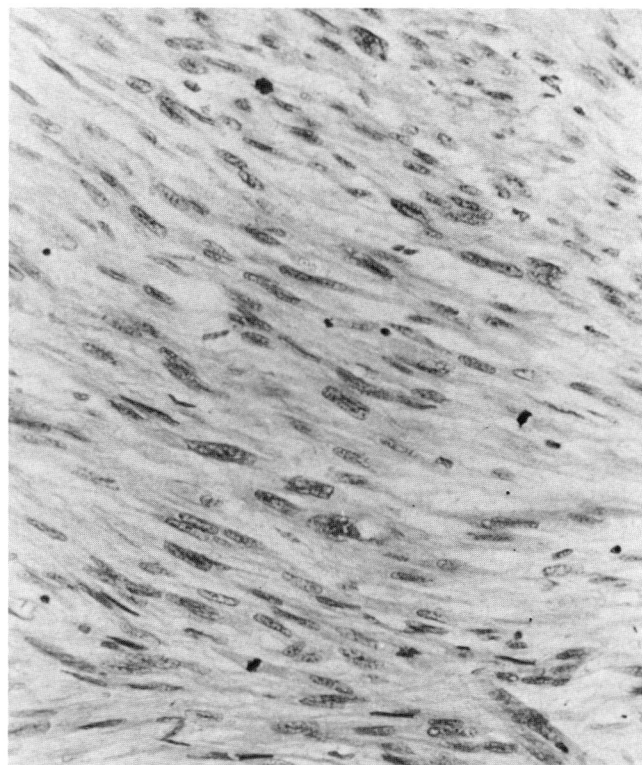

FIG. 21.2. Primary ovarian leiomyosarcoma. Higher magnification of tumor shown in Fig. 21.1. Note brisk mitotic activity and cellular and nuclear pleomorphism.

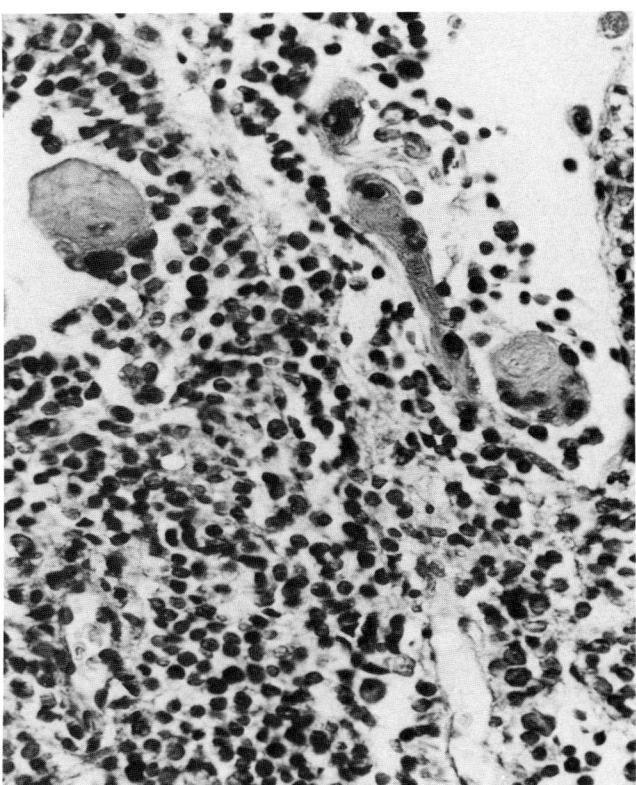

FIG. 21.3. Primary rhabdomyosarcoma of ovary of embryonal type. Most tumor cells are of small round type, but occasional large rhabdomyoblasts, some exhibiting cross-striations, are seen.

rhabdomyosarcoma usually have symptoms associated with the presence of a large, usually rapidly growing, abdominal mass, frequently associated with hemorrhagic ascites. Metastases frequently are seen at presentation.

Macroscopically, the tumors are unilateral, but metastatic involvement of the contralateral ovary may be present and should be differentiated from bilateral involvement. The tumors usually are large, exceeding 10 cm in diameter. They are solid, soft, fleshy, and gray-pink to yellow-tan, with areas of hemorrhage and necrosis that may be prominent.

Microscopically, the tumors are composed entirely of rhabdomyoblasts, either of the embryonal type (Figs. 21.3, 21.4) admixed with the alveolar (Fig. 21.5) or botryoid types, or of the pleomorphic type. Tumors composed of the former types occur in children and young adults, whereas those of the pleomorphic type are observed in older women. Whereas the diagnosis of pleomorphic rhabdomyosarcoma should not present undue difficulty, because of the presence of at least some typical rhabdomyoblasts showing cross-striation, the diagnosis of embryonal rhabdomyosarcoma is much more difficult because the tumor cells are poorly differentiated, making rhabdomyoblastic differentiation discernible only with difficulty. Furthermore, it is necessary to recognize the distinctive alveolar (Fig. 21.5) or botryoid patterns, which may not be easy. The embryonal rhabdomyosarcoma is composed of rhabdomyoblasts in various stages of differentiation (Figs. 21.3, 21.4) and is composed at least partly of collections of small round cells having a narrow rim of cytoplasm (Fig. 21.3) that are poorly differentiated. Therefore, the lesion is difficult to distinguish from poorly differentiated small cell carcinoma, malignant lymphoma, or even neuroblastoma or leukemia.[76] Among the small round cells, there are scattered occasional better-differentiated cells with bright eosinophilic cytoplasm and eccentric nuclei (Fig. 21.4). Occasionally, large, more typical rhabdomyoblasts are seen. The presence of cross-striations is not necessary for diagnosis, but the cells comprising the tumor may be well enough differentiated to exhibit cross-striations (Fig. 21.3). Demonstration of Z bands or their precursors by electron microscopy is helpful in making the diagnosis.[40] Immunocytochemical demonstration of myoglobin and desmin also is helpful in this respect. The tumor frequently is affected by edema, hemorrhage, and necrosis, making the diagnosis even more difficult. Therefore, thorough examination and sampling of the tumor are essential to make the correct diagnosis. The tumor may be more common than has been

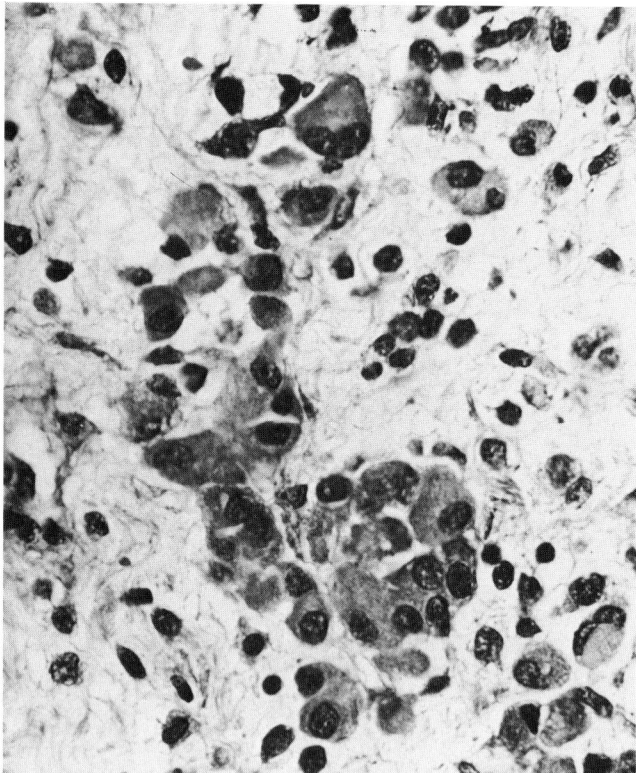

FIG. 21.4. Primary rhabdomyosarcoma of ovary of embryonal type. The tumor is composed of primitive rhabdomyoblasts with ample amount of bright eosinophilic cytoplasm and eccentric nuclei.

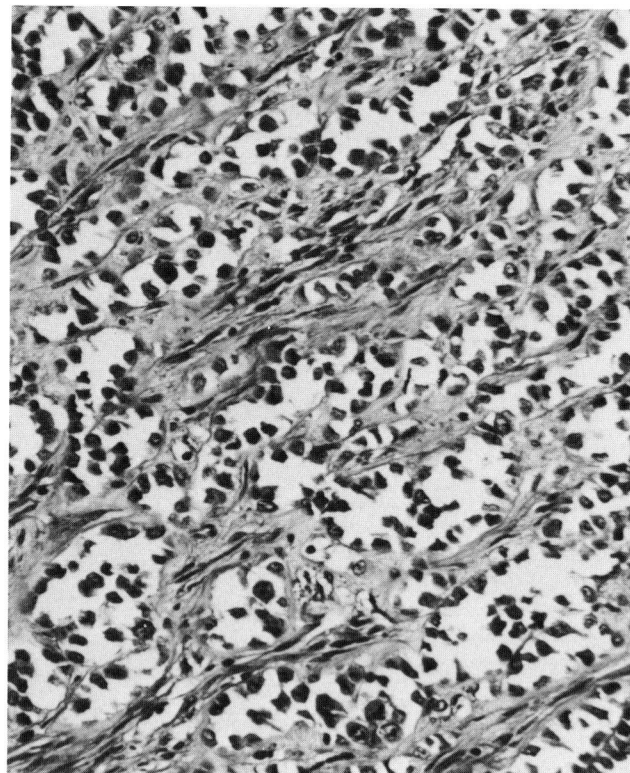

FIG. 21.5. Primary rhabdomyosarcoma of ovary. The tumor has a pronounced alveolar pattern.

hitherto believed, but because of its poor differentiation, it may have been either assigned to the group of undifferentiated ovarian tumors or misdiagnosed. It is therefore emphasized that embryonal rhabdomyosarcoma must be considered in the differential diagnosis of *undifferentiated small round cell tumor* of the ovary in a young patient. The presence of other neoplastic elements always must be excluded when making this diagnosis.

The importance of making the correct diagnosis is not only academic but practical, in view of the advances that have been made in the therapy of embryonal rhabdomyosarcoma during the last two decades. In the past, the prognosis was considered poor, and in most reported cases, the patients died of extensive metastatic disease within 1 year of diagnosis. Recently, two patients with embryonal rhabdomyosarcoma, one of whom had metastases, are well and disease-free after surgery, chemotherapy, and radiotherapy. The combination chemotherapy advocated in such patients consists of dactinomycin, vincristine, and cyclophosphamide. The addition of methotrexate with folinic acid rescue and doxorubicin to this combination also may be of value.

Tumors of Vascular and Lymphatic Origin

Hemangioma

Hemangioma is found only occasionally in the ovary; the number of well-documented cases does not exceed 40. Although some cases may not have been recognized or recorded, all investigators consider ovarian hemangioma rare.[27,38,39,55,102] This is somewhat surprising, since the ovary has a very rich and complex vasculature.

The origin of ovarian hemangioma in common with hemangioma in general is a matter of controversy; it is considered either a hamartomatous malformation[108] or a true neoplasm.[30] It is likely that both modes of origin are responsible for their formation. The age of patients with ovarian hemangioma ranges from 4 months to 63 years[35,102] and does not show a predominance in any decade. In most patients, ovarian hemangioma has been noted as an incidental finding at operation or autopsy.[35,102] In a few cases, the lesion was large and the patient had abdominal enlargement because of the presence of an ovarian mass[27,38,65,95] or had acute abdominal pain associated with torsion of the tumor.[61,94] In one case, there was as-

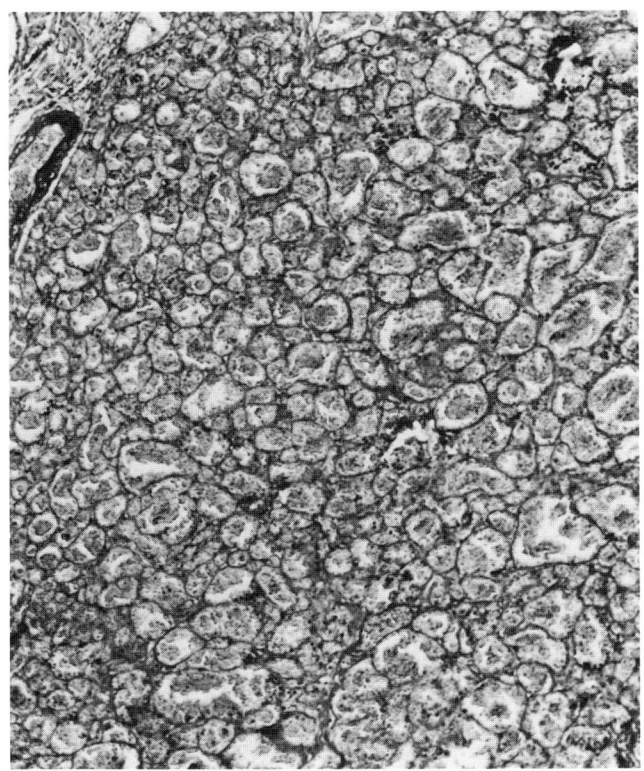

FIG. 21.6. Hemangioma of the ovary. The tumor is composed of numerous small vascular spaces lined by a single layer of endothelial cells. Elastic van Gieson.

cites.[65] The lesions usually are unilateral, although in four patients they were bilateral.[11,37,55,98] Ovarian hemangiomas have been noted in patients with generalized hemangiomatosis[55,98] and in patients with hemangiomas in other parts of the genital tract.[55,102] One patient with bilateral ovarian hemangiomas and diffuse abdominopelvic hemangiomatosis had thrombocytopenia. The platelet count returned to normal after excision of the affected ovaries.[55]

Macroscopically, the lesions are small, red or purple, round or oval nodules, measuring from a few millimeters to 1.5 cm in diameter. Larger lesions also have been encountered measuring up to 11.5 cm in the largest diameter.[61] On cut section, they usually are spongy and show a honeycomb appearance. Although they have been found in different parts of the ovary, the medulla and the hilar region appear to be the most common sites.[102]

Microscopically, ovarian hemangioma is of the cavernous or mixed capillary–cavernous type. It consists of collections of vascular spaces, which may vary in size but usually are small, lined by a single layer of endothelial cells, and usually contain red blood cells in their lumen (Fig. 21.6). Occasionally, thrombosis may be seen. A small amount of connective tissue may be present within the lesion.

Hemangioma must be differentiated from proliferations of dilated blood vessels, frequently seen in the hilar region of the ovary. Although a very small hemangioma may not be easily distinguished from such vascular proliferations, the hemangioma usually forms a nodule or a small mass; the presence of a circumscribed nodule composed of vascular spaces tends to distinguish hemangioma from vascular proliferations, which usually are smaller and more diffuse. The presence of numerous blood cells within the vascular spaces and the absence of pale eosinophilic homogeneous material usually distinguish hemangioma from lymphangioma. Hemangioma also must be distinguished from teratoma with a prominent vascular component. In such cases, careful sampling will detect other teratomatous elements, the presence of which will distinguish the lesions from a hemangioma.

The treatment of choice is oophorectomy or adnexectomy, which results in a complete cure.

Hemangioendothelial Sarcoma (Hemangioendothelioma, Hemangiosarcoma, Angiosarcoma)

Hemangioendothelial sarcoma is a very rare ovarian neoplasm: only nine examples have been recorded.[35,80,83] Five unreported cases have been seen by me. The age of the patients varies from 19 to 77 years. The statement that it usually occurs in childhood and adolescence[49] is incorrect and may indicate the inclusion of immature teratomas with a prominent vascular component. The tumor usually is unilateral, but one case of bilateral tumors has been recorded.[35] Bilaterality must be differentiated from metastatic spread to the contralateral ovary, which was seen in one personally observed case. The histogenesis of the tumor is uncertain, but it may originate from the vascular tissue present in the ovary, or as a one-sided development of a teratoma. Patients usually have symptoms related to the presence of a lower abdominal mass, which may be associated with torsion and rupture of the tumor and hemorrhage.

Macroscopically, the tumors usually are large, blue-brown, hemorrhagic, soft, and friable. They may be confined to the ovary but also are associated with invasion of the surrounding structures.

Microscopically, they are composed of vascular spaces of varying size and appearance, lined by endothelial cells that usually are large, showing atypical appearance, bizarre nuclei, and mitotic activity (Figs. 21.7, 21.8). In some areas, the tumor may contain a considerable amount of connective tissue interspersed between the vascular spaces (Fig. 21.7). The tumor invades locally and metastasizes via the bloodstream. Prognosis is poor, especially in patients who have metastases at the time of presentation. Hemangioendothelial sarcoma of the ovary must be distinguished from immature teratomatous neoplasms with a prominent

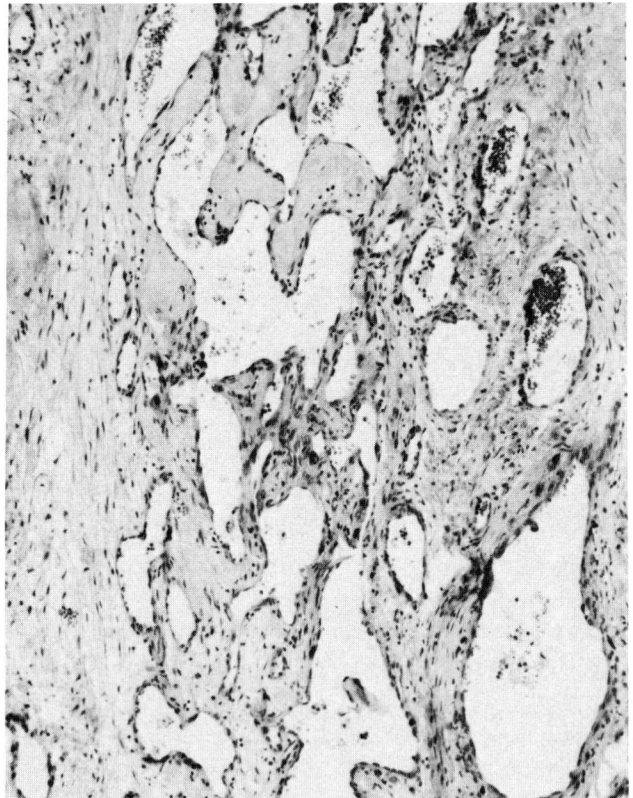

FIG. 21.7. Primary hemangioendothelial sarcoma of ovary. The tumor is composed of vascular spaces surrounded by connective tissue.

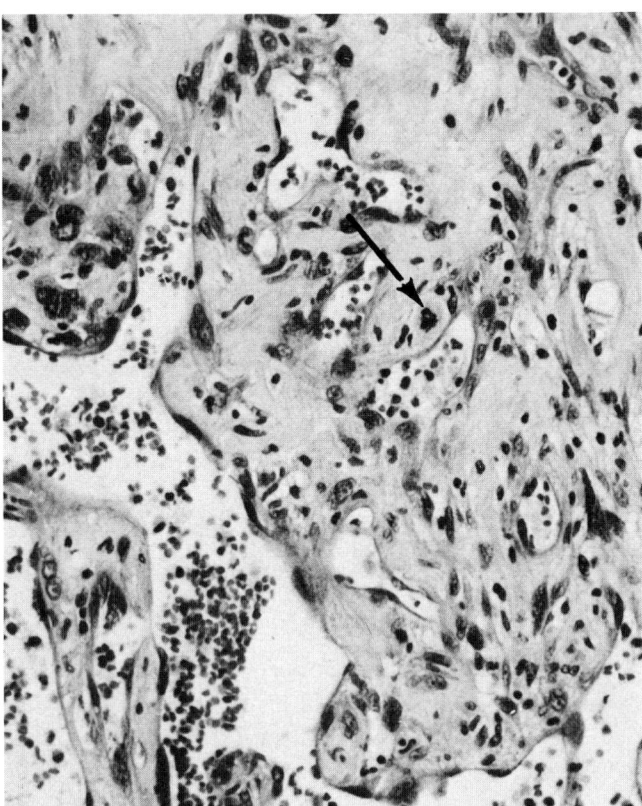

FIG. 21.8. Primary hemangioendothelial sarcoma of ovary. Note the large endothelial cells lining vascular spaces. Large abnormal mitosis is seen to right of center (*arrow*).

vascular component. The presence of other neoplastic germ cell elements distinguishes teratoma from primary hemangioendothelial sarcoma. It also must be distinguished from the occasional lymphangiosarcoma, which is composed of lymphatic and not of blood vessels, as well as from malignant hemangiopericytoma, which is composed of a proliferation of pericytes and shows a different histological pattern. Hemangiopericytoma can be distinguished further from hemangioendothelial sarcoma with the help of reticulum stains.

Lymphangioma

Lymphangioma of the ovary is very rare, with fewer than 10 documented cases reported.[35] I have seen two cases. In both cases, the tumor was small and was found incidentally. Macroscopically, the tumor is unilateral and small, having a smooth, gray surface. On cut section, it is yellow, honeycombed, and composed of numerous small cystic spaces exuding clear yellow fluid.

Microscopically, lymphangioma of the ovary is composed of closely packed, thin-walled vascular spaces lined with flattened endothelial cells and containing pale homogeneous eosinophilic fluid. As in the case of hemangioma,

the histogenesis is a matter of controversy. Some investigators consider these lesions as malformations or hamartomas[108] and some as neoplasms.[30]

Lymphangioma is differentiated from a teratoma with a prominent vascular component by the absence of other germ cell elements. Lymphangioma also must be distinguished from hemangioma and an adenomatoid tumor that contains thin-walled, vessel-like spaces. In contrast to hemangioma, lymphangioma does not contain blood cells in the vascular spaces. The adenomatoid tumor has solid areas, and the cells lining the vessel-like spaces stain positively with periodic acid–Schiff (PAS) and alcian blue stains.

Lymphangiosarcoma

Only one case of lymphangiosarcoma of the ovary has been reported.[88] The tumor, which measured 15 cm in diameter, was found in a 31-year-old woman who had symptoms of a rapidly enlarging abdominal mass. The tumor was composed of proliferating, closely packed lymphatic vessels that, in one area, showed cellular and nuclear atypia. There was extensive necrosis and hemorrhage. The patient died 1 year after diagnosis of extensive metastatic disease.[88]

Hemangiopericytoma

No well-documented case of ovarian hemangiopericytoma has been recorded.

Tumors of Cartilage Origin

Chondroma

Only a few reports of ovarian chondroma are available, and documentation in most cases is unsatisfactory. A well-documented case considered to originate from the ovarian stroma has been reported.[75] The tumor, which measured 4 × 3 × 3 cm and was composed entirely of mature cartilage, was found incidentally. Although chondroma may originate from the connective tissue of the ovary by a process of metaplasia, it is more likely that most ovarian tumors described as chondroma were either fibromas showing cartilaginous metaplasia or teratomas having a prominent cartilaginous component.[35]

Chondrosarcoma

A single example of pure chondrosarcoma of the ovary has been reported[103] (Fig. 21.9). A 61-year-old woman had an abdominal mass that, on extensive microscopic examina-

tion, proved to be a pure, well-differentiated chondrosarcoma (Figs. 21.10, 21.11). The patient was well and disease-free 6 years after one-sided adnexectomy. The histogenesis of this tumor is uncertain, but the age of the patient and the histological appearances of the tumor point to an origin in a dermoid cyst with malignant transformation and overgrowth by the malignant cartilaginous component.[103] A well-documented case of mature cystic teratoma (dermoid cyst) with malignant transformation of the cartilaginous element has been reported; the patient died of extensive metastatic disease.[20]

Tumors of Bone Origin

Osteoma

Few documented examples of osteoma occurring in the ovary exist, and although an origin from ovarian stroma is possible, most such lesions probably were examples of osseous metaplasia occurring in fibromas or leiomyomas,[49] or possibly examples of metaplasia or heterotopia and not neoplasia occurring in the connective tissue of the ovary.[96] The lesions usually are small but may be large and are histologically composed of dense cortical bone.[49]

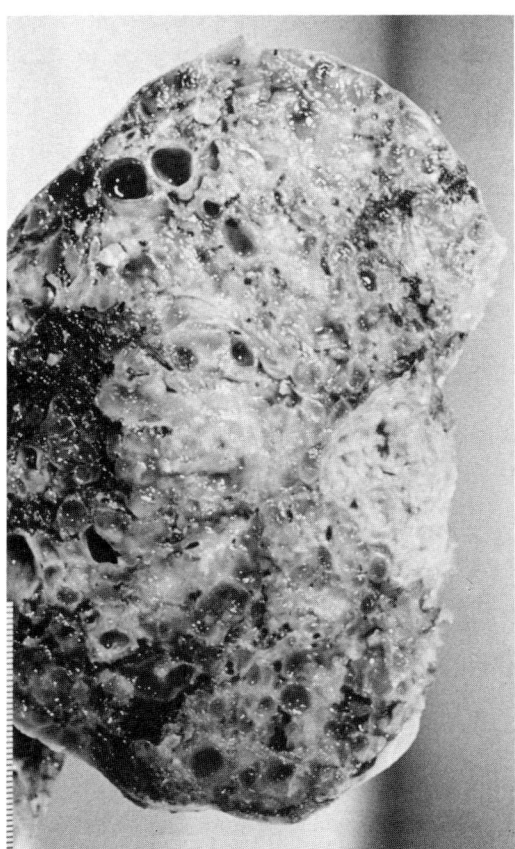

FIG. 21.9. Primary ovarian chondrosarcoma. The tumor was large, solid, hard, and gray-white.

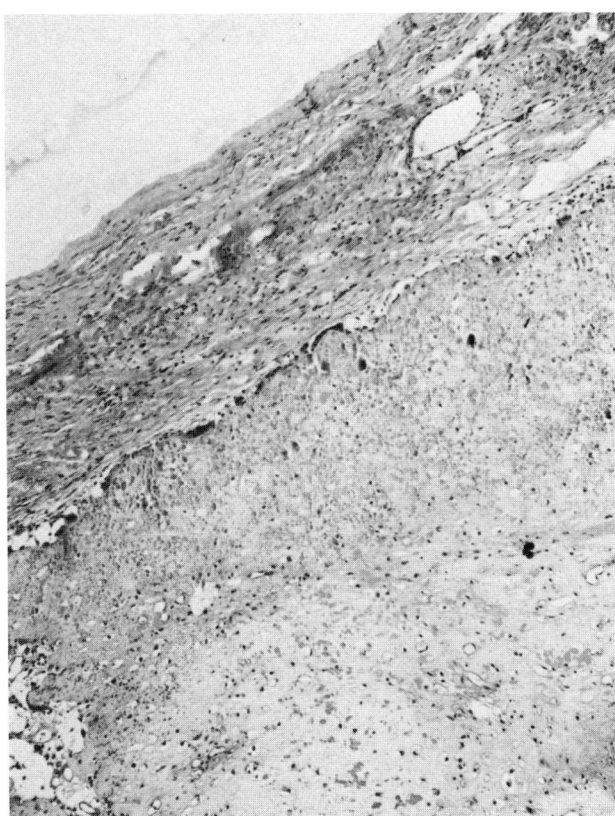

FIG. 21.10. Primary ovarian chondrosarcoma. Tumor is seen beneath normal ovarian cortex.

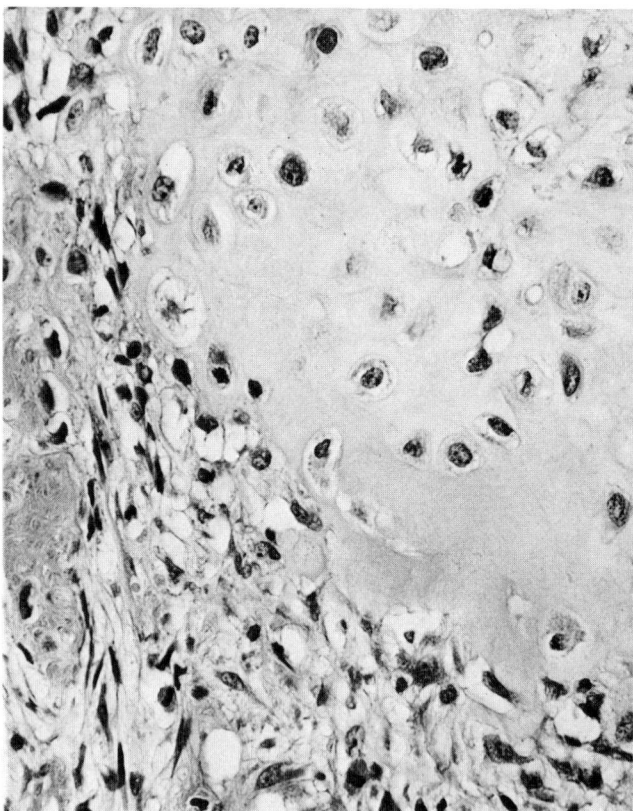

FIG. 21.11. Primary ovarian chondrosarcoma. Higher magnification showing well-differentiated tumor.

Osteosarcoma

Only one example of pure osteosarcoma of the ovary has been reported.[2] The tumor occurred in a 41-year-old woman in whom there was associated metastatic disease. The patient died 5 months after diagnosis. Histologically, the tumor showed typical appearances of osteosarcoma occurring in the skeleton. Although it was believed that the tumor originated directly from ovarian stroma, the histogenesis of this tumor is uncertain. Occasional cases of osteosarcoma originating in ovarian teratoma have been recorded,[101] but such cases should not be confused with pure ovarian osteosarcoma, nor should cases of MMMT with a prominent osteosarcomatous component.

Giant Cell Tumor of the Ovary

A single case of giant cell tumor of the ovary histologically indistinguishable from a giant cell tumor of bone has been reported.[57] The tumor was found incidentally in an ovary of a 31-year-old woman. It was composed of small ovoid or spindle-shaped stromal cells admixed with multinucleated giant cells, many of which contained between 50 and 100 small hyperchromatic nuclei. In places, there was brisk mitotic activity. The patient was well and disease-free 4½ years after excision of the affected adnexa.

Tumors of Neural Tissue Origin

Ovarian tumors originating from neural tissue are rare. The presenting symptoms usually are related to the presence of an intraabdominal mass. The tumors are solid and usually are small. The histogenesis is uncertain and probably is similar to that of other mesenchymal tumors of the ovary.

Neurofibroma

Two cases of neurofibroma of the ovary have been reported in patients with generalized neurofibromatosis (von Recklinghausen's disease),[43,97] one as an incidental finding.[97] Histologically the tumors showed appearances similar to those of a neurofibroma occuring elsewhere.

Neurofibrosarcoma

One case of neurofibrosarcoma occurring in a 38-year-old woman with generalized neurofibromatosis (von Recklinghausen's disease) has been described.[25] The tumor was an incidental finding and had replaced the ovary. It was solid and histologically showed typical appearances of a neurofibrosarcoma with a moderate degree of cellular and nuclear pleomorphism and mitotic activity. There was no evidence of metastases, and the patient was well and disease-free 1 year after diagnosis.[25]

Neurilemmoma

Three cases of ovarian neurilemmoma (schwannoma) have been reported.[21,66,70] In one case, the tumor was large.[70] The tumors were solid and the patients were well and disease-free after the excision of the tumor. Histologically, the tumors showed the typical appearances of a neurilemmoma occurring in other locations.

Malignant Neurilemmoma (Schwannoma)

One case of malignant neurilemmoma (Schwannoma) of the ovary has been reported.[99] The affected patient, a 71-year-old, nulliparous woman was admitted for evaluation of lower abdominal enlargement and pain. There were no stigmata of generalized neurofibromatosis.[99] At laparotomy a 15-cm, firm, somewhat hemorrhagic tumor was found arising from the left ovary. There were numerous tumor deposits involving the peritoneal cavity. A debulking procedure was performed and the ovarian tumor was excised together with the omentum.[99] Histological and ultrastructural examinations revealed that the tumor was a malignant neurilemmoma (Schwannoma).[99] After surgery the patient was treated with combination chemotherapy consisting of doxorubicin and cyclophosphamide, but the disease progressed and she died 5 months after surgery with extensive intraabdominal metastatic disease.[99]

Ganglioneuroma

A single case of ovarian ganglioneuroma occurring in a 4-year-old girl has been reported.[91] The child had abdominal enlargement. The tumor was solid, weighing 200 g, and replaced nearly the whole ovary. Histologically, the tumor was composed of well-differentiated ganglion cells. There was a recurrence after the excision of the tumor. True ganglioneuroma must be differentiated from teratomas showing prominence of ganglion cells and from proliferations of ganglion cells occasionally seen in the hilar region of the ovary; the latter are nonneoplastic and probably hamartomatous in nature.

Pheochromocytoma

A single case of ovarian pheochromocytoma occurring in a 15-year-old girl has been reported.[32] The patient had hypertension, convulsions, and a large, left-sided abdominal tumor mass. The tumor had undergone torsion and weighed 970 g. It was solid, and microscopic examination showed typical appearances of pheochromocytoma. Epinephrine and norepinephrine were extracted from tumor tissue. The symptoms disappeared after excision of the tumor, and the patient was well and disease-free 15 months after the operation.[32]

Primitive Neuroectodermal Tumors

These tumors are described in Chapter 20, Germ Cell Tumors of the Ovary.

Tumors of Adipose Tissue Origin

There are no well-documented cases of tumors of adipose tissue origin in the ovary. Some reports relating to the presence of both benign and malignant neoplasms composed of adipose tissue in the ovary exist, but they are not well substantiated. Collections of adipose cells forming islands of fatty tissue that are not encapsulated are seen occasionally within ovarian tissue and are attributed to metaplasia of connective tissue of the ovary. These collections have been described as adipose prosoplasia.[41] Benign adipose tissue seen in the ovary may be part of a teratoma with a prominent adipose tissue component. Malignant adipose tissue may be a part of a MMMT with a prominent liposarcomatous component, or it may represent metastases from a liposarcoma occurring at another location.[35]

Tumors of Mesothelial Origin

Adenomatoid Tumor

The adenomatoid tumor, which in the female is found most frequently in the fallopian tubes and broad ligament and occasionally in the uterus near the serosal surface, is found only rarely in the ovary (see Chapter 13, Mesenchymal Tumors of the Uterus, and Chapter 14, Diseases of the Fallopian Tube). Although its histogenesis was long disputed, it is now considered to be of mesothelial origin. This is supported by morphologic, histochemical, and ultrastructural observations.[33,105] Adenomatoid tumor is benign and, therefore, is considered a benign mesothelioma.

Six cases of ovarian adenomatoid tumor have been recorded, most of which occurred in patients in the third and fourth decades. The lesions, which are small, round or oval, and measuring from 0.5 to 1.5 cm in diameter, usually are found in the hilus of the ovary as incidental findings. Histologically they show similar appearances to adenomatoid tumors occurring in other locations and are composed of clefts and spaces lined by cuboidal, low columnar, or flattened epithelial-like cells (Fig. 21.12) and of solid aggregates of similar cells surrounded by connective tissue that varies from loose and edematous to dense and hyalinized. The epithelial-like cells may exhibit marked vacuolation. They exhibit positive staining with alcian blue, which is digestible with hyaluronidase, and similarly staining material is present in the clefts and spaces. Occasionally, the cells may show weak PAS staining. Ultrastructural observations support the mesothelial origin of this lesion and show an abundance of microvilli, bundles of cytoplasmic filaments, tight junctional complexes, and intercellular spaces (Fig. 21.13). The lesion is benign, and its excision results in a complete cure.

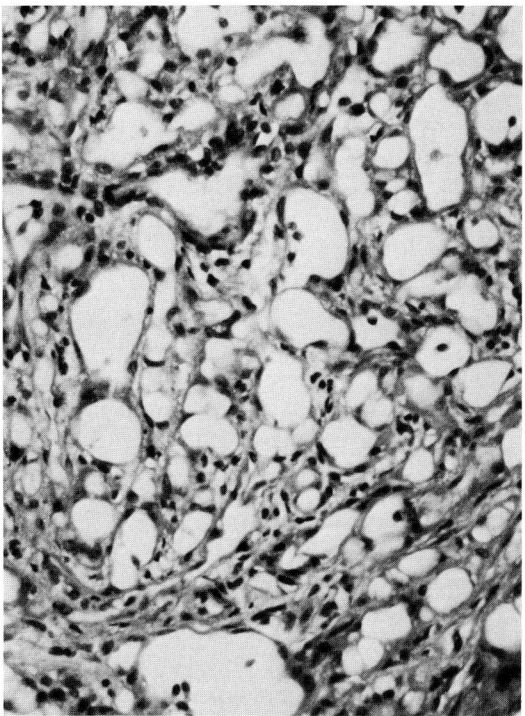

Fig. 21.12. **Adenomatoid tumor.** The tumor has numerous clefts and spaces lined by a single layer of flattened endothelial-like or low cuboid cells.

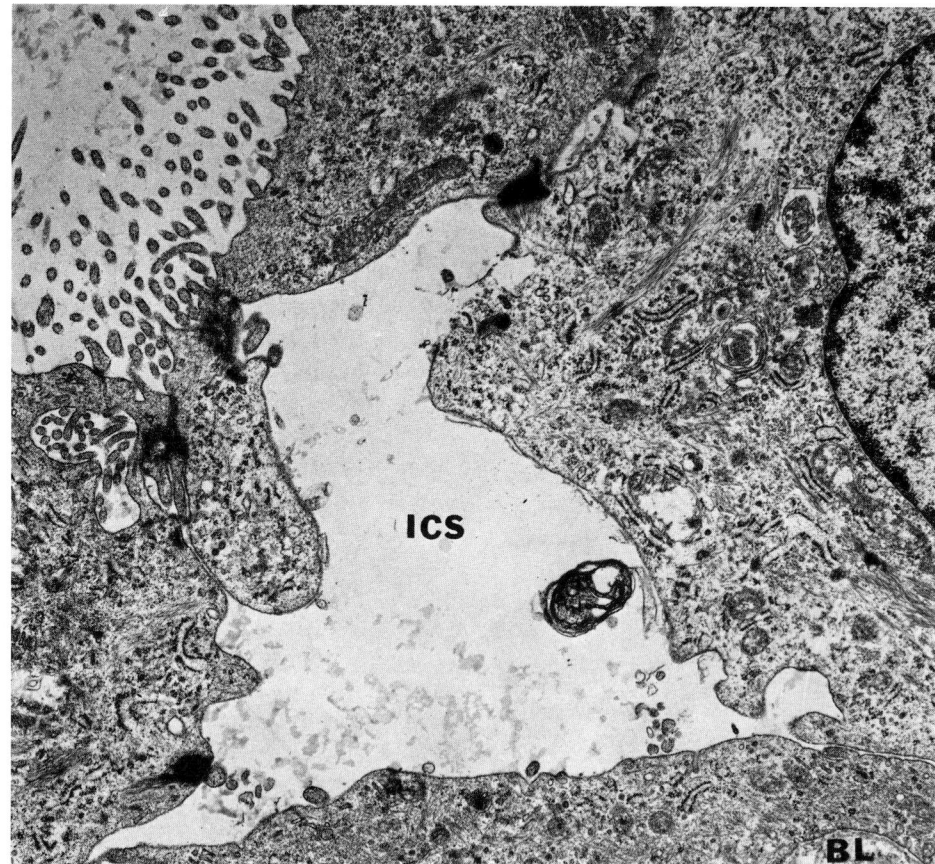

FIG. 21.13. Electron micrograph of an ovarian mesothelioma. Intercellular spaces (*ICS*) with apical tight junctional complexes are shown. ×16,000. (Reprinted by permission of Ferenczy et al., ref. 25.)

Peritoneal Mesothelioma

Occasionally, peritoneal mesothelioma may involve the surface of the ovary (see Chapter 17, Diseases of the Peritoneum). When the tumor affects the ovary, confusion with primary ovarian neoplasms or benign conditions may occur.[104] The histological pattern, ultrastructural and immunohistochemical observations, and behavior and distribution of the lesion are helpful in making the correct diagnosis.[52,104,107] Most patients with malignant peritoneal mesothelioma are middle-aged or elderly adults, and the tumor shows a considerable male predominance.[52] Very rarely, it may occur in children.[104]

Other Mesenchymal Tumors

Other mesenchymal tumors occurring in the ovary include the sclerosing stromal tumor of the ovary described in detail in Chapter 19. Sex Cord–Stromal, Steroid Cell, and Other Ovarian Tumors with Endocrine, Paraendocrine, and Paraneoplastic Manifestations. Tumors of teratomatous origin containing mesenchymal tissue are described in Chapter 20. Germ Cell Tumors of the Ovary, and MMMTs, carcinosarcomas, endometrial stromal sarcomas, and adenosarcoma are discussed in Chapter 18, Surface Epithelial–Stromal Tumors of the Ovary.

Undifferentiated Sarcomas

Some ovarian tumors are poorly differentiated, and although a diagnosis of sarcoma can be made, the tumor does not exhibit further differentiation beyond showing its mesenchymal origin. Careful and extensive histological examination in such cases is helpful and may result in finding better-differentiated areas, which will yield a more accurate diagnosis. It is always worthwhile to undertake such an examination, although for some cases a more precise diagnosis cannot be made despite extensive sampling.

Tumors of Hematopoietic Origin

Malignant Lymphoma

Malignant lymphoma affecting the ovary can be divided into two types: *primary malignant lymphoma* of the ovary, and *disseminated malignant lymphoma* affecting the ovary.

Primary malignant lymphoma of the ovary is rare and, in turn, can be divided further into two categories: (1) manifestation of generalized malignant lymphoma and (2) localized extranodal malignant lymphoma. *Disseminated malignant lymphoma* is far more common than the primary type. It too can be divided into two categories: (1) the ovarian tumor being either the initial or predominant presenting manifestation of the disease and (2) ovarian involvement occurring during the course of the disseminated disease, only discovered histologically after surgery or autopsy.

One specific type of malignant lymphoma, that is, *Burkitt's lymphoma*, frequently affects the ovary—which is the second most common site after the jaws. The ovary may be the site of primary disease as well as of disseminated disease, and the manifestations of Burkitt's lymphoma may accord with any of the specific types described for both primary and disseminated disease. Patients with primary disease localized to the ovary and with disseminated disease discovered only by histological examination at surgery or autopsy are uncommon. Consequently, Burkitt's lymphoma is the most common malignant lymphoma in which involvement of the ovary manifests itself clinically and is an important feature of the disease.

Other hematopoietic neoplasms affecting the ovary, such as leukemia, myelomatosis, or plasmacytoma, also can be classified in a similar manner to malignant lymphoma. It should be noted, however, that their primary manifestation in the ovary is rare, even when compared with primary malignant lymphoma, which is itself very uncommon.

Primary Extranodal Malignant Lymphoma of the Ovary

Before the diagnosis of primary extranodal malignant lymphoma can be made, the presence of lymph node, as well as blood and bone marrow involvement by the disease, must be carefully excluded, and the involvement of the affected organ must be the first manifestation of the disease. This is of considerable importance because there is now good evidence that primary extranodal malignant lymphoma tends to run a less aggressive course than does malignant lymphoma affecting the lymph nodes. Although primary extranodal malignant lymphoma is not uncommon, the ovary is an infrequent site, and the number of well-documented cases reported in the literature is fewer than 70.[18,34,36,71,81,82,89]

The diagnosis of primary malignant lymphoma of the ovary can be made only if, in addition to the general criteria for the diagnosis of extranodal malignant lymphoma mentioned earlier, the tumor is confined to the ovary at the time of diagnosis. If, in addition to the ovarian involvement, only the lymph nodes immediately draining the ovary are affected or if local spread from the ovary to the adjacent structures is present, this should not preclude the diagnosis. Primary malignant lymphoma of the ovary shows a wide age range but tends to occur more frequently before

menopause. The most common symptoms are abdominal enlargement or abdominal pain. Primary malignant lymphoma of the ovary also has been noted as an incidental finding. On examination, ovarian enlargement is nearly always present and often is bilateral. The tumors range in size from 3.5 to 27 cm.[18,34,36,71,81,82] They usually are soft, white to gray-white, with a lobulated or nodular external surface, and solid and white to gray-pink on cut section, with evidence of hemorrhage and necrosis.

Microscopically, the ovarian tissue is replaced almost completely by a diffuse proliferation of malignant lymphoma cells forming a diffuse pattern, although occasionally a nodular (follicular) pattern, which may be pure or associated with the diffuse pattern, also is seen.[71,82] Normal ovarian structures, for example, corpora lutea and corpora albicantia, sometimes are present and are surrounded by the neoplastic cells, which may invade them.[18,34,36,71,81,82,89] Acute inflammatory cells, plasma cells, and normal lymphocytes may be admixed with the tumor cells, causing diagnostic difficulties. The malignant lymphoma usually is of a poorly differentiated type and may be difficult to classify (Fig. 21.14). It usually

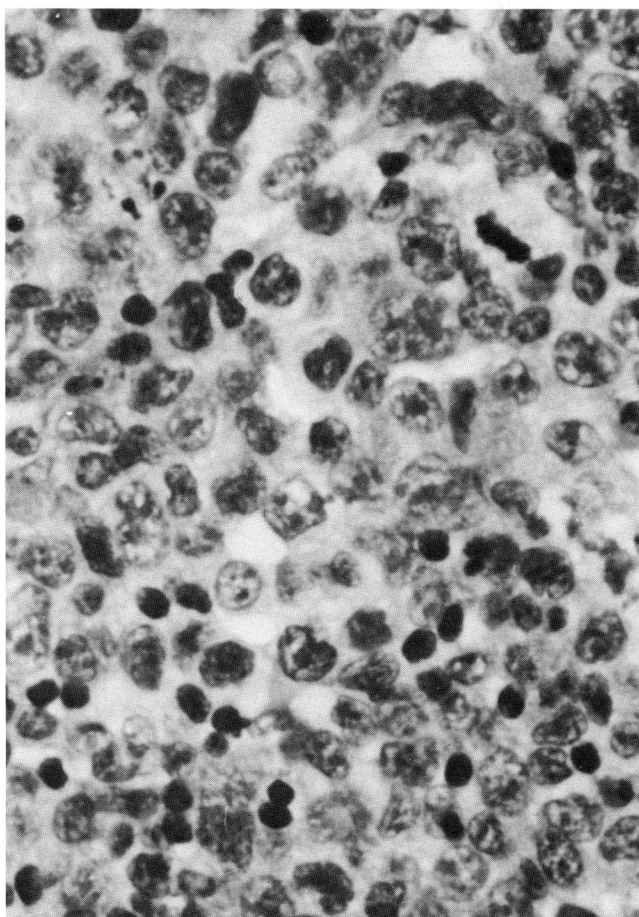

FIG. 21.14. **Primary malignant lymphoma of ovary, poorly differentiated type.** Note brisk mitotic activity and infiltration by inflammatory cells.

is of the lymphoblastic or histiocytic type[86] of the large cleaved or noncleaved type.[58,81] Using recent nomenclature, most tumors are classified as of the diffuse large cell type, or diffuse mixed large and small cell type, and the great majority are B-cell tumors.[34,71]

Malignant lymphoma of the ovary must be distinguished from other small round tumors composed of diffuse or nodular proliferations of small uniform tumor cells. Malignant lymphoma, especially of the lymphoblastic or poorly differentiated lymphocytic (small cell and large cell cleaved) types, must be distinguished from poorly differentiated metastatic carcinoma, most frequently of mammary origin. The carcinoma cells tend to be less uniform, show usually less marked mitotic activity, may be associated with evidence of fibroblastic reaction, and in places may exhibit an attempt at acinar formation. Malignant lymphoma also must be distinguished from primary or metastatic small (oat) cell carcinoma (see below).

The presence of positive immunocytochemical staining for leukocyte common antigen (LCA) distinguishes malignant lymphoma from neoplasms that are not composed of lymphoreticular cells and is the most valuable diagnostic aid in this context. Further immunocytochemical typing with large panels of antibodies for light and heavy chains, and various B- and T-marker antibodies, are recommended in LCA-positive cases. Molecular studies, including gene rearrangement, also can be performed if fresh frozen tissue is available.

Histochemical demonstration of mucin and positive immunocytochemical staining for cytokeratin, which indicate carcinoma, also are helpful in distinguishing between these two entities. The presence of occasional, better-differentiated rhabdomyoblasts and of rosette formation helps to distinguish embryonal rhabdomyosarcoma and metastatic neuroblastoma, respectively, from malignant lymphoma.

Malignant lymphoma also must be distinguished from ovarian involvement by leukemia, and in such cases, blood and bone marrow studies obviously are helpful. The presence of red granular staining in the cytoplasm of the tumor cells when using naphthol-AS-D-chloroacetate esterase (Leder's stain) distinguishes malignant lymphoma cells, which do not stain by this method, from myeloid series cells, which stain positively.

Malignant lymphoma also must be distinguished from granulosa cell tumors showing diffuse pattern, but other patterns seen in granulosa cell tumor may be evident, at least in some parts of the tumor. Mitotic activity is less brisk in granulosa cell tumor, and the cellular and nuclear appearances are different. Malignant lymphoma of the histiocytic (large cell noncleaved) type, which sometimes contains normal lymphocytes, must be distinguished from dysgerminoma. The dysgerminoma cells are more uniform in size and appearance and usually contain larger amounts of cytoplasm, which tends to be clear or pale and granular. The cytoplasm typically contains abundant glycogen, which stains positively with PAS stain and is removed by

diastase digestion. The nuclei of dysgerminoma cells are more uniform and do not display the marked variation in shape and size seen in the nuclei of the malignant lymphoma cells.

The course of the disease of patients with primary malignant lymphoma of the ovary is variable. Whereas generalized disease develops in most patients within a few months of the excision of the ovarian neoplasm, in some patients generalized disease does not develop for years. An occasional patient does not show any further involvement, and in some patients the only further involvement is enlargement of para-aortic and parailiac lymph nodes, the lymph nodes that provide lymphatic drainage of the ovary. Although some patients in whom generalized disease develops might not have been examined carefully enough to detect the presence of further disease, on presentation there is little doubt that in some patients with malignant lymphoma confined to the ovary generalized disease will develop within a few months. Unfortunately, at present it is not possible to determine which patients will and which will not develop generalized disease. Therefore, all patients should be staged properly and given adequate therapy, which should include radiation to the regional lymph nodes and the most efficacious combination chemotherapy. Occasional cases have been reported[18,34,36,71,81,82,89] in which patients were well and disease-free for periods of 2–5 years after initial treatment; some further unreported cases are known as well.

Hodgkin's Disease Localized to the Ovary

Two cases of Hodgkin's disease localized to the ovary have been reported.[6,56] In both cases, the tumor was unilateral. Microscopically, the ovary was replaced by a malignant cellular infiltrate consisting of lymphocytes, eosinophils, plasma cells, atypical histiocytic cells, and typical Sternberg–Reed cells. Fibrosis and necrosis also were evident. Both patients were well and disease-free for periods of 2 and 6 years after diagnosis. Although it is difficult to draw any conclusions from only two cases, it appears that Hodgkin's disease, when localized to the ovary, has a better prognosis than does primary non-Hodgkin's lymphoma of the ovary.

Disseminated Malignant Lymphoma Affecting the Ovary

As mentioned earlier, this entity must be divided into two categories: (1) the ovarian tumor being either the initial or predominant presenting manifestation of the disease and (2) ovarian involvement occurring during the course of the disease and being noted at surgery or autopsy, either grossly or microscopically.

The first type of disseminated malignant tumor is uncommon. Although it is more common than primary malignant lymphoma of the ovary, with more than 100 examples recorded.[34,36,71,73,81,89,109] The second type is common and is becoming even more so because of the longer survival of patients with malignant lymphoma as a result of recent therapy.

The age of patients in whom the ovarian involvement is the presenting sign of malignant lymphoma ranges from childhood to old age, but most are 20–50 years of age.[34,36,71,73,81,89,109] The symptoms in these patients are largely similar to those observed in patients with primary malignant lymphoma of the ovary, the most common being abdominal enlargement often associated with abdominal pain. In contrast to women with primary malignant lymphoma of the ovary, these patients frequently complain of malaise, weight loss, pallor, and fatigue. On physical examination, in addition to the finding of an adnexal mass, which is frequently bilateral, lymph node enlargement—either widespread or localized—may be noted. There may be enlargement of the spleen and the liver. The blood count may show anemia. A leukemic blood picture or pancytopenia may be observed. The macroscopic and microscopic appearances of the ovarian tumor are similar to those described in cases of malignant lymphoma localized to the ovary. The malignant lymphoma usually is of a poorly differentiated B-cell type, either lymphoblastic, poorly differentiated lymphocytic, or reticulum cell sarcoma,[86] or large or small cleaved or noncleaved type,[58,81] diffuse large cell, or diffuse mixed large and small cell type.[71]

It is extremely uncommon for generalized Hodgkin's disease to present in this manner. The course of the disease and the prognosis are similar to those observed in patients with generalized non-Hodgkin's malignant lymphoma of the poorly differentiated cell type, which are, at best, very guarded despite recent advances in treatment of these conditions.

Ovarian involvement is observed nowadays in up to 50% of cases of disseminated malignant lymphoma examined at autopsy, but it occurs rarely in patients with disseminated Hodgkin's disease. Patients with malignant lymphoma live longer with the disease because of the improved therapy, and this contributes to the wider dissemination once response to therapy is lost. In such cases, the lymphoma affects many sites that did not become affected in the past, when patients died earlier, with the disease involving mainly the lymphoreticular system. The involvement of the ovaries usually is bilateral, and the ovaries may be of normal size or only slightly enlarged. Microscopically, extensive infiltration by malignant lymphoma cells usually is present, but sometimes the infiltration may be slight.

These patients should be treated according to the most effective current protocols used for treating patients with disseminated malignant lymphoma.

Burkitt's Lymphoma

Burkitt's lymphoma is a specific type of malignant lymphoma showing a typical age prevalence, clinical and histological picture, and having a specific geographic distribution. It is observed primarily in East and West Africa south of the Sahara desert and in Papua and New Guinea.[7,14] These are considered the endemic areas, where the tumor is common. The tumor also occurs sporadically outside the endemic areas.[24,71,78]

Burkitt's lymphoma is a poorly differentiated malignant lymphoma, showing multicentric or multifocal origin. Clinically, it is seen affecting the jaw, ovary, orbit, kidney, thyroid, testis, and other sites, with involvement of the lymph nodes a minor feature. Frequent ovarian involvement by the disease was first noted in West Africa[12] and also was found in the East African cases.[14,77] Relatively frequent involvement of the ovary also is observed in cases from outside the endemic areas.[24,71,78]

Abdominal pain and swelling caused by ovarian enlargement represent the principal symptoms in 38% of patients with Burkitt's lymphoma. Burkitt's lymphoma occurs mainly in children, with a peak incidence at 4–7 years. Young adults also are affected. Occasionally, the tumor is localized to the ovary without involvement of other sites.[93]

Macroscopically, ovarian involvement by Burkitt's lymphoma usually is bilateral. The ovarian tumors are large, white, and solid with a slightly lobulated surface and on cut section have a solid, white, firm surface that can be altered by the presence of necrosis and hemorrhage.

Microscopically, the ovary is completely or nearly completely replaced by proliferation of primitive lymphoreticular cells (Figs. 21.15, 21.16) that appear round, oval, or indented with a narrow rim of basophilic cytoplasm, exhibiting strong pyroninophilia. The nuclei are large, prominent, and usually round but sometimes oval or reniform (Fig. 21.16). The nuclear membrane is sharp and well defined, and the chromatin is coarse, containing a few small nucleoli. Mitotic activity is brisk. The cytoplasm of the tumor cells contains numerous small vacuoles that contain lipid material. This is more obvious in imprint preparations from the tumor, a procedure that should always be undertaken, since it provides a very good diagnostic aid. Interspersed among the tumor cells are numerous nonneoplastic macrophages (histiocytes) containing phagocytosed material that stains positively with PAS and lipid stains. It is the presence of these macrophages scattered between the tumor cells that gives the tumor its typical *starry sky* appearance (Fig. 21.15). It should be noted that this starry sky appearance is not pathognomonic of Burkitt's lymphoma and may be observed in other types of poorly differentiated neoplasms. The histological appearance of the cells and the histochemical reactions mentioned earlier are the main features leading to the diagnosis of Burkitt's lymphoma.

Burkitt's lymphoma progresses quickly and, in the absence of therapy, is rapidly fatal. It responds dramatically to chemotherapy with antimetabolites and alkylating agents, leading to long remissions, and to complete cure in approximately 20% of cases. Radiotherapy can be used in conjunction with chemotherapy. The behavior of the tu-

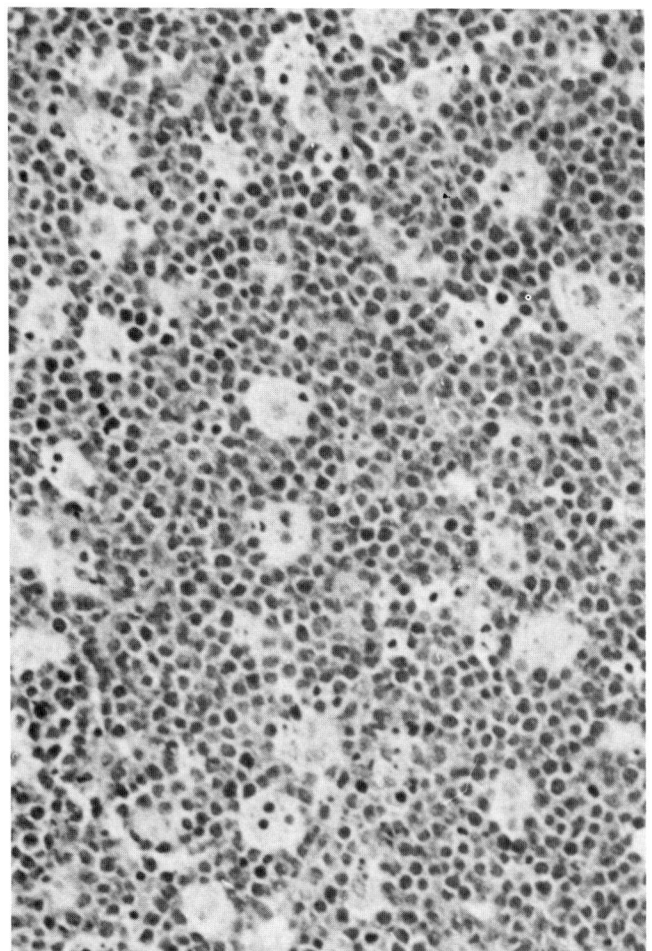

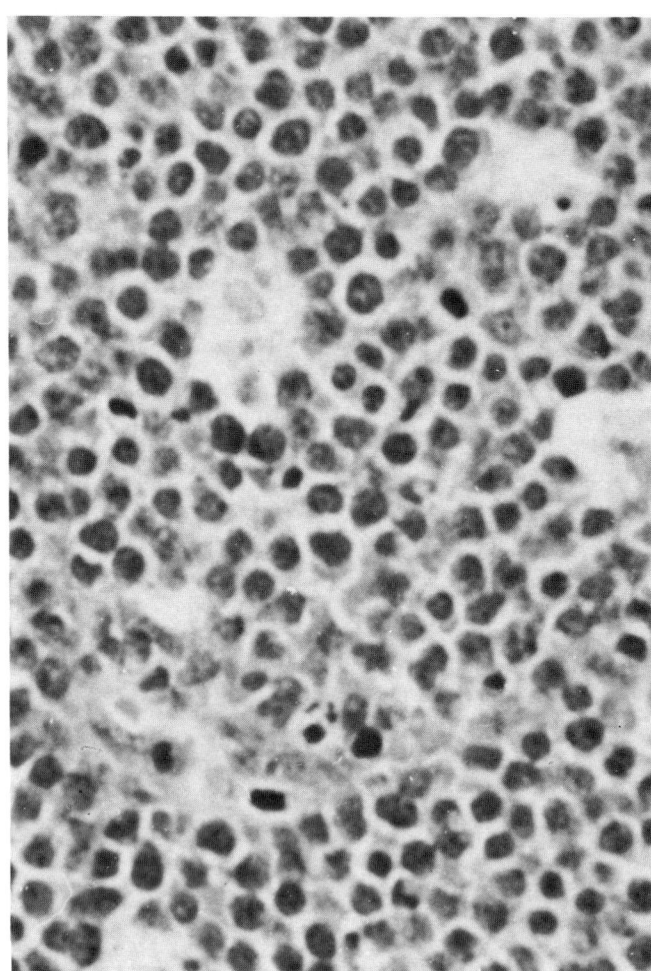

Fig. 21.15. Burkitt's lymphoma affecting ovary. The tumor has a typical starry sky appearance.

Fig. 21.16. Burkitt's lymphoma affecting ovary. Higher magnification of tumor shown in Fig. 21.15.

mor and its response to therapy are similar, whether it is encountered in the endemic or nonendemic areas.[114]

Involvement of the Ovary by Leukemia

Ovarian involvement by leukemia as seen at autopsy is common and is observed in 30–50% of cases. Recent reports indicate more frequent involvement than earlier studies. This may be due to longer containment of the disease by chemotherapy and radiotherapy, such as that observed in malignant lymphoma of the non-Hodgkin's type.

Lymphocytic and Granulocytic Leukemia

Occasionally, the ovary has been found to be the site of a relapse of childhood acute lymphocytic leukemia, although this course of events is by far not as common as in the case of the testes.[15] At times, ovarian enlargement may be the first sign of granulocytic leukemia, the ovarian tumor being

designated *ovarian granulocytic sarcoma* or *chloroma*, the latter term due to the green color of the tumor mass. Such cases usually are observed in children[4,72,81] but occasionally are seen in adults.[18] On examination, the peripheral blood or the bone marrow usually shows evidence of leukemia. Occasionally, the presence of an ovarian mass precedes the leukemia by a number of months.[4,72,81] The tumors frequently are bilateral, although one ovary may be larger than the other.

Microscopically, the tumor may resemble malignant lymphoma, especially if it is composed of early and primitive hematopoietic cells (Figs. 21.17, 21.18). The presence of myeloblasts and better differentiated cells (Fig. 21.18) that may be seen in places is helpful in making the diagnosis. The application of naphthol-AS-D-chloroacetate esterase (Leder's) stain confirms the diagnosis. Electron microscopy also is helpful in making the diagnosis. The prognosis of the patients is generally poor, but some patients survive a few years.[18] The treatment of choice in patients with granulocytic sarcoma is the combination che-

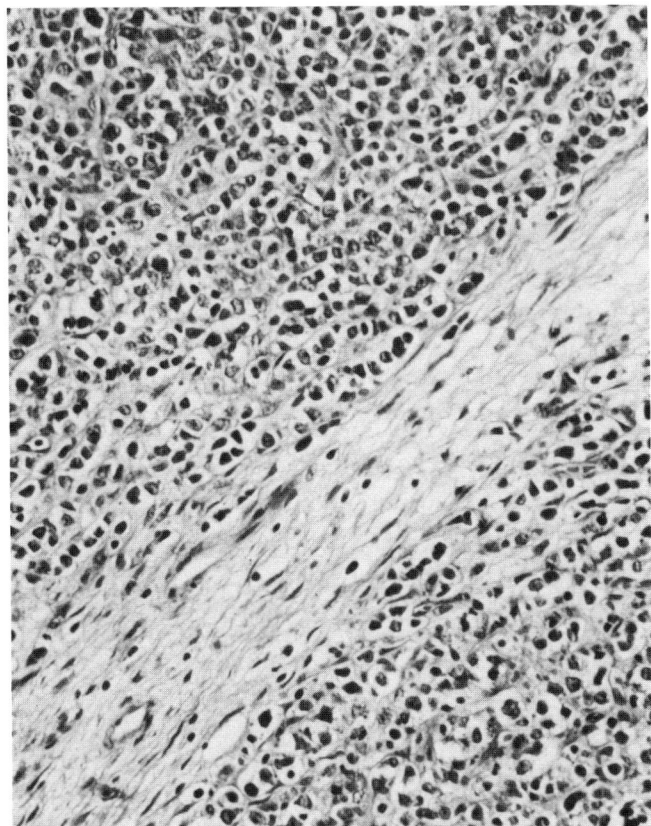

FIG. 21.17. Myelocytic sarcoma of ovary. Tumor is composed of collections of small round cells separated by bands of unaffected connective tissue.

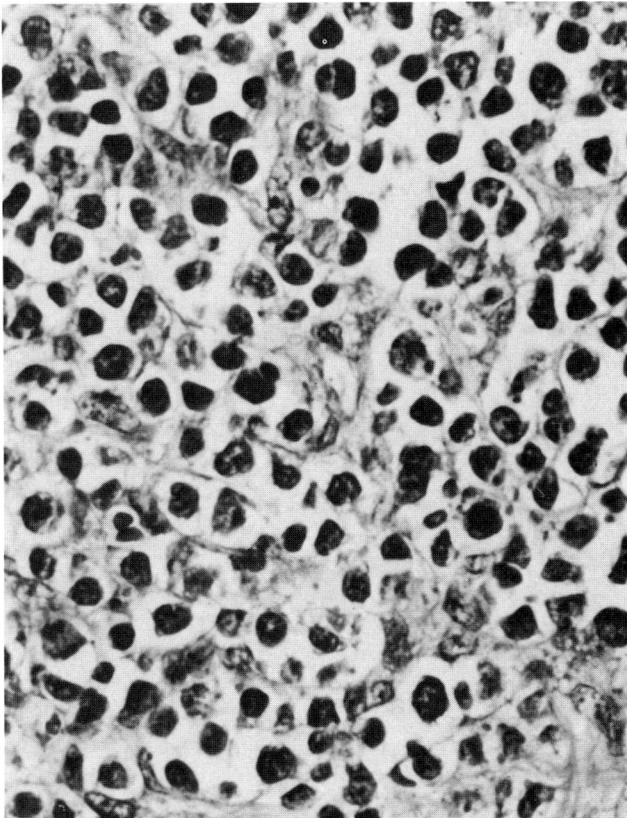

FIG. 21.18. Myelocytic sarcoma of ovary. Tumor is composed of primitive myeloid series cells. In places, slightly better differentiation indicates the myelocytic nature of the lesion.

motherapy used in patients with acute or subacute myelocytic leukemia.

Plasma Cell Dyscrasia

Involvement of the ovary by malignant disorders of plasma cells is very rare. It can manifest itself either as involvement of the ovary by multiple myeloma, usually observed at autopsy, although one case in a 44-year-old living woman has been reported,[5] or rarely as a primary extranodal plasmacytoma similar to primary malignant lymphoma of the ovary. One such case, which I observed, occurred in a 35-year-old woman, who had a painful lower abdominal mass. The tumor was unilateral, solid, firm, and gray-white. It measured 15 × 12 × 9 cm and showed ovarian tissue replaced by diffuse proliferation of plasma cells, including many immature forms. There was no evidence of biochemical abnormalities, including monoclonal gammopathy, and no evidence of bone or bone marrow involvement. The patient was well and disease-free 9 months after the operation, when she was lost to follow-up. Two similar cases have been reported in the literature.[42,106] Plasmacytoma must be differentiated from malignant lymphoma affecting the ovary as well as from granulocytic sarcoma.

The appearance of the tumor cells, aided by special stains, such as methyl green–pyronin, and electron microscopy are helpful in differentiating these lesions. Biochemical studies including electrophoresis, full blood, and radiologic examinations are necessary to differentiate between the disseminated disease and primary plasmacytoma. Because of the rarity of primary plasmacytoma of the ovary, it is possible only to speculate about the prognosis, but in common with extramedullary plasmacytoma found in other locations, it probably is better than in cases of multiple myeloma. The treatment of choice is excision of the lesion and careful follow-up of the patient. Chemotherapy used in cases of multiple myeloma may be administered prophylactically.

Tumors of Probable Wolffian Origin

Ovarian Tumor of Probable Wolffian Origin

In the original report describing tumors of this type,[53] all the tumors were located within the leaves of the broad ligament or were attached to it or to the fallopian tube. This also applied to subsequent reports dealing with this entity. Subsequently, 12 ovarian tumors of probable wolffian origin were reported,[45,110] indicating that tumors of this type also occur in the ovary. The age of the patients ranged from 28 to 79 years. Five patients had abdominal enlargement, and in the remaining seven patients, the tumor was found on physical examination.[45,110] At laparotomy, all the tumors were found to be unilateral. In 11 patients, they were confined to the ovary, and in the remaining patient, there were metastatic deposits in the abdominal cavity.[45,110] In the latter case, the tumor contained foci of undifferentiated carcinoma.[110]

The tumors range in size from 2 to 20 cm in the largest diameter. They are smooth and often lobulated and are either solid or solid and cystic. The cysts vary in size and may range up to 11 cm.[110] Microscopically, the tumor is composed of relatively uniform epithelial cells that line cysts and tubules, sometimes forming a sieve-like pattern (Fig. 21.19). The tumor cells also may form closely packed tubules (Fig. 21.20), grow in a diffuse pattern, or fill tubules or tubular spaces. They have uniform round or oval nuclei, and there is low mitotic activity. The tumor cells do not contain mucin but occasionally may contain glycogen. The amount of intervening connective tissue varies from imperceptible to considerable, forming fibrous bands separating the islands of tumor cells and producing a lobular

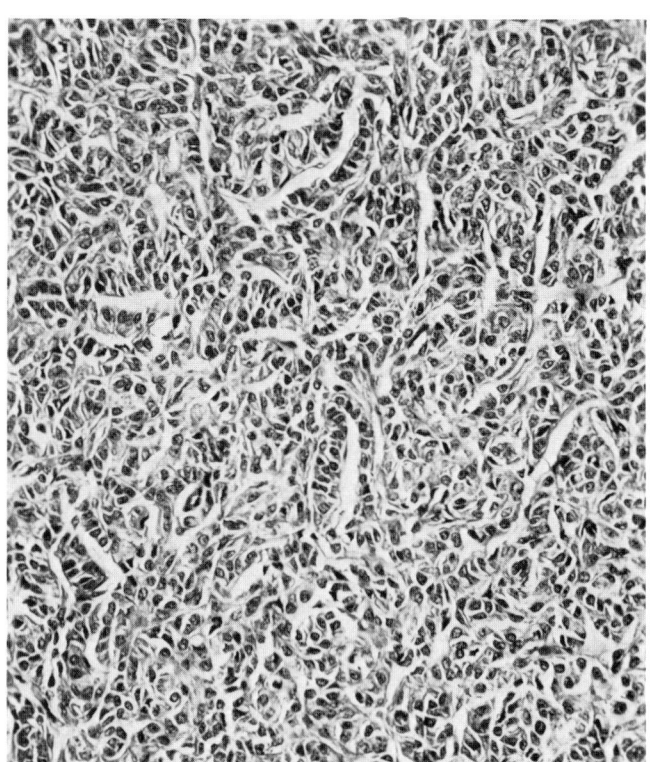

FIG. 21.20. Ovarian tumor of probable wolffian origin. The tumor is composed of closely packed tubules with compressed lumens and is lined by cuboid epithelial cells. (Reprinted by permission of Young and Scully, ref. 88.)

pattern.[110] In two patients in whom the tumors were associated with aggressive behavior, there was brisk mitotic activity with 10 or more mitoses/10 high power fields (HPF), and in one of the these patients, there was cellular and nuclear pleomorphism.

Two patients have subsequently developed metastases.[110] Eight patients were known to be alive and disease-free from 1 to 15 years postoperatively, and one was lost to follow-up,[110] indicating that in most cases the tumor is not associated with an aggressive course. It is also of note that there is a good correlation between the mitotic activity and the behavior of this neoplasm. Ovarian tumor of probable wolffian origin may be confused with sex cord–stromal tumors, especially various types of Sertoli–Leydig cell tumors and common epithelial tumors from which it must be differentiated (see Chapter 19, Sex Cord–Stromal, Steroid Cell, and Other Ovarian Tumors with Endocrine, Paraendocrine, and Paraneoplastic Manifestations). The presence of the typical features of this tumor described above and the absence of the various patterns observed in Sertoli–Leydig cell tumors differentiate it from the latter. The tumor of probable wolffian origin is distinguished from the various common epithelial tumors of the ovary by the absence of cellular and nuclear pleomorphism, a papillary pattern, and intraluminal and intracellular mucin.

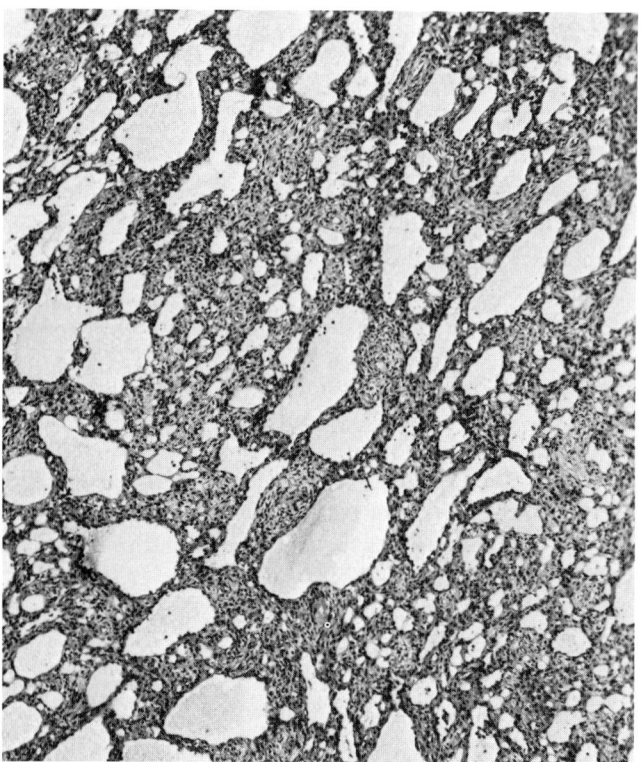

FIG. 21.19. Ovarian tumor of probable wolffian origin. The tumor shows a sieve-like pattern. The tumor cells line clefts and spaces and form solid aggregates. (Reprinted by permission of Young and Scully, ref. 88.)

Tumors of Uncertain Histogenesis

Hepatoid Carcinoma of the Ovary

In 1987, Ishikura and Scully[46] described five cases of ovarian carcinoma with hepatoid features, three of them primary and two probably primary. The age of the patients ranged from 42 to 78 years and thus differed considerably from patients with yolk sac tumor with a hepatoid pattern, which is invariably seen in children, adolescents, and young women. The age range, as well as the histological appearances of the tumors, showed considerable similarity to gastric carcinomas with hepatic features described some years earlier.[47,48]

Unlike yolk sac tumor with a hepatoid pattern, which may be pure, mixed with other yolk sac tumor patterns, or combined with other germ cell tumors, hepatoid carcinoma of the ovary occurs in pure form, and is not associated with other types of ovarian tumors.[46] Hepatoid carcinoma of the ovary,[46] like yolk sac tumor with hepatoid pattern and gastric adenocarcinoma with hepatoid features,[47,48] is associated with alpha-fetoprotein (AFP) secretion and AFP can be demonstrated within the tumor cells by immunohistochemical techniques. In a case known to the author, occurring in a 67-year-old woman, very high levels of serum AFP were noted, and serum AFP is being used to monitor the disease activity. Clinically, patients present with symptoms and signs related to the presence of an adnexal mass. Abdominal enlargement, which may be associated with pain, malaise, and weight loss, is the main presenting sign.[46]

Hepatoid carcinomas of the ovary are large and are associated with metastatic tumor deposits within the abdominal cavity (stage III) in most cases.[46] Histologically, the tumor shows a close resemblance to hepatocellular carcinoma, and is composed of solid sheets or aggregates of uniform cells with moderate or abundant eosinophilic cytoplasm, distinct cell borders, and centrally located nuclei with prominent nucleoli (Fig. 21.21).[46] Mitotic activity generally is brisk and abnormal forms are seen. In some parts of the tumor there may be a considerable degree of cellular and nuclear pleomorphism and multinucleated giant cells may be seen.[46] PAS-positive diastase-resistant hyaline globules may be seen, and glycogen can be demonstrated within the cytoplasm of the tumor cells. Histological patterns seen in germ cell tumors or surface epithelial stromal tumors are not detectable and the tumor is seen only in pure form.[46] Immunohistochemical studies demonstrate the presence of AFP in a considerable number of tumor cells. In addition the tumor cells are immunoreactive for albumin, alpha$_1$-antitrypsin, and alpha$_1$-antichymotrypsin. Focal positive immunostaining for carcinoembryonic antigen (CEA) also is seen.[46]

Hepatoid carcinoma of the ovary is a highly malignant neoplasm.[46] Most patients present with disseminated dis-

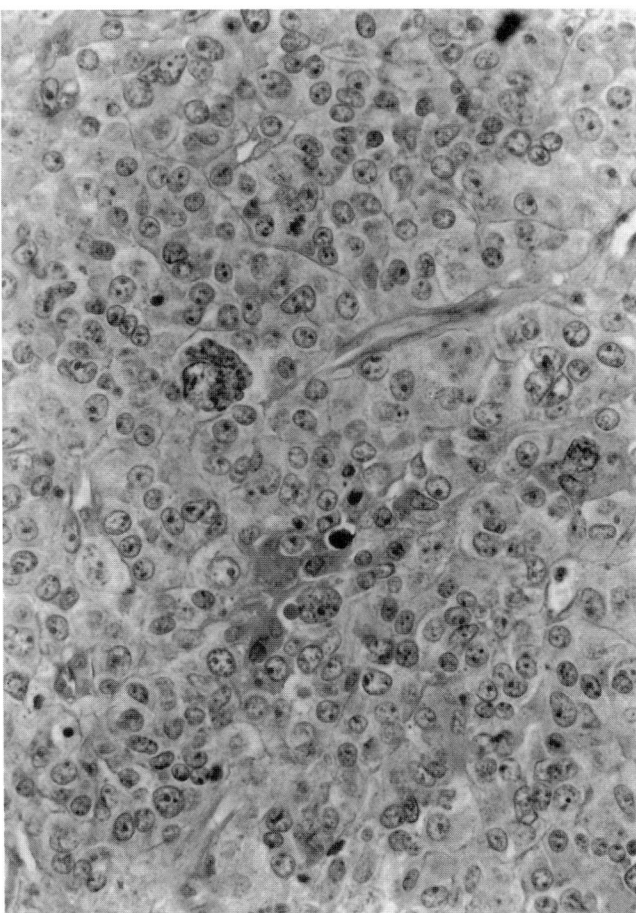

Fig. 21.21. Hepatoid carcinoma of the ovary. Note the close resemblance to hepatocellular carcinoma. Occasional giant cells are seen, and help to differentiate this tumor from yolk sac tumor with hepatoid pattern. (Courtesy of R. E. Scully, M.D., Boston, MA.)

ease and die of the disease within a few years of diagnosis. One patient is well and disease-free for 2 years after pelvic irradiation.[46] One patient is alive with evidence of disease 2 years after surgery and combination chemotherapy. She is at present being treated with Taxol and appears to be responding as evidenced by some decrease in the serum AFP level.

The histogenesis of hepatoid carcinoma of the ovary has not been established. Unlike yolk sac tumor with hepatoid pattern, it is not of germ cell origin, as it occurs in older patients, is not associated with other neoplastic germ cell elements, and is not found in patients with gonadal dysgenesis. Because of the age distribution and the possibility that it may be a metaplastic tumor, it has been suggested that it may represent a variant of a surface epithelial stromal tumor.[46]

Hepatoid carcinoma of the ovary must be distinguished from yolk sac tumor with hepatoid pattern. It can be distinguished clinically by its occurrence in older, usually postmenopausal patients and by its presentation in a more advanced clinical stage, usually in stage III. Histologically, hepatoid carcinoma shows a greater degree of cellular and nuclear pleomorphism and tumor giant cells are much more frequently seen.

Demonstration of positive immunocytochemical staining for AFP in the tumor cells and elevated levels of serum AFP differentiate hepatoid carcinoma from other ovarian tumors like undifferentiated adenocarcinomas, endometrioid adenocarcinomas with marked squamous differentiation and steroid cell tumors.[46] Primary hepatoid carcinoma of the ovary also must be differentiated from primary hepatocellular carcinoma, metastatic to the ovary. Although the latter is uncommon, this possibility must be carefully excluded before the diagnosis of primary hepatoid carcinoma of the ovary is made.

Primary Ovarian Small Cell Carcinoma with Pulmonary Differentiation

Recently Eichhorn et al.[29] reported 11 primary ovarian tumors that resembled small cell carcinoma of the lung and differed both clinically and histologically from primary small cell carcinoma of the ovary, usually associated with hypercalcemia.[22,113] The age of the patients ranged from 28 to 85 years.[29] Most patients presented with abdominal enlargement. Six of the tumors were unilateral, and five were bilateral. Spread beyond the ovary was noted in seven tumors. None of the patients had distant metastases at presentation.[29] The tumors measured from 4.5 to 26 cm in the greatest dimension. They were mostly solid with a variable minor cystic component.[29]

Histologically, the tumor was composed of small to medium-sized round to spindle-shaped cells with scanty cytoplasm, hyperchromatic nuclei, and inconspicuous nucleoli forming sheets, large aggregates, and closely packed nests (Fig. 21.22). Sometimes an insular or a trabecular pattern was seen.[29] In four tumors there was a component of endometrioid carcinoma present, one tumor showed focal squamous differentiation, two tumors were associated with Brenner tumor, and one contained a cyst lined by atypical mucinous cells.[29] In two of six tumors, argyrophil granules were demonstrated. In nine cases immunocytochemical studies were performed that demonstrated positive staining for cytokeratin in six cases, for epithelial membrane antigen (EMA) in five, for neuron-specific enolase (NSE) in seven, for chromogranin in two, and for Leu-7 in a single case. All nine tumors were vimentin negative.[29] Flow cytometric studies performed on eight tumors showed that five tumors were aneuploid and three were diploid.[29]

The tumors were aggressive and of the nine patients with known follow-up, five died of the disease 1–13 months after diagnosis, one died after an unknown interval, and two had recurrent disease 6 and 8 months after surgery. One patient was alive without evidence of disease 7.5 years after surgery.[29] Five of the patients with stage III tumors

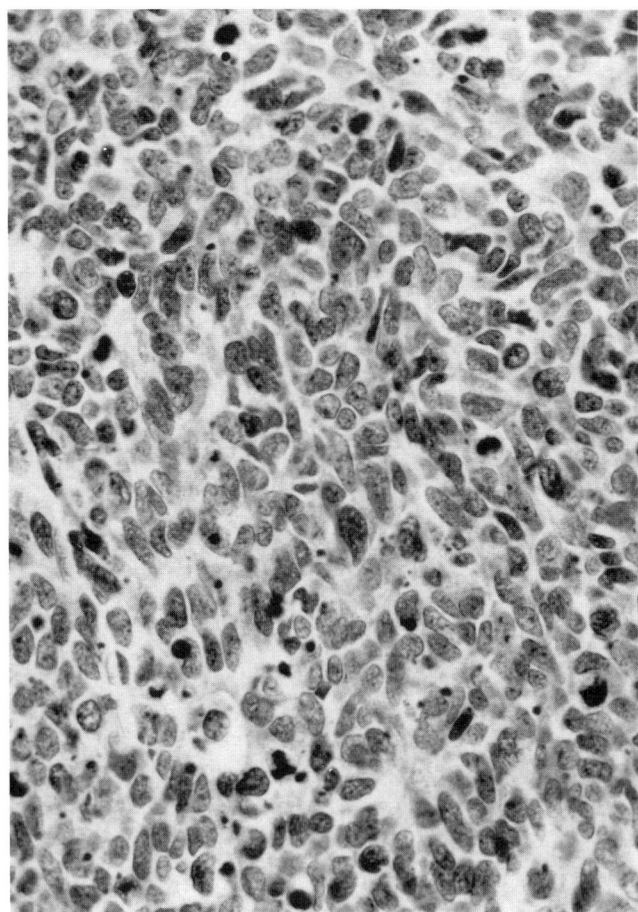

FIG. 21.22. Small cell carcinoma of the ovary with pulmonary differentiation. Note the ovoid and spindle shape of the nuclei, the finely dispersed chromatin, and inconspicuous nucleoli. (Courtesy of R. E. Scully, M.D., Boston, MA.)

and two with stage I tumors were treated with combination chemotherapy, which included cisplatin in all cases and doxorubicin in most cases. One of these treated patients is the 7.5-year survivor.[29] Aggressive treatment with agents effective in treating small cell pulmonary carcinoma appears to be the treatment of choice. Primary ovarian small cell carcinoma with pulmonary differentiation must be distinguished from pulmonary small cell carcinoma metastatic to the ovary, which shows both clinical and pathological differences.[112] It also must be differentiated from primary ovarian small cell carcinoma, usually associated with hypercalcemia (see Chapter 19, Sex Cord–Stromal, Steroid Cell, and Other Ovarian Tumors With Endocrine, Paraendocrine, and Paraneoplastic Manifestations).[22,113] The patients with primary ovarian small cell carcinoma with pulmonary differentiation are older. The tumor is seen either in perimenopausal or postmenopausal women.[29] Hypercalcemia is absent. The tumors are bilateral in 45% of cases, whereas in the hypercalcemic type, this is seen only rarely (1% of cases).[29] Histologically the cells of primary ovarian small cell carcinoma with pulmonary differentiation differ from those of the hypercalcemic type in having finely dispersed chromatin and inconspicuous nucleoli, whereas the latter is composed of cells with nuclei showing clumped chromatin and prominent nucleoli, as well as showing the presence of larger cells with abundant eosinophilic cytoplasm in 40% of cases.[29] Folliculoid spaces are always seen in the hypercalcemic type and virtually absent in the pulmonary type of small cell carcinoma.[29] Endometrioid and Brenner tumor components are present in more than half of the small cell carcinomas with pulmonary differentiation, and are absent in the hypercalcemic type.[29] The former also tend to be more frequently aneuploid.[29]

Although the histogenesis of the primary ovarian small cell carcinoma with pulmonary differentiation has not been established, the frequent association with endometrioid and Brenner tumors points toward a surface epithelial stromal origin. This is supported further by the age range of the patients.[29]

References

1. Abell MR, Holtz F (1965) Ovarian neoplasms in childhood and adolescence. 2. Tumors of non-germ cell origin. Am J Obstet Gynecol 93: 850

2. Azoury RS, Woodruff JD (1971) Primary ovarian sarcomas. Report of 43 cases from the Emil Novak Ovarian Tumor Registry. Obstet Gynecol 37: 920

3. Balaton A, Vaury P, Imbert MC, Mussy MA (1987) Primary leiomyosarcoma of the ovary. A histological and immunocytochemical study. Gynecol Oncol 28: 116

4. Ballon SC, Donaldson RC, Berman ML, Swanson GA, Byron RL (1978) Myeloblastoma (granulocytic sarcoma) of the ovary. Arch Pathol Lab Med 102: 474

5. Bambirra EA, Miranda D, Magalhaes GMC (1982) Plasma cell myeloma simulating Krukenberg's tumor. South Med J 75: 511

6. Bare WW, McCloskey JF (1961) Primary Hodgkin's disease of the ovary. Obstet Gynecol 17: 447

7. Berard C, O'Conor GT, Thomas LB, Torloni H (1969) Histopathological classification of Burkitt's tumour. Bull WHO 40: 601

8. Biggart JH, Macafee CHG (1955) Tumours of ovarian mesenchyme. A clinico-pathological survey. J Obstet Gynaecol Br Emp 62: 829

9. Bower JF, Erikson ER (1967) Bilateral ovarian fibroma in a 5 year old. Am J Obstet Gynecol 99: 880

10. Brady K, Page DV, Benn LE, de las Morenas A, O'Brien M (1987). Ovarian myxoma. Am J Obstet Gynecol 156: 1240

11. Braithwaite J (1894) On atrophy with collapse (cirrhosis), fibroid degeneration, angioma of the ovaries. Trans Obstet Soc London 36: 235

12. Brew DS, Jackson JG (1960) Lymphosarcoma of the ovary in young African girls. Br J Cancer 14: 621

13. Burket RL, Rauh JL (1976) Gorlin's syndrome. Ovarian fibromas at adolescence. Obstet Gynecol 47: 43S

14. Burkitt DP, Wright DH (1970) Burkitt's lymphoma. Edinburgh, Livingstone.

15. Cecalupo AJ, Frankel LS, Sullivan MP (1982) Pelvic and ovarian extramedullary leukemic relapse in young girls. A report of four cases and review of the literature. Cancer 50: 587

16. Chan YF, Leung CS, Ma L (1989) Primary embryonal rhabdomyosarcoma of the ovary in a 4-year-old girl. Histopathology 15: 211

17. Charache H (1959) Ovarian tumors in childhood. Arch Surg 79: 573

18. Chorlton I, Norris HJ, King FM (1974) Malignant reticuloendothelial disease involving the ovary as a primary manifestation. A series of 19 lymphomas and 1 granulocytic sarcoma. Cancer 34: 397

19. Clendenning WE, Herdt JR, Black JB (1963) Ovarian fibromas and mesenteric cysts. Their association with hereditary basal cell cancer of the skin. Am J Obstet Gynecol 87: 1008

20. Climie AR, Heath LP (1968) Malignant degeneration of benign cystic teratoma of the ovary. Review of the literature and report of a chondrosarcoma and a carcinoid tumor. Cancer 22: 824

21. De Franchis M, Galliani F (1964) Nurinoma del ovario. Riv Patol Clin 19: 567

22. Dickersin GR, Kline IW, Scully RE (1982) Small cell carcinoma of the ovary with hypercalcemia. A report of eleven cases. Cancer 49: 188

23. Dockerty MB, Masson JC (1944) Ovarian fibromas: A clinical and pathologic study of two hundred eighty three cases. Am J Obstet Gynecol 47: 741

24. Dorfman FR (1965) Childhood lymphoma in St. Louis, Missouri, clinically and histologically resembling Burkitt's tumor. Cancer 18: 418

25. Dover H (1950) Neurofibrosarcoma of the ovary, associated with neurofibromatosis. Can Med Assoc J 63: 488

26. Dutz W, Stout AP (1961) The myxoma in childhood. Cancer 14: 629

27. Ebrahimi T, Goldsmith JW, Okagaki T (1971) Hemangioma of the ovary. A case report. Obstet Gynecol 38: 677

28. Eichhorn JH, Scully RE (1991). Ovarian myxoma. Clinicopathologic and immunocytologic analysis of five cases and a review of the literature. Int J Gynecol Pathol 10: 156

29. Eichhorn JH, Young RH, Scully RE (1992). Primary ovarian small cell carcinoma of pulmonary type. A clinicopathologic, immunohistologic and flow cytometric analysis of 11 cases. Am J Surg Pathol 16: 926

30. Ewing J (1940) Neoplastic diseases, 4th ed. Philadelphia, Saunders

31. Fallahzadeh H, Dockerty MB, Lee RA (1972) Leiomyoma of the ovary. Report of five cases and review of the literature. Am J Obstet Gynecol 113: 394

32. Fawcett FJ, Kimbell NKB (1971) Phaeochromocytoma of the ovary. J Obstet Gynaecol Br Commonw 78: 458

33. Ferenczy A, Fenoglio CM, Richart RM (1972) Observations on benign mesothelioma of the genital tract (adenomatoid tumor). Cancer 30: 244

34. Ferry JA, Young RH (1991) Malignant lymphoma, pseudolymphoma and hematopoietic disorders of the female genital tract. Pathol Annu 26: 227

35. Fox H, Langley FA (1976) Tumours of the ovary. London, William Heinemann

36. Fox H, Langley FA, Govan ADT, Hill AS, Bennett MM (1988) Malignant lymphoma presenting as an ovarian tumor. A clinicopathologic analysis of 34 cases. Br J Obstet Gynecol 95: 386

37. Fundaro P (1969) Emangioma cavernoso bilaterale dell ovaia: Presentazione di un caso e rassegna della literatura. Folia Hered Patol 18: 45

38. Gay RM, Janovski NA (1969) Cavernous hemangioma of the ovary. Gynaecologia 168: 248

39. Gerbie AB, Hirsch MR, Greene RR (1955) Vascular tumors of the female genital tract. Obstet Gynecol 6: 499

40. Guérard MJ, Arguelles MA, Ferenczy A (1983) Rhabdomyosarcoma of the ovary. Ultrastructural study of a case and review of the literature. Gynecol Oncol 15: 325

41. Hart WR, Abell MR (1970) Adipose prosoplasia of the ovary. Am J Obstet Gynecol 106: 929

42. Hautzer NW (1984) Primary plasmacytoma of ovary. Gynecol Oncol 18: 115

43. Hegg CA, Flint A (1990) Neurofibroma of the ovary. Gynecol Oncol 37: 437

44. Howell CG, Rogers DA, Gable DS, Falls GD (1990) Bilateral ovarian fibromas in children. J Pediatr Surg 25: 690

45. Hughesdon PE (1982) Ovarian tumors of wolffian or allied nature. Their place in ovarian oncology. J Clin Pathol 35: 526

46. Ishikura H, Scully RE (1987) Hepatoid carcinoma of the ovary. A newly described tumor. Cancer 60: 2775

47. Ishikura H, Fukasawa Y, Ogasawara K, Natori T, Tsukada Y, Aizawa M (1985) An AFP-producing gastric carcinoma with featurs of hepatoid differentiation. A case report. Cancer 56: 840

48. Ishikura H, Kirimoto K, Shamoto M, et al (1986) Hepatoid adenocarcinomas of the stomach. An analysis of seven cases. Cancer 58: 119

49. Janovski NA, Paramanandhan TL (1973) Ovarian tumors. Tumors and tumor-like conditions of the ovaries, fallopian tubes, and ligaments of the uterus. Philadelphia, W B Saunders

50. Kalstone CE, Jaffe RB, Abell MR (1969) Massive edema of the ovary simulating fibroma. Obstet Gynecol 34: 564

51. Kandalaft PL, Esteban JM (1992) Bilateral massive ovarian leiomyomata in a young woman. A case report with review of the literature. Mod Pathol 5: 586

52. Kannerstein M, Churg J (1977) Peritoneal mesothelioma. Hum Pathol 8: 83

53. Kariminejad MH, Scully RE (1973) Female adnexal tumor of probable wolffian origin. Cancer 31: 671

54. Kraemer BB, Silva EG, Sneige N (1984) Fibrosarcoma of the ovary. A new component in the nevoid basal-cell carcinoma syndrome. Am J Surg Pathol 8: 231

55. Lawhead RA, Copeland LJ, Edwards CL (1985) Bilateral ovarian hemangiomas associated with diffuse abdominopelvic hemangiomatosis. Obstet Gynecol 65: 597

56. Long JP, Patchefsky AS (1971) Primary Hodgkin's disease of the ovary. Obstet Gynecol 38: 680

57. Lorentzen M (1980) Giant cell tumor of the ovary. Virch Arch [Pathol Anat] 388: 113

58. Lukes RJ, Collins RD (1974) Immunologic characterization of human malignant lymphomas. Cancer 34: 1488

59. Lyday RO (1952) Fibroma of the ovary with abdominal implants. Am J Surg 84: 737

60. Majmudar B, Kapernick PS, Phillips RS (1978) Ovarian myxoma. Hum Pathol 9: 723

61. Mann LS, Metrick S (1961) Hemangioma of the ovary. Report of a case. J Int Coll Surg 36: 500

62. Martins SM, Klinger OJ (1964) Bilateral ovarian fibromas before the menarche. Am J Obstet Gynecol 87: 386

63. Masubuchi K, Kimura M, Suzuki H, Suzuki P, Aoki M (1970) Case of ovarian myxoma. Jpn J Cancer Clin 16: 156

64. Matamala MF, Nogales FF, Aneiros J, Heraiz MA, Caracuel MD (1988) Leiomyomas of the ovary. Int J Gynecol Pathol 7: 190

65. McBurney RC, Trumbull M (1955) Hemangioma of the ovary with ascites. Miss Doct 32: 271

66. Meyer R (1943) Nerve tumors of the female genitals and pelvis. Arch Pathol 36: 437

67. Michael CA (1966) Pelvic fibroma causing recurrent attacks of hypoglycaemia in a post-menopausal patient. Proc Roy Soc Med 59: 835

68. Miles PA, Kiley KC, Mena H (1985) Giant fibrosarcoma of the ovary. Int J Gynecol Pathol 4: 83

69. Mira JL (1991) Lipoleiomyoma of the ovary. Report of a case and review of the English literature. Int J Gynecol Pathol 10: 198

70. Mishura VI (1963) Report of large benign tumor—report of three cases. Vopr Onkol 9: 103

71. Monterosso V, Jaffe ES, Merino MJ, Medeiros LJ (1993). Malignant lymphomas involving the ovary. A clinicopathologic analysis of 39 cases. Am J Surg Pathol 17: 154

72. Morgan ER, Labotka RJ, Gonzalez-Crussi F, Wiederhold M, Sherman JO (1981) Ovarian granulocytic sarcoma as a primary manifestation of acute infantile myelomonocytic leukemia. Cancer 48: 1819

73. Nelson GA, Dockerty MB, Pratt JH, Re-Mine WH (1958) Malignant lymphoma involving the ovaries. Am J Obstet Gynecol 76: 861

74. Nieminen U, von Numers C, Purola E (1969) Primary sarcoma of the ovary. Acta Obstet Gynecol Scand 48: 423

75. Nogales FF (1982) Primary chondroma of the ovary. Histopathology 6: 376

76. Nunez C, Abboud SL, Lemon NC, Kemp JA (1983) Ovarian rhabdomyosarcoma presenting as leukemia. Case report. Cancer 52: 297

77. O'Conor GT (1961) Malignant lymphoma in African children. II. A pathological entity. Cancer 14: 270

78. O'Conor GT, Rappaport H, Smith EB (1965) Childhood lymphoma resembling "Burkitt tumor" in the United States. Cancer 18: 411

79. Okamura H, Virutamasen P, Wright KH, Wallach EE (1972) Ovarian smooth muscle in the human being, rabbit, and cat: Histochemical and electron microscopic study. Am J Obstet Gynecol 112: 183

80. Ongkasuwan C, Taylor JE, Tang CK, Prempree T (1982) Angiosarcomas of the uterus and ovary. Clinicopathologic report. Cancer 49: 1469

81. Osborne BM, Robboy SJ (1983) Lymphomas or leukemia presenting as ovarian tumors. An analysis of 42 cases. Cancer 52: 1933

82. Paladugu RR, Bearman RM, Rappaport H (1980) Malignant lymphoma with primary manifestation in the gonad. A clinicopathologic study of 38 patients. Cancer 45: 561

83. Prat J (1979) Sarcomas of the ovary. Pathol Res Pract 165: 146

84. Prat J, Scully RE (1981) Cellular fibromas and fibrosarcomas of the ovary. A comparative clinicopathologic analysis of seventeen cases. Cancer 47: 2663

85. Prayson RS, Hart WR (1992) Primary smooth muscle tumors of the ovary. A clinicopathologic study of four leiomyomas and two mitotically active leiomyomas. Arch Pathol Lab Med 116: 1068

86. Rappaport H (1966) Tumors of the hematopoietic system. Atlas of tumor pathology, Sect 3, Vol. 8. Washington, D.C., Armed Forces Institute of Pathology

87. Raggio M, Kaplan AL, Harberg JF (1983) Recurrent ovarian fibromas with basal cell nevus syndrome (Gorlin syndrome). Obstet Gynecol 61: 95S

88. Rice M, Pearson B, Treadwell WB (1943) Malignant lymphangioma of the ovary. Am J Obstet Gynecol 45: 884

89. Rotmensch J, Woodruff JD (1982) Lymphoma of the ovary. Report of twenty new cases and update of previous series. Am J Obstet Gynecol 143: 870

90. Sandison AT (1955) Rhabdomyosarcoma of the ovary. J Pathol Bacteriol 70:433

91. Schmeisser HC, Anderson WAD (1938) Ganglioneuroma of the ovary. JAMA 111: 2005

92. Scully RE (1979) Tumors of the ovary and maldeveloped gonads. Vol 16, 2nd ser. Washington, D.C., Armed Forces Institute of Pathology

93. Seed PG (1966) Burkitt's tumour in Britain. J Obstet Gynecol Br Commonw 73: 808

94. Shaeffer MD, Cancelmo JJ (1939) Cavernous hemangioma of the ovary in a girl twelve years of age. Am J Obstet Gynecol 38: 722

95. Shearer JP (1935) Hemangioma of the ovary. Reported in a child 3½ years of age. Med Ann DC 4: 223

96. Shipton EA, Meares SD (1965) Heterotopic bone formation in the ovary. Aust NZ J Obstet Gynecol 5: 100

97. Smith FR (1931) Neurofibroma of the ovary associated with Recklinghausen's disease. Am J Cancer 15: 859

98. Stamm C (1891) Beitrag zur Lehre von Blutgefassgeschwulsten. Thesis. University of Gottingen

99. Stone GC, Bell DA, Fuller A, Dickersin GR, Scully RE

(1986) Malignant Schwannoma of the ovary. Report of a case. Cancer 58: 1575

100. Stout AP (1948) Myxoma, tumor of primitive mesenchyme. Ann Surg 127: 706

101. Stowe LM, Watt JY (1952) Osteogenic sarcoma of the ovary. Am J Obstet Gynecol 64: 422

102. Talerman A (1967) Hemangiomas of the ovary and the uterine cervix. Obstet Gynecol 30: 108

103. Talerman A, Auerbach WM, Van Meurs AJ (1981) Primary chondrosarcoma of the ovary. Histopathology 5: 319

104. Talerman A, Montero JR, Chilcote RR, Okagaki T (1985) Diffuse malignant peritoneal mesothelioma in a 13-year-old girl. Am J Surg Pathol 9: 73

105. Taxy JB, Battifora H, Oyasu R (1974) Adenomatoid tumors. A light microscopic, histochemical and ultrastructural study. Cancer 34: 306

106. Voegt H (1938) Extramedullary plasmacytoma. Virch Arch [Pathol Anat] 302: 497

107. Warhol MJ, Hunter NJ, Carson JM (1982) An ultrastructural comparison of mesotheliomas and adenocarcinomas of ovary and endometrium. Int J Gynecol Pathol 1: 125

108. Willis RA (1967) Pathology of tumours, 4th ed. London, Butterworths

109. Woodruff JD, Noll Castillo RD, Novak ER (1963) Lymphoma of the ovary. Am J Obstet Gynecol 85: 912

110. Young RH, Scully RE (1983) Ovarian tumors of probable wolffian origin. A report of 11 cases. Am J Surg Pathol 7: 125

111. Young RH, Scully RE (1984) Fibromatosis and massive edema of the ovary, possibly related entities. A report of 14 cases of fibromatosis and 11 cases of massive edema. Int J Gynecol Pathol 3: 153

112. Young RH, Scully RE (1985) Ovarian metastases from cancer of the lung. Problems in interpretation. A report of seven cases. Gynecol Oncol 21: 337

113. Young RH, Dickersin GR, Scully RE (1987) Small cell carcinoma of the ovary. An analysis of 75 cases of a distinctive ovarian tumor commonly associated with hypercalcemia. (Abstract) Lab Invest 56: 89A

114. Ziegler JL (1977) Treatment results of 54 American patients with Burkitt's lymphoma are similar to the African experience. N Engl J Med 297: 75

22

Metastatic Tumors of the Ovary

Robert H. Young, M.D., F.R.C. Path., and Robert E. Scully, M.D.

Metastatic tumors are an important group of ovarian neoplasms because the misinterpretation of those cases encountered as surgical pathology specimens may have im-

portant adverse consequences for the patient. Tumors may metastasize to the ovary from numerous organs and tissues outside the female genital tract but neoplasms arising in the intestines, stomach, and breast and hematopoietic tumors (rare examples of which are also primary in the ovary) are the most common forms encountered by the pathologist.* Hematopoietic tumors are discussed in Chapter 21 (Nonspecific Tumors of the Ovary, Including Mesenchymal Tumors and Malignant Lymphoma), and will not be considered further here. Tumors that extend to the ovary directly from adjacent organs or tissues also are included in the broad category of secondary tumors; determination of the origin of the tumor in such cases may be impossible when both ovarian and extraovarian involvement is extensive.

Recognition of the metastatic nature of an ovarian tumor depends on several factors: (1) an awareness of the frequency with which metastases occur and simulate a variety of primary tumors, (2) a detailed clinical history, (3) a thorough clinical and operative search by the gynecologist for a primary tumor outside the ovary and for other sites of tumor spread, and (4) a careful evaluation of the gross and microscopic features of the ovarian tumor by the pathologist. It is surprising how often the diagnosis of a metastatic tumor is missed by the pathologist because the existence of a present or prior tumor in another organ is either not known or, if known, disregarded. The surgical and pathological findings from previous operations should be reviewed if there is any possibility that they could be related

---

*Refs. 33,62,65,69,83,102,126,127,136.

to the ovarian tumor being evaluated. In some cases a search for an extraovarian primary tumor must be conducted postoperatively on the basis of the suspicion of the pathologist that the ovarian tumor is metastatic. Even if an extraovarian primary tumor is not detected, a diagnosis of ovarian metastasis must be strongly considered if the distribution of the metastatic disease is atypical for primary ovarian cancer or if pathological examination is highly suggestive of metastasis. For example, the presence of pulmonary or hepatic metastases in the absence of extensive peritoneal spread would be unusual for an ovarian cancer, but not for certain other tumors that are prone to metastasize to the ovary. The mere presence of tumor outside the ovaries should lead to the serious consideration of a metastasis in certain situations. For example, if a well-differentiated ovarian mucinous tumor is associated with extensive mucinous adenocarcinoma in the omentum and on the peritoneal surfaces, the possibility of spread to the ovary from, for example, the pancreas or biliary tract should be entertained. Additionally, certain tumors, such as Sertoli cell tumors or primary carcinoid tumors, which are almost always benign, should be diagnosed with caution in cases in which there also is extraovarian tumor. In cases of these types the putative Sertoli cell tumor may prove to be a metastatic tumor that is mimicking it, for example, a tubular Krukenberg tumor,[15] and the carcinoid tumor probably is metastatic[104] rather than primary in the ovary. It also must be emphasized that an association of an ovarian tumor with clinical or pathological evidence of excess estrogens, androgens, or progesterone does not exclude the diagnosis of a metastatic tumor, which may have a functioning stroma (see Chapter 19, Sex Cord–Stromal, Steroid Cell, and Other Ovarian Tumors with Endocrine, Paraendocrine, and Paraneoplastic Manifestations).

For a variety of reasons it is difficult to establish accurately the frequency of metastatic tumors among all ovarian tumors from the available literature. Some studies have been based on autopsy findings, others on surgical specimens, and still others on both. In addition, some series have included clinically silent metastases such as breast carcinoma found in prophylactic or therapeutic oophorectomy specimens and small metastases detected incidentally during operations for gastric or intestinal carcinoma. In contrast, other series have been restricted to metastatic tumors that presented clinically as pelvic or abdominal masses. Finally, some investigations have included as metastases ovarian carcinomas associated with uterine cancers of similar histologic type, whereas in many cases the ovarian tumors are independent primary tumors.

The frequency of metastases to the ovary also varies from one country to another because of wide differences in the prevalence of the various cancers that are associated with high rates of ovarian spread. For example, metastatic carcinoma was reported to account for approximately 40% of all ovarian cancers in one series from Japan, where gastric carcinoma is common, but for fewer than 3% in a series from Uganda, where this form of cancer is relatively rare.[64] The frequency of metastases also has varied greatly in series in which differences in the prevalence of the primary tumors do not adequately explain the discrepant results. For example, in an autopsy study from Brazil[79] metastases to the ovary were found in 29% of cancer patients, whereas in a similar investigation from the United States the frequency was only 5%.[130] Such variations may be related, in part, to the frequency and thoroughness of microscopic examination of the ovaries, since gross inspection may not reveal evidence of involvement in from one-third to one-half the cases. The figure for the frequency of ovarian metastases that is most meaningful to the gynecologist is one that expresses the probability that an ovarian neoplasm found on exploration of a pelvic or abdominal mass is metastatic; this figure was about 6% in the experience of Santesson and Kottmeier[108] and 7% in the series of Ulbright et al.[127]

The age distribution of patients with ovarian metastases depends to a great extent on that of the corresponding primary tumors, but for each of the most common types (intestinal, gastric, and breast) the average age of the patients with ovarian involvement is significantly lower than that of those without ovarian spread. This indicates that the richly vascularized ovaries of young women are more receptive to metastases than are those of older patients.

Tumors spread to the ovary by several routes. Direct spread is an important pathway for carcinomas of the fallopian tube and uterus, for mesotheliomas, and for occasional colonic carcinomas and retroperitoneal sarcomas. A second mechanism of spread of genital tract carcinomas is through the lumen of the fallopian tube and onto the surface of the ovary; this route is taken most often by carcinomas of the uterine corpus.[28] Spread from more distant sites is mainly via blood vessels and lymphatics. The frequent association of ovarian metastases with other blood-borne metastases, the common finding of tumor within ovarian blood vessels on microscopic examination in cases of metastasis, and the higher frequency of ovarian metastases in young patients are consistent with the important role of hematogenous spread. Retrograde flow within lymphatics is an unlikely route of spread except in the presence of extensive involvement of the lymph nodes draining the ovaries. Such a mechanism of spread also seems inconsistent with the sporadic reports of prolonged survival after a primary tumor and its apparently solitary ovarian metastatic tumor have been removed. Finally, transcoelomic dissemination with surface implantation is an important route by which intraabdominal cancers spread to the ovary. This is supported by the common association of ovarian involvement with generalized peritoneal spread. Also, the pathologist often encounters foci of metastatic carcinoma on the surface of the ovary, or so superficially located within its cortex that any explanation other than implantation seems improbable. It is possible that ovulation, by creating a defect in the ovarian surface, provides a portal of entry for cancer cells floating in the peritoneal cavity in premenopausal patients.

The gross features of tumors metastatic to the ovary vary greatly, and may resemble those of a variety of primary ovarian tumors. Because of the relatively high frequency with which metastases are bilateral (Fig. 22.1) (two-thirds to three-quarters of the cases), the possibility of metastasis should be considered particularly in evaluating bilateral tumors other than serous and undifferentiated carcinomas, which also are commonly bilateral. Endometrioid and mucinous carcinomas, in contrast, are bilateral in less than 15% of the cases and bilateral tumors with endometrioid-like and mucinous features merit more serious consideration for possibly being metastatic.[151] Although metastatic tumors often are bilateral, many metastatic tumors are unilateral and if the microscopic features of a tumor suggest metastasis, unilaterality should not be considered a significant argument against it. In general, almost 10% of bilateral ovarian cancers presenting as adnexal masses prove to be metastatic on careful evaluation. Two other gross findings that are highly suggestive, but not pathognomonic, of metastasis are the presence of multiple nodules (Fig. 22.1) and the location of nodules on the surface of the ovary (Fig. 22.2), sometimes without significant involvement of the underlying parenchyma. Conversely, a gross feature of some metastatic tumors, which should not be regarded as establishing the primary nature of the tumor, is

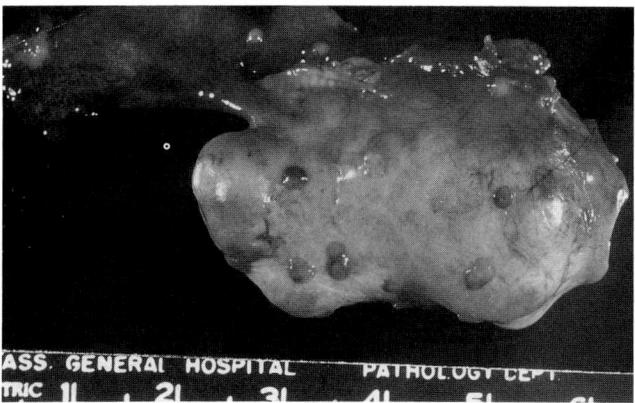

FIG. 22.2. Metastatic carcinoma from the breast. Several discrete nodules of tumor are present on the external aspect of the ovary. (Reproduced by permission of ref. 151.)

the presence of cysts, which often are large and occasionally thin-walled, despite the absence of cysts in the primary neoplasm (Fig. 22.3).

The microscopic appearance of a metastatic tumor obviously varies with the appearance of the primary neoplasm.

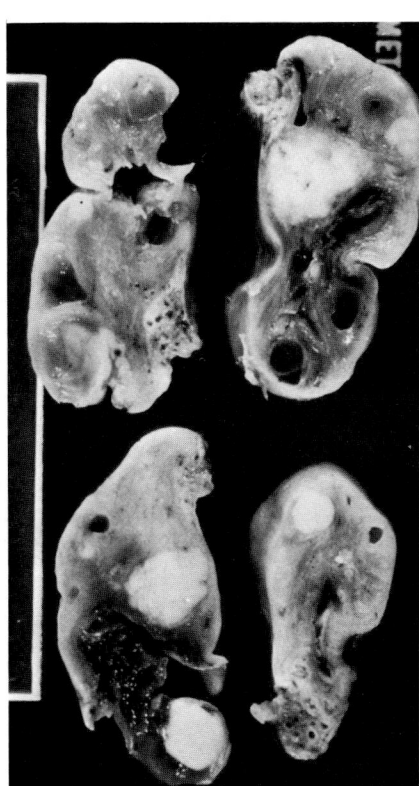

FIG. 22.1. Metastatic carcinoma from the breast. Multiple nodules are seen on the sectioned surfaces of both ovaries.

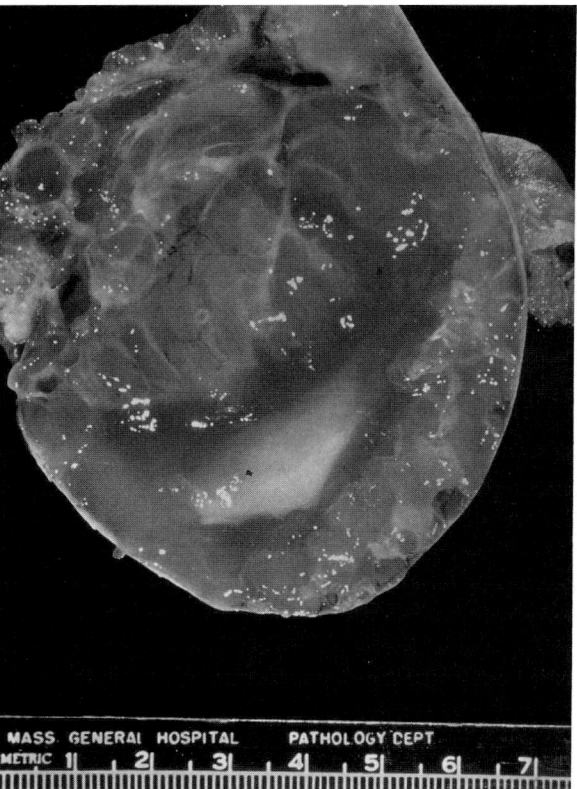

FIG. 22.3. Metastatic carcinoma from the cecum. The tumor is indistinguishable on gross examination from a primary mucinous cystic tumor from the ovary. (Reproduced by permission of ref. 151.)

In addition to the presence of specific features of various primary tumors, the presence of implants on the surface of the ovary (Fig. 22.4), growth in the form of multiple nodules (Fig. 22.5), and lymphatic or blood vessel invasion (Fig. 22.6) strongly suggest metastasis. The surface implants typically are focal, often projecting above the surface of the adjacent cortex, and characteristically are imbedded in desmoplastic or hyalinized fibrous tissue (Fig. 22.4), unlike the generally typical ovarian stroma found elsewhere in the tumor. The presence of surface implants in cases of metastasis sometimes correlates with the presence of excrescences on the external surface of the ovary that may be detected on careful gross inspection. A confusing microscopic feature of some metastatic tumors is the presence of cysts, some of which simulate follicles (Fig. 22.7). These follicle-like spaces[151] may be encountered in a variety of metastatic tumors including gastric and intestinal carcinomas, carcinoids, small cell carcinomas from various sites (Fig. 22.7), and malignant melanomas. A wide variety of other patterns and cell types in metastatic tumors suggest diverse possible primary sites, as discussed in detail elsewhere.[151]

Female Genital Tract Tumors

Tubal Carcinoma

The ovary is involved secondarily in approximately 13% of tubal carcinomas, usually by direct extension, sometimes via tuboovarian inflammatory adhesions, and at other times by surface implantation on the ipsilateral or contralateral

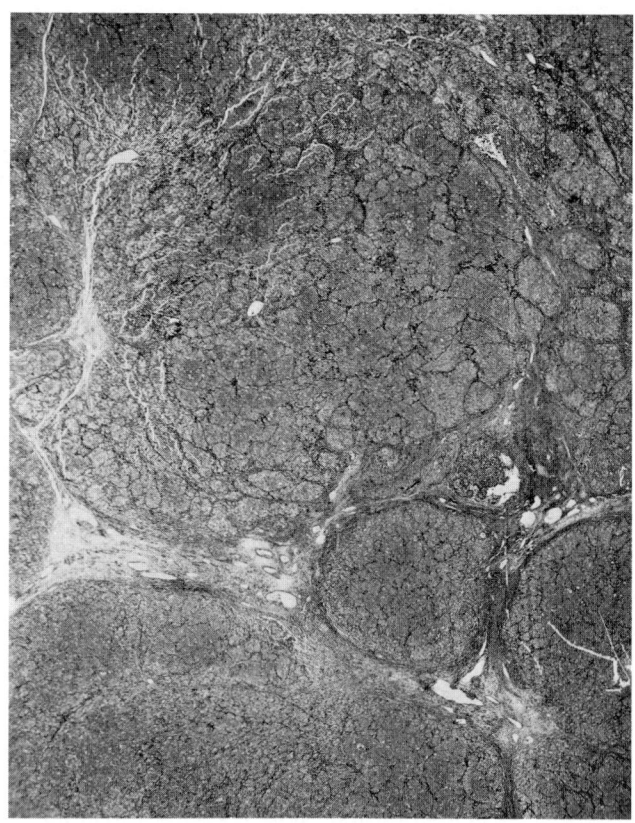

FIG. 22.5. **Metastatic carcinoma from the lung.** The tumor is growing in the form of multiple nodules.

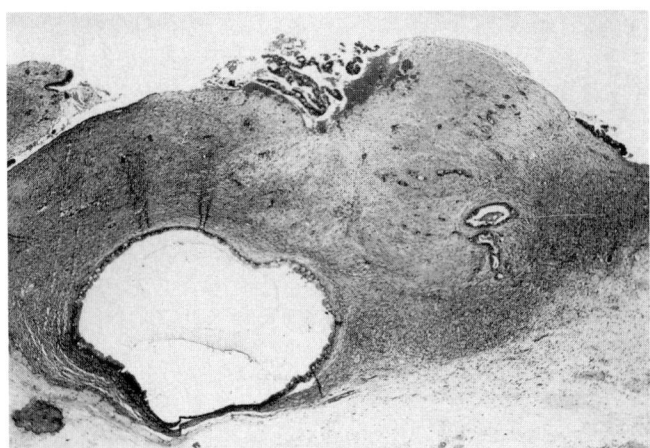

FIG. 22.4. **Metastatic carcinoma from the pancreas.** Tumor is present on the external aspect of the specimen (*top center*) and is associated with an underlying desmoplastic stromal reaction in the superficial cortex. One neoplastic gland has become cystic in the deeper portion of the ovary (*lower left*). (Reproduced by permission of ref. 151.)

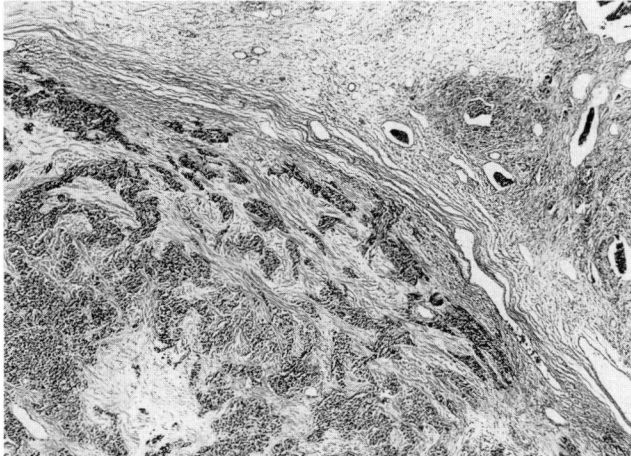

FIG. 22.6. **Metastatic carcinoma from the breast.** Vascular channels at the periphery of the tumor (*upper right*) contain metastatic tumor. (Reproduced by permission of ref. 151.)

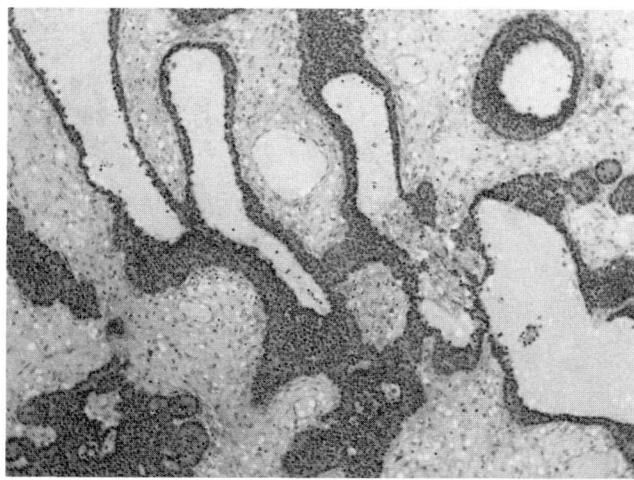

FIG. 22.7. Metastatic small cell carcinoma from the cervix. The tumor contains many follicle-like spaces.

ovary.[112] In some cases, there is clinical or pathological evidence of salpingitis and salpingo-oophoritis, but often it is unclear whether the inflammatory process preceded or followed the development of the carcinoma. If the involvement of the tube and the ovary is extensive, the primary site of the tumor may not be established with certainty; the term *tuboovarian carcinoma* has been suggested for these cases. Green and Scully[48] encountered six such tumors in an investigation of 24 carcinomas initially considered to be of tubal origin. The tuboovarian carcinomas formed solid and/or cystic masses; at least one of the cystic tumors appeared to have developed in a postinflammatory tuboovarian cyst.

Since most tubal carcinomas closely resemble serous or undifferentiated carcinomas of the ovary, microscopic examination often fails to establish whether a carcinoma involving both organs is primary in one or the other. Because of the great rarity of primary mucinous, endometrioid, and clear cell carcinomas of the fallopian tube, a tumor of any of these cell types involving both organs usually is considered primary in the ovary. It should be emphasized that surface growth within the tube may be seen as a result of implantation from an ovarian carcinoma and does not necessarily indicate that a tumor is primary in the tube.

Endometrial Carcinoma

Ovarian involvement in cases in which a diagnosis of endometrial carcinoma has been made has been reported in 34–40% of autopsy cases,[8,16] and 5–15% of hysterectomy and bilateral salpingo-oophorectomy specimens (see Chapter 12, Endometrial Carcinoma). Conversely, in approximately one-third of the cases in which a diagnosis of endometrioid carcinoma of the ovary has been made an endometrial carcinoma also has been found. When the uterine corpus and the ovary are both involved by carcinomas, the question arises whether both cancers are primary or one is metastatic from the other. A number of studies, many of them relatively recent, have addressed this issue.[26,38,63,107,125,135,158] If the endometrial carcinoma extends deeply into the myometrium with lymphatic or vascular invasion, if tumor is present in the lumen of the fallopian tube, or if tumor is on the ovarian surface or within its lymphatics or blood vessels, it is usually reasonable to conclude that the ovarian involvement is secondary. On the other hand, if lymphatic or hematogenous spread is absent, if the corpus carcinoma is small and limited to the endometrium or superficial myometrium, if it arises on a background of atypical hyperplasia, and if there is a centrally located ovarian tumor, sometimes arising on a background of endometriosis, the tumors probably are independent primaries. Criteria that are helpful in the determination of primary versus metastatic concomitant ovarian and endometrial carcinomas are presented in Table 22.1. Although the ovarian and uterine tumors are of the endometrioid type in most cases, occasionally they are similar but of other cell types, and rarely the histological type of tumor is different in the two organs.[38] When the tumors are of serous, clear cell, or small cell type, there is a greater likelihood that the ovarian tumors are metastatic.

In some cases of combined involvement it is impossible to establish the site of origin even after consideration of the features described above and listed in Table 22.1. In our experience and that of most series, most synchronous ovarian and corpus carcinomas are independent primary tumors; in one study, however, the ovarian tumors were interpreted as metastatic from the corpus in most of the cases[125] and other valid cases of metastasis are present in the literature.[103] An independent-primary explanation for most concomitant ovarian and corpus carcinomas is supported by the survival rates associated with this combination of tumors, which have generally been high. These results would be surprising if either the ovarian or corpus carcinoma was metastatic in most of the cases.

Rarely, ovarian spread from an adenoacarcinoma of the uterine corpus with squamous differentiation takes the form of deposits of keratin or degenerated mature squamous cells associated with a foreign-body giant cell response on the serosal surface of one or both ovaries.[24,71] If no viable-appearing tumor cells can be identified in these deposits on careful sampling, this finding does not appear to worsen the prognosis even when the granulomas are also found elsewhere on the peritoneum (see Chapter 17, Diseases of the Peritoneum).

Cervical Carcinoma

Ovarian spread of cervical carcinomas of all types generally has been considered rare. There has been considerable recent interest in this topic, however, stimulated in part by

Table 22.1. Criteria for interpretations of nature of concomitant uterine corpus and ovarian carcinomas

Corpus primary ovarian metastasis	Ovarian primary corpus metastasis	Ovarian primary corpus primary	Ovarian metastasis corpus metastasis	Uncertain primary
Direct extension to ovary from large corpus tumor	Direct extension to corpus from large ovarian primary	No direct extension of either tumor	Usually no direct extension of tumors	Massive involvement of both organs or conflicting findings listed in first four columns
Deep myometrial invasion from endometrium	Myometrial invasion from serosal surface	Myometrial invasion usually absent or superficial	Tumor characteristically in endometrial stroma. Myometrial invasion may be present	
Lymphatic or blood vessel invasion in corpus, ovary, or both	Lymphatic or blood vessel invasion in corpus, ovary, or both	No lymphatic or blood vessel invasion	Lymphatic or blood vessel invasion frequent in ovary and corpus	
Atypical hyperplasia of endometrium frequent	Atypical hyperplasia of endometrium usually absent	Atypical hyperplasia of endometrium frequent	Atypical hyperplasia of endometrium absent	
Tumor present in fallopian tube	Tumor present on peritoneal surfaces and sometimes in fallopian tube	Usually both tumors confined to primary sites or have spread minimally	Tumor usually evident outside female genital tract	
Tumor predominant on surface of ovary	Tumor predominant within ovary	Tumor predominant within ovary and endometrium	Ovarian tumor usually bilateral—ovarian surface involvement frequent	
Usually no endometriosis in ovary	Endometriosis sometimes present in ovary	Endometriosis sometimes present in ovary	Endometriosis absent	
Histological types uniform and consistent with corpus primary	Histological types uniform and consistent with ovarian primary	Histological types uniform or dissimilar	Type of tumor inconsistent with or unusual for either organ	

observations suggesting that it is more common in cases of adenocarcinoma than in cases of squamous cell carcinoma and raising the question of whether or not ovarian conservation is justified in patients with cervical adenocarcinoma. In addition, occasional patients with cervical carcinomas of diverse types have had clinically significant ovarian metastases.[143]

One of the most detailed studies of ovarian spread of cervical carcinoma is that of Tabata et al.[120] In their autopsy series ovarian metastases were detected in 104 of 597 (17%) cases of squamous cell carcinoma and in 22 of 77 (28.6%) cases of adenocarcinoma. The frequency of ovarian metastases of squamous cell carcinoma at autopsy in their series is much higher than the 3% frequency in the prior literature. Ovarian metastases discovered during life are much rarer. In their series of 318 patients with Stage IA cervical carcinoma treated by hysterectomy with ovarian preservation, Tabata et al.[120] found no examples of subsequent ovarian metastasis during follow-up periods that were over 5 years in more than half the cases. In cases of Stage IB, II, and III carcinoma in their series there were no ovarian metastases in 278 cases of squamous cell carcinoma in contrast to 6 ovarian metastases out of 48 (12.5%) cases of adenocarcinoma. In another series there were

three cases of microscopic ovarian metastasis in 185 cases of Stage IIB cervical carcinoma[122]; in the same series there were no metastases in 335 cases of Stage IB disease, 71 cases of Stage IIA disease, and 6 cases of Stage IIIB disease[122]; one of the ovarian metastases was from a squamous cell carcinoma (0.2% of all squamous cell carcinomas) whereas two were adenocarcinomas (5.5% of these tumors). The cervical carcinomas in these three cases had invaded the uterine corpus and vascular spaces. Tabata et al.[120] also found that ovarian metastasis was much more common when a cervical carcinoma had invaded the uterine corpus.

There are only seven well-documented examples of clinically significant ovarian metastases from squamous cell carcinomas.[143] The youngest patient was 30 years old, and the oldest 59 years. The ovarian and cervical tumors were discovered at essentially the same time in three of the patients. In three others the ovarian metastases occurred 18 months to 10 years after the cervical primary tumor had been treated. In the seventh case the cervical tumor was not discovered until autopsy 7 months after the patient had been treated for a squamous cell carcinoma involving the left ovary. The cervical tumor in that case was invasive only to 3.8 mm, whereas in the other cases there appears to have been deep infiltration of the cervical wall with frequent extrauterine extension of the neoplasm.[143] The ovarian tumors, two of which were bilateral, ranged from 5 to 17 cm in greatest dimension. Three of the nine tumors in these patients were solid, three solid and cystic, and three cystic. Microscopic examination has shown the typical features of squamous cell carcinoma except that many of the tumors had striking cystification within the squamous nests. In one additional unusual case a cervical squamous cell carcinoma that was invasive to only 1.2 mm extended in an in situ manner to involve the endometrium and involved the surface and inclusion glands and cysts within one ovary, tumor cells presumably having spread there via the tubal lumen.[143] The differential diagnosis in these cases with squamous cell carcinoma primary in the ovary usually has been aided by the knowledge of the presence of a cervical tumor but in the one case in which the cervical tumor was not detected until autopsy and some of the others, there were major problems in diagnosis.[143] Before the diagnosis of primary squamous cell carcinoma of the ovary is made, the possibility of spread of a cervical tumor, even one that is occult, should be considered. As most squamous cell carcinomas of the ovary arise on the background of a preexistent neoplasm such as a dermoid cyst, thorough sampling to identify such a component is crucial in determining the primary nature of the neoplasm. Although the evidence strongly points to the ovarian tumors being metastatic when both organs have been involved by squamous cell carcinoma, the rare association of squamous cell carcinoma of the ovary with squamous cell carcinoma in situ of the cervix leaves open the possibility of independent primary neoplasms in some cases.

In a series from Armed Forces Institute of Pathology 10% of mucinous adenocarcinomas of the cervix were reported to metastasize to the ovary[68] and occasional other examples have been reported.[152] When a cervical mucinous adenocarcinoma and an ovarian mucinous adenocarcinoma co-exist, however, difficulties may be encountered in deciding whether they are independent primary tumors[78] or metastatic from one organ to the other. Two adenosquamous carcinomas and two glassy cell carcinomas with ovarian metastases have been reported.[143] Both metastatic adenosquamous carcinomas were discovered at the same time as the cervical primary tumors. The ovarian tumors were bilateral in both cases and the cervical tumors were deeply invasive with extracervical extension, findings facilitating the diagnosis in these cases. In one of the cases of glassy cell carcinoma the ovarian involvement was a microscopic finding; in the other the ovarian involvement was grossly evident but the ovary was not enlarged.

Four cases have been reported in detail in which cervical small cell carcinomas or mixed tumors with a component of adenocarcinoma and small cell carcinoma or poorly differentiated carcinoid have been associated with ovarian metastases. In each of these four cases the ovarian spread

was manifest clinically[113] (Fig. 22.7). In one of them the patient had evidence of the carcinoid syndrome. The four patients were from 23 to 34 years of age. The cervical tumors and ovarian tumors were synchronous findings in two of them. In the other two the ovarian tumors were discovered 10 months and 3 years after the cervical tumors.

In one final case a cervical transitional cell carcinoma metastasized to the ovary and was detected before the cervical tumor, which was not discovered until pathological examination.[143] The ovarian metastatic tumor in this case was a large cystic mass that was indistinguishable microscopically from a primary transitional cell carcinoma of the ovary but was associated with prominent vascular space invasion, suggesting its metastatic nature.

Uterine Sarcomas

In our experience and that in the literature, endometrial stromal sarcomas metastasize to the ovary more frequently than leiomyosarcomas.[155] In our series of 11 uterine sarcomas that metastasized to the ovary (none of them autopsy findings), 8 were endometrial stromal sarcomas and 3 leiomyosarcomas.[155] The patients with endometrial stromal sarcomas ranged from 33 to 79 (average 50) years of age; five of them were less than 50 years old. The ovarian metastases accounted for the clinical presentation in three of the patients. In two of these patients the primary uterine tumors were not discovered until 7 months and 10 months after bilateral ovarian tumors had been resected. In four of the other cases the ovarian and uterine tumors were found synchronously and in the remaining two the ovarian metastases occurred 4 to 9 years after the uterine neoplasms had been discovered. The ovarian tumors were bilateral in six of the cases and ranged up to 17 cm in greatest dimension. These tumors usually are solid (Fig. 22.8) or solid and cystic, but rarely are they cystic.

The major problem with the interpretation of these tumors on microscopic examination is that when growing in the ovary, the tongue-like pattern of infiltration characteristic of this neoplasm often is inconspicuous. Other problems result from the presence in some of the tumors of large fibromatous areas that may contain hyaline plaques, a finding not typical of the uterine primary tumor. Yu et al.[157] described the case of a 24-year-old woman with an ovarian metastatic endometrial stroma sarcoma that was misinterpreted initially as a thecoma. In other cases the ovarian tumors have a diffuse pattern (Fig. 22.9) and in areas their characteristic content of small arteries resembling the spiral arteries of the endometrium is inconspicuous, resulting in a resemblance to a diffuse granulosa cell tumor. Confusion with sex cord–stromal tumors may be heightened by the occasional presence of areas of sex cord–like differentiation in metastatic endometrial stromal sarcomas. However, high-power examination does not show the typical nuclear features of granulosa cell tumors

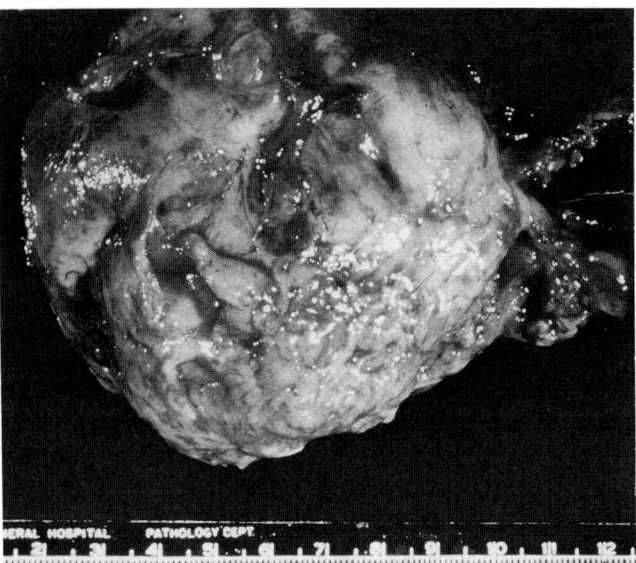

FIG. 22.8. Metastatic endometrial stromal sarcoma from the uterus. Several worm-like foci of tumor are visible.

and careful examination usually shows, at least focally, the typical vascular pattern of endometrial stromal tumors (Fig. 22.9). Reticulum stains often are helpful in the differential diagnosis showing individual cell investment by fibrils in the endometrial stromal sarcoma and only small amounts, mainly perivascular, in the granulosa cell tumor. Bilaterality also is far more common in the former than the latter as is the presence of extraovarian tumor, examination of which often shows the distinctive growth pattern of the endometrial stromal sarcoma.

Metastatic endometrial stromal sarcomas in the ovary must be distinguished from primary endometrioid stromal sarcomas.[148] An association of the tumor with endometriosis is evidence of an ovarian origin; bilaterality favors me-

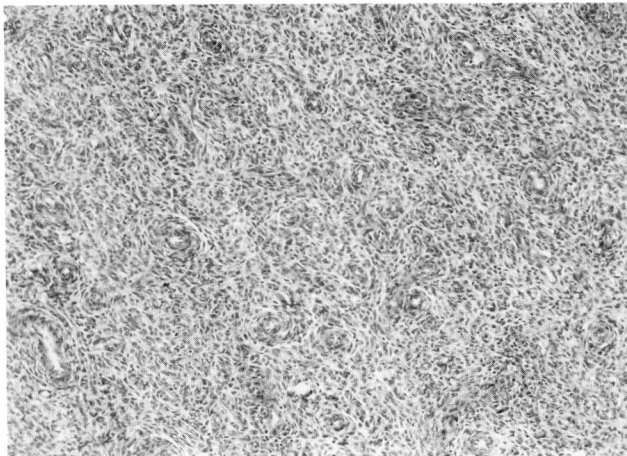

FIG. 22.9. Metastatic endometrial stromal sarcoma from the uterus. The tumor has a diffuse pattern. Note the presence of many characteristic small arterioles.

tastasis. When both organs are involved it is possible that the tumors may be independent primary tumors. Six of 38 uterine and ovarian cancers that were thought to be independent primary tumors in the series of Woodruff and Julian[135] were of endometrial stromal type.

Leiomyosarcomas of the uterus with ovarian metastases probably are more common than the rare reports in the literature suggest, particularly in patients with widespread disease. The three leiomyosarcomas with ovarian metastases in our series of sarcomas metastatic to the ovary occurred in patients 35, 44, and 49 years of age.[155] In the first patient a large ovarian metastatic tumor became symptomatic 14 months after hysterectomy. In the second patient the ovarian metastatic tumor was in the setting of widespread disease. In the third case the ovarian involvement was only microscopic. In two reports seven of nine metastatic "sarcomas" to the ovary were malignant mixed müllerian tumors.[25,106] Ovarian involvement in cases of müllerian adenosarcoma of the uterus is uncommon and in some cases may be an independent primary.

Trophoblastic Tumors

The frequency of spread of choriocarcinoma of the uterus to the ovary has varied from one series to another. In an autopsy study of 44 patients Ober et al.[90] found no examples of ovarian metastasis; however, in other series the frequency has ranged from 6% to 22%.[2,96,132] Although a choriocarcinoma that develops in a prepubertal girl obviously is of germ cell origin, the occurrence of a similar tumor in a woman of child-bearing age that is not clearly metastatic from a uterine or tubal choriocarcinoma requires thorough sampling in an attempt to demonstrate the presence of teratomatous elements, thereby establishing the germ cell origin of the tumor. If such elements are not found it may be difficult or impossible to differentiate between a primary choriocarcinoma of the ovary of either gestational or germ cell origin and a metastatic tumor from a choriocarcinoma of the uterus that has regressed. Invasive hydatidiform mole also has been documented to spread to the ovary[132] and at least two placental site trophoblastic tumors have spread through the uterine wall to involve an ovary.[1]

Vulvar and Vaginal Tumors

Only rare vulvar and vaginal carcinomas with ovarian spread have been reported.[79] Occasional vaginal clear cell adenocarcinomas have metastasized to the ovary, in most cases associated with extensive pelvic spread.

Breast Carcinoma

The frequency of ovarian involvement at autopsy in cases of breast cancer has ranged from 6% to 40%[51,79,129]; the average figure from the literature is about 10%. In one study metastatic breast carcinoma accounted for 29% of all ovarian metastases at autopsy.[79] Metastases from the breast are bilateral at autopsy in approximately 80% of the cases and in approximately two-thirds of all cases, autopsy and surgical combined.[45]

Most surgical pathological experience with ovarian metastases of mammary carcinoma has resulted from examination of ovaries removed to decrease the estrogen level in patients with known spread of the tumor.[76,101] In such cases, ovarian involvement has been reported in from 25% to almost 50% of the cases,[70,80,99,124] with bilateral involvement in approximately 60%.[99] About two-thirds of the affected ovaries were considered normal on gross examination in one series.[80] In contrast, only 2–11% of ovaries obtained by prophylactic oophorectomy for breast cancer (oophorectomy done in the absence of clinical evidence of distant spread) contain metastases.[12,65]

It is unusual for metastatic carcinoma of the breast to produce signs or symptoms of an ovarian tumor and only rarely is the ovarian metastasis evident before the primary tumor is detected.[70,127,140] In a series of 79 ovarian metastases presenting as pelvic or abdominal masses, Johansson[65] found 11 (14%) to be of mammary origin. The ovarian involvement was discovered before diagnosis of the primary tumor in only 1 case; in the remaining 10 cases in that series the ovarian tumors became evident clinically at subsequent intervals ranging from less than 1 year to 16 years.[65] Death occurred within 1 year of the detection of ovarian involvement in all but 1 of the 11 patients. In contrast, Osborne and Pitts[95] recorded a mean survival of more than 20 months after the diagnosis of metastasis in therapeutic oophorectomy specimens. In one large series breast metastases accounted for almost 40% of all metastases, being slightly more common than gastrointestinal tract metastases.[45] However, 22 of the 59 cases of breast metastasis were autopsy findings and 28 were incidental findings in therapeutic oophorectomy specimens. In four of the remaining nine cases the ovarian metastases were incidental findings during an operation for another indication; in the remaining five patients, however, the ovarian metastases caused a mass of sufficient size to be the clinical indication for operation. The ovarian metastatic tumor was detected before the breast cancer in only one case. This patient presented with hepatic and ovarian tumors and did not have her primary breast cancer identified until 15 months later. The median interval between the diagnosis of breast cancer and the ovarian metastasis was 11.5 months and was related to the stage of the breast cancer. The median survival after the diagnosis of ovarian metastasis was 16 months. One patient with metastatic breast carcinoma in the ovaries presented 10 years after initial treatment of the breast cancer, as a result of virilization caused by stromal luteinization associated with the ovarian metastasis.[19] Although ovarian metastases of breast cancer usually are accompanied by other foci of abdominal spread, isolated ovarian metastases occasionally are en-

countered. In one series the metastasis was limited to the ovary in 8 of 59 cases.[45] Lobular carcinomas, including those of signet-ring cell type, spread to the ovary more frequently than those of ductal type; in an autopsy study 36% of the former metastasized to the ovaries in contrast to only 2.6% of the latter.[51]

GROSS FINDINGS

On gross examination, the visibly involved ovaries often have irregular, nodular surfaces and typically contain firm or gritty, white nodules of various sizes (Fig. 22.1). When the organ is replaced by tumor, it is transformed into a smooth surfaced or bosselated mass; exceptionally, it contains cysts and very rarely it is entirely cystic. When all cases are considered tumors larger than 5 cm are uncommon, accounting for only 15% of the cases in one large study.[45]

MICROSCOPIC FINDINGS

Microscopic examination reveals the same variety of patterns and cell types that are observed in primary breast carcinomas (Figs. 22.10–22.12). In early examples, small cords and clusters of cells may be found in the ovarian cortex. In premenopausal women, small deposits often are

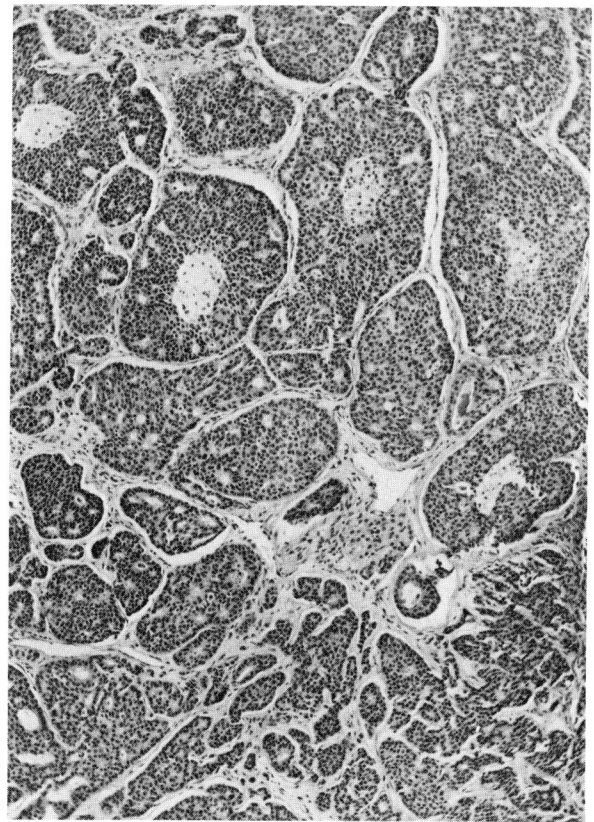

FIG. 22.10. Metastatic ductal carcinoma from the breast. A cribriform pattern is present.

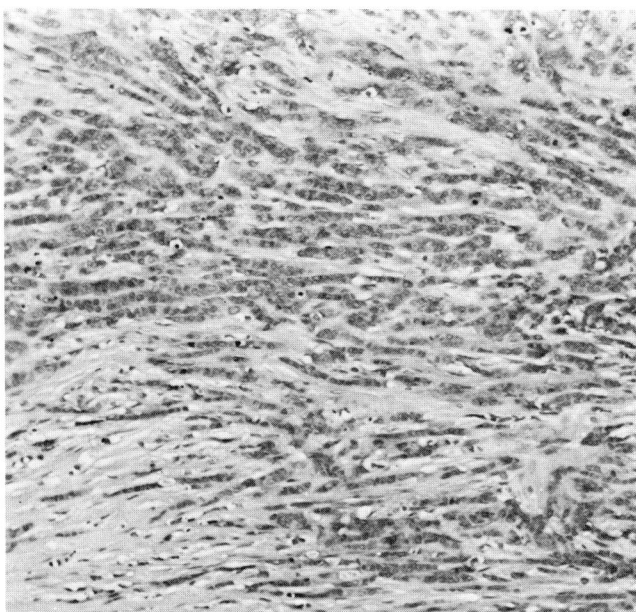

FIG. 22.11. Metastatic lobular carcinoma from the breast.
An Indian-file pattern is present.

situated in the highly vascular theca interna of a graafian follicle or in the granulosa or theca layer of a corpus luteum. In larger metastatic foci a pattern of tubular glands and nests similar to that of ductal carcinoma is common (Fig. 22.10), as is an Indian-file pattern such as that of lobular carcinoma (Fig. 22.11): such patterns were seen in 42% and 32% of the cases, respectively, in one series.[45] A pure cribriform pattern is infrequent but focal cribriform areas are relatively common. Finally, in approximately 10% of the cases, there is a diffuse pattern and occasionally the tumor cells grow as single cells or in clusters.[45] Admixtures of these various patterns may be seen. Signet cells usually

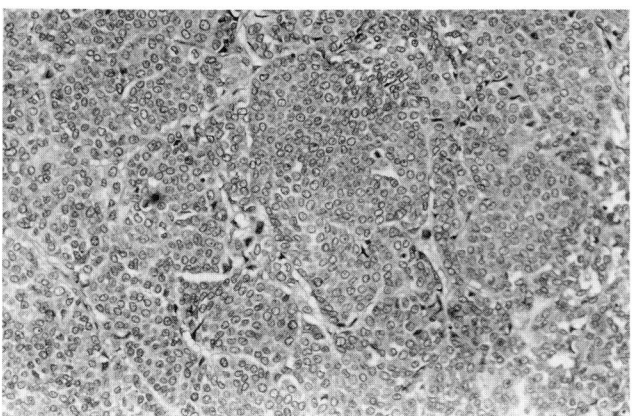

FIG. 22.12. Metastatic lobular carcinoma from the breast.
An insular growth of small cells with pale nuclei superficially resembles an insular granulosa cell tumor.

are not a conspicuous feature of metastatic breast carcinoma unless the primary tumor is of the relatively uncommon signet-ring type but, rarely, the features of a metastatic breast cancer are those of a typical Krukenberg tumor,[80] as described below; 1.8% of Krukenberg tumors in one series were of breast origin.[138] The stroma of the tumor varies from sparse to abundant; it rarely shows luteinization, no examples in one series of 59 cases,[45] in contrast to the stroma of metastatic carcinomas of intestinal origin. Rare tumors with a Krukenberg pattern have been associated with luteinization and evidence of virilization. Lymphatic invasion was seen in 15% of the cases in one series.[45]

DIFFERENTIAL DIAGNOSIS

The differential diagnosis of metastatic breast carcinoma may be difficult, particularly if the primary tumor is remote, or not apparent, or if its existence is not known by the pathologist. Rare, predominantly glandular, tumors may resemble surface epithelial tumors, particularly those of endometrioid type, and the insular pattern may mimic a carcinoid tumor (Fig. 22.10). Exceptionally, a tumor with a diffuse pattern or one with an Indian-file arrangement of the cells simulates a lymphoma or granulocytic sarcoma (chloroma).[40] Metastatic breast carcinomas also have been misinterpreted as granulosa cell tumors (Fig. 22.12). The growth patterns and characteristics of the neoplastic cells and the clinical features, however, almost always permit their distinction from these and other tumors, but this is occasionally difficult on the evaluation of routinely stained sections alone. It should be remembered that patients with breast cancer have an increased frequency of ovarian carcinoma, and rarely ovarian carcinoma metastasizes to the breast. A recent study has shown that staining of an ovarian neoplasm immunohistochemically for gross cystic disease fluid protein-15 (GCDFP-15) may be helpful in distinguishing a metastasis from the breast (Fig. 22.13) from a primary ovarian carcinoma.[87] In that study, 11 of 14 cases (71%) of ovarian metastatic tumors from the breast exhibited strong cytoplasmic staining, usually in a paranuclear pattern; in contrast, seven ovarian metastases of other tumors and 32 primary ovarian carcinomas failed to stain. Finally, in cases of ovarian involvement by the intraabdominal desmoplastic small round cell tumor,[141] the diagnosis of metastatic breast cancer may be suggested in areas. However, these patients usually are in their teens, when breast cancer is rare, and other more characteristic foci of the tumor and the typical immunohistochemical profile of the former tumor facilitate the interpretation. We have seen one case in which this tumor involved the breast, confusing the picture, but the breast involvement suggested metastasis and the tumor exhibited the characteristic immunohistochemical staining of the desmoplastic small round cell tumor.

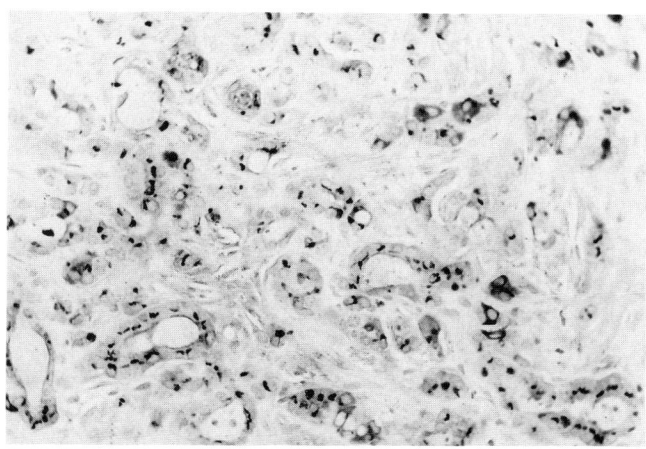

FIG. 22.13. **Metastatic ductal carcinoma from the breast.** A section of the tumor has been stained by the immunohistochemical technique for gross cystic disease fluid protein-15 and is strongly positive.

Carcinoma of the Stomach, Including Krukenberg Tumor

The great majority of metastatic gastric carcinomas to the ovary are Krukenberg tumors,[34,49,59,137] which are defined as tumors characterized by the presence of mucin-filled signet-ring cells, typically lying within a cellular stroma derived from the ovarian stroma. The source of Krukenberg tumors in from 70% to 100% of the reported cases is a gastric carcinoma, usually arising in the pylorus. Carcinomas of the large intestine, appendix, and breast are the next most common primary sites; the gallbladder, biliary tract, pancreas, cervix, and urinary bladder are rare sources of these tumors. Saphir[109] demonstrated in an autopsy study that signet-ring cell carcinomas of various organs are associated more often with ovarian metastasis than carcinomas of other histologic types by a ratio of about 4:1. More recent studies have supported his observation; gastric signet-ring cell carcinomas metastasize to the ovary in 41% of the cases whereas intestinal-type carcinomas of the stomach do so in only 17%[35]; signet-ring cell carcinoma of the colon also metastasizes to the ovaries more frequently than does the usual colonic adenocarcinoma.[4]

The frequency of the Krukenberg tumor varies with that of gastric carcinoma in the population analyzed. At the Radiumhemmett, 39% of ovarian metastases presenting as ovarian tumors were of gastric origin, although not specified to be of the Krukenberg type.[65] In a similar series, Krukenberg tumors of gastric origin accounted for approximately 30% of clinically apparent ovarian metastases.[110] In countries such as Japan, with a high prevalence of gastric carcinoma and a low prevalence of primary ovarian carcinoma, the Krukenberg tumor accounts for a large proportion of all ovarian cancers.[138] The average age of

patients with Krukenberg tumors is about 45 years. From one-quarter to almost one-half the patients have been under 40 years, and only slightly more than 10% of them have been over 60 years of age. This age distribution is related in part to the disproportionate frequency of gastric signet-ring cell carcinomas in young women as well as the greater vascularity of the ovary in young women. In one study 10% of women 35 years or younger with this tumor had ovarian metastases at presentation.[123]

Almost 90% of patients with Krukenberg tumors have symptoms related to ovarian involvement, the most common of which are abdominal pain and swelling; occasionally, there is abnormal uterine bleeding and rarely overt signs of excess hormone production such as virilization (see Chapter 19, Sex Cord–Stromal, Steroid Cell, and Other Ovarian Tumors with Endocrine, Paraendocrine, and Paraneoplastic Manifestations). The remainder of the patients have gastrointestinal or miscellaneous symptoms, or are asymptomatic. A history of prior carcinoma of the stomach or, rarely, another organ can be obtained in 20–30% of the cases.[49,65] The interval between the diagnosis of a gastric carcinoma and the subsequent discovery of ovarian involvement usually is six months or less,[65] but periods as long as 12 years have been reported.[49] In most cases, the diagnosis of the gastric carcinoma is made preoperatively, during the operation for the ovarian metastasis, or within a few months thereafter. Often, the primary tumor is too small to be detected at operation,[59] and radiographic examination of the upper gastrointestinal tract also may fail to reveal evidence of a tumor even after the diagnosis of Krukenberg tumor has been established. Rarely, the gastric carcinoma may not be detected until 5 or more years after discovery of the ovarian metastatic tumor.

Almost all the patients die within a year of the diagnosis of ovarian metastasis, with an average duration of 7 months from diagnosis to death,[49] but a rare patient has survived, apparently free of tumor, for as long as 6 years after gastrectomy and bilateral oophorectomy.[59] Such a result, even though exceptional, justifies removal of both the stomach and the ovarian metastases for possible cure in cases in which the tumor appears limited to those organs. It also is prudent for the surgeon to remove the ovaries routinely in menopausal and postmenopausal women who have a gastric resection for carcinoma so as to prevent the later complication of ovarian metastasis and avoid another operation.

Almost all tumors with microscopic features of the Krukenberg tumor are metastatic, but very rare examples may be primary. Joshi[67] accepted as primary 18 reported cases, including 11 in which autopsy examination revealed no evidence of an extraovarian source, and 7 in which the patient survived for 5 to 13 years after the removal of the ovarian tumor. These tumors occurred in patients ranging in age from 16 to 61 years, with an average of 38 years. Although a primary Krukenberg tumor probably exists, one should exercise considerable caution before making such a diagnosis or accepting reported cases as valid. Primary carcinomas, particularly those arising in the breast and stomach, may be very small, requiring exhaustive sectioning to detect them, despite the presence of metastases in some cases. It is possible that tiny primary tumors were missed in these or other organs in the reported autopsied cases of "primary" Krukenberg tumors. Ulbright and Roth[126] cited a case observed by Kraus in which a primary tumor in the stomach was detected only after microscopic sections prepared from 200 blocks had been examined. Also, it is well known that mammary and gastric carcinomas may remain silent for many years. We have seen one case of a Krukenberg tumor in which a primary gastric carcinoma did not become apparent until 5½ years after the ovarian tumor had been removed. Thus, clinical dormancy of the primary tumor probably accounts for some of the cases of Krukenberg tumor with long survival. As poorly differentiated primary mucinous carcinoids of the ovary may have extensive foci of signet-ring cell proliferation, it is possible that some of the "primary Krukenberg" tumors in the literature may be in that category.

Gross Findings

Krukenberg tumors typically form rounded or reniform, firm, white masses that may be bosselated and may attain a large size. The sectioned surfaces usually are yellow or white (Fig. 22.14) but areas of purple, red, or brown discoloration and extensive hemorrhage also are encountered (Fig. 22.15). The consistency is characteristically firm but fleshy, gelatinous, or spongy areas are common. Occasionally, the gross presentation is atypical with large, thin-walled cysts containing mucinous or watery fluid, separated by relatively small amounts of solid tissue. Both ovaries are involved in 80% or more of the cases. The

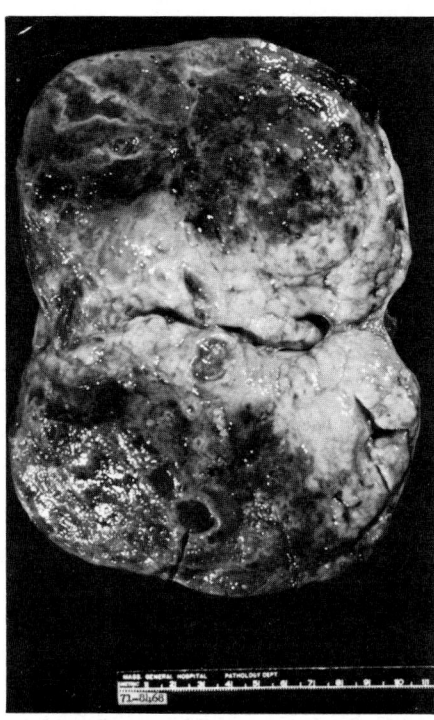

FIG. 22.15. **Krukenberg tumor.** There is extensive hemorrhagic necrosis.

occasional metastatic gastric carcinoma that is not a Krukenberg tumor may be predominantly solid or predominantly cystic (Fig. 22.16).

Microscopic Findings

Microscopic examination of a Krukenberg tumor reveals mucin-laden, signet-ring cells strewn individually and in small clusters within a cellular ovarian stroma (Figs. 22.17,

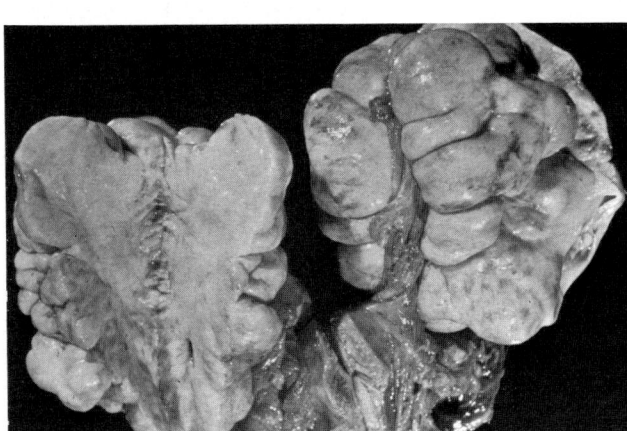

FIG. 22.14. **Krukenberg tumor.** Bilateral bosselated masses are composed of solid white tissue.

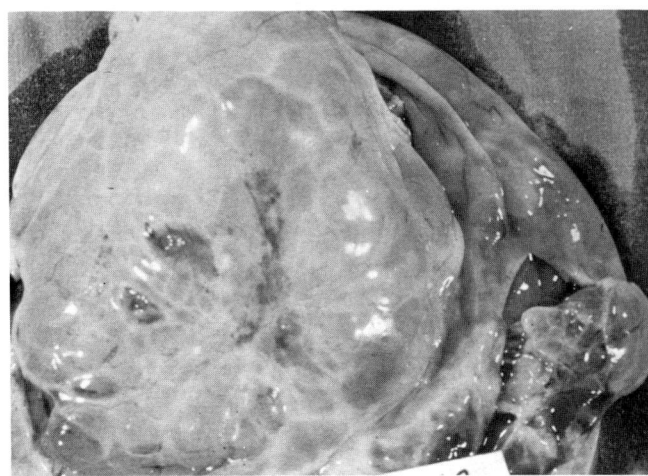

FIG. 22.16. **Metastatic carcinoma from the stomach.** Multiloculated cystic neoplasm simulating a mucinous cystadenoma.

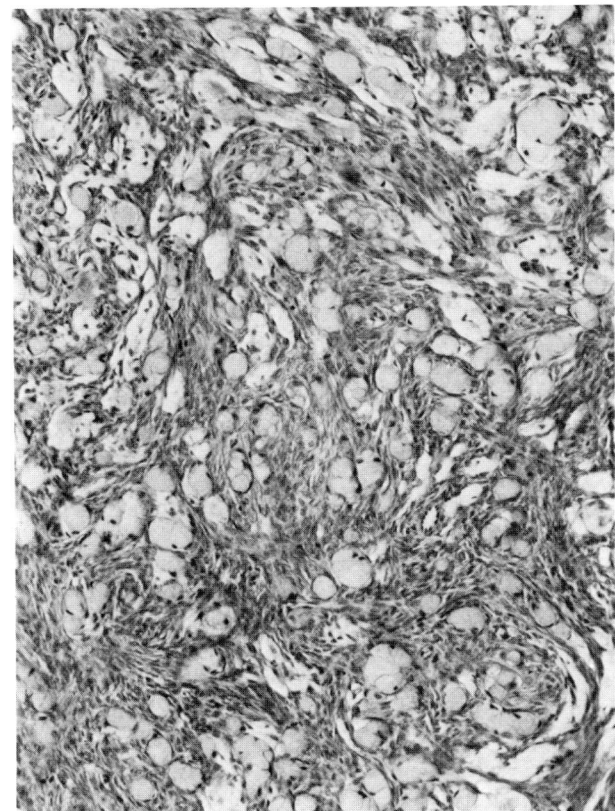

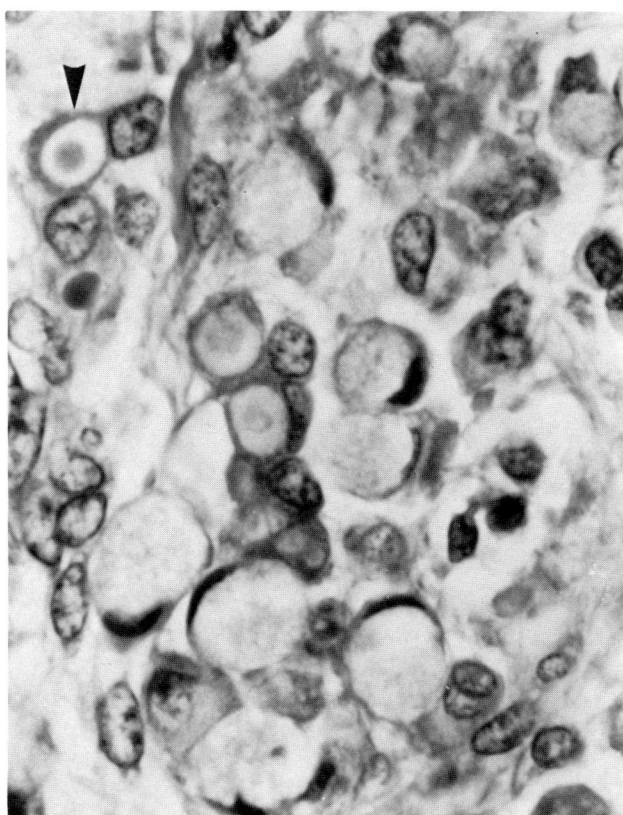

FIG. 22.17. **Krukenberg tumor.** Numerous signet-ring cells are present within a cellular stroma.

FIG. 22.18. **Krukenberg tumor.** Signet-ring cells with eccentric nuclei and abundant pale cytoplasm. In one cell a droplet of mucin with a targetoid appearance is present (*arrow*). (Reprinted by permission of Scully RE (1979) Tumors of the ovary and maldeveloped gonads. In: Atlas of Tumor Pathology, second series, fascicle 16, Washington D.C., Armed Forces Institute of Pathology.)

22.18); occasionally the stroma has a storiform pattern. Frequent variations from the classical appearance include small glands, a prominent tubular architecture[15] (Fig. 22.19), mucin-poor tumor cells in trabeculae, and large masses, abundant collagen formation, marked stromal edema (Fig.22.20), and cell-free pools of mucin in the stroma. Occasionally, small or large cysts lined by minimally atypical-appearing mucinous epithelium forms a conspicuous component of the tumor, with more characteristic areas lying between the cysts. The cytoplasm of the signet-ring cells occasionally is granular and eosinophilic rather than pale and vacuolated; the cytoplasm sometimes has a bull's-eye appearance, containing a large vacuole with a central eosinophilic body (Fig. 22.18). As with metastases in general, blood vessel and lymphatic invasion is common. Lutein cells occasionally are present in the stroma, particularly if the patient is pregnant (see Chapter 19).

Although most metastatic gastric carcinomas to the ovary have the characteristics of a Krukenberg tumor, occasional examples do not and may be composed of glands of intestinal type in varying degrees of differentiation (Fig. 22.21) that occasionally are cystically dilated (Fig. 22.22), as well as sheets and irregular aggregates of poorly differentiated carcinoma cells.

DIFFERENTIAL DIAGNOSIS

The Krukenberg tumor may resemble a fibroma or any other type of solid ovarian tumor on gross examination. Its appearance also occasionally may be deceptive on frozen section or low-power examination[87] (Fig. 22.23) but should be readily diagnosable on high-power microscopic examination, especially with the aid of mucin stains. A frequent misdiagnosis is a Sertoli–Leydig cell tumor, particularly when a prominent tubular component and luteinization of the stroma are encountered in a Krukenberg tumor[15]; signet-ring cells, however, are not a feature of Sertoli–Leydig cell tumors except for occasional tumors of heterologous type (see Chapter 19). The sclerosing stromal tumor may contain cells resembling signet cells as well as a proliferating fibroblastic component, but such cells contain lipid rather than mucin. The rare signet-ring stromal tumor also may enter the differential diagnosis (see Chapter 19), but the signet-ring cells in that tumor also fail to react with mucin stains. In clear cell carcinomas, the clear cells contain glycogen; mucin, when present, is typically luminal

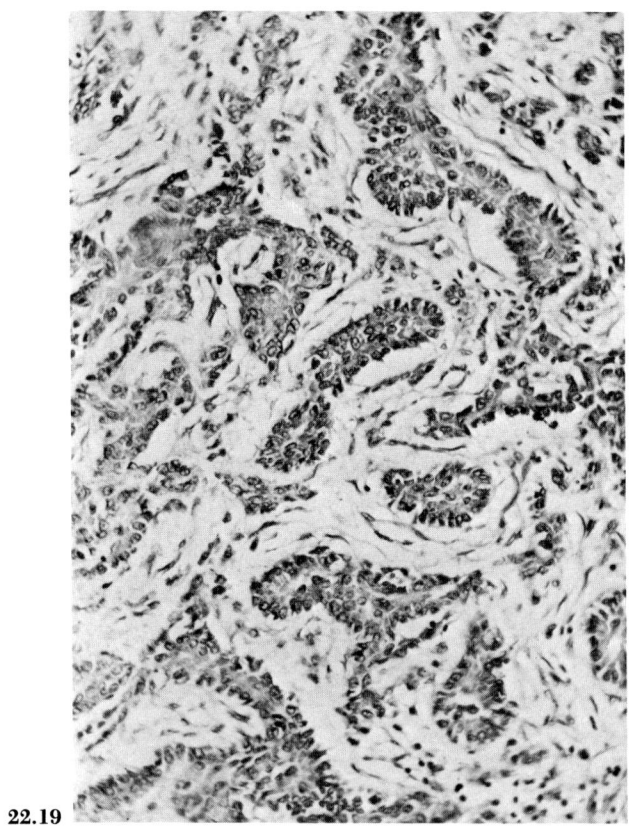

22.19

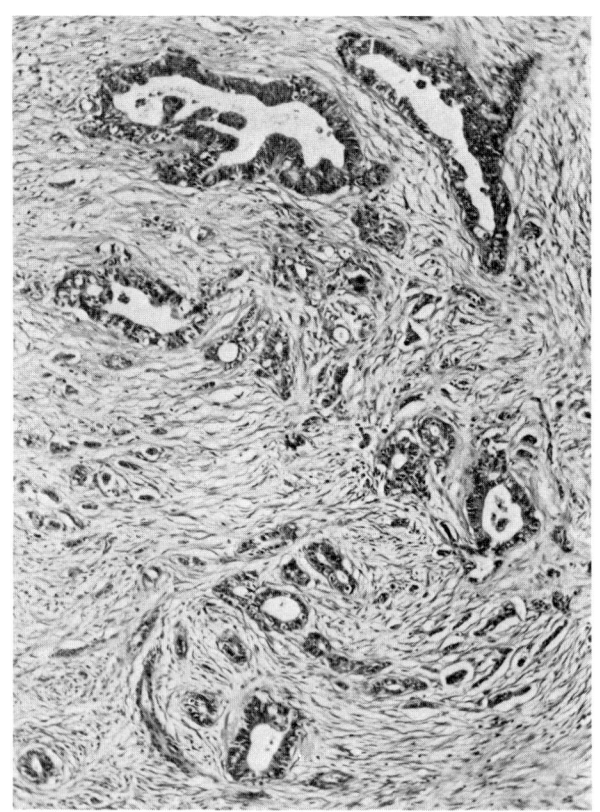

22.21

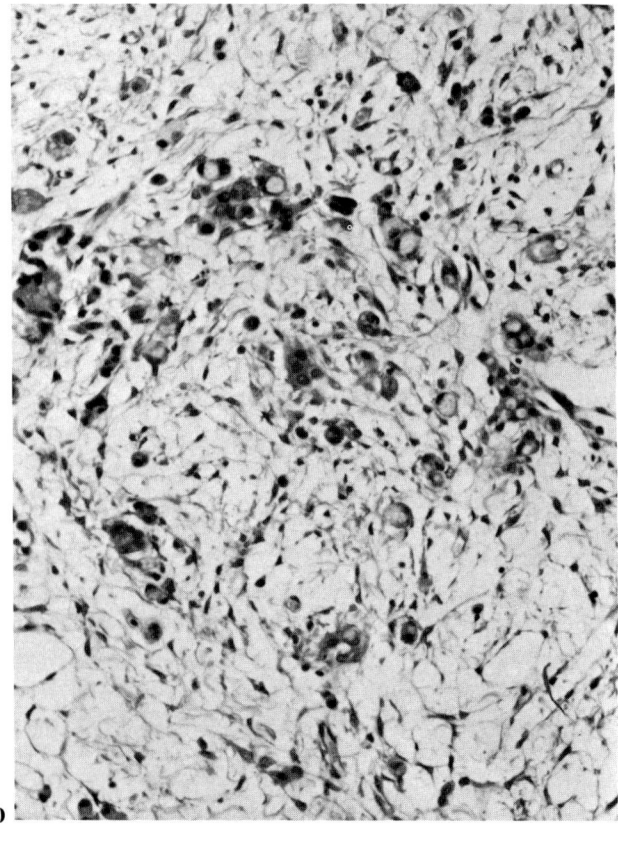

22.20

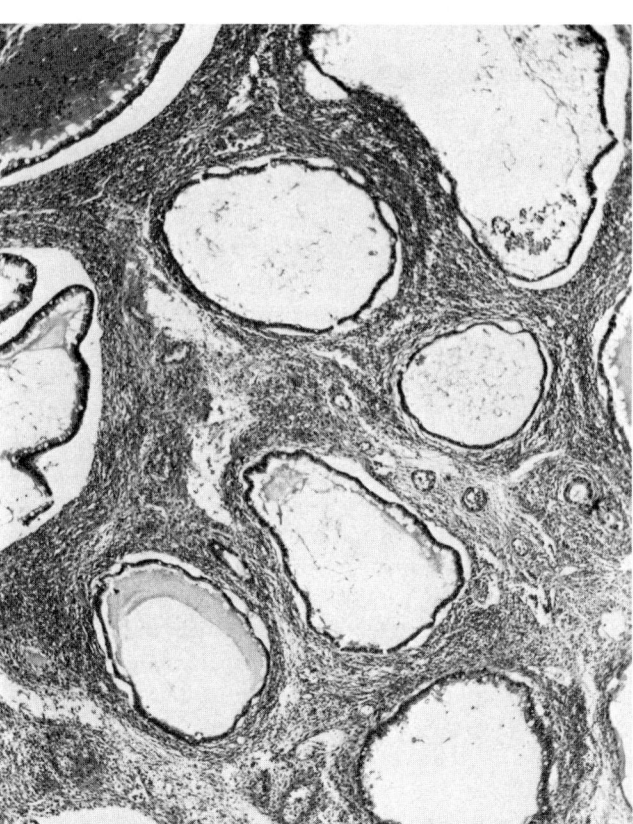

22.22

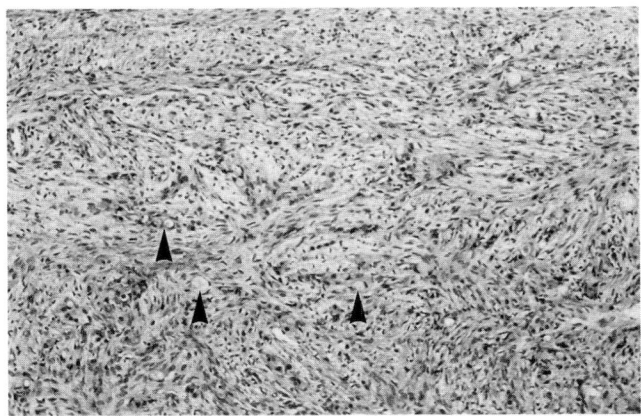

FIG. 22.23. Krukenberg tumor. At this magnification the appearance is similar to that of an ovarian fibroma, but occasional signet-ring cells are evident on careful inspection. (Reproduced by permission of ref. 151.)

and extracellular. In rare cases portions of the tumor contain aggregates of signet-ring cells but the presence of other characteristic features of this tumor permit its identification. Mucinous carcinoid tumors that contain large numbers of signet-ring cells are distinguished from Krukenberg tumors by their additional component of carcinoid, the presence of which can be confirmed by argyrophil staining. These tumors are discussed further in the section on metastatic carcinoid tumor. Finally, the rare nonneoplastic lesion, mucinocarminophilic histiocytosis,[74] which is caused by injection of substances containing polyvinylpyrrolidine, is characterized by signet ring–like cells and may involve numerous tissues and organs including the ovaries. Although these cells are stained by mucicarmine, they are periodic acid-Schiff (PAS)-negative.

Intestinal Carcinoma

Most metastatic ovarian tumors of intestinal origin are from the large intestine, with occasional examples of small intestinal derivation.[65] Ovarian metastases from intestinal carcinomas have been reported to be less common than

◁ ─────────────────────────

FIG. 22.19. Tubular Krukenberg tumor. The tubules simulate those of a Sertoli–Leydig cell tumor. Signet-ring cells are not evident in this illustration.
FIG. 22.20. Krukenberg tumor. Signet-ring cells are dispersed in an edematous stroma.
FIG. 22.21. Metastatic carcinoma from the stomach. Glands of varying sizes and shapes and small clusters of tumor cells lie in a fibrous stroma.
FIG. 22.22. Metastatic carcinoma from the stomach. Cystic glands are separated by stroma lacking tumor cells (×50). Same case as Figure 22.21.

those from gastric carcinomas at autopsy, 14% versus 38%, respectively,[109] but when malignant ovarian tumors encountered at the time of operation are evaluated metastases from intestinal carcinomas are almost five times as frequent as those from gastric carcinomas.[65,110,131,134] Lash and Hart[75] have estimated that up to 45% of large intestinal metastases to the ovary are thought clinically to be primary ovarian tumors and many are misinterpreted as such on pathological examination, even when there is a known intestinal cancer.

Approximately 4% of women with intestinal cancer have ovarian metastases at some time during the course of their disease,[10,17,29,47,50,91,116] but in one study this figure was as high as 10% when the ovaries were cut into 2-mm slices.[47] Four of the six metastatic ovarian tumors in that series of 58 cases were not recognized on gross examination. Metastases from the large intestine to the ovary occur relatively more frequently in women under 40 years of age (in 18–27% of the patients in this age group).[18,92,98] The mean age of the patients with carcinoma of the large intestine at the Memorial Sloan–Kettering Cancer Center in whom ovarian metastases developed was 51 years in contrast to 62 years for all the patients with large intestinal carcinoma.[88] The mean age in another large recent series was 57 years, with a range of 42 to 76 years.[75] In that series 32% of the intestinal tumors were Duke's Stage B and 68% Stage C.

From a clinical viewpoint patients with this type of metastatic carcinoma fall into three categories: (1) patients who present with an intestinal carcinoma (50–75% of the cases),[55,65,88,91] which antedates diagnosis of the ovarian tumor by up to 3 years in 90% of the cases, (2) patients in whom ovarian involvement is found unexpectedly during an operation for resection of an intestinal carcinoma, and (3) patients whose initial manifestations are those of an ovarian tumor (3–20% of the cases).[50,56,73] Ovarian metastases have been found in up to 8% of patients who have bilateral prophylactic oophorectomy because of intestinal carcinoma.[81,100,115] It has been estimated that routine preoperative barium x-ray examination of the large intestine in women suspected of having an ovarian tumor would be positive for carcinoma in approximately 1 to 2 of 1000 cases. In one study 77% of the intestinal primary tumors were in the rectum or sigmoid colon, 5% in the descending colon, 9% in the ascending colon, and 9% in the cecum.[75] Occasional patients with an intestinal metastasis have endocrine symptoms because of the presence of luteinized stromal cells in the ovarian tumor.[20,21] The symptoms usually are related to elevated estrogens or androgens but an elevated serum progesterone level also has been documented.[66]

Almost all patients with intestinal carcinoma metastatic to the ovary die within 3 years of detection of the ovarian involvement[11,55,65] and more than half of them within 1 year.[65] The mean survival in one series was 16 months.[88] Webb et al.[131] reported a 5-year survival of 5% after treatment of ovarian metastases from gastrointestinal carcinomas, and a survival of 9% if the primary tumor was grade 1 or 2; 6 of 169 patients (4%) were still alive at 10 years. These results justify removal of both the primary tumor and the metastases whenever feasible. Routine removal of the ovaries in menopausal and postmenopausal women having intestinal resections for carcinoma also is indicated to prevent the later development of symptoms of ovarian metastasis and avoid another operation, which has been necessary in from 1% to 7% of these patients in various series.[10,11,73,88] In some patients, even a third operation has been necessary when only a unilateral oophorectomy has been performed during the second operation.[88] There is no evidence, however, that prophylactic oophorectomy enhances the overall survival rate of patients with intestinal carcinoma.[115] Because young women are more likely to have ovarian metastases than older women, an argument could be made for oophorectomy in these patients as well, but other factors such as the patient's desire to retain her reproductive capacity and avoid the necessity for estrogen replacement therapy make the decision difficult and one that must be made on an individual basis.

We have seen two unpublished cases in which clear cell adenocarcinoma of the colon has exhibited ovarian spread, and three cases of intestinal small cell carcinoma with ovarian metastases have been reported.[36] Signet-ring cell carcinomas of the colon may form typical Krukenberg tumors; 5.4% of the latter tumors in one large series originated in the sigmoid colon.[138]

Gross Findings

Metastatic ovarian carcinomas of large intestinal origin, which are bilateral in approximately 60% of the cases, may form solid masses (Fig. 22.24), but are more often predominantly cystic (Figs. 22.3, 22.24, 22.25); frequently they are large, with a median largest dimension in one series of 11 cm,[75] and may simulate closely primary carcinomas of the ovary (Fig. 22.3). They may be much larger than the small primary tumor in the intestine. Sectioning typically reveals friable or mushy yellow, red, or gray tissue with cystic compartments that contain necrotic tumor (Fig. 22.25), mucinous or clear fluid, or fresh or old blood. Approximately 10% of the tumors rupture spontaneously, during pelvic examination or removal. An occasional example is composed of multiple, thin-walled cysts filled with mucinous or clear fluid[125] (Fig. 22.3).

Microscopic Findings

The neoplastic cells characteristically grow in patterns similar to those of primary intestinal carcinomas (Figs. 22.26, 22.27), typically forming small or large glands with a frequent cribriform pattern; mucin-containing goblet cells may be scattered among the mucin-free cells. Cystic glands lined by well-differentiated mucin-rich neoplastic cells

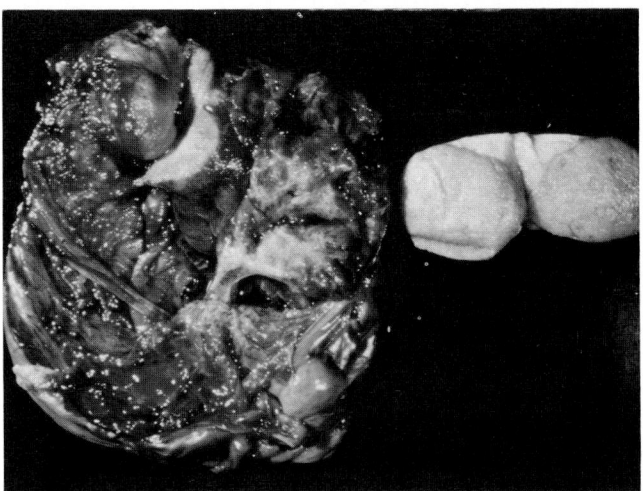

Fig. 22.24. Metastatic carcinoma from the colon. The smaller tumor is solid and buff-colored. The larger tumor is cystic with extensive hemorrhage and necrosis. (Reprinted by permission of Scully RE (1979) Tumors of the ovary and maldeveloped gonads. In: Atlas of Tumor Pathology, second series, fascicle 16, Washington, D.C., Armed Forces Institute of Pathology.)

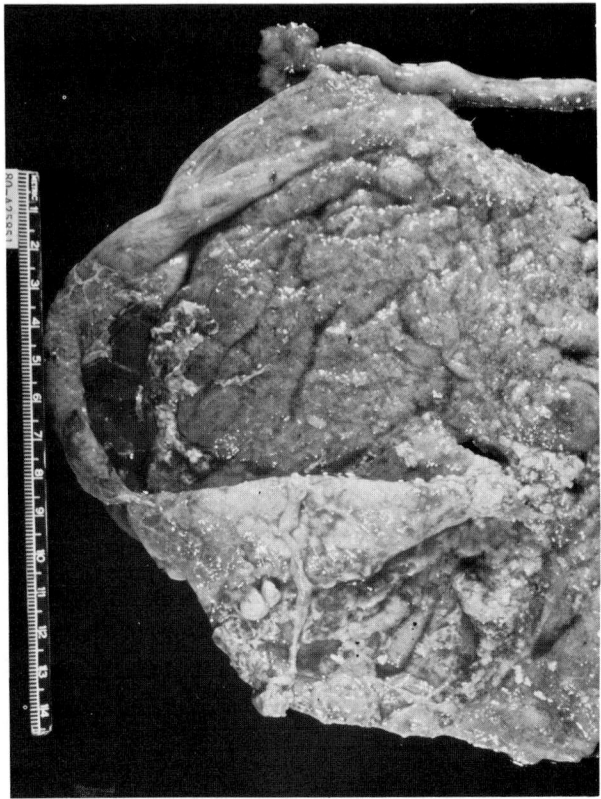

Fig. 22.25. Cystic metastatic carcinoma from the colon. The cyst is lined by shaggy necrotic tumor tissue.

formed a prominent component of the tumor in almost 20% of the cases in one series[75] (Fig. 22.28) and occasionally the tumor has the pattern of colloid carcinoma. Necrosis is common and often extensive, forming striking eosinophilic masses containing nuclear debris within the lumens (Fig. 22.26); this feature has been referred to as *dirty necrosis* and was present in all the cases in one series.[75] Two other features of the tumor, the frequent disposition of glands in a ring at the edge of the necrotic material (likened to a garland) and focal segmental necrosis of the glandular epithelium were emphasized by Lash and Hart.[75] The stroma varies from negligible to abundant; it may be desmoplastic, edematous, or mucoid, but often resembles ovarian stroma, containing cells resembling theca externa cells or theca-lutein cells in one-quarter to one-third of the cases.[75,127]

DIFFERENTIAL DIAGNOSIS

In one series more than two-thirds of the cases of metastatic intestinal carcinoma were misinterpreted initially as primary ovarian adenocarcinomas.[127] The most difficult tumors to exclude on microscopic examination are primary endometrioid and mucinous adenocarcinomas. In the series of 22 metastatic intestinal cancers described by Lash and Hart,[75] 19 mimicked endometrioid carcinoma, two mucinous carcinoma, and one a mixed endometrioid and mucinous carcinoma. Aside from clinical clues, gross features may be helpful in the differential diagnosis. The usual bilaterality of metastatic intestinal carcinomas contrasts with the less than 15% frequency of bilateral involve-

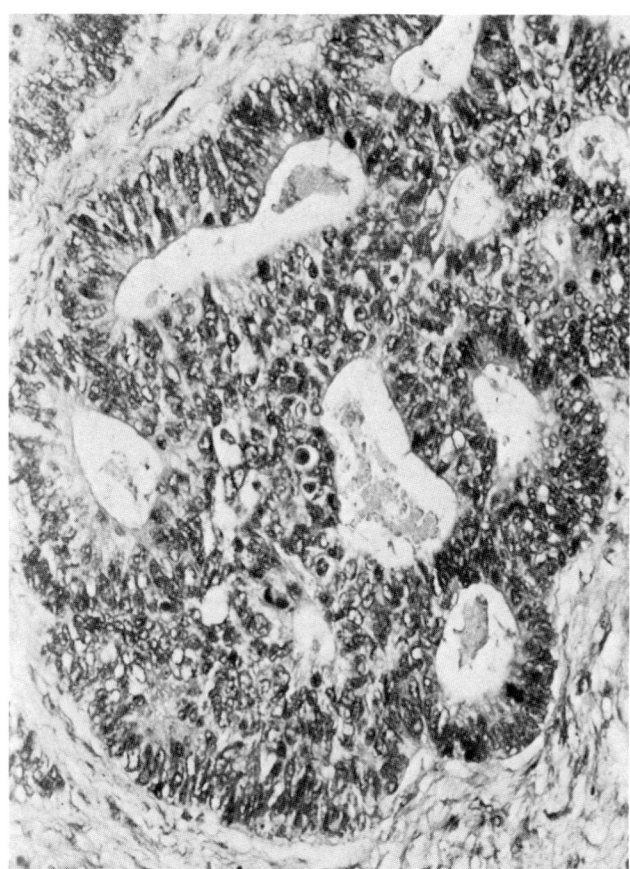

FIG. 22.27. Metastatic carcinoma from the colon. The shape of the glands suggests an endometrioid adenocarcinoma but they are lined by more poorly differentiated stratified epithelial cells than usually seen in gland-forming endometrioid tumors.

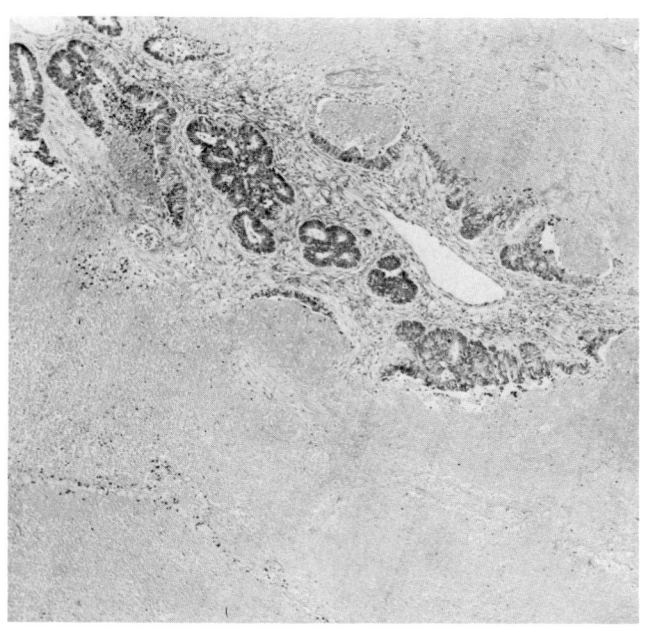

FIG. 22.26. Metastatic carcinoma from the colon. There is extensive necrosis.

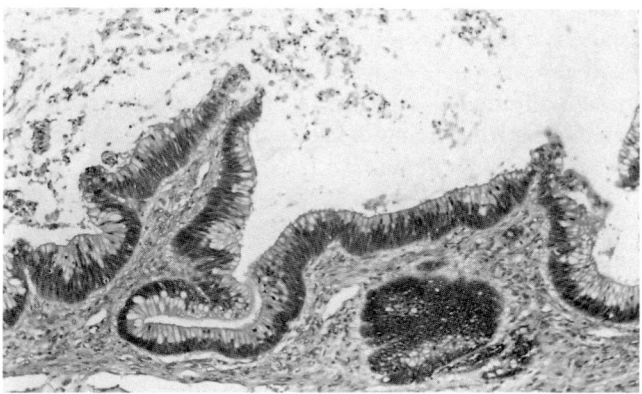

FIG. 22.28. Metastatic carcinoma from the colon. The mucinous epithelium in this illustration is indistinguishable from that of a primary mucinous borderline tumor. (Reproduced by permission of ref. 151.)

ment in cases of primary endometrioid and mucinous carcinomas. A confusing gross feature of metastatic intestinal carcinomas is the presence of solid masses and cysts lined by necrotic debris, and thin-walled cysts with smooth linings. These cysts occasionally are so numerous as to suggest a primary benign or borderline mucinous cystic tumor (Fig. 22.3). Endometrioid adenocarcinomas often are cystic but the cysts are sometimes filled with chocolate material, the presence of which is generally related to a background of endometriosis and a more homogeneous, less often necrotic, solid component usually is present. With regard to the microscopic differential diagnosis of metastatic intestinal adenocarcinoma and endometrioid adenocarcinoma, the glands of the former typically are lined by more poorly differentiated cells with greater degrees of nuclear hyperchromatism and loss of polarity (Fig. 22.27) than those of endometrioid adenocarcinomas with similar degrees of glandular differentiation. In addition, extensive confluent necrosis is common in metastatic intestinal carcinomas (Fig. 22.26), being present in 50% of the tumors in the series of Lash and Hart,[75] but uncommon in gland-forming endometrioid carcinomas. A similar comment pertains to so-called dirty necrosis within gland lumens, but it should be emphasized that this and the other features correctly emphasized by Lash and Hart[75] as typical of metastatic intestinal carcinoma, such as focal segmental necrosis of glandular lining epithelium, may be seen in rare cases of endometrioid carcinoma. Foci of squamous differentiation are frequent in endometrioid carcinomas, but extremely rare in intestinal carcinomas, and an adjacent adenofibromatous component or endometriosis strongly favors endometrioid carcinoma. The frequent presence of glands and cysts lined by endocervical-type mucinous cells with basal nuclei favors a primary ovarian carcinoma, although as mentioned above, differentiated glands and cysts are encountered in some metastatic intestinal carcinomas. Although goblet cells are encountered more commonly in primary mucinous carcinomas, they also may be seen in metastatic mucinous tumors. Other typical features of metastatic disease in the ovary already discussed are helpful in many cases but in occasional cases it may be impossible to make a differential diagnosis of metastatic versus primary mucinous adenocarcinoma on the basis of examination of the ovarian tumor alone.

In the occasional cases in which consideration of the above criteria for the distinction of a primary endometrioid or mucinous carcinoma from a metastatic carcinoma of the large intestine do not yield a confident diagnosis, confirmatory evidence may be obtained by the use of immunohistochemical techniques. HAM 56, a monoclonal antibody prepared against human alveolar macrophages, stains approximately 90% of primary ovarian cancers in the above categories and only 10% of colonic carcinomas. The antibodies COL 1 and COL 4 stain colon carcinomas more frequently and more extensively than ovarian primary carcinomas; the reverse is true for OM 1, a monoclonal antibody prepared against sebaceous glands, and OC 125, but these antibodies are not as selective as HAM 56 in distinguishing these two categories of carcinoma (Cheung AN, Thor AD, Scully RE: personal observations).

Tumors of the Appendix

Ovarian metastases from appendiceal tumors may be seen in cases of frankly invasive intestinal type adenocarcinomas including colloid and signet-ring cell carcinomas, carcinoids, almost always of mucinous type (adenocarcinoids), and finally, in cases of low-grade mucinous epithelial tumors that typically have the gross features of a so-called mucocele. The largest proportion of cases of spread of tumor from the appendix to ovary are in the last category but some interpret the ovarian tumor in such cases as an independent primary tumor; in the literature the relation between the ovarian and mucinous tumors has been controversial, as discussed below. If these low-grade appendiceal tumors are excluded, only about 30 appendiceal tumors with ovarian metastases have been reported.[23,85] In about one-third of the cases the ovarian involvement accounted for the presenting symptom. Approximately one-quarter of the tumors have been mucinous carcinoids (goblet cell carcinoids, adenocarcinoids). This type of tumor has been associated with metastasis in 20 of 55 reported cases, with ovarian involvement in 18 of them.[23] In 13 of the cases the ovarian metastatic tumor was found at presentation and in 11 of these cases the patient presented with an ovarian mass; in three cases the ovary was the only known site of metastasis. In five patients ovarian spread occurred after disease-free intervals of 6 months to 8 years. The 32% frequency of ovarian spread of appendiceal mucinous carcinoids exceeds the figure of 8% for appendiceal adenocarcinomas.[42] In cases of metastatic mucinous carcinoid the distinction from a primary mucinous carcinoid may be difficult and criteria similar to those discussed below are helpful in the differential diagnosis. Only very rare pure carcinoids of the appendix have been reported to spread to the ovary.[60]

An unknown, but probably relatively large, percentage of patients with low-grade mucinous tumors of the appendix, which typically appear as mucoceles on gross examination, have similar tumors in one or both ovaries, accompanied by pseudomyxoma peritonei.[18,84,98a,113] The relation between the ovarian and appendiceal tumors in these cases is controversial. Some writers have favored metastasis from the ovary to the appendix,[98a,144] whereas others have favored an independent origin for the tumors.[112a] In a recent study of 22 cases of this type the evidence suggested that the ovarian involvement was secondary to the appendiceal neoplasm.[144] The patients in that series ranged from 23 to 83 (average 49) years of age and usually presented with increasing abdominal girth. The appendiceal and ovarian tumors were synchronous in all but one of the cases. Laparotomy typically disclosed cystic ovarian tumors that averaged 16 cm in diameter and usually were multilocular (Fig. 22.29), an appendix that usually was dilated and covered with mucus, and abundant intraabdominal mucus. Seven of the ovarian tumors were bilateral. The ovarian and appendiceal tumors were typically similar, having histological features similar to those of mucinous cystadenomas (Fig. 22.30) and cystic tumors of borderline malignancy. In many of the ovarian tumors mucin dissected into the ovarian stroma (pseudomyxoma ovarii) and the mucinous cells typically were taller than those seen in ovarian mucinous tumors encountered in women without pseudomyxoma peritonei. The authors concluded that the ovarian involvement probably was secondary because of the typical synchronous presentation of the ovarian and appendiceal tumors, their histological similarity, the 32% frequency of bilaterality of the ovarian tumors (primary mucinous tumors are bilateral in less than 10% of the cases), and the predominance of right-sided ovarian involvement.[144] A problem in the conclusion reached was a failure to detect rupture of the appendiceal tumor in many of the cases. It has been shown, however, that the site of rupture of an appendiceal tumor of this type may be very small and require extensive sectioning to demonstrate; such examinations have not been performed in most of the cases in which a site of rupture has not been identified. An argu-

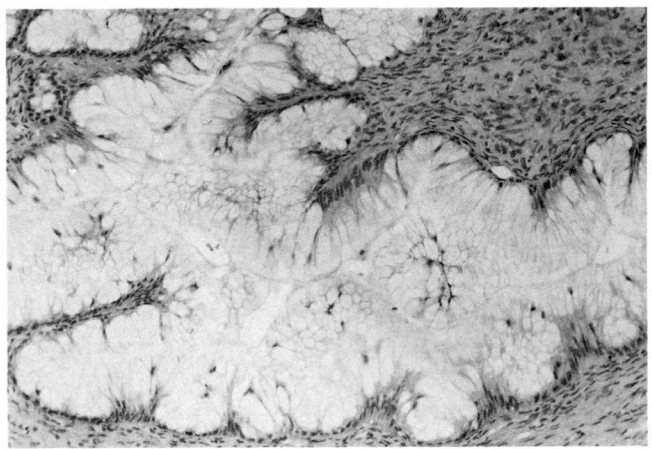

FIG. 22.30. **Mucinous cystic tumor of ovary in patient with borderline mucinous cystadenoma of appendix.** The tumor is characterized by tall, stratified mucinous cells with minimal atypia.

ment against independent primary tumors in the appendix and ovary is the infrequency of their co-existence in the absence of pseudomyxoma peritonei. Finally, in rare cases of pseudomyxoma peritonei, the appendix has been thoroughly studied and found to be negative, indicating that the pseudomyxoma is a complication of a primary ovarian tumor; cases in which the ovarian mucinous tumor has a component of dermoid cyst, suggesting a primary germ cell origin, probably also belong in this category. It is important in cases of pseudomyxoma peritonei for the pathologist to examine carefully specimens of peritoneal mucin for the presence of tumor cells since the prognosis appears to be better in their absence.

Seidman and his associates[112a] reviewed 25 cases of co-existent ovarian and appendiceal lesions and presented the following evidence for an independent primary origin of the tumors: In six of their cases the tumors co-existed in the absence of pseudomyxoma peritonei; in 13 cases the tumor in one organ appeared to be of a different degree of malignancy than that in the other organ; and in two-thirds of the cases there was a lack of complete concordance of immunocytochemical staining of the ovarian and appendiceal tumors for four antigens.

The evidence for and against the metastatic nature of the ovarian tumors in cases with appendiceal involvement suggests that in some cases the ovarian tumor is metastatic and in other cases, independently primary. Molecular genetic analysis of the two tumors in a series of cases may be necessary to solve the mystery of this perplexing disease.

Carcinoid Tumors

Carcinoid tumors account for approximately 2% of metastases that form ovarian masses; although most of these tumors are of small intestinal origin, rarely the primary

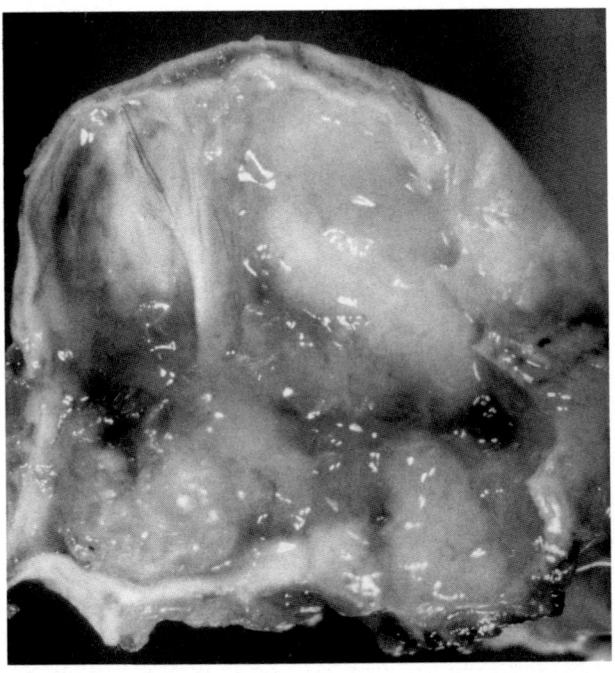

FIG. 22.29. **Mucinous cystic tumor of ovary in patient with borderline mucinous cystadenoma of appendix.** The thin-walled cyst is filled with jelly-like material. (Reproduced by permission of ref. 144.)

tumor originates in the colon, stomach, pancreas, or lung.[9,14,104,127,147,153] From another viewpoint, about 2% of small intestinal carcinoids greater than 1 cm in diameter spread to the ovary. In the largest series of carcinoids metastatic to the ovary the age of the 35 patients ranged from 21 to 82 years, with a median of 57 years; almost all of them were older than 40 years.[104] Ten of the tumors in that series were not diagnosed until autopsy. Forty percent of the women whose metastases were discovered at operation had preoperative manifestations of the carcinoid syndrome. Some of them also had signs and symptoms referrable to intestinal or ovarian involvement. Extraovarian metastases were found in at least 90% of the cases, a figure that contrasts with the rarity of similar spread of primary ovarian carcinoids. The primary site usually was in the ileum but the cecum, jejunum, appendix, and pancreas were sources in occasional cases.[104] One-third of the patients died within 1 year, and three-fourths of them within 5 years after unilateral or bilateral salpingo-oophorectomy, which was accompanied by a hysterectomy and an intestinal operation in some of the cases. Six of the 25 patients, however, were asymptomatic for a median period of 5 years postoperatively; all four patients with the carcinoid syndrome had postoperative relief, two for periods of more than 3 years after the removal of the ovarian tumors. Almost all metastatic mucinous carcinoids originate in the appendix.

In view of the occasional complications of ovarian metastasis, menopausal or postmenopausal patients with gastrointestinal carcinoids should have a bilateral oophorectomy even in the absence of obvious ovarian involvement to prevent the subsequent growth of occult metastases or the appearance of new metastases. Whenever bilateral ovarian carcinoids are detected, a careful search for an extraovarian primary tumor should be instituted. Both the metastases and the primary tumor, if found, should be excised whenever feasible. In a young woman with a unilateral neoplasm, careful examination of the intestine and its mesentery and other organs for a primary tumor, biopsy of the opposite ovary if enlarged, a thorough search for teratomatous elements in the tumor, and postoperative radiologic studies and measurement of 5-hydroxyindole acetic acid in the urine may be necessary before a determination of the primary or metastatic nature of the tumor and selection of appropriate therapy is made. Since the primary tumor in the intestine may be very small, it may not be detected by radiologic studies for a year or more after the diagnosis of the ovarian metastasis.

GROSS FINDINGS

Metastatic carcinoids may be large and typically are predominantly solid, with smooth or bosselated surfaces (Fig. 22.31). Sectioning reveals single or confluent firm, white or yellow nodules, which may resemble ovarian fi-

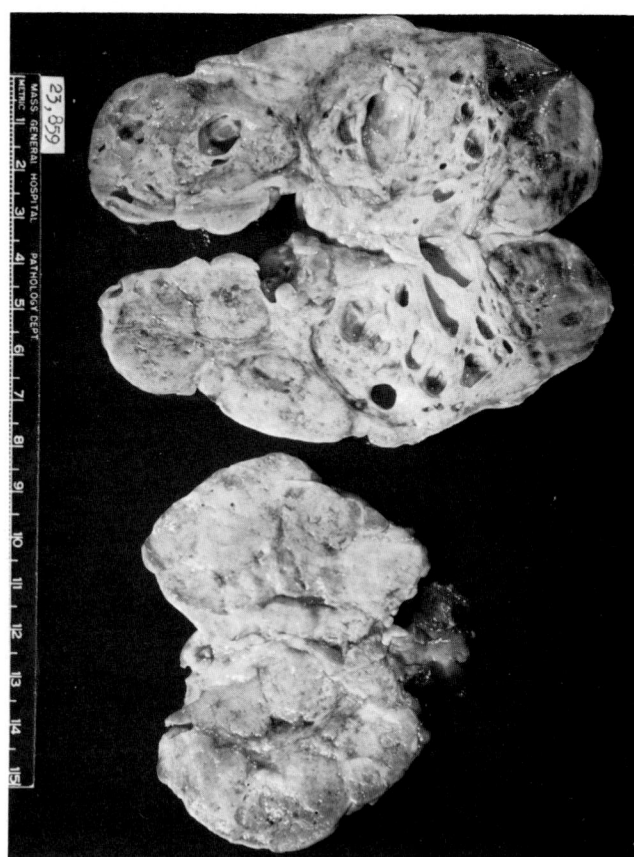

FIG. 22.31. Metastatic carcinoid. The larger tumor contains multiple cysts simulating a cystadenofibroma. (Reprinted by permission of Scully RE (1979) Tumors of the ovary and maldeveloped gonads. In: Atlas of Tumor of Pathology, second series, fascicle 16, Washington, D.C., Armed Forces Institute of Pathology.)

bromas or thecomas; cysts of varying size (Fig. 22.32) occasionally are present and typically are filled with clear, watery fluid, resulting in a gross appearance similar to that of a cystadenofibroma (Fig. 22.31); focal necrosis and hemorrhage may occur (Fig. 22.32). Most of these tumors are bilateral in contrast to primary ovarian carcinoids, which are almost always unilateral.

MICROSCOPIC FINDINGS

The microscopic features of metastatic carcinoids are similar to those of primary ovarian carcinoids except that teratomatous elements are not encountered, multinodularity often is prominent, and vascular invasion occasionally is observed. An insular pattern is most common (Figs. 22.33, 22.34) but trabecular, mixed, and rarely solid tubular patterns (Fig. 22.35) also are encountered. Acini, which typically are uniformly small and round, are common (Fig. 22.33); they often contain a homogeneous eosinophilic secretion that may undergo calcification (Fig. 22.34),

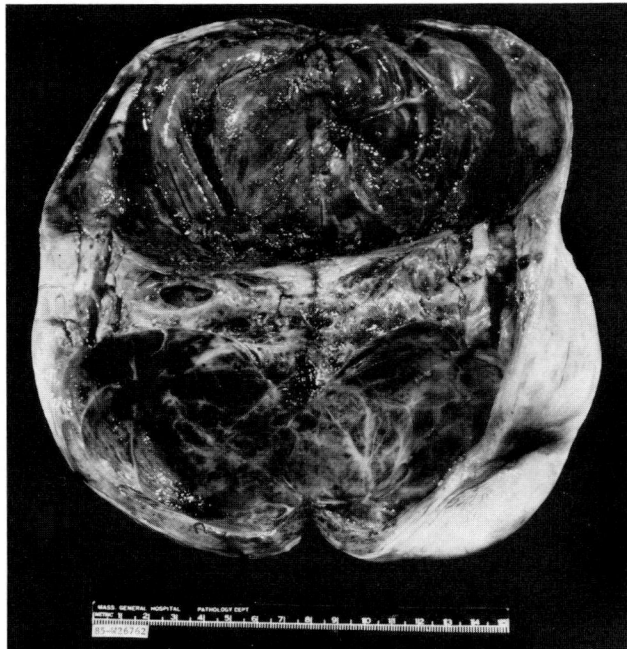

Fig. 22.32. Metastatic carcinoid. The tumor is predominantly cystic with extensive hemorrhage.

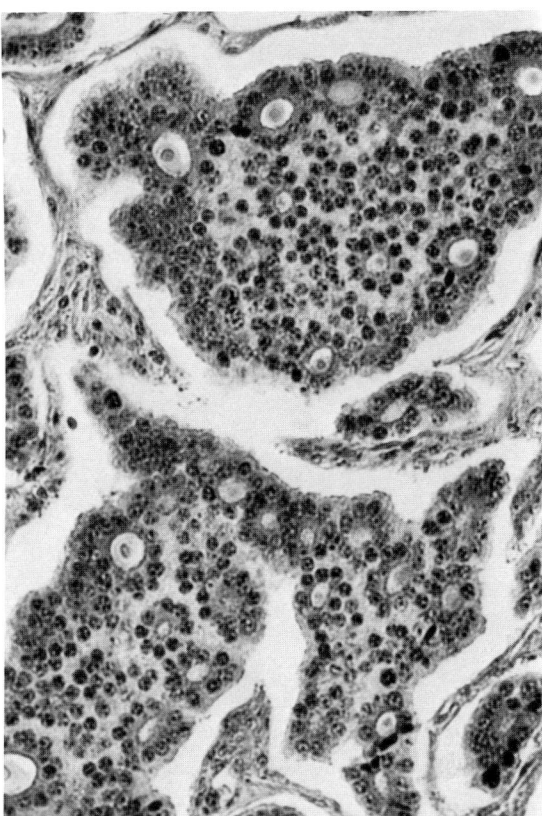

Fig. 22.33. Metastatic insular carcinoid. The gland lumens have smooth, rounded outlines; the nuclei are round with evenly distributed, coarse chromatin.

sometimes in the form of psammoma bodies. Large glands and cysts lined by one or a few layers of neoplastic cells sometimes are seen (Fig. 22.36). With rare exceptions the carcinoid is the only ovarian metastatic tumor that elicits an extensive stromal proliferation that closely resembles an ovarian fibroma; occasionally this stroma becomes extensively hyalinized (Fig. 22.37). A final microscopic pattern of metastatic carcinoid is that of a mucinous or goblet cell carcinoid (adenocarcinoid), almost always of appendiceal origin (see above), in which rounded nests containing goblet cells and argentaffin or argyrophil cells are present (Fig. 22.38). These tumors also may have foci resembling a Krukenberg tumor as well as cystic glands filled with mucin.

DIFFERENTIAL DIAGNOSIS

Metastatic carcinoids may be confused with a number of tumors other than primary carcinoid tumors, including granulosa cell tumors, Sertoli or Sertoli–Leydig cell tumors, Brenner tumors, adenofibromas and cystadenofibromas, benign, borderline, and malignant, and adenocarcinomas of various types. The microfollicular granulosa cell tumor often is confused with a metastatic carcinoid. The Call–Exner body of the granulosa cell tumor may resemble the acinus of the carcinoid when it is filled with eosinophilic dense basement membrane material, but it often differs by containing watery, eosinophilic fluid and shrunken nuclei in its lumen. Examination of the neoplastic cells is the most helpful clue to the correct diagnosis.

The cells of a microfollicular granulosa cell tumor usually have scanty cytoplasm, and ovoid, angular, or round nuclei that typically are pale and grooved. The cells typically are haphazardly oriented with respect to one another and the cavities of the Call–Exner bodies. In contrast, the cells of carcinoid tumors characteristically have round nuclei with coarse chromatin and their cytoplasm often contains prominent red or red-brown argentaffin granules. The sex cord–like formations of Sertoli–Leydig cell tumors may resemble the ribbons of the trabecular carcinoid but the latter usually are longer and thicker and have a more orderly architecture. The tubules of Sertoli or Sertoli–Leydig cell tumors may simulate the acini of insular carcinoids. Further confusion may be caused by the presence of a carcinoid component, which typically is minor in extent, in a Sertoli–Leydig cell tumor with heterologous elements. The presence of other distinctive patterns of Sertoli–Leydig cell tumor and attention to the characteristic cytologic features of carcinoid cells, however, should enable one to make the correct diagnosis.

The fibromatous stroma of a Brenner tumor often is indistinguishable from that of a carcinoid but the epithelial nests of the former contain cells of urothelial type with oval, pale, grooved nuclei rather than cells with the charac-

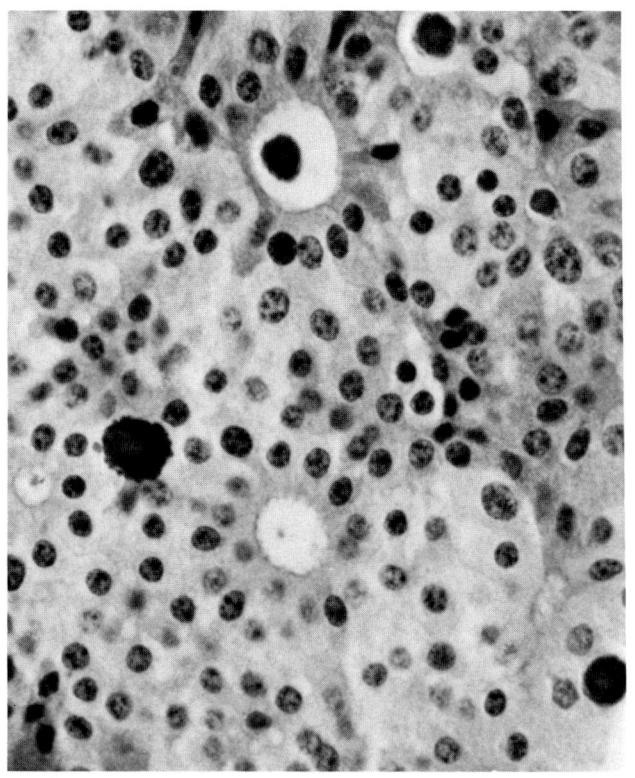

22.34

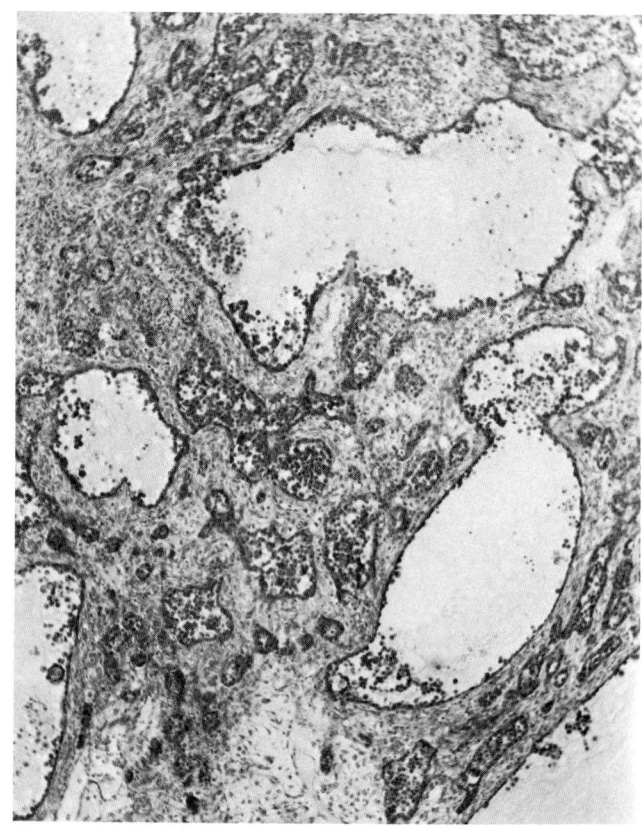

22.36

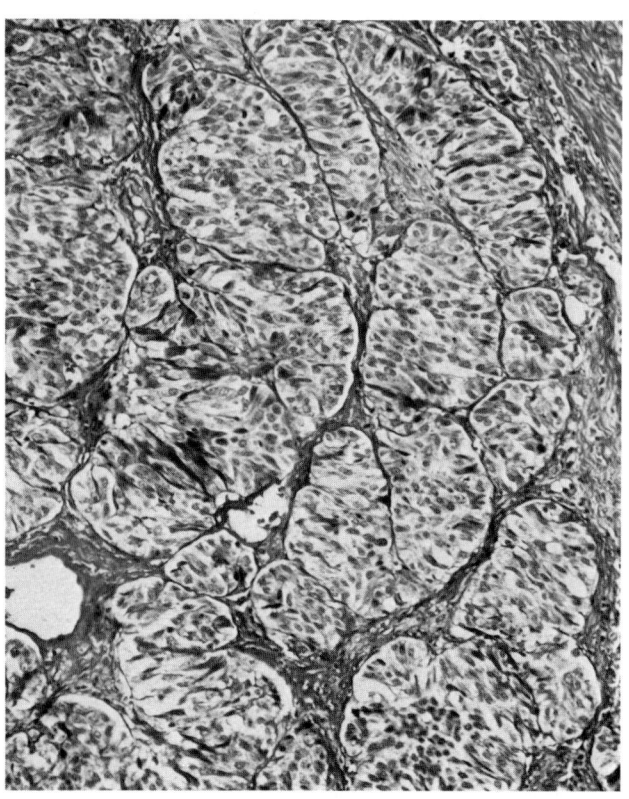

22.35

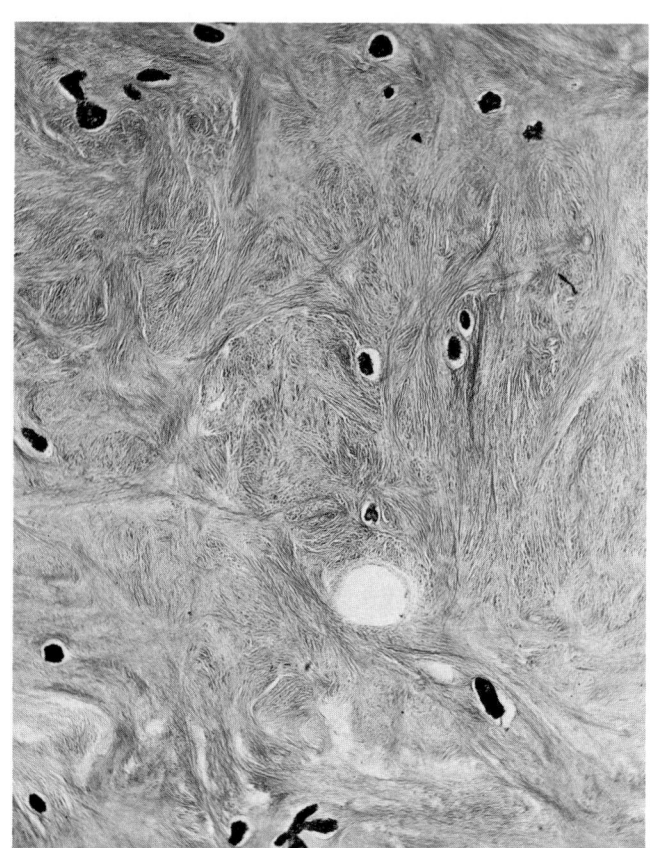

22.37

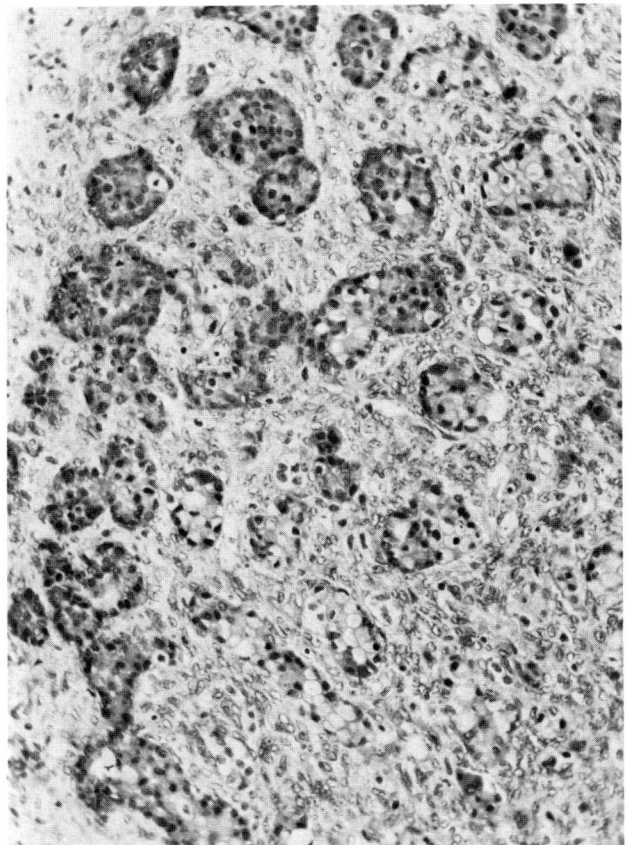

Fig. 22.38. Metastatic mucinous carcinoid. Nests containing cells with dense cytoplasm, which contained argentaffin granules and signet-ring cells.

teristic features of carcinoid tumors. Benign and malignant adenofibromatous tumors and endometrioid adenocarcinomas containing small tubules and acini are generally readily distinguished from carcinoids by recognition of the differing patterns and cytological features of these tumors. As mentioned earlier, a metastatic breast carcinoma with a prominent insular pattern may simulate a carcinoid tumor (Fig. 22.10). We have seen one case of microadenocarcinoma of the pancreas that metastasized to the ovary and, in the absence of a known pancreatic primary tumor,

◁ ————————————————————————

Fig. 22.34. Metastatic insular carcinoid. Several lumens contain dark calcified secretion.
Fig. 22.35. Metastatic carcinoid. A solid tubular pattern simulates a Sertoli cell tumor.
Fig. 22.36. Metastatic carcinoid. Cysts are lined by one or a few layers of neoplastic cells.
Fig. 22.37. Metastatic carcinoid. There is abundant hyalinized stroma.

prompted an initial diagnosis of probable metastatic carcinoid. If the diagnosis of a carcinoid tumor is difficult, more thorough sampling, histochemical staining for argentaffin and argyrophil granules, immunohistochemical staining for chromogranin, neuron-specific enolase, peptide hormones and serotonin, and electron microscopy for dense-core granules should resolve the differential diagnosis. It must be emphasized, however, that some of the other tumors mentioned above on occasion may contain scattered cells that stain for these substances and contain dense-core granules.

Metastatic mucinous carcinoids may contain foci of adenocarcinoma and be difficult to distinguish from pure metastatic adenocarcinomas unless the characteristic pattern of the mucinous carcinoid is recognized and the presence of argentaffin or argyrophil cells is confirmed by special staining. Adenocarcinomas of the stomach, intestine, and ovary may contain scattered argentaffin or argyrophil cells and the diagnosis of mucinous carcinoid should be reserved for cases in which the distinctive pattern of that tumor is present. Distinction of a metastatic mucinous carcinoid from the rare primary mucinous carcinoid of the ovary may be difficult and depends on knowledge of the distribution of disease and the presence or absence of teratomatous elements; bilaterality and extraovarian spread strongly favor a metastasis.

Tumors of the Pancreas

Although spread of pancreatic carcinoma to the ovary has generally been considered uncommon, seven pancreatic adenocarcinomas that spread to the ovary and mimicked primary mucinous tumors of the ovary recently have been reported in detail.[145] The patients were 29 to 87 (average, 63) years of age. The ovarian and pancreatic tumors were discovered synchronously in five patients. In two patients, the pancreatic tumor preceded the ovarian tumor by 9 months and 8.5 years, respectively. The clinical presentation simulated that of primary ovarian carcinoma in four patients. The ovarian tumors were typically large, cystic, and multiloculated (Fig. 22.39); six of them were bilateral and the status of the contralateral ovary was not known in the remaining case. Microscopic examination showed varying degrees of differentiation, but usually contained foci resembling mucinous cystadenoma (Fig. 22.40), mucinous cystic tumor of borderline malignancy, and well-differentiated mucinous cystadenocarcinoma (Fig. 22.41). The pancreatic tumors were typical ductal adenocarcinomas in six cases and mucinous cystadenocarcinoma in the seventh. A number of features were helpful in distinguishing between a primary and metastatic mucinous tumor in these cases. The bilaterality of the ovarian tumors in all but one case strongly favored metastasis. A finding that was helpful in

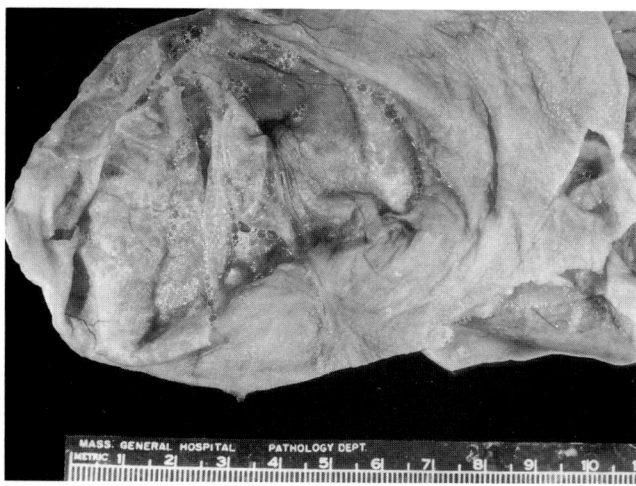

FIG. 22.39. **Metastatic carcinoma from the pancreas.** The multiloculated cystic ovarian tumor is indistinguishable from a primary mucinous cystic tumor.

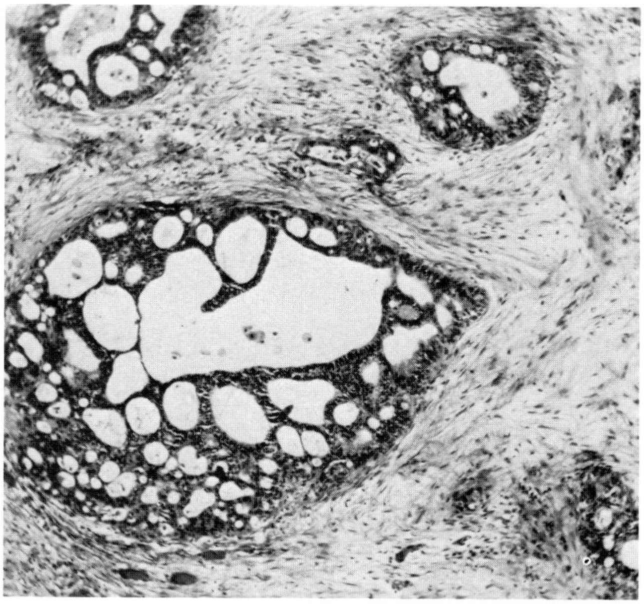

FIG. 22.41. **Metastatic carcinoma from the pancreas.** There is a prominent cribriform pattern.

many cases was the presence of desmoplastic implants of carcinoma on the ovarian surface and in the superficial ovarian cortex.

A probable example of islet cell carcinoma metastatic to the ovaries has been reported.[133] We also have seen two microadenocarcinomas of the pancreas with ovarian metastases (Fig. 22.42), one of which accounted for the clinical presentation. These tumors, as noted above, may mimic a carcinoid tumor, primary or metastatic, but are negative with silver stains. Most series of Krukenberg tumors do not

contain any of pancreatic origin but 6% of these tumors in one series were primary in the pancreas.[138]

Tumors of the Gallbladder and Bile Ducts

Ovarian metastases of biliary tumors occasionally are clinically significant. Seven such cases have recently been reported.[74a,154] The patients ranged from 33 to 72 (aver-

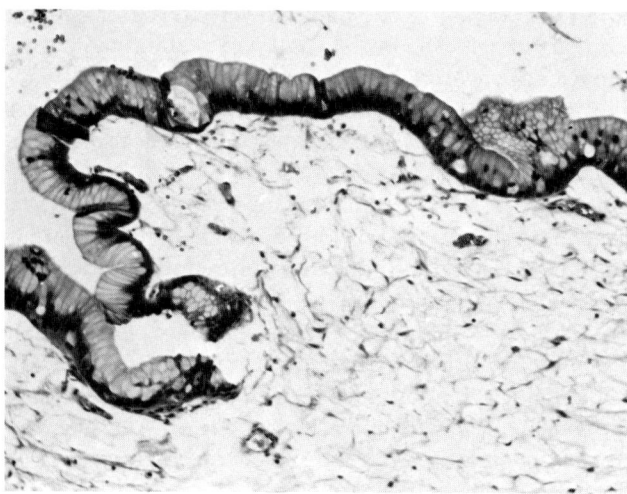

FIG. 22.40. **Metastatic carcinoma from the pancreas.** Cysts lined by only slightly atypical mucinous epithelium were a prominent component of this neoplasm. Same neoplasm as that in Figure 22.41.

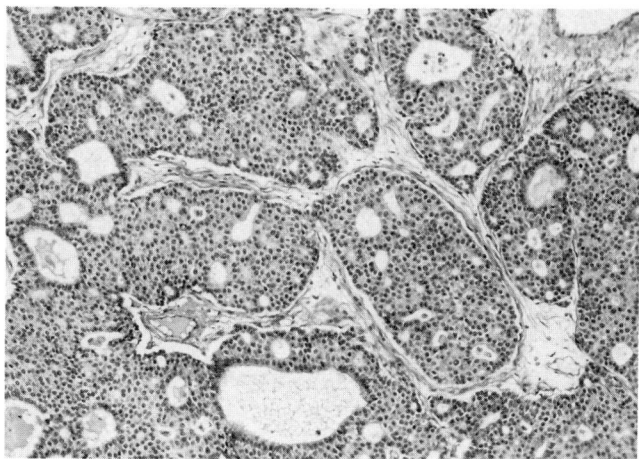

FIG. 22.42. **Metastatic microadenocarcinoma from the pancreas.** Islands of tumor cells contain numerous small acini. The tumor mimics a carcinoid tumor. (Reproduced by permission of ref. 151.)

age, 55) years of age. In one case the ovarian tumor was discovered 5 weeks before a gallbladder carcinoma was detected; in four cases the gallbladder tumors and ovarian metastases were discovered simultaneously, and in two cases the ovarian metastases were recognized 1 and 2 years after the biliary tumors, respectively. The ovarian tumors were bilateral in six cases and in one case the metastatic tumor was a large multiloculated cystic tumor, simulating a primary mucinous tumor of the ovary and in another case the ovarian tumors were "cystic masses" (74a). The remaining neoplasms were uniformly or predominantly solid, usually had lobulated external surfaces, and often were multinodular on section. The ovarian tumors in three of these cases posed problems in differential diagnosis. One of them closely simulated an endometrioid carcinoma; the neoplasm that simulated a mucinous tumor grossly also was similar on microscopic examination (Fig. 22.43) and, finally, one neoplasm initially raised the question of a Sertoli–Leydig cell tumor. The general features of metastatic involvement of the ovaries were helpful in the evaluation of these cases.

Tumors of the Liver

Spread of hepatocellular carcinoma to the ovary is even rarer than that of pancreatic and biliary tumors, but four clinically important cases recently have been reported.[93,142] The patients ranged from 31 to 67 (average, 43) years of age. One patient had bilateral ovarian tumors discovered at the same time as the liver tumor. In another patient the liver tumor was discovered by radiologic investigation after bilateral ovarian tumors had been removed. In the other two cases unilateral ovarian tumors were dis-

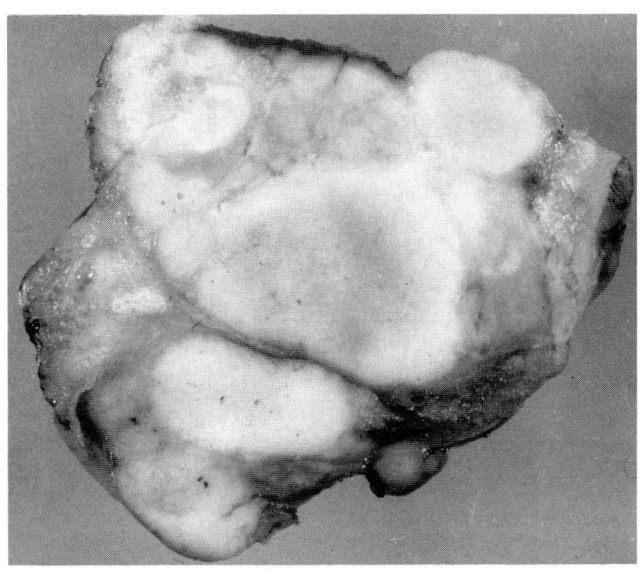

FIG. 22.44. Metastatic hepatocellular carcinoma. Multiple nodules are visible on the sectioned surface of a tumor that was yellow-green in the fresh state. (Reproduced by permission of ref. 142.)

covered 3 and 7 months, respectively, after the liver tumors had been detected. The ovarian neoplasms ranged from 4 to 11 cm in diameter and three of them were solid (Fig. 22.44). Microscopic examination has shown features characteristic of hepatocellular carcinoma (Fig. 22.45) except for one case, in which cysts were prominent.

The major differential diagnosis in these cases involves both primary and metastatic hepatoid tumors of the ovary.[142] In most cases of hepatoid yolk sac tumor the finding of foci of more typical yolk sac neoplasia or of other

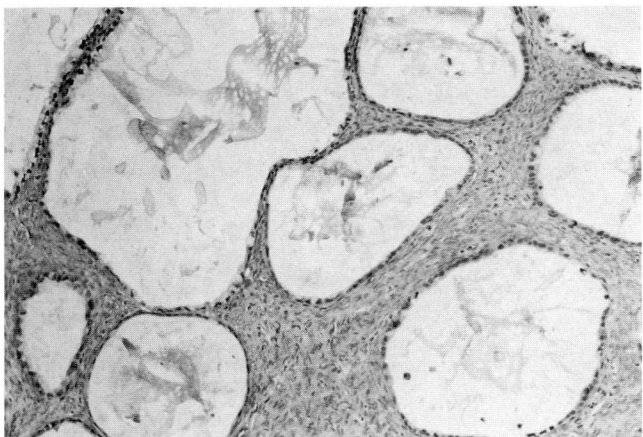

FIG. 22.43. Metastatic carcinoma from the gallbladder. In this field there are many cystically dilated glands lined by slightly atypical epithelium imparting a resemblance to a cystadenoma of the ovary. (Reproduced by permission of ref. 151.)

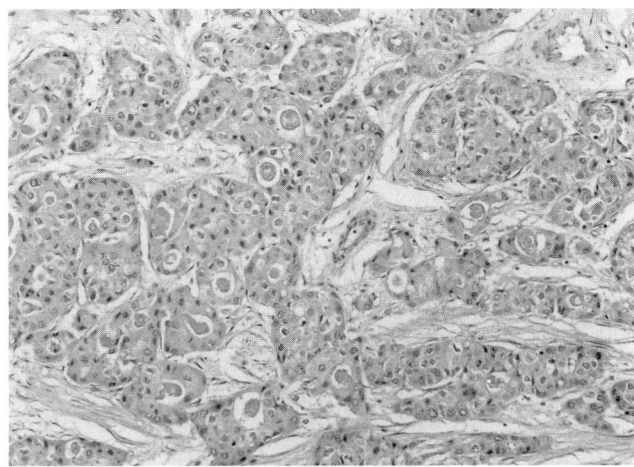

FIG. 22.45. Metastatic hepatocellular carcinoma. Tumor cells with abundant cytoplasm are arranged in trabeculae punctuated by occasional small glands.

germ cell elements exclude the diagnosis of metastatic hepatocellular carcinoma and the young age of the patient will argue against the latter diagnosis. In a postmenopausal patient the differential diagnosis involves hepatoid carcinoma rather than a hepatoid yolk sac tumor. In this situation, bilaterality and other characteristic findings of metastatic spread to the ovary may be helpful in indicating the metastatic nature of the tumor. Hepatoid carcinomas may arise outside the ovary, for example in the stomach and lung, and may metastasize to the ovary. There is one report in the literature of a cholangiocarcinoma that metastasized to the ovaries[69] and we have seen an additional example. A hepatoblastoma that occurred in a 19-year-old woman and was associated with bilateral ovarian metastases at presentation has recently been reported.[48a]

Renal Tumors

Renal cell carcinoma rarely spreads to the ovary, with only nine cases of clinically detectable ovarian metastatic tumors reported in detail.[146] In five of the nine cases, the ovarian tumor was discovered first, leading to the initial misdiagnosis of primary ovarian clear cell carcinoma in two cases. The renal tumors usually were detected within a short period of time in these patients but in one the renal primary was not detected until 8 years later. In the other four cases the ovarian tumor was detected 5 months to 11 years after the renal tumors had been removed. The nine patients were from 39 to 64 (average, 52) years of age. The ovarian tumors, two of which were bilateral, were 7 to 18 (average, 12.5) cm in greatest dimension and were either solid or solid and cystic (Fig. 22.46), with one cystic tumor

being unilocular and containing a 2.5-cm solid nodule in one area. The solid components of the tumors were either uniformly or focally yellow. With one possible exception the renal tumors were well-differentiated clear cell adenocarcinomas; microscopic examination showed a relatively uniform picture of diffuse sheets of clear cells or tubules lined by similar cells and containing eosinophilic material or blood (Fig. 22.47); a prominent sinusoidal vascular pattern was almost always present. It is helpful from the viewpoint of the differential diagnosis that primary clear cell carcinomas of the ovary have a tubulocystic and papillary component, or both, hobnail cells, and intraluminal mucin in the greater majority of cases. Hobnail cells and conspicuous mucin production, in contrast, are exceptional in renal cell carcinomas. In addition, the typical sinusoidal vascular framework of renal cell carcinoma is not a feature of ovarian clear cell carcinoma. In cases of pure clear cell carcinoma of the ovary without hobnail cells or mucin secretion, radiologic evaluation of the kidney may be necessary to exclude a renal cell carcinoma. Renal transitional cell tumors rarely spread to the ovary,[33] but in one case a patient with a renal pelvic tumor of this type had an ovarian metastasis at the time of presentation.[61]

Ovarian metastases from Wilms' tumor of the kidney must be very rare as no examples are present in several large series of this neoplasm. In one remarkable case, a

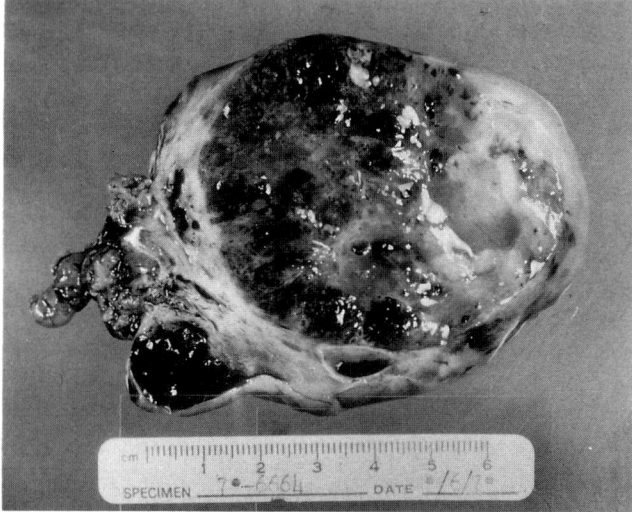

FIG. 22.46. Metastatic renal cell carcinoma. The tumor has a solid and cystic sectioned surface. (Reproduced by permission of Buller RE, et al. (1983) Renal-cell carcinoma metastatic to the ovary. A case report. J Reprod Med 28: 217–220.)

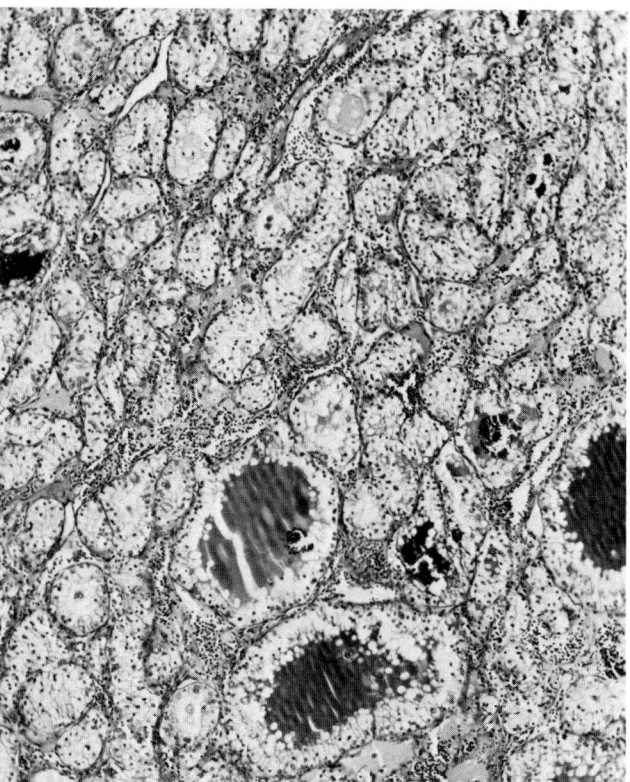

FIG. 22.47. Metastatic renal cell carcinoma, clear cell type. The primary tumor in this case was not diagnosed until 8 years after the removal of the metastasis.

patient with a rhabdoid tumor of the kidney presented with an ovarian metastasis, initially misinterpreted as a granulosa cell tumor, the primary renal tumor being undiscovered until autopsy.[147]

Tumors of the Urinary Bladder, Ureter, and Urethra

Tumors from these sites uncommonly metastasize to the ovaries. In two combined autopsy studies only 1 of 42 women with bladder cancer had ovarian metastases,[6,72] and in an older review of the literature on the spread of bladder cancer no cases of ovarian involvement were recorded.[41] Three signet-ring cell carcinomas metastatic from the bladder have had the appearance of a Krukenberg tumor.[27,105,156] In one of them the ovarian tumor was an autopsy finding and in another the ovarian involvement was an incidental finding on microscopic examination. In the third case the ovarian metastatic tumor, which was symptomatic, was not discovered until 7 years after the primary bladder tumor had been resected. Another case of ovarian metastasis of an adenocarcinoma of the bladder has been documented.[52] There is little information about the spread to the ovary of ureteral and urethral cancers. In one study 2 of 12 women with ureteral cancer had ovarian metastases[7] and occasional other examples have been recorded.[69] Only isolated examples of ovarian metastasis of urethral cancer have been reported in the literature.[156]

In many cases of possible transitional cell carcinoma metastatic to the ovary it is difficult to distinguish between a metastatic tumor and a borderline or malignant Brenner tumor or independent primary transitional cell carcinoma of the ovary.[5,44,118,156] In almost all borderline or malignant Brenner tumors, however, foci of typical benign Brenner tumor also can be found and the presence of associated benign mucinous elements also favors the diagnosis of a Brenner tumor. The extent of invasion of the primary extraovarian tumor, and the general features of metastatic involvement of the ovary, all have to be considered in the evaluation of these cases. The metastatic transitional cell carcinoma in the series of Ulbright et al.[127] was cystic, exemplifying the great propensity of ovarian metastases from various sites to undergo cystic change.

Adrenal Gland Tumors

Neuroblastoma spreads to the ovary more frequently than other tumors of the adrenal gland. From 25% to 50% of females with neuroblastoma have ovarian involvement at autopsy[57,86] and the literature suggests that this is the childhood tumor that spreads to the ovary most frequently.[147] Although usually an autopsy finding of clinically significant metastases occasionally are seen. In one

reported case there was bilateral ovarian involvement at presentation[86] and in two others ovarian metastatic tumor caused the clinical presentation.[117,147] Rarely neuroblastoma is primary in the ovary[3,72a] and such tumors must be distinguished from metastatic neuroblastomas.[147] The unilaterality of the primary tumors, their occasional association with a teratoma, and the absence of a known primary tumor elsewhere are helpful in the differential diagnosis in individual cases. The prominent fibrillary background of neuroblastoma and the presence of pseudorosettes should aid in the distinction of metastatic neuroblastoma from other metastatic small cell tumors; immunohistochemical staining also may help in a case in which routine stains are not diagnostic.

Adrenal cortical carcinomas metastasize to the ovary rarely even at autopsy. We are not aware of a case in which an ovarian metastatic tumor from the adrenal cortex was the presenting manifestation of the disease. Pheochromocytomas spread to the ovary even less commonly; a review of the literature has failed to disclose a documented case. Very rarely a pheochromocytoma is primary in the ovary.[39]

Malignant Melanoma

Autopsies of patients who died of malignant melanoma have revealed ovarian involvement in 18% of the cases; 95% of these tumors were bilateral.[30] Most of them have originated in the skin, but occasional examples have arisen in the choroid or elsewhere. Occasionally ovarian involvement is clinically symptomatic, as exemplified by many of the cases in two relatively large series of melanomas metastatic to the ovary published since the prior edition of this book.[43,150] In the first, 7 of the 10 patients had their ovarian tumors discovered during life.[43] The patients ranged from 29 to 55 (average, 38) years of age and had symptoms attributable to the ovarian metastases. Five of them had a known history of malignant melanoma and most of them also had extraovarian metastases as well. The tumors were bilateral in three of the seven cases and had an average diameter of 11.4 cm. In the second study[150] none of the tumors were autopsy findings. The 20 patients ranged from 21 to 60 (average, 37.5) years of age and typically presented because of abdominal swelling or pain. In 75% of the cases there was a history of removal of a cutaneous malignant melanoma or "pigmented lesion." The history of melanoma was more than 5 years previously (7–13 years) in three of the patients. Laparotomy disclosed unilateral ovarian tumors in 11 cases and bilateral tumors in 9. Approximately 50% of the patients also had metastatic tumor outside the ovary, usually within the pelvis and upper abdomen. The ovarian tumors averaged 10.5 cm in diameter; only 30% of them were noted to be black or brown (Fig. 22.48). On low-power examination a feature suggesting the metastatic nature in a number of the cases was growth of the tumor in the form of multiple nodules. The

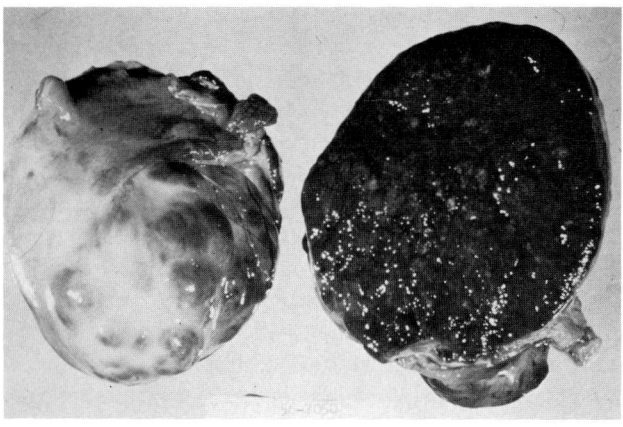

FIG. 22.48. Metastatic malignant melanoma. The tumor has a bosselated external surface; the sectioned surface is black.

most common microscopic appearance in one series was the presence of large cells with abundant eosinophilic cytoplasm.[150] Occasional tumors were characterized by small cells with scanty cytoplasm and in five tumors spindle cells were present. In the other series small cells with scanty cytoplasm predominated in most of the cases, often suggesting a sex cord–stromal tumor.[43] Metastatic melanoma may mimic closely a juvenile granulosa cells tumor[77] because of the presence of cells with abundant eosinophilic cytoplasm and follicle-like spaces, which are seen in approximately 40% of the cases[150] (Fig. 22.49). A helpful diagnostic feature of many metastatic melanomas is the presence of discrete rounded aggregates with a nevoid

appearance (Fig. 22.50). In our series of metastatic melanomas prominent nucleoli were seen in 65% of the cases and cytoplasmic pseudoinclusions in many nuclei in 25%.[150] The presence of melanin pigment is an obvious clue to the nature of the tumor in these cases but melanin was inconspicuous or absent in approximately half the cases in the two series just summarized.[43,150]

Metastatic melanoma must be distinguished from the rare primary melanoma that usually arises in the wall of a dermoid cyst, and sometimes is accompanied by junctional activity beneath the squamous lining of the cyst or is associated with another teratomatous component such as a struma ovarii. Since recognition of teratomatous elements is important in establishing the primary nature of a melanoma, the pathologist should sample the specimen extensively. In cases of apparently pure ovarian melanoma without obvious evidence of a primary tumor elsewhere, a meticulous search for an occult primary tumor should be conducted. If there is no evidence of a primary tumor elsewhere, it is possible that a primary cutaneous melanoma that has regressed was the source of the ovarian tumor. In these cases bilaterality and/or growth of the ovarian tumor in the form of multiple nodules strongly suggests metastasis even in the absence of a known primary tumor. In some cases removal of a primary melanoma may be remote, for example, as long as 14 and 25 years in two cases,[31,32] and possibly not considered relevant by the patient or known by the clinician.

Metastatic melanoma, particularly if it is amelanotic, may resemble closely a lipid-poor steroid cell tumor or, if it is found during pregnancy, a pregnancy luteoma. Melanin can be misinterpreted as lipochrome pigment, the presence of which may be a feature of steroid cell tumors and impart a dark green-brown or almost black color to the neoplastic tissue. The presence of follicle-like spaces in metastatic melanomas (Fig. 22.49) has resulted in their confusion

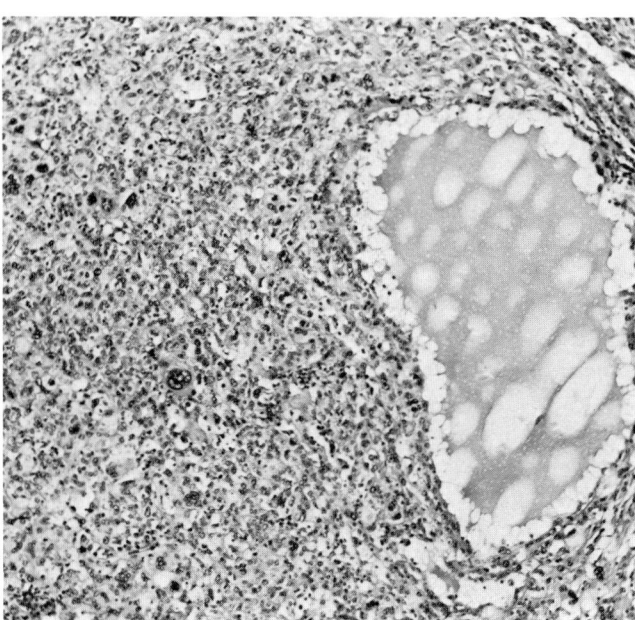

FIG. 22.49. Metastatic malignant melanoma. A follicle-like space is present adjacent to sheets of cells exhibiting conspicuous nuclear atypicality.

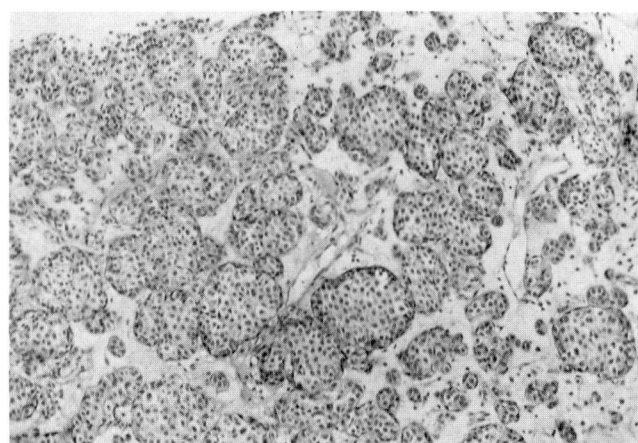

FIG. 22.50. Metastatic malignant melanoma. Nests of cells have a nevoid appearance.

with small cell carcinomas of the hypercalcemic type[119] as well as juvenile granulosa cell tumors. The diagnosis of metastatic melanoma to the ovary may be confirmed in problem cases by the immunohistochemical demonstration of S-100 protein and HMB-45 (Fig. 22.51) and negative staining for keratin and other antigens characteristic of other neoplasms that may be in the differential diagnosis.

Lung Tumors

Only approximately 5% of women with lung cancer have ovarian metastases at autopsy and the surgical pathologist uncommonly encounters an ovarian tumor of this type.[83,88a,153] Exceptionally an ovarian metastatic tumor either precedes the discovery of a pulmonary tumor or is found simultaneously.[82,153] In our series of seven cases of pulmonary tumors metastatic to the ovary, the ovarian tumors were discovered first in three cases, the ovarian and pulmonary tumors were synchronous in three cases, and in the final case the ovarian tumor was found less than 1 year after the pulmonary tumor.[153] In the first category a pulmonary neoplasm was detected 2, 4, and 26 months after the ovarian metastasis. The seven patients ranged from 26 to 66 (average, 42) years of age. Four of them were heavy smokers and one had scleroderma with diffuse interstitial

pulmonary fibrosis. Six patients had symptoms referable to the presence of an ovarian mass. The ovarian metastasis was not associated with other foci of intraabdominal spread in any of the cases, indicating the propensity for isolated ovarian spread of neoplasms to occur occasionally. Only one of the ovarian tumors was bilateral. On microscopic examination three tumors were small cell undifferentiated carcinomas, two large cell undifferentiated carcinomas, one a poorly differentiated adenocarcinoma, and one an atypical spindle cell carcinoid. In our experience since the time of publication of our paper on this subject the small cell carcinoma has been the most commonly encountered type.

When a patient has a pulmonary and ovarian neoplasm it can be difficult to decide which tumor is primary. When the histological features are typical of a lung carcinoma (Figs. 22.52, 22.53), a pulmonary origin can be assumed with possible rare exceptions. It should be mentioned that small cell carcinomas of pulmonary type may be primary in the ovary but in our series of such cases there was no pulmonary involvement facilitating the diagnosis of an ovarian primary.[37] The focal presence of a surface epithelial tumor is sometimes helpful in excluding a metastasis in these cases. In the absence of such a finding and in the presence of tumor in the lung it may be impossible to decide whether an ovarian small cell carcinoma of pulmonary type is primary or metastatic. It is worth pointing out

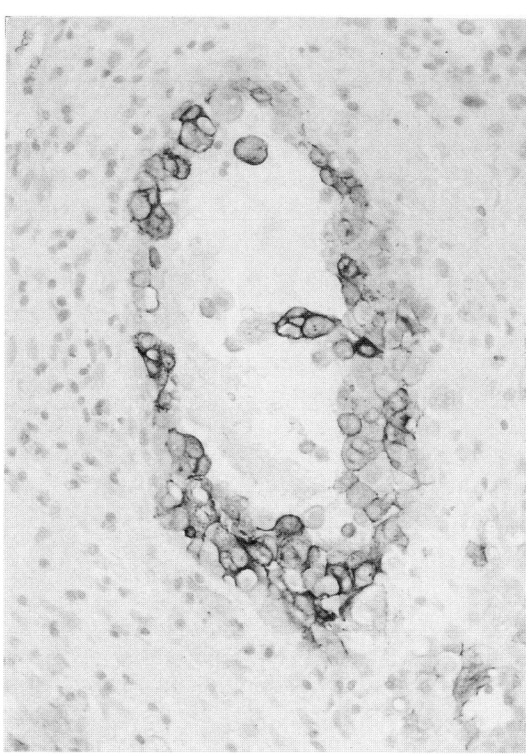

FIG. 22.51. Metastatic malignant melanoma. The cells surrounding a follicle-like space are positive for HMB-45. (Reproduced by permission of ref. 151.)

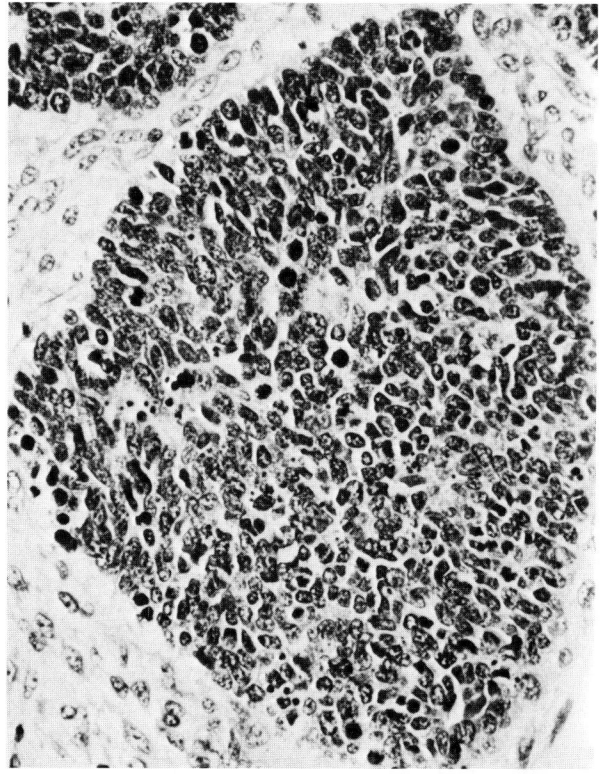

FIG. 22.52. Metastatic small cell carcinoma from the lung. (Reprinted by permission of Young and Scully, ref. 153.)

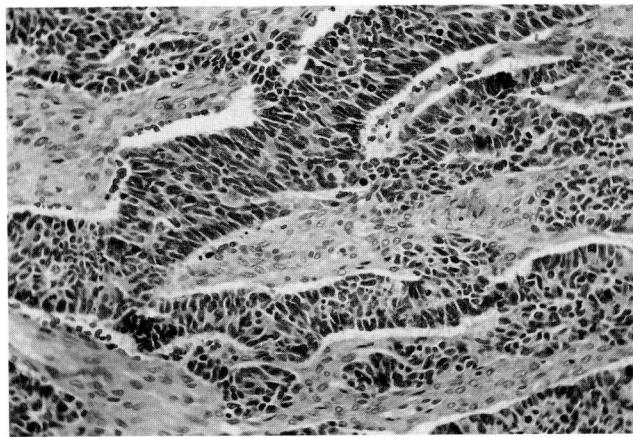

FIG. 22.53. Metastatic small cell carcinoma from the lung. The tumor cells are growing in trabeculae.

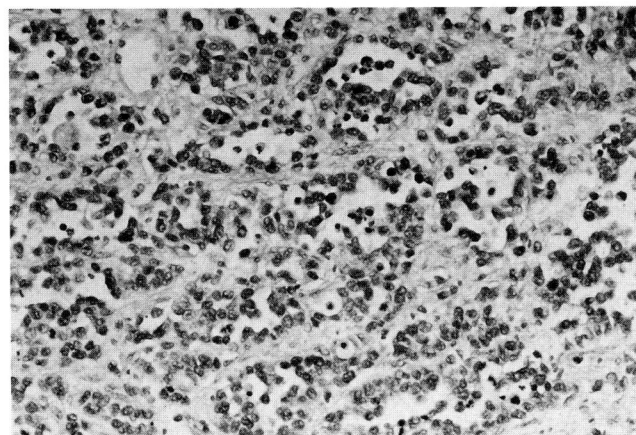

FIG. 22.54. Metastatic alveolar rhabdomyosarcoma. (Reproduced by permission of ref. 151.)

here that, as noted elsewhere in this chapter, metastatic small cell carcinomas in the ovary may originate in sites other than the lung.[36]

Mediastinal Tumors

Three patients with mediastinal small cell carcinomas, apparently of thymic origin, and ovarian metastases at the time of presentation have been reported.[36] One neuroblastoma primary in the posterior mediastinum metastasized to the ovary.[147] Thymomas have involved the ovary rarely.[13,139]

Extragenital Sarcomas

Extragenital sarcomas, whether from the viscera or the soft tissues, uncommonly metastasize to the ovary except in late stages of the disease. Eleven rhabdomyosarcomas metastatic to the ovary (Fig. 22.54) have now been reported in patients 6 to 27 years of age.[149] Six tumors were alveolar rhabdomyosarcomas, three embryonal, one mixed embryonal and alveolar rhabdomyosarcoma, and one of unstated subtype. In most of the cases, the ovarian spread was a late manifestation of disease. The ovarian tumors were symptomatic in only two patients, in whom the ovarian involvement was detected within a few weeks of discovery of a soft tissue mass by the patient. The ovarian tumors were bilateral in two cases. In cases of embryonal rhabdomyosarcoma metastatic to the ovary, the diagnosis of rhabdomyosarcoma usually is evident because of the presence of strap cells and the tumor must be distinguished from a primary embryonal rhabdomyosarcoma, which is the most common subtype of primary malignant striated muscle tumor of the ovary. Since a primary alveolar rhabdomyosarcoma of the ovary has not been reported to the best of our knowledge, metastatic alveolar rhabdomyosarcoma more commonly

raises the question of other primary and metastatic small cell tumors of the ovary in young women. Two other cases in which the ovary was involved by rhabdomyosarcoma have occurred in patients with a clinical picture that simulated acute leukemia.[53,89]

In our study of 21 metastatic sarcomas, other than rhabdomyosarcoma, 10 were extragenital and all of them were clinically significant.[155] These tumors included three leiomyosarcomas, one primary in the stomach and two in the small intestine, and single examples of retrovesical leiomyosarcoma, fibrosarcoma of the anterior abdominal wall, sarcoma of the mesentery of smooth muscle or neural type, hemangiosarcoma probably primary in the heart, osteosarcoma of the maxilla, chondrosarcoma of the rib, and Ewing's sarcoma of a pubic bone. Three other cases of hemangiosarcoma that metastasized to the ovaries have been documented,[22,54,111] as have two other cases of Ewing's sarcoma.[136,147] The only tumor in our series that caused major difficulty in diagnosis was the tumor that was primary in the stomach. The leiomyosarcoma in that case was epithelioid and a unilateral ovarian metastasis accounted for the clinical presentation. The primary tumor was not noted at the initial operation and not discovered until 4 months later.

Ovarian Involvement by Peritoneal Tumors

Although ovarian involvement in cases of malignant mesothelioma and malignant serous tumors of the peritoneum is secondary in most of the cases, this subject is generally not included in discussions of secondary tumors of the ovary as the ovarian involvement is only one part of widespread peritoneal disease. Criteria for the differential diagnosis of peritoneal serous neoplasia and serous neoplasms of the ovary with peritoneal spread are beyond the scope of this chapter and are covered elsewhere in this book.

One recently described peritoneal tumor that may involve the ovary, however, merits discussion here because the ovarian manifestations may be a major component of the clinical presentation, and the differential diagnosis of this tumor, the so-called intraabdominal desmoplastic small round cell tumor with divergent differentiation (see Chapter 17, Diseases of the Peritoneum), with other small cell tumors of the ovary may be difficult. Three examples of this tumor with ovarian involvement at presentation recently have been described in three girls, one 14, and two 15 years of age.[141] In two cases the ovarian tumor initially was thought to be the primary neoplasm. In all the cases there was extensive extraovarian tumor at the time of presentation. The ovarian involvement was bilateral in two cases and unilateral in the third. Microscopic examination of the ovarian tumors showed nodules composed predominantly of small cells with hyperchromatic nuclei and scanty cytoplasm surrounded by a prominent desmoplastic stroma (Fig. 22.55). The neoplasms exhibited the characteristic immunohistochemical staining profile, with many of the tumor cells staining for cytokeratin, epithelial membrane antigen, desmin, and vimentin. The differential diagnosis in these cases was extensive and included a number of small cell tumors that may involve the ovary, either primarily or secondarily in young females.

Miscellaneous Rare Ovarian Metastases

Metastases to the ovary other than those discussed above are of great rarity and generally only of relevance to autopsy pathology. Carcinomas of the thyroid only exceptionally spread to the ovary; rare examples of spread at autopsy in cases of follicular, medullary, and anaplastic carcinoma are mentioned in the literature.[146a] We are not aware of a

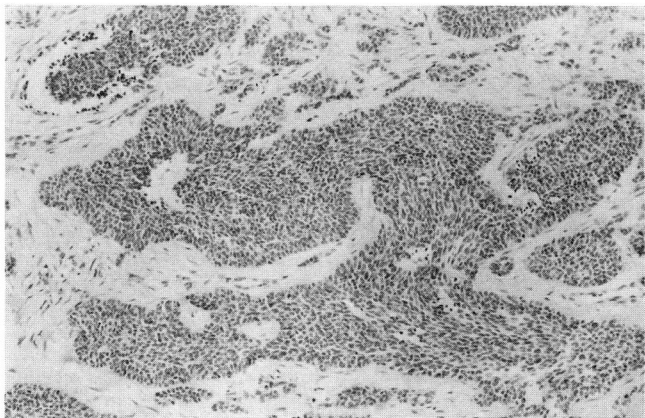

FIG. 22.55. Ovarian involvement by intraabdominal desmoplastic small round cell tumor. Nests of small cells with scanty cytoplasm are embedded in a desmoplastic stroma.

documented case of ovarian spread of papillary carcinoma. There is only one case in which ovarian spread of thyroid carcinoma is documented to have caused some diagnostic difficulty.[146a] In that case a 29-year-old woman had a 17-cm right ovarian tumor 12 years after undergoing a partial thyroidectomy for follicular carcinoma. The tumor also had spread to the brain and one adrenal gland by the time the ovarian tumor was discovered. Initial consideration was given to the diagnosis of a malignant struma ovarii in this case because of the interval since the thyroid tumor and also because it was only the existence of the ovarian tumor that prompted review of the thyroid neoplasm and its reinterpretation as carcinoma, a diagnosis not made initially. A review of the literature on parathyroid carcinoma has not disclosed any examples of ovarian metastasis.

Rare examples of head and neck carcinoma metastatic to the ovary are documented[94] and we have seen one case in which the primary tumor was an undifferentiated carcinoma of the ethmoid sinus. Salivary gland tumors also spread to the ovary with extreme rarity. We have seen a case of a young woman who had an adenoid cystic carcinoma of the parotid gland excised at the age of 12 years followed by local recurrence, lung metastasis, and bilateral symptomatic ovarian metastases 11 years after presentation. This case emphasizes that a history of neoplasia of any type, even relatively remote, may be relevant in the evaluation of an unusual ovarian tumor. We are unaware of a well-documented case of esophageal cancer that has spread to the ovary. In one report "gonadal" spread is mentioned in 2 of 73 patients who came to autopsy.[121]

There are only two reports to our knowledge in which ovarian spread of tumors of the central nervous system and cranium is mentioned. One was a case of metastatic meningioma[69] and the other was a metastatic medulloblastoma in a 4-year-old girl, in whose ovary "a cleft near the hilum was full of tumor cells."[97] Tumors of the skin, other than malignant melanoma, rarely spread to the ovary; Eichhorn et al.[36] have reported a case of Merkel cell tumor primary in the skin of the groin that metastasized to the ovary, producing a large, symptomatic mass; a similar case has been reported.[46] Finally, one chordoma has metastasized to the ovary.[159]

Rarely a metastatic tumor involves an ovary that contains a primary ovarian neoplasm; two of these metastatic tumors were of gastric origin and involved dermoid cysts[138]; one was a breast carcinoma and another a cystosarcoma phyllodes, both metastatic to a Brenner tumor[58,114]; additionally we have seen one Krukenberg tumor of gastric origin in an ovary containing a granulosa cell tumor and another involving an ovarian fibroma.

References

1. Abdul-Hafeez M, Akhtar M, Aqeel HS Ba, Kidess EA (1987) Placental site trophoblastic tumor: Report of a case with review of literature. Ann Saudi Med 7: 340–344

2. Acosta-Sison H (1958) The relative frequency of various anatomic sites as the point of first metastasis in 32 cases of chorionephithelioma. Am J Obstet Gynecol 75: 1149–1152

3. Aguirre P, Scully RE (1982) Malignant neuroectodermal tumor of the ovary, a distinctive form of monodermal teratoma. Report of five cases. Am J Surg Pathol 6: 283–292

4. Amorn Y, Knight WA (1978) Primary linitis plastica of the colon: Report of two cases and review of the literature. Cancer 41: 2420–2425

5. Andriole GL, Garnick MB, Richie JP (1985) Unusual behavior of low-grade, low-stage transitional cell carcinoma of bladder. Urology 25: 524–526

6. Babaian RJ, Johnson DE, Llamas L, Ayala AG (1980) Metastases from transitional cell carcinoma of urinary bladder. Urology 16: 142–144

7. Batata MA, Whitmore WF, Hilaris BS, Tokita N, Grabstald H (1975) Primary carcinoma of the ureter: A prognostic study. Cancer 35: 1616–1632

8. Beck RP, Latour JPA (1963) Necropsy reports on 36 cases of endometrial carcinoma. Am J Obstet Gynecol 85: 307–311

9. Berardi RS (1986) Carcinoid tumors of the colon (exclusive of the rectum): Review of the literature. Dis Colon Rectum 29: 767–771

10. Birnkrant A, Sampson J, Sugarbaker PH (1986) Ovarian metastasis from colorectal cancer. Dis Colon Rectum 29: 767–771

11. Blamey SL, McDermott FT, Pihl E, Hughes SR (1981) Resected ovarian recurrence from colorectal adenocarcinoma: A study of 13 cases. Dis Colon Rectum 24: 272–275

12. Brickman M, Ferreira B (1967) Metastasis of breast carcinoma to the ovaries—incidence, significance, and relationship to survival. A preliminary study. Grace Hosp Bull 45: 44–49

13. Briese VV, Rohde E (1984) Ovarielle metastasierung eines thymoms. Zbl Gynakol 106: 473–476

14. Brown BL, Scharifker DA, Gordon R, Deppe GG, Cohen CJ (1980) Bronchial carcinoid tumor with ovarian metastasis. A light microscopic and ultrastructural study. Cancer 46: 543–546

15. Bullon A, Arseneau J, Prat J, Young RH, Scully RE (1981) Tubular Krukenberg tumor. A problem in histopathologic diagnosis. Am J Surg Pathol 5: 225–232

16. Bunker ML (1959) The terminal findings in endometrial carcinoma. Am J Obstet Gynecol 77: 530–538

17. Burt CAV (1951) Prophylactic oophorectomy with resection of the large bowel for cancer. Am J Surg 82: 572–577

18. Campbell JS, Lou P, Ferguson JP, Krongold I, Kemeny T, Mitton DM, Allan N (1973) Pseudomyoxoma peritonei et ovarii with occult neoplasms of appendix. Obstet Gynecol 42: 897–902

19. Caron P, Roche H, Gorguet B, Martel P, Bennet A, Carton M (1990) Mammary ovarian metastases with stromal cell hyperplasia and postmenopausal virilization. Cancer 66: 1221–1224

20. Case Records of the Massachusetts General Hospital (1967) (Case 10-1967). N Engl J Med 276: 519–523

21. Case records of the Massachusetts General Hospital (1975) (Case 10-1975). N Engl J Med 292: 521–526

22. Case Records of the Massachusetts General Hospital (1975) (Case 35-1975). N Engl J Med 293: 494–499

23. Chen KTK (1990) Appendiceal adenocarcinoid with ovarian metastasis. Gynecol Oncol 38: 286–288

24. Chen KTK, Kostich ND, Rosai J (1978) Peritoneal foreign body granulomas to keratin in uterine adenoacanthoma. Arch Pathol Lab Med 102: 174–177

25. Chen SS (1989) Propensity of retroperitoneal lymph node metastases in patients with Stage I sarcoma of the uterus. Gynecol Oncol 32: 215–217

26. Choo YC, Naylor B (1982) Multiple primary neoplasms of the ovary and uterus. Int J Gynaecol Obstet 20: 327–334

27. Corwin S, Tassy F, Malament M, Grady H (1971) Rare signet-ring variant of mucinous adenocarcinoma of the bladder. J Urol 106: 697–700

28. Creasman WT, Lukeman J (1972) Role of the fallopian tube in dissemination of malignant cells in corpus cancer. Cancer 20: 456–457

29. Cutait R, Lesser ML, Enker WE (1983) Prophylactic oophorectomy in surgery for large-bowel cancer. Dis Colon Rectum 26: 6–11

30. Das Gupta T, Brasfield R (1964) Metastatic melanoma: A clinicopathological study. Cancer 17: 1323–1339

31. David MB, Feldberg D, Dicker D, Kessler H, Goldman JA (1984) Ovarian melanoma. An interesting case. Int J Gynaecol Obstet 22: 77–79

32. Dawson HGW (1922) Melanotic sarcoma of choroid and ovary. Br Med J 2: 757–758

33. Demopoulos RI, Touger L, Dubin N (1987) Secondary ovarian carcinoma: A clinical and pathological evaluation. Int J Gynecol Pathol 6: 166–175

34. Diddle AW (1955) Krukenberg tumors: Diagnostic problem. Cancer 8: 1026–1034

35. Duarte I, Llanos O (1981) Patterns of metastases in intestinal and diffuse types of carcinoma of the stomach. Hum Pathol 12: 237–242

36. Eichhorn JH, Young RH, Scully RE (1993) Non-pulmonary small cell carcinomas of extragenital origin metastatic to the ovary: A report of seven cases. Cancer 71: 177–186

37. Eichhorn JH, Young RH, Scully RE (1992) Primary ovarian small cell carcinoma of pulmonary type: A clinicopathologic immunohistologic and flow cytometric analysis of 11 cases. Am J Surg Pathol 16: 926–938

38. Eifel P, Hendrickson M, Ross J, Ballon S, Martinez A, Kempson R (1982) Simultaneous presentation of carcinoma involving the ovary and the uterine corpus. Cancer 50: 163–170

39. Fawcett FJ, Kimbell NKB (1971) Phaeochromocytoma of the ovary. J Obstet Gynaecol Br Commonw 78: 458–459

40. Ferry JA, Young RH (1991) Malignant lymphoma, pseudolymphoma, and hematopoietic disorders of the female genital tract. Path Annu 26(pt I): 227–263

41. Fetter TR, Bogaev JH, McCuskey B, Seres JL (1959) Carcinoma of the bladder: Sites of metastases. J Urol 81: 746–748

42. Fichera A, Petty NM, Park RC, Muir PW (1976) Primary adenocarcinoma of the vermiform appendix in gynecologic patient. Am J Obstet Gynecol 124: 663–664

43. Fitzgibbons PL, Martin SE, Simmons TJ (1987) Malignant melanoma metastatic to the ovary. Am J Surg Pathol 11: 959–964

44. Fossa SD, Schjølseth SA, Miller A (1977) Multiple urothelial tumours with metastases to uterus and left ovary. A case report. Scand J Urol Nephrol 11: 81–84

45. Gagnon Y, Tetu B (1989) Ovarian metastases of breast carcinoma. A clinicopathologic study of 59 cases. Cancer 64: 892–898

46. George TK, di Sant'Agnese PA, Bennett JM (1985) Chemotherapy for metastatic Merkel cell carcinoma. Cancer 56: 1034–1038

47. Graffner HOL, Alm POA, Oscarson JEA (1983) Prophylactic oophorectomy in colorectal carcinoma. Am J Surg 146: 233–235

48. Green TH Jr, Scully RE (1962) Tumors of the fallopian tube. Clin Obstet Gynecol 5: 886–906

48a. Green LK, Silva EG (1989) Hepatoblastoma in an adult with metastasis to the ovaries. Am J Clin Pathol 92: 110–115

49. Hale RW (1968) Krukenberg tumor of the ovaries. A review of 81 records. Obstet Gynecol 32: 221–225

50. Harcourt KF, Dennis DL (1968) Laparotomy for "ovarian tumors" in unsuspected carcinoma of the colon. Cancer 21: 1244–1246

51. Harris M, Howell A, Chrissohou M, Swindell RIC, Hudson M, Sellwood RA (1984) A comparison of the metastatic pattern of infiltrating lobular carcinoma and infiltrating duct carcinoma of the breast. Br J Cancer 50: 23–30

52. Hasegawa S, Ohshima S, Kinukawa T, et al (1988) Adenocarcinoma of the bladder 29 years after ileocystoplasty. Br J Urol 61: 162

53. Hayashi Y, Kikuchi F, Oka T, et al (1988) Rhabdomyosarcoma with bone marrow metastasis simulating acute leukemia. Report of two cases. Acta Pathol Jpn 38: 789–798

54. Hermann GG, Fogh J, Graem N, Hansen OP, Hippe E (1984) Primary hemangiosarcoma of the spleen with angioscintigraphic demonstration of metastases. Cancer 53: 1682–1685

55. Herrera LO, Ledesma EJ, Natarajan N, Lopez GE, Tsukada Y, Mittelman A (1982) Metachronous ovarian metastases from adenocarcinoma of the colon and rectum. Surg Gynecol Obstet 154: 531–533

56. Herrera-Ornelas L, Natarajan N, Tsukada Y, et al (1983) Adenocarcinoma of the colon masquerading as primary ovarian neoplasia. An analysis of ten cases. Dis Colon Rectum 26: 377–380

57. Himelstein-Braw R, Peters H, Faber M (1977) Influence of irradiation and chemotherapy on the ovaries of children with abdominal tumors. Br J Cancer 36: 269–275

58. Hines JR, Gordon RT, Widger C, et al (1976) Cystosarcoma phyllodes metastatic to a Brenner tumor of the ovary. Arch Surg 111: 299–300

59. Holtz F, Hart WR (1982) Krukenberg tumors of the ovary. A clinicopathologic analysis of 27 cases. Cancer 50: 2438–2447

60. Hopping RA, Dockerty MB, Masson JC (1942) Carcinoid tumor of the appendix. Report of a case in which extensive intra-abdominal metastases occurred, including involvement of the right ovary. Arch Surg 45: 613–622

61. Hsiu J-G, Kemp GM, Singer GA, Rawls WH, Siddiky MA (1991) Transitional cell carcinoma of the renal pelvis with ovarian metastasis. Gynecol Oncol 41: 178–181

62. Israel SL, Helsel EV, Hausman DH (1965) The challenge of metastatic ovarian carcinoma. Am J Obstet Gynecol 93: 1094–1101

63. Jambhekar NA, Sampat MB (1988) Simultaneous endometrioid carcinoma of the uterine corpus and ovary: A clinicopathologic study of 15 cases. J Surg Oncol 37: 20–23

64. James PD, Taylor CW, Templeton AC (1973) Tumors of the female genitalia. In: Templeton AC (ed) Tumours in a Tropical Country. New York, Springer–Verlag

65. Johansson H (1960) Clinical aspects of metastatic ovarian cancer of extragenital origin. Acta Obstet Gynecol Scand 39: 681–697

66. Jolles CJ, Beeson JH, Abbott T (1985) Progesterone production in adenocarcinoma metastatic to the ovaries. Obstet Gynecol 65: 853–857

67. Joshi VV (1968) Primary Krukenberg tumor of ovary. Review of literature and case report. Cancer 22: 1199–1207

68. Kaminski PF, Norris HJ (1984) Coexistence of ovarian neoplasms and endocervical adenocarcinoma. Obstet Gynecol 64: 553–556

69. Karsh J (1951) Secondary malignant disease of the ovaries. A study of 72 autopsies. Am J Obstet Gynecol 61: 154–160

70. Kasilag FB Jr, Rutledge FN (1957) Metastatic breast carcinoma in ovary. Am J Obstet Gynecol 74: 989–992

71. Kim K-R, Scully RE (1990) Peritoneal keratin granulomas with carcinomas of endometrium and ovary and atypical polypoid adenomyoma of endometrium. A clinicopathological analysis of 22 cases. Am J Surg Pathol 14: 925–932

72. Kishi K, Hirota T, Matsumoto K, Kakizo ET, Murase T, Fujita J (1981) Carcinoma of the bladder: A clinical and pathological analysis of 87 autopsy cases. J Urol 125: 36–39

72a. Kleinman GM, Young RH, Scully RE (1993) Primary neuroectodermal tumors of the ovary. A report of 25 cases. Am J Surg Pathol 17: 764–778

73. Knoepp LF, Ray JE, Overby I (1973) Ovarian metastases from colorectal carcinoma. Dis Colon Rectum 16: 305–311

74. Kuo T-T, Hsueh S (1984) Mucicarminophilic histiocytosis. A polyvinylpyrrolidone (PVP) storage disease simulating signet-ring cell carcinoma. Am J Surg Pathol 8: 419–428

74a. Lashgari M, Behmaram B, Hoffman JS, Garcia J (1992) Primary biliary carcinoma with metastasis to the ovary. Gynecol Oncol 47: 272–274

75. Lash RH, Hart WR (1987) Intestinal adenocarcinomas metastatic to the ovaries. A clinicopathological evaluation of 22 cases. Am J Surg Pathol 11: 114–121

76. Lee YN, Hori JM (1971) Significance of ovarian metastases in therapeutic oophorectomy for advanced breast cancer. Cancer 27: 1374–1378

77. Listrom MB, Foucar CE (1990) Letter to the editor. Am J Clin Pathol 94: 803–804

78. LiVolsi VA, Merino MJ, Schwartz PE (1983) Coexistent endocervical adenocarcinoma and mucinous adenocarcinoma of ovary: A clinicopathological study of four cases. Int J Gynecol Pathol 1: 391–402

79. Luisi A (1968) Metastatic ovarian tumours. In: Gentil F, Junqueira AC, (eds) In: UICC Monograph Series, Vol. 11, Ovarian Cancer. Berlin, Heidelberg, New York, Springer–Verlag, pp 87–104

80. Lumb G, Mackenzie DH (1959) The incidence of me-

tastases in adrenal glands and ovaries removed for carcinoma of the breast. Cancer 12: 521–526

81. MacKeigan JM, Ferguson JA (1979) Prophylactic oophorectomy and colorectal cancer in premenopausal patients. Dis Colon Rectum 22: 401–405

82. Malviya VK, Bansal M, Chahinian P, Deppe G, Lauresen N, Gordon RE (1982) Small cell anaplastic lung cancer presenting as an ovarian metastasis. Int J Gynaecol Obstet 20: 487–493

83. Mazur MT, Hsueh S, Gersell DJ (1984) Metastases to the female genital tract. Analysis of 325 cases. Cancer 53: 1978–1984

84. McKenna H, Ritchie G, Monks P (1978) Pseudomyxoma peritonei et ovarii with an occult neoplasm of appendix: Case report. Pathology 10: 157–160

85. Merino MJ, Edmonds P, LiVolsi V (1985) Appendiceal carcinoma metastatic to the ovaries and mimicking primary ovarian tumors. Int J Gynecol Pathol 4: 110–120

86. Meyer WH, Yu GW, Milvenan ES, Jeffs RD, Kaizer H, Leventhal BG (1979) Ovarian involvement in neuroblastoma. Med Pediatr Oncol 7: 49–54

87. Monteagudo C, Merino MJ, Laporte N, Neumann RD (1991) Value of gross cystic disease fluid protein-15 in distinguishing metastatic breast carcinomas among poorly differentiated neoplasms involving the ovary. Hum Pathol 22: 368–372

88. Morrow M, Enker WE (1984) Late ovarian metastases in carcinoma of the colon and rectum. Arch Surg 119: 1385–1388

88a. Nelson BE, Carcangiu ML, Chambers JT (1992) Intraabdominal hemorrhage with pulmonary large cell carcinoma metastatic to the ovary. Gynecol Oncol 47: 377–381

89. Nunez C, Abboud SL, Lemon NC, Kemp JA. Ovarian rhabdomyosarcoma presenting as leukemia. Case report. Cancer 52: 297–300

90. Ober WB, Edgcomb JH, Price EB Jr (1970) The pathology of choriocarcinoma. Ann NY Acad Sci 172: 299–426

91. O'Brien PH, Newton BB, Metcalf JS, Rittenbury MS (1981) Oophorectomy in women with carcinoma of the colon and rectum. Surg Gynecol Obstet 153: 827–830

92. Odone V, Chang L, Caces J, George SL, Pratt CB (1982) The natural history of colorectal carcinoma in adolescents. Cancer 49: 1716–1720

93. Oortman EH, Elliott JP (1983) Hepatocellular carcinoma metastatic to the ovary: A case report. Am J Obstet Gynecol 146: 715–718

94. Orr JW, Grizzle WE, Huddleston JF (1982) Squamous cell carcinoma metastatic to placenta and ovary. Obstet Gynecol 59: 81S–83S

95. Osborne MP, Pitts RM (1961) Therapeutic oophorectomy for advanced breast cancer. The significance of metastases to the ovary and of ovarian cortical stromal hyperplasia. Cancer 14: 126–130

96. Park WLH, Lees JC (1950) Choriocarcinoma. A general review, with an analysis of five hundred and sixteen cases. Arch Pathol 49: 205–241

97. Paterson E (1961) Distant metastases from medulloblastoma of the cerebellum. Brain 84: 301–309

98. Pitluk H, Poticha SM (1983) Carcinoma of the colon and rectum in patients less than 40 years of age. Surg Gynecol Obstet 157: 335–337

98a. Prayson RA, Hart WR, Petras RE (in press) Pseudomyxoma peritonei. A clinicopathologic study of 19 cases with emphasis on site of origin and nature of associated ovarian tumors. Am J Surg Pathol

99. Puga FJ, Gibbs CP, Williams TJ (1973) Castrating operations associated with metastatic lesions of the breast. Obstet Gynecol 41: 713–719

100. Rendelman DF, Gilchrist RK (1959) Indications for oophorectomy in carcinoma of the gastrointestinal tract. Surg Gynecol Obstet 109: 364–366

101. Resta L, De Benedictis G, Colucci GA, Cimmino A, Borraccino V, Milillo F (1989) Secondary tumors of the ovary II: Breast carcinoma. J Exp Clin Cancer Res 8: 147–151

102. Resta L, De Benedictis G, Colucci GA, et al (1992) Secondary tumors of the ovary. III. Tumors of the gastrointestinal tract and other sites. Eur J Gynaec Oncol 11: 289–298

103. Resta L, De Benedictis G, Colucci GA, Napoli A, Borraccino V, Milillo F (1989) Secondary tumors of the ovary. I: Tumors of the female genital tract. J Exp Clin Cancer Res 8: 87–94

104. Robboy SJ, Scully RE, Norris HJ (1974) Carcinoid metastatic to the ovary. A clinicopathologic analysis of 35 cases. Cancer 33: 798–811

105. Rosas-Uribe A, Luna M (1969) Primary signet-ring cell carcinoma of the urinary bladder. Arch Path 88: 294–297

106. Rose PG, Piver MS, Tsukada Y, Lau T (1989) Patterns of metastasis in uterine sarcoma. An autopsy study. Cancer 63: 935–938

107. Russell P, Bannatyne PM, Solomon HJ, Stoddard LD, Tattersall MHN (1985) Multifocal tumorigenesis in the upper female genital tract—implications for staging and management. Int J Gynecol Pathol 4: 192–210

108. Santesson L, Kottmeier HL (1968) General classification of ovarian tumours. In: Gentil F, Junqueira AC (eds) UICC Monograph Series, Vol. 11, Ovarian Cancer. Berlin, Heidelberg, New York, Springer–Verlag, pp 1–8

109. Saphir O (1951) Signet-ring cell carcinoma. Mil Surg 109: 360–369

110. Scully RE, Richardson GS (1961) Luteinization of the stroma of metastatic cancer involving the ovary and its endocrine significance. Cancer 14: 827–840

111. Sedgely MG, Ostor AG, Fortune DW (1985) Angiosarcoma of breast metastatic to the ovary and placenta. Aust NZ J Obstet Gynaecol 25: 299–302

112. Sedlis A (1961) Primary carcinoma of the fallopian tube. Obstet Gynecol Surv 16: 209–226

112a. Seidman JD, Elsayed AM, Sobin LH, Tavassoli FA (1993) Association of mucinous tumors of the ovary and appendix. A clinicopathologic study of 25 cases. Am J Surg Pathol. 17: 22–34

113. Shanks HGI (1961) Pseudomyxoma peritonei. J Obstet Gynaecol Br Commonw 68: 212–224

114. Smale L (1980) Metastatic breast adenocarcinoma to Brenner Tumors. Gynecol Oncol 9: 251–253

115. Spratt JS (1983) What to do about ovarian metastases from colonic adenocarcinomas. Am J Surg 146: 286

116. Stearns MW, Deddish MR (1959) Five-year results of abdominal pelvic lymph node dissection for carcinoma of the rectum. Dis Colon Rectum 2: 169–172

117. Sty JR, Kun LE, Casper JT (1980) Bone scintigraphy in neuroblastoma with ovarian metastasis. Wis Med J 79: 28–29

118. Svenes KB, Eide J (1984) Proliferative Brenner tumor or ovarian metastases? A case report. Cancer 53: 2692–2697

119. Swanson PE, Dehner LP (1990) Letter to the editor. Am J Clin Pathol 94: 805

120. Tabata M, Ichinoe K, Sakuragi N, Shina Y, Yamaguchi T, Mabuchi Y (1987) Incidence of ovarian metastasis in patients with cancer of the uterine cervix. Gynecol Oncol 28: 255–261

121. Takita H, Vincent RG, Caicedo V, Gutierrez AC (1977) Squamous cell carcinoma of the esophagus: A study of 153 cases. J Surg Oncol 9: 547–554

122. Toki N, Tsukamoto N, Kaku T, et al (1991) Microscopic ovarian metastasis of the uterine cervical cancer. Gynecol Oncol 41: 46–51

123. Tso PL, Bringaze III WL, Dauterive AH, Correa P, Cohn Jr I (1987) Gastric carcinoma in the young. Cancer 59: 1362–1365

124. Turksoy N (1960) Ovarian metastasis of breast carcinoma. A surgical surprise. Obstet Gynecol 15: 573–578

125. Ulbright TM, Roth LM (1985) Metastatic and independent cancers of the endometrium and ovary: A clinicopathologic study of 34 cases. Hum Pathol 16: 28–34

126. Ulbright TM, Roth LM (1985) Secondary tumors of the ovary. In: Roth LM, Czernobilsky B (eds) Tumors and Tumor-like Conditions of the Ovary, pp. 129–152. Contemporary Issues in Surgical Pathology No. 6. New York, Churchill-Livingstone

127. Ulbright TM, Roth LM, Stehman FB (1984) Secondary ovarian neoplasia. A clinicopathologic study of 35 cases. Cancer 53: 1164–1174

128. Van der Weiden RMF, Gratama S (1987) Proliferative and malignant Brenner tumors (BT) and their differentiation from metastatic transitional cell carcinoma of the bladder: A case report and review of the literature. Eur J Obstet Gynecol Reprod Biol 26: 251–260

129. Viadana E, Bross IDJ, Pickren JW (1973) An autopsy study of some routes of dissemination of cancer of the breast. Br J Cancer 27: 336–340

130. Warren S, Macomber WB (1935) Tumor metastasis. VI. Ovarian metastasis of carcinoma. Arch Pathol 19: 75–82

131. Webb MJ, Decker DG, Mussey E (1975) Cancer metastatic to the ovary. Factors influencing survival. Obstet Gynecol 45: 391–396

132. Wei P-Y, Ouyang P-C (1963) Trophoblastic disease in Taiwan. A review of 157 cases in a 10 year period. Am J Obstet Gynecol 85: 844–849

133. Weitberg AB, Weitzman SA (1983) Metastatic islet cell carcinoma: A potentially treatable cause of "carcinoma of unknown origin." CA—Cancer J Clin 33: 167–171

134. Wheelock MC, Putong P (1959) Ovarian metastases from adenocarcinomas of colon and rectum. Obstet Gynecol 14: 291–295

135. Woodruff JD, Julian CG (1969) Multiple malignancy in the upper genital canal. Am J Obstet Gynecol 103: 810–822

136. Woodruff JD, Murthy YS, Bhaskar TN, Bordbar F, Tseng S-S (1970) Metastatic ovarian tumors. Am J Obstet Gynecol 107: 202–209

137. Woodruff JD, Novak ER (1960) The Krukenberg tumor. Study of 48 cases from the Ovarian Tumor Registry. Obstet Gynecol 15: 351–360

138. Yakushiji M, Tazaki T, Nishimura H, Kato T (1987) Krukenberg tumors of the ovary: A clinicopathologic analysis of 112 cases. Acta Obstet Gynaecol Jpn 39: 479–485

139. Yoshida A, Shigematsu T, Mori H, Yoshida H, Fukunishi R (1981) Non-invasive thymoma with widespread blood-borne metastasis. Virchows Arch (Path Anat) 390: 121–126

140. Young RH, Carey RW, Robboy SJ (1981) Breast carcinoma masquerading as a primary ovarian neoplasm. Cancer 48: 210–212

141. Young RH, Eichhorn JH, Dickersin GR, Scully RE (1992) Ovarian involvement by the intra-abdominal desmoplastic small round cell tumor with divergent differentiation. A report of three cases. Hum Pathol 23: 454–464

142. Young RH, Gersell DJ, Clement PB, Scully RE (1992) Hepatocellular carcinoma metastatic to the ovary: A report of three cases discovered during life with discussion of the differential diagnosis of hepatoid tumors of the ovary. Hum Pathol 23: 574–580

143. Young RH, Gersell DJ, Roth LM, Scully RE (1993) Ovarian metastases from cervical carcinomas other than pure adenocarcinomas: A report of 12 cases. Cancer 71: 407–418

144. Young RH, Gilks CB, Scully RE (1991) Mucinous tumors of the appendix associated with mucinous tumors of the ovary and pseudomyxoma peritonei: A clinicopathological analysis of 22 cases supporting an origin in the appendix. Am J Surg Pathol 15: 415–429

145. Young RH, Hart WR (1989) Metastases from carcinomas of the pancreas simulating primary mucinous tumors of the ovary: A report of seven cases. Am J Surg Pathol 13: 748–756

146. Young RH, Hart WR (1992) Renal cell carcinoma metastatic to the ovary: a report of three cases emphasizing possible confusion with ovarian clear cell adenocarcinoma. Int J Gynecol Pathol 11: 96–104

146a. Young RH, Jackson A, Wells M (1994) Ovarian metastasis from thyroid carcinoma twelve years after partial thyroidectomy mimicking struma ovarii. Report of a case. Int J Gynecol Pathol 13: 181–185

147. Young RH, Kozakewich HPW, Scully RE (1993) Metastatic ovarian tumors in children: A report of 14 cases and review of the literature. Int J Gynecol Pathol 12: 8–19

148. Young RH, Prat J, Scully RE (1984) Endometrial stromal sarcomas of the ovary. A clinicopathologic analysis of 23 cases. Cancer 53: 1143–1155

149. Young RH, Scully RE (1989) Alveolar rhabdomyosarcoma metastatic to the ovary. A report of two cases and discussion of the differential diagnosis of small cell malignant tumors of the ovary. Cancer 64: 899–904

150. Young RH, Scully RE (1991) Malignant melanoma metastatic to the ovary: A clinicopathologic analysis of 20 cases. Am J Surg Pathol 15: 849–860

151. Young RH, Scully RE (1991) Metastatic tumors in the ovary: A problem-oriented approach and review of the recent literature. Semin Diagn Pathol 8: 250–276

152. Young RH, Scully RE (1988) Mucinous tumors of the ovary associated with mucinous adenocarcinomas of the cervix. A clinicopathological analysis of 16 cases. Int J Gynecol Pathol 7: 99–111

153. Young RH, Scully RE (1985) Ovarian metastases from cancer of the lung: Problems in interpretation—a report of seven cases. Gynecol Oncol 21: 337–350

154. Young RH, Scully RE (1990) Ovarian metastases from carcinoma of the gallbladder and extrahepatic bile ducts simulating primary tumors of the ovary: A report of six cases. Int J Gynecol Pathol 9: 60–72

155. Young RH, Scully RE (1990) Sarcomas metastatic to the ovary. A report of 21 cases. Int J Gynecol Pathol 9: 231–252

156. Young RH, Scully RE (1988) Urothelial and ovarian carcinomas of identical cell types: Problems in interpretation. A report of three cases and review of the literature. Int J Gynecol Pathol 7: 197–211

157. Yu TJ, Iwasaki I, Horie H, Tamaru J, Takahashi A (1986) Endolymphatic stromal myosis of the uterus with metastasis to ovary and recurrence in vagina. Acta Pathol Jpn 36: 301–308

158. Zaino RJ, Unger ER, Whitney C (1984) Synchronous carcinomas of the uterine corpus and ovary. Gynecol Oncol 19: 329–335

159. Zukerberg LR, Young RH (1990) Chordoma metastatic to the ovary: Report of a case. Arch Path Lab Med 114: 208–210

23

Diseases of the Placenta

Deborah J. Gersell, M.D., and Frederick T. Kraus, M.D.

Development and Anatomy

The importance of placental examination, unfortunately, is often underestimated, not only by gynecologists and pediatricians but by pathologists as well. The evaluation of a diseased or dead fetus is inadequate without the examination of its most accessible organ, the placenta. Examination of the placenta is complicated by the fact that during intrauterine life, the mother, fetus, umbilical cord, membranes, and placenta are all components of a single system, and disease in any one part may profoundly affect the others. Opportunities for examination of the maternal component are limited because maternal tissue is scant, consisting of only a thin layer of decidua adherent to the fetal membranes or basal plate. Small as it is, this layer is important because it contains the terminal portion of the spiral arteries, which are extremely important in the evaluation of many maternal diseases. The placenta is readily available for study, and its examination may provide significant information relating to intrauterine or perinatal death, intrauterine growth retardation, malformations, infections, and the effects of maternal disease on fetal growth and development. As in any organ, appreciation of pathological changes demands a sound knowledge of normal structure and development. Unlike more static tissues, the placenta undergoes a series of profound morphologic changes during its short life span, making an understanding of the normal somewhat more difficult.

Development

Among the many excellent treatises devoted to the description of implantation and the various stages in the development of the placenta, the monograph by Boyd and Hamilton[65] provides thorough coverage and exhaustive and detailed illustrations of the stages of human implantation.

The ovum is fertilized in the fallopian tube. Rapid cellular proliferation results in the development of the blastocyst. The outer cell layer of the blastocyst differentiates into the trophoblast, which completely envelopes the previllous blastocyst. The embryo ultimately will be derived from only a few cells in the inner cell mass. The trophoblast attaches to and penetrates the endometrium on the 6th to 7th postovulatory day. By the 10th to 11th day, the ovum is totally embedded in the endometrial stroma, and the superficial endometrial epithelium has reestablished its continuity. The trophoblast differentiates into an inner layer of cytotrophoblast, characterized by uniform cells with clear cytoplasm, distinct cell membranes, and vesicular nuclei, and an outer layer of syncytiotrophoblast, a syncytium with multiple, dense pyknotic nuclei suspended in abundant amphophilic cytoplasm. Admixed with the cytotrophoblast and syncytiotrophoblast are intermediate trophoblastic cells, which have some features of both cytotrophoblast and syncytiotrophoblast[208] (see Chapter 24, Gestational Trophoblastic Disease and Related Lesions).

Between the 8th and 13th postovulatory day, blood-filled lacunae form within the rapidly growing syncytiotrophoblast and separate it into trabecular columns (Fig. 23.1). Thereafter (14th–20th day), the syncytiotrophoblast of the columns becomes radially oriented around central, solid cores of cytotrophoblast. The cytotrophoblast continues to grow peripherally and, at the same time, is penetrated by extraembryonic mesenchyme within which small blood vessels form. By 21 days, the placenta is a vascularized, villous organ. These vessels eventually establish continuity with other blood vessels forming in the inner chorionic mesenchyme and body stalk. Early in the 5th week, a complete fetoplacental circulation is established. Growth of new villi from the primary villous stems follows the same sequence, syncytiotrophoblastic sprouting, intrusion of a cytotrophoblastic core, ingrowth of mesenchyme, and eventual vascularization, throughout gestation.[333]

The most peripheral portions of the primary stem villi consist of solid aggregates of cytotrophoblast and intermediate trophoblast, which anchor the villi to the basal plate (Fig. 23.2). The masses of intermediate and cytotrophoblast grow laterally and circumferentially to form a complete shell, which continues to expand and enlarge the intervillous space (Fig. 23.3). The decidua and myometrium at the placental site are infiltrated diffusely by trophoblast. This mingling of trophoblast and decidua is so intimate that it may be difficult to characterize any particular cell as being maternal or fetal by conventional light microscopy. Intermediate trophoblast is the predominant form of trophoblast in the implantation site. In this location, intermediate trophoblastic cells vary greatly in appearance. Most are mononucleate, but bi-, tri- and multinucleate forms occur. They may be round, polyhedral, or spindle-shaped, and have abundant eosinophilic to amphophilic cytoplasm and irregular, hyperchromatic nuclei with coarsely granular chromatin.

The intermediate trophoblast is responsible for a remarkable sequence of structural modifications that occurs in the maternal circulation in pregnancy. These physiological alterations have been described and illustrated in the work of Robertson et al.[103,312,313] In the early weeks of normal pregnancy, intermediate trophoblast invades and alters the intradecidual portions of the spiral arteries. The maternal endothelium and the muscular and elastic tissue of the media are replaced by fibrinoid material composed of a complex of fibrin, plasma constituents, and proteinaceous substances produced by the trophoblast (Fig. 23.4). As pregnancy advances, the intermediate trophoblast infiltrates the inner myometrium. Between 14 and 20 weeks, a retrograde wave of endovascular trophoblast moves from the decidual segments into the myometrial segments of the spiral arteries, where the same alterations (destruction and fibrinoid replacement of the arterial intima and media) occur. There is some evidence that adaptations in the myometrial segments of the spiral arteries are necessary be-

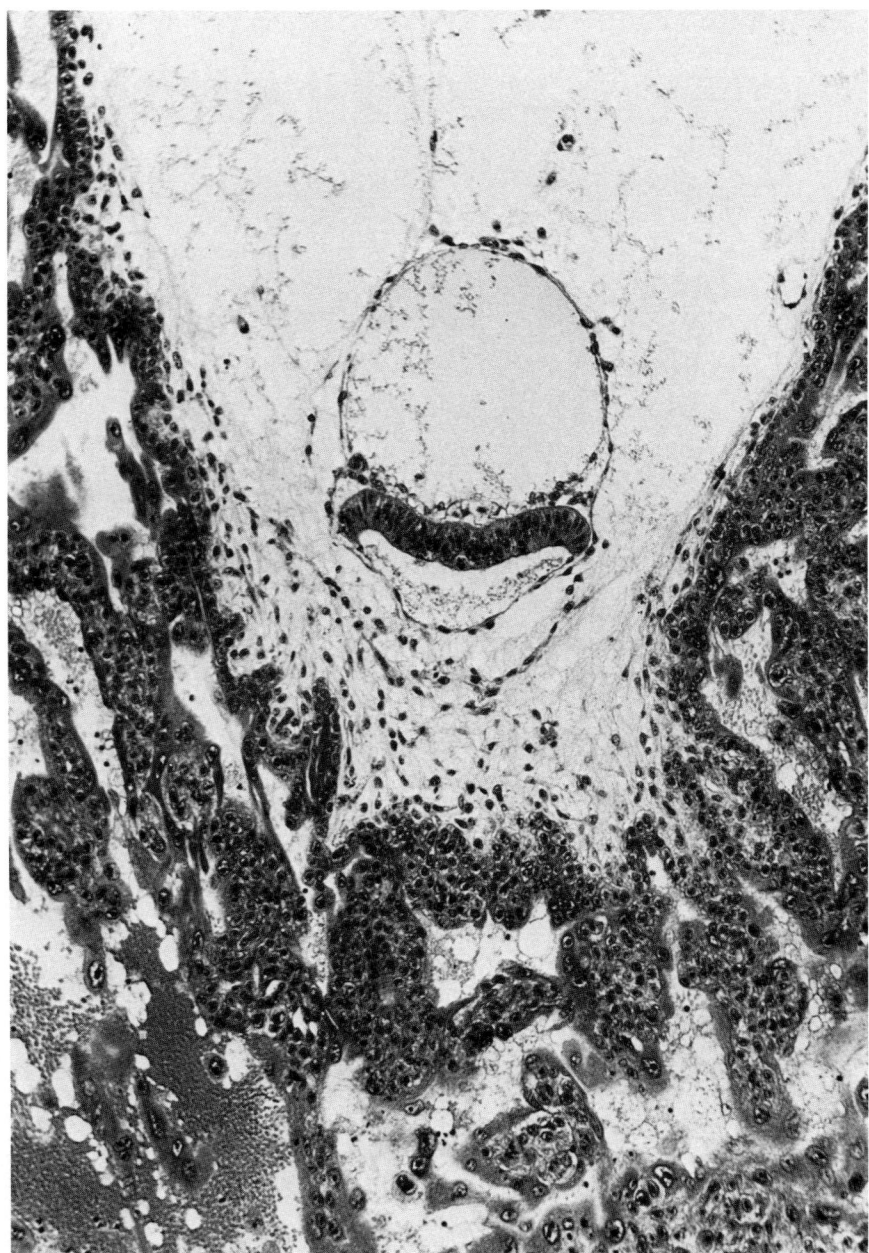

Fig. 23.1. Implantation at 13 days. Trophoblast has differentiated into inner (cytotrophoblast) and outer (syncytiotrophoblast) layers. Focally, the cytotrophoblast has proliferated to form projections, the forerunners of the primary villi. The germ disc is located near the center. (Reprinted courtesy of Department of Embryology, Davis Division, Carnegie Institute of Washington.)

fore endovascular trophoblastic migration can occur. As detailed by Pijnenborg et al.,[289] these changes may be effected by the migrating intermediate trophoblast.

The vessels affected by these physiologic changes undergo progressive distention to funnel-shaped channels that augment the blood flow to the implantation site from 100 ml/min in the nonpregnant uterus to >500 ml/min in the uterus at term. The vascular dilatation that occurs as a consequence of these alterations also results in a considerable fall in blood pressure. The physiologic changes that occur in the spiral arteries during pregnancy originally were attributed to cytotrophoblast. More recent evidence indicates that the cells currently referred to as intermediate trophoblast actually play this key role in implantation and establishment of the uteroplacental circulation.[208]

Continued growth and enlargement of the chorion result in eventual obliteration of the uterine cavity through fusion of the decidua capsularis and the decidua vera of the opposite uterine wall. This usually is achieved by 20 weeks. During this time, the villi oriented toward the uterine cavity undergo progressive atrophy to form the chorion

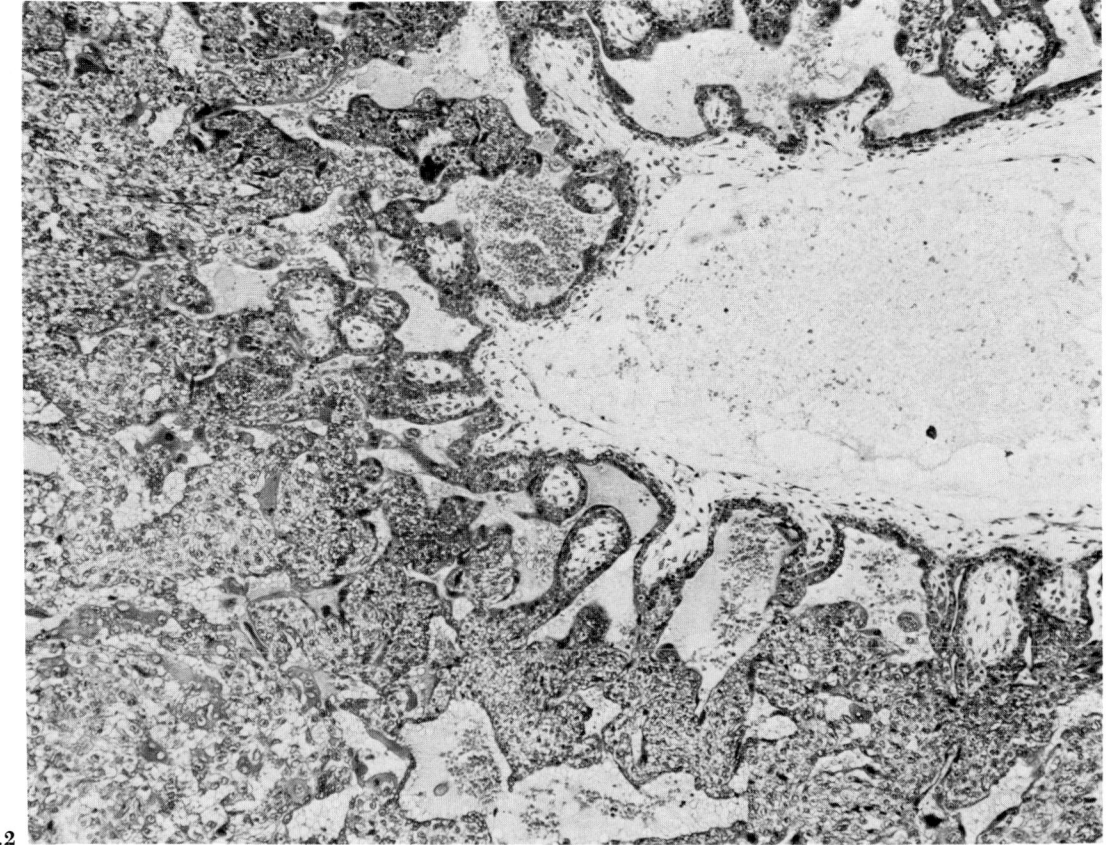

23.2

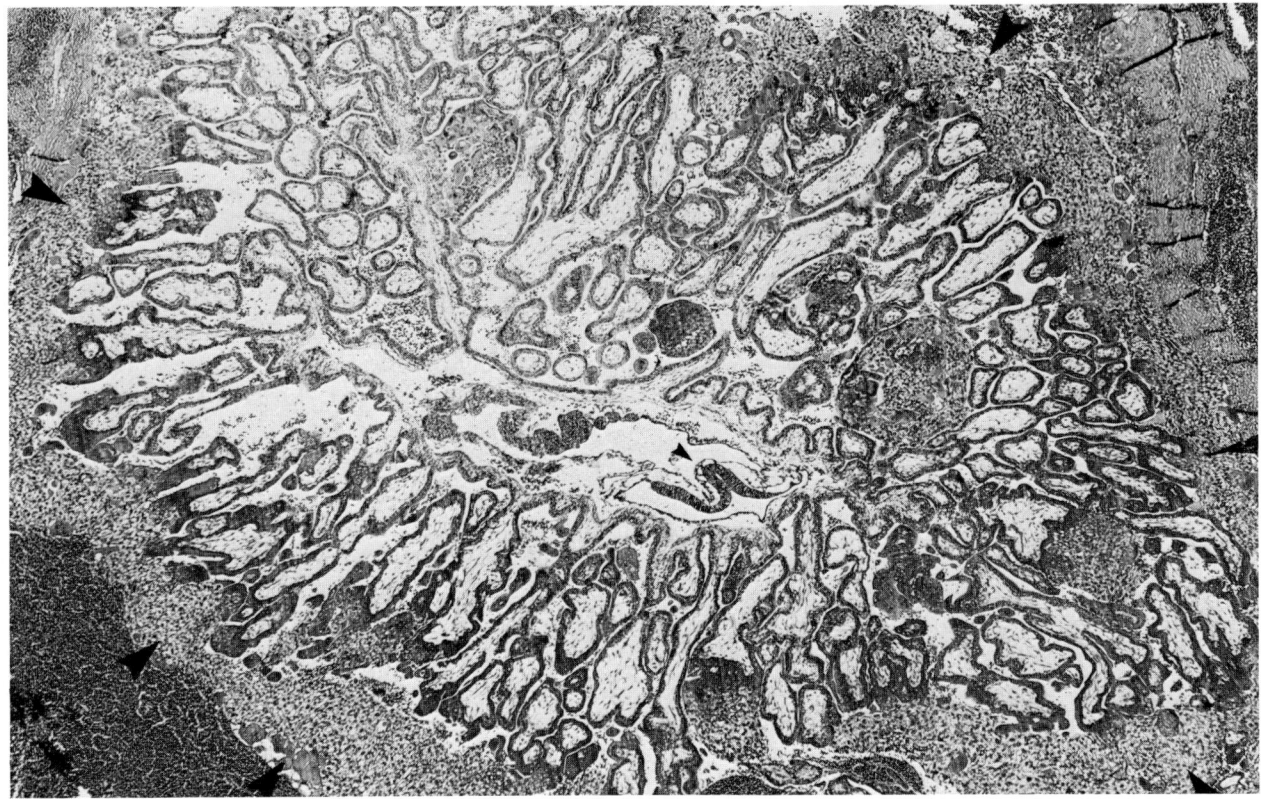

23.3

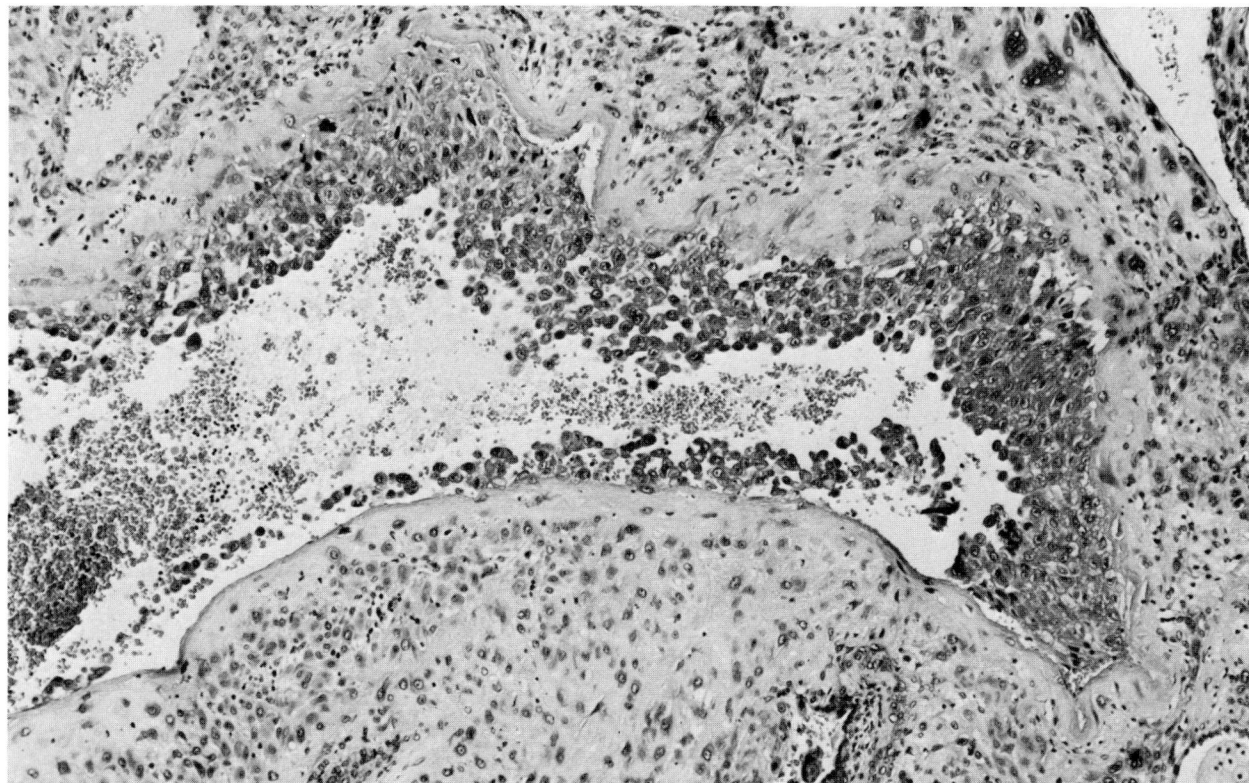

FIG. 23.4. Normal physiologic changes in a spiral artery. The replacement of maternal endothelium by intermediate trophoblast and destruction of the media with deposition of fibrinoid material result in marked vascular dilatation. (Reproduced by permission from Kraus, Frederick T: Female Genitalia. In: Kissane JM (ed) Anderson's Pathology, ed. 8, St. Louis, 1985, The C.V. Mosby Co.)

laeve (smooth chorion). Remnants of these atrophic villi are still apparent in sections of the extraplacental membranes of the mature placenta (Fig. 23.5). The chorion frondosum, those villi on the embryonic aspect of the chorion that directly contact the decidua basalis, continue to proliferate and form the definitive placenta. Departure from this orderly process of growth and regression is thought to result in some of the abnormal forms of placentation described below. In time, the chorionic cavity also is obliterated by progressive enlargement of the amnion.

Septae appear in the placenta at about 3 months. These are composed of irregular folds of the basal plate that are drawn into the intervillous space by the relatively slow growth of the anchoring villi. The cells islands in the septae have been referred to as X cells, but more recently have

FIG. 23.2. Secondary villi. Solid cytotrophoblastic cores are penetrated by mesenchyme. (Reproduced by permission from Kraus, Frederick T: Female Genitalia. In: Kissane JM (ed) Anderson's Pathology, ed. 8, St. Louis, 1985, The C.V. Mosby Co.)

FIG. 23.3. Cytotrophoblastic shelf. Complete cytotrophoblastic shell (*large arrows*) surrounds the entire conceptus. Portions of the germ disk and yolk sac are present at center (*small arrow*).

been identified as intermediate trophoblast. The septae partition the maternal surface incompletely and irregularly into 15 to 20 divisions that have no physiologic significance.

The identification and immunocytochemical localization of pregnancy-specific [human chorionic gonadotropin (hCG), human placental lactogen (hPL), pregnancy-specific beta 1-glycoprotein (SP$_1$)] and pregnancy-associated [pregnancy-associated plasma protein A (PAPP-A)] hormones have resulted in some interesting observations about the process of normal development and maturation of the placenta.[174,208,209,335,388] Not only have these studies confirmed the unique, biochemical, and functional features of the intermediate trophoblast, but they also have defined a changing ratio and pattern of distribution of these hormones in various stages of development, suggesting a linkage between hormone biosynthesis and degree of trophoblastic differentiation.[174,208] In normal placentas, all hormones (hCG, hPL, and SP$_1$) are distributed most widely in the syncytiotrophoblast. The intermediate trophoblast, however, contains a considerable amount of both hPL and SP$_1$ throughout pregnancy as well as a small amount of hCG early in gestation. After the first trimester, there is a marked diminution of hCG in both the syncytiotrophoblast and intermediate trophoblast. In contrast, both hPL and SP$_1$ increase during the second and third

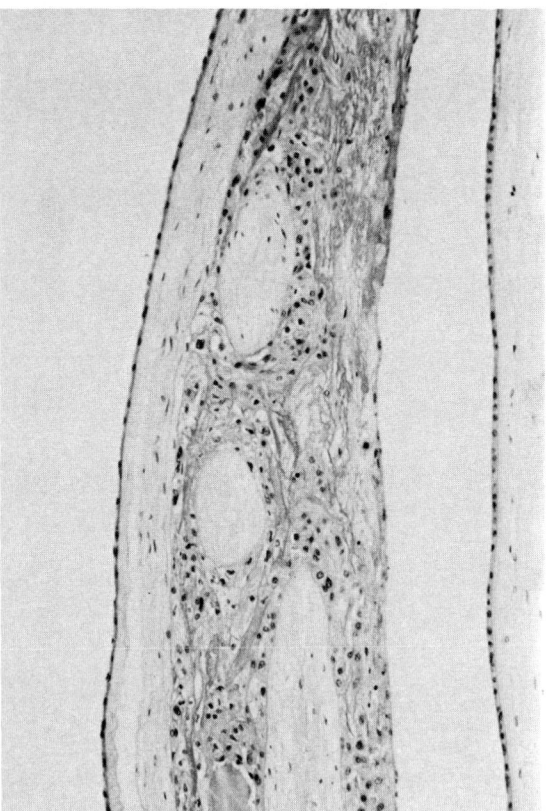

FIG. 23.5. **Chrion laeve.** Remnants of atrophic villi in the fetal membranes of a normal term gestation.

trimesters. None of these hormones is localized in the cytotrophoblast. Similar studies of hormone expression and distribution have been extended to some types of abnormal gestations (diabetes mellitus,[205] preeclampsia[108]) and trophoblastic disease.[68,174,209]

Anatomy and Circulation

The primary stem villi divide into secondary stem villi, which in turn give rise to the tertiary stem villi. These grow downward, insert onto the basal plate, and then reenter the intervillous space, where they branch to form the terminal villi. A smaller number of terminal villi may originate from the tertiary stem villi as they course toward the basal plate. The functional subunit referred to as a *lobule* is composed of villous parenchyma derived from a single secondary stem villus. The aggregate of villi derived from a primary stem villus defines the fetal cotyledon.

Deoxygenated fetal blood reaches the placenta through the two arteries of the umbilical cord. These branch and redivide in the stem villi until they ultimately terminate in the complex anastomosing capillary network of the terminal villi. It is at this interface, across capillary endothelium and attenuated trophoblast, that gas and nutrient exchange occurs. Oxygenated blood returns via venous tributaries to the umbilical vein.

Maternal blood enters the intervillous space through arterial inlets in the basal plate. The maternal blood flows toward the chorionic plate, disperses laterally, percolates around the villi, and exits through venous outlets in the placental floor. The exact anatomic relationship between the maternal arterial inlets in the basal plate and the fetal placental lobules is a matter of debate.

Maturation

The structure of the villi changes dramatically over the course of a normal gestation, but little is known about factors that influence placental maturation. Immature first trimester villi are large (170 μm in diameter) and are covered by two distinct layers of trophoblast, an inner layer of cytotrophoblast and an outer layer of syncytiotrophoblast. The villous stroma is very loose, and Hofbauer cells, the placental macrophages, are numerous. Blood vessels are small and centrally placed (Fig. 23.6).

Second trimester villi average 70 μm in diameter. The syncytiotrophoblastic layer is thinner, and the nuclei are less evenly dispersed. The cytotrophoblast does not form a continuous layer and is, in fact, difficult to identify with the light microscope after 16 weeks. The villous stroma is more compact and collagenized. Hofbauer cells are less conspicuous. Villous capillaries are larger, more numerous, and are peripherally located (Fig. 23.7).

Third trimester, mature, terminal villi are smaller still (average 40 μm in diameter). The syncytiotrophoblastic nuclei are irregularly aggregated to form knots, leaving between them stretches of anucleated and attenuated syncytiotrophoblastic cytoplasm (Fig. 23.8). Syncytial knots normally are found in about 30% of mature terminal villi. The stroma of the terminal villus is reduced to thin strands compressed between numerous dilated capillaries. The fetal capillaries protrude beneath and fuse with the overlying thinned syncytiotrophoblast, forming vasculosyncytial membranes (Fig. 23.9). It is in these areas that the closest approximation of fetal and maternal circulations occurs.

FIG. 23.6. **Large, immature first trimester villi (8 weeks).** The villous stroma is loose, Hofbauer cells are numerous, and the villous vessels are small and central in location. Two distinct layers of trophoblast are apparent.

FIG. 23.7. **Smaller, second trimester villi.** The villous stroma is more compact. Villous capillaries are larger and more numerous. The syncytiotrophoblastic nuclei are less evenly dispersed, and the cytotrophoblast is inconspicuous.

FIG. 23.8. **Third trimester villi.** In cross-section, third trimester villi are composed primarily of fetal capillaries with only a small amount of compressed intervening stroma.

FIG. 23.9. **Third trimester villi, vasculosyncytial membranes.** Syncytiotrophoblastic nuclei aggregate to form knots. Fetal capillaries protrude beneath and fuse with the anucleate syncytiotrophoblast to form vasculosyncytial membranes (*arrows*).

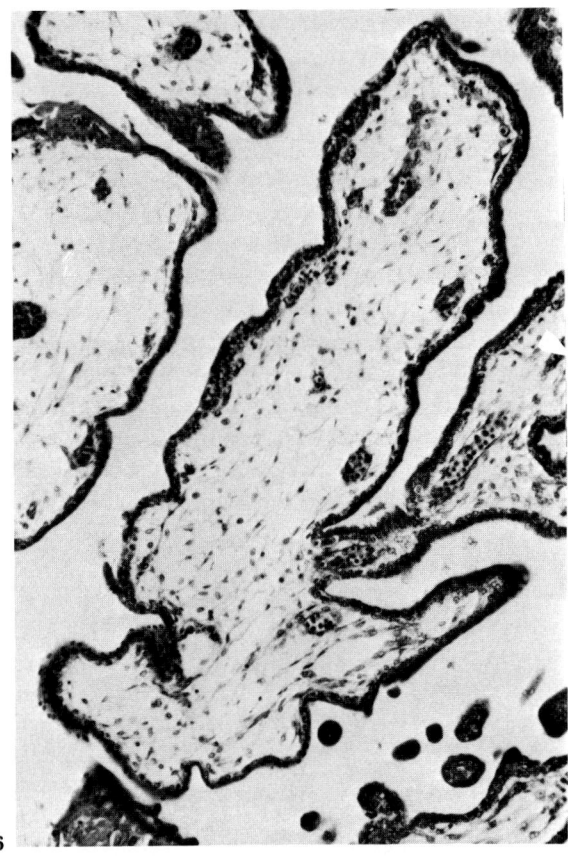

23.6

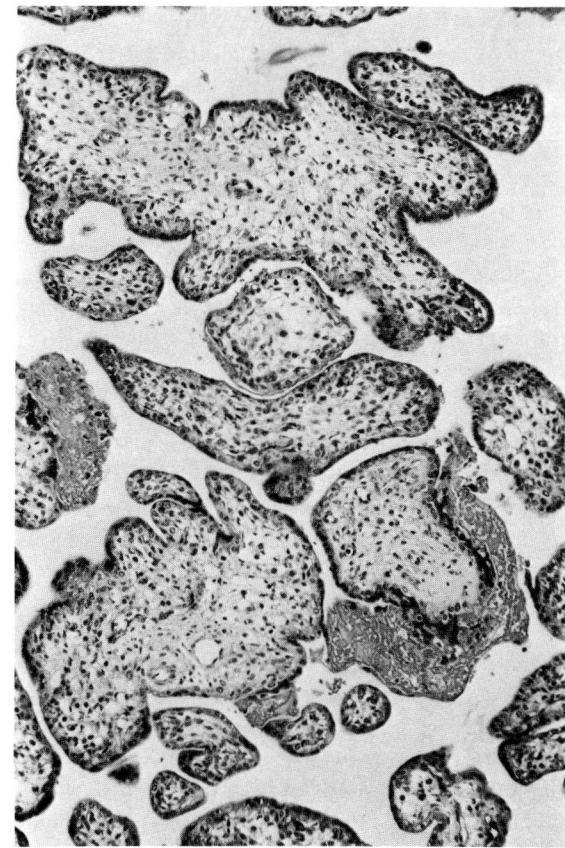

23.7

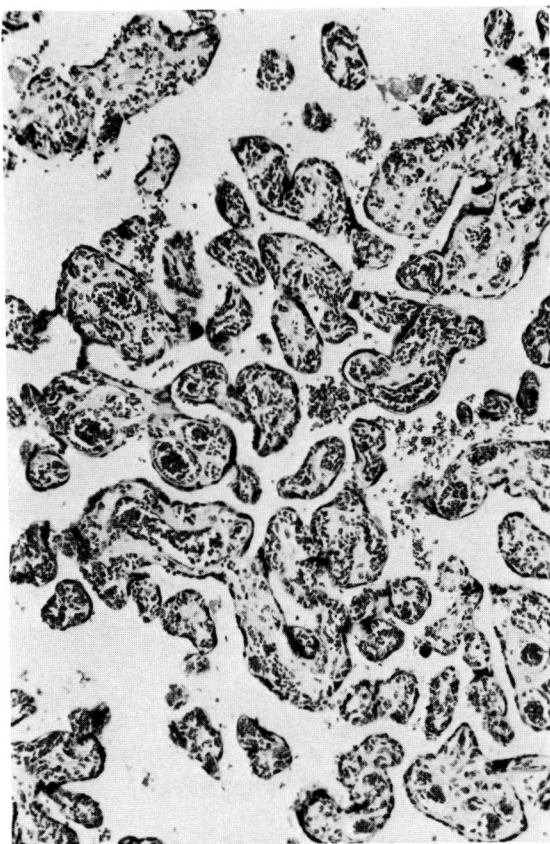

23.8

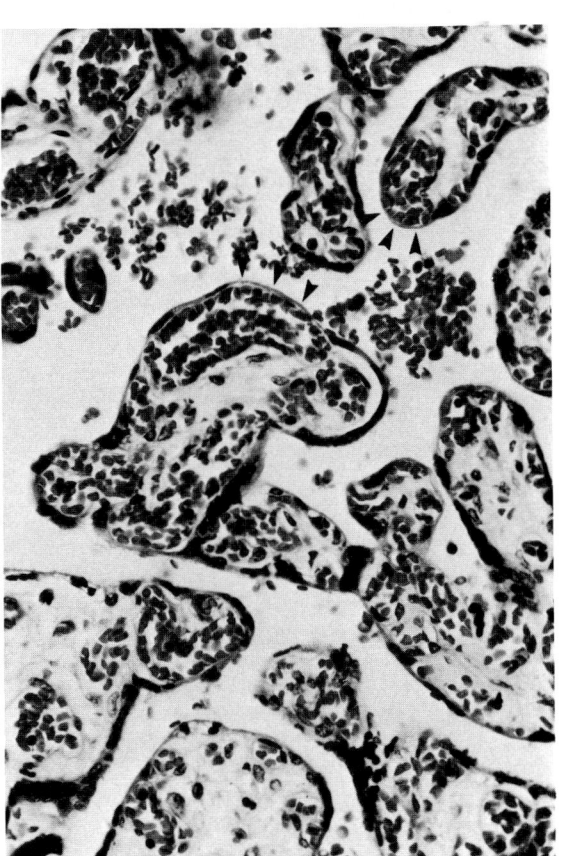

23.9

The maturation process, then, combines a reduction in thickness of syncytiotrophoblast, a diminution in cytotrophoblast, a decrease in mean villous diameter, and apposition of fetal capillaries to the villous surface, all of which reduce the barrier between maternal and fetal circulations.

The villi within any placenta are not completely homogeneous in appearance. The peripheral villi and those located near the chorionic plate tend to be smaller, with more collagenous stroma and a thicker trophoblastic basement membrane. The villi located in the central portion of the fetal lobule tend to look less mature than those at the periphery.

Abnormalities of Placentation

Anomalous Shapes

Occasionally, the placenta may deviate from its usual round or oval discoid shape. The pathogenesis of these variations in shape is not understood. Among the many theories proposed is that these anomalies reflect a focal failure or disturbance of the normal process of orderly villous atrophy that occurs early in gestation.

One of the most common of these variations is the *accessory* or *succenturiate lobe*, a condition in which usually one mass but occasionally multiple discrete masses of placental tissue are separated from the main placenta (Fig. 23.10). The accessory lobe may be attached to the main placenta by a narrow isthmus of chorionic tissue or may be separated from it by only fetal membranes. The umbilical cord generally inserts into the main placental mass. The vascular supply to the accessory lobe runs on the fetal surface, in many cases through fetal membranes unsupported by any

underlying villous parenchyma. If these large intramembranous vessels are traumatized during delivery, severe fetal hemorrhage may result. Thrombosis of the intramembranous vessels may result in fetal thromboemboli and multiple brain infarcts (Fig. 23.11).[302] Occasionally, the accessory lobe may present as placenta previa or be retained in utero after delivery, resulting in postpartum bleeding or infection. Succenturiate lobes tend to infarct. The reported frequency of the accessory lobe is variable; Fox estimates that it occurs in about 3% of placentas.[132]

The *bilobate* or *bipartite* placenta consists of two equally sized placental lobes that may be separated by fetal membranes or connected to each other by a narrow isthmus of placental tissue. The umbilical cord usually inserts centrally between the lobes, either into the placental bridge or into the membranes. The clinical significance of this abnormality has not been extensively studied. Fugikura et al.[141] have noted that bilobate placentas occur more

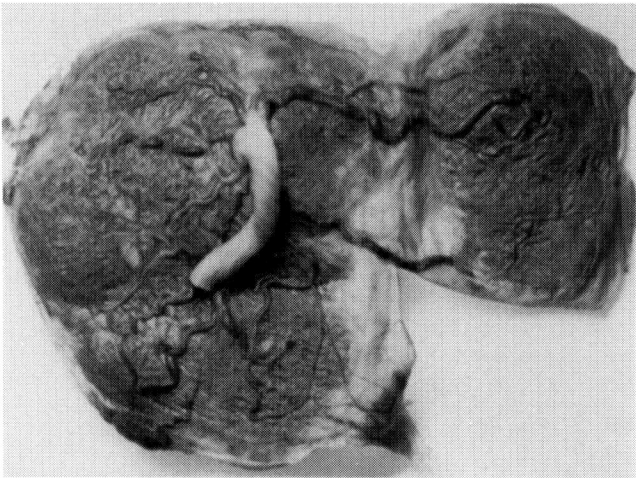

FIG. 23.10. Accessory (succenturiate) lobe. Discrete mass of placental tissue attached to the main placental mass by fetal membranes. Vascular supply to the accessory lobe must traverse unsupported membranes.

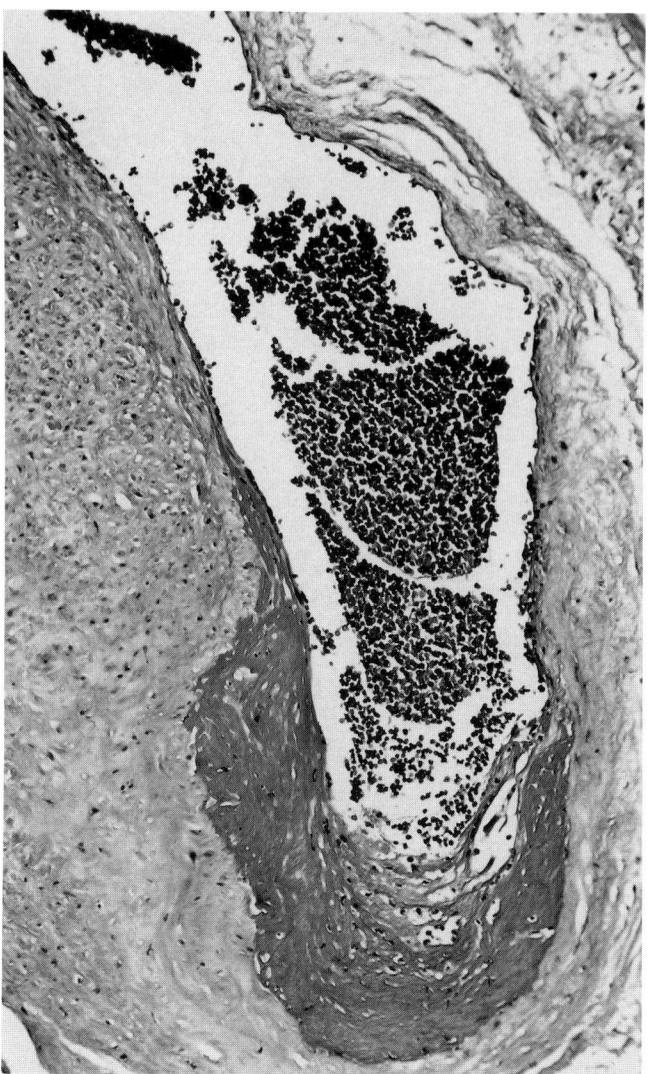

FIG. 23.11. Succenturiale lobe. This large membranous vessel supplying a succenturiate lobe contains a mural thrombus.

frequently in older women of high gravidity and in patients with a history of infertility. They also found a higher frequency of first trimester bleeding and undue placental adherence requiring manual extraction in association with bipartite placentation.

A variety of other anomalous shapes occur, but these are uncommon and are rarely encountered. The *multilobate* placenta is one consisting of three or more lobes of roughly equal size. *Placenta membranacea* is a large, thin placenta in which functional chorionic villi diffusely cover the entire gestational sac. The placental tissue may vary in thickness, but only exceptionally is there a dominant area resembling a placental disk. In the human, the placenta normally assumes this configuration in the first few weeks of development, but ultimately the villi oriented toward the uterine cavity atrophy (chorion laeve), leaving the chorion frondosum as the definitive placenta. In some animal species, the placenta is normally of this membranous type. Placenta membranacea in humans is extremely rare. In the few cases reported, obstetric complications, such as antepartum bleeding, have been frequent, undoubtedly relating to the obligate placenta previa that accompanies this form of placentation. *Ring-shaped placenta* also is a rare occurrence, in which the placenta is annular or cylindrical in shape. A *fenestrate placenta* is distinguished by a focal absence of villous parenchyma in the center of the placenta. The resulting defect may be a through-and-through hole, or the chorionic plate may remain intact over the parenchymal defect.

Circummarginate and Circumvallate Placenta (Extrachorial Placenta)

Circummarginate and circumvallate placenta is a common gross structural deviation in which the chorionic plate of the placenta is smaller than its basal plate. The transition from membranous to villous chorion occurs not at the placental margin as in a normal placenta but inside its circumference, some distance from the peripheral edge of the placenta. A ring of bare placental tissue (extrachorial portion) extends submerged into the decidua beyond the limits of the chorionic plate (Fig. 23.12).

CLINICAL FEATURES

The many theories attempting to explain the etiology and pathogenesis of extrachorial placentation have been summarized by Scott.[340] Estimates of the frequency of the condition vary widely (presumably because the terms are not used uniformly).

GROSS FINDINGS

The two types of extrachorial placenta, circummarginate and circumvallate, are categorized based on the nature of the transition from the membranous to the villous chorion.

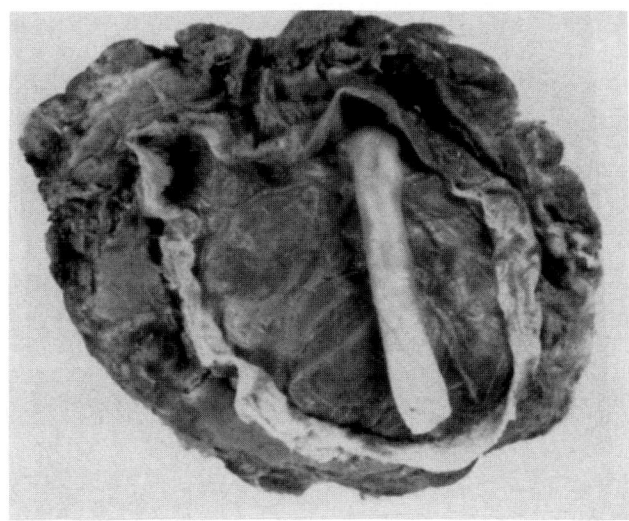

FIG. 23.12. Extrachorial placenta. The fetal membranes do not extend to the peripheral margin of the placenta, leaving a ring of placental tissue extending beyond the chorionic plate. (Reproduced by permission from Kraus, Frederick T: Gynecologic Pathology, St. Louis, 1967, The C.V. Mosby Co.)

Grossly, in circummarginate placentas, the transition is flat, whereas in circumvallate placentas, the marginal membrane ring is folded or rolled back on itself (Fig. 23.13). Variable amounts of fibrin and recent and old blood clot are found frequently at the margin. In both varieties, the fetal vessels appear to terminate at the margin of the chorionic plate (Fig. 23.14) but actually continue their course peripherally in the deeper villous tissue. These

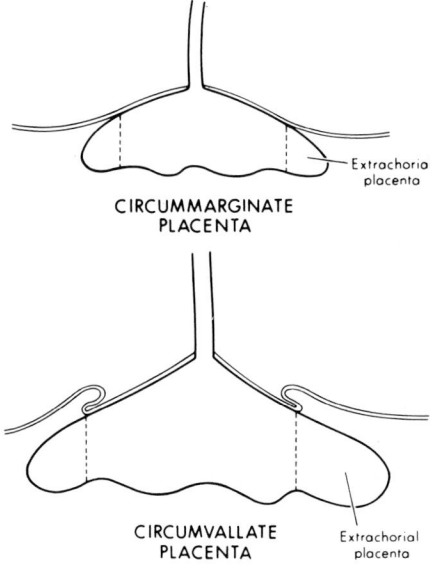

FIG. 23.13. Extrachorial placenta. Diagram comparing the rolled membrane ring in the circumvallate placenta to the flat transition in the circummarginate placenta. (After Fox, ref. 132.)

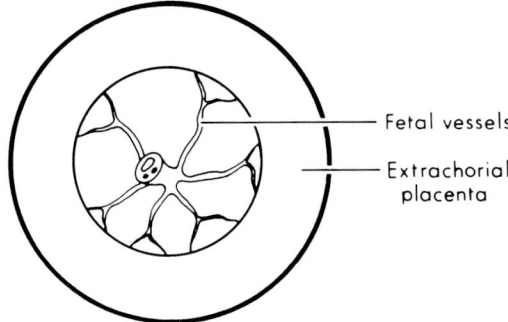

FIG. 23.14. Diagram of an extrachorial placenta, fetal side. Vessels appear to terminate at the margin of the chorionic plate but actually continue peripherally in the extrachorial portion. (After Fox, ref. 132.)

two forms of extrachorial placentas may be partial or complete (circumferential) and may occur in combination with one another.

CLINICAL BEHAVIOR AND TREATMENT

There is considerable disagreement concerning the clinical relevance of extrachorial placentation. Most agree that extrachorial placentas are more common in multigravidas.[46,134,402] An increased frequency of antepartum bleeding, premature labor, fetal hypoxia, and perinatal mortality has been reported in circumvallate placenta.[46,134,213,271,340,416] Both partial and complete forms of circumvallate placentas are associated with an unduly high proportion of low birth weight babies.[134,318] Recurrence of circumvallate placentation in successive pregnancies has been reported.[408]

Placenta Accreta, Increta, and Percreta

Placenta accreta, increta, and percreta are defined clinically as an abnormal adherence of the placenta to the uterine wall so that separation does not occur after delivery of the newborn. In these abnormal forms of implantation, placental villi adhere directly to (placenta accreta), invade into (placenta increta), or penetrate through (placenta percreta) the myometrium. Commonly, the degree of placental invasiveness is not uniform, and as a practical matter, the term *placenta accreta* is used often to encompass all degrees of abnormal placental adherence or invasiveness. The condition may be total (involving the entire placenta), partial (involving one or more cotyledons), or focal (involving isolated foci of the placenta).

CLINICAL FEATURES

The true frequency of placenta accreta is difficult to determine. Reported figures have varied widely from 1 in 1667

to 1 in 70,000 pregnancies.[67] In studying a large number of cases reported in the literature, Fox emphasized the particular tendency for placenta accreta to occur in multigravid and obstetrically elderly women.[131] There is frequent reference to previous placental retention requiring manual removal in these patients. A number of predisposing factors have been related to this condition; the two most significant are placenta previa and previous cesarean section (Fig. 23.15). As many as 64% of patients with placenta accreta have had associated placenta previa in some reports,[67] and many placenta previa accretas occur in cesarean section scars.[250,372] In some cases of partial placenta accreta, only that portion of the placenta implanted over the lower uterine segment or cesarean section scar has been abnormally adherent.[387] A smaller number of patients have a history of previous uterine curettage,[146] uterine sepsis, previous manual removal of the placenta, cornual implantation, leiomyomas, or uterine malformation. The common end point in all these conditions is presumably a deficiency in or absence of the decidua. Alternatively, some authors have suggested that placenta accreta is due to an abnormal invasiveness of the placenta rather than to an inadequate decidua.

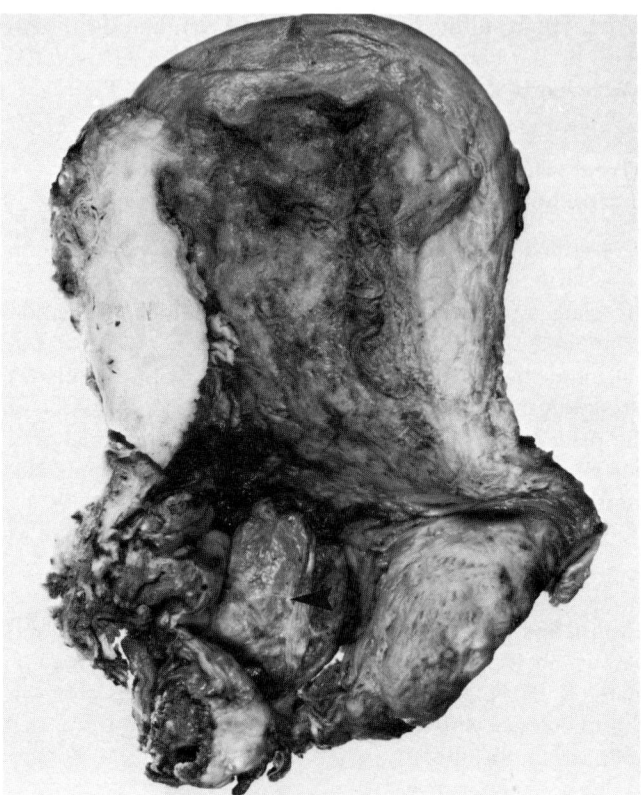

FIG. 23.15. Placenta percreta. Penetration of the placenta through the myometrium at the site of three previous cesarean sections (*lower left* portion of the specimen). A portion of the chorionic plate is indicated by the *arrowhead*.

MICROSCOPIC FINDINGS

Microscopically, the cardinal feature is partial or complete absence of the decidua basalis.[236] The region normally occupied by decidua is replaced by loose connective tissue. The decidua parietalis may be normal but is commonly absent as well. Placental villi adhere directly to or actually invade the myometrium without intervening decidua (Fig. 23.16). The villi usually are separated partially from focally hyalinized myometrial smooth muscle cells by a layer of fibrin. Abnormalities in the pattern of physiologic changes in the uteroplacental vasculature have been reported in placenta accreta.[53,199] The diagnosis is made most often in a hysterectomy specimen but rarely may be confirmed by examining the placenta itself. In either situation, evaluation is difficult, since the specimen usually is distorted markedly by the disruptive effects of attempts to remove the adherent placenta at the time of delivery.

CLINICAL BEHAVIOR AND TREATMENT

Clinically, the condition is compatible with normal fetal development and most commonly is suspected only after delivery. Failure of separation of the placenta in the third stage of labor and postpartum bleeding, often life-threat-ening, are the cardinal clinical signs of placenta accreta. Antepartum bleeding and premature labor also are common; these are due principally to the high frequency of associated placenta previa. Uterine rupture may occur at any stage of pregnancy or during labor.[63,372] The overall maternal mortality has dropped from 37%[179] to 2–3% in more recent series.[67,250] Hysterectomy may be necessary, although conservative treatment has been successful in some cases.[234,387]

Multiple Pregnancy

There are a number of excellent and detailed accounts describing various aspects of multiple pregnancy.[5,41–44] These are recommended to supplement the abbreviated coverage of the subject presented here.

Twin Gestation

Twins may arise from the fertilization of two separate ova (dizygotic or fraternal twins) or from the division of a single fertilized ovum (monozygotic or identical twins). Monozygotic twins are genetically and almost always phenotypically identical, but occasionally they may be phenotypically

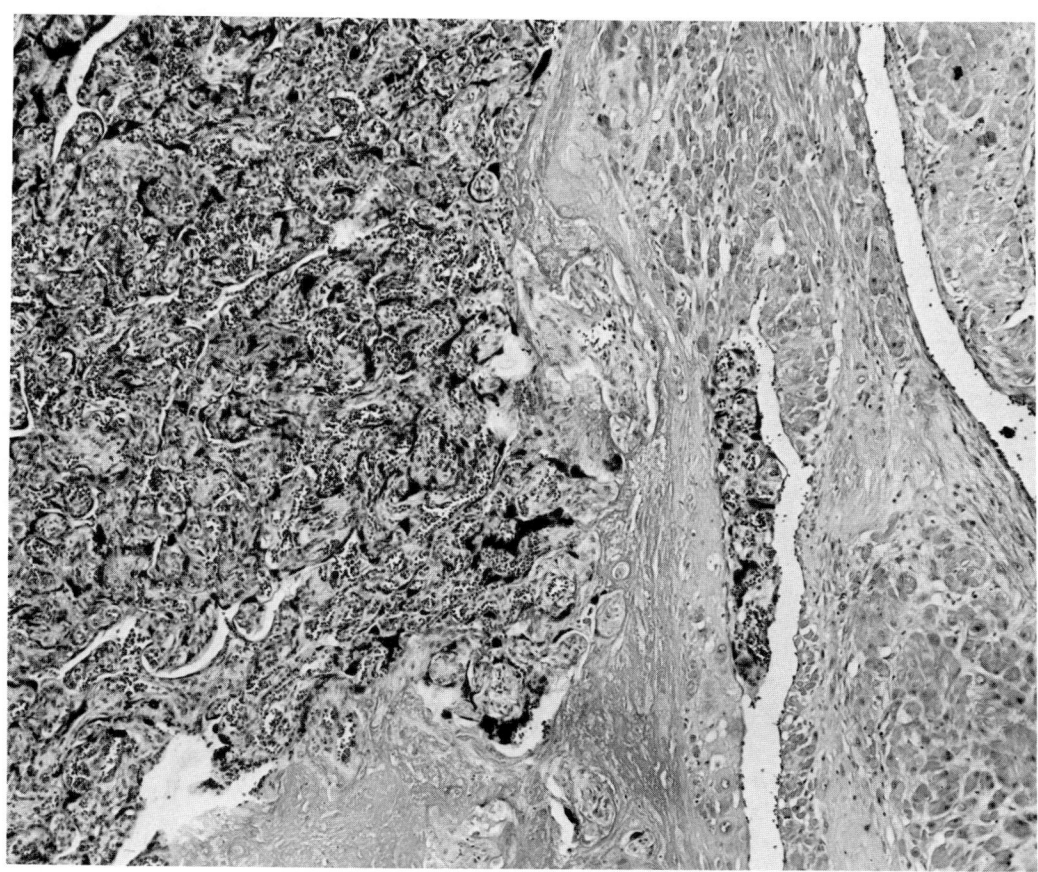

FIG. 23.16. Placenta accreta. Chorionic villi adherent to myometrium without intervening decidua.

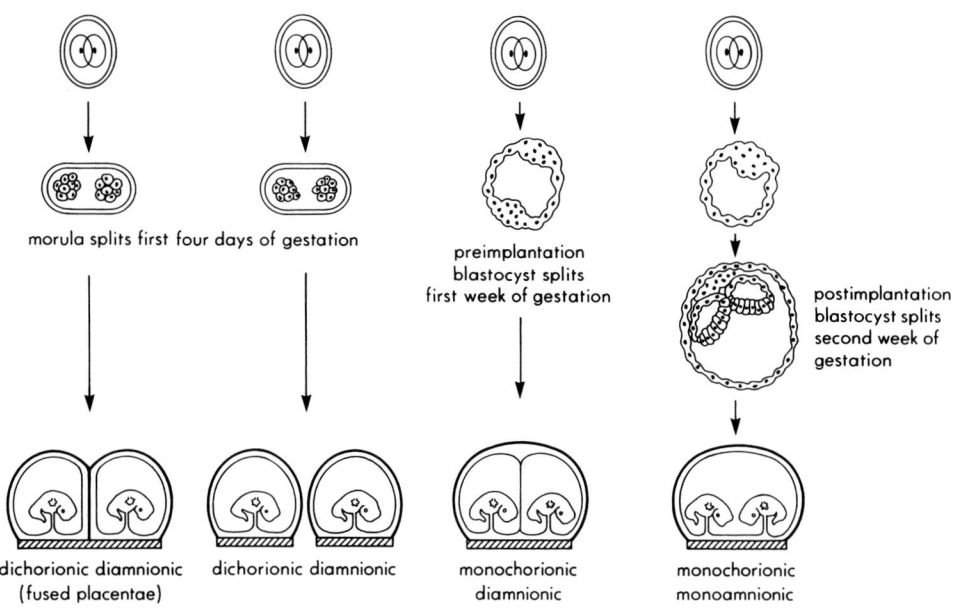

Fig. 23.17. Diagrammatic representation of the placentation of monochorionic twins. (Adapted from Fox H (1978) Pathology of the Placenta, Philadelphia: WB Saunders, ref. 132.)

quite discordant.[158,183] Dizygotic twins are no more genetically similar than other singleton siblings.

The frequency of monozygous twinning is relatively constant worldwide (about 3.5 in 1000 pregnancies). The marked geographical differences in total twinning rate reflect the greater predisposition for multiple ovulation in some populations and families than in others. There is a strong hereditary element in dizygous twinning, and there is some evidence that this may be related to increased endogenous levels of follicle-stimulating hormone (FSH). Multiple ovulation also may be induced by the administration of clomiphene or a combination of FSH with luteinizing hormone (LH) or hCG. The occurrence of twins in Caucasians in the United States is about 1 in 80 pregnancies, and about one-third of these are monozygotic.

There are basically two types of placentas in twin gestations, monochorionic and dichorionic. All dizygotic twins have dichorionic placentas; in double ovulation, two blastocysts implant, each generating a separate placenta with chorion and amnion [diamnionic–dichorionic (DiDi)] (Fig. 23.17). If these implantations occur close together, varying degrees of fusion are common (DiDi fused). Otherwise, DiDi placentas are entirely separate. Monozygotic twins may show any type of placentation depending on when division occurs (Fig. 23.17). If the single fertilized ovum divides very early, before differentiation of the chorion (first 2 or 3 days), two separate embryos, each with its own placenta (DiDi), will develop. If splitting occurs in the blastocyst stage, after formation of the chorion but before formation of the amnion (3rd–8th day after fertilization), the twins will develop a single placenta with two amnionic sacs [diamnionic–monochorionic (DiMo)]. A

split between the 8th and 13th days after fertilization will result in one placenta and only one amnionic cavity [monoamnionic–monochorionic (MoMo)]. Later splitting will result in conjoined twins.

All twins with a monochorionic placenta are monozygotic. Dichorionic placentation, however, may result from either dizygous or monozygous twinning. Obviously, different fetal sex establishes a dizygous relation. Blood group analysis, HLA typing, or other modes of investigation may be necessary to determine zygosity in like-sex dichorionic twins. The frequency of different types of twin placentation in a study of 250 consecutive twin deliveries is summarized in Table 23.1.[41]

Establishment of the type of placentation is important, not only as the initial step in the determination of zygosity but also because of its significant impact on perinatal morbidity and mortality. Perinatal mortality is much higher in twins than in single pregnancies. An overall mortality of 14% was documented in one study of 250 consecutive twin births.[41] In the same study, twins with monochorionic placentation had a higher perinatal mortality (25.9%) than those with dichorionic placentas (8.9%). The most impor-

Table 23.1. Frequency of different types of placentation in 250 consecutive twin deliveries

77 Monochorionic (31%)	173 Dichorionic (69%) by blood group analysis
3 MoMo (1%)	33 Monozygotic (13%)
74 DiMo (30%)	140 Dizygotic (56%)

Reprinted by permission of Benirschke and Driscoll, ref. 41.

tant factor contributing to this increased death rate is premature onset of labor and delivery. An increased frequency of hydramnios, maternal hypertension, twin-twin transfusion syndrome, and congenital fetal anomalies also contribute to the excessive perinatal death rate in twin gestations. Monoamnionic placentation is associated with highest rate of fetal mortality.[42,284,385,406] Reported perinatal mortality rates range from 33% to nearly 70%.[406] A significant factor in this mortality rate is the high frequency of cord complications. Twisting and knotting of the two umbilical cords is a very common occurrence.[284,385]

In examining the twin placenta, the pathologist should attempt to (1) define the type of placentation (dichorionic vs. monochorionic) and (2) demonstrate the type and number of vascular anastomoses if they are present (see below). If two entirely separate placentas are delivered, they obviously are dichorionic, and each requires routine examination. Practically speaking, the principal task for the pathologist is to distinguish between a DiMo placenta and a DiDi fused placenta. In dichorionic placentas, chorionic tissue is present in the septum between the amnionic cavities. This is absent in the DiMo placenta. Grossly, the chorionic tissue makes the septum appear opaque (DiDi fused); in its absence, the septum appears more translucent (DiMo). Histological examination of a roll of the membranous septum will show two layers of amnion separated by two layers of chorion in dichorionic placentas (Fig. 23.18). The septum will consist solely of two layers of amnion in monochorionic placentas (Fig. 23.19). Identical information may be obtained by examination of a section including the T zone, that portion of the placenta where the septum meets the fetal surface. This is an alternative method for examining the septum in cases in which the septal membranes have been torn or otherwise distorted and cannot be rolled (see Chapter 30, Gross Description, Processing, and Reporting of Gynecologic and Obstetric Specimens).

When the dividing membranes are peeled apart, the two amnions are readily stripped from one another in the DiMo placenta, leaving no trace of the T zone on the fetal surface. On the other hand, there is always a separate layer of chorion inserting at the base of the septum in the DiDi fused placenta that persists after the amnions are stripped away.

The distribution of the fetal vessels also is helpful in distinguishing DiDi fused from DiMo placentas. In dichorionic placentas, fetal vessels on the chorionic plate approach, but do not cross, the area of fusion (Fig. 23.20). In most DiMo placentas, the two vascular districts are imperceptibly merged, and portions are shared by both fetuses (Fig. 23.21).

An important feature of monochorionic placentas is the presence of vascular communications between the two fetal circulations. Although estimates of the frequency of this phenomenon differ somewhat, it is generally agreed that they occur in essentially all monochorionic placentas.

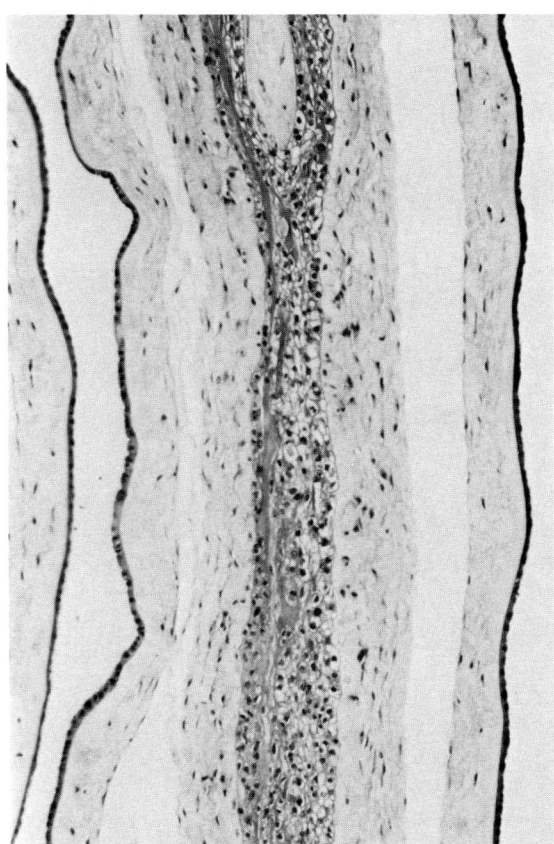

FIG. 23.18. DiDi fused twin placenta. Histologic section of the septal membranes shows separation of the two amnions by a central layer of chorionic tissue.

These vascular communications may be superficial, between the large vessels on the fetal surface or deep within the placental substance. Most superficial anastomoses are between the arteries (Fig. 23.21). Vein-to-vein anastomoses are much less common. Of greater physiologic importance are the arteriovenous anastomoses that occur deep within the capillary bed of a shared cotyledon. Arteriovenous anastomoses are very common, but the physiologic consequences of these communications vary greatly depending on their size, number, and overall balance of blood flow. Vascular communications in DiDi fused placentas are absent as a rule, although vascular anastomoses of various types have been reported rarely.[78,215,300,311]

To demonstrate the possible presence of vascular communications, the amnionic membranes should be stripped from the placenta. This facilitates the study of vessels on the fetal surface. The distribution of the fetal blood vessels does not necessarily conform to the division of placental tissue indicated by the line of insertion of the dividing membranes. Anastomoses, therefore, do not always lie directly beneath the insertion of the septal membranes. Large, superficial anastomoses often are easily identified

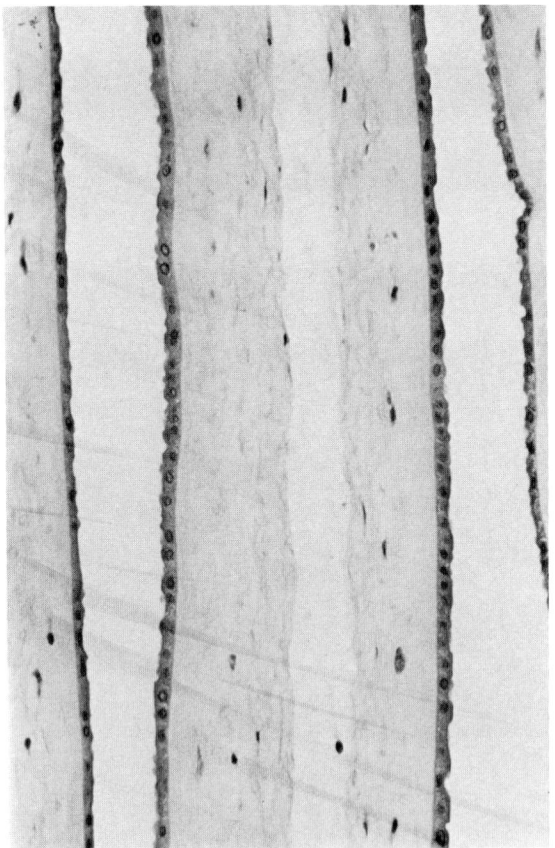

FIG. 23.19. DiMo twin placenta. Septal membranes are composed of only two amnions without intervening chorionic tissue.

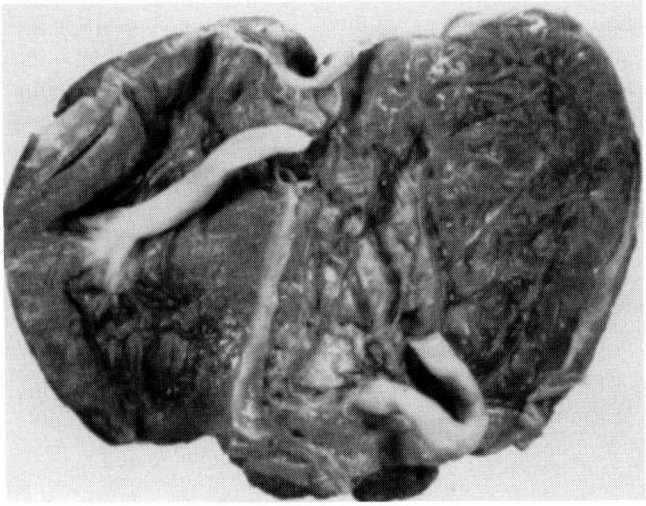

FIG. 23.20. DiDi fused twin placenta. The two placental masses are fused but discrete. Fetal vessels do not approach or cross the area of fusion.

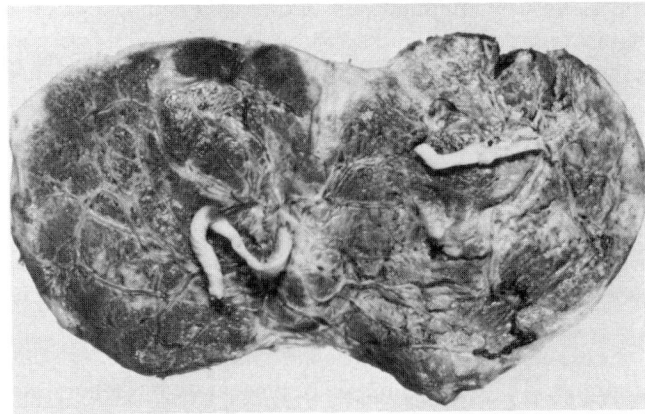

FIG. 23.21. DiMo twin placenta. Central merging of the two vascular districts with anastomoses of superficial vessels. (Reproduced by permission from Kraus, Frederick T: Gynecologic Pathology, St. Louis, 1967, The C.V. Mosby Co.)

grossly on the fetal surface and can be highlighted by the injection of milk or colored dye. Identification of the deep arteriovenous anastomoses is more important and more difficult. These anastomoses cannot be identified on gross examination. Various methods have been used to document arteriovenous communications, including radiologic examination after the vascular injection of radiopaque dye[78] or injection of colored plastic followed by preparation of a corrosion specimen. These techniques are relatively difficult and time consuming. A simpler method is to inject colored saline, milk, or a colloidal dye solution[311] into an arterial branch of one twin's vascular territory and to determine whether it returns to the same infant or to its co-twin. This procedure can be repeated at multiple sites in an attempt to document the nature and number of anastomoses. Unfortunately, areas of villous disruption will cause leakage of fluid and compromise the usefulness of this technique. The perfusion pressure also is important. False positive anastomoses may be created by unphysiologically high perfusion pressure, whereas lower pressures may fail to demonstrate existing communications.[311] It should be emphasized that such studies are merely qualitative and do not necessarily reflect the physiologic significance of the anastomoses in vivo.

TWIN–TWIN TRANSFUSION SYNDROME

A major cause of perinatal mortality in monochorionic twins is the twin–twin transfusion syndrome.[300] Schatz proposed the now widely accepted concept that the twin–twin transfusion syndrome results when there is an unbalanced flow of blood from the donor twin to the recipient twin through arteriovenous anastomoses deep within shared placental lobules (the "third circulation"). Arteriovenous anastomoses may be multiple and may proceed in opposite directions, creating a complex hemodynamic state with great variation in clinical expression.[42]

CLINICAL FEATURES AND PATHOLOGIC FINDINGS

Typically, the twin–twin transfusion syndrome manifests itself in the second trimester with acute hydramnios and growth discrepancy between the twins. Unidirectional diversion of significant amounts of blood results in relative deprivation and growth retardation of the donor as compared to the larger recipient. Hydramnios, usually associated with the recipient, may become sufficiently severe to cause maternal discomfort or respiratory embarrassment. The donor twin frequently exhibits oligohydramnios and decreased movement, and is sometimes referred to as the "stuck twin."

Postnatally, there is a marked discrepancy in the size and appearance of the infants and their corresponding placental segments. The donor twin is smaller, pale, and anemic, whereas the recipient is heavier, edematous, plethoric, and polycythemic. Either twin may be hydropic. Classically, there is marked discordance in the size and weight of the fetal organs, the organs of the recipient being larger and heavier than those of the donor. In the recipient twin, the heart is grossly enlarged and microscopically, there is myocardial hypertrophy involving all chambers, as well as increased smooth muscle mass in the media of the pulmonary and systemic arteries and arterioles. The heart of the donor twin usually is subnormal in size, and the arterial muscle mass is decreased. Glomeruli are enlarged, up to twice normal size, in the recipient twin, and they are either reduced or normal in size in the donor.[257]

The placental territories of the donor and recipient twins also may be quite discrepant.[3,327] The donor portion of the placenta greatly resembles the placenta in Rh incompatibility both grossly and microscopically. It is large, bulky, and pale (Fig. 23.22). The villi are large and edematous, with numerous Hofbauer cells and small capillaries containing nucleated red blood cells (Fig. 23.23). The recipient placental territory is generally smaller, firm, and deep red. The villous capillaries are somewhat dilated and intensely congested, and the villi are more mature. (Fig. 23.23)[5,88] When there is oligohydramnios, amnion nodosum may be found in the sac of the donor member.

The clinical definition of the syndrome is not precise.[92] A combination of hematologic and anatomic criteria is generally used. A difference in hemoglobin concentration of greater than 5 g/100 ml between the twins was considered valid for definitive diagnosis by Rausen et al.[300] Others require a weight difference of 15–20%.[60] The diagnosis is difficult because monochorionic twins may show asymmetric growth for reasons other than the twin–twin transfusion syndrome. Furthermore, plethora of one twin and anemia of the other do not always signify the chronic twin–twin

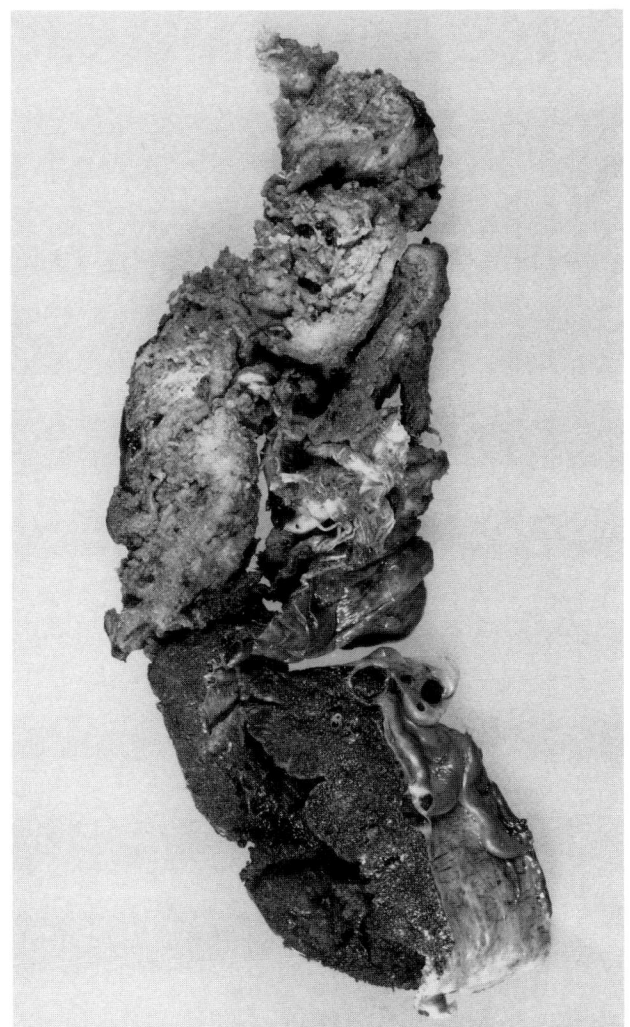

FIG. 23.22. Placenta, twin-twin transfusion syndrome. The donor portion (*top*) of this twin gestation complicated by the twin–twin transfusion syndrome is pale in comparison to the congested, darker recipient portion (*bottom*). Only a portion of the donor's placental territory, which was approximately three times the size of the recipient's territory, is included in this photograph.

transfusion syndrome, but instead sometimes reflect acute shifts of blood through large superficial anastomoses that may occur when pressure relations change at the time of delivery. The classic expression of a chronic twin–twin transfusion, then, may be greatly complicated or obscured by the superimposition of an acute transfusion.[35] The concomitant presence of superficial large vessel anastomoses may modify or compensate for the hemodynamic imbalance created by deep arteriovenous anastomoses.

The difficulty in establishing a uniform, clear definition of the twin–twin transfusion syndrome explains, in part, the discrepancies in frequency with which the twin–twin transfusion syndrome is reported to complicate DiMo pla-

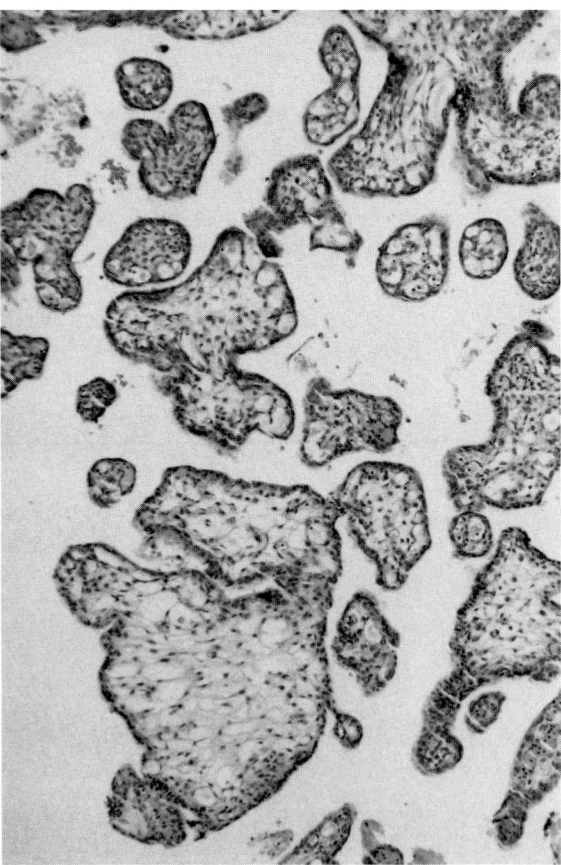

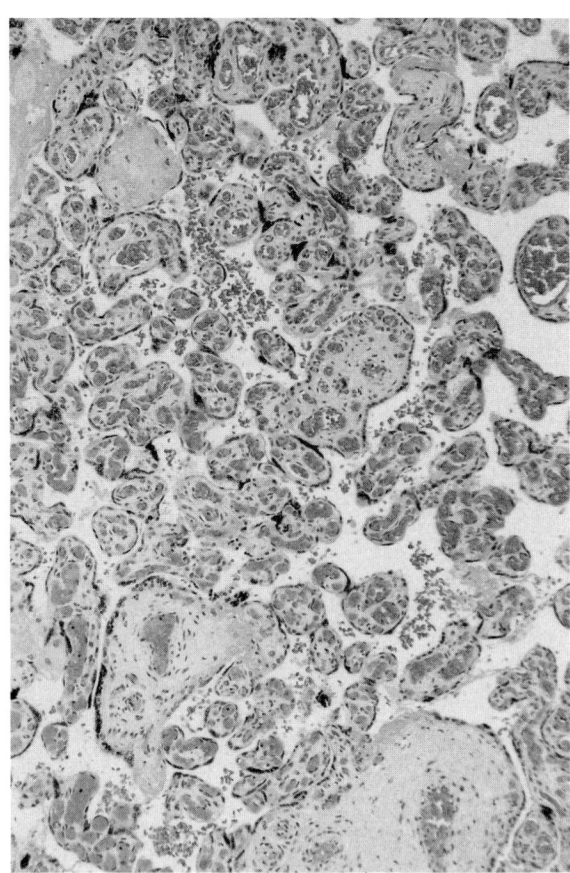

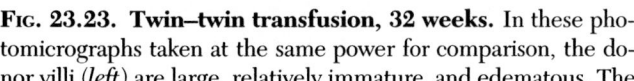

Fig. 23.23. Twin–twin transfusion, 32 weeks. In these photomicrographs taken at the same power for comparison, the donor villi (*left*) are large, relatively immature, and edematous. The

fetal capillaries contain numerous red blood cells precursors. The recipient villi (*right*) are more mature and congested.

centation; estimates vary from 15% to 30%.[300,371] Whatever the true frequency, the twin–twin transfusion syndrome obviously does not occur as often as one would anticipate given the universal presence of vascular communications in monochorionic twin pregnancies. The twin–twin transfusion syndrome is not a significant cause of fetal mortality in monoamnionic twins.[406]

CLINICAL BEHAVIOR AND TREATMENT

The consequences of the twin–twin transfusion syndrome are grave. Mortality rates may be as high as 70–100%, depending on the gestational age at diagnosis and delivery.[33,153,345] When the condition develops in the second trimester, it is usually associated with preterm labor and death of one or both fetuses before viability or significant morbidity if the neonates survive. Both twins are at great risk. The recipient twin is subject to cardiac failure, hemolytic jaundice, kernicterus, and thrombosis due to hemoconcentration. The donor twin may be severely anemic or hypoglycemic.

If one twin dies in utero, the transfusion may cease and the situation may resolve. Alternatively, the surviving twin may nearly exsanguinate acutely into the suddenly relaxed circulatory system of the dead twin.[221] In addition, multiorgan necrotic lesions may occur in the surviving twin after death of a co-twin in utero.[80,91,92,117,189,377,413] It has been suggested that these lesions result from tissue thromboplastins or thromboemboli crossing from the dead twin to the survivor via vascular anastomoses,[34,175] although antenatal necrosis of cerebral white matter also may occur when neither twin dies. Multiple placental vascular connections may result in altered hemodynamics associated with transitory cardiovascular compromise or hyperfibrinogenemia and thromboembolism resulting in damage to one or both twins.

Management options are limited and frequently unsuccessful. Serial amniocenteses, maternal digoxin treatment, intrauterine ligation of one umbilical cord, and selected feticide have been attempted in severe cases.[29,110] A successful outcome has been reported in a few cases of severe twin–twin transfusion syndrome following Yag laser ablation of vascular communications[96] or inadvertent puncture of the vessels.[394] Doppler studies may be helpful in evaluating the results of intervention in the twin–twin transfusion syndrome.[122,148,296]

ACARDIA

The development of acardiac fetuses (monsters) is another complication of monochorionic implantation involving a particular type of vascular anastomosis. This anomaly occurs in about 1% of monozygotic twin gestations. The acardius is a bizarre and grossly malformed fetus that lacks a functioning heart and is perfused and sustained entirely by its normal twin (Fig. 23.24).[62,150,276,344,409] It may be small or large (up to 3500 g) and is attached to the placenta by an umbilical cord, usually containing one artery and one vein. These fetuses differ greatly in gross appearance and degree of organogenesis; some are amorphous, shapeless masses, others have rudimentary trunk and limb development, and still others are remarkably well developed. Elements of myocardial tissue may or may not be present providing the basis for the subdivision of acardiacs into two categories: (1) holoacardius—denoting complete absence of myocardial elements, and (2) hemiacardius—indicating the presence of some myocardial tissue.

Regardless of the state of cardiac and bodily development, circulation to all acardiacs is accomplished by the co-twin. Blood flows to the acardius in a reverse course, from the heart of the normal twin, through a large placental artery–artery anastomosis, and into the umbilical artery of the acardius. After coursing through the acardius, blood returns via its umbilical vein and into the circulatory system of the normal twin through a large placental vein–vein anastomosis.

There are two main theories of pathogenesis: (1) the reversal of the circulation is responsible for regression or resorption of a previously formed heart in the acardiac, or (2) the anomaly results from primary agenesis of the heart, the acardiac fetus surviving only when maintained by these very specific types of vascular anastomoses with a twin. When karyotyped, the acardius and its co-twin have been isosexual. Chromosomal abnormalities have been documented in some acardiacs, all of whom have been associated with a genotypically normal co-twin.[19,95]

FETUS PAPYRACEUS

Fetus papyraceus results from the early intrauterine death of one twin that is compressed against the membranes by the growth of the other twin. The dead fetus shrinks and flattens, eventually resembling amorphous necrotic tissue (Fig. 23.25). Its size and shape depend on the time of death and, undoubtedly, many are overlooked. Fetus papyracei occur in both monochorial and dichorial placentation and may result from the twin–twin transfusion syndrome. The frequency with which twin pregnancies are converted to single pregnancies by the death of one twin is unknown.

Higher Multiple Births

The principles of monozygotic and dizygotic placentation apply equally to triplet, quadruplet, and other higher multiple births. For example, triplets may be trizygotic, dizygotic, or monozygotic. Trizygotic triplets have trichorionic-triamnionic placentation but may be separate or variably fused. Dizygotic triplets may be dichorionic or trichorionic. Monozygotic triplets may be monochorionic, dichorionic, or trichorionic.

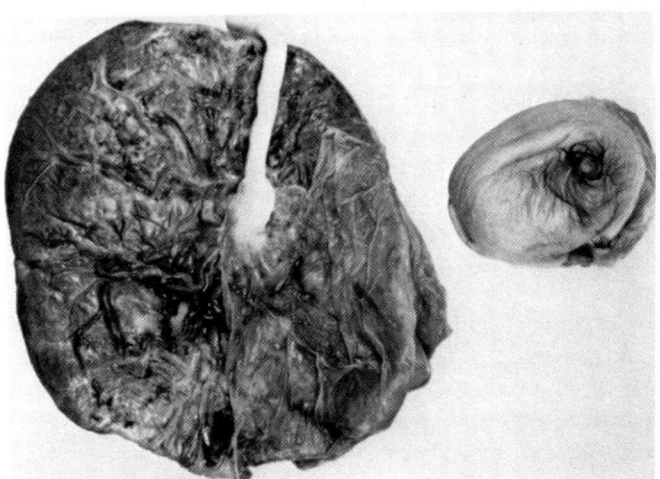

FIG. 23.24. **Acardiac fetus.** Holoacardius (amorphous).

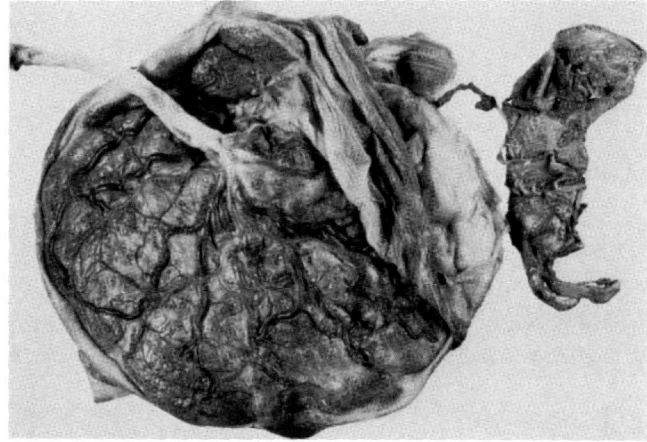

FIG. 23.25. **Fetus papyraceus.** Necrotic fetus compressed by the growth of its normal twin.

Placental Inflammation and Intrauterine Infections

Inflammation and infection of the placenta and fetus are important but controversial subjects. Debate has centered on the definition of inflammation, its etiologic relation to infectious agents, and the clinical relevance of the histologic findings. A great deal of attention has been focused on the consequences of intrauterine and intrapartum infections. At worst, some well-defined infections can result in abortion, stillbirth, prematurity, or multiply handicapped, severely disabled children who are mentally retarded, blind, deaf or suffer from numerous other congenital malformations. In addition to the obvious and identified toll, many more subtle, late sequelae, including learning disabilities, school failure, and especially deafness, are being identified in children whose infections were asymptomatic at birth. The social and financial burden posed by the support of these children is enormous, not to mention the long-term grief and emotional cost to the families involved.

The placenta and fetus are infected via two major pathways: (1) the ascending, amniotic (transcervical) route and (2) the hematogenous (transplacental) route. Combinations of these pathways (i.e., ascending deciduoplacentofetal) or other pathways (transfallopian, transuterine via amniocentesis or intrauterine transfusion) have been described or proposed, but for practical purposes, only the first two are of major importance. The pattern of the inflammatory response in the placenta is entirely different for these two entities. In ascending infections, microorganisms produce an acute inflammatory reaction in the fetal membranes (chorioamnionitis), the umbilical cord (funisitis), and ultimately in the fetus itself. The etiologic agents usually are bacterial, but fungi and possibly viruses occasionally are involved. In hematogenous infections, the infectious agent produces an inflammatory response in the villi (villitis) and intervillous space. Viruses are believed to be the most common agents involved, but some bacteria (spirochetes, *Listeria*) and protozoa (*Toxoplasma gondii*) also infect the placenta in this manner. A third important route by which infectious agents may reach the fetus is during passage through an infected birth canal (intrapartum infection). The placenta, of course, is not involved in this process.

Ascending Infection and Chorioamnionitis

Chorioamnionitis, the pattern of inflammation associated with ascending infection, is by far the most common form of placental inflammation in humans.

CLINICAL FEATURES

The exact frequency varies depending on the population studied. The incidence of chorioamnionitis is increased in patients of low socioeconomic status and in black women.[265,270,319] Naeye has emphasized the role of coitus in increasing the frequency and severity of ascending amniotic infection.[255,267] The role of the incompetent cervix has been stressed by Russell.[320]

The etiology and pathogenesis of chorioamnionitis are only partially understood. Certainly, there is a consistent and well-documented relationship between chorioamnionitis and prolonged rupture of membranes: the longer the membranes have been ruptured, the greater the likelihood that amniotic infection will occur.[87,151] This sequence of events, membrane rupture followed by infection, seems to be operative in term gestations, and in these circumstances the threat of infection is universally recognized. However, it is not correct to ascribe chorioamnionitis solely to rupture of membranes. The same histological findings, culture data, and clinical syndromes can be seen in the absence of membrane rupture.[121,237,266,267] In this situation, the cause and effect relationship between membrane rupture and chorioamnionitis actually may be reversed, chorioamnionitis preceding and being the cause, rather than a complication, of ruptured membranes.

Microorganisms, especially bacteria, have been cultured from the amniotic surface and amniotic fluid in many cases of chorioamnionitis. This fact, in addition to the experimental production of chorioamnionitis and congenital pneumonia in animals receiving intraamniotic injections of bacteria, support the widespread although not universal view that chorioamnionitis is caused by amniotic contamination with bacteria and other microorganisms. Similar injections of sterile exogenous irritants, such as gastric juice, acid, or India ink, do not result in chorioamnionitis.[218] A perplexing observation has been the relatively high frequency of negative bacterial cultures when there are obvious histological changes of chorioamnionitis.[232,282,418] This may be explained by the inability of routine culture techniques to detect mycoplasmas, chlamydiae, viruses, or even some organisms, such as *Listeria monocytogenes* or *Clostridium difficile*.[106,207,230,253,352,378] In fact, when specifically sought, genital mycoplasmas are emerging with significant regularity in association with chorioamnionitis.[77,109,171,298] The demonstrated antibacterial effect of amniotic fluid itself may interfere with growth in culture.[24,27,334,383] Many studies have ignored the so-called saprophytic or nonpathogenic organisms, which may in fact be relatively nonpathogenic for the fetus but are able to produce an inflammatory reaction in the fetal membranes. Bacteria and inflammatory cells release phospholipid leading to the production of prostaglandins, which are thought to initiate cervical dilatation and uterine contractions.[42] There is some evidence that bacteria, bacterial products, and inflammation in the umbilical cord and chorionic plate may alter umbilical vascular reactivity and fetal heart patterns.[178,328] The relationship of vasoconstriction to fetal hypoperfusion and its importance as a factor in chorioamnionitis-related fetal morbidity and mortality remains to be determined. The possibility that many cases of chorioamnionitis are actually noninfective in nature has been cogently disputed by Fox.[132]

Gross Findings

In most cases of chorioamnionitis, the placenta and fetal membranes are macroscopically normal. Occasionally, the membranes may be opaque, friable, or foul smelling in cases of particularly severe, long-standing bacterial infection. In rare instances of *Candida* infection, tiny white foci of colonization, 2 to 3 mm in size, may be seen on the amniotic surface of the umbilical cord.

Microscopic Findings

Histologically, there is evidence of maternal and usually fetal response to amniotic infection.[51,56,57,132] The earliest reaction is maternal and is manifested by an accumulation of neutrophils in the decidua at the lower pole of the amniotic sac, either at the site of membrane rupture or where intact membranes are exposed by the dilating cervix. These leukocytes come from maternal decidual vessels and migrate progressively through the chorion, amnion, and into the amnionic fluid in response to chemotactic factors released by the infecting agent or cells in the inflammatory exudate (Fig. 23.26). Various terms, including *membranous deciduitis*, *membranous chorionitis*, and *membranous chorioamnionitis*, have been applied to distinguish these stages in the progression of the inflammatory response (Fig. 23.27). Maternal polymorphonuclear leukocytes also migrate out of the intervillous space of the placenta early in the course of the infection and accumulate immediately beneath the chorionic plate, often in a deposit of subchorionic fibrin (Fig. 23.28). These neutrophils eventually extend across the chorionic plate, migrating toward the amniotic cavity in response to the same leukotactic stimuli.

The fetus also may respond to the amniotic infection. The fetal reaction is less marked and somewhat delayed when compared with the maternal response. In the chorionic plate of the placenta and in the umbilical cord, fetal leukocytes first marginate against vascular endothelium and then migrate through the walls of the large chorionic and umbilical arteries and veins into the chorionic plate or Wharton's jelly. The migration of inflammatory cells in this vasculitis is crescent shaped, oriented toward the source of infection in the amniotic cavity (Figs. 23.29, 23.30, 29.31). Inflammation of the umbilical cord tends to be segmental, perhaps reflecting proximity to the cervical os, and may be found, therefore, in only one of multiple sections of umbilical cord in this circumstance.

Amniotic infection, then, is a unique situation in which two individuals, mother and fetus, respond to the same infectious stimulus. The overwhelming majority of leukocytes that participate in this process are maternal. This is not unexpected given the great discrepancy in surface area

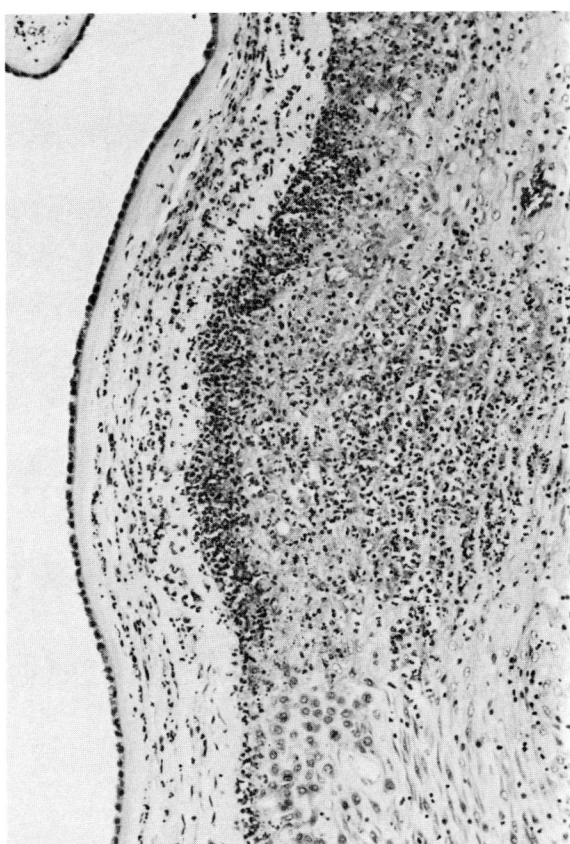

Fig. 23.26. Ascending infection, extraplacental membranes. Maternal neutrophils migrate from decidual vessels through the chorion and amnion toward the source of infection in the amnionic cavity.

available for stimulation and migration of maternal (free membranes and chorionic plate) versus fetal (chorionic plate, umbilical cord) leukocytes and has been confirmed by analyzing the sex chromatin of the inflammatory cells in the amnionic exudate.[56] The fetal leukocytic response is often absent in gestations of less than 19 to 20 weeks (fetal weight less than 500 g). Therefore, in very early abortions, the inflammatory response may be solely maternal. If infection occurs after fetal death, the fetal component will be absent. The time course for the inflammatory reaction in ascending infection is poorly defined.

In ascending infection, the inflammatory process is characteristically confined to the fetal membranes, chorionic plate, and umbilical cord. Villous tissue is not involved unless fetal infection and bacteremia result secondarily in villitis, an expression of inflammation that may occur in any other fetal organ under these circumstances. The character of the inflammatory infiltrate usually is not specific enough to identify a particular offending agent. In fact, it is relatively unusual to find bacteria in histological sections even when they have been demonstrated on smears of the amnion. Notable exceptions to this include infections with group B β-hemolytic streptococci, in which colonies of the

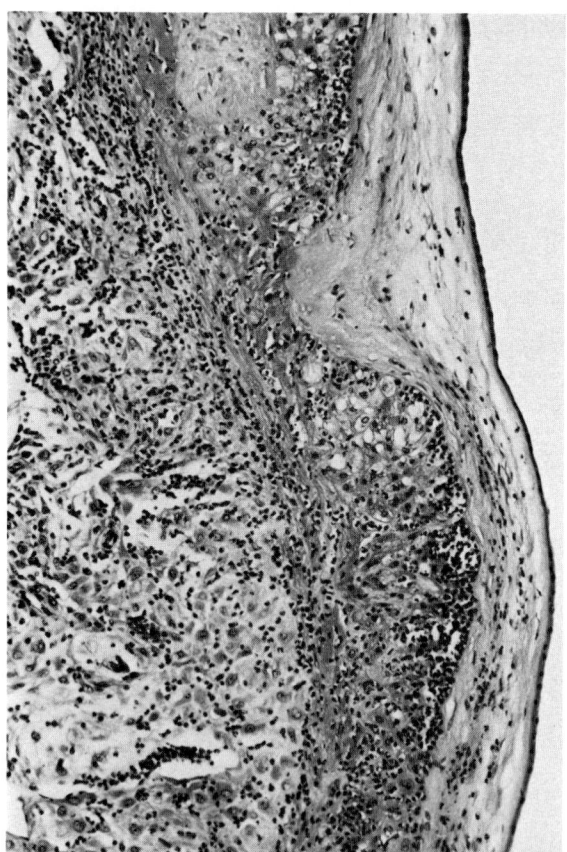

FIG. 23.27. **Ascending infection, extraplacental membranes.** The progression of the inflammatory response is illustrated here. Neutrophilic infiltration that involves the decidua and chorion on the *top* has extended into the amnion on the *bottom* as well.

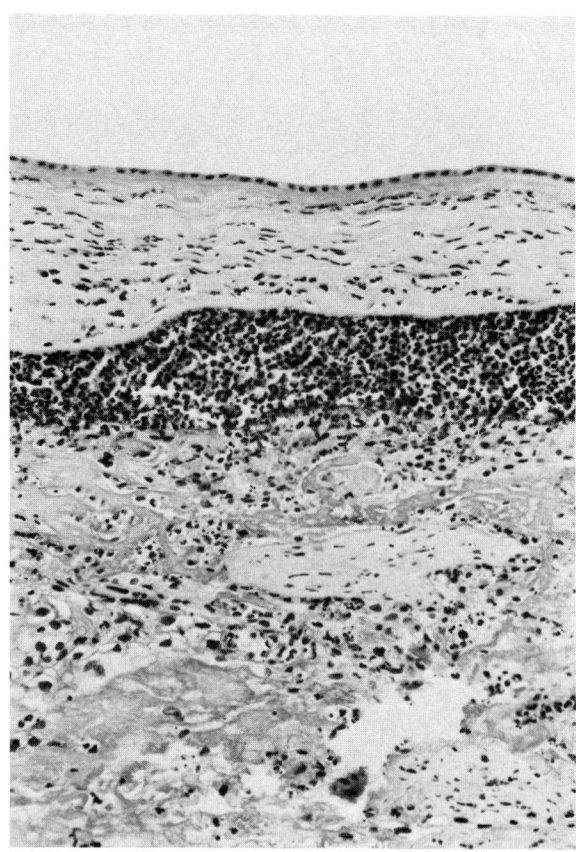

FIG. 23.28. **Ascending infection, chorionic plate.** Maternal neutrophils migrate out of the blood in the intervillous space and accumulate beneath the chorionic plate.

organism are frequently found without difficulty (Fig. 23.32). This type of infection may occur so rapidly that histological evidence of chorioamnionitis may be absent even when bacterial colonies are numerous.[57] Fusobacterial infection usually is associated with very severe inflammation, often with necrosis. The faintly basophilic, wavy organisms may be seen on the amniotic surface and stain with Brown and Hopp's or silver stains. Hyphal and yeast forms of *Candida* also may be identified, characteristically in small, superficial, crescentic microabscesses under the amniotic surface of the umbilical cord (Fig. 23.33).[172] The rarity of ascending candidal infection is surprising in view of the frequency with which it is found in the vagina. Natural defenses against *Candida* may help control its spread.[27]

The bacteria recovered from the amniotic fluid, fetal membranes, fetal tissues, and cord blood include a variety of anaerobes and aerobes, frequently as mixed flora. The most commonly recovered bacteria are *Escherichia coli*, coagulase-positive staphylococci, streptococci, *Proteus mirabilis, Klebsiella,* and *Pseudomonas*. These bacteria, in-

habitants or contaminants of the vagina and cervix, are thought to ascend into the amniotic cavity, a process facilitated by membrane rupture.

CLINICAL BEHAVIOR AND TREATMENT

Although there are maternal hazards associated with chorioamnionitis (maternal sepsis), the principal clinical impact of chorioamnionitis is the potential spread of infection to the fetus, which greatly outweighs any risk to the mother. Actually, in most cases of chorioamnionitis, neither mother nor neonate is overtly ill. Nevertheless, neonatal infection and sepsis are the leading cause of perinatal death in the United States as well as in developing countries,[254,256,320] and such serious neonatal infection often is associated with chorioamnionitis.[114,320,418]

Chorioamnionitis implies only that the fetus has been exposed to infection, not necessarily that the fetus is infected. In cases of chorioamnionitis, the exposed fetus may be infected in one of two ways: by orificial or hematogenous spread. Microorganisms may gain access to the respi-

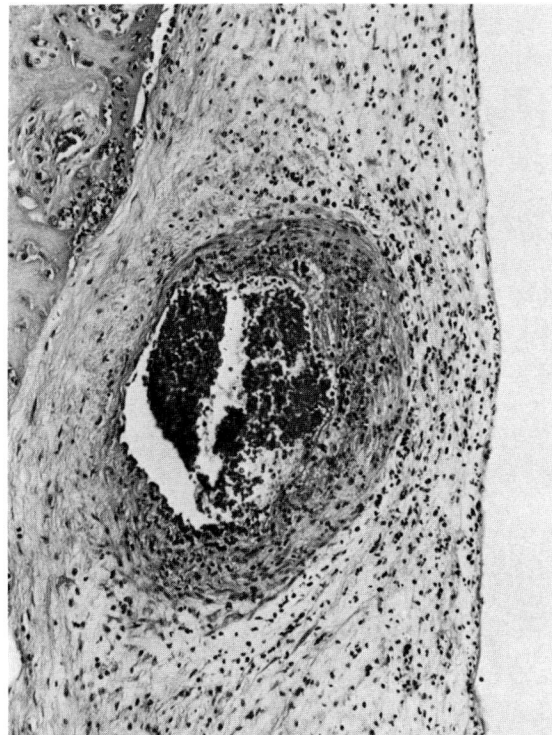

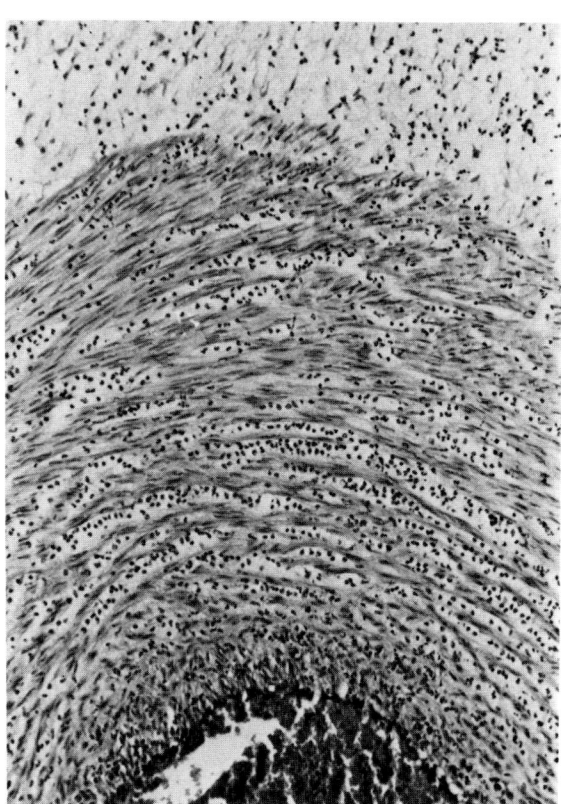

FIG. 23.29. Ascending infection, chorionic plate. Fetal neutrophils migrate through large fetal vessels of the chorionic plate. Orientation toward the source of infection in the amnionic cavity results in crescentic migration pattern.

FIG. 23.31. Ascending infection, umbilical cord. Migration of fetal leukocytes from the umbilical artery.

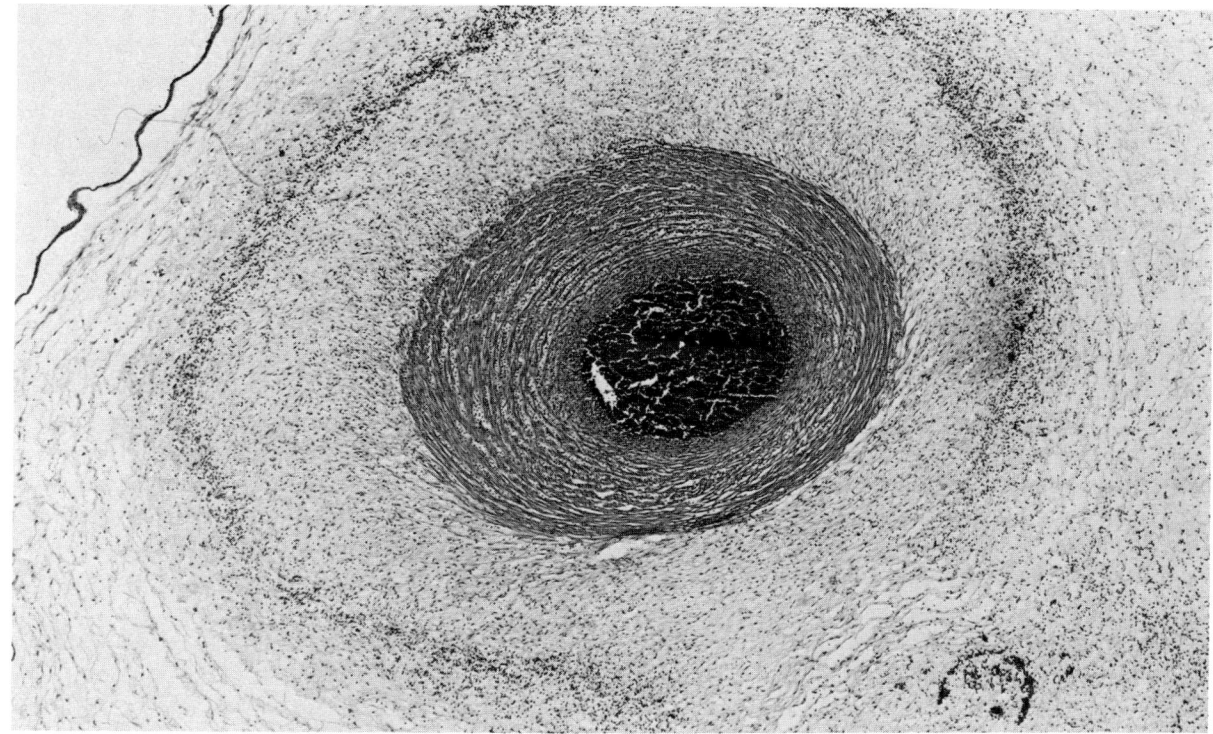

FIG. 23.30. Ascending infection, umbilical cord. Prominent crescentic band of leukocytes is accompanied by continued migration of neutrophils from the umbilical artery. This particular pattern of inflammation has been called *subacute necrotizing (healed) funisitis* and is thought to result from prolonged low-grade or spontaneously healed amnionic infection.

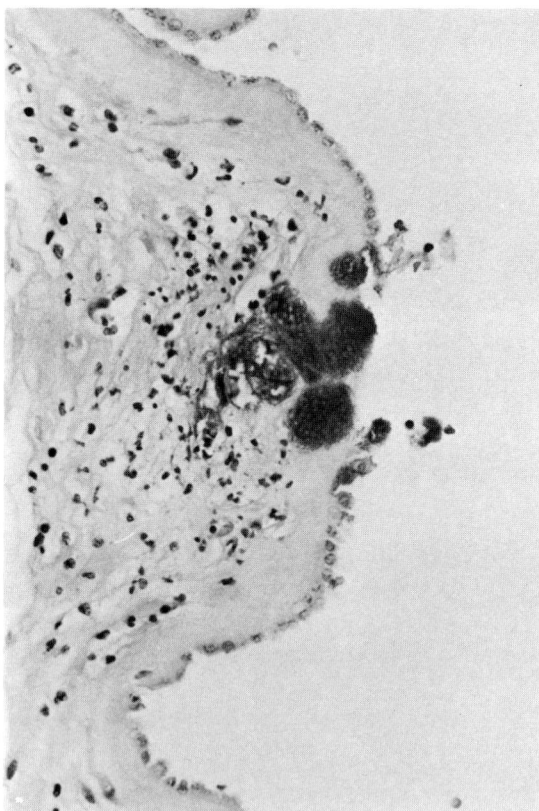

FIG. 23.32. **Ascending infection.** Colonies of group B β-he-molytic streptococci in amnion.

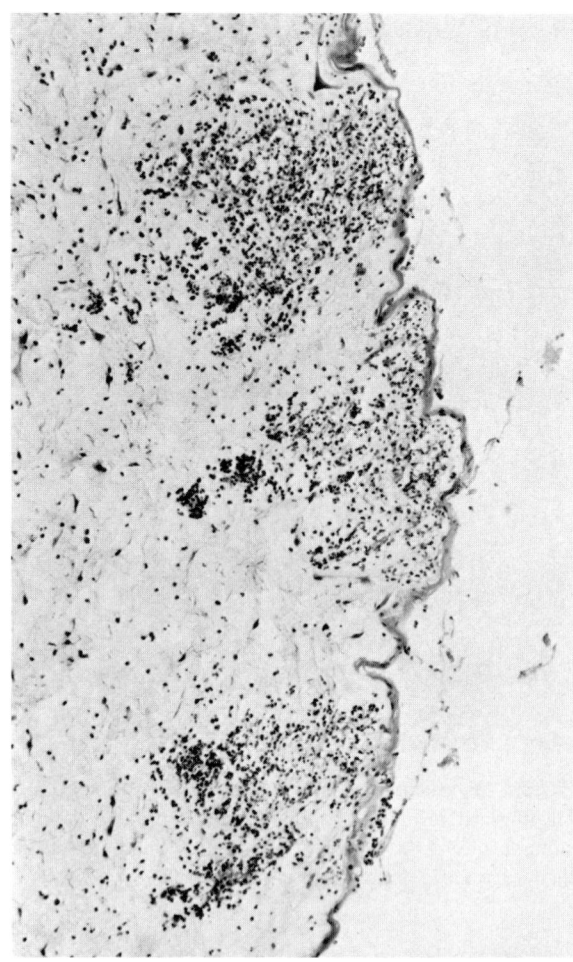

FIG. 23.33. *Candida* **infection of umbilical cord.** Small can-didal microabscesses beneath the amnion of the umbilical cord. Gomori methenamine silver stain showed yeast and hyphae.

ratory or gastrointestinal tracts via aspiration or swallowing of infected amniotic fluid. A distinction should be made between aspiration of amniotic exudate and true pneumonia. In the former, the bronchioles and alveoli contain a mixture of amniotic elements, including neutrophils, many degenerating. These are confined to the bronchoalveolar tree, and there is no evidence of fetal response to infection (Fig. 23.34). True congenital pneumonia differs in that there is a definite pulmonary interstitial leukocytic infiltrate characteristic of bronchopneumonia. Swallowing of infected amniotic fluid may result in gastritis, ileitis, or gastrointestinal perforation with peritonitis. Orificial contamination of the fetus does occur in a significant number of caes of chorioamnionitis.[51,268] The fetal skin, eyes, or ear canals also may be contaminated by direct contact with infected amniotic fluid. Hematogenous spread of organisms from the infected amniotic fluid directly to the fetal circulation via the superficial chorionic vessels is another possible mechanism of fetal infection. The relative importance of orificial versus direct spread of microorganisms to fetal chorionic vessels has not yet been clarified.

A combination of histological and clinical parameters may be used to predict fetal outcome in cases of chorioamnionitis. The absence of chorioamnionitis is an important finding. This virtually excludes intrauterine ascending infection and significant clinical sepsis in the first 48 hours of

life.[320] Infants whose placentas show evidence of chorioamnionitis are at increased risk to develop sepsis and die in the neonatal period.[196,298,418] The magnitude of the risk has been correlated with the severity of the inflammatory reaction. Neonatal morbidity and mortality are significantly greater when the inflammatory response is graded moderate or severe than when it is mild in degree.[109,263,418] The frequency of positive cultures also increases with the severity of the inflammatory response, although the histological identification of moderate to severe chorioamnionitis alone, even in the absence of a positive culture, is a useful indicator of infection in both the mother and the newborn.[320,418] Naeye et al.[269] noted that placental villous edema correlated strongly with morbidity and mortality in neonates with chorioamnionitis. The chief morphologic alteration is the presence of open spaces in the interstitium of the villi (Fig. 23.35). Villous edema also occurs in association with maternal hypertension, diabetes mellitus, premature rupture of membranes, abruption, and other states associated with fetal hypoxia. In many instances, no disorder has been identified.

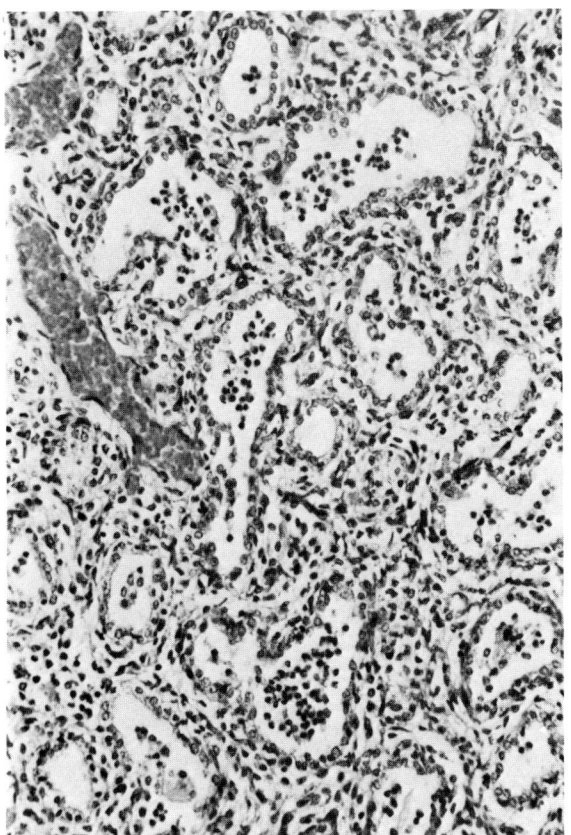

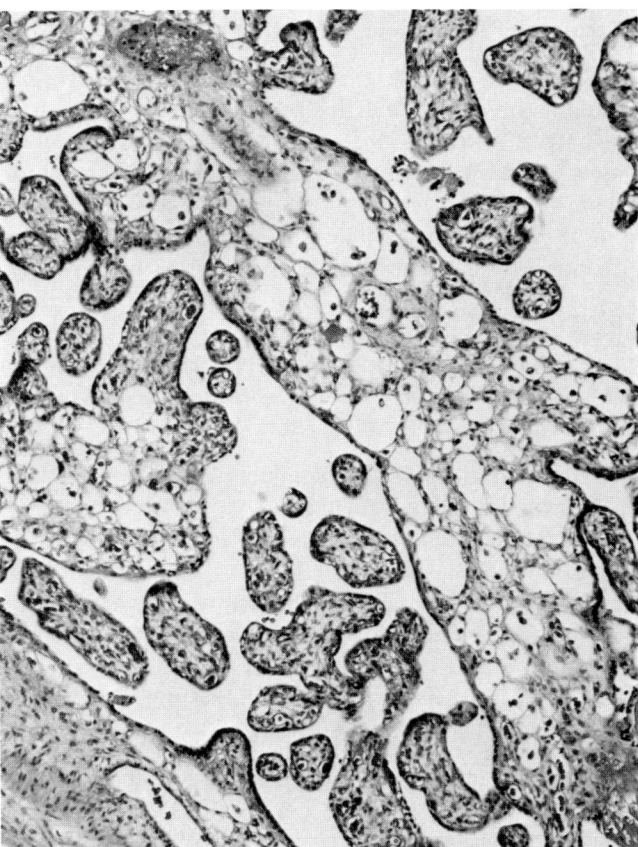

FIG. 23.34. Chorioamnionitis, fetal lung. Neutrophils aspirated from amnionic fluid are accumulated in the fetal bronchoalveolar tree. True fetal pneumonia is not present.

FIG. 23.35. Villous edema. Clusters of open spaces are delimited by attenuated strands of stromal cells and collagen. When associated with amnionitis, the clinical severity is much greater and mortality is more likely.

Acute chorioamnionitis is strongly correlated with prematurity; its occurrence is inversely proportional to gestational age.[171,320] This association between chorioamnionitis and preterm labor and delivery is well known, and the combination of chorioamnionitis and prematurity is definitely associated with a high frequency of perinatal death.

Several methods have been proposed to permit a rapid diagnosis of chorioamnionitis and potential infection of the exposed fetus. These include (1) cytology of a gastric aspirate or ear canal fluid, (2) smear of chorion or amnion, (3) whole mount of amnion, and (4) frozen section of the umbilical cord. These techniques attempt to document an inflammatory infiltrate and the presence and type of microorganisms involved. Since many cases of chorioamnionitis are associated with normal healthy neonates, these techniques serve only to alert the clinician to the potential for infection in an exposed neonate.

Hematogenous Infection

In hematogenous infections of the placenta, infectious agents reach the placenta through the maternal blood.

CLINICAL FEATURES

In contrast to chorioamnionitis, which is a purely local infection, placental involvement in hematogenous infection usually is only one manifestation of maternal systemic disease. The hallmark of this type of infection is villitis, inflammation of the villous parenchyma itself. When a specific etiologic agent is identified, it is usually viral, although some bacteria and protozoa reach the placenta hematogenously. The vast majority of villitides, however, are of unknown etiology. Serologic studies of the mother and infant may, on occasion, provide information about etiology.

GROSS FINDINGS

Villitis usually is discovered incidentally on microscopic exam. Typically there is neither clinical suspicion of, nor gross pathological clue, to the underlying inflammatory process. In some cases, there may be subtle gross abnormalities including placental enlargement, pallor, or edema, or scattered, minute necrotic foci.

MICROSCOPIC FINDINGS

Histologically, the essential feature of villitis is a villous inflammatory infiltrate with a predilection for vascular involvement. Morphologically, the villitides may be subdivided based on the nature of the inflammatory infiltrate (acute or chronic), type of inflammatory cell involved (lymphocyte, histiocyte, plasma cell, neutrophil), distribution of lesions (focal, diffuse, basal), and severity (mild, moderate, severe).[13,57,132,133,322] Frequently the villitides exhibit all degrees of active inflammation, resolution, and complete repair in the same placenta. These stages of evolution are the basis for the following classification of villitides proposed by Altshuler and Russell.[16]

1. *Proliferative villitis:* Inflammatory cells are present in the villi, but there is no necrosis.
2. *Necrotizing villitis:* Inflammatory cells and necrosis are present in the villi.
3. *Reparative villitis:* The inflammatory process is resolving with granulation tissue and fibroblastic proliferation.
4. *Stromal fibrosis:* The villi are fibrotic but do not show evidence of active inflammation.

Practically speaking, villitis is typically a focal process and, therefore, may be entirely overlooked if a considerable number of sections are not examined.[203]

There is some correlation between the morphologic features of villitis and the etiologic agent, but the differences are subtle. Available information is based on a relatively small number of cases in which a specific agent has been identified by light or electron microscopy or has been cultured from the placental or fetal tissue.

Viral Infection

Cytomegalovirus

The pathology of cytomegalovirus (CMV) placentitis is the prototype for all viral villitides.[16,45,55,57,132,133,248] The placenta may be normal in size, small in cases of fetal growth retardation, or large and edematous when associated with fetal anemia. Histologically, the villi may exhibit any or all of a wide spectrum of changes including acute necrotizing villitis, a villous infiltrate that is especially rich in plasma cells, or complete villous fibrosis (Figs. 23.36, 23.37). Vasculitis and stromal hemosiderin deposition are very characteristic (Fig. 23.38). In old lesions, only the remnants of occluded vessels may remain (Fig. 23.39). Villous histiocytes and stromal cells usually are increased, and foci of stromal calcification may be found. The typical, large, intranuclear and intracytoplasmic eosinophilic inclusions may be found in endothelial cells, Hofbauer cells, or trophoblast (Fig. 23.40). When found, they are diagnostic, but unfortunately they usually are scarce and seldom identified, even after diligent search. In practical terms, a multi-

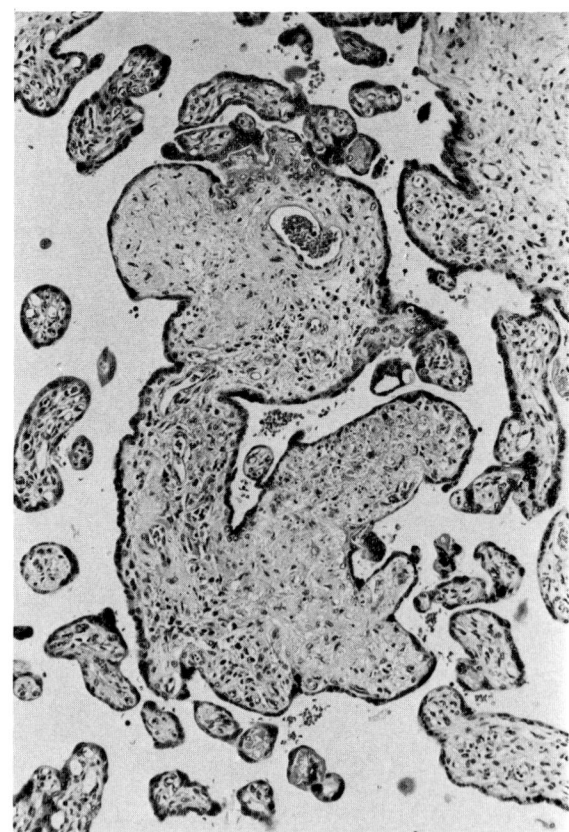

FIG. 23.36. Villitis, cytomegalovirus infection. Lymphoplasmacytic villous infiltrate and focal villous necrosis.

focal lymphoplasmacytic villitis with vasculitis and stromal hemosiderin in the United States is probably a CMV infection. Relative villous immaturity and edema are nonspecific changes related to the fetal anemia in some cases.

CMV placentitis is the most commonly identified of all viral placental infections. The prevalence of congenital infection ranges from 0.2% to 2.2% among all live births. CMVs are common and readily infect the fetus and newborn. They are unique in their ability to cause both acute infection and chronic subtle disease that may not manifest itself for months or years. At this time, CMV is the most commonly recognized infectious cause of developmental impairments.

The natural history of CMV infection in pregnancy is complex and not completely understood.° Epidemiologic data indicate that (1) transmission to the offspring may occur in utero, at birth, or postnatally, (2) intrauterine infection may result from either primary or recurrent maternal infection, the latter despite substantial humoral immunity, (3) infection may be symptomatic at birth (hepatosplenomegaly, microcephaly, petechiae), but in the

---

°Refs. 6,7,9,157,229,275,308,362,364–366.

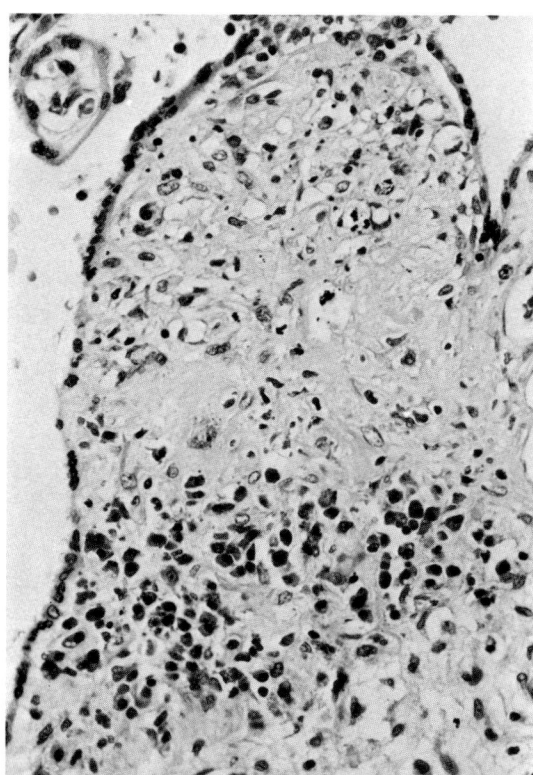

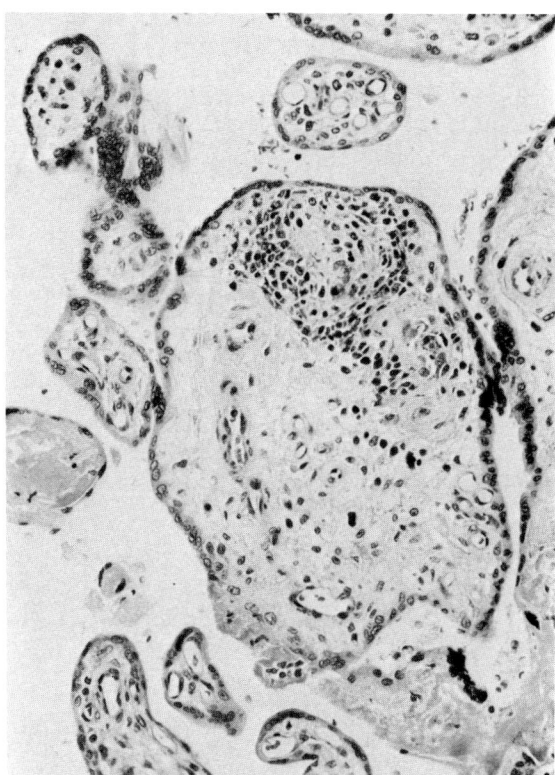

FIG. 23.37. Villitis, CMV infection. Villous inflammatory infiltrate, especially rich in plasma cells, is associated with focal necrosis and fibrosis, *top*.

FIG. 23.38. Villitis, CMV infection. Segmental vasculitis.

vast majority of infants, is subclinical, (4) late complications, including mental retardation, chorioretinitis, seizures, learning disabilities, and especially neurosensory hearing loss, are most common among the survivors of symptomatic congenital infection but may also occur later in children with no clinical manifestations at birth, and (5) congenital infections resulting from reactivation of latent virus are less likely to produce fetal damage and late sequelae than those resulting from primary maternal infections. Some authors have found a "fairly good" correlation between the severity of the placental lesions and the clinical outcome.[55]

Rubella

The pathological findings associated with rubella infection have been described mainly in placentas from first and second trimester abortions[113,281,386] but in a few term deliveries as well.[41,143,281] In placental tissue examined shortly after the acute clinical infection, there may be focal necrotizing villitis and vasculitis that vary markedly in severity and extent. Some villi exhibit only focal trophoblastic necrosis, whereas in others, totally necrotic trophoblast is associated with perivillous fibrin and acute inflammation. Endothelial necrosis, often associated with fragmentation of fetal red cells, probably is the most characteristic find-

ing. There may be an associated chronic perivascular infiltrate. Eosinophilic cytoplasmic viral inclusion bodies may be found in endothelial cells, Hofbauer cells, villous stromal cells, and trophoblast. Identical viral inclusions and perivascular chronic inflammatory infiltrates have been reported in the decidua in some cases.[281] A mild, focal chronic inflammatory infiltrate occurs infrequently in the membranes and cord.[143] Placentas delivered and examined after the acute stage of the maternal disease may show only scattered, shrunken, avascular villi. In some cases, these healed lesions co-exist with more acute changes, as described above. Such placentas may be very small for gestational age. The combination of severe hypoplasia and vascular change is characteristic of rubella infection. A number of placentas from which rubella virus has been isolated do not show any inflammatory changes or other morphologic abnormality.[132,281]

The consequences of rubella infection during pregnancy include spontaneous abortion, fetal death, intrauterine growth retardation, congenital malformations, active neonatal infection, and such delayed manifestations as deafness and mental retardation. Fortunately, these are now limited to rare sporadic cases since epidemics of rubella have been controlled by immunization. The exact frequency of fetal damage from maternal rubella infection is unknown, but infection during the first trimester appears

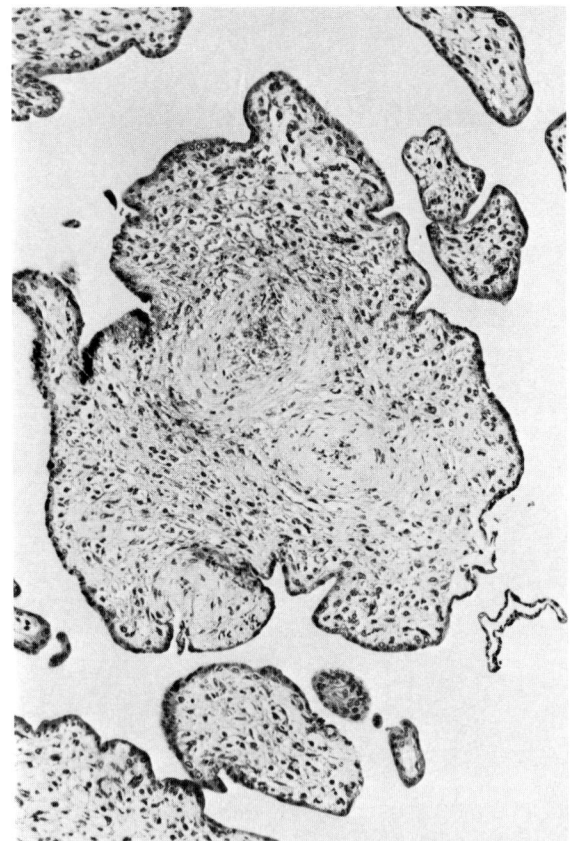

Fig. 23.39. Villitis, CMV infection. Villi showing remnants of hyalinized, obliterated vessels.

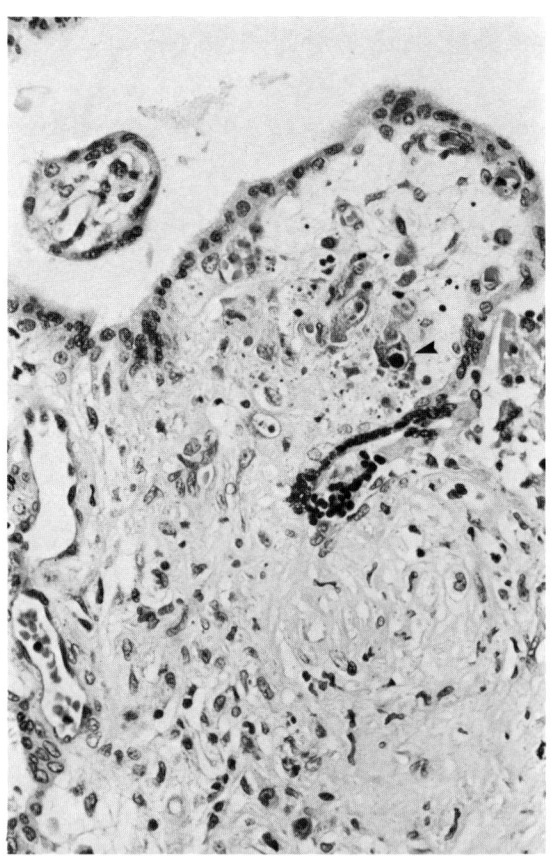

Fig. 23.40. Villitis, CMV infection. Typical CMV intranuclear inclusion bodies (*arrow*) associated with focal villous necrosis.

to present the greatest risk to the fetus. During past rubella epidemics, microscopic abnormalities have been documented in 33–68% of fetuses infected and aborted in the first trimester, although gross malformations were not evident in these fetuses.[281,386] However, gross abnormalities, usually multiple, were found in half of the fetuses infected in the first trimester and not aborted until 5 to 6 months.[281] These involve primarily the eyes (cataract), cardiovascular system (patent ductus arteriosus, ventricular septal defect), and central nervous system (microcephaly) and are postulated to result from a combination of viral inhibition of cell growth, cytolysis, and interference with blood supply.[264] Survivors of congenital rubella infection also can suffer from late sequelae, including panencephalitis[286,400] and diabetes mellitus.[126,182,235]

Herpes Simplex Virus

Disseminated herpes simplex virus infection, once a rare occurrence, has become an increasingly common cause of devastating disease and death in the newborn. Intrapartum transmission of virus from the maternal genital tract is by far the most common mode of fetal infection.[363] In only a very few cases has there been histological documentation of ascending[12,57] or transplacental dissemination[57,411] or

both of the herpes simplex virus. Foci of villous necrosis, agglutination of villi, and fibrinoid necrosis of villous vessels have been documented in the rare cases of hematogenous infection. Chorioamnionitis, of both the necrotizing and chronic lymphoplasmacytic types, has been described in a few cases of ascending infection. An increased frequency of spontaneous abortion and congenital malformation has been reported in patients with primary infection in the first 20 weeks of pregnancy.[*]

Parvovirus B19

Human parvovirus B19 is the agent of "fifth disease," or erythema infectiosum, a mild, acute, exanthematous disease mainly of children. In adults, most infections are asymptomatic. Self-limited polyarthropathy is a common complication, especially in women, and aplastic crises occur in individuals with chronic hemolytic anemias.[82] Parvovirus B19 only recently has been added to the growing list of viruses that may cross the placenta and result in fetal infection, morbidity, and mortality.[20,82,135,297,330,351] Hydrops fetalis is a consistent finding in the parvovirus-in-

---

[*]Refs. 125,161,249,272–274,359,363.

fected fetus. Grossly, the placenta is typically large, pale, and friable. Microscopically, there is a uniform pattern of relative villous immaturity and stromal edema. Numerous erythroblasts, some containing intranuclear eosinophilic inclusions with peripheral chromatin condensation characteristic of parvovirus infection, are present in the villous vessels (Fig. 23.41).[351] In situ hybridization may be used to confirm the diagnosis and is somewhat more sensitive than conventional microscopy in identifying infected cells.[292,337] Unlike most other congenital hematogenous infections, there is no villous inflammatory reaction in parvovirus infection.

Parvovirus B19 preferentially infects actively replicating cells, especially erythroblasts. As targets in infection, erythroblasts are destroyed and, therefore, the pathophysiology of parvovirus hydrops is similar to that of the hemoglobinopathies and hemolytic anemias (see discussion of Rh incompatibility).

Studies to date would indicate that most fetuses are spared the adverse consequences of an acute maternal parvovirus B19 infection.[200] The risk of fetal loss is estimated to be less than 10%,[82] with most abortions occurring between the 10th and 28th weeks of pregnancy.[82,337] To date, the most commonly recognized consequence of fetal parvovirus infection is nonimmune hydrops and fetal

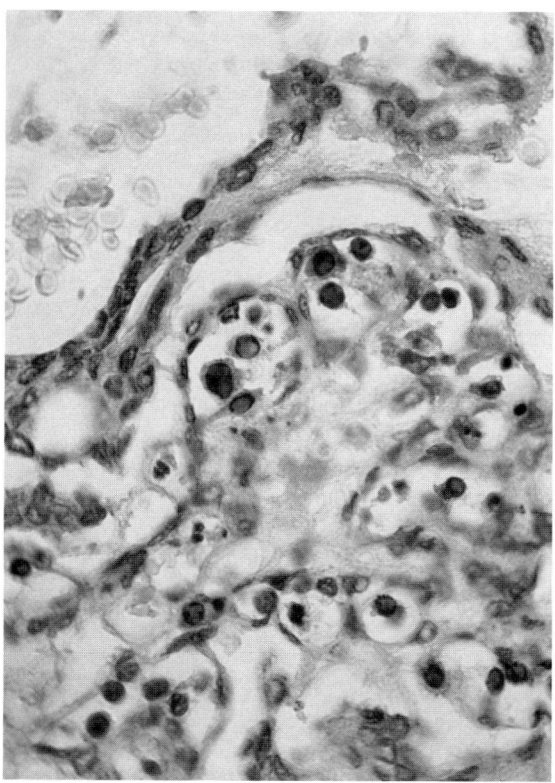

FIG. 23.41. Parvovirus infection. Erythroblasts in the villous capillaries show central nuclear eosinophilic inclusions with peripheral chromatin condensation.

death, but neonatal anemia also has been observed in infants infected in the third trimester.[86,351] Malformations reminiscent of ocular rubella embryopathy have been reported only rarely.[164,401]

Human Immunodeficiency Virus

Evidence suggests that human immunodeficiency virus (HIV) may be transmitted to the fetus transplacentally, at the time of delivery, or through breast feeding.[58,317,326,361] The exact proportion of cases attributable to these various modes of transmission is unknown. The polymerase chain reaction (PCR) technique has been adapted to detect HIV in peripheral blood mononuclear cells of neonates. With this technique, it may be possible to discriminate between infants infected in utero and those infected intrapartum or after birth.[317] In some studies but not all, seropositive mothers have been more likely to deliver prematurely and to produce infants with relatively low birth weights.[244,326]

No histopathological lesions directly attributable to HIV have been described in the placenta.[83,180] Specifically, there have been no reports of villitis. Placentas from seropositive mothers have demonstrated an increased incidence of chorioamnionitis.[83,180,231] Immunohistochemical studies of placentas from HIV-seropositive pregnancies have produced contradictory data. HIV antigens have been variably expressed in amnionic and fetal cells,[181,361] trophoblast,[83,220] and macrophages.[181,220,231] The distribution of HIV antigen may vary with gestational age. Immunohistochemical demonstration of HIV has not correlated perfectly with culture status.[231] In one small study, there was no obvious correlation between immunohistochemical localization of HIV antigen or recovery of HIV in cell culture from the placenta and fetal HIV infection.[231] Ultrastructurally, retrovirus-like particles have been detected in syncytiotrophoblast, villous fibroblasts, and endothelial cells.[180]

Other Viruses

Pathological findings in the few placentas with documented infection by other viruses, such as vaccinia, variola, varicella, Coxsackie B, and hepatitis B virus, have been detailed by Fox,[132,133] Blanc,[55,57] and Altshuler and Russell.[16] Unfortunately, the potential effects of many of the most common viruses that must be encountered frequently during pregnancy (enteroviruses, adenoviruses, influenza viruses) are not well known.

Bacterial Infection

Treponema pallidum

Once a major cause of abortion and stillbirth, congenital syphilis has shown a dramatic increase in incidence recently. Grossly, infected placentas tend to be large and bulky. Histologically, the villi are large and relatively immature but not markedly edematous (Fig. 23.42). Villous vessels exhibit subendothelial and perivascular fibrosis, resulting in luminal narrowing and occlusion (Figs. 23.43, 23.44). A lymphoplasmacytic villous infiltrate and increased numbers of Hofbauer cells may be seen focally (Fig. 23.44). The histological changes in the placenta are not diagnostic but are highly suggestive, especially in conjunction with the characteristic lesions that occur in the fetal organs (pneumonia alba, pancreatic fibrosis, cirrhosis, osteitis). Definitive diagnosis depends on demonstration of spirochetes in the placental or fetal tissue, which may be accomplished by a Warthin–Starry or Levaditi stain.[323]

The traditional view that congenital syphilis occurs only after infection in the second half of pregnancy has now been disproved. Transplacental transmission of circulating spirochetes may occur at any time during pregnancy.[57,162] Morphologic expression of the placental and fetal lesions of congenital syphilis, however, seems to depend on the fetal inflammatory response, which is not yet developed in the very immature fetus.[37,357]

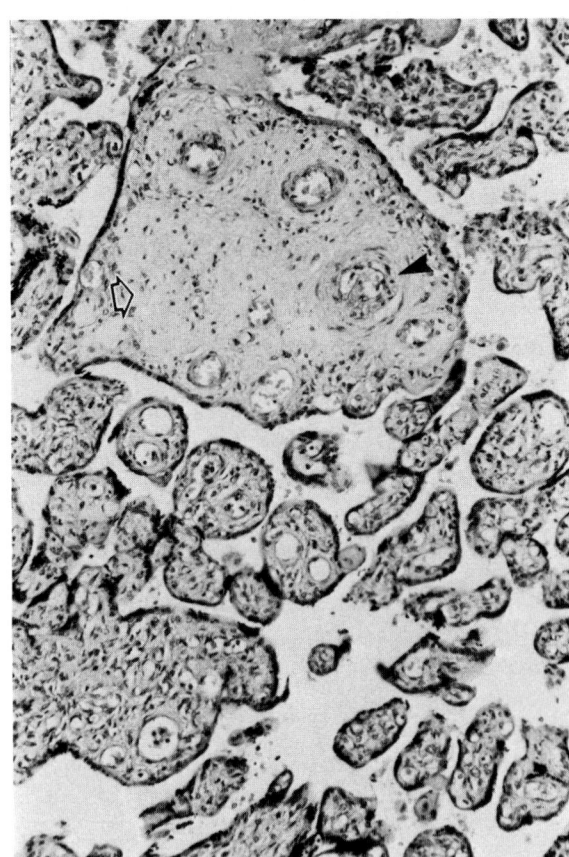

FIG. 23.43. Congenital syphilis at term in a liveborn infant. Perivascular and subendothelial fibrosis resulting in partial (*black arrow*) and complete (*open arrow*) vascular obliteration in a stem villus.

Listeria monocytogenes

L. monocytogenes is a significant cause of intrauterine infection, spontaneous abortion, prematurity, neonatal sepsis, morbidity, and death.[21,160,173, 288,301,417] Although *L. monocytogenes* is a well-recognized cause of septic abortion in animals, reports incriminating it as a possible cause of habitual abortion in humans are conflicting.[155,219,299] The epidemiology, mode of spread, and pathogenesis of *L. monocytogenes* infection are still obscure.[173]

Grossly, the placenta may appear normal or, on careful inspection, contain minute, yellow-white necrotic foci that correspond histologically to small foci of purulent villitis in which groups of acutely inflamed villi are enmeshed in fibrin and an acute perivillous and intervillous inflammatory infiltrate. These abscesses may be surrounded by a rim of palisaded histiocytes and occasional giant cells (Fig. 23.45). Occasionally, extensive spread into the intervillous space may cause infarction, in which case macroscopic abscesses may be present.[367] The earliest lesion, a ring of neutrophils localized between the trophoblast and villous stroma, may be found in scattered, individual villi.

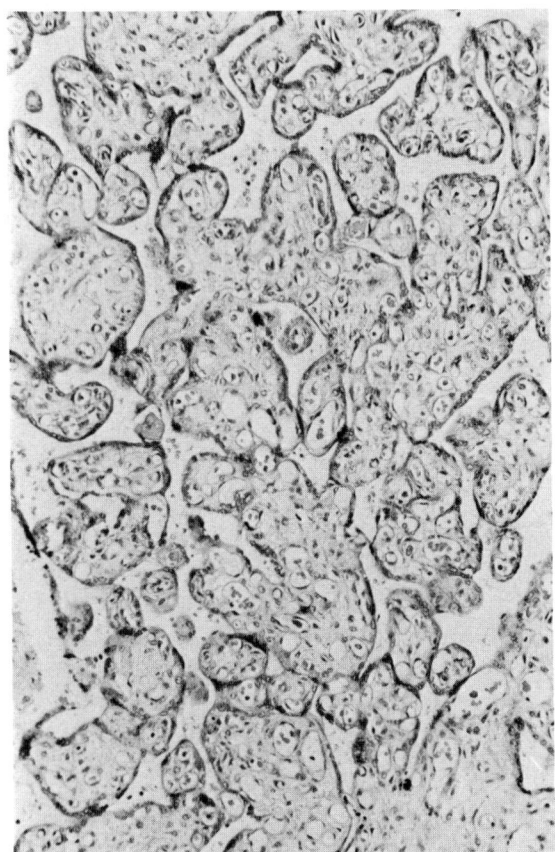

FIG. 23.42. Congenital syphilis at term in a liveborn infant. Large, immature, actively budding villi with pronounced increase in vascularity. Erythroblasts are present in villous capillaries.

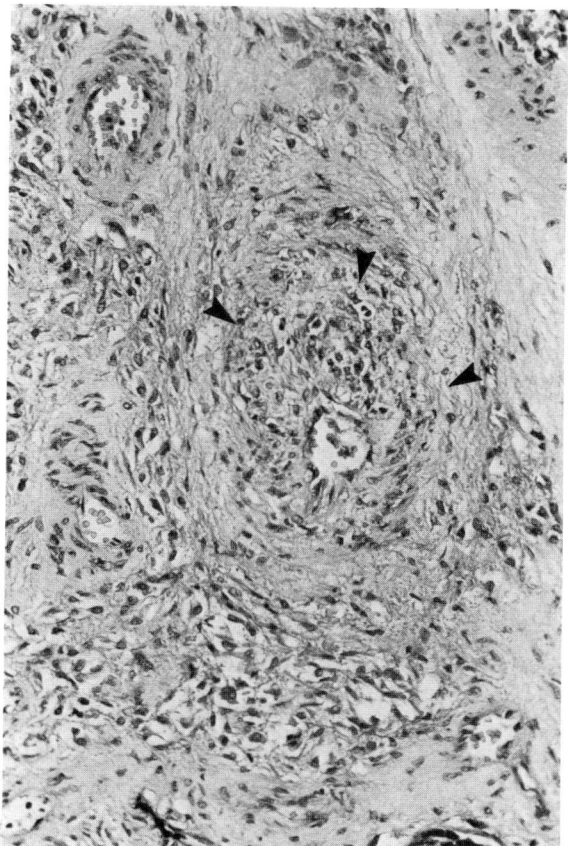

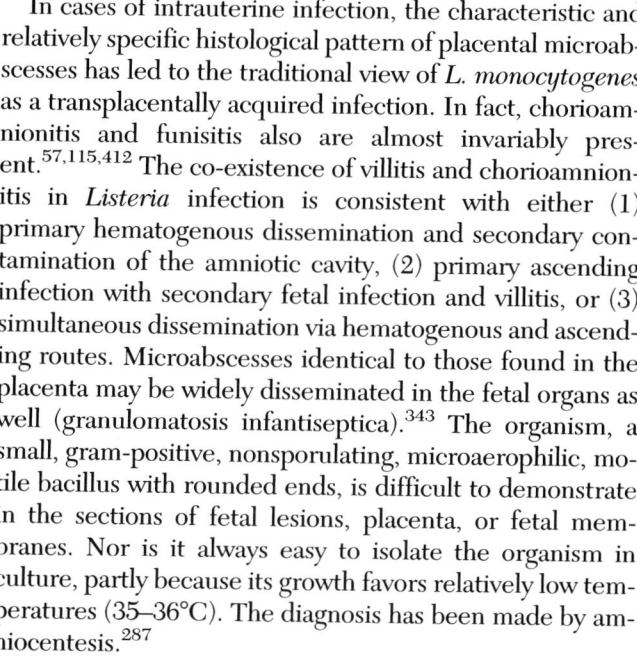

FIG. 23.44. Congenital syphilis at term in a liveborn infant. Stem villus with a lymphohistiocytic infiltrate and vasculitis. *Arrows* indicate a vessel infiltrated by lymphocytes.

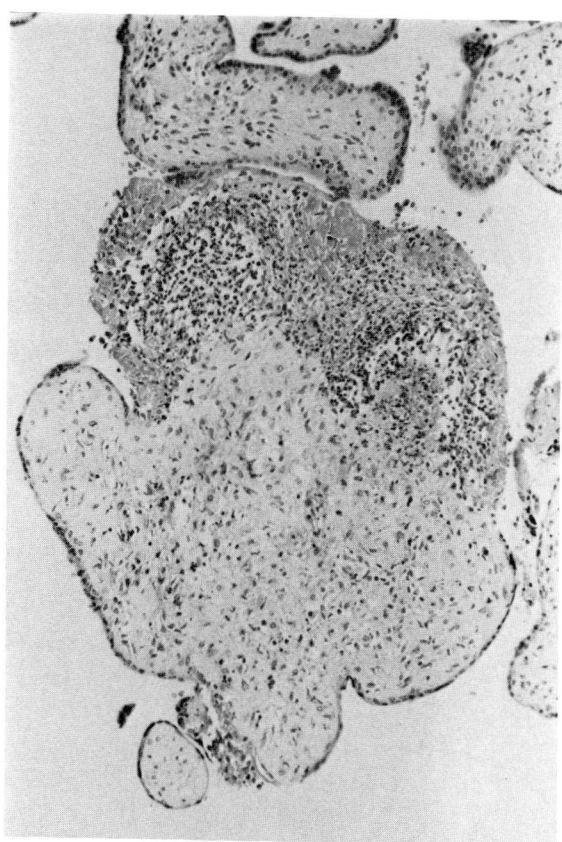

FIG. 23.45. Congenital listeriosis. Massive subtrophoblastic acute villitis with necrosis.

In cases of intrauterine infection, the characteristic and relatively specific histological pattern of placental microabscesses has led to the traditional view of *L. monocytogenes* as a transplacentally acquired infection. In fact, chorioamnionitis and funisitis also are almost invariably present.[57,115,412] The co-existence of villitis and chorioamnionitis in *Listeria* infection is consistent with either (1) primary hematogenous dissemination and secondary contamination of the amniotic cavity, (2) primary ascending infection with secondary fetal infection and villitis, or (3) simultaneous dissemination via hematogenous and ascending routes. Microabscesses identical to those found in the placenta may be widely disseminated in the fetal organs as well (granulomatosis infantiseptica).[343] The organism, a small, gram-positive, nonsporulating, microaerophilic, motile bacillus with rounded ends, is difficult to demonstrate in the sections of fetal lesions, placenta, or fetal membranes. Nor is it always easy to isolate the organism in culture, partly because its growth favors relatively low temperatures (35–36°C). The diagnosis has been made by amniocentesis.[287]

Other Bacteria

Hematogenous dissemination of other bacteria to the placenta occurs but is uncommon. The placental lesions in the few documented cases of hematogenous spread of organisms such as pyogenic and enteric bacteria, *Francisella tularensis*, *Brucella*, Vibrio fetus, *Mycobacterium tuberculosis*, and *Mycobacterium leprae*, are detailed in the treatises by Fox[132] and Blanc.[57]

Protozoan and Parasitic Infection

Toxoplasma gondii

The placenta infected with *T. gondii* may be grossly normal but is commonly large and edematous, resembling the hydropic placenta of severe Rh incompatibility.[11,28] Microscopically, there is a low-grade chronic villitis in which a predominantly lymphocytic infiltrate involves scattered villi. Endarteritis, focal villous necrosis, or fibrosis are less commonly seen (Fig. 23.46).[119] A chronic inflammatory

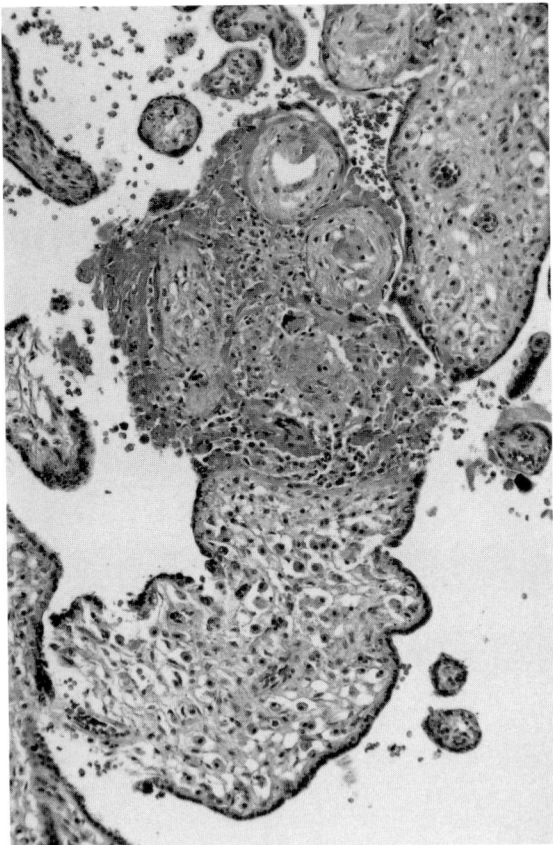

FIG. 23.46. Toxoplasma villitis. Villous necrosis and granulomatous inflammation.

infiltrate has been reported in the umbilical cord.[278] The organism, usually in the encysted form, is identified rarely, usually in the fetal membranes or chorionic plate, if found at all. It is typically unassociated with any inflammation.[11,41,119] In instances of perinatal death, organisms can be identified readily in the fetal brain.

The epidemiology, clinical features, and laboratory diagnosis of toxoplasma have been reviewed in several articles.[99,136] Congenital infection appears to result mainly from maternal infection acquired for the first time early in pregnancy, usually by ingesting undercooked meat or by contact with cat feces. The risk of fetal infection in these circumstances is less than 50%. The clinical spectrum of fetal involvement ranges from severe damage to the central nervous system and eyes to completely asymptomatic infection, recognized only by the development of chorioretinitis after months or years of follow-up. Antibiotic treatment during pregnancy seems to reduce the frequency of congenital infection.[407] Infection acquired later in pregnancy is less likely to cause overt disease in the newborn, presumably because of the resistance offered by a more mature immune system. In the presence of maternal antibodies from past infections, fetal lesions, with rare exception, do not occur.[99]

Villitis of Unknown Etiology

Although potentially catastrophic, fetoplacental infections caused by the agents detailed previously (CMV, rubella, *T. gondii*, *T. pallidum*) are infrequent. Far more commonly, a focal chronic villitis, for which no etiology can be established, is discovered incidentally in sections of the placenta. Estimates of this phenomenon vary greatly, but Russell identified chronic villitis of unknown etiology (VUE) in 7.6% of more than 7500 consecutively examined single placentas.[321] Knox and Fox identified the same lesion in 13.6% of 1000 randomly selected patients.[203]

The infant associated with such placental changes generally is unaffected, although Russell and others have presented convincing evidence that VUE is associated with intrauterine growth retardation and that the severity of the villitis correlates directly with the degree of growth retardation and the perinatal mortality rate.[203,210,303,321,322] VUE has a considerable tendency to recur,[303,321,322,324] but its potential role in repeated pregnancy loss is unknown, since routine histological examination of the placenta is not performed in most institutions.

The lesions are always found incidentally in histological sections of the placenta; there are no macroscopic abnormalities. Histologically, the villitis may resemble any of the previously described morphologic varieties, with predominance of any one, or combination of, cell types. Russell has subdivided cases of VUE into two groups, lymphocytic and histiocytic, but has shown no difference in clinical significance between the two.[321] A chronic inflammatory infiltrate has been identified in the fetal membranes in some cases of VUE.[147]

Because of the histological similarity between these lesions and those caused by known infectious agents, VUE is presumed to be infectious. Attempts to identify a causative agent by microscopic, serologic, or morphologic techniques have, by definition, failed. The possibility that VUE might represent an immunologic response has been presented.[212,303]

Circulatory Disorders

Infarct

An infarct in the placenta, as in any other organ, is an area of ischemic necrosis resulting from obstruction of its blood supply.

GENERAL FEATURES

Because of the unique, dual vasculature of the placenta, there has been some controversy historically about whether infarction is a result of obstruction of the fetal or the maternal circulatory system or both. It is now clear that the villi are sustained by the oxygen and nutrients supplied by the maternal blood in the intervillous space and that most infarcts are due to occlusion of maternal uteroplacental vessels. A retroplacental hematoma also may result in an infarct by physically separating the placenta from its maternal blood supply. It may be conceptually difficult to imagine how villi immersed in a pool of blood supplied by numerous maternal arterioles can become ischemic after the occlusion of a single or even a few maternal vessels. Hemodynamically, however, there does not appear to be any significant amount of mixing of blood from the various maternal inflow streams, despite the fact that these are not defined by actual anatomic channels. The streams or jets of blood from the maternal spiral arteries, then, function as any other end arteriole.

CLINICAL FEATURES

Infarcts are common; they occur in about 25% of otherwise normal term placentas.[128] In this situation, they are small, generally involving less than 5% of the villous parenchyma. The finding of a small infarct in an otherwise normal placenta is of no clinical significance. Multiple or large infarcts or infarcts in the first or second trimester are indicative of significant, underlying maternal vascular disease. In women with hypertension (preeclampsia and essential hypertension), the frequency and extent of infarction are increased in proportion to the severity of the underlying maternal disease.[128] Extensive placental infarction also has been documented in the condition of the circulating lupus anticoagulant.[104,279,355]

GROSS FINDINGS

Infarcts may occur in any portion of the placenta but are most common at its periphery. They often are triangular in shape with the base abutting the basal plate (Fig. 23.47). The gross appearance of a placental infarct changes with age. Fresh infarcts are red and might be difficult to distinguish from the surrounding normal placenta were it not for their firm consistency. Infarcts grow progressively firmer and change in color from red to brown and then to yellow or white.

MICROSCOPIC FINDINGS

The histological appearance of an infarct also changes with age. In early infarcts, the villi are crowded together, with extreme narrowing or obliteration of the intervillous space (Fig. 23.48). Small amounts of fibrin may accumulate in the intervillous space. The villous vessels are dilated and congested (Fig. 23.49). The syncytiotrophoblast, vascular endothelium, and villous stroma undergo progressive necrosis until eventually the infarct consists of crowded, ghost-like remnants of necrotic villi. A perivillous rim of acidophilic material is all that remains of the syncytiotro-

phoblast (Fig. 23.50). Eventually, the fetal stem arteries supplying the infarcted villi undergo fibromuscular sclerosis. There may be an acute inflammatory response to the infarct, which is peripheral, generally mild, and does not actually involve the villous parenchyma. Infarcts in the placenta are not phagocytized or organized as they are in other organs.

CLINICAL BEHAVIOR AND TREATMENT

Extensive placental infarction is associated with fetal hypoxia, intrauterine growth retardation, and fetal death in utero.[128] These ill effects on the fetus probably are not due simply to the destruction of villous tissue but are the result of the superimposition of infarction on a placenta already compromised by a pathologically altered maternal vascular tree and low uteroplacental blood flow (see Preeclampsia (Toxemia of Pregnancy) and Eclampsia).

Maternal Floor Infarct

Maternal floor infarction is a disorder characterized by heavy deposition of fibrin in the decidua basalis. The fibrin extends into the intervillous space where it envelops villi that become avascular and sclerotic. Grossly the maternal surface of the placenta is thickened, firm, and pale yellow. The lesion often is diffuse but, on occasion, may not involve the entire floor.

The reported frequency of maternal floor infarction ranges from 0.09% to 5%.[23,260] The entity has been associ-

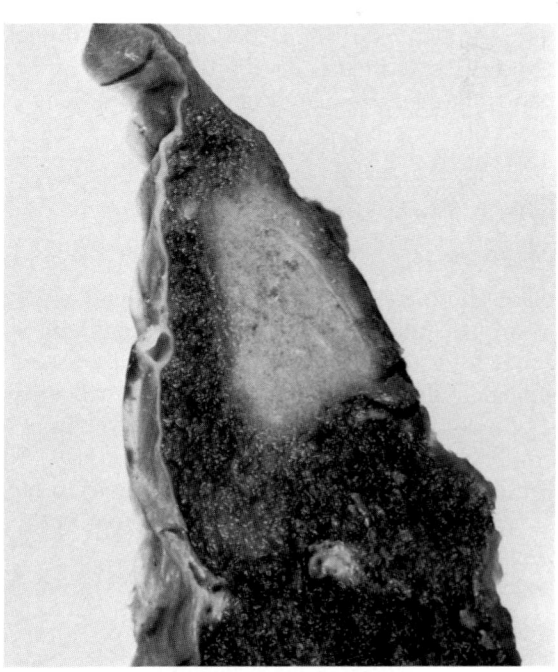

FIG. 23.47. Infarct. Triangular, white infarct with base abutting the basal plate.

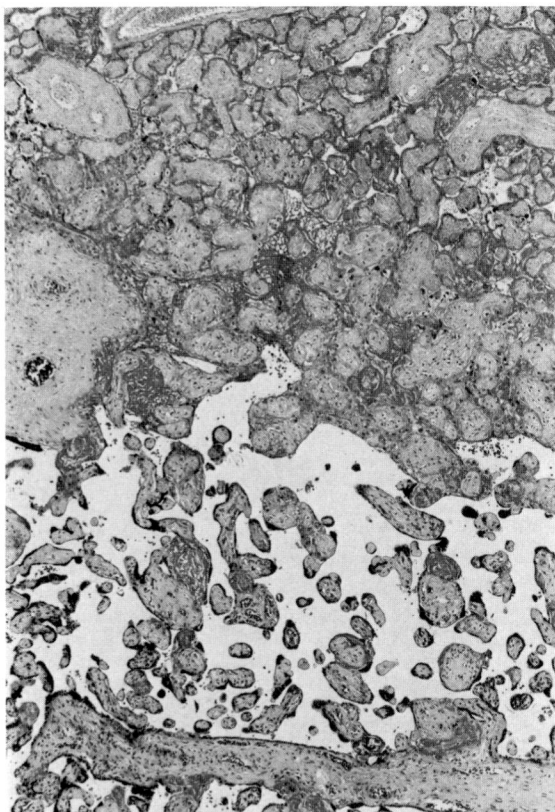

FIG. 23.48. Placental infarct (*top*). Aggregation of villi and obliteration of the intervillous space. Adjacent normal placenta is on the *bottom*.

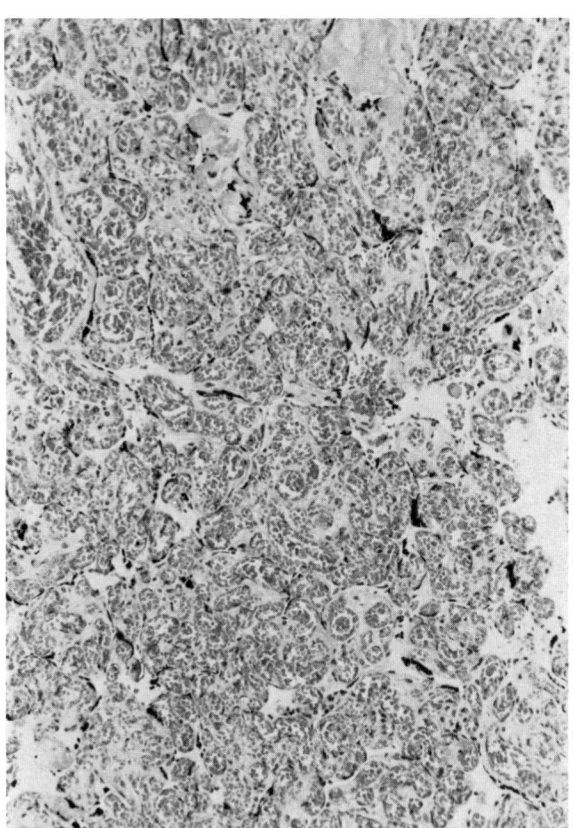

FIG. 23.49. Very early placental infarct. The villous vessels are markedly dilated and congested, but there is little evidence of necrosis.

ated with a high rate of fetal mortality (17–40%) and intrauterine growth retardation (51%). The pathophysiologic basis for the lesion and its complications is unclear. Maternal floor infarction frequently recurs in successive pregnancies.[23,85]

Perivillous Fibrin Deposition

CLINICAL FEATURES

Perivillous fibrin deposition is a regular finding in the normal term placenta. The etiology of this condition is unknown, but it is thought to result from localized stasis and thrombosis of the maternal blood in the intervillous space. The fibrin deposition isolates the entrapped villi from their maternal blood supply and they undergo sclerosis. Fox[127] has presented evidence that the process seems to require good maternal blood flow and is less frequent in the placentas of women with preeclampsia.[127]

GROSS FINDINGS

When the process is extensive enough to result in a grossly visible lesion, it usually is seen as irregular white mottling. Occasionally, it may form a hard, white, well-defined

plaque, often located peripherally in the marginal angle of the placenta, which may be difficult to distinguish from an infarct or an old intervillous thrombohematoma.

MICROSCOPIC FINDINGS

Microscopically, the intervillous space is distended and obliterated by fibrin, which widely separates the entrapped, fibrotic, avascular villi (Fig. 23.51). These villi lose their syncytiotrophoblastic covering, but the cytotrophoblast proliferates markedly, forming prominent mantles around the villi and extending into the surrounding fibrin.

CLINICAL BEHAVIOR

Perivillous fibrin deposition, in general, seems to have no adverse clinical effects, even when relatively large sectors of the villous parenchyma are rendered nonfunctional by this process. Specifically, there is no relationship between the occurrence of perivillous fibrin deposition and decreased fetal weight, fetal distress, or intrauterine fetal death.[127] This emphasizes the considerable functional reserve of the placenta under normal conditions. In contrast, when large true infarcts result in the inactivation of a

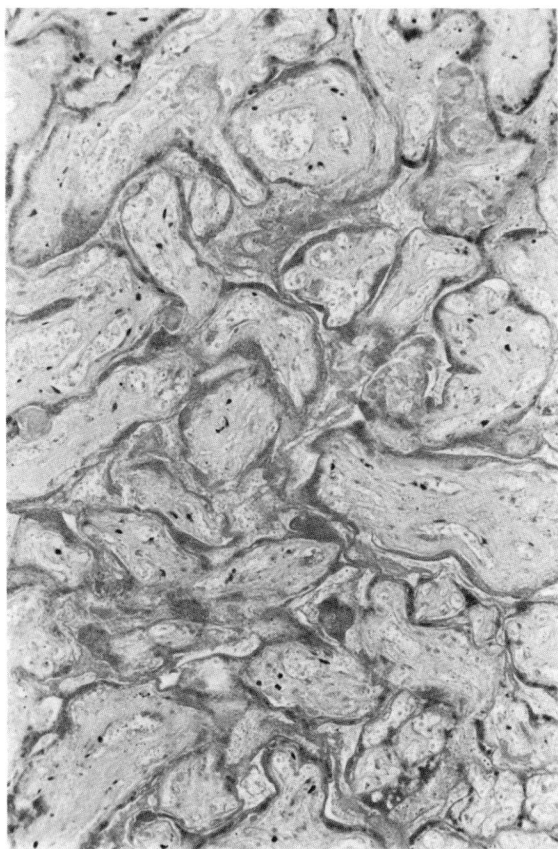

FIG. 23.50. **Placental infarct.** The villi in this old infarct are ghost-like. A perivillous eosinophilic rim is all that remains of the completely necrotic trophoblast.

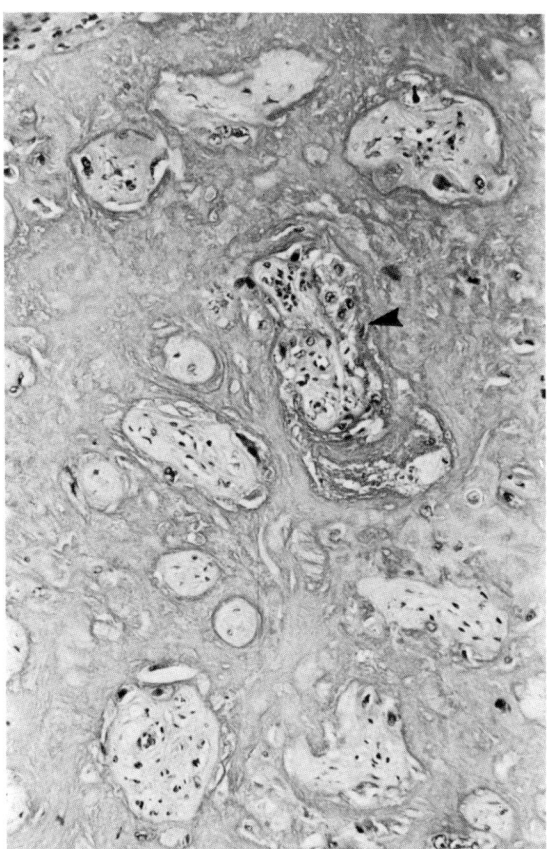

FIG. 23.51. **Perivillous fibrin deposition.** Villi are separated by and enmeshed in dense perivillous fibrin plaque. The cytotrophoblast proliferates around villi (*arrow*) and extends into surrounding fibrin.

similar or even lesser number of villi, fetal anoxia or growth retardation is much more likely. The difference may be explained by the differing background from which the two lesions arise, placental ischemia and uteroplacental vascular disease in the case of infarction as opposed to healthy maternal vessels and good blood supply in perivillous fibrin deposition. Massive perivillous fibrin deposition, sometimes referred to as *gitter infarct*, occasionally may accompany maternal floor infarction, in which case it may be associated with intrauterine growth retardation or stillbirth.[42]

Subchorionic Fibrin

Fibrin plaques similar to perivillous fibrin deposits normally are distributed beneath the chorionic plate of the term placenta. They are thought to have the same pathogenesis as perivillous fibrin deposition, that is, thrombosis of maternal blood in the subchorionic space. The amount of subchorionic fibrin and its distribution varies considerably but, in general, it seems to increase with gestational age. One recent study has linked the absence of subchorionic fibrin with markers of fetal hypoactivity.[262]

Massive Subchorial Thrombosis (Breus' Mole)

The massive subchorial thrombohematoma has been defined as coagulated blood, at least 1 cm in thickness, which separates the chorionic plate from the underlying villi over much of its area (Fig. 23.52).[346] These generally are rela-

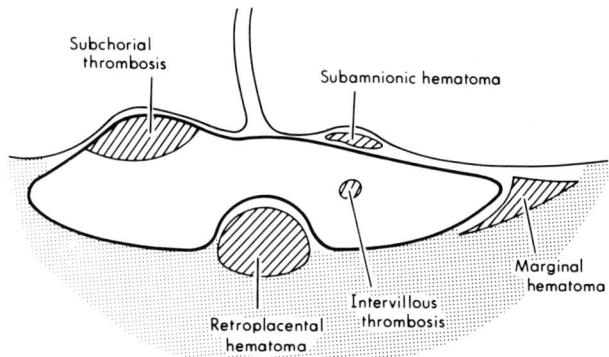

FIG. 23.52. **Diagrammatic representation of various placental thrombi and hematomas.** (After Fox, ref. 132.)

tively fresh, red thrombi that distort the chorionic plate and protrude as nodular or tuberous masses into the amnionic cavity. They may dissect into the chorionic plate itself or extend into the intervillous space, sometimes as far as the basal plate. Histologically, they consist of laminated thrombus devoid of villi.

A massive thrombohematoma in the subchorionic region is a rare event. The incidence of massive subchorial thrombohematoma was estimated to be 0.53 per 1000 deliveries in one large study.[346] The etiology and pathogenesis of the lesion are unknown. The original description by Breus and subsequent reports by others indicated that these thrombi are found mainly in abortions and, therefore, may be a consequence of fetal death. However, the demonstration of massive subchorial thrombohematomas in mature placentas associated with live births refutes the view that fetal death is necessarily the primary event.[346] Rather, it is possible that the hematoma may cause fetal death by distortion and compression of the chorionic plate and fetal vessels. Most authors agree that the thrombi are maternal in origin.[41,132,346]

Retroplacental Hematoma

A retroplacental hematoma is located between the basal plate of the placenta and the uterine wall (Fig. 23.53).

GENERAL FEATURES

The etiology and pathogenesis of retroplacental bleeding are uncertain. The overall prevalence of retroplacental hematoma is reportedly about 4.5%,[132] but it is considerably increased in the placentas of women with preeclampsia. Rupture of a spiral artery weakened by the pathological alterations that occur in preeclampsia is the usual explanation, but since retroplacental hematomas are by no means confined to women with preeclampsia, other factors must be involved. Alternative theories include venous rupture following thrombosis of decidual arterioles and decidual necrosis, venous outflow obstruction, or primary placental separation. A deficiency of folic acid has been proposed as one factor predisposing to abnormal placental separation.[169] Other factors associated with retroplacental hematoma include trauma, cigarette smoking, acute chorioamnionitis,[93] cocaine abuse, and previous abruption.[195]

CLINICAL FEATURES

Retroplacental hematoma, the pathological lesion, should be distinguished from placental abruption (abruptio placenta), the acute clinical syndrome characterized by pain, uterine tetany, fetal distress, and sometimes disseminated intravascular coagulation. Although the two frequently are associated, clinical abruption often is not associated with any discernible placental abnormality and, conversely, ret-

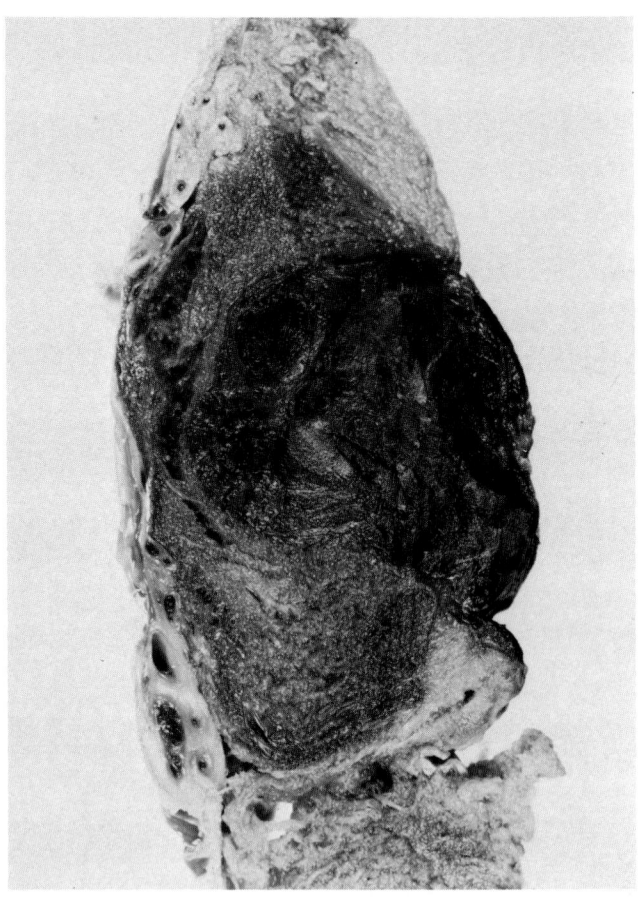

FIG. 23.53. Retroplacental hematoma. Characteristic compression and infarction of the placental parenchyma overlying a large retroplacental hematoma. The surrounding, lighter, normal placenta contrasts with the darker, infarcted tissue.

roplacental hematomas may be found in the absence of clinical signs or symptoms. In fact, Gruenwald et al. have shown that each of these conditions is present more frequently without than with the other.[159] Placental abruption is an acute clinical situation followed rapidly by delivery. It is not surprising that the authentic clinical syndrome may be associated with a placenta that lacks the expected pathological changes. A retroplacental hematoma must have been present for some period of time to be recognizable as such. The frequent association of the two conditions may be explained by postulating that retroplacental hematomas and premature separation may occur in several stages, finally resulting in the clinical syndrome of placental abruption in some patients.

GROSS FINDINGS

When confined, a retroplacental hematoma compresses the overlying placental parenchyma, which is often, but not always, infarcted (Fig. 23.54). This characteristic depression in the maternal surface permits gross recognition and

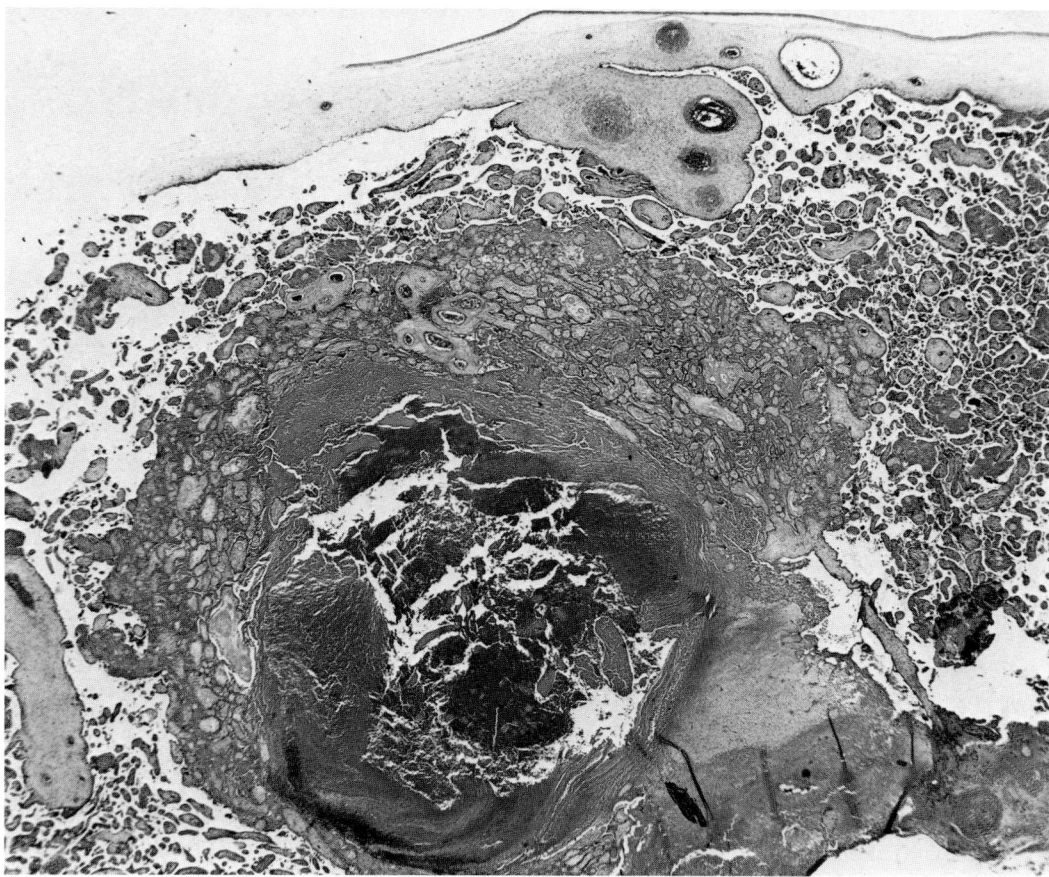

Fig. 23.54. Retroplacental hematoma. Histological appearance of a retroplacental hematoma showing elevation of the basal plate and infarction of the adjacent placenta.

diagnosis of the pathological process, even when the hematoma itself has been detached from the placenta during delivery. As the name indicates, retroplacental hematomas originate behind the placenta. A large retroperitoneal hematoma, however, may extend to the placental margin, in which case it may decompress, resulting in vaginal bleeding. In this circumstance, the overlying placenta may not be depressed. If the pregnancy continues, the devascularized villous tissue eventually will infarct, but the placenta delivered immediately after the development of symptoms and signs of abruption may show little or no histological change.

MICROSCOPIC FINDINGS

Microscopically, retroplacental hematomas consist of red cells and fibrin, the proportion of fibrin increasing as the lesion ages and the red cells degenerate. The time course of the evolution of retroplacental hematomas is unknown. The overlying basal plate may be normal but is more commonly necrotic. An acute inflammatory infiltrate and hemosiderin deposits often are present. Retroplacental hematomas are composed predominantly of maternal blood, but in some cases there may be a significant fetal component as well.[79]

The infarcted placenta overlying the hematoma is microscopically identical to the infarcts described above. Blanc[54] has described an additional, somewhat different pattern in some infarcts associated with retroplacental hematoma. These so-called divergent infarcts are characterized by necrotic villi that are widely separated by a markedly enlarged and congested intervillous space. This particular infarction pattern has been attributed to interruption of both venous and arterial circulations in contrast to true or convergent infarcts, which are secondary to pure maternal artery occlusion.

CLINICAL BEHAVIOR

Both abruption and retroplacental hematoma have serious implications for fetal well-being. Individually, each carries a high risk of premature birth and perinatal mortality. The significance of a retroplacental hematoma appears to be related to size.[132] In separating a portion of the placenta from its maternal blood supply, a retroplacental hematoma is responsible for an infarct. The larger the infarct, the more likely it will be to exceed the functional reserve capability of the placenta. When complicated by disseminated intravascular coagulation, abruption also is responsible for high maternal morbidity and mortality.

Marginal Hematoma

A marginal hematoma occurs where the external, or lateral, margin of the placenta joins the fetal membranes (Fig. 23.52). Grossly, the marginal hematoma forms a crescent-shaped clot adherent to the lateral margin of the placenta. It may extend beneath the adjacent fetal membranes or for some distance onto the maternal aspect of the placenta, but in contrast to retroplacental hematoma, it does not cause depression of the basal plate or infarction of overlying villous parenchyma. On cut section, the clot is triangular in shape, the apex of the triangle being formed by the junction of the membranous and villous chorion.

Microscopically, the blood clot often is accompanied by an acute inflammatory infiltrate and hemosiderin deposition. The clot usually lies entirely outside the placental disk but occasionally may involve the intervillous space. With this exception, the presence of a marginal hematoma has no effect on the adjacent villi.

Marginal hematomas are thought to result from rupture of uteroplacental veins at the margin of a low-lying placenta. The hematoma invariably is found at the margin of the placenta closest to the site of membrane rupture, which usually is only a few centimeters from the placental margin.[132] A marginal hematoma is associated with antepartum maternal hemorrhage but does not have any untoward affects on the fetus.

Intervillous Thrombus

Intervillous thrombi are round or oval blood clots that may occur anywhere in the intervillous space but are most common midway between the chorionic and basal plates. They begin as red, fluid, or semifluid blood (Kline's hemorrhage) and become progressively laminated and depigmented with age (Fig. 23.55). They may be single, although multiple lesions are very common. Most are 1 to 3 cm in diameter. Microscopically, the thrombi consist of erythrocytes and fibrin, the proportion of fibrin increasing with the age of the lesion (Fig. 23.56). The villi are displaced to the margins of the clot. Nucleated red blood cells have been identified in these thrombi.[100,132,194]

Recent studies have confirmed that intervillous thrombi do contain a proportion of fetal erythrocytes,[194] although maternal erythrocytes seem to comprise most of the lesion. Fetal bleeding into the intervillous space is thought to occur through rupture of the attenuated vasculosyncytial membrane. Factors cited as potential causes of villous damage resulting in fetomaternal transfusion include

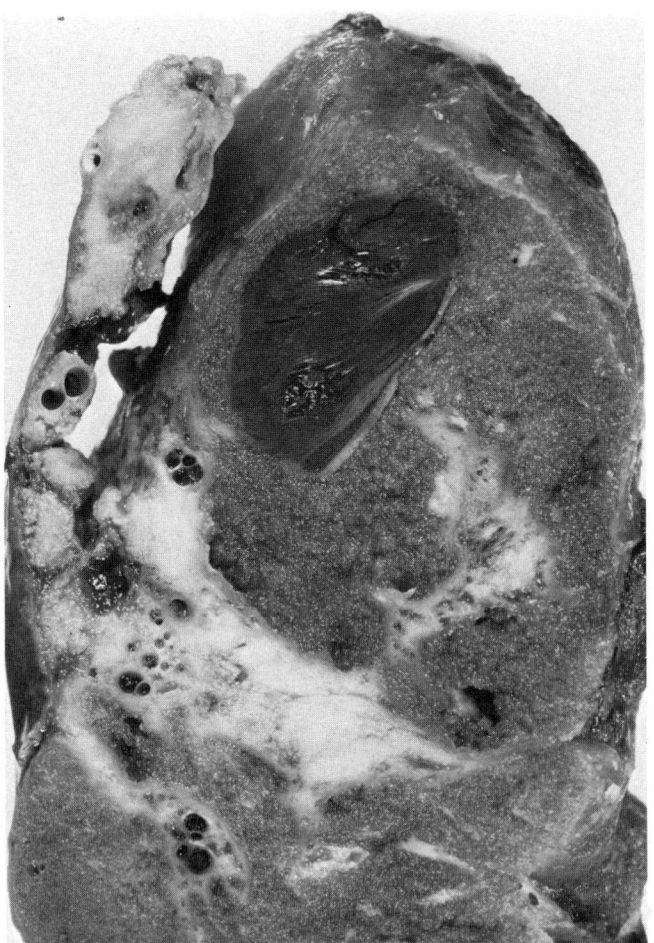

FIG. 23.55. Intervillous thrombus. Intervillous thrombi become laminated as they age.

trauma, amniocentesis, and external version.[306] The mechanism of coagulation is unknown. There does not appear to be a link between intervillous thrombi and maternofetal ABO incompatibility.[32]

An intervillous thrombus is significant in that it marks the site of hemorrhage from the fetal to the maternal circulation. Fetomaternal hemorrhages, as assessed by the Kleihauer–Betke technique, are relatively common in the third trimester of pregnancy, occurring in 15–30% of cases. Intervillous thrombi also are found with increasing frequency in the third trimester. There appears to be good correlation between the number of fetal cells in the maternal circulation and the number of intervillous thrombi.[100,405] The same relationship applies in some other placental lesions, including retroplacental hematomas and infarct.[405]

Fetomaternal hemorrhage, when massive, may be a cause of fetal anemia or intrauterine demise.[306] Smaller fetomaternal transfusions may initiate the production of maternal antibodies to fetal cells, resulting in hemolytic disease in the fetus.

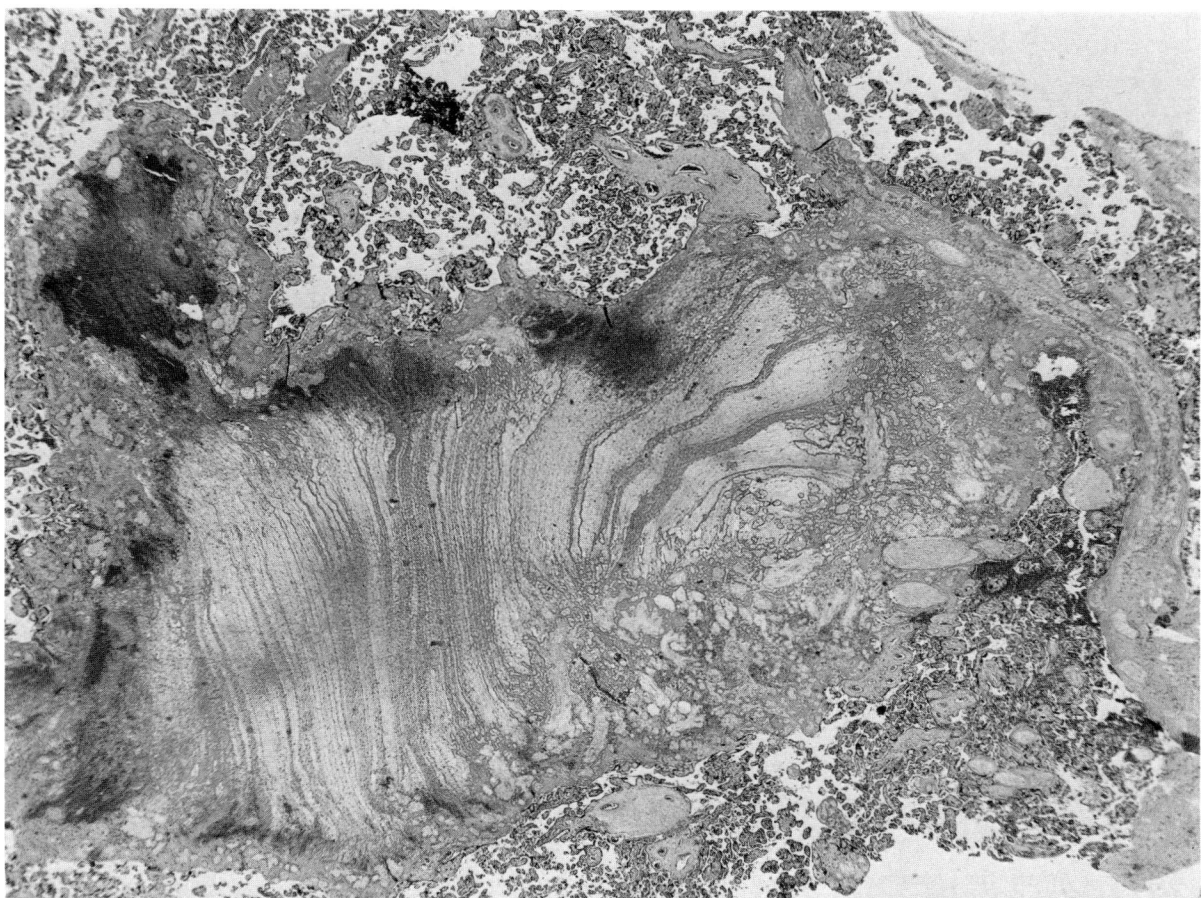

FIG. 23.56. **Intervillous thrombus.** Histological appearance of laminated fibrin and erythrocytes in an intervillous thrombus.

Subamnionic Hematoma

A subamnionic hematoma lies between the amnion and chorion on the fetal surface of the placenta (Fig. 23.52). Very recent lesions are thought to result from trauma to the chorionic veins during delivery, especially after excessive traction on the umbilical cord. Older chorionic fibrin clots, of unknown pathogenesis, form dome-shaped blisters and contain a mixture of brown-tinged fluid and fibrin. Neither lesion has significant implications for the fetus.

Fetal Artery Thrombosis

Occlusion of a fetal stem artery results in villous avascularity distally. Grossly, the lesion produced is a well-delineated area of pallor without any marked change in consistency as compared to the surrounding normal parenchyma. Microscopically, the villi are avascular, the villous stroma is hyalinized and fibrotic, and the syncytiotrophoblast nuclei cluster extensively to form prominent syncytial knots (Fig. 23.57). The intervillous space is normally patent. The thrombosed fetal stem artery may show some degree of recanalization. There usually is marked fibromuscular sclerosis in the vessels of stem villi distal to the thrombosis.

Isolated thrombosis of a fetal stem artery is uncommon; it occurs in about 4.5% of full-term placentas.[132] The lesion is seen with increased frequency in diabetes mellitus.[111,132] The pathogenesis of fetal artery thrombosis is not always apparent, but it has been seen in association with thrombi in velamentous blood vessels and in placentas associated with maternal hypercoagulable states, including protein C deficiency and the lupus anticoagulant.[342,350]

Hemorrhagic Endovasculitis and Villitis

Hemorrhagic endovasculitis (HEV) is a distinctive lesion involving the fetal blood vessels of the placenta.[331] As described by Sander in 1980, HEV is characterized by a constellation of histological findings including vascular necrosis, thrombi in various stages of organization, endothelial proliferation, recanalization of vessels, fragmentation and diapedesis of red cells, and villous stromal hemorrhage and hemosiderin deposition (Figs. 23.58, 23.59). In most cases, the lesion involves all segments of the fetal vascular tree, but occasionally it may be confined to vessels of one caliber. Associated placental findings have included decreased placental weight, umbilical cord abnormalities, meconium staining, VUE, and erythroblastosis.[332]

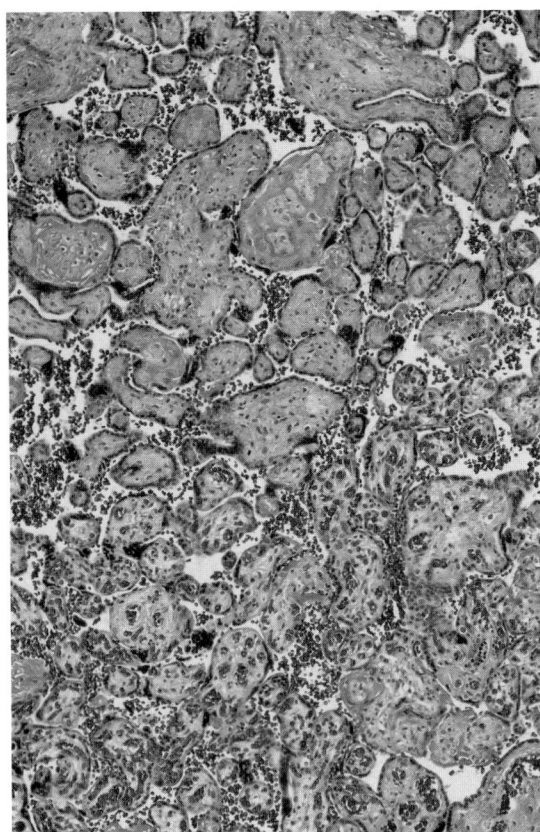

FIG. 23.57. Fetal artery thrombosis. The avascular villi (*upper*) reflect the changes associated with fetal artery thrombosis and contrast with the functional villi (*lower*) in this placenta from a liveborn baby.

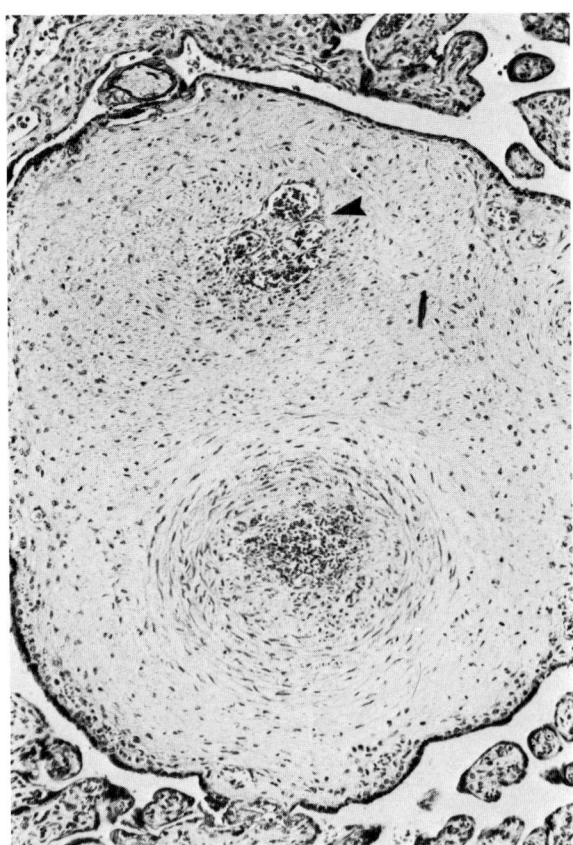

FIG. 23.58. Hemorrhagic endovasculitis. Thrombi in various stages of organization in vessels of stem villi. Recanalized channels are apparent (*arrow*).

The reported prevalence of HEV is highly variable; Sander diagnosed the lesion in 19.5% of placentas submitted to the Michigan Placental Tissue Registry, but Shen-Schwartz and others found it in the placentas of only 0.67% of unselected pregnancies.[331,347] Clinically, the lesion has been significantly associated with stillbirth, intrauterine growth retardation, long-term developmental delay, maternal hypertension or preeclampsia, post-term gestation, and the presence of a nuchal cord during delivery.[332,347] HEV has recurred in successive pregnancies in some patients.[332]

The etiology and pathogenesis of HEV are not clear. Its reported association with chronic villitis and the identification of viral and mycoplasma-like structures ultrastructurally have been cited as support for the hypothesis that HEV is infection related.[332] The finding of localized HEV adjacent to venous thrombi, its frequent association with nuchal cord, and the identification of an HEV-like lesion in human chorionic villous organ culture have led others to postulate that HEV results from regional compromise of villous perfusion and hypoxia.[347,354] An HEV-like lesion also has been reported in a patient with protein C deficiency and thrombotic lesions in the mother and fetus.[206]

Spiral Artery Thrombosis

Recurrent pregnancy loss is a well-recognized complication in women with circulating antiphospholipid antibody (lupus anticoagulant).[104,206] The same problem occurs with other maternal coagulation disorders such as deficiencies of protein C, protein S, and antithrombin III.[206] Some patients have experienced multiple abortions occurring late in the second or early in the third trimester, and some have had unexplained intrauterine growth retardation in previous gestations. In these conditions, both acute and organizing thrombi may occur in spiral arteries (Fig. 23.60), and infarcts are common.[302] Thrombi also may occur in the fetal circulation, evident in the placenta as fetal artery thrombosis or in the newborn as catastrophic large vessel thrombi.[342,350]

Chorangiosis

Chorangiosis refers to the occurrence of numerous greatly enlarged, highly vascular villi throughout the placenta. The villous stroma usually is abundant and is interspersed diffusely with the numerous capillaries (Fig. 23.61). As defined by Altshuler, there should be more than 10 villi in clusters that contain more than 10 capillaries per villus, oc-

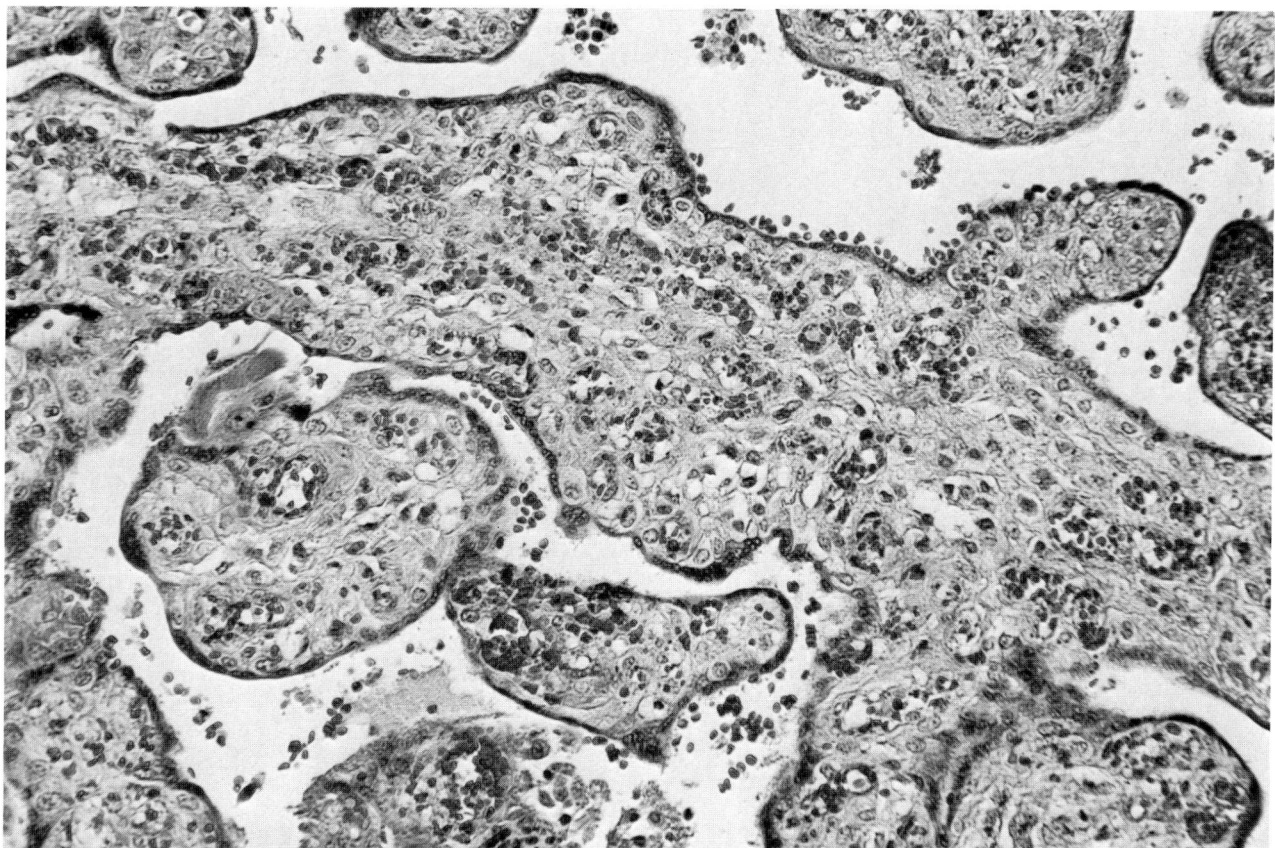

FIG. 23.59. **Hemorrhagic endovasculitis.** Fragmented red blood cells and nuclear debris are present in the terminal villi. Many of the vessels of these terminal villi have been destroyed.

curring in multiple areas (at least three) in multiple sections of the placenta.[14] Chorangiosis appears to be a nonspecific change related to a variety of conditions including gestational diabetes, hypertension, infections, anomalies, intrauterine fetal death, and growth retardation.[14,360]

In one large study, chorangiosis occurred in 3% of 1614 deliveries and was associated with placental lesions including infarcts, chronic villitis, fetal artery thrombi, and spiral artery thrombi.[360] The pathogenesis of chorangiosis is unknown, and its functional significance has not been studied directly. The central location of most of the capillaries might suggest the possibility of a shunt, comparable to hemangioma, that could become clinically significant if sufficient numbers of villi are affected; hence, the importance of the quantitative criteria recommended by Altshuler.[14] The finding of occasional villi with these features seems to have no clinical significance.

The Placenta in Maternal and Fetal Disorders

Placentas in pregnancies complicated by any maternal disease should be submitted routinely for pathological examination with the goal of defining what morphologic effect such diseases have had on the placenta and fetus. Although many studies have focused on these very issues, there is, unfortunately, a great deal of disagreement and direct contradiction about the nature and significance of the lesions or alterations described.

Preeclampsia (Toxemia of Pregnancy) and Eclampsia

Preeclampsia has been defined traditionally as the development of hypertension in pregnancy with proteinuria or generalized edema or both after 20 weeks of gestation. In a recent classification of the hypertensive disorders of pregnancy, preeclampsia has been designated gestational proteinuric hypertension.[94] Eclampsia signifies the occurrence of convulsions in a patient with preeclampsia.

CLINICAL FEATURES

Preeclampsia is a major cause of morbidity and mortality in both the mother and fetus. The etiology and pathogenesis of preeclampsia is unknown, but reduced choriodecidual blood flow and uteroplacental ischemia are constant features.[72,73,107,224] Doppler-derived patterns of vascular re-

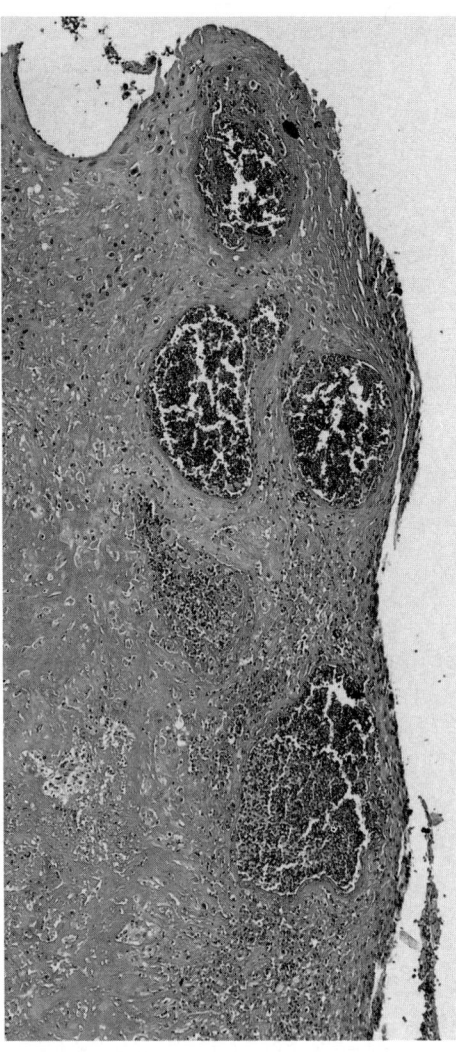

FIG. 23.60. Spiral artery thrombosis. The spiral arteries show thrombi in various stages of development in this patient with the lupus anticoagulant.

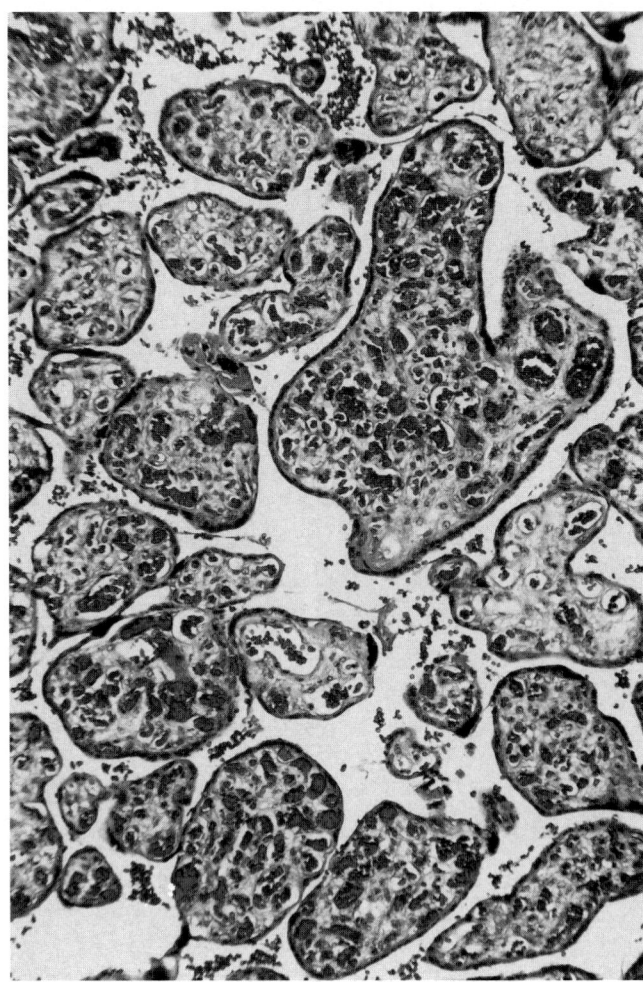

FIG. 23.61. Choriangiosis. Greatly increased numbers of villous capillaries in choriangiosis.

sistance in umbilical and uterine arteries appear to correlate with perinatal outcome in women with preeclampsia and other forms of hypertension.[116] Umbilical artery blood flow and vascular resistance as determined by Doppler velocimetry have been related to placental microvascular anatomy.[149] The possibility that preeclampsia is an immune-mediated disorder has long been considered.[338] Immunoglobulins and complement have been demonstrated in spiral arteries showing acute atherosis, but this is neither a specific nor a constant finding in preeclampsia.[201] Attention also has been focused on the cellular reaction at the maternal–fetal interface but, as yet, there is no clear immunological explanation for preeclampsia. There is a growing body of evidence relating preeclampsia to an imbalance in prostacyclin and thromboxane.[137,384] These observations have led to some successful preventive efforts.[384,395] At present, it is uncertain which of the derangements seen in preeclampsia are primary and which represent secondary phenomena.

GROSS FINDINGS

There is an extensive but conflicting literature dealing with the placental lesions associated with preeclampsia. Most investigators agree that, overall, infarcts are more numerous and larger in placentas from preeclamptic women than in uncomplicated pregnancy.[132,403] The extent of infarction is related directly to the severity of the preeclampsia. Extensive placental infarction is a cardinal sign of preeclampsia, but it is neither specific for nor invariable in that condition. Placental infarcts are common, and their significance in preeclampsia is a quantitative distinction. Retroplacental hematoma is the other gross lesion identified with undue frequency (12–15%) in preeclamptic women.[132] This, of course, is an added factor in the increased frequency of infarction in these placentas. The placenta in preeclampsia tends to be smaller on average than the placenta from an uncomplicated pregnancy.[132]

MICROSCOPIC FINDINGS

Histologically, the infarcts may be old or recent, but there is some indication that recent infarcts are particularly characteristic of the placenta of severe preeclampsia.[31,403] There are no distinctive microscopic features of the infarcts or retroplacental hematomas associated with preeclampsia. The villi in preeclampsia show subtle but consistent microscopic changes, which include cytotrophoblastic proliferation, thickening and alteration of the trophoblastic basement membrane, small, inconspicuous fetal capillaries, and increased prominence of the villous stroma.[261,310] The villi may be exceedingly small, and villous syncytial knots are increased ("Tenney-Parker" change) (Fig. 23.62).[216,217,261,382] There is narrowing and

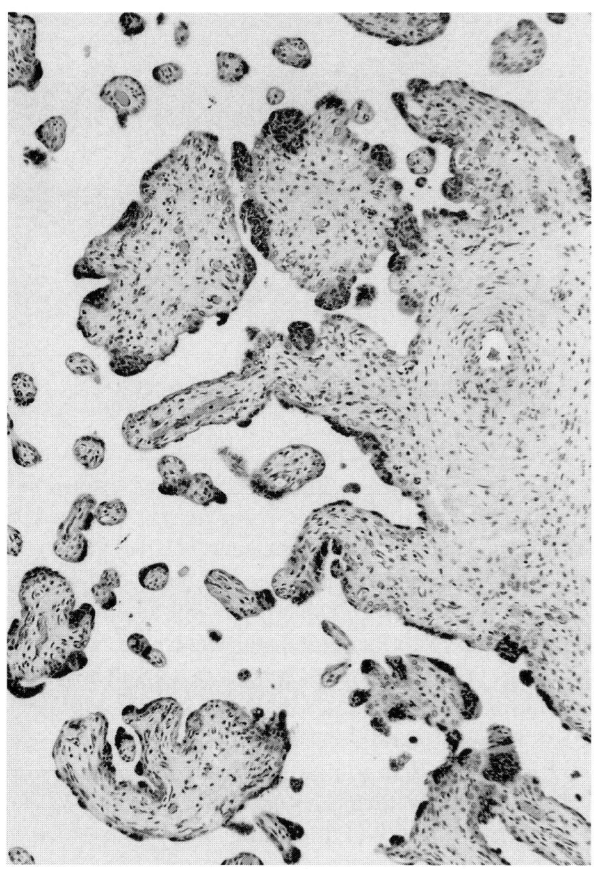

FIG. 23.62. Villi in preeclampsia. The villous changes in this placenta from a pregnancy complicated by severe preeclampsia at 17 weeks include markedly accelerated maturation and increased syncytial knots (Tenney–Parker change).

ultimate obliteration of the lumina of the fetal stem arteries.[217,393] Ultrastructural studies have confirmed all these changes and have emphasized the additional finding of focal syncytiotrophoblastic necrosis, not appreciated at the light microscopic level.[187] These changes have been attributed to placental ischemia, and they occur in villi cultured under conditions of low oxygen tension[130,226] as well as in the placentas of pregnant animals in whom toxemia has been produced experimentally.[1,2] Hypoxia also has been associated with three-dimensional deformation in the shape of the terminal villi, which have been characterized as short, knob-like, and multiply indented.[42]

In addition, well-described, distinctive morphologic abnormalities occur in the maternal arteries of the placental bed in preeclampsia. These arteries differ from their normal counterparts in two important respects: (1) the adaptive and physiologic changes that take place routinely in the vessels of the placental bed are decreased in degree and extent, and (2) some of the vessels exhibit an acute necrotizing arteriopathy termed *acute atherosis*. The identification and characterization of pathologic lesions in the uteroplacental arteries is greatly complicated by the marked morphologic changes that occur in these vessels during the course of normal pregnancy.

In women with preeclampsia, it appears that the second wave of intravascular trophoblastic migration does not occur. The intramyometrial segments of the spiral arteries retain their musculoelastic media and do not dilate. The physiologic vascular changes that accompany normal implantation, therefore, are incomplete in women with preeclampsia. In some cases of growth-retarded or small-for-gestational-age babies, the physiologic changes of the placental bed·spiral arteries also may be limited to their decidual segments.[10,70,348]

A dramatic vascular lesion termed *acute atherosis* also occurs in the spiral arteries of women with preeclampsia and is characterized by fibrinoid necrosis of vessel walls, accumulation of lipid-containing macrophages, and a perivascular mononuclear infiltrate (Fig. 23.63).[415] The evolution of the lesion, as defined in ultrastructural studies, begins with lipid accumulation in the muscle cells of the intima and media. These cells undergo necrosis and release lipid, which is engulfed by macrophages that accumulate in the damaged vessel wall.[102] Spiral artery thrombosis is commonly associated with acute atherosis but may be difficult to demonstrate unless the pathologist searches carefully for spiral arteries in the thin layer of attached maternal decidua. Placental infarction is thought to be the direct result of the vascular lesions in preeclamptics (Fig. 23.63).[69]

Acute atherosis is thought by some to be a specific feature of preeclampsia with a characteristic distribution. According to Robertson, acute atherosis is a lesion limited to those vessels that have not been altered by the normal adaptive processes of implantation, namely, the decidual

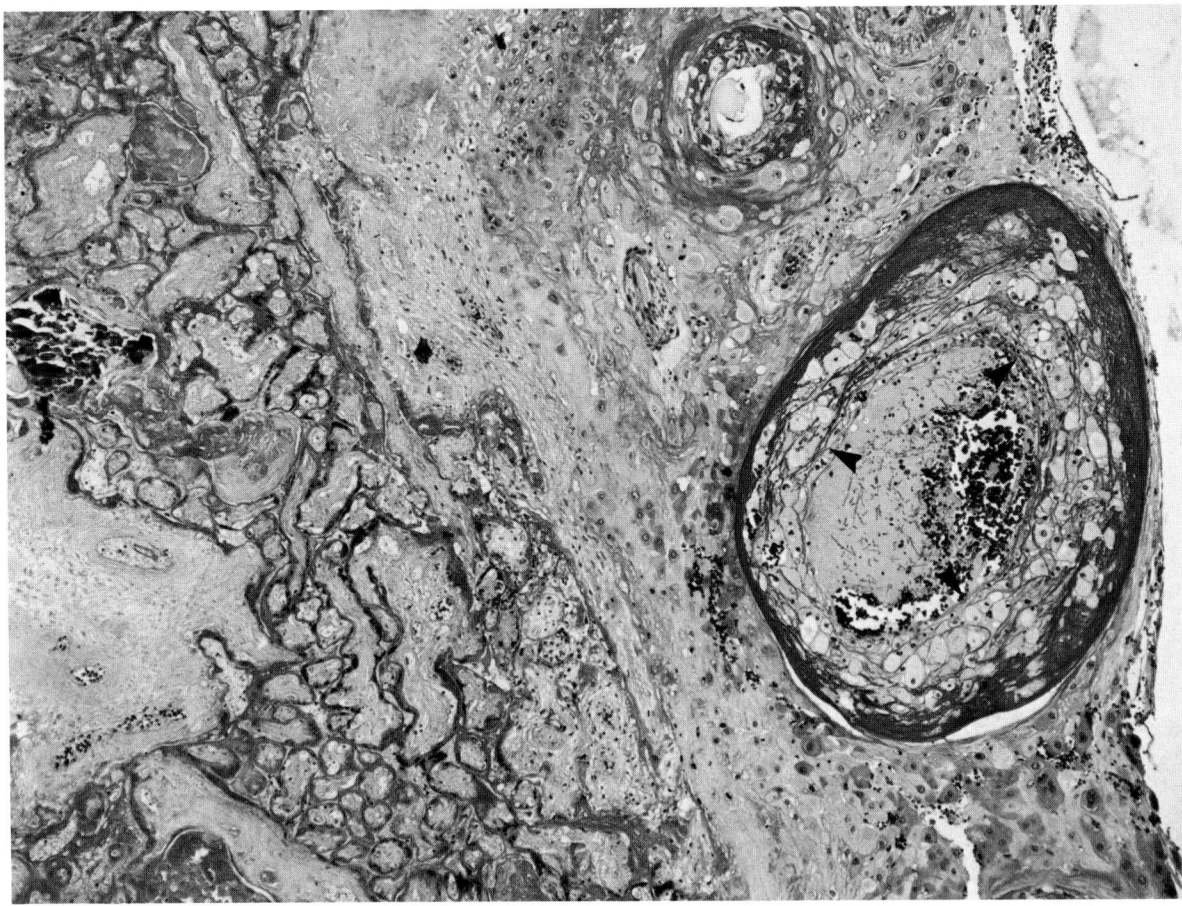

FIG. 23.63. Acute atherosis, preeclampsia. The spiral arteries are distorted by fibrinoid necrosis of the vessel wall and accumulation of lipid-containing macrophages (*arrows*). The largest artery is thrombosed, and there is infarction of the overlying placenta (*left*).

segments of spiral arteries outside the placental bed, the basal arteries, and the myometrial segments of the spiral arteries in the placental bed that have not undergone physiologic adaptations.[312] In fact, the lesions may be seen best outside the placental bed in the decidua vera or decidua capsularis. Acute atherosis, however, also has been described in placentas from pregnancies complicated by diabetes, systemic lupus erythematosus, and the lupus anticoagulant even in the absence of hypertension and albuminuria.[4,104,202] In addition, the lesion has been observed in the spiral arteries of the placental bed in normotensive women with intrauterine growth retardation.[101,348] What relation the acute atherosis of preeclampsia has to that seen in intrauterine growth retardation and various maternal disorders other than preeclampsia remains to be determined.[101,314] How the multitude of pathological changes occurring in preeclampsia relate etiologically to the reduced choriodecidual blood flow, biochemical abnormalities,[97,137,384] and clinical manifestations[339] is unknown.

Essential Hypertension

The pathology of the placenta in essential hypertension has received little attention. A few studies have shown that morphologic changes in the placenta in this disease are qualitatively very similar to those found in preeclampsia (increased frequency and extent of infarcts, cytotrophoblastic hyperplasia, trophoblastic basement membrane thickening). The similarities extend to the ultrastructural level, although the extent and degree of pathological changes are less marked in placentas from cases of essential hypertension than in preeclampsia.[188] A maternal vascular abnormality, termed *hyperplastic arteriosclerosis*, characterized by marked thickening of all coats of the vessel wall, intimal hyperplasia, and luminal narrowing, has been described in women with essential hypertension.[312,313,349] These changes are most conspicuous in the myometrial segments of the spiral arteries. When preeclampsia complicates essential hypertension, there may be superimposition of acute atherosis on hyperplastic arteriosclerosis. Surprisingly, the placental changes (presumably reflecting ischemic damage) in cases of essential hypertension complicated by preeclampsia are less marked than those found in the placentas of previously normotensive women who develop preeclampsia of comparable severity.[188]

Diabetes Mellitus

Reports on the pathology of the placenta in diabetes mellitus are numerous but often contradictory. The inconsistency may be explained, in part, by the inclusion of cases with superimposed hypertension or fetal death in utero. Moreover, the category of diabetic pregnant women is not homogeneous. Many women are diabetic before pregnancy (overt diabetes), whereas others become diabetic during pregnancy. In the latter group, the diabetes may persist (early diabetes) or regress (gestational diabetes) after pregnancy. Furthermore, a number of normal women may give birth to infants resembling those born to women with established diabetes. When followed, some of these mothers may become diabetic and, in retrospect, may be considered to have had prediabetes during pregnancy.

The placentas from diabetic women are, on the average, heavier than normal controls of the same gestational age.[132,165,280] Some, however, may be of normal weight or even small if the patient is suffering from diabetic vascular disease. Grossly, the placenta may appear to be bulky and edematous. The umbilical cord may be increased in diameter, and there is an increased likelihood of finding a single umbilical artery (3–5%) as compared with the general population (1%).[111,165] Most agree that infarcts are not increased in extent or frequency in the placentas of diabetics, but there has been some debate on this point.[258]

Histologically, there are no specific features allowing absolute distinction of the diabetic placenta from any other. There are, however, a constellation of abnormalities that, when taken together, are fairly characteristic. Some degree of villous immaturity is common, although villous maturation sometimes may be normal or even accelerated. Villous edema is common. Cytotrophoblastic cells are numerous and may contain mitotic figures. The trophoblastic basement membrane often shows focal, marked thickening. Villous vascularity is variable; the villi may be hypovascular, normovascular, or show diffuse hypervascularity (chorangiosis).[14,111] Proliferative endarteritis and fetal artery thrombosis have been reported.[111,132] Villi showing fibrinoid necrosis, the deposition of fibrinoid material between the trophoblast and basement membrane, are unduly frequent.[184] Extramedullary hematopoiesis in the villous stroma has been described,[111] although we have not encountered it. Some diabetic placentas have significantly more parenchymal and villous tissue than normal placentas when studied by morphometric techniques.[379]

The status of the uteroplacental vasculature in diabetic women is debated. Some investigators have found no morphologic abnormalities in the maternal vessels.[132,290] Driscoll, however, has described two types of vascular lesions in the decidual vessels: (1) arteriolar medial hypertrophy, hyalinization, and onion skinning in 50% of diabetics, and (2) acute atherosis identical to that described in preeclamptic women.[111] The latter change has been reported both in diabetics with superimposed preeclampsia and in normotensive diabetic women.[202]

Ultrastructural studies have confirmed the light microscopic observations.[165,185] Patchy focal trophoblastic necrosis, usually involving only the syncytiotrophoblast but occasionally also the cytotrophoblast, is an ultrastructural feature. Enlargement and immaturity of the endothelial cells with protrusion into and reduction in the size of the capillary lumen also has been emphasized in ultrastructural studies.[185]

Light and electron microscopic changes qualitatively identical to those found in placentas from women with well-established, overt diabetes mellitus have been documented in women with well-controlled gestational diabetes.[8,185] Although these changes tend to be less marked and occur with less frequency in the group with gestational diabetes, there is considerable overlap between the pathological findings in overt and gestational diabetics.[184,185] Correlation between the severity of the diabetes or degree of metabolic control and the extent of placental changes is poor.[50,380,381]

So far, there has been no good correlation between the presence or extent of the pathological changes in the placenta and the well-documented increase in congenital fetal malformations, neonatal morbidity, or fetal macrosomia in diabetic pregnancies.[165,176,277,286]

Sickle-Cell Trait/Disease

The placenta is a very sensitive detector of sickle cells.[61,140] The maternal erythrocytes in the intervillous space undergo sickling, and careful placental examination can uncover unsuspected or undiagnosed sickle cell trait in some patients (Fig. 23.64). Other placental abnormalities have not been described. The significance of sickle-cell trait in pregnancy outcome is a matter of debate. Reports range from those showing no evidence of adverse clinical sequelae[59] to others that document increased rates of maternal pyelonephritis, refractory anemia,[309] premature rupture of membranes, prematurity,[309] and increased perinatal mortality[291] in pregnancies associated with sickle-cell trait. Lethal maternal complications are rare.[283]

In contrast, pregnant patients with sickle-cell disease experience increased maternal morbidity and mortality. Reported complications include urinary tract infections, pneumonia, painful crises, and worsening anemia. Sickle cell disease also is associated with a high rate of spontaneous abortion, stillbirth, premature delivery, and fetal growth retardation.[22,84,124,204,242,295] Meticulous care and

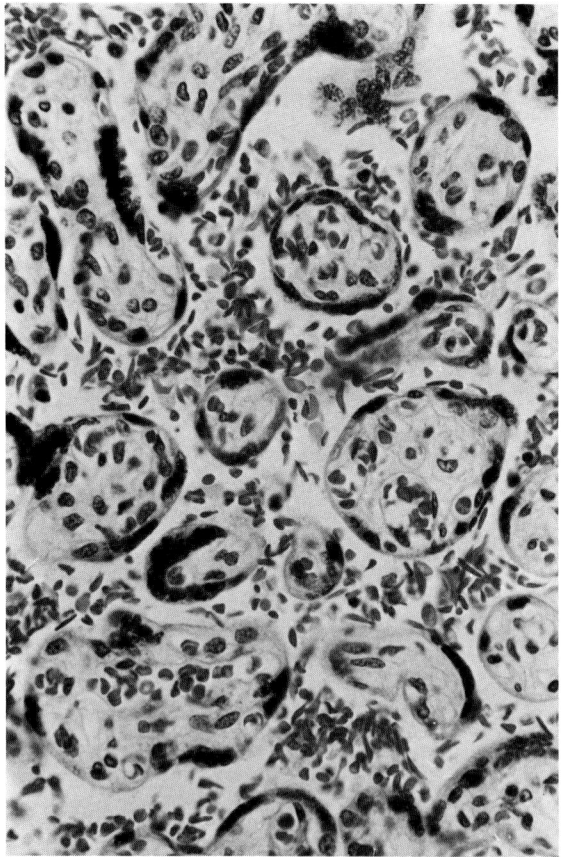

FIG. 23.64. Placenta from a patient with sickle-cell trait. Maternal erythrocytes in the intervillous space show marked sickling.

close hematologic monitoring have resulted in a significant reduction in maternal and fetal mortality. Prophylactic transfusion reduces the frequency of painful crises but does not appear to influence fetal outcome.[204]

The placenta in patients with sickle-cell disease invariably shows sickled maternal erythrocytes in the intervillous space. Additional reported findings include infarction and thrombosis of the maternal sinuses.[204,295]

Maternofetal Rhesus Incompatibility

Maternofetal Rh incompatibility is a condition caused by maternal antibodies directed against the Rh (D) antigens in fetal red blood cells.

CLINICAL FEATURES

Before the advent of prevention programs in the 1960s, maternofetal Rh incompatibility was a significant cause of fetal compromise. The pathological findings in this condition have been well characterized.[404] Commonly associated with fetal edema (hydrops fetalis), the placental changes have been considered part of a generalized ex-

pression of fluid accumulation in the fetus. Anemia, decreased plasma oncotic pressure, and congestive heart failure, together, are the pathophysiologic factors involved in the development of fetoplacental hydrops.

GROSS FINDINGS

Classically, these placentas are enlarged, bulky, edematous, and strikingly pale, although a proportion may be grossly normal in all respects. Intervillous thrombosis is the only gross lesion that occurs with undue frequency; such thrombi are present in almost 50% of placentas and often are multiple. Septal cysts are more common in edematous placentas and, therefore, are found frequently in cases of maternofetal Rh incompatibility.

MICROSCOPIC FINDINGS

Histologically, the villi typically exhibit a combination of nonspecific but characteristic changes. There is a generalized delay in villous maturation, and clumps of markedly immature villi are scattered throughout the placenta. Cytotrophoblastic cells, many containing mitoses, are conspicuous, and there is some degree of thickening of the trophoblastic basement membrane (Fig. 23.65). The vil-

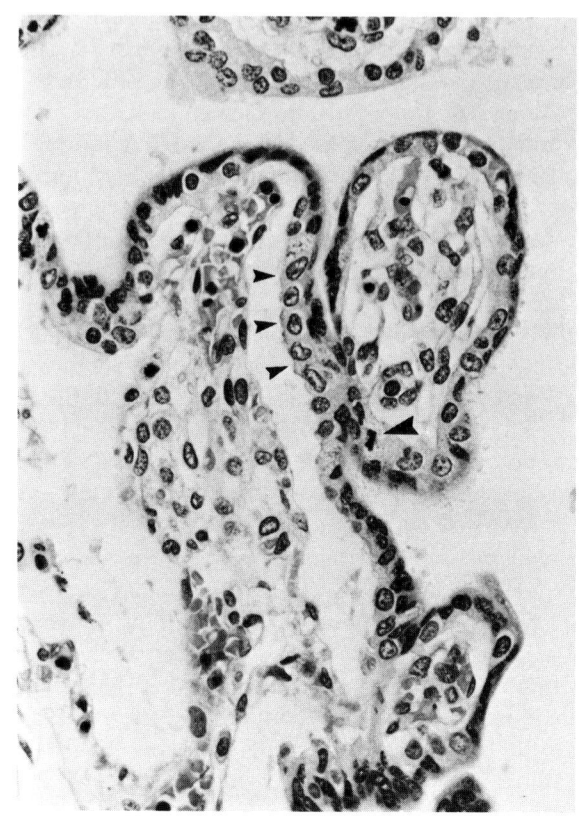

FIG. 23.65. Maternofetal Rh incompatibility, placenta at term. Immature villi with conspicuous cytotrophoblast (*small black arrows*), showing some mitotic activity (*large black arrow*).

lous stroma is edematous and abundant. Hofbauer cells are numerous and prominent. One of the characteristic features of the placenta in Rh incompatibility is the wide variance in the appearance of the villi even in the same field of examination (Fig. 23.66). Nucleated red blood cells and erythroblasts are present within the fetal capillaries (Fig. 23.67). This finding is indicative of fetal anemia and, therefore, is characteristic of maternofetal Rh incompatibility but may be found in any other situation resulting in severe fetal anemia. There is some evidence that placental hyperplasia may contribute to the increased bulk of the placenta.[90] It also has been demonstrated that the intervillous space is reduced.[18] An ultrastructural study of placentas in Rh incompatibility has shown no evidence of immune-mediated damage.[186]

The classic constellation of gross and microscopic findings, including placental enlargement and pallor, villous dysmaturity and edema, cytotrophoblastic hyperplasia, and erythroblastosis, is common and represents an end-stage picture of variable etiology. In addition to Rh incompatibility, isoimmunization against other blood group antigens (ABO, Kell antigens), red cell enzyme defects, alpha-thalassemia, cardiac failure (malformations, endocardial fibroelastosis, large arteriovenous shunts), hypoproteinemia (congenital nephrotic syndrome, defects in hepatic protein synthesis), congenital malformations, congenital infections, fetal blood loss (fetomaternal hemorrhage), and other miscellaneous disorders (Gaucher disease, sacrococcygeal teratoma) may result in identical gross and microscopic changes.[112,120,225,227,251] With the marked decline in Rh incompatibility–associated hydrops, nonimmune hydrops is encountered relatively more commonly. It is estimated that 1:4000 to 1:5000 pregnancies are complicated by the latter disorders. When none of these immunologic or nonimmunologic causative factors is identified, the hydrops is considered to be idiopathic. Idiopathic fetoplacental hydrops has been reported to recur in successive pregnancies.[356]

Pathology of the Membranes

Squamous Metaplasia

Foci of squamous metaplasia may be found on the amnionic surface of the fetal membranes and umbilical cord. Grossly, these foci are slightly elevated, pearly white macules that tend to be most numerous at the site of cord

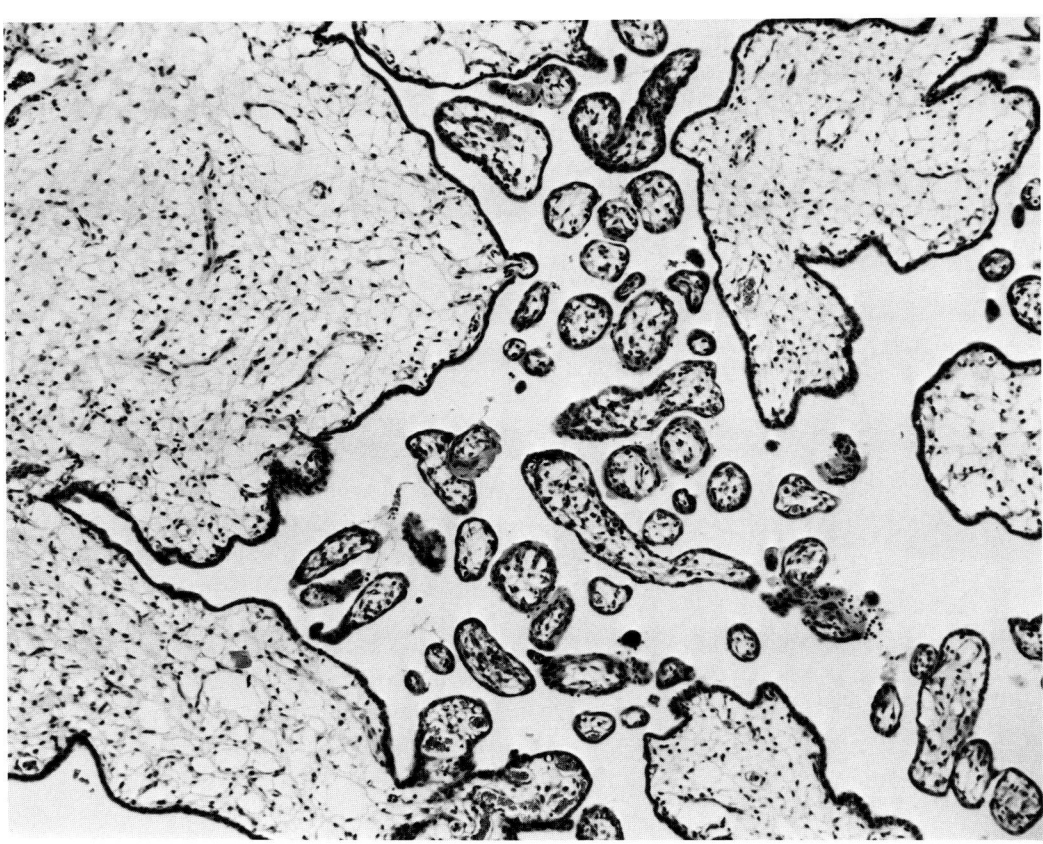

FIG. 23.66. Maternofetal Rh incompatibility, placenta at term. Pronounced variability in villous appearance characterized by markedly immature (*large*) villi interspersed among normal, mature villi.

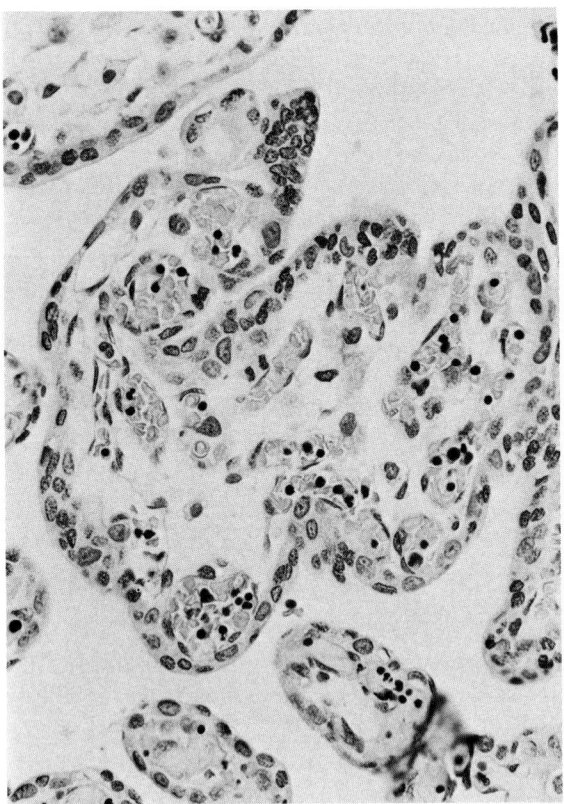

Fig. 23.67. Maternofetal Rh incompatibility, placenta at term. Fetal capillaries are filled with normoblasts and erythroblasts.

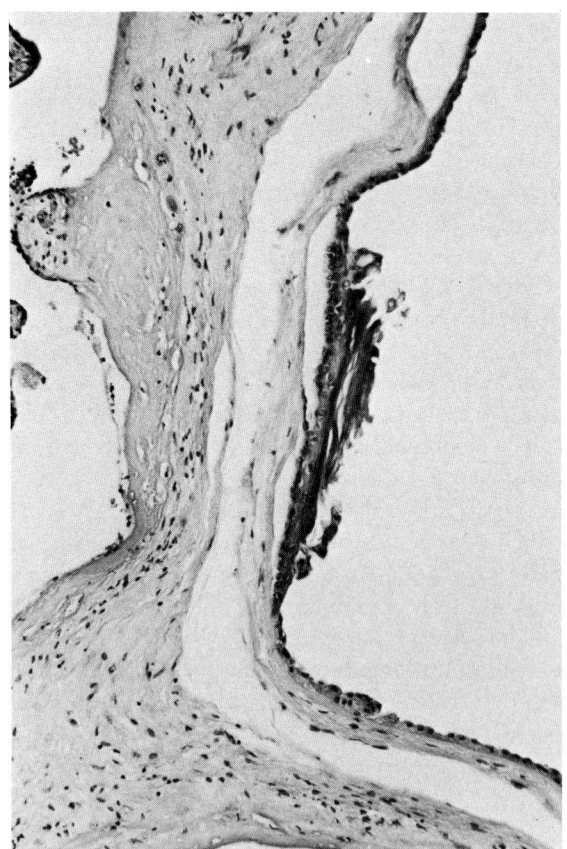

Fig. 23.69. Squamous metaplasia of amnion. Small focus of squamous metaplasia showing keratinization.

insertion (Fig. 23.68). Although they are generally very small, measuring no more than a few millimeters in diameter, they may rarely form larger plaques. Histologically, the foci consist of stratified squamous epithelium, with or without superficial keratinization, that has a sharp transition from the surrounding normal amnion (Fig. 23.69). The frequency of squamous metaplasia is a matter of some

dispute. According to Benirschke and Driscoll, it may be found in most placentas if specifically sought.[42] Squamous metaplasia has no clinical significance, and it is not known to be associated with any particular pathological event. Its only importance is in distinguishing it from amnion nodosum pathologically.

Amnion Nodosum

Amnion nodosum is a relatively rare condition in which the surface of the amnion is studded with small (1–5 mm), yellowish, elevated nodules (Fig. 23.70). These are concentrated generally on the chorionic plate, particularly around the insertion of the umbilical cord, although they may occur on the extraplacental amnion as well. The nodules are composed of amorphous, eosinophilic, and granular material containing scattered cells, degenerating cell fragments, and fragments of hair (Fig. 23.71, 23.72). On conventional microscopy, the amnionic epithelium may be totally preserved, partially persistent, or totally absent beneath the nodules (Fig. 23.72). A layer of amnion is commonly present over the surface of the nodule. The relationship of the nodule to the amnionic epithelium, basement membrane, and underlying connective tissue is a matter of

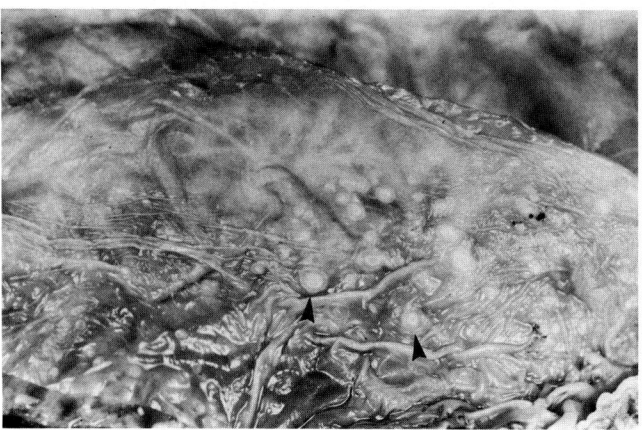

Fig. 23.68. Squamous metaplasia of amnion. Elevated white macules of squamous metaplasia (*arrows*).

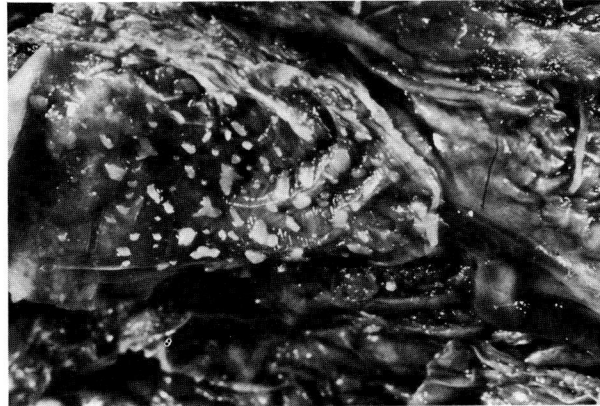

FIG. 23.70. **Amnion nodosum.** Elevated, irregular nodules on the fetal surface of the placenta.

some dispute. According to Blanc, the nodules may be infiltrated by the underlying connective tissue cells.[52] In one ultrastructural study of two cases, however, the nodules were separated from the underlying stroma by a well-defined, although often multilaminated, basement membrane.[329] A distinct cell type thought to represent amnionic epithelium was found lying on the basement

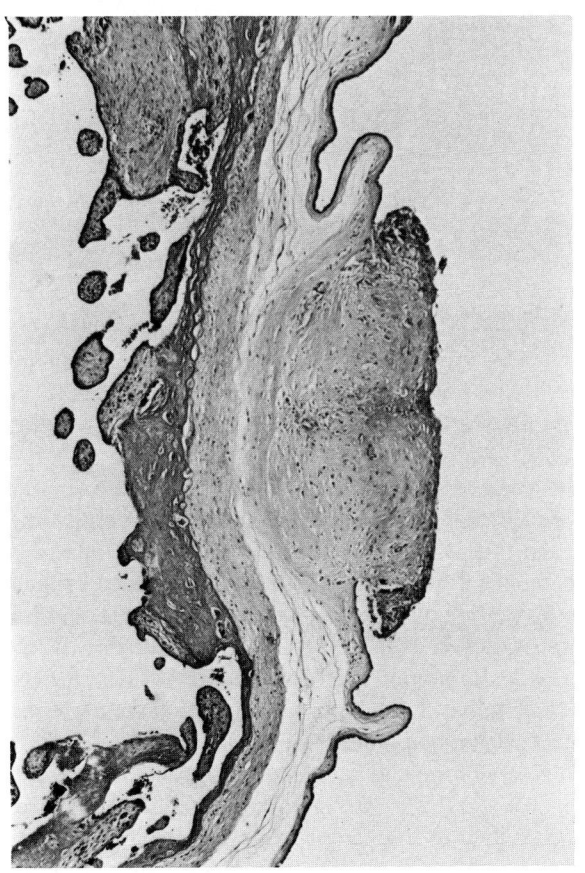

FIG. 23.71. **Amnion nodosum.** Nodular deposit on the amnionic surface of the placenta.

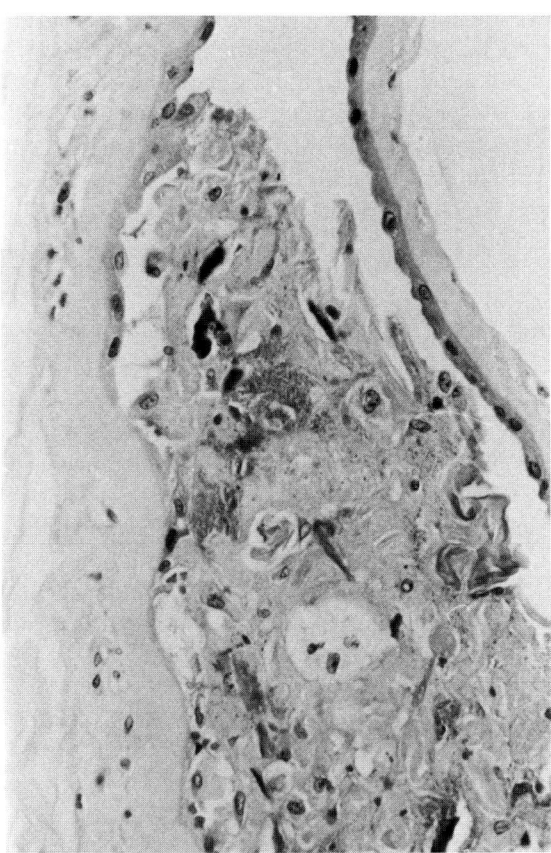

FIG. 23.72. **Amnion nodosum.** Nodular deposits are composed of degenerating cell fragments and hair embedded in amorphous granular material. Amnionic epithelium is preserved under a portion of this nodule.

membrane beneath the nodules. The electron-dense fibrillar material that forms the major component of the nodules is believed by Salazar and Kanbour to resemble the material that constitutes the vernix caseosum.[329] Most of the cells and cell fragments studied ultrastructurally have been epithelial, consistent with fetal skin origin.[329]

Amnion nodosum is clearly associated with oligohydramnios. Presumably, desquamated elements from the fetal epidermis, oral cavity, urinary and gastrointestinal tracts, or amnion itself are abnormally concentrated when amnionic fluid is scant and are deposited nonspecifically on the amnionic surface. Whether the process requires a primary abnormality of the amnion, antecedent trauma to the amnion, or direct contact and transfer of squamous cells, vernix, and lanugo hair from the fetal skin to the amnion are debated issues.[41,183]

The underlying cause of the oligohydramnios varies. In many cases, a fetal renal urinary tract abnormality (renal agenesis, urethral obstruction) is responsible for diminished fetal urine and the resulting decreased amnionic fluid. Prolonged amnionic fluid loss or the oligohydramnios associated with an acardiac fetus or the donor twin in the twin–twin transfusion syndrome also may be accompanied by amnion nodosum.[257] Although amnion nodosum is not invariably present in cases of oligohydramnios,[71] it is a reliable, if not totally absolute, indication of oligohydramnios. This finding should alert the pediatrician to the possibility of fetal abnormalities known to accompany oligohydramnios including those in the urinary tract and lungs (pulmonary hypoplasia).

Amnionic Bands

Amnionic bands, strings, and adhesions have been associated with a wide variety of fetal deformities. These vary in distribution and severity from constriction and amputation defects of the limbs and digits to major craniofacial and visceral abnormalities. The bands and strings are thought to result from amnionic rupture early in pregnancy. The ruptured amnion becomes partially or totally detached from the chorion and may fragment, shred, or shrink down to form a collar around the insertion of the umbilical cord. The mesoblastic tissue of the amnion and exposed chorion may form thin fibrous strands that encircle the fetal limbs, digits, neck, or umbilical cord, causing constriction, pseudosyndactyly, or amputation (Fig. 23.73). Malformations also may result when a band interferes with the normal sequence of embryonic development, as when interruption of fusion of the facial processes results in irregular clefts. Adhesions may form between the placenta and fetus.

Some babies with amnionic band defects have structural anomalies that are not easily explained by the amnionic bands alone. These abnormalities, usually severe, include major limb deficiencies, body wall defects, clubfeet, open cranial defects, and short umbilical cord.° This spectrum of defects, termed the *limb body wall complex*, is commonly associated with internal defects in a number of organ systems.[163,222,392] The amnion is continuous with the skin of the body wall defect in most of these cases.

Torpin strongly espoused the concept that amnionic bands cause the structural defects.[389] The more severe (craniofacial and body wall) defects are thought to be the result of oligohydramnios and fetal compression that presumably follow amnionic rupture. This hypothesis is supported by experimental studies in which puncture of the amnion of rats during early gestation produces an identical array of defects.[98,197,198,223,293,391] The widely variable nature and extent of the defects are presumed to be due to the timing of amnionic rupture.[170] Early rupture is thought to result in severe, multiple system defects, whereas characteristic limb involvement is thought to be the consequence of amnionic rupture later in gestation. Kalousek, however, suggests that the specific type of fetal involvement is as dependent on the extent of amnionic bands as

---

°Refs. 48,167,168,214,239,341,369.

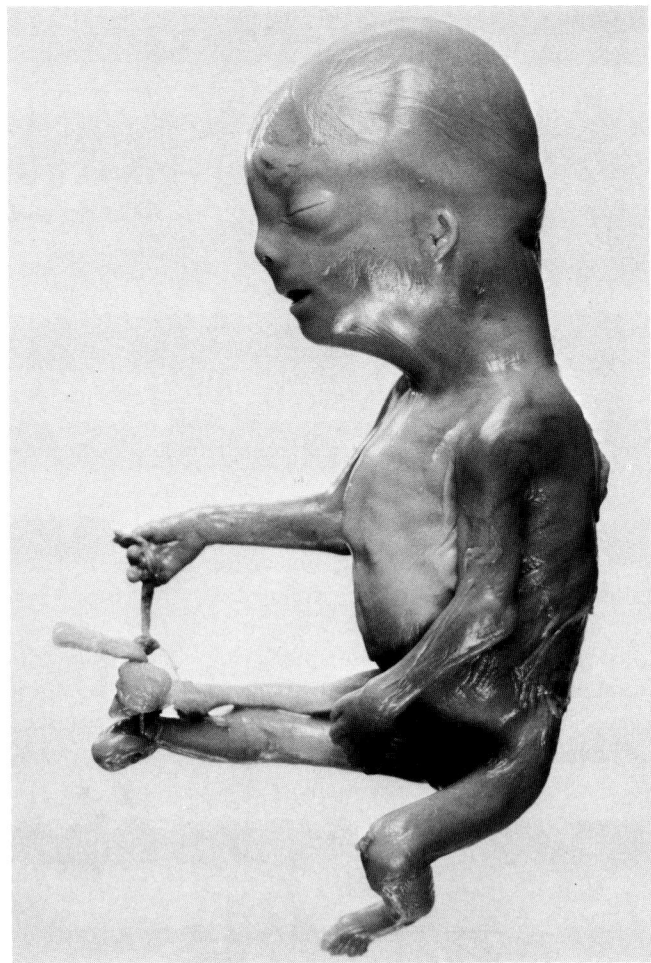

FIG. 23.73. Amnionic bands. Thin fibrous bands encircle and deform the leg and digits of this fetus.

on the stage of development when amnionic bands occur.[193] The etiology of amnionic rupture early in pregnancy is unknown, although amnionic bands have been noted rarely after trauma, amniocentesis, and in connective tissue disorders.[26,245,305,414]

The absence of amnionic bands and presence of internal abnormalities in some cases of the limb body wall complex have led other authors to postulate that the more severe fetal abnormalities are the result of vascular disruption or a primary embryologic defect and that the amnionic bands are secondary.[163,167,222,369,392] The relationship between the classical amnionic band syndrome with constrictions and amputations of the limbs and digits and the more severe craniofacial and body wall defects remains controversial.

The recognition and correct diagnosis of amnion rupture and its consequences are important in counseling parents, since the risk of recurrence in this event is negligible. Major craniofacial and body wall defects may be difficult to diagnose unless accompanied by ring constrictions and amputations. When this syndrome is suspected, submersion of the placenta in water facilitates recognition of the thin, delicate fibrous strands. Histological examination of the placental surface will show absence or necrosis of the amnion and chorionic fibrosis.

Meconium Stain

The passage of meconium may result in degenerative changes in the amnion evidenced by heaping, pseudostratification, and nuclear pyknosis of the epithelial cells. When exposure to meconium is prolonged, the amnionic epithelium may undergo complete necrosis. After some time has elapsed, macrophages in the compact layer of the amnion may engulf the meconium and become distended with granular, greenish yellow pigment (Fig. 23.74). The time course of these changes as described in one in vitro study may or may not reflect the situation in vivo.[241] There is some evidence that meconium may cause umbilical and placental vascular necrosis and vasoconstriction.[15] Meconium should be distinguished from hemosiderin, which is yellowish, crystalline, slightly refractile, and forms larger granules.

Gastroschisis

Gastroschisis is associated with an alteration in the amnionic epithelial cells characterized by extensive fine, uniform vacuolization (Fig. 23.75).[25] Ultrastructural studies confirm that the vacuoles contain lipid, but the origin of the lipid is obscure.[154] These amnionic changes have not been noted in cases of omphalocoele.

Pathology of the Umbilical Cord

Vestigial Remnants

The normal umbilical cord contains two arteries and one vein surrounded by Wharton's jelly, a loosely structured myxomatous tissue. The cord is covered by a layer of amnion. No other vessels, specifically vasa vasorum, or lymphatics are found in the cord. Occasionally, remnants of the allantoic or omphalomesenteric ducts may be apparent on microscopic examination. Traces of the omphalomesenteric duct are infrequent. This duct connects the fetal ileum and the yolk sac in the early embryo. Its remnants

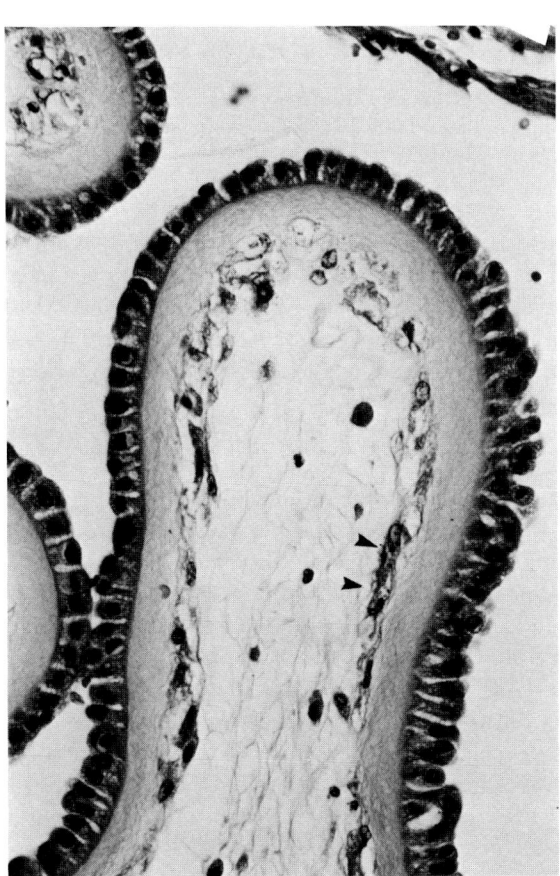

FIG. 23.74. **Meconium stain.** Accumulation of granular meconium pigment in the amnionic macrophages (*arrows*).

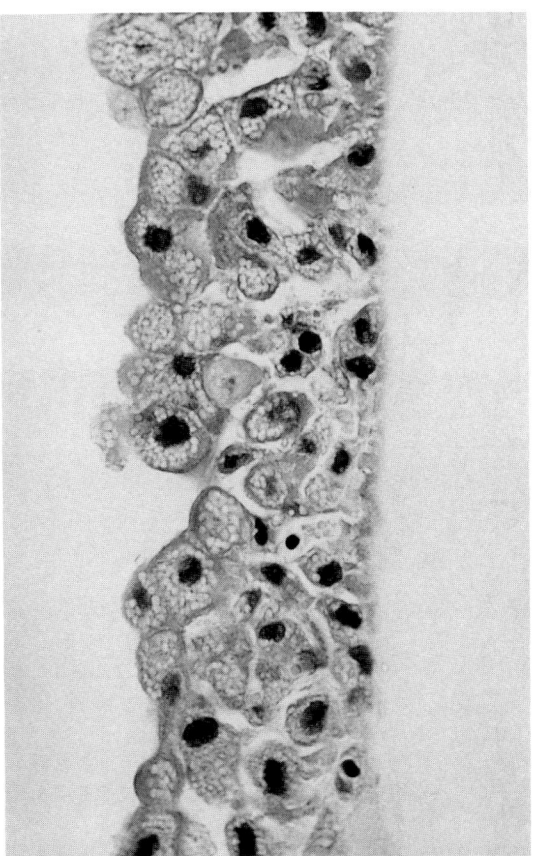

FIG. 23.75. **Amnion, gstroschisis.** The amnionic epithelium in this case of gastroschisis shows the typical fine vacuolation. The epithelial stratification is a result of meconium passage.

usually are discontinuous, are located peripherally beneath the amnionic surface, and may be lined by either nondescript flat or columnar epithelium. Frequently, the lining resembles intestinal epithelium (Fig. 23.76). Rarely, omphalomesenteric remnants have been reported to show remarkable differentiation to gastric or small intestinal mucosa or pancreas. If found at all, the remainder of the original yolk sac, usually only a tiny, yellow-white nodule, is present beneath the amnion at the periphery of the placenta. Histologically, this consists of an amorphous, subamnionic, basophilic mass.

Remnants of the allantoic duct are more frequently recognized. This duct, the connection between the bladder via the urachus and rudimentary allantois, is lined by flat or cuboidal cells often reminiscent of transitional epithelium (Fig. 23.77). A lumen may or may not be present. Allantoic duct remnants are located regularly between the umbilical arteries.

Insertion of the Cord

The umbilical cord generally inserts into the placenta either centrally or at some distance from the center (eccentric insertion). Insertion onto the peripheral margin of the

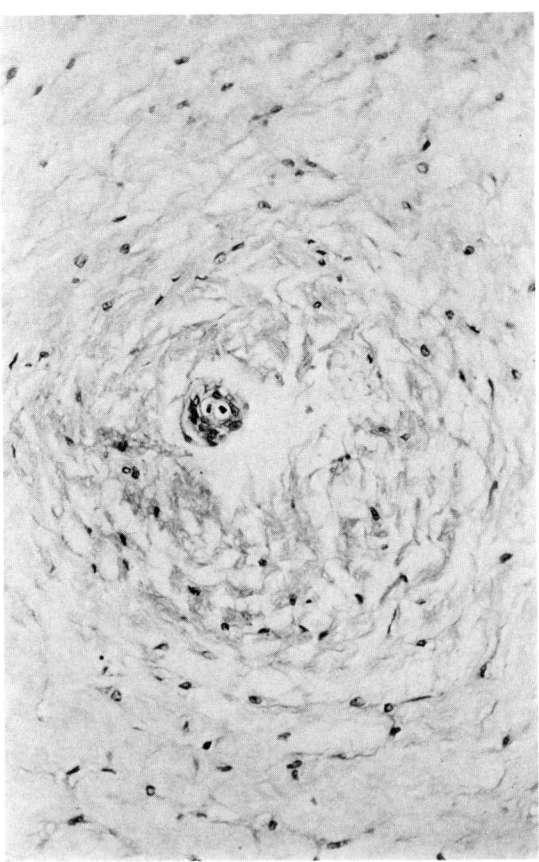

FIG. 23.77. Allantoic duct remnant, umbilical cord. Allantoic duct remnant lined by transitional type cuboidal cells.

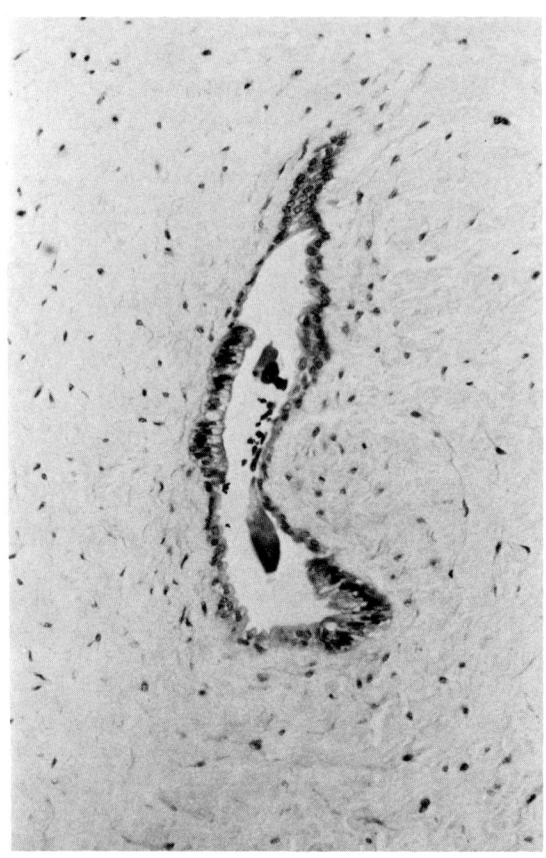

FIG. 23.76. Omphalomesenteric duct remnant, umbilical cord. This omphalomesenteric duct remnant is lined by columnar, mucin-containing epithelium.

placenta (*marginal*, or *battledore*, insertion) is less common than either central or eccentric insertion, but its reported frequency varies greatly. The significance of a marginal insertion is debated. It has been reported to occur with increased frequency in abortions, with malformed fetuses, and in association with neonatal asphyxia and premature labor. Fox[132] could not confirm any of the reported associations.

In approximately 1% of all deliveries, the cord inserts into the fetal membranes at some distance from the edge of the placenta (*velamentous insertion*). The umbilical vessels run in the chorion from the point of insertion to the main placental mass. During their course, they are unprotected by the connective tissue of the umbilical cord or underlying villous parenchyma. These vessels are injured easily during labor and delivery, especially if they traverse the internal os (vasa previa). If one or more of these vessels is torn, rapid fetal exsanguination may result.

The frequency of velamentous insertion is definitely increased in multiple pregnancies. Other conditions that have been reported to be associated with velamentous insertion include extrachorial placentation and single umbilical artery. Velamentous insertion has been correlated with an increased frequency of fetal structural defects.[247,315] Theories of pathogenesis of velamentous insertion include abnormal primary implantation and trophotropism.

Two rare forms of cord insertion are *furcate insertion*, in which the umbilical vessels separate, losing Wharton's jelly before reaching the placental surface, and *interpositio velamentosa*, in which the cord runs in the fetal membranes to the placental surface.

Cord Length

The length of the umbilical cord varies considerably but averages between 54 and 61 cm. Occurrence of longer than average cords is more frequent in series of infants in whom the cord is wound about the neck. Excessive cord length has been associated with knots, torsion, partial or complete vascular occlusion, and cord prolapse during delivery. Abnormally short umbilical cords may predispose to intrauterine distress, neonatal asphyxia, cord rupture and hemorrhage, abruptio placenta, and uterine inversion. In cases of acordia (total absence of the umbilical cord), the umbilical region of the fetus, often malformed, merges with the placenta. This anomaly usually is found in abortions or stillbirths.

Interest in cord length has been directly mainly toward the potential adverse affects of extremes of length; relatively little attention has been focused on factors that influence cord growth. There is some evidence that linear cord growth is influenced by tensile forces and depends on both fetal motor activity and the space available for movement.[238,240,246] Conditions restricting fetal mobility (amnionic bands/oligohydramnios) often are associated with short umbilical cords. Whether or not fetal activity and cord length reflect prenatal central nervous system status remains to be determined.[259]

Single Umbilical Artery

The presence of a single umbilical artery (SUA) is a common anomaly that frequently is associated with other congenital malformations (Fig. 23.78). The reported frequency of SUA varies depending on the type of study. In neonatal autopsies and spontaneous abortions, SUA occurs in about 2.5–3.0%.[166] In prospective studies of consecutive deliveries, the frequency is consistently somewhat less than 1%.[39,74,138] Other factors influence the prevalence of this abnormality. SUA is more common in white infants than in blacks and Asians.[138,285] There is an excess of SUA in babies of diabetic mothers.[138] Some authors have reported that SUAs are found more commonly in multiple pregnancies,[39,358] but this has been disputed in other series, in which the frequency has not been greater and has even been somewhat less in twins.[74,285] There is no association with maternal age or parity.

There is a definite and well-documented association between fetal malformations and SUA.[39–41,74,138,166,358] The severity of these malformations varies tremendously, and

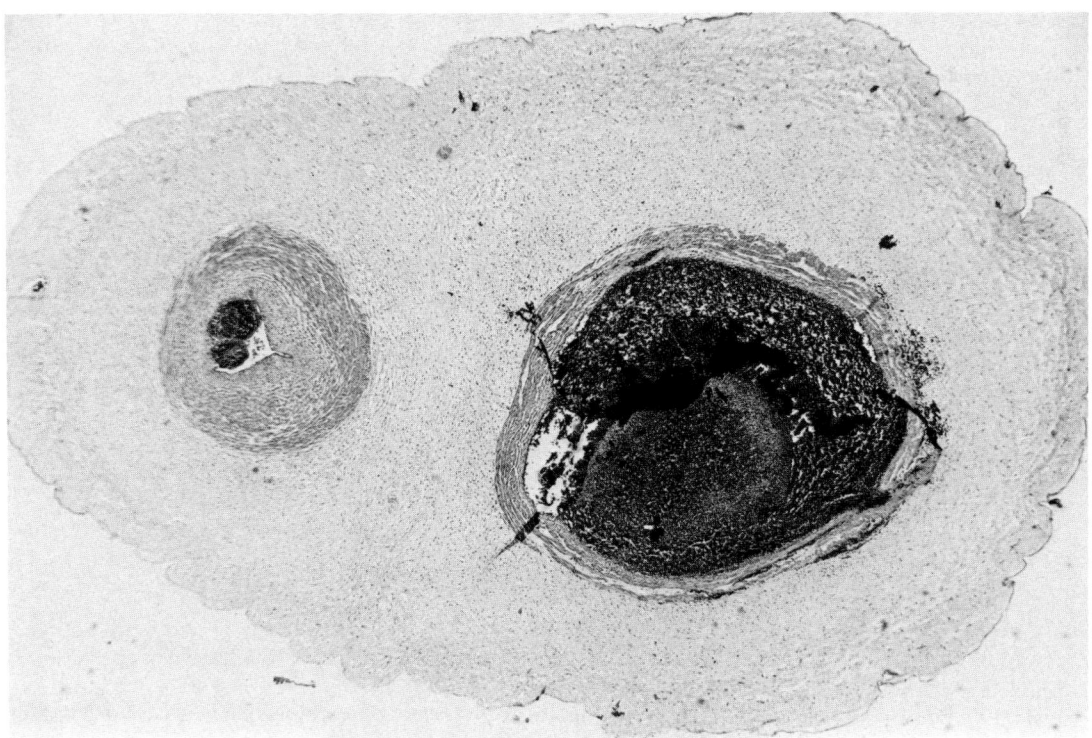

FIG. 23.78. Single umbilical artery; on *left*, umbilical cord.

there is no particular organ or specific abnormality characterizing this association. Any organ system may be involved. Genitourinary, musculoskeletal, cardiovascular, central nervous system, and gastrointestinal malformations are encountered most frequently,[74,138,139,358] and malformations often are multiple. The frequency with which these malformations are reported to occur in association with SUA varies considerably, from 17.5% to 97%.[358] This discrepancy largely reflects the much higher malformation rate found in autopsied SUA infants when compared with infants having SUA who survive. This is emphasized in one study in which 52.8% of autopsied infants with SUA had associated malformations compared with only 4.1% of SUA survivors.[139] Furthermore, the most severe malformations are found predominantly in stillborn fetuses and in infants dying in the first weeks of life.[74,75,138,139] Major malformations are much less common in babies surviving the neonatal period. This suggests that SUA infants with severe abnormalities tend to die in utero or early in the perinatal period. One follow-up study of SUA infants who survived the neonatal period with no clinically detectable malformation at birth showed only an unexplained increase in inguinal hernia.[139] Bryan and Kohler[75] reported the subsequent discovery of malformations in 10 of 98 infants in whom anomalies had not been apparent at birth. These were much less severe than those documented at birth.

The overall perinatal mortality rate of infants with SUA is greatly increased (11–41%). The occurrence of major malformations is the most significant factor in the high perinatal mortality rate, although an increased mortality rate also has been reported among the normal infants with SUA.[74] SUA also is associated with a tendency toward low birth weight. This relationship persists even when infants with major malformations are excluded from analysis.[74,165] A remarkable frequency of SUA in chromosomal abnormalities, especially trisomies, has been reported.[358] In some series, SUA has been associated with velamentous insertion of the cord and low placental weight.[138,166]

There has been considerable debate whether a single umbilical artery is due to primary aplasia or secondary atrophy. Certainly, histological evidence of portions or remnants of a vessel may be documented in the umbilical cord in some cases of SUA, providing support for the theory of secondary atrophy of a formerly present vessel (Figs. 23.79, 23.80). Evidence of such atrophy was found in 19 of 48 cases of SUA in a study that specifically investigated this point.[17] Whether the SUA actually causes the associated fetal malformations or is just another manifestation of them is a matter of conjecture.

The practical point is that it is important for the pathologist to recognize and document the occurrence of SUA. Gross examination of a fresh cord is not sufficient, since a

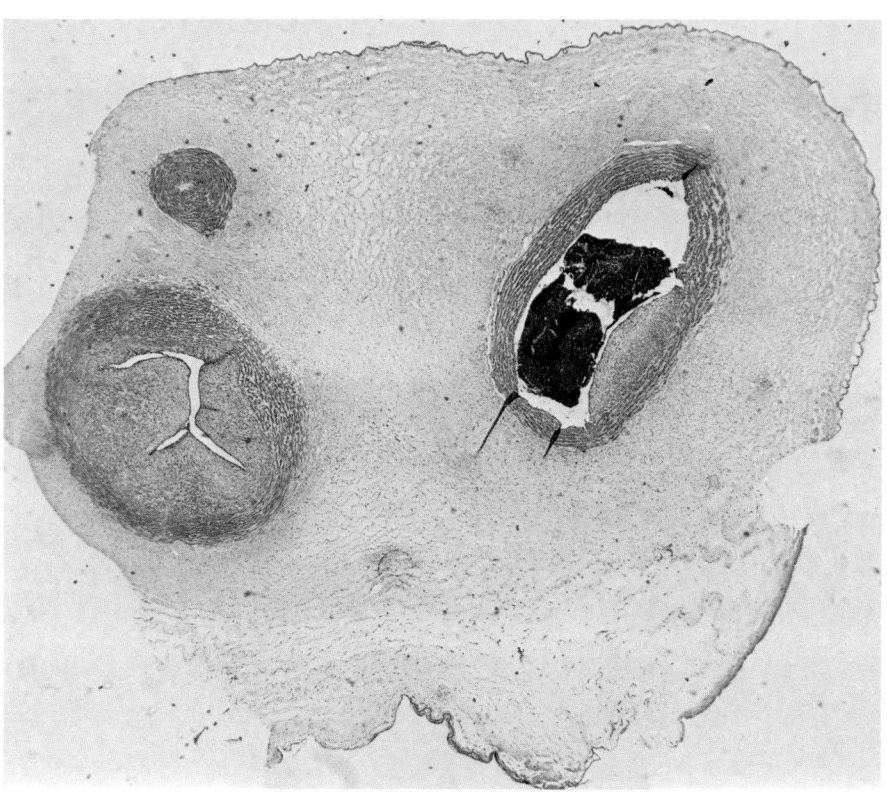

FIG. 23.79. Marked hypoplasia of one umbilical artery. This anomaly was found in conjunction with several congenital malformations in a fetus dying shortly after birth.

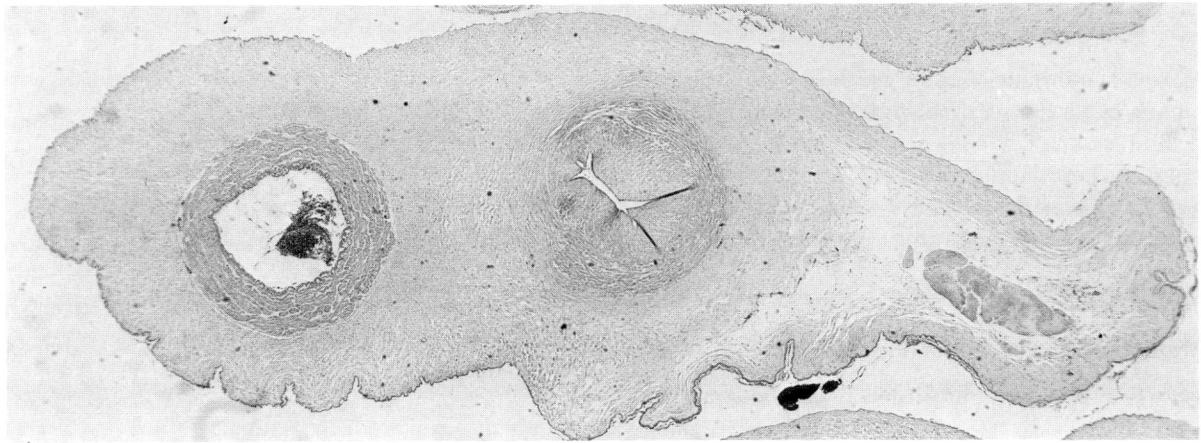

FIG. 23.80. **Amorphous remnant of one umbilical artery (*right*).**

significant number of cases of SUA will be missed. Fixation does aid in gross examination, but sections of the cord should be examined microscopically. If the umbilical cord is sectioned close to the chorionic plate, fusion of the two umbilical arteries, which often occurs normally in this location, may be misinterpreted as SUA. This source of error may be obviated by taking an additional section at a different level of the cord.

Knots

True knots in the umbilical cord (Fig. 23.81) sometimes are confused with, and must be distinguished from, false knots resulting from focal accentuation of the vascular spiral, a varicosity, or excess Wharton's jelly. True knots are found in fewer than 1% of all deliveries. They usually are a complication of an excessively long umbilical cord. An increased perinatal mortality rate in the range of 8–11% is associated with the presence of true knots, presumably due to obstruction of the fetal circulation through a tight knot. The criteria for distinguishing a long-standing knot from one that has undergone acute tightening during labor and delivery include compression and a definite groove at the

site of the knot, loss of Wharton's jelly, and persistence of these structural changes after the knot is untied. Knots that have been acutely tightened show edema, venous stasis and congestion distal to the knot, and occlusive thrombi in the vessels. Either an acutely tightened or long-standing knot may be responsible for intrauterine or intrapartum fetal death.

Torsion and Stricture

The normal spiraling of vessels in the umbilical cord creates the impression of twisting. Occasionally, however, excessive torsion of the cord occurs, characteristically at its fetal end. Associated congestion, edema, and vascular thrombi provide evidence that this anomaly may result in interruption of blood flow and fetal death. Strictures of the umbilical cord are rare and often are complicated by torsion. Strictures usually are single, sharply defined, short segments located most commonly at the fetal end of the cord.[399] Microscopically, there may be contraction of the vessels, loss of Wharton's jelly, or fibrosis in the area of the constriction. This anomaly usually is described in stillborn babies.

Hematoma

Hematomas of the umbilical cord are a rare complication of pregnancy.[105,325,336] They usually are confined to the cord but occasionally may rupture into the amnionic cavity. Grossly, hematomas appear as a red-purple, fusiform swelling of the cord, most often near its fetal end. In some cases, the hemorrhage may be demonstrated to originate from the umbilical vein and much less commonly from an umbilical artery. In most cases, an obvious source of the hemorrhage is not apparent.

The etiology of such hemorrhage is unknown. Included among the possible causes are rupture of a varix, trauma,

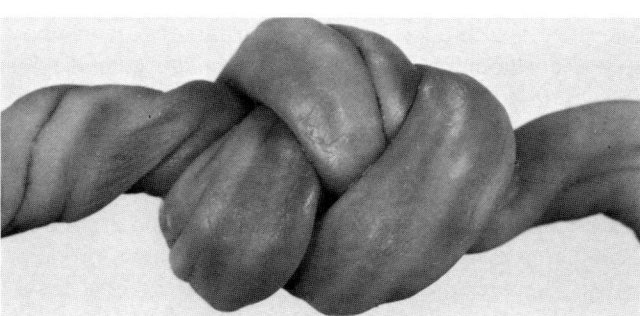

FIG. 23.81. **True knot of umbilical cord.** This true knot occurred in a normal liveborn infant.

structural anomalies of the vessel wall, mechanical damage due to traction on a short cord, and inflammation.

The perinatal mortality of infants with an umbilical cord hematoma is in the range of 40–50%. The nature of the relationship between this high perinatal mortality and the occurrence of a cord hematoma is unclear, but it has been theorized that the hematoma may result in compression and thrombosis of fetal vessels with cessation of fetal blood flow.

Ulceration/Absence of Wharton's Jelly

Linear ulceration of Wharton's jelly over the umbilical vessels has been associated with severe intraamnionic hemorrhage, profound fetal anemia, and fetal death in utero.[36] Microscopically, the Wharton's jelly overlying the vessels is necrotic and replaced by amorphous debris. The vessels may show focal myonecrosis and aneurysmal dilation (Fig. 23.82). These findings have been reported to occur in conjunction with fetal intestinal atresia, but the nature of the relationship between these two phenomena is unknown. Rarely, Wharton's jelly may be completely absent around the umbilical arteries. This anomaly also has been associated with fetal death in utero.[211]

Cysts

Cysts within the umbilical cord may be of several types. Probably the most common type is not a true cyst at all but rather a cavity resulting from degeneration of Wharton's jelly. These lack an epithelial lining. Remnants of either an omphalomesenteric or allantoic duct may undergo cystic dilatation. These sometimes can be distinguished by their resemblance to gastrointestinal-type or transitional-type epithelium. They generally are small and inconsequential. Cystic inclusions of the amnion are uncommon.

Edema

The umbilical cord occasionally appears enlarged and swollen with very loose, edematous Wharton's jelly. Edema has been specifically defined as a visibly edematous cord with a cross-sectional area of 1.3 cm^2 or greater.[89] Edema of the cord is not uncommon in maternal diabetes, Rh incompatibility, or fetal death in utero.

Abortion

Abortion is defined as the spontaneous or operative termination of pregnancy before fetal viability. The legal definition of viability varies from one location to another and may not correspond to the medical definition of viability. Spontaneous abortions are common, and their exact incidence is difficult to assess, since many are clinically inap-

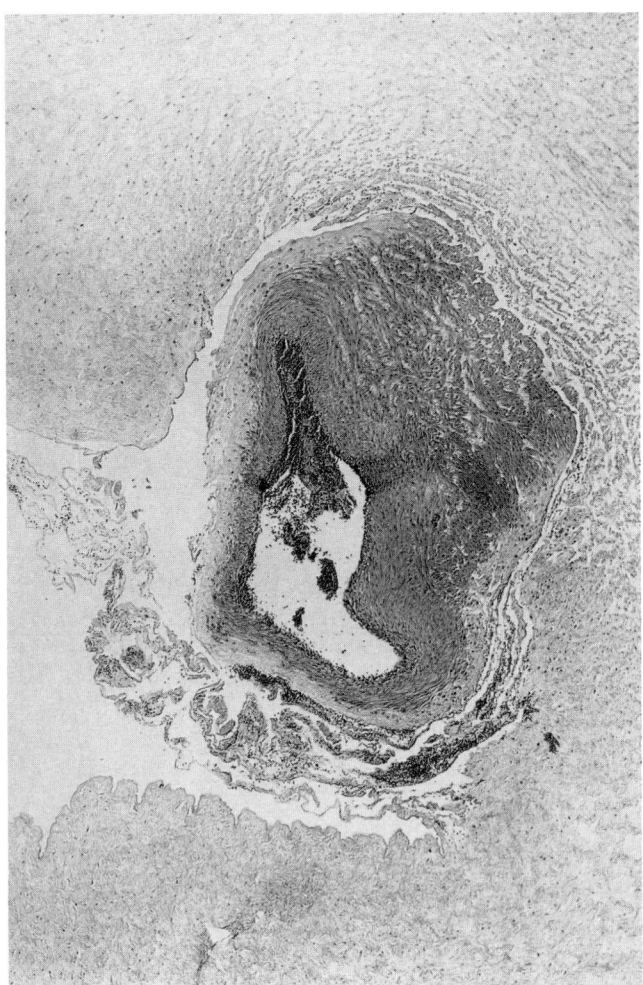

Fig. 23.82. Wharton's jelly, ulceration. Wharton's jelly is completely necrotic over the umbilical artery, which is markedly thinned and focally necrotic. This pregnancy was complicated by massive intraamnionic hemorrhage and fetal death in utero.

parent. It has been estimated that as many as 50% of conceptions fail to complete their development. The etiology of spontaneous abortion is diverse and may result from either fetal or maternal factors. In general, the factors associated with early abortion are fetal, primarily chromosomal abnormalities and an ill-defined group of immunologic incompatibilities. Maternal factors (cervical incompetence, developmental abnormalities in the genital tract, infection) are associated more often with midtrimester abortions.

Products of conception submitted for pathological examination consist of a combination of placental, fetal, and maternal elements, in any state of organization or disarray. Early in pregnancy, the decidual component predominates. Thereafter, the placental and then the fetal tissues are most conspicuous. Intrauterine pregnancy should be documented in any putative early abortion specimen. This requires the definite identification of trophoblast, which usually is found in association with villi but is sometimes limited to a few isolated cell clumps in clotted blood or to the trophoblastic elements infiltrating the endometrium or myometrium at the implantation site. The presence of decidua or gestational endometrium does not constitute adequate documentation of intrauterine pregnancy since this change may be associated with ectopic pregnancy or hormonal manipulation. When trophoblastic elements are not found in the initial sections, the entire specimen should be examined microscopically. If trophoblast is still not identified, the clinician should be alerted to the possibility of an ectopic gestation. It should be recognized that no combination of findings in the endometrium, including villi, can exclude an ectopic pregnancy. There are numerous reports of simultaneous intrauterine and tubal pregnancy.[410]

The villi, if present, may be normal or show characteristic pathological changes known to be associated with fetal death in utero. A constellation of morphologic alterations in the villi begins about 24 hours after fetal death and is fully established within 5 to 6 days.[129,177] These changes include sclerosis and obliteration of fetal stem arteries and villous capillaries, progressive villous stromal fibrosis, increased numbers of syncytial knots, increased numbers of cytotrophoblastic cells, and thickening of the trophoblastic basement membrane (Fig. 23.83). Vascular changes in the placenta may be useful in establishing the time of death in stillborn fetuses.[145]

Genetic Defects

The defects responsible for most early spontaneous abortions appear to be genetically determined, and many can be identified by karyotyping fetal or placental tissue.[233] The most common abnormal karyotypes are trisomies, triploidy, and 45 XO (Table 23.2).[64] In much smaller numbers, tetraploidy and a variety of mosaics have been documented. Earlier abortions, occurring before the 8th week of gestation, have the highest percentage of aneuploidy (about 66%), whereas later abortions (23% aneuploid) are more likely to have other causes.

Morphologic correlations, although not absolute, can be distinctive enough in some instances to suggest an abnormal karyotype. Certain combinations can be extremely useful in suggesting specific abnormal karyotypes when cytogenetic studies cannot be performed, for instance, in specimens already fixed at the time of examination (Figs. 23.84, 23.85).[192] These observations are important because they may carry serious implications for repeated abortion or malformations in subsequent pregnancies.

The fetus or embryo, when present, deserves careful study. Morphologic recognition of embryonic growth disorganization points to a high probability of a chromosomal anomaly.[190–192] Localized developmental defects such as fusion defects in the face, ocular anomalies, limb bud de-

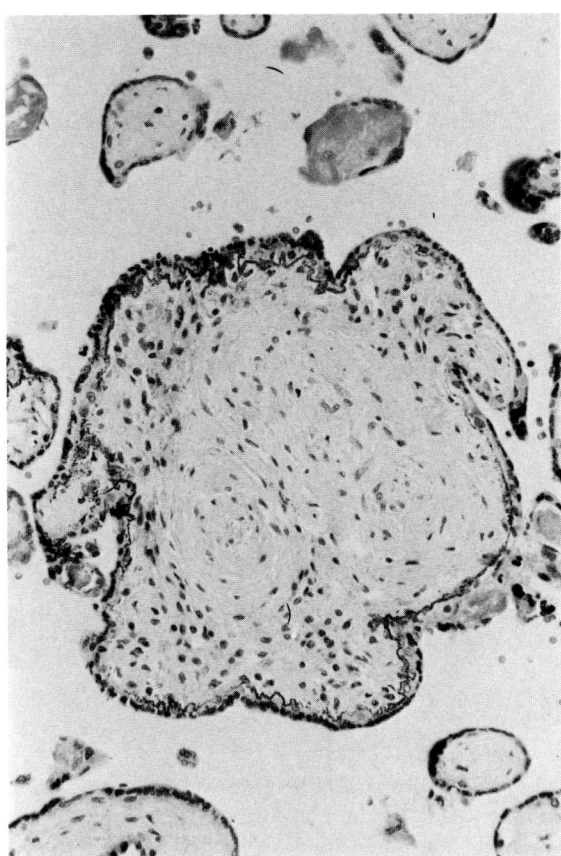

FIG. 23.83. **Fetal death in utero.** The villous alterations resulting from fetal death in utero include sclerosis and obliteration of the fetal vessels, stromal fibrosis, and prominence of the cytotrophoblast.

formities, neural tube defects, and cervical edema also are commonly genetically determined. Localized defects, however, have several pathogenetic mechanisms, and the risk of recurrence is related to the pathogenesis.[190–192] Specific morphologic defects may be difficult to identify in the early embryo and may require the use of a dissecting microscope. The finding of a well-developed, normal embryo in an abortion specimen also is important. This

Table 23.2. Proportions of abnormal karyotypes in 1500 spontaneous abortions

Karyotype abnormality	Approximate percentage
Trisomies	52
Triploidy	20
XO	15
Tetraploidy	6
Translocations	4
Double trisomy	2
Mosaics	1

From data of Boue and Boue, modified after Benirschke, ref. 64.

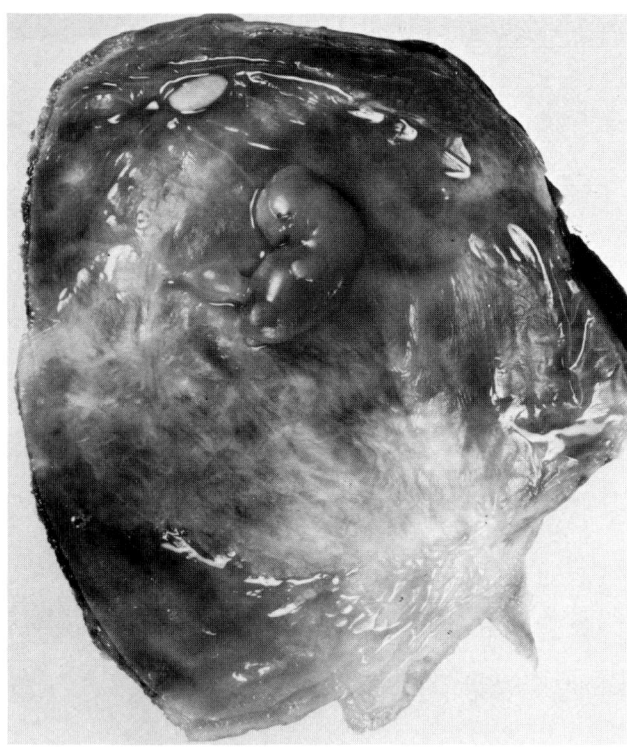

FIG. 23.84. Spontaneous abortion with intact amnion and deformed embryo. The bulbous, amorphous limb buds, distorted facial clefts, constricted body stalk (umbilical cord), and greatly distended amnion all suggest abnormal karyotype, probably a trisomy.

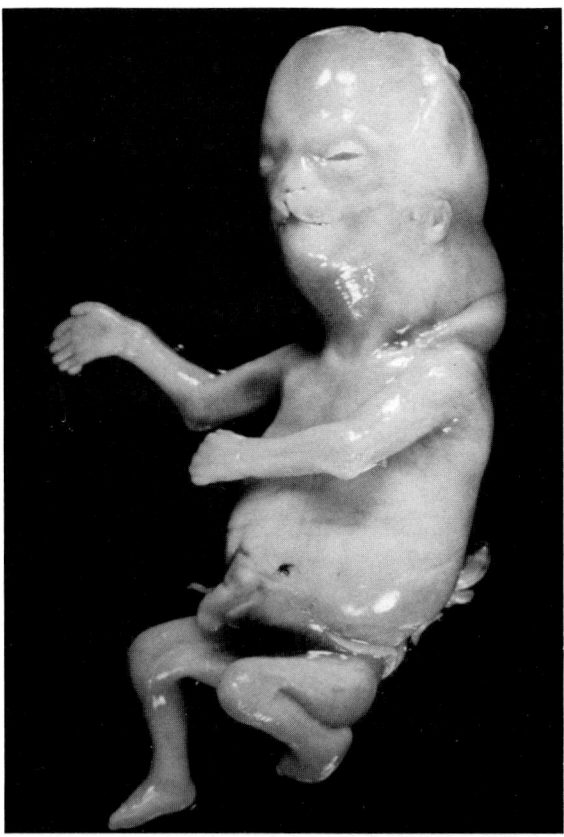

FIG. 23.85. Aborted 47 XX (trisomy 13) fetus. Note supernumerary digits, facial fusion defect, cervical swelling, low-set ears, and ventral hernia. (Karyotype courtesy of P. Monteleone, M.D., St. Louis, Missouri.)

strongly suggests a maternal causative factor, some of which are treatable.

There is, then, a fairly good correlation between phenotypic expression in the embryo/fetus and cytogenetic findings. Many aborted specimens, however, are curetted and are received as multiple dissociated fragments. Gross evaluation of the fetal tissue, if recognizable at all, is obviously suboptimal. For this reason, there have been numerous attempts to correlate specific chromosomal abnormalities with morphologic features of the placenta. Whereas some early work suggests that assessment of placental histology is a fairly accurate way to predict karyotype, three recent studies conclude that the appearance of the placenta is not sufficient to discriminate normal from abnormal karyotypes or to define a specific karyotype.[243,304,398] There are, however, some definite trends.

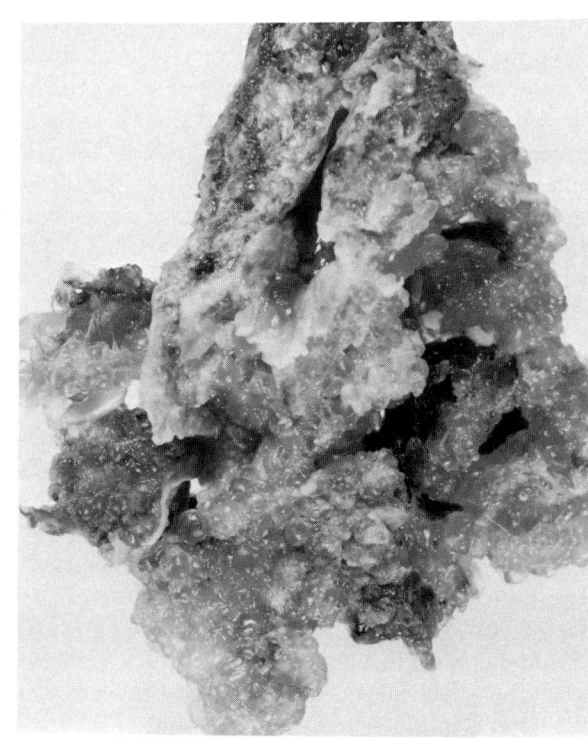

FIG. 23.86. Partial mole. Empty amnionic sac is at *top center*. Many villi are swollen and hydropic (at *bottom*) but many others (at *top*) are nearly normal. Total mass, in contrast to true hydatidiform mole, is approximately the size of other spontaneous abortions. (Reproduced by permission from Kraus, Frederick T: Gynecologic Pathology, St. Louis, 1967, The C.V. Mosby Co.)

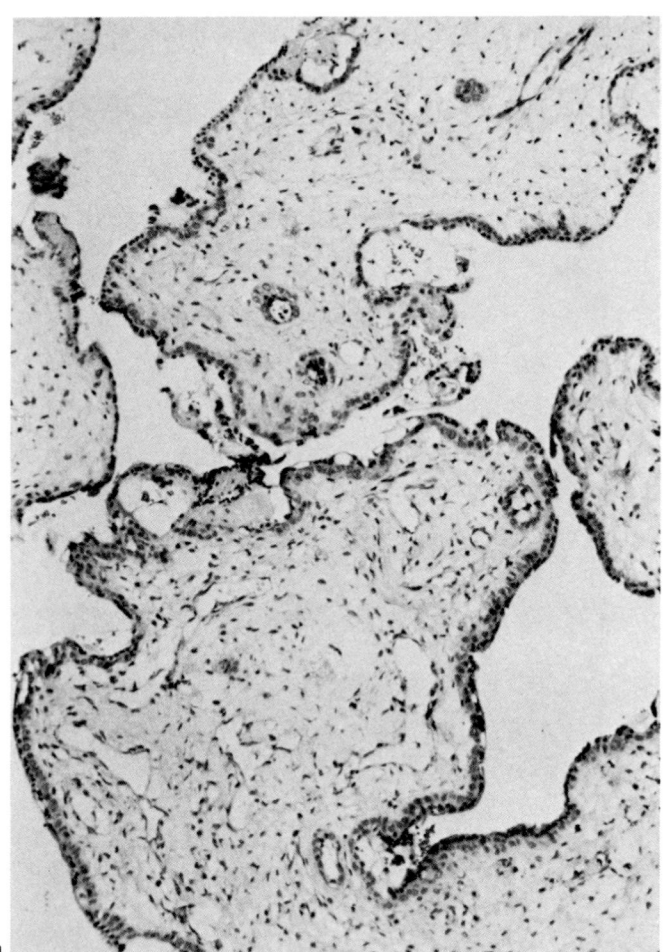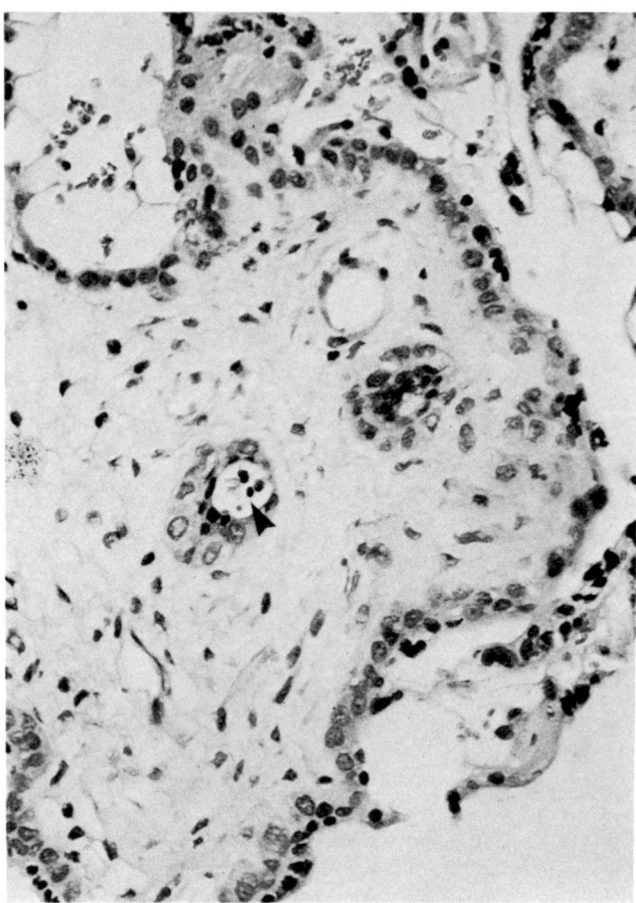

Fig. 23.87. Partial mole (69 XXY). a. Distinctive features are trophoblastic invaginations that appear circular in cross-section (villus at *top center*), the scalloped, irregular margins, and empty endothelium-lined vascular sinusoids (villus at *bottom*). (Karyo-

type courtesy of K. Taysi, M.D., St. Louis, Missouri). **b:** Higher magnification of trophoblastic invaginations. Note the peripheral, pale-staining, larger cytotrophoblast cells and the more central, darker, syncytiotrophoblast nuclei. The central space (*arrow*) communicates with the maternal intervillous space.

All agree that *triploid* abortions have the most distinctive morphologic features. About 86% have the gross and microscopic characteristics of partial mole (see Chapter 24, Gestational Trophoblastic Disease and Related Lesions).[374,375] Numerous villi are grossly hydropic (not all as in hydatidiform mole) (Fig. 23.86). The typical histological features include villi with trophoblastic invaginations, cisterns or empty spaces in the villous stroma, and extremely irregular surfaces, often covered by hyperplastic, vacuolated syncytiotrophoblast (Fig. 23.87a).[376] The trophoblastic invaginations form a target-like arrangement of central space, syncytiotrophoblast, and peripheral cytotrophoblast cells (Fig. 23.87b). Fetal membranes or fetal tissue may be identified. The fetuses, when present, have external dysmorphic features that include hypertelorism, micrognathia, low-set ears, camptodactyly, 3–4 syndactyly, and adrenal hypoplasia. Triploid abortions are sporadic, unlikely to be repeated, and not related to abnormal parental karyotypes. The presence of hydropic villi and the ex-

pression, mole, seem to cast an ominous shadow on the potential for aggressive trophoblastic disease after triploid partial moles.[47] It is desirable to emphasize, therefore, that morphologically diagnosed invasive mole and choriocarcinoma have been recorded only rarely in this setting[142,144] and that the chromosomes of a hydatidiform mole (usually 46 XX, all paternally derived) are different from partial mole, which is nearly always 69 XXY or 69 XXX[374] (see Chapter 24).

The villi in *autosomal trisomies* also are frequently swollen and avascular, but they are smaller than in partial mole, and cisterns usually are absent. Trophoblast invaginations occur but less commonly. The most characteristic histological feature may be large, mononuclear cells infiltrating into the villous stroma (Fig. 23.88). These cells are generally believed to represent migratory cytotrophoblast,[192] but altered Hofbauer cells represent a possible alternative.[38] In our experience, some, at least, react with antibodies to human placental lactogen, suggesting tropho-

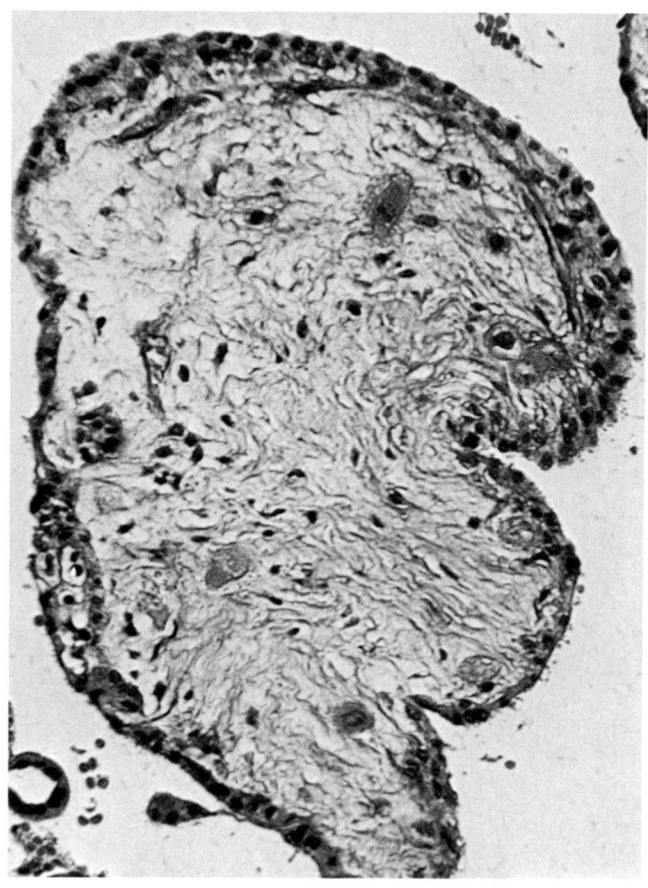

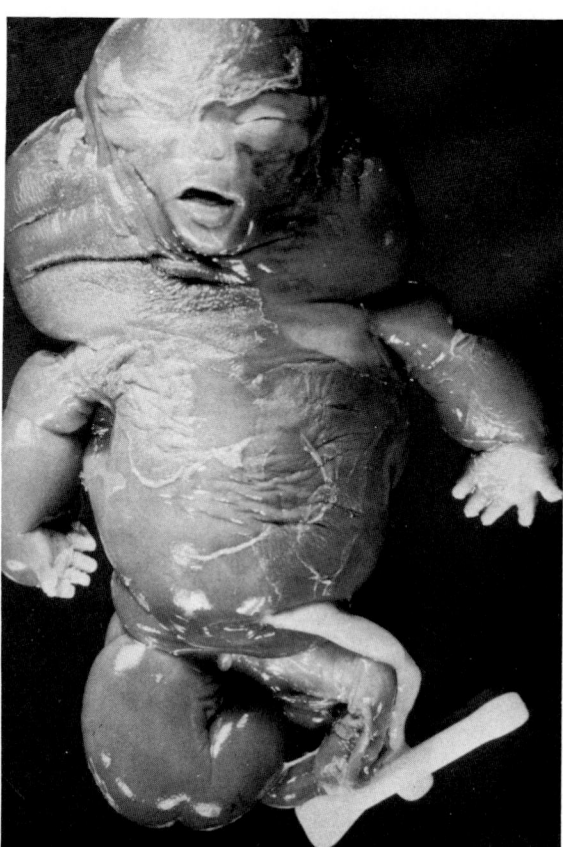

FIG. 23.88. Villus from D-trisomy spontaneous abortion. A few large, irregular cells resembling cytotrophoblast extend into the villous stroma at *top, center*, and *bottom center*.

FIG. 23.90. Aborted 45 XO fetus. The large, symmetrical cervical swellings and generalized edema are characteristic features. Cardiovascular anomalies are also common, as in Turner syndrome. (Karyotype courtesy of K. Taysi, M.D., St. Louis, Missouri.)

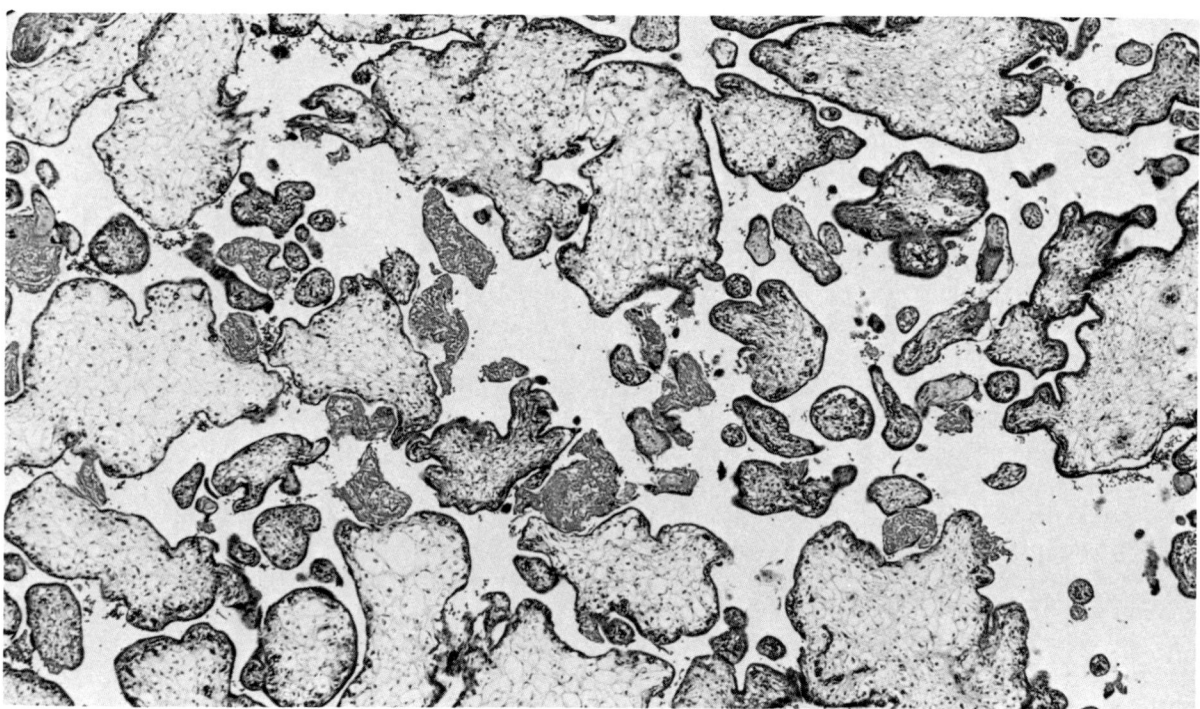

FIG. 23.89. Placenta, 45 XO. Immature, enlarged villi from a 45XO spontaneous abortion similar to the fetus shown in Figure 23.81, but of longer (26 weeks) gestation. Patchy clusters of larger immature villi with abundant stroma are not specific but suggestive of this and other abnormal placental genotypes, including trisomies. (Karyotype courtesy of K. Taysi, M.D., St. Louis, Missouri.)

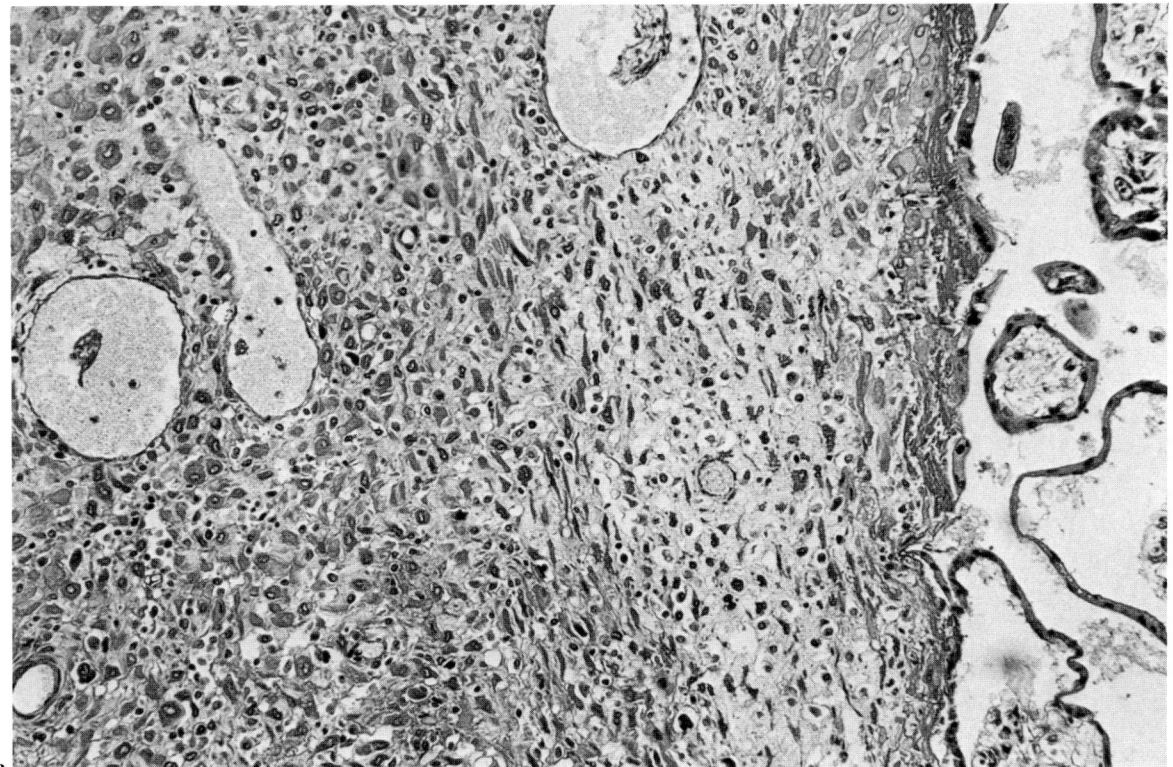

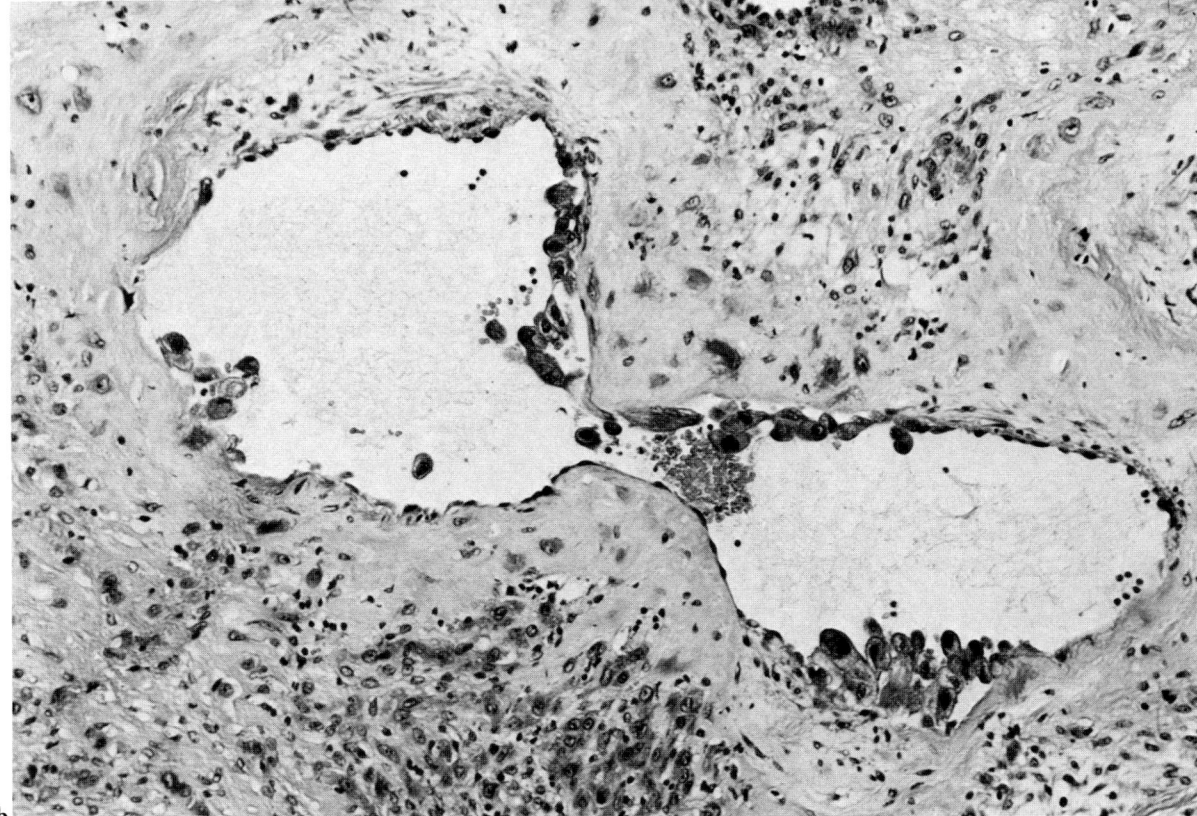

FIG. 23.91. a: **Implantation site of spontaneous abortion.** Placental site intermediate trophoblast cells are markedly deficient in size and numbers. b: **Normal appearance of intermediate trophoblast at implantation site.** Numerous trophoblast cells replace intima, infiltrate the wall of the large spiral artery at *center*, and cluster irregularly in the surrounding decidua, especially at *bottom center*.

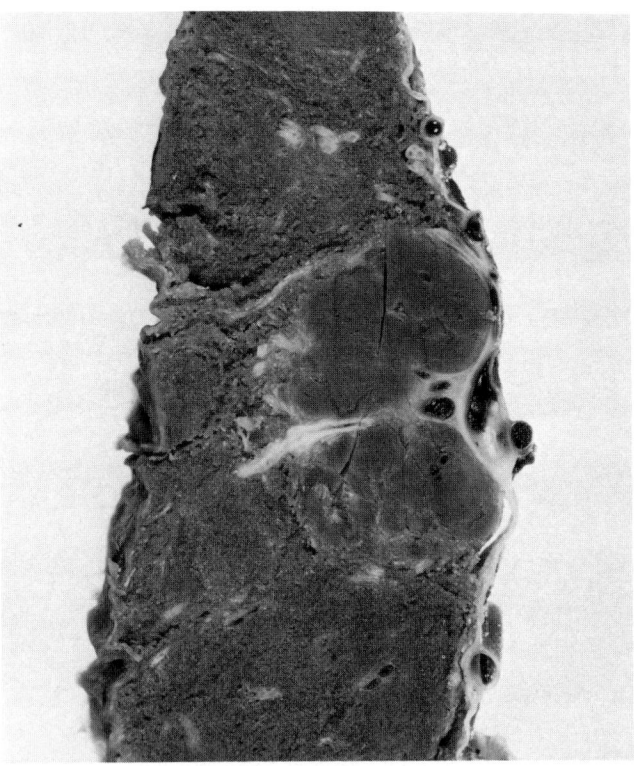

FIG. 23.92. Placental hemangioma. Firm, red hemangioma, well demarcated from the surrounding placental parenchyma.

blastic derivation. Trisomies may result from parental chromosomal anomalies, mostly balanced translocations. When abnormal parental karyotypes are demonstrated, the prospects for future anomalous conceptions are much greater.

The villi of abortions with *45 XO* (monosomy X) karyotype are extremely variable. There may be focal, slight villous swelling in early abortions, scattered large immature villi in later abortions, or marked villous edema with cisterns (Fig. 23.89), but the most distinctive morphological changes affect the fetus itself. Massive edema of the entire fetus is common. Most are dead and macerated, but most characteristic is the pronounced dorsal and lateral swelling of the neck, which may triple the size of the fetal head (Fig. 23.90). Monosomy X conceptions usually are not repeated, and they seem to be associated more commonly with young maternal age.[397] The phenotype in those who survive is that of Turner syndrome.

The histological features described above are more frequent and more marked in abortions with abnormal karyotypes. The same abnormalities, however, may be seen in abortions with normal karyotypes. Chromosomal analysis remains the only definitive means of determining the abortion karyotype, but it is expensive and time-consuming and practically cannot be performed on all abortion specimens. Flow cytometric analysis may provide useful information in

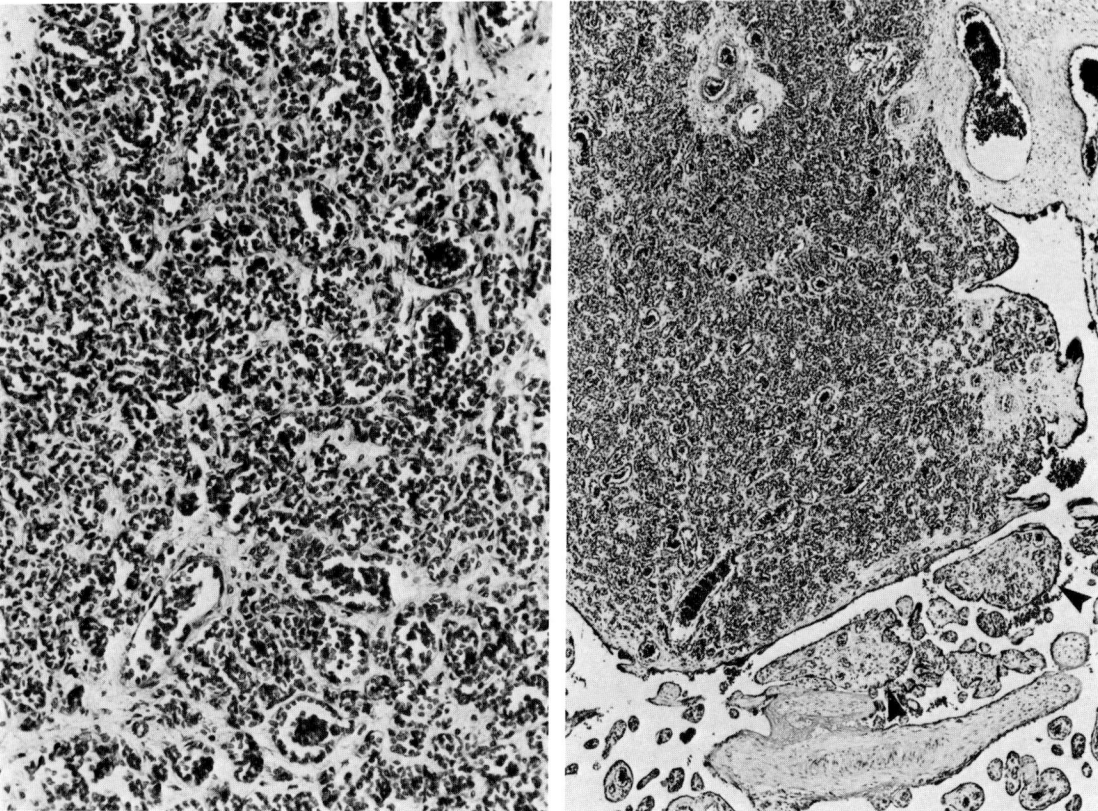

FIG. 23.93. Placental hemangioma. Angiomatous type characterized by numerous capillary-sized vessels separated by inconspicuous stroma (*left*). Adjacent villi show telangiectatic change (*arrowheads, right*).

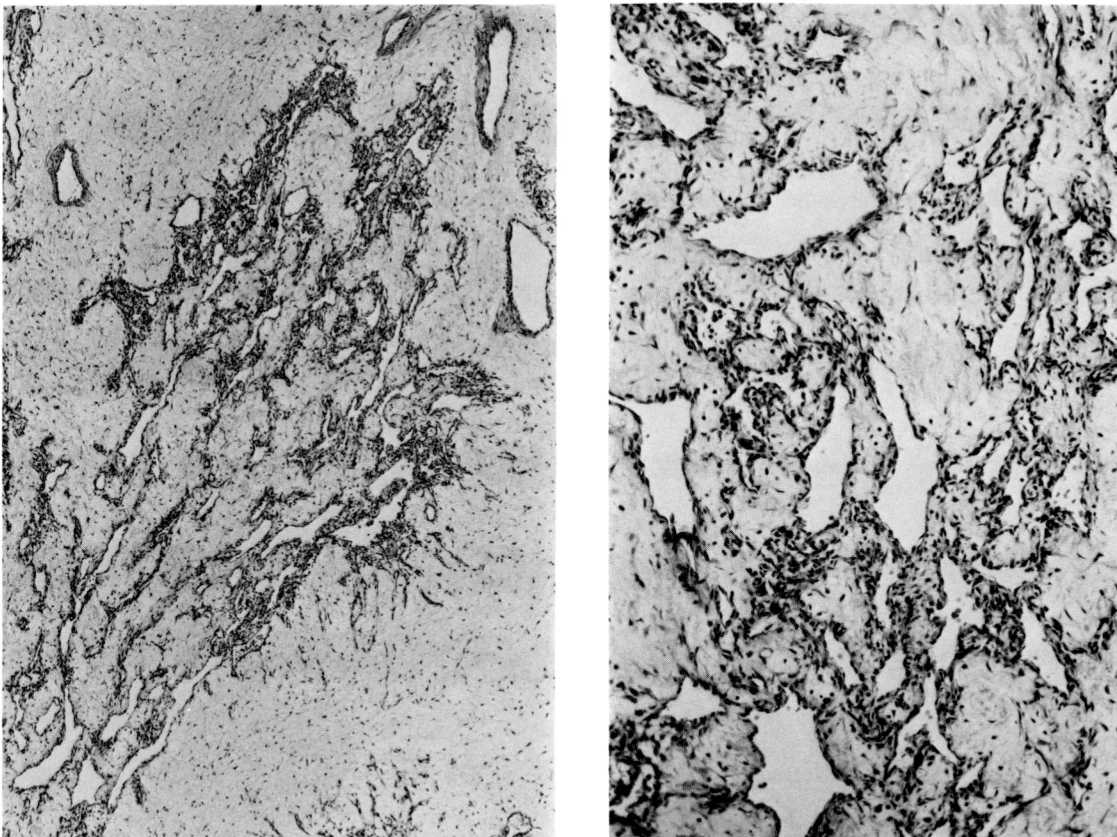

FIG. 23.94. **Hemangioma of umbilical cord.** Large, cavernous vessels suspended in abundant, myxoid stroma. *Left:* Low power. *Right:* High power.

some cases, but cannot distinguish the trisomies from a normal DNA complement. Some abnormalities, especially trisomies when they occur repeatedly, may reflect chromosomal anomalies in the parents. Karyotyping may be clinically useful in the evaluation of couples distressed by repeated spontaneous abortion.[368] Balanced translocations are the most common parental karyotypic defects and may represent the basis for repeated abortion in such cases.[368] Although these are not currently treatable, they are of immense importance in genetic counseling as the prospects for future pregnancies are evaluated.

Immunologic Factors

Some immunologic problems are associated with repeated abortions and life-threatening thrombotic problems in the mother. Rocklin et al.[316] identified a maternal immunoglobulin G (IgG) antibody in normal multigravid women that is absent in some women who experience repeated abortion. The presence of this serum-blocking factor is be-

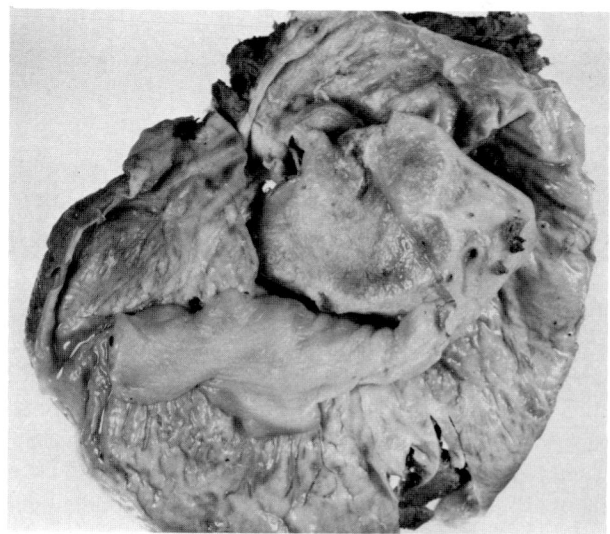

FIG. 23.95. **Hemangioma of umbilical cord in a liveborn normal infant.** Large hemangioma is located near cord insertion.

lieved to support the fetus and placenta as an allograft. Morphologic changes at the implantation site in these abortions have not been correlated with the immunologic findings. It would be interesting and desirable to see if placental site trophoblast is altered or absent in women who experience habitual abortion. The absence of vessel changes and intermediate trophoblast is an easily recognized pattern variation in some abortions, but clinical correlations with this deficit are lacking (Fig. 23.91).

The circulating lupus anticoagulant, an immunoglobulin (usually IgG but sometimes IgM) that inhibits coagulation, derives its name (a misnomer) from the circumstances of its first identification in patients with lupus erythematosus. It has been implicated as a clinical marker for recurrent first trimester spontaneous abortion and for fetal death in later trimesters as well. It prolongs phospholipid-dependent coagulation times but paradoxically is associated with an increased risk of thrombotic disease in the mother.[66,118,123,152] Limited morphologic studies of the placenta associated with this condition have shown changes indistinguishable from those of preeclampsia.[104,279,355]

Nontrophoblastic Tumors

Hemangioma (Chorangioma)

GROSS FINDINGS

Hemangiomas occur in about 1% of placentas.[396] They usually are small and entirely intraplacental and are not obvious on simple external examination. These tumors may be brown, yellow, tan, red, or white and usually are firm and well demarcated from the surrounding parenchyma (Fig. 23.92). Large tumors are rare and either may project above the chorionic plate of the placenta or be visible on the maternal surface. Rarely, a hemangioma is attached to the placenta by a thin pedicle. Usually hemangiomas are solitary, but they may be multiple or, rarely, involve the placenta diffusely.

MICROSCOPIC FINDINGS

The microscopic appearance of placental hemangiomas varies depending on the degree of differentiation and distribution of the vascular elements and on the amount of degeneration. Three microscopic types have been described: (1) angiomatous (vascular, mature)—composed of numerous blood vessels, usually capillary but occasionally cavernous in type, supported by inconspicuous, loose stroma (Fig. 23.93), (2) cellular (immature)—compact arrangement of primitive cells, presumably endothelial, and (3) degenerate—with prominent myxoid change, hyalinization, necrosis, or calcification (Fig. 23.94). Many tumors have a variable appearance, with gradual transition between the different histological patterns. Localized groups

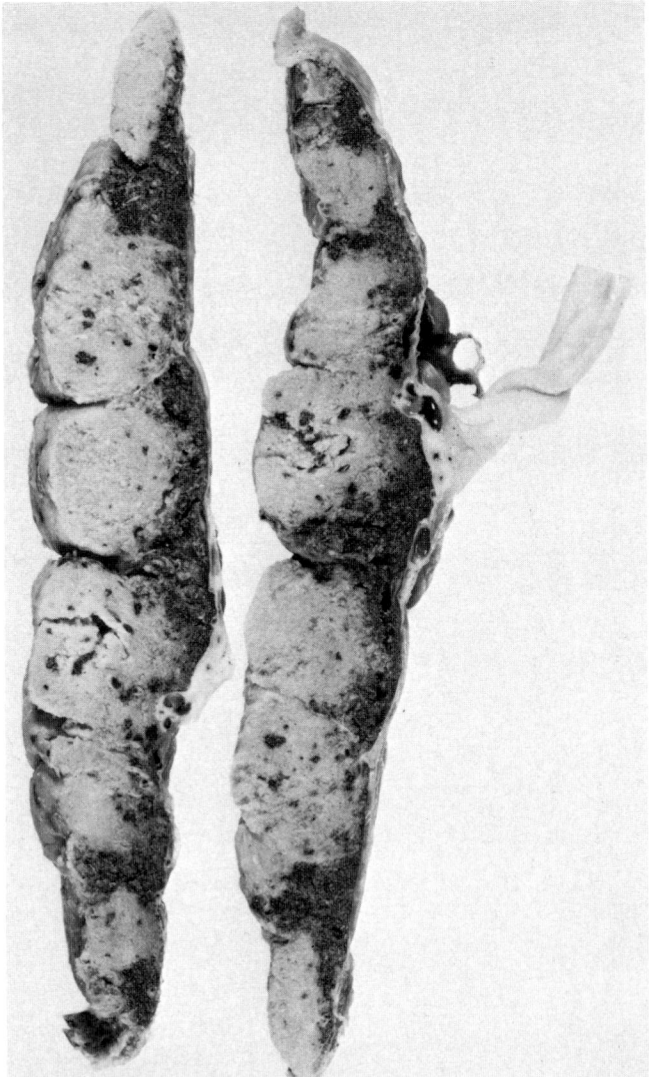

FIG. 23.96. Metastatic malignant melanoma of placenta. Dark areas represent metastatic deposits of malignant melanoma.

of large telangiectatic villi often are identified adjacent to the tumor (Fig. 23.93). Although mitotic figures and some degree of nuclear atypicality may be found in occasional tumors,[228] there has yet to be a proven case of angiosarcoma arising in the placenta. The tumor cells have been demonstrated to contain factor VIII antigen[228] and to resemble endothelial cells ultrastructurally.[81] Whether these tumors represent hamartomas or true neoplasms is a subject of debate. Hemangiomas of identical gross and microscopic appearance also may occur in the umbilical cord (Fig. 23.95).[30]

CLINICAL BEHAVIOR

Various clinical complications have been reported in association with hemangiomas of the placenta.[76,81,353,396] The most significant of these are hydramnios and premature

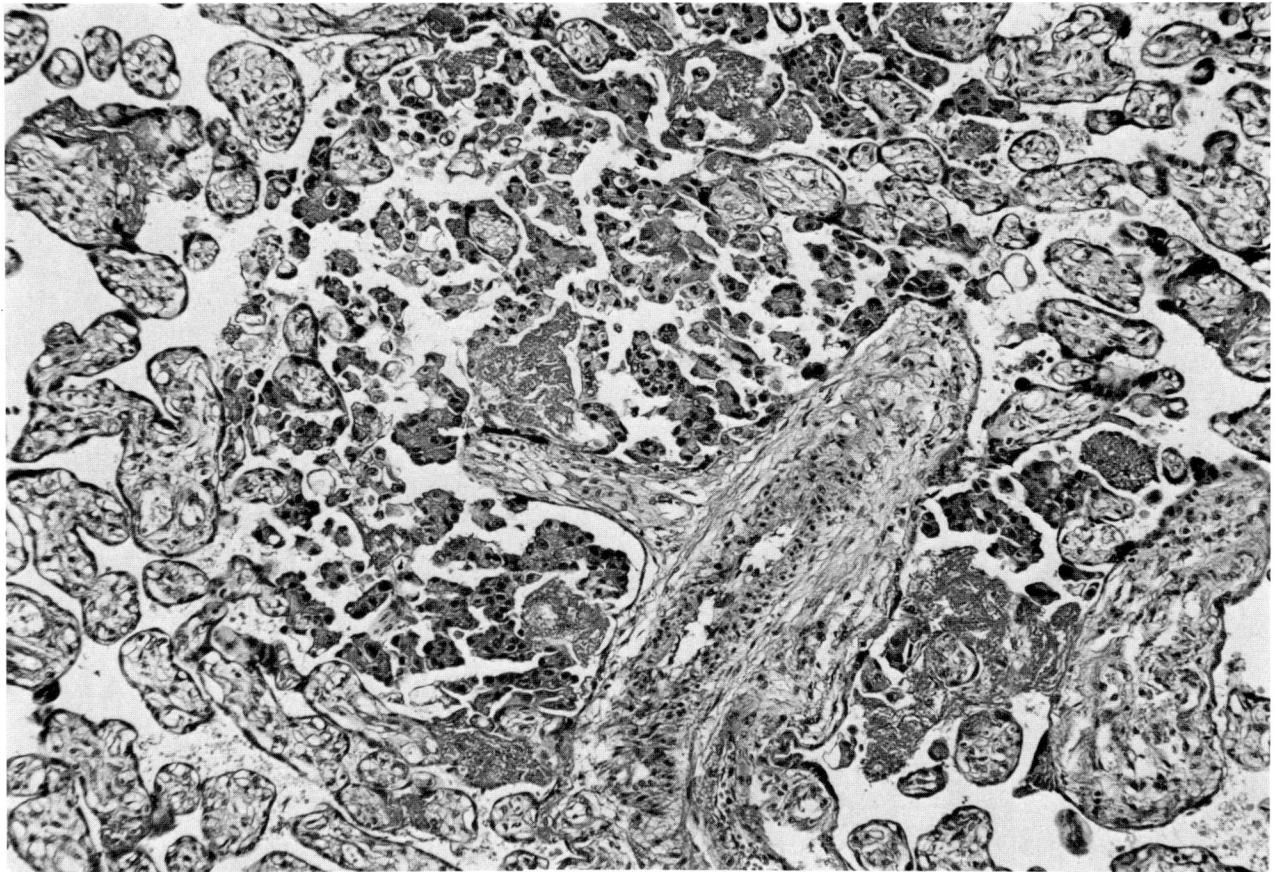

Fig. 23.97. Metastatic breast carcinoma of placenta. Metastatic breast carcinoma is confined to the intervillous space. There is no villous invasion.

delivery; the latter appears to be a consequence of the former. Hydramnios is always associated with larger tumors. Fetal cardiomegaly and congestive heart failure have been attributed to shunting of blood through the hemangioma. Growth retardation may occur if the hemangioma produces a significant shunt in the placental circulation.[252] Other transitory fetal complications have included edema, anemia, and thrombocytopenia. Skin angiomas have been reported in a few babies with placental hemangiomas.

Teratoma

Placental teratomas are rare. The few tumors reported have been located between the amnion and chorion, usually on the placental surface. Teratomas have been found in the umbilical cord as well. Histologically, they have the usual features of a mature teratoma. They are distinguished from an acardiac fetus by the lack of an umbilical cord and the total disorganization of the component tissues.

Placental Metastases

Metastases to the placenta from either maternal or fetal neoplasms are very rare. Although carcinomas of the cervix and breast are the most frequently encountered malignancies in pregnant women, malignant melanoma is by far most common maternal tumor to metastasize to the placenta or spread to the fetus.[294,307,373]

Placentas harboring metastases usually are normal on gross inspection. Tumor deposits may be seen in cases of metastatic melanoma (Fig. 23.96) and have been reported in one recent case of metastatic Ewing's sarcoma.[156] Microscopically, nests of malignant cells usually are confined to the intervillous space. Villous or fetal vascular invasion is very uncommon (Fig. 23.97).

A few cases of dissemination of congenital malignant tumors to the placenta have been reported. There are well-documented cases of placental metastases from neuroblastoma.[49,370] Grossly, these placentas have been pale and bulky, resembling the hydropic placentas of Rh incompatibility. Fetal vessels plugged by clumps of neuroblastoma cells have been found microscopically. Rare cases of

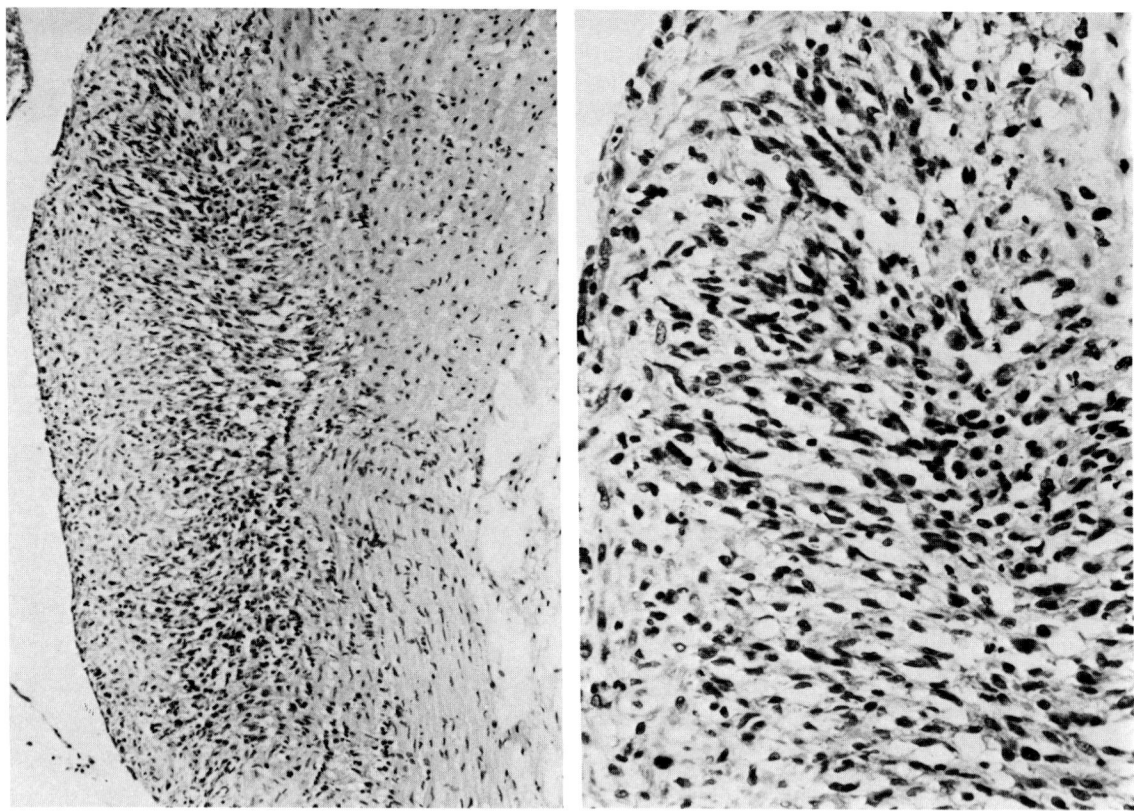

FIG. 23.98. **Umbilical artery.** Disseminated histiocytosis in subendothelial location. *Left:* Low power. *Right:* High power.

fetal leukemic involvement of the placenta also have been illustrated.[41] Disseminated histiocytosis involving the vessels of the umbilical cord may occur (Fig. 23.98).

References

1. Abitbol MM, Driscoll SG, Ober WB (1976) Placental lesions in experimental toxemia in the rabbit. Am J Obstet Gynecol 125: 942–948
2. Abitbol MM, Pirani CL, Ober WB, et al (1976) Production of experimental toxemia in the pregnant dog. Obstet Gynecol 48: 537–548
3. Abraham JM (1967) Intrauterine feto-fetal transfusion syndrome. Clinical observations and speculations on pathogenesis. Clin Pediatr 6: 405–410
4. Abramowsky CR, Vegas ME, Swinehart G, Gyves MT (1980) Decidual vasculopathy of the placenta in lupus erythematosus. N Engl J Med 303: 668–672
5. Aherne W, Strong SJ, Corney G (1968) The structure of the placenta in the twin transfusion syndrome. Biol Neonate 12: 121–135
6. Ahlfors K, Forsgren M, Ivarsson S-A, et al (1983) Congenital cytomegalovirus infection: On the relation between type and time of maternal infection and infant's symptoms. Scand J Infect Dis 15: 129–138
7. Ahlfors K, Ivarsson S-A, Harris S, et al (1984) Congenital cytomegalovirus infection and disease in Sweden and the

relative importance of primary and secondary maternal infections. Scand J Infect Dis 16: 129–137
8. Aladjem S (1967) Morphologic aspects of the placenta in gestational diabetes seen by phase-contrast microscopy. An anatomicroclinical correlation. Am J Obstet Gynecol 99: 341–349
9. Alford CA, Stagno S, Pass RF (1980) Natural history of perinatal cytomegaloviral infection. Excerpta Medica Ciba Foundation Symposium 77: 125–147
10. Althabe O, LaBarrere C, Telenta M (1985) Maternal vascular lesions in placentae of small-for-gestational-age infants. Placenta 6: 265–276
11. Altshuler G (1973) Toxoplasmosis as a cause of hydranencephaly. Am J Dis Child 125: 251–252
12. Altshuler G (1974) Pathogenesis of congenital herpesvirus infection. Am J Dis Child 127: 427–429
13. Altshuler G (1977) Placentitis, with a new light on and old torch. Obstet Gynecol Annu 6: 197–221
14. Altshuler G (1984) Chorangiosis. Arch Pathol Lab Med 108: 71–74
15. Altshuler G, Hyde S (1989) Meconium-induced vasoconstriction: A potential cause of cerebral and other fetal hypoperfusion and of poor pregnancy outcome. J Child Neurol 4: 137–142
16. Altshuler G, Russell P (1975) The human placental villitides. A review of chronic intrauterine infection. Curr Top Pathol 60: 63–112
17. Altshuler G, Tsang RC, Ermocilla R (1975) Single umbilical

artery. Correlation of clinical status and umbilical cord histology. Am J Dis Child 129: 697–700

18. Alvarez H, Sala MA, Benedetti WL (1972) Intervillous space reduction in the edematous placenta. Am J Obstet Gynecol 112: 819–820

19. Amatuzio JC, Gorlin RJ (1981) Conjoined acardiac monsters. Arch Pathol 105: 253–255

20. Anand A, Gray ES, Brown T, et al (1987) Human parvovirus infection in pregnancy and hydrops fetalis. N Engl J Med 316: 183–6

21. Anderson GD (1975) Listeria monocytogenes septicemia in pregnancy. Obstet Gynecol 46: 102–104

22. Anderson M, Went LN, MacIver JE, Dixon HG (1960) Sickle-cell disease in pregnancy. Lancet 2: 516–521

23. Andres RL, Kuyper W, Resnik R, et al (1990) The association of maternal floor infarction of the placenta with adverse perinatal outcome. Am J Obstet Gynecol 163: 935–938

24. Appelbaum PC, Shulman G, Chambers NL, et al (1980) Studies on the growth-inhibiting property of amniotic fluids from two United States population groups. Am J Obstet Gynecol 137: 579–582

25. Ariel IB, Landing BH (1985) A possibly distinctive vacuolar change of the amniotic epithelium associated with gastroschisis. Pediatr Pathol 2: 283–289

26. Ashkenazy M, Borenstein R, Katz Z, Segal M (1982) Constriction of the umbilical cord by an amniotic band after midtrimester amniocentesis. Acta Obstet Gynecol Scand 61: 89–91

27. Auger P, Marquis G, Dallaire L, et al (1980) Natural occurrence of a humoral response to Candida in human amniotic fluid. Am J Obstet Gynecol 136: 1075–1079

28. Bain AD, Bowie JH, Flint WF, et al (1956) Congenital toxoplasmosis simulating haemolytic disease of the newborn. J Obstet Gynaecol Br Emp 63: 826–832

29. Baldwin VJ, Wittmann BK (1990) Pathology of intragestational intervention in twin-to-twin transfusion syndrome. Pediatr Pathol 10: 79–93

30. Barry FE, McCoy CP, Callahan, Jr WP (1951) Hemangioma of the umbilical cord. Am J Obstet Gynecol 62: 675–680

31. Bartholomew RA, Colvin ED, Grimes WH Jr, et al (1961) Criteria by which toxemia of pregnancy may be diagnosed from unlabeled formalin-fixed placentas. Am J Obstet Gynecol 82: 277–290

32. Batcup G, Tovey LAD, Longster G (1983) Fetomaternal blood group incompatibility studies in placental intervillous thrombosis. Placenta 4: 449–454

33. Bebbington MW, Wittmann BK (1989) Fetal transfusion syndrome: Antenatal factors predicting outcome. Am J Obstet Gynecol 160: 913–915

34. Bejar R, Vigliocco G, Gramajo H, et al (1990) Antenatal origin of neurologic damage in new born infants. II. Multiple gestations. Am J Obstet Gynecol 162: 1230–1236

35. Bendon RW, Siddiqi (1989) Clinical pathology conference: Acute twin-to-twin in utero transfusion. Pediatr Pathol 9: 591–598

36. Bendon RW, Tyson RW, Baldwin VJ, et al (1991) Umbilical cord ulceration and intestinal atresia: A new association? Am J Obstet Gynecol 164: 582–586

37. Benirschke K (1974) Syphilis—the placenta and the fetus. Am J Dis Child 128: 142–143

38. Benirschke K (1981) Abortions and moles. In: Naeye RL, Kissane JM, Kaufman N (eds) Perinatal Diseases, International Academy of Pathology Monograph, Baltimore, Williams & Wilkins

39. Benirschke K, Bourne GL (1960) The incidence and prognostic implication of congenital absence of one umbilical artery. Am J Obstet Gynecol 79: 251–254

40. Benirschke K, Brown WH (1955) A vascular anomaly of the umbilical cord: The absence of one umbilical artery in the umbilical cords of normal and abnormal fetuses. Obstet Gynecol 6: 399–404

41. Benirschke K, Driscoll SG (1967) The Pathology of the Human Placenta. New York, Springer–Verlag

42. Benirschke K, Kaufmann P (1990) Pathology of the Human Placenta, 2nd ed, New York, Springer–Verlag

43. Benirschke K, Kim CK (1973) Multiple pregnancy (first of two parts). N Engl J Med 288: 1276–1284

44. Benirschke K, Kim CK (1973) Multiple pregnancy (second of two parts). N Engl J Med 288: 1329–1335

45. Benirschke K, Mendoza GR, Bazely PL (1974) Placental and fetal manifestations of cytomegalovirus infection. Virch Arch [B Cell Pathol] 16: 121–139

46. Benson RC, Fujikura T (1969) Circumvallate and circummarginate placenta. Obstet Gynecol 34: 799–804

47. Berkowitz RS, Goldstein DP, Bernstein MR (1983) Natural history of partial molar pregnancy. Obstet Gynecol 66: 677–681

48. Beyth Y, Perlman M, Ornoy A (1977) Amniogenic bands associated with facial dysplasia and paresis. J Reprod Med 18: 83–86

49. Birner WF (1961) Neuroblastoma as a cause of antenatal death. Am J Obstet Gynecol 82: 1388–1391

50. Bjork O, Persson B (1982) Placental changes in relation to the degree of metabolic control in diabetes mellitus. Placenta 3: 367–378

51. Blanc WA (1959) Amniotic infection syndrome. Pathogenesis, morphology, and significance in circumnatal mortality. Clin Obstet Gynaecol 2: 705–734

52. Blanc WA (1961) Vernix granulomatosis of amnion ("amnion nodosum") in oligohydramnios. Lesion associated with urinary abnormalities, retention of dead fetuses, and prolonged leakage of amniotic fluid. NY State J Med 61: 1492–1496

53. Blanc WA (1976) Pathology of placenta accreta. Verh Deutsch Ges Pathol 60: 393–399

54. Blanc WA (1976) Circulatory lesions of the human placenta in abruptio. Verh Deutsch Ges Pathol 60: 386–392

55. Blanc WA (1978) Pathology of the placenta and cord in some viral infections. In: Hanshan JB, Dregeon JA (eds). Viral Diseases of the Fetus and Newborn. Major Problems in Clinical Pediatrics, Vol. 17. Philadelphia, WB Saunders

56. Blanc WA (1980) Pathology of the placenta and cord in ascending and in haematogenous infection. Excerpta Medica Ciba Foundation Symposium 77: 17–38

57. Blanc WA (1981) Pathology of the placenta, membranes, and umbilical cord in bacterial, fungal and viral infections in man. In: Naeye RL, Kissane JM, Kaufman N (eds) Perinatal Diseases. International Academy of Pathology Monograph. Baltimore, Williams & Wilkins

58. Blanche S, Rouzioux C, Moscata M-LG, et al (1989) A

prospective study of infants born to women seropositive for human immunodeficiency virus Type I. N Engl J Med 320: 1643–1648

59. Blattner P, Dar H, Nitowsky HM (1977) Pregnancy outcome in women with sickle cell trait. JAMA 238: 1392–1394

60. Blickstein I (1990) The twin-twin transfusion syndrome. Obstet Gynecol 76: 714–722

61. Bloomfield RD, Suarez JR, Malangit AC (1978) The placenta: A diagnostic tool in sickle cell disorders. J Natl Med Assoc 70: 87–88

62. Boronow RC, West RH (1964) Monster acardius parasiticus. Am J Obstet Gynecol 88: 233–237

63. Botha MC (1969) Spontaneous rupture of the uterus due to placenta percreta. South Afr Med J 43: 39–41

64. Boue J, Phillipe E, Girond A, Boue A (1976) Phenotypic expression of lethal chromosomal anomalies in human abortuses. Teratology 14: 3–20

65. Boyd JD, Hamilton WJ (1970) The Human Placenta. Cambridge, W Heffer and Sons

66. Branch DW, Scott JR, Kochenour NK, Hershgold E (1985) Obstetric complications associated with the lupus anticoagulant. N Engl J Med 313: 1322–1326

67. Breen JL, Neubecker R, Gregori CA, Franklin JE (1977) Placenta accreta, increta and percreta. Obstet Gynecol 49: 43–47

68. Brescia RJ, Kurman RJ, Main C, et al (1987) The immunocytochemical localization of human chorionic gonadotropin, human placental lactogen and placental alkaline phosphatase in the diagnosis of complete and partial hydatidiform moles. Int J Gynecol Pathol 6: 213–29

69. Brosens I, Renaer M (1972) On the pathogenesis of placental infarcts in preeclampsia. J Obstet Gynaecol Br Commonw 79: 794–799

70. Brosens I, Dixon HG, Robertson WB (1977) Fetal growth retardation and the arteries of the placental bed. Br J Obstet Gynaecol 84: 656–663

71. Brown DR, Doshi N, Taylor PM (1978) Oligohydramnios and fatal pulmonary hyperplasia without amnion nodosum. J Reprod Med 20: 293–296

72. Browne JC (1958) The uterine circulation in toxemia. Clin Obstet Gynaecol 1: 341–348

73. Browne JC, Veall N (1953) The maternal placental blood flow in normotensive and hypertensive women. J Obstet Gynaecol Br Emp 60: 141–147

74. Bryan EM, Kohler HG (1974) The missing umbilical artery. I. Prospective study based on a maternity unit. Arch Dis Child 49: 844–852

75. Bryan EM, Kohler HG (1975) The missing umbilical artery. II. Paediatric follow-up. Arch Dis Child 50: 714–718

76. Burrows S, Gaines JL, Hughes FJ (1973) Giant chorioangioma. Am J Obstet Gynecol 115: 579–580

77. Butany J, Quinn PA (1986) Correlation between chorioamnionitis and evidence of infection during pregnancy. Lab Invest 54: 8A

78. Cameron AH (1968) The Birmingham twin survey. Proc Roy Soc Med 61: 229–234

79. Cardwell MS (1987) Ultrasound diagnosis of abruptio placentae with fetomaternal hemorrhage. Am J Obstet Gynecol 157: 358–359

80. Carlson NJ, Towers CV (1989) Multiple gestation compli-

cated by the death of one fetus. Obstet Gynecol 73: 685–689

81. Cash JB, Powell DE (1980) Placental chorioangioma. Presentation of a case with electron microscopic and immunochemical studies. Am J Surg Pathol 4: 87–92

82. Centers for Disease Control (1989) Risks associated with human parvovirus B19 infection. MMWR 38: 81–97

83. Chandwani S, Greco MA, Mittal K, et al (1991) Pathology and human immunodeficiency virus expression in placentas of seropositive women. J Infect Dis 163: 1134–1138

84. Charache S, Scott J, Niebyl J, Bonds D (1980) Management of sickle cell disease in pregnant patients. Obstet Gynecol 55: 407–410

85. Clewell WH, Manchester DK (1983) Recurrent maternal floor infarction: A preventable cause of fetal death. Am J Obstet Gynecol 147: 346–347

86. Committee on Infectious Diseases, American Academy of Pediatrics. Parvovirus, erythema infectiosum, and pregnancy. Pediatrics 85: 131

87. Cooperman NR, Kasim M, Rajashekaraiah KR (1980) Clinical significance of amniotic fluid, amniotic membranes, and endometrial biopsy cultures at the time of cesarean section. Am J Obstet Gynecol 137: 536–542

88. Corney G, Aherne W (1965) The placental transfusion syndrome in monozygous twins. Arch Dis Child 40: 264–270

89. Coulter JBS, Scott JM, Jordan MM (1975) Oedema of the umbilical cord and respiratory distress in the newborn. Br J Obstet Gynaecol 82: 453–459

90. Crawford JM (1959) A study of human placental growth with observations on the placenta in erythroblastosis foetalis. J Obstet Gynaecol Br Emp 66: 885–896

91. Cruikshank SH, Granados JL (1988) Increased amniotic acetylcholinesterase activity with a fetus papyraceus and aplasia cutis congenita. Obstet Gynecol 71: 997–999

92. Danskin FH, Neilson JP (1989) Twin-to-twin transfusion syndrome: What are appropriate diagnostic criteria? Am J Obstet Gynecol 161: 365–369

93. Darby MJ, Caritis SN, Shen-Schwarz S (1989) Placental abruption in the preterm gestation: An association with chorioamnionitis. Obstet Gynecol 74: 88–92

94. Davey DA, MacGillivray I (1988) The classification and definition of the hypertensive disorders of pregnancy. Am J Obstet Gynecol 158: 892–898

95. Deacon JS, Machin GA, Martin JME, et al (1980) Investigation of acephalus. Am J Med Genet 5: 85–99

96. DeLia JE, Cruikshank DP, Keye WR (1990) Fetoscopic neodymium:Yag laser occlusion of placental vessels in severe twin-twin transfusion syndrome. Obstet Gynecol 75: 1046–1053

97. Demers LM, Gabbe SG (1976) Placental prostaglandin levels in pre-eclampsia. Am J Obstet Gynecol 126: 137–139

98. DeMyer W, Baird I (1969) Mortality and skeletal malformations from amniocentesis and oligohydramnios in rats: Cleft palate, clubfoot, microstomia, and adactyly. Teratology 2: 33–38

99. Desmonts G, Couvreur J (1974) Congenital toxoplasmosis. A prospective study of 378 pregnancies. N Engl J Med 290: 1110–1116

100. Devi B, Jennison RF, Langley FA (1968) Significance of

placental pathology in transplacental haemorrhage. J Clin Pathol 21: 322–331

101. DeWolf F, Brosens I, Renaer M (1980) Fetal growth retardation and the maternal arterial supply of the human placenta in the absence of sustained hypertension. Br J Obstet Gynaecol 87: 678–685

102. DeWolf F, Robertson WB, Brosens I (1975) The ultrastructure of acute atherosis in hypertensive pregnancy. Am J Obstet Gynecol 123: 164–174

103. DeWolf F, DeWolf-Peeters C, Brosens I, Robertson WB (1980) The human placental bed: Electron microscopic study of trophoblastic invasion of spiral arteries. Am J Obstet Gynecol 137: 58–70

104. DeWolf F, Carreras LO, Moerman P, et al (1982) Decidual vasculopathy and extensive placental infarction in a patient with repeated thromboembolic accidents, recurrent fetal loss, and a lupus anticoagulant. Am J Obstet Gynecol 142: 829–834

105. Dippel AL (1940) Hematomas of the umbilical cord. Surg Gynecol Obstet 70: 51–57

106. Dische MR, Quinn PA, Czegledy-Nagy E, Sturgess JM (1979) Genital mycoplasma infection. Am J Clin Pathol 72: 167–174

107. Dixon HG, Browne JCM, Davey DA (1963) Choriodecidual and myometrial blood-flow. Lancet 2: 369–373

108. Dobashi K, Ajika K, Ohkawa T, et al (1984) Immunohistochemical localization of pregnancy-associated plasma protein A (PAPP-A) in placentae form normal and pre-eclamptic pregnancies. Placenta 5: 205–212

109. Dong Y, St. Clair PJ, Ramzy I, et al (1987) A microbiologic and clinical study of placental inflammation at term. Obstet Gynecol 70: 175–182

110. Donnenfeld AE, Glazerman LR, Cutillo DM, et al (1989) Fetal exsanguination following intrauterine angiographic assessment and selective termination of a hydrocephalic, monozygotic co-twin. Prenatal Diag 9: 301–308

111. Driscoll SG (1965) The pathology of pregnancy complicated by diabetes mellitus. Med Clin North Am 49: 1053–1067

112. Driscoll SG (1966) Current concepts. Hydrops fetalis. N Engl J Med 275: 1432–1434

113. Driscoll SG (1969) Histopathology of gestational rubella. Am J Dis Child 118: 49–53

114. Driscoll SG (1979) Significance of acute chorioamnionitis. Clin Obstet Gynecol 22: 339–349

115. Driscoll SG, Gorbach A, Feldman D (1962) Congenital listeriosis: Diagnosis from placental studies. Obstet Gynecol 20: 216–220

116. Ducey J, Schulman H, Farmakides G, et al (1987) A classification of hypertension in pregnancy based on Doppler velocimetry. Am J Obstet Gynecol 157: 680–685

117. Dudley DKL, D'Alton ME (1986) Single fetal death in twin gestation. Sem Perinatol 10: 65–72

118. Elias M, Eldor A (1984) Thromboembolism in patients with the 'Lupus'-type circulating anticoagulant. Arch Intern Med 144: 510–515

119. Elliott WG (1970) Placental toxoplasmosis: Report of a case. Am J Clin Pathol 53: 413–417

120. Etches PC, Lemons JA (1979) Nonimmune hydrops fetalis: Report of 22 cases including three siblings. Pediatrics 64: 326–332

121. Evaldson GR, Malmborg AS, Nord CE (1982) Premature rupture of the membranes and ascending infection. Br J Obstet Gynaecol 89: 793–801

122. Farmakides G, Schulman H, Saldana LR, et al (1985) Surveillance of twin pregnancy with umbilical arterial velocimetry. Obstet Gynecol 153: 789–792

123. Feinstein DI (1985) Lupus anticoagulant, thrombosis, and fetal loss. N Engl J Med 313: 1348–1350

124. Fiakpui EZ, Moran EM (1973) Pregnancy in the sickle hemoglobinopathies. J Reprod Med 11: 28–34

125. Florman AL, Gershon AA, Blackett PR, Nahmias AJ (1973) Intrauterine infection with herpes simplex virus. Resultant congenital malformations. JAMA 225: 129–132

126. Forrest JM, Menser MA, Burgess JA (1971) High frequency of diabetes mellitus in young adults with congenital rubella. Lancet 2: 332–334

127. Fox H (1967) Perivillous fibrin deposition in the human placenta. Am J Obstet Gynecol 98: 245–251

128. Fox H (1967) The significance of placental infarction in perinatal morbidity and mortality. Biol Neonate 11: 87–105

129. Fox H (1968) Morphological changes in the human placenta following fetal death. J Obstet Gynaecol Br Commonw 75: 839–843

130. Fox H (1970) Effect of hypoxia on trophoblast in organ culture. A morphologic and autoradiographic study. Am J Obstet Gynecol 107: 1058–1064

131. Fox H (1972) Placenta accreta, 1945–1969. Obstet Gynecol 27: 475–486

132. Fox H (1978) Pathology of the Placenta. Major Problems in Pathology, Vol 7. Philadelphia, WB Saunders

133. Fox H (1981) Placental involvement in maternal systemic infection. In: Rosenberg HS, Bernstein J (eds) Perspectives in Pediatric Pathology. Infectious Diseases, Vol 6. New York, Masson

134. Fox H, Sen DK (1972) Placenta extrachorialis. A clinicopathologic study. J Obstet Gynaecol Br Commonw 79: 32–35

135. Franciosi RA, Tattersall P (1988) Fetal infection with human parvovirus B19. Hum Pathol 19: 489–491

136. Frenkel JK (1971) Toxoplasmosis. Mechanisms of infection, laboratory diagnosis and management. Curr Top Pathol 54: 28–75

137. Friedman SA (1988) Preeclampsia: A review of the role of prostaglandins. Obstet Gynecol 71: 122–137

138. Froehlich LA, Fujikura T (1966) Significance of a single umbilical artery. Report from the collaborative study of cerebral palsy. Am J Obstet Gynecol 94: 274–279

139. Froehlich LA, Fujikura T (1973) Follow-up of infants with single umbilical artery. Pediatrics 52: 22–29

140. Fujikura T, Froehlich L (1968) Diagnosis of sickling by placental examination. Geographic differences in incidence. Am J Obstet Gynecol 100: 1122–1124

141. Fujikura T, Benson RC, Driscoll SG (1970) The bipartite placenta and its clinical features. Am J Obstet Gynecol 107: 1013–1017

142. Gaber LW, Redline RW, Moustoufi-Zadeh M, Driscoll SG (1986) Invasive partial mole. Am J Clin Pathol 85: 722–724

143. Garcia AGP, Marques RLS, Lobato YY, et al (1985) Placental pathology in congenital rubella. Placenta 6: 281–295

144. Gardner H and Lage JM (1992) Choriocarcinoma following

a partial hydatidiform mole: A case report. Hum Pathol 23: 468–471

145. Genest DR (1992) Estimating the time of death in stillborn fetuses: II. Histologic evaluation of the placenta; a study of 71 stillborns. Obstet Gynecol 80: 585–592

146. Georgakopoulos P (1974) Placental accreta following lysis of uterine synechiae (Asherman's syndrome). J Obstet Gynaecol Br Commonw 81: 730–733

147. Gersell DJ, Phillips NJ, Beckerman K (1991) Chronic chorioamnionitis: A clinicopathologic study of 17 cases. Int J Gynecol Pathol 10: 217–229

148. Gerson AG, Wallace DM, Bridgens NK, et al (1987) Duplex Doppler ultrasound in the evaluation of growth in twin pregnancies. Obstet Gynecol 70: 419–423

149. Giles WB, Trudinger BJ, Baird PJ (1985) Fetal umbilical artery flow velocity waveforms and placental resistance: Pathological correlation. Br J Obstet Gynaecol 92: 31–38

150. Gillim DL, Hendricks CH (1953) Holoacardius. Review of the literature and case report. Obstet Gynecol 2: 647–653

151. Gilstrap LC III, Cunningham FG (1979) The bacterial pathogenesis of infection following cesarean section. Obstet Gynecol 53: 545–549

152. Gleicher N, Friberg J (1985) IgM gammopathy and the lupus anticoagulant syndrome in habitual aborters. JAMA 253: 3278–3281

153. Gonsoulin W, Moise KJ, Kirshon B, et al (1990) Outcome of twin-twin transfusion diagnosed before 28 weeks of gestation. Obstet Gynecol 75: 214–216

154. Grafe MR, Benirschke K (1990) Ultrastructural study of the amniotic epithelium in a case of gastroschisis. Pediatr Pathol 10: 95–101

155. Gray ML (1960) Genital listeriosis as a cause of repeated abortion. Lancet 2: 315–317

156. Greenberg P, Collins JD, Voet RL, Jariwala L (1982) Ewing's Sarcoma metastatic to placenta. Placenta 3: 191–196

157. Griffiths PD, Baboonian C (1984) A prospective study of primary cytomegalovirus infection during pregnancy: Final report. Br J Obstet Gynaecol 91: 307–315

158. Gruenwald P (1970) Environmental influences on twins apparent at birth. Biol Neonate 15: 79–93

159. Gruenwald P, Levin H, Yousem H (1968) Abruption and premature separation of the placenta. The clinical and the pathologic entity. Am J Obstet Gynecol 102: 604–610

160. Halliday HL, Hirata T (1979) Perinatal listeriosis—a review of twelve patients. Am J Obstet Gynecol 133: 405–410

161. Hanshaw JB (1973) Herpesvirus hominis infections in the fetus and the newborn. Am J Dis Child 126: 546–555

162. Harter CA, Benirschke K (1976) Fetal syphilis in the first trimester. Am J Obstet Gynecol 124: 705–711

163. Hartwig NG, Vermeij-Keers C, DeVries HE, et al (1989) Limb body wall malformation complex: An embryologic etiology? Hum Pathol 20: 1071–1077

164. Hartwig NG, Vermeij-Keers C, Van Elsacker-Neile VE, Fleuren GF (1989) Embryonic malformations in a case of intrauterine parvovirus B19 infection. Teratology 39: 295–302

165. Haust MD (1981) Maternal diabetes mellitus—effects on the fetus and placenta. In: Perinatal Diseases, Naeye RL, Kissane JM, Kaufman N (eds). International Academy of Pathology monograph No. 22. Baltimore, Williams & Wilkins, pp 201–285

166. Heifetz SA (1984) Single umbilical artery: A statistical analysis of 237 autopsy cases and review of the literature. Perspect Pediatr Pathol 8: 345–378

167. Herva R, Karkinen-Jaaskelainen M (1984) Amnionic adhesion malformation syndrome: Fetal and placental pathology. Teratology 29: 11–19

168. Herva R, Rapola J, Rosti J, Karlson H (1980) Cluster of severe amniotic adhesion malformations in Finland. Lancet 1: 818–819

169. Hibbard BM, Jeffcoate TNA (1966) Abruptio placentae. Obstet Gynecol 27: 155–167

170. Higginbottom MC, Jones KL, Hall BD, Smith DW (1979) The amniotic band disruption complex: Timing of amniotic rupture and variable spectra of consequent defects. J Pediatr 95: 544–549

171. Hillier SL, Martius J, Krohn M, et al (1988) A case-control study of chorioamnionic infection and histologic chorioamnionitis in prematurity. N Engl J Med 319: 972–978

172. Hood IC, Desa DJ, Whyte RK (1983) The inflammatory response in candidal chorioamnionitis. Hum Pathol 14: 984–990

173. Hood M (1961) Listeriosis as an infection of pregnancy manifested in the newborn. Pediatrics 27: 390–396

174. Hoshina M, Boothby M, Hussa R, et al (1985) Linkage of human chorionic gonadotrophin and placental lactogen biosynthesis to trophoblast differentiation and tumorigenesis. Placenta 6: 163–172

175. Hoyme HE, Higginbottom MC, Jones KL (1981) Vascular etiology of disruptive structural defects in monozygotic twins. Pediatrics 67: 288–291

176. Hubbell JP, Muirhead DM, Drorbaugh JE (1965) The newborn infant of the diabetic mother. Med Clin North Am 49: 1035–1052

177. Hustin J, Gaspard U (1977) Comparison of histological changes seen in placental tissue cultures and in placentae obtained after fetal death. Br J Obstet Gynaecol 84: 210–215

178. Hyde S, Smotherman J, Moore JI, Altshuler G (1989) A model of bacterially induced umbilical vein spasm, relevant to fetal hypoperfusion. Obstet Gynecol 73: 996–970

179. Irving FL, Hertig AT (1937) A study of placenta accreta. Surg Gynecol Obstet 64: 178

180. Jauniaux E, Nessman C, Imbert C, et al (1988) Morphological aspects of the placenta in HIV pregnancies. Placenta 9: 633–642

181. Jimenes E, Unger M, Eitelbach F, et al (1989) Demonstration of HIV-antigens in birth placentae and therapeutic abortions. Placenta 10: 467

182. Johnson GM, Tudor RB (1970) Diabetes mellitus and congenital rubella infection. Am J Dis Child 120: 453–455

183. Johnstone BH, Benirschke K (1975) Monozygotic twins discordant for urinary tract anomalies and presenting as hydramnios. Obstet Gynecol 47: 610–615

184. Jones CJP, Fox H (1976) Placental changes in gestational diabetes. An ultrastructural study. Obstet Gynecol 48: 274–280

185. Jones CJP, Fox H (1976) An ultrastructural and ultrahistochemical study of the placenta of the diabetic woman. J Pathol 119: 91–99

186. Jones CJP, Fox H (1978) An ultrastructural study of the

placenta in matero-fetal Rhesus incompatibility. Virch Arch [A Pathol Anat] 379: 229–241

187. Jones CJP, Fox H (1980) An ultrastructural and ultrahistochemical study of the human placenta in maternal pre-eclampsia. Placenta 1: 61–76

188. Jones CJP, Fox H (1981) An ultrastructural and ultrahistochemical study of the human placenta in maternal essential hypertension. Placenta 2: 193–204

189. Jones KL, Benirschke K (1983) The developmental pathogenesis of structural defects: the contribution of monozygotic twins. Semin Perinatol 7: 239–243

190. Kalousek DK (1987) Anatomic and chromosomal anomalies in specimens of early spontaneous abortion: Seven years experience. Birth Defects 23: 153–168

191. Kalousek DK (1991) Pathology of abortion. In: Kraus FT, Danjanov I, Kaufman N (eds) Pathology of Reproductive Failure. Baltimore, Williams & Wilkins, pp 228–256

192. Kalousek D, Poland BJ (1984) Embryonic and fetal pathology of abortion. In: Perrin EDVK (ed) Pathology of the Placenta. New York, Churchill–Livingstone

193. Kalousek DK, Bamforth S (1988) Amnion rupture sequence in previable fetuses. Am J Med Genet 31: 63–73

194. Kaplan C, Blanc WA, Elias J (1982) Indentification of erythrocytes in intervillous thrombi. A study using immunoperoxidase identification of hemoglobins. Hum Pathol 13: 554–557

195. Karegard M, Gennser G (1986) Incidence and recurrence rate of abruptio placentae in Sweden. Obstet Gynecol 67: 523–528

196. Keenan WJ, Steichen JJ, Mahmood K, Altshuler G (1977) Placental pathology compared with clinical outcome. Am J Dis Child 131: 1224–1227

197. Kendrick FJ, Feild LE (1967) Congenital anomalies induced in normal and adrenalectomized by rats by amniocentesis. Anat Rec 159: 353–356

198. Kennedy LA, Persaud TVN (1977) Pathogenesis of developmental defects induced in the rat by amniotic sac puncture. Acta Anat 97: 23–35

199. Khong TY, Robertson WB (1987) Placenta creta and placenta praevia creta. Placenta 8: 399–409

200. Kinney JS, Anderson LJ, Farrar J, et al (1988) Risk of adverse outcome after human parvovirus B19 infection. J Infect Dis 157: 663–667

201. Kitzmiller JL, Benirschke K (1973) Immunofluorescent study of placental bed vessels in pre-eclampsia of pregnancy. Am J Obstet Gynecol 115: 248–251

202. Kitzmiller JL, Watt N, Driscoll SG (1981) Decidual arteriopathy in hypertension and diabetes in pregnancy: Immunofluorescent studies. Am J Obstet Gynecol 141: 733–779

203. Knox WF, Fox H (1984) Villitis of unknown aetiology: Its incidence and significance in placentae from a British population. Placenta 5: 395–402

204. Koshy M, Burd L, Wallace D, et al (1988) Prophylactic red-cell transfusions in pregnant patients with sickle cell disease. N Engl J Med 319: 1447–1452

205. Kraemer BB, Kraus FT, Sheldon G (1985) Expression of pregnancy-specific proteins in maternal diabetes. An immunocytochemical study of placental bed biopsies and placental tissues. Lab Invest 52: 37A

206. Kraus FT (1991) Role of the pathologist in evaluation of infertility: Current practice and future developments. In: Kraus FT, Damjanov I, Kaufman N (eds) Pathology of Reproductive Failure. Baltimore, Williams & Wilkins, pp 339

207. Kundsin RB, Driscoll SG, Monson RR, et al (1984) Association of Ureaplasma urealyticum in the placenta with perinatal morbidity and mortality. N Engl J Med 310: 941–945

208. Kurman RJ, Main CS, Chen H-C (1984) Intermediate trophoblast: A distinctive form of trophoblast with specific morphological, biochemical and functional features. Placenta 5: 349–370

209. Kurman RJ, Young RH, Norris HJ, et al (1984) Immunocytochemical localization of placental lactogen and chorionic gonadotropin in the normal placenta and trophoblastic tumors, with emphasis on intermediate trophoblast and the placental site trophoblastic tumor. Int J Gynecol Pathol 3: 101–121

210. LaBarrere C, Althabe O, Telenta M (1982) Chronic villitis of unknown aetiology in placentae of idiopathic small for gestational age infants. Placenta 3: 309–318

211. Labarrere C, Sebastiani M, Siminovich M, et al (1985) Absence of Wharton's jelly around the umbilical arteries: an unusual cause of perinatal mortality. Placenta 6: 555–559

212. LaBarrere C, McIntyre JA, Faulk WP (1990) Immunohistologic evidence that villitis in human normal term placentas is an immunologic lesion. Am J Obstet Gynecol 162: 515–522

213. Lademacher DS, Vermeulen RCW, Harten JJ, Arts NF (1981) Circumvallate placenta and congenital malformation. Lancet 1: 732

214. Lage JM, VanMarter LJ, Bieber FR (1988) Questionable role of amniocentesis in the etiology of amniotic band formation. J Reprod Med 33: 71–73

215. Lage JM, Vanmarter LJ, Mikhail E (1989) Vascular anastomoses in fused, dichorionic twin placentas resulting in twin transfusion syndrome. Placenta 10: 55–59

216. Las Heras J, Harding P, Haust MD (1980) The morphology of third order fetal arteries in normal and "toxemic" placentas. Lab Invest 40: 260

217. Las Heras J, Baskerville JC, Harding PGR, Haust MD (1985) Morphometric studies of fetal placental stem arteries in hypertensive disorders ("toxaemia") of pregnancy. Placenta 6: 217–228

218. Lauweryns J, Bernat R, Lerut A, Detournay G (1973) Intrauterine pneumonia. An experimental study. Biol Neonate 22: 301–318

219. Lawler FC, Wood WS, King S, Metzger W (1964) Listeria monocytogenes as a cause of fetal loss. Am J Obstet Gynecol 89: 915–923

220. Lewis SH, Reynolds-Kohler C, Fox HE, Nelson JA (1990) HIV-1 in trophoblastic and villous Hofbauer cells, and haematologic precursors in eight-week fetuses. Lancet 1: 565–568

221. Liu S, Benirschke K, Scioscia AL, Maunino FL (1992) Intrauterine death in multiple gestation. Acta Genet Med Gemellol 41:5–26

222. Lockwood C, Ghidini A, Romero R, Hobbins JC (1989) Amniotic band syndrome: Reevaluation of its pathogenesis. Am J Obstet Gynecol 160: 1030–1033

223. Love AM, Vickers TH (1972) Amniocentesis dysmelia in rats. Br J Exp Pathol 53: 435–444

224. Lunell NO, Nylund LE, Lewander R, et al (1982) Uteroplacental blood flow in pre-eclampsia measurements with indium-113m and a computer-linked gamma camera. Clin Exper Hyper-Hyper Preg B1(1): 105–117

225. Machin GA (1981) Differential diagnosis of hydrops fetalis. Am J Med Genet 9: 341–350

226. MacLennan AH, Sharp F, Shaw-Dunn J (1972) The ultrastructure of human trophoblast in spontaneous and induced hypoxia using a system of organ culture. A comparison with ultrastructural changes in pre-eclampsia and placental insufficiency. J Obstet Gynaecol Br Commonw 79: 113–121

227. Maidman JE, Yeager C, Anderson V, et al (1980) Prenatal diagnosis and management of nonimmunologic hydrops fetalis. Obstet Gynecol 56: 571–576

228. Majlessi HF, Wagner KM, Brooks JJ (1983) Atypical cellular chorangioma of the placenta. Int J Gynecol Pathol 1: 403–408

229. Mar JL (1975) Cytomegalovirus: A major cause of birth defects. Science 190: 1184–1186

230. Martin DH, Koutsky L, Eschenbach DA, et al (1982) Prematurity and perinatal mortality in pregnancies complicated by maternal *Chlamydia trachomatis* infections. JAMA 247: 1585–1588

231. Mattern CFT, Murray K, Jensen A, et al (1992) Localization of human immunodeficiency virus core antigen in term human placentas. Pediatrics 89: 207–209

232. Maudsley RF, Brix GA, Hinton NA, et al (1966) Placental inflammation and infection. A prospective bacteriologic and histologic study. Am J Obstet Gynecol 95: 648–659

233. McConnell HD, Carr DH (1975) Recent advances in the cytogenetic study of human spontaneous abortions. Obstet Gynecol 45: 547–552

234. McKeogh RP, D'Errico E (1951) Placenta accreta: Clinical manifestations and conservative management. N Engl J Med 245: 159–165

235. Menser MA, Forrest JM, Bransby RD (1978) Rubella infection and diabetes mellitus. Lancet 1: 57–60

236. Meyer B (1955) Placenta accreta. An analysis based on an unusual case. Acta Obstet Gynecol Scand 34: 189–201

237. Miller JM, Pupkin MJ, Hill GB (1980) Bacterial colonization of amniotic fluid from intact fetal membranes. Am J Obstet Gynecol 136: 796–804

238. Miller ME, Higginbottom M, Smith DW (1981) Short umbilical cord: Its origin and relevance. Pediatrics 67: 618–621

239. Miller ME, Graham JM Jr, Higginbottom MC, Smith DW (1981) Compression-related defects from early amnion rupture: Evidence for mechanical teratogenesis. J Pediatr 98: 292–297

240. Miller ME, Jones MC, Smith DW (1982) Tension: The basis of umbilical cord growth. J Pediatr 101: 844

241. Miller PW, Coen RW, Benirschke K (1985) Dating the time interval from meconium passage to birth. Obstet Gynecol 66: 459–462

242. Milner PF, Jones BR, Dobler J (1980) Outcome of pregnancy in sickle cell anemia and sickle cell-hemoglobin C disease. An analysis of 181 pregnancies in 98 patients, and a review of the literature. Am J Obstet Gynecol 138: 239–245

243. Minguillon C, Eiben B, Bahr-Porsch S, et al (1989) The predictive value of chorionic villus histology for identifying chromosomally normal and abnormal spontaneous abortions. Hum Genet 82: 373–376

244. Minkoff H, Nanda D, Menez R, Fikrig S (1987) Pregnancies resulting in infants with acquired immunodeficiency syndrome or AIDS-related complex. Obstet Gynecol 69: 285–287

245. Moessinger AC, Blanc WA, Byrne J, et al (1981) Amniotic band syndrome associated with amniocentesis. Am J Obstet Gynecol 141: 588–591

246. Moessinger AC, Blanc WA, Marone PS, Polsen DC (1982) Umbilical cord length as an index of fetal activity: Experimental study and clinical implications. Pediatr Res 16: 109–112

247. Monie IW (1965) Velamentous insertion of the cord in early pregnancy. Am J Obstet Gynecol 93: 276–281

248. Monif GRG, Dische RM (1972) Viral placentitis in congenital cytomegalovirus infection. Am J Clin Pathol 58: 445–449

249. Montgomery JR, Flanders RW, Yow MD (1973) Congenital anomalies and herpesvirus infection. Am J Dis Child 126: 364–366

250. Morison JE (1978) Placenta accreta: A clinicopathologic review of 67 cases. Obstet Gynecol Annu 7: 107–123

251. Mostoufi-Zadeh M, Weiss LM, Driscoll SG (1985) Nonimmune hydrops fetalis. A challenge in perinatal pathology. Hum Pathol 16: 785–789

252. Mucitelli DR, Charles EZ, Kraus FT (1990): Chorangiomas of intermediate size and intrauterine growth retardation. Pathol Res Pract 186: 455–458, 1990.

253. Naeye RL (1975) Causes and consequences of chorioamnionitis. N Engl J Med 293: 40–41

254. Naeye RL (1977) Causes of perinatal mortality in the U.S. Collaborative Perinatal Project. JAMA 238: 228–229

255. Naeye RL (1979) Coitus and associated amniotic-fluid infections. N Engl J Med 301: 1198–1200

256. Naeye RL (1980) Factors in the mother/infant dyad that influence the development of infections before and after birth. Excerpta Medica Ciba Foundation Symposium 77: 3–16

257. Naeye RL (1963) Human intrauterine parabiotic syndrome and its complications. N Engl J Med 268: 804–809

258. Naeye RL (1979) The outcome of diabetic pregnancies: A prospective study. In: Pregnancy, metabolism, diabetes and the fetus. Ciba Foundation Symposium 63: 227–241

259. Naeye RL (1985) Umbilical cord length: Clinical significance. J Pediatr 107: 278–281

260. Naeye RL (1985) Maternal floor infarction. Hum Pathol 16: 823–828

261. Naeye RL (1989) Pregnancy hypertension, placental evidence of low uteroplacental blood flow, and spontaneous premature delivery. Hum Pathol 20: 441–444

262. Naeye RL (1990) The clinical significance of absent subchorionic fibrin in the placenta. Am J Clin Pathol 94: 196–198

263. Naeye RL (1991) Acute chorioamnionitis and the disorders that produce placental insufficiency. In: Kraus FT, Damjanov I, Kaufman N (eds) Pathology of Reproductive Failure. Baltimore, Williams and Wilkins, pp 293

264. Naeye RL, Blanc W (1965) Pathogenesis of congenital rubella. JAMA 194: 109–115

265. Naeye RL, Blanc WL (1970) Relation of poverty and race to antenatal infection. N Engl J Med 283: 555–560

266. Naeye RL, Peters EC (1978) Amniotic fluid infections with intact membranes leading to perinatal death: a prospective study. Pediatrics 61: 171–177

267. Naeye RL, Peters EC (1980) Causes and consequences of premature rupture of fetal membranes. Lancet 1: 192–194

268. Naeye RL, Dellinger WS, Blanc WA (1971) Fetal and maternal features of antenatal bacterial infections. J Pediatr 79: 733–739

269. Naeye RL, Maisels J, Lorenz RP, Botti JJ (1983) The clinical significance of placental villous edema. Pediatrics 71: 588–594

270. Naeye RL, Tafari N, Judge D, et al (1977) Amniotic fluid infections in an African city. J Pediatr 90: 965–970

271. Naftolin F, Khudr G, Benirschke K, Hutchinson DL (1973) The syndrome of chronic abruptio placentae, hydrorrhea, and circumvallate placenta. Am J Obstet Gynecol 116: 347–350

272. Nahmias AJ, Alford CA, Korones SB (1970) Infection of the newborn with herpesvirus hominis. Adv Pediatr 17: 185–226

273. Nahmias AJ, Josey WE, Naib ZM, et al (1971) Perinatal risk associated with maternal genital herpes simplex virus infection. Am J Obstet Gynecol 110: 825–837

274. Naib ZM, Nahmias AJ, Josey WE, Wheeler JH (1970) Association of maternal genital herpetic infection with spontaneous abortion. Obstet Gynecol 35: 260–263

275. Nankervis GA, Kumar ML, Cox FE, Gold E (1984) A prospective study of maternal cytomegalovirus infection and its effect on the fetus. Am J Obstet Gynecol 149: 435–440

276. Napolitani FD, Schreiber I (1960) The acardiac monster. A review of the world literature and presentation of 2 cases. Am J Obstet Gynecol 80: 582–589

277. Navarrete VN, Torres IH, Rivera IR, et al (1967) Maternal carbohydrate disorder and congenital malformations. Diabetes 16: 127–130

278. Navarro C, Blanc WA (1977) Chronic viral funistis. J Pediatr 91: 967–973

279. Nilsson IM, Astedt B, Hedner U, Berezin D (1975) Intrauterine death and circulating anticoagulant ("antithromboplastin"). Acta Med Scand 197: 153–159

280. Nummi S (1972) Relative weight of the placenta and perinatal mortality. A retrospective clinical and statistical analysis. Acta Obstet Gynecol Scand 17(suppl): 1–69

281. Ornoy A, Segal S, Nishmi M, et al (1973) Fetal and placental pathology in gestational rubella. Am J Obstet Gynecol 116: 949–956

282. Pankuch GA, Applebaum PC, Lorenz RP, et al (1983) Placental microbiology in the diagnosis of chorioamnionitis. Abstracts of the Annual Meeting of American Society for Microbiology. Am Soc Microbiol p 319

283. Pastorek JG II, Seiler B (1985) Maternal death associated with sickle cell trait. Am J Obstet Gynecol 152: 295–297

284. Pauls F (1969) Monoamniotic twin pregnancy: A review of the world literature and a report of two new cases. Can Med Assoc J 100: 254–256

285. Peckham CH, Yerushalmy J (1965) Aplasia of one umbilical artery: Incidence by race and certain obstetric factors. Obstet Gynecol 26: 359–366

286. Pedersen LM, Tygstrup I, Pedersen J (1964) Congenital malformations in newborn infants of diabetic women. Correlation with maternal diabetic vascular complications. Lancet 1: 1124–1126

287. Petrilli ES, D'Ablaing G, Ledger WJ (1980) Listeria monocytogenes chorioamnionitis: Diagnosis by transabdominal amniocentesis. Obstet Gynecol 55s: 5–8

288. Pezeshkian R, Fernando N, Carne CA, Simanowita MD (1984) Listeriosis in mother and fetus during the first trimester of pregnancy. Case report. Br J Obstet Gynaecol 91: 85–86

289. Pijnenborg R, Bland JM, Robertson WB, Brosens I (1983) Uteroplacental arterial changes related to interstitial trophoblast migration in early human pregnancy. Placenta 4: 397–414

290. Pinkerton JHM (1963) The placental bed arterioles in diabetes. Proc Roy Soc Med 56: 1021–1022

291. Platt HS (1971) Effect of maternal sickle cell trait on perinatal mortality. Br Med J 4: 334–336

292. Porter HJ, Khong TY, Evans MF, et al (1988) Parvovirus as a cause of hydrops fetalis: detection by in situ DNA hybridisation. J Clin Pathol 41: 381–383

293. Poswillo D (1966) Observations of fetal posture and causal mechanisms of congenital deformity of palate, mandible, and limbs. J Dent Res 45(suppl): 584–596

294. Potter JF, Schoeneman M (1970) Metastasis of maternal cancer to the placenta and fetus. Cancer 25: 380–388

295. Powars DR, Sandhu M, Niland-Weiss J, et al (1986) Pregnancy in sickle cell disease. Obstet Gynecol 67: 217–228

296. Pretorius DH, Manchester D, Barkin S, et al (1988) Doppler ultrasound of twin transfusion syndrome. J Ultrasound Med 7: 117–124

297. Public Health Laboratory Service Working Party on Fifth Disease (1990) Prospective study of human parvovirus (B19) infection in pregnancy. Br Med J 300: 1166–1170

298. Quinn PA, Butany J, Taylor J, Hannah W (1987) Chorioamnionitis: Its association with pregnancy outcome and microbial infection. Am J Obstet Gynecol 156: 379–387

299. Rappaport F, Rabinovitz M, Toaff R, Krochik N (1960) Genital listeriosis as a cause of repeated abortion. Lancet 1: 1273–1275

300. Rausen AR, Seki M, Strauss L (1965) Twin transfusion syndrome. A review of 19 cases studied at one institution. J Pediatr 66: 613–628

301. Ray CG, Wedgwood RJ (1964) Neonatal listeriosis. Six case reports and a review of the literature. Pediatrics 34: 378–392

302. Rayne SC, Kraus FT (1993): Placental thrombi and other vascular lesions. Classification, morphology, and clinical correlations. Pathol Res Pract 189:2–17

303. Redline RW, Abramowsky CR (1985) Clinical and pathologic aspects of recurrent placental villitis. Hum Pathol 16: 727–731

304. Rehder H, Coerdt W, Eggers R, et al (1989) Is there a correlation between morphological and cytogenetic findings in placental tissue from early missed abortions. Hum Genet 82: 337–385

305. Rehder H, Weitzel H (1978) Intrauterine amputations after amniocentesis. Lancet 1: 382

306. Ranaer M, Van de Putte I, Vermylen C (1976) Massive fetomaternal hemorrhage as a cause of perinatal mortality and morbidity. Eur J Obstet Gynecol Reprod Biol 6: 125–140

307. Rewell RE, Whitehouse WL (1966) Malignant metastasis to the placenta from carcinoma of the breast. J Pathol 91: 255–256

308. Reynolds DW, Stagno S, Stubbs KG, et al (1974) Inapparent congenital cytomegalovirus infection with elevated cord IgM levels. N Engl J Med 290: 291–296

309. Rimer BA (1975) Sickle-cell trait and pregnancy: A review of a community hospital experience. Am J Obstet Gynecol 123: 6–11

310. Risteli J, Foidart JM, Risteli L, et al (1984) The basement membrane proteins laminin and type IV collagen in isolated villi in pre-eclampsia. Placenta 5: 541–550

311. Robertson EG, Neer KJ (1983) Placental injection studies in twin gestation. Am J Obstet Gynecol 147: 170–174

312. Robertson WG (1976) Uteroplacental vasculature. J Clin Pathol 10(suppl): 9–17

313. Robertson WB, Brosens I, Dixon G (1975) Uteroplacental vascular pathology. Eur J Obstet Gynecol Reprod Biol 5: 47–65

314. Robertson WB, Khong TY, Brosen I, et al (1986) The placental bed biopsy: Review from three European centers. Am J Obstet Gynecol 155: 401–412

315. Robinson LK, Jones KL, Benirschke K (1983) The nature of structural defects associated with velamentous and marginal insertion of the umbilical cord. Am J Obstet Gynecol 146: 191–193

316. Rocklin RE, Kitzmiller VL, Carpenter CB, et al (1976) Maternal-fetal relation. Absence of an immunologic blocking factor from the serum of women with chronic abortions. N Engl J Med 295: 1209–1213

317. Rogers MF, Ou C-Y, Rayfield M, et al (1989) Use of the polymerase chain reaction for early detection of the proviral sequences of human immunodeficiency virus in infants born to seropositive mothers. N Engl J Med 320: 1649–1654

318. Rolschau J (1978) Circumvallate placenta and intrauterine growth retardation. Acta Obstet Gynecol Scand 72: 11–14

319. Ross SM, MacPherson T, Wallace J, et al (1978) Unsuccessful pregnancies—Report on 200 perinatal postmortems. South Afr Med J 53: 828–829

320. Russell P (1979) Inflammatory lesions of the human placenta I. Am J Diagn Gynecol Obstet 1: 127–137

321. Russell P (1979) Inflammatory lesions of the human placenta II. Villitis of unknown etiology in perspective. Am J Diagn Gynecol Obstet 1: 339–346

322. Russell P (1980) Inflammatory lesions of the human placenta. III. The histopathology of villitis of unknown etiology. Placenta 1: 227–244

323. Russell P, Altshuler G (1974) Placental abnormalities of congenital syphilis. A neglected aid to diagnosis. Am J Dis Child 128: 160–163

324. Russell P, Atkinson K, Krishnan L (1980) Recurrent reproductive failure due to severe placental villitis of unknown etiology. J Reprod Med 24: 93–98

325. Ruvinsky ED, Wiley TL, Morrison JC, Blake PG (1981) In utero diagnosis of umbilical cord hematoma by ultrasonography. Am J Obstet Gynecol 140: 833–834

326. Ryder RW, Hassig SE, Behets F, et al (1989) Perinatal transmission of the human immunodeficiency virus type I to infants of seropositive women in Zaire. N Engl J Med 320: 1637–1642

327. Sala MA, Matheus M (1989) Placental characteristics in twin transfusion syndrome. Arch Gynecol Obstet 246: 51–56

328. Salafia CM, Mangam HE, Weigl CA, et al (1989) Abnormal fetal heart rate patterns and placental inflammation. Am J Obstet Gynecol 160: 140–147

329. Salazar H, Kanbour AI (1974) Amnion nodosum. Ultrastructure and histopathogenesis. Arch Pathol 98: 39–46

330. Samra JS, Obhrai MS, Constantine G (1989) Parvovirus infection in pregnancy. Obstet Gynecol 73: 832–834

331. Sander CH (1980) Hemorrhagic endovasculitis and hemorrhagic villitis of the placenta. Arch Pathol Lab Med 104: 371–373

332. Sander CH, Kinnane L, Stevens NG, Echt R (1986) Haemorrhagic endovasculitis of the placenta: A review with clinical correlation. Placenta 7: 551–574

333. Sands J, Dobbing J (1985) Continuing growth and development of the third-trimester human placenta. Placenta 6: 13–22

334. Schlievert P, Johnson W, Galask RP (1976) Bacterial growth inhibition by amniotic fluid. VI. Evidence for a zinc-peptide antibacterial system. Am J Obstet Gynecol 125: 906–910

335. Schindler A-M, Bordignon P, Bischop P (1984) Immunohistochemical localization of pregnancy-associated plasma protein A in decidua and trophoblast: Comparison with human chorionic gonadotropin and fibrin. Placenta 5: 227–236

336. Schreier R, Brown S (1962) Hematoma of the umbilical cord. Report of a case. Obstet Gynecol 20: 798–800

337. Schwarz TF, Nerlich A, Hottentrager B, et al (1991) Parvovirus B19 infection of the fetus. Histology and in situ hybridization. Am J Clin Pathol 96: 121–126

338. Scott JR, Beer AA (1976) Immunologic aspects of preeclampsia. Am J Obstet Gynecol 125: 418–427

339. Scott JS (1958) Pregnancy toxaemia associated with hydrops foetalis, hydatidiform mole and hydramnios. J Obstet Gynaecol Br Emp 65: 689–701

340. Scott JS (1960) Placenta extrachorialis (placenta marginata and placenta circumvallata). A factor in antepartum hemorrhage. J Obstet Gynaecol Br Emp 67: 904–918

341. Seidman JD, Abbondanzo SL, Watkin WG, et al (1989) Amniotic band syndrome. Arch Pathol Lab Med 113: 891–897

342. Seligsohn U, Berger A, Abend M, et al (1984): Homozygous protein C deficiency manifested by massive venous thrombosis in the newborn. N Engl J Med 310: 559–562

343. Sepp AH, Roy TE (1963) *Listeria monocytogenes* infections in metropolitan Toronto. Can Med Assoc J 88: 549–561

344. Severn CB, Holyoke EA (1973) Human acardiac anomalies. Am J Obstet Gynecol 116: 358–365

345. Shah DM, Chaffin D (1989) Perinatal outcome in very preterm births with twin-twin transfusion syndrome. Am J Obstet Gynecol 161: 1111–1113

346. Shanklin DR, Scott JS (1975) Massive subchorial thrombohaematoma (Breus' mole). Br J Obstet Gynaecol 82: 476–487

347. Shen-Schwarz S, Macpherson TA, Mueller-Heubach E (1988) The clinical significance of hemorrhagic endovasculitis of the placenta. Am J Obstet Gynecol 159: 48–51

348. Sheppard BL, Bonnar J (1976) The ultrastructure of the

arterial supply of the human placenta in pregnancy complicated by fetal growth retardation. Br J Obstet Gynaecol 83: 948–959

349. Sheppard BL, Bonnar J (1980) Uteroplacental arteries and hypertensive pregnancy. In: Bonnar J, McGilliray I, Symonds E (eds) Pregnancy Hypertension. Lancaster, MTP Press, pp 213–219

350. Sheridan-Pereira M, Porreco RP, Hayes T, Shannon Burke MS (1988) Neonatal aortic thrombosis associated with the lupus anticoagulant. Obstet Gynecol 71: 1016–1018

351. Shmoys S, Kaplan C (1990) Parvovirus and pregnancy. Clin Obstet Gynecol 33: 268–275

352. Shurin PA, Alpert S, Rosner B, et al (1975) Chorioamnionitis and colonization of the newborn infant with genital mycoplasmas. N Engl J Med 293: 5–8

353. Sieracki JC, Panke TW, Horvat BL, et al (1975) Chorioangiomas. Obstet Gynecol 46: 155–159

354. Silver MM, Yeger H, Lines LD (1988) Hemorrhagic endovasculitis-like lesion induced in placenta organ culture. Hum Pathol 19: 251–256

355. Silver MM (1988) Massive placental infarction due to the lupus anticoagulant. Mod Pathol 1: 85A

356. Silverstein AJ, Kanbour AI (1981) Repetitive idiopathic fetal hydrops. Obstet Gynecol 57(suppl): 18s–21s

357. Silverstein AM (1962) Congenital syphilis and the timing of immunogenesis in the human foetus. Nature 194: 196–197

358. Soma H (1979) Single umbilical artery with congenital malformations. Curr Top Pathol 66: 159–173

359. South MA, Tompkins WAF, Morris CR, Rawls WE (1969) Congenital malformation of the central nervous system associated with genital type (type 2) herpesvirus. J Pediatr 75: 13–18

360. Spencer GD, Kraus FT (1992) Placental chorangiosis: A nonspecific marker of abnormal gestation. Unpublished observations.

361. Sprecher S, Soumenkoff G, Puissant F, Degueldre M (1986) Vertical transmission of HIV in 15-week fetus. Lancet 2: 288

362. Stagno S, Whitley RJ (1985) Herpesvirus infections of pregnancy. Part I. Cytomegalovirus and Epstein-Barr virus infections. N Engl J Med 313: 1270–1274

363. Stagno S, Whitley RJ (1985) Herpesvirus infections of pregnancy. Part II. Herpes simplex virus and varicella zoster infections. N Engl J Med 313: 1327–1330

364. Stagno S, Pass RF, Dworsky ME, Alford CA (1983) Congenital and perinatal cytomegalovirus infections. Semin Pathol 7: 31–42

365. Stagno S, Reynolds DW, Huang E-S, et al (1977) Congenital cytomegalovirus infection. Occurrence in an immune population. N Engl J Med 296: 1254–1258

366. Stagno S, Pass RF, Dworsky ME, et al (1982) Congenital cytomegalovirus infection. The relative importance of primary and recurrent maternal infection. N Engl J Med 306: 945–949

367. Steele PE, Jacobs DS (1979) *Listeria monocytogenes* macroabscesses of placenta. Obstet Gynecol 53: 124–127

368. Stenchever MA, Parks KA, Daines TL, et al (1977) Cytogenetics of habitual abortion and other reproductive wastage. Am J Obstet Gynecol 127: 143–150

369. Stock RJ, Stock ME (1979) Congenital annular contrictions

370. Strauss L, Driscoll SG (1964) Congenital neuroblastoma involving the placenta. Pediatrics 34: 23–31

371. Strong SJ, Corney G (1967) The Placenta in Twin Pregnancy. Oxford, Pergamon

372. Sumawong V, Nondasuta A, Thanapath S, Budthimedhee V (1966) Placenta accreta. A review of the literature and a summary of 10 cases. Obstet Gynecol 27: 511–516

373. Sweet LK, Connerty HV (1941) Congenital melanoma. Report of a case in which antenatal metastasis occurred. Am J Dis Child 62: 1029–1040

374. Szulman AE, Surti U (1978) The syndromes of hydatidiform mole. I. Cytogenetic and morphologic correlations. Am J Obstet Gynecol 131: 665–671

375. Szulman AE, Surti U (1978) The syndromes of hydatidiform mole. II. Morphologic evolution of the complete and partial mole. Am J Obstet Gynecol 132: 20–27

376. Szulman AE, Philippe E, Boue JG, Boue A (1981) Human tripoloidy: Association with partial hydatidiform moles and non-molar conceptuses. Hum Pathol 12: 1016–1021

377. Szymonowicz W, Preston H, Yu VYH (1986) The surviving monozygotic twin. Arch Dis Child 61: 454–458

378. Tafari N, Ross S, Naeye RL, et al (1976) Mycoplasma T strains and perinatal death. Lancet 1: 108–109

379. Teasdale F (1981) Histomorphometry of the placenta of the diabetic woman: Class A diabetes mellitus. Placenta 2: 241–252

380. Teasdale F (1983) Histomorphometry of the human placenta in class B diabetes mellitus. Placenta 4: 1–12

381. Teasdale F (1985) Histomorphometry of the human placenta in class C diabetes mellitus. Placenta 6: 69–82

382. Tenney B, Parker F (1940) The placenta in toxemia of pregnancy. Am J Obstet Gynecol 39: 1000–1005

383. Thadepalli H, Appleman MD, Maidman JE, et al (1977) Antimicrobial effect of amniotic fluid against anaerobic bacteria. Am J Obstet Gynecol 127: 250–254

384. Thorp JA, Walsh SW, Brath PC (1988) Low-dose aspirin inhibits thromboxane, but not prostacyclin, production by human placental arteries. Am J Obstet Gynecol 159: 1381–1384

385. Timmons JD, de Alvarez RR (1963) Monoamniotic twin pregnancy. Am J Obstet Gynecol 86: 875–881

386. Tondury G, Smith DW (1966) Fetal rubella pathology. J Pediatr 68: 867–879

387. Torbet TE, Tsoutsoplides GC (1968) Placenta praevia accreta: Conservative management. J Obstet Gynaecol Br Commonw 75: 737–740

388. Tornehave D, Chemnitz J, Teisner B, et al (1984) Immunohistochemical demonstration of pregnancy-associated plasma protein A (PAPP-A) in the syncytiotrophoblast of the normal placenta at different gestational ages. Placenta 5: 427–432

389. Torpin R (1965) Amniochorionic mesoblastic fibrous strings and amnionic bands: Associated contricting fetal malformations of fetal death. Am J Obstet Gynecol 91: 65–75

390. Townsend JJ, Baringer JR, Wolinsky JS, et al (1975) Progressive rubella panencephalitis. N Engl J Med 292: 990–993

391. Trasler DG, Walker BE, Fraser FC (1956) Congenital mal-

formations produced by amnionic sac puncture. Science 124: 439

392. Van Allen MI, Curry C, Gallagher L (1987) Limb body wall complex: I. Pathogenesis. Am J Med Genet 28: 529–548

393. Van Der Veen F, Walker S, Fox H (1982) Endarteritis obliterans of the fetal stem arteries of the human placenta: An electron microscopic study. Placenta 3: 181–190

394. Vetter K, Schneider KTM (1988) Iatrogenic remission of twin transfusion syndrome. Am J Obstet Gynecol 158: 221

395. Wallenburg HCS, Makovitz JW, Dekker GA, Rotmans P (1986) Low-dose aspirin prevents pregnancy-induced hypertension and pre-eclampsia in angiotensin-sensitive primigravidae. Lancet 1:1–3

396. Wallenburg HCS (1971) Chorioangioma of the placenta. Obstet Gynecol Surv 26: 411–425

397. Warburton D, Kline J, Stein Z, Susser M (1980) Monosomy X: A chromosomal anomaly associated with young maternal age. Lancet 1: 167–169

398. Warren CT, Kraus FT, Taysi K, et al (1990) Histologic-karyotypic correlations in spontaneous abortions. Mod Pathol 3: 105A

399. Weber J (1963) Constriction of the umbilical cord as a cause of fetal death. Acta Obstet Gynecol Scand 42: 259–268

400. Weil ML, Itabashi HH, Cremer NE, et al (1975) Chronic progressive panencephalitis due to rubella virus simulating subacute sclerosing panencephalitis. N Engl J Med 292: 994–998

401. Weiland HT, Vermey-Keers C, Salimans MMM, et al (1987) Parvovirus B19 associated with fetal abnormality. Lancet 1: 682–683

402. Wentworth P (1968) Circumvallate and circummarginate placentas. Am J Obstet Gynecol 102: 44–47

403. Wentworth P (1967) Placental infarction and toxemia of pregnancy. Am J Obstet Gynecol 99: 318–326

404. Wentworth P (1967) The placenta in cases of hemolytic disease of the newborn. Am J Obstet Gynecol 98: 283–289

405. Wentworth P (1964) A placental lesion to account for feotal

406. Wharton B, Edwards JH, Cameron AH (1968) Monoamniotic twins. J Obstet Gynaecol Br Commow 75: 158–163

407. Wilson CB, Remington JS (1980) What can be done to prevent congenital toxoplasmosis? Am J Obstet Gynecol 138: 357–363

408. Wilson D, Paalman J (1967) Clinical significance of circumvallate placenta. Obstet Gynecol 29: 774–778

409. Wilson EA (1972) Holoacardius. Obstet Gynecol 40: 740–748

410. Winer AE, Bergman WD, Fields C (1957) Combined intra- and extrauterine pregnancy. Am J Obstet Gynecol 74: 170–178

411. Witzleben CL, Driscoll SG (1965) Possible transplacental transmission of herpes simplex infection. Pediatrics 36: 192–199

412. Yamazaki K, Price JT, Altshuler G (1977) A placental view of the diagnosis and pathogenesis of congenital listeriosis. Am J Obstet Gynecol 129: 703–705

413. Yoshioka H, Kadomoto Y, Mino M, et al (1979) Multicystic encephalomalacia in liveborn twin with a stillborn macerated co-twin. J Pediatr 95: 798–800

414. Young ID, Lindenbaum RH, Thompson EM, Pembrey ME (1985) Amniotic bands in connective tissue disorders. Arch Dis Child 60: 1061–1063

415. Zeek PM, Assali NS (1950) Vascular changes in the decidua associated with eclamptogenic toxemia of pregnancy. Am J Clin Pathol 20: 1099–1109

416. Ziel H (1963) Circumvallate placenta, a cause of antepartum bleeding, premature delivery, and perinatal mortality. Obstet Gynecol 22: 798–802

417. Zervoudakis IA, Cederqvist LL (1977) Effect of *Listeria monocytogenes* septicemia during pregnancy on the offspring. Am J Obstet Gynecol 129: 465–467

418. Zhang J, Kraus FT, Aquino (1985) Chorioamnionitis: A comparative histologic, bacteriologic, and clinical study. Int J Gynecol Pathol 4: 1–10

24

Gestational Trophoblastic Disease and Related Lesions

Michael T. Mazur, M.D., and Robert J. Kurman, M.D.

Gestational trophoblastic disease (GTD) encompasses a heterogeneous group of lesions, including hydatidiform mole, invasive mole, choriocarcinoma, and placental site trophoblastic tumor, that are characterized by an abnormal proliferation of trophoblastic tissue. Some of these lesions are true neoplasms, whereas others represent abnormally formed placentas with a predisposition for neoplastic transformation of the trophoblast. The literature on this subject is extensive but sometimes confusing because of inconsistencies in classification and terminology. In fact, the necessity of a morphologic classification has been questioned, since current management is largely medical and in the case of trophoblastic disease following a mole, often conducted in the absence of a histological diagnosis. Thus, all trophoblastic lesions are frequently combined under the rubric of GTD without applying specific pathological terms. Recent cytogenetic and immunocytochemical studies demonstrate profound differences in the etiology, morphology, and clinical behavior of various forms of the disease, however. These studies underscore the importance of a uniform histological classification to facilitate standardized reporting of data and to ensure appropriate clinical management. Nonetheless, the term GTD has clinical utility, since the principles of human chorionic gonadotropin (hCG) monitoring in follow-up and the chemotherapy of metastatic or persistent disease are similar for all these entities.[147]

This chapter discusses the clinical and pathological features of each specific form of GTD. In addition, the morphologic and functional characteristics of the three types of trophoblastic cells, cytotrophoblast, syncytiotrophoblast, and intermediate trophoblast, are reviewed. Awareness of the biologic properties of these trophoblastic cells is essential for understanding the pathological and clinical aspects of the various forms of GTD. Sections on epidemiology, risk factors, behavior, and management of GTD are included to correlate with the pathology, not to provide a comprehensive review of these subjects.

General Features

The pathogenesis of trophoblastic tumors is not known. Two mechanisms have been proposed for the development of hydatidiform moles: (1) failure of developement of the fetal circulation with resultant hydropic swelling of the villi[101] and (2) overgrowth of the villous trophoblast with secondary hydropic swelling.[197] Neither mechanism adequately explains why moles arise only in a small percentage of abortions, even those with failure of developement of the embryo. The etiology of choriocarcinoma also is enigmatic. The trophoblast of a normal gestation grows rapidly after implantation, but this growth is limited and contained. In gestational choriocarcinoma, trophoblast escapes these normal growth and control mechanisms. Although the causes of GTD are not known, epidemiologic and cytogenetic studies offer some clues to its developement (see Chapter 29, Epidemiology).

Age

Both hydatidiform mole and choriocarcinoma are disorders of the reproductive years. Women who are sexually active are at risk for developing GTD, but the incidence is substantially higher in older women. Women over the age of 30 years[20] and especially those over 40 years are at increased risk for GTD,* but the absolute number of cases of mole or choriocarcinoma in women over 40 years is smaller because of their lower fertility. There also is a higher rate of occurrence of hydatidiform mole in teenagers. Thus, there appears to be an increased risk of having a complete mole at both extremes of reproductive age. In contrast, maternal age has no effect on the risk of partial mole.[115,163,164] Paternal age does not seem to have an effect on the risk of developing a hydatidiform mole. Malignant sequelae for hydatidiform mole occur more frequently in older patients.[15,247,248]

Incidence and Geographic Distribution

The reported incidence of hydatidiform mole and choriocarcinoma varies widely throughout the world, being greatest in Asia, Africa, and Latin America and substantially lower in North America, Europe, and Australia (Table 24.1).[27,42,92,259] The incidence rates are difficult to compare, however, because of limitations in the methodology of these studies.[27,92] Among these limitations, failure to define clearly the disease entities, that is, complete versus partial mole, and lack of consistent diagnostic criteria are common shortcomings.[118]

Some studies of incidence rates have used hospital-based rather than population-based figures, which proba-

*Refs. 14,27,98,162,164,179,227,277.

Table 24.1. Selected incidences of hydatidiform mole to show geographic variation

Region	Rate per 1000[a]
Indonesia	9.9 (pregnancies)
Taiwan	8.3 (deliveries)
Philippines	5.0 (deliveries)
Mexico	4.6 (pregnancies)
Nigeria	2.6 (deliveries)
Japan	1.9 (pregnancies)
Australia	1.4 (pregnancies)
United States	1.1 (pregnancies)
Israel	0.8 (live births)
Sweden	0.6 (pregnancies)
Paraguay	0.2 (pregnancies)

[a] Data include populuation-based and hospital-based studies.
Adapted with permission of Bracken et al., ref. 27.

bly results in overreporting.[92] This is especially true of data from less well-developed countries, where uncomplicated deliveries tend to occur at home and patients with abnormal pregnancies, such as hydatiform mole, are more likely to receive hospital care. Finally, different denominators, such as the total number of pregnancies, deliveries, or live births, have been used to determine incidence rates in different studies (Table 24.1). The incidence rate based on the number of pregnancies would best estimate the risk of GTD in a population, but this figure is extremely difficult to determine, especially in countries in which there is less consistent obstetrical care. In addition, since incidence rates by country are not age adjusted, countries with high age-specific pregnancy rates in young and older women, as occurs in underdeveloped countries, have higher crude rates of hydatidiform mole.[42]

The incidence rate for hydatidiform mole in the United States and Europe is between 1 in 1000 and 1 in 2000 pregnancies.[5,42,67,98,206,269,277] In some other geographic regions, especially Asia, the incidence is as high as 1 in 500 pregnancies.[27,67,92] The striking variability in incidence rates even within geographic regions is illustrated by the low incidence of hydatidiform mole in Paraguay (1 in 5000 pregnancies)[208] compared with the high incidence in Mexico (25 in 5000 pregnancies).[160]

Choriocarcinoma occurs with a frequency of 1 in 20,000 to 1 in 40,000 pregnancies in the United States and Europe.[27,67,92,206,277] Estimates for the incidence in Asia, Africa, and Latin America generally are higher, and incidence rates as high as 1 in 500 to 1000 pregnancies have been reported,[27,67,92,160,201] although marked regional variations occur.[209] In Nigeria, choriocarcinoma is the third most common malignant tumor in women at one institution, ranking behind breast and cervical carcinoma.[123] Thus, despite methodologic problems it appears that choriocarcinoma occurs at a substantially higher rate in developing countries than it does in North America and Europe. These differences suggest that low socioeconomic conditions or dietary factors may contribute to the development of GTD. One case-control study suggested that dietary deficiency of carotene, a vitamin A precursor, may predispose to molar pregnancy.[20] Definitive evidence linking possible etiologic factors with GTD is lacking.

Previous Obstetrical History

Several studies find that a history of prior spontaneous abortions is more common in patients with hydatidiform mole and choriocarcinoma.[14,168,194] Furthermore, women who have had one hydatidiform mole are at greatly increased risk of having another.[21,162,277] Conversely, term pregnancy and live births have a protective effect, with GTD less common in patients who are parous.[194] The protective effect appears to increase with an increased number of live births.

Blood Groups

An association has been reported between ABO blood groups and the occurrence of choriocarcinoma but not hydatidiform mole. Blood group A is more frequent and group O less common in patients with choriocarcinoma. This association is particularly strong with blood group A women whose husbands are group O and, conversely, for group O women whose husbands are group A.[8,12,49] Patients of blood group B or AB have a worse prognosis, however.[8,49] The significance of these data is difficult to assess, since the children of the gestation associated with the choriocarcinoma show no trend in blood group distribution.[8] Furthermore, some studies have found no association or even a decrease in the frequency of group A among patients with malignant GTD.[172,214] In contrast to ABO blood group interactions, there has been no consistent pattern in human leukocyte antigen (HLA) distribution between women with choriocarcinoma and their consorts.[8,172,276]

Cytogenetics

Cytogenetic studies of complete and partial hydatidiform mole show that chromosomal abnormalities play a role in the developement of molar gestations.[57,237] Furthermore, the karyotype patterns of the two types of moles are generally different. Most complete hydatidiform moles have a normal complement at 46XX,[237,256] but both X chromosomes are androgenic, that is, of paternal origin[126,262] (Fig. 24.1). This 46XX karyotype results from duplication of a haploid sperm (23 chromosomes) pronucleus in an empty ovum that lacks functional maternal DNA.[117,263] Duplication of a 23Y sperm results in a nonviable 46YY cell. A smaller proportion (3–13%) of complete moles have

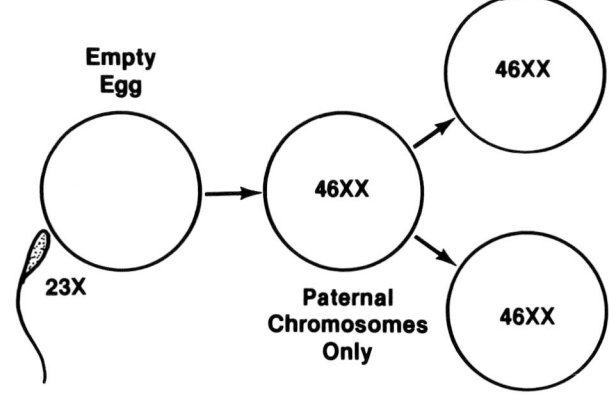

FIG. 24.1. **Chromosomal origin of a complete hydatidiform mole.** A single sperm fertilizes an empty egg. Reduplication of its 23X set gives a completely homozygous diploid genome of 46XX. A similar process follows fertilization of an empty egg by two sperms with two independently drawn sets of 23X or 23Y. Note that both karyotypes 46XX and 46XY can ensue. (Adapted by permission of Szulman AE (1984) Syndromes of hydatidiform moles. Partial vs. complete. J Reprod Med 29: 788.)

a 46XY chromosome complement, but in these moles, too, the chromosomes are androgenic.[125,198,229,230] In this instance, the 46XY-complete mole is believed to form by dispermy, that is, fertilization of an empty ovum by two sperm pronuclei, one with the X and the other with the Y chromosome.[191,230] The complete mole, being paternally derived, constitutes a total allograft in the mother.

The karyotypes of partial mole most frequently show triploidy (69 chromosomes)[237] (Fig. 24.2) with a maternal chromosome complement.[11,57] Conversely, most (86%) triploid conceptuses have histological features of partial mole.[236] Rarely, however, partial mole with an identifiable fetus have a 46XX karyotype,[115,237] and even tetraploidy has been reported.[141,231] When triploidy is present in partial mole, the chromosomal complement usually is 69XXY or 69XXX and rarely is 69XYY.[237] These abnormal conceptuses result from the fertilization of an egg with a haploid set of chromosomes by either two sperms, each with a set of haploid chromosomes, or by a single sperm with a diploid genome of 46XY.[116] This condition is known as *diandric* (paternally derived) triploidy. A conceptus with a diploid 46XX maternal genome due to failure of the first meiotic division and a haploid paternal set of chromosomes results in an abnormal, triploid (69XXX or 69XXY) fetus yet generally a nonmolar pregnancy. This is referred to as a *digynic* (maternally derived) conceptus and is believed to account for only 15–20% of cases of triploidy.[115] Thus, most well-documented partial moles are triploid, but not all triploid conceptuses are associated with partial moles. Partial molar pregnancies may have a grossly identifiable embryo or fetus with congenital anomalies.[237]

Although many partial moles do have a triploid karyotype and evidence of an embryo or fetus, there is no con-

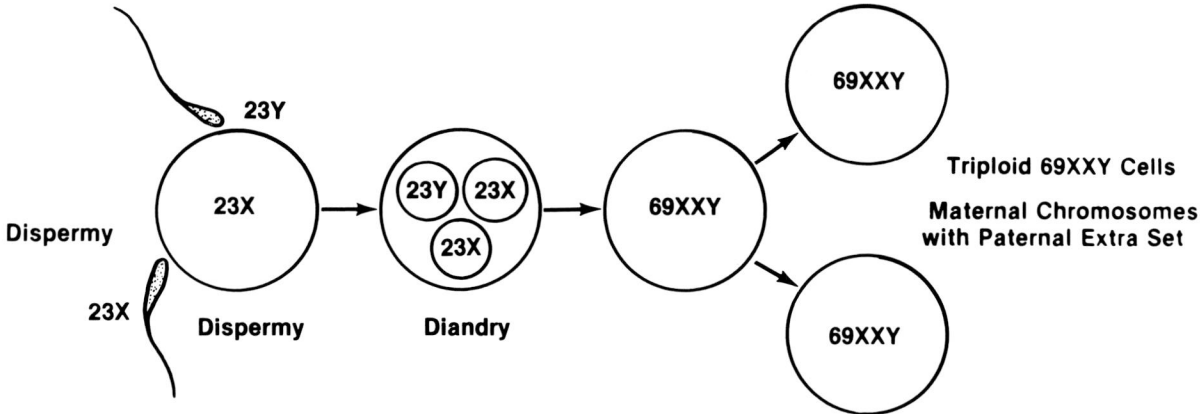

FIG. 24.2. Chromosomal origin of the triploid, partial hydatidiform mole. A normal egg with a 23X haploid set is fertilized by two sperm that carry either sex chromosome, to give a total of 69 chromosomes with a sex configuration of XXY, XXX, or XYY. A similar result can be obtained by fertilization of a sperm carrying the unreduced paternal genome 46XY (resulting sex complement, XXY only). (Adapted by permission of Szulman AE (1984) Syndromes of hydatidiform moles. Partial vs. complete. J Reprod Med 29: 788.)

sensus yet that all partial moles have these features. Flow cytometry studies show that some partial moles may be diploid, tetraploid, polyploid, and aneuploid.[47,139,141,145] Likewise, not all molar pregnancies with evidence of fetal development need be regarded as partial moles, since fetal development rarely occurs in complete moles.[26,101,115]

The cytogenetic findings indicate that abnormal fertilization plays a key role in the evolution of both complete and partial hydatidiform moles. Although it is not known why these chromosomal aberrations lead to the formation of a molar pregnancy, experimental studies in mice suggest a relationship between the molar phenotype and the ratio of paternal/maternal haploid sets of chromosomes. Development of a mole appears to be associated with an excess of paternal compared with maternal haploid contributions.[231] The higher the ratio of paternal/maternal chromosomes, the greater the molar change. Complete moles show a 2:0 paternal/maternal ratio, whereas partial moles show a 2:1 ratio. This hypothesis is supported by experimental evidence in mice in which enucleated eggs are implanted with male or female pronuclei. In a conceptus with two maternal sets of chromosomes, the embryo develops, albeit not beyond a certain stage, but the trophoblast is stunted. In contrast, in a conceptus with two paternal sets of chromosomes, there is much greater trophoblastic developement, and the embryo dies earlier.[228]

The chromosomal complements of invasive mole and choriocarcinoma have not been as well studied. In a retrospective analysis, Davis et al.[48] evaluated the presence of Y chromatin using quinacrine fluorescent staining. Fourteen (73%) of 19 choriocarcinomas and two (50%) of four invasive moles were Y chromatin positive, whereas only 9% of 182 hydatidiform moles contained a Y chromosome.

Morphology and Immunohistochemistry of Normal Trophoblast

The abnormal trophoblastic tissue in GTD recapitulates the trophoblast present in the early developing placenta and the implantation site. In normal placentation, the trophoblast growing in association with chorionic villi is referred to as *villous trophoblast*, whereas the trophoblast in all other locations is termed *extravillous trophoblast*. Three distinct types of trophoblastic cells have been recognized: cytotrophoblast (CT), syncytiotrophoblast (ST), and intermediate trophoblast (IT). Villous trophoblast is composed, for the most part, of CT and ST with small amounts of IT. In contrast, extravillous trophoblast that infiltrates the decidua, myometrium, and spiral arteries of the placental site is composed mostly of IT with a minor component of CT and ST. This area is also known as the *implantation site* or the *placental bed*.

The CT or Langhans' cell is the germinative trophoblastic cell, whereas the ST is the highly differentiated cell that interfaces with the maternal circulation and produces most of the placental hormones. The IT is a distinct form of trophoblastic cell that shares some of the morphologic and functional features of both CT and ST.[134] Each type of trophoblastic cell has specific microscopic, ultrastructural, and immunohistochemical features.

Light Microscopy

In normal gestation, CT is composed of primitive epithelial cells that are uniform and polygonal to oval in shape. Cytotrophoblastic cells have a single nucleus, clear to granular cytoplasm, and well-defined cell borders (Fig. 24.3a).

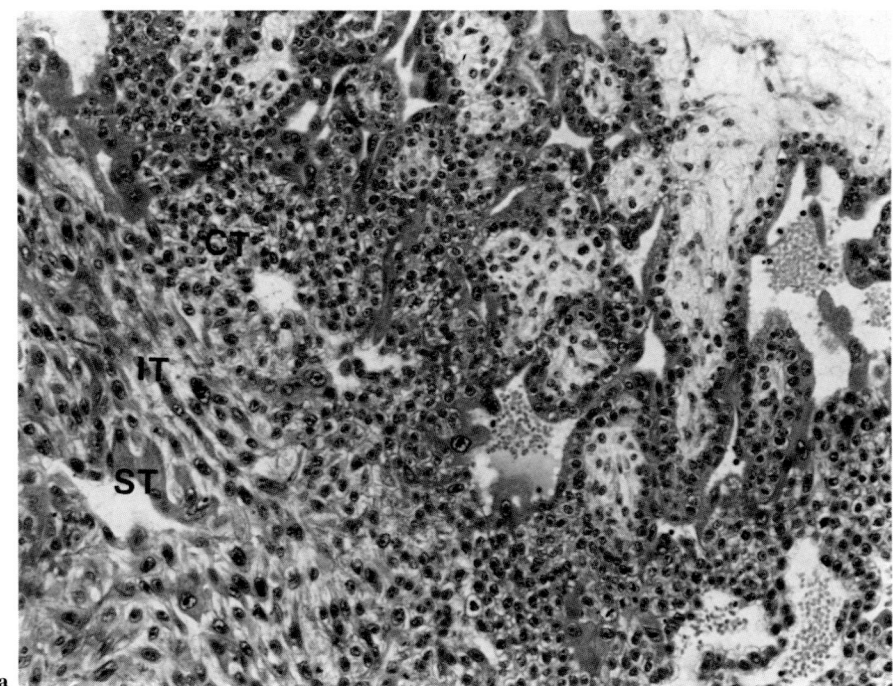

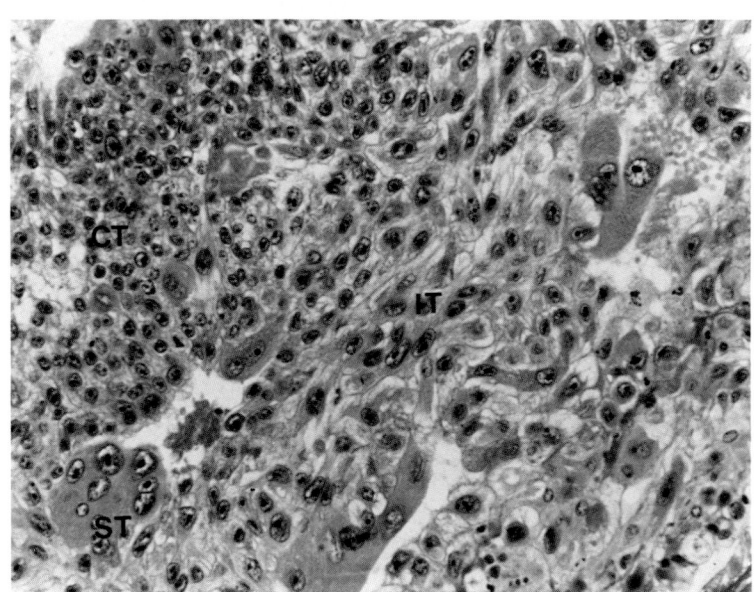

FIG. 24.3. **Villous and extravillous trophoblast of a 16-day blastocyst. a:** Cytotrophoblast (*CT*), intermediate trophoblast (*IT*), and syncytiotrophoblast (*ST*). **b:** Cytotrophoblast (*CT*) is characterized by small, uniform, mononucleate cells with distinct cell membranes, intermediate trophoblast (*IT*) by larger cells that are mononucleate but show greater pleomorphism, and syncytiotrophoblast (*ST*) by multinucleate giant cells with much larger nuclei.

Mitotic activity is clearly evident. Syncytiotrophoblast is composed of large, multinucleate cells with dense amphophilic cytoplasm containing multiple vacuoles that vary in size, some of which form lacunae (Fig. 24.3). A distinct brush order often lines the cell membrane. The ST nuclei are dark and often appear pyknotic. They do not show mitotic activity.

The cells of IT generally are mononucleate but cells with several nuclei can be present.[132] IT cells vary in shape, ranging from round to polyhedral cells to spindle-shaped, bipolar cells with attenuated cytoplasmic processes. Cytoplasm is abundant and is eosinophilic to amphophilic (Fig. 24.3). Scattered small vacuoles may be present in the IT cytoplasm. The nuclear morphology of these cells is most characteristic. Nuclei of IT have highly irregular nuclear outlines and hyperchromatic, coarsely granular chromatin. Often the nuclei are lobulated or show multiple deep nuclear clefts.[264] Nucleoli are smaller and less prominent than those seen in CT. Cytoplasmic nuclear invaginations may be seen. The cytological features that distinguish IT from CT include their larger size, more abundant amphophilic or clear cytoplasm, and coarse, granular chromatin with irregular nuclear membranes.

IT, particularly in extravillous locations, show infiltrative growth into decidua, myometrium, and blood vessels, dissecting between the normal cells. Intermediate trophoblastic cells characteristically invade the wall of large vascular channels until the wall is entirely replaced. This highly infiltrative growth pattern is a prominent feature of IT. Eosinophilic fibrinoid material often is deposited around IT.

The IT is the predominant cell of the placental site trophoblastic tumor and the exaggerated placental site, and the cytological and growth patterns of these cells are illustrated in more detail in those sections.

Immunohistochemistry

A large number of protein hormones, steroid hormones, and enzymes such as hCG, human placental lactogen (hPL), pregnancy-specific beta-$_1$-glycoprotein (SP-1), placental protein 5, pregnancy-associated plasma protein A, estradiol, progesterone, and placental alkaline phosphatase have been localized in the placenta during various stages of development by immunohistochemical techniques. Most of these products are confined to the ST. In particular, the localization of hCG and hPL gives a more complete characterization of the various types of trophoblast.[134,136]

The immunohistochemical localization of hCG and hPL in the normal placenta according to the gestational age is shown in Table 24.2. Intermediate trophoblast contains abundant hPL, which appears as early as 12 days and reaches a peak at 11–15 weeks of gestation (Fig. 24.4).[134] In contrast, hCG is present only focally in IT (Fig. 24.4), appearing as early as 12 days and remaining until 6 weeks, after which it disappears. Cytotrophoblast does not appear to contain either hCG or hPL. Syncytiotrophoblast contains abundant hCG from at least 12 days of gestation until approximately 8–10 weeks, after which it diminishes. By 40 weeks it is present only focally (Fig. 24.5). Placental lactogen also is localized in ST at 12 days but increases steadily thereafter. From late in the second trimester to term, hPL is diffusely distributed in the ST overlying the chorionic villi (Fig. 24.5).[134]

At the placental site, immunohistochemical reactions for hPL aid in distinguishing IT from decidual and smooth muscle cells because the hormone is not present in either decidua or smooth muscle (Fig. 24.6). The binucleate and trinucleate cells show the same pattern of staining as the mononucleate form of IT.[136] In contrast, although some multinucleate IT contain hPL, a larger proportion of them contain hCG in the first trimester. During the second and third trimesters, hCG progressively decreases in these cells, whereas hPL is present through the second trimester and diminishes in the last trimester. The IT cells that invade the spiral arteries show the same pattern of staining as those within the decidua and myometrium. Typically, they contain hPL and little if any hCG (Fig. 24.7). These findings indicate that the invasive property of trophoblast in normal placentation appears to reside in IT, which plays a key role in the development of the uteroplacental circulation.[134,136]

Since the trophoblastic cells are all epithelial, immunohistochemistry for keratin also helps identify this tissue. All forms of trophoblast react intensely for keratin when broad-spectrum antibodies are used.[182] Keratin immunostains are especially useful for demonstrating intermediate trophoblastic cells at the placental site. These cells stand out well amid nonreactive stromal decidual cells; the keratin stain shows multiple, randomly dispersed single cells or small clusters of cells within decidua.[50,132,187]

Table 24.2. Localization of chorionic gonadotropin beta-subunit and placental lactogen in different types of trophoblastic cells in the placenta and the placental site throughout gestation

Trophoblastic cell type	First trimester		Second trimester		Third trimester	
	hCG	hPL	hCG	hPL	hCG	hPL
Cytotrophoblast	−	−	−	−	−	−
Intermediate trophoblast	+	+ +	−/+	+ + +	+	+/+ +
Syncytiotrophoblast	+ + + +	+	+ +	+ + +	+	+ + + +

− → + + + + denotes semiquantitative scoring of the proportion of cells showing a positive reaction: +, 1–24%, + +, 25–49%, + + +, 50–74%, + + + +, 75–100%.
hCG, human chorionic gonadotropin; hPL, human placental lactogen.

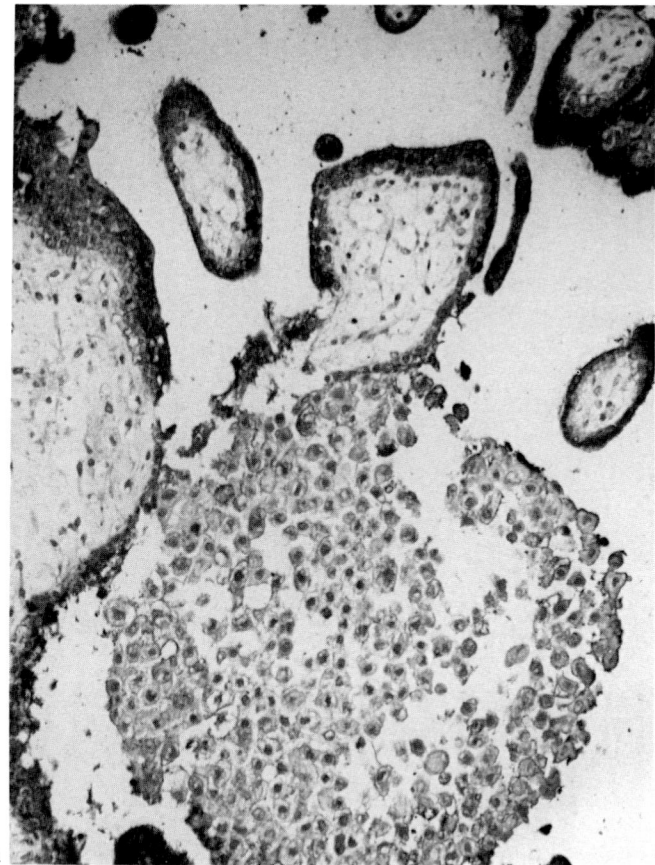
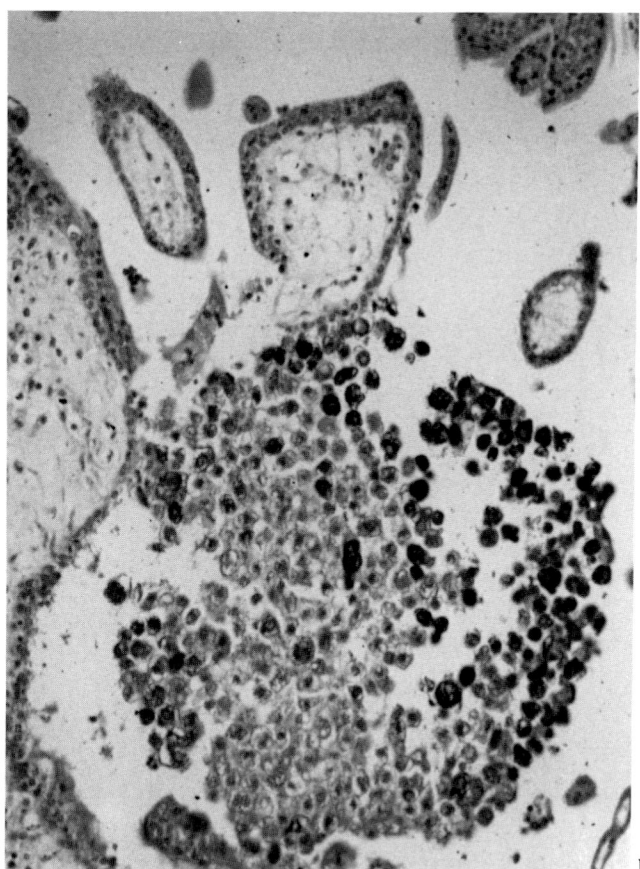

FIG. 24.4. Chorionic villus from a 4-week gestation. a: Localization of hPL (*black deposit*) within the cytoplasm of intermediate trophoblastic cells sprouting from a chorionic villus. Note absence of hPL in syncytiotrophoblast. **b:** Localization of hCG (*black deposit*) within the cytoplasm of syncytiotrophoblast. Note absence of hCG in intermediate trophoblast. (Reprinted by permission of Kurman et al., ref. 134.)

Classification of Gestational Trophoblastic Disease and Related Lesions

The classification of GTD and related lesions has been revised recently by the World Health Organization (WHO) in conjunction with the International Society of Gynecological Pathologists (Table 24.3).[218,222,272]

Clinicopathological Features and Behavior

Hydatidiform Mole

A hydatidiform mole is a lesion of the placenta characterized by enlarged, edematous, and vesicular chorionic villi accompanied by a variable amount of proliferative trophoblast. This entity is subdivided into complete hydatidiform mole and partial hydatidiform mole. The two types of moles have characteristic morphologic, cytogenetic, and clinicopathological features.

Complete Hydatidiform Mole

Complete mole is hydatidiform mole in which there is hydropic swelling of the majority of villi, associated with a variable degree of trophoblastic proliferation. Fetal tissue usually is not present. Most complete hydatidiform moles have a 46XX karyotype.

CLINICAL FEATURES

Complete hydatidiform mole, also known as *classic hydatidiform mole*, is the most frequent form of molar pregnancy and GTD. This disorder typically develops between the 11th and 25th weeks of pregnancy, with a mean gestational age of about 18 weeks.[44,101,173] Patients often have vaginal bleeding or excessive uterine enlargement for the gestational age.[21,44,86,173] In approximately one-third of patients, however, the uterus is small for dates.[44] Occasion-

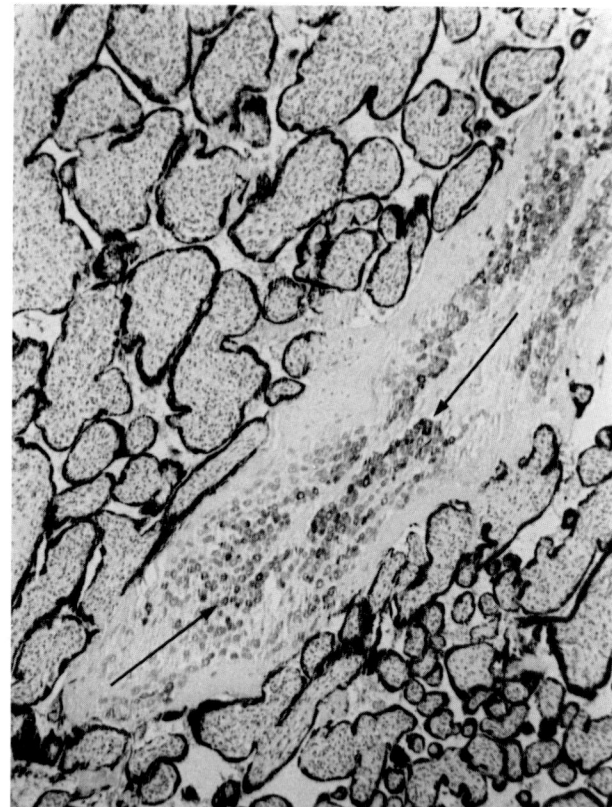

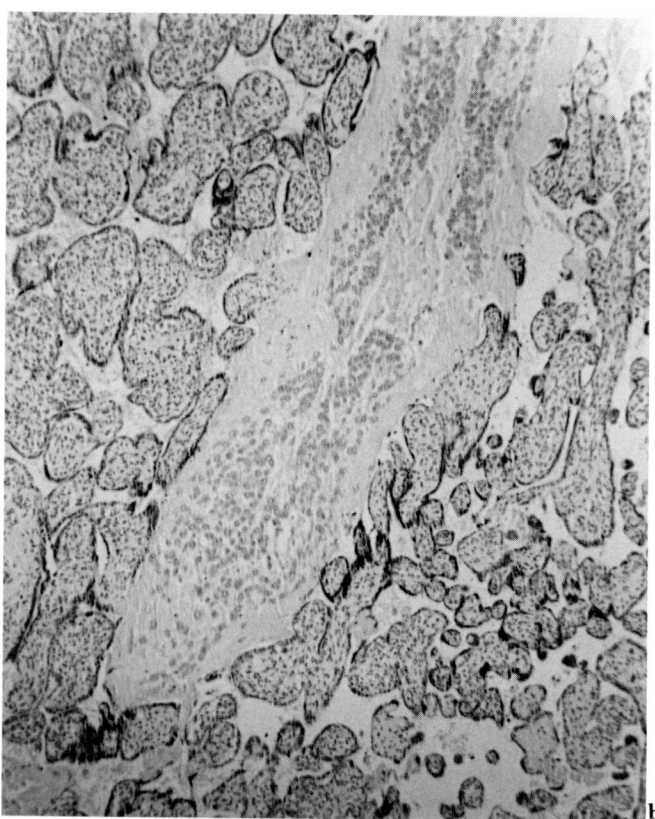

FIG. 24.5. Chorionic villi in a 27-week placenta. a: Diffuse distribution of hPL in syncytiotrophoblast overlying chorionic villi. hPL also is present in intermediate trophoblast (*arrows*) within a trophoblastic column. **b:** hCG is focally distributed in syncytiotrophoblast and is absent in intermediate trophoblast.

ally, the initial clinical manifestation is sudden passage of molar vesicles. Preeclampsia (pregnancy-induced hypertension with edema and proteinuria) occurs in up to one-fourth of patients with complete mole.[86] In contrast to nonmolar gestations in which preeclampsia occurs typically in the last trimester, in molar gestations preeclampsia occurs in the first trimester. Thus, early onset of preeclampsia, especially when coupled with excessive uterine enlargement, suggests the presence of a molar pregnancy. Additional clinical signs of molar pregnancy include hyperemesis gravidarum, occurring in a quarter of patients, and hyperthyroidism in 7%.[86] The cause of hyperthyroidism is not fully known. Intrinsic thyroid-stimulating activity of hCG is one possible mechanism,[86,184] but some investigators suggest that trophoblast produces other undefined substances that cause thyrotoxicosis.[2] Pulmonary embolization of trophoblast and massive ovarian enlargement due to benign theca-lutein cysts (hyperreactio luteinalis) (see Chapter 16, Nonneoplastic Lesions of the Ovary) are other possible clinical manifestations of a hydatidiform mole. Usually with complete mole the hCG titer is markedly elevated. Pelvic ultrasonic examination often discloses a diagnostic snowstorm pattern. This pattern, especially when associated with a markedly elevated hCG level, can be clinically diagnostic of molar pregnancy.[210]

Although these clinical signs and symptoms permit the diagnosis of a molar pregnancy before evacuation, the clinical presentation is quite variable. Many moles are not recognized before curettage,[115,237] and up to 80% of cases are first diagnosed by histological study of spontaneously passed or operatively evacuated tissue.[44] Hydatidiform moles also can be found unexpectedly in elective abortion specimens of asymptomatic patients.[281] In one study, almost 1 in 600 consecutive elective abortions revealed hydatidiform mole, and a quarter of these were not apparent on gross examination.[39]

GROSS FINDINGS

Massively enlarged, edematous villi give the classic grape-like appearance to the placenta (Fig. 24.8). The swollen villi may range from a few millimeters to as large as 3.0 cm in diameter but usually average about 1.5 cm. Rarely, fetal development may occur in complete mole (Fig. 24.9). After suction curettage, a large amount of bloody tissue may obscure the edematous villi, especially if a mole is ex-

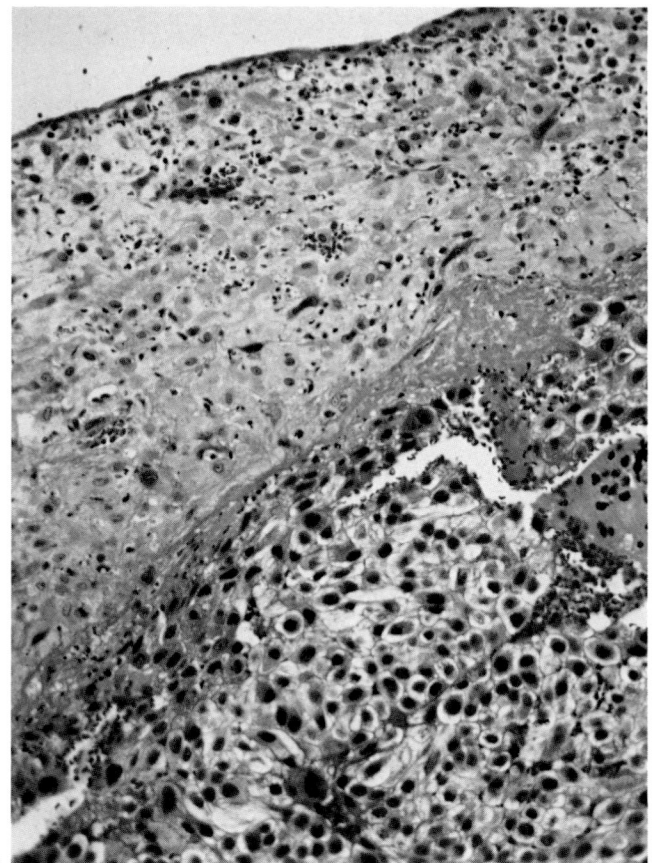

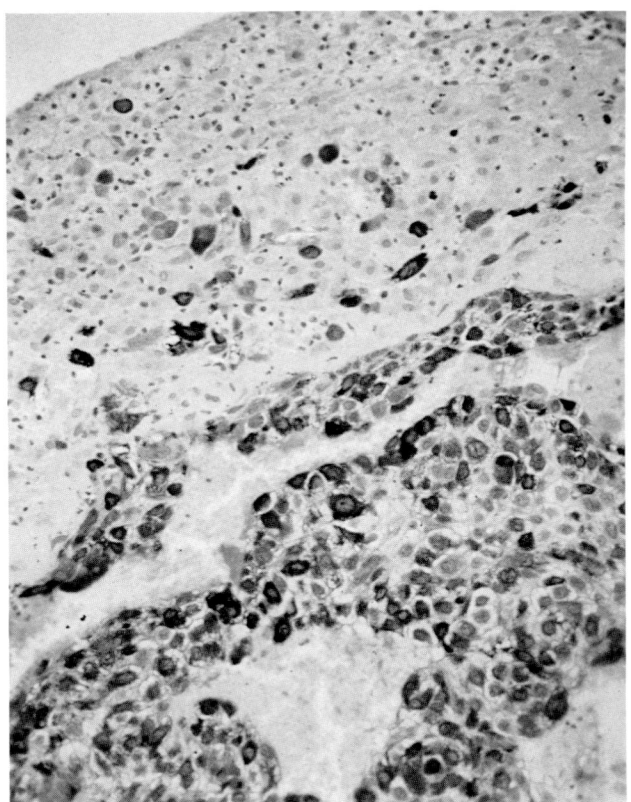

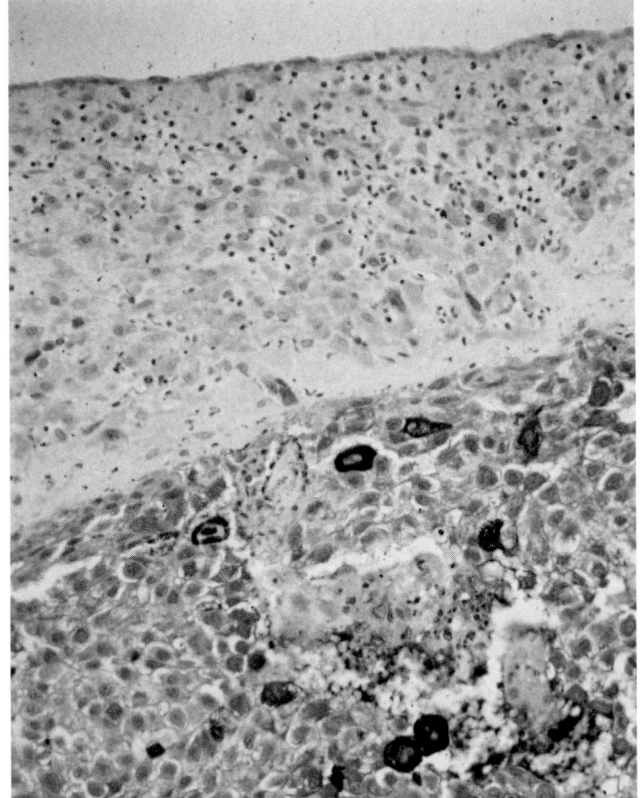

FIG. 24.6. A 12-day blastocyst. a: The decidua in the upper part of the field contains numerous intermediate trophoblastic cells with enlarged nuclei. These cells may be difficult to distinguish from decidua. b: The intermediate trophoblastic cells in the trophoblastic shell (*lower half of field*) and those infiltrating the decidua contain hPL, but decidual cells do not. c: A few intermediate trophoblastic cells in the trophoblastic shell are positive for hCG, but those in the decidua are negative. (Reprinted by permission of Kurman et al., ref. 136.)

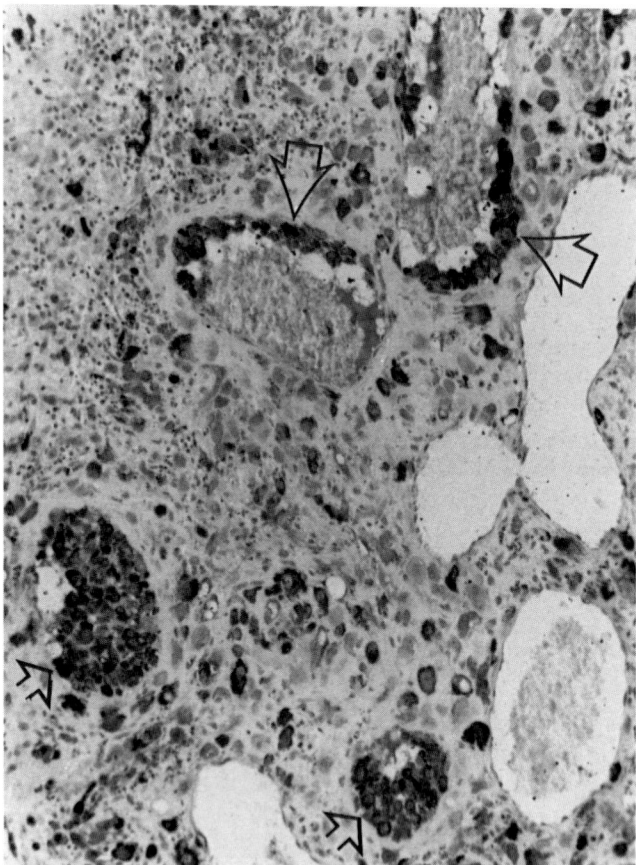

FIG. 24.7. Placental site at 11 weeks' gestation. Numerous intermediate trophoblastic cells containing hPL (*black deposit*) infiltrate the decidua and invade spiral arteries. Two arteries are completely plugged with intermediate trophoblast (*small arrows*), and two have the intimal surface partially lined by intermediate trophoblast (*large arrows*).

Table 24.3. Modified World Health Organization Histopathological Classification of Gestational Trophoblastic Disease

Hydatidiform mole
  Complete
  Partial
Invasive mole
Choriocarcinoma
Epithelioid trophoblastic tumor
Placental site trophoblastic tumor
Trophoblastic lesions, miscellaneous
    Exaggerated placental site
    Placental site nodule or plaque
Unclassified trophoblastic lesions

Typically, patchy villous calcification is present. All hydatidiform moles display some degree of trophoblastic proliferation on the villous surface. This trophoblastic proliferation in hydatidiform mole is haphazard and circumferential around the villus. Columns and streamers of cells composed of a mixture of CT, ST, and IT project randomly from the villous surface (Figs. 24.11, 24.12). Frequently, the trophoblast shows cytological atypia similar to that seen in choriocarcinoma (see below, Choriocarcinoma) (Fig. 24.13). The amount of proliferative trophoblast in moles varies greatly. It may be marked, affecting most villi, or it may be subtle and only focally present, emphasizing the need for thorough sampling.[81] Large sheets of trophoblast including IT that appear to be unattached to villi also may be present (Fig. 24.14). These latter trophoblast result from tangential sectioning, or they represent detached fragments of the trophoblast from the implantation site.

Differential Diagnosis

See below, Partial Mole.

Clinical Behavior

Between 2% and 12% of patients experience severe respiratory distress immediately after uterine evacuation of a hydatidiform mole.[86,130,173] This phenomenon usually is attributed to massive deportation of trophoblast to lungs,[130,261] an exaggeration of a physiologic process occurring in normal pregnancy.[59] Other factors, including fluid overload, dilutional edema, preeclampsia, and hyperthyroidism, also may contribute to the pathogenesis of the respiratory distress.[41,250]

The greatest threat from hydatidiform mole is the risk of persistent or metastatic GTD. Postmolar trophoblastic disease may represent persistent mole in the uterine cavity or

tracted early in pregnancy when villous enlargement is less striking. Suction curettage also distorts molar villi by causing them to collapse. In this instance, there may be no gross evidence of molar enlargement. Histological evaluation of the tissue adherent to the gauze that collects suctioned uterine contents is necessary to establish the diagnosis. Immersing the gross tissue in water can resuspend collapsed villi.[40]

Microscopic Findings

Complete moles have two key features: trophoblastic proliferation and villous edema. Many villi display central cistern formation characterized by a prominent central space that is entirely acellular (Fig. 24.10). A few smaller villi usually are present but these, too, are edematous. The villi usually are avascular, although occasionally attenuated vascular spaces that may contain necrotic debris are found.

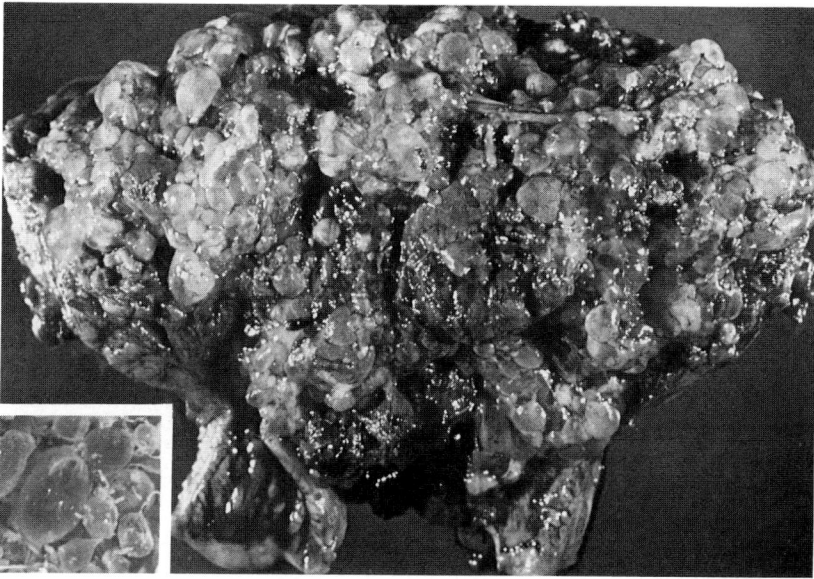

FIG. 24.8. Complete hydatidiform mole. Hysterectomy specimen shows an enlarged uterus with molar placental tissue protruding from the opened specimen. *Inset:* The hydropic villi range from a few millimeters to more than 1 cm in diameter.

it may be invasive mole or choriocarcinoma. A number of clinical and pathological features have been analyzed in an attempt to identify patients who are at increased risk of developing persistent GTD after uterine evacuation of a mole, but most studies have not distinguished complete from partial moles. Important clinical risk factors in more

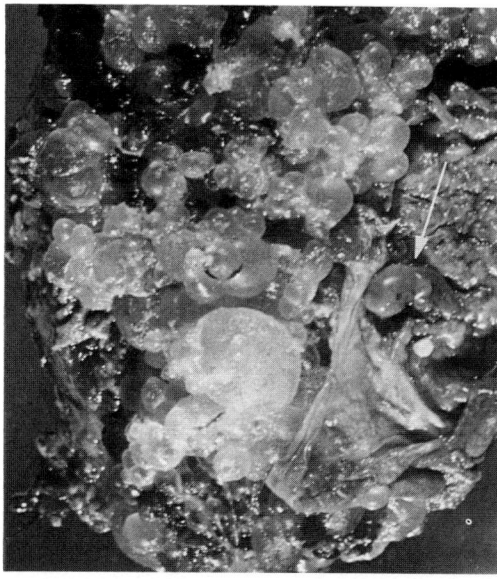

FIG. 24.9. Complete hydatidiform mole. Specimen contains a small, 2.0-cm embryo (*arrow*). Histologically, the villi showed generalized edema, and there was marked proliferation of the trophoblast.

than 60% of patients who have required subsequent chemotherapy, however, included large-for-dates uteri and ovarian enlargement due to theca-lutein cysts.[44,173]

Morphologic studies have tried to predict the prognosis of moles based on the degree of trophoblastic proliferation and atypia,[61,103,104] but at present it appears that grading of moles has little predictive value, because moles with little trophoblastic proliferation may still develop postmolar disease requiring therapy.[81] Conversely, not all patients with proliferative and atypical trophoblast in moles require therapy.[44,70,245] Part of the difficulty in grading may be due to the marked variation of the trophoblastic proliferation and atypia in microscopic sections.[81] Although evaluation of the amount of trophoblastic hyperplasia and atypia is worthy of recording to give a general assessment of the status of the trophoblast, meticulous follow-up with serial serum hCG titers using sensitive assays is used to direct therapy.

The frequency with which invasive mole or choriocarcinoma occurs after diagnosis of a mole depends on the sensitivity of the follow-up hCG assay, length of follow-up, type of primary therapy, and terminology used in reporting sequelae.[35] Hertig and Sheldon,[35,104] in an early study performed before sensitive assays for hCG and cytotoxic chemotherapy were available, reported that 16% of hydatidiform moles developed into invasive moles and 2.5% into choriocarcinomas. About 8–30% of patients with hydatidiform mole will require chemotherapy sometime after primary evacuation.[13,44,155,179] The wide range in percentage of treated patients reflects the different criteria for persistent disease among investigators as well as variations in compliance for follow-up between patient populations.

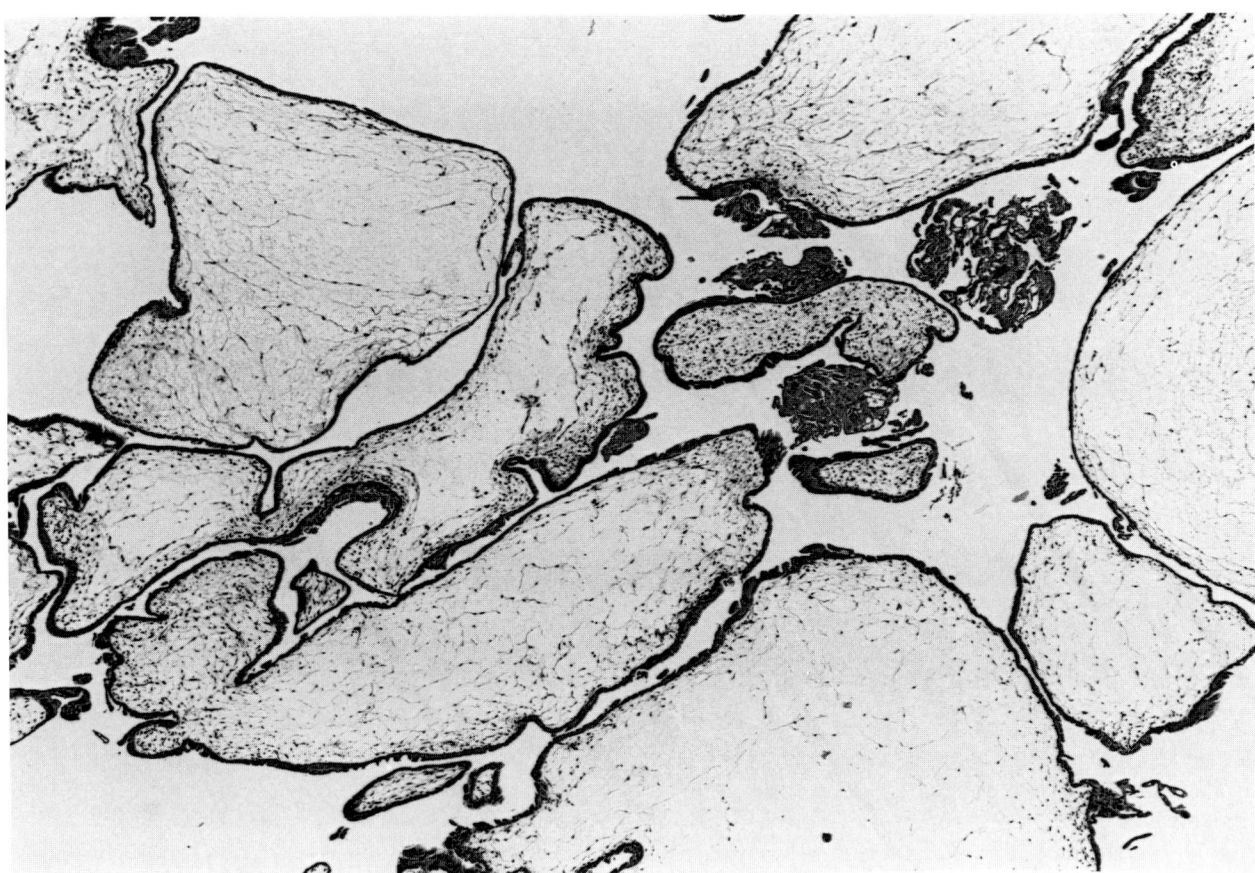

24.10

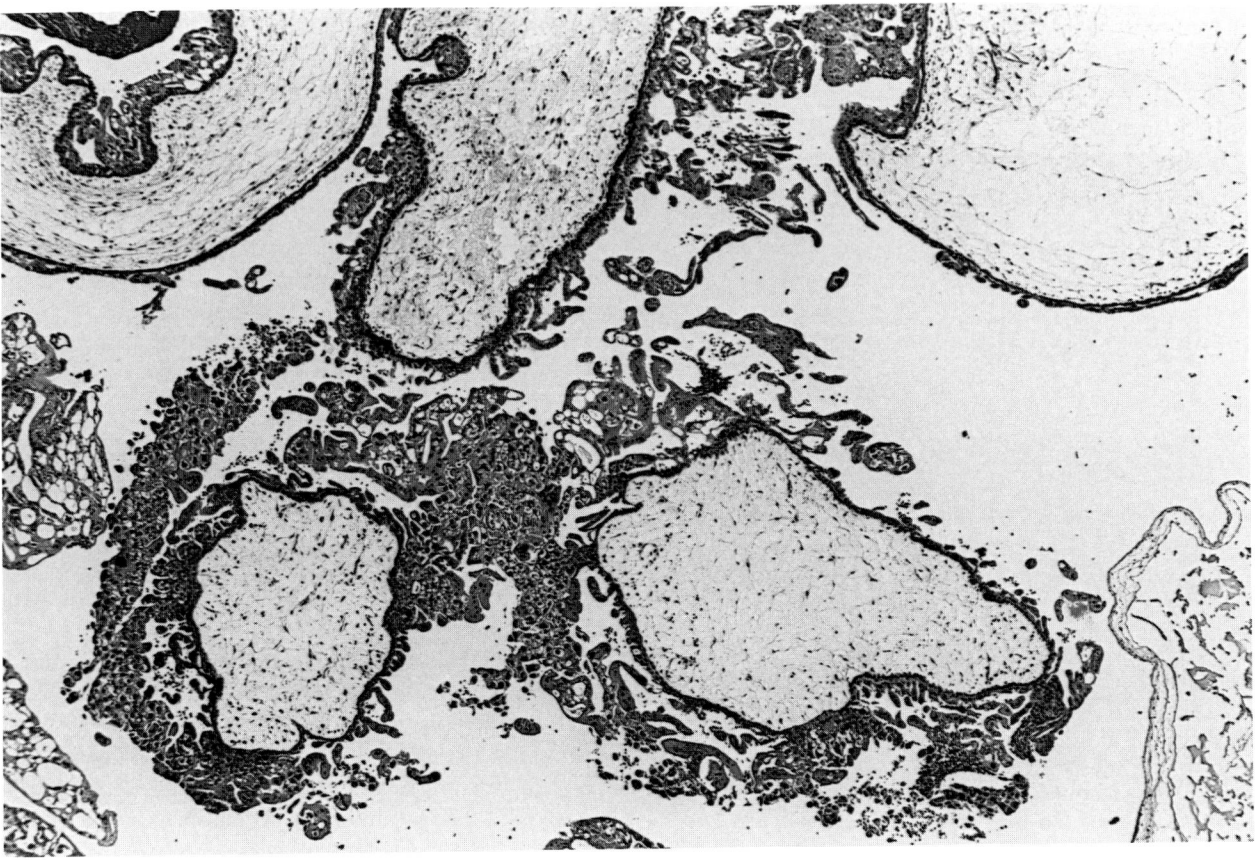

24.11

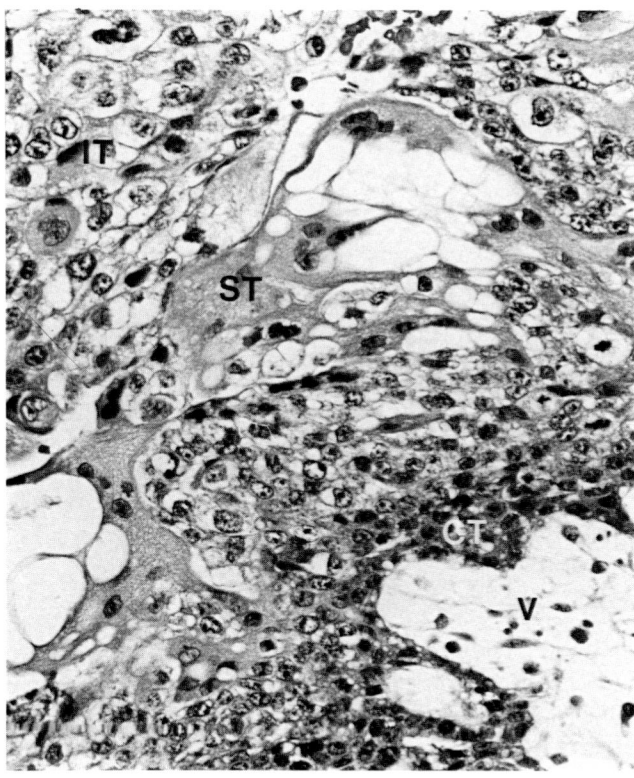

FIG. 24.12. Trophoblast in a complete mole. A mixture of cytotrophoblast (*CT*), intermediate trophoblast (*IT*), and syncytiotrophoblast (*ST*) grows from the surface of a villus (*V*).

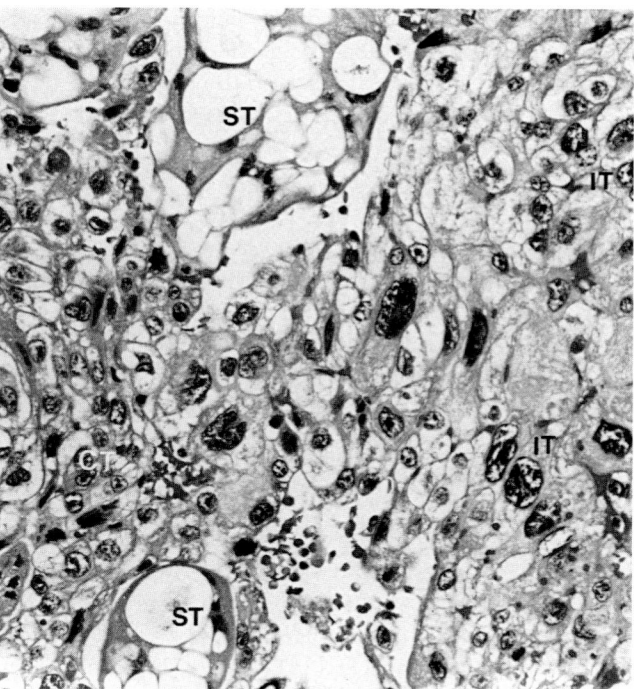

FIG. 24.13. Trophoblast of a complete mole. Note cytologic atypia. The intermediate trophoblast (*IT*) in the *center* and the *right side* of the field has enlarged, irregular nuclei. Cytotrophoblast (*CT*) is present on the *left*, and vacuolated syncytiotrophoblast (*ST*) is present in the *upper* and *lower portions* of the micrograph.

DNA ploidy analysis is not an independent factor for predicting persistence of hydatidiform mole,[139] although one study suggested that aneuploidy was a risk factor for persistent disease in complete moles.[161] Regardless of ploidy status, all patients with hydatidiform mole require close follow-up with serum hCG titers to identify cases that may persist or metastasize. Although it has been suggested that this feature may play some role in the behavior of GTD, such as spontaneous remission, a recent study did not demonstrate an increased risk for metastasis in complete moles with a Y chromosome compared with those with an XX karyotype[176] (see below).

Between 0.6% and 1.5% of patients who have had a complete hydatidiform mole are at risk of having recurrent molar pregnancies.[74,158] As many as nine consecutive molar pregnancies have been reported.[273] Some reports sug-

◁————————————————————

FIG. 24.10. Complete hydatidiform mole. Villi have extensive stromal edema with central cisterns. There is a minimal amount of proliferative trophoblast in this field.

FIG. 24.11. Complete hydatidiform mole. Enlarged villi have a circumferential proliferation of trophoblast from the surface of several villi. A portion of a necrotic villus is seen in the *right lower corner*.

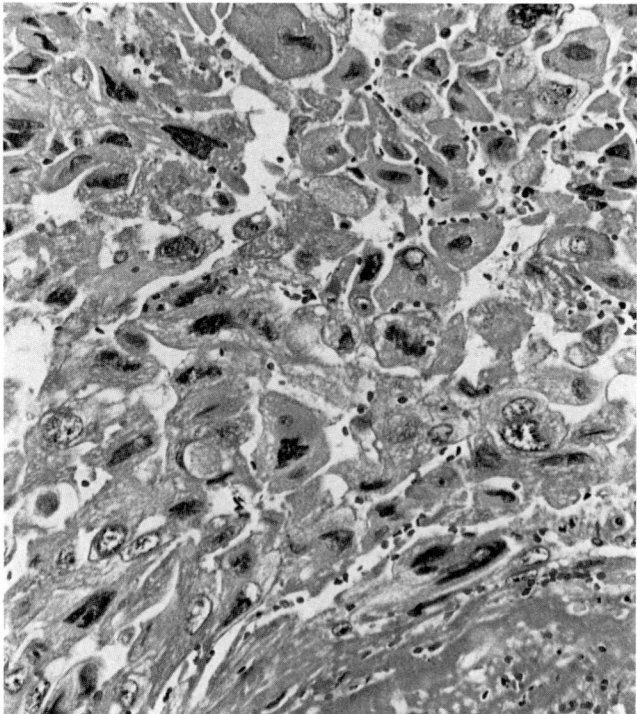

FIG. 24.14. Intermediate trophoblast in a complete hydatidiform mole. The mononucleate cells are pleomorphic with abundant amphophilic cytoplasm.

gest that recurrent molar pregnancy may show more proliferative trophoblast and that the likelihood of the need for chemotherapy is greater than with the first molar gestation.[74] Successful term pregnancies may occur after recurrent disease, however.[158]

Partial Hydatidiform Mole

A partial hydatidiform mole has an intimate admixture of two populations of villi: enlarged, edematous villi and normal-sized, fibrotic villi. Evidence of fetal development often is present in partial moles. Most partial moles have a triploid karyotype.

CLINICAL FEATURES

Partial moles account for 25–74% of all molar pregnancies and occur between the 9th and 34th weeks of pregnancy.[45,118a,239,271] Patients with partial moles may have signs and symptoms similar to those seen in complete moles, but usually this is less likely.[24,45,239] Uterine size is generally small for dates. Enlargement in excess of that expected for the gestational age is uncommon.[24,118a,239] Frequently, patients with partial mole appear to have a missed abortion. Preeclampsia tends to occur later than in complete mole but can be equally severe with partial mole.[239] Serum hCG levels often are in the low or normal range for gestational age.[24,223] Only a few patients with partial mole show markedly elevated hCG titers such as those seen in complete mole.[45] Table 24.4 compares the clinical features of partial and complete moles.

GROSS FINDINGS

The volume of tissue is generally small, less than 100 or 200 ml. The villi frequently are enlarged grossly and recognizable as molar, yet are smaller than those found in complete mole.[237,238] (Fig. 24.15). Fragments of more normal placental tissue also may be seen. In some cases a fetus or

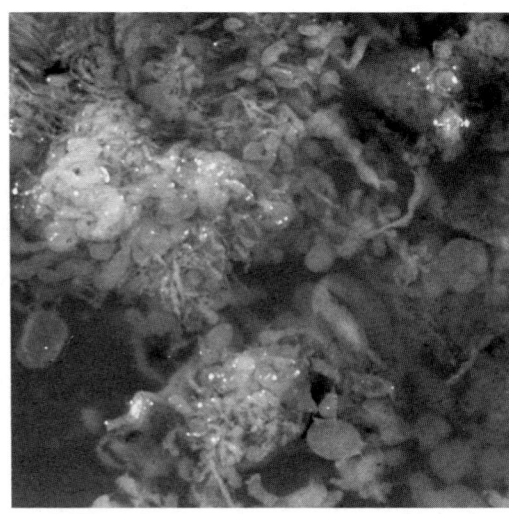

FIG. 24.15. **Partial hydatidiform mole.** Hydropic villi mixed with smaller villi.

fetal membranes is present (Fig. 24.16). When a fetus is found, it often shows gross congenital anomalies.[237]

MICROSCOPIC FINDINGS

Partial mole shows features in some villi that are similar to those seen in complete moles, but the molar change is focal[237,238] (Fig. 24.17). By definition, there should be a mixture of edematous villi and small, relatively normal-sized villi.[45,237,238] Central cisterns are less conspicuous than in complete moles. Smaller villi usually show stromal fibrosis similar to that seen in missed abortions (Fig. 24.18). Trophoblastic hyperplasia is less marked than in

Table 24.4. Clinical features of complete and partial moles

Feature	Complete	Partial
Clinical presentation	Spontaneous abortion	Missed or spontaneous abortion
Uterine size	Often large for dates	Often small for dates
Serum hCG	++++	++
Behavior	10–30% develop persistent GTD	4–12% develop persistent GTD

hCG, human chorionic gonadotropin; GTD, gestational trophoblastic disease.

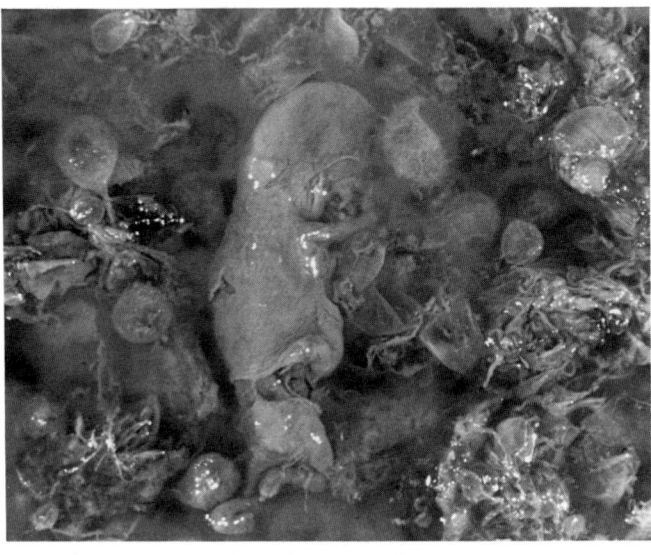

FIG. 24.16. **Partial hydatidiform mole.** A macerated fetus surrounded by villi with visible hydropic change. Often, the fetus in partial mole shows congenital abnormalities.

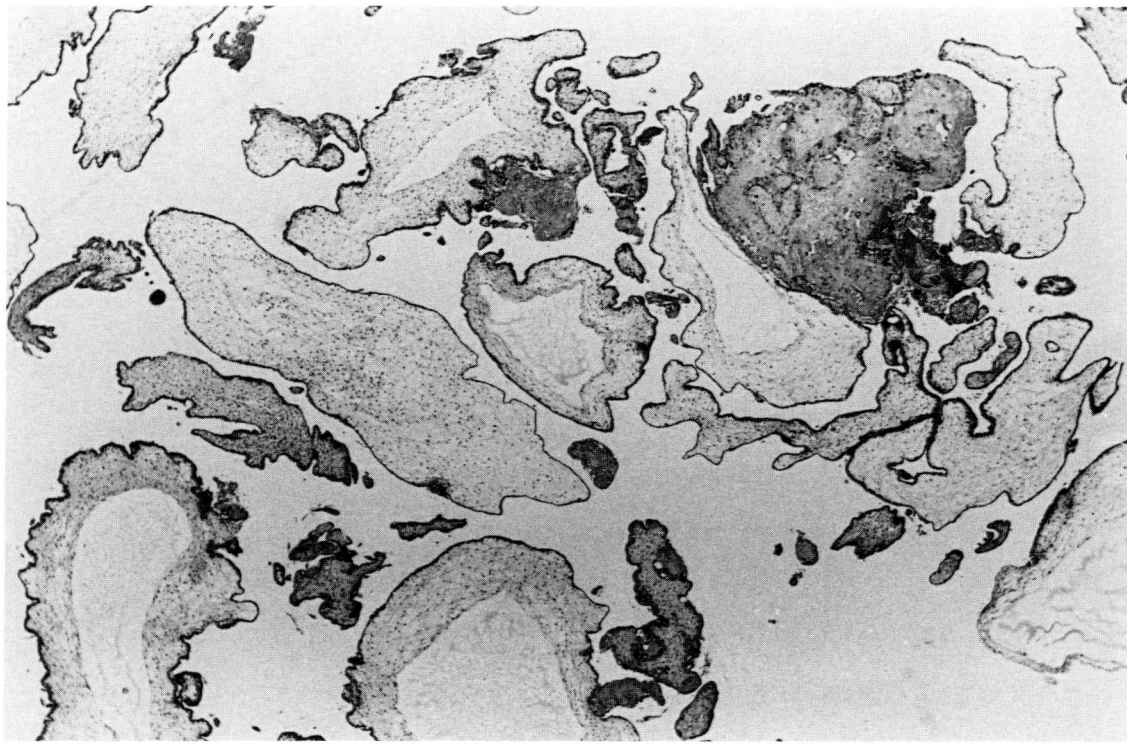

FIG. 24.17. **Partial hydatidiform mole.** A mixture of enlarged villi with cisterns and small, normal-sized villi. A small degenerating fetus was present.

complete mole. Generally it is focal and shows little, if any, atypia. Another feature commonly encountered in partial mole is invaginations of trophoblast into the villous stroma, which results in the molar villi having a scalloped appearance.[238] When the invaginations do not show continuity with the surface trophoblast, they appear as inclusions within the stroma (Fig. 24.18). Invaginations are not exclusive for partial moles and may, on occasion, be found in other conditions including complete mole.

Partial moles with triploid chromosomes are associated with the presence of a fetus or its amniotic covering, in contrast to the absence of fetal structures in most complete moles. Fetal demise with subsequent degeneration of fetal structures may make identification of fetal development more difficult, however. A subtle clue is the presence of a functioning villous circulation containing nucleated red cells, a feature that requires fetal development.[238] In contrast, the embryo associated with a complete mole usually dies before organogenesis and, therefore, fetal structures are not present in the specimen and fetal erythrocytes are not present within placental vessels. One concern in the diagnosis of an apparent partial mole is that the specimen represents a twin gestation with a fetus and a complete mole. Such twin pregnancies may occur[17,139,258] but probably are an infrequent occurrence relative to singleton gestations of a partial mole.

DIFFERENTIAL DIAGNOSIS

Most hydatidiform moles, complete and partial, are readily identifiable and present little diagnostic difficulty, but some may be extremely difficult to distinguish. The pathological features of partial as compared with complete moles are shown in Table 24.5. When there is evidence of a fetus or embryo as well, the diagnosis of partial mole usually is readily apparent. In the absence of fetal tissues, the other morphologic criteria, most importantly the amount of villous involvement, must be evaluated carefully to render the appropriate diagnosis.

Distinction of a mole from an abortus with hydropic villi may be a problem.[66] Spontaneous abortions often are associated with failure of development or early demise of the embryo, the so-called blighted ovum or hydropic abortus. These specimens show some villous edema with hydropic swelling and an absence of villous blood vessels, features shared with molar placentas. The hydropic abortus usually is a smaller specimen, however.[40] The villi in a hydropic abortus are enlarged only slightly and do not assume the large dimensions found in molar gestations, complete or partial. A few cisterns do occur in nonmolar abortions but they are focal. Clearly, there is a point when a developing gestation evolves into a molar pregnancy as "the missed abortion of a pathologic ovum,"[101] and the exact point at

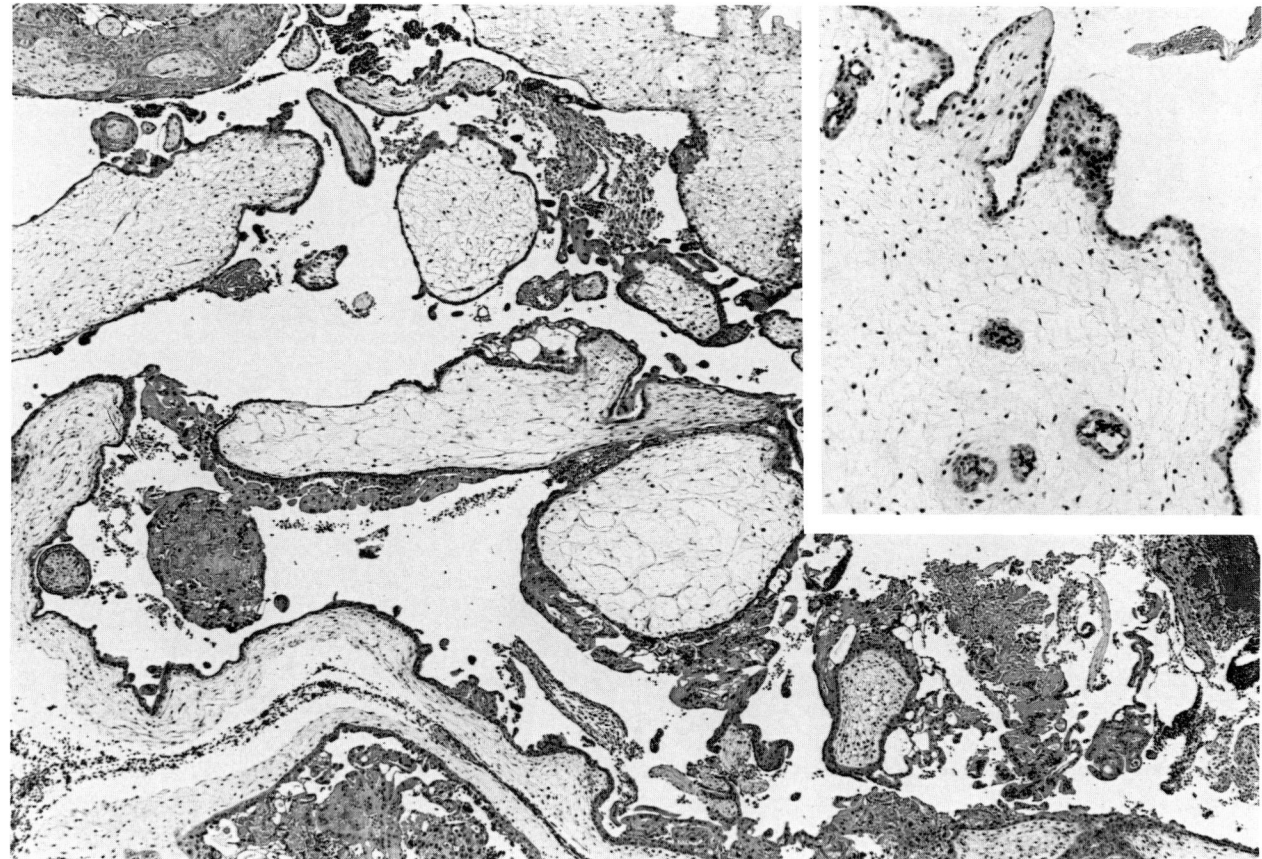

FIG. 24.18. Partial hydatidiform mole. Proliferative tropho-blast projecting randomly from the villus surface. Normal-sized, fibrotic villi are present in the left upper corner. This specimen consisted of 50 ml of tissue. There was no evidence of a fetus. *Inset:* Scalloped villous surface with trophoblast infolding form-ing inclusions.

which the transformation is sufficient to warrant a diagno-sis of molar pregnancy is not known. For practical pur-poses, however, if an abortion specimen shows villous edema that is only evident microscopically and has minimal to no cistern formation, it should not be considered a molar pregnancy.

The proliferative trophoblast of early pregnancy also must be distinguished from the trophoblastic hyperplasia of molar pregnancy.[66,69] In very early gestation, masses of ST and CT normally are present at the implantation site. Characteristically, the trophoblast proliferating from the villous surface shows polarity, and is localized to the distal end of the villus that implants into decidua. This direc-tional orientation contrasts with the irregular, circumfer-ential proliferation of molar trophoblast. In later preg-nancy, however, trophoblastic growth associated with villi is limited, and at this time sheets of trophoblast should be viewed as abnormal. If the villi are not molar, the rare possibility of choriocarcinoma originating within a placenta should be considered.[31,32,60]

When large aggregates of atypical or proliferating tro-phoblast are encountered without any villi, the differential

Table 24.5. Pathological features of complete and partial moles

	Complete mole	*Partial mole*
Karyotype	46XX, 46XY	Triploid
Embryo/fetus	Absent	Present
Villous outline	Round	Scalloped
Hydropic swelling	Marked	Less pronounced
	Cisterns present	Cisterns less prominent
	All villi involved	Focal villous involvement
		Villous fibrosis
Trophoblastic proliferation	Circumferential	Focal
	Variable, may be marked	Minimal
Trophoblastic atypia	Often present	Absent
Immunocytochemistry		
hCG	++++	+
PLAP	+	++++

hCG, human chorionic gonadotropin; PLAP, placental alkaline phos-phatase.
Adapted and reprinted with permission of World Health Organization, ref. 272.

diagnosis should include choriocarcinoma or placental site trophoblastic tumor but not hydatidiform mole. Care must be taken to be certain that sampling is adequate. Limited examination of a uterine, vaginal, or pulmonary lesion may show only trophoblast, but further sectioning might reveal the presence of molar villi.[268]

Studies indicate that there is no single criterion that allows distinction between complete mole, partial mole, and hydropic abortus.[40] Volume of tissue, size of hydropic villi, degree of microscopic villous swelling, distribution of trophoblast, amount of trophoblast proliferation, and presence or absence of fetal tissue all must be taken into account in the differential diagnosis. There can be significant interobserver variability in the diagnosis of hydatidiform mole.[78,118,169] DNA ploidy analysis of molar tissue may be helpful in classifying cases that do not clearly fall into the complete or partial category by morphologic features alone,[40,118a,138] and this can help predict behavior because complete mole is more likely to develop persistent GTD.

The distribution of hCG and human placental alkaline phosphatase (PLAP) also may aid in the distribution of complete and partial moles and hydropic abortuses. In complete moles, there is a much greater distribution of hCG compared with PLAP, whereas in partial moles the reverse is found.[29] In placentas with hydropic change, there is only focal staining for PLAP, whereas in partial moles, the staining is significantly more.[29]

CLINICAL BEHAVIOR

The behavior of partial mole is becoming understood better as more cases are recognized and followed. The risk of persistent or metastatic GTD is less after a partial mole than after a complete mole. Several series have reported that only about 5% of patients with partial mole will have persistent or metastatic GTD that requires chemotherapy,[45,87,239] although few studies have found that more patients, up to 12%, with partial mole require chemotherapy.[24,139,175,271] One study identified a few diploid partial moles that were less sensitive to single-agent chemotherapy than compared with triploid partial moles.[137]

Invasive mole[79,235] and metastatic pulmonary lesions[226,271] have occurred in association with partial mole. Only a rare case of well-documented partial mole has been followed by choriocarcinoma.[80] A few other reports of hydatidiform mole with a fetus interpreted as partial mole were followed by invasive mole and choriocarcinoma, but these reports did not give histological verification of true partial molar change to the villi.[151,242] These cases emphasize the necessity of applying strict morphologic criteria for a diagnosis of partial mole to ensure exclusion of rare cases of complete mole with a fetus in clinicopathological studies. Nonetheless, there is a decreased risk of persistent GTD requiring treatment in partial mole. The magnitude

of the risk of repeated partial moles is not known, although repetitive partial mole does occur.[205]

Invasive Mole

Invasive mole is a hydatidiform mole in which hydropic villi invade the myometrium or blood vessels or, more rarely, are deported to extrauterine sites.

CLINICAL FEATURES

Invasive mole is a possible sequela of hydatidiform mole, complete or partial. It is unusual for invasive mole to present primarily, although invasive mole may occur simultaneously with intracavitary molar pregnancy.[110] Pathological diagnosis requires demonstration of molar villi invading the myometrium or deported to extrauterine sites. When metastases occur they generally are found in the lungs, vagina, vulva, or broad ligament.[1,110,120,243,268] The diagnosis usually is made on a hysterectomy specimen. Since hysterectomy is rarely performed in patients with persistent hCG titers after removal of an intrauterine mole and since metastatic lesions of GTD usually are treated successfully with cytotoxic chemotherapy without biopsy, invasive mole is rarely confirmed histologically.[52,240]

GROSS FINDINGS

In the uterus, invasive mole is an erosive, hemorrhagic lesion extending from the uterine cavity into the myometrium (Fig. 24.19). Invasion can range from superficial penetration to extension through the wall, with perforation or involvement of the broad ligament. Molar vesicles often are grossly apparent.

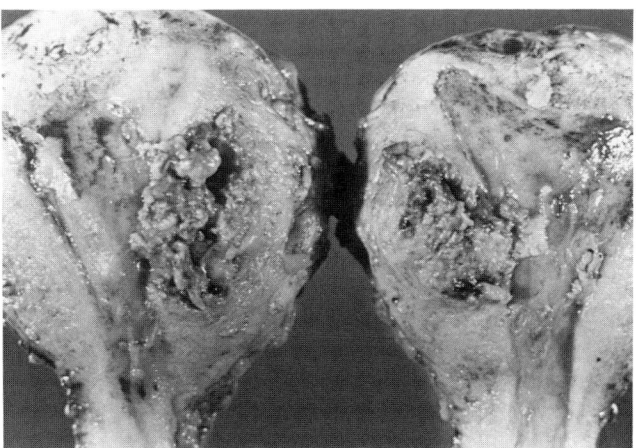

FIG. 24.19. **Invasive mole.** The lesion infiltrates deeply into the myometrium, forming a ragged, irregular mass.

Microscopic Findings

Microscopically, the diagnostic feature is the presence of molar villi along with trophoblast in the myometrium or at an extrauterine site (Fig. 24.20). Trophoblastic proliferation with atypia invariably accompanies the enlarged villi and is as variable as in noninvasive mole, ranging from slightly proliferative or atypical trophoblast to marked trophoblastic proliferation with extreme atypia (Fig. 24.21). Hydropic swelling tends not to be as marked as in noninvasive mole. Molar villi usually are no more than 4–5 mm in diameter. In metastatic sites, the diagnosis is based on the presence of villi. Careful searching may be necessary to identify villi within a lesion seemingly composed entirely of highly proliferative trophoblast. Lesions at distant sites usually are composed of molar villi confined within blood vessels without invasion into adjacent tissue. Some authors regard this as deportation rather than metastasis.

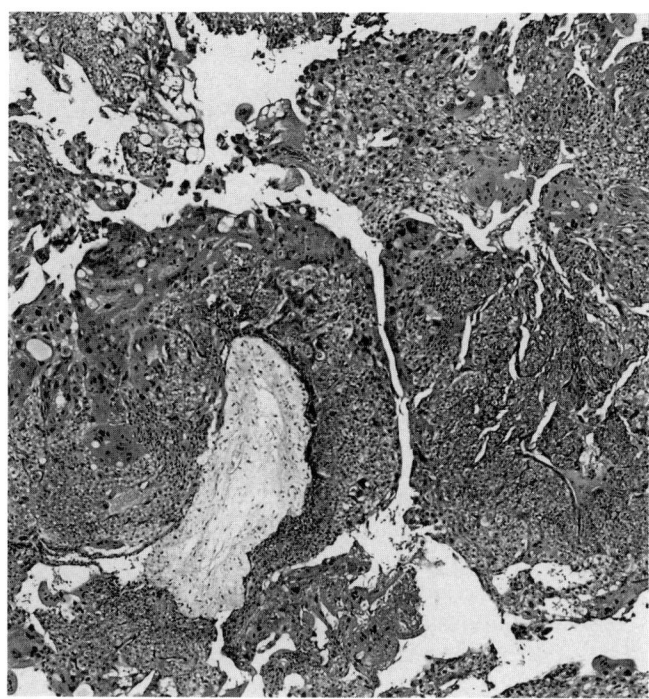

Fig. 24.21. Invasive mole. A single hydropic villus with marked trophoblastic hyperplasia is found in a biopsy of the uterine serosa. The lesion perforated the uterus and formed multiple hemorrhagic nodules on the serosa several months after abortion of a complete mole.

Differential Diagnosis

Since the pathological diagnosis of invasive moles requires identification of molar villi and trophoblast either within the myometrium or at an extrauterine site, there are few lesions that enter into the differential. Recurettage of the endometrium after diagnosis of a mole may show proliferative trophoblast with villi but this does not represent an invasive mole unless myometrial invasion is found. If post–mole curettage yields only trophoblast, the diagnosis of invasive mole is not established. Two forms of placenta accreta, specifically placenta increta or percreta, represent normal placenta that has implanted without an intervening decidual layer and invaded myometrium. In contrast to invasive mole, however, the villi in accreta are not hydropic and the trophoblast does not show the proliferative activity found in a mole.

Invasive mole must be discriminated from choriocarcinoma. Both invasive mole and choriocarcinoma after a hydatidiform mole are manifested by a plateau or elevation in the hCG titer. Furthermore, both can give rise to metastatic lesions. Consequently, it is often not possible clinically to distinguish between these lesions.[268] A repeat curettage may yield more molar tissue, obvious choriocar-

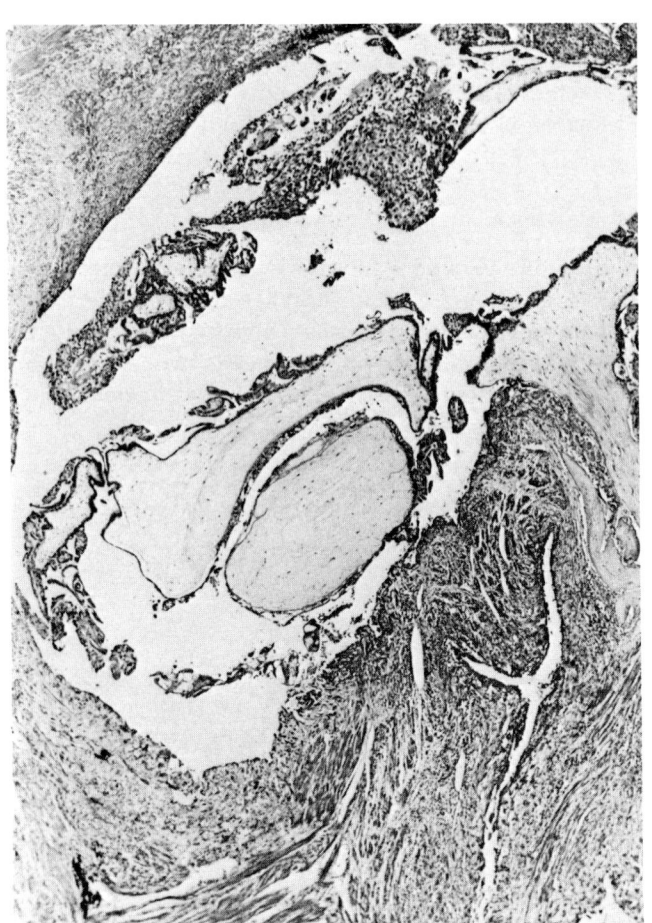

Fig. 24.20. Invasive mole. A hydropic villus within a large vein deep within the myometrium. Proliferative trophoblast accompanies the villi.

cinoma, or scant fragments of trophoblast unaccompanied by villi but lacking unequivocal features of choriocarcinoma (Fig. 24.22). In this instance a diagnosis of *atypical trophoblast* is appropriate, accompanied by a description and the reasons why a diagnosis of residual mole of choriocarcinoma was not made. When more molar tissue is found, a diagnosis of persistent hydatidiform mole is made.

CLINICAL BEHAVIOR

Invasive mole is the most common form of persistent or metastatic GTD after hydatidiform mole, occurring 6–10 times more frequently than choriocarcinoma.[35,104,155,240] In histologically verified cases, the lesion most often is confined to the uterus, with metastases occurring in 20–40% of cases.[67] Metastasis typically involves the lungs, and may be multiple or localized. Spread to the vagina, vulva, and broad ligament is well recognized.[1,91,268] Metastasis to other sites is unusual, but there are rare examples of histologically verified metastases to regions such as the paraspinal soft tissue.[53,113] Using modern chemotherapy, death from invasive mole is unusual.[30,154] Before cytotoxic chemotherapy, 4–15% of patients with invasive mole died of disease.[34,67,68,91] Mortality usually was due to local compli-

cations, such as uterine perforation with intraperitoneal hemorrhage.[67,68] Death from metastasis was less frequent. Most patients, even those with metastases, survived, and untreated metastases frequently regressed spontaneously.[201,243,268] The risk of progression to choriocarcinoma is no greater than that after complete mole.[189,195]

Invasive mole is the clinical diagnosis given to many patients with metastases or abnormally persistent hCG titers after molar pregnancy and no residual hydatidiform mole within the uterine cavity.[30,154,240] In such instances, there is, however, a possibility that persistent hCG levels may, however, be due to choriocarcinoma. In these cases, the clinical term *persistent GTD* or *gestational trophoblastic neoplasia*[129] is used without attempting to discriminate between invasive mole and choriocarcinoma.

Choriocarcinoma

Choriocarcinoma is a highly malignant epithelial tumor arising from the trophoblast of any type of gestational event, most often a hydatidiform mole. It consists predominantly of a biphasic proliferation of cytotrophoblast and syncytiotrophoblast that recapitulates the primitive trophoblast of the implanting blastocyst. Chorionic villi are not a component of this tumor.

CLINICAL FEATURES

This highly aggressive neoplasm of trophoblast may be associated with any form of gestation. Theoretically, choriocarcinoma may arise in the trophoblast of the primitive blastocyst before implantation, but most cases of choriocarcinoma appear to follow a recognizable gestational event. The more abnormal the pregnancy, the more likely that choriocarcinoma may supervene. Hertig and Mansell found an incidence of 1 in 160,000 normal gestations, 1 in 15,386 abortions, 1 in 5333 ectopic pregnancies, and 1 in 40 molar pregnancies.[103] In that series, one-half of the cases of choriocarcinoma were preceded by hydatidiform mole, with 25% following abortion, 22.5% following normal pregnancy, and 2.5% following ectopic pregnancy.[103] Other studies have generally confirmed these figures.[154]

The signs and symptoms of choriocarcinoma are protean, whether it occurs in association with a molar or nonmolar pregnancy.[95,189,192] Abnormal uterine bleeding is one of the most frequent presentations of choriocarcinoma[192] (Fig. 24.23), but uterine lesions may be restricted to the myometrium and remain asymptomatic (Fig. 24.24). Not all patients will have a demonstrable lesion in the uterus after an intrauterine gestation. Many examples of metastatic choriocarcinoma with no uterine tumor have been described.[35,109,123,167] Apparently the neoplasm undergoes regression in the uterus.[35,109,197]

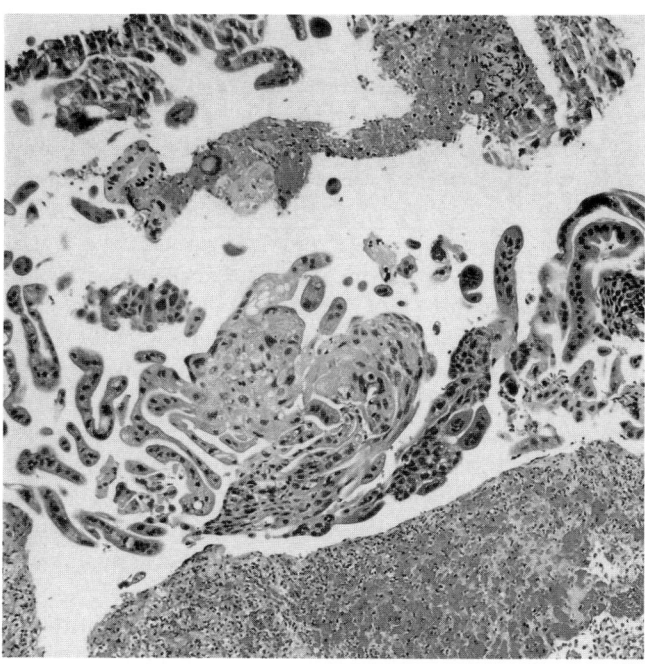

FIG. 24.22. Atypical trophoblast after hydatidiform mole. Small fragments of trophoblast in a curettage specimen several weeks after evacuation of a complete hydatidiform mole. No villi are present, yet the amount of tissue is insufficient for unequivocal choriocarcinoma. A definitive diagnosis cannot be made.

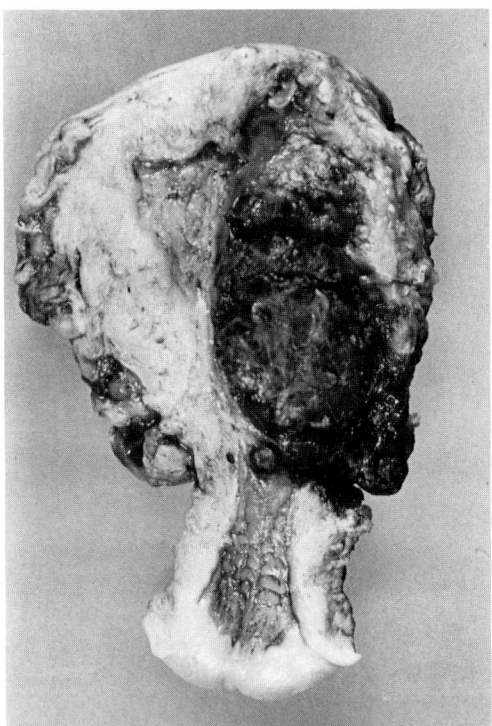

Fig. 24.23. Choriocarcinoma. The tumor forms a large, hemorrhagic mass that involves the endometrium and myometrium.

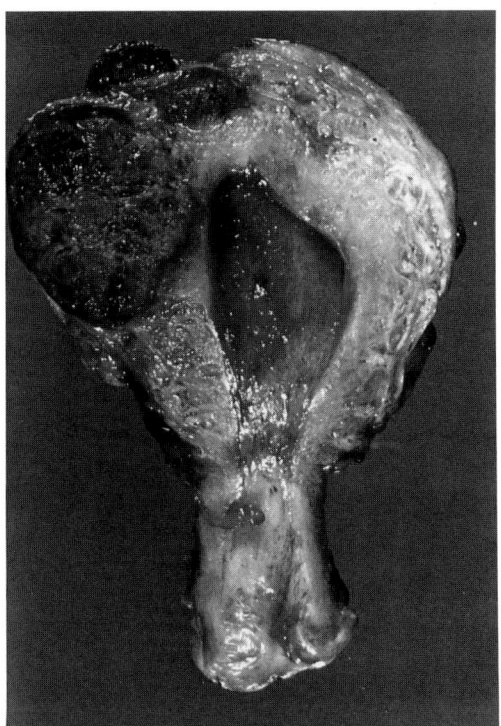

Fig. 24.24. Choriocarcinoma. The tumor forms a circumscribed mass within the myometrium that does not involve the endometrium. Lesions such as this may be asymptomatic because of their location.

Sometimes, symptoms related to metastases are the first indication that choriocarcinoma is present.[38,249] The lungs are the most frequent site for blood-borne lesions,[150,167,189] and a patient may present with hemoptysis.[246] Symptomatology related to hemorrhagic events in the central nervous system, liver, and gastrointestinal or urinary tracts also occurs[55,90,254] (Figs. 24.25, 24.26). Choriocarcinoma may have an unusually long latent period,[93,143,197] becoming manifest 10 or more years after hysterectomy or tubal ligation. There are rare examples of choriocarcinoma in postmenopausal women.[58] Thyrotoxicosis may occur in choriocarcinoma.[184]

Gross Findings

Uterine choriocarcinoma generally is a dark red, hemorrhagic mass with a shaggy, irregular surface[67,68,185,189] (Figs. 24.23, 24.24). Occasionally, a lesion may lack significant hemorrhage and appear as a fleshy, tan-gray mass with necrosis. The size of uterine lesions varies greatly, ringing from tiny, microscopic foci to huge, necrotic tumors. Metastases beyond the uterus appear well circumscribed and hemorrhagic[189] (Figs. 24.25, 24.26). Ill-defined, infiltrative growth is unusual because of the rapid proliferation with hemorrhage and necrosis that characterize the neoplasm.

Microscopic Findings

Choriocarcinoma is characterized by masses and sheets of trophoblastic cells without chorionic villi that invade surrounding tissue and permeate vascular spaces (Figs. 24.27–24.29). Central hemorrhage and necrosis with viable tumor constituting only a thin peripheral rim is a characteristic feature. The interface with normal tissue, if preserved, is circumscribed and appears expansile (Fig. 24.27).

An intimate mixture of CT, IT, and ST forms the cellular population of choriocarcinoma (Fig. 24.28). The CT and IT (Fig. 24.29) tend to grow in clusters and sheets, separated by ST (Fig. 24.28). The latter lines large, angular spaces containing red cells. A network of ST intimately admixed with CT and IT comprises the plexiform pattern of trophoblast in many trophoblastic lesions. The patterns of growth recapitulate the relationship of the trophoblast to the maternal–placental circulation of the early implanting previllous blastocyst.

There may be considerable cytological atypia in the IT and ST with pleomorphic enlarged nuclei, abnormal mitotic figures, and bizarre cellular configurations. Nuclear chromatin is coarsely granular, with an uneven distribution, and multiple nucleoli may be present. Enlarged, IT with two or several nuclei also occur, and they are distinguished from ST by their cytoplasm, which lacks the dense eosinophilia and vacuolization (Fig. 24.29).

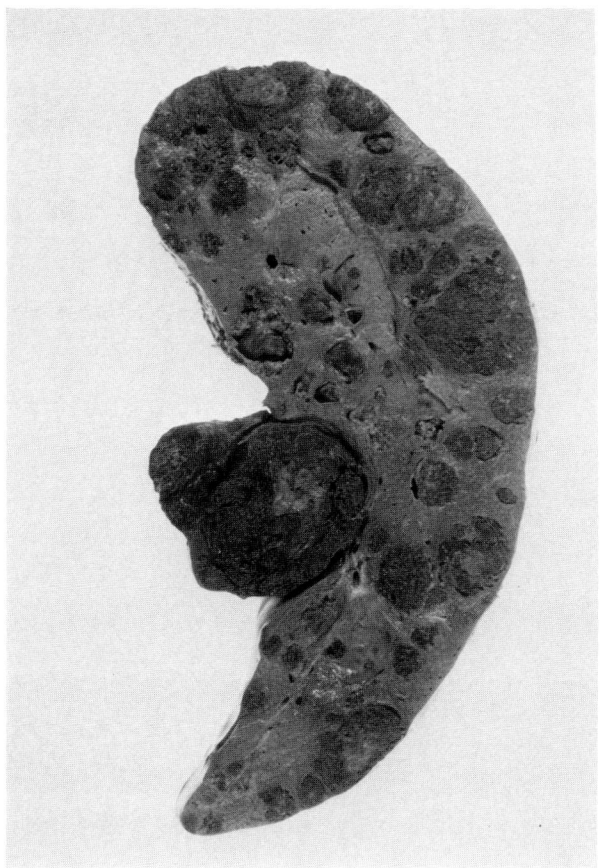

FIG. 24.25. **Liver metastases from choriocarcinoma.** Multiple, circumscribed, hemorrhagic masses are evident.

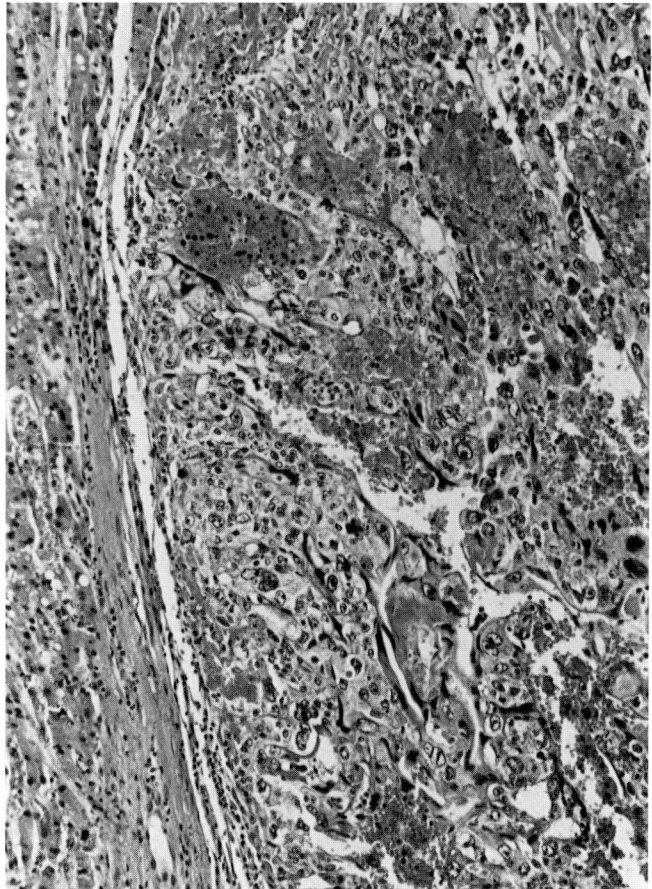

FIG. 24.27. **Metastatic choriocarcinoma in the liver.** Syncytiotrophoblast, cytotrophoblast, and intermediate trophoblast are present. On the *left*, the boundary with preserved liver is circumscribed.

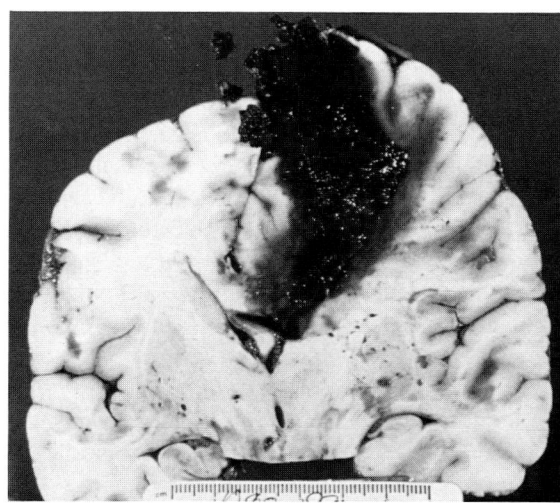

FIG. 24.26. **Metastatic choriocarcinoma to the brain.** Extensive hemorrhage caused death. At autopsy, the patient had metastases in multiple organs.

The tumor can undergo sufficient necrosis so that little or no viable tissue is identified in a lesion. Diagnosis may require extensive sectioning to identify the typical pattern of choriocarcinoma. Generally, choriocarcinoma has no intrinsic vascular stroma, the tumor receiving its vascular supply by syncytial cells permeating and replacing host vessels.[52,61,189] Infiltrative growth of normal tissues and blood vessels, however, can add an apparent vascular framework to the pattern.[167]

Histological features that reportedly correlate with response to treatment and clinical outcome include a marked lymphoid infiltrate, high mitotic activity, nuclear atypia, vascular invasion, and a compact growth pattern showing minimal differentiation into ST.[54,71,114,124,167,183] These observations may have prognostic value but are based on a small number of cases, and therefore further study is needed to determine their significance.

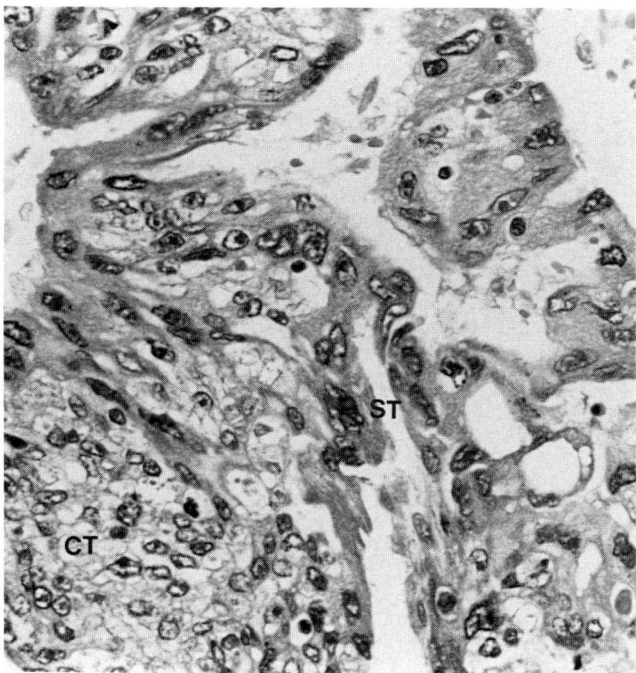

FIG. 24.28. **Trophoblast in choriocarcinoma.** Syncytiotrophoblast (*ST*) lining vascular spaces and capping cytotrophoblast (*CT*).

ULTRASTRUCTURAL FINDINGS

The fine structure of the trophoblastic cells of choriocarcinoma correlates with their functional and light microscopic features.[51,63,67,68,142] These cells have features similar to trophoblast in the normally developing placenta and in hydatidiform mole. The CT are closely apposed with polygonal outlines (Fig. 24.30). The most striking feature is their simplicity, with electron-lucent cytoplasm containing numerous free cytoplasmic ribosomes and aggregates of particulate glycogen. Others organelles are sparse. Mitochondria, scattered strands of rough endoplasmic reticulum (RER), and Golgi complexes are the other components. A few small electron-dense lysosomes, vesicles, and lipid droplets may be found, but cytoplasmic filaments are not present. The nuclei have smooth, round to oval contours and contain a prominent nucleolus. The cells are joined by widely separated, well-formed desmosomes.

The ST contrasts markedly with CT.[51,63,67,68,142] These highly developed epithelial cells have a complex cytoplasm and cell membrane structure. Often, ST is joined directly to CT by desmosomes, and here the distinction between the two cell types is immediately apparent (Fig. 24.31). In addition to the multiple nuclei, ST demonstrate an electron-dense cytoplasm because of the presence of multiple organelles (Fig. 24.32). RER is abundant and often dilated, giving an appearance of multiple tiny vacuoles within the cytoplasm. In addition, the cytoplasm contains abundant

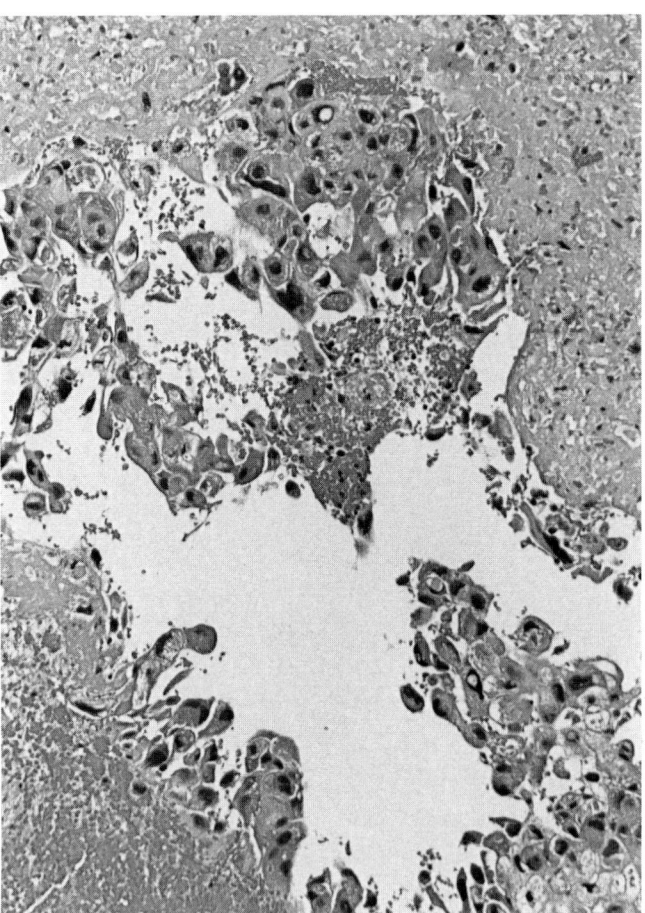

FIG. 24.29. **Intermediate trophoblast in choriocarcinoma.** Intermediate trophoblast is composed largely of mononucleate and binucleate cells with amphophilic cytoplasm. In other areas, this tumor showed biphasic cytotrophoblast and syncytiotrophoblast.

free cytoplasmic ribosomes, many prominent lipid droplets, vesicles, and lysosomes. Another important cytoplasmic constituent is thick bundles of tonofilaments scattered throughout the cell. The ST cell surface is covered with many long microvilli. Infolding of the microvillous surface into the cytoplasm forms interconnecting lacunae and gives an appearance of multiple intracytoplasmic lumens when viewed in cross-section. Well-formed desmosomes connect the cells. The ST nuclei tend to have highly irregular outlines and coarsely clumped chromatin, which further contribute to the cellular complexity.

Since ST forms by coalescence of CT, transition forms can be found ultrastructurally that share features of both CT and ST.[63,166,200,275] These cells correspond to IT and may have one or more nuclei in a cytoplasm that is more dense and complex than that of CT but less well developed than ST cytoplasm. Occasional aggregates of intracytoplasmic desmosomes can be found where fusion of cell membranes has taken place.

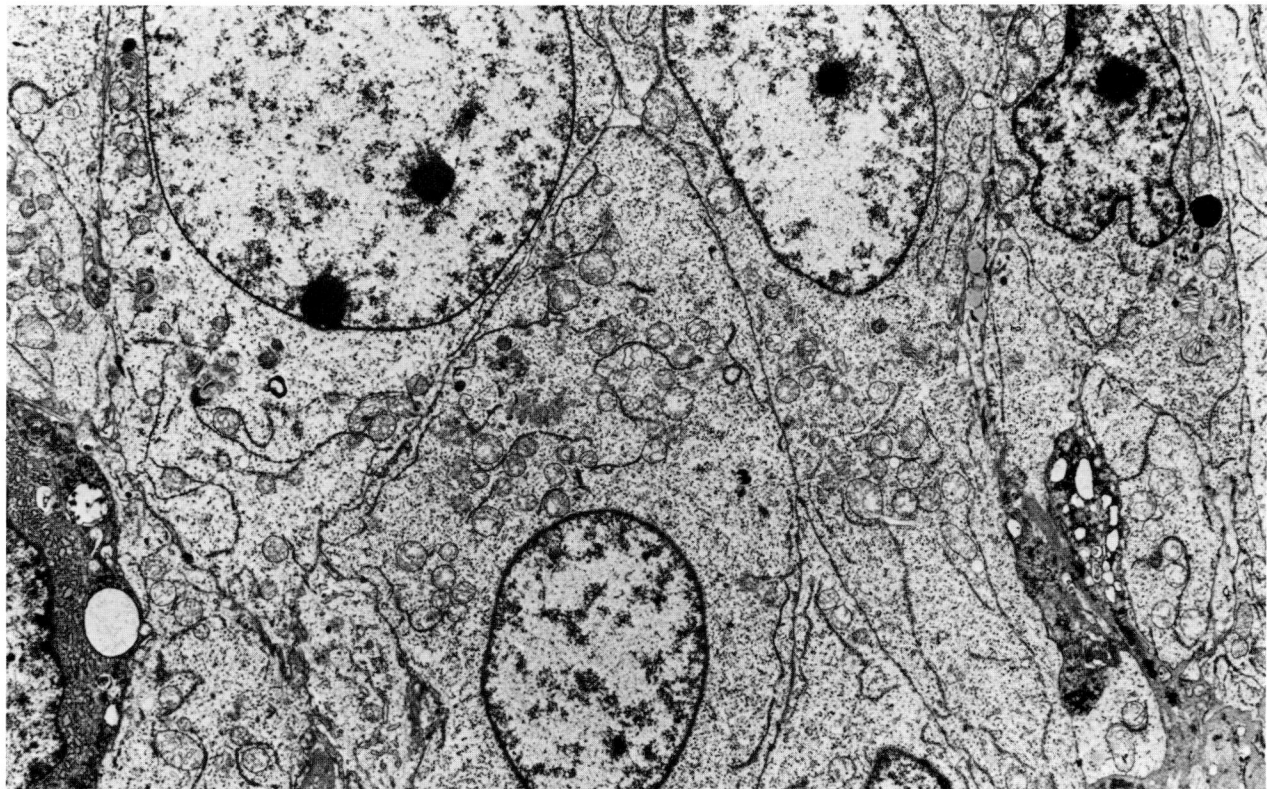

Fig. 24.30. Choriocarcinoma. Cytotrophoblastic cells have simple cytoplasm with few organelles except RER and mitochondria. Occasional desmosomes join cells. Nuclei are round to oval. ×4000.

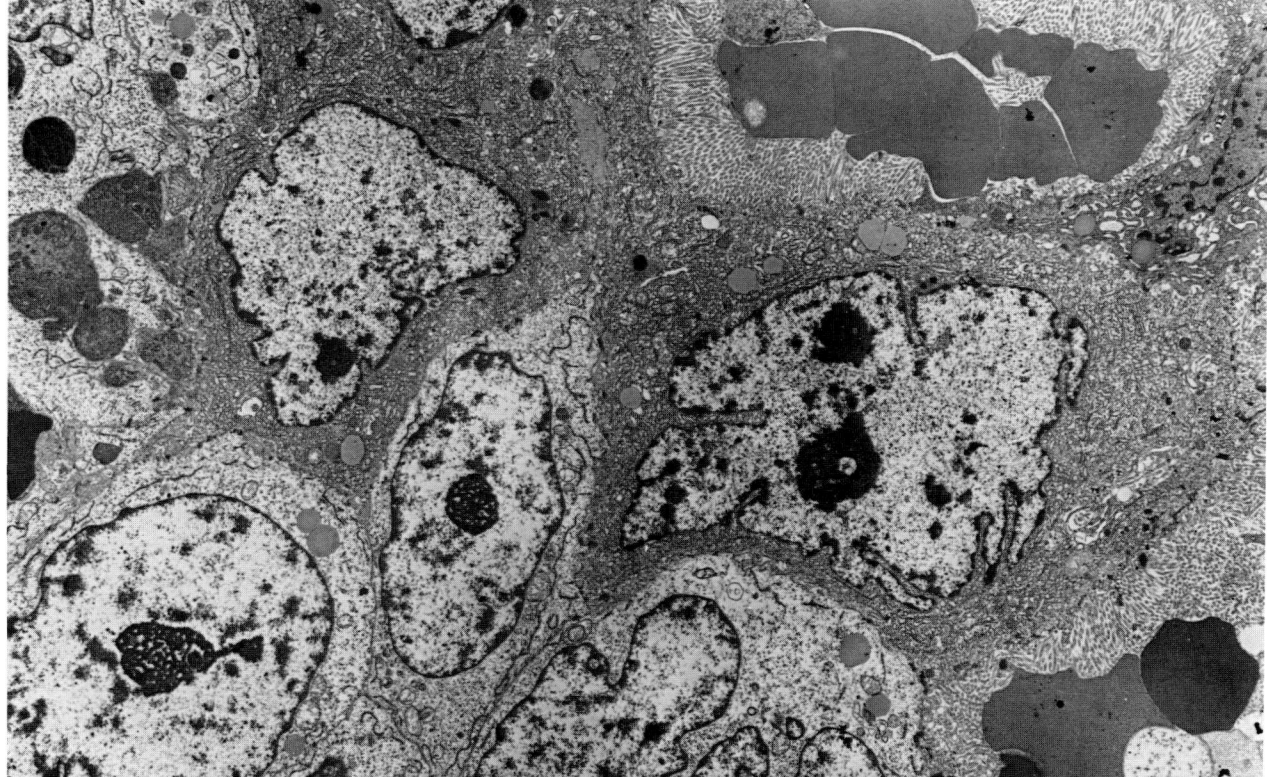

Fig. 24.31. Electron micrograph of trophoblast in chorio-carcinoma. Syncytiotrophoblast in *right upper portion*, with dense, complex cytoplasm and multiple nuclei. A vascular lacuna containing red blood cells is present in the *right upper portion*. In contrast, the cytotrophoblast at the *left lower portion* of the micrograph has electron-lucent cytoplasm. ×4000.

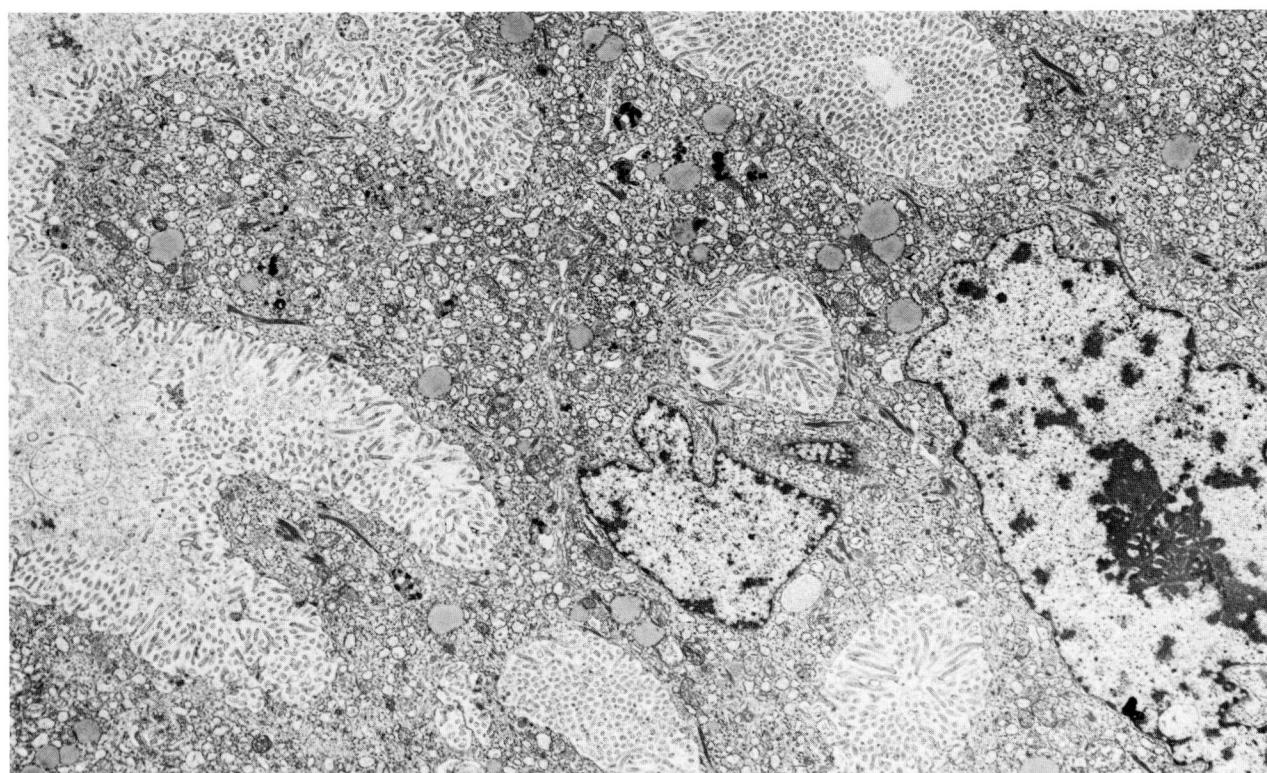

Fɪɢ. 24.32. Syncytiotrophoblast in choriocarcinoma. Multiple lacunae lined by slender microvilli. The complex cytoplasm contains dilated RER, lipid vacuoles, and dark granules. The nuclei have irregular contours and clumped chromatin. ×4500.

DIFFERENTIAL DIAGNOSIS

Choriocarcinoma must be distinguished from the normal trophoblast of early gestations, from molar pregnancies, from placental site trophoblastic tumor, and from other forms of epithelial malignancy.[69] Occasionally, normal trophoblast of an early gestation will be found in curettings without associated villi. In this circumstance, the trophoblast should be present only in small quantities. Normal trophoblast of an early gestation, although proliferative, does not show atypical features with the marked cellular enlargement and nuclear abnormalities found in choriocarcinoma. Also, fragments of normal trophoblast in curettings do not show tumor necrosis or destructive invasion. Large amounts of trophoblast showing atypia and no associated villi should be viewed suspiciously for choriocarcinoma. If the diagnosis is in doubt, a chest radiograph and careful monitoring of beta-hCG levels should resolve the problem.

As a general rule, choriocarcinoma should not be diagnosed in the presence of villi.[185] Proliferative trophoblast in association with villi usually indicates either an abortion or hydatidiform mole. The differential diagnosis of these lesions is discussed under Hydatidiform Mole. Rarely, gestational choriocarcinoma arises within normally developing placenta, with the neoplasm intimately associated with well-formed, mature nonmolar villi[31,32,60,140,193,249] (Fig. 24.33).

Discriminating choriocarcinoma from other carcinomas either within the uterus or at other sites usually is not a problem, but on occasion a biopsy of choriocarcinoma may show a few ST cells, and the pattern can mimic a poorly differentiated carcinoma (Fig. 24.34).[167] When this differential diagnosis arises, the clinical history may reveal a previous molar pregnancy or another suspicious pregnancy event that can clarify the diagnosis. Serum hCG levels and immunohistochemical localization of hCG are extremely helpful.

CLINICAL BEHAVIOR

In the past, gestational choriocarcinoma usually was fatal.[189] Before cytotoxic chemotherapy was available, hysterectomy and, in some instances, irradiation were the only forms of treatment. The absolute 5-year survival for patients treated by hysterectomy before the chemotherapy era was 32%.[33] If metastases were not evident at the time of surgery, the survival rate was 41%, whereas if metastases were present, the survival rate was 19%. More than 90% of patients with extrauterine gestational choriocarcinoma have lung metastases.[109,123,150,167,189,197] The frequency of involvement of other sites is somewhat variable, depending on whether the data represent autopsy studies or whether the patients have received chemotherapy. Brain and liver metastases are frequent, occurring in 20–60% of pa-

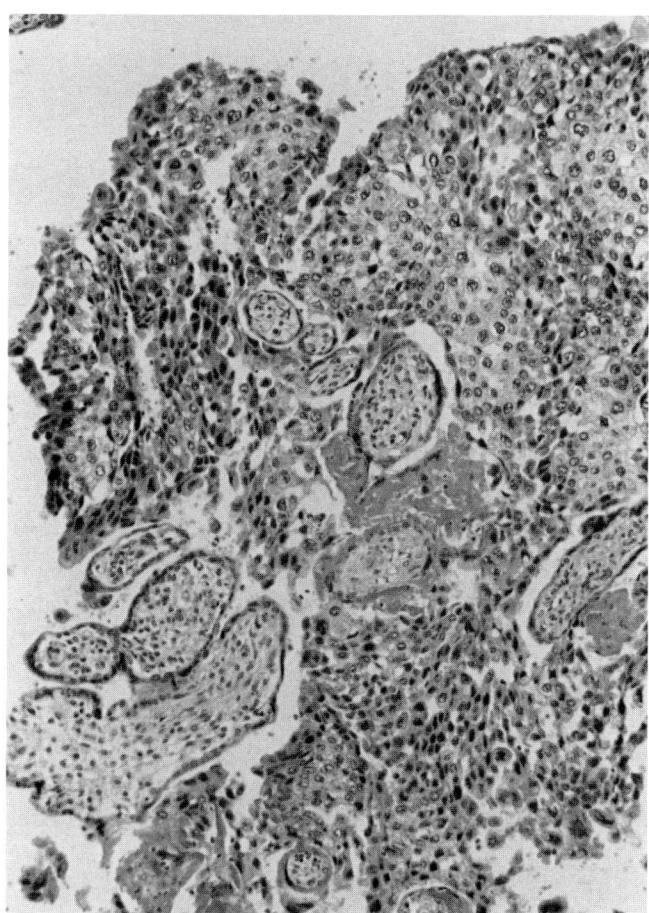

FIG. 24.33. **Choriocarcinoma arising in a placenta.** Malignant trophoblast arising from the surface of normally formed villi.

tients.[67,123,167,189] Kidney and abdomen, including intestinal tract, are the other common sites of spread, but almost any organ, including the skin, may be involved.[72,167,189] Lymph nodes contain tumor on occasion, often as tertiary metastatic lesions from other organs.[167,189] Vaginal involvement has been reported in 16–32% of patients.[123,167,185,189] There have been a few isolated reports of metastatic choriocarcinoma occurring in the mother and child of a term pregnancy.[3,46,75] Usually, the infant is disease-free.

Survival rates have improved dramatically since the introduction of cytotoxic chemotherapy combined with accurate and sensitive assays for hCG to monitor the course of the disease (see below, Management). The overall survival now for persistent and metastatic GTD is about 90%.[148,154] With a morphologic diagnosis of choriocarcinoma, however, the survival rate declines to 81% of all patients and 71% of patients with metastatic choriocarcinoma.[154]

Death from choriocarcinoma most commonly results from hemorrhage or pulmonary insufficiency.[21,153,167] Fatal hemorrhage usually occurs in the central nervous system or lungs, but intraperitoneal and gastrointestinal hemorrhage also can cause death.[21,167] Exsanguination may

occur after biopsy of a vaginal metastasis.[35] Pulmonary insufficiency can be due either to a large tumor burden or to the effects of irradiation and cytotoxic chemotherapy.[167]

Epithelioid Trophoblastic Tumor

We are tentatively proposing the term *epithelioid trophoblastic tumor* to describe a specific type of trophoblastic tumor that does not appear to have identified previously by earlier investigators. This tumor is related to choriocarcinoma and was observed initially in lung metastases of a few patients with persistent tumors after intensive chemotherapy for documented choriocarcinoma.[122,166] In these cases the therapy appears to have eradicated the typical dimorphic choriocarcinoma, leaving only residual tumor with an unusual morphology. Subsequently, we have observed similar tumors in the uterus in which there was no history of prior chemotherapy for choriocarcinoma.[133] In at least two cases we have seen this tumor merge imperceptibly with typical choriocarcinoma. This lesion also has been found in the uterus adjacent to placental site nodules after hydatidiform mole.[221]

These tumors are associated with elevated serum hCG levels and are composed predominantly of highly atypical mononucleate trophoblastic cells and indistinct syncytiotrophoblast (Fig. 24.35). The predominant cells are relatively uniform in size and are mononucleate. They are enlarged relative to cytotrophoblast but smaller than intermediate trophoblast (Fig. 24.36). The tumor has a striking epithelioid appearance both in its cytological features and its pattern of invasion. The latter is characterized by diffusely infiltrating cords and nests of cells typically surrounded by a dense eosinophilic hyaline material (Fig. 24.37). The mononucleate trophoblastic cells have single, convoluted, and slightly vesicular nuclei with a moderate amount of eosinophilic cytoplasm. They show ultrastructural features that are transitional between cytotrophoblast and syncytiotrophoblast but differ from intermediate trophoblast of the placental site trophoblastic tumor.[166]

The epithelioid trophoblastic tumor invades in an expansile fashion similar to choriocarcinoma, lacking the permeative type of infiltrative growth manifested by placental site trophoblastic tumors (see below, Placental Site Trophoblastic Tumor). Unlike choriocarcinoma, however, this lesion is not associated with extensive central hemorrhage and necrosis. The cells tend to form small nests that often contain dense central hyaline material and necrotic debris. The hyaline material and necrotic debris simulate keratin and therefore these tumors may be confused easily with a poorly differentiated squamous carcinoma, particularly since the syncytiotrophoblastic component is indistinct. Immunohistochemistry for hCG is helpful in identifying syncytiotrophoblast in these tumors.

Because we have seen only a few cases, it is difficult to draw conclusions concerning the biologic behavior of these

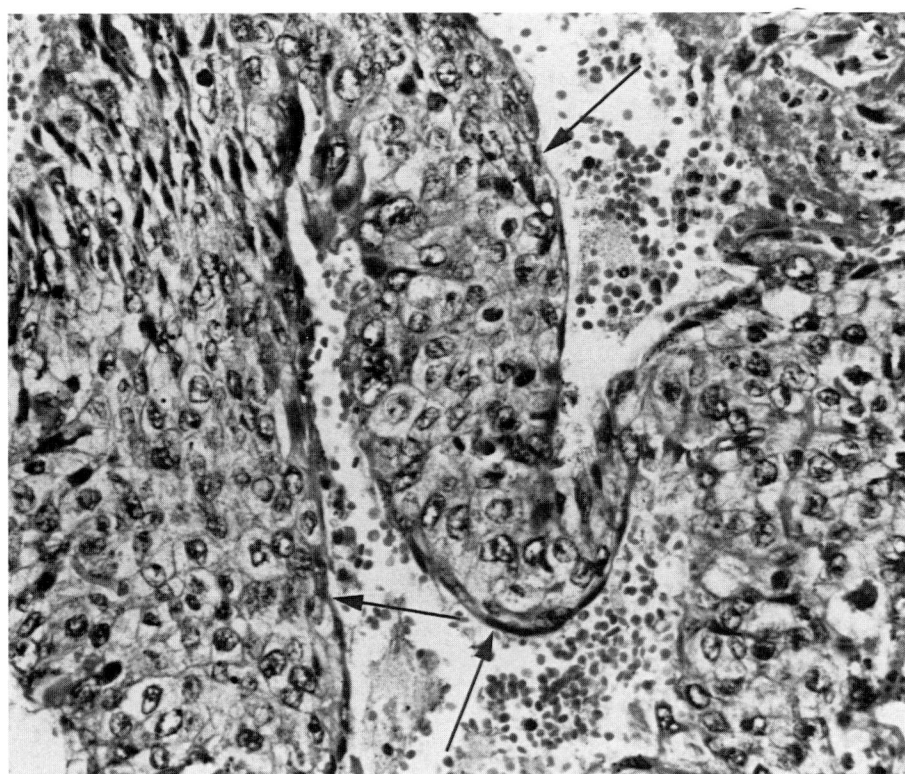

FIG. 24.34. Choriocarcinoma. Most of the cells are cytotrophoblast and may simulate a poorly differentiated carcinoma. Syncytiotrophoblast (*arrows*) is attenuated, forming a thin layer between the cytotrophoblast and vascular spaces.

neoplasms, although they appear to have a somewhat more favorable prognosis than the usual dimorphic choriocarcinoma. Patients with pulmonary metastases have had longstanding remissions after surgical removal of the tumors. The term *epithelioid trophoblastic tumor* seems appropriate for this lesion because its distinctive epithelioid appearance sets it apart from the choriocarcinoma or placental site trophoblastic tumors.

Placental Site Trophoblastic Tumor

The placental site trophoblastic tumor (PSTT) is a neoplasm composed predominantly of intermediate trophoblast. It is generally benign but may be highly malignant. It resembles the trophoblastic infiltration of the endometrium and myometrium of the placental bed. The neoplasm lacks the biphasic pattern of trophoblast seen in choriocarcinoma.

The PSTT of the uterus is the rarest from of GTD. The tumor originally was termed *atypical chorioepithelioma* by Marchand in 1895,[159] but because of its rarity, it took many years before it was recognized as a separate entity distinct from choriocarcinoma. In the century after its initial description, it was periodically rediscovered and renamed. Terms that have been used include *atypical choriocarcinoma*,[196] *syncytioma*,[73] *chorioepitheliosis*,[217,253] and *trophoblastic pseudotumor*,[135] but these are no longer consid-

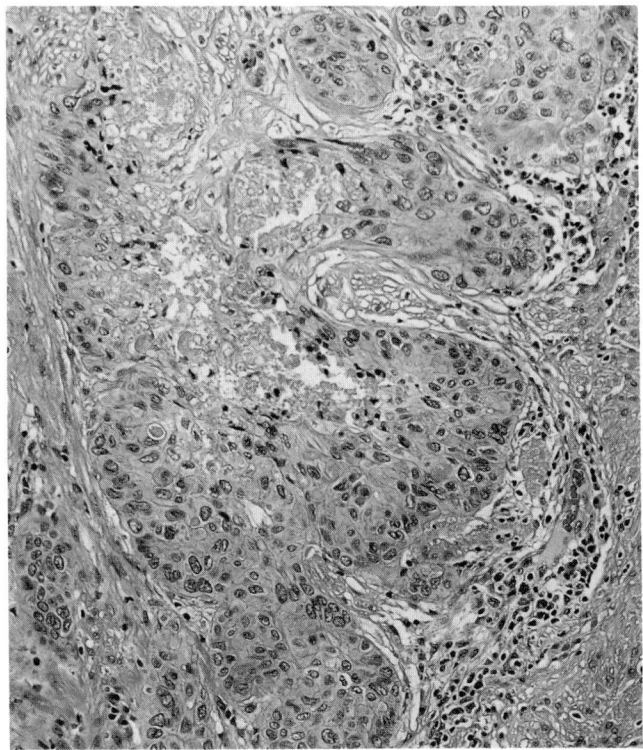

FIG. 24.35. Epithelioid trophoblastic tumor. Tumor in hysterectomy shows nests of atypical mononucleate trophoblastic cells. The tumor lacks the typical dimorphic pattern of choriocarcinoma.

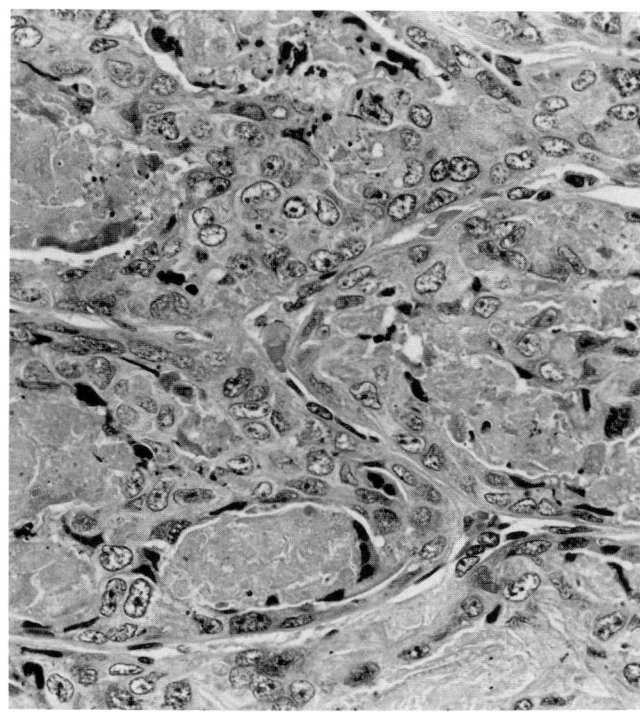

FIG. 24.36. **Epithelioid trophoblastic tumor.** Solitary lung metastasis after chemotherapy for typical dimorphic choriocarcinoma shows a rim of enlarged, mononucleate trophoblast surrounding dense eosinophilic debris. ST is subtle.

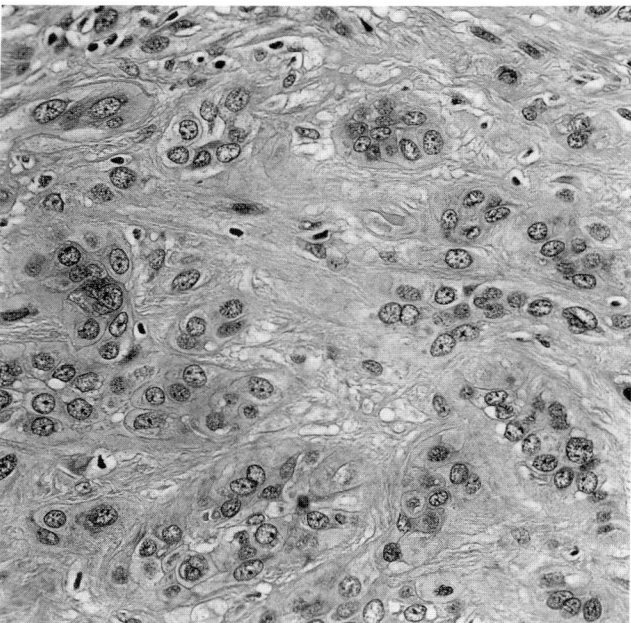

FIG. 24.37. **Epithelioid trophoblastic tumor.** Tumor in uterus shows infiltrating cords and nests of cells surrounded by dense hyaline material. Cells have single nuclei with vesicular chromatin and a moderate amount of finely granular cytoplasm.

ered appropriate.[219] Occasionally, the tumor has been mistaken for a sarcoma.[84,102,188]

CLINICAL FEATURES

Patients are in the reproductive age group and can have either amenorrhea or abnormal bleeding, often accompanied by uterine enlargement.[64,84,135] These women frequently are thought to be pregnant. If progressive uterine enlargement ceases, the diagnosis of a missed abortion is made.[135] The results of pregnancy tests depend on the type of test used, but with a sensitive immunologic assay, they are almost always positive. Rarely, PSTT is associated with virilization.[177,178] The clinical features of PSTT as compared with choriocarcinoma are shown in Table 24.6.

GROSS FINDINGS

The lesion varies from one that is just grossly visible to a diffuse nodular enlargement of the myometrium. Most of the tumors are well circumscribed but sometimes they are ill-defined. The PSTT may be polypoid, projecting into the uterine cavity or predominantly involve the myometrium (Fig. 24.38). The sectioned surface is soft and tan and contains only focal areas of hemorrhage or necrosis. Invasion frequently extends to the uterine serosa and, in rare instances, to the adnexal structures.

MICROSCOPIC FINDINGS

The predominant cell in PSTT is IT.[134,136] Most of the cellular population is monomorphic in contrast to the mixture of cell types in choriocarcinoma (Figs. 24.39–24.42). PSTT also contains scattered syncytiotrophoblastic giant cells. In most cases the ST is a minor component, but occasionally multinucleated ST are present.

Table 24.6. Clinical features of placental site trophoblastic tumor (PSTT) choriocarcinoma

Feature	PSTT	Choriocarcinoma
Clinical presentation	Missed abortion	Persistent GTD after hydatidiform mole
Serum hCG	Low	High
Behavior	Self-limited, persistent, or highly aggressive	Highly aggressive
Response to chemotherapy	Poor	Good
Treatment	Surgery (hysterectomy)	Chemotherapy

GTD, gestational trophoblastic disease; hCG, human chorionic gonadotropin.

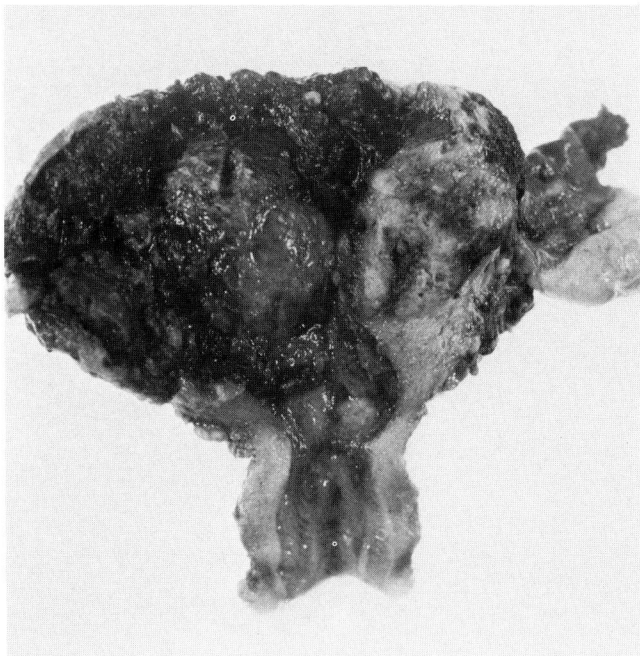

FIG. 24.38. **Placental site trophoblastic tumor.** Opened uterus showing a large, erosive tumor involving most of the fundus with invasion to the serosal surface. The uterus was perforated at curettage.

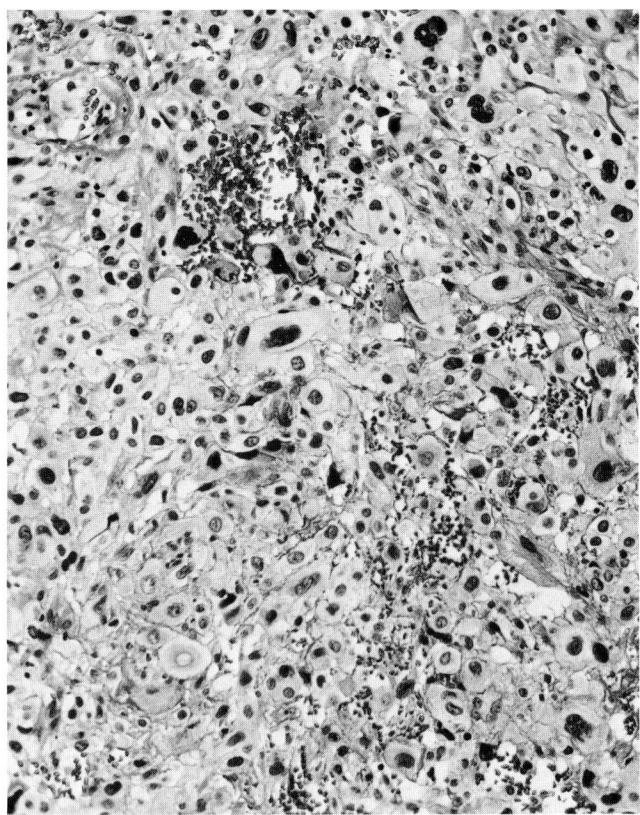

FIG. 24.39. **Placental site trophoblastic tumor.** Sheets of intermediate trophoblast characterized by large polyhedral cells with pleomorphic nuclei. (Reprinted by permission of Kurman et al., ref. 135.)

The IT cells invade singly or in cords and sheets, characteristically separating individual muscle fibers and groups of fibers. Although some tumors appear to cause relatively little tissue destruction, others are associated with extensive necrosis. This is an ominous feature (see below). Many of the intermediate trophoblastic cells assume a spindle shape (Fig. 24.42) and are closely apposed to myometrial cells (Fig. 24.40). The intermediate trophoblastic cells have irregular, hyperchromatic nuclei and dense eosinophilic to amphophilic cytoplasm with occasional vacuoles. As in the normal placental implantation site, abundant extracellular eosinophilic fibrinoid is present in the tumor. The neoplasm has a characteristic form of vascular invasion in which the blood vessel wall is extensively replaced by trophoblastic cells and fibrinoid material, as observed near the placental site (Figs. 24.43, 24.44). Decidua or an Arias–Stella reaction may be present in the adjacent, uninvolved endometrium. Villi are only rarely present.

Rarely a trophoblastic tumor will show histological features of both choriocarcinoma and PSTT, and these are termed *mixed choriocarcinoma and PSTT*. Too few of these mixed cases have been studied to define their clinical behavior. One such case known to us had approximately 50% choriocarcinoma and 50% PSTT in the uterus but a lymph node me-

tastasis showed choriocarcinoma. Extensive lung metastases developed but the serum hCG titer was relatively low. The patient subsequently died of disease.[133]

ULTRASTRUCTURAL FINDINGS

The ultrastructural morphology of IT is best demonstrated in the PSTT, where specific patterns of fine structure have emerged from isolated case reports.[19,63,84,107,251] Intermediate trophoblastic cells are large and have abundant cytoplasm. When they are closely apposed, their cell outlines are polygonal, and they are joined by well-formed desmosomes (Fig. 24.45). Free surfaces show microvilli that are less numerous and more blunt than the microvilli of ST. The cytoplasm of IT is electron-dense and contains numerous organelles, although lacking the overall complexity of ST cytoplasm. Typically, moderate numbers of mitochondria, dilated RER, scattered single strands of RER, and free ribosomes are present. Some cells contain vesicles of smooth endoplasmic reticulum, Golgi complexes, and pools of glycogen. One feature described in most of the reported cases is the presence of large bundles of paranuclear intermediate filaments that are apparently distinctive for IT as compared with ST or CT.

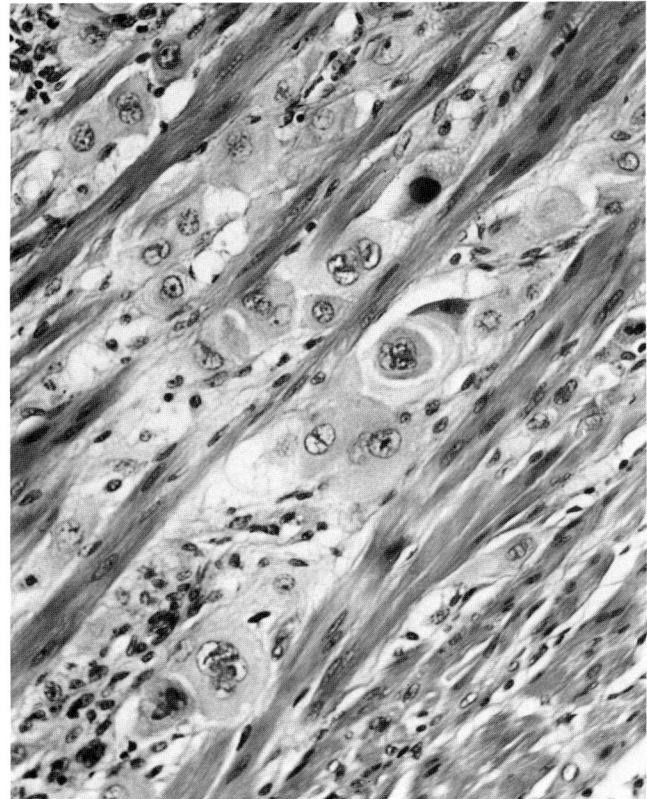

FIG. 24.40. **Placental site trophoblastic tumor.** The intermediate trophoblastic cells characteristically separate muscle bundles as they invade myometrium. (Reprinted by permission of Kurman et al., ref. 135.)

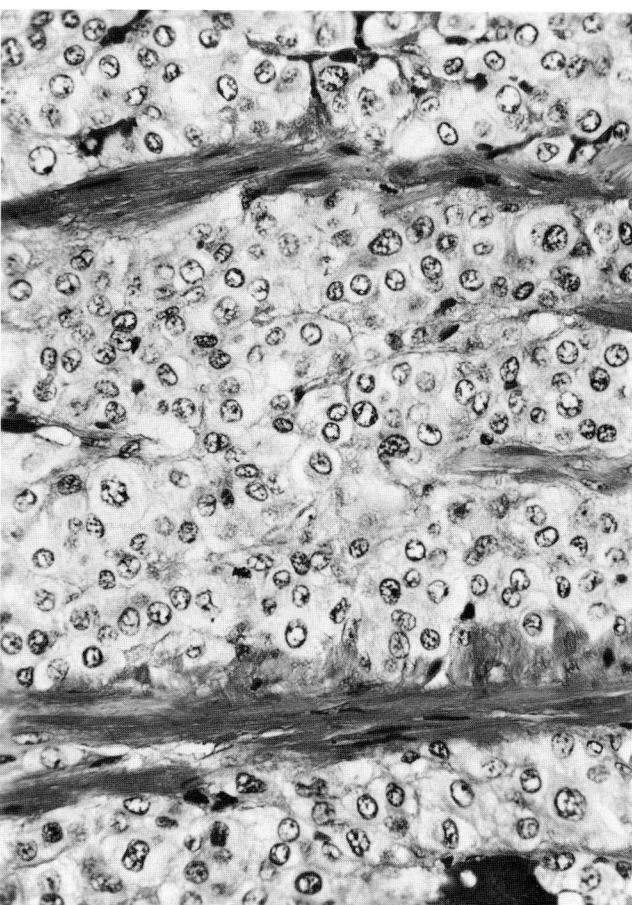

FIG. 24.41. **Placental site trophoblastic tumor.** Tumor is composed of a monomorphic population of intermediate trophoblast in contrast to the mixture of cytotrophoblast, syncytiotrophoblast, and intermediate trophoblast in choriocarcinoma.

DIFFERENTIAL DIAGNOSIS

The PSTT must be distinguished from choriocarcinoma. In contrast to the biphasic cell pattern of choriocarcinoma, PSTT is composed of a relatively monomorphic cell population (Table 24.7). Other neoplasms in the differential diagnosis include sarcomas, especially epithelioid leiomyosarcoma because of the infiltrative pattern within the myometrium, poorly differentiated carcinoma, or even metastatic melanoma because many of the cells have a distinct epithelial appearance. The pattern of prominent blood vessel invasion (Figs. 24.43, 24.44), characteristic myometrial invasion (Fig. 24.40), and extensive deposition of fibrinoid material (Fig. 24.43) are key diagnostic features of PSTT. Immunohistochemical stains for hPL, hCG, and keratin assist in the differential diagnosis.[136] Stains for hPL typically are diffusely positive within PSTT and only focally positive for hCG, whereas the reverse staining pattern is seen in choriocarcinoma (Figs. 24.46–24.49). Localization of hPL and hCG also helps to distinguish this tumor from sarcomas and other malignant tumors (Fig. 24.49). Like all

trophoblastic cells, the IT are epithelial, and therefore immunostains for keratin are intensely positive in PSTT.

The PSTT also must be differentiated from an exaggerated placental site (see below).

CLINICAL BEHAVIOR

These tumors often invade through the myometrium to the serosa, causing perforation.[135] Curettage of the lesion also may result in perforation when there is deep myometrial invasion.[135,251] In several cases, the tumor invaded into the broad ligament and ovary.[64,135] The clinical behavior of PSTT is enigmatic. Despite deep myometrial invasion, most cases of PSTT are self-limited,[19,84,135,178,181,211] some patients being cured by curettage only. Some cases show malignant behavior,[64,65,83,107,219,251] however, and patients have died despite intensive multiagent chemotherapy. There are at least 20 deaths[128] among 90 cases, which corresponds to a mortality rate of about 15–20% since benign cases generally are not reported. The overtly malig-

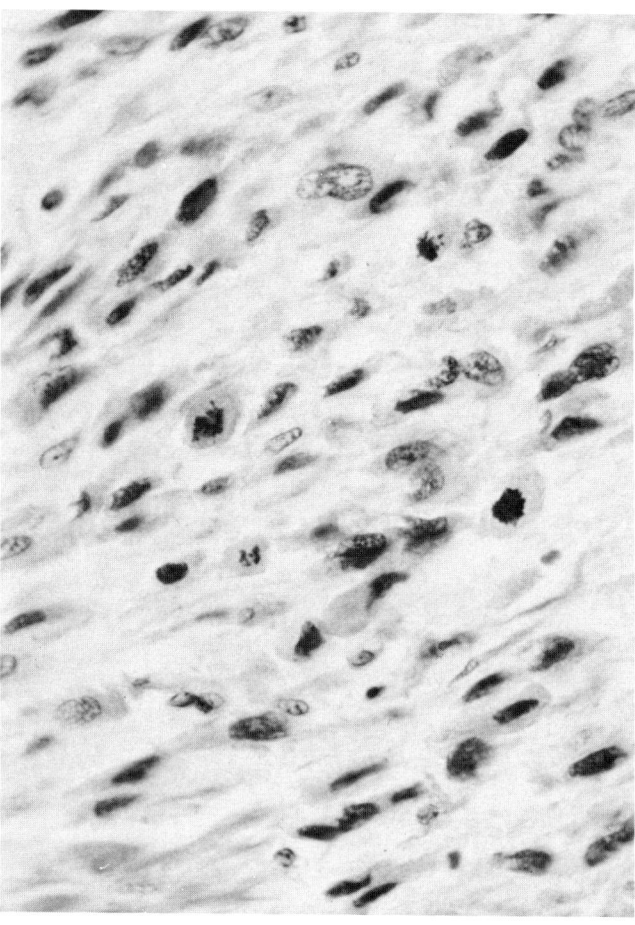

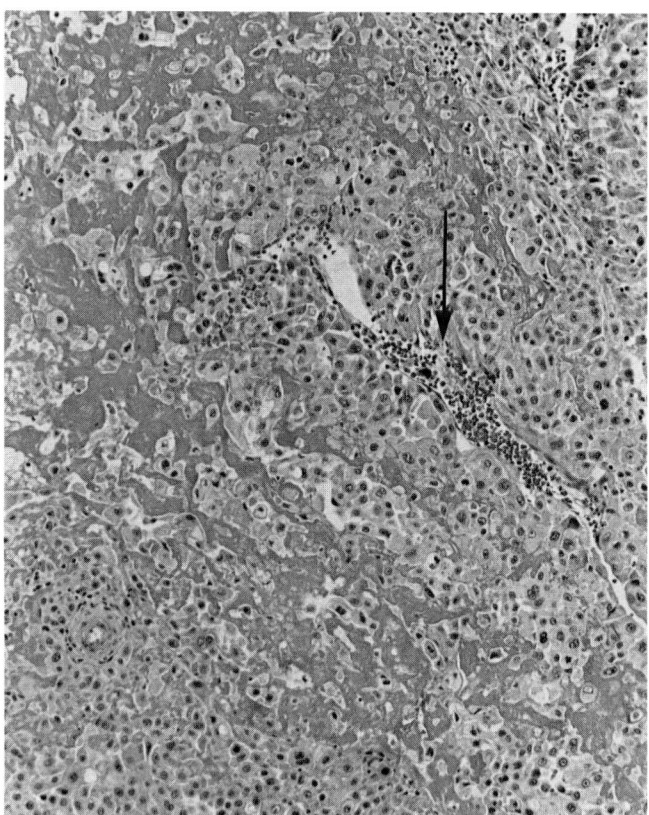

FIG. 24.43. Placental site trophoblastic tumor. Fibrin and intermediate trophoblast replace the wall of a uterine blood vessel. The vessel lumen (*arrow*) still contains red cells.

FIG. 24.42. Placental site trophoblastic tumor. Intermediate trophoblastic cells may assume spindle-shape and may, therefore, be confused with leiomyosarcoma. Four mitotic figures are in center of field. (Reprinted by permission from Kurman et al., ref. 135.)

nant cases have had widely disseminated metastases resembling choriocarcinoma in their distribution with lung, liver, abdominal cavity, and brain involved. Metastases have the same histological appearance as the primary tumor and may develop rapidly after initial diagnosis, but one fatal case recurred 5 years after hysterectomy that was thought to be curative.[83] Generally, metastatic PSTTs have not responded to multiagent chemotherapy[64,65,83,107,251] but, recently, three patients with metastases limited to the lungs apparently have been cured with multiagent chemotherapy.[56,128] Because these tumors are composed of neoplastic IT that contain only small amounts of hCG, the serum levels of hCG are much lower than with choriocarcinoma, which is composed predominantly of CT and ST.

It is difficult to predict with certainty the behavior of PSTTs. Compared with benign cases, malignant PSTTs generally are composed of larger masses and sheets of cells, many with clear instead of amphophilic cytoplasm. They have more extensive necrosis and higher mitotic activity.[219,279] In general, PSTTs with a mitotic rate of 2

mitotic figures (MF) or less/10 high power fields (HPF) have behaved in a benign fashion.[219,279] In two fatal cases, however, the mean mitotic rate was 2 MF/10 HPF[76,83] and in another case in which the patient developed pulmonary metastasis the mitotic count was 0.4 MF/10 HPF.[128] The latter patient was cured with multiagent chemotherapy. Abnormal mitotic figures can be found in benign or malignant tumors. Flow cytometric DNA analysis of six cases of PSTT revealed a diploid DNA stemline with S-phase fractions ranging from 6% to 19% and one case that was tetraploid.[76,131] In summary, at the present time there are no reliable histological, immunohistochemical, or DNA ploidy features that predict prognosis.

An apparently unique form of renal disease has occurred in a few patients with PSTT.[64,280] These patients had severe proteinuria and, in one patient, hematuria. These women were thought to have the nephrotic syndrome. Renal biopsies showed glomerular lesions with prominent eosinophilic deposits in the capillary lumens that stained for fibrinogen and IgM. This lesion has been found in 3 and possibly 4 of more than 90 patients with PSTT, suggesting that the lesion is specific and not fortuitous.[280] However, its pathogenesis in unknown. Nephrotic syndrome is not observed in association with other forms of GTD.[9]

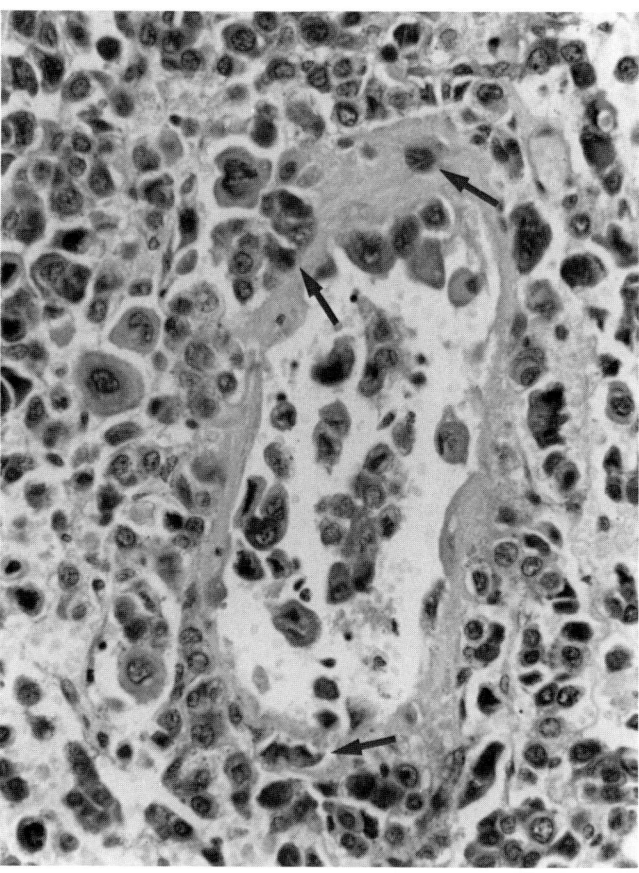

FIG. 24.44. Placental site trophoblastic tumor. Vascular invasion by intermediate trophoblast resembles that of the normal inplantation site (compare with Fig. 24.20). The neoplastic cells surround and invade (*arrows*) a blood vessel, extending into the vascular lumen. The vessel wall has been replaced by fibrin. The tissue is immunostained for hPL, and all the neoplastic cells in this field contain hPL. (Reprinted by permission of Kurman et al., ref. 136).

Unclassified Trophoblastic Lesions

The term unclassified trophoblastic lesion is reserved for those unusual cases that cannot be placed clearly in one of the defined subgroups of GTD or suspected GTD.

Nonneoplastic Trophoblastic Lesions

Exaggerated Placental Site

This lesion is an exuberant infiltration of the endometrium and myometrium at the implantation site by trophoblastic cells most of which are IT and syncytial trophoblastic giant cells (Fig. 24.50).[222] In the past the lesion has been termed *syncytial endometritis*, but this designation is no longer used since the process is neither inflammatory, confined to the endometrium, or composed mainly of ST (Fig. 24.51). The exaggerated placental site can occur in normal pregnancy or an abortion and is invariably associated with all types of hydatidiform mole. Despite the extensive infiltration by trophoblastic cells, the overall architecture of the placental site is not disturbed. Endometrial glands and spiral arteries may be surrounded by trophoblasts but there is no necrosis. Generally, the nuclei of the intermediate trophoblastic cells are hyperchromatic and irregular in size and shape. Mitotic activity is absent or rare. This is physiologic process that resolved spontaneously after pregnancy.

Distinction of an exaggerated placental site from a PSTT in curettings at times can be difficult. In the placental site the intermediate trophoblastic cells do not form confluent masses, there is no necrosis, and there is little or no mitotic activity. In addition, other components associated with pregnancy, including decidua, villi, thickened spiral arteries, CT, and ST will be present in normal implantations but not in PSTT.

Placental Site Nodule

Placental site nodules are small, localized, circumscribed aggregates of intermediate trophoblast that may be found in uterine curettings or hysterectomy specimens.[278] They also are known as *hyalinized implantation sites*, and they have been mistakenly called decidua in the past. In reported cases patients range in age from 20 to 47 years with their last gestational event ranging from 6 to 108 months before diagnosis.[111] The lesions usually are microscopic abnormalities found at curettage performed for abnormal bleeding, and they often are admixed with proliferative or secretory endometrium. They represent benign retention of small areas of placental implantation site from remote gestations. An inordinate number of cases have occurred several years after tubal ligation, suggesting that there may be more than a coincidental association. The nodules and plaques are circumscribed, microscopic foci of hyalin material that contain intermediate trophoblast (Fig. 24.52). Often these nodules have a thin rim of chronic inflammatory cells. The IT in the placental site nodule appear degenerate; their nuclei have granular chromatin and they lack defined cytoplasmic borders (Fig. 24.53). The cells react with antibodies against keratin, epithelial membrane antigen (EMA), pregnancy-specific SP-1, and placental alkaline phosphatase (PLAP), which can assist in their diagnosis.[111,220] Their microscopic size, circumscription, and extensive hyalinization are features that separate them from PSTT.

Gestational Trophoblastic Disease at Ectopic Sites

Hydatidiform mole, choriocarcioma, and PSTT rarely arise at ectopic sites, since GTD can arise wherever a gestation implants. Hydatidiform mole may occur in the fallopian tube[88,267] and ovary.[119,225] Primary mole of the adnexa should be discriminated from the hydropic change that is

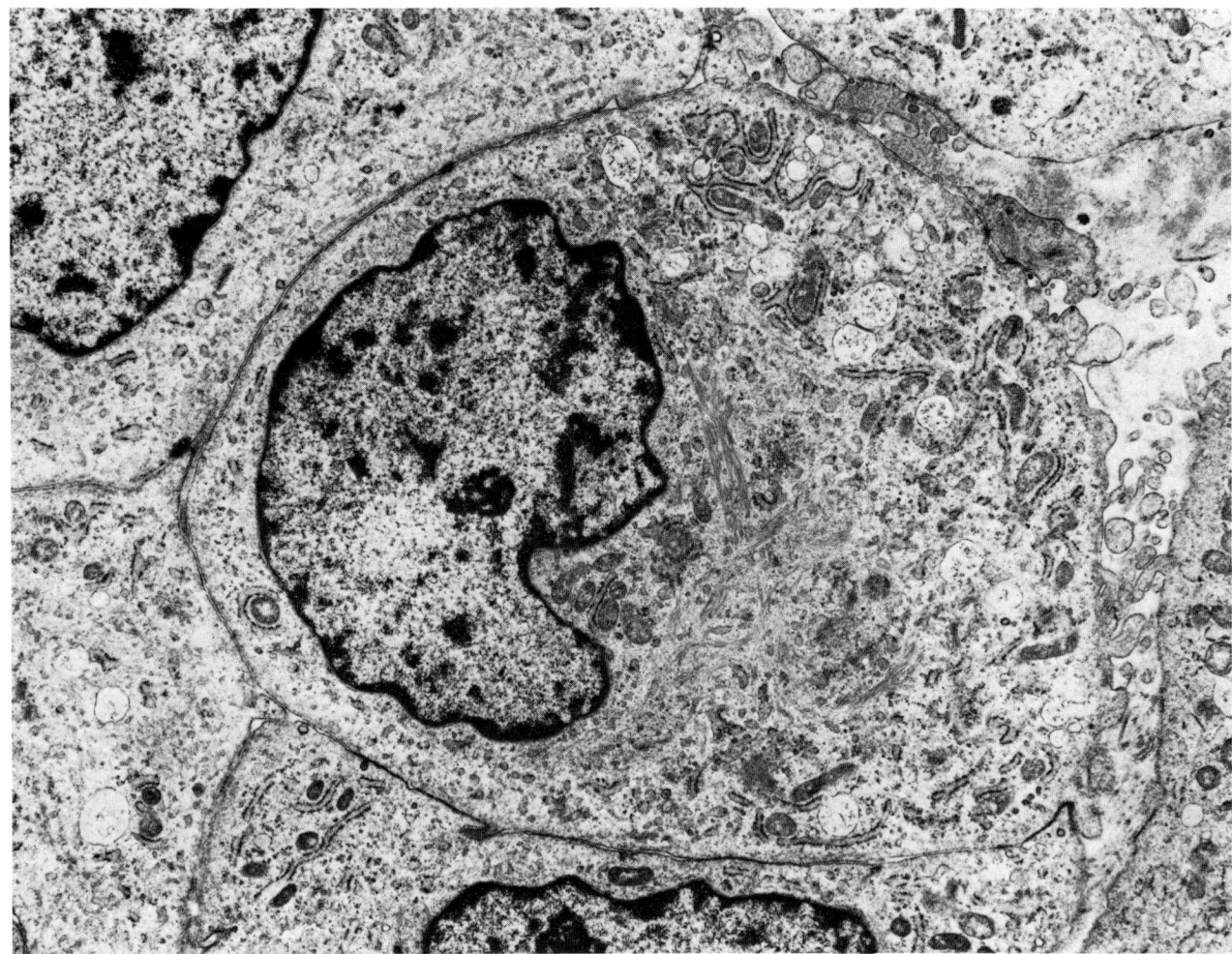

Fig. 24.45. Electron micrograph of intermediate trophoblast. The cells have abundant cytoplasm containing RER, mitochondria, and perinuclear filament bundles. The cell surface to the right contains blunt microvilli. ×6000.

Table 24.7. Pathological features of placental site trophoblastic tumor (PSTT) and choriocarcinoma

Feature	PSTT	Choriocarcinoma
Cellular population	Monomorphic; intermediate trophoblastic	Dimorphic; mainly cytotrophoblast and syncytiotrophoblast
Margin	Infiltrating	Circumscribed
Hemorrhage	Focal and haphazard	Massive and central
Vascular invasion	From periphery to lumen	From lumen to periphery
Fibrinoid change	Present	Absent
Immunocytochemistry		
hCG	+	++++
hPL	++++	+

hCG, human chorionic gonadotropin; hPL, human placental lactogen.

frequent in aborting ectopic pregnancy and from invasive mole with extension to the broad ligament.

Gestational choriocarcinoma also may be primary in the fallopian tube,[127,190,199] and in this instance, the tumor probably is a sequela to an ectopic pregnancy.[157] These tumors usually cause symptoms suggesting an ectopic pregnancy or appear as an adnexal mass that mimics an ovarian tumor.[190] With proper diagnosis and therapy, survival rates are similar to those of choriocarcinoma arising from an intrauterine gestation. Primary gestational choriocarcinoma of the ovary is difficult to document but does occur.[18,43,199,260] Most examples of ovarian choriocarcinoma represent metastases from uterine primaries or are germ cell tumors.[6,82,255] In primary germ cell tumors, sufficient sampling often reveals other germ cell elements, thus establishing a diagnosis of mixed germ cell tumor.

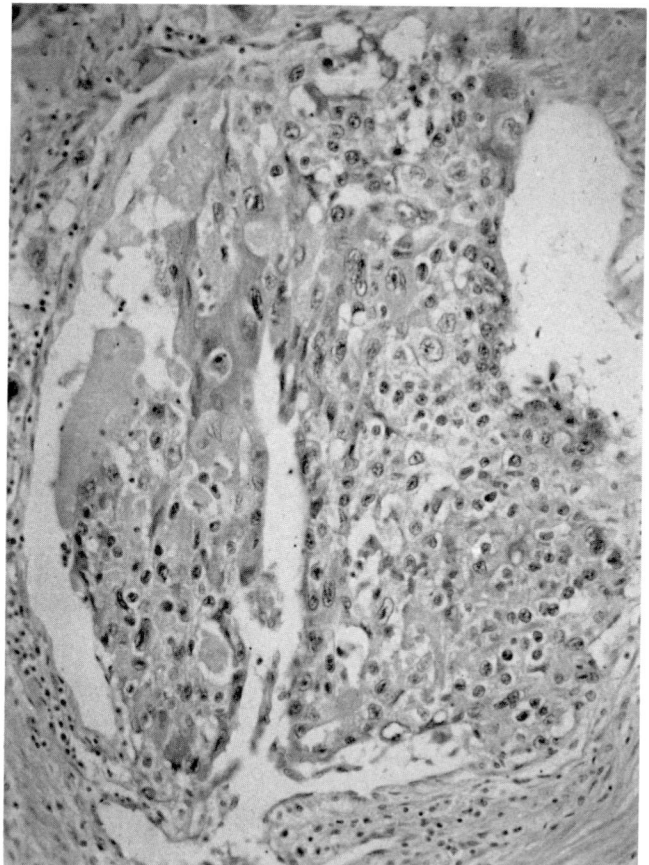
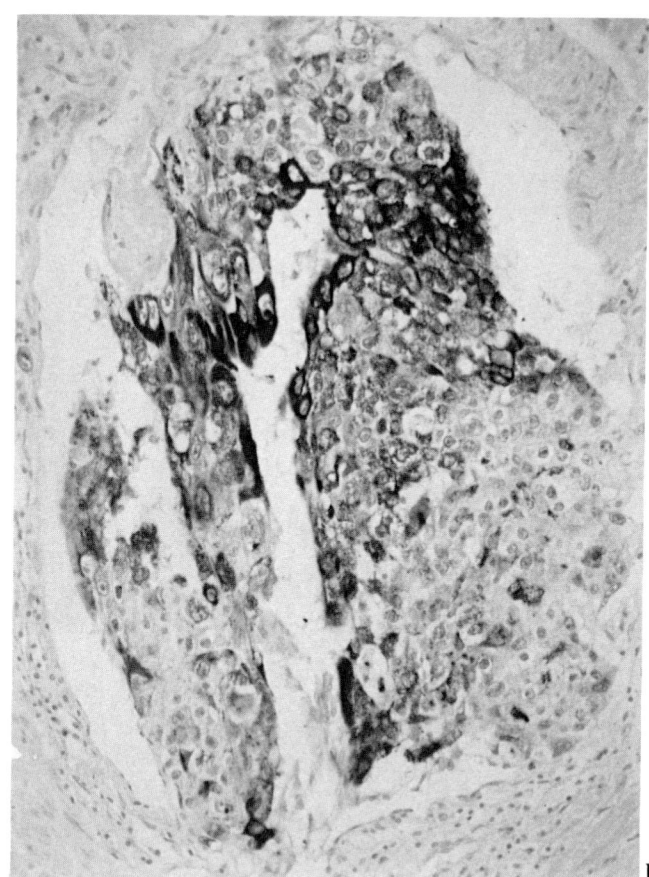

FIG. 24.46. **Choriocarcinoma. a:** No staining for hPL. **b:** Diffuse staining for hCG in syncytiotrophoblast. Compare with Figs. 24.48 and 24.49. (Reprinted by permission of Kurman et al., ref. 136.)

When pure choriocarcinoma is present in the ovary, the principles of hCG monitoring and chemotherapy remain the same whether it is a gestational or germ cell neoplasm.[6,82]

Choriocarcinoma has been described as a primary tumor arising in a number of different sites besides the uterus and gonads.[99,165] In women of reproductive age, however, pure choriocarcinoma that appears to be an extrauterine primary tumor probably represents gestational choriocarcinoma in which the index pregnancy was undetected. True primary choriocarcinoma at an unusual site may be an extragonadal germ cell tumor, or it may be derived from dedifferentiation of an ordinary carcinoma.[77,274] Primary somatic tumors of the gastrointestinal tract, bladder, breast, lung, or endometrium rarely show choriocarcinomatous differentiation, and these show transitions from ordinary carcinoma to the trophoblastic component.° Since somatic tumors also may produce hCG without showing choriocarcinoma histology,[100,106] the classic biphasic growth pattern of should be present before accepting the diagnosis of choriocarcinoma.

°Refs. 37,77,89,171,202,204,215,274.

Although PSTT is a rare neoplasm even in the uterus, we are aware of one case that occurred in the groin after a cesarean section for a full-term infant. After biopsy the mass disappeared spontaneously.[133] In another case a small periurethral vaginal mass was excised at the time of delivery of a full-term infant. In this patient the lesion did not recur and the hCG levels rapidly fell to normal after delivery. These cases may represent deported benign intermediate trophoblast rather than a true neoplasm, but more cases must be identified and studied to determine the significance of these lesions.

Management

Chorionic Gonadotropin and Other Tumor Markers

In GTD, hCG has proved to be an ideal tumor marker and a prototype for all other tumor markers. Produced mainly by ST,[136] it is almost invariably present when trophoblastic tissue exists, and it can be measured at extremely low levels in the serum. For these reasons, its presence or absence is

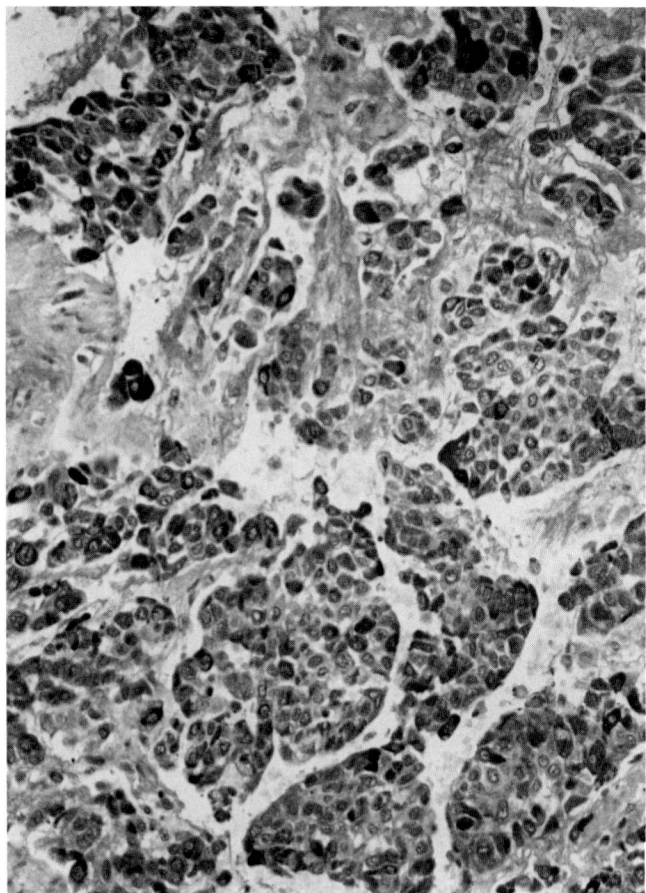

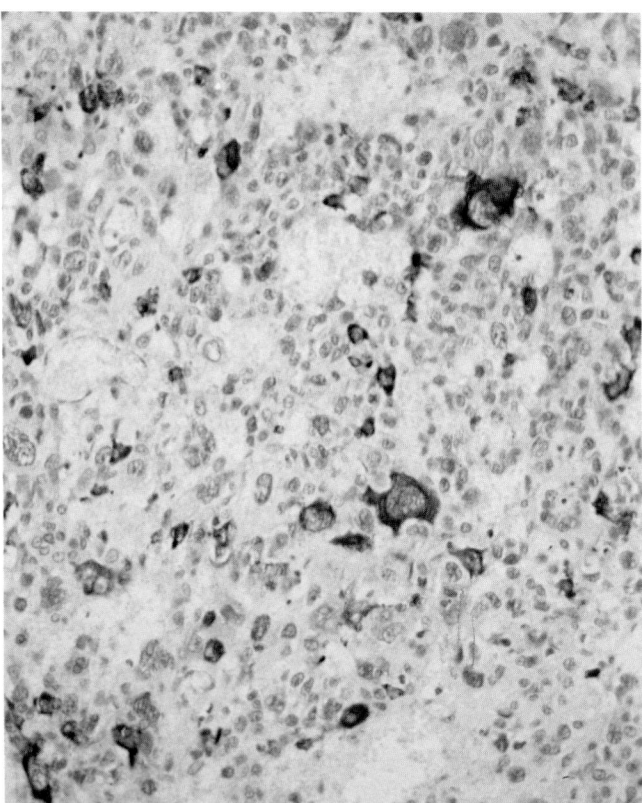

FIG. 24.48. Placental site trophoblastic tumor. Focal staining for hCG.

FIG. 24.47. Placental site trophoblastic tumor. Diffuse staining for hPL.

a critical factor in the diagnosis, follow-up, and therapy of GTD.

Human chorionic gonadotropin is a glycoprotein composed of two polypeptide chains, alpha and beta, attached to a carbohydrate moiety. There is a high content of sialic acid in the molecule.[86,212] The configuration of hCG is similar to other gonadotropins, particularly luteinizing hormone (LH). The alpha-polypeptide chain in all these hormones is identical; it is the difference in the beta chain that gives the hormones their unique immunologic specificity and biologic function.

In normal pregnancy, hCG reaches a peak level of 50,000–100,000 mIU/ml at about 10 weeks' gestation and decreases to 10,000–20,000 mIU/ml by 20 weeks, remaining at that level until term.[28,53] Levels as high as 600,000 mIU/ml in early pregnancy have been reported.[53] In molar gestations, hCG levels at diagnosis are variable, but most show a markedly elevated hCG titer, which is a useful diagnostic feature.[34,53] Levels greater tha 2 million mIU/ml have been reported. Markedly elevated hCG titers are more common in complete as compared with partial molar pregnancies.[45,223,239]

It has been possible to assess the presence of hCG qual-

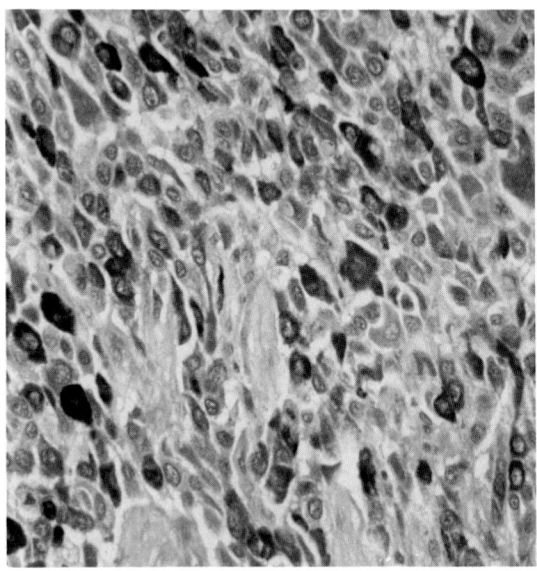

FIG. 24.49. Placental site trophoblastic tumor. The intermediate trophoblastic cells are spindle-shaped. The diffuse staining for hPL (*gray and black intracytoplasmic deposit*) is useful in distinguishing the tumor from a sarcoma, which is negative. (Reprinted by permission of Kurman et al., ref. 136.)

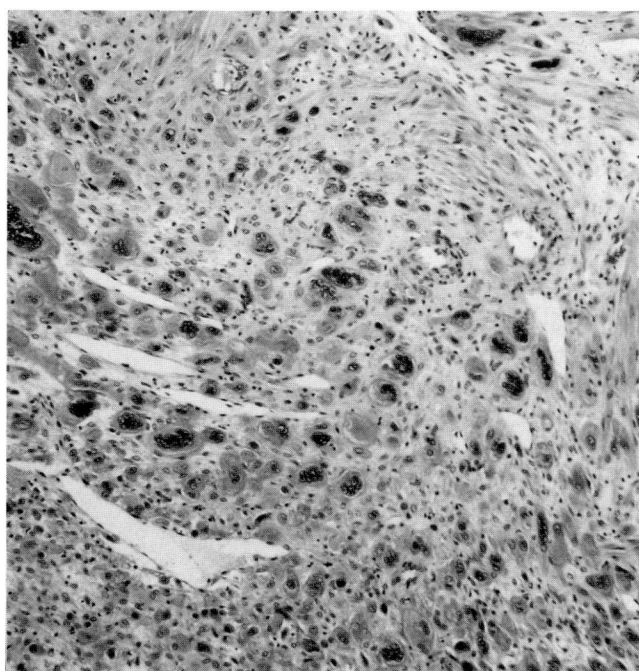

FIG. 24.50. **Exaggerated placental implantation site.** Numerous IT and syncytial trophoblastic giant cells infiltrate decidua and myometrium. The trophoblastic cells are widely spaced, lacking confluent growth or necrosis.

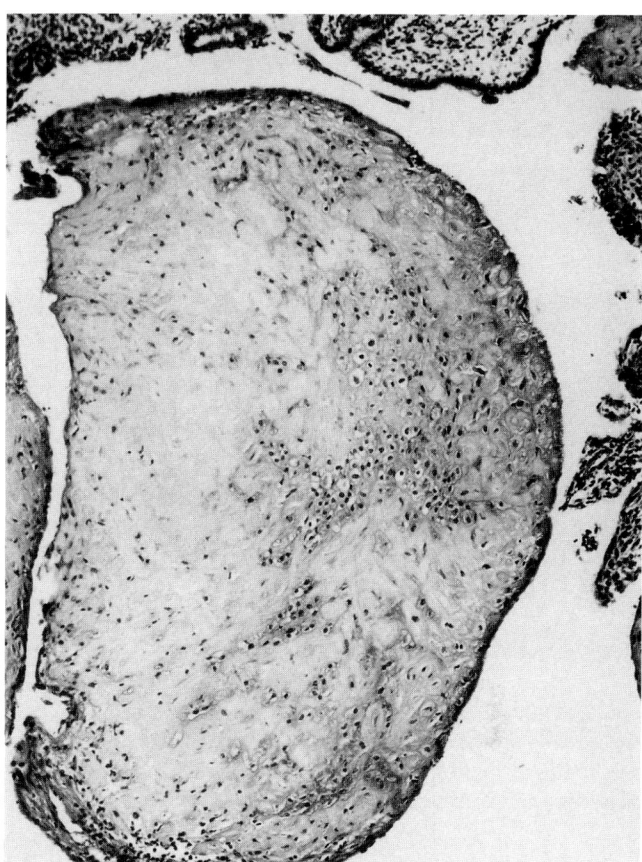

FIG. 24.52. **Placental site nodule.** The nodule is composed of hyalin material that contains scattered IT. The remainder of the endometrium had a proliferative phase pattern. (Reprinted by permission of Silverberg and Kurman, ref. 222.)

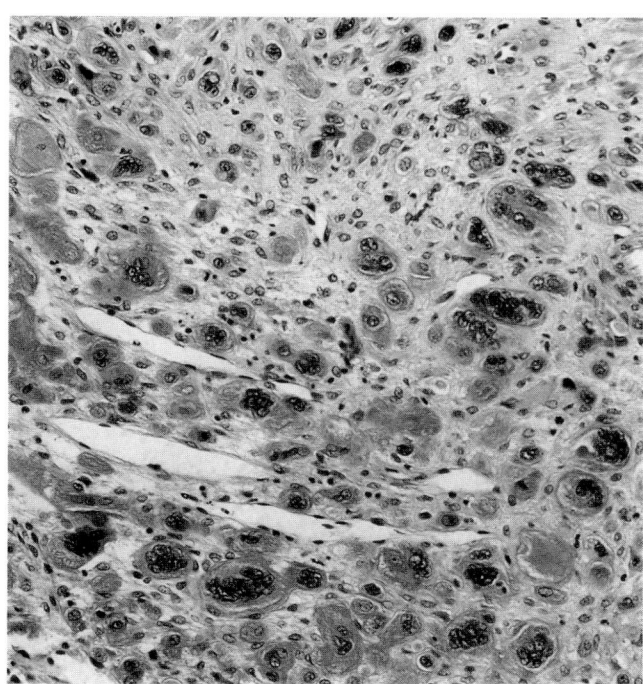

FIG. 24.51. **Exaggerated placental site.** Mixture of IT and multinucleated trophoblast. The cells show no mitotic activity.

itatively and semiquantitatively for many years using bioassays[35,36,53] and immunoassays.[86,144] These methods were sufficient to detect hCG at higher concentrations but lacked sensitivity to detect hCG at lower concentrations and were not specific, measuring LH as well. The development of the radioimmunoassay (RIA) lowered the sensitivity to the normal level of LH but still did not discriminate between LH and hCG.[13]

A RIA for the beta-subunit of hCG was developed in 1972,[252] which was sufficiently sensitive and specific to permit follow-up to complete disappearance of trophoblastic tissue. Disappearance of hCG from the serum as measured by half-life shows two components, one with a half-life of 6 hours and a slower component with a half-life of about 30 hours.[207,212] With the serum RIA for beta-hCG, it is possible to measure hCG to a level of 1.6–5 mIU/ml, depending on the lowest level of sensitivity measured in the laboratory performing the test. Normally, the values do not reach zero. The assay is sufficiently sensitive to determine hCG production from as few as 1000 trophoblast cells.[86] Rarely, however, choriocarcinoma may be associ-

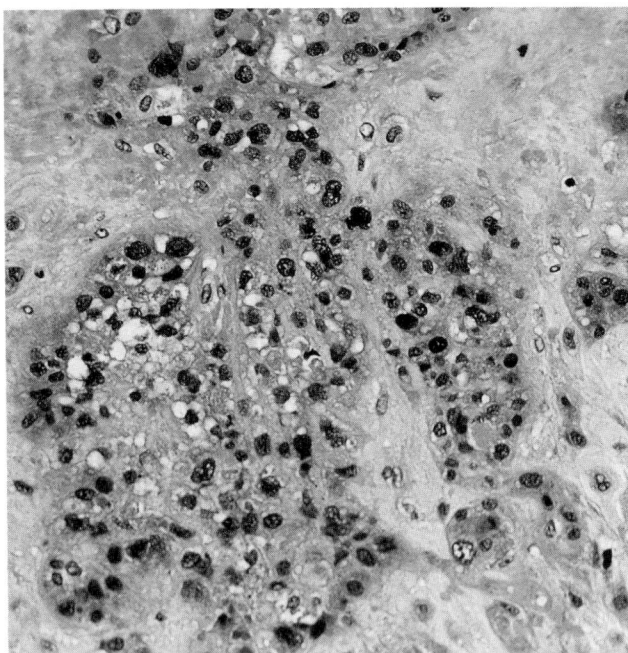

FIG. 24.53. **Placental site nodule.** Intermediate trophoblast appear degenerate with smudged nuclei and indistinct cell borders. Mitotic figures are absent. (Reprinted by permission of Silverberg and Kurman, ref. 222.)

Table 24.8. International Federation of Gynecology and Obstetrics (FIGO) staging of gestational trophoblastic disease

Stage	Definition
I	Confined to uterine corpus
II	Metastases to pelvis and vagina
III	Metastases to lung
IV	Distant metastases

ated plasma protein-A (PAPP-A), appear to offer no advantages over monitoring hCG.[108,112]

Staging and Prognostic Factors

The International Federation of Gynecology and Obstetrics (FIGO) uses an anatomic staging system for GTD (Table 24.8). Recognition of important prognostic factors has led to a clinical classification of GTD that is useful in predicting outcome of an individual case (Table 24.9). Four factors are especially important for determining successful therapy of GTD: (1) level of hCG elevation before therapy, (2) duration of disease before initiation of chemotherapy, (3) absence of CNS and hepatic metastases, and (4) proper administration of chemotherapy.

Further studies have shown that in a carefully managed program of care for patients with GTD, the only patients who have died had a clinicopathological diagnosis of choriocarcinoma. In addition to the diagnosis of choriocarcinoma, poor prognostic factors include advanced disease at diagnosis, cerebral or hepatic metastases, symptoms of the disease for more than 4 months, failure of prior chemotherapy, and a pretreatment serum beta-hCG titer of more than 100,000 mIU/ml.[8,62,94,147,152,174] More recently, the critical hCG level has been reduced to 40,000 mIU/ml by some investigators.[232,233,265] Metastatic disease limited to the lungs or vagina is not a poor prognostic sign. In contrast, although it is difficult to assess precisely the prognostic significance of extrapulmonary metastases, patients with CNS metastases have an approximately 50% remission rate compared with other visceral organs.[4,10,266] Development of CNS metastases during the course of treatment has an even worse prognosis.[4,10,154] Patients with hepatic metastases also have a poor prognosis,[16] but multiagent chemotherapy appears to increase the survival rate.[270]

Choriocarcinoma after term gestation has a generally worse prognosis than that after a mole. These patients have lower cure rates than other poor prognosis patients, the decreased survival attributed to delay in treatment and metastases beyond the lungs and vagina.[23,170,192]

Multivariate analysis using these various prognostic factors helps to predict the outcome of GTD.[156] Several different scoring systems for prognosis have evolved, and the WHO scoring system has received the greatest acceptance (Table 24.10).

ated with undetectable levels of hCG.[146] Cerebral spinal fluid also can be assayed for the presence of hCG in patients at risk of central nervous system (CNS) involvement by choriocarcinoma. A serum to cerebral spinal fluid ratio of less than 60 usually is suggestive but not diagnostic of CNS metastases.[10,25,224]

Measurement of other pregnancy-specific proteins in conjunction with hCG may be useful in the follow-up of patients with GTD. Measurement of the alpha-hCG subunit helps identify patients at risk of recurrences after successful initial chemotherapy.[203] Human placental lactogen has a rapid half-life and, therefore, may be undetectable in the serum despite the presence of metastases.[108] Goldstein reported that hPL levels are inversely correlated with the histological grade of hydatidiform moles, suggesting that patients with low hPL levels along with high hCG levels represents a high-risk group.[85] Furthermore, since most cells in the PSTT contain hPL, as compared with hCG, hPL may be useful as a marker for this neoplasm.[136]

Pregnancy-specific SP-1 often is present in GTD.[108,241] This protein is less sensitive than hCG in monitoring GTD, but in a few patients with recurrent disease, elevated levels of SP-1 have been present when hCG was undetectable.[241] It also is suggested that the ratio between SP-1 and beta-hCG may reflect the degree of differentiation of trophoblastic cells, lower levels being found in choriocarcinoma than in hydatidiform mole.[108,186,213] Other markers, including placental protein 5 (PP5) and pregnancy-associ-

Table 24.9. Clinical classification of malignant trophoblastic disease

Nonmetastatic GTD
Metastatic GTD
  Good prognosis
    Low hCG level (<40,000 mIU/ml serum β-hCG)
    Symptoms present for less than 4 months
    No brain or liver metastases
    No prior chemotherapy
    Pregnancy event is not term delivery (i.e., mole, ectopic, or spontaneous abortion)
  Poor prognosis
    High pretreatment hCG level (>40,000 mIU/ml serum β-hCG)
    Symptoms present for over 4 months
    Brain or liver metastases
    Prior chemotherapeutic failure
    Antecedent term pregnancy

GTD, gestational trophoblastic disease; hCG, human chorionic gonadotropin.

Treatment

The basic principles of treatment of GTD include identifying, when possible, the specific histological type of GTD, monitoring serum hCG titers, and instituting chemotherapy when appropriate.[44,96,148] Molar pregnancy, complete or partial, generally is treated first by suction curettage of the uterus. In patients in whom preservation of fertility is not a consideration, abdominal hysterectomy is an effective alternative initial treatment of molar pregnancy, but careful follow-up is mandatory.[86] Regardless of the initial method of removal of the hydatidiform mole, a chest radiograph before treatment and 4 weeks later should be performed to exclude metastases.

In the follow-up of GTD, serial hCG titers are mandatory until titers fall and remain within the normal range.[22,155] A typical regimen for follow-up of a molar pregnancy is a baseline hCG level within 48 hours of evacuation and weekly hCG titers until the levels fall to normal. A plateau or rise in titers can be the first sign of persistent GTD. The titers should fall to normal between 10 and 170 days after evacuation of a mole, and most patients will have normal titers by 60 days postevacuation.[155] After hCG levels reach normal values, monthly assays are performed for 6 months, and pregnancy must be avoided.[86,155] If the values remain normal, chances of recurrence are slight. Occasional late recurrences of GTD more than 1 year after therapy have been reported, however.[121,234,257]

Persistent GTD after molar pregnancy is heralded by plateauing hCG titers for 2–4 weeks, rising hCG titers, persistent uterine disease, or evidence of metastases.[86,129] Depending on clinical criteria for treatment, between 8% and 30% of patients with mole who are carefully followed require therapy.[13,35,36,44,155,179] Either invasive mole or choriocarcinoma may be present, but in the absence of histological confirmation, the disorder is regarded clinically as post–molar GTD. When disease appears confined to the uterus, hysterectomy may be curative in patients who do not wish to preserve fertility. All other patients with persistent or metastatic GTD after moles require chemotherapy. In addition, hCG monitoring is necessary until titers fall to normal whether patients are treated surgically or medically. Thereafter, titers are followed weekly for 3 consecutive weeks and then monthly for at least 12 months to ensure no recurrence.[86] Contraception is necessary during the entire follow-up period.

Methotrexate, a folic acid antagonist, was the first drug used successfully in the therapy of choriocarcinoma.[105,149] Subsequently, numerous other chemotherapeutic agents have been used, especially dactinomycin and an alkylating agent (cyclophosphamide or chlorambucil).[152] Initial therapy for persistent disease after a molar pregnancy usually consists of methotrexate or dactinomycin or a combination of the two.[86,154] Some patients with high-risk GTD (see

Table 24.10. World Health Organization scoring system based on prognostic factors[a]

Prognostic factors	Score			
	0	1	2	4
Age (years)	≤39	>39		
Antecedent pregnancy	Mole	Abortion	Term	
Interval[b]	4	4–6	7–12	>12
hCG (IU/L)	<10³	10³–10⁴	10⁴–10⁵	>10⁵
ABO groups (female × male)		O × A	B	
		A × O	AB	
Largest tumor (including uterine tumor)		3–5 cm	>5 cm	
Site of metastases		Spleen, kidney	GI tract, liver	Brain
No. of metastases identified		1–4	4–8	>8
Prior chemotherapy			Single drug	2 or more drugs

[a] The total score for a patient is obtained by adding the individual scores for each prognostic factor. Total score ≤4, low risk; 5–7, middle risk; and ≥8, high risk.
[b] Interval time (months) between end of antecedent pregnancy and start of chemotherapy.
hCG, human chorionic gonadotropin; GI tract, gastrointestinal tract.

above, Staging) are treated with a combination of dactino-mycin, methotrexate, and an alkylating agent (MAC).[154] Triple-agent therapy is not adequate for treating patients with metastases and a high-risk score, however. Therefore, multiagent chemotherapy programs that include etoposide (VP-16) have been developed[7,180,216] that offer an increased rate of sustained remissions for very high-risk patients and for those who have not benefited from other conventional forms of chemotherapy.[233,265]

GTD without a preceding molar pregnancy represents choriocarcinoma or, rarely, PSTT. The principles of management of choriocarcinoma are similar to those for GTD after hydatidiform mole; hCG monitoring and chemotherapy are essential.[32,154] Hysterectomy can reduce hospitalization and the amount of chemotherapy needed to induce remission.[97] Resection of pulmonary metastases may have therapeutic value in patients with persistent but limited pulmonary disease, if there is no evidence of tumor at other sites and the hCG titer is low.[122,244] When the histology reveals the pattern of a postchemotherapy choriocarcinoma (see above, Epithelioid Trophoblastic Tumor), the prognosis is especially favorable.[122,166] Irradiation combined with chemotherapy will give a 50% remission rate for cerebral metastases,[4,266] but irradiation to other sites generally is not useful.[154]

Once the diagnosis of a PSTT is established microscopically, continued close surveillance with frequent serologic measurements of the hCG level using an RIA specific for the beta-subunit is essential. Curettage may be therapeutic, but if uterine disease persists, as evidenced by persistently elevated serum hCG levels, hysterectomy is indicated to remove the tumor.[135,279] Limited experience with clinically malignant tumors suggests that they may secrete relatively low levels of hCG and are not as responsive to the usual chemotherapeutic agents that have proved successful with other forms of trophoblastic disease.[219] Immunocytochemical staining in some of the aggressive tumors has shown a reversal of the usual hPL/hCG ratio, with hCG predominating,[136,282] suggesting that serum measurement of hPL along with hCG may prove to be valuable in monitoring these tumors. However, more cases must be studied.

References

1. Acosta-Sison H (1960) Chorioadenoma destruens. A report of 41 cases. Am J Obstet Gynecol 80: 176
2. Amir SM, Osathanondh R, Berkowitz RS, Goldstein DP (1984) Human chorionic gonadotropin and thyroid function in patients with hydatidiform mole. Am J Obstet Gynecol 150: 723
3. Aozasa K, Ito H, Kohro T, Ha K, et al (1981) Choriocarcinoma in infant and mother. Acta Pathol Jpn 31: 317–322
4. Athanassiou A, Begent RHJ, Newlands ES, Parker D, et al (1983) Central nervous system metastases of choriocarcinoma. Cancer 52: 1728–1735

5. Atrash HK, Hogue CJR, Grimes DA (1986) Epidemiology of hydatidiform mole during early gestation. Am J Obstet Gynecol 154: 906
6. Axe SR, Klein VR, Woodruff JD (1985) Choriocarcinoma of the ovary. Obstet Gynecol 66: 111–114
7. Bagshawe KD (1976) Treatment of trophoblastic tumors. Ann Acac Med 5: 273
8. Bagshawe KD (1976) Risk and prognostic factors in trophoblastic neoplasia. Cancer 38: 1373–1385
9. Bagshawe KD (1992) Personal communication.
10. Bagshawe KD, Harland S (1976) Immunodiagnosis and monitoring of gonadotrophin-producing metastases in the central nervous system. Cancer 38: 112–118
11. Bagshawe KD, Lawler SD (1982) Unmasking moles. Br J Obstet Gynaecol 89: 255
12. Bagshawe KD, Rawlins GJ, Pike MC, Lawler SD (1971) ABO blood groups in trophoblastic neoplasia. Lancet 1: 553–557
13. Bagshawe KD, Wilson H, Dublon P, Smith A, et al (1973) Follow-up after hydatidiform mole: Studies using radioimmunoassay for urinary human chorionic gonadotrophin (hCG). J Obstet Gynaecol Br Commonw 80: 461–468
14. Baltazar JC (1976) Epidemiological features of choriocarcinoma. Bull WHO 54: 523–532
15. Bandy LC, Clarke-Pearson DL, Hammond CB (1984) Malignant potential of gestational trophoblastic disease at the extreme ages of reproductive life. Obstet Gynecol 64: 395
16. Barnard DE, Woodward KT, Yancy SG, Weed JC, et al (1986) Hepatic metastases of choriocarcinoma: A report of 15 patients. Gynecol Oncol 25: 73
17. Beischer NA, Fortune DW (1968) Significance of chromatin patterns in cases of hydatidiform mole with an associated fetus. Am J Obstet Gynecol 100: 276
18. Benjamin F, Rorat E (1978) Primary gestational choriocarcinoma of the ovary. Am J Obstet Gynecol 131: 343–345
19. Berger V, Verbaere J, Feroldi J (1984) Placental site trophoblastic tumor of the uterus: An ultrastructural and immunohistochemical study. Ultrastruct Pathol 6: 319–329
20. Berkowitz RS, Cramer DW, Bernstein MR, Cassells S, et al (1985) Risk factors for complete molar pregnancy from a case-control study. Am J Obstet Gynecol 152: 1016
21. Berkowitz RS, Goldstein DP (1981) Pathogenesis of gestational trophoblastic neoplasms. Pathobiol Annu 11: 391–411
22. Berkowitz RS, Goldstein DP (1988) Diagnosis and management of primary hydatidiform mole. Obstet Gynecol Clin North Am 15: 491–503
23. Berkowitz RS, Goldstein DP, Bernstein MR (1984) Choriocarcinoma following term gestation. Gynecol Oncol 17: 52–57
24. Berkowitz RS, Goldstein DP, Bernstein MR (1985) Natural history of partial molar pregnancy. Obstet Gynecol 66: 677–681
25. Berkowitz RS, Osathanondh R, Goldstein DP, Martin PM, et al (1981) Cerebrospinal fluid human chorionic gonadotropin levels in normal pregnancy and choriocarcinoma. Surg Gynecol Obstet 153: 687–689
26. Block MF, Merrill JA (1982) Hydatidiform mole with coexistent fetus. Obstet Gynecol 60: 130

27. Bracken MB, Brinton LA, Hayashi K (1984) Epidemiology of hydatidiform mole and choriocarcinoma. Epidemiol Rev 6: 52–75

28. Braunstein GD, Rasor J, Adler D, Danzer H, et al (1976) Serum human chorionic gonadotropin levels throughout normal pregnancy. Am J Obstet Gynecol 126: 678

29. Brescia RJ, Kurman RJ, Main C, Surti U, et al (1987) Immunocytochemical localization of chorionic gonadotropin, placental lactogen, and placental alkaline phosphatase in the diagnosis of complete and partial hydatidiform moles. Int J Gynecol Pathol 6: 213–229

30. Brewer JI, Eckman TR, Dolkart RE, Torok EE, et al (1971) Gestational trophoblastic disease. A comparative study of the results of therapy in patients with invasive mole and with choriocarcinoma. Am J Obstet Gynecol 109: 335

31. Brewer JI, Gerbie AL (1966) Early development of choriocarcinoma. Am J Obstet Gynecol 94: 692–710

32. Brewer JI, Mazur MT (1981) Gestational choriocarcinoma: Its origin in the placenta during seemingly normal pregnancy. Am J Surg Pathol 5: 267–277

33. Brewer JI, Smith RT, Pratt GB (1963) Choriocarcinoma. Absolute 5-year survival rates of 122 patients treated by hysterectomy. Am J Obstet Gynecol 85: 841–843

34. Brewer JI, Tamimi HK (1976) Gestational trophoblastic disease. Obstet Gynecol Annu 5: 367–397

35. Brewer JI, Torok EE, Kahan BD, Shanhope CR, et al (1978) Gestational trophoblastic disease: Origin of choriocarcinoma, invasive mole and choriocarcinoma associated with hydatidiform mole, and some immunologic aspects. Adv Cancer Res 27: 89–147

36. Brewer JI, Torok EE, Webster A, Dolkart RE (1968) Hydatidiform mole. A follow-up regimen for identification of invasive mole and choriocarcinoma and for selection of patients for treatment. Am J Obstet Gynecol 101: 557

37. Campo E, Algaba R, Palacin A, Germa R, et al (1989) Placental proteins in high-grade urothelial neoplasms. An immunohistochemical study of human chorionic gonadotropin, human placental lactogen, and pregnancy-specific beta-1-glycoprotein. Cancer 63: 2497–2504

38. Carlson JA, Day TG Jr, Kuhns JG, Howell RS, et al (1984) Endoarterial pulmonary metastasis of malignant trophoblast associated with a term intrauterine pregnancy. Gynecol Oncol 17: 241–248

39. Cohen BA, Burkman RT, Rosenshein NB, Antienza MF, et al (1979) Gestational trophoblastic disease within an elective abortion population. Am J Obstet Gynecol 135: 452–455

40. Conran RM, Hitchcock CL, Popek EJ, Norris HJ, et al (1993) Diagnostic considerations in molar gestations. Hum Pathol 24: 41–48

41. Cotton DB, Bernstein SG, Read JA, Benedetti TJ, et al (1980) Hemodynamic observations in evacuation of molar pregnancy. Am J Obstet Gynecol 138: 6

42. Craighill MC, Cramer DW (1984) Epidemiology of complete molar pregnancy. J Reprod Med 29: 784–787

43. Cunanan RG, Jr., Lippes J, Tancinco PA (1980) Choriocarcinoma of the ovary with coexisting normal pregnancy. Obstet Gynecol 55: 669–672

44. Curry SL, Hammond CB, Tyrey L, Creasman WT, et al (1975) Hydatidiform mole: Diagnosis, management, and long-term follow-up of 347 patients. Obstet Gynecol 45: 1–8

45. Czernobilsky B, Barash A, Lancet M (1982) Partial moles: A clinicopathologic study of 25 cases. Obstet Gynecol 59: 75–77

46. Daamen CBF, Bloem GWD, Westerbeek AJ (1961) Chorionepithelioma in mother and child. J Obstet Gynecol Br Commonwlth 68: 144–149

47. Davis JR, Kerrigan DP, Way DL, Weiner SA (1987) Partial hydatidiform moles: Deoxyribonucleic acid content and course. Am J Obstet Gynecol 157: 969–973

48. Davis JR, Surwit EA, Garay JP, Fortier KJ (1984) Sex assignment in gestational trophoblastic neoplasia. Am J Obstet Gynecol 148: 722–725

49. Dawood MY, Teoh ES, Ratnam SG (1971) ABO blood group in trophoblastic disease. J Obstet Gynaecol Br Commonw 78: 918–923

50. Daya D, Sabet L (1991) The use of cytokeratin as a sensitive and reliable marker for trophoblastic tissue. Am J Clin Pathol 95: 137–141

51. Dearden L, Ockleford CD, Gupta M (1983) Structure of human trophoblast: Correlation with function. In: Luke YW, Whyte A (eds) Biology of trophoblast. New York, Elsevier, pp 70–110

52. Dehner LP (1980) Gestational and nongestational trophoblastic neoplasia. A historic and pathobiologic surgery. Am J Surg Pathol 4: 43–58

53. Delfs E (1957) Quantitative chorionic gonadotrophin: Prognostic value in hydatidiform mole and chorionepithelioma. Obstet Gynecol 9: 1–24

54. Deligdisch L, Driscoll SG, Goldstein DP (1978) Gestational trophoblastic neoplasms: Morphologic correlates of therapeutic response. Am J Obstet Gynecol 130: 801–806

55. Deligdisch L, Waxman J (1984) Metastatic gestational trophoblastic neoplasm. A study of two cases in unusual clinical settings and review of the literature. Gynecol Oncol 19: 323–328

56. Dessau R, Rustin GJS, Dent J, Paradinas FJ, et al (1990) Surgery and chemotherapy in the management of placental site tumor. Gynecol Oncol 39: 56–59

57. Dodson MG (1983) New concepts and questions in gestational trophoblastic disease. J Reprod Med 28: 741

58. Dougherty CM, Cunningham C, Mickal A (1978) Choriocarcinoma with metastasis in a postmenopausal woman. Am J Obstet Gynecol 132: 700–701

59. Douglas GW, Thomas L, Carr M, Cullen NM, et al (1959) Trophoblast in the circulating blood during pregnancy. Am J Obstet Gynecol 78: 960

60. Driscoll SG (1963) Choriocarcinoma: An "incidental finding" within a term placenta. Obstet Gynecol 21: 96–101

61. Driscoll SG (1977) Gestational trophoblastic neoplasms: Morphologic considerations. Hum Pathol 8: 529–539

62. DuBeshter B, Berkowitz RS, Goldstein DP, Cramer DW, et al (1987) Metastatic gestational trophoblastic disease: Experience at the New England Trophoblastic Disease Center, 1965 to 1985. Obstet Gynecol 69(3): 390–395

63. Duncan DA, Mazur MT (1989) Trophoblastic tumors. Ultrastructural comparison of choriocarcinoma and placental-site trophoblastic tumor. Hum Pathol 20: 370–381

64. Eckstein RP, Paradinas FJ, Bagshawe KD (1982) Placental site trophoblastic tumour (trophoblastic pseudotumour): A study of four cases requiring hysterectomy, including one fatal case. Histopathology 6: 211–226

65. Eckstein RP, Russell P, Friedlander ML, Tattersall MHN, et al (1983) Metastasizing placental site trophoblastic tumor: A case study. Hum Pathol 16: 632–636

66. Elston CW (1976) The histopathology of trophoblastic tumors. J Clin Pathol 29 [Suppl] (Roy Coll Pathol) 10: 111–131

67. Elston CW (1978) Trophoblastic tumors of the placenta. In: Fox H (ed) Pathology of the placenta. Philadelphia, WB Saunders, pp 368–425

68. Elston CW (1983) Development and structure of trophoblastic neoplasms. In: Luke YW, Whyte A (eds) Biology of trophoblast. New York, Elsevier, pp 188–232

69. Elston CW, Bagshawe KD (1972) The diagnosis of trophoblastic tumours from uterine curettings. J Clin Pathol 25: 111–118

70. Elston CW, Bagshawe KD (1972) The value of histological grading in the management of hydatidiform mole. J Obstet Gynaecol Br Commonw 79: 717

71. Elston CW, Bagshawe KD (1973) Cellular reaction in trophoblastic tumours. Br J Cancer 28: 245–256

72. Ertungealp E, Axelrod J, Stanek A, Boyce A, et al (1982) Skin metastases from malignant gestational trophoblastic disease: Report of two cases. Am J Obstet Gynecol 143: 843–846

73. Ewing J (1910) Chorioma. Surg Gynecol Obstet 10: 366–392

74. Federschneider JM, Goldstein DP, Berkowitz RS, Marean AR, et al (1980) Natural history of recurrent molar pregnancy. Obstet Gynecol 55: 457

75. Fraser GC, Blair GK, Hemming A, Murphy JJ, et al (1992) The Treatment of Simultaneous Choriocarcinoma in Mother and Baby. J Pediatr Surg 27: 1318–1319

76. Fukanaga M (1993) Metastasizing placental site trophoblastic tumor. An immunohistochemical and flow cytometric analysis of two cases. Am J Surg Pathol (in press)

77. Fukuda Y, Sakurai M, Matsuura N (1985) Primary gastric choriocarcinoma. Report of an autopsy case with immunohistochemical study. Acta Pathol Jpn 35: 655–666

78. Fukunaga M, Ushigome S, Sugishita M (1993) Application of flow cytometry in diagnosis of hydatidiform moles. Mod Pathol 6: 353–359

79. Gaber LW, Redline RW, Mostoufi-Zadeh M, Driscoll SG (1986) Invasive partial mole. Am J Clin Pathol 85: 722–724

80. Gardner HAR, Lage JM (1992) Choriocarcinoma following a partial hydatidiform mole—a case report. Hum Pathol 23: 468–471

81. Genest DR, Laborde O, Berkowitz RS, Goldstein DP, et al (1991) A clinicopathologic study of 153 cases of complete hydatidiform mole (1980–1990)—histologic grade lacks prognostic significance. Obstet Gynecol 78: 402–409

82. Gerbie MV, Brewer JI, Tamimi H (1975) Primary choriocarcinoma of the ovary. Obstet Gynecol 46: 720–723

83. Gloor E, Dialdas J, Hurlimann J, Ribolzi J, et al (1983) Placental site trophoblastic tumor (trophoblastic pseudotumor) of the uterus with metastases and fatal outcome. Am J Surg Pathol 7: 483–486

84. Gloor E, Hurlimann J (1981) Trophoblastic pseudotumor of the uterus. Clinicopathologic report with immunohistochemical and ultrastructural studies. Am J Surg Pathol 5: 5–13

85. Goldstein DP (1979) Gestational neoplasms. In: DeGroot LJ, Cahill GF, Martini L, et al (eds) Endocrinology, vol. 3. New York, Grune & Stratton, pp 1629–1648

86. Goldstein DP, Berkowitz RS (1982) Gestational trophoblastic neoplasms. Clinical principles of diagnosis and management. Philadelphia, WB Saunders

87. Goto S, Yamada A, Ishizuka T, Tomoda Y (1993) Development of postmolar trophoblastic disease after partial molar pregnancy. Gynecol Oncol 48: 165–170

88. Govender NSK, Goldstein DP (1977) Metastatic tubal mole and coexisting intrauterine pregnancy. Obstet Gynecol 49(suppl): 67s

89. Grammatico D, Grignon DJ, Eberwein P, Shepherd RR, et al (1993) Transitional cell carcinoma of the renal pelvis with choriocarcinomatous differentiation—immunohistochemical and immunoelectron microscopic assessment of human chorionic gonadotropin production by transitional cell carcinoma of the urinary bladder. Cancer 71: 1835–1841

90. Greene JB, McCue SA (1978) Choriocarcinoma with cerebral metastases coexistent with a first pregnancy. Am J Obstet Gynecol 131: 253–254

91. Greene RR (1959) Chorioadenoma destruens. Ann NY Acad Sci 80: 143

92. Grimes DA (1984) Epidemiology of gestational trophoblastic disease. Am J Obstet Gynecol 150: 309–318

93. Guvener S, Kazancigil A, Erez S (1972) Long latent development of trophoblastic disease. Am J Obstet Gynecol 114: 679–684

94. Hammond CB, Borchert LG, Tyrey L, Creasman WT, et al (1973) Treatment of metastatic trophoblastic disease. Good and poor prognosis. Am J Obstet Gynecol 115: 451–457

95. Hammond CB, Hertz R, Ross GT, Lipsett MB, et al (1967) Diagnostic problems of choriocarcinoma and related trophoblastic neoplasms. Obstet Gynecol 29: 224–229

96. Hammond CB, Parker RT (1970) Diagnosis and treatment of trophoblastic disease. A report from the Southeastern Regional Center. Obstet Gynecol 35: 132

97. Hammond CB, Weed JC, Currie JL (1980) The role of operation in the current therapy of gestational trophoblastic disease. Am J Obstet Gynecol 136: 844

98. Hayashi K, Bracken MB, Freeman DH, Hellenbrand K (1982) Hydatidiform mole in the United States (1970–1977): A statistical and theoretical analysis. Am J Epidemiol 115: 67

99. Heaton GE, Matthews TH, Christopherson WM (1986) Malignant trophoblastic tumors with massive hemorrhage presenting as liver primary. A report of two cases. Am J Surg Pathol 10: 342–347

100. Heitz PU, vonHerbay G, Kloppel G, Komminoth P, et al (1987) The expression of subunits of human chorionic gonadotropin (hCG) by nontrophoblastic, nonendocrine, and endocrine tumors. Am J Clin Pathol 88(4): 467–472

101. Hertig AT, Edmonds HW (1940) Genesis of hydatidiform mole. Arch Pathol 30: 260

102. Hertig AT, Gore H (1960) Tumors of the female sex organs, Part 2, Tumors of the vulva, vagina and uterus. In: Atlas of tumor pathology, Section IX, Fascicle 33. Washington, D.C., Armed Forces Institute of Pathology, pp 329–333

103. Hertig AT, Mansell (1956) Tumors of the female sex organs. Part 1. Hydatidiform mole and choriocarcinoma. In: Atlas of Tumor Pathology, Section 9, Fascicle 33. Washington, D.C., Armed Forces Institute of Pathology

104. Hertig AT, Sheldon WH (1947) Hydatidiform mole. A pathologicoclinical correlation of 200 cases. Am J Obstet Gynecol 53: 1–36

105. Hertz R, Lewis J Jr, Lipsett MB (1961) Five years' experience with the chemotherapy of metastatic choriocarcinoma and related trophoblastic tumors in women. Am J Obstet Gynecol 82: 631

106. Heyderman E, Chapman DV, Richardson TC, Calvert I, et al (1985) Human chorionic gonadotropin and human placental lactogen in extragonadal tumors: An immunoperoxidase study of ten non-germ cell neoplasm. Cancer 56: 2674–2682

107. Hopkins M, Nunez C, Murphy JR, Wentz WB (1985) Malignant placental site trophoblastic tumor. Obstet Gynecol 66: 95S–100S

108. Horne CHW, Rankin R, Bremner RD (1984) Pregnancy-specific proteins as markers for gestational trophoblastic disease. Int J Gynecol Pathol 3: 27–40

109. Hou PC, Pang SC (1956) Chorionepithelioma: An analytical study of 28 necropsied cases with special reference to the possibility of spontaneous retrogression. J Pathol Bacteriol 72: 95–104

110. Hsu CT, Huang LC, Chen TY (1962) Metastases in benign hydatidiform mole and chorioadenoma destruens. Am J Obstet Gynecol 84: 1412

111. Huettner PC, Gersell DJ (1993) Placental site nodules: An analysis of 40 cases. (Abstract) Mod Pathol 6: 74A

112. Inaba N, Ishige H, Ijichi M, Satoh N, et al (1982) Possible new markers in trophoblastic diseases. Am J Obstet Gynecol 143: 973–974

113. Ishizuka N (1967) Chemotherapy of chorionic tumors. In: Holland JF, Hreshchyshyn MM (eds) Choriocarcinoma, UICC Monograph Series, vol. 3. New York, Springer-Verlag, pp 116–118

114. Ito H, Sekine T, Komuro N, Tanaka T, et al (1981) Histologic stromal reaction of the host with gestational choriocarcinoma and its relation to clinical stage classification and prognosis. Am J Obstet Gynecol 140: 781–786

115. Jacobs PA, Hunt PA, Matsuura JS, Wilson CC, et al (1982) Complete and partial hydatidiform mole in Hawaii: Cytogenetics, morphology and epidemiology. Br J Obstet Gynaecol 89: 258–266

116. Jacobs PA, Szulman AE, Funkhouser J, Matsuura JS, et al (1982) Human triploidy: Relationship between parental origin of the additional haploid complement and development of partial hydatidiform mole. Ann Hum Genet 46: 223–231

117. Jacobs PA, Wilson CM, Sprenkle JA, Rosenshein NB, et al (1980) Mechanism of origin of complete hydatidiform moles. Nature 286: 714

118. Javey H, Borazjani G, Behmard S, Langley FA (1979) Discrepancies in the histological diagnosis of hydatidiform mole. Br J Obstet Gynaecol 86: 480

118a. Jeffers MD, O'Dwyer P, Curran B, Leader M, Gillan JE (1993) Partial hydatidiform mole: A common but under-diagnosed condition. A 3-year retrospective clinicopatho-

logic and DNA flow cytometric analysis. Int J Gynecol Pathol 12: 315–323

119. Jock DE, Schwartz PE, Portnoy L (1981) Primary ovarian hydatidiform mole: Addition of a sixth case to the literature. Obstet Gynecol 58: 657

120. Johnson TR, Comstock CH, Anderson DG (1979) Benign gestational trophoblastic disease metastatic to pleura: Unusual case of hemothorax. Obstet Gynecol 53: 509

121. Jones WB, Lewis JL (1985) Late recurrence of gestational trophoblastic disease. Gynecol Oncol 20: 83

122. Jones WB, Romain K, Erlandson RA, Burt ME, et al (1993) Thoracotomy in the management of gestational choriocarcinoma: A clinicopathologic study. Cancer 72: 2175–2181

123. Junaid TA, de V Hendrickse JP, Oladiran B, Edington GM, et al (1974) Choriocarcinoma in Ibadan, Nigeria: Epidemiologic aspects. J Natl Cancer Inst 53: 1597–1599

124. Junaid TA, de V Hendrickse JP, Williams AO, Osunkoya BO (1976) Choriocarcinoma in Ibadan: Clinicopathologic studies. Hum Pathol 7: 215

125. Kajii T, Kurashige H, Ohama K, Uchino F (1984) XY and XX complete moles: Clinical and morphologic correlations. Am J Obstet Gynecol 150: 57–64

126. Kajii T, Ohama K (1977) Androgenetic origin of hydatidiform mole. Nature (Lond) 268: 633–634

127. Kay S, Schneider V, Litt J (1983) Choriocarcinoma of the mesosalpinx masquerading as congestive heart failure: Ultrastructural observations of the tumor. Int J Gynecol Pathol 2: 72–87

128. King LA, Okagaki T, Twiggs LB (1992) Resolution of pulmonary metastases with chemotherapy in a patient with a placental site trophoblastic tumor. Int J Gynecol Cancer 2: 328–331

129. Kohorn EI (1993) Evaluation of the criteria used to make the diagnosis of nonmetastatic gestational trophoblastic neoplasia. Gynecol Oncol 48: 139–147

130. Kohorn EI, McGinn RC, Gee JBL, Goldstein DP, et al (1978) Pulmonary embolization of trophoblastic tissue in molar pregnancy. Obstet Gynecol 51(suppl): 16S

131. Kotylo PK, Michael H, Davis TE, Sutton GP, et al (1992) Flow cytometric DNA analysis of placental site trophoblastic tumors. Int J Gynecol Pathol 11: 245–252

132. Kurman RJ (1991) The morphology, biology, and pathology of intermediate trophoblast—a look back to the present. Hum Pathol 22: 847–855

133. Kurman RJ (1993) Personal observation.

134. Kurman RJ, Main CS, Chen HC (1984) Intermediate trophoblast: A distinctive form of trophoblast with specific morphological, biochemical and functional features. Placenta 5: 349–370

135. Kurman RJ, Scully RE, Norris HJ (1976) Trophoblastic pseudotumor of the uterus. An exaggerated form of "syncytial endometritis" simulating a malignant tumor. Cancer 38: 1214–1226

136. Kurman RJ, Young RH, Norris HJ, Main CS, et al (1984) Immunocytochemical localization of placental lactogen and chorionic gonadotropin in the normal placenta and trophoblastic tumors, with emphasis on intermediate trophoblast and the placental site trophoblastic tumor. Int J Gynecol Pathol 3: 101–121

137. Lage JM, Berkowitz RS, Rice LW, Goldstein DP, et al (1991) Flow cytometric analysis of DNA content in partial hydatidiform moles with persistent gestational trophoblastic tumor. Obstet Gynecol 77: 111–115

138. Lage JM, Driscoll SG, Yavner DL, Olivier AP, et al (1988) Hydatidiform moles. Application of flow cytometry in diagnosis. Am J Clin Pathol 89: 596–600

139. Lage JM, Mark SD, Roberts DJ, Goldstein DP, et al (1992) A flow cytometric study of 137 fresh hydropic placentas: Correlation between types of hydatidiform moles and nuclear DNA ploidy. Obstet Gynecol 79: 403–410

140. Lage JM, Roberts DJ (1993) Choriocarcinoma in a term placenta: Pathologic diagnosis of tumor in an asymptomatic patient with metastatic disease. Int J Gynecol Pathol 12: 80–85

141. Lage JM, Weinberg DS, Yavner DL, Bieber FR (1989) The biology of tetraploid hydatidiform moles: Histopathology, cytogenetics, and flow cytometry. Hum Pathol 20: 419–425

142. Larsen JF (1973) Ultrastructure of abnormal human trophoblast. Acta Anat 86(suppl 1): 47

143. Lathrop JC, Wachtel TJ, Meissner GF (1978) Uterine choriocarcinoma fourteen years following bilateral tubal ligation. Obstet Gynecol 51: 477–482

144. Lau HL, Jones GS, Schwartz CM (1965) Immunoassay of serum human chorionic gonadotropin by quantitative complement fixation and its comparison with Delfs bioassay and two international standard preparations. Am J Obstet Gynecol 92: 483

145. Lawler SD, Fisher RA, Dent J (1991) A prospective genetic study of complete and partial hydatidiform moles. Am J Obstet Gynecol 164: 1270–1277

146. Lemonnier M-C, Glezerman M, Vauclair R, Audet-Lapointe P (1986) Choriocarcinoma associated with undetectable levels of human chorionic gonadotropin. Gynecol Oncol 25: 48

147. Lewis JL (1979) Classification of trophoblastic neoplasia. Ann Clin Lab Sci 9: 387–392

148. Lewis JL (1980) Treatment of metastatic gestational trophoblastic neoplasms. A brief review of developments in the years 1968 to 1978. Am J Obstet Gynecol 136: 163

149. Li MC, Hertz R, Spencer DB (1956) Effect of methotrexate therapy upon choriocarcinoma and chorioadenoma. Proc Soc Exp Biol Med 93: 361

150. Libshitz HI, Baber CE, Hammond CB (1977) The pulmonary metastases of choriocarcinoma. Obstet Gynecol 49: 412–416

151. Looi LM, Sivanesaratnam V (1981) Malignant evolution with fatal outcome in a patient with partial hydatidiform mole. Aust NZ J Obstet Gynaecol 21: 51

152. Lurain JR, Brewer JI (1985) Treatment of high-risk gestational trophoblastic disease with methotrexate, actinomycin D, and cyclophosphamide chemotherapy. Obstet Gynecol 65: 830–836

153. Lurain JR, Brewer JI, Mazur MT, Torok EE (1982) Fetal gestational trophoblastic disease: An analysis of treatment failures. Am J Obstet Gynecol 144: 391–395

154. Lurain JR, Brewer JI, Torok EE, Halpern B (1982) Gestational trophoblastic disease: Treatment results at the Brewer Trophoblastic Disease Center. Obstet Gynecol 60: 354–360

155. Lurain JR, Brewer JI, Torok EE, Halpern B (1983) Natural history of hydatidiform mole after primary evacuation. Am J Obstet Gynecol 145: 591–595

156. Lurain JR, Casanova LA, Miller DS, Rademaker AW (1991) Prognostic factors in gestational trophoblastic tumors: A proposed new scoring system based on multivariate analysis. Am J Obstet Gynecol 164(2): 611–616

157. Lurain JR, Sand PK, Brewer JI (1986) Choriocarcinoma associated with ectopic pregnancy. Obstet Gynecol 68: 286

158. Lurain JR, Sand PK, Carson SA, Brewer JI (1982) Pregnancy outcome subsequent to consecutive hydatidiform moles. Am J Obstet Gynecol 142: 1060

159. Marchand F (1895) Uber die sogenannten "decidualen" Geschwulste im Anschloss an normale Geburt, Abort, Blasenmole, und Extrauterin Schwangerschaft. Monatsschr Geburtshilfe Gynaekol 1: 419

160. Marquez-Monter H, De La Vega GA, Ridaura C, Robles M (1968) Gestational choriocarcinoma in the general hospital of Mexico. Cancer 22: 91–98

161. Martin DA, Sutton GP, Ulbright TM, Sledge GW, et al (1989) DNA content as a prognostic index in gestational trophoblastic neoplasia. Gynecol Oncol 34: 383–388

162. Matalon M, Modan B (1972) Epidemiologic aspects of hydatidiform mole in Israel. Am J Obstet Gynecol 112: 107

163. Matsurra J, Chin D, Jacobs PA, et al (1984) Complete hydatidiform mole in Hawaii: An epidemiologic study. Genet Epidemiol 1: 271

164. Matsuura J, Chin D, Jacobs PA, Szulman AE (1984) Complete hydatidiform mole in Hawaii: An epidemiologic study. Genet Epidemiol 1: 271–284

165. Matthews TH, Heaton GE, Christopherson WM (1986) Primary duodenal choriocarcinoma. Arch Pathol Lab Med 110: 550–552

166. Mazur MT (1989) Metastatic gestational choriocarcinoma. Unusual pathologic variant following theapy. Cancer 63: 1370–1377

167. Mazur MT, Lurain JR, Brewer JI (1982) Fetal gestational choriocarcinoma. Clinicopathologic study of patients treated at a trophoblastic disease center. Cancer 50: 1833–1846

168. Messerli ML, Lilienfeld AM, Parmley T, Woodruff JD, et al (1985) Risk factors for gestational trophoblastic neoplasia. Am J Obstet Gynecol 153: 294–300

169. Messerli ML, Parmley T, Woodruff JD, Lilienfeld AM, et al (1987) Inter- and intra-pathologist variability in the diagnosis of gestational trophoblastic neoplasia. Obstet Gynecol 69(4): 622–626

170. Miller JM, Surwit EA, Hammond CB (1979) Choriocarcinoma following term pregnancy. Obstet Gynecol 53: 207–212

171. Millis RR (1990) Choriocarcinomatous features in mammary mucoid carcinoma. Histopathology 17: 486–487

172. Mittal KK, Kachru RB, Brewer JI (1975) The HL-A and ABO antigens in trophoblastic disease. Tissue Antigens 6: 57–69

173. Morrow CP, Kletzky OA, Disaia PJ, Townsend DE, et al (1977) Clinical and laboratory correlates of molar pregnancy and trophoblastic disease. Am J Obstet Gynecol 128: 424

174. Mortakis AE, Braga CA (1990) "Poor prognosis" metastatic gestational trophoblastic disease: The prognostic signifi-

cance of the scoring system in predicting chemotherapy failures. Obstet Gynecol 76(2): 272–277

175. Mostoufi M, Driscoll SG (1987) Persistence of partial mole. (Abstract) Am J Clin Pathol 87: 377–380

176. Mutter GL, Pomponio RJ, Berkowitz RS, Genest DR (1993) Sex chromosome composition of complete hydatidiform moles: relationship to metastasis. Am J Obstet Gynecol 168: 1547–1551

177. Nagamani M, Kaspar HG, Dinh TV, Hannigan EV, et al (1990) Hyperthecosis of the ovaries in a woman with a placental site trophoblastic tumor. Obstet Gynecol 76: 931–935

178. Nagelberg SB, Rosen SW (1985) Clinical and laboratory investigation of a virilized woman with placental site trophoblastic tumor. Obstet Gynecol 65: 527–534

179. Nakano R, Sasaki K, Yamoto M, Hata H (1980) Trophoblastic disease: Analysis of 342 patients. Gynecol Obstet Invest 11: 237–242

180. Newlands ES, Bagshawe KD, Begenet RHJ, Rustin GJS, et al (1993) Results with the EMA/CO (etoposide, methotrexate, actinomycin D, cyclophosphamide, vincristine) regimen in high-risk gestational trophoblastic tumors 1979 to 1989. Br J Obstet Gynaecol

181. Nickels J, Risberg B, Melander S (1978) Trophoblastic pseudotumor of the uterus. (Abstract) Acta Pathol Microbiol Immunol Scand 86: 14–16

182. Niehans GA, Manivel JC, Copland GT, Scheithauer BW, et al (1988) Immunohistochemistry of germ cell and trophoblastic neoplasms. Cancer 62: 1113–1123

183. Nishikawa Y, Kaseki S, Tomoda Y, Ishizuka T, et al (1985) Histopathologic classification of uterine choriocarcinoma. Cancer 55: 1044–1051

184. Nisula BC, Taliadoruros GS (1980) Thyroid function in gestational trophoblastic neoplasia: Evidence that the thyrotropic activity of chorionic gonadotropin mediates the thyrotoxicosis of choriocarcinoma. Am J Obstet Gynecol 138: 77–85

185. Novak E, Seah CS (1954) Choriocarcinoma of the uterus. A study of 74 cases from the Mathieu Memorial Chorionepithelioma Registry. Am J Obstet Gynecol 67: 933–961

186. O'Brien TJ, Engvall E, Schlaerth JB, Morrow CP (1980) Trophoblastic disease monitoring: Evaluation of pregnancy-specific β_1-glycoprotein. Am J Obstet Gynecol 138: 313–320

187. O'Connor DM, Kurman RJ (1988) Intermediate trophoblast in uterine curettings in the diagnosis of ectopic pregnancy. Obstet Gynecol 72: 665–670

188. Ober WB (1970) Gestational choriocarcinma. Immunologic aspects, diagnosis and treatment. In: Gynecological oncology—a comprehensive review and evaluation. Proceedings of the Lenox Hill Hospital Symposium, New York, May 19–23, 1969. Excerpta Medica International Congress Series No. 203. Amsterdam, New York, Excerpta Medica Foundation, pp 304–315

189. Ober WB, Edgcomb JH, Price EB (1971) The pathology of choriocarcinoma. Ann NY Acad Sci 179: 299–321

190. Ober WB, Maier RC (1981) Gestational choriocarcinoma of the fallopian tube. Diagn Gynecol Obstet 3: 213–231

191. Ohama K, Kajii T, Okamoto E, Fukuda Y, et al (1981) Dispermic origin of XY hydatidiform moles. Nature 292: 551

192. Olive DL, Lurain JR, Brewer JI (1984) Choriocarcinoma associated with term gestation. Am J Obstet Gynecol 148: 711–716

193. Ollendorff DA, Goldberg JM, Abu-Jawdeh GM, Lurain JR (1990) Markedly elevated maternal serum alpha-fetoprotein associated with a normal fetus and choriocarcinoma of the placenta. Obstet Gynecol 76(3): 494–497

194. Parazzini F, LaVecchia C, Pampallona S, Franceschi S (1985) Reproductive patterns and the risk of gestational trophoblastic disease. Am J Obstet Gynecol 152: 866–870

195. Park WW (1971) Choriocarcinoma. A study of its pathology. Philadelphia, Davis

196. Park WW (1981) Pathology and classification of trophoblastic tumors. In: Coppleson W (ed) Gynecologic oncology, Edinburgh, Churchill-Livingstone, pp 745–756

197. Park WW, Lees JC (1936) Choriocarcinoma. A general review with an analysis of 516 cases. Arch Pathol 160: 205–241

198. Pattillo RA, Sasaki S, Katayama KP, Roesler M, et al (1981) Genesis of 46, XY hydatidiform mole. Am J Obstet Gynecol 141: 104

199. Patton GW, Goldstein DP (1973) Gestational choriocarcinoma of the tube and ovary. Surg Gynecol Obstet 137: 608

200. Pierce GB Jr, Midgley AR Jr. (1963) The origin and function of human syncytiotrophoblastic giant cells. Am J Pathol 43: 153

201. Poen HJ, Djojopranoto M (1965) The possible etiologic factors of hydatidiform mole and choriocarcinoma. Am J Obstet Gynecol 92: 510–513

202. Pushchak MJ, Farhi DC (1987) Primary choriocarcinoma of the lung. Arch Pathol Lab Med 111: 477–479

203. Quigley MM, Tyrey L, Hammond CB (1980) Utility of assay of alpha-subunit of human chorionic gonadotropin in managemet of gestational trophoblastic malignancies. Am J Obstet Gynecol 138: 545–549

204. Ramponi A, Angeli G, Arceci F, Pozzuoli R (1986) Gastric choriocarcinoma: An immunohistochemical study. Pathol Res Pract 181: 390–396

205. Rice LW, Lage JM, Berkowitz RS, Goldstein DP, et al (1989) Repetitive complete and partial hydatidiform mole. Obstet Gynecol 74: 217–219

206. Ringertz N (1970) Hydatidiform mole, invasive mole and choriocarcinoma in Sweden 1958–1965. Acta Obstet Gynecol Scand 49: 195–203

207. Rizkallah T, Gurpide E, Van de Wiele RL (1969) Metabolism of hCG in man. J Clin Endocrinol 29: 92–100

208. Rolon PA, de Lopez BH (1977) Epidemiological aspects of hydatidiform mole in the Republic of Paraguay (South America). Br J Obstet Gynaecol 84: 862

209. Rolon PA, de Lopez BH (1979) Malignant trophoblastic disease in Paraguay. J Reprod Med 23: 94–96

210. Romero R, Horgan JG, Kohorn EI, Kadar N, et al (1985) New criteria for the diagnosis of gestational trophoblastic disease. Obstet Gynecol 66: 553

211. Rosenshein NB, Wijnen H, Woodruff JD (1980) Clinical importance of the diagnosis of trophoblastic pseudotumors. Am J Obstet Gynecol 136: 635–638

212. Ross GT (1977) Clinical relevance of research on the structure of human chorionic gonadotropin. Am J Obstet Gynecol 129: 795

213. Sakuragi N (1982) Serum SPI and hCG B-subunit (hCG-B) levels in choriocarcinoma, invasive mole and hydatidiform mole—clinical significance of SPI/hCG-B ratio. Gynecol Oncol 13: 393–398

214. Sasaki K, Hata H, Nakano R (1985) ABO blood group in patients with malignant trophoblastic disease. Gynecol Obstet Invest 20: 23–26

215. Savage J, Subby W, Okagaki T (1987) Adenocarcinoma of the endometrium with trophoblastic differentiation and metastases as choriocarcinoma: A case report. Gynecol Oncol 26: 257–262

216. Schink JC, Singh DK, Rademaker AW, Miller DS, et al (1992) Etoposide, methotrexate, actinomycin-D, cyclophosphamide, and vincristine for the treatment of metastatic, high-risk gestational trophoblastic disease. Obstet Gynecol 80: 817–820

217. Schopper W, Pliess G (1949) Uber chorioepitheliosis. Ein beitrag zur genese, diagnostik und bewertung ektopischer chorionepithelialer wurcherungen. Virch Arch (Pathol Anat) 317: 347–384

218. Scully RE, Poulsen H, Sobin LH (1994) International histological classification and typing of female genital tract tumours. Berlin, Springer-Verlag (in press)

219. Scully RE, Young RH (1981) Trophoblastic pseudotumor. (Editorial) Am J Surg Pathol 5: 75–76

220. Shitabata PK, Rutgers JL (1993) The placental site nodule. An immunohistochemical study. (Abstract) Mod Pathol 6: 78A

221. Silva EG, Tornos C, Lage J, Ordonez NG, et al (1993) Multiple nodules of intermediate trophoblast following hydatidiform moles. Int J Gynecol Pathol 12: 324–332

222. Silverberg SG, Kurman RJ (1992) Tumors of the uterine corpus and gestational trophoblastic disease. Atlas of tumor pathology, 3rd series, fascicle 3. Washington, D.C., Armed Forces Institute of Pathology

223. Smith EB, Szulman AE, Hinsaw W, Tyrey L, et al (1984) Human chorionic gonadotropin levels in complete and partial hydatidiform moles and in nonmolar abortuses. Am J Obstet Gynecol 149: 129–132

224. Soma H, Takayama M, Tokoro K, Kikuchi K, et al (1980) Radioimmunoassay of hCG as an early diagnosis of cerebral metastases in choriocarcinoma patients. Acta Obstet Gynecol Scand 59: 445–448

225. Stanhope CR, Stuart GCE, Curtis KL (1983) Primary ovarian hydatidiform mole: Review of the literature and report of a case. Am J Obstet Gynecol 145: 886

226. Stone M, Bagshawe KD (1976) Hydatidiform mole: Two entities. Lancet 1: 535

227. Stone M, Bagshawe KD (1979) An analysis of the influence of maternal age, gestational age, contraceptive method, and the mode of primary treatment of patients with hydatidiform moles on the incidence of subsequent chemotherapy. Br J Obstet Gynaecol 86: 782–792

228. Surani MAH, Barton SC, Norris ML (1984) Development of reconstituted mouse eggs suggests imprinting of the genome during gametogenesis. Nature 308: 548

229. Surti U, Szulman AE, O'Brien S (1979) Complete (classic) hydatidiform mole with 46,XY karyotype of paternal origin. Hum Genet 51: 153

230. Surti U, Szulman AE, O'Brien S (1982) Dispermic origin and clinical outcome of three complete hydatidiform moles with 46,XY karyotype. Am J Obstet Gynecol 144: 84–87

231. Surti U, Szulman AE, Wagner K, et al (1986) Tetraploid partial moles: Two cases with a triple paternal contribution and a 92,XXXY karyotype. Hum Genet 72: 15

232. Surwit EA, Alberts DS, Christian CD, Graham VE (1984) Poor-prognosis gestational trophoblastic disease: An update. Obstet Gynecol 64: 21–26

233. Surwit EA, Hammond CB (1980) Treatment of metastatic trophoblastic disease with poor prognosis. Obstet Gynecol 55: 565–570

234. Surwit EA, Hammond CB (1981) Recurrent gestational trophoblastic disease. Gynecol Oncol 12: 177

235. Szulman AE, Ma HK, Wong LC, Hsu C (1981) Residual trophoblastic disease in association with partial hydatidiform mole. Obstet Gynecol 57: 392–394

236. Szulman AE, Philippe E, Boue JG, Boue A (1981) Human triploidy: Association with partial hydatidiform moles and nonmolar conceptuses. Hum Pathol 12: 1016

237. Szulman AE, Surti U (1978) The syndromes of hydatidiform mole. I. Cytogenetic and morphologic correlations. Am J Obstet Gynecol 131: 665–671

238. Szulman AE, Surti U (1978) The syndromes of hydatidiform mole. II. Morphologic evolution of the complete and partial mole. Am J Obstet Gynecol 132: 20–27

239. Szulman AE, Surti U (1982) The clinicopathologic profile of the partial hydatidiform mole. Obstet Gynecol 59: 597–602

240. Takeuchi S (1982) Nature of invasive mole and its rational treatment. Semin Oncol 9: 181–186

241. Tatarinov YS, Sokolov AV (1977) Development of a radioimmunoassay for pregnancy-specific beta-globulin and its measurement in serum of patients with trophoblastic and non-trophoblastic tumors. Int J Cancer 19: 161–169

242. Teng NNH, Ballon SC (1984) Partial hydatidiform mole with diploid karyotype: Report of three cases. Am J Obstet Gynecol 150: 961

243. Thiele RA, de Alvarez RR (1962) Metastasizing benign trophoblastic tumors. Am J Obstet Gynecol 84: 1395

244. Tomoda Y, Arii Y, Kaseki S, Asai Y, et al (1980) Surgical indications for resection in pulmonary metastasis of choriocarcinoma. Cancer 46: 2723

245. Tow WSH, Yung RH (1967) The value of histological grading in the prognostication of hydatidiform mole. J Obstet Gynaecol Br Commow 74: 292

246. Tsao MS, Schraufnagel D, Wang NS (1981) Pulmonary metastasis of choriocarcinoma with a miliary roentgenographic pattern. (Letter to the Editor) Arch Pathol Lab Med 105: 557

247. Tsuji K, Yagi S, Nakano R (1981) Increased risk of malignant transformation of hydatidiform moles in older gravidas: A cytogenetic study. Obstet Gynecol 58: 351–355

248. Tsukamoto N, Iwasaka T, Kashimura Y, Uchino H, et al (1985) Gestational trophoblastic disease in women aged 50 or more. Gynecol Oncol 20: 53

249. Tsukamoto N, Kashimura Y, Sano M, et al (1981) Choriocarcinma occurring within the normal placenta with breast metastasis. Gynecol Oncol 11: 348

250. Twiggs LB, Morrow CP, Schlaerth JB (1979) Acute pul-

monary complications of molar pregnancy. Am J Obstet Gynecol 135: 189

251. Twiggs LB, Okagaki T, Phillips GL, Stroemer JR, et al (1981) Trophoblastic pseudotumor—evidence of malignant disease potential. Gynecol Oncol 12: 238–248

252. Vaitukaitis JL, Braunstein GD, Ross GT (1972) A radioimmunoassay which specifically measures human chorionic gonadotropin in the presence of human luteinizing hormone. Am J Obstet Gynecol 113: 751–758

253. Van Bogaert L-J, Staguet J-P (1977) Chorionepitheliosis: A rare benign trophoblastic disease. Acta Obstet Gynecol Scand 56: 69–73

254. Van Der Werf AJM, Broeders GHB, Vooys GP, Mastboom JL (1970) Metastatic choriocarcinoma as a complication of pregnancy. Obstet Gynecol 35: 78–88

255. Vance RD, Geisinger KR (1985) Pure nongestational choriocarcinoma of the ovary. Report of a case. Cancer 56: 2321

256. Vassilakos P, Riotton G, Kajii T (1977) Hydatidiform mole: Two entities. A morphologic and cytogenetic study with some clinical considerations. Am J Obstet Gynecol 127: 167–170

257. Vaughn TC, Surwit EA, Hammond CB (1980) Late recurrences of gestational trophoblastic neoplasia. Am J Obstet Gynecol 138: 73

258. Vejerslev LD, Dueholm M, Hassing N (1986) Hydatidiform mole: Cytogenetic marker analysis in twin gestation. Report of two cases. Am J Obstet Gynecol 155: 614

259. Vejerslev LO, Fisher RA, Surti U, Walka N (1987) Hydatidiform mole: Cytogenetically unusual cases and their implications for the present classification. Am J Obstet Gynecol 157: 180–184

260. Veridiano NP, Gal D, Delke I, Rosen Y, et al (1980) Gestational choriocarcinoma of the ovary. Gynecol Oncol 10: 235–240

261. Wagner D (1967) Trophoblastic cells in the blood stream in normal and abnormal pregnancy. Acta Cytol 12: 137

262. Wake N, Takagi N, Sasaki M (1978) Androgenesis as a cause of hydatidiform mole. J Natl Cancer Inst 60: 51–57

263. Wallace DC, Surti U, Adams CW, Szulman AE (1982) Complete moles have paternal chromosomes but maternal mitochondrial DNA. Hum Genet 61: 145

264. Wan SK, Lam PWY, Pau MY, Chan JKC (1992) Multiclefted nuclei. A helpful feature for indentification of intermediate trophoblastic cells in uterine curetting specimens. Am J Surg Pathol 16: 1226–1232

265. Weed JC Jr, Barnard DE, Currie JL, Clayton LA, et al (1982) Chemotherapy with the modified Bagshawe protocol for poor prognosis metastatic trophoblastic disease. Obstet Gynecol 59: 377–380

266. Weed JC Jr, Hammond CB (1980) Cerebral metastatic choriocarcinoma: Intensive therapy and prognosis. Obstet Gynecol 55: 89–94

267. Westerhout FC (1964) Ruptured tubal hydatidiform mole. Report of a case. Obstet Gynecol 23: 138

268. Wilson RB, Hunter JS Jr, Dockerty MB (1961) Chorioadenoma destruens. Am J Obstet Gynecol 81: 546–559

269. Womack C, Elston W (1985) Hydatidiform mole in Nottingham: A 12-year retrospective epidemiological and morphological study. Placenta 6: 93–106

270. Wong LC, Choo YC, Ma HK (1986) Hepatic metastases in gestational trophoblastic disease. Obstet Gynecol 67: 107

271. Wong LC, Ma HK (1984) The syndrome of partial mole. Arch Gynecol 234: 161–166

272. World Health Organization Scientific Group on Gestational Trophoblastic Disease (1983) Gestational trophoblastic diseases. In: Technical Report Series 692. Geneva, WHO

273. Wu FYW (1973) Recurrent hydatidiform mole: A case report of nine consecutive molar pregnancies. Obstet Gynecol 41: 200

274. Wurzel J, Brooks JJ (1981) Primary gastric choriocarcinoma: Immunohistochemistry, postmortem documentation and hormonal effects in a postmenopausal female. Cancer 48: 2756–2761

275. Wynn RM (1972) Cytotrophoblastic specializations: An ultrastructural study of the human placenta. Am J Obstet Gynecol 114: 339

276. Yamashita K, Nakamura T, Shimizu T (1984) Absence of major histocompatibility complex antigens in choriocarcinoma. Am J Obstet Gynecol 150: 896–897

277. Yen S, MacMahon B (1968) Epidemiologic features of trophoblastic disease. Am J Obstet Gynecol 101: 126–132

278. Young RH, Kurman RJ, Scully RE (1990) Placental site nodules and plaques—a clinicopathologic analysis of 20 cases. Am J Surg Pathol 14: 1001–1009

279. Young RH, Scully RE (1984) Placental-site trophoblastic tumor: Current status. Clin Obstet Gynecol 27: 248

280. Young RH, Scully RE, McCluskey RT (1985) A distinctive glomerular lesion complicating placental site trophoblastic tumor: Report of two cases. Hum Pathol 16: 35–42

281. Yuen BH, Callegari PB (1986) Occurrence of molar pregnancy in patients undergoing elective abortion: Comparison with other clinical presentations. Am J Obstet Gynecol 154: 273–276

282. Zhang J, Kraus FT (1986) Placental site trophoblastic tumor. Immunocytochemical correlations. Lab Invest 54: 73A

II

Adjunctive Techniques in Gynecologic Pathology

25

Cytopathology

Mark E. Sherman, M.D.

In the last four decades, cytopathology has become an essential technique in the detection and management of gynecological disease. Most notably, the success of cytological screening for cervical cancer has made the Pap smear a routine procedure. More recently, the diagnosis of fluids and fine-needle aspirates has been formally recognized in the staging of endometrial and ovarian cancer. Cytopathology practice continues to evolve, shaped by biological and clinical advances. Data establishing a causal relationship between human papillomavirus (HPV) infection and cervical cancer[86] and the introduction of The Bethesda System[108,109] have altered the diagnostic approach to cervical smears. The increasing incidence of cervical adenocarcinoma has fostered the development of more accurate cytological criteria for the diagnosis of this tumor and increased interest in its early detection.* In addition, growing reliance on laparoscopic examination and aspiration techniques to evaluate ovarian cysts has provided cytopatholo-

gists with the challenge of diagnosing lesions never before sampled.

Changes in clinical practice have increased the need for close consultation between surgical pathologists, cytopathologists, and gynecologists. Cytological diagnoses rendered without knowledge of a patient's menstrual history, preceding disorders, and treatments often are compromised. Review of serial smears obtained over time may provide information about disease progression necessary for choosing treatment options. Finally, formal reference to relevant clinical and histological correlations in cytopathology reports often is the best vehicle for providing gynecologists with an integrated picture of a patient's health.

The extensive literature in gynecological cytology precludes a detailed summary in this chapter. Excellent comprehensive discussions are available elsewhere. This chapter provides a problem-oriented discussion of gynecological cytopathology, including issues related to the interpretation of cervical/vaginal smears, fluid specimens, and ovarian cyst aspirates.

The Bethesda System

The Bethesda System (TBS) for reporting cervical/vaginal cytological diagnoses was developed to provide uniform guidelines for reviewing and reporting gynecological smears.[108,109] The system was designed to be clinically relevant and reflect our current understanding of the biology of cervical disease. A central aspect of TBS is that

---

*Refs. 6,7,12,18,29,73,83,84,90,117,173.

cytopathological diagnoses should include an assessment of specimen adequacy and an unambiguous descriptive diagnosis. TBS is intended to be a flexible classification that is updated periodically to reflect new advances in the field. The version resulting from the 1991 workshop, presented in Table 25.1, serves as an outline for the first part of this chapter.

Specimen Adequacy

Effective cytological screening for cervical carcinoma and its precursors requires optimally prepared and stained specimens that adequately reflect the status of the cervix, including the transformation zone. Ensuring that preparations meet the standards for specimen adequacy as proposed in TBS[109] should reduce the rate of false-negative cytological diagnoses. Under TBS guidelines, preparations in which 75% of the epithelial cells are obscured by blood, inflammation, or artifacts are considered unsatisfactory. Smears in which 50% of the material is uninterpretable are categorized as satisfactory for evaluation but limited by the presence of obscuring elements as specified. In addition, adequate smears must contain a sufficient number of epithelial cells to cover at least 10% of the surface of the slide. The Bethesda guidelines represent the minimum requirements for specimen adequacy. Smears that meet these criteria may be considered unsatisfactory in patients who have a history of cervical disease or inconsistent follow-up. Knowledge of the patient's gynecological history is indispensable in assessing the adequacy of marginal specimens.

Under the original Bethesda System guidelines,[108] smears obtained from premenopausal women lacking endocervical cells, metaplastic squamous cells, or cellular cervical mucus were categorized as less than optimal. Under the revised guidelines, the category of less than optimal has been eliminated. Adequate transformation zone sampling is defined in a women of any age as the presence of two clusters of endocervical or metaplastic squamous cells with a cluster containing a minimum of five cells. Smears lacking these elements are considered satisfactory for evaluation but limited by the absence of these elements. Since recognition of metaplastic squamous cells is unreliable in atrophic smears, the absence of transformation zone elements is not reported in these specimens. The effect of TBS on the reproducibility of determinations of specimen adequacy is unknown. Before the development of TBS, Yobs et al.[173] found that interlaboratory agreement in classifying specimens as unsatisfactory was poor. In a recent study, the assessment of transformation zone sampling by three pathologists within a single institution using the original Bethesda guidelines was reproducible.[147]

The College of American Pathologists (CAP) estimates that TBS eventually will be implemented in approximately 90% of the laboratories in the United States.[174] In a survey of 544 institutions employing the original Bethesda System

Table 25.1. The 1991 Bethesda System

Adequacy of the specimen
Satisfactory for evaluation
Satisfactory for evaluation but limited by . . . (specify reason)
Unsatisfactory for evaluation . . . (specify reason)
General categorization (optional)
Within normal limits
Benign cellular changes: see descriptive diagnosis
Epithelial cell abnormality: see descriptive diagnosis
Descriptive diagnoses
  Benign cellular changes
  Infection
    Trichomonas vaginalis
    Fungal organisms morphologically consistent with
      Candida spp
    Predominance of coccobacilli consistent with shift in
      vaginal flora
    Bacteria morphologically consistent with *Actinomyces* spp
    Cellular changes associated with herpes simplex virus
    Other[a]
  Reactive changes
    Reactive cellular changes associated with:
    Inflammation (includes typical repair)
    Atrophy with inflammation ("atrophic vaginalis")
    Radiation
    Intrauterine contraceptive device (IUD)
    Other
  Epithelial cell abnormalities
  Squamous cell
    Atypical squamous cells of undetermined significance:
      qualify[b]
    Low-grade squamous intraepithelial lesion (LSIL)
      encompassing: HPV,[a] mild dysplasia/CIN 1
    High-grade squamous intraepithelial lesion (HSIL)
      encompassing: moderate and severe dysplasia, CIS/CIN
      2 and CIN 3
    Squamous cell carcinoma
  Glandular cell
    Endometrial cells, cytologically benign in a
      postmenopausal woman
    Atypical glandular cells of undetermined significance:
      qualify[b]
    Endocervical adenocarcinoma
    Endometrial adenocarcinoma
    Extrauterine adenocarcinoma
    Adenocarcinoma, NOS
  Other malignant neoplasms: Specify
  Hormonal evaluation (applies to vaginal smears only)
    Hormonal pattern compatible with age and history
    Hormonal pattern incompatible with age and history: specify
    Hormonal evaluation not possible due to: specify

[a] Cellular changes of human papillomovirus (HPV), previously termed *koilocytosis, koilocytotic atypia,* and *condylomatous atypia,* are included in the category of LSIL.
[b] Atypical squamous or glandular cells of undetermined significance should be qualified further, if possible, as to whether a reactive or premalignant/malignant process is favored.
NOS, including adenocarcinoma of uncertain origin.

criteria, the CAP reported a less than optimal rate of 5.7% and an unsatisfactory rate of 0.7%. Forty-six percent of less than optimal specimens were due to the absence of an endocervical component (and currently would be classified as satisfactory but limited by the absence of transformation zone elements) and 45% of unsatisfactory smears lacked sufficient cellularity.

The reliability of cervical smears lacking transformation zone elements has been debated. Studies demonstrate that smears containing endocervical cells detect more abnormalities than those that lack endocervical cells.° Weid et al. reported that the endocervical component of smears contained more diagnostic cells than the ectocervical component in patients with carcinoma in situ.[166] Mitchell et al. reported that only 11.9% of 143 smears obtained from patients who subsequently developed invasive squamous carcinoma were negative on rescreening and lacked both endocervical and metaplastic squamous cells.[103] Thus, the possibility of sampling error appears to be reduced in specimens containing an endocervical component, but not eliminated. Paradoxically, recent studies failed to identify a significant number of squamous intraepithelial lesions (SILs) in repeat smears obtained after smears that were negative but lacked transformation zone elements.[76,104] Issues related to the significance of identifying transformation zone elements in cervical smears have been summarized expertly by Mitchell and Medley.[105] The decision to obtain a repeat specimen immediately after one that is negative and lacks transformation zone cells is best decided on individual case basis by a gynecologist who is familiar with the patient's history.

The number of endocervical cells present in smears is related to age, parity, inflammation, menses, douching, and pregnancy.[164] Patients whose smears lack an endocervical component[76,147,163] or have undergone cone biopsy[147] are likely to lack transformation zone cells in future specimens. Use of an endocervical brush improves endocervical sampling in patients of all ages[14,20,68,126,160,161] and especially in women who have undergone cone biopsy.[81,147] Unfortunately, specimens obtained by vigorous brushing may display crowded sheets of crushed cells that are difficult to interpret. Boon et al.[17] identified such artifacts in approximately 0.5% of cases and developed a technique of plastic embedding and thin sectioning to improve the interpretability of endocervical brush preparations obtained from women whose smears displayed thick fragments. Using this method, 28% of specimens containing uninterpretable fragments were diagnosed as high-grade SILs, squamous or adenocarcinoma. Thus, the presence of crowded sheets of cells in cytobrush preparations should never be dismissed as artifact without further investigation. To compound matters, these lesions may be located in the endocervical canal where they cannot be visualized colposcopically. A diagnosis of atypical squamous cells of undetermined significance (ASCUS); rule out a high-grade squamous intraepithelial lesion (HSIL) may be appropriate for cases displaying sheets of crowded small cells that cannot be reliably assessed. A recommendation to perform

colposcopy and biopsy is appropriate in circumstances in which clinicians desire this type of information.

Descriptive Diagnosis

Reactive Changes

INFLAMMATORY CHANGES AND REPAIR

Smears displaying reactive cellular changes should be reported as negative for atypia. Inflammatory changes are commonly appreciated in smears displaying infectious agents, during menses, and for 3 months after gynecological procedures. The distinction between inflammatory changes and significant atypia is based on the appearance of the nuclei and the ratio of the nuclear/cytoplasmic area. These evaluations are subjective, but accumulated experience enhanced by frequent histological correlation and follow-up of patients is important in refining diagnostic criteria. The most frequent errors are overestimating the significance of minor cytological changes in mature squamous cells and underestimating the importance of small cells with increased nuclear/cytoplasmic ratios.

Mature squamous cells displaying reactive changes contain pale-staining nuclei that are enlarged two to three times and possess even chromatin and smooth contours (Fig. 25.1). Chromocenters and slight hyperchromasia may be present. Degenerative nuclear changes such as pyknosis and karyorrhexis are of no significance. Degenerated cells often show frayed edges and vacuolization of the nucleus and cytoplasm. Small, thin-walled perinuclear halos may be present.

Highly reactive endocervical cells and a variety of specific benign conditions may resemble endocervical adenocarcinoma. Reactive endocervical cells often display nuclear enlargement and prominent nucleoli, but generally lack the increased ratio of nuclear/cytoplasmic area and nuclear hyperchromasia of endocervical adenocarcinomas (Fig. 25.2). More significantly, reactive endocervical cells

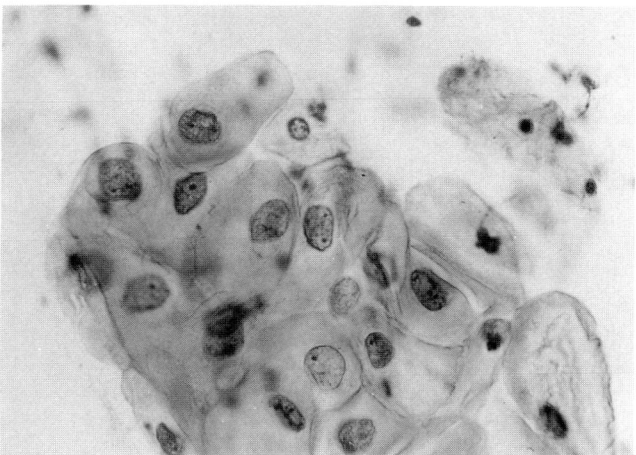

FIG. 25.1. **Reactive squamous cells.** Cells display enlarged, pale nuclei with minimally clumped chromatin.

°Refs. 37,72,78,89,99,131,162,163.

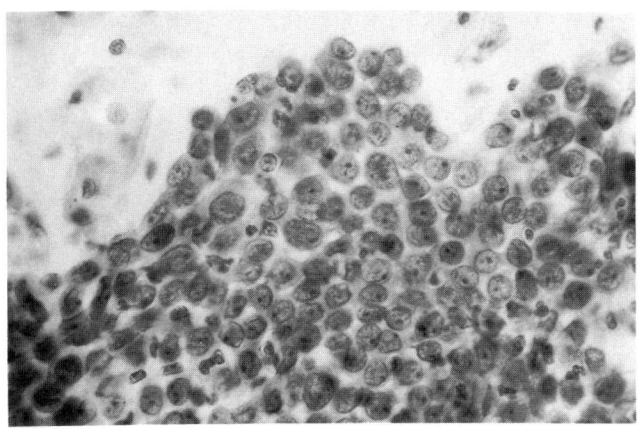

FIG. 25.2. Reactive endocervical cells. Cells are slightly crowded with nuclear enlargement and nucleoli. Chromatin pattern is uniform.

usually maintain a honeycomb configuration with only slight cellular crowding. Formation of rosettes, feathering, and nuclear pseudostratification are not typical of reactive changes.

Reparative squamous epithelium sheds cohesive sheets of cells with indistinct cytoplasmic membranes and large vesicular nuclei with prominent nucleoli (Fig. 25.3). Spindle-shaped cells may predominate at the margins of the groups. In rare cases, cellular overlapping and anisocytosis are evident. The monotony of the chromatin pattern, regularity of the nuclear membranes, and the presence of nucleoli characterize these lesions.

ATROPHIC VAGINITIS

The cytological pattern of atrophic vaginitis reflects two major effects: (1) loss of mucosal thickness and maturation

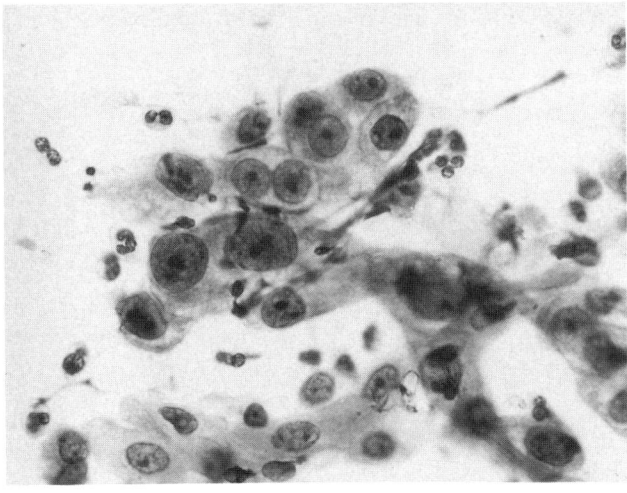

FIG. 25.3. Reparative epithelium. Sheets of cohesive cells with prominent nucleoli and indistinct cell membranes are present in an inflammatory background.

attributable to the loss of the trophic effects of estrogen and (2) mucosal breakdown with degeneration of squamous cells, inflammation, and blood. Single round or oval parabasal cells with nuclear/cytoplasmic ratios approaching 50% predominate. Parabasal cells in sheets often lack distinct cytoplasmic borders and may display a spindled appearance. Densely staining, homogeneous blue globules ("blue blobs") representing either degenerated naked nuclei or inspissated mucus may cause undue concern if interpreted out of context.[79] Sheets of cells that appear to be undergoing active repair and a background of blood and inflammation are typical.

RADIATION THERAPY

Cellular degeneration is the major finding immediately after radiation. In contrast to other treatments, radiation may produce alterations that persist for years after cessation of therapy. Cytological features that have been ascribed to radiation include cytomegaly, characterized by proportionate cellular and nuclear enlargement, nuclear wrinkling, nuclear and cytoplasmic vacuolization, multinucleation, bizarre shape changes, and irregular cytoplasmic staining[111] (Fig. 25.4). Often these findings are accompanied by severe atrophy, air-drying artifact, and fresh blood. Application of topical estrogen to induce maturation facilitates interpretation. Koss emphasizes that grading SIL after radiation therapy (postradiation dysplasia) is unreliable and that all patients with definite squamous abnormalities require thorough investigation.[79]

INTRAUTERINE DEVICES

Smears obtained from patients wearing intrauterine devices (IUDs) often display glandular and squamous atypias that mimic SIL or carcinoma.[50] Vacuolated glandular cells arranged in papillary or acinar structures with enlarged hyperchromatic nuclei may falsely suggest adenocarcinoma. Since IUD users shed endometrial cells in the luteal phase of the menstrual cycle, unwarranted concerns about the presence of an endometrial lesion may be raised in patients for whom a history of IUD use is lacking. In most cases, few atypical clusters of columnar cells are present and these display nuclei that are clearly degenerated. In some patients, an unequivocal evaluation is impossible despite a history of IUD use and atypical glandular cells of undetermined significance must be reported. Small cells displaying degenerated hyperchromatic nuclei resembling high-grade SIL and bizarre tadpole-shaped cells simulating invasive squamous cell carcinoma also are found in smears obtained from IUD wearers (Fig. 25.5). The paucity of the cells, their degenerated appearance, and the absence of low-grade SIL are clues to correct interpretation. A diagnosis of ASCUS may be warranted in difficult cases.

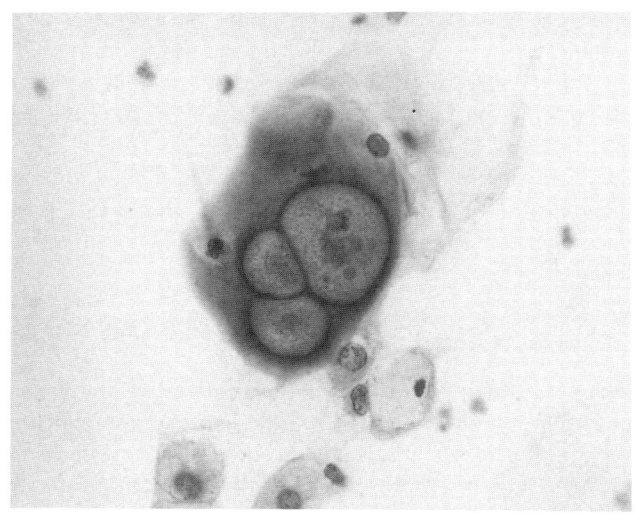

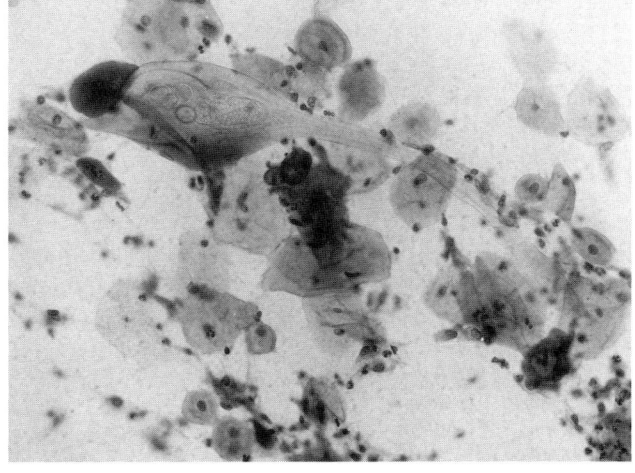

FIG. 25.4. Radiation changes. a: Cell showing prominent cytomegaly and degenerative vacuolization. **b:** Bizarre radiated cell assuming tadpole shape mimicking squamous carcinoma. The absence of a tumor diathesis and preserved cells with nuclear abnormalities distinguishes cells with radiation changes from carcinoma.

EFFECTS OF ABLATIVE THERAPY ON GYNECOLOGICAL SMEARS

In the weeks immediately after ablative therapy for SIL, smears reveal changes related to cellular destruction and mucosal repair.[79] Evidence of cellular damage includes nuclear hyperchromasia, smudged chromatin, pyknosis and fragmentation, and cytoplasmic vacuolization.

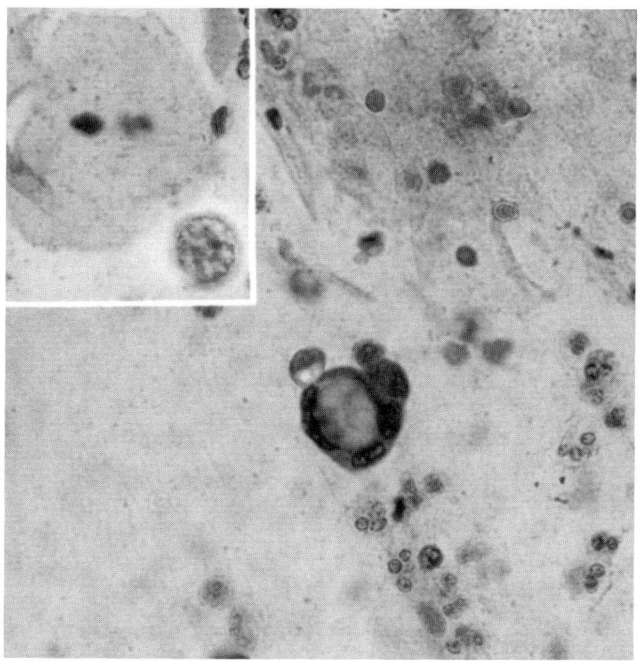

FIG. 25.5. Changes associated with IUDs. Degenerated glandular cells surround a large vacuole. *Inset:* Isolated small squamous cells resembling HSIL (CIN 3) also were present.

Changes related to therapy usually disappear within 3 months and SIL is readily detectable 6 months after ineffective ablative therapy. In cytological samples obtained within 3 months of therapy, it may be impossible to distinguish treatment-related effects from significant atypia. Since inconclusive reports raise the spector of inadequately treated disease, it is ill-advised to obtain smears until 3 months after treatment of SIL. The rate of adequate transformation zone sampling is not reduced after laser or cryotherapy, but is significantly increased after cone biopsy.

HYPERKERATOSIS AND PARAKERATOSIS

Squamous cells with orangeophilic or yellow cytoplasm that are anucleate or display a faintly stained nuclear ghost surrounded by a halo are indicative of hyperkeratosis. SILs and invasive squamous carcinoma may be associated with surface keratinization, but hyperkeratosis is more frequently related to benign conditions including uterine prolapse, prior cryosurgery or electrocautery, exposure to diethylstilbestrol (DES), long-standing chronic cervicitis, and use of a pessary. Therefore, hyperkeratosis is considered a reactive cellular change and smears displaying this finding should be considered negative. Hyperkeratosis was identified in 0.47% of smears examined in a large laboratory and was found repeatedly in 15.4% of these patients.[70] Follow-up smears and biopsies obtained after a smear showing hyperkeratosis revealed ASCUS or SIL in 4.3% of women compared with 1.69% of all women screened during the same period. The author concluded that identification of hyperkeratosis provides marginal evidence of a cervical abnormality in routine cancer screening, but may indicate the presence of disease in patients with a history of lower genital tract lesions.

Parakeratotic cells are miniature squamous cells that may display variable degrees of flattening or keratinization. Parakeratotic cells possess small, dense, hyperchromatic nuclei similar to those of superficial cells. Parakeratosis is commonly identified in women infected with HPV, but also is identified in a similar spectrum of benign conditions such as hyperkeratosis. Consequently, parakeratosis may be mentioned as part of a descriptive diagnosis, but smears displaying only parakeratosis should be classified as negative.

CYTOLOGY OF PREGNANCY AND THE PUERPERIUM

Smears obtained during pregnancy or in the postpartum period are interpreted in the same manner as specimens obtained from nongravid patients. The two most critical cytological diagnoses during pregnancy are herpes simplex virus infection and invasive carcinoma. Recognition of the former does not pose specific problems, whereas diagnosis of the latter may be more difficult in pregnant women because of the tendency of engorged cervical tissue to bleed, mimicking the hemorrhage of a tumor diathesis. Smears obtained from pregnant women may contain decidual cells that appear as large single cells with nuclear degeneration and nucleoli. When numerous, decidual cells may simulate SIL or invasive squamous carcinoma. In general, decidual cells possess more abundant cytoplasm than most SILs or carcinomas and are less numerous. Multinucleated trophoblasts appearing as large-cell single cells with vacuolated cytoplasm and many uniform nuclei occasionally are identified in smears obtained during pregnancy but are rarely numerous enough to cause confusion (Fig. 25.6).

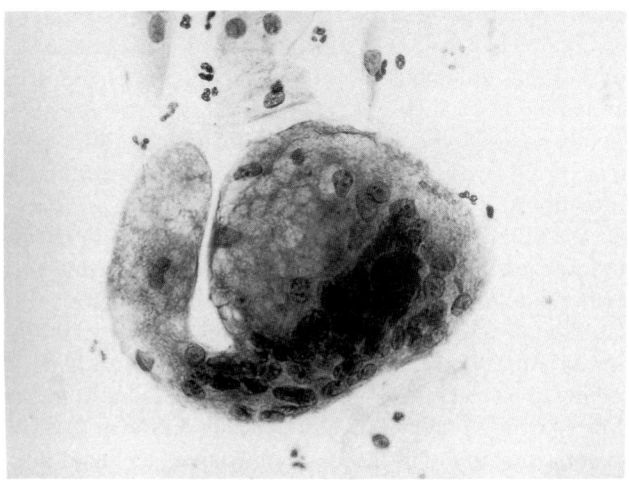

FIG. 25.6. Trophoblast. Giant multinucleated cell consistent with syncytial trophoblast in a postpartum smear.

Smears obtained in the postpartum period often show variable degrees of parabasal atrophy. The duration of atrophic changes is prolonged in women who breast feed and in some patients who fail to develop normal menses after delivery. Interpretation of atrophic specimens in the postpartum period may present similar problems to those encountered in postmenopausal women. In general, postpartum smears should not be obtained until 6 months after delivery.

Infectious Agents

Cervical cytology is a relatively insensitive but highly specific technique for identifying pathogenic microorganisms. Recognition of infectious agents in cervical smears facilitates therapy of symptomatic infections and, more importantly, aids the cytopathologist in distinguishing reactive changes from significant atypia. Smears obtained from patients with infections often are bloody, highly inflamed, and display reactive changes that may mimic or mask the presence of SILs. A repeat smear after treatment of a specific infection is suitable follow-up for patients with atypical squamous cells of undetermined significance (ASCUS) that are probably reactive; however, colposcopy may be indicated in patients with more worrisome abnormalities.

TRICHOMONAS VAGINALIS

Trichomonas vaginalis occurs singly or in small aggregates that coat the surface of mature squamous cells. Most trichomonas are intermediate in size between an inflammatory cell and a parabasal cell, but large forms occur. The organisms are oval or pear-shaped, with a faintly staining vesicular nucleus and eosinophilic intracytoplasmic granules. Rarely, an apical flagellum is identifiable in well-preserved specimens. Thin filamentous bacteria of the genus Leptothrix are accompanied by *Trichomonas* in 95% of cases. Coating of squamous cells with numerous neutrophils, referred to as *cannonballs*, pseudoeosinophilia, increased maturation, and pronounced reactive changes often are found. Squamous cells displaying nuclear degeneration and perinuclear cytoplasmic halos are distinguished from koilocytosis by the lack of diagnostic nuclear changes and the small, ill-defined appearance of the halos.

CANDIDA

In cervical smears, *Candida albicans* appears as oval eosinophilic yeast forms displaying a central clear zone and budding. Linear pseudohyphal fragments usually are present. The spores of *Candida glabrata* are smaller than those of *C. albicans* and do not form pseudohyphae. Squamous cells in patients with monilial infections often stick together, forming thick mats containing partially obscured fungal forms. Yeasts engulfed by phagocytes or located within the cytoplasm of epithelial cells often are surrounded by a halo. The presence of hyperkeratosis, pseudoparakeratosis, and reactive changes may mimic low-grade SIL. Since *Candida* is difficult to recognize in cervical biopsies without fungal stains, cytological identification of these organisms can provide an explanation for nonspecific colposcopic and histological findings.

BACTERIAL VAGINOSIS

Bacterial vaginosis results from replacement of the normal *Lactobacillus*-rich vaginal flora by a mixture of *Gardnerella vaginalis* and anaerobes, including cocci and curved bacilli of the species *Mobiluncus*.[134] Microscopically, the large rods of Lactobacilli are inconspicuous and many small cocci and bacilli are found. Squamous cells heavily covered by small bacilli, known as *clue cells*, are the hallmark of this disorder. In contrast to nonpecific adherence of bacteria to squamous cells, clue cells are more heavily coated at the edge of cell, imparting a "beard-like" or fringed appearance. Clue cells previously were attributed entirely to *Gardnerella* species, which was erroneously identified as the primary etiologic agent of bacterial vaginosis. More recent work indicates that clue cells are related to several bacterial species, including *Mobiluncus*, and that bacterial vaginosis is a polymicrobial disease. In TBS, smears displaying the pattern characteristic of bacterial vaginosis are reported as "shift in bacterial flora—predominance of coccobacilli."

HERPES VIRUS

Squamous cells infected with herpes simplex virus display finely granular or optically clear nuclei, reflecting effacement of the normal chromatin structure, multinucleation with nuclear molding, eosinophilic inclusions surrounded by halos, and formation of giant cells. Bizarre forms of virally infected cells and severe reactive and reparative changes related to ulceration may mimic invasive squamous cell carcinoma. Cells infected with herpes must be distinguished from trophoblastic cells, foreign body giant cells, and multinucleated cells occurring in atrophic smears. Rarely, nonspecific cellular degeneration may produce an effaced chromatin pattern resembling herpes infection. In these specimens, the other findings typical of herpes are absent.

Cytomegalovirus, another member of the Herpes family of viruses, has been rarely identified in smears of both immunosuppressed and immunocompetent women.[57] Endocervical cells displaying cytomegaly and deeply hematoxyphilic nuclear inclusions surrounded by large halos are diagnostic. Smaller satellite inclusions beneath the nuclear membrane and intracytoplasmic particles also are found. The nuclear inclusions of cytomegalovirus are basophilic in contrast to those of herpes simplex, which are eosinophilic

(Fig. 25.7). Adenovirus produces cytological findings that are easily distinguished from those of herpes. Adenovirus produces dense basophilic nuclear inclusions surrounded by halos associated with margination of chromatin beneath the nuclear membrane.[106]

ACTINOMYCES

Actinomyces usually are identified in endocervical mucus as dense aggregates of purple or blue filamentous bacteria radiating from a central core.[50] The organisms often are beaded and display acute angle branching and bulbous tips. The aggregates sometimes are ill-defined or arranged in a spherical or linear configuration (Fig. 25.8). The bacteria generally are surrounded by inflammatory cells including neutrophils, macrophages, and occasionally foreign body giant cells. Smears also may contain refractile fragments of plastic or metal derived from degenerating IUDs and psammoma bodies. Up to 1% of women with *Actinomyces* also are infected with *Entameba gingivalis*, an irregularly shaped 15-μm to 60-μm protozoan that displays a 4-μm vesicular nucleus containing a prominent endosome. The cytoplasm of the entamebae is granular and may contain engulfed leukocytes, but not erythrocytes.

Distinguishing *Actinomyces* from other microorganisms and artifacts is sometimes challenging. *C. albicans* may superficially resemble *Actinomyces*, but the pseudohyphae of *Candida* are thicker, associated with budding spores, and they do not form dense aggregates. *Aspergillus* rarely appears in smears as a contaminant characterized by large, thick segmented hyphae. Leptothrix and nocardia also may mimic *Actinomyces*. The former is thinner, nonbranching, and rarely appears in clumps; the latter displays right-angle

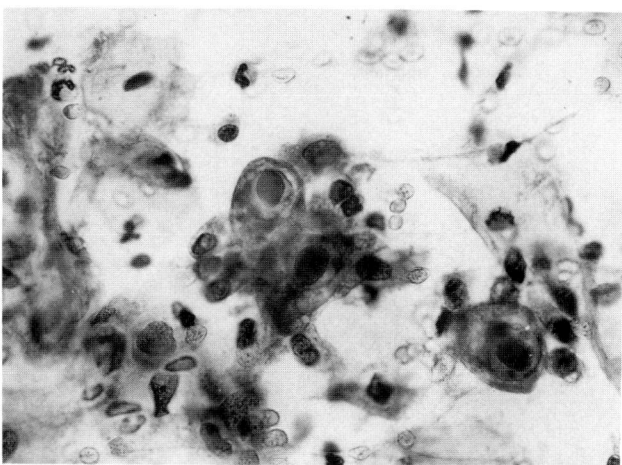

FIG. 25.7. **Cytomegalovirus.** Endocervical cells containing basophilic nuclear inclusions surrounded by halos typical of cytomegalovirus. Note large size of infected cells compared with normal-appearing endocervical cells.

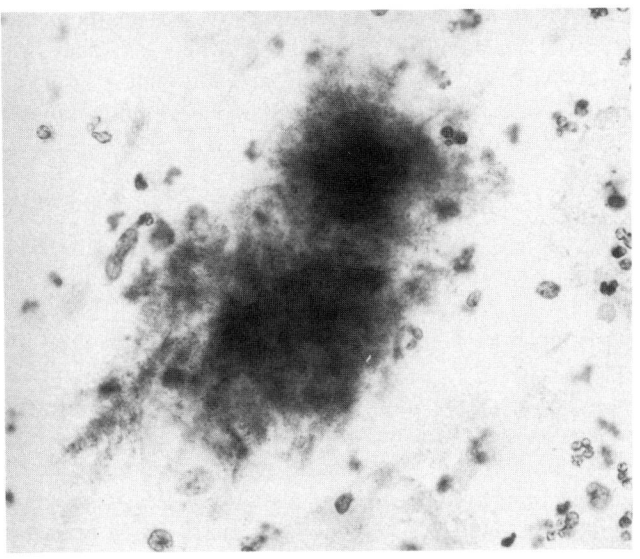

FIG. 25.8. *Actinomyces*. Dense mats of filamentous bacteria consistent with *Actinomyces*.

branching. Other structures resembling *Actinomyces* include fibrin and mucus threads, which appear more amorphous and tampon strings, which are birefringent and polarizable. Patients receiving antibiotic therapy occasionally form sulfa crystals that display radiating filaments reminiscent of *Actinomyces* (Fig. 25.9). The highly regular internal structure and contour of the crystals usually is distinctive. Staining artifacts, foreign material, and other microorganisms occasionally also may pose diagnostic difficulty.

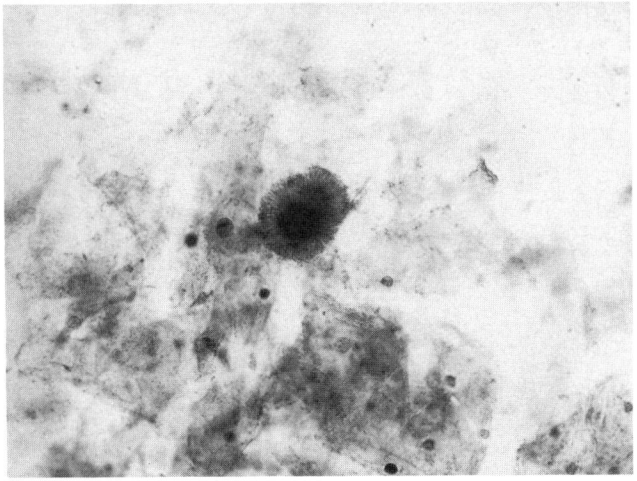

FIG. 25.9. Crystal resembling *Actinomyces*. Crystal with dense crystal core related to antibiotic use.

CHLAMYDIA

Although early reports proposed a wide range of cytological criteria for the diagnosis of chlamydia cervicitis,* the sensitivity and specificity of these criteria have not been substantiated in most carefully controlled investigations. Although endocervical or metaplastic squamous cells containing cytoplasmic vacuoles or inclusions have been described in *C. trachomatis* infections, diagnostic patterns cannot be reliably identified. Cytoplasmic vacuoles containing mucin or debris related to cellular degeneration often mimic chlamydial inclusions and lead to a high rate of false-positive diagnoses. In addition, many patients with proven chlamydial infections have unremarkable smears. Therefore it is best to avoid suggesting a diagnosis of *Chlamydia* in most instances.

Smears of patients who harbor *C. trachomatis* often reveal severe mucopurulent cervicitis. The presence of transformed lymphocytes and more than 30 histiocytes per 400× field in three fields is a typical finding.[75] Fully developed follicular cervicitis manifested by the presence of polymorphous lymphocytes and tingible macrophages surrounding thin-walled blood vessels also may be identified, although no inflammatory pattern is diagnostic of chlamydial infection.

Chlamydial infections have been associated with squamous atypias characterized by nuclear enlargement, hyperchromasia, and multinucleation. Since chlamydia cervicitis and SIL share similar demographics and frequently co-exist, atypias identified in patients with chlamydia cervicitis may be associated with HPV infection.

Squamous Epithelial Cell Abnormalities

Diagnoses of cervical smears and colposcopically directed biopsies agree within one grade in approximately 75% of patients.[65,66,96,136,137,152,167] Cytological diagnoses of high-grade SIL (HSIL) are confirmed more frequently than those of low-grade SIL (LSIL) when all patients diagnosed cytologically with SIL are routinely referred for colposcopy. Older reports in the literature suggest that up to a third of patients with a cytological diagnosis of LSIL prove to have HSIL histologically. In more recent studies, only 10–15% of patients demonstrated HSIL on biopsy.[53] The number of atypical cells present in a smear showing LSIL appears to represent the best cytological predictor of biopsy confirmation. This suggests that failure to confirm histologically a cytological diagnosis of LSIL is related to the small size of the lesion or regression in many cases.

---

*Refs. 11,27,43,46,51,56,93,122,129,141,148.

Patients referred for colposcopy because of a cytological abnormality may have negative repeat smears at the time of colposcopy despite the presence of biopsy-confirmed lesions.[53] Snyder et al.[151] reported that repeat smears obtained within 8 weeks of an abnormal initial smear often were falsely negative. Nonetheless, smears procured before colposcopy occasionally demonstrate a more severe lesion than preceding smears and the corresponding biopsies. The critical point in patient management is that colposcopically directed biopsies must account for the most severe cytological abnormality revealed by any preceding smear. In particular, patients whose smears reveal HSIL or invasive carcinoma that are histologically unconfirmed require further clinical evaluation. Four percent of squamous carcinomas in situ and 2% of invasive carcinomas measuring less than 4 mm in greatest dimension were missed by colposcopy in one study.[167] Rarely, clinically occult vaginal or vulvar intraepithelial neoplasia may shed suspicious squamous cells in cervical smears, resulting in a scenario in which patients have persistently abnormal cytology and repeatedly normal colposcopic examinations.

ATYPICAL SQUAMOUS CELLS OF UNDETERMINED SIGNIFICANCE

In TBS, ASCUS is defined as "cellular abnormalities that are more marked than those attributable to reactive changes but that quantitatively or qualitatively fall short of a SIL. Because the cellular changes in the ASCUS category may reflect an exuberant benign change or a potentially serious lesion which can not be unequivocally classified, they are interpreted as being of "undetermined significance."[109] The distinction between ASCUS and LSIL may be subtle and nonreproducible. Slight nuclear enlargement or irregularity, chromatin clumping, and cytoplasmic clearing may suggest LSIL, but are insufficient for a definitive diagnosis (Fig. 25.10). Similarly, large sheets of slightly pleomorphic keratinized squamous cells also should be classified as ASCUS if diagnostic nuclear atypia is lacking. Uterine prolapse, monilial infection, and other reactive processes may produce parakeratosis and hyperkeratosis, which resembles these changes. In addition, metaplasia, glycogen accumulation, and degeneration produce cytoplasmic vacuolization mimicking koilocytotic cavitation, but the absence of nuclear abnormalities distinguishes these changes from SIL. HPV DNA is present in the cervical lavages of most patients with ASCUS, although many of these patients have occult HPV infections and are colposcopically normal.[146]

The cytological diagnosis of ASCUS also may be applied to smears in which the differential diagnosis includes repair, atrophy, squamous metaplasia, reactive endocervical cells, and HSIL. In these cases, it is important to emphasize that a high-grade lesion cannot be excluded and to direct further investigations to the endocervical canal if appropriate. In atrophic vaginitis, degenerated cells with extremely large hyperchromatic, smudgy nuclei may be present in a bloody, inflammatory background. The patient's age and the lack of well-preserved abnormal cells distinguishes these cases from those diagnostic of HSIL. A repeat smear after a course of topical estrogen often will clarify the patient's diagnosis and should always precede colposcopy and biopsy in postmenopausal patients with worrisome smears. Failure to induce mucosal maturation with hormonal therapy can compromise colposcopic examination and yield biopsy specimens that do not resolve the distinction between atrophy and HSIL. In addition, nuclear pyknosis in biopsy specimens may be misinterpreted as mitoses, leading to an erroneous diagnosis and unnecessary treatment.

Metaplastic squamous cells are small and present a nuclear/cytoplasmic ratio that approaches that of SIL. Linearly arranged metaplastic squamous cells may resemble HSIL on low power. If inflammatory or degenerative changes are present, a suspicion of HSIL may result. Ultimately, the distinction of metaplasia from SIL is based on the benign appearance of the nuclei. In some patients, examination of biopsies and smears in isolation is insufficient to resolve the differential diagnosis; final classification requires a comparison of the cytological features in the smears with those in the biopsy (Fig. 25.11).

Although nucleoli are unusual in SIL, microinvasive and invasive squamous carcinomas may occur in sheets that resemble repair (Fig. 25.12). Inconclusive cases may be designated as "ASCUS with findings suggestive of carcinoma."

Accurate cytological diagnosis of cervical lesions is achieved most readily when smears reveal a pattern of consistent changes that point to a single diagnosis. However, some smears contain a few severely abnormal cells in an otherwise unremarkable background. Smears containing rare, highly abnormal cells should be reported as "ASCUS; findings suggestive of HSIL" and should prompt colposcopy and biopsy in addition to a repeat smear. Underestimation of an abnormality is especially likely to occur in smears obscured by blood or inflammation or in cases in which an endocervical component is absent. Since HSILs often involve the endocervical canal, these lesions tend to be inadequately sampled. In contrast, specimens that contain rare atypical cells of minimal concern are best diagnosed as ASCUS, probably reactive. These patients may require only routine follow-up.

LOW-GRADE SQUAMOUS INTRAEPITHELIAL LESIONS

LSIL encompasses lesions previously diagnosed as CIN 1, mild dysplasia, and cellular changes consistent with HPV infection.[109] CIN 1 usually appears as loose aggregates of flat polygonal cells displaying eosinophilic or cyanophilic

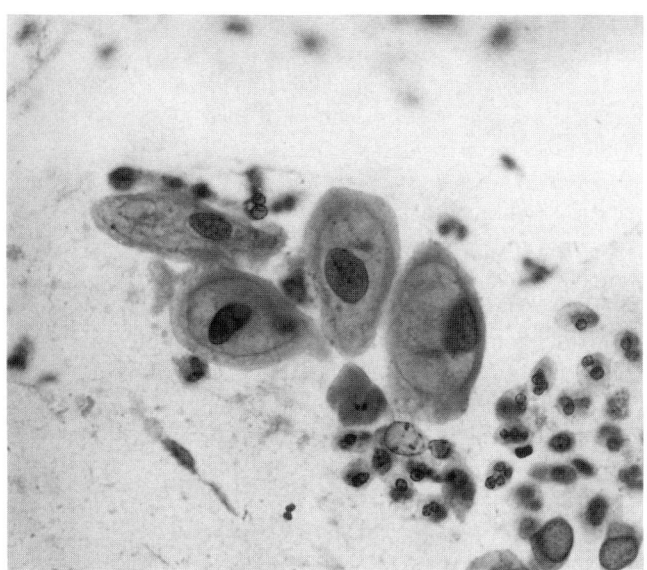

a

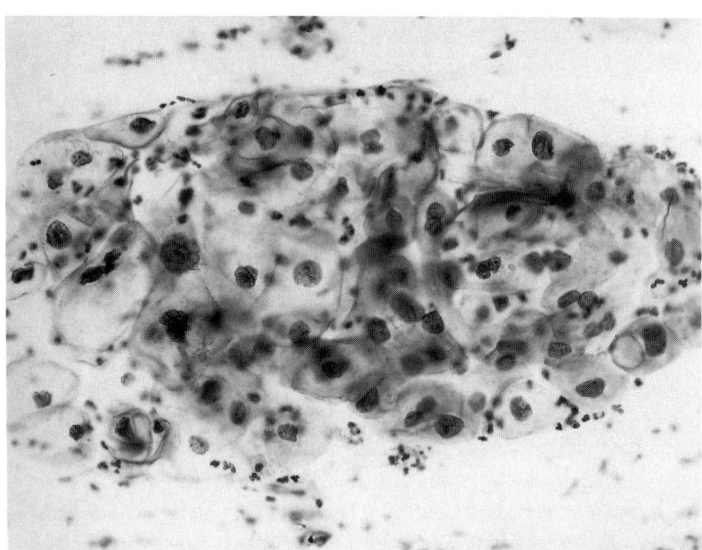

b

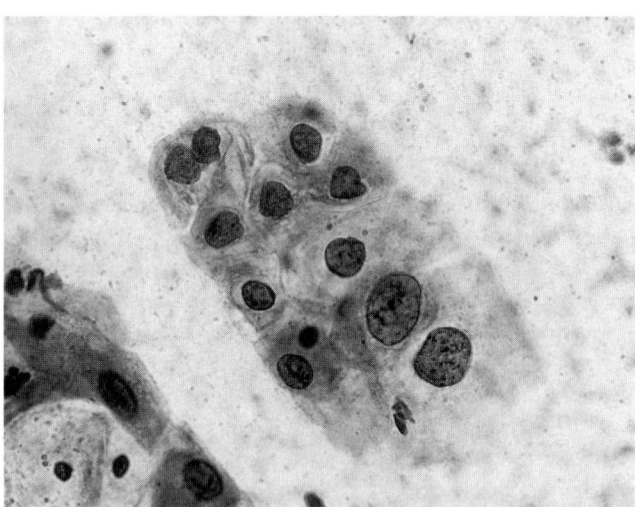

c

FIG. 25.10. Atypical squamous cells of undetermined significance (ASCUS) a: Cells display slightly enlarged, eccentrically placed nuclei lacking the hyperchromasia and chromatin irregularity characteristic of LSIL. **b:** Squamous cells with slight nuclear hyperchromasia, irregular outlines, and multinucleation are present in an inflammatory background. The cells may be reported as suggestive of LSIL, but would be considered as ASCUS unless additional cellular changes are identified elsewhere in the smear. **c:** Nuclei are enlarged with irregular contours and clumped chromatin. Changes closely approach those necessary for a diagnosis of LSIL.

cytoplasm. The cells of CIN 1 are approximately the size of intermediate cells but the nuclei are enlarged two to four times, resulting in an increased nuclear/cytoplasmic ratio. The nuclei of LSILs are mildly hyperchromatic and display variable degrees of chromatin clumping and irregularity (Fig. 25.13). Koilocytes have perinuclear cavitations surrounded by a dense rim of cytoplasm but otherwise have nuclear abnormalities similar to CIN 1 cells (Fig. 25.14). Some koilocytes display minimally enlarged nuclei that are extremely hyperchromatic, wrinkled, and have smudged chromatin. Sheets of keratinized cells with dense, waxy orange cytoplasm and atypical pleomorphic nuclei also are indicative of LSIL. Although, bi- and multinucleation, parakeratosis keratohyaline granules, and spindle-shaped cells may be found in smears displaying LSIL, these findings are nonspecific and do not by themselves indicate the presence of SIL.

Most smears that show well-developed LSILs contain a mixture of cell types and are not readily classified as either koilocytotic atypia or CIN 1. Since CIN 1 and koilocytotic atypia cannot be morphologically distinguished reliably[38,145] and are identical from an epidemiologic clinical and biologic perspective,[67,107,132,133,156,168] it is unnecessary to distinguish them cytologically. Studies indicate that only 15% of LSILs progress to high-grade lesions* and that one-fourth to one-half of LSILs are not histologically confirmed. Consequently, the diagnosis of LSIL should be rendered only when unequivocal nuclear abnormalities are present. Smears displaying marginal diagnostic findings are better classified as ASCUS.

_____

*Refs. 53,65,66,96,136,152,167.

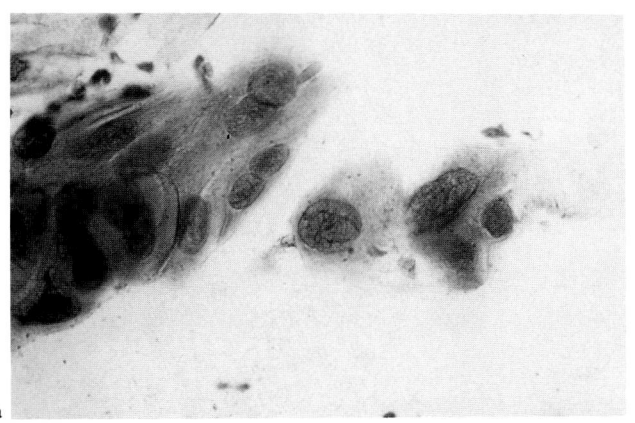

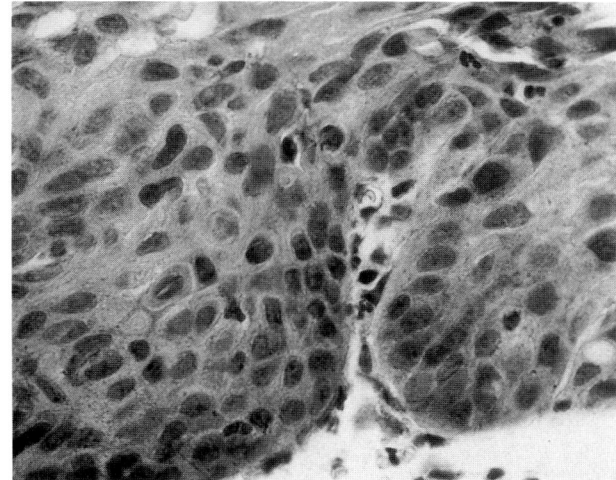

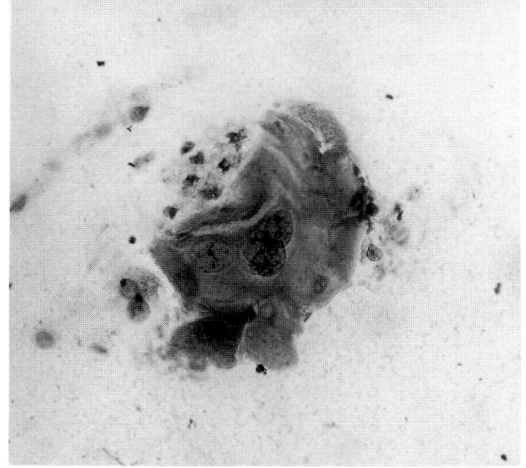

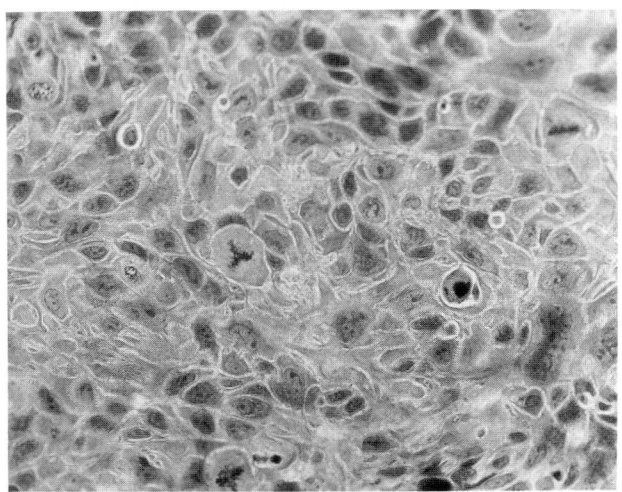

FIG. 25.11. **a: ASCUS, rule out HSIL.** Metaplastic squamous cells showing nuclear enlargement and anisocytosis. **b: Atypical squamous metaplasia.** Biopsy demonstrates squamous metaplasia with reactive and degenerative changes. **c: ASCUS, rule out HSIL.** Metaplastic squamous cells containing slightly enlarged nuclei with clumped chromatin. **d: HSIL.** Poorly oriented fragments of HSIL with tripolar mitosis.

HIGH-GRADE SQUAMOUS INTRAEPITHELIAL LESIONS

The designation HSIL subsumes CIN 2, CIN 3, moderate dysplasia, severe dysplasia, and carcinoma in situ. Criteria for CIN 3 are well established, but criteria for the diagnosis of CIN 2 are inexact. CIN 3 is characterized by loose aggregates of round or oval cells, about the size of parabasal cells, which display a ratio of nuclear/cytoplasmic area exceeding 50%. Pronounced nuclear aberrations are the rule (Fig. 25.15). The cells usually are numerous, but poorly sampled lesions in the endocervical canal often shed few cells that are easily overlooked because of their small size. In endocervical brush specimens, CIN 3 may appear as fragments of crowded cells with irregularly shaped, hyperchromatic nuclei. Sheets of severely abnormal squamous cells with indistinct cytoplasmic borders were previously designated as carcinoma in situ. Sometimes the cells composing fragments of CIN 3 are crushed and difficult to interpret. Identification of single cells diagnostic of HSIL usually is possible, but in smears containing atypical cells only within fragments, the distinction between HSIL, endocervical neoplasia, and reactive endocervical cells may be difficult. Examination of the edge of the fragments is the best strategy to assess the appearance of the nucleus and determine whether the cytoplasm displays the delicate texture and columnar shape of glandular cells or the denser cytoplasm and polygonal shape of squamous cells. When SIL involves endocervical glands, the squamous cells may be admixed with benign endocervical cells or acquire columnar features further complicating interpretation (Fig. 25.16). Since the cytological distinction between severe dysplasia and carcinoma in situ is not reproducible

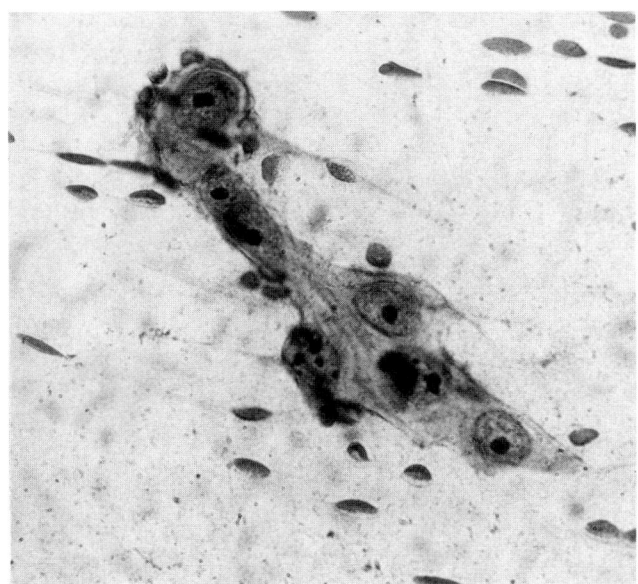

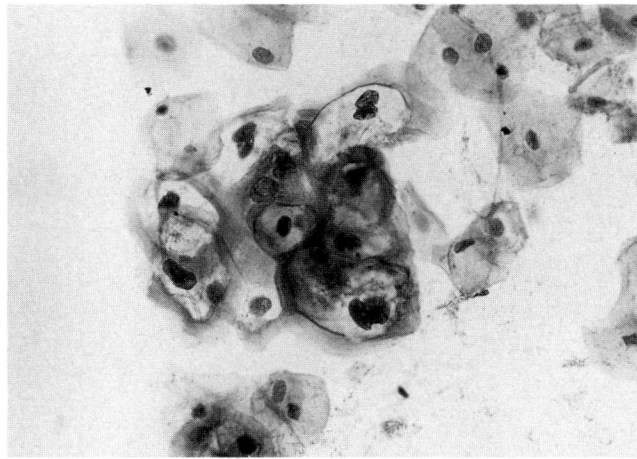

FIG. 25.14. LSIL (koilocytotic atypia). Cells display nuclear hyperchromasia, binucleation, and cytoplasmic cavities surrounded by dense rim of cytoplasm.

FIG. 25.12. ASCUS, rule out squamous carcinoma. Bloody smear containing rare sheets of overlapping squamous cells with hyperchromatic nuclei containing nucleoli. Smear was diagnosed as ASCUS; cannot distinguish repair from carcinoma. Biopsy revealed squamous carcinoma.

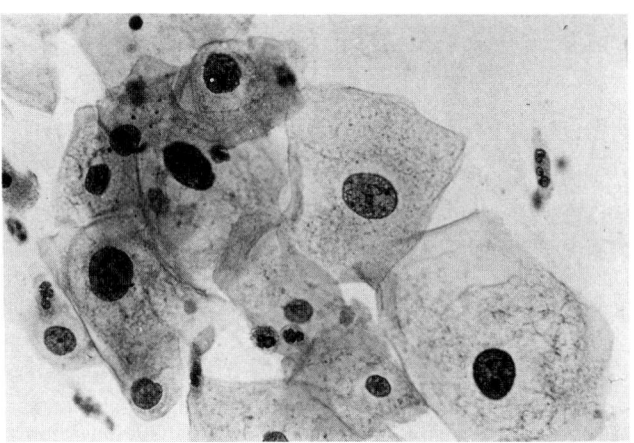

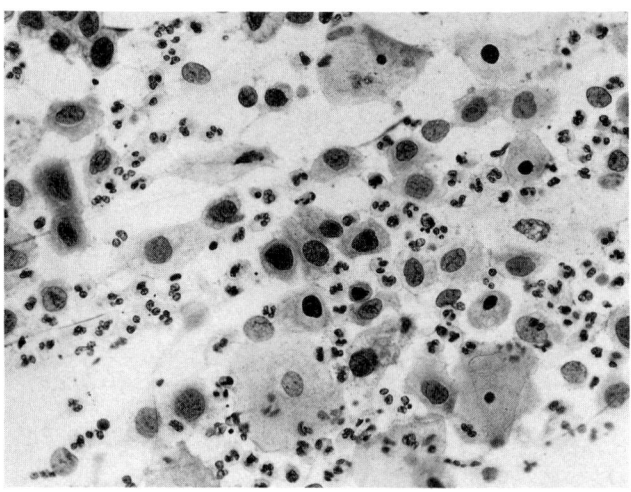

25-15a

FIG. 25.13. LSIL (CIN 1). Note the presence of nuclear hyperchromasia and clumped chromatin.

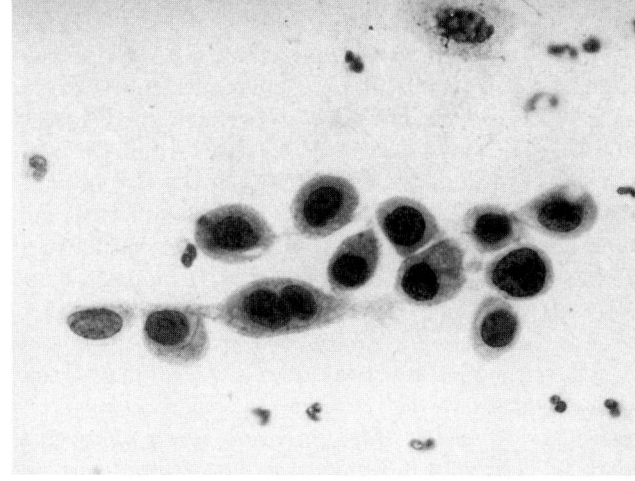

FIG. 25.15. HSIL. a: Many small cells with hyperchromatic nuclei and scant cytoplasm. **b:** Nuclei are hyperchromatic with clumped chromatin and irregular outlines.

25-15

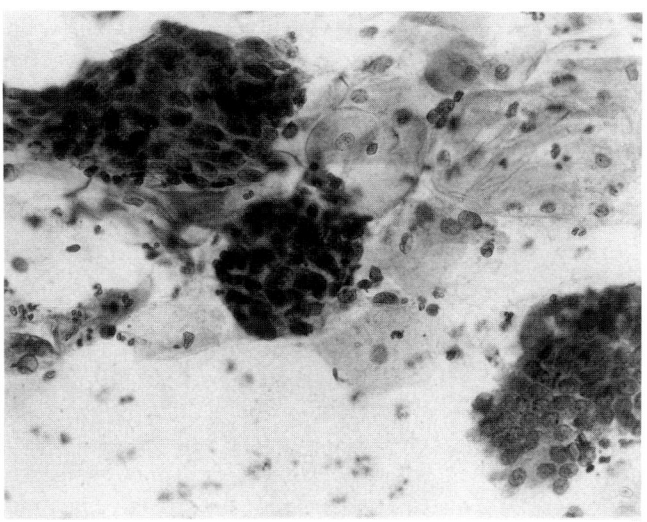

Fig. 25.16. HSIL. Two clusters of HSIL with rounded contours suggestive of endocervical involvement. Contrast the crowding and nuclear hyperchromasia of the HSIL with the evenly spaced reactive endocervical cells (*lower right*).

and lacks biologic significance, it has been eliminated (see Chapter 7, Precancerous Lesions of the Cervix). Cells with severely atypical nuclei and a ratio of nuclear/cytoplasmic area approaching 50% are designated as CIN 2 (Fig. 25.17). Biopsies of CIN 2 often display a proliferation of atypical cells extending from the basement membrane into the middle of the epithelium associated with variable degrees of surface maturation or koilocytotic atypia. Some cases consist of polygonal cells with dense cytoplasm resembling metaplastic cells. The distinction between atypical immature squamous metaplasia and HSIL may be difficult. Cells displaying significant nuclear hyperchromasia and irregular nuclear contours are best classified as HSIL. The nuclei of immature metaplasia generally are more vesicular and display nucleoli, a feature rarely found in SIL. Biopsies of SIL reveal cellular disorientation, overlapping, and crowding whereas immature metaplasia is characterized by a regular arrangement of the cells. Mitoses may be present in both lesions. Review of the smears in conjunction with the biopsies is useful in reaching a final diagnosis in these cases.

Progression of HSIL to invasive squamous carcinoma has been reported in approximately 10–25% of cases.[101] In contrast with LSIL, most experts agree that all HSILs require treatment. Consequently, cytological diagnoses of HSIL have important therapeutic implications.

GRADING SIL

The main purpose of grading SILs is to facilitate correlation of smears and biopsies. The best method for excluding a biopsy sampling error is to compare the appearance of the cells in the smears and the biopsies. Since correlation of all cytological and histological specimens is impractical, only cases with highly discrepant reports must be reviewed. Specifically, smears demonstrating HSIL or carcinoma that are unconfirmed histologically require correlation. Cytological grading of SIL also is important for estimating the biologic potential of lesions and may be used to monitor progression of disease in untreated patients. Although there is disagreement among gynecologists as to whether all women with LSIL require treatment, there is widespread agreement that all women with HSIL require treatment. Finally, comparison of cytological and histological grading is important for quality assurance purposes.

The rationale for classifying SILs into low-grade and high-grade disease in TBS is based on pathological, clinical, and virologic data.* Many studies using three- or four-grade classification systems have shown poor diagnostic reproducibility,[33,58,77,87,140,173] suggesting that elaborate grading schemes do not provide additional information. Although natural history studies of SIL indicate that lesions of any severity may regress, it appears that most LSILs regress, whereas HSILs display a greater tendency to persist or progress. In addition, both oncogenic and nononcogenic HPV types are identified in both LSIL and HISL, but oncogenic types are relatively more frequent in HSIL (see Chapter 7, Precancerous Lesions of the Cervix). To date, the treatment of SIL has been based primarily on the size and distribution of histologically confirmed lesions and not the pathologic grade. The development of strategies to manage LSIL conservatively may render the dis-

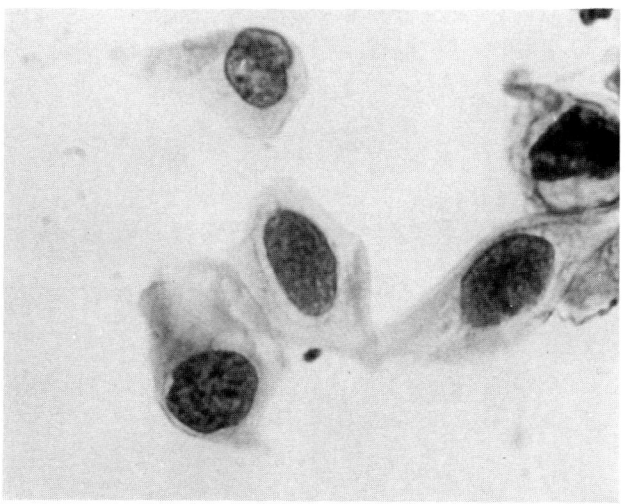

Fig. 25.17. HSIL (CIN 2). Cells display severe nuclear hyperchromasia and clumped chromatin, but possess more cytoplasm than those of CIN 3.

---

*Refs. 38,67,107,132,133,145,156,168.

tinction between LSIL and HSIL of greater clinical significance. Based on reproducibility studies, we currently report LSILs without qualification and subclassify HSILs as CIN 2 or CIN 3 for academic purposes.

Cytological grading is based primarily on the pattern of the entire smear. HSILs generally shed more cells than LSILs. The cells of HSILs usually are smaller and display a higher ratio of nuclear/cytoplasmic area and greater nuclear abnormalities than those of LSILs. Cells indicative of LSIL are sometimes present in smears classified as HSIL. When SIL cells are found primarily in endocervical brush material or in a background of cervical mucus, a lesion within the endocervical canal should be suspected. The presence of smooth, rounded groups of abnormal cells also may reflect an origin in the canal. Some smears revealing SIL are difficult to grade because of hyperkeratosis, poor preservation, a paucity of diagnostic cells or obscuring blood, inflammation, or air drying. A diagnosis of SIL of indeterminate degree is appropriate in these cases.

SQUAMOUS CARCINOMA

More than 50% of women developing invasive cervical carcinoma have not been screened within 5 years of diagnosis.[28] Nonetheless, the reported false-negative rate for the cytological detection of cervical squamous carcinoma ranges from 17% to 86%.* The vast majority of these missed diagnoses reflect failure to recognize rare, poorly preserved tumor cells in smears obscured by blood and inflammation. Some cases may be due to rapidly developing carcinomas,[34,103] but designation of carcinomas as rapidly developing based on a single negative smear is questionable.[143] Since cervical smears are relatively insensitive in detecting carcinoma, all visible cervical lesions should be biopsied.

The reliability of cytology in diagnosing microinvasive squamous carcinoma has been debated. Microinvasive carcinoma was accurately diagnosed cytologically in most patients in two series,[114,115] but was recognized less accurately in other reports.[30,155] More than half the patients with early invasion are asymptomatic and have normal-appearing cervices; consequently, it is important to suggest the possibility of invasion in these women to ensure adequate evaluation. Ng et al.[114] described four criteria that suggest microinvasion: (1) a tumor diathesis, (2) arrangement of most malignant cells in aggregates resembling syncytia, (3) irregular chromatin distribution in the tumor cells, and (4) the presence of prominent nucleoli in approximately 20% of the cells. Since HSIL developing in the setting of severe inflammation and repair can display some of these features, it is preferable to suggest rather than unequivocally diagnose microinvasion in most cases. Comparison of smears and biopsies is required in all patients in whom a cytological diagnosis of possible microinvasion is histologically unconfirmed to ensure that a lesion in the endocervical canal has not been missed. Rarely tumors in the vagina may be the source of undetected invasive carcinomas.

The cytological diagnosis of invasive squamous carcinoma is based on both the appearance of the abnormal squamous cells and the background.[111] The tumor cells occur singly or in loosely cohesive sheets displaying loss of polarity and indistinct cell membranes. The background typically reveals a tumor diathesis consisting of fresh and lysed blood, acute inflammation, and necrotic debris. Cells indicative of HSIL and LSIL are present in some specimens, but may be absent. Unaffected squamous cells usually are of superficial and intermediate type. Squamous carcinoma cells generally are larger than cells of HSIL and display a ratio of nuclear/cytoplasmic area that ranges from moderately to markedly increased (Fig. 25.18). Keratinized squamous carcinomas often shed spindle-shaped cells with dense orange cytoplasm and black, irregularly shaped nuclei. Cells may resemble tadpoles or contain cytoplasmic fibers termed *herxheimer spirals* (Fig. 25.19). Squamous pearls consisting of rounded structures formed from concentric layering of tumor cells and keratinaceous debris are characteristic. Large cell nonkeratinizing squamous carcinomas are more difficult to recognize than their keratinized counterparts. These tumors exfoliate cells with dense cyanophilic cytoplasm arranged singly or in round aggregates or sheets. The nuclei are hyperchromatic with variable degrees of chromatin clumping and clearing,

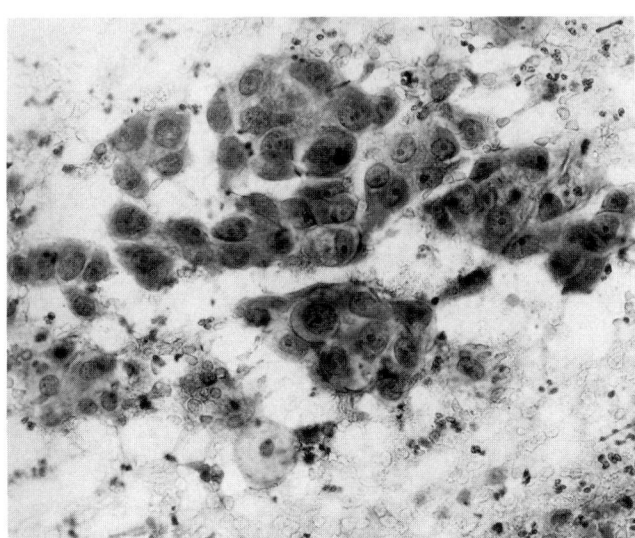

FIG. 25.18. **Invasive squamous carcinoma.** Malignant squamous cells displaying irregularly shaped nuclei with thickened rims and prominent nucleoli. Note tumor diathesis.

*Refs. 5,8,10,22,34,82,98,103,118,131,143.

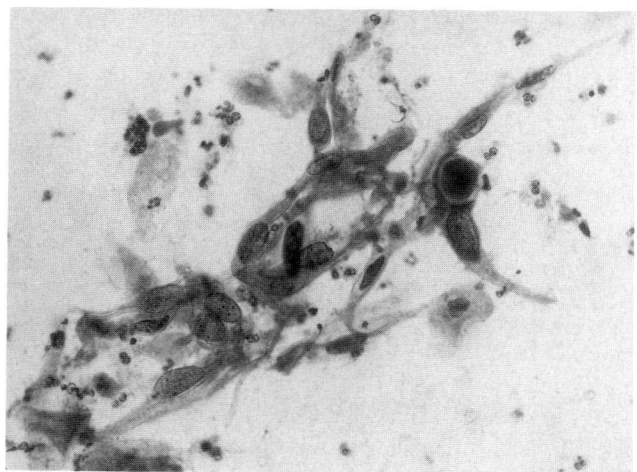

FIG. 25.19. **Squamous carcinoma.** Malignant spindle cells of squamous carcinoma. Note the presence of acellular, dense keratinaceous debris.

which may impart a vesicular appearance. Cells often display a high nuclear/cytoplasmic ratio and macronucleoli. Small cell carcinomas of squamous and neuroendocrine types are not easily separated cytologically. These neoplasms shed cells that are smaller than parabasal cells and are characterized by a high nuclear/cytoplasmic ratio and hyperchromatic nuclei with clumped chromatin and small or absent nucleoli. Nuclear molding and mitotic figures usually are evident.

The differential diagnosis of invasive squamous carcinoma includes both preneoplastic and nonneoplastic conditions. Invasive carcinomas are distinguished from SIL by the presence of greater pleomorphism, macronucleoli, and a tumor diathesis. SIL may shed cells displaying nucleoli or bizarre multinucleation, but this is rare. Some keratinized carcinomas shed plaques of dyskeratotic cells that resemble the findings associated with HPV infection. Sheets of reparative epithelium typically contain cells that display one or more macronucleoli, but the cells are cohesive, uniform in appearance, and do not display clumped chromatin. Scrapes obtained from ulcerated lesions of herpes simplex virus may contain cells that display Cowdry type A intranuclear inclusions resembling nucleoli and sheets of reparative epithelium that together simulate carcinoma. Hyperchromatic degenerated nuclei in smears revealing atrophic vaginitis also may raise a suspicion of carcinoma. In atrophy well-preserved malignant cells are lacking. In general, squamous carcinoma should be diagnosed cautiously in atrophic smears. Recommending a repeat smear, colposcopy, and biopsy after a course of topical estrogen is preferrable. Large degenerated decidual cells containing nucleoli may cause diagnostic confusion and provoke unnecessary procedures in pregnant women. Decidual cells usually are rare and occur singly, but may be numerous in

patients with decidual polyps. Well-preserved malignant cells and SIL are not found in these smears.

Small cell carcinomas are the most difficult tumor to diagnose. Aggregates of tumor cells in a bloody background are readily misinterpreted as endometrial cells in menstruating women or as endometrial carcinoma in postmenopausal patients. The presence of nuclear abnormalities distinguishes the small cell carcinoma cells from normal endometrial cells. The arrangement of small cell carcinomas mainly in sheets instead of three-dimensional clusters contrasts with the appearance of endometrial adenocarcinoma. Finally, adenosquamous carcinomas and squamous carcinomas that contain columnar-shaped cells resembling endocervical adenocarcinoma may be difficult to distinguish, but all of these diagnoses point to a malignant lesion in the cervix; consequently these differences are of little clinical importance.

Endocervical Cell Abnormalities

ATYPICAL GLANDULAR (ENDOCERVICAL) CELLS OF UNCERTAIN SIGNIFICANCE

Sheets of columnar cells displaying nuclear enlargement, hyperchromasia, and overlapping may not be classifiable as reactive or neoplastic (Fig. 25.20). In addition, SIL involving the endocervix may masquerade as an endocervical glandular atypia. Endocervical atypias were reported in 0.46% of smears in a recent study.[47] Cervical lesions were histologically demonstrated in half these patients, but three-fourths of these were SIL. If biopsies and curettages are negative in a patient receiving a cytological diagnosis of glandular atypia, the smears and biopsies must be compared to determine whether the source of the cytologically atypical cells has been identified. Cone biopsy may be indicated to conclusively exclude carcinoma in some patients.

Despite caution, several nonneoplastic conditions may mimic endocervical adenocarcinoma cytologically. Pacey et al.[117] reported three cases diagnosed cytologically as adenocarcinoma that proved to represent benign lesions: endometriosis, glandular atypia after a cone biopsy, and tubal metaplasia. The authors observed that after a cone biopsy, the mucosa may be regenerated by ingrowth of cells from the lower uterine segment, resulting in exfoliation of endometrial-type cells with reactive changes in smears. Tubal metaplasia is recognized easily when columnar cells display well-preserved terminal bars and cilia. However, cilia may become unrecognizable in air-dried smears and ciliated endocervical cells may be found in smears obtained from patients with endocervical adenocarcinoma. Tubal metaplasia was found in 66% of cone biopsies and hysterectomy specimens and 90% of cervical biopsies and endocervical curettages after a cytologic diagnosis of endocervical atypia.[116] Microglandular hyperplasia

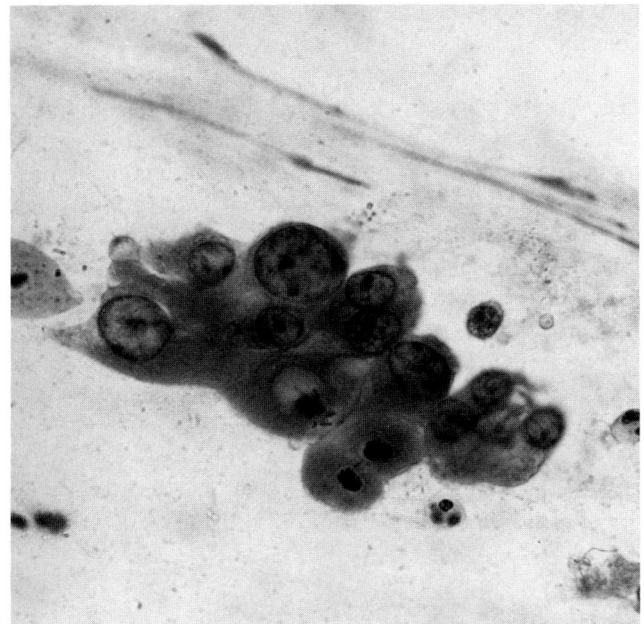

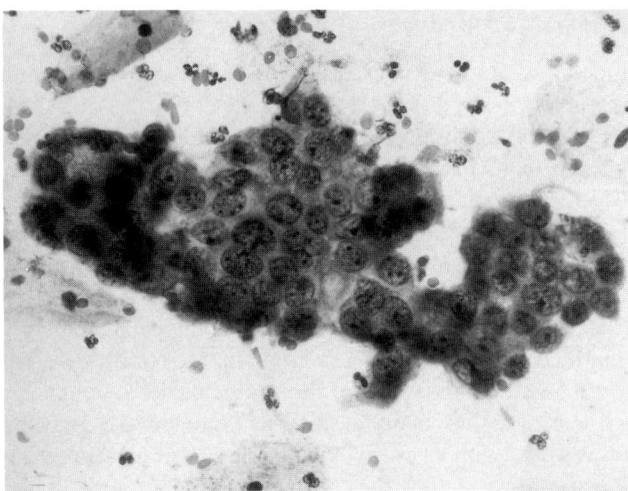

FIG. 25.20. a: AGUS, favor-reactive endocervical cells. Glandular cells display marked anisokaryosis and mitotic figures. Follow-up studies have been negative. **b: AGUS, rule out endocervical adenocarcinoma.** Crowded sheet of endocervical cells with coarse chromatin and nucleoli. Biopsy revealed endocervical adenocarcinoma.

(MGH) also has been recognized as a source of false suspicious cytological diagnoses of adenocarcinoma.[171] Microglandular hyperplasia may display nuclear enlargement and nucleoli similar to reactive endocervical epithelium, but usually lacks the severe nuclear and architectural atypia characteristic of adenocarcinoma. Repair and inflammation often are present in cases of MGH showing cytological atypia and mitoses may be seen. A diagnosis of AGUS rule out adenocarcinoma in situ is rendered in about 10% of women who are subsequently shown to have

MGH on subsequent histological examination. In the setting of oral contraceptives or hormone use, glandular lesions should be cautiously assessed.

ENDOCERVICAL ADENOCARCINOMA

Adenocarcinoma in situ (AIS) usually is asymptomatic and undetectable by colposcopy; therefore, responsibility for the early diagnosis of AIS rests solely with the cytopathologist. In two early studies of cervical adenocarcinoma, the ratio of invasive squamous carcinoma to invasive adenocarcinoma was 1:12 and 1:15, whereas the ratio of squamous carcinoma in situ of the cervix to AIS was 1:26 and 1:239.[15,26] Based on these findings, the authors concluded that AIS is an underdiagnosed disease. In addition, more than half the cases of AIS reported in older series were incidental findings in patients investigated for abnormal bleeding or SIL. The development of better cytological criteria for the diagnosis of AIS should result in improved cytological detection. Ayer et al.[7] reported 78.5% sensitivity in the diagnosis of adenocarcinoma and concluded that 98.5% of cases were diagnosable on review. Growing emphasis on the importance of sampling the endocervical canal and the widespread use of devices to ensure endocervical sampling undoubtedly will increase the cytological detection of AIS and glandular atypias. Cytological diagnoses of AIS are significant because cone biopsy may be required if punch biopsies and curettages are nondiagnostic. Recognition of endocervical adenocarcinoma in the setting of SIL is important because treatment of SIL is never adequate to eradicate invasive endocervical adenocarcinoma.

The cytological diagnosis of AIS is based on architectural and nuclear features.° AIS usually sheds sheets of columnar cells with crowding and overlapping and strips of cells displaying palisading and pseudostratification. Fragments resembling the honeycomb arrangement of benign endocervix, but with loss of polarity and architectural disarray, may be present. The cytoplasm of the tumor cells is finely vacuolated and the nuclei are eccentrically placed. The cells may be enlarged or normal in size and the nuclear/cytoplasmic ratio usually is increased to about twice that found in normal endocervical cells. Strips of columnar cells with palisaded, hyperchromatic naked nuclei protruding from the edge of the groups, referred to as *feathering*, and formation of rosettes is typical (Fig. 25.21). Ayer et al.[7] described two variants of AIS based on the appearance of the nuclei. The more common pattern of AIS displays oval, hyperchromatic nuclei possessing granular chromatin measuring less than 15 μM. Small to medium-sized nucleoli are present in half these cases, but are masked by the heavily stained chromatin. In the other variant of AIS, cells possess round, vesicular nuclei exceeding 15 μM in diam-

---

°Refs. 6,7,12,15,18,29,73,83,84,90,117.

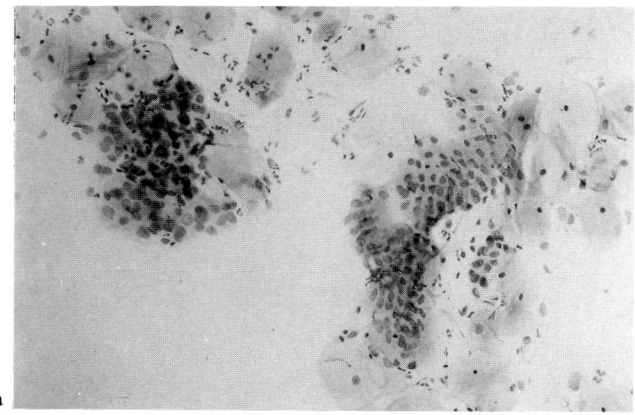

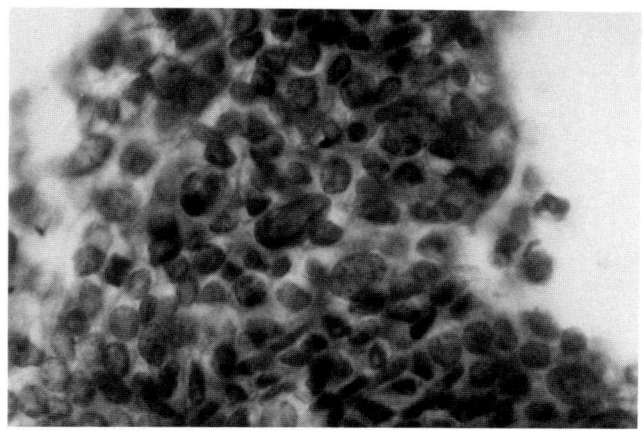

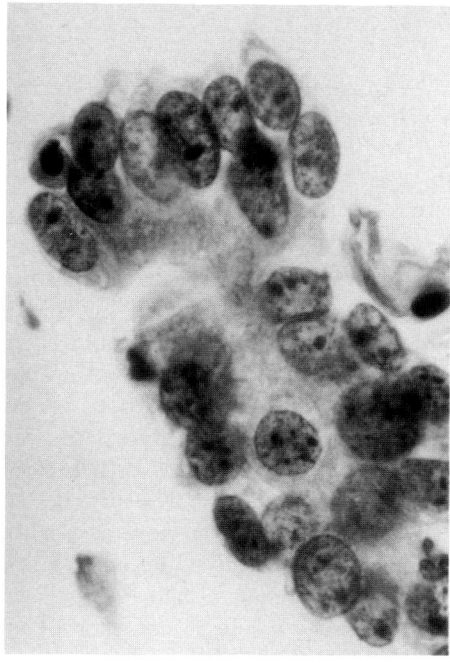

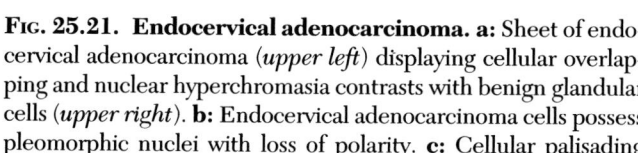

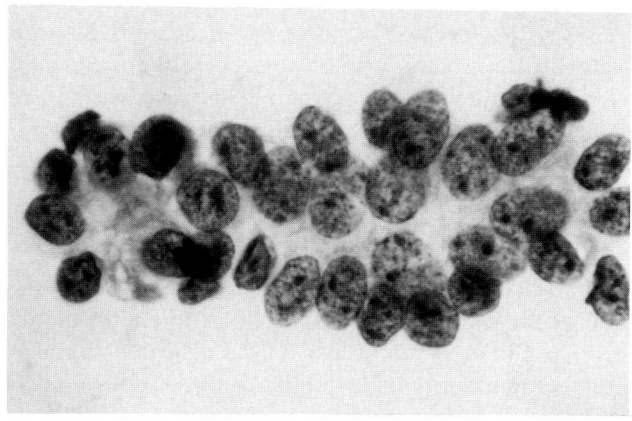

FIG. 25.21. Endocervical adenocarcinoma. a: Sheet of endocervical adenocarcinoma (*upper left*) displaying cellular overlapping and nuclear hyperchromasia contrasts with benign glandular cells (*upper right*). **b:** Endocervical adenocarcinoma cells possess pleomorphic nuclei with loss of polarity. **c:** Cellular palisading typical of endocervical adenocarcinoma. Cells have prominent nucleoli which are partially observed by dense chromatin. **d:** Nuclei appear to extend beyond edge of fragment (*feathering*). Poorly formed rosette is present. (Figs. **a, c,** and **d** courtesy of Bruce Werness, M.D., Washington, D.C.)

eter that show peripheral margination of the chromatin beneath the nuclear membrane. Macronucleoli are characteristic of this pattern of AIS.

Features to distinguish invasive endocervical adenocarcinoma from AIS have been described,[6,84] but it is unlikely that these entities can be separated in all cases. Generally, invasive adenocarcinomas are more pleomorphic and may be accompanied by a tumor diathesis consisting of necrotic cells, blood, and inflammation. The nuclei tend to be vesicular and contain macronucleoli. Consequently, one variant of AIS described by Ayer resembles invasive adenocarcinoma. Other features that have been suggested as predict-

ing invasion are syncytial-like groupings, small cells in supercrowded sheets, papillary clusters, and dense cytoplasm displaying squamous-like features. Mucosal ulceration and necrosis may result in smears obscured by blood and inflammation. A careful search for malignant glandular cells often is required in smears displaying a suspicious background.

Minimal deviation adenocarcinoma displays only focal cytological atypia in histological sections, but limited data suggest that most of these cases may be diagnosed or suspected cytologically.[159] One report described the absence of squamous metaplasia and repair and the presence of

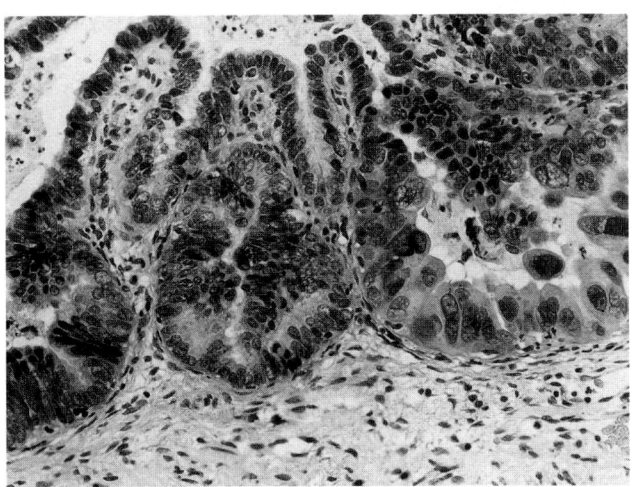

Fig. 25.22. Endocervical adenocarcinoma. Typical pattern of AIS (*left*) involving surface mucosa merging with polygonal cells (*lower right*) containing abundant, dense cytoplasm suggestive of squamous differentiation.

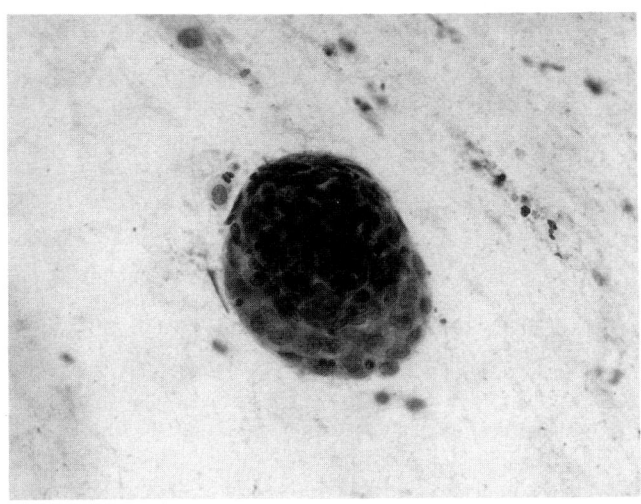

Fig. 25.23. Endometrial stromal breakdown. Smooth ball of small glandular cells enveloping endometrial stroma. Appearance resembles that of endometrial stromal breakdown in curettage specimens.

mitoses in three cases of adenoma malignum. Biopsies obtained from women with obvious cervical enlargement that reveal only benign-appearing endocervical glands should suggest the possibility of minimal deviation adenocarcinoma. Definite diagnosis requires a cone biopsy (see Chapter 8, Carcinoma and Other Tumors of the Cervix).

The cytological distinction between endocervical and endometrial carcinoma often is impossible. Costa et al.[29] reported that only 18% of 39 adenocarcinomas diagnosed cytologically were localized correctly as to site of origin. This is not unexpected in light of the similar patterns of differentiation displayed by tumors of these sites. In addition, endocervical adenocarcinomas sometimes display a mixture of cells that may suggest both glandular and squamous differentiation (Fig. 25.22). Although some endocervical adenocarcinomas may be specifically diagnosed cytologically, fractional curettage and sometimes cone biopsy are necessary to identify the site of the primary tumor.

Endometrial Cell Abnormalities

ABNORMAL SHEDDING OF NORMAL-APPEARING ENDOMETRIAL CELLS

Endometrial cells typically possess a scant amount of delicate cytoplasm and eccentrically located, round nuclei with dense chromatin and smooth contours, similar in size to an intermediate squamous cell nucleus. The ratio of the nuclear/cytoplasmic area of cells shed from proliferative or atrophic endometrium generally is above 50%. Stromal cells appear as loose aggregates of spindle-shaped cells possessing a scant amount of delicate cytoplasm and oval or round nuclei with delicate chromatin (Fig. 25.23).

In women with regular cycles, endometrial epithelial and stromal cells are identified in 21% of smears obtained during the first 10 days of the menstrual cycle and in only 2% of smears obtained at other times.[95] However, endometrial cells are identified after day 10 in 14.8% of women who have abnormal bleeding.[165] The presence of endometrial cells in a smear obtained from a postmenopausal woman is always considered abnormal. The presence of endometrial cells in smears obtained after day 10 of the menstrual cycle rarely results in detection of an endometrial lesion in women under 40 years of age.[113] In contrast, Gondos and King[48] identified 33 (22%) endometrial lesions among 147 patients over age 40 years who shed endometrial cells after day 10 or during the menopause. Ng et al.[113] reported that polyps were the most common cause of endometrial shedding after day 10 at all ages and that the likelihood of discovering a carcinoma was correlated with the age of the patient. Adenocarcinomas were discovered in 2.1% of patients in the fifth decade, 4.2% in the sixth decade, and 13.2% in the seventh decade of life among women who shed morphologically normal-appearing endometrial cells after day 10 or in the postmenopausal period. Endometrial hyperplasia was found in an additional 18.4% of patients over 60 years in this series. Exfoliation of large fragments of endometrial tissue from the lower uterine segment occurs when an endocervical brush is placed above the endocervical canal, but the appearance of the cells is easily distinguished from that of naturally shed cells (Fig. 25.24).

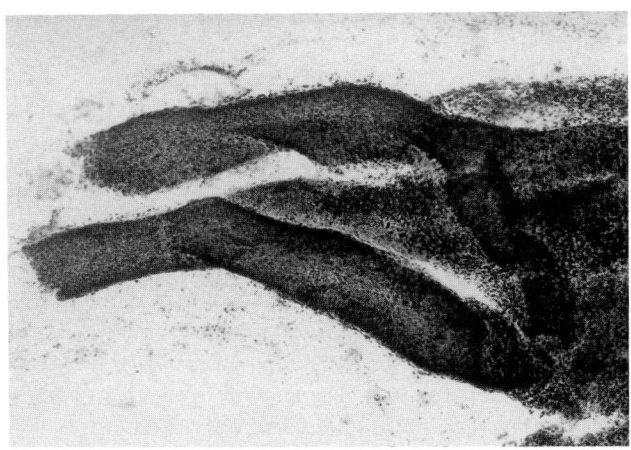

FIG. 25.24. Fragments of endometrial tissue removed with cytobrush. Intact endometrial glands and stroma, which were dislodged with an endocervical brush.

ATYPICAL GLANDULAR (ENDOMETRIAL) CELLS OF UNDETERMINED SIGNIFICANCE

The diagnosis of atypical glandular cells of undetermined significance (AGUS) is employed most frequently in postmenopausal women whose smears contain atypical endometrial cells that lack features diagnostic of adenocarcinoma. These smears are reported as "AGUS suspicious for adenocarcinoma" and tissue studies are recommended. Features that suggest that endometrial cells are abnormal include cellular and nuclear enlargement, abnormal nuclear shapes, hyperchromasia irregular chromatin clumping and clearing, and the presence of nucleoli.[112] Since the nuclei of well-differentiated adenocarcinomas may be only one and a half to two times normal, they are easily missed. Nucleoli are identified in 73% of invasive carcinomas and 32% of adenocarcinoma precursors, but are rare in normal endometrial cells. The number of abnormal cells per smear, the cellular and nuclear area, the severity of chromatin irregularities, and the presence of cells with nucleoli are found more frequently in adenocarcinoma than complex hyperplasia and least frequently in simple hyperplasia.

The diagnosis of AGUS also is applied appropriately to smears that contain atypical glandular cells of uncertain origin. Normal and neoplastic endocervical cells usually are larger than endometrial cells and differ in their shape and arrangement. Endocervical cells are generally columnar, whereas endometrial cells are cuboidal. Endocervical cells tend to exfoliate in sheets displaying a honeycomb arrangement or palisades. Endometrial cells usually occur in round fragments. The cytoplasm of individual endometrial cells is indiscernible when endometrial cells shed in clusters, whereas the more abundant cytoplasm of endocervical cells is easily appreciated.

Endometritis and endocervicitis also may result in shedding of atypical glandular cells showing nuclear enlargement, prominent nucleoli, and overlapping. Since cytoplasmic vacuolization with engulfment of neutrophils may be present in endometritis (Fig. 25.25) and in one fifth of endometrial carcinoma, a diagnosis of endometrial carcinoma should not be made solely on the basis of this finding. The most useful features in avoiding a false-positive diagnosis in these conditions is to note the relative cohesiveness of the cells, the absence of variability in nuclear size, shape, and chromatin pattern, and the regularity of the nuclear contours. Rarely, an endometrial curettage performed on a patient with adenocarcinoma reveals only endometritis; therefore, the smears and biopsies must be compared before dismissing a suspicious cytological diagnosis. Endometrial polyps and hyperplasia also may shed cells classifiable as AGUS. If a smear displays findings suspicious for endometrial adenocarcinoma and a concurrent biopsy reveals only a polyp, a curettage is necessary to exclude the presence of carcinoma within or adjacent to the polyp unless the cells in the smear and biopsy are identical. Reports of negative biopsies or curettings in patients whose smears were suspicious for an endometrial abnormality should state whether the histological findings account for the cytologic abnormality originally reported.

ENDOMETRIAL ADENOCARCINOMA

The impact of cytological screening on the morbidity and mortality related to endometrial adenocarcinoma has been limited. Vuopala[165] reported that the sensitivity of Papanicolaou smears in the detection of endometrial adenocarci-

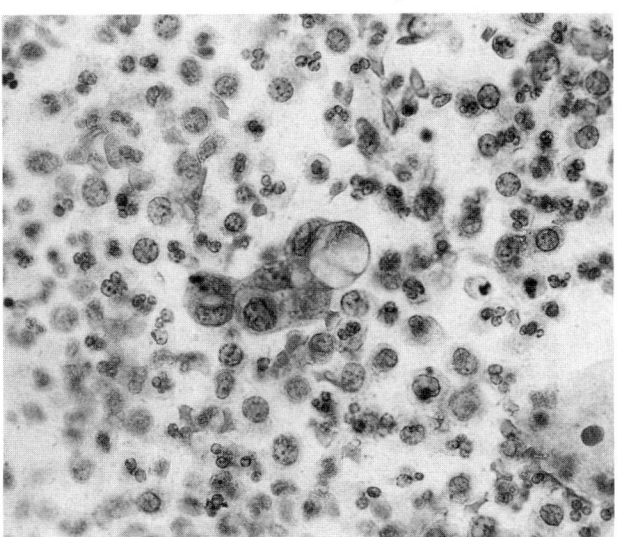

FIG. 25.25. Endometritis. Degenerated endometrial cells with cytoplasmic vacuoles shed in a case of endometritis. Smear reported as AGUS; rule out an endometrial lesion.

noma ranges from 18% to 94%, but most studies have achieved only 50% sensitivity. The variability in these data reflects differences in patient populations, criteria for false negatives, and, possibly, changing patterns of disease and other factors. Although 80% of patients are symptomatic at diagnosis, cytological detection of asymptomatic endometrial carcinoma may improve the prognosis of the remaining 20% by facilitating the detection of minimally or noninvasive tumors.[80]

The high false-negative rate of routine cytology in the detection of endometrial lesions has many explanations.[165] The cells of most low-grade carcinomas and hyperplasias are cohesive and, therefore, may not exfoliate. Cervical stenosis, which is not infrequently associated with endometrial adenocarcinoma, prevents tumor cells from reaching the lower genital tract or results in sporadic shedding. Many endometrial carcinomas exfoliate only a few cells that are degenerated and obscured by blood and inflammation. Most endometrial carcinomas are well differentiated and the cells that exfoliate are difficult to recognize (Fig. 25.26). In one report, 12% of endometrial carcinomas shed cells that were morphologically unremarkable.[165] Detection of endometrial cells is especially problematic in atrophic smears with poor cellular preservation. In premenopausal patients, endometrial carcinoma cells may be mistaken for normal endometrial exfoliation occurring during the first 10 days of the menstrual cycle. In contrast, tumors that display papillary or polypoid architecture, grade 2 or 3 histopathology, endocervical involvement, squamous, serous or clear cell differentiation, and large surface area are more frequently detected cytologically than typical low-grade endometrial carcinomas.[97,135]

Cytopathology contributes to the diagnosis of endome-

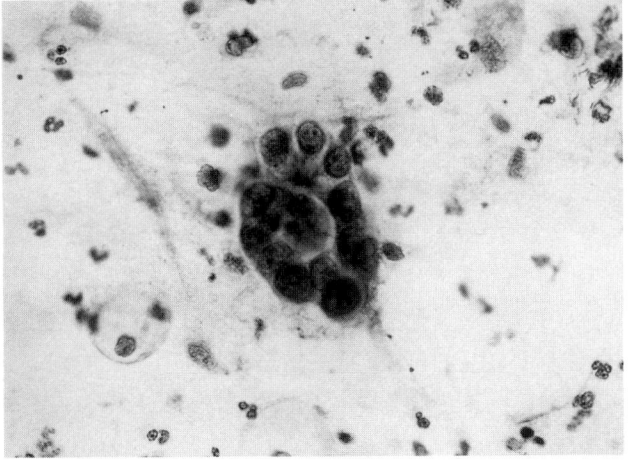

FIG. 25.26. Endometrioid adenocarcinoma, grade 1. Endometrial cells displaying minimal nuclear enlargement and small nucleoli identified in a postmenopausal smear of a patient with well-differentiated endometrioid adenocarcinoma.

trial carcinomas by facilitating detection of clinically unsuspected lesions and suggesting an endometrial primary in patients with symptoms suggestive of a gynecological tumor. It is important to compare the appearance of smears and histological samples in patients with suspicious or positive cytological findings and negative biopsies since lesions that are small or located within the cornua or polyps may be missed by endometrial biopsy or curettage (Fig. 25.27). In light of the 50% false-negative rate of cytological examination, histological examination is mandatory whenever a smear suggests an endometrial abnormality. It is never appropriate to evaluate a suspected endometrial abnormality with serial smears. Histological examination is mandatory whenever a smear suggests an endometrial abnormality.

The ideal specimen for detecting endometrial neoplasms has been debated. Vuopala found that the sensitivity of cervical scrapes, endocervical aspirates, and vaginal pool specimens reported in the literature was approximately equal.[165] Ng[110] advocated the use of endocervical aspirates to detect endometrial lesions, whereas Berg and Durfee[9] favor the use of vaginal pool specimens. Vaginal pool material is most easily interpretable because problems related to the distinction of reactive endocervical cells from endometrial cells and reactive inflammatory changes are minimized. The cytological manifestations of endometrial carcinoma includes the presence of morphologically unremarkable endometrial cells after day 10 of the menstrual cycle in premenopausal women or at any time in postmenopausal women, findings indicative of abnormal bleeding such as lysed erythrocytes or hemosiderin and the presence of atypical endometrial cells (Fig. 25.28).

Lipid-laden cells possessing dense degenerated pyknotic nuclei and abundant foamy cytoplasm ("histiocyte-like" cells) often are present.[40] True histiocytes may be present as well. Koss[79] has emphasized that only recognition of mononucleated histiocytes in vaginal smears has value in detecting endometrial lesions. Multinucleated histiocytes are an inconsequential finding in postmenopausal patients. In postmenopausal women when the criteria of five or more histiocytes per high power field and the identification of endometrial cells was used, the sensitivity of vaginal cytology increased from 61% to 82% in one report. However, the positive predictive value of smears displaying histiocytes alone was only 23%.[13] Although smears obtained from postmenopausal women containing histiocytes suggest abnormal endometrial shedding, few patients prove to have an endometrial carcinoma unless blood or endometrial cells also are present.

The presence of old blood should prompt a search for evidence of abnormal endometrial shedding. If only old blood is present, this finding should be reported with a note attesting to the uncertain significance of this finding in the setting of atrophy. After radiation therapy for endometrial carcinoma, smears are obtained routinely to rule out a recurrence. Atypical cells in this setting are inter-

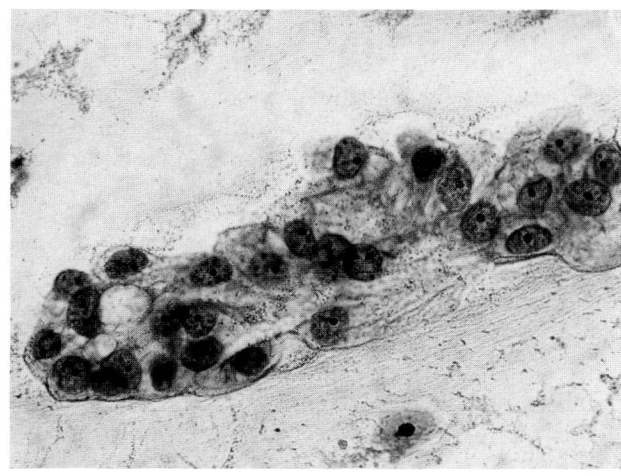

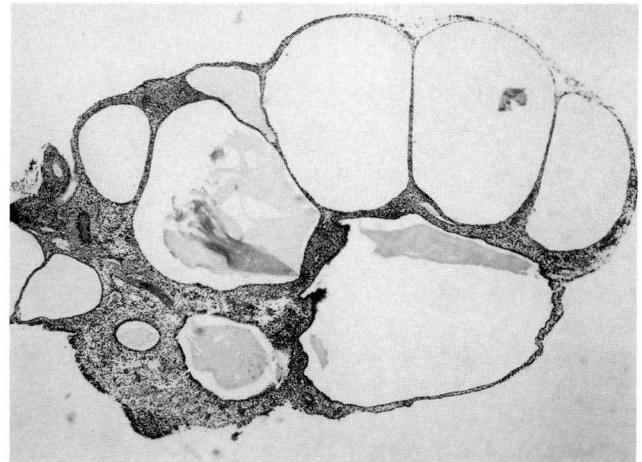

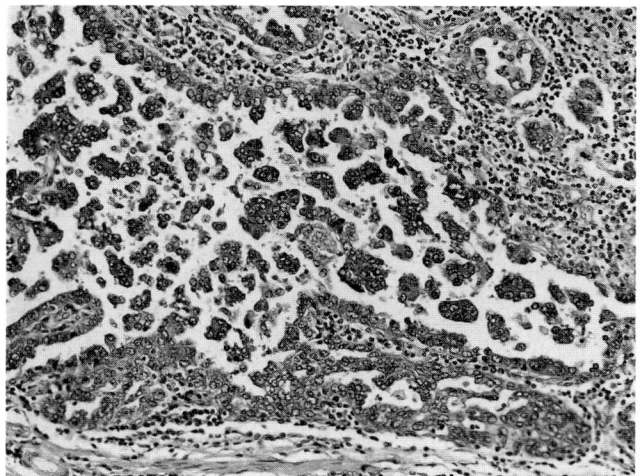

FIG. 25.27. a: **Endometrial adenocarcinoma.** Smear revealing glandular cells with large nuclei and macronucleoli diagnostic of adenocarcinoma. b: **Benign endometrial polyp.** Concurrent biopsy demonstrating a benign endometrial polyp. c: **Endometrial serous carcinoma.** Further investigation demonstrated that an endometrial serous carcinoma was the source of the malignant cells present in the smear.

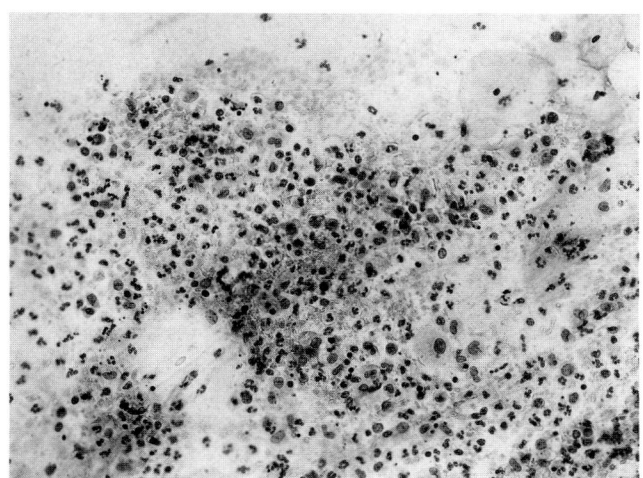

FIG. 25.28. **Appearance of background in endometrial carcinoma.** Lysed blood and inflammatory cells in a postmenopausal smear suggesting an endometrial lesion.

preted using the usual cytological criteria for malignancy. Comparison of the atypical cells in the smears with the tissue of the resected carcinoma may be useful in excluding a recurrence.

High-grade endometrioid, serous and clear cell adenocarcinomas are easily recognized as malignant. Smears reveal many cells possessing large vesicular nuclei with macronucleoli in a background of old blood and debris (Fig. 25.29). Most of these patients present with advanced stage disease and clinical findings indicative of malignancy including pain, bleeding, pelvic mass, or evidence of metastasis.

Vaginal Maturation—Estrogen Effect in the Menopause

Studies attempting to define the association between the presence of superficial squamous cells in vaginal smears and the risk of endometrial adenocarcinoma have yielded conflicting results. An estrogenic effect has been detected

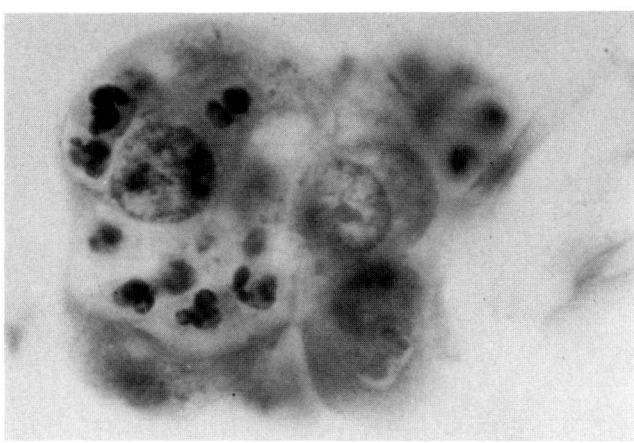

FIG. 25.29. Endometrial adenocarcinoma, grade 3. Malignant glandular cells displaying prominent nucleoli and engulfment of neutrophils typical of grade 3 endometrial adenocarcinoma.

2 to 15 times more frequently in smears containing carcinoma than in controls by some investigators,[9,23,35,49,127] whereas others report that up to 80% of patients with endometrial adenocarcinoma have atrophic smears.[94] Chang and Craig[24] found that the mean percentage of superficial cells was higher in carcinoma patients than controls, but that the difference was not statistically significant because of the extremely wide variation in the percentage of superficial cells in both groups. A prospective study of 507 patients followed for 10 years revealed that 3.6% of postmenopausal patients with estrogen effect in their smears developed endometrial carcinoma compared with 0.7% of women with atrophic specimens. Lin and So-Bosita emphasized that pseudoeosinophilia, infection, and misinterpretation frequently led to overreporting of superficial cells in postmenopausal patients.[92] Although the prevalence of atrophic smears increases with age, the level of squamous maturation observed cytologically varies over time in individual patients and 5–10% of normal women display a pronounced estrogen effect 20 years after menopause.[102] Koss[79] has emphasized that patients and physicians often fail to recognize that certain medications and cosmetics may produce an estrogen effect on vaginal epithelium. Since postmenopausal patients with evidence of abnormal maturation may be at increased risk for the development of endometrial adenocarcinoma, the presence of 20% superficial cells in postmenopausal women should be reported. However, use of tamoxifen, digoxin, other medications, beauty products, and peripheral conversion in obese women frequently are the cause of this finding. We report the presence of estrogen effect in postmenopausal patients, but never advocate tissue studies unless endometrial cells or old blood are present.

Metastatic Tumors in Gynecological Smears

Metastatic carcinoma can reach the lower genital tract via blood vessels and lymphatics by direct growth from contiguous anatomic sites and through the fallopian tube and endocervix. Aspiration of fluid from the posterior vaginal fornix (vaginal pool) is generally considered the most sensitive technique to detect metastases, but these lesions also may be detected in cervical and endocervical samples.

Cervical or vaginal smears in which tumor cells appear in a clean background containing relatively little blood and inflammation suggest a metastasis from an extrauterine tumor (Fig. 25.30). Carcinomas of the breast, fallopian tube, and ovary often produce this pattern. However, large necrotic metastases may result in a bloody, inflammatory background. Metastases from colorectal primaries often undergo necrosis and are associated with blood, debris, and inflammation.

Most metastases detected in gynecological smears occur in patients in whom the primary site is known. Review of pathological material from the primary tumor is helpful in confirming the metastatic nature of the tumor. In addition, certain tumors display morphologic appearances that suggest an extrauterine primary. Signet-cell adenocarcinomas, for example, are highly unusual in the gynecological tract and suggest a breast, gastric, or pancreatic primary (Fig. 25.31). Colorectal adenocarcinomas often display tall columnar cells with hyperchromatic, elongated, cigar-shaped nuclei arranged in sheets and strips. The background may contain mucin, debris, and inflammatory cells. Papillary serous carcinomas often shed three-dimensional clusters of cells containing psammoma bodies. The cells have large vesicular nuclei and macronucleoli, sometimes surrounded by a halo. Such tumors may arise from the

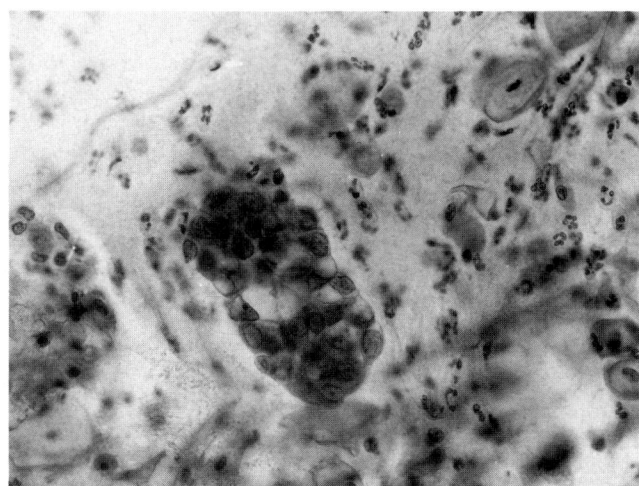

FIG. 25.30. Ovarian carcinoma. Clusters of cells with smooth contours in a clean background shed from a papillary serous carcinoma of the ovary.

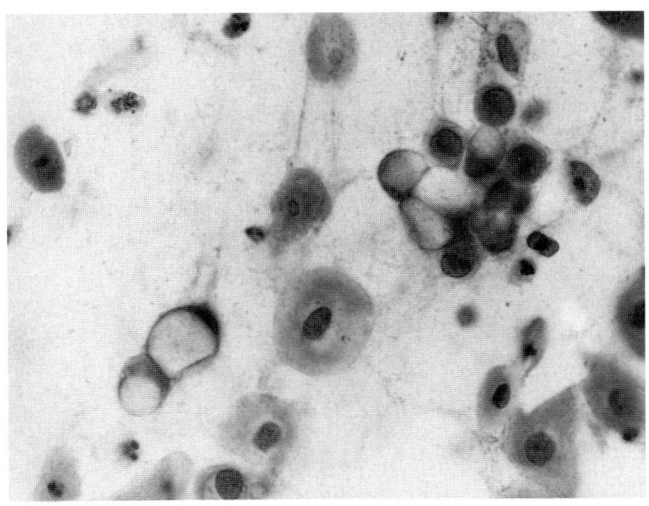

FIG. 25.31. **Breast carcinoma.** Vacuolated tumor cells representing metastatic breast adenocarcinoma.

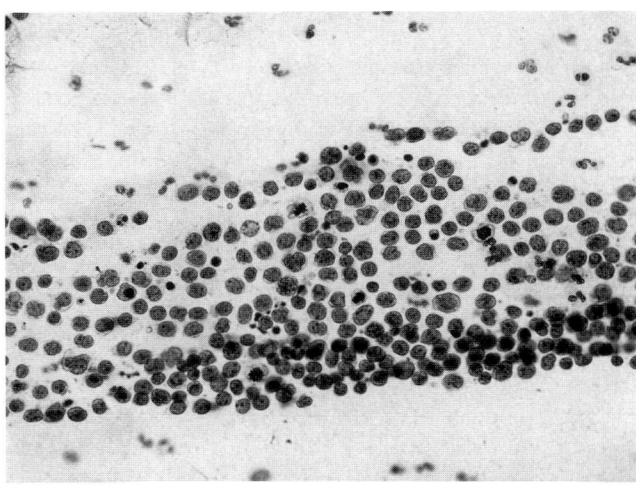

FIG. 25.32. **Lymphoma.** Lymphoblastic lymphoma presenting in smear as a streak of atypical mononuclear cells with convoluted nuclei and numerous mitoses.

ovary, fallopian tube, peritoneum, and endometrium. Urothelial carcinomas also are encountered in gynecological smears, but generally lack specific identifying features. Both metastatic and primary malignant melanomas of the gynecological tract are highly distinctive. These tumors exfoliate as polygonal and spindle-shaped cells present singly or in loosely cohesive sheets. The cells have large eccentric nuclei displaying nucleoli and pseudoinclusions. Fine brown melanin pigment, if present, is pathognomonic. Paget's disease and hematologic malignancies also tend to shed single cells. The glandular characteristics of Paget's disease and the high ratio of nuclear/cytoplasmic area lymphomas and leukemias are useful in differential diagnosis (Fig. 25.32).

Other Findings in Cytological Smears

PSAMMOMA BODIES

Psammoma bodies are well-defined, concentrically laminated structures that appear cyanophilic or basophilic in Papanicolaou-stained material and may demonstrate cracking or shattering. The discrete appearance of psammoma bodies contrasts with the more amorphous appearance of inspissated mucus, crystals, pollen, and other contaminants. Kern[69] identified only seven smears containing psammoma bodies among 234,318 cases screened in a 3-year period. In reviewing 30 cases reported in the literature, the author noted that most smears containing psammoma bodies are obtained from patients with papillary serous carcinoma of the ovary, endometrium, or other gynecological organs. However, psammoma bodies have been recognized increasingly in benign conditions including

tuberculous endometritis, tuboovarian abscess, endosalpingiosis, benign ovarian cysts and neoplasms, and in the setting of oral contraceptive use. Smears obtained from patients with carcinomas generally display malignant tumor cells, whereas those from patients with benign lesions often reveal calcifications surrounded by bland-appearing cuboidal cells (Fig. 25.33). Consequently, follow-up of young patients whose smears contain psammoma bodies but not atypical cells should be conservative. An endometrial biopsy and radiologic studies of the pelvis may be adequate to evaluate these patients.

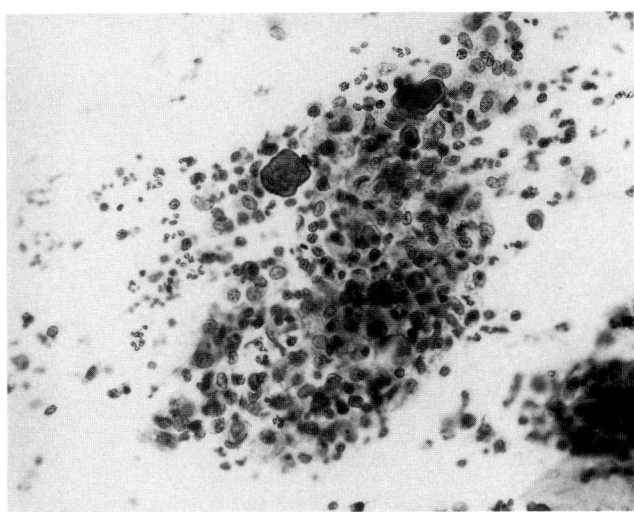

FIG. 25.33. **Psammoma bodies.** Numerous psammoma bodies surrounded by histiocytes suggestive of an endometrial lesion reported as AGUS. Biopsy revealed an endometrial polyp.

GLANDULAR CELLS IN THE ABSENCE OF A UTERUS

The presence of columnar cells in a smear from a woman who has undergone a hysterectomy should be reported. Verification that the smear was properly labeled and that the patient in question has undergone a hysterectomy is a logical initial step. In patients who have undergone a hysterectomy in the remote past, confirmation that the cervix was removed is necessary because the patient may have undergone a supracervical hysterectomy. Parabasal cells that assume a columnar shape may lead to erroneous reporting of glandular cells in a woman who has had a hysterectomy. Parabasal cells contain dense cytoplasm more typical of squamous than glandular cells, lack cytoplasmic vacuoles, and resemble recognizable parabasal cells elsewhere in the smear.

Benign sources of exfoliated glandular cells in patients having undergone a hysterectomy include endometriosis, mesonephric remnants, Bartholin glands, and adenosis. Patients who develop rectovaginal fistulas may have colonic epithelium and bowel contents in their smears. The atypia of the colonic epithelium in these highly inflamed specimens may raise a question of adenocarcinoma. Glandular cells also may be detected in patients who have a neovagina constructed from intestinal mucosa. Finally, the cells of ovarian neoplasms of low malignant potential and the columnar epithelium of pseudomyxoma peritonei exhibit minimal cytological atypia and may be recognizable only because they appear as glandular epithelium in vaginal smears of women who have undergone hysterectomy (Fig. 25.34).

Vaginal Intraepithelial Neoplasia

In TBS, vaginal intraepithelial neoplasia (VAIN) is subdivided into low- and high-grade SIL. Based on the poor correlation between smears diagnosed as VAIN2 and corresponding biopsies, it appears that including VAIN2 and VAIN3 under the heading of high-grade SIL is justifiable.[144] In contrast with cervical SIL, most patients who develop vaginal SIL are postmenopausal. Many of the patients have a history of CIN or cervical carcinoma. Consequently, some gynecologists advocate yearly vaginal cytology in women who have undergone a recent hysterectomy for cervical neoplasia.[39,45,74] Less frequent sampling is advocated for women treated for benign disease. Others have emphasized that a significant percentage of patients without a history of cervical disease develop vaginal SIL and that all women should have regular vaginal cytological examinations after hysterectomy.[130,131] Stuart et al.[154] reported that women who develop vaginal neoplasia after a hysterectomy for benign disease usually were identified because of symptoms related to invasive carcinoma and 5 (42%) of 12 patients died. In contrast, patients who underwent a hysterectomy for cervical neoplasia were closely followed cytologically and none of 17 died of invasive carcinoma.

Atrophy[21,25] and changes related to radiation[25] complicate the cytological detection of vaginal SIL. In addition, vaginal cuff cysts[60] that form at suture lines after hysterectomy may contain SIL or carcinoma that exfoliates few diagnostic cells. Vaginal smears diagnosed as SIL underestimate the grade of subsequent biopsies in one-third of cases and overestimate the severity of disease in an equal number.[144] Biopsies that demonstrate a higher grade of SIL than was diagnosed cytologically frequently display severe hyperkeratosis, which prevents the exfoliation of representative cells. The failure to confirm histologically a cytological diagnosis of vaginal SIL usually reflects biopsy sampling error. Obtaining smears from designated areas of the vagina may help localize the lesion.

Fine-needle Aspiration of Ovarian Cysts

The indications for performing a fine-needle aspiration (FNA) of an ovarian cyst are controversial. Arguments against the use of FNA include spillage of malignant cells into the abdominal cavity leading to dissemination of tumor, infection, and misdiagnosis related to sampling errors and misinterpretation.[153] We have encountered a single case in which tumor apparently implanted in a needle tract after FNA. In contrast, the use of FNA is supported by several studies demonstrating that approximately 90% of ovarian cysts were accurately diagnosed cytologically without complications.[4,44] Most cysts in premenopausal women are self-limited functional cysts. The risk of malignancy in young women who have unilocular cysts measuring 5 cm or less by ultrasound that are free of solid areas, thick septations, and irregularities is exceptionally low. If aspiration of

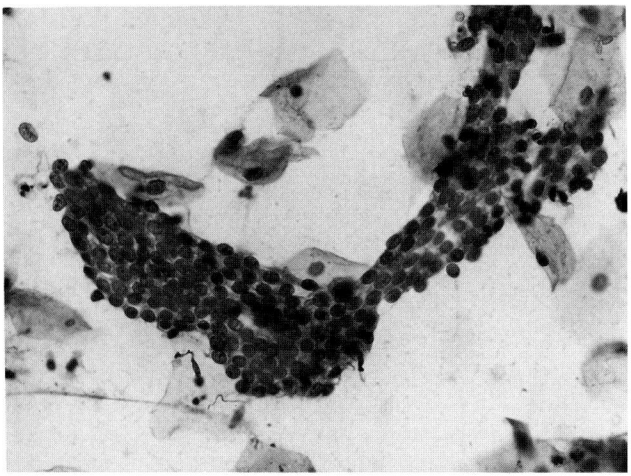

FIG. 25.34. **Pseudomyxoma peritoneii.** Vaginal smear containing sheets of small glandular cells in a honeycomb arrangement consistent with recurrent pseudomyxoma peritoneii.

these cysts yields clear fluid that does not contain atypical cells, fenestration performed under laparoscopic guidance may be curative and an unnecessary surgical procedure is avoided.[55,71,88] FNA also may be used in diagnosing ovarian cysts in patients who clinically appear to have inoperable cancer.

Follicular cysts are the most commonly aspirated ovarian lesion in most reports. Specimens from follicular cysts contain varying numbers of granulosa cells in a thin, watery background.[124,138] The granulosa cells may be present in sheets or in rosettes corresponding to Call–Exner bodies. Granulosa cells have round or oval nuclei with fine uniform chromatin surrounded by a scant amount of cytoplasm. Grooves and mitoses may be evident. Sheets of granulosa cells that display intercellular spaces may resemble aggregates of mesothelial cells, but granulosa cells are smaller. Stanley et al.[153] described three atypical follicular cysts that cytologically suggested low-grade neoplasms. FNAs performed on these cysts displayed many granulosa cells with a high ratio of nuclear/cytoplasmic area, nuclear hyperchromasia, and nucleoli. The presence of three-dimensional cell clusters, loosely cohesive pseudopapillary fragments, and cellular degeneration added to the diagnostic confusion. The appearance of these FNAs may be cytologically indistinguishable from papillary serous neoplasms of low malignant potential and grade 1 carcinomas. Antibodies to cytokeratins AE-1/AE-3 may help distinguish granulosa cells from mesothelial cells because the latter are reactive whereas granulosa cells generally do not stain.[153] Elevated estrogen-17β levels in cyst aspirates favor a diagnosis of a follicular cyst, although some stromal lesions may contain estrogen-rich fluid.[44] After an inconclusive FNA, the decision as to whether to excise an ovarian cyst usually is based on the radiologic appearance of the lesion and the clinical findings.

Luteinized granulosa cells of corpus luteum cysts are larger than their nonluteinized counterparts and have abundant vacuolated cytoplasm and nuclei with nucleoli[124,138] (Fig. 25.35). Luteinized cells may be difficult to distinguish from histiocytes. Selvaggi[139] described three cyst fluids containing cytologically atypical cells obtained 6 to 8 months postpartum that were compatible with luteinized follicular cysts of pregnancy and the puerperium. These cysts contained atypical granulosa cells with nuclear atypia and nucleoli in addition to groups of unremarkable granulosa cells. Recognition that the atypical cells are morphologically similar to unremarkable granulosa cells and the clinical setting argue against a diagnosis of malignancy. FNAs of a hemorrhagic corpus luteum and endometriotic cysts typically contain hemosiderin-laden macrophages, hematoidin, and fibrin. A definitive diagnosis of endometriosis requires the unequivocal identification of endometrial cells. Khaw et al.[71] described two FNAs misdiagnosed as endometriosis in patients presenting with ovarian cysts that proved to represent an adenocarcinoma and a

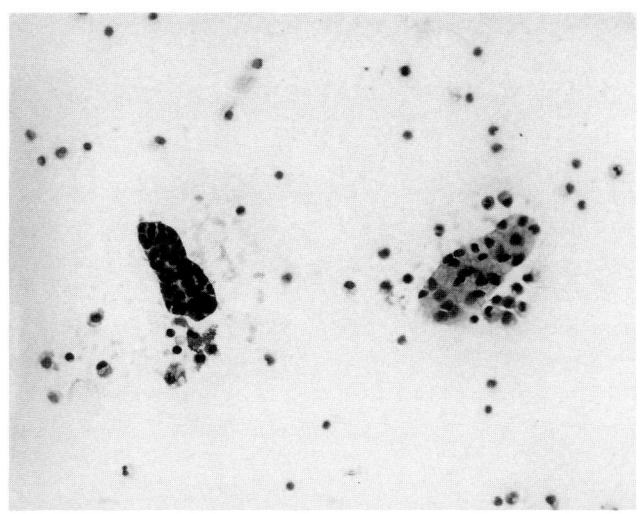

FIG. 25.35. **Corpus luteum.** Aspirate of luteinized follicular cyst containing fragments of small tightly packed granulosa cells and luteinized cells with more abundant foamy cytoplasm. Background contains histiocytes.

mucinous cystadenoma. Classification of hemorrhagic cysts is based on the appearance of the epithelial cells; the presence of hemosiderin in a cyst fluid is not diagnostic of endometriosis.

Granulosa cell tumors contain numerous small monomorphous granulosa cells arranged in trabeculae, follicles, and solid sheets.[36,41] The arrangement of the cells in granulosa cell tumors distinguishes them from follicular cysts. Brenner tumors, like granulosa cell tumors, are composed of cells with nuclear folds and grooves, but the cells of Brenner tumors are larger and may be associated with eosinophilic bodies.

FNAs of dermoid cysts may display squamous cells, sebaceous cells, sebum, and hair.[124] Identification of multiple cell and tissue types is pathognomonic (Fig. 25.36). Since aspirates obtained transvaginally normally contain squamous cells, the presence of squamous cells alone is insufficient for a diagnosis of a benign cystic teratoma.

FNAs of most carcinomas are highly cellular and contain cytologically malignant cells.[4,123] Angstrom et al.[111] reported that a malignant tumor was diagnosed or suspected in 109 (94%) of 116 patients who underwent an FNA of an ovarian lesion that was resected and proved to represent carcinoma. Accurate classification of ovarian tumors may be impossible based on cytological examination alone. In particular, the distinction between low-grade carcinoma and a neoplasm of low malignant potential requires microscopic assessment of tissue sections to determine the presence or absence of invasion (Fig. 25.37). Mucinous tumors are distinguished from serous tumors by the more columnar shape of the cells and the presence of the large cytoplasmic vacuoles and mucin (Fig. 25.38). Pinto et al.[119]

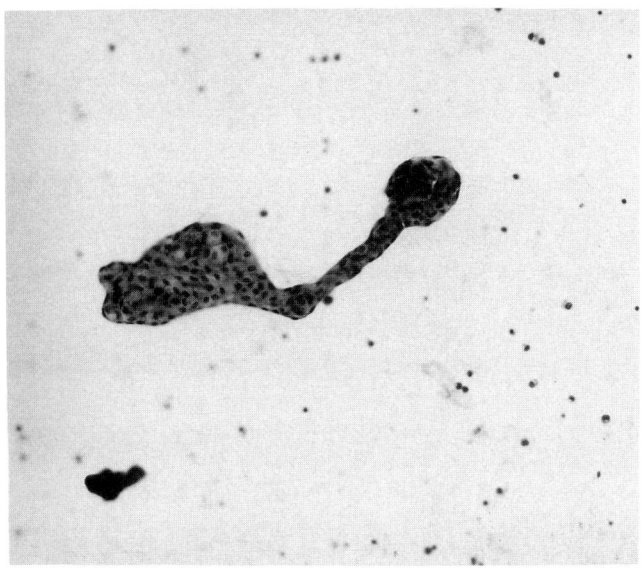

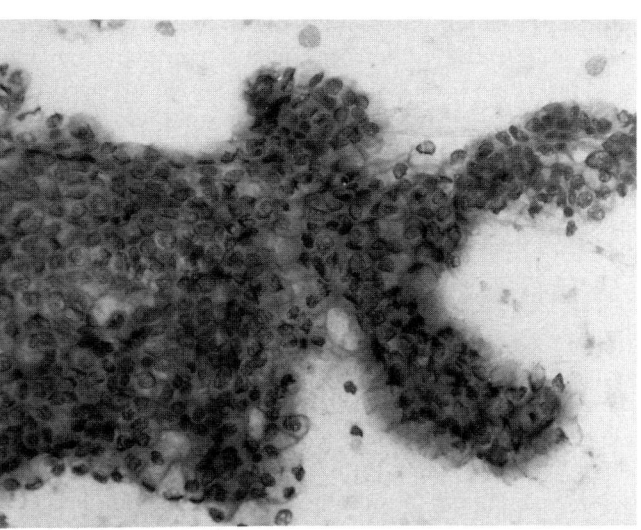

FIG. 25.38. Papillary mucinous neoplasm of low malignant potential. Papillary fragments of columnar cells containing apical mucin aspirated from an ovarian mucinous tumor of low malignant potential.

FIG. 25.36. Dermoid cyst. Fine needle aspirate of ovary demonstrating hair appendage diagnostic of dermoid cyst. Few squames were present.

reported that elevated fluid levels of CA125 are characteristic of ovarian neoplasms and that CEA levels are increased in fluids obtained from mucinous tumors. Fragments of rectal mucosa are distinguished from mucinous neoplasms by the benign appearance of the glandular cells, identification of smooth muscle, ganglion cells or luminal contents, and overall smear pattern. Endometrioid and serous carcinomas, however, are not always reliably separated. FNAs of serous carcinomas prepared as cell blocks

often demonstrate unequivocal fibrovascular cores indicative of papillary growth, which contrasts with the gland-forming architecture of endometrioid carcinomas. The presence of psammoma bodies favors a serous neoplasm, whereas the cells of endometrioid carcinomas tend to be more elongated than those of serous tumors. Clear cell carcinomas consist of large cells with abundant, frothy cytoplasm and prominent nucleoli. The cells of clear cell carcinoma may resemble benign mucinous cells or histiocytes, but the nuclear abnormalities of the cells should allow correct interpretation (Fig. 25.39).

Examination of Specimens Obtained with the Cavitron Ultrasonic Aspirator

The Cavitron ultrasonic aspirator (CUSA) is a device that employs a rapidly vibrating probe to fragment and remove tissue. The CUSA has been used for intraabdominal debulking of gynecological tumors and treatment of lower genital tract lesions. The fragmented tissue is aspirated into a trap and can be processed for cytological and histological diagnosis. Since the device spares collagen-rich tissues such as blood vessels, hemorrhage and intraoperative complications are minimized.

Pathological material obtained with the CUSA includes tissue fragments and cellular fluid. Tissue is best prepared as cell blocks for histological examination, whereas fluid may be processed similarly to effusions. Diagnostic mate-

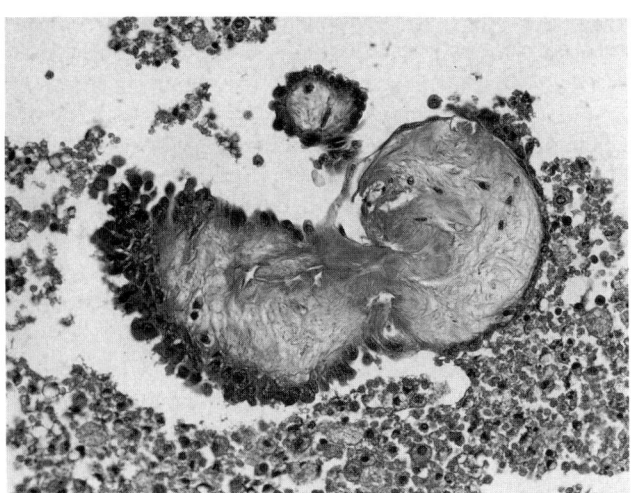

FIG. 25.37. Papillary serous neoplasm of low malignant potential. Cell block containing fibrotic papillary structure lined by serous-type epithelial cells. Oophorectomy demonstrated a papillary serous neoplasm of low malignant potential.

Peritoneal Cytology

Peritoneal samples are obtained routinely during staging laparotomies for ovarian and endometrial carcinomas and at second-look procedures performed to rule out recurrences in patients with these malignancies. The specimens usually are obtained by instilling normal saline into the abdominal cavity immediately after the peritoneal cavity is entered and then aspirating the fluid. Specimens often are submitted from patients undergoing exploration for undiagnosed benign pelvic masses.

Cytological examination of peritoneal fluids has a false-negative rate of less than 15% in patients undergoing a primary exploration for ovarian carcinoma,[178] but the false-negative rate is two to four times higher at second-look procedures.[121,130] Cytology is more sensitive in detecting ovarian carcinoma in ascites than in peritoneal washes, in patients whose tumors measure more than 0.5 cm, and in clear as compared with bloody specimens. Stage, grade, histological type, and fluid volume appear unrelated to the sensitivity of cytological diagnosis. Peritoneal fluid cytology is the only indicator of extraovarian spread in approximately 3–10% of patients. The results of peritoneal cytology are used in the International Federation of Gynecology and Obstetrics (FIGO) Staging System.[3] Malignant fluid cytology increases the stage of tumors histologically confined to the ovaries to IC and that of tumors limited to the pelvis to IIC.

Malignant cells are present in peritoneal fluid specimens in approximately 10–20% of women with endometrial carcinoma.[19,31,54,59,62,63,100,172] Most studies demonstrate that fluid cytology has prognostic value in endometrial cancer patients, although a few reports have failed to confirm these data. Accordingly, the results of peritoneal cytology are included in the FIGO Staging System for these neoplasms.[2] Endometrial carcinomas associated with positive pelvic washes are stage IIIA. The results of a large mutivariate analysis of prognostic factors in endometrial carcinoma indicated that peritoneal fluid cytology had greater prognostic value than depth of myometrial invasion or adnexal spread, but less utility than stage, grade, and patient age.[54] Malignant peritoneal cytology correlates with other recognized prognostic indicators including stage, grade, depth of myometrial invasion, involvement of the lower uterine segment and endocervix, lymph node metastases, and adnexal spread in several studies.[31,62,63] Fluid cytology provided the only evidence of peritoneal spread in 6–16% of patients reported in the literature and was positive in 43% of patients in the absence of gross disease in one study.

Malignant fluid cytology has been reported in more than 50% of patients with serous carcinoma of the endometrium and was present in the absence of myometrial invasion in some patients.[142] One-quarter of endometrial cancer patients with malignant cells in washes and negative perito-

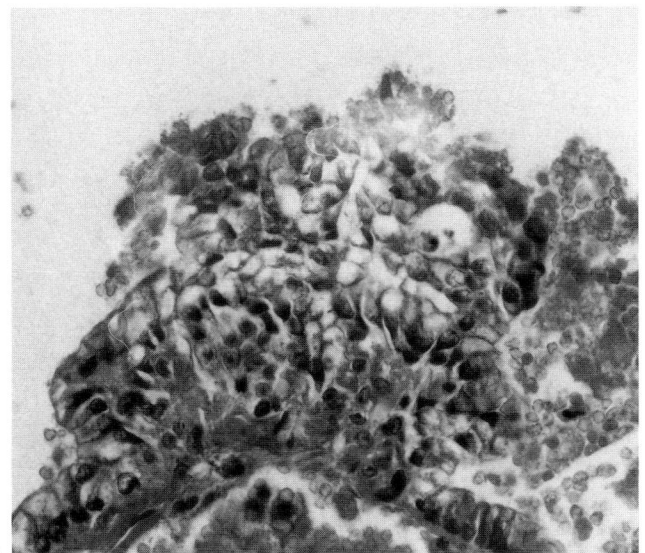

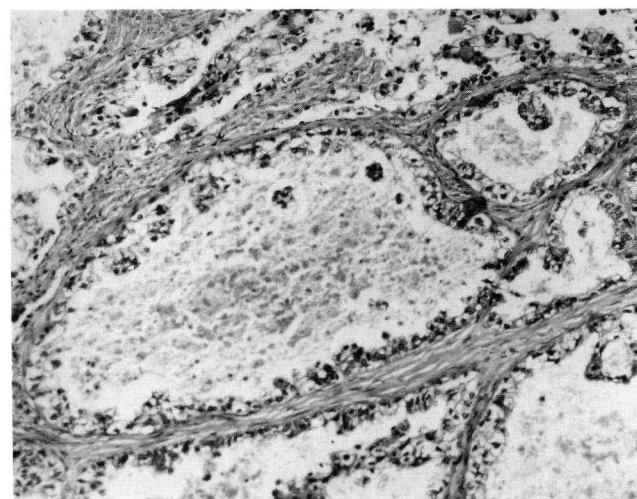

FIG. 25.39. **Clear cell adenocarcinoma. a:** Fragment of cuboidal and columnar shaped tumor cells present in a background of blood and debris diagnosed as adenocarcinoma with clear cell features. **b:** Oophorectomy revealing clear cell carcinoma with prominent cystic growth pattern.

rial is present in more than 90% of specimens obtained by intraabdominal tumor debulking or ablation of lower genital tract disease prepared in this manner.[170] Thermal artifact and the fragmentation of the tissue hampers exact grading of SIL; and therefore the distinction between SIL and invasive carcinoma in specimens obtained from the lower genital tract may at times be difficult. Since the CUSA is used primarily to remove lesions that have been previously diagnosed by conventional biopsy, the main purpose of pathological examination is to confirm the successful removal of lesional tissue.

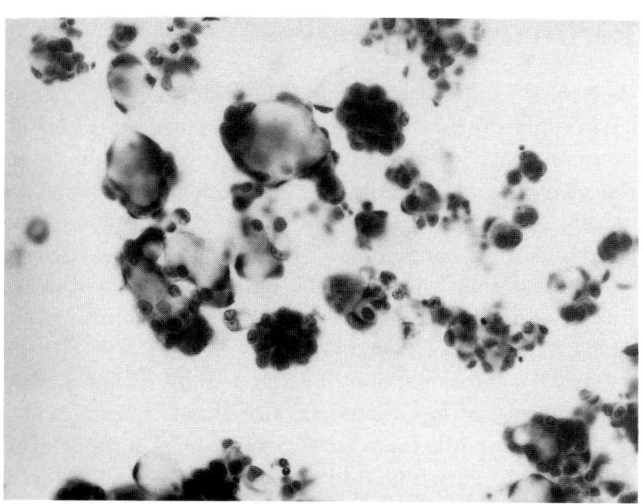

Fig. 25.40. Ovarian adenocarcinoma. Three-dimensional clusters of adenocarcinoma displaying hyperdistended vacuoles typically found in ovarian tumors.

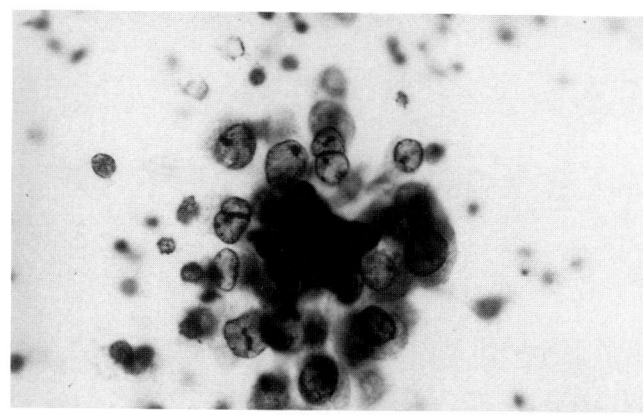

Fig. 25.41. Endosalpingiosis. Cells with slight nuclear enlargement and nucleoli are loosely adherent to a psammoma body.

neal biopsies developed recurrences in one report.[100] In another study, 6 (46%) of 13 patients with positive washes and negative peritoneal biopsies died of disease.[59] Patients with more than 1000 tumor cells/ml of peritoneal fluid may recur more quickly than those with smaller tumor burdens.[158]

Peritoneal washes do not appear to represent an independent prognostic factor in patients with cervical carcinoma.[1,128,176] Positive washes in cervical cancer patients correlate with retroperitoneal lymph node metastases and advanced disease. Cells derived from nonkeratinized squamous cell carcinoma may be misinterpreted as mesothelial cells because the cytoplasm appears similar. Adenocarcinomas and adenosquamous carcinomas may shed cells in washes four times more frequently than pure squamous carcinomas,[176] but the value of peritoneal washes in staging these tumors has not been extensively studied.

Mesothelial cells arranged singly and in sheets are the main component of benign peritoneal washes. In Papanicolaou stains, mesothelial cells appear as round or polygonal cells with dense, cyanophilic cytoplasm and centrally placed, round nuclei with smooth contours and finely granular chromatin. Reactive or degenerated mesothelial cells may display fine or coarse cytoplasmic vacuolization and a lightly stained perinuclear zone (endoplasm) surrounded by a darker staining peripheral zone (ectoplasm).

Useful criteria in the diagnosis of malignant cells in peritoneal washes include the presence of classic nuclear abnormalities indicative of malignancy (such as hyperchromasia, irregular chromatin distribution, nuclear contours, etc.), morphologic similarity between the cells in the fluid and the histology of the tumor, and an appearance that is distinct from the mesothelial cells in the sample (Fig. 25.40). The primary cause of false-negative washes in patients with ovarian carcinoma is sampling error. Bloody

and degenerated specimens also compromise interpretation and reduce diagnostic sensitivity.

Immunoperoxidase staining occasionally is useful in distinguishing tumor cells from reactive mesothelial cells, but its application frequently is limited by the paucity of cellular material available. Staining for epithelial membrane antigen and Leu M-1 may be valuable in the diagnosis of serous neoplasms.[52] Most mucinous tumors are decorated with antibodies to carcinoembryonic antigen and stain for mucin.[32] Reactive mesothelial cells, particularly those associated with chronic effusions, tuboovarian abscesses, and ectopic pregnancies, may closely simulate carcinoma.[125,175,177] Reactive mesothelial cells may show nuclear enlargement with formation of chromocenters or nucleoli. In mesothelial hyperplasia, cells may assume three-dimensional arrangements that mimic adenocarcinoma. The cardinal feature that distinguishes mesothelial groups from carcinoma is the presence of spaces between the cells, sometimes referred to as *windows*. In cell block material, mesothelial cells appear as single cells, long strips, and clusters.

In addition, several benign conditions shed cells in fluids that resemble low-grade carcinomas. Endosalpingiosis may present as three-dimensional clusters and gland-like formations composed of small cells with a high nuclear/cytoplasmic ratio.[150] The cells often display slightly coarse chromatin with chromocenters or nucleoli (Fig. 25.41). Psammoma bodies and round spherical structures composed of densely staining cyanophilic material, referred to as *collagen balls*, frequently are evident.[169] Recognition of cilia, the benign nuclear features of the cells, and knowledge of the patient's age and clinical history aid in diagnosis. Serous tumors of low malignant potential (LMP) resemble endosalpingiosis, but display slightly more nuclear atypia and generally are arranged in larger, more complex

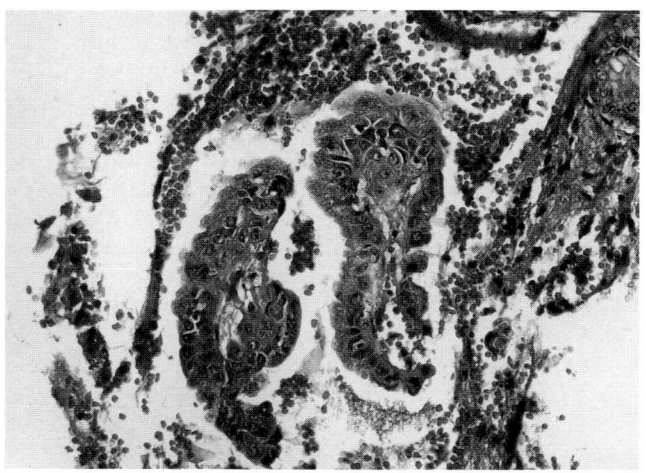

FIG. 25.42. **Peritoneal fluid contaminant.** Peritoneal fluid cell block containing two papillary fragments with squamous metaplasia. Patient had undergone prior hysteroscopy and biopsy of an atypical polypoid adenomyoma.

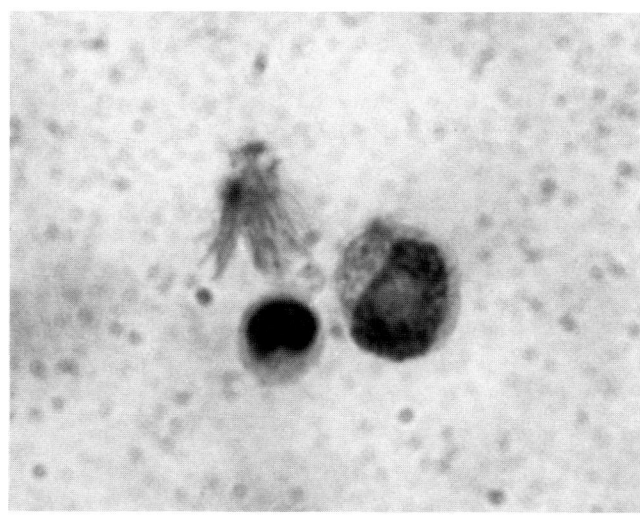

FIG. 25.43. **Detached ciliary tuft.** Minute fragment of epithelial cytoplasm with attached cilia.

fragments.[64] Cell block preparations demonstrate the true papillary nature of LMP neoplasms. The distinction between carcinomas and LMP neoplasms is based on the larger and smoother fragments of the latter, which are composed of cells that are smaller, more uniform, less vacuolated, and possess smaller nucleoli. Benign cystic tumors that rupture or involve the surface of the ovary may cause diagnostic confusion, but are recognizable by the lack of nuclear atypia and knowledge of the patient's history.

Benign endometrial tissue and cells may be detected in the peritoneal cavity. These cells are derived from endometrial tissue that has been expelled through the fallopian tube into the peritoneal cavity after hysteroscopy or rupture of an endometriotic cyst[85] (Fig. 25.42). The latter occasionally may yield endometrial cells with significant cytological atypia. The young age of the patient and a history of pain and a suddenly enlarging mass are clues to the diagnosis. Epithelial cells arranged in a honeycomb pattern and tight clusters or syncytial-like sheets of cells in combination with spindle-shaped stromal cells and hemosiderin-laden macrophages suggest endometriosis. A curious finding in fluids obtained during the luteal phase is the presence of detached ciliary tufts, which represent anucleate fragments of fallopian tube cytoplasm[120,149] (Fig. 25.43). Detached ciliary tufts are best seen in airdried Diff-Quik–stained smears and also are found in ethanol-fixed Papanicolaou-stained preparations.

Future Directions

The development of cervical sampling devices that simultaneously exfoliate cells from the ectocervix and endocervix promises to streamline the process of obtaining a cervi-

cal smear. Preliminary data suggest that using devices such as the Cervex brush may provide sensitivity similar to that obtained by using the Ayre spatula and cytobrush in combination.[15,61a,89,157] It is hoped that newer devices will produce less traumatic bleeding and fewer artifacts than currently used instrument without loss of diagnostic sensitivity.

The Cytyc monolayer system offers a novel approach to slide preparation. Cellular samples are suspended in a vial containing fixative and reagents that reduce the amount of blood and debris in the specimen. The vials are placed on a machine that disburses the cells on standard glass slides in a monolayer. One vial contains sufficient cells to prepare multiple slides and the specimens may be stored for use in ancillary studies. Early studies using Cytyc monolayers suggest that the sensitivity of this method is comparable to standard smears.[61]

Computer-assisted image analysis represents another cervical cancer screening technique designed to extend the capacity of human observers to assess the cervix morphologically. This technology has several possible applications in cervical cytology: automated screening, rescreening samples that were normal by routine light microscopy for quality assurance purposes, and measurement of morphologic parameters and ploidy analysis. The utility of commercially available computer-assisted imaging systems are currently the subject of active investigation.

References

1. Abu-Ghazaleh S, Johnston W, Creasman WT (1984) The significance of peritoneal cytology in patients with carcinoma of the cervix. Gynecol Oncol 17: 139–148
2. American College of Obstetricians and Gynecologists Clas-

sification and Staging of Malignant Tumors in the Female Pelvis, Chicago Technical Bulletin No. 47, 1977

3. American Joint Committee for Cancer Staging and End Result Reporting: Manual for Staging of Cancer. Chicago, American Joint Committee for Cancer Staging and End Result Reporting, 1978

4. Ångström T, Kjellgren O, Bergman F (1972) The cytologic diagnosis of ovarian tumors by means of aspiration biopsy. Acta Cytol 26: 336–341

5. Attwood ME, Woodman CBJ, Luesley D, Jordan JA (1985) Previous cytology in patients with invasive carcinoma of the cervix. Acta Cytol 29: 108–110

6. Ayer B, Pacey F, Greenberg M (1988) The cytologic diagnosis of adenocarcinoma in situ of the cervix uteri and related lesions. II. Microinvasive adenocarcinoma. Acta Cytol 32: 318–324

7. Ayer B, Pacey F, Greenberg M, Bousfield L (1987) The cytologic diagnosis of adenocarcinoma in situ of the cervix uteri and related lesions. I. Adenocarcinoma in situ. Acta Cytol 31: 397–411

8. Benoit AG, Krepart GV, Kotocki RJ (1984) Results of prior cytologic screening in patients with a diagnosis of Stage I carcinoma of the cervix. Am J Obstet Gynecol 148: 690–694

9. Berg JW, Durfee GR (1958) The cytological presentation of endometrial carcinoma. Cancer 11: 158–172

10. Berkely AS, LiVolsi V, Schwartz PE (1980) Advanced squamous cell carcinoma of the cervix with recent normal Papanicolaou tests. Lancet 2: 375–376

11. Bernal JN, Martinez MA, Dabancens A (1989) Evaluation of proposed cytomorphologic criteria for the diagnosis of chlamydia in trachomatis in Papanicolaou smears. Acta Cytol 33: 309–313

12. Betsill WL, Clark AH (1986) Early endocervical glandular neoplasia. I. Histomorphology and cytomorphology. Acta Cytol 30: 115–126

13. Blumenfeld W, Holly EA, Mansur DL, King EB (1985) Histiocytes and the detection of endometrial adenocarcinoma. Acta Cytol 29: 317–322

14. Boon ME, Alons-van Kordelaar JJM, Rietveld-Scheffers PEM (1986) Consequences of the introduction of combined spatula and cytobrush sampling for cervical cytology. Improvements in smear quality and detection rates. Acta Cytol 30: 264–270

15. Boon ME, Kirk RS, Rietveld-Scheffers PEM (1981) The morphogenesis of adenocarcinoma of the cervix—a complex pathological entity. Histopathology 5: 564–577

16. Boon ME, de Graaff Guilloud JC, Rietveld WJ (1989) Analysis of five sampling methods for the preparation of cervical smears. Acta Cytol 33: 843–848

17. Boon ME, Zeppa P, Ouwerkerk-Noordam E, Kok LP (1991) Exploiting the "toothpick effect" of the cytobrush by plastic embedding of cervical samples. Acta Cytol 35: 57–63

18. Bousfield L, Pacey F, Young Q, et al (1980) Expanded cytologic criteria for the diagnosis of adenocarcinoma in situ of the cervix and related lesions. Acta Cytol 24: 283–296

19. Brewington KC, Hughes RR, Coleman S (1989) Peritoneal cytology as a prognostic indicator in endometrial carcinoma. J Reprod Med 34: 824–826

20. Brink AL, DuToit JP, Deale CJC (1989) In search of more representative cervical cytology. A preliminary prospective study. South Afr Med J 76: 55–57

21. Caglar H, Hertzog RW, Hreshchyshyn MM (1981) Topical 5-fluorouracil treatment of vaginal intraepithelial neoplasia. Obstet Gynecol 58: 580–583

22. Carmichael JA, Jeffrey JF, Steele HD, Ohlke ID (1984) The cytologic history of 245 patients developing invasive cervical carcinoma. Am J Obstet Gynecol 148: 685–690

23. Cassano PA, Saigo PE, Hajdu SI (1986) Comparison of cytohormonal status of postmenopausal women with cancer to age-matched controls. Acta Cytol 30: 93–98

24. Chang YC, Craig JM (1963) Vaginal-smear assessment of estrogen activity in endometrial carcinoma. Obstet Gynecol 21: 170–174

25. Choo YG, Anderson DG (1982) Neoplasms of the vagina following cervical carcinoma. Gynecol Oncol 14: 125–132

26. Christopherson WM, Nealon N, Gray LA (1979) Non invasive precursor lesions of adenocarcinoma and mixed adenosquamous carcinoma of the cervix uteri. Cancer 44: 975–983

27. Clark RB, Schneider V, Gentile FG, et al (1985) Cervical chlamydial infections: Diagnostic accuracy of the Papanicolaou smear. South Med J 78: 1301–1303

28. Clarke AE, Anderson TW (1979) Does screening by "Pap" smears help prevent cervical cancer? Lancet ii: 1–4

29. Costa MJ, Kenny MB, Naib ZM (1991) Cervicovaginal cytology in uterine adenocarcinoma and adenosquamous carcinoma. Comparison of cytologic and histologic findings. Acta Cytol 35: 127–134

30. Covell JL, Frierson HF (1992) Intraepithelial neoplasia mimicking microinvasive squamous cell carcinoma in endocervical brushings. Diagn Cytopathol 8: 18–22

31. Creasman WT, Disaia PJ, Blessing J, et al (1981) Prognostic significance of peritoneal cytology in patients with endometrial cancer and preliminary data concerning therapy with intraperitoneal radiopharmaceuticals. Am J Obstet Gynecol 141: 921–929

32. Czernobilsky B (1987) Common epithelial tumors of the ovary, Chapter 18. In: Kurman RJ (ed) Blaustein's Pathology of The Female Genital Tract, 3rd ed. New York, Springer-Verlag, pp 599–600

33. Duca P, Braga M, Chiappa L, et al (1988) Intralaboratory reproducibility of interpretation of pap smears: Results of an experiment. Tumori 74: 737–744

34. Dunn JE, Schweitzer V (1981) The relationship of cervical cytology to the incidence of invasive cervical cancer and mortality in Alameda County, California, 1969 to 1974. Am J Obstet Gynecol 139: 868–876

35. Efstratiades M, Tamvakopoulou E, Papatheodorou B, Batrinos M (1982) Postmenopausal vaginal cytohormonal pattern in 597 healthy women and 301 patients with genital cancer. Acta Cytol 26: 126–130

36. Ehya H, Lang WR (1986) Cytology of granulosa cell tumor of the ovary. Am J Clin Pathol 85: 402–405

37. Elias A, Linthrost G, Bekker B, Vooijs PG (1983) The significance of endocervical cells in the diagnosis of cervical epithelial changes. Acta Cytol 27: 225–229

38. Evans DMD, Hudson EA, Brown CL, et al (1986) Review article: Terminology in gynecological cytopathology: Report of the Working Party of the British Society for Clinical Cytology. J Clin Pathol 39: 933–944

39. Fawdry RDS (1984) Carcinoma in situ of the cervix: Is post-hysterectomy cytology worthwhile? Br J Obstet Gynaecol 91: 67–72

40. Fechner RE, Bossart MI, Spjut HJ (1979) Ultrastructure of endometrial stromal foam cells. Am J Clin Pathol 72: 628–633

41. Fidler WJ (1982) Recurrent granulosa-cell tumor. Aspiration cytology findings. Acta Cytol 26: 688–690

42. Gallup DG, Morley GW (1975) Carcinoma in situ of the vagina: A study and review. Obstet Gynecol 46: 334–340

43. Geerling S, Nettum JA, Lindner LE, et al (1985) Sensitivity and specificity of the Papanicolaou-stained cervical smear in the diagnosis of chlamydia trachomatis infection. Acta Cytol 29: 671–675

44. Geier GR, Strecker JR (1981) Aspiration cytology and E_2 content in ovarian tumors. Acta Cytol 25: 400–406

45. Gemmell J, Holmes DM, Duncan ID (1990) How frequently need vaginal smears be taken after hysterectomy for cervical intraepithelial neoplasia? Br J Obstet Gynaecol 97: 58–61

46. Ghirardini C, Ghinosi P, Raisi O, et al (1991) Detection of chlamydia trachomatis in Papanicolaou-stained cervical smears: Control study by in situ hybridization. Diagn Cytopathol 7: 211–214

47. Goff BA, Atanasoff P, Brown E, et al (1992) Endocervical glandular atypia in Papanicolaou smears. Obstet Gynecol 79: 101–104

48. Gondos B, King EB (1977) Significance of endometrial cells in cervicovaginal smears. Ann Clin Lab Sci 7: 486–490

49. Grönroos M, Tyrkkö J, Siiteri PK, et al (1986) Cytolysis and karyopyknosis in postmenopausal vaginal smears as markers of endometrial cancer, diabetes and obesity. Studies based on a ten-year follow-up. Acta Cytol 30: 628–632

50. Gupta PK (1982) Intrauterine contraceptive devices. Vaginal cytology, pathologic changes and clinical implications. Acta Cytol 26: 571–613

51. Gupta PK, Shurbaji MS, Minto LJ, et al (1988) Cytopathologic detection of chlamydia trachomatis in vaginopancervical (fast) smear. Diagn Cytopathol 4: 224–229

52. Guzman J, Hilgarth M, Bross KJ, et al (1988) Malignant ascites of serous papillary ovarian adenocarcinoma. An immunocytochemical study of the tumor cells. Acta Cytol 32: 519–522

53. Hall S, Wu TC, Soudi N, Sherman ME (in press) Low-grade squamous intraepithelial lesions: Cytologic predictors of biopsy confirmation. Diagn Cytopathol

54. Harouny VR, Sutton GP, Clark SA, et al (1988) The importance of peritoneal cytology in endometrial carcinoma. Obstet Gynecol 72: 394–398

55. Hasson HM (1990) Laparoscopic management of ovarian cysts. J Reprod Med 35: 863–867

56. Henry MR, de Mesy Jensen KL, Skoglund CD, Armstrong DW (1993) Chlamydia trachomatis in routine cervical smears. A microscopic and ultrastructural analysis. Acta Cytol 37: 343–352

57. Henry-Stanley MJ, Stanley MW, Horwitz CA (1992) Cytologic diagnosis of cytomegalovirus in cervical smears (abst). Acta Cytol 36: 604–605

58. Hicklin MD, Uatts JC, Plott AE, et al (1984) Retrospective evaluation of gynecologic cytodiagnosis, I: Reproducibility using an experimental diagnostic scale. Acta Cytol 28: 58–71

59. Hirai Y, Fujimoto I, Yamauchi K, et al (1989) Peritoneal fluid cytology and prognosis in patients with endometrial carcinoma. Obstet Gynecol 73: 335–338

60. Hoffman MS, Roberts WS, LaPolla JP, et al (1989) Neoplasia in vaginal cuff epithelial inclusion cysts after hysterectomy. J Reprod Med 34:412–414

61. Hutchinson ML, Agarwal P, Denaulty T, et al (1992) A new look at cervical cytology. Thin prep multicenter trial results. Acta Cytol 36: 499–504

61a. Hutchinson M, Fertitta L, Goldbaum B, et al (1991) Cervex-brush and cytobrush. Comparison of their ability to sample abnormal cells for cervical smears. J Reprod Med 36: 581–586

62. Ide P (1984) Prognostic value of peritoneal fluid cytology in patients with endometrial cancer stage I. Eur J Obstet Gynecol Reprod Biol 18: 343–347

63. Imachi M, Tsukamoto N, Matsuyama T, Nakano H (1988) Peritoneal cytology in patients with endometrial carcinoma. Gynecol Oncol 30: 76–86

64. Johnson TL, Kumar NB, Hopkins M, Hughes JD (1988) Cytologic features of ovarian tumors of low malignant potential in peritoneal fluids. Acta Cytol 32: 513–518

65. Jones DED, Creasman WT, Dombroski RA, et al (1987) Evaluation of the atypical pap smear. Am J Obstet Gynecol 157: 544–549

66. Joseph MG, Cragg F, Wright VC, et al (1991) Cyto-histological correlates in a colposcopic clinic: A 1-year prospective study. Diagn Cytopathol 7: 477–481

67. Kataja V, Syrjänen K, Mäntyjärvi R, et al (1989) Prospective follow-up of cervical HPV infections: Life-table analysis of histopathological, cytological and colposcopic data. Eur J Epidemiol 8: 1–7

68. Kawaguchi K, Nogi M, Ohya M, et al (1987) The value of the cytobrush for obtaining cells from the uterine cervix. Diagn Cytopathol 3: 262–267

69. Kern SB (1991) Prevalence of psammoma bodies in Papanicolaou-stained cervicovaginal smears. Acta Cytol 35: 81–88

70. Kern SB (1991) Significance of anucleate squames in Papanicolaou-stained cervicovaginal smears. Acta Cytol 35: 89–93

71. Khaw KT, Walker WJ (1990) Ultrasound guided fine needle aspiration of ovarian cysts: Diagnosis and treatment in pregnant and non-pregnant women. Clin Radiol 41: 105–108

72. Killough BW, Clark AH, Garvin JB (1988) Correlation between cytodiagnosis and the presence of endocervical or squamous metaplastic cells in gynecologic smears. Acta Cytol 32: 758

73. Kim H-S, Underwood D (1991) Adenocarcinomas in the cervicovaginal Papanicolaou smear: Analysis of a 12-year experience. Diagn Cytopathol 7: 119–124

74. Kirkup W, Singer A, Hill AS (1979) Follow-up of women treated for cervical precancer. An argument for a more rational approach. Lancet ii: 22–24

75. Kiviat NB, Paavonen JA, Brockway J, et al (1985) Cytologic manifestations of cervical and vaginal infections. I. Epithelial and inflammatory cellular changes. JAMA 253: 989–996

76. Kivlahan C, Ingram E (1986) Papanicolaou smears without endocervical cells: Are they inadequate? Acta Cytol 30: 258–260, 1986

77. Klinkhamer PJJM, Vooijs GP, deHaan AFJ (1988) Intraobserver and interobserver variability in the diagnosis of epithelial abnormalities in cervical smears. Acta Cytol 32: 794–800

78. Klinkhamer PJJM, Vooijs GP, de Haan AFJ (1989) Intraobserver and interobserver variability in the quality assessment of cervical smears. Acta Cytol 33: 215–218

79. Koss LG (1992) The normal female genital tract, Chapter 8, pp 251–204, Proliferative disorders and carcinoma of the endometrium, Chapter 14, pp 535–587, Effect of irradiation on cervical and vaginal epithelia, Chapter 18, pp 663–686. In: Koss LG (ed) Diagnostic Cytology and its Histopathologic Bases. Philadelphia, Lippincott

80. Koss LG, Durfee GR (1962) Cytologic diagnosis of endometrial carcinoma. Result of ten years of experience. Acta Cytol 6: 519–531

81. Kristensen GB, Jensen LK, Ejersbo D, Holund B (1989) The efficiency of the cytobrush and cotton swab in obtaining endocervical cells in smears taken after conization of the cervix. Arch Gynecol Obstet 246: 207–210

82. Kristensen GB, Skyggebjerg KD, Holund B, et al (1991) Analysis of cervical smears obtained within three years of the diagnosis of invasive cervical cancer. Acta Cytol 35: 47–50

83. Krumins I, Young Q, Pacey F, et al (1977) The cytologic diagnosis of adenocarcinoma in situ of the cervix uteri. Acta Cytol 21: 320–329

84. Kudo R, Sagae S, Hayakawa O, et al (1991) Morphology of adenocarcinoma in situ and microinvasive adenocarcinoma of the uterine cervix. A cytologic and ultrastructural study. Acta Cytol 35: 109–116

85. Kumar PV, Esfahani FN (1988) Cytopathology of peritoneal endometriosis caused by ruptured ovarian cysts. Acta Cytol 32: 523–526

86. Kurman RJ, Norris HJ, Wilkinson E (1992) Human papillomaviruses and cancer of the lower female genital tract in Atlas of tumor pathology. Tumors of the cervix, vagina, and vulva. Third series. Fascicle 4. Armed Forces Institute of Pathology, Washington, DC, pp 23–25

87. Lambourne A, Lederer H (1973) Effects of observer variation in population screening for cervical carcinoma. J Clin Pathol 26: 564–569

88. Larsen JF, Pedersen OD, Gregersen E (1986) Ovarian cyst fenestration via the laparoscope. A laparoscopic method for treatment of non-neoplastic ovarian cysts. Acta Obstet Gynecol Scand 65: 539–542

89. Laverty CR, Farnsworth A, Thurlow JK, Bowditch RC (1989) The importance of the cell sample in cervical cytology: A controlled trial of a new sampling device. Med J Aust 150: 432–436

90. Lee KR, Manna EA, Jones MA (1991) Comparative cytologic features of adenocarcinoma in situ of the uterine cervix. Acta Cytol 35: 117–126

91. Lenehan PM, Meffe F, Lickrish GM (1986) Vaginal intraepithelial neoplasia: Biologic aspects and management. Obstet Gynecol 68: 333–337

92. Lin TJ, So-Bosita JL (1972) Pitfalls in the interpretation of estrogenic effect in postmenopausal women. Am J Obstet Gynecol 114: 929–931

93. Lindner LE, Geerling S, Nettum JA, et al (1985) The cytologic features of chlamydial cervicitis. Acta Cytol 29: 676–682

94. Liu W (1970) Hypoestrogenism and endometrial carcinoma. Acta Cytol 14: 583–585

95. Liu W, Barrow MJ, Spitler MF, Kochis AF (1963) Normal exfoliation of endometrial cells in premenopausal women. Acta Cytol 7: 211–214

96. Lozowski MS, Mishriki Y, Talebian F, Solitare G (1982) The combined use of cytology and colposcopy in enhancing diagnostic accuracy in preclinical lesions of the uterine cervix. Acta Cytol 26: 285–291

97. Lozowski MS, Mishriki Y, Solitare GB (1986) Factors determining the degree of endometrial exfoliation and their diagnostic implications in endometrial adenocarcinoma. Acta Cytol 30: 623–627

98. Martin PL (1972) How preventable is invasive cervical cancer? A community study of preventable factors. Am J Obstet Gynecol 113: 541–548

99. Mauney M, Eide D, Sotham J (1990) Rates of condyloma and dysplasia in Papanicolaou smears with and without endocervical cells. Diagn Cytopathol 6: 18–21

100. Mazurka JL, Krepart GV, Lotocki RJ (1988) Prognostic significance of positive peritoneal cytology in endometrial carcinoma. Am J Obstet Gynecol 158: 303–306

101. McIndoe WA, McLean MR, Jones RW, Mullins PR (1984) The invasive potential of carcinoma in situ of the cervix. Obstet Gynecol 64: 451–458

102. Meisels A (1966) The menopause: A cytohormonal study. Acta Cytol 10: 49–55

103. Mitchell H, Medley G, Giles G (1990) Cervical cancers diagnosed after negative results on cervical cytology. Perspective in the 1980s. Br Med J 300: 1622–1626

104. Mitchell H, Medley G (1991) Longitudinal study of women with negative cervical smears according to endocervical status. Lancet 337: 265–267

105. Mitchell H, Medley G (1992) Influence of endocervical status on the cytologic prediction of cervical intraepithelial neoplasia. Acta Cytol 36: 875–880

106. Naib ZM (1966) Exfoliative cytology of viral cervico-vaginitis. Acta Cytol 10: 126–129

107. Nasiell K, Roger V, Nasiell M (1986) Behavior of mild cervical dysplasia during long-term follow-up. Obstet Gynecol 67: 665–669

108. National Cancer Institute Workshop (1989) The 1988 Bethesda System for reporting cervical/vaginal cytologic diagnoses. JAMA 262: 931–934

109. National Cancer Institute Workshop (1991) The revised Bethesda System for reporting cervical/vaginal cytologic diagnoses: Report of the 1991 Bethesda Workshop. JAMA 267: 1892

110. Ng ABP (1974) The cellular detection of endometrial carcinoma and its precursors. Gynecol Oncol 2: 162–179

111. Ng ABP, Reagan JW (1988) The pathology and cytopathology of squamous cell carcinoma of the uterine cervix, pp 123–131, Boschann HW Radiation changes in benign cells, pp 254–266, Angstrom T Aspiration cytology of ovarian tumors, pp 507–512. In: Weid GL, Keebler CM, Loss LG, Reagan JW (eds) The Tutorials of Cytology, Chicago, IL, Compendium on Diagnostic Cytology, 6th ed.

112. Ng ABP, Reagan JW, Cechner RL (1973) The precursors of

endometrial cancer: A study of their cellular manifestations. Acta Cytol 17: 439–448

113. Ng ABP, Reagan JW, Hawliczek S, Wentz BW (1974) Significance of endometrial cells in the detection of endometrial carcinoma and its precursors. Acta Cytol 18: 356–361

114. Ng ABP, Reagan JW, Linder EA (1972) The cellular manifestations of microinvasive squamous cell carcinoma of the cervix. Acta Cytol 16: 5–13

115. Nguyen GK (1984) Exfoliative cytology of microinvasive squamous cell carcinoma of the uterine cervix. Acta Cytol 28: 457–460

116. Novotny DB, Maygarden SJ, Johnson DE, Frable WJ (1992) Tubal metaplasia. A frequent potential pitfall in the cytologic diagnosis of endocervical glandular dysplasia on cervical smears. Acta Cytol 36: 1–10

117. Pacey F, Ayer B, Greenberg M (1988) The cytologic diagnosis of adenocarcinoma in situ of the cervix uteri and related lesions. III. Pitfalls in diagnosis. Acta Cytol 32: 325–330

118. Paterson MEL, Peel KR, Joslin CAF (1984) Cervical smear histories of 500 women with invasive cervical cancer in Yorkshire. Br Med J 289: 896–898

119. Pinto MM, Bernstein LH, Brogan DA, et al (1990) Measurement of CA 125, carcinoembryonic antigen, and alpha-fetoprotein in ovarian cyst fluid: Diagnostic adjunct to cytology. Diagn Cytopathol 6: 160–163

120. Poropatich C, Ehya H (1986) Detached ciliary tufts in pouch of douglas fluid. Acta Cytol 30: 442–444

121. Pretorius RG, Lee KR, Papillo J, et al (1986) False-negative peritoneal cytology in metastatic ovarian carcinoma. Obstet Gynecol 68: 619–623

122. Quinn TC, Gupta PK, Burkman RT, et al (1987) Detection of chlamydia trachomatis cervical infection: A comparison of Papanicolaou and immunofluorescent staining with cell culture. Am J Obstet Gynecol 157: 394–399

123. Ramzy I, Delaney M (1979) Fine needle aspiration of ovarian masses. I. Correlative cytologic and histologic study of celomic epithelial neoplasms. Acta Cytol 23: 97–104

124. Ramzy I, Delaney M, Rose P (1979) Fine needle aspiration of ovarian masses. II. Correlative cytologic and histologic study of nonneoplastic cysts and noncelomic epithelial neoplasms. Acta Cytol 23: 185–193

125. Ravinsky E (1986) Cytology of peritoneal washings in gynecologic patients. Diagnostic criteria and pitfalls. Acta Cytol 30: 8–16

126. Reissman SE (1988) Comparison of two Papanicolaou smear techniques in a family practice setting. J Fam Pract 26: 525–529

127. Ritchie DA (1965) The vaginal maturation index and endometrial carcinoma. Am J Obstet Gynecol 91: 578–580

128. Roberts WS, Bryson SCP, Cavanagh D, et al (1986) Peritoneal cytology and invasive carcinoma of the cervix. Gynecol Oncol 24: 331–336

129. Roongpisuthipong A, Grimes DA, Hadgu A (1987) Is the Papanicolaou smear useful for diagnosing sexually transmitted diseases? Obstet Gynecol 69: 820–824

130. Rubin SC, Dulaney ED, Markman M, et al (1988) Peritoneal cytology as an indicator of disease in patients with residual ovarian carcinoma. Obstet Gynecol 71: 851–853

131. Rylander E (1977) Negative smears in women developing invasive cervical cancer. Acta Obstet Gynecol Scand 56: 115–118

132. Schiffman MH, Bauer HM, Lorincz AT, et al (1991) Comparison of Southern blot hybridization and polymerase chain reaction methods for the detection of human papillomavirus DNA. J Clin Microbiol 29: 573–577

133. Schiffman MH, Kurman R, Barnes W, Lancaster W (1990) HPV infection and early cervical cytological abnormalities in 3175 Washington, DC women. In: Howley DM, Broker TR (eds) Papillomaviruses. New York, Wiley-Liss

134. Schnadig VJ, Davie KD, Shafer SK, et al (1989) The cytologist and bacterioses of the vaginal-ectocervical area: Clues, commas and confusion. Acta Cytol 33: 287–297

135. Schneider ML, Wortmann M, Weigel A (1986) Influence of the histologic and cytologic grade and the clinical and post-surgical stage on the rate of endometrial carcinoma detection by cervical cytology. Acta Cytol 30: 616–622

136. Sedlis A (1991) Histology/cytology correlates using both Bethesda and traditional systems. Data presented at the 1991 Bethesda System Conference

137. Selvaggi SM (1986) Cytologic detection of condylomas and cervical intraepithelial neoplasia of the uterine cervix with histologic correlation. Cancer 58: 2076–2081

138. Selvaggi SM (1990) Cytology of nonneoplastic cysts of the ovary. Diagn Cytopathol 6: 77–85

139. Selvaggi SM (1991) Fine-needle aspiration cytology of ovarian follicle cysts with cellular atypia from reproductive-age patients. Diagn Cytopathol 7: 189–192

140. Seybolt JF, Johnston WD (1971) Cervical cytodiagnostic problems: A survey. Am J Obstet Gynecol 109: 1089–1103

141. Shafer M-A, Chew KL, Kromhout LK, et al (1985) Chlamydial endocervical infections and cytologic findings in sexually active female adolescents. Am J Obstet Gynecol 151: 765–771

142. Sherman ME, Bitterman P, Rosenshein NB, et al (1992) Uterine serous carcinoma. A morphologically diverse neoplasm with unifying clinicopathologic features. Am J Surg Pathol 16: 600–610

143. Sherman ME, Kelly D (1992) High-grade squamous intraepithelial lesions and invasive carcinoma following the report of three negative Papanicolaou smears: Screening failures or rapid progression? Mod Pathol 5: 337–342

144. Sherman ME, Paull G (1993) Vaginal intraepithelial neoplasia: Reproducibility of pathologic diagnosis and correlation of smears and biopsies. Acta Cytol 37:699–704

145. Sherman ME, Schiffman MH, Erozan YS, et al (1992) The Bethesda System. A proposal for reporting abnormal cervical smears based on the reproducibility of cytopathologic diagnoses. Arch Pathol Lab Med 116: 1155–1158

146. Sherman ME, Schiffman MH, Lorincz AT, et al (in press) Towards objective quality assurance in cervical cytopathology: Correlation of cytopathologic diagnoses with detection of high-risk HPV types. Am J Clin Pathol

147. Sherman ME, Weinstein M, Sughayer M, et al (1993) The Bethesda System. Impact on reporting cervicovaginal specimens and reproducibility of criteria for assessing endocervical sampling. Acta Cytol 37: 55–60

148. Shiina Y (1985) Cytomorphologic and immunocytochemical studies of chlamydial infections in cervical smears. Acta Cytol 29: 683–691

149. Sidaway MK, Chandra P, Oertel YC (1987) Detached ciliary tufts in female peritoneal washings. A common finding. Acta Cytol 31: 841–844

150. Sneige N, Fernandez T, Copeland LJ, Kata RL (1986) Müllerian inclusions in peritoneal washings. Potential source of error in cytologic diagnosis. Acta Cytol 30: 271–276

151. Snyder RA, Ortiz Y, Samona W, Cove JKJ (1976) Dysplasia and carcinoma in situ of the uterine cervix: Prevalence in very young women (under age 22). Am J Obstet Gynecol 124: 751–756

152. Soutter WP, Wisdom S, Brough AK, Monaghan JM (1986) Should patients with mild atypia in a cervical smear be referred for colposcopy? Br J Obstet Gynecol 93: 70–74

153. Stanley MW, Horwitz CA, Frable WJ (1991) Cellular follicular cyst of the ovary: Fluid cytology mimicking malignancy. Diagn Cytopathol 7: 48–52

154. Stuart GCE, Allen HH, Anderson RJ (1981) Squamous cell carcinoma of the vagina following hysterectomy. Am J Obstet Gynecol 139:311–315, 1981

155. Sugimori H, Iwasaka T, Yoshimura T, Tsukamoto N (1987) Cytology of microinvasive squamous cell carcinoma of the uterine cervix. Acta Cytol 28: 457–460

156. Syrjänen K, Mäntyjärvi R, Saarikoski E, et al (1988) Factors associated with progression of cervical human papillomavirus (HPV) infections into carcinoma in situ during a long-term prospective follow-up. Br J Obstet Gynecol 95: 1096–1102

157. Szarewski A, Cuzick J, Nayagam M, Thin RN (1990) A comparison of four cytologic sampling techniques in a genitourinary medicine clinic. Genitourin Med 66: 439–443

158. Szpak CA, Creasman WT, Vollmer RT, Johnston WW (1981) Prognostic value of cytologic examination of peritoneal washings in patients with endometrial carcinoma. Acta Cytol 25: 640–646

159. Szyfelbein WM, Young RG, Scully RE (1984) Adenoma malignum of the cervix. Cytologic findings. Acta Cytol 28: 691–698

160. Taylor PT, Andersen WA, Barber SR, et al (1987) The screening Papanicolaou smear: Contribution of the endocervical brush. Obstet Gynecol 70:734–737

161. van Erp EJM, Dersjant-Roorda MC, Arentz NPW, et al (1989) Should the cytobrush® be used in routine screening for cervical pathology? Int J Gynecol Obstet 30: 139–144

162. Vooijs GP, Elias A, van der Graaf Y, Poelen-van de Berg M (1986) The influence of sample takers on the cellular composition of cervical smears. Acta Cytol 30: 251–257

163. Vooijs PC, Elias A, van der Graaf Y, Veling S (1985) Relationship between the diagnosis of epithelial abnormalities and the composition of cervical smears. Acta Cytol 29: 323–328

164. Vooijs GP, van der Graaf Y, Elias AG (1987) Cellular composition of cervical smears in relation to the day of the menstrual cycle and the method of contraception. Acta Cytol 31: 417–426

165. Vuopala S (1977) Diagnostic accuracy and clinical applicability of cytological and histological methods for investigating endometrial carcinoma. Acta Obstet Gynecol Scand 70(suppl): 1–72

166. Weid GL, Bartels PH, Bibbo M, Keebler CM (1981) Frequency and reliability of diagnostic cytology of the female genital tract. Acta Cytol 25: 543–549

167. Wetrich DW (1986) An analysis of the factors involved in the colposcopic evaluation of 2194 patients with abnormal Papanicolaou smears. Am J Obstet Gynecol 1986; 154: 1339–1349

168. Willet GD, Kurman RJ, Reid R, et al (1989) Correlation of the histologic appearance of intraepithelial neoplasia of the cervix with human papillomavirus types. Int J Gynecol Pathol 8: 18–25

169. Wojcik EM, Naylor B (1992) "Collagen balls" in peritoneal washings. Prevalence, morphology, origin and significance. Acta Cytol 36: 466–470

170. Wu AY, Sherman ME, Rosenshein NB, Erozan YS (1992) Pathologic evaluation of gynecologic specimens obtained with the cavitron ultrasonic surgical aspirator (CUSA). Gynecol Oncol 44: 28–32

171. Yahr LJ, Lee KR (1991) Cytologic findings in microglandular hyperplasia of the cervix. Diagn Cytopathol 7: 248–251

172. Yazugu R, Piver MS, Blumenson L (1983) Malignant peritoneal cytology as prognostic indicator in stage I endometrial cancer. Obstet Gynecol 62: 359–362

173. Yobs AR, Plott AE, Hicklin MD, et al (1987) Retrospective evaluation of gynecologic cytodiagnosis. II. Interlaboratory reproducibility as shown in rescreening large consecutive samples of reported cases. Acta Cytol 31: 900–910

174. Zarbo RJ (1991) How labs are defining specimen adequacy. CAP Today 5: 12

175. Ziselamn EM, Harkavy SE, Hogan M, et al (1984) Peritoneal washing cytology. Uses and diagnostic criteria in gynecologic neoplasms. Acta Cytol 28: 105–110

176. Zuna RE, Hansen K, Mann W (1990) Peritoneal washing cytology in cervical carcinoma. Analysis of 109 patients. Acta Cytol 34: 645–651

177. Zuna RE, Mitchell ML (1988) Cytologic findings in peritoneal washings associated with benign gynecologic disease. Acta Cytol 32: 139–147

178. Zuna RE, Mitchell ML, Mulick KA, Weijchert WM (1989) Cytohistologic correlation of peritoneal washing cytology in gynecologic disease. Acta Cytol 33: 327–336

Immunohistochemistry

Norio Azumi, M.D., Ph.D., and Bernard Czernobilsky, M.D.

In recent years, immunohistochemistry has largely replaced "special stains" and electron microscopy as an adjunctive method to assist in the differential diagnosis of tumors and in the identification of infectious agents. This technique permits visualization of immunologically detectable markers (antigens) in tissue sections; thus, the pathologist can observe both the morphology and immunophenotype of a given tissue or neoplasm. To exploit this technique fully, the pathologist must be acquainted not only with the distribution of various antigens in different tumors and tissue, but also must have sufficient knowledge of the methodology to avoid pitfalls in interpretation. Accordingly, this chapter is divided into a section describing various aspects of the methodology of this technique and a section describing the application of immunohistochemistry in the identification of a variety of antigens, including intermediate filaments, hormone receptors, oncofetal antigens, and gene products, which can be useful in the differential diagnosis and prognosis of tumors of the female genital tract. This latter section is organized by antigens and is intended to complement the individual (organ) chapters. Table 26.1 can assist the reader in selecting which antibodies are useful in the differential diagnosis of various lesions. Appropriate page numbers also are included in the table.

Methodology

Because an antigen is morphologically not identifiable, it is necessary to visualize and localize the antigen in tissue sections. There are two major techniques that can accomplish this: the *immunoenzyme technique* (immunohistochemistry) and *immunofluorescence.*

The contemporary immunoenzyme technique has two major components: (1) a primary antibody and (2) a detection system to identify the resulting antigen-antibody complex. The detection system uses a secondary or bridging antibody and an enzyme such as peroxidase or alkaline phosphatase that converts a chromogen, which is colorless, to a visible product in the presence of an appropriate substrate. This technique is used most commonly for diagnostic purposes and is discussed in more detail.

In the immunofluorescent technique, a fluoresceinated compound, such as fluorescein isothiocyanate or tetramethylrhodamin isothiocyanate, is used that emits light when excited by light (excitatory light). Because the emitted light is always longer in wavelength than that of the excitatory light, the emitted light can be detected using a fluorescent microscope equipped with an appropriate barrier filter. The simplest application of this technique is to directly conjugate a fluoresceinated compound with an antibody that is then applied to the tissue section. The immunofluorescent technique has several limitations: (1) precise evaluation of morphology is difficult, (2) a fluorescent microscope is required, (3) immunostained slides are not permanent, and (4) fixed tissue has considerable autofluorescence that precludes interpretation. The advantages of this technique are its simplicity and fine resolution of positive patterns that allow distinction between "granular," "smooth," "fibrillary," and "linear." For these reasons, the immunofluorescent technique is not commonly used in diagnostic surgical pathology; it is limited almost exclusively to the evaluation of kidney biopsies.

Antigens

Antigens are usually proteins, although other substances such as carbohydrates can also be antigens. Antibodies react with a part (in case of monoclonal antibodies) or parts (in case of polyclonal antibodies) of antigens, which are called *epitopes.* An antigen usually has multiple potential epitopes that can be detected by antibodies. Fixation and embedding may alter the structure of an epitope to such a degree that it is not recognized by the antibody. To overcome this problem, a mixture (cocktail) of multiple antibodies that detect the same antigen but recognize different epitopes are used for more sensitive detection of antigens. Because some epitopes are more resistant to routine tissue processing, it is possible to select antibodies that detect an epitope that is resistant to fixation. When tissue is fixed in cross-linking fixatives, pretreatment by proteolytic enzymes (enzyme digestion) such as trypsin, pepsin, and pronase may recover or "unmask" epitopes. Keratin, factor VIII, laminin, collagen type IV, neurofilament, desmin, estrogen receptors, and CA125 are among the antigens that benefit from enzyme digestion. The length of enzymatic digestion required to unmask epitopes is roughly proportional to the duration of formalin fixation.[8] For certain antigens such as vimentin, enzyme digestion does not help recover antigenecity. Recently, a new antigen retrieval method that uses microwave irradiation in a heavy metal salt solution such as lead thiocyanate and zinc sulfate has been proposed.[170] The efficacy of this method is comparable to that of enzyme digestion with the additional antigen recovery of vimentin and a few other antigens. The method is cumbersome, however, and may possibly create personal and environmental contamination. Coagulative fixatives preserve many antigens better than formalin, especially the antigenecity of intermediate filaments.[5] A few exceptions are estrogen and progesterone receptors and S-100 protein, in which the antigenicity is better preserved in cross-linking than in coagulative fixative. Enzyme digestion is detrimental to non–formalin-fixed tissue.

Antibodies

Although any subclass of immunoglobulin can be used in immunohistochemistry, the majority that are used belong to either the IgG or, less frequently, the IgM class. Antibodies that react with antigens are called *primary antibodies.* Depending on how these antibodies are produced, two kinds of antibodies are available: polyclonal and monoclonal antibodies.

Polyclonal antibodies are produced by immunization of an animal with a specific antigen. Because the immunized animal produces antisera that include a variety of antibodies to the specific antigen as well as other nonspecific antibodies, it may be necessary to purify the antisera by removing unwanted antibodies. Affinity purification is a process in which antisera are passed through a column with beads containing the purified antigen. After all irrelevant antibodies have been washed away, the antibodies that specifically reacted with the purified antigen on the beads are extracted, thus producing affinity-purified antisera. Although a polyclonal antibody may react with a specific antigen, it recognizes multiple different and overlapping epitopes of the same antigen. Polyclonal antibodies are easier to produce and often more sensitive as compared with monoclonal antibodies, probably because of the larger and multiple epitopes that they recognize. Polyclonal antibodies, however, have several significant disadvantages: (1) even after affinity purification, polyclonal antibodies may include antibodies that may nonspecifically react with unwanted antigens, (2) there is a tendency to produce high background staining, and (3) there is a batch-to-batch variation, which makes interlaboratory comparison impossible. Because of these shortcomings, highly specific monoclonal antibodies have largely replaced polyclonal antibodies, although certain polyclonal antibodies are still in use for diagnostic immunohistochemistry because of their superb sensitivity or difficulty in obtaining monoclonal antibodies.

Monoclonal antibodies are produced by a hybridoma, which is a hybrid of mouse plasmacytoma cells and splenic B lymphocytes from the immunized animal (mouse or rat). Resulting numerous hybridoma clones are then screened against the antigen to find a clone (or clones) that produced the specific antibody. These clones are selected and propagated in tissue culture or in ascites. Because the antibody is produced by a single clone of hybridoma cells, a pure antibody that recognizes a single epitope (monospecific) is obtained. Although creation and screening of hybridoma are extremely labor intensive, the hybridoma cells provide a constant and almost infinite supply of exactly the same antibody. The sensitivity of monoclonal antibodies is usually less and fixation may affect its reactivity more frequently as compared with the equivalent polyclonal antibody. By immunizing with fixed antigens and by careful screening of antibodies, it is possible to develop monoclonal antibodies that are as sensitive as polyclonal antibodies and that recognize epitopes even after fixation. In addition, monoclonal antibody cocktails (mixtures of monoclonal antibodies that react with the same antigen but each of which detects different epitopes) provide sensitivity surpassing that of polyclonal antibodies without sacrificing specificity. Some monoclonal antibody cocktails are commercially available (e.g., antikeratin antibody cocktails such as AE1/AE3 combination).

Detection System

Because an antigen–antibody complex is invisible by conventional light microscopy, a detection system by which a visible product is developed at the site of the antigen–antibody reaction must be used. The detection system is composed of two components: (1) a secondary or bridging antibody and (2) a color development system. Because the secondary antibody must connect (bridge) the primary antibody to the color development system, it is an antibody against the immunoglobulin of the primary antibody (e.g., if the primary antibody is mouse IgG, the secondary antibody is rabbit or goat anti-mouse IgG). In the Avidin–Biotin–Complex method (ABC) and Streptavidin methods, the secondary antibody is biotinylated. The color development system consists of an enzyme, substrate, and chromogen. The enzyme must first bind to the secondary antibody by an antigen–antibody reaction (in peroxidase-antiperoxidase and alkaline–phosphatase–antialkaline phosphatase methods) or by chemical binding of avidin and biotin (in ABC and Streptavidin methods). An appropriate substrate for the enzyme is then added. The colorless chromogen is then converted to a visible product that permits identification of the antigen by the light microscopy.

Two enzymes are most commonly used in modern immunoenzyme techniques: (1) horseradish peroxidase and (2) alkaline phosphatase. *Horseradish peroxidase* is an enzyme that reduces hydrogen peroxide (substrate) to water and oxidizes the chromogen to a visible product. Two of the most commonly used chromogens for peroxidase are diaminobenzidine (DAB) and 3-amino-9-ethylcarbazole (AEC). DAB forms a brown, nonsoluble product that can be dehydrated and cover-slipped for permanent storage. To enhance the contrast further, metallic ions can be added such as copper or nickel, which produce a darker, almost black, reaction product. AEC forms a red color product that is soluble in organic solvents (such as alcohol). Special aqueous mounting medium is needed and the color fades after long storage. The main disadvantage of DAB is its known carcinogenicity. In addition, the brown reaction product may be difficult to differentiate from other naturally occurring pigments such as melanin and hemosiderin. Many normal tissues do have endogenous peroxidase activity that results in nonspecific positivity. In many tissues, the endogenous peroxidase activity is totally suppressed after formalin fixation. For example, epithelial cells of breast and secretory endometrium do not show endogenous peroxidase activity after fixation; however, neutrophils, eosinophils, basophils, histiocytes, and red blood cells may show endogenous peroxidase activity that survives the conventional fixation process. When endogenous peroxidase activity interferes with interpretation such as when a heavy acute inflammatory infiltrate is present, it can be suppressed by incubating sections with a 0.5% H_2O_2 in absolute methanol for 30 minutes. It is difficult, however, to suppress completely the endogenous peroxidase activity without adversely affecting preservation of the antigenicity. *Alkaline phosphatase* uses naphthol AS-MX phosphate as a substrate and converts fast red TR and fast blue BB salts to visible products (red and blue, respectively). This method is particularly useful in double immunostaining. Unlike DAB, the color products are soluble in organic solvents, which makes it necessary to use aqueous mounting media. Endogenous alkaline phosphatase activity is present in many tissues and especially intense in vascular endothelial cells, bladder epithelium, renal tubules, small intestinal epithelium, trophoblastic tissue, neutrophils, and mast cells. After formalin fixation, most of the endogenous alkaline phosphatase activity diminishes to a degree that it does not pose a problem. Although levamisol is known to suppress nonintestinal-type alkaline phosphatase activity, suppression of the endogenous alkaline phosphatase is rarely needed or practical.

Specific Techniques

PEROXIDASE-ANTIPEROXIDASE (PAP) TECHNIQUE

This method was widely used recently because of its superior sensitivity as compared with the direct method; however, newer detection systems such as the ABC method largely replaced the PAP technique. The main innovation of the PAP technique is the PAP complex. Using the antigenic property of peroxidase, the antiperoxidase antibody is raised in the same species in which the primary antibody was raised. Peroxidase and antiperoxidase antibodies are then mixed to form the PAP complex. A secondary antibody that reacts with both the primary and antiperoxidase antibodies bridges the primary antibody and the PAP complex. After addition of a chromogen such as DAB or AEC, the antigen is localized.

ALKALINE PHOSPHATASE AND ANTIALKALINE PHOSPHATASE (APAAP) TECHNIQUE

The principal of this method is exactly the same as the PAP method except that the antibodies are raised against alkaline phosphatase and instead of the PAP complex, APAAP complex is formed. Diazonium salts are used as chromogens.

AVIDIN-BIOTIN-COMPLEX (ABC) TECHNIQUE

Avidin is a glycoprotein contained in egg-white, which shows strong affinity to biotin (much stronger than antigen–antibody reaction). Biotin can be chemically attached to antibodies or enzymes to produce biotinylated antibodies and enzymes. The ABC method exploits these properties of avidin and biotin. In the ABC method, the secondary antibody is biotinylated. The ABC, which is a mixture of avidin and biotinylated peroxidase or biotinylated alkaline phophatase, is used as a color development system. Because avidin has free binding sites available after forming the ABC, it binds with the biotinylated secondary antibody. Although egg-white avidin is most commonly used, because of its carbohydrate side chains it may react with pectin-like substances found in normal tissue such as kidney, liver, brain, and mast cells. The ABC method using peroxidase as the enzyme and DAB as the chromogen is the method used most commonly in diagnostic immunohistochemistry because of its sensitivity, antibody efficiency, good contrast, and permanent preparation.

BIOTIN-STREPTAVIDIN AMPLIFIED TECHNIQUE

This technique uses a type of avidin produced by a bacterium *Streptomyces avidinii*. Streptavidin does not have carbohydrate side chains and has a more neutral isoelectric point as compared with egg-white avidin. When streptavidin is used instead of egg-white avidin, theoretically it produces less nonspecific staining. Although streptavidin may be used to replace egg-white avidin in the ABC method, in some of the commercially available detection kits, streptavidin is directly conjugated to the enzyme, thus producing a stable reagent. This eliminates the need of preparing the ABC complex just before use (biotin–streptavidin amplified technique).

Tissue Fixation and Embedding

Fixation is necessary for better morphologic preservation of the tissue and for preventing antigens from leaching out of tissues. Alteration of antigenicity by chemicals and heat, however, is inevitable during tissue processing. It would be ideal if all the diagnostic immunohistochemistry could be performed on routinely processed formalin-fixed paraffin-embedded tissue; however, certain antigens are detectable only in frozen tissue. Therefore, it is most desirable to obtain additional tissue samples snap-frozen (both naked and embedded in supporting medium such as OCT) and fixed in an alcohol-based fixative whenever possible for future immunohistochemical investigation and additional studies.

FROZEN

This is the method that alters the tissue the least and is suited for investigation of very fragile antigens and of new antigens. After sections are cut in a cryostat, they are briefly fixed in cold acetone or other mild fixatives before proceeding with immunostaining. Detection of most lymphoma and leukemia markers requires frozen sections. Recently, increasing numbers of newly developed antibodies in conjunction with antigen retrieval methods allow detection of many additional antigens in paraffin sections that were detectable only in frozen sections in the past. The disadvantages of using frozen sections, besides the requirement of fresh tissue, snap freezing equipment, a deep freezer, and a cryostat, are poor preservation of morphology, diffusion of antigens, and strong endogenous enzyme activity.

FORMALIN, B5, BOUIN, ALCOHOL, MICROWAVE

Formalin is by far the most widely used fixative. Although formalin fixation is a rather slow process that acts by cross-linking proteins, it provides good tissue penetration and adequate morphologic preservation at a light microscopic level; however, it is not an ideal fixative for immunohistochemistry. Some epitopes may be "masked" or destroyed. This masking effect becomes more pronounced when the fixation time exceeds 24 hours. Because formalin has been and continues to be the fixative that is universally used in diagnostic pathology, it is most useful and practical to develop antibodies and/or antigen recovery systems that allow detection of antigens in formalin-fixed paraffin-embedded tissues.

B5 is both a coagulative and cross-linking fixative; it is a mixture of formalin and mercuric chloride and is used mainly for hematopathology specimens because it provides better definition of nuclear detail. In general, B5 is similar in antigen preservation to formalin; however, added mercuric salt occasionally may produce background staining in some antibodies such as antikeratin antibodies.

Alcohol is coagulative fixative that is good for antigen preservation; intermediate filaments especially show far superior antigen preservation in alcohol-fixed tissue compared with formalin-fixed tissues. Alcohol fixation, however, is not suited for detection of estrogen and progesterone receptors and S-100 protein. In these instances, formalin-fixation provides better results. Poor penetration and a tendency to harden tissues are shortcomings.

Microwave irradiation is reported to facilitate fixation and staining. Special solutions such as Karnovsky's and commercially available solutions are used with microwave irradiation. This technique requires precise control of the temperature and duration of the irradiation. Total loss of antigenicity beyond recovery may ensure if this technique is performed under poorly controlled conditions which makes this technique not feasible in busy laboratories. Advantages of microwave fixation over alcohol-base fixative are not significant and in view of the potential of destruction of antigens, it is not recommended as a routine method.[7]

PLASTIC EMBEDDING

Plastic embedding using methacrylates and epoxy resins allows extremely thin sectioning. Besides its use in electron microscopy, thin sectioning of tissues provides better cytological detail. Although many of the conventional plastic embedding materials have an adverse effect on antigen preservation, some of the newly developed polymers such as LR White and Lowicryl preserve antigenicity better. A special plastic embedding kit using these polymers for immunohistochemistry is commercially available. Although immunohistochemistry can be performed when these specially designed embedding media are used, a much higher concentration of primary antibody is necessary. The sensitivity tends to be much less than paraffin-embedded tissue. Although for hematopathology specimens, plastic embedding has practical merit, no specific advantage is present in gynecological immunohistochemistry; therefore, this method should be reserved for special investigational purposes only.

Pitfalls in Interpretation

Besides knowing the antigen expression of different lesions, the pathologist must be aware of false-positive and false-negative results to avoid misinterpretation. Causes of false-positive results (nonspecific staining) are multiple and may occur at different stages of the immunostaining procedure. False-negative results may be due to loss of activity of the primary antibodies or loss of antigenicity because of tissue processing (especially fixation). Using appropriate controls and multiple antibodies (a "panel") rather than a single antibody will reduce the chance of misinterpretation.

PRIMARY ANTIBODIES

When a primary antibody is not specific for the antigen of interest, immunologic nonspecific binding will ensue. This phenomenon is especially common in polyclonal antibodies because they may contain a mixture of several antibodies that recognize large and/or multiple epitopes. One of these epitopes may be shared by other unwanted antigens. Even quality controlled commercial antibodies may have this problem. Contaminating antibodies may be removed by affinity purification as previously discussed (see above). Among the markers used frequently in gynecological pathology, commercially available polyclonal anticarcinoembryonic antigen (CEA) antibodies may cross-react with nonspecific cross-reacting antigen (NCA) contained in polymorphonuclear leukocytes. Monoclonal antibodies are much less likely to have this problem.

Antibodies may become denatured depending on how diluted they are and how long they have been stored. As a rule, primary antibodies should be freshly prepared the day these antibodies are used. Stock antibodies should be immediately aliquotted into multiple vials when they are received. Commercially available concentrated antibodies tend to be stable, with a shelf-life of approximately 1 year at 4°C. Frozen or lyophilized antibodies may have a much longer shelf-life, although some antibodies cannot be frozen and multiple freeze-thaw cycles may destroy antibody activity. Addition of proteins such as normal calf serum to diluted antibodies may prolong their shelf-life. To ensure proper antibody activity, it is essential to use a positive control for every run of immunostaining.

TISSUES

Antibodies may bind to other proteins in a nonimmunological fashion. This phenomenon is secondary to excessive concentration of primary antibodies and/or certain types of tissue. For example, collagenous tissue and tissue fixed with a heavy metal salt solution (such as in B5 and the antigen retrieval method) tend to show background staining because of the nonimmunological and nonspecific binding. Covering the tissue section with a blocking serum such as normal horse serum before applying the primary antibodies as well as appropriate titration of the primary antibodies reduces this type of nonspecific (background) staining.

Tissue processing at high temperature and/or fixation may produce a loss of antigenicity. Vimentin is well known to be sensitive to prolonged formalin fixation and can be used as a general indicator of antigen loss with the formalin fixation. Some antigens such as p53 protein may be heat sensitive and processing tissues and baking slides at the high temperature may have to be avoided. Because the effect of fixation, processing, and antigen retrieval differs from tissue to tissue, the only sure way of knowing that the antigenicity was properly preserved or recovered is to check so-called built-in, intrinsic controls. Intrinsic controls are tissue components in the section to be immunostained that are expected to be positive for a particular antibody such as squamous epithelium for keratin and peripheral nerve for S-100 protein. When intrinsic controls are not present and there is no immunostaining in the lesion, it cannot be determined whether this is a "true" negative immunostain or a false negative.

ENZYMES AND LABELS

Enzymes used in the color development system may be present in the tissue itself (endogenous activity). Although fixation usually suppresses most of the endogenous peroxidase activity, it may remain in macrophages, red blood cells, and polymorphonuclear leukocytes. When these endogenous peroxidase activities interfere with the interpretation, incubation with hydrogen peroxide–alcohol solution can be used. Alkaline phosphatase activity may be also seen in macrophages even after fixation. In frozen sections, bladder mucosa and vascular endothelial cells may show strong positivity because of endogenous alkaline phosphatase activity. Levamisol suppresses certain types of endogenous alkaline phosphatase activity; however, suppression of alkaline phosphatase activity usually cannot be effectively performed. In systems using avidin and biotin, the presence of biotin and/or cross-reactivity of avidin with lectin-like substances in tissues such as liver theoretically may cause false-positive staining; however, in practice, this type of nonspecific reaction produces only weak background staining in fixed tissue.

CONTROLS USED TO AVOID MISINTERPRETATION

It is important to use appropriate negative and positive controls for validating the specificity of immunostaining. For a negative control, the primary antibody should be replaced with an irrelevant antibody of the same animal species and of the same immunoglobulin class as the primary antibody. In practice, separate negative controls may not be necessary because a panel of antibodies should always be used in diagnostic immunohistochemistry and these different antibodies act as negative controls to each other. For example, if the differential diagnosis includes carcinoma and lymphoma, a panel of antibodies consisting of keratin and leukocyte common antigen (LCA) should be used. If the tumor is a carcinoma, LCA will serve as a negative control for keratin. As a positive control, one should use tissue that is positive in the best of conditions (i.e., positive when your system is most sensitive). This will allow detection of the slightest decrease in sensitivity of the immunohistochemical method. For this purpose, multitumor or multitissue blocks are useful.[9] Multiple tumor tissues that show various degrees of positivity could be in-

cluded and the disappearance of some of the weakly positive samples may be an indication of deterioration of the sensitivity in your immunostaining system. In addition, it is important to check internal controls as discussed earlier. Because the internal positive controls are subjected to the exact same tissue fixation, processing, and immunostaining as the lesion under investigation, the presence of positive staining in the internal control is the best assurance of the validity of the immunostaining.

Markers Useful in Gynecological Pathology

Although immunohistochemical markers, especially lineage-specific markers, are useful in establishing the diagnosis, it cannot be overemphasized that diagnostic immunohistochemistry should be used to differentiate a narrow morphologic differential diagnosis. The pathologist must know aberrant expression of certain markers, such as keratin (epithelial marker) expression in normal myometrium and uterine smooth muscle tumors. Furthermore, it must be understood that no marker is completely specific and therefore diagnostic immunohistochemistry must be employed in conjunction with the morphologic and clinical findings. The diagnostic application of immunophenotyping is based on the same premise, specifically that neoplastic tissues largely preserve the immunophenotype of the putative parent normal tissue. Table 26.1 lists suggested panels of antibodies that are useful in the differential diagnosis of various lesions in the female genital tract. The table also includes the pages in the text where a detailed discussion of the use of the antibodies as they relate to specific diagnostic problems can be found.

Tissue, Cellular, and Lineage-specific Markers

Examples in this category include intermediate filaments (IFs), which are composed of five classes, each of which is specific for a distinct group of cells: (1) keratins are characteristic of epithelial cells, (2) vimentin occurs in mesenchymal cells, (3) desmin decorates myogenic cells, (4) neurofilaments are found in neurons, and (5) glial fibrillary acidic proteins (GFAP) are present in glial cells.[174] Although the tissue specificity of IFs is extremely helpful in establishing the diagnosis, caution has to be exercised because aberrant expression of IFs and co-expression of multiple IFs in the same tumor cells have been reported. Others tissue-specific markers that are discussed in more detail are *actin* and *myoglobin* (for muscle tissue), *chromogranin* and *neuron-specific enolase* (for neuroendocrine tissue), *S-100 protein* and *HMB45* (for melanocytes), *human chorionic gonadotropin* (hCG) and *human placental lactogen* (hPL) (for

Table 26.1. Immunohistochemical markers[a] useful or relevant in the differential diagnosis of gynecological lesions

			Antibodies (pages discussed)
Vulva and cervix			
Paget's disease	vs.	Superficial spreading melanoma	CAM5.2 (1138, 1145), S-100 (1145), HMB45 (1145)
Cervical intraepithelial neoplasia	vs.	Invasive carcinoma	CAM5.2 (1139), SMA (1144), collagen type IV (1147), CEA (1149)
Minimal deviation endocervical adenocarcinoma	vs.	Benign endocervical glands	Blood-group antigens (1152)
Endocervical adenocarcinoma	vs.	Endocervical microglandular hyperplasia	HMFG-1 (1149)
Endocervical adenocarcinoma	vs.	Endometrial adenocarcinoma	GFAP (1140), keratin (1140, 1142), vimentin (1142), CEA (1149), S-100 (1145)
Uterine corpus			
Endometrial carcinoma	vs.	Atypical hyperplasia	HMFG-1,2 (1149), blood-group–related antigens (1152)
Endometrial carcinoma, poorly differentiated	vs.	Malignant mixed mesodermal tumor	Keratin (1142), MSA, SMA (1144), myoglobin (1144)
Endometrial carcinoma, poorly differentiated	vs.	Stromal sarcoma	Keratin, vimentin (1141), GFAP (1144), CA125 (1148), CEA (1149)
Stromal sarcoma	vs.	Leiomyosarcoma	Keratin, vimentin (1141), MSA, SMA, desmin (1144)
Ovary			
Surface-epithelial carcinoma	vs.	Granulosa cell tumor	Vimentin (1143), keratin (1141)
Nonmucinous carcinoma	vs.	Mucinous carcinoma	Keratin, vimentin (1143), GFAP (1144), CA125 (1148), CEA (1149), S-100 (1145), EMA (1149)
Germ cell tumor	vs.	Carcinoma	hPLAP (1147)
Dysgerminoma	vs.	Embryonal carcinoma	Keratin (1142), AFP (1150)
Yolk sac tumor	vs.	Clear cell carcinoma	AFP (1150), LeuM1 (1150)
Thecoma-fibroma	vs.	Leiomyoma	Vimentin, MSA, SMA (1144)
Metastatic gastrointestinal carcinoma	vs.	Primary mucinous carcinoma	Keratin (1142), CEA (1149), GFAP (1144)
Placenta			
Partial mole	vs.	Complete mole	hCG (1146), hPL (1146), hPLAP (1147)
Trophoblast	vs.	Decidual cell	Keratin (1142), hPL, hCG (1147)
Cytology			
Carcinoma cells	vs.	Mesothelial cells	B72.3 (1148)
Benign cervical squamous cells	vs.	High-grade cervical intraepithelial neoplasia	Blood-group antigens (1152)

CEA, carcinoembryonic antigen: GFAP, glial fibrillary acidic protein: MSA, muscle-specific actin; SMA, α smooth muscle actin; EMA, epithelial membrane antigen; hPLAP, human placental alkaline phosphatase; AFP, alpha-fetoprotein; hCG, human chorionic gonadotropin; hPL, human placental lactogen.
[a] All are commercially available and can be applied to routinely processed paraffin sections.

trophoblastic tissue), *placental alkaline phosphatase* (PLAP) (for germ cells), and *LCA* (for hematolymphoid cells).

EPITHELIAL MARKERS

Markers specific to epithelial cells include keratins and epithelial membrane antigen (EMA). Although there are many conflicting reports comparing the sensitivity and specificity of keratins and EMA as epithelial markers, keratins are by far the most specific and useful epithelial marker. Keratins are complex fibrillary proteins. At least 19 subtypes differing in their isoelectric pH values and their molecular weights[132,137] have been characterized.

Numbering of the keratins in this chapter is according to the classification of Moll et al.[132] Some antikeratin antibodies detect a wide range of keratin subtypes and some a very narrow range or just one keratin type. Because expression of the keratin subtype(s) differs in different types of epithelia, it is possible to come up with a "keratin profile" by using multiple narrow-spectrum antikeratin antibodies (Fig. 26.1). The keratin profiles may be helpful in arriving at more specific diagnoses in epithelial tumors, especially poorly differentiated neoplasms. Antikeratin antibodies that are the most widely used and ones relevant to the following discussion are listed in Table 26.2 with keratin classes that they detect. The antibodies to the keratins and other intermediate filaments that are discussed in this

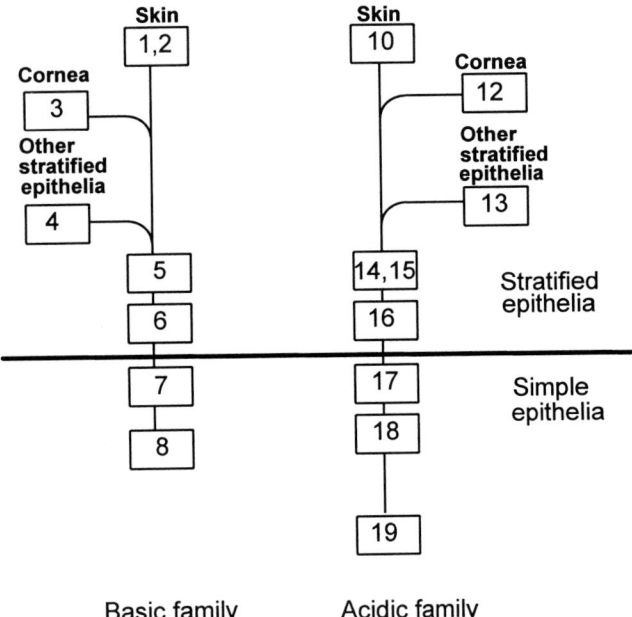

Fig. 26.1. **A unifying model of keratin expression.** The numbers denote Moll's classification of keratin (see also Table 26.2).

chapter are commercially available and most can be used on formalin-fixed, paraffin-embedded tissue.

Vulva

The major keratins identified in the normal epidermis of the labia majora are keratins 1, 5, 10, and 14.[134] This pattern is essentially the same as that present in the epidermis of other locations.[133] Distinctive differences in the keratin profile, especially AE1, AE2, and AE3 of the normal vulva, nonneoplastic disorders, vulvar intraepithelial neoplasia (VIN),[54] and squamous cell carcinoma[20] are reported (Table 26.3). Among VIN, there were differences in the keratin expression in so-called warty and basaloid VIN 3 lesions (Table 26.3) (Fig. 26.2). In the squamous cell carcinoma, expression of keratin 10 (recognized by the antibody DE-K10[85]) may have prognostic significance. Keratin 10 is expressed in the mature keratinizing squamous cells in normal epidermis (Fig. 26.1) and also in well-differentiated keratinizing squamous cell carcinoma. Occasionally it may be expressed in nonkeratinizing portion of squamous cell carcinoma. In one study, among 26 vulvar squamous cell carcinomas of clinical stages II and III, 21 tumors that expressed keratin 10 did not recur, whereas the remaining 5 that did not express keratin 10 did recur, which suggested that this antibody might be a helpful prognostic factor in this neoplasm.[85] Verrucous carcinoma expresses keratins detected by AE1 and AE3 in a uniform and homogeneous manner whereas in typical squamous cell carcinoma, the positivity is disorganized and patchy (Table 26.2 and Fig. 26.3).

Cells of Paget disease express keratins 7, 8, 18, and 19, which are characteristic of simple epithelia, including apocrine and eccrine sweat glands and not keratinocytes.[131] Poorly differentiated adenocarcinoma without skin involvement also expressed keratins 7, 8, 18, and 19.[89] Among the various keratin antibodies, CAM5.2, which detects low molecular weight keratins (keratin 8, 18, and 19), is most useful because it highlights Paget cells

Table 26.2. Classes of keratins and reactivity of antikeratin antibodies

			Antibodies					
pI^a	Moll	Mol Wt	AE1	AE2	AE3	CAM5.2	DE-K10	DE-SCK
Basic	1	65		X	X			X
	2	67		X	X			
	3	64			X			
	4	59			X			
	5	58			X			
	6	56			X			
	7	54			X			
	8	52			X	X		
Acidic	9	64						
	10	56.5	X	X			X	X
	11	56						
	12	55						
	13	51	X					
	14	50	X					
	15	50	X					
	16	48						
	17	46						
	18	45				X		
	19	40	X			X		

Moll, Moll's classification of keratin; Mol Wt, molecular weight, (kDa).
^{a} Isoelectric pH.

Table 26.3. Keratin expression in vulvar lesions

Antibodies	AE1	AE2	AE3	CAM5.2
Normal vulva	Basal	Granular, horny layers	All layers	Negative
Squamous cell hyperplasia	Suprabasal	Granular and horny layers	All layers	Negative
Lichen sclerosis	Suprabasal or all layers	Granular and horny layers or suprabasal	supra basal or all layers	Negative
VIN1,2	Superficial mature layers	Granular and horny layers	All layers	Negative
VIN3, basaloid	All layers (patchy)	Negative	All layers (patchy)	Focally positive
VIN3, warty	All layers (patchy)	All layers (patchy)	All layers (patchy)	Negative
Squamous cell carcinoma	All layers (patchy)	Negative	All layers (patchy)	Negative
Verrucous carcinoma[a]	All layers (homogeneous and uniform)		All layers (homogeneous and uniform)	

Summarized from a study by Esquius et al., ref. 54.
[a] By Brisigotti et al., ref. 20.

but does not react with the surrounding squamous cells. In the differential diagnosis of superficial-spreading melanoma and Paget disease, a panel of CAM5.2, S-100 protein and HMB45 helpful (Paget disease CAM5.2+, S-100−, HMB45−, and melanoma CAM5.2−, S-100+, HMB45+). One caution is that malignant melanoma cells may rarely express low molecular weight keratins.[127] In terms of the keratin profile, mammary and extramammary Paget cells are identical, suggesting a similar histogenesis.[143]

Cervix and Vagina

Because the major keratins detected in the normal exocervix (keratins 1, 4, 5, 6, 13, 14, and 15) are also present in the normal vaginal epithelium,[134] both vaginal and cervical intraepithelial neoplasia (VAIN and CIN, respectively) and invasive squamous cell carcinoma are expected to express a similar keratin profile. Normal endocervical columnar epithelium expresses keratins commonly found in the simple epithelia[65] (keratins 7, 8, 18, and 19). Keratin profiles of the

endocervical subcolumnar reserve cells are complex, showing expression at least of keratins 5, 14, 17, and 19.[65,86,105,178,179] Metaplastic squamous epithelium in the endocervix was accompanied by the expression of keratin 13 and by a reduced expression of keratin 18. Keratins 5, 14, 17,[177] and 19[65,159] are also found throughout the entire thickness of immature metaplasia. These results support the hypothesis of a reserve cell origin of the immature metaplasia[157] (Fig. 26.4).

In CIN, the keratin expression of immature squamous metaplasia is partly conserved.[86,177–179] Similar keratin profiles among the subcolumnar reserve cells, immature metaplasia, and CIN suggest their histogenic relationship. Although similarities of the keratin patterns in CIN 3 and invasive carcinoma[207] is reported, some differences in keratin expression are also noted. For example, CAM5.2 is positive in invasive squamous cell carcinoma but rarely so in CIN 3 and not in CIN 1 and 2.[159]

Invasive cervical squamous cell carcinoma expresses many keratins encompassing almost the entire spectrum of

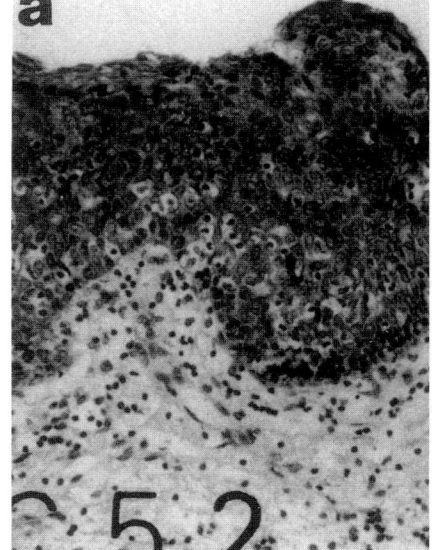
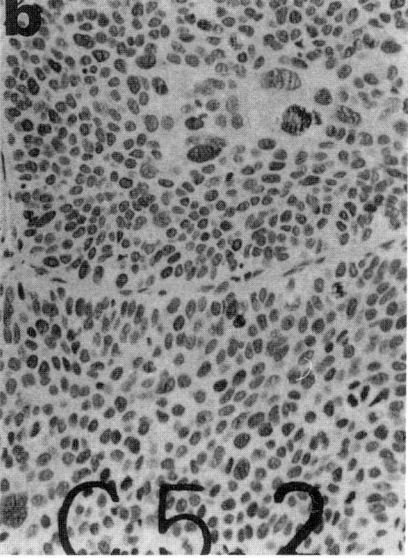

Fig. 26.2. a: VIN3, basaloid type. There is positive keratin staining with CAM 5.2. b: VIN3, warty type. Staining for keratin with CAM 5.2 is negative (antibody to keratins 8, 18, and 19). (Reprinted by permission of Esquius et al., ref. 54.)

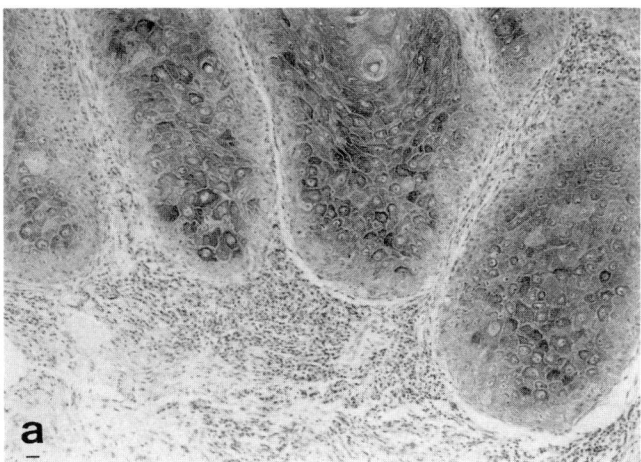

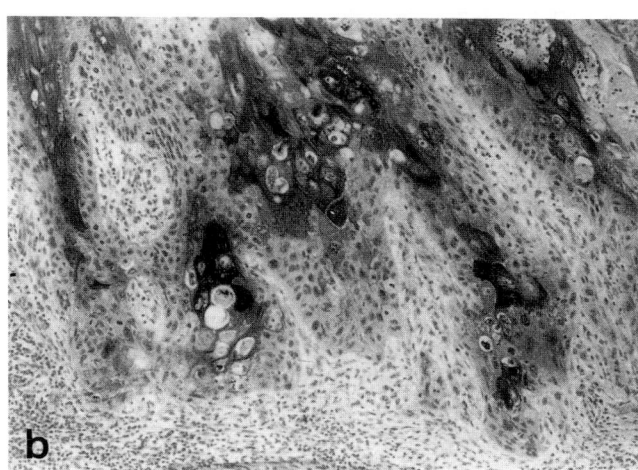

FIG. 26.3. a: Verrucous carcinoma of the vulva. Immunostaining for keratin with AE1 shows a homogeneous staining pattern. **b: Squamous cell carcinoma of the vulva.** Immuno-

staining with AE1 demonstrates disorganized and patchy positive reaction. (Reprinted by permission of Brisigotti et al., ref. 20.)

basic and acidic keratin isotypes.[134,178] Differences in keratin profile between keratinizing and nonkeratinizing squamous cell carcinoma is also reported.[86] Keratinizing carcinomas tend to express keratins 4, 10, and 17, which are expressed only rarely by the nonkeratinizing squamous cell carcinomas in contrast to CIN or squamous metaplasia. Cervical carcinomas have been subdivided into squamous and reserve cell types by means of their keratins expression. The former contain keratins 13, 14, and 16 whereas the latter, which are more aggressive, show, in addition, keratins 8 and CEA and are usually associated with the presence of HPV 16 and 18.[46]

Endocervical adenocarcinoma expresses primarily the same keratins as the normal columnar cells, namely keratins 7, 8, 18, and 19.[134] In addition, a small amount of keratin 17[134] as well as keratins 4[86] and 14[178] have also been detected. These keratin phenotypes may be useful in the distinction between nonkeratinizing squamous cell carcinoma and poorly differentiated adenocarcinoma because the latter does not express keratins 5 and 6. The relatively common presence of GFAP[136] and co-expression of keratins and vimentin in endometrial adenocarcinoma and the negative vimentin and positive CEA in endocervical adenocarcinoma may serve as a useful diagnostic tool in the differential diagnosis between these two neoplasms.[45]

FIG. 26.4. Schematic diagram showing different patterns of staining by various antikeratin antibodies in the uterine cervix. Positive reactivity is indicated by shaded areas. The occasional faint labeling obtained with KS 18.18 is marked by partial shading. EX, exocervix; M, metaplasia; EN, endocervix. (Reprinted by permission of Gigi-Leitner et al., ref. 65.)

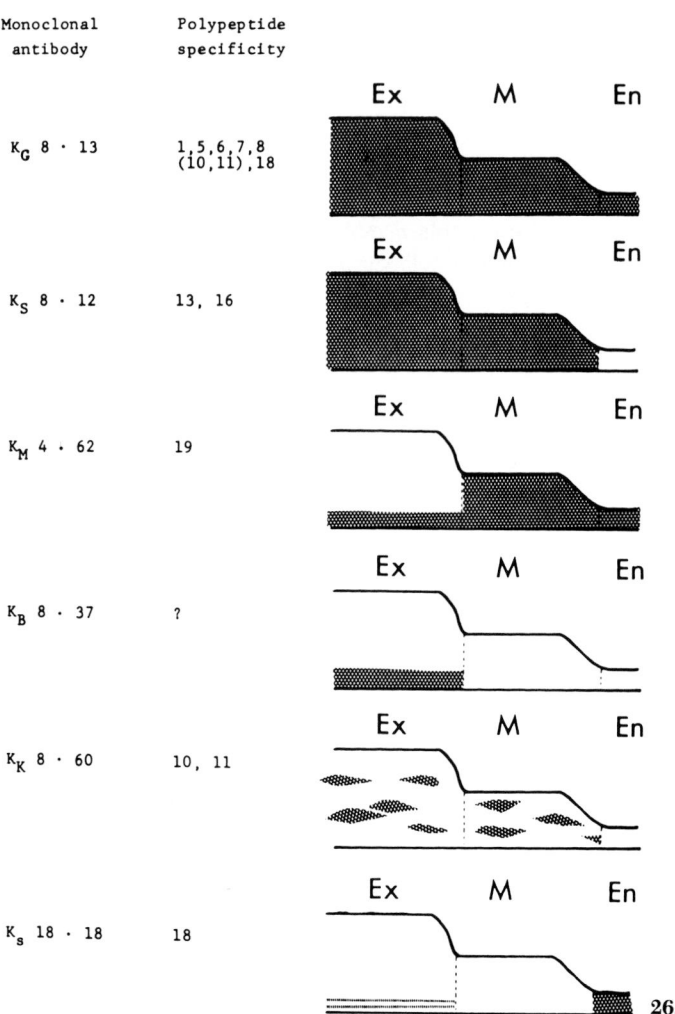

Monoclonal antibody	Polypeptide specificity
K_G 8 · 13	1,5,6,7,8 (10,11),18
K_S 8 · 12	13, 16
K_M 4 · 62	19
K_B 8 · 37	?
K_K 8 · 60	10, 11
K_S 18 · 18	18

26.4

Uterine Corpus

Like simple epithelium in other sites, normal endometrial glands and endometrial adenocarcinoma react with broad-spectrum keratin antibodies and expresses keratins 7, 8, 18, and 19.[41,134] Co-expression of keratin and vimentin is well documented in normal proliferative endometrium and many endometrial carcinomas,[124,137,156] regardless of degree of differentiation. Keratin 5, 6, 10, 11, 13, 14, 16, and 17 (stratification-related keratins) are also present in endometrial adenocarcinoma in various combinations and in irregular patterns that are most prominent in areas of squamous differentiation, but they can also be consistently detected in isolated nonsquamous epithelium.[136] These findings suggest that endometrial adenocarcinomas have a general development potential for squamous differentiation even if the latter is not morphologically evident. Stratification-related keratins, especially keratin 5, which are prominent in endometrial adenocarcinoma, are usually absent in gastrointestinal, renal, and breast adenocarcinoma and may help in the differential diagnosis of a primary endometrial carcinoma versus a metastasis. Keratin 7 can also be used in differentiating endometrial from gastrointestinal neoplasms in metastases since it is present in the former[136] and absent in the latter.[161]

Endometrial stromal sarcoma, however, may show rare keratin-positive individual tumor cells, especially low molecular weight keratins, identified by CAM5.2.[55,60] Normal endometrial stromal cells in a proliferative and secretory phase are negative for keratins. Although IFs, especially keratin and vimentin, are useful in differentiating endometrial stromal sarcomas from anaplastic carcinomas because the former shows mostly expression of vimentin and the latter shows more extensive expression of keratins, caution should be exercised because focal keratin or vimentin positivity does not necessarily exclude the diagnosis of an endometrial stroma sarcoma and anaplastic carcinoma, respectively.[107]

In malignant mixed mesodermal tumors (MMMT), the mesodermal component may be overlooked by routine H&E staining.[156] Especially in the homologous-type MMMT, immunoreactive patterns are helpful in making an accurate distinction between the carcinomatous and sarcomatous components.[16,156,160,162] In these cases the carcinomatous areas express mainly keratins whereas vimentin is the dominant intermediate filament in the sarcomatous component. Careful correlation with the morphologic findings is necessary, however, because vimentin and keratin co-expression in the carcinoma and focal keratin positivity in the stromal sarcoma may occur.

Leiomyosarcomas, leiomyomas, and normal myometrium may express keratin immunoreactivity, especially keratins 8 and 18.[22,149,192] This finding, which was regarded at first as cross-reactivity, has now been shown to represent a true expression of keratin by the smooth muscle cells.[95,104] Although at first disturbing, the presence of keratins in occasional cells of a soft tissue tumor does not diminish the diagnostic usefulness of IF typing in these neoplasms because most tumor cells in the latter continue to express vimentin or other relevant mesenchymal specific markers.

Ovary

All ovarian epithelial neoplasms are positive with broad-spectrum antikeratin antibodies and are positive for simple epithelium-type keratins (keratins 7, 8, 19),[41,59,128,134,142,156,203] which is helpful in the differential diagnosis between poorly differentiated epithelial tumors, sarcomas, and MMMT[156] (Fig. 26.5). Antibodies against stratification-related keratins (keratins 4, 5, and 13) can be used to confirm or detect early squamous differentiation, which may not be easily identifiable on routine H&E stains. Detection of squamous differentiation may be particularly helpful in the differential diagnosis of endometrioid carcinoma from serous carcinoma.[136] Keratins 10 and 11, which are markers for keratinizing squamous epithelia, are identified in squamous nests as well as in individual cells within transitional epithelium nests of a Brenner tumor, suggesting a potential of the latter to transform into squamous-type epithelium.[108]

The distinction of a primary ovarian carcinoma from a

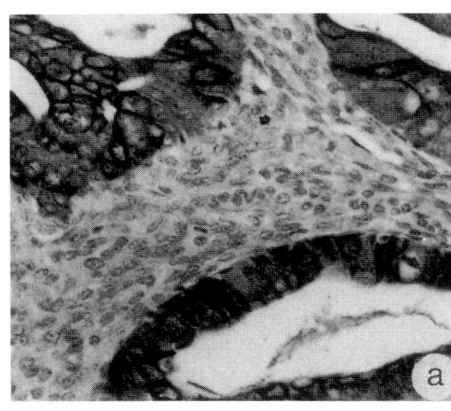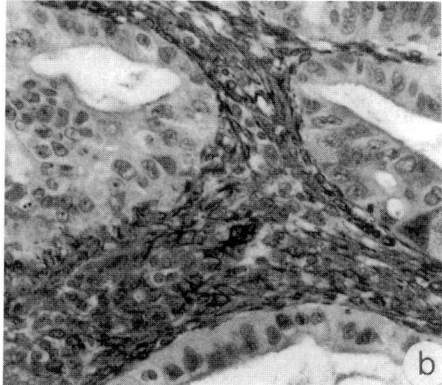

FIG. 26.5. Ovarian MMMT. a: There is positive staining of glands with a broad-spectrum antikeratin antibody. b: Positive vimentin staining of the stromal elements. (Reprinted by permission of Puts et al., ref. 156.)

metastatic gastrointestinal carcinoma can be aided by the detection of keratins 7 and 10.[136,161] Keratin 7 is positive in primary ovarian carcinomas but negative in gastrointestinal carcinomas. In contrast, keratin 10 is sparse or absent in nonmucinous ovarian epithelial carcinomas but is consistently expressed in colonic adenocarcinoma.[135–137]

Granulosa cell tumors generally do not show keratin on fixed tissue.[129,130] However, keratins 8 and 18 may be detected in the tumors showing trabecular (focally) and follicular patterns on frozen tissue. Keratins are absent in tumors with sarcomatoid and watered-silk patterns.[42] Thus, keratin expression is useful in the differential of the so-called anaplastic or sarcomatoid variety of granulosa cell tumors and poorly differentiated carcinoma, which almost always express keratins. In granulosa–theca cell tumors, the thecal elements are found to express keratins[200] as well as vimentin. These results suggest an origin of granulosa cell tumors from normal granulosa cells, which present a similar keratin pattern.[43]

Other sex cord–stromal tumors such as thecoma–fibroma predominantly express vimentin[69,129]; however, keratins 7, 8, 18, and 19[200] may be present. In Sertoli–Leydig cell tumors, keratins were reported to be detected in the epithelial-like (Sertoli) cells of this neoplasm.[130] The stromal elements are positive for vimentin. Similar results have been reported in one case of gynandroblastoma.[130] In the sex cord tumor with annular tubules, isolated cells show keratin positivity.[130]

Ovarian germ cell tumors have not been studied extensively, in contrast to testicular germ cell tumors. The latter reveal a complex, heterogeneous IF profile in both seminomatous[58] and nonseminomatous tumors,[110] indicative of the differentiation potential inherent in these neoplasms. In the absence of detailed studies in ovarian germ cell tumors, it is possible with due reservations only to extrapolate the results from testicular tumors.

Dysgerminomas, as a rule, do not express keratin,[129,130] a situation similar to seminomas.[129] Although one report[200] also demonstrated keratins 7, 8, and 18, marked, keratin positivity in a germ cell tumor may indicate the presence of nondygerminomatous component. Embryonal carcinoma is positive with broad-spectrum antikeratin antibody.[130] Endodermal sinus tumor expresses keratins,[130] especially keratins 7, 8, 18, and 19,[200] with weak expression of keratin 4 and 10. Choriocarcinoma strongly expresses simple epithelium-type keratins[130] and epidermal keratins weakly, which is an immunophenotype similar to normal trophoblast. In teratoma, each tissue present expresses its appropriate intermediate filaments.[128,200] An investigation of the keratin patterns in the epidermis of mature cystic teratoma reveals that histological maturity in these tumors is not necessarily expressed by the keratin pattern, which reflects the state of molecular rather than histological differentiation.[40] Since prognosis in germ cell tumors is usually related to the degree of tissue maturation, the above observa-

tion may eventually prove to be of prognostic value in some of these teratomas.

Placenta and Trophoblast

Studies using cultured cells and amniotic fluid[10,92] showed that all trophoblastic cells (syncytial, cyto-, and intermediate) react with antikeratin antibodies to the simple epithelium type keratins (keratins 8, 18, and 19). Because trophoblastic cells are positive and decidual cells are negative for keratin,[92] keratin expression is useful in distinguishing these two types of cells. Amniotic epithelium expresses keratins proteins 5, 6, 7, 8, 14, 17, 18, and 19 (with the addition of keratin 4 and the disappearance of keratin 7 at the 16th week of pregnancy).[38] Amniotic epithelial cells in culture continue to express their characteristic keratins, whereas cells in amnion fluid cultures usually synthesize a different, simpler set of keratins. Based on these findings, it has been suggested that cells in the amnion fluid cultures are not derived from amniotic epithelium, but probably from simple epithelial cells of the fetus.[164] This could have important implications in prenatal diagnosis. A subset of fetal mesenchymal cells of the amniochorion and chorionic villi are reported to express not only vimentin but also keratin and desmin, suggesting that these cells are in a unique indeterminate stage of differentiation showing multipotential characteristics.[92] The trophoblast of hydatidiform moles and choriocarcinoma express low molecular keratins[27,130,166] (keratins 7, 8, and 18[38]).

Chorangioma of the placenta reveals that the blood vessels of this lesion are not only positive for vimentin and alpha-smooth muscle actin but also for keratins 18 in areas.[109] Because blood vessels within the chorionic plate, anchoring villi,[109] and in the stem villi[10,199] also express keratin 18,[109] whereas those of the terminal villi show no staining for keratins. Chorangiomas most likely originate from blood vessels of the chorionic plate and anchoring villi.

MESENCHYMAL MARKERS

Vimentin, which is one of the five IFs, is expressed predominantly by normal mesenchymal cells and tumors of mesenchymal derivation. Because vimentin antigenicity is sensitive to fixation, the most sensitive demonstration of vimentin is accomplished with frozen or alcohol-fixed tissues. Unlike keratin, enzyme digestion of formalin-fixed tissues does not recover vimentin antigenicity. With the use of more sensitive antibodies and better fixed tissues, increasing numbers of epithelial neoplasms are reported to express vimentin in addition to keratin.[5] Thus, although still useful in certain circumstances especially as a part of the panel of antibodies, vimentin is not a specific mesenchymal marker.

Cervix

Endocervical adenocarcinoma is negative for vimentin and positive for CEA. This can serve as a useful tool in the differential diagnosis between cervical and endometrial adenocarcinoma (see below).

Uterine Corpus

Endometrial adenocarcinomas co-express keratin and vimentin.[124,136,156] Normal proliferative endometrial glands also co-express both of these markers. Normal endometrial stromal cells express primarily vimentin.

Ovary

Epithelial ovarian neoplasms[124,136,203] generally co-express vimentin and keratin. Most ovarian serous and clear cell carcinomas and some endometrioid carcinomas express both markers, but mucinous and Brenner tumors do not[203] (Fig. 26.6). This phenomenon is comparable to keratin and vimentin expression by endocervical and endometrial cells. Vimentin tends to be positive more frequently in the better differentiated cases.[203] These findings correspond to the co-expression of keratins and vimentin in normal ovarian coelomic surface epithelium from which the above neoplasms originate.[136]

Granulosa cell tumors predominantly express vimentin,[129,130] but co-expression of keratins and vimentin is also reported.[69,200] Granulosa cell tumors also contain desmo-plakins in addition to vimentin.[42] Vimentin filaments rather than keratin filaments insert to desmoplakin-positive plaques of desmosomes much like in meningeal cells and meningiomas. In so-called granulosa–theca cell tumors, the thecal elements express vimentin as well as keratins.[200] Thecoma–fibroma also predominantly express vimentin.[69,129] In addition to vimentin, keratins 7, 8, 18, and 19 and desmin are reported to be present in some of these neoplasms.[200] Leydig cell tumors express only vimentin but not keratin.[130] In sex cord tumors with annular tubules, the tumor cells in the islands with annular tubules show distinct vimentin positivity, which is also observed in the stromal cells. Between these cellular islands, isolated cells show keratin positivity.[130]

Placenta

In the full-term placenta, vimentin is demonstrated not only in mesenchymal cells of the amnion connective tissue, but also in groups of cells in the epithelial layer.[10,38,92]

MUSCLE MARKERS

There are several markers specific for muscle differentiation. Desmin, one of the IFs, is expressed by both skeletal and smooth muscle tissues.[49] Actin is a ubiquitous fibrillary protein thinner than desmin and present in many epithelial and nonepithelial cells as a cytoskeletal protein. Actin is a heterodimer that is composed of combination of α, β, and

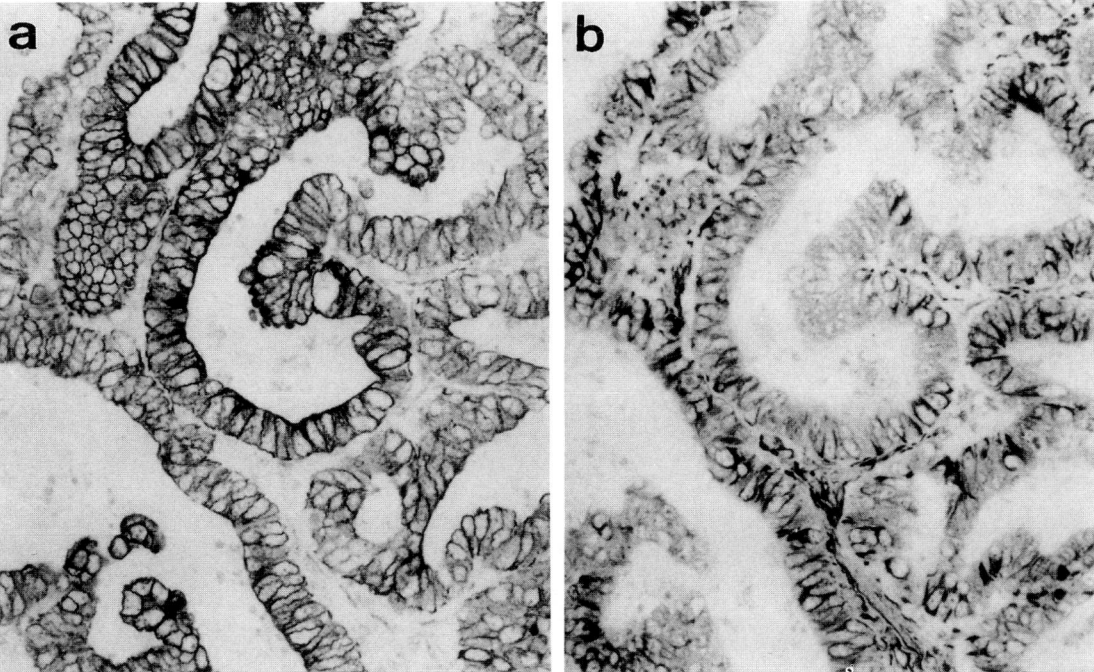

FIG. 26.6. Endometrioid adenocarcinoma of the ovary. a: Immunostaining of keratin (broad-spectrum antibody). **b:** Co-expression of vimentin in glandular epithelium. (Reprinted by permission of Viale et al., ref. 203.)

δ chains. α and δ chains are specific to muscle cells. Two antiactin antibodies that are specific for muscle differentiation are most useful in diagnostic immunohistochemistry: muscle-specific actin (MSA; HHF-35)[196] and α-smooth muscle actin (SMA).[168] MSA recognizes α and δ chains and reacts with both skeletal and smooth muscle cells, whereas α-SMA is specific for smooth muscle tissue. In addition to normal smooth and skeletal muscle tissue, myoepithelial cells and myofibroblasts also express actin especially detectable by SMA and, to a lesser extent, by MSA and desmin.[66] Myofibroblasts are postulated to be induced from mesenchymal stem cells or fibroblasts in reparative or reactive processes such as granulation tissue and nodular fasciitis and are believed to contribute to contraction of the scar tissue. Myoglobin is oxygen-binding protein and is specific for the skeletal muscle tissue; however, because it is present only in the well-differentiated skeletal muscle cells, its utility in the diagnosis of rhabdomyosarcoma is limited.

Cervix

Normal cervical stromal cells are negative for α-SMA; however, actin may be expressed in reactive processes. In microinvasive squamous cells carcinoma and high-grade CIN, the stromal cells express α-SMA.[37]

Uterine Corpus

Normal endometrial stroma expresses vimentin, desmin, MSA, and α-SMA with more pronounced reactivity in the secretory phase stroma.[60] Endometrial stromal nodules show an immunophenotype similar to that of the normal endometrial stromal cells. Although detectable muscle differentiation is usually focal in stromal sarcoma and the sarcomatous component of MMMT, MSA and α-SMA may occasionally show diffuse staining. In the heterologous MMMT, specific elements such as rhabdosarcomatous cells can be identified by positive actin, desmin, and myoglobin.[3]

Leiomyosarcomas stain diffusely for MSA, α-SMA, and desmin.[6] In contrast, stromal sarcomas express mostly vimentin with focal positivity for the muscle markers. These differences may assist in differential diagnosis. Normal myometrium expresses MSA, α-SMA, vimentin, and to a lesser degree desmin. The similar immunophenotype is found in leiomyomas and leiomyosarcomas.[156]

Ovary

Normal stromal cells are negative for α-SMA except in the inner cortex and around corpora lutea and albicans. In stromal hyperplasia, the stromal cells including ones showing luteinization are negative. Strong expression of α-SMA in the stromal cells around epithelial cells such as in primary ovarian and metastatic carcinoma suggests an induc-

tive effect of smooth muscle differentiation by the epithelial cells.[44] Tumors of the thecoma–fibroma group are negative for α-SMA in contrast to the rare ovarian leiomyomas, which are α-SMA positive.[44]

Glial Markers

One of the intermediate proteins, GFAP is a major component of cytoplasmic protein in glial cells and is composed of a 51-kDa polypeptide. Although GFAP is expressed most frequently in astrocytes, ependymal cells, Schwann cells, and satellite cells of human sensory ganglia, GFAP expression in other nonglial tissues and tumors has been observed. Among gynecological tumors, rare true glial tumors, glial components of teratoma, and peritoneal gliomatosis express GFAP as expected. For example, "glial polyps (or gliomas)" of the uterine cervix[114] and uterine corpus[106] show GFAP expression. Additionally, nonglial müllerian-derived tumors express seemingly ectopic expression of GFAP. For example, occasional examples of endometrial adenocarcinoma show positive GFAP in scattered tumor cells that otherwise are morphologically indistinguishable from adjacent GFAP-negative carcinoma cells.[136] In MMMT, GFAP positivity is observed in the sarcomatous component showing high-grade stromal sarcoma-like appearance as well as in occasional epithelial tumor cells.[106]

In ovarian carcinomas, GFAP may be present in small subpopulations of tumor cells of occasional serous (ovarian and extraovarian) and endometrioid adenocarcinomas (Fig. 25.7), but not in mucinous or clear cell carcinomas.[136] Thus, the presence of GFAP in a metastatic adenocarcinoma might warrant the consideration of a müllerian duct–derived primary tumor, since in no other carcinomas, with the exception of an occasional renal cell carcinoma and

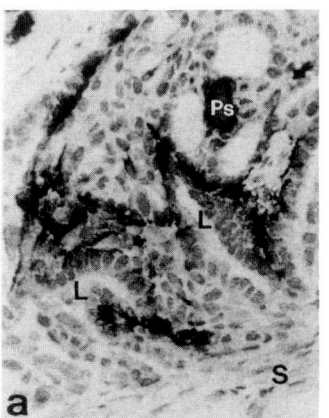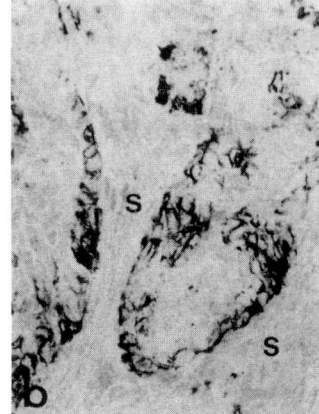

FIG. 26.7. a: **Serous carcinoma of the ovary.** Focal and strong GFAP positivity. b: **Endometrioid adenocarcinoma of the ovary.** GFAP positivity. S, stroma; L, lumen, Ps, psammoma body. (Reprinted by permission of Moll et al., ref. 136.)

and endometrial stromal neoplasms. Evidence for smooth muscle differentiation. Am J Surg Pathol 15: 861–870

61. Garcia E, Bouchard P, De Brux J, et al (1988) Use of immunocytochemistry of progesterone and estrogen receptors for endometrial dating. J Clin Endocrinol Metab 67: 80–87

62. Geisinger KR, Marshall RB, Kute TE, Homesley HD (1986) Correlation of female sex steroid hormone receptors with histologic and ultrastructural differentiation in adenocarcinoma of the endometrium. Cancer 58: 1506–1517

63. Ghazizadeh M, Oguro T, Sasaki Y, Aihara K, Araki T, Springer GF (1990) Immunohistochemical and ultratructural localization of T antigen in ovarian tumors. Am J Clin Pathol 93: 315–321

64. Giancotti FR, Dorsett BH, Kim KT, Ioachim HL, Barber HR (1990) Immunohistochemical characterization of a monoclonal antibody detecting an endometrioid ovarian cancer-associated antigen. Int J Gynecol Pathol 9: 253–262

65. Gigi-Leitner O, Geiger B, Levy R, Czernobilsky B (1986) Cytokeratin expression in squamous metasplasia of the human uterine cervix. Differentiation 31: 191–205

66. Gilks CB, Taylor GP, Clement PB (1987) Inflammatory pseudotumor of the uterus. Int J Gynecol Pathol 6: 275–286

67. Girling A, Bartkova J, Burchell J, Gendler S, Gillett C, Taylor-Papadimitriou J (1989) A core protein epitope of the polymorphic epithelial mucin detected by the monoclonal antibody SM-3 is selectively exposed in a range of primary carcinomas. Int J Cancer 43: 1072–1076

68. Glasgow BJ, Wen DR, Al-Jitawi S, Cochran AJ (1987) Antibody to S-100 protein aids the separation of pagetoid melanoma from mammary and extramammary Paget's disease. J Cutan Pathol 14: 223–226

69. Gown AM, Vogel AM (1985) Monoclonal antibodies to human intermediate filament proteins III. Analysis of tumors. Am J Clin Pathol 84: 413–424

70. Hachisuga T, Fukuda K, Hayashi Y, Iwasaka T, Sugimori H (1989) Immunohistochemical demonstration of histiocytes in normal ectocervical epithelium and epithelial lesions of the uterine cervix. Gynecol Oncol 33: 273–278

71. Haldane JS, Hird V, Huges CM, Gullick WJ (1990) c-erbB-2 oncogene expression in ovarian cancer. J Pathol 162: 231–237

72. Hamilton-Dutoit SJ, Lou H, Pallesen G (1990) The expression of placental alkaline phosphatase (PLAP) and PLAP-like enzymes in normal and neoplastic human tissues. An immunohistological survey using monoclonal antibodies. APMIS 98: 797–811

73. Hammond RH, Bates D, Clarke DG, et al (1991) The immunoperoxidase localization of tumour markers in ovarian cancer: The value of CEA, EMA, cytokeratin and DD9. Br J Obstet Gynaecol 98: 73–83

74. Harding M, Cowan S, Hole D, et al (1990) Estrogen and progesterone receptors in ovarian cancer. Cancer 65: 486–491

75. Harms D, Janig U (1986) Germ cell tumours of childhood. Report of 170 cases including 59 pure and partial yolk-sac tumours. Virch Arch [A] 409: 223–239

76. Henry RJ, Goodman JD, Godley M, Raju KS, Coffer AI, King RJ (1988) Immunohistochemical study of cytoplasmic oestradiol receptor in normal, dysplastic and malignant cervical tissue. Br J Obstet Gynaecol 95: 927–932

77. Heyderman E, Steele K, Ormerod MG (1979) A new antigen on epithelial membrane: Its immunoperoxidase location in normal and neoplastic tissue. J Clin Pathol 32: 35–39

78. Himes TR, Ernst CS, Koprowska I (1986) Loss of blood isoantigens in exfoliated cells during the progression of CIN demonstrated by monoclonal antibody staining. Acta Cytol 30: 461–469

79. Hung MC, Zhang X, Yan DH, et al (1992) Aberrant expression of the c-erbB-2/neu protooncogene in ovarian cancer. Cancer Lett 61: 95–103

80. Iemura K, Sonoda T, Hayakawa A, et al (1991) Small cell carcinoma of the uterine cervix showing Cushing's syndrome caused by ectopic adrenocorticotropin hormone production. Jpn J Clin Oncol 21: 293–298

81. Ingram SS, Rosenman J, Heath R, Morgan TM, Moore D, Varia M (1989) The predictive value of progesterone receptor levels in endometrial cancer. Int J Radiat Oncol Biol Phys 17: 21–27

82. Inoue M, DeLellis RA, Scully RE (1986) Immunohistochemical demonstration of chromogranin in endometrial carcinomas with argyrophil cells. Hum Pathol 17: 841–847

83. Ishikura H, Scully RE (1987) Hepatoid carcinoma of the ovary. A newly described tumor. Cancer 60: 2775–2784

84. Isola J, Kallioniemi OP, Korte JM, et al (1990) Steroid receptors and Ki-67 reactivity in ovarian cancer and in normal ovary: Correlation with DNA flow cytometry, biochemical receptor assay, and patient survival. J Pathol 162:295–301

85. Ivanyi D, Ansink A, Groeneveld E, Hageman PC, Mooi WJ, Heintz AP (1989) New monoclonal antibodies recognizing epidermal differentiation-associated keratins in formalin-fixed, paraffin-embedded tissue. Keratin 10 expression in carcinoma of the vulva. J Pathol 159: 7–12

86. Ivanyi D, Groeneveld E, Van Doornewaard G, Mooi WJ, Hageman PC (1990) Keratin subtypes in carcinomas of the uterine cervix: Implications for histogenesis and differential diagnosis. Cancer Res 50: 5143–5152

87. Iversen OE, Skaarland E, Utaaker E (1986) Steroid receptor content in human ovarian tumors: survival of patients with ovarian carcinoma related to steroid receptor content. Gynecol Oncol 23: 65–76

88. Iwamori M, Sakayori M, Nozawa S, et al (1989) Monoclonal antibody-defined antigen of human uterine endometrial carcinomas is Leb. J Biochem (Tokyo) 105: 718–722

89. Kerner H, Gal D, Friedman M, Moll R (1988) An immunohistochemical and biochemical study of cytokeratin polypeptides in a non-Paget type adenocarcinoma of the vulva. J Obstet Gynecol 8: 294–298

90. Kerns BJ, Jordan PA, Moore MB, et al (1992) p53 overexpression in formalin-fixed, paraffin-embedded tissue detected by immunohistochemistry. J Histochem Cytochem 40: 1047–1051

91. Khalifa MA, Sesterhenn IA (1990) Tumor markers of epithelial ovarian neoplasms. Int J Gynecol Pathol 9: 217–230

92. Khong TY, Lane EB, Robertson WB (1986) An immunocytochemical study of fetal cells at the maternal-placental interface using monoclonal antibodies to keratins, vimentin and desmin. Cell Tissue Res 246: 189–195

93. Kiguchi K, Takamatsu K, Tanaka J, Nozawa S, Iwamori M, Nagai Y (1992) Glycosphingolipids of various human ova-

rian tumors: A significantly high expression of I3SO3GalCer and Lewis antigen in mucinous cystadenocarcinoma. Cancer Res 52: 416–421

94. Kleine W, Maier T, Geyer H, Pfleiderer A (1990) Estrogen and progesterone receptors in endometrial cancer and their prognostic relevance. Gynecol Oncol 38: 59–65

95. Knapp AC, Franke WW (1989) Spontaneous loss of control of cytokeratin gene expression in transformed, non-epithelial human cells occurring at different levels of regulation. Cell 59: 67–79

96. Kommoss F, Franklin WA, Talerman A (1989) Estrogen and progesterone receptors in endodermal sinus (yolk sac) tumor. Evaluation of immunocytochemical and biochemical methods. J Reprod Med 34: 943–945

97. Konishi I, Fujii S, Kataoka N, et al (1988) Ovarian mucinous cystadenocarcinoma producing alpha-fetoprotein. Int J Gynecol Pathol 7: 182–189

98. Konishi I, Fujii S, Nonogaki H, Nanbu Y, Iwai T, Mori T (1991) Immunohistochemical analysis of estrogen receptors, progesterone receptors, Ki-67 antigen, and human papillomavirus DNA in normal and neoplastic epithelium of the uterine cervix. Cancer 68: 1340–1350

99. Koprowski H, Steplewski Z, Mitchell K, et al (1979) Colorectal carcinoma antigens detected by hybridoma antibodies. Somat Cell Genet 5: 957–972

100. Kuhnel R, Rao BR, Stolk JG, van Kessel H, Seldenrijk CA, Willig AP (1987) Estrogen synthesizing rare malignant Brenner tumor of the ovary with the presence of progesterone and androgen receptors in the absence of estrogen receptors. Gynecol Oncol 26: 263–269

101. Kupryja'nczyk J, Moller P (1988) estrogen receptor distribution in the normal and pathologically changed human cervix uteri: An immunohistochemical study with use of monoclonal anti-ER antibody. Int J Gynecol Pathol 7: 75–85

102. Kurman RJ, Young RH, Norris HJ, Main CS, et al (1984) Immunohistochemical localization of placental lactogen and chorionic gonadotropin in the normal placenta and trophoblastic tumors, with emphasis on intermediate trophoblast and the placental site trophoblastic tumor. Int J Gynecol Pathol 3: 101–121

103. Kurrasch RH, Rutherford AV, Rick ME, et al (1989) Characterization of a monoclonal antibody, OVB1, which binds to a unique determinant in human ovarian carcinomas and myeloid cells. J Histochem Cytochem 37: 57–67

104. Kuruc N, Franke WW (1988) Transient coexpression of desmin and cytokeratins 8 and 18 in developing myocardial cells. Differentiation 38: 177–193

105. Levy R, Czernobilsky B, Geiger B (1988) Subtyping of epithelial cells of normal and metaplastic human uterine cervix, using polypeptide-specific cytokeratin antibodies. Differentiation 39: 186–196

106. Liao SY, Choi BH (1986) Expression of glial fibrillary acidic protein by neoplastic cells of müllerian origin. Virch Arch B Cell Pathol 52: 185–193

107. Lifschitz-Mercer B, Czernobilsky B, Dgani R, Dallenbach-Hellweg G, Moll R, Franke WW (1987) Immunocytochemical study of an endometrial diffuse clear cell stromal sarcoma an dother endometrial stromal sarcomas. Cancer 59: 1494–1499

108. Lifschitz-Mercer B, Czernobilsky B, Shezen E, Dgani P,

Leitner O, Geiger B (1988) Selective expression of cytokeratin polypeptides in various epithelia of human Brenner tumor. Hum Pathol 19: 640–650

109. Lifschitz-Mercer B, Fogel M, Kushnir I, Czernobilsky B (1989) Chorangioma. A cytoskeletal profile. Int J Gynecol Pathol 8: 349–356

110. Lifschitz-Mercer B, Fogel M, Moll R, et al (1991) Intermediate filament protein profiles of human testicular nonseminomatous germ cell tumors: Correlation of cytokeratin synthesis to cell differentiation. Differentiation 48: 191–198

111. Lin M, Hanai J, Wada A, et al (1991) S-100 protein in ovarian tumors. A comparative immunohistochemical study of 135 cases. Acta Pathol Jpn 41: 233–239

112. Lidngren J, Vesterinen E, Purola E, Wahlstrom T (1986) Prognostic significance of tissue carcinoembryonic antigen in mild dysplasia of the uterine cervix. Tumour Biol 6: 465–470

113. Loy TS, Darkow VD (1993) Distribution of colon-ovarian tumor antigen in adenocarcinomas. An immunohistochemical study of 501 cases. Am J Clin Pathol 99: 207–210

114. Luevano-Flores E, Sotelo J, Tena-Suck M (1985) Glial polyp (glioma) of the uterine cervix, report of a case with demonstration of glial fibrillary acidic protein. Gynecol Oncol 21: 385–390

115. Mainguene C, Aillet G, Kremer M, Chatal JF (1986) Immunohistochemical study of ovarian tumors using the OC 125 monoclonal antibody as a basis for potential in vivo and in vitro applications. J Nucl Med Allied Sci 30: 19–22

116. Manivel C, Wick MR, Sibley RK (1986) Neuroendocrine differentiation in müllerian neoplasms. An immunohistochemical study of a "pure" endometrial small-cell carcinoma and a mixed müllerian tumor containing small-cell carcinoma. Am J Clin Pathol 86: 438–443

117. Marks JR, Davidoff AM, Kerns BJ, et al (1991) Overexpression and mutation of p53 in epithelial ovarian cancer. Cancer Res 51: 2979–2984

118. Martin JD, Hahnel R, McCartney AJ, De Klerk N (1986) The influence of estrogen and progesterone receptors on survival in patients with carcinoma of the uterine cervix. Gynecol Oncol 23: 329–335

119. Masood S (1988) Use of monoclonal antibodies in immunocytochemical localization of estrogen receptors in ovarian cancer. Cancer Detect Prev 12: 283–290

120. Masood S, Hosein I, Pitcher M, Graf W (1990) Potential value of immunoperoxidase technique in assessment of genital herpes. J Fla Med Assoc 77: 516–519

121. Matsukuma K, Tsukamoto N (1988) Alpha-fetoprotein producing endometrial adenocarcinoma: Report of a case. Gynecol Oncol 29: 370–377

122. McDicken IW, Rainey M (1983) The immunohistological demonstration of carcinoembryonic antigen in intra-epithelial and invasive squamous carcinoma of the cervix. Histopathology 7: 475–485

123. McLaughlin PJ, Warne PH, Hutchinson GE, Johnson PM, Tucker DF (1987) Placental-type alkaline phosphatase in cervical neoplasia. Br J Cancer 55: 197–201

124. McNutt M, Bolen JW, Gown AM, Hammar SP, Vogel AM (1985) Coexpression of intermediate filaments in human epithelial neoplasms. Ultrastruct Pathol 9: 31–43

125. Metoki R, Kakudo K, Tsuji Y, Teng N, Clausen H, Hako-

mori S (1989) Deletion of histo-blood group A and B antigens and expression of incompatible A antigen in ovarian cancer. J Natl Cancer Inst 81: 1151–1157

126. Mettler L, Radzun HJ, Salmassi A, Kochling W, Parwaresch MR (1990) Six new monoclonal antibodies to serous, mucinous, and poorly differentiated ovarian adenocarcinomas. Cancer 65: 1525–1532

127. Miettinen A, Franssila K (1989) Immunohistochemical spectrum of malignant melanoma. The common presence of keratins. Lab Invest 6: 623–628

128. Miettinen M, Lehto VP, Bradley R, Virtanen I (1982) expression of intermediate filaments in soft tissue sarcomas. Int J Cancer 30: 545–546

129. Miettinen M, Lehto VP, Virtanen I (1983) Expression of intermediate filaments in normal ovaries and ovarian epithelial, sex-cord-stromal, and germinal tumours. Int J Gynecol Pathol 2: 64–71

130. Miettinen M, Wahlstrom T, Virtanen I, Talerman A, Astengo-Osuna C (1985) Cellular differentiation in ovarian sex-cord stromal and germ cell tumors studied with antibodies to intermediate filament proteins. Am J Surg Pathol 9: 640–651

131. Moll I, Moll R (1985) Cells of extramammary Paget's disease express cytokeratins different from those of epidermal cells. J Invest Dermatol 84: 3–8

132. Moll R, Franke WW, Schiller DL, Geiger B, Krepler R (1982) The catalog of human cytokeratins: Patterns of expression in normal epithelia, tumors and cultured cells. Cell 31: 11–24

133. Moll R, Franke WW, Volc-Platzer B, Krepler R (1982) Different keratin polypeptides in epidermis and other epithelia of human skin: A specific cytokeratin of molecular weight 46,000 in epithelial of the pilosebaceous tract and basal cell epithelioma. J Cell Biol 95: 285–295

134. Moll R, Levy R, Czernobilsky B, Hohlweg-Majert P, Dallenbach-Hellweg G, Franke WW (1983) Cytokeratins of normal epithelia and some neoplasms of the female genital tract. Lab Invest 49: 599–610

135. Moll R, Lowe A, Laufer J, Franke WW (1992) Cytokeratin 20 in human carcinoma. Am J Pathol 140: 1–2

136. Moll R, Pitz S, Levy R, Weikel W, Franke WW, Czernobilsky B (1991) Complexity of expression of intermediate filament proteins, including glial filament protein, in endometrial and ovarian adenocarcinomas. Hum Pathol 22: 989–1001

137. Moll R, Schiller DL, Franke WW (1990) Identification of protein IT of the intestinal cytoskeleton as a novel type I cytokeratin with unusual properties and expression patterns. J Cell Biol 111: 567–580

138. Monsonego J, Magdelenat H, Catalan F, Coscas Y, Zerat L, Sastre X (1991) Estrogen and progesterone receptors in cervical human papillomavirus related lesions. Int J Cancer 48: 533–539

139. Morris WP, Griffin NR, Wells M (1989) Patterns of reactivity with the monoclonal antibodies HMFG1 and HMFG2 in normal endometrium, endometrial hyperplasia and adenocarcinoma. Histopathology 15: 179–186

140. Mosny DS, Herholz J, Degen W, Bender HG (1989) Immunohistochemical investigations of steroid receptors in normal and neoplastic squamous epithelium of the uterine cervix. Gynecol Oncol 35: 373–377

141. Mutch DG, Soper JT, Budwit-Novotny DA, et al (1987) Endometrial adenocarcinoma estrogen receptor content: Association of clinicopathologic features with immunohistochemical analysis compared with standard biochemical methods. Am J Obstet Gynecol 157: 924–931

142. Nagle RB, Clark VA, McDaniel KM, Davis JR (1983) Immunohistochemical demonstration of keratins in human ovarian neoplasms. A comparative method. J Histochem Cytochem 31: 1010–1014

143. Nagle RB, Lucas DO, McDaniel KM, Clark VA, Schmalzel GM (1985) New evidence linking mammary and extramammary Paget cells to a commoncell phenotype. Am J Clin Pathol 83: 431–438

144. Navarro D, Cabrera JJ, Falcon O, et al (1989) Monoclonal antibody characterization of progesterone receptors, estrogen receptors and the stress-responsive protein of 27 kDa (SRP27) in human utrine leiomyoma. J Steroid Biochem 34: 491–498

145. Navarro D, Cabrera JJ, Leon L, et al (1992) Endometrial stromal sarcoma expression of estrogen receptors, progesterone receptors and estrogen-induced srp27 (24K) suggests hormone responsiveness. J Steroid Biochem Mol Biol 41: 589–596

146. Neunteufel W, Breitenecker G (1989) Tissue expression of CA 125 in benign and malignant lesions of ovary and fallopian tube: A comparison with CA 19-9 and CEA. Gynecol Oncol 32: 297–302

147. Neunteufel W, Breitenecker G (1989) CA 19-9, CA 125 and CEA in the endometrial mucosa during the menstrual cycle, in atypical hyperplasia and endometrial carcinoma. Cancer Lett 48: 77–83

148. Nonogaki H, Fujii S, Konishi I, et al (1990) Estrogen receptor localization in normal and neoplastic epithelium of the uterine cervix. Cancer 66: 2620–2627

149. Norton AJ, Thomas JA, Isaacson PG (1987) Cytokeratin-specific antibodies are reactive with tumours of smooth muscle derivation. An immunohistochemical and biochemical study using antibodies to intermediate filament cytoskeletal proteins. Histopathology 11: 487–499

150. Notohara K, Hsueh CL, Awai M (1990) Glial fibrillary acidic protein immunoreactivity of chondrocytes in immature and mature teratomas. Acta Pathol Jpn 40: 335–342

151. Nozawa S, Yajima M, Sasaki H, et al (1991) A new CA125-like antigen (CA602) recognized by two monoclonal antibodies against a newly established ovarian clear cell carcinoma cell line (RMG-II). Jpn J Cancer Res 82: 854–861

152. Okamoto A, Sameshima Y, Yamada Y, et al (1991) Allelic loss on chromosome 17p and p53 mutations in human endometrial carcinoma of the uterus. Cancer Res 51: 5632–5635

153. Ordoñez NG, Freedman RS, Herlyn M (1987) Lewis and related tumor-associated determinants on ovarian carcinoma. Gynecol Oncol 26: 1–10

154. Pertschuk LP, Beddoe AM, Gorelic LS, Shain SA (1986) Immunocytochemical assay of estrogen receptors in endometrial carcinoma with monoclonal antibodies. Comparison with biochemical assay. Cancer 57: 1000–1004

155. Poels LG, Peters D, van Megen Y, et al (1986) Monoclonal antibody against human ovarian tumor-associated antigens. J Natl Cancer Inst 76: 781–791

156. Puts JJG, Moesker O, Aldeweireldt J, Vooijs GP, Ramaekers F (1987) Application of antibodies to intermediate filament proteins in simple and complex tumors of the female genital tract. Int J Gynecol Pathol 6: 257–274

157. Puts JJG, Moesker O, Kenemans P, Vooijs GP, Ramaekers F (1985) Expression of cytokeratins in early neoplastic epithelial lesions of the uterine cervix. Int J Gynecol Pathol 4: 300–313

158. Quinn MA, Rome RM, Cauchi M, Fortune DW (1988) Steroid receptors and ovarian tumors: Variation within primary tumors and between primary tumors and metastases. Gynecol Oncol 31: 424–429

159. Raju GC (1988) Expression of the cytokeratin marker CAM 5.2 in cervical neoplasia. Histopathology 12: 437–443

160. Ramaekers F, Puts J, Kenemans P, Vooijs GP (1985) Use of intermediate filament antibodies in the differential diagnosis of gynecological neoplasia. Eur J Obstet Gynecol Reprod Biol 19: 347–353

161. Ramaekers F, van Niekerk C, Poels L, et al (1990) Use of monoclonal antibodies to keratin 7 in the differential diagnosis of adenocarcinomas. Am J Pathol 136: 641–655

162. Ramaekers F, Verheijen R, Moesker O, Kant A, Vooijs GP, Herman CY (1983) Mesodermal mixed tumors. Diagnosis by analysis of intermediate filament proteins. Am J Surg Pathol 7: 381–385

163. Ravn V, Jensen H, Hilgers J (1989) Human milk-fat globule membrane antigens (Mam-3 group) in normal cycling endometrium and endometrial carcinomas–an immunohistochemical study. A preliminary report. APMIS 97: 452–458

164. Regauer S, Franke WW, Virtanen S (1985) Intermediate filament cytoskeleton of amnion epithelium and cultured amnion epithelial cells. Expression of epidermal cytokeratins in cells of a simple epithelium. J Cell Biol 100: 997–1009

165. Runowicz CD, Nuchtern LM, Braunstein JD, Jones JG (1990) Heterogeneity in hormone receptor status in primary and metastatic endometrial cancer. Gynecol Oncol 38: 437–441

166. Sasagawa M, Watanabe S, Ohmomo Y, Honma S, Kanazawa K, Takeuchi S (1986) Reactivity of two monoclonal antibodies (Troma 1 and CAM 5.2) on human tissue sections: Analysis of their usefulness as a histological trophoblast marker in normal pregnancy and trophoblastic disease. Int J Gynecol Pathol 5: 345–356

167. Scambia G, Panici PB, Baiocchi G, et al (1990) Steroid hormone receptors in carcinoma of the cervix: Lack of response to an antiestrogen. Gynecol Oncol 37: 323–326

168. Schruch W, Skalli O, Seemayer TA, Gabbiani G (1987) Intermediate filament proteins and actin isoforms as markers for soft tissue tumor differentiation and origin. I. Smooth muscle tumors. Am J Pathol 128: 91–103

169. Setzu A, Puligheddu P, Marcello C, et al (1987) Immunoperoxidase localization of HSV2 antigens in cervical dysplasia and carcinoma. Eur J Gynaecol Oncol 8: 616–618

170. Shi SR, Key ME, Kalra KL (1991) Antigen retrieval in formalin-fixed, paraffin-embedded tissues: An enhancement method for immunohistochemical staining based on microwave oven heating of tissue sections. J Histochem Cytochem 39: 741–748

171. Shiozawa T, Tsukahara Y, Nakayama J, Ishii K, Katsuyama

T (1991) Immunohistochemical localization of blood group substances in normal and neoplastic endometrial tissues— with special reference to type 1 core chain expression. Gynecol Obstet Invest 32: 185–188

172. Shishi J, Ghazizadeh M, Oguro T, Aihara K, Araki T (1986) Immunohistochemical localization of CA 125 antigen in formalin-fixed paraffin sections of ovarian tumors with the use of Pronase. Am J Clin Pathol 85: 595–598

173. Silcocks PB, Herbert A, Wright DH (1986) Evaluation of PAS-diastase and carcinoembryonic antigen staining in the differential diagnosis of malignant mesothelioma and papillary serous carcinoma of the ovary. J Pathol 149: 133–141

174. Skalli O, Gabbiani G (1990) Expression, organization, and involvement of intermediate filaments in disease processes. In: DeLellis RA (ed) Advances in Immunohistochemistry. Paris, Masson Publishing, pp 89–109

175. Slamon DJ, Godolphin W, Jones LA, et al (1989) Studies of the HER-2/neu proto-oncogene in human breast and ovarian cancer. Science 244: 707–712

176. Slotman BJ, Nauta JJ, Rao BR (1990) Survival of patients with ovarian cancer. Apart from stage and grade, tumor progesterone receptor content is a prognostic indicator. Cancer 66: 740–744

177. Smedts F, Ramaekers F, Robben H, et al (1992) Changing patterns of keratin expression during progression of cervical intraepithelial neoplasia. Am J Pathol 140: 601–612

178. Smedts F, Ramaekers F, Troyanovsky S, et al (1992) Keratin expression in cervical cancer. Am J Pathol 141: 497–511

179. Smedts F, Ramaekers F, Troyanovsky S, et al (1992) Basal-cell keratins in cervical reserve cells and a comparison to their expression in cervical intraepithelial neoplasia. Am J Pathol 140: 601–612

180. Soisson AP, Berchuck A, Lessey BA, et al (1989) Immunohistochemical expression of TAG-72 in normal and malignant endometrium: Correlation of antigen expression with estrogen receptor and progesterone receptor levels. Am J Obstet Gynecol 161: 1258–1263

181. Soper JT, Christensen CW (1986) Steroid receptors and endometrial cancer. Clin Obstet Gynaecol 13: 825–842

182. Steeper TA, Wick MR (1986) Minimal deviation adenocarcinoma of the uterine cervix ("adenoma malignum"). An immunohistochemical comparison with microglandular endocervical hyperplasia and conventional endocervical adenocarcinoma. Cancer 58: 1131–1138

183. Sterrett GF, Alessandri LM, Pixley E, Kulski JK (1987) Assessment of precancerous lesions of the uterine cervix for evidence of human papillomavirus infection: A histological and immunohistochemical study. Pathology 19: 84–90

184. Sutton GP, Senior MB, Strauss JF, Mikuta JJ (1986) Estrogen and progesterone receptors in epithelial ovarian malignancies. Gynecol Oncol 23: 176–182

185. Sweeney EC, Barry-Walsh C, Robinson A (1983) Sertoli-Leydig cell tumor of the ovary with heterologous elements and carcinoid: An immunohistochemical and ultrastructural study. Ultrastruct Pathol 5: 185–194

186. Szpak CA, Soper JT, Thor A, Schlom J, Johnston WW (1989) Detection of adenocarcinoma in peritoneal washings by staining with monoclonal antibody B72.3. Acta Cytol 33: 205–214

187. Tay SK, Jenkins D (1989) Langerhans cell population in

early invasive squamous cell carcinoma of the uterine cervix. Aust NZ J Obstet Gynaecol 29: 38–40

188. Tay SK, Jenkins D, Singer A (1987) Natural killer cells in cervical intraepithelial neoplasia and human pappilomavirus infection. Br J Obstet Gynaecol 94: 901–906

189. Thomas P, Battifora H, Manderino GL, Patrick J (1987) A monoclonal antibody against neuron-specific enolase. Immunohistochemical comparison with a polyclonal antiserum. Am J Clin Pathol 88: 146–152

190. Thor A, Ohuchi N, Szpak CA, Johnston WW, Schlom J (1986) Distribution of oncofetal antigen tumor-associated glycoprotein-72 defined by monoclonal antibody B72.3. Cancer Res 46: 3118–3124

191. Thor A, Viglione MJ, Muraro R, Ohuchi N, Schlom J, Gorstein F (1987) Monoclonal antibody B72.3 reactivity with human endometrium: A study of normal and malignant tissues. Int J Gynecol Pathol 6: 235–247

192. Tippers D (1988) Smooth m uscle cells can express cytokeratins of "simple" epithelium. Am J Pathol 132: 223–232

193. Tohya T, Iwamasa T, Maeyama M (1986) Biochemical and immunohistochemical studies on carcinoembryonic antigen of ovarian mucinous and serous tumors. Gynecol Oncol 23: 291–303

194. Tosi P, Sforza V, Santopietro R (1989) Estrogen receptor content, immunohistochemically determined by monoclonal antibodies, in endometrial stromal sarcoma. Obstet Gynecol 73: 75–78

195. Tsao SW, Mok CH, Oike K, et al (1991) Involvement of p53 gene in the allelic deletion of chromosome 17p in human ovarian tumors. Anticancer Res 11: 1975–1982

196. Tsukada T, Tippens D, Gordon D, Ross R, Gown AM (1987) HHF35, a muscle-actin-specific monoclonal antibody. I. Immunocytochemical and biochemical characterization. Am J Pathol 126: 51–60

197. Tsukazaki K, Sakayori M, Arai H, Yamaoka K, Kurihara S, Nozawa S (1991) Abnormal expression of blood group-related antigens in uterine endometrial cancers. Jpn J Cancer Res 82: 934–941

198. Ueda G, Yamasaki M (1992) Neuroendocrine carcinoma of the uterus. Curr Top Pathol 85: 309–335

199. van Muijen G, Ruiter DY, Warnaar SO (1987) Coexpression of intermediate filament polypeptides in human fetal and adult tissues. Lab Invest 57: 359–369

200. van Niekerk CC, Ramaekers F, Hanselaar AG, Aldeweireldt J, Poels LG (1993) Changes in expression of differentiation markers between normal ovarian cells and derived tumors. Am J Pathol 142: 157–177

201. Veggian R, Fasolato S, Menard S, et al (1989) Immunohistochemical reactivity of a monoclonal antibody prepared against human ovarian carcinoma on normal and pathological female genital tissues. Tumori 75: 510–513

202. Vengerov YY, Gudima SO, Voronov AV, Votrin II (1988) Immunochemical studies of human placental alkaline phosphatase in normal and neoplastic tissues. Adv Enzyme Regul 27: 345–354

203. Viale G, Gambacorta M, Dell'Orto P, Coggi G (1988) Coexpression of cytokeratins and vimentin in common epithelial tumours of the ovary: An immunocytochemical study of eighty-three cases. Virch Arch A (Pathol Anat) 413: 91–101

204. Vogel HP, Mendelsohn G (1987) Laminin immunostaining in hyperplastic, dysplastic, and neoplastic lesions of the endometrium and uterine cervix. Obstet Gynecol 69: 794–799

205. Ward BG, Lowe DG, Shepherd JH (1987) Patterns of expression of a tumor associated antigen, defined by the monoclonal antibody HMFG2, in human epithelial ovarian carcinoma. Comparison with expression of the HMFG1, AUA1 and F36/22 antigens. Cancer 60: 787–793

206. Weiner SA, Alberts DS, Surwit EA, Davis J, Grosso D (1987) Tamoxifen therapy in recurrent epithelial ovarian carcinoma. Gynecol Oncol 27: 208–213

207. Whitaker JR, Samy AMJ, Sunter JP, Sinha DP, Monaghan JH (1989) Cytokeratin expression in cervical epithelium: An immunohistochemical study of normal, wart virus-infected and neoplastic tissue. Histopathology 14: 151–160

208. Wolber RA, Dupuis BA, Wick MR (1991) Expression of c-erbB-2 oncoprotein in mammary and extramammary Paget's disease. Am J Clin Pathol 96: 243–247

209. Yamashita K, Nakamura T, Shimizu T, Ohno H (1986) Monoclonal antibodies to human choriocarcinoma. Am J Reprod Immunol Microbiol 11: 130–134

210. Yang GC, Rotterdam H (1991) Mixed (composite) glandular-endocrine cell carcinoma of the stomach. Report of a case and review of literature. Am J Surg Pathol 15: 592–598

211. Yavner DL, Dwyer IM, Hancock WW, Ehrmann RL (1990) Basement membrane of cervical adenocarcinoma: An immunoperoxidase study of laminin and type IV collagen. Obstet Gynecol 76: 1014–1019

212. Yokoyama S, Hayashida Y, Nagahama J, Nakayama I, Kashima K, Ogata J (1992) Primary and metaplastic choriocarcinoma of the bladder. A report of two cases. Acta Cytol 36: 176–182

213. Young RH, Prat J, Scully RE (1982) Ovarian Sertoli-Leydig cell tumors with heterologous elements. I Gastrointestinal epithelium and carcinoid: A clinicopathologic analysis of thirty-six cases. Cancer 50: 2448–2456

214. Zaino RJ, Clarke CL, Mortel R, Satyaswaroop PG (1988) Heterogeneity of progesterone receptor distribution in human endometrial adenocarcinoma. Cancer Res 48: 1889–1895

215. Zirker TA, Silva EG, Morris M, Ordoñez NG (1989) Immunohistochemical differentiation of clear-cell carcinoma of the female genital tract and endodermal sinus tumor with the use of alpha-fetoprotein and Leu-M1. Am J Clin Pathol 91: 511–514

27

Flow Cytometry

Debra A. Bell, M.D.

Flow cytometry is a technique that optoelectronically measures the relative intensities of fluorescence of various dyes bound to many individual cells or particles in a rapid period of time. This technique may be used to measure DNA content, analyze cell cycle events, or measure the p.esence of various antigens such as hematopoietic cell surface markers.[11,17,20] Most work using flow cytometry in investigations of the female genital tract have focused on the diagnostic or prognostic significance of DNA ploidy analysis or cell cycle analysis in tumors, particularly epithelial carcinomas of the ovary[11] and uterine gestational trophoblastic disease.[68] The first part of this chapter discusses technical issues of DNA analysis and the second part reviews the clinically or diagnostically important applications of DNA ploidy and cell cycle analysis in neoplasms of the female genital tract.

Flow Cytometric DNA Analysis

The steps involved in performing DNA analysis flow cytometrically are summarized in Table 27.1[11,17,20,64]; each step is discussed in detail in this section.

Tissue Acquisition

Cells or nuclei may be obtained either from fresh or paraffin-embedded specimens.[41] Fresh specimens are directly disaggregated whereas paraffin-embedded specimens are disaggregated enzymatically after deparaffinization and rehydration.[39,40] The advantages and disadvantages of fresh as compared with fixed specimens are summarized in Table 27.2.[20,39]

Tissue Disaggregation

Fresh solid tumors may be disaggregated by mechanical, detergent, or enzymatic methods. A common mechanical method involves syringing the specimen across a small-caliber needle.[64] The enzymatic methods usually involve treatment of the tissue with pepsin, trypsin, or collagenase and the detergent methods use reagents such as Triton-X-100 or Nonidet P-40.[75] These methods yield either individual intact cells or individual nuclei. Unfortunately, the optimal method of disaggregation of fresh material is highly tissue dependent and must be individualized based on specimen type.

Formalin-fixed paraffin embedded tissue is processed by first cutting 50-μm sections that are then deparaffinized

Table 27.1. Summary of flow cytometric DNA analysis

1. Tissue acquired
2. Disaggregation of tumor into individual cells or particles
3. Staining with fluorescent antibody to DNA
4. Detection of fluorescence of each particle
5. Data for each particle recorded
6. Generation of data
7. Data analysis

in xylene, rehydrated in graded alcohols, and enzymatically digested with pepsin or trypsin.[39,40] This process results in free nuclei devoid of cytoplasm.

Staining Methods

After disaggregation, the cells or nuclei are stained with a fluorescent dye that binds stoichiometrically or proportionally with DNA. Several types of dyes are available; the most commonly used ones are propidium iodide (PI), ethidium bromide (EB), and diamidinophenylindole (DAPI).[17,64,75] PI and EB bind to RNA, so the specimens stained with these dyes must be pretreated with ribonuclease.

Flow Cytometer Function

In the flow cytometer, single cells or nuclei pass through a beam of light (usually an argon laser using a 488-nm line) suspended in single file in a sheath of fluid. The cells or nuclei pass through the beam that excites the fluorescent

Table 27.2. Comparison of fresh and deparaffinized tissue

Fresh tissue
Advantages:
1. External standards with known ploidy may be used to determine the DNA index of the tumor population
2. Less debris is present, resulting in better histogram resolution
3. Whole cells may be analyzed, allowing identification of cytoplasmic and plasma membrane antigens in addition to DNA content analysis
Disadvantages:
1. Tissue must be obtained prospectively
2. Histological localization of specific regions of interest is not possible
Deparaffinized tissue
Advantages:
1. May be analyzed retrospectively
2. Histologic examination of tissue sections allows specific sampling of small lesions by trimming the paraffin block
Disadvantages:
1. External ploidy standards cannot be used due to a variable reduction in DNA fluorescence secondary to fixation; normal inflammatory and stromal cells in the block are used as the diploid "normal" population
2. Cutting sections from the paraffin block results in debris, which decreases the histogram resolution
3. Only bare nuclei are obtained

molecules bound to the particle. Detectors measure the relative intensity of this fluorescence as well as other data, such as the amount of light transmitted in a forward direction (forward angle scatter, which is proportional to cell size) and that reflected at an angle (90°C angle scatter or side scatter, which is related to the granularity of the particle).[17,20] These data are recorded for each cell in a computer.

Data Presentation

DNA content data usually are presented as a DNA histogram or frequency distribution of the relative DNA fluorescence intensities of the particles. The fluorescence intensity of each particle is assigned a relative value compared with the intensities of the other particles and is expressed as arbitrary units or channel numbers. The DNA histogram is a graphic representation of the number of cells or nuclei with each fluorescent intensity on the y-axis and the relative fluorescent intensities or channel numbers on the x-axis (Fig. 27.1). In general, 10,000 cells or nuclei are analyzed per specimen.

Data Analysis

ANALYSIS OF PLOIDY

The normal cell cycle is divided into three phases, *G0/G1*, in which the cells have a diploid or 2N quantity of DNA, *S*, in which cycling cells are synthesizing DNA and have a quantity of DNA between 2N and 4N in amount, and *G2/M*, in which the cells are about to divide and have double the normal quantity (4N) of DNA.[64] In normal

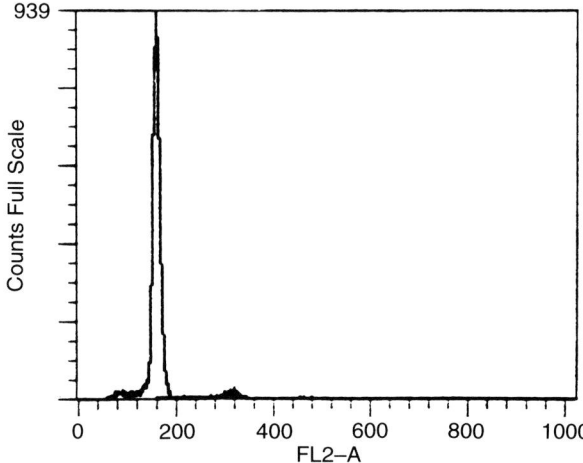

Fig. 27.1. DNA diploid histogram. Note the large G0/G1 peak at channel 160 and a smaller G2M peak with twice the relative fluorescence of the G0/G1 peak at channel 320 (y-axis: number of nuclei; x-axis relative fluorescence intensity in channel numbers, which are arbitrary units.)

tissue or a DNA diploid tumor, the great majority of cells are in G0 or G1 and have a diploid DNA content. This is reflected in the DNA histogram, which shows a single large peak of cells, the G0/G1 peak, with a 2N DNA content. In most specimens, a smaller peak of cells in G2 and M is present at a channel number two times that of the G0/G1 peak (4N). Cells in S-phase are present in the region between the large G0/G1 and smaller G2M peaks. As shown in Figure 27.1, if the G0/G1 peak is located at channel 160, the G2M peak will be located at approximately channel 320.

In a specimen that contains abnormal populations (or stem lines) with a DNA content different from that of normal cells, one or more additional peaks are present, representing the cells in the abnormal population in G0 or G1 (Figs. 27.2, 27.3). Often these abnormal populations are cycling and have G2M peaks with the twice the fluorescence intensity (twice the channel number) of the abnormal G0/G1 peak. The amount the abnormal stem line differs from a diploid or 2N quantity of DNA is expressed as the *DNA index*, which is defined as the mean or modal channel number of the G0/G1 peak of the abnormal population divided by the mean or modal channel number of the diploid G0/G1 peak.[46] Thus, as shown in Figure 27.2, if the abnormal G0/G1 peak is located at channel 310 and the diploid G0/G1 peak is at channel 200, the DNA index of the abnormal population is 1.55. Specimens with a diploid DNA content have a DNA index of 1.0 (Fig. 27.1).

The quality of the histogram is determined by the ability to resolve abnormal peaks near the normal G0/G1 peak (peridiploid aneuploid peaks) within it. This is dependent on the width of the curve—the wider the peak, the more likely it will obscure a peak nearby. The width or spread of the curve is judged by the co-efficient of variation, or CV,

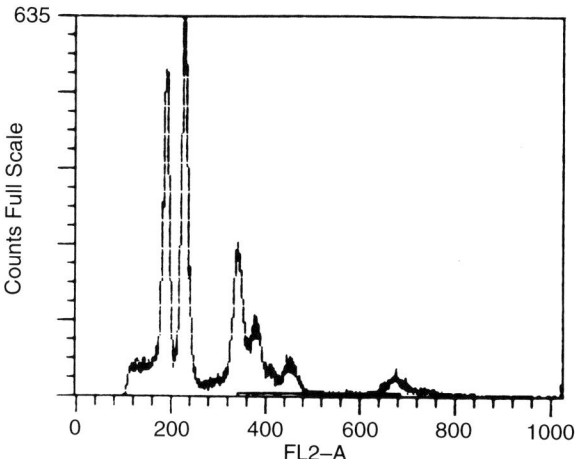

FIG. 27.3. DNA multiploid histogram. Several additional discrete aneuploid peaks are present with corresponding G2M populations.

or the diploid of G0/G1 peak, which is defined as the mean channel number of the G0/G1 peak divided by its standard deviation expressed as a percent. CVs of 2–3% are reported from most laboratories for specimens of lymphocytes, which are often used to calibrate the flow cytometer or as controls; most laboratories report CVs in the range of 4–6% for tumor cell populations. CVs of larger than 8% or 10% generally are considered to be unacceptably large, in that peridiploid aneuploid peaks may be easily obscured in such a wide diploid peak.[64]

CLASSIFICATION OF DNA HISTOGRAMS

DNA histograms generally are classified as DNA diploid or DNA aneuploid. *Diploid* and *aneuploid* are qualified by the prefix DNA to distinguish flow cytometric from cytogenetically determined ploidy.[46] The most conservative definition of DNA aneuploidy is the presence of one or more peaks distinct from the normal G0/G1 peak and separated from the normal G0/G1 peak by 10% or more of its mean DNA content[39,40] (Fig. 27.2). This "10%" criterion is necessary because it has been shown that the measurement of the DNA content of some diploid normal cells, such as lymphocytes, may vary up to ±10% of the mean DNA content of other normal diploid cells. It has been speculated that this difference is due to chromatin packing, variable dye uptake, or differences in processing.[46,51,89] Regardless of the cause, this difference may be minimized by using normal epithelial cells similar to the tumor type being analyzed (such as normal endometrial cells when analyzing an endometrial carcinoma), rather than lymphocytes, as the diploid control.[51] Aneuploid tumors may contain more than one abnormal stem line (Fig. 27.3); these tumors are classified as *multiploid*. Although this definition of aneuploidy is the most commonly used, many other

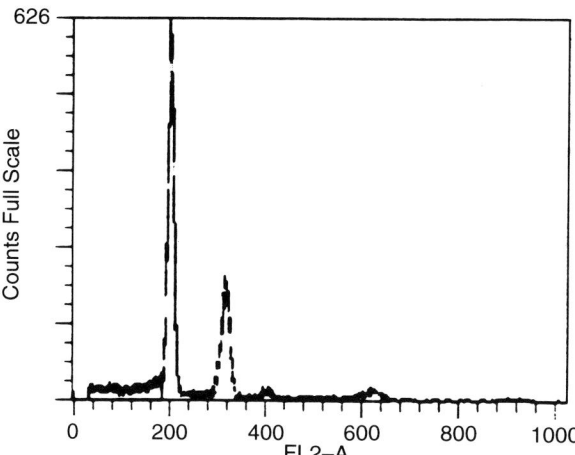

FIG. 27.2. DNA aneuploid histogram. An additional discrete large G0/G1 peak is present at channel 310 (DNA index, 1.55). Note the G2M of the diploid population at channel 400 and the G2M of the abnormal peak at channel 620.

criteria for aneuploidy have been proposed (Table 27.3). These additional criteria are not used in most laboratories because although they increase the detection of aneuploid populations, they also increase the number of falsely aneuploid specimens.

It should be emphasized that histograms with the CVs generally produced in most laboratories can detect only relatively large genetic abnormalities, equivalent to greater or equal than two to three chromosomes. For this reason, although single peak histograms are classified as DNA diploid, they are in reality "near diploid" and karyotypic analysis of these tumors may reveal deletion or addition of several chromosomes.

CELL CYCLE ANALYSIS

The percentage of cells or nuclei in each cell cycle compartment may be calculated by mathematically determining the area beneath the curve in each region of the histogram.[6] Two of the most widely used methods of determining the percentage of cells in S-phase approximate the area in the S region by fitting either a polynomial function[23] or a trapezoidal or broadened rectangle beneath the S portion of the curve.[6,7] The percentage of cells in each region is generally issued in list form by the computer with a notation as to the calculation method used such as:

Cell cycle statistics:

Phase	Percent
G0/G1:	95.0
S:	2.5
G2$^+$M:	2.5

In a cycling population of normal cells, more than 90% of the cells are found in the G0/G1 portion of the cell cycle. The main reason this information is of interest in the analysis of neoplasms is that the percent of cells in S and G2M may reflect the proliferation rate of the tumor and thus be a measure of its biological aggressiveness. The proliferation rate usually is expressed as the S-phase fraction (SPF) (percentage of cells in S phase) or the proliferative index, which is defined as the percentage of cells in S and G2M. The results of such calculations have been shown to be less

Table 27.3. Definitions of DNA aneuploidy

1. Presence of two or more discrete G0/G1 peaks
2. DNA index greater than 1.1[83] in fresh tissue when compared with an external diploid standard
3. A single broad G1 peak[74]
4. More than 20% of total number of cells in the region of the diploid G2M peak (4N) with a corresponding G2M peak in the 8N location (DNA tetraploid)[14]
5. Diploid tumors with a G2/M two times greater than SPF and more than 15% of total cell count (DNA tetraploid)[60]
6. "Peak" in the diploid G2/M region (4N) with another peak at 8N location[62,74]

reproducible than the presence of DNA aneuploidy and the DNA index.

Technical and Interpretation Problems

DNA PLOIDY ANALYSIS

A variety of technical and interpretation errors at each step of DNA analysis may result in inaccurate findings. During tissue disaggregation, many neoplasms, particularly those with dense, fibrous stroma, may result in too few cells for analysis (Fig. 27.4). When analyzing deparaffinized material, it is imperative to examine the microscopic slides to assure that a substantial amount of normal tissue is present to provide the normal internal diploid control; insufficient diploid tissue may result in falsely diploid samples. When fresh tissue is used, it is necessary to determine that the tissue in question is appropriately sampled. When tissue is disaggregated, partial digestion of RNA may result in artifactual small aneuploid peaks; however, these peaks are not associated with a G2M component and are not present on careful repeat evaluation. When the particles pass through the flow cytometer, cells or particles may clump together, giving false aneuploid peaks at 4N, 6N, and 8N (Fig. 27.5).

The nature of the tumor or tissue analyzed also may affect the accuracy of DNA analysis. It has been shown that considerable heterogeneity in DNA content is present in most neoplasms; approximately 20% of tumors of various types have been shown to contain differing DNA content if multiple samples from different sites or different blocks are obtained.[8,33,58,93] It is thus recommended that multiple samples (generally three or more) from a neoplasm be examined. Samples containing necrosis should be avoided or trimmed from the paraffin block, since such areas have been shown to result in false aneuploid peaks.[55] Formalin has been shown to be the optimal fixative for paraffin-

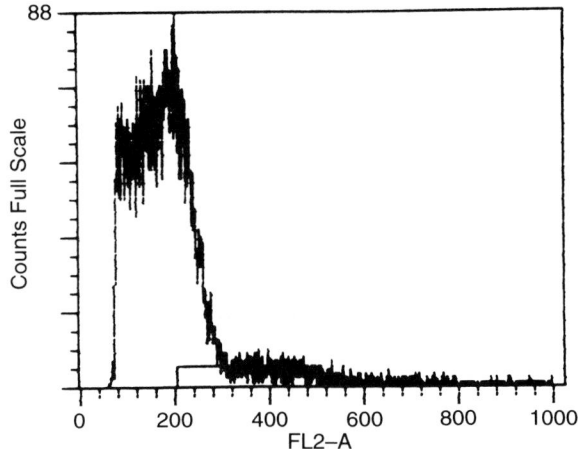

FIG. 27.4. Unsatisfactory histogram showing few cells and extensive debris.

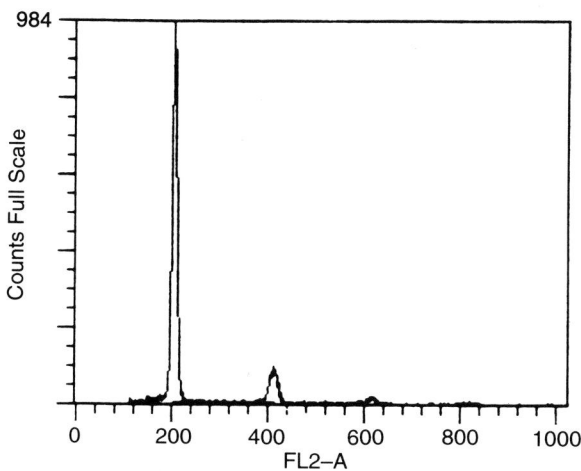

FIG. 27.5. DNA histogram from a normal lymphocyte control specimen. Artifactual peaks due to particle clumping at channels 200 (2N), 400 (4N), 600 (6N), and 800 (8N) are present.

confirm DNA aneuploidy as would comparison with the amount of tumor in the original sample. Analysis of another specimen from elsewhere in the neoplasm also might confirm the presence of an abnormal stem line with the same DNA index.

Finally, it has been suggested that an increase in the number of cells in the G2M region above a certain value (10, 15, or 20%) should be considered DNA aneuploid. The safest means to determine if a peak in this region (with a DNA index of 2.0) is definitively aneuploid is to identify a corresponding G2M with an 8N DNA content. In the absence of a G2M peak, a number of samples with this finding will be falsely considered DNA aneuploid. Thus, in most cases problems in histogram interpretation can be solved by (1) eliminating areas of necrosis or autolysis from samples and reanalyzing the specimen, (2) sampling other areas of the tumor, and (3) identification of a G2M component of the abnormal stem line.

embedded samples; specimens fixed in solutions containing heavy metals, such as Zenker's solution, Bouin's fixative, or Omnifix, produce specimens with broad CVs and abundant debris[34,39,44] that may, in our experience, cause false aneuploid peaks.

HISTOGRAM INTERPRETATION

Although interpretation of DNA histograms often is straightforward, substantial disagreement in classification has been documented among experts experienced in the field,[56] emphasizing the subjectivity of their interpretation. These factors and the absence of standardized criteria for histogram "diagnosis" lead to differences in laboratory results on individual specimens and most probably account in part for the variations in DNA ploidy results for the same types of tumors that have been reported in the literature. The most common problems that arise in histogram classification include the presence of a single wide peak, asymmetrical peaks, small peaks, and an increased number of cells in the G2M region. The approach to resolving these problems in our laboratory is as follows.

When a wide single peak is present the specimen is examined for excessive debris or tissue necrosis. If present, such areas are trimmed from the paraffin block and the specimen rerun. Asymmetrical single peaks with a "shoulder" or flattening of the right side of the peak may be confirmed as aneuploid if a more distinct peak is present on reanalysis of the specimen or if a corresponding G2M peak is present. If neither is apparent, these histograms are classified as suspicious for aneuploidy in our laboratory. Small peaks containing less than 5–10% of the cell population may be due to excessive debris, necrosis, or a small aneuploid population. The presence of a G2M peak would

CELL CYCLE ANALYSIS

Cell cycle analysis may be less reproducible than DNA ploidy analysis because of the many different software programs used to analyze the results. These programs use different cutoff points for delimiting the overlap between the G0/G1 area, S area, and G2M areas of the histogram, and they use different mathematical methods for approximating the area under the curve in each compartment. There are several additional causes of faulty S-phase determinations. The presence of excessive debris in a specimen may result in an inaccurate assessment of the true fraction of cells in S phase. Debris subtraction software programs that correct the S-phase calculation to eliminate the contribution from debris are now available and may alleviate this problem somewhat. Insufficient RNAse digestion may result in skewing of the G0/G1 peak, rendering it unsuitable for analysis by the mathematical models. Clumping of cells may artifactually increase the percentage of cells in G2M[36,37] (Fig. 27.5). Cell clumping can be detected by pulse processing circuitry that allows resolution of clumps of G0/G1 cells from the larger cells in G2M.[85]

Characteristics of the tissue also may affect the accuracy of S-phase calculations. Since it is not possible to separate inflammatory cells from tumor cells in a single parameter histogram, measurements of S-phase fraction may be elevated because of the contributions of cycling inflammatory cells. Inflammatory cell and tumor cell S phases may be distinguished in fresh tissue by simultaneous multiparameter analysis of cytokeratin and DNA staining using fluorescent molecules of different wavelengths.[28,49] Overlap of diploid and aneuploid populations in a sample also renders S-phase analysis more difficult and less reproducible. Although software that mathematically estimates the contribution of each population is now available, the accuracy of such determinations is at present poorly defined.

Controls and Quality Assurance

Uniform quality assurance procedures in laboratories performing DNA flow cytometry theoretically would improve consistency of results from cell to cell in the same run and allow comparisons of data between runs in the same laboratory and between laboratories; unfortunately, such standards have not been established. Quality assurance methods performed daily in most laboratories include calibration of instrument alignment, fluorescence intensity, and the signal processing circuitry for fluorescence linearity.[48]

Controls are widely used in each analysis session to assess the quality of sample processing. Commonly used controls include human lymphocytes in fresh specimens and normal lymph node in deparaffinized tissue. These controls are stained and processed in parallel with the samples in each run, to assess reagent stability, preparation procedures and instrument optimization.[34,48]

Several studies of interlaboratory variability in DNA flow cytometry have demonstrated that determination of aneuploidy and DNA index are in general quite reproducible.[19,47,94] Determinations of the percentage of aneuploid cells or hyperdiploid fraction[94] or the S-phase fraction,[59] however, are much less reproducible, indicating that comparisons of these parameters between laboratories are not feasible at the present time, and that each laboratory must establish its own standards for elevation of SPF or proliferative index.[34]

Applications in Gynecological Pathology

The most extensive work on the clinical usefulness of DNA flow cytometry in gynecological pathology has been in the relationship of DNA ploidy and S-phase fraction to the prognosis of epithelial carcinomas of the ovary and in the differential diagnosis and prognosis of possible molar gestations.

Ovarian Surface Epithelial Tumors

Carcinomas

Although advances in therapy have resulted in prolonged disease-free survivals in women with ovarian carcinoma, these intensive treatments are associated with substantial side effects and most women with advanced stage disease eventually die of their tumor despite therapy.[9] These factors have resulted in a search for features that would permit greater prognostic accuracy and tailoring of treatment regimens to the biological behavior of the tumor in an individual patient. Numerous investigations of the prognostic significance of DNA content and cell cycle analysis

as possibly more objective and reproducible indicators of tumor behavior have been performed in the last decade. Numerous studies reporting the results of flow cytometric DNA analysis in ovarian carcinomas from several thousand patients have shown DNA aneuploidy in most (50–80%) tumors. These studies have generally examined the relation of DNA content to either survival or clinicopathological features previously shown to be of probable prognostic significance.

There is general agreement that the most important clinical prognostic factors in surface epithelial carcinoma are stage and extent of residual tumor after debulking surgery.[24] A number of studies have examined the relation of DNA ploidy and staging in detail.[*] Although several failed to show a relationship, most of the studies found a greater frequency of DNA aneuploidy in stage III or IV (from 50–80%) than stage I or II carcinomas (from 8–80%).[10,32,38,50,71] The few studies that analyzed the relation of SPF and stage all showed an increased percentage of cells in the SPF with increasing stage. The findings were not statistically significant in one study[10] and were of marginal statistical significance in another.[62] In the third study the statistical significance of the data was not reported,[59] and only advanced stage tumors were compared in the fourth study.[91] Most studies also have demonstrated a statistically significant association between DNA aneuploidy and bulky postoperative residual disease.[10,14,25,38,61,62,78] One study found an elevation of SPF with a large amount of residual tumor,[10] but another found no association between these factors.[62]

A number of studies have suggested that the histological type and degree of differentiation of surface epithelial carcinomas are important prognostic features[1,86]; however, others have been unable to confirm these findings. Although most studies have concluded that there is no clear relationship between DNA ploidy and histological type,[†] it is apparent that most serous and undifferentiated carcinomas are DNA aneuploid and the frequency of aneuploidy in the other cell types is highly variable. These latter results may reflect the substantial intra- and interobserver variation in histological subtyping that has been amply documented in the literature.[2-4,21,45] Only a small number of articles have included data on unusual types of surface epithelial carcinomas. Of the 23 cases of transitional cell carcinoma reported, 13 were DNA aneuploid, 6 were DNA tetraploid, and the remainder were DNA diploid.[35,72,77] Six of the nine malignant Brenner tumors were DNA aneuploid.[42,66,72,88] Twenty-six (71%) of the 36 cases of serous surface carcinoma were DNA aneuploid.[15,71,82] The small number of studies that have examined SPF and

---

*Refs. 10,14,15,16,32,38,50,53,60,62,63,74.
†Refs. 10,11,14,15,27,30,32,33,35,38,42,52,53,59,62,63,65,71,74, 90,92.

histological type have demonstrated a relatively low SPF among mucinous and endometrioid carcinomas[10,59,62,66] when compared with other histological types.

Many studies have examined the relation of DNA content to grade as determined by various methods. Most of these studies have shown an increased frequency of DNA aneuploidy and an elevated SPF with increasing grade as determined by various methods* when all surface epithelial carcinoma types were combined in the analysis. The two studies that examined this feature in serous carcinoma only did not find an association between ploidy and grade.[63,92] Several studies have analyzed the relation of DNA ploidy to the interval to first recurrence with conflicting results. Two studies[10,38] were unable to document a difference in length of disease-free survival between patients with DNA aneuploid and DNA diploid tumors, whereas other groups[61,74,78] found a significantly longer time to first recurrence in patients with diploid rather than aneuploid tumors. Barnabei and co-workers[10] also noted that an SPF of less than 18% was associated with a longer disease-free survival than a larger SPF. Other studies did not examine this feature.

The major emphasis of most of the studies in this area has been the relation of DNA analysis and overall survival. Many large studies have noted a statistically significant shorter median survival time or a smaller percentage of survivors among patients with DNA aneuploid tumors rather than DNA diploid ones in tumors of all stages, advanced stage and early stage.† In a few studies the differences in survival were most marked during the first several years of follow-up.[14,38] A few studies failed to demonstrate a difference in prognosis between ploidy groups in tumors of all epithelial types[25,81] or in serous carcinomas only.[63] Most studies that examined the association between SPF and survival found a shorter median survival time or smaller percentage of survivors among those patients whose tumors had a high rather than low SPF of marginal statistical significance.[10,60,62,65,66,81,91]

Of the numerous studies that examined the independent prognostic significance of DNA ploidy by multivariate analysis,‡ more than half[14,29,60,65,79] found that DNA ploidy was a major, independent prognostic factor in surface epithelial ovarian carcinomas. Some groups did not document this association[5,10,25,62]; however, Klemi and co-workers[62] noted that a DNA index of greater than or less than 1.3 was independently associated with prognosis. The divergent results in the series by Erba and co-workers[25,26] may be secondary to the inclusion of cases in which the DNA content was determined on ascites only. No obvious explanation for the conflicting results of the other

groups[5,10] is apparent. Two of the three studies that included SPF in the multivariate analysis found that it was an independent prognostic indicator.[10,62] The divergent results of the third study may be because of the inclusion of SPF data on ascites samples as previously noted.[25]

Two groups have examined the relation of DNA content and response to therapy. Brescia and co-workers[15] found that DNA ploidy may identify patients with negative second-look laparotomies who are at greater risk of recurrence. Friedlander and colleagues[29] also noted a higher "true response rate" at second-look laparotomy among patients with DNA diploid tumors. Friedlander et al.[29] also have shown that flow cytometry may identify a group of patients with advanced stage diploid carcinomas that have a good prognosis regardless of the type of treatment in whom the initial use of relatively nontoxic therapy may be considered. These findings also strongly support randomization of patients according to DNA content in prospective clinical trials.[29]

It has been suggested that determination of the DNA index may aid in distinguishing independent primary neoplasms from metastases in simultaneous carcinomas of the endometrium and ovary.[75a]

BORDERLINE TUMORS

Much less data is available on the DNA content of borderline tumors and its biological significance. Results of DNA analysis have been reported from more than 100 stage I–III serous borderline tumors. Although the great majority of tumors were DNA diploid,[12,31,42,50,63,66,92] the rate of DNA aneuploidy varied with the tissue source; none of the cases derived from fresh tissue were DNA aneuploid,[50,66,71] but 15–33% were DNA aneuploid in tissue obtained from paraffin-embedded material.[11,57,63,67] Several studies have suggested that DNA aneuploidy is associated with an adverse clinical outcome,[31,57] whereas others have not demonstrated such a striking difference.[11,63] There is a suggestion that DNA aneuploidy is associated with advanced stage disease.[11,31] Therefore, DNA content analysis has not been definitively established as a prognostic factor independent of stage. Interestingly, two patients with DNA aneuploid ovarian tumors on further histopathological investigation were found to have invasive peritoneal implants.[31]

The DNA content of a smaller number of mucinous borderline tumors has been reported; most studies reported DNA diploid results,[31,42,50,66] and all of these patients in whom follow-up data were available were living without tumor.[31,66] One study that examined the DNA content of a group of patients with fatal tumors and compared the findings with matched controls reported a rate of DNA aneuploidy of 47% in ovarian mucinous borderline tumors and also found a strong relation of DNA aneuploidy

---

*Refs. 10,14,15,25,32,50,59,62,71,79,81.

†Refs. 5,10,14,15,29,35,38,60–62,74,76,78,84,91.

‡Refs. 5,14,25,29,30,60,62,63,78,79,80.

with an adverse outcome.[57] DNA analysis has been reported from small numbers of borderline endometrioid and borderline Brenner tumors; all were stage I and DNA diploid.[31,88] These data indicate that the prognostic significance of DNA aneuploidy in borderline tumors has yet to be definitively established.

Benign Tumors

A few articles have analyzed the DNA content and SPF of benign tumors of the ovary. Sixty-five benign serous cystadenomas or cystadenofibromas have been analyzed[42,50,63]; four of them were DNA aneuploid.[63,71] Follow-up data were given on three aneuploid cases; one woman died without tumor at autopsy 9 years postoperatively, and two were living without evidence of tumor for 10 months and 14 years, respectively.[63] Three simple cysts,[42] 15 mucinous cystadenomas,[42,50,71] and 22 benign Brenner tumors[50,72,88] reported were all DNA diploid. Thus, although DNA aneuploidy may occur in benign tumors, it is a rare finding.

Gestational Trophoblastic Disease

As discussed in detail later in this text (see Chapter 24, Gestational Trophoblastic Disease and Related Lesions), gestations showing villous swelling are classified as complete hydatidiform mole, partial hydatidiform mole, and hydropic abortus.[54,71] It is important to distinguish between these entities because of their differing cytogenetic and clinicopathological features. To summarize briefly, complete hydatidiform moles are characterized microscopically by generalized villous swelling, villous cistern formation, and diffuse trophoblastic hyperplasia. They are generally diploid and the chromosomal content is paternally derived. Persistent trophoblastic disease develops in approximately 20% of patients. Partial hydatidiform moles are characterized microscopically by focal villous swelling (two populations of villi, one normal and one swollen), and focal trophoblastic hyperplasia. Cytogenetically, they usually are triploid, with the extra haploid set of chromosomes being paternally derived. Persistent trophoblastic disease is noted in these patients much less frequently than in those with complete moles, at a rate of about 5%. Hydropic abortuses show villous swelling without trophoblastic hyperplasia, are usually diploid or near-diploid, and have a benign clinical course.[69a]

Although these entities may be distinguished on routine microscopic examination in many cases, substantial interpathologist disagreement has been reported.[18,54] It has been shown that flow cytometry of either fresh or paraffin-embedded hydropic placentas can accurately distinguish between DNA diploid specimens and those that are DNA triploid,[18,69] and that correlation of the flow cytometry data with the gross and microscopic features increases interpathologist agreement.[18] Thus, DNA content determined by flow cytometry coupled with the histological features of a hydropic gestation may aid in distinguishing complete from partial hydatidiform moles and partial moles from hydropic abortuses.[13,18,69]

Flow cytometric examination of molar specimens also has resulted in documentation of greater heterogeneity of DNA content in molar gestations with histological features of complete and partial mole than had been recognized previously.[18,43,69,69a,73] Although most specimens with the histological features of complete mole are DNA diploid or near diploid, and most specimens with the histological features of partial hydatidiform mole are triploid, conceptuses with diploid, triploid, aneuploid, and tetraploid DNA content have been noted in both groups.[43,69] It has been suggested that DNA diploid partial moles may have a greater likelihood of development of persistent gestational trophoblastic disease[22]; however, the large number of DNA diploid partial moles in that study (83%) raises the possibility that a number of the cases may have been either complete moles or hydropic abortuses. When DNA diploidy is documented in a partial mole, review of the slides should be performed to rule out the co-existence of a complete mole and a twin gestation.[71] It has been suggested in one study[73] that aneuploidy in complete moles is associated with persistent gestational trophoblastic disease. The criteria for aneuploidy in that study (more than 10% of cells in the G2M region) were less stringent than those of several other studies that failed to document such an association.[43,69a] A small number of triploid complete moles have been reported; cytogenetic analysis of at least one of these cases revealed a completely androgenic origin, possibly explaining its morphologic expression as a complete mole.[87] DNA tetraploid complete and partial moles have been described as well, but their biological significance remains unclear because of the small number of cases reported.[70]

References

1. Aure JC, Hoeg K, Kolstad P (1971) Clinical and histologic studies of ovarian carcinoma: Long term follow-up of 900 cases. Obstet Gynecol 37: 1–9
2. Baak JPA, Delemarre JFM, Langley FA, Talerman A (1986) Grading ovarian tumors. Evaluation of decision making by different pathologists. Anal Quant Cytol Histol 8: 349–353
3. Baak JPA, Langley FA, Talerman A, Delemarre JFM (1986) Interpathologist and intrapathologist disagreement in ovarian tumor grading and typing. Anal Quant Cytol Histol 8: 354–357
4. Baak JPA, Langley FA, Talerman A, Delemarre JFM (1987) The prognostic variability of ovarian tumor grading by different pathologists. Gynecol Oncol 27: 166–172
5. Baak JPA, Schipper NW, Wisse-Brekelmans ECM, et al (1988) The prognostic value of morphometrical features and cellular DNA content in cis-platin treated late ovarian cancer patients. Br J Cancer 57: 503–508

6. Baisch H, Beck H-P, Christensen JJ, et al (1982) A comparison of mathematical methods for the analysis of DNA histograms obtained by flow cytometry. Cell Tissue Kinet 15: 235–249

7. Baisch H, Gohde W, Linden W (1975) Analysis of PCP-data to determine the fraction of cells in the various phases of the cell cycle. Radiat Environ Biophys 12: 31–39

8. Baker VV, Haskill S, Fowler WC, Walton LA, Currie JL (1987) Cellular DNA content and CA-125 antigen expression in ovarian carcinomas. Oncology 44: 283–186

9. Ball HG, Bell DA, Griffin TW (1990) Cancer of the ovary. In: Osteen RT (ed) Cancer Manual, 8th ed. American Cancer Society Massachusetts Division, Boston, pp 266–270

10. Barnabei UM, Miller PS, Bauer ED, Murad TM, Rademaker AW, Lurain JR (1990) Flow cytometric evaluation of epithelial ovarian cancer. Am J Obstet Gynecol 162: 1584–1592

11. Bell DA (1992) Flow cytometry of ovarian neoplasms. Curr Topics Pathol 85: 337–356

12. Bell DA, Pastel-Levy C, Flotte TJ (1988) DNA content in serous borderline tumors. Lab Invest 58: 8A

13. Benirschke K (1989) Flow cytometry for all mole-like abortion specimens. Hum Pathol 20: 403–404

14. Blumenfeld D, Braly PS, Ben-Ezra J, Klevecz RR (1987) Tumor DNA content as a prognostic feature in advanced epithelial ovarian carcinoma. Gynecol Oncol 27: 389–398

15. Bresica RJ, Barakat RA, Beller U, et al (1990) The prognostic significance of nuclear DNA content in malignant epithelial tumors of the ovary. Cancer 65: 141–147

16. Christov K, Vassilev N (1987) Flow cytometric analysis of DNA and cell proliferation in ovarian tumors. Cancer 60: 121–125

17. Colvin RB, Preffer FI (1987) New technologies in cell analysis by flow cytometry. Arch Pathol Lab Med 111: 628–632

18. Conran RM, Hitchcock CL, Popek EJ, et al (1993) Diagnostic considerations in molar gestations. Hum Pathol 24: 41–48

19. Coon JS, Deitch AD, de Vere White RW, et al (1988) Interinstitutional variability in DNA flow cytometric analysis of tumors. The National Cancer Institute's flow cytometry network experience. Cancer 61: 126–130

20. Coon JS, Landay AL, Weinstein RS (1987) Advances in flow cytometry for diagnostic pathology. Lab Invest 47: 453–479

21. Cramer SF, Roth LM, Ulbright TN, et al (1987) Evaluation of the reproducibility of the World Health Organization classification of common ovarian cancers. With emphasis on methodology. Arch Pathol Lab Med 111: 819–829

22. Davis JR, Kerrigan DP, Way DL, Weiner SA (1987) Partial hydatidiform moles: Deoxyribonucleic acid content and course. Am J Obstet Gynecol 157: 969–973

23. Dean PN, Jett JH (1974) Mathematical analysis of DNA distributions derived from flow microfluoremetry. J Cell Biol 60: 523–527

24. DiSaia PJ, Creasman WT (1989) Clinical Gynecologic Oncology, 3rd ed. St. Louis, C V Mosby Co, p 349

25. Erba E, Ubezio P, Pepe S, et al (1989) Flow cytometric analysis of DNA content in human ovarian cancers. Br J Cancer 60: 45–50

26. Erba E, Vaghi M, Pepe S, et al (1985) DNA index of ovarian carcinomas from 56 patients: in vivo in vitro studies. Br J Cancer 52: 565–573

27. Feichter GE, Kuhn W, Czernobilsky B, et al (1985) DNA flow cytometry of ovarian tumors with correlation to histopathology. Int J Gynecol Pathol 4: 336–345

28. Feitz WFJ, Beck HLM, Smeets AWGB, et al (1985) Tissue-specific markers in flow cytometry of urological cancers: Cytokeratins in bladder carcinoma. Int J Cancer 36: 349–356

29. Friedlander ML, Hedley DW, Swanson C, Russell P (1988) Prediction of long-term survival by flow cytometric analysis of cellular DNA content in patients with advanced ovarian cancer. J Clin Oncol 6: 282–290

30. Friedlander ML, Hedley DW, Taylor IW, Russell P, Coates AS, Tattersall MHN (1984) Influence of cellular DNA content on survival in advanced ovarian cancer. Cancer Res 44: 397–400

31. Friedlander ML, Russell P, Taylor IW, Hedley DW, Tattersall HN (1984) Flow cytometric analysis of cellular DNA content as an adjunct to the diagnosis of ovarian tumours of borderline malignancy. Pathology 16: 301–306

32. Friedlander ML, Taylor IW, Russell P, Musgrove EA, Hedley DH, Tattersall MHN (1983) Ploidy as a prognostic factor in ovarian cancer. Int J Gynecol Pathol 2: 55–63

33. Friedlander ML, Taylor IW, Russell P, Tattersall MKN (1984) Cellular DNA content—a stable feature in epithelial ovarian cancer. Br J Cancer 49: 173–179

34. Frierson HF (1991) The need for improvement in flow cytometric analysis of ploidy and S-phase fraction. Am J Clin Pathol 95: 439–441

35. Gajewski WH, Fuller AF, Pastel-Levy C, Flotte TJ, Bell DA (in press) Prognostic significance of DNA content in epithelial ovarian cancer. Gynecol Oncol

36. Gonchoroff NJ, Ryan JJ, Kimlinger TK, et al (1990) Effect of sonication on paraffin-embedded tissue preparation for DNA flow cytometry. Cytometry 11: 642–646

37. Gray JW, Dolbeare F, Pallavicini MG (1990) Quantitative cell-cycle analysis. In: Melamed MR, Lindmo T, Mendelsohn ML (eds) Flow Cytometry and Sorting, 2nd ed. New York, Wiley-Liss, pp 445–467

38. Hamaguchi K, Nishimura H, Miyoshi T, et al (1990) Flow cytometric analysis of cellular DNA content in ovarian cancer. Gynecol Oncol 37: 219–223

39. Hedley DW (1989) Flow cytometry using paraffin-embedded tissue: Five years on. Cytometry 10: 229–241

40. Hedley DW Friedlander ML, Taylor IW, et al (1983) Method for analysis of cellular DNA content of paraffin-embedded pathological material using flow cytometry. Histochem Cytochem 31: 1333–1335

41. Hedley DW, Friedlander ML, Taylor IW (1985) Application of DNA flow cytometry to paraffin-embedded archival material for the study of aneuploidy and its clinical significance. Cytometry 6: 327–333

42. Heinonen PK, Morsky P, Aine R, Koivula T, Pystynen P (1988) Hormonal activity of epithelial ovarian tumours in postmenopausal women. Maturitas 9: 325–338

43. Hemming JD, Quirke P, Womack C, Wells M, Elston CW, Bird CC (1987) Diagnosis of molar pregnancy and persistent trophoblastic disease by flow cytometry. J Clin Pathol 40: 615–620

44. Herbert DJ, Nishiyama RH, Bagwell CB, et al (1989) Effects of several commonly used fixatives on DNA and total nuclear protein analysis by flow cytometry. Am J Clin Pathol 91: 535–541

45. Hernandez E, Bhagavan BS, Parmley TH, Rosenshein NB (1984) Interobserver variability in the interpretation of epithelial ovarian cancer. Gynecol Oncol 17: 117–123

46. Hiddeman W, Schumann J, Andreeff M, et al (1984) Convention on nomenclature for DNA cytometry. Cytometry 5: 445–446

47. Homburger HA, McCarthy R, Deodhar S (1989) Assessment of interlaboratory variability in analytical cytology. Results of the College of American Pathologists Flow Cytometry Study. Arch Pathol Lab Med 113: 667–670

48. Horan PK, Muirhead KA, Slezak E (1990) Standards and controls in flow cytometry. In: Melamed MR, Lindmo T, Mendelsohn ML (eds) Flow Cytometry and Sorting, 2nd ed. New York, Wiley-Liss, pp 397–414

49. Huffman JL, Garin-Chesa P, Gay H, Whitmore Jr WF, Melamed MR (1986) Flow cytometric identifications of human bladder cells using a cytokeratin monoclonal antibody. Ann NY Acad Sci 468: 302–315

50. Iversen O-E, Skaarland E (1987) Ploidy assessment of benign and malignant ovarian tumors by flow cytometry. A clinicopathological study. Cancer 60: 82–87

51. Iversen OE, Laerum OD (1987) Trout and salmon erythrocytes and human leukocytes as internal standards for ploidy control in flow cytometry. Cytometry 8: 190–196

52. Jakobsen A, Bichel P (1989) Ploidy level, histopathological differentiation and response to chemotherapy in serous ovarian cancer. Eur J Cancer Clin Oncol 25: 1589–1593

53. Jakobsen A, Hansen V, Poulsen HS (1988) DNA profile and steroid receptor content of human ovarian cancer. Eur J Gynaecol Oncol 6: 461–463

54. Javey H, Borazjani G, Behmard S, Langley FA (1979) Discrepancies in the histological diagnosis of hydatidiform mole. Br J Obstet Gynaecol 86: 480–483

55. Joensuu H, Alanen KA, Klemi PJ, Aine R (1990) Evidence for false aneuploid peaks in flow cytometric analysis of paraffin-embedded tissue. Cytometry 11: 421–437

56. Joensuu H, Kallioniemi O-P (1989) Different opinions on classification of DNA histograms produced from paraffin-embedded tissue. Cytometry 10: 711–717

57. Kaerns J, Trope C, Kjorstad KE, Abeler V, Pettersen EO (1990) Cellular DNA content as a new prognostic tool in patients with borderline tumors of the ovary. Gynecol Oncol 38: 452–457

58. Kallioniemi O-P (1988) Comparison of fresh and paraffin-embedded tissue as starting material for DNA flow cytometry and evaluation of intratumor heterogeneity. Cytometry 9: 164–169

59. Kallioniemi OP, Mattila J, Punnonen R, Koivula T (1988) DNA ploidy level and cell cycle distribution in ovarian cancer: relation to histopathological features of the tumor. Int J Gynecol Pathol 7: 1–11

60. Kallioniemi O-P, Punnonen R, Mattila J, Lehtinen M, Koivula T (1988b) Prognostic significance of DNA index, multiploidy, and S-phase fraction in ovarian cancer. Cancer 61: 334–339

61. Khoo SK, Hurst T, Kearsley J, et al (1990) Prognostic significance of tumor ploidy in patients with advanced ovarian carcinoma. Gynecol Oncol 39: 284–288

62. Klemi PJ, Joensuu H, Mäenpää J, Kiiolholma P (1989) Influence of cellular DNA content on survival in ovarian carcinoma. Obstet Gynecol 74: 200–204

63. Klemi PJ, Joensuu H, Kiilholma P, Maenpaa J (1988) Clinical significance of abnormal nuclear DNA content in serous ovarian tumors. Cancer 62: 2005–2010

64. Koss LG (1992) Flow cytometry. In: Diagnostic Cytology and Its Histopathologic Bases, 4th ed. Philadelphia, J B Lippincott, pp 1613–1641

65. Kuhn W, Kaufmann M, Feichter GE, Schmid H, Hanke J, Rummel HH (1988) Psammoma body content and DNA-flow cytometric results as prognostic factors in advanced ovarian carcinoma. Eur J Gynaecol Oncol 9: 234–241

66. Kuhn W, Kaufmann M, Feichter GE, Rummel HH, Schmid H, Heberling D (1989) DNA flow cytometry, clinical and morphological parameters as prognostic factors for advanced malignant and borderline ovarian tumors. Gynecol Oncol 33: 360–367

67. Kotylo PK, Michael H, Fineberg N, Sutton G, Roth LM (1992) Flow cytometric analysis of DNA content and RAS P21 oncoprotein expression in ovarian neoplasms (1992) Int J Gynecol Pathol 11: 30–37

68. Lage J (1991) Flow cytometric analysis of nuclear DNA content in gestational trophoblastic disease. J Reprod Med 36: 31–35

69. Lage JM, Driscoll SG, Yavner DL, Oliview AP, Mark SD, Weinberg DS (1988) Hydatidiform moles. Application of flow cytometry in diagnosis. Am J Clin Pathol 89: 596–600

69a. Lage JM, Mark SD, Roberts DJ, Goldstein DP, Bernstein MR, Berkowitz RS (1992) A flow cytometric study of 137 fresh hydropic placentas: Correlation between types of hydatidiform moles and nuclear DNA ploidy. Obstet Gynecol 79: 403–410

70. Lage JM, Weinberg DS, Yavner DL, Bieber FR (1989) The biology of tetraploid hydatidiform moles: Histopathology, cytogenetics, and flow cytometry. Hum Pathol 20: 419–425

71. Lage JM, Weinberg DS, Huettner PC, Mark SD (1992) Flow cytometric analysis of nuclear DNA content in ovarian tumors. Association of ploidy with tumor type, histologic grade, and clinical stage. Cancer 69: 2668–2675

72. Martin AR, Kotylo PK, Kennedy JC, Fineberg NS, Roth LM (1992) Flow cytometric DNA analysis of ovarian Brenner tumors and transitional cell carcinomas. Int J Gynecol Pathol 11: 188–196

73. Martin DA, Sutton GP, Ulbright TM, Sledge GW, Stehman FB, Ehrlich CE (1989) DNA content as a prognostic index in gestational trophoblastic neoplasia. Gynecol Oncol 34: 383–388

74. Murray K, Hopwood L, Volk D, Wilson JF (1989) Cytofluorometric analysis of the DNA content in ovarian carcinoma and its relationship to patient survival. Cancer 63: 2456–2460

75. Pallavicini MG, Taylor IW, Vindelov LL (1990) Preparation of cell/nuclei suspensions from solid tumors for flow cytometry. In: Melamed MR, Lindmo T, Mendelsohn ML (eds) Flow Cytometry and Sorting, 2nd ed. New York, Wiley-Liss, pp 187–194

75a. Prat J, Matias-Guiu X, Barreto J (1991) Simultaneous carcinoma involving the endometrium and the ovary. A clinicopathologic, immunohistochemical, and DNA flow cytometric study of 18 cases. Cancer 68: 2455–2459

76. Punnonen R, Kallioniemi O-P, Mattila J, Koivula T (1989) Prognostic assessment in Stage I ovarian cancer using a

discriminant analysis with clinicopathological and DNA flow cytometric data. Gynecol Obstet Invest 27: 213–216

77. Robey SS, Silva EG, Gershenson DM, McLemore D, El-Naggar A, Ordonez NC (1989) Transitional cell carcinoma in high-grade high-stage ovarian carcinoma. An indicator of favorable response to chemotherapy. Cancer 63: 839–847

78. Rodenburg CJ, Cornelisse CJ, Heintz PAM, Hermans J, Fleuren GJ (1987) Tumor ploidy as a major prognostic factor in advanced ovarian cancer. Cancer 59: 317–323

79. Rodenburg CJ, Cornelisse CJ, Hermans J, Fleuren GJ (1988) DNA flow cytometry and morphometry as prognostic indicators in advanced ovarian cancer: a step forward in predicting the clinical outcome. Gynecol Oncol 29: 176–187

80. Rodenburg CJ, Ploem-Zaaijer JJ, Cornelisse CJ, et al (1987) Use of DNA image cytometry in addition to flow cytometry for the study of patients with advanced ovarian cancer. Cancer Res 47: 3938–3941

81. Rutgers DH, Wils IS, Schaap AHP, van Lindert ACM (1987) DNA flow cytometry, histological grade, stage, and age as prognostic factors in human epithelial ovarian carcinomas. Path Res Pract 182: 207–213

82. Rutledge ML, Silva EG, McLemore D, El-Naggar A (1989) Serous surface carcinoma of the ovary and peritoneum. A flow cytometry study. Pathol Ann 24(2): 227–236

83. Sahni K, Tribukait B, Einhorn N (1989) Flow cytometric measurement of ploidy and proliferation in effusions of ovarian carcinoma and their possible prognostic significance. Gynecol Oncol 35: 240–245

84. Schueler JA, Cornelisse CJ, Jermans J, Trimbos JB, van der Burg MEL, Fleuren GJ (1993) Prognostic factors in well-differentiated early-stage epithelial ovarian cancer. Cancer 71: 787–795

85. Sharpless T, Traganos F, Darzynkiewicz Z, Melamed MR (1975) Flow cytofluorimetry: discrimination between single cells and cell aggregates by direct size measurements. Acta Cytol 19: 577–581

86. Sobre B, Frankendal B, Veress B (1982) Importance of histologic grading in the prognosis of epithelial ovarian carcinoma. Obstet Gynecol 59: 567–582

87. Sunde L, Vejerslev LO, Larsen JK, et al (1989) Genetically different cell subpopulations in hydatidiform moles. A study of three cases by RFLP, flow cytometric, cytogenetic, HLA, and morphologic analyses. Cancer Genet Cytogenet 37: 179–192

88. Trebeck CE, Friedlander ML, Russell P, Baird PJ (1987) Brenner tumours of the ovary: A study of the histology, immunohistochemistry and cellular DNA content in benign, borderline and malignant ovarian tumours. Pathology 19: 241–246

89. Vindelov LL, Christensen IJ, Jensen G, et al (1983) Limits of detection of nuclear DNA abnormalities by flow cytometric DNA analysis. Cytometry 3: 332–339

90. Volm M, Bruggemann A, Gunther M, Kleine W, Pfleiderer A, Vogt-Schaden M (1985) Prognostic relevance of ploidy, proliferation, and resistance-predictive tests in ovarian carcinoma. Cancer Res 45: 5180–5185

91. Volm M, Kleine W, Pfleiderer A (1989) Flow-cytometric prognostic factors for the survival of patients with ovarian carcinoma: A 5-year follow-up study. Gynecol Oncol 35: 84–89

92. Watson JV, Curling ON, Munn CF, Hudson CN (1987) Oncogene expression in ovarian cancer: a pilot study of c-myc oncoprotein in serous papillary ovarian cancer. Gynecol Oncol 28: 137–150

93. Wersto RP, Liblit RL, Deitch D, Koss LG (1991) Variability in DNA measurements in multiple tumor samples of human colonic carcinoma. Cancer 67: 106–115

94. Wheeless LL, Coon JS, Cox C, et al (1991) Precision of DNA flow cytometry in inter-institutional analyses. Cytometry 12: 405–412

28

Molecular Biology

Kathleen R. Cho, M.D. and Lora Hedrick, M.D.

Understanding the etiology and pathogenesis of human tumors has been a goal actively pursued by investigators in diverse fields including pathology, oncology, virology, radiation biology, and many others. These various avenues of research have provided significant insights into the properties of neoplastic cells and have laid the foundation for our current understanding and future investigations of human tumorigenesis. Most recently, the application of molecular biological techniques to cancer research has added a new dimension to our knowledge of the neoplastic process. These molecular tools have made it possible to address directly the mechanisms that lead to the altered properties of neoplastic cells. Over the past two decades molecular biology has confirmed many well-accepted hypotheses of

tumorigenesis, revealed many new facts about tumor cells, and opened the door to a more thorough understanding of the pathogenesis of human cancer. It is now clear that molecular biology will not only greatly enhance our basic understanding of tumorigenesis, but will have a huge impact on the manner in which we diagnose and treat cancer patients. The aims of this chapter are threefold. First, we provide a brief discussion of basic molecular biological principals and techniques to build a framework with which to understand molecular studies of human tumorigenesis. Second, we review a molecular model of colorectal tumorigenesis that highlights the major concepts of our current understanding of the molecular pathogenesis of human tumors. Third, we have compiled what is currently known about the specific genetic alterations associated with common gynecological malignancies. To assist the reader's understanding of unfamiliar terms, a glossary appears at the end of the chapter. Terms within the text indicated in boldface are defined in the glossary.

Basic Principles of Molecular Biology

Cells have the capacity to synthesize simultaneously thousands of molecules required for normal cellular function. These molecules include deoxyribonucleic and ribonucleic acids (DNA and RNA), which encode genetic information, and proteins, which are the primary effector molecules within cells. Nucleic acids are constructed from smaller building blocks called *nucleotides*, which are linked end to end through phosphodiester bonds. The arrangement of

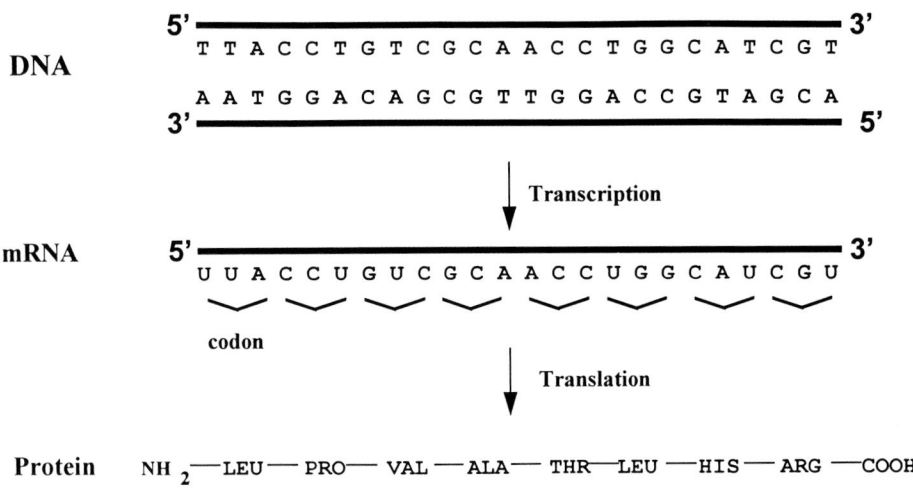

FIG. 28.1. The genetic code. DNA encodes the primary genetic information. DNA is a double-stranded molecule formed by complementary base pairing between nucleotides on strands of opposite orientation. An RNA copy of the coding DNA strand is synthesized by a process known as *transcription*. Triplets of nucleotides (called *codons*) specify individual amino acids that are joined together to form proteins in the process known as *translation*. DNA, RNA, and protein are synthesized in a unidirectional fashion; DNA and RNA in the 5′ to 3′ direction, and protein from the amino (NH₂) to carboxyl (COOH) terminus.

these nucleotides in various sequences is ultimately responsible for the tremendous variety of proteins encoded by the nucleic acids of a given organism. Human chromosomes are composed of two major components: DNA and small basic proteins called *histones*. Although the DNA within a given chromosome encodes only a subset of the estimated 10^5 genes represented in the human genome, it is important to keep in mind that, on average, each chromosome or chromosomal arm encodes several thousand genes. Furthermore, individual genes are distributed throughout the genome, separated by large expanses of DNA that do not contain genes. Thus, identification of specific genes altered in various tumor types can be a monumental task.

The primary genetic information is encoded by DNA, a double helical molecule formed by two intertwined DNA strands joined by hydrogen bonds between complementary nucleotide base pairs (Fig. 28.1). Adenine (A) can pair only with thymine (T), and cytosine (C) can pair only with guanine (G). On each strand, nucleotides are joined end to end by covalent linkage of a phosphate group connecting the 5′ carbon atom of the sugar residue on one nucleotide to the 3′ carbon atom of the sugar residue in the adjacent nucleotide. This 5′–3′ linkage is responsible for setting the direction of the nucleic acid chains such that each strand has a 5′ end and a 3′ end. All nucleic acid chains are extended in the 5′–3′ direction. In a double-stranded DNA molecule, the two strands are complementary and of opposite orientation. The sequence of nucleotides in DNA is critical, as the coding regions (**open reading frames°**) of genes are read in sequential groups of three base pairs known as **codons,** which ultimately specify the order of amino acids in proteins encoded by specific genes. It follows that critically placed nucleotide substitutions at the

DNA level (i.e., **point mutations**) can lead to changes in the amino acid sequence of the protein encoded by that DNA. These substitutions can have grave consequences on protein function. Although chromosomal DNA is contained within the cell nucleus, protein synthesis takes place in the cell cytoplasm. One form of RNA serves as an intermediate molecule that transports genetic information from the nucleus to the cytoplasmic machinery responsible for the synthesis of proteins. Signals for starting and stopping the synthesis of specific RNA molecules also are encoded within DNA sequences. RNA is synthesized by enzymes called *RNA polymerases*, which bind to sequences in the DNA upstream (toward the 5′ end) of coding regions called **promoters.** The synthesis of RNA from the DNA template occurs by a process known as **transcription** (Fig. 28.1), in which an RNA copy of the coding DNA strand of a gene is created by linking ribonucleotides end to end (using the noncoding strand as a template). The sequence of nucleotides in this initial form of RNA (**heteronuclear RNA**) is identical to that of the coding DNA strand except that ribonucleotides rather than deoxyribonucleotides form the chain and RNA-specific uracil (U) residues are substituted for thymine residues. The heteronuclear RNA subsequently undergoes several modifications, including **capping, polyadenylation,** and **splicing,** which result in **messenger RNA or mRNA** (Fig. 28.2). After transcription, eukaryotic mRNAs are "capped" by the addition of 7-methyl guanosine residues joined by triphosphate linkages to the 5′ end of the RNA molecules. The 5′ cap is believed to guide the translation machinery to the correct translation initiation codon. In addition, long runs of (A) residues are added to the 3′ ends of mRNAs in a process known as *polyadenylation*. The poly(A) sequence is not coded in the DNA, but is added to the RNA after transcription. Although the function of the poly(A) tail is not understood completely, it may help protect mRNA from RNA-degrading enzymes. In the process known as *splicing*, the **exons,** or coding portions of genes, are

---

°Terms within text indicated in boldfaced type are defined in the Glossary at the end of the chapter.

FIG. 28.2. **RNA synthesis and processing.** Genes are composed of alternating exons and introns. After transcription, introns are removed from the heteronuclear RNA by a process called *splicing* to produce messenger RNA (mRNA). The splicing machinery is directed by sequences surrounding the junctions of the exon–intron boundaries. Most eukaryotic mRNAs are modified further at the 5′ end by addition of 7-methyl guanosine residues (called a *cap*) and at the 3′ end by addition of several adenosine residues (*polyadenylation*).

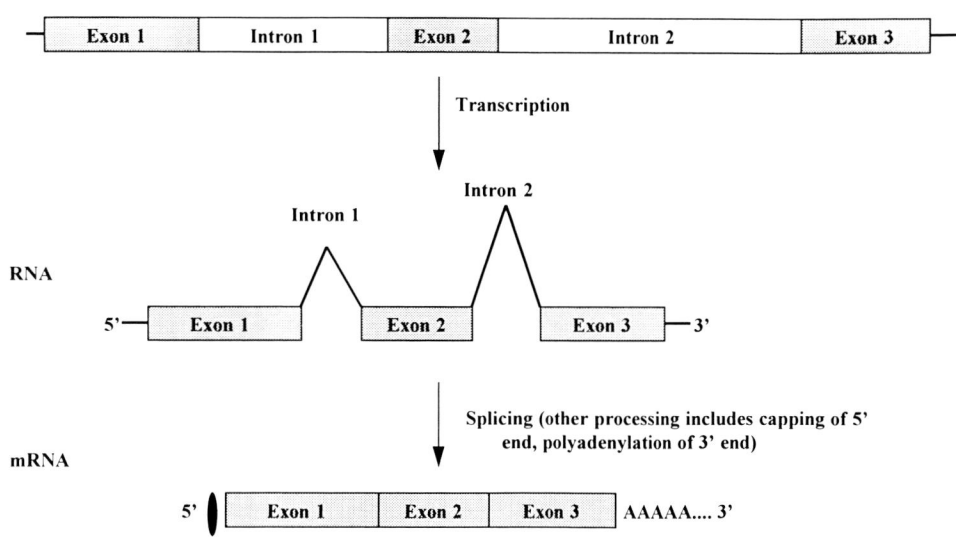

joined together, and intervening noncoding regions called **introns** are spliced out and removed. The mature spliced RNA (messenger RNA or mRNA) is transported to the cytoplasm, where it serves as a template to order amino acids during the process of protein synthesis known as **translation** (Fig. 28.1). One end of a newly translated protein has an amino acid with a free amino group, whereas the other end bears an amino acid with a free carboxyl group. Translation starts with the amino-terminal residue and ends with the carboxyl-terminal residue.

Clearly, only a small portion of the genome is ultimately expressed as mRNA or protein. Although cells from virtually every tissue within an individual contain the same DNA, specific genes are expressed variably in different tissues. Tissue-specific **gene expression** can be controlled at the level of transcription, such that DNA is not transcribed to RNA, or at the level of RNA translation to protein. A thorough discussion of these control mechanisms is beyond the scope of this chapter; however, it is important to emphasize that many tumors develop and progress, at least in part, as a result of alterations of gene expression in tumor cells in comparison to their normal counterparts. Many of the molecular biological techniques used in cancer research laboratories today are aimed at studying gross and subtle alterations of DNA, changes in gene expression at the RNA and protein levels, and alterations of protein function within tumor cells.

Commonly Used Molecular Biological Techniques

The human genome is extremely complex, containing approximately 3×10^9 base pairs. This complexity poses significant problems for investigators interested in studying individual genes or even smaller portions of the genome. The development and progression of many human cancers involves alterations of specific genes at the DNA level. Many different types of alterations have been identified, including (1) **gene amplification,** in which tumor cells contain multiple copies of a gene normally present in only two copies per somatic cell, (2) **gene rearrangement,** in which a gene is broken and one or both segments are joined to other parts of the genome, (3) **gene deletions,** in which part or all of a gene is deleted from tumor cells, (4) **insertions,** in which new genetic material is inserted into a gene, and (5) *point mutations,* in which single nucleotide substitutions at the DNA level result in proteins with amino acid substitutions (**missense mutations**) or truncated proteins (**nonsense mutations**). These genetic alterations typically alter gene expression. Gene amplification results most commonly in overexpression; underexpression is the usual consequence of gene deletions or insertions. Rearrangements and point mutations may cause either overexpression or underexpression of the target gene depending on the specific nature of the genetic lesion. Several laboratory tools have been developed that allow detection of these abnormalities in DNA isolated from tumor cells.

Methods of DNA Analysis

SOUTHERN BLOTTING

This technique, developed in 1975 by E.M. Southern,[93] is an extremely powerful tool with which to analyze gene structure (Fig. 28.3). First, genomic DNA is cut with one or more **restriction endonucleases,** enzymes that cut the DNA at specific recognition sequences distributed randomly throughout the genome. The resultant DNA frag-

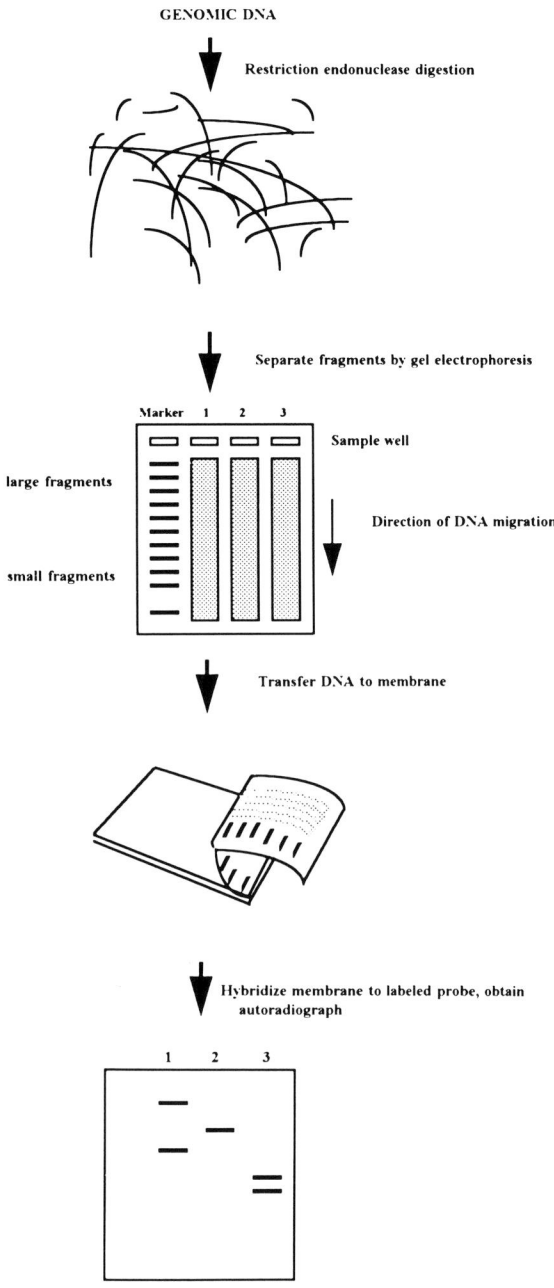

GENOMIC DNA

Restriction endonuclease digestion

Separate fragments by gel electrophoresis

Marker 1   2   3

Sample well

large fragments

Direction of DNA migration

small fragments

Transfer DNA to membrane

Hybridize membrane to labeled probe, obtain autoradiograph

1   2   3

FIG. 28.3. Southern blot. This powerful technique is used frequently to detect structural alterations of genes in human tumors. High molecular weight genomic DNA is cut with a restriction endonuclease and the resultant DNA fragments are size fractionated by gel electrophoresis. The DNA is denatured in alkali, transferred from the gel, and bound to a nylon membrane. The DNA on the membrane is hybridized to a radiolabeled probe under conditions that allow complementary sequences to stick to each other. Autoradiography yields a discrete pattern of bands whose pattern, number, and size confer information about the status of a particular gene in each sample. Southern blotting can be used to detect gene amplification, gene insertions, gene deletions, and gene rearrangements, and for RFLP analysis (see Fig. 28.4).

ments range in size from very small (a few base pairs) to very large (several thousand or more base pairs). These fragments subsequently are separated according to size by electrophoresis through an agarose gel such that smaller molecules migrate faster. The DNA in the gel is denatured in alkali to separate the strands of the double helix, then the gel is overlaid with a solid substrate (usually nylon membrane) and an appropriate buffer is used to transport DNA out of the gel toward the membrane. The DNA fragments bind to the membrane, resulting in transfer of the DNA from the gel to the membrane. A radiolabeled probe, specific for the gene under study, is then hybridized to the DNA on the membrane under conditions that allow complementary sequences to stick to each other. Autoradiography of the membrane results in discrete bands whose pattern, number, and size confer information about the status of the evaluated gene in that particular sample. The size of the bands is altered if there is a change in the position of the restriction endonuclease sites relative to one another. This can occur if one of the restriction endonuclease recognition sites within or around the region of interest is changed such that the endonuclease no longer cleaves the DNA at that site, thereby changing the distance between intact recognition sites. The distance between restriction endonuclease sites also can be affected by DNA rearrangement, or insertions or small deletions of DNA sequences in or around the gene under study. Therefore, when compared with the same patient's nontumor DNA, size alterations of one or more bands in tumor DNA usually indicate gene rearrangement, insertions, or small deletions; increased intensity of bands represents gene amplification; and loss of bands indicates gene deletion. Southern hybridization to probes detecting **restriction fragment length polymorphisms (RFLPs)** is used frequently to detect **losses of heterozygosity** (LOH) or losses of specific chromosomal regions in tumor DNA. The term *RFLP* refers to single base pair substitutions in the germline DNA of different individuals that either destroy or create new cutting sites for a given restriction enzyme. Most of these changes are without consequence because most do not affect gene products in any way. Normal cells contain two copies of each chromosome, one inherited from each parent. If the paternal and maternal copies of a given **locus** can be distinguished by RFLP analysis of DNA from normal cells, that individual is considered *heterozygous* (or **informative**) at that locus. If the two chromosomes cannot be distinguished from one another, the individual is referred to as *homozygous* (or **uninformative**) at that locus. Therefore, if the specific chromosomal region containing that locus is lost in an individual's tumor cells, RFLP analysis will detect this loss because the individual's DNA from normal cells will be heterozygous at that locus but the tumor cell DNA will be homozygous (Fig. 28.4). Thus, the tumor cells have undergone LOH for the region of the chromosome detected by the probe. As an example,

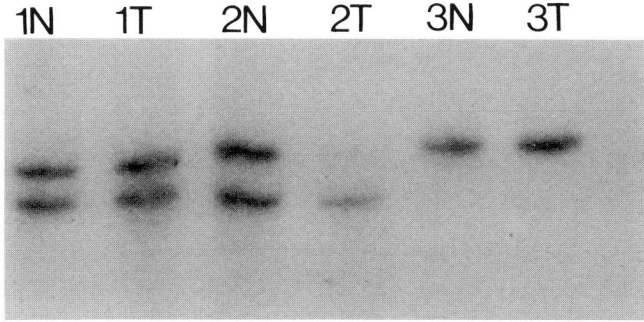

FIG. 28.4. RFLP analysis. Southern blot hybridization of paired normal and endometrial carcinoma DNAs to a RFLP probe is shown. Each case is represented by the patient's normal DNA (*N*) in the left lane and tumor DNA (*T*) in the right lane. Case 1 is informative (heterozygous), because two bands are distinguishable in the normal DNA lane. The tumor shows no loss of heterozygosity at the locus detected by the probe because both bands are retained. Case 3 is uninformative (homozygous) because only one band is present in the normal DNA lane. In Case 2, the larger band is missing in the tumor DNA, i.e., the tumor has undergone loss of heterozygosity at this locus.

the recognition site for the restriction enzyme *EcoRI* is (. . . G-A-A-T-T-C . . .). Although the maternally derived copy of an individual's DNA may contain this sequence at a given locus, the paternally inherited **allele** may have substituted a (T) residue for an (A) residue, such that this copy of the DNA will contain the sequence (. . . G-A-T-T-T-C . . .) at the same locus. When this individual's DNA is cut with *EcoRI,* one allele will cut at this site and the other will not, resulting in two distinguishable bands following Southern hybridization to a probe detecting the region containing the polymorphic *EcoRI* restriction site. When the patient's tumor DNA is compared with his or her own normal DNA, a loss of heterozygosity at the locus detected by the probe shows up as a loss of one of the bands detected in the normal DNA. Clearly, the success of such efforts depends largely on the isolation of tumor DNA from tumors that are relatively free of contaminating normal tissue, which can mask allelic loss events. Although an individual patient may be uninformative at the locus detected by one probe, it does not render their DNA samples useless for further study because they may be informative at other loci. In addition, the development of probes detecting highly polymorphic regions in human DNA has made LOH studies substantially less difficult by improving the percentage of individuals informative at the loci detected by the probes. LOH analysis with probes distributed throughout the genome can be used to look for regions of chromosomes that are frequently and specifically deleted in various tumor types.

DNA CLONING

DNA isolated from primary tumors and normal tissues usually is available in only limited quantities. It is frequently desirable to obtain large amounts of specific portions of these DNAs. One method used to generate unlimited quantities of specific DNA fragments is called **cloning.** Cleavage of DNA with restriction endonucleases generates cut ends of DNA that can later be resealed with enzymes known as *DNA ligases.* DNA fragments with specific cohesive ends can be ligated to **vectors** cut in a fashion generating complementary cohesive ends (Fig. 28.5). The vector containing the inserted DNA can then be introduced into bacteria by a process known as **bacterial transformation.** Using the bacterial hosts' replication machinery, the recombinant vector can be propagated in essentially unlimited quantities. The cloned insert DNA subsequently can be excised and separated from the vector DNA using appropriate restriction enzymes. The most commonly used cloning vectors are plasmids (circular autonomously replicating bacterial minichromosomes) and bacteriophage (small viruses that replicate in bacteria).

THE POLYMERASE CHAIN REACTION

Although cloning is an extremely effective method to generate large quantities of specific DNA fragments, the process is quite time consuming, tedious, and often difficult. In the mid-1980s, Kary Mullis developed a technique called the *polymerase chain reaction* (PCR).[84] This technique has revolutionized molecular genetics and spawned the development of numerous new approaches for the identification and characterization of genes involved in tumorigenesis. PCR allows production of large quantities of specific DNA sequences in a single tube within a few hours. The reaction exploits several features of DNA replication (Fig. 28.6). The template for synthesis of a new complementary DNA strand is a single-stranded DNA molecule. Single-stranded templates can be generated simply by heating double-stranded DNA to near boiling temperatures (95°C). DNA polymerases require a small section of double-stranded DNA to initiate or "prime" synthesis of the new strand. New DNA synthesis is unidirectional, incorporating nucleotides in the 5'–3' direction on the new strand. Consequently, the starting point for new DNA synthesis can be specified by choosing a short complementary oligonucleotide (usually 15–25 base pairs) that, at lower temperatures, anneals to the single-stranded DNA template at the specific initiation site. Since both strands of the melted double-stranded DNA can serve as templates for new DNA synthesis, **primers** can be chosen such that new double-stranded DNA molecules are formed in the region of DNA between the two oligonucleotide primers. These new double-stranded molecules can

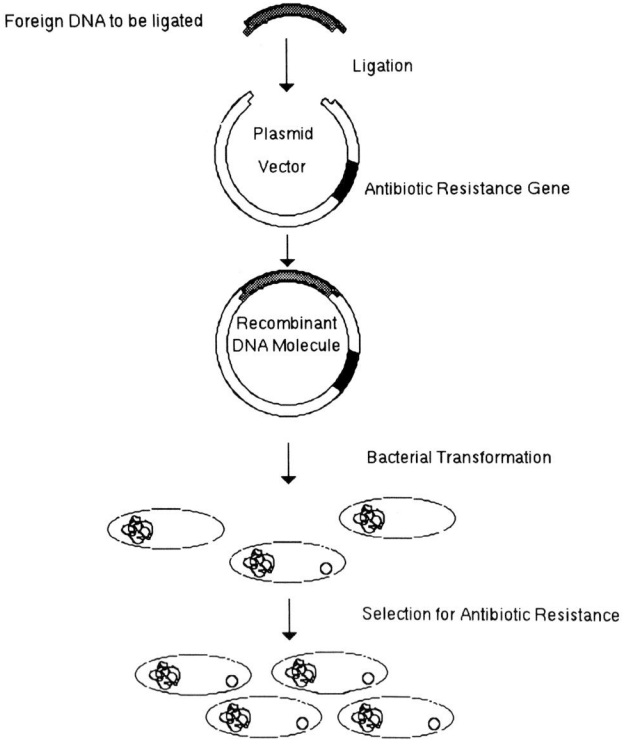

Foreign DNA to be ligated

Ligation

Plasmid
Vector

Antibiotic Resistance Gene

Recombinant
DNA Molecule

Bacterial Transformation

Selection for Antibiotic Resistance

Fig. 28.5. DNA cloning. A process known as *cloning* allows the generation of essentially unlimited quantities of specific DNA fragments. Several different types of cloning vectors are available, each capable of accommodating DNA of specific size ranges. As an example, plasmid vectors are used typically to clone DNA fragments no larger than several kilobase pairs. First, the selected DNA fragment is joined to the plasmid vector using specialized enzymes called *DNA ligases*. Often, the ligation is facilitated by the presence of complementary cohesive ends on the vector and foreign fragment to be ligated. After ligation, the recombinant DNA molecule is introduced as a circular plasmid into a host strain of bacteria by a process known as *bacterial transformation*. Inside the bacteria, the plasmid replicates independently from the bacterial DNA. Since the plasmids contain a selectable marker (antibiotic resistance gene), bacteria that have received the plasmid can be selected for with the appropriate antibiotic, allowing growth only of transformants. Large quantities of plasmid DNA can then be isolated from the transformed bacteria and the foreign fragment re-excised from the vector.

be melted with high temperature and the cycle repeated, such that the specific segment of DNA is synthesized in an exponential fashion. In other words, the net result of PCR is that at the end of n cycles, the reaction tube will contain a theoretical maximum of 2^n double-stranded molecules representing copies of the sequence specified by the two primers. Identification of heat stable DNA polymerases, such as the *Taq* polymerase isolated from the bacterium *Thermus aquaticus*, greatly simplified PCR because it eliminated the need to add additional polymerase during

the synthesis of each new DNA strand. As with other techniques, PCR is not without some drawbacks. These include (1) limitation of the size of the amplified products to a maximum of a few thousand base pairs, (2) occasional incorporation of incorrect nucleotides into the newly synthesized DNA, (3) nonspecific priming from regions of DNA complementary to the PCR primers, and (4) extreme sensitivity often resulting in sample to sample contamination. Nevertheless, PCR has opened the door to a myriad of new lines of laboratory investigation, certainly not limited to studies of tumor genetics. Of particular relevance to pathologists is that template DNA for PCR can be obtained from a variety of sources, including fresh and frozen tissues, blood and body fluids containing cellular material (e.g., urine, ascites, cerebrospinal fluid, etc.), and even fixed, paraffin-embedded archival material. PCR also obviates the need for large quantities of template DNA. Even DNA from single cells can serve as a template to generate essentially unlimited quantities of a target sequence.

DNA Sequencing

Some genetic alterations that occur during tumorigenesis are subtle, involving only single nucleotide substitutions at critical positions within a gene. Such mutations may occur in the coding region (missense and nonsense mutations), whereas others affect sequences that direct splicing of the initial RNA transcript (**splice site mutations**) or portions of the gene that regulate transcription. Both oncogenes (e.g., K-*ras*) and tumor suppressor genes (e.g., p53, Rb, WT-1) can be altered by point mutations, and it is often desirable to characterize the specific mutations that occur within tumors. To sequence the region of interest, large quantities of the specific region are first generated through cloning or with PCR. The most commonly used sequencing method today is that of Sanger.[85] This method capitalizes on several of the same features of DNA replication described above for PCR. Again, double-stranded DNA is melted to single strands under the appropriate conditions, followed by annealing of a specific oligonucleotide primer to the strand to be sequenced. DNA polymerase is then added to the reaction and allowed to incorporate radiolabeled nucleotides into the newly synthesized strand in the 5'–3' direction. However, in contrast to PCR, the nucleotides in a single reaction tube include small quantities of individual modified nucleotides (di-deoxy A,C,G, or T) that terminate DNA chain elongation at the corresponding nucleotide. Upon inactivation of the polymerase, the reaction tube will contain a series of radiolabeled DNA strands terminated at various positions along the DNA template determined by the specific chain terminator chosen. For example, a reaction containing di-deoxy ATPs will contain a distribution of newly synthesized strands of varying lengths, each terminated at different (A) residues. For every template, the products of four separate reactions,

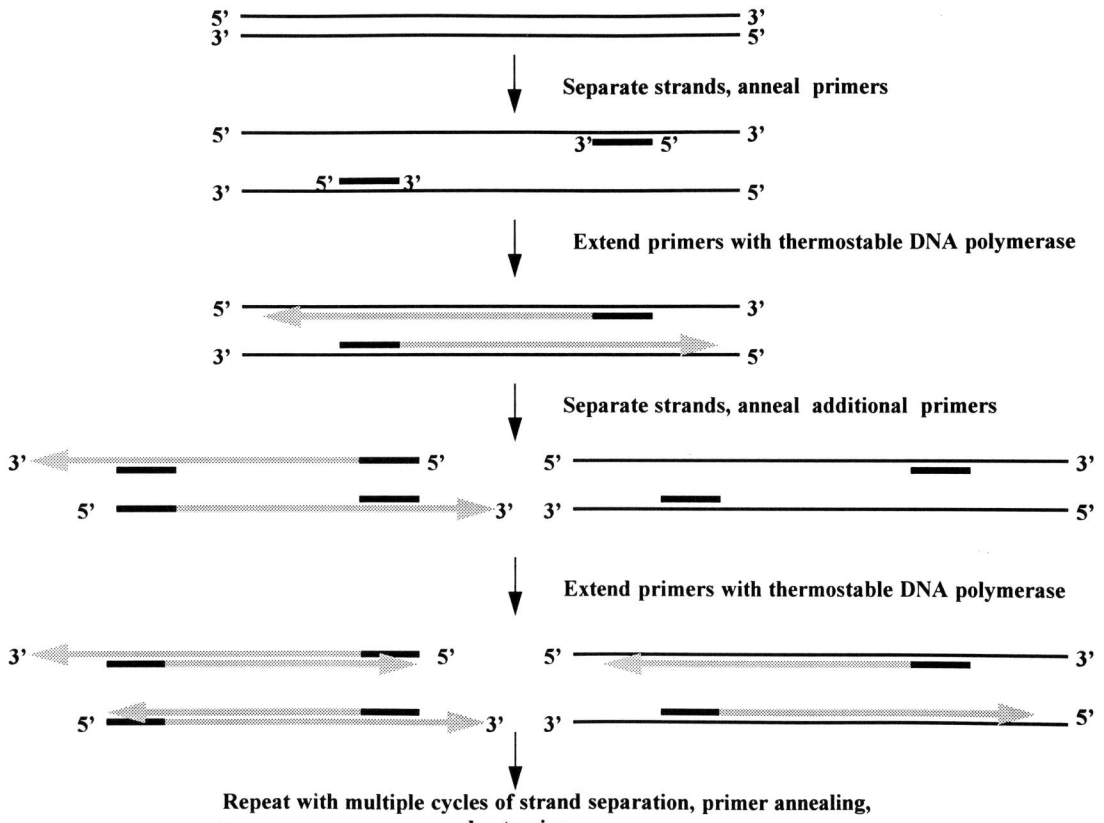

FIG. 28.6. The polymerase chain reaction. The PCR provides another method with which to generate essentially unlimited quantities of specific DNA fragments. In a basic PCR experiment, the DNA template is denatured by heating at near boiling temperature to separate the two strands. The temperature of the reaction in then reduced to allow short oligonucleotide primers (15–25 nucleotides) to anneal to each individual strand through complementary base pairing. The primers must be of opposite orientation with their 3' ends facing each other. A thermostable DNA polymerase is then used to extend the DNA sequence from each primer in the 5' to 3' direction. The newly synthesized double-stranded DNA molecules can then be denatured again and subjected to multiple cycles of PCR, such that the desired DNA fragment is synthesized in an exponential fashion.

each containing a different di-deoxy nucleotide, can be analyzed on high resolution polyacrylamide gels. After autoradiography, a ladder of bands will be identified that displays the DNA sequence of the original template read from bottom to top (Fig. 28.7, *right panel*). When analyzing gene mutations in DNA isolated from primary tumors, it is important to keep in mind that unlike cultured tumor cell lines, primary tumors are invariably "contaminated" with normal cells. In addition, an individual gene mutation usually affects only one of the two alleles present in a given tumor cell. The other allele may be wild type, may be deleted, or may have sustained a separate independent mutation. An individual clone of a segment of DNA can, by definition, represent only one allele. For example, if the original sample contains 80% tumor cells and 20% normal cells, and only one allele of the target gene is mutated in the tumor cells, only 40% of the target sequence clones will be derived from mutant alleles. Thus, most sequence analyses are performed on templates that reflect the relative contribution of all alleles in a given sample (e.g., PCR products or pools of cloned products) (Fig. 28-7, *left panel*) rather than on individual clones, which may have been derived from normal rather than mutant alleles.

Methods of RNA Analysis

Mutations in the DNA of tumor cells are meaningful only if they affect the function of the proteins encoded by the mutant genes. Many gene mutations lead to alterations of gene expression reflected at the RNA as well as protein level. For example, amplification of the HER-2/*neu* oncogene frequently identified in ovarian carcinomas results in overexpression with increases in both Her-2/*neu* RNA and protein levels.[91] In contrast, deletions of the DCC gene in many colorectal carcinomas is associated with marked reduction of DCC RNA levels in the tumor cells.[27] Several techniques have been developed with which to analyze RNA levels in normal and neoplastic tissues. A few commonly used methods are described below.

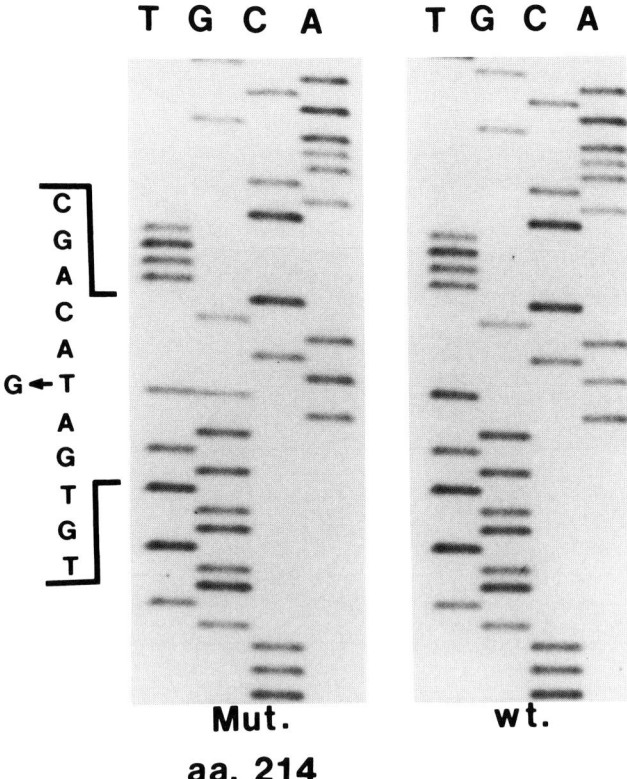

FIG. 28.7. DNA sequencing (Sanger method). DNA sequence analysis is used often to detect subtle gene mutations in human tumors. Most mutations are acquired somatically (are not present in the patient's normal/germline DNA). **Right panel** (wild type; *wt*): Sequence of the p53 gene in DNA isolated from the patient's normal myometrium. **Left panel** (mutant; *mt*): Sequence of the p53 gene in DNA isolated from the same patient's cervical carcinoma. In addition to the band in the "T" lane seen in normal DNA, the tumor DNA contains a new parallel band in the "G" lane, indicating a T to G point mutation at codon 214 of the p53 gene. The residual band in the "T" lane may represent the contribution of DNA from normal cells contaminating the original sample, and/or from the wild-type copy of p53 in the tumor cells. (Reprinted with permission from the American Journal of Pathology, ref. 48).

NORTHERN BLOTTING

Using straightforward extraction techniques, total cellular RNA can be isolated from the tissues to be studied. Total cellular RNA consists of ribosomal, transfer, and messenger RNA and only 2–5% of total RNA is mRNA. Therefore, it may be desirable to enrich the RNA sample for mRNA. This enrichment may be accomplished by selection for RNA molecules with polyadenylated 3′ ends [poly(A) RNA], which are added only to mRNA molecules after transcription. The total cellular or poly(A) RNA is then size-separated by electrophoresis through agarose gels. As in a Southern blot, the RNA is transferred from the

gel to a solid matrix such as nylon membrane, then hybridized to a gene-specific probe (DNA, RNA, or oligonucleotide). Autoradiography results in bands whose relative intensity reflects levels of RNA specific for the gene detected by the probe (Fig. 28.8). When comparing signal intensity between two or more samples, it is important that equal quantities of total RNA are loaded in each lane. To control for equal loading, Northern blot analyses often include hybridization to probes detecting genes such as actin or glyceraldehyde phosphate dehydrogenase (GDPH), whose expression remains relatively constant, regardless of tissue type or other factors.

REVERSE-TRANSCRIPTASE PCR

Northern blotting is an effective method to study expression of specific genes. However, the technique is limited to analysis of genes with relatively high expression levels and requires fairly large quantities of fresh tissue as a source of intact, undegraded RNA. Again, the discovery of PCR has led to the development of gene expression assays that capitalize on PCR's great sensitivity and applicability to even minute tissue samples. The reverse-transcriptase PCR (RT-PCR) method takes advantage of normal mRNA processing. As discussed above, the initial RNA transcript is an RNA copy of the DNA coding strand. However, gene-specific expression is reflected in RNA molecules that have undergone splicing (joining of exons with removal of intronic sequences). Using an enzyme called *reverse transcriptase* isolated from certain RNA tumor viruses, DNA copies (**complementary DNAs or cDNAs**) of the RNA molecules present in total RNA can be synthesized in vitro. This cDNA can be used as a template for PCR using primers specific for the gene of interest. If primers are chosen from two different exons within the target gene, the size of the PCR product generated by amplification of spliced templates (expressed sequences) will be smaller than that generated from unspliced templates or from genomic DNA. In fact, primers may be spread out so far on genomic DNA that amplification cannot occur at all (Fig. 28.9). As with Northern blotting, it is helpful to include primers detecting genes with little variation of gene expression, in order to control for equal starting material as well as for integrity of the amplified product.

IN SITU HYBRIDIZATION

When applied to the study of primary tissues, Northern blotting and RT-PCR evaluate specific gene expression in pools of cells that usually reflect some combination of tumor cells and bystanding normal cells. Furthermore, these methods are not easily applied to studying variations of gene expression within a given lesion or within different cell types of a tissue sample. A method called *in situ hybridization* allows detection of specific gene expression in

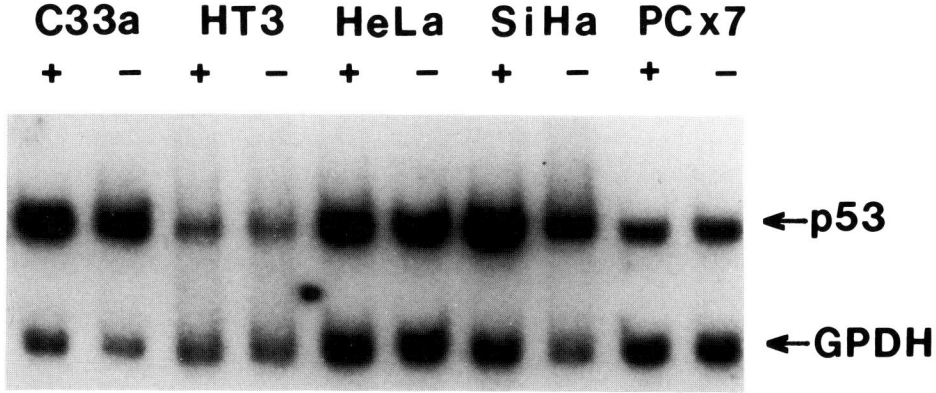

FIG. 28.8. Northern blot. Northern blot analysis is a method used to analyze gene expression and alterations of gene expression in tumor cells. An example is shown in which a blot of total RNA isolated from several cervical carcinoma cell lines has been hybridized to a radiolabeled p53 gene probe and a GPDH (glyceraldehyde phosphate dehydrogenase) gene control probe. Lanes labeled (+) represent RNA from irradiated tumor cells, whereas lanes labeled (−) represent RNA from untreated cells. Irradiation does not appear to alter p53 gene expression at the RNA level because the intensity of bands detected by the p53 probe is the same in the irradiated and untreated samples when normalized to the intensity of the signal from the control probe.

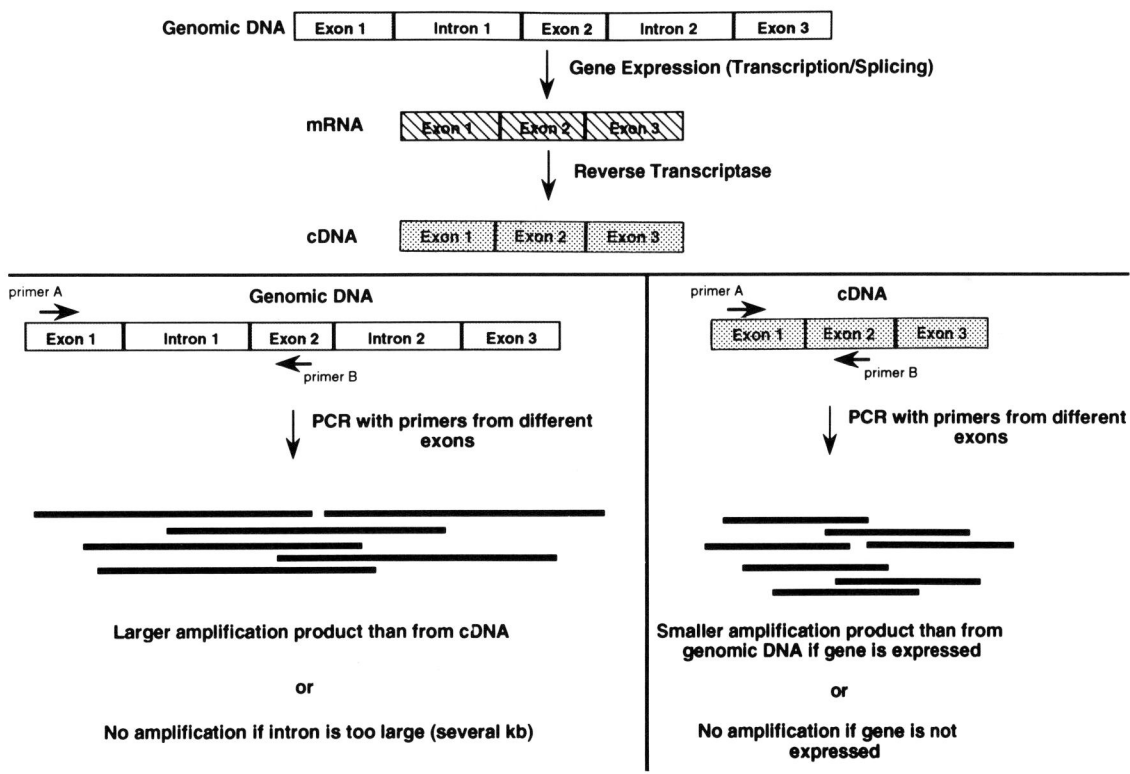

FIG. 28.9. Reverse transcriptase PCR. RT-PCR is an extremely sensitive assay for gene expression. After transcription of a gene, the initial RNA transcript undergoes splicing. Thus, in mRNA, exons are spliced together and intronic sequences are excluded. A complementary DNA molecule (cDNA) can be synthesized by the enzyme reverse transcriptase, using mRNA as the template. This cDNA, which also excludes introns, can then be used as a template for PCR in which primers are chosen from within different exons. If the gene is expressed, the two exons should be close enough together in the cDNA to allow amplification of a sequence of predicted size. Since genomic DNA contains introns, the PCR product will be longer than that from cDNA. Alternatively, the primers may be spread so far apart (introns can be several hundred kilobases or more) that amplification cannot occur at all. The size of the PCR products can be determined by gel electrophoresis.

individual cells within the context of the tissue as a whole. The principles of this method are straightforward. Sections of the tissue to be studied are cut and mounted on microscope slides. The sections are then hybridized to labeled RNA probes specific for the gene being studied, under conditions that allow the probes to anneal to complementary mRNA anywhere in the tissue section. Subsequent detection of hybridized probes (autoradiography for radiolabeled probes or colorimetric detection for nonradioactive probes) with counterstaining of the tissue sample allows localization of the signal to individual cells. The in situ hybridization method also can be used to detect DNA in tissues, if genomic DNA rather than RNA is used as a probe. For example, type-specific DNA probes can be used to detect human papillomavirus DNA in cervical biopsies and exfoliated cervical cells.

Methods of Protein Analysis

Gene mutations and alterations of RNA expression in tumor cells achieve significance only through their effects on the function of the proteins that they encode. As a result of genetic alterations, proteins may be overexpressed, underexpressed, or expressed as mutant forms with aberrant function. Several laboratory techniques have been developed that allow detection of specific proteins in neoplastic and normal cells. Essentially all of these techniques use antibodies directed at the target protein as part of the detection scheme.

IMMUNOHISTOCHEMISTRY

To most pathologists, immunohistochemical staining (discussed in detail in Chapter 26, Immunohistochemistry) is the most familiar assay of protein detection in tissues. Immunohistochemistry is used widely as a diagnostic and research tool. Like in situ hybridization, immunohistochemistry allows detection of specific proteins in individual cells within the context of the tissue as a whole as well as their subcellular localization (e.g., nuclear, cytoplasmic, or membrane bound). Furthermore, it does not require the use of radioactive reagents. However, the technique is not without limitations, often related to the quality and availability of antibodies targeted at the proteins of interest. Thus, some assays may lack sensitivity or specificity, or may be applicable to only fresh-frozen rather than formalin-fixed tissues. In these cases, other methods of protein detection may be more appropriate.

IMMUNOBLOTTING (WESTERN BLOTTING)

This technique combines the specificity of immunochemical detection with the resolution of gel electrophoresis. Immunoblotting can be used to determine the presence, quantity, and size of a target protein. Thus, tumors can be analyzed for changes in protein levels or the presence of mutant (e.g., truncated) forms. Typically, an unlabeled solution of proteins (usually an extract of cells or tissue) is prepared in gel electrophoresis sample buffer. The proteins are then size fractionated by electrophoresis through a polyacrylamide gel followed by electrophoretic transfer of the proteins to a membrane. Nonspecific binding sites are first blocked, then the location of specific antigens is determined using a labeled antibody specific for the target. In some cases, specific protein is detected with unlabeled primary antibody followed by incubation with radiolabeled secondary antibody or secondary antibody conjugated to moieties allowing nonradioactive colorimetric or chemical detection. These latter methods often result in signal amplification and enhanced detection sensitivity. The major factor determining the success of an immunoblotting assay is the nature of the epitopes recognized by the antibodies. The high resolution gel electrophoresis techniques required to separate proteins typically involve denaturation of the proteins in the sample. Thus, only epitopes resistant to denaturation will be recognized by the antibodies. In addition, the target protein must be present in sufficient quantities (approximately one part per 150,000).[36]

IMMUNOPRECIPITATION

This method also combines the specificity of the antigen–antibody interaction with the resolution of gel electrophoresis. Both immunoblotting and immunoprecipitation evaluate protein expression in pools of cells rather than in individual cells. Typically, the target protein is radioactively labeled in vivo by growing cells in the presence of a labeled precursor such as a radioactive amino acid. The labeled antigen is then extracted from cells in an appropriate buffer and incubated with specific antibodies under conditions which allow formation of immune complexes. A solid phase matrix containing staphylococcal protein A (which binds the Fc portion of antibodies) is added and allowed to adsorb the immune complexes. Unbound proteins are removed by washing the solid phase, leaving the purified antibody–antigen complex bound to the matrix. The purified complexes can be eluted from the matrix, then analyzed by gel electrophoresis to determine protein presence, size, and quantity. This method also may be used to study the rate of synthesis or degradation of specific proteins, interactions with other cellular macromolecules, and the presence or absence of some post-translational modifications.

The appropriate choice of protein detection methods is determined by several factors, including the type of information sought, the nature of the specific antigen–antibody interaction, and availability of reagents. In practice, the best method of analyzing specific proteins in specific cell types often is determined empirically.

Transferring Genes into Mammalian Cells (Transfection)

Research on the genetic basis of cancer has led to the identification and cloning of several cancer-related genes, including numerous oncogenes and tumor suppressor genes. However, many studies aimed at determining the function of altered genes and their normal counterparts require introduction of these genes into living cells. For instance, the effects of activated oncogene expression in normal cells and tumor suppressor gene expression in tumor cells can be studied with gene transfer experiments. Several techniques have been developed that allow expression of exogenous genes in living cells maintained in cell culture. More recently, sophisticated methods have been devised that permit investigators to introduce new genes or alter existing genes in intact animals. These advances have greatly enhanced our ability to model numerous human diseases in the laboratory.

The most common means of introducing exogenous genes into mammalian cells involves cloning the gene of interest into a plasmid vector that is then delivered into the cytoplasm of recipient cells using any of several techniques. Alternatively, viral vectors containing the gene of interest are used to infect host cells. Most vectors contain a selectable marker such as antibiotic resistance, which allows efficient selection of cells that have received the exogenous construct. Expression of the cloned gene typically is driven by an upstream promoter present in the vector. Depending on the transfection method used, type of vector, and type of recipient cells, exogenous DNA can be introduced into a large percentage of host cells. However, for most vectors, only a few (1 in 10^3–10^6) transfected cells incorporate the exogenous DNA stably into the host genome. The remaining cells fail to integrate the DNA, which disappears from these cells in a matter of days. During this period, the transfected cells transiently express the exogenous gene using the host's transcriptional machinery. Selection for appropriate antibiotic resistance yields clones of cells that have stably integrated the expression construct and that are capable of expressing the exogenous gene indefinitely.

Genetic Linkage and Mapping

Inherited predispositions to particular tumor types result from germline mutations in specific genes. For example, the genes responsible for some forms of neurofibromatosis, retinoblastoma, Wilms' tumor, and adenomatous polyposis coli already have been identified and cloned. Active searches are underway for the genes responsible for familial ovarian and endometrial carcinomas (discussed in greater detail later in this chapter). To localize disease genes to particular chromosomes, researchers often study families with an inherited predisposition to that disease

using a method called *linkage analysis.* Linkage describes the tendency of genetic loci to be inherited together as a result of their location on the same chromosome. When homologous chromosomes pair during meiosis, they exchange segments in a process called *recombination.* The farther apart two loci are, the greater the chance that recombination will occur between them. In contrast, if two loci are close together recombination between them will be rare. Loci on different chromosomes would be expected to segregate independently. As part of a linkage analysis, co-inheritance of polymorphic markers (determined by Southern blot analysis) and disease genes (manifested by the phenotype of individuals) are followed within a family, and the odds of their being inherited separately (unlinked or not on the same chromosome) versus together (linked or on the same chromosome) are calculated. Although a thorough discussion of linkage analyses is well beyond the scope of this chapter, suffice it to say that evaluation of the inheritance patterns of multiple polymorphic markers with respect to each other and to disease phenotype can allow assignment of disease genes to particular chromosomes and generate a map of marker order along that chromosome. Identification of markers more and more closely linked to a disease phenotype can lead ultimately to localization of genes responsible for specific diseases. The DNA of individuals affected by the particular disease can then be examined for the presence of germline mutations in the disease gene.

A Molecular Model of Human Carcinogenesis

There are two fundamental properties of human tumors that are inextricably linked. First, tumors develop and progress through a multistep process and second, they evolve from the clonal expansion of a single cell. Many lines of evidence have clearly demonstrated that human cancers arise through a series of independent events. Early epidemiologic studies of age-dependent tumor incidence indicated that the kinetics were dependent on the fifth or sixth power of elapsed time, suggesting that the tumors arose secondary to five or six independent and successive rate-limiting steps.[35] However, the nature of the biologic events underlying this multistep process was unclear. Not only did these studies highlight that multiple events were necessary to produce neoplastic growth, but they also hinted at the second fundamental feature of human tumors, clonality. These important features of tumors can be understood easily if an assumption is made about the growth of normal cells. The assumption is that cells must have multiple regulatory mechanisms to ensure normal cell growth. Therefore, it is likely that each of these mechanisms may have to be overcome in an individual cell to manifest the transformed phenotype. Thus, the cell that accumulates the multiple changes would be selected for because it has obtained the capacity to proliferate and ultimately form a tumor mass (Fig. 28.10). Over the past decade molecular studies have confirmed both of these hypotheses through direct experimental approaches. Furthermore, such studies have led to the finding that specific mutant proteins, encoded by mutated genes, are responsible for the altered growth properties of the tumor cells.

Recently, molecular studies of colorectal tumorigenesis have established a model for the molecular basis of the multistep theory.[26] Several factors make colorectal tumorigenesis particularly attractive for molecular analyses. Pathologists made the important observation that most color-

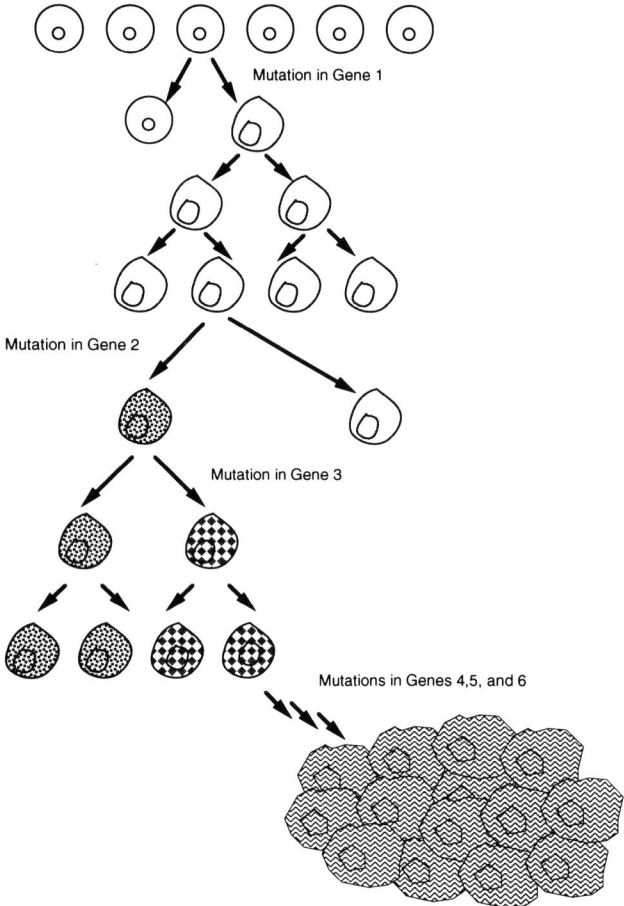

FIG. 28.10. **Accumulation of genetic alterations and clonal selection during tumorigenesis.** A single normal cell sustains a mutation in a gene that gives it a growth advantage over its normal counterparts. This cell continues to divide and one of its progeny undergoes a mutation in a second gene, which provides a further growth advantage. In a subsequent cell division, one of the daughter cells sustains a third mutation. Each mutation may confer a different type of selective advantage such as increased growth rate, loss of contact inhibition, ability to invade, etc. The mutational process continues until a subpopulation of cells accumulates enough mutations in oncogenes and tumor suppressor genes to result in the fully transformed phenotype.

ectal cancers develop along a continuum via several histopathologically distinct stages, from normal colonic epithelium through benign lesions (adenomas) of increasing size and cytological atypia, to frankly invasive carcinomas.[97] For this reason, it was thought that the progressive development of colorectal cancer might provide an in vivo model system for the multistep theory of tumorigenesis. Furthermore, colorectal cancer is common and tissue is accessible, either by colonoscopic biopsy or surgical resection, from all the lesions in the continuum. Consequently, each lesion in the progression can be studied at the molecular level. Using molecular genetic techniques, investigators have identified several genes that are responsible, at least in part, for the development of colorectal cancer. In addition, studies of the colorectal system have demonstrated that the number of genes altered during tumorigenesis accumulates with the progression of the disease.[102] As mentioned earlier, progeny of the cell that has overcome the numerous growth regulatory controls present in normal cells will be selected for and ultimately predominate. The genes identified in colorectal cancer development fall into two major categories: **oncogenes** and **tumor suppressor genes.** Alterations in these two types of genes are now thought to be involved in the development of the vast majority of human tumors. Recently, a third class of genes involved in colorectal tumorigenesis has been identified. These genes, termed mutator genes, are believed to increase the frequency of mutations at other genetic loci in tumor cells and their progenitors. Some of these mutations, if they occur in oncogenes or tumor suppressor genes, will confer a growth advantage and be selected for in affected cells. Therefore, understanding the normal function of the proteins encoded by these three classes of genes and how they go awry in neoplasia, is critical to unraveling the etiology and pathogenesis of cancer.

For historical reasons, oncogenes will be discussed first, as they were the first genes identified to play a role in the pathogenesis of human tumors. To date, many more oncogenes have been identified than tumor suppressor genes, with a current total of approximately 50–60.[10] They were first identified as the normal cellular counterparts of the transforming genes of "oncogenic" viruses. The genes from the oncogenic viruses that were responsible for the transforming capabilities of the virus were termed oncogenes. Subsequently, normal human cells were found to contain genes that were very similar in sequence to the viral oncogenes. These cellular genes are referred to as **proto-oncogenes,** because they are not capable of transforming cells in their normal or **wild-type** state. The proteins encoded by proto-oncogenes are thought to be involved in controlling normal cell growth and proliferation in a positive manner. Typically, these genes cycle "on" and "off" in such a manner that the "on" state promotes growth and proliferation. These genes play a role in tumorigenesis when they are "activated" by a mutational event that alters the function of the gene product. When they are mutated to an active form they become oncogenes. The most common molecular mechanisms for activating proto-oncogenes are gene amplification, point mutation, and gene rearrangement. The activating mutations basically lead to the constant "on" state of the gene product, which provides the constant proliferative stimulus necessary in tumorigenesis. For this reason, oncogenes tend to behave in a "dominant" fashion, requiring the activation of only one copy of the gene while leaving the other copy of the gene in its wild-type state. Both amplification and rearrangement of oncogenes often lead to an increase in the amount of their protein products with a concomitant increase in the proteins' functional activity. Gene amplification is created by over-replication of a specific portion of a chromosome such that multiple copies of the amplified gene are either retained on the chromosome or as extrachromosomal fragments. Gene amplification thus results in numerous copies of the proto-oncogene from which the product can be expressed. Chromosomal rearrangements increase gene expression by different mechanisms than gene amplification. For example, a chromosomal rearrangement can alter the expression of a proto-oncogene by replacing its normal regulatory region with one from a gene that is highly expressed, leading to increased expression of the proto-oncogene. In addition, chromosomal rearrangements can join the coding portions of two genes together, resulting in a hybrid product that is functionally overactive. Point mutations also can create products that are constitutively active by causing substitutions in critical amino acids of the protein.

Proto-oncogenes have been found to encode proteins that fall into four major classes based on their functions. These include **growth factors, growth factor receptors, cytoplasmic signal transduction molecules,** and **nuclear transcription factors.** Growth factors are secreted molecules that interact with growth factor receptors that are expressed on the cell surface. The interaction of these molecules sets in motion the transmission of a signal that reaches the cell nucleus and ultimately results in cellular proliferation. Therefore, the signal must involve molecules in the cytoplasm (cytoplasmic signal transduction molecules) to send the appropriate message to nuclear proteins that control the nuclear functions necessary for DNA synthesis. For any one of these classes it is possible to imagine how aberrations that lead to a constitutively active product would influence cellular proliferation. This classification also emphasizes the fact that normal cells have a variety of mechanisms operative throughout the cell to ensure control of proliferation. In the final section of this chapter individual oncogenes will be discussed as they pertain to the specific gynecological tumors.

Tumor suppressor genes, the second category of genes involved in tumorigenesis, have been defined as genes whose gene products normally regulate cell growth and differentiation in a negative manner. Therefore, it is loss of the normal function of their gene products that allows cells to escape growth regulation. To date, less than a dozen tumor suppressor genes have been identified and cloned.[10] Before tumor suppressor genes were identified, their possible existence was proposed based on the results of numerous experiments in which tumor cells were fused with normal cells.[37,95] These studies demonstrated that tumor-normal hybrid cells lost many features of the transformed cells, suggesting that the normal cells provided functions that the tumor cells had lost. In addition, epidemiologic studies of retinoblastoma, a childhood eye tumor, led Knudson to propose what is now known as the "two hit hypothesis."[51,52] He suggested that the development of retinoblastoma required two separate mutational events. Subsequent cytogenetic studies of retinoblastomas revealed a consistent loss of genetic material on the long arm of chromosome 13.[30,59,73] Therefore, the commonly deleted region of chromosome 13q was used as an indication for the presence of the gene responsible for the development of retinoblastoma. This region was analyzed carefully and a specific gene from within the deleted region was identified and named the retinoblastoma (Rb) gene.[56] Further molecular studies showed that the second "hit" was the inactivation of the remaining normal copy of Rb,[19] such that the other Rb allele is not lost by gross chromosomal deletion but is "functionally lost" by mutations that inactivate the gene product. It is now recognized that deletion of the Rb-containing region of chromosome 13 is actually the second hit and the first hit is the inactivation of the other allele by intragenic mutation. Thus, the loss event typically follows rather than precedes the mutation. Furthermore, patients with early onset and/or bilateral retinoblastomas have Rb gene mutations in their germline DNA.[19] This finding correlates with Knudson's two hit hypothesis. Patients who inherit one mutant and one wild-type copy of Rb, present in every cell of the body, require only one additional hit in the cell that will ultimately give rise to the tumor. In contrast, the development of sporadic tumors requires two hits in a single cell, which is statistically much less likely, explaining the early onset and bilaterality of retinoblastoma in the inherited form of the disease. Thus, patients who inherit a mutant copy of the Rb gene inherit a predisposition to retinoblastoma. In any event, the finding that the target of the "second hit" was the other copy of the Rb gene correlated with the cell fusion studies that had suggested that some genes important in tumor development behaved in a "recessive" manner, implying that both copies of the gene must be inactivated for the effects of the mutations to be manifested. Since the identification of the Rb gene, experimental studies have shown that its gene product plays a role in the regulation of the cell cycle.[34] Therefore, the loss of normal Rb function may allow cells to proliferate in an uncontrolled manner, an important feature of neoplastic cells. These molecular studies thus validated Knudson's hypothesis and provided important evidence for the existence of a class of genes whose "loss of function" contributes to the neoplastic phenotype. In addition, these experiments provided a paradigm that could be used to search for other candidate tumor suppressor genes.

As mentioned above, during the development of retinoblastomas, one copy of the Rb gene typically is inactivated through deletion of a portion of chromosome 13, which contains the Rb gene. The example provided by retinoblastomas suggests that such regions of loss would target the location of tumor suppressor genes. In other words, identification of chromosomal regions frequently deleted in a specific tumor type presumably would allow localization of suppressor gene candidates important in the development of those tumors. Such an approach was taken by researchers interested in identifying the genetic alterations responsible for colorectal tumorigenesis. Investigators examined numerous colorectal tumors for chromosomal losses by comparing the DNA from the same individual's normal cells with DNA from their tumor cells. This resulted in a landmark study uncovering four chromosomal regions that undergo frequent and consistent losses in colorectal cancers.[101] Since the initial discovery of these regions of chromosomal loss, tumor suppressor genes have been identified that reside within three of the commonly deleted regions: (1) the *adenomatous polyposis coli* (APC) gene on chromosome 5q,[50,69] (2) a gene on the long arm of chromosome 18 called the *deleted in colorectal carcinoma* (DCC) gene,[27] and (3) the p53 gene, which is located on chromosome 17p.[5] A short discussion of each of the genes and their gene products follows.

The APC gene is the gene responsible for the hereditary disease known as familial adenomatous polyposis. This disease accounts for approximately 1% of colorectal cancers and is characterized by numerous colorectal polyps and an early age of onset of colorectal cancer. The most frequent type of mutations in the APC gene are nonsense mutations, creating truncated proteins.[92] The normal APC protein has been shown to be located primarily in the cytoplasm. At present the function of the APC protein is unknown. However, immunohistochemical studies have suggested that it is expressed in the nonproliferating epithelial cells of the colonic crypt.[92] This finding is consistent with a gene whose loss of function may contribute to tumorigenesis, as its expression may be inversely correlated with proliferation. Studies currently are underway to uncover the normal function of the APC gene product.

The gene on chromosome 18q, DCC, encodes a transmembrane protein with an extracellular domain with significant homology to a class of molecules involved in cell adhesion. Although DCC has not been shown experimentally to be responsible for cell adhesion, this possibility is intriguing. Many experimental studies have demonstrated that neoplastic cells have altered adhesive properties. Furthermore, in vitro studies have suggested that loss of adhesion may be important in the development of the invasive capability of tumor cells. The DCC gene is expressed in normal colon but its expression is lost in most colorectal cell lines and primary colorectal cancers.[27] This finding suggests that the loss of DCC expression contributes to the neoplastic phenotype and is in keeping with the idea that loss of adhesion may be critical in the development of malignant tumors.

The other tumor suppressor gene identified was p53, which is located on the short arm of chromosome 17. The p53 gene has become one of the most well studied tumor suppressor genes because, to date, it is the most commonly mutated gene in human cancer.[40] Besides its involvement in colorectal tumorigenesis, it is mutated in a wide variety of human cancers including common malignancies such as breast and lung carcinomas. As will become clear later, p53 alterations also are important in the pathogenesis of many gynecological tumors.

The p53 gene encodes a protein that is located in the nucleus and binds specific DNA sequences.[46] Studies of p53 suggest that, through its DNA binding, it regulates the expression of other genes that ultimately control cell proliferation. Therefore, the loss of p53 function leads to abnormalities in growth control by releasing the normal regulation of numerous other genes. As with Rb, one copy of the p53 gene usually is inactivated by intragenic point mutations that typically lead to amino acid substitutions in the p53 protein.[40] Most of the mutant proteins lose their ability to bind to the specific DNA sequences.[46] Consequently, they also lose their ability to regulate gene expression. Inactivation of the remaining copy of p53 gene occurs through subsequent chromosomal loss events.[6] The story of p53 gets slightly more complicated because it normally functions as a homodimer, meaning that two molecules of p53 form a complex and function as a unit. Consequently, mutations in one copy of p53 can have an effect on the function of the p53 protein expressed by the remaining wild-type gene through formation of a complex containing one mutant protein and one wild type protein. This mutant/wild-type complex is no longer capable of normal function. In this context the p53 gene is not truly recessive, because mutation of only one allele has phenotypic consequences. On the other hand, p53 is not behaving in a classically dominant manner either, because the remaining wild-type gene produces some normal protein that can still form homodimers and maintain some residual normal function. Therefore, the term "dominant negative" has been coined to describe this type of function. Presumably, inactivation of the second wild-type allele must confer yet an additional growth advantage, since most tumors contain only mutant p53. Further information on the function of p53 and its role in tumorigenesis will be presented in the cervical tumor section of the chapter.

The third class of genes, mutator genes, has only recently been recognized. These genes were identified based on a phenotype of colorectal tumor cells removed from patients with hereditary nonpolyposis colorectal cancer (HNPCC). DNA extracted from these tumor cells revealed instability of microsatellite DNA sequences. Microsatellite DNA sequences are short tandem repeats made up of di- or trinucleotides that are distributed throughout the human genome. Through an elegant series of experiments, mutator genes have been shown to be responsible for microsatellite instability.[27a,54a] These genes encode proteins involved in DNA mismatch repair. Alterations of these genes interfere with the ability of affected cells to repair mistakes generated during DNA replication. Thus, cells with altered mutator genes replicate DNA errors more frequently than normal cells, allowing fixation of such alterations in daughter cells.

The application of molecular biological techniques to the investigation of human tumorigenesis has rapidly elevated our level of understanding of this complex process. Over the past two decades molecular studies have provided keen insights into the cellular mechanisms responsible for characteristics of neoplastic cells that had long been observed in vivo and in vitro. An in-depth study of colorectal tumorigenesis uncovered the molecular basis of the multistep theory of tumorigenesis. This model system demonstrates that it is the accumulation of genetic alterations in both oncogenes and tumor suppressor genes that underlies the progression of the neoplastic phenotype. Further molecular studies undoubtedly will result in the discovery of additional target genes and a greater understanding of how alterations in these genes contribute to the development of human cancer.

Molecular Biology of Gynecological Tumors

The identification and characterization of genetic alterations in gynecological tumors are just beginning. Although previous cytogenetic studies have identified a few consistent chromosomal abnormalities in certain gynecological tumors (e.g., rearrangements involving chromosomes 7, 12, and 14 in uterine leiomyomas),[39,68] relatively little is known about the specific genes involved in the development and progression of female genital tract neoplasms. However, the development of powerful molecular biological tools has led to a virtual explosion of studies aimed at elucidating the molecular pathogenesis of these tumors. Most current research is directed at the more common malignancies, namely epithelial tumors of the cervix/vulva, endometrium, and ovary. Therefore, only studies pertaining to these tumor types will be reviewed in this chapter.

Cervical Cancer

Most cervical cancers are squamous, and are preceded by *s*quamous *i*ntraepithelial *l*esions (SIL, also known as *c*ervical *i*ntraepithelial *n*eoplasia, or CIN). The incidence and death rate from cervical cancer have decreased markedly, largely as a result of cytological screening and treatment of putative precursor lesions. Although the death rate from cervical cancer is relatively low in the United States, cervical cancer is one of the most common types of cancer and a major cause of cancer-related deaths in women in developing countries.[74]

Epidemiologic studies have consistently implicated a sexually transmitted agent as an important risk factor in cervical tumorigenesis. In the 1960s and 1970s, DNA viruses such as herpes simplex virus (HSV) and in the 1980s, human papillomavirus (HPV) have been examined extensively as candidate etiologic agents. Early attention focused on HSV-2 because serologic studies found a strong association between HSV-2 infection and cervical neoplasia. More recent molecular studies have failed to demonstrate this association convincingly and at least one large scale prospective epidemiologic study failed to demonstrate a role for HSV-2 infection in the development of cervical cancer.[103] Thus, interest in HSV as a causative agent has waned.

In 1976, zur Hausen proposed that certain types of HPV were likely candidates for sexually transmissible agents that contribute to cervical tumorigenesis.[113] The past few years have seen a remarkable convergence of several lines of investigation implicating involvement of HPV in the development of cervical carcinoma. Although initial suspicions were aroused primarily by molecular biological and immunohistochemical studies, epidemiologic data have provided convincing corroborating evidence supporting this association. More recent molecular studies also have provided insight into probable mechanisms by which oncogenic HPVs contribute to cervical neoplasia. As a result, there is now sufficient evidence to implicate HPV infection as a major risk factor in cervical carcinogenesis.

Papillomaviruses are small DNA viruses composed of an approximately 8-kb double-stranded circular genome enclosed by a 55-nm viral capsid. More than 60 different HPV types have been characterized on the basis of differences in DNA sequence, and a single host may be infected by multiple types of HPVs. Based on extensive examination of the association of different types of HPV with exophytic condylomas, SIL, and cervical cancers, genital HPVs can be classified broadly into two groups: those associated with benign lesions (primarily HPVs 6, 11, 30, 34, 40, 42, 43, 44, and 57) and those associated with invasive carcinomas (primarily HPVs 16, 18, 31, 33, 35, 39, 45, 51, 52, 56, and 58). This classification into low risk (non–cancer associated) and high risk (cancer associated) types is reflected in vitro by the ability of cloned DNA of only the high-risk types to efficiently immortalize primary human keratinocytes.[21,77] "Oncogenic" or high-risk HPV types are detected in 90–95% of invasive squamous cervical cancers,[80] depending on the detection method used. In condylomas and in all grades of SIL, the HPV genome usually is maintained as an episome (free circular molecule), whereas in most invasive tumors and tumor cell lines, the viral genome is stably integrated into the host cell DNA.[15] Although several studies have failed to find a common point of integration in the host genome, at least two groups have found HPV sequences integrated near cellular oncogenes (specifically c-*myc* and n-*myc*) in at least a few cervical cancer cell lines.[11,20] Interruption of the oncogenes' regulatory sequences potentially could lead to oncogene overexpression/activation. Although there may be variation in the point of viral integration into the host genome, the site where the viral genome breaks is remarkably consistent. The viral genome contains several open reading frames (ORFs) encoding both "early" and "late" proteins. In almost all cases, integration interrupts the E1 and/or E2 ORFs but leaves the E6 and E7 ORFs intact. Integration may serve to release E6 and E7 from normal transcriptional regulation by virally encoded regulatory proteins such as E2. Together, the proteins encoded by E6 and E7 of oncogenic HPVs can efficiently immortalize primary keratinocytes.[9]

Although the association of high-risk HPV infection with invasive cervical cancer provides compelling evidence for HPV as a causative factor, several lines of evidence suggest that HPV infection alone is insufficient to bring about the fully malignant phenotype. First, although high-risk HPV E6 and E7 can efficiently immortalize primary cells, a fully transformed phenotype rarely appears until after numerous passages.[38,66] Second, although infection with high-risk HPV type is quite common,[109] only a small percentage of infected women develop invasive cervical cancer. Third, those who develop cancer generally do so long after initial infection with HPV (20 or more years in most cases). Taken together, these findings suggest that in addition to high-risk HPV infection, other events are required for the development of cervical cancer. This requirement for other genetic alterations is consistent with the multistep model of tumorigenesis discussed earlier in this chapter. Studies implicating involvement of both oncogenes and tumor suppressor genes in cervical tumorigenesis are accumulating. Data suggesting alterations of specific oncogenes are summarized in Table 28.1.

Although these findings are largely preliminary, they provide considerable evidence supporting oncogene activation in the development of at least some cervical carcinomas. Losses of heterozygosity of the short arm of chromosome 3[108] and of the short arm of 17[4] have been found with high frequency in cervical carcinomas, suggesting involvement of suppressor genes in these regions. More extensive allelic loss analyses are likely to implicate involvement of even more tumor suppressor genes.

As discussed earlier in this chapter, tumor suppressor genes may be inactivated through any of several genetic mechanisms including rearrangement, deletions, and point mutations. In addition, tumor suppressors may be inactivated at the protein level as well. Recent experiments pro-

Table 28.1. Summary of oncogene abnormalities in cervical carcinomas

Oncogene	Summary of results	Reference
ras group	Increased staining by immunohistochemistry in 39–57% of invasive squamous carcinomas, depending on type (170 cases evaluated)	Sagae et al.[83]
	Increased staining in 7/7 invasive carcinomas	Agnantis et al.[2]
c-Ha-*ras*	Loss of one allele in 10/28 informative cases, mutations in 7/29 advanced stage carcinomas	Riou et al.[79]
c-*myc*	Increased staining by immunohistochemistry in 8/17 early and 8/14 late stage carcinomas; overexpression correlated with poor prognosis	Sowani et al.[94]
c-*myc*	Increased staining by immunohistochemistry in 2/7 high-grade CIN and in 2/4 invasive carcinomas	Di Luca et al.[17]
c-*myc*	Amplification without structural gene rearrangement in 14/44 invasive carcinomas	Baker et al[8]
c-*myc*	Amplification and/or gene rearrangement in nearly 90% of 35 invasive carcinomas	Ocadiz etal.[70]

CIN, cervical intraepithelial lesion.

vide evidence for direct interaction between HPV oncoproteins and tumor suppressor gene products. Specifically, the E6 oncoprotein of the high-risk HPV types 16 and 18 has been shown to bind the tumor suppressor protein p53 with higher affinity than those of the low-risk types 6 and 11, and this binding appears to promote degradation of p53.[90,104] Similarly, the HPV16 E7 protein has been shown to bind the tumor suppressor protein Rb,[22] which may serve to inactivate Rb's suppressor function. As both p53 and Rb play important roles in cell cycle regulation, it follows that cells infected with high-risk HPVs may have a selective growth advantage over uninfected cells. Based on these observations, it was hypothesized that tumors lacking HPV DNA might harbor p53 and/or Rb gene mutations, whereas those containing HPV sequences might inactivate wild-type copies of these suppressor genes by binding their protein products. Recent studies of Scheffner et al.[89] and Crook et al.[14] support this hypothesis. Point mutations in the p53 and Rb genes were found only in cervical carcinoma cell lines that did not contain HPV whereas HPV-positive cell lines contained wild-type copies of these genes. However, evaluation of primary cervical carcinomas has yielded less straightforward results. In one recent study, tumors containing large copy numbers of oncogenic HPVs lacked p53 gene mutations as expected, but HPV-negative tumors similarly lacked p53 gene mutations.[31] In another study of 35 primary cervical tumors,[48] one HPV16-positive carcinoma was found to contain a missense mutation in p53. Again, all HPV-negative tumors lacked p53 gene mutations. These studies suggest that HPV infection and p53 gene mutation are not mutually exclusive and that many HPV-negative carcinomas may arise via a pathway independent of p53 inactivation. Nevertheless, p53 is an important target of inactivation in most cervical carcinomas and p53 gene mutation may play a role in the progression of at least some cervical tumors. Recently, Crook and Vousden identified p53 point mutations in metastases arising from HPV-positive cervical carcinomas.[13] Presumably, these mutations confer an additional growth advantage to cells containing HPV sequences, perhaps via a mechanism in which the mutant p53 protein escapes targeted degradation mediated by E6.

The molecular basis for variation in oncogenic potential between the high-risk and low-risk types of HPVs remains unclear. However, recent studies partially mapping functional domains of the E6 and E7 protein provide some insight. Münger et al.[67] have shown that some biochemical and biologic differences between E7 proteins of low-risk viruses such as HPV-6 and high-risk viruses such as HPV16 are determined by amino terminal sequences. Specifically, the amino-terminal half of E7 was found to determine transformation properties and affinity for binding to Rb. Furthermore, the DNA binding properties of the Rb gene product were found to be inhibited by HPV16 E7,[96] suggesting a mechanism through which E7-Rb interactions may contribute to tumor progression. Crook et al. have found that a C-terminal region of E6 conserved among all HPV types is important for p53 binding, whereas an N-terminal domain conserved only among oncogenic HPV types mediates p53 degradation.[12]

Several recent studies suggest that p53 may be functioning as an "emergency brake" in cells that have sustained damage to DNA.[45,53] Cells damaged by irradiation or DNA strand-breaking drugs arrest in the G1-S portion of the cell cycle, presumably allowing the cells to undertake DNA repair and avoid the accumulation of genetic lesions. This cell cycle arrest is temporally associated with increases in wild-type p53 and is not seen in cells containing mutant p53 genes. Kessis et al. hypothesized that oncogenic HPV E6 expression may similarly disrupt this p53-mediated cellular response to DNA damage. When HPV16 E6 was transfected into cells exhibiting the normal DNA damage response, p53 protein levels were essentially undetectable and the cell cycle arrest after DNA damage was abolished.[49] Thus, it appears infection with HPV16 may promote genomic instability, leading to the acquisition of additional genetic changes required for cervical tumorigenesis. The molecular mechanism through which this occurs may involve the inactivation of p53 mediated by the HPV E6 protein.

The preceding discussion pertains not only to squamous carcinomas of the cervix, but to all cell types that can be infected by high-risk HPVs. HPV sequences frequently are identified in cervical adenocarcinomas as well as in its precursor lesion, adenocarcinoma in situ. As with squamous cancers, invasive adenocarcinomas typically contain the HPV genome integrated into host genomic DNA.[61] Most studies have shown that HPV18 predominates in invasive endocervical adenocarcinomas,[18] in contrast to the squamous carcinomas in which HPV16 sequences are more common. Although the various high-risk HPV types presumably contribute to tumor development and progression through similar molecular mechanisms, the molecular basis for variation in oncogenic potential between different types remains unclear and may be a consequence of differences in the way the viral oncoproteins interact with cellular tumor suppressors. Whether or not cervical adenocarcinomas and squamous carcinomas will share other molecular steps in the carcinogenesis pathway in addition to HPV infection has yet to be determined.

Vulvar Cancer

Like cervical cancer, invasive vulvar carcinomas are associated with intraepithelial precursor lesions (vulvar intraepithelial neoplasia, or VIN). Based on epidemiologic evidence, a sexually transmitted agent also has been thought to play a role in the pathogenesis of vulvar cancer, but since vulvar cancer is less common than cervical cancer, thorough investigation of the role of HPV in vulvar tumorigenesis has lagged behind that of the cervix. Recent studies, using in situ hybridization and PCR, identified HPV16 or 18 in nearly all cases of VIN found adjacent to invasive squamous carcinomas as well as in the associated invasive tumors.[100] These tumors appeared to be of specific histological subtypes characterized as "basaloid" or "warty." However, other invasive squamous carcinomas were not associated with VIN. These cancers were designated "typical" or "keratinizing" squamous carcinomas and generally did not contain HPV sequences. "Typical" squamous carcinomas tended to occur in older women (mean age, 77 years) whereas the HPV-associated "basaloid" and "warty" carcinomas tended to occur in younger women (mean age, 55 years). These findings suggest that the molecular pathogenesis of vulvar cancer in these two groups may be different, or may share only some steps. A recent cytogenetic study of six vulvar squamous carcinomas found that these tumors are genetically complex but tend to contain certain consistent chromosomal abnormalities, including losses of chromosomes 3p, 8p, 22q, and the short arm of the inactive X as well as gains of 3q and 11q. Interestingly, losses of 10q and 18q were found only in cases that exhibited biologically aggressive behavior.[107] Larger studies are needed to determine the significance of these findings. As with cervical cancer, HPV infection may set the course of the molecular "pathway" by which a normal cell ultimately gives rise to a tumor. In one preliminary study of 21 vulvar carcinomas, four of nine HPV-negative tumors were found to contain p53 gene mutations, whereas only 1 of 12 HPV-positive tumors had mutated p53.[105] Although vulvar cancers in younger women (HPV related) may share several genetic alterations with squamous carcinomas of the cervix, the molecular pathogenesis of vulvar cancer in older women may be quite different.

Endometrial Cancer

Endometrial carcinogenesis is believed to progress along a continuum from normal proliferative endometrium through endometrial hyperplasia showing increasingly severe degrees of architectural and cytological atypia until, ultimately, an invasive cancer develops. Unopposed estrogen, either exogenous or endogenous, provides the stimulus to proliferate in many cases and little is known about the genetic changes accompanying tumor development and progression. Several small studies have identified some molecular alterations of oncogenes that may play a role in the development of endometrial adenocarcinoma (summarized in Table 28.2). Alterations of several of these genes have correlated with presentation at advanced stage, high histological grade, and/or poor prognosis. Suppressor gene alterations also are likely to play a role in endometrial carcinogenesis. Okamoto et al. evaluated 24 endometrial carcinomas for allelic losses using polymorphic probes

Table 28.2. Summary of oncogene abnormalities in endometrial carcinomas

Oncogene	Summary of results	Reference
ras group	Increased staining by immunohistochemistry in 6/12 endometrial hyperplasias and 17/17 invasive carcinomas	Agnantis et al.[2]
	Increased staining in 1/4 atypical endometrial hyperplasias, 2/11 grade 1, and 21/22 grade 2 or 3 adenocarcinomas	Long et al.[60]
K-*ras*	Mutant K-*ras* in 2/9 endometrial adenocarcinomas	Enomoto et al.[25]
	Mutant K-*ras* in 3/30 endometrial adenocarcinomas	Ignartrowbridge et al.[41]
c-*fms*	*Fms* overexpression by *in situ* hybridization in 13/13 endometrial adenocarcinomas; level of overexpression increased in parallel with grade, stage, and degree of invasiveness	Kacinski et al.[42]
	Fms RNA expression in 53 benign and malignant endometria studied by Northern blot analysis; *fms* overexpression highest in endometrial carcinomas, lowest in secretory endometria, and intermediate in proliferative and hyperplastic endometria	Leiserowitz et al.[57]
c-*erb*-1	Rearrangement of 5′ end of *erb*B-1 in one endometrial adenocarcinoma	Zhang et al.[111]

spanning all 23 chromosome pairs.[71] Losses of heterozygosity were identified in seven cases, five of which lost loci on 17p, which harbors the p53 gene. In at least three of these cases, the retained copy of p53 was mutated. Another study of 21 endometrial carcinomas found p53 gene point mutations in three cases (14%).[81] In addition, endometrial carcinoma frequently occurs in patients with hereditary nonpolyposis colorectal cancer (HNPCC or Lynch syndrome II), suggesting that inactivation of a common gene may participate in the development of both endometrial and colonic carcinomas. Recently, linkage studies have mapped a gene responsible for at least some cases of HNPCC to chromosome 2.[76] Alterations of this gene appear to predispose certain cell types (e.g., colonic epithelial cells) of affected patients to widespread instability of short repeated sequences in their genomes, suggesting that many replication errors had occurred during tumor development.[1] The human homolog (hMSH2) of a microbial DNA mismatch repair gene has recently been identified. hMSH2 is located on chromosome 2 and, as predicted, alterations of this gene have been found in germline and tumor DNA from those patients with HNPCC linked to chromosome 2. Two groups of investigators have shown similar replication errors (microsatellite instability) in approximately 20% of presumably sporadic endometrial carcinomas[10a,81a]. Studies are currently in progress to determine whether mutations in hMSH2 or related genes are associated with microsatellite instability in endometrial carcinomas. If mutations in hMSH2 are identified in any of the endometrial carcinomas, DNA extracted from the same patient's normal tissue will reveal if the mutations are inherited or acquired somatically. Clearly, more numerous and larger studies will be required to determine how often alterations of specific oncogenes, tumor suppressor genes, and mutator genes are involved in endometrial cancer development.

Ovarian Cancer

Ovarian carcinomas are responsible for more cancer deaths than any other type of gynecological malignancy. Unfortunately, ovarian epithelial tumors have several characteristics that present difficult problems not only for the diagnosis and management of this disease, but also for research aimed at understanding the molecular pathogenesis of these aggressive tumors.

First, ovarian epithelial tumors are notorious for the diversity of their histopathological appearance. Many of the molecular studies completed to date have combined several subtypes as ovarian "cancer" as if they represented a single disease; a few have even combined epithelial, stromal, and/or germ cell neoplasms. The fact that tumors within different histopathological subsets tend to exhibit distinctive clinical behaviors suggests that the genetic alterations underlying the development and progression of tumors within each group may not be comparable. Ideally, then, studies should be undertaken that take these issues into account, correlating specific molecular markers with histological subtype and appropriate clinical parameters.

Second, ovarian carcinomas typically have an insidious presentation, such that most patients are diagnosed with advanced stage disease. Furthermore, compared with other portions of the genital tract, ovarian tumor tissue is relatively inaccessible and tumor sampling requires invasive procedures. Thus, it is extremely difficult to obtain "early" ovarian carcinomas or premalignant lesions, or even to obtain tumor tissue at all.

Third, whereas SIL and atypical endometrial hyperplasia are accepted precursors of cervical and endometrial carcinomas, respectively, the precursor lesions leading to ovarian carcinoma are poorly understood and remain controversial. Most investigators believe that ovarian epithelial tumors are derived from the epithelium or mesothelium covering the ovarian surface. However, evidence supporting tumor progression via benign cysts or low malignant potential (LMP) tumors is limited. Puls et al. recently examined a series of 94 serous and mucinous carcinomas and LMP tumors for the presence of benign epithelium and areas of histological transition from benign to LMP or malignant epithelium.[78] Histologically benign epithelium was identified in 100% of LMP tumors and in 56% and 90% of serous and mucinous carcinomas, respectively. Furthermore, "transition" areas were identified in 79% of LMP tumors and in 27% of carcinomas. Although these findings are consistent with the hypothesis that malignant tumors typically arise from pre-existing benign neoplasms, this study was unable to exclude the possibility that benign and malignant epithelial lesions frequently co-exist in the same patient or that regions designated as "transition" areas simply reflect extension of malignant cells into a pre-existing benign lesion. In a recent review of the pathology of early malignant change in the ovary, Fox emphasized further that the presence of benign epithelium in a malignant tumor does not in itself indicate evolution from a pre-existing adenoma, as areas of apparently benign epithelium are observed frequently even in metastatic carcinomas to the ovary.[28] Certainly, many investigators' reluctance to embrace the "transition" theory stems, in part, from our increased understanding of the biologic behavior of LMP tumors. Although some studies indicate a 30–40% mortality for advanced stage LMP tumors, a recent review by Kurman[54] disclosed that the great majority of these deaths could be attributed to "benign" complications of the disease or to complications of therapy. Only 0.7% of the 953 cases reviewed appeared to have undergone malignant transformation. This percentage is roughly equivalent to the general incidence of ovarian carcinoma, such that women with LMP tumors appear to be no more likely to develop ovarian cancer than women without these lesions. We now have the molecular tools with which to address this issue more definitively. For example, it is theoretically possible to show that the carcinoma and putative precursor lesion (i.e., cystadenoma or LMP tumor) are derived from the same clone of cells, assuming, of course, that the precursor lesion is a clonal process.

Fourth, there has been a long-standing debate whether the tendency of ovarian carcinoma to involve multiple peritoneal sites reflects multifocal origin in a "field" of susceptible cells[106] or unifocal origin with widespread metastases. The occurrence of occasional cases of well-documented extraovarian papillary serous neoplasia[29,33] as well as synchronous uterine endometrial carcinomas with endometrioid carcinoma of the ovary[110] support the concept of multifocal origin of at least some ovarian carcinomas. Investigators have already begun to apply molecular biological techniques toward answering this question. In one study,[64] Mok et al. showed that in nine cases with widespread disease the mutational pattern of the p53 gene was identical in cancer cells from different sites in the same patient, suggesting that these tumors were of unifocal origin. In a related study by the same group of investigators, Tsao et al.[98] used a different molecular marker (X-chromosome inactivation) to arrive at the same conclusion. Although these early studies certainly suggest that many high-stage ovarian carcinomas reflect widespread metastasis from a single primary, they may have been biased in that they mainly evaluated aggressive tumors involving numerous sites. It would be interesting to examine more limited multifocal tumors (e.g., bilateral ovarian or synchronous ovarian and endometrial) in a similar fashion.

Despite these difficulties, significant progress has been made in identifying at least some of the molecular events that appear to play a role in ovarian tumorigenesis. The recent literature contains numerous reports of activation of different oncogenes in ovarian malignancies. Overexpression of erbB-2 (also known as HER-2neu) both with and without gene amplification has been reported by several groups.[44,91,112] The protein encoded by this proto-oncogene is a transmembrane molecule with structural similarities to the epidermal growth factor receptor. Receptor proteins of this type are believed to transduce signals (e.g., growth stimuli) from the outside to the inside of the cell. The extracytoplasmic portion of these transmembrane receptors includes a domain that specifically binds the receptor's ligand. Ligand binding typically activates an enzymatic function in the intracytoplasmic portion of the receptor, which, in the case of erbB-2, is a tyrosine kinase. The activated tyrosine kinase can then specifically phosphorylate other intracytoplasmic molecules that can continue to transmit the signal in a cascade-like fashion. Putative ligands for the erbB-2 receptor have recently been reported.[75] Increased levels of erbB-2 protein are believed to be involved in the pathogenesis of both breast and ovarian cancer. Using Southern blot analysis, Slamon et al.[91] found erbB-2 amplification in 26% of 120 primary ovarian malignancies studied. Increased levels of erbB-2 RNA and protein was seen in every case with gene amplification that was comprehensively studied. In addition, 12% of cases showed *erb*B-2 overexpression without evidence of gene amplification. Overexpression of *erb*B-2 correlated significantly with poor clinical outcome, suggesting that evaluation of expression levels of this gene eventually may become useful in predicting prognosis and determining appropriate therapy for ovarian cancer patients.

Like *erb*B-2, *fms* belongs to a family of oncogenes that transduce signals via tyrosine kinase activity. Kacinski et al. have shown overexpression of *fms* protein (CSF-1) in all types of ovarian carcinomas studied (including mucinous, serous, clear cell, endometrioid, and undifferentiated) in comparison with benign and borderline (LMP) lesions.[43]

The *myc* gene family encodes proteins that localize to the nucleus and affect transcription of growth-related genes by binding to specific DNA sequences. C-*myc* gene amplification has been reported in both hematopoietic and solid tumors and is associated with more biologically aggressive behavior in some neoplasms. Baker et al. reported c-*myc* amplification in 29% of ovarian carcinomas.[7] In another study, c-*myc* amplification was reported in 50% of ovarian carcinomas.[87] Six of seven cases with amplification of this gene were of serous differentiation whereas none of four cases of mucinous adenocarcinoma had this change. C-*myc* amplification was not detected in normal ovarian tissue, benign adenomas, or LMP tumors. These data support the hypothesis that different genetic alterations may be associated with and/or be responsible for the development of benign versus malignant ovarian tumors.

Abnormalities of other oncogenes, such as *ras* gene deletion, amplification, and point mutation, and *fos* gene overexpression also have been reported. The biologic and clinical significance of these findings remains unclear.

The pathogenesis of ovarian neoplasia also is likely to involve inactivation of several tumor suppressor genes. The specific genes altered in different types of tumors have yet to be identified. Several investigators have recently found allelic loss events at nonrandom frequencies in ovarian carcinomas. The results of these studies are summarized in Table 28.3. The series of Sato et al. probably is most illustrative.[88] These investigators studied 37 ovarian tumors with a set of polymorphic DNA probes spanning all of the nonacrocentric chromosomal arms. When their data were analyzed by tumor type, allelic losses on 6q, 13q, and 19q were observed exclusively in serous carcinomas. In addition, the average number of allelic losses seen in mucinous tumors (corrected for the number of informative cases) was significantly lower than that of other types, including serous and clear cell tumors, which tend to have a worse prognosis. These findings suggest that (1) alterations of several suppressor genes are likely to play a role in ovarian cancer development, and that (2) losses of different chromosomal regions, presumably harboring specific suppressor genes, may be responsible in part for the variable histopathological appearance as well as biologic behavior of different tumor types.

A few studies have evaluated the status of known tumor suppressor genes in ovarian epithelial tumors. Homozygous deletion (loss of both copies) of the Rb gene was found in 1 of 24 ovarian carcinomas.[86] In another analysis, p53 gene mutations were identified in 36% of 34 ovarian carcinomas, with the mutations clustered in exons 5 and 7.[63] In at least one tumor, both copies of p53 were independently mutated, whereas in other cases mutation of one allele was accompanied by loss of the other. Several matched sets of primary tumor and metastasis also were studied. In these cases, the same mutation was identified

Table 28.3. Summary of losses of heterozygosity in ovarian carcinoma

Chromosomal arms with LOH	Additional comments	Reference
11p	Loss of one c-Ha-*ras* allele in 5/10 informative cases; losses occurred in 4 "adenocarcinomas" and 1 MMMT	Lee et al.[55]
17p (69%), 17q (77%)	16 carcinomas evaluated (12 SA, 2 MA, 2 EA)	Eccles et al.[23]
3p, 6q, 11p	12 carcinomas evaluated (7 SA, 1 mixed MA/SA, 4 EA)	Ehlen and Dubeau[24]
6q (64%), 17p (75%), 11p (46%)	19 tumors evaluated (4 "adenocarcinomas," 2 müllerian adenocarcinomas, 1 TCC, 7 SA, 2 EA, 2 CCA, 1 MMMT)	Lee et al.[58]
17p (31%), 17q (77%)	19 tumors evaluated (7 SA, 7 EA, 2 mucinous LMP, 1 mucinous cystadenoma, 1 serous cystadenoma, 1 cystic teratoma)	Russell et al.[82]
3p, 6p, 6q, 11p	30 grades 1–3 tumors evaluated; losses on chromosomes 3 or 11 were not seen in low-grade lesions	Zheng[112]
17p (67%), 11p (53%), 13q (58%)	Included 24 carcinomas, 4 benign and 5 LMP tumors; 11p losses identified only in invasive tumors	Gallion et al.[32]
4p (42%), 6p (50%), 7p (43%), 8q (31%), 12p (38%), 12q (33%), 16p (33%), 16q (38%), 17p (46%), 17q (39%), 19p (34%)	37 tumors evaluated (included 16 SA, 8 MA, 5 CCA, and 2 EA); 6q, 13q, and 19q losses seen only in serous carcinomas; mucinous carcinomas typically had fewer losses than other histological subtypes	Sato et al.[88]

LOH, losses of heterozygosity; MMMT, malignant mixed mesodermal tumor; SA, serous adenocarcinoma; MA, mucinous adenocarcinoma; EA, endometrioid adenocarcinoma; CCA, clear cell adenocarcinoma; TCC, transitional cell carcinoma.

in tumor from both sites, suggesting that p53 gene mutation precedes metastasis. Marks et al. examined p53 gene expression in more than 100 ovarian carcinomas using immunohistochemical techniques.[62a] Previous investigators have shown that many mutant p53 proteins, although incapable of normal function, have prolonged half-lives and accumulate in cells at higher steady-state levels than in most cells containing wild-type p53. Increased levels of mutant p53 protein can be detected by routine immunohistochemical staining with appropriate anti-p53 antibodies. The concordance between overexpression of p53 protein by immunohistochemical staining and the presence of an actual p53 gene mutation is on the order of 80%.[16] In Marks' study, high levels of p53 protein were detected in 50% of ovarian carcinomas whereas p53 was undetectable in several benign gynecological tissue samples. As in other tumors, overexpression of p53 protein was found to correlate closely with the presence of p53 gene mutation in the tumors. These and other similar studies[47,72,99] provide strong evidence that inactivation of the p53 gene through deletion and/or point mutation plays a role in the development or progression of a significant number of ovarian cancers.

Most of the above discussion pertains to genetic alterations that occur in somatic cells during tumor development and progression. However, primary genetic factors (germline changes) account for an unknown proportion of ovarian cancer cases. Hereditary ovarian cancer has been primarily observed in three types of families: (1) apparently site-specific ovarian cancer families, (2) breast–ovarian cancer families, and (3) hereditary nonpolyposis colorectal cancer (Lynch syndrome II) families. Recent studies have found significant heterogeneity in the age at diagnosis of ovarian cancer among patients with these different ovarian cancer-prone syndromes, suggesting that they may not share the same pathogenesis.[3,62] The familial breast–ovarian cancer locus recently has been mapped to chromosome 17q12–q23, although the target gene has not been identified and cloned. The intensive study of kindreds affected with these syndromes is likely to pinpoint candidate genes in the near future. It can then be determined if somatic alterations of these genes are playing a role in the development of sporadic ovarian cancers.

Summary

Many long-standing questions concerning the molecular pathogenesis of gynecological tumors can now be addressed using recently developed molecular tools. Many, if not most, of the experimental methods routinely employed in molecular biology laboratories today are straightforward and potentially accessible to many research laboratories. Despite the routine availability of these powerful techniques, the importance of clinicians' and pathologists' contributions cannot be overemphasized. Simply stated, the quality of the results are only as good as the question asked and the materials and methods used. For example, LOH analyses rely on the comparison of normal and tumor DNA from the same patient. Losses of heterozygosity can easily be concealed in tumor samples heavily contaminated with normal cells. Degraded DNA obtained from necrotic cells also might yield misleading results.

Ultimately, the knowledge gained from many of these molecular biological studies will be applicable to improving the care and management of patients with gynecological malignancies. Identification of specific genetic alterations in these tumors could potentially form the basis of new screening programs to detect early, and therefore curable, cancers. Patients with strong family histories of endometrial or ovarian cancer could be screened for inherited mutations in relevant tumor suppressor genes. Finally, this type of knowledge could be exploited in the development of new and more effective treatment strategies for cancer patients. Possible examples include gene therapy to replace defective copies of tumor suppressor genes, development of drugs that interfere with the interaction of viral oncoproteins with cellular tumor suppressor proteins, and reagents such as "antisense" oligonucleotides, which can specifically reduce expression of overexpressed oncogenes.

Like many other solid tumors, the common gynecological malignancies appear to develop and progress, at least in part, as a result of activational mutation of oncogenes coupled with inactivation of tumor suppressor genes. Over the next several years, many of the specific genetic alterations within these genes will be characterized. It is important for clinicians to stay aware of the studies emerging from basic science laboratories, since many are likely to impact heavily on the diagnosis and management of cancer patients in the near future.

Glossary

Allele: Alternative forms of the same gene. These alternative forms are not considered mutant genes because they are found in normal individuals and encode proteins with normal function.

Bacterial transformation: A method to introduce foreign DNA into bacterial cells, usually for the purposes of **cloning.**

Capping: The addition of 7-methylguanosine residues to the 5′ end of most eukaryotic **mRNAs.**

Cloning: An in vivo (in living cells) method to produce unlimited quantities of specific DNA fragments from as little as a single DNA molecule.

Codons: A group of three nucleotides within an **open reading frame** that specify either the amino acid to be incorporated into the protein or a translation termination signal.

Complementary DNA (cDNA): DNA synthesized from a **mRNA** template such that the DNA sequence is complementary to the mRNA.

Cytoplasmic signal transduction molecules: Proteins within the cytoplasm of cells responsible for transmitting signals from one event to the next event.

Exons: The coding portion of genes. After transcription, portions of **heteronuclear RNA** encoded by **exons** are joined together by **splicing** to produce **mRNA.**

Gene amplification: The presence of multiple copies of a gene within a cell that is normally present in only two copies per somatic cell.

Gene deletion: The deletion of part or all of a gene through removal of DNA sequences by any of several molecular mechanisms.

Gene expression: The active **transcription** of a gene into an RNA molecule followed by **translation** of the protein product.

Gene rearrangement: The process by which part or all of a gene is moved from its normal location in the genome to another site within the genome.

Growth factors: Proteins that act on cells to promote cell growth.

Growth factor receptors: Proteins that interact with **growth factors** and transmit the growth signal to the cell.

Heteronuclear RNA: A form of RNA, a pre-**mRNA,** that exists before splicing and consists of both **introns** and **exons.**

Informative: A term used to describe the situation when the two homologous chromosomes from an individual can be distinguished from one another at a given **locus;** *heterozygous* is an alternative term.

Insertions: The addition of DNA sequence into the genome.

Introns: Portions of genomic DNA that are interspersed between **exons** and are transcribed along with the **exons** into **heteronuclear RNA.** After transcription, the **introns** are removed during splicing such that they are not represented in **mRNA.**

Locus: A general term to describe a defined chromosomal region.

Loss of heterozygosity: Losses of specific regions of DNA from one copy of a given chromosome that can be distinguished from the region retained on the other chromosome.

Messenger RNA (mRNA): The mature form of processed RNA used as a template for directing **translation** of proteins.

Missense mutations: A nucleotide substitution (**point mutation**) in a **codon** of the **open reading frame** of a gene that results in the replacement of one amino acid for another in the protein product.

Nonsense mutations: A nucleotide substitution that results in a truncated protein product by generating a stop codon specifying premature cessation of **translation** within an **open reading frame.**

Nuclear transcription factors: Proteins involved in regulating the expression of genes by controlling **transcription.** Some factors enhance and others repress **gene expression** and others can do both, depending on the intracellular environment.

Oncogenes: Genes that regulate cell growth in a positive fashion, i.e., to promote cell growth. Oncogenes include transforming genes of viruses and normal cellular genes (**proto-oncogenes**) that are activated by mutations to promote cell growth.

Open reading frame: A sequence of DNA, representing at least some of the coding portion of a gene, that is **transcribed** and subsequently **translated** into a protein because it does not contain any internal translation termination **codons.**

Point mutation: The replacement of one nucleotide in the DNA sequence of the **wild-type** gene with another nucleotide.

Polyadenylation: A process by which a stretch of adenosine residues are added to the 3′ end of most eukaryotic **mRNA** molecules.

Primers: Short DNA sequences (oligonucleotides) that are complementary to portions of specific DNA sequences.

Promoter: The DNA sequence of a gene to which RNA polymerase binds and initiates **transcription.** This sequence usually is found 5′ to the coding portion of the gene and is responsible for regulating the expression of the gene at the transcriptional level.

Proto-oncogenes: Cellular genes that are the normal counterparts of transforming viral **oncogenes.**

Restriction endonucleases: Enzymes that cleave DNA at specific DNA sequences.

Restriction fragment length polymorphism (RFLP): Variations in the DNA of different individuals that create or destroy cleavage sites for a given **restriction endonuclease.**

Splice site mutations: Nucleotide substitutions that occur in the sequences adjacent to **intron–exon** boundaries of genes. These mutations result in aberrant RNA **splic-**

ing, which in turn results in aberrant (or nonexistent) protein products.

Splicing: The process by which **introns** are removed from **heteronuclear RNA** and the exons are joined together to maintain the **open reading frame** of the **mRNA.**

Transcription: The process by which RNA is synthesized from the DNA template.

Translation: The process by which specific amino acids are incorporated into a protein as dictated by the sequence of the **mRNA** template.

Tumor suppressor genes: Normal cellular genes that encode proteins thought to normally regulate growth in a negative fashion.

Uninformative: The term used to describe the situation when the two homologous chromosomes from an individual cannot be distinguished from one another at a given **locus;** *homozygous* is an alternative term.

Vectors: A DNA vehicle that can be propagated in living cells (e.g., bacteria and yeast) into which foreign DNA can be inserted and propagated with the vector DNA. Examples of vectors include bacterial plasmids, cosmids, bacteriophage, and, most recently, yeast artificial chromosomes.

Wild-type: The term used to describe the normal gene or gene product. In contrast, a gene that has had its DNA sequence altered is referred to as a *mutant gene* and its resultant product is a *mutant protein.*

References

1. Aaltonen L, Peltomaki P, Leach F, et al (1993) Clues to the pathogenesis of familial colorectal cancer. Science 260: 812–816
2. Agnantis NJ, Spandidos DA, Mahera H, et al (1988) Immunohistochemical study of ras oncogene expression in endometrial and cervical human lesions. Eur J Gynaecol Oncol 9: 360–365
3. Amos CI, Shaw GL, Tucker MA, Hartge P (1992) Age at onset for familial epithelial ovarian cancer. JAMA 268: 1896–1899
4. Atkin NB, Baker MC (1989) Chromosome 17p loss in carcinoma of the cervix uteri. Cancer Genet Cytogenet 37: 229–233
5. Baker S, Fearon E, Nigro J, et al (1989) Chromosome 17 deletions and p53 gene mutations in colorectal carcinomas. Science 244: 217–221
6. Baker S, Preisinger A, Jessup J, et al (1990) p53 gene mutations occur in combination with 17p allelic deletions as late events in colorectal tumorgenesis. Cancer Res 50: 7717–7722
7. Baker VV, Borst MP, Dixon D, Hatch KD, Shingleton HM, Miller D (1990) c-myc amplification in ovarian cancer. Gynecol Oncol 38: 340–342
8. Baker V, Hatch K, Shingleton H (1988) Amplification of the c-myc proto-oncogene in cervical carcinoma. J Surg Oncol 39: 225–228
9. Barbosa MS, Schlegel R (1989) The E6 and E7 genes of HPV-18 are sufficient for inducing two-stage in vitro transformation of human keratinocytes. Oncogene 4: 1529–1532
10. Bishop JM (1991) Molecular themes in oncogenesis. Cell 64: 235–248
10a. Burks RT, Kessis TD, Cho KR, Hedrick L (1994) Microsatellite instability in endometrial carcinoma. Oncogene 9: 1163–1166
11. Couturier J, Sastre-Garau X, Schneider-Maunoury S, Labib A, Orth G (1991) Integration of papillomavirus DNA near myc genes in genital carcinomas and its consequences for proto-oncogene expression. J Virol 65: 4534–4538
12. Crook T, Tidy JA, Vousden KH (1991) Degradation of p53 can be targeted by HPV E6 sequences distinct from those required for p53 binding and trans-activation. Cell 67: 547–556
13. Crook T, Vousden KH (1992) Properties of p53 mutations detected in primary and secondary cervical cancers suggest mechanisms of metastasis and involvement of environmental carcinogens. EMBO J 11: 3935–3940
14. Crook T, Wrede D, Vousden KH (1991) p53 point mutation in HPV negative human cervical carcinoma cell lines. Oncogene 6: 873–875
15. Cullen AP, Reid R, Campion M, Lörincz AT (1991) Analysis of the physical state of different human papillomavirus DNAs in intraepithelial and invasive cervical neoplasm. J Virol 65: 606–612
16. Cunningham J, Lust JA, Schaid DJ, et al (1992) Expression of p53 and 17p allelic loss in colorectal carcinoma. Cancer Res 52: 1974–1980
17. Di Luca D, Costa S, Monini P, et al (1989) Search for human papillomavirus, herpes simplex virus and c-myc oncogene in human genital tumors. Int J Cancer 43: 570–577
18. Duggan MA, Benoit JL, McGregor SE, Nation JG, Inoue M, Stuart GCE (1993) The human papillomavirus status of 114 endocervical adenocarcinoma cases by dot blot hybridization. Hum Pathol 24: 121–125
19. Dunn JM, Phillips RA, Becker AJ, Gallie BL (1988) Identification of germline and somatic mutations affecting the retinoblastoma gene. Science 241: 1797–1800
20. Durst M, Croce C, Gissmann L, Schwarz E, Huebner K (1987) Papillomavirus sequences integrate near cellular oncogenes in some cervical carcinomas. Proc Natl Acad Sci USA 80: 3812–3815
21. Durst M, Dzarlieva-Petrusevska R, Boukamp P, Fusenig N, Gissman L (1987) Molecular and cytogenetic analysis of immortalized human primary keratinocytes obtained after transfection with human papillomavirus type 16 DNA. Oncogene 1: 251–256
22. Dyson N, Howley P, Münger K, Harlow E (1989) The human papillomavirus-16 E7 oncoprotein is able to bind to the retinoblastoma gene product. Science 243: 934–937
23. Eccles DM, Cranston G, Steel CM, Nakamura Y, Leonard RC (1990) Allele losses on chromosome 17 in human epithelial ovarian carcinoma. Oncogene 5: 1599–1601

24. Ehlen T, Dubeau L (1990) Loss of heterozygosity on chromosomal segments 3p, 6q and 11p in human ovarian carcinomas. Oncogene 5: 219–223

25. Enomoto T, Inoue M, Perantoni AO, Terakawa N, Tanizawa O, Rice JM (1990) K-ras activation in neoplasms of the human female reproductive tract. Cancer Res 50: 6139–6145

26. Fearon E, Vogelstein B (1990) A genetic model for colorectal tumorigenesis. Cell 61: 759–767

27. Fearon ER, Cho KR, Nigro JM, et al (1990) Identification of a chromosome 18q gene that is altered in colorectal cancers. Science 247: 49–56

27a. Fishel R, Lescoe MK, Rao MRS, et al. (1993) The human mutator gene homolog MSH2 and its association with hereditary nonpolyposis colon cancer. Cell 75: 1027–1038

28. Fox H (1993) Pathology of early malignant change in the ovary. Int J Gynecol Pathol 12: 153–155

29. Foyle A, Al-Jabi M, McCaughey W (1992) Papillary peritoneal tumors in women. Am J Surg Pathol 5: 241–249

30. Francke U (1976) Retinoblastoma and chromosome 13. Cytogenet Cell Genet 16: 131–134

31. Fujita M, Inoue M, Tanizawa O, Iwamoto S, Enomoto T (1992) Alterations of terations of the p53 gene in human primary cervical carcinoma with and without human papillomavirus infection. Cancer Res 52: 5323–5328

32. Gallion H, Powell D, Morrow J, et al (1992) Molecular genetic changes in human epithelial ovarian malignancies. Gynecol Oncol 47: 137–142

33. Genadry R, Poliakoff S, Rotmensch J, Rosenshein N, Parmley T, Woodruff J (1981) Primary, papillary peritoneal neoplasia. Obstet Gynecol 58: 730–734

34. Hamel P, Gallie B, Phillips R (1992) The retinoblastoma protein and cell cycle regulation. TIG 8: 180–185

35. Hansen MF, Cavanee WK (1987) Genetics of cancer predisposition. Cancer Res 47: 5518–5527

36. Harlow E, Lane D (1988) Antibodies: A laboratory manual. Cold Spring Harbor, New York, Cold Spring Harbor Laboratory

37. Harris H (1988) The analysis of malignancy in cell fusion: The position in 1988. Cancer Res 48: 3302–3306

38. Hawley-Nelson P, Vousden KH, Hubbert NL, Lowy DR, Schiller JT (1989) HPV16 E6 and E7 proteins cooperate to immortalize human foreskin keratinocytes. EMBO J 8: 3905–3910

39. Heim S, Nilbert M, Vanni R, et al (1988) A specific translocation, t(12;14)(q14-15;q23-24), characterized a subgroup of uterine leiomyomas. Cancer Genet Cytogenet 32: 13–17

40. Hollstein M, Sidransky D, Vogelstein B, Harris C (1991) p53 mutations in human cancers. Science 253: 49–53

41. Ignartrowbridge D, Risinger JI, Dent GA, et al (1992) Mutations of the Ki-ras oncogene in endometrial carcinoma. Am J Obstet Gynecol 167: 227–232

42. Kacinski BM, Carter D, Mittal K, et al (1983) High level expression of fms proto-oncogene mRNA is observed in clinically aggressive human endometrial adenocarcinomas. Int J Rad Oncol Biol Phys 15: 823–829

43. Kacinski BM, Carter D, Mittal K, et al (1990) Ovarian adenocarcinomas express fms-complementary transcripts and fms antigen, often with coexpression of CSF-1. Am J Pathol 137: 135–147

44. Kacinski BM, Mayer AG, King BL, Carter D, Chambers SK (1992) Neu protein overexpression in benign, borderline, and malignant ovarian neoplasms. Gynecol Oncol 44: 245–253

45. Kastan MB, Onyekwere O, Sidransky D, Vogelstein B, Craig RW (1991) Participation of p53 protein in the cellular response to DNA damage. Cancer Res 51: 6304–6311

46. Kern SE, Kinzler KW, Bruskin A, et al (1991) Identification of p53 as a sequence-specific DNA-binding protein. Science 252: 1708–1711

47. Kerns BJ, Jordan PA, Moore MB, et al (1992) p53 overexpression in formalin-fixed, paraffin-embedded tissue detected by immunohistochemistry. J Histochem Cytochem 40: 1047–1051

48. Kessis T, Slebos R, Han S, et al (1993) p53 gene mutations and mdm2 amplification are uncommon in primary carcinomas of the uterine cervix. Am J Pathol 143: 1398–1405

49. Kessis T, Slebos R, Nelson W, et al (1993) Human papillomavirus 16 E6 disrupts the p53 mediated cellular response to DNA damage. Proc Natl Acad Sci USA 90: 3988–3992

50. Kinzler K, Nilbert M, Su L, et al (1991) Identification of FAP locus genes from chromosome 5q21. Science 253: 661–665

51. Knudson A (1985) Hereditary cancer, oncogenes, and antioncogenes. Cancer Res 45: 1437–1443

52. Knudson A (1971) Mutation and cancer: Statistical study of retinoblastoma. Proc Natl Acad Sci USA 68: 820–823

53. Kuerbitz S, Plunkett B, Walsh W, Kastan M (1992) Wildtype p53 is a cell cycle checkpoint determinant following irradiation. Proc Natl Acad Sci USA 51: 7491–7495

54. Kurman R, Trimble C (1993) The behavior of serous tumors of low malignant potential: Are they ever malignant? Int J Gynecol Pathol 12: 120–127

54a. Leach FS, Nicolaides NC, Papadopoulos N, et al. (1993) Mutations of a mutS homolog in hereditary nonpolyposis colorectal cancer. Cell 75: 1215–1226

55. Lee JH, Kavanagh JJ, Wharton JT, Wildrick DM, Blick M (1989) Allele loss at the c-Ha-ras1 locus in human ovarian cancer. Cancer Res 49: 1220–1222

56. Lee W, Bookstein R, Hong F, Young L, Shew J, Lee E (1987) Human retinoblastoma susceptibility gene: Cloning, identification, and sequence. Science 235: 1394–1399

57. Leiserowitz G, Harris S, Subramaniam M, Keeney G, Podratz K, Spelsberg T (1993) The proto-oncogene c-fms is overexpressed in endometrial cancer. Gynecol Oncol 49: 190–196

58. Lee JH, Kavanagh JJ, Wildrick DM, Wharton JT, Blick M (1990) Frequent loss of heterozygosity on chromosomes 6q, 11, and 17 in human ovarian carcinomas. Cancer Res 50: 2724–2728

59. Lele KP, Penrose LS, Stallard HB (1963) Chromosome deletion in a case of retinoblastoma. Ann Hum Genet 27: 171–174

60. Long CA, O'Brien TJ, Sanders MM, Bard DS, Quirk GJ Jr (1988) ras oncogene is expressed in adenocarcinoma of the endometrium. Am J Obstet Gynecol 159: 1512–1516

61. Low SH, Thong TW, Ho TH, et al (1990) Prevalence of human papillomavirus types 16 and 18 in cervical carcinomas: A study by dot and Southern blot hybridization and the polymerase chain reaction. Jap J Cancer Res 81: 1118–1123

62. Lynch HT, Watson P, Bewtra C, et al (1991) Hereditary ovarian cancer. Heterogeneity in age at diagnosis. Cancer 67: 1460–1466

62a. Marks JR, Davidoff AM, Kerns BJ, et al. (1991) Overexpression and mutation of p53 in epithelial ovarian cancer. Cancer Res 51: 2979–2984

63. Mazars R, Pujol P, Maudelonde T, Jeanteur P, Theillet C (1991) p53 mutations in ovarian cancer: A late event? Oncogene 6: 1685–1690

64. Mok CH, Tsao SW, Knapp RC, Fishbaugh PM, Lau CC (1992) Unifocal origin of advanced human epithelial ovarian cancers. Cancer Res 52: 5119–5122

65. Mullis K, Faloona F (1987) Specific synthesis of DNA in vitro via a polymerase catalyzed chain reaction. Meth Enzymol 55: 335–350

66. Münger K, Phelps W, Bubb V, Howley P, Schlegel R (1989) The E6 and E7 genes of human papillomavirus type 16 together are necessary and sufficient for transformation of primary human keratinocytes. J Virol 63: 4417–4421

67. Münger K, Yee CL, Phelps WC, Pietenpol JA, Moses HL, Howley PM (1991) Biochemical and biological differences between E7 oncoproteins of the high- and low-risk human papillomavirus types are determined by amino-terminal sequences. J Virol 65: 3943–3948

68. Nilbert M, Heim S, Mandahl N, Floderus U, Willen H, Mitelman F (1989) Different karyotypic abnormalities, t(1;6) and del(7), in two uterine leiomyomas from the same patient. Cancer Genet Cytogenet 42: 51–53

69. Nishisho I, Nakamura Y, Miyoshi Y, et al (1991) Mutations of chromosome 5q21 genes in FAP and colorectal cancer patients. Science 253: 665–669

70. Ocadiz R, Sauceda R, Cruz M, Graef A, Gariglio P (1987) High correlation between molecular alterations of the c-myc oncogene and carcinoma of the uterine cervix. Cancer Res 47: 4173–4177

71. Okamoto A, Sameshima Y, Yamada Y, et al (1991) Allelic loss on chromosome 17p and p53 mutations in human endometrial carcinoma of the uterus. Cancer Res 51: 5632–5635

72. Okamoto A, Sameshima Y, Yokoyama S, et al (1991) Frequent allelic losses and mutations of the p53 gene in human ovarian cancer. Cancer Res 51: 5171–5176

73. Orye E, Delbeke MJ, Vandenabeele B (1974) Retinoblastoma and long arm deletion at chromosome 13: Attempts to define the deleted segment. Clin Genet 5: 457–464

74. Parkin DM, Läärä E, Muir CS (1988) Estimates of the worldwide frequency of sixteen major cancers in 1980. Int J Cancer 41: 184–197

75. Peles E, Bacus SS, Koski RA, et al (1992) Isolation of the neu/HER-2 stimulatory ligand: A 44 kd glycoprotein that induces differentiation of mammary tumor cells. Cell 69: 205–216

76. Peltomaki P, Aaltonen L, Sistonen P, et al (1993) Genetic mapping of a locus predisposing to human colorectal cancer. Science 260: 810–812

77. Pirisi L, Yasumoto S, Feller M, Doniger J, DiPaolo J (1987) Transformation of human fibroblasts and keratinocytes with human papillomavirus type 16 DNA. J Virol 61: 1061–1066

78. Puls LE, Powell DE, Depriest PD, et al (1992) Transition from benign to malignant epithelium in mucinous and serous ovarian cystadenocarcinoma. Gynecol Oncol 47: 53–57

79. Riou G, Barrois M, Sheng ZM, Duvillard P, Lhomme C (1988) Somatic deletions and mutations of c-Ha-ras gene in human cervical cancers. Oncogene 3: 329–333

80. Riou G, Favre M, Jeannel D, Bourhis J, LeDoussal V, Orth G (1990) Association between poor prognosis in early-stage invasive cervical carcinomas and non-detection of HPV DNA. Lancet 335: 1171–1174

81. Risinger JI, Dent GA, Ignartrowbridge D, et al (1992) p53 gene mutations in human endometrial carcinoma. Mol Carcino 5: 250–253

81a. Risinger JI, Berchuck A, Kohler MF, et al. (1993) Genetic instability of microsatellites in endometrial carcinoma. Cancer Res 53: 1–4

82. Russell SE, Hickey GI, Lowry WS, White P, Atkinson RJ (1990) Allele loss from chromosome 17 in ovarian cancer. Oncogene 5: 1581–1583

83. Sagae S, Kudo R, Kuzumaki N, et al (1990) Ras oncogene expression and progression in intraepithelial neoplasia of the uterine cervix. Cancer 66: 295–301

84. Saiki R, Scharf S, Faloona F, et al (1985) Enzymatic amplification of beta-globin sequences and restriction site analysis for diagnosis of sickle cell anemia. Science 230: 1350–1354

85. Sanger F, Nicklen S, Coulson AR (1977) DNA sequencing with chain-terminating inhibitors. Proc Natl Acad Sci USA 74: 5463–5467

86. Sasano H, Comerford J, Silverberg SG, Garrett CT (1990) An analysis of abnormalities of the retinoblastoma gene in human ovarian and endometrial carcinoma. Cancer 66: 2150–2154

87. Sasano H, Garrett CT, Wilkinson DS, Silverberg S, Comerford J, Hyde J (1990) Protooncogene amplification and tumor ploidy in human ovarian neoplasms. Hum Pathol 21: 382–391

88. Sato T, Saito H, Morita R, Koi S, Lee JH, Nakamura Y (1991) Allelotype of human ovarian cancer. Cancer Res 51: 5118–5122

89. Scheffner M, Münger K, Myrne JC, Howley PM (1991) The state of the p53 and retinoblastoma genes in human cervical carcinoma cell lines. Proc Natl Acad Sci USA 88: 5523–5527

90. Scheffner M, Werness BA, Huibregtse JM, Levine AJ, Howley PM (1990) The E6 oncoprotein encoded by human papillomavirus types 16 and 18 promotes the degradation of p53. Cell 63: 1129–1136

91. Slamon DJ, Godolphin W, Jones LA, et al (1989) Studies of the HER-2/neu proto-oncogene in human breast and ovarian cancer. Science 244: 707–712

92. Smith K, Johnson K, Bryan R, et al (1993) The APC gene product in normal and tumor cells. Proc Natl Acad Sci USA 90: 2846–2850

93. Southern E (1975) Detection of specific sequences among DNA fragments separated by gel electrophoresis. J Mol Bio 98: 503–506

94. Sowani A, Ong G, Dische S, et al (1989) c-myc oncogene expression and clinical outcome in carcinoma of the cervix. Mol Cell Probes 3: 117–123

95. Stanbridge EJ, Cavanee WK (1989) Heritable cancer and tumor suppressor genes: A tentative connection. In: Weinberg RA (ed) Oncogenes and the molecular origins of cancer. Cold Spring Harbor, New York, Cold Spring Harbor Laboratory, pp 281–306

96. Stirdivant S, Huber H, Patrick D, et al (1992) Human papillomavirus type 16 E7 protein inhibits DNA binding by the retinoblastoma gene product. Mol Cell Biol 12: 1905–1914

97. Sugarbaker JP, Gunderson LL, Wittes RE (1985) Colorectal cancer. In: DeVita VT, Hellman S, Rosenberg SA (eds) Cancer: Principles and practices of oncology. Philadelphia, J.B. Lippincott, pp 800–803

98. Tsao S, Mok C, Knapp R, et al (1993) Molecular genetic evidence of a unifocal origin for human serous ovarian carcinomas. Gynecol Oncol 48: 5–10

99. Tsao SW, Mok CH, Oike K, et al (1991) Involvement of p53 gene in the allelic deletion of chromosome 17p in human ovarian tumors. Anticancer Res 11: 1975–1982

100. Toki T, Kurman RJ, Park JS, Kessis T, Daniel RW, Shah KV (1991) Probable nonpapillomavirus etiology of squamous cell carcinoma of the vulva in older women: A clinicopathologic study using in situ hybridization and polymerase chain reaction. Int J Gynecol Pathol 10: 107–125

101. Vogelstein B, Fearon E, Kern S, et al (1989) Allelotype of colorectal carcinomas. Science 244: 207–211

102. Vogelstein B, Fearon E, Hamilton S, et al (1988) Genetic alterations during colorectal-tumor development. N Engl J Med 319: 525–532

103. Vonka V, Kanka J, Jelinek J, et al (1984) Prospective study on the relationship between cervical neoplasia and herpes simplex type-2 virus. I. Epidemiological characteristics. Int J Cancer 33: 49–60

104. Werness B, Levine A, Howley P (1990) Association of human papillomavirus types 16 and 18 E6 proteins with p53. Science 248: 76–79

105. Wilczynski S, Lee Y, Paquette R, Koeffler P (1992) p53 mutations in cervical and vulvar squamous cell carcinomas. 11th International Papillomavirus Workshop, 136 (Abstract)

106. Woodruff J, TeLinde R (1976) The histology and histogenesis of ovarian neoplasia. Cancer 38: 411–413

107. Worsham MJ, Van Dyke DL, Grenman SE, et al (1991) Consistent chromosome abnormalities in squamous cell carcinoma of the vulva. Genes Chrom Cancer 3: 420–432

108. Yokota J, Tsukada Y, Nakajima T, et al (1989) Loss of heterozygosity on the short arm of chromosome 3 in carcinoma of the uterine cervix. Cancer Res 49: 3598–3601

109. Young L, Bevan I, Johnson M, et al (1989) The polymerase chain reaction: A new epidemiological tool for investigating cervical human papillomavirus infection. Br Med J 298: 14–18

110. Zaino R, Unger E, Whitney C (1984) Synchronous carcinomas of the uterine corpus and ovary. Gynecol Oncol 19: 329–335

111. Zhang X, Silva E, Gershenson D, Hung MC (1989) Amplification and rearrangement of c-erb B proto-oncogenes in cancer of human female genital tract. Oncogene 4: 985–989

112. Zheng JP, Robinson WR, Ehlen T, Yu MC, Debeau L (1991) Distinction of low grade from high grade human ovarian carcinomas on the basis of losses of heterozygosity on chromosomes 3, 6, and 11 and HER-2/neu gene amplification. Cancer Res 51: 4045–4051

113. zur Hausen H (1976) Condylomata acuminata and human genital cancer. Cancer Res 36: 794

29

Epidemiology

Mark H. Schiffman, M.D., and Louise A. Brinton, Ph.D.

Most pathologists are part-time epidemiologists as well. The two medical disciplines are more closely allied than most realize. Epidemiologists study the distribution and determinants of diseases in human populations. In current medical practice, diseases often are defined by histopathological diagnoses or by clinical pathological test values. Thus, whenever a pathologist shifts intellectually from the level of the individual slide or specimen to thinking about a group of diagnoses, an informal epidemiologic question is being raised. For example, "How common is this diagnosis?" is a question of prevalence or incidence. "Why am I seeing so many cases of this type of tumor?" is a question of time trends. "How would my colleague interpret these slides compared with me?" is a question of interpathologist agreement. "What causes this disease I am seeing every week?" is a question of etiology that can be addressed by pathologists working as epidemiologists, or with them.

This chapter is meant to introduce the major epidemiologic concepts of greatest use to pathologists who are considering a research project or who wish to think more formally, at the population level, about their case material or diagnostic criteria. The review is certainly not exhaustive; rather, it is meant to be informal and readable, and to encourage the pathologist to pursue epidemiologic projects and collaborations. The first section, accordingly, is organized around types of possible epidemiologic studies that a pathologist might wish to pursue. The next section outlines nonmathematically a few basics of statistical thinking that pathologists need to know if they wish to do more formal epidemiologic research. The third section discusses a few problem issues that often emerge when epidemiologists and pathologists work together. The final section summarizes what is known about the epidemiology of the major gynecological cancers.

Applications of Epidemiology to Pathology

This section illustrates the types of epidemiologic projects that a pathologist may undertake, either informally or formally. The examples are drawn mainly from etiologic and screening studies of gynecological neoplasia, especially cervical neoplasia.

Throughout this section, epidemiologic terms are introduced and simply defined. There is a useful dictionary of epidemiology for readers interested in learning more terminology.[104] For a more complete understanding of basic epidemiologic concepts, the reader is referred to one of several introductory texts.[109,114,119] For readers with some statistical training, a brief text summarizing the basic methods of epidemiology also is available.[84]

Prevalence, Incidence, and Mortality Rates of Disease

One of the first questions that an expert or novice epidemiologist is likely to ask about a disease under study is "How common is it?" The pathologist at the microscope is interested in how common various conditions are, as one element of differential diagnosis (witness the maxims, "Rare diseases occur rarely," and "If you hear hoofbeats, think of a horse not a zebra.")

For the pathologist considering a research study, the frequency of disease occurrence is crucial for two reasons: On the practical level, very rare conditions are difficult to study epidemiologically. The statistical principles underlying epidemiology require moderately large numbers in order to deal with chance, which is the unavoidable and defining characteristic of observational studies in humans.

More importantly, the amount of disease in a population is the starting point for epidemiologic thought, leading to all of the major epidemiologic comparisons, such as "How much disease occurs in Population A compared with Population B, and what does the difference tell us? Why is the amount of disease changing over time? What risk factors are associated with groups having the most disease?"

Because measuring the occurrence of disease is so important to epidemiologists, they find it important, like skiers discussing snow, to define terms carefully using a resultant epidemiologic jargon. A few key terms related to the frequency of disease occurrence are essential and worth memorizing by anyone interested in epidemiology.

The *prevalence* of a disease is the number of occurrences of the disease in a given population at a given time, for example, "Twenty percent of the patients seen in this clinic have at least reactive changes on their Papanicolaou smears." Often, prevalence is discussed with reference to a single point in time, as in a screening program, yielding a *point prevalence*: "Two percent of the screening smears last month showed changes suggestive of CIN."

The *incidence* of disease is the number of new cases that develop in a given time period. Accordingly, *incident disease* refers to new disease, whereas *prevalent disease* refers to all the cases in the population, whether new or chronic. The connection between prevalence and incidence is the *duration* of the condition (Prevalence = Incidence × Duration); thus, the prevalence of rabies in a given week is close to the incidence because duration is unfortunately short, whereas the prevalence of a long-duration disease such as rheumatoid arthritis much exceeds the incidence for any time period.

Incidence is defined most often as a yearly rate, as in "13,500 incident cases of cervical cancer were diagnosed in the United States in 1993." However, *lifetime cumulative incidence* also is an intuitively useful term, meaning the estimated risk of occurrence of a disease over a woman's life: "About 1% of women in the United States will develop cervical cancer in their lifetime." For chronic diseases such as cancer, endometriosis, or genital herpes, incidence usually is thought of as a one-time phenomenon, for example, second primaries rarely occur. (Recurrences of the same disease imply that it is prevalent, not incident). For acute, self-limited, or curable conditions, such as gonorrhea, incidence must be defined over a fairly narrow range of time if one wishes to avoid counting twice the same patients in a population.

Rates of death from a disease are measured as the *mortality rate*. The connection between incidence and mortality is, of course, survival, measured often by the *case/fatality ratio*.

In sum, the epidemiologist is interested in the prevalence, incidence, and mortality rates of a disease as the fundamental basis of further study. These terms can be applied to any study population, whether that population is a single gynecological practice or hospital, a city, country, or the world.

National incidence and mortality data are cited most often when discussing the scope of a medical problem. Where can national data be obtained? In the United States, most pathologists probably are aware that mortality rates from all causes are compiled and available from a variety of sources, most notably and simply from the National Center for Health Statistics (6525 Belcrest Road, Room 1064, Hyattsville, MD 20784; 301-436-8500). Despite the problems of death certificates as the source of the mortality data, with the obvious uncertainties and errors in ascribing causes of death, mortality rates for often-fatal diseases usually are the most reliable gauge of disease occurrence, when comparing different populations or time periods (except when the case/fatality ratio has been altered sharply by improved treatment).

If a condition is not often fatal, mortality rates may not be useful for disease surveillance. It is often more difficult to obtain reliable incidence data, and the researcher must rely on data from voluntary registries, published surveys, or occasionally government-mandated registries. For cancer, fortunately, careful and complete incidence rates for a (nonrandom but stable) 10% sample of the U.S. population are compiled by the National Cancer Institute's Surveillance, Epidemiology, and End Results (SEER) Program. The most accessible source of SEER cancer incidence and survival data (as well as national cancer mortality data) is *CA—A Cancer Journal for Clinicians*, published annually by the American Cancer Society and mailed free to physicians. More detailed cancer data can be obtained from other American Cancer Society publications, such as *Cancer Facts and Figures*, or from the SEER program itself (EPN 343 National Cancer Institute, Bethesda, MD 20892;301-496-8510).

Geographic Differences and Time Trends in Disease Occurrence

Pathologists may wish to go beyond descriptions of disease occurrence at a place and time, to compare rates between geographic areas or over time. The usual hope is that the comparisons may yield clues to etiology and pathogenesis. A cautious approach is critical because of the omnipresent effects of chance on observational data. How can one tell if the amount of disease in one place or time is truly different from the amount found earlier or elsewhere? Disease rates fluctuate over time and place. Many geographic differences and temporal trends do not persist over time, appearing random (to the limit of our understanding!).

Hence, the need for statistics as one of the disciplines underlying epidemiology. Distinguishing chance differences from true differences requires statistical thinking and an appreciation of the types of differences that arise by chance. This point is important because overinterpretation of chance differences is one of most common errors that novice epidemiologists make when comparing disease rates from one place or time with another. For example, many cancer "outbreaks" in which several neighbors get similar tumors turn out to be quite explainable as chance clusterings of events, expected for common malignancies like breast cancer. A good bit of advice might be to treat health statistics like the monthly economic news: it takes a long-term trend or a persistent difference to trust that something important is happening.

When comparing place to place or analyzing time trends, the cardinal rule is to make sure that the comparison is valid. A checklist of common-sense questions should be asked:

1. Are the rates being compared truly comparable (incidence, prevalence, mortality)? In particular, are the sources of data comparable (e.g., a mandatory registry cannot be compared with a voluntary reporting system because of differences in the completeness of reporting).
2. Are the diagnostic criteria the same in both comparison groups? This particular problem has plagued the interpretation of time trend data regarding minor cervical cytological abnormalities because increased recognition by pathologists of subtle koilocytotic changes cannot be distinguished easily from increased incidence of koilocytotic atypia.
3. Are the two populations comparable in age and other factors affecting risk of disease? No one would think of comparing the prevalence of CIN in a gynecological referral practice to the prevalence in a screening clinic because, of course, the prevalence would be higher in the referral clinic. But some researchers make the analogous mistake of comparing populations that differ with regard to age, socioeconomic status, or other more subtle characteristics related to the risk of disease (called *confounding variables* in epidemiologic jargon). Most importantly, almost all diseases vary in incidence and prevalence by age; thus, almost all comparisons should take age into account. The section on error and bias below mentions simple methods of adjustment for age and other confounding variables. The statistical bases of making geographic and temporal comparisons are covered below in the sections on descriptive data and measures of risk.

Validating New (or Old) Histopathologic Diagnostic Distinctions

The creation and refinement of pathological classifications can be aided by epidemiologic corroboration. For example, the Bethesda System of cervical cytology combines koilocytotic atypia and CIN 1 as low grade squamous intraepithelial lesion (LSIL). This combination was supported by epidemiologic data. The two diagnoses, which are not reliably distinguishable on morphologic grounds, share the same epidemiologic profiles of younger average

age and varied human papillomavirus (HPV) types as compared with the older average age and restricted HPV types found in higher grade lesions. As another example, a recent pathological study of squamous vulvar cancer, which proposed new pathological subtypes, was strengthened by a separate epidemiologic analysis showing that the new subtypes had different epidemiologic characteristics. Pathologists and epidemiologists can work iteratively to refine disease classifications, asking each other "Do categories X and Y look the same or different from your point of view?"

Judging Intra- or Interpathologist Agreement

Pathology agreement studies have been motivated by the needs of both disciplines. Pathologists obviously are concerned with the reliability of the diagnoses they make. Epidemiologists are concerned with uniform case definition in their studies. When comparisons of intra- and interpathologist agreement are performed, the epidemiologist can serve the role of scientific organizer, ensuring independence of the reviews by *masking* the reviewers (also called *blinding*) to each others' diagnoses until after the data are complete. It is the widespread opinion of epidemiologists that unmasked comparisons, in which reviewers have access to each others' diagnoses, have limited scientific value. Like all human beings, pathologists tend to agree much more in public than in private, and masking provides a guarantee that a comparison rather than a consensus is being achieved. In the area of cervical pathology, the diagnosis of CIN by either cytology or histology has proved much more variable among experts when masked comparisons were performed than initially expected.

Epidemiologic Studies of Disease Etiology

Epidemiologists attempt to find the determinants of disease by statistically correlating the presence or absence of possible *exposures* (often called *risk factors*) with the presence or absence of disease. Epidemiologic studies attempting to relate exposures and disease are called *analytic studies*, as distinguished from *descriptive studies* that yield rates of disease without explicitly addressing etiology.

A description of the many types of analytic studies is beyond the scope of this chapter. At the simplest level, *prospective* or *cohort studies* start with the measurement of an exposure, then proceed to compare incidence rates or *absolute risk* of disease in the exposed versus the unexposed groups. The ratio of the incidence rate in exposed subjects divided by the incidence rate in the unexposed is called the *incidence rate ratio*. The reader might correctly expect that there are as many types of rate ratios as there are types of rates (e.g., *prevalence rate ratio*, *lifetime cu-*

mulative risk ratio). Many epidemiologists casually refer to the entire group as the *relative risk* of exposed versus nonexposed subjects, and use the abbreviation *RR* as a general shorthand.

Prospective studies are the most appealing type of analytic study because they determine most directly how commonly disease occurs in exposed versus unexposed individuals. The relative risk, measured directly, is an intuitively clear answer to the question: "If a woman has this characteristic (the exposure), how much more likely is she to develop the disease, compared with a similar unexposed woman?" The absolute risk translates as "How likely to get disease is an exposed woman?" (see below, Measures of Risk). The problem with prospective studies is that they are expensive, usually take years to organize and complete, and must be very large to generate enough occurrences of disease for reliable estimates of risk, unless the disease is extraordinarily common.

Other analytic study designs try, in general, to estimate the relative risk that might be observed in the ideal prospective study while saving time and money. Analytic studies that start by collecting a series of *cases* (women diagnosed with a given disease) and appropriate *controls* (women without that disease who are measured for comparison) are called *case-control* studies. The exposures of interest are ascertained for both groups and the relative risk (RR) of disease among the exposed versus the unexposed is estimated by calculating the ratio of the odds of exposure in cases versus controls (for more explanation, see the the statistical section on measures of risk).

The estimation of the prospective relative risk by the case-control *odds ratio* (*OR*) is one of the most important statistical concepts in epidemiology, and one of the most subtle. For this statistical approximation to be valid, incident cases and controls must be chosen to be strictly comparable. The control group must represent the group of subjects at risk of developing disease at the time the incident case was diagnosed, otherwise the estimation of the relative risk can be grossly mistaken because of *bias* (a nonrandom or systematic error in estimation of a statistic, to be distingushed from *random error*).

In practice, it is difficult to define and recruit an unbiased sample of the general population that gave rise to the cases appearing in one hospital or clinic. Thus, all kinds of compromises of convenience and practicality must be made, and it becomes difficult to avoid bias in choosing controls. For example, smoking causes or worsens so many kinds of illness that it is very difficult to use hospitalized controls to estimate the relative risk of a disease in smokers compared with nonsmokers. The exposure to smoking in the hospitalized controls is elevated compared with the general at-risk population; thus, the odds ratio obtained in a naively conducted hospital-based study tends to provide too low an estimate of the relative risk.

Because case-control studies are used so commonly as an analytic design, choosing proper controls is one of the two most important aspects of epidemiology. The other is assuring proper measurements of exposure and disease. The mark of a good epidemiologist is a dedicated attention to control selection, whereas many novices tend to focus more on the cases while relying on a *convenience sample* of whichever controls are most easily available.

Besides prospective and case-control studies, another common analytic study design is the *cross-sectional* study, in which exposure and disease status are ascertained concurrently for a study population. An example would be a screening study of HPV infection and abnormal cervical cytology, in which all women attending a clinic are tested for viral DNA at the same time the cytological smear is taken. The analysis of a cross-sectional study is somewhat similar to that of a case-control study, but the researcher must be careful because the cases are a combination of incident and prevalent disease. The odds ratio computed in a cross-sectional study is a good estimation of the prospective relative risk only if certain conditions are met, including an assumption that the disease under study is rare (an assumption not met for cervical cytological abnormalities in many clinics).

The pathologist collaborator should play a key role in all analytic studies of diseases whose definitions rely on nonroutine pathological expertise. Misclassification of disease status can be damaging to a study because the effect of misclassification on correlative statistics such as the relative risk and odds ratio is, generally, to reduce the apparent strength of the association between disease and exposure. If the disease is poorly defined, no epidemiologic risk factors may be found even if they exist. Moreover, it is often very difficult to measure the risk factors (exposures) without substantial error, whether laboratory testing or interviews are being used. The combination of multiple errors in measuring both exposure and disease can literally make a study worthless. For example, early studies correlating HPV DNA detection and CIN revealed only a moderate association, in that less than 50% of cases were found to be HPV positive.[148] Moreover, HPV infection was not apparently associated with sexual activity, an established strong risk factor for CIN. These weak associations were due to misclassification. Subsequent studies with better HPV tests and expert review of pathology revealed that virtually all cases of CIN contain HPV DNA,[153] and that HPV is the sexually transmitted agent explaining the association of sexual activity and risk of CIN.[148]

As the result of the strong, damaging effects of misclassification on epidemiologic studies, epidemiologists pay careful attention to the pathological classifications that define their study cases and controls, and often establish formal collaborations with reviewing pathologists as part of epidemiologic studies.

Follow-up Studies of Patients with the Same Pathological Diagnosis

Clinicians, pathologists, and epidemiologists are all interested in learning what happens to patients diagnosed with a given disease. For a possibly fatal disease, survival rates are critical, whereas for other chronic diseases, progression rates or recurrence rates often are estimated. It is often of interest to divide the patients into groups to determine whether subtypes of disease follow different courses, or whether different treatments influence outcome. The *randomized clinical trial* is a specialized version of such a follow-up study, in which subjects are randomly assigned to various treatment groups to maximize the comparability of the groups. The hope is that the randomization will minimize differences in both known and unknown confounding variables that could bias the comparison.

Follow-up studies almost invariably involve the concept of *time to an event*. In other words, it is important when death or recurrence or progression occur, not just if they occur. Clearly, all participants in any clinical trial eventually die, the question is when (and why). A good treatment prolongs time to death, a bad type of disease shortens it.

Because of the critical notion of "time to event" in epidemiologic follow-up studies, they depend heavily on actuarial methods, like survival curves and life-table analyses, when comparing exposed to unexposed patients or treated to untreated patients. The central statistical concept in such studies is a kind of rate called a *hazard*, which refers to the risk of disease occurring in a unit of follow-up time. A hazard is computed as the number of *events* (e.g., death, cure, progression) divided by the amount of *person-time* of follow-up. One thousand women followed for a year or 100 women followed for 10 years both yield 1000 person-years of follow-up time. Two cancers arising during that follow-up would yield a hazard of two cases per 1000 person-years.

A hazard is a special kind of rate because it is conceived of as the rate of disease at a single moment in time, as the mathematical "limit" of the rate as time "goes to zero." Accordingly, the hazard of disease can change from moment to moment as conditions change. A woman lights up a cigarette and her hazard for lung cancer increases. She quits smoking the next day and her hazard decreases.

Moreover, the computation of the denominator of hazards, person-time, of follow-up requires some training and thought. For each successive time interval during followup, the denominator of women at risk for an event changes. For example, women are lost to follow-up as they drop out of the study, or they die for other reasons, or they experience the event itself (since one can develop a disease for the first time only once). Thus, computing the proper amount of person-time during which the events occurred requires some knowledge of *censoring*, which is the proper deletion of irrelevant follow-up time during which the subject was not truly at risk of diagnosis of the event.

Usually, researchers are not content to describe the simple survival curve of a disease, which represents the hazard of death over time after diagnosis. They wish to determine which factors affect the hazard, that is, what the relative or *proportional hazard* of death, etc., might be for women in different groups defined by pathological differences or treatment types. The proportional hazard is almost identical to the incident rate ratio discussed above, but the denominator is person-time of follow-up, not just time. Proportional hazard analyses are too complex to be described here, and pathologists performing follow-up studies might consider consulting an epidemiologist or biostatistician early in the design phase of such projects. Data collection must be organized carefully to permit a correct determination of person-time.

Screening for Gynecological Malignancies

Screening is inherently epidemiologic, thus, the pathologist involved in screening programs (e.g., cervical cytological screening or CA125 testing) needs to understand the interrelated concepts of sensitivity, specificity, and predictive value. The basics are outlined below in a statistical section on screening.

A common mistake in evaluating the results of a screening trial is to ignore the clinical setting. The *sensitivity* of a screening technique (percentage of diseased women who test positive) and its *specificity* (percentage of disease-free women who test negative) theoretically do not change when the test is taken out of a high-risk hospital clinic to be applied to the general population. But most clinicians are more interested in the *positive predictive value* and *negative predictive value*, two statistics that are highly dependent on the clinical setting. For example, the positive predictive value is the percentage of women testing positive who truly have disease. Given the same sensitivity and specificity, positive predictive value decreases sharply as the prevalence of the disease decreases. Therefore, the same screening test that looks promising because of high sensitivity in a high-risk clinic often will perform poorly in the general population, producing so many false positives compared with the disease yield that the costs outweigh the benefits. As a general rule, specificity is the prime requirement of a screening test. A screening test such as a tumor marker must be highly specific (negative in virtually all nondiseased women, certainly more than 95%) to be cost effective for general population screening.

Basic Statistical Concepts

Hopefully, the preceding discussion has firmly established the relevance of epidemiology to gynecological pathology research and even daily practice. Epidemiologic work re-

quires an understanding of biostatistics. This section mentions the bare basics of what the author believes pathologists collaborating in epidemiologic research might wish to know about biostatistical methods. Introductory biostatistics texts are available and easy to read for the pathologists wishing to work independently, or for those who want computational formulae for chi-square or other commonly used tests.

Variability as a Fundamental Principle of Pathology

Virtually all measurements that one could make about a human population are variable. Height, weight, fine points of anatomy, metabolic patterns, serum levels of hormones, and nutrients are all commonly recognized to be variable. The same variability is seen by pathologists at the tissue and cellular levels, and by research pathologists at the molecular biological level (e.g., varying tissue levels of DNA adducts given equivalent carcinogenic exposures, genetic polymorphisms in human genes, and varying molecular responses to infection with viral DNA). Even the intricate, multistep molecular pathways to cancer demonstrate substantial variability between individuals who develop the same type of malignancy.[171]

Variability in pathology is mainly described by *categorical* or *discrete* data and statistics, as compared with *continuous* data and statistics (the province of the mean, median, and standard deviation). Similar (but not identical) histological and cytological appearances are categorized and named. More attention is paid to the borderlines and overlaps of the categories, rather than subtler differences within the categories (unless splitting into finer categories is being considered). Categorical data analysis relies on *contingency tables*, which are discussed in a section below. Contingency tables, like the common 2×2 *table*, are frequency counts of categorical data, for example, how many (not what percent of) CIN 2 lesions demonstrated aneuploidy or not, compared with how many CIN 3 lesions demonstrated aneuploidy or not.

The variability in categorical data such as pathology categories shows up in diagnostic error (i.e., the misassignment of a patient to the wrong category). In general, error cannot be avoided. To the epidemiologist, categorization of variable biological continuua virtually dictates that there will be error. If two categories blend into each other with regard to a characteristic (even one as complex and general as microscopic appearance), they cannot be perfectly separated based on that characteristic. Thus, pathologists search for additional characteristics to discriminate difficult-to-distinguish indeterminate cases, such as immunocytochemistry, but these ancillary measurements also have error and overlap. There is a field of statistics called *discriminant analysis*, in which the goal is to determine how many characteristics must be measured to maximize correct assignment to overlapping categories. This complicated set of statistical methods underlies the development of computer-assisted cytology screening.

Error Versus Bias

Error is inevitable, but epidemiologists hope that it is mainly random, not systematically pushing the data in one way or the other. *Random error* reduces the *reliability* of repeated measurements, affecting their *precision*, and reduces the perceived strength of correlations, but the average measured value still becomes increasingly true or *accurate* as the study size increases. Systematic error, called *bias*, impacts directly on the accuracy of the measurement; no matter how large a study based on biased measurements is, the answer will be wrong. Thus, epidemiologists struggle to reduce random measurement error, but they have an even stronger dislike of biased measurements. If the exact direction and magnitude of a fixed bias were known, the data could be adjusted (like a scale that always reads three pounds heavy), but adjustments for bias usually are not possible.

Epidemiologists combat error and bias in a few standard ways. To quantify and reduce random error, reliability is measured by repeating data collection, whether that involves re-asking a question, re-running an assay, or submitting a pathology slide for re-review.

For continuous variables, statistics of reliability include the *variance* (sum of the squared deviations of the measurements from their arithmetic average or *mean*, divided by the number of data points minus one), the *standard deviation* (the square root of the variance) of the raw data or of the mean (called the *standard error* of the mean), and the *coefficient of variation* (the ratio of the standard deviation to the mean).

For categorical variables, statistics of reliability include the simple percentage of agreement and more complicated statistics mentioned below in the section on measures of interpathologist agreement.

To reduce bias, epidemiologists would like to compare the study measurement to a reference standard of truth, but such reference standards virtually never exist. Certainly, there is no source of absolute truth in pathology, only advancing degrees of expertise correlated with decreasing amounts of diagnostic error. Therefore, to reduce bias in pathology, researchers are limited to the comparison of different experts. To the extent that truly independent experts agree (without consideration of each other's opinion), the possibility that either one is biased is reduced.

Of course, experts can share or even teach each other the same biases, destroying the notion of independence and reducing the possibility of identifying the biases. Hence the value to epidemiologists of outspoken pathologists, who point out beliefs in pathology that might be changing.

Also to reduce the possibility of bias, epidemiologists try to ensure that all study measurements are made independent of each other, so that knowledge of one variable cannot bias a decision about another. The difficulties of masking are discussed in a section below.

Descriptive Data

The terms used most often to describe and summarize descriptive data, such as prevalence and incidence, are defined in the section on geographic differences and time trends above, and are not repeated. A few additional statistical concepts critical to the interpretation of descriptive data are mentioned.

First, there is an important choice of scale in the plotting of descriptive data. The scale of the y or vertical axis greatly affects the appearance of the data, and must always be noted when examining plotted data. A log scale flattens curves and reduces the apparent strength of trends and differences, whereas an arithmetic scale does the opposite. On a log scale, an increasing, straight-line trend implies an exponential, not linear, rate of increase.

A common error in inference when interpreting descriptive data is the *ecologic fallacy*, the attribution of causality to an association seen only in descriptive data. For example, the international risk of colon cancer (mortality rates for each country plotted on a graph) correlates with the average dietary intake of those countries for fat, meat, and sugar, and with the average amount of sunlight (the major determinant of vitamin D levels). To assume that all four variables are true risk factors for colon cancer at the level of the individual would be an example of the ecologic fallacy, confusing descriptive data for analytic (individual level) data.

In the interpretation of time trend data, the possibility of a *cohort effect* must be kept in mind. A cohort effect, familiar by analogy to anyone who studies the sociology of baby-boomers, is the variation in disease occurrence that occurs in a population over time, as successive birth cohorts (persons of the same age) experience the unique environment that typifies their life course. For example, based on cross-sectional prevalence data compiled in 1991, the prevalence rates of koilocytotic atypia of the cervix decrease sharply with increasing age, from a peak at about age 20 to 25 years. This age trend might represent a biological phenomenon, the result of immunity, with many women becoming infected with HPV at the time of initiation of sexual intercourse, then becoming increasingly immune and having fewer new sexual partners as they age. Or, the age trend also could reflect a cohort effect, with changing sexual practices and increasing prevalence of HPV infection over the past decades placing younger women today at higher risk for koilocytotic changes compared with their older sisters and mothers.

To distinguish cohort effects from simple age trends requires a *cohort analysis*, a type of descriptive graphing in

Table 29.1. The basic contingency table

	Disease	No disease	Total
Exposed or test positive	a	b	a + b
Unexposed or test negative	c	d	c + d
Total	a + c	b + d	a + b + c + d = n

which the age- specific prevalence rates are graphed separately for each birth cohort. These analyses usually are difficult enough in interpretation to merit a statistical consultation.

The Basic Contingency Table

The pathology slide of epidemiology is the contingency table, the basic form of which is the 2×2 table (Table 29.1).

Most important epidemiologic findings, relating an exposure to risk of a disease, have been derived and can be expressed in this simple form. Extension of the table to more rows or columns does not change the concepts, only the statistical complexity.

The most common statistics computed from a contingency table are simple percentages, which can then be compared: "Ninety percent of the group with disease were smokers $[(a/ a + c) = 0.90]$ compared with 20% of the nondiseased $[(b/ b + d) = 0.20]$. These proportions could be compared statistically using the well-known t test or another test of the difference between independent proportions. More often, the *chi-square statistic* is computed, which gives equivalent interpretations but has a slightly different intent.

The chi-square test is meant to determine whether the disease categories and the exposure categories are associated or independent (i.e., does being exposed affect the probability of having disease?). Chi-square values are derived by comparing the expected counts of a, b, c, and d to the values that would be expected if disease and exposure were totally independent. For example, the expected value of a is the cross-product of $(a + b) \times (a + c)$ divided by n. The divergence of observed from expected values for all of the *cells* of the table (a, b, c, d) are summed to derive the chi-square statistic. The larger the statistic, summarizing how much observed counts differ from expected, the more likely disease and exposure are associated by more than chance.

The chi-square statistic obtained is compared with the tabled values of the *chi-square distribution* to yield a p value, the probability of observing such a chi-square value if disease and exposure are not related. If the p value is less than 0.05 or 0.01, then convention dictates that chance is unlikely to explain the degree of association seen in the table, and the association is considered *statistically significant*.

Thanks to many recent published cautions, most clinicians and researchers know that a strict dependence on p values is incorrect, because the magnitude of the p value depends on the size of the study. Smaller studies require stronger associations to achieve the same level of statistical significance; thus, a p value of 0.06 in a small study by no means rules out a true exposure-disease association whereas a highly statistically significant difference from a huge study may be so small as to be clinically irrelevant.

Contingency tables larger than 2×2 should be analyzed in a methodical and hierarchical fashion, not restricting the analysis to the most "significant-looking" internal comparisons. First, the evidence for association in the full table should be assessed and, if there is none, then the analysis should stop. A common mistake some novices make is to look at a large contingency table, choosing the most interesting difference seen, then testing the significance of that extracted comparison. Given a large enough contingency table, some subtables will yield statistically significant results by chance alone. Permitting a prescreening of the data before applying a statistical test to the most divergent data points is wrong. If one wishes to define the likely source of the association when the overall contingency table indicates statistical significance, the proper approach is to analyze smaller subtables in a complete and hierarchical manner. A formal description of the proper approach to contingency table analyses can be found in standard biostatistics texts.

When the number of study subjects is very small, such that the expected count in any cell is less than about five, then chi-square analyses are unreliable and should be replaced by a test called *Fisher's exact test*. Of course, if the study is too small, no result will be statistically significant.

One other key point about contingency tables is that the two measurements (disease status and exposure, for example) must be assumed to be independent, as one embarks on statistical testing. Although a significant chi-square statistic indicates that the measurements are not independent, the initial or *null hypothesis* of independence is what the test is designed to reject. Thus, standard chi-square analyses should not be performed to test tables in which the measurements are explicitly correlated, as in interpathologist agreement studies, or comparisons of the efficacy of two cell collection techniques used in the same group of patients. For *paired-sample comparisons*, the Mc-Nemar's test is easy to use. The test ignores the points of agreement of the two measurements and tests the statistical significance of the amount of divergence.

Measures of Risk (Absolute, Relative, and Attributable Risks)

The chi-square provides limited information regarding the strength of an association (yes/no). Therefore, epidemiologists often prefer instead to compute the more informative statistic, the relative risk (or odds ratio estimate of the relative risk). These key terms are defined in the section on epidemiologic studies of disease etiology. In this section, the relation of the terms to the contingency table are explained, with a brief discussion of ancillary topics such as statistical adjustment of confounding variables, interaction, and confidence intervals.

Suppose a prospective study started by defining an exposed group and an unexposed group of women, then followed the two groups for disease occurrence. The absolute risk of disease following exposure can be represented as an incidence rate $a/(a + b)$. (See Table 29.1.) The time period for this incidence rate is implicitly the duration of follow-up. The absolute risk of disease in the unexposed group, analogously, would be the incidence rate $c/(c + d)$. The ratio of these absolute risks would be the relative risk (specifically, the incidence rate ratio) in exposed versus nonexposed women, $a/(a + b)$ divided by $c/(c + d)$. A relative risk above 1.0 implies an increased risk. For example, a relative risk of 2.0 means that the risk of disease in exposed women is twice that of unexposed women. In contrast, a relative risk between 0.0 and 1.0 indicates a protective association (a relative risk of 0.5 implies a halving of risk associated with the exposure). A relative risk of approximately 1.0 implies the exposure is not related to risk of the disease.

Prospective studies permit the computational directness and intuitive quality of the relative risk calculation and the ability to decompose the relative risk into the absolute risks among the exposed and unexposed groups.

In contrast, absolute risks usually cannot be calculated in case-control studies because the true numbers of exposed women $(a + b)$ and unexposed women $(c + d)$ are not known. In fact, in 2×2 tables from case-control studies the values $a + b$ and $c + d$ are meaningless and should never be computed. The numbers of cases $(a + c)$ and controls $(b + d)$ are chosen first, and not in proportion to the true ratio of cases to controls in the population. Cases are almost always sampled in excess; in fact, oversampling cases to overcome the limitation of rarity is the major reason to perform a case-control analysis.

As mentioned earlier, although case-control data do not permit direct calculation of the relative risk, the odds ratio provides a valid estimate if the cases and controls represent an unbiased sample of all women with and without disease in the population, and if the disease in question is very rare (if the cases are all incident, the rare disease assumption is not as important, unless the disease is so common that a nonnegligible percentage of the population is developing it at any given time).

To understand the concept of the odds ratio, again consider a prospective study. The odds of disease in exposed women is a/b, very close to the risk of disease $a/(a + b)$ if a, the occurrence of disease among the exposed, is very infrequent. Similarly, the odds of disease in nonexposed women

is c/d, close to the risk of the disease if uncommon in the nonexposed women, $c/(c + d)$.

With a little algebra, it is easy to see that the relative odds or odds ratio for a rare disease (a/b divided by c/d, often computed as the cross-product ad/bc) is quite close to the relative risk.

The important point is that the cross-product ad/bc can be computed from a case-control study without knowing the total number of exposed and unexposed women. As long as the odds a/c and b/d are unbiased with regard to the entire population, then a/c divided by b/d equals ad/bc equals the prospective odds ratio of a/b divided by c/d. The key is to select an unbiased sample of cases and controls. Because epidemiologists usually try to recruit all cases occurring in a population, bias among cases usually is not an issue unless participation rates are poor. The place where bias is a major concern is among the controls. Epidemiologists spend most of their intellectual energy attempting to ensure that the ratio b/d in controls (also thought of as the percentage of controls exposed to the risk factor) is unbiased compared with the same ratio in the whole population that gave rise to the cases. Without the elimination of bias, the odds ratio does not estimate the relative risk, and the case-control design will yield a false result.

Confounding is the type of bias that concerns epidemiologists the most, particularly when they are conducting case-control studies or nonrandomized prospective studies. *Confounding variables* are factors that influence both the risk of disease and the likelihood of exposure to a risk factor under study. The relationship between exposures, confounding variables, and disease outcome is illustrated in Figure 29.1.

When assessing whether an exposure such as smoking causes cervical cancer, the researcher must consider and adjust for the confounding influence of sexual activity leading to HPV infection, a central cause of cervical cancer. Women who smoke tend to have more sexual partners and, consequently, are more likely to be HPV infected (i.e., the confounding variable is linked to the likelihood of the study exposure). HPV is a cause of cervical cancer. The apparent influence of smoking on risk of cervical cancer is reduced by statistically adjusting for HPV infection status. A residual association between smoking and cervical cancer risk

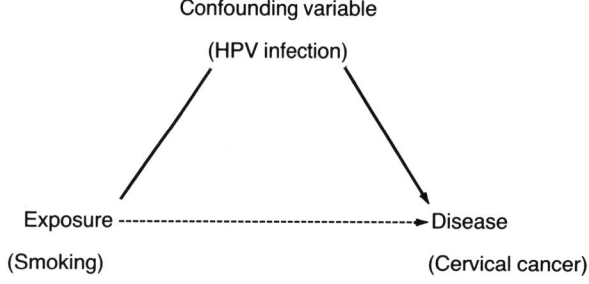

FIG. 29.1. **Confounding.** Confounding variables are risk factors for diseases correlated with the exposure under study.

may still exist, as mentioned later in the chapter, but the true strength of the association is only estimated, correcting when adjusted for confounding. In summary of this important point, epidemiologic analyses must adjust statistically for the influence of confounding factors to generate unbiased risk estimates.

Adjustment for confounding is commonly undertaken by one of three methods: *exclusion, stratification,* or *regression modeling.* Exclusion is exemplified in the example above by restricting the analysis to women known to be infected with HPV, or to virgins (limiting the exposure to HPV). Using stratification, one could analyze either of the two "strata" defined on HPV status, eliminating the possibility of confounding (if HPV infection status could be defined perfectly). Rather than excluding any subjects, the association of smoking with cervical cancer could be examined separately in each of the two strata (HPV −/ HPV +), providing two unconfounded estimates akin to those derived by exclusion. The risk estimates could then be pooled to obtain a global estimate for the risk of smoking adjusted for HPV. This kind of stratified analysis is commonly performed using a group of procedures called a *Mantel–Haenszel analysis* in recognition of its developers.

A more conceptually difficult approach that is widely used is *logistic regression analysis,* a multivariable regression technique available in the major statistical software packages such as SAS and BMDP. This is especially well suited to calculation of the odds ratio as an estimate of the relative risk in case-control studies. This technique permits the simultaneous estimation of the relative risks for multiple risk factors, adjusted for each others' confounding influences. A discussion of this technique, its uses and misuses, is beyond the scope of the chapter. The commercially available statistical packages offer multivariable regression packages in a seductively simple format that might inspire some novice epidemiologists to perform complicated analyses. However, to master the art of multivariable regression analysis takes statistical training and apprenticeship. Moreover, the results cannot be "checked" easily. It is wise both to avoid and distrust complicated analyses, especially because the bulk of what can be learned from most data sets can be expressed using simple tables and intuitively approachable statistics.

Adjustment for confounding often is not perfectly achieved, particularly when the confounding variable cannot be measured well or when variables under study are highly correlated. In fact, it is sometimes virtually impossible using statistical methods to adjust for the confounding influences of correlated variables. For example, the most conceptually difficult areas of chronic disease epidemiology relate to time. In all data analyses involving time, the correlated effects of age at first exposure, duration of exposure, and latency (time since first exposure) are among the most difficult to figure out.

Sometimes the risk of an exposure is modified by levels of another variable. For example, the risk of esophageal cancer associated with smoking is much higher among alcohol drinkers than among nondrinkers. This effect modification, often called *interaction,* is different from confounding in that no global adjustment to arrive at a single correct risk estimate for the exposure is possible. The proper approach is to present the risk estimates for the exposure separately for each level of the effect modifier.

It is common to place *confidence intervals* around relative risk estimates to indicate the likely range of the true risk that we are trying to estimate. Confidence intervals take into account only random error, not bias, and are conceptually somewhat similar to p values although more informative. Thus, a 95% confidence interval and a p value of 0.05 are both commonly chosen as standard, and have analogous interpretations. For example, if the relative risk of an exposure for a disease is 1.8 with a 95% confidence interval of 1.1 to 3.0, this implies that given random error, the true relative risk has a 95% chance of falling within that range. If the confidence interval for a relative risk excludes 1.0, the result is conventionally considered statistically significant. A relative risk with confidence intervals including 1.0 indicates no statistically significant association between exposure and disease. As with p values, confidence intervals should be used as a guide but not followed slavishly in interpreting data.

Most analytic epidemiologic research centers around estimation of relative risks. Another useful concept, especially for public health applications of epidemiologic results, is the *attributable risk,* also known as the *attributable proportion,* or *etiologic fraction.* These terms subsume several computational forms and subtle differences in meaning, but the general meaning is clear: how much of the disease is due to the exposure and would theoretically disappear if the exposure were eliminated (from 0 to 100%). One useful computational formula for the attributable risk, using the notation in Table 29.1, is: Attributable risk $= [(a/a + c) \times (1 - 1/RR)] \times 100\%$. In words, the fraction of disease attributable to the risk factor is equal to the percentage of cases of the disease who are exposed, adjusted for the strength of the estimated relative risk. Although the formula may appear a bit complicated, it is easy to use. The adjustment part of the formula, $(1 - 1/RR)$, goes to zero as the relative risk goes to 1.0, and goes to 1 as the relative risk goes to infinity. Thus, even if all cases are exposed, the attributable risk will be 0% if all controls also are exposed, because the RR is 1.0 and the adjustment term is 0.

Measures of Interpathologist Agreement

Simply put, there is no universally accepted statistical measure of interrater agreement. The problem is adjustment for the influence of chance agreement, which varies with the numbers of categories and the composition of the study population. All currently available statistical methods have limitations and, therefore, it is best when possible to present the actual data to the reader, in addition to any percentage or statistic.

Consider a study of interpathologist agreement for the categories of the Bethesda System of cervical cytology. A group of 100 smears was given to two pathologists, who were asked to rate them as normal or benign reactive changes, atypical squamous cells of undetermined significance (ASCUS), LSIL, or HSIL. The trouble with simply calculating percent agreement is not only that some agreement is expected by chance, but the results are strongly dependent on how the smears are chosen. If mainly normal smears were submitted, the percentage of agreement would be high. If a wide range of changes were equally represented, then agreement undoubtedly would decrease. In general, the most information is obtained by choosing a wide range of smears, oversampling the rarer grades to achieve a balanced study group.

The most widely used, more sophisticated statistic of agreement of use to pathologists is the *kappa statistic*. Its limitations are discussed in a worthwhile review.[112] The kappa statistic computes the proportion of agreement in excess of the expected chance agreement. Kappa values can range from 1.0 (perfect agreement) to less than 0.0 (zero implies only chance agreement). The interpretation of kappa values is not clear cut, in that researchers disagree as to what good agreement is. According to one group, values greater than 0.75 represent excellent agreement beyond chance, 0.40 to 0.75 is fair to good, and less than 0.40 indicates poor agreement beyond chance.[60]

Screening Terms

Screening is a special area of epidemiology distinct from descriptive or analytic studies. It is rare to find a useful screening test. Finding a strong risk factor for a disease does not imply that we should screen for that risk factor, because the factor often is too common in the general population to permit its use as a trigger for clinical action.

Screening terms have exact meanings, which may vary from other common uses of the same terms. In Table 29.1 above, the women in cell "a" have *true-positive* screening tests, in that they have the disease and tested positive. The women in cell "c" have *false-negative* results because they have the disease but tested negative. The *sensitivity* of a test, also called the true positive rate, is the percentage of diseased women who test positive [a/(a + c) in Table 29.1]. The screening sensitivity must be clearly distinguished from the analytic sensitivity of a laboratory assay, which has a different meaning.

The *true-negative* results are in cell "d"; the *false-negative* results are in cell c. The *specificity*, also called the true negative rate, is the percentage of women without the

disease who test negative [d/(b+ d)]. The concept of specificity is more important in screening than most realize. Because the overwhelming majority of women in a population do not have the disease under study, as the specificity percentage falls even slightly, the absolute numbers of false-positive screening tests rise dramatically in comparison to the number of true positives.

Therefore, decreased specificity leads to low *positive predictive value*, the percentage of women with a positive test who truly have the disease [a/(a + b)]. Positive predictive value is, for many diseases, the major screening statistic of interest. Clinicians ask: If a woman tests positive, what is the likelihood that she will have disease confirmed on referral to the next clinical step (e.g., colposcopically directed biopsy, laparoscopy, or more major surgery). Low positive predictive value leads to overreferral and overtreatment.

For grave diseases, in which overtreatment of normal women is less of a concern than not missing any cases, the *negative predictive value* is an important concept. The negative predictive value is the percentage of women who test negative who are truly disease-free [d/(c + d)]. A clinician may ask, accordingly, "If the test is negative, what is the percentage assurance that the disease is not present, and that I can safely stop the diagnostic workup?" The sensitivity of the test usually is the key determinant of negative predictive value.

Some of the current controversy regarding the proper clinical management of inconclusive cervical cytological smears centers around the competing needs for good negative predictive value (assurance that we are not missing any high-grade disease) and good positive predictive value (desire not to overtreat). This problem highlights an inescapable feature of screening (or more fundamentally of trying to categorize overlapping distributions): increased sensitivity virtually always leads to decreased specificity and, as a corollary, increasingly reassuring negative predictive value can be obtained only at the price of decreased positive predictive value.

There is a formal method for choosing the proper screening *cutpoint* (e.g., level of a serologic assay, degree of atypia meriting the diagnosis of LSIL) to achieve an optimal compromise between sensitivity and specificity. The technique is called the *receiver operating characteristic (ROC)*, because the approach was developed to test how well an electronic receiver could distinguish signals from electrical noise. The concepts are easy to understand, useful, and well explained in one key article that is recommended to anyone wishing to evaluate a screening test.[79]

When screening is mentioned, there is always an implicit notion of a *reference standard* or *gold standard* of disease. The performance of screening tests is described statistically in relation to this reference standard and if it is flawed, then the screening statistics will be flawed. For example, colposcopically directed biopsy with pathological diagnosis often is taken as the reference standard of cervical intraepithelial neoplasia, but the colposcopic biopsy may be misdirected or the histopathological diagnosis may be in error. Thus, the true performance of screening tests such as cytology, cervicography, or HPV testing may be misinterpreted when compared with the results of colposopically directed biopsies.

Screening tests may detect prevalent disease or predict the future diagnosis of disease, and the two time frames may be confused. If some type of HPV test could truly predict incipient cervical neoplasia, even when biopsies were still negative, it would be misleading to compare the HPV screening result only to prevalent (same-day) disease defined by biopsies.

Another mistake is the following: Researchers who wish to compare the sensitivity of two screening tests double-test a research population, referring for a definitive diagnostic procedure those women who are positive for either screening test. If they then compute and report the "sensitivity" of each test, an error of circular reasoning has been made. Because both screening tests could have missed disease (double false-negatives), the true sensitivity of either test cannot be known without referring all women in the study population for the definitive work-up. Sometimes, in large studies it suffices to refer a random sample of the women who screen negative on both tests as a way of correcting (or of verifying, to think optimistically) the estimates of sensitivity.

The point of this discussion is that, when screening terms such sensitivity or specificity are mentioned, then the reference standard must be explicitly stated and, if necessary, questioned.

Problem Areas

The major goal of including an introduction to epidemiology in a textbook on gynecological pathology is to encourage pathologists to do epidemiologic studies, and to work with epidemiologists. Accordingly, it may be worth alerting the pathologist to recurrent problem areas that exist at the juncture of the two disciplines. This section informally catalogs a few practical problems that appear to arise most commonly.

Dividing a Spectrum of Disease into Categories

Unfortunately, some epidemiologists may seek out pathologists to perform a service function of "making sure the cases are right," without understanding much about pathology (just as pathologists might seek out statisticians to do a rote data analysis or to figure "how many cases are needed for statistical significance?"). Providing rote pathology review may prove a difficult collaboration, because epidemiologists are prompted by their statistical methods to seek overly simplistic and discrete categorization of disease outcomes. Because the statistical methods for considering a spectrum of disease are difficult to perform and understand, epidemiologists tend to simplify disease measurements into a few (ideally two) reliably distinguished categories, such as "invasive cervical cancer" versus "normal." But as the example of cervical neoplasia demonstrates, diseases may exist as a spectrum of changes that are impossible to divide perfectly into a few categories.

When an epidemiologist asks a pathologist to state whether a slide shows disease (i.e., defines a case) or not (i.e., rejects the case), an uncertain or heavily qualified diagnosis is difficult to force into the study dichotomy. Often, the epidemiologist must subsequently exclude the uncertain diagnoses from the analyses. It is possible to perform a "malicious analysis" in which the uncertain cases are added to the analysis as cases, then reanalyzed as controls, in order to see whether the uncertainty in pathological definition affects the comparisons being made. But too large a proportion of uncertain diagnoses can make an analytic study unreliable.

The collaborating epidemiologist must be willing to understand diagnostic error as a fact of nature and not a failing of pathologists. The pathologist must be willing to sacrifice absolute truth in order to simplify the statistical data to the point of understanding. The limitations of epidemiology should be recognized. As a great physician–epidemiologist once said: "Epidemiology is a butcher shop, don't try to use a scalpel." In other words, epidemiology can only study strong risk associations, because even strong associations are made to appear weak by unavoidable measurement errors and biases. Truly weak associations probably will be missed by all but the largest and luckiest studies. With this in mind, the routine use of pathological qualifiers such as "consistent with" and "cannot exclude" should be abandoned in epidemiologic studies, with the recognition that diagnostic errors will exist (the extent of which should be measured by reliability studies and reported).

The Need for Masking

Epidemiologists tend to mask all data collection as an automatic part of good research technique, to avoid the influence of possible subtle biases that could distort risk estimates. Thus, they do not routinely tell interviewers the disease status of the subjects to minimize bias in questioning, they do not tell laboratory collaborators the identity of specimens until the results are obtained, and they ask pathologists to make their diagnoses with a minimum of information regarding the patients. Epidemiologists are seeking a completely independent decision from pathologists, without influence from previous diagnoses or clinical tests, which often are being studied as risk factors for the current condition. All common statistical tests assume that the study measurements are completely independent of each other; thus, using any data to influence a decision on another piece of data is wrong.

Pathologists, however, realize that diagnoses are best made in the context of complete information regarding the patient, and that asking for a microscopic diagnosis out of context, as one would demand a lab result from a machine, risks error. Some pathologists incorrectly view the request for masking as a sign of distrust of their intellectual integrity or ability to make an independent decision. The request actually is a sign of epidemiologists' belief that everyone is biased about every decision unless masked. As a revealing example, an epidemiologist's wine tasting group in Maryland covers all labels from the bottles before tasting, and unmasks the results only after the "data" (opinions) are in. Fortunately, it is usually easy for good collaborators to achieve a balance between automatic demands for complete masking, and the kind of complete disclosure of study information that could lead to serious biases.

Standardization of the Scientific Art of Pathology

A more thorny problem arises when epidemiologists challenge the accuracy and reliability of pathologic diagnoses, either as part of a formal pathology agreement study or as part of a larger epidemiologic project. This challenge takes the form of calculation and publication of rates of (dis)agreement between experts, or between the expert and him/herself on different days. The epidemiologist is trained to believe that all biological phenomena are variable and that all measurements of biological phenomena are prone to random error. The pathologist has the weighty daily task of being the final arbiter of disease definition, a responsibility that does not mesh well with error.

The epidemiologist authors have learned something about the world of gynecological pathology only because of the intellectual humility of expert gynecological pathologists (responsible for several of the chapters in this text) whose curiosity outweighed their urges to preserve their national reputations for infallibility. Most of the comparisons performed have related to the cytopathology and histopathology of cervical intrepithelial neoplasia and benign "look-alikes." Agreement rates between expert pathologists have been only fair at best, but have led to a greatly increased understanding of the diagnoses.

If a pathologist ever feels irritated at the demands for reliability studies from new epidemiologist colleagues, it should suffice to ask them when the last time was that they performed a masked logistic regression data analysis in parallel with other epidemiologists, then published the agreement obtained for the relative risk estimates. Since such painful comparative exercises are almost never perpetrated by epidemiologists on themselves, mutual humility and curiosity should reign.

Specimen Adequacy Versus the Bias of Convenience Samples

Epidemiologists seeking to minimize bias are loathe to permit exclusions from a complete series. They suspect that the excluded members of the set will differ from those included in a systematic (biased), rather than random, way. Thus, epidemiologists working with pathologists wish to start their analyses by considering the entire collection of pathological specimens available, winnowing down as needed to usable specimens but always with an eye to possible biases of exclusion that could affect the general applicability of the results. Epidemiologists distrust *convenience samples*, groups of specimens that happen to be available for testing or for review. Pathologists may view the task of defining and retrieving all relevant specimens from their center to be unnecessary. It may be difficult to decide in advance when a convenience sample is sufficient and when a more definitive collection is required. In general, convenience samples are useful for preliminary methodologic work, as in checking if genomic DNA can be amplified from the paraffin blocks available, but such studies cannot be used to reach definitive, generalizable conclusions.

Deciding How Large a Study to Do: Statistical Significance Versus Practicality

Bigger is better for the epidemiologist. It is not much more difficult to do a statistical analysis of 1000 patients than 100; in fact, it is methodologically easier because the numbers are clearly sufficient. But the pathologist collaborator may view it differently. The question of study size is almost always negotiable, in that bigger studies permit the detection of smaller differences, but the critical difference that needs to be detected usually is open to discussion.

There are minimum numbers of subjects that permit epidemiologic analyses. It is impossible to generate a statistically significant result with fewer than five subjects, regardless of how strong an association is. Thirty subjects is another breakpoint. One M.D. epidemiologist's wife reports that when she asked her husband about her rash, he replied: "Give me 30 of them, with the right controls, and I'll venture a guess at what it is." Thirty subjects is a common minimum number in that common statistics such as means start to "behave" more reliably when there are about 30 or more data points. About 200 cases and 200 controls are needed to find reliably a relative risk of about 2.0 (a doubling of risk), given typical prevalences of common exposures. Case-control studies of more than 1000 subjects are relatively rare. Cohort studies, however, often require thousands or even tens of thousands of subjects to generate enough disease end points for analysis. Clinical trials range from small (20 subjects) to large (thousands of subjects) based on the size of the difference being sought.

In general, small studies miss weak associations, do not permit adequate adjustment for confounding, and generate less reliable estimates of risk. Still, many landmark studies of new topics have been small.

The key to defining the proper size of the study is to agree on the hypothesis and the range of expected results. Sample size calculations are very assumption-dependent, and usually demand information not available until the study is completed. Most epidemiologists choose a reasonable number based on cost and time available, then compute the *statistical power* of such a study to detect associations of various strengths. It is standard to require the study to have an 80% or greater chance of finding (as statistically significant) the key disease-exposure association under study, assuming the association truly exists.

Epidemiologic Features of the Major Gynecological Cancers

There have been a number of investigations focusing on the etiology of the major gynecological cancers, with a number of risk factors identified. Both cervical and endometrial cancers have been intensively studied, and for both there have been important recent insights regarding possible mechanisms of action of many of the previously identified risk factors. Fewer advances have been made with respect to ovarian cancer, although several etiologic clues have emerged from recent studies. Less is known about the etiology of cancers of the vulva and vagina and of trophoblastic disease, mainly because their rarity renders epidemiologic investigations difficult.

Cervical Cancer

An estimated 13,500 new cases of cervical cancer were diagnosed in the United States in 1993.[14] The average annual age-adjusted incidence in all SEER areas was 8.8 per 100,000 women for 1990, with a corresponding age-adjusted mortality rate of 3.0. The 5-year survival rate for cervical cancer is 67%, with the rate rising to 88% for cancers diagnosed at early stages.[1]

Substantial decreases in the incidence of invasive cervical cancer have occurred over time in the United States. Among whites, the incidence per 100,000 women declined 75% from 32.6 in the late 1940s to 8.3 in the early 1980s.[53] The decline in incidence in blacks started later than that for whites.

There is about a twofold difference in age-adjusted incidence for invasive cervical cancer for blacks as compared with whites. This differential, although previously observed for all ages, now appears restricted to older women. The incidence also is approximately two times higher for Hispanics and even higher for American Indians. Racial differences also exist in survival experience, with blacks having a 59% 5-year survival rate compared with a 67% 5-year survival rate among whites.

At least some of the racial differences can be explained by strong inverse associations observed between cervical cancer rates and socioeconomic indicators, such as education and income. These relationships prevail among both whites and blacks. When adjustment is made for socioeconomic differences, the excess risk of cervical cancer among blacks is substantially reduced from more than 70% to less than 30%.[51]

There is considerable geographic diversity in cervical cancer rates, with the highest rates having been reported from certain Latin American countries, where rates exceed those of the United States by approximately sixfold.[124] Although rates in the United States are among the lowest in the world, mortality rates are higher in certain Southern areas, particularly in Appalachia.

Recent upturns in incidence and mortality rates among young women have been observed in a number of countries, including Canada, Great Britain, New Zealand, and Australia. Similar increases may be slower to appear in the United States because of the effectiveness of cytology screening programs. The greatest evidence of increased incidence in the United States is for cervical adenocarcinomas among white women 35 to 54 years of age.[54]

Cervical cancer is believed to result from the progression of milder epithelial abnormalities, that is, dysplasia or cervical intraepithelial neoplasia. Support for a continuum of disease is provided by the observations that cervical dysplasia is diagnosed most often among women in their 20s, carcinoma in situ in women in their 30s, and invasive cancer after age 40 years. Because of this presumed continuum, there is little doubt that exfoliative cytology or the Pap smear can have profound effects on morbidity and mortality. The eradication of precursor lesions has preceded significant declines in cervical cancer incidence and mortality in areas where screening has been widespread, such as Kentucky and British Columbia.[16,40] The rates for cervical cancer have not declined in regions with limited screening programs.[88] Case-control studies that have evaluated the role of screening in preventing invasive cervical cancer have found relative risks ranging from 0.2 to 0.4 associated with screening within the last 3 to 5 years.[41,100] In a Finnish study, even patients who had been screened more than 5 years previously had a relative risk of 0.7 compared with those who had never been screened.[128]

Risk factors for cervical cancer are shown in Table 29.2. It is well established that women with either early ages at first sexual intercourse or multiple sexual partners are at an elevated risk.[15,22,77,91,143,166] Although several studies have attempted to determine the independence of these two risk factors (since they usually are highly correlated), both appear to be important predictors. Early age at first intercourse is thought to support a notion of increased suscepti-

Table 29.2. Risk factors for cervical cancers

Factors influencing risk	Estimated relative risk[a]
Older ages	2
Residence in certain parts of Latin America, Asia, or Africa	2–6
Lower levels of education or income	2–3
Black, Hispanic, or American Indian	2
Multiparity	2–4
Early ages at first sexual intercourse	2–4
Multiple sexual partners	2–5
Previous episodes of sexually transmitted disease, especially genital herpes and warts	2–10
Long-term smoking	2–4
Long-term oral contraceptive use	1.5–2
No prior regular Pap smear screening	2–6
Diets low in carotene, vitamin C	2–3
Human papillomavirus infection	>20

[a] Relative risks depend on the study and referent group employed.

bility of the cervix during adolescence, and the effect of multiple partners is postulated to operate through an infectious mechanism, in particular HPV infection. In contrast, most investigations have failed to find any influence on risk of frequency of intercourse after adjusting for the effects of these other sexual factors.[15,22,143,166]

Although most attention has focused on the role of female sexual behavior, there has been recent interest in the contribution of the male factor in the etiology of cervical cancer, especially given geographic clusters of cervical and penile cancer rates[62] and elevated rates of cervical cancer among the wives of men with penile cancer.[64,118,160] Several case-control studies have examined the sexual behavior of the husbands of women with cervical cancer, finding that the husbands of these women report more sexual partners than the husbands of controls.[30,33,92,190] The husbands of affected women also were more likely to report prior venereal diseases, early sexual experiences, affairs during marriage, and visits to prostitutes.[33] In contrast, there appears to be no effect on risk of circumcision status of the partner.[15,30,143]

Although there is little evidence that the character of menses affects cervical cancer risk,[15,22,143] there is increasing support for the role of reproductive factors. A number of studies indicate that women with multiple births are at elevated risk.[29,91,131] Possible explanations for the association include cervical trauma during parturition, hormonal or nutritional influences of pregnancy, or an immunologic effect on HPV infection.

The epidemiologic association of cervical neoplasia with sexual risk factors motivated the search for a venereally transmitted agent. Among the agents most widely investigated have been herpes simplex virus type 2 (HSV-2) and HPV. An etiologic role for HSV-2 was suggested on the basis of laboratory findings that HSV-2 can transform cells in culture, that HSV-2 proteins and integrated DNA can be found in some cervical cancers, and that the prevalence of antibody to HSV-2 was generally greater among cervical cancer patients than controls.[120] However, several follow-up studies[106,172] have cast doubt on the association because of the failure to demonstrate significantly increased risks of cervical neoplasia related to HSV-2 serology. Thus, more recent studies have focused on an etiologic role for HPV.

There is now extensive laboratory evidence for the oncogenic potential of HPV.[137] Initial studies demonstrated the presence of viral particles in cervical tissues by electron microscopy and of structural proteins by immunocytochemistry. However, these techniques are relatively insensitive and, because serologic techniques were not available to permit assessment of past exposure to HPV, it was not until the application of DNA hybridization methods that the frequent presence of venereal HPV infection among cervical neoplasia patients was fully recognized. Approximately 85–90% of squamous cervical carcinomas have been found to contain HPV, mainly types 16 and 18.

Only recently have analytic epidemiologic investigations been undertaken to estimate the relative risk of cervical neoplasia associated with HPV infection after adjustment for known risk factors. One of the first studies, which used filter in situ hybridization to test for HPV (a method now generally considered fairly insensitive and nonspecific) found a ninefold increased risk associated with high levels of HPV types 16 and 18 after controlling for other risk factors.[136] In more recent studies, which have used the more valid polymerase chain reaction (PCR) test to assess HPV infection, the estimates have been found to be considerably higher—more than 20.[126,145] The more recent studies, in contradiction to early studies, also support the notion that HPV detection correlates with most suspected risk factors for cervical cancer, including number of sexual partners, use of oral contraceptives, and race.[108] In one recent study, these factors failed to persist as risk predictors after adjustment for HPV, supporting the view that HPV is a central causal factor.[145]

Despite the central etiologic role of HPV in cervical cancer, an effect of other infections as independent or supporting factors has not been dismissed. Most recently, infection with the human immunodeficiency virus (HIV) has been correlated with the detection of HPV-related cytological changes.[116]

In recent years, there have been an increasing number of reports linking cigarette smoking to an elevated risk of both preinvasive and invasive cervical cancer.[184] Although initially the association was thought to reflect the influence of correlated factors, such as increased sexual activity and greater use of oral contraceptives, studies now seem to support an independent role for smoking.[7,27,42,98,157] It is notable that the recent Surgeons' General Report noted cervical cancer as a likely consequence of smoking. In most studies, a history of smoking is associated with about a twofold elevation in risk, with stronger relationships observed among women who report either high intensity or long durations of smoking. The association with smoking is most apparent for squamous cell tumors.[27] Further supporting a biologic mechanism are studies that have demonstrated high levels of smoke-derived nicotine and cotinine in the cervical mucus of smokers.[146] However, the immunosuppressive effects of smoking also should be considered,[8] particularly as an enhancement to the effects of infectious agents (e.g., HPV).

Oral contraceptive use also has emerged recently as a predictor of cervical cancer, particularly invasive disease. Issues of study design and analysis have been complex, generating questions about confounding factors, especially sexual behavior.[18] Even after considering correlated effects, most studies show some evidence of an increased risk, rising to approximately twofold for users of 5 or more years.[24,28] In several studies, higher risks have been observed for adenocarcinomas, in line with descriptive surveys showing increasing rates of this cell type among young women.[39,151]

In a number of studies, users of barrier methods of contraception have been shown to be at a low risk of developing cervical cancer.[15,185] This association usually is attributed to the prevention of spread of infectious agents.

A number of recent studies have suggested a role for dietary factors in the etiology of cervical cancer. Micronutrients associated with protection include vitamin A, beta-carotene, vitamin C, and vitamin E.[9,32,95,117,156,170,174] In addition, it has been suggested that folate deficiency may increase risk, possibly by acting as a cocarcinogen with HPV.[35] Although case-control studies do not generally support an effect of folates on risk,[32,189] the hypothesis deserves further attention, particularly as an explanation to the high risks associated with parity.

Vulvar Cancer

Carcinoma of the vulva is a rare genital neoplasm, with an average annual age-adjusted incidence in all SEER areas during 1985 to 1989 of 1.6 per 100,000 women. The disease occurs primarily in older women.

Cancers of the vulva occur significantly more frequently among women with primary cancers of the cervix, and the two diseases often occur simultaneously.[82,139] Approximately 15–20% of women with vulvar cancer have a second primary cancer occurring simultaneously or nonsimultaneously in the cervix, vagina, or anogenital area. Many patients with vulvar cancer have multifocal genital lesions, commonly including a mixture of condyloma acuminatum and intraepithelial neoplasia, with evidence that these multifocal lesions are HPV-related.[94,124]

Given synchronous occurrences of vulvar and cervical cancers, there has been interest in determining whether cervical cancer risk factors are predictive of vulvar cancer risk. In one study, there appeared to be a strong relation-

ship between the number of reported sexual partners and risk, with women reporting five or more partners being at a two- to threefold excess risk compared with sexually monogamous women.[25] A sexual etiology for vulvar carcinoma derives further support from serologic findings of antibodies against HSV-2 in vulvar cancer patients and identification of HSV-2 in vulvar tumor tissue.[87] More recently, interest has focused on the role of HPV, with a number of studies showing that certain types of vulvar cancers contain HPV DNA whereas other types do not.[2,94,167] This may explain recent time trends in the occurrence of the disease, with rates of in situ vulvar cancer having nearly doubled while rates of invasive disease having remained relatively stable.[164] Several studies suggest that a history of vulvar warts is associated with an elevated risk of vulvar cancer, with the relative risks ranging from 15 to 23.[25,49] In one study, a particularly high risk was associated with multiple episodes of genital warts,[25] possibly reflecting poor immunologic response among these women.

Other suggested, although unconfirmed, risk factors for vulvar cancer include low socioeconomic status, nulliparity and/or late ages at first birth, diabetes, obesity, and hypertension. A more consistently observed risk factor is cigarette smoking,[25,111,127] with one study showing particularly high risks for current smokers.[25] Smokers with a history of genital warts were at especially high risk, possibly supporting the suggestion that the effects of HPV depend on the presence of co-factors.[191] An excess risk of vulvar cancer among users of oral contraceptives was found in one study,[25] but not in another.[127]

Vaginal Cancer

Cancer of the vagina is rare, with an average annual age-adjusted incidence of 0.7 per 100,000 women in the SEER areas for the period from 1985 to 1989. The incidence is approximately three times higher for blacks than for whites, but the reasons for the discrepancy are unknown. About 1000 new cases and 350 deaths from vaginal cancer occur each year in the United States.[1] The average 5-year survival rate is 46% for whites.

Vaginal cancer is primarily a disease of older women, with almost 60% occurring among women 60 years or older. In the past, carcinoma of the vagina was only rarely reported in young girls, but starting in the late 1960s cases of clear cell adenocarcinoma of the vagina, an uncommon cancer at any age, began to be observed with much greater frequency than expected among women between 15 and 22 years of age. Most of these cases have been related to prenatal exposure to diethylstilbestrol (DES).[75]

There are few etiologic clues regarding vaginal cancer, and most clues for this cancer derive from clinical studies. Among factors that have been suggested, trauma to the vagina has received the most attention. Injury to the vagina from wearing ring pessaries (i.e., to support the uterus or rectum or as a contraceptive device) has been mentioned as a possible carcinogen.[150] The one case-control study of vaginal cancer, based on relatively few cases (n=41), found associations of risk with low socioeconomic status, histories of genital warts or other genital irritation, and previous abnormal Pap smears.[26] Women who had a previous hysterectomy were at high risk, consistent with several clinical observations,[10,163] but in contrast with one analytic study, in which vaginal cancer cases were matched to controls on history of previous dysplasia or neoplasia of the cervix.[76]

Vaginal cancer is found frequently as a synchronous or a metachronous neoplasm with cervical cancer.[139] This has led to the suggestion that there may be shared etiologic features between vaginal and cervical cancers. Recent reports of the co-existence of condylomatous lesions with vaginal cancer and the existence of HPV antigens and DNA in preinvasive and invasive vaginal tumors provide further support to this notion.

Endometrial Cancer

Cancer of the endometrium is the most common invasive gynecological cancer and the fourth most frequently diagnosed cancer among American women today. An estimated 31,000 new cases were diagnosed in the United States in 1993.[14] The average annual age-adjusted incidence for corpus and not otherwise specified uterine cancers from the SEER Program, was 21.5 per 100,000 women for 1990; the age-adjusted mortality rate for corpus cancers was 3.5 per 100,000, reflecting the relatively good prognosis for this cancer.

Endometrial cancer rates are highest in North America and Northern Europe; intermediate in Israel, Southern Europe, and Latin America; and lowest in Asia and Africa.[124] The disease is rare before the age of 45 years, but the risk rises sharply among women in their late 40s to middle 60s. The age-adjusted incidence for whites is approximately twice as high as for nonwhites, with reasons for the discrepancy largely undefined. Within the last several decades in the United States, a dramatic change in the incidence pattern for endometrial cancer has occurred, characterized by a marked increase that peaked about 1975.[173] This rise and fall has been linked with the widespread use of estrogen replacement therapy in the late 1960s and early 1970s. Recent reports show a continued decline in endometrial cancer incidence rates since 1979, despite an upswing in the use of menopausal estrogens to prevent osteoporosis and cardiovascular disease.[134] This may reflect the increased use since 1980 of progestins with estrogen replacement therapy to offset the adverse effects of unopposed estrogens.

Table 29.3 shows the variety of the risk factors and the range of magnitude of relative risks that have been identified for endometrial cancer. Many of these risk factors support a central role for estrogenic factors in the etiology

Table 29.3. Risk factors for endometrial cancers

Factors influencing risk	Estimated relative risk[a]
Older ages	2–3
Residence in North America, Northern Europe	3–18
Higher levels of education or income	1.5–2
White race	2
Nulliparity	3
History of infertility	2–3
Menstrual irregularities	2
Early ages at menarche	1.5–2
Late ages at natural menopause	2–3
Long-term use or use of high doses of menopausal estrogens	10–20
Use of oral contraceptives	0.3–0.5
Stein–Leventhal disease or estrogen-producing tumors	>5
Histories of diabetes, hypertension, gallbladder disease, or thyroid disease	1.5–3
Cigarette smoking	0.5

[a] Relative risks depend on the study and referent group employed.

of the disease. Apart from age and residency in North America or Europe, the most consistent and strongest risk factors include nulliparity, menstrual irregularities (including late ages at menopause), and obesity. Most studies demonstrate approximately a threefold or greater excess risk for nulliparous than parous women, and decreases in risk with increasing parity.[57,74,101] There is some indication that the association with nulliparity may reflect prolonged periods of infertility,[59,74,169] especially if anovulation was involved.[59] Although early ages at menarche have been inconsistently related to endometrial cancer risk,[58,74,88,169] several studies have noted associations with various measures of menstrual irregularity, including amenorrhea and heavy bleeding.[20,74,187] Most endometrial cancers are diagnosed postmenopausally, and among these women late ages at natural menopause are associated with increased risk, on the order of a twofold greater risk for those with menopause after the age of 52 as compared with before age 49.[115] Obesity also is a well-recognized risk factor for endometrial cancer, with as much as 25% of the disease possibly explained by this factor.[57,81,89,96,178] Obesity (as measured either by total weight or a measure of weight adjusted for height) appears to affect both premenopausal as well as postmenopausal onset disease, and there is some indication that very heavy women appear to have a disproportionately high risk.[20,187] Although one study has suggested that adolescent obesity might be the most important risk factor,[12] other studies indicate that weight gain later in life is the stronger predictor.[74,154,187] In addition, recent interest has focused on the distribution of body fat, with several studies showing that those whose fat distributes on either the trunk or upper body are at highest risk.[5,55,154]

Despite the fact that obesity has been consistently related to endometrial cancer risk, few studies have focused on the etiologic role of dietary factors. Geographic correlations between per capita fat intake and endometrial cancer incidence[4] have raised interest in this dietary effect, with there being some support from analytic studies for the association.[96] Studies in vegetarians suggest that dietary factors may affect endometrial cancer risk through modifications in hormone metabolism.[3] Alterations in endogenous hormones also have been offered as the explanation for the reduced risk of endometrial cancer observed among regular consumers of alcoholic beverages,[175] although this association has not been consistently observed.[96]

Endometrial cancer also has been noted to be elevated in women with histories of certain diseases (e.g., diabetes, hypertension, thyroid disease),[57,115] but until recently the extent to which the association might reflect correlations with obesity was unclear. Of interest therefore was a recent study[20] that showed that associations with most diseases did not persist after adjustment for body mass; the relationship with diabetes, however, did appear independent, possibly reflecting the role of associated hormonal alterations.

As previously noted, use of menopausal estrogens has been found associated with a 2- to 12-fold elevation in risk.[23,65,81,113,144,152,179] In most investigations, the increased risk was not observed until the drugs were used for at least 2 to 3 years, and longer use of estrogens was generally associated with higher risk.[23,65,81,144,179] The highest relative risks have been observed after 10 years of use, reaching risks of approximately 10 to 20. In most studies, cessation of use appears associated with a relatively rapid decrease in risk, continuous use is associated with higher risks than cyclic administration, and use of preparations with higher estrogen doses imparts the highest risks, although these relationships have not been consistently observed.[23,65,113,144,152,179]

Studies also have attempted to identify whether certain subgroups of estrogen users may be more adversely affected, with there being some evidence that effects are strongest among women who are thin, nondiabetic, or normotensive.[81,113,159] In addition, a recent study showed that cigarette smokers may be more adversely affected by estrogen use than nonsmokers.[23] These findings suggest that estrogen metabolism differs in these groups of women. Alternatively, risk already may be high enough in obese, hypertensive, or diabetic women that exposure to exogenous estrogens has only a small additional effect. Furthermore, it has been shown that estrogen use predisposes toward tumors that demonstrate favorable characteristics, including earlier stages at diagnosis, lower grade, and fewer instances of myometrial invasion.[65,81,89,113,144] Estrogen users also tend to be younger at diagnosis than patients who have not used estrogens, and the tumors are accompanied more frequently by hyperplasia or adenomyosis.[57,159]

Further evidence for the role of exogenous hormones in the pathogenesis of endometrial cancer derives from studies that have demonstrated significantly high risks in users of sequential oral contraceptives (i.e., containing a high dose of estrogen and a weak progestin)[74,178] and significantly low risks of endometrial cancer in women using estrogen-progestin combination pills.[37,80,86,178] Users of combination oral contraceptives experience about half the risk of nonusers, and long-term users have even further reductions in risk. Recent evidence suggests that the reduced risk associated with use of oral contraceptives relates more to the dose of the progestin rather than to the dose of the estrogen in the oral contraceptives.[142] The extent to which reduced risk persists after discontinuation remains an area of controversy.[86,178] In several studies, the protective effect of the pill appears greatest among nulliparous women, nonobese subjects or those who have not used menopausal estrogens.[37,74,178]

Several recent studies suggest that smokers are at a reduced risk of endometrial cancer.[7,19,105,107,169] In most of these studies, a gradient of decreasing risk with increasing amounts smoked has not been observed, but current smokers are at the lowest risk, leading to the suggestion that smoking may affect risk through an alteration in the absorption, distribution or metabolism of hormones.[19]

Women of upper socioeconomic status also have been reported to be a higher risk of endometrial cancer.[58,89] Findings related to socioeconomic status may be partially explained by other endometrial cancer risk factors correlated with affluence (e.g., overnutrition or use of replacement estrogens).

Genetic factors also may explain a small proportion of endometrial cancer, since some women present with Lynch syndrome II, a familial aggregation of endometrial, ovarian, and colon cancers.[110]

Ovarian Cancer

Ovarian cancer accounts for 4% of all cancers in women, with approximately 1 in 70 American women developing the disease in their lifetimes.[1] The average annual age-adjusted incidence for all SEER areas during 1990 was 14.9 per 100,000 women, with an estimated 22,000 new cases having been diagnosed in 1993. A relative survival of 85% can be achieved if ovarian cancer is diagnosed early, but usually the disease is not detected until it has reached an advanced stage, which imposes a high fatality rate (38% 5-year survival rate).

Ovarian cancer rates are high in North America and Northern Europe and low in Japan.[124] White women had considerably higher rates of ovarian cancer than blacks, but there is evidence that this difference may be narrowing.[52]

Table 29.4 shows the identified risk factors for ovarian cancer. Although the incidence of ovarian cancer increases with age, there is a marked flattening in the age-specific

Table 29.4. Risk factors for ovarian cancers

Factors influencing risk	Estimated relative risk[a]
Older ages	3
Residence in North America, Northern Europe	2–5
Higher levels of education or income	1.5–2
White race	1.5
Nulligravidity	2–3
History of infertility or use of infertility drugs	2–5
Early ages at menarche	1.5
Late ages at natural menopause	1.5–2
History of a hysterectomy	0.5–0.7
Use of oral contraceptives	0.3–0.5
Perineal talc exposure	1.5–2
Female relative with ovarian cancer	3–4

[a] Relative risks depend on the study and referent group employed.

incidence curves shortly after menopause. Fewer risk factors have been identified for ovarian cancer than for endometrial cancer, although nulligravidity and infertility have been fairly consistent predictors.[13,73,83,180,186] Compared with nulligravidous women, women with a single pregnancy have a relative risk of 0.6 to 0.8, with each additional pregnancy lowering risk by about 10–15%. This derives primarily from associations with number of full-term births, although in several studies, risk also has been found to decrease with increasing number of incomplete pregnancies. In most studies that have adjusted effects of age at first pregnancy by number of pregnancies, no residual effect of age at first pregnancy persisted.[73,78,83,186] There is, however, support from several recent studies for a reduced risk of ovarian cancer for women who breast feed for extended periods.[13,66,73,180]

The extent to which the relationship of risk to pregnancy history reflects a hazardous role for infertility or a protective role for pregnancy remains unresolved. Studies appear to support a role for infertility in the etiology of ovarian cancer.[13,73,83,181] In a recent combined analysis of data from multiple studies, the relationship with infertility was linked to use of infertility drugs.[180] Although provocative because of the fact that many of the drugs used in the treatment for infertility stimulate ovulation, the relationship requires confirmation from additional studies.

Several studies have reported early ages at menarche and late ages at menopause as ovarian cancer risk factors, although these patterns have not always been observed.[13,61,78,130,186] Numerous studies have noted a reduced risk of ovarian cancer associated with hysterectomy, with the apparent protective effect ranging from 30% to 40%.[13,45,61,71,83,182] This may reflect the opportunity for visualization and removal of abnormal ovaries during surgery, although it is also possible that hysterectomy compromises ovarian function through reduced blood supply to the ovaries.[56]

Similar to endometrial cancer, oral contraceptive use

has been linked with a reduced risk of ovarian cancer. A reduction in risk is apparent after only a few months' use, but the apparent protection is greatest among long-term users.[38,141,177,183,186] The reduction in risk appears to persist for a number of years after discontinuation and applies to all histological types of ovarian cancer.

Most studies that have examined the effect of menopausal estrogens on ovarian cancer risk have not found an association.[13,45,61,73,78,85,186] However, in one study, a threefold excess risk of endometrioid ovarian cancers was linked with estrogen use.[176] This relationship was not confirmed in another study.[85]

The role of dietary factors in the etiology of ovarian cancer only recently has been given attention. International data correlating ovarian cancer incidence and per capital fat availability[3] and the increased incidence of ovarian cancer among Japanese migrants to the United States[68] has stimulated interest in the role of dietary fat. Several follow-up studies support an association,[135,138,161] although the relationship has not been consistently observed.[90] Similarly, several case-control studies show a greater consumption of a variety of indicators of fat consumption among cases than controls.[46,97,155] However, other studies do not support the association, but rather show that risk is more dependent on low consumption of fruits and vegetables and foods containing either beta-carotene or vitamin A.[36,158] Cramer and others[43,44] found a high risk of ovarian cancer associated with consumption of lactose-rich dairy products. This association was restricted to women with low levels of galactose-1-phosphate uridyl transferase activity, an enzyme linked with hypergonadotropic hypogonadism.

Familial clusters of ovarian cancer suggest a genetic component. Case-control studies have attempted to estimate the magnitude of the genetic contribution,[93,133,149] with the largest of the studies showing estimated relative risks of 3.6 and 2.9 associated with having a first- and second-degree relative with ovarian cancer, respectively.[149]

Other suggested factors afffecting ovarian cancer risk include talc exposure, a history of mumps infection, and alcohol consumption. Talc exposure, which has been related to an excess risk of ovarian cancer in a number of case-control studies,[47,69,70,182] is of interest biologically in that ovarian cancer is thought to arise from the mesothelium that lines the peritoneal cavity. Ovarian cancer may be analogous, therefore, to pleural mesothelioma, which has been shown to be caused by asbestos, a chemical similar to talc. Mumps infection, which usually has been assessed by history, has been shown to correlate poorly with mumps serology, raising questions about the biological reality of infection history as a true predictor.[121,147] Smoking has not been related to ovarian cancer in most investigations. Some studies have shown slightly lower risks of ovarian cancer among alcohol drinkers.[36,63,67] Coffee drinking, linked to an excess risk of ovarian cancer in several studies, has not been confirmed as a risk factor in other investigations.[72,99,123,168,182]

Gestational Trophoblastic Disease

Choriocarcinoma is a rare malignancy in the United States, with a recent incidence in all SEER areas of 0.2 per 100,000 women, or approximately 1 per 22,623 live-births.[21] Hydatidiform mole occurs about once in every 1000 pregnancies, and approximately one of six occurrences results in invasion. Trophoblastic disease has been reported to be more common in certain parts of the world, although part of the differences may be due to a variety of selection biases.[17] The epidemiologic study of choriocarcinoma has been complicated by its relative infrequency. Most studies have focused on defining risk factors for hydatidiform or invasive mole, and it is uncertain the extent to which these findings can be extrapolated to choriocarcinoma.

Apart from a history of hydatidiform mole, the most clearly established risk factor for choriocarcinoma and hydatidiform mole is late maternal age. In one study, a 24-fold increased incidence of choriocarcinoma was found for women with a pregnancy after 45 years as compared with those with a pregnancy between 20 and 39 years.[165] Rates of trophoblastic disease also appear to be considerably higher in Asian and African countries, but the true extent of difference from Western rates is difficult to decipher because of variations in reporting practices. One incidence survey in the United States showed that, even after adjustment for birth distribution effects, blacks and other nonwhite races had 2.1- and 1.8-fold greater risks, respectively, than whites.[21]

An association between blood group A and choriocarcinoma has been found in two studies, and the combination of mother's group A and father's group O was considerably higher than expected (10.4-fold risk).[6,50] Blood groups A and AB were associated with elevated risks of hydatidiform mole in one study, although blood group was not predictive of risk in two others.[122,129,165]

In several studies that have adjusted for effects of later maternal age, parous women have remained at substantially reduced risk of hydatidiform mole compared with nulliparous women, with some evidence of further reductions in risk with multiple births.[31,122,132] Several studies found an increased risk associated with the occurrence of a prior spontaneous abortion, although this has not been consistently observed.[31,102] An increased risk of hydatidiform mole was associated with induced abortions, although information was not available on reasons for the terminations.[31] A history of infertility has been suggested in one study, although other studies do not confirm the association.[31,102,132] In one study, Chinese patients reporting use of herbal medicines during the first trimester of a previous pregnancy were at elevated risk.[31]

Low body mass, unrelated to dieting or exercise, has been reported as a risk factor for choriocarcinoma in one study.[34] Patients also had later onset of menarche and lighter menstrual periods than controls, possibly reflecting lower estrogen levels.

Although several studies have found an increased risk of trophoblastic diseases associated with long-term use of oral contraceptives,[11,31,140] others have found no such influence.[102,122] Others have suggested that oral contraceptives may increase the risk of malignant sequelae after mole evacuation through a tumor-stimulating effect.[162,188] In one study, this effect was restricted to users of high-dose estrogens, although in others, there were no such effects.[11,48,188]

Late paternal age has been suggested in one study as a risk factor for trophoblastic disease,[103] although other studies have failed to confirm this.[31,122] Cigarette smoking also has been linked with the occurrence of trophoblastic disease.[102] One study suggested that low carotene intake affected the risk of hydatidiform mole,[11] but no specific dietary associations were observed in another study.[31]

References

1. American Cancer Society (1991): Cancer Facts and Figures
2. Anderson WA, Franquemont DW, Williams J, Taylor PT, Crum CP (1991): Vulvar squamous cell carcinoma and papillomaviruses: Two separate entities. Am J Obstet Gynecol 16S: 329–336
3. Armstrong BK, Brown JB, Clarke HT, et al (1981): Diet and reproductive hormones: A study of vegetarian and non-vegetarian postmenopausal women. JNCI 67: 761–767
4. Armstrong B, Doll R (1975): Environmental factors and cancer incidence and mortality in different countries, with special reference to dietary practices. Int J Cancer 15: 617–631
5. Austin H, Austin MJ Jr, Partridge EE, et al (1991): Endometrial cancer, obesity, and body fat distribution. Cancer Res 51: 568–572
6. Bagshawe KD, Rawlins G, Pike MC, et al (1971): ABO blood groups in trophoblastic neoplasia. Lancet 1: 553–557
7. Baron JA, Byers T, Greenberg ER, et al (1986): Cigarette smoking in women with cancers of the breast and reproductive organs. JNCI 77: 677–680
8. Barton SE, Jenkins D, Cuzick J, et al (1988): Effect of cigarette smoking on cervical epithelial immunity: A mechanism for neoplastic change? Lancet 2: 652–654
9. Basu J, Palan P, Vermund S, et al (1991): Plasma ascorbic acid and beta-carotene levels in women evaluated for HPV infection, smoking, and cervix dysplasia. Cancer Detection Prev 15: 165–170
10. Bell J, Sevin B, Averette H, et al (1984) Vaginal cancer after hysterectomy for benign disease: Value of cytologic screening. Obstet Gynecol 54: 699–701
11. Berkowitz RS, Cramer DW, Bernstein MR, et al (1985) Risk factors for complete molar pregnancy from a case-control study. Am J Obstet Gynecol 152: 1016–1020
12. Blitzer PH, Blitzer EC, Rimm AA (1976): Association be-

tween teen-age obesity and cancer in 56,111 women: All cancers and endometrial carcinoma. Prev Med 5: 20–31

13. Booth M, Beral V, Smith P (1989) Risk factors for ovarian cancer: A case-control study. Br J Cancer 60: 592–598

14. Boring CC, Squires TS, Tong T (1993): Cancer statistics, 1993. CA-A Ca J for Clin 43: 7–26

15. Boyd JT, Doll R (1964): A study of the aetiology of carcinoma of the cervix uteri. Br J Cancer 18: 419–434

16. Boyes DA (1981) The value of a pap smear program and suggestions for its implementation. Cancer 48: 613–621

17. Bracken MB, Brinton LA, Hayashi K (1984): Epidemiology of hydatidiform mole and choriocarcinoma. Epidemiol Rev 6: 52–75

18. Brinton LA (1991): Oral contraceptives and cervical neoplasia. Contraception 43: 581–595

19. Brinton LA, Barrett RJ, Berman ML, et al (1993): Cigarette smoking and the risk of endometrial cancer. Am J Epidemiol 137: 281–291

20. Brinton LA, Berman ML, Mortel R, et al (1992): Reproductive, menstrual, and medical risk factors for endometrial cancer: Results from a case-control study. Am J Obstet Gynecol 167: 1317–1325

21. Brinton LA, Bracken MB, Connelly RR (1986): Choriocarcinoma incidence in the United States. Am J Epidemiol 123: 1094–1100

22. Brinton LA, Hamman RF, Huggins GR, et al (1987): Sexual and reproductive risk factors for invasive squamous cell cervical cancer. JNCI 79: 23–30

23. Brinton LA, Hoover RN, and the Endometrial Cancer Collaborative Group (1993) Estrogen replacement therapy and endometrial cancer risk: Unresolved issues. Obstet Gynecol 81: 265–271

24. Brinton LA, Huggins GR, Lehman HF, et al (1986): Long-term use of oral contraceptives and risk of invasive cervical cancer. Int J Cancer 38: 339–344

25. Brinton LA, Nasca PC, Mallin K, et al (1990): Case-control study of cancer of the vulva. Obstet Gynecol 75: 859–866

26. Brinton LA, Nasca PC, Mallin K, et al (1990): Case-control study of in situ and invasive carcinoma of the vagina. Gynecol Oncol 38: 49–54

27. Brinton LA, Schairer C, Haenszel W, et al (1986): Cigarette smoking and invasive cervical cancer. JAMA 255: 3265–3269

28. Brinton LA, Reeves WC, Brenes MM, et al (1990): Oral contraceptive use and risk of invasive cervical cancer. Int J Epidemiol 19: 4–11

29. Brinton LA, Reeves WC, Brenes MM, et al (1989): Parity as a risk factor for cervical cancer. Am J Epidemiol 130: 486–496

30. Brinton LA, Reeves WC, Brenes MM, et al (1989) The male factor in the etiology of cervical cancer among sexually monogamous women. Int J Cancer 44: 199–203

31. Brinton LA, Wu B, Wang W, et al (1989) Gestational trophoblastic disease: A case-control study from the People's Republic of China. Am J Obstet Gynecol 161: 121–127

32. Brock KE, Berry G, Mock PA, et al (1988) Nutrients in diet and plasma and risk of in situ cervical cancer. JNCI 80: 580–585

33. Buckley JD, Harris RWC, Doll R, et al (1981) Case-control study of the husbands of women with dysplasia or carcinoma of the cervix uteri. Lancet 2: 1010–1015

34. Buckley JD, Henderson BE, Morrow CP, et al (1988): Case-control study of gestational choriocarcinoma. Cancer Res 48: 1004–1010

35. Butterworth CE Jr, Hatch KD, Soong S-J, et al (1992): Oral folic acid supplementation for cervical dysplasia: A clinical intervention trial. Am J Obstet Gynecol 166: 803–809

36. Byers T, Marshall J, Graham S, et al (1983): A case-control study of dietary and nondietary factors in ovarian cancer. JNCI 71: 681–686

37. Cancer and Steroid Hormone Study of the Centers for Disease Control and the National Institute of Child Health and Human Development (1987): Combination oral contraceptive use and the risk of endometrial cancer. JAMA 257: 796–800

38. Cancer and Steroid Hormone Study of the Centers for Disease Control and the National Institute of Child Health and Human Development (1987) The reduction in risk of ovarian cancer associated with oral contraceptive use. N Engl J Med 316: 650–655

39. Chilvers C, Mant D, Pike MC (1987): Cervical adenocarcinoma and oral contraceptives. Br Med J 295: 1446–1447

40. Christopherson WM, Parker JE, Mendez WM, et al (1970): Cervix cancer death rates and mass cytologic screening. Cancer 26: 808–811

41. Clarke EA, Anderson TW (1979): Does screening by "pap" smears help prevent cervical cancer? A case-control study. Lancet 2: 1–4

42. Clarke EA, Morgan RW, Newman AM (1982): Smoking as a risk factor in cancer of the cervix: Additional evidence from a case-control study. Am J Epidemiol 115: 59–66

43. Cramer DW (1989): Lactase persistence and milk consumption as determinants of ovarian cancer risk. Am J Epidemiol 130: 904–910

44. Cramer DW, Harlow BL, Willett WC, et al (1989): Galactose consumption and metabolism in relation to the risk of ovarian cancer. Lancet 2: 66–71

45. Cramer DW, Hutchison GB, Welch WR, et al (1983): Determinants of ovarian cancer risk. I. Reproductive experiences and family history. JNCI 71: 711–716

46. Cramer DW, Welch WR, Hutchison BG, et al (1984) Dietary animal fat in relation to ovarian cancer risk. Obstet Gynecol 63: 833–838

47. Cramer DW, Welch WR, Scully RE, et al (1982) Ovarian cancer and talc. A case-control study. Cancer 50: 372–376

48. Curry SL, Schlaerth JB, Kohorn EI, et al (1989) Hormonal contraception and trophoblastic sequelae after hydatidiform mole (a Gynecologic Oncology Group study). Am J Obstet Gynecol 160: 805–811

49. Daling JR, Chu J, Weiss NS, et al (1984): The association of condylomata acuminata and squamous carcinoma of the vulva. Br J Cancer 50: 533–535

50. Dawood MY, Teoh ES, Ratnam SS (1971): ABO blood group in trophoblastic diseases. J Obstet Gynaecol Br Commonw 78: 918–923

51. Devesa SS, Diamond EL (1980): Association of breast cancer and cervical cancer incidences with income and education among whites and blacks. JNCI 65: 515–528

52. Devesa SS, Silverman DT (1978) Cancer incidence and mortality trends in the United States: 1935–74. JNCI 60: 545–571

53. Devesa SS, Silverman DT, Young JL Jr, et al (1987) Cancer incidence and mortality trends among whites in the Unites States, 1947–84. JNCI 79: 701–770

54. Devesa SS, Young JL Jr, Brinton LA, et al (1989) Recent trends in cervix uteri cancer. Cancer 64: 2184–2190

55. Elliott EA, Matanowski GM Rosenshein NB, et al (1990) Body fat patterning in women with endometrial cancer. Gynecol Oncol 39: 253–258

56. Ellsworth LR, Allen HH, Nisker JA (1983): Ovarian function after radical hysterectomy for stage IB carcinoma of the cervix. Am J Obstet Gynecol 145: 185–188

57. Elwood JM, Boyes DA (1980) Clinical and pathological features and survival of endometrial cancer patients in relation to prior use of estrogens. Gynecol Oncol 10: 173–187

58. Elwood JM, Cole P, Rothman KJ, et al (1977): Epidemiology of endometrial cancer. JNCI 59: 1055–1060

59. Escobedo LG, Lee NC, Peterson HB, et al (1991) Infertility-associated endometrial cancer risk may be limited to specific subgroups of infertile women. Obstet Gynecol 77: 124–128

60. Fleiss JL (1981): *Statistical Methods for Rates and Proportions, 2nd ed.* New York, John Wiley and Sons

61. Franceschi S, La Vecchia C, Helmrich SP, et al (1982): Risk factors for epithelial ovarian cancer in Italy. Am J Epidemiol 115: 715–719

62. Franco EL, Filho NC, Villa LL, et al (1988): Correlation patterns of cancer relative frequencies with some socioeconomic and demographic indicators in Brazil: An ecologic study. Int J Cancer 41: 24–29

63. Franks AL, Lee NC, Kendrick JS, et al (1987) Cigarette smoking and the risk of epithelial ovarian cancer. Am J Epidemiol 126: 112–117

64. Graham S, Priore R, Graham M, et al (1979): Genital cancer in wives of penile cancer patients. Cancer 44: 1870–1874

65. Gray LA, Christopherson WM, Hoover RN (1977): Estrogens and endometrial carcinoma. Obstet Gynecol 49: 385–389

66. Gwinn ML, Lee NC, Rhodes PH, et al (1990) Pregnancy, breast feeding, and oral contraceptives and the risk of epithelial ovarian cancer. J Clin Epidemiol 43: 559–568

67. Gwinn ML, Webster LA, Lee NC, et al (1986): Alcohol consumption and ovarian cancer risk. Am J Epidemiol 123: 759–766

68. Haenszel W, Kurihara M (1968) Studies of Japanese migrants. I. Mortality from cancer and other diseases among Japanese in the United States. JNCI 40: 43–68

69. Harlow BL, Cramer DW, Bell DA, et al (1992): Perineal exposure to talc and ovarian cancer risk. Obstet Gynecol 80: 19–26

70. Hartge P, Hoover R, Lesher LP, et al (1983): Talc and ovarian cancer (Letter). JAMA 250: 1844

71. Hartge P, Hoover R, McGowan L, et al (1988): Menopause and ovarian cancer. Am J Epidemiol 127: 990–998

72. Hartge P, Lesher LP, McGowan L, et al (1982): Coffee and ovarian cancer (Letter). Int J Cancer 30: 531

73. Hartge P, Schiffman MH, Hoover R, et al (1989): A case-control study of epithelial ovarian cancer. Am J Obstet Gynecol 161: 10–16

74. Henderson BE, Casagrande JT, Pike MC, et al (1983): The epidemiology of endometrial cancer in young women. Br J Cancer 47: 749–756

75. Herbst AL, Anderson S, Hubby MM, et al (1986): Risk factors for the development of diethylstilbestrol-associated clear cell adenocarcinoma: A case-control study. Am J Obstet Gynecol 154: 814–822

76. Herman JM, Homelsey HD, Dignan MB (1986): Is hysterectomy a risk factor for vaginal cancer? JAMA 256: 601–603

77. Herrero R, Brinton LA, Reeves WC, et al (1990) Sexual behavior, venereal diseases, hygiene practices, and invasive cervical cancer in a high- risk population. Cancer 65: 380–386

78. Hildreth NG, Kelsey JL, LiVolsi VA, et al (1981): An epidemiologic study of epithelial carcinoma of the ovary. Am J Epidemiol 114: 398–405

79. Hsiao JK, Bartko JJ, and Potter WZ (1989): Diagnosing diagnoses: Receiver operating characteristic methods and psychiatry. Arch Gen Psychiatry 46:664–667

80. Hulka BS, Chambless LE, Kaufman DG, et al (1982) Protection against endometrial carcinoma by combination-product oral contraceptives. JAMA 247: 475–477

81. Hulka BS, Fowler WC, Kaufam DG, et al (1980): Estrogen and endometrial cancer: Cases and two control groups from North Carolina. Am J Obstet Gynecol 137: 92–101

82. Jimerson GK, Merrill JA (1970): Multicentric squamous malignancy involving both cervix and vulva. Cancer 26: 150–153

83. Joly DJ, Lilienfeld AM, Diamond EL, et al (1974): An epidemiologic study of the relationship of reproductive experience to cancer of the ovary. Am J Epidemiol 99: 190–209

84. Kahn HA (1983): *An Introduction to Epidemiologic Methods.* New York, Oxford University Press

85. Kaufman DW, Kelly JP, Welch WR, et al (1989): Noncontraceptive estrogen use and epithelial ovarian cancer. Am J Epidemiol 130: 1142–1151

86. Kaufman DW, Shapiro S, Slone D, et al (1980): Decreased risk of endometrial cancer among oral-contraceptive users. N Engl J Med 303: 1045–1047

87. Kaufman RH, Bornsteing J, Adam E, et al (1988): Human papillomavirus and herpes simplex virus in vulvar squamous cell carcinoma in situ. Am J Obstet Gynecol 158: 862–871

88. Kelsey JL, Hildreth NG (eds) (1983): Breast and Gynecologic Cancer Epidemiology. Boca Raton, FL, CRC Press

89. Kelsey JL, LiVolsi VA, Holford TR, et al (1982): A case-control study of cancer of the endometrium. Am J Epidemiol 116: 333–342

90. Kinlen LJ (1982): Meat and fat consumption and cancer mortality: A study of strict religious orders in Britain. Lancet 1: 946–949

91. Kjaer SK, Dahl C, Engholm G, et al (1992) Case-control study of risk factors for cervical neoplasia in Denmark. II. Role of sexual activity, reproductive factors, and venereal infections. Cancer Causes Control 3: 339–348

92. Kjaer SK, de Villiers E-M, Dahl C, et al (1991) Case-control study of risk factors for cervical neoplasia in Denmark: I. Role of the 'male factor' in women with one lifetime sexual partner. Int J Cancer 48: 39–44

93. Koch M, Gaedke H, Jenkins H (1989) Family history of ovarian cancer patients: A case-control study. Int J Epidemiol 18: 782–785

94. Kurman RJ, Toki T, Schiffman MH (1993) Basaloid and

warty carcinomas of the vulva. Am J Surg Pathol 17: 133–145

95. La Vecchia C, Decarli A, Fasoli M, et al (1988) Dietary vitamin A and the risk of intraepithelial and invasive neoplasia. Gynecol Oncol 30: 187–195

96. La Vecchia C, Decarli A, Fasoli M, et al (1986) Nutrition and diet in the etiology of endometrial cancer. Cancer 57: 1248–1253

97. La Vecchia C, Decarli A, Negri E, et al (1987): Dietary factors and the risk of epithelial ovarian cancer. JNCI 79: 663–669

98. La Vecchia C, Franceschi S, Decarli A, et al (1986) Cigarette smoking and the risk of cervical neoplasia. Am J Epidemiol 123: 22–29

99. La Vecchia C Franceschi S, Decarli A, et al (1984): Coffee drinking and the risk of epithelial ovarian cancer. Int J Cancer 33: 559–562

100. La Vecchia C, Franceschi S, Decarli A, et al (1984) "Pap" smear and the risk of cervical neoplasia. Quantitative estimates from a case- control study. Lancet 2: 779–782

101. La Vecchia C, Franceschi S, Decarli A, et al (1984) Risk factors for endometrial cancer at different ages. JNCI 73: 667–671

102. La Vecchia C, Franceschi S, Parazzini F, et al (1985) Risk factors for gestational trophoblastic disease in Italy. Am J Epidemiol 121: 457–464

103. La Vecchia C, Parazzini F, Decarli A, et al (1984) Age of parents and risk of gestational trophoblastic disease. JNCI 73: 639–642

104. Last JM, Abramson JH, Greenland S, et al (1983): A Dictionary of Epidemiology. New York, Oxford University Press

105. Lawrence C, Tessaro I, Durgerian S, et al (1987): Smoking, body weight, and early-stage endometrial cancer. Cancer 49: 1665–1669

106. Lehtinen M, Hakama M, Aaran R-K, et al (1992) Herpes simplex virus type 2 infection and cervical cancer: A prospective study of 12 years of follow-up in Finland. Cancer Causes Control 3: 333–338

107. Lesko SM, Rosenberg L, Kaufman DW, et al (1985) Cigarette smoking and the risk of endometrial cancer. N Engl J Med 313: 593–596

108. Ley C, Bauer HM, Reingold R, et al (1991): Determinants of genital human papillomavirus infection in young women. J Natl Cancer Inst 83: 997–1003

109. Lilienfeld AM, Lilienfeld DE (1980): Foundations of Epidemiology, 2 ed. New York, Oxford University Press

110. Lynch HT, Cavalieri RJ, Lynch JF, et al (1992): Gynecologic cancer clues to Lynch syndrome II diagnosis: A family report. Gynecol Oncol 44: 198–203

111. Mabuchi K, Bross DS, Kessler II (1985): Epidemiology of cancer of the vulva. A case-control study. Cancer 55: 1843–1848

112. Maclure M and Willett WC (1987): Misinterpretation and misuse of the kappa statistic. Am J Epidemiol 126: 161–169

113. Mack TM, Pike MC, Henderson BE, et al (1976): Estrogens and endometrial cancer in a retirement community. N Engl J Med 294: 1262–1267

114. MacMahon B and Pugh TF (1970): Epidemiology: Principles and Methods. Boston, Little, Brown, and Co

115. MacMahon B (1974) Risk factors for endometrial cancer: Gynecol Oncol 2: 122–129

116. Mandelblatt JS, Fahs M, Garibaldi K, et al (1992) Association between HIV infection and cervical neoplasia: Implications for clinical care of women at risk of both conditions. AIDS 6: 173–178

117. Marshall JR, Graham S, Byers T, et al (1983) Diet and smoking in the epidemiology of cancer of the cervix. JNCI 70: 847–851

118. Martinez I (1969) Relationship of squamous cell carcinoma of the cervix uteri to squamous cell carcinoma of the penis among Puerto Rican women married to men with penile carcinoma. Cancer 24: 777–780

119. Mausner AK, Bahn JS (1974): Epidemiology: An Introductory Text. Philadelphia, W. B. Saunders

120. McDougall JK, Beckmann AM, Galloway DA (1986): The enigma of viral nucleic acids in genital neoplasia. In Peto R, zur Hausen H (eds): Viral Etiology of Cervical Cancer. Banbury Report 21, pp 199–210. New York, Cold Spring Harbor Laboratory

121. Menczer J, Modan M, Ranon L, et al (1979) Possible role of mumps virus in the etiology of ovarian cancer. Cancer 43: 1375–1379

122. Messerli ML, Lilienfeld AM, Parmley T, et al (1985) Risk factors for gestational trophoblastic neoplasia. Am J Obstet Gynecol 153: 294–300

123. Miller DR, Rosenberg L, Kaufman DW, et al (1987) Epithelial ovarian cancer and coffee drinking. Int J Epidemiol 16: 13–17

124. Mitchell MF, Prasad CJ, Silva EG, et al (1993) Second genital primary squamous neoplasms in vulvar carcinoma: Viral and histopathologic correlates. Obstet Gynecol 81: 13–18

125. Muir C, Waterhouse J, Mack T, et al (eds) (1987) Cancer Incidence in Five Continents, Vol V. Lyon, France, IARC Scientific Publication 88

126. Munoz N, Bosch FX, Sanjose S, et al (1992) The causal link between human papillomavirus and invasive cervical cancer: A population-based case-control study in Colombia and Spain. Int J Cancer 52: 743–749

127. Newcomb PA, Weiss NS, Daling J (1984): Incidence of vulvar carcinoma in relation to menstrual, reproductive, and medical factors. JNCI 73: 391–396

128. Olesen F (1988) A case-control study of cervical cytology before diagnosis of cervical cancer in Denmark. Int J Epidemiol 17: 501–508

129. Parazzini F, La Vecchia C, Franceschi S, et al (1985) ABO blood groups and the risk of gestational trophoblastic disease. Tumori 71: 123–126

130. Parazzini F, La Vecchia C, Negri E, et al (1989) Menstrual factors and the risk of epithelial ovarian cancer. J Clin Epidemiol 42: 443–448

131. Parazzini F, La Vecchia C, Negri E, et al (1989) Reproductive factors and the risk of invasive and intraepithelial cervical neoplasia. Br J Cancer 59: 805–809

132. Parazzini F, La Vecchia C, Pampallona S, et al (1985) Reproductive patterns and the risk of gestational trophoblastic disease. Am J Obstet Gynecol 152; 866–870

133. Parazzini F, Negri E, La Vecchia C, et al (1992) Family history of reproductive cancers and ovarian cancer risk: An Italian case-control study. Am J Epidemiol 135: 35–40

134. Persky V, Davis F, Barrett R, et al (1990) Recent time trends in uterine cancer. Am J Public Health 80: 935–939

135. Phillips RL, Garfinkel L, Kuzma JW, et al (1980) Mortality among California Seventh-Day Adventists for selected cancer sites. JNCI 65: 1097–1107

136. Reeves WC, Brinton LA, Garcia M, et al (1989) Human papillomavirus (HPV) infection and cervical cancer in Latin America. N Engl J Med 320: 1436–1441

137. Reeves WC, Rawls WE, Brinton LA (1989): Epidemiology of genital papillomaviruses and cervical cancer. Rev Infect Dis 11: 426–439

138. Rose DP, Boyar AP (1985) Diet and ovarian cancer. JAMA 254: 2553

139. Rose PG, Herterick EE, Boutselis JG, et al (1987) Multiple primary gynecologic neoplasms. Am J Obstet Gynecol 157: 261–267

140. Rosenberg L, Shapiro S, Slone D, et al (1989) Gestational trophoblastic disease and use of oral contraceptives (Letter). Am J Obstet Gynecol 161: 1087–1088

141. Rosenberg L, Shapiro S, Slone D, et al (1982) Epithelial ovarian cancer and combination oral contraceptives. JAMA 247: 3210–3212

142. Rosenblatt KA, Thomas DB, and the WHO Collaborative Study of Neoplasia and Steroid Contraceptives (1991) Hormonal content of combined oral contraceptives in relation to the reduced risk of endometrial carcinoma. The WHO Collaborative Study of Neoplasia and Steroid Contraceptives. Int J Cancer 49: 870–874

143. Rotkin ID (1967) Adolescent coitus and cervical cancer: Associations of related events with increased risk. Cancer Res 27: 603–617

144. Rubin GL, Peterson HB, Lee NC, et al (1990) Estrogen replacement therapy and the risk of endometrial cancer: Remaining controversies. Am J Obstet Gynecol 162: 148–154

145. Schiffman MH, Bauer HM, Hoover RN, et al (1993) Epidemiologic evidence showing that human papillomavirus infection causes most cervical intraepithelial neoplasia. JNCI 85: 958–964

146. Schiffman MH, Haley NJ, Felton JS, et al (1987) Biochemical epidemiology of cervical neoplasia: Measuring cigarette smoke constitutents in the cervix. Cancer Res 47: 3886–3888

147. Schiffman MH, Hartge P, Lesher LP, et al (1985) Mumps and postmenopausal ovarian cancer (Letter). Am J Obstet Gynecol 152: 116–117

148. Schiffman MH, Schatzkin A (1994) Test reliability is critically important to molecular epidemiology: An example from studies of HPV infection and cervical neoplasia. Cancer Res

149. Schildkraut JM, Thompson WD (1988) Familial ovarian cancer: A population-based case-control study. Am J Epidemiol 128: 456–466

150. Schraub S, Sun XS, Maingon PH, et al (1992) Cervical and vaginal cancer associated with pessary use. Cancer 69: 2505–2509

151. Schwartz SM, Weiss NS (1986) Increased incidence of adenocarcinoma of the cervix in young women in the United States. Am J Epidemiol 124: 1045–1047

152. Shapiro S, Kaufman DW, Slone D, et al (1980) Recent and past use of conjugated estrogens in relation to adenocarcinoma of the endometrium. N Engl J Med 303: 485–489

153. Sherman ME, Schiffman MH, Lorincz AT, et al (1994) Towards objective quality assurance in cervical cytopathology: correlation of cytopathologic diagnoses with detection of high-risk HPV types. J Clin Pathol, Aug

154. Shu XO, Brinton LA, Zheng W, et al (1992) Relation of obesity and body fat distribution to endometrial cancer in Shanghai, China. Cancer Res 52: 3865–3870

155. Shu XO, Gao GT, Yuan JM, et al (1989) Dietary factors and epithelial ovarian cancer. Br J Cancer 59: 92–96

156. Slattery ML, Abbott TM, Overall JC Jr, et al (1990) Dietary vitamins A, C, and E and selenium as risk factors for cervical cancer. Epidemiology 1: 8–15

157. Slattery ML, Robison LM, Schuman KL, et al (1989) Cigarette smoking and exposure to passive smoke are risk factors for cervical cancer. JAMA 261: 1593–1598

158. Slattery ML, Schuman KL, West DW, et al (1989) Nutrient intake and ovarian cancer. Am J Epidemiol 130: 497–501

159. Smith DC, Prentice R, Thompson DJ, et al (1975) Association of exogenous estrogen and endometrial carcinoma. N Engl J Med 293: 1164–1167

160. Smith PG, Kinlen LJ, White GC, et al (1980) Mortality of wives of men dying with cancer of the penis. Br J Cancer 41: 442–448

161. Snowdon DA (1985) Diet and ovarian cancer (Letter). JAMA 254: 356–357

162. Stone M, Dent J, Karana A, et al (1976) Relationship of oral contraception to development of trophoblastic tumour after evacuation of a hydatidiform mole. Br J Obstet Gynaecol 83: 913–916

163. Stuart GC, Allen HH, Anderson RJ (1981) Squamous cell carcinoma of the vagina following hysterectomy. Am J Obstet Gynecol 139: 311–315

164. Sturgeon SR, Brinton LA, Devesa SS (1992): In situ and invasive vulvar cancer incidence trends (1973 to 1987). Am J Obstet Gynecol 166: 1482–1485

165. Teoh ES, Dawood My, Ratnam SS (1972) Observations on choriocarcinoma in Singapore. Obstet Gynecol 40: 519–524

166. Terris M, Wilson F, Smith H, et al (1967) The relationship of coitus to carcinoma of the cervix. Am J Public Health 57: 840–847

167. Toki T, Kurman RJ, Park JP, Kessis T, Daniel RW, Shah K (1991) Probable nonpapillomavirus etiology of squamous cell carcinoma of the vulva in older women: A clinicopathologic study using in situ hybridization and polymerase chain reaction. Int J Gynecol Pathol 10: 107–125

168. Trichopoulos D, Papapostolou M, Polychronopoulou A (1981): Coffee and ovarian cancer. Int J Cancer 28: 691–693

169. Tyler CW Jr, Webster LA, Ory HW, et al (1985): Endometrial cancer: How does cigarette smoking influence the risk of women under age 55 years having this tumor? Am J Obstet Gynecol 151: 899–905

170. Verreault R, Chu J, Mandelson M, et al (1989): A case-control study of diet and invasive cervical cancer. Int J Cancer 43: 1050–1054

171. Vogelstein B, Fearon ER, Hamilton SR, et al (1988): Genetic alterations during colorectal-tumor development. N Engl J Med 319: 525–532

172. Vonka V, Kanka J, Hirsch I, et al (1984) Prospective study on the relationship between cervical neoplasia and herpes simplex type–2 virus. II. Herpes simplex type–2 antibody presence in sera taken at enrollment. Int J Cancer 33: 61–66

173. Walker AM, Jick H (1980): Declining rates of endometrial cancer. Obstet Gynecol 56: 733–736

174. Wassertheil-Smoller S, Romney SL, Wylie-Rosett J, et al (1981) Dietary vitamin C and uterine cervical dysplasia. Am J Epidemiol 114: 714–724

175. Webster LA, Weiss NS, the Cancer and Steroid Hormone Study Group (1989) Alcoholic beverage consumption and the risk of endometrial cancer. Int J Epidemiol 18: 786–791

176. Weiss NS, Lyon JL, Krishnamurthy S, et al (1982) Non-contraceptive estrogen use and the occurrence of ovarian cancer. JNCI 68: 95–98

177. Weiss NS, Lyon JL, Liff JM, et al (1981) Incidence of ovarian cancer in relation to the use of oral contraceptives. Int J Cancer 28: 669–671

178. Weiss NS, Sayvetz TA (1980) Incidence of endometrial cancer in relation to the use of oral contraceptives. N Engl J Med 302: 551–554

179. Weiss NS, Szekely DR, English DR, et al (1979): Endometrial cancer in relation to patterns of menopausal estrogen use. JAMA 242: 261–264

180. Whittemore AS, Harris R, Itnyre J, et al (1992) Characteristics relating to ovarian cancer risk: Collaborative analysis of 12 US case-control studies. Am J Epidemiol 136: 1184–1203

181. Whittemore AS, Wu ML, Paffenbarger RS, et al (1989) Epithelial ovarian cancer and the ability to conceive. Cancer Res 49: 4047–4052

182. Whittemore AS, Wu ML, Paffenbarger RS, et al (1988): Personal and environmental characteristics related to epithelial ovarian cancer. II. Exposures to talcum powder, tobacco, alcohol and coffee. Am J Epidemiol 128: 1228–1240

183. WHO Collaborative Study of Neoplasia and Steroid Contraceptives (1989) Epithelial ovarian cancer and combined oral contraceptives. Int J Epidemiol 18: 538–545

184. Winkelstein W Jr (1990) Smoking and cervical cancer—current status: A review. Am J Epidemiol 131: 945–957

185. Wright NH, Vessey MP, Kenward B, et al (1978) Neoplasia and dysplasia of the cervix uteri and contraception: A possible protective effect of the diaphragm. Br J Cancer 38: 273–279

186. Wu ML, Whittemore AS, Paffenbarger RS Jr, et al (1988) Personal and environmental characterics related to epithelial ovarian cancer. I. Reproductive and menstrual events and oral contraceptive use. Am J Epidemiol 128: 1216–1227

187. Wynder EL, Escher GC, Mantel N (1966) An epidemiologic investigation of cancer of the endometrium. Cancer 19: 489–520

188. Yuen BH, Burch P (1983) Relationship of oral contraceptives and the intrauterine contraceptive devices to the regression of concentrations of the beta subunit of human chorionic gonadotropin and invasive complications after molar pregnancy. Am J Obstet Gynecol 145: 214–217

189. Ziegler RG, Brinton, Hamman RF, et al (1990) Diet and the risk of invasive cervical cancer among white women in the United States. Am J Epidemiol 132: 432–435

190. Zunzunegui MV, King MC, Coria CF, et al (1986) Male influences on cervical cancer risk. Am J Epidemiol 123: 302–307

191. zur Hausen H (1982) Human genital cancer: Synergism between two virus infections or synergism between a virus infection and initiating event? Lancet 2: 1370–1372

30

Gross Description, Processing, and Reporting of Gynecologic and Obstetric Specimens

Stanley J. Robboy, M.D., Frederick T. Kraus, M.D., and Robert J. Kurman, M.D.

The surgical pathology report provides the histopathological diagnosis and specific information relating to prognosis and treatment. Accordingly, the surgical pathologist must have sufficient familiarity with the management of gynecologic and obstetric disorders to assure that a major focus of the report is to communicate the clinically relevant information. This chapter provides an approach to the processing of gynecologic and obstetric tissue specimens. The techniques of the gross examination and the method of reporting the pathological findings are guided by the clinical principles on which patient management is based.

The types of gynecologic tissue specimens that are submitted to the surgical pathology laboratory can be divided into two categories: biopsy specimens and therapeutic resections. Obstetric tissue specimens include placentas and sometimes uterine curettings. The main purpose of the biopsy is to provide a histological diagnosis that will guide management. Biopsy specimens should, therefore, be pro-cessed expeditiously. The gross description must be precise and brief. There should be correlation between the microscopic tissue section and the gross specimen with regard to the number of specimens and the approximate site of each or aggregate site of the total. This is especially important when it appears that a slide or block may have been mislabeled. Two examples of appropriate description are "3 ovoid fragments 2 to 4 mm in diameter" and "multiple shreds of tissue 5 cm in aggregate diameter."

For operative specimens, particularly those containing a tumor, information in the surgical pathology report should include a description of the extent of the tumor and specific features that are related to prognosis. The adequacy of the surgical treatment as well as the need for additional therapy depend on these findings. Since the gynecologic surgeon has seen the pathology in vivo, it is important that he communicate the operative findings, since these will bear directly on how the pathologist processes the specimen. For example, adequacy of resection margins requires an appreciation of the orientation of the specimen to certain anatomic landmarks that are obvious to the surgeon but cannot always be reconstructed by the pathologist in the laboratory.

The gross description and final diagnosis must be clearly written. A good gross description enables the reader to reconstruct an image that corresponds to the specimen and its lesion. Since the histological diagnosis for many tumors has been made by biopsy before the operative procedure, the gross description of the specimen should focus on the site and extent of the lesion and its relationship to adjacent structures. In this sense the gross description is analogous to the provisional anatomic diagnosis of a postmortem examination in which the microscopic examination confirms the gross anatomic findings. It should be uncommon to have significant findings discovered unexpectedly on the microscopic examination. A careful gross examination and description are mandatory to ensure that the appropriate microscopic sections are obtained.

The final diagnosis of a tumor should include its cell type, grade, location, and extent as well as the adequacy of the resection margins, presence of lymphatic or vascular invasion, and status of the regional lymph nodes. It is one thing to report an "endometrial adenocarcinoma" but far better to report "serous carcinoma of the endometrium with vascular invasion, penetrating to within 0.2 mm of the margin, with metastases to 2 of 24 lymph nodes" with a detailed listing to follow of which lymph nodes, and how many in each group, are involved. The former merely reaffirms what was known before the operation, whereas the latter presents information that helps to predict prognosis and plan further treatment.

General Procedures

Gross Description

Specimens received in the fresh state should be described before fixation, since formalin alters the natural color and consistency of tissue. The opening sentence of the gross description should indicate whether the tissue is received fresh or fixed and how it is labeled. Note whether the specimen received corresponds with how it is labeled. For example, "Received fresh is a specimen labeled 'uterus, tubes, and ovaries'; however, only the uterus and right ovary and tube are identified." The overall measurements and weight of the entire specimen are useful, but those of the individual components are critical.

The gross description should proceed in an orderly fashion, with the focus on the primary lesion. For example, in a radical hysterectomy, the cervical cancer should be described before the normal ovaries, incidentally removed appendix, and multiple lymph nodes. Emphasize the pathology and avoid elaborate descriptions of normal anatomy. For example, a normal appendix can be described as "5 cm long" and "normal" rather than as a "5 cm long, 4 mm in diameter, vermiform appendix with a tan, unremarkable serosa, a 1-mm thick wall, and a lumen without identifiable abnormality." The gross description, especially of small specimens, should conclude with a statement of whether all of the tissue has been processed for microscopic examination or whether tissue remains. All descriptions should include an inventory listing the number of blocks sampled and from where they were obtained.

Drawings and Photographs

The description of a specimen with complicated relationships may be simplified by including a drawing or photo-graph as part of the surgical pathology report. This permits orientation of the tumor to the remainder of the specimen, especially surgical resection margins, and visual identification of section codes.

Synoptic Checklists

Checklists are being used with increasing frequency in recording and evaluating the details of operative and pathological findings. The checklists we have developed for each organ and which detail areas of importance are included in an appendix at the end of this chapter. Although the checklists useful, it is important they be employed with care and full understanding of their purpose. They help highlight features that are of known importance or are being currently investigated as of potential import, thus serving as an aid to foster issuance of more complete reports. In particular, they should not be slavishly adopted, for "pigeonholing" according to the checklist may hinder rather than foster open-mindedness as specimens are examined.

Sections Codes

Several section code systems are in common use. These include assigning each specimen/container received with a unique letter, e.g., A . . . Each block sampled from that specimen/container then receives a sequential number, e.g., A1, A2, . . . An. A second method is to label blocks consecutively in alphabetical order. After Z, proceed to AA. After AZ, proceed to BA and continue in this way. A third is to label organs with letters, e.g., RO and LO for right and left ovaries. Although this method has the advantage of providing a readily apparent link to the organ that was sampled, it may lead to ambiguities when dealing with margins and relations with other organs, and sometimes leads to overly complex lettering schemes.

A key at the end of the gross description is used more often and clearly seen than a key included in the text of the gross description. However, inclusion of the key, or at least portions of the key within the text of the gross description, often leads to greater clarity. For example, it is easier in describing a probable leiomyosarcoma to state that the borders in one region are irregular (Block B10) and in another area appear to blend into the surrounding myometrium (Block B11) than to repeat the finding in detail in the key summary.

Formalin Fixation

Neutral buffered formalin is generally the most practical and commonly used fixative. A specimen to be submitted for microscopic examination should be cut into blocks no more than 3 mm in thickness. Thicker specimens will autolyze at the center. It is much easier and efficient to cut blocks from tissue that have been fixed for several hours instead of attempting to cut 3-mm blocks directly from the fresh specimen. Large specimens should be bread-loafed or alternatively cut into slabs, ~1 cm in thickness, to permit adequate penetration by formalin and then trimmed to 3-mm blocks after ~3 hours of fixation. For large specimens, e.g., uteri removed for leiomyomata, fixation is facilitated by allowing the tissue blocks that have been placed into cassettes (with all labeling complete) to fix for an extra 24 hours.

Other Types of Fixatives

Bouin fixative provides superior cellular detail and is practical for the fixation of biopsies and curettings. In endometrial biopsies, stromal edema is appreciated much more easily with Bouin fixative than with formalin. Bouin fixative, however, also has distinct disadvantages for which reasons it is not often used routinely. Both polymerase chain reaction (PCR) and in situ hybridization techniques work poorly with Bouin fixed tissue. Also, Bouin fixative penetrates tissues slowly, requiring meticulous handling of large specimens. As a result, the entire process becomes more labor-intensive and time-consuming. For these reasons, Bouin fixative is not recommended.

Although not always feasible in a busy surgical pathology laboratory, it is useful to fix some tissue from all tumors in glutaraldehyde for possible electron microscopic examination. A portion of tumor also should be snap frozen for immunocytochemical analysis, since some antibodies do not bind to antigens that have been altered by formalin fixation, e.g., monoclonal antibodies to estrogen receptor protein and immunoglobulin antibodies to lymphomas.

Specific Procedures

Biopsies and Curettings

Vulvar Biopsy

Excisional biopsies should be handled like skin biopsies. Several methods are in common use to assess both deep as well as lateral resection margins. Orientation is aided if the surgeon places a suture for orientation. In one method, India ink is used to facilitate their recognition on microscopic examination. Sections should be perpendicular to the surface and should be obtained from the longitudinal axis and perpendicular to it across the shorter axis. A second method uses two ink colors, commonly black and alcian blue. Black is used on one lateral margin and alcian blue on the other lateral and entire deep margin. Sections are then taken sequentially from the cranial to caudal end of the specimen. In each method, the color code used needs to be recorded in the section on Gross Description.

Small punch biopsies are submitted totally. Specimens large enough to bisect may be cut perpendicular to the mucosal surface, and the cut surface inked. It is useful also to request at the time of submission that the paraffin block be cut at multiple levels. This shortens the turnaround time, since small biopsies frequently are sectioned inadequately the first time they are cut. Remounting the block and cutting again takes more time than obtaining multiple levels at the outset, and not infrequently exhausts the specimen.

Vaginal Biopsy

Most vaginal biopsies are small punch biopsies and should be handled in a manner similar to vulvar punch biopsies.

Cervical Punch Biopsy

Colposcopically directed punch biopsies should be handled in the same manner as small vulvar and vaginal biopsies. A technique to facilitate orientation is to sandwich the biopsy specimen between blue Gelfoam sponges that fit into the cassette. Another effective technique is to have the gynecologist place the biopsy on its side on a piece of paper towel and then place the specimen and attached paper into fixative (Fig. 30.1). The paper must be removed by the surgical pathologist before processing.

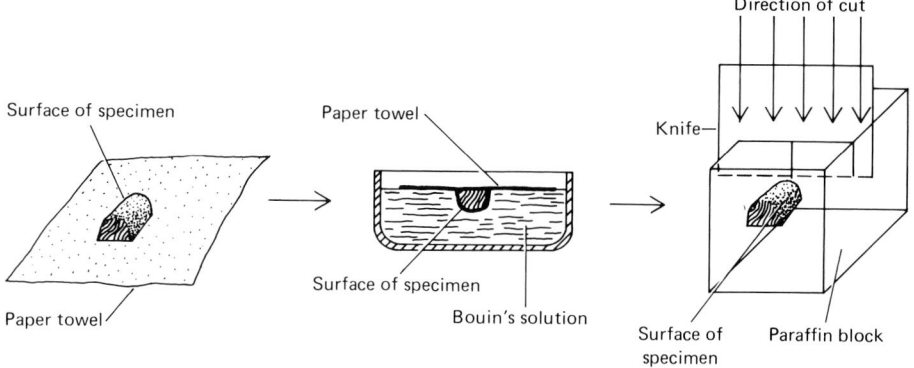

Fig. 30.1. Cervical punch biopsy. Orientation, fixation, and microtome sectioning of a cervical punch biopsy. (Courtesy of Alex Ferenczy, M.D., Montreal, Quebec, Canada.)

ENDOCERVICAL CURETTINGS

The endocervical curettage is performed to evaluate the presence of endocervical neoplasms, cervical neoplasia in the endocervical canal, or to determine whether endometrial carcinoma has spread into the cervix. Clinical management depends on the presence or absence of disease in the curettings and, therefore, considerable care must be exercised in handling these specimens, which are typically scant and composed mostly of blood and mucus.

The specimen should be transferred directly from the curette by the gynecologist to a Telfa pad. Sponges should be avoided, since tissue becomes enmeshed in the sponge and is difficult to retrieve. After the curettage is completed, the curette can be passed through the fixative to dislodge small fragments of tissue that otherwise might remain adherent to the curette. In the laboratory, the entire specimen should be wrapped in a Shandon mesh bag or a tea bag before placing it into a cassette so as to avoid losing small fragments of tissue during processing. Filter paper should be avoided as it is difficult to handle.

CERVICAL CONE BIOPSY AND LOOP ELECTROSURGICAL EXCISION PROCEDURE (LEEP)

This procedure can be diagnostic or therapeutic. In either case, the information desired is the microscopic diagnosis, depth of invasion if microinvasive cancer is present, and status of margins.

The gynecologist should remove the cone biopsy intact, if possible. If a laser is used, the endocervical margin should be resected with scissors so that the tissue at this crucial site can be evaluated microscopically in the absence of cautery artifact. Another method to assess the endocervical margin is to amputate the endocervical margin and send it as a separate specimen labeled "apical margin." Avoid manipulation of the surface epithelium, since it is easily denuded. The specimen, wrapped in saline-soaked gauze, should be transported immediately to the surgical pathology laboratory.

The surgical pathologist can limit the gross description to the measurements of the specimen and any obvious lesion. The endocervical margin is marked with alcian blue ink, and pinned on a corkboard with the mucosa facing up (Fig. 30.2). Three hours of fixation before cutting is adequate. The specimen should be sectioned serially at 1- to 3-mm intervals. Each block should be marked with India ink or eosin to orient embedding. Serially cut blocks should be submitted in separate cassettes numbered consecutively, and the entire specimen should be submitted. When there are many blocks, and especially if the blocks are small, it is often more convenient and economical to place two to three blocks in each cassette.

The LEEP biopsy uses a low-voltage diathermy loop to excise a lesion or the entire transformation zone. The spec-

imen should be serially sectioned at 1 to 3 mm intervals as with a cone biopsy. The cautery artifact that results from the procedure is comparable to that of the laser. Surgical margins may be difficult to evaluate.

ENDOMETRIAL BIOPSY AND CURETTINGS

All tissues should be submitted from diagnostic procedures, whereas selected samples should be submitted from therapeutic procedures in which a large volume of tissue is received, e.g., curettage performed to remove products of conception. Endometrial biopsies and diagnostic curettings should be processed in the same manner as endocervical curettings. The gross description should include a measurement of the aggregate specimen. The specimen should be wrapped in fine Shandon mesh bads or tea bags and submitted in its entirety.

For abortion specimens, evaluate the completeness of removal of the fetus and placenta when possible. Single small samples of fetal parts and placenta should suffice for sectioning. If fetal parts are not identified grossly, then particular attention should be given to find the feathery papillations diagnostic of chorionic villi. A dissecting scope or hand lens may be helpful in this regard. Soft, tan, solid tissue often is decidua, and in itself is insufficient to diagnose the presence of an intrauterine pregnancy. When a fetus or fetal parts can be identified grossly, microscopic sampling of the specimen is not necessary if there is no gross abnormality. Note the length of the fetus and, if possible, obtain the weight. If microscopic examination does not reveal any tissues of fetal origin, only then should additional tissue be processed. In contrast to an ectopic pregnancy in the fallopian tube where blood clots typically contain chorionic villi, blood clots from intrauterine pregnancies rarely contain chorionic villi, and therefore generally are not sampled. If no tissues of fetal origin are found after examination of all tissues, it is important that the clinician be notified immediately about the possibility of an ectopic pregnancy. In the appropriate clinical setting, for example, habitual abortion or previous newborn with multiple congenital malformations, some tissue should be transported to a cytogenetics laboratory in the appropriate transfer medium (see section on Placental Examination).

Curettings from a hydatidiform mole come in two parts: the suction curettage and the sharp curettage. The former should be examined carefully for the presence of fetal parts. Tissue from the sharp curettage should be processed entirely, since it must be evaluated for the presence of myometrial invasion.

Large Operative Specimens

WIDE LOCAL EXCISION AND SUPERFICIAL VULVECTOMY

Most specimens are highly variable in their composition, since these procedures are tailored to the extent of the

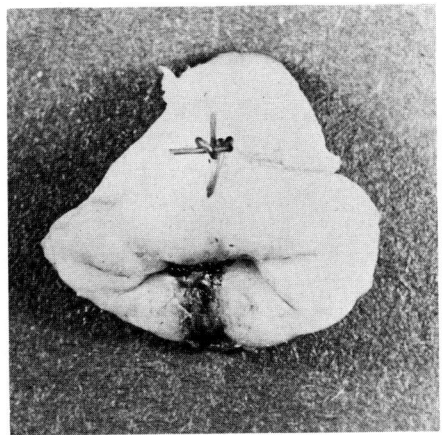

Cone of cervix

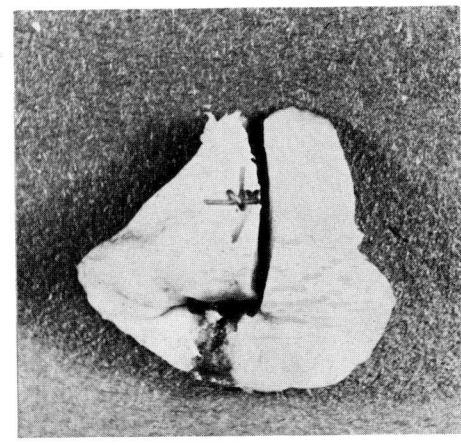

Incised at 12 o'clock

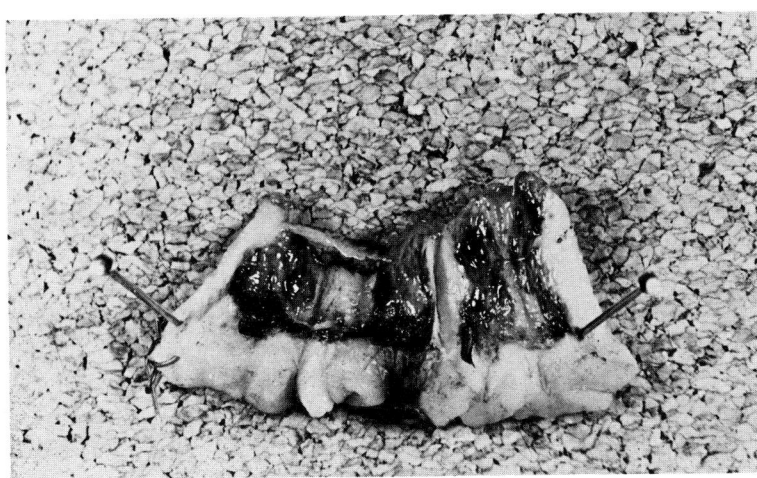

Opened cervix

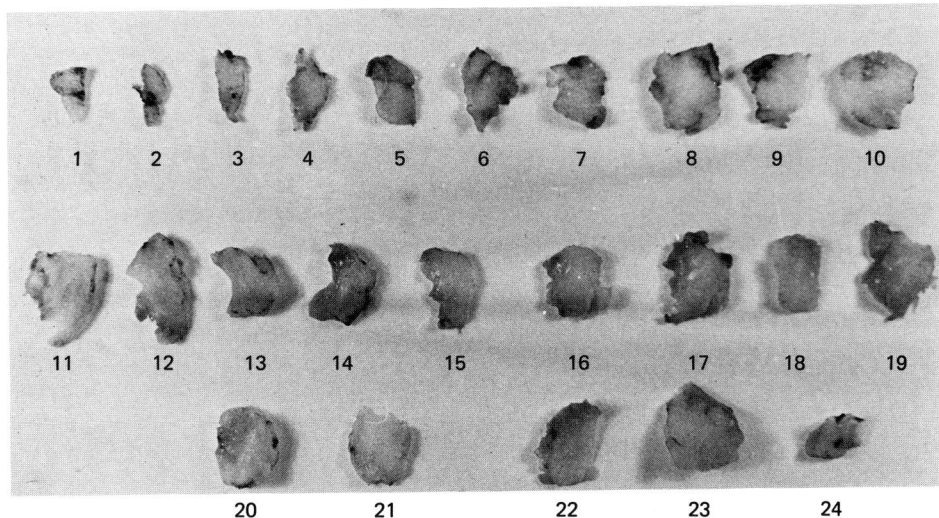

Fixation

FIG. 30.2. Method of sectioning a cone biopsy of the cervix. In this case the specimen has been opened at 12 o'clock.

lesion. Recently, wide local excision has been performed for superficially (<1 mm) invasive tumors, whereas laser techniques often are used to treat vulvar intraepithelial neoplasia (VIN-3). The operative specimens include the labia minora, labia majora, clitoris, perineal body, and perianal tissue without subcutaneous fat.

The gross description should specify the features and extent of the lesion as well as the anatomic structures involved. Since intraepithelial lesions are subtle, careful attention must be paid to coloration and surface texture. The lesions typically are red, brown, or white and often are roughened. They should be measured, and distances from the lesion to the resection margin should be recorded.

Because the disease process often is multifocal and difficult to discern with the naked eye, all surgical resection margins must be examined microscopically. This requires sections through all obvious lesions to rule out invasive carcinoma and sections from all the lateral resection margins. Sections parallel to the surgical margins (shave biopsies) often are taken to evaluate the excision lines, a method that uses fewer sections than those taken perpendicular to the line of resection. Multiple perpendicular sections, however, have the advantage that the central lesion, margin, and intervening areas can be included in one slide and tumor "close to" the margin is much easier to evaluate. To facilitate sectioning, pin the specimen on a corkboard or a block of paraffin and fix for 2–3 hours before sectioning.

The surgical pathology report should include the microscopic diagnosis, extent of the involvement, and adequacy of the surgical resection margins.

Total Vulvectomy (Appendix, Table 30.1)

The specimen includes the entire vulva and subcutaneous fat, since the surgical dissection is carried down to the deep fascia. This procedure usually is performed only for vulvar Paget disease.

The gross description is similar to that outlined for the superficial vulvectomy. Although Paget disease of the vulva usually is an intraepithelial lesion, at times it may be invasive or associated with an underlying sweat gland or anal carcinoma and, therefore, the underlying subcutaneous tissue is removed. The specimen should be pinned, fixed, and then sectioned at approximately 0.5-cm intervals in order to evaluate adequately the underlying dermis for an invasive carcinoma. Typically, microscopic involvement of Paget disease exceeds the visible extent of the lesion on gross examination. Occult foci of Paget disease also may be present within normal-appearing skin, and consequently the entire deep and lateral resection margins must be thoroughly evaluated in a similar manner as that described for the superficial vulvectomy specimen.

The surgical pathology report should include the microscopic diagnosis, extent of involvement, adequacy of the

resection margins, and whether an underlying carcinoma is present.

Radical Vulvectomy, with Lymphadenectomy (Appendix, Table 30.1)

The specimen consists of the vulva, inguinal skin, subcutaneous tissue, femoral and inguinal lymph nodes, and portions of the saphenous veins. The procedure is performed for invasive squamous carcinoma.

The gross description should include the size, location, and depth of penetration of the primary lesion, and all resection margins, including the perirectal and vaginal margins. Examination often is aided if the specimen is first pinned out and fixed for a short period. Sections should include the tumor, showing the maximum depth of invasion, labia majora and minora, clitoris, resection margins including the vaginal margin, and all lymph nodes. Sections should evaluate the status of the skin immediately adjacent to the primary lesion, as preinvasive disease often is present. Separation of lymph nodes into superficial and deep groups requires communication with the gynecologic surgeon. Invasive vulvar neoplasms, in contrast to intraepithelial lesions, tend to be solitary and, consequently, evaluation of resection margins can be limited to the margins near the tumor. Because the specimen contains a considerable amount of fatty tissue, identification of lymph nodes may be difficult. In the fresh state, lymph nodes are recognized by palpation. Alternatively, Bouin's fixation or xerography[4] (Fig. 30.3) may assist in locating lymph nodes. The fatty tissue should be bread loafed at 1- to 2-cm intervals to allow adequate penetration of the fixation. After a few hours in Bouin's fixation, fat remains yellow but lymph nodes appear white. Location of lymph nodes is facilitated by an understanding of the lymphatic drainage of the vulva (Fig. 30.4).

The surgical pathology report should include the microscopic diagnosis, tumor grade, dimensions, location and maximum depth of invasion, presence of lymphatic invasion, number and location of the involved lymph nodes, and status of resection margins.

Vaginectomy and Pelvic Exenteration

The vaginectomy specimen consists of the vagina as well as the cervix and uterus, since the procedure is an en bloc resection for invasive carcinoma of the vagina. Depending on the location and extent of the tumor, the urinary bladder and rectum also may be removed. The procedure is termed an *anterior exenteration* if the urinary bladder is included and a posterior exenteration if the rectum is included. Pelvic exenteration is performed infrequently today. The most common indication is for a central recurrence of a cervical carcinoma.

The vagina should be opened longitudinally on the side opposite the tumor. The total length of the vagina is measured and the distances between the tumor, the cervix, and

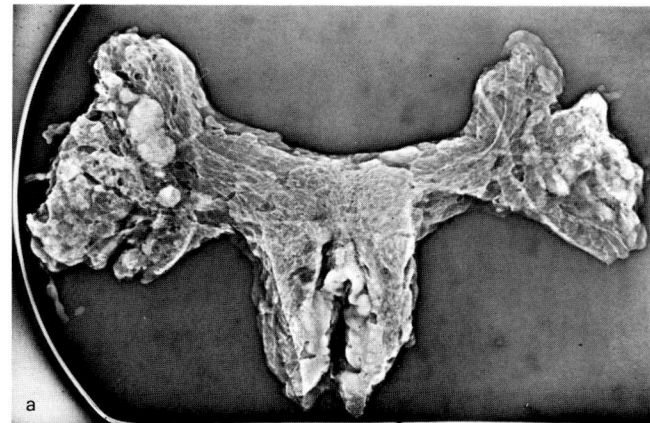

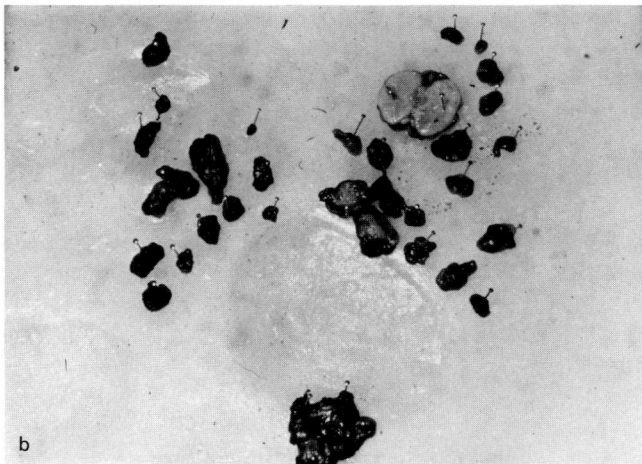

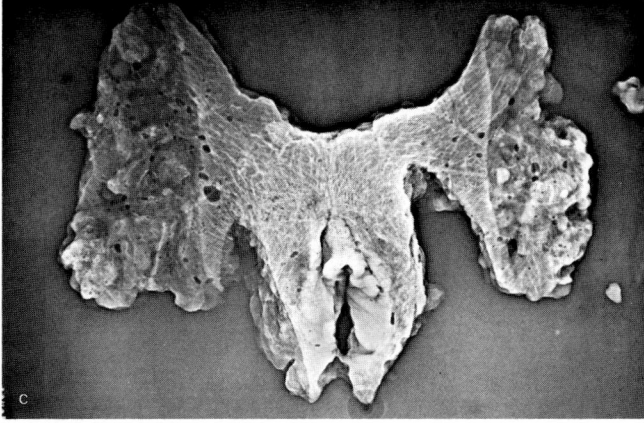

FIG. 30.3. Lymph nodes in vulvar cancers. a: Xerogram of radical vulvectomy specimen before dissection. Nodes can be clearly seen. **b:** Lymph nodes dissected from specimen. **c:** Xerogram of postdissection specimen. (Courtesy of J. Milbrath, M.D., and Edward J. Wilkinson, M.D., Gainesville, FL.)

the resection margins are recorded. The tumor mass should be described and measured and the maximum depth of invasion noted. The extent of involvement should be described, in particular, the relationship of the tumor to the cervix and the urinary bladder or rectum if the latter organs have been removed. To evaluate these features, the

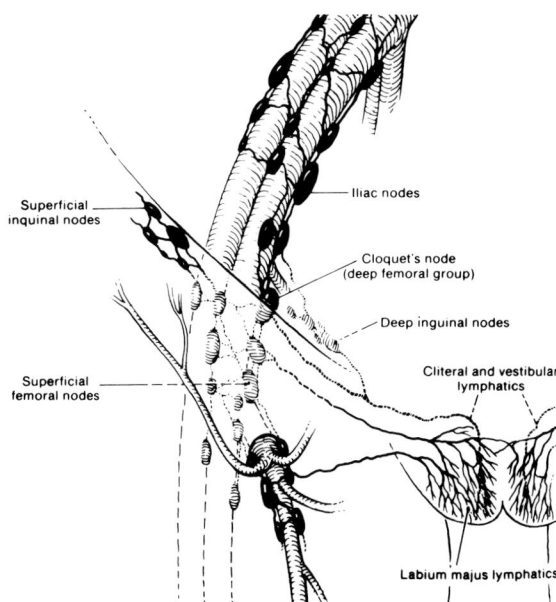

FIG. 30.4. Lymphatics of the vulva. (Reprinted by permission of Schmidt, WA (1983) Principles and Techniques of Surgical Pathology. Butterworth-Heinemann, Stoneham, MA.)

rectum and bladder must be opened, the specimen fixed, and sections taken perpendicular to the mucosa directly overlying the tumor in the vagina. A good method that provides excellent orientation of the tumor to adjacent structures for exenteration specimens is to inflate the urinary bladder and rectum with formalin and fix the specimen for several hours. The entire specimen can then be hemisected through the neoplasm, and the appropriate sections can be obtained (Fig. 30.5). Sections from the surgical resection margins and any lymph nodes identified in the attached soft tissue should be obtained. India ink marking of all resection margins and a diagram describing the specimen, tumor, and section code is useful for orientation and correlation of the microscopic sections and the gross findings.

The surgical pathology report should include the microscopic diagnosis, tumor grade, dimensions, location and relationship to adjacent structures, presence of lymphatic invasion, number of involved lymph nodes, and adequacy of the surgical resection margins.

TOTAL HYSTERECTOMY

The total hysterectomy specimen consists of the cervix and the uterine corpus. Supracervical hysterectomy, a procedure in which the uterus is amputated at the internal cervical os, is now rarely performed. Removal of the cervix and uterus is treatment for a variety of benign and malignant diseases. Because of the diverse nature of the disease processes for which a hysterectomy is performed, the approach to processing the specimen as well as the hysterectomy procedure itself vary accordingly. The different

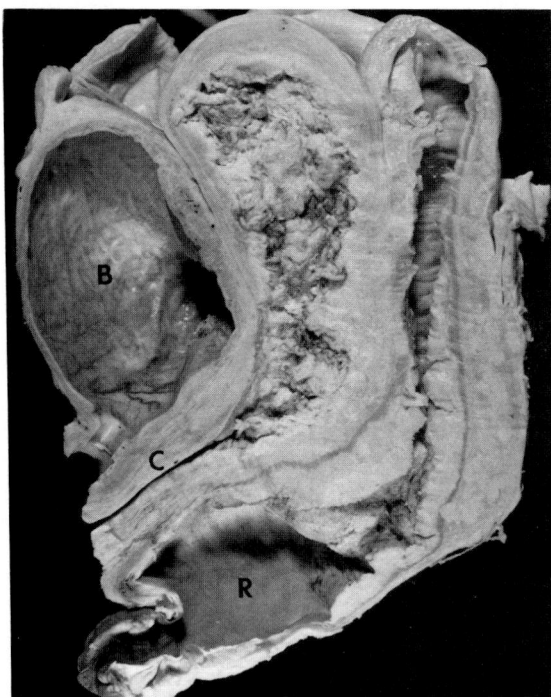

FIG. 30.5. Pelvic exenteration for cervical cancer. Hemisection of bladder (**B**), uterus with cervix (**C**), rectum (**B**), and sigmoid colon. (Courtesy of Dennis O'Connor, M. D., Washington, D. C.)

pathological techniques used, therefore, are considered according to the surgical indication.

HYSTERECTOMY FOR BENIGN FUNCTIONAL UTERINE DISEASE

Included in this category are hysterectomies for persistent abnormal bleeding, uterine prolapse, or intractable pelvic pain. The last sometimes may be due to unrecognized organic causes, such as adenomyosis or endometriosis, that are recognized only after thorough pathological examination.

Begin the description by listing the specimens received, including whether the cervix or adnexae are attached or separate. The specimen is oriented (Fig. 30.6) by identifying the round ligaments that insert anterior to the fallopian tubes. In addition, on the posterior surface of the uterus the peritoneum covers a larger area and extends farther down toward the cervix than anteriorly, where it is reflected high over the bladder (Fig. 30.7). The specimen should then be weighed after the adnexae have been removed. The parous uterus is heavier (premenopausal adult 75–100 g) than the nulliparous uterus (premenopausal adult 30–40 g), and weight increases with increasing parity. After eight pregnancies a weight of 240 g is normal.[3] The postmenopausal uterus, because of the diminished amount of muscle, weighs 20 to 40 g. The following measurements should be taken: (1) top of the fundus to the exocervix (premenopausal adult 5–8 cm), (2) cornu to cornu (premenopausal adult 3–5 cm), (3) thickness from anterior to posterior surface (premenopausal adult 2–4 cm), and (4) length and diameter of the cervix (premenopausal adult 3 cm each).

The uterine serosa, particularly the posterior surface, should be examined carefully for adhesions and brown hemosiderin deposits, so-called powder burns, if endometriosis is suspected. The exocervix should be examined for lacerations, scarring, ulcerations, and cysts.

Before opening of the uterus, the cervical canal and endometrial cavity should be probed. This establishes the patency of the endocervical canal and facilitates opening the uterus. An incision is made with a scalpel or scissors along the probe extending from the cervical os to the cornu along one lateral margin to the fundus and then along the other lateral margin (Fig. 30.8). The average thickness of the endometrium should be measured and a statement made whether it is atrophic, polypoid, or hemorrhagic. Polyps should be measured and their location specified. The myometrium is evaluated with sections through the full thickness of the anterior and posterior walls. The maximum thickness of the myometrium should be measured. A thickened myometrium showing small cystic or focal areas of hemorrhage is suggestive of adenomyosis. If the cervix is normal, a section including the endocervix and portio is adequate. The section of the cervix should include the entire wall to involve the endocervix, squamocolumnar junction, and exocervix. The section through the endometrium, if the lesion is benign, should be up to 2 cm long and should include the full thickness of the endometrium and a wedge of myometrium. In routine cases, two microscopic sections, one each from the anterior or posterior cervix and one from the anterior or posterior endomyometrium, suffice.

Hysterectomy for Benign Organic Uterine Disease

This includes hysterectomies performed for leiomyomas and endometrial hyperplasia. In addition to the routine processing described previously, more detailed examination is required in these cases.

In a specimen removed for leiomyomas, the number of leiomyomas present, their location (submucosal, intramural, subserosal) and size (e.g., "ten less than 1 cm and two measuring 13 and 18 cm in diameter") should be noted. If submucous, whether the tumor distorts the endometrial cavity or whether it protrudes into the lower uterine canal or cervix should be stated. Each leiomyoma should be sectioned and examined grossly but not necessarily microscopically. Usually one to two blocks are sufficient if all the leiomyomas are small, white, firm, whorled, have well-circumscribed margins, and do not contain areas that are soft, necrotic, or hemorrhagic. Since leiomyomas under 5 cm in size virtually never metastasize regardless of microscopic appearance, routine microscopic examination of every typical leiomyoma is considered unnecessary. Conversely, as leiomyomas tend to be multiple and

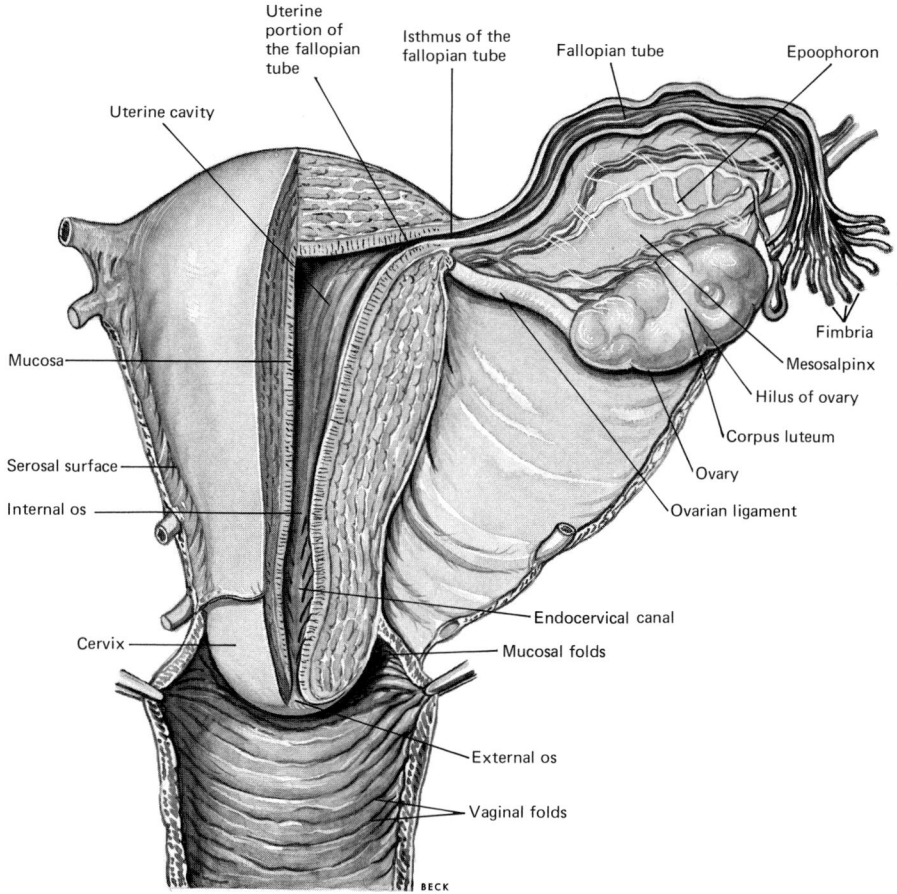

FIG. 30.6. The uterus, vagina, and adnexa. (Modified from Gray's Anatomy, 30th ed. (C. D. Clemente, ed.), 1985. Courtesy of Lea & Febiger.)

leiomyosarcomas single, solitary tumors that are soft, degenerating, or in any way suspicious must be sampled thoroughly. As a general rule, one microscopic section per centimeter of the greatest tumor diameter is recommended if the lesion is suspicious. Sections taken for variation of color, soft or hemorrhagic areas, or some other specific finding yield much greater information than "random" sections. For myomectomy specimens, each leiomyoma should be transected and a section taken from each. Additional sections should be taken if suspicious areas are present.

Uteri removed for endometrial hyperplasia should have multiple full-thickness sections of the endomyometrium to rule out the presence of carcinoma. Four sections (two sections, each 2 cm long, of each wall) should adequately sample the endometrium in most cases.

HYSTERECTOMY FOR MALIGNANT CERVICAL DISEASE
(APPENDIX, TABLE 30.2)

For intraepithelial neoplasms, a simple hysterectomy often with a vaginal cuff is performed. For microinvasive

squamous carcinoma, a simple hysterectomy or a modified radical hysterectomy (inclusion of some paracervical soft tissue) is performed depending on the depth of invasion and the institutional criteria, which vary. For stage I squamous carcinomas, depending on size and configuration of the tumor in the endocervical canal, and for stage IIa tumors, depending on the extent of vaginal involvement, a radical hysterectomy (Wertheim hysterectomy) and pelvic lymphadenectomy is performed. Para-aortic lymph nodes also are frequently sampled.

For uteri removed for intraepithelial neoplasms, the cervix should be amputated no less than 0.5 cm above the level of the external os and processed as a cone biopsy. Preferably the amputation should include the maximum amount of endocervix that will fit into the cassette. If a vaginal cuff has been submitted, the distance from the exocervix to the line of resection should be measured. Sections should be obtained from the surgical resection line to determine the adequacy of the margin. As with the vulva, sections may be circumferential or perpendicular as long as the blocking process is thorough and complete. Sections perpendicular to the line of resection, as stated above, permit assessment of the cervical lesion and margins together

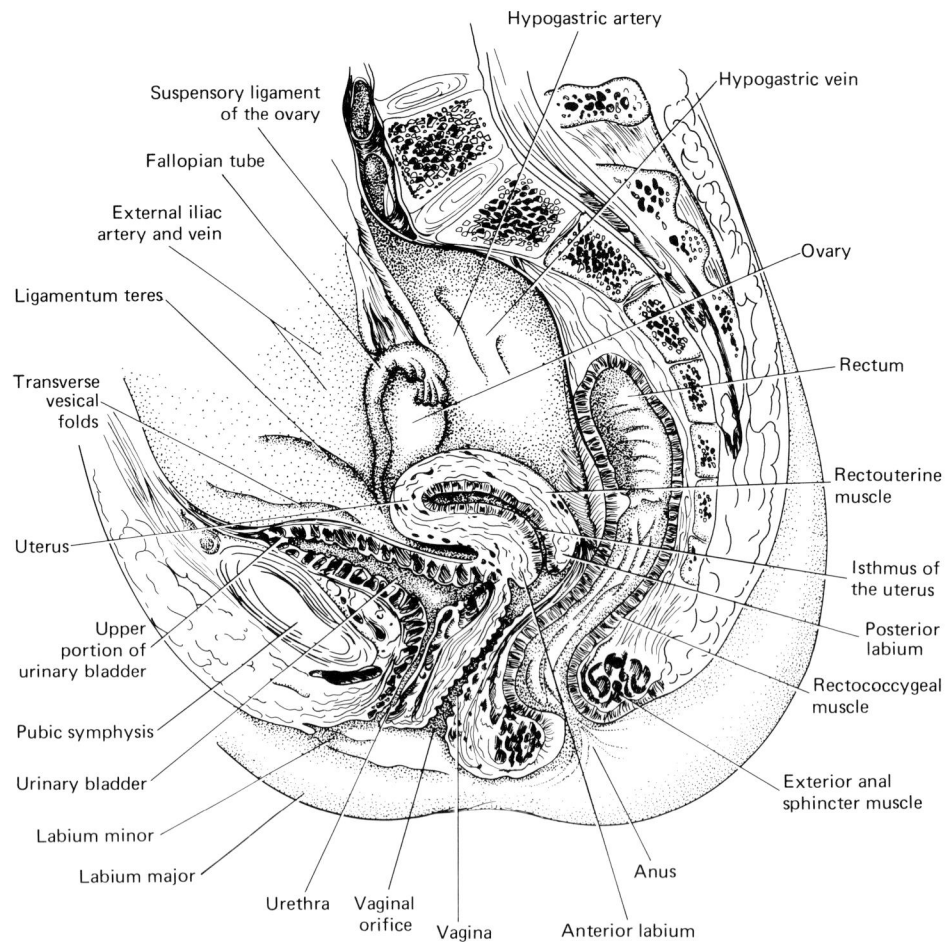

FIG. 30.7. Sagittal section through the pelvis illustrating the anterior and posterior peritoneal reflections on the uterus. (Modified from Gray's Anatomy, 30th ed. (C. D. Clemente, ed.), 1985. Courtesy of Lea & Febiger.)

in context. This information, along with the microscopic diagnosis, should appear in the surgical pathology report.

A radical hysterectomy differs from a simple hysterectomy by virtue of the presence of attached paracervical tissues, which extend to the ureter and iliac artery and vein. Accompanying the specimen is a cuff of vagina and pelvic lymph nodes. The gross description should include the dimensions of the tumor, its location, relation to the vaginal margin, depth of invasion, and an impression of whether the lymph nodes appear normal or contain metastases. The cervix can be processed either as a cone biopsy or selectively sampled to demonstrate the maximum depth of invasion and relationship to the surgical margins. The vaginal resection margin is evaluated as described previously. In addition, since the lymphatic drainage of the uterus is lateral toward the parametrium, these areas are especially important in defining the spread of disease. The parametrial tissue should be completely processed, since this represents the lateral and most significant resection margin. The outer surface of the cervix overlying the tumor anteriorly and posteriorly should

be marked with India ink to delineate the extent of the tumor in relationship to the bladder and rectum. Lymph nodes should be grouped according to areas. Right and left should be separated and internal iliac, external iliac, obturator, and so on should be separately grouped. Lymph nodes often can be evaluated better when they are fresh, at which time they are firm and nodular. Alternatively, Bouin's fixation, by turning lymph nodes white (whereas fat remains yellow) can be used to facilitate their detection.

The surgical pathology report should include the microscopic diagnosis, maximum size, location, extension, and depth of invasion of the tumor. In addition, the presence of lymphatic invasion, number of involved lymph nodes, and adequacy of the resection margins, especially lateral margins, adjacent to the uterine arteries should be noted.

HYSTERECTOMY FOR MALIGNANT UTERINE DISEASE
(APPENDIX, TABLE 30.3)

This includes uteri removed for endometrial carcinoma and sarcomas of the uterus. Hysterectomy specimens re-

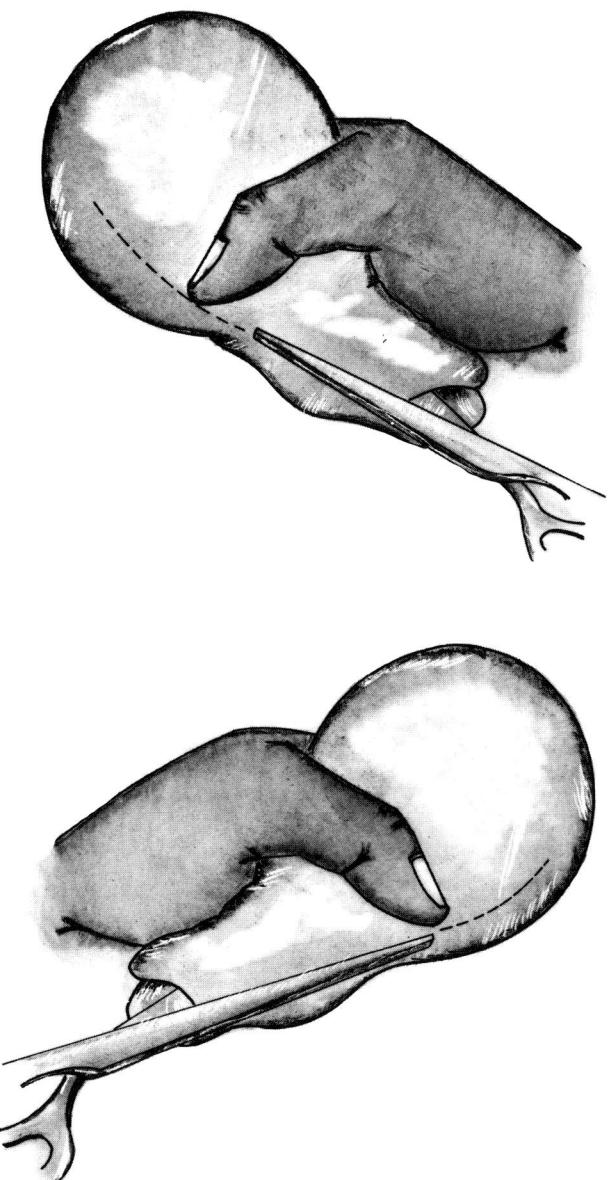

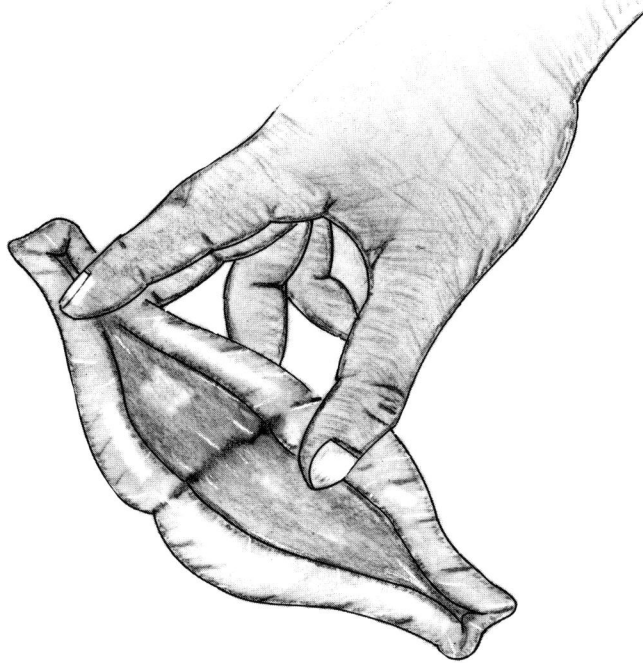

Fig. 30.8. Bivalve opening of the uterus. The specimen is opened to best demonstrate the uterine lesion present.

ceived with a preoperative diagnosis of carcinoma or sarcoma must be evaluated for residual tumor. The gross evaluation should be the same as for uteri removed for benign organic disease. In addition, the description should include whether the tumor is focal or diffuse, sessile or polypoid. The uninvolved endometrium should be described and sampled microscopically. The dimensions and location of the tumor including involvement of the cervix should be noted, and the gross depth of myometrial invasion recorded. The sounding depth from the external os to the inside of the top of the fundus (premenopausal adult 7–8 cm) is optional as it is no longer included in the FIGO staging system. Microscopic sections should be obtained to determine the maximum depth of myometrial invasion and involvement of the cervix.

The surgical pathology report should include the microscopic diagnosis, tumor grade, depth of myometrial invasion, involvement of the cervix, presence of vascular invasion, and the number of positive lymph nodes with their location specified, that is, pelvic or para-aortic.

Hysterectomy Performed During Obstetrical Procedures

Hysterectomy at the time of delivery is performed for intractable hemorrhage, placenta accreta, uterine rupture, or cervical neoplasia. For the last, processing of the specimen should be as described previously. For the other conditions, the gross description and sectioning should focus on the relationship of the placenta and membranes to the uterus. Lacerations should be described carefully as to location, extent, and depth of penetration. Sections should be obtained from these sites. If the patient has had a previous cesarean section, the old scar, usually in the anterior lower uterine segment, should be sampled. In instances of placenta previa, the zone of the internal os should be sampled carefully to identify associated placenta accreta.

SALPINGECTOMY

Removal of the fallopian tube (salpingectomy) often accompanies removal of the ovary (oophorectomy). Removal of both fallopian tubes and ovaries (bilateral salpingo-oophorectomy) often is performed in conjunction with a hysterectomy, especially in older women in whom it is no longer necessary to preserve fertility. In these cases, there is typically no pathological condition in the fallopian tubes, and the gross examination and sampling are routine. The overall length and diameter of the tube should be measured. The patency of the fimbriated end can be determined with a blunt-tipped probe. If a lesion is present, it should be measured, its location (cornual, isthmic, infundibular, or ampullary) noted, and its relationship to the lumen and serosa described. If no lesion is present, transverse sections from the isthmic, infundibular, and ampullary portions of the tube can be placed into one cassette and labeled "right" or "left" (Fig. 30.9).

TOTAL OR PARTIAL SALPINGECTOMY FOR TUBAL ECTOPIC PREGNANCY OR STERILIZATION

If the tubal pregnancy is apparent, its site and location should be noted as described previously. A rupture site if present should be described and sampled. If the ectopic pregnancy is not obvious, a focal enlargement or swelling of the tube should be searched for. Blood distending the lumen of the fallopian tube is so unlikely to result from any other cause that it is worth documenting. It may be necessary to section the area extensively. Even a tubal abortion leaves foci of trophoblast at the

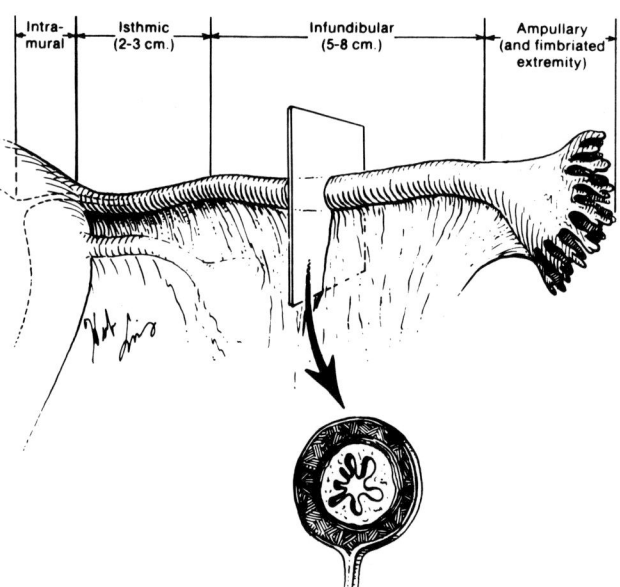

FIG. 30.9. **Technique for sectioning the fallopian tube in the absence of abnormalities.** Representative transverse sections are obtained from the isthmic, infundibular, and ampullary regions. (Reprinted by permission of Schmidt WA (1983) Principles and Techniques of Surgical Pathology. Butterworth-Heinemann, Stoneham, MA.)

implantation site. Blood clot in the tube, sometimes submitted as a separate specimen, should be examined carefully for gray-white tissue and sampled for microscopic examination to identify trophoblastic cells or chorionic villi.

Segments of fallopian tube removed for sterilization should be received labeled "right" and "left," measured and maintained separately throughout processing. If submitted whole for processing, the histotechnologist should be instructed to cut and orient the specimen before embedding, a process that greatly facilitates proper orientation. Alternatively, transverse sections can be obtained from each side and submitted to confirm that the specimen represents a segment from the fallopian tube. Epithelium needs to be present to confirm the presence of fallopian tube.

SALPINGECTOMY FOR A TUBAL NEOPLASM

Tubal carcinoma is rare, and its behavior and management are similar to ovarian carcinoma. Typically, a total abdominal hysterectomy and bilateral salpingo-oophorectomy are performed. The size of the tumor, location, and extent, with reference to other pelvic structures, should be described. Transverse sections through the full thickness of the tube permit determination of the depth of penetration. All of this information as well as the grade of the tumor should be included in the microscopic diagnosis of the surgical pathology report.

OOPHORECTOMY

The ovaries, like the fallopian tubes, frequently are removed at the time of hysterectomy in older women even if there is no apparent pathology. Routine processing of this type of specimen includes weighing and measuring the ovary in three dimensions. The normal ovary in the reproductive years weighs approximately ~12 g, is ovoid, and measures approximately $4 \times 2.5 \times 1.5$ cm. The external surface should be inspected for stigmata of ovulation, adhesions, excrescences hemorrhage, or hemosiderin (powder burns), indicative of possible endometriosis. The hilus and broad ligament should be examined, and any suspicious lesion should be submitted for microscopic examination. Each ovary should be sectioned sagittally through its greatest dimension to include the hilus and submitted in a single cassette labeled "right" or "left" (Fig. 30.10).

CYSTECTOMY OR OOPHORECTOMY FOR A NEOPLASM

Cystectomy usually is performed for a dermoid cyst. After weighing and measuring the specimen in three dimensions, the external surface should be examined and the cyst opened. The sebum within the cyst can be removed by washing with hot water. The water must be hot to liquefy the sebum. Short exposure to hot water does not destroy

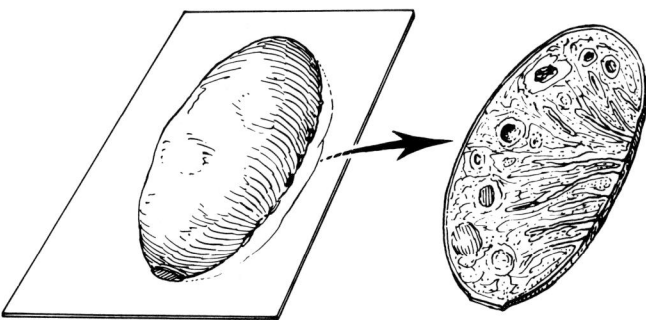

FIG. 30.10. **Technique for sectioning the ovary in the absence of abnormalities.** The cross-section, contains cortex, medulla, and hilum. (Reprinted by permission of Schmidt WA (1983) Principles and Techniques of Surgical Pathology. Butterworth-Heinemann, Stoneham, MA.)

the epithelial lining. Identify and serially block the knobby protuberance in the wall, so-called Rokitansky's tubercle, teat, or mammilla, and any other areas where the wall is thickened.

Except for obvious benign paraovarian and functional ovarian cysts, all other cystic and solid ovarian neoplasms are treated by a unilateral salpingooophorectomy or a hysterectomy and bilateral salpingo-oophorectomy. The hysterectomy specimen and normal-appearing contralateral ovary and fallopian tube should be processed and reported as described previously. The ovarian tumor should be weighed and measured in three dimensions. The fallopian tube generally is removed with the ovary but may be draped over the tumor and difficult to identify. If present, it should be measured and its relationship to the ovary noted. Similarly, if a tumor appears to have largely replaced the ovary, any residual ovary should be identified and its relationship to the tumor noted. Not uncommonly, the only portion of residual ovary in a tumor is that portion of the gonad immediately adjacent to the fallopian tube. Therefore, it is useful to take sections transversely through the fallopian tube to include a wedge of ovary.

The gross description should state whether the specimen is received intact or fragmented. The capsule should be examined for rents, adhesions, implants, or extension and penetration of the underlying tumor. The tumor is then hemisected, and the cut surfaces are examined. Each cyst of a cystic tumor should be examined for papillary excrescences and solid foci, since these may reveal areas of low malignant potential or frankly malignant tumor on microscopic examination. In about 5% of mucinous tumors, evidence of a dermoid cyst, e.g., hair, will be found in a mucinous locule. If a solid ovarian tumor is small, identify it if its location is cortical, medullary, or hilar.

Microscopic sections should be obtained from the external surface of the neoplasm, especially in areas of adhesions, to document whether tumor involves the surface or if the adherence is the result simply of a chemical reaction.

In particular, penetration of underlying tumor through the surface should be documented, since this plays a role in staging. Surgeons should be asked to place a stitch in the adhesions noted during the operative procedure. It is important to demonstrate invasion microscopically. Blocks cut to show the interface between the tumor and the adjacent tube are especially useful. All solid and hemorrhagic areas should be sampled thoroughly. It is commonly stated that the pathologist should submit a minimum of one block per 1–2 cm of the greatest tumor dimension. However, this dictum is clearly to be applied with judgment. For example, serous tumors tend to be relatively uniform throughout. Other tumors, in contrast, e.g., mucinous tumors, vary greatly such that large areas may appear grossly and microscopically benign, whereas only a few areas are typically of borderline or frank malignancy. Solid areas need to be more thoroughly sought grossly, and those sampled extensively microscopically. Unilocular cysts with a smooth lining of the inner wall, in contrast, may be large, but require fewer sections for microscopical examination. The microscopic diagnosis should include the cell type and, for epithelial tumors, whether benign, of low malignant potential, or frankly malignant. For frankly malignant tumors, include tumor grade, whether the surface is involved, the extent of the tumor, and the site and number of involved lymph nodes.

Placental Examination

ROUTINE PROCESSING

Since most newborns and their mothers are normal and healthy, detailed pathological examination of all placentas is not warranted. The obstetrician must select for examination those placentas that may help in the diagnosis of illness in parent or newborn. The pathologist must respond with an informative report.[2]

Examination of the placenta can provide information useful in patient management, especially infections, and identify instances in which karyotyping is indicated. Furthermore, in the current litigious environment, placental examination may define types of birth injury that lie outside the control of the obstetrician. Documentation of twinning relationships may be useful in later life, for example, in patients evaluated for organ transplantation.

Placentas selected for examination should be sent fresh to the laboratory with a requisition that states the questions the pathologist is requested to answer. Placentas not selected can be labeled and stored in plastic bags, either frozen or refrigerated, for retrieval if problems develop in the neonatal period.

Indications for placental examination and a format suitable for transmission of the placenta and necessary data to the laboratory are listed in Table 30.5 (see Appendix.) The list begins with the mother's name and age. It can be used as a checklist sufficient to provide the pathologist with enough clinical data to start the examination. The membrane of the specimen should be translucent and the fetal surface should be shiny, dark purple. Reconstruct the membranous sac, noting its narrowest margin between placental edge and site of rupture. The absence of a margin may explain bleeding; any margin excludes placenta previa. Record tears or bands. Cut a strip of membrane about 5 cm wide, roll it toward the placental margin, and affix it with a pin (Fig. 30.11). Cut away the rest of the membranes from the rest of the placental margin with scissors. Next, examine the fetal surface. Note exudate, discoloration (green-brown) from meconium staining, and adherent extraneous material that does not easily wipe away. The umbilical cord must be carefully examined and measured. Record knots, hemorrhages, and number of vessels on cross-section cut away from the placenta near the fetal surface. Insertion of the cord near the narrowest membrane margin may be a cause of intrapartum fetal distress (vasa previa). The inspection should conclude with an examination of the maternal surface. Cotyledons should be intact. Note any adherent clot, especially clots that compress the placenta or have become indurated and laminated.

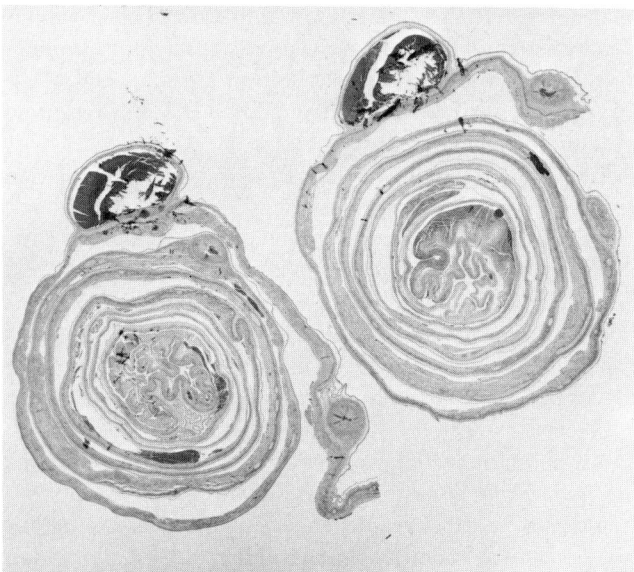

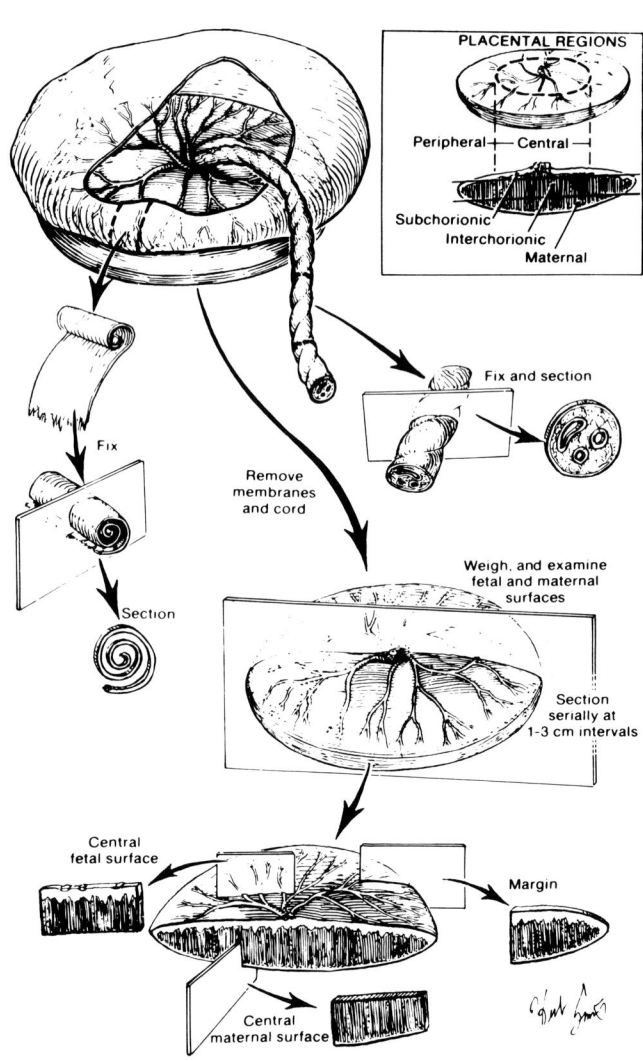

FIG. 30.11. Placental examination. *Top:* A placenta with membrane roll attached at top before fixation. The resulting spiral in cassette retains its tight coil after the block has been processed. *Bottom:* Margin of membrane opening is always at the center of the spiral. This consistent orientation helps demonstrate the ascending route of infections.

FIG. 30.12. Placental examination. Adequate sampling for histologic study includes membrane roll, cross-section of cord, and specific placental regions, specifically cut to display fetal and maternal surfaces. (Reprinted by permission of Schmidt WA (1983) Principles and Techniques of Surgical Pathology. Butterworth-Heinemann, Stoneham, MA.)

Weigh the placenta and record the maximum dimensions. Cut sections at 1- to 20-cm intervals with a sharp knife; this is accomplished most easily with the maternal surface up. The cut surface should have a uniform granular surface and a bright red color. Record clots, infarcts, and other lesions.

After the specimen has been fixed for several hours in 10% buffered neutral formalin, blocks can be cut for histological sections (Fig. 30.12) to include a cross-section of the cord, membrane roll, fetal surface with amnion attached, and lesions identified on cross-section.

TWINS AND OTHER MULTIPLE GESTATIONS

The amnionic septum between two amnionic cavities serves to define identical or fraternal relationships insofar as placental examination allows. The dividing membrane of dichorionic placentas is thicker and opaque because of the intervening chorionic tissue. Attach a roll of this membrane as described for single placentas, affixing it to the placental surface with a pin. After fixation, cut a cross-section from this roll and the T zone, where it attaches to the fetal surface of the placenta (Fig. 30.13). When both amnions are stripped away, a ridge or layer of chorion persists in fused dichorionic twin placentas. In monochorionic twin placentas the septal site vanishes, and the only visible traces are vascular connections on the fetal surface.

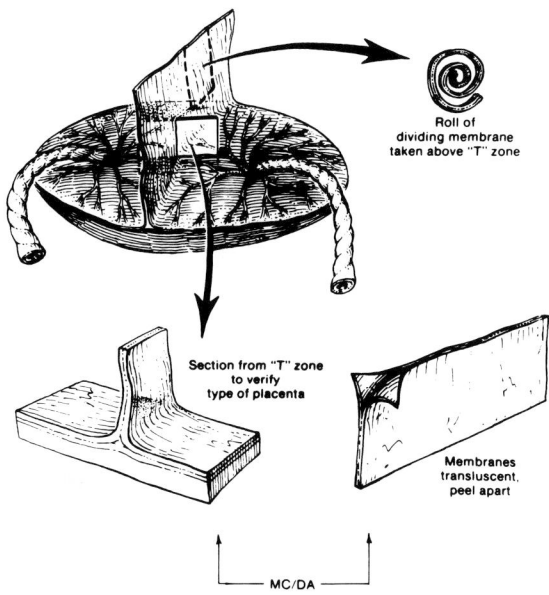

FIG. 30.13. Examination of placenta of twins. Sampling of a twin placenta includes a section of septal membrane dividing the amnionic cavities, cut to display the T zone, where the septal membrane attaches to the placental surface. (Reprinted by permission of Schmidt WA (1983) Principles and Techniques of Surgical Pathology. Butterworth-Heinemann, Stoneham, MA.)

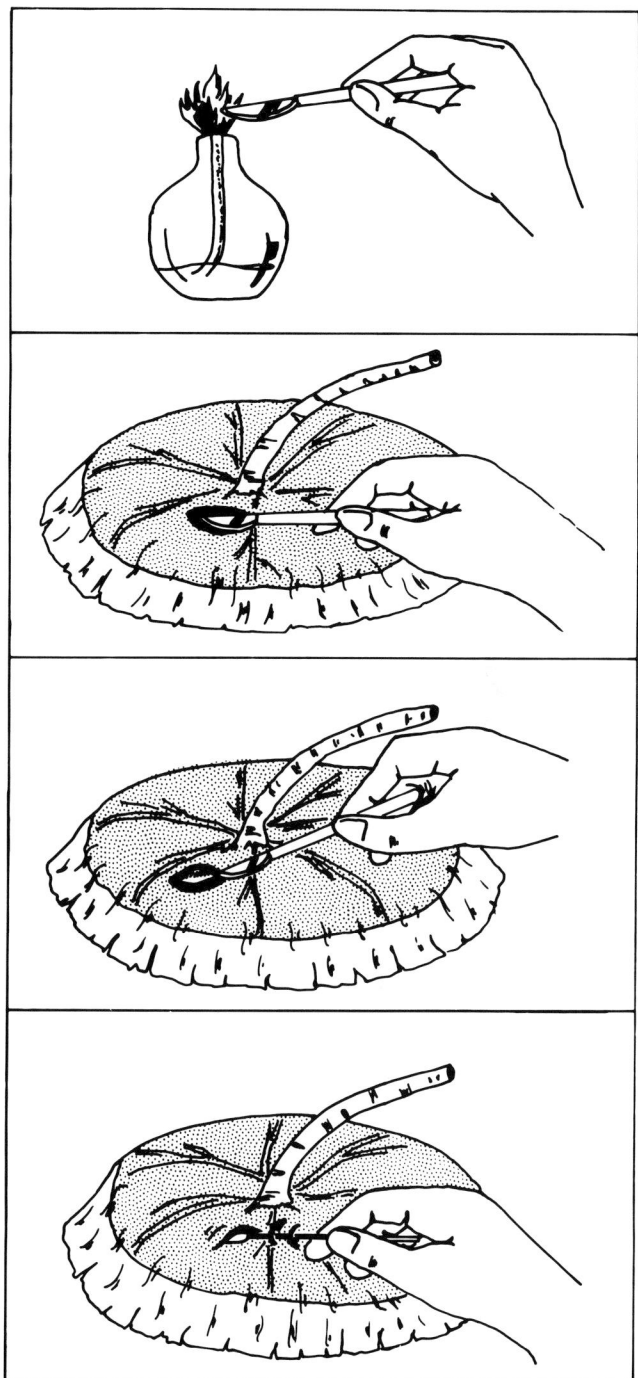

FIG. 30.14. Culture technique to sample subchorionic fibrin layer. This method reduces surface contamination.

CULTURE METHODS

Aerobic and anaerobic bacterial cultures, when performed by swabbing the fetal surface, introduce so many contaminants that the procedure has little value. To reduce the frequency of contaminants the subchorionic zone is best cultured with a swab after the surface has been seared and incised with a heated or sterile scalpel[1] (Fig. 30.14).

Cytogenetic Studies

These studies require a fragment of villous tissue or skin or pericardium if perinatal death has occurred. Death of the fetus does not necessarily preclude successful culture. The tissue should be placed in sterile media containers provided by the cytogenetics laboratory. Tissue obtained properly may be shipped to a distant facility if desired. (See Table 30.6 in the Appendix for directions for preparation and transmission of tissue.)

Dissecting Microscope

A dissecting microscope should be available for adequate study of many small abortuses. Some anomalies, including fusion defects of the facial clefts, fused or supernumerary digits, partial limb reduction, and such ocular defects as coloboma, are too minute to evaluate adequately with the unaided eye, but alone or in combination they may be sufficiently suggestive of trisomy to indicate the need for karyotypes of the conceptus and possibly the parents.

Appendix

Table 30.1. Vulvar carcinoma

Operative Procedure: _____ CASE: _____

Diagnosis:
VULVA: _____ (histology), measuring ___ × ___ × ___ cm depth
    with extension into _____
    and metastases to _____ lymph nodes
    and _____ (other sites).
    Resection margins _____ .

1 Degree of differentiation Squamous cell	Well, moderately, poorly differentiated
2 Size of tumor	___ × ___ cm
Tumor thickness:	___ mm (Fm granular layer (surface if no keratin to deepest point of invasion))

Depth of invasion:	___ mm (Fm epithelial stromal junction of
	    adjacent most supfl dermal papillae
	    to deepest point of invasion)

Uninvolved zone to deep margin:	___ mm
3 Location & Gross configuration	Unifocal Multifocal Left Right Cross_Midline Labia: Minora Majora Ant Post Clitoral PeriUrethral PeriVaginal Bartholin Gland Post Fourchette PeriAnal Perineum

4 Margins, distance to:
  Surface margin
  Deep margin
	If uninvolved, closest distance ___ mm
	Involved, which: Ant Post L_Lat R_lat
	Involved

5 Depth invasion		Invasive
For melanoma	Levels	in -mm
	1 (In epidermis/ In situ)	0 mm
	2 (Into papillary dermis)	<1 mm
	3 (To pap/reticular interface)	1–2 mm
	4 (Into reticular dermis)	>2 mm
	5 (Into subcutaneous fat)	In fat

6 Extravulvar tumor:
  Anus:
  Rectum:
  Vagina:
  Urethra:
  Bladder:
  Pelvic bone attachment:
  Other
	
	No Wall Mucosa
	No Wall Mucosa
	No Wall Mucosa Lower Upper
	No Wall Mucosa Lower Upper
	No Wall Mucosa
	No Yes
	_____ where

7 Vascular involvement:	No Yes_type Uncertain Lymphatics Blood_vessel Both

8 Associated changes
  Squamous
  Appendages involved
	
	None VIN-I II III
	No Yes

9 Special studies:
  DNA ploidy:
  HPV type:
	
	Euploid Tetraploid Aneuploid
	6/11 16/18 31/33/35

10 Non-neoplastic changes
  Lichen sclerosus
  Hyperplasia
  Hyperkeratosis
  Koilocytosis
  Other:
	
	No Yes
	No Yes
	No Yes
	No Yes
	Yes, _____ Specify

11 Lymph nodes: NOS	None ___ of ___ contain metastases

	Left		Right	
Inguinal, NOS	None ___/___	w Mets	None ___/___	w Mets
Superficial	None ___/___	w Mets	None ___/___	w Mets
Deep	None ___/___	w Mets	None ___/___	w Mets
Pelvic, NOS	None ___/___	w Mets	None ___/___	w Mets
External iliac	None ___/___	w Mets	None ___/___	w Mets
Obturator (Med Ext Iliac)	None ___/___	w Mets	None ___/___	w Mets
Internal iliac (Hypogastr)	None ___/___	w Mets	None ___/___	w Mets
Aortic, NOS	None ___/___	w Mets	None ___/___	w Mets

Adapted from
INTERNATIONAL SOCIETY OF
GYNECOLOGICAL PATHOLOGISTS

Squamous Lesions
Squamous cell carcinoma
Basaloid carcinoma
Verrucous carcinoma
Basal cell carcinoma

Glandular Lesions
Paget disease
Bartholin gland tumors
Breast ca & others ectopic origin
Carcinomas of sweat gland origin
Other adenocarcinomas

Mesenchymal Tumors
Embry rhabdomyosarc (sarc botryoid)
Aggressive angiomyxoma
Leiomyosarcoma
Dermatofibrosarcoma protuberans
Malignant fibrous histiocytoma
Epithelioid sarcoma
Malignant rhabdoid tumor
Malignant schwannoma
Angiosarcoma
Kaposi sarcoma
Hemangiopericytoma
Liposarcoma
Alveolar soft-part sarcoma

Miscellaneous Tumors
Malignant melanoma
Malignant lymphoma
Tumors of germ cell type
  Yolk sac (endodermal sinus tumor)
Neurectodermal tumors
  Merkel cell tumor

Reprinted by permission of Robboy et al., ref. 5.

Table 30.2. Cervical carcinoma

Operative Procedure: CASE: _____

Diagnosis:

CERVIX: _____ (histology)

    FIGO grade ___ , measuring ___ × ___ × ___ cm depth

    with extension into _____

    and metastases to _____ lymph nodes

    and _____ (other sites).

    Resection margins _____ .

1 Grade

  If Squamous cell   Non-keratinizing; Keratinizing

  If glandular

  Architectural grade: G1- Well differentiated (5% or less solid growth)

  (% solid growth)   G2- Moderately differentiated (6–50% solid growth)

                 G3- Poorly differentiated (over 50% solid growth)

  .Solid excludes squamous growth

2 Size of tumor   ___ × ___ cm (length/width)

  Depth invasion: ___ mm

  Uninvolved zone

    to deep margin: ___ mm

3 Location: Left   Right

                      Ant   Post

                      Exocervix SQ junction Endocervix

                      Confined to polyp Parametrium

4 Shape of cervix: Normal, Cylindrical, Barrel shaped (>4 cm)

5 Extracervical tumor: No _____ (where)

  Uterine corpus: No Yes Lower uter segment Endomet Myomet

  Vagina: No Upper 2/3rds Lower 3rd Mucosa Wall

  Parauterine: No Yes Left Right

  Ureter: No Yes L/R Hydronephrosis Non-function kidney

  Bone Pelvic Side wall: No Yes L/R

  Bladder: No Wall Mucosa

  Rectum: No Wall Mucosa

  Abdomen/peritoneum: No Yes

  Liver: No Yes

6 Vascular involvement: No Yes type Uncertain

                      Lymphatics Blood vessel Both

7 Associated premalignant changes

  Squamous   None CIN-I II III

  Glandular   None AIN-I/Atyp II III/In-situ

  If involved   Multifocal

8 Margins, distance to: If uninvolved, closest distance ___ mm

  Surface margins: Involved, which: Cranial Caudal L_Lat R_lat

  Depth: Involved:

9 Special studies:

  DNA ploidy: Euploid Tetraploid Aneuploid

  HPV type: 6/11 16/18 31/33/35

10 Non-Neoplastic cervix

  Koilocytosis (Condyloma) No Yes

  Other: Yes, _____ Specify

11 Lymph nodes: NOS   None ___ of ___ contain metastases

	Left	Right
Parauterine	None ___/___ w Mets	None ___/___ w Mets
Obturator (Med Ext Iliac)	None ___/___ w Mets	None ___/___ w Mets
External iliac	None ___/___ w Mets	None ___/___ w Mets
Sacral	None ___/___ w Mets	None ___/___ w Mets
Internal iliac (Hypogastric)	None ___/___ w Mets	None ___/___ w Mets
Common Iliac	None ___/___ w Mets	None ___/___ w Mets
Pelvic, NOS	None ___/___ w Mets	None ___/___ w Mets
Aortic, NOS	None ___/___ w Mets	None ___/___ w Mets
Inguinal, NOS	None ___/___ w Mets	None ___/___ w Mets

Adapted from
INTERNATIONAL SOCIETY OF
GYNECOLOGICAL PATHOLOGISTS

Squamous lesions
Squamous cell carcinoma
  Keratinizing   Non-keratinizing
Verrucous
Warty (condylomatous)
Papillary (transitional)
Lymphoepithelioma-like

Glandular lesions
Adenocarcinoma
Mucinous adenocarcinoma
Clear-cell adenocarcinoma
Minimal deviation (adenoma malignum)
Villoglandular adenocarcinoma

Other epithelial tumors
Adenosquamous carcinoma
Glassy cell carcinoma
Adenoid basal carcinoma
Adenoid cystic carcinoma
Carcinoid tumor
Small cell carcinoma
Wollfian duct (mesonephric)

Mesenchymal Tumors
Leiomyosarcoma
Endocervical stromal sarcoma
Sarc botryoides (embry rhabdomyosarc)
Alveolar soft-part sarcoma
Osteosarcoma

Mixed Epithelial & Mesenchymal Tumors
Adenosarcoma
Malig mixed mesodermal tumor (MMMT)
Wilms tumor

Miscellaneous Tumors
Malignant melanoma
Lymphoma and leukemia
Germ cell type
  Yolk sac tumor

Table 30.3. Endometrial cancer[a]

Operative Procedure: _____   CASE: _____

Diagnosis:

UTERUS: _____ (histology) (___ % each major cell type)

    FIGO grade ___ , measuring ___ × ___ × ___ cm

    with extension into _____

    and metastases to _____ lymph nodes

    and _____ (other sites).

    Tumor penetrates _____ mm into _____ thick myometrium.

1 Architectural grade: G1-Well differentiated (5% or less solid growth)

    % solid growth)   G2-Moderately differentiated (6–50% solid growth)

                  G3-Poorly differentiated (over 50% solid growth)

  .Solid excludes squamous growth

  .Notable nuclear atypia, inappropriate for architectural grade,

    raises the nuclear grade by 1.

  .Nuclear grade takes precedence for clear cell, squamous & serous CA.

2 Special Attributes

    Nuclear grade: 1 (Uniform nuclei, small nucleoli, rare mitoses)

    (glandular)   2 (More variability, larger nucleoli, more mitoses)

    (controversial)   3 (Pleomorphic, many mitoses)

    Squamous differentiation ___ % total neoplasm

3 Size of uterus: Weight ___ gm; ___ × ___ × ___ cm

    Size of tumor   ___ × ___ cm (length/width)

    Thickness of myometrium: ___ mm

    Deepest invasion: None ___ mm Serosa involved

4 Location: Unifocal Multifocal

                  Ant Post Cornua

                  Fundus Body Lower uterine segment

                  Polyp (involves limited to)

5 Extrauterine tumor:

    Ovary: No Left Right Histology: _____

                  Synchronous v metastasis

    Fallopian tube: No Left Right

    Broad Ligament: No Left Right

    Cervix: No Yes Supfl/glands Wall/stroma

                  Endocervix Exocervix

    If endocervix curetted: No Tumor only (No stroma) EC with implant

                  EC with invasion into stroma

    Parauterine: No Yes Left Right

    Vagina: No Yes

    Pelvic Peritoneum: No Yes

    Cul-de-sac: No Yes

    Omentum: No Yes

    Large Intestine: No Yes

    Other: No _____ (where)

6 Vascular involvement: No Yes type Uncertain

                  Lymphatics Blood vessel Both

7 Tissues adjacent to cancer

    Non-hyperplastic   Prolif Secretory Atrophy Disordered prolif

    Hyperplasia   Simple Complex Atypical

8 Ascites (>100cc)   Absent Neg Pos

    Pelvic washing: Neg Pos

9 Special studies:

    DNA ploidy: Euploid Tetraploid Aneuploid

    Estrogen-receptor: Neg Pos

    Progesterone-receptor: Neg Pos

    S-Phase fraction:

    Other: Yes, _____ Specify

10 Non-Neoplastic endometrium/uterine

    Metaplasia:

                  Squamous Mucinous Ciliary Clear cell

                  Eosinophilic cell Surface syncytial

    Adenomyosis   Papillary Other, Specify

    Arias-Stella: No Yes W tumor

    Other: No Yes

                  Yes, _____ Specify

11 Lymph nodes: NOS   None _____ of _____ contain metastases

	Left			Right		
Parauterine	None ____/____ w Mets			None ____/____ w Mets		
Internal iliac (Hypogastric)	None ____/____ w Mets			None ____/____ w Mets		
Obturator (Med Ext Iliac)	None ____/____ w Mets			None ____/____ w Mets		
External iliac	None ____/____ w Mets			None ____/____ w Mets		
Common Iliac	None ____/____ w Mets			None ____/____ w Mets		
Pelvic, NOS	None ____/____ w Mets			None ____/____ w Mets		
Aortic, NOS	None ____/____ w Mets			None ____/____ w Mets		
Inguinal, NOS	None ____/____ w Mets			None ____/____ w Mets		

12 Serum blood levels

    CA-125

Adapted from
INTERNATIONAL SOCIETY OF
GYNECOLOGICAL PATHOLOGISTS

Epithelial tumors
Adenocarcinoma (endometrioid)
  Secretory   Ciliated cell
Adenoca with Squamous differentiation
    Adenoacanthoma Adenosquamous_ca
Serous adenocarcinoma
Clear cell adenocarcinoma
Mucinous adenocarcinoma
Squamous cell carcinoma
Mixed
Undifferentiated

Reprinted by permission of Robboy et al., ref. 5.

[a] FIGO staging incorporates pathological findings.

Table 30.4. Ovarian carcinoma[a]

Operative Procedure: _____   CASE: _____

Adapted from
WORLD HEALTH ORGANIZATION

Diagnosis:
OVARY: _____ (histology) (___ % each major cell type)
    FIGO grade ___ , measuring ___ × ___ × ___ cm
    with extension into _____
    and metastases to _____ lymph nodes
    and _____ (other sites).

1 Architectural grade: G1-Well differentiated (5% or less solid growth)
    (% solid growth)   G2-Moderately differentiated (6–50% solid growth)
    (Common epith tumors) G3-Poorly differentiated (over 50% solid growth)

2 Size of tumor   Left: ___ gm; ___ × ___ × ___ cm (___ Check if normal)
    & Location   Right: ___ gm; ___ × ___ × ___ cm (___ Check if normal)

3 Tumor characteristics
    Capsule
      Adhesions   Inflammatory Tumor
      Ruptured   Spontaneous Surgically
      Surface tumor   Benign Borderline Malig
      Implants on ovary No Yes
    Parenchyma
      Solid   None Minimal (<10%) Extensive All
      Necrosis   None Minimal (<10%) Extensive All
      Cysts/locules   None Single Rare (<5) Many Hundreds

4 Staging bx, Peritoneum:
    Under diaphragm: Neg Pos
    Liver: Neg Supfl Parenchymal
    Stomach: Neg Pos
    Omentum: Neg Invasive Non-invasive
    Abdominal peritoneum: Neg Invasive Non-invasive
    Gutter: Neg Pos
    Pelvic peritoneum: Neg Pos
    Side-wall: Neg Pos
    Cul-de-sac, Ant Post: Neg Pos
    Falciform ligament: Neg Pos
    Uterosacral ligament: Neg Pos
    Serosal bowel implants: Neg Pos
      Mesentery: Neg Pos
      Small: Neg Pos
      Large: Neg Pos
      Rectosigmoid: Neg Pos
    Appendix: Neg Pos
    Vagina, apex: Neg Pos
    Misc _____

    Pelvis: staging
    Fallopian tube: No Yes L/R Mucosa Wall Serosa/Mesosalpinx
    Uterus: Neg Pos Serosa Endocervix Endometrium
    Broad ligament: Neg Pos Left Right
    Retroperitoneum: No Yes _____ (where)

5 Possible 2nd primary: No Yes _____ (where)
    Possible synchronous primary
    If endometrium involved _____ Histology, _____ Grade
    If myometrium involved Invade from Endomet Invade from Serosa
    Possible peritoneal primary
    If peritoneum involved If borderline: _____ Type & Locations
                      If carcinoma: _____ Type & Locations

6 Effusions/fluids:
    Ascites (>100cc)   Absent Neg Pos
    Washing, peritoneal, NOS Neg Pos
    Washing, diaphragm   Neg Pos
    Washing, left abdomen Neg Pos
    Washing, right abdomen Neg Pos
    Washing, pelvis   Neg Pos
    Scraping (Pap) diaphragm Neg Pos
    Pleural: Absent Neg Pos

7 Vascular involvement: No Yes_type Uncertain
                     Lymphatics Blood_vessel Both

8 Non-neoplastic changes
    Stromal luteinization No Yes
    Endometriosis: Ovary Elsewhere (_____ sites)
    Endometrium: Atrophy Prolif Secretory Hyperplasia Carcinoma
    Peritoneum: Common epithelial changes:
                   Benign ("endosalpingiosis"): _____ Locations

9 Lymph nodes: NOS None _____ of _____ contain metastases

	Left		Right	
External iliac	None _____/_____	w Mets	None _____/_____	w Mets
Obturator (Med Ext Iliac)	None _____/_____	w Mets	None _____/_____	w Mets
Common Iliac	None _____/_____	w Mets	None _____/_____	w Mets
Pelvic, NOS	None _____/_____	w Mets	None _____/_____	w Mets
Aortic, NOS	None _____/_____	w Mets	None _____/_____	w Mets
Inguinal, NOS	None _____/_____	w Mets	None _____/_____	w Mets

10 Special studies:
    DNA ploidy: Euploid Tetraploid Aneuploid
    Oncogenes   _____ Specify
    Receptors   _____ Specify
    Other: _____ Specify

11 Serum blood levels
    CA-125

Common epithelial tumor
Serous
  Borderline malignancy (LMP)
    Cystadenoma/papillary cystadenoma
    Surface papilloma
    Adenofibroma and cystadenofibroma
  Malignant
    Adenocarcinoma
    Surface papillary carcinoma
    Malignant adeno/cystadenofibroma
Mucinous
  Borderline malignancy (LMP)
    Cystadenoma
    Adenofibroma and cystadenofibroma
  Malignant
    Adeno/cystadenocarcinoma
    Malignant adeno/cystadenofibroma
Endometrioid
  Borderline malignancy (LMP)
    Cystadenoma
    Adenofibroma and cystadenofibroma
  Malignant
    Carcinoma
      Adenocarcinoma
        W squamous differentiation
      Malignant adenofibroma
    Endometrioid stromal sarcoma
    Mesodermal (mullerian) mixed tum
Clear-cell
  Of borderline malignancy (LMP)
  Malignant
Brenner
  Prolif (borderline malignancy)
  Malignant
  Transitional cell
Undifferentiated carcinoma
Mixed (specify)

Sex-cord-stroma
Granulosa-cell tumor
  Adult
  Juvenile
Tumors in thecoma-fibroma group
  Fibroma-fibrosarcoma
    Cellular fibroma
    Fibrosarcoma
  Sertoli-stromal cell tumors
Sertoli-Leydig cell tumor
  Gynandroblastoma
  Sex-cord tumor with annular tubules

Steroid (lipid-lipoid)-cell tumors
  Leydig-cell tumor
  Steroid-cell tumor, NOS

Tumors of rete ovarii

Tumors of uncertain cell type
  Of probable wolffian origin
  Small cell carcinoma

Reprinted by permission of Robboy et al., ref. 5.
[a] FIGO staging incorporates pathological findings.

Table 30.5. Request for placental examination

Circle appropriate indications
Mother's name _____ Age _____ M.D. _____
Cesarean section/vaginal delivery
 1. Specific maternal disease: Diagnosis _____
 2. High-risk pregnancy: Diagnosis _____
 3. Death: Antepartum Intrapartum Neonatal
 4. Baby small for date: Baby anemic
 5. Postmature
 6. Premature rupture of membranes
 7. Possible intrauterine infection: viral (specify) _____
    toxoplasma _____ chorioamnionitis _____ other _____
 8. Isoimmunization: Rh _____ Other _____
 9. Malformations of baby or placenta _____ Single umbilical artery _____
10. Evaluate antepartum intrauterine procedures (specify) _____
11. Gestational bleeding: 1st 2nd 3rd trimester _____
12. Placenta previa-vasa previa _____
13. Premature separation _____
14. Toxemia, eclampsia _____
15. Maternal diabetes mellitus _____
16. Maternal anemias (sickle cell, megaloblastic, other)
17. Other disease _____
18. History of habitual abortion _____
19. Cord entanglements, amniotic bands, or adhesions. Membrane tears, defects

Table 30.6. Cytogenetic studies for curetted and miscarried material

Curettings

1. Call laboratory for sterile media containers and to notify that a specimen is coming.
2. Cytogenetics needs 2–3 cm of sterile material for culture. Put the material into the bottle, cap tightly, label and send to the laboratory with the appropriate request form.

Miscarriage

1. Call laboratory for two sterile media and two sodium heparin Vacutainers. Also notify the laboratory that a specimen is coming.
2. If the miscarriage is small, put the material into the containers and cap tightly. Draw maternal blood into sodium heparin Vacutainer and send with miscarriage material and the appropriate forms to the laboratory.
3. If the miscarriage is term (stillborn baby) and large:
    a. Cut a skin sample and/or pericardium and put into one media container (sterile).
    b. Draw fetal blood (intracardiac puncture with heparinized syringe) and put into sodium heparin Vacutainer.
    c. Cut a small piece of placenta and put into second media bottle.
    d. Draw maternal blood into a sodium heparin Vacutainer.
4. Label all specimens and send to the laboratory with the appropriate form.

Cytogenetics Lab, St. John's Mercy Medical Center.

References

1. Aquino TI, Zhang J, Kraus FT, et al. (1984) Subshorionic fibrin cultures for bacteriologic study of the placenta. Am J Clin Pathol 81: 482
2. Benirschke K, Driscoll SG (1967) The Pathology of the Human Placenta. New York, Springer-Verlag
3. Langlois PL (1970) The size of the normal uterus. J Reprod Med 4: 220
4. Milbrath JR, Wilkinson EJ, Friedrich EG (1975) Xerographic evaluation of radical vulvectomy specimens. AJR 125: 486
5. Robboy SJ, Bentley RC, Krigman H, Silverberg SG, Norris HJ, Zaino RJ (1994) Synoptic reports in gynecologic pathology. Int J Gynecol Pathol 13: 161–174
6. Schmidt WA (1983) Principles and Techniques of Surgical Pathology. Butterworth-Heinemann, Stoneham, Massachusetts.

Index

ISBN 0-387-94166-5